Quick Table of Contents

PATHOPHYSIOLOGY
Concepts of Altered Health States

EIGHTH EDITION

Carol Mattson Porth, RN, MSN, PhD (Physiology)
Professor Emerita
College of Nursing
University of Wisconsin—Milwaukee
Milwaukee, Wisconsin

Glenn Matfin, BSc (Hons), MB ChB, DGM, FFPM, FACE, FACP, FRCP
Clinical Associate Professor of Medicine, Department of Endocrinology
School of Medicine
New York University
New York, New York

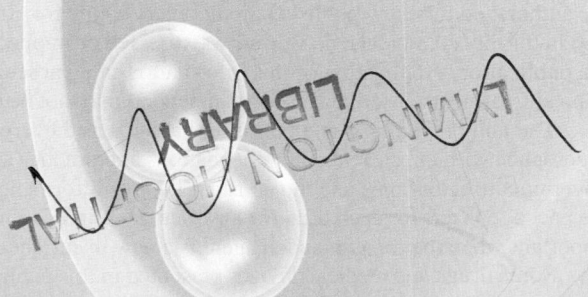

Senior Acquisitions Editor: Hilarie Surrena
Senior Managing Editor: Helen Kogut
Editorial Assistant: Brandi Spade
Senior Production Editor: Debra Schiff
Director of Nursing Production: Helen Ewan
Senior Managing Editor/Production: Erika Kors
Senior Designer: Joan Wendt
Senior Designer, Illustration: Brett MacNaughton
Manufacturing Coordinator: Karin Duffield
Indexer: Cassar Technical Services
Compositor: Circle Graphics

8th Edition

Copyright © 2009 Wolters Kluwer Health | Lippincott Williams & Wilkins.

9 8 7 6 5 4 3

Printed in China

ISBN: 978-16054-7390-1
Not authorized for sale in North America.

Care has been taken to confirm the accuracy of the information presented and to describe generally accepted practices. However, the authors, editors, and publisher are not responsible for errors or omissions or for any consequences from application of the information in this book and make no warranty, expressed or implied, with respect to the currency, completeness, or accuracy of the contents of the publication. Application of this information in a particular situation remains the professional responsibility of the practitioner; the clinical treatments described and recommended may not be considered absolute and universal recommendations.

The authors, editors, and publisher have exerted every effort to ensure that drug selection and dosage set forth in this text are in accordance with the current recommendations and practice at the time of publication. However, in view of ongoing research, changes in government regulations, and the constant flow of information relating to drug therapy and drug reactions, the reader is urged to check the package insert for each drug for any change in indications and dosage and for added warnings and precautions. This is particularly important when the recommended agent is a new or infrequently employed drug.

Some drugs and medical devices presented in this publication have Food and Drug Administration (FDA) clearance for limited use in restricted research settings. It is the responsibility of the health care provider to ascertain the FDA status of each drug or device planned for use in his or her clinical practice.

This book is dedicated to
My family: Rick, Susan, Tom, Cody, and Noah

—Carol Mattson Porth

To my wife Marcia
and my parents, Enid and Sid
I also dedicate it to my mentor, Professor Harold Adelman, Tampa, Florida

—Glenn Matfin

Consultants

Kathryn J. Gaspard, PhD
Clinical Associate Professor Emerita
College of Nursing
University of Wisconsin—Milwaukee
Milwaukee, Wisconsin

Kim Litwack, RN, PhD, FAAN, APNP
Associate Professor
College of Nursing
University of Wisconsin—Milwaukee
Milwaukee, Wisconsin

Contributors

Judith A. Aberg, MD
Principal Investigator, AIDS Clinical Trials Unit
Director of HIV, Bellevue Hospital Center
Associate Professor of Medicine
New York University School of Medicine
(Chapter 20)

Toni Balistrieri, RN, MSN, CCNS
Clinical Nurse Specialist, Critical Care
Zablocki Veterans Affairs Medical Center
Milwaukee, Wisconsin
(Chapter 24)

Anna Barkman, RN, BN, MN
Mount Royal College
School of Nursing
Faculty of Health & Community Studies
Calgary, Alberta, Canada
(Chapter 26)

Diane S. Book, MD
Assistant Professor of Neurology
Medical College of Wisconsin
Milwaukee, Wisconsin
(Chapter 51)

Edward W. Carroll, MS, PhD
Clinical Assistant Professor
Department of Biomedical Sciences, College of Health Sciences
Marquette University
Milwaukee, Wisconsin
(Chapters 4, 6, 48, 54)

Robin Curtis, PhD
Professor, Retired
Department of Cellular Biology, Neurobiology, and Anatomy
Medical College of Wisconsin
Milwaukee, Wisconsin
(Chapters 48, 54)

W. Michael Dunne Jr., PhD
Professor of Pathology, Immunology, and Molecular Microbiology
Washington University School of Medicine
Medical Director of Microbiology
Barnes-Jewish Hospital
St. Louis, Missouri
(Chapter 16)

Jason Faulhaber, MD, Fellow
Division of Infectious Diseases and Immunology
New York University School of Medicine
New York, New York
(Chapter 20)

Susan A. Fontana, PhD, APRN-BC
Associate Professor and Family Nurse Practitioner
College of Nursing
University of Wisconsin-Milwaukee
Milwaukee, Wisconsin
(Chapter 55)

Kathryn J. Gaspard, PhD
Clinical Associate Professor Emerita
College of Nursing
University of Wisconsin-Milwaukee
Milwaukee, Wisconsin
(Chapters 12, 13, 14)

Kathleen E. Gunta, MSN, RN, OCNS-C
Clinical Nurse Specialist
Aurora St. Luke's Medical Center
Milwaukee, Wisconsin
(Chapters 57, 58)

Safak Guven, MD, MBA, FACE, FACP
Las Vegas, Nevada
(Chapter 42)

Serena W. Hung, MD
Assistant Professor, Department of Neurology
Medical College of Wisconsin
Milwaukee, Wisconsin
(Chapter 50)

Scott A. Jens, OD, FAAO
Doctor of Optometry
Isthmus Eye Care, SC
Middleton, Wisconsin
(Chapter 54)

Mary Kay Jiricka, RN, MSN, CCRN, APN-BC
Staff Nurse, Cardiac Intensive Care Unit
Aurora St. Luke's Medical Center
Milwaukee, Wisconsin
(Chapter 11)

Julie A. Kuenzi, RN, MSN, CDE
Manager–Diabetes and Endocrine Center
Froedtert Hospital and Medical College of Wisconsin
Milwaukee, Wisconsin
(*Chapter 42*)

Mary Pat Kunert, RN, PhD
Associate Professor
College of Nursing
University of Wisconsin-Milwaukee
Milwaukee, Wisconsin
(*Chapters 9, 10*)

Nathan A. Ledeboer, PhD
Assistant Professor of Pathology
Medical College of Wisconsin
Director, Clinical Microbiology
DynaCare Laboratories
Milwaukee, Wisconsin
(*Chapter 16*)

Kim Litwack, RN, PhD, FAAN, APNP
Associate Professor
College of Nursing
University of Wisconsin-Milwaukee
Milwaukee, Wisconsin
(*Chapters 27, 32, 49*)

Judy Wright Lott, RNC, DSN, FAAN
Dean and Professor of Nursing
Louise Herrington School of Nursing
Baylor University
Waco, Texas
(*Chapter 2*)

Patricia McCowen Mehring, RNC, MSN, WHNP
Nurse Practitioner, Department of OB-GYN
Medical College of Wisconsin
Milwaukee, Wisconsin
(*Chapters 45, 46, 47*)

Carrie J. Merkle, RN, PhD, FAAN
Associate Professor
College of Nursing
University of Arizona
Tucson, Arizona
(*Chapters 5, 8*)

Kathleen Mussatto, RN, PhD(C)
Research Manager
Herma Heart Center
Children's Hospital of Wisconsin
Milwaukee, Wisconsin
(*Chapter 24*)

Sandra Kawczynski Pasch, RN, MS, MA
Assistant Professor
Columbia College of Nursing
Milwaukee, Wisconsin
(*Chapter 53*)

Janice Kuiper Pikna, RN, MSN, CS
Clinical Nurse Specialist–Gerontology
Froedtert Hospital
Milwaukee, Wisconsin
(*Chapter 3*)

Joan Pleuss, RD, MS, CDE, CD
Program Manager/Bionutrition Core
General Clinical Research Center (GCRC)
Medical College of Wisconsin
Milwaukee, Wisconsin
(*Chapter 39*)

Charlotte Pooler, RN, BScN, MN, PhD (Nursing), CNCC(C), CNC(C)
Director, Baccalaureate Nursing Program
Faculty of Health and Community Studies
Grant MacEwan College
Edmonton, Alberta, Canada
(*Chapters 26, 29*)

Debra Bancroft Rizzo, RN, MSN, FNP-C
Nurse Practitioner
Rheumatic Disease Center
Glendale, Wisconsin
(*Chapter 59*)

Gladys Simandl, RN, PhD
Professor
Columbia College of Nursing
Milwaukee, Wisconsin
(*Chapters 60, 61*)

Cynthia Sommer, PhD, MT (ASCP)
Associate Professor Emerita, Department of Biological Sciences
University of Wisconsin-Milwaukee
Milwaukee, Wisconsin
(*Chapters 17, 18*)

Jill Winters, RN, PhD
Director of Research and Scholarship; Associate Professor
Marquette University College of Nursing
Milwaukee, Wisconsin
(*Chapter 25*)

Reviewers

Sally Aboelela, PhD
Assistant Professor
Columbia University
New York, New York

Joann Acierno, RN, BSN, MSN
Assistant Professor
Clarkson College
Omaha, Nebraska

Karen Bailey, RN, MSN, BC-FNP
Assistant Professor; Family Nurse
   Practitioner
Marshall University; Valley Health
Huntington, West Virginia

Joseph Balatbat, MD
Vice President of Academic Affairs
Sanford-Brown Institute NYC
New York, New York

Susan Blakey, RN, MS
Assistant Professor
Georgia Baptist College of Nursing
Atlanta, Georgia

Carey Bosold, RN, MSN, APN, FNP
Assistant Professor
Arkansas Tech University
Russellville, Arkansas

Donna Bowles, RN, MSN, EdD
Associate Professor of Nursing
Indiana University Southeast
New Albany, Indiana

Carolyn M. Burger, RN, MSN, BC, AOCN
Associate Professor
Miami University Middletown
Middletown, Ohio

Wanda Emberley Burke, RN, BN, MEd, PCNP
Faculty (Nurse Practitioner Program)
Centre for Nursing Studies
St. John's, Newfoundland and Labrador,
   Canada

Connie Lorette Calvin, CRNA, ARNP, MS, Doctoral Fellow
Associate Clinical Coordinator
Northeastern University
Boston, Massachusetts

Jackie Carnegie, PhD, MEd
Assistant Professor, Department of Cellular
   and Molecular Medicine
University of Ottawa
Ottawa, Ontario, Canada

Margaret Christensen, RN, PhD
Associate Professor
Northeastern University
Boston, Massachusetts

Elizabeth Cohn, RN, NP, ACNP, DNSc
Assistant Professor
Adelphi University
Garden City, New York

Christine Colella, MSN, CS, CNP
Associate Professor of Clinical Nursing;
   Adult Nurse Practitioner
University of Cincinnati
Cincinnati, Ohio

Cathleen A. Collins, RN, MSN
Assistant Professor
Texas Tech University
Lubbock, Texas

David Derrico, RN, MSN
Assistant Clinical Professor
University of Florida
Gainesville, Florida

Dare Domico, RN, DSN
Professor
Mercer University-Atlanta
Atlanta, Georgia

Crystal Donlevy, EdD
Professor
Cincinnati State Technical
   and Community College
Cincinnati, Ohio

Patricia A. Dunn, PhD, RNC
Associate Professor
Holy Family University
Philadelphia, Pennsylvania

Margaret Fink, RN, EdD, BC
Assistant Professor
Dominican University of California
San Rafael, California

Cindy Fitzgerald, RN, PhD(c), ARNP
Assistant Professor and Coordinator,
   Family Nurse Practitioner Program
Gonzaga University
Spokane, Washington

Jamie Flower, RN, MS
Assistant Professor
University of Arkansas-Fort Smith
Fort Smith, Arkansas

Joyce S. Fontana, RN, PhD
Assistant Professor of Nursing
St. Joseph College-W. Hartford
West Hartford, Connecticut

Dorothy Ann Fraser, MSN, FNP-C
Lecturer
University of California-Davis
Davis, California

Susan K. Frazier, RN, PhD
Associate Professor
University of Kentucky
Lexington, Kentucky

Laura M. Freidhoff, MD
Assistant Professor
Michigan State University College
   of Nursing
Lansing, Michigan

Louise Glover, RN, BA, A-EMCA
Professor and Coordinator
College Boreal
Sudbury, Ontario, Canada

James Hampton, PhD
Professor
Medical College of Ohio
Toledo, Ohio

Sharon R. Haymaker, PhD, CRNP
Associate Professor
Bloomsburg University
Bloomsburg, Pennsylvania

Judy Hembd, RN, MSN
Assistant Professor
Montana State University Northern
Havre, Montana

Lori Hendrickx, RN, EdD, CCRN
Associate Professor
South Dakota State University
Brookings, South Dakota

Leslie Higgins, PhD, APRN, BC
Associate Professor and Director,
    Graduate Nursing Program
Belmont University
Nashville, Tennessee

Lisa Hight, EdD
Associate Professor, Biology
Baptist Memorial College of Health Sciences
Memphis, Tennessee

Kathleen J. Holbrook, BS
Vice President and Director
Andrews and Holbrook Training Corporation
Latham, New York

Patricia C. Hunt, DO, MHA
Adjunct Professor
Pace University
New York, New York

Joanne Itano, RN, PhD, OCN
Interim Vice Chancellor; Director of
    Academic Plan and Policy
University of Hawaii
Honolulu, Hawaii

Frances Jackson, RN, PhD
Associate Professor of Nursing
Oakland University
Rochester, Michigan

Nadine T. James, RN, BSN, MSN, PhD
Assistant Professor
University of Southern Mississippi
Hattiesburg, Mississippi

Judy Jezierski, RN, MSN
Chair, Department of Nursing
Saint Joseph's College
West Hartford, Connecticut

Ritamarie John, DrNP, CPNP
PNP/NNP Program Director
Columbia University School of Nursing
New York, New York

Brenda P. Johnson, RN, PhD
Associate Professor
Southeast Missouri State University
Cape Girardeau, Missouri

Jennifer Johnson, MSN
Assistant Professor, Department of Nursing
University of NC-Pembroke
Pembroke, North Carolina

Brian Kipp, PhD
Assistant Professor
Grand Valley State University
Allendale, Michigan

Lori Knight, CCHRA(c)
Instructor, Health Information
    Management Program
SIAST Wascana Campus
Regina, Saskatchewan, Canada

Therese M. Lahnstein, RN, MSN, CCRN
Assistant Professor
Columbus State University
Columbus, Georgia

Brigitte Lalonde, ACP
Coordinator/Professor
La Cite Collegiale
Ottawa, Ontario, Canada

Gemme Langor, BN, Med
Professor
Centre for Nursing Studies
St. John's, Newfoundland and Labrador,
    Canada

Ramona Lazenby, EdD, CRNP
Assistant Dean and Associate Professor
    of Nursing
Auburn University-Montgomery
Montgomery, Alabama

Edna Johnson Lewis, MS, RN, CCRN, CS
Clinical Assistant Professor
Downstate Medical Center,
    College of Nursing
Brooklyn, New York

Linda Linc, RN, PhD, CNS
Professor
University of Akron
Akron, Ohio

Anne Lincoln, DVM
Associate Professor, Biology
North Country Community College
Saranac Lake, New York

Suzanne E. Lindley, PhD, MS
Associate Professor, Biology
Limestone College
Gaffney, South Carolina

Wendy B. Loren, MS, LMT
Faculty
Lane Community College
Eugene, Oregon

Eve Main, ARNP
Assistant Professor
Western Kentucky University
Bowling Green, Kentucky

Maria E. Main, MSN, ARNP, MSN
Assistant Professor
Western Kentucky University
Bowling Green, Kentucky

Brenda Mason, MSN, APRN, FNP-BC
Assistant Professor of Nursing
Alderson-Broadus College
Philippi, West Virginia

Timothy Maze, PhD
Assistant Professor
Lander University
Greenwood, South Carolina

Sharon McCleave, BS, MEd
Professor
Seneca College
Toronto, Ontario, Canada

Leigh Ann McInnis, PhD, APRN, BC, FNP
Instructor
Belmont University
Nashville, Tennessee

Rhonda M. McLain, RN, DSN
Assistant Professor
Clayton College and State University
Atlanta, Georgia

Thomas McNeilis, PhD, DO
Associate Professor, Biology
Dixie State College
St. George, Utah

James A. Metcalf, PhD
Professor
George Mason University
Fairfax, Virginia

Anita Mills, RN, MSN
4th Semester Lead Faculty
Butler County Community College-El Dorado
El Dorado, Kansas

Robert Moldenhauer, MS
Professor
St. Clair County Community College
Port Huron, Michigan

Donna Moralejo, RN, PhD
Memorial University School of Nursing
St. John's, New Foundland and Labrador,
 Canada

Mary Moran
Clinical Instructor
Columbia University
New York, New York

Mary Morehouse, DO
Faculty
Drury University
Springfield, Missouri

Marguerite Murphy, MS, RN
Assistant Professor
Medical College of Georgia
Augusta, Georgia

Joan Nelson, DNP
Assistant Professor
University of Colorado Denver Health
 Sciences Center
Denver, Colorado

Janet Nieveen, RN, PhD
Assistant Professor
University of Nebraska Medical Center
Omaha, Nebraska

Amy Obringer, PhD
Assistant Professor, Biology
University of St. Frances-Ft. Wayne
Fort Wayne, Indiana

Thomas Lon Owen, PhD
Professor
Northern Arizona University
Flagstaff, Arizona

Frank Paladino, BA, MA, PhD
Professor
Indiana Purdue University, Ft. Wayne
Fort Wayne, Indiana

Davonya J. Person, MS
Instructor/Laboratory Coordinator
Auburn University
Auburn, Alabama

Paul Pillitteri, PhD
Assistant Professor of Biology
Southern Utah University
Cedar City, Utah

Lori Ploutz-Snyder, PhD
Associate Professor and Chair
 of Exercise Science
Syracuse University
Syracuse, New York

Harry Plummer, RN, PhD
Professor
University of Calgary
Calgary, Alberta, Canada

Deborah Pool, RN, MS, CCRN
Instructor, Department of Nursing
Glendale Community College
Glendale, Arizona

Debbie Pringnitz, PhD
Professor, Biology
University of Maine-Fort Kent
Fort Kent, Maine

Heidi Putman, RN, DNSc
Assistant Professor
West Virginia University
Morgantown, West Virginia

Micki S. Raber, MSN, FNP-BC, PNP-BC
Assistant Clinical Professor
University of Southern Alabama
Mobile, Alabama

Shirlee Rankin, RMT, BA
Lead Instructor, Massage Therapy
 Programme
CDI College
Ottawa, Ontario, Canada

Carl A. Ross, RN, PhD, CRNP, BC, CNE
Professor of Nursing
Robert Morris University School of Nursing
 and Allied Health
Moon Township, Pennsylvania

Christine Ruff, RN, MS, WHNP
Assistant Professor
University of Arkansas at Monticello
Monticello, Arkansas

Jo-Ann Sawatzky, RN, MN, PhD
Assistant Professor
University of Manitoba
Winnipeg, Manitoba, Canada

Claire Schuster, RN, MSN, CNS,
 ARNP, CWS
Professor; Family Nurse Practitioner;
 Clinical and Wound Care Specialist
Berea College
Berea, Kentucky

Jane Shelby, RN, MSN
Director of Undergraduate Studies
Belmont University
Nashville, Tennessee

Frederick Slone, MD
Visiting Assistant Professor;
 Program Director
 for Basic Disaster Life Support
University of South Florida College
 of Nursing
Tampa, Florida

Rachel Smetanka, PhD
Assistant Professor, Biology
Southern Utah University
Cedar City, Utah

Melissa Smith, RN, MSN, FNP
Clinical Instructor
University of Missouri-Kansas City
Kansas City, Missouri

Nan Smith-Blair, RN, PhD
Assistant Professor
University of Arkansas-Fayetteville
Fayetteville, Arkansas

Janet Squires, RN, BN, MNC
Memorial University School of Nursing
St. John's, Newfoundland and Labrador,
 Canada

Mary Stanley, RN, MA
Assistant Professor
University of Nebraska Medical Center
 College of Nursing
Omaha, Nebraska

Gail Starich, BS, MS, PhD
Dean, School of Health Sciences
Brenau University
Decatur, Georgia

Elaine E. Steinke, RN, PhD
Professor
Wichita State University
Wichita, Kansas

Barbara Steuble, RN, MS
Assistant Professor
Samuel Merritt College
Oakland, California

Jill Steuer, RN, PhD
Associate Professor
Capital University
Columbus, Ohio

Lachel Story, RN, MSN
Instructor
University of Southern Mississippi
Hattiesburg, Mississippi

Cheryl Swallow, RN, MSN
Professor
St. Louis Community College-Forest Park
Forest Park, Missouri

Costellia Talley, BSN, MSN, PhD
Assistant Professor
Michigan State University
East Lansing, Michigan

Stephenie Thibodeaux, MSN
Instructor
Lamar State College-Orange
Orange, Texas

Donna Thompson, RN, MSN
Professor
Salt Lake Community College
Salt Lake City, Utah

Ann Tritak, RN, BS, MA, EdD
Associate Director RN-BSN Program;
    Associate Professor of Nursing
Farleigh Dickinson University-Teaneck
Teaneck, New Jersey

Jo Voss, RN, PhD, CNS
Associate Professor
South Dakota State University
Brookings, South Dakota

Laura Jean Waight, RN, MSN
Instructor of Nursing
West Texas A&M University
Canyon, Texas

Annette Ward, RN, MSN
Instructor
Lower Columbia College
Longview, Washington

A. Denyce Watties-Daniels, MS, RN
Assistant Professor
Coppin State University
Baltimore, Maryland

Dorie Weaver, RN, MSN, FNP,
    APRN, BC
Instructor
DeSales University
Center Valley, Pennsylvania

Karen S. Webber, RN, MN
Associate Professor
Memorial University of Newfoundland
St. John's, Newfoundland and Labrador,
    Canada

Michelina Eva Weicker, MD, MBA
Professor
Alvernia College
Reading, Pennsylvania

Keeta Wilborn, RN, PhD
Department of Nursing Chair
Brenau University
Decatur, Georgia

Linda Wilson, MSN, PhD
Professor
Middle Tennessee State University
Murfreesboro, Tennessee

Sheryl Winn, BSN, MSN
Assistant Professor
Macon State College
Macon, Georgia

K. Mark Wooden, BS, PhD
Associate Dean, CLAS; Department Chair,
    Math and Science
Grand Canyon University
Phoenix, Arizona

Nicholas P. Ziats, PhD
Associate Professor of Pathology
Case Western Reserve University
Cleveland, Ohio

Astatkie Zikarge, BS, MS, MD, MPH
Associate Professor of Environmental Health
    and Toxicology
Texas Southern University
Houston, Texas

Preface

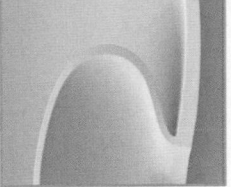

The preparation of this edition has been both challenging and humbling. Challenging to incorporate the myriad of new information; humbling to realize that despite the advances in science and technology, illness and disease continue to occur and take their toll in terms of the physiologic as well as the social, psychological, and economic well-being of individuals, their families and communities, and the world.

As the others before it, the eighth edition has been carefully reviewed and critiqued, reorganized, updated, and revised. Careful attention has been given to the incorporation of the most recent advances from the fields of genetics, immunity, and molecular biology. This edition maintains many of the features of the previous edition, including chapters on health and disease, sleep and sleep disorders, and neurobiology of thought and mood disorders. In addition there is added content on obesity and the metabolic syndrome.

This edition, as no other, typifies a saying among scientists that "you can't pick a flower without jiggling a star." The forging of communications, travel and migration, and trade on a global scale has established links that have forever changed the understanding and application of scientific information and health care practices. The isolation of peoples and information is no longer possible or beneficial. As the borders and boundaries of individuals, countries, and continents have become more permeable, there has been an increased focus on exploring issues and incorporating practices relative to the world community. Within this text, the efforts of the world community in the expansion of scientific knowledge and the advances in health care technology are presented through the inclusion of international studies, WHO guidelines, and the health variants of diverse populations. In line with the greater international focus, this edition has added Dr. Glenn Matfin, who has roots in the United Kingdom, as coauthor and has also added two new contributing authors from Canada, Charlotte Pooler, RN, PhD, and Anna Barkman, RN, MN.

The integration of full color into the design and illustrations has continued. Over 200 of the illustrations that appear in this edition are new or have been extensively modified. The illustrations have been carefully chosen to support the concepts that are presented in the text, while maintaining a balance between line drawings of anatomic structures and pathophysiologic processes, flow charts, and photographic illustrations of disease states. This offers not only visual appeal but also enhances conceptual learning, linking text content to illustration content. Two new features have heightened the synergism of text and illustration. The first, a feature called "Understanding," focuses on the key physiologic processes and phenomena of a disorder. A process is broken down into its consecutive parts, which are presented in a sequential manner, to provide an insight into the many opportunities for disease processes to disrupt the sequence. The second new element, the "clinical feature," uses illustration to depict the clinical manifestations of selected disease states.

This edition also retains the list of suffixes and prefixes, the glossary, and the table of normal laboratory values that were in the seventh edition. The table of laboratory values includes both conventional and SI units, as well as Internet addresses for conversion resources. Objectives continue to appear at the beginning of each major section in a chapter, and summary statements appear at the end. The key concept boxes have been retained within each chapter. They are intended to help the reader retain and use text information by providing a mechanism to incorporate the information into a larger conceptual unit as opposed to merely memorizing a string of related and unrelated facts. Review exercises appear at the end of each chapter and assist the reader in using the conceptual approach to solving problems related to chapter content.

Despite the extensive changes and revision, every attempt has been made to present content in a manner that is logical, understandable, and that inspires reader interest. The content has been arranged so that concepts build on one another. Words are defined as content is presented. Concepts from physiology, biochemistry, physics, and other sciences are reviewed as deemed appropriate. A conceptual model that integrates the developmental and preventative aspects of health has been used. Selection of content was based on common health problems, including the special needs of children and elderly persons. Although intended as a course textbook, it also is designed to serve as a reference book that students can take with them and use in their practice once the course is finished.

And finally, as a nurse-physiologist, my major emphasis with each revision has been to relate normal body functioning to the physiologic changes that participate in disease production and occur as a result of disease, as well as the body's remarkable ability to compensate for these changes. The beauty of physiology is that it integrates all of the aspects of human genetics, molecular and cellular biology, and organ anatomy and physiology into a functional whole that can be used to explain both the physical and psychological aspects of altered health. Indeed, it has been my philosophy to share the beauty of the human body and to emphasize that in disease as in health, there is more "going right" in the body than is "going wrong." This book is an extension of my career and, as such, of my philosophy. It is my hope that readers will learn to appreciate the marvelous potential of the body, incorporating it into their own philosophy and ultimately sharing it with their clients.

Carol Mattson Porth

To the Reader

This book was written with the intent of making the subject of pathophysiology an exciting exploration that relates normal body functioning to the physiologic changes that occur as a result of disease, as well as the body's remarkable ability to compensate for these changes. Indeed, it is these changes that represent the signs and symptoms of disease.

Using a book such as this can be simplified by taking time out to find what is in the book and how to locate information when it is needed. The *table of contents* at the beginning of the book provides an overall view of the organization and content of the book. It also provides clues as to the relationships among areas of content. For example, the location of the chapter on neoplasia within the unit on cell function and growth indicates that neoplasms are products of altered cell growth. The *index,* which appears at the end of the book, can be viewed as a road map for locating content. It can be used to quickly locate related content in different chapters of the book or to answer questions that come up in other courses.

ORGANIZATION

The book is organized into units and chapters. The *units* identify broad areas of content, such as alterations in the circulatory system. Many of the units have an introductory chapter that contains essential information about the structure and function of the body systems that are being discussed in the unit. These chapters provide the foundation for understanding the pathophysiology content presented in the subsequent chapters. The *chapters* focus on specific areas of content, such as heart failure and circulatory shock. The *chapter outline* that appears at the beginning of each chapter provides an overall view of the chapter content and organization. *Icons* identify specific content related to infants and children , pregnant women , and older adults .

READING AND LEARNING AIDS

In an ever-expanding world of information you will not be able to read, let alone remember, everything that is in this book, or in any book, for that matter. With this in mind, we have developed a number of special features that will help you focus on and master the essential content for your current as well as future needs.

The *objectives* that appear at the beginning of each major area of content provide a focus for your study. After you have finished each of these areas of content, you may want to go back and make sure that you have met each of the objectives.

> *After completing this section of the chapter, you should be able to meet the following objectives:*
>
> ■ Define the term *orthostatic hypotension.*
> ■ Describe the cardiovascular, neurohumoral, and muscular responses that serve to maintain blood pressure when moving from the supine to standing position.

It is essential for any professional to use and understand the vocabulary of his or her profession. Throughout the text, you will encounter terms in *italics*. This is a signal that a word and the ideas associated with it are important to learn. In addition, two aids are provided to help you expand your vocabulary and improve your comprehension of what you are reading: the glossary and the list of prefixes and suffixes.

The *glossary* contains concise definitions of frequently encountered terms. If you are unsure of the meaning of a term you encounter in your reading, check the glossary in the back of the book before proceeding.

The *list of prefixes and suffixes* is a tool to help you derive the meaning of words you may be unfamiliar with and increase your vocabulary. Many disciplines establish a vocabulary by affixing one or more letters to the beginning or end of a word or base to form a derivative word. Prefixes are added to the beginning of a word or base, and suffixes are added to the end. If you know the meanings of common prefixes and suffixes, you can usually derive the meaning of a word, even if you have never encountered it before. A list of prefixes and suffixes can be found on the inside back cover.

BOXES

Boxes are used throughout the text to summarize and highlight key information. You will frequently encounter two types of boxes: Key Concept Boxes and Summary Boxes.

One of the ways to approach learning is to focus on the major ideas or concepts rather than trying to memorize a list of related and unrelated bits of information. As you have probably already discovered, it is impossible to memorize everything that is in a particular section or chapter of the book. Not only does your brain have a difficult time trying to figure out where to store all the different bits of information, your brain doesn't know how to retrieve the information when you need it. Most important of all, memorized lists of content can seldom, if ever, be applied directly to an actual clinical situation. The *Key Concept Boxes* guide you in identifying the major ideas or concepts that form the foundation for truly understanding the major areas of content. When you understand the concepts in the Key Concept Boxes, you will have a framework for remembering and using the facts given in the text.

PRIMARY IMMUNODEFICIENCY DISORDERS

- Primary immunodeficiency disorders are congenital or inherited abnormalities of immune function that render a person susceptible to diseases normally prevented by an intact immune system.
- Disorders of B-cell function impair the ability to produce antibodies and defend against microorganisms and toxins that circulate in body fluids (IgM and IgG) or enter the body through the mucosal surface of the respiratory or gastrointestinal tract (IgA). Persons with primary B-cell immunodeficiency are particularly prone to pyogenic infections due to encapsulated organisms.

The *Summary Boxes* at the end of each section provide a review and a reinforcement of the main content that has been covered. Use the summaries to assure that you have covered and understand what you have read.

IN SUMMARY, CKD results from the destructive effects of many forms of renal disease. Regardless of the cause, the consequences of nephron destruction in CKD are alterations in the filtration, reabsorption, and endocrine functions of the kidneys. Chronic disease is defined as either diagnosed kidney damage or GFR of less than 60 mL/min/1.73 m² for 3 months or more, and kidney failure as a GFR of less than 15 mL/min/1.73 m², usually accompanied by most of the signs and symptoms of uremia, or a need to start renal replacement therapy.

CKD affects almost every body system. It causes an accumulation of nitrogenous wastes (*i.e.,* azotemia), alters sodium and water excretion, and alters regulation of body levels of potassium, phosphate, calcium, and magnesium. It also causes skeletal disorders, anemia, cardiovascular disorders, neurologic disturbances, gastrointestinal dysfunction, and discomforting skin changes.

TABLES AND CHARTS

Tables and charts are designed to present complex information in a format that makes it more meaningful and easier to remember. Tables have two or more columns, and are often used for the purpose of comparing or contrasting information. Charts have one column and are used to summarize information.

TABLE 31-2 Sources of Body Water Gains and Losses in the Adult

GAINS		LOSSES	
Oral intake		Urine	1500 mL
As water	1000 mL	Insensible losses	
In food	1300 mL	Lungs	300 mL
Water of oxidation	200 mL	Skin	500 mL
		Feces	200 mL
Total	2500 mL	Total	2500 mL

CHART 22-1 RISK FACTORS IN CORONARY HEART DISEASE OTHER THAN LOW-DENSITY LIPOPROTEINS

Positive Risk Factors
Age
  Men: ≥45 years
  Women: ≥55 years or premature menopause without estrogen replacement therapy
Family history of premature coronary heart disease (definite myocardial infarction or sudden death before 55 years of age in father or other male first-degree relative, or before 65 years of age in mother or other female first-degree relative)
Current cigarette smoking
Hypertension (≥140/90 mm Hg* or on antihypertensive medication)

ILLUSTRATIONS AND PHOTOS

The full-color illustrations will help you to build your own mental image of the content that is being presented. Each drawing has been developed to fully support and build upon the ideas in the text. Some illustrations are used to help you picture the complex interactions of the multiple phenomena that are involved in the development of a particular disease; others can help you to visualize normal function or understand the mechanisms whereby the disease processes exert their effects. In addition, photographs of pathologic processes and lesions provide a realistic view of selected pathologic processes and lesions.

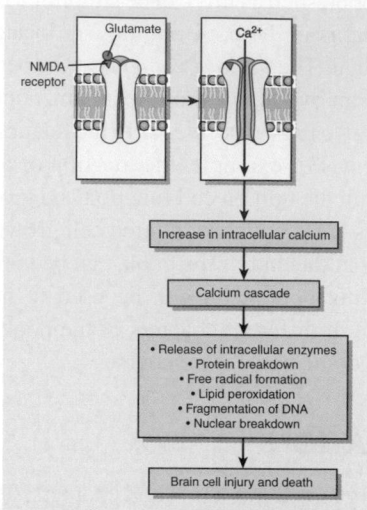

FIGURE 51-2 • The role of the glutamate-NMDA receptor in brain cell injury.

CLINICAL FEATURES

New to this edition is a new type of illustration that depicts the clinical features of persons with selected diseases. This feature is designed to help you visualize the entire spectrum of clinical manifestations that are associated with these disease states.

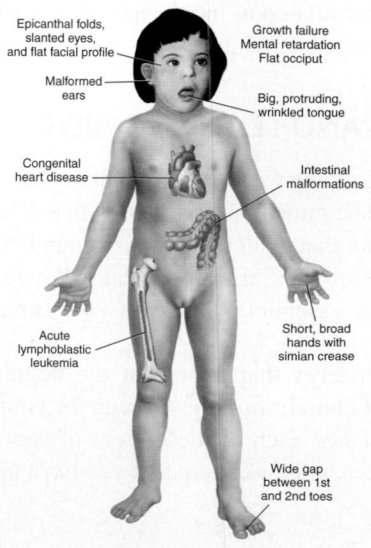

FIGURE 7-9 • Clinical features of a child with Down syndrome.

UNDERSTANDING PHYSIOLOGIC PROCESSES

Also new to this edition is a feature called "Understanding" that focuses on the physiologic processes and phenomenon that form the basis for understanding disorders presented in the text. This feature breaks a process or phenomena down into its component parts and presents them in a sequential manner, providing an insight into the many opportunities for disease processes to disrupt the sequence.

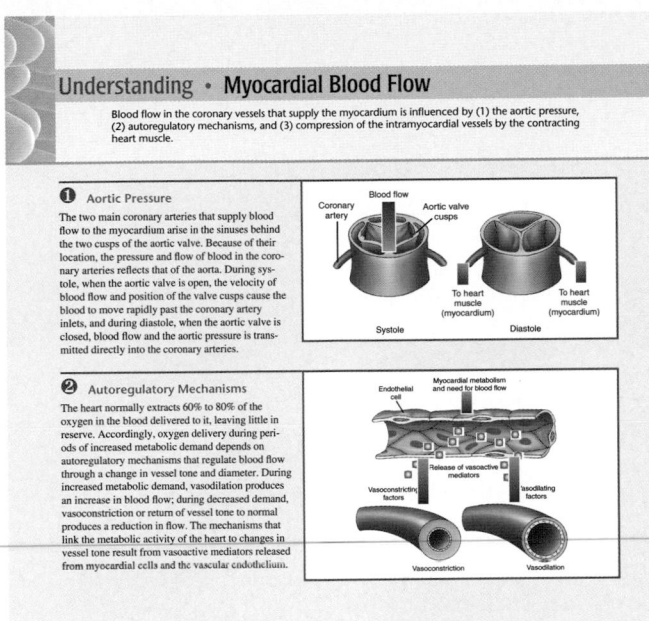

MATERIAL FOR REVIEW

An important feature has been built into the text to help you verify your understanding of the material presented. After you have finished reading and studying the chapter, work on answering the *review exercises* at the end of the chapter. They are designed to help you integrate and synthesize material. If you are unable to answer a question, reread the relevant section in the chapter.

Review Exercises

1. A 34-year-old woman with diabetes is admitted to the emergency department in a stuporous state. Her skin is flushed and warm, her breath has a sweet odor, her pulse is rapid and weak, and her respirations are rapid and deep. Her initial laboratory tests indicate a blood sugar of 320 mg/dL, serum HCO_3^- of 12 mEq/L (normal, 24 to 27 mEq/L), and a pH of 7.1 (normal, 7.35 to 7.45).

   A. *What is the most likely cause of her lowered pH and bicarbonate levels?*

   B. *How would you account for her rapid and deep respirations?*

   C. *Using the Henderson-Hasselbalch equation and the solubility coefficient for CO_2 given in this chapter, what would you expect her PCO_2 to be?*

   D. *How would you explain her warm, flushed skin and stuporous mental state?*

APPENDICES

Your book contains two appendices. Appendix A, *Lab Values,* provides rapid access to normal values for many laboratory tests, as well as a description of the prefixes, symbols, and factors (*e.g.,* micro, μ, 10^{-6}) used for describing these values. Knowledge of normal values can help you to put abnormal values in context. Appendix B contains tables of dietary reference for carbohydrates, fats, proteins, fiber, vitamins, and minerals.

We hope that this guide has given you a clear picture of how to use this book. Good luck and enjoy the journey!

STUDENT AND INSTRUCTOR RESOURCES

A variety of ancillary materials are available to support students and instructors alike.

Resources for Students

- **Student Resource CD-ROM.** This free CD-ROM is found in the front of the book, and contains
  - **Animations** of selected pathophysiologic processes
  - **Links** to relevant **journal articles**
- thePoint.*. Even **more animations** are available online at thePoint.LWW.com along with **Student Review Questions** for every chapter.
- *Study Guide for Porth's Pathophysiology: Concepts of Altered Health States.* This study guide reinforces and complements the text by helping you assess and apply your knowledge through **case studies** and a **variety of questions styles**, including multiple choice, fill-in-the-blank, matching, short answer, and figure-labeling exercises that will help you **practice for the NCLEX**.

Resources for Instructors

Instructor's Resource DVD. This comprehensive resource includes the following:

- A **Test Generator**, containing more than 800 multiple-choice questions.
- **Guided Lecture Notes** that walk you though the chapter learning objective by learning objective with integrated references to the PowerPoint presentations.
- **PowerPoint** presentations.
- **Student Assignments (written, group, clinical, and web)** and **Discussion Topics** that can be implemented in the classroom or online.
- An **Image Bank**, containing approximately 300 images from the text in formats suitable for printing, projecting, and incorporating into web sites.
- **WebCT- and Blackboard-ready materials**, for use with your institution's Learning Management system.
- **Case Studies with critical-thinking/discussion questions.**

---

*thePoint is a trademark of Wolters Kluwer Health.

Acknowledgments

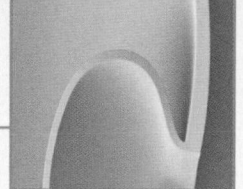

As in past editions, many persons participated in the creation of this work. The contributing authors deserve a special mention, for they worked long hours preparing the content for the eighth edition of *Pathophysiology: Concepts of Altered Health States.* This edition is particularly meaningful since it marks over a quarter of a century since the first edition was published in 1982, and many of these authors have been with the book during this time and have played an essential role in the development of this edition.

I would also like to acknowledge Dr. Glenn Matfin, who joined me as coauthor for this edition. His expertise contributed greatly to the development of this edition. I would also like to acknowledge Dr. Kathryn Gaspard and Dr. Kim Litwack for their consultation. Kathryn spent endless hours proofreading manuscripts and page proofs and tirelessly assisted in the development and modification of illustrations. Several other persons deserve special recognition. Georgianne Heymann assisted in editing the manuscript. As with previous editions, she provided not only excellent editorial assistance, but also encouragement and support when the tasks associated with manuscript preparation became most frustrating.

Sara Krause deserves recognition for her work in coordinating the development and modification of illustrations in the book. Sarah, along with Wendy Beth Jackelow and Anne Rains, are acknowledged for their talent in creating the many new illustrations and modifying the old illustrations for the book. I would also like to recognize the efforts of the editorial and production staff at Lippincott Williams & Wilkins that were directed by Margaret Zuccarini and Hilarie Surrena, Senior Acquisitions Editors. I particularly want to thank Helen Kogut, who served as Managing Editor; and Debra Schiff for her dedication as Production Editor.

The students in the classes I have taught also deserve a special salute, for they provided the inspiration upon which this book is founded. They provided the questions, suggestions, and contact with the "real world" of patient care that have directed the organization and selection of content for the book.

And last, but not least, I would like to acknowledge my family, my friends, and my colleagues for their patience, their understanding, and their encouragement throughout the entire process.

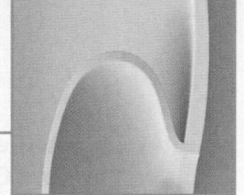

Index of Specified Content
Child 👋, Pregnancy 🤰, Elderly 🍃

Contents

CHAPTER 5

Cellular Adaptation, Injury, and Death   94

Carrie J. Merkle

CHAPTER 6

Genetic Control of Cell Function and Inheritance   112

Edward W. Carroll

CHAPTER 7

Genetic and Congenital Disorders   133

Carol M. Porth

CHAPTER 8

Neoplasia   156

Carrie J. Merkle

UNIT · III
DISORDERS OF INTEGRATIVE FUNCTION   197

CHAPTER 9

Stress and Adaptation   198
Mary Pat Kunert

CHAPTER 10

Alterations in Temperature Regulation   214
Mary Pat Kunert

CHAPTER 11

Activity Tolerance and Fatigue   231
Mary Kay Jiricka

UNIT · IV
DISORDERS OF THE HEMATOPOIETIC SYSTEM   253

CHAPTER 12

Blood Cells and the Hematopoietic System   254
Kathryn J. Gaspard

UNIT · VI

DISORDERS OF CARDIOVASCULAR FUNCTION   449

CHAPTER 25

CHAPTER 26

CHAPTER 27

CHAPTER 28

xxx   Contents

UNIT · IX

DISORDERS OF GASTROINTESTINAL FUNCTION   893

CHAPTER 36

Structure and Function of the Gastrointestinal System   894

Carol M. Porth

CHAPTER 37

Disorders of Gastrointestinal Function   916

Carol M. Porth

CHAPTER 38

Disorders of Hepatobiliary and Exocrine Pancreas Function   949

Carol M. Porth

UNIT • XIII
DISORDERS OF SPECIAL SENSORY FUNCTION   1387

CHAPTER 54

Disorders of Visual Function   1388
Edward W. Carroll, Scott A. Jens, and Robin Curtis

CHAPTER 55

Disorders of Hearing and Vestibular Function   1427
Susan A. Fontana and Carol M. Porth

UNIT • XIV
DISORDERS OF MUSCULOSKELETAL AND INTEGUMENTARY FUNCTION   1453

CHAPTER 56

Structure and Function of the Musculoskeletal System   1454
Carol M. Porth

Concepts of Health and Disease

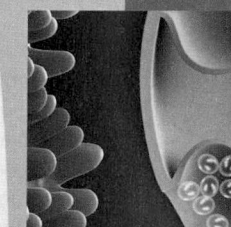

Early peoples were considered long-lived if they reached 30 years of age—that is, if they survived infancy. For many centuries, infant mortality was so great that large families became the tradition; many children in a family ensured that at least some would survive. Life expectancy has increased over the centuries, and today an individual in a developed country can expect to live about 71 to 79 years. Although life expectancy has increased radically since ancient times, human longevity has remained fundamentally unchanged.

The quest to solve the mystery of human longevity, which appears to be genetically programmed, began with Gregor Mendel (1822–1884), an Augustinian monk. Mendel laid the foundation of modern genetics with the pea experiments he performed in a monastery garden. Today, geneticists search for the determinant, or determinants, of the human life span. Up to this time, scientists have failed to identify an aging gene that would account for a limited life span. However, they have found that cells have a finite reproductive capacity. As they age, genes are increasingly unable to perform their functions. The cells become poorer and poorer at making the substances they need for their own special tasks or even for their own maintenance. Free radicals, mutation in a cell's DNA, and the process of programmed cell death are some of the factors that work together to affect a cell's functioning.

Concepts of Health and Disease

CAROL M. PORTH

➤ The term *pathophysiology,* which is the focus of this book, may be defined as the physiology of altered health. The term combines the words *pathology* and *physiology.* Pathology (from the Greek *pathos,* meaning "disease") deals with the study of the structural and functional changes in cells, tissues, and organs of the body that cause or are caused by disease. Physiology deals with the functions of the human body. Thus, pathophysiology deals not only with the cellular and organ changes that occur with disease, but with the effects that these changes have on total body function. Pathophysiology also focuses on the mechanisms of the underlying disease and provides the background for preventive as well as therapeutic health care measures and practices. This chapter is intended to orient the reader to the concepts of health and disease, various terms that are used throughout the book, the sources of data and what they mean, and the broader aspects of pathophysiology in terms of the health and well-being of populations.

CONCEPTS OF HEALTH AND DISEASE

After completing this section of the chapter, you should be able to meet the following objectives:

- State the World Health Organization definition of health.
- State a definition of pathophysiology.
- Characterize the disease process in terms of etiology, pathogenesis, morphology, clinical manifestations, and prognosis.
- Explain the meaning of reliability, validity, sensitivity, specificity, and predictive value as it relates to observations and tests used in the diagnosis of disease.

What constitutes health and disease often is difficult to determine because of the way different people view the topic. What is defined as health is determined by many factors, including heredity, age and sex, cultural and ethnic differences, as well as individual, group, and governmental expectations.

Health

In 1948, the Preamble to the Constitution of the World Health Organization (WHO) defined health as a "state of complete physical, mental, and social well-being and not merely the absence of disease and infirmity," a definition that has not been amended since that time.[1] Although ideal for many people, this was an unrealistic goal. At the World Health Assembly in 1977, representatives of the member governments of WHO agreed that their goal was to have all citizens of the world reach a level of health by the year 2000 that allows them to live a socially and economically productive life.[1] The U.S. Department of Health and Human Services in *Healthy People 2010* described the determinants of health as an interaction between an individual's biology and behavior, physical and social environments, government policies and interventions, and access to quality health care.[2]

Disease

A *disease* has been defined as an interruption, cessation, or disorder of a body system or organ structure that is characterized usually by a recognized etiologic agent or agents, an identifiable group of signs and symptoms, or consistent anatomic alterations.[3] The aspects of the disease process include etiology, pathogenesis, morphologic changes, clinical manifestations, diagnosis, and clinical course.

Etiology

The causes of disease are known as *etiologic factors*. Among the recognized etiologic agents are biologic agents (*e.g.,* bacteria, viruses), physical forces (*e.g.,* trauma, burns, radiation), chemical agents (*e.g.,* poisons, alcohol), and nutritional excesses or deficits. At the molecular level, it is important to distinguish between abnormal molecules and molecules that cause disease.[4] This is true of diseases such as cystic fibrosis, sickle cell anemia, and familial hypercholesterolemia, in which the genetic abnormality of a single amino acid, transporter molecule, or receptor protein produces widespread effects on health.

Most disease-causing agents are nonspecific, and many different agents can cause disease of a single organ. On the other hand, a single agent or traumatic event can lead to disease of a number of organs or systems. Although a disease agent can affect more than a single organ and a number of disease agents can affect the same organ, most disease states do not have a single cause. Instead, the majority of diseases are multifactorial in origin. This is particularly true of diseases such as cancer, heart disease, and diabetes. The multiple factors that predispose to a particular disease often are referred to as *risk factors.*

One way to view the factors that cause disease is to group them into categories according to whether they were present at birth or acquired later in life. *Congenital conditions* are defects that are present at birth, although they may not be evident until later in life. Congenital conditions may be caused by genetic influences, environmental factors (*e.g.,* viral infections in the mother, maternal drug use, irradiation, or intrauterine crowding), or a combination of genetic and environmental factors. *Acquired defects* are those that are caused by events that occur after birth. These include injury, exposure to infectious agents, inadequate nutrition, lack of oxygen, inappropriate immune

responses, and neoplasia. Many diseases are thought to be the result of a genetic predisposition and an environmental event or events that serve as a trigger to initiate disease development.

Pathogenesis

Pathogenesis is the sequence of cellular and tissue events that take place from the time of initial contact with an etiologic agent until the ultimate expression of a disease. Etiology describes what sets the disease process in motion, and pathogenesis, how the disease process evolves. Although the two terms often are used interchangeably, their meanings are quite different. For example, atherosclerosis often is cited as the cause or etiology of coronary heart disease. In reality, the progression from fatty streak to the occlusive vessel lesion seen in persons with coronary heart disease represents the pathogenesis of the disorder. The true etiology of atherosclerosis remains largely uncertain.

Morphology

Morphology refers to the fundamental structure or form of cells or tissues. *Morphologic changes* are concerned with both the gross anatomic and microscopic changes that are characteristic of a disease. *Histology* deals with the study of the cells and extracellular matrix of body tissues. The most common method used in the study of tissues is the preparation of histologic sections—thin, translucent sections of human tissues and organs—that can be examined with the aid of a microscope. Histologic sections play an important role in the diagnosis of many types of cancer. A *lesion* represents a pathologic or traumatic discontinuity of a body organ or tissue. Descriptions of lesion size and characteristics often can be obtained through the use of radiographs, ultrasonography, and other imaging methods. Lesions also may be sampled by biopsy and the tissue samples subjected to histologic study.

Clinical Manifestations

Diseases can manifest in a number of ways. Sometimes the condition produces manifestations, such as fever, that make it evident that the person is sick. In other cases, the condition is silent at the onset and is detected during examination for other purposes or after the disease is far advanced.

Signs and *symptoms* are terms used to describe the structural and functional changes that accompany a disease. A *symptom* is a subjective complaint that is noted by the person with a disorder, whereas a *sign* is a manifestation that is noted by an observer. Pain, difficulty in breathing, and dizziness are symptoms of a disease. An elevated temperature, a swollen extremity, and changes in pupil size are objective signs that can be observed by someone other than the person with the disease. Signs and symptoms may be related to the primary disorder or they may represent the body's attempt to compensate for the altered function caused by the pathologic condition. Many pathologic states are not observed directly—one cannot see a sick heart or a failing kidney. Instead, what can be observed is the body's attempt to compensate for changes in function brought about by the disease, such as the tachycardia that accompanies blood loss or the increased respiratory rate that occurs with pneumonia.

A *syndrome* is a compilation of signs and symptoms (*e.g.*, chronic fatigue syndrome) that are characteristic of a specific disease state. *Complications* are possible adverse extensions of a disease or outcomes from treatment. *Sequelae* are lesions or impairments that follow or are caused by a disease.

Diagnosis

A *diagnosis* is the designation as to the nature or cause of a health problem (*e.g.*, bacterial pneumonia or hemorrhagic stroke). The diagnostic process usually requires a careful history and physical examination. The history is used to obtain a person's account of his or her symptoms and their progression, and the factors that contribute to a diagnosis. The physical examination is done to observe for signs of altered body structure or function.

The development of a diagnosis involves weighing competing possibilities and selecting the most likely one from among the conditions that might be responsible for the person's clinical presentation. The clinical probability of a given disease in a person of a given age, sex, race, lifestyle, and locality often is influential in arrival at a presumptive diagnosis. Laboratory tests, radiologic studies, computed tomography (CT) scans, and other tests often are used to confirm a diagnosis.

An important factor when interpreting diagnostic test results is the determination of whether they are normal or abnormal. Is a blood count above normal, within the normal range, or below normal? What is termed a *normal* value for a laboratory test is established statistically from test results obtained from a selected sample of people. The normal values refer to the 95% distribution (mean plus or minus two standard deviations [mean ± 2 SD]) of test results for the reference population.[5,6] Thus, the normal levels for serum sodium (136 to 145 mEq/L) represent the mean serum level for the reference population ± 2 SD. The normal values for some laboratory tests are adjusted for sex or age. For example, the normal hemoglobin range for women is 12.0 to 16.0 g/dL, and for men, 14.0 to 17.4 g/dL.[7] Serum creatinine level often is adjusted for age in the elderly, and normal values for serum phosphate differ between adults and children.

The quality of data on which a diagnosis is based may be judged for their validity, reliability, sensitivity, specificity, and predictive value.[8,9] *Validity* refers to the extent to which a measurement tool measures what it is intended to measure. This often is assessed by comparing a measurement method with the best possible method of measure that is available. For example, the validity of blood pressure measurements obtained by a sphygmomanometer might be compared with those obtained by intra-arterial measurements. *Reliability* refers to the extent to which an observation, if repeated, gives the same result. A poorly calibrated blood pressure machine may give inconsistent measurements of blood pressure, particularly of pressures in either the high or low range. Reliability also depends on the persons making the measurements. For example, blood pressure measurements may vary from one observer to another because of the technique that is used (*e.g.*, different observers may deflate the cuff at a different rate, thus obtaining different

values), the way the numbers on the manometer are read, or differences in hearing acuity.

In the field of clinical laboratory measurements, *standardization* is aimed at increasing the trueness and reliability of measured values. Standardization relies on the use of written standards, reference measurement procedures, and reference materials.[10] In the United States, the Food and Drug Administration (FDA) regulates in vitro diagnostic devices, including clinical laboratory instruments, test kits, and reagents. Manufacturers who propose to market new diagnostic devices must submit information on their instrument, test kit, or reagent to the FDA, as required by existing statutes and regulations. The FDA reviews this information to decide whether the product may be marketed in the United States.

Measures of sensitivity and specificity are concerned with determining how likely or how well the test or observation will identify people with the disease and people without the disease[11] (Fig. 1-1). *Sensitivity* refers to the proportion of people with a disease who are positive for that disease on a given test or observation (called a *true-positive* result). If the result of a very sensitive test is negative, it tells us the person does not have the disease and the disease has been excluded or "ruled out." *Specificity* refers to the proportion of people without the disease who are negative on a given test or observation (called a *true-negative* result). Specificity can be calculated only from among people who do not have the disease. A test that is 95% specific correctly identifies 95 of 100 normal people. The other 5% are *false-positive* results. A false-positive test result can be unduly stressful for the person being tested, whereas a *false-negative* test result can delay diagnosis and jeopardize the outcome of treatment.

Predictive value is the extent to which an observation or test result is able to predict the presence of a given disease or condition.[11,12] A *positive predictive value* refers to the proportion of true-positive results that occurs in a given population. In a group of women found to have "suspect breast nodules" in a cancer screening program, the proportion later determined to have breast cancer would constitute the positive predictive value. A *negative predictive value* refers to the true-negative

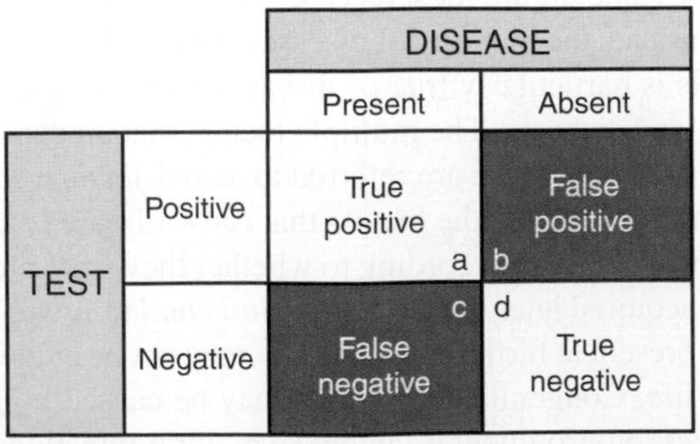

		DISEASE	
		Present	Absent
TEST	Positive	True positive a	False positive b
	Negative	False negative c	True negative d

FIGURE 1-1 • The relationship between a diagnostic test result and the occurrence of disease. There are two possibilities for the test result to be correct (true positive and true negative) and two possibilities for the result to be incorrect (false positive and false negative). (From Fletcher R. H., Fletcher S. W. [2005]. *Clinical epidemiology: The essentials* [4th ed., p. 36]. Philadelphia: Lippincott Williams & Wilkins.)

observations in a population. In a screening test for breast cancer, the negative predictive value represents the proportion of women without suspect nodules who do not have breast cancer. Although predictive values rely in part on sensitivity and specificity, they depend more heavily on the prevalence of the condition in the population. Despite unchanging sensitivity and specificity, the positive predictive value of an observation rises with prevalence, whereas the negative predictive value falls.

Clinical Course

The clinical course describes the evolution of a disease. A disease can have an acute, subacute, or chronic course. An *acute disorder* is one that is relatively severe, but self-limiting. *Chronic disease* implies a continuous, long-term process. A chronic disease can run a continuous course or can present with exacerbations (aggravation of symptoms and severity of the disease) and remissions (a period during which there is a decrease in severity and symptoms). *Subacute disease* is intermediate or between acute and chronic: it is not as severe as an acute disease and not as prolonged as a chronic disease.

The spectrum of disease severity for infectious diseases, such as hepatitis B, can range from preclinical to persistent chronic infection. During the *preclinical stage,* the disease is not clinically evident but is destined to progress to clinical disease. As with hepatitis B, it is possible to transmit a virus during the preclinical stage. *Subclinical disease* is not clinically apparent and is not destined to become clinically apparent. It is diagnosed with antibody or culture tests. Most cases of tuberculosis are not clinically apparent, and evidence of their presence is established by skin tests. *Clinical disease* is manifested by signs and symptoms. A persistent chronic infectious disease persists for years, sometimes for life. *Carrier status* refers to an individual who harbors an organism but is not infected, as evidenced by antibody response or clinical manifestations. This person still can infect others. Carrier status may be of limited duration or it may be chronic, lasting for months or years.

IN SUMMARY,   the term *pathophysiology,* which is the focus of this book, may be defined as the physiology of altered health. A *disease* has been defined as any deviation from or interruption of the normal structure or function of any part, organ, or system of the body that is manifested by a characteristic set of symptoms or signs and whose etiology, pathology, and prognosis may be known or unknown. The causes of disease are known as *etiologic factors. Pathogenesis* describes how the disease process evolves. *Morphology* refers to the structure or form of cells or tissues; *morphologic changes* are changes in structure or form that are characteristic of a disease.

A disease can manifest in a number ways. A *symptom* is a subjective complaint, such as pain or dizziness, whereas a *sign* is an observable manifestation, such as an elevated temperature or a reddened, sore throat. A *syndrome* is a compilation of signs and symptoms that are characteristic of a specific disease state.

A *diagnosis* is the designation as to the nature and cause of a health problem. The diagnostic process requires a careful history and physical examination. Laboratory tests, radiologic studies (*e.g.,* CT scans), and other tests are used to confirm a diagnosis. The value of many tests is based on their reliability and validity, as well as their sensitivity and specificity.

The *clinical course* of a disease describes its evolution. It can be acute (relatively severe, but self-limiting), chronic (continuous or episodic, but taking place over a long period), or subacute (not as severe as acute or as prolonged as chronic). Within the disease spectrum, a disease can be designated preclinical, or not clinically evident; subclinical, not clinically apparent and not destined to become clinically apparent; or clinical, characterized by signs and symptoms. ∎

HEALTH AND DISEASE IN POPULATIONS

After completing this section of the chapter, you should be able to meet the following objectives:

- Define the term *epidemiology.*
- Compare the meaning of the terms *incidence* and *prevalence* as they relate to measures of disease frequency.
- Compare the sources of information and limitations of mortality and morbidity statistics.
- Characterize the natural history of a disease.
- Differentiate primary, secondary, and tertiary levels of prevention.
- Propose ways in which practice guidelines can be used to improve health care.

The health of individuals is closely linked to the health of the community and to the population it encompasses. The ability to traverse continents in a matter of hours has opened the world to issues of populations at a global level. Diseases that once were confined to local areas of the world now pose a threat to populations throughout the world.

As we move through the 21st century, we are continually reminded that the health care system and the services it delivers are targeted to particular populations. Managed care systems are focused on a population-based approach to planning, delivering, providing, and evaluating health care. The focus of health care also has begun to emerge as a partnership in which individuals are asked to assume greater responsibility for their own health.

Epidemiology and Patterns of Disease

Epidemiology is the study of disease occurrence in human populations.[11] It was initially developed to explain the spread of infectious diseases during epidemics and has emerged as a science to study risk factors for multifactorial diseases, such as heart disease and cancer. Epidemiology looks for patterns of persons affected with a particular disorder, such as age, race, dietary habits, lifestyle, or geographic location. In contrast to biomedical researchers, who seek to elucidate the mechanisms of disease production, epidemiologists are more concerned with whether something happens than how it happens. For example, the epidemiologist is more concerned with whether smoking itself is related to cardiovascular disease and whether the risk of heart disease decreases when smoking ceases. On the other hand, the biomedical researcher is more concerned about the causative agent in cigarette smoke and the pathway by which it contributes to heart disease.

Much of our knowledge about disease comes from epidemiologic studies. Epidemiologic methods are used to determine how a disease is spread, how to control it, how to prevent it, and how to eliminate it. Epidemiologic methods also are used to study the natural history of disease, to evaluate new preventative and treatment strategies, to explore the impact of different patterns of health care delivery, and to predict future health care needs. As such, epidemiologic studies serve as a basis for clinical decision making, allocation of health care dollars, and development of policies related to public health issues.

Prevalence and Incidence

Measures of disease frequency are an important aspect of epidemiology. They establish a means for predicting what diseases are present in a population and provide an indication of the rate at which they are increasing or decreasing. A *disease case* can be either an existing case or the number of new episodes of a particular illness that is diagnosed within a given period. *Incidence* reflects the number of new cases arising in a population at risk during a specified time. The population at risk is considered to be persons without the disease but who are at risk for developing it. It is determined by dividing the number of new cases of a disease by the population at risk for development of the disease during the same period (*e.g.,* new cases per 1000 or 100,000 persons in the population who are at risk). The cumulative incidence estimates the risk of developing the disease during that period of time. *Prevalence* is a measure of existing disease in a population at a given point in time (*e.g.,* number of existing cases divided by the current population).[11] The prevalence is not an estimate of risk of developing a disease because it is a function of both new cases and how long the cases remain in the population. Incidence and prevalence are always reported as rates (*e.g.,* cases per 100 or cases per 100,000).

Morbidity and Mortality

Morbidity and mortality statistics provide information about the functional effects (morbidity) and death-producing (mortality) characteristics of a disease. These statistics are useful in terms of anticipating health care needs, planning of public education programs, directing health research efforts, and allocating health care dollars.

Mortality statistics provide information about the causes of death in a given population. In most countries, people are legally required to record certain facts such as age, sex, and cause of death on a death certificate. Internationally agreed on classification procedures (the International Classification of Diseases [ICD] by the WHO) are used for coding the cause of death, and the data are expressed as death rates.[1] Crude mortality rates (*i.e.,* number of deaths in a given period) do not account for age, sex, race, socioeconomic status, and other factors. For this reason, mortality often is expressed as death rates for a specific population, such as the infant mortality rate. Mortality also can be described in terms of the leading causes of death according to age, sex, race, and ethnicity. Among all persons 65 years of age and older, the five leading causes of death in the United States are heart disease, malignant disease, cerebrovascular disease, chronic lower respiratory disease, and Alzheimer disease.[13]

Morbidity describes the effects an illness has on a person's life. Many diseases, such as arthritis, have low death rates but a significant impact on a person's life. Morbidity is concerned not only with the occurrence or incidence of a disease but with persistence and the long-term consequences of the disease.

Determination of Risk Factors

Conditions suspected of contributing to the development of a disease are called *risk factors*. They may be inherent to the person (high blood pressure or overweight) or external (smoking or drinking alcohol). There are different types of studies used to determine risk factors, including cross-sectional studies, case-control studies, and cohort studies.

Cross-Sectional and Case-Control Studies

Cross-sectional studies use the simultaneous collection of information necessary for classification of exposure and outcome status. They can be used to compare the prevalence of a disease in those with the factor (or exposure) with the prevalence of a disease in those who are unexposed to the factor, such as the prevalence of coronary heart disease in smokers and nonsmokers. *Case-control studies* are designed to compare persons known to have the outcome of interest (*cases*) and those known not to have the outcome of interest (*controls*).[11] Information on exposures or characteristics of interest is then collected from persons in both groups. For example, the characteristics of maternal alcohol consumption in infants born with fetal alcohol syndrome (cases) can be compared with those in infants born without the syndrome (controls).

Cohort Studies

A *cohort* is a group of persons who were born at approximately the same time or share some characteristics of interest.[11] Persons enrolled in a cohort study (also called a *longitudinal study*) are followed over a period of time to observe a specific health outcome. A cohort may consist of a single group of persons chosen because they have or have not been exposed to suspected risk factors; two groups specifically selected because one has been exposed and the other has not; or a single exposed group in which the results are compared with the general population.

Framingham Study. One of the best-known examples of a cohort study is the Framingham Study, which was carried out in Framingham, Massachusetts.[14] Framingham was selected because of the size of the population, the relative ease with which the people could be contacted, and the stability of the population in terms of moving into and out of the area. This longitudinal study, which began in 1950, was set up by the U.S. Public Health Service to study the characteristics of people who would later develop coronary heart disease. The study consisted of 5000 persons, aged 30 to 59 years, selected at random and followed for an initial period of 20 years, during which time it was predicted that 1500 of them would develop coronary heart disease. The advantage of such a study is that it can explore a number of risk factors at the same time and determine the relative importance of each. Another advantage is that the risk factors can be related later to other diseases such as stroke. Chart 1-1 describes some of the significant milestones from the Framingham Study.

CHART 1-1   FRAMINGHAM STUDY: SIGNIFICANT MILESTONES

- 1960—Cigarette smoking found to increase risk of heart disease
- 1961—Cholesterol level, blood pressure, and electrocardiogram abnormalities found to increase risk of heart disease
- 1967—Physical activity found to reduce risk of heart disease and obesity to increase risk of heart disease
- 1970—High blood pressure found to increase risk of stroke
- 1976—Menopause found to increase risk of heart disease
- 1977—Effects of triglycerides and low-density lipoprotein (LDL) and high-density lipoprotein (HDL) cholesterol noted
- 1978—Psychosocial factors found to affect heart disease
- 1986—First report on dementia
- 1988—High levels of HDL cholesterol found to reduce risk of death
- 1994—Enlarged left ventricle shown to increase risk of stroke
- 1996—Progression from hypertension to heart failure described
- 1997—Report of cumulative effects of smoking and high cholesterol on the risk of atherosclerosis

(Abstracted from Framingham Heart Study. [2001]. Research milestones. [Online.] Available: http://www.nhlbi.nih.gov/about/framingham.)

Nurses' Health Study. A second well-known cohort study is the Nurses' Health Study, which was developed by Harvard University and Brigham and Women's Hospital. The study began in 1976 with a cohort of 121,700 female nurses, 30 to 55 years of age, living in the United States.[15] Initially designed to explore the relationship between oral contraceptives and breast cancer, nurses in the study have provided answers to detailed questions about their menstrual cycle, smoking habits, diet, weight and waist measurements, activity patterns, health problems, and medication use. They have collected urine and blood samples, and even provided researchers with their toenail clippings. In selecting the cohort, it was reasoned that nurses would be well organized, accurate, and observant in their responses, and that physiologically they would be no different from other groups of women. It also was anticipated that their childbearing, eating, and smoking patterns would be similar to those of other working women.

Natural History

The *natural history* of a disease refers to the progression and projected outcome of the disease without medical intervention. By studying the patterns of a disease over time in populations, epidemiologists can better understand its natural history. Knowledge of the natural history can be used to determine disease outcome, establish priorities for health care services, determine the effects of screening and early detection programs on disease outcome, and compare the results of new treatments with the expected outcome without treatment.

There are some diseases for which there are no effective treatment methods available, or the current treatment measures are effective only in certain people. In this case, the natural history of the disease can be used as a predictor of outcome. For example, the natural history of hepatitis C indicates that 80% of people who become infected with the virus fail to clear the virus and progress to chronic infection.[16] Information about the natural history of a disease and the availability of effective treatment methods provides directions for preventive measures. In the case of hepatitis C, careful screening of blood donations and education of intravenous drug abusers can be used to prevent transfer of the virus. At the same time, scientists are striving to develop a vaccine that will prevent infection in persons exposed to the virus. The development of vaccines to prevent the spread of infectious diseases such as polio and hepatitis B undoubtedly has been motivated by knowledge about the natural history of these diseases and the lack of effective intervention measures. With other diseases, such as breast cancer, early detection through use of breast self-examination and mammography increases the chances for a cure.

Prognosis refers to the probable outcome and prospect of recovery from a disease. It can be designated as chances for full recovery, possibility of complications, or anticipated survival time. Prognosis often is presented in relation to treatment options—that is, the expected outcomes or chances for survival with or without a certain type of treatment. The prognosis associated with a given type of treatment usually is presented along with the risk associated with the treatment.

Levels of Prevention

Basically, leading a healthy life contributes to the prevention of disease. There are three fundamental types of prevention: primary prevention, secondary prevention, and tertiary prevention[11,17] (Fig. 1-2). It is important to note that all three levels are aimed at prevention.

Primary prevention is directed at keeping disease from occurring by removing all risk factors. Examples of primary prevention include the administration of folic acid to pregnant women and women who may become pregnant to prevent fetal neural tube defects, giving immunizations to children to prevent communicable disease, and counseling people to adopt healthy lifestyles as a means of preventing heart disease.[11] Primary prevention is often accomplished outside the health care system at the community level. Some primary prevention measures are mandated by law (*e.g.,* wearing seat belts in automobiles and helmet use on motorcycles). Other primary prevention activities (*e.g.,* use of ear plugs or dust masks) occur in specific occupations.

Secondary prevention detects disease early when it is still asymptomatic and treatment measures can effect a cure or stop it from progressing. The use of a Papanicolaou (Pap) smear for early detection of cervical cancer is an example of secondary prevention. Screening also includes history taking (asking if a person smokes), physical examination (blood pressure measurement), laboratory tests (cholesterol level determination), and other procedures (colonoscopy) that can be "applied reasonably rapidly to asymptomatic people."[11] Most secondary prevention is done in clinical settings. All types of health care professionals (*e.g.,* physicians, nurses, dentists, audiologists, optometrists) participate in secondary prevention.

Tertiary prevention is directed at clinical interventions that prevent further deterioration or reduce the complications of a disease once it has been diagnosed. An example is the use of β-adrenergic drugs to reduce the risk of death in persons

who have had a heart attack. The boundaries of tertiary prevention go beyond treating the problem with which the person presents. In persons with diabetes, for example, tertiary prevention requires more than good glucose control—it includes provision for regular ophthalmologic examinations for early detection of retinopathy, education for good foot care, and treatment for other cardiovascular risk factors such as hyperlipidemia.[11] Tertiary prevention measures also include measures to limit physical impairment and the social consequences of an illness. Most tertiary prevention programs are located within health care systems and involve the services of a number of different types of health care professionals.

Evidence-Based Practice and Practice Guidelines

Evidence-based practice and evidence-based practice guidelines have recently gained popularity with clinicians, public health practitioners, health care organizations, and the public as a means of improving the quality and efficiency of health care.[18] Their development has been prompted, at least in part, by the enormous amount of published information about diagnostic and treatment measures for various disease conditions, as well as demands for better and more cost-effective health care.

Evidence-based practice has been defined as "the conscientious, explicit, and judicious use of current best evidence in making decisions about the care of individual patients."[18] It is based on the integration of the individual expertise of the practitioner with the best external clinical evidence from systematic research.[18] The term *clinical expertise* implies the proficiency and judgment that individual clinicians gain through clinical experience and clinical practice. The best external clinical evidence relies on the identification of clinically relevant research, often from the basic sciences, but especially from patient-centered clinical studies that focus on the accuracy and precision of diagnostic tests and methods, the power of prognostic indicators, and the effectiveness and safety of therapeutic, rehabilitative, and preventive regimens.

Clinical practice guidelines are systematically developed statements intended to inform practitioners and clients in making decisions about health care for specific clinical circumstances.[19,20] They not only should review but must weigh various outcomes, both positive and negative, and make recommendations. Guidelines are different from systematic reviews. They can take the form of algorithms, which are step-by-step methods for solving a problem, written directives for care, or a combination thereof.

The development of evidence-based practice guidelines often uses methods such as meta-analysis to combine evidence from different studies to produce a more precise estimate of the accuracy of a diagnostic method or the effects of an intervention method.[21] It also requires review: by practitioners with expertise in clinical content, who can verify the completeness of the literature review and ensure clinical sensibility; from experts in guideline development who can examine the method

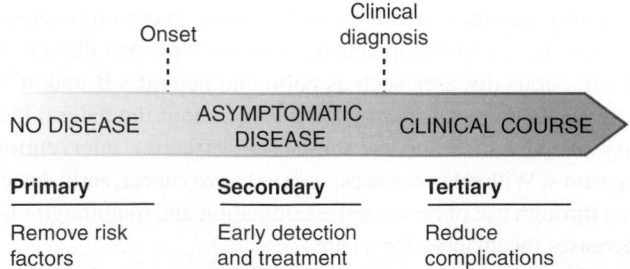

FIGURE 1-2 • Levels of prevention. Primary prevention prevents disease from occurring. Secondary prevention detects and cures disease in the asymptomatic phase. Tertiary prevention reduces complications of disease. (From Fletcher R. H., Fletcher S. W. [2005]. *Clinical epidemiology: The essentials* [4th ed., p. 149]. Philadelphia: Lippincott Williams & Wilkins.)

by which the guideline was developed; and by potential users of the guideline.[19]

Once developed, practice guidelines must be continually reviewed and changed to keep pace with new research findings and new diagnostic and treatment methods. For example, the Guidelines for the Prevention, Evaluation, and Treatment of High Blood Pressure (see Chapter 23), first developed in 1972 by the Joint National Committee, have been revised seven times, and the Guidelines for the Diagnosis and Management of Asthma (see Chapter 29), first developed in 1991 by the Expert Panel, have undergone three revisions.

Evidence-based practice guidelines, which are intended to direct client care, are also important in directing research into the best methods of diagnosing and treating specific health problems. This is because health care providers use the same criteria for diagnosing the extent and severity of a particular condition such as hypertension, and because they use the same protocols for treatment.

ible research studies. Practice guidelines may take the form of algorithms, which are step-by-step methods for solving a problem, written directives, or a combination thereof. ■

CONCEPTSin action **ANIMATION**

References

1. World Health Organization. (2007). About WHO: Definition of health; disease eradication/elimination goals. [Online.] Available: www.who.int/about/definition/en/. Accessed September 16, 2007.
2. U.S. Department Health and Human Services. (2000). Healthy people 2010. National Health Information Center. [Online.] Available: www.healthypeople.gov. Accessed September 16, 2007.
3. *Stedman's medical dictionary.* (2006). (28th ed., p. 855). Philadelphia: Lippincott Williams & Wilkins.
4. Waldenstrom J. (1989). Sick molecules and our concepts of illness. *Journal of Internal Medicine* 225, 221–227.
5. Brigden M. L., Heathcote J. C. (2000). Problems with interpreting laboratory tests. *Postgraduate Medicine* 107(7), 145–162.
6. Mayer D. (2004). *Essentials of evidence-based medicine.* New York: Cambridge University Press.
7. Fischbach F. (2004). *A manual of laboratory and diagnostic tests* (7th ed., p. 74, 964). Philadelphia: Lippincott Williams & Wilkins.
8. Bickley L. (2003). *Bates' guide to physical assessment and history taking* (6th ed., pp. 641–642). Philadelphia: J. B. Lippincott.
9. Dawson B., Trapp R. G., Trapp R. (2004). *Basic and clinical biostatistics.* New York: Lange Medical Books/McGraw-Hill.
10. Michaud G. Y. (2005). The role of standards in the development and implementation of clinical laboratory tests: A domestic and global perspective. *Cancer Biomarkers* 1, 209–216.
11. Fletcher R. H., Fletcher S. W. (2005). *Clinical epidemiology: The essentials* (4th ed.). Philadelphia: Lippincott Williams & Wilkins.
12. Montori V. M., Wyer P., Newman T. B., et al. (2005). Tips for learning of evidence-based medicine: 5. The effect of spectrum of disease on performance of diagnostic tests. *Canadian Medical Association Journal* 173, 385–390.
13. Centers for Disease Control and Prevention. (2003). Death, percent of deaths, and death rates for 15 leading causes of death in selected age groups by race and sex: United States 1999. [Online]. Available: www.cdc.gov/nchs/data/hestat/preliminarydeaths05_tables.pdf#C. Accessed September 16, 2007.
14. Framingham Heart Study. (2001). Framingham Heart Study: Design, rationale, objectives, and research milestones. [Online]. Available: www.nhlbi.nih.gov/about/framingham/design.htm. Accessed September 16, 2007.
15. Channing Laboratory. (2007). Nurses' Health Study. [Online]. Available: www.channing.harvard.edu/nhs/publications/2005.shtml. Accessed September 16, 2007.
16. Liang J., Reherman B., Seeff L. B., et al. (2000). Pathogenesis, natural history, treatment, and prevention of hepatitis C. *Annals of Internal Medicine* 132, 296–305.
17. Stanhope M., Lancaster J. (2000). *Community and public health nursing* (5th ed., p. 43). St. Louis: Mosby.
18. Sackett D. L. (1996). Evidence based medicine: What it is and what it isn't. *British Medical Journal* 312, 71–72.
19. Shekelle P. G., Woolff S. H., Eccles M., et al. (1999). Developing guidelines. *British Medical Journal* 318, 593–596.
20. Natsch S., van der Meer J. W. M. (2003). The role of clinical guidelines, policies, and stewardship. *Journal of Hospital Infection* 53, 172–176.
21. Acton G. J. (2001). Meta-analysis: A tool for evidence-based practice. *AACN Clinical Issues* 12, 539–545.

IN SUMMARY, *epidemiology* refers to the study of disease in populations. It looks for patterns such as age, race, and dietary habits of persons who are affected with a particular disorder to determine under what circumstances the particular disorder will occur. *Incidence* is the number of new cases arising in a given population during a specified time. *Prevalence* is the number of people in a population who have a particular disease at a given point in time or period. Incidence and prevalence are reported as proportions or rates (*e.g.,* cases per 100 or 100,000 population). *Mortality* or death statistics provide information about the trends in the health of a population, whereas *morbidity* describes the effects an illness has on a person's life. It is concerned with the incidence of disease as well as its persistence and long-term consequences.

Conditions suspected of contributing to the development of a disease are called *risk factors*. Studies used to determine risk factors include cross-sectional studies, case-control studies, and cohort studies. The *natural history* refers to the progression and projected outcome of a disease without medical intervention. *Prognosis* is the term used to designate the probable outcome and prospect of recovery from a disease.

The three fundamental types of prevention are primary prevention, secondary prevention, and tertiary prevention. *Primary prevention,* such as immunizations, is directed at removing risk factors so disease does not occur. *Secondary prevention,* such as a Pap smear, detects disease when it still is asymptomatic and curable with treatment. *Tertiary prevention,* such as use of β-adrenergic drugs to reduce the risk of death in persons who have had a heart attack, focuses on clinical interventions that prevent further deterioration or reduce the complications of a disease.

Evidence-based practice and *evidence-based practice guidelines* are mechanisms that use the current best evidence to make decisions about the health care of individuals. They are based on the expertise of the individual practitioner integrated with the best clinical evidence from systematic review of credible

Visit the**Point** http://thePoint.lww.com for animations, journal articles, and more!

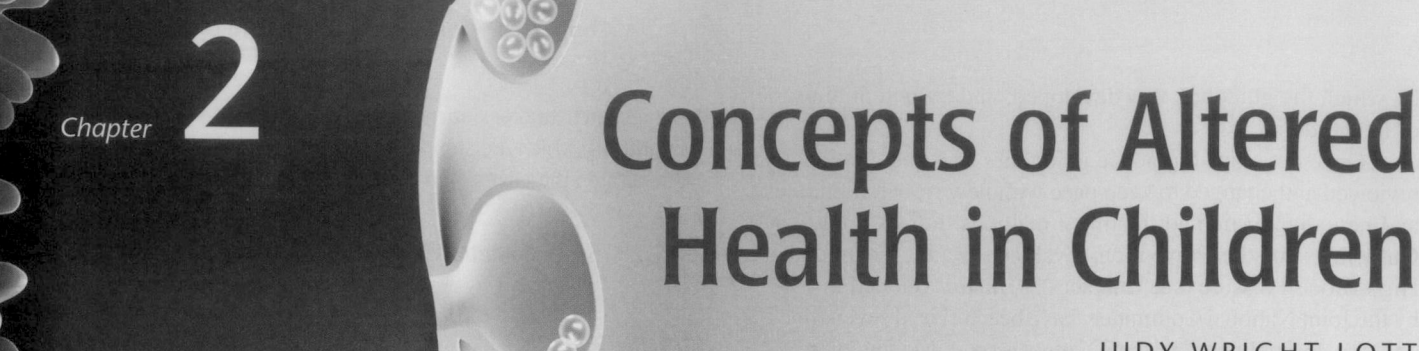

Chapter 2

Concepts of Altered Health in Children

JUDY WRIGHT LOTT

➤ Children are not miniature adults. Physical and psychological maturation and development strongly influence the type of illnesses children experience and their responses to these illnesses. Although many signs and symptoms are the same in persons of all ages, some diseases and complications are more likely to occur in the child. This chapter provides an overview of the developmental stages of childhood and the related health care needs of children. Specific diseases are presented in the different chapters throughout the book.

At the beginning of the 20th century the infant mortality rate was 200 deaths per 1000 live births.[1] Infectious diseases were rampant, and children, with their immature and inexperienced immune systems and their frequent exposure to other infected children, were especially vulnerable. With the introduction of antimicrobial agents, infectious disease control, and nutritional and technologic advances, infant mortality decreased dramatically. Although infant mortality in the United States has declined over past decades, the record low of 6.8 infant deaths per 1000 live births in 2004 was higher than that of many other industrialized countries in the world.[2] Also of concern is the difference in mortality rates for white and nonwhite infants. Black non-Hispanic and American Indian/Alaska Native infants have consistently had a higher mortality rate than those of other racial or ethnic groups. The greatest disparity exists for black non-Hispanics, whose infant death rate was 13.6 per 1000 in 2004.[2]

One of the more perplexing causes of infant mortality is the incidence of preterm birth among women of all races and classes. Despite continued, gradual declines in the overall infant mortality rate during the latter part of the 20th century, the incidence of premature births continues to present a challenge to reducing the racial disparities in infant mortality rates, as well as the overall incidence of infant mortality. The percentage of infants born with very low birth weight (<1500 g) has increased gradually in recent years. One reason for the increase in children born with low birth weight is that the number of twin, triplet, and higher-order multiple births has increased.[2]

GROWTH AND DEVELOPMENT

After completing this section of the chapter, you should be able to meet the following objectives:

■ Characterize the use of percentiles to describe growth and development during infancy and childhood.

■ Describe the major events that occur during prenatal development from fertilization to birth.

■ Define the terms *low birth weight, small for gestational age,* and *large for gestational age.*

■ Identify reasons for abnormal intrauterine growth.

■ Describe assessment methods for determination of gestational age.

The terms *growth* and *development* describe a process whereby a fertilized ovum becomes an adult person. *Physical growth* describes changes in the body as a whole or in its individual parts. *Development,* on the other hand, embraces other aspects of growth, such as changes in body function and psychosocial behaviors.

The first year of life is a period of rapid growth demonstrated by lengthening of the trunk and deposition of subcutaneous fat.[3] After the first year until the onset of puberty, the legs grow more rapidly than any other part of the body. The onset of puberty is marked by significant alterations in body proportions because of the effects of the pubertal growth spurt. The feet and hands are the first to grow. Because the trunk grows faster than the legs, at adolescence a large portion of the increase in height is a result of trunk growth.[4]

Normal children follow a trajectory of increasing linear growth and body weight. Linear growth is a result of skeletal growth. After maturation of the skeleton is complete, linear growth is complete. By 2 years of age, the length is 50% of the adult height. Beginning with the third year, the growth rate is 5 to 6 cm for the next 9 years. A growth spurt during adolescence is necessary for adult height to be reached. Males add approximately 20 cm and females 16 cm to height during this time. Weight rapidly increases after birth. Generally by 6 months of age the birth weight has doubled, and by 1 year of age it has tripled. The average weight increase is 2 to 2.75 kg per year until the adolescent growth spurt begins.[3] The head also increases in size, reflecting brain growth. A child achieves 50% of his or her brain size by 1 year of age and 90% by 5 years.[3] Growth charts provide an overview of the normal growth trajectory of children, thus alerting parents and health professionals to what is atypical or disturbed[5] (Fig. 2-1).

Growth and development encompass a complex interaction between genetic and environmental influences. The experience of each child is unique, and the patterns of growth and development may be profoundly different for individual children within the context of what is considered *normal.* Because of the wide variability, these norms often can be expressed only in statistical terms.

Evaluation of growth and development requires comparison of an individual's growth and development with a standard. Statistics are calculations derived from measurements that are used to describe the sample measured or to make predictions about the rest of the population represented by the sample. Because all individuals grow and develop at different rates, the standard must somehow take this individual variation into account. The standard typically is derived from measurements made on a sample of individuals deemed representative of the total population. When multiple measurements of biologic variables such as height, weight, head circumference, and blood pressure are made, most values fall around the center or middle of all the values. Plotting the data on a graph yields a bell-shaped curve, which depicts the normal distribution of these continuously variable values.

The mean and standard deviation are common statistics used in describing the characteristics of a population. The mean represents the average of the measurements; it is the sum of the values divided by the number of values. A normal bell-shaped curve is symmetric, with the mean falling in the center of the curve and one half of the values falling on either side of the mean. The standard deviation determines how far a value varies or deviates from the mean. The points one standard deviation above and below the mean include 68% of all values, two standard deviations 95% of all values, and three standard deviations 99.7% of all values.[3] If a child's height is within one standard deviation of the mean, he or she is as tall as 68% of children in the population. If a child's height is greater than three standard deviations above the mean, he or she is taller than 99.7% of children in the population.

The bell-shaped curve can also be marked by percentiles, which are useful for comparison of an individual's values with other values. When quantitative data are arranged in ascending and descending order, a middle value called the *median* can be described, with one half (50%) of the values falling on either side. The values can be further divided into percentiles. A percentile is a number that indicates the percentage of values for the population that are equal to or below the number. Percentiles are used most often to compare an individual's value with a set of norms. They are used extensively to develop and interpret physical growth charts and measurements of ability and intelligence.

Prenatal Growth and Development

Human development is considered to begin with fertilization, the union of sperm and ovum resulting in a zygote (Fig. 2-2). The process begins with the intermingling of a haploid number of paternal (23, X or Y) and maternal (23, X) chromosomes in the ampulla of the oviduct that fuse to form a zygote.[6,7] Within 24 hours, the unicellular organism becomes a two-cell organism and, within 72 hours, a 16-cell organism called a *morula.* This series of mitotic divisions is called *cleavage.* During cleavage, the rapidly developing cell mass travels down the oviduct to the uterus by a series of peristaltic movements. Shortly after entering the uterus (about 4 days after fertilization), the morula is separated into two parts by fluid from the

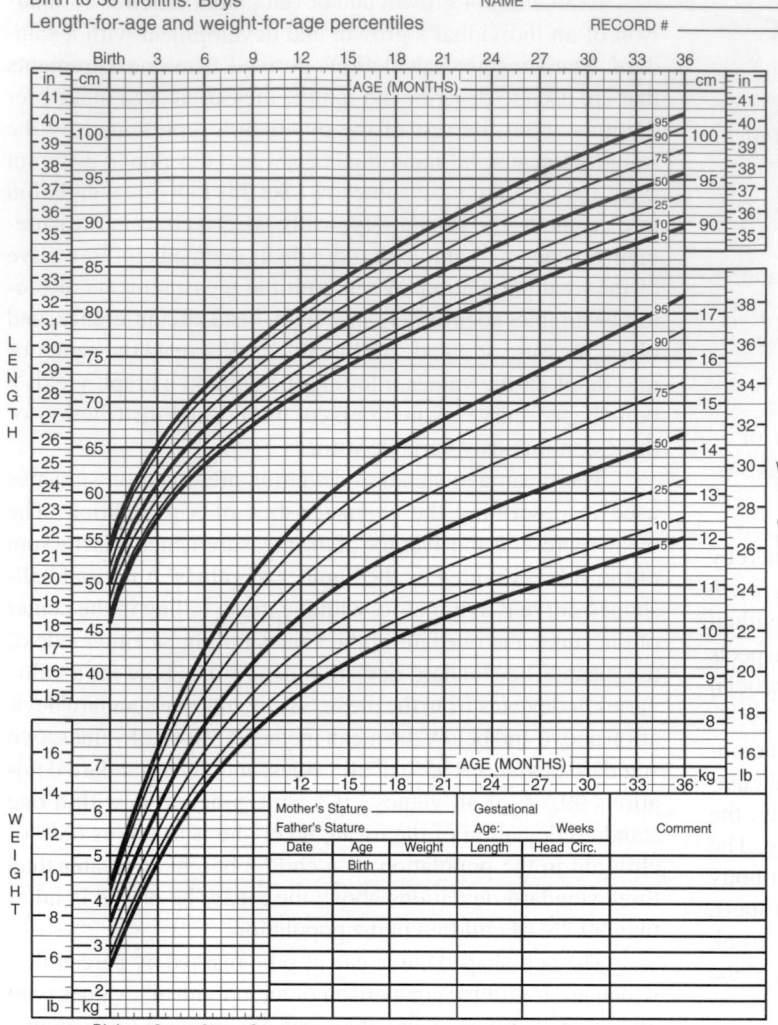

Birth to 36 months: Boys
Length-for-age and weight-for-age percentiles

NAME _____

RECORD # _____

FIGURE 2-1 • Percentile standards for length and weight in boys, birth to age 36 months. Similar charts are available for girls, for head circumference, and for different ages. (From Centers for Disease Control and Prevention. [Online.] Available: www.cdc.gov/growthcharts/.)

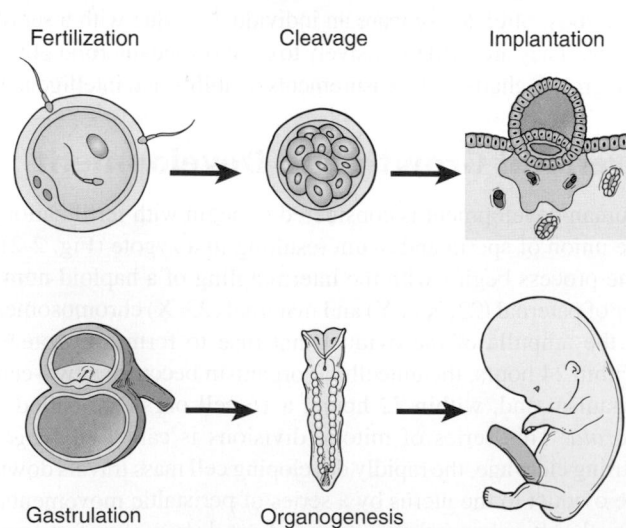

FIGURE 2-2 • Milestones in embryonic development.

uterus. The outer layer gives rise to the placenta (trophoblast), and the inner layer gives rise to the embryo (embryoblast). The structure is now called a *blastocyst*. By the sixth day the blastocyst attaches to the endometrium. This is the beginning of *implantation,* and it is completed during the second week of development.[8]

Prenatal development is divided into two main periods. The first, or *embryonic period,* begins during the second week and continues through the eighth week after fertilization.[7,8] During the embryonic period, the main organ systems are developed and many function at a minimal level (see Chapter 4). The second, or *fetal period,* begins during the ninth week. During the fetal period, the growth and differentiation of the body and organ systems occur.

Embryonic Development

Embryonic development progresses through three stages.[6] During the first stage, growth occurs through an increase in cell numbers and the elaboration of cell products. The second stage is one of morphogenesis (development of form), which includes massive cell movement. During this stage, the movement of cells allows them to interact with each other in the formation of tissues and organs. The third stage is the stage of differentiation or maturation of physiologic processes. Completion of differentiation results in organs that are capable of performing specialized functions.

Embryonic development begins during the second week of gestation with implantation of the *blastocyst*. As implantation of the blastocyst progresses, a small space appears in the embryoblast, which is the primordium of the amniotic cavity. Concurrently, morphologic changes occur in the embryoblast that result in formation of a flat, almost circular bilaminar plate of cells called the *embryonic disk*. The embryonic disk, which forms the embryo proper, gives rise to all three germ layers of the embryo (*i.e.,* ectoderm, mesoderm, endoderm). The third week is a period of rapid development, noted for the conversion of the bilaminar embryonic disk into a trilaminar embryonic disk through a process called *gastrulation*[6-8] (see Fig. 2-2). The ectoderm differentiates into the epidermis and nervous system, and the endoderm gives rise to the epithelial linings of the respiratory passages, digestive tract, and glandular cells of organs such as the liver and pancreas (see Chapter 4, Fig. 4-16). The mesoderm becomes smooth muscle tissue, connective tissue, blood vessels, blood cells, bone marrow, skeletal tissue, striated muscle tissue, and reproductive and excretory organs.

The notochord, which is the primitive axis about which the axial skeleton forms, is also formed during the third week (see Chapter 48, Fig. 48-7). The neurologic system begins its development during this period. *Neurulation,* a process that involves formation of the neural plate, neural folds, and their closure, is completed by the fourth week.[6,7] Disturbances during this period can result in brain and spinal defects such as spina bifida (see Fig. 48-9). The cardiovascular system is the first functional organ system to develop. The primitive heart, which beats and circulates blood, develops during this period (see Chapter 24, Fig. 24-22).

By the fourth week, the neural tube is formed. The embryo begins to curve and fold into a characteristic "C"-shaped structure. The limb buds are visible, as are the otic pits (*i.e.,* primordia of the internal ears) and the lens placodes (primordia of the crystalline lenses). The fifth week is notable for the rapid growth of the head secondary to brain growth.

During the sixth week, the upper limbs are formed by fusion of the swellings around the branchial groove. In the seventh week, there is the beginning of the digits, and the intestines enter the umbilical cord (umbilical herniation). By the eighth week, the embryo is human-like in appearance—eyes are open, and eyelids and ear auricles are easily identified.

Fetal Development

The fetal period extends from the ninth week to birth.[6-8] During the 9th to 12th weeks, fetal head growth slows, whereas body length growth is greatly accelerated. By the 11th week, the intestines in the proximal portion of the cord have returned to the abdomen. The primary ossification centers are present in the

skull and long bones, and maturation of the fetal external genitalia is established by the 12th week. During the fetal period, the liver is the major site of red blood cell formation (*i.e.,* erythropoiesis); at 12 weeks, this activity has decreased and erythropoiesis begins in the spleen. Urine begins to form during the 9th to 12th weeks and is excreted into the amniotic fluid.[8]

The 13th through 16th weeks are notable for ossification of the skeleton, scalp hair patterning, and differentiation of the ovaries in female fetuses.[6] By the 17th through 20th week, growth has slowed. The fetal skin is covered with a fine hair called *lanugo* and a white, cheeselike material called *vernix caseosa.* Eyebrows and head hair are visible. In male fetuses, the testes begin to descend, and in female fetuses, the uterus is formed. Brown fat, which is a specialized type of adipose tissue that produces heat by oxidizing fatty acids, also forms during this period. It is found near the heart and blood vessels that supply the brain and kidneys and is thought to play a role in maintaining the temperature of these organs during exposure to environmental changes that occur after birth.

During the 21st through 25th weeks, significant fetal weight gain occurs. At 21 weeks rapid eye movements begin, and blink-startle reflexes have been reported at 22 to 23 weeks after application of a vibroacoustic noise source to the mother's abdomen.[6] The type II alveolar cells of the lung begin to secrete surfactant (see Chapter 27). The pulmonary system becomes more mature and able to support respiration during the 26th through 29th weeks. Breathing movements are present as a result of central nervous system (CNS) maturation. At this age a fetus can survive if born prematurely and given intensive care. There is substantial weight gain during this time. Although still somewhat lean, the fetus is better proportioned.

The 30th through 34th weeks are significant for an increasing amount of white fat (8% of body weight), which gives the fetal limbs an almost chubby appearance.[6] During the 35th week, grasp and the pupillary light reflex are present. If a normal-weight fetus is born during this period, it is premature by "date" as opposed to premature by "weight."[7]

Expected time of birth is 266 days, or 38 weeks after fertilization, or 40 weeks after the last menstrual period (LMP).[7] At this time, the neurologic, cardiovascular, and pulmonary systems are developed enough for the infant to make the transition to extrauterine life. The survival of the newborn depends on this adaptation after the placenta is removed.

Birth Weight and Gestational Age

Development during the fetal period is primarily concerned with rapid growth and differentiation of tissues, organs, and systems. Fetal weight gain is linear from 20 weeks' gestation through 38 weeks' gestation. In the last half of pregnancy, the fetus gains 85% of birth weight. After 38 weeks of gestation, the rate of growth declines, probably related to the constraint of uterine size and decreased placental function. After birth, weight gain resumes at a rate similar to intrauterine rates.

At birth, the average weight of the full-term newborn is 3000 to 4000 g. Infants weighing 2500 g or less at birth are classified as low birth weight (LBW). LBW is further broken down into very low birth weight (VLBW) and extremely low birth weight (ELBW). VLBW is defined as a birth weight less than 1500 g, and ELBW as a birth weight less than 1000 g.[9]

An infant is considered term when born between the beginning of the 38th week and completion of the 41st week. An infant is considered premature when born before the end of the 37th week and postmature when born after the end of the 41st week. The lowest mortality rates occur among newborns with weights between 3000 and 4000 g and gestational ages of 38 to 42 weeks.[10,11]

Abnormal Intrauterine Growth

Growth of the fetus in the uterus depends on a multitude of intrinsic and extrinsic factors. Optimal fetal growth depends on efficient placental function, adequate provision of energy and growth substrates, appropriate hormonal environment, and adequate room in the uterus. Birth weight variability in a population is primarily determined by genetic factors, fetal sex, maternal health and nutrition, intrinsic fetal growth potential, and environmental factors. Abnormal growth, which can occur at any time during fetal development, can have immediate and long-term consequences.

Lubchenco and Battaglia established standards for birth weight, gestational age, and intrauterine growth in the United States in the 1960s[12,13] (Fig. 2-3). With these standards, gestational age can be assessed and normal and abnormal growth can be identified. The Colorado Growth Curve places newborns into

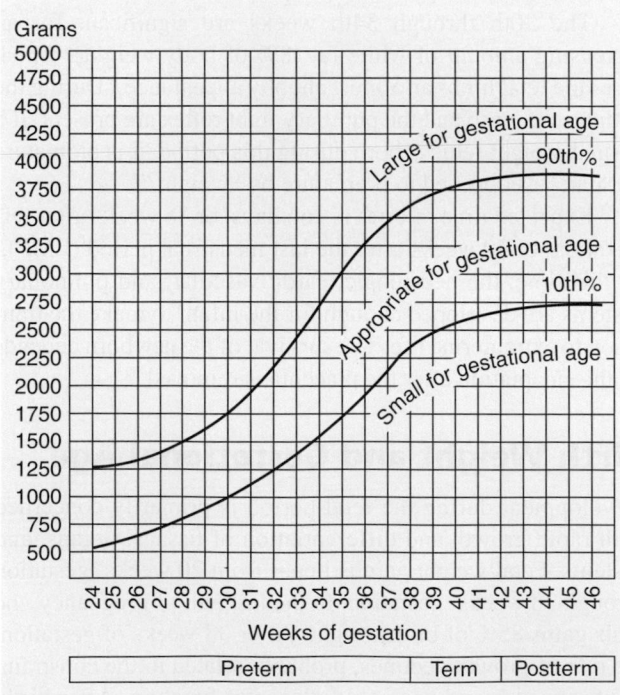

FIGURE 2-3 • Classification of newborns by birth weight and gestational age. (Redrawn from Battaglia F. C., Lubchenco L. O. [1967]. A practical classification of newborn infants by weight and gestational age. *Journal of Pediatrics* 71, 159.)

percentiles.[12] The 10th through 90th percentiles of intrauterine growth encompass 80% of births.[14] Growth is considered abnormal when a newborn falls above or below the 90th and 10th percentiles, respectively.

Small for Gestational Age. *Small for gestational age* (SGA) is a term that denotes fetal undergrowth. SGA is defined as a birth weight less than two standard deviations below the mean for gestational age, or below the 10th percentile. The terms *small for gestational age* and *intrauterine growth retardation* (IUGR) are used interchangeably, but are not synonymous. IUGR refers to a process that causes a reduction in an expected pattern of growth. SGA refers to an infant with a birth weight lower than the predetermined cutoff point.[15]

IUGR can occur at any time during fetal development. Depending on the time of insult, the infant can have symmetric or proportional growth retardation or asymmetric or disproportional growth retardation.[9,15] Impaired growth that occurs early in pregnancy during the hyperplastic phase of growth results in a symmetric growth retardation, and there is a proportionate decrease in length, weight, and head size for gestational age.[15] This is irreversible postnatally. Causes of proportional IUGR include chromosomal abnormalities, congenital infections, and exposure to environmental toxins. Impaired growth that occurs later in pregnancy during the hypertrophic phase of growth results in asymmetric growth retardation.[10] Infants with IUGR due to intrauterine malnutrition often have weight reduction out of proportion to length or head circumference but are spared impairment of head and brain growth. Tissues and organs are small because of decreased cell size, not decreased cell numbers. Postnatally, the impairment may be partially corrected with good nutrition.

Gestational growth can be affected by maternal, placental, and fetal factors. The maternal environment can have a drastic effect on birth weight and size.[15] Underweight mothers are more likely to give birth to small-weight infants. Maternal nutrition and weight gain are influenced by many factors. Women at risk for poor nutrition and poor fetal growth include adolescents, women of low economic status, women with short interpregnancy intervals, women with unusual or stringent diet restrictions, and women who do heavy physical work during pregnancy.[15] Various maternal diseases have been associated with restricted fetal growth, including prepregnancy hypertension, diabetes mellitus, and chronic maternal illnesses and infections. Growth retardation in the fetus may be related to maternal exposure to environmental agents such as recreational drugs (drugs of abuse), therapeutic drugs, and environmental hazards. Tobacco in the form of cigarette smoking during pregnancy reduces birth weight; and the reduction is related to the number of cigarettes smoked. Occupational exposure to agents such as industrial solvents used as thinners in paint, glue, and varnishes can pose a threat to the pregnant mother and fetus.[15] Abnormal placentation comprises a broad range of pathologic processes that compromise uteroplacental blood flow and fetal growth. Fetal factors include chromosomal and gene abnormalities. There is also a progressive decrease in placental and fetal weight as the number of fetuses increase in multiple-fetus gestations. Infants of twin and triplet gestations tend to weigh less than those of singlet gestations.[15]

The perinatal mortality rate among infants with IUGR is 10 to 20 times that among infants whose size and weight are appropriate for gestational age.[15] The causes of this mortality are primarily hypoxia and congenital anomalies. Other complications include polycythemia, hyperbilirubinemia, and hypoglycemia. Compared with infants who are appropriate for gestational age, SGA infants have a larger plasma volume and circulating red cell mass, most likely the result of fetal hypoxia and subsequent erythropoietin production.[15] SGA infants also are more prone to fasting hypoglycemia during the first days of life, probably as the result of depleted hepatic glycogen stores.[15]

The long-term effects of growth retardation depend on the timing and severity of the insult. Many of these infants have developmental disabilities on follow-up examination, especially if the growth retardation is symmetric. They may remain small, especially if the insult occurred early. If the insult occurred later because of placental insufficiency or uterine restraint, with good nutrition catch-up growth can occur and the infant may attain appropriate growth goals.

Large for Gestational Age. *Large for gestational age* (LGA) is a term that denotes fetal overgrowth and a birth weight above the 90th percentile.[10,15] The excessive growth may result from maternal or fetal factors. Maternal factors include maternal body size and diabetes. Fetal factors consist primarily of gene and chromosome disorders. Maternal size has long been recognized as a factor that influences birth weight—heavy women tend to have LGA infants. Women with diabetes also tend to have LGA infants, especially if the diabetes was poorly controlled during pregnancy.[15]

Complications when an infant is LGA include birth asphyxia and trauma due to mechanical difficulties during the birth process, hypoglycemia, and polycythemia.[15] Maternal hyperglycemia exposes the fetus to increased levels of glucose, which stimulate fetal pancreatic islet hyperplasia and increased insulin secretion. Insulin increases fat deposition and the result is a macrosomic (large body size) infant. Infants with macrosomia have enlarged viscera and are large and plump because of an increase in body fat. Fetal hyperinsulinemia is associated with fetal hypoxia and erythropoietin-induced polycythemia. Infants with polycythemia are at direct risk for hyperbilirubinemia. LGA infants and infants of diabetic mothers are also at risk for hypoglycemia (to be discussed).

Assessment Methods

Gestational age assessment can be divided into two categories: prenatal assessment and postnatal assessment. *Prenatal assessment* of gestational age most commonly includes careful menstrual history, physical milestones during pregnancy (*e.g.,* uterine size, detection of fetal heart rate and movements), and prenatal tests for maturity (*e.g.,* ultrasonography, amniotic fluid studies). The Nägele rule uses the first day of the LMP to calculate the day of labor by adding 7 days to the LMP and counting back 3 months.[6] This method may be inaccurate if the mother is not a good historian or has a history of irregular menses, which interferes with identification of a normal cycle.

Postnatal assessment of gestational age is done by examination of external physical and neuromuscular characteristics alone or in combination. Assessment of gestational age should be a part of every initial newborn examination. Accurate assessment of gestational age facilitates risk assessment and identification of abnormalities and allows for earlier interventions. Dubowitz and Ballard developed the most common methods used in nurseries today. The Dubowitz method is comprehensive and includes 21 criteria using external physical (11) and neuromuscular (10) signs.[16] The estimate of gestational age is best done within 12 hours of birth and is accurate within 1 week. The method is less accurate for infants born at less than 30 weeks' gestational age. The Ballard method is an abbreviated Dubowitz method that includes 12 criteria, using 6 external physical and 6 neuromuscular signs (Fig. 2-4). The New Ballard Score (NBS) was updated and modified to include newborns at gestational ages of 20 to 44 weeks and is the most commonly used method.[14]

IN SUMMARY, growth and development begin with union of ovum and sperm and are ongoing throughout a child's life to adulthood. Abnormalities during this process can have profound effects on the individual. Prenatal development is composed of two periods, the embryonic period and the fetal period. During these periods, the zygote becomes the newborn with the organ maturity to make the adjustments necessary for extrauterine life. An infant is considered term when born between the beginning of the 38th week and completion of the 41st week. An infant is considered premature when born before the end of the 37th week and postmature when born after the end of the 41st week.

At birth, the average weight of the full-term newborn is 3000 to 4000 g. Infants weighing 2500 g or less at birth are classified as being low birth weight. Low birth weight is further broken down into very low birth weight (<1500 g) and extremely low birth weight (<1000 g). Infants with a birth weight above the 90th percentile are considered large for gestational age. The lowest mortality rates occur among newborns with weights between 3000 and 4000 g and gestational ages of 38 to 42 weeks. ∎

INFANCY

After completing this section of the chapter, you should be able to meet the following objectives:

- Describe the use of the Apgar score in evaluating infant well-being at birth.
- Describe the causes and manifestations of neonatal hypoglycemia.

(objectives continue)

Neuromuscular maturity

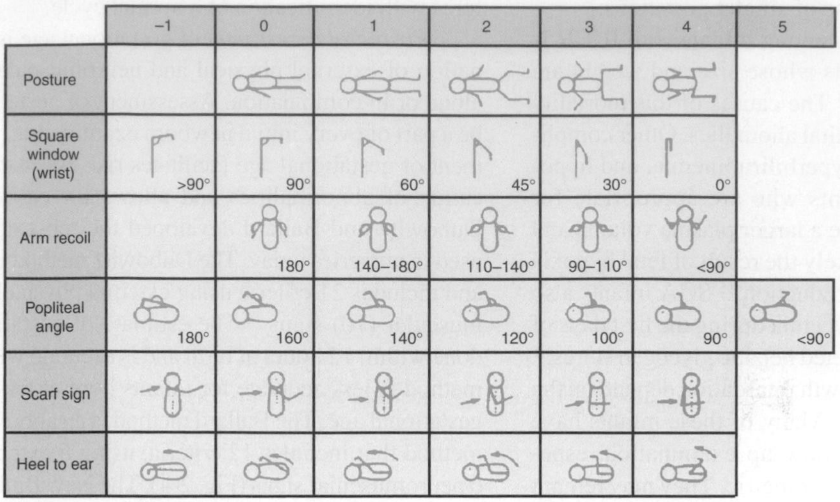

	−1	0	1	2	3	4	5
Posture							
Square window (wrist)	>90°	90°	60°	45°	30°	0°	
Arm recoil		180°	140–180°	110–140°	90–110°	<90°	
Popliteal angle	180°	160°	140°	120°	100°	90°	<90°
Scarf sign							
Heel to ear							

Physical maturity

Skin	Sticky, friable, transparent	Gelatinous, red, translucent	Smooth, pink; visible veins	Superficial peeling and/or rash, few veins	Cracking pale areas, rare veins	Parchment, deep cracking, no vessels	Leathery, cracked, wrinkled
Lanugo	None	Sparse	Abundant	Thinning	Bald areas	Mostly bald	
Plantar surface	Heel–toe 40–50 mm: −1 <40 mm: −2	>50 mm No crease	Faint red marks	Anterior transverse crease only	Creases anterior 2/3	Creases over entire sole	
Breast	Imperceptible	Barely perceptible	Flat areola, no bud	Stippled areola 1–2 mm bud	Raised areola 3–4 mm bud	Full areola 5–10 mm bud	
Eye/ear	Lids fused loosely: −1 tightly: −2	Lids open; pinna flat, stays folded	Slightly curved pinna; soft; slow recoil	Well-curved pinna; soft but ready recoil	Formed and firm, instant recoil	Thick cartilage, ear stiff	
Genitals: male	Scrotum flat, smooth	Scrotum empty, faint rugae	Testes in upper canal, rare rugae	Testes descending, few rugae	Testes down, good rugae	Testes pendulous, deep rugae	
Genitals: female	Clitoris prominent, labia flat	Prominent clitoris, small labia minora	Prominent clitoris, enlarging minora	Majora and minora equally prominent	Majora large, minora small	Majora cover clitoris and minora	

Maturity rating

Score	Weeks
−10	20
−5	22
0	24
5	26
10	28
15	30
20	32
25	34
30	36
35	38
40	40
45	42
50	44

FIGURE 2-4 • Ballard scoring system for determining gestational age in weeks. (From Ballard J. L., Khoury J. C., Wedig K., et al. [1991]. New Ballard Score, expanded to include extremely premature infants. *Journal of Pediatrics,* 119, 417.)

- List three injuries that can occur during the birth process.
- Describe physical growth and organ development during the first year of life.
- Explain how the common health care needs of the premature infant differ from the health care needs of the term newborn or infant.
- Differentiate between organic and nonorganic failure to thrive syndrome.

Infancy is defined as the time from birth to approximately 18 months of age, the first 4 weeks of which are designated as the newborn or neonatal period. This is a period of rapid phys-

ical growth and maturation. The infant begins life as a relatively helpless organism and, through a process of progressive development, gains the skills to interact and cope with the environment. The infant begins life with a number of primitive reflexes and little body control. By 18 months, a child is able to run, grasp and manipulate objects, feed himself or herself, play with toys, and communicate with others.

Growth and Development

The average length of a full-term infant is 50 cm, with a range of 48 to 53 cm.[6,10] During the first 6 months, height increases by 2.5 cm per month. By 1 year, the increase in length is approxi-

🔑 INFANCY

- Infancy, which is the time from birth to 18 months of age, is a period of rapid physical growth and maturation.

- From an average birth weight of 3000 to 4000 g in the full-term infant and a median height of 49.9 cm for girls and 50.5 cm for boys, the infant manages to triple its weight and increase its length by 50% at 1 year of age.

- Developmentally, the infant begins life with a number of primitive reflexes and little body control. By 18 months, a child is able to run, grasp and manipulate objects, feed himself/herself, play with toys, and communicate with others.

- Basic trust, the first of Erikson's psychosocial stages, develops as infants learn that basic needs are met regularly.

- At the age of 18 months or the end of the infancy period, the emergence of symbolic thought causes a reorganization of behaviors with implications for the many developmental domains that lie ahead as the child moves to the early childhood stage of development.

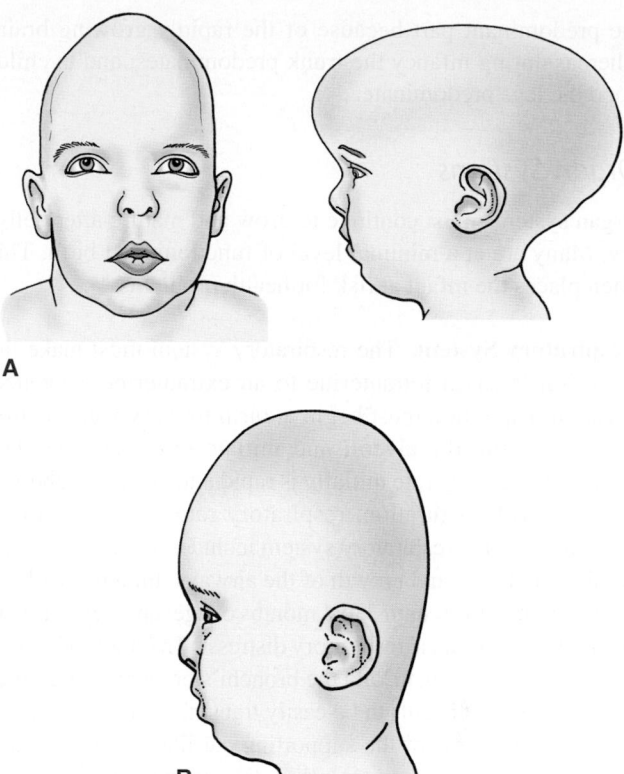

A

B

FIGURE 2-5 • Craniosynostosis. **(A)** Scaphocephaly due to closure of the sagittal suture, in which the anterior fontanel is small or absent, results in a long, narrow, wedge-shaped cranium. **(B)** Oxycephaly due to premature closure of the coronal suture results in a high, tower-like cranium. (Adapted from Moore K. L., Dalley A. F. [2006]. *Clinically oriented anatomy* [5th ed., p. 905]. Philadelphia: Lippincott Williams & Wilkins.)

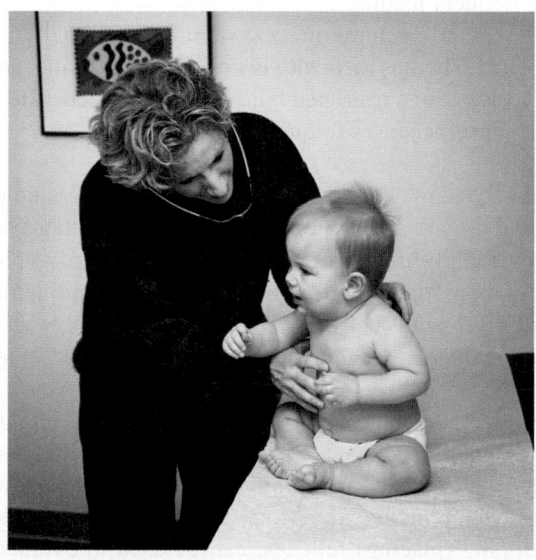

mately 50% of the birth length. This increase is primarily in trunk growth.

The skull bones of newborn infants are incomplete and are connected by bands of connective tissue called *sutures*. At the junction of the sutures are wider spaces of unossified membranous tissue called *fontanels*. The larger anterior fontanel is palpable until about 18 months to 2 years of age; the smaller ones are replaced by bone by the end of the first year. The soft-

ness of the cranial bones and loose connections of the sutures and fontanels enable the shape of the infant's head to change (mold) during the birth process. The fibrous sutures of the infant's skull also permit the cranium to enlarge during infancy and childhood. The increase in head size is greatest during the first 2 years, the period of most rapid brain development. Premature closure of any suture in the skull is called *craniosynostosis*. The cause of primary craniosynostosis is unknown, but genetic factors appear to be important. These malformations are more common in boys than girls and are often associated with other skeletal abnormalities. The closed suture prevents growth from occurring in the affected area, but growth continues in the unaffected sutures, resulting in an abnormally shaped head. The clinical consequences of premature suture closure depend on which suture is affected[17] (Fig. 2-5).

Chest circumference at birth is smaller than head circumference. By 1 year, the head and chest are approximately equal in circumference; after 1 year, chest circumference exceeds head circumference.[6] After birth, most organ systems continue to grow and mature in an orderly fashion. Variations in growth and development are responsible for the differences in body proportions. For example, during the fetal period, the head is the predominant part because of the rapidly growing brain, whereas during infancy the trunk predominates, and in childhood the legs predominate.

Organ Systems

Organ systems must continue to grow and mature after delivery. Many are at a minimal level of functioning at birth. This often places the infant at risk for health problems.

Respiratory System. The respiratory system must make the transition from an intrauterine to an extrauterine existence. Onset of respiration must begin at birth for survival. The first breaths expand the alveoli and initiate gas exchange. The infant's respiratory rate initially is rapid and primarily abdominal, but with maturation, respiratory rate gradually slows. Maturation of the respiratory system includes an increase in the number of alveoli and growth of the airways. Infants are obligatory nose breathers until 3 to 4 months of age; any upper airway obstruction may cause respiratory distress.[4] The trachea is small and close to the bronchi, and the bronchi's branching structures enable infectious agents to be easily transmitted throughout the lungs. The softness of the supporting cartilage in the trachea, along with its small diameter, places the infant at risk for airway obstruction. The auditory (eustachian) tube is short and straight and closely communicates with the ear, putting the infant at risk for middle ear infections (see Chapter 55).

Cardiovascular System. Birth initiates major changes in the cardiovascular system. The fetal shunts, the foramen ovale and ductus arteriosus, begin to close and the circulation of blood changes from series to parallel circuits (see Chapter 24). At birth, the size of the heart is large in relation to the chest cavity. The size and weight of the heart double the first year. Initially, the right ventricle is more muscular than the left ventricle, but this reverses in infancy. The heart rate gradually slows, and systolic blood pressure rises.

Thermoregulation. Maintaining a stable body temperature is a function of heat production and conservation coupled with heat loss. Heat production in response to cold stress can occur through voluntary muscle activity, involuntary muscle activity (shivering), and nonshivering thermogenesis, which relies heavily on heat liberated from brown fat stores.[18] Newborns generate heat primarily through the last three mechanisms, which is very limited in the preterm infant.

Heat loss to the environment can occur through the following mechanisms: (1) radiation, or transfer of heat from a warmer to cooler area that is not in contact with the body; (2) convection, transfer of heat to the surrounding environment, influenced by air currents; (3) conduction transfer of heat to a cooler surface that is in direct contact with the body; and (4) evaporation, cooling secondary to water loss from the skin (see Chapter 10). Heat loss in the preterm infant is accelerated because of the higher ratio of surface area to body mass, reduced insulation of subcutaneous tissue, and water loss through immature skin.

The thermal environment of the preterm infant must be regulated carefully. Ideally, the infant should be kept in a neutral environment to maintain a stable core body temperature with minimal need for metabolic heat production through oxygen consumption. The neutral thermal environment for a given infant depends on size, gestational age, and postnatal age. In general, when infants reach a weight of 1700 to 1800 g, they can maintain temperature when bundled in an open crib.[18]

Gastrointestinal and Genitourinary Systems. The infant's gastrointestinal system is immature, and most digestive processes are poorly functioning until approximately 3 months of age. Solid food may pass incompletely digested and be evident in the stool. The newborn's first stool is called *meconium* and is composed of amniotic fluid, intestinal secretions, shed mucosal cells, and sometimes blood from ingested maternal blood or minor bleeding of intestinal tract vessels. Passage of meconium should occur within the first 24 to 48 hours in healthy term newborns, but may be delayed for up to 7 days in preterm newborns or in newborns who do not receive enteral nutrition because of illness.

At birth, sucking may be poor and require several days to become effective. The tongue thrust reflex is present and aids in sucking, but it disappears at approximately 6 months of age. Stomach capacity increases rapidly in the first months, but because of the limited capacity and rapid emptying, infants require frequent feeding.[4]

The infant's genitourinary system is functionally immature at birth. There is difficulty in concentrating urine, and the ability to adjust to a restricted fluid intake is limited. The small bladder capacity causes frequent voiding.

Nervous System. The nervous system undergoes rapid maturation and growth during infancy. In contrast to other systems that grow rapidly after birth, the nervous system grows proportionately more rapidly before birth. The most rapid period of fetal brain growth is between 15 and 20 weeks of gestation, at which time there is a significant increase in neurons. A second increase occurs between 30 weeks' gestation and 1 year of age.

At birth, the nervous system is incompletely integrated, but sufficiently developed to sustain extrauterine life. Most of the neurologic reflexes are primitive reflexes. Normal newborn reflexes, which include the Moro (startle), rooting (sucking), and stepping (placing) reflexes, can be used to evaluate the newborn and infant's developing CNS.

The maturation of the nervous system includes an increase in the size of neurons, size and number of glial cells, and number of interneuron connections and branching of axons and dendrites. As this maturation progresses, the level of infant functioning increases from simple to complex and from primitive reflexes to purposeful movement. Cortical control of motor functions is closely associated with myelination of nerve fibers. Myelination of the various nerve tracts progresses rapidly after birth and follows a cephalocaudad and proximodistal direction sequence, beginning with myelination of the spinal cord and cranial nerves and followed by the brain stem and corticospinal tracts.[4] In general, sensory pathways become myelinated before motor pathways. The acquisition of fine and gross motor skills depends on this myelination and maturation.

The first year of life also is filled with psychosocial developmental milestones for the infant. Basic needs must be met before the infant can accomplish these developmental tasks. Erikson described the development of a sense of trust as the task of the first stage.[19] If trust is not acquired, the infant becomes mistrustful of others and frustrated with his or her inability to control the surrounding environment.

Health Problems of the Neonate

The most profound physiologic changes required of the newborn occur at the time of transition from intrauterine to extrauterine life. Onset of respiration must begin at birth for survival. The fetal shunts (i.e., foramen ovale and ductus arteriosus) begin to close and the circulation of blood changes from a serial to parallel circuitry. Heat regulation is a response critical to the infant's survival. The newborn's large surface area and lack of subcutaneous fat predispose to excessive heat loss. Blood glucose concentration in the fetus is approximately 15 mg/dL less than maternal glucose concentrations and can drop to hypoglycemic levels in certain high-risk groups.

Distress at Birth and the Apgar Score

The Apgar score, devised by Dr. Virginia Apgar, is a scoring system that evaluates infant well-being at birth.[20] The system addresses five categories (i.e., heart rate, respiratory effort, muscle tone, reflex irritability, and color) with a total score ranging from 0 to 10, depending on the degree to which these functions are presented (Table 2-1). Evaluations are performed at 1 minute and 5 minutes after delivery. A score of 0 to 3 is indicative of severe distress, 4 to 6 of moderate distress, and 7 to 10 of mild to no distress. Most infants score 6 to 7 at 1 minute and 8 to 9 at 5 minutes. If the score is 7 or less, the evaluation should be repeated every 5 minutes until a score of 7 or greater is obtained. An abnormal score at 5 minutes is more predictive of problems with survival and neurologic outcome than at 1 minute.[10]

Neonatal Hypoglycemia

Glucose concentration normally decreases in the immediate postnatal period, with levels below 40 to 45 mg/dL considered indicative of hypoglycemia.[18] By 3 hours, the glucose concentration in normal-term infants stabilizes between 50 and 80 mg/dL. After the first hours of life, concentrations below 40 to 45 mg/dL should be considered abnormal. In neonates, there is not always a correlation between blood glucose and the classic clinical manifestations of hypoglycemia.[21] Instead, the signs of hypoglycemia include cyanosis, apnea, hypothermia, hypotonia, poor feeding, lethargy, and seizures. Some of the symptoms may be so mild they are missed. The absence of symptoms does not mean that that the glucose concentration is normal and has not fallen below that needed for maintaining normal brain metabolism. Furthermore, there is evidence that hypoxemia and ischemia may potentiate the role of hypoglycemia in causing permanent brain damage.[21] Newborn infants who are at particular risk for neonatal hypoglycemia are infants of diabetic mothers (IDMs) and premature and SGA newborns. Blood glucose can be measured by heel stick using a glucometer. All infants should be screened, including IDMs, SGA infants, premature infants, and any infant with signs that could be due to hypoglycemia.

Hypoglycemia in IDMs is mostly related to hyperinsulinemia and partly related to diminished glucagon secretion (see Chapter 42 for a discussion of blood glucose regulation, and diabetes in pregnant women). Glucose readily crosses the placenta and consequently IDMs are exposed to elevated blood glucose levels, a condition that stimulates islet cell hypertrophy and hyperplasia. Infants of diabetic mothers also have a subnormal surge in plasma glucagon immediately after birth, a subnormal glucagon response to hypoglycemic stimuli, and, initially, excessive sympathetic activity that may lead to adrenomedullary exhaustion, as evidenced by decreased urinary excretion of epinephrine. Newborns with hyperinsulinemia are often LGA. Mothers whose diabetes is well controlled during pregnancy, labor, and delivery generally have infants of near-normal size who are less likely to experience neonatal hypoglycemia.[21]

TABLE 2-1 Apgar Score Assessment

CRITERION	SCORE* 0	1	2
Heart rate	Absent	<100	>100
Respiratory effort	Absent	Weak, irregular	Crying
Muscle tone	Limp	Some flexion	Well flexed
Reflex irritability	No response	Grimace	Cry, gag
Color	Pale	Cyanotic	Pink
Total	0	5	10

*The Apgar score should be assigned at 1 minute and 5 minutes after birth, using a timer. Each criterion is assessed and assigned a 0, 1, or 2. The total score is the assigned Apgar score. If resuscitation is required beyond the 5 minutes, additional Apgar scores also may be assigned as a method to document the response of the newborn to the resuscitation.[20]

Premature and SGA infants are also vulnerable to hypoglycemia. The factors responsible for this vulnerability include inadequate stores of liver glycogen, muscle protein, and body fat needed to sustain the substrates required to meet energy needs. These infants are small by virtue of prematurity and impaired placental transfer of nutrients. Their enzyme systems for gluconeogenesis may not be fully developed. In addition, infants with perinatal asphyxia and some SGA newborns may have transient hyperinsulinemia, which promotes hypoglycemia.

Neonatal Jaundice

Jaundice or a yellow-orange hue to the skin is a common problem affecting over half of all full-term and most preterm infants (Fig. 2-6). The color usually results from excessive circulating levels of unconjugated, lipid-soluble bilirubin that accumulates in the skin.[22] A newborn infant's metabolism of bilirubin is in transition from the fetal stage, during which the placenta is the principal route of elimination of lipid-soluble bilirubin, to the postnatal stage, during which the water-soluble conjugated form is excreted from hepatic cells into the biliary system and then into the gastrointestinal tract (see Chapter 14). Bilirubin is formed from the breakdown of hemoglobin in red blood cells. Red blood cells live only for 70 to 90 days in the newborn, unlike the older child, in whom red blood cells live for 120 days.[22] Normally, about two thirds of the unconjugated bilirubin produced by a term newborn can be effectively cleared by the liver. However, the relative immaturity of the newborn liver and the shortened life span of the fetal red blood cells may predispose the term newborn to hyperbilirubinemia. With the establishment of sufficient enteral nutrition, regular bowel elimination, and nor-

mal fluid volume, the liver is usually able to clear the excess bilirubin.

Physiologic jaundice refers to jaundice in the immediate neonatal period without signs of illness. Under normal circumstances, the level of unconjugated or indirect-reacting bilirubin in umbilical cord blood is 1 to 3 mg/dL.[23] This level rises to less than 5 mg/dL per 24 hours, usually peaking between the second and fourth days of life and decreasing to below 2 mg/dL between 5 and 7 days of life.[23] Jaundice and its underlying hyperbilirubinemia are considered pathologic if their time of appearance, duration, and pattern of appearance vary significantly from those of physiologic jaundice. The greatest risk associated with hyperbilirubinemia is the development of kernicterus or bilirubin encephalopathy, a neurologic syndrome resulting from deposition of unconjugated bilirubin in the basal ganglia and brain stem nuclei. Kernicterus develops at lower bilirubin levels in preterm infants. The exact level at which bilirubin levels are harmful to infants with LBW is unclear.

Regardless of the cause, the goal of therapy is to prevent the concentration of bilirubin in the blood from reaching neurotoxic levels.[22,23] Treatment measures include frequent breast-feeding to prevent dehydration, phototherapy using overhead or fiberoptic pads, and, in severe cases, exchange blood transfusions (see Chapter 14). Phototherapy uses a special artificial blue light to alter bilirubin so it may be more readily excreted in the urine and stool. Exchange transfusion is seldom used but is indicated when bilirubin levels reach 25 to 30 mg/dL, and to correct anemia in infants severely affected by the hemolytic process.[22]

Jaundice and elevated unconjugated bilirubin levels can also occur in breast-fed infants (breast milk jaundice), but is uncommon. It occurs after the seventh day of life, with maximal concentrations as high as 10 to 12 mg/dL reached during the second to third week.[23] Cessation of breast-feeding for 1 to 2 days is recommended and substitution of formula usually results in a rapid decline in serum bilirubin, after which breast-feeding can usually be resumed without return of hyperbilirubinemia.

Birth Injuries

Injuries sustained during the birth process are responsible for a significant amount of neonatal mortality and morbidity. Predisposing factors for birth injuries include macrosomia, prematurity, forceps delivery, abnormal fetal presentation, cephalopelvic disproportion, prolonged labor, and precipitous delivery.[23,24]

Cranial Injuries. The contour of the head of the newborn often reflects the effects of the delivery presentation. The softness of the cranial bones in infants and their loose connections at the sutures and fontanels allow the shape of head to mold during birth. In a vertex (head-first) delivery, the head is usually flattened at the forehead with the apex rising and forming a plane at the end of the parietal bones and the posterior skull or occiput dropping abruptly (Fig. 2-7). By one to two days of age, the head has taken on a more oval shape.[17] Such molding does not occur in infants born by breech presentation or cesarean section.

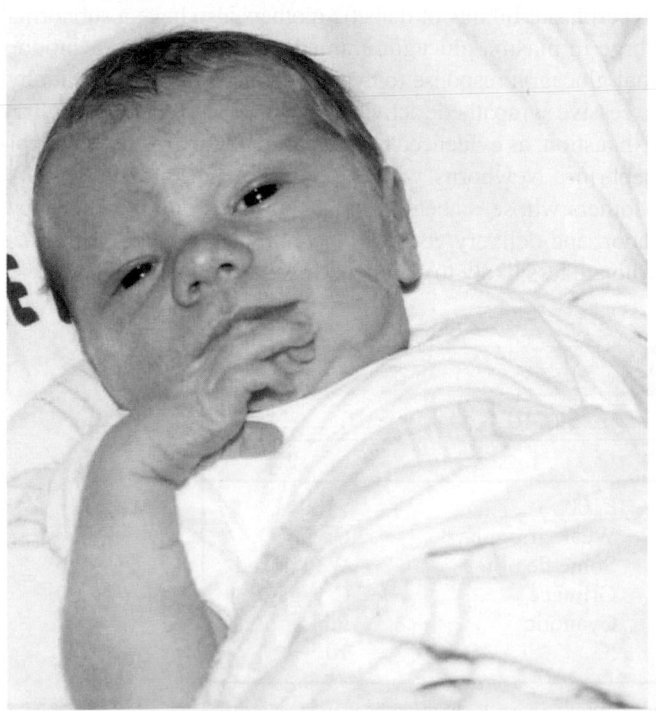

FIGURE 2-6 • A newborn infant with jaundice.

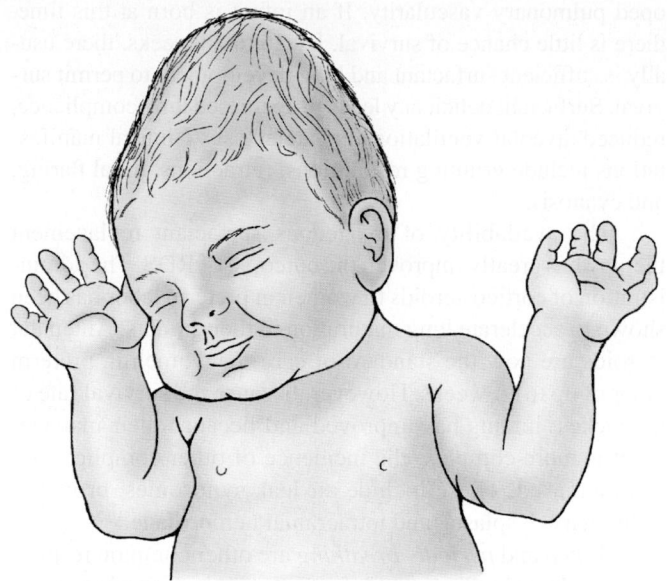

FIGURE 2-7 • Molding of the calvaria or posterior portion of the skull in a newborn infant. (From Moore K. L., Dalley A. F. [2006]. *Clinically oriented anatomy* [5th ed., p. 903]. Philadelphia: Lippincott Williams & Wilkins.)

Caput succedaneum is a localized area of scalp edema caused by sustained pressure of the presenting part against the cervix.[23 25] The caput succedaneum may extend across suture lines and have overlying petechiae, purpura, or ecchymosis. No treatment is needed, and it usually resolves over the first week of life. *Cephalhematoma* is a subperiosteal collection of blood from ruptured blood vessels.[23–25] The margins are sharply delineated and do not cross suture lines. It usually is unilateral, but it may be bilateral, and it usually occurs over the parietal area. The subperiosteal bleeding may be slow and therefore not apparent for 24 to 48 hours. The overlying skin is not discolored. Skull fractures may be present. Usually the fractures are linear, nondepressed, and do not require treatment. Infants with cephalhematomas are usually asymptomatic. Management includes monitoring for hyperbilirubinemia. Resolution usually occurs over a period of 2 weeks to 3 months. Rarely, a cephalhematoma may develop complications. Large cephalhematomas may result in significant blood loss, causing anemia and hyperbilirubinemia. In rare cases, an infant may develop a subdural or subarachnoid hemorrhage. Calcium deposits occasionally develop, and the swelling may remain for the first year.

Fractures. Skull fractures are uncommon because the infant's compressible skull is able to mold to fit the contours of the birth canal. However, fractures can occur and more often follow a forceps delivery or severe contraction of the pelvis associated with prolonged, difficult labor. Skull fractures may be linear or depressed. Uncomplicated linear fractures often are asymptomatic and do not require treatment. Depressed skull fractures are observable by the palpable indentation of the infant's head. They require surgical intervention if there is compression of underlying brain tissue. A simple linear fracture usually heals within several months.[23–25]

The clavicle is the most frequently fractured bone during the birth process.[24] It is more common in LGA infants and occurs when delivery of the shoulders is difficult in vertex (*i.e.,* head-first) or breech presentations. The infant may or may not demonstrate restricted motion of the upper extremities, but passive motion elicits pain. There may be discoloration or deformity and, on palpation, crepitus (*i.e.,* a crackling sound from bones rubbing together), and irregularity may be found. Treatment of complete fractures consists of immobilizing the arm and shoulder and providing pain relief.

Peripheral Nerve Injuries. The brachial plexuses are situated above the clavicles in the anterolateral bases of the neck. They are composed of the ventral rami of the fifth cervical (C5) through the first thoracic (T1) nerves. During vertex deliveries, excessive lateral traction of the head and neck away from the shoulders may cause a stretch injury to the brachial plexus on that side. In a breech presentation, excessive lateral traction on the trunk before delivery of the head may tear the lower roots of the cervical cord. If the breech presentation includes delivery with the arms overhead, an injury to the fifth and sixth cervical roots may result. When injury to the brachial plexus occurs, it causes paralysis of the upper extremity. The paralysis often is incomplete.[23–25]

Brachial plexus injuries include three types: Erb palsy (*i.e.,* upper arm), Klumpke palsy (*i.e.,* lower arm), and paralysis of the entire arm. Risk factors include an LGA infant and a difficult, traumatic delivery. Erb palsy or upper plexus injury involving C5 to C7 accounts for approximately 90% of plexus injuries.[24] It manifests with variable degrees of paralysis of the shoulder and arm. The affected arm is held in the "waiter's tip position," with adduction and internal rotation of shoulder, extension at the elbow, pronation of the forearm, and flexion of the wrist and fingers[23,24] (Fig. 2-8). When the infant is lifted, the affected extremity is limp. The Moro reflex is impaired or absent, but the grasp reflex is present. Klumpke palsy or lower plexus injury at C5 to T1 is rare and presents with paralysis of the hand.[23,24] The infant has wrist drop, the fingers are relaxed, and the grasp reflex is absent. The Moro reflex is impaired, with the upper extremity extending and abducting normally while the wrist and fingers remain flaccid.[23]

Treatment of brachial plexus injuries includes immobilization, appropriate positioning, and an exercise program. Most infants recover in 3 to 6 months. If paralysis persists beyond this time, surgical repair (*i.e.,* neuroplasty, end-to-end anastomosis, nerve grafting) may be done.[23]

Health Problems of the Premature Infant

Infants born before 37 weeks' gestation are considered premature. They often fall into the LBW category, with most weighing less than 2500 g, and many weighing less than 1500 g. Mortality and morbidity are increased in the premature population, with their rates inversely proportional to the length of

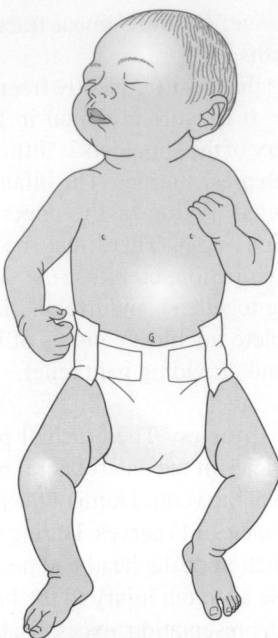

FIGURE 2-8 • Position of the right arm in an infant with Erb palsy. After partial upper arm paralysis, the upper arm is held in a "waiter's tip" position with adduction and internal rotation of the shoulder, extension of the elbow with pronation of the forearm, and flexion of the wrist and fingers.

gestation. Despite the advances in obstetric management since the late 1960s, the rate of premature delivery has not significantly changed. The percentage of infants born with VLBW (<1500 g) has increased gradually in recent years. In 2005, 1.49% of infants were VLBW, compared with 1.26% in 1989.[2] One reason for the recent increase is that the number of twin, triplet, and higher-order multiple births has increased.[2]

The premature infant is poorly equipped to withstand the rigors of extrauterine transition. The organ systems are immature and may not be able to sustain life. The respiratory system may not be able to support gas exchange; the skin may be thin and gelatinous and easily damaged; the immune system is compromised and may not effectively fight infection; and the lack of subcutaneous fat puts the infant at risk for temperature instability. Complications of prematurity include respiratory distress syndrome, pulmonary hemorrhage, transient tachypnea, congenital pneumonia, pulmonary air leaks, bronchopulmonary dysplasia, recurrent apnea, glucose instability, hypocalcemia, hyperbilirubinemia, anemia, intraventricular hemorrhage, necrotizing enterocolitis, circulatory instability, hypothermia, bacterial or viral infection, retinopathy of prematurity, and disseminated intravascular coagulopathies.

Respiratory Problems. The *respiratory distress syndrome* (RDS) is the most common complication of prematurity. The primary cause of RDS is the lack of surfactant in the lungs (see section on Respiratory Distress Syndrome, Chapter 28). At 24 weeks' gestation, there are small amounts of surfactant and few terminal air sacs (*i.e.*, primitive alveoli), with underdevel-

oped pulmonary vascularity. If an infant is born at this time, there is little chance of survival. By 26 to 28 weeks, there usually is sufficient surfactant and lung development to permit survival. Surfactant deficiency leads to decreased lung compliance, reduced alveolar ventilation, and atelectasis. Clinical manifestations include grunting respirations, retractions, nasal flaring, and cyanosis.

The availability of exogenous surfactant replacement therapy has greatly improved the outcome of RDS. The administration of corticosteroids to women in preterm labor has been shown to accelerate lung maturation in their infants. Antenatal steroids are now the standard of care for women in preterm labor of up to 34 weeks. However, because the survival rate of the sickest infants has improved and because their management is more complex, the incidence of other complications has increased. These include air leak syndromes, bronchopulmonary dysplasia, and intracranial hemorrhage.[10,26]

Apnea and *periodic breathing* are other common respiratory problems in premature infants. *Apnea* is defined as cessation of breathing; it is characterized by failure to breathe for 20 seconds or more and often is accompanied by bradycardia or cyanosis. Because the respiratory center in the medulla oblongata is underdeveloped in the premature infant, the ability for sustained ventilatory drive often is impaired. In contrast to adults, infants respond to hypoxemia with only a brief period of increased ventilation followed by hypoventilation or apnea. Among infants weighing less than 1.5 kg, 50% require intervention for significant apneic spells.[10,26] *Periodic breathing* commonly occurs in those infants weighing less than 1800 g. It is an intermittent failure to breathe for periods lasting less than 10 to 15 seconds.

Management of apnea and periodic breathing includes use of medications or ventilatory support until the CNS is developed and able to sustain adequate ventilatory drive.[10,26] Prompt tactile stimulation is often sufficient to abort mild episodes of apnea. Infants with apneic episodes accompanied by profound bradycardia need prompt attention to their immediate needs and more aggressive diagnostic and therapeutic interventions. The methylxanthines (*e.g.*, caffeine, theophylline) are often used in the treatment of apnea. These drugs appear to exert a central stimulatory effect on brain stem respiratory neurons and often markedly decrease the frequency and severity of the apneic attacks.

Intraventricular Hemorrhage. Intraventricular hemorrhage (IVH), or hemorrhage into the germinal matrix tissues, with possible rupture of the ventricular septum and tissue of the developing brain, is a major problem almost exclusive to preterm infants[27] (Fig. 2-9). Bleeding is thought to result from alterations in cerebral blood flow to damaged vessels in the germinal matrix, an early developmental structure that contains a fragile vascular bed that is poorly supported by connective tissue. Because the germinal matrix begins to involute after 34 weeks of gestation, germinal matrix hemorrhages (GMHs) and IVHs are lesions of preterm infants. The incidence of IVH increases with decreasing birth weight and gestational age: 60%

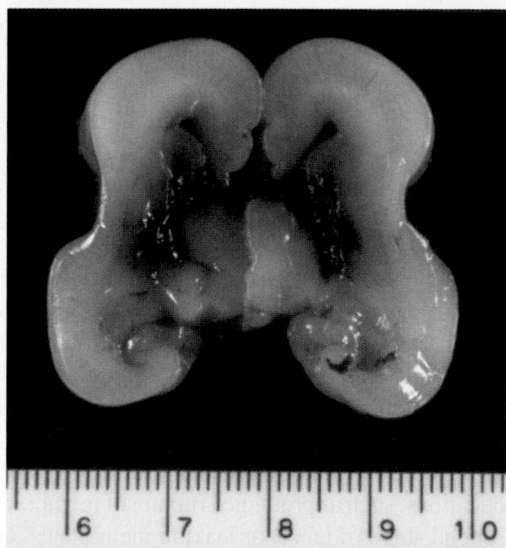

FIGURE 2-9 • Intraventricular hemorrhage in a premature infant. (From Rubin R., Strayer D. S. [Eds.]. [2008]. *Rubin's pathophysiology: Clinicopathologic foundations of medicine* [5th ed., p. 223]. Philadelphia: Lippincott Williams & Wilkins.)

to 70% for 500- to 750-g infants, and 10% to 20% for 1000- to 1500-g infants.[27] New-onset IVH is rare after the first month of life regardless of birth weight or gestational age.

Risk factors for GMH/IVH include prematurity, RDS, hypoxic–ischemic injury, hypotension or hypertension, increased or decreased cerebral blood flow, pneumothorax, and hypervolemia.[27] Cranial ultrasonography is the method of choice for diagnosis of GMH/IVH. A standard grading system using cranial ultrasonography has been adopted for evaluation of GMH/IVH, with grade I lesions describing GMH; grade II, blood within but not distending the lateral ventricular system; grade III, blood within and distending the ventricular system; and grade IV brain tissue (parenchymal) involvement with or without grade I, II, or III manifestations.[27] Clinical manifestations are determined by the level (grade) of involvement. The most common symptoms are diminished or absent Moro reflex, poor muscle tone, lethargy, apnea, and somnolence.[27] In some cases (grades I and II), no clinical manifestations may be seen. Most hemorrhages resolve, but the more severe hemorrhages may obstruct the flow of cerebrospinal fluid, causing a progressive hydrocephalus.

Necrotizing Enterocolitis. Necrotizing enterocolitis (NEC) is an acquired life-threatening emergency of the gastrointestinal system in the newborn period. The disorder is characterized by various degrees of mucosal and transmural necrosis of the intestine. The incidence is 1% to 5% of admissions to the neonatal intensive care unit.[27] Both the incidence and case fatality increase with decreasing birth weight and gestational age. The disorder is rare in term infants.

The etiology and pathogenesis of NEC are largely unknown. At present, a triad of intestinal ischemia, oral feedings (metabolic substrate), and bacterial flora of the intestine have been linked to NEC. The greatest risk for NEC is prematurity.

Although no proven cause has been documented, the disorder probably results from an interaction between mucosal damage caused by a variety of factors (*i.e.,* intestinal ischemia, infection) and the infant's response to the injury (circulatory, immunologic, inflammatory).[27,28] The selective bowel ischemia is really an asphyxiation mechanism that protects the heart and brain by shunting blood away from the kidney, gastrointestinal tract, and peripheral vascular bed. Asphyxiated infants and those suffering from respiratory compromise are the most commonly affected. The clustering of cases also suggests a primary role for infectious agents, including various viral and bacterial agents. Colonization of the intestine is a postnatal event. An infant's gastrointestinal tract, which is sterile in utero, becomes seeded with a variety of organisms during the birth process and subsequent contact with the surrounding environment. These organisms then multiply and spread with enteral feedings. NEC rarely occurs before enteral feeding is initiated and is more common in infants fed human breast milk.

Any portion of the bowel may be affected, but the distal part of the ileum and proximal segment of the colon are involved most frequently. The necrosis of the intestine may be superficial, affecting only the mucosa or submucosa, or may extend through the entire intestinal wall (Fig. 2-10). If the full thickness of the intestinal wall is damaged, perforation can result.[23,29] NEC usually has its onset in the second week, but it may occur as late as the third month in VLBW infants.[29] Age of onset is inversely related to gestational age. Manifestations of NEC are variable, but the first signs are usually abdominal distention with gastric retention. Obvious bloody stools are seen in 25% of affected infants.[29] Because of the nonspecific signs, sepsis may be suspected before an intestinal lesion is suspected. The spectrum of illness is broad and ranges from mild disease to severe illness with bowel perforation, peritonitis, systemic inflammatory response, shock, and death.

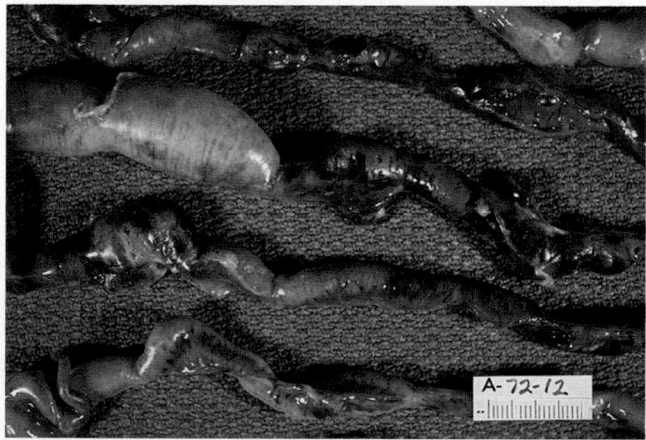

FIGURE 2-10 • Neonatal necrotizing enterocolitis. Autopsy photograph of the intestine of an infant who died of necrotizing enterocolitis shows necrosis and pneumatosis of the intestine. (From Centers for Disease Control and Prevention. [2008]. Public Health Image Library. ID #857 [Online.] Available: http://phil.cdc.gov/phil/home.asp.)

Clinical diagnosis is primarily radiographic. The radiographic hallmark of NEC is pneumatosis intestinalis or intramural air. Pneumoperitoneum is indicative of intestinal perforation. A large, stationary, distended loop of intestine on repeated radiographs may indicate gangrene, and a gasless abdomen may indicate peritonitis.[23]

Treatment includes cessation of feedings, stomach decompression, broad-spectrum antibiotic coverage, and supportive treatment. Intestinal perforation requires surgical intervention. Intestinal resection of dead intestine with a diverting ostomy is the procedure of choice.[29]

Infection and Sepsis. Sepsis is a major cause of neonatal morbidity and mortality in the neonate. Preterm infants are particularly at risk, having a 3- to 10-fold higher incidence of infection than full-term infants with normal birth weight.[30] There are a number of possible factors that contribute to the high incidence of infection in the preterm infant, including maternal genitourinary tract infections, which are thought to be a cause of preterm labor with an increased risk of vertical transmission to the infant.[30] Preterm infants are also at increased risk of infection because of the immaturity and relative inexperience of their immune system. The majority of maternal antibodies (immunoglobulin [Ig] G) are transferred during the later weeks of gestation; in preterm infants, cord immunoglobulin levels are directly proportional to gestational age[30] (see Chapter 17, Fig. 17-16). In addition, preterm infants often require invasive treatments that further increase their susceptibility to microbial invasion.

Maternal factors that increase the likelihood of infection in the preterm infant include prolonged rupture of membranes, foul-smelling amniotic fluid, maternal fever, maternal colonization with group B *Streptococcus* (GBS), and presence of a urinary tract infection.[31] Neonatal factors associated with the development of infection include antenatal or intrapartal asphyxia, congenital abnormalities, invasive diagnostic or therapeutic procedures, and administration of medications that alter normal microbial flora.[31]

Bacterial sepsis is characterized by signs of systemic infection in the presence of bacteria in the bloodstream. The incidence of bacterial sepsis in the newborn is about 1 to 8 newborns per every 1000 live births and 160 to 300 per 1000 newborns weighing less than 1500 g (VLBW).[32,33] Almost 30% of infants admitted to neonatal intensive care units may have positive blood cultures. Because of the severe consequences of untreated bacterial sepsis and the association of infection as the cause of preterm labor, preterm infants often are treated for sepsis despite the absence of a confirmatory positive blood culture. The mortality rate due to neonatal bacterial sepsis is about 25% despite the use of potent antibacterial agents and supportive care.[33]

The microorganisms responsible for newborn infection and sepsis have changed over the past decades.[32,33] Because there are significant regional variations, it is necessary to know the specific microorganisms and antibacterial agent susceptibilities in specific institutions, as well as the general predominant bacterial patterns. In this way, early therapy can be selected for the most likely bacteria when sepsis is suspected. GBS and

Escherichia coli account for 70% to 80% of positive blood cultures in the neonatal population.[33] Other bacteria such as *Listeria monocytogenes,* enterococci, and gram-negative enteric bacilli (other than *E. coli*) are seen less commonly, but must be considered.

The terms *early onset* and *late onset* are often used to describe an infant's age at the onset of infection. Early-onset infections are typically defined as those acquired before or during delivery and late-onset as those acquired after delivery in the newborn nursery, neonatal intensive care unit, or the community.[30] *Early-onset infection* is a severe, rapidly progressive multiorgan system illness that occurs within the first few days of life. The microorganisms causing early-onset infection are those that are usually found in the mother's genital tract (*e.g.,* GBS, *L. monocytogenes,* and *E. coli*). There may be a history of obstetric complications, such as prolonged rupture of membranes, prolonged second stage of labor, or leaking membranes. GBS are the most common bacteria causing early-onset bacterial sepsis in newborns, especially preterm newborns. Early-onset GBS disease typically presents with respiratory distress, hypotension, and other signs characteristic of sepsis. Signs of neurologic involvement are more common in late-onset infection.

Late-onset infections have a slower progression than early-onset infections and usually have a focal site. Meningitis is seen more often with late-onset infection than early-onset. In addition to those microorganisms responsible for early onset infection, *Staphylococcus aureus, Staphylococcus epidermidis,* other enterobacteria, as well as pseudomonads are implicated in late-onset infections.

The manifestations of bacterial infection in the newborn result from two sources: the effects of the bacterial invasion of the microorganism and the response of the infant's immune system to the invasion. Bacteria release endotoxins and other vasoactive substances, causing central vasodilation, peripheral vasoconstriction, and systemic hypovolemia. The immune response to the endotoxins leads to hemodynamic, metabolic, respiratory, CNS, gastrointestinal, and dermatologic changes. The signs of bacterial sepsis in a newborn, which can occur in all body systems, are generally nonspecific and are not easily distinguished from other causes. Therefore, it is important to have a high index of suspicion for sepsis in the newborn, especially the preterm newborn. The observation that there has been a subtle change in an infant's general condition, often marked by the nursing assessment that the infant "is not doing right," may be the first indication of infection. However, as the septicemia progresses, the signs become more severe and more specific

Optimal prognosis depends on early diagnosis and implementation of appropriate therapy; thus, frequent and careful assessment and evaluation of the infant's physical condition can have a significant impact on outcome. Administration of antimicrobial agents to mothers during the intrapartal period or to newborns immediately postpartum has been shown to reduce the risk of early-onset GBS infection. The Centers for Disease Control and Prevention (CDC) in collaboration with the American College of Obstetricians and Gynecologists and the American Academy of Pediatrics developed guidelines for prevention of neonatal GBS disease in 1996.[34,35] GBS disease continues to be a threat to the newborn because of the high mortality and morbidity rates associated with the disease and the increased survival of smaller and more preterm newborns with a higher risk for GBS disease.

Health Problems of the Infant

Infants are prone to numerous health problems during the first year of life, which may become serious if not recognized and treated appropriately. Many of them may be precipitated by the relative immaturity of the organ systems. Infants are prone to nutritional disturbances, feeding difficulties, irritable infant syndrome or colic, and failure to thrive. Injuries, the major cause of death during infancy, are caused by events such as aspiration of foreign objects, suffocation, motor vehicle accidents, falls, and poisoning. Childhood diseases may be a problem if the infant is not adequately immunized.

Nutrition

Good nutrition is important during infancy because of rapid growth. Human milk or commercial infant formulas form the basis for the early nutritional needs of the newborn and young infant. The American Academy of Pediatrics recommends breast-feeding for the first 12 months of life. Human milk from a well-nourished mother is easily digested, provides sufficient nutrients and calories for normal growth and development, and has the added benefit of offering some immune protection. Fluoride is recommended for breast-fed infants and those receiving formula made with unfluorinated water. Dietary or supplemental iron is added at approximately 6 months of age, when the fetal iron stores are depleted.

Mothers who do not choose to breast-feed their child or who are unable to breast-feed may choose from a variety of commercial formulas designed to closely match the nutrition of human milk. Several companies produce infant formulas that contain the essential nutrients for infants. Although there are some minor differences, most infant formulas are similar, regardless of which company produces the formula.

Some infants may experience difficulties in consuming mother's milk or infant formulas that are based on cow's milk because of lactase deficiency. Lactase is an enzyme that breaks down lactose, the carbohydrate found in human milk and cow's milk. Some infant formulas contain carbohydrates other than lactose. These formulas are made from soybeans. Other feeding intolerances also may occur. Treatment of any milk or formula intolerance depends on identification of the specific offender and elimination of it from the diet. Newborns and infants frequently exhibit "spitting up" or regurgitation of formula, despite the absence of a formula intolerance. In general, cow's milk–based formulas are preferable to soy-based formulas, and changing to a soy-based formula should be undertaken only when there is a proven case of intolerance. It is important that all claims of formula intolerance be thoroughly investigated before an infant is changed to a soy-based formula. Education of the parents about the signs and symptoms of intolerance and reassurance that spitting up formula is normal may be all that is required. An infant that is gaining weight, appears alert and well-nourished, has adequate stools, and demonstrates normal hunger is unlikely to have a formula intolerance.

One area of infant nutrition that is still the subject of much controversy is the introduction of solid foods. There is great variation in advice regarding when to start solid foods and what solid foods to introduce. In general, human milk or iron-fortified infant formulas should supply most infant nutrition during the first year of life. However, solid foods usually are introduced beginning at 6 months. When solid foods are being introduced, they should be considered as supplemental to the total nutrition and not as the main component of nutrition. Bland infant cereals, such as rice cereal, usually are introduced first. Slow progression to the addition of individual vegetables, fruits, and, finally, meats occurs as the infant learns to chew and swallow food. Infants also become able to drink from a cup rather than a bottle during this time.

Sometime between 9 and 12 months, the infant's intake of solid foods and formula increases, and the infant can be weaned from the breast or bottle. Much anxiety can accompany weaning, so it should be done gradually. Mothers may need reassurance that their infant is progressing normally at that time.

Irritable Infant Syndrome or Colic

Colic is usually defined as paroxysmal abdominal pain or cramping in an infant and usually is manifested by loud crying, drawing up of the legs to the abdomen, and extreme irritability.[36,37] Episodes of colic may last from several minutes to several hours a day. During this time, most efforts to soothe the infant or relieve the distress are unsuccessful. Colic is most common in infants younger than 3 months of age but can persist up to 9 months of age.

"Colic has often been described by the *rule of three:* crying for more than three hours a day, for more than three days a week, and for longer than three weeks in well-fed and healthy infants."[37] When parents seek advice about a colicky baby, their concerns should be substantiated by their health care provider. Because there may be an underlying organic cause, a careful history and physical examination should be performed. A history of apnea, cyanosis, or struggling to breathe may suggest previously undiagnosed pulmonary or cardiac conditions.[37] Tilting of the head and arching of the back may be indicative of gastroesophageal reflux (see Chapter 37).

There is no single etiologic factor that causes colic; therefore, the treatment of colic is not precise. Many nonmedical techniques and pharmacologic preparations such as antispasmodics, sedatives, and antiflatulents have been tried. Because the incidence of colic in breast-fed and bottle-fed infants is similar, mothers should be encouraged to continue breast-feeding. Early termination would deny the infant the beneficial effects of breast-feeding without relieving colic symptoms.[37] Nonpharmacologic interventions should be attempted before administration of drugs. Support of the parents is probably the single most important factor in the treatment of colic. Many times the mother (or primary care provider) may be afraid to state just how frustrated she is with her inability to console the infant. An open discussion of this frustration can help the mothers or care providers recognize that their feelings of frustration are normal; frequently, this gives them the added support needed to deal with their infant.

Failure to Thrive

Failure to thrive is a term that refers to inadequate growth of the child due to the inability to obtain or use essential nutrients. Failure to thrive may be organic or nonorganic. Organic failure to thrive is the result of a physiologic cause that prevents the infant from obtaining or using nutrients appropriately. An example of organic failure to thrive is inadequate growth of an infant with deficient energy reserve because of a congenital defect that makes sucking and feeding difficult. Nonorganic failure to thrive is the result of psychological factors that prevent adequate intake of nutrition. An example of nonorganic failure to thrive is inadequate weight gain due to inadequate intake of nutrients because of parental neglect.

Diagnosis of the type of failure to thrive depends on careful examination and history of the infant and serial follow-up evaluations. An individual infant's growth can be compared with the standards for normal growth and development. Cases of organic failure to thrive usually are easier to diagnose than cases of nonorganic failure to thrive. Diagnosis of nonorganic failure to thrive requires extensive investigation of history, family situation, relationship of the care provider to the infant, and evaluation of feeding practices. The nonorganic basis should be considered early in every case of failure to thrive.

Therapy for failure to thrive depends on the cause. Because long-term nutritional deficiencies can result in impaired physical and intellectual growth, provision of optimal nutrition is essential. Methods to increase nutritional intake by adjusting caloric density of the formula or by parenteral nutrition may be required in cases of organic failure to thrive.

Sudden Infant Death Syndrome

Sudden infant death syndrome (SIDS) is defined as death of an infant younger than 1 year of age that remains unexplained after autopsy, investigation of the death scene, and review of the history.[38,39] SIDS is rare during the first month of life, increases to a peak between 2 and 3 months of life, and then declines. Although its incidence has decreased since the "back to sleep" campaign was initiated in the United States in 1994, SIDS continues to account for more infant deaths beyond the neonatal period than any other cause.[40,41] This campaign advocated that infants be laid down to sleep in the supine position.

Factors associated with an increased risk of SIDS include sleeping in the prone position, prematurity and LBW, African American or Native American race, and exposure to environmental cigarette smoke; as well as young age of the mother, lack of or inadequate prenatal care, and smoking or substance use during pregnancy.[38,39] Sleeping prone has consistently been

shown to increase the risk of SIDS. Originally, the American Academy of Pediatrics identified any nonprone position (*i.e.*, side or back) as being optimum for reducing the risk of SIDS. The American Academy of Pediatrics now recommends that placing infants on their backs confers the lowest risk and is the preferred position.[39] Soft sleep surfaces on beds, such as comforters and pillows, also increase the risk of SIDS, as does bed sharing between infants and adults.

The exact cause of SIDS is unknown. Theories focus on brain stem abnormality, which prevents effective cardiorespiratory control.[38] Features of SIDS include prolonged sleep apnea, increased frequency of brief inspiratory pauses, excessive periodic breathing, and impaired response to increased carbon dioxide or decreased oxygen. A diagnosis of SIDS can be made only if an autopsy is performed to exclude other causes of death. Differentiation of child abuse from SIDS is an important consideration, and each case of SIDS must be subjected to careful examination.

Support of family members of an infant who dies of SIDS is crucial. Parents frequently feel guilty or inadequate as parents. The fact that there must be close scrutiny to differentiate a SIDS death from a death by child abuse adds to the guilt and disappointment felt by the family. After a diagnosis of SIDS is made, it is important that the parents and other family members receive information about SIDS. Health care providers need to be fully aware of resources available to families with a SIDS death. The siblings of the child who died of SIDS also need information and support to get through the grief process.

Injuries

Injuries are the major cause of death in infants 6 to 12 months of age. Aspiration of foreign objects, suffocation, falls, poisonings, drowning, burns, and other bodily damage may occur because of the infant's increasing ability to investigate the environment.[42] Childproofing the environment can be an important precaution to prevent injuries. No home or environment can be completely childproofed, and close supervision of the child by a competent care provider is essential to prevent injury.

Motor vehicle accidents are responsible for a significant number of infant deaths. After 1 year of age, motor vehicle accidents become the number one cause of accidental death. Most states require that infants be placed in an approved infant safety restraint while riding in a vehicle. The middle of the back seat is considered the safest place for the infant to ride. Many hospitals do not discharge an infant unless there is a safety restraint system in the car. If a family cannot afford a restraint system, programs are available that donate or loan the family a restraint. Health care providers must be involved in educating the public about the dangers of carrying infants in vehicles without taking proper precautions to protect them.

Infectious Diseases

One of the most dramatic improvements in infant health has been related to widespread immunization for the major childhood communicable diseases, including diphtheria, pertussis, tetanus, polio, measles, mumps, rubella, hepatitis B, and *Haemophilus influenzae* type B infection. Immunizations to these infectious diseases have greatly reduced morbidity and mortality in infants and young children. These immunizations are given at standard times as part of health promotion in infants and children. However, although they have lowered their prevalence, immunization programs have not completely eradicated these diseases. Immunization programs are effective only if all children receive the immunizations. Although most immunizations can be received through local health departments at no or low cost, many infants or young children do not routinely receive immunizations or do not receive the full regimen of immunizations. Methods to improve compliance and access to immunizations are needed. Immunization recommendations are subject to change as research leads to development of improved vaccines or greater understanding of the microorganisms.

IN SUMMARY, infancy is defined as that period from birth to 18 months of age. During this time, growth and development are ongoing. The relative immaturity of many of the organ systems places the infant at risk for a variety of illnesses. Birth initiates many changes in the organ systems as a means of adjusting to postnatal life. The birth process is a critical event, and maladjustments and injuries during the birth process are a major cause of death or disability. Premature delivery is a significant health problem in the United States. The premature infant is at risk for numerous health problems because of the interruption of intrauterine growth and immaturity of organ systems. ■

EARLY CHILDHOOD

After completing this section of the chapter, you should be able to meet the following objectives:

■ Define *early childhood*.
■ Describe the growth and development of early childhood.
■ Discuss the common health problems of early childhood.

Early childhood is considered the period of 18 months through 5 years of age. During this time, the child passes through the stages of toddler (*i.e.,* 18 months to 3 years) and preschooler (*i.e.,* 3 to 5 years). There are many changes as the child moves from infancy through the toddler and preschool years. The major achievements are the development and refinement of locomotion and language, which take place as children progress from dependence to independence.

EARLY CHILDHOOD

■ Early childhood, which encompasses the period from 18 months through 5 years of age, is a period of continued growth and development.
■ During this time, the child passes through the stages of toddler (*i.e.,* 18 months to 3 years) and preschooler (*i.e.,* 3 years through 5 years).
■ The major achievements are the development and refinement of locomotion and language, which take place as children progress from dependence to independence.
■ During early childhood, the child begins to develop independence. The toddler must acquire a sense of autonomy while overcoming a sense of doubt and shame. The preschooler must acquire a sense of initiative and develop a conscience.
■ Learning is ongoing and progressive and includes interactions with others, appropriate social behavior, and sex role functions.

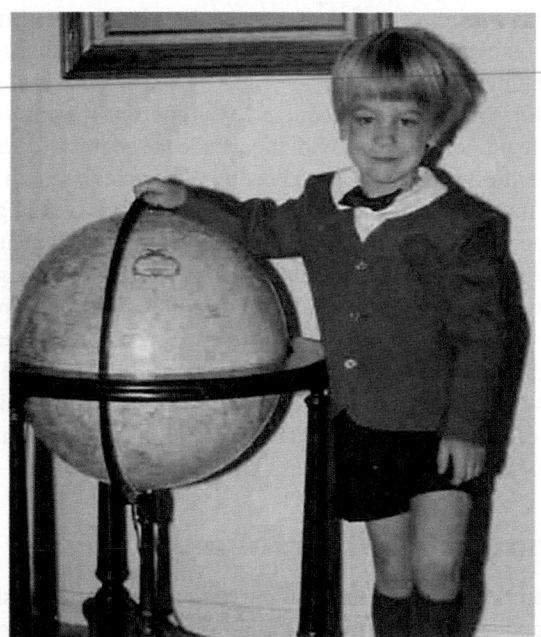

Growth and Development

Early childhood is a period of continued physical growth and maturation. Compared with infancy, physical growth is not as dramatic. Between the ages of 2 and 5 years, the average child gains approximately 2 kg in weight and 7 cm in height each year. The toddler's abdomen flattens, and the body becomes leaner. Physical energy peaks and the need for sleep declines to 11 to 13 hours a day, usually including one nap. Visual acuity reaches 20/30 by age 3 years and 20/20 by 4 years. All 20 primary teeth have erupted by 3 years of age.[3]

The maturation of organ systems is ongoing during early childhood. The respiratory system continues its growth and maturation, but because of the relative immaturity of the airway structures, otitis media and respiratory infections are common. The barrel-shaped chest that is characteristic of infancy has begun to change to a more adult shape. The respiratory rate of infancy has slowed and averages 20 to 30 breaths per minute. Respirations remain abdominal until 7 years of age.[4]

Neural growth remains rapid during early childhood. Growth is primarily hypertrophic. The brain is 90% of adult size by 2 years of age. The cephalocaudad, proximodistal principle is followed as myelinization of the cortex, brain stem, and spinal cord is completed. The spinal cord is usually completely myelinated by 2 years of age. At that time, control of anal and urethral sphincters and the motor skills of locomotion can be achieved and mastered. The continuing maturation of the neuromuscular system is increasingly evident as complex gross and fine motor skills are acquired throughout early childhood.

Growth and maturation in the musculoskeletal system continue with ossification of the skeletal system, growth of the legs, and changes in muscle and fat proportions. Legs grow faster than the trunk in early childhood; after the first year of life, approximately two thirds of the increase in height is leg growth. Muscle growth is balanced by a corresponding decrease in adipose tissue accumulation.

During early childhood, many important psychosocial tasks are mastered by the child. Independence begins to develop, and the child is on the way to becoming a social being in control of the environment. Development and refinement of gross and fine motor abilities allow involvement with a potentially infinite number of tasks and activities. Learning is ongoing and progressive and includes interactions with others, appropriate social behavior, and sex role functions. Erikson described the tasks that must be accomplished in early childhood. The toddler must acquire a sense of autonomy while overcoming a sense of doubt and shame. The preschooler must acquire a sense of initiative and develop a conscience.[19]

Common Health Problems

The early childhood years can pose significant health risks to the growing and maturing child. Injuries are the leading cause of death in children between the ages of 1 and 4 years; only adolescents experience more injuries. Locomotion, together with a lack of awareness of danger, places toddlers and preschoolers at special risk for injuries. Motor vehicle accidents are responsible for almost 50% of all accidental deaths in this group.[42] Many of the injuries and deaths can be prevented by appropriate seat belts and restraints in car seats. Other major causes of injuries include drowning, burns, poisoning, falls, aspiration and suffocation, and bodily damage.[4]

Infectious diseases can be a problem for children during early childhood owing to the immaturity of their immune system. This also may be the time when children first enter day care, which increases their exposure to other children and infectious diseases. The major disorders include the communicable childhood diseases (*e.g.,* common cold, influenza, varicella [chicken pox], gastrointestinal tract infections, and otitis media).[4]

Child maltreatment is an increasing problem in the United States. Although the numbers vary according to the methods and definitions used, the best estimates indicate that approximately 1.4 million children in the United States undergo some form of abuse.[43] Child maltreatment includes physical and emotional neglect, physical abuse, and sexual abuse. Neglect is the most common type of maltreatment and can take the form of deprivation of basic necessities or failure to meet the child's emotional needs. It is often attributed to poor parenting skills. Physical abuse is the deliberate infliction of injury. The cause is probably multifactorial, with predisposing factors that include the parent, child, and environment. Sexual abuse is on the rise and includes a spectrum of types. The typical abuser is male. Children often do not report the abuse because they are afraid of not being believed.[4,43]

IN SUMMARY, early childhood is defined as the period from 18 months to 5 years of age—the toddler and preschool years. Growth and development continue but are not as dramatic as during the prenatal and infancy periods. Early childhood is a time when most organ systems reach maturity and the child becomes an independent, mobile being. There continue to be significant health risks during this period, especially from infectious diseases and injuries. Injuries are the leading cause of death during this period. Child abuse is rapidly increasing as a major health problem. ■

MIDDLE TO LATE CHILDHOOD

After completing this section of the chapter, you should be able to meet the following objectives:

■ Define *middle to late childhood.*
■ Characterize the growth and development that occurs during the early school years.
■ Discuss the common health problems of middle to late childhood.

In this text, middle to late childhood is defined as the period in which a child begins school through the beginning of adolescence. These 6 years, from 6 to 12 years of age, involve a great deal of change; when one recollects "childhood," these are the years most often remembered. The experiences of this period have a profound effect on the physical, cognitive, and psychosocial development of the child and contribute greatly to the adult that the child will become.

🔑 MIDDLE TO LATE CHILDHOOD

- Middle to late childhood years (6 to 12 years) are those during which the child begins school through the beginning of adolescence.

- Growth during this period averages 3 to 3.5 kg and 6 cm per year, and occurs in approximately three to four bursts per year that last for approximately 8 weeks.

- Muscular strength, coordination, and stamina increase progressively, as does the ability to perform complex movements such as shooting basketballs, playing the piano, and dancing.

- During this stage, the child develops the cognitive skills that are needed to consider several factors simultaneously and to evaluate oneself and perceive others' evaluations.

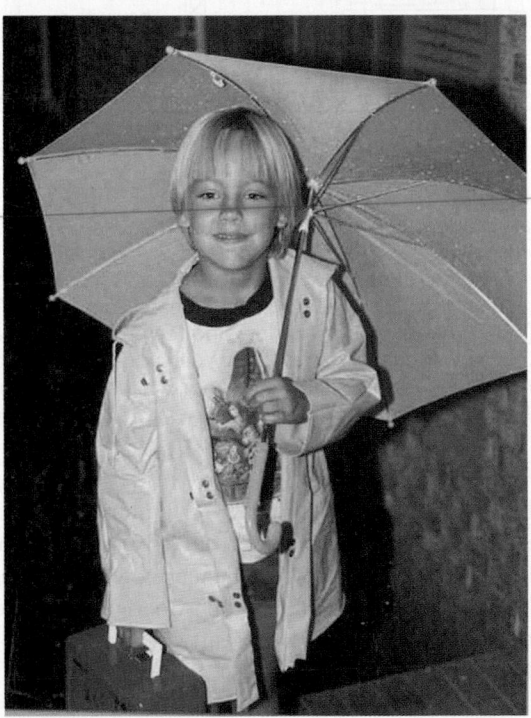

Growth and Development

Although physical growth is steady throughout middle childhood, it is slower than in the previous periods and the adolescent period to follow. During late childhood, children typically gain approximately 3 to 3.5 kg and grow an average of 6 cm per year.[3] Growth occurs discontinuously, in three to six irregularly timed spurts each year.

During late childhood, a child's legs grow longer, posture improves, and his or her center of gravity descends to a lower point. These changes make children more graceful and help

them to be successful at climbing, bike riding, roller skating, and other physical activities. Body fat distribution decreases and, in combination with the lengthening skeleton, gives the child a thinner appearance. As body fat decreases, lean muscle mass increases. By 12 years of age, boys and girls have doubled their body strength and physical capabilities. Although muscular strength increases, the muscles are still relatively immature and injury from over strenuous activities, such as difficult sports, can occur. With the gains in length, the head circumference decreases in relation to height, waist circumference decreases in relation to height, and leg length increases in relation to height.

The head grows only 2 to 3 cm during this period, indicating slower brain growth; myelination is complete by 7 years of age. Facial proportions change as the face grows faster in relation to the rest of the cranium. Primary teeth are lost and replaced by permanent teeth. When the permanent teeth first appear, they may appear to be too big for the mouth and face. This is a temporary imbalance that is alleviated as the face grows.

Caloric requirements usually are lower compared with previous periods and with the adolescent period to follow. Cardiac growth is slow. Heart rate and respiratory rates continue to decrease, and blood pressure gradually rises. Growth of the eye continues, and the normal farsightedness of the preschool child is gradually converted to 20/20 vision by approximately 11 to 12 years. Frequent vision assessment is recommended during late childhood as part of normal routine health screenings.[4]

Bone ossification and mineralization continue. Children's bones cannot resist muscle pressure and pull as well as mature bones. Precautions should be taken to prevent alterations in bone structure, such as providing properly fitting shoes and adequate desks to prevent poor posture. Children should be checked routinely and often for scoliosis (see Chapter 58) during this period.

Toward the end of late childhood, the physical differences between the two sexes become apparent. Girls usually enter pubescence approximately 2 years before boys, resulting in noticeable differences in height, weight, and development of secondary sex characteristics. There is much individual variation among children of the same sex. These differences can be extremely difficult for children to cope with.

Entry into the school setting has a major impact on the psychosocial development of the child at this age. The child begins to develop relationships with other children, forming groups. Peers become more important as the child moves out of the security of the family and into the bigger world. Usually during this period, children begin to form closer bonds with individual "best friends." However, the best friend relationships may frequently change. The personality of the child begins to appear. Although the personality is still developing, the basic temperament and approach to life become apparent. Although changes in personality occur with maturity, the basic elements may not change. The major task of this stage, as identified by Erikson, is the development of industry or accomplishment.[19] Failure to meet this task results in a sense of inferiority or incompetence, which can impede further progress.

Common Health Problems

Because of the high level of immune system competence in late childhood, these children have an immunologic advantage over earlier years. Respiratory infections are the leading cause of illness at this time, followed by gastrointestinal disorders. The chief cause of mortality is accidents, primarily motor vehicle accidents. Immunization against the major communicable diseases of childhood has greatly improved the health of children in their middle childhood years.

Health promotion includes appropriate dental care. The incidence of dental caries has decreased since the addition of fluoride to most water systems in the United States. There is a high incidence of dental caries during late childhood that is related to inadequate dental care and a high amount of dietary sugar. Children at the early part of this stage may not be as effective in brushing their teeth and may require adult assistance, but they may be reluctant to allow parental help.

Infections with bacterial and fungal agents are a common problem in childhood. These infections commonly occur as respiratory, gastrointestinal, or skin diseases. Infections of the skin occur more frequently in this age group than in any other, probably related to increased exposure to skin lesions. Other acute or chronic health problems may surface for the first time. Asthma, caused by allergic reactions, frequently manifests for the first time during middle childhood (see Chapter 29). Epilepsy also may be first diagnosed during this period. Many childhood cancers also may appear. Developmental disabilities or specific learning disabilities may become apparent as the child enters school.

Overweight and Obesity

Overweight and obesity is becoming an increasingly common problem that begins in childhood[44-47] (see discussion of childhood obesity in Chapter 39). Overweight and obesity in children and adolescents is defined by body mass index (weight in kilograms divided by the square of height in meters) at or above the 95th percentile for children of the same age and gender[47] (Fig. 2-11). Data for two National Health and Nutrition Examination Surveys (NHANES; 1976 to 1980 and 2003 to 2004) show that the prevalence of over-

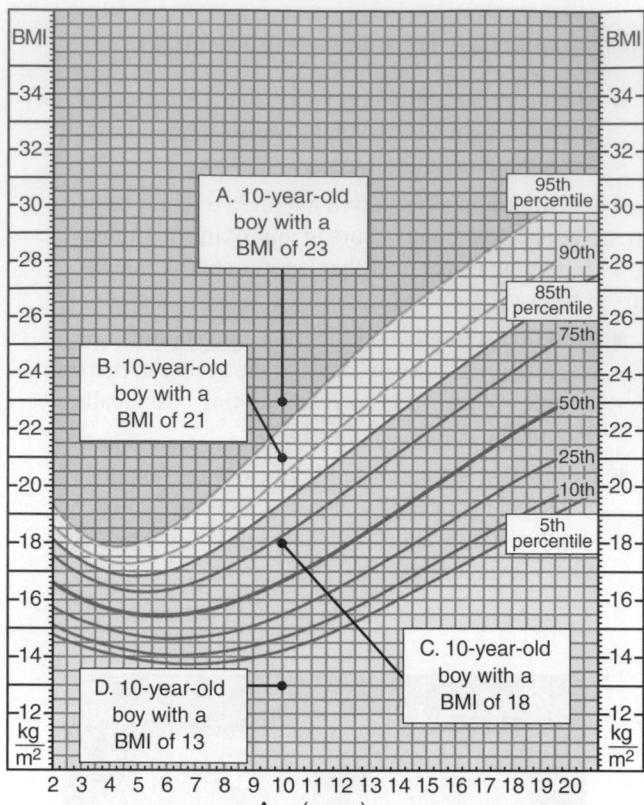

FIGURE 2-11 • Body mass index-for-age percentiles for boys 2 to 20 years of age. Overweight in children and adolescents is defined by body mass index (weight in kilograms divided by the square of height in meters) at or above the 95th percentile for children of the same age and sex. (From Centers for Disease Control and Prevention. [2007]. About BMI in children and teens. [Online.] Available: www.cdc.gov/nccdphp/dnpa/obesity/defining.htm. Calculator for determining BMI available at http://apps.nccd.cdc.gov/dnpabmi/Calculator.aspx.)

weight for children is increasing: for children 6 to 11 years of age, the prevalence increased from 6.5% to 18.8%, and for those 12 to 19 years, the prevalence increased from 5.0% to 17.4%[46,47] (Table 2-2). African American and Mexican American children and adolescents are disproportionately affected.

AGE (YEARS)	NHANES I 1971–1974	NHANES II 1976–1980	NHANES III 1988–1994	NHANES IV 2003–2004
2–5	5%	5%	7.2%	13.9%
6–11	4%	6.5%	11.3%	18.8%
12–19	6.1%	5%	10.5%	17.4%

TABLE 2-2 Prevalence of Overweight* Among U.S. Children and Adolescents (Aged 2 to 19 Years): Data From National Health and Nutrition Examination Surveys (NHANES)

*Sex- and age-specific body mass index >95th percentile based on Centers for Disease Control and Prevention growth charts.
Data available online: http://cdc.gov/nccdphp/dnpa/obesity/childhood/index.htm.

The causes of childhood overweight are undoubtedly multifactorial, but ultimately reflect an imbalance between the amount of calories the child consumes in food and beverages and the calories that the child uses to support growth and development, metabolism, and physical activity.[44] Evidence is limited on specific foods or dietary patterns that contribute to excessive energy intake in children; however, large portion sizes for food and beverages, eating meals away from home, frequent snacking and consumption of energy-dense foods, and consuming beverages with added calories are often hypothesized as contributing to excessive energy intake. Participating in physical activity is important for children because of its beneficial effects not only on weight, but on blood pressure and bone strength. Media use, and specifically television viewing, may displace time children spend in physical activity. It may also contribute to increased energy consumption through excessive snacking and eating meals in front of the television. Genetic factors may increase a child's susceptibility to become overweight. However, this genetic susceptibility may need to exist in conjunction with other contributing factors such as a high-calorie food intake and minimal physical activity.[44]

Pediatric obesity is not just a cosmetic issue, but is associated with a significant burden of ill health both in obese children and for adults who were obese as children.[44] Approximately 60% of overweight children have at least one additional risk factor for cardiovascular disorders, such as hypertension, hyperlipidemia, or hyperinsulinemia; and more than 25% have two risk factors.[44] Overweight and obesity also predisposes to type 2 diabetes mellitus. It has been estimated that type 2 diabetes accounts for anywhere from 8% to 45% of all new cases of diabetes in children and adolescents.[44]

IN SUMMARY, middle to late childhood is defined as that period from beginning school through adolescence. During these 6 years, growth is steady but much slower than in the previous periods. Entry into school begins the formation of relationships with peers and has a major impact on psychological development. This is a wonderful period of relatively good health secondary to an immunologic advantage, but respiratory disease poses a leading cause of illness, and motor vehicle accidents are the major cause of death. Several chronic health problems such as asthma, epilepsy, and childhood cancers may surface during this time.

Overweight and obesity, defined by body mass index (weight in kilograms divided by the square of height in meters) at or above the 95th percentile for children of the same age and sex, is becoming an increasingly common problem that begins in childhood. The causes of childhood overweight are undoubtedly multifactorial, but ultimately reflect an imbalance between the amount of calories the child consumes in food and beverages and the calories that the child uses to support growth and development, metabolism, and physical activity. ∎

ADOLESCENCE

After completing this section of the chapter, you should be able to meet the following objectives:

- Define what is meant by the period known as *adolescence*.
- Characterize the physical and psychosocial changes that occur during adolescence.
- Cite the developmental tasks that adolescents need to fulfill.
- Describe common concerns of parents regarding their adolescent child.
- Discuss how the changes that occur during adolescence can influence the health care needs of the adolescent.

Adolescence is a transitional period between childhood and adulthood. It is a period of physical, emotional, and cognitive growth. The changes of adolescence do not occur on a strict timeline; instead, they occur at different times according to a unique internal calendar. For definition's sake, adolescence is considered to begin with the development of secondary sex characteristics, around 11 or 12 years of age, and to end with the completion of somatic growth from approximately 18 to 20 years of age. Girls usually begin and end adolescence earlier than boys. The adolescent period is conveniently referred to as the *teenaged years*, from 13 through 19 years of age.

ADOLESCENT PERIOD

- The adolescent period, which extends from 13 through 19 years of age, is a time of rapid changes in body size and shape, and physical, psychological, and social functioning.
- Adolescence is a time when hormones and sexual maturation interact with social structures in fostering the transition from childhood to adulthood.
- The developmental tasks of adolescence include achieving independence from parents, adopting peer codes and making personal lifestyle choices, forming or revising individual body image, and coming to terms with one's body image.

Several "tasks" that adolescents need to fulfill have been identified. These tasks include achieving independence from parents, adopting peer codes and making personal lifestyle choices, forming or revising individual body image and coming to terms with one's body image if it is not "perfect," and establishing sexual, ego, vocational, and moral identities.

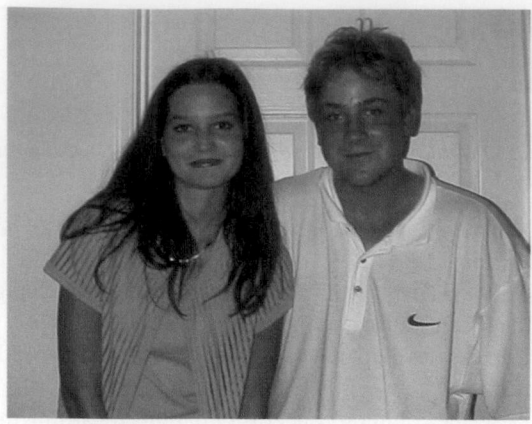

Growth and Development

Adolescence is influenced by CNS-mediated hormonal activity. Physical growth occurs simultaneously with sexual maturation.[3,48] Adolescents typically experience gains of 20% to 25% in linear growth. An adolescent growth spurt lasting approximately 24 to 36 months accounts for most of this somatic growth. The age at onset, duration, and extent of the growth vary between boys and girls and among individuals. In girls, the growth spurt usually begins around 10 to 14 years of age. It begins earlier in girls than in boys and ends earlier, with less dramatic changes in weight and height. Girls usually gain approximately 5 to 20 cm in height and 7 to 25 kg in weight. Most girls have completed their growth spurt by 16 or 17 years of age. Boys begin their growth spurt later, but it usually is more pronounced, with an increase in height of 10 to 30 cm and an increase in weight of 7 to 30 kg. Boys may continue to gain in height until 18 to 20 years of age. Increases in height are possible until approximately 25 years of age.[48]

The changes in physical body size have a characteristic pattern. Growth in arms, legs, hands, feet, and neck is followed by increases in hip and chest size and several months later by increases in shoulder width and depth and trunk length.[3] The period of these rapid and dramatic changes may be difficult for the adolescent and parents. Shoe size may change several times over several months. Although brain size is not significantly increased during adolescence, the size and shape of the skull and facial bones change, making the features of the face appear to be out of proportion until full adult growth is attained.[4,48] Muscle mass and strength also increase during adolescence. Sometimes, there may be a discrepancy between the growth of bone and muscle mass, creating a temporary dysfunction with slower or less smooth movements resulting from the mismatch of bone and muscle. Body proportions undergo typical changes during adolescence. In boys, the thorax becomes broader, and the pelvis remains narrow. In girls, the opposite occurs: the thorax remains narrow, and the pelvis widens.

Organ systems also undergo changes in function, and some have changes in structure. The heart increases in size as the result of increased muscle cell size. Heart rate decreases to normal adult rates, whereas blood pressure increases rapidly to adult rates. Circulating blood volume and hemoglobin concentration increase. Boys demonstrate greater changes in blood volume and higher hemoglobin concentrations because of the influence of testosterone and their relatively greater muscle mass.

Skin becomes thicker and additional hair growth occurs in both sexes. Sebaceous and sweat gland activity increases. Adrenal androgens stimulate the sebaceous glands, promoting the development of acne (see Chapter 61). Increased sweat gland activity results in perspiration and body odor. Voice changes are of significant importance during adolescence for both sexes; however, the change is more pronounced in boys. The voice change results from growth of the larynx, pharynx, and lungs.[3] There is more growth of the larynx in boys than in girls. The paranasal sinuses reach adult proportions, which increases the resonance of the voice, adding to the adult sound of the voice.[4,48] Dental changes include jaw growth, loss of the final deciduous teeth, and eruption of the permanent cuspids, premolars, and molars.[3] Orthodontic appliances may be needed.

Changes in the endocrine system are of great importance in the initiation and continuation of the adolescent growth spurt. The hormones involved include growth hormone (GH), thyroid hormones, adrenal hormones, insulin, and the gonadotropic hormones. GH regulates growth in childhood but is essentially replaced by sex hormones as the primary impetus for growth during adolescence. The exact role of GH in the adolescent growth spurt is unclear. Thyroid hormone, a significant hormone in the regulation of metabolism during childhood, continues to be important during adolescence. The relation of thyroid hormone to the other hormones and its role in the adolescent growth spurt is unclear. The thyroid gland becomes larger during adolescence, and it is believed that production of thyroid hormones is increased during this period. Insulin is necessary for appropriate growth at all stages, including adolescence. Insulin must be present for GH to be effective. The pancreatic islets of Langerhans increase in size during adolescence.[48]

The anterior pituitary gland produces the gonadotropic hormones, follicle-stimulating hormone and luteinizing hormone. These hormones influence target organs to secrete sex hormones. The ovaries respond by secreting estrogens and progesterone, and the testes respond by producing androgens, resulting in the maturation of the primary sex characteristics and the appearance of secondary sex characteristics. Primary sex characteristics are those involved in reproductive function (*i.e.,* internal and external genitalia). The secondary sex characteristics are the physical signs that signal the presence of sexual maturity but are not directly involved in reproduction (*e.g.,* pubic and axillary hair). Androgens initiate the beginning of the growth spurt. Sex hormones, including androgens, also conclude growth in height by triggering bone maturity, epiphyseal closure of bones, and discontinuation of skeletal growth.

The dramatic and extensive physical changes that occur during the transition from child to adult are matched only by the psychosocial changes that occur during the adolescent period. It is not possible to develop one guide that adequately describes and explains the tremendous changes that occur during adolescence because the experience is unique for each adolescent. There are, fortunately, some commonalities within the process that can be used to facilitate understanding of these changes. The transition from child to adult is not a smooth, continuous, or uniform process. There are frequent periods of rapid change, followed by brief plateaus. These periods can change with little or no warning, which makes living with an adolescent difficult at times.

There is one thing that persons who deal with adolescents must remember: no matter how rocky the transition from child to adult, adolescence is not a permanent disability. Eighty percent of adolescents go through adolescence with few or no lasting difficulties. Health care professionals who care for adolescents may need to offer support to worried parents that the difficulties their adolescent is experiencing, and that the entire family is experiencing as a result, may be normal. The adolescent also may need reassurance that his or her feelings are not abnormal.[48]

Common concerns of adolescents include conflicts with parents, conflicts with siblings, concerns about school, and concerns about peers and peer relationships. Personal identity is an overwhelming concern expressed by adolescents. Common health problems experienced by adolescents include headache, stomachache, and insomnia. These disorders may be psychosomatic in origin. Adolescents also may exhibit situational anxiety and mild depression. The health care worker may need to refer adolescents for specialized counseling or medical care if any of these health care concerns are exaggerated.

Parents of adolescents also may have concerns about their child. Common concerns related to the adolescent's behavior include rebelliousness, wasting time, risk-taking behaviors, mood swings, drug experimentation, school problems, psychosomatic complaints, and sexual activity.[48] Adolescence is a period of transition from childhood to adulthood and it is often filled with conflicts as the adolescent attempts to take on an adult role. Open communication between the adolescent and family can help make the transition less stressful; however, communication between parents and adolescents can be difficult.

Common Health Problems

Adolescence is considered to be a relatively healthy period; however, significant morbidity and mortality do occur. Health promotion is of extreme importance during the adolescent period. There are fewer actual physical health problems during this period, but there is a greater risk of morbidity and mortality from other causes, such as accidents, homicide, or suicide.[48-51]

Cancer is the fourth leading cause of death in adolescents, but it is the leading cause of death from nonviolent sources. There is an increased incidence of certain types of cancer during adolescence, including lymphomas, and bone and genital tumors.[48]

Several factors contribute to the risk for injury during adolescence. The adolescent often is unable to recognize potentially dangerous situations, possibly because of a discrepancy between physical maturity and cognitive and emotional

development. Certain behavioral and developmental characteristics of the adolescent exaggerate this problem. Adolescents typically feel the need to challenge parental or other authority. They also have a strong desire to "fit in" with the peer group. Adolescents exhibit a type of magical thinking and have a need to experiment with potentially dangerous situations or behaviors. They believe that bad things will not happen to them, despite engaging in risky behaviors.

The leading causes of adolescent mortality are motor vehicle crashes and other accidents, homicide, and suicide.[48] Many of the accidental injuries are preventable with the use of simple safety measures, including automobile seat belts and bicycle and motorcycle helmets. Although the number of adolescents reporting suicidal thoughts has decreased in the past decade, the number of suicide attempts has remained constant.[49] Risk factors for suicide in adolescents include substance abuse, personal or family history of depression, problems at school, problems communicating with parents, current legal problems, and family ownership of a handgun. Suicide attempts are often associated with drug or alcohol abuse.

Additional types of behavior that contribute to the leading causes of death and disability among adolescents include risky sexual behaviors, drug and alcohol abuse, and tobacco use.[48-51] The increasing prevalence of sexual activity among adolescents has created unique health problems. These include adolescent pregnancy, sexually transmitted infections, and human immunodeficiency virus (HIV) transmission. Associated problems include substance abuse, such as alcohol, tobacco, inhalants, and other illicit drugs. Health care providers must not neglect discussing sexual activity with the adolescent. Nonjudgmental, open, factual communication is essential for dealing with an adolescent's sexual practices. Discussion of sexual activity frequently is difficult for the adolescent and the adolescent's family. If a relationship exists between the adolescent and the health care provider, this may provide a valuable forum for the adolescent to get accurate information about safe sex, including contraception and avoidance of high-risk behaviors for acquiring sexually transmitted infections or acquired immunodeficiency syndrome (AIDS).

Pregnancy has become a major problem of the teen years. Approximately 1 million adolescents in the United States become pregnant each year.[2] Four of every 10 female teenagers become pregnant before reaching 20 years of age. One fifth of all pregnancies occur within the first month after beginning sexual activity; one half occur within the first 6 months of sexual activity. Of the slightly more than 1 million pregnant adolescents, 47% delivered, 40% had therapeutic abortions, and 13% had spontaneous abortions.[4]

Adolescent pregnancy poses significant risks to the mother and to the fetus or newborn. The topic of adolescent pregnancy involves issues related to physical and biologic maturity of the adolescent, growth requirements of the adolescent and fetus, and unique prenatal care requirements of the pregnant adolescent. Emotional responses and psychological issues regarding relationships of the adolescent in her family and with the father of the infant, as well as how the pregnancy will affect the adolescent's future, must be considered.

Substance abuse among adolescents increased rapidly during the 1960s and 1970s but has declined since that time. However, substance abuse still is prevalent in the adolescent age group. Health care workers must be knowledgeable about the symptoms of drug abuse, the consequences of drug abuse, and the appropriate management of adolescents with substance abuse problems. Substance abuse among adolescents includes the use of tobacco products, particularly cigarettes and "smokeless" tobacco (*e.g.,* snuff, chewing tobacco). Other substances include alcohol, marijuana, stimulants, inhalants, cocaine, hallucinogens, tranquilizers, and sedatives. Adolescents are at high risk for succumbing to the peer pressure to participate in substance abuse. They have a strong desire to fit in and be accepted by their peer group. It is difficult for them to "just say no." Magical thinking leads adolescents to believe that they will not get "hooked" or that the bad consequences will not happen to them. Adolescents and the rest of society are constantly bombarded with the glamorous side of substance use. Television shows, movies, and magazine advertisements are filled with beautiful, healthy, successful, happy, and popular persons who are smoking cigarettes or drinking beer or other alcoholic beverages. Adolescents are trying to achieve the lifestyle depicted in those ads, and it takes tremendous willpower to resist that temptation. It is important that adolescents be provided with "the rest of the story" through education and constant communication.[4,48]

IN SUMMARY, adolescence is a transitional period between childhood and adulthood. It begins with development of secondary sex characteristics (11 to 12 years) and ends with cessation of somatic growth (18 to 20 years). This is the period of a major growth spurt, which is more pronounced in boys. The endocrine system is of great importance, with its numerous hormonal changes and their initiation and continuation of the growth spurt. Psychosocial changes are equally dramatic during this period and often place tremendous pressure on relationships between adults and the adolescent. Adolescence is a relatively healthy period, but significant morbidity and mortality exist as a result of accidents, homicide, and suicide. The prevalence of sexual activity and substance abuse places the adolescent at risk for HIV infection; alcohol, tobacco, and other drug abuse; and adolescent pregnancy. ■

Review Exercises

1. The vital signs of a full-term, 1-day-old newborn are temperature 101.4°F (axillary), heart rate 188 beats/minute, respirations 70 breaths/minute, blood pressure 56/36 mm Hg.

   A. *What laboratory test(s) should be performed?*

   B. *What information could be obtained from review of the maternal record that may be helpful in*

   establishing a differential diagnosis for this infant?

   C. *What other clinical signs should be assessed?*

2. A preterm newborn, approximately 30 weeks' gestation, is admitted to the neonatal intensive care unit. The infant exhibits respiratory distress, including tachypnea, retractions, and expiratory grunting.

   A. *Identify the two most common causes for respiratory distress in such an infant.*

   B. *Explain the etiology for the two causes identified.*

3. A 10-year-old boy is seen in the clinic for a routine physical examination. His weight is 50 kg and his height is 149 cm. His mother complains that he is constantly watching television or playing video games and seems to have no interest in riding his bike or participating in physical sports. Furthermore, he is constantly snacking and drinking sugar-sweetened cola drinks.

   A. *Use the CDC's online child and teen body mass index (BMI) calculator (http://apps.nccd.cdc.gov/dnpabmi/Calculator.aspx) to calculate this boy's BMI and determine whether he is overweight.*

   B. *What suggestions might you provide for this boy and his mother?*

4. An adolescent boy is seen in the health clinic for a routine sports examination. The nurse practitioner notes that the adolescent has a mild to moderate case of facial acne. The nurse practitioner discusses the causes, prevention, and treatment of acne with the young man.

   A. *What physiologic changes contribute to the development of acne in adolescents?*

   B. *What other physical changes also occur during adolescence?*

   C. *What are common health problems in adolescents?*

References

1. U.S. Department of Health and Human Services. (2000). *Healthy children 2000.* Washington, DC: Author.
2. Federal Interagency Forum on Child and Family Statistics. (2007). *America's children: Key national indicators of well-being.* [Online.] Available: http://childstats.gov/americaschildren/health2.asp. Accessed April 20, 2008.
3. Needlman R. D. (2004). Growth and development. In Behrman R. E., Kliegman R. M., Jenson H. B. (Eds.), *Nelson textbook of pediatrics* (17th ed., pp. 23–64). Philadelphia: Elsevier Saunders.
4. Zitelli B. J., Davis H. J. (2002). *Atlas of pediatric physical diagnosis* (4th ed.). St. Louis: Mosby-Year Book.
5. Centers for Disease Control and Prevention (CDC), National Center for Health Statistics. (2000). CDC growth charts United States. [Online.] Available: www.cdc.gov/growthcharts/.

6. Moore K. L., Persaud T. V. N., Chabner D. E. B. (2003). *The developing human: Clinically oriented embryology* (7th ed.). Philadelphia: W. B. Saunders.

7. Lott J. W. (2007). Fetal development: Environmental influences and critical periods. In Kerner C., Lott J. W. (Eds.). *Comprehensive neonatal care: An interdisciplinary approach* (4th ed., pp. 625–647). Philadelphia: Elsevier Saunders.

8. O'Brien P. (2003). *Langman's medical embryology* (9th ed.). Philadelphia: Lippincott Williams & Wilkins.

9. Bowers B. (2007). Prenatal, antenatal, and postnatal risk factors. In Kenner C., Lott J. W. (Eds.), *Comprehensive neonatal nursing: A physiologic perspective* (4th ed., pp. 648–665). Philadelphia: Elsevier Saunders.

10. Sansoucie D. A., Calvaliere T. A. (2007). Newborn and infant assessment. In Kenner C., Lott J. W. (Eds.), *Comprehensive neonatal nursing: A physiologic perspective* (4th ed., pp. 677–718). Philadelphia: Elsevier Saunders.

11. Barnes F. L. (2000). The effects of the early uterine environment on the subsequent development of embryo and fetus [review]. *Theriogenology* 53, 649–658.

12. Lubchenco L. O., Hansman C., Dressler M., et al. (1963). Intrauterine growth as estimated from liveborn birthweight data at 24 to 42 weeks of gestation. *Pediatrics* 32, 793–800.

13. Battaglia F. C., Lubchenco L. O. (1967). A practical classification of newborn infants by weight and gestational age. *Journal of Pediatrics* 71, 748–758.

14. Ballard J. L., Khoury J. C., Wedig K., et al. (1991). New Ballard score, expanded to include extremely premature infants. *Journal of Pediatrics* 119, 417–423.

15. Das U. G., Sysyn G. D. (2004). Abnormal fetal growth: Intrauterine growth retardation, small for gestational age, large for gestational age. *Pediatric Clinics of North America* 51, 639–654.

16. Dubowitz L. M., Dubowitz V., Goldberg C. (1970). Clinical assessment of gestational age in the newborn infant. *Journal of Pediatrics* 77, 1–10.

17. Moore K. L., Dalley A. F. (2006). *Clinically oriented anatomy* (5th ed., pp. 904–905). Philadelphia: Lippincott Williams & Wilkins.

18. Thilo E. H., Rosenberg A. A. (2003). The newborn infant. In Hay W. W., Hayward A. R., Levin M., et al. (Eds.), *Current pediatric diagnosis and treatment* (16th ed., pp. 1–63). New York: McGraw-Hill Medical.

19. Erikson E. (1963). *Childhood and society.* New York: W. W. Norton.

20. Apgar V. (1953). A proposal for a new method of evaluation of the newborn infant. *Current Research in Anesthesia and Analgesia* 32, 260.

21. Sperling M. A. (2004). Hypoglycemia. In Behrman R. E., Kliegman R. M., Jenson H. B. (Eds.), *Nelson textbook of pediatrics* (17th ed., pp. 505–518). Philadelphia: Elsevier Saunders.

22. Cohen S. M. (2006). Jaundice in the full-term newborn. *Pediatric Nursing* 32, 202–208.

23. Stoll B. J., Kliegman R. M. (2004). The fetus and neonatal infant. In Behrman R. E., Kliegman R. M., Jenson H. B. (Eds.), *Nelson textbook of pediatrics* (17th ed., pp. 561–566, 590–599). Philadelphia: Elsevier Saunders.

24. Blackburn S. T., Ditzenberger G. R. (2003). Neurologic system. In Kenner C., Lott J. W. (Eds.), *Comprehensive neonatal nursing: A multidisciplinary approach* (4th ed., pp. 624–660). Philadelphia: Elsevier Saunders.

25. Uhing M. R. (2004). Management of birth injuries. *Pediatric Clinics of North America* 51, 1169–1186.

26. Cifuentes J., Segars A. H., Ross M., et al. (2007). Respiratory system. In Kenner C., Lott J. W. (Eds.), *Comprehensive neonatal nursing: An interdisciplinary approach* (4th ed., pp. 1–31). Philadelphia: Elsevier Saunders.

27. Crocetti M., Barone M. A. (2004). *Oski's essential pediatrics* (2nd ed., pp. 61–64). Philadelphia: Lippincott Williams & Wilkins.

28. Papile L. S., Burstein J., Burstein R., et al. (1978). Incidence and evolution of the subependymal intraventricular hemorrhage: A study of infants weighing less than 1500 grams. *Journal of Pediatrics* 92, 529–534.

29. Thigpen J. (2007). Assessment and management of gastrointestinal dysfunction. In Kenner C., Lott J. W. (Eds.), *Comprehensive neonatal nursing: A multidisciplinary approach* (pp. 92–133). Philadelphia: Elsevier Saunders.

30. Stoll B. J. (2004). Infections in the neonatal infant. In Behrman R. E., Kliegman R. M., Jenson H. B. (Eds.), *Nelson textbook of pediatrics* (17th ed., pp. 623–640). Philadelphia: Elsevier Saunders.

31. Gerdes J. S. (2004). Diagnosis and management of bacterial infections in the neonate. *Pediatric Clinics of North America* 51, 939–959.

32. Baltimore S., Huie S., Meek J., et al. (2001). Early-onset neonatal sepsis in the era of group B streptococcal prevention. *Pediatrics* 108, 1094–1098.

33. Klein J., Remington J. S. (2001). Current concepts of infections of the fetus and newborn infant. In Remington J. S., Klein J. O. (Eds.), *Infectious disease in the fetus and newborn infant* (5th ed., pp. 1–23). Philadelphia: W. B. Saunders.

34. Edwards M., Baker C. (2001). Group B streptococcal infections. In Remington J. S., Klein J. O. (Eds.), *Infectious disease in the fetus and newborn infant* (5th ed., pp. 1091–1156). Philadelphia: W. B. Saunders.

35. Rosenstein N. E., Sucuchat A., for the Neonatal Group B Study Group. (1997). Opportunities for prevention of perinatal group B streptococcal disease: A multi-state analysis. *Obstetrics and Gynecology* 90, 901–906.

36. Rogovik A. L., Goldman R. D. (2005). Treating infants' colic. *Canadian Family Physician* 51, 1209–1211.

37. Roberts D. M., Ostapchuk M., O'Brien J. G. (2004). Infantile colic. *American Family Physician* 70, 735–740.

38. Hunt C., Hauck F. R. (2004). Sudden infant death syndrome. In Behrman R. E., Kliegman R. M., Jenson H. B. (Eds.), *Nelson textbook of pediatrics* (17th ed., pp. 1380–1385). Philadelphia: Elsevier Saunders.

39. America Academy of Pediatrics Task Force on Sudden Infant Death Syndrome. (2005). The changing concept of sudden infant death syndrome: Diagnostic coding shifts, controversies regarding sleeping environment, and new variables to consider in reducing risk. *Pediatrics* 116, 1245–1255.

40. Pastore G., Guala A., Zaffaroni M. (2003). Back to sleep: Risk factors for SIDS as targets for public health campaigns. *Journal of Pediatrics* 142, 453–454.

41. Hunt C. E., Lesko S. M., Vezina R. M., et al. (2003). Infant sleep position and associated health outcomes. *Archives of Pediatric and Adolescent Medicine* 157, 469–474.

42. Rivara F. P., Grossman D. (2004). Injury control. In Behrman R. E., Kliegman R. M., Jenson H. B. (Eds.), *Nelson textbook of pediatrics* (17th ed., pp. 256–263). Philadelphia: Elsevier Saunders.

43. Leventhal J. M. (2003). The field of child maltreatment enters its fifth decade. *Child Abuse and Neglect* 27, 1–4.

44. Dietz W. H. (2004). Overweight in childhood and adolescence. *New England Journal of Medicine* 350, 855–857.

45. Reilly J. J. (2006). Obesity in childhood and adolescence: Evidence based clinical and public health perspectives. *Postgraduate Medicine* 82, 429–437.

46. Ogden C. L., Carroll M. D., Curtin L. R., et al. (2006). Prevalence of overweight and obesity in the United States, 1999–2004. *Journal of the American Medical Association* 295, 1549–1555.

47. Centers for Disease Control and Prevention. (2007). Childhood overweight. [Online.] Available: www.cdc.gov/nccdphp/dnpa/bmi/. Accessed April 20, 2008.

48. Lopez R. I., Kelly K. (2002). *The teen health book: A parents' guide to adolescent health and well-being* (pp. 3–37, 561–575). New York: W. W. Norton.

49. Department of Health and Human Services, Centers for Disease Control and Prevention. (2006). Youth risk behavior surveillance—United States, 2005. *Morbidity and Mortality Weekly Report* 55(SS-5), 1–30.

50. Jenkins R. R. (2004). Special health problems during adolescence. In Behrman R. E., Kliegman R. M., Jenson H. B. (Eds.), *Nelson textbook of pediatrics* (17th ed., pp. 641–680). Philadelphia: Elsevier Saunders.

51. Stephens M. A. (2006). Preventative health counseling for adolescents. *American Family Physician* 74, 1151–1156.

Visit thePoint **http://thePoint.lww.com for animations, journal articles, and more!**

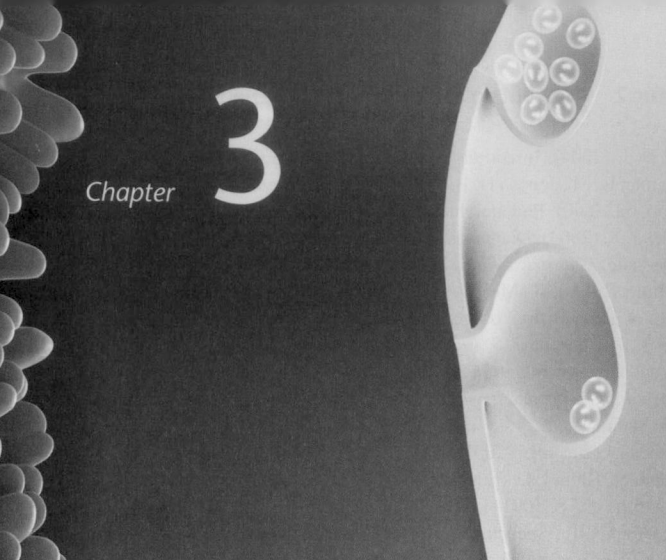

Chapter 3

Concepts of Altered Health in Older Adults

JANICE KUIPER PIKNA

For age is opportunity no less than youth, itself, though in another dress. And as the evening twilight fades away the sky is filled with stars, invisible by day.

—HENRY WADSWORTH LONGFELLOW

➤ Aging is a natural, lifelong process that brings with it unique biopsychosocial changes. For many older adults there are changes in bodily function, physical appearance, cognitive abilities, family structure, and social environment. *Gerontology* is the discipline that studies aging and the aged from biologic, psychological, and sociologic perspectives. It explores the dynamic processes of complex physical changes, adjustments in psychological functioning, and alterations in social identities.

An important first distinction is that aging and disease are not synonymous. Unfortunately, a common assumption is that growing older is inevitably accompanied by illness, disability, and overall decline in function. The fact is that the aging body can accomplish most, if not all, of the functions of its youth; the difference is that they may take longer, require greater motivation, and be less precise. But as in youth, maintenance of physiologic function occurs through continued use.

THE ELDERLY AND THEORIES OF AGING

After completing this section of the chapter, you should be able to meet the following objectives:

- State a definition for *young-old, middle-old,* and *old-old,* and characterize the changing trend in the elderly population.
- State a philosophy of aging that incorporates the positive aspects of the aging process.
- Discuss theories of biologic aging.

Who Are the Elderly?

The older adult population is typically defined in chronologic terms and includes individuals 65 years of age and older. This age was chosen somewhat arbitrarily, and historically it is linked to the Social Security Act of 1935. With this Act, the first national pension system in the United States, which designated 65 years as the pensionable age, was developed. Since then, the expression *old age* has been understood to apply to anyone older than 65 years. Because there is considerable heterogeneity among this group, older adults often are subgrouped into young-old (65 to 74 years), middle-old (75 to 84 years), and old-old (85+ years) to reflect more accurately the changes in function that occur. Age parameters, however, are somewhat irrelevant because chronologic age is a poor predictor of biologic function. However, chronologic age does help to quantify the number of individuals in a group and allows predictions to be made for the future.

In the year 2004, nearly 13% of the total U.S. population (36.3 million) was 65 years of age or older. The proportion of older adults declined for the first time in the 1990s, partly because of the relatively low number of births in the late 1920s and early 1930s. This trend is not expected to continue, however, as the "baby boomers" (*i.e.,* people born from 1946 to 1964) reach age 65.

The older adult population itself is getting older. Average life expectancy has increased as a result of overall advances in health care technology, improved nutrition, and improved sanitation. In 2004, the 65- to 74-year-old age group (18.5 million) was over 8 times larger than in 1900, whereas the 75- to 84-year-old group (13.0 million) was 17 times larger and the 85-year-old and over group (4.9 million) was nearly 40 times larger. The entire population of older adults is expected to grow to about 72 million by the year 2030 (Fig. 3-1). Women who are now 65 years of age can expect to live an additional 19.8 years (84.8 years of age), and men an additional 16 years (81.8 years of age).[1,2]

Women tend to outlive men throughout the aging process. In 2003, there was a sex ratio of 139 women for every 100 men older than 65 years in the United States. This ratio increases to as high as 222 women for every 100 men in the 85 years and

older age group. Marital status also changes with advancing age. In 2004, almost half of all older women living in the community were widows, and there were four times as many widows as there were widowers.[1,2]

Although about 5 million older adults were in the workforce in 2004 (*i.e.,* working or actively seeking work), most were retired.[1] Retirement represents a significant role change for older adults. Attitudes and adjustment to retirement are influenced by preretirement lifestyles and values. Individuals with leisure pursuits during their work life seem to adjust better to retirement than those whose lives were dominated by work. For many of today's cohort of older adults, especially the old-old, the work ethic of the Great Depression remains profoundly ingrained as the central purpose in life. When work is gone, a significant loss is felt, and something must be substituted in its place. Because leisure has not always been a highly valued activity, older adults may have difficulty learning to engage in meaningful leisure pursuits.

THE ELDERLY

- The older population, which is subgrouped into the young-old (65 to 74 years), the middle-old (75 to 84 years), and the old-old (85+ years), has increased dramatically during the past century and is expected to continue to grow as the result of overall advances in health care technology, improved nutrition, and improved sanitation.

- As the result of increased years, many older adults are confronted with retirement, changes in lifestyle, loss of significant others, and a decline in physical functioning.

- Although aging brings with it a unique set of biophysiologic changes, it is not synonymous with disease and disability. Most older adults can perform most or all of the activities they performed in earlier years, although they often take longer and require greater motivation.

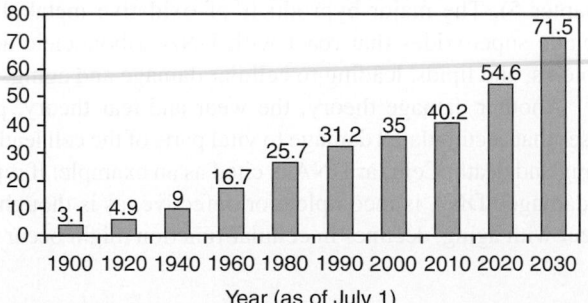

Number of Persons 65+:
1900 to 2030 (numbers in millions)

FIGURE 3-1 • Number of people 65 years of age and older, 1990 to 2030 (numbers in millions). Note: increments in years are uneven. Based on U.S. Bureau of Census. (Sources: Projections of the population by age are taken from the January 2004 Census Internet Release. Historical data are taken from "65+ in the United States," Current Population Reports, Special Studies, P23-190. Data for 2000 are from the 2000 Census and 2005 data are taken from Census estimates for 2004. [Online.] Available: http://assets.aarp.org/rgcenter/general/profile_2005.pdf. Accessed April 20, 2008.)

Loss of productive work is just one of many losses that can accompany the aging process. Loss of a spouse is a highly significant life event that commonly has negative implications for the survivor. Experts cite an increased mortality rate among recently bereaved older adults (especially men); an increased incidence of depression, psychological distress, and loneliness; and higher rates of chronic illness. Loss of physical health and loss of independence are other changes that can affect the psychosocial aspects of aging, as can relocation, loss of friends and relatives, and changes in the family structure.

Poverty is common among the elderly population. In 2004, 9.8% of those 65 years of age and older lived below the poverty line, and another 6.7% were classified as "near poor" (income between the poverty level and 125% of this level). Poverty rates vary among elderly subgroups, with 23.9% of elderly African American, 18.7% of elderly Hispanics, and 7.5% of elderly whites being at the poverty level in 2003. The main sources of income for older persons in 2003 were Social Security (90% of older persons), income from assets (56%), public and private pensions (30%), and earnings (23%).[1,2]

Contrary to popular belief, most older adults live in community settings. Most live in some type of family setting, with a spouse, their children, or other relatives, and approximately 30% live alone. Only 4.5% of all individuals 65 years of age and older reside in long-term care facilities or nursing homes. However, this number increases to 18.2% for persons 85 years of age or older. In addition, about 5% of older adults live in other various types of senior housing, many of which have supportive services available to their residents.[1,2]

Older adults are the largest consumers of health care. In 1997, more than half of the population reported having one or more disabilities. One third had at least one severe disability and approximately one sixth had difficulties with activities of daily living (ADLs). Almost half of all adult hospital beds are filled with patients 65 years of age and older.[2]

Theories of Aging

Multiple theories have attempted to explain the biology of aging through a variety of scientific observations at the molecular, cellular, organ, and system levels. In general, these theories can be divided into either intrinsic (developmental–genetic) or extrinsic (stochastic) theories. *Developmental–genetic theories* propose that the changes that occur with aging are genetically programmed, whereas *stochastic theories* maintain that the changes result from an accumulation of random events or damage from environmental agents or influences.[3] In reality, evidence suggests that the process of aging and longevity is multifaceted, with both genetics and environmental factors playing a role. In animal studies, genetics accounted for less than 35% of the effects of aging, whereas environmental influences accounted for over 65% of the effects.[4] In humans, a very long life, to beyond 90 years of age, appears to have a stronger genetic basis, which explains why centenarians and near-centenarians tend to cluster in families.[5]

Developmental–Genetic Theories

The developmental–genetic theories focus on the genetic influences that determine physical condition, occurrence of disease, age of death, cause of death, and other factors contributing to longevity.[3,6] At the cellular level, Hayflick and Moorhead observed more than 40 years ago that cultured human fibroblasts have a limited ability to replicate (approximately 50 population doublings) and then die.[7] Before achieving this maximum, they slow their rate of division and manifest identifiable and predictable morphologic changes characteristic of senescent cells.

Another explanation of cellular aging resides with an enzyme called *telomerase* that is believed to govern chromosomal aging through its action on telomeres, the outermost

extremities of the chromosome arms. With each cell division, a small segment of telomeric deoxyribonucleic acid (DNA) is lost, unless a cell has a constant supply of telomerase. In the absence of telomerase, the telomeres shorten, resulting in senescence-associated gene expression and inhibition of cell replication. It is thought that in certain cells, such as cancer cells, telomerase maintains telomere length, thereby enhancing cell replication.

However, many genes that are associated with the human life span are not "longevity genes," per se. For example, because mutations in the tumor suppressor genes *BRAC1* and *BRAC2* increase mortality rates associated with breast and ovarian cancer, they are rare among long-lived women.[5] Conversely, genes that reduce the risk of atherosclerosis may be more common in long-lived individuals. Genetic studies of biologic aging have explored the involvement of allelic variants in genes encoding apolipoproteins, in particular, that of apolipoprotein E (apoE). The presence of apoE4 is associated with an increased incidence of cardiovascular diseases and neurodegenerative diseases, thereby shortening the life span through disease processes.[3,8]

Stochastic Theories

The stochastic theories propose that aging is caused by random damage to vital cell molecules (*e.g.,* mitochondrial DNA damage, oxygen radical accumulation, nuclear DNA cross-linking).[3] The damage eventually accumulates to a level sufficient to result in the physiologic decline associated with aging.

The somatic mutation theory of aging states that the longevity and function of cells in various tissues of the body are determined by the double-stranded DNA molecule and its specific repair enzymes. DNA undergoes continuous change in response both to exogenous agents and intrinsic processes. Aging may result from conditions that produce mutations in DNA or deficits in DNA repair mechanisms.

The oxidative free radical theory is another stochastic idea in which aging is thought to result partially from oxidative metabolism and the effects of free radical damage (see Chapter 5). The major byproducts of oxidative metabolism include superoxides that react with DNA, ribonucleic acid, proteins, and lipids, leading to cellular damage and aging.

Another damage theory, the wear-and-tear theory, proposes that accumulated damage to vital parts of the cell leads to aging and death. Cellular DNA is cited as an example. If repair to damaged DNA is incomplete or defective, as is thought to occur with aging, declines in cellular function might occur.[3,6]

IN SUMMARY, aging is a natural, lifelong process that brings with it unique biopsychosocial changes. Aging is not synonymous with disease or ill health. The aging body can accomplish most or all of the functions of its youth, although they may take longer, require greater motivation, and be less precise.

The older adult population is typically defined in chronologic terms as individuals 65 years of age and older, and can be further defined as young-old (65 to 74 years), middle-old (75 to 84 years), and old-old (85+ years). The number of older persons has increased and is expected to continue to grow in the future, with an anticipated 72 million Americans older than 65 years of age by the year 2030.

There are two main types of theories used to explain the biologic changes that occur with aging: developmental–genetic theories, which propose that aging changes are genetically programmed, and stochastic theories, which maintain that aging changes result from an accumulation of random events or damage from environmental hazards. ■

PHYSIOLOGIC CHANGES OF AGING

After completing this section of the chapter, you should be able to meet the following objectives:

- Describe common skin changes that occur with aging.
- Explain how muscle changes that occur with aging affect high-speed performance and endurance.
- Describe the process of bone loss that occurs with aging.
- State the common changes in blood pressure regulation that occur with aging.
- List the changes in respiratory function that occur with aging.
- Relate aging changes in neural function to the overall function of the body.
- Briefly discuss the effects of aging on vision, hearing, taste, and smell.
- Describe changes that occur in the gastrointestinal tract with aging.
- State the significance of decreased lean body mass on interpretation of the glomerular filtration rate using serum creatinine levels.

The physiologic changes seen in the elderly reflect not only the aging process, but the effects of years of exposure to environmental agents such as sunlight and cigarette smoke, and disease processes such as diabetes mellitus or arthritis. Overall, there is a general decline in the structure and function of the body with advancing age (Fig. 3-2). The decline results in a decreased reserve capacity of the various organ systems that consequently produce reduced homeostatic capabilities, making the older adult more vulnerable to stressors such as illness, trauma, surgery, medications, and environmental changes.

Research to identify true age-related changes as opposed to disease states is difficult. Studies using cross-sectional methodologies are the easiest to perform; however, mortality can confound the results. Although longitudinal studies tend to be more precise, they require years to perform and may not be able to account for numerous variables that enter into the aging equation, such as environment, occupation, and diet. However, it is important to differentiate, as much as possible, those changes that occur in the body as a result of aging from those that occur owing to disease. This distinction allows for more accurate diagnosis and treatment of disease conditions and helps to avoid inappropriate labeling of aging changes.

Regardless of the difficulty in defining normal aging as it relates to the various organ systems, there is a pattern of gradual loss that occurs. Many of these losses begin in early adulthood, but because of the large physiologic reserve of most organ systems, the decrement does not become functionally significant until the loss reaches a certain level. Some changes, such as those that affect the skin and posture, are more visible, whereas others, such as those affecting the kidney, may go unnoticed until the person is challenged with situations such as eliminating medications.

Integumentary Changes

Changes in the skin more obviously reflect the aging process than do changes in other organ systems (see Chapter 61). Aging can impinge on the primary functions of the skin: protection from the environment, temperature regulation, fluid and electrolyte balance, sensory function, and excretion of metabolic wastes. Exposure to sunlight and harsh weather accelerates aging of the skin.

With aging, the skin becomes wrinkled and dry and develops uneven pigmentation. The thickness of the dermis, or middle layer of skin, decreases by approximately 20%, which gives the skin an overall thin and transparent quality. This is especially true for areas exposed to sunlight. Dermal collagen fibers rearrange and degenerate, resulting in decreased skin strength and elasticity. Cellularity and vascularity of the dermis decrease with advancing age and can cause vascular fragility, leading to senile purpura (*i.e.*, skin hemorrhages) and slow skin healing. Delayed wound healing may be influenced by other factors such as poor nutrition and circulation and by changes in immune function.[9–11] The function of the sebaceous glands diminishes with age and leads to a decrease in sebum secretion. The decrease in size, number, and activity of the eccrine sweat glands causes a decrease in their capacity to produce sweat. Fingernails and toenails become dull, brittle, and thick, mostly as a result of decreased vascularity of the nail beds.

Age-related changes in hair occur as well. Owing to a decline in melanin production by the hair follicle, approximately one half of the population older than 50 years of age has at least 50% gray hair, regardless of sex or original hair color. Changes in hair growth and distribution also are seen.[9,10] Hair on the scalp, axillae, and pubis becomes more sparse, and the hairs of the ears and nostril coarsen. Skin disorders are common among the older adult population and can include skin cancers, keratoses (*i.e.*, warty lesions), xerosis (*i.e.*, excessive dryness), dermatitis, and pruritus (*i.e.*, generalized itching).

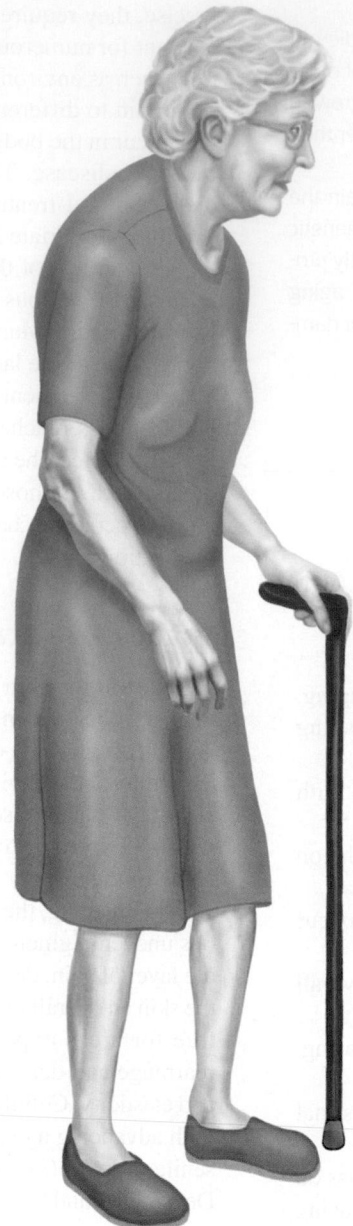

Neuromuscular function
• Loss of neurons, atrophy of
  neuronal dendrites, impaired
  synaptic connections
• Declined motor strength,
  slowed reaction time,
  diminished reflexes
• Decrease in proprioceptor
  function that controls balance

Cardiovascular function
• Increased stiffness of
  blood vessels
• Decreased responsiveness
  to catecholamines
• Decrease in exercise
  heart rate
• Decrease in diastolic
  ventricular relaxation

Immune function
• Altered function of
  helper T cells
• Diminished immune
  response

**Stature and musculoskeletal
changes**
• Decrease in height
• Loss of bone mass
• Decrease in muscle strength
• Skeletal bone loss

Integumentary function
• Thin, dry skin
• Decreased sebum and sweat
• Thick and brittle nails
• Sparse, gray hair

Special senses
• Decline in visual acuity
• Hearing loss
• Decline in smell

Respiratory function
• Decrease in $\dot{V}O_2$max
• Progressive loss of elastic
  recoil in lungs and chest wall
• Decrease in PO_2

Gastrointestinal function
• Dental problems
• Dry mouth
• Mucosal atrophy
• Constipation

Renal function
• Decrease in functional glomeruli
• Decline in renal blood flow
• Decreased glomerular filtration rate
• Decreased urine concentration ability

Genitourinary function
• Decreased bladder capacity,
  incomplete emptying
• Increased incidence of incontinence
• Decreased serum testosterone levels
  in men
• Increased vaginal dryness in women
• Decreased sexual response

FIGURE 3-2 • Clinical manifestations of aging.

Stature and Musculoskeletal Function

Aging is accompanied by a progressive decline in height, especially among older women. This decline in height is attributed mainly to compression of the vertebral column. Body composition changes as well. The amount of fat increases, and lean body mass and total body water decrease with advancing age.

With aging, there is a reduction in muscle size and strength that is related to a loss of muscle fibers and a reduction in the size of the existing fibers. Although the decline in strength that occurs with aging cannot be halted, its progress

can be slowed with exercise. There is a decline in high-speed performance and reaction time because of a decrease in type II muscle fibers.[12] Impairments in the nervous system also can cause movements to slow. However, type I muscle fibers, which offer endurance, are thought to remain consistent with age (see Chapter 11).

Numerous studies have reported a loss of bone mass with aging, regardless of sex, race, or body size (see Chapter 58). With aging, the process of bone formation (*i.e.,* renewal) is slowed in relation to bone resorption (*i.e.,* breakdown), resulting in a loss of bone mass and weakened bone structure. This is especially true for postmenopausal women. By

65 years of age, most women have lost two thirds of their skeletal mass owing to a decrease in estrogen production.[12] Skeletal bone loss is not a uniform process. At approximately 30 years of age, bone loss begins, predominantly in the trabecular bone (*i.e.,* fine network of bony struts and braces in the medullary cavity) of the heads of the femora and radii and vertebral bodies.[12,13] By 80 years of age, women have lost nearly 43% of their trabecular bone, and men have lost 27%. This process becomes pathologic (*i.e.,* osteoporosis) when it significantly increases the predisposition to fracture and associated complications (see Chapter 58).

The prevalence of joint disease is increased among the elderly. By age 65 years, 80% of the population has some articular disease. Osteoarthritis is so common among the elderly that it is often incorrectly assumed to be a normal age-related change rather than a disease. The synovial joints ultimately are affected by osteoarthritis, most commonly the joints of the hands, feet, knees, hips, and shoulders. It is characterized by cartilage loss and new bone formation, accounting for a distortion in articulation, limited range of motion, and joint instability (see Chapter 59). Age is the single greatest risk factor for development of osteoarthritis, in part because of the mechanical impact on joints over time, but it also is related to injury, altered physical condition of the articular cartilage, obesity (*e.g.,* knee), congenital deformity (*e.g.,* hip), crystal deposition in articular cartilage (*e.g.,* knee), and heredity. Pain, immobility, and joint inflammation often ensue. Treatment is aimed at minimizing risk factors, weight loss if indicated, exercise to increase muscle strength, and pain relief measures.

Cardiovascular Function

Cardiovascular disease remains the leading cause of morbidity and mortality in older adults. It often is difficult to separate true age-related changes in the cardiovascular system from disease processes. The aorta and arteries tend to become stiffer and less distensible with age, the heart becomes less responsive to the catecholamines, the maximal exercise heart rate declines, and there is a decreased rate of left ventricular diastolic relaxation.

Blood Pressure

The relationship between blood pressure and risk of cardiovascular disease is continuous, consistent, and independent of other risk factors. Numerous studies have shown that systolic blood pressure progressively increases with age, whereas increases in diastolic blood pressure tend to plateau and even decline after age 50.[14] As a result, there is a sharp increase in what is known as *systolic hypertension* among older adults, which occurs as a consequence of increased arterial stiffness (see Chapter 23).

An elevation in systolic blood pressure accompanied by a normotensive diastolic pressure causes a dramatic increase in pulse pressure. This is a known prognostic indicator for future coronary events. Thus aggressive treatment of systolic hypertension is recommended and has been shown to demonstrate a reduction in stroke, heart failure, kidney disease, and other complications.[14–16] Individuals who are normotensive at 55 years of age have a 90% lifetime risk for development of hypertension. There is now a push to intervene when individuals are prehypertensive (*i.e.,* systolic blood pressure of 120 to 139 mm Hg or diastolic blood pressure of 80 to 89 mm Hg) with lifestyle modification strategies to prevent hypertension.[14,17]

Orthostatic hypotension, or a significant drop in systolic pressure on assumption of the upright position, is more common among the elderly (see Chapter 23). Compensatory cardiovascular mechanisms often are delayed or insufficient, so that a drop in blood pressure due to position change or consumption of a meal is also common.[18] Even in the absence of orthostatic hypotension, the elderly respond to postural stress with diminished changes in heart rate and diastolic pressure. This altered response to orthostatic stress is thought to result from changes in autonomic nervous system function, inadequate functioning of the circulatory system, or both.[16]

Cardiac Function

Multiple factors determine the effect of aging on cardiac function in healthy older adults. With aging, there is an increase in left ventricular wall thickness; a delay in early left ventricular filling; a decrease in responsiveness to β-adrenergic stimulation and circulating catecholamines; a decrease in the maximal heart rate and maximal cardiac output; and an increase in systemic vascular resistance and left ventricular afterload. The afterload (*i.e.,* opposition to left ventricular ejection) rises steadily with age as the ascending aorta becomes more rigid and the resistance in peripheral arterial vessels increases.[19,20] Although the overall size of the heart does not increase, the thickness of the left ventricular wall may increase with age, in part responding to the increased afterload that develops because of blood vessel changes.[19]

Both left ventricular diastolic and systolic function are affected by aging. Although early diastolic filling decreases by approximately 50% between 20 and 80 years of age, more filling occurs in late diastole, in part because of more vigorous atrial contraction.[19] The augmented atrial contraction is accompanied by atrial hypertrophy and enlargement. Despite a decrease in the age-associated changes in the diastolic filling pattern in older persons, their left ventricular end-diastolic volume in the supine position does not substantially differ from that of younger persons. However, it is reduced to a lesser extent in older persons than in younger persons during postural change (moving from the supine to seated position) and during graded upright exercise. Furthermore, the maximum left ventricular ejection fraction (*i.e.,* percentage of the left ventricular end-diastolic volume that is ejected during systole) that can be achieved during maximal exercise decreases with age—in this case because of a lesser decrease in left ventricular end-systolic volume. An age-associated decline in myocardial contractility is thought to contribute to this defect in end-systolic volume regulation.

The supine resting heart rate remains unchanged or decreases only slightly with age; however, the maximum heart rate that can be achieved during maximal exercise is decreased. The magnitude of this age-associated reduction in peak heart rate is about 30% between 20 and 85 years of age.[19] The reduction in heart rate is the reason why the maximum cardiac output reserve decreases in healthy older adults.

Despite aging changes and cardiovascular disease, overall cardiovascular function at rest in most healthy elderly persons is considered adequate to meet the body's needs. Cardiac output is essentially maintained in healthy older adults (men more than women) during exercise despite the decreased heart rate response, apparently because of a greater stroke volume resulting from increased end-diastolic volume during exercise.[17,21]

Respiratory Function

As lung function changes with age, it often is difficult to differentiate the effects of age from those of environmental and disease factors. Maximal oxygen consumption ($\dot{V}O_2max$), a measure used to determine overall cardiopulmonary function, declines with age. Numerous studies have indicated that $\dot{V}O_2max$ can improve significantly with exercise and that the $\dot{V}O_2max$ of older adult master athletes can meet that of their younger counterparts.

A progressive loss of elastic recoil in the lung is caused by changes in the amount of elastin and composition of collagen fibers. Calcification of the soft tissues of the chest wall causes increased stiffness and thus increases the workload of the respiratory muscles. There is a loss of alveolar structure that decreases the surface area of gas exchange. Although the total lung capacity remains constant, the consequences of these changes result in an increased residual lung volume, increased functional reserve capacity, and a decline in vital capacity. There is a linear decrease in arterial oxygen tension (PO_2) of approximately 20 mm Hg from 20 to 70 years of age. This is thought to result primarily from the ventilation–perfusion mismatching of the aging lung.[22,23]

Neurologic Function

Changes at the structural, chemical, and functional levels of the nervous system occur with normal aging, but overall they do not interfere with day-to-day routines unless specific neurologic diseases come into play. The weight of the brain decreases with age, and there is a loss of neurons in the brain and spinal cord. Neuron loss is most pronounced in the cerebral cortex, especially in the superior temporal area. Additional changes take place in the neurons and supporting cells. Atrophy of the neuronal dendrites results in impaired synaptic connections, diminished electrochemical reactions, and neural dysfunction. Synaptic transmissions also are affected by changes in the chemical neurotransmitters dopamine, acetylcholine, and serotonin. As a result, many neural processes slow. Lipofuscin deposits (*i.e.,* yellow, insoluble intracellular material) are found in greater amounts in the aged brain.[24–26]

Sensorimotor changes show a decline in motor strength, slowed reaction time, diminished reflexes (especially in the ankles), and proprioception changes. These changes can cause the balance problems and slower, more deliberate movements that are frequently seen in older individuals.[25]

Even though changes in the brain are associated with aging, overall cognitive abilities remain intact. Although language skills and attention are not altered with advanced age, performance and constructional task abilities can decline, as can short-term memory and immediate recall. A change in personality or significant cognitive deficits is considered unusual with normal aging, and if either occurs, evaluation is in order. Dementia or depression can frequently be the cause.

Special Sensory Function

Sensory changes with aging can greatly affect the older adult's level of functioning and quality of life. Vision and hearing impairments due to disease states, for example, can interfere with communication and may lead to social isolation and depression.

Vision

There is a general decline in visual acuity with age, and nearly all individuals older than 55 years of age require vision correction for reading or distance. The decline occurs as a result of a smaller pupil diameter, loss of refractive power of the lens, and an increase in the scattering of light. The most common visual problem among older adults is presbyopia, or difficulty focusing on near objects. It is caused mainly by decreased elasticity of the lens and atrophy of the ciliary muscle (see Chapter 54).

Glare and abrupt changes in light pose particular problems for older adults. Both are reasons why the elderly frequently give up night driving; they also increase their risk for falls and injury. Color discrimination changes also take place with aging. In particular, older adults have more difficulty identifying blues and greens. This is thought to be related to problems associated with filtering short wavelengths of light (*i.e.,* violet, blue, green) through a yellowed, opaque lens. Corneal sensitivity also may diminish with age, so that older adults may be less aware of injury or infection.[27,28]

Ophthalmologic diseases and disorders are common in the elderly. Cataracts, glaucoma, and macular degeneration are frequently seen and can greatly impair vision and function. Both medical and surgical interventions can restore or improve vision problems that occur as a result of disease states of the eye. Low-vision aids, such as special magnifiers and high-intensity lighting that mimics sunlight, can assist in optimizing vision in otherwise uncorrectable ophthalmologic problems.

Hearing

Hearing loss is common among older adults, and some degree of impairment is almost inevitable with advancing age. It has been reported that 40% of independent individuals older than 65 and about half of those older than 85 years of age have a hearing impairment.[29–31]

Presbycusis, or the hearing loss of old age, is largely considered multifactorial in etiology. It occurs as a result of aging combined with auditory stressors, trauma, environmental influences, and otologic diseases, as well as genetic factors. It is characterized by a gradual, progressive onset of bilateral and symmetric sensorineural hearing loss of high-frequency tones (see Chapter 55). The hearing deficit often has both a peripheral and a central component. Speech discrimination, or the ability to distinguish among words that are near-homonyms or distinguish words spoken by several different speakers, often is impaired. Accelerated speech and shouting can increase distortion and further compound the problem. When speaking to hearing-impaired older adults, it is helpful to face them directly so they can observe lip movements and facial expressions. Speech should be slow and direct. Loudness can be irritating. Rephrasing misunderstood messages also can improve understanding of the spoken word. Hearing deficits with age are not always limited to an increased detection threshold, but can include other aspects of hearing, such as sound, comprehension of speech, and noise discrimination, as noted previously.

Hearing aids can be effective for various levels of hearing loss and may greatly improve the ability to hear and communicate. Cochlear implants may be indicated for individuals with severe hearing loss not helped by hearing aids. Research in the area of hearing restoration by regeneration of cochlear hair cells as well as gene therapy holds promise.[29,30]

Cerumen (i.e., earwax) impaction in the external auditory canal also is commonly seen in older adults and can impair hearing. The cerumen glands, which are modified apocrine sweat glands, atrophy and produce drier cerumen. This may be partially responsible for more frequent cerumen impactions in the older adult population.[28]

Taste and Smell

Olfaction, or the sense of smell, declines with aging, possibly as a result of generalized atrophy of the olfactory bulbs and a moderate loss of olfactory neurons. Smell is a protective mechanism, and persons who cannot smell may be at risk for exposure to environmental hazards. For example, people who cannot smell smoke would be at particular risk if a fire broke out.

The sense of taste decreases with aging, but it is believed to be less affected than olfaction. In fact, in many cases what is perceived to be a decline in ability to taste is actually a defect in olfaction. Because taste and smell are necessary for the enjoyment of food flavor, older adults may not enjoy eating as much as in their youth. Drugs and disease also may affect taste. Alterations in taste and smell, along with other factors such as eating alone, decreased ability to purchase and prepare food, and the high cost of some foods, may account for poor nutritional intake in some older adults. Conversely, the lack of sensory feedback may lead the person to eat more and gain weight. A decline in taste is more pronounced among older adults with Alzheimer disease, presumably because of the neuropathologic changes in the brain.[32]

Immune Function

A functional immune system is a vital component in surviving microorganism infection and damage caused by other pathogens. Immunosenescence, or age-related changes in the immune system, can pose an increased risk for some infections in the elderly. Involution of the thymus gland is complete by approximately 45 to 50 years of age, and although the total number of T cells remains unchanged, there are changes in the function of helper T cells that alter the cellular immune response of older adults. There also is evidence of an increase in various autoantibodies (e.g., rheumatoid factor) as a person ages, increasing the risk of autoimmune disorders.

Extensive studies show that although changes in immunity occur with aging, it is the compounding effects of age-related diseases and external conditions that result in an overall state of dysfunctional immunity that are responsible for the increased risk and severity of common infections in older adults. Hence, immunosenescence is a predisposing condition, but its contribution to infection risk likely is small until immunity is impaired further as a result of chronic disease, external circumstances, or repeated or chronic infections.[33,34] This is different from the changes related to immunosuppression resulting from certain conditions such as human immunodeficiency virus infection or immunosuppressive medications that result in unusual opportunistic infections.[35] However, older adults are more susceptible to urinary tract infections, respiratory tract infections, wound infections, and nosocomial infections. The mortality rate from influenza and bronchopneumonia is increased in this population.

Early detection of infections is more difficult in older adults because the typical symptoms, such as fever and elevated white blood cell count, often are absent.[36] A change in mental status or decline in function often is the only presenting sign. It has been reported that frank delirium occurs in 50% of older adults with infections. Thus, infections in the elderly may be far advanced at the time of diagnosis.

Gastrointestinal Function

The gastrointestinal tract shows less age-associated change in function than many other organ systems. Although tooth loss is common and approximately 40% to 50% of the older adult population is edentulous, it is not considered part of the normal aging process. Poor dental hygiene with associated caries and periodontal disease is the main reason for the loss. *Edentia,* or toothlessness, can lead to dietary changes and can be associated with malnutrition. Use of dentures can enhance mastication; however, taste sensation is inhibited. Because of improved dental technology and the fluoridated water supply, more persons are able to keep their teeth into their later years. *Xerostomia,* or dry mouth, also is common, but it is not universal among older adults and typically occurs as a result of decreased salivary secretions. Other causes of dry mouth can include medications, such as anticholinergics and tranquilizers, radiation therapy, and obstructive nasal diseases that induce mouth breathing.

Soergel and colleagues (1964) coined the term *presby-esophagus* to denote changes in esophageal function, such as decreased motility and inadequate relaxation of the lower esophageal sphincter, that occur with aging.[37] However, in studies that controlled for disease states such as diabetes mellitus and neuropathies, no increase in abnormal motility was observed. In general, the physiologic function of the esophagus appears to remain intact with advancing age.

Atrophy of the gastric mucosa and a decrease in gastric secretions can occur in older adults. Achlorhydria (*i.e.,* decrease in hydrochloric acid secretion) occurs, probably as a result of a loss of parietal cells. Although not universal, achlorhydria is more prevalent among older adults and can cause impaired gastric absorption of substances requiring an acidic environment.

Atrophic gastritis and decreased secretion of intrinsic factor are more common with aging and can result in a malabsorption of vitamin B_{12}. Because vitamin B_{12} is necessary for the maturation of red blood cells, a deficiency can lead to a type of macrocytic anemia called *pernicious anemia.* Vitamin B_{12} deficiency also can cause neurologic abnormalities such as peripheral neuropathy, ataxia, and even dementia. Treatment consists of regular periodic vitamin B_{12} replacement therapy through injection because the oral form is not absorbed owing to a lack of intrinsic factor.[38]

The small intestine shows some age-related morphologic changes, such as mucosal atrophy; however, absorption of most nutrients and other functions appear to remain intact. Absorption of calcium, however, decreases with aging and may reflect decreased intestinal absorption along with other factors, such as reduced intake of vitamin D, decreased formation of vitamin D_3 by the skin because of reduced sun exposure, and decreased activation of vitamin D_3 by the liver and kidney.

Diverticula of the colon are common among older adults, with more than 50% of individuals older than 80 years having diverticular disease. The high incidence appears to result mainly from a low-fiber diet. Constipation, or infrequent passage of hard stool, is another frequently occurring phenomenon. It often is attributed to immobility and decreased physical activity, a low-fiber diet, decreased fluid intake, and medications; malignancies and other disease states also can be responsible. Complications of constipation can include fecal impaction or obstruction, megacolon, rectal prolapse, hemorrhoids, and laxative abuse.

Renal Function

Although age-related anatomic and physiologic changes occur, the aging kidney remains capable of maintaining fluid and electrolyte balance remarkably well. Aging changes result in a decreased reserve capacity, which may alter the kidney's ability to maintain homeostasis in the face of illnesses or stressors. Overall, there is a general decline in kidney mass with aging, predominantly in the renal cortex. The number of functional glomeruli decreases by 30% to 50%, with an increased percentage of sclerotic or abnormal glomeruli.[39]

Numerous cross-sectional and longitudinal studies have documented a steady, age-related decline in total renal blood flow of approximately 10% per decade after 20 years of age, so that the renal blood flow of an 80-year-old person averages approximately 300 mL/minute, compared with 600 mL/minute in a younger adult. The major decline in blood flow occurs in the cortical area of the kidney, causing a progressive, age-related decrease in the glomerular filtration rate (GFR). Serum creatinine, a byproduct of muscle metabolism, often is used as a measure of GFR. The decline in GFR that occurs with aging is not accompanied by an equivalent increase in serum creatinine levels because the production of creatinine is reduced as muscle mass declines with age.[39] Serum creatinine levels often are used as an index of kidney function when prescribing and calculating drug doses for medications that are eliminated through the kidneys; this has important implications for older adults. If not carefully addressed, improper drug dosing can lead to an excess accumulation of circulating drugs and result in toxicity. A formula that adjusts for age-related changes in serum creatinine for individuals 40 through 80 years of age is available (see Chapter 34).

Renal tubular function declines with advancing age, and the ability to concentrate and dilute urine in response to fluid and electrolyte impairments is diminished. The aging kidney's ability to conserve sodium in response to sodium depletion is impaired and can result in hyponatremia. A decreased ability to concentrate urine, an age-related decrease in responsiveness to antidiuretic hormone, and an impaired thirst mechanism may account for the older adult's greater predisposition to dehydration during periods of stress and illness. Older adults also are more prone to hyperkalemia and hypokalemia when stressed than are younger individuals. An elevated serum potassium may result from a decreased GFR, lower renin and aldosterone levels, and changes in tubular function. Low potassium levels, on the other hand, are more commonly caused by gastrointestinal disorders or diuretic use. Neither is the result of aging.[40]

Genitourinary Function

Both men and women undergo changes in genitourinary function as a result of the aging process. There are changes in bladder structure and function, decreases in steroid sex hormones, and changes in genital structures.

Changes in the bladder structure that occur because of the aging process can result in a decline in function. Overall, the smooth muscle and supportive elastic tissue are replaced with fibrous connective tissue. This can cause incomplete bladder emptying and a diminished force of urine stream. Bladder capacity also decreases with age, whereas the frequency of urination increases. As elastic tissue and muscles weaken, stress incontinence becomes more prevalent.

In aging women, atrophy of perineal structures can cause the urethral meatus to recede along the vaginal wall. Atrophy of other pelvic organs occurs in the aging woman because of diminished estrogen production after menopause: vaginal secretions diminish; the vaginal lining is thinner, drier, less elastic, and more easily traumatized; and normal flora are altered. These changes can result in vaginal infections, pruritus, and painful intercourse.[41]

In aging men, benign prostatic hyperplasia (BPH) is very common (See Chapter 44). The incidence progressively increases to approximately 80% of men by 80 years of age. The condition often is asymptomatic until approximately 50 years of age. Thereafter, the incidence and severity of symptoms increase with age. BPH can cause obstructive symptoms such as urinary hesitancy, diminished force of stream, retention, and postvoid dribbling; it also can cause irritative symptoms such as frequency, nocturia, urgency, and even urge incontinence.[42,43]

Serum testosterone levels are known to decline as men age, although the definition of and treatment for hypogonadism remain somewhat controversial. Symptoms associated with androgen deficiency in the aging man can include diminished muscle strength, stamina, and energy; loss of muscle mass; low libido (with or without erectile dysfunction); irritable mood; osteoporosis; and testicular atrophy (see Chapter 43). Although some guidelines for androgen replacement therapy for older men have been developed by several groups, there is a general lack of consensus on whether to treat.[44]

Sexual activity remains possible into late life for men and women. In general, the duration and intensity of the sexual response cycle are diminished in both sexes.[43] Women take longer to experience the physiologic changes of vaginal expansion and lubrication during the excitement phase. Penile erection in aging men takes longer to develop because of changes in neural innervation and vascular supply. Social factors affecting sexual behavior include the desire to remain sexually active, access to a sexually functioning partner, and availability of a conducive environment.

IN SUMMARY, there is a general decline in the structure and function of the body with advancing age, resulting in a decreased reserve capacity of the various organ systems, including the integumentary, musculoskeletal, cardiorespiratory, nervous, sensory, immune, gastrointestinal, and genitourinary systems (see Fig. 3-2). This results in a reduction of homeostatic capabilities, making the older adult more vulnerable to stressors such as illness, trauma, surgery, medication administration, and environmental changes. ■

FUNCTIONAL PROBLEMS ASSOCIATED WITH AGING

After completing this section of the chapter, you should be able to meet the following objectives:

- Compare information obtained from functional assessment with that obtained from a physical examination used to arrive at a medical diagnosis.
- Cite the differences between chronic and transient urinary incontinence.
- State four risk factors for falls in older individuals.
- List five symptoms of depression in older adults.
- Name a tool that can be used for assessing cognitive function.
- State the difference between delirium and dementia.

Although aging is not synonymous with disease, the aging process does lend itself to an increased incidence of illness. As chronologic age increases, so does the probability of having multiple chronic diseases. The vast majority of older adults have at least one chronic condition, and most actually have more than one. The extent of these problems is described in Table 3-1. Older adults are more likely to experience a decline in overall health and function because of the increased incidence of chronic illness that occurs with advancing age. Because aging also brings with it a decreased ability to maintain homeostasis, illnesses often manifest in an atypical manner. For example, myocardial infarction may occur without chest pain or other presenting symptoms. Sepsis without fever is common, and pneumonia may present with acute confusion but lack the prodromal symptom of cough.

In addition to chronic illnesses, older adults suffer disproportionately from functional disabilities, or the inability to perform the necessary ADLs. It is most likely that the decrements in health that can accompany the aging process are responsible for these functional disabilities. Among the more common

TABLE 3-1 **Common Health Problems in the Elderly**	
HEALTH PROBLEMS	**PERCENTAGE WITH PROBLEMS**
Hypertension	51
Arthritis	48
Heart disease	31
Any cancer	21
Diabetes	16
Sinusitis	14

Data from American Association of Retired Persons. (2005). A profile of older Americans. [Online.] Available: www.aarp.org.

functional problems of the older adult are urinary incontinence, instability and falls, sensory impairment, and depression and cognitive impairment.

Functional Assessment

Evaluation of the older adult's functional abilities is a key component of gerontologic health care. Medical diagnoses alone are incomplete without an assessment of function. Two older adults with similar medical diagnoses of arthritis, hypertension, and osteoporosis, for example, can be at opposite ends of the spectrum of functional abilities.

Assessing functional status can be done in many different ways, using a variety of methods. Measures of function should attempt systematically and objectively to evaluate the level at which an individual is functioning in a variety of areas, including biologic, psychological, and social health.

Selection of a screening tool to measure function depends on the purpose of data collection, the individual or target population to be assessed, availability and applicability of the instruments, reliability and validity of the screening tools, and the setting or environment. An issue that arises when assessing function is the question of capability versus performance. For example, an older adult may be able to bathe without supervision; however, the long-term care facility where the person resides may discourage it for safety reasons. Among the more commonly used assessment tools are those that measure the ability to perform ADLs and the patient's cognitive function.

When evaluating levels of function, determination of the older adult's ability to perform ADLs and instrumental ADLs (IADLs) should be included. ADLs are basic self-care tasks, such as bathing, dressing, grooming, ambulating, transferring (*e.g.,* from a chair to bed), feeding, and communicating. IADLs are more complex tasks that are necessary to function in society, such as writing, reading, cooking, cleaning, shopping, laundering, climbing stairs, using the telephone, managing money, managing medications, and using transportation. The IADL tasks indirectly examine cognitive abilities as well because they require a certain level of cognitive skill to complete.

Several tools are available for measuring functional status. One of the more commonly used tools is the Index of Activities of Daily Living. Developed by Katz in 1963 and revised in 1970, it summarizes performance in six functions: bathing, dressing, toileting, transferring, continence, and feeding. It is used as an assessment tool to determine the need for care and the appropriateness of treatment, and as a teaching aid in rehabilitation settings. Through questioning and observation, the rater forms a mental picture of the older adult's functional status as it existed during a 2-week period preceding the evaluation, using the most dependent degree of performance.[45,46] Numerous studies using the Katz Index tool show significant validity and reliability. The advantage of the tool is that it is easy to administer and provides a "snapshot" of the older adult's level of physical functioning. The disadvantage is that it does not include IADL categories that are of equal importance, especially for older adults living in the community.

Urinary Incontinence

Urinary incontinence, or involuntary loss of urine, plagues over 30% of community-living individuals older than 60 years of age, 50% of hospitalized older adults, and 60% of residents in long-term care facilities. These estimates may be low because individuals often fail to report symptoms of urinary incontinence, perhaps owing to the attached social stigma. Health care professionals often neglect to elicit such information as well.

Incontinence is an expensive problem. A conservative estimate of cost for direct care of adults with incontinence is over $16 billion annually.[47] Urinary incontinence can have deleterious consequences, such as social isolation and embarrassment, depression and dependency, skin rashes and pressure sores, and financial hardship. Although urinary incontinence is a common disorder, it is not considered a normal aspect of aging. Studies reveal that 60% to 70% of community-dwelling older adults with urinary incontinence can be successfully treated and even cured.[47]

Changes in the micturition cycle that accompany the aging process make the older adult prone to urinary incontinence. A decrease in bladder capacity, in bladder and sphincter tone, and in the ability to inhibit detrusor (*i.e.,* bladder muscle) contractions, combined with the nervous system's increased variability in interpreting bladder signals, can cause incontinence (see Chapter 35). Impaired mobility and a slower reaction time also can aggravate incontinence.

The causes of incontinence can be divided into two categories: transient and chronic. Of particular importance is the role of pharmaceuticals as a cause of transient urinary incontinence. Numerous medications, such as long-acting sedatives and hypnotics, psychotropics, and diuretics, can induce incontinence. Treatment of transient urinary incontinence is aimed at ameliorating or relieving the cause on the assumption that the incontinence will resolve.

Chronic, or established, urinary incontinence occurs as a failure of the bladder to store urine or a failure to empty urine.

Failure to store urine can occur as a result of detrusor muscle overactivity with inappropriate bladder contractions (*i.e.,* urge incontinence). There is an inability to delay voiding after the sensation of bladder fullness is perceived. Urge incontinence is typically characterized by large-volume leakage episodes occurring at various times of day. Urethral incompetence (*i.e.,* stress incontinence) also causes a bladder storage problem. The bladder pressure overcomes the resistance of the urethra and results in urine leakage. Stress incontinence causes an involuntary loss of small amounts of urine with activities that increase intra-abdominal pressure, such as coughing, sneezing, laughing, or exercising.[48–50]

Failure of the bladder to empty urine can occur because of detrusor instability, resulting in urine retention and overflow incontinence. Also called *neurogenic incontinence,* this type of incontinence can be seen with neurologic damage from conditions such as diabetes mellitus and spinal cord injury. Outlet obstruction, as with prostate enlargement and urethral stricture, also can cause urinary retention with overflow incontinence. Functional incontinence, or urine leakage due to toileting problems, occurs because cognitive, physical, or environmental barriers impair appropriate use of the toilet.[49,50]

After a specific diagnosis of urinary incontinence is established, treatment is aimed at correcting or ameliorating the problem. Probably the most effective interventions for older adults with incontinence are behavioral techniques. These strategies involve educating the individual and providing reinforcement for effort and progress. Techniques include bladder training, timed voiding or habit training, prompted voiding, pelvic floor muscle (*i.e.,* Kegel) exercises, and dietary modifications. Biofeedback, a training technique to teach pelvic floor muscle exercises, uses computerized instruments to relay information to individuals about their physiologic functions. Biofeedback can be helpful when used with other behavioral treatment techniques. Use of pads or other absorbent products should be seen as a temporary measure and not as a cure. Numerous types of products are available to meet many different consumer needs.

Pharmacologic intervention may be helpful for some individuals. Estrogen replacement therapy in postmenopausal women, for example, was thought to help relieve stress incontinence. However, it is no longer recommended as a treatment approach in light of newer information about the cardiovascular side effects and increased cancer risks that estrogen can pose. Drugs with anticholinergic and antimuscarinic properties (*e.g.,* oxybutynin, tolterodine, darifenacin) may help with urge incontinence. These medications are not without side effects, however, and their use must be carefully weighed against the possible benefits, which are limited at best.

Surgical intervention may help to relieve urinary incontinence symptoms in appropriate patients. Bladder neck suspension may assist with stress incontinence unrelieved by other interventions, and prostatectomy may be appropriate for men with overflow incontinence due to an enlarged prostate. However, older adults may have medical conditions that preclude surgery. Other treatments include intermittent self-catheterization for some types of overflow incontinence.

Instability and Falls

Unstable gait and falls are a common source of concern for the older adult population. The literature reveals that 30% of community-dwelling individuals older than 65 years of age and 50% of nursing home residents fall each year. Most falls do not result in serious injury, but the potential for serious complications and even death is real. Accidents are the fifth leading cause of death among older adults, with falls ranking first in this category. Worldwide, more than 8 million fractures occur annually among individuals 60 years of age and older, with falls as the most common cause.

The way in which a person falls can often determine the type of injury that occurs. Wrist fractures are common and frequently sustained from forward or backward falls onto an outstretched hand. Hip fractures can result from a sideways fall and are one of the most feared complications from a fall. Hip fractures predominate in the 75 years and older age group. Significant morbidity ensues from a hip fracture. The literature varies, but as much as 50% of older adults who sustain a hip fracture are reported to require nursing home care for at least 1 year, and up to 20% die in the year after a hip fracture.[51] The problem of falls in the older adult population is an issue of high incidence combined with a high potential for injury, owing to the high prevalence of medical problems along with physiologic changes that occur with advancing age. In addition, recovery from a fall-related injury can be lengthy and result in deconditioning, weakness and abnormality of gait, further potentiating the risk of subsequent falls.[51] An individual's activity may be restricted because of fear on the individual's or caregiver's part about possible falling. These anxieties may lead to unnecessary restrictions in independence and mobility and commonly are mentioned as a reason for institutionalization.

Although some falls have a single, obvious cause, such as a slip on a wet or icy surface, most are the result of several factors. Risk factors that predispose to falling include a combination of age-related biopsychosocial changes, chronic illnesses, and situational and environmental hazards. Table 3-2 summarizes the possible causes of falls.

Gait and stability require the integration of information from the special senses, the nervous system, and the musculoskeletal system. Changes in gait and posture that occur in healthy aged individuals also contribute to the problem of falls. The older person's stride shortens; the elbows, trunk, and knees become more flexed; toe and heel lift decrease while walking; and sway while standing increases. Muscle strength and postural control of balance decrease, proprioception input diminishes, and righting reflexes slow.[51–53] Because the central nervous system integrates sensory input and sends signals to the effector components of the musculoskeletal system, any alteration in neural function can predispose to falls. For this reason, falls have been associated with strokes, Parkinson disease, and normal-pressure hydrocephalus. Similarly, diseases or disabilities that affect the musculoskeletal system, such as arthritis, muscle weakness, or foot deformities, are associated with an increase in the incidence of falls.

TABLE 3-2 Risk Factors for Falls

CATEGORY OF RISK FACTORS	EXAMPLES
Accidents and environmental hazards	Slips, trips Clutter, cords, throw rugs
Age-related functional changes	Decreased muscle strength, slowed reaction time, decreased proprioception, impaired righting reflexes, increased postural sway, altered gait, impaired visual and hearing function
Cardiovascular disorders	Aortic stenosis, cardiac arrhythmias, autonomic nervous system dysfunction, hypovolemia, orthostatic hypotension, carotid sinus syncope, vertebrobasilar insufficiency
Gastrointestinal disorders	Diarrhea, postprandial syncope, vasovagal response
Genitourinary disorders	Urinary incontinence, urinary urgency/frequency, nocturia
Medication use	Alcohol, antihypertensives, cardiac medications, diuretics, narcotics, oral hypoglycemic agents, psychotropic medications, drug–drug interactions, polypharmacy
Metabolic disorders	Anemia, dehydration, electrolyte imbalance, hypothyroidism
Musculoskeletal disorders	Osteoarthritis, rheumatoid arthritis, myopathy
Neurologic disorders	Balance/gait disorders, cerebellar dysfunction, stroke with residual effects, cervical spondylosis, central nervous system lesions, delirium, dementia, normal-pressure hydrocephalus, peripheral neuropathy, Parkinson disease, seizure disorders, transient ischemic attack
Prolonged bed rest	Hypovolemia, muscle weakness from disuse and deconditioning
Respiratory disorders	Hypoxia, pneumonia
Sensory impairments	Decreased visual acuity, cataract, glaucoma, macular degeneration, hearing impairment, vestibular disorders

Age- and disease-related alterations in vision and hearing can impair sensory input, increasing the risk for falls. Vestibular system alterations such as benign positional vertigo or Ménière disease cause balance problems that can result in falls (see Chapter 55). Input from the cardiovascular and respiratory systems influences function and ambulation. Syncope, a type of dizziness, is a transient global cerebral hypoperfusion stemming from cardiovascular symptoms. Syncope occurs fairly rapidly and usually results in falling. Syncope is common among older adults, with higher incidences among those aged 80 years and older.[54] Cognitive impairments such as dementia have been associated with an increased risk of falling, most likely because of impaired judgment and problem-solving abilities.[51–53]

Medications are an important and potentially correctable cause of instability and falls. Central-acting medications, such as sedatives and hypnotics, have been associated with an increase in the risk of falling and injury. Diuretics can cause volume depletion, electrolyte disturbances, and fatigue, predisposing to falls. Antihypertensive drugs can cause fatigue, orthostatic hypotension, and impaired alertness, contributing to the risk of falls.[51–53]

Environmental hazards play a significant role in falling. Most falls occur in the home and often involve objects that are tripped over, such as cords, scatter rugs, and small items left on the floor. Poor lighting, ill-fitting shoes, surfaces with glare, and improper use of ambulatory devices such as canes or walkers also contribute to the problem.[52]

Preventing falls is the key to controlling the potential complications that can result. Because multiple factors usually contribute to falling, the aim of the clinical evaluation is to identify risk factors that can be modified. Assessment of sensory, neurologic, and musculoskeletal systems; direct observation of gait and balance; and a careful medication inventory can help identify possible causes. Preventive measures can include a variety of interventions, such as surgery for cataracts or cerumen removal for hearing impairment related to excessive earwax accumulation. Other interventions may include podiatric care, discontinuation or alteration of the medication regimen, exercise programs, physical therapy, and appropriate adaptive devices. The home also should be assessed by an appropriate health care professional (e.g., occupational therapist) and recommendations made regarding modifications to promote safety. Simple changes such as removing scatter rugs, improving the lighting, and installing grab bars in the bathtub can help prevent falling.

Use of specially designed external hip protector pads in high-risk older adults has demonstrated a dramatic reduction in hip fractures occurring after a fall. The impacting force and energy caused by the fall are weakened and diverted away from the greater trochanteric region by use of the pad. Compliance is somewhat problematic, however, because individuals may be reluctant to wear the pads.[52] Vitamin D supplementation has also shown promising results and may have an independent role in the prevention of falls. Use of vitamin D is credited with improvement in functional strength and dynamic muscle performance, thereby reducing fall risk.[55] A meta-analysis of vitamin D supplementation concluded that fall risks were reduced by 22% among both community-dwelling and institutionalized older adults.[56]

Sensory Impairment

Although sensory impairments are not imminently life-threatening, their impact on health can be substantial. Hearing impairment is associated with decreased quality of life, depression, isolation, and dementia. Visual impairment is related to increased risk of falls, hip fractures, physical disability, and depression. Nursing home residents with visual impairment are more likely to require assistance with ADLs and can be at risk for falls and hip fractures. Visual impairment also appears to increase mortality rates.[27,28,57,58]

Sensory impairment results not only from deficits in peripheral sensory structures but from the central processing of sensory information. The older person's difficulty in processing multisensory information is seen most strikingly when there is a rapid fluctuation in the nature of the information that is received from the environment.[27,28]

Lack of sensory information can predispose to psychological symptoms. Charles Bonnet syndrome is an organic disorder occurring in the elderly that is characterized by complex visual hallucinations. It is associated with ocular disease and, strictly speaking, is seen in older adults with preserved intellectual functions.[59] Estimates of incidence vary, but up to 14% of those with severe visual impairments may experience visual hallucinations. Those who obtain insight into the problem generally only need reassurance that their hallucinations do no represent mental illness. For those who have limited insight and are distressed by the symptom, antipsychotics may afford some relief.[59] Both auditory and visual impairment can have important psychological effects in association with dementia. Delusions have been associated with hearing impairment. In one study that used a case-control method, elderly persons with late-life psychosis with paranoid symptomatology were four times more likely to have hearing impairments than control subjects.[59]

Depression and Cognitive Impairment

Depression

Depression is a significant health problem affecting the older adult population. Estimates of the prevalence of depression in the elderly vary widely; however, there is a consensus that the size of the problem is underestimated owing to misdiagnosis and mistreatment. Up to 25% of community-dwelling older adults are thought to have depressive symptoms. The estimate drops to approximately 1% to 2% when diagnosis is restricted to major depression. Depressive symptoms are even more common in nursing home residents.[60]

The term *depression* is used to describe a symptom, syndrome, or disease. As listed in the fourth edition of the American Psychiatric Association's *Diagnostic and Statistical Manual of Mental Disorders* (*DSM-IV-TR*), the criteria for the diagnosis and treatment of a major depression include at least five of the following symptoms during the same 2-week period, with at least one of the symptoms being depressed mood or anhedonia (*i.e.,* loss of interest or pleasure): depressed or irritable mood; loss of interest or pleasure in usual activities; appetite and weight changes; sleep disturbance; psychomotor agitation or retardation; fatigue and loss of energy; feelings of worthlessness, self-reproach, or excessive guilt; diminished ability to think or concentrate; and suicidal ideation, plan, or attempt.[61] Depressive symptomatology can be incorrectly attributed to the aging process, making recognition and diagnosis difficult. Depressed mood, the signature symptom of depression, may be less prominent in the older adult, and more somatic complaints and increased anxiety are reported, confusing the diagnosis. Symptoms of cognitive impairment can be seen in the depressed older adult. Although a thorough investigation is necessary to discern whether the symptoms are a result of depression versus dementia, evidence now shows that depression can be a prodromal symptom of dementia.[62]

Physical illnesses can complicate the diagnosis as well. Depression can be a symptom of a medical condition, such as pancreatic cancer, hypothyroidism or hyperthyroidism, pneumonia and other infections, congestive heart failure, dementia, and stroke. In fact, major depression is a common consequence of stroke and occurs in about one third of all patients with ischemic stroke. Hypertension is also possibly associated with increased risk of major depression.[62-64] Medications such as sedatives, hypnotics, steroids, antihypertensives, and analgesics also can induce a depressive state. Numerous confounding social problems, such as bereavement, loss of job or income, and loss of social support, can contribute to the diagnosis.[62-64]

The course of depression in older adults is similar to that in younger persons. As much as 40% experience recurrences. Suicide rates are highest among the elderly. There is a linear increase in suicide with age, most notably among white men older than 60 years of age. Although the exact reasons are unclear, it may be caused by the emotional alienation that can accompany the aging process, combined with complex biopsychosocial losses.[62-65]

Because diagnosis of depression can be difficult, use of a screening tool may help to measure affective functioning objectively. The Geriatric Depression Scale, an instrument of known reliability and validity, was developed to measure depression specifically in the noninstitutionalized older adult population. The 30-item dichotomous scale elicits information on topics relevant to symptoms of depression among older adults, such as memory loss and anxiety.[66] Many other screening tools, each with its own advantages and disadvantages, exist to evaluate the older adult's level of psychological functioning, in its entirety or as specific, separate components of function.

Treatment goals for older adults with depression are to decrease the symptoms of depression, improve the quality of life, reduce the risk of recurrences, improve health status, decrease health care costs, and decrease mortality. Pharmacotherapy (*i.e.,* use of antidepressants) is an effective treatment approach for the depressed older adult. The selection of a particular medication depends on a variety of factors, such as a prior positive or negative response, history of first-degree relatives responding to medication, concurrent medical illnesses that may interfere with medication use, concomitant use of nonpsychotropic medications that may alter the metabolism or increase the side effect profile, likelihood of adherence, patient preference, and cost. Selective serotonin reuptake inhibitors (SSRIs), a class of antidepressants (*e.g.*, sertraline, citalopram, escitalopram), provide high specificity by blocking or slowing serotonin reuptake without the antagonism of neurotransmitter receptors or direct cardiac effects. Because of this, they are an attractive first choice for pharmacotherapy. Dosing is usually once per day, creating ease of administration. They also are less lethal in overdose than other types of antidepressants, such as the tricyclics, an important consideration because of the high suicide rate among older adults. The anticholinergic and cardiovascular side effects that can be problematic with tricyclic antidepressants (*e.g.*, nortriptyline, desipramine, amitriptyline) are minimal with SSRIs. Regardless of the classification, psychotropic medications should be given in low doses initially and gradually titrated according to response and side effects. Response to antidepressants usually requires 4 to 6 weeks at therapeutic dose levels. For a single episode of major depression, drug therapy usually should continue for a minimum of 6 months to 1 year, and 2 to 5 years for recurrent depression, to prevent relapse.[60,62,64]

Electroconvulsive therapy (ECT) may be the treatment of choice for older adults with severe, pharmacologically resistant major depressive episodes. Studies indicate that individuals older than 60 years of age are the largest group of patients who receive ECT. Despite the negative publicity that has been associated with ECT, the evidence for its efficacy in the treatment of depression is strong. Unfortunately, relapse after ECT is common, and alternative treatment strategies, including maintenance ECT or maintenance antidepressants after ECT, are being used.[67]

"Talking therapy," such as supportive counseling or psychotherapy, is considered to be an important part of the treatment regimen, alone or in combination with pharmacotherapy or ECT. Alterations in life roles, lack of social support, and chronic medical illnesses are just a few examples of life event changes that may require psychosocial support and new coping skills. Counseling in the older adult population requires special considerations. Individuals with significant vision, hearing, or cognitive impairments may require special approaches. Many elderly persons do not see themselves as depressed and reject referrals to mental health professionals. Special efforts are needed to engage these individuals in treatment. Family therapy can be beneficial as a way to help the family understand more about depression and its complexities and as an important source of support for the older adult. Although depression can impose great risks for older adults, it is thought to be the most treatable psychiatric disorder in late life and therefore warrants aggressive case finding and intervention.

Dementia

Dementia is a complex and devastating problem that is a major cause of disability in the older adult population. Estimates vary, but indicate the prevalence of dementia in the United States is 5% to 10% in older adults, with the rate increasing with advancing age.

Although there can be a decline in intellectual function with aging, dementia, sometimes called *senility,* is not a normal aging process. Dementia is a syndrome of acquired, persistent impairment in several domains of intellectual function, including memory, language, visuospatial ability, and cognition (*i.e.,* abstraction, calculation, judgment, and problem solving). Mood disturbances and changes in personality and behavior often accompany the intellectual deterioration.[61]

Dementia or cognitive dysfunction can result from a wide variety of conditions, including degenerative, vascular, neoplastic, demyelinating, infectious, inflammatory, toxic, metabolic, and psychiatric disorders. Up to 70% of older adults with dementia (4.5 million Americans and 15 million people worldwide) are thought to have Alzheimer disease, a chronic, progressive neurologic disorder of unknown cause. Two microscopic changes occur in the brain of persons with Alzheimer disease: senile plaques that develop between neurons, and neurofibrillary tangles that develop within neurons.[62] Researchers have speculated that inflammation around plaques destroys neighboring neurons. Involvement of cholinergic neurons causes levels of acetylcholine in synapses to decline. Levels of acetylcholinesterase also drop, perhaps to compensate for the loss of acetylcholine. Vascular dementia is the second most common disorder and risk factors include ischemic stroke, hemorrhagic stroke, hypertension, hyperlipidemia, heart disease, tobacco use, and diabetes mellitus.[68,69] Chapter 53 provides an additional discussion of cognitive disorders.

Diagnostic Methods. Currently there are no specific diagnostic tests to determine the presence of Alzheimer disease, and the diagnosis is made by excluding other possible causes of the dementia symptoms. More recently, use of positron emission tomography (PET) scans of the brain using a newer imaging molecule has proved to be of value in diagnosis. Research has shown that it can help differentiate the diagnosis by determining regional cerebral patterns of amyloid plaques and tau neurofibrillary tangles.[71]

A commonly used measure of cognitive function is the Mini-Mental State Examination (MMSE), developed by Folstein and colleagues in 1975.[72] This tool provides a brief, objective measure of cognitive functioning and has been widely used. The MMSE, which can be administered in 5 to 10 minutes, consists of a variety of questions that cover memory, orientation, attention, and constructional abilities. The test has been studied and found to fulfill its original goal of providing a brief screening tool that quantifies cognitive impairments and documents cognitive changes over time. However, it has been cautioned that this examination should not be used by itself as a diagnostic tool to identify dementia.

Pharmacologic Treatment. Several medications have become available over the past decade to help halt further cognitive decline in Alzheimer disease. At present, four drugs (tacrine, donepezil, rivastigmine, and galantamine) are available in the therapeutic category of cognitive-enhancing agents, although tacrine is no longer marketed in the United States.[73–75] All four medications are acetylcholinesterase inhibitors whose action elevates acetylcholine concentrations in the cerebral cortex by slowing degradation of acetylcholine released by still-intact neurons. The magnitude of tacrine's cognitive-enhancing effects, the first-released drug in this category, has been modest and associated with significant side effects that generally preclude its use. Donepezil has been shown to be a more potent, specific inhibitor of acetylcholinesterase with minimal side effects.[73] The newer agents, rivastigmine and galantamine, are thought to be more selective in the binding and inactivation of acetylcholinesterase; however, adverse reactions, especially gastrointestinal symptoms, can impede therapeutic dosing. Although there still is no cure for dementia, acetylcholinesterase inhibitors are considered efficacious as antidementia drugs on the basis of improvements seen on standardized cognitive tests, as well as a slower decline in loss of function due to the disease process. Evidence suggest that the cognitive-enhancing drugs are also beneficial in individuals with vascular dementia.[73]

Memantine, a moderate-affinity, uncompetitive N-methyl-D-aspartate (NMDA) receptor antagonist, is a newer agent that has consistently demonstrated safe and efficacious use in dementia. Glutamate is a neurotransmitter that potentially overexcites NMDA receptors, and excessive release of glutamate is believed to contribute to the neurodegeneration associated with Alzheimer disease. Memantine has known clinical efficacy in treating patients with moderate to severe Alzheimer disease. It is also safe and well tolerated in individuals with mild to moderate Alzheimer disease.[75,76] Newer evidence suggests that memantine could have a neuroprotective action in Alzheimer disease.[73,74]

There has also been interest in other neuroprotective drugs that may delay the onset or progression of Alzheimer disease. Nonsteroidal anti-inflammatory drugs (NSAIDs) are thought to decrease the inflammatory response to inflammatory mediators released from injured or degenerating nerve cells, although study results are somewhat inconclusive. Because of these general concerns about lack of efficacy, combined with potential side effects, NSAIDs are not considered a standard treatment for Alzheimer disease. Vitamin E may also play a role in Alzheimer disease prevention. Vitamin E, a fat-soluble vitamin, interacts with cell membranes, traps free radicals, and may interrupt chain reactions that damage cells.[74] Although earlier studies were promising, more recent investigation of the long-term use of vitamin E did not demonstrate cognitive benefits, although the dose was markedly diminished.[77] Elevated plasma homocysteine concentrations have been linked as a vascular risk factor in the development of dementia and can be lowered by folic acid supplementation. A recent longitudinal, prospective, randomized, double-blind, controlled study on cognitive function in older adults who took folic acid for elevated homocysteine levels showed significant improvement in cognitive functioning.[78]

Nonpharmacologic Treatment Methods. Studies have also shown that certain mental exercises can offset some of the expected cognitive changes that can occur with aging. One study investigating long-term effects of cognitive training on everyday functional outcomes in community-dwelling older adults demonstrated less decline in function over time compared with a control group. This was especially true for subjects exposed to "reasoning training" (inductive reasoning). The training roughly counteracted the degree of decline in cognitive performance that would be expected over a 7- to 14-year period in older adults without dementia.[79] This may have applicability to individuals with dementia, and current therapies include enrollment in cognitive training programs. Likewise, physical exercise, such as aerobics or weight training, may have the potential for delaying functional decline in individuals with Alzheimer disease and may even help to delay the onset of dementing disorders.[80]

In more advanced cases of dementia, ensuring that the individual's physical needs, such as hygiene, bowel and bladder elimination, safety, and nutrition are met can help prevent catastrophic reactions. Providing a consistent routine in familiar surroundings also helps to alleviate stress. Matching the cognitive needs of the older adult by avoiding understimulation and overstimulation often helps in preventing behavior problems.

The work of Hall has shown positive results in the care of older adults with Alzheimer disease.[81] Hall's conceptual model, progressively lowered stress threshold (PLST), proposes that the demented individual's ability to tolerate any type of stress progressively declines as the disease advances. Interventions for the older adult with dementia therefore center on eliminating and avoiding stressors as a way to prevent dysfunctional behaviors. These stressors include fatigue, change of routine, excessive demands, overwhelming stimuli, and physical stressors. Hall's work with the PLST model has shown that individuals tend to awaken less at night, use less sedatives and hypnotics, eat better, socialize more, function at a higher level, and experience fewer episodes of anxiety, agitation, and other dysfunctional behaviors. Further work has shown that family caregivers trained using the PLST model improved their abilities to provide care to loved ones with dementia and lowered their own stress levels.[82]

Management of older adults with Alzheimer disease and other dementias usually involves assuming increasing responsibility for and supplying increasing care to individuals as the illness renders them incapable. Impaired judgment and cognition can prevent the older adult from making reasonable decisions and choices and eventually threatens their overall well-being. Family members often assume the monumental task of caring for older adults with dementia until the burden becomes too great, at which time many older adults may be relocated to long-term care facilities.

Delirium

It is important to differentiate dementia from delirium, also referred to as *acute confusional state*. The demented older adult is far more likely to become delirious. The onset of delirium in the demented individual may be mistaken as an exacerbation of the dementia and consequently not treated.[83]

Delirium is an acute disorder developing over a period of hours to days and is seen frequently in hospitalized elderly patients. Prevalence rates range from 6% to 56% of hospitalized older adults, up to 53% of older adults after surgery, and up to 87% of those in intensive care.[83–85] Delirium is defined by the *DSM-IV-TR* as an organic mental syndrome featuring a global cognitive impairment, disturbances of attention, reduced level of consciousness, increased or decreased psychomotor activity, and a disorganized sleep–wake cycle.[61] The severity of the symptoms tends to fluctuate unpredictably, but often is more pronounced at night.

Delirium can be a presenting feature of a physical illness and may be seen with disorders such as myocardial infarction, pneumonia and other infections, cancer, and hypothyroidism. Patients with drug toxicities may present with delirium. Malnutrition, use of physical restraints, and iatrogenic events also can precipitate delirium.

The exact reason why delirium occurs is unclear. It is speculated that the decreased central nervous system capacity in older adults may precipitate delirium. Other possible contributing factors include vision and hearing impairments, psychological stress, and diseases of other organ systems. Delirium has a high mortality rate, ranging between 20% and 40%.[83-86] Agitation, disorientation, and fearfulness—the key symptoms of delirium—place the individual at high risk for injuries such as fracture from a fall.[83–85]

Diagnosis of delirium involves recognition of the syndrome and identification of its causes. Management involves treatment of the underlying disease condition and symptomatic relief through supportive therapy, including good nutrition and hydration, rest, comfort measures, and emotional support. Prevention of delirium is the overall goal. Avoidance of the devastating and life-threatening acute confusional state is often the key to successful management and treatment.[82–85]

IN SUMMARY, health care for older adults requires unique considerations, taking into account age-related physiologic changes and specific disease states common in this population. Although aging is not synonymous with disease, the aging process does lend itself to an increased incidence of illness. The overall goal is to assist the older adult in maximizing independence and functional capabilities and minimizing disabilities that can result from various acute and chronic illnesses.

The evaluation of the older adult's functional abilities is a key component in gerontologic health care. Medical diagnoses alone are incomplete without an assessment of function. When evaluating levels of function, determination of the older adult's ability to perform ADLs and IADLs should be included.

Among the functional disorders that are common in the older population are urinary incontinence, instability and falls, sensory impairment, and depression, dementia, and delirium. The older adult is especially prone to urinary incontinence because of changes in the micturition cycle that accompany the aging process. Behavioral techniques can be an effective way

to treat incontinence problems in the older adult population. Falls are a common source of concern for the older adult population. Although most falls do not result in serious injury, the potential for serious complications and even death is real. Most falls are the result of several risk factors, including age-related biopsychosocial changes, chronic illness, and situational and environmental hazards. Both hearing and visual impairment, which are common in the elderly, contribute to communication problems, depression, and social isolation.

Depression is a significant but treatable health problem that often is misdiagnosed and mistreated in the older adult population. Dementia is a syndrome of acquired, persistent impairment in several domains of intellectual function, including memory, language, visuospatial ability, and cognition (*i.e.,* abstraction, calculation, judgment, and problem solving). Although there can be a slight decline in intellectual function with aging, dementia is not a normal aging process. Delirium is an acute confusional disorder developing over a period of hours to days and often is seen as a presenting feature of a physical illness or drug toxicity. ■

DRUG THERAPY IN THE OLDER ADULT

After completing this section of the chapter, you should be able to meet the following objectives:

- Characterize drug therapy in the older adult population.
- List five factors that contribute to adverse drug reactions in the elderly.
- Cite cautions to be used in prescribing medications for the elderly.

Drug therapy in the older adult population is a complex phenomenon influenced by numerous biopsychosocial factors. The elderly are the largest group of consumers of prescription and over-the-counter drugs. Although the older population comprises only about 13% of the U.S. population, they consume one third of all prescription drugs and 50% of all over-the-counter medications. The incidence of adverse drug reactions in the elderly is two to three times that found in young adults. This is considered to be a conservative estimate because drug reactions are less well recognized in older adults and reactions often can mimic symptoms of specific disease states.

Errors in the administration of medications and compliance are common among the older adult population, with a prevalence estimated by several authorities at 25% to 50% for community-dwelling elderly. Reasons for this high rate of errors are numerous. Poor manual dexterity, failing eyesight, lack of understanding about the treatment regimen, attitudes and beliefs about medication use, mistrust of health care providers, and forgetfulness or confusion are but a few factors that can affect the adherence to medication regimens. The role of the health care provider also can contribute to improper medication use. There can be a tendency to treat symptoms with drugs rather than fully investigate the cause of those symptoms. To compound matters, accurate diagnosis of specific disease states can be difficult because older adults tend to underreport symptoms and because presenting symptoms are often atypical.[87–90]

Age-related physiologic changes also account for adverse effects of medications. In general, the absorption of orally ingested drugs remains essentially unchanged with age, even though the gastric pH is known to rise and gastric emptying time can be delayed. Changes in drug distribution, however, are clinically significant. Because lean body mass and total body water decrease with advancing age, water-soluble drugs such as digoxin and propranolol tend to have a smaller volume of distribution, resulting in higher plasma concentrations for a given dose and increased likelihood of a toxic reaction. Conversely, fat-soluble drugs such as diazepam are more widely distributed and accumulate in fatty tissue owing to an increase in adipose tissue with aging. This can cause a delay in elimination and accumulation of the drug over time (*i.e.*, prolonged half-life) with multiple doses of the same drug. Drug metabolism through the liver is thought to be altered owing to the decrease in hepatic blood flow seen in the older adult. Renal excretion controls the elimination of drugs from the body, and because kidney function declines with age, the rate of drug excretion decreases. This can result in an increased half-life of drugs and is why estimates of creatinine clearance are recommended to determine drug dosing.[87,88]

Drug use for older adults warrants a cautious approach. "Start low and go slow" is the adage governing drug prescription in geriatric pharmacology. Older adults often can achieve therapeutic results on small doses of medications. If necessary, dosing can then be titrated slowly according to response.

Further complicating matters is the issue of polypharmacy in older adults, who often have multiple disorders that may require multiple drug therapies. Polypharmacy increases the risk of drug interactions and adverse drug reactions, and decreases compliance. Drugs and disease states also can interact, causing adverse effects. For example, psychotropic drugs administered to older adults with dementia may cause a worsening of confusion; β-adrenergic blocking agents administered to an individual with chronic obstructive pulmonary disease may induce bronchoconstriction; and NSAIDs given to an older adult with hypertension can raise blood pressure further.

The use of certain types of medications carries a high risk for older adults and should be avoided if possible. In general, long-acting drugs or drugs with prolonged half-lives can be problematic. Many sedatives and hypnotics fit into this category, and drugs such as diazepam and flurazepam should be avoided. Other classes of drugs, such as antidepressants and anxiolytics, may provide the necessary symptomatic relief and may be more appropriate for older adults than sedatives and hypnotics. Use of these agents warrants caution, however, with consideration for the unique pharmacokinetic changes that accompany aging. Drugs that possess anticholinergic properties should also be used with caution. Anticholinergics are used for a variety of conditions; however, side effects such as dry mouth and eyes, blurred vision, and constipation are common. These drugs can also cause more serious side effects, such as confusion, urinary retention, and orthostatic hypotension. Agents that enter the central nervous system, including narcotics and alcohol, can cause a variety of problems, most notably delirium. These problems most likely occur as a result of a decreased central nervous system reserve capacity.[87–91]

Because of the serious implications of medication use in the elderly, strategies need to be used to enhance therapeutic effects and prevent harm. Careful evaluation of the need for the medication by the health care provider is the first step. Once decided, analysis of the individual's current medication regimen and disease state is necessary to prevent drug–drug interactions, drug–disease interactions, and adverse responses. Dosing should be at the low end, and frequency of drug administration should be kept to a minimum to simplify the routine and enhance compliance. Timing the dose to a specific activity (*e.g.*, "take with breakfast") can also improve compliance, as can special packaging devices such as pill boxes and blister packs. The cost of medications is another important factor for older adults on reduced, fixed incomes. Choosing less expensive products of equal efficacy can increase compliance. The importance of educating the individual about the medication cannot be overemphasized. Health care professionals need to provide verbal and written information on the principles of medication use and on the specific medications being used. This facilitates active, involved participation by the older adult and enhances the individual's ability to make informed decisions.

IN SUMMARY, drug therapy in the older adult population is a complex phenomenon influenced by numerous biopsychosocial factors. Alterations in pharmacokinetics occur with advancing age and increase the likelihood of toxic reactions. "Start low and go slow" is the adage governing geriatric pharmacology. Centrally acting drugs and drugs with long half-lives should be avoided when possible. Drug–drug interactions, drug–disease interactions, and adverse reactions are increased in the elderly population. Educating the older adult about drug use is an important factor in ensuring compliance and accurate medication administration. ∎

Review Exercises

1. It is said that the aging body can accomplish most, if not all, of the functions of its youth; the difference is that they may take longer, require greater motivation, and be less precise.

   A. *Explain how this concept might contribute to falls in the elderly.*

2. Nocturia or the need to urinate during the night is a common problem of the elderly.

  A. *Explain the rationale for this complaint.*

3. Errors of administration and adverse drug reactions are a continual threat for the elderly.

  A. *Explain common causes of inappropriate medication use in the elderly.*

References

1. U.S. Census Bureau. (2000). The 65 years and older population. [Online.] Available: www.census.gov/population/www/socdemo/age.html#older. Accessed April 20, 2008.
2. American Association of Retired Persons. (2005). A profile of older Americans. [Online.] Available: http://assets.aarp.org/rgcenter/general/profile_2005. pdf. Accessed April 20, 2008.
3. Troen B. R. (2003). The biology of aging. *Mount Sinai Journal of Medicine* 70, 3–22.
4. Hayflick L. (2007). Biological aging is no longer an unsolved problem. *Annals of the New York Academy of Sciences* 1100, 1–13.
5. Browner W. S., Kahn A. J., Ziv E., et al. (2004). The genetics of human longevity. *American Journal of Medicine* 117, 851–860.
6. Salvioli S., Olivieri F., Marchegiani F., et al. (2006). Genes, ageing and longevity in humans: Problems, advantages and perspectives. *Free Radical Research* 40, 1303–1323.
7. Hayflick L., Moorehead P. S. (1965). The limited in vitro lifetime of human diploid cell strains. *Experimental Cell Research* 37, 614–636.
8. Vijg J., Suh Y. (2005). Genetics of longevity and aging. *Annual Review of Medicine* 56, 193–212.
9. Timiras M. L. (2003). The skin. In Timiras P. S. (Ed.), *Physiological basis of aging and geriatrics* (3rd ed., pp. 397–404). Boca Raton, FL: CRC Press.
10. Smith E. S., Fleishcer A. B. Jr., Feldman S. R. (2001). Demographics of aging and skin disease. *Clinics in Geriatric Medicine* 17, 631–641.
11. Waller J. M., Maibach H. I. (2006). Age and skin structure and function, a quantitative approach (II): Protein, glycosaminoglycan, water, and lipid content and structure. *Skin Research and Technology* 12(3), 145–154.
12. Timiras P. S. (2003). The skeleton, joints, and skeletal and cardiac muscles. In Timiras P. S. (Ed.), *Physiological basis of aging and geriatrics* (3rd ed., pp. 375–395). Boca Raton, FL: CRC Press.
13. Loeser R. F., Delbono O. (2003). Aging of the muscles and joints. In Hazzard W. R., Blass J. P., Halter J. B., et al. (Eds.), *Principles of geriatric medicine and gerontology* (5th ed., pp. 905–918). New York: McGraw-Hill.
14. Joint National Committee. (2003). *The seventh report of the Joint National Committee on Prevention, Detection, Evaluation, and Treatment of High Blood Pressure.* NIH publication no. 03-5233. Bethesda, MD: National Institutes of Health.
15. Franklin S. S. (2004). Systolic blood pressure. *American Journal of Hypertension* 17(Suppl. 1), S49–S54.
16. Pinto E. (2007). Blood pressure and ageing. *Postgraduate Medical Journal* 83, 109–114.
17. Taffet G. E., Lakatta E. (2003). Aging of the cardiovascular system. In Hazzard W. R., Blass J. P., Halter J. B., et al. (Eds.), *Principles of geriatric medicine and gerontology* (5th ed., pp. 403–421). New York: McGraw-Hill.
18. Smith N. L., Psaty B. M., Rutan G. H., et al. (2003). The association between time since last meal and blood pressure in older adults: The Cardiovascular Health Study. *Journal of the American Geriatrics Society* 51, 824–828.
19. Lakatta E. G., Levy D. (2003). Arterial and cardiac aging: Major shareholders in cardiovascular disease enterprises. Part II: The aging heart in health; Links to heart disease. *Circulation* 107, 346–354.
20. Lakatta E. G. (2002). Age-associated cardiovascular changes in health: Impact on cardiovascular disease in older persons. *Heart Failure Reviews* 7, 29–49.
21. Schwartz R. S., Kohrt W. M. (2003). Exercise in elderly people: Physiologic and functional effects. In Hazzard W. R., Blass J. P., Ouslander J. G., et al. (Eds.), *Principles of geriatric medicine and gerontology* (5th ed., pp. 931–946). New York: McGraw-Hill.
22. Timiras P. S. (2003). Pulmonary respiration, hematopoiesis and erythrocytes. In Timiras P. S. (Ed.), *Physiological basis of aging and geriatrics* (3rd ed., pp. 319–336). Boca Raton, FL: CRC Press.
23. Zelnick J. (2003). Normative aging of the respiratory system. *Clinics in Geriatric Medicine* 19, 1–18.
24. Timiras P. S. (2003). Aging of the nervous system: Structural and biochemical changes. In Timiras P. S. (Ed.), *Physiological basis of aging and geriatrics* (3rd. ed., pp. 99–117). Boca Raton, FL: CRC Press.
25. Timiras P. S. (2003). The nervous system: Functional changes. In Timiras P. S. (Ed.), *Physiological basis of aging and geriatrics* (3rd ed., pp. 119–140). Boca Raton, FL: CRC Press.
26. Peters R. (2006). Ageing and the brain. *Postgraduate Medical Journal* 82, 84–88.
27. Schneck M. E., Haegerstrom-Portnoy G. (2003). Practical assessment of vision in the elderly. *Ophthalmology Clinics of North America* 16, 269–287.
28. Meisani E., Brown C., Emerle H. (2003). Sensory systems: Normal aging, disorder, and treatment of vision and hearing in humans. In Timiras P. S. (Ed.), *Physiological basis of aging and geriatrics* (3rd ed., pp. 141–165). Boca Raton, FL: CRC Press.
29. Gates G. A., Mills J. H. (2005). Presbycusis. *Lancet* 366, 1111–1120.
30. Howarth A., Shone G. R. (2006). Ageing and the auditory system. *Postgraduate Medical Journal* 82, 166–171.
31. Mills J. A. (2003). Age-related changes in the auditory system. In Hazzard W. R., Blass J. P., Ouslander J. G., et al. (Eds.), *Principles of geriatric medicine and gerontology* (5th ed., pp. 1239–1251). New York: McGraw-Hill.
32. Boyce J. M., Shone G. R. (2006). Effects of ageing on smell and taste. *Postgraduate Medical Journal* 82, 239–241.
33. Ginaldi L., Strennberg H. (2003). The immune system. In Timiras P. S. (Ed.), *Physiological basis of aging and geriatrics* (3rd ed., pp. 265–283). Boca Raton, FL: CRC Press.
34. Aw D., Silver A. B., Palmer D. (2007). Immunosenescence: Emerging challenges for an ageing population. *Immunology* 120, 435–446.
35. Castle S. C., Uyemura K., Fulop T., et al. (2007). Host resistance and immune responses in advanced age. *Clinics in Geriatric Medicine* 23, 463–479.
36. Liang S. Y., Mackowiak P. A. (2007). Infections in the elderly. *Clinics in Geriatric Medicine* 23, 441–456.
37. Soergel K. H., Zboralske F. E., Amberg J. R. (1964). Presbyesophagus: Esophageal motility in nonagenarians. *Journal of Clinical Investigation* 43, 1472–1476.
38. Hall K. E. (2003). Effects of aging on the gastrointestinal function. In Hazzard W. R., Blass J. P., Ouslander J. G. (Eds.), *Principles of geriatric medicine and gerontology* (5th ed., pp. 593–600). New York: McGraw-Hill.
39. Patel S. R., Wiggins J. (2007). Renal and electrolyte disorders. In Duthie E. H. Jr., Katz P. R., Malone M. L. (Eds.), *Practice of geriatrics* (4th ed., pp. 631–644). Philadelphia: Elsevier Saunders.
40. Wiggins J. (2003). Changes in renal function. In Hazzard W. R., Blass J. P., Ouslander J. G., et al. (Eds.), *Principles of geriatric medicine and gerontology* (5th ed., pp. 543–549). New York: McGraw-Hill.
41. Amin S. H., Kuhle C. L., Fitzpatrick L. A. (2007). Comprehensive evaluation of the older woman. *Mayo Clinic Proceedings* 78, 1157–1185.
42. DuBeau C. (2003). Benign prostate disorders. In Hazzard W. R., Blass J. P., Ouslander J. G., et al. (Eds.), *Principles of geriatric medicine and gerontology* (5th ed., pp. 1303–1310). New York: McGraw-Hill.
43. Ginsberg T. B. (2006). Aging and sexuality. *Medical Clinics of North America* 90, 1025–1036.
44. Wald M., Meacham R. B., Ross L. S., et al. (2006). Testosterone replacement therapy for older men. *Journal of Andrology* 27, 126–132.

45. Katz S., Ford A. B., Jackson B. A., et al. (1963). Studies of illness in the aged: The Index of ADL. *Journal of the American Medical Association* 185, 914–919.

46. Katz S., Downs T. D., Cash H. R., et al. (1970). Progress in development of the Index of ADL. *Gerontologist* 10, 20–30.

47. Wilson L., Brown J. S., Shin G. P., et al. (2001). Annual direct costs of urinary incontinence. *Obstetrics and Gynecology* 98, 398–406.

48. Cohan M. E., Kuiper Pikna J., Duecy E. (2007). Urinary incontinence. In Duthie E. H. Jr., Katz P. R., Malone M. L. (Eds.), *Practice of geriatrics* (4th ed., pp. 187–194). Philadelphia: Elsevier Saunders.

49. Norton P., Brubaker L. (2006). Urinary incontinence in women. *Lancet* 367, 57–67.

50. Kane R. L., Ouslander J. G., Abrass I. B. (2004). *Essentials of clinical geriatrics* (5th ed.). New York: McGraw-Hill.

51. Rubenstein L. Z. (2006). Falls in older people: Epidemiology, risk factors and strategies for prevention. *Age and Ageing* 35(Suppl. 2), ii37–ii41.

52. Kannus P., Uusi-Rasi K., Palvanen M., et al. (2005). Non-pharmacological means to prevent fractures among older adults. *Annals of Medicine* 37, 303–310.

53. Hile E. S., Studenski S. A. (2007). Instability and falls. In Duthie E. H. Jr., Katz P. R., Malone M. L. (Eds.), *Practice of geriatrics* (4th ed., pp. 195–218). Philadelphia: Elsevier Saunders.

54. Brignole M. (2006). Distinguishing syncopal from non-syncopal causes of falls in older people. *Age and Ageing* 35(Suppl. 2), ii46–ii50.

55. Bischoff H. A., Stahelin H. B., Dick W., et al. (2003). Effects of vitamin D and calcium supplementation on falls: A randomized control trial. *Journal of Bone and Mineral Research* 18, 43–51.

56. Bischoff-Ferrari H. A., Dawson-Hughes B., Willett W. C., et al. (2004). Effect of vitamin D on falls: A meta-analysis. *Journal of the American Medical Association* 291, 1999–2006.

57. Medwetsky L. (2007). Hearing loss. In Duthie E. H. Jr., Katz P. R., Malone M. L. (Eds.), *Practice of geriatrics* (4th ed., pp. 285–300). Philadelphia: Elsevier Saunders.

58. Sterns G. K., McCormick G. J. (2007). Ophthalmologic disorders. In Duthie E. H. Jr., Katz P. R., Malone M. L. (Eds.), *Practice of geriatrics* (4th ed., pp. 301–316). Philadelphia: Elsevier Saunders.

59. Rovner B. W. (2006). The Charles Bonnet syndrome: A review of recent research. *Current Opinions in Ophthalmology* 17, 275–277.

60. Lebowitz B. D., Olin J. T. (2005). Older Americans and mental illness. In Salzman C. (Ed.), *Clinical geriatric psychopharmacology* (4th ed., pp. 3–21). Philadelphia: Lippincott Williams & Wilkins.

61. American Psychiatric Association. (2000). *Diagnostic and statistical manual of mental disorders* (4th ed., text revision). Washington, DC: Author.

62. Alexopoulos G. S. (2005). Depression in the elderly. *Lancet* 365, 1961–1970.

63. Barnes D. E., Alexopoulos G. S., Lopez O. L., et al. (2006). Depressive symptoms, vascular disease, and mild cognitive impairment. *Archives of General Psychiatry* 63, 273–280.

64. Privitere M. R., Lyness J. M. (2007). Depression. In Duthie E. H. Jr., Katz P. R., Malone M. L. (Eds.), *Practice of geriatrics* (4th ed., pp. 345–358). Philadelphia: Elsevier Saunders.

65. National Institute of Mental Health. (2007). Older adults: Depression and suicide facts. [Online.] Available: www.nih.gov/publicat/elderlydep suicide.cfm.

66. Yesavage J. A., Brink T. L., Rose T. L., et al. (1983). Development and validation of a geriatric depression scale: A preliminary report. *Journal of Psychiatric Research* 17, 37–49.

67. Greenberg R. M., Kellner C. H. (2005). Electroconvulsive therapy. *American Journal of Geriatric Psychiatry* 13, 268–281.

68. Frosch M. P., Anthony D. C., DeGirolami U. (2005). The central nervous system. In Kumar V., Abbas A. K., Fausto N. (Eds.), *Robbins and Cotran pathologic basis of medicine* (5th ed., pp. 1386–1389). Philadelphia: Elsevier Saunders.

69. Aggarwal N. T., DeCarli C. (2007). Vascular dementia: Emerging trends. *Seminars in Neurology* 27, 66–77.

70. Nelson N. W. (2007). Differential diagnosis of Alzheimer's dementia and vascular dementia. *Disease-a-Month* 53, 148–151.

71. Small G. W., Kepe V., Ercoli L. M., et al. (2006). PET of brain amyloid and tau in mild cognitive impairment. *New England Journal of Medicine* 355, 2652–2663.

72. Folstein M. F., Folstein B. E., McHugh P. R. (1975). "Mini-Mental State": A practical method for grading the cognitive state of patients for the clinician. *Journal of Psychiatric Research* 12, 189–198.

73. Malay S., Wilson B., Santhi K., et al. (2006). Alzheimer's disease and its management: A review. *American Journal of Therapeutics* 13, 516–526.

74. Mari E., Hashimoto M., Krishnan R., et al. (2006). What constitutes clinical evidence for neuroprotection in Alzheimer's disease: Support for the cholinesterase inhibitor? *Alzheimer's Disease and Associated Disorders* 20(Suppl. 1), S19–S26.

75. Farlow M. R., Cummings J. L. (2007). Effective pharmacologic management of Alzheimer's disease. *American Journal of Medicine* 120, 388–397.

76. Robinson D. M., Keating G. M. (2006). Memantine: A review of its use in Alzheimer's disease. *Drugs* 66, 1515–1534.

77. Kang J. H., Cook N., Manson J., et al. (2006). A randomized trial of vitamin E supplementation and cognitive function in women. *Archives of Internal Medicine* 166, 2462–2468.

78. Durga J., VanBoxtel M. P. J., Schouten E. G., et al. (2007). Effects of 3-year folic acid supplementation on cognitive function in older adults in the FACIT trial: A randomized, double blind, controlled trial. *Lancet* 369, 208–216.

79. Willis S. L., Tennstedt S. L., Marsiske M., et al. (2006). Long-term effects of cognitive training on everyday functional outcomes in older adults. *Journal of the American Medical Association* 296, 2805–2814.

80. Yu F., Kolanowski A. M., Strumpf N. E., et al. (2006). Improving cognitive functioning through exercise intervention in Alzheimer's disease. *Journal of Nursing Scholarship* 38, 358–65.

81. Smith M., Gerdner L. A., Hall G. R., et al. (2004). History, development and future of the progressively lowered stress threshold: A conceptual model for dementia care. *Journal of the American Geriatrics Society* 52, 1755–1760.

82. Smith M., Hall G. R., Buckwalter K. C. (2006). Application of the progressively lowered stress threshold model across the continuum of care. *Nursing Clinics of North America* 41, 57–81, vi.

83. Inouye S. K. (2006). Delirium in older person. *New England Journal of Medicine* 354, 1157–65.

84. Farley A., McLafferty E. (2007). Delirium part one: Clinical features, risk factors and assessment. *Nursing Standard* 21(29), 35–40.

85. Maraga A. V., Rodrigues-Pascuel C. (2007). Accurate diagnosis of delirium in elderly patients. *Current Opinions in Psychiatry* 20, 262–267.

86. McLafferty E., Farley A. (2007). Delirium part two: Clinical features, risk factors and assessment. *Nursing Standard* 21(30), 42–46.

87. Beyth R. J., Shorr R. I. (2007). Medication use. In Duthie E. H. Jr., Katz P. R., Malone M. L. (Eds.), *Practice of geriatrics* (4th ed., pp. 17–32). Philadelphia: Elsevier Saunders.

88. Katzung B. G. (2007). Special aspects of geriatric pharmacology. In Katzung B. G. (Ed.), *Basic and clinical pharmacology* (10th ed., pp. 983–990). New York: McGraw-Hill Medical.

89. Aspinall S., Sevick M. A., Donoue J., et al. (2007). Medication errors in older adults. *American Journal of Geriatric Pharmacotherapy* 5, 75–84.

90. Timiras M. L., Luxenberg J. (2003). Pharmacology and drug management in the elderly. In Timiras P. S. (Ed.), *Physiological basis of aging and geriatrics* (3rd ed., pp. 407–414). Boca Raton, FL: CRC Press.

91. McLean A. J., LeCarteur D. G. (2004). Aging biology and geriatric clinical pharmacology. *Pharmacological Reviews* 56, 163–184.

Visit the**Point** http://thePoint.lww.com for animations, journal articles, and more!

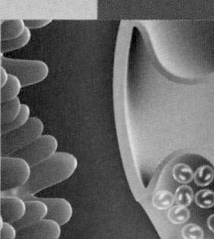

Cell Function and Growth

With its elegant structure and astonishing range of functions, the living cell is an object of wonder. It is the basic unit of all living organisms. There are more than 300 trillion cells in the human body, and every second of every day, more than 10 million die and are replaced.

In 1665, these impressive structures were named. While examining a thin slice of cork, Robert Hooke (1635–1703), an English scientist and pioneer microscopist, noted that it was made up of tiny boxlike units. The units reminded him of the small enclosures in which monks lived, and he named the microscopic spaces "cells," from the Latin word cells, meaning "small enclosures."

Although Hooke, as well as other scientists, intently studied microscopic life, few guessed the significance of the cells. That would be delayed until microscopes were advanced enough to yield more detailed information. It was with the work of Anton van Leeuwenhoek (1632–1723), a Dutch biologist and microscopist, that the mysteries and importance of the cell were revealed. He ground a single lens to such perfection that he was able to produce a microscope with great resolving power—one that was capable of magnifying a specimen from approximately 50 to 300 times in diameter. Van Leeuwenhoek's work, which included constructing an aquatic microscope that he used to study red blood cells and their flow through the body, was responsible for helping scientists investigate human tissue in ways that once they only dreamed of.

Chapter 4

Cell and Tissue Characteristics

EDWARD W. CARROLL

➤ In most organisms, the *cell* is the smallest functional unit that can retain the characteristics necessary for life. Cells are organized into larger functional units called *tissues* based on their embryonic origin. These tissues, in turn, combine to form the various body structures and organs. Although the cells of different tissues and organs vary in structure and function, certain characteristics are common to all cells. Cells are remarkably similar in their ability to exchange materials with their immediate environment, obtain energy from organic nutrients, synthesize complex molecules, and replicate themselves. Because most disease processes are initiated at the cellular level, an understanding of cell function is crucial to understanding the disease process. Some diseases affect the cells of a single organ, others affect the cells of a particular tissue type, and still others affect the cells of the entire organism. This chapter discusses the structural and functional components of the cell, integration of cell function and growth, movement of molecules such as ions across the cell membrane, and tissue types.

FUNCTIONAL COMPONENTS OF THE CELL

After completing this section of the chapter, you should be able to meet the following objectives:

■ State why the nucleus is called the "control center" of the cell.
■ List the cellular organelles and state their functions.
■ State four functions of the cell membrane.

Although diverse in their organization, all eukaryotic cells have in common structures that perform unique functions. When seen under a light microscope, three major components of the cell become evident: the nucleus, the cytoplasm, and the cell membrane (Fig. 4-1).

Protoplasm

Biologists call the internal matrix of the cell *protoplasm.* Protoplasm is composed of water, proteins, lipids, carbohydrates, and electrolytes. Two distinct regions of protoplasm

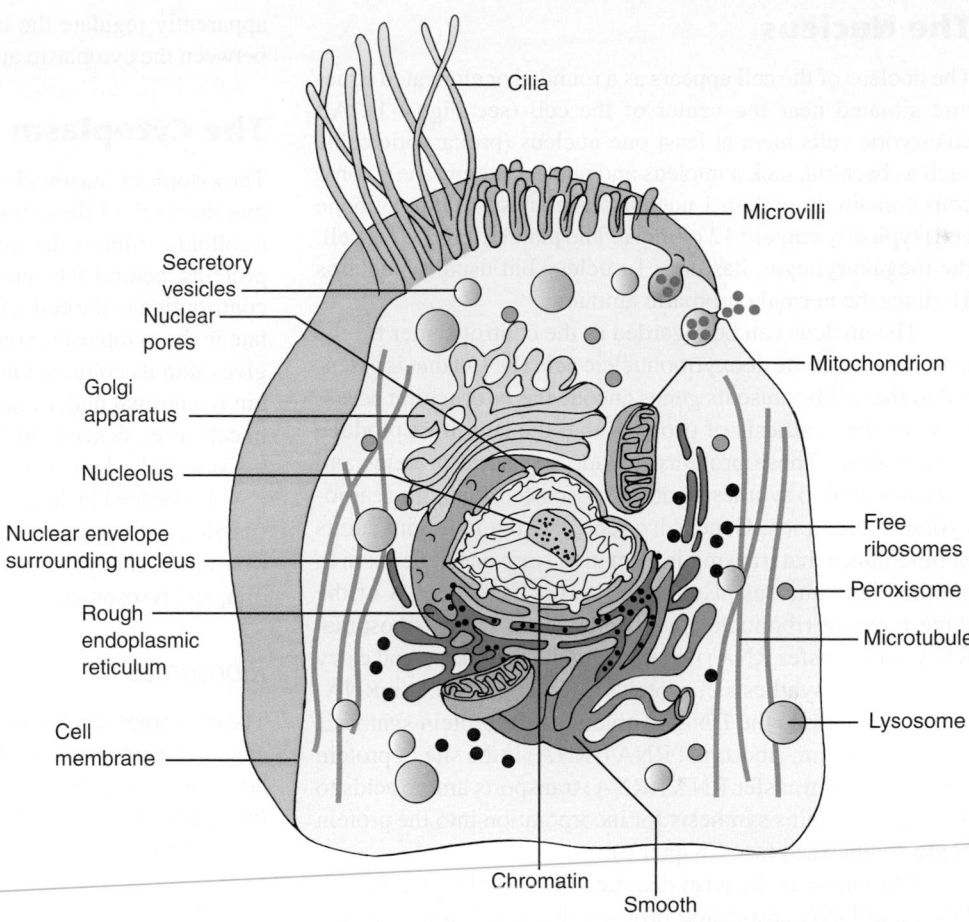

Cilia

Microvilli

Secretory
vesicles

Nuclear
pores

Golgi
apparatus

Nucleolus

Nuclear envelope
surrounding nucleus

Rough
endoplasmic
reticulum

Cell
membrane

Mitochondrion

Free
ribosomes

Peroxisome

Microtubule

Lysosome

Chromatin

Smooth
endoplasmic reticulum

FIGURE 4-1 • Composite cell designed to show in one cell all of the various components of the nucleus and cytoplasm.

exist in the cell: the *cytoplasm,* which lies outside the nucleus, and the *karyoplasm* or *nucleoplasm,* which lies inside the nucleus.

Water makes up 70% to 85% of the cell's protoplasm. The second most abundant constituents (10% to 20%) of protoplasm are the cell proteins, which form cell structures and the enzymes necessary for cellular reactions. Proteins can be bound to other compounds to form nucleoproteins, glycoproteins, and lipoproteins. Lipids comprise 2% to 3% of most cells. The most important lipids are the phospholipids and cholesterol, which are mainly insoluble in water; they combine with proteins to form the cell membrane and the membranous barriers that separate different cell compartments. Some cells also contain large quantities of triglycerides. In fat cells, triglycerides can comprise up to 95% of the total cell mass. This fat represents stored energy, which can be mobilized and used wherever it is needed in the body. Only a few carbohydrates are found in the cell and these serve primarily as a rapid source of energy. Potassium, magnesium, phosphate, sulfate, and bicarbonate ions are the major intracellular electrolytes. Small quantities of sodium, chloride, and calcium ions are also present in the cell. These electrolytes participate in reactions that are necessary for the cell's metabolism and they help in the generation and transmission of electrochemical impulses in nerve and muscle cells.

THE FUNCTIONAL ORGANIZATION OF THE CELL

- Cells are the smallest functional unit of the body. They contain structures that are strikingly similar to those needed to maintain total body function.

- The nucleus is the control center for the cell. It also contains most of the hereditary material.

- The organelles, which are analogous to the organs of the body, are contained in the cytoplasm. They include the mitochondria, which supply the energy needs of the cell; the ribosomes, which synthesize proteins and other materials needed for cell function; and the lysosomes and proteosomes, which function as the cell's digestive system.

- The cell membrane encloses the cell and provides for intracellular and intercellular communication, transport of materials into and out of the cell, and maintenance of the electrical activities that power cell function.

The Nucleus

The nucleus of the cell appears as a rounded or elongated structure situated near the center of the cell (see Fig. 4-1). All eukaryotic cells have at least one nucleus (prokaryotic cells, such as bacteria, lack a nucleus and nuclear membrane). Some cells contain more than 1 nucleus; osteoclasts (a type of bone cell) typically contain 12 or more. The platelet-producing cell, the megakaryocyte, has only 1 nucleus but usually contains 16 times the normal chromatin amount.

The nucleus can be regarded as the control center for the cell. It contains the deoxyribonucleic acid (DNA) that is essential to the cell because its genes encode the information necessary for the synthesis of proteins that the cell must produce to stay alive. These proteins include structural proteins and enzymes used to synthesize other substances, including carbohydrates and lipids. Genes also represent the individual units of inheritance that transmit information from one generation to another. The nucleus also is the site for the synthesis of the three types of ribonucleic acid (messenger RNA, ribosomal RNA, and transfer RNA) that move to the cytoplasm and carry out the actual synthesis of proteins. Messenger RNA (mRNA) copies and carries the DNA instructions for protein synthesis to the cytoplasm; ribosomal RNA (rRNA) is the site of protein synthesis; and transfer RNA (tRNA) transports amino acids to the site of proteins synthesis for incorporation into the protein being synthesized (see Chapter 6).

Chromatin is the term denoting the complex structure of DNA and DNA-associated proteins dispersed in the nuclear matrix. Depending on its transcriptional activity, chromatin may be condensed as an inactive form of chromatin called *heterochromatin* or extended as a more active form called *euchromatin*. Because heterochromatic regions of the nucleus stain more intensely than regions consisting of euchromatin, nuclear staining can be a guide to cell activity. The nucleus also contains the darkly stained round body called the *nucleolus*. Although nucleoli were first described in 1781, their function was unknown until the early 1960s, when it was determined that the processing of rRNA and its assembly into ribosomes occurs exclusively in the nucleolus. Nucleoli are structures composed of regions from five different chromosomes, each with a part of the genetic code needed for the synthesis of rRNA. Euchromatic nuclei and prominent nucleoli are characteristic of cells that are actively synthesizing proteins.

Surrounding the nucleus is the *nuclear envelope* formed by two (outer and inner) nuclear membranes containing a perinuclear cisternal space between them. The inner nuclear membrane is supported by a rigid network of protein filaments that bind to chromosomes and secure their position in the nucleus. The outer nuclear membrane resembles the membrane of the endoplasmic reticulum and is continuous with it. The nuclear envelope contains many structurally complex circular pores where the two membranes fuse to form a gap filled with a thin protein diaphragm. Many classes of molecules, including fluids, electrolytes, RNA, some proteins, and hormones, can move in both directions through the nuclear pores. Nuclear pores apparently regulate the bidirectional exchange of molecules between the cytoplasm and the nucleus.

The Cytoplasm and Its Organelles

The cytoplasm surrounds the nucleus, and it is in the cytoplasm that the work of the cell takes place. Cytoplasm is essentially a colloidal solution that contains water, electrolytes, suspended proteins, neutral fats, and glycogen molecules. Although not contributing to the cell's function, pigments may also accumulate in the cytoplasm. Some pigments, such as melanin, which gives skin its color, are normal constituents of the cell. Bilirubin is a normal major pigment of bile; its excess accumulation in cells is evidenced clinically by a yellowish discoloration of the skin and sclera, a condition called *jaundice*.

Embedded in the cytoplasm are various *organelles*, which function as the organs of the cell. These organelles include the ribosomes, endoplasmic reticulum, Golgi complex, mitochondria, and lysosomes.

Ribosomes

The ribosomes serve as sites of protein synthesis in the cell. They are small particles of nucleoproteins (rRNA and proteins) that are held together by a strand of mRNA to form polyribosomes (also called *polysomes*). Polyribosomes exist as isolated clusters of free ribosomes within the cytoplasm (Fig. 4-2) or attached to

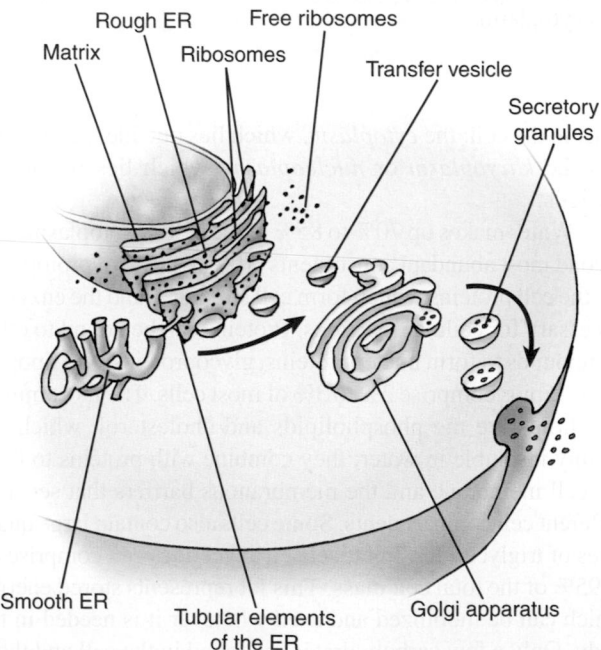

FIGURE 4-2 • Three-dimensional view of the rough and smooth endoplasmic reticulum (ER) and the Golgi apparatus. The ER functions as a tubular communication system through which substances can be transported from one part of the cell to another and as the site of protein (rough ER), carbohydrate, and lipid (smooth ER) synthesis. Most of the proteins synthesized by the rough ER are sealed into transfer vesicles and transported to the Golgi apparatus, where they are modified and packaged into secretory granules.

the membrane of the endoplasmic reticulum. Whereas free ribosomes are involved in the synthesis of proteins, mainly enzymes that aid in the control of cell function, those attached to the endoplasmic reticulum translate mRNAs that code for proteins secreted from the cell or stored within the cell (*e.g.*, granules in white blood cells).

Endoplasmic Reticulum

The endoplasmic reticulum (ER) is an extensive system of paired membranes and flat vesicles that connect various parts of the inner cell (see Fig. 4-2). Between the paired ER membranes is a fluid-filled space called the *matrix*. The matrix connects the space between the two membranes of the nuclear envelope, the cell membrane, and various cytoplasmic organelles. It functions as a tubular communication system for transporting various substances from one part of the cell to another. A large surface area and multiple enzyme systems attached to the ER membranes also provide the machinery for a major share of the cell's metabolic functions.

Two forms of ER exist in cells: rough and smooth. *Rough ER* is studded with ribosomes attached to specific binding sites on the membrane. Proteins produced by the rough ER are usually destined to become components of lysosomes or other organelles, incorporated into cell membranes, or leave the cell as a secretory protein. The rough ER segregates these proteins from other components of the cytoplasm and modifies their structure for a specific function. For example, the synthesis of both digestive enzymes by pancreatic acinar cells and plasma proteins by liver cells takes place in the rough ER. All cells require a rough ER for the synthesis of lysosomal enzymes.

The *smooth ER* is free of ribosomes and is continuous with the rough ER. It does not participate in protein synthesis; instead, its enzymes are involved in the synthesis of lipid molecules, regulation of intracellular calcium, and metabolism and detoxification of certain hormones and drugs. It is the site of lipid, lipoprotein, and steroid hormone synthesis. The sarcoplasmic reticulum of skeletal and cardiac muscle cells is a form of smooth ER. Calcium ions needed for muscle contraction are stored and released from cisternae of the sarcoplasmic reticulum. The smooth ER of the liver is involved in glycogen storage and metabolism of lipid-soluble drugs.

Golgi Complex

The Golgi apparatus, sometimes called the *Golgi complex,* consists of stacks of thin, flattened vesicles or sacs (see Fig. 4-2). These Golgi bodies are found near the nucleus and function in association with the ER. Substances produced in the ER are carried to the Golgi complex in small, membrane-covered transfer vesicles. Many cells synthesize proteins that are larger than the active product. The Golgi complex modifies these substances and packages them into secretory granules or vesicles. Insulin, for example, is synthesized as a large, inactive proinsulin molecule that is cut apart to produce a smaller, active insulin molecule within the Golgi complex of the beta cells in

the pancreas. In addition to producing secretory granules, the Golgi complex is thought to produce large carbohydrate molecules that combine with proteins produced in the rough ER to form glycoproteins. Recent data suggest that the Golgi apparatus has yet another function: it can receive proteins and other substances from the cell surface by a retrograde transport mechanism. This retrograde pathway has been exploited by several bacterial toxins, such as Shiga and cholera toxins, and plant toxins, such as ricin, that have cytoplasmic targets.

Lysosomes and Peroxisomes

Lysosomes can be viewed as the digestive system of the cell. These small, membrane-enclosed sacs contain powerful hydrolytic enzymes. These enzymes can break down excess and worn-out cell parts as well as foreign substances that are taken into the cell. All of the lysosomal enzymes are acid hydrolases, which means that they require an acidic environment. The lysosomes provide this environment by maintaining a pH of approximately 5 in their interior. The pH of the cytoplasm, which is approximately 7.2, serves to protect other cellular structures from this acidity. *Primary lysosomes* are membrane-bound intracellular organelles that contain a variety of hydrolytic enzymes that have not yet entered the digestive process. They receive their enzymes as well as their membranes from the Golgi apparatus. Primary lysosomes become *secondary lysosomes* after they fuse with membrane-bound vacuoles that contain material to be digested. Lysosomes breakdown phagocytosed material by either heterophagy or autophagy (Fig. 4-3).

Heterophagy refers to digestion of an exogenous substance phagocytosed from the cell's external environment. An infolding of the cell membrane takes external materials into the cell to form a surrounding phagocytic vesicle, or *phagosome*. Primary lysosomes then fuse with phagosomes to form secondary

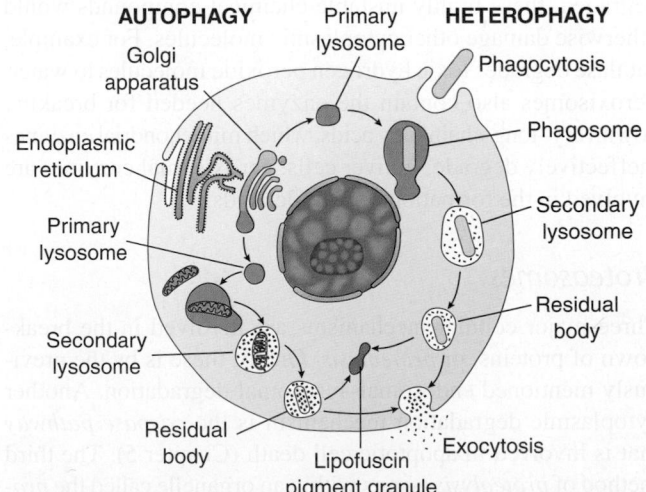

FIGURE 4-3 • The processes of autophagy and heterophagy, showing the primary and secondary lysosomes, residual bodies, extrusion of residual body contents from the cell, and lipofuscin-containing residual bodies.

lysosomes. Heterophagocytosis is most common in phagocytic white blood cells such as neutrophils and macrophages. *Autophagy* involves the segregation and disposal of damaged cellular organelles, such as mitochondria or ER, that the lysosomes must remove if the cell's normal function is to continue. Autophagocytosis is most pronounced in cells undergoing atrophy. Although enzymes in the secondary lysosomes can break down most proteins, carbohydrates, and lipids to their basic constituents, some materials remain undigested. These undigested materials may remain in the cytoplasm as *residual bodies* or are extruded from the cell by exocytosis. In some long-lived cells, such as neurons and heart muscle cells, large quantities of residual bodies accumulate as lipofuscin granules or age pigment. Other indigestible pigments, such as inhaled carbon particles and tattoo pigments, also accumulate and may persist in residual bodies for decades.

Lysosomes play an important role in the normal metabolism of certain substances in the body. In some inherited diseases known as *lysosomal storage diseases,* a specific lysosomal enzyme is absent or inactive, in which case the digestion of certain cellular substances (*e.g.,* glucocerebrosides, gangliosides, sphingomyelin) does not occur. As a result, these substances accumulate in the cell. In Tay-Sachs disease, an autosomal recessive disorder, hexosaminidase A, which is the lysosomal enzyme needed for degrading the GM_2 ganglioside found in nerve cell membranes, is deficient. Although GM_2 ganglioside accumulates in many tissues, such as the heart, liver, and spleen, its accumulation in the nervous system and retina of the eye causes the most damage (see Chapter 7).

Smaller than lysosomes, spherical membrane-bound organelles called *peroxisomes* contain a special enzyme that degrades peroxides (*e.g.,* hydrogen peroxide). Unlike lysosomes, peroxisomes are not formed by the Golgi apparatus. Peroxisomes are self-replicating like mitochondria and are initially formed by proteins produced by free ribosomes. Peroxisomes function in the control of free radicals (see Chapter 5). Unless degraded, these highly unstable chemical compounds would otherwise damage other cytoplasmic molecules. For example, catalase degrades toxic hydrogen peroxide molecules to water. Peroxisomes also contain the enzymes needed for breaking down very–long-chain fatty acids, which mitochondrial enzymes ineffectively degrade. In liver cells, peroxisomal enzymes are involved in the formation of the bile acids.

Proteasomes

Three major cellular mechanisms are involved in the breakdown of proteins, or *proteolysis.* One of these is by the previously mentioned endosomal–lysosomal degradation. Another cytoplasmic degradation mechanism is the *caspase pathway* that is involved in apoptotic cell death (Chapter 5). The third method of *proteolysis* occurs within an organelle called the *proteasome.* Proteasomes are small organelles composed of protein complexes that are thought to be present in both the cytoplasm and the nucleus. This organelle recognizes misformed and misfolded proteins that have been targeted for degradation, includ-

ing transcription factors and the cyclins that are important in controlling the cell cycle. It has been suggested that as much as one third of the newly formed polypeptide chains are selected for proteasome degradation because of quality-control mechanisms in the cell.

Mitochondria

The mitochondria are literally the "power plants" of the cell because they transform organic compounds into energy that is easily accessible to the cell. They do not make energy, but extract it from organic compounds. Mitochondria contain the enzymes needed for capturing most of the energy in foodstuffs and converting it into cellular energy. This multistep process is often referred to as *cellular respiration* because it requires oxygen. Cells store most of this energy as high-energy phosphate bonds in compounds such as adenosine triphosphate (ATP), using it to power the various cellular activities. Mitochondria are found close to the site of energy consumption in the cell (*e.g.,* near the myofibrils in muscle cells). The number of mitochondria in a given cell type varies by the type of activity the cell performs and the energy needed to undertake this activity. For example, a dramatic increase in mitochondria occurs in skeletal muscle repeatedly stimulated to contract.

Mitochondria are composed of two membranes: an outer membrane that encloses the periphery of the mitochondrion and an inner membrane that forms shelflike projections, called *cristae* (Fig. 4-4). The narrow space between the outer and inner membranes is called the *intermembrane space,* whereas the large space enclosed by the inner membrane is termed the *matrix space.* The outer mitochondrial membrane contains a large number of transmembrane porins, through which water-soluble molecules may pass. Because this membrane is relatively permeable to small molecules, including proteins, the contents of the intermembrane space resembles that of the cytoplasm. The inner membrane contains the respiratory chain

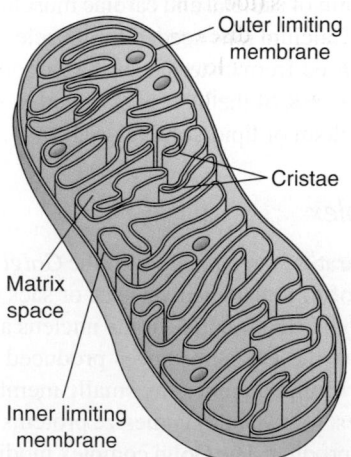

FIGURE 4-4 • Mitochondrion. The inner membrane forms transverse folds called *cristae,* where the enzymes needed for the final step in adenosine triphosphate (ATP) production (*i.e.,* oxidative phosphorylation) are located.

enzymes and transport proteins needed for the synthesis of ATP. In certain regions, the outer and inner membranes contact each other, these contact points serve as pathways for proteins and small molecules to enter and leave the matrix space.

Mitochondria contain their own DNA and ribosomes and are self-replicating. Mitochondrial DNA (mtDNA) is found in the mitochondrial matrix and is distinct from the chromosomal DNA found in the nucleus. Also known as the "other human genome," mtDNA is a double-stranded, circular molecule that encodes the rRNA and tRNA required for intramitochondrial synthesis of the proteins needed for the energy-generating functions of the mitochondria. Although mtDNA directs the synthesis of 13 of the proteins required for mitochondrial function, the DNA of the nucleus encodes the structural proteins of the mitochondria and other proteins needed to carry out cellular respiration.

Mitochondrial DNA is inherited matrilineally (*i.e.,* from the mother), thus providing a basis for familial lineage studies. Mutations have been found in each of the mitochondrial genes, and an understanding of the role of mtDNA in certain diseases is beginning to emerge (see Chapter 7). Most tissues in the body depend to some extent on oxidative metabolism and can therefore be affected by mtDNA mutations.

Mitochondria also function as key regulators of apoptosis or programmed cell death (see Chapter 5). The initiation of the mitochondrial pathway for apoptosis results from an increase in mitochondrial permeability and the subsequent release of proapoptotic molecules into the cytoplasm. One of these proapoptotic molecules is cytochrome c, well known for its role in mitochondrial respiration. In the cytosol, cytochrome c binds to a protein called *apoptosis activating factor-1,* initiating the molecular events involved in the apoptosis cascade. Other apoptotic proteins also enter the cytoplasm, where they bind to and neutralize the various apoptotic inhibitors, whose normal function is to block the apoptotic cascade. Both the formation of reactive oxygen species (*e.g.,* peroxide) and the activation of the *p53* tumor suppressor gene by DNA damage or other means initiate apoptotic signaling through the mitochondria. Dysregulated apoptosis (too little or too much) has been implicated in a wide range of diseases, including cancer, in which there is an inappropriately low rate of apoptosis, and neurodegenerative diseases, in which there is an increased or excessive rate of apoptosis.

The Cytoskeleton

Besides its organelles, the cytoplasm contains a network of microtubules, microfilaments, intermediate filaments, and thick filaments (Fig. 4-5). Because they control cell shape and movement, these structures are a major component of the structural elements called the *cytoskeleton*. The cytoskeleton also participates in the movement of entire cells.

Microtubules

Microtubules are formed from protein subunits called *tubulin*. They are long, stiff, hollow, cylindrical structures, 25 nm in

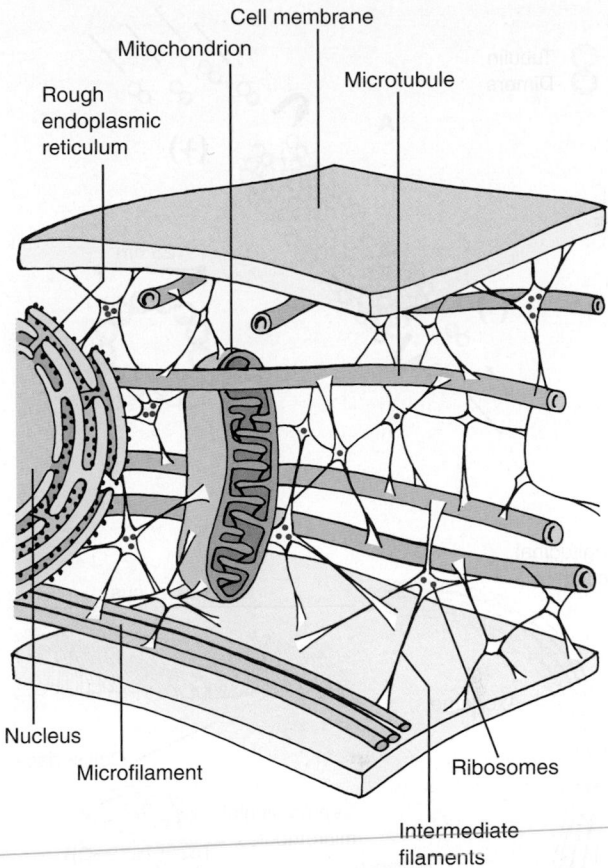

FIGURE 4-5 • Microtubules and microfilaments of the cell. The microfilaments are associated with the inner surface of the cell and aid in cell motility. The microtubules form the cytoskeleton and maintain the position of the organelles.

outer diameter with a lumen 15 nm in diameter (Fig. 4-6A and B). Each microtubule consists of parallel protofilaments, each composed of α- and β-tubulin dimers. Microtubules are dynamic structures that can rapidly disassemble in one location and reassemble in another. During the reassembly process the tubulin dimers polymerize in an end-to-end fashion to form protofilaments. As a result of the polymerization process, each microtubule possesses a nongrowing "minus" end and a rapidly growing "plus" end. During the disassembly process, the tubulin dimers dissociate from the protofilaments and form a pool of free tubulin in the cytoplasm. This pool is used in the polymerization process for reassembly of the protofilaments.

Microtubules function in many ways, including the development and maintenance of cell form. They participate in intracellular transport mechanisms, including axoplasmic transport in neurons and melanin dispersion in pigment cells of the skin. Other functions include formation of the basic structure for several complex cytoplasmic organelles, including the centrioles, basal bodies, cilia, and flagella.

The plant alkaloid *colchicine* binds to tubulin molecules and prevents the assembly of microtubules. This compound stops cell mitosis by interfering with formation of the mitotic spindle and is often used for cytogenetic (chromosome) studies.

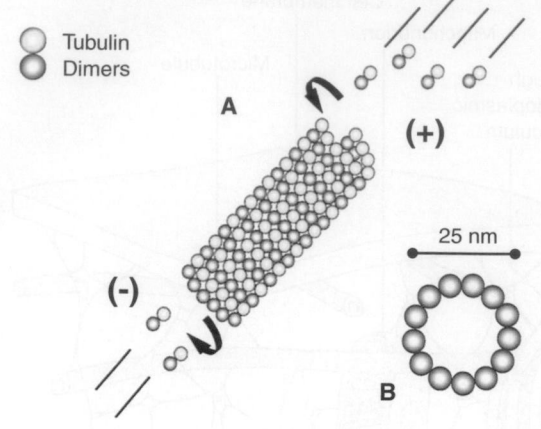

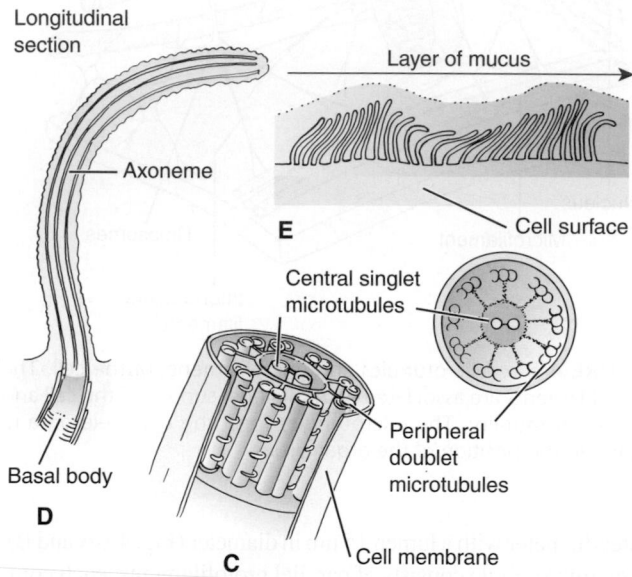

FIGURE 4-6 • **(A)** The formation of a microtubule from tubulin dimers is indicated, showing the faster-growing end (+) and the slower-growing end (–). **(B)** A cross-sectional view of a microtubule showing the 13 columns of spherical protofilaments. **(C)** Structure of cilium, showing the nine sets of doublet microtubules surrounding a central pair of singlet microtubules. **(D)** All of the microtubules are anchored to a basal body that is responsible for the formation of a core structure called the *axoneme*. **(E)** The sweeping movements of cilia move the mucous layer of the respiratory tract. **(A and B** courtesy of Edward W. Carroll.)

It is also used in treating gout to prevent migration of neutrophils and to lower their ability to respond to urate crystals in the tissues. The vinca alkaloid drugs (*e.g.,* vinblastine and vincristine), which are used in the treatment of cancer, also bind to microtubules and inhibit formation of the mitotic spindle, which is essential for cell proliferation (see Chapter 8).

Centrioles and Basal Bodies. Centrioles and basal bodies are structurally identical organelles composed of highly organized microtubules. Internally, centrioles and basal bodies have an

amorphous central core surrounded by clusters formed of triplet sets of microtubules.

Centrioles are small, cylindrical structures composed of an array of highly organized microtubules. Usually they are paired structures, arranged perpendicular to each other. In dividing cells, the two cylindrical centrioles are initially found in the vicinity of the Golgi apparatus in a region of the cell called the *centrosome.* During cell division, centrioles form the mitotic spindle that aids in the separation and movement of the chromosomes.

Basal bodies are more numerous than centrioles and are found near the cell membrane in association with cilia and flagella (see Fig. 4-6D). They are responsible for the formation of the highly organized core of microtubules found in cilia and flagella.

Cilia and Flagella. Cilia and flagella are microtubule-filled cellular extensions whose enclosing membrane is continuous with the cell membrane. Ciliated cells typically possess a large number of cilia, whereas flagellated cells have only one flagellum. In humans, the spermatozoa are the only cell type with flagella. Cilia are found on the apical (luminal) surfaces of many epithelial linings, including the nasal sinuses or passages such as the upper respiratory system. They also play a prominent role in sensory tissues such as the photoreceptor proteins in the eye, the odorant receptors of the olfactory epithelium, and the kinocilium on the hair cells in the inner ear. Cilia also act in sensory roles at critical stages of embryonic development, and they are essential for the normal functioning of many tissues, including the kidney, during postnatal life. Recent research has linked the pathogenesis of a condition called *polycystic kidney disease* to a genetic defect in the cilia of the renal tubular cells (see Chapter 33).

A motile cilium contains nine sets of doublet microtubules that form a hollow cylinder surrounding a central pair of singlet microtubules (see Fig. 4-6C). The outer doublet microtubules contain ATP motor–driven complexes that cause the adjacent microtubule doublets to slide past each other. All of these microtubules and their associated proteins are anchored to a *basal body* that is responsible for the formation of a core structure called the *axoneme* (see Fig. 4-6D). The axoneme serves as the internal framework that supports the cilium and provides a structure on which mechanical movement is generated. Recent evidence suggests that not all cilia contain this internal structure, and some may be missing the central pair of microtubules. Cilia lacking the central core of microtubules are often called *primary cilia,* and are immotile.

Cilia and flagella are assembled through a process called *intraflagellar transport,* during which large protein complexes are transported along the ciliary microtubules from the basal body to the ciliary tip and then back to the basal body. These protein complexes are thought to carry ciliary precursors from their site of synthesis in the cytoplasm to their site of assembly at the tip of the cilium. Genetic defects can result in improper ciliary assembly and, as a result, the cilia may be nonfunctional. One of these disorders, the *immobile cilia syndrome,* impairs sperm motility, causing male sterility while also immobilizing the cilia of the respiratory tract, thus interfering with clearance of inhaled bacteria, leading to a chronic lung disease called *bronchiectasis* (see Chapter 29).

Microfilaments

Microfilaments are thin, threadlike cytoplasmic structures. Three classes of microfilaments exist: thin microfilaments, which are equivalent to the thin actin filaments in muscle; intermediate filaments, which are a heterogeneous group of filaments with diameter sizes between those of the thick and thin filaments; and thick myosin filaments, which are present in muscle cells, but may also exist temporarily in other cells.

Muscle contraction depends on the interaction between the thin actin filaments and thick myosin filaments. Microfilaments are present in the superficial zone of the cytoplasm in most cells. Contractile activities involving the microfilaments and associated thick myosin filaments contribute to the movement of the cytoplasm and cell membrane during endocytosis and exocytosis. Microfilaments are also present in the microvilli of the intestine. The intermediate filaments assist in supporting and maintaining the asymmetric shape of cells. Examples of intermediate filaments are the keratin filaments that are found anchored to the cell membrane of epidermal keratinocytes of the skin and the glial filaments that are found in astrocytes and other glial cells of the nervous system. The *neurofibrillary tangle* found in the brain in Alzheimer disease contains microtubule-associated proteins and neurofilaments, evidence of a disrupted neuronal cytoskeleton (see Chapter 53).

The Cell (Plasma) Membrane

The cell is enclosed in a thin membrane that separates the intracellular contents from the extracellular environment. To differentiate it from the other cell membranes, such as the mitochondrial or nuclear membranes, the cell membrane is often called the *plasma membrane*. In many respects, the plasma membrane is one of the most important parts of the cell. It acts as a semipermeable structure that separates the intracellular and extracellular environments. It provides receptors for hormones and other biologically active substances, participates in the electrical events that occur in nerve and muscle cells, and aids in the regulation of cell growth and proliferation.

The cell membrane is a dynamic and fluid structure consisting of an organized arrangement of lipids, carbohydrates, and proteins (Fig. 4-7). A main structural component of the membrane is its lipid bilayer. It is a bimolecular layer that consists primarily of phospholipids, with glycolipids and cholesterol. This lipid bilayer provides the basic fluid structure of the membrane and serves as a relatively impermeable barrier to all but lipid-soluble substances. Approximately 75% of the lipids are phospholipids, each with a hydrophilic (water-soluble) head and a hydrophobic (water-insoluble) tail. Phospholipid molecules along with the glycolipids are aligned such that their hydrophilic heads face outward on each side of the membrane and their hydrophobic tails project toward the middle of the membrane. The hydrophilic heads retain water and help cells stick to each other. At normal body temperature, the viscosity of the lipid component of the membrane is equivalent to that of olive oil. The presence of cholesterol stiffens the membrane.

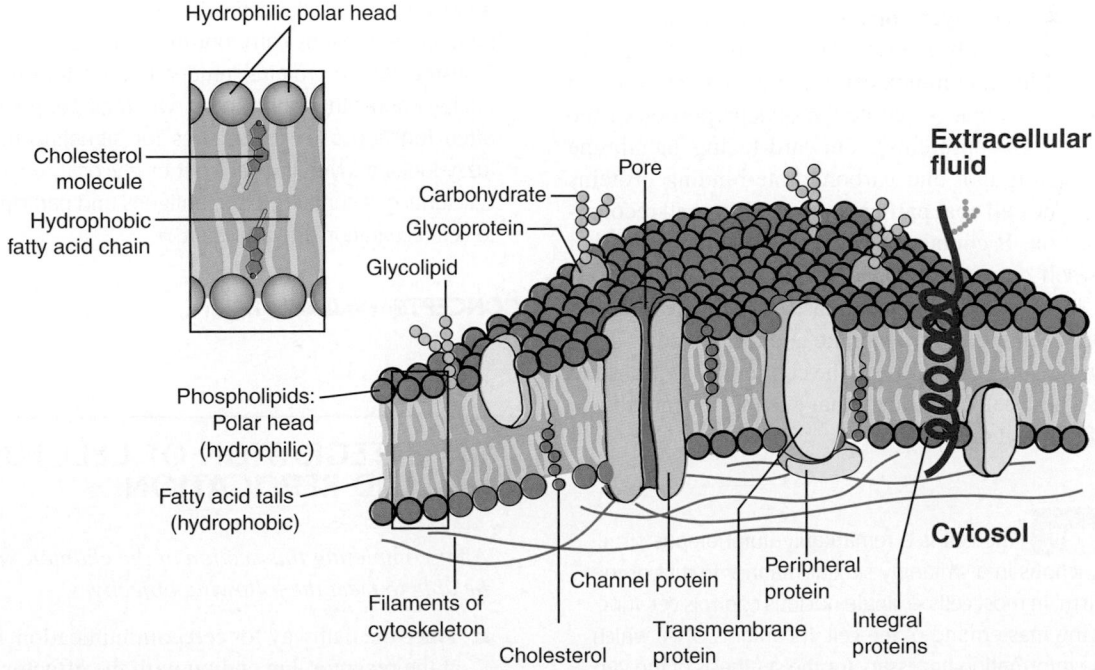

FIGURE 4-7 • Structure of the cell membrane showing the hydrophilic (polar) heads and the hydrophobic (fatty acid) tails (*inset*) and the position of the integral and peripheral proteins in relation to the interior and exterior of the cell.

Although the lipid bilayer provides the basic structure of the cell membrane, proteins carry out most of the specific functions. The *integral proteins* span the entire lipid bilayer and are essentially part of the membrane. Because most of the integral proteins pass directly through the membrane, they are also referred to as *transmembrane proteins*. A second type of protein, the *peripheral proteins*, is bound to one or the other side of the membrane and does not pass into the lipid bilayer. Removal of peripheral proteins from the membrane surface usually causes damage to the membrane.

The manner in which proteins are associated with the cell membrane often determines their function. Thus, peripheral proteins are associated with functions involving the inner or outer side of the membrane where they are found. Several peripheral proteins serve as receptors or are involved in intracellular signaling systems. By contrast, only the transmembrane proteins can function on both sides of the membrane or transport molecules across it.

Many integral transmembrane proteins form the ion channels found on the cell surface. These channel proteins have a complex morphology and are selective with respect to the substances they transmit. Mutations in these channel proteins, often called *channelopathies*, are responsible for a host of genetic disorders. For example, in *cystic fibrosis*, the primary defect resides in an abnormal chloride channel, which results in increased sodium and water reabsorption that causes respiratory tract secretions to thicken and occlude the airways (see Chapter 29). A recent discovery showed that there are specific water channels or pores called *aquaporins* in the plasma membrane. It is now known that aquaporin disorders are responsible for a number of diseases, including nephrogenic diabetes insipidus (see Chapter 31).

A fuzzy-looking layer surrounding the cell surface is called the *cell coat*, or *glycocalyx*. The structure of the glycocalyx consists of long, complex carbohydrate chains attached to protein molecules that penetrate the outside portion of the membrane (*i.e.*, glycoproteins); outward-facing membrane lipids (*i.e.*, glycolipids); and carbohydrate-binding proteins called *lectins*. The cell coat participates in cell-to-cell recognition and adhesion. It contains tissue transplant antigens that label cells as self or nonself. The cell coat of a red blood cell contains the ABO blood group antigens. An intimate relationship exists between the cell membrane and the cell coat. If the cell coat is enzymatically removed, the cell remains viable and can generate a new cell coat, but damage to the cell membrane usually results in cell death.

IN SUMMARY, the cell is a remarkably autonomous structure that functions in a strikingly similar manner to that of the total organism. In most cells, a single nucleus controls cell function and is the mastermind of the cell. It contains DNA, which provides the information necessary for the synthesis of the various proteins that the cell must produce to stay alive and to transmit information from one generation to another. The

nucleus also is the site for the synthesis of the three types of RNA (mRNA, rRNA, tRNA) that move to the cytoplasm and carry out the actual synthesis of proteins.

The cytoplasm contains the cell's organelles and cytoskeleton. Ribosomes serve as sites for protein synthesis in the cell. The ER functions as a tubular communication system that transports substances from one part of the cell to another and as the site of protein (rough ER), carbohydrate, and lipid (smooth ER) synthesis. Golgi bodies modify materials synthesized in the ER and package them into secretory granules for transport within the cell or for export from the cell. Lysosomes, which are viewed as the digestive system of the cell, contain hydrolytic enzymes that digest worn-out cell parts and foreign materials. They are membranous structures formed in the Golgi complex from hydrolytic enzymes synthesized in the rough ER. Another organelle, the proteasome, digests misformed and misfolded proteins. The mitochondria serve as power plants for the cell because they transform food energy into ATP, to power cell activities. Mitochondria contain their own extrachromosomal DNA, important in the synthesis of mitochondrial RNAs and proteins used in oxidative metabolism. Besides its organelles, the cytoplasm contains a network of microtubules, microfilaments, intermediate filaments, and thick filaments. Microtubules are slender, stiff tubular structures that influence cell shape, provide a means of moving organelles through the cytoplasm, and effect movement of the cilia and of chromosomes during cell division. Microfilaments, which are thin, threadlike cytoplasmic structures, include the actin and myosin filaments that participate in muscle contraction.

The plasma membrane is a lipid bilayer that surrounds the cell and separates it from its surrounding external environment. Although the lipid bilayer provides the basic structure of the cell membrane, proteins carry out most of the specific functions. Transmembrane proteins frequently form transport channels for ions and other substances, whereas peripheral proteins often function as receptor sites for signaling molecules. A fuzzy-looking layer, the cell coat or glycocalyx, surrounds the cell surface. It contains tissue antigens and participates in cell-to-cell recognition and adhesion. ■

CONCEPTSin action**ANIMATI**◯**N**

INTEGRATION OF CELL FUNCTION AND REPLICATION

After completing this section of the chapter, you should be able to meet the following objectives:

■ Trace the pathway for cell communication, beginning at the receptor and ending with the effector response, and explain why the process is often referred to as *signal transduction*.

■ Compare the functions of G-protein–linked, ion-channel–linked, and enzyme-linked cell surface receptors.
■ Describe the phases of mitotic cell division.
■ Relate the function of ATP to cell metabolism.
■ Compare the processes involved in anaerobic and aerobic metabolism.

Cell Communication

Cells in multicellular organisms need to communicate with one another to coordinate their function and control their growth. The human body has several means of transmitting information between cells. These mechanisms include direct communication between adjacent cells through gap junctions, autocrine and paracrine signaling, and endocrine or synaptic signaling. *Autocrine signaling* occurs when a cell releases a chemical into the extracellular fluid that affects its own activity (Fig. 4-8). With *paracrine signaling,* enzymes rapidly metabolize the chemical mediators, and therefore they act mainly on nearby cells. *Endocrine signaling* relies on hormones carried in the bloodstream to cells throughout the body. *Synaptic signaling* occurs in the nervous system, where neurotransmitters act only on adjacent

nerve cells through special contact areas called *synapses.* In some parts of the body, the same chemical messenger can function as a neurotransmitter, a paracrine mediator, and a hormone secreted by neurons into the bloodstream.

CELL COMMUNICATION

■ Cells communicate with each other and with the internal and external environments by a number of mechanisms, including electrical and chemical signaling systems that control electrical potentials, the overall function of a cell, and gene activity needed for cell division and cell replication.
■ Chemical messengers exert their effects by binding to cell membrane proteins or receptors that convert the chemical signal into signals within the cell, in a process called *signal transduction.*
■ Cells can regulate their responses to chemical messengers by increasing or decreasing the number of active receptors on their surface.

Cell Receptors

Signaling systems consist of receptors that reside either in the cell membrane (surface receptors) or within the cells (intracellular receptors). Receptors are activated by a variety of extracellular signals or *first messengers,* including neurotransmitters, protein hormones and growth factors, steroids, and other chemical messengers. Some lipid-soluble chemical messengers move through the membrane and bind to cytoplasmic or nuclear receptors to exert their physiologic effects. Signaling systems also include transducers and effectors that are involved in conversion of the signal into a physiologic response. The pathway may include additional intracellular mechanisms, called *second messengers.* Many molecules involved in signal transduction are proteins. A unique property of proteins that allows them to function in this way is their ability to change their shape or conformation, thereby changing their function and consequently the functions of the cell. Proteins often accomplish these conformational changes through enzymes called *protein kinases* that catalyze the phosphorylation of amino acids in the protein structure.

Cell Surface Receptors

Each cell type in the body contains a distinctive set of surface receptors that enable it to respond to a complementary set of signaling molecules in a specific, preprogrammed way. These proteins are not static components of the cell membrane; they increase or decrease in number according to the needs of the cell. When excess chemical messengers are present, the number of active receptors decreases in a process called *down-regulation;*

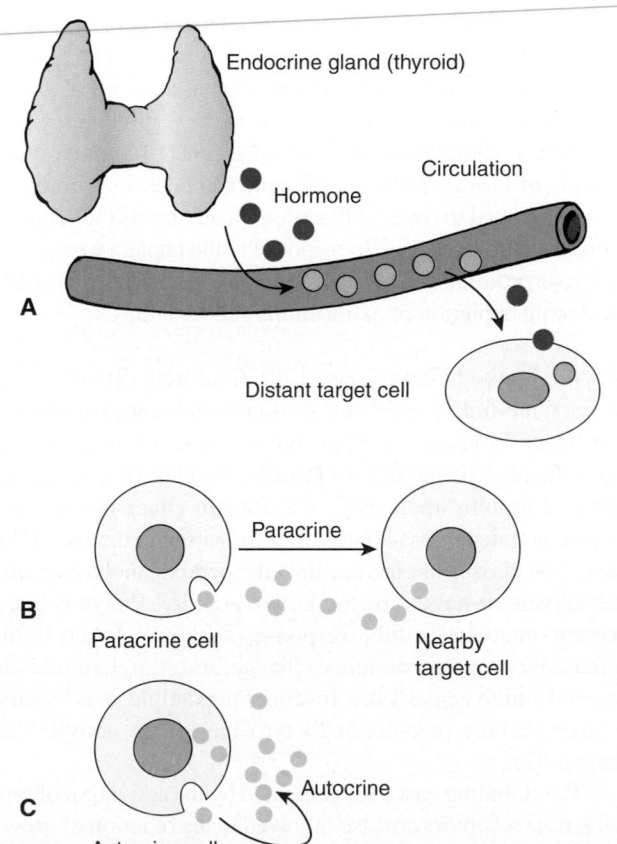

FIGURE 4-8 • Examples of endocrine (**A**), paracrine (**B**), and autocrine (**C**) secretions.

when there is a deficiency of the messenger, the number of active receptors increases through *up-regulation*. Three known classes of cell surface receptor proteins exist: G-protein–linked, ion-channel–linked, and enzyme-linked.

G-Protein–Linked Receptors. With more than a 1000 members, G-protein–linked receptors are the largest family of cell surface receptors. Although many intercellular messengers exist, they rely on the intermediary activity of a separate class of membrane-bound regulatory proteins to convert external signals (first messengers) into internal signals (second messengers). Because these regulatory proteins bind to guanine nucleotides such as guanine diphosphate (GDP) and guanine triphosphate (GTP), they are called *G proteins*. G-protein–linked receptors mediate cellular responses for numerous types of first messengers, including proteins, small peptides, amino acids, and fatty acid derivatives such as the prostaglandins.

Although there are differences among the G-protein–linked receptors, all share a number of features. They all have a ligand-binding extracellular receptor component, which functions as a signal discriminator by recognizing a specific first messenger, and they all undergo conformational changes with receptor binding that activates the G protein (Fig. 4-9). All G pro-

teins are found on the cytoplasmic side of the cell membrane, and all incorporate the *GTPase cycle*, which functions as a molecular switch that exists in two states. In its activated (on) state, the G protein has a high affinity for GTP, and in its inactivated (off) state, it binds GDP.

At the molecular level, G proteins are heterotrimeric (*i.e.*, they have three subunits) proteins (see Fig. 4-9). The three subunits are designated alpha (α), beta (β), and gamma (γ). The α subunit can bind either GDP or GTP and contains the GTPase activity. GTPase is an enzyme that converts GTP with its three phosphate groups to GDP with its two phosphate groups.

When GDP is bound to the α subunit, the G protein is inactive; when GTP is bound, it is active. The activated G protein has GTPase activity, so eventually the bound GTP is hydrolyzed to GDP, and the G protein reverts to its inactive state. Receptor activation causes the α subunit to dissociate from the receptor and the β and γ subunits and transmit the signal from the first messenger to its effector protein. Often, the effector is an enzyme that converts an inactive precursor molecule into a second messenger, which diffuses into the cytoplasm and carries the signal beyond the cell membrane. A common second messenger is cyclic adenosine monophosphate (cAMP). It is activated by the enzyme *adenylyl cyclase,* which generates cAMP by transferring phosphate groups from ATP to other proteins. This transfer changes the conformation and function of these proteins. Such changes eventually produce the cell response to the first messenger, whether it is a secretion, muscle contraction or relaxation, or a change in metabolism. Sometimes, it is the opening of membrane channels involved in calcium or potassium influx.

Certain bacterial toxins can bind to the G proteins, causing inhibition or stimulation of their signal function. For example, the toxin of *Vibrio cholerae* binds and activates the stimulatory G protein linked to the cAMP system that controls the secretion of fluid into the intestine. In response to the cholera toxin, these cells overproduce fluid, leading to severe diarrhea and life-threatening depletion of extracellular fluid volume.

Enzyme-Linked Receptors. Like G-protein–linked receptors, enzyme-linked receptors are transmembrane proteins with their ligand-binding site on the outer surface of the cell membrane. Instead of having a cytosolic domain that associates with a G protein, their cytosolic domain either has intrinsic enzyme activity or associates directly with an enzyme. There are several classes of enzyme-linked receptors, including those that activate or have tyrosine kinase activity. Enzyme-linked receptors mediate cellular responses such as calcium influx, increased sodium–potassium exchange, and stimulation of glucose and amino acid uptake. Insulin, for example, acts by binding to a surface receptor with tyrosine kinase activity (see Chapter 42).

The signaling cascades generated by the activation of tyrosine kinase receptors are also involved in the function of growth factors. As their name implies, many growth factors are important messengers in signaling cell replacement and cell growth. Most of the growth factors belong to one of three groups: fac-

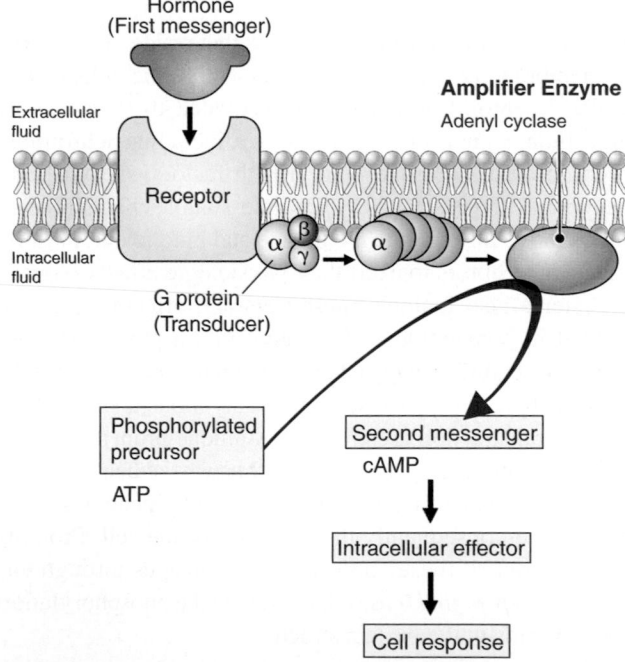

FIGURE 4-9 • Activation of a G-protein–linked receptor and production of cyclic adenosine monophosphate (cAMP). Binding of a hormone (the first messenger) causes the activated receptor to interact with the inactive, guanine diphosphate (GDP)–bound G protein. This results in activation of the G protein and dissociation of the G protein α, β, and γ subunits. The activated α subunit of the G protein can then interact with and activate the membrane protein adenyl cyclase to catalyze the conversion of adenosine triphosphate (ATP) to the second messenger cAMP. The second messenger then activates an internal effector, which leads to the cell response.

tors that foster the multiplication and development of various cell types (*e.g.*, epidermal growth factor and vascular endothelial growth factor); cytokines, which are important in the regulation of the immune system (see Chapter 17); and colony-stimulating factors, which regulate the proliferation and maturation of white and red blood cells (see Chapter 12). All growth factors function by binding to specific receptors that deliver signals to target cells. These signals have two general effects: they stimulate the transcription of many genes that were silent in resting cells, and they regulate the entry of cells into the cell cycle and their passage through the cell cycle.

Ion-Channel–Linked Receptors. Ion-channel–linked receptors are involved in the rapid synaptic signaling between electrically excitable cells. Many neurotransmitters mediate this type of signaling by transiently opening or closing ion channels formed by integral proteins in the cell membrane (to be discussed). This type of signaling is involved in the transmission of impulses in nerve and muscle cells.

Intracellular Receptors

Some messengers, such as thyroid hormone and steroid hormones, do not bind to membrane receptors but move directly across the lipid layer of the cell membrane and are carried to the cell nucleus, where they influence DNA activity. Many of these hormones bind to a cytoplasmic receptor, and the receptor–hormone complex is carried to the nucleus. In the nucleus, the receptor–hormone complex binds to DNA, thereby increasing transcription of mRNA (see Chapter 6). The mRNAs are translated in the ribosomes, with the production of increased amounts of proteins that alter cell function.

The Cell Cycle and Cell Division

The life cycle of a cell is called the *cell cycle*. It is usually divided into five phases: G_0, G_1, S, G_2, and M (Fig. 4-10). G_0 is the stage when the cell may leave the cell cycle and either remain in a state of inactivity or reenter the cell cycle at another time. G_1 is the stage during which the cell begins to prepare for mitosis through DNA and protein synthesis and an increase in organelle and cytoskeletal elements. The S phase is the synthesis phase, during which DNA replication occurs and the centrioles begin to replicate. G_2 is the premitotic phase and is similar to G_1 in terms of RNA activity and protein synthesis. The M phase is the phase during which cell mitosis occurs. Tissues may be composed primarily of quiescent cells in G_0, but most tissues contain a combination of cells that are continuously moving through the cell cycle and quiescent cells that occasionally enter the cell cycle. Nondividing cells, such as neurons and skeletal and cardiac muscle cells, have left the cell cycle and are not capable of mitotic division in postnatal life.

Cell division, or *mitosis,* is the process during which a parent cell divides and each daughter cell receives a chromosomal karyotype identical to the parent cell. Cell division gives the body a means of replacing cells that have a limited life span

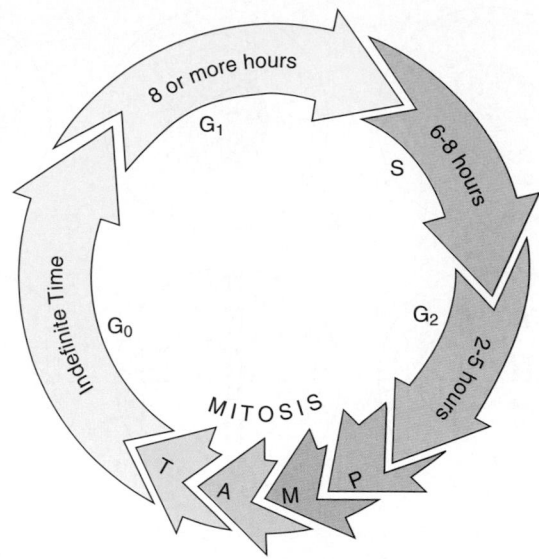

FIGURE 4-10 • The cell cycle. G_0, nondividing cell; G_1, cell growth; S, DNA replication; G_2, protein synthesis; and mitosis, which lasts for 1 to 3 hours and is followed by cytokinesis or cell division. T, telophase; A, anaphase; M, metaphase; P, prophase.

such as skin and blood cells, increasing tissue mass during periods of growth, and providing for tissue repair and wound healing.

Mitosis, which is a dynamic and continuous process, usually lasts from 1 to 1½ hours. It is divided into four stages: prophase, metaphase, anaphase, and telophase (Fig. 4-11). The phase during which the cell is not undergoing division is called *interphase.* During *prophase,* the chromosomes become visible because of increased coiling of the DNA, the two centrioles replicate, and a pair moves to each side of the cell. Simultaneously, the microtubules of the mitotic spindle appear between the two pairs of centrioles. Later in prophase, the nuclear envelope and nucleolus disappear. *Metaphase* involves the organization of the chromosome pairs in the midline of the cell and the formation of a mitotic spindle composed of microtubules. *Anaphase* is the period during which separation of the chromosome pairs occurs, with the microtubules pulling one member of each pair of 46 chromosomes toward the opposite cell pole. Cell division or *cytokinesis* is completed after *telophase,* the stage during which the mitotic spindle vanishes and a new nuclear membrane develops and encloses each complete set of chromosomes.

Cell division is controlled by changes in the concentrations and activity of three major groups of intracellular proteins: (1) cyclins, (2) cyclin-dependent kinases (CDKs), and (3) anaphase-promoting complex (see Chapter 8). The central components of the cell cycle control system are the CDKs, whose activity depends on their association with the regulatory units called *cyclins.* Oscillations in the activity of the various CDKs lead to initiation of the different phases of the cell cycle. Cell division is also controlled by several external factors, including the presence of cytokines, various growth factors, or

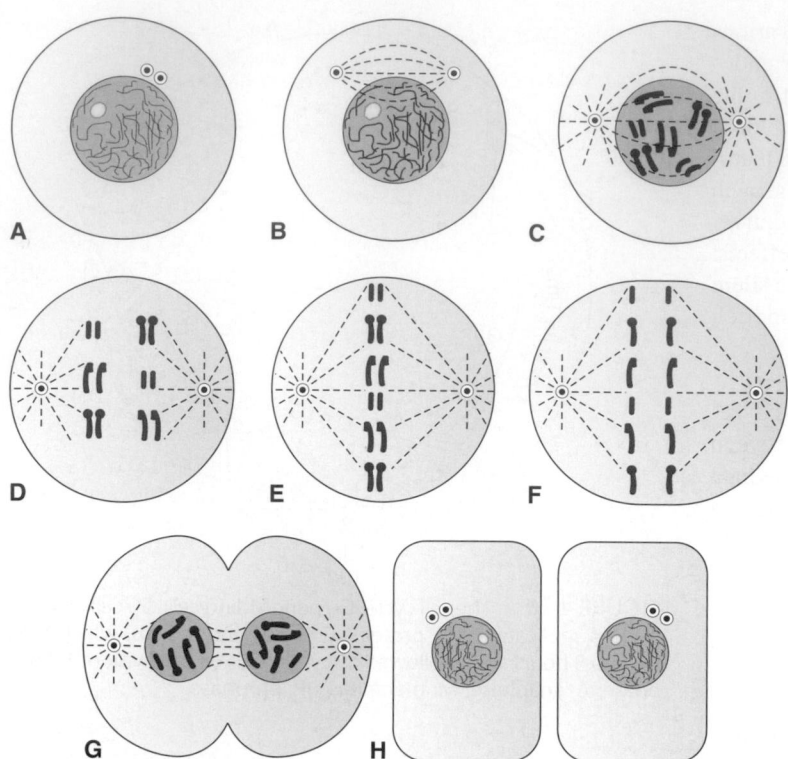

FIGURE 4-11 • Cell mitosis. *A* and *H* represent the nondividing cell; *B, C,* and *D* represent prophase; *E* represents metaphase; *F* represents anaphase; and *G* represents telophase.

even adhesion factors when the cell is associated with other cells in a tissue.

Cell Metabolism and Energy Sources

Energy is the ability to do work. Cells use oxygen to transform the breakdown products of the foods we eat into the energy needed for muscle contraction; the transport of ions and other molecules across cell membranes; and the synthesis of enzymes, hormones, and other macromolecules. *Energy metabolism* refers to the processes by which fats, proteins, and carbohydrates from the foods we eat are converted into energy or complex energy sources in the cell. Catabolism and anabolism are the two phases of metabolism. *Catabolism* consists of breaking down stored nutrients and body tissues to produce energy. *Anabolism* is a constructive process in which more complex molecules are formed from simpler ones.

The special carrier for cellular energy is ATP. ATP molecules consist of adenosine, a nitrogenous base; ribose, a five-carbon sugar; and three phosphate groups (Fig. 4-12). The phosphate groups are attached by two high-energy bonds. Large amounts of free energy are released when ATP is hydrolyzed to form adenosine diphosphate (ADP), an adenosine molecule that contains two phosphate groups. The free energy liberated from the hydrolysis of ATP is used to drive reactions that require free energy. Energy from foodstuffs is used to convert ADP back to ATP. Because energy can be "saved or

spent" using ATP, ATP is often called the *energy currency* of the cell.

Energy transformation takes place within the cell through two types of energy production: the *anaerobic (i.e.,* without oxygen) glycolytic pathway, occurring in the cytoplasm, and the *aerobic (i.e.,* with oxygen) pathway, occurring in the mitochondria. The anaerobic glycolytic pathway serves as an important prelude to the aerobic pathway. Both pathways involve oxidation-reduction reactions involving an electron donor, which is oxidized in the reaction, and an electron acceptor, which is reduced in the reaction. In energy metabolism, the breakdown products of carbohydrate, fat, and protein metabolism donate electrons and are oxidized, and the coenzymes nicotinamide adenine dinucleotide (NAD^+) and flavin adenine dinucleotide (FAD) accept electrons and are reduced.

Anaerobic Metabolism

Glycolysis is the process by which energy is liberated from glucose. It is an important energy provider for cells that lack mitochondria, the cell organelle in which aerobic metabolism occurs. This process also provides energy in situations when delivery of oxygen to the cell is delayed or impaired. Glycolysis involves a sequence of reactions that convert glucose to pyruvate, with the concomitant production of ATP from ADP. The net gain of energy from the glycolysis of one molecule of glucose is two ATP molecules. Although comparatively inefficient as to energy yield, the glycolytic pathway is important during periods of

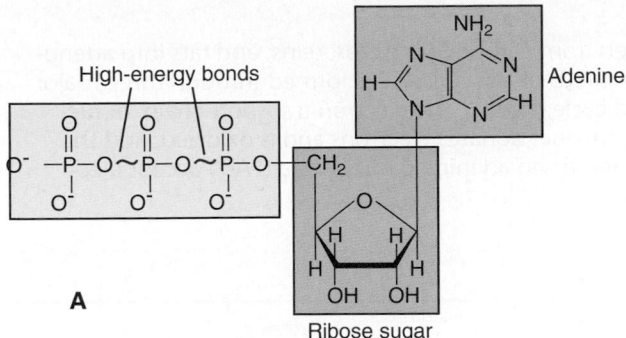

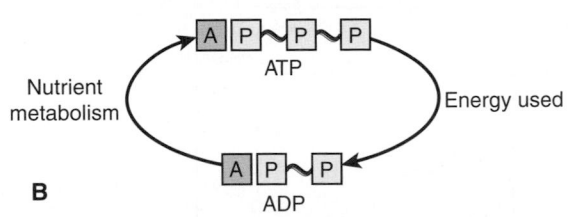

FIGURE 4-12 • Adenosine triphosphate (ATP) is the major source of cellular energy. **(A)** Each molecule of ATP contains two high-energy bonds, each containing about 12 kcal of potential energy. **(B)** The high-energy ATP bonds are in constant flux. They are generated by substrate (glucose, amino acid, and fat) metabolism and are consumed as the energy is expended.

decreased oxygen delivery, as occurs in skeletal muscle during the first few minutes of exercise.

Glycolysis requires the presence of NAD^+. Important end products of glycolysis are pyruvate and NADH (the reduced form of NAD^+) plus H^+. When oxygen is present, pyruvate moves into the aerobic mitochondrial pathway, and NADH + H^+ delivers its electron and proton (H^+) to the oxidative electron transport system. Transfer of electrons from NADH + H^+ to the electron transport system allows the glycolytic process to continue by facilitating the regeneration of NAD^+. Under anaerobic conditions, such as cardiac arrest or circulatory shock, pyruvate is converted to lactic acid, which diffuses out of the cells into the extracellular fluid. Conversion of pyruvate to lactic acid is reversible, and after the oxygen supply has been restored, lactic acid is converted back to pyruvate and used directly for energy or to synthesize glucose.

Much of the conversion of lactic acid occurs in the liver, but a small amount can occur in other tissues. The liver removes lactic acid from the bloodstream and converts it to glucose in a process called *gluconeogenesis.* This glucose is released into the bloodstream to be used again by the muscles or by the central nervous system. Heart muscle is also efficient in converting lactic acid to pyruvic acid and then using the pyruvic acid for fuel. Pyruvic acid is a particularly important source of fuel for the heart during heavy exercise when the skeletal muscles are producing large amounts of lactic acid and releasing it into the bloodstream.

Aerobic Metabolism

Aerobic metabolism occurs in the cell's mitochondria and involves the citric acid cycle and the electron transport chain. It is here that the carbon compounds from the fats, proteins, and carbohydrates in our diet are broken down and their electrons combined with molecular oxygen to form carbon dioxide and water as energy is released. Unlike lactic acid, which is an end product of anaerobic metabolism, carbon dioxide and water are generally harmless and easily eliminated from the body. In a 24-hour period, oxidative metabolism produces 300 to 500 mL of water.

The citric acid cycle, sometimes called the *tricarboxylic acid* (TCA) or *Krebs cycle,* provides the final common pathway for the metabolism of nutrients. In the citric acid cycle, which takes place in the matrix of the mitochondria, an activated two-carbon molecule of acetyl-coenzyme A (acetyl-CoA) condenses with a four-carbon molecule of oxaloacetic acid and moves through a series of enzyme-mediated steps. This process produces hydrogen atoms and carbon dioxide. As hydrogen is generated, it combines with NAD^+ or FAD for transfer to the electron transport system. In the citric acid cycle, each of the two pyruvate molecules formed in the cytoplasm from one molecule of glucose yields another molecule of ATP along with two molecules of carbon dioxide and eight electrons that that end up in three molecules of NADH + H^+ and one of $FADH_2$. Besides pyruvate from the glycolysis of glucose, products of amino acid and fatty acid degradation enter the citric acid cycle and contribute to the generation of ATP.

Oxidative metabolism, which supplies 90% of the body's energy needs, takes place in the electron transport chain in the mitochondria. The electron transport chain oxidizes NADH + H^+ and $FADH_2$ and donates the electrons to oxygen, which is reduced to water. Energy from reduction of oxygen is used for phosphorylation of ADP to ATP. Because the formation of ATP involves the addition of a high-energy phosphate bond to ADP, the process is sometimes called *oxidative phosphorylation.*

Among the members of the electron transport chain are several iron-containing molecules called *cytochromes.* Each cytochrome is a protein that contains a heme structure similar to that of hemoglobin. The last cytochrome complex is cytochrome oxidase, which passes electrons from cytochrome c to oxygen. Cytochrome oxidase has a lower binding affinity for oxygen than myoglobin (the intracellular heme-containing oxygen carrier) or hemoglobin (the heme-containing oxygen transporter in erythrocytes in the blood). Thus, oxygen is pulled from erythrocytes to myoglobin and from myoglobin to cytochrome oxidase, where it is reduced to H_2O. Although iron-deficiency anemia (discussed in Chapter 14) is characterized by decreased levels of hemoglobin, the iron-containing cytochromes in the electron transport chain in tissues such as skeletal muscle are affected as well. Thus, the fatigue that develops in iron-deficiency anemia results, in part, from impaired function of the electron transport chain.

Understanding • Cell Metabolism

Cell metabolism is the process that converts dietary fuels from carbohydrates, proteins, and fats into adenosine triphosphate (ATP), which provides for the energy needs of the cell. ATP is formed through three major pathways: (1) the glycolytic pathway, (2) the citric acid cycle, and (3) the electron transport chain. In fuel metabolism, which is an oxidation–reduction reaction, the fuel donates electrons and is oxidized, and the coenzymes nicotinamide adenine dinucleotide (NAD) and flavin adenine dinucleotide (FAD) accept electrons and are reduced.

❶ Glycolytic Pathway

Glycolysis, which occurs in the cytoplasm of the cell, involves the splitting of the six-carbon glucose molecule into two three-carbon molecules of pyruvic acid. Because the reaction that splits glucose requires two molecules of ATP, there is a net gain of only two molecules of ATP from each molecule of glucose that is metabolized. The process is anaerobic and does not require oxygen (O_2) or produce carbon dioxide (CO_2). When O_2 is present, pyruvic acid moves into the mitochondria, where it enters the aerobic citric acid cycle. Under anaerobic conditions, pyruvate is converted to lactic acid, allowing glycolysis to continue as a means of supplying cells with ATP when O_2 is lacking.

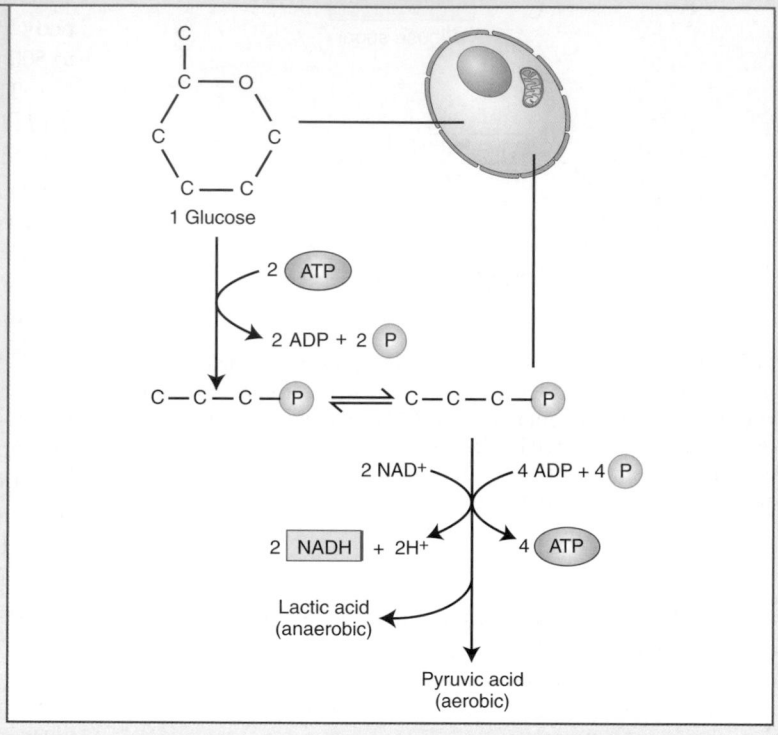

❷ Citric Acid Cycle

Under aerobic conditions, both of the pyruvic acid molecules formed by the glycolytic pathway enter the mitochondria, where each combines with acetyl-coenzyme to form acetyl-coenzyme A (acetyl-CoA). The formation of acetyl-CoA begins the reactions that occur in the citric acid cycle. Some reactions release CO_2 and some transfer electrons from the hydrogen atom to NADH or FADH. In addition to pyruvic acid from the glycolysis of glucose, fatty acid and amino acid breakdown products can also enter the citric acid cycle. Fatty acids, which are the major source of fuel in the body, are oxidized by a process called *beta oxidation* to acetyl-CoA for entry into the citric acid cycle.

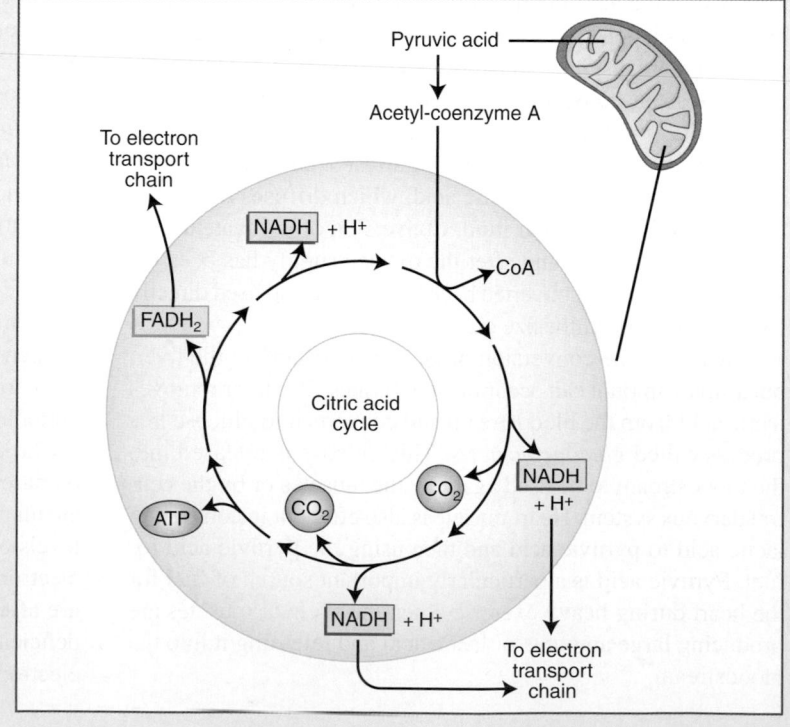

❸ Electron Transport Chain

At the completion of the citric acid cycle, each glucose molecule has yielded only four new molecules of ATP (two from glycolysis and two from the citric acid cycle). In fact, the principal function of these earlier stages is to make the electrons (e^-) from glucose and other food substrates available for oxidation. Oxidation of the electrons carried by NADH and $FADH_2$ is accomplished through a series of enzymatically catalyzed reactions in the mitochondrial electron transport chain. During these reactions, protons (H^+) combine with O_2 to form water (H_2O), and large amounts of energy are released and used to add a high-energy phosphate bond to adenosine diphosphate (ADP), converting it to ATP. There is a net yield of 36 molecules of ATP from 1 molecule of glucose (2 from glycolysis, 2 from the citric acid cycle, and 32 from the electron transport chain). In general, the net amount of ATP formed from each gram of protein that is metabolized is less than for glucose, whereas that obtained from fat is greater (*e.g.*, each 16-carbon fatty acid molecule yields about 129 molecules of ATP).

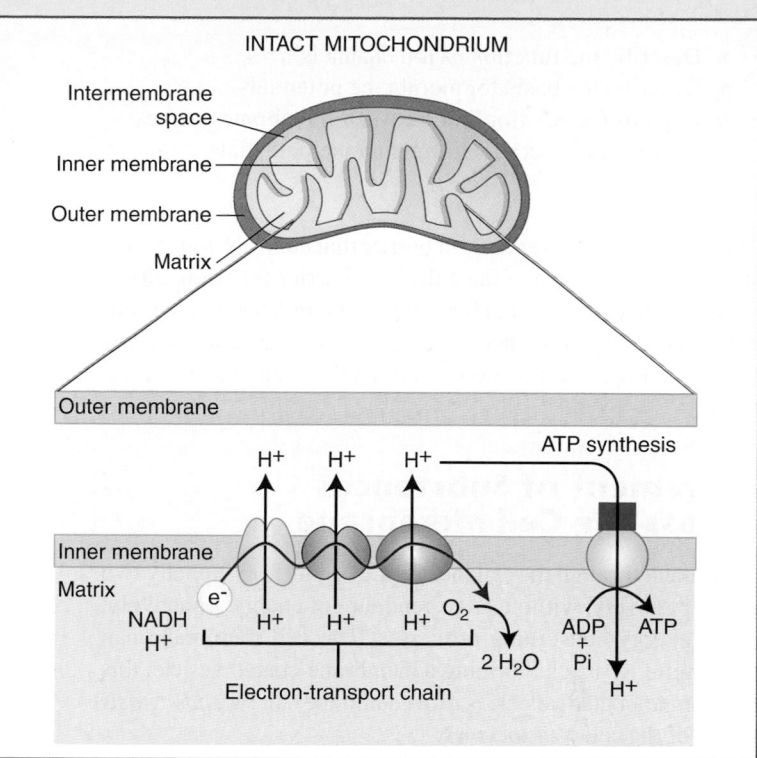

IN SUMMARY, cells communicate with each other by chemical messenger systems. In some tissues, chemical messengers move from cell to cell through gap junctions without entering the extracellular fluid. Other types of chemical messengers bind to receptors on or near the cell surface. Three classes of cell surface receptor proteins are known: G-protein–linked, ion-channel–linked, and enzyme-linked. G-protein–linked receptors rely on a class of molecules called *G proteins* that function as an on–off switch to convert external signals (first messengers) into internal signals (second messengers). Ion-channel–linked signaling is mediated by neurotransmitters that transiently open or close ion channels formed by integral proteins in the cell membrane. Enzyme-linked receptors interact with certain peptide hormones, such as insulin and growth factors, and directly initiate the activity of the intracellular protein–tyrosine kinase enzyme.

The life cycle of a cell is called the *cell cycle*. It is usually divided into five phases: G_0, or the resting phase; G_1, during which the cell begins to prepare for division through DNA and protein synthesis; the S or synthetic phase, during which DNA replication occurs; G_2, which is the premitotic phase and is similar to G_1 regarding RNA and protein synthesis; and the M phase, during which cell division occurs. Cell division, or mitosis, is the process during which a parent cell divides into two daughter cells, each receiving an identical pair of chromosomes. The process of mitosis is dynamic and continuous and is divided into four stages: prophase, metaphase, anaphase, and telophase.

Metabolism is the process whereby carbohydrates, fats, and proteins from the foods we eat are broken down and subsequently converted into the energy needed for cell function. Energy is converted to ATP, the energy currency of the cell. Two sites of energy conversion are present in cells: the anaerobic glycolytic pathway in the cytoplasm, and the aerobic pathways in the mitochondria. The most efficient of these pathways is the aerobic citric acid cycle and electron transport chain in the mitochondria. This pathway requires oxygen and produces carbon dioxide and water as end products. The glycolytic pathway in the cytoplasm involves the breakdown of glucose to form ATP. This pathway can function without oxygen by producing lactic acid. ■

MOVEMENT ACROSS THE CELL MEMBRANE AND MEMBRANE POTENTIALS

After completing this section of the chapter, you should be able to meet the following objectives:

■ Discuss the mechanisms of membrane transport associated with diffusion, osmosis, endocytosis, and exocytosis and compare them with active transport mechanisms.

(objectives continue)

- Describe the function of ion channels.
- Describe the basis for membrane potentials.
- Explain the relationship between membrane permeability and generation of membrane potentials.

The cell membrane serves as a barrier that controls which substances enter and leave the cell. This barrier function allows materials that are essential for cellular function to enter the cell, while excluding those that are harmful. It is responsible for differences in the composition of intracellular and extracellular fluids.

Movement of Substances Across the Cell Membrane

Movement through the cell membrane occurs in essentially two ways: passively, without an expenditure of energy, or actively, using energy-consuming processes. The cell membrane can also engulf a particle, forming a membrane-coated vesicle; this membrane-coated vesicle is moved into the cell by *endocytosis* or out of the cell by *exocytosis.*

Passive Movement

Passive movement of particles or ions across the cell membrane is directly influenced by chemical or electrical gradients and does not require an expenditure of energy. A difference in the number of particles on either side of the membrane creates a chemical gradient and a difference in charged particle or ions creates an electrical gradient. Chemical and electrical gradients are often linked and are called *electrochemical gradients.*

Diffusion. Diffusion refers to the process by which molecules and other particles in a solution become widely dispersed and reach a uniform concentration because of energy created by their spontaneous kinetic movements (Fig. 4-13A). Electrolytes and other substances move from an area of higher to an area of lower concentration. With ions, diffusion is affected by energy supplied by their electrical charge. Lipid-soluble molecules such as oxygen, carbon dioxide, alcohol, and fatty acids become dissolved in the lipid matrix of the cell membrane and diffuse through the membrane in the same manner that diffusion occurs in water. Other substances diffuse through minute pores of the cell membrane. The rate of movement depends on how many particles are available for diffusion and the velocity of the kinetic movement of the particles. The number of openings in the cell membrane through which the particles can move also determines transfer rates. Temperature changes the motion of the particles; the greater the temperature, the greater is the thermal motion of the molecules. Thus, diffusion increases in proportion to increased temperature.

Osmosis. Most cell membranes are semipermeable in that they are permeable to water but not to all solute particles. Water

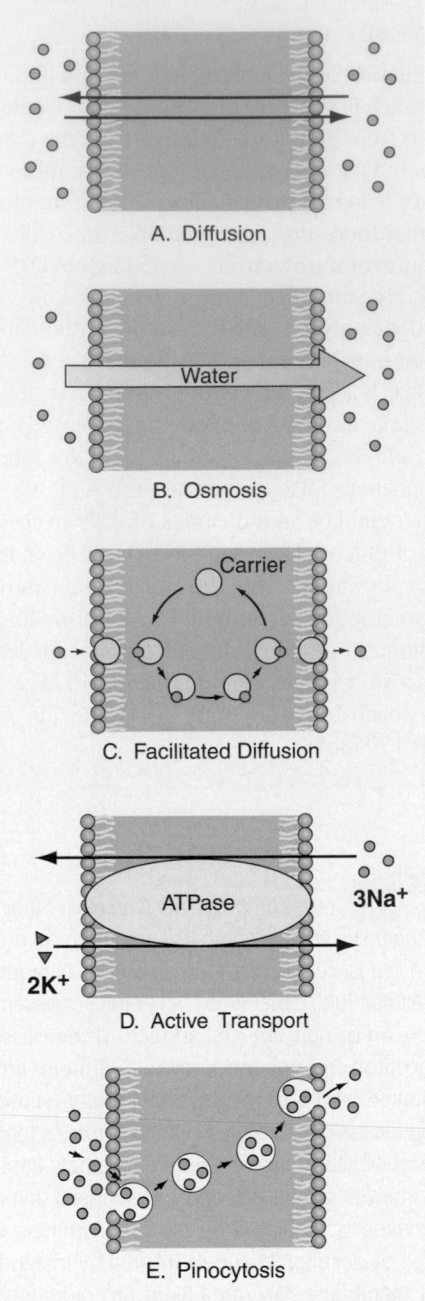

FIGURE 4-13 • Mechanisms of membrane transport. **(A)** In diffusion, particles move freely to become equally distributed across the membrane. **(B)** In osmosis, osmotically active particles regulate the flow of water. **(C)** Facilitated diffusion uses a carrier system. **(D)** In active transport, selected molecules are transported across the membrane using the energy-driven (Na^+/K^+ ATPase) pump. **(E)** In pinocytosis, the membrane forms a vesicle that engulfs the particle and transports it across the membrane, where it is released.

moves through water channels (aquaporins) in a semipermeable membrane along a concentration gradient, moving from an area of higher to one of lower concentration (see Fig. 4-13B). This process is called *osmosis,* and the pressure that water generates as it moves through the membrane is called *osmotic pressure.*

Osmosis is regulated by the concentration of nondiffusible particles on either side of a semipermeable membrane. When there is a difference in the concentration of particles, water moves from the side with the lower concentration of particles and higher concentration of water to the side with the higher concentration of particles and lower concentration of water. The movement of water continues until the concentration of particles on both sides of the membrane is equally diluted or until the hydrostatic (osmotic) pressure created by the movement of water opposes its flow.

Facilitated Diffusion. Facilitated diffusion occurs through a transport protein that is not linked to metabolic energy (see Fig. 4-13C). Some substances, such as glucose, cannot pass unassisted through the cell membrane because they are not lipid soluble or are too large to pass through the membrane's pores. These substances combine with special transport proteins at the membrane's outer surface, are carried across the membrane attached to the transporter, and then released on the inside of the membrane. In facilitated diffusion, a substance can move only from an area of higher concentration to one of lower concentration. The rate at which a substance moves across the membrane because of facilitated diffusion depends on the difference in concentration between the two sides of the membrane. Also important are the availability of transport proteins and the rapidity with which they can bind and release the substance being transported. It is thought that insulin, which facilitates the movement of glucose into cells, acts by increasing the availability of glucose transporters in the cell membrane (see Chapter 42).

Active Transport and Cotransport

Active transport mechanisms involve the expenditure of energy. The process of diffusion describes particle movement from an area of higher concentration to one of lower concentration, resulting in an equal distribution across the cell membrane. Sometimes, however, different concentrations of a substance are needed in the intracellular and extracellular fluids. For example, to function, a cell requires a much higher intracellular concentration of potassium ions than is present in the extracellular fluid, while maintaining a much lower intracellular concentration of sodium ions than the extracellular fluid. In these situations, energy is required to pump the ions "uphill" or against their concentration gradient. When cells use energy to move ions against an electrical or chemical gradient, the process is called *active transport.*

The active transport system studied in the greatest detail is the sodium-potassium (Na^+/K^+)-ATPase pump (see Fig. 4-13D). This pump moves sodium from inside the cell to the extracellular region, where its concentration is approximately 14 times greater than inside; the pump also returns potassium to the inside, where its concentration is approximately 35 times greater than it is outside the cell. Energy used to pump sodium out of the cell and potassium into the cell is obtained by splitting and releasing energy from the high-energy phosphate bond in ATP by the enzyme ATPase. Were it not for the activity of the Na^+/K^+-ATPase pump, the osmotically active sodium particles would accumulate in the cell, causing cellular swelling because of an accompanying influx of water (see Chapter 5).

Two types of active transport systems exist: primary active transport and secondary active transport. In *primary active transport,* the source of energy (*e.g.,* ATP) is used directly in the transport of a substance. *Secondary active transport* mechanisms harness the energy derived from the primary active transport of one substance, usually sodium, for the cotransport of a second substance. For example, when sodium ions are actively transported out of a cell by primary active transport, a large concentration gradient develops (*i.e.,* high concentration on the outside and low on the inside). This concentration gradient represents a large storehouse of energy because sodium ions are always attempting to diffuse into the cell. Similar to facilitated diffusion, secondary transport mechanisms use membrane transport proteins. These proteins have two binding sites, one for sodium and the other for the substance undergoing secondary transport. Secondary transport systems are classified into two groups: *cotransport* or *symport* systems, in which the sodium ion and the solute are transported in the same direction, and *countertransport* or *antiport* systems, in which the sodium ion and the solute are transported in the opposite direction (Fig. 4-14). An example of cotransport occurs in the

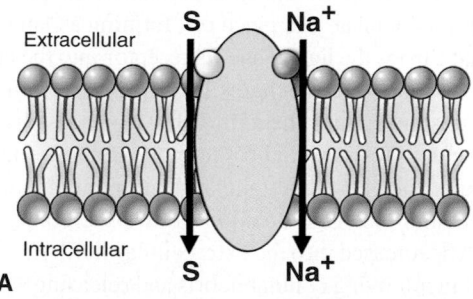

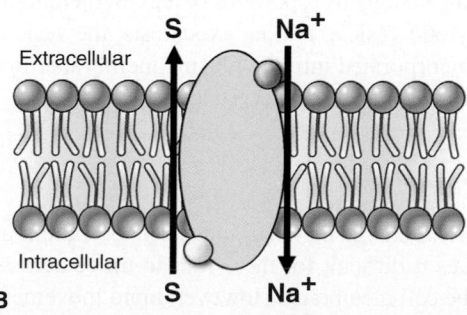

FIGURE 4-14 • Secondary active transport systems. **(A)** Symport or cotransport carries the transported solute (S) in the same direction as the sodium (Na^+) ion. **(B)** Antiport or countertransport carries the solute and Na^+ in the opposite direction.

intestine, where the absorption of glucose and amino acids is coupled with sodium transport.

Endocytosis and Exocytosis

Endocytosis is the process by which cells engulf materials from their surroundings. It includes pinocytosis and phagocytosis. *Pinocytosis* involves the ingestion of small solid or fluid particles. The particles are engulfed into small, membrane-surrounded vesicles for movement into the cytoplasm. The process of pinocytosis is important in the transport of proteins and strong solutions of electrolytes (see Fig. 4-13E).

Phagocytosis literally means "cell eating" and can be compared with pinocytosis, which means "cell drinking." It involves the engulfment and subsequent killing or degradation of microorganisms or other particulate matter. During phagocytosis, a particle contacts the cell surface and is surrounded on all sides by the cell membrane, forming a phagocytic vesicle or phagosome. Once formed, the phagosome breaks away from the cell membrane and moves into the cytoplasm, where it eventually fuses with a lysosome, allowing the ingested material to be degraded by lysosomal enzymes. Certain cells, such as macrophages and polymorphonuclear leukocytes (neutrophils), are adept at engulfing and disposing of invading organisms, damaged cells, and unneeded extracellular constituents.

Receptor-mediated endocytosis involves the binding of substances such as low-density lipoproteins to a receptor on the cell surface. Binding of a ligand (*i.e.,* a substance with a high affinity for a receptor) to its receptor normally causes widely distributed receptors to accumulate in clathrin-coated pits. An aggregation of special proteins on the cytoplasmic side of the pit causes the coated pit to invaginate and pinch off, forming a clathrin-coated vesicle that carries the ligand and its receptor into the cell.

Exocytosis is the mechanism for the secretion of intracellular substances into the extracellular spaces. It is the reverse of endocytosis in that a secretory granule fuses to the inner side of the cell membrane and an opening is created in the cell membrane. This opening allows the contents of the granule to be released into the extracellular fluid. Exocytosis is important in removing cellular debris and releasing substances, such as hormones, synthesized in the cell.

During endocytosis, portions of the cell membrane become an endocytotic vesicle. During exocytosis, the vesicular membrane is incorporated into the plasma membrane. In this way, cell membranes can be conserved and reused.

Ion Channels

The electrical charge on small ions such as sodium and potassium makes it difficult for these ions to move across the lipid layer of the cell membrane. However, rapid movement of these ions is required for many types of cell functions, such as nerve activity. This is accomplished by facilitated diffusion through selective ion channels. Ion channels are integral proteins that span the width of the cell membrane and are normally composed of several polypeptides or protein subunits that form a gating system. Specific stimuli cause the protein subunits to undergo conformational changes to form an open channel or gate through which the ions can move (Fig. 4-15). In this way, ions do not need to cross the lipid-soluble portion of the membrane but can remain in the aqueous solution that fills the ion channel. Ion channels are highly selective; some channels allow only for passage of sodium ions, and others are selective for potassium, calcium, or chloride ions. Specific interactions between the ions and the sides of the channel can produce an extremely rapid rate of ion movement. For example, ion channels can become negatively charged, promoting the rapid movement of positively charged ions.

The plasma membrane contains two basic groups of ion channels: leakage channels and gated channels. Leakage channels are open even in the unstimulated state, whereas gated channels open and close in response to specific stimuli. Three main types of gated channels are present in the plasma membrane: *voltage-gated channels,* which have electrically operated channels that open when the membrane potential changes beyond a certain point; *ligand-gated channels,* which are chemically operated and respond to specific receptor-bound ligands, such as the neurotransmitter acetylcholine; and *mechanically gated channels,* which open or close in response to such mechanical stimulations as vibrations, tissue stretching, or pressure (see Fig. 4-15).

Membrane Potentials

Electrical potentials exist across the membranes of most cells in the body. Because these potentials occur at the level of the cell membrane, they are called *membrane potentials.* In excitable tissues, such as nerve or muscle cells, changes in the membrane potential are necessary for generation and conduction of nerve impulses and muscle contraction. In other types of cells, such as glandular cells, changes in the membrane potential contribute to hormone secretion and other functions.

Electrical potentials, measured in volts (V), describe the ability of separated electrical charges of opposite polarity (+ and −) to do work. The potential difference is the difference between the separated charges. The terms *potential difference* and *voltage* are synonymous. Voltage is always measured with respect to two points in a system. For example, the voltage in a car battery (6- or 12-V) is the potential difference between the two battery terminals. Because the total amount of charge that can be separated by a biologic membrane is small, the potential differences are small and are measured in millivolts (mV), or 1/1000 of a volt. Potential differences across the cell membrane can be measured by inserting a very fine electrode into the cell and another into the extracellular fluid surrounding the cell and connecting the two electrodes to a voltmeter. The movement of charge between two points is called *current.* It occurs when a potential difference has been established and a connection is made such that the charged particles can move between the two points.

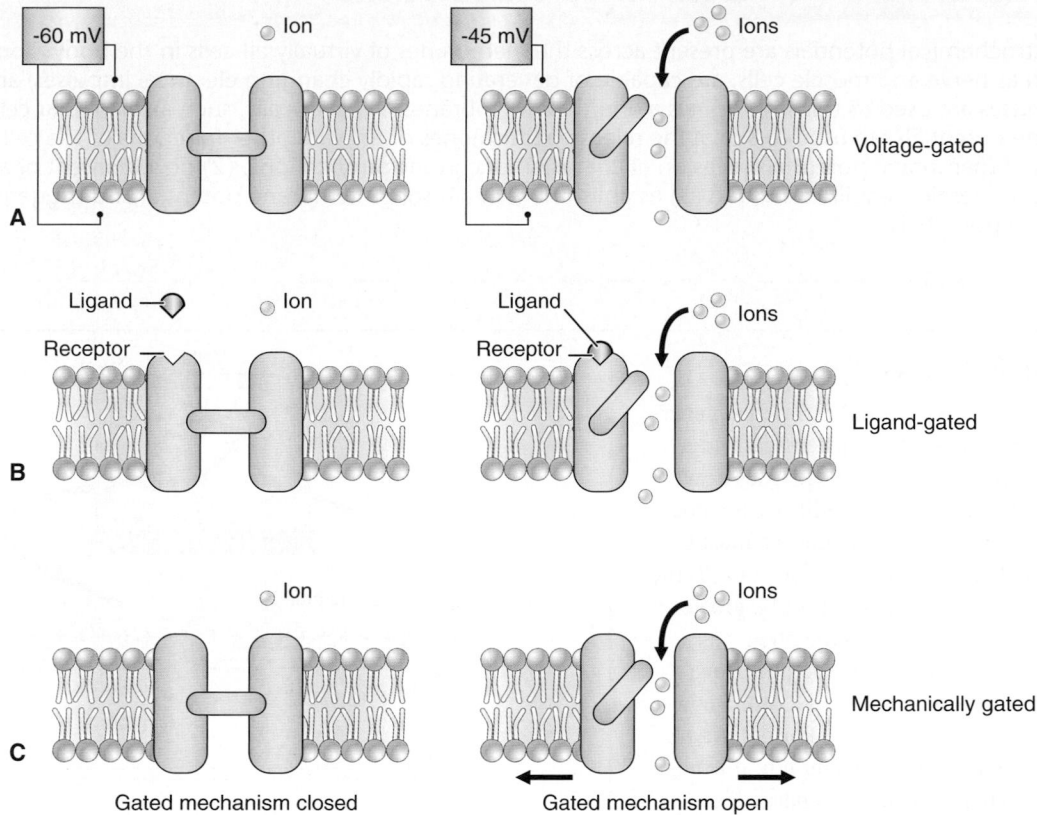

FIGURE 4-15 • Gated ion channels that open in response to a specific stimuli. (**A**) Voltage-gated channels are controlled by a change in membrane potential. (**B**) Ligand-gated channels are controlled by binding of a ligand to a receptor. (**C**) Mechanically gated channels, which are controlled by mechanical stimuli such as stretching, often have links that connect to the cytoskeleton.

Extracellular and intracellular fluids are electrolyte solutions containing approximately 150 to 160 mmol/L of positively charged ions and an equal concentration of negatively charged ions. These current-carrying ions are responsible for generating and conducting membrane potentials. Usually, a small excess of charged ions exists at the outer surface of the cell membrane. This is represented as positive charges on the outside of the membrane and is balanced by an equal number of negative charges on the inside of the membrane. Because of the extreme thinness of the cell membrane, the accumulation of these ions at the surfaces of the membrane contributes to the establishment of a *resting membrane potential.*

A *diffusion potential* describes the voltage generated by ions that diffuse across the cell membrane. Two conditions are necessary for a membrane potential to occur by diffusion: the membrane must be selectively permeable, allowing a single type of ion to diffuse through membrane pores, and the concentration of the diffusible ion must be greater on one side of the membrane than on the other. An *equilibrium potential* is one in which no net movement of ions occurs because the diffusion and electrical forces are exactly balanced.

When using this formula, it is generally assumed that the potential in the extracellular fluid outside the membrane remains at zero potential and the Nernst potential is inside the membrane. The sign of the potential is negative (–) if a positive ion diffuses from the inside of the membrane to the outside and it is positive (+) if a positively charged ion diffuses from the outside to the inside of the membrane.

In the resting or unexcited state, when the membrane is highly permeable to potassium, the concentration of potassium ions inside the cell is approximately 35 times greater than outside. Because of the large concentration gradient existing across the cell membrane, potassium ions tend to diffuse outward. As they do so, they carry their positive charges with them, causing the inside to become negative in relation to the outside. This new potential difference repels further outward movement of the positively charged potassium ion. The membrane is said to be *polarized* during this stage because of the negative membrane potential that is present. The same phenomenon occurs during an *action potential* (discussed in Chapter 49), when the membrane becomes highly permeable to sodium, allowing the positively charged ion to diffuse to the interior of the cell. The inflowing sodium ions produce a reversal in the normal resting membrane potential to one of the opposite polarity (positive on the inside and negative on the outside). This is called *depolarization.*

(text continues on page 80)

Understanding • Membrane Potentials

Electrochemical potentials are present across the membranes of virtually all cells in the body. Some cells, such as nerve and muscle cells, are capable of generating rapidly changing electrical impulses, and these impulses are used to transmit signals along their membranes. In other cells, such as glandular cells, membrane potentials are used to signal the release of hormones or activate other functions of the cell. Generation of membrane potentials relies on (1) diffusion of current-carrying ions, (2) development of an electrochemical equilibrium, and (3) establishment of a resting membrane potential and triggering of action potentials.

❶ Diffusion Potentials

A diffusion potential is a potential difference generated across a membrane when a current-carrying ion, such as the potassium (K^+) ion, diffuses down its concentration gradient. Two conditions are necessary for this to occur: (1) the membrane must be selectively permeable to a particular ion, and (2) the concentration of the diffusible ion must be greater on one side of the membrane than the other.

The magnitude of the diffusion potential, measured in millivolts, depends on the size of the concentration gradient. The sign (+ or −) or polarity of the potential depends on the diffusing ion. It is negative on the inside when a positively charged ion such as K^+ diffuses from the inside to the outside of the membrane, carrying its charge with it.

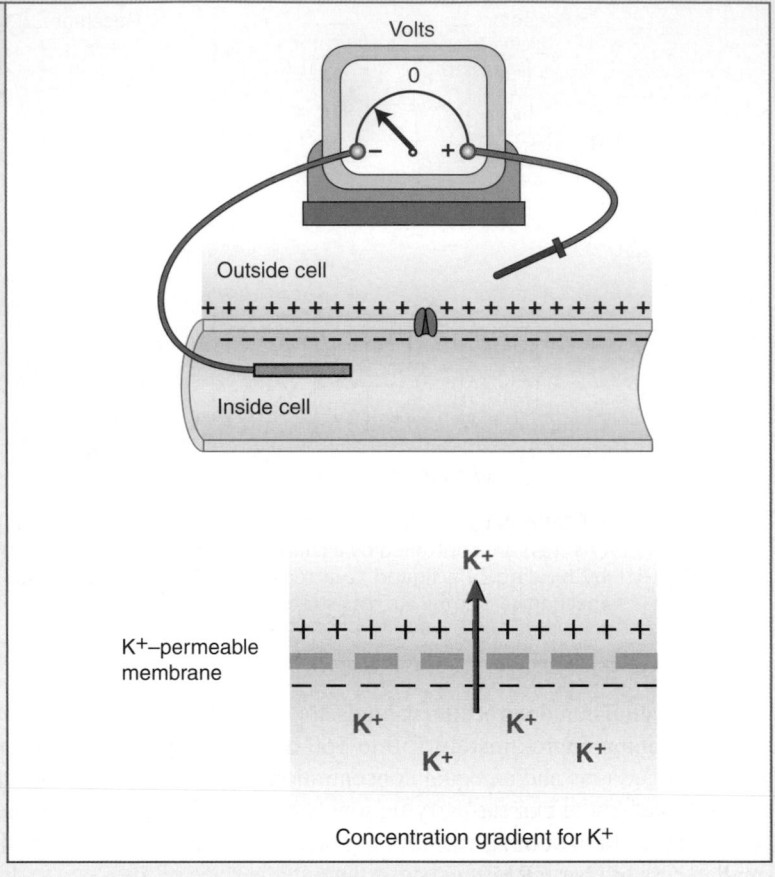

Concentration gradient for K^+

❷ Equilibrium Potentials

An equilibrium potential is the membrane potential that exactly balances and opposes the net diffusion of an ion down its concentration gradient. As a cation diffuses down its concentration gradient, it carries its positive charge across the membrane, thereby generating an electrical force that will eventually retard and stop its diffusion. An electrochemical equilibrium is one in which the *chemical forces driving* diffusion and the *repelling electrical forces* are exactly balanced so that no further diffusion occurs. The equilibrium potential (EMF, electromotive force) can be calculated by inserting the inside and outside ion concentrations into the Nernst equation.

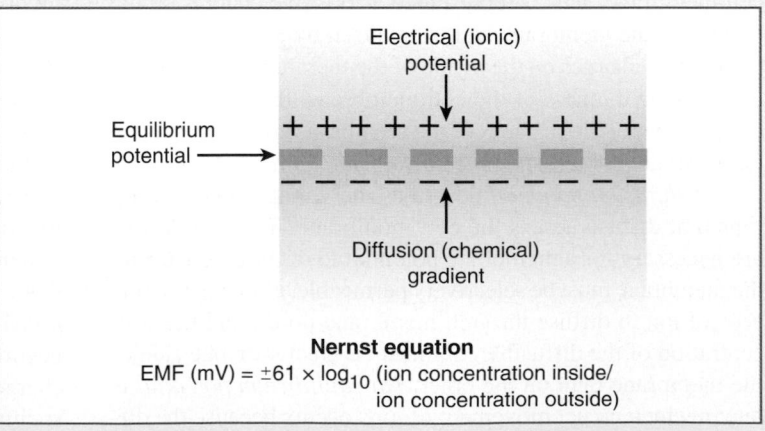

Nernst equation
EMF (mV) = $\pm 61 \times \log_{10}$ (ion concentration inside/ion concentration outside)

❸ Resting Membrane Potential (RMP)

The RMP, which is necessary for electrical excitability, is present when the cell is not transmitting impulses. Because the resting membrane is permeable to K⁺, it is essentially a K⁺ equilibrium potential. This can be explained in terms of the large K⁺ concentration gradient (*e.g.,* 140 mEq/L inside and 4 mEq/L outside), which causes the positively charged K⁺ to diffuse outward, leaving the nondiffusible, negatively charged intracellular anions (A⁻) behind. This causes the membrane to become polarized, with negative charges aligned along the inside and positive charges along the outside. The Na⁺/K⁺ membrane pump, which removes three Na⁺ from inside while returning only two K⁺ to the inside, contributes to the maintenance of the RMP.

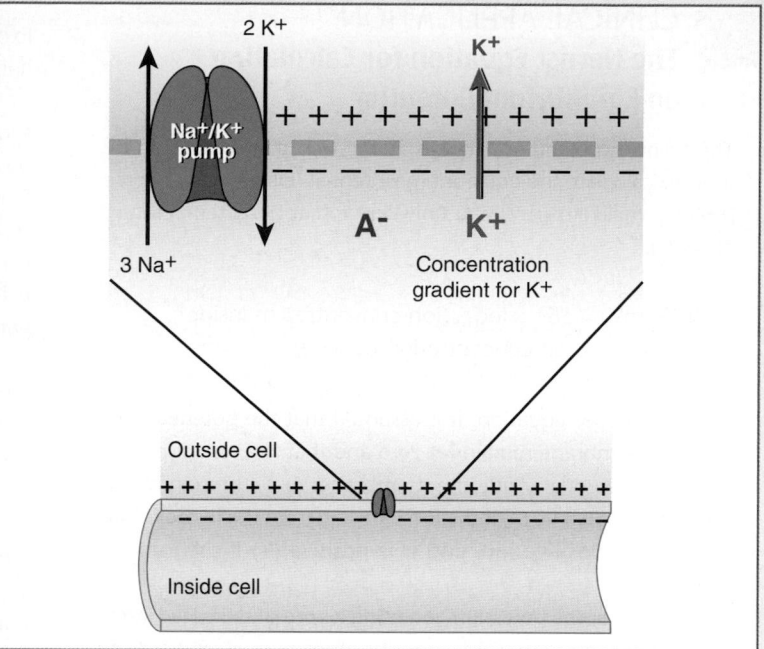

❹ Action Potentials

Action potentials involve rapid changes in the membrane potential. Each action potential begins with a sudden change from the negative RMP to a positive threshold potential, causing an opening of the membrane channels for Na⁺ (or other ions of the action potential). Opening of the Na⁺ channels allows large amounts of the positively charged Na⁺ ions to diffuse to the interior of the cell, causing the membrane potential to undergo depolarization or a rapid change to positive on the inside and negative on the outside. This is rapidly followed by closing of Na⁺ channels and opening of the K⁺ channels, which leads to a rapid efflux of K⁺ from the cell and reestablishment of the RMP.

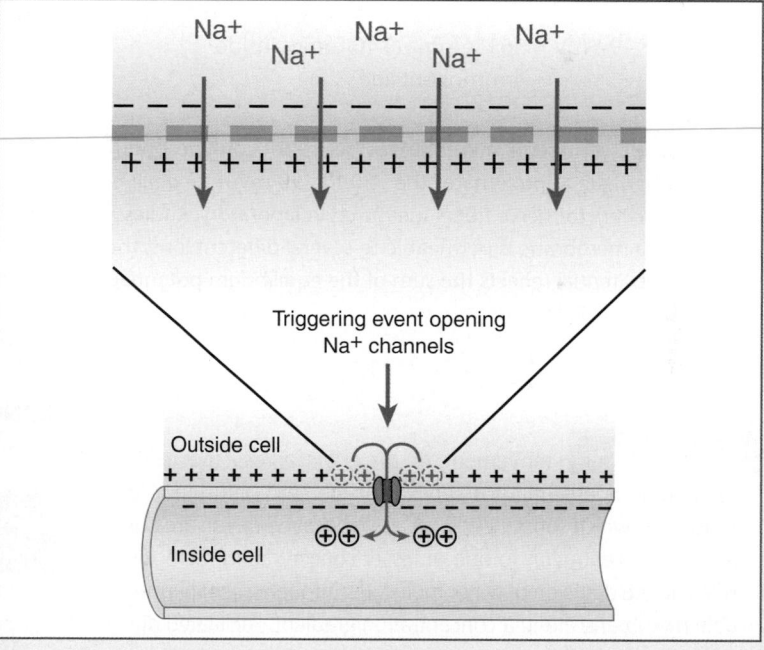

CLINICAL APPLICATION
The Nernst Equation for Calculating an Equilibrium Potential

The following equation, known as the *Nernst equation,* can be used to calculate the equilibrium potential (electromotive force [EMF] in millivolts [mV] of a univalent ion at body temperature of 37°C).

$$EMF\ (mV) = \pm 61 \times \log_{10}\ (\text{ion concentration inside/ion concentration outside})$$

When using the equation, it is assumed that the potential outside the membrane remains at zero and that the Nernst potential is the potential inside the membrane. Also, the sign of the potential is negative (–) if the ion diffusing from the inside to the outside is a positive ion, and it is positive (+) if the ion is a negative.

The EMF for the potassium ion using a normal estimated intracellular concentration of 140 mmol/L and a normal extracellular concentration of 4 mmol/L is –94 mV:

$$-94\ mV = \pm 61 \times \log_{10}\ (140\ mmol\ inside/\ 4\ mmol\ outside)$$

This value assumes the membrane is permeable only to potassium. This value approximates the –70 to –90 mV *resting membrane potential* for nerve fibers measured in laboratory studies.

When a membrane is permeable to several different ions, the diffusion potential reflects the sum of the equilibrium potentials for each of the ions.

Exocytosis involves the removal of large particles from the cell and is essentially the reverse of endocytosis.

Ion channels are integral transmembrane proteins that span the width of the cell membrane and are normally composed of polypeptide or protein subunits that form a gating system. Many ions can diffuse through the cell membrane only if conformational changes occur in the membrane proteins that comprise the ion channel. Two basic groups of ion channels exist: leakage channels and ligand-, voltage-, and mechanically gated channels.

Electrochemical potentials exist across the membranes of most cells in the body. The resting membrane potential results from the selective permeability of the cell membrane to potassium; the presence of nondiffusible anions inside the cell membrane; and the activity of the Na^+/K^+-ATPase membrane pump, which extrudes sodium ions from inside the membrane and returns potassium ions to the inside.

There are two main factors that contribute to the generation of membrane potentials: a difference in the concentration of ions inside and outside the membrane, and the permeability of the membrane. An equilibrium or diffusion potential is one in which no net movement of ions occurs because the diffusion and electrical forces are exactly balanced. The resting membrane potential (negative on the inside and positive on the outside) is essentially a potassium equilibrium potential that results from the selective permeability of the membrane to potassium and the large difference in potassium ion concentration that exists between the intracellular and extracellular compartments. During an action potential, the cell membrane becomes highly permeable to sodium, causing it to depolarize and reverse its polarity, becoming positive on the inside and negative on the outside. ■

CONCEPTS in action **ANIMATION**

IN SUMMARY, movement of materials across the cell's membrane is essential for survival of the cell. Diffusion is a process by which substances such as ions move from an area of greater concentration to one of lesser concentration. Osmosis refers to the diffusion of water molecules through a semipermeable membrane along a concentration gradient. Facilitated diffusion is a passive process, in which molecules that cannot normally pass through the cell's membrane do so with the assistance of a carrier molecule. Another type of transport, called *active transport,* requires the cell to expend energy in moving ions against a concentration gradient. Two types of active transport exist, primary and secondary, both of which require carrier proteins. The Na^+/K^+-ATPase pump is the best-known mechanism of active transport. Endocytosis is a process by which cells engulf materials from the surrounding medium. Small particles are ingested by a process called *pinocytosis* and larger particles by *phagocytosis.* Some particles require bonding with a ligand, and the process is called *receptor-mediated endocytosis.*

BODY TISSUES

After completing this section of the chapter, you should be able to meet the following objectives:

- Explain the process of cell differentiation in terms of development of organ systems in the embryo and the continued regeneration of tissues in postnatal life.
- Explain the function of stem cells.
- Describe the characteristics of the four different tissue types.
- Explain the function of intercellular adhesions and junctions.
- Characterize the composition and functions of the extracellular components of tissue.

In the preceding sections, we discussed the individual cell, its metabolic processes, and mechanisms of communication and replication. Although cells are similar, their structure and function vary according to the special needs of the body. For example, muscle cells perform different functions from skin cells or nerve cells. Groups of cells that are closely associated in structure and have common or similar functions are called *tissues.* Four categories of tissue exist: (1) epithelium, (2) connective (supportive) tissue, (3) muscle, and (4) nerve. These tissues do not exist in isolated units, but in association with each other and in variable proportions, forming different structures and organs of the body. This section provides a brief overview of the cells in each of these four tissue types, the structures that hold these cells together, and the extracellular matrix in which they live.

Cell Differentiation

After conception, the fertilized ovum undergoes a series of divisions, ultimately forming approximately 200 different cell types. The formation of different types of cells and the disposition of these cells into tissue types is called *cell differentiation,* a process controlled by a system that switches genes on and off. Embryonic cells must become different to develop into all of the various organ systems, and they must remain different after the signal that initiated cell diversification has disappeared. The process of cell differentiation is controlled by cell memory, which is maintained through regulatory proteins contained in the individual members of a particular cell type. Cell differentiation also involves the sequential activation of multiple genes and their protein products. This means that after differentiation has occurred, the tissue type does not revert to an earlier stage of differentiation. The process of cell differentiation normally moves forward, producing cells that are more specialized than their predecessors. Usually, highly differentiated cell types, such as skeletal muscle and nervous tissue, lose their ability to undergo cell division in postnatal life.

Although most cells differentiate into specialized cell types, many tissues contain a few *stem cells* that apparently are only partially differentiated. These stem cells are still capable of cell division and serve as a reserve source for specialized cells throughout the life of the organism. They are the major source of cells that make regeneration possible in some tissues. Stem cells have varying abilities to differentiate. Some tissues, such as skeletal muscle tissue, lack sufficient numbers of undifferentiated cells and have limited regenerative capacity. Stem cells of the hematopoietic (blood) system have the greatest potential for differentiation. These cells can potentially reconstitute the entire blood-producing and immune systems. They are the major ingredient in bone marrow transplants. Other stem cells, such as those that replenish the mucosal surface of the gastrointestinal tract, are less general but can still differentiate.

🔑 ORGANIZATION OF CELLS INTO TISSUES

- Cells with a similar embryonic origin or function are often organized into larger functional units called *tissues,* and these tissues in turn associate with other, dissimilar tissues to form the various organs of the body.

- Epithelial tissue forms sheets that cover the body's outer surface, lines internal surfaces, and forms glandular tissue. It is supported by a basement membrane, is avascular, and must receive nourishment from capillaries in supporting connective tissues.

- Connective tissue is the most abundant tissue of the body. It is found in a variety of forms, ranging from solid bone to blood cells that circulate in the vascular system.

- Muscle tissue contains actin and myosin filaments that allow it to contract and provide locomotion and movement of skeletal structures (skeletal muscle), pumping of blood through the heart (cardiac muscle), and contraction of blood vessels and visceral organs (smooth muscle).

- Nervous tissue, which consists of two cell types, nerve cells or neurons and glial or supporting cells, is distributed throughout the body, and serves as the body's communication system. The nervous system is divided anatomically into the central nervous system (CNS), which consists of the brain and spinal cord, and the peripheral nervous system (PNS), which is composed of nerve tissue outside the CNS.

Embryonic Origin of Tissue Types

All of the approximately 200 different types of body cells can be classified into four basic or primary tissue types: epithelial, connective, muscle, and nervous (Table 4-1). These basic tissue types are often described by their embryonic origin. The embryo is essentially a three-layered tubular structure (Fig. 4-16). The outer layer of the tube is called the *ectoderm;* the middle layer, the *mesoderm;* and the inner layer, the *endoderm.* All of the adult body tissues originate from these three cellular layers. Epithelium has its origin in all three embryonic layers, connective tissue and muscle develop mainly from the mesoderm, and nervous tissue develops from the ectoderm.

Epithelial Tissue

Epithelial tissue covers the body's outer surface and lines the internal closed cavities (including blood vessels) and body tubes that communicate with the exterior (gastrointestinal, res-

TABLE 4-1 Classification of Tissue Types

TISSUE TYPE	LOCATION
Epithelial Tissue	
Covering and lining of body surfaces	
Simple epithelium	
Squamous	Lining of blood vessels, body cavities, alveoli of lungs
Cuboidal	Collecting tubules of kidney; covering of ovaries
Columnar	Lining of intestine and gallbladder
Stratified epithelium	
Squamous keratinized	Skin
Squamous nonkeratinized	Mucous membranes of mouth, esophagus, and vagina
Cuboidal	Ducts of sweat glands
Columnar	Large ducts of salivary and mammary glands; also found in conjunctiva
Transitional	Bladder, ureters, renal pelvis
Pseudostratified	Tracheal and respiratory passages
Glandular	
Endocrine	Pituitary gland, thyroid gland, adrenal and other glands
Exocrine	Sweat glands and glands in gastrointestinal tract
Neuroepithelium	Olfactory mucosa, retina, tongue
Reproductive epithelium	Seminiferous tubules of testis; cortical portion of ovary
Connective Tissue	
Embryonic connective tissue	
Mesenchymal	Embryonic mesoderm
Mucous	Umbilical cord (Wharton jelly)
Adult connective tissue	
Loose or areolar	Subcutaneous areas
Dense regular	Tendons and ligaments
Dense irregular	Dermis of skin
Adipose	Fat pads, subcutaneous layers
Reticular	Framework of lymphoid organs, bone marrow, liver
Specialized connective tissue	
Bone	Long bones, flat bones
Cartilage	Tracheal rings, external ear, articular surfaces
Hematopoietic	Blood cells, myeloid tissue (bone marrow)
Muscle Tissue	
Skeletal	Skeletal muscles
Cardiac	Heart muscles
Smooth	Gastrointestinal tract, blood vessels, bronchi, bladder, and others
Nervous Tissue	
Neurons	Central and peripheral neurons and nerve fibers
Supporting cells	Glial and ependymal cells in central nervous system; Schwann and satellite cells in peripheral nervous system

piratory, and genitourinary tracts). Epithelium also forms the secretory portion of glands and their ducts, and the receptors for the special senses (taste, touch, hearing, and vision).

Origin and Characteristics

Epithelial tissue is derived from all three embryonic layers. Most epithelia of the skin, mouth, nose, and anus are derived from the ectoderm. Linings of the respiratory tract, gastrointestinal tract, and glands of the digestive system are of endodermal origin. The endothelial lining of blood vessels originates from the mesoderm. Many types of epithelial tissue retain the ability to differentiate and undergo rapid proliferation for replacing injured cells.

The cells that make up epithelium have three general characteristics: (1) they are characterized by three distinct surfaces: a free surface or apical surface, a lateral surface, and a basal surface; (2) they are closely apposed and joined by cell-to-cell adhesion molecules, which form specialized cell junctions; and (3) their basal surface is attached to an underlying basement membrane (Fig. 4-17). The characteristics and geometric arrangement of the cells in the epithelium determine their function. The free or apical surface is always directed toward the exterior surface or lumen of an enclosed cavity or tube, the lateral surface communicates with adjacent cells and is characterized by specialized attachment areas, and the basal surface rests on the basement membrane anchoring the cell to the surrounding connective tissue.

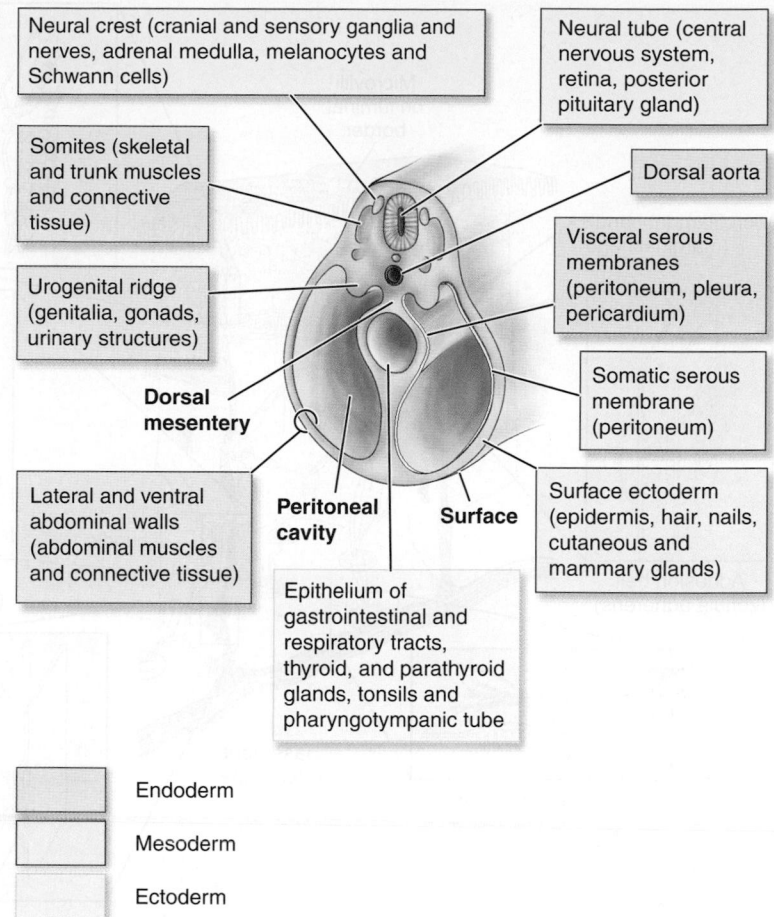

FIGURE 4-16 • Cross-section of human embryo illustrating the development of the somatic and visceral structures.

Epithelial tissue is avascular (*i.e.,* without blood vessels) and must therefore receive oxygen and nutrients from the capillaries of the connective tissue on which the epithelial tissue rests (see Fig. 4-17). To survive, epithelial tissue must be kept moist. Even the seemingly dry skin epithelium is kept moist by

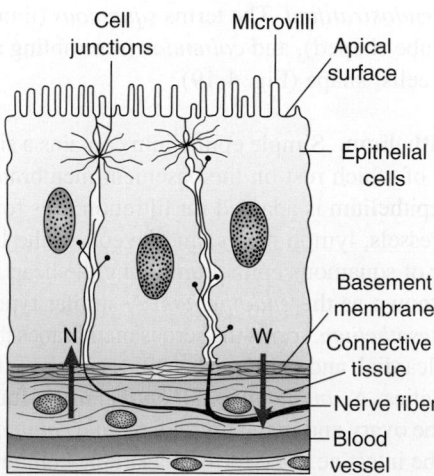

FIGURE 4-17 • Typical arrangement of epithelial cells in relation to underlying tissues and blood supply. Epithelial tissue has no blood supply of its own but relies on the blood vessels in the underlying connective tissue for nutrition (N) and elimination of wastes (W).

a nonvitalized, waterproof layer of superficial skin cells called *keratin,* which prevents evaporation of moisture from the deeper living cells.

Basement Membrane. Underneath all types of epithelial tissue is an extracellular matrix, called the *basement membrane.* A basement membrane consists of the basal lamina and an underlying reticular layer. The terms *basal lamina* and *basement membrane* are often used interchangeably. Epithelial cells have strong intracellular protein filaments (*i.e.,* cytoskeleton) that are important in transmitting mechanical stresses from one cell to another.

Cell Junctions and Cell-to-Cell Adhesions. Cells of epithelial tissue are tightly bound together by specialized junctions. These specialized junctions enable the cells to form barriers to the movement of water, solutes, and cells from one body compartment to the next. Three basic types of intercellular junctions are observed in epithelial tissues: continuous tight junctions, adhering junctions, and gap junctions (Fig. 4-18).

Continuous tight or *occluding junctions* (*i.e.,* zonula occludens), which are found only in epithelial tissue, seal the surface membranes of adjacent cells together. This type of intercellular junction prevents materials such as macromolecules in the intestinal contents from entering the intercellular space.

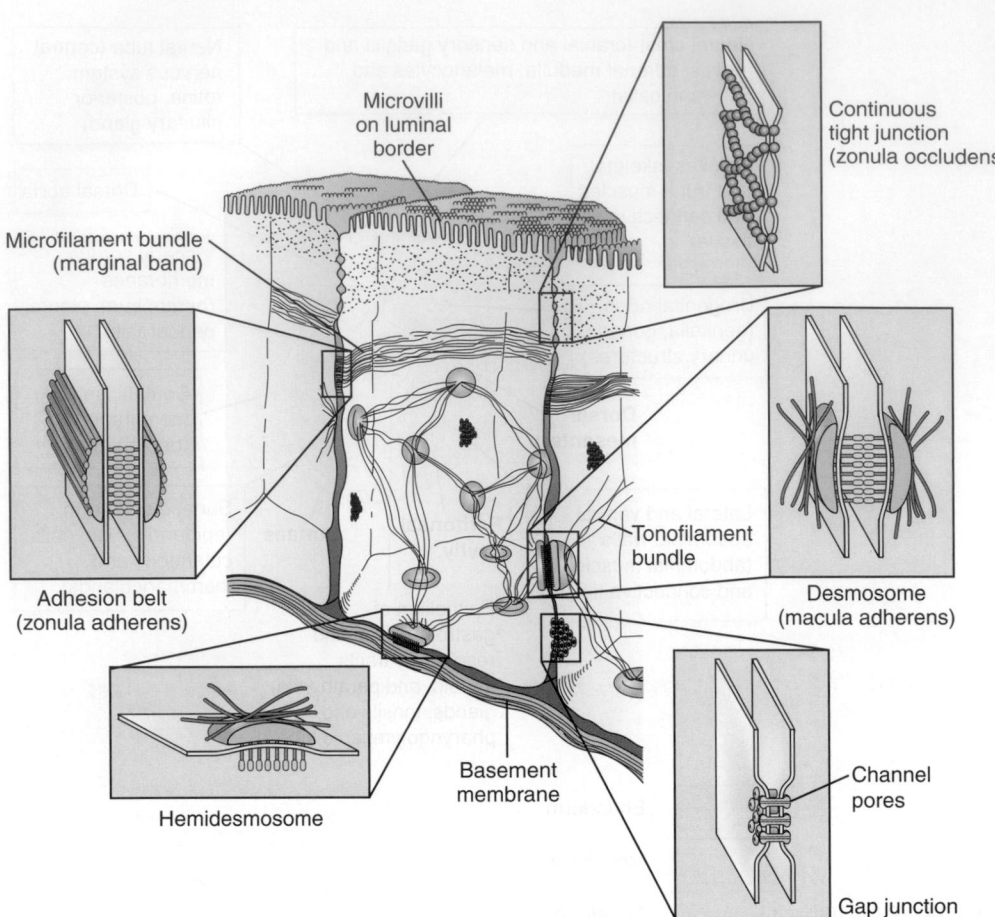

FIGURE 4-18 • Three types of intercellular junctions found in epithelial tissue: the continuous tight junction (zonula occludens); the adhering junction, which includes the adhesion belt (zonula adherens), desmosomes (macula adherens), and hemidesmosomes; and the gap junction.

Adhering junctions represent sites of strong adhesion between cells. The primary role of adhering junctions may be that of preventing cell separation. Adhering junctions are not restricted to epithelial tissue; they provide adherence between adjacent cardiac muscle cells as well. Adhering junctions are found as continuous, beltlike adhesive junctions (*i.e.,* zonula adherens) or scattered, spotlike adhesive junctions, called *desmosomes* (*i.e.,* macula adherens). A special feature of the adhesion belt junction is that it provides an anchoring site to the cell membrane for microfilaments. In epithelial desmosomes, bundles of keratin-containing intermediate filaments (*i.e.,* tonofilaments) are anchored to the junction on the cytoplasmic area of the cell membrane. A primary disease of desmosomes is pemphigus, which is caused by a buildup of antibodies to desmosome proteins. Affected persons have skin and mucous membrane blistering. *Hemidesmosomes,* which resemble a half-desmosome, are another type of junction. They are found at the base of epithelial cells and help attach the epithelial cell to the underlying connective tissue.

Gap or *nexus junctions* involve the close adherence of adjoining cell membranes with the formation of channels that link the cytoplasm of the two cells. Gap junctions are not unique to epithelial tissue; they play an essential role in many types of cell-to-cell communication. Because they are low-resistance channels, gap junctions are important in cell-to-cell conduction of electrical signals (*e.g.,* between cells in sheets of smooth muscle or between adjacent cardiac muscle cells, where they function as electrical synapses). These multiple communication channels also enable ions and small molecules to pass directly from one cell to another.

Types of Epithelium

Epithelial tissues are classified according to the shape of the cells and the number of layers that are present: *simple, stratified,* and *pseudostratified.* The terms *squamous* (thin and flat), *cuboidal* (cube shaped), and *columnar* (resembling a column) refer to the cells' shape (Fig. 4-19).

Simple Epithelium. Simple epithelium contains a single layer of cells, all of which rest on the basement membrane. Simple squamous epithelium is adapted for filtration; it is found lining the blood vessels, lymph nodes, and alveoli of the lungs. The single layer of squamous epithelium lining the heart and blood vessels is known as the *endothelium.* A similar type of layer, called the *mesothelium,* forms the serous membranes that line the pleural, pericardial, and peritoneal cavities and cover the organs of these cavities. A *simple cuboidal epithelium* is found on the surface of the ovary and in the thyroid. *Simple columnar epithelium* lines the intestine. One form of a simple columnar epithelium has hairlike projections called *cilia,* often with specialized mucus-secreting cells called *goblet cells.* This form of simple columnar epithelium lines the airways of the respiratory tract.

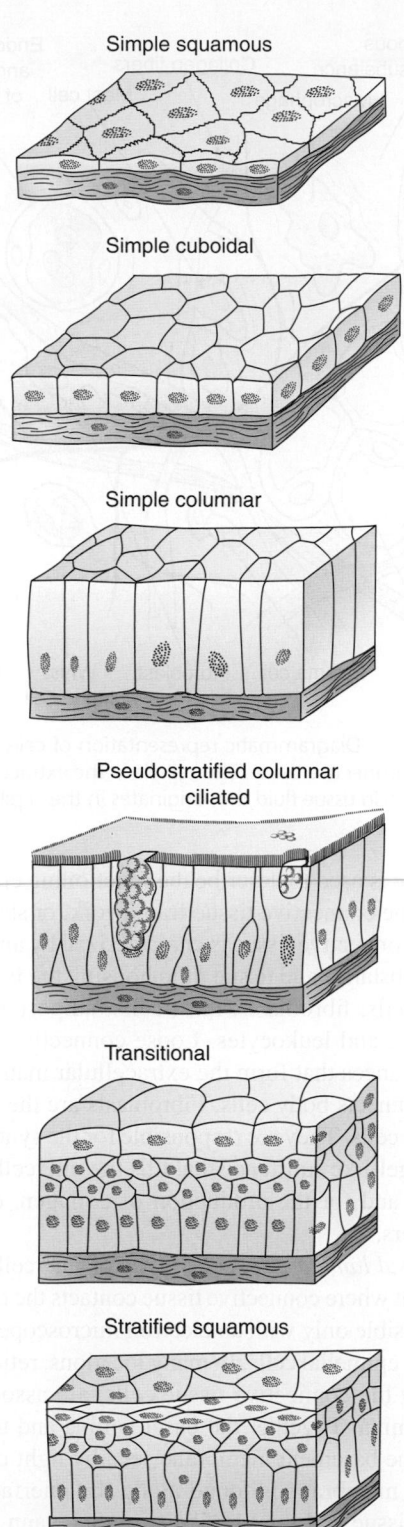

Simple squamous

Simple cuboidal

Simple columnar

Pseudostratified columnar ciliated

Transitional

Stratified squamous

FIGURE 4-19 • The various epithelial tissue types.

Stratified and Pseudostratified Epithelia. Stratified epithelium contains more than one layer of cells, with only the deepest layer resting on the basement membrane. It is designed to protect the body surface. *Stratified squamous keratinized* epithelium makes up the epidermis of the skin. *Keratin* is a tough,

fibrous protein found as filaments in the outer cells of skin. A stratified squamous keratinized epithelium is made up of many layers. The layers closest to the underlying tissues are cuboidal or columnar. The cells become more irregular and thinner as they move closer to the surface. Surface cells become totally filled with keratin and die, are sloughed off, and then replaced by the deeper cells. A stratified squamous nonkeratinized epithelium is found on moist surfaces such as the mouth and tongue. Stratified cuboidal and columnar epithelia are found in the ducts of salivary glands and the larger ducts of the mammary glands. In smokers, the normal columnar ciliated epithelial cells of the trachea and bronchi are often replaced with stratified squamous epithelium cells that are better able to withstand the irritating effects of cigarette smoke.

Pseudostratified epithelium is a type of epithelium in which all of the cells are in contact with the underlying intercellular matrix, but some do not extend to the surface. A pseudostratified ciliated columnar epithelium with goblet cells forms the lining of most of the upper respiratory tract. All of the tall cells reaching the surface of this type of epithelium are either ciliated cells or mucus-producing goblet cells. The basal cells that do not reach the surface serve as stem cells for ciliated and goblet cells. *Transitional epithelium* is a stratified epithelium characterized by cells that can change shape and become thinner when the tissue is stretched. Such tissue can be stretched without pulling the superficial cells apart. Transitional epithelium is well adapted for the lining of organs that are constantly changing their volume, such as the urinary bladder.

Glandular Epithelium. Glandular epithelial tissue is formed by cells specialized to produce a fluid secretion. This process is usually accompanied by the intracellular synthesis of macromolecules. The chemical nature of these macromolecules is variable. The macromolecules typically are stored in the cells in small, membrane-bound vesicles called *secretory granules.* For example, glandular epithelia can synthesize, store, and secrete proteins (*e.g.,* insulin), lipids (*e.g.,* adrenocortical hormones, secretions of the sebaceous glands), and complexes of carbohydrates and proteins (*e.g.,* saliva). Less common are secretions that require minimal synthetic activity, such as those produced by the sweat glands.

All glandular cells arise from surface epithelia by means of cell proliferation and invasion of the underlying connective tissue, and all release their contents or secretions into the extracellular compartment. *Exocrine glands,* such as the sweat glands and lactating mammary glands, retain their connection with the surface epithelium from which they originated. This connection takes the form of epithelium-lined tubular ducts through which the secretions pass to reach the surface. Exocrine glands are often classified according to the way secretory products are released by their cells. In *holocrine*-type cells (*e.g.,* sebaceous glands), the glandular cell ruptures, releasing its entire content into the duct system. New generations of cells are replaced by mitosis of basal cells. *Merocrine*- or *eccrine*-type glands (*e.g.,* salivary glands, exocrine glands of the pancreas) release their glandular products by exocytosis. In *apocrine* secretions (*e.g.,* mammary glands, certain sweat glands), the apical portion of the cell, along with small portions of the cytoplasm, is pinched off the glandular cell. *Endocrine glands* are epithelial structures that have had their connection with the surface obliterated during development. These glands are ductless and produce secretions (*i.e.,* hormones) that move directly into the bloodstream.

Connective or Supportive Tissue

Connective or supportive tissue is the most abundant tissue in the body. As its name suggests, it connects and binds or supports the various tissues. Connective tissue is unique in that its cells produce the extracellular matrix that supports and holds tissues together. The capsules that surround organs of the body are composed of connective tissue. Bone, adipose tissue, and cartilage are specialized types of connective tissue that function to support the soft tissues of the body and store fat. The proximity of the extracellular matrix to blood vessels allows it to function as an exchange medium through which nutrients and metabolic wastes pass.

Origin and Characteristics

Most connective tissue is derived from the embryonic mesoderm, but some is derived from the neural crest, a derivative of the ectoderm. During embryonic development, mesodermal cells migrate from their site of origin and then surround and penetrate the developing organ. These cells are called *mesenchymal cells,* and the tissue they form is called *mesenchyme.* Tissues derived from embryonic mesenchymal cells include bone, cartilage, and adipose (fat) cells. Besides providing the source or origin of most connective tissues, mesenchyme develops into other structures such as blood cells and blood vessels. Connective tissue cells include fibroblasts, chondroblasts, osteoblasts, hematopoietic stem cells, blood cells, macrophages, mast cells, and adipocytes. The matrix of the umbilical cord is composed of a second type of embryonic mesoderm called *mucous connective tissue* or *Wharton jelly.*

Types of Connective Tissue

Adult connective tissue can be divided into two types: connective tissue proper, which is the focus of the discussion in this chapter, and specialized connective tissue (cartilage, bone, and blood cells), which is discussed in other chapters. There are four recognized types of connective tissue proper: loose (areolar), adipose, reticular, and dense connective tissue.

Loose Connective Tissue. Loose connective tissue, also known as *areolar tissue,* is soft and pliable. It fills spaces between muscle sheaths and forms a layer that encases blood and lymphatic vessels (Fig. 4-20). Areolar connective tissue supports the epithelial tissues and provides the means by which these tissues are nourished. In an organ containing functioning epithelial tissue and supporting connective tissue, the term *paren-*

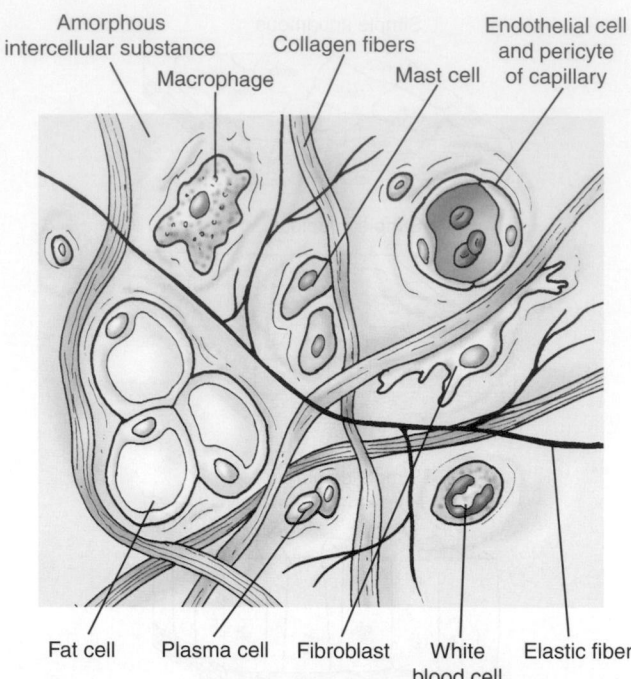

FIGURE 4-20 • Diagrammatic representation of cells that may be seen in loose connective tissue. The cells lie in the extracellular matrix, which is bathed in tissue fluid that originates in the capillaries.

chymal tissue is used to describe the functioning epithelium as opposed to the connective tissue framework, or stroma.

Loose connective tissue is characterized by an abundance of ground substance and tissue fluid housing the fixed connective tissue cells: fibroblasts, mast cells, adipose or fat cells, macrophages, and leukocytes. Loose connective tissue cells secrete substances that form the extracellular matrix that supports and connects body cells. Fibroblasts are the most abundant of these cells. They are responsible for the synthesis of the fibrous and gel-like substance that fills the intercellular spaces of the body and for the production of collagen, elastic, and reticular fibers.

The *basal lamina* is a special type of intercellular matrix that is present where connective tissue contacts the tissue it supports. It is visible only with an electron microscope and is produced by the epithelial cells. In many locations, reticular fibers, produced by the connective tissue cells, are associated with the basal lamina. Together the basal lamina and the reticular layer form the basement membrane seen by light microscopy. A basement membrane is found along the interface between connective tissue and muscle fibers, on Schwann cells of the peripheral nervous system, on the basal surface of endothelial cells, and on fat cells. These basement membranes bond cells to the underlying or surrounding connective tissues, serve as selective filters for particles that pass between connective tissue and other cells, and contribute to cell regeneration and repair.

Adipose Tissue. Adipose tissue is a special form of connective tissue in which adipocytes predominate. Adipocytes do not generate an extracellular matrix but maintain a large intracellular space. These cells store large quantities of triglycerides and are the largest repository of energy in the body. Adipose tissue helps fill spaces between tissues and helps to keep organs in place. The subcutaneous fat helps to shape the body. Because fat is a poor conductor of heat, adipose tissue serves as thermal insulation for the body. Adipose tissue exists in two forms: unilocular and multilocular. Unilocular (white) adipose tissue is composed of cells in which the fat is contained in a single, large droplet in the cytoplasm. Multilocular (brown) adipose tissue is composed of cells that contain multiple droplets of fat and numerous mitochondria. These two types of fat are discussed in Chapter 39.

Reticular Connective Tissue. *Reticular tissue* is characterized by a network of fibers interspersed with fibroblasts and macrophages. The fibroblasts synthesize type III collagen fibers. Reticular tissue forms the architecture of liver sinusoids, adipose tissue, bone marrow, and lymphoid tissues such as the spleen.

Dense Connective Tissue. Dense connective tissue exists in two forms: dense irregular and dense regular. Dense irregular connective tissue consists of the same components found in loose connective tissue, but exhibits a predominance of collagen fibers and fewer cells. This type of tissue can be found in the dermis of the skin (*i.e.*, reticular layer), the fibrous capsules of many organs, and the fibrous sheaths of cartilage (*i.e.*, perichondrium) and bone (*i.e.*, periosteum). It also forms the fascia that invests muscles and organs. Dense regular connective tissues are rich in collagen fibers and form the tendons and aponeuroses that join muscles to bone or other muscles and the ligaments that join bone to bone.

Muscle Tissue

Muscle tissue, whose primary function is contraction, is responsible for movement of the body and its parts and for changes in the size and shape of internal organs. Muscle tissue contains two types of fibers that are responsible for contraction: thin and thick filaments. The thin filaments are composed primarily of actin, whereas the thick filaments are composed of myosin. The two types of myofilaments occupy the bulk of the cytoplasm, which in muscle cells is called the *sarcoplasm.*

There are three types of muscle tissues: *skeletal, cardiac,* and *smooth.* Skeletal and cardiac muscles are striated muscles, in which the actin and myosin filaments are arranged in large, parallel arrays in bundles, giving the muscle fibers a striped or striated appearance when observed with a microscope. *Smooth muscle* lacks striations and is found in the iris of the eye, the walls of blood vessels, hollow organs such as the stomach and urinary bladder, and hollow tubes, such as the ureters and common bile duct, that connect internal organs.

Neither skeletal nor cardiac muscle can undergo the mitotic activity needed to replace injured cells. Smooth muscle, however, may proliferate and undergo mitotic activity. Some increases in smooth muscle are physiologic, as occurs in the uterus during pregnancy. Other increases, such as the increase

in smooth muscle that occurs in the arteries of persons with chronic hypertension, are pathologic.

Although the three types of muscle tissue differ significantly in structure, contractile properties, and control mechanisms, they have many similarities. In the following section, the structural properties of skeletal muscle are presented as the prototype of striated muscle tissue. Smooth muscle and the ways in which it differs from skeletal muscle are also discussed. Cardiac muscle is described in Chapter 21.

Skeletal Muscle

Skeletal muscle is the most abundant tissue in the body, accounting for 40% to 45% of the total body weight. Most skeletal muscles are attached to bones, and their contractions are responsible for movements of the skeleton. Each skeletal muscle is a discrete organ made up of hundreds or thousands of muscle fibers. At the periphery of skeletal muscle fibers, randomly scattered satellite cells are found. They represent a source of undifferentiated myoblast cells that may be involved in the limited regeneration capabilities of skeletal muscle. Although muscle fibers predominate, substantial amounts of connective tissue, blood vessels, and nerve fibers are also present.

Organization and Structure. In an intact muscle, the individual muscle fibers are held together by several different layers of connective tissue. Skeletal muscles such as the biceps brachii are surrounded by a dense, irregular connective tissue covering called the *epimysium* (Fig. 4-21A). Each muscle is subdivided into smaller bundles called *fascicles,* which are surrounded by a connective tissue covering called the *perimysium.* The number of fascicles and their size vary among muscles. Fascicles consist of many elongated structures called *muscle fibers,* each of which is surrounded by connective tissue called the *endomysium.* Skeletal muscles are syncytial or multinucleated structures, meaning there are no true cell boundaries within a skeletal muscle fiber.

The sarcoplasm of the muscle fiber is contained within the sarcolemma, which represents the cell membrane. Embedded throughout the sarcoplasm are the contractile elements actin and myosin, which are arranged in parallel bundles called *myofibrils.* The thin, lighter-staining myofilaments are composed of actin, and the thicker, darker-staining myofilaments are composed of myosin. Each myofibril consists of regularly repeating units along the length of the myofibril, called *sarcomeres* (see Fig. 4-21B).

Sarcomeres are the structural and functional units of cardiac and skeletal muscle. A sarcomere extends from one Z-line to another Z-line. Within the sarcomere are alternating light and dark bands. The central portion of the sarcomere contains the dark band (A-band) consisting mainly of myosin filaments, with some overlap with actin filaments. Straddling the Z-line, the lighter I-band contains only actin filaments; therefore, it takes two sarcomeres to complete an I-band. An H-zone is found in the middle of the A-band and represents the region where only myosin filaments are found. In the center of the H-zone is a thin,

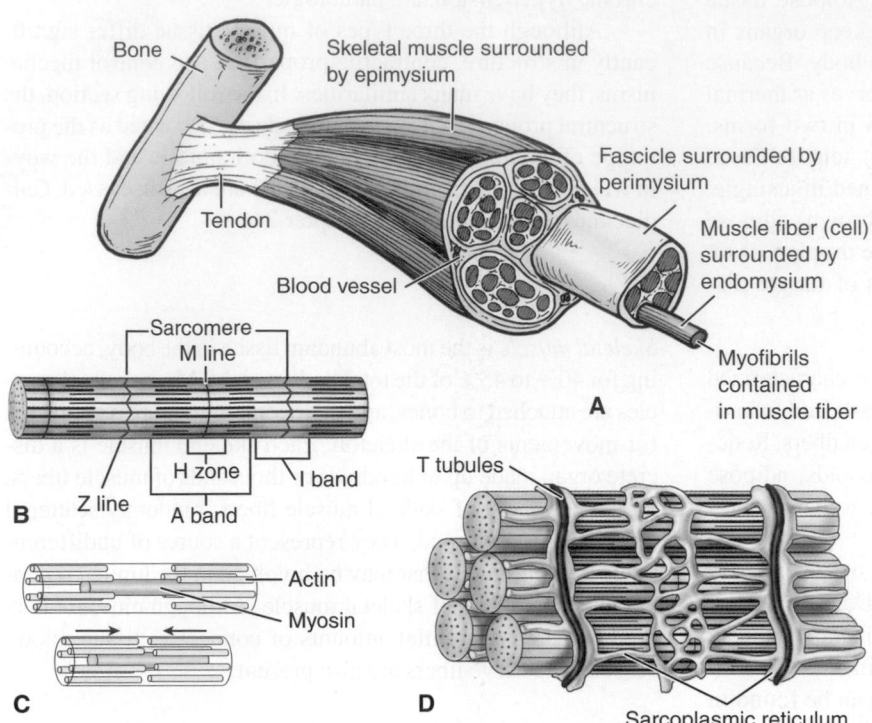

FIGURE 4-21 • Connective tissue components of a skeletal muscle (**A**). Striations of the myofibril showing the overlap of contractile proteins and the A and I bands, the H zone, and the Z and M lines (**B**). The relaxed and contracted states of the myofibril showing the position of actin filaments (blue) between the myosin filaments (pink) in the relaxed muscle (*top*) and pulling of the Z membranes toward each other (*bottom*) as the muscle contracts (**C**). The sarcoplasmic reticulum with T tubules (**D**).

dark band, the M-band or M-line, produced by linkages between the myosin filaments. Z-lines consist of short elements that interconnect and provide the thin actin filaments from two adjoining sarcomeres with an anchoring point.

The *sarcoplasmic reticulum,* which is comparable to the smooth ER, is composed of longitudinal tubules that run parallel to the muscle fiber and surround each myofibril (see Fig. 4-21D). This network ends in enlarged, saclike regions called the *lateral sacs* or *terminal cisternae.* These sacs store calcium that is released during muscle contraction. A binding protein called *calsequestrin* found in the terminal cisternae enables a high concentration of calcium ions to be sequestered in the cisternae. Concentration levels of calcium ions in the cisternae are 10,000 times higher than in the sarcoplasm.

A second system of tubules consists of the *transverse* or *T tubules,* which are extensions of the plasma membrane and run perpendicular to the muscle fiber. The hollow portion or lumen of the transverse tubule is continuous with the extracellular fluid compartment. Action potentials, which are rapidly conducted over the surface of the muscle fiber, are in turn propagated by the T tubules into the sarcoplasmic reticulum. As the action potential moves through the lateral sacs, the sacs release calcium, initiating muscle contraction. The membrane of the sarcoplasmic reticulum also has an active transport mechanism for pumping calcium back into the reticulum. This prevents interactions between calcium ions and the actin and myosin myofilaments after cessation of a muscle contraction.

Skeletal Muscle Contraction. During muscle contraction, the thick myosin and thin actin filaments slide over each other,

causing shortening of the muscle fiber, although the length of the individual thick and thin filaments remains unchanged (see Fig. 4-21C). The structures that produce the sliding of the filaments are the myosin heads that form cross-bridges with the thin actin filaments (Fig. 4-22). When activated by ATP, the cross-bridges swivel in a fixed arc, much like the oars of a boat, as they become attached to the actin filament. During contraction, each cross-bridge undergoes its own cycle of movement, forming a bridge attachment and releasing it, and moving to another site where the same sequence of movement occurs. This pulls the thin and thick filaments past each other.

Myosin is the chief constituent of the thick filament. It consists of a thin tail, which provides the structural backbone for the filament, and a globular head. Each globular head contains a binding site able to bind to a complementary site on the actin molecule. Besides the binding site for actin, each myosin head has a separate active site that catalyzes the breakdown of ATP to provide the energy needed to activate the myosin head so that it can form a cross-bridge with actin. After contraction, myosin also binds ATP, thus breaking the linkage between actin and myosin. Myosin molecules are bundled together side by side in the thick filaments such that one half have their heads toward one end of the filament and their tails toward the other end; the other half are arranged in the opposite manner.

The thin filaments are composed mainly of actin, a globular protein lined up in two rows that coil around each other to form a long helical strand. Associated with each actin filament are two regulatory proteins, tropomyosin and troponin (see Fig. 4-22A). *Tropomyosin,* which lies in grooves of the actin strand, provides the site for attachment of the globular

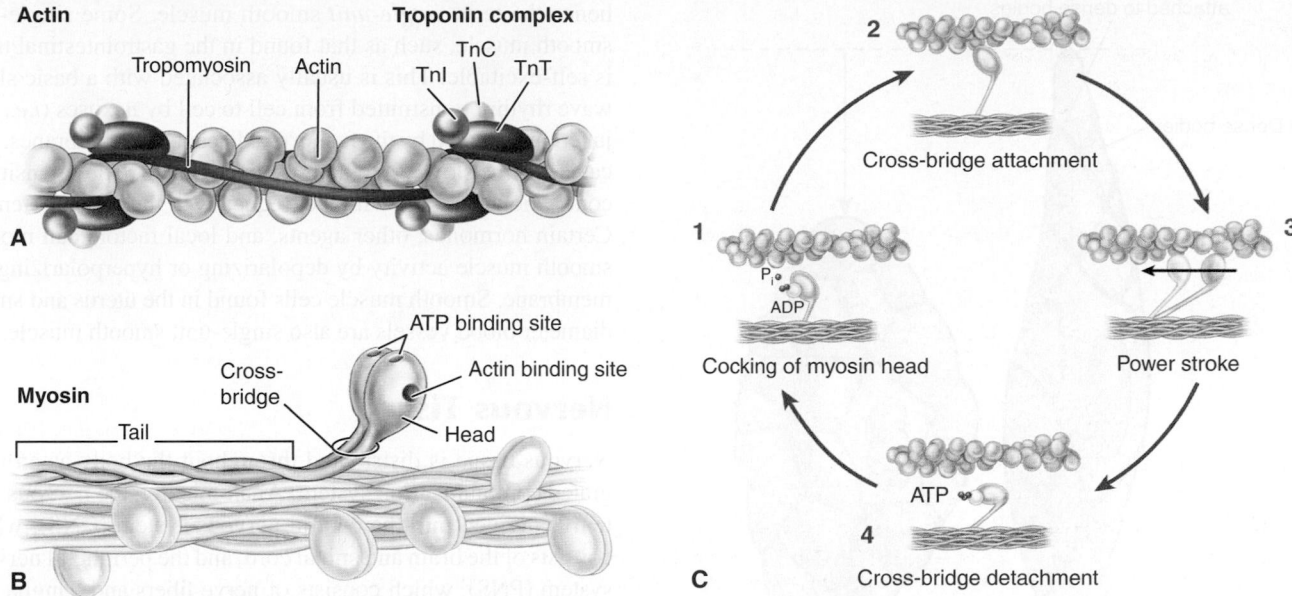

FIGURE 4-22 • Molecular structure of the thin actin filament (**A**) and the thicker myosin filament (**B**) of striated muscle. The thin filament is a double-stranded helix of actin molecules with tropomyosin and troponin molecules lying along the grooves of the actin strands. (**C**) Sequence of events involved in sliding of adjacent actin and myosin filaments: (1) cocking of the myosin head occurs as ATP is split to ADP, (2) cross-bridge attachment, (3) power stroke during which the myosin head bends as it moves the actin forward, and (4) cross-bridge detachment occurs as a new ATP attaches to the myosin head.

heads of the myosin filament. In the noncontracted state, *troponin* covers the tropomyosin binding sites and prevents formation of cross-bridges between the actin and myosin. During an action potential, calcium ions released from the sarcoplasmic reticulum diffuse to the adjacent myofibrils, where they bind to troponin. Binding of calcium to troponin uncovers the tropomyosin binding sites such that the myosin heads can attach and form cross-bridges. Energy from ATP is used to break the actin and myosin cross-bridges, stopping the muscle contraction. After the linkage between actin and myosin is broken, the concentration of calcium around the myofibrils decreases as calcium is actively transported into the sarcoplasmic reticulum by a membrane pump that uses energy derived from ATP.

The basis of *rigor mortis* can be explained by the binding of actin and myosin. As the muscle begins to degenerate after death, the sarcoplasmic cisternae release their calcium ions, which enable the myosin heads to combine with their sites on the actin molecule. As ATP supplies diminish, no energy source is available to start the normal interaction between actin and myosin, and the muscle is in a state of rigor until further degeneration destroys the cross-bridges between actin and myosin.

Smooth Muscle

Smooth muscle is often called *involuntary muscle* because its activity arises spontaneously or through activity of the autonomic nervous system. Smooth muscle contractions are slower and more sustained than skeletal or cardiac muscle contractions.

Organization and Structure. Smooth muscle cells are spindle shaped and smaller than skeletal muscle fibers. Each smooth muscle cell has one centrally positioned nucleus. Z-lines and M-lines are not present in smooth muscle fibers, and cross-striations are absent because the bundles of filaments are not parallel but crisscross obliquely through the cell. Instead, the actin filaments are attached to structures called *dense bodies* (Fig. 4-23). Some dense bodies are attached to the cell membrane, and others are dispersed in the cell and linked together by structural proteins.

The lack of Z-lines and the regular overlapping of contractile elements provide a greater range of tension development. This is important in hollow organs that undergo changes in volume, with consequent changes in the length of the smooth muscle fibers in their walls. Even with the distention of a hollow organ, the smooth muscle fiber retains some ability to develop tension, whereas such distention would stretch skeletal muscle beyond the area where the thick and thin filaments overlap.

Smooth muscle is usually arranged in sheets or bundles. In hollow organs, such as the intestines, the bundles are organized into the two-layered muscularis externa consisting of an outer, longitudinal layer and an inner, circular layer. A thinner muscularis mucosae often lies between the muscularis externa and the endothelium. In blood vessels, the bundles are arranged circularly or helically around the vessel wall.

Smooth Muscle Contraction. As with cardiac and skeletal muscle, smooth muscle contraction is initiated by an increase in intracellular calcium. However, smooth muscle differs from skeletal muscle in the way its cross-bridges are formed. The

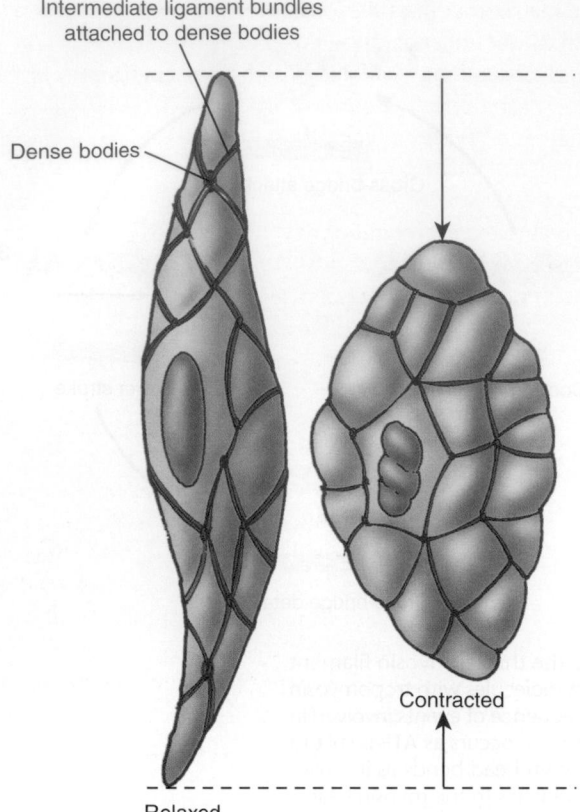

Intermediate ligament bundles attached to dense bodies

Dense bodies

Contracted

Relaxed

FIGURE 4-23 • Structure of smooth muscle showing the dense bodies. In smooth muscle, the force of contraction is transmitted to the cell membrane by bundles of intermediate fibers.

sarcoplasmic reticulum of smooth muscle is less developed than in skeletal muscle, and no transverse tubules are present. Smooth muscle relies on the entrance of extracellular calcium and its release from the sarcoplasmic reticulum for muscle contraction. This dependence on movement of extracellular calcium across the cell membrane during muscle contraction is the basis for the action of calcium-blocking drugs used in the treatment of cardiovascular disease.

Smooth muscle also lacks troponin, the calcium-binding regulatory protein found in skeletal and cardiac muscle. Instead, it relies on another calcium-binding protein called *calmodulin.* The calcium–calmodulin complex binds to and activates the myosin-containing thick filaments, which interact with actin.

Types of Smooth Muscle. Smooth muscle may be divided into two broad categories according to the mode of activation: multiunit and single-unit smooth muscle. In *multiunit* smooth muscle, each unit operates almost independently of the others and is often enervated by a single nerve, such as occurs in skeletal muscle. It has little or no inherent activity and depends on the autonomic nervous system for its activation. This type of smooth muscle is found in the iris, in the walls of the vas deferens, and attached to hairs in the skin. The fibers in *single-unit* smooth muscle are in close contact with each other and can contract spontaneously without nerve or hormonal stimulation.

Normally, most of the muscle fibers contract synchronously, hence the term *single-unit* smooth muscle. Some single-unit smooth muscle, such as that found in the gastrointestinal tract, is self-excitable. This is usually associated with a basic slow-wave rhythm transmitted from cell to cell by nexuses (*i.e.,* gap junctions) formed by the fusion of adjacent cell membranes. The cause of this slow-wave activity is unknown. The intensity of contraction increases with the frequency of the action potential. Certain hormones, other agents, and local factors can modify smooth muscle activity by depolarizing or hyperpolarizing the membrane. Smooth muscle cells found in the uterus and small-diameter blood vessels are also single-unit smooth muscle.

Nervous Tissue

Nervous tissue is distributed throughout the body as an integrated communication system. Anatomically, the nervous system is divided into the central nervous system (CNS), which consists of the brain and spinal cord, and the peripheral nervous system (PNS), which consists of nerve fibers and ganglia that exist outside the CNS. Nerve cells develop from the embryonic ectoderm. Nerve cells are highly differentiated and therefore incapable of regeneration in postnatal life. Embryonic development of the nervous system and the structure and functions of the nervous system are discussed more fully in Chapter 48.

Structurally, nervous tissue consists of two cell types: nerve cells or neurons and glial or supporting cells. Most nerve cells consist of three parts: the soma or cell body, dendrites, and the axon. The cytoplasm-filled dendrites, which are multiple elongated processes, receive and carry stimuli from the environment, from sensory epithelial cells, and from other neurons to the cell. The axon, which is a single cytoplasm-filled process, is specialized for generating and conducting nerve impulses away from the cell body to other nerve cells, muscle cells, and glandular cells.

Neurons can be classified as afferent and efferent neurons according to their function. Afferent or sensory neurons carry information toward the CNS; they are involved in the reception of sensory information from the external environment and from within the body. Efferent or motor neurons carry information away from the CNS; they are needed for control of muscle fibers and endocrine and exocrine glands.

Communication between neurons and effector organs, such as muscle cells, occurs at specialized structures called *synapses.* At the synapse, chemical messengers (*i.e.,* neurotransmitters) alter the membrane potential to conduct impulses from one nerve to another or from a neuron to an effector cell. In addition, electrical synapses exist in which nerve cells are linked through gap junctions that permit the passage of ions from one cell to another.

Neuroglia (*glia* means "glue") are the cells that support neurons, form myelin, and have trophic and phagocytic functions. Four types of neuroglia are found in the CNS: astrocytes, oligodendrocytes, microglia, and ependymal cells. Astrocytes are the most abundant of the neuroglia. They have many long processes that surround blood vessels in the CNS. They provide structural support for the neurons, and their extensions form a sealed barrier that protects the CNS. The oligodendrocytes provide myelination of neuronal processes in the CNS. The microglia are phagocytic cells that represent the mononuclear phagocytic system in the nervous system. Ependymal cells line the cavities of the brain and spinal cord and are in contact with the cerebrospinal fluid. In the PNS, supporting cells consist of the Schwann and satellite cells. The Schwann cells provide myelination of the axons and dendrites, and the satellite cells enclose and protect the dorsal root ganglia and autonomic ganglion cells.

Extracellular Tissue Components

The discussion thus far has focused on the cellular components of the different tissue types. Within tissues, cells are held together by cell junctions; the space between cells is filled with an extracellular matrix; and adhesion molecules form intercellular contacts.

Extracellular Matrix

Tissues are not made up solely of cells. A large part of their volume is made up of an extracellular matrix. This matrix is composed of a variety of proteins and polysaccharides (*i.e.,* a molecule made up of many sugars). These proteins and polysaccharides are secreted locally and are organized into a supporting meshwork in close association with the cells that produced them. The amount and composition of the matrix vary with the different tissues and their function. In bone, for example, the matrix is more plentiful than the cells that surround it; in the brain, the cells are much more abundant and the matrix is only a minor constituent.

Two main classes of extracellular macromolecules make up the extracellular matrix. The first is composed of polysaccharide chains of a class called *glycosaminoglycans* (GAGs), which are usually found linked to protein as proteoglycans. The second type consists of the fibrous proteins (*i.e.,* collagen and elastin) and the fibrous adhesive proteins (*i.e.,* fibronectin and laminin) that are found in the basement membrane. Members of each of these two classes of extracellular macromolecules come in a variety of shapes and sizes.

The proteoglycan and GAG molecules in connective tissue form a highly hydrated, gel-like substance, or tissue gel, in which the fibrous proteins are embedded. The polysaccharide gel resists compressive forces, the collagen fibers strengthen and help organize the matrix, the rubber-like elastin adds resilience, and the adhesive proteins help cells attach to the appropriate part of the matrix. Polysaccharides in the tissue gel are highly hydrophilic, and they form gels even at low concentrations. They also accumulate a negative charge that attracts cations such as sodium, which are osmotically active, causing large amounts of water to be sucked into the matrix. This creates a swelling pressure, or turgor, that enables the matrix to withstand extensive compressive forces. This is in contrast to collagen, which resists stretching forces. For example, the car-

tilage matrix that lines the knee joint can support pressures of hundreds of atmospheres by this mechanism.

Glycosaminoglycan and proteoglycan molecules in connective tissue usually constitute less than 10% by weight of fibrous tissue. Because they form a hydrated gel, the molecules fill most of the extracellular space, providing mechanical support to the tissues while ensuring rapid diffusion of water and electrolytes and the migration of cells. One GAG, hyaluronan or hyaluronic acid, is thought to play an important role as a space-filler during embryonic development. It creates a cell-free space into which cells subsequently migrate. When cell migration and organ development are complete, the excess hyaluronan is degraded by the enzyme hyaluronidase. Hyaluronan is also important in directing the cell replacement that occurs during wound repair (see Chapter 18).

Three types of fibers are found in the extracellular space: collagen, elastin, and reticular fibers. *Collagen* is the most common protein in the body. It is a tough, nonliving, white fiber that serves as the structural framework for skin, ligaments, tendons, and many other structures. *Elastin* acts like a rubber band; it can be stretched and then returns to its original form. Elastin fibers are abundant in structures subjected to frequent stretching, such as the aorta and some ligaments. *Reticular fibers* are extremely thin fibers that create a flexible network in organs subjected to changes in form or volume, such as the spleen, liver, uterus, or intestinal muscle layer.

Adhesion Molecules

Important classes of extracellular macromolecules are the cell adhesion molecules (CAMs). CAMs can be cell-to-cell or cell-to-matrix adhesion molecules. There are four main classes of CAMs: cadherins, selectins, integrins, and the immunoglobulin (Ig) superfamily of proteins. Cadherins, selectins, and integrins all depend on extracellular calcium ions (or magnesium for some integrins) to function. The calcium-independent cell-to-cell adhesion molecules belong to the Ig superfamily of proteins.

Cadherins. Cadherins link parts of the internal cytoskeleton (actin and structures called *catenins*) with extracellular cadherins of an adjacent cell. This type of linkage is called *homophilic,* meaning that molecules on one cell bind to other molecules of the same type on adjacent cells (Fig. 4-24A). More than 40 different types of cadherins are known, and they are found in such intercellular junctions as the zonula and macula adherens.

Selectins. Selectins bind carbohydrates present on the ligands of an adjacent cell in a *heterophilic* type of interaction (see Fig. 4-24B). In heterophilic interactions, the molecules on one cell bind to molecules of a different type on adjacent cells. Selectins are found on activated endothelial cells of blood vessels, on leukocytes, and on platelets. They, together with integrins and immunoglobulins, participate in leukocyte movement through the endothelial lining of blood vessels during inflammation.

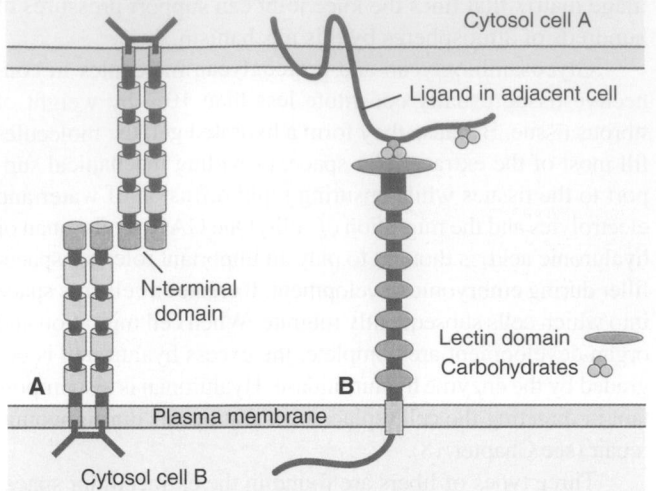

Cytosol cell A

Ligand in adjacent cell

N-terminal domain

Lectin domain

Carbohydrates

A

B

Plasma membrane

Cytosol cell B

FIGURE 4-24 • Examples of homophilic and heterophilic intercellular adhesion. **(A)** Homophilic adhesion can be accomplished by two identical cadherin dimer molecules joined at their N-terminal domains. **(B)** Binding of the lectin domain of an integrin with the carbohydrate portions of a ligand is an example of heterophilic binding. (Courtesy of Edward W. Carroll.)

Integrins. Integrins usually assist in attaching epithelial cells to the underlying basement membrane. Unlike other CAMs, they are heterodimers consisting of α and β subunits. Extracellularly, they are attached to fibronectin and laminin, the two major components of the basement membrane. Like the cadherins, their intracellular portion is linked to actin (see Fig. 4-24). One group of integrins is associated with hemidesmosomes, whereas others are associated with the surface of white blood cells, macrophages, and platelets. Integrins usually have a weak affinity for their ligands unless they are associated with cellular focal contacts and hemidesmosomes. This allows some movement between cells except where a firm attachment is required to attach epithelial cells to the underlying connective tissue.

Certain integrins play an important role in allowing white blood cells to pass through the vessel wall, a process called *transmigration*. Persons affected with leukocyte adhesion deficiency are unable to synthesize appropriate integrin molecules. As a result, they experience repeated bacterial infections because their white blood cells are unable to transmigrate through vessel walls.

Immunoglobulin Superfamily. The Ig superfamily proteins consist of groups of one or more Ig-like adhesion proteins that are structurally similar to antibody molecules. The best-studied example of Ig superfamily proteins are the neural cell adhesion molecules (NCAMs), which are expressed in a variety of cells, including most nerve cells. All are calcium ion independent but, unlike other CAMs, they may participate in homophilic or heterophilic interactions. Heterophilic attachments are to other members of the superfamily such as intracellular adhesion molecules (ICAMs). During early development of the CNS, cells at the roof of the neural tube express high levels of NCAM on their cell surface and are unable to move because of intercellu-

lar adhesions. Future neural crest cells lose their NCAM and begin migrating to various areas of the body. Members of the Ig superfamily also play a role in the homing process of leukocytes during inflammation.

IN SUMMARY, body cells are organized into four basic tissue types: epithelial, connective, muscle, and nervous. The epithelium covers and lines the body surfaces and forms the functional components of glandular structures. Epithelial tissue is classified into three types according to the shape of the cells and the number of layers that are present: simple, stratified, and pseudostratified. The cells in epithelial tissue are held together by three types of intercellular junctions: tight, adhering, and gap. They are attached to the underlying tissue by hemidesmosomes.

Connective tissue supports and connects body structures; it forms the bones and skeletal system, joint structures, blood cells, and intercellular substances. Connective tissue proper can be divided into four types: loose or areolar, which fills body spaces and is characterized by an abundance of ground substance; adipose, which stores fat; reticular, which forms the architectural framework in many structures of the body; and dense, regular and irregular, which forms structures such as tendons and ligaments (regular) and the dermis of the skin (irregular).

Muscle tissue is a specialized tissue designed for contractility. Three types of muscle tissue exist: skeletal, cardiac, and smooth. Actin and myosin filaments interact to produce muscle shortening, a process activated by the presence of calcium. In skeletal muscle, calcium is released from the sarcoplasmic reticulum in response to an action potential. Smooth muscle is often called *involuntary muscle* because it contracts spontaneously or through activity of the autonomic nervous system. It differs from skeletal muscle in that its sarcoplasmic reticulum is less defined and it depends on the entry of extracellular calcium ions for muscle contraction.

Nervous tissue is designed for communication purposes and includes the neurons, the supporting neural structures, and the ependymal cells that line the ventricles of the brain and the spinal canal.

The extracellular matrix is made up of a variety of proteins and polysaccharides. These proteins and polysaccharides are secreted locally and are organized into a supporting meshwork in close association with the cells that produced them. The amount and composition of matrix vary with the different tissues and their function. Extracellular fibers include collagen fibers, which comprise tendons and ligaments; elastic fibers, found in large arteries and some ligaments; and thin reticular fibers, which are plentiful in organs that are subject to a change in volume (*e.g.,* spleen and liver). Important classes of extracellular macromolecules are the adhesion molecules that maintain intercellular contacts. There are three classes of adhesion molecules that depend on extracellular calcium to function in cell adhesion: *cadherins,* which link parts of the internal cytoskeleton with the extracellular cadherins of an adjacent cell; *selectins,* which bind carbohydrates present on the ligands of adjacent cells; and *integrins* (some of which are magnesium dependent), which assist in attaching epithelial cells to the underlying basement membrane. The Ig superfamily of proteins are calcium-independent adhesion molecules that bind cells, such as those of the nervous system, together. ∎

Review Exercises

1. Tattoos consist of pigments that have been injected into the skin.
   A. *Explain what happens to the dye once it has been injected and why it does not eventually wash away.*

2. Persons who drink sufficient amounts of alcohol display rapid changes in central nervous system function, including both motor and behavioral changes, and the odor of alcohol can be detected on their breath.
   A. *Use the concepts related to the lipid bilayer structure of the cell membrane to explain these observations.*

3. The absorption of glucose from the intestine involves a cotransport mechanism in which the active primary transport of sodium ions is used to provide for the secondary transport of glucose.
   A. *Hypothesize how this information might be used to design an oral rehydration solution for someone who is suffering from diarrhea.*

Bibliography

Alberts B., Johnson A., Lewis J., et al. (2002). *Molecular biology of the cell* (4th ed., pp. 129–188, 583–614, 771–792, 852–870, 1065–1126). New York: Garland Science.

Antonin W., Mattaj I. W. (2005). Nuclear pore complexes: Round the bend? *Nature Cell Biology* 7, 10–12.

Ashcroft F. M. (2000). *Ion channels and disease* (pp. 67–96, 95–133, 211–229). San Diego: Academic Press.

Badano J. L., Teslovich T. M., Katsanis N. (2005). The centrosome in human genetic disease. *Nature Review of Genetics* 6, 194–205.

Baserga R. (1999). Introduction to the cell cycle. In Stein G. S., Baserga R., Giordano A., et al. (Eds.), *The molecular basis of cell cycle and growth control* (pp. 1–14). New York: Wiley-Liss.

Bonifacino J. S., Rojas R. (2006). Retrograde transport from endosomes to the trans-Golgi network. *Nature Review of Molecular Cell Biology* 7, 568–579.

Chatterjee A., Mambo E., Sidransky D. (2006). Mitochondrial DNA mutations in human cancer. *Oncogene* 25, 4663–4674.

Davis B. (2005). A peek at the pore. *The Scientist* 19(8), 18–19.

Dubyak G. R. (2004). Ion homeostasis, channels, and transporters: An update on cellular mechanisms. *Advances in Physiological Education* 28, 143–154.

Fontenay M., Cathelin S., Aminot M., et al. (2006). Mitochondria in hematopoiesis and hematological diseases. *Oncogene* 25, 4757–4767.

Gartner L. P., Hiatt J. L. (2001). *Color textbook of histology* (2nd ed.). Philadelphia: W. B. Saunders.

Goldberg A. L., Elledge S. J., Harper J. W. (2001). The cellular chamber of doom. *Scientific American* 284(1), 68–73.

Gottlieb E. (2006). OPA1 and PARL keep a lid on apoptosis. *Cell* 126, 27–29.

Guyton A. C., Hall J. E. (2006). *Textbook of medical physiology* (11th ed., pp. 11–24). Philadelphia: Elsevier Saunders.

Joachim F. (1998). How the ribosome works. *American Scientist* 86, 428–439.

Kerr J. B. (1999). *Atlas of functional histology* (pp. 1–24, 25–37, 81–106). London: Mosby.

Kierszenbaum A. L. (2007). *Histology and cell biology: An introduction to pathology* (2nd ed., pp. 67–75, 101–102). St. Louis: Mosby.

Lodish H., Berk A., Matsudaria P. (2004). *Molecular cell biology* (5th ed., pp. 147–231, 779, 817–897). New York: W. H. Freeman.

Moore K. L., Persaud T. V. N. (2003). *The developing human: Clinically oriented embryology* (7th ed., pp. 15–42). Philadelphia: W. B. Saunders.

Pan J., Wang Q., Snell W. J. (2005). Cilium-generated signaling and cilia-related disorders. *Laboratory Investigation* 85, 452–463.

Rhoades R. A., Tanner G. A. (2003). *Medical physiology* (2nd ed.). Philadelphia: Lippincott Williams & Wilkins.

Ross M. H., Kaye G. I., Pawlina W. (2003). *Histology: A text and atlas* (4th ed.). Philadelphia: Lippincott Williams & Wilkins.

Smith C., Marks A. D., Lieberman M. (2005). *Marks' basic medical biochemistry: A clinical approach* (2nd ed.). Philadelphia: Lippincott Williams & Wilkins.

Thiry M., Goessens G. (1996). Historical overview. In *The nucleolus during the cell cycle* (pp. 1–11). Molecular Biology Intelligence Unit. Georgetown, TX: RG Landes.

Tortora G. J., Derrickson B. (2009). *Principles of anatomy and physiology* (11th ed., pp. 61–103, 301–332, 415–454). New York: John Wiley & Sons.

United Mitochondrial Disease Foundation. (2001). Mitochondrial disease: Basis of disease. [Online.] Available: http://www.umdf.org/mitodisease. Accessed June 20, 2001.

Voeltz G. V., Rolls M. M., Rapoport T. A. (2002). Structural organization of the endoplasmic reticulum. *EMBO Reports* 3, 944–950.

Visit thePoint **http://thePoint.lww.com for animations, journal articles, and more!**

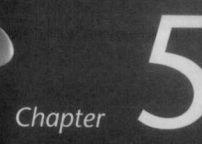

Chapter **5**

Cellular Adaptation, Injury, and Death

CARRIE J. MERKLE

> When confronted with stresses that endanger its normal structure and function, the cell undergoes adaptive changes that permit survival and maintenance of function. It is only when the stress is overwhelming or adaptation is ineffective that cell injury and death occur. This chapter focuses on cellular adaptation, injury, and death.

CELLULAR ADAPTATION

After completing this section of the chapter, you should be able to meet the following objectives:

■ Cite the general purpose of changes in cell structure and function that occur as the result of normal adaptive processes.
■ Describe cell changes that occur with atrophy, hypertrophy, hyperplasia, metaplasia, and dysplasia and state general conditions under which the changes occur.
■ Cite three sources of intracellular accumulations.
■ Compare the pathogenesis and effects of dystrophic and metastatic calcifications.

Cells adapt to changes in the internal environment, just as the total organism adapts to changes in the external environment. Cells may adapt by undergoing changes in size, number, and type. These changes, occurring singly or in combination, may lead to atrophy, hypertrophy, hyperplasia, metaplasia, and dysplasia (Fig. 5-1). Adaptive cellular responses also include intracellular accumulations and storage of products in abnormal amounts.[1,2]

There are numerous molecular mechanisms mediating cellular adaptation, including factors produced by other cells or by the cells themselves. These mechanisms depend largely on signals transmitted by chemical messengers that exert their effects by altering gene function. In general, the genes expressed in all cells fall into two categories: "housekeeping" genes that are necessary for normal function of a cell, and genes that determine the differentiating characteristics of a particular cell type. In many adaptive cellular responses, the expression of the differentiation genes is altered, whereas that of the housekeeping genes remains unaffected. Thus, a cell is able to change size or form without

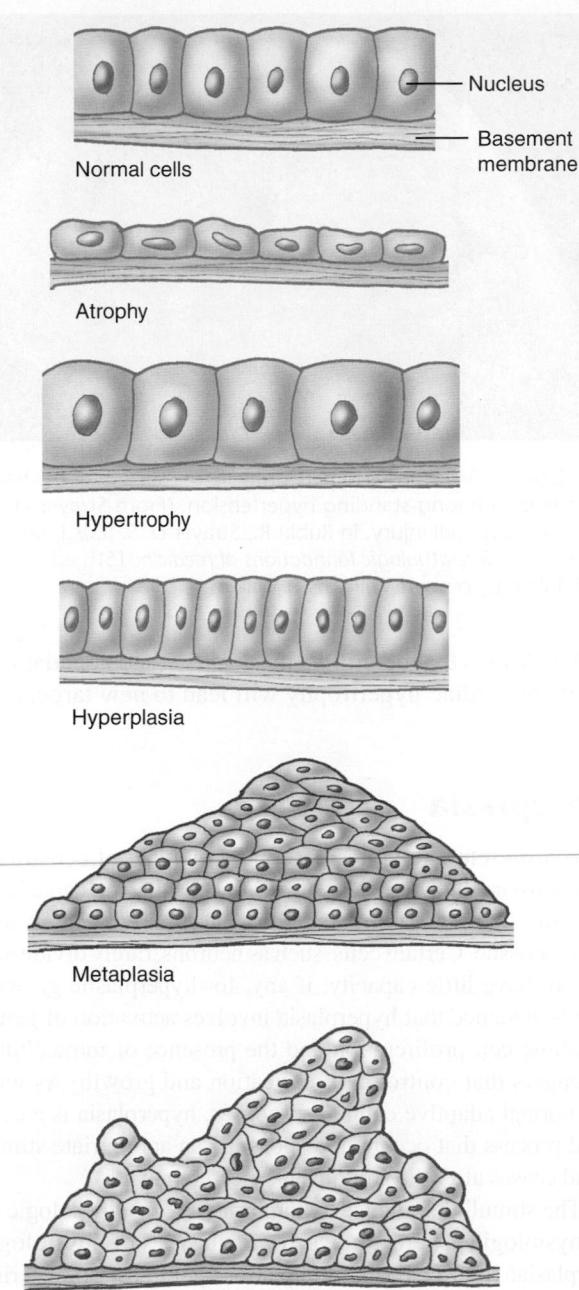

Normal cells

— Nucleus

— Basement membrane

Atrophy

Hypertrophy

Hyperplasia

Metaplasia

Dysplasia

FIGURE 5-1 • Adaptive cell and tissue responses involving a change in cell size (atrophy and hypertrophy), number (hyperplasia), cell type (metaplasia), or size, shape, and organization (dysplasia). (From Anatomical Chart Company. [2002]. *Atlas of pathophysiology* [p. 4]. Springhouse, PA: Springhouse.)

compromising its normal function. Once the stimulus for adaptation is removed, the effect on expression of the differentiating genes is removed and the cell resumes its previous state of specialized function. Whether adaptive cellular changes are normal or abnormal depends on whether the response was mediated by an appropriate stimulus. Normal adaptive responses occur in response to need and an appropriate stimulus. After the need has been removed, the adaptive response ceases.

CELLULAR ADAPTATIONS

- Cells are able to adapt to increased work demands or threats to survival by changing their size (atrophy and hypertrophy), number (hyperplasia), and form (metaplasia).
- Normal cellular adaptation occurs in response to an appropriate stimulus and ceases once the need for adaptation has ceased.

Atrophy

When confronted with a decrease in work demands or adverse environmental conditions, most cells are able to revert to a smaller size and a lower and more efficient level of functioning that is compatible with survival. This decrease in cell size is called *atrophy*. Cells that are atrophied reduce their oxygen consumption and other cellular functions by decreasing the number and size of their organelles and other structures. There are fewer mitochondria, myofilaments, and endoplasmic reticulum structures. When a sufficient number of cells are involved, the entire tissue or muscle atrophies.

Cell size, particularly in muscle tissue, is related to workload. As the workload of a cell declines, oxygen consumption and protein synthesis decrease. Furthermore, proper muscle mass is maintained by sufficient levels of insulin and insulin-like growth factor-1 (IGF-1). When insulin and IGF-1 levels are low or catabolic signals are present, muscle atrophy occurs by mechanisms that include reduced synthetic processes, increased proteolysis by the ubiquitin-proteasome system, and apoptosis or programmed cell death (to be discussed).[3] In the ubiquitin-proteasome system, intracellular proteins destined for destruction are covalently bonded to a small protein called *ubiquitin* and then degraded by small cytoplasmic organelles called *proteasomes* (discussed in Chapter 4).

The general causes of atrophy can be grouped into five categories: (1) disuse, (2) denervation, (3) loss of endocrine stimulation, (4) inadequate nutrition, and (5) ischemia or decreased blood flow. Disuse atrophy occurs when there is a reduction in skeletal muscle use. An extreme example of disuse atrophy is seen in the muscles of extremities that have been encased in plaster casts. Because atrophy is adaptive and reversible, muscle size is restored after the cast is removed and muscle use is resumed. Denervation atrophy is a form of disuse atrophy that occurs in the muscles of paralyzed limbs. Lack of endocrine stimulation produces a form of disuse atrophy. In women, the loss of estrogen stimulation during menopause results in atrophic changes in the reproductive organs. With malnutrition and decreased blood flow, cells decrease their size and energy requirements as a means of survival.

Hypertrophy

Hypertrophy represents an increase in cell size and with it an increase in the amount of functioning tissue mass. It results from an increased workload imposed on an organ or body part and is commonly seen in cardiac and skeletal muscle tissue, which cannot adapt to an increase in workload through mitotic division and formation of more cells. Hypertrophy involves an increase in the functional components of the cell that allows it to achieve equilibrium between demand and functional capacity. For example, as muscle cells hypertrophy, additional actin and myosin filaments, cell enzymes, and adenosine triphosphate (ATP) are synthesized.

Hypertrophy may occur as the result of normal physiologic or abnormal pathologic conditions. The increase in muscle mass associated with exercise is an example of physiologic hypertrophy. Pathologic hypertrophy occurs as the result of disease conditions and may be adaptive or compensatory. Examples of adaptive hypertrophy are the thickening of the urinary bladder from long-continued obstruction of urinary outflow and the myocardial hypertrophy that results from valvular heart disease or hypertension. Compensatory hypertrophy is the enlargement of a remaining organ or tissue after a portion has been surgically removed or rendered inactive. For instance, if one kidney is removed, the remaining kidney enlarges to compensate for the loss.

The initiating signals for hypertrophy appear to be complex and related to ATP depletion, mechanical forces such as stretching of the muscle fibers, activation of cell degradation products, and hormonal factors. In the case of the heart, initiating signals can be divided into two broad categories: (1) biomechanical and stretch-sensitive mechanisms; and (2) neurohumoral mechanisms that are associated with the release of hormones, growth factors, cytokines, and chemokines.[4] Internal stretch-sensitive receptors for the biochemical signals and an array of membrane-bound receptors for the specific neurohumoral ligands, such as IGF-1 and epidermal growth factor (EGF), activate specific signal transduction pathways. These pathways control myocardial growth by altering gene expression to increase protein synthesis and reduce protein degradation, thereby causing hypertrophic enlargement of the heart. A limit is eventually reached beyond which further enlargement of the tissue mass can no longer compensate for the increased work demands. The limiting factors for continued hypertrophy might be related to limitations in blood flow. In hypertension, for example, the increased workload required to pump blood against an elevated arterial pressure results in a progressive increase in left ventricular muscle mass and need for coronary blood flow (Fig. 5-2).

There continues to be interest in the signaling pathways that control the arrangement of contractile elements in myocardial hypertrophy. Research suggests that certain signal molecules can alter gene expression controlling the size and assembly of the contractile proteins in hypertrophied myocardial cells. For example, the hypertrophied myocardial cells of well-trained athletes have proportional increases in width and length. This is in contrast to the hypertrophy that develops in dilated cardiomyopathy, in which the hypertrophied cells have a relatively greater increase in length than width. In pressure overload, as occurs with hypertension, the hypertrophied cells have greater width than length.[5] It is anticipated that further elucidation of the

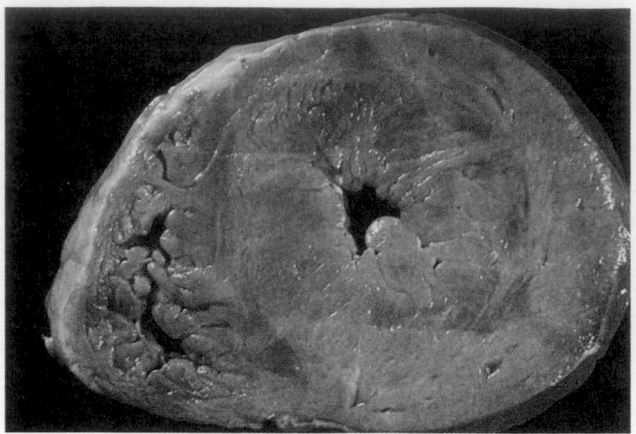

FIGURE 5-2 • Myocardial hypertrophy. Cross-section of the heart in a patient with long-standing hypertension. (From Strayer D. S., Rubin E. [2008]. Cell injury. In Rubin R., Strayer D. S. [Eds.], *Rubin's pathology: Clinicopathologic foundations of medicine* [5th ed., p. 5]. Philadelphia: Lippincott Williams & Wilkins.)

signal pathways that determine the adaptive and nonadaptive features of cardiac hypertrophy will lead to new targets for treatment.

Hyperplasia

Hyperplasia refers to an increase in the number of cells in an organ or tissue. It occurs in tissues with cells that are capable of mitotic division, such as the epidermis, intestinal epithelium, and glandular tissue. Certain cells, such as neurons, rarely divide and therefore have little capacity, if any, for hyperplastic growth. There is evidence that hyperplasia involves activation of genes controlling cell proliferation and the presence of intracellular messengers that control cell replication and growth. As with other normal adaptive cellular responses, hyperplasia is a controlled process that occurs in response to an appropriate stimulus and ceases after the stimulus has been removed.

The stimuli that induce hyperplasia may be physiologic or nonphysiologic. There are two common types of physiologic hyperplasia: hormonal and compensatory. Breast and uterine enlargements during pregnancy are examples of a physiologic hyperplasia that results from estrogen stimulation. The regeneration of the liver that occurs after partial hepatectomy (*i.e.,* partial removal of the liver) is an example of compensatory hyperplasia. Hyperplasia is also an important response of connective tissue in wound healing, during which proliferating fibroblasts and blood vessels contribute to wound repair. Although hypertrophy and hyperplasia are two distinct processes, they may occur together and are often triggered by the same mechanism.[1] For example, the pregnant uterus undergoes both hypertrophy and hyperplasia as the result of estrogen stimulation.

Most forms of nonphysiologic hyperplasia are due to excessive hormonal stimulation or the effects of growth factors on target tissues.[2] Excessive estrogen production can cause endometrial hyperplasia and abnormal menstrual bleeding (see Chapter 46). Benign prostatic hyperplasia, which is a common disorder of men older than 50 years of age, is thought to be related to the action of androgens (see Chapter 44). Skin warts are an example of hyperplasia caused by growth factors produced by certain viruses, such as the papillomaviruses.

Metaplasia

Metaplasia represents a reversible change in which one adult cell type (epithelial or mesenchymal) is replaced by another adult cell type. Metaplasia is thought to involve the reprogramming of undifferentiated stem cells that are present in the tissue undergoing the metaplastic changes.

Metaplasia usually occurs in response to chronic irritation and inflammation and allows for substitution of cells that are better able to survive under circumstances in which a more fragile cell type might succumb. However, the conversion of cell types never oversteps the boundaries of the primary tissue type (*e.g.,* one type of epithelial cell may be converted to another type of epithelial cell, but not to a connective tissue cell). An example of metaplasia is the adaptive substitution of stratified squamous epithelial cells for the ciliated columnar epithelial cells in the trachea and large airways of a habitual cigarette smoker. Although the squamous epithelium is better able to survive in these situations, the protective function that the ciliated epithelium provides for the respiratory tract is lost. Also, continued exposure to the influences that cause metaplasia may predispose to cancerous transformation of the metaplastic epithelium.

Dysplasia

Dysplasia is characterized by deranged cell growth of a specific tissue that results in cells that vary in size, shape, and organization. Minor degrees of dysplasia are associated with chronic irritation or inflammation. The pattern is most frequently encountered in areas of metaplastic squamous epithelium of the respiratory tract and uterine cervix. Although dysplasia is abnormal, it is adaptive in that it is potentially reversible after the irritating cause has been removed. Dysplasia is strongly implicated as a precursor of cancer. In cancers of the respiratory tract and the uterine cervix, dysplastic changes have been found adjacent to the foci of cancerous transformation. Through the use of the Papanicolaou (Pap) smear, it has been documented that cancer of the uterine cervix develops in a series of incremental epithelial changes ranging from severe dysplasia to invasive cancer. However, dysplasia is an adaptive process and as such does not necessarily lead to cancer. In many cases, the dysplastic cells revert to their former structure and function.

Intracellular Accumulations

Intracellular accumulations represent the buildup of substances that cells cannot immediately use or eliminate. The substances may accumulate in the cytoplasm (frequently in the lysosomes) or in the nucleus. In some cases the accumulation may be an abnormal substance that the cell has pro-

duced, and in other cases the cell may be storing exogenous materials or products of pathologic processes occurring elsewhere in the body. These substances can be grouped into three categories: (1) normal body substances, such as lipids, proteins, carbohydrates, melanin, and bilirubin, that are present in abnormally large amounts; (2) abnormal endogenous products, such as those resulting from inborn errors of metabolism; and (3) exogenous products, such as environmental agents and pigments that cannot be broken down by the cell.[2] These substances may accumulate transiently or permanently, and they may be harmless or, in some cases, toxic.

The accumulation of normal cellular constituents occurs when a substance is produced at a rate that exceeds its metabolism or removal. An example of this type of process is fatty changes in the liver due to intracellular accumulation of triglycerides. Liver cells normally contain some fat, which is either oxidized and used for energy or converted to triglycerides. This fat is derived from free fatty acids released from adipose tissue. Abnormal accumulation occurs when the delivery of free fatty acids to the liver is increased, as in starvation and diabetes mellitus, or when the intrahepatic metabolism of lipids is disturbed, as in alcoholism.

Intracellular accumulation can result from genetic disorders that disrupt the metabolism of selected substances. A normal enzyme may be replaced with an abnormal one, resulting in the formation of a substance that cannot be used or eliminated from the cell, or an enzyme may be missing, so that an intermediate product accumulates in the cell. For example, there are at least 10 genetic disorders that affect glycogen metabolism, most of which lead to the accumulation of intracellular glycogen stores. In the most common form of this disorder, von Gierke disease, large amounts of glycogen accumulate in the liver and kidneys because of a deficiency of the enzyme glucose-6-phosphatase. Without this enzyme, glycogen cannot be broken down to form glucose. The disorder leads not only to an accumulation of glycogen but to a reduction in blood glucose levels. In Tay-Sachs disease, another genetic disorder, abnormal lipids accumulate in the brain and other tissues, causing motor and mental deterioration beginning at approximately 6 months of age, followed by death at 2 to 5 years of age. In a similar manner, other enzyme defects lead to the accumulation of other substances.

Pigments are colored substances that may accumulate in cells. They can be endogenous (*i.e.,* arising from within the body) or exogenous (*i.e.,* arising from outside the body). Icterus, also called *jaundice,* is characterized by a yellow discoloration of tissue due to the retention of bilirubin, an endogenous bile pigment. This condition may result from increased bilirubin production from red blood cell destruction, obstruction of bile passage into the intestine, or toxic diseases that affect the liver's ability to remove bilirubin from the blood. Lipofuscin is a yellow-brown pigment that results from the accumulation of the indigestible residues produced during normal turnover of cell structures (Fig. 5-3). The accumulation of lipofuscin increases with age and is sometimes referred to as the *wear-and-tear pigment.* It is more common in heart, nerve, and liver cells than

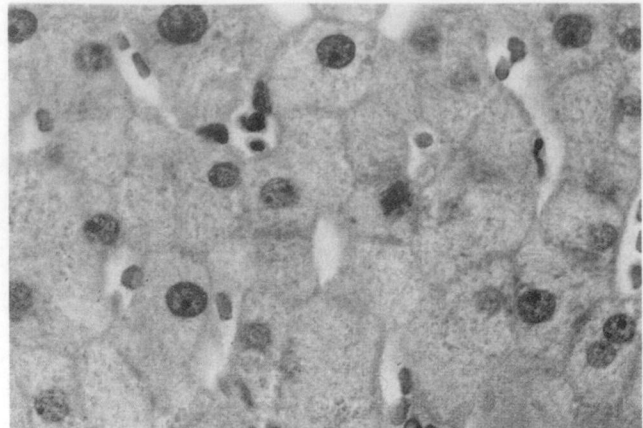

FIGURE 5-3 • Accumulation of intracellular lipofuscin. A photomicrograph of the liver of an 80-year-old man shows golden cytoplasmic granules, which represent lysosomal storage of lipofuscin. (From Rubin E., Farber J. L. [Eds.]. [1999]. *Pathology* [3rd ed., p. 13]. Philadelphia: Lippincott Williams & Wilkins.)

other tissues and is seen more often in conditions associated with atrophy of an organ.

One of the most common exogenous pigments is carbon in the form of coal dust. In coal miners or persons exposed to heavily polluted environments, the accumulation of carbon dust blackens the lung tissue and may cause serious lung disease. The formation of a blue lead line along the margins of the gum is one of the diagnostic features of lead poisoning. Tattoos are the result of insoluble pigments introduced into the skin, where they are engulfed by macrophages and persist for a lifetime.

The significance of intracellular accumulations depends on the cause and severity of the condition. Many accumulations, such as lipofuscin and mild fatty change, have no effect on cell function. Some conditions, such as the hyperbilirubinemia that causes jaundice, are reversible. Other disorders, such as glycogen storage diseases, produce accumulations that result in organ dysfunction and other alterations in physiologic function.

Pathologic Calcifications

Pathologic calcification involves the abnormal tissue deposition of calcium salts, together with smaller amounts of iron, magnesium, and other minerals. It is known as *dystrophic calcification* when it occurs in dead or dying tissue and as *metastatic calcification* when it occurs in normal tissue.

Dystrophic Calcification

Dystrophic calcification represents the macroscopic deposition of calcium salts in injured tissue. It is often visible to the naked eye as deposits that range from gritty, sandlike grains to firm, hard rock material. The pathogenesis of dystrophic calcification involves the intracellular or extracellular formation of crystalline calcium phosphate. The components of the calcium deposits are derived from the bodies of dead or dying cells as well as from the circulation and interstitial fluid.

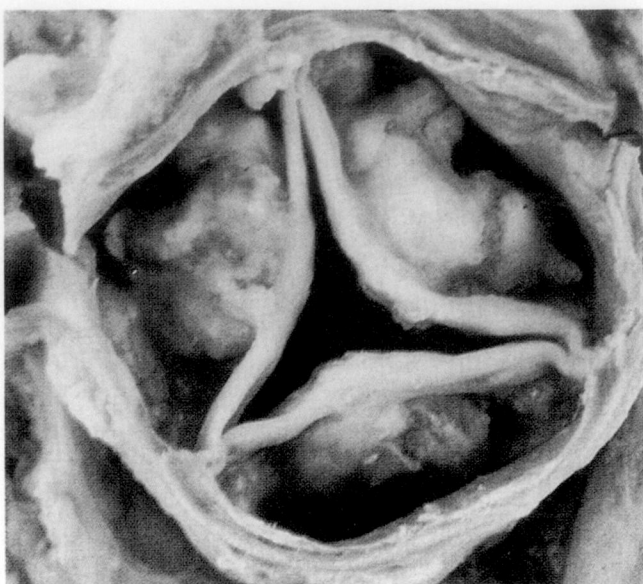

FIGURE 5-4 • Calcific aortic stenosis. Large deposits of calcium salts are evident in the cusps and free margins of the thickened aortic valve as viewed from above. (From Strayer D. S., Rubin E. [2008]. Cell injury. In Rubin R., Strayer D. S. [Eds.], *Rubin's pathology: Clinicopathologic foundations of medicine* [5th ed., p. 8]. Philadelphia: Lippincott Williams & Wilkins.)

Dystrophic calcification is commonly seen in atheromatous lesions of advanced atherosclerosis, areas of injury in the aorta and large blood vessels, and damaged heart valves. Although the presence of calcification may only indicate the presence of previous cell injury, as in healed tuberculosis lesions, it is also a frequent cause of organ dysfunction. For example, calcification of the aortic valve is a frequent cause of aortic stenosis in the elderly (Fig. 5-4).

Metastatic Calcification

In contrast to dystrophic calcification, which occurs in injured tissues, metastatic calcification occurs in normal tissues as the result of increased serum calcium levels (hypercalcemia). Almost any condition that increases the serum calcium level can lead to calcification in inappropriate sites such as the lung, renal tubules, and blood vessels. The major causes of hypercalcemia are hyperparathyroidism, either primary or secondary to phosphate retention in renal failure; increased mobilization of calcium from bone as in Paget disease, cancer with metastatic bone lesions, or immobilization; and vitamin D intoxication.

IN SUMMARY, cells adapt to changes in their environment and in their work demands by changing their size, number, and characteristics. These adaptive changes are consistent with the needs of the cell and occur in response to an appropriate stimulus. The changes are usually reversed after the stimulus has been withdrawn.

When confronted with a decrease in work demands or adverse environmental conditions, cells atrophy or reduce their size and revert to a lower and more efficient level of functioning. Hypertrophy results from an increase in work demands and is characterized by an increase in tissue size brought about by an increase in cell size and functional intracellular components. An increase in the number of cells in an organ or tissue that is still capable of mitotic division is called *hyperplasia.* Metaplasia occurs in response to chronic irritation and represents the substitution of cells of a type that is better able to survive under circumstances in which a more fragile cell type might succumb. Dysplasia is characterized by deranged cell growth of a specific tissue that results in cells that vary in size, shape, and appearance. It is often a precursor of cancer.

Under some circumstances, cells may accumulate abnormal amounts of various substances. If the accumulation reflects a correctable systemic disorder, such as the hyperbilirubinemia that causes jaundice, the accumulation is reversible. If the disorder cannot be corrected, as often occurs in many inborn errors of metabolism, the cells become overloaded, causing cell injury and death.

Pathologic calcification involves the abnormal tissue deposition of calcium salts. Dystrophic calcification occurs in dead or dying tissue. Although the presence of dystrophic calcification may only indicate the presence of previous cell injury, it is also a frequent cause of organ dysfunction (*e.q.,* when it affects the heart valves). Metastatic calcification occurs in normal tissues as the result of elevated serum calcium levels. Almost any condition that increases the serum calcium level can lead to calcification in inappropriate sites such as the lung, renal tubules, and blood vessels. ■

CELL INJURY AND DEATH

After completing this section of the chapter, you should be able to meet the following objectives:

- Describe the mechanisms whereby physical agents such as blunt trauma, electrical forces, and extremes of temperature produce cell injury.
- Differentiate between the effects of ionizing and nonionizing radiation in terms of their ability to cause cell injury.
- Explain how the injurious effects of biologic agents differ from those produced by physical and chemical agents.
- State the mechanisms and manifestations of cell injury associated with lead poisoning.
- Identify the causes and outcomes of mercury toxicity.
- State how nutritional imbalances contribute to cell injury.

- Describe three types of reversible cell changes that can occur with cell injury.
- Define *free radical* and *reactive oxygen species.*
- Relate free radical formation and oxidative stress to cell injury and death.
- Describe cell changes that occur with ischemic and hypoxic cell injury.
- Relate the effects of impaired calcium homeostasis to cell injury and death.
- Differentiate cell death associated with necrosis and apoptosis.
- Cite the reasons for the changes that occur with the wet and dry forms of gangrene.

Cells can be injured in many ways. The extent to which any injurious agent can cause cell injury and death depends in large measure on the intensity and duration of the injury and the type of cell that is involved. Cell injury is usually reversible up to a certain point, after which irreversible cell injury and death occur. Whether a specific stress causes irreversible or reversible cell injury depends on the severity of the insult and on variables such as blood supply, nutritional status, and regenerative capacity. Cell injury and death are ongoing processes, and in the healthy state, they are balanced by cell renewal.

CELL INJURY

- Cells can be damaged in a number of ways, including physical trauma, extremes of temperature, electrical injury, exposure to damaging chemicals, radiation damage, injury from biologic agents, and nutritional factors.
- Most injurious agents exert their damaging effects through uncontrolled free radical production, impaired oxygen delivery or utilization, or the destructive effects of uncontrolled intracellular calcium release.
- Cell injury can be reversible, allowing the cell to recover, or it can be irreversible, causing cell death and necrosis.
- In contrast to necrosis, which results from tissue injury, apoptosis is a normal physiologic process designed to remove injured or worn-out cells.

Causes of Cell Injury

Cell damage can occur in many ways. For purposes of discussion, the ways by which cells are injured have been grouped into five categories: (1) injury from physical agents, (2) radiation injury, (3) chemical injury, (4) injury from biologic agents, and (5) injury from nutritional imbalances.

Injury From Physical Agents

Physical agents responsible for cell and tissue injury include mechanical forces, extremes of temperature, and electrical forces. They are common causes of injuries due to environmental exposure, occupational and transportation accidents, and physical violence and assault.

Mechanical Forces.   Injury or trauma due to mechanical forces occurs as the result of body impact with another object. The body or the mass can be in motion or, as sometimes happens, both can be in motion at the time of impact. These types of injuries split and tear tissue, fracture bones, injure blood vessels, and disrupt blood flow.

Extremes of Temperature.   Extremes of heat and cold cause damage to the cell, its organelles, and its enzyme systems. Exposure to low-intensity heat (43° to 46°C), such as occurs with partial-thickness burns and severe heat stroke, causes cell injury by inducing vascular injury, accelerating cell metabolism, inactivating temperature-sensitive enzymes, and disrupting the cell membrane. With more intense heat, coagulation of blood vessels and tissue proteins occurs. Exposure to cold increases blood viscosity and induces vasoconstriction by direct action on blood vessels and through reflex activity of the sympathetic nervous system. The resultant decrease in blood flow may lead to hypoxic tissue injury, depending on the degree and duration of cold exposure. Injury from freezing probably results from a combination of ice crystal formation and vasoconstriction. The decreased blood flow leads to capillary stasis and arteriolar and capillary thrombosis. Edema results from increased capillary permeability.

Electrical Injuries.   Electrical injuries can affect the body through extensive tissue injury and disruption of neural and cardiac impulses. The effect of electricity on the body is mainly determined by its voltage, the type of current (*i.e.,* direct or alternating), its amperage, the resistance of the intervening tissue, the pathway of the current, and the duration of exposure.[6]

Lightning and high-voltage wires that carry several thousand volts produce the most severe damage.[2] Alternating current (AC) is usually more dangerous than direct current (DC) because it causes violent muscle contractions, preventing the person from releasing the electrical source and sometimes resulting in fractures and dislocations. In electrical injuries, the body acts as a conductor of the electrical current. The current enters the body from an electrical source, such as an exposed wire, and passes through the body and exits to another conductor, such as the moisture on the ground or a piece of metal the person is holding. The pathway that a current takes is critical because the electrical energy disrupts impulses in excitable tissues. Current flow through the brain may interrupt impulses from respiratory centers in the brain stem, and current flow through the chest may cause fatal cardiac arrhythmias.

The resistance to the flow of current in electrical circuits transforms electrical energy into heat. This is why the elements in electrical heating devices are made of highly resistive metals. Much of the tissue damage produced by electrical injuries is caused by heat production in tissues that have the highest electrical resistance. Resistance to electrical current varies from the greatest to the least in bone, fat, tendons, skin, muscles, blood, and nerves. The most severe tissue injury usually occurs at the skin sites where the current enters and leaves the body (Fig. 5-5). After electricity has penetrated the skin, it passes rapidly through the body along the lines of least resistance—through body fluids and nerves. Degeneration of vessel walls may occur, and thrombi may form as current flows along the blood vessels. This can cause extensive muscle and deep tissue injury. Thick, dry skin is more resistant to the flow of electricity than thin, wet skin. It is generally believed that the greater the skin resistance, the greater is the amount of local skin burn, and the less the resistance, the greater are the deep and systemic effects.

Radiation Injury

Electromagnetic radiation comprises a wide spectrum of wave-propagated energy, ranging from ionizing gamma rays to radiofrequency waves (Fig. 5-6). A photon is a particle of radiation energy. Radiation energy above the ultraviolet (UV) range is called *ionizing radiation* because the photons have enough energy to knock electrons off atoms and molecules. *Nonionizing radiation* refers to radiation energy at frequencies below those of visible light. *UV radiation* represents the portion of the spectrum of electromagnetic radiation just above the visible range. It contains increasingly energetic rays that are powerful enough to disrupt intracellular bonds and cause sunburn.

Ionizing Radiation.   Ionizing radiation affects cells by causing ionization of molecules and atoms in the cell, by directly

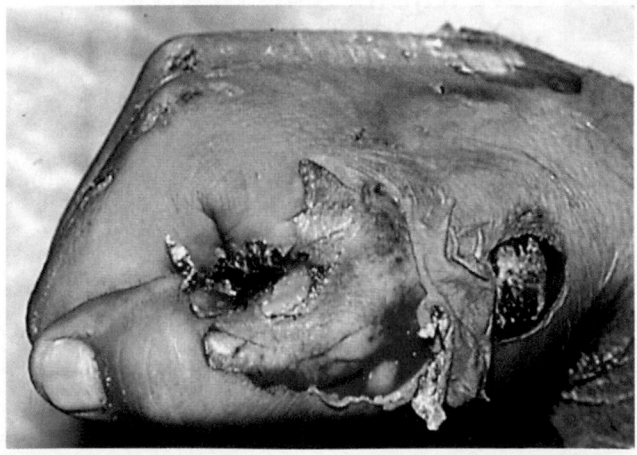

FIGURE 5-5 • Electrical burn of the skin. The victim was electrocuted after attempting to stop a fall from a ladder by grasping a high-voltage line. (From Strayer D. S., Rubin E. [2008]. Environmental and nutritional pathology. In Rubin R., Strayer D. S. [Eds.], *Rubin's pathology: Clinicopathologic foundations of medicine* [5th ed., p. 272]. Philadelphia: Lippincott Williams & Wilkins.)

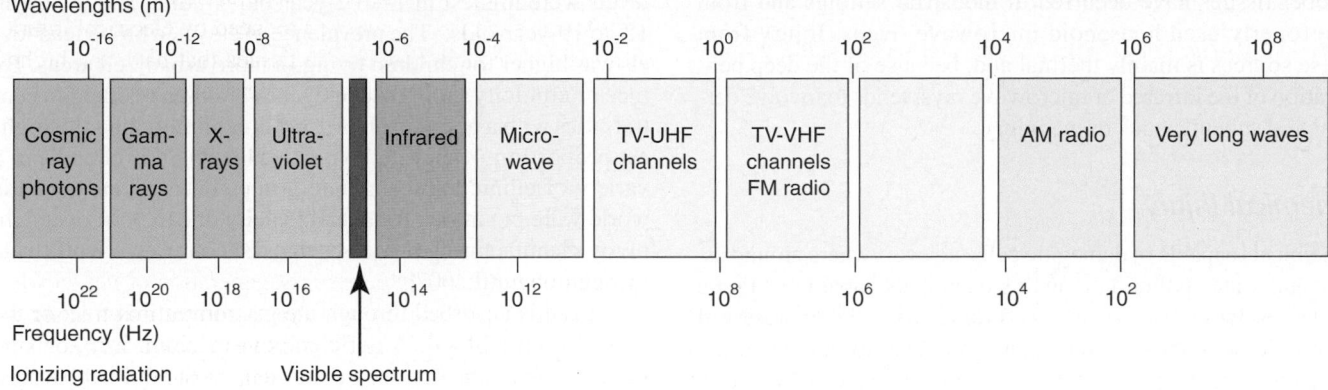

FIGURE 5-6 • Spectrum of electromagnetic radiation.

hitting the target molecules in the cell, or by producing free radicals that interact with critical cell components.[1,2,7] It can immediately kill cells, interrupt cell replication, or cause a variety of genetic mutations, which may or may not be lethal. Most radiation injury is caused by localized irradiation that is used in the treatment of cancer (see Chapter 8). Except for unusual circumstances such as the use of high-dose irradiation that precedes bone marrow transplantation, exposure to whole-body irradiation is rare.

The injurious effects of ionizing radiation vary with the dose, dose rate (a single dose can cause greater injury than divided or fractionated doses), and the differential sensitivity of the exposed tissue to radiation injury. Because of the effect on deoxyribonucleic acid (DNA) synthesis and interference with mitosis, rapidly dividing cells of the bone marrow and intestine are much more vulnerable to radiation injury than tissues such as bone and skeletal muscle. Over time, occupational and accidental exposure to ionizing radiation can result in increased risk for the development of various types of cancers, including skin cancers, leukemia, osteogenic sarcomas, and lung cancer.

Many of the clinical manifestations of radiation injury result from acute cell injury, dose-dependent changes in the blood vessels that supply the irradiated tissues, and fibrotic tissue replacement. The cell's initial response to radiation injury involves swelling, disruption of the mitochondria and other organelles, alterations in the cell membrane, and marked changes in the nucleus. The endothelial cells in blood vessels are particularly sensitive to irradiation. During the immediate postirradiation period, only vessel dilatation is apparent (*e.g.*, the initial erythema of the skin after radiation therapy). Later or with higher levels of radiation, destructive changes occur in small blood vessels such as the capillaries and venules. Acute reversible necrosis is represented by such disorders as radiation cystitis, dermatitis, and diarrhea from enteritis. More persistent damage can be attributed to acute necrosis of tissue cells that are not capable of regeneration and chronic ischemia. Chronic effects of radiation damage are characterized by fibrosis and scarring of tissues and organs in the irradiated area

(*e.g.*, interstitial fibrosis of the heart and lungs after irradiation of the chest). Because the radiation delivered in radiation therapy inevitably travels through the skin, radiation dermatitis is common. There may be necrosis of the skin, impaired wound healing, and chronic radiation dermatitis.

Ultraviolet Radiation. Ultraviolet radiation causes sunburn and increases the risk of skin cancers (see Chapter 61). The degree of risk depends on the type of UV rays, the intensity of exposure, and the amount of protective melanin pigment in the skin. Skin damage produced by UV radiation is thought to be caused by reactive oxygen species and by damage to melanin-producing processes in the skin. UV radiation also damages DNA, resulting in the formation of pyrimidine dimers (*i.e.*, the insertion of two identical pyrimidine bases into replicating DNA instead of one). Other forms of DNA damage include the production of single-stranded breaks and formation of DNA–protein cross-links. Normally, errors that occur during DNA replication are repaired by enzymes that remove the faulty section of DNA and repair the damage. The importance of DNA repair in protecting against UV radiation injury is evidenced by the vulnerability of persons who lack the enzymes needed to repair UV-induced DNA damage. In a genetic disorder called *xeroderma pigmentosum*, an enzyme needed to repair sunlight-induced DNA damage is lacking. This autosomal recessive disorder is characterized by extreme photosensitivity and a 2000-fold increased risk of skin cancer in sun-exposed skin.[2]

Nonionizing Radiation. Nonionizing radiation includes infrared light, ultrasound, microwaves, and laser energy. Unlike ionizing radiation, which can directly break chemical bonds, nonionizing radiation exerts its effects by causing vibration and rotation of atoms and molecules. All of this vibrational and rotational energy is eventually converted to thermal energy. Low-frequency nonionizing radiation is used widely in radar, television, industrial operations (*e.g.*, heating, welding, melting of metals, processing of wood and plastic), household appliances (*e.g.*, microwave ovens), and medical applications (*e.g.*, diathermy). Isolated cases of skin burns and thermal injury to deeper tissues have occurred in industrial settings and from improperly used household microwave ovens. Injury from these sources is mainly thermal and, because of the deep penetration of the infrared or microwave rays, tends to involve dermal and subcutaneous tissue injury.

Chemical Injury

Chemicals capable of damaging cells are everywhere around us. Air and water pollution contains chemicals capable of tissue injury, as does tobacco smoke and some processed or preserved foods. Some of the most damaging chemicals exist in our environment, including gases such as carbon monoxide, insecticides, and trace metals such as lead.

Chemical agents can injure the cell membrane and other cell structures, block enzymatic pathways, coagulate cell proteins, and disrupt the osmotic and ionic balance of the cell. Corrosive substances such as strong acids and bases destroy cells as the substances come into contact with the body. Other chemicals may injure cells in the process of metabolism or elimination. Carbon tetrachloride (CCl_4), for example, causes little damage until it is metabolized by liver enzymes to a highly reactive free radical (CCl_3·). Carbon tetrachloride is extremely toxic to liver cells.

Drugs. Many drugs—alcohol, prescription drugs, over-the-counter drugs, and street drugs—are capable of directly or indirectly damaging tissues. Ethyl alcohol can harm the gastric mucosa, liver (see Chapter 37), developing fetus (see Chapter 7), and other organs. Antineoplastic (anticancer) and immunosuppressant drugs can directly injure cells. Other drugs produce metabolic end-products that are toxic to cells. Acetaminophen, a commonly used over-the-counter analgesic drug, is detoxified in the liver, where small amounts of the drug are converted to a highly toxic metabolite. This metabolite is detoxified by a metabolic pathway that uses a substance (*i.e.,* glutathione) normally present in the liver. When large amounts of the drug are ingested, this pathway becomes overwhelmed and toxic metabolites accumulate, causing massive liver necrosis.

Lead Toxicity. Lead is a particularly toxic metal. Small amounts accumulate to reach toxic levels. There are innumerable sources of lead in the environment, including flaking paint, lead-contaminated dust and soil, lead-contaminated root vegetables, lead water pipes or soldered joints, pottery glazes, newsprint, and toys made in foreign countries. Adults often encounter lead through occupational exposure. Lead and other metal smelters, miners, welders, storage battery workers, and pottery makers are particularly at risk.[1,8] Children are exposed to lead through ingestion of peeling lead paint, by breathing dust from lead paint (*e.g.,* during remodeling), or from playing in contaminated soil. There has been a substantial decline in blood lead levels of the entire population since the removal of lead from gasoline and from soldered food cans.[9] High lead blood levels continue to be a problem, however, particularly among children. In the Third National Health and Nutrition Examination Survey (NHANES III, 1988 to 1991), blood lead levels were highest in 1- to 2-year-old children and lowest in 12- to 19-year-olds.[9] The prevalence of elevated blood lead levels was higher for children living in more urbanized areas. By race or ethnicity, non-Hispanic black children residing in central cities with a population of 1 million or more had the highest proportion of elevated blood lead levels. Children from a variety of ethnic and economic groups in many areas of the world were put at risk for a lead toxicity due to poor oversight of toy manufacturing processes that did not receive worldwide recognition until 2007.[10]

Lead is absorbed through the gastrointestinal tract or the lungs into the blood. A deficiency in calcium, iron, or zinc increases lead absorption. In children, most lead is absorbed through the lungs. Although children may have the same or a lower intake of lead, the absorption in infants and children is greater; thus, they are more vulnerable to lead toxicity.[2] Lead crosses the placenta, exposing the fetus to levels of lead that are comparable with those of the mother. Lead is stored in bone and eliminated by the kidneys. Approximately 85% of absorbed lead is stored in bone (and teeth of young children), 5% to 10% remains in the blood, and the remainder accumulates in soft tissue deposits. Although the half-life of lead is hours to days, bone deposits serve as a repository from which blood levels are maintained. In a sense, bone protects other tissues, but the slow turnover maintains blood levels for months to years.

The toxicity of lead is related to its multiple biochemical effects.[2] It has the ability to inactivate enzymes, compete with calcium for incorporation into bone, and interfere with nerve transmission and brain development. The major targets of lead toxicity are the red blood cells, the gastrointestinal tract, the kidneys, and the nervous system.

Anemia is a cardinal sign of lead toxicity. Lead competes with the enzymes required for hemoglobin synthesis and with the membrane-associated enzymes that prevent hemolysis of red blood cells. The resulting red cells are coarsely stippled and hypochromic, resembling those seen in iron-deficiency anemia. The life span of the red cell is also decreased. The gastrointestinal tract is the main source of symptoms in the adult. This is characterized by "lead colic," a severe and poorly localized form of acute abdominal pain. A lead line formed by precipitated lead sulfite may appear along the gingival margins. The lead line is seldom seen in children. The kidneys are the major route for excretion of lead. Lead can cause diffuse kidney damage, eventually leading to renal failure. Even without overt signs of kidney damage, lead toxicity leads to hypertension.

In the nervous system, lead toxicity is characterized by demyelination of cerebral and cerebellar white matter and death of cortical cells. When this occurs in early childhood, it can affect neurobehavioral development and result in lower IQ levels and poorer classroom performance.[11] Peripheral demyelinating neuropathy may occur in adults. The most serious manifestation of lead poisoning is acute encephalopathy. It is manifested by persistent vomiting, ataxia, seizures, papilledema, impaired consciousness, and coma. Acute encephalopathy may manifest suddenly, or it may be preceded by other signs of lead toxicity such as behavioral changes or abdominal complaints.

Because of the long-term neurobehavioral and cognitive deficits that occur in children with even moderately elevated lead levels, the Centers for Disease Control and Prevention and the American Academy of Pediatrics have issued recommendations for childhood lead screening.[12–14] A safe blood level of lead is still uncertain. At one time, 25 µg/dL was considered safe. Surveys have shown abnormally low IQs in children with levels as low as 10 to 15 µg/dL; in 1991, the safe level was lowered to 10 µg/dL.[15] Recent research suggests that even levels below 10 µg/dL are associated with declines in children's IQ at 3 to 5 years of age.[16]

Screening for lead toxicity involves use of capillary blood obtained from a finger stick to measure free erythrocyte protoporphyrin (EP). Elevated levels of EP result from the inhibition by lead of the enzymes required for heme synthesis in red blood cells. The EP test is useful in detecting high lead levels but usually does not detect levels below 20 to 25 µg/dL. Thus, capillary screening test values greater than 10 µg/dL should be confirmed with those from a venous blood sample. This test also reflects the effects of iron deficiency, a condition that increases lead absorption.[15]

Because the symptoms of lead toxicity usually are vague, diagnosis is often delayed. Anemia may provide the first clues to the disorder. Laboratory tests are necessary to establish a diagnosis. Measurement of lead levels in venous blood is usually used. Treatment involves removal of the lead source and, in cases of severe toxicity, administration of a chelating agent. Asymptomatic children with blood levels of 45 to 69 µg/dL usually are treated. A public health team should evaluate the source of lead because meticulous removal is needed.

Mercury Toxicity. Mercury has been used for industrial and medical purposes for hundreds of years. Mercury is toxic, and the hazards of mercury-associated occupational and accidental exposures are well known. In recent times, the primary concern of the general public to the potential hazards of mercury has focused on exposure from eating certain fish, amalgams used in dentistry, and vaccines.[17] Mercury is toxic in four primary forms: mercury vapor, inorganic divalent mercury, methyl mercury, and ethyl mercury.[17] Depending on the form of mercury exposure, toxicity involving the central nervous system and kidney can occur.

In the case of dental fillings, the concern involves mercury vapor being released into the mouth. However, the amount of mercury vapor released from fillings is very small. There is no clear evidence supporting health risk from this type of exposure, and removal of amalgams may temporarily increase blood levels of mercury.[17] The main source of methyl mercury exposure is from consumption of long-lived fish, such as tuna and swordfish. Fish concentrate mercury from sediment in the water. Only certain types of fish pose potential risk, however, and types such as salmon have miniscule amounts or no mercury. Because the developing brain is more susceptible to mercury-induced damage, it is recommended that young children and pregnant and nursing women avoid consumption of fish known to contain high mercury content. Thimerosal is an ethyl mercury–containing preservative that helps prevent microorganism growth in vaccines. Concern about potential adverse effects have led to the making of single-dose vials that eliminate the need for thimerosal.[17] In the United States, most vaccines are either free of thimerosal or contain trace amounts.

Injury From Biologic Agents

Biologic agents differ from other injurious agents in that they are able to replicate and can continue to produce their injurious effects. These agents range from submicroscopic viruses to the larger parasites. Biologic agents injure cells by diverse mechanisms. Viruses enter the cell and become incorporated into its DNA synthetic machinery. Certain bacteria elaborate exotoxins that interfere with cellular production of ATP. Other bacteria, such as the gram-negative bacilli, release endotoxins that cause cell injury and increased capillary permeability.

Injury From Nutritional Imbalances

Nutritional excesses and nutritional deficiencies predispose cells to injury. Obesity and diets high in saturated fats are thought to predispose persons to atherosclerosis. The body requires more than 60 organic and inorganic substances in amounts ranging from micrograms to grams. These nutrients include minerals, vitamins, certain fatty acids, and specific amino acids. Dietary deficiencies can occur in the form of starvation, in which there is a deficiency of all nutrients and vitamins, or because of a selective deficiency of a single nutrient or vitamin. Iron-deficiency anemia, scurvy, beriberi, and pellagra are examples of injury caused by the lack of specific vitamins or minerals. The protein and calorie deficiencies that occur with starvation cause widespread tissue damage.

Mechanisms of Cell Injury

The mechanisms by which injurious agents cause cell injury and death are complex. Some agents, such as heat, produce direct cell injury; other factors, such as genetic derangements, produce their effects indirectly through metabolic disturbances and altered immune responses. There seem to be at least three major mechanisms whereby most injurious agents exert their effects: free radical formation, hypoxia and ATP depletion, and disruption of intracellular calcium homeostasis (Fig. 5-7).

Free Radical Injury

Many injurious agents exert damaging effects through reactive chemical species known as *free radicals*.[1,2,18–20] Free radicals are highly reactive chemical species with an unpaired electron in the outer orbit (valence shell) of the molecule. In the literature, the unpaired electron is denoted by a dot, for example ·NO. The unpaired electron causes free radicals to be unstable and highly reactive, so that they react nonspecifically with molecules in the vicinity. Moreover, free radicals can establish chain reactions consisting of many events that generate new

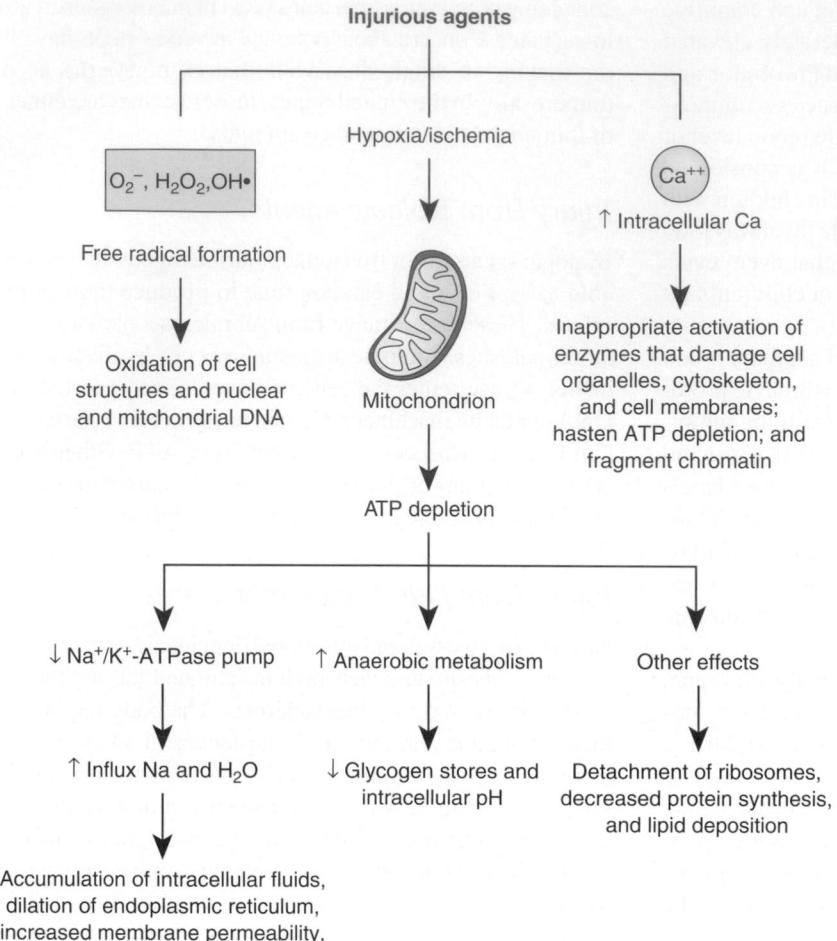

Injurious agents

$O_2^-, H_2O_2, OH\bullet$

Hypoxia/ischemia

Ca^{++}

↑ Intracellular Ca

Free radical formation

Oxidation of cell structures and nuclear and mitchondrial DNA

Mitochondrion

Inappropriate activation of enzymes that damage cell organelles, cytoskeleton, and cell membranes; hasten ATP depletion; and fragment chromatin

ATP depletion

↓ Na$^+$/K$^+$-ATPase pump

↑ Anaerobic metabolism

Other effects

↑ Influx Na and H$_2$O

↓ Glycogen stores and intracellular pH

Detachment of ribosomes, decreased protein synthesis, and lipid deposition

Accumulation of intracellular fluids, dilation of endoplasmic reticulum, increased membrane permeability, decreased mitochondrial function

FIGURE 5-7 • Mechanisms of cell injury.

free radicals. In cells and tissues, free radicals react with proteins, lipids, and carbohydrates, thereby damaging cell membranes; inactivate enzymes; and damage nucleic acids that make up DNA. The actions of free radicals may disrupt and damage cells and tissues.

Reactive oxygen species (ROS) are oxygen-containing molecules that include free radicals such as superoxide (O_2^-) and hydroxyl radical (OH·), and nonradicals such as hydrogen peroxide (H_2O_2). These molecules are produced endogenously by normal metabolic processes or cell activities, such as the metabolic burst that accompanies phagocytosis. However, exogenous causes, including ionizing and UV radiation, can cause ROS production in the body. *Oxidative stress* is a condition that occurs when the generation of ROS exceeds the ability of the body to neutralize and eliminate ROS. Oxidative stress can lead to oxidation of cell components, activation of signal transduction pathways, and changes in gene and protein expression. DNA modification and damage can occur as a result of oxidative stress. In addition to focusing on genomic DNA as a target of oxidative injury, current studies are investigating mitochondrial DNA as a target of oxidation and subsequent cause of mitochondrial dysfunction.[21] Although ROS and oxidative stress are clearly associated with cell and tissue

damage, recent evidence shows that ROS do not always act in a random and damaging manner. Current studies have found that ROS are also important signaling molecules that are used in healthy cells to regulate and maintain normal activities and functions such as vascular tone, insulin and vascular endothelial growth factor signaling, and even a preconditioning function to protect cells from injury due to high levels of ROS.[22]

Antioxidants are natural and synthetic molecules that inhibit the reactions of ROS with biologic structures or prevent the uncontrolled formation of ROS. Antioxidants include enzymatic and nonenzymatic compounds. Enzymes known to function as antioxidants include superoxide dismutase (SOD), catalase, glutathione peroxidase, and thioreductase. SOD forms hydrogen peroxide from superoxide. Catalase can catalyze the reaction that forms water from hydrogen peroxide. Nonenzymatic antioxidants include carotenes (*e.g.,* vitamin A), tocopherols (*e.g.,* vitamin E), ascorbate (vitamin C), glutathione, and flavonoids, as well as micronutrients such as selenium and zinc.[23] Nonenzymatic antioxidants often directly react with oxidants to "disarm" them. For example, vitamin C directly scavenges superoxide and hydroxyl radicals.[24]

Oxidative damage has been implicated in many diseases. Mutations in the gene for SOD are associated with amyotrophic lateral sclerosis (ALS; so-called Lou Gehrig disease).[25] Oxidative stress is thought to play an important role in the development of cancer.[26] Reestablishment of blood flow after loss of perfusion, as occurs during heart attack and stroke, is associated with oxidative injury to vital organs. The endothelial dysfunction that contributes to the development, progression, and prognosis of cardiovascular disease is thought to be caused in part by oxidative stress.[27] In addition to the many diseases and altered health conditions associated with oxidative damage, oxidative stress has been linked with the age-related functional declines that underlie the process of aging.[28]

Hypoxic Cell Injury

Hypoxia deprives the cell of oxygen and interrupts oxidative metabolism and the generation of ATP. The actual time necessary to produce irreversible cell damage depends on the degree of oxygen deprivation and the metabolic needs of the cell. Some cells, such as those in the heart, brain, and kidney, require large amounts of oxygen to provide energy to perform their functions. Brain cells, for example, begin to undergo permanent damage after 4 to 6 minutes of oxygen deprivation. A thin margin can exist between the time involved in reversible and irreversible cell damage. A classic study found that the epithelial cells of the proximal tubule of the kidney in the rat could survive 20 but not 30 minutes of ischemia.[29] Recent work has identified a group of proteins called *hypoxia-inducible factors* (HIFs). During hypoxic conditions, HIFs cause the expression of genes that stimulate red blood cell formation, manufacture glycolytic enzymes that produce ATP in the absence of oxygen, and increase angiogenesis[30] (*i.e.,* the formation of new blood vessels).

Hypoxia can result from an inadequate amount of oxygen in the air, respiratory disease, ischemia (*i.e.,* decreased blood flow due to vasoconstriction or vascular obstruction), anemia, edema, or inability of the cells to use oxygen. Ischemia is characterized by impaired oxygen delivery and impaired removal of metabolic end products such as lactic acid. In contrast to pure hypoxia, which depends on the oxygen content of the blood and affects all cells in the body, ischemia commonly affects blood flow through limited numbers of blood vessels and produces local tissue injury. In some cases of edema, the distance for diffusion of oxygen may become a limiting factor in the delivery of oxygen. In hypermetabolic states, cells may require more oxygen than can be supplied by normal respiratory function and oxygen transport. Hypoxia also serves as the ultimate cause of cell death in other injuries. For example, a physical agent such as cold temperature can cause severe vasoconstriction and impair blood flow.

Hypoxia causes a power failure in the cell, with widespread effects on the cell's structural and functional components. As oxygen tension in the cell falls, oxidative metabolism ceases and the cell reverts to anaerobic metabolism, using its limited glycogen stores in an attempt to maintain vital cell functions. Cellular pH falls as lactic acid accumulates in the cell. This reduction in pH can have adverse effects on intracellular structures and biochemical reactions. Low pH can alter cell membranes and cause chromatin clumping and cell shrinkage.

One important effect of reduced ATP is acute cell swelling caused by failure of the energy-dependent sodium/potassium (Na^+/K^+)-ATPase membrane pump, which extrudes sodium from and returns potassium to the cell. With impaired function of this pump, intracellular potassium levels decrease and sodium and water accumulate in the cell. The movement of water and ions into the cell is associated with dilation of the endoplasmic reticulum, increased membrane permeability, and decreased mitochondrial function.[2] To a point, the cellular changes due to ischemia are reversible if oxygenation is restored. If the oxygen supply is not restored, however, there is a continued loss of enzymes, proteins, and ribonucleic acid through the hyperpermeable cell membrane. Injury to the lysosomal membranes results in the leakage of destructive lysosomal enzymes into the cytoplasm and enzymatic digestion of cell components. Leakage of intracellular enzymes through the permeable cell membrane into the extracellular fluid provides an important clinical indicator of cell injury and death. These enzymes enter the blood and can be measured by laboratory tests.

Impaired Calcium Homeostasis

Calcium functions as an important second messenger and cytosolic signal for many cell responses. Various calcium-binding proteins, such as troponin and calmodulin, act as transducers for the cytosolic calcium signal. Calcium/calmodulin–dependent kinases indirectly mediate the effects of calcium on responses such as smooth muscle contraction and glycogen breakdown. Normally, intracellular calcium ion levels are kept extremely low compared with extracellular levels. These low intracellular levels are maintained by energy-dependent membrane-associated calcium/magnesium (Ca^{2+}/Mg^{2+})-ATPase exchange systems and sequestration of calcium ions within organelles[2] such as the mitochondria and smooth endoplasmic reticulum. Ischemia and certain toxins lead to an increase in cytosolic calcium because of increased influx across the cell membrane and the release of calcium from intracellular stores. The increased calcium level may inappropriately activate a number of enzymes with potentially damaging effects. These enzymes include the phospholipases, responsible for damaging the cell membrane; proteases that damage the cytoskeleton and membrane proteins; ATPases that break down ATP and hasten its depletion; and endonucleases that fragment chromatin. Although it is known that injured cells accumulate calcium, it is unknown whether this is the ultimate cause of irreversible cell injury.

Reversible Cell Injury and Cell Death

The mechanisms of cell injury can produce sublethal and reversible cellular damage or lead to irreversible injury with cell destruction or death (Fig. 5-8). Cell destruction and removal can involve one of two mechanisms: apoptosis, which is designed to remove injured or worn-out cells, or cell death or necrosis, which occurs in irreversibly damaged cells.

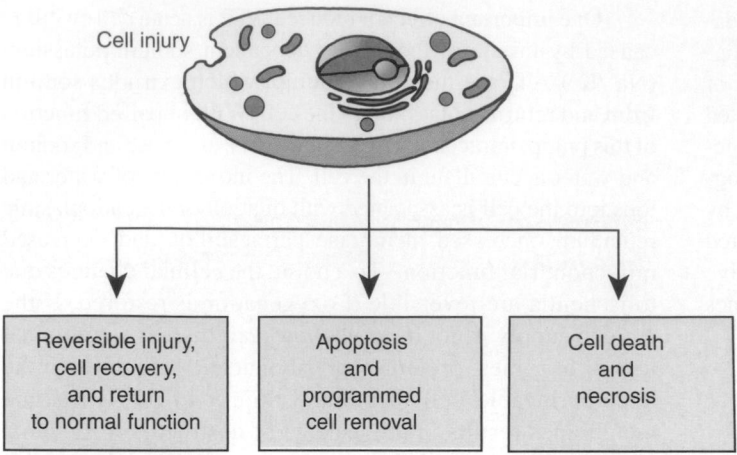

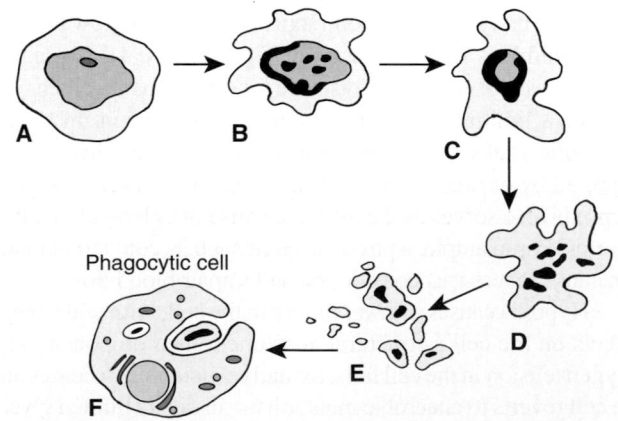

FIGURE 5-8 • Outcomes of cell injury: reversible cell injury, apoptosis and programmed cell removal, cell death and necrosis.

Reversible Cell Injury

Reversible cell injury, although impairing cell function, does not result in cell death. Two patterns of reversible cell injury can be observed under the microscope: cellular swelling and fatty change. Cellular swelling occurs with impairment of the energy-dependent Na^+/K^+-ATPase membrane pump, usually as the result of hypoxic cell injury.

Fatty changes are linked to intracellular accumulation of fat. When fatty changes occur, small vacuoles of fat disperse throughout the cytoplasm. The process is usually more ominous than cellular swelling, and although it is reversible, it usually indicates severe injury. These fatty changes may occur because normal cells are presented with an increased fat load or because injured cells are unable to metabolize the fat properly. In obese persons, fatty infiltrates often occur within and between the cells of the liver and heart because of an increased fat load. Pathways for fat metabolism may be impaired during cell injury, and fat may accumulate in the cell as production exceeds use and export. The liver, where most fats are synthesized and metabolized, is particularly susceptible to fatty change, but fatty changes may also occur in the kidney, the heart, and other organs.

Programmed Cell Death

In most normal nontumor cells, the number of cells in tissues is regulated by balancing cell proliferation and cell death. Cell death occurs by necrosis or a form of programmed cell death called *apoptosis.*

Apoptosis, from the Greek *apo* for "apart" and *ptosis* for "fallen," means "fallen apart." Apoptosis was discovered in 1972 and continues to be one of the most investigated processes in biologic and pathobiologic research.[31] Apoptosis is a highly selective process that eliminates injured and aged cells, thereby controlling tissue regeneration. Cells undergoing apoptosis have characteristic morphologic features as well as biochemical changes. As shown in Figure 5-9, shrinking and condensation of the nucleus and cytoplasm occur. The chromatin aggregates at the nuclear envelope, and DNA fragmentation occurs. Then,

the cell becomes fragmented into multiple apoptotic bodies in a manner that maintains the integrity of the plasma membrane and does not initiate inflammation. Changes in the plasma membrane induce phagocytosis of the apoptotic bodies by macrophages and other cells, thereby completing the degradation process.

Apoptosis is thought to be responsible for several normal physiologic processes, including the programmed destruction of cells during embryonic development, hormone-dependent involution of tissues, death of immune cells, cell death by cytotoxic T cells, and cell death in proliferating cell populations. During embryogenesis, in the development of a number of organs such as the heart, which begins as a pulsating tube and is gradually modified to become a four-chambered pump, apoptotic cell death allows for the next stage of organ development. It also separates the webbed fingers and toes of the developing embryo (Fig. 5-10). Apoptotic cell death occurs in the hormone-dependent involution of endometrial cells during the menstrual cycle and in the regression of breast tissue after weaning from breast-feeding. The control of immune cell numbers and

FIGURE 5-9 • Apoptotic cell removal: shrinking of the cell structures (**A**), condensation and fragmentation of the nuclear chromatin (**B** and **C**), separation of nuclear fragments and cytoplasmic organelles into apoptotic bodies (**D** and **E**), and engulfment of apoptotic fragments by phagocytic cell (**F**).

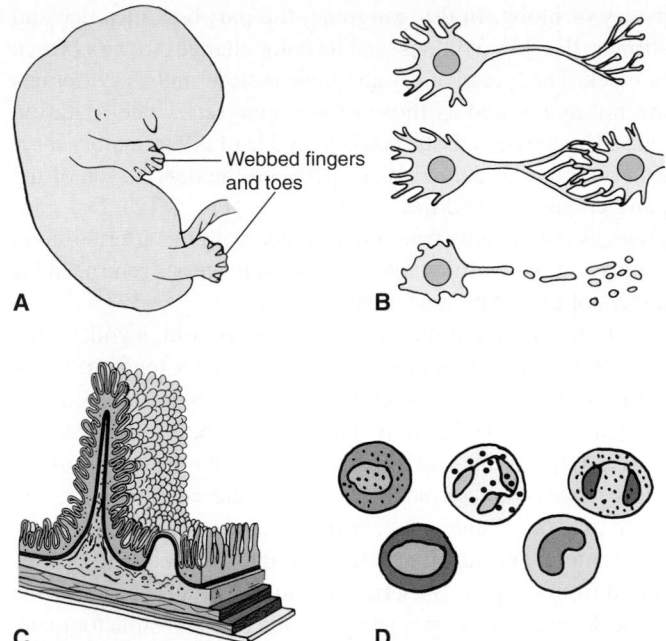

FIGURE 5-10 • Examples of apoptosis: **(A)** separation of webbed fingers and toes in embryo; **(B)** development of neural connections; neurons that do not establish synaptic connections and receive survival factors may be induced to undergo apoptosis; **(C)** removal of cells from intestinal villi; new epithelial cells continuously form in the crypt, migrate to the villus tip as they age, and undergo apoptosis at the tip at the end of their life span; and **(D)** removal of senescent blood cells.

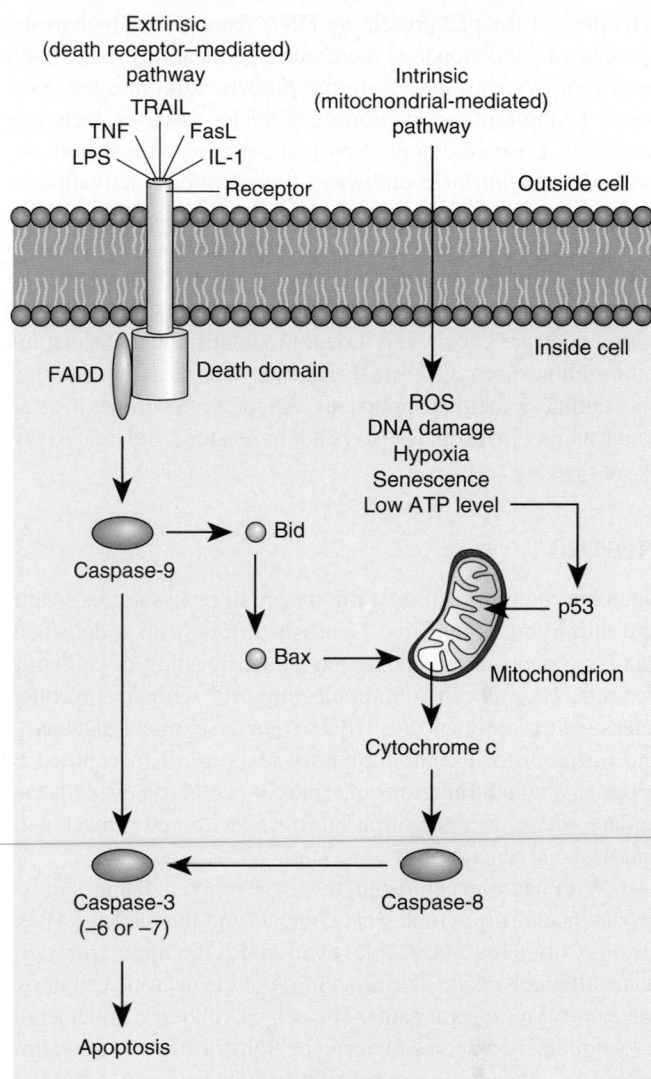

FIGURE 5-11 • Extrinsic and intrinsic pathways of apoptosis. The extrinsic pathway is activated by signals such as Fas ligand (FasL) that, on binding to the Fas receptor, form a death-inducing complex by joining the Fas-associated death domain (FADD) to the death domain of the Fas receptor. The intrinsic pathway is activated by signals, such as reactive oxygen species (ROS) and DNA damage, that induce the release of cytochrome c from mitochondria into the cytoplasm. Both pathways activate caspases to execute apoptosis.

destruction of autoreactive T cells in the thymus have been credited to apoptosis. Cytotoxic T cells and natural killer cells are thought to destroy target cells by inducing apoptotic cell death.

Apoptosis is linked to many pathologic processes and diseases. For example, interference with apoptosis is known to be a mechanism that contributes to carcinogenesis.[32] Apoptosis is also known to be involved in the cell death associated with viral infections, such as hepatitis B and C.[33,34] Apoptosis may also be implicated in neurodegenerative disorders such as Alzheimer disease, Parkinson disease, and ALS. However, the exact mechanisms involved in these diseases remain under investigation.

Two basic pathways for apoptosis have been described (Fig. 5-11). These are the extrinsic pathway, which is death receptor dependent, and the intrinsic pathway, which is death receptor independent. The execution phase of both pathways is carried out by proteolytic enzymes called *caspases,* which are present in the cell as *procaspases* and are activated by cleavage of an inhibitory portion of their polypeptide chain.

The *extrinsic pathway* involves the activation of receptors such as tumor necrosis factor (TNF) receptors and the Fas ligand receptor. Fas ligand may be expressed on the surface of certain cells such as cytotoxic T cells, or appear in a soluble form. When Fas ligand binds to its receptor, proteins congregate at the cytoplasmic end of the Fas receptor to form a death-initiating complex. The complex then converts procaspase-8 to

caspase-8. Caspase-8, in turn, activates a cascade of caspases that execute the process of apoptosis. The end result includes activation of endonucleases that cause fragmentation of DNA and cell death. In addition to TNF and Fas ligand, primary signaling molecules known to activate the extrinsic pathway include TNF-related apoptosis-inducing ligand (TRAIL); the cytokine interleukin-1 (IL-1); and lipopolysaccharide (LPS), the endotoxin found in the outer cell membrane of gram-negative bacteria.

The *intrinsic pathway,* or *mitochondrion-induced pathway,* of apoptosis is activated by conditions such as DNA damage, ROS, hypoxia, decreased ATP levels, cellular senescence, and activation of the p53 protein by DNA damage. It involves the opening of mitochondrial membrane permeability pores with release of cytochrome c from the mitochondria into the cytoplasm. Cytoplasmic cytochrome c activates caspases, including caspase-3. Caspase-3 activation is a common step to both the extrinsic and intrinsic pathways. Furthermore, activation or increased levels of proapoptotic proteins, such as Bid and Bax, after caspase-8 activation in the extrinsic pathway can lead to mitochondrial release of cytochrome c, thereby bridging the two pathways for apoptosis. Many inhibitors of apoptosis within cells are known and thought to contribute to cancer and autoimmune diseases.[35] The therapeutic actions of certain drugs may induce or facilitate apoptosis. Apoptosis continues to be an active area of investigation to better understand and treat a variety of diseases.

Necrosis

Necrosis refers to cell death in an organ or tissue that is still part of a living organism.[36] Necrosis differs from apoptosis in that it involves unregulated enzymatic digestion of cell components, loss of cell membrane integrity with uncontrolled release of the products of cell death into the extracellular space, and initiation of the inflammatory response.[37] In contrast to apoptosis, which functions in removing cells so new cells can replace them, necrosis often interferes with cell replacement and tissue regeneration.

With necrotic cell death, there are marked changes in the appearance of the cytoplasmic contents and the nucleus. These changes often are not visible, even under the microscope, for hours after cell death. The dissolution of the necrotic cell or tissue can follow several paths. The cell can undergo liquefaction (*i.e.,* liquefaction necrosis); it can be transformed to a gray, firm mass (*i.e.,* coagulation necrosis); or it can be converted to a cheesy material by infiltration of fatlike substances (*i.e.,* caseous necrosis). *Liquefaction necrosis* occurs when some of the cells die but their catalytic enzymes are not destroyed. An example of liquefaction necrosis is the softening of the center of an abscess with discharge of its contents. During *coagulation necrosis,* acidosis develops and denatures the enzymatic and structural proteins of the cell. This type of necrosis is characteristic of hypoxic injury and is seen in infarcted areas. *Infarction (i.e.,* tissue death) occurs when an artery supplying an organ or part of the body becomes occluded and no other source of blood supply exists. As a rule, the shape of the infarction is conical and corresponds to the distribution of the artery and its branches. An artery may be occluded by an embolus, a thrombus, disease of the arterial wall, or pressure from outside the vessel.

Caseous necrosis is a distinctive form of coagulation necrosis in which the dead cells persist indefinitely as soft, cheeselike debris.[1] It is most commonly found in the center of tuberculosis granulomas, or tubercles, and is thought to result from immune mechanisms (see Chapter 28).

Gangrene. The term *gangrene* is applied when a considerable mass of tissue undergoes necrosis. Gangrene may be classified as dry or moist. In dry gangrene, the part becomes dry and shrinks, the skin wrinkles, and its color changes to dark brown or black. The spread of dry gangrene is slow, and its symptoms are not as marked as those of wet gangrene. The irritation caused by the dead tissue produces a line of inflammatory reaction (*i.e.,* line of demarcation) between the dead tissue of the gangrenous area and the healthy tissue (Fig. 5-12). Dry gangrene usually results from interference with the arterial blood supply to a part without interference with venous return, and is a form of coagulation necrosis.

In moist or wet gangrene, the area is cold, swollen, and pulseless. The skin is moist, black, and under tension. Blebs form on the surface, liquefaction occurs, and a foul odor is caused by bacterial action. There is no line of demarcation between the normal and diseased tissues, and the spread of tissue damage is rapid. Systemic symptoms are usually severe, and death may occur unless the condition can be arrested. Moist or wet gangrene primarily results from interference with venous return from the part. Bacterial invasion plays an important role in the development of wet gangrene and is responsible for many of its prominent symptoms. Dry gangrene is confined almost exclusively to the extremities, but moist gangrene may affect the internal organs or the extremities. If bacteria invade the necrotic tissue, dry gangrene may be converted to wet gangrene.

Gas gangrene is a special type of gangrene that results from infection of devitalized tissues by one of several *Clostridium* bacteria, most commonly *Clostridium perfringens.* These anaerobic and spore-forming organisms are widespread in nature, particularly in soil; gas gangrene is prone to occur in trauma and compound fractures in which dirt and debris are embedded. Some species have been isolated in the stomach, gallbladder, intestine, vagina, and skin of healthy persons. The bacteria produce toxins that dissolve cell membranes, causing death of muscle cells, massive spreading edema, hemolysis of red blood cells, hemolytic anemia, hemoglobinuria, and renal failure.[37] Characteristic of this disorder are the bubbles of hydrogen sulfide gas that form in the muscle. Gas

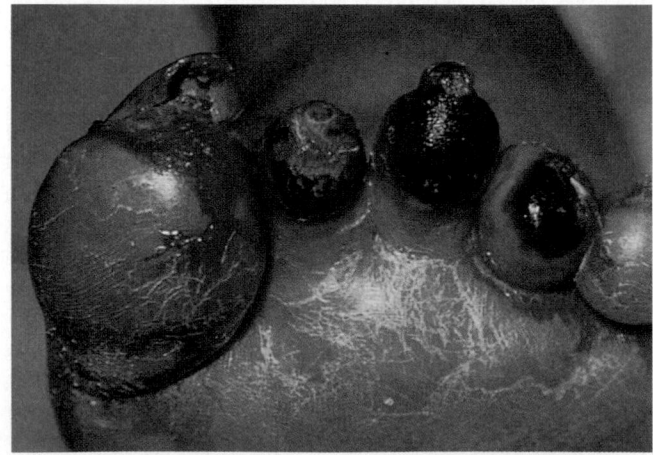

FIGURE 5-12 • Gangrenous toes. (Biomedical Communications Group, Southern Illinois University School of Medicine, Springfield, IL.)

gangrene is a serious and potentially fatal disease. Antibiotics are used to treat the infection and surgical methods are used to remove the infected tissue. Amputation may be required to prevent spreading infection involving a limb. Hyperbaric oxygen therapy has been used, but clinical data supporting its efficacy have not been rigorously assessed.

Cellular Aging

Like adaptation and injury, aging is a process that involves the cells and tissues of the body. A number of theories have been proposed to explain the cause of aging. These theories are not mutually exclusive, and aging is most likely complex with multiple causes. The main theories of aging can be categorized based on evolutionary, molecular, cellular, and systems-level explanations.[38]

The *evolutionary theories* focus on genetic variation and reproductive success. After the reproductive years have passed, it is not clear that continued longevity contributes to the fitness of the species. Thus, "antiaging" genes would not necessarily be selected, preserved, and prevalent in the gene pool.

The *molecular theories* of cellular aging focus more on mutations or changes in gene expression. Because the appearance, properties, and function of cells depend on gene expression, this aspect is likely to be involved in aging at some level. Recent attention is being given to the so-called aging genes identified in model systems.

There are a number of *cellular theories of senescence* that are currently under investigation, including those that focus on telomere shortening, free radical injury, and apoptosis. It has been known since the mid-1960s that many cells in culture exhibit a limit in replicative capacity, the so-called Hayflick limit of about 50 population doublings. This limit seems to be related to the length of the telomeres, which are DNA sequences at the ends of chromosomes. Each time a cell divides, the telomeres shorten until a critical minimal length is attained, senescence ensues, and further cell replication does not occur. Some cells have telomerase, an enzyme that "rebuilds" telomeres and lessens or prevents shortening. Cancer cells have high levels of telomerase, which prevents senescence and contributes to the cellular immortality that characterizes cancer. Telomere shortening appears to be related to other theories of cellular causes of aging. For example, free radicals and oxidative damage can kill cells and hasten telomere shortening. Caloric restriction, which appears to increase longevity, may be related to reduced mitochondrial free radical generation owing to reduced methionine or other dietary amino acid intake.[39]

Systems-level theories center on a decline in the integrative functions of organ systems such as the immunologic and neuroendocrine systems, which are necessary for overall control of other body systems. The immune system may decline with age and be less effective in protecting the body from infection or cancer. In addition, mutations and manipulations of genes such as *daf*-2, which is similar to human insulin/IGF-1 receptor genes, in the aging worm model *Caenorhabditis elegans* cause significant changes in longevity.[40] Pathways related to *daf*-2 may be responsible for relationships between caloric restriction and prolonged life span in rodents and other animals. The mechanisms that regulate aging are likely to be complex and multifactorial, as will be any interventions to prolong aging.

IN SUMMARY, cell injury can be caused by a number of agents, including physical agents, chemicals, biologic agents, and nutritional factors. Among the physical agents that generate cell injury are mechanical forces that produce tissue trauma, extremes of temperature, electricity, radiation, and nutritional disorders. Chemical agents can cause cell injury through several mechanisms: they can block enzymatic pathways, cause coagulation of tissues, or disrupt the osmotic or ionic balance of the cell. Biologic agents differ from other injurious agents in that they are able to replicate and continue to produce injury. Among the nutritional factors that contribute to cell injury are excesses and deficiencies of nutrients, vitamins, and minerals.

Injurious agents exert their effects largely through generation of free radicals, production of cell hypoxia, or dysregulation of intracellular calcium levels. Partially reduced oxygen species called *free radicals* are important mediators of cell injury in many pathologic conditions. They are an important cause of cell injury in hypoxia and after exposure to radiation and certain chemical agents. Lack of oxygen underlies the pathogenesis of cell injury in hypoxia and ischemia. Hypoxia can result from inadequate oxygen in the air, cardiorespiratory disease, anemia, or the inability of the cells to use oxygen. Increased intracellular calcium activates a number of enzymes with potentially damaging effects.

Injurious agents may produce sublethal and reversible cellular damage or may lead to irreversible cell injury and death. Cell death can involve two mechanisms: apoptosis or necrosis. Apoptosis involves controlled cell destruction and is the means by which the body removes and replaces cells that have been produced in excess, developed improperly, have genetic damage, or are worn out. Necrosis refers to cell death that is characterized by cell swelling, rupture of the cell membrane, and inflammation.

Like adaptation and injury, aging is a process that involves the cells and tissues of the body. A number of theories have been proposed to explain the complex causes of aging, including those based on evolutionary mechanisms that explain aging as a consequence of natural selection, in which traits that maximize the reproductive capacity of an individual are selected over those that maximize longevity; molecular theories, such as those that explain aging as a result of changes in gene expression; cellular theories that explain cellular senescence in relation to telomere length or molecular events, free radical damage, accumulated wear-and-tear, or apoptosis; and systems theories that attribute cellular aging to a decline in the integrative functions of organ systems such as the neuroendocrine and immunologic systems. ■

CONCEPTS in action **ANIMATION**

Review Exercises

1. A 30-year-old man sustained a fracture of his leg 2 months ago. The leg has been encased in a cast and he has just had it removed. He is amazed at the degree to which the muscles in his leg have shrunk.

   A. *Would you consider this to be a normal adaptive response? Explain.*

   B. *Will these changes have an immediate and/or long-term effect on the function of the leg?*

   C. *What types of measures can be taken to restore full function to the leg?*

2. A 45-year-old woman has been receiving radiation therapy for breast cancer.

   A. *Explain the effects of ionizing radiation in eradicating the tumor cells.*

   B. *Why is the radiation treatment given in smaller divided, or fractionated, doses rather than as a single large dose?*

   C. *Part way through the treatment schedule, the woman notices that her skin over the irradiated area has become reddened and irritated. What is the reason for this?*

3. People who have had a heart attack may experience additional damage once blood flow has been restored, a phenomenon referred to as *reperfusion injury.*

   A. *What is the proposed mechanism underlying reperfusion injury?*

   B. *What factors might influence this mechanism?*

4. Every day blood cells in our body become senescent and die without producing signs of inflammation, yet massive injury or destruction of tissue, such as occurs with a heart attack, produces significant signs of inflammation.

   A. *Explain.*

References

1. Rubin E., Strayer D. S. (2005). Cell injury. In Rubin E., Gorstein F., Rubin R., et al. (Eds.), *Rubin's pathology: Clinicopathologic foundations of medicine* (4th ed., pp. 3–39). Philadelphia: Lippincott Williams & Wilkins.
2. Kumar V., Abbas A. K., Fausto N. (2005). Cellular adaptations, cell injury, and cell death. In Kumar V., Abbas A. K., Fausto N. (Eds.), *Robbins and Cotran pathologic basis of disease* (7th ed., pp. 3–46). Philadelphia: Elsevier Saunders.
3. Heszele M. F. C., Price S. R. (2004). Insulin-like growth factor 1: The yin and yang of muscle atrophy. *Endocrinology* 145, 4803–4805.
4. Heineke J., Molkentin J. D. (2006). Regulation of cardiac hypertrophy by intracellular signalling pathways. *Nature Reviews: Molecular Cell Biology* 7, 589–600.
5. Hunter J. J., Chien K. R. (1999). Signaling pathways in cardiac hypertrophy and failure. *New England Journal of Medicine* 341, 1276–1283.
6. Anastassios C., Koumbourlis M. D. (2002). Electrical injuries. *Critical Care Medicine* 30(Suppl.), S424–S430.
7. Hahn S. M., Glatstein E. (2001). Radiation injury. In Braunwald E., Fauci A., Kasper D. L., et al. (Eds.), *Harrison's principles of internal medicine* (15th ed., pp. 2585–2590). New York: McGraw-Hill.
8. Landrigan P. J., Todd A. C. (1994). Lead poisoning. *Western Journal of Medicine* 161, 153–156.
9. Brody D. J., Pirkle J. L., Kramer R. A. (1994). Blood lead levels in the US population: Phase I of the Third National Health and Nutrition Examination Survey (NHANES III, 1988–1991). *Journal of the American Medical Association* 272, 277–283.
10. Centers for Disease Control and Prevention. (2007). Toys and lead exposure. [Online.] Available: http://www.cdc.gov/nceh/lead/faq/toys.htm. Accessed February 4, 2008.
11. Markowitz M. (2004). Lead poisoning. In Behrman R. E., Kliegman R. M., Jenson H. B. (Eds.), *Nelson textbook of pediatrics* (17th ed., pp. 2358–2362). Philadelphia: WB Saunders.
12. Ellis M. R., Kane K. Y. (2000). Lightening the lead load in children. *American Family Physician* 62, 545–554, 559–560.
13. Centers for Disease Control and Prevention. (1997). *Screening young children for lead poisoning: Guidance for state and local health officials.* Atlanta: Centers for Disease Control and Prevention, National Center for Environmental Health, U.S. Department of Health and Human Services, Public Health Service.
14. American Academy of Pediatrics Committee on Environmental Health. (1998). Screening for elevated blood levels. *Pediatrics* 101, 1072–1078.
15. Centers for Disease Control. (1991). *Preventing lead poisoning in young children: A statement by the Centers for Disease Control.* Atlanta: U.S. Department of Health and Human Services, Public Health Service.
16. Canfield R. L., Henderson C. R., Jr., Cory-Slechta D. A., et al. (2003). Intellectual impairment in children with blood lead concentrations below 10 μg per deciliter. *New England Journal of Medicine* 348, 1517–1526.
17. Clarkson T. W., Magos L., Myers G. J. (2003). The toxicity of mercury: Current exposures and clinical manifestations. *New England Journal of Medicine* 349, 1731–1737.
18. McCord J. M. (2000). The evolution of free radicals and oxidative stress. *American Journal of Medicine* 108, 652–659.
19. Kerr M. E., Bender C. M., Monti E. J. (1996). An introduction to oxygen free radicals. *Heart and Lung* 25, 200–209.
20. Chuyanyu C. L., Jackson R. M. (2002). Reactive species mechanisms of cellular hypoxia-reoxygenation injury. *American Journal of Physiology: Cell Physiology* 282, C227–C241.
21. Van Houten B., Woshner V., Santos J. H. (2006). Role of mitochondrial DNA in toxic responses to oxidative stress. *DNA Repair* 5, 145–152.
22. Finkel T. (2003). Oxidant signals and oxidative stress. *Current Opinion in Cell Biology* 15, 247–254.
23. Brenneistein P., Steinbrenner H., Seis H. (2005). Selenium, oxidative stress, and health aspects. *Molecular Aspects of Medicine* 26, 256–267.
24. Comhair S. A, Erzuum S. C. (2005). The regulation and role of extracellular glutathione peroxidase. *Antioxidants and Redox Signaling* 7, 72–79.
25. Johnson F., Giulivi C. (2005). Superoxide dismutases and their impact upon human health. *Molecular Aspects of Medicine* 26, 340–352.
26. Klaunig J. E., Kamendulis L. M. (2004). The role of oxidative stress in carcinogenesis. *Annual Review of Pharmacology and Toxicology* 44, 239–267.
27. Fenster B. E., Tsao P. S., Rockson S. G. (2003). Endothelial dysfunction: Clinical strategies for treating oxidant stress. *American Heart Journal* 146, 218–226.
28. Martin I., Grotewiel M. S. (2006). Oxidative damage and age-related functional declines. *Mechanisms of Ageing and Development* 127, 411–423.
29. Vogt M. T., Farber E. (1968). On the molecular pathology of ischemic renal cell death: Reversible and irreversible cellular and mitochondrial metabolic alterations. *American Journal of Pathology* 53, 1–26.
30. Marx J. (2004). How cells endure low oxygen. *Science* 303, 1454–1456.
31. Skikumar P., Dong Z., Mikhailov V., et al. (1999). Apoptosis: Definitions, mechanisms, and relevance to disease. *American Journal of Medicine* 107, 490–505.

32. Vermeulen K., Van Bockstaele D. R., Berneman Z. N. (2005). Apoptosis: Mechanisms and relevance in cancer. *Annals of Hematology* 84, 627–639.

33. Cruise M. W., Lukens J. R., Nguyen A. P., et al. (2006). Fas ligand is responsible for CXCR3 chemokine induction in CD4+ T cell-dependent liver damage. *Journal of Immunology* 176, 6235–6244.

34. Malhi H., Gores G. J., Lemasters J. J. (2006). Apoptosis and necrosis in the liver: A tale of two deaths? *Hepatology* 43(2, Suppl. 1), S31–S44.

35. Dorner T., Lipsky P. E. (2006). Signalling pathways in B cells: Implications for autoimmunity. *Current Topics in Microbiology and Immunology* 305, 213–240.

36. Proskuryakov S. Y., Konoplyannikov A. G., Gabai V. L. (2003). Necrosis: A specific form of programmed cell death. *Experimental Cell Research* 283, 1–16.

37. Kasper D. L., Zaleznik D. F. (2001). Gas gangrene, antibiotic-associated colitis, and other clostridial infections. In Braunwald E., Fauci A., Kasper D. L., et al. (Eds.). *Harrison's principles of internal medicine* (15th ed., pp. 922–927). New York: McGraw-Hill.

38. Weinert B. T., Timiras P. S. (2003). Invited review: Theories of aging. *Journal of Applied Physiology* 95, 1706–1716.

39. Sanz A., Caro P., Ayala V., et al. (2006). Methionine restriction decreases mitochondrial oxygen radical generation and leak as well as oxidative damage to mitochondrial DNA and proteins. *FASEB Journal* 20, 1064–1073.

40. Halaschek-Wiener J., Khattra J. S., Pouzyrev A., et al. (2005). Analysis of long-lived *C. elegans* daf-2 mutants using serial analysis of gene expression. *Genome Research* 15, 603–615.

Visit thePoint **http://thePoint.lww.com for animations, journal articles, and more!**

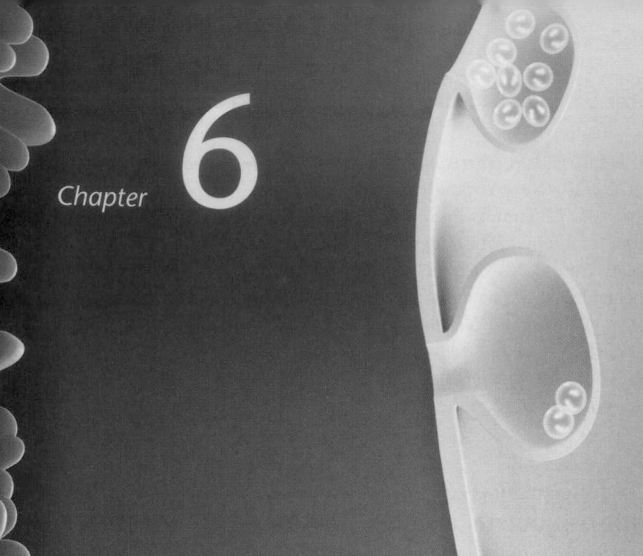

Chapter 6

Genetic Control of Cell Function and Inheritance

EDWARD W. CARROLL

➤ Our genetic information is stored in the structure of *deoxyribonucleic acid* (DNA), an extremely stable macromolecule. Genetic information directs the function of our body cells, determines our appearance and how we respond to our environment, and serves as the unit of inheritance passed on from generation to generation. Genes also determine our disease susceptibility and how we react to drugs.

An understanding of the role that genetics plays in pathogenesis of disease has expanded greatly over the past century. It is now apparent that many diseases, including cancer, diabetes, and cardiovascular diseases, have a genetic component. In the case of cancer, recent genetic advances have led to new methods for early detection and more effective treatment. Advances in immunogenetics have made compatible blood transfusion and organ transplants a reality, and recombinant DNA technology has provided the methods for producing human insulin, growth hormone, and clotting factors. Perhaps the most extensive use of gene technology involved the Human Genome Project, begun in 1990 and completed in 2003, in which the entire human genetic complement (the genome) has been sequenced. Some of what was discovered was quite unexpected, including the revelation that humans have a mere 30,000 genes, rather than the predicted 100,000; and that on an average any two individuals share 99.9% of their DNA sequence, indicating that the remarkable diversity among individuals is vested in about 0.1% of our DNA.

This chapter includes discussions of genetic control of cell function, chromosomes, patterns of inheritance, and gene technology.

GENETIC CONTROL OF CELL FUNCTION

After completing this section of the chapter, you should be able to meet the following objectives:

■ Describe the structure and function of DNA.
■ Relate the mechanisms of DNA repair to the development of a gene mutation.

- Describe the function of messenger RNA, ribosomal RNA, and transfer RNA as they relate to protein synthesis.
- Cite the effects of post-translational processing on protein structure and function.
- Explain the role of transcription factors in regulating gene activity.

The DNA that contains our genetic information is an extremely stable molecule. Because of its stable structure, the genetic information carried in DNA can survive the many stages of cell division and the day-to-day process of cell renewal and tissue growth. Its stable structure also allows the information to survive the many processes of reduction division involved in gamete (*i.e.,* ovum and sperm) formation, the fertilization process, and the mitotic cell divisions involved in the formation of a new organism from the single-celled fertilized ovum called the *zygote*.

FUNCTION OF DNA IN CONTROLLING CELL FUNCTION

- The information needed for the control of cell structure and function is embedded in the genetic information encoded in the stable DNA molecule.
- Although every cell in the body contains the same genetic information, each cell type uses only a portion of the information, depending on its structure and function.
- The production of the proteins that control cell function is accomplished by (1) the transcription of the DNA code for assembly of the protein onto messenger RNA, (2) the translation of the code from messenger RNA and assembly of the protein by ribosomal RNA in the cytoplasm, and (3) the delivery of the amino acids needed for protein synthesis to ribosomal RNA by transfer RNA.

A second type of nucleic acid, *ribonucleic acid* (RNA), is involved in the actual synthesis of cellular proteins. The information contained in a given gene is first transcribed into an RNA molecule that, after being processed in the nucleus, carries the information to the cytoplasm, where it is translated and used in synthesizing proteins.

Although DNA and RNA have received a lot of attention, it is the proteins that the genes encode that make up the majority of cellular structures and perform most life functions. Proteins are responsible for the functional diversity of cells, they perform most biologic functions, and it is at their level that many regulatory processes take place, many disease

processes occur, and most drug targets are found. The term *proteome* is a relatively new term, created to define the complete set of proteins encoded by a genome. *Proteomics,* the study of the proteome, uses highly sophisticated technological methods to examine the molecular and biochemical events in a cell.

DNA Structure and Function

The DNA molecule that stores the genetic information in the nucleus is a long, double-stranded, helical structure. DNA is composed of *nucleotides,* which consist of phosphoric acid, a five-carbon sugar called *deoxyribose,* and one of four nitrogenous bases (Fig. 6-1). These nitrogenous bases carry the genetic information and are divided into two groups: the *pyrimidine bases,* thymine (T) and cytosine (C), which have one nitrogen ring, and the *purine bases,* adenine (A) and guanine (G), which have two. The backbone of DNA consists of alternating groups of sugar and phosphoric acid, with the paired bases projecting inward from the sides of the sugar molecule.

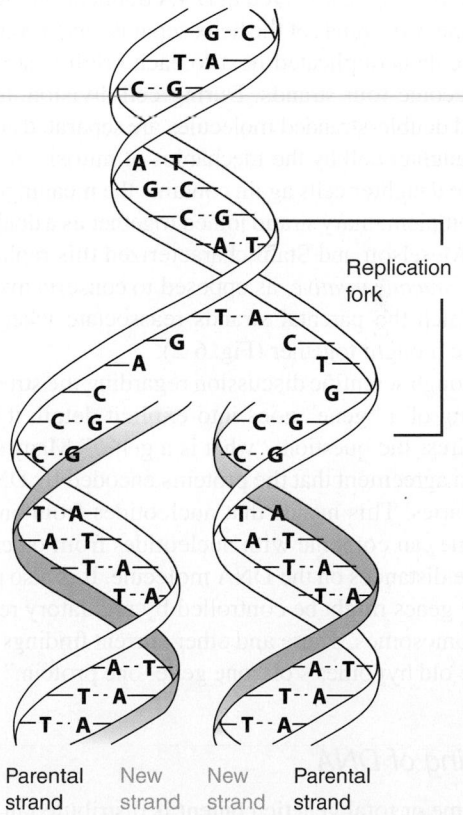

FIGURE 6-1 • A replicating DNA helix. The parental strands separate at the replication fork. Each parental strand serves as a template for the synthesis of a new strand. DNA consists of a sugar–phosphate backbone with paired pyrimidine bases (thymine [T] and cytosine [C]) and purine bases (adenine [A] and guanine [G]) projecting inward. (From Smith C., Marks A. D., Lieberman M. [2005]. *Marks' basic medical biochemistry* [2nd ed., p. 222]. Philadelphia: Lippincott Williams & Wilkins.)

Double Helix and Base-Pairing

The native structure of DNA, as elucidated by James Watson and Frances Crick in 1953, is that of a spiral staircase, with the paired bases representing the steps (see Fig. 6-1). A precise complementary pairing of purine and pyrimidine bases occurs in the double-stranded DNA molecule in which A is paired with T and G is paired with C. Each nucleotide in a pair is on one strand of the DNA molecule, with the bases on opposite DNA strands bound together by hydrogen bonds that are extremely stable under normal conditions. The double-stranded structure of DNA molecules allows them to replicate precisely by separation of the two strands, followed by synthesis of two new complementary strands. Similarly, the base complementary pairing allows for efficient and correct repair of damaged DNA molecules.

Several hundred to almost one million base pairs can represent a gene, the size being proportional to the protein product it encodes. Of the two DNA strands, only one is used in transcribing the information for the cell's protein-building machinery. The genetic information of one strand is meaningful and is used as a template for transcription; the complementary code of the other strand does not make sense and is ignored. Both strands, however, are involved in DNA duplication. Before cell division, the two strands of the helix separate and a complementary molecule is duplicated next to each original strand. Two strands become four strands. During cell division, the newly duplicated double-stranded molecules are separated and placed in each daughter cell by the mechanics of mitosis. As a result, each of the daughter cells again contains the meaningful strand and the complementary strand joined together as a double helix. In 1958, Meselson and Stahl characterized this replication of DNA as *semiconservative,* as opposed to conservative replication in which the parental strands reassociate when the two strands are brought together (Fig. 6-2).

Although scientific discussion regarding the structure and functioning of a "gene" goes into explicit detail, it does not really address the question, "what is a gene?" Many scientists are now in agreement that the proteins encoded by DNA know no boundaries. This means that nucleotides from one part of the genome can combine with nucleotides from other regions at extreme distances on the DNA molecule. It is also proposed that some genes might be controlled by regulatory regions on other chromosomes. These and other current findings have put to rest the old hypothesis of "one gene–one protein."

Packaging of DNA

The genome or total genetic content is distributed in chromosomes. Each human somatic cell (cells other than the gametes [sperm and ovum]) has 23 pairs of different chromosomes, one pair derived from the individual's mother and the other from the father. One of the chromosome pairs consists of the sex chromosomes. Genes are arranged linearly along each chromosome. Each chromosome contains one continuous, linear DNA helix. The DNA in the longest chromosome is more than 7 cm

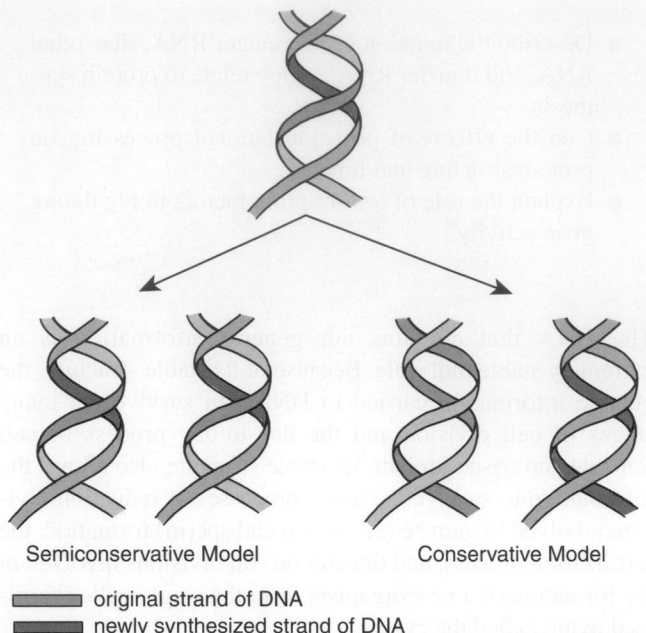

original strand of DNA
newly synthesized strand of DNA

FIGURE 6-2 • Semiconservative versus conservative models of DNA replication as proposed by Meselson and Stahl in 1958. In semiconservative DNA replication, the two original strands of DNA unwind and a complementary strand is formed along each original strand.

in length. If the DNA of all 46 chromosomes were placed end-to-end, the total DNA would span a distance of about 2 m (more than 6 feet).

Because of their large size, DNA molecules are combined with several types of protein and small amounts of RNA into a coiled structure known as *chromatin.* The organization of DNA into chromatin is essential for controlling transcription and for packaging the molecule. Some DNA-associated proteins form binding sites for repressor molecules and hormones that regulate genetic transcription; others may block genetic transcription by preventing access of nucleotides to the surface of the DNA molecule. A specific group of proteins called *histones* is thought to control the folding of the DNA strands. Each double-stranded DNA molecule periodically coils around histones, forming regularly spaced spherical structures called *nucleosomes* that resemble beads on a string (Fig. 6-3). This string of beads further winds into filaments that make up the structure of chromatin.

Although solving the structural problem of how to fit a huge amount of DNA into the nucleus, the chromatin fiber, when complexed with histones and folded into various levels of compaction, makes the DNA inaccessible during the processes of replication and gene expression. To accommodate these processes, chromatin must be induced to change its structure, a process called *chromatin remodeling.* Several chemical interactions are now known to affect this process. One of these involves the acetylation of a histone amino acids group that is linked to the opening of the chromatin fiber and gene activation. Another important chemical modification involves the methylation of histone amino acids, which is correlated with gene inactivation.

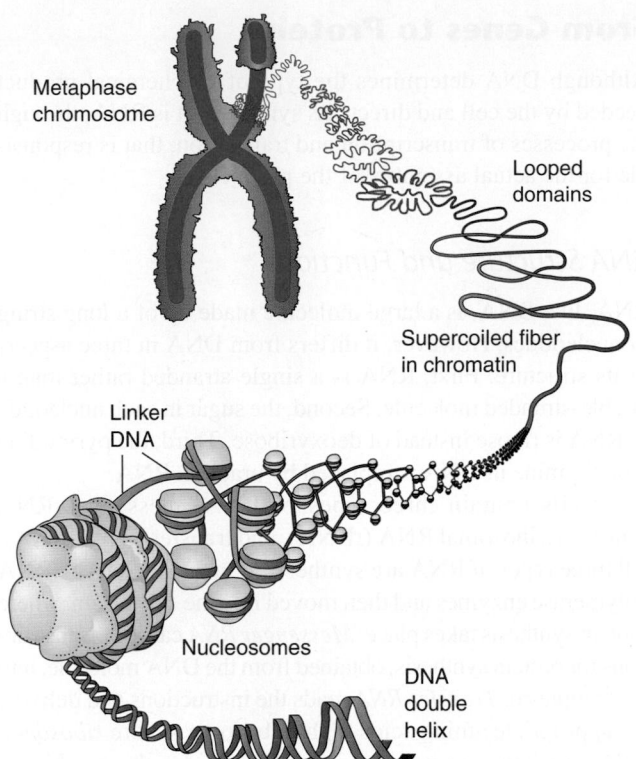

Metaphase
chromosome

Looped
domains

Supercoiled fiber
in chromatin

Linker
DNA

Nucleosomes

DNA
double
helix

FIGURE 6-3 • Increasing orders of DNA compaction in chromatin and mitotic chromosomes. (From Cormack D. H. [1993]. *Essential histology.* Philadelphia: JB Lippincott.)

Genetic Code

Four bases—guanine, adenine, cytosine, and thymine (uracil is substituted for thymine in RNA)—make up the alphabet of the genetic code. A sequence of three of these bases forms the fundamental triplet code used in transmitting the genetic information needed for protein synthesis. This triplet code is called a *codon* (Table 6-1). An example is the nucleotide sequence UGG (uracil, guanine, guanine), which is the triplet RNA code for the amino acid tryptophan. The genetic code is a universal language used by most living cells (*i.e.,* the code for the amino acid tryptophan is the same in a bacterium, a plant, and a human being). *Stop codes,* which signal the end of a protein molecule, are also present. Mathematically, the 4 bases can be arranged in 64 different combinations. Sixty-one of the triplets correspond to particular amino acids, and three are stop signals. Only 20 amino acids are used in protein synthesis in humans. Several triplets code for the same amino acid; therefore, the genetic code is said to be *redundant* or *degenerate*. For example, AUG is a part of the initiation or start signal as well as the codon for the amino acid methionine. Codons that specify the same amino acid are called *synonyms.* Synonyms usually have the same first two bases but differ in the third base.

DNA Repair

Rarely, accidental errors in duplication of DNA occur. These errors are called *mutations*. Mutations result from the substitution of one base pair for another, the loss or addition of one or more base pairs, or rearrangements of base pairs. Many of these

TABLE 6-1 **Triplet Codes for Amino Acids**					
AMINO ACID	**RNA CODONS**				
Alanine	GCU	GCC	GCA	GCG	
Arginine	CGU	CGC	CGA	CGG	AGA	AGG
Asparagine	AAU	AAC			
Aspartic acid	GAU	GAC			
Cysteine	UGU	UGC			
Glutamic acid	GAA	GAG			
Glutamine	CAA	CAG			
Glycine	GGU	GGC	GGA	GGG	
Histidine	CAU	CAC			
Isoleucine	AUU	AUC	AUA		
Leucine	CUU	CUC	CUA	CUG	UUA	UUG
Lysine	AAA	AAG			
Methionine	AUG				
Phenylalanine	UUU	UUC			
Proline	CCU	CCC	CCA	CCG	
Serine	UCU	UCC	UCA	UCG	AGC	AGU
Threonine	ACU	ACC	ACA	ACG	
Tryptophan	UGG				
Tyrosine	UAU	UAC			
Valine	GUU	GUC	GUA	GUG	
Start (CI)	AUG				
Stop (CT)	UAA	UAG	UGA		

mutations occur spontaneously, whereas others occur because of environmental agents, chemicals, and radiation. Mutations may arise in somatic cells or in germ cells. Only those DNA changes that occur in germ cells can be inherited.

Considering the millions of base pairs that must be duplicated in each cell division, it is not surprising that random changes in replication occur. Most of these defects are corrected by DNA repair mechanisms. Several repair mechanisms exist, and each depends on specific enzymes called *endonucleases* that recognize local distortions of the DNA helix, cleave the abnormal chain, and remove the distorted region. The gap is then filled when the correct deoxyribonucleotides, created by a DNA polymerase using the intact complementary strand as a template, are added to the cleaved DNA. The newly synthesized end of the segment is then joined to the remainder of the DNA strand by a DNA ligase. The normal regulation of these gene repair mechanisms is under the control of DNA repair genes. Loss of these gene functions renders the DNA susceptible to accumulation of mutations; when these affect proto-oncogenes or tumor suppressor genes, cancer may result (discussed in Chapter 8).

Genetic Variability

As the Human Genome Project was progressing, it became evident that the human genome sequence is almost exactly (99.9%) the same in all people. It is the small variation (0.01%) in gene sequence (termed a *haplotype*) that is thought to account for the individual differences in physical traits, behaviors, and disease susceptibility. These variations are sometimes referred to as *polymorphisms* (from the existence of more than one morphologic or body form in a population). An international effort has been organized to develop a map (HapMap) of these variations with the intent of providing a link between genetic variations and common complex diseases such as cancer, heart disease, diabetes, and some forms of mental disease (discussed in the section on Gene Technology, later).

Mitochondrial DNA

In addition to nuclear DNA, part of the DNA of a cell resides in the mitochondria. Mitochondrial DNA is inherited from the mother by her offspring (*i.e.,* matrilineal inheritance). It is a double-stranded closed circle, containing 37 genes, 24 of which are needed for mitochondrial DNA translation and 13 of which encode enzymes needed for oxidative metabolism. Replication of mitochondrial DNA depends on enzymes encoded by nuclear DNA. Thus, the protein-synthesizing apparatus and molecular components for oxidative metabolism are jointly derived from nuclear and mitochondrial genes. Genetic disorders of mitochondrial DNA, although rare, commonly affect tissues such as those of the neuromuscular system that have a high requirement for oxidative metabolism (discussed in Chapter 7).

From Genes to Proteins

Although DNA determines the type of biochemical product needed by the cell and directs its synthesis, it is RNA, through the processes of transcription and translation, that is responsible for the actual assembly of the products.

RNA Structure and Function

RNA, like DNA, is a large molecule made up of a long string of nucleotides. However, it differs from DNA in three aspects of its structure. First, RNA is a single-stranded rather than a double-stranded molecule. Second, the sugar in each nucleotide of RNA is ribose instead of deoxyribose. Third, the pyrimidine base thymine in DNA is replaced by uracil in RNA.

Cells contain three types of RNA: messenger RNA (mRNA), ribosomal RNA (rRNA), and transfer RNA (tRNA). All three types of RNA are synthesized in the nucleus by RNA polymerase enzymes and then moved into the cytoplasm, where protein synthesis takes place. *Messenger RNA* carries the instructions for protein synthesis, obtained from the DNA molecule, into the cytoplasm. *Transfer RNA* reads the instructions and delivers the appropriate amino acids to the ribosome, where *ribosomal RNA* translates the instructions and provides the machinery needed for protein synthesis.

Messenger RNA. Messenger RNA is the template for protein synthesis. It is a long molecule containing several hundred to several thousand nucleotides. Each group of three nucleotides forms a codon that is exactly complementary to a nucleotide triplet of the DNA molecule. Messenger RNA is formed by a process called *transcription*. In this process, the weak hydrogen bonds of DNA are broken so that free RNA nucleotides can pair with their exposed DNA counterparts on the meaningful strand of the DNA molecule (see Fig. 6-4). As with the base pairing of the DNA strands, complementary RNA bases pair with the DNA bases. In RNA, uracil (U) replaces thymine and pairs with adenine.

Ribosomal RNA. The ribosome is the physical structure in the cytoplasm where protein synthesis takes place. Ribosomal RNA forms 60% of the ribosome, with the remainder of the ribosome composed of the structural proteins and enzymes needed for protein synthesis. As with the other types of RNA, rRNA is synthesized in the nucleus. Unlike the two other types of RNA, rRNA is produced in a specialized nuclear structure called the *nucleolus*. The formed rRNA combines with ribosomal proteins in the nucleus to produce the ribosome, which is then transported into the cytoplasm. On reaching the cytoplasm, most ribosomes become attached to the endoplasmic reticulum and begin the task of protein synthesis.

Transfer RNA. *Transfer RNA* is a clover-shaped molecule containing only 80 nucleotides, making it the smallest RNA molecule. Its function is to deliver the activated form of an amino acid

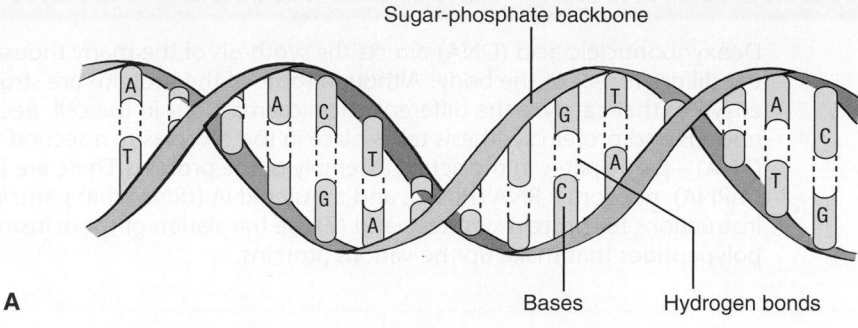

Sugar-phosphate backbone

A

Bases Hydrogen bonds

Transcription

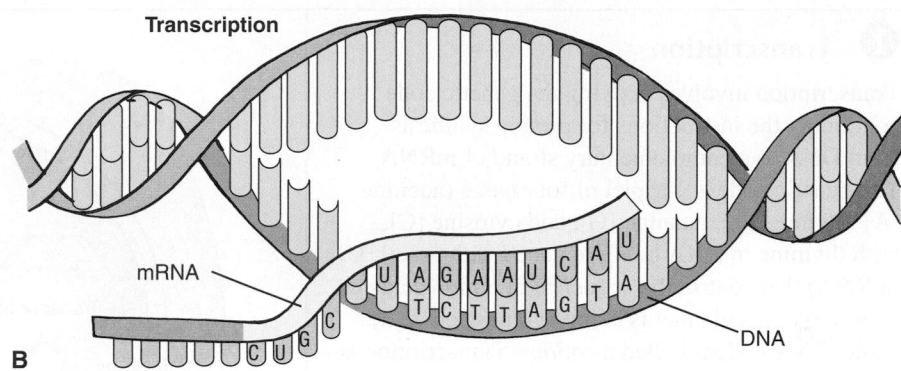

mRNA

DNA

B

FIGURE 6-4 • The DNA double helix and transcription of messenger RNA (mRNA). The top panel (**A**) shows the sequence of four bases (adenine [A], cytosine [C], guanine [G], and thymine [T]) that determines the specificity of genetic information. The bases face inward from the sugar–phosphate backbone and form pairs (*dashed lines*) with complementary bases on the opposing strand. In the bottom panel (**B**), transcription creates a complementary mRNA copy from one of the DNA strands in the double helix.

to the protein that is being synthesized in the ribosomes. At least 20 different types of tRNA are known, each of which recognizes and binds to only one type of amino acid. Each tRNA molecule has two recognition sites: the first is complementary for the mRNA codon, the second for the amino acid itself. Each type of tRNA carries its own specific amino acid to the ribosomes, where protein synthesis is taking place; there it recognizes the appropriate codon on the mRNA and delivers the amino acid to the newly forming protein molecule.

Transcription

Transcription occurs in the cell nucleus and involves the synthesis of RNA from a DNA template (Fig. 6-4). Genes are transcribed by enzymes called *RNA polymerases* that generate a single-stranded RNA identical in sequence (with the exception of U in place of T) to one of the strands of DNA. It is initiated by the assembly of a transcription complex composed of RNA polymerase and other associated factors. This complex binds to the double-stranded DNA at a specific site called the *promoter region.* Within the promoter region the so-called TATA box is located. The TATA box contains the crucial thymine-adenine-thymine-adenine (TATA) nucleotide sequence that RNA polymerase recognizes and binds to (Fig. 6-5). This binding also requires transcription factors, a transcription initiation site, and other proteins. Transcription continues to copy the meaningful strand into a single strand of RNA as it travels along the length of the gene, stopping only when it reaches a termination site with a stop codon (see Fig. 6-5). On reaching the stop signal, the RNA polymerase enzyme leaves

the gene and releases the RNA strand. The RNA strand then is processed.

Processing involves the addition of certain nucleic acids at the ends of the RNA strand and cutting and splicing of certain internal sequences. Splicing often involves the removal of stretches of RNA (Fig. 6-6). Because of the splicing process, the final mRNA sequence is different from the original DNA template. The retained protein-coding regions of the mRNA sequences are called *exons* and the regions between exons are called *introns.* The functions of the introns are unknown. They are thought to be involved in the activation or deactivation of genes during various stages of development.

Splicing permits a cell to produce a variety of mRNA molecules from a single gene. By varying the splicing segments of the initial mRNA, different mRNA molecules are formed. For example, in a muscle cell, the original tropomyosin mRNA is spliced in as many as 10 different ways, yielding distinctly different protein products. This permits different proteins to be expressed from a single gene and reduces how much DNA must be contained in the genome.

Translation

Translation occurs in the cytoplasm of the cell and involves the synthesis of a protein using its mRNA template. Proteins are made from a standard set of amino acids, which are joined end-to-end to form the long polypeptide chains of protein molecules. Each polypeptide chain may have as many as 100 to more than 300 amino acids in it. Besides rRNA, translation requires

Understanding • DNA-Directed Protein Synthesis

Deoxyribonucleic acid (DNA) directs the synthesis of the many thousands of proteins that are contained in the different cells of the body. Although some of the proteins are structural proteins, the majority are enzymes that catalyze the different chemical reactions in the cell. Because DNA is located in the cell's nucleus and protein synthesis takes place in the cytoplasm, a second type of nucleic acid—ribonucleic acid (RNA)—participates in the actual assembly of the proteins. There are three types of RNA: messenger RNA (mRNA), ribosomal RNA (rRNA), and transfer RNA (tRNA) that participate in (1) the transcription of the DNA instructions for protein synthesis and (2) the translation of those instructions into the assembly of the polypeptides that make up the various proteins.

❶ Transcription

Transcription involves copying the genetic code containing the instructions for protein synthesis from DNA to a complementary strand of mRNA. The genetic code is a triplet of four bases (adenine [A], thymine [T], guanine [G], and cytosine [C], with thymine in DNA being replaced with uracil [U] in RNA) that control the sequence of amino acids in a protein molecule that is being synthesized. (The triplet RNA code is called a *codon*.) Transcription is initiated by an enzyme called *RNA polymerase,* which binds to a promoter site on DNA. Many other proteins, including transcription factors, function to increase or decrease transcriptional activity of the genes. After mRNA has been transcribed, it detaches from DNA and is processed by cutting, removing, and splicing the internal RNA sequences to produce a variety of mRNA molecules from a single gene. Once mRNA has been processed, it diffuses through the nuclear pores into the cytoplasm, where it controls protein synthesis.

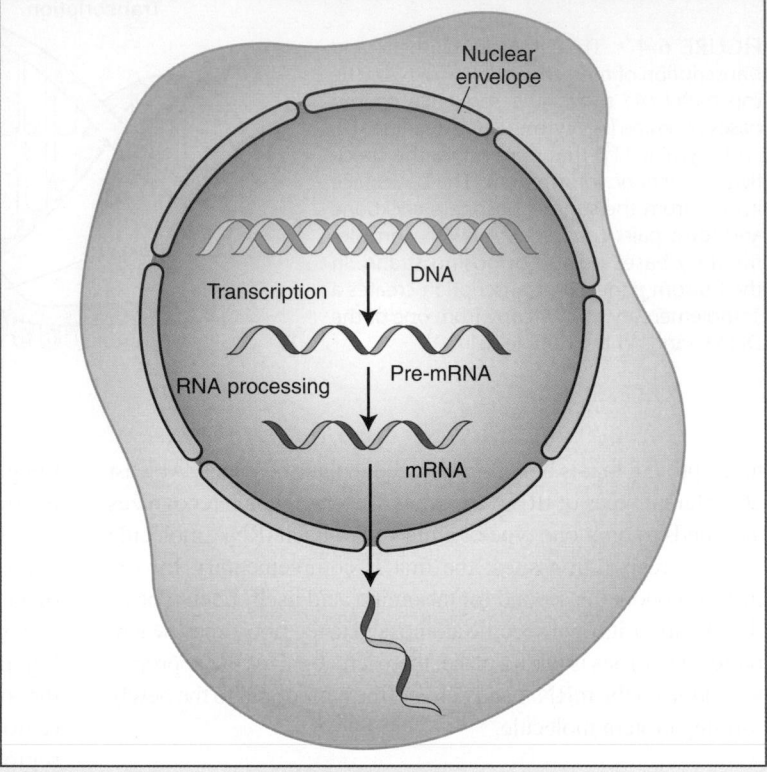

the coordinated actions of mRNA and tRNA (Fig. 6-7). Each of the 20 different tRNA molecules transports its specific amino acid to the ribosome for incorporation into the developing protein molecule. Messenger RNA provides the information needed for placing the amino acids in their proper order for each specific type of protein. During protein synthesis, mRNA contacts and passes through the ribosome, during which it "reads" the directions for protein synthesis. As mRNA passes through the ribosome, tRNA delivers the appropriate amino acids for attachment to the growing polypeptide chain. The long mRNA molecule usually travels through and directs protein synthesis in more than one ribosome at a time. After the first part of the mRNA is read by the first ribosome, it moves onto a second and a third. As a result, ribosomes that are actively involved in protein synthesis are often found in clusters called *polyribosomes.*

The process of translation is not over when the genetic code has been used to create the sequence of amino acids that constitute a protein. To be useful to a cell, this new polypeptide chain must fold up into its unique three-dimensional conformation. The folding of many proteins is made more efficient by special classes of proteins called *molecular chaperones.* Typically the function of a chaperone is to assist a newly synthesized polypeptide chain to attain a functional conformation as a new protein and then to assist the protein's arrival at the site in the cell where the protein carries out its function. Molecular chaperones also assist in preventing the misfolding of existing proteins. Disruption of chaperoning mechanisms causes intracellular molecules to become denatured and insoluble. These denatured proteins tend to stick to one another, precipitate, and form inclusion bodies. The development of inclusion bodies is a common

❷   Translation

The process of translation involves taking the instructions transcribed from DNA to mRNA and transferring them to the rRNA of ribosomes located in the cytoplasm. When the mRNA carrying the instructions for a particular protein comes in contact with a ribosome, it binds to a small subunit of the rRNA. It then travels through the ribosome where the transcribed instructions are communicated to the tRNA, which delivers and transfers the correct amino acid to its proper position on the growing peptide chain. There are 20 types of tRNA, one for each of the 20 different types of amino acid. Each type of tRNA carries an anticodon complementary to the mRNA codon calling for the amino acid carried by the tRNA, and it is the recognition of the mRNA codon by the tRNA anticodon that ensures the proper sequence of amino acids in a synthesized protein.

In order to be functional, the newly synthesized protein must be folded into its functional form, modified further, and then routed to its final position in the cell.

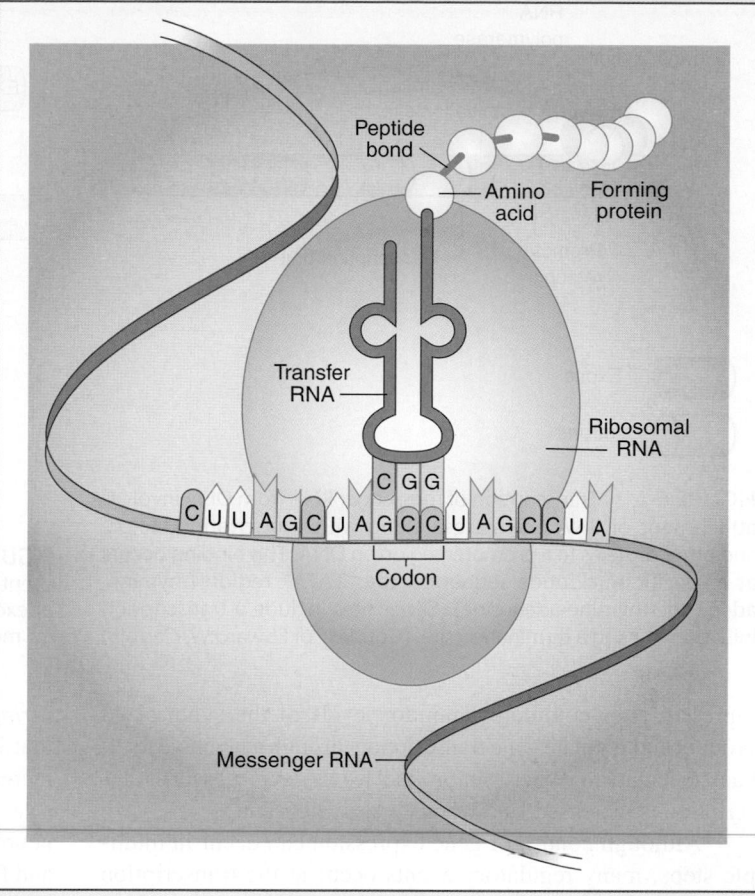

pathologic process in Parkinson, Alzheimer, and Huntington diseases.

A newly synthesized polypeptide chain may also need to combine with one or more polypeptide chains from the same or an adjacent chromosome, bind small cofactors for its activity, or undergo appropriate enzyme modification. During the post-translation process, two or more peptide chains may combine to form a single product. For example, two α-globin chains and two β-globin chains combine to form the $\alpha_2\beta_2$-hemoglobin molecule (see Chapter 14). The protein products may also be modified chemically by the addition of various types of functional groups. For example, fatty acids may be added, providing hydrophobic regions for attachment to cell membranes. Other modifications may involve cleavage of the protein, either to remove a specific amino acid sequence or to split the molecule into smaller chains. As an example, the two chains that make up the circulating active insulin molecule, one containing 21 and the other 30 amino acids, were originally part of an 82-amino-acid proinsulin molecule.

Regulation of Gene Expression

Only about 2% of the genome encodes instructions for synthesis of proteins; the remainder consists of noncoding regions that serve to determine where, when, and in what quantity proteins are made. The degree to which a gene or particular group of genes is active is called *gene expression*. A phenomenon termed *induction* is an important process by which gene expression is increased. *Gene repression* is a process by which a regulatory gene acts to reduce or prevent gene expression. Activator and

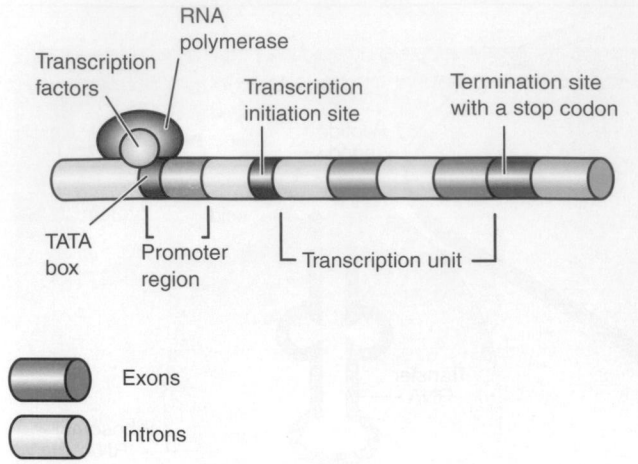

FIGURE 6-5 • Transcription of messenger RNA from DNA involves attachment of RNA polymerase along with transcription factors and other proteins to a promoter region on DNA. This binding occurs at a specific nucleotide sequence, the "TATA" region (thymine-adenosine-thymine-adenosine). Other sites include a transcription initiation site and a termination site. (Courtesy of Edward W. Carroll.)

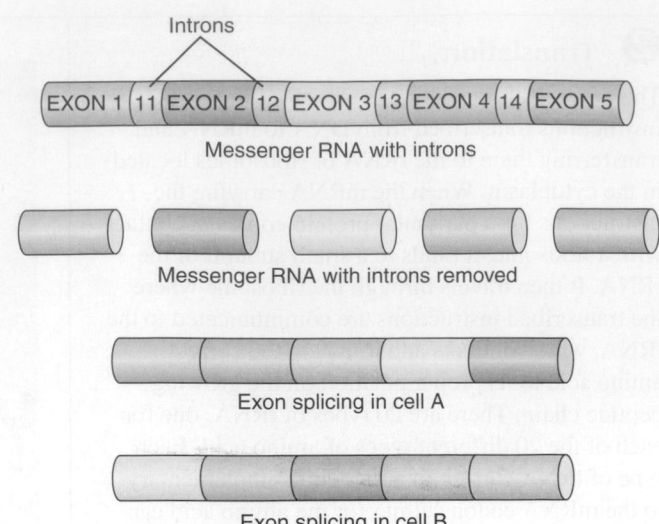

FIGURE 6-6 • RNA processing. In different cells, an RNA strand may eventually produce different proteins depending on the sequencing of exons during gene splicing. This variation allows a gene to code for more than one protein. (Courtesy of Edward W. Carroll.)

repressor sites commonly monitor levels of the synthesized product and regulate gene transcription through a negative feedback mechanism. Whenever product levels decrease, gene transcription is increased, and when levels increase, it is repressed.

Although control of gene expression can occur in multiple steps, many regulatory events occur at the transcription level. The initiation and regulation of transcription require the collaboration of a battery of proteins, collectively termed *tran-*

scription factors. Transcription factors are a class of proteins that bind to their own specific DNA region and function to increase or decrease transcriptional activity of the genes. The role of transcription factors in gene expression explains why neurons and liver cells have completely different structures and functions although all the nucleated cells in a person contain the same DNA and thus the same genetic information. Some, referred to as *general transcription factors,* are required

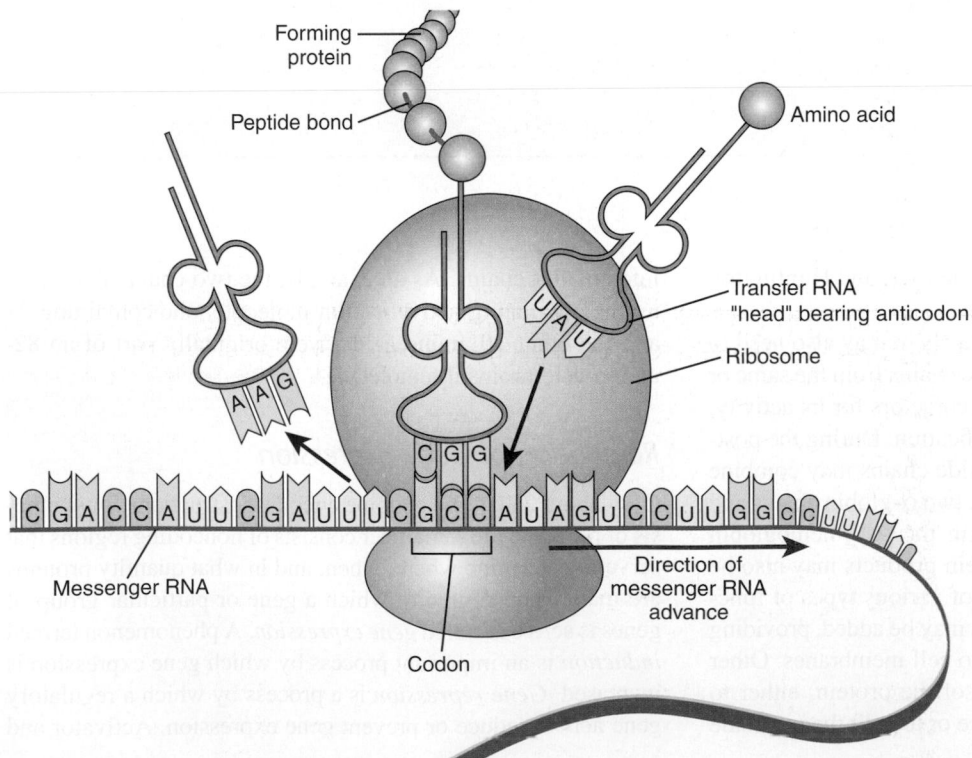

FIGURE 6-7 • Protein synthesis. A messenger RNA (mRNA) strand is shown moving along a small ribosomal subunit in the cytoplasm. As the mRNA codon passes along the ribosome, a new amino acid is added to the growing peptide chain by the transfer RNA (tRNA) bearing the anticodon for the mRNA-designated amino acid. As each amino acid is bound to the next by a peptide bond, its tRNA is released.

for transcription of all structural genes. Others, termed *specific transcription factors,* have more specialized roles, activating genes only at specific stages of development. For example, the PAX family of transcription factors is involved in the development of such embryonic tissues as the eye and portions of the nervous system.

Genetic Mediators of Embryonic Development

Regulation of gene expression also plays an essential role in the developing embryo. During embryonic development, many thousands of genes are expressed to control axial specification (*i.e.,* ventral/dorsal, anterior/posterior/medial/lateral, left/right), pattern formation (spatial arrangement of differentiated cells in body tissues and organs), and organogenesis (development of the different body organs). Many of these genes code transcription factors that produce signaling molecules, two examples being *sonic hedgehog* and *fibroblast growth factor.* Signaling molecules bind to cells and are transported to the nucleus, where they initiate changes in gene expression. Depending on the embryonic tissue, these transcription factors and signaling molecules are produced temporally at various times during embryonic development.

Sonic hedgehog signaling is involved in many key developmental events at multiple times during embryogenesis. It participates in such diverse developmental steps as establishment of the left-to-right axis responsible for the rostral–caudal orientation of the nervous system (see Chapter 48), the separation of the brain into two cerebral hemispheres, right and left eye orientation, and the separation and development of the correct number of fingers and toes. Fibroblast growth factors participate in a wide variety of developmental processes, including cell migration, growth, and differentiation. They are widely expressed in developing bone, and many autosomal dominant disorders of bone growth are mutations of fibroblast growth factor receptor genes. The most prevalent of these is a condition called *achondroplasia,* which is characterized by short stature with limbs that are disproportionately shorter than the trunk and macrocephaly (large head).

IN SUMMARY, genes are the fundamental unit of information storage in the cell. They determine the types of proteins and enzymes made by the cell and therefore control inheritance and day-to-day cell function. Genetic information is stored in a stable macromolecule called *DNA.* Genes transmit information contained in the DNA molecule as a triplet code. The genetic code is determined by the arrangement of the nitrogenous bases of the four nucleotides (*i.e.,* adenine, guanine, thymine [or uracil in RNA], and cytosine). Gene mutations represent accidental errors in duplication, rearrangement, or deletion of parts of the genetic code. Fortunately, most mutations are corrected by DNA repair mechanisms in the cell.

The transfer of stored information from DNA into production of cell products is accomplished through a second type of nucleotide called *RNA.* Messenger RNA transcribes the instructions for product synthesis from the DNA molecule and carries it into the cell's cytoplasm, where ribosomal RNA uses the information to direct protein synthesis. Transcription is initiated by RNA polymerase and other associated factors that bind to the double-stranded DNA at a specific site called the *promoter region.* Transfer RNA acts as a carrier system for delivering the appropriate amino acids to the ribosomes.

The degree to which a gene or particular group of genes is active is called *gene expression.* Gene expression involves a set of complex interrelationships among different levels of control, including RNA transcription and post-translational processing. The initiation and regulation of RNA transcription are controlled by *transcription factors* that bind to specific DNA regions and function to regulate gene expression of the many different types of cells in the body. Post-translational processing involves the proper folding of the newly synthesized polypeptide chain into its unique three-dimensional conformation. Special classes of proteins called *molecular chaperones* make the folding of many proteins more efficient. Post-translational processing may also involve the combination of polypeptide chains from the same or an adjacent chromosome, the binding of small cofactors, or enzyme modification. ■

CHROMOSOMES

After completing this section of the chapter, you should be able to meet the following objectives:

- Define the terms *autosomes, chromatin, meiosis,* and *mitosis.*
- List the steps in constructing a karyotype using cytogenetic studies.
- Explain the significance of the Barr body.

Most genetic information of a cell is organized, stored, and retrieved in small intracellular structures called *chromosomes.* Although the chromosomes are visible only in dividing cells, they retain their integrity between cell divisions. The chromosomes are arranged in pairs; one member of the pair is inherited from the father, the other from the mother. Each species has a characteristic number of chromosomes. In the human, 46 single or 23 pairs of chromosomes are present. Of the 23 pairs of human chromosomes, 22 are called *autosomes* and are alike in both males and females. Each of the 22 pairs of autosomes has the same appearance in all individuals, and each has been given a numeric designation for classification purposes (Fig. 6-8).

In the diploid cell, each of the 22 autosomal chromosomes has a homolog. Homologous chromosomes contain a similar series of genes; that is, they have similar sequences. They are not identical, however, because one homolog comes from the

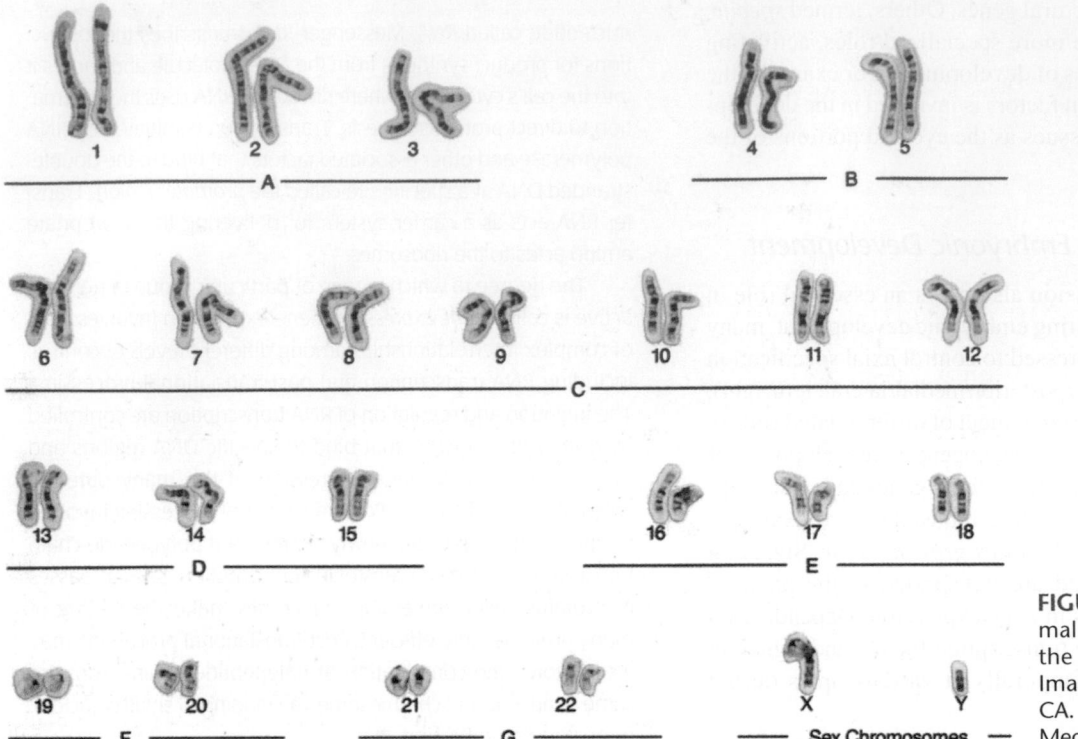

FIGURE 6-8 • Karyotype of normal human boy. (Courtesy of the Prenatal Diagnostic and Imaging Center, Sacramento, CA. Frederick W. Hansen, MD, Medical Director.)

haploid sperm of the father and one from the haploid ovum of the mother. The sex chromosomes, which make up the 23rd pair of chromosomes, determine the sex of a person. All males have an X and Y chromosome (*i.e.,* an X chromosome from the mother and a Y chromosome from the father); all females have two X chromosomes (*i.e.,* one from each parent). The much smaller Y chromosome contains the *male-specific region* (MSY) that determines sex. This region comprises more than 90% of the length of the Y chromosome.

CHROMOSOME STRUCTURE

- The DNA that stores genetic material is organized into 23 pairs of chromosomes. There are 22 pairs of autosomes, which are alike for males and females, and one pair of sex chromosomes, with XX pairing in females and XY pairing in males.
- Cell division involves the duplication of the chromosomes. Duplication of chromosomes in somatic cell lines involves mitosis, in which each daughter cell receives a pair of 23 chromosomes. Meiosis is limited to replicating germ cells and results in formation of a single set of 23 chromosomes.

Only one X chromosome in the female is active in controlling the expression of genetic traits; however, both X chromosomes are activated during gametogenesis. In the female, the active X chromosome is invisible, but the inactive X chromosome can be visualized with appropriate nuclear staining. Inac-

tivation is thought to involve the addition of a methyl group to the X chromosome. This inactive chromatin mass is seen as the *Barr body* in epithelial cells or as the drumstick body in the chromatin of neutrophils. The genetic sex of a child can be determined by microscopic study of cell or tissue samples. The total number of X chromosomes is equal to the number of Barr bodies plus one (*i.e.,* an inactive plus an active X chromosome). For example, the cells of a normal female have one Barr body and therefore a total of two X chromosomes. A normal male has no Barr bodies. Males with Klinefelter syndrome, who have one Y and two X chromosomes (one active and one inactive), exhibit one Barr body (discussed in Chapter 7). In the female, whether the active X chromosome is derived from the mother or father is determined within a few days after conception, the selection being random for each postmitotic cell line. Thus, the tissues of normal women have on average 50% maternally derived and 50% paternally derived active X chromosomes. This is called the *Lyon principle*, after Mary Lyon, the British geneticist who described it.

Cell Division

Two types of cell division occur in humans and many other animals: mitosis and meiosis. Mitosis involves duplication of somatic cells in the body and is represented by the cell cycle (see Chapter 4). *Meiosis* is limited to replicating germ cells and takes place only once in a cell line. It results in the formation of gametes or reproductive cells (*i.e.,* ovum and sperm), each of which has only a single set of 23 chromosomes. Meiosis is typically divided into two distinct phases, meiosis I and meiosis II. Similar to mitosis, cells about to undergo the first meiotic division replicate their DNA during interphase (Fig. 6-9). During

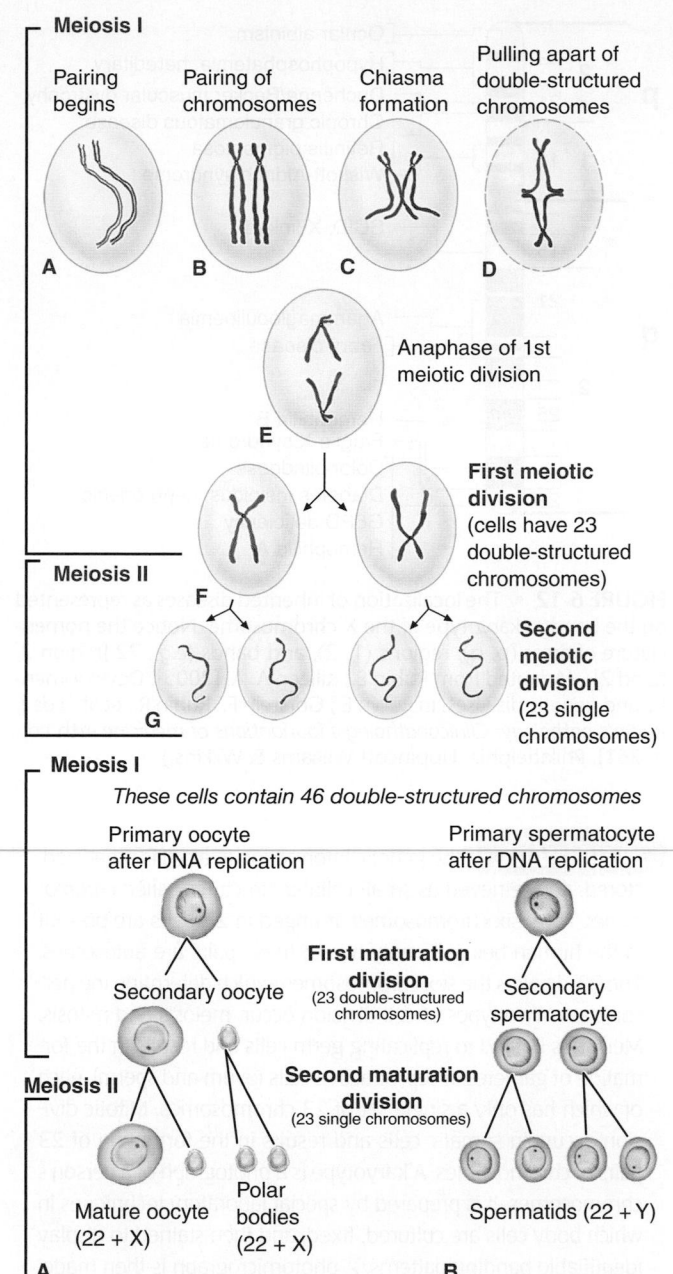

Meiosis I

Pairing begins | Pairing of chromosomes | Chiasma formation | Pulling apart of double-structured chromosomes

A   B   C   D

Anaphase of 1st meiotic division

E

First meiotic division (cells have 23 double-structured chromosomes)

Meiosis II

F

Second meiotic division (23 single chromosomes)

G

Meiosis I

These cells contain 46 double-structured chromosomes

Primary oocyte after DNA replication | Primary spermatocyte after DNA replication

First maturation division (23 double-structured chromosomes)

Secondary oocyte | Secondary spermatocyte

Meiosis II

Second maturation division (23 single chromosomes)

Mature oocyte (22 + X) | Polar bodies (22 + X) | Spermatids (22 + Y)

A   B

FIGURE 6-9 • First and second meiotic divisions. **(Top)** Meiosis I, during which homologous chromosomes (A) approach each other and (B) pair; (C) intimately paired homologous chromosomes interchange chromatid fragments (crossing over); and (D) double-structured chromosomes pull apart. (E) Anaphase of first meiotic division. During meiosis II (F, G), the double-structured chromosomes pull apart at the centromere to form four single-stranded chromosomes (reduction division). **(Bottom)** Events occurring during meiosis I and II in female and male gametes. (A) The primitive female germ cell (oocyte) produces only one mature gamete, the mature oocyte. (B) The primitive male germ cell (primary spermatocyte) produces four spermatids, all of which develop into spermatozoa. (Adapted from Sadler R. W. [2006]. *Langman's medical embryology* [10th ed., p. 14]. Philadelphia: Lippincott Williams & Wilkins.)

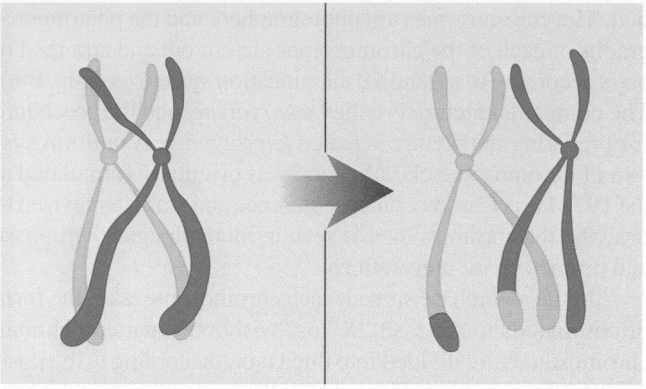

FIGURE 6-10 • Crossing over of DNA at the time of meiosis.

metaphase I, homologous autosomal chromosomes pair up, forming a synapsis or tetrad (two chromatids per chromosome). They are sometimes called *bivalents.* They do, however, pair up in several regions. The X and Y chromosomes are not homologs and do not form bivalents. While in metaphase I, an interchange of chromatid segments can occur. This process is called *crossing over* (Fig. 6-10). Crossing over allows for new combinations of genes, increasing genetic variability. After telophase I, each of the two daughter cells contains one member of each homologous pair of chromosomes and a sex chromosome (23 double-stranded chromosomes). No DNA synthesis occurs before meiotic division II. During anaphase II, the 23 double-stranded chromosomes (two chromatids) of each of the two daughter cells from meiosis I divide at their centromeres. Each subsequent daughter cell receives 23 single-stranded chromatids. Thus, a total of four daughter cells are formed by a meiotic division of one cell.

Meiosis, occurring only in the gamete-producing cells found in the testes or ovaries, has a different outcome in males and females. In males, meiosis (spermatogenesis) results in four viable daughter cells called *spermatids* that differentiate into sperm cells. In females, gamete formation or oogenesis is quite different. After the first meiotic division of a primary oocyte, a secondary oocyte and another structure called a *polar body* are formed. This small polar body contains little cytoplasm, but it may undergo a second meiotic division, resulting in two polar bodies. The secondary oocyte undergoes its second meiotic division, producing one mature oocyte and another polar body. Four viable sperm cells are produced during spermatogenesis, but only one ovum from oogenesis.

Chromosome Structure

Cytogenetics is the study of the structure and numeric characteristics of the cell's chromosomes. Chromosome studies can be done on any tissue or cell that grows and divides in culture. Lymphocytes from venous blood are frequently used for this purpose. After the cells have been cultured, a drug called *colchicine* is used to arrest mitosis in metaphase. A chromosome spread is prepared by fixing and spreading the chromosomes on a slide. Subsequently, appropriate staining techniques show the chromosomal banding patterns so they can be identified. The chromosomes are photographed, and the photomicrographs of each of the chromosomes are cut out and arranged in pairs according to a standard classification system (see Fig. 6-8). The completed picture is called a *karyotype,* and the procedure for preparing the picture is called *karyotyping.* A uniform system of chromosome classification was originally formulated at the 1971 Paris Chromosome Conference and was later revised to describe the chromosomes as seen in more elongated prophase and prometaphase preparations.

In the metaphase spread, each chromosome takes the form of chromatids to form an "X" or "wishbone" pattern. Human chromosomes are divided into three types according to the position of the centromere (Fig. 6-11). If the centromere is in the center and the arms are of approximately the same length, the chromosome is said to be *metacentric;* if it is not centered and the arms are of clearly different lengths, it is *submetacentric;* and if it is near one end, it is *acrocentric.* The short arm of the chromosome is designated as "p" for "petite," and the long arm is designated as "q" for no other reason than that it is the next letter of the alphabet. The arms of the chromosome are indicated by the chromosome number followed by the p or q designation (*e.g.,* 15p). Chromosomes 13, 14, 15, 21, and 22 have small masses of chromatin called *satellites* attached to their short arms by narrow stalks. At the ends of each chromosome are special DNA sequences called *telomeres.* Telomeres allow the end of the DNA molecule to be replicated completely.

The banding patterns of a chromosome are used in describing the position of a gene on a chromosome. Each arm of a chromosome is divided into regions, which are numbered from the centromere outward (*e.g.,* 1, 2) The regions are further divided into bands, which are also numbered (Fig. 6-12). These numbers are used in designating the position of a gene on a chromosome. For example, Xp22 refers to band 2, region 2 of the short arm (p) of the X chromosome.

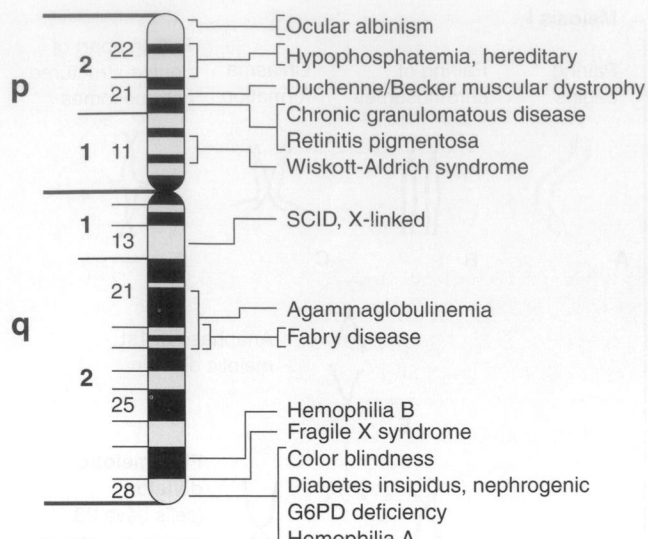

FIGURE 6-12 • The localization of inherited diseases as represented on the banded karyotype of the X chromosome. Notice the nomenclature of arms (p, q), regions (1, 2), and bands (*e.g.,* 22 [region 2, band 2]). (Adapted from Rubin E., Killeen A. A. [2005]. Developmental and genetic diseases. In Rubin E., Gorstein F., Rubin R., et al. [Eds.], *Rubin's pathology: Clinicopathologic foundations of medicine* [4th ed., p. 261]. Philadelphia: Lippincott Williams & Wilkins.)

IN SUMMARY,   the genetic information in a cell is organized, stored, and retrieved as small cellular structures called *chromosomes.* Forty-six chromosomes arranged in 23 pairs are present in the human being. Twenty-two of these pairs are autosomes. The 23rd pair is the sex chromosomes, which determine the person's sex. Two types of cell division occur, meiosis and mitosis. Meiosis is limited to replicating germ cells and results in the formation of gametes or reproductive cells (ovum and sperm), each of which has only a single set of 23 chromosomes. Mitotic division occurs in somatic cells and results in the formation of 23 pairs of chromosomes. A karyotype is a photograph of a person's chromosomes. It is prepared by special laboratory techniques in which body cells are cultured, fixed, and then stained to display identifiable banding patterns. A photomicrograph is then made. Often the photomicrographs of individual chromosomes are cut out and regrouped according to chromosome number. ■

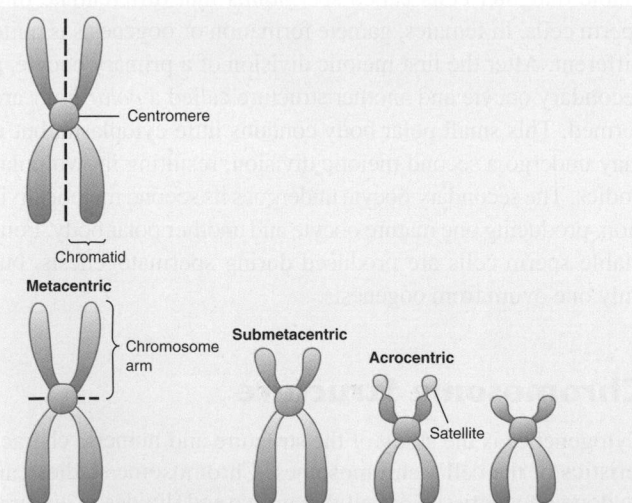

FIGURE 6-11 • Three basic shapes and the component parts of human metaphase chromosomes. The relative size of the satellite on the acrocentric chromosome is exaggerated for visibility (Adapted from Cormack D. H. [1993]. *Essential histology.* Philadelphia: JB Lippincott.)

PATTERNS OF INHERITANCE

After completing this section of the chapter, you should be able to meet the following objectives:

■ Construct a hypothetical pedigree for a recessive and dominant trait according to Mendel's laws.
■ Contrast genotype and phenotype.
■ Define the terms *allele, locus, expressivity,* and *penetrance.*

The characteristics inherited from a person's parents are inscribed in gene pairs found along the length of the chromosomes. Alternate forms of the same gene are possible (*i.e.*, one inherited from the mother and the other from the father), and each may produce a different aspect of a trait.

Definitions

Genetics has its own set of definitions. The *genotype* of a person is the genetic information stored in the base sequence triplet code. The *phenotype* refers to the recognizable traits, physical or biochemical, associated with a specific genotype. Often, the genotype is not evident by available detection methods. More than one genotype may have the same phenotype. Some brown-eyed persons are carriers of the code for blue eyes, and other brown-eyed persons are not. Phenotypically, these two types of brown-eyed persons are the same, but genotypically they are different.

TRANSMISSION OF GENETIC INFORMATION

- The transmission of information from one generation to the next is vested in genetic material transferred from each parent at the time of conception.
- Alleles are the alternate forms of a gene (one from each parent), and the locus is the position that they occupy on the chromosome.
- The genotype of a person represents the sum total of the genetic information in the cells, and the phenotype the physical manifestations of that information.
- Penetrance is the percentage in a population with a particular genotype in which that genotype is phenotypically manifested, whereas expressivity is the manner in which the gene is expressed.
- Mendelian, or single-gene, patterns of inheritance include autosomal dominant and recessive traits that are transmitted from parents to their offspring in a predictable manner. Polygenic inheritance, which involves multiple genes, and multifactorial inheritance, which involves multiple genes as well as environmental factors, are less predictable.

With regard to a genetic disorder, not all persons with a mutant gene are affected to the same extent. *Expressivity* refers to the manner in which the gene is expressed in the phenotype, which can range from mild to severe. *Penetrance* represents the ability of a gene to express its function. Seventy-five percent penetrance means 75% of persons of a particular genotype present with a recognizable phenotype. Syndactyly and blue sclera are genetic mutations that often do not exhibit 100% penetrance.

The position of a gene on a chromosome is called its *locus,* and alternate forms of a gene at the same locus are called *alleles.* When only one pair of genes is involved in the transmission of information, the term *single-gene trait* is used. Single-gene traits follow the mendelian laws of inheritance (to be discussed).

Polygenic inheritance involves multiple genes at different loci, with each gene exerting a small additive effect in determining a trait. Most human traits are determined by multiple pairs of genes, many with alternate codes, accounting for some dissimilar forms that occur with certain genetic disorders. Polygenic traits are predictable, but with less reliability than single-gene traits. *Multifactorial* inheritance is similar to polygenic inheritance in that multiple alleles at different loci affect the outcome; the difference is that multifactorial inheritance includes environmental effects on the genes.

Many other gene–gene interactions are known. These include *epistasis,* in which one gene masks the phenotypic effects of another, nonallelic gene; *multiple alleles,* in which more than one allele affects the same trait (*e.g.,* ABO blood types); *complementary genes,* in which each gene is mutually dependent on the other; and *collaborative genes,* in which two different genes influencing the same trait interact to produce a phenotype neither gene alone could produce.

Genetic Imprinting

Besides autosomal and sex-linked genes and mitochondrial inheritance, it was found that certain genes exhibit a "parent of origin" type of transmission in which the parental genomes do not always contribute equally in the development of an individual (Fig. 6-13). The transmission of this phenomenon was given the name *genomic imprinting* by Helen Crouse in 1960. Although rare, it is estimated that approximately 100 genes exhibit genomic, or genetic, imprinting. Evidence suggests a genetic conflict occurs in the developing embryo: the male genome attempts to establish larger offspring, whereas the female prefers smaller offspring to conserve her energy for the current and subsequent pregnancies.

It was the pathologic analysis of ovarian teratomas (tumors made up of various cell types derived from an undifferentiated germ cell) and hydatidiform moles (gestational tumors made up of trophoblastic tissue) that yielded the first evidence of genetic imprinting. All ovarian teratomas were found to have a 46,XX karyotype. The results of detailed chromosomal polymorphism analysis confirmed that these tumors developed without the paternally derived genome. Conversely, analysis of hydatidiform moles suggested that they were tumors of paternal origin.

Well-known examples of genomic imprinting are the transmission of the mutations in Prader-Willi and Angelman syndromes. Both syndromes exhibit mental retardation as a common feature. It was also found that both disorders had the same deletion in chromosome 15. When the deletion is inherited from the mother, the infant presents with Angelman ("happy puppet") syndrome; when the same deletion is inherited from the father, Prader-Willi syndrome results.

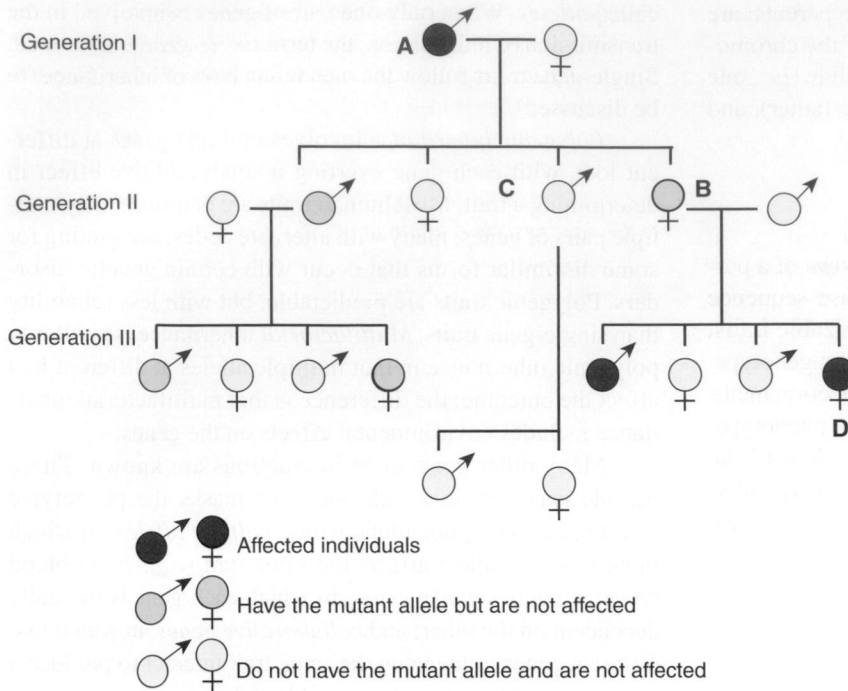

FIGURE 6-13 • Pedigree of genetic imprinting. In generation I, male **A** has inherited a mutant allele from his affected mother (not shown); the gene is "turned off" during spermatogenesis, and therefore none of his offspring (generation II) will express the mutant allele, regardless of whether they are carriers. However, the gene will be "turned on" again during oogenesis in any of his daughters (**B**) who inherit the allele. All offspring (generation III) who inherit the mutant allele will be affected. All offspring of normal children (**C**) will produce normal offspring. Children of female **D** will all express the mutation if they inherit the allele.

A related chromosomal disorder is *uniparental disomy.* This occurs when two chromosomes of the same number are inherited from one parent. Normally, this is not a problem except in cases where a chromosome has been imprinted by a parent. If an allele is inactivated by imprinting, the offspring will have only one working copy of the chromosome, resulting in possible problems.

Mendel's Laws

A main feature of inheritance is predictability: given certain conditions, the likelihood of the occurrence or recurrence of a specific trait is remarkably predictable. The units of inheritance are the genes, and the pattern of single-gene expression can often be predicted using Mendel's laws of genetic transmission. Techniques and discoveries since Gregor Mendel's original work was published in 1865 have led to some modification of the original laws.

Mendel discovered the basic pattern of inheritance by conducting carefully planned experiments with simple garden peas. Experimenting with several phenotypic traits in peas, Mendel proposed that inherited traits are transmitted from parents to offspring by means of independently inherited factors—now known as genes—and that these factors are transmitted as recessive and dominant traits. Mendel labeled dominant factors (his round peas) "A" and recessive factors (his wrinkled peas) "a." Geneticists continue to use capital letters to designate dominant traits and lowercase letters to identify recessive traits. The possible combinations that can occur with transmission of single-gene dominant and recessive traits can be described by constructing a figure called a *Punnett square* using capital and lowercase letters (Fig. 6-14).

The observable traits of single-gene inheritance are inherited by the offspring from the parents. During maturation, the primordial germ cells (*i.e.,* sperm and ovum) of both parents undergo meiosis, or reduction division, in which the number of chromosomes is divided in half (from 46 to 23). At this time, the two alleles from a gene locus separate so that each germ cell

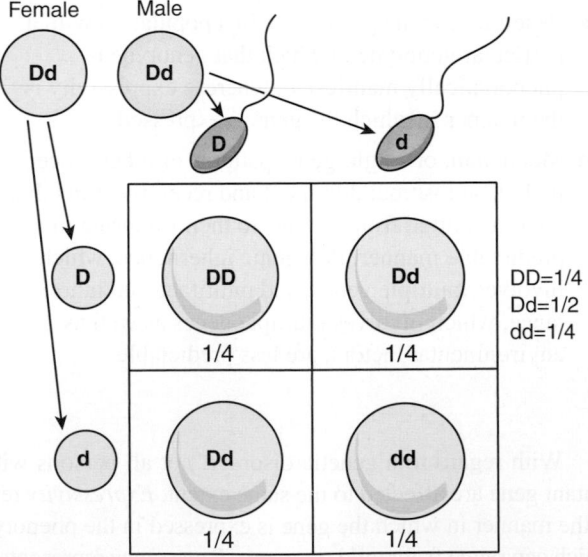

FIGURE 6-14 • The Punnett square showing all possible combinations for transmission of a single gene trait (dimpled cheeks). The example shown is when both parents are heterozygous (Dd) for the trait. The alleles carried by the mother are on the left and those carried by the father are on the top. The D allele is dominant and the d allele is recessive. The DD and Dd offspring have dimples and the dd offspring does not.

receives only one allele from each pair (*i.e.,* Mendel's first law). According to Mendel's second law, the alleles from the different gene loci segregate independently and recombine randomly in the zygote. Persons in whom the two alleles of a given pair are the same (AA or aa) are called *homozygotes. Heterozygotes* have different alleles (Aa) at a gene locus. A *recessive trait* is one expressed only in a homozygous pairing; a *dominant trait* is one expressed in either a homozygous or a heterozygous pairing. All persons with a dominant allele (depending on the penetrance of the genes) manifest that trait. A *carrier* is a person who is heterozygous for a recessive trait and does not manifest the trait. For example, the genes for blond hair are recessive and those for brown hair are dominant. Therefore, only persons with a genotype having two alleles for blond hair would be blond; persons with either one or two brown alleles would have dark hair.

Pedigree

A pedigree is a graphic method for portraying a family history of an inherited trait. It is constructed from a carefully obtained family history and is useful for tracing the pattern of inheritance for a particular trait.

> **IN SUMMARY,** inheritance represents the likelihood of the occurrence or recurrence of a specific genetic trait. The genotype refers to information stored in the genetic code of a person, whereas the phenotype represents the recognizable traits, physical and biochemical, associated with the genotype. Expressivity refers to the expression of a gene in the phenotype, and penetrance is the ability of a gene to express its function. The point on the DNA molecule that controls the inheritance of a particular trait is called a *gene locus.* Alternate forms of a gene at a gene locus are called *alleles.* The alleles at a gene locus may carry recessive or dominant traits. A recessive trait is one expressed only when two copies (homozygous) of the recessive allele are present. Dominant traits are expressed with either homozygous or heterozygous pairing of the alleles. A pedigree is a graphic method for portraying a family history of an inherited trait. ■

GENE TECHNOLOGY

After completing this section of the chapter, you should be able to meet the following objectives:

- Differentiate between genetic and physical genomic maps.
- Briefly describe the methods used in linkage studies, dosage studies, and hybridization studies.
- Describe the goals of the International HapMap Project.
- Describe the process of recombinant DNA technology.
- Characterize the process of RNA interference.

The past several decades have seen phenomenal advances in the field of genetics. These advances have included the assembly of physical and genetic maps through the Human Genome Project; the establishment of the International HapMap Project to map the haplotypes of the many closely related single-nucleotide polymorphisms in the human genome; and the development of methods for applying the technology of these projects to the diagnosis and treatment of disease.

Genetic Mapping

Genetic mapping is the assignment of genes to specific chromosomes or parts of the chromosome. Another type of mapping strategy, the haplotype map, focuses on identifying the slight variations in the human genome that affect an individual's susceptibility to disease and responses to environmental factors such as microbes, toxins, and drugs.

There are two types of gene maps: genetic maps and physical maps. Genetic maps are like highway maps. They use linkage studies (*e.g.,* dosage, hybridization) to estimate the distances between chromosomal landmarks (*i.e.,* gene markers). Physical maps are similar to a surveyor's map. They make use of cytogenetic and molecular techniques to determine the actual, physical locations of genes on chromosomes. Genetic maps and physical maps have been refined over the decades. The earliest mapping efforts localized genes on the X chromosome. The initial assignment of a gene to a particular chromosome was made in 1911 for the color blindness gene inherited from the mother (*i.e.,* following the X-linked pattern of inheritance). In 1968, the specific location of the Duffy blood group on the long arm of chromosome 1 was determined.

The Human Genome Project

The Human Genome Project, initiated in 1990, sought to identify all the genes in the human genome. The international project was charged with developing genetic and physical maps that allowed the precise location of genes and with exploring technologies that would enable the sequencing of large amounts of DNA with high accuracy and low cost. One of the surprising findings of the 2003 final report of the project was that humans have only 30,000 to 35,000 genes, much less than the previously estimated 80,000 to 150,000 genes.

To date, the locations of more than 25,000 genes have been mapped to a specific chromosome, and most of them to a specific region on the chromosome. However, genetic mapping is continuing so rapidly that these numbers are constantly being updated. An excellent source of articles regarding specific chromosome sequencing in humans is the National Center for Biotechnology Information (NCBI) (www.ncbi.nlm.nih.gov/index.html). Another source is the Genome Data Base, a central database for mapped genes and an international repository for most mapping information.

Genetic Mapping Methods

Many methods have been used for developing genetic maps. The most important ones are family linkage studies, gene dosage methods, and hybridization studies. Often, the specific assignment of a gene is made using information from several mapping techniques.

Linkage Studies. Linkage studies assume that genes occur in a linear array along the chromosomes. During meiosis, the paired chromosomes of the diploid germ cell exchange genetic material because of the crossing-over phenomenon (see Fig. 6-10). This exchange usually involves more than one gene; large blocks of genes (representing large portions of the chromosome) are usually exchanged. Although the point at which one block separates from another occurs randomly, the closer together two genes are on the same chromosome, the greater the chance is that they will be passed on together to the offspring. When two inherited traits occur together at a rate greater than would occur by chance alone, they are said to be *linked.*

Several methods take advantage of the crossing over and recombination of genes to map a particular gene. In one method, any gene that is already assigned to a chromosome can be used as a marker to assign other linked genes. For example, it was found that an extra long chromosome 1 and the Duffy blood group were inherited as a dominant trait, placing the position of the blood group gene close to the extra material on chromosome 1. Color blindness has been linked to classic hemophilia A (*i.e.,* lack of factor VIII) in some pedigrees; hemophilia A has been linked to glucose-6-phosphate dehydrogenase deficiency in others; and color blindness has been linked to glucose-6-phosphate dehydrogenase deficiency in still others. Because the gene for color blindness is found on the X chromosome, all three genes must be found in a small section of the X chromosome. Linkage analysis can be used clinically to identify affected persons in a family with a known genetic defect. Males, because they have one X and one Y chromosome, are said to be *hemizygous* for sex-linked traits. Females can be homozygous (normal or mutant) or heterozygous for sex-linked traits. Heterozygous females are known as *carriers* for X-linked defects.

One autosomal recessive disorder that has been successfully diagnosed prenatally by linkage studies using amniocentesis is congenital adrenal hyperplasia (due to 21-hydroxylase deficiency), which is linked to an immune response gene (human leukocyte antigen [HLA]) type. Postnatal linkage studies have been used in diagnosing hemochromatosis, which is closely linked to another HLA type. Persons with this disorder are unable to metabolize iron, and it accumulates in the liver and other organs. It cannot be diagnosed by conventional means until irreversible damage has been done. Given a family history of the disorder, HLA typing can determine if the gene is present, and if it is present, dietary restriction of iron intake may be used to prevent organ damage.

Gene Dosage Studies. Dosage studies involve measuring enzyme activity. Autosomal genes are normally arranged in pairs, and normally both are expressed. If both alleles are present and both are expressed, the activity of the enzyme should be 100%. If one member of the gene pair is missing, only 50% of the enzyme activity is present, reflecting the activity of the remaining normal allele.

Hybridization Studies. A recent biologic discovery revealed that two somatic cells from different species, when grown together in the same culture, occasionally fuse to form a new hybrid cell. Two types of hybridization methods are used in genomic studies: somatic cell hybridization and in situ hybridization.

Somatic cell hybridization involves the fusion of human somatic cells with those of a different species (typically, the mouse) to yield a cell containing the chromosomes of both species. Because these hybrid cells are unstable, they begin to lose chromosomes of both species during subsequent cell divisions. This makes it possible to obtain cells with different partial combinations of human chromosomes. The enzymes of these cells are then studied with the understanding that for an enzyme to be produced, a certain chromosome must be present and, therefore, the coding for the enzyme must be located on that chromosome.

In situ hybridization involves the use of specific sequences of DNA or RNA to locate genes that do not express themselves in cell culture. DNA and RNA can be chemically tagged with radioactive or fluorescent markers. These chemically tagged DNA or RNA sequences are used as probes to detect gene location. The probe is added to a chromosome spread after the DNA strands have been separated. If the probe matches the complementary DNA of a chromosome segment, it hybridizes and remains at the precise location (therefore the term *in situ*) on a chromosome. Radioactive or fluorescent markers are used to find the location of the probe.

Haplotype Mapping

As work on the Human Genome Project progressed, many researchers reasoned that identifying the common patterns of DNA sequence variations in the human genome would be possible. An international project, known as the *International HapMap Project,* was organized with the intent of developing a haplotype map of these variations. One of the findings of the Human Genome Project was that the genome sequence was 99.9% identical for all people. It is anticipated that the 0.1% variation may greatly affect an individual's response to drugs, toxins, and predisposition to various diseases. Sites in the DNA sequence where individuals differ at a single DNA base are called *single nucleotide polymorphisms* (SNPs, pronounced "snips"). A haplotype consists of the many closely linked SNPs on a single chromosome that generally are passed as a block from one generation to another in a particular population (Fig. 6-15). One of the motivating factors behind the HapMap Project was the realization that the identification of a few SNPs was enough to uniquely identify the haplotypes in a block. The specific SNPs that identify the haplotypes are called *tag SNPs.* A HapMap is a map of these haplotype blocks and their tag SNPs. This approach should prove useful in reducing the number of SNPs required to examine an entire genome and make genome scanning methods much more efficient in finding regions with genes that contribute to disease development.

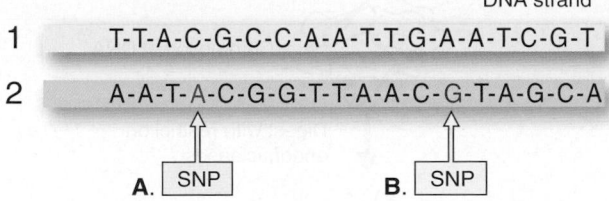

DNA strand

1   T-T-A-C-G-C-C-A-A-T-T-G-A-A-T-C-G-T

2   A-A-T-A-C-G-G-T-T-A-A-C-G-T-A-G-C-A

A. SNP   **B.** SNP

FIGURE 6-15 • Two single nucleotide substitutions (SNPs) along DNA strand 2. At **A**, the SNP replaces adenine (A) for guanine, whereas at **B**, guanine (G) is substituted for thymine. SNPs occur on average every 1200 bases along the DNA molecule. It is estimated that a human genome contains about 10,000 SNPs. (Courtesy of Edward W. Carroll.)

It is anticipated that the HapMap Project will provide a useful tool for disease diagnosis and management. Much attention has focused on the use of SNPs to decide whether a genetic variant is associated with a higher risk of disease susceptibility in one population versus another. Pharmacogenetics addresses the variability of drug response due to inherited characteristics in individuals. With the availability of SNPs, it may soon be possible to identify persons who can be expected to respond favorably to a drug and those who can be expected to experience adverse reactions. This would result in safer, more effective, and more cost-efficient use of medications.

Recombinant DNA Technology

The term *recombinant DNA* refers to a combination of DNA molecules that are not found together in nature. Recombinant DNA technology makes it possible to identify the DNA sequence in a gene and produce the protein product encoded by a gene. The specific nucleotide sequence of a DNA fragment can often be identified by analyzing the amino acid sequence and mRNA codon of its protein product. Short sequences of base pairs can be synthesized, radioactively labeled, and subsequently used to identify their complementary sequence. In this way, identifying normal and abnormal gene structures is possible.

Tests of DNA sequences are particularly useful in identifying polymorphisms, including the previously discussed SNPs, that are associated with various diseases. Because genetic variations are so distinctive, DNA fingerprinting (analysis of DNA sequence differences) can be used to determine family relationships or help identify persons involved in criminal acts. The methods of recombinant DNA technology can also be used in the treatment of disease. For example, recombinant DNA technology is used in the manufacture of human insulin that is used to treat diabetes mellitus.

Gene Isolation and Cloning

The gene isolation and cloning methods used in recombinant DNA technology rely on the fact that the genes of all organisms, from bacteria through mammals, are based on a similar molecular organization. Gene cloning requires cutting a DNA molecule apart, modifying and reassembling its fragments, and producing copies of the modified DNA, its mRNA, and its gene product. The DNA molecule is cut apart by using a bacterial enzyme, called a *restriction enzyme,* that binds to DNA wherever a particular short sequence of base pairs is found and cleaves the molecule at a specific nucleotide site. In this way, a long DNA molecule can be broken down into smaller, discrete fragments, one of which presumably contains the gene of interest. Many restriction enzymes are commercially available that cut DNA at different recognition sites.

The restrictive fragments of DNA can often be replicated through insertion into a unicellular organism, such as a bacterium (Fig. 6-16). To do this, a cloning vector such as a bacterial virus or a small DNA circle that is found in most bacteria,

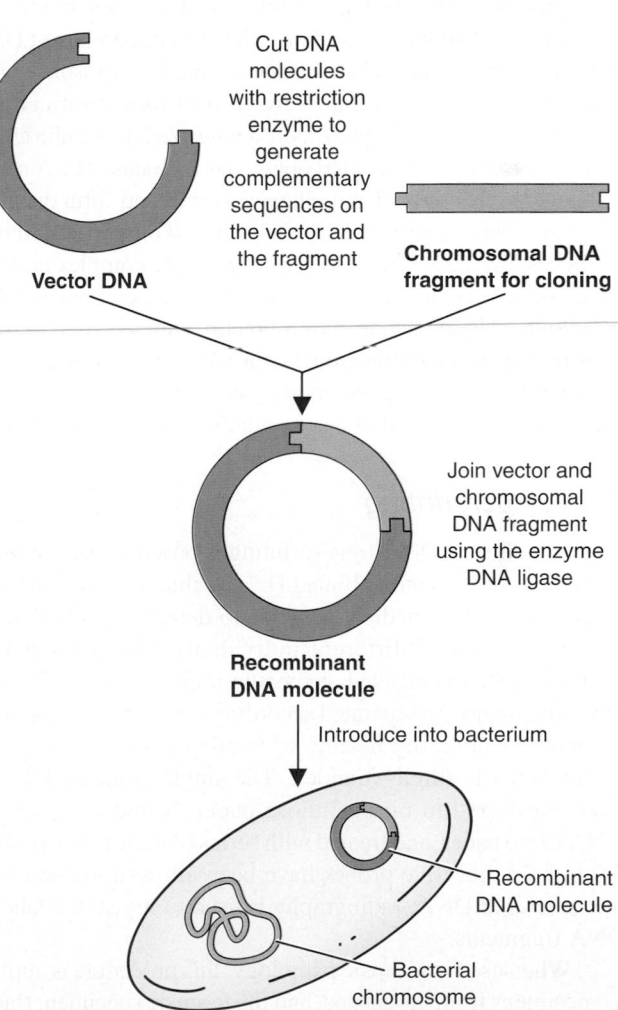

Cut DNA molecules with restriction enzyme to generate complementary sequences on the vector and the fragment

Vector DNA

Chromosomal DNA fragment for cloning

Join vector and chromosomal DNA fragment using the enzyme DNA ligase

Recombinant DNA molecule

Introduce into bacterium

Recombinant DNA molecule

Bacterial chromosome

FIGURE 6-16 • Recombinant DNA technology. By fragmenting DNA of any origin and inserting it in the DNA of rapidly reproducing foreign cells, billions of copies of a single gene can be produced in a short time. DNA to clone is inserted into a plasmid (a small, self-replicating circular molecule of DNA) that is separate from chromosomal DNA. When the recombinant plasmid is introduced into bacteria, the newly inserted segment will be replicated along with the rest of the plasmid. (From the U.S. Department of Energy Genomic Image Gallery.)

called a *plasmid,* is used. Viral and plasmid vectors replicate autonomously in the host bacterial cell. During gene cloning, a bacterial vector and the DNA fragment are mixed and joined by a special enzyme called a *DNA ligase.* The recombinant vectors formed are then introduced into a suitable culture of bacteria, and the bacteria are allowed to replicate and express the recombinant vector gene. Sometimes, mRNA taken from a tissue that expresses a high level of the gene is used to produce a complementary DNA molecule that can be used in the cloning process. Because the fragments of the entire DNA molecule are used in the cloning process, additional steps are taken to identify and separate the clone that contains the gene of interest.

Pharmaceutical Applications

Recombinant DNA technology has also made it possible to produce proteins that have therapeutic properties. One of the first products to be produced was human insulin. Recombinant DNA corresponding to the A chain of human insulin was isolated and inserted into plasmids that were in turn used to transform *Escherichia coli.* The bacteria then synthesized the insulin chain. A similar method was used to obtain the B chains. The A and B chains were then mixed and allowed to fold and form disulfide bonds, producing active insulin molecules. Human growth hormone has also been produced in *E. coli.* More complex proteins are produced in mammalian cell culture using recombinant DNA techniques. These include erythropoietin, which is used to stimulate red blood cell production; factor VIII, which is used to treat hemophilia; and tissue plasminogen activator (tPA), which is frequently administered after a heart attack to dissolve thrombi.

DNA Fingerprinting

The technique of DNA fingerprinting is based in part on those techniques used in recombinant DNA technology and on those originally used in medical genetics to detect slight variations in the genomes of different individuals. Using restriction enzymes, DNA is cleaved at specific regions (Fig. 6-17). The DNA fragments are separated according to size by electrophoresis and denatured (by heating or treating chemically) so that all the DNA is single stranded. The single-stranded DNA is then transferred to nitrocellulose paper, baked to attach the DNA to the paper, and treated with series of radioactive probes. After the radioactive probes have been allowed to bond with the denatured DNA, radiography is used to reveal the labeled DNA fragments.

When used in forensic pathology, this procedure is applied to specimens from the suspect and the forensic specimen. Banding patterns are then analyzed to see if they match. With conventional methods of analysis of blood and serum enzymes, a 1 in 100 to 1000 chance exists that the two specimens match because of chance. With DNA fingerprinting, these odds are 1 in 100,000 to 1 million.

When necessary, the polymerase chain reaction (PCR) can be used to amplify specific segments of DNA (see Chapter 16). It is particularly suited for amplifying regions of DNA for clin-

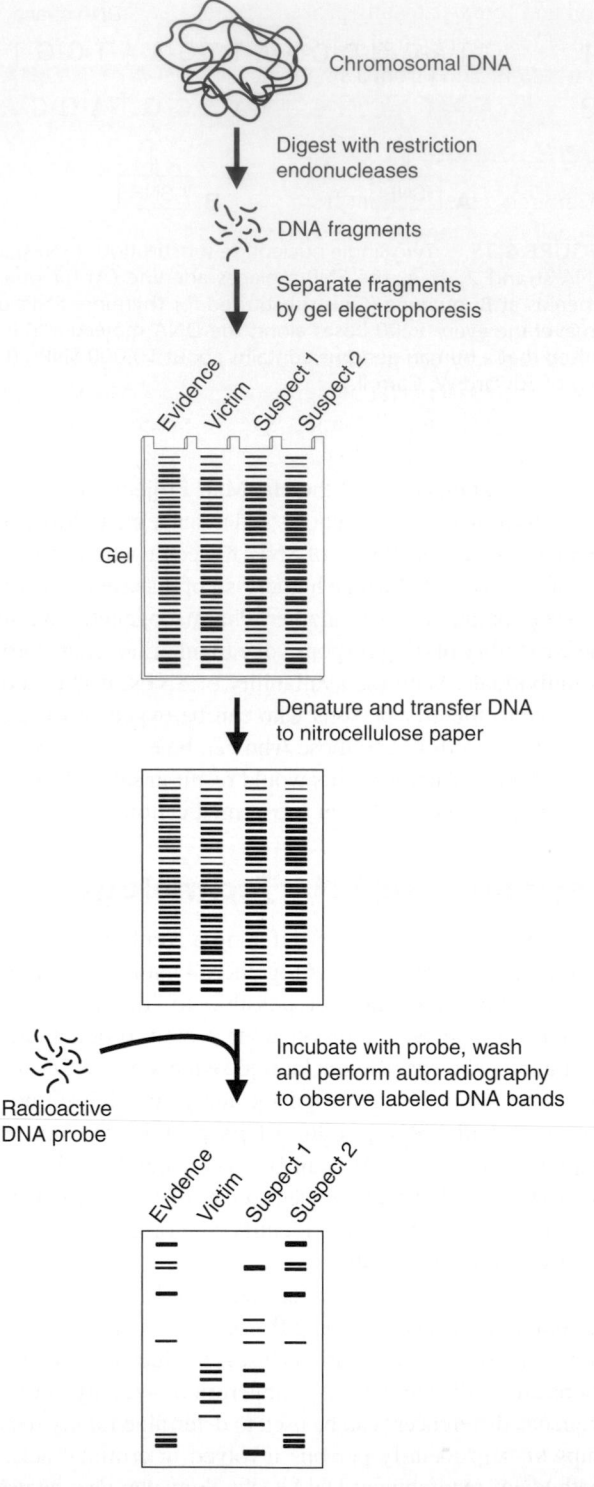

FIGURE 6-17 • DNA fingerprinting. Restrictive enzymes are used to break chromosomal DNA into fragments, which are then separated by gel electrophoresis, denatured, and transferred to nitrocellulose paper; the DNA bands are labeled with a radioactive probe and observed using autoradiography. (Modified from Smith C., Marks A. D., Lieberman M. [2005]. *Marks' basic medical biochemistry* [2nd ed., p. 309]. Philadelphia: Lippincott Williams & Wilkins.)

ical and forensic testing procedures because only a small sample of DNA is required as the starting material. Regions of DNA can be amplified from a single hair or drop of blood or saliva.

Gene Therapy

Although quite different from inserting genetic material into a unicellular organism such as bacteria, techniques are available for inserting genes into the genome of intact multicellular plants and animals. Promising delivery vehicles for these genes are the adenoviruses. These viruses are ideal vehicles because their DNA does not become integrated into the host genome; however, repeated inoculations are often needed because the body's immune system usually targets cells expressing adenovirus proteins. Sterically stable liposomes also show promise as DNA delivery mechanisms. This type of therapy is one of the more promising methods for the treatment of genetic disorders such as cystic fibrosis, certain cancers, and many infectious diseases.

Two main approaches are used in gene therapy: transferred genes can replace defective genes or they can selectively inhibit deleterious genes. Cloned DNA sequences are usually the compounds used in gene therapy. However, the introduction of the cloned gene into the multicellular organism can influence only the few cells that get the gene. An answer to this problem would be the insertion of the gene into a sperm or ovum; after fertilization, the gene would be replicated in all of the differentiating cell types. Even so, techniques for cell insertion are limited. Not only are moral and ethical issues involved, but these techniques cannot direct the inserted DNA to attach to a particular chromosome or supplant an existing gene by knocking it out of its place.

To date, gene therapy has been used successfully to treat children with severe combined immunodeficiency disease (see Chapter 20), and in a suicide gene transfer to facilitate treatment of graft-versus-host disease after donor lymphocyte infusion.

RNA Interference Technology

One approach of gene therapy focuses on the previously described replacement of missing or defective genes. However, several genetic disorders are not due to missing genes, but to faulty gene activity. With this in mind, some scientists are approaching the problem by using *RNA interference* (RNAi) to stop genes from making unwanted disease proteins. RNAi is a naturally occurring process in which small pieces of double-stranded RNA (small interfering RNA [siRNA]) suppress gene expression. Scientists believe that RNAi may have originated as a defense against viral infections and potentially harmful genomic invaders. In viral infections, RNAi would serve to control the infection by preventing the synthesis of viral proteins.

With the continued refinement of techniques to silence genes, RNAi has already had a major impact on molecular biology. For example, it has given scientists the ability to practice reverse genomics, in which a gene's function can be inferred through silencing its expression. Increasingly, pharmaceutical companies are using RNAi to identify disease-related drug targets. There also is considerable interest in harnessing RNAi

for therapeutic purposes, including the treatment of human immunodeficiency virus (HIV) infection and hepatitis C. Before this can occur, however, the therapeutic methods must be shown to be safe and effective, and obstacles to delivering the RNAi into targeted cells must be overcome. It is difficult for RNA to cross the cell membrane, and it is quickly broken down by enzymes in the blood.

IN SUMMARY, the genome is the gene complement of an organism. Genomic mapping is a method used to assign genes to particular chromosomes or parts of a chromosome. The most important ones used are family linkage studies, gene dosage methods, and hybridization studies. Often the specific assignment of a gene is determined by using information from several mapping techniques. Linkage studies assign a chromosome location to genes based on their close association with other genes of known location. Recombinant DNA studies involve the extraction of specific types of mRNA used in synthesis of complementary DNA strands. The complementary DNA strands, labeled with a radioisotope, bind with the genes for which they are complementary and are used as gene probes. A haplotype consists of the many closely linked SNPs on a single chromosome that generally are passed as a block from one generation to another in a particular population. The International HapMap Project has been developed to map the SNPs on the human genome with the anticipation that it may be useful in the prediction and management of disease.

Genetic engineering has provided the methods for manipulating nucleic acids and recombining genes (recombinant DNA) into hybrid molecules that can be inserted into unicellular organisms and reproduced many times over. As a result, proteins that formerly were available only in small amounts can now be made in large quantities once their respective genes have been isolated. DNA fingerprinting, which relies on recombinant DNA technologies and those of genetic mapping, is often used in forensic investigations. A newer strategy for management of genetic disorders focuses on gene silencing by using RNAi to stop genes from making unwanted disease proteins. ∎

Review Exercises

1. The human genome project has revealed that humans have only 30,000 to 35,000 genes. Only about 2% of the genome encodes instructions for protein synthesis, whereas 50% consists of repeat sequences that do not code proteins.

   A. *Use this information to explain how this small number of protein-encoding genes is able to produce the vast array of proteins needed for organ and structural development in the embryo, as well as those needed for normal function of the body in postnatal life.*

2. A child about to undergo surgery is typed for possible blood transfusions. His parents are told that he is type O positive. Both his mother and father are type A positive.

   A. *How would you explain this variation in blood type to the parents?*

3. The post-translational folding of proteins is essential to their proper functioning and degradation.

   A. *Hypothesize how age-related changes in the folding of proteins in the central nervous system could contribute to the development of the neurofibrillary tangles that are characteristic of Alzheimer disease.*

4. More than 100,000 people die of adverse drug reactions each year; another 2.2 million experience serious reactions, whereas others fail to respond at all to the therapeutic actions of drugs.

   A. *Explain how the use of information about single nucleotide polymorphisms (SNPs) might be used to map individual variations in drug responses.*

5. Human insulin, prepared by recombinant DNA technology, is now available for the treatment of diabetes mellitus.

   A. *Explain the techniques used for the production of a human hormone with this technology.*

Bibliography

Alberts B., Johnson A., Lewis J., et al. (2008). *Molecular biology of the cell* (5th ed., pp. 195–233, 386–387). New York: Garland Science.

Agrawal N., Dasaradhi P. V. N., Mohmmed A., et al. (2003). RNA interference: Biology, mechanism, and applications. *Microbiology and Molecular Biology Reviews* 67, 657–685.

Aparicio S. A. J. R. (2000). How to count human genes. *Nature Genetics* 25, 129–130.

Cheng J., Kapranov P., Drenkow J., et al. (2005). Transcriptional maps of 10 human chromosomes at 5-nucleotide resolution. *Science* 308, 1149–1154.

Choi C. Q. (2005). A new view of translational control: How P-bodies, stress granules, and other cytoplasmic foci manage the cellular currency. *The Scientist* 19(23), 20–22.

Fischer A., Cavazzana-Clavo M. (2006). Wither gene therapy? *The Scientist* 20(2), 36–40.

Gibbs R. (2005). Deeper into the genome. *Nature* 437, 1233–1234.

Gibson G., Muse S. V. (2004). *A primer of genome science.* Sunderland, MA: Sinauer Associates.

Hawley R. S., Mori C. A. (1999). *The human genome: A user's guide.* San Diego: Harcourt Academic Press.

Izaurralde E. (2005). Post-transcriptional regulation of gene expression. *EMBL Research Reports*, 82–84.

Jegalian K., Lahn B. T. (2001). Why the Y is so weird. *Scientific American* 282(2), 56–61.

Jorde L. B., Carey J. C., Bamshad M. J., et al. (2006). *Medical genetics* (3rd ed.). St. Louis: Mosby.

Kierszenbaum A. L. (2003). *Histology and cell biology: An introduction to pathology* (pp. 87–88). St. Louis: Mosby.

Klug W. S., Cummings M. R. (2005). *Essentials of genetics* (5th ed.). Upper Saddle River, NJ: Pearson Prentice Hall.

Marcario A. J. L., deMarario C. (2005). Sick chaperones, cellular stress, and disease. *New England Journal of Medicine* 353, 1489–1501.

MacFarlane W. M. (2000). Demystified: Transcription. *Journal of Clinical Pathology: Molecular Pathology* 53, 1–7.

Marieb E. N., Hoehn K. (2007). *Human anatomy and physiology* (7th ed., pp. 1146–1159). San Francisco: Pearson-Benjamin Cummings.

Martini F. H. (2006). *Fundamentals of anatomy and physiology* (7th ed., pp. 1098–1109). San Francisco: Pearson-Benjamin Cummings.

McElheny V. K. (2006). The human genome project. *The Scientist* 20(2), 42–48.

Moore K. L., Persaud T. V. N. (2003). *The developing human: Clinically orientated embryology* (7th ed., pp. 157–185). Philadelphia: WB Saunders.

Myers S., Bottolo L., Freeman C., et al. (2005). A fine-scale map of recombination rates and hotspots across the human genome. *Science* 310, 321–324.

National Human Genome Project. All about the Human Genome Project. [Online]. Available: www.genome.gov/10001772. Accessed September 1, 2006.

National Center for Biotechnology Information (NCBI). (2006). NCBI human genome resources site, including site for Human Genome Map. [On-line]. Available: www.ncbi.nlm.nih.gov/projects/genome/guide/human//. Accessed September 1, 2006.

Phimister E. G. (2005). Genomic cartography: Presenting the HapMap. *New England Journal of Medicine* 353, 1766–1768.

Sadler R. W. (2003). *Langman's medical embryology* (9th ed., pp. 3–30). Philadelphia: Lippincott Williams & Wilkins.

Sapienza C. (1990). Parenteral imprinting of genes. *Scientific American* 263(4), 52–60.

Selkirk S. M. (2004). Gene therapy in clinical medicine. *Postgraduate Medicine* 80, 560–570.

Shankar P., Manjunath N., Lieberman J. (2005). The prospect of silencing disease using RNA interference. *Journal of the American Medical Association* 293, 1367–1373.

Skaletsky H., Kuroda-Kawaguchi T., Minx P. J., et al. (2003). The male-specific region of the Y chromosome is a mosaic of discrete sequence classes. *Nature* 423, 825–837.

Smith C., Marks A. D., Lieberman M. (2005). *Marks' basic biochemistry: A clinical approach* (2nd ed., pp. 205–316). Philadelphia: Lippincott Williams & Wilkins.

Snustad D. P., Simmons J. M. (Eds.). (2000). *Principles of genetics* (2nd ed., pp. 3–21, 52–71, 91–115, 665–669). New York: John Wiley & Sons.

Stevenson M. (2004). Therapeutic potential of RNA interference. *New England Journal of Medicine* 351, 1772–1777.

Tuteja N., Tuteja R. (2001). Unraveling DNA repair in humans: Molecular mechanisms and consequences of repair defect. *Critical Review in Biochemistry and Molecular Biology* 36, 261–290.

Villard J. (2004). Transcription regulation and human disease. *Swiss Medicine Weekly* 124, 571–579.

Visit the**Point** http://thePoint.lww.com for **animations, journal articles, and more!**

Genetic and Congenital Disorders

CAROL M. PORTH

➤ Congenital defects, sometime called *birth defects,* are abnormalities of a body structure, function, or metabolism that are present at birth. They affect more than 120,000 (1 in 33) infants in the United States each year and are the leading cause of infant death.[1] Birth defects may be caused by genetic factors (*i.e.,* single-gene or multifactorial inheritance or chromosomal aberrations) or environmental factors that are active during embryonic or fetal development (*e.g.,* maternal disease, infections, or drugs taken during pregnancy). Although congenital defects are present at birth, genetic disorders may make their appearance later in life. This chapter provides an overview of genetic and congenital disorders and is divided into three parts: (1) genetic and chromosomal disorders, (2) disorders due to environmental agents, and (3) diagnosis and counseling.

GENETIC AND CHROMOSOMAL DISORDERS

After completing this section of the chapter, you should be able to meet the following objectives:

- Define the terms *congenital, allele, gene locus, gene mutation, genotype, phenotype, homozygous, heterozygous, polymorphism, gene penetrance,* and *gene expression.*
- Describe three types of single-gene disorders and their patterns of inheritance.
- Explain the genetic abnormality responsible for the fragile X syndrome.
- Contrast disorders due to multifactorial inheritance with those caused by single-gene inheritance.
- Describe three patterns of chromosomal breakage and rearrangement.
- Trace the events that occur during meiosis and explain the events that lead to trisomy or monosomy.
- Describe the chromosomal and major clinical characteristics of Down, Turner, and Klinefelter syndromes.
- State the primary mechanism of altered body function in mitochondrial gene disorders and relate it to the frequent involvement of neural and muscular tissues.

A genetic disorder can be described as a discrete event that affects gene expression in a group of cells related to each other by gene linkage. Most genetic disorders are caused by changes in the deoxyribonucleic acid (DNA) sequence that alters the synthesis of a single gene product. However, some genetic disorders are caused by chromosomal rearrangements that result in deletion or duplication of a group of closely linked genes, or by an abnormal number of chromosomes resulting from mistakes that occur during meiosis or mitosis.[2]

The genes on each chromosome are arranged in pairs and in strict order, with each gene occupying a specific location or *locus.* The two members of a gene pair, one inherited from the mother and the other from the father, are called *alleles.* If the members of a gene pair are identical (*i.e.,* code the exact same gene product), the person is *homozygous,* and if the two members are different, the person is *heterozygous.* The genetic composition of a person is called a *genotype,* whereas the *phenotype* is the observable expression of a genotype in terms of morphologic, biochemical, or molecular traits. If the trait is expressed in the heterozygote (one member of the gene pair codes for the trait), it is said to be *dominant;* if it is expressed only in the homozygote (both members of the gene pair code for the trait), it is *recessive.*

GENETIC AND CHROMOSOMAL DISORDERS

- Genetic disorders are inherited as autosomal dominant disorders, in which each child has a 50% chance of inheriting the disorder, or as autosomal recessive disorders, in which each child has a 25% chance of being affected, a 50% chance of being a carrier, and a 25% chance of being unaffected.

- Sex-linked disorders almost always are associated with the X chromosome and are predominantly recessive.

- Chromosomal disorders reflect events that occur at the time of meiosis and result from defective movement of an entire chromosome or from breakage of a chromosome with loss or translocation of genetic material.

Although gene expression usually follows a dominant or recessive pattern, it is possible for both alleles (members) of a gene pair to be fully expressed in the heterozygote, a condition called *codominance.* Many genes have only one normal version, which geneticists call the *wild-type* allele. Other genes have more than one normal allele (alternate forms) at the same locus. This is called *polymorphism.* Blood group inheritance (*e.g.,* AO, BO, AB) is an example of codominance and polymorphism (see Chapter 14).

A gene *mutation* is a biochemical event such as nucleotide change, deletion, or insertion that produces a new allele. A single mutant gene may be expressed in many different parts of the body. Marfan syndrome, for example, is a defect in a connective tissue protein that has widespread effects involving skeletal, eye, and cardiovascular structures. In other single-gene disorders, the same defect can be caused by mutations at several different loci. Childhood deafness can result from at least 16 different types of autosomal recessive mutations.

Genetic disorders can involve a single-gene trait, multifactorial inheritance, a chromosomal abnormality, or a mitochondrial gene disorder. The disorder may be inherited as a family trait or arise as a sporadic case due to a new mutation.

 Single-Gene Disorders

Single-gene disorders are caused by a defective or mutant allele at a single gene locus and follow mendelian patterns of inheritance described in Chapter 6. Single-gene disorders are primarily disorders of the pediatric age group. Less than 10% manifest after puberty, and only 1% after the reproductive years.[3]

Single-gene disorders are characterized by their patterns of transmission, which usually are obtained through a family genetic history. The patterns of inheritance depend on whether the phenotype is dominant or recessive and whether the gene is located on an autosomal or sex chromosome. In addition to disorders caused by mutations of genes located on the chromosomes located within the nucleus, another class of disorders with a maternal pattern of inheritance involves the mitochondrial genome.

Virtually all single-gene disorders lead to formation of an abnormal protein or decreased production of a gene product. The disorder can result in a defective enzyme or decreased amounts of an enzyme, defects in receptor proteins and their function, alterations in nonenzyme proteins, or mutations resulting in unusual reactions to drugs. Table 7-1 lists some of the common single-gene disorders and their manifestations.

Autosomal Dominant Disorders

In autosomal dominant disorders, a single mutant allele from an affected parent is transmitted to an offspring regardless of sex. The affected parent has a 50% chance of transmitting the disorder to each offspring (Fig. 7-1). The unaffected relatives of the parent or unaffected siblings of the offspring do not transmit the disorder. In many conditions, the age of onset is delayed, and the signs and symptoms of the disorder do not appear until later in life, as in Huntington chorea (see Chapter 53).

Autosomal dominant disorders also may manifest as a new mutation. Whether the mutation is passed on to the next generation depends on the affected person's reproductive capacity. Many new autosomal dominant mutations are accompanied by reduced reproductive capacity; therefore, the defect is not perpetuated in future generations. If an autosomal defect is accompanied by a total inability to reproduce, essentially all new cases of the disorder will be due to new mutations. If the defect does not affect reproductive capacity, it is more likely to be inherited.

TABLE 7-1 Some Disorders of Mendelian or Single-Gene Inheritance and Their Significance

DISORDER	SIGNIFICANCE
Autosomal Dominant	
Achondroplasia	Short-limb dwarfism
Adult polycystic kidney disease	Chronic kidney disease
Huntington chorea	Neurodegenerative disorder
Familial hypercholesterolemia	Premature atherosclerosis
Marfan syndrome	Connective tissue disorder with abnormalities in the skeletal, ocular, cardiovascular systems
Neurofibromatosis (NF)	Neurogenic tumors: fibromatous skin tumors, pigmented skin lesions, and ocular nodules in NF-1; bilateral acoustic neuromas in NF-2
Osteogenesis imperfecta	Brittle bone disease due to defects in collagen synthesis
Spherocytosis	Disorder of red blood cells
von Willebrand disease	Bleeding disorder
Autosomal Recessive	
Cystic fibrosis	Disorder of membrane transport of chloride ions in exocrine glands causing lung and pancreatic disease
Glycogen storage diseases	Excess accumulation of glycogen in the liver and hypoglycemia (von Gierke disease); glycogen accumulation in striated muscle in myopathic forms
Oculocutaneous albinism	Hypopigmentation of skin, hair, eyes as a result of inability to synthesize melanin
Phenylketonuria (PKU)	Lack of phenylalanine hydroxylase with hyperphenylalaninemia and impaired brain development
Sickle cell disease	Red blood cell defect
Tay-Sachs disease	Deficiency of hexosaminidase A; severe mental and physical deterioration beginning in infancy
X-Linked Recessive	
Bruton-type hypogammaglobulinemia	Immunodeficiency
Hemophilia A	Bleeding disorder
Duchenne dystrophy	Muscular dystrophy
Fragile X syndrome	Mental retardation

Although there is a 50% chance of inheriting a dominant genetic disorder from an affected parent, there can be wide variation in gene penetration and expression. When a person inherits a dominant mutant gene but fails to express it, the trait is described as having *reduced penetrance.* Penetrance is expressed in mathematical terms: a 50% penetrance indicates that a person who inherits the defective gene has a 50% chance of expressing the disorder. The person who has a mutant gene but does not express it is an important exception to the rule that unaffected persons do not transmit an autosomal dominant trait. These persons can transmit the gene to their descendants and so produce a skipped generation. Autosomal dominant disorders also can display *variable expressivity,* meaning that they can be expressed differently among individuals. Polydactyly or supernumerary digits, for example, may be expressed in either the fingers or the toes.

The gene products of autosomal dominant disorders usually are regulatory proteins involved in rate-limiting components of complex metabolic pathways or key components of structural proteins such as collagen.[4,5] Two disorders of autosomal inheritance, Marfan syndrome and neurofibromatosis (NF), are described in this chapter.

Marfan Syndrome. Marfan syndrome is an autosomal dominant disorder of the connective tissue, which gives shape and structure to other tissues in the body and holds them in place. The basic biochemical abnormality in Marfan syndrome affects *fibrillin I,* a major component of microfibrils found in the

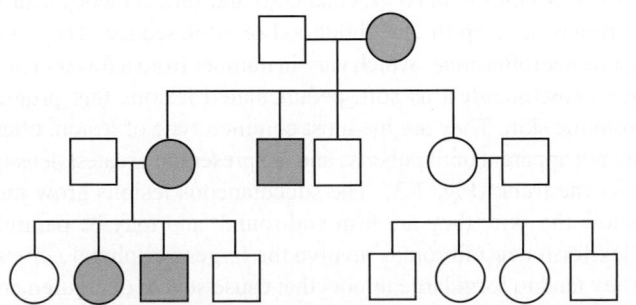

FIGURE 7-1 • Simple pedigree for inheritance of an autosomal dominant trait. The colored circle or square represents an affected parent with a mutant gene. An affected parent with an autosomal dominant trait has a 50% chance of passing the mutant gene on to each child regardless of sex.

extracellular matrix.[5] These microfibrils form the scaffolding for the deposition of elastin and are considered integral components of elastic fibers. Fibrillin I is coded by the *FBNI* gene, which maps to chromosome 15q21. Over 100 mutations in the *FBNI* gene have been found, making genetic diagnosis unfeasible. The prevalence of Marfan syndrome is estimated to be 1 per 5000. Approximately 70% to 80% of cases are familial and the remainder are sporadic, arising from new mutations in the germ cells of the parents.[5]

Marfan syndrome affects several organ systems, including the ocular system (eyes), the cardiovascular system (heart and blood vessels), and the skeletal system (bones and joints).[5–8] There is a wide range of variation in the expression of the disorder. Persons may have abnormalities of one or all three systems. The skeletal deformities, which are the most obvious features of the disorder, include a long, thin body with exceptionally long extremities and long, tapering fingers, sometimes called *arachnodactyly* or *spider fingers;* hyperextensible joints; and a variety of spinal deformities, including kyphosis and scoliosis (Fig. 7-2).

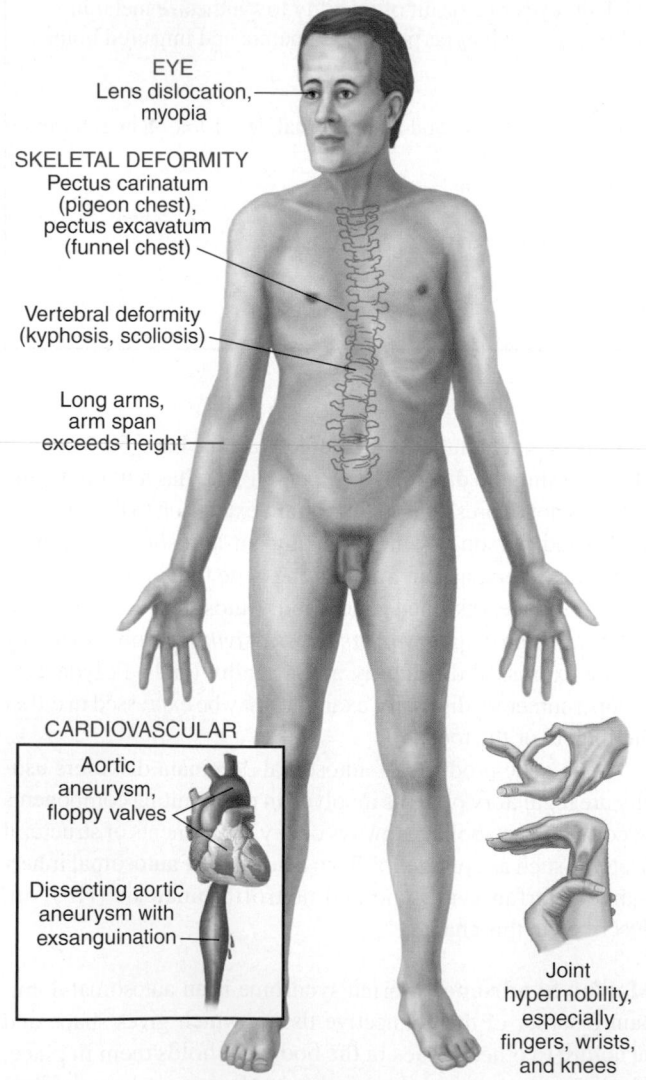

EYE
Lens dislocation, myopia

SKELETAL DEFORMITY
Pectus carinatum (pigeon chest), pectus excavatum (funnel chest)

Vertebral deformity (kyphosis, scoliosis)

Long arms, arm span exceeds height

CARDIOVASCULAR
Aortic aneurysm, floppy valves

Dissecting aortic aneurysm with exsanguination

Joint hypermobility, especially fingers, wrists, and knees

FIGURE 7-2 • Clinical features of Marfan syndrome.

Chest deformities, pectus excavatum (*i.e.,* deeply depressed sternum), or pigeon chest deformity, often are present and may require surgery. The most common eye disorder is bilateral dislocation of the lens due to weakness of the suspensory ligaments. Myopia and predisposition to retinal detachment also are common, the result of increased optic globe length due to altered connective tissue support of ocular structures. However, the most life-threatening aspects of the disorder are the cardiovascular defects, which include mitral valve prolapse, progressive dilation of the aortic valve ring, and weakness of the aorta and other arteries. Dissection and rupture of the aorta may lead to premature death. In women, the risk of aortic dissection is increased in pregnancy.

The diagnosis of Marfan syndrome is based on major and minor diagnostic criteria that include skeletal, cardiovascular, and ocular deformities. There is no cure for Marfan syndrome; treatment plans include echocardiograms and electrocardiograms to assess the status of the cardiovascular system, periodic eye examinations, and evaluation of the skeletal system, especially in children and adolescents. The risks associated with participation in sports depend on which organ systems are involved. Low to moderate activity levels are usually well tolerated. Strenuous activities such as contact sports, weight training, high-impact aerobics, and scuba diving should usually be avoided. Surgical treatment may become necessary in cases of progressive aortic dilation or acute aortic dissection.

Neurofibromatosis. Neurofibromatosis is a condition involving benign neurogenic tumors that arise from Schwann cells and other elements of the peripheral nervous system.[4,5,9,10] There are at least two genetically and clinically distinct forms of the disorder: type 1 NF (NF-1), also known as *von Recklinghausen disease,* and type 2 bilateral acoustic NF (NF-2). Both of these disorders result from a genetic defect in a tumor suppressor gene that regulates cell differentiation and growth. The gene for NF-1 has been mapped to chromosome 17, and the gene for NF-2 to chromosome 22.

Type 1 NF is a relatively common disorder, with a frequency of 1 in 3500.[5] Approximately 50% of cases have a family history of autosomal dominant transmission, and the remaining 50% appear to represent a new mutation. In more than 90% of persons with NF-1, cutaneous and subcutaneous neurofibromas develop in late childhood or adolescence. The cutaneous neurofibromas, which vary in number from a few to many hundreds, manifest as soft, pedunculated lesions that project from the skin. They are the most common type of lesion, often are not apparent until puberty, and are present in greatest density over the trunk (Fig. 7-3). The subcutaneous lesions grow just below the skin; they are firm and round, and may be painful. Plexiform neurofibromas involve the larger peripheral nerves. They tend to form large tumors that cause severe disfigurement of the face, overgrowth of an extremity, or skeletal deformities such as scoliosis. Pigmented nodules of the iris (Lisch nodules), which are specific for NF-1, usually are present after 6 years of age. They do not present any clinical problem but are useful in establishing a diagnosis.

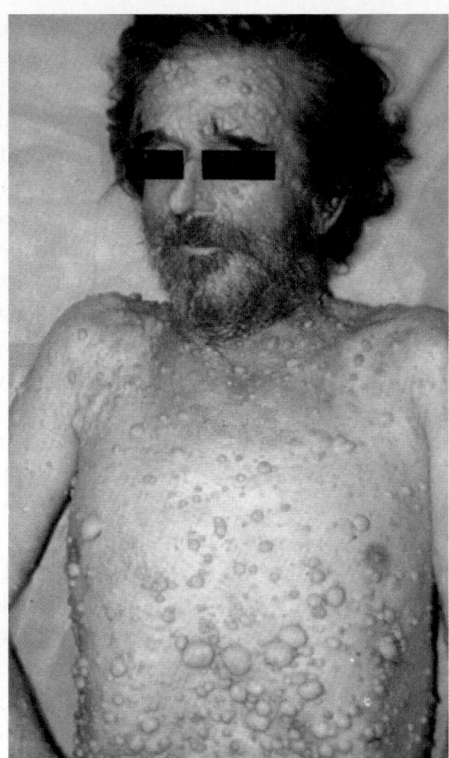

FIGURE 7-3 • Neurofibromatosis type 1. Multiple cutaneous neurofibromas are noted on the face and trunk. (From Rubin E., Killeen A. A., Strayer D. S. [2008]. Developmental and genetic diseases. In Rubin R., Strayer D. S. [Eds.], *Rubin's pathology: Clinicopathologic foundations of medicine* [5th ed., p. 201]. Philadelphia: Lippincott Williams & Wilkins.)

A second major component of NF-1 is the presence of large (usually ≥15 mm in diameter), flat cutaneous pigmentations, known as *café au lait spots.* They are usually a uniform light brown in whites and darker brown in persons of color, with sharply demarcated edges. Although small single lesions may be found in normal children, larger lesions or six or more spots larger than 1.5 cm in diameter suggest NF-1. The skin pigmentations become more evident with age as the melanosomes in the epidermal cells accumulate melanin.

Children with NF-1 are also susceptible to neurologic complications. There is an increased incidence of learning disabilities, attention deficit disorders, and abnormalities of speech among affected children. Complex partial and generalized tonic-clonic seizures are a frequent complication. Malignant neoplasms are also a significant problem in persons with NF-1. One of the major complications of NF-1, occurring in 3% to 5% of persons, is the appearance of a neurofibrosarcoma in a neurofibroma, usually a larger plexiform neurofibroma.[4] NF-1 is also associated with increased incidence of other neurogenic tumors, including meningiomas, optic gliomas, and pheochromocytomas.

Type 2 NF is characterized by tumors of the acoustic nerve. Most often, the disorder is asymptomatic through the first 15 years of life. The most frequent symptoms are headaches, hearing loss, and tinnitus (*i.e.,* ringing in the ears). There may be associated intracranial and spinal meningiomas. The condition is often made worse by pregnancy, and oral contraceptives may increase the growth and symptoms of the tumors. Persons with the disorder should be warned that severe disorientation may occur during diving or swimming underwater, and drowning may result. Surgery may be indicated for debulking or removal of the tumors.

Autosomal Recessive Disorders

Autosomal recessive disorders are manifested only when both members of the gene pair are affected. In this case, both parents may be unaffected but are carriers of the defective gene. Autosomal recessive disorders affect both sexes. The occurrence risks in each pregnancy are one in four for an affected child, two in four for a carrier child, and one in four for a normal (noncarrier, unaffected), homozygous child (Fig. 7-4). *Consanguineous mating* (mating of two related individuals), or inbreeding, increases the chance that two people who mate will be carriers of an autosomal recessive disorder.[3]

With autosomal recessive disorders, the age of onset is frequently early in life; the symptomatology tends to be more uniform than with autosomal dominant disorders; and the disorders are characteristically caused by loss-of-function mutations, many of which impair or eliminate the function of an enzyme. In the case of a heterozygous carrier, the presence of a mutant gene usually does not produce symptoms because equal amounts of normal and defective enzymes are synthesized. This "margin of safety" ensures that cells with half their usual amount of enzyme function normally. By contrast, the inactivation of both alleles in a homozygote results in complete loss of enzyme activity. Autosomal recessive disorders include almost all inborn errors of metabolism. Enzyme disorders that impair catabolic pathways result in an accumulation of dietary substances (*e.g.,* phenylketonuria) or cellular constituents (*e.g.,* lysosomal storage diseases). Other disorders result from a defect in the enzyme-mediated synthesis of an essential protein (*e.g.,* the cystic fibrosis transmembrane conductance regulator in cystic

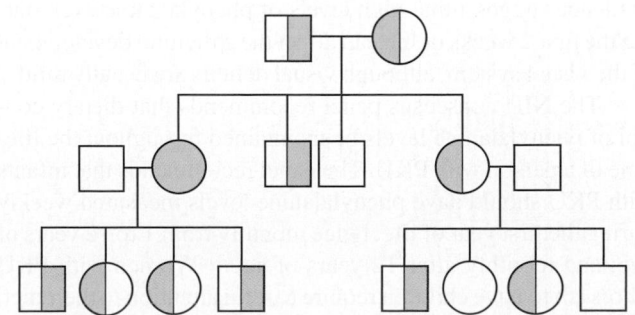

FIGURE 7-4 • Simple pedigree for inheritance of an autosomal recessive trait. The half-colored circle and square represent a mutant gene. When both parents are carriers of a mutant gene, there is a 25% chance of having an affected child (full-colored circle or square), a 50% chance of a carrier child, and a 25% chance of a nonaffected or noncarrier child, regardless of sex. All children (100%) of an affected parent are carriers.

fibrosis [see Chapter 29]). Two examples of autosomal recessive disorders that are not covered elsewhere in this book are phenylketonuria and Tay-Sachs disease.

Phenylketonuria. Phenylketonuria (PKU) is a rare metabolic disorder that affects approximately 1 in every 15,000 infants in the United States and Canada.[11,12] The disorder, which is inherited as a recessive trait, is caused by a deficiency of the liver enzyme phenylalanine hydroxylase. As a result of this deficiency, toxic levels of the amino acid phenylalanine accumulate in the blood and other tissues.[11] If untreated, the disorder results in mental retardation, microcephaly, delayed speech, and other signs of impaired neurologic development.

Because the symptoms of untreated PKU develop gradually and would often go undetected until irreversible mental retardation had occurred, newborn infants are routinely screened for abnormal levels of serum phenylalanine.[11,12] It is important that blood samples for PKU screening be obtained at least 12 hours after birth to ensure accuracy. It also is possible to identify carriers of the trait by subjecting them to a phenylalanine test, in which a large dose of phenylalanine is administered orally and the rate at which it disappears from the bloodstream is measured.

In 2000, the National Institutes of Health (NIH) released a consensus statement on the screening and management of PKU.[11] This statement emphasized the need for a universal approach to newborn screening that includes appropriate specimen collection; specimen tracking; laboratory analysis; data collection and analysis; locating and notifying families with abnormal results; diagnosis; treatment; and long-term management, including psychological, nursing, and social services, nutritional therapy, and genetic and family counseling.[13]

Infants with the disorder are treated with a special diet that restricts phenylalanine intake. The results of dietary therapy of children with PKU have been impressive. The diet can prevent mental retardation as well as other neurodegenerative effects of untreated PKU. However, dietary treatment must be started early in neonatal life to prevent brain damage. Infants with elevated phenylalanine levels (>10 mg/dL) should begin treatment by 7 to 10 days of age, indicating the need for early diagnosis. Evidence suggests that high levels of phenylalanine even during the first 2 weeks of life can affect the structural development of the visual system, although visual deficits are usually mild.[13]

The NIH consensus panel recommends that dietary control of phenylalanine levels be maintained throughout the lifetime of a person with PKU. The panel recommends that infants with PKU should have phenylalanine levels measured weekly during the first year of life; twice monthly from 1 to 12 years of age; and monthly after 12 years of age.[11] Women with PKU who wish to have children require careful attention to their diet, both before conception and during pregnancy, as a means of controlling their phenylalanine levels.[11]

Tay-Sachs Disease. Tay-Sachs disease is a variant of a class of lysosomal storage diseases, known as the *gangliosidoses,* in which there is failure to break down the GM2 gangliosides of cell membranes. Tay-Sachs disease is inherited as an autosomal

recessive trait and is predominantly a disorder of Eastern European (Ashkenazi) Jews, in which a carrier rate of 1 in 30 has been reported.[4,5]

The GM2 ganglioside accumulates in the lysosomes of all organs in Tay-Sachs disease, but is most prominent in the brain neurons and retina.[4,5] Microscopic examination reveals neurons ballooned with cytoplasmic vacuoles, each of which constitutes a markedly distended lysosome filled with gangliosides. In time, there is progressive destruction of neurons within the brain substance, including the cerebellum, basal ganglia, brain stem, spinal cord, and autonomic nervous system. Involvement of the retina is detected by ophthalmoscopy as a cherry-red spot on the macula.

Infants with Tay-Sachs disease appear normal at birth but begin to manifest progressive weakness, muscle flaccidity, and decreased attentiveness at approximately 6 to 10 months of age. This is followed by rapid deterioration of motor and mental function, often with development of generalized seizures. Retinal involvement leads to visual impairment and eventual blindness. Death usually occurs before 4 to 5 years of age. Although there is no cure for the disease, analysis of the blood serum for the lysosomal enzyme, hexosaminidase A, which is deficient in Tay-Sachs disease, allows for accurate identification of genetic carriers for the disease.

X-Linked Disorders

Sex-linked disorders are almost always associated with the X, or female, chromosome, and the inheritance pattern is predominantly recessive. Because of the presence of a normal paired gene, female heterozygotes rarely experience the effects of a defective gene, whereas all males who receive the gene are typically affected. The common pattern of inheritance is one in which an unaffected mother carries one normal and one mutant allele on the X chromosome. This means that she has a 50% chance of transmitting the defective gene to her sons, and her daughters have a 50% chance of being carriers of the mutant gene (Fig. 7-5). When the affected son procreates, he transmits the defective gene to all of his daughters, who become carriers of the mutant gene. Because the genes of the Y chromosome are unaffected, the affected male does not transmit the defect to any of his sons, and they will not be carriers or transmit the disorder to their children. X-linked recessive disorders include glucose-6-phosphate dehydrogenase deficiency (see Chapter 14), hemophilia A (see Chapter 13), and X-linked agammaglobulinemia (see Chapter 19).

Fragile X Syndrome

Fragile X syndrome is a single-gene disorder in which the mutation is characterized by a long repeating sequence of three nucleotides within the fragile X gene.[14] The disorder, which affects approximately 1 in 4000 males and 1 in 6000 females, is the most common form of inherited mental retardation.[15] It is second only to Down syndrome as an identifiable cause of mental retardation.

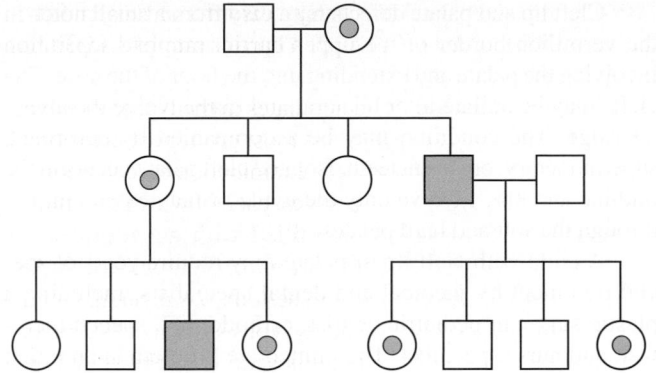

FIGURE 7-5 • Simple pedigree for inheritance of an X-linked recessive trait. X-linked recessive traits are expressed phenotypically in the male offspring. A small colored circle represents the X chromosome with the defective gene, and the larger colored square the affected male. The affected male passes the mutant gene to all of his daughters, who become carriers of the trait and have a 50% chance of passing the gene; her sons and her daughters have a 50% chance of being carriers of the gene (remember that their father has a normal X).

As with other X-linked disorders, fragile X syndrome affects boys more often than girls. Affected boys are mentally retarded and share a common physical phenotype that includes a long face with large mandible and large, everted ears. Hyperextensible joints, a high-arched palate, and mitral valve prolapse, which are observed in some cases, mimic a connective tissue disorder. Some physical abnormalities may be subtle or absent. The most distinctive feature, which is present in 90% of prepubertal boys, is macroorchidism or large testes.[2,14–17] Because girls have two X chromosomes, they are more likely to have relatively normal cognitive development, or they may show a learning disability in a particular area, such as mathematics. Women with the disorder may also experience premature ovarian failure or begin menopause earlier than women who are not affected by fragile X syndrome.[14]

The fragile X gene has been mapped to a small area on the long arm of the X chromosome, now designated the *FMR1* (fragile X mental retardation 1) site.[4,5] The gene product, the fragile X mental retardation protein (FMRP), is a widely expressed cytoplasmic protein. It is most abundant in the brain and testis, the organs most affected by the disorder. Although the function of FMRP has not been fully established, researchers believe that it may regulate communication between cells.[14] As discussed in Chapter 6, each gene contains an introduction or promoter region and an instruction region that carries the directions for protein synthesis. The promoter region of the *FMR1* gene contains repeats of a specific CGG (cytosine, guanine, guanine) triplet code that, when normal, controls gene activity. The mechanism by which the normal *FMR1* gene is converted to an altered, or mutant, gene capable of producing disease symptoms involves an increase in the number of CGG repeats in the promoter region of the gene. Once the repeat exceeds a threshold length, no FMRP is produced, resulting in the fragile X phenotype. People without fragile X syndrome have between 6 and 40 repeats. A gene with 55 to 200 repeats is generally considered a permutation, and one with more than 200 repeats, a full mutation.[5,17]

The inheritance of the *FMR1* gene follows the pattern of X-linked traits, with the father passing the gene on to all his daughters but not his sons. Approximately 20% of males who have been shown to carry the fragile X mutation are clinically and cytogenetically normal. Because these male carriers transmit the trait through all their daughters (who are phenotypically normal) to affected grandchildren, they are called *transmitting males*.

In fragile X families, the probability of being affected with the disorder is related to the position in the pedigree. Later generations are more likely to be affected than earlier generations. For example, brothers of transmitting males are at a 9% risk of having mental retardation, whereas grandsons of transmitting males are at a 40% risk.[5] The increase in occurrence of the disorder in successive generations is referred to as *genetic anticipation*.[5] In the case of the fragile X syndrome, genetic anticipation is caused by the progressive expansion of the CCG triplet repeat.

Diagnosis of fragile X syndrome is based on mental and physical characteristics. DNA molecular tests can be done to confirm the presence of an abnormal *FMR1* gene. Because the manifestations of fragile X syndrome may resemble those of other learning disorders, it is recommended that persons with mental retardation of unknown cause, developmental delay, learning disabilities, autism, or autism-like behaviors be evaluated for the disorder.[14]

 **Multifactoral Inheritance Disorders**

Multifactorial inheritance disorders are caused by multiple genes and, in many cases, environmental factors. The exact number of genes contributing to multifactorial traits is not known, and these traits do not follow the same clear-cut pattern of inheritance as do single-gene disorders. Multifactorial inheritance has been described as a threshold phenomenon in which the factors contributing to the trait can be compared with water filling a glass.[18] Using this analogy, one might say that expression of the disorder occurs when the glass overflows. Disorders of multifactorial inheritance can be expressed during fetal life and be present at birth, or they may be expressed later in life. Congenital disorders that are thought to arise through multifactorial inheritance include cleft lip or palate, clubfoot, congenital dislocation of the hip, congenital heart disease, pyloric stenosis, and urinary tract malformation. Environmental factors are thought to play a greater role in disorders of multifactorial inheritance that develop in adult life, such as coronary artery disease, diabetes mellitus, hypertension, cancer, and common psychiatric disorders such as bipolar disorder and schizophrenia.

Although multifactorial traits cannot be predicted with the same degree of accuracy as mendelian single-gene mutations, characteristic patterns exist. First, multifactorial congenital malformations tend to involve a single organ or tissue derived from the same embryonic developmental field. Second, the risk of recurrence in future pregnancies is for the same or a similar defect. This means that parents of a child with a cleft palate defect have an increased risk of having another child with a cleft palate, but not with spina bifida. Third, the increased risk (compared with the general population) among first-degree relatives of the affected person is 2% to 7%, and among second-degree relatives, it is approximately one half that amount.[4] The risk increases with increasing incidence of the defect among relatives. This means that the risk is greatly increased when a second child with the defect is born to a couple. The risk also increases with severity of the disorder and when the defect occurs in the sex not usually affected by the disorder.

Cleft Lip and Cleft Palate

Cleft lip with or without cleft palate is one of the most common birth defects. It is also one of the more conspicuous birth defects, resulting in an abnormal facial appearance and defective speech. The incidence varies among ethnic groups, ranging from 3.6 per 1000 live births among Native Americans to 2.0 per 1000 among Asians, 1.0 per 1000 among people of European ancestry, to 0.3 per 1000 among Africans.[19] Cleft lip with or without cleft palate is more frequent among boys, whereas isolated cleft palate is twice as common among girls.

Developmentally, the defect has its origin at about the 35th day of gestation when the frontal prominences of the craniofacial structures fuse with the maxillary process to form the upper lip.[4] This process is under the control of many genes, and disturbances in gene expression (hereditary or environmental) at this time may result in cleft lip with or without cleft palate (Fig. 7-6). The defect may also be caused by teratogens (*e.g.,* rubella, anticonvulsant drugs) and is often encountered in children with chromosomal abnormalities.

Cleft lip and palate defects may vary from a small notch in the vermilion border of the upper lip to complete separation involving the palate and extending into the floor of the nose. The clefts may be unilateral or bilateral and may involve the alveolar ridge. The condition may be accompanied by deformed, supernumerary, or absent teeth. Isolated cleft palate occurs in the midline and may involve only the uvula or may extend into or through the soft and hard palates.

A child with cleft lip or palate may require years of special treatment by medical and dental specialists, including a plastic surgeon, pediatric dentist, orthodontist, speech therapist, and nurse specialist. The immediate problem in an infant with cleft palate is feeding. Nursing at the breast or nipple depends on suction developed by pressing the nipple against the hard palate with the tongue. Although infants with cleft lip usually have no problems with feeding, those with cleft palate usually require specially constructed, soft artificial nipples with large openings and a squeezable bottle. A specially constructed plastic obturator that fits over the palate defect may be used to facilitate sucking for some infants.[20]

Major advances in the care of children born with cleft lip and palate have occurred within the last quarter of the 20th century.[21] Surgical closure of the lip is usually performed by 3 months of age, with closure of the palate usually done before 1 year of age. Depending on the extent of the defect, additional surgery may be required as the child grows. Displacement of the maxillary arches and malposition of the teeth usually require orthodontic correction.

Cleft lip and palate can also cause speech defects. The muscles of the soft palate and the lateral and posterior walls of the nasopharynx constitute a valve that separates the nasopharynx from the oropharynx during swallowing and in the production of certain sounds. If the valve does not function properly, it is difficult to build up sufficient pressure in the mouth to make explosive sounds such as *p, b, d, t, h,* and *y,* or the sibilants *s, sh,* and *ch.*[20] Although speech therapy is usually needed, early and more effective surgical procedures help to reduce the extent of the problem.

Chromosomal Disorders

Chromosomal disorders form a major category of genetic disease, accounting for a large proportion of reproductive wastage (early gestational abortions), congenital malformations, and mental retardation. Specific chromosomal abnormalities can be linked to more than 60 identifiable syndromes that are present in 0.7% of all live births, 2% of all pregnancies in women older than 35 years of age, and 50% of all first-term abortions.[4]

During cell division (*i.e.,* mitosis) in nongerm cells, the chromosomes replicate so that each cell receives a full diploid number. In germ cells, a different form of division (*i.e.,* meiosis) takes place (see Chapter 6). During meiosis, the double sets of 22 autosomes and the 2 sex chromosomes (normal diploid number) are reduced to single sets (haploid number) in each gamete. At the time of conception, the haploid number in the ovum and that in the sperm join and restore the diploid number of chromosomes.

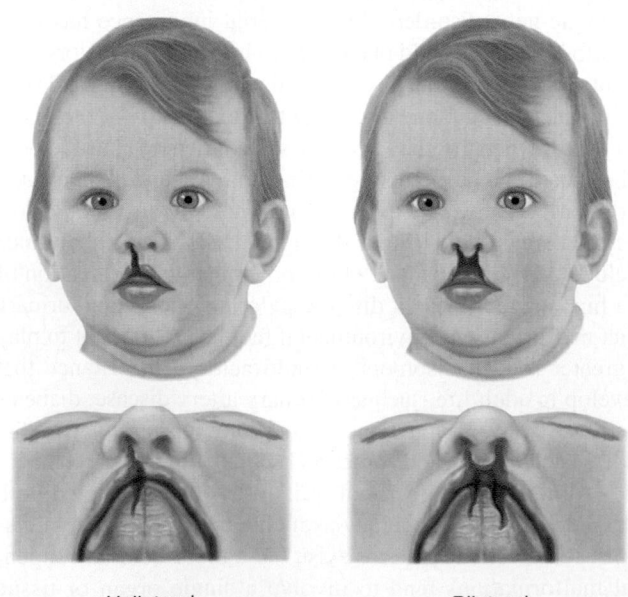

Unilateral   Bilateral

FIGURE 7-6 • Cleft lip and cleft palate.

Chromosomal abnormalities are commonly described according to the shorthand description of the karyotype. In this system, the total number of chromosomes is given first, followed by the sex chromosome complement, and then the description of any abnormality. For example, a male with trisomy 21 is designated 47,XY,+21.

The aberrations underlying chromosomal disorders may take the form of alterations in the structure of one or more chromosomes, or an abnormal number of chromosomes. Occasionally, mitotic errors in early development give rise to two or more cell lines characterized by distinctive karyotypes, a condition referred to as *mosaicism*. Mosaicism can result from mitotic errors during cleavage of the fertilized ovum or in somatic cells. Sometimes, mosaicism consists of an abnormal karyotype and a normal one, in which case the physical deformities caused by the abnormal cell line usually are less severe.

Structural Chromosomal Abnormalities

Structural changes in chromosomes usually result from breakage in one or more of the chromosomes followed by rearrangement or deletion of the chromosome parts. Among the factors believed to cause chromosome breakage are exposure to radiation sources, such as x-rays; influence of certain chemicals; extreme changes in the cellular environment; and viral infections.

Several patterns of chromosome breakage and rearrangement can occur (Fig. 7-7). There can be a *deletion* of the broken portion of the chromosome. When one chromosome is involved, the broken parts may be *inverted. Isochromosome formation* occurs when the centromere, or central portion, of the chromosome separates horizontally instead of vertically. *Ring formation* results when deletion is followed by uniting of the chromatids to form a ring. *Translocation* occurs when there are simultaneous breaks in two chromosomes from different pairs, with exchange of chromosome parts. With a balanced reciprocal translocation, no genetic information is lost; therefore, persons with translocations usually are normal. However, these persons are translocation carriers and may have normal or abnormal children.

A special form of translocation called a *centric fusion* or *robertsonian translocation* involves two acrocentric chromosomes in which the centromere is near the end, most commonly chromosomes 13 and 14 or 14 and 21. Typically, the break occurs near the centromere affecting the short arm in one chromosome and the long arm in the other. Transfer of the chromosome fragments leads to one long and one extremely short fragment. The short fragment is usually lost during subsequent divisions. In this case, the person has only 45 chromosomes, but the amount of genetic material that is lost is so small that it often goes unnoticed. Difficulty, however, arises during meiosis; the result is gametes with an unbalanced number of chromosomes. The chief clinical importance of this type of translocation is that carriers of a robertsonian translocation involving chromosome 21 are at risk for producing a child with Down syndrome (to be discussed).

The manifestations of aberrations in chromosome structure depend to a great extent on the amount of genetic mater-

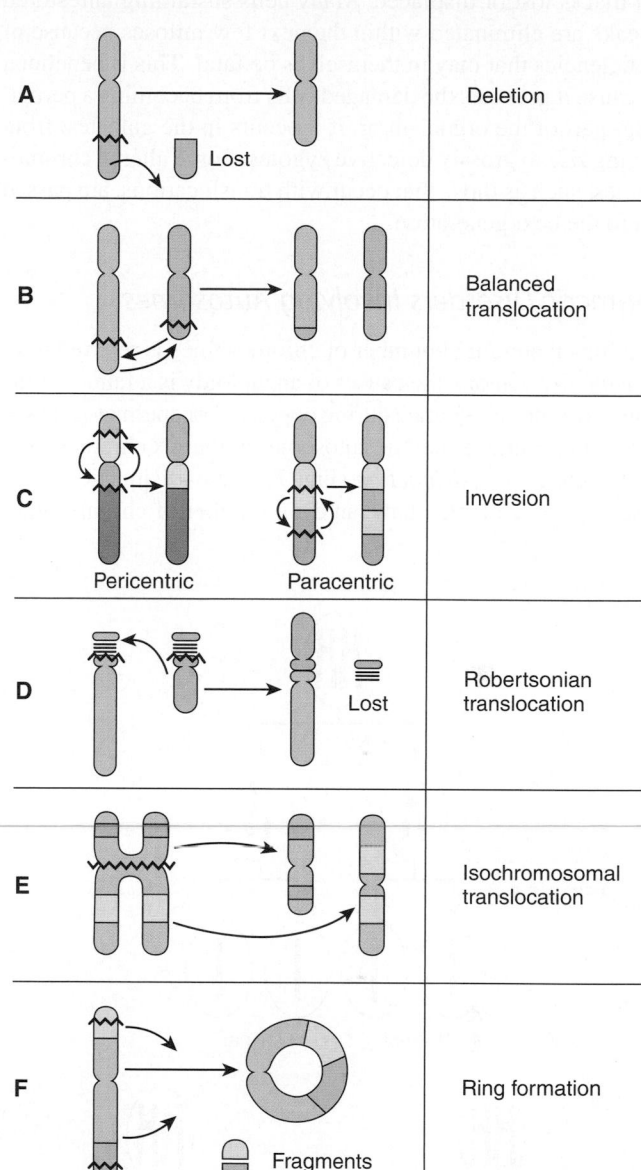

FIGURE 7-7 • Structural abnormalities in the human chromosome. (**A**) Deletion of part of a chromosome leads to loss of genetic material and shortening of the chromosome. (**B**) A reciprocal translocation involves two nonhomologous chromosomes, with exchange of the acentric segment. (**C**) Inversion requires two breaks in a single chromosome, with inversion to the opposite side of the centromere (pericentric) or with the fragment inverting but remaining on the same arm (paracentric). (**D**) In robertsonian translocation, two nonhomologous acrocentric chromosomes break near their centromeres, after which the long arms fuse to form one large metacentric chromosome. (**E**) Isochromosomes arise from faulty centromere division, which leads to duplication of the long arm and deletion of the short arm, or the reverse. (**F**) A ring chromosome forms with breaks in both telomeric portions of a chromosome, deletion of the acentric fragments, and fusion of the remaining centric portion. (Adapted from Killeen A. A., Rubin E., Strayer D. S. [2008]. Developmental and genetic diseases. In Rubin R., Strayer D. S. [Eds.], *Rubin's pathology: Clinicopathologic foundations of medicine* [5th ed., p. 187]. Philadelphia: Lippincott Williams & Wilkins.)

ial that is lost or displaced. Many cells sustaining unrestored breaks are eliminated within the next few mitoses because of deficiencies that may in themselves be fatal. This is beneficial because it prevents the damaged cells from becoming a permanent part of the organism or, if it occurs in the gametes, from giving rise to grossly defective zygotes. Some altered chromosomes, such as those that occur with translocations, are passed on to the next generation.

Numeric Disorders Involving Autosomes

Having an abnormal number of chromosomes is referred to as *aneuploidy.* Among the causes of aneuploidy is a failure of the chromosomes to separate during oogenesis or spermatogenesis. This can occur in either the autosomes or the sex chromosomes and is called *nondisjunction* (Fig. 7-8). Nondisjunction gives rise to germ cells that have an even number of chromosomes

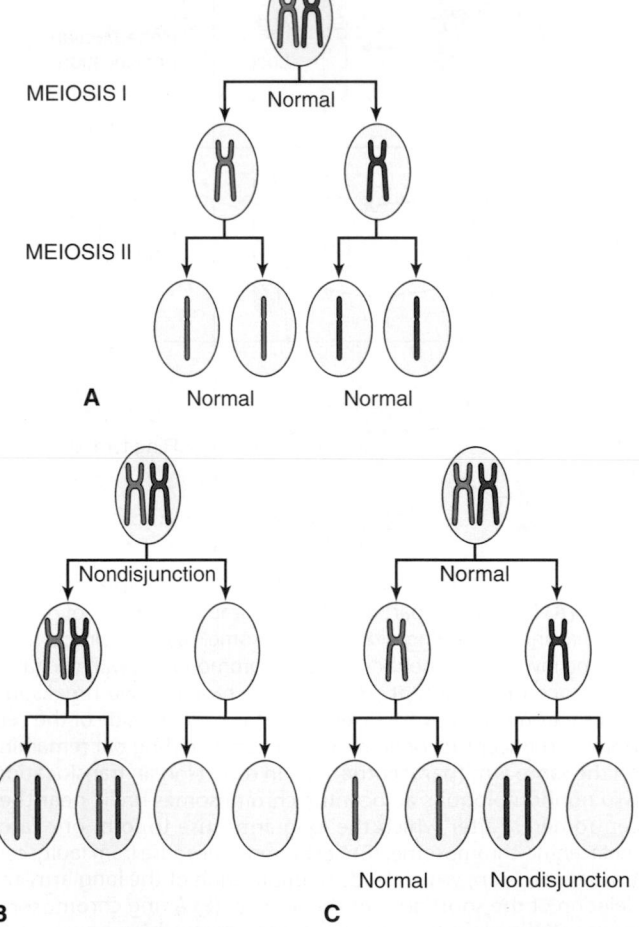

FIGURE 7-8 • Nondisjunction as a cause of disorders of chromosomal numbers. **(A)** Normal distribution of chromosomes during meiosis I and II. **(B)** If nondisjunction occurs at meiosis I, the gametes contain either a pair of chromosomes or a lack of chromosomes. **(C)** If nondisjunction occurs at meiosis II, the affected gametes contain two of copies of one parenteral chromosome or a lack of chromosomes.

(22 or 24). The products of conception formed from this even number of chromosomes have an uneven number of chromosomes, 45 or 47. *Monosomy* refers to the presence of only one member of a chromosome pair. The defects associated with monosomy of the autosomes are severe and usually cause abortion. Monosomy of the X chromosome (45,X), or Turner syndrome, causes less severe defects.

Polysomy, or the presence of more than two chromosomes to a set, occurs when a germ cell containing more than 23 chromosomes is involved in conception. A variety of trisomies involving autosomal chromosomes 8, 9, 12, 18, and 22 have been described.[4,5] Trisomy 18 (Edwards syndrome) and trisomy 13 (Patau syndrome) share several karyotypic and clinical features with trisomy 21 (Down syndrome). In contrast to Down syndrome, however, the malformations are much more severe and wide-ranging. As a result, these infants rarely survive beyond the first years of life.[5]

Down Syndrome. First described in 1866 by John Langdon Down, trisomy 21, or Down syndrome, causes a combination of birth defects including some degree of mental retardation, characteristic facial features, and other health problems. According to the National Down Syndrome Association, it is the most common chromosomal disorder, occurring approximately once in every 800 to 1000 births.

Approximately 95% of cases of Down syndrome are caused by nondisjunction or an error in cell division during meiosis, resulting in a trisomy of chromosome 21. A rare form of Down syndrome can occur in the offspring of persons in whom there has been a robertsonian translocation (see Fig. 7-7) involving the long arm of chromosome 21q and the long arm of one of the acrocentric chromosomes (most often 14 or 22). The translocation adds to the normal long arm of chromosome 21; therefore, the person with this type of Down syndrome has 46 chromosomes, but essentially a trisomy of 21q.[4–6]

The risk of having a child with Down syndrome increases with maternal age—it is 1 in 1250 at 25 years of age, 1 in 400 at 35 years, and 1 in 100 at 45 years of age.[22] The reason for the correlation between maternal age and nondisjunction is unknown, but is thought to reflect some aspect of aging of the oocyte. Although men continue to produce sperm throughout their reproductive life, women are born with all the oocytes they ever will have. These oocytes may change as a result of the aging process. With increasing age, there is a greater chance of a woman having been exposed to damaging environmental agents such as drugs, chemicals, and radiation. Unlike trisomy 21, Down syndrome due to a chromosome (21;14) translocation shows no relation to maternal age but has a relatively high recurrence risk in families when a parent, particularly the mother, is a carrier.

The physical features of a child with Down syndrome are distinctive, and therefore the condition usually is apparent at birth.[4,5,23,24] These features include growth failure and a small and rather square head. There is a flat facial profile, with a small nose and somewhat depressed nasal bridge; small folds on the inner corners of the eyes (epicanthal folds) and upward slanting of the eyes; small, low-set, and malformed ears; a fat pad at the back of the neck; an open mouth; and a large, protruding tongue (Fig. 7-9). The child's hands usually are short and stubby, with fingers that curl inward, and there usually is only a single palmar (*i.e.,* simian) crease. There is excessive space between the large and second toes. Hypotonia and joint laxity also are present in infants and young children. There often are accompanying congenital heart defects and an increased risk of gastrointestinal malformations. Approximately 1% of persons with trisomy 21 Down syndrome have mosaicism (*i.e.,* cell populations with the normal chromosome number and trisomy 21); these persons may be less severely affected. Of particular concern is the much greater risk of development of acute leukemia among children with Down syndrome—10 to 20 times greater than that of other children.[5] With increased life expectancy due to improved health care, it has also been found that there is an increased risk of Alzheimer disease among older persons with Down syndrome.

There are several prenatal screening tests that can be done to determine the risk of having a child with Down syndrome.[23–25] The most commonly used are blood tests that measure maternal serum levels of α-fetoprotein, human chorionic gonadotropin (hCG), unconjugated estriol, inhibin

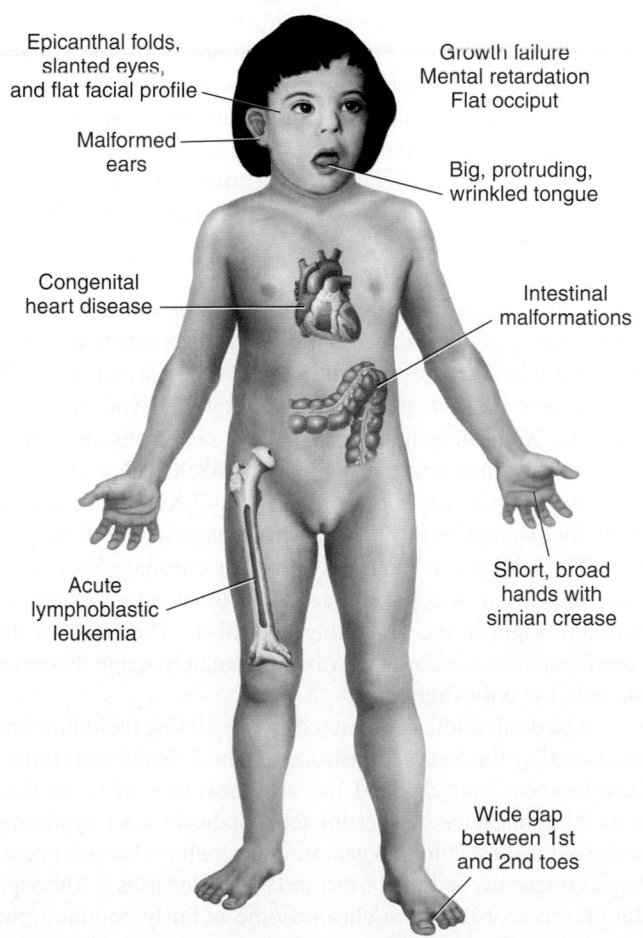

FIGURE 7-9 • Clinical features of a child with Down syndrome.

A, and pregnancy-associated plasma protein A (PAPP-A; see section on Diagnosis and Counseling). The results of three or four of these tests, together with the woman's age, often are used to determine the probability of a pregnant woman having a child with Down syndrome. Another test, fetal nuchal translucency (sonolucent space on the back of the fetal neck), uses ultrasonography and can be performed between 10 and 13 weeks' gestation.[25] The fetus with Down syndrome tends to have a greater area of translucency compared with a chromosomally normal infant. The nuchal transparency test is usually used in combination with other screening tests. The only way to accurately determine the presence of Down syndrome in the fetus is through chromosome analysis using chorionic villus sampling, amniocentesis, or percutaneous umbilical blood sampling.

Numeric Disorders Involving Sex Chromosomes

Chromosomal disorders associated with the sex chromosomes are much more common than those related to the autosomes, save for trisomy 21. Furthermore, imbalances (excess or deletions) are much better tolerated than those involving the autosomes. This is related in a large part to two factors that are peculiar to the sex chromosomes: (1) the inactivation of all but one X chromosome, and (2) the modest amount of genetic material that is carried on the Y chromosome.

Although girls normally receive both a paternal and a maternal X chromosome, the clinical manifestations of X chromosome abnormalities can be quite variable because of the process of X inactivation (see discussion of the Lyon principle in Chapter 6). In somatic cells of females, only one X chromosome is transcriptionally active. The other chromosome is inactive. The process of X inactivation, which is random, occurs early in embryonic life and is usually complete at about the end of the first week of development. After one X chromosome has become inactivated in a cell, all cells descended from that cell have the same inactivated X chromosome. Although much of one X chromosome is inactivated in females, several regions contain genes that escape inactivation and continue to be expressed by both X chromosomes. These genes may explain some of the variations in clinical symptoms seen in cases of numeric abnormalities of the X chromosome, such as Turner syndrome.

It is well known that the Y chromosome determines the male sex. The gene that dictates testicular development (*Sry:* sex-determining region Y gene) has been located on its distal short arm.[5] Recent studies of the Y chromosome have yielded additional information about gene families in the so-called "male-specific Y" or MSY region. All of these are believed to be involved in spermatogenesis. A few additional genes with homologs on the X chromosome have been mapped to the Y chromosome, but to date, no disorders resulting from mutations in these genes have been described.

Turner Syndrome. Turner syndrome describes an absence of all (45,X/0) or part of the X chromosome.[26–28] Some women with Turner syndrome may have part of the X chromosome and some may display a mosaicism with one or more additional cells lines. This disorder affects approximately 1 of every 2500 live births, and it has been estimated that almost all fetuses with the 45,X/0 karyotype are spontaneously aborted during the first trimester.[4]

Characteristically, the girl with Turner syndrome is short in stature, but her body proportions are normal (Fig. 7-10). Because of the absence of the ovaries, she does not menstruate and shows no signs of secondary sex characteristics. There are variations in the syndrome, with abnormalities ranging from essentially none to webbing of the neck with redundant skin folds, nonpitting lymphedema of the hands and feet, and congenital heart defects, particularly coarctation of the aorta and bicuspid aortic valve.[26–29] There also may be abnormalities in kidney development (i.e., abnormal location, abnormal vascular supply, or double collecting system). There may be other abnormalities, such as changes in nail growth, high-arched palate, short fourth metacarpal, and strabismus. Although most women with Turner syndrome have normal intelligence, they may have problems with visuospatial organization (e.g., difficulty in driving, nonverbal problem-solving tasks such as mathematics, and psychomotor skills) and attention deficit disorders.[26,27]

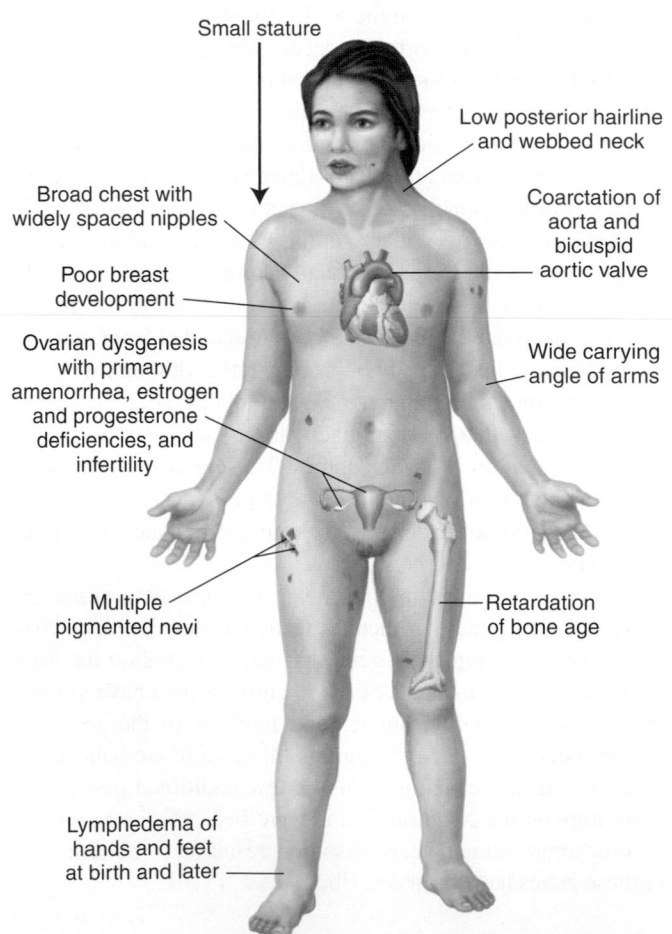

Small stature

Low posterior hairline and webbed neck

Broad chest with widely spaced nipples

Coarctation of aorta and bicuspid aortic valve

Poor breast development

Ovarian dysgenesis with primary amenorrhea, estrogen and progesterone deficiencies, and infertility

Wide carrying angle of arms

Multiple pigmented nevi

Retardation of bone age

Lymphedema of hands and feet at birth and later

FIGURE 7-10 • Clinical features of Turner syndrome.

The diagnosis of Turner syndrome often is delayed until late childhood or early adolescence in girls who do not present with the classic features of the syndrome. Only about 20% to 33% of affected girls receive a diagnosis as a newborn because of puffy hands and feet or redundant nuchal skin; another 33% are diagnosed in mid-childhood because of short stature; and the rest are mainly diagnosed in adolescence when they fail to enter puberty.[26] Early diagnosis is an important aspect of treatment for Turner syndrome.[29] It allows for counseling about the phenotypic characteristics of the disorder; screening for cardiac, renal, thyroid, and other abnormalities; and provision of emotional support for the girl and her family. Because of the potential for delay in diagnosis, it has been recommended that girls with unexplained short stature (height below the fifth percentile), webbed neck, peripheral lymphedema, coarctation of the aorta, or delayed puberty have chromosomal studies done.[30]

The management of Turner syndrome begins during childhood and requires ongoing assessment and treatment. Growth hormone therapy is now standard treatment and can result in a gain of 6 to 10 cm in final height. Estrogen therapy, which is instituted around the normal age of puberty, is used to promote development and maintenance of secondary sexual characteristics.[26–29]

There also are health concerns for adult women with Turner syndrome.[30,31] Until recently, girls with Turner syndrome received intensive medical care during childhood, but were discharged from specialty clinics after induction of puberty and attainment of final height. It is now known that women with Turner syndrome have increased morbidity owing to cardiovascular disease and gastrointestinal, renal, and various endocrine disorders. Adults with Turner syndrome continue to have reduced bone mass, which has been associated with increased risk of fractures.

Klinefelter Syndrome. Klinefelter syndrome is a condition of testicular dysgenesis accompanied by the presence of one or more extra X chromosomes in excess of the normal male XY complement.[4,32–34] Most males with Klinefelter syndrome have one extra X chromosome (47,XXY). In rare cases, there may be more than one extra X chromosome (48,XXXY). The presence of the extra X chromosome in the 47,XXY male results from nondisjunction during meiotic division in one of the parents. The additional X chromosome (or chromosomes) is of maternal origin in approximately two thirds of cases and of paternal origin in the remaining one third.[5] The cause of the nondisjunction is unknown. Advanced maternal age increases the risk, but only slightly.

Based on studies conducted in the 1970s, including one sponsored by the National Institute of Child Health and Human Development that checked the chromosomes of more than 40,000 infants, it has been estimated that the 47,XXY syndrome is one of the most common genetic abnormalities known, occurring as frequently as 1 in 500 to 1 in 1000 male births.[32] Although the presence of the extra chromosome is fairly common, the syndrome with its accompanying signs and symptoms that may result from the extra chromosome is uncommon. Many men live their lives without being aware that they have an additional chromosome. For this reason, it has been suggested that the term *Klinefelter syndrome* be replaced with *47,XXY male.*[32]

Klinefelter syndrome is characterized by enlarged breasts, sparse facial and body hair, small testes, and the inability to produce sperm[33,34] (Fig. 7-11). Regardless of the number of X chromosomes present, the male phenotype is retained. The condition often goes undetected at birth. The infant usually has normal male genitalia, with a small penis and small, firm testicles. At puberty, the intrinsically abnormal testes do not respond to stimulation from the gonadotropins and undergo degeneration. This leads to a tall stature with abnormal body proportions in which the lower part of the body is longer than the upper part. Later in life, the body build may become heavy, with a female distribution of subcutaneous fat and variable degrees of breast enlargement. There may be deficient secondary male sex characteristics,

such as a voice that remains feminine in pitch and sparse beard and pubic hair. Although the intellect usually is normal, most 47,XXY males have some degree of language impairment. They often learn to talk later than other children and often have trouble learning to read and write.

Adequate management of Klinefelter syndrome requires a comprehensive neurodevelopmental evaluation. In infancy and early childhood, this often includes a multidisciplinary approach to determine appropriate treatments such as physical therapy, infant stimulation programs, and speech therapy.[34] Men with Klinefelter syndrome have congenital hypogonadism, which results in an inability to produce normal amounts of testosterone accompanied by an increase in hypothalamic gonadotrophic hormones (see Chapter 43). Androgen therapy is usually initiated when there is evidence of a testosterone deficit. This may begin as early as 12 to 14 years of age.[34] Because gynecomastia predisposes to breast cancer, breast self-examination should be encouraged for men with Klinefelter syndrome. Infertility is common in men with Klinefelter syndrome because of a decreased sperm count. If sperm are present, cryopreservation may be useful for future family planning. However, genetic counseling is advised because of the increased risk of autosomal and sex chromosomal abnormalities.

Mitochondrial Gene Disorders

The mitochondria contain their own DNA, which is distinct from the DNA contained in the cell nucleus. An understanding of the role of mitochondrial DNA (mtDNA) has evolved since 1988, when the first mutation of mtDNA was discovered.[35] Since then, more than 100 different disease-related rearrangements and point mutations have been identified.[3]

Mitochondrial DNA, which is packaged in a double-stranded circular chromosome located inside the mitochondria, is often referred to as the "other human genome."[35–38] Mitochondrial DNA contains 37 genes: two ribosomal RNA (rRNA) genes; 22 transfer RNA (tRNA) genes; and 13 structural genes encoding subunits of the mitochondrial respiratory chain enzymes, which participate in oxidative phosphorylation and generation of adenosine triphosphate (see Chapter 4).

In contrast to the mendelian pattern of inheritance of nuclear DNA, disorders of mtDNA are inherited on the maternal line. This can be explained by the fact that ova contain numerous mitochondria in their abundant cytoplasm, whereas spermatozoa contain few, if any, mitochondria. Thus, the mtDNA in the zygote is derived solely from the mother. The zygote and its daughter cells have many mitochondria, each of which contains multiple copies of the maternally derived mtDNA. During growth of the fetus or later, it is likely that some cells will contain only normal or mutant mtDNA (a situation called *homoplasmy*), whereas others receive a mixture of normal and mutant DNA (*heteroplasmy*). In turn, the clinical expression of a disease produced by a given mutation of mtDNA depends on the total content of mitochondrial genes and the proportion that is mutant. The fraction of mutant mtDNA must exceed a critical value for a mitochondrial disease

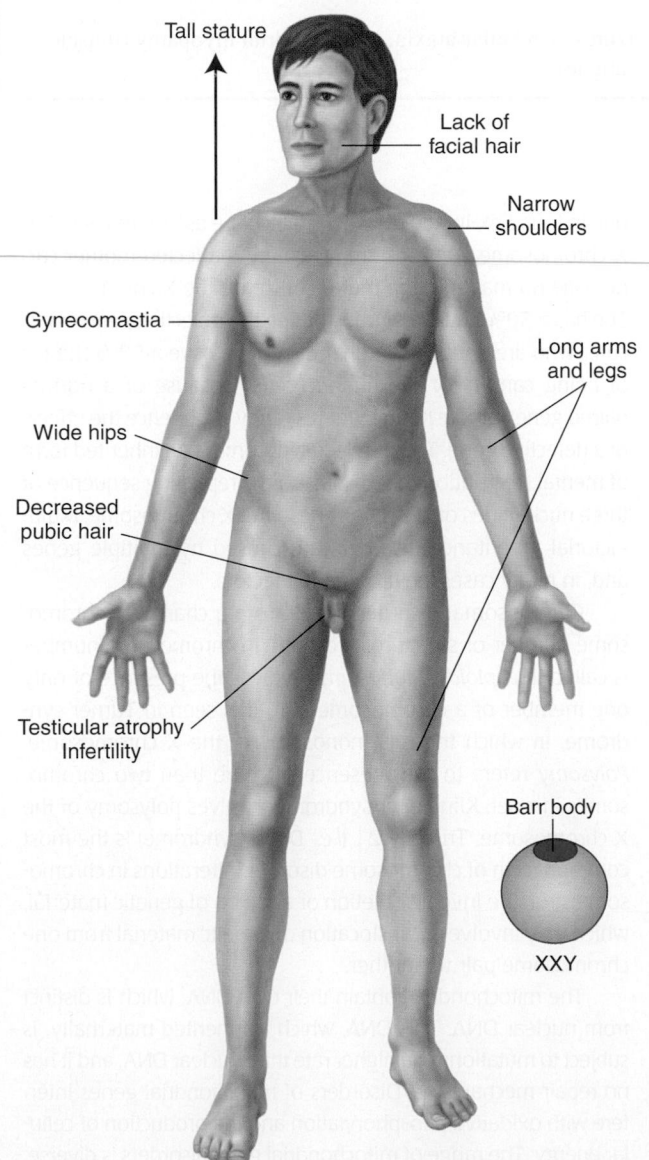

Tall stature

Lack of facial hair

Narrow shoulders

Gynecomastia

Long arms and legs

Wide hips

Decreased pubic hair

Testicular atrophy Infertility

Barr body

XXY

FIGURE 7-11 • Clinical features of Klinefelter syndrome.

TABLE 7-2 Some Disorders of Organ Systems Associated With Mitochondrial DNA Mutations

DISORDER	MANIFESTATIONS
Chronic progressive external ophthalmoplegia	Progressive weakness of the extraocular muscles
Deafness	Progressive sensorineural deafness, often associated with aminoglycoside antibiotics
Kearns-Sayre syndrome	Progressive weakness of the extraocular muscles of early onset with heart block, retinal pigmentation
Leber hereditary optic neuropathy	Painless, subacute, bilateral visual loss, with central blind spots (scotomas) and abnormal color vision
Leigh disease	Proximal muscle weakness, sensory neuropathy, developmental delay, ataxia, seizures, dementia, and visual impairment due to retinal pigment degeneration
MELAS	_M_itochondrial _E_ncephalomyopathy (cerebral structural changes), _L_actic _A_cidosis, and _S_trokelike syndrome, seizures, and other clinical and laboratory abnormalities; may manifest only as diabetes mellitus
MERRF	_M_yoclonic _E_pilepsy, _R_agged _R_ed _F_ibers in muscle, ataxia, sensorineural deafness
Myoclonic epilepsy with ragged red fibers	Myoclonic seizures, cerebellar ataxia, mitochondrial myopathy (muscle weakness, fatigue)

to become symptomatic. This threshold varies in different organs and is presumably related to the energy requirements of the cells.

Mitochondrial DNA mutations generally affect tissues that are dependent on oxidative phosphorylation to meet their high needs for metabolic energy. Thus, mtDNA mutations frequently affect the neuromuscular system and produce disorders such as encephalopathies, myopathies, retinal degeneration, loss of extraocular muscle function, and deafness.[37–39] The mitochondrial myopathies are often associated with the so-called _ragged red fibers,_ a histologic phenotype resulting from degeneration of muscle fibers and massive accumulation of abnormal mitochondria.[5] The range of mitochondrial diseases is broad, however, and may include liver dysfunction, bone marrow failure, and pancreatic islet cell dysfunction and diabetes, among other disorders. Table 7-2 describes representative examples of disorders due to mutations in mtDNA.

IN SUMMARY, genetic disorders can affect a single gene (mendelian inheritance) or several genes (polygenic inheritance). Single-gene disorders may be present on an autosome or on the X chromosome, and they may be expressed as a dominant or recessive trait. In autosomal dominant disorders, a single mutant allele from an affected parent is transmitted to an offspring regardless of sex. The affected parent has a 50% chance of transmitting the disorder to each offspring. Autosomal recessive disorders are manifested only when both members of the gene pair are affected. Usually, both parents are unaffected but are carriers of the defective gene. Their chances of having an affected child are one in four; of having a carrier child, two in four; and of having a noncarrier, unaffected child,

one in four. Sex-linked disorders, which are associated with the X chromosome, are those in which an unaffected mother carries one normal and one mutant allele on the X chromosome. She has a 50% chance of transmitting the defective gene to her sons, who are affected, and her daughters have a 50% chance of being carriers of the mutant gene. Because of a normal paired gene, female heterozygotes rarely experience the effects of a defective gene. The fragile X syndrome is an inherited form of mental retardation that results from a repeating sequence of three nucleotides on a single gene in the X chromosome. Multifactorial inheritance disorders are caused by multiple genes and, in many cases, environmental factors.

Chromosomal disorders result from a change in chromosome number or structure. A change in chromosome number is called _aneuploidy. Monosomy_ involves the presence of only one member of a chromosome pair; it is seen in Turner syndrome, in which there is monosomy of the X chromosome. _Polysomy_ refers to the presence of more than two chromosomes in a set. Klinefelter syndrome involves polysomy of the X chromosome. Trisomy 21 (_i.e.,_ Down syndrome) is the most common form of chromosome disorder. Alterations in chromosome structure involve deletion or addition of genetic material, which may involve a translocation of genetic material from one chromosome pair to another.

The mitochondria contain their own DNA, which is distinct from nuclear DNA. This DNA, which is inherited maternally, is subject to mutations at a higher rate than nuclear DNA, and it has no repair mechanisms. Disorders of mitochondrial genes interfere with oxidative phosphorylation and the production of cellular energy. The range of mitochondrial gene disorders is diverse, with neuromuscular disorders predominating. ■

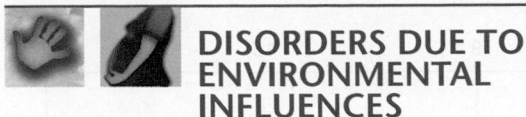

DISORDERS DUE TO ENVIRONMENTAL INFLUENCES

After completing this section of the chapter, you should be able to meet the following objectives:

- Cite the most susceptible period of intrauterine life for development of defects due to environmental agents.
- State the cautions that should be observed when considering use of drugs during pregnancy, including the possible effects of alcohol abuse, vitamin A derivatives, and folic acid deficiency on fetal development.
- List four infectious agents that cause congenital defects.

The developing embryo is subject to many nongenetic influences. After conception, development is influenced by the environmental factors that the embryo shares with the mother. The physiologic status of the mother—her hormone balance, her general state of health, her nutritional status, and the drugs she takes—undoubtedly influences the development of the unborn child. For example, diabetes mellitus is associated with increased risk of congenital anomalies. Smoking is associated with lower-than-normal neonatal weight. Alcohol, in the context of chronic alcoholism, is known to cause fetal abnormalities. Some agents cause early abortion. Measles and other infectious agents cause congenital malformations. Other agents, such as radiation, can cause chromosomal and genetic defects and produce developmental disorders.

Period of Vulnerability

The embryo's development is most easily disturbed during the period when differentiation and development of the organs are taking place. This time interval, which is often referred to as the period of *organogenesis,* extends from day 15 to day 60 after conception. Environmental influences during the first 2 weeks after fertilization may interfere with implantation and result in abortion or early resorption of the products of conception. Each organ has a critical period during which it is highly susceptible to environmental derangements[4,40] (Fig. 7-12). Often, the effect is expressed at the biochemical level just before the organ begins to develop. The same agent may affect different organ systems that are developing at the same time.

Teratogenic Agents

A teratogenic agent is a chemical, physical, or biologic agent that produces abnormalities during embryonic or fetal development. Maternal disease or altered metabolic state also can affect the development of the embryo or fetus. Theoretically, teratogenic agents can cause birth defects in three ways: by direct exposure of the pregnant woman and the embryo or fetus to the agent;

through exposure of the soon-to-be-pregnant woman to an agent that has a slow clearance rate such that a teratogenic dose is retained during early pregnancy; or as a result of mutagenic effects of an environmental agent that occur before pregnancy, causing permanent damage to a woman's (or a man's) reproductive cells. For discussion purposes, teratogenic agents have been divided into three groups: radiation, drugs and chemical substances, and infectious agents. Chart 7-1 lists commonly identified agents in each of these groups.

Radiation

Heavy doses of ionizing radiation have been shown to cause microcephaly, skeletal malformations, and mental retardation. There is no evidence that diagnostic levels of radiation cause congenital abnormalities. Because the question of safety remains, however, many agencies require that the day of a woman's last menstrual period be noted on all radiologic requisitions. Other institutions may require a pregnancy test before any extensive diagnostic x-ray studies are performed. Radiation is teratogenic and mutagenic, and has the capacity to effect inheritable changes in genetic materials. Administration of therapeutic doses of radioactive iodine (^{131}I) during the 13th week of gestation, the time when the fetal thyroid is beginning to concentrate iodine, has been shown to interfere with thyroid development.

Chemicals and Drugs

Environmental chemicals and drugs can cross the placenta and cause damage to the developing embryo and fetus. It has been estimated that only 2% to 3% of developmental defects have a known drug or environmental origin. Some of the best-documented environmental teratogens are the organic mercurials, which cause neurologic deficits and blindness. Sources of exposure to mercury include contaminated food (fish) and water.[41] The precise mechanisms by which chemicals and drugs exert their teratogenic effects are largely unknown. They may produce cytotoxic (cell-killing), antimetabolic, or growth-inhibiting effects. Often their effects depend on the time of exposure (in terms of embryonic and fetal development) and extent of exposure (dosage).[40]

Drugs top the list of chemical teratogens, probably because they are regularly used at elevated doses. Many drugs can cross the placenta and expose the fetus to both the pharmacologic and teratogenic effects. Factors that affect placental drug transfer and drug effects on the fetus include the rate at which the drug crosses the placenta, the duration of exposure, and the stage of placental and fetal development at the time of exposure.[42] Lipid-soluble drugs tend to cross the placenta more readily and enter the fetal circulation. The molecular weight of a drug also influences the rate and amount of drug transferred across the placenta. Drugs with a molecular weight of less than 500 can cross the placenta easily, depending on lipid solubility and degree of ionization; those with a molecular weight of 500 to 1000 cross the placenta with more difficulty;

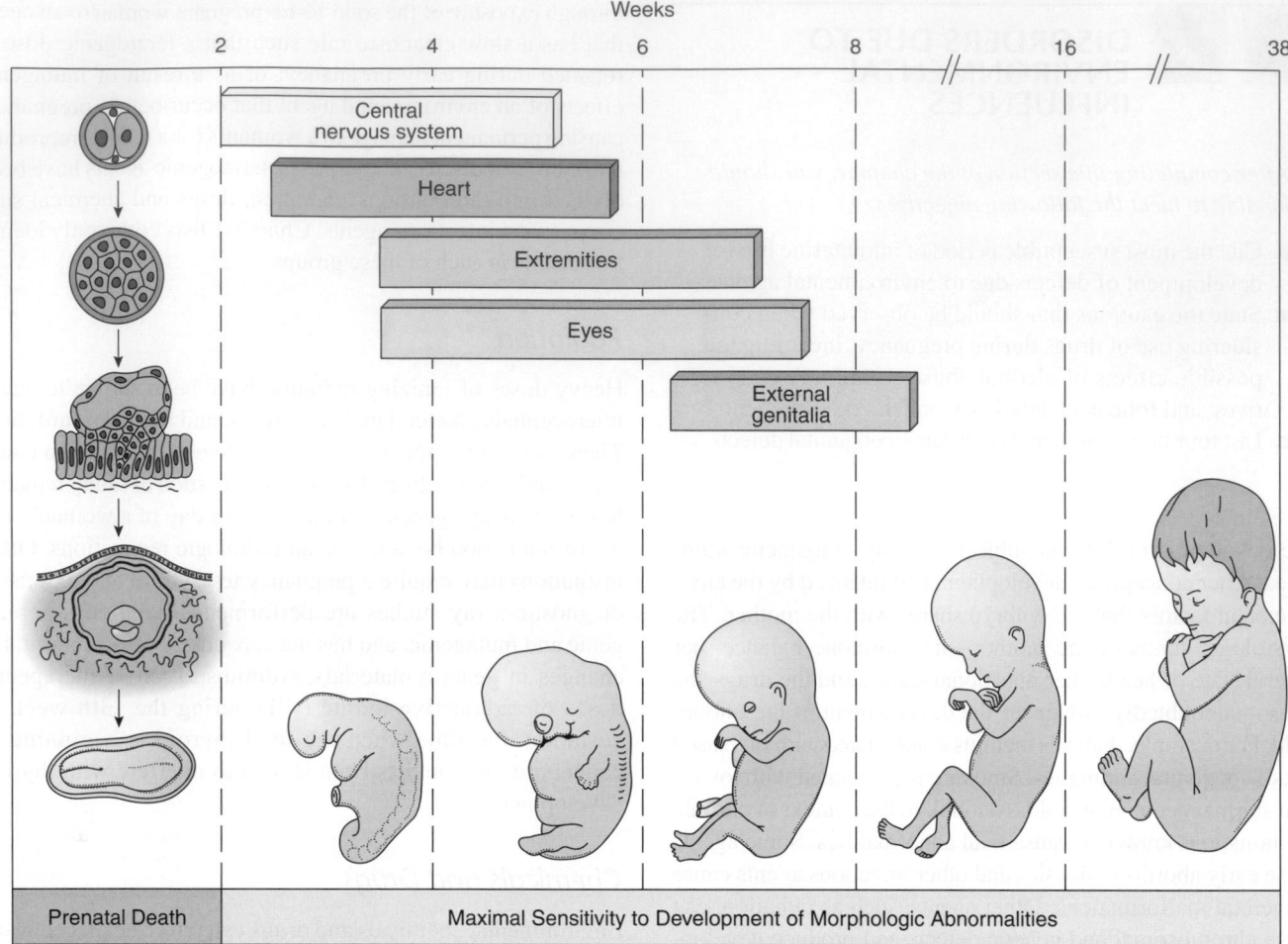

Weeks

FIGURE 7-12 • Sensitivity of specific organs to teratogenic agents at critical periods in embryogenesis. Exposure to adverse influences in the preimplantation and early postimplantation stages of development (*far left*) leads to prenatal death. Periods of maximal sensitivity to teratogens (*horizontal bars*) vary for different organ systems, but overall are limited to the first 8 weeks of pregnancy. (From Killeen A. A., Rubin E., Strayer D.S. [2008]. Development and genetics. In Rubin R., Strayer D. S. [Eds.], *Rubin's pathology: Clinicopathologic foundations of medicine* [5th ed., p. 179]. Philadelphia: Lippincott Williams & Wilkins.)

and those with molecular weights of more than 1000 cross very poorly.[42]

A number of drugs are suspected of being teratogens, but only a few have been identified with certainty.[43] Perhaps the best known of these drugs is thalidomide, which has been shown to give rise to a full range of malformations, including phocomelia (*i.e.,* short, flipper-like appendages) of all four extremities. Other drugs known to cause fetal abnormalities are the antimetabolites used in the treatment of cancer, the anticoagulant drug warfarin, several of the anticonvulsant drugs, ethyl alcohol, and cocaine. Some drugs affect a single developing structure; for example, propylthiouracil can impair thyroid development and tetracycline can interfere with the mineralization phase of tooth development. More recently, vitamin A and its derivatives (the retinoids) have been targeted for concern because of their teratogenic potential. Concern over the teratogenic effects of vitamin A derivatives arose with the introduction of the acne drug isotretinoin (Accutane). Fetal abnormalities such as cleft palate, heart defects, retinal and optic nerve abnormalities, and central nervous system (CNS) malformations were observed with women ingesting therapeutic doses of the drug during the first trimester of pregnancy.[44] There also is concern about the teratogenic effects when a woman consumes high doses of vitamin A, such as those contained in some dietary supplements or vitamin pills. It is currently recommended that doses greater than 10,000 IU should be avoided.[45]

In 1983, the U.S. Food and Drug Administration established a system for classifying drugs according to probable risks to the fetus. According to this system, drugs are put into five categories: A, B, C, D, and X. Drugs in category A are the least dangerous, and categories B, C, and D are increasingly more dangerous. Those in category X are contraindicated during pregnancy because of proven teratogenicity.[42] The law does not require classification of drugs that were in use before 1983.

CHART 7-1 TERATOGENIC AGENTS*

Radiation
Drugs and Chemical Substances
Alcohol
Anticoagulants
 Warfarin
Anticonvulsants
Cancer drugs
 Aminopterin
 Methotrexate
 6-Mercaptopurine
Isotretinoin (Accutane)
Propylthiouracil
Tetracycline
Thalidomide

Infectious Agents
Viruses
 Cytomegalovirus
 Herpes simplex virus
 Measles (rubella)
 Mumps
 Varicella-zoster virus (chickenpox)
Nonviral factors
 Syphilis
 Toxoplasmosis

* Not inclusive.

Because many drugs are suspected of causing fetal abnormalities, and even those that were once thought to be safe are now being viewed critically, it is recommended that women in their childbearing years avoid unnecessary use of drugs. This pertains to nonpregnant women as well as pregnant women because many developmental defects occur early in pregnancy. As happened with thalidomide, the damage to the embryo may occur before pregnancy is suspected or confirmed. A drug that is often abused and can have deleterious effects on the fetus is alcohol.

🔑 TERATOGENIC AGENTS

- Teratogenic agents such as radiation, chemicals and drugs, and infectious organisms are agents that produce abnormalities in the developing embryo.

- The stage of development of the embryo determines the susceptibility to teratogens. The period during which the embryo is most susceptible to teratogenic agents is the time during which rapid differentiation and development of body organs and tissues are taking place, usually from days 15 to 60 postconception.

Fetal Alcohol Syndrome. The term *fetal alcohol syndrome* (FAS) refers to a constellation of physical, behavioral, and cognitive abnormalities resulting from maternal alcohol consumption.[46–49] It has been estimated that among the 4 million infants born each year, 1000 to 6000 will be born with FAS.[46] Alcohol, which is lipid soluble and has a molecular weight between 600 and 1000, passes freely across the placental barrier; concentrations of alcohol in the fetus are at least as high as in the mother. Unlike other teratogens, the harmful effects of alcohol are not restricted to the sensitive period of early gestation but extend throughout pregnancy.

Alcohol has widely variable effects on fetal development, ranging from minor abnormalities to FAS. There may be prenatal or postnatal growth retardation; CNS involvement, including neurologic abnormalities, developmental delays, behavioral dysfunction, intellectual impairment, and skull and brain malformation; and a characteristic set of facial features that include small palpebral fissures (*i.e.,* eye openings), a thin vermilion border (upper lip), and an elongated, flattened midface and philtrum (*i.e.,* the groove in the middle of the upper lip)[46–49] (Fig. 7-13). The facial features of FAS may not be as apparent in the newborn but become more prominent as the infant develops. As the children grow into adulthood, the facial features become more subtle, making diagnosis of FAS in older individuals more difficult. Each of these defects can vary in severity, probably reflecting the timing of alcohol consumption in terms of the period of fetal development, amount of alcohol consumed, and hereditary and environmental influences.

In 2004, the National Task Force on Fetal Alcohol Syndrome and Fetal Alcohol Effect published guidelines for the referral and diagnosis of FAS.[46] The criteria for FAS diagnosis require the documented presence of three of the following findings: (1) three facial abnormalities (smooth philtrum, thin vermilion border on the upper lip, and small palpebral fissures);

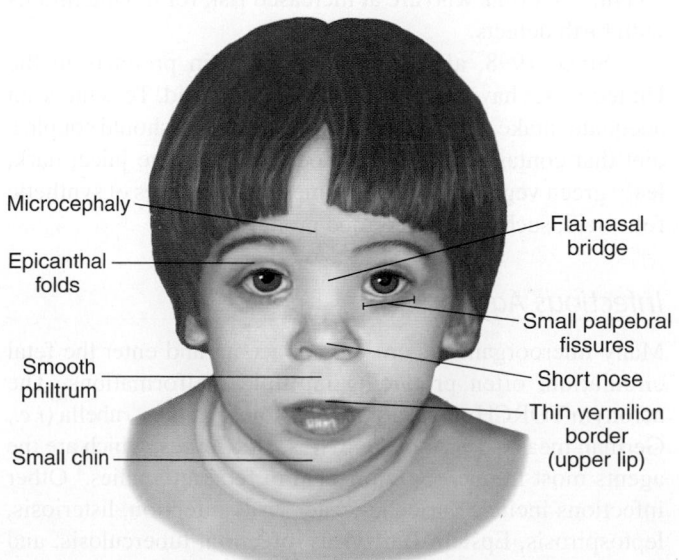

FIGURE 7-13 • Clinical features of fetal alcohol syndrome.

Microcephaly

Epicanthal folds

Smooth philtrum

Small chin

Flat nasal bridge

Small palpebral fissures

Short nose

Thin vermilion border (upper lip)

(2) growth deficits (prenatal or postnatal height or weight, or both, below the 10th percentile); and (3) CNS abnormalities (*e.g.,* head circumference below the 10th percentile, global cognitive or intellectual deficits, motor functioning delays, problems with attention or hyperactivity).

The amount of alcohol that can be safely consumed during pregnancy is unknown. Even small amounts of alcohol consumed during critical periods of fetal development may be teratogenic. For example, if alcohol is consumed during the period of organogenesis, a variety of skeletal and organ defects may result. If alcohol is consumed later in gestation, when the brain is undergoing rapid development, there may be behavioral and cognitive disorders in the absence of physical abnormalities. Chronic alcohol consumption throughout pregnancy may result in a variety of effects, ranging from physical abnormalities to growth retardation and compromised CNS functioning. Evidence suggests that short-lived high concentrations of alcohol, such as those that occur with binge drinking, may be particularly significant, with abnormalities being unique to the period of exposure. Because of the possible effect on the fetus, it recommended that women abstain from alcohol during pregnancy.

Folic Acid Deficiency. Although most birth defects are related to exposure to a teratogenic agent, deficiencies of nutrients and vitamins also may be a factor. Folic acid deficiency has been implicated in the development of neural tube defects (*e.g.,* anencephaly, spina bifida, encephalocele). Studies have shown a reduction in neural tube defects when folic acid was taken before conception and continued during the first trimester of pregnancy.[50–52] Therefore, it is recommended that all women of childbearing age receive 400 micrograms of folic acid daily. These recommendations are particularly important for women who have previously had an affected pregnancy, for couples with a close relative with the disorder, and for women with diabetes mellitus and those taking anticonvulsant drugs who are at increased risk for having infants with birth defects.

Since 1998, all enriched cereal grain products in the United States have been fortified with folic acid. To achieve an adequate intake of folic acid, pregnant women should couple a diet that contains folate-rich foods (*e.g.,* orange juice; dark, leafy green vegetables; and legumes) with sources of synthetic folic acid, such as fortified food products.[52]

Infectious Agents

Many microorganisms cross the placenta and enter the fetal circulation, often producing multiple malformations. The acronym TORCH stands for *t*oxoplasmosis, *o*ther, *r*ubella (*i.e.,* German measles), *c*ytomegalovirus, and *h*erpes, which are the agents most frequently implicated in fetal anomalies.[4] Other infections include varicella-zoster virus infection, listeriosis, leptospirosis, Epstein-Barr virus infection, tuberculosis, and syphilis. Human immunodeficiency virus (HIV) and human parvovirus (B19) have been suggested as additions to the list.

The TORCH screening test examines the infant's serum for the presence of antibodies to these agents. However, the titers for serum antibodies against the TORCH agents in the mother and newborn usually are not diagnostic, and the precise cause of the disorder often remains uncertain.

Infections with the TORCH agents are reported to occur in 1% to 5% of newborn infants and are among the major causes of neonatal morbidity and mortality.[4] Common clinical and pathologic manifestations include growth retardation and abnormalities of the brain (microcephaly, hydrocephalus), eye, ear, liver, hematopoietic system (anemia, thrombocytopenia), lungs (pneumonitis), and heart (myocarditis, congenital heart disorders).[4] These manifestations vary among symptomatic newborns, however, and only a few present with multisystem abnormalities.

Toxoplasmosis is a protozoal infection caused by *Toxoplasma gondii.* The infection can be contracted by eating raw or inadequately cooked meat or food that has come in contact with infected meat.[53] The domestic cat can carry the organism, excreting the protozoa in its feces. It has been suggested that pregnant women should avoid contact with excrement from the family cat. The introduction of the rubella vaccine has virtually eliminated the congenital rubella syndrome in most developed countries. Rubella remains endemic in many developing countries, however, where it is the major preventable cause of hearing impairment, blindness, and adverse neurodevelopmental outcome. The epidemiology of cytomegalovirus infection is largely unknown. Some infants are severely affected at birth, and others, although having evidence of the infection, have no symptoms. In some symptom-free infants, brain damage becomes evident over a span of several years. There also is evidence that some infants contract the infection during the first year of life, and in some of them the infection leads to retardation a year or two later. Herpes simplex virus type 2 infection is considered to be a genital infection and usually is transmitted through sexual contact. The infant acquires this infection in utero or in passage through the birth canal.

IN SUMMARY, a teratogenic agent is one that produces abnormalities during embryonic or fetal life. It is during the early part of pregnancy (15 to 60 days after conception) that environmental agents are most apt to produce their deleterious effects on the developing embryo. A number of environmental agents can be damaging to the unborn child, including radiation, drugs and chemicals, and infectious agents. FAS is a risk for infants of women who regularly consume alcohol during pregnancy. Because many drugs have the potential for causing fetal abnormalities, often at an early stage of pregnancy, it is recommended that women of childbearing age avoid unnecessary use of drugs. It also has been shown that folic acid deficiency can contribute to neural tube defects. The acronym TORCH stands for *t*oxoplasmosis, *o*ther, *r*ubella, *c*ytomegalovirus, and *h*erpes, which are the infectious agents most frequently implicated in fetal anomalies. ∎

DIAGNOSIS AND COUNSELING

After completing this section of the chapter, you should be able to meet the following objectives:

- Describe the process of genetic assessment.
- Cite the rationale for prenatal diagnosis.
- Describe methods used in arriving at a prenatal diagnosis, including ultrasonography, amniocentesis, chorionic villus sampling, percutaneous umbilical fetal blood sampling, and laboratory methods to determine the biochemical and genetic makeup of the fetus.

The birth of a defective child is a traumatic event in any parent's life. Usually two issues must be resolved. The first deals with the immediate and future care of the affected child, and the second with the possibility of future children in the family having a similar defect. Genetic assessment and counseling can help to determine whether the defect was inherited and the risk of recurrence. Prenatal diagnosis provides a means of determining whether the unborn child has certain types of abnormalities.

Genetic Assessment

Effective genetic counseling involves accurate diagnosis and communication of the findings and of the risks of recurrence to the parents and other family members who need such information. Counseling may be provided after the birth of an affected child, or it may be offered to persons at risk for having defective children (*i.e.,* siblings of persons with birth defects). A team of trained counselors can help the family to understand the problem and can support their decisions about having more children.

Assessment of genetic risk and prognosis usually is directed by a clinical geneticist, often with the aid of laboratory and clinical specialists. A detailed family history (*i.e.,* pedigree), a pregnancy history, and detailed accounts of the birth process and postnatal health and development are included. A careful physical examination of the affected child and often of the parents and siblings usually is needed. Laboratory tests, including chromosomal analysis and biochemical studies, often precede a definitive diagnosis.

Prenatal Screening and Diagnosis

The purpose of prenatal screening and diagnosis is not just to detect fetal abnormalities. Rather, it has the following objectives: to provide parents with information needed to make an informed choice about having a child with an abnormality; to provide reassurance and reduce anxiety among high-risk groups; and to allow parents at risk for having a child with a specific defect, who might otherwise forgo having a child, to begin a

pregnancy with the assurance that knowledge about the presence or absence of the disorder in the fetus can be confirmed by testing.[3] Prenatal screening cannot be used to rule out all possible fetal abnormalities. It is limited to determining whether the fetus has (or probably has) designated conditions indicated by late maternal age, family history, or well-defined risk factors.

Among the methods used for fetal diagnosis are ultrasonography, maternal serum (blood) screening tests, amniocentesis, chorionic villus sampling, and percutaneous umbilical fetal blood sampling[3,25,54] (Fig. 7-14). Termination of pregnancy is indicated only in a small number of cases; in the rest, the fetus is normal and the procedure provides reassurance for the parents. Prenatal diagnosis can also provide the information needed for prescribing prenatal treatment for the fetus. For example, if congenital adrenal hyperplasia is diagnosed, the mother can be treated with adrenal cortical hormones to prevent masculinization of a female fetus.

Ultrasonography

Ultrasonography is a noninvasive diagnostic method that uses reflections of high-frequency sound waves to visualize soft tissue structures. Since its introduction in 1958, it has been used during pregnancy to determine number of fetuses, fetal size and position, amount of amniotic fluid, and placental location. It also is possible to assess fetal movement, breathing movements, and heart pattern. There is also good evidence that early ultrasonography (*i.e.,* before 14 weeks) accurately determines gestational age.

Improved resolution and real-time units have enhanced the ability of ultrasound scanners to detect congenital anomalies. With this more sophisticated equipment, it is possible to obtain information such as measurements of hourly urine output in a high-risk fetus. Ultrasonography makes possible the in utero diagnosis of hydrocephalus, spina bifida, facial defects, congenital heart defects, congenital diaphragmatic hernias, disorders of the gastrointestinal tract, and skeletal anomalies. Cardiovascular abnormalities are the most commonly missed malformation. A four-chamber view of the fetal heart improves the detection of cardiac malformations. Intrauterine diagnosis of congenital abnormalities permits planning of surgical correction shortly after birth, preterm delivery for early correction, selection of cesarean section to reduce fetal injury, and, in some cases, intrauterine therapy. When a congenital abnormality is suspected, a diagnosis made using ultrasonography usually can be obtained by weeks 16 to 18 of gestation.

Maternal Serum Markers

Maternal blood testing began in the early 1980s with the test for α-fetoprotein (AFP). Since that time, a number of serum factors have been studied as screening tests for fetal anomalies. Current maternal testing uses three distinct tests (AFP, human chorionic gonadotropin [hCG], and unconjugated estriol) to screen for trisomy syndromes in high-risk women, while incorporating the detection of neural tube defects. The combined

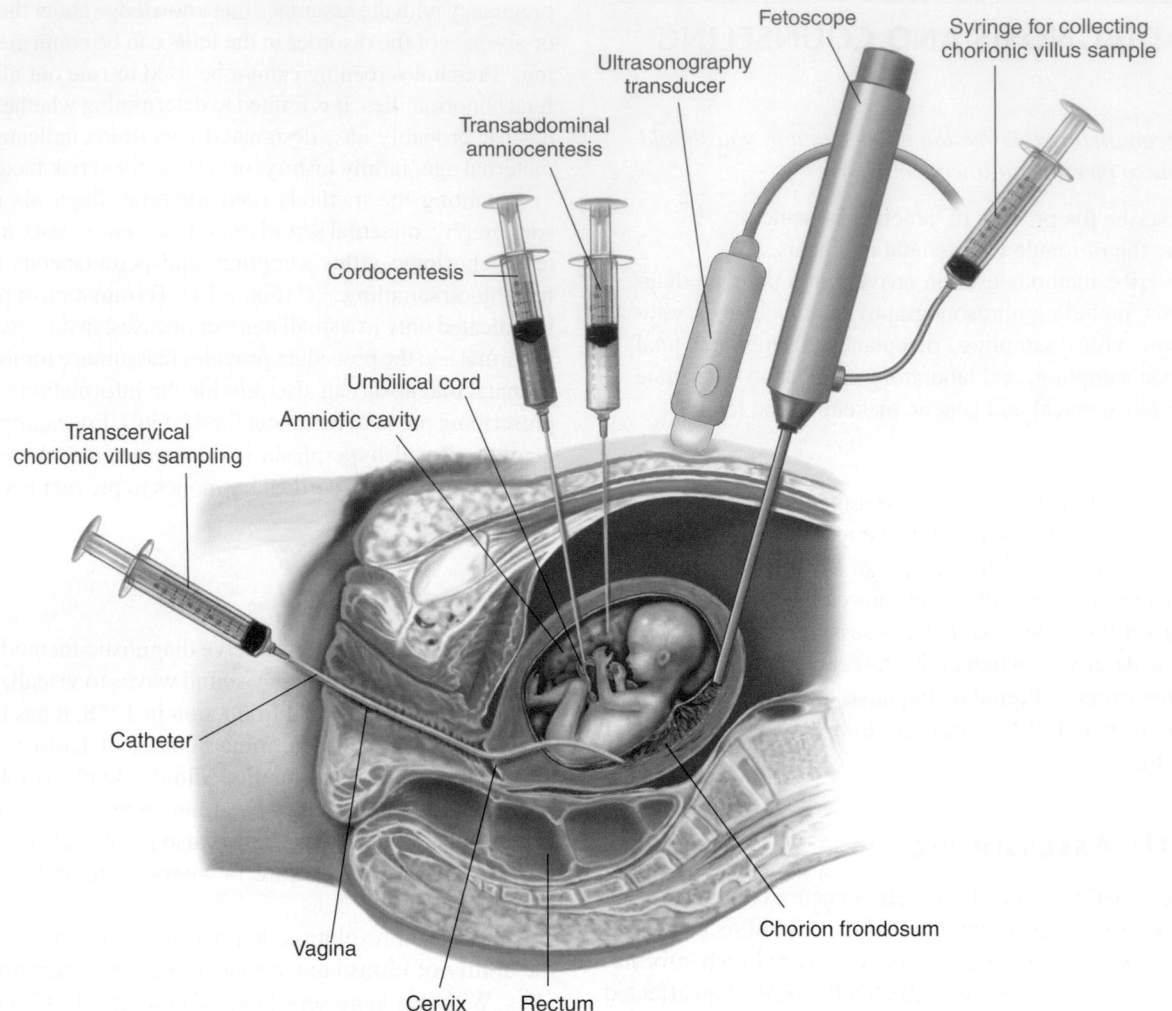

FIGURE 7-14 • Methods of prenatal screening.

use of the three maternal serum markers between 15 and 22 weeks of pregnancy has been shown to detect as much as 60% of Down syndrome pregnancies.[3] The use of ultrasonography to verify fetal age can reduce the number of false-positive tests with this screening method.

AFP is a major fetal plasma protein and has a structure similar to the albumin found in postnatal life. AFP is made initially by the yolk sac, gastrointestinal tract, and liver. Fetal plasma levels peak at approximately 10 to 13 weeks' gestation and then decline progressively until term, whereas maternal levels peak in the third trimester.[55] Maternal and amniotic fluid levels of AFP are elevated in pregnancies where the fetus has a neural tube defect (*i.e.,* anencephaly and open spina bifida) or certain other malformations such as an anterior abdominal wall defect in which the fetal integument is not intact. Screening of maternal blood samples usually is done between weeks 16 and 18 of gestation.[3,55] Although neural tube defects have been associated with elevated levels of AFP, decreased levels have been associated with Down syndrome.

A complex glycoprotein, hCG is produced exclusively by the outer layer of the trophoblast shortly after implantation in the uterine wall. It increases rapidly in the first 8 weeks of gestation, declines steadily until 20 weeks, and then plateaus. The single maternal serum marker that yields the highest detection rate for Down syndrome is an elevated level of hCG. Unconjugated estriol is produced by the placenta from precursors provided by the fetal adrenal glands and liver. It increases steadily throughout pregnancy to a higher level than that normally produced by the liver. Unconjugated estriol levels are decreased in Down syndrome and trisomy 18.

Other maternal serum markers include pregnancy-associated plasma protein A (PAPP-A) and inhibin A. PAPP-A, which is secreted by the placenta, has been shown to play an important role in promoting cell differentiation and proliferation in various body systems. In complicated pregnancies, the PAPP-A concentration increases with gestational age until term. Decreased PAPP-A levels in the first trimester (between 10 and 13 weeks) have been shown to be associated with Down syndrome. When used along with maternal age, free β-hCG, and ultrasonographic measurement of nuchal translucency, serum PAPP-A levels can reportedly detect 85% to 95% of affected pregnancies with a false-positive rate of approximately 5%.[56] Inhibin A, which is secreted by the corpus luteum and fetoplacental unit, is also a maternal serum marker for fetal Down syndrome.[57]

Amniocentesis

Amniocentesis involves the withdrawal of a sample of amniotic fluid from the pregnant uterus using either a transabdominal or transcervical approach (see Fig. 7-14). The procedure is useful in women older than 35 years of age, who have an increased risk of giving birth to an infant with Down syndrome; in parents who have another child with chromosomal abnormalities; and in situations in which a parent is known to be a carrier of an inherited disease. Ultrasonography is used to gain additional information and to guide the placement of the amniocentesis needle. The amniotic fluid and cells that have been shed by the fetus are studied. Amniocentesis is performed on an outpatient basis typically at the 15th to 16th week after the first day of the last menstrual period.[3] For chromosomal analysis, the fetal cells are grown in culture and the result is available in 10 to 14 days. The amniotic fluid also can be tested using various biochemical tests.

Chorionic Villus Sampling

Sampling of the chorionic villi usually is done after 10 weeks of gestation.[58] Doing the test before that time is not recommended because of the danger of limb reduction defects in the fetus. The chorionic villi are the site of exchange of nutrients between the maternal blood and the embryo—the chorionic sac encloses the early amniotic sac and fetus, and the villi are the primitive blood vessels that develop into the placenta. The sampling procedure can be performed using either a transabdominal or transcervical approach (see Fig. 7-14). The tissue that is obtained can be used for fetal chromosome studies, DNA analysis, and biochemical studies. The fetal tissue does not have to be cultured, and fetal chromosome analysis can be made available in 24 hours. DNA analysis and biochemical tests can be completed within 1 to 2 weeks.[58]

Percutaneous Umbilical Cord Blood Sampling

Percutaneous umbilical cord blood sampling involves the transcutaneous insertion of a needle through the uterine wall and into the umbilical artery. It is performed under ultrasonographic guidance and can be done any time after 16 weeks of gestation. It is used for prenatal diagnosis of hemoglobinopathies, coagulation disorders, metabolic and cytogenetic disorders, and immunodeficiencies. Fetal infections such as rubella and toxoplasmosis can be detected through measurement of immunoglobulin M antibodies or direct blood cultures. Results from cytogenetic studies usually are available within 48 to 72 hours. Because the procedure carries a greater risk of pregnancy loss than amniocentesis, it usually is reserved for situations in which rapid cytogenetic analysis is needed or in which diagnostic information cannot be obtained by other methods.

Fetal Biopsy

Fetal biopsy is done with a fetoscope under ultrasonographic guidance. It is used to detect certain genetic skin defects that cannot be diagnosed with DNA analysis. It also may be done to obtain muscle tissue for use in the diagnosis of Duchenne muscular dystrophy.

Cytogenetic and Biochemical Analyses

Amniocentesis and chorionic villus sampling yield cells that can be used for cytogenetic and DNA analyses. Biochemical analyses can be used to detect abnormal levels of AFP and abnormal biochemical products in the maternal blood and in specimens of amniotic fluid and fetal blood.

Cytogenetic studies are used for fetal karyotyping to determine the chromosomal makeup of the fetus. They are done to detect abnormalities of chromosome number and structure. Karyotyping also reveals the sex of the fetus. This may be useful when an inherited defect is known to affect only one sex.

Analysis of DNA is done on cells extracted from the amniotic fluid, chorionic villi, or fetal blood from percutaneous umbilical sampling to detect genetic defects such as inborn errors of metabolism. The defect may be established through direct demonstration of the molecular defect or through methods that break the DNA into fragments that can be studied to determine the presence of an abnormal gene. Direct demonstration of the molecular defect is done by growing the amniotic fluid cells in culture and measuring the enzymes that the cultured cells produce. Many of the enzymes are expressed in the chorionic villi; this permits earlier prenatal diagnosis because the cells do not need to be subjected to prior culture. DNA studies are used to detect genetic defects that cause inborn errors of metabolism, such as Tay-Sachs disease, glycogen storage diseases, and familial hypercholesterolemia. Prenatal diagnoses are possible for more than 70 inborn errors of metabolism.

IN SUMMARY, genetic and prenatal diagnosis and counseling are done in an effort to determine the risk of having a child with a genetic or chromosomal disorder. They often involve a detailed family history (*i.e.*, pedigree), examination of any affected and other family members, and laboratory studies including chromosomal analysis and biochemical studies. They usually are done by a genetic counselor and a specially prepared team of health care professionals. Prenatal screening and diagnosis are used to detect fetal abnormalities. Ultrasonography is used for fetal anatomic imaging. It is used for determination of fetal size and position and for the presence of structural anomalies. Maternal serum screening is used to identify pregnancies that are at increased risk of adverse outcomes such as Down syndrome and neural tube defects. Amniocentesis and chorionic villus sampling may be used to obtain specimens for cytogenetic and biochemical studies. ■

Review Exercises

1. A 23-year-old woman with sickle cell disease and her husband want to have a child, but worry that the child will be born with the disease.

   A. *What is the mother's genotype in terms of the sickle cell gene? Is she heterozygous or homozygous?*

   B. *If the husband is found not to have the sickle cell gene, what is the probability of their child having the disease or being a carrier of the sickle cell trait?*

2. A couple has a child who was born with a congenital heart disease.

   A. *Would you consider the defect to be the result of a single gene or a polygenic trait?*

   B. *Would these parents be at greater risk of having another child with a heart defect or would they be at equal risk of having a child with a defect in another organ system, such as cleft palate?*

3. A couple has been informed that their newborn child has the features of Down syndrome and it is suggested that genetic studies be performed.

   A. *The child is found to have trisomy 21. Use Figure 7-7, which describes the events that occur during meiosis, to explain the origin of the third chromosome.*

   B. *If the child had been found to have the robertsonian chromosome, how would you explain the origin of the abnormal chromosome?*

4. An 8-year-old boy has been diagnosed with mitochondrial myopathy. His major complaints are those of muscle weakness and exercise intolerance. His mother gives a report of similar symptoms, but to a much lesser degree.

   A. *Explain the cause of this boy's symptoms.*

   B. *Mitochondrial disorders follow a nonmendelian pattern of inheritance. Explain. Define the terms* homoplasmy *and* heteroplasmy *in relation to the diversity of tissue involvement and symptoms in persons with mitochondrial disorders.*

5. A 26-year-old woman is planning to become pregnant.

   A. *What information would you give her regarding the effects of medications and drugs on the fetus? What stage of fetal development is associated with the greatest risk?*

   B. *What is the rationale for ensuring that she has an adequate intake of folic acid before conception?*

   C. *She and her husband have an indoor cat. What precautions should she use in caring for the cat?*

References

1. March of Dimes Foundation. (2006). Birth defects information. [On-line]. Available: www.marchofdimes.com/pnhec/4439.asp.
2. Barsch G. (2002). Genetic diseases. In McPhee S. J., Lingappa V. R., Ganong W. F. (Eds.), *Pathology of disease: An introduction to clinical medicine* (4th ed., pp. 2–27). New York: McGraw-Hill.
3. Nussbaum R. L., McInnes R. R., Willard H. F. (2007). *Thompson & Thompson genetics in medicine* (7th ed., pp. 115–146, 382–387, 443–458, 485–490). Philadelphia: Elsevier Saunders.
4. Rubin E., Killeen A. A. (2006). Developmental and genetic diseases. In Rubin E., Gorstein F., Rubin R., et al. (Eds.), *Pathology: Clinicopathologic foundations of medicine* (4th ed., pp. 214–279). Philadelphia: Lippincott Williams & Wilkins.
5. Kumar V., Abbas A. K., Fausto N. (2006). Genetic disorders. In *Robbins and Cotran pathologic basis of disease* (7th ed., pp. 145–192). Philadelphia: Elsevier Saunders.
6. Dean J. C. S. (2002). Management of Marfan syndrome. *Heart* 88, 97–103.
7. Ryan-Krause P. (2002). Identify and manage Marfan syndrome in children. *Nurse Practitioner* 27(10), 26–36.
8. Milewicz D. M., Dietz H. C., Miller C. (2005). Treatment of aortic disease in patients with Marfan syndrome. *Circulation* 111, e150–e157.
9. Theos A., Korf B. R. (2006). Pathophysiology of neurofibromatosis type I. *Annals of Internal Medicine* 144, 842–849.
10. Yohay K. (2006). Neurofibromatosis type 1 and 2. *Neurologist* 12, 86–93.
11. National Institutes of Health Consensus Development Panel. (2001). National Institutes of Health Consensus Development Conference Statement. Phenylketonuria: Screening and management, October 16–18, 2000. *Pediatrics* 108, 972–982.
12. Hanley W.B. (2005). Newborn screening in Canada—Are we out of step? *Paediatric Child Health* 10(4), 203–207.
13. Hellekson K. L. (2001). Practice guidelines: NIH consensus statement on phenylketonuria. *American Family Physician* 63, 1430–1432.
14. National Institutes of Health. (2003). Families and fragile X syndrome. U.S. Department of Health and Human Services, Public Health Services, NIH Publication no. 96-3402. [On-line.] Available: www.nichd.nih.gov/publications/pubs/fragileX/sub22.htm.
15. Oostra B. A., Chiurazzi P. (2001). The fragile X gene and its function. *Clinical Genetics* 60, 399–408.
16. O'Donnell W. T., Warren S. T. (2002). A decade of molecular studies of fragile X syndrome. *Annual Review of Neuroscience* 25, 315–338.
17. Hagerman P. J., Hagerman R. J. (2004). The fragile-X permutation: A maturing perspective. *American Journal of Human Genetics* 74, 805–816.
18. Riccardi V. M. (1977). *The genetic approach to human disease* (p. 92). New York: Oxford University Press.
19. Schutte B. C., Murray J. C. (1999). The many faces and factors of orofacial clefts. *Human Molecular Genetics* 10, 1853–1859.
20. Tinanoff N. (2004). Cleft lip and palate. In Behrman R. E., Kliegman R. M., Jenson H. B. (Eds.), *Nelson textbook of pediatrics* (17th ed., pp. 1207–1208). Philadelphia: Elsevier Saunders.
21. Mulliken J. B. (2004). The changing faces of children with cleft lip and palate. *New England Journal of Medicine* 351, 745–747.
22. March of Dimes Foundation. (2006). Down syndrome. [On-line]. Available: www.marchofdimes.com/pnhec/4439_1214.asp.
23. Roizen N. J., Patterson D. (2003). Down syndrome. *Lancet* 361, 1281–1289.
24. Newberger D. S. (2000). Down syndrome: Prenatal risk assessment and diagnosis. *American Family Physician* 62, 825–832, 837–838.
25. Cunniff C., American Academy of Pediatrics Committee on Genetics. (2004). Prenatal screening and diagnosis for pediatricians. *Pediatrics* 114, 889–894.
26. Sybert V. P., McCauley E. (2004). Turner's syndrome. *New England Journal of Medicine* 351, 1227–1238.
27. Ranke M. R. (2001). Turner syndrome. *Lancet* 358, 309–314.
28. Gravholt C. H. (2004). Epidemiological, endocrine and metabolic features in Turner syndrome. *European Journal of Endocrinology* 151, 657–687.
29. American Academy of Pediatrics Clinical Report. (2005). Health supervision of children with Turner syndrome. *Pediatrics* 111, 691–702.

30. Elsheikh M., Dunger D. B., Conway G. S., et al. (2002). Turner syndrome in adulthood. *Endocrine Reviews* 21, 120–140.

31. Frías J. L., Davenport M. L., American Academy of Pediatrics Committee on Genetics, Section on Endocrinology. (2005). Health supervision of children with Turner syndrome. *Pediatrics* 111, 692–702.

32. National Institute of Child Health and Human Development. (2000). A guide for XXY males and their family. [On-line]. Available: www.nichd.nih.gov/publications/pubs/klinefelter.htm.

33. Lanfranco F., Kamischke A., Zitzmann M., et al. (2004). Klinefelter syndrome. *Lancet* 364, 273–283.

34. Wattendorf D. J., Muenke M. (2005). Klinefelter syndrome. *American Family Physician* 72, 2259–2262.

35. Johns D. R. (1995). Mitochondrial DNA and disease. *New England Journal of Medicine* 333, 638–644.

36. Johnston M. V. (2004). Mitochondrial encephalomyopathies. In Behrman R. E., Kliegman R. M., Jenson H. B. (Eds.), *Nelson textbook of pediatrics* (17th ed., pp. 2025–2027). Philadelphia: Elsevier Saunders.

37. Dimauro S., Schon E. A. (2003). Mitochondrial respiratory chain disease. *New England Journal of Medicine* 348, 2656–2668.

38. Dimauro S., Davidzon G. (2005). Mitochondrial DNA and disease. *Annals of Medicine* 37, 222–232.

39. Chaturvedi S., Bala K., Thakur G., et al. (2005). Mitochondrial encephalomyopathies: Advances in understanding. *Medical Science Monitor* 11, RA238–RA246.

40. Brent R. L. (2004). Environmental causes of congenital malformations: The pediatrician's role in dealing with these complex clinical problems caused by a multiplicity of environmental and genetic factors. *Pediatrics* 113, 957–968.

41. Steurerwald U., Weibe P., Jorgensen P. J., et al. (2000). Maternal seafood diet, methylmercury exposure, and neonatal neurologic function. *Journal of Pediatrics* 136, 599–605.

42. Young V. S. L. (2005). Teratogenicity and drugs in breast milk. In Koda-Kimble M. A., Young L. Y., Kradjan W. A. (Eds.), *Applied therapeutics: The clinical use of drugs* (8th ed., pp. 47-1–47 15). Philadelphia: Lippincott Williams & Wilkins.

43. Koren G., Pstuszak A., Ito S. (1998). Drugs in pregnancy. *New England Journal of Medicine* 338, 1128–1137.

44. Ross S. A., McCaffery P. J., Drager U. C., et al. (2000). Retinoids in embryonal development. *Physiological Reviews* 80, 1021–1055.

45. Oakley G. P., Erickson J. D. (1995). Vitamin A and birth defects. *New England Journal of Medicine* 333, 1414–1415.

46. Bertrand J., Floyd R. L., Weber M. K., et al., National Task Force on Fetal Alcohol and Fetal Alcohol Effects. (2004). *Fetal alcohol syndromes: Guidelines for referral and diagnosis.* Atlanta: Centers for Disease Control and Prevention.

47. Sokol R. J., Delaney-Black V., Nordstrom B. (2003). Fetal alcohol syndrome. *Journal of the American Medical Association* 290, 2996–2999.

48. Wattendorf D. J., Muenke M. (2005). Fetal alcohol spectrum disorders. *American Family Physician* 72, 279–285.

49. Riley E. P., McGee C. L. (2005). Fetal alcohol spectrum disorders: An overview with emphasis on changes in brain and behavior. *Experimental Biology and Medicine* 230, 357–365.

50. Centers for Disease Control and Prevention. (1992). Recommendations for use of folic acid to reduce the number of cases of spina bifida and other neural tube defects. *Morbidity and Mortality Weekly Report* 41, 1–8.

51. Scholl T. O., Johnson W. G. (2000). Folic acid: Influence on outcome of pregnancy. *American Journal of Clinical Nutrition* 71(Suppl.), 1295S–1303S.

52. Bailey L. B. (2000). New standard for dietary folate intake in pregnant women. *American Journal of Clinical Nutrition* 71(Suppl.), 1304S–1307S.

53. Jones J., Lopez A., Wilson M. (2003). Congenital toxoplasmosis. *American Family Physician* 67, 2131–2138.

54. Kirkham C., Harris S., Grzybowski S. (2005). Evidence-based prenatal care: Part I. General prenatal care and counseling issues. *American Family Physician* 71, 1307–1316.

55. Graves J. C., Miller K. E. (2002). Maternal serum triple analyte screening in pregnancy. *American Family Physician* 65, 915–920.

56. Qin Q.-P., Christiansen M., Pettersson K. (2002). Point of care time-resolved immunofluorometric assay of human pregnancy-associated plasma protein A: Use in first-trimester screening for Down syndrome. *Clinical Chemistry* 48, 473–483.

57. Lambert-Messerlian G. M., Canick J. A. (2004). Clinical application of inhibin a measurement. Prenatal serum screening for Down syndrome. *Seminars in Reproductive Medicine* 22, 235–242.

58. Wilson R. D. (2000). Amniocentesis and chorionic villus sampling. *Current Opinion in Obstetrics and Gynecology* 12, 81–86.

Visit the Point. **http://thePoint.lww.com for animations, journal articles, and more!**

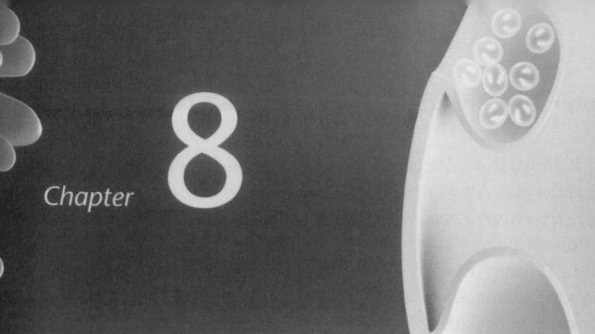

Chapter 8

Neoplasia

CARRIE J. MERKLE

➤ Cancer is the second leading cause of death in the United States. For the year 2007, it was estimated that 1.45 million people in the United States would be newly diagnosed with cancer and 559,650 people would die of the disease.[1] During the same period, it was estimated that 159,000 new cases of cancer would be diagnosed and 72,700 deaths from cancer would occur in Canada.[2] Trends in cancer survival demonstrate that relative 5-year survival rates have improved since the early 1960s. Although the mortality rate has decreased, the number of cancer deaths has increased due to the aging and expanding population. According to the Canadian Cancer Society, 44% of new cancer cases and 60% of deaths occur among people who are at least 70 years of age.[2]

Cancer is not a single disease. It can originate in almost any organ, with skin cancers being the most common site in persons in the United States. Excluding skin cancers, the prostate is the most common site in men and the breast is the most common site in women (Fig. 8-1). The ability to cure cancer varies considerably and depends on the type of cancer and the extent of the disease at time of diagnosis. Cancers such as acute lymphoblastic leukemia, Hodgkin disease, testicular cancer, and osteosarcoma, which only a few decades ago had poor prognoses, are today cured in many cases. However, lung cancer, which is the leading cause of death in men and women in the United States and Canada,[1,2] is resistant to therapy, and although some progress has been made in its treatment, mortality rates remain high.

This chapter is divided into six sections: concepts of cell differentiation and growth, characteristics of benign and malignant neoplasms, etiology of cancer, clinical manifestations, diagnosis and treatment, and childhood cancers. Hematologic malignancies (lymphomas and leukemias) are presented in Chapter 15.

CONCEPTS OF CELL DIFFERENTIATION AND GROWTH

After completing this section of the chapter, you should be able to meet the following objectives:

- Define *neoplasm* and explain how neoplastic growth differs from the normal adaptive changes seen in atrophy, hypertrophy, and hyperplasia.
- Distinguish between cell proliferation and differentiation.
- Describe the phases of the cell cycle.
- Explain the function of cyclins, cyclin-dependent kinases, and cyclin-dependent kinase inhibitors in terms of regulating the cell cycle.
- Describe the properties of stem cells.

Estimated New Cases	
Prostate (29%)	Breast (26%)
Lung and bronchus (15%)	Lung and bronchus (15%)
Colon and rectum (10%)	Colon and rectum (11%)
Urinary bladder (7%)	Uterine corpus (6%)
Non-Hodgkin lymphoma (4%)	Non-Hodgkin lymphoma (4%)
Melanoma of the skin (4%)	Melanoma of the skin (4%)
Kidney and renal pelvis (4%)	Thyroid (4%)
Leukemia (3%)	Ovary (3%)
Oral cavity and pharynx (3%)	Kidney and renal pelvis (3%)
Pancreas (2%)	Leukemia (3%)
All other sites (19%)	All other sites (21%)

Estimated Deaths	
Lung and bronchus (31%)	Lung and bronchus (26%)
Prostate (9%)	Breast (15%)
Colon and rectum (9%)	Colon and rectum (10%)
Pancreas (6%)	Pancreas (6%)
Leukemia (4%)	Ovary (6%)
Liver and intrahepatic bile duct (4%)	Leukemia (4%)
Esophagus (4%)	Non-Hodgkin lymphoma (3%)
Urinary bladder (3%)	Uterine corpus (3%)
Non-Hodgkin lymphoma (3%)	Brain and other nervous system (2%)
Kidney and renal pelvis (3%)	Liver and intrahepatic bile duct (2%)
All other sites (24%)	All other sites (23%)

*Excludes basal and squamous cell skin cancers and in situ carcinomas except urinary bladder.
Note: Percentages may not total 100 percent due to rounding.

FIGURE 8-1 • Cancer incidence and mortality by site and sex. (Adapted from Jemal A., Seigel R., Ward E., et al. [2007]. Cancer statistics, 2007. *CA: A Cancer Journal for Clinicians* 57, 47.)

Cancer is a disorder of altered cell differentiation and growth. The resulting process is called *neoplasia,* meaning "new growth," and the new growth is called a *neoplasm.* Unlike changes in tissue growth that occur with hypertrophy and hyperplasia, the growth of a neoplasm tends to be uncoordinated and relatively autonomous in that it lacks normal regulatory controls over cell growth and division. Neoplasms tend to increase in size and continue to grow after the stimulus that evoked the change has ceased or the needs of the organism have been met.

Normal tissue renewal and repair involves two components: cell proliferation and differentiation. *Proliferation,* or the process of cell division, is an inherent adaptive mechanism for cell replacement when old cells die or additional cells are needed. *Differentiation* is the process whereby cells become increasingly more specialized with each mitotic division. Apoptosis, which is discussed in Chapter 5, is a form of programmed cell death that eliminates senescent cells, cells with deoxyribonucleic acid (DNA) damage, or unwanted cells. In a given tissue, the size of a population of cells is determined by the rates of cell proliferation and cell death, such as loss by apoptosis.[3]

CELL PROLIFERATION AND GROWTH

- Tissue growth and repair involve cell proliferation, differentiation, and apoptosis.
- Cell proliferation is the process whereby tissues acquire new or replacement cells through mitotic cell division.
- Cell differentiation is the orderly process in which proliferating cells are transformed into different and more specialized cell types. It determines the microscopic characteristics of the cell, its functions, and its life span. Cells that are fully differentiated often have reduced rates of proliferation.
- Apoptosis is a form of programmed cell death that eliminates senescent and some types of injured cells (*e.g.,* those with DNA damage or hydrogen peroxide-induced injury).

The Cell Cycle

The cell cycle is an orderly sequence of events that occur as a cell duplicates its contents and divides. During the cell cycle, genetic information is duplicated and the duplicated chromosomes are appropriately aligned for distribution between two genetically identical daughter cells.

The cell cycle is divided into four distinct phases, referred to as G_1, S, G_2, and M. G_1 (*gap 1*) is the postmitotic phase during which DNA synthesis ceases while ribonucleic acid (RNA) and protein synthesis and cell growth take place.[3,4] During the *S phase,* DNA synthesis occurs, giving rise to two separate sets of chromosomes, one for each daughter cell. G_2 (*gap 2*) is the premitotic phase and is similar to G_1 in that DNA synthesis ceases while RNA and protein synthesis continue. Collectively G_1, S, and G_2 are referred to as *interphase.* The *M phase* is the phase of nuclear division, or mitosis, and cytokinesis or cytoplasmic division. Continually dividing cells, such as the stratified squamous epithelium of the skin, continue to cycle from one mitotic division to the next. When environmental conditions are adverse, such as nutrient or growth factor unavailability, or when cells are highly specialized, cells may exit the cell cycle, becoming mitotically quiescent, and reside in a special resting state known as G_0. Cells in G_0 may reenter the cell cycle in response to extracellular nutrients, growth factors, hormones, and other signals such as blood loss or tissue injury that trigger cell renewal.[5] Highly specialized and terminally differentiated cells, such as neurons, may permanently stay in G_0.

Within the cell cycle are checkpoints where pauses or arrests can be made if the specific events in the phases of the cell cycle have not been completed. Mitosis is prevented until DNA is properly replicated. Chromosome separation in mitosis is delayed until all spindle fibers have properly attached to the chromosomes. There are also opportunities for ensuring the accuracy of DNA replication. These DNA damage checkpoints allow for any defects to be edited and repaired, thereby ensuring

Understanding • The Cell Cycle

A cell reproduces by performing an orderly sequence of events called the *cell cycle*. The cell cycle is divided into four phases of unequal duration that include the (1) synthesis (S) and mitosis (M) phases that are separated by (2) two gaps (G_1 and G_2). There is also (3) a dormant phase (G_0) during which the cell may leave the cell cycle. Movement through each of these phases is mediated at (4) specific checkpoints that are controlled by specific enzymes and proteins called *cyclins*.

❶ Synthesis and Mitosis

Synthesis (S) and mitosis (M) represent the two major phases of the cell cycle. The S phase, which takes about 10 to 12 hours, is the period of DNA synthesis and replication of the chromosomes. The M phase, which usually takes less than an hour, involves formation of the mitotic spindle and cell division with formation of two daughter cells.

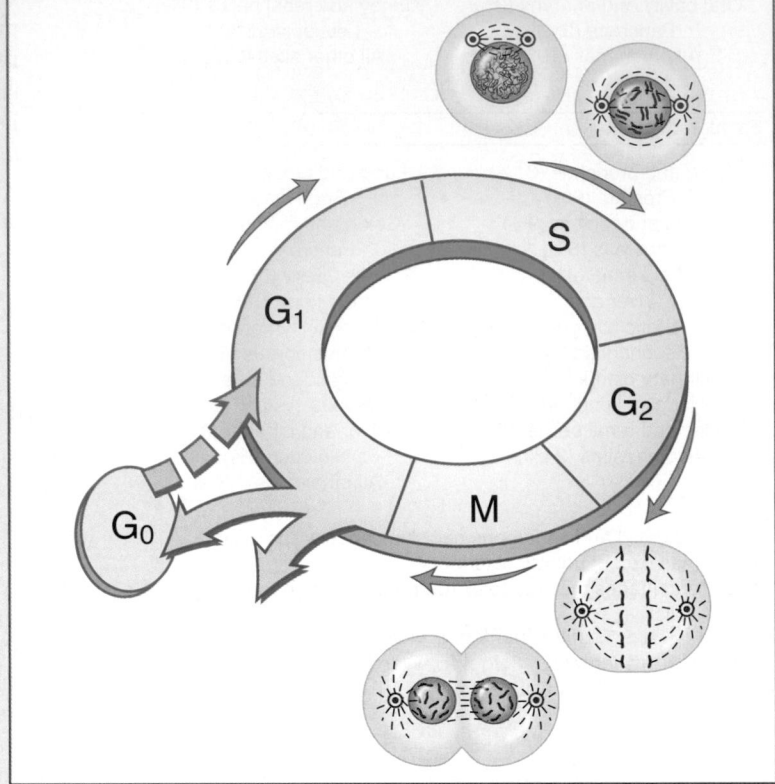

❷ Gaps 1 and 2

Because most cells require time to grow and double their mass of proteins and organelles, extra gaps (G) are inserted into the cell cycle. G_1 is the stage during which the cell is starting to prepare for DNA replication and mitosis through protein synthesis and an increase in organelle and cytoskeletal elements. G_2 is the premitotic phase. During this phase, enzymes and other proteins needed for cell division are synthesized and moved to their proper sites.

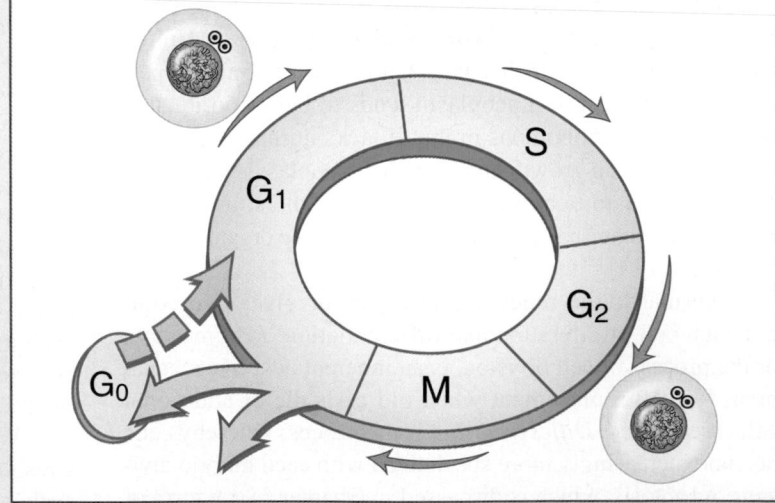

❸ Gap 0

G₀ is the stage after mitosis during which a cell may leave the cell cycle and either remain in a state of inactivity or reenter the cell cycle at another time. Labile cells, such as blood cells and those that line the gastrointestinal tract, do not enter G₀ but continue cycling. Stable cells, such as hepatocytes, enter G₀ after mitosis but can reenter the cell cycle when stimulated by the loss of other cells. Permanent cells, such as neurons that become terminally differentiated after mitosis, leave the cell cycle and are no longer capable of cell renewal.

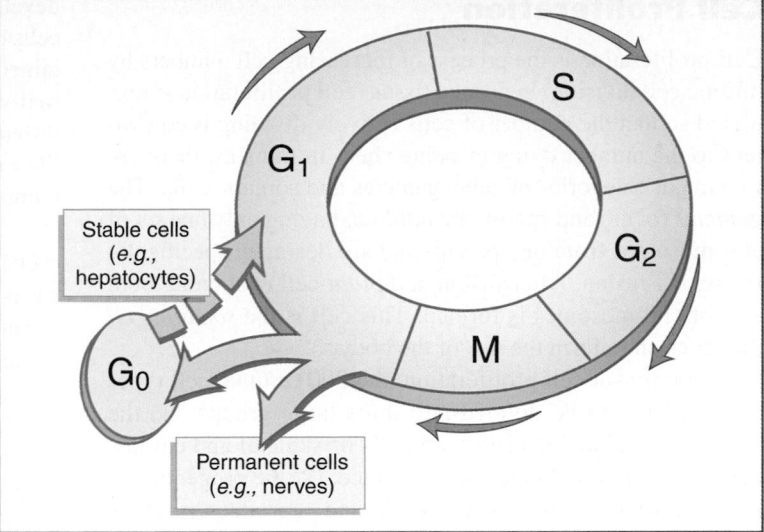

❹ Checkpoints and Cyclins

In most cells there are several checkpoints in the cell cycle, at which time the cycle can be arrested if previous events have not been completed. For example, the G₁/S checkpoint monitors whether the DNA in the chromosomes is damaged by radiation or chemicals, and the G₂/M checkpoint prevents entry into mitosis if DNA replication is not complete.

The cyclins are a family of proteins that control entry and progression of cells through the cell cycle. They function by activating proteins called *cyclin-dependent kinases* (CDKs). Different combinations of cyclins and CDKs are associated with each stage of the cell cycle. In addition to the synthesis and degradation of the cyclins, the cyclin-CDK complexes are regulated by the binding of CDK inhibitors. The CDK inhibitors are particularly important in regulating cell cycle checkpoints during which mistakes in DNA replication are repaired.

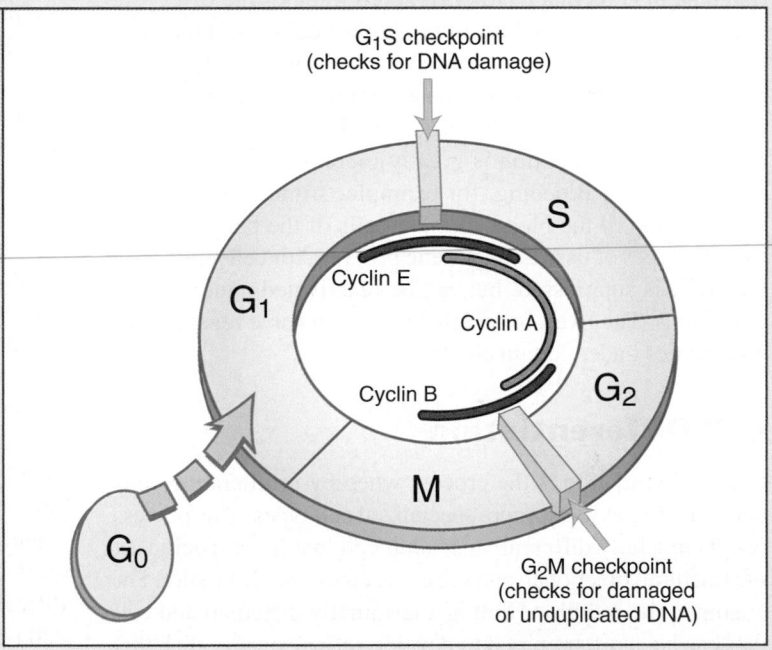

that each daughter cell receives a full complement of genetic information, identical to that of the parent cell.[3,4]

The cyclins are a family of proteins that control the entry and progression of cells through the cell cycle. Cyclins bind to (thereby activating) proteins called *cyclin-dependent kinases* (CDKs). Kinases are enzymes that phosphorylate proteins. The CDKs phosphorylate specific target proteins and are expressed continuously during the cell cycle but in an inactive form, whereas the cyclins are synthesized during specific phases of the cell cycle and then degraded by ubiquitation once their task is completed.[6] Different arrangements of cyclins and CDKs are associated with each stage of the cell cycle. For example, cyclin B and CDK1 control the transition from G₂ to M. As the cell moves into G₂, cyclin B is synthesized and binds to CDK1. The cyclin B–CDK1 complex then directs the events leading to mitosis, including DNA replication and assembly of the mitotic spindle. Although each phase of the cell cycle is monitored carefully, the transition from G₂ to M is believed to be one of the most important checkpoints in the cell cycle. In addition to the synthesis and degradation of the cyclins, the cyclin–CDK complexes are regulated by the binding of CDK inhibitors. The CDK inhibitors are particularly important in regulating cell cycle checkpoints during which mistakes in DNA replication are repaired. Manipulation of cyclins, CDKs, and CDK inhibitors serves as the basis for development of newer forms of drug therapy that can be used in cancer treatment.[7]

Cell Proliferation

Cell proliferation is the process of increasing cell numbers by mitotic cell division. In normal tissue, cell proliferation is regulated so that the number of cells actively dividing is equivalent to the number dying or being shed. In humans, there are two major categories of cells: gametes and somatic cells. The *gametes* (ovum and sperm) are *haploid,* having only one set of chromosomes from one parent, and are designed specifically for sexual fusion. After fusion, a *diploid* cell containing both sets of chromosomes is formed. This cell is the *somatic cell* that goes on to form the rest of the body.

In terms of cell proliferation, the 200 or more cell types of the body can be divided into three large groups: (1) the well-differentiated neurons and cells of skeletal and cardiac muscle that rarely divide and reproduce; (2) the progenitor or parent cells that continue to divide and reproduce, such as blood cells, skin cells, and liver cells; and (3) the undifferentiated stem cells that can be triggered to enter the cell cycle and produce large numbers of progenitor cells when the need arises. The rates of reproduction of cells vary greatly. White blood cells and cells that line the gastrointestinal tract live several days and must be replaced constantly. In most tissues, the rate of cell reproduction is greatly increased when tissue is injured or lost. Bleeding, for example, stimulates the rapid reproduction of the blood-forming cells of the bone marrow. In some types of tissue, the genetic program for cell replication normally is suppressed, but can be reactivated under certain conditions. The liver, for example, has extensive regenerative capabilities under certain conditions.

Cell Differentiation

Cell differentiation is the process whereby proliferating cells become progressively more specialized cell types. This process results in a fully differentiated, adult cell that has a specific set of structural, functional, and life expectancy characteristics. For example, the red blood cell is a terminally differentiated cell that has been programmed to develop into a concave disk that functions as a vehicle for oxygen transport and lives approximately 120 days.

All of the different cell types of the body originate from a single cell—the fertilized ovum. As the embryonic cells increase in number, they engage in an orderly and coordinated process of differentiation that is necessary for the development of all the various organs of the body. The process of differentiation is regulated by a combination of internal processes involving the expression of specific genes and external stimuli provided by neighboring cells, the extracellular matrix, exposure to substances in the maternal circulation, and growth factors, cytokines, oxygen, and nutrients.

What make the cells of one organ different from those of another organ are the specific genes that are expressed and the particular pattern of gene expression. Although all cells have the same complement of genes, only a small number of these genes are expressed in postnatal life. When cells, such as those of the developing embryo, differentiate and give rise to committed cells of a particular tissue type, the appropriate genes are maintained in an active state, while the rest remain inactive. Normally, the rate of cell reproduction and the process of cell differentiation are precisely controlled in prenatal and postnatal life so that both of these mechanisms cease once the appropriate numbers and types of cells are formed.

The process of differentiation occurs in orderly steps; with each progressive step, increased specialization is exchanged for a loss of ability to develop different cell characteristics and different cell types. As a cell becomes more highly specialized, the stimuli that are able to induce mitosis become more limited. Neurons, which are highly specialized cells, lose their ability to divide and reproduce once development of the nervous system is complete. More importantly, there are very few remaining precursor cells to direct their replacement. However, appropriate numbers of these cell types are generated in the embryo such that loss of a certain percentage of cells does not affect the total cell population and specific functions.

In some tissues, such as the skin and mucosal lining of the gastrointestinal tract, a high degree of cell renewal continues throughout life. Even in these continuously renewing cell populations, the more specialized cells are unable to divide. These cell populations rely on *progenitor* or *parent cells* of the same lineage that have not yet differentiated to the extent that they have lost their ability to divide. These cells are sufficiently differentiated so that their daughter cells are limited to the same cell line, but they are insufficiently differentiated to preclude the potential for active proliferation. However, their cell renewal properties are restricted by growth factors required for cell division.

Another type of cell, called a *stem cell,* remains incompletely differentiated throughout life. Stem cells are reserve cells that remain quiescent until there is a need for cell replenishment, in which case they divide, producing other stem cells and cells that can carry out the functions of the differentiated cell. When a stem cell divides, one daughter cell retains the stem cell characteristics, and the other daughter cell becomes a progenitor cell that proceeds through a process that leads to terminal differentiation (Fig. 8-2). The progeny of each progenitor cell follow more restricted genetic programs, with the differentiating cells undergoing multiple mitotic divisions in the process of becoming a mature cell type and with each generation of cells becoming more specialized. In this way, a single stem cell can give rise to the many cells needed for normal tissue repair or blood cell production. When the dividing cells become fully differentiated, the rate of mitotic division is reduced. In the immune system, for example, appropriately stimulated B lymphocytes become progressively more differentiated as they undergo successive mitotic divisions, until they become mature plasma cells that no longer can divide but are capable of secreting large amounts of antibody.

Stem cells have two important properties, that of self-renewal and potency. *Self-renewal* means that the stem cells

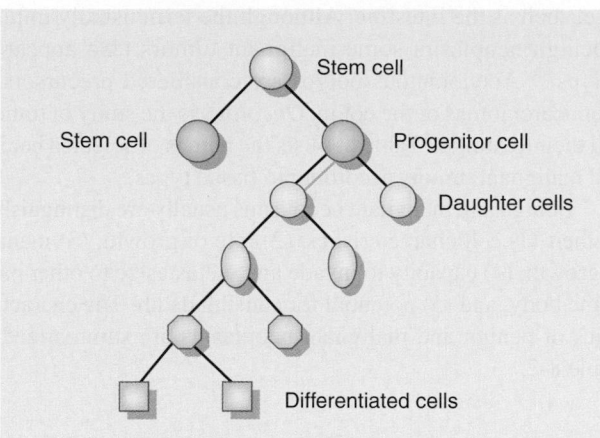

FIGURE 8-2 • Mechanism of stem cell–mediated cell replacement. Division of a stem cell with an unlimited potential for proliferation results in one daughter cell, which retains the characteristics of a stem cell, and a second daughter cell that differentiates into a progenitor or parent cell, with a limited potential for differentiation and proliferation. As the daughter cells of the progenitor cell proliferate they become more differentiated, until they reach the stage where they are fully differentiated.

can undergo numerous mitotic divisions while maintaining an undifferentiated state.[3] The term *potency* is used to define the differentiation potential of stem cells. *Totipotent stem cells* are those produced by fertilization of the egg. The first few cells produced after fertilization are totipotent and can differentiate into embryonic and extraembryonic cells. Totipotent stem cells give rise to *pluripotent stem cells* that can differentiate into the three germ layers of the embryo. *Multipotent stem cells* are cells such as hematopoietic stem cells that give rise to only a few cell types. Finally, *unipotent stem cells* produce only one cell type but retain the property of self-renewal.

It has become useful to categorize stem cells into two basic categories: embryonic stem cells and adult stem cells (sometimes called *somatic stem cells*).[3] *Embryonic stem cells* are pluripotent cells derived from the inner cell mass of the blastocyst stage of the embryo. These give rise to the three embryonic germ cell layers. As development progresses, the embryo forms germline stem cells for reproduction and somatic stem cells for organogenesis. Both the germline stem cells and the somatic stem cells retain the property of self-renewal. *Adult stem cells* reside in specialized microenvironments that differ depending on tissue type. These stem cells have important roles in homeostasis as they contribute to tissue regeneration and replacement of cells lost to cell death.[8]

Recently, an important role of stem cells in the pathogenesis of cancer was identified, and it continues to be elucidated. Cancer stem cells (called *tumor-initiating cells* [T-ICs]) have been identified in breast, prostate, acute myeloid leukemia, and other cancers. T-ICs constitute less than 2% of cells in breast tumors and 0.1% of cells in acute leukemia.[3] To maintain their self-renewing properties, these stem cells express cell cycle inhibitors. There is also strong experimental support for the notion that, in certain cancers, cancer stem cells are the initial target for malignant transformation. If confirmed, these findings could have important implications for cancer treatment aimed at the elimination of proliferating cells.

IN SUMMARY, the term *neoplasm* refers to an abnormal mass of tissue in which the growth exceeds and is uncoordinated with that of the normal tissues. Unlike normal cellular adaptive processes such as hypertrophy and hyperplasia, neoplasms do not obey the laws of normal cell growth. They serve no useful purpose, they do not occur in response to an appropriate stimulus, and they continue to grow at the expense of the host.

The process of cell growth and division is called the *cell cycle.* It is divided into four phases: G_1, the postmitotic phase, during which DNA synthesis ceases while RNA and protein synthesis and cell growth take place; S, the phase during which DNA synthesis occurs, giving rise to two separate sets of chromosomes; G_2, the premitotic phase, during which RNA and protein synthesis continues; and M, the phase of cell mitosis or cell division. The G_0 phase is a resting or quiescent phase in which nondividing cells reside. The entry into and progression through the various stages of the cell cycle are controlled by cyclins, cyclin-dependent kinases, and cyclin-dependent kinase inhibitors.

Normal tissue renewal and repair involves cell proliferation, differentiation, and apoptosis. Proliferation, or the process of cell division, is an inherent adaptive mechanism for cell replacement when old cells die or additional cells are needed. Differentiation is the process of specialization whereby new cells acquire the structure and function of the cells they replace. Apoptosis is a form of programmed cell death that eliminates senescent cells, cells with damaged DNA, or unwanted cells. Body cells can be divided into two large groups: the well-differentiated neurons and cells of skeletal and cardiac muscle that rarely divide and reproduce, and the progenitor or parent cells that continue to divide and reproduce, such as blood cells, skin cells, and liver cells.

A third category of cells are the stem cells that remain quiescent until there is a need for cell replenishment, in which case they divide, producing other stem cells and cells that can carry out the functions of differentiated cells. Stem cells have two important properties, those of self-renewal and potency. Self-renewal means that the stem cells can undergo numerous mitotic divisions while maintaining an undifferentiated state. The term *potency* is used to define the differentiation potential of stem cells. There are two main categories of stem cells. Embryonic stem cells are pluripotent cells derived from the inner cell mass of the blastocyst stage of the embryo. Adult stem cells reside in specialized microenvironments and have important roles in homeostasis as they contribute to tissue regeneration and replacement of cells lost to apoptosis. Recently, cancer stem cells were identified in breast, prostate, acute myeloid leukemia, and other cancers. ■

CONCEPTSin action **ANIMATI** ⬤ **N**

CHARACTERISTICS OF BENIGN AND MALIGNANT NEOPLASMS

After completing this section of the chapter, you should be able to meet the following objectives:

- Cite the method used for naming benign and malignant neoplasms.
- State at least five ways in which benign and malignant neoplasms differ.
- Relate the properties of cell differentiation to the development of a cancer cell clone and the behavior of the tumor.
- Trace the pathway for hematologic spread of a metastatic cancer cell.
- Use the concepts of growth fraction and doubling time to explain the growth of cancerous tissue.

Body organs are composed of two types of tissue: parenchymal tissue and stromal or supporting tissue. The *parenchymal tissue cells* represent the functional components of an organ. The parenchymal cells of a tumor determine its behavior and are the component for which a tumor is named. The *supporting tissue* includes the extracellular matrix and connective tissue that surround the parenchymal cells. It contains the lymphatic vessels and blood vessels that provide nourishment and support for the parenchymal cells.

Terminology

Traditionally, by definition a *tumor* is a swelling that can be caused by a number of conditions, including inflammation and trauma, but more recently the term has been used to define a mass of cells that arises because of overgrowth. Although not synonymous, the terms *tumor* and *neoplasm* often are used interchangeably. Neoplasms usually are classified as benign or malignant. Neoplasms that contain well-differentiated cells that are clustered together in a single mass are considered to be *benign.* These tumors usually do not cause death unless their location or size interferes with vital functions. In contrast, malignant neoplasms are less well differentiated and have the ability to break loose, enter the circulatory or lymphatic system, and form secondary malignant tumors at other sites. *Malignant neoplasms* frequently cause suffering and death if untreated or uncontrolled.

Tumors usually are named by adding the suffix *-oma* to the parenchymal tissue type from which the growth originated.[3,9] Thus, a benign tumor of glandular epithelial tissue is called an *adenoma,* and a benign tumor of bone tissue is called an *osteoma.* The term *carcinoma* is used to designate a malignant tumor of epithelial tissue origin. In the case of a malignant tumor of glandular epithelial tissue, the term *adenocarcinoma* is used. Malignant tumors of mesenchymal origin are called *sarcomas* (*e.g.,* osteosarcoma). *Papillomas* are benign, microscopic or macroscopic finger-like projections that grow on any surface. A *polyp* is a growth that projects from a mucosal surface, such as the intestine. Although the term usually implies a benign neoplasm, some malignant tumors also appear as polyps.[3,9] Adenomatous polyps are considered precursors to adenocarcinomas of the colon. *Oncology* is the study of tumors and their treatment. Table 8-1 lists the names of selected benign and malignant tumors according to tissue types.

Benign and malignant neoplasms usually are distinguished by their (1) cell characteristics, (2) rate of growth, (3) manner of growth, (4) capacity to invade and metastasize to other parts of the body, and (5) potential for causing death. The characteristics of benign and malignant neoplasms are summarized in Table 8-2.

BENIGN AND MALIGNANT NEOPLASMS

- A neoplasm, benign or malignant, represents a new growth.
- Benign neoplasms are well-differentiated tumors that resemble the tissues of origin but have lost the ability to control cell proliferation. They grow by expansion, are enclosed in a fibrous capsule, and do not cause death unless their location is such that it interrupts vital body functions.
- Malignant neoplasms are less well-differentiated tumors that have lost the ability to control both cell proliferation and differentiation. They grow in a disorganized and uncontrolled manner to invade surrounding tissues, have cells that break loose and travel to distant sites to form metastases, and inevitably cause suffering and death unless their growth can be controlled through treatment.

Benign Neoplasms

Benign tumors are composed of well-differentiated cells that resemble the cells of the tissues of origin and are characterized by a slow, progressive rate of growth that may come to a standstill or regress. For unknown reasons, benign tumors have lost the ability to suppress the genetic program for cell proliferation but have retained the program for normal cell differentiation. They grow by expansion and remain localized to their site of origin, lacking the capacity to infiltrate, invade, or metastasize to distant sites. Because they expand slowly, they develop a surrounding rim of compressed connective tissue called a *fibrous capsule.*[3] The capsule is responsible for a sharp line of demarcation between the benign tumor and the adjacent tissues, a factor that facilitates surgical removal.

Benign tumors are usually much less of a threat to health and well-being than malignant tumors, and they usually do not cause death unless they interfere with vital functions because of their location. For instance, a benign tumor growing in the cranial cavity can eventually cause death by compressing brain

TABLE 8-1 Names of Selected Benign and Malignant Tumors According to Tissue Types

TISSUE TYPE	BENIGN TUMORS	MALIGNANT TUMORS
Epithelial		
Surface	Papilloma	Squamous cell carcinoma
Glandular	Adenoma	Adenocarcinoma
Connective		
Fibrous	Fibroma	Fibrosarcoma
Adipose	Lipoma	Liposarcoma
Cartilage	Chondroma	Chondrosarcoma
Bone	Osteoma	Osteosarcoma
Blood vessels	Hemangioma	Hemangiosarcoma
Lymph vessels	Lymphangioma	Lymphangiosarcoma
Lymph tissue		Lymphosarcoma
Muscle		
Smooth	Leiomyoma	Leiomyosarcoma
Striated	Rhabdomyoma	Rhabdomyosarcoma
Neural Tissue		
Nerve cell	Neuroma	Neuroblastoma
Glial tissue	Glioma	Glioblastoma, astrocytoma, medullo-blastoma, oligodendroglioma
Nerve sheaths	Neurilemmoma	Neurilemmal sarcoma
Meninges	Meningioma	Meningeal sarcoma
Hematologic		
Granulocytic		Myelocytic leukemia
Erythrocytic		Erythrocytic leukemia
Plasma cells		Multiple myeloma
Lymphocytic		Lymphocytic leukemia or lymphoma
Monocytic		Monocytic leukemia
Endothelial Tissue		
Blood vessels	Hemangioma	Hemangiosarcoma
Lymph vessels	Lymphangioma	Lymphangiosarcoma

structures. Benign tumors also can cause disturbances in the function of adjacent or distant structures by producing pressure on tissues, blood vessels, or nerves. Some benign tumors are also known for their ability to cause alterations in body function by abnormally producing hormones.

Malignant Neoplasms

Malignant neoplasms, which invade and destroy nearby tissue and spread to other parts of the body, tend to grow rapidly and spread widely, and have the potential to cause death. Because

TABLE 8-2 Characteristics of Benign and Malignant Neoplasms

CHARACTERISTICS	BENIGN	MALIGNANT
Cell characteristics	Well-differentiated cells that resemble cells in the tissue of origin	Cells are undifferentiated, with anaplasia and atypical structure that often bears little resemblance to cells in the tissue of origin
Rate of growth	Usually progressive and slow; may come to a standstill or regress	Variable and depends on level of differentiation; the more undifferentiated the cells, the more rapid the rate of growth
Mode of growth	Grows by expansion without invading the surrounding tissues; usually encapsulated	Grows by invasion, sending out processes that infiltrate the surrounding tissues
Metastasis	Does not spread by metastasis	Gains access to blood and lymph channels to metastasize to other areas of the body

of their rapid rate of growth, malignant tumors may compress blood vessels and outgrow their blood supply, causing ischemia and tissue injury. Some malignancies secrete hormones or cytokines, liberate enzymes and toxins, or induce an inflammatory response that injures normal tissue as well as the tumor itself. A number of malignancies secrete vascular endothelial cell growth factor (VEGF), which increases the blood supply to the tumor and facilitates more rapid growth.

There are two categories of malignant neoplasms—solid tumors and hematologic cancers. Solid tumors initially are confined to a specific tissue or organ. As the growth of the primary solid tumor progresses, cells detach from the original tumor mass, invade the surrounding tissue, and enter the blood and lymph systems to spread to distant sites, a process termed *metastasis*. Hematologic cancers involve cells normally found in the blood and lymph, thereby making them disseminated diseases from the beginning.

Carcinoma in situ is a localized preinvasive lesion. As an example, in breast ductal carcinoma in situ, the cells have not crossed the basement membrane. Depending on its location, in situ lesions usually can be removed surgically or treated so that the chances of recurrence are small. For example, carcinoma in situ of the cervix is essentially 100% curable.

Cancer Cell Characteristics

Cancer cells are characterized by two main features: (1) abnormal and rapid proliferation; and (2) loss of differentiation so that they do not exhibit normal features and properties of differentiated cells, and hence are more similar to embryonic cells.

The term *anaplasia* describes the loss of cell differentiation in cancerous tissue.[3,9] Undifferentiated cancer cells are marked by a number of morphologic changes. Both the cells and nuclei display variations in size and shape, a condition referred to as *pleomorphism*. Their nuclei are variable in size and bizarre in shape, their chromatin is coarse and clumped, and their nucleoli are often considerably larger than normal (Fig. 8-3A). Frequently, the nuclei contain an abnormal number of chromosomes (aneuploidy). The cells of undifferentiated tumors usually display greater numbers of cells in mitosis due to their high rate of proliferation. They also display atypical, bizarre mitotic figures, sometimes producing tripolar, tetrapolar, or multipolar spindles (Fig. 8-3B). Highly anaplastic cancer cells, whatever their tissue of origin, begin to resemble undifferentiated or embryonic cells more than they do their tissue of origin. Some cancers display only slight anaplasia, whereas others display marked anaplasia. The cytologic/histologic grading of tumors is based on the degree of differentiation and the number of proliferating cells. The closer the tumor cells resemble comparable normal tissue cells, both morphologically and functionally, the lower the grade. Accordingly, on a scale ranging from grades I to IV, grade I neoplasms are well differentiated and grade IV are poorly differentiated and display marked anaplasia.[3]

The characteristics of altered proliferation and differentiation are associated with a number of other changes in cell

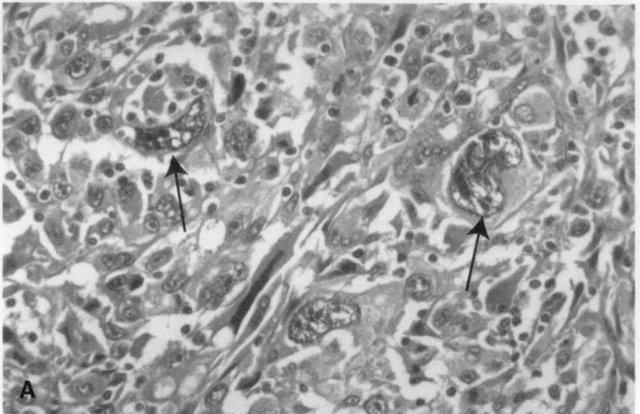

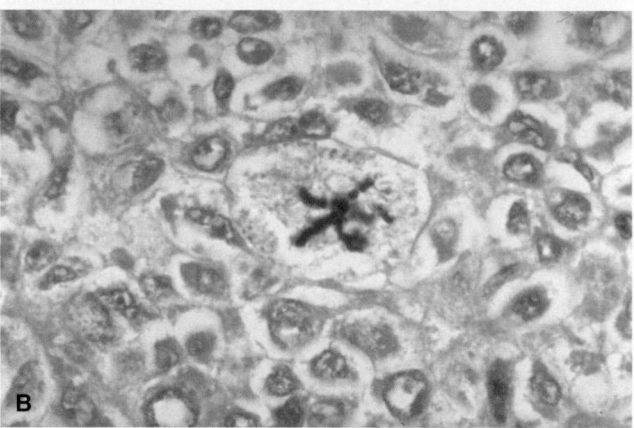

FIGURE 8-3 • Anaplastic features of malignant tumors. **(A)** The cells of this anaplastic carcinoma are highly pleomorphic (*i.e.,* they vary in size and shape). The nuclei are hyperchromatic and are large relative to the cytoplasm. Multinucleated tumor giant cells are present (*arrows*). **(B)** A malignant cell in metaphase exhibits an abnormal mitotic figure. (From Giordano A., De Falco G., Rubin E., et al. [2008]. Neoplasia. In Rubin R., Strayer D. S. [Eds.], *Rubin's pathology: Clinicopathologic foundations of medicine* (5th ed., p. 141). Philadelphia: Lippincott Williams & Wilkins.)

characteristics and function that distinguish cancer cells from their normally differentiated counterparts. These changes, which are listed in Table 8-3, include (1) genetic instability; (2) growth factor independence; (3) loss of cell density–dependent inhibition; (4) loss of cohesiveness and adhesion; (5) loss of anchorage dependence; (6) faulty cell-to-cell communication; (7) indefinite cell life span (immortality); (8) expression of altered tissue antigens; (9) abnormal secretion of degradative enzymes that enable invasion and metastatic spread, or ectopic production of hormones, and (10) abnormal cytoskeletal characteristics.

Genetic Instability. Most cancer cells exhibit a characteristic called *genetic instability* that is often considered to be a hallmark of cancer. The concept arose after the realization that uncorrected mutations in normal cells are rare because of the numerous cellular mechanisms to prevent them. To account for the high frequency of mutations in cancer cells, it is thought that cancer cells have a "mutation phenotype" with genetic

TABLE 8-3 Comparison of Normal Cell Characteristics With Those of Cancer Cells

CHARACTERISTIC	NORMAL CELLS	CANCER CELLS
Growth	Regulated	Unregulated
Differentiation	High	Low
Genetic stability	Stable	Unstable
Growth factor dependence	Dependent	Independent
Density-dependent inhibition	High	Low
Cell-to-cell adhesion	High	Low
Anchorage dependence	High	Low
Cell-to-cell communication	High	Low
Cell life span	Limited	Unlimited
Antigen expression	Absent	May be present
Substance production (e.g., proteases, hormones)	Normal	Abnormal
Cytoskeletal composition and arrangement	Normal	Abnormal

instability that contributes to the development and progression of cancer.[10] Characteristics of genetic instability include aneuploidy, in which chromosomes are lost or gained; intrachromosomal instability, which includes insertions, deletions, and amplifications; microsatellite instability, which involves short, repetitive sequences of DNA; and point mutations.

Growth Factor Independence. Another characteristic of cancer cells is the ability to proliferate even in the absence of growth factors. This characteristic is often observed when cancer cells are propagated in cell culture—the addition of serum, which is rich in growth factors, is unnecessary for the cancers to proliferate. Normal cells grown in culture often die without serum or growth factor addition. In some cases, this is because the cancer cells can rapidly divide without growth factor binding to its receptor. Breast cancer cells that do not express estrogen receptors are an example. These cancer cells grow even in the absence of estrogen, which is the normal growth stimulus for breast duct epithelial cells. Some cancer cells may produce their own growth factors and secrete them into the culture medium, whereas others have abnormal receptors or signaling proteins that may inappropriately activate growth signaling pathways in the cells.

Cell Density–Dependent Inhibition. Cancer cells often lose *cell density–dependent inhibition,* which is the cessation of growth after cells reach a particular density. This is sometimes referred to as *contact inhibition* because cells often stop growing when they come into contact with each other. In wound healing, contact inhibition causes tissue growth to

cease at the point where the edges of the wound come together. Cancer cells, however, tend to grow rampantly without regard for adjacent tissue. Possible explanations for cancer cell loss of density–dependent contact inhibition include growth factor independence, oxidative mechanisms,[11] and alterations in interactions between cell adhesion and cell growth signaling pathways (*e.g.,* surface integrin receptors, mitogen-activated protein [MAP] kinase, and focal adhesion kinase [FAK] phosphorylation).[12]

Cell Cohesiveness and Adhesion. The reduced tendency of cancer cells to stick together (*i.e.,* loss of cohesiveness and adhesiveness) permits shedding of the tumor's surface cells; these cells appear in the surrounding body fluids or secretions and often can be detected using cytologic methods. As discussed in Chapter 4, cadherins are adhesion molecules that link one cell with adjacent cells. Extracellularly, the cadherins of one cell bind to cadherins of adjacent cells, causing cell-to-cell attachment. Intracellularly, cadherins are connected to the actin cytoskeleton through protein intermediates, including the catenins. The cadherin–catenin–actin complex, acting with other proteins, has been proposed to be involved with cell migration, apoptosis, and cell cycle regulation. In some cancers, the cell adhesion molecule E-cadherin appears to play an important role in the lack of cohesiveness of cancer cells and the increased tendency for cancer cells to break free and migrate into the surrounding tissues. E-cadherin is reduced at the cell surface, whereas its partner protein β-catenin accumulates within the cancer cells and associates with the actin cytoskeletal-binding protein actinin-4. It has been postulated that the resulting β-catenin interaction with actinin-4 in the absence of E-cadherin may be the "switch" that shuts off cancer cell-to-cell adhesion and activates cancer cell motility and other mechanisms that facilitate invasion and metastasis.[13]

Anchorage Dependence. Cancer cells also differ from their normal counterparts in attaining anchorage independence. Normal epithelial cells must be anchored to either neighboring cells or the underlying extracellular matrix to live and grow. If normal cells become detached, they often undergo a type of apoptosis known as *anoikis,* a term from the Greek for "homeless." Normal epithelial cells must be attached to either other cells or extracellular matrix to stay alive. Cancer cells, however, frequently remain viable and multiply without normal attachments to other cells and the extracellular matrix. Cancer cells often survive in microenvironments different from those of normal cells. Although the process of anchorage independence is complex and incompletely understood, recent studies have made progress in understanding the genes and mechanistic pathways involved.[14]

Cell-to-Cell Communication. Another characteristic of cancer cells is faulty cell-to-cell communication, a feature that may in turn contribute to other characteristics of cancer cells. Impaired cell-to-cell communication may interfere with formation of intercellular connections and responsiveness to membrane-derived signals. For example, changes in gap junction proteins, which enable cytoplasmic continuity and communication between cells, have been described in some types of cancer.[15]

Life Span. Cancer cells differ from normal cells by being *immortal,* with an unlimited life span. If normal, noncancerous cells are harvested from the body and grown under culture conditions, most cells divide a limited number of times, usually about 50 population doublings, then become senescent and fail to divide further. In contrast to the limited life span of normal cells, cancer cells may divide an infinite number of times, hence achieving immortality. Telomeres are short, repetitive nucleotide sequences at outermost extremities of chromosome arms (see Chapter 3). Telomeres shorten with each cell division. When length is diminished sufficiently, chromosomes can no longer replicate, and cell division will not occur. Most cancer cells maintain high levels of telomerase, an enzyme that prevents telomere shortening; this keeps telomeres from aging and attaining the critically short length that is associated with cellular replicative senescence.

Antigen Expression. Cancer cells also express a number of cell surface molecules or antigens that are immunologically identified as foreign. These *tissue antigens* are coded by the genes of a cell. Many transformed cancer cells revert to embryonic patterns of gene expression and produce antigens that are immunologically distinct from the antigens that are expressed by cells of the well-differentiated tissue from which the cancer originated. Some cancers express fetal antigens that are not produced by comparable cells in the adult. Tumor antigens may be clinically useful as markers to indicate the presence, recurrence, or progressive growth of a cancer (to be discussed).

Production of Enzymes, Hormones, and Other Substances. Cancer cells may produce substances that normal cells of the tissue of origin either do not produce or secrete in lesser amounts. They may also secrete degradative enzymes that enable invasion and metastatic spread. Cancer cells may also assume hormone synthesis or production and secretion of procoagulant substances that affect clotting mechanisms.

Cytoskeletal Changes. Finally, cancer cells may show cytoskeletal changes and abnormalities. These may involve the appearance of abnormal intermediate filament types or changes in actin filaments and microtubules that facilitate invasion and metastasis. Actin, microtubules, and their regulatory proteins remain the focus of many cancer-related investigations.

Invasion and Metastasis

Unlike benign tumors, which grow by expansion and usually are surrounded by a capsule, cancer spreads by direct invasion and extension, seeding of cancer cells in body cavities, and metastatic spread through the blood or lymph pathways. The word *cancer* is derived from the Latin word meaning "crablike" because cancers grow and spread by sending crablike projections into the surrounding tissues. Most cancers synthe-

size and secrete enzymes that break down proteins and contribute to the infiltration, invasion, and penetration of the surrounding tissues. The lack of a sharp line of demarcation separating them from the surrounding tissue makes the complete surgical removal of malignant tumors more difficult than removal of benign tumors. Often it is necessary for the surgeon to excise portions of seemingly normal tissue bordering the tumor for the pathologist to establish that cancer-free margins are present around the excised tumor and to ensure that the remaining tissue is cancer free.

The *seeding* of cancer cells into body cavities occurs when a tumor sheds cells into these spaces. Most often, the peritoneal cavity is involved, but other spaces such as the pleural cavity, pericardial cavity, and joint spaces may be involved. Seeding into the peritoneal cavity is particularly common with ovarian cancers. Similar to tissue culture, tumors in these sites grow in masses and are often associated with fluid accumulation (*e.g.,* ascites, pleural effusion).[9] The seeding of cancers is often a concern during the surgical removal of cancers where it is possible inadvertently to introduce free cancer cells into a body cavity such as the peritoneal cavity.[16]

The term *metastasis* is used to describe the development of a secondary tumor in a location distant from the primary tumor.[3,9,17] Because metastatic tumors frequently retain many of the characteristics of the primary tumor from which they were derived, it usually is possible to determine the site of the primary tumor from the cellular characteristics of the metastatic tumor. Some tumors tend to metastasize early in their developmental course, whereas others do not metastasize until later. Occasionally, a metastatic tumor will be found far advanced before the primary tumor becomes clinically detectable. Malignant tumors of the kidney, for example, may go completely undetected and be asymptomatic until a metastatic lesion is found in the lung.

Metastasis occurs through the lymph channels (*i.e.,* lymphatic spread) and the blood vessels (*i.e.,* hematogenic spread).[3,17] In many types of cancer, the first evidence of disseminated disease is the presence of tumor cells in the lymph nodes that drain the tumor area. When metastasis occurs by the lymphatic route, the tumor cells lodge first in the initial lymph node that receives drainage from the tumor site. Once in this lymph node, the cells may die because of the lack of a proper environment, grow into a discernible mass, or remain dormant for unknown reasons. If they survive and grow, the cancer cells may spread from more distant lymph nodes to the thoracic duct, and then gain access to the vasculature. Cancer cells also may gain access to the vasculature from the initial node and more distant lymph nodes through tumor-associated blood vessels infiltrating the tumor mass.[18]

The term *sentinel node* is used to describe the initial lymph node to which the primary tumor drains.[19] Because the initial metastasis in breast cancer is almost always lymphatic, lymphatic spread and therefore extent of disease may be determined through lymphatic mapping and sentinel lymph node biopsy. This is done by injecting a radioactive tracer and/or blue dye into the tumor to determine the first lymph node in the route of lymph drainage from the cancer. Once the sentinel lymph node has been identified, it is examined to determine the presence or absence of cancer cells. The procedure is also used to map the spread of melanoma and other cancers that have their initial metastatic spread through the lymphatic system.

With hematologic spread, the blood-borne cancer cells may enter the venous flow that drains the site of the primary neoplasm. Cancer cells may also enter tumor-associated blood vessels that either infiltrate the tumor or are found at the periphery of the tumor. Before entering the general circulation, venous blood from the gastrointestinal tract, pancreas, and spleen is routed through the portal vein to the liver. The liver is therefore a common site for metastatic spread of cancers that originate in these organs. Although the site of hematologic spread usually is related to vascular drainage of the primary tumor, some tumors metastasize to distant and unrelated sites. One explanation is that cells of different tumors tend to metastasize to specific target organs that provide suitable microenvironments containing substances such as cytokines or growth factors that are needed for their survival.[3] For example, transferrin, a growth-promoting substance isolated from lung tissue, has been found to stimulate the growth of malignant cells that typically metastasize to the lungs. Other organs that are preferential sites for metastasis contain particular cytokines, growth factors, and other microenvironmental characteristics that facilitate metastatic tumor survival and growth.

The selective nature of hematologic spread indicates that metastasis is a finely orchestrated, multistep process, and only a small, select clone of cancer cells has the right combination of gene products to perform all of the steps needed for establishment of a secondary tumor (Fig. 8-4). It has been estimated that fewer than 1 in 10,000 tumor cells that leave a primary tumor survives to start a secondary tumor.[20] To metastasize, a cancer cell must be able to break loose from the primary tumor, invade the surrounding extracellular matrix, gain access to a blood vessel, survive its passage in the bloodstream, emerge from the bloodstream at a favorable location, invade the surrounding tissue, begin to grow, and establish a blood supply. However, there is also growing evidence for the significant role of the tumor microenvironment—which includes but is not limited to the extracellular matrix, myoepithelial cells, endothelial cells, and macrophages—in enabling cancer cells to establish metastatic sites.[21]

Considerable evidence suggests that cancer cells capable of metastasis secrete enzymes that break down the surrounding extracellular matrix, allowing them to move through the degraded matrix and gain access to a blood vessel. Once in the circulation, the tumor cells are vulnerable to destruction by host immune cells. Some tumor cells gain protection from the antitumor host cells by aggregating and adhering to circulating blood components, particularly platelets, to form tumor emboli. Tumor cells that survive their travel in the circulation must be able to halt their passage by adhering to the vessel wall. Tumor cells express various cell surface attachment factors such as laminin receptors that facilitate their anchoring to laminin in the basement membrane. After attachment, the tumor cells secrete proteolytic enzymes such as type IV collagenase that degrade the basement membrane and facilitate the migration of the tumor cells through the capillary membrane into the interstitial area, where they subsequently establish growth of a secondary tumor.

Once in the distant tissue site, the process of metastatic tumor development depends on the establishment of blood vessels and specific growth factors that promote proliferation of the tumor cells. Tumor cells as well as other cells in the microenvironment secrete factors that enable the development of new blood vessels within the tumor, a process termed *angiogenesis*.[17] The presence of stimulatory or inhibitor growth factors correlates with the site-specific pattern of metastasis. For example, a potent growth-stimulating factor has been isolated from lung tissue, and stromal cells in bone have been shown to produce a factor that stimulates growth of prostatic cancer cells.[17]

Tumor Growth

Once cells have an adequate blood supply, the rate of tissue growth in normal and cancerous tissue depends on three factors: (1) the number of cells that are actively dividing or moving through the cell cycle, (2) the duration of the cell cycle, and (3) the number of cells that are being lost relative to the number of new cells being produced. One of the reasons cancerous tumors often seem to grow so rapidly relates to the size of the cell pool that is actively engaged in cycling. It has been shown that the cell cycle time of cancerous tissue cells is not necessarily shorter than that of normal cells. Rather, cancer cells do not die on schedule and growth factors prevent cells from exiting the cycle cell and entering the G_0 phase. Thus, a greater percentage of cells are actively engaged in cycling than occurs in normal tissue.

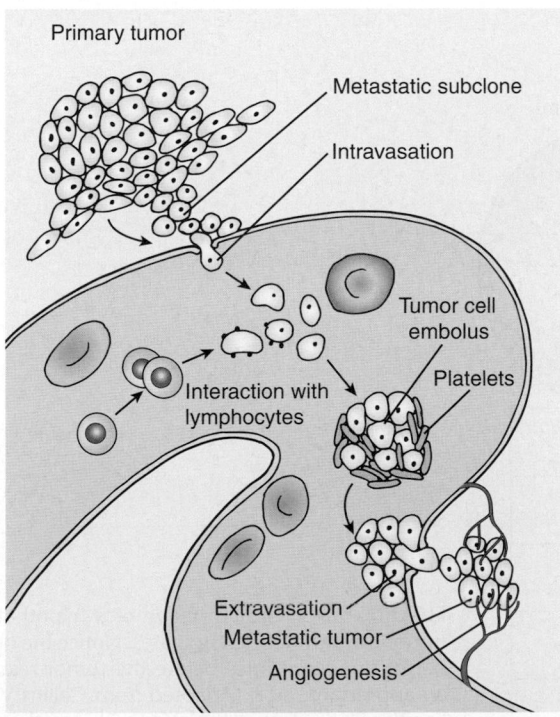

FIGURE 8-4 • The pathogenesis of metastasis. (Adapted from Kumar V., Abbas A. K., Fausto N. [Eds.]. [2005]. *Robbins and Cotran pathologic basis of disease* [7th ed., p. 311]. Philadelphia: Elsevier Saunders.)

The ratio of dividing cells to resting cells in a tissue mass is called the *growth fraction*. The *doubling time* is the length of time it takes for the total mass of cells in a tumor to double. As the growth fraction increases, the doubling time decreases. When normal tissues reach their adult size, equilibrium between cell birth and cell death is reached. Cancer cells, however, continue to divide until limitations in blood supply and nutrients inhibit their growth. When this happens, the doubling time for cancer cells decreases. If tumor growth is plotted against time on a semilogarithmic scale, the initial growth rate is exponential and then tends to decrease or flatten out over time. This characterization of tumor growth is called the *Gompertzian model.*[22]

By conventional radiographic methods, a tumor usually is undetectable until it has doubled 30 times and contains more than 1 billion (10^9) cells. At this point, it is approximately 1 cm in size (Fig. 8-5). Methods to identify tumors at smaller sizes are under investigation; in some cases, the application of ultrasonography and magnetic resonance imaging (MRI) enable detection of tumors smaller than 1 cm. After 35 doublings, the mass contains more than 1 trillion (10^{12}) cells, which is a sufficient number to kill the host.

IN SUMMARY, neoplasms may be either benign or malignant. Benign and malignant tumors differ in terms of cell characteristics, manner of growth, rate of growth, potential for metastasis, ability to produce generalized effects, tendency to cause tissue destruction, and capacity to cause death. The growth of a benign tumor is restricted to the site of origin, and the tumor

usually does not cause death unless it interferes with vital functions. Malignant neoplasms grow in a poorly controlled fashion that lacks normal organization, spreads to distant parts of the body, and causes death unless tumor growth and metastasis are inhibited or stopped by treatment. There are two basic types of cancer: solid tumors and hematologic tumors. In solid tumors, the primary tumor is initially confined to a specific organ or tissue, whereas hematologic cancers are disseminated from the onset.

Cancer is a disorder of cell proliferation and differentiation. The term *anaplasia* is used to describe the loss of cell differentiation in cancerous tissue. Undifferentiated cancer cells are marked by a number of morphologic changes, including variations in size and shape, a condition referred to a *pleomorphism*. The characteristics of altered proliferation and differentiation are associated with a number of other changes in cell characteristics and cell function, including genetic instability; growth factor independence; loss of cell density–dependent inhibition, cohesiveness and adhesion, and anchorage dependence; faulty cell-to-cell communication; indefinite cell life span (immortality); expression of altered tissue antigens; abnormal secretion of degradative enzymes that enable invasion and metastatic spread, or ectopic production of hormones; and abnormal cytoskeletal characteristics.

The spread of cancer occurs through three pathways: direct invasion and extension, seeding of cancer cells in body cavities, and metastatic spread through vascular or lymphatic pathways. Only a proportionately small clone of cancer cells is capable of metastasis. To metastasize, a cancer cell must be able to break loose from the primary tumor, invade the surrounding extracellular matrix, gain access to a blood vessel, survive its pas-

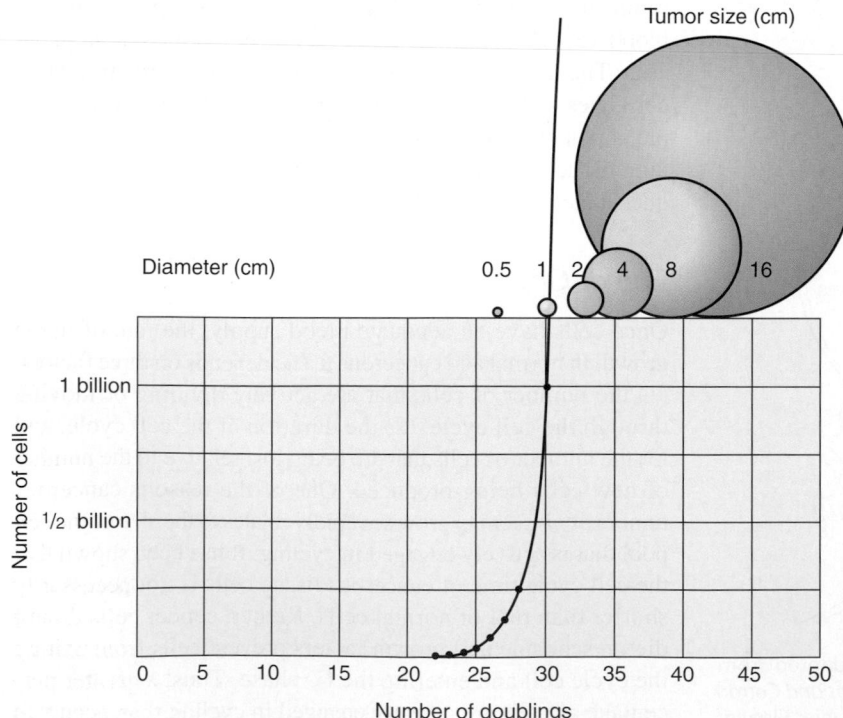

FIGURE 8-5 • Growth curve of a hypothetical tumor on arithmetic coordinates. Notice the number of doubling times before the tumor reaches an appreciable size. (Adapted from Collins V. P., Loeffler R. K., Tivey H. [1956]. Observations of growth rates of human tumors. *American Journal of Roentgenology, Radium Therapy and Nuclear Medicine* 76, 988.)

sage in the bloodstream, emerge from the bloodstream at a favorable location, invade the surrounding tissue, and begin to grow. The rate of growth of cancerous tissue depends on the ratio of dividing to resting cells (growth fraction) and the time it takes for the total cells in the tumor to double (doubling time). A tumor is usually undetectable until it has doubled 30 times and contains more than 1 billion cells. ■

ETIOLOGY OF CANCER

After completing this section of the chapter, you should be able to meet the following objectives:

- Describe various types of cancer-associated genes and cancer-associated cellular and molecular pathways.
- Describe genetic events and epigenetic factors that are important in tumorigenesis.
- State the importance of cancer stem cells, angiogenesis, and the cell microenvironment in cancer growth and metastasis.
- Explain how host factors such as heredity, levels of endogenous hormones, and immune system function increase the risk for development of selected cancers.
- Relate the effects of environmental factors such as chemical carcinogens, radiation, and oncogenic viruses to the risk of cancer development.
- Identify concepts and hypotheses that may explain the processes by which normal cells are transformed into cancer cells by carcinogens.

The causes of cancers are very diverse and complex. It is useful to discuss causation in terms of (1) the genetic and molecular mechanisms that are involved and that characterize the transformation of normal cells to cancer cells; and (2) the external and more contextual factors such as age, heredity, and environmental agents that contribute to the development and progression of cancer. Together, both mechanisms contribute to a multidimensional web of causation by which cancers develop and progress over time.

Genetic and Molecular Basis of Cancer

The molecular pathogenesis of most cancers is thought to originate with genetic damage or mutation with resultant changes in cell physiology that transform a normally functioning cell into a cancer cell. Epigenetic factors that involve silencing of a gene or genes may also be involved in the molecular pathogenesis of cancer. In recent years, an important role of cancer stem cells in the pathogenesis of cancer has been identified, and it continues to be elucidated. Finally, the cellular microenvironment, which involves multiple cell types, the complex milieu of cytokines

and growth factors, and the extracellular matrix, is now recognized as an important contributor to cancer development, growth, and progression.

Cancer-Associated Genes

Most cancer-associated genes can be classified into two broad categories based on whether gene overactivity or underactivity increases the risk for cancer. The category associated with gene overactivity involves *proto-oncogenes,* which are normal genes that become cancer-causing oncogenes if mutated. Proto-oncogenes encode for normal cell proteins such as growth factors, growth factor receptors, growth factor signaling molecules, and transcription factors that promote cell growth or increase growth factor–dependent signaling. The category associated with gene underactivity comprises the *tumor suppressor genes,* which, by being less active, create an environment in which cancer is promoted. Tumor suppressor genes include the retinoblastoma (*RB*) gene, which normally prevents cell division, and the *TP53* gene, which normally becomes activated in DNA-damaged cells to initiate apoptosis.[3,9] Loss of *RB* activity may accelerate the cell cycle and lead to increased cell proliferation, whereas inactivity of *TP53* may increase the survival of DNA-damaged cells. There are a number of genetic events that can lead to oncogene formation or loss of tumor suppressor gene function.

Genetic Events Leading to Oncogene Formation or Activation. There are a number of genetic events that create or activate oncogenes. A common event is a point mutation in which there is a single nucleotide base change due to an insertion, deletion, or substitution. An example of an oncogene caused by point mutations is the *ras* oncogene, which has been found in many cancers. Members of the *ras* proto-oncogene family are important signal-relaying proteins that transmit growth signals to the nucleus. Hence, activation of the *ras* oncogene can increase cell proliferation.

Chromosomal translocations have traditionally been associated with cancers such as Burkitt lymphoma and chronic myelogenous leukemia (CML). In Burkitt lymphoma, the *myc* proto-oncogene, which encodes a growth signal protein, is translocated from its normal position on chromosome 8 to chromosome 14, placing it at the site of an immunoglobulin gene.[3] The outcome of the translocation in CML is the appearance of the so-called *Philadelphia chromosome* involving chromosomes 9 and 22 and the formation of an abnormal fusion protein that promotes cell proliferation (see Chapter 15, Fig. 15-8). Recent advances in biotechnology and genomics are enabling the identification of gene translocations and an increased understanding of how these translocations, even within the same chromosome, contribute to tumorigenesis by the creation of abnormal fusion proteins that promote cell proliferation.

Another genetic event common in cancer is gene amplification. Multiple copies of certain genes may lead to overexpression, with higher-than-normal levels of proteins that increase cell proliferation. For example, the human epidermal growth factor receptor-2 (*HER-2/neu*) gene is amplified in up to 30% of breast cancers; its presence indicates an aggressive tumor with a poor prognosis.[23] One of the agents used in treatment of *HER-2/neu*–overexpressing breast cancers is trastuzumab (Herceptin), a monoclonal antibody that selectively binds to HER-2, thereby inhibiting the proliferation of tumor cells that overexpress HER-2.

Genetic Events Leading to Loss of Tumor Suppressor Gene Function. Tumor suppressor genes inhibit the proliferation of cells in a tumor. When this type of gene is inactivated, a genetic signal that normally inhibits cell proliferation is removed, thereby causing unregulated growth to begin. Numerous tumor suppressor genes have been identified and linked to inherited and sporadic forms of cancer.[3] Of particular interest in this group is the *TP53* gene. Located on the short arm of chromosome 17, it codes for the p53 protein, which functions as a suppressor of tumor growth. Mutations in the *TP53* gene have been implicated in the development of lung, breast, and colon cancer—the three leading causes of cancer death.[3] The *TP53* gene also appears to initiate apoptosis in radiation- and chemotherapy-damaged tumor cells. Thus, tumors that retain normal *TP53* function are more likely to respond to such therapy than tumors that carry a defective *TP53* gene.[3]

Although a single mutation may play an important role in oncogene activation, the malfunction of tumor suppressor genes may require "two hits" to contribute to total loss of function, as suggested by the *two-hit hypothesis* of carcinogenesis[3,9,24] (Fig. 8-6). The first "hit" may be a point mutation in an allele of a particular chromosome; later, a second "hit" occurs that involves the companion allele of the gene. In hereditary cases, the first hit is inherited from an affected parent and is therefore present in all somatic cells of the body. In retinoblastoma, the second hit occurs in one of many retinal cells (all of which already carry the mutated gene). In sporadic (noninherited) cases, both mutations (hits) occur in a single somatic cell, whose progeny then form the cancer. In persons carrying an inherited mutation, such as a mutated *RB* allele, all somatic cells are perfectly normal, except for the increased risk of developing cancer. That person is said to be *heterozygous* at the gene locus. Cancer develops when a person becomes homozygous for the mutant allele, a condition referred to as *loss of heterozygosity*.[3] For example, loss of heterozygosity is known to occur in hereditary cancers, in which a mutated gene is inherited from a parent, and other conditions (*e.g.,* radiation

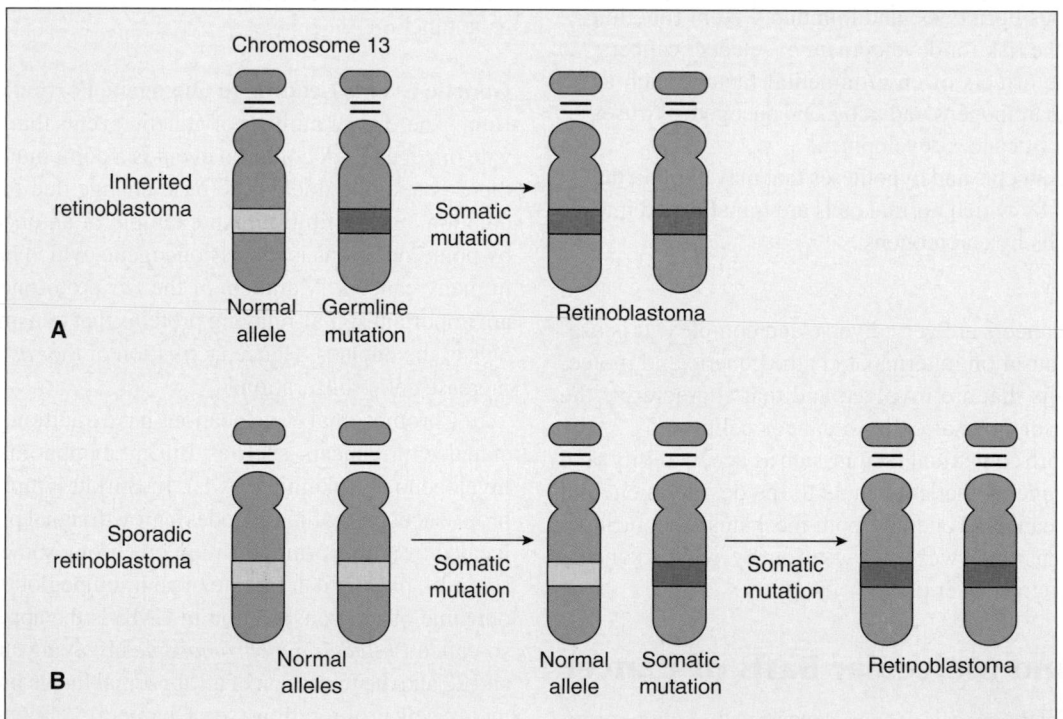

FIGURE 8-6 • The "two-hit" origin of retinoblastoma. **(A)** A child with an inherited form of retinoblastoma is born with a germline mutation in one allele of the retinoblastoma (*RB*) gene located on the long arm of chromosome 13. A second somatic mutation in the retina leads to inactivation of the normally functioning *RB* allele and subsequent development of retinoblastoma. **(B)** In sporadic (noninherited) cases of retinoblastoma, the child is born with two normal *RB* alleles. It requires two independent somatic mutations to inactivate *RB* gene function and allow for the appearance of a neoplastic clone. (From Rubin E., Rubin R., Aaronson S. [2005]. Neoplasia. In Rubin E., Gorstein F., Rubin R., et al. [Eds.], *Rubin's pathology: Clinicopathologic foundations of medicine* [4th ed., p. 171]. Philadelphia: Lippincott Williams & Wilkins.)

exposure) are present that make individuals more susceptible to cancer.

Epigenetic Mechanisms

In addition to mechanisms that involve DNA and chromosomal structural changes, there are molecular and cellular mechanisms, termed *epigenetic mechanisms,* that involve changes in the patterns of gene expression without a change in the DNA. Epigenetic mechanisms may "silence" genes, such as tumor suppressor genes, so that even though the gene is present, it is not expressed and a cancer-suppressing protein is not made. One such mechanism of epigenetic silencing is by methylation of the promoter region of the gene, a change that prevents transcription and causes gene inactivity. Genes silenced by hypermethylation can be inherited, and epigenetic silencing of genes can be considered a first "hit" in the two-hit hypothesis described previously.[25] The epigenetic mechanisms that alter expression of genes associated with cancer are under intensive investigation, as are hypomethylating drugs to prevent or treat cancer.

Molecular and Cellular Pathways

There are numerous molecular and cellular mechanisms with a myriad of associated pathways and genes that are known or suspected to facilitate the development of cancer. Genes that increase susceptibility to cancer or facilitate cancer include defects in DNA repair mechanisms, defects in growth factor signaling pathways, evasion of apoptosis, avoidance of cellular senescence, development of sustained angiogenesis, and metastasis and invasion. In addition, associated genetic mutations are involved that enable invasion of and survival in neighboring tissue, as well as evasion of immune detection and attack.

DNA Repair Defects. Genetic mechanisms that regulate repair of damaged DNA have been implicated in the process of onco-genesis (Fig. 8-7). The DNA repair genes affect cell proliferation and survival indirectly through their ability to repair nonlethal damage in proto-oncogenes, tumor suppressor genes, and the genes that control apoptosis.[3] These genes have been implicated as the principal targets of genetic damage occurring during the development of a cancer cell.[26] Such genetic damage may be caused by the action of chemicals, radiation, or viruses, or it may be inherited in the germline. Significantly, it appears that the acquisition of a single-gene mutation is not sufficient to transform normal cells into cancer cells. Instead, cancerous transformation appears to require the activation of multiple independently mutated genes.

Defects in Growth Factor Signaling Pathways. A relatively common way in which cancer cells gain autonomous growth is through mutations in genes that control growth factor signaling pathways. These signaling pathways couple growth factor receptors to their nuclear targets.[3] Under normal conditions, cell proliferation involves the binding of a growth factor to its

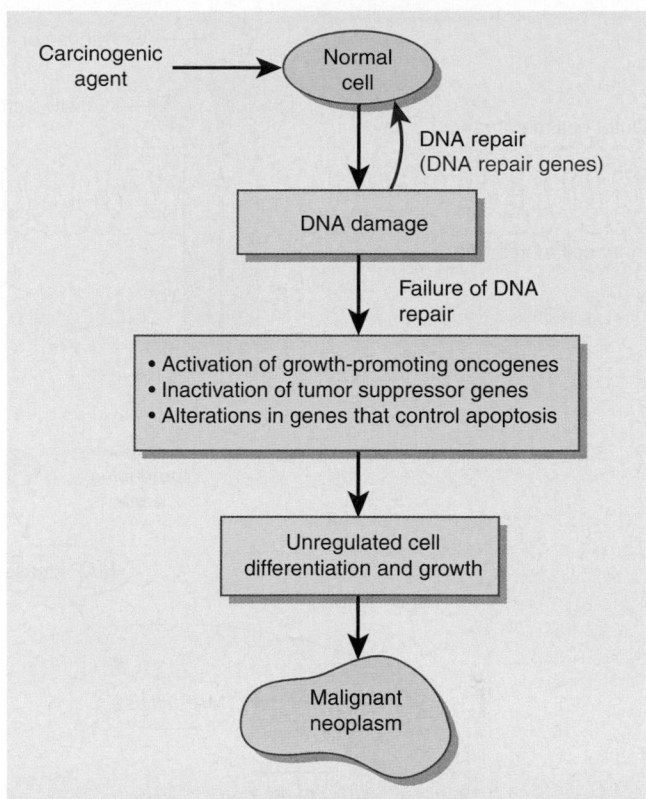

FIGURE 8-7 • Flow chart depicting the stages in the development of a malignant neoplasm resulting from exposure to an oncogenic agent that produces DNA damage. When DNA repair genes are present (*red arrow*), the DNA is repaired and gene mutation does not occur.

receptor on the cell membrane, activation of the growth factor receptor on the inner surface of the cell membrane, transfer of the signal across the cytosol to the nucleus by signal-transducing proteins that function as second messengers, induction and activation of regulatory factors that initiate DNA transcription, and entry of the cell into the cell cycle (Fig. 8-8). Many of the proteins involved in the signaling pathways that control the action of growth factors exert their effects through *kinases,* enzymes that phosphorylate proteins. In some types of cancer such as CML, mutation in a proto-oncogene controlling tyrosine kinase activity occurs, causing unregulated cell growth and proliferation.

Evasion of Apoptosis. Faulty apoptotic mechanisms have an important role in cancer. The failure of cancer cells to undergo apoptosis in a normal manner may be due to a number of problems. There may be altered cell survival signaling, overly active Ras proteins, *TP53* mutations, down-regulation of death receptors (*e.g.,* TRAIL), stabilization of the mitochondria, inactivation of proapoptotic proteins (*e.g.,* methylation of caspase-8), overactivity of nuclear factor kappa B (NF-κB), heat-shock protein production, or failure of immune cells to induce cell death.[27] Alterations in apoptotic and antiapoptotic pathways, genes, and proteins have been found in many cancers. One

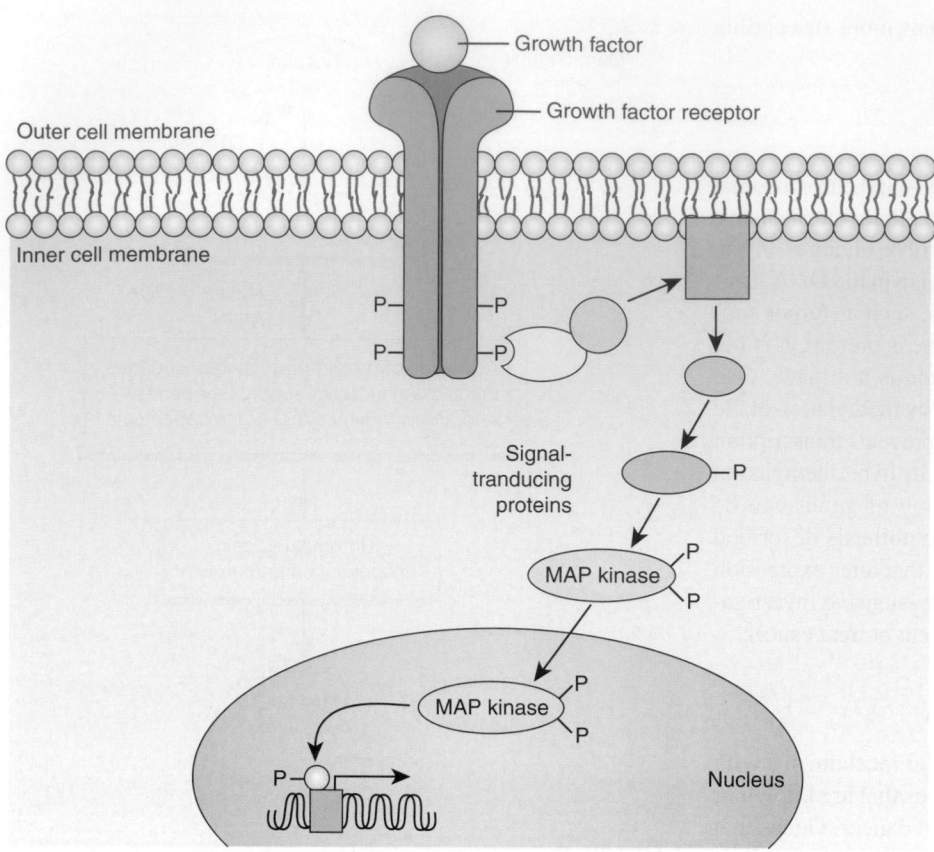

FIGURE 8-8 • Pathway for genes regulating cell growth and replication. Stimulation of a normal cell by a growth factor results in activation of the growth factor receptor and signaling proteins that transmit the growth-promoting signal to the nucleus, where it modulates gene transcription and progression through the cell cycle. Many of these signaling proteins exert their effects through enzymes called *kinases* that phosphorylate proteins. MAP, mitogen-activated protein.

example is the high levels of the antiapoptotic protein Bcl-2 that occur secondary to a chromosomal translocation in certain B-cell lymphomas. The mitochondrial membrane is a key regulator of the balance between cell death and survival. Proteins in the Bcl-2 family reside in the inner mitochondrial membrane and are either proapoptotic or antiapoptotic. Because apoptosis is considered a normal cellular response to DNA damage, loss of normal apoptotic pathways may contribute to cancer by enabling DNA-damaged cells to survive.

Evasion of Cellular Senescence. Another normal cell response to DNA damage is cellular senescence. As stated earlier, cancer cells are characterized by immortality due to high levels of telomerase that prevent cell aging and senescence (see Chapter 3). High levels of telomerase and prevention of telomere shortening may also contribute to cancer and its progression because senescence is considered to be a normal response to DNA damage in cells as well as a tumor suppressor mechanism, and in model systems, short telomeres limit cancer growth.[28,29]

Development of Sustained Angiogenesis. Even with all the aforementioned genetic abnormalities, tumors cannot enlarge unless angiogenesis occurs and supplies them with the blood vessels necessary for survival. Angiogenesis is required not only for continued tumor growth but for metastasis. The molecular basis for the angiogenic switch is unknown, but it appears to involve increased production of angiogenic factors or loss of angiogenic inhibitors. The normal *TP53* gene seems to in-

hibit angiogenesis by inducing the synthesis of an antiangiogenic molecule called *thrombospondin-1*.[3] With mutational inactivation of both *TP53* alleles (as occurs in many cancers), the levels of thrombospondin-1 drop precipitously, tilting the balance in favor of angiogenic factors. Angiogenesis is also influenced by hypoxia and release of proteases that are involved in regulating the balance between angiogenic and antiangiogenic factors. Because of the crucial role of angiogenic factors in tumor growth, much interest is focused on the development of antiangiogenesis therapy. Antiangiogenesis therapy is showing synergistic antitumor actions when combined with conventional forms of chemotherapy in the treatment of certain cancers.

Furthermore, antiangiogenesis therapy may have more broad-based actions. For example, it is now thought that cancer cells are a heterogeneous population of cells that include a cancer stem cell population characterized by mitotic quiescence and an increased ability to survive chemotherapy agents, which make cancer stem cells particularly difficult to treat. Cancer stem cells may reside close to blood vessels, where they receive signals for self-renewal. Use of antiangiogenesis therapy appears to destroy the niche where these stem cells reside.[30]

Invasion and Metastasis. Finally, multiple genes and molecular and cellular pathways are known to be involved in invasion and metastasis. There is evidence that cancer cells with invasive properties are actually members of the cancer stem cell population discussed previously. This evidence suggests that genetic programs that are normally operative in stem cells during embryonic development may become operative in cancer stem cells, enabling them to detach, cross tissue boundaries, escape death by anoikis, and colonize new tissues.[31] The *MET* proto-oncogene, which is expressed in both stem cells and cancer cells, is a key regulator of invasive growth. Recent findings suggest that adverse conditions such as tissue hypoxia, which are commonly present in cancerous tumors, trigger this invasive behavior by activating the MET tyrosine kinase receptor.

Role of the Microenvironment

Traditionally, the molecular and cellular biology of cancer has focused on the cancer itself. More recently, the important role of the microenvironment in the development of cancer and metastasis has been elucidated. The microenvironment of the cancer cell consists of multiple cell types, including macrophages, fibroblasts, endothelial cells, and a variety of immune and inflammatory cells; the extracellular matrix; and the primary signaling substances such as cytokines, chemokines, and hormones. For example, signaling of the cytokine transforming growth factor-beta (TGF-β) is known to be important in the cellular pathway leading to cancer cell formation or suppression.[32] The ability of TGF-β to cause the cancer to progress and metastasize, however, depends on the microenvironment of various cell types and crosstalk of signals among the cell types. In some cases, the phenotype of a cancer cell can actually normalize when it is removed from the tumor microenvironment and placed in a normal environment, and vice versa. Finally, essential steps needed for tumor growth and metastasis, such as angiogenesis and metastatic tumor survival, depend on the microenvironment.

Carcinogenesis

The process by which carcinogenic (cancer-causing) agents cause normal cells to become cancer cells is hypothesized to be a multistep mechanism that can be divided into three stages: initiation, promotion, and progression (Fig. 8-9). *Initiation* involves the exposure of cells to appropriate doses of a carcinogenic agent that makes them susceptible to malignant transformation.[3] The carcinogenic agents can be chemical, physical, or biologic, and produce irreversible changes in the genome of a previously normal cell. Because the effects of initiating agents are irreversible, multiple divided doses may achieve the same effects as a single exposure to the same total dose or to small amounts of highly carcinogenic substances. The cells most susceptible to mutagenic alterations are those that are actively synthesizing DNA.

Promotion involves the induction of unregulated accelerated growth in already initiated cells by various chemicals and growth factors.[3] Promotion is reversible if the promoter substance is removed. Cells that have been irreversibly initiated may be promoted even after long latency periods. The latency period varies with the type of agent, the dosage, and the characteristics of the target cells. Many chemical carcinogens are called *complete carcinogens* because they can initiate and

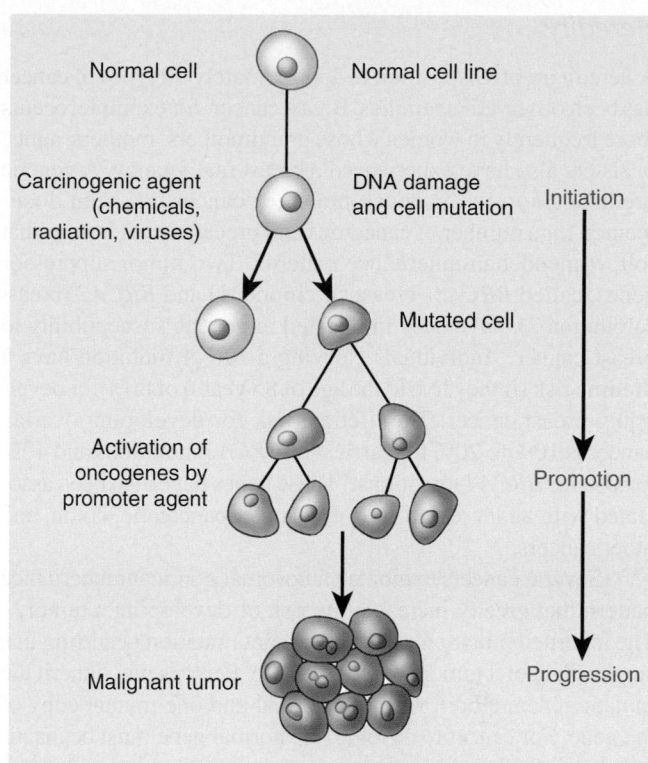

FIGURE 8-9 • The processes of initiation, promotion, and progression in the clonal evolution of malignant tumors. Initiation involves the exposure of cells to appropriate doses of a carcinogenic agent; promotion, the unregulated and accelerated growth of the mutated cells; and progression, the acquisition of malignant characteristics by the tumor cells.

promote neoplastic transformation. *Progression* is the process whereby tumor cells acquire malignant phenotypic changes that promote invasiveness, metastatic competence, autonomous growth tendencies, and increased karyotypic instability.

Host and Environmental Factors

Because cancer is not a single disease, it is reasonable to assume that it does not have a single cause. More likely, cancer occurs because of interactions among multiple risk factors or repeated exposure to a single carcinogenic agent. Among the traditional risk factors that have been linked to cancer are heredity, hormonal factors, immunologic mechanisms, and environmental agents such as chemicals, radiation, and cancer-causing viruses. More recently, there has been interest in obesity as a risk factor for cancer. A strong and consistent relationship has been reported between obesity and mortality from all cancers among men and women.[33] Obese persons tend to produce increased amounts of androgens, a portion of which is converted to the active form of estrogen in adipose tissue, causing a functional state of hyperestrogenism. Because of the association of estrogen with postmenopausal breast cancer and endometrial cancer (see Chapter 46), the relation is stronger among women than among men.[33]

Heredity

A hereditary predisposition to approximately 50 types of cancer has been observed in families. Breast cancer, for example, occurs more frequently in women whose grandmothers, mothers, aunts, or sisters also have experienced a breast malignancy. A genetic predisposition to the development of cancer has been documented for a number of cancerous and precancerous lesions that follow mendelian inheritance patterns. Two tumor suppressor genes, called *BRCA1* (breast carcinoma 1) and *BRCA2* (breast carcinoma 2), have been implicated in genetic susceptibility to breast cancer.[3] Individuals carrying a *BRCA* mutation have a lifetime risk (if they live to the age of 85 years) of 80% for developing breast cancer. The lifetime risk for developing ovarian cancer is 10% to 20% for carriers of *BRCA2* mutations and 40% to 60% for *BRCA1* mutations.[3] These genes have also been associated with an increased risk of prostate, pancreatic, colon, and other cancers.

Several cancers exhibit an autosomal dominant inheritance pattern that greatly increases the risk of developing a tumor.[3,9] The inherited mutation is usually a point mutation occurring in a single allele of a tumor suppressor gene. Persons who inherit the mutant gene are born with one normal and one mutant copy of the gene. For cancer to develop, the normal gene must be inactivated, usually through a somatic mutation. Retinoblastoma, a rare childhood tumor of the retina, is an example of a cancer that follows an autosomal dominant inheritance pattern. Approximately 40% of retinoblastomas are inherited, and carriers of the mutant *RB* tumor suppressor gene have a 10,000-fold increased risk for developing retinoblastoma, usually with bilateral involvement.[9] Familial adenomatous polyposis of the colon also follows an autosomal dominant inheritance pattern. It is caused by mutation of another tumor suppressor gene, the *APC* gene.[9] In people who inherit this gene, hundreds of adenomatous polyps may develop, some of which inevitably become malignant.[3]

Hormones

Hormones have received considerable research attention with respect to cancer of the breast, ovary, and endometrium in women and of the prostate and testis in men. Although the link between hormones and the development of cancer is unclear, it has been suggested that it may reside with the ability of hormones to drive the cell division of a malignant phenotype. Because of the evidence that endogenous hormones affect the risk of these cancers, concern exists regarding the effects on cancer risk if the same or closely related hormones are administered for therapeutic purposes.

Immunologic Mechanisms

There is substantial evidence for the immune system's participation in resistance against the progression and spread of cancer. The central concept, known as the *immune surveillance hypothesis,* first proposed by Paul Ehrlich in 1909, postulates that the immune system plays a central role in resistance against the development of tumors.[34] In addition to cancer–host inter-

actions as a mechanism of cancer development, immunologic mechanisms provide a means for the detection, classification, and prognostic evaluation of cancers and as a potential method of treatment. *Immunotherapy* (discussed later in this chapter) is a cancer treatment modality designed to heighten the patient's general immune responses to increase tumor destruction.

It has been suggested that the development of cancer might be associated with impairment or decline in the surveillance capacity of the immune system. For example, increases in cancer incidence have been observed in people with immunodeficiency diseases and in those with organ transplants who are receiving immunosuppressant drugs. The incidence of cancer also is increased in the elderly, in whom there is a known decrease in immune activity. The association of Kaposi sarcoma with acquired immunodeficiency syndrome (AIDS) further emphasizes the role of the immune system in preventing malignant cell proliferation.

It has been shown that most tumor cells have molecular configurations that can be specifically recognized by immune T cells or by antibodies and hence are termed *tumor antigens.* The most relevant tumor antigens fall into two categories: unique, tumor-specific antigens found only on tumor cells, and tumor-associated antigens found on tumor cells and normal cells. Quantitative and qualitative differences permit the use of tumor-associated antigens to distinguish cancer cells from normal cells.[3]

Virtually all of the components of the immune system have the potential for eradicating cancer cells, including T lymphocytes, B lymphocytes and antibodies, macrophages, and natural killer (NK) cells (see Chapter 17). The T-cell response is undoubtedly one of the most important host responses for controlling the growth of antigenic tumor cells; it is responsible for direct killing of tumor cells and for activation of other components of the immune system. The T-cell immunity to cancer cells reflects the function of two subsets of T cells: the CD4+ helper T cells and CD8+ cytotoxic T cells. The finding of tumor-reactive antibodies in the serum of people with cancer supports the role of the B cell as a member of the immune surveillance team. Antibodies can destroy cancer cells through complement-mediated mechanisms or through antibody-dependent cellular cytotoxicity, in which the antibody binds the cancer cell to another effector cell, such as the NK cell, that does the actual killing of the cancer cell. NK cells do not require antigen recognition and can lyse a wide variety of target cells. The cytotoxic activity of NK cells can be augmented by the cytokines interleukin (IL)-2 and interferon, and its activity can be amplified by immune T-cell responses. Macrophages are important in tumor immunity as antigen-presenting cells to initiate the immune response and as potential effector cells to participate in tumor cell lysis.

Chemical Carcinogens

A carcinogen is an agent capable of causing cancer. The role of environmental agents in causation of cancer was first noted in 1775 by Sir Percivall Pott, who related the high incidence of scrotal cancer in chimney sweeps to their exposure to coal soot.[3] A few year later, based on this observation, the Danish Chimney Guild ruled that its members must bathe daily. Few public health measures since that time have so successfully controlled a form of cancer.[3] Over the next two centuries, many chemicals have been shown to transform cells in the laboratory and to be carcinogenic in animals (Chart 8-1). These agents include both natural (*e.g.,* aflatoxin B_1) and artificial products (*e.g.,* vinyl chloride).

Chemical carcinogens can be divided into two groups: (1) direct-reacting agents, which do not require activation in the body to become carcinogenic; and (2) indirect-reacting agents, called *procarcinogens or initiators,* which become active only after metabolic conversion. Direct- and indirect-acting initiators form highly reactive species (*i.e.,* electrophiles and free radicals) that bind with the nucleophilic residues on DNA, RNA, or cellular proteins. The action of these reactive species tends to cause cell mutation or alteration in synthesis of cell enzymes and structural proteins in a manner that alters cell replication and interferes with cell regulatory controls. The carcinogenicity of some chemicals is augmented by agents called *promoters* that, by themselves, have little or no cancer-causing ability. It is believed that promoters exert their effect by changing the expression of genetic material in a cell, increasing DNA synthesis, enhancing gene amplification (*i.e.,* number of gene copies that are made), and altering intercellular communication.

Exposure to many chemical carcinogens is associated with lifestyle risk factors, such as smoking, dietary factors, and alcohol consumption. Cigarette smoke contains both procarcinogens and promoters. It is directly associated with lung and laryngeal cancer and has been linked with cancers of the mouth, nasal cavities, pharynx, esophagus, pancreas, liver, kidney, uterus, cervix, and bladder, and with myeloid leukemias.[35] Chewing tobacco or tobacco products increases the risk of cancers of the oral cavity and esophagus. It has been estimated that 30% of all cancer deaths and 87% of lung cancer deaths in the United States are related to tobacco.[36] Not only is the smoker at risk, but others passively exposed to cigarette smoke are at risk. Environmental tobacco smoke has been classified as a "group A" carcinogen based on the U.S. Environmental Protection Agency's system of carcinogen classification. Each year, about 3000 non-smoking adults die of lung cancer as a result of environmental tobacco smoke.[36]

There is strong evidence that certain elements in the diet contain chemicals that contribute to cancer risk. Most known dietary carcinogens occur either naturally in plants (*e.g.,* aflatoxins) or are produced during food preparation.[37] For example, benzo[*a*]pyrene and other polycyclic hydrocarbons are converted to carcinogens when foods are fried in fat that has been reused multiple times. Among the most potent of the procarcinogens are the polycyclic aromatic hydrocarbons. The polycyclic aromatic hydrocarbons are of particular interest because they are produced from animal fat in the process of charcoal-broiling meats and are present in smoked meats and fish. They also are produced in the combustion of tobacco and are present in cigarette smoke. Nitrosamines, which are powerful carcinogens, are formed in foods that are smoked, salted, cured, or pickled using nitrites or nitrates as preservatives.[37] Formation of nitrosamines may be inhibited by the presence of antioxidants such as vitamin C, found in fruits and vegetables. Cancer of the colon has been associated with high dietary intake of fat and red meat and a low intake of dietary fiber. A high-fat diet was thought to be carcinogenic because it increases the flow of primary bile acids that are converted to secondary bile acids in the presence of anaerobic bacteria in the colon, producing carcinogens or promoters. Recent studies have identified obesity and lowered physical activity with an increased risk of colon cancer.[37]

Alcohol is associated with a variety of cancers; the causative mechanisms are very complex. The first and most toxic metabolite of ethanol is acetaldehyde, which is a known carcinogen that interferes with DNA synthesis and repair and causes point mutations in some cells.[38] In addition, ethanol can alter DNA methylation and interfere with retinoid metabolism, which is important in antioxidant mechanisms. The carcinogenic effect of cigarette smoke can be enhanced by concomitant consumption of alcohol; persons who smoke and drink considerable amounts of alcohol are at increased risk for development of cancer of the oral cavity, larynx, and esophagus.

The effects of carcinogenic agents usually are dose dependent—the larger the dose or the longer the duration of exposure, the greater the risk that cancer will develop. Some chemical carcinogens may act in concert with other carcinogenic influences, such as viruses or radiation, to induce neoplasia. There usually is a time delay ranging from 5 to 30 years from

---

| CHART 8-1 | **CHEMICAL AND ENVIRONMENTAL AGENTS KNOWN TO BE CARCINOGENIC IN HUMANS** |

Polycyclic Hydrocarbons
Soots, tars, and oils
Cigarette smoke

Industrial Agents
Aniline and azo dyes
Arsenic compounds
Asbestos
β-Naphthylamine
Benzene
Benzo[*a*]pyrene
Carbon tetrachloride
Insecticides, fungicides
Nickel and chromium compounds
Polychlorinated biphenyls
Vinyl chloride

Food and Drugs
Smoked foods
Nitrosamines
Aflatoxin B_1
Diethylstilbestrol
Anticancer drugs (*e.g.,* alkylating agents, cyclophosphamide, chlorambucil, nitrosourea)

the time of chemical carcinogen exposure to the development of overt cancer. This is unfortunate because many people may have been exposed to the agent and its carcinogenic effects before the association was recognized. This occurred, for example, with the use of diethylstilbestrol, which was widely used in the United States from the mid-1940s to 1970 to prevent miscarriages. But it was not until the late 1960s that many cases of vaginal adenosis and adenocarcinoma in young women were found to be the result of their exposure in utero to diethylstilbestrol.[39]

Radiation

The effects of *ionizing radiation* in carcinogenesis have been well documented in atomic bomb survivors, in patients diagnostically exposed, and in industrial workers, scientists, and physicians who were exposed during employment. Malignant epitheliomas of the skin and leukemia were significantly elevated in these populations. Between 1950 and 1970, the death rate from leukemia alone in the most heavily exposed population groups of atomic bomb survivors in Hiroshima and Nagasaki was 147 per 100,000 persons, 30 times the expected rate.[40]

The type of cancer that developed depended on the dose of radiation, the sex of the person, and the age at which exposure occurred. For instance, approximately 25 to 30 years after total-body or trunk irradiation, there were increased incidences of leukemia and cancers of the breast, lung, stomach, thyroid, salivary gland, gastrointestinal system, and lymphoid tissues. The length of time between exposure and the onset of cancer is related to the age of the individual. For example, children exposed to ionizing radiation in utero have an increased risk for developing leukemias and childhood tumors, particularly 2 to 3 years after birth. This latency period for leukemia extends to 5 to 10 years if the child was exposed after birth and to 20 years for certain solid tumors.[41] As another example, the latency period for the development of thyroid cancer in infants and small children who received radiation to the head and neck to decrease the size of the tonsils or thymus was as long as 35 years after exposure.

The association between sunlight and the development of skin cancer (see Chapter 61) has been reported for more than 100 years. *Ultraviolet radiation* consists of relatively low-energy rays that do not deeply penetrate the skin. The evidence supporting the role of ultraviolet radiation in the cause of skin cancer includes skin cancer that develops primarily on the areas of skin more frequently exposed to sunlight (*e.g.,* the head and neck, arms, hands, and legs), a higher incidence in light-complexioned individuals who lack the ultraviolet-filtering skin pigment melanin, and the fact that the intensity of ultraviolet exposure is directly related to the incidence of skin cancer, as evidenced by higher rates occurring in Australia and the American Southwest.[41] There also are studies that suggest intense, episodic exposure to sunlight, particularly during childhood, is more important in the development of melanoma than prolonged, low-intensity exposure. As with other carcinogens, the effects of ultraviolet radiation usually are additive, and there usually is a long delay between the time of exposure and detection of the cancer.

Oncogenic Viruses

An oncogenic virus is one that can induce cancer. It has been suspected for some time that viruses play an important role in the development of certain forms of cancer, particularly leukemia and lymphoma. Ellermann in 1908 and Rous in 1911 were the first to describe the transmissibility of avian leukemia and sarcoma, respectively.[42] Interest in the field of viral oncology, particularly in human populations, has burgeoned with the discovery of reverse transcriptase and the development of recombinant DNA technology, and more recently with the discovery of oncogenes and tumor suppressor genes.

Viruses, which are small particles containing genetic material (DNA or RNA), enter a host cell and become incorporated into its chromosomal DNA, taking control of the cell's machinery for the purpose of producing viral proteins. A large number of DNA and RNA viruses (*i.e.,* retroviruses) have been shown to be oncogenic in animals. However, only a few viruses have been linked to cancer in humans.

Four DNA viruses have been implicated in human cancers: the human papillomavirus (HPV), Epstein-Barr virus (EBV), hepatitis B virus (HBV), and human herpesvirus-8 (HHV-8).[3] HHV-8, which causes Kaposi sarcoma in persons with AIDS, is discussed in Chapter 20. There are over 60 genetically different types of HPV. Some types (*i.e.,* types 1, 2, 4, 7) have been shown to cause benign squamous papillomas (*i.e.,* warts). HPVs also have been implicated in squamous cell carcinoma of the cervix and anogenital region. HPV types 16 and 18 and, less commonly, HPV types 31, 33, 35, and 51 are found in approximately 85% of squamous cell carcinomas of the cervix and presumed precursors (*i.e.,* severe cervical dysplasia and carcinoma in situ).[3] A quadrivalent vaccine to protect against HPV types 6, 11, 16, and 18 is now available, and vaccination of 9- to 26-year-old girls/women is being encouraged as a means of preventing cervical cancer[43] (see Chapter 47).

EBV is a member of the herpesvirus family. It has been implicated in the pathogenesis of four human cancers: Burkitt lymphoma, nasopharyngeal cancer, B-cell lymphomas in immunosuppressed individuals such as those with AIDS, and in some cases of Hodgkin lymphoma. Burkitt lymphoma, a tumor of B lymphocytes, is endemic in parts of East Africa and occurs sporadically in other areas worldwide. In persons with normal immune function, the EBV-driven B-cell proliferation is readily controlled and the person becomes asymptomatic or experiences a self-limited episode of infectious mononucleosis (see Chapter 15). In regions of the world where Burkitt lymphoma is endemic, concurrent malaria or other infections cause impaired immune function, allowing sustained B-lymphocyte proliferation. The incidence of nasopharyngeal cancer is high in some areas of China, particularly southern China, and in the Cantonese population in Singapore. An increased risk of B-cell lymphomas is seen in individuals with drug-suppressed immune systems, such as individuals with transplanted organs.

HBV is the etiologic agent in the development of hepatitis B, cirrhosis, and hepatocellular carcinoma. There is a significant correlation between elevated rates of hepatocellular carcinoma worldwide and the prevalence of HBV carriers.[3] Other etiologic factors also may contribute to the development of liver cancer. Ingestion of aflatoxin and infection with HCV, the hepatitis C virus, have been implicated.[3] The precise mechanism by which HBV induces hepatocellular cancer has not been determined, although it has been suggested that it may be the result of prolonged HBV-induced liver damage and regeneration.

Although there are a number of retroviruses (RNA viruses) that cause cancer in animals, human T-cell leukemia virus-1 (HTLV-1) is only known retrovirus to cause cancer in humans. HTLV-1 is associated with a form of T-cell leukemia that is endemic in parts of Japan and some areas of the Caribbean and Africa, and is found sporadically elsewhere, including the United States and Europe.[3] Similar to the human immunodeficiency virus (HIV) responsible for AIDS, HTLV-1 is attracted to CD4+ T cells, and this subset of T cells is therefore the major target for cancerous transformation. The virus requires transmission of infected T cells through sexual intercourse, infected blood, or breast milk.

IN SUMMARY, the causes of cancer are highly complex and can be viewed from two perspectives: (1) the molecular and cellular origins and mechanisms; and (2) the external and contextual causative factors, including age, heredity, and environmental agents, that influence its inception and growth. In most cases, the molecular pathogenesis of cancer is thought to have its origin in genetic damage or mutation that changes cell physiology and transforms a normally functioning cell into a cancer cell. However, the complexity of the causation and pathogenesis of cancer is becoming increasingly apparent as more is learned about the roles of epigenetic mechanisms, cancer stem cells, and the microenvironment in tumorigenesis.

The types of genes involved in cancer are numerous, with the two main categories being the proto-oncogenes, which control cell growth and replication, and tumor suppressor genes, which are growth-inhibiting regulatory genes. Genetic and molecular mechanisms that increase susceptibility to cancer or facilitate cancer include defects in DNA repair mechanisms, defects in growth factor signaling pathways, evasion of apoptosis, avoidance of antiaging and senescence mechanisms, development of sustained angiogenesis, and invasion and metastasis. Because cancer is not a single disease, it is likely that multiple factors interact at the molecular and cellular levels to transform normal cells into cancer cells. Genetic and epigenetic damage may be the result of interactions between multiple risk factors or repeated exposure to a single carcinogenic (cancer-producing) agent. Among the risk factors that have been linked to cancer are heredity, hormonal factors, immunologic mechanisms, and environmental agents such as chemicals, radiation, and cancer-causing viruses. ■

CLINICAL MANIFESTATIONS

After completing this section of the chapter, you should be able to meet the following objectives:

- Describe the many possible ways by which cancer acts to disrupt organ function.
- Characterize the mechanisms involved in the anorexia and cachexia, fatigue and sleep disorders, anemia, and venous thrombosis experienced by patients with cancer.
- Define the term *paraneoplastic syndrome* and explain its pathogenesis and manifestations.

There probably is not a single body function left unaffected by the presence of cancer. Because tumor cells replace normally functioning parenchymal tissue, the initial manifestations of cancer usually reflect the primary site of involvement. For example, cancer of the lung initially produces impairment of respiratory function; as the tumor grows and metastasizes, other body structures become affected. Cancer also produces generalized manifestations such as fatigue, anorexia and cachexia, anemia, decreased resistance to infections, and symptoms unrelated to the tumor site (paraneoplastic syndromes). Many of these manifestations are compounded by the side effects of methods used to treat the disease. In its late stages, cancer often causes pain (see Chapter 49). Pain is one of the most dreaded aspects of cancer, and pain management is one of the major treatment concerns for persons with incurable cancers.

Tissue Integrity

Cancer disrupts tissue integrity. As cancers grow, they compress and erode blood vessels, causing ulceration and necrosis along with frank bleeding and sometimes hemorrhage. One of the early warning signals of colorectal cancer is blood in the stool. Cancer cells also may produce enzymes and metabolic toxins that are destructive to the surrounding tissues. Usually, tissue damaged by cancerous growth does not heal normally. Instead, the damaged area persists and often continues to grow; a sore that does not heal is another warning signal of cancer. Cancer has no regard for normal anatomic boundaries; as it grows, it invades and compresses adjacent structures. Abdominal cancer, for example, may compress the viscera and cause bowel obstruction.

The development of effusions (*i.e.,* fluid) in the pleural, pericardial, or peritoneal spaces may be the presenting sign of some tumors.[44] Direct involvement of the serous surface seems to be the most significant inciting factor, although many other mechanisms, such as obstruction of lymphatic flow, may play a role. It has been reported that almost 50% of undiagnosed effusions in persons not known to have cancer turn out to be due to malignancy. Lung cancers, breast cancers, and lymphomas account for about 75% of malignant pleural effusions.[44] Most persons with pleural effusions are symptomatic at presentation, with chest pain, shortness of breath, and cough. More than any other malignant neoplasms, ovarian cancers are associated with the accumulation of fluid in the peritoneal cavity. Complaints of abdominal discomfort, swelling and a feeling of heaviness, and increase in abdominal girth, which reflect the presence of peritoneal effusions or ascites, are the most common presenting symptoms in ovarian cancer, occurring in up to 65% of women with the disease.[45]

Systemic Manifestations

Many of the manifestations of cancer, including anorexia and cachexia, fatigue and sleep disorders, and anemia, are not directly related to the presence of a tumor mass but to altered metabolic pathways and the presence of circulating cytokines and other mediators. Although research has produced amazing insights into the causes and cures for cancer, only recently have efforts focused on the associated side effects of the disease.[46]

Anorexia and Cachexia

Many cancers are associated with weight loss and wasting of body fat and muscle tissue, accompanied by profound weakness, anorexia, and anemia. This wasting syndrome is often referred to as the *cancer anorexia–cachexia syndrome*.[46–50] It is a common manifestation of most solid tumors, with the exception of breast cancer. It has been estimated that it is a significant cause of morbidity and mortality in 80% of persons with advanced cancer, and responsible for death in up to 20% of cases.[46] The condition is more common in children and elderly persons and becomes more pronounced as the disease progresses. Persons with cancer cachexia also respond less well to chemotherapy and are more prone to toxic side effects.

Although anorexia, reduced food intake, and abnormalities of taste are common in people with cancer and often are accentuated by treatment methods, the extent of weight loss and protein wasting cannot be explained in terms of diminished food intake alone. In contrast to starvation due to lack of food intake, where weight is preferentially lost from the fat compartment, in cachexia, it is lost from both the fat and skeletal muscle compartments.[49] Furthermore, the protein loss that occurs with starvation is divided equally between skeletal muscle and visceral proteins, whereas in cachexia, visceral proteins are relatively well preserved. Thus, there is a loss of liver mass in starvation, but an increase in cachectic persons because of hepatic recycling of nutrients and the acute-phase response. Finally, and more important, weight loss that occurs with starvation is usually reversed by refeeding, whereas oral or parenteral nutritional supplementation does not reverse cachexia. It has been suggested that the altered metabolism and weight loss seen in cancer cachexia more closely resembles that seen in persons suffering from severe sepsis or trauma rather than starvation.[49]

The mechanisms of cancer cachexia appear to reside in a hypermetabolic state and altered nutrient metabolism that are specific to the tumor-bearing state. Tumors tend to consume large amounts of glucose, with a resultant increase in lactate formation because the tumor oxygen levels are too low to support the citric acid cycle and mitochondrial oxidative phospho-

rylation (see Chapter 4, Understanding Cell Metabolism). The lactate that is produced then circulates to the liver, where it is converted back to glucose. The production of glucose (gluconeogenesis) from lactate uses adenosine triphosphate (ATP) and is very energy inefficient, contributing to the hypermetabolic state of cachectic patients. Another mechanism for the increasing energy expenditure in cachectic persons is the increased expression of mitochondrial uncoupling proteins that uncouple the oxidative phosphorylation process, so that energy is lost as heat. Abnormalities in fat and protein metabolism have also been reported. During starvation in persons without cancer, ketones derived from fat replace the glucose normally used by the brain, leading to decreased gluconeogenesis from amino acids with conservation of muscle mass, whereas in persons with cancer cachexia, amino acids are not spared and there is depletion of lean body mass, a condition thought to contribute to decreased survival time.

Although the mechanisms of the cancer anorexia–cachexia syndrome remain incompletely understood, they are probably multifactorial, resulting from a persistent inflammatory response in conjunction with production of specific cytokines and catabolic factors by the tumor. The syndrome shows similarities to that of the acute-phase response seen with tissue injury, infection, or inflammation, in which liver protein synthesis changes from synthesis of albumin to acute-phase proteins such as C-reactive protein, fibrinogen, and α_1-antitrypsin (see Chapter 18). The acute-phase response is known to be activated by cytokines such as tumor necrosis factor-α (TNF-α) and IL-1 and IL-6, suggesting that they may also play a role in cancer cachexia.[46–50] High serum levels of these cytokines have been observed in persons with cancer, and their levels appear to correlate with progression of the tumor. TNF-α, secreted primarily by macrophages in response to tumor cell growth or gram-negative bacterial infections, was the first cytokine associated with cachexia and wasting to be identified. It causes anorexia by suppressing satiety centers in the hypothalamus and increasing the synthesis of lipoprotein lipase, an enzyme that facilitates the release of fatty acids from lipoproteins so that they can be used by tissues. IL-1 and IL-6 share many of the features of TNF-α in terms of the ability to initiate cachexia.

Fatigue and Sleep Disorders

Fatigue and sleep disturbances are two of the most frequent side effects experienced by persons with cancer.[51–54] Cancer-related fatigue is characterized by feelings of tiredness, weakness, and lack of energy, and is distinct from the normal tiredness experienced by healthy individuals in that it is not relieved by rest or sleep. It occurs both as a consequence of the cancer itself and as a side effect of cancer treatment. Cancer-related fatigue may be an early symptom of malignant disease and has been reported by as many as 40% of patients at the time of diagnosis.[53] Furthermore, the symptom often remains for months or even years after treatment.

The cause of cancer-related fatigue is largely unknown, but is probably multifactorial and involves the dysregulation of several interrelated physiologic, biochemical, and psychological systems. The basic mechanisms of fatigue have been broadly categorized into two components: peripheral and central.[52] Peripheral fatigue, which occurs in the neuromuscular junctions and muscles, results from the inability of the peripheral neuromuscular apparatus to perform a task in response to central stimulation. Mechanisms implicated in peripheral fatigue include a lack of ATP and the buildup of metabolic byproducts such as lactic acid. Central fatigue arises in the central nervous system (CNS) and is often described as difficulty in initiating or maintaining voluntary activities. One hypothesis proposed to explain cancer-related fatigue is that cancer and cancer treatments result in dysregulation of brain serotonin (5-hydroxytryptamine [5-HT]) levels or function. There is evidence that proinflammatory cytokines, such as TNF-α, can influence 5-HT metabolism.[52]

Although cancer-related fatigue and sleep disorders are distinct conditions, they are closely linked in terms of prevalence and symptoms.[54] Persons with cancer report poor sleep quality, disturbed initiation and maintenance of sleep, insufficient sleep, nighttime awakening, and restless sleep (see Chapter 52 for a discussion of sleep disorders). As with fatigue, precipitating factors include the diagnosis of cancer, type and stage of cancer, pain, and side effects of treatment (e.g., nausea, vomiting). Once it begins, insomnia is often self-perpetuating because of the natural tendency to compensate for sleep loss by napping, going to bed earlier, and getting out of bed later. It may also be that the fatigue that occurs with cancer or anticancer therapy may, in fact, prompt persons to extend their sleep opportunity and thus becomes a contributing factor to ongoing insomnia. Correlations have also been noted between fatigue and daytime symptoms of sleep problems, such as daytime sleepiness and napping.

Anemia

Anemia is common in persons with various types of cancers. It may be related to blood loss, hemolysis, impaired red blood cell production, or treatment effects.[55,56] For example, drugs used in treatment of cancer are cytotoxic and can decrease red blood cell production. Also, there are many mechanisms through which erythrocyte production can be impaired in persons with malignancies, including nutritional deficiencies, bone marrow failure, and a blunted erythropoietin response to hypoxia. Inflammatory cytokines generated in response to tumors decrease erythropoietin production, resulting in a decrease in erythrocyte production.

Cancer-related anemia is associated with reduced treatment effectiveness, increased mortality, increased transfusion requirements, and reduced performance and quality of life. Hypoxia, a characteristic feature of advanced solid tumors, has been recognized as a critical factor in promoting tumor resistance to radiation therapy and some chemotherapeutic agents. Severe anemia may delay surgical interventions when preoperative transfusions are required. Similarly, low hemoglobin levels before or during chemotherapy may require dose reductions or delays in administration, resulting in a decrease in overall treatment effectiveness. Cancer-related anemia is often treated with recombinant human erythropoietin (rHuEPO, epoetin alfa) (see Chapter 14).

Paraneoplastic Syndromes

In addition to signs and symptoms at the sites of primary and metastatic disease, cancer can produce manifestations in sites that are not directly affected by the disease. Such manifestations are collectively referred to as *paraneoplastic syndromes.*[57,58] Some of these manifestations are caused by the elaboration of hormones by cancer cells, and others from the production of circulating factors that produce hematopoietic, neurologic, and dermatologic syndromes (Table 8-4). These syndromes are most commonly associated with lung, breast, and hematologic malignancies.[3]

A variety of peptide hormones are produced by both benign and malignant tumors. Although not normally expressed, the biochemical pathways for the synthesis and release of

TABLE 8-4 Common Paraneoplastic Syndromes

TYPE OF SYNDROME	ASSOCIATED TUMOR TYPE	PROPOSED MECHANISM
Endocrinologic		
Syndrome of inappropriate ADH	Small cell lung cancer, others	Production and release of ADH by tumor
Cushing syndrome	Small cell lung cancer, bronchial carcinoid cancers	Production and release of ACTH by tumor
Hypercalcemia	Squamous cell cancers of the lung, head, neck, ovary	Production and release of polypeptide factor with close relationship to PTH
Hematologic		
Venous thrombosis	Pancreatic, lung, other cancers	Production of procoagulation factors
Nonbacterial thrombolytic endocarditis	Advanced cancers	
Neurologic		
Eaton-Lambert syndrome	Small cell lung cancer	Autoimmune production of antibodies to motor end-plate structures
Myasthenia gravis	Thymoma	
Dermatologic		
Acanthosis nigricans	Gastric carcinoma	Possibly caused by production of growth factors (epidermal) by tumor cells

ADH, antidiuretic hormone; ACTH, adrenocorticotropic hormone; PTH, parathyroid hormone.

peptide hormones (*e.g.*, antidiuretic [ADH], adrenocorticotropic [ACTH], and parathyroid [PTH] hormones) are present in most cells.[59] Thus, the three most common endocrine syndromes associated with cancer are the syndrome of inappropriate ADH secretion (see Chapter 31), Cushing syndrome due to ectopic ACTH production (see Chapter 41), and hypercalcemia[58,59] (see Chapter 31). Hypercalcemia of malignancy does not appear to be related to PTH but to a PTH-related protein that shares several biologic actions with PTH. Hypercalcemia also can be caused by osteolytic processes induced by cancers such as multiple myeloma or bony metastases from other cancers.

Some paraneoplastic syndromes are associated with the production of circulating mediators that produce hematologic complications.[58] For example, a variety of cancers may produce procoagulation factors that contribute to an increased risk for venous thrombosis and nonbacterial thrombotic endocarditis. Sometimes, unexplained thrombotic events are the first indication of an undiagnosed malignancy. The precise relationship between coagulation disorders and cancer is still unknown. Several malignancies, such as mucin-producing adenocarcinomas, release thromboplastin and other substances that activate the clotting system.

The symptomatic paraneoplastic neurologic disorders are relatively rare, with the exception of the Lambert-Eaton myasthenic syndrome, which affects about 3% of persons with small cell lung cancer; and myasthenia gravis, which affects about 15% of people with thymoma.[60] The *Lambert-Eaton syndrome*, or reverse myasthenia gravis, is seen almost exclusively in small cell lung cancer. It produces muscle weakness in the limbs rather than the initial bulbar and ocular muscle weakness seen in myasthenia gravis. The origin of paraneoplastic neurologic disorders is thought to be immune mediated.[60,61] The altered immune response is initiated by the production of onconeural antigens (*e.g.*, antigens normally expressed in the nervous system) by the cancer cells. The immune system, in turn, recognizes the onconeural antigens as foreign and mounts an immune response. In many cases, the immune attack controls the growth of the cancer. The antibodies and cytotoxic T cells are not sufficient to cause neurologic disease unless they cross the blood-brain barrier and react with neurons expressing the onconeural antigen.[60]

A wide variety of cutaneous syndromes is associated with malignancies and may precede, be concurrent with, or follow the discovery of cancer. Among the paraneoplastic dermatologic disorders is *acanthosis nigricans,* characterized by pigmented hyperkeratoses consisting of symmetric, verrucous and papillary lesions that occur in skin flexures, particularly the axillary and perineal areas.[58] The lesions are usually symmetric and may be accompanied by pruritus. The condition is usually associated with adenocarcinomas of the gastrointestinal tract, particularly gastric carcinoma, but may be associated with a variety of adenocarcinomas, including lung, breast, ovarian, and even hematologic cancers. The pathogenesis of these lesions is uncertain.

The paraneoplastic syndromes may be the earliest indication that a person has cancer, and should be regarded as such.[57]

They may also represent significant clinical problems, may be potentially lethal in persons with cancer, and may mimic metastatic disease and confound treatment. Diagnostic methods focus on both identifying the cause of the disorder and on locating the malignancy responsible. Techniques for precise identification of minute amounts of polypeptides may allow for early diagnosis of curable malignancies in asymptomatic individuals.[58] The treatment of paraneoplastic syndromes involves concurrent treatment of the underlying cancer and suppression of the mediator causing the syndrome.

IN SUMMARY,   there probably is no single body function left unaffected by the presence of cancer. Because tumor cells replace normally functioning parenchymal tissue, the initial manifestations of cancer usually reflect the primary site of involvement. Cancer compresses blood vessels, obstructs lymph flow, disrupts tissue integrity, invades serous cavities, and compresses visceral organs. It may result in development of effusion (*i.e.*, fluid) in the pleural, pericardial, or peritoneal spaces, and generalized manifestations such as anorexia and cachexia, fatigue and sleep disorders, and anemia. It may also produce paraneoplastic syndromes that arise from the ability of neoplasms to elaborate hormones and other chemical mediators to produce endocrine, hematopoietic, neurologic, and dermatologic syndromes. Many of these manifestations are compounded by the side effects of methods used to treat the disease. ■

SCREENING, DIAGNOSIS, AND TREATMENT

After completing this section of the chapter, you should be able to meet the following objectives:

- Cite three characteristics of an ideal screening test for cancer.
- Describe the four methods that are used in the diagnosis of cancer.
- Differentiate between the methods used for grading and staging of cancers.
- Explain the mechanism by which radiation exerts its beneficial effects in the treatment of cancer.
- Describe the adverse effects of radiation therapy.
- Differentiate between the action of direct DNA-interacting and indirect DNA-interacting chemotherapeutic agents and cell cycle–specific and cell cycle–independent drugs.
- Describe the three mechanisms whereby biotherapy exerts its effects.
- Describe three examples of targeted therapy used in the treatment of cancer.

Screening

Screening represents a secondary prevention measure for the early recognition of cancer in an otherwise asymptomatic population.[62,63] Screening can be achieved through observation (*e.g.,* skin, mouth, external genitalia), palpation (*e.g.,* breast, thyroid, rectum and anus, prostate, lymph nodes), and laboratory tests and procedures (*e.g.,* Papanicolaou [Pap] smear, colonoscopy, mammography). It requires a test that will specifically detect early cancers or premalignancies, is cost effective, and results in improved therapeutic outcomes.[63] For most cancers, stage at presentation is related to curability, with the highest rates reported when the tumor is small and there is no evidence of metastasis. For some tumors, however, metastasis tends to occur early, even from a small primary tumor. For other cancers, such as cancer of the pancreas, no screening methods are currently available. More sensitive screening methods such as tumor markers are being developed for these forms of cancer.

Cancers for which current screening or early detection has led to improvement in outcomes include cancers of the breast (breast self-examination and mammography, discussed in Chapter 46), cervix (Pap smear, Chapter 46), colon and rectum (rectal examination, fecal occult blood test, and flexible sigmoidoscopy and colonoscopy, Chapter 37), prostate (prostate-specific antigen [PSA] testing and transrectal ultrasonography, Chapter 44), and malignant melanoma (self-examination, Chapter 61). Although not as clearly defined, it is recommended that screening for other types of cancers such as cancers of the thyroid, testicles, ovaries, lymph nodes, and oral cavity be done at the time of periodic health examinations.

Diagnostic Methods

The methods used in the diagnosis and staging of cancer are determined largely by the location and type of cancer suspected. A number of procedures are used in the diagnosis of cancer, including blood tests for tumor markers, cytologic studies and tissue biopsy, endoscopic examinations, ultrasonography, x-ray studies, MRI, computed tomography (CT), and positron emission tomography (PET).

Tumor Markers

Tumor markers are antigens expressed on the surface of tumor cells or substances released from normal cells in response to the presence of tumor.[3,64] Some substances, such as hormones and enzymes, that are produced normally by the involved tissue become overexpressed as a result of cancer. Other tumor markers, such as oncofetal proteins, are produced during fetal development and are induced to reappear later in life as a result of benign and malignant neoplasms. Tumor markers are used for screening, establishing prognosis, monitoring treatment, and detecting recurrent disease. Table 8-5 identifies some of the more commonly used tumor markers and summarizes their source and the cancers associated with them.

The serum markers that have proved most useful in clinical practice are human chorionic gonadotropin (hCG), CA-125,

PSA, α-fetoprotein (AFP), carcinoembryonic antigen (CEA), and CD blood cell antigens.[9] A hormone normally produced by the placenta, hCG is used as a marker for diagnosing, prescribing treatment, and following the disease course in persons with high-risk gestational trophoblastic tumors. PSA is used as a marker in prostate cancer, and CA-125 is used as a marker in ovarian cancer. Markers for leukemia and lymphomas are grouped by so-called *cluster of differentiation* (CD) antigens (see Chapter 15). The CD antigens help to distinguish among T and B lymphocytes, monocytes, granulocytes, and NK cells, and immature variants of these cells.[3,9]

Some cancers express fetal antigens that are normally present only during embryonal development.[3] The two that have proved most useful as tumor markers are AFP and CEA. AFP is synthesized by the fetal liver, yolk sac, and gastrointestinal tract and is the major serum protein in the fetus. Elevated levels are encountered in people with primary liver cancers and have also been observed in some testicular, ovarian, pancreatic, and stomach cancers. CEA normally is produced by embryonic tissue in the gut, pancreas, and liver and is elaborated by a number of different cancers. Depending on the serum level adopted for significant elevation, CEA is elevated in approximately 60% to 90% of colorectal carcinomas, 50% to 80% of pancreatic cancers, and 25% to 50% of gastric and breast tumors.[3] As with most other tumor markers, elevated levels of CEA and AFP are found in other, noncancerous conditions, and elevated levels of both depend on tumor size, so that neither is useful as an early screening test for cancer.

As diagnostic tools, tumor markers have limitations. Nearly all markers can be elevated in benign conditions, and most are not elevated in the early stages of malignancy. Hence, tumor markers have limited value as screening tests. Furthermore, they are not in themselves specific enough to permit a diagnosis of a malignancy, but once a malignancy has been diagnosed and shown to be associated with elevated levels of a tumor marker, the marker can be used to assess response to therapy. Extremely elevated levels of a tumor marker can indicate a poor prognosis or the need for more aggressive treatment. Perhaps the greatest value of tumor markers is in monitoring therapy in people with widespread cancer. The level of most cancer markers tends to decrease with successful treatment and increase with recurrence or spread of the tumor.

Cytologic and Histologic Methods

Histologic and cytologic studies are laboratory methods used to examine tissues and cells. Several sampling approaches are available, including cytologic smears, tissue biopsies, and needle aspiration.[3]

Papanicolaou Test. The Pap test is a cytologic method used for detecting cancer cells. It consists of a microscopic examination of a properly prepared slide by a cytotechnologist or pathologist for the purpose of detecting the presence of abnormal cells. The usefulness of the Pap test relies on the fact that the cancer cells lack the cohesive properties and intercellular junctions that are

TABLE 8-5 Tumor Markers

MARKER	SOURCE	ASSOCIATED CANCERS
Oncofetal Antigens		
α-Fetoprotein (AFP)	Fetal yolk sac and gastrointestinal structures early in fetal life	Primary liver cancers; germ cell cancer of the testis
Carcinoembryonic antigen (CEA)	Embryonic tissues in gut, pancreas, and liver	Colorectal cancer and cancers of the pancreas, lung, and stomach
Hormones		
Human chorionic gonadotropin (hCG)	Hormone normally produced by placenta	Gestational trophoblastic tumors; germ cell cancer of testis
Calcitonin	Hormone produced by thyroid parafollicular cells	Thyroid cancer
Catecholamines (epinephrine, norepinephrine) and metabolites	Hormones produced by chromaffin cells of the adrenal gland	Pheochromocytoma and related tumors
Specific Proteins		
Monoclonal immunoglobulin	Abnormal immunoglobulin produced by neoplastic cells	Multiple myeloma
Prostate-specific antigen (PSA)	Produced by the epithelial cells lining the acini and ducts of the prostate	Prostate cancer
Mucins and Other Glycoproteins		
CA-125	Produced by müllerian cells of ovary	Ovarian cancer
CA-19-9	Produced by alimentary tract epithelium	Cancer of the pancreas, colon
Cluster of Differentiation		
CD antigens	Present on leukocytes	Used to determine the type and level of differentiation of leukocytes involved in different types of leukemia and lymphoma

characteristic of normal tissue; without these characteristics, cancer cells tend to exfoliate and become mixed with secretions surrounding the tumor growth. Although the Pap test is widely used as a screening test for cervical cancer, it can be performed on other body secretions, including nipple drainage, pleural or peritoneal fluid, and gastric washings.

Tissue Biopsy. Tissue biopsy, which is of critical importance in designing the treatment plan should cancer cells be found, involves the removal of a tissue specimen for microscopic study. Biopsies are obtained in a number of ways, including needle biopsy; endoscopic methods, such as bronchoscopy or cystoscopy, which involve the passage of an endoscope through an orifice and into the involved structure; or laparoscopic methods. In some instances, a surgical incision is made from which biopsy specimens are obtained. Excisional biopsies are those in which the entire tumor is removed. The tumors usually are small, solid, palpable masses. If the tumor is too large to be completely removed, a wedge of tissue from the mass can be excised for examination. Appropriate preservation of the specimen includes prompt immersion in a fixative solution such as formalin, with preservation of a portion of the specimen in a special fixative for electron microscopy, or prompt refrigeration to permit optimal hormone, receptor, and other types of molecular analysis. A quick frozen section may be done to determine the nature of

a mass lesion or evaluate the margins of an excised tumor to ascertain that the entire neoplasm has been removed.[9]

Fine-needle aspiration is another approach that is widely used. The procedure involves aspirating cells and attendant fluid with a small-bore needle. The method is most commonly used for assessment of readily palpable lesions in sites such as the thyroid, breast, and lymph nodes. Modern imaging techniques have also enabled the method to be extended to deeper structures such as the pelvic lymph nodes and pancreas.

Immunohistochemistry. Immunohistochemistry involves the use of antibodies to facilitate the identification of cell products or surface markers.[9] For example, certain anaplastic carcinomas, malignant lymphomas, melanomas, and sarcomas look very similar under the microscope, but must be accurately identified because their treatment and prognosis are quite different. Antibodies against intermediate filaments have proved useful in such cases because tumor cells often contain intermediate filaments characteristic of their tissue of origin.[9] Immunohistochemistry can also be used to determine the site of origin of metastatic tumors. Many patients with cancer present with metastasis. In cases in which the origin of the metastasis is obscure, immunochemical detection of tissue-specific or organ-specific antigens can often help to identify the tumor source. Immunohistochemistry can also be used to detect molecules that have prognostic or therapeutic significance. For example, detection of estrogen receptors on breast cancer cells is of prognostic and therapeutic significance because these tumors respond to antiestrogen therapy.

Microarray Technology. Microarray technology uses "gene chips" that can simultaneously perform miniature assays to detect and quantify the expression of large numbers of genes.[3] The advantage of microarray technology is the ability to analyze a large number of changes in cancer cells to determine overall patterns of behavior that could not be assessed by conventional means. DNA arrays are now commercially available to assist in making clinical decisions regarding breast cancer treatment. In addition to identifying tumor types, microarrays have been used for predicting prognosis and response to therapy, examining tumor changes after therapy, and classifying hereditary tumors.[3]

Staging and Grading of Tumors

The two basic methods for classifying cancers are *grading* according to the histologic or cellular characteristics of the tumor and *staging* according to the clinical spread of the disease. Both methods are used to determine the course of the disease and aid in selecting an appropriate treatment or management plan. Grading of tumors involves the microscopic examination of cancer cells to determine their level of differentiation and the number of mitoses. Cancers are classified as grades I, II, III, and IV with increasing anaplasia or lack of differentiation. Staging of cancers uses methods to determine the extent and spread of the disease. Surgery may be used to determine tumor size and lymph node involvement.

The clinical staging of cancer is intended to group patients according to the extent of their disease. It is useful in determining the choice of treatment for individual patients, estimating prognosis, and comparing the results of different treatment regimens. The TNM system of the American Joint Committee on Cancer (AJCC) is used by most cancer facilities.[65] This system, which is briefly described in Chart 8-2, classifies the disease into stages using three tumor components: *T* stands for the size and local spread of the primary tumor, *N* refers to the involvement of the regional lymph nodes, and *M* describes the extent of the metastatic involvement. The time of staging is indicated as clinical–diagnostic staging (cTNM), postsurgical resection–pathologic staging (pTNM), surgical–evaluative staging (sTNM), retreatment staging (rTNM), and autopsy staging (aTNM).[65]

Cancer Treatment

The goals of cancer treatment methods fall into three categories: curative, control, and palliative. The most common modalities are surgery, radiation therapy, chemotherapy, hormonal therapy, and biotherapy. The treatment of cancer involves the use of a carefully planned program that combines the benefits of multiple treatment modalities and the expertise of an interdisciplinary team of specialists, including medical, surgical,

CHART 8-2	TNM CLASSIFICATION SYSTEM

T (tumor)
Tx   Tumor cannot be adequately assessed
T0   No evidence of primary tumor
Tis   Carcinoma in situ
T1–4 Progressive increase in tumor size or involvement

N (nodes)
Nx   Regional lymph nodes cannot be assessed
N0   No evidence of regional node metastasis
N1–3 Increasing involvement of regional lymph nodes

M (metastasis)
Mx   Not assessed
M0   No distant metastasis
M1   Distant metastasis present, specify sites

and radiation oncologists; clinical nurse specialists; nurse practitioners; pharmacists; and a variety of ancillary personnel.

Surgery

Surgery is the oldest treatment for cancer and, until recently, the only treatment that could cure persons with cancer. Surgery is now used for diagnosis, staging of cancer, tumor removal, and palliation (*i.e.,* relief of symptoms) when a cure cannot be achieved. The type of surgery to be used is determined by the extent of the disease, the location and structures involved, the tumor growth rate and invasiveness, the surgical risk to the patient, and the quality of life the patient will experience after the surgery. Surgery is often thought of as the first line of treatment for solid tumors.[67] If the tumor is small and has well-defined margins, the entire tumor often can be removed. If, however, the tumor is large or involves vital tissues, surgical removal may be difficult, if not impossible.

Surgery provides several approaches for cancer treatment. For example, it can be the primary, curative treatment for cancers that are locally or regionally contained, have not metastasized, or have not invaded major organs. It also is used as a component of adjuvant therapy in combination with chemotherapy or radiation therapy in other types of cancers. Surgical techniques also may be used to control oncologic emergencies such as gastrointestinal hemorrhages. Another approach includes using surgical techniques for cancer prophylaxis in families that have a high genetically confirmed risk for developing cancer. For instance, a total colectomy may be suggested for an individual with familial adenomatous polyposis coli because of the increased risk for developing cancer by 40 years of age.

Surgical techniques have expanded to include cryosurgery, chemosurgery, laser surgery, and laparoscopic surgery. *Cryosurgery* involves the instillation of liquid nitrogen into the tumor through a probe. It is used in treating cancers of the liver and prostate. *Chemosurgery* is used in skin cancers. It involves the use of a corrosive paste in combination with multiple frozen sections to ensure complete removal of the tumor. *Laser surgery* uses a laser beam to resect a tumor. It has been used effectively in retinal and vocal cord surgery. *Laparoscopic surgery* involves the performance of abdominal surgery through two small incisions—one for viewing within the cavity and the other for insertion of the instruments to perform the surgery.

Cooperative efforts among cancer centers throughout the world have helped to standardize and improve surgical procedures, determine which cancers benefit from surgical intervention, and establish in what order surgical and other treatment modalities should be used. Increased emphasis also has been placed on the development of surgical techniques that preserve body image and form without compromising essential function. Nerve-sparing prostatectomy and limb-salvage surgery for soft tissue tumors preserve functional abilities while permitting complete removal of the tumor.[67]

Radiation Therapy

Radiation therapy is one of the most commonly used methods of cancer treatment.[68,69] It can be used alone as a primary method of therapy or as an adjuvant treatment with surgery, chemotherapy, or both. It can also be used as a palliative treatment to reduce symptoms such as bone pain resulting from metastasis in persons with advanced cancers. Radiation is used to treat oncologic emergencies such as superior vena cava syndrome, spinal cord compression, or bronchial obstruction.

Radiation therapy uses high-energy particles or waves to destroy or damage cancer cells. The absorption of energy from radiation in tissue leads to the ionization of molecules or creation of free radicals. Radiation can also produce effects indirectly by interacting with water (which makes up approximately 80% of a cell's volume) to produce free radicals, which damage cell structures (see Chapter 5). Radiation can immediately kill cells, delay or halt cell cycle progression, or, at dose levels commonly used in radiation therapy, produce damage to the cell's DNA, resulting in cell death after replication.[69] Radiation must produce double-stranded breaks in DNA to kill a cell, owing to the high capacity of cells for repairing single-stranded breaks.

The therapeutic effects of radiation therapy derive from the fact that the rapidly proliferating and poorly differentiated cells of a cancerous tumor are more likely to be injured than are the more slowly proliferating cells of normal tissue. To some extent, however, radiation is injurious to all rapidly proliferating cells, including those of the bone marrow and the mucosal lining of the gastrointestinal tract. Normal tissue usually is able to recover from radiation damage more readily than cancerous tissue. In addition to its lethal effects, radiation also produces sublethal injury. Recovery from sublethal doses of radiation occurs in the interval between the first dose of radiation and subsequent doses.[69,70] This is why large total doses of radiation can be tolerated when they are divided into multiple, smaller fractionated doses.[68-70]

The radiation dose that is chosen for treatment of a particular cancer is determined by factors such as the radiosensitiv-

ity of the tumor type, the size of the tumor, and, more important, the tolerance of the surrounding tissues.[69,70] The term *radiosensitivity* describes the inherent properties of a tumor that determine its responsiveness to radiation. It varies widely among the different types of cancers and is thought to vary as a function of their position in the cell cycle. Fast-growing cancers have cells that typically are more radiosensitive than slow-growing cancers. The combination of selected cytotoxic drugs with radiation has demonstrated a radiosensitizing effect on tumor cells by altering the cell cycle distribution, increasing DNA damage, and decreasing DNA repair. Radiosensitizers include 5-fluorouracil, capecitabine, paclitaxel, gemcitabine, and cisplatin.[71]

Radiation responsiveness describes the manner in which a radiosensitive tumor responds to irradiation. One of the major determinants of radiation responsiveness is tumor oxygenation because oxygen is a rich source of free radicals that form and destroy essential cell components during irradiation.[70] Many rapidly growing tumors outgrow their blood supply and become deprived of oxygen. The hypoxic cells of these tumors are more resistant to radiation than normal or well-oxygenated tumor cells. Methods of ensuring adequate oxygen delivery, such as adequate hemoglobin levels, are important.

Dose–response curves, which express the extent of lethal tissue injury in relation to the dose of radiation, are determined by the number of cells that survive graded, fractional doses of radiation. The use of more frequent fractionated doses increases the likelihood that the cancer cells will be dividing and in the vulnerable period of the cell cycle during radiation administration. This type of dose also allows time for normal tissues to repair the radiation damage. An important focus of research has been the search for drugs to reduce the biologic effects of radiation on normal tissue. These drugs, known as *radioprotectants,* would preferentially protect normal cells from the cytotoxic effects of radiation. One drug, amifostine, is approved by the U.S. Food and Drug Administration (FDA) to reduce the incidence of dryness of the mouth (*i.e.,* xerostomia) due to the effects of radiation on salivary gland function in patients undergoing radiation therapy for head and neck cancers.[71]

Administration. Therapeutic radiation can be delivered in one of three ways: external beam or teletherapy, with beams generated at a distance and aimed at the tumor in a patient; brachytherapy, in which a sealed radioactive source is placed close to or directly in the tumor site; and systemic therapy, in which radioisotopes with a short half-life are given by mouth or injected into the tumor site.[69] Radiation from any source decreases in intensity as a function of the square of the distance from the source. Teletherapy, which is the most commonly used form of radiation therapy, maintains intensity over a large volume of tissue by increasing the source-to-surface distance. In brachytherapy, the source-to-surface distance is small; therefore, the effective treatment volume is small.

External-beam radiation is commonly delivered by a linear accelerator or a cobalt-60 machine.[69] The linear accelerator is the preferred machine because of its versatility and precision of dose distribution, as well as the speed with which treatment can be given. Linear accelerators produce ionizing radiation through a process in which electrons are accelerated at a very high rate, strike a target, and produce high-energy x-rays (photons). The linear accelerator can vary the level of radiation energy that is delivered so that different depths can be treated. Various beam-modifying approaches are used to define and shape the beam, thereby increasing the radiation damage to the tumor site while sparing the normal surrounding tissues. Three-dimensional conformal radiation therapy (3-D CRT) uses CT scans or MRI to construct an image of the tumor.[72,73] The patient is fitted with a plastic mold or cast to keep the body still, while radiation beams are delivered to the body from several directions. Intensity-modulated radiation therapy (IMRT) is another advanced form of external radiation therapy. As with 3-D CRT, computer imaging techniques are used to calculate the most efficient dosages and combinations of radiation treatment. This precise mapping of the tumor allows for the delivery of radiation beams that conform to the contours of the tumor, reducing the dose and therefore the toxicity to adjacent normal tissue. Because of its precision, it is even more important that the patient remain in the right place and perfectly still during the treatment. This usually requires fabricating a special cast or mold before treatment to keep the body in place.

Brachytherapy involves the insertion of sealed radioactive sources into a body cavity (intracavitary) or directly into body tissues (interstitial). The term *brachytherapy* means "short therapy," implying that the radiation effect is limited to areas close to the radiation source.[74] Brachytherapy can be subdivided into high-dose radiation (HDR) and low-dose radiation (LDR) according to the rate at which the radiation is delivered. HDR uses a single highly radioactive source that is attached to a cable and housed in a robotic machine referred to as an HDR remote afterloader. When the treatment is delivered, the radiation source is pushed from the remote afterloader through a tube to a location near the tumor site. Remote afterloading machines make it possible to insert a radioactive material (*e.g.,* cesium-137, iridium-192) into a tumor area for a specific time and remove it while oncology personnel are outside the treatment room. This minimizes staff radiation exposure and decreases treatment times by allowing use of intermediate- and high-dose radioactive sources.[74] In contrast, the radiation source for LDR brachytherapy may be packed into catheter devices or sealed radiation sources (*e.g.,* beads, seeds) and placed directly in or near the area being treated. LDR therapy can be temporary or permanent. Temporary LDR brachytherapy can be accomplished as an inpatient procedure, with radiation applicators and sources remaining in the patient for a few days. Radioactive materials with a relatively short half-life, such as iodine-125 or palladium-103, are commonly encapsulated and used in permanent implants (*e.g.,* seed implants used to treat prostate cancer).

Unsealed internal radiation sources are injected intravenously or administered by mouth. Iodine-131, which is given by mouth, is used in the treatment of thyroid cancer. Strontium-89, administered intravenously, is given to control bone pain due to multiple skeletal metastases in patients with advanced breast, lung, or prostate cancer.[69] Stereotactic radiosurgery is a method of destroying brain tumors and brain metastases by delivering a single large dose of radiation through stereotactically directed narrow beams. Gamma knife radiosurgery allows the application of focused radiation for limited brain metastasis and is associated with fewer long-term complications, such as cognitive dysfunction, than whole-brain radiation.

Adverse Effects. Radiation cannot distinguish between malignant cells and rapidly proliferating cells of normal tissue.[69] During radiation treatment, injury to normal cells can produce adverse effects. Tissues within the treatment fields that are most frequently affected are the skin, the mucosal lining of the gastrointestinal tract, and the bone marrow. Anorexia, nausea, emesis, and diarrhea are common with abdominal and pelvic irradiation. These symptoms are usually controlled by medication and dietary measures. The primary systemic effect is fatigue. Most of these side effects are temporary and reversible.

Radiation can also cause bone marrow suppression, particularly when it is delivered to the bone marrow in skeletal sites. Subsequently, the complete blood count is affected, resulting in an initial decrease in the number of the leukocytes, followed by a decrease in thrombocytes (platelets) and, finally, red blood cells. This predisposes the individual to infection, bleeding, and anemia, respectively. Frequent blood counts are used during radiation therapy to monitor bone marrow function.

External-beam radiation must first penetrate the skin and, depending on the total dose and type of radiation used, skin reactions may develop. With moderate doses of radiation, the hair falls out spontaneously or when being combed after the 10th to the 14th day. With larger doses, erythema develops (much like sunburn) and may turn brown; and, at higher doses, patches of dry or moist desquamation may develop. Fortunately, reepithelialization takes place after the treatments have been stopped. Mucositis or desquamation of the oral and pharyngeal mucous membranes, which sometimes may be severe, may occur as a predictable side effect in people receiving head and neck irradiation. Pain and difficulty eating and drinking can negatively affect the individual's nutritional status. Pelvic radiation can cause impotence or erectile dysfunction in men and vaginal irritation, dryness, and discharge, dyspareunia, and, as a late effect, vaginal stenosis in women.

Chemotherapy

Cancer chemotherapy has evolved as one of the major systemic treatment modalities for cancer. Unlike surgery and radiation, chemotherapy is a systemic treatment that enables drugs to reach the site of the tumor as well as other distant sites. Chemotherapeutic drugs may be the primary form of treatment, or they may be used as part of a multimodal treatment plan. It is the primary treatment for most hematologic and some solid tumors, including choriocarcinoma, testicular cancer, acute and chronic leukemia, non-Hodgkin and Hodgkin lymphomas, and multiple myeloma. In persons with widespread disseminated disease, chemotherapy provides only palliative rather than curative therapy at present.

Cancer chemotherapeutic drugs exert their effects through several mechanisms. At the cellular level, they exert their lethal action by targeting processes that prevent cell growth and replication. These mechanisms include disrupting the production of essential enzymes; inhibiting DNA, RNA, and protein synthesis; and preventing cell mitosis.[75–77] Under ideal conditions, anticancer drugs would eradicate cancer cells without damaging normal tissues. Unfortunately, no cancer agents currently available are completely without toxic effects, and their clinical use involves weighing their beneficial effects against their toxicity.

For most chemotherapy drugs, the relationship between tumor cell survival and drug dose is exponential, with the number of cells surviving being proportional to the drug dose, and the number of cells at risk for exposure being proportional to the destructive action of the drug. Chemotherapeutic drugs are most effective in treating tumors that have a high growth fraction because of their ability to kill rapidly dividing cells. Exponential killing implies that a proportion or percentage of tumor cells is killed, rather than an absolute number[75] (Fig. 8-10).

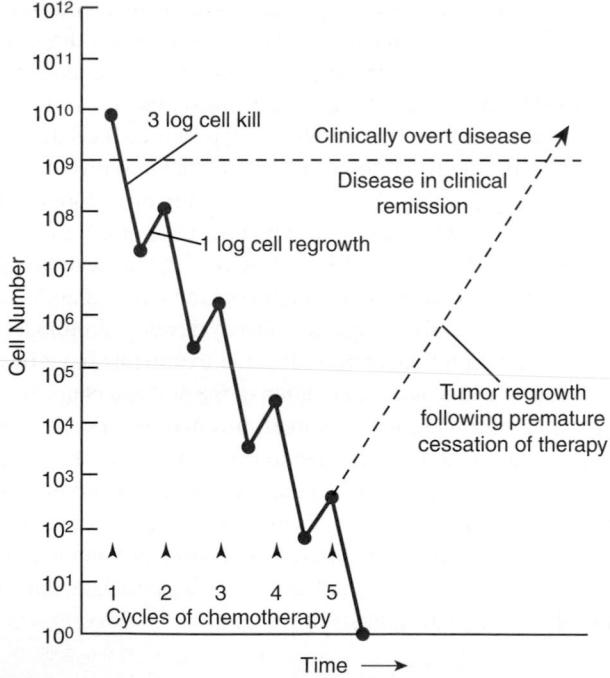

FIGURE 8-10 • Relationship between tumor cell survival and administration of chemotherapy. The exponential relationship between drug dose and tumor cell survival dictates that a constant proportion, not number, of tumor cells is killed with each treatment cycle. In this example, each cycle of drug administration results in a 99.9% (3 log) cell kill, and 1 log of cell growth occurs between cycles. The *broken line* indicates what would occur if the last cycle of therapy were omitted: despite complete clinical remission of disease, the tumor ultimately would recur. (From Cooper M. R., Cooper M. R. [2001]. Basis for current major therapies for cancer: Systemic therapy. In Lenhard R. E., Osteen R. T., Gansler T. [Eds.], *The American Cancer Society's Clinical Oncology* [p. 181]. Atlanta: American Cancer Society.)

This proportion is a constant percentage of the total number of cells. For this reason, multiple courses of treatment are needed if the tumor is to be eradicated.

A major problem in cancer chemotherapy is the development of cellular resistance. Acquired resistance develops in a number of drug-sensitive tumor types.[76] Experimentally, drug resistance can be highly specific to a single agent and is usually based on genetic changes in a given tumor cell. In other instances, a multidrug-resistant phenomenon encompassing anticancer drugs with differing structures occurs. This type of resistance often involves the increased expression of transmembrane transporter genes involved in drug efflux.

Chemotherapy drugs are commonly classified according to their site and mechanism of action. Chemotherapy drugs that have similar structures and effects on cell function usually are grouped together, and these drugs usually have similar side effect profiles. The major classifications of chemotherapy drugs are the direct DNA-interacting and indirect DNA-interacting agents.[76] Other systemic agents include hormonal and molecularly targeted agents. Cancer chemotherapy drugs may also be classified as either cell cycle specific or cell cycle nonspecific. Drugs are cell cycle specific if they exert their action during a specific phase of the cell cycle. For example, methotrexate, an antimetabolite, acts by interfering with DNA synthesis and thereby interrupts the S phase of the cell cycle. Drugs that are cell cycle nonspecific exert their effects throughout all phases of the cell cycle. The alkylating agents are cell cycle nonspecific and act by disrupting DNA when the cells are in the resting state as well as when they are dividing. Because chemotherapy drugs differ in their mechanisms of action, cell cycle–specific and cell cycle–nonspecific agents are often combined to treat cancer.

Direct DNA-Interacting Agents. The direct DNA-interacting agents include the alkylating agents, antitumor antibiotics, and topoisomerase inhibitors. As a class, the alkylating agents exert their cytotoxic effects by transfer of their alkyl group to various cellular constituents.[76,77] Alkylation of DNA within the cell nucleus is probably the major interaction that causes cell death. Alkylating agents have direct vesicant effects and can damage tissues at the site of injection as well as produce systemic toxicity. Toxicities are generally dose related and occur particularly in rapidly proliferating tissues such as bone marrow, the gastrointestinal tract, and reproductive tissues.

The *antitumor antibiotics* are substances produced by bacteria that in nature appear to provide protection against hostile microorganisms. As a class they bind directly to DNA and frequently undergo electron transfer reactions to generate free radicals in close proximity to DNA, resulting in DNA damage in the form of single breaks or cross-links. All of the anticancer antibiotics now in clinical use are produced by the soil microbe *Streptomyces*. These include the anthracyclines, dactinomycin, bleomycin, and mitomycin. The anthracycline antibiotics (*e.g.*, doxorubicin and daunorubicin) are among the most widely used cytotoxic cancer drugs.[76] The main dose-limiting toxicity of all anthracyclines is cardiotoxicity and myelosuppression, with neutropenia more commonly observed than thrombocytopenia. Two forms of cardiotoxicity can occur—acute and chronic. The acute form occurs within the first 2 to 3 days of therapy and presents with arrhythmias, conduction disorders, other electrocardiographic changes, pericarditis, and myocarditis.[76] This form is usually transient and in most cases asymptomatic. The chronic form of cardiotoxicity results in a dose-dependent dilated cardiomyopathy (see Chapter 24). Efforts to minimize the toxicity profile of the antitumor antibiotics have resulted in the development of analog compounds (*e.g.,* idarubicin, epirubicin). Liposome technology has been used with two antitumor antibiotics (*i.e.,* doxorubicin and daunorubicin) to develop chemotherapy drugs that are encapsulated by coated liposomes. These drugs (*i.e.,* Doxil, Caelyx [doxorubicin], and DaunoXome [daunorubicin]) have been found to distribute more chemotherapy to the desired site with fewer side effects.[78]

The DNA *topoisomerase inhibitors* block cell division by interfering with the action of the topoisomerase enzymes that break and rejoin phosphodiester bonds in the DNA strands to prevent them from tangling during separation and unwinding of the double helix.[76,77] Topoisomerase I produces single-strand breaks (nicks) and topoisomerase II, double-strand breaks. The epipodophyllotoxins (etoposide and teniposide) are topoisomerase II inhibitors that block cell division in the late S-G2 phase of the cell cycle. The camptothecins (topotecan, irinotecan) inhibit the action of topoisomerase I, the enzyme responsible for cutting and rejoining single DNA strands. Inhibition of this enzyme interferes with resealing of the breaks and DNA damage.

Indirect DNA-Interacting Agents. The indirect DNA-interacting agents include the antimetabolites and mitotic spindle inhibitors. The antimetabolites (folic acid antagonists and purine and pyrimidine antagonists) interrupt the biochemical pathways relating to nucleotide and nucleic acid synthesis (see Chapter 6). Antimetabolites can cause DNA damage indirectly through misincorporation into DNA, abnormal timing or progression of DNA synthesis, or altered function of purine and pyrimidine biosynthetic enzymes.[75,76] They tend to convey their greatest effect during the S phase of the cell cycle. Because of their S-phase specificity, the antimetabolites have been shown to be more effective when given as a prolonged infusion. Common side effects include stomatitis, diarrhea, and myelosuppression.

The plant alkaloids, including the vinca alkaloids and taxanes, are drugs affecting the microtubule structures required for formation of the cytoskeleton and mitotic spindle[76,77] (see Chapter 4). Although each group of drugs affects the microtubule, their mechanism of action differs. The vinca alkaloids (*e.g.,* vinblastine, vincristine) inhibit tubulin polymerization, which disrupts assembly of microtubules. This inhibitory effect results in mitotic arrest in metaphase, bringing cell division to a stop, which then leads to cell death. Vinblastine is a potent vesicant and care must be taken in its administration. Toxicities include nausea and vomiting, bone marrow suppression, and alopecia. Despite similarities in their mechanisms of action, vincristine has a different spectrum of actions and toxicities than vinblastine. The main dose-limiting toxicity is neurotoxicity, usually expressed as a peripheral sensory neuropathy, although autonomic nervous system dysfunction (*e.g.,* orthostatic hypotension, sphincter problems, paralytic ileus), cranial nerve palsies, ataxia, seizures, and coma have been observed. The taxanes (*e.g.,* paclitaxel, docetaxel) differ from the vinca alkaloids in that they stabilize the microtubules against depolymerization. The stabilized microtubules are unable to undergo the normal changes necessary for cell cycle completion. These drugs are administered intravenously and require the use of a vehicle that can cause hypersensitivity reactions. In addition to hypersensitivity reactions, their side effect profile includes myelosuppression and peripheral neurotoxicity in the form of glove-and-stocking numbness, and paresthesia.

Combination Chemotherapy. Combination chemotherapy has been found to be more effective than treatment with a single drug. Combination chemotherapy creates a more hostile environment for tumor cell growth through higher drug concentrations and prevents the development of resistant clones of cancer cells. With this method, several drugs with different mechanisms of action, metabolic pathways, times of onset of action and recovery, side effects, and times of onset of side effects are used. Drugs used in combination must be individually effective against the tumor and may be synergistic with each other. Routes of administration and dosage schedules are carefully designed to ensure optimal delivery of the active forms of the drugs to a tumor during the sensitive phase of the cell cycle.

Administration. Many of the cancer chemotherapy drugs are administered intravenously. Venous access devices (VADs) often are used for people with poor venous access and those who require frequent or continuous intravenous therapy. The VAD can be used for home administration of chemotherapy drugs, blood sampling, and administration of blood components. These systems access the venous circulation either through an externalized catheter or an implanted catheter with access ports. In some cases, the drugs are administered by continuous infusion using an ambulatory infusion pump that allows the person to remain at home and maintain his or her activities. Newer drugs (*e.g.,* capecitabine, a pyrimidine antagonist) have been formulated for the oral route. Although adherence to a dosing schedule and reimbursement for oral drugs are a challenge, these drugs provide a more convenient administration form for the patient.

Adverse Effects. Chemotherapy is administered on a dose–response basis (*i.e.,* the more drug administered, the greater the number of cancer cells killed). Chemotherapeutic drugs affect neoplastic cells and the rapidly proliferating cells of normal tissue. The nadir (*i.e.,* lowest point) is the point of maximal toxicity for a given adverse effect of a drug and is stated in the time it takes to reach that point. Because many toxic effects of chemotherapeutic drugs persist for some time after the drug is discontinued, the nadir times and recovery rates are useful guides in evaluating the effects of cancer therapy. Some side effects appear immediately or after a few days (acute), some within a few weeks (intermediate), and others months to years after chemotherapy administration (long-term).

Most chemotherapeutic drugs suppress bone marrow function and formation of blood cells, leading to anemia, neutropenia, and thrombocytopenia.[77] With neutropenia, there is risk for developing serious infections, whereas thrombocytopenia increases the risk for bleeding. The availability of hematopoietic growth factors (*e.g.,* granulocyte colony-stimulating factor [G-CSF]; erythropoietin, which stimulates red blood production; and IL-11, which stimulates platelet production) has shortened the period of myelosuppression, thereby reducing the need for hospitalizations due to infection and decreasing the need for blood products.

Anorexia, nausea, and vomiting are common problems associated with cancer chemotherapy.[77,79] The severity of the vomiting is related to the emetic potential of the particular drug. These symptoms can occur within minutes or hours of drug administration and are thought to be due to stimulation of the chemoreceptor trigger zone in the medulla that initiates vomiting (see Chapter 36). The chemoreceptor trigger zone responds to levels of chemicals circulating in the blood. The acute symptoms usually subside within 24 to 48 hours and often can be relieved by antiemetics. The pharmacologic approaches to prevent chemotherapy-induced nausea and vomiting have greatly improved over the past several decades. The development of serotonin receptor ($5-HT_3$) antagonists (*e.g.,* ondansetron, granisetron, dolasetron, palonosetron) has facilitated the use of highly emetic chemotherapy drugs by more effectively reducing the nausea and vomiting induced by these drugs. These antiemetics are effective when given by both the oral and intravenous routes. Aprepitant, a selective high-affinity antagonist of substance P/neurokinin-1 receptors, has recently been approved by the FDA for use in treatment of nausea and vomiting associated with cancer chemotherapy.[77] The drug, which is given orally, has been shown to inhibit both the acute and chronic phases of chemotherapy-induced nausea and vomiting.

Alopecia or hair loss results from impaired proliferation of the hair follicles and is a side effect of a number of cancer drugs; it usually is temporary, and the hair tends to regrow when treatment is stopped. The rapidly proliferating structures of the reproductive system are particularly sensitive to the action of cancer drugs. Women may experience changes in menstrual flow or have amenorrhea. Men may have a decreased sperm count (*i.e.,* oligospermia) or absence of sperm (*i.e.,* azoospermia). Many chemotherapeutic agents also may have teratogenic or mutagenic effects leading to fetal abnormalities.[80]

Chemotherapy drugs are toxic to all cells. The mutagenic, carcinogenic, and teratogenic potential of these drugs has been strongly supported by both animal and human studies. Because of these potential risks, special care is required when handling or administering the drugs. Drugs, drug containers, and administration equipment require special disposal as hazardous waste. Several organizations, including the Occupational Safety and Health Administration (OSHA), the Oncology Nursing Society (ONS), and the American Society of Hospital Pharmacists (ASHP), have developed special guidelines for the safe handling and disposal of antineoplastic drugs as well as for accidental spills and exposure.[79–82]

Epidemiologic studies have shown an increased risk for second malignancies such as acute leukemia after long-term use of alkylating agents, particularly procarbazine, for treatment of various forms of cancer.[76] These second malignancies are thought to result from direct cellular changes produced by the drug or from suppression of the immune response.

Hormonal Therapy

Hormonal therapy consists of administration of drugs designed to disrupt the hormonal environment of cancer cells. It is used for cancers that are responsive to or dependent on hormones for growth.[76,77] The actions of hormones and antihormones depend on the presence of specific receptors in the tumor. Among the tumors that are known to be responsive to hormonal manipulation are those of the breast, prostate, and endometrium. Other cancers, such as Kaposi sarcoma and renal, liver, ovarian, and pancreatic cancer, are also responsive to hormonal manipulation, but to a lesser degree.[83] The theory behind the majority of hormone-based cancer treatments is to deprive the cancer cells of the hormonal signals that otherwise would stimulate them to divide.

The therapeutic options for altering the hormonal environment in the woman with breast cancer or the man with prostate cancer include surgical and pharmacologic measures. Surgery involves the removal of the organ responsible for the hormone production that is stimulating the target tissue (*e.g.,* oophorectomy in women or orchiectomy in men). Pharmacologic methods focus largely on reducing circulating hormone levels or changing the hormone receptors so that they no longer respond to the hormone.

Pharmacologic suppression of circulating hormone levels can be effected through pituitary desensitization, as with the administration of androgens, or through the administration of *gonadotropin-releasing hormone* (GnRH) analogs that act at the level of the hypothalamus to inhibit gonadotropin production and release. Another class of drugs, the *aromatase inhibitors,* is used to treat breast cancer; these drugs act by interrupting the biochemical processes that convert the adrenal androgen androstenedione to estrone.[75,84] Aromatization of an androgenic precursor into an estrogen occurs in body fat. Because estrogen promotes the growth of breast cancer, estrogen synthesis in adipose tissue can be an important factor in breast cancer growth in postmenopausal women.

Hormone receptor function can be altered by the administration of pharmacologic doses of exogenous hormones that act by producing a decrease in hormone receptors, or by antihormone drugs (*i.e.,* antiestrogens [tamoxifen, fulvestrant] and antiandrogens [flutamide, bicalutamide, nilutamide]) that bind to hormone receptors, making them inaccessible to hormone stimulation. Initially, patients often respond favorably to hormonal treatments, but eventually the cancer becomes resistant to hormonal manipulation, and other approaches must be sought to control the disease.

Biotherapy

Biotherapy involves the use of immunotherapy and biologic response modifiers as a means of changing the person's own immune response to cancer.[76,85] The major mechanisms by which biotherapy exerts its effects are modifications of host responses or tumor cell biology.

Immunotherapy. Immunotherapy techniques include active and passive, or adoptive immunotherapy. *Active immunotherapy* involves nonspecific treatments such as bacille Calmette-Guérin (BCG). BCG is an attenuated strain of the bacterium that causes bovine tuberculosis. It acts as a nonspecific stimulant of the immune system and is instilled into the bladder as a means of treating superficial bladder cancer. *Passive* or *adoptive immunotherapy* involves the transfer of cultured immune cells into a tumor-bearing host. Early research efforts with adoptive immunotherapy involved the transfer of sensitized NK cells or T lymphocytes, combined with cytokines, to the tumor-bearing host in an attempt to augment the host's immune response. However, randomized clinical trials demonstrated no benefit from the addition of the cellular component beyond the benefit from the cytokines alone. Further research has focused on using antigen-presenting dendritic cells as delivery vehicles for tumor antigens. Dendritic cells are efficient at activating not only CD4+ helper T cells and CD8+ killer T cells but B cells and innate effectors such as NK cells.[85]

Biologic Response Modifiers. Biologic response modifiers can be grouped into three types: cytokines, which include the interferons and interleukins; monoclonal antibodies; and hematopoietic growth factors. Some agents, such as interferons, have more than one biologic function, including antiviral, immunomodulatory, and antiproliferative actions. The *interferons* are endogenous polypeptides that are synthesized by a number of cells in response to a variety of cellular or viral stimuli. The three major types of interferons are alpha (α), beta (β), and gamma (γ), each group differing in terms of their cell surface receptors.[86] The interferons appear to inhibit viral replication and also may be involved in inhibiting tumor protein synthesis and in prolonging the cell cycle, increasing the percentage of cells in the G_0 phase. Interferons stimulate NK cells and T-lymphocyte killer cells. Interferon-γ has been approved for the treatment of hairy cell leukemia, AIDS-related Kaposi sarcoma, and CML, and as adjuvant therapy for patients at high risk for recurrent melanoma.[86] Interferon-α has been used to treat some solid tumors (*e.g.,* renal cell carcinoma, colorectal cancer, carcinoid tumors, ovarian cancer) and hematologic neoplasms (e.g., B-cell and T-cell lymphomas, cutaneous T-cell lymphoma, and multiple myeloma).[86] Research now is focusing on combining interferons with other forms of cancer therapy and establishing optimal doses and treatment protocols.

The *interleukins* are cytokines that effect communication between cells by binding to receptor sites on the cell surface membranes of the target cells. Of the 18 known interleukins (see Chapter 17), IL-2 has been the most widely studied. A recombinant human IL-2 (rIL-2, aldesleukin) has been approved by the FDA and is currently being used for the treatment of metastatic renal cell carcinoma and metastatic melanoma.[87]

Monoclonal antibodies (MoAbs) are highly specific antibodies (*e.g.,* IgG, which is the most commonly used immunoglobulin) derived from cloned cells or hybridomas.[88,89] Scientists have developed methods for producing large quantities of MoAbs that are specific for tumor cells. For a MoAb to be therapeutic as a cancer treatment modality, a specific target antigen should be present on cancer cells only. There are four types of therapeutic MoAbs that are grouped according to their origin: murine (mouse), chimeric (mixed mouse and human), humanized, and human.[88] Chimeric antibodies essentially splice light- and heavy-chain regions of the murine antibody to human IgG, making a molecule that is 75% human and 25% murine IgG, whereas in a humanized antibody, the short segment of murine antibody that determines its specificity is grafted onto human IgG, making a molecule that is 5% murine.[88] A fully human IgG can be isolated from transgenic mice bred to produce human IgG. There has been recent interest in the development of technology for generating recombinant polyclonal antibodies capable of the multitargeting of tumor cells.[92]

Therapeutic monoclonal antibodies can be unconjugated (*i.e.,* "naked"), conjugated, or combined with a toxin, chemotherapy drug, or radioisotope.[88,90] A number of unconjugated MoAbs are available, including alemtuzumab, a humanized MoAb that targets the CD52 antigen of human B cells, T cells, NK cells, and monocyte-macrophages; rituximab, an anti-CD20 chimeric MoAb; and trastuzumab, a humanized MoAb that binds to the HER-2 receptor (a member of a family of receptor tyrosine kinases).[88,90] Several conjugated MoABs also have FDA approval, including gemtuzumab ozogamicin, a humanized antibody combined with an antitumor antibiotic; ibritumomab tiuxetan, a murine MoAb combined with a radioisotope; and tositumomab, a murine anti-CD20 MoAb bonded to radioactive iodine-131.[88,91]

Targeted Therapy

Targeted cancer therapy uses drugs that selectively attack malignant cells while leaving normal cells unharmed.[88] It focuses on altered molecules and signaling pathways that allow cancer cells to grow and spread in an uncontrolled manner. The first targeted therapies were the MoAbs.

Other targeted therapies include small molecules that block specific enzymes and growth factors involved in cancer cell growth. The protein tyrosine kinases are intrinsic components of the signaling pathways for growth factors involved in the proliferation of lymphocytes and other cell types. Imatinib mesylate (Gleevac) is a protein tyrosine kinase inhibitor indicated in the treatment of CML (see Chapter 15). The epidermal growth factor receptor signaling pathway is an important mediator of cancer cell oncogenesis, proliferation, maintenance, and survival.[89] For this reason, it has long been proposed as a target for an anticancer drug. In the past several years, two agents, gefitinib and erlotinib, have made a significant impact on the understanding of non–small cell lung cancer and treatment options for persons with the neoplasm.[89] Angiogenesis is also being explored as a target for targeted cancer therapy.[88] One of the newly developed antiangiogenic agents, bevacizumab, targets and blocks vascular endothelial growth factor, which is released by many cancers to stimulate proliferation of new blood vessels. The combination of bevacizumab and chemotherapy was found to increase objective responses, median time to progression, and survival time of persons with metastatic colorectal cancer, compared with chemotherapy alone.[88]

Another class of drugs, the apoptosis-inducing drugs, causes cancer cells to undergo apoptosis by interfering with proteins involved the process. Bortezomib is approved by the FDA to treat multiple myeloma that has not responded to other treatments.[88] It causes cancer cells to die by blocking enzymes known as proteosomes, which help regulate cell function and growth.

IN SUMMARY, the methods used in the diagnosis of cancer vary with the type of cancer and its location. Because many cancers are curable if diagnosed early, health care practices designed to promote early detection are important. Histologic studies are done in the laboratory using cells or tissue specimens. There are two basic methods of classifying tumors: grading according to the histologic or tissue characteristics and clinical staging according to spread of the disease. The TNM system for clinical staging of cancer takes into account tumor size, lymph node involvement, and presence of metastasis.

Treatment plans that use more than one type of therapy, often in combination, are providing cures for a number of cancers that a few decades ago had a poor prognosis, and are increasing the life expectancy in other types of cancer. Surgical procedures are more precise and less invasive, preserving organ function and resulting in better quality-of-life outcomes. Newer radiation equipment and novel radiation techniques permit greater and more controlled destruction of cancer cells while sparing normal tissues. Cancer chemotherapy has evolved as one of the major systemic treatment modalities for cancer. Unlike surgery and radiation, chemotherapy is a systemic treatment that enables drugs to reach the site of the tumor as well as other distant sites. The major classifications of chemotherapy drugs are the direct DNA-interacting (alkylating agents, antitumor antibiotics, and topoisomerase inhibitors) and indirect DNA-interacting agents (antimetabolites and mitotic spindle inhibitors). Cancer chemotherapeutic drugs may also be classified as either cell cycle specific or cell cycle nonspecific depending on whether they exert their action during a specific phase of the cell cycle. Other systemic agents include hormonal and molecularly targeted agents that block specific enzymes and growth factors involved in cancer cell growth. ■

CHILDHOOD CANCERS

After completing this section of the chapter, you should be able to meet the following objectives:

- Cite the most common types of cancer affecting infants, children, and adolescents.
- Describe how cancers that affect children differ from those that affect adults.
- Discuss possible long-term effects of radiation therapy and chemotherapy on adult survivors of childhood cancer.

Cancer in children is relatively rare, accounting for about 1% of all malignancies in the United States and Canada.[1,2] Despite progressively improved 5-year survival rates, from 56% in 1974 to 75% in 2000, cancer remains the second leading cause of death among children 1 to 14 years of age in the United States.[1] Leukemia (discussed in Chapter 15) accounts for 30% of the cases of childhood cancer and one third of the expected deaths.[1] Other forms of cancer that occur in children include non-Hodgkin and Hodgkin lymphomas (discussed in Chapter 15), and bone cancers (osteosarcoma and Ewing sarcoma, discussed in Chapter 57).

Incidence and Types

The spectrum of cancers that affect children differs markedly from those that affect adults. Although most adult cancers are of epithelial cell origin (*e.g.,* lung cancer, breast cancer, colorectal cancers), childhood cancers usually involve the hematopoietic system, nervous system, soft tissues, bone, and kidneys.[93] Histologically, many of the childhood cancers tend to have "a more primitive (embryonal) rather than pleomorphic-anaplastic microscopic appearance, are often characterized by sheets of

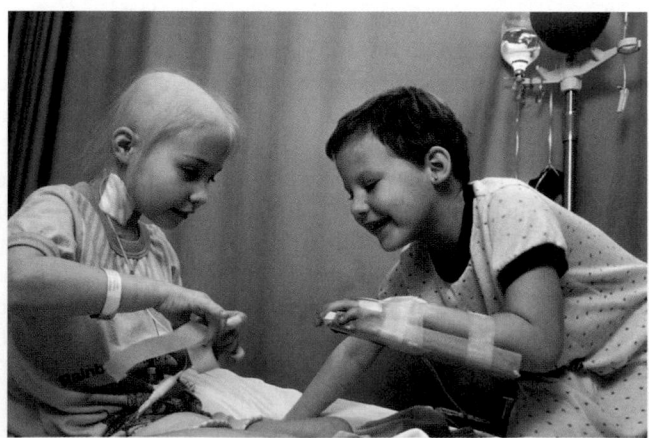

Two young girls with acute lymphocytic leukemia are receiving chemotherapy. (From National Cancer Institute Visuals Online. Available: http://visualsonline.cancer.gov.)

cells, with small round nuclei, and frequently exhibit features of organogenesis specific to the site of origin."[3]

The incidence of childhood cancers is greatest during the first years of life, decreases during middle childhood, and then increases during puberty and adolescence[92–94] (Fig. 8-11). During the first year of life, embryonal tumors such as Wilms tumor, retinoblastoma, and neuroblastoma are among the most common types of tumors. Embryonal tumors along with acute leukemia, non-Hodgkin lymphoma, and gliomas have a peak incidence in children 2 to 5 years of age. As children age, especially after they pass puberty, bone malignancies, Hodgkin lymphoma, gonadal germ cell tumors (testicular and ovarian carcinomas), and various carcinomas such as thyroid cancer and malignant melanoma increase in incidence.

Embryonal Tumors

A number of the tumors of infancy and early childhood are embryonal in origin, meaning that they exhibit features of organogenesis similar to that of embryonic development. Because of this characteristic, these tumors are frequently designated with the suffix "blastoma" (*e.g.,* nephroblastoma [Wilms tumor], retinoblastoma, neuroblastoma).[3] Wilms tumor (discussed in Chapter 33) and neuroblastoma are particularly illustrative of this type of childhood tumor.

Neuroblastoma. Neuroblastomas arise from the primordial neural crest tissue (see Chapter 48) of the sympathetic ganglia and adrenal medulla.[3,92] It is the second most common solid malignancy in childhood after brain tumors, accounting for 7% to 10% of pediatric malignancies and as much as 50% of neoplasms in infancy.[3] About 40% of neuroblastomas arise in the adrenal gland, with the remainder occurring anywhere along the sympathetic chain, most commonly in the paravertebral region

of the abdomen and posterior mediastinum. Tumors may arise in numerous other sites, including the pelvis, neck, and within the brain. Clinical manifestations vary with the primary site and neuroendocrine function of the tumor. In children younger than 2 years of age, neuroblastoma generally presents with large abdominal masses, fever, and possibly weight loss. Bone pain suggests metastatic disease. In neonates, disseminated neuroblastoma may present as multiple cutaneous metastases with deep blue discoloration (sometimes designated as the "blueberry muffin baby").[3,93] About 90% of the tumors, regardless of location, secrete catecholamines, which is an important diagnostic feature (*i.e.,* elevated blood levels of catecholamines and elevated urine levels of catecholamine metabolites).[3]

As a group, these tumors demonstrate certain characteristics such as spontaneous or therapy-induced regression or differentiation to benign tumors.[3,92] Unfortunately, neuroblastoma is also an extremely malignant neoplasm, particularly in children with advanced disease. Although the 5-year survival rate has improved from 25% in the early 1960s to 55% in the mid-1990s, neuroblastoma continues to account for at least 15% of all childhood cancer deaths.[3] Infants tend to have a better prognosis than older children.

Biology of Childhood Cancers

As with adult cancers, there probably is no single cause of childhood cancer. Although a number of genetic conditions are associated with childhood cancer, such conditions are relatively rare, suggesting an interaction between genetic susceptibility and environmental exposures. The most notable heritable conditions that impart susceptibility to childhood cancer include Down syndrome (20- to 30-fold increased risk of acute lymphoblastic leukemia [ALL]),[1] neurofibromatosis (NF) type 1 (neurofibromas, optic gliomas, brain tumors), NF type 2 (acoustic

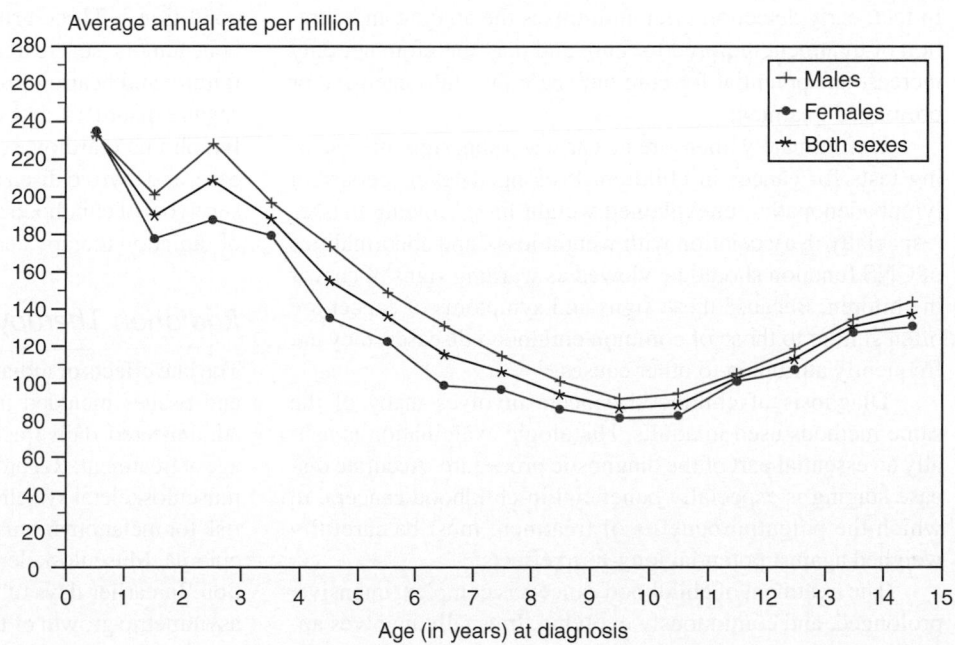

FIGURE 8-11 • Total childhood cancer age-specific incidence rates by sex, all races; data from the Surveillance, Epidemiology and End Results (SEER) Program, 1976–1984 and 1986–1994 combined. (From Gurney J. G., Smith M. A., Rose J. A. *Cancer among infants.* SEER Pediatric Monograph. Bethesda, MD: National Cancer Institute.)

neuroma, meningiomas), xeroderma pigmentosum (skin cancer), ataxia-telangiectasia (lymphoma, leukemia), and the Beckwith-Wiedemann syndrome (Wilms tumor).[3,93]

Although constituting only a small percentage of childhood cancers, the biology of a number of these tumors illustrates several important biologic aspects of neoplasms, such as the two-hit theory of recessive tumor suppressor genes (*e.g., RB* gene mutation in retinoblastoma); defects in DNA repair; and the histologic similarities between organogenesis and oncogenesis. Syndromes associated with defects in DNA repair include xeroderma pigmentosa, in which there is increased risk of skin cancers owing to defects in repair of DNA damaged by ultraviolet light. The development of childhood cancers has also been linked to genomic imprinting, which is characterized by selective inactivation of one of the two alleles of a certain gene.[93] The inactivation is determined by whether the gene is inherited from the mother or father (see Chapter 6). For example, the maternal allele for the insulin-like growth factor-2 (IGF-2) gene normally is inactivated (imprinted). In some Wilms tumors, loss of imprinting (re-expression of the maternal allele) can be demonstrated by overexpression of the IGF-2 protein, which is an embryonal growth factor.[92] The Beckwith-Wiedemann syndrome is an overgrowth syndrome characterized by organomegaly, macroglossia (enlargement of the tongue), hemihypertrophy (muscular or osseous hypertrophy of one side of the body or face), renal abnormalities, and enlarged adrenal cells.[3,93] The syndrome, which reflects changes in the imprinting of IGF-2 genes located on chromosome 11, is also associated with increased risk of Wilms tumor, hepatoblastoma, rhabdomyosarcoma, and adrenal cortical carcinoma.

Diagnosis and Treatment

Because most childhood cancers are curable, early detection is imperative. In addition, there are several types of cancer for which less therapy is indicated than for more advanced disease. In fact, early detection often minimizes the amount and duration of treatment required for cure and may therefore not only increase the potential for cure but spare the child intensive or prolonged treatment.

Unfortunately, there are no early warning signs or screening tests for cancer in children. Prolonged fever, persistent lymphadenopathy, unexplained weight loss, growing masses (especially in association with weight loss), and abnormalities of CNS function should be viewed as warning signs of cancer in children. Because these signs and symptoms of cancer are often similar to those of common childhood diseases, they are frequently attributed to other causes.[93]

Diagnosis of childhood cancers involves many of the same methods used in adults. Histologic examination is usually an essential part of the diagnostic procedure. Accurate disease staging is especially beneficial in childhood cancers, in which the potential benefits of treatment must be carefully weighed against potential long-term effects.

The treatment of childhood cancers is complex, intensive, prolonged, and continuously evolving. It usually involves appropriate multidisciplinary and multimodal therapies, as well as the evaluation for recurrent disease and late effects of the disease and therapies used in its treatment. The treatment program should include specialized teams of health care providers with expertise in pediatric cancer care, such as pediatric oncologists, pathologists, radiologists, surgeons, nurses, and support staff, including nutritionists, social workers, psychologists, pharmacists, and other specialists.[93]

Two modalities are frequently used in the treatment of childhood cancer, with chemotherapy being the most widely used, followed, in order of use, by surgery, radiation therapy, and biologic agent therapy. Chemotherapy is more widely used in treatment of children with cancer than in adults because children better tolerate the acute adverse effects and, in general, pediatric tumors are more responsive to chemotherapy than adult cancers.[92] Radiation therapy tends to be used sparingly in children because they are more vulnerable to the late adverse effects.[93] As with care of adults, adequate pain management is critical.

Adult Survivors of Childhood and Adolescent Cancer

With improvement in treatment methods, the number of children who survive childhood cancer continues to increase. As a result of cancer treatment, almost 80% of children and adolescents with a diagnosis of cancer become long-term survivors.[1] Unfortunately, therapy may produce late sequelae, such as impaired growth, neurologic dysfunction, hormonal dysfunction, cardiomyopathy, pulmonary fibrosis, and risk for second malignancies. Thus, one of the growing challenges is providing appropriate health care to survivors of childhood and adolescent cancers.

In a large, retrospective cohort study that tracked the health status of 10,397 adult survivors of childhood cancer who were treated in the 1970s and 1980s and compared the results with 3034 of their siblings, it was found that 62% had at least one chronic health problem and 28% had a severe or life-threatening condition.[95] Three groups were at highest risk: survivors of bone tumors (severe musculoskeletal problems, congestive heart failure, and hearing loss), CNS tumors (cognitive impairment, seizure disorders, and various endocrinopathies), and Hodgkin lymphoma (cardiovascular disease, second cancers, lung disease, and thyroid disease). Many of the health problems of adult survivors of childhood cancer can be attributed to the late effects of radiation therapy and chemotherapy.

Radiation Therapy

The late effects of radiation therapy are influenced by the organs and tissues included in the treatment field, type of radiation administered, daily fractional and cumulative radiation dose, and age at treatment. Regardless of the region irradiated, the skin and musculoskeletal system are often involved.[96] There is increased risk for melanoma, squamous cell carcinoma, and basal cell carcinoma. Musculoskeletal changes are also common after radiation. In earlier days of radiation therapy, this often resulted in asymmetric growth of the spine and other structures. Even with current methods, survivors may have changes leading to pain and altered musculoskeletal function.

Cranial radiation therapy (CRT) has been used to treat brain tumors, ALL, head and neck soft tissue tumors, and retinoblastoma. The most common late effect of moderate- to high-dose whole-brain radiation is diminished intellectual function.[95] Brain tumor survivors treated at a younger age are particularly susceptible. Cranial radiation is also associated with neuroendocrine disorders, particularly growth hormone deficiency. Thus, children reaching adulthood after CRT may have reduced physical stature. The younger the age and the higher the radiation dose, the greater the deviation from normal growth. Growth hormone deficiency in adults is associated with increased prevalence of dyslipidemia, insulin resistance, and cardiovascular mortality. Moderate doses of CRT are also associated with obesity, particularly in female patients.[95] For many years, whole-brain radiation or CRT was the primary method of preventing CNS relapse in children with ALL. Recognition of cognitive dysfunction associated with CRT has led to the use of other methods of CNS prophylaxis.[95]

Radiation to the chest or mantle field (lymph nodes of neck, subclavicular, axillary, and mediastinal areas) is often used in treatment of Hodgkin and non-Hodgkin lymphomas and metastases to the lung. This field exposes the developing breast tissue, heart, and lungs to ionizing radiation. Female survivors who were treated with this type of radiation face significant risk for development of breast cancer.[95] Much of the heart is exposed in chest and mantle radiation fields, resulting in subsequent premature coronary artery, valvular, and pericardial disease. Exposure of the lungs to radiation therapy can result in a reduction in pulmonary function. Thyroid disease, particularly hypothyroidism, is common after mantle or neck radiation.

Childhood cancer survivors treated with abdominal or pelvic radiation are also at risk for a variety of late health problems involving the gastrointestinal tract, liver, spleen, kidneys, and genitourinary tract structures, including the gonads.[95] Gastrointestinal tract complications include chronic mucosal inflammation that interferes with absorption and digestion of nutrients. Chronic radiation injury to the kidneys may interfere with glomerular or tubular function, and fibrosis from pelvic radiation may adversely affect bladder capacity and function. The adverse effects of radiation on gonadal function vary by age, sex, and cumulative dose. Delayed sexual maturation in boys and girls can result from irradiation of the gonads. In boys, sperm production is reduced in a dose-dependent manner. In girls, radiation to the abdomen, pelvis, and spine is associated with increased risk of ovarian failure, especially if the ovaries are in the treatment field.

Chemotherapy

Chemotherapy also poses the risk of long-term effects for survivors of childhood cancer. Potential late effects of alkylating agents include dose-related gonadal injury (hypogonadism, infertility, and early menopause).[95] Alkylating agent therapy has also been linked to dose-related secondary acute myelogenous leukemia, pulmonary fibrosis, kidney disease, and bladder dis-

orders. Anthracyclines, including doxorubicin and daunomycin, which are widely used in treatment of childhood cancers, can result in cardiomyopathy and eventual congestive heart failure.[95] The late effects of cisplatin and carboplatin, the most frequently used nonclassic alkylators, are nephrotoxicity, ototoxicity, and neurotoxicity. Although combination chemotherapy increases the effectiveness of treatment, it may also be associated with increased risk of side effects if the agents have a similar spectrum of toxicity. Intrathecal combination chemotherapy to prevent relapse of ALL in the CNS, which is a sanctuary for ALL cells, is known to cause significant and persistent cognitive impairment in many children.

IN SUMMARY, although most adult cancers are of epithelial cell origin, most childhood cancers usually involve the hematopoietic system, nervous system, or connective tissue. Heritable forms of cancer tend to have an earlier age of onset, a higher frequency of multifocal lesions in a single organ, and bilateral involvement of paired organs or multiple primary tumors. The early diagnosis of childhood cancers often is missed because the signs and symptoms mimic those of other childhood diseases. With improvement in treatment methods, the number of children who survive childhood cancer is continuing to increase. As these children approach adulthood, there is continued concern that the life-saving therapy they received during childhood may produce late effects, such as impaired growth, cognitive dysfunction, hormonal dysfunction, cardiomyopathy, pulmonary fibrosis, and risk for second malignancies. ■

Review Exercises

1. A 30-year-old woman has experienced heavy menstrual bleeding and is told she has a uterine tumor called a *leiomyoma*. She is worried she has cancer.

   A. *What is the difference between a leiomyoma and leiomyosarcoma?*

   B. *How would you explain the difference to her?*

2. Among the characteristics of cancer cells are lack of cell differentiation, impaired cell-to-cell adhesion, and loss of anchorage dependence.

   A. *Explain how each of these characteristics contributes to the usefulness of the Pap smear as a screening test for cervical cancer.*

3. A 12-year-old boy is seen at the pediatric cancer clinic with osteosarcoma. His medical history reveals that his father had been successfully treated for retinoblastoma as an infant.

   A. *Relate the genetics of the RB gene and the "two-hit" hypothesis to the development of osteosarcoma in this boy.*

4. A 48-year-old man presents at his health care clinic with complaints of leg weakness. He is a heavy smoker and has had a productive cough for years. Subsequent diagnostic tests reveal he has a small cell lung cancer with brain metastasis. His proposed plan of treatment includes chemotherapy and radiation therapy.

   A. *What is the probable cause of the leg weakness, and is it related to the lung cancer?*

   B. *Relate this man's smoking history to the development of lung cancer.*

   C. *Explain the mechanism of cancer metastasis.*

   D. *Explain the mechanisms whereby chemotherapy and irradiation are able to destroy cancer cells while having a lesser or no effect on normal cells.*

5. A 17-year-old-girl is seen by a guidance counselor at her high school because of problems in keeping up with assignments in her math and science courses. She tells the counselor that she had leukemia when she was 2 years old and was given radiation treatment to the brain. She confides that she has always had more trouble with learning than her classmates and thinks it might be due to the radiation. She also relates that she is shorter than her classmates, and this has been bothering her.

   A. *Explain the relationship between cranial radiation therapy and decreased cognitive function and short stature.*

   B. *What other neuroendocrine problems might this girl have as a result of the radiation treatment?*

References

1. Jemal A., Siegel R., Ward E., et al. (2007). Cancer statistics, 2007. *CA: A Cancer Journal for Clinicians* 57, 43–66.

2. Marrett L., Logan H., Les Mery M., et al. (2007). *Canadian cancer statistics—2007.* Toronto, Canada: Canadian Cancer Society/National Cancer Institute of Canada.

3. Kumar V., Abbas A. K., Fausto N. (Eds.). (2005). *Robbins and Cotran pathologic basis of disease* (7th ed., pp. 11–20, 87–111, 269–342, 499–506, 1136–1137). Philadelphia: Elsevier Saunders.

4. Reed S. I. (2005). Molecular targets in cancer: The cell cycle. In DeVita V. T. Jr., Hellman S., Rosenberg S. A. (Eds.), *Cancer: Principles and practice of oncology* (7th ed., pp. 83–94). Philadelphia: Lippincott Williams & Wilkins.

5. Lee W. M. F., Dang C. V. (2000). Control of cell growth and differentiation. In Hoffman R., Benz E. K., Shattil S. J., et al. (Eds.), *Hematology: Basic principles and practice* (3rd ed., pp. 57–71). New York: Churchill Livingstone.

6. Fung T. K., Poon R. Y. C. (2005). A roller coaster ride with the mitotic cyclins. *Seminars in Cell and Developmental Biology* 16, 335–342.

7. Fischer P. M., Gianella-Borradori A. (2005). Recent progress in the discovery and development of cyclin-dependent kinase inhibitors. *Expert Opinion on Investigational Drugs* 14, 457–477.

8. Li L., Xie T. (2005). Stem cell niche: Structure and function. *Annual Review of Cell and Developmental Biology* 21, 605–631.

9. Giordano A., De Falco G., Rubin E., et al. (2008). Neoplasia. In Rubin R., Strayer D. S. (Eds.), *Rubin's pathology: Clinicopathologic foundations of medicine* (5th ed., pp. 137–176). Philadelphia: Lippincott Williams & Wilkins.

10. Loeb K. R., Loeb L. A. (1999). Genetic instability and the mutator phenotype: Studies in ulcerative colitis. *American Journal of Pathology* 154, 1621–1626.

11. Pani G., Colavitti R., Bedogni B., et al. (2000). A redox signaling mechanism for density-dependent inhibition of cell growth. *Journal of Biological Chemistry* 49, 38891–38899.

12. Zhang L., Bewick M., Lafrenie R. M. (2002). Role of Raf-1 and FAK in cell density-dependent regulation of integrin-dependent activation of MAP kinase. *Carcinogenesis* 23, 1251–1258.

13. Hayashida Y., Honda K., Idogawa M., et al. (2005). E-cadherin regulates the association between β-catenin and actinin-4. *Cancer Research* 65, 8836–8845.

14. Shen Y., Jia Z., Nagele R. G., et al. (2006). Src uses Cas to suppress Fhl1 in order to promote nonanchored growth and migration of tumor cells. *Cancer Research* 66, 1543–1552.

15. Carruba G., Webber M. M., Quader S. T. A., et al. (2002). Regulation of cell-to-cell communication in non-tumorigenic and malignant human prostate epithelial cells. *The Prostate* 50, 73–82.

16. Marutsuka T., Shimada S., Shiomori K., et al. (2003). Mechanisms of peritoneal metastasis after operation for non-serosa-invasive gastric carcinoma: An ultrarapid detection system for intraperitoneal free cancer cells and a prophylactic strategy for peritoneal metastasis. *Clinical Cancer Research* 9, 678–685.

17. Stetler-Stevenson W. G. (2005). Molecular biology of cancer: Invasion and metastasis. In DeVita V. T. Jr., Hellman S., Rosenberg S. A. (Eds.), *Cancer: Principles and practice of oncology* (7th ed., pp. 113–126). Philadelphia: Lippincott Williams & Wilkins.

18. Tobler N. E., Detmar M. (2006). Tumor and lymph node lymphangiogenesis: Impact on cancer metastasis. *Journal of Leukocyte Biology* 8, 691–696.

19. Chen S. L., Iddings D. M., Scheri R., et al. (2006). Lymphatic mapping and sentinel node analysis: Current concepts and applications. *CA: Cancer Journal for Clinicians* 56, 292–307.

20. Liotta L. A. (1992). Cancer cell invasion and metastasis. *Scientific American* 266(2), 54–63.

21. Allinen M., Beroukhim R., Cai L., et al. (2004). Molecular characterization of the tumor microenvironment in breast cancer. *Cancer Cell* 6, 17–32.

22. Yaeger T. E., Brady L. W. (2001). Basis for current major therapies in cancer. In Lenhard R. E., Osteen R. T., Gansler T. (Eds.), *The American Cancer Society's clinical oncology* (pp. 159–229). Atlanta: American Cancer Society.

23. Zhou B. P., Hung M. C. (2003). Dysregulation of cellular signaling by HER2/neu in breast cancer. *Seminars in Oncology* 30(5 Suppl. 16), 38–48.

24. Knudson A. G. (2001). Two genetic hits (more or less). *Nature Reviews Cancer* 1, 157–162.

25. Baylin S. B. (2005). DNA methylation and gene silencing in cancer. *Nature Clinical Practice Oncology* 2, S4–S11.

26. Heath C. W., Fontham E. T. (2001). Cancer etiology. In Lenhard R. E., Osteen R. T., Gansler T. (Eds.), *American Cancer Society's clinical oncology* (9th ed., pp. 38–54). Atlanta: American Cancer Society.

27. Schulze-Bergkamen H., Krammer P. H. (2004). Apoptosis in cancer: Implications for therapy. *Seminars in Oncology* 31, 90–119.

28. Feldser D. M., Grieder C. W. (2007). Short telomeres limit tumor progression in vivo by inducing senescence. *Cancer Cell* 11, 461–469.

29. Sedivy J. M. (2007). Telomeres limit cancer growth by inducing senescence: Long-sought in vivo evidence obtained. *Cancer Cell* 11, 389–391.

30. Yang Z.-J., Wechsler-Reya R. J. (2007). Hit 'em where they live: Targeting the cancer stem cell. *Cancer Cell* 11, 3–5.

31. Boccaccio C., Comoglio P. M. (2006). Invasive growth: A MET-driven genetic programme for cancer and stem cells. *Nature Reviews Cancer* 6, 637–645.

32. Bierie B., Moses H. L. (2006). TGFβ: The molecular Jekyll and Hyde. *Nature Reviews Cancer* 6, 506–520.

33. Colditz G., Wolin K. Y. (2005). Physical activity and body weight. In DeVita V. T. Jr., Hellman S., Rosenberg S. A. (Eds.), *Cancer: Principles and practice of oncology* (7th ed., pp. 549–554). Philadelphia: Lippincott Williams & Wilkins.

34. Burnett F. M. (1967). Immunologic aspects of malignant disease. *Lancet* 1, 1171.

35. Stellman J. M., Stellman S. D. (1996). Cancer and the workplace. *CA: A Cancer Journal for Clinicians* 46, 70–92.

36. American Cancer Society. (2003). *American Cancer Society facts and figures: 2003*. Atlanta: Author.

37. Willett W. C. (2001). Cancer prevention: Diet and chemopreventive agents. In DeVita V. T. Jr., Hellman S., Rosenberg S. A. (Eds.), *Cancer: Principles and practice of oncology* (6th ed., pp. 561–614). Philadelphia: Lippincott Williams & Wilkins.

38. Seitz H. K., Stickel F. (2007). Molecular mechanisms of alcohol-mediated carcinogenesis. *Nature Reviews Cancer* 7, 599–612.

39. Poskanzer D. C., Herbst A. (1977). Epidemiology of vaginal adenosis and adenocarcinoma associated with exposure to stilbestrol in utero. *Cancer* 39, 1892–1895.

40. Jablon S., Kato H. (1972). Studies of the mortality of A-bomb survivors: 5. Radiation dose and mortality, 1950–1970. *Radiation Research* 50, 649–698.

41. Ruddon R. W. (Ed.). (1995). *Cancer biology* (pp. 3–60, 141–276). New York: Oxford University Press.

42. Howley P. M., Ganem D., Kieff E. (2005). Etiology of cancer: Viruses. In DeVita V. T. Jr., Hellman S., Rosenberg S. A. (Eds.), *Cancer: Principles and practice of oncology* (7th ed., pp. 173–183). Philadelphia: Lippincott Williams & Wilkins.

43. Centers for Disease Control and Prevention. (2006). HPV vaccine questions and answers. [Online.] Available: www.cdc.gov/std/hpv/STDFact-HPV-vaccine.htm#hpvvac1. Accessed April 25, 2008.

44. Rugo H. S. (2007). Cancer. In McPhee S. J., Papadakis M. A., Tierney L. M. Jr. (Eds.), *Current medical diagnosis and treatment* (46th ed., pp. 1670–1766). New York: McGraw-Hill.

45. Davidson B., Risberg B., Reich R., et al. (2003). Effusion cytology in ovarian cancer: New molecular methods as aids to diagnosis and prognosis. *Clinics in Laboratory Medicine* 23, 729–754.

46. Imui A. (2002). Cancer anorexia-cachexia syndrome: Current issues in research and management. *CA: Cancer Journal for Clinicians* 52, 72–91.

47. Lagman R. L., Davis M. P., LeGrand S. B., et al. (2005). Common symptoms of advanced cancer. *Surgical Clinics of North America* 85, 237–255.

48. Rubin H. (2003). Cancer cachexia: Its correlations and causes. *Proceedings of the National Academy of Science* 100, 5384–5389.

49. Gordon J. N., Green S. R., Goggin P. M. (2005). Cancer cachexia. *Quarterly Journal of Medicine* 98, 779–788.

50. Tisdale M. J. (2005). Molecular pathways leading to cancer cachexia. *Physiology* 20, 340–348.

51. Patrick D. L., Ferketich S. L., Frame P. S., et al., National Institutes of Health State-of-the-Science Panel. (2004). National Institutes of Health State-of-the Science Conference Statement: Symptom management in cancer: pain, depression, and fatigue, July 15–17, 2002. *Journal of the National Cancer Institute* 95, 1110–1117.

52. Ryan J. L., Carroll J. K., Ryan E. P., et al. (2007). Mechanisms of cancer-related fatigue. *Oncologist* 12(Suppl. 1), 22–34.

53. Hofman M., Ryan J. L., Comar D., et al. (2007). Cancer-related fatigue: The scale of the problem. *Oncologist* 12(Suppl. 1), 4–10.

54. Roscoe J. A., Kaufman M. E., Matteson-Rusby S. E., et al. (2007). Cancer-related fatigue and sleep disorders. *Oncologist* 12(Suppl. 1), 35–42.

55. Knight K., Wade S., Balducci L. (2004). Prevalence and outcomes of anemia in cancer: A systematic review of the literature. *American Journal of Medicine* 116(Suppl. 7A), 11S–26S.

56. Hurter B., Bush N. J. (2007). Cancer-related anemia: Clinical review and management update. *Clinical Journal of Oncology Nursing* 11, 349–359.

57. Arnold S. M., Lieberman F. S., Foon K. A. (2005). Paraneoplastic syndromes. In DeVita V. T. Jr., Hellman S., Rosenberg S. A. (Eds.), *Cancer: Principles and practice of oncology* (7th ed., pp. 2191–2210). Philadelphia: Lippincott Williams & Wilkins.

58. Rosenthal P. E. (2001). Paraneoplastic and endocrine syndromes. In Lenhard R. E., Osteen R. T., Gansler T. (Eds.), *The American Cancer Society's clinical oncology* (pp. 721–732). Atlanta: American Cancer Society.

59. Shoback D., Funk J. (2004). Humoral manifestations of malignancy. In Greenspan F. S., Gardner D. G. (Eds.), *Basic and clinical endocrinology* (7th ed., 814–841). New York: McGraw-Hill.

60. Darnell R. B., Posner J. B. (2003). Paraneoplastic syndromes involving the nervous system. *New England Journal of Medicine* 349, 1543–1554.

61. de Beukelarr J. W., Smitt P. A. S. (2006). Managing paraneoplastic neurologic disorders. *Oncologist* 11, 292–305.

62. Miser W. F. (2007). Cancer screening in the primary care setting. *Primary Care Clinics in Office Practice* 34, 137–167.

63. Smith R. A., Eyre H. J. (2007). Cancer screening in the United States, 2007: A review of current guidelines. *CA: Cancer Journal for Clinicians* 57, 90–104.

64. Pfiefer J. D., Wick M. R. (2001). Pathologic evaluation of neoplastic diseases. In Lenhard R. E., Osteen R. T., Gansler T. (Eds.), *The American Cancer Society's clinical oncology* (pp. 123–147). Atlanta: American Cancer Society.

65. Green F. L., Page D. L., Fleming I. D. (2002). *AJCC cancer staging manual* (6th ed). New York: Springer-Verlag.

66. Rosenberg S. A. (2005). Cancer management: Principles of surgical oncology. In DeVita V. T. Jr., Hellman S., Rosenberg S. A. (Eds.), *Cancer: Principles and practice of oncology* (7th ed., pp. 243–252). Philadelphia: Lippincott Williams & Wilkins.

67. Bland K. B. (1997). Quality-of-life management for cancer patients. *CA: Cancer Journal for Clinicians* 47, 194–197.

68. Jeremic B. (2004). Radiation therapy. *Hematology/Oncology Clinics of North America* 18, 1–12.

69. Hahn S. M., Gladstein E. (2005). Principles of radiation therapy. In Kasper D. L., Fauci A. S., Longo D. L., et al. (eds.), *Harrison's principles of internal medicine* (16th ed. pp. 482–489). New York: McGraw-Hill.

70. Willers H., Held K. D. (2006). Introduction to clinical radiation biology. *Hematology/Oncology Clinics of North America* 20, 1–24.

71. Thomas C. T., Ammar A., Farrell J. J., et al. (2006). Radiation modifiers: Treatment overview and future investigations. *Hematology/Oncology Clinics of North America* 20, 119–139.

72. Smith R. P., Heron D. E., Huq M. S., et al. (2006). Modern radiation therapy: Treatment planning and delivery—From Röntgen to real time. *Hematology/Oncology Clinics of North America* 20, 45–62.

73. Bucci M. K., Bevan A., Roach M. III. (2005). Advances in radiation therapy: Conventional to 3D, to IMRT, to 4D, and beyond. *CA: Cancer Journal for Clinicians* 55, 117–134.

74. Patel R. R., Arthur D. W. (2006). The emergence of advanced brachytherapy techniques for common malignancies. *Hematology/Oncology Clinics of North America* 20, 97–118.

75. Cooper M. R., Cooper M. R. (2001). Basis for current major therapies for cancer: Systemic therapy. In Lenhard R. E., Osteen R. T., Gansler T (Eds.), *The American Cancer Society's clinical oncology* (pp. 175–215). Atlanta: American Cancer Society.

76. Chu E., Sartorelli A. C. (2007). Cancer chemotherapy. In Katzung B. G. (Ed.), *Basic and clinical pharmacology* (10th ed., pp. 878–907). New York: McGraw-Hill.

77. Sausville E. A., Longo D. L. (2005). Principles of cancer treatment: Surgery, chemotherapy, and biologic therapy. In Kasper D. L., Fauci A. S., Longo D. L., et al. (Eds.), *Harrison's principles of internal medicine* (16th ed., pp. 464–482). New York: McGraw-Hill.

78. Torchilin V. P. (2007). Targeted pharmaceutical nanocarriers for cancer therapy and imaging. *AAPS Journal* 9(2), E128–E146.

79. Schnell F. M. (2003). Chemotherapy-induced nausea and vomiting: The importance of acute antiemetic control. *Oncologist* 8, 187–198.

80. Lindley C. (2005). Neoplastic disorders. In Koda-Kimble M. A., Young L. Y., Kradjan W. A., et al. (Eds.), *Applied therapeutics: The clinical use of drugs* (8th ed., pp.. 88-31–88-33, 89-1–89-40). Philadelphia: Lippincott Williams & Wilkins.

81. U.S. Department of Labor, Office of Occupational Medicine, Occupational Safety and Health Administration (OSHA). (1986). *Work practice guidelines for personnel dealing with cytotoxic (antineoplastic) drugs.* Publication no. 8-1.1. Washington, DC: Author.

82. Polovich M. (2003). *Safe handling of hazardous drugs.* Pittsburgh: Oncology Nursing Society.

83. Hawkins R. (2002). Hormone therapy in cancer. *Oncology Nursing Updates* 9(3), 1–16.

84. Altundag K., Ibrahim N. K. (2006). Aromatase inhibitors in breast cancer: An overview. *Oncologist* 11, 553–562.

85. Reiger P. T. (2001). Biotherapy: An overview. In Reiger P. T. (Ed.), *Biotherapy: A comprehensive overview* (2nd ed., pp. 3–37) Sudbury, MA: Jones and Bartlett.

86. Sondak V. K., Redman B. G. (2005). Interferons. In DeVita V. T. Jr., Hellman S., Rosenberg S. A. (Eds.), *Cancer: Principles and practice of oncology* (7th ed., pp. 423–430). Philadelphia: Lippincott Williams & Wilkins.

87. Mier J. W., Atkins M. B. (2005). Interleukin-2. In DeVita V. T. Jr., Hellman S., Rosenberg S. A. (Eds.), *Cancer: Principles and practice of oncology* (7th ed., pp. 431–438). Philadelphia: Lippincott Williams & Wilkins.

88. Sharkey R. M., Goldenberg D. M. (2006). Targeted therapy of cancer: New prospects for antibodies and immunoconjugates. *CA: Cancer Journal for Clinicians* 56, 226–243.

89. Marshall J. (2006). Clinical implications of the mechanism of epidermal growth factor receptor inhibitors. *Cancer* 107, 1207–1218.

90. Von Mehren M., Adams G. P., Weiner L. M. (2003). Monoclonal antibody therapy for cancer. *Annual Review of Medicine* 54, 343–369.

91. Schmidt K. V., Wood B. A. (2003). Trends in cancer therapy: Role of monoclonal antibodies. *Seminars in Oncology Nursing* 19, 169–179.

92. Sharon J., Liebman M. A., Williams B. R. (2005). Recombinant polyclonal antibodies for cancer treatment. *Journal of Cell Biochemistry* 96(2), 305–313.

93. Behrman R. E., Kliegman R. M., Jenson H. B. (Eds.). (2004). *Nelson textbook of pediatrics* (17th ed., pp. 1679–1693, 1709–1711). Philadelphia: Elsevier Saunders.

94. Ries L. A. G., Smith M. A., Gurney J. G., et al. (Eds.). (1999). Cancer incidence and survival among children and adolescents: United States SEER program 1975–1995. Bethesda, MD: National Cancer Institute, SEER Program. [Online.] Available: http://seer.cancer.gov/publications/childhood/. Accessed April 25, 2008.

95. Oeffinger K. C., Mertens A. C., Sklar C. A., et al. (2006). Chronic health conditions in adult survivors of childhood cancer. *New England Journal of Medicine* 355, 1572–1582.

96. Oeffinger K. C., Hudson M. M. (2004). Long-term complications following childhood and adolescent cancer: Foundations for providing risk-based health care for survivors. *CA: Cancer Journal for Clinicians* 54, 208–236.

Visit thePoint **http://thePoint.lww.com for animations, journal articles, and more!**

Disorders of Integrative Function

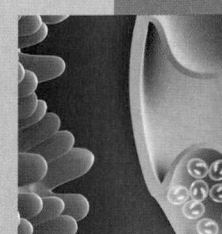

French physiologist Claude Bernard (1813–1878) was the first to theorize that, in a closely orchestrated process, the body strives to achieve and maintain a steady state. In the middle of the 19th century, Bernard proposed his concept of the *milieu intérieur*, or the stable internal environment, regulated by a multitude of interacting control mechanisms geared to maintain the body's chemical and physical status. He proposed that internal secretions functioned as a part of the body's regulatory mechanism, maintaining a balance in response to a range of changing conditions imposed by the external environment.

Through his experiments, Bernard discovered a number of mechanisms that were dedicated to maintaining homeostasis. One of his discoveries was the process by which internal temperature is kept constant. He was able to show that the nervous system responds to internal cold by sending chemical messages to the blood vessels to constrict in order to conserve body heat. The product of his considerable work is the classic *Introduction to the Study of Experimental Medicine* (1865).

9

Stress and Adaptation

MARY PAT KUNERT

➤ Stress has become an increasingly discussed topic in today's world. The concept is discussed extensively in the health care fields, and it is found as well in economics, political science, business, and education. In the popular press, the physiologic response to stress is often implicated as a contributor to a variety of individual physical and mental challenges and societal problems.

Whether stress is more prevalent today than it was in centuries past is uncertain. Certainly, the pressures that existed in the past were equally challenging, although of a different type. Social psychologists Richard Lazarus and Susan Folkman related that as early as the 14th century the term was used to indicate hardship, straits, adversity, or affliction.[1] In the 17th century, *stress* and related terms appeared in the context of physical sciences: *load* was defined as an external force, *stress* as the ratio of internal force created by the load to the area over which the force acted, and *strain* was the deformation or distortion of the object.[1] These concepts are still used in engineering today.

The concepts of stress and strain survived, and throughout the 19th and early 20th centuries, stress and strain were thought to be the cause of "ill health" and "mental disease."[2] By the 20th century, stress had drawn considerable attention both as a health concern and as a research focus. In 1910, when Sir William Osler delivered his Lumleian Lectures on "Angina Pectoris," he described the relationship of stress and strain to angina pectoris.[3] Approximately 15 years later, Walter Cannon, well known for his work in physiology, began to use the word *stress* in relation to his laboratory experiments on the "fight-or-flight" response. It seems possible that the term emerged from his work on the homeostatic features of living organisms and their tendency to "bound back" and "resist disruption" when acted on by an "external force."[4] At about the same time, Hans Selye, who became known for his research and publications on stress, began using the term *stress* in a very special way to mean an orchestrated set of bodily responses to any form of noxious stimulus.[5]

The content in this chapter has been organized into three sections: homeostasis, the stress response and adaptation to stress, and disorders of the stress response.

HOMEOSTASIS

After completing this section of the chapter, you should be able to meet the following objectives:

- Cite Cannon's four features of homeostasis.
- Describe the components of a control system, including the function of a negative feedback system.

The concepts of stress and adaptation have their origin in the complexity of the human body and the interactions between the body cells and its many organ systems. These interactions require that a level of homeostasis or constancy be maintained during the many changes that occur in the internal and external environments. In effecting a state of constancy, homeostasis requires feedback control systems that regulate cellular function and integrate the function of the different body systems.

HOMEOSTASIS

- Homeostasis is the purposeful maintenance of a stable internal environment by coordinated physiologic processes that oppose change.
- The physiologic control systems that oppose change operate by negative feedback mechanisms consisting of a sensor that detects a change, an integrator/comparator that sums and compares incoming data with a set point, and an effector system that returns the sensed function to within the range of the set point.

Constancy of the Internal Environment

The environment in which body cells live is not the external environment that surrounds the organism, but rather the local fluid environment that surrounds each cell. Claude Bernard, a 19th century physiologist, was the first to describe clearly the central importance of a stable internal environment, which he termed the *milieu intérieur.* Bernard recognized that body fluids surrounding the cells and the various organ systems provide the means for exchange between the external and the internal environments. It is from this internal environment that body cells receive their nourishment, and it is into this fluid that they secrete their wastes. Even the contents of the gastrointestinal tract and lungs do not become part of the internal environment until they have been absorbed into the extracellular fluid. A multicellular organism is able to survive only as long as the composition of the internal environment is compatible with the survival needs of the individual cells. For example, even a small change in the pH of the body fluids can disrupt the metabolic processes of the individual cells.

The concept of a stable internal environment was supported by Walter B. Cannon, who proposed that this kind of stability, which he called *homeostasis,* was achieved through a system of carefully coordinated physiologic processes that oppose change.[6] Cannon pointed out that these processes were largely automatic and emphasized that homeostasis involves resistance to both internal and external disturbances (Box 9-1).

In his book *Wisdom of the Body,* published in 1939, Cannon presented four tentative propositions to describe the general features of homeostasis.[6] With this set of propositions, Cannon emphasized that when a factor is known to shift homeostasis in one direction, it is reasonable to expect the existence of mechanisms that have the opposite effect. In the homeostatic regulation of blood sugar, for example, mechanisms that both raise and lower blood sugar would be expected to play a part. As long as the responding mechanism to the initiating disturbance can recover homeostasis, the integrity of the body and the status of normality are retained.

Control Systems

The ability of the body to function and maintain homeostasis under conditions of change in the internal and external environment depends on the thousands of physiologic *control systems* that regulate body function. A homeostatic control system consists of a collection of interconnected components that

---

BOX 9-1 CONSTANCY OF THE INTERNAL ENVIRONMENT

1. Constancy in an open system, such as our bodies represent, requires mechanisms that act to maintain this constancy. Cannon based this proposition on insights into the ways by which steady states such as glucose concentrations, body temperature, and acid-base balance were regulated.
2. Steady-state conditions require that any tendency toward change automatically meets with factors that resist change. An increase in blood sugar results in thirst as the body attempts to dilute the concentration of sugar in the extracellular fluid.
3. The regulating system that determines the homeostatic state consists of a number of cooperating mechanisms acting simultaneously or successively. Blood sugar is regulated by insulin, glucagon, and other hormones that control its release from the liver or its uptake by the tissues.
4. Homeostasis does not occur by chance, but is the result of organized self-government.

(Cannon W. B. [1932]. *The wisdom of the body* (pp. 299–300). New York: W.W. Norton)

function to keep a physical or chemical parameter of the body relatively constant. The body's control systems regulate cellular function, control life processes, and integrate functions of the different organ systems.

Of recent interest have been the neuroendocrine control systems that influence behavior. Biochemical messengers that exist in our brain serve to control nerve activity, regulate information flow, and, ultimately, influence behavior.[7] These control systems mediate the physical, emotional, and behavioral reactions to stressors that, taken together, are called the *stress response.*

Feedback Systems

Most control systems in the body operate by *negative feedback mechanisms,* which function in a manner similar to the thermostat on a heating system. When the monitored function or value decreases below the set point of the system, the feedback mechanism causes the function or value to increase; and when the function or value is increased above the set point, the feedback mechanism causes it to decrease (Fig. 9-1). For example, in the negative feedback mechanism that controls blood glucose levels, an increase in blood glucose stimulates an increase in insulin, which enhances the removal of glucose from the blood. When glucose has been taken up by cells and blood glucose levels fall, insulin secretion is inhibited and glucagon and other counter-regulatory mechanisms stimulate the release of glucose from the liver, which causes the blood glucose to return to normal.

The reason most physiologic control systems function under negative rather than *positive feedback mechanisms* is that a positive feedback mechanism interjects instability rather than stability into a system. It produces a cycle in which the initiating stimulus produces more of the same. For example, in a positive feedback system, exposure to an increase in environmental temperature would invoke compensatory mechanisms designed to increase rather than decrease body temperature.

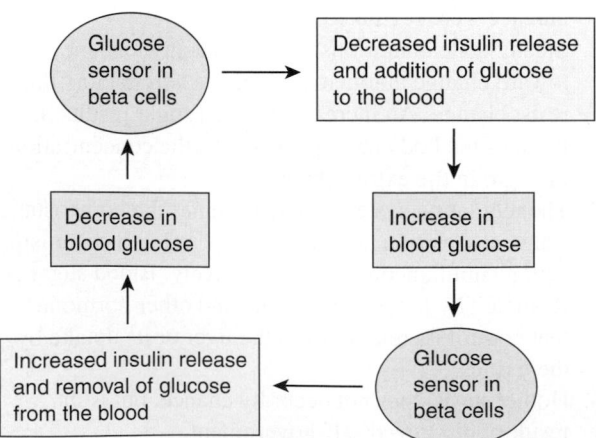

FIGURE 9-1 • Illustration of negative feedback control mechanisms using blood glucose as an example.

IN SUMMARY, physiologic and psychological adaptation involves the ability to maintain the constancy of the internal environment (homeostasis) and behavior in the face of a wide range of changes in the internal and external environments. It involves negative feedback control systems that regulate cellular function, control life's processes, regulate behavior, and integrate the function of the different body systems. ■

STRESS AND ADAPTATION

After completing this section of the chapter, you should be able to meet the following objectives:

- State Selye's definition of stress.
- Define *stressor.*
- Cite two factors that influence the nature of the stress response.
- Explain the interactions among components of the nervous system in mediating the stress response.
- Describe the stress responses of the autonomic nervous system, the endocrine system, the immune system, and the musculoskeletal system.
- Explain the purpose of adaptation.
- List at least six factors that influence a person's adaptive capacity.
- Relate experience and previous learning to the process of adaptation.
- Contrast anatomic and physiologic reserve.
- Propose a way by which social support may serve to buffer challenges to adaptation.

The increased focus on health promotion has heightened interest in the roles of stress and biobehavioral stress responses in the development of disease.[8] Stress may contribute directly to the production or exacerbation of a disease, or it may contribute to the development of behaviors such as smoking, overeating, and drug abuse that increase the risk of disease.[9]

The Stress Response

In the early 1930s, the world-renowned endocrinologist Hans Selye was the first to describe a group of specific anatomic changes that occurred in rats that were exposed to a variety of different experimental stimuli. He came to an understanding that these changes were manifestations of the body's attempt to adapt to stimuli. Selye described *stress* as "a state manifested by a specific syndrome of the body developed in response to any stimuli that made an intense systemic demand on it."[10] As a young medical student, Selye noticed that patients with diverse disease conditions had many signs and symptoms in common. He observed that "whether a man suffers from a loss of blood, an infectious disease, or advanced cancer, he loses his appetite, his muscular strength, and his ambition to accomplish anything; usually the patient also loses weight and even his facial expression betrays that he is ill."[11] Selye referred to this as the "syndrome of just being sick."

In his early career as an experimental scientist, Selye noted that a triad of adrenal enlargement, thymic atrophy, and gastric ulcers appeared in rats he was using for his studies. These same three changes developed in response to many different or nonspecific experimental challenges. He assumed that the hypothalamic-pituitary-adrenal (HPA) axis played a pivotal role in the development of this response. To Selye, the response to stressors was a process that enabled the rats to resist the experimental challenge by using the function of the system best able to respond to it. He labeled the response the *general adaptation syndrome* (GAS): *general* because the effect was a general systemic reaction, *adaptive* because the response was in reaction to a stressor, and *syndrome* because the physical manifestations were coordinated and dependent on each other.[10]

According to Selye, the GAS involves three stages: the alarm stage, the resistance stage, and the exhaustion stage. The *alarm stage* is characterized by a generalized stimulation of the sympathetic nervous system and the HPA axis, resulting in the release of catecholamines and cortisol. During the *resistance stage,* the body selects the most effective and economic channels of defense. During this stage, the increased cortisol levels that were present during the first stage drop because they are no longer needed. If the stressor is prolonged or overwhelms the ability of the body to defend itself, the *exhaustion stage* ensues, during which resources are depleted and signs of "wear and tear" or systemic damage appear.[12] Selye contended that many ailments, such as various emotional disturbances, mildly annoying headaches, insomnia, upset stomach, gastric and duodenal ulcers, certain types of rheumatic disorders, and cardiovascular and kidney diseases appear to be initiated or encouraged by the "body itself because of its faulty adaptive reactions to potentially injurious agents."[11]

The events or environmental agents responsible for initiating the stress response were called *stressors.* According to Selye, stressors could be endogenous, arising from within the body, or exogenous, arising from outside the body.[11] In explaining the stress response, Selye proposed that two factors determine the nature of the stress response: the properties of the stressor and the conditioning of the person being stressed. Selye indicated that not all stress was detrimental; hence, he coined the terms *eustress* and *distress.*[12] He suggested that mild, brief, and controllable periods of stress could be perceived as positive stimuli to emotional and intellectual growth and development. It is the severe, protracted, and uncontrolled situations of psychological and physical distress that are disruptive of health.[11] For example, the joy of becoming a new parent and the sorrow of losing a parent are completely different experiences, yet their stressor effect—the nonspecific demand for adjustment to a new situation—can be similar.

It is becoming increasingly clear that the physiologic stress response is far more complicated than can be explained fully by a classic stimulus–response mechanism. Stressors tend to produce different responses in different persons or in the same person at different times, indicating the influence of the adaptive capacity of the person, or what Selye called *conditioning factors.* These conditioning factors may be internal (*e.g.,* genetic predisposition, age, sex) or external (*e.g.,* exposure to environmental agents, life experiences, dietary factors, level of social support).[11] The relative risk for development of a stress-related pathologic process seems, at least in part, to depend on these factors.

Richard Lazarus, a well-respected psychologist who devoted his career to the study of stress and emotions, considered "meanings and values to be at the center of human life and to represent the essence of stress, emotion and adaptation."[13] Others describe a "cognitive activation theory of stress" based on the belief that the stress response depends on what a person expects to happen in a given situation given previous learning experiences.[14] In other words, stimuli are filtered or evaluated before they reach a response system. Furthermore, there is evidence that the hypothalamic-pituitary-adrenocortical axis, the adrenomedullary hormonal system, and the sympathetic nervous system are differentially activated depending on the type and intensity of the stressor.[15]

Neuroendocrine Responses

The manifestations of the stress response are strongly influenced by both the nervous and endocrine systems. The neuroendocrine systems integrate signals received along neurosensory pathways and from circulating mediators that are carried in the bloodstream. In addition, the immune system both affects and is affected by the stress response. Table 9-1 summarizes the action of hormones involved in the neuroendocrine responses to stress. The results of the coordinated release of these neurohormones include the mobilization of energy, a sharpened focus and awareness, increased cerebral blood flow and glucose utilization, enhanced cardiovascular and respiratory functioning, redistribution of blood flow to the brain and muscles, modulation of the immune response, inhibition of reproductive function, and a decrease in appetite.[16]

The stress response is a normal, coordinated physiologic system meant to increase the probability of survival, but importantly also designed to be an acute response—turned on when necessary to bring the body back to a stable state and turned off when the challenge to homeostasis abates. Therefore, under normal circumstances, the neural responses and the hormones that are released during the response do not persist long enough to cause damage to vital tissues. Since the early 1980s, the term *allostasis* has been used by some investigators to describe the physiologic changes in the neuroendocrine, autonomic, and immune systems that occur in response to either real or perceived challenges to homeostasis. The persistence or accumulation of these allostatic changes (*e.g.,* immunosuppression, activation of the sympathetic nervous and renin-angiotensin-aldosterone systems) has been called an *allostatic load,* and this concept has been used to measure the cumulative effects of stress on humans.[17,18]

TABLE 9-1 Hormones Involved in the Neuroendocrine Responses to Stress

HORMONES ASSOCIATED WITH THE STRESS RESPONSE	SOURCE OF THE HORMONE	PHYSIOLOGIC EFFECTS
Catecholamines (norepinephrine, epinephrine)	Locus ceruleus, adrenal medulla	Produces a decrease in insulin release and an increase in glucagon release resulting in increased glycogenolysis, gluconeogenesis, lipolysis, proteolysis, and decreased glucose uptake by the peripheral tissues; an increase in heart rate, cardiac contractility, and vascular smooth muscle contraction; and relaxation of bronchial smooth muscle
Corticotropin-releasing factor (CRF)	Hypothalamus	Stimulates ACTH release from the anterior pituitary and increased activity of the locus ceruleus neurons
Adrenocorticotropic hormone (ACTH)	Anterior pituitary	Stimulates the synthesis and release of cortisol
Glucocorticoid hormones (e.g., cortisol)	Adrenal cortex	Potentiates the actions of epinephrine and glucagon; inhibits the release and/or actions of the reproductive hormones and thyroid-stimulating hormone; and produces a decrease in immune cells and inflammatory mediators
Mineralocorticoid hormones (e.g., aldosterone)	Adrenal cortex	Increases sodium absorption by the kidney
Antidiuretic hormone (ADH, vasopressin)	Hypothalamus, posterior pituitary	Increases water absorption by the kidney; produces vasoconstriction of blood vessels; and stimulates the release of ACTH

The integration of the components of the stress response, which occurs at the level of the central nervous system (CNS), is complex and not completely understood. It relies on communication along neuronal pathways of the cerebral cortex, the limbic system, the thalamus, the hypothalamus, the pituitary gland, and the reticular activating system (RAS; Fig. 9-2). The cerebral cortex is involved with vigilance, cognition, and focused attention, and the limbic system with the emotional components (e.g., fear, excitement, rage, anger) of the stress response. The thalamus functions as the relay center and is important in receiving, sorting out, and distributing sensory input. The hypothalamus coordinates the responses of the endocrine and autonomic nervous systems (ANS). The RAS modulates mental alertness, ANS activity, and skeletal muscle tone, using input from other neural structures. The musculoskeletal tension that occurs during the stress response reflects increased activity of the RAS and its influence on the reflex circuits that control muscle tone. Adding to the complexity of this system is the fact that the individual brain circuits that participate in the mediation of the stress response interact and regulate the activity of each other. For example, reciprocal connections exist between neurons in the hypothalamus that initiate release of corticotropin-releasing factor (CRF), and neurons in the locus ceruleus associated with release of norepinephrine. Thus, norepinephrine stimulates the secretion of CRF, and CRF stimulates the release of norepinephrine.[16]

Locus Ceruleus. Central to the neural component of the neuroendocrine response to stress is an area of the brain stem called the *locus ceruleus* (LC).[16,19] The LC is densely populated with neurons that produce norepinephrine (NE), and is thought to be the central integrating site for the ANS response to stressful stimuli (Fig. 9-3). The LC-NE system has afferent pathways to the hypothalamus, the limbic system, the hippocampus, and the cerebral cortex.

The LC-NE system confers an adaptive advantage during a stressful situation. The sympathetic nervous system manifestation of the stress reaction has been called the *fight-or-flight response*. This is the most rapid of the stress responses and represents the basic survival response of our primitive ancestors when confronted with the perils of the wilderness and its inhabitants. The increase in sympathetic activity in the brain increases attention and arousal and thus probably intensifies memory. The heart and respiratory rates increase, the hands and feet become moist, the pupils dilate, the mouth becomes dry, and the activity of the gastrointestinal tract decreases.

Corticotropin-Releasing Factor. CRF is central to the endocrine component of the neuroendocrine response to stress (see Fig. 9-3). CRF is a small peptide hormone found in both the hypothalamus and in extrahypothalamic structures, such as the limbic system and the brain stem. It is both an important endocrine regulator of pituitary and adrenal activity and a neurotransmitter involved in ANS activity, metabolism, and behavior.[9,16,20,21] Receptors for CRF are distributed throughout the brain as well as many peripheral sites. CRF from the hypothalamus induces secretion of adrenocorticotropic hormone (ACTH) from the anterior pituitary gland. ACTH, in turn, stim-

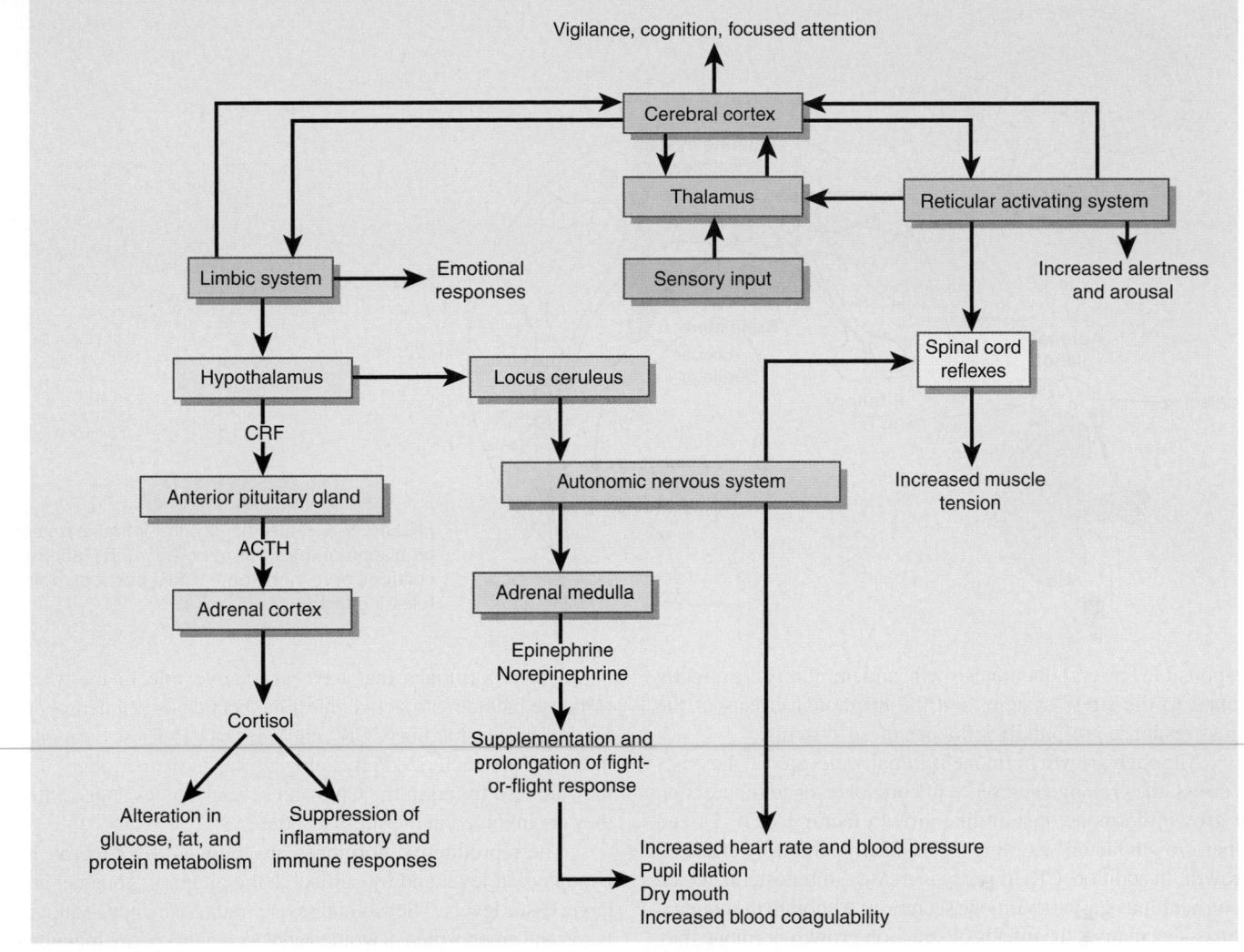

FIGURE 9-2 • Neuroendocrine pathways and physiologic responses to stress. ACTH, adrenocorticotropic hormone; CRF, corticotropin-releasing factor.

ulates the adrenal gland to synthesize and secrete the glucocorticoid hormones (*e.g.*, cortisol).

The glucocorticoid hormones have a number of direct or indirect physiologic effects that mediate the stress response, enhance the action of other stress hormones, or suppress other components of the stress system. In this regard, cortisol acts not only as a mediator of the stress response but as an inhibitor, such that overactivation of the stress response does not occur.[22,23] Cortisol maintains blood glucose levels by antagonizing the effects of insulin and enhances the effect of catecholamines on the cardiovascular system. It also suppresses osteoblast activity, hematopoiesis, protein and collagen synthesis, and immune responses. All of these functions are meant to protect the organism against the effects of a stressor and to focus energy on regaining balance in the face of an acute challenge to homeostasis.

Angiotensin II. Stimulation of the sympathetic nervous system also activates the peripheral renin-angiotensin-aldosterone system (RAAS), which mediates a peripheral increase in vascular tone and renal retention of sodium and water (see Chapter 23). These changes contribute to the physiologic changes that occur with the stress response and, if prolonged, may contribute to pathologic changes. Angiotensin II, peripherally delivered or locally produced, also has CNS effects; angiotensin II type 1 (AT$_1$) receptors are widely distributed in the hypothalamus and locus ceruleus. Through these receptors, angiotensin II enhances CRF formation and release, contributes to the release of ACTH from the pituitary, enhances stress-induced release of vasopressin from the posterior pituitary, and stimulates the release of norepinephrine from the locus ceruleus. Studies in animals of the effect of AT$_1$ receptor blockade suggest that receptor antagonists attenuate the activation of the stress response and may be an effective treatment for the effects of chronic stimulation of the stress response.[16]

Other Hormones. A wide variety of other hormones, including growth hormone, thyroid hormone, and the reproductive hormones, also are responsive to stressful situations. Systems

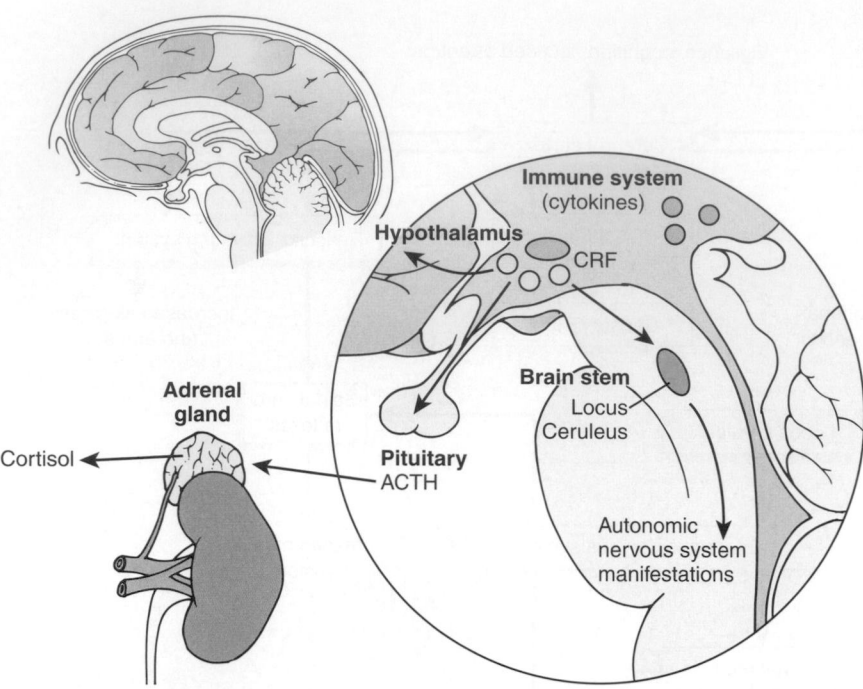

FIGURE 9-3 • Neuroendocrine–immune system regulation of the stress response. ACTH, adrenocorticotropic hormone; CRF, corticotropin-releasing factor.

responsible for reproduction, growth, and immunity are directly linked to the stress system, and the hormonal effects of the stress response profoundly influence these systems.

Although growth hormone is initially elevated at the onset of stress, the prolonged presence of cortisol leads to suppression of growth hormone, insulin-like growth factor 1 (IGF-1), and other growth factors, exerting a chronically inhibitory effect on growth. In addition, CRF directly increases somatostatin, which in turn inhibits growth hormone secretion. Although the connection is speculative, the effects of stress on growth hormone may provide one of the vital links to understanding failure to thrive in children.

Stress-induced cortisol secretion also is associated with decreased levels of thyroid-stimulating hormone and inhibition of conversion of thyroxine (T_4) to the more biologically active triiodothyronine (T_3) in peripheral tissues (see Chapter 41). Both changes may serve as a means to conserve energy at times of stress.

Antidiuretic hormone (ADH) released from the posterior pituitary is also involved in the stress response, particularly in hypotensive stress or stress due to fluid volume loss. ADH, also known as *vasopressin,* increases water retention by the kidneys and produces vasoconstriction of blood vessels. In addition, vasopressin synthesized in parvicellular neurons of the hypothalamus and transported to the anterior pituitary appears to synergize the capacity of CRF to stimulate the release of ACTH.

The neurotransmitter serotonin or 5-hydroxytryptamine (5-HT) probably also plays a role in the stress response through neurons that innervate the hypothalamus, amygdala, and other limbic structures. Administration of 5-HT receptor agonists to laboratory animals was shown to increase the secretion of several stress hormones. In addition, it has been demonstrated that CRF inhibits the firing of serotonergic neurons.[16]

Other hormones that have a putative role in the stress response include vasoactive intestinal peptide (VIP), neuropeptide Y, cholecystokinin (CCK), and substance P. These hormones have well-characterized physiologic roles in the periphery, but they are also found in the CNS and several studies suggest that they are involved in the stress response.[16]

The reproductive hormones are inhibited by CRF at the hypophyseal level and by cortisol at the pituitary, gonadal, and target tissue levels.[11] Sepsis and severe trauma can induce anovulation and amenorrhea in women and decreased spermatogenesis and decreased levels of testosterone in men.

Immune Responses

The hallmark of the stress response, as first described by Selye, are the endocrine–immune interactions (*i.e.,* increased corticosteroid production and atrophy of the thymus) that are known to suppress the immune response. In concert, these two components of the stress system, through endocrine and neurotransmitter pathways, produce the physical and behavioral changes designed to adapt to acute stress. Much of the literature regarding stress and the immune response focuses on the causal role of stress in immune-related diseases. It has also been suggested that the reverse may occur; emotional and psychological manifestations of the stress response may be a reflection of alterations in the CNS resulting from the immune response (see Fig. 9-3). Immune cells such as monocytes and lymphocytes can penetrate the blood-brain barrier and take up residence in the brain, where they secrete chemical messengers called *cytokines* that influence the stress response. In the case of cancer, this could mean that the subjective feelings of helplessness and hopelessness that have been repeatedly related to the onset and progression of cancers may arise secondary to the CNS effects of products released by immune cells during the early stage of the disease.[24,25]

The exact mechanism by which stress produces its effect on the immune response is unknown and probably varies from person to person, depending on genetic endowment and environmental factors. The most significant arguments for interaction between the neuroendocrine and immune systems derive from evidence that the immune and neuroendocrine systems share common signal pathways (*i.e.,* messenger molecules and receptors), that hormones and neuropeptides can alter the function of immune cells, and that the immune system and its mediators can modulate neuroendocrine function.[26] Receptors for a number of CNS-controlled hormones and neuromediators reportedly have been found on lymphocytes. Among these are receptors for glucocorticoids, insulin, testosterone, prolactin, catecholamines, estrogens, acetylcholine, and growth hormone, suggesting that these hormones and neuromediators influence lymphocyte function. For example, cortisol is known to suppress immune function, and pharmacologic doses of cortisol are used clinically to suppress the immune response. There is evidence that the immune system, in turn, influences neuroendocrine function.[27] For example, it has been observed that the HPA axis is activated by cytokines such as interleukin-1, interleukin-6, and tumor necrosis factor that are released from immune cells (see Chapter 17).

A second possible route for neuroendocrine regulation of immune function is through the sympathetic nervous system and the release of catecholamines. The lymph nodes, thymus, and spleen are supplied with ANS nerve fibers. Centrally acting CRF activates the ANS through multisynaptic descending pathways, and circulating epinephrine acts synergistically with CRF and cortisol to inhibit the function of the immune system.

Not only is the quantity of immune expression changed because of stress, but the quality of the response is changed. Stress hormones differentially stimulate the proliferation of subtypes of T-lymphocyte helper cells. Because these T-helper cell subtypes secrete different cytokines, they stimulate different aspects of the immune response. One subtype tends to stimulate T lymphocytes and the cellular-mediated immune response, whereas a second type tends to activate B lymphocytes and humoral-mediated immune responses.[7]

Coping and Adaptation to Stress

The ability to adapt to a wide range of environments and stressors is not peculiar to humans. According to René Dubos (a microbiologist noted for his study of human responses to the total environment), "adaptability is found throughout life and is perhaps the one attribute that distinguishes most clearly the world of life from the world of inanimate matter."[28] Living organisms, no matter how primitive, do not submit passively to the impact of environmental forces. They attempt to respond adaptively, each in its own unique and most suitable manner. The higher the organism is on the evolutionary scale, the larger its repertoire of adaptive mechanisms and its ability to select and limit aspects of the environment to which it responds. The most fully evolved mechanisms are the social responses through which individuals

> ### ⚷ STRESS AND ADAPTATION
>
> - Stress is a state manifested by symptoms that arise from the coordinated activation of the neuroendocrine and immune systems, which Selye called the general adaptation syndrome.
>
> - The hormones and neurotransmitters (catecholamines and cortisol) that are released during the stress response function to alert the individual to a threat or challenge to homeostasis, to enhance cardiovascular and metabolic activity in order to manage the stressor, and to focus the energy of the body by suppressing the activity of other systems that are not immediately needed.
>
> - Adaptation is the ability to respond to challenges of physical or psychological homeostasis and to return to a balanced state.
>
> - The ability to adapt is influenced by previous learning, physiologic reserve, time, genetic endowment, age, health status and nutrition, sleep–wake cycles, and psychosocial factors.

or groups modify their environments, their habits, or both to achieve a way of life that is best suited to their needs.

Adaptation

Human beings, because of their highly developed nervous system and intellect, usually have alternative mechanisms for adapting and have the ability to control many aspects of their environment. Air conditioning and central heating limit the need to adapt to extreme changes in environmental temperature. The availability of antiseptic agents, immunizations, and antibiotics eliminates the need to respond to common infectious agents. At the same time, modern technology creates new challenges for adaptation and provides new sources of stress, such as increased noise, air pollution, exposure to harmful chemicals, and changes in biologic rhythms imposed by shift work and transcontinental air travel.

Of particular interest are the differences in the body's response to events that threaten the integrity of the body's physiologic environment and those that threaten the integrity of the person's psychosocial environment. Many of the body's responses to physiologic disturbances are controlled on a moment-by-moment basis by feedback mechanisms that limit their application and duration of action. For example, the baroreflex-mediated rise in heart rate that occurs when a person moves from the recumbent to the standing position is almost instantaneous and subsides within seconds. Furthermore, the response to physiologic disturbances that threaten the integrity of the internal environment is specific to the threat; the body usually does not raise the body temperature when an increase in heart rate is needed. In contrast, the response to psychological disturbances is not regulated with the same degree of specificity and feedback control; instead, the effect may be inappropriate and sustained.

Factors Affecting the Ability to Adapt

Adaptation implies that an individual has successfully created a new balance between the stressor and the ability to deal with it. The means used to attain this balance are called *coping strategies* or *coping mechanisms*. Coping mechanisms are the emotional and behavioral responses used to manage threats to our physiologic and psychological homeostasis. According to Lazarus, how we cope with stressful events depends on how we perceive and interpret the event.[29] Is the event perceived as a threat of harm or loss? Is the event perceived as a challenge rather than a threat? Physiologic reserve, time, genetic endowment and age, health status, nutrition, sleep–wake cycles, hardiness, and psychosocial factors influence a person's appraisal of a stressor and the coping mechanisms used to adapt to the new situation (Fig. 9-4).

Physiologic and Anatomic Reserve. The trained athlete is able to increase cardiac output six- to sevenfold during exercise. The safety margin for adaptation of most body systems is considerably greater than that needed for normal activities. The red blood cells carry more oxygen than the tissues can use, the liver and fat cells store excess nutrients, and bone tissue stores calcium in excess of that needed for normal neuromuscular function. The ability of body systems to increase their function given the need to adapt is known as the *physiologic reserve*. Many of the body organs, such as the lungs, kidneys, and adrenals, are paired to provide anatomic reserve as well. Both organs are not needed to ensure the continued existence and maintenance of the internal environment. Many persons function normally with only one lung or one kidney. In kidney disease, for example, signs of renal failure do not occur until

approximately 90% of the functioning nephrons have been destroyed.

Time. Adaptation is most efficient when changes occur gradually rather than suddenly. It is possible, for instance, to lose a liter or more of blood through chronic gastrointestinal bleeding over a week without manifesting signs of shock. However, a sudden hemorrhage that causes rapid loss of an equal amount of blood is likely to cause hypotension and shock.

Genetic Endowment. Adaptation is further affected by the availability of adaptive responses and flexibility in selecting the most appropriate and economical response. The greater the number of available responses, the more effective is the capacity to adapt.

Genetic endowment can ensure that the systems that are essential to adaptation function adequately. Even a gene that has deleterious effects may prove adaptive in some environments. In Africa, the gene for sickle cell anemia persists in some populations because it provides some resistance to infection with the parasite that causes malaria.

Age. The capacity to adapt is decreased at the extremes of age. The ability to adapt is impaired by the immaturity of an infant, much as it is by the decline in functional reserve that occurs with age. For example, the infant has difficulty concentrating urine because of immature renal structures and therefore is less able than an adult to cope with decreased water intake or exaggerated water losses. A similar situation exists in the elderly owing to age-related changes in renal function.

Gender. Within the last decade, primarily because females have been included in basic science and clinical investigations, differences between the sexes in cardiovascular, respiratory, endocrine, renal, and neurophysiologic function have been found, and it has been hypothesized that sex hormones are the basis of these biologic differences. Technological advances in cellular and molecular biology have made it clear, however, that there are fundamental differences in the locale and regulation of individual genes in the male and female genome that can account at a very basic level for the differences in physiologic function and disease manifestation.[30] These differences have general implications for the prevention, diagnosis, and treatment of disease and specific implications for our understanding of the sex-based differences in response to life's stressors.

Given the nature of sex-based differences, it is not surprising that there are differences in the physiologic stress response in both the HPA axis and in the ANS. For example, the male hypothalamus produces more CRF and more ACTH than the premenopausal female hypothalamus in response to a psychological stressor (*i.e.,* public speaking).[31] However, the secretion of arginine vasopressin (AVP), a hormone that has cardiovascular and renal effects and potentiates the release of ACTH, is greater in the female. Premenopausal women also tend to have a lower activation of the sympathetic nervous system than men in response to stressors. The phase of menstruation (luteal vs. follicular) as well as menopausal status can alter these

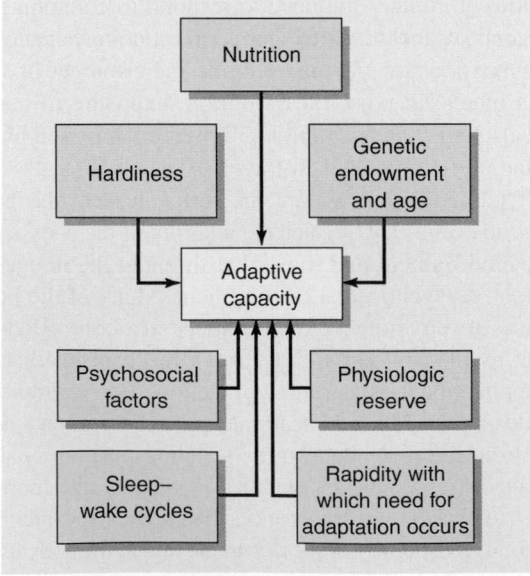

FIGURE 9-4 • Factors affecting adaptation.

responses and need to be taken into account when studying these responses.[31] These sex-based differences in activation of the stress response may partially explain differences in susceptibility to diseases in which the stress response may play a causal role. These research results are not definitive but are intriguing and can serve as a springboard for further research.

Health Status. Physical and mental health status determines physiologic and psychological reserves and is a strong determinant of the ability to adapt. For example, persons with heart disease are less able to adjust to stresses that require the recruitment of cardiovascular responses. Severe emotional stress often produces disruption of physiologic function and limits the ability to make appropriate choices related to long-term adaptive needs. Those who have worked with acutely ill persons know that the will to live often has a profound influence on survival during life-threatening illnesses.

Nutrition. There are 50 to 60 essential nutrients, including minerals, lipids, certain fatty acids, vitamins, and specific amino acids. Deficiencies or excesses of any of these nutrients can alter a person's health status and impair the ability to adapt. The importance of nutrition to enzyme function, immune response, and wound healing is well known. On a worldwide basis, malnutrition may be one of the most common causes of immunodeficiency.

Among the problems associated with dietary excess are obesity and alcohol abuse. Obesity is a common problem. It predisposes an individual to a number of health problems, including atherosclerosis and hypertension. Alcohol is commonly used in excess. It acutely affects brain function and, with long-term use, can seriously impair the function of the liver, brain, and other vital structures.

Sleep–Wake Cycles. Sleep is considered to be a restorative function in which energy is restored and tissues are regenerated.[32] Sleep occurs in a cyclic manner, alternating with periods of wakefulness and increased energy use (see Chapter 52). Biologic rhythms play an important role in adaptation to stress, development of illness, and response to medical treatment. Many rhythms such as rest and activity, work and leisure, and eating and drinking oscillate with a frequency similar to that of the 24-hour light–dark solar day. The term *circadian,* from the Latin *circa* ("about") and *dies* ("day"), is used to describe these 24-hour diurnal rhythms.

Sleep disorders and alterations in the sleep–wake cycle have been shown to alter immune function, the normal circadian pattern of hormone secretion, and physical and psychological functioning.[33] The two most common manifestations of an alteration in the sleep–wake cycle are insomnia and sleep deprivation or increased somnolence. In some persons, stress may produce sleep disorders, and in others, sleep disorders may lead to stress. Acute stress and environmental disturbances, loss of a loved one, recovery from surgery, and pain are common causes of transient and short-term insomnia. Air travel and jet lag constitute additional causes of altered sleep–wake cycles, as does shift work. In persons with chronic insomnia, the bed often acquires many unpleasant secondary associations and becomes a place of stress and worry rather than a place of rest.[34]

Hardiness. Studies by social psychologists have focused on individuals' emotional reactions to stressful situations and their coping mechanisms to determine those characteristics that help some people remain healthy despite being challenged by high levels of stressors. For example, the concept of *hardiness* describes a personality characteristic that includes a sense of having control over the environment, a sense of having a purpose in life, and an ability to conceptualize stressors as a challenge rather than a threat.[35] Many studies by nurses and social psychologists suggest that hardiness is correlated with positive health outcomes.[35]

Psychosocial Factors. Several studies have related social factors and life events to illness. Scientific interest in the social environment as a cause of stress has gradually broadened to include the social environment as a resource that modulates the relation between stress and health. Presumably, persons who can mobilize strong supportive resources from within their social relationships are better able to withstand the negative effects of stress on their health. Studies suggest that social support has direct and indirect positive effects on health status and serves as a buffer or modifier of the physical and psychosocial effects of stress.[36]

Social networks contribute in a number of ways to a person's psychosocial and physical integrity. The configuration of significant others that constitutes this network functions to mobilize the resources of the person; these friends, colleagues, and family members share the person's tasks and provide monetary support, materials and tools, and guidance in improving problem-solving capabilities.[36] Persons with ample social networks are not as likely to experience many types of stress-producing situations, such as homelessness or loneliness.[9] There is also evidence that persons who have social supports or social assets may live longer and have a lower incidence of somatic illness.[37]

Social support has been viewed in terms of the number of relationships a person has and the person's perception of these relationships.[38] Close relationships with others can involve positive effects as well as the potential for conflict and may, in some situations, leave the person less able to cope with life stressors.

IN SUMMARY, the stress response involves the activation of several physiologic systems (sympathetic nervous system, the HPA axis, and the immune system) that work in a coordinated fashion to protect the body against damage from the intense demands made on it. Selye called this response the *general adaptation syndrome.* The stress response is divided into three stages: the *alarm stage,* with activation of the sympathetic nervous system and the HPA axis; the *resistance stage,* during which the body selects the most effective defenses; and the *exhaustion stage,* during which physiologic resources are depleted and signs of systemic damage appear.

The activation and control of the stress response are mediated by the combined efforts of the nervous and endocrine systems. The neuroendocrine systems integrate signals received along neurosensory pathways and from circulating mediators that are carried in the bloodstream. In addition, the immune system both affects and is affected by the stress response.

Adaptation is affected by a number of factors, including experience and previous learning, the rapidity with which the need to adapt occurs, genetic endowment and age, health status, nutrition, sleep–wake cycles, hardiness, and psychosocial factors. ■

DISORDERS OF THE STRESS RESPONSE

After completing this section of the chapter, you should be able to meet the following objectives:

■ Describe the physiologic and psychological effects of a chronic stress response.
■ Describe the three states characteristic of post-traumatic stress disorder.
■ List five nonpharmacologic methods of treating stress.

For the most part, the stress response is meant to be acute and time limited. The time-limited nature of the process renders the accompanying catabolic and immunosuppressive effects advantageous. It is the chronicity of the response that is thought to be disruptive to physical and mental health.

Stressors can assume a number of patterns in relation to time. They may be classified as acute time-limited, chronic intermittent, or chronic sustained. An acute time-limited stressor is one that occurs over a short time and does not recur; a chronic intermittent stressor is one to which a person is chronically exposed. The frequency or chronicity of circumstances to which the body is asked to respond often determines the availability and efficiency of the stress responses. The response of the immune system, for example, is more rapid and efficient on second exposure to a pathogen than it is on first exposure, but chronic exposure to a stressor can fatigue the system and impair its effectiveness.

Effects of Acute Stress

The reactions to acute stress are those associated with the ANS, the fight-or-flight response. The manifestations of the stress response—a pounding headache, cold, moist skin, a stiff neck—are all part of the acute stress response. Centrally, there is facilitation of neural pathways mediating arousal, alertness, vigilance, cognition, and focused attention, as well as appropriate aggression. The acute stress response can result from either psychologically or physiologically threatening

events. In situations of life-threatening trauma, these acute responses may be lifesaving in that they divert blood from less essential to more essential body functions. Increased alertness and cognitive functioning enable rapid processing of information and arrival at the most appropriate solution to the threatening situation.

However, for persons with limited coping abilities, either because of physical or mental health, the acute stress response may be detrimental. This is true of persons with preexisting heart disease in whom the overwhelming sympathetic behaviors associated with the stress response can lead to arrhythmias. For people with other chronic health problems, such as headache disorder, acute stress may precipitate a recurrence. In healthy individuals, the acute stress response can redirect attention from behaviors that promote health, such as attention to proper meals and getting adequate sleep. For those with health problems, it can interrupt compliance with medication regimens and exercise programs. In some situations, the acute arousal state actually can be life-threatening, physically immobilizing the person when movement would avert catastrophe (*e.g.,* moving out of the way of a speeding car).

Effects of Chronic Stress

The stress response is designed to be an acute self-limited response in which activation of the ANS and the HPA axis is controlled in a negative feedback manner. As with all negative feedback systems, pathophysiologic changes can occur in the stress response system. Function can be altered in several ways, including when a component of the system fails; when the neural and hormonal connections among the components of the system are dysfunctional; and when the original stimulus for the activation of the system is prolonged or of such magnitude that it overwhelms the ability of the system to respond appropriately. In these cases, the system may become overactive or underactive.

Chronicity and excessive activation of the stress response can result from chronic illnesses as well as contribute to the development of long-term health problems. Chronic activation of the stress response is an important public health issue from both a health and a cost perspective. The National Institute for Occupational Safety and Health declared stress a hazard of the workplace.[39]

It is linked to a myriad of health disorders, such as diseases of the cardiovascular, gastrointestinal, immune, and neurologic systems, as well as depression, chronic alcoholism and drug abuse, eating disorders, accidents, and suicide.

Occurrence of the oral disease acute necrotizing gingivitis, in which the normal bacterial flora of the mouth become invasive, is known by dentists to be associated with acute stress, such as final examinations.[40] Similarly, herpes simplex virus type 1 infection (*i.e.,* cold sores) often develops during periods of inadequate rest, fever, ultraviolet radiation, and emotional upset. The resident herpesvirus is kept in check by body defenses, probably T lymphocytes, until a stressful event occurs that causes suppression of the immune system. Psychological stress is associated in a dose–response manner with an increased risk for development of the common cold, and this risk is attributable to increased rates of infection rather than frequency of symptoms after infection.[41]

In a study in which participants were infected with the influenza virus, those persons who reported the greatest amount of premorbid stress also reported the most intense influenza symptoms and had a statistically greater production of interleukin-6, a cytokine that acts as a chemotactic agent for immune cells.[42] Elderly caregivers of a spouse with dementia had a significantly higher score for emotional distress and higher salivary cortisol than matched control subjects. The higher stress was correlated with a decreased immune response to the influenza vaccine.[43] The experience of stress also has been associated with delays in wound healing.[44]

Post-traumatic Stress Disorder

Post-traumatic stress disorder (PTSD) is an example of chronic activation of the stress response as a result of experiencing a significant traumatic event.[45,46] A traumatic event has been defined as its capacity to provoke fear, helplessness, or horror in response to the threat of injury or death.[45] It was formerly called *battle fatigue* or *shell shock* because it was first characterized in men and women returning from combat. Although war is still a significant cause of PTSD, other major catastrophic events, such as weather-related disasters (hurricanes and floods), airplane crashes, terrorist bombings, and rape or child abuse, also may result in development of the disorder. People who are exposed to such events are also at risk for development of major depression, panic disorder, generalized anxiety disorder, and substance abuse.[45] They may also have bodily symptoms and physical illnesses, particularly hypertension, asthma, and chronic pain syndromes. PTSD became an official psychiatric diagnosis in 1980 in the third edition of the American Psychiatric Association's *Diagnostic and Statistical Manual of Mental Disorders (DSM-III)*.[46]

PTSD is characterized by a constellation of symptoms that are experienced as states of intrusion, avoidance, and hyperarousal. *Intrusion* refers to the occurrence of "flashbacks" during waking hours or nightmares in which the past traumatic event is relived, often in vivid and frightening detail. *Avoidance* refers to the emotional numbing that accompanies this disorder and disrupts important personal relationships. Because a person with PTSD has not been able to resolve the painful feelings associated with the trauma, depression is commonly a part of the clinical picture. Survivor guilt also may be a product of traumatic situations in which the person survived the disaster but loved ones did not. *Hyperarousal* refers to the presence of increased irritability, difficulty concentrating, an exaggerated startle reflex, and increased vigilance and concern over safety. In addition, memory problems, sleep disturbances, and excessive anxiety are commonly experienced by persons with PTSD.

For a diagnosis of PTSD to be made, the person must have experienced, witnessed, or confronted an event that threatened death or serious injury to themselves or others, with the person's response involving intense fear, helplessness or horror.[47] The triad of symptoms of intrusion, avoidance, and hyperarousal that characterize PTSD must be present together for at least 1 month and the disorder must have caused clinically significant distress or impairment in social, occupational, and other areas of functioning.[47]

Although the pathophysiology of PTSD is not completely understood, the revelation of physiologic changes related to the disorder has shed light on why some people recover from the disorder, whereas others do not. It has been hypothesized that the intrusive symptoms of PTSD may arise from exaggerated sympathetic nervous system activation in response to the traumatic event. Persons with chronic PTSD have been shown to have increased levels of norepinephrine and increased activity of α_2-adrenergic receptors.[45] The increase in catecholamines, in tandem with increased thyroid hormone levels in persons with PTSD, is thought to explain some of the intrusive and somatic symptoms of the disorder.[45,48]

Recent neuroanatomic studies have identified alterations in two brain structures (the amygdala and hippocampus). Positron emission tomography and functional magnetic resonance imaging have shown increased reactivity of the amygdala and hippocampus and decreased reactivity of the anterior cingulate and orbitofrontal areas. These areas of the brain are involved in fear responses. The hippocampus also functions in memory processes. Differences in hippocampal function and memory processes suggest a neuroanatomic basis for the intrusive recollections and other cognitive problems that characterize PTSD.[45]

Importantly, the observed neuroanatomic changes in persons with PTSD do not uniformly resemble those seen with other types of stress.[49] For example, persons with PTSD demonstrate decreased cortisol levels, increased sensitivity of cortisol receptors, and an enhanced negative feedback inhibition of cortisol release with the dexamethasone suppression test. Dexamethasone is a synthetic glucocorticoid that mimics the effects of cortisol and directly inhibits the action of CRF and ACTH. This is in contrast to patients with major depression, who have a decreased sensitivity of glucocorticoid receptors, a high plasma level of cortisol, and decreased dexamethasone suppression.[49] The hypersuppression of cortisol observed with the dexamethasone test suggests that persons with PTSD do not exhibit a classic stress response as described by Selye. Because this hypersuppression has not been described in other psychiatric disorders, it may serve as a relatively specific marker for PTSD.

Little is known about the risk factors that predispose people to the development of PTSD. It is important to note that less than half of all people who are exposed to a traumatic event develop PTSD. For example, only 15% to 30% of soldiers exposed to combat develop the disorder.[50] It also has been found that children exposed to violent events but who have strong family relationships rarely develop PTSD.[51] Statistics indicate there is a need for studies to determine risk factors for PTSD as a means of targeting individuals who may need intensive therapeutic measures after a life-threatening event. Research also is needed to determine the mechanisms by which the disorder develops so that it can be prevented or, if that is not possible, so that treatment methods can be developed to decrease the devastating effects of this disorder on affected individuals and their families.[48]

Health care professionals need to be aware that clients who present with symptoms of depression, anxiety, and alcohol or drug abuse may in fact be suffering from PTSD. The client history should include questions concerning the occurrence of violence, major loss, or traumatic events in the person's life. The results of the U.S. National Comorbidity Survey (National Institute of Mental Health, 1995) suggest that these incidents are very common; over 50% of the respondents experienced at least one traumatic event, men more than women.[52] In addition, there was a sex-based difference in the type of trauma experienced. Women reported childhood physical and sexual abuse whereas men reported combat or physical attacks, and women are twice as likely to develop PTSD after exposure to a traumatic event than men. Symptoms in women with a history of abuse might include, in addition to the previously mentioned symptoms, chronic pelvic pain, gastrointestinal disorders, intractable back pain, and chronic headache.[52] The cause for this sex-based difference is unclear but it is surmised that the element of powerlessness in the event plays a role. In this regard, a concept from cognitive psychology, helplessness, defined as a perception by an individual that he or she had no control over the outcome of an event, may provide a context for understanding the differences in activation of the HPA axis in PTSD (increased) versus depression (inhibited).[14]

Debriefing, or talking about the traumatic event at the time it happens, often is an effective therapeutic tool. Crisis teams are often among the first people to attend to the emotional needs of those caught in catastrophic events. Some people may need continued individual or group therapy. Often concurrent pharmacotherapy with antidepressant and antianxiety agents is useful and helps the individual participate more fully in therapy.

Most important, the person with PTSD should not be made to feel responsible for the disorder or that it is evidence of a so-called character flaw. It is not uncommon for persons with this disorder to be told to "get over it" or "just get on with it, because others have." There is ample evidence to suggest that there is a biologic basis for the individual differences in responses to traumatic events, and these differences need to be taken into account.

Treatment and Research of Stress Disorders

Treatment

The treatment of stress should be directed toward helping people avoid coping behaviors that impose a risk to their health and providing them with alternative stress-reducing strategies. Purposeful priority setting and problem solving can be used by

persons who are overwhelmed by the number of life stressors to which they have been exposed. Other nonpharmacologic methods used for stress reduction are relaxation techniques, guided imagery, music therapy, massage, and biofeedback.

Relaxation. Practices for evoking the relaxation response are numerous. They are found in virtually every culture and are credited with producing a generalized decrease in sympathetic system activity and musculoskeletal tension. According to Herbert Benson, a physician who worked in developing the technique, four elements are integral to the various relaxation techniques: a repetitive mental device, a passive attitude, decreased mental tonus, and a quiet environment.[53] Benson developed a noncultural method that is commonly used for achieving relaxation (Box 9-2).

Progressive muscle relaxation, originally developed by Edmund Jacobson, who did extensive research on the muscle correlates of anxiety and tension, is another method of relieving tension. He observed that tension can be defined physiologically as the inappropriate contraction of muscle fibers. His procedure, which has been modified by a number of therapists, consists of systematic contraction and relaxation of major muscle groups.[54] As the person learns to relax, the various muscle groups are combined. Eventually, the person learns to relax individual muscle groups without first contracting them.

Imagery. Guided imagery is another technique that can be used to achieve relaxation. One method is scene visualization, in which the person is asked to sit back, close the eyes, and concentrate on a scene narrated by the therapist. Whenever possible, all five senses are involved: the person attempts to see, feel, hear, smell, and taste aspects of the visual experience. Other types of imagery involve imagining the appearance of each of the major muscle groups and how they feel during tension and relaxation.

BOX 9-2 THE RELAXATION RESPONSE

- Sit quietly in a comfortable position.
- Deeply relax all your muscles, beginning at your feet and progressing up to your face.
- Breathe through your nose. Become aware of your breathing. As you breathe out, say the word "one" silently to yourself. Continue for 20 minutes. When you have finished, sit quietly for several minutes, first with your eyes closed and then with them open.
- Do not worry about whether you are successful in achieving a deep level of relaxation. Maintain a positive attitude and permit the relaxation to occur at its own rate. Expect distracting thoughts, ignore them, and continue repeating "one" as you breathe out.

(Modified from Benson H. [1977]. Systemic hypertension and the relaxation response. *New England Journal of Medicine* 296, 1152.)

Music Therapy. Music therapy is used for both its physiologic and psychological effects. It involves listening to selected pieces of music as a means of ameliorating anxiety or stress, reducing pain, decreasing feelings of loneliness and isolation, buffering noise, and facilitating expression of emotion. Music is defined as having three components: rhythm, melody, and harmony.[55,56] Rhythm is the order in the movement of the music. Rhythm is the most dynamic aspect of music, and particular pieces of music often are selected because they harmonize with body rhythms such as heart rhythm, respiratory rhythm, or gait. The melody is created by the musical pitch and the distance (or interval) between the musical tones. The melody contributes to the listener's emotional response to the music. The harmony results from the way pitches are blended together, with the combination of sounds described as consonant or dissonant by the listener. Music usually is selected based on a person's musical preference and past experiences with music. Depending on the setting, headphones may be used to screen out other distracting noises. Radio and television music is inappropriate for music therapy because of the inability to control the selection of pieces that are played, the interruptions that occur (*e.g.,* commercials and announcements), and the quality of the reception.

Massage Therapies. Massage is the manipulation of the soft tissues of the body to promote relaxation and relief of muscle tension. The technique that is used may involve a gentle stroking along the length of a muscle (effleurage), application of pressure across the width of a muscle (petrissage), deep massage movements applied by a circular motion of the thumbs or fingertips (friction), squeezing across the width of a muscle (kneading), or use of light slaps or chopping actions (hacking).[57] Massage may be administered by practitioners who have received special training in its use or by less-prepared persons such as parents of small children[58,59] or caregivers of confused elders.[60] It often is used as a means of physiologic relaxation and stress relief in critically ill patients.[61]

Biofeedback. Biofeedback is a technique in which an individual learns to control physiologic functioning. It involves electronic monitoring of one or more physiologic responses to stress with immediate feedback of the specific response to the person undergoing treatment. Several types of responses are used: electromyographic (EMG), electrothermal, and electrodermal.[62] The EMG response involves the measurement of electrical potentials from muscles, usually the forearm extensor or frontalis. This is used to gain control over the contraction of skeletal muscles that occurs with anxiety and tension. The electrodermal sensors monitor skin temperature in the fingers or toes. The sympathetic nervous system exerts significant control over blood flow in the distal parts of the body such as the digits of the hands and feet. Consequently, anxiety often is manifested by a decrease in skin temperature in the fingers and toes. Electrodermal sensors measure conductivity of skin (usually the hands) in response to anxiety. Fearful and anxious people often have cold and clammy hands, which lead to a decrease in conductivity.

Research

Research in stress has focused on personal reports of the stress situation and the physiologic responses to stress. A number of interview guides and written instruments are available for measuring the personal responses to stress and coping in adults[63,64] and children.[65]

There are fewer methods available for measuring the physiologic responses to stress in humans because much of the research in the field of stress has been accomplished using animal models. There are some good reasons for this. First, the human experience of stress varies among individuals based on previous life experiences and availability of adaptive resources; therefore, it is difficult to find a stimulus that produces equivalent stress in all subjects in a study. Second, suitable methods for measuring the components of the stress response in humans are limited. Some methods require invasive procedures, many demand expensive equipment, and all require investigator competency in their use.[66] In addition, many measurement methods, such as venipuncture, can introduce additional stress to the experimental condition.

Some of the current methods for studying the physiologic manifestations of the stress response include electrocardiographic recording of heart rate, blood pressure measurement, electrodermal measurement of skin resistance associated with sweating, and biochemical analyses of hormone levels.[66] Measurements of urinary and plasma catecholamines can be used as an index of ANS activation. Cortisol levels can be obtained from salivary samples. The effect of the stress response on the immune system can be studied through the use of blood tests to obtain immune cell (lymphocyte) counts and antibody levels.

Research that attempts to establish a link between the stress response and disease needs to be interpreted with caution owing to the influence that individual differences have in the way people respond to stress. Not everyone who experiences stressful life events develops a disease. The evidence for a link between the stress response system and the development of disease in susceptible persons is compelling but not conclusive. No study has established a direct cause-and-effect relationship between the stress response and disease occurrence. For example, depressive illness often is associated with an increase in both plasma cortisol and cerebrospinal fluid concentrations of CRF. The question that arises is whether this increased plasma cortisol is a cause or an effect of the depressive state. Although health care professionals continue to question the role of stressors and coping skills in the pathogenesis of disease states, we must resist the temptation to suggest that any disease is due to excessive stress or poor coping skills.

IN SUMMARY, stress in itself is neither negative nor deleterious to health. The stress response is designed to be time limited and protective, but in situations of prolonged activation of the response because of overwhelming or chronic stressors, it could be damaging to health. PTSD is an example of chronic activation of the stress response as a result of experiencing a severe trauma. In this disorder, memory of the traumatic event seems to be enhanced. Flashbacks of the event are accompanied by intense activation of the neuroendocrine system.

Treatment of stress should be aimed at helping people avoid coping behaviors that can adversely affect their health and providing them with other ways to reduce stress. Nonpharmacologic methods used in the treatment of stress include relaxation techniques, guided imagery, music therapy, massage techniques, and biofeedback.

Research in stress has focused on personal reports of the stress situation and the physiologic responses to stress. A number of interview guides and written instruments are available for measuring the personal responses to acute and chronic stressors. Methods used for studying the physiologic manifestations of the stress response include electrocardiographic recording of heart rate, blood pressure measurement, electrodermal measurement of skin resistance associated with sweating, and biochemical analyses of hormone levels. ■

Review Exercises

1. A 21-year-old college student notices that she frequently develops "cold sores" during the stressful final exam week.

   A. *What is the association between stress and the immune system?*

   B. *One of her classmates suggests that she listen to music or try relaxation exercises as a means of relieving stress. Explain how these interventions might work in relieving stress.*

2. A 75-year-old woman with congestive heart failure complains that her condition gets worse when she worries and is under a lot of stress.

   A. *Relate the effects stress has on the neuroendocrine control of cardiovascular function and its possible relationship to a worsening of the woman's congestive heart failure.*

   B. *She tells you that she dealt with much worse stresses when she was younger and never had any problems. How would you explain this?*

3. A 30-year-old woman who was rescued from a collapsed building has been having nightmares recalling the event, excessive anxiety, and loss of appetite, and is afraid to leave her home for fear something will happen.

   A. *Given her history and symptoms, what is the likely diagnosis?*

   B. *How might she be treated?*

References

1. Lazarus R. S., Folkman S. (1984). *Stress, appraisal, and coping.* New York: Springer.
2. Hinkle L. E. (1977). The concept of "stress" in the biological and social sciences. In Lipowskin Z. J., Lipsitt D. R., Whybrow P. C. (Eds.), *Psychosomatic medicine* (pp. 27–49). New York: Oxford University Press.
3. Osler W. (1910). The Lumleian lectures in angina pectoris. *Lancet* 1, 696–700, 839–844, 974–977.
4. Cannon W. B. (1935). Stresses and strains of homeostasis. *American Journal of Medical Science* 189, 1–5.
5. Selye H. (1946). The general adaptation syndrome and diseases of adaptation. *Journal of Clinical Endocrinology* 6, 117–124.
6. Cannon W. B. (1939). *The wisdom of the body* (pp. 299–300). New York: WW Norton.
7. Wilcox R. E., Gonzales R. A. (1995). Introduction to neurotransmitters, receptors, signal transduction, and second messengers. In Schatzberg A. F., Nemeroff C. B. (Eds.), *Textbook of psychopharmacology* (pp. 3–29). Washington, DC: American Psychiatric Press.
8. Elenkov I. J., Webster E. L., Torpy D. J., et al. (1999). Stress, corticotrophin-releasing hormone, glucocorticoids, and the immune/inflammatory response: Acute and chronic effects. *Annals of the New York Academy of Sciences* 876, 1–11.
9. Chrousos G. P. (1998). Stressors, stress, and neuroendocrine integration of the adaptive response. *Annals of the New York Academy of Sciences* 851, 311–335.
10. Selye H. (1976). *The stress of life* (rev. ed.). New York: McGraw-Hill.
11. Selye H. (1973). The evolution of the stress concept. *American Scientist* 61, 692–699.
12. Selye H. (1974). *Stress without distress* (p. 6). New York: New American Library.
13. Lazarus R. (1999). *Stress and emotion: A new synthesis* (p. 6). New York: Springer.
14. Ursin H., Eriksen H. R. (2004). The cognitive-activation theory of stress. *Psychoneuroendocrinology* 29, 567–592.
15. Goldstein D. S. (2003). Catecholamines and stress. *Endocrine Regulations* 37, 69–80.
16. Carrasco G. A., Van de Kar L. D. (2003). Neuroendocrine pharmacology of stress. *European Journal of Pharmacology* 463, 235–272.
17. Motzer S. A., Hertig V. (2004). Stress, stress response, and health. *Nursing Clinics of North America* 39, 1–17.
18. Stewart J. A. (2006). The detrimental effects of allostasis: Allostatic load as a measure of cumulative stress. *Journal of Physiologic Anthropology* 25(1), 133–145.
19. Lopez J. F., Akil H., Watson S. J. (1999). Neural circuits mediating stress. *Biological Psychiatry* 46, 1461–1471.
20. Koob G. F. (1999). Corticotropin-releasing factor, norepinephrine, and stress. *Biological Psychiatry* 46, 1167–1180.
21. Lehnert H., Schulz C., Dieterich K. (1998). Physiological and neurochemical aspects of corticotrophin-releasing factor actions in the brain: The role of the locus ceruleus. *Neurochemical Research* 23, 1039–1052.
22. Sapolsky R. M., Romero L. M., Munck A. U. (2000). How do glucocorticoids influence stress responses? Integrating permissive, suppressive, stimulatory, and preparative actions. *Endocrine Reviews* 21, 55–89.
23. de Kloet E. R. (2003). Hormones, brain and stress. *Endocrine Regulations* 37, 51–68.
24. Sternberg E. M. (2006). Neural regulation of innate immunity: A coordinated nonspecific host response to pathogens. *Nature Reviews: Immunology* 6, 318–328.
25. Dantzer R., Kelley K. W. (1989). Stress and immunity: An integrated view of relationships between the brain and immune system. *Life Sciences* 44, 1995–2008.
26. Falaschi P., Martocchia A., Proietti A., et al. (1994). Immune system and the hypothalamus-pituitary-adrenal axis. *Annals of the New York Academy of Sciences* 741, 223–231.
27. Woiciechowsky C., Schoning F., Lanksch W. R., et al. (1999). Mechanisms of brain mediated systemic anti-inflammatory syndrome causing immunodepression. *Journal of Molecular Medicine* 77, 769–780.

28. Dubos R. (1965). *Man adapting* (pp. 256, 258, 261, 264). New Haven, CT: Yale University Press.

29. Lazarus R. (2000). Evolution of a model of stress, coping, and discrete emotions. In Rice V. H. (Ed.), *Handbook of stress, coping, and health* (pp. 195–222). Thousand Oaks, CA: Sage.

30. Wizemann T. M., Pardue M. L. (Eds.). (2001). *Exploring the biological contributions to human health: Does sex matter?* Committee on Understanding the Biology of Sex and Gender Differences. Board on Health Sciences Policy, Institute of Medicine. Washington, DC: National Academy Press.

31. Kajantie E., Phillips D. I. (2006). The effects of sex and hormonal status on the physiological response to acute psychosocial stress. *Psychoneuroendocrinology* 31, 151–178.

32. Adams K., Oswold I. (1983). Protein synthesis, bodily renewal and sleep-wake cycle. *Clinical Science* 65, 561–567.

33. Gillin J. C., Byerley W. F. (1990). The diagnosis and management of insomnia. *New England Journal of Medicine* 322, 239–248.

34. Moldofsky H., Lue F. A., Davidson J. R., et al. (1989). Effects of sleep deprivation on human immune functions. *FASEB Journal* 3, 1972–1977.

35. Ford-Gilboe M., Cohen J. A. (2000). Hardiness: A model of commitment, challenge, and control. In Rice V. H. (Ed.), *Handbook of stress, coping, and health* (pp. 425–436). Thousand Oaks, CA: Sage.

36. Broadhead W. E., Kaplan B. H., James S. A., et al. (1983). The epidemiologic evidence for a relationship between social support and health. *American Journal of Epidemiology* 117, 521–537.

37. Greenblatt M., Becerra R. M., Serafetinides E. A. (1982). Social networks and mental health: An overview. *American Journal of Psychiatry* 139, 977–984.

38. Tilden V. P., Weinert C. (1987). Social support and the chronically ill individual. *Nursing Clinics of North America* 33, 613–620.

39. National Institute for Occupational Safety and Health. (1999). *Stress at work* (pp. 1–26). Publication no. 99-101, HE 20.7102: ST 8/4. Bethesda, MD: U.S. Department of Health and Human Services.

40. Dworkin S. F. (1969). Psychosomatic concepts and dentistry: Some perspectives. *Journal of Periodontology* 40, 647.

41. Cohen S., Tyrrell D. A. J., Smith A. P. (1991). Psychological stress and susceptibility to the common cold. *New England Journal of Medicine* 325, 606–612.

42. Cohen S., Doyle W. J., Skoner D. P. (1999). Psychological stress, cytokine production, and severity of upper respiratory illness. *Psychosomatic Medicine* 61, 175–180.

43. Vedhara K., Wilcock G. K., Lightman S. L., et al. (1999). Chronic stress in elderly carers of dementia patients and antibody response to influenza vaccination. *Lancet* 353, 627–631.

44. Rozlog L. A., Kiecolt-Glaser J. K., Marucha P. T., et al. (1999). Stress and immunity: Implication for viral disease and wound healing. *Journal of Periodontology* 70, 786–792.

45. Yehuda R. (2002). Post-traumatic stress disorder. *New England Journal of Medicine* 346, 108–114.

46. Galea S., Nandi A., Viahov D. (2005). The epidemiology of post-traumatic stress disorder after disasters. *Epidemiologic Reviews* 27, 78–91.

47. American Psychiatric Association. (2000). *Diagnostic and statistical manual of mental disorders* (4th ed., text revision, pp. 467–468). Washington, DC: Author.

48. Yehuda R. (2000). Biology of posttraumatic stress disorder. *Journal of Clinical Psychiatry* 61(Suppl. 7), 14–21.

49. Yehuda R. (1998). Psychoneuroendocrinology of posttraumatic stress disorder. *Psychiatric Clinics of North America* 21, 359–379.

50. Sapolsky R. (1999). Stress and your shrinking brain (posttraumatic stress disorder's effect on the brain). *Discover* 20(3), 116.

51. McCloskey L. A. (2000). Posttraumatic stress in children exposed to family violence and single event trauma. *Journal of the American Academy of Child and Adolescent Psychiatry* 39, 108–115.

52. Hegedoren K. M., Lasiuk G. C., Coupland N. J. (2006). Posttraumatic stress disorder, part III: Health effects of interpersonal violence among women. *Perspectives in Psychiatric Care* 42(3), 163–173.

53. Benson H. (1977). Systemic hypertension and the relaxation response. *New England Journal of Medicine* 296, 1152–1154.

54. Jacobson E. (1958). *Progressive relaxation.* Chicago: University of Chicago Press.

55. Chlan L., Tracy M. F. (1999). Music therapy in critical care: Indications and guidelines for intervention. *Critical Care Nurse* 19(3), 35–41.

56. White J. M. (1999). Effects of relaxing music on cardiac autonomic balance and anxiety after acute myocardial infarction. *American Journal of Critical Care* 8, 220–230.

57. Vickers A., Zollman C. (1999). ABC of complementary therapies: Massage therapies. *British Medical Journal* 319, 1254–1257.

58. Rusy L. M., Weisman S. J. (2000). Complementary therapies for acute pediatric pain management. *Pediatric Clinics of North America* 47, 589–599.

59. Huhtala V., Lehtonen L., Heinonen R., et al. (2000). Infant massage compared with crib vibrator in treatment of colicky infants. *Pediatrics* 105, E84.

60. Rowe M., Alfred D. (1999). The effectiveness of slow-stroke massage in diffusing agitated behaviors in individuals with Alzheimer's disease. *Journal of Gerontological Nursing* 25(6), 22–34.

61. Richards K. C. (1998). Effect of back massage and relaxation intervention on sleep in critically ill patients. *American Journal of Critical Care* 7, 288–299.

62. Fischer-Williams M., Nigl A. J., Sovine D. L. (1986). *A textbook of biological feedback.* New York: Human Sciences Press.

63. Wimbush F. B., Nelson M. L. (2000). Stress, psychosomatic illness, and health. In Rice V. H. (Ed.), *Handbook of stress, coping, and health* (pp. 143–194). Thousand Oaks, CA: Sage.

64. Backer J. H., Bakas T., Bennett S. J., et al. (2000). Coping with stress: Programs of nursing research. In Rice V. H. (Ed.), *Handbook of stress, coping, and health* (pp. 223–263). Thousand Oaks, CA: Sage.

65. Ryan-Wenger N. A., Sharrer V. W., Wynd C. A. (2000). Stress, coping, and health in children. In Rice V. H. (Ed.), *Handbook of stress, coping, and health* (pp. 265–293). Thousand Oaks, CA: Sage.

66. White J. M., Porth C. M. (2000). Physiological measurement of the stress response. In Rice V. H. (Ed.), *Handbook of stress, coping, and health* (pp. 69–94). Thousand Oaks, CA: Sage.

Visit thePoint **http://thePoint.lww.com for animations, journal articles, and more!**

Chapter 10

Alterations in Temperature Regulation

MARY PAT KUNERT

➤ Body temperature, at any given point in time, represents a balance between heat gain and heat loss. Body heat is generated in the core tissues of the body, transferred to the skin surface by the blood, and then released into the environment surrounding the body. Body temperature rises in fever because of cytokine-mediated changes in the set-point of the temperature-regulating center in the hypothalamus, and in hyperthermia because of excessive heat production, inadequate heat dissipation, or a failure of thermoregulatory mechanisms. It falls during hypothermia caused by exposure to cold. This chapter is organized into three sections: body temperature regulation, increased body temperature (fever and hyperthermia), and decreased body temperature (hypothermia).

BODY TEMPERATURE REGULATION

After completing this section of the chapter, you should be able to meet the following objectives:

- Differentiate between body core temperature and skin temperature and relate the differences to methods used for measuring body temperature.
- Describe the physiologic mechanisms that control the gain and loss of heat from the body.
- Define the terms *conduction, radiation, convection,* and *evaporation,* and relate them to the mechanisms for gain and loss of heat from the body.

Virtually all biochemical processes in the body are affected by changes in temperature. Metabolic processes speed up or slow down depending on whether body temperature is rising or falling. *Core body temperature (i.e.,* intracranial, intrathoracic, and intra-abdominal) normally is maintained within a range of 36.0°C to 37.5°C (97.0°F to 99.5°F).[1–3] Within this range, there are individual differences and diurnal variations; internal core temperatures reach their highest point in late afternoon and evening and their lowest point in the early morning hours (Fig. 10-1).

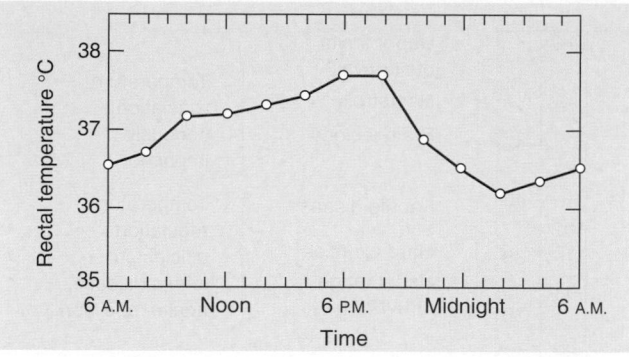

FIGURE 10-1 • Normal diurnal variations in body temperature.

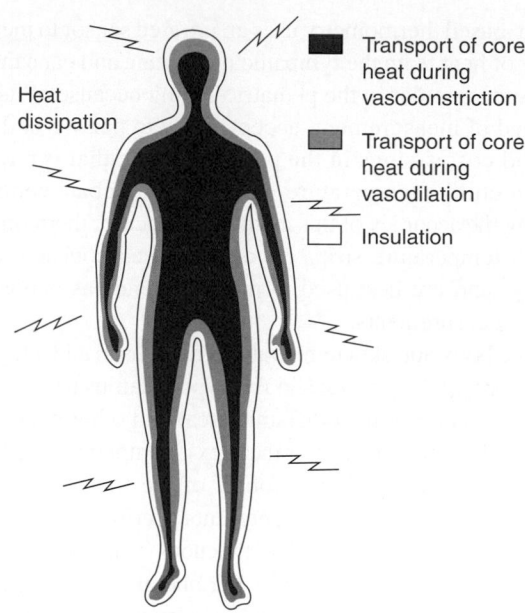

FIGURE 10-2 • Control of heat loss. Body heat is produced in the deeper core tissues of the body, which is insulated by the subcutaneous tissues and skin to protect against heat loss. During vasodilation, circulating blood transports heat to the skin surface, where it dissipates into the surrounding environment. Vasoconstriction decreases the transport of core heat to the skin surface, and vasodilation increases transport.

Body temperature reflects the difference between heat production and heat loss and varies with exercise and extremes of environmental temperature. Properly protected, the body can function in environmental conditions that range from −50°C (−58°F) to +50°C (+122°F). Individual body cells, however, cannot tolerate such a wide range of temperatures: at −1°C (+30°F) ice crystals form, and at +45°C (+113°F), cell proteins coagulate.[4]

THERMOREGULATION

■ Core body temperature is a reflection of the balance between heat gain and heat loss by the body. Metabolic processes produce heat, which must be dissipated.

■ The hypothalamus is the thermal control center for the body, receives information from peripheral and central thermoreceptors, and compares that information with its temperature set point.

■ Heat loss occurs through transfer of body core heat to the surface through the circulation. Heat is lost from the skin through radiation, conduction, convection, and evaporation.

■ An increase in core temperature is effected by vasoconstriction and shivering, a decrease in temperature by vasodilation and sweating.

Most of the body's heat is produced by the deeper core tissues (*i.e.,* muscles and viscera), which are insulated from the environment and protected against heat loss by an outer shell of subcutaneous tissues and skin (Fig. 10-2). Because the shell lies between the core and the environment, all heat leaving the body core, with the exception of that lost through the respiratory tract, must pass through the outer shell.[2] The thickness of the shell depends on blood flow. In a warm environment, blood flow is increased and the thickness of the outer shell is decreased, allowing for greater dissipation of heat. In a cold environment, the

vessels supplying blood flow to the skin and underlying tissues, including those of the limbs and more superficial muscles of the neck and trunk, constrict. This increases the thickness of the shell and helps to minimize the loss of core heat for the body. The subcutaneous fat layer contributes to the insulation value of the outer shell because of its thickness and because it conducts heat only about one third as effectively as other tissues.

Temperatures differ in various parts of the body, with core temperatures being higher than those at the skin surface. In general, the rectal temperature is used as a measure of core temperature. Rectal temperatures usually range from 37.3°C (99.1°F) to 37.6°C (99.6°F).[3] Core temperatures may also be obtained from the esophagus using a flexible thermometer, from a pulmonary artery catheter that is used for thermodilution measurement of cardiac output, or from a urinary catheter with a thermosensor that measures the temperature of urine in the bladder. Because of location, pulmonary artery and esophageal temperatures closely reflect the temperatures of the heart and thoracic organs. This is the preferred measurement when body temperatures are changing rapidly and need to be followed reliably.[3]

The oral temperature, taken sublingually, is usually 0.2°C (0.36°F) to 0.51°C (0.9°F) lower than the rectal temperature; however, it usually follows changes in core temperature closely. The axillary temperature also can be used as an estimate of core temperature. However, the parts of the axillary fossa must be pressed closely together for an extended period (5 to 10 minutes for a glass thermometer) because this method requires considerable heat to accumulate before the final temperature is reached.

Ear-based thermometry uses an infrared sensor to measure the flow of heat from the tympanic membrane and ear canal.[5] It has become popular in the pediatric setting because of its ease and speed of measurement, acceptability to parents and children, and cost savings in the personnel time that is required to take a child's temperature.[6] However, a debate continues regarding the accuracy of this method.[5,7,8] Pacifier thermometers and skin temperature strips have also raised concerns about accuracy, and are best used to monitor trends as opposed to absolute measurements.

Core body and skin temperatures are sensed and integrated by thermoregulatory regions in the hypothalamus (particularly, the preoptic-anterior hypothalamic area) and other brain structures (*i.e.,* thalamus and cerebral cortex). Temperature-sensitive ion channels, identified as a subset of the transient receptor potential family (thermoTRPs), present in peripheral and central sensory neurons are activated by innocuous (warm and cool) and noxious (hot and cold) stimuli.[9] Peripheral signals regarding temperature are initiated by changes in local membrane potentials that are transmitted to the brain through dorsal root ganglia.[9] The *set-point* of the hypothalamic thermoregulatory center is set so that the temperature of the body core is regulated within the normal range of 36.0°C (96.8°F) to 37.5°C (99.5°F). When body temperature begins to rise above the set-point, the hypothalamus signals the central and peripheral nervous systems to initiate heat-dissipating behaviors. Likewise, when the temperature falls below the set-point, signals from the hypothalamus elicit physiologic behaviors that increase heat conservation and production. Core temperatures above 41°C (105.8°F) or below 34°C (93.2°F) usually mean that the body's ability to thermoregulate has been impaired (Fig. 10-3). Body responses that produce, conserve, and dissipate heat are described in Table 10-1. Spinal cord injuries that transect the cord at T6 or above can seriously impair temperature regulation because the thermoregulatory centers in the hypothalamus can no longer control skin blood flow and sweating.

In addition to reflexive and automatic thermoregulatory mechanisms, humans engage in voluntary behaviors to help regulate body temperature based on their conscious sensation of being too hot or too cold. These behaviors include the selection of proper clothing and regulation of environmental temperature through heating systems and air conditioning. Body positions that hold the extremities close to the body prevent heat loss and are commonly assumed in cold weather.

Mechanisms of Heat Production

Metabolism is the body's main source of heat production. There is a 0.55°C (1°F) increase in body temperature for every 7% increase in metabolism. The sympathetic neurotransmitters, epinephrine and norepinephrine, which are released when an increase in body temperature is needed, act at the cellular level to shift body metabolism to heat production rather than energy generation. This may be one of the reasons fever tends to produce feelings of weakness and fatigue. Thyroid hormone

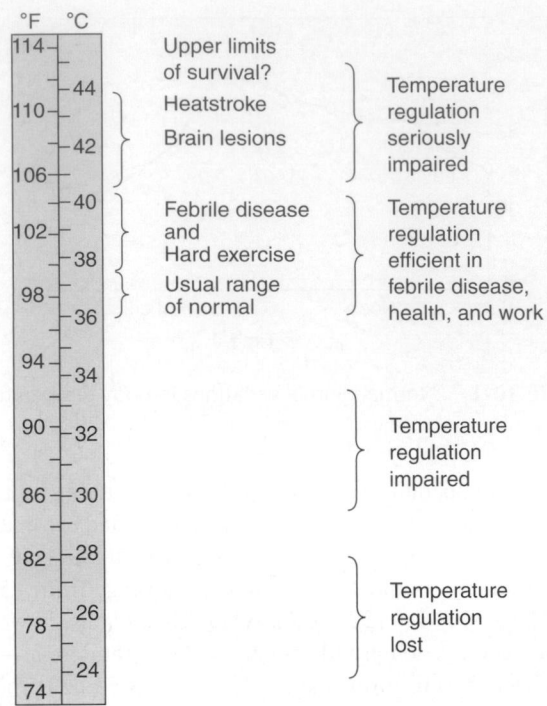

FIGURE 10-3 • Body temperatures under different conditions. (From Dubois E. F. [1948]. *Fever and the regulation of body temperature.* Springfield, IL: Charles C Thomas.)

increases cellular metabolism, but this response usually requires several weeks to reach maximal effectiveness. The metabolic rate is typically 45% or more above normal in hyperthyroidism.[2]

Fine involuntary actions such as shivering and chattering of the teeth can produce a three- to fivefold increase in body temperature. *Shivering* is initiated by impulses from the hypothalamus. The first muscle change that occurs with shivering is a general increase in muscle tone, followed by an oscillating rhythmic tremor involving the spinal-level reflex that controls muscle tone. Because no external work is performed, all the energy liberated by the metabolic processes from shivering is in the form of heat.[10] Physical exertion increases body temperature. Muscles convert most of the energy in the fuels they consume into heat rather than mechanical work. With strenuous exercise, more than three fourths of the increased metabolism resulting from muscle activity appears as heat within the body, and the remainder appears as mechanical work.

Mechanisms of Heat Loss

Most of the body's heat losses occur at the skin surface as heat from the blood moves to the skin and from there into the surrounding environment. There are numerous arteriovenous (AV) shunts under the skin surface that allow blood to move directly from the arterial to the venous system[1] (Fig. 10-4). These AV shunts are much like the radiators in a heating system. When the shunts are open, body heat is freely dissipated to the skin and surrounding environment; when the shunts are closed, heat

TABLE 10-1 **Heat Gain and Heat Loss Responses Used in Regulation of Body Temperature**			
HEAT GAIN		**HEAT LOSS**	
Body Response	Mechanism of Action	Body Response	Mechanism of Action
Vasoconstriction of the superficial blood vessels	Confines blood flow to the inner core of the body, with the skin and subcutaneous tissues acting as insulation to prevent loss of core heat	Dilatation of the superficial blood vessels	Delivers blood containing core heat to the periphery where it is dissipated through radiation, conduction, and convection
Contraction of the pilomotor muscles that surround the hairs on the skin	Reduces the heat loss surface of the skin	Sweating	Increases heat loss through evaporation
Assumption of the huddle position with the extremities held close to the body	Reduces the area for heat loss		
Shivering	Increases heat production by the muscles		
Increased production of epinephrine	Increases the heat production associated with metabolism		
Increased production of thyroid hormone	Is a long-term mechanism that increases metabolism and heat production		

is retained in the body. The blood flow in the AV shunts is controlled almost exclusively by the sympathetic nervous system in response to changes in core temperature and environmental temperature. Contraction of the *pilomotor muscles* of the skin, which raises skin hairs and produces goose bumps, also aids in heat conservation by reducing the surface area available for heat loss.

Heat is lost from the body through radiation, conduction, and convection from the skin surface; through the evaporation of sweat and insensible perspiration; through the exhalation of air that has been warmed and humidified; and through heat lost in urine and feces. Of these mechanisms, only heat losses that occur at the skin surface are directly under hypothalamic control.

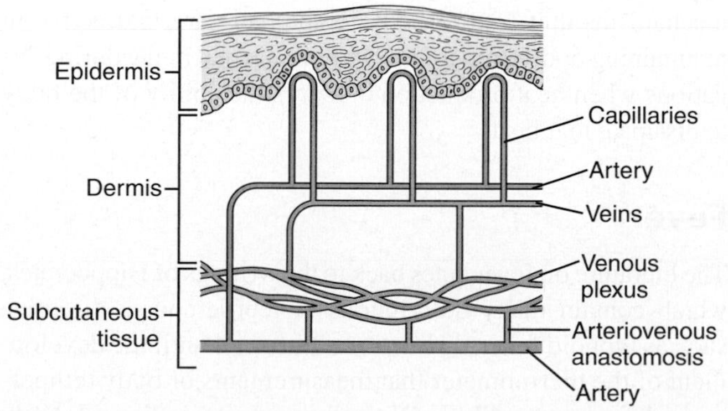

Radiation

Radiation is the transfer of heat through air or a vacuum. Heat from the sun is carried by radiation. Heat loss by radiation varies with the temperature of the environment. Environmental temperature must be less than that of the body for heat loss to occur. In a nude person sitting inside a normal-temperature room, approximately 60% of body heat typically is dissipated by radiation.[1]

Conduction

Conduction is the direct transfer of heat from one molecule to another. Blood carries, or conducts, heat from the inner core of the body to the skin surface. Normally only a small amount of body heat is lost through conduction to a cooler surface. Cooling blankets or mattresses that are used for reducing fever rely on conduction of heat from the skin to the cool surface of the mattress. Heat also can be conducted in the opposite direction—from the external environment to the body surface. For instance, body temperature may rise slightly after a hot bath.

Water has a specific heat several times greater than air, so water absorbs far greater amounts of heat than air does. The loss of body heat can be excessive and life-threatening in situations of cold water immersion or cold exposure in damp or wet clothing.

FIGURE 10-4 • Skin circulation with arteriovenous shunts and venous plexuses that participate in transfer of core heat to the skin. (Adapted from Guyton A., Hall J. E. [2000]. *Textbook of medical physiology* [10th ed., p. 823]. Philadelphia: WB Saunders, with permission from Elsevier Science.)

Epidermis —

Dermis —

Subcutaneous tissue —

Capillaries

Artery

Veins

Venous plexus

Arteriovenous anastomosis

Artery

The conduction of heat to the body's surface is influenced by blood volume. In hot weather, the body compensates by increasing blood volume as a means of dissipating heat. A mild swelling of the ankles during hot weather (called *heat edema*) provides evidence of blood volume expansion. Exposure to cold produces a cold diuresis and a reduction in blood volume as a means of controlling the transfer of heat to the body's surface.

Convection

Convection refers to heat transfer through the circulation of air currents. Normally, a layer of warm air tends to remain near the body's surface; convection causes continual removal of the warm layer and replacement with air from the surrounding environment. The wind-chill factor that often is included in the weather report combines the effect of convection due to wind with the still-air temperature.

Evaporation

Evaporation involves the use of body heat to convert water on the skin to water vapor. Water that diffuses through the skin independent of sweating is called *insensible perspiration.* Insensible perspiration losses are greatest in a dry environment. Sweating occurs through the sweat glands and is controlled by the sympathetic nervous system. Unlike other sympathetically mediated functions, in which the catecholamines serve as neuromediators, sweating is mediated by acetylcholine. This means that anticholinergic drugs, such as atropine, can interfere with heat loss by interrupting sweating.

Evaporative heat losses involve insensible perspiration and sweating, with 0.58 calorie being lost for each gram of water that is evaporated.[1] As long as body temperature is greater than the atmospheric temperature, heat is lost through radiation. However, when the temperature of the surrounding environment becomes greater than skin temperature, evaporation is the only way the body can rid itself of heat. Any condition that prevents evaporative heat losses causes the body temperature to rise.

IN SUMMARY, core body temperature is normally maintained within a range of 36.0°C to 37.5°C (97.0°F to 99.5°F). Core body and skin temperature are sensed and integrated by thermoregulatory regions in the hypothalamus and other brain structures that function to modify heat production and heat loss as a means of regulating body temperature. Most of the body's heat is produced by metabolic processes that occur within deeper core structures (*i.e.,* muscles and viscera) of the body. The sympathetic neurotransmitters (epinephrine and norepinephrine) and thyroid hormone act at the cellular level to shift body metabolism to heat production, whereas shivering and chattering of the teeth use the heat liberated from involuntary muscle movements to increase body temperature. Most of the body's

heat losses occur at the skin surface as heat from the blood moves through the skin and from there into the surrounding environment. Heat is lost from the skin through radiation, conduction, convection, and evaporation of perspiration and sweat. Contraction of the *pilomotor muscles* of the skin aids in heat conservation by reducing the surface area available for heat loss. ■

INCREASED BODY TEMPERATURE

After completing this section of the chapter, you should be able to meet the following objectives:

- Characterize the physiology of fever.
- Describe the four stages of fever.
- Explain what is meant by intermittent, remittent, sustained, and relapsing fevers.
- State the relation between body temperature and heart rate.
- Differentiate between the physiologic mechanisms involved in fever and hyperthermia.
- State the definition of fever of unknown source in children 0 to 36 months of age.
- State the definition for fever in the elderly and cite possible mechanisms for altered febrile response in the elderly.
- Compare the characteristics of fevers caused by infectious agents and drug-related fevers.
- Compare the mechanisms of malignant hyperthermia and neuroleptic malignant syndrome.

Both fever and hyperthermia describe conditions in which body temperature is higher than the normal range. Fever is due to an upward displacement of the thermostatic set-point of the thermoregulatory center in the hypothalamus. This is in contrast to hyperthermia, in which the set-point is unchanged, but the mechanisms that control body temperature are ineffective in maintaining body temperature within a normal range during situations when heat production outpaces the ability of the body to dissipate that heat.

Fever

The literature on fever dates back to the writings of Hippocrates, which contain many descriptions of febrile-course diseases, such as typhoid fever.[11] However, it was not until the development of the thermometer that measurements of body temperature became possible. One of the first studies of body temperature was reported in 1868 by the German physician Carl Wunderlich. During a 20-year period, Wunderlich studied the body temperature of 25,000 patients with observations made twice daily with a foot-long thermometer held in the axilla for 20 minutes.[12] Wunderlich observed that the thermometer was a useful instrument for providing insight into the condition of the ill person. Today, temperature is one of the most frequent physiologic responses to be monitored during illness.

🔑 FEVER

- Fever represents an increase in body temperature that results from a cytokine-induced increase in the set-point of the thermostatic center in the hypothalamus.

- Fever is a nonspecific response that is mediated by endogenous pyrogens released from host cells in response to infectious or noninfectious disorders.

- The development of fever involves a prodrome, a chill during which the temperature rises until it reaches the new hypothalamic set-point, a flush during which the skin vessels dilate and the temperature begins to fall, and a period of defervescence that is marked by sweating.

- Fever is resolved when the condition causing the increase in the set-point of the thermostatic center in the hypothalamus is resolved.

Mechanisms

Fever, or *pyrexia,* describes an elevation in body temperature that is caused by an upward displacement of the thermostatic set-point of the hypothalamic thermoregulatory center. Many proteins, breakdown products of proteins, and certain other substances released from bacterial cell membranes can cause a change in the set-point to rise. Fever is resolved or "broken" when the condition that caused the increase in the set-point is removed. Fevers that are regulated by the hypothalamus usually do not rise above 41°C (105.8°F), suggesting a built-in thermostatic safety mechanism. Temperatures above that level are usually the result of superimposed activity, such as convulsions, hyperthermic states, or direct impairment of the temperature control center.

Pyrogens are exogenous or endogenous substances that produce fever. *Exogenous pyrogens* are derived from outside the body and include such substances as bacterial products, bacterial toxins, or whole microorganisms. Exogenous pyrogens induce host cells to produce fever-producing mediators called *endogenous pyrogens.* When bacteria or breakdown products of bacteria are present in blood or tissues, they are engulfed by phagocytic cells of the immune system (see Chapter 17). These phagocytic cells digest the bacterial products and then release pyrogenic cytokines, principally interleukin-1 (IL-1), interleukin-6 (IL-6), and tumor necrosis factor-α (TNF-α), into the bloodstream for transport to the hypothalamus, where they exert their action.[13] Prostaglandin E_2 (PGE$_2$), which is a metabolite of arachidonic acid (an intramembrane fatty acid), is considered to be the final fever mediator in the hypothalamus, induced by these cytokines. PGE$_2$ binds to receptors in the hypothalamus to induce changes in its set-point through the second messenger cyclic adenosine monophosphate (cAMP).[14] In response to the increase in its thermostatic set-point, the hypothalamus initiates shivering and vasoconstriction that raise the body's core temperature to the new set-point, and fever is established.

Although the central role of PGE$_2$ in raising the set-point of the hypothalamic thermoregulatory center and producing fever is not questioned, recent research suggests that the febrile response to invading gram-negative bacteria and their products (mainly endotoxic lipopolysaccharides) is mediated by peripherally rather than centrally produced PGE$_2$.[15,16] These pathogens are thought to activate the alternative pathway of the complement system, which in turn stimulates Kupffer cells (*i.e.,* phagocytic cells found on luminal surface of hepatic sinusoids) in the liver to produce an almost instantaneous release of PGE$_2$. The PGE$_2$ produced by the Kupffer cells is thought to cause an immediate rise in temperature by activating vagal afferents in the liver that project to the hypothalamus or by being carried directly to the hypothalamus by the circulation.[15,16] The pyrogenic cytokines (IL-1, IL-2, TNF-α) are produced later and contribute to the continued rise in temperature.

In addition to their fever-producing actions, the endogenous pyrogens mediate a number of other responses. For example, IL-1 and TNF-α are inflammatory mediators that produce other signs of inflammation such as leukocytosis, anorexia, and malaise (see Chapter 18). Many noninfectious disorders, such as myocardial infarction, pulmonary emboli, and neoplasms, produce fever. In these conditions, the injured or abnormal cells incite the production of endogenous pyrogens. For example, trauma and surgery can be associated with up to 3 days of fever. Some malignant cells, such as those of leukemia and Hodgkin disease, secrete chemical mediators that function as endogenous pyrogens.

A fever that has its origin in the central nervous system is sometimes referred to as a *neurogenic fever.* It usually is caused by damage to the hypothalamus due to central nervous system trauma, intracerebral bleeding, or an increase in intracranial pressure. Neurogenic fevers are characterized by a high temperature that is resistant to antipyretic therapy and is not associated with sweating.

Purpose

The purpose of fever is not completely understood. However, from a purely practical standpoint, fever is a valuable index to health status. For many, fever signals the presence of an infection and may legitimize the need for medical treatment. In ancient times, fever was thought to "cook" the poisons that caused the illness. With the availability of antipyretic drugs in the late 19th century, the belief that fever was useful began to wane, probably because most antipyretic drugs also had analgesic effects.

There is little research to support the belief that fever is harmful unless the temperature rises above 40°C (104°F). Animal studies have demonstrated a clear survival advantage in infected members with fever compared with animals that were unable to produce a fever. It has been shown that small elevations in temperature such as those that occur with fever enhance immune function. There is increased motility and activity of the white blood cells, stimulation of interferon production, and activation of T cells.[13,17] Many of the microbial agents that cause infection grow best at normal body temperatures, and their growth is inhibited by temperatures in the fever range. For example, the rhinoviruses responsible for the common cold are cultured best at 33°C (91.4°F), which is close to the temperature in the nasopharynx; temperature-sensitive mutants of the virus that cannot grow at temperatures above 37.5°C (99.5°F) produce fewer signs and symptoms.[18]

Patterns

The patterns of temperature change in persons with fever vary and may provide information about the nature of the causative agent.[19–21] These patterns can be described as intermittent, remittent, sustained, or relapsing (Fig. 10-5). An *intermittent fever* is one in which temperature returns to normal at least once every 24 hours. In a *remittent fever,* the temperature does not return to normal and varies a few degrees in either direction. In a *sustained* or *continuous fever,* the temperature remains above normal with minimal variations (usually less than 0.55°C or 1°F). A *recurrent* or *relapsing fever* is one in which there is one or more episodes of fever, each as long as several days, with one or more days of normal temperature between episodes.

Critical to the analysis of a fever pattern is the relation of heart rate to the level of temperature elevation. Normally, a 1°C rise in temperature produces a 15 beats/minute increase in heart rate (1°F, 10 beats/minute).[19] Most persons respond to an increase in temperature with an appropriate increase in heart rate. The observation that a rise in temperature is not accompanied by the anticipated change in heart rate can provide useful information about the cause of the fever. For example, a heart rate that is slower than would be anticipated can occur with Legionnaire's disease and drug fever, and a heart rate that is more rapid than anticipated can be symptomatic of hyperthyroidism and pulmonary emboli.

Manifestations

The physiologic behaviors that occur during the development of fever can be divided into four successive stages: a prodrome; a chill, during which the temperature rises; a flush; and defervescence (Fig. 10-6). During the *first* or *prodromal* period, there are nonspecific complaints such as mild headache and fatigue, general malaise, and fleeting aches and pains. During the *second stage* or *chill,* there is the uncomfortable sensation of being chilled and the onset of generalized shaking, although the temperature is rising. Vasoconstriction and piloerection usually precede the onset of shivering. At this point, the skin is pale and covered with goose flesh. There is a feeling of being cold and an urge to put on more clothing or covering and to curl up in a position that conserves body heat. When the shivering has caused the body temperature to reach the new set-point of the temperature control center, the shivering ceases, and a sensation of warmth develops. At this point, the *third stage* or *flush* begins, during which cutaneous vasodilation occurs and the skin becomes warm and flushed. The *fourth,* or *defervescence,* stage of the febrile response is marked by the initiation of sweating. Not all persons proceed through the four stages of fever development.

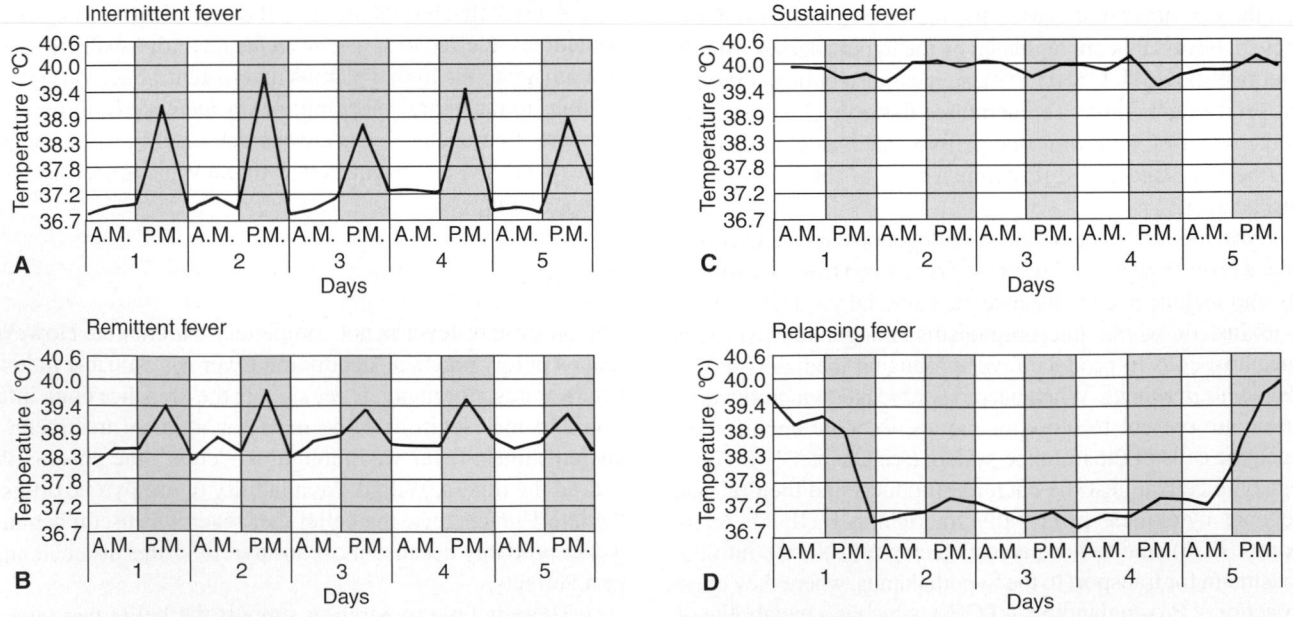

FIGURE 10-5 • Schematic representation of fever patterns: **(A)** intermittent, **(B)** remittent, **(C)** sustained, and **(D)** recurrent or relapsing.

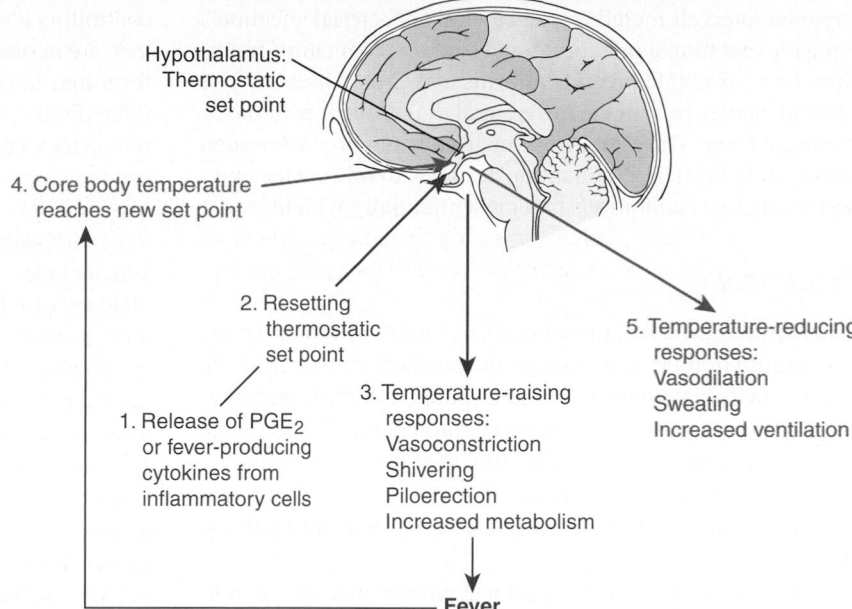

FIGURE 10-6 • Mechanisms of fever. (1) Release of prostaglandin E₂ (PGE₂) or fever-producing cytokines from inflammatory cells; (2) resetting of the thermostatic set-point in the hypothalamus to a higher level (prodrome); (3) generation of hypothalamus-mediated responses that raise body temperature (chill); (4) development of fever with elevation of body to new thermostatic set-point; and (5) production of temperature-lowering responses (flush and defervescence) and return of body temperature to a lower level.

Sweating may be absent, and fever may develop gradually with no indication of a chill or shivering.

Common manifestations of fever are anorexia, myalgia, arthralgia, and fatigue. These discomforts are worse when the temperature rises rapidly or exceeds 39.5°C (103.1°F). Respiration is increased, and the heart rate usually is elevated. Dehydration occurs because of sweating and the increased vapor losses due to the rapid respiratory rate. The occurrence of chills commonly coincides with the introduction of pyrogen into the circulation. Many of the manifestations of fever are related to the increases in the metabolic rate, increases in oxygen demands, and use of body proteins as an energy source. During fever, the body switches from using glucose (an excellent medium for bacterial growth) to metabolism based on protein and fat breakdown.[22] With prolonged fever, there is an increased breakdown of endogenous fat stores. If fat breakdown is rapid, metabolic acidosis may result (see Chapter 32).

Headache is a common accompaniment of fever and is thought to result from the vasodilation of cerebral vessels occurring with fever. Delirium is possible when the temperature exceeds 40°C (104°F). In the elderly, confusion and delirium may follow moderate elevations in temperature. Owing to increasingly poor oxygen uptake by the aging lung, pulmonary function may prove to be a limiting factor in the hypermetabolism that accompanies fever in older persons. Confusion, incoordination, and agitation commonly reflect cerebral hypoxemia. Febrile convulsions can occur in some children.[23] They usually occur with rapidly rising temperatures or at a threshold temperature that differs with each child.

The herpetic lesions, or fever blisters, that develop in some persons during fever are caused by a separate infection by the type 1 herpes simplex virus that established latency in the regional ganglia and is reactivated by a rise in body temperature.

Differential Diagnosis

Most febrile illnesses are due to common infections and are relatively easy to diagnose. In certain instances, however, it is difficult to establish the cause of a fever. A prolonged fever for which the cause is difficult to ascertain is often referred to as *fever of unknown origin* (FUO). FUO is defined as a temperature elevation of 38.3°C (101°F) or higher that is present for 3 weeks or longer.[24] Among the causes of FUO are malignancies (*i.e.,* lymphomas, metastases to the liver and central nervous system); infections such as human immunodeficiency virus or tuberculosis, or abscessed infections; and drug fever. Malignancies, particularly non-Hodgkin lymphoma, are important causes of FUO in the elderly. Cirrhosis of the liver is another cause of FUO.

Recurrent or periodic fevers may occur in predictable intervals or without any discernible time pattern. They may be associated with no discernible cause or they can be the presenting symptom of several serious illnesses, often preceding the other symptoms of those diseases by weeks or months. The PFAPA syndrome, which is characterized by *p*eriodic *f*ever, *a*phthous (small ulcerative) stomatitis, *p*haryngitis, and cervical *a*denopathy occurring every 21 to 28 days, is the most common cause of recurrent fevers in children younger than 5 years of age.[25] Other conditions in which recurrent fevers occur but do not follow a strictly periodic pattern include genetic disorders such as familial Mediterranean fever.[26] Familial Mediterranean fever, an autosomal recessive disease, is characterized by an early age of onset (<20 years) of acute episodic bouts of peritonitis and high fever with an average duration of less than 2 days. In some cases pleuritis, pericarditis, and arthritis are present. The primary chronic complication is the presence of serum antibodies that can result in kidney or heart failure. This complication can be prevented by treatment with colchicine.[26]

Conditions that present with recurrent fevers occurring at irregular intervals include repeated viral or bacterial infections, parasitic and fungal infections, and some inflammatory conditions (*e.g.,* systemic juvenile arthritis and Crohn disease). The clinical challenge is in the differential diagnosis of periodic or recurrent fever. The initial work-up usually requires a thorough history and physical examination designed to rule out the more serious medical conditions that present initially with fever.

Treatment

The methods of fever treatment focus on modifications of the external environment intended to increase heat transfer from the internal to the external environment, support of the hypermetabolic state that accompanies fever, protection of vulnerable body organs and systems, and treatment of the infection or condition causing the fever. Because fever is a disease symptom, its manifestation suggests the need for diagnosis and treatment of the primary cause.

Modification of the environment ensures that the environmental temperature facilitates heat transfer away from the body. Sponge baths with cool water or an alcohol solution can be used to increase evaporative heat losses. More profound cooling can be accomplished through the use of a cooling mattress, which facilitates the conduction of heat from the body into the coolant solution that circulates through the mattress. Care must be taken so that the cooling method does not produce vasoconstriction and shivering that decrease heat loss and increase heat production.

Adequate fluids and sufficient amounts of simple carbohydrates are needed to support the hypermetabolic state and prevent the tissue breakdown that is characteristic of fever. Additional fluids are needed for sweating and to balance the insensible water losses from the lungs that accompany an increase in respiratory rate. Fluids also are needed to maintain an adequate vascular volume for heat transport to the skin surface.

Antipyretic drugs, such as aspirin, ibuprofen, and acetaminophen, often are used to alleviate the discomforts of fever and protect vulnerable organs, such as the brain, from extreme elevations in body temperature. These drugs act by resetting the set-point of the temperature-regulating center in the hypothalamus to a lower level, presumably by blocking the activity of cyclooxygenase, an enzyme that is required for the conversion of arachidonic acid to PGE_2.[27] Because of the risk of Reye syndrome, the Centers for Disease Control and Prevention, U.S. Food and Drug Administration, and American Academy of Pediatrics Committee on Infectious Diseases advise against the use of aspirin and other salicylates in children with influenza or chickenpox.

 ## Fever in Children

Fever occurs frequently in infants and young children (*i.e.,* 1 day to 3 years of age) and is a common reason for visits to the clinic or emergency department.[28–32] Infants and young children have decreased immunologic function and are more commonly infected with virulent organisms. Also, the mechanisms for controlling temperature are not as well developed in infants as they are in older children and adults. Even though infants with fever may not appear ill, this does not imply an absence of bacterial disease. In infants younger than 3 months, a mild elevation in temperature (*i.e.,* rectal temperature of 38°C [100.4°F]) can indicate serious infection that requires immediate medical attention.[28–30]

Although the differential diagnosis of fever is quite broad and includes both infectious and noninfectious causes, the majority of febrile children have an underlying infection. The most common causes are minor or more serious infections of the respiratory system, gastrointestinal tract, urinary tract, or central nervous system. The epidemiology of serious bacterial disease has changed dramatically with the introduction of the *Haemophilus influenzae* and *Streptococcus pneumoniae* vaccines in developed countries.[30,31] *H. influenzae* type b has been nearly eliminated, and the incidence of pneumococcal disease caused by vaccine and cross-reactive vaccine serotypes has declined substantially.

Although most children have identifiable causes for their fevers, many have fever without an apparent source. The American College of Emergency Physicians has developed clinical guidelines for use in the treatment of previously healthy infants and children 1 day to 3 years of age with fever without a source.[31,32] The guidelines define fever in this age group as an elevation in rectal temperature of at least 38°C (100.4°F). The reliability of other methods of temperature measurements is lower and must be considered when making decisions about the seriousness of the fever.[30] In addition, bundling of infants may raise the skin temperature but not the rectal temperature.[29]

Fever in infants and children can be classified as low risk or high risk, depending on the probability of the infection progressing to bacteremia or meningitis and signs of toxicity. Infants between the ages of 1 and 28 days with a fever should be considered to have a bacterial infection that can cause bacteremia or meningitis. Signs of toxicity include lethargy, poor feeding, hypoventilation, poor tissue oxygenation, and cyanosis. The response to antipyretic medications does not change the likelihood of the child having a serious bacterial infection and should not be used as an indicator of infection severity.[30,31] A white blood cell count and blood cultures usually are done in high-risk infants and children to determine the cause of fever. A lumbar puncture is usually performed on febrile neonates to rule out meningitis.[30]

A chest radiograph should be obtained in febrile infants younger than 3 months of age with at least one sign of a respiratory illness (*e.g.,* tachypnea, crackles, decreased breath sounds, wheezing, coughing).[31] Febrile children who are younger than 1 year of age and girls between 1 and 2 years of age should be considered at risk for a urinary tract infection (see Chapter 33).[31] Because of the significant sequelae associated with undiagnosed and untreated urinary tract infections, urine cultures are recommended for children aged younger than 2 years.[31] Although various options for rapid testing for urinary tract infections are available, no rapid test detects all cases of urinary tract infection.[30]

The approach to treatment of the young child who has a fever without source varies depending on the age of the child. Because of the high rates of serious bacterial infections, febrile infants usually receive antibiotics.[30] High-risk infants and infants who are younger than 28 days are often hospitalized for evaluation of their fever and treatment.[30] Of children aged 3 to 36 months with fever without source, 1.5% to 2% will have occult bacteremia and only a small percentage will go on to develop serious sequelae.[31] Antibiotic therapy should be considered if the fever of 39.0°C (102.2°F) or greater is accompanied by a white blood cell count of 15,000/mm³ or higher.[31]

Fever in the Elderly

In the elderly, even slight elevations in temperature may indicate serious infection or disease. This is because the elderly often have a lower baseline temperature, and although they increase their temperature during an infection, it may fail to reach a level that is equated with significant fever.[33–35]

Normal body temperature and the circadian pattern of temperature variation often are altered in the elderly. Elderly persons are reported to have a lower basal temperature (36.4°C [97.6°F] in one study) than younger persons.[36] It has been recommended that the definition of fever in the elderly be expanded to include an elevation of temperature of at least 1.1°C (2°F) above baseline values.[35]

It has been suggested that 20% to 30% of elders with serious infections present with an absent or blunted febrile response.[35] When fever is present in the elderly, it usually indicates the presence of serious infection, most often caused by bacteria. The absence of fever may delay diagnosis and initiation of antimicrobial treatment. Unexplained changes in functional capacity, worsening of mental status, weakness and fatigue, and weight loss are signs of infection in the elderly. They should be viewed as possible signs of infection and sepsis when fever is absent. A thorough history and physical examination are critically important. The probable mechanisms for the blunted fever response include a disturbance in sensing of temperature by the thermoregulatory center in the hypothalamus, alterations in release of endogenous pyrogens, and the failure to elicit responses such as vasoconstriction of skin vessels, increased heat production, and shivering that increase body temperature during a febrile response.

Another factor that may delay recognition of fever in the elderly is the method of temperature measurement. Oral temperature remains the most commonly used method for measuring temperature in the elderly. It has been suggested that rectal and tympanic membrane methods are more effective in detecting fever in the elderly. This is because conditions such as mouth breathing, tongue tremors, and agitation often make it difficult to obtain accurate oral temperatures in the elderly.

Hyperthermia

Hyperthermia describes an increase in body temperature that occurs without a change in the set-point of the hypothalamic thermoregulatory center. It occurs when the thermoregulatory mechanisms are overwhelmed by heat production, excessive environmental heat, or impaired dissipation of heat.[37] It includes (in order of increasing severity) heat cramps, heat exhaustion, and heatstroke. Malignant hyperthermia describes a rare genetic disorder of anesthetic-related hyperthermia. Hyperthermia also may occur as the result of a drug reaction.

 HYPERTHERMIA

- Hyperthermia is a pathologic increase in core body temperature without a change in the hypothalamic set point. The thermoregulatory center is overwhelmed by either excess heat production, impaired heat loss, or excessive environmental heat.

- Malignant hyperthermia is an autosomal dominant disorder in which an abnormal release of intracellular stores of calcium causes uncontrolled skeletal muscle contractions, resulting in a rapid increase in core body temperature. This usually is in response to an anesthetic.

A number of factors predispose to hyperthermia. If muscle exertion is continued for long periods in warm weather, as often happens with athletes, military recruits, and laborers, excessive heat loads are generated.[37] Because adequate circulatory function is essential for heat dissipation, elderly persons and those with cardiovascular disease are at increased risk for hyperthermia. Drugs that increase muscle tone and metabolism or reduce heat loss (*e.g.*, diuretics, neuroleptics, drugs with anticholinergic action) can impair thermoregulation. Infants and small children who are left in a closed car for even short periods in hot weather are potential victims of hyperthermia.

The best approach to heat-related disorders is prevention, primarily by avoiding activity in hot environments, increasing fluid intake, and wearing climate- and activity-appropriate clothing. The ability to tolerate a hot environment depends on both temperature and humidity. A high relative humidity retards heat loss through sweating and evaporation and decreases the body's cooling ability. The *heat index* is the temperature that the body senses when both the temperature and humidity are combined. The Heat Index/Heat Disorder Table, produced by the National Weather Service, provides a useful guide for determining when to avoid outside activity (Table 10-2).

Heat Cramps

Heat cramps are slow, painful, skeletal muscle cramps and spasms, usually occurring in the muscles that are most heavily

TABLE 10-2 Heat Index Values Associated With Possible Heat Disorders

HEAT INDEX (Combination of Heat and Humidity Effects)	POSSIBLE HEAT DISORDER
26.6°C–32.2°C (80°F–90°F)	Fatigue possible with prolonged exposure and physical activity
32.2°C–40.6°C (90°F–105°F)	Sunstroke, heat cramps, and heat exhaustion possible
40.6°C–54.4°C (105°F–130°F)	Sunstroke, heat cramps, and heat exhaustion likely, and heatstroke possible
54.4°C (130°F) or greater	Heatstroke highly likely with continued exposure

Data from www.crh.noaa.gov/pub/heat.htm (U.S. National Weather Service).

used and lasting for 1 to 3 minutes. Cramping results from salt depletion that occurs when fluid losses from heavy sweating are replaced by water alone. The muscles are tender, and the skin usually is moist. Body temperature may be normal or slightly elevated. There almost always is a history of vigorous activity preceding the onset of symptoms.

Treatment consists of drinking an oral saline solution (commercially prepared electrolyte solutions or 1 tsp of salt in 500 mL of water), stretching the affected muscles, and resting in a cool environment.[38] Because absorption is slow and unpredictable, salt tablets are not recommended. Salt tablets also can cause gastric irritation, vomiting, and cerebral edema. Strenuous physical activity should be avoided for several days, while dietary sodium replacement is continued.

Heat Exhaustion

Heat exhaustion is related to a gradual loss of salt and water, usually after prolonged and heavy exertion in a hot environment. The symptoms include thirst, fatigue, nausea, oliguria, giddiness, and finally delirium. Gastrointestinal flulike symptoms are common. Hyperventilation in association with heat exhaustion may contribute to heat cramps and tetany by causing respiratory alkalosis (see Chapter 32). The skin is moist, the rectal temperature usually is higher than 37.8°C (100°F) but below 40°C (104°F), and the heart rate is elevated, usually by more than half again the normal resting rate. Signs of heat cramps may accompany heat exhaustion.

Like heat cramps, heat exhaustion is treated by rest in a cool environment, the provision of adequate hydration, and salt replacement. Intravenous fluids are administered when adequate oral intake cannot be achieved. If the individual has water-depleted heat exhaustion and is hypernatremic, rehydration needs to occur at a regulated rate to reduce the development of iatrogenic cerebral edema (see Chapter 31).[37]

Heatstroke

Heatstroke is a severe, life-threatening failure of thermoregulatory mechanisms resulting in an excessive rise in body temperature—a core temperature greater than 40°C (104°F), a hot, dry skin, absence of sweating, and central nervous system abnormalities such as delirium, convulsions, and loss of consciousness.[38–41] The risk of developing heatstroke in re-

sponse to heat stress is increased in conditions (*i.e.,* alcoholism, obesity, diabetes mellitus, and chronic cardiac, renal, or mental disease) and with drugs (*i.e.,* alcohol, anticholinergics, beta blockers, or tricyclic antidepressants) that impair vasodilation and sweating.[38,39]

The pathophysiology of heatstroke is thought to result from the direct effect of heat on body cells and the release of cytokines (*e.g.,* interleukins, TNF-α, and interferon) from heat-stressed endothelial cells, leukocytes, and epithelial cells that protect against tissue injury. The net result is a combination of local and systemic inflammatory responses that may result in acute respiratory distress syndrome, acute renal failure, disseminated intravascular coagulation, multiorgan dysfunction, and rhabdomyolysis.[39] Hyperthermia is also known to cause edema and microhemorrhages in the brain.[42]

Heatstroke may be designated as *classic* or *nonexertional* when it arises as a consequence of exposure to high environmental temperatures or as *exertional* when it arises as a consequence of strenuous exercise.[38,39] The reported incidence of heatstroke in the United States varies from 17.6 to 26.5/100,000 persons.[39,41] However, data on the incidence of heatstroke are imprecise because many heat-related illnesses and deaths are unrecognized as such and because heat-related deaths are not a reportable condition in all states.[41]

The classic or nonexertional form of heatstroke is seen most commonly at the extremes of age. Infants and small children (younger than 5 years of age) lack sufficient body surface area to dissipate excess heat, have a lower rate of sweating, and a slower rate of acclimatization.[38] In the elderly, the problem often is one of impaired heat loss and failure of homeostatic mechanisms, such that body temperature rises with any increase in environmental temperature.[41] Elderly persons with a decreased ability to perceive changes in environmental temperature or decreased mobility are at particular risk because they also may be unable to take appropriate measures such as removing clothing, moving to a cooler environment, and increasing fluid intake. This is particularly true of elderly persons who live alone in small and poorly ventilated housing units and who may be too confused or weak to complain or seek help at the onset of symptoms.

Exertional heatstroke occurs most often in summer and mainly affects athletes and laborers who are exposed to high-temperature environments. Persons with exertional heatstroke often continue to perspire, a factor that often results in a delay in diagnosis. In addition, rhabdomyolysis and its complications (hyperkalemia, hyperphosphatemia, hypocalcemia, and myo-globinuria) contribute to the morbidity and mortality associated with the disorder.[38]

The symptoms of heatstroke include tachycardia, hyperventilation, dizziness, weakness, emotional lability, nausea and vomiting, confusion, delirium, blurred vision, convulsions, collapse, and coma. The skin is hot and usually dry, and the pulse is typically strong initially. The blood pressure may be elevated at first, but hypotension develops as the condition progresses. As vascular collapse occurs, the skin becomes cool. Associated abnormalities include electrocardiographic changes consistent with heart damage, blood coagulation disorders, potassium and sodium depletion, and signs of liver damage.

Early recognition and aggressive treatment of heatstroke are critical to reduce the morbidity and mortality associated with cellular injury due to direct heat and the effects of inflammatory mediators.[38-40] Treatment consists of measures to support the function of vital organs while instituting cooling procedures aimed at producing a rapid reduction in core temperature. Care must be taken that the cooling methods used do not produce vasoconstriction or shivering and thereby decrease the cooling rate or induce heat production. Two methods of cooling are generally used. One method involves submersion in cold water or application of ice packs, and the other involves spraying the body with tepid water while a fan is used to enhance heat loss through evaporation and convection. Whatever method is used, it is important that the temperature of vital structures, such as the brain, heart, and liver, be reduced rapidly because tissue damage ensues when core temperatures rise above 43°C (109.4°F). Selective brain cooling has reportedly been achieved by fanning the face during hyperthermia.[38] Blood flows from the emissary venous pathways of the skin on the head through the bones of the skull to the brain. In hyperthermia, face fanning is thought to cool the venous blood that flows through these emissary veins and thereby produce brain cooling by enhancing heat exchange between the hot arterial blood and the surface-cooled venous blood in the intracranial venous spaces. Because reducing the body temperature may not modulate the inflammatory or coagulation responses elicited in response to heat stress, new pharmacologic interventions to inhibit or attenuate these responses are being investigated.[39]

Drug Fever

Drug fever has been defined as fever coinciding with the administration of a drug and disappearing after the drug has been discontinued.[43-45] Drugs can induce fever by several mechanisms. They can interfere with heat dissipation; they can alter temperature regulation by the hypothalamic centers; they can act as direct pyrogens; they can injure tissues directly; or they can induce an immune response.

Exogenous thyroid hormone increases the metabolic rate and can increase heat production and body temperature. Peripheral heat dissipation can be impaired by atropine and anticholinergic drugs, antihistamines, phenothiazine antipsychotic drugs, and tricyclic antidepressants, which decrease sweating; or by

amphetamines (especially ecstasy), cocaine, and sympathomimetic drugs, which produce peripheral vasoconstriction.[46] Bleomycin (an anticancer drug), amphotericin B (an antifungal drug), and vaccines that contain bacterial and viral products all can act to induce the release of pyrogens. Intravenously administered drugs can lead to infusion-related phlebitis with production of cellular pyrogens that produce fever. Treatment with anticancer drugs can cause the release of endogenous pyrogen from the cancer cells that are destroyed. Overdoses of serotonin reuptake inhibitors or use in persons taking monoamine oxidase (MOA) inhibitors can cause agitation, hyperactivity, and hyperthermia (serotonin syndrome).[46]

The most common cause of drug fever is a *hypersensitivity reaction.* Hypersensitivity drug fevers develop after several weeks of exposure to the drug, cannot be explained in terms of the drug's pharmacologic action, are not related to drug dose, disappear when the drug is stopped, and reappear when the drug is readministered. The fever pattern is typically spiking in nature and exhibits a normal diurnal rhythm. Persons with drug fevers often experience other signs of hypersensitivity reactions, such as arthralgias, urticaria, myalgias, gastrointestinal discomfort, and rashes.

Temperatures of 38.9°C to 40.0°C (101.8°F to 104.0°F) are common in drug fever. The person may be unaware of the fever and appear to be well for the degree of fever that is present. The absence of an appropriate increase in heart rate for the degree of temperature elevation is an important clue to the diagnosis of drug fever. A fever often precedes other, more serious effects of a drug reaction; for this reason, the early recognition of drug fever is important. Drug fever should be suspected whenever the temperature elevation is unexpected and occurs despite improvement in the condition for which the drug was prescribed.

Malignant Hyperthermia

Malignant hyperthermia is an autosomal dominant metabolic disorder in which heat generated by uncontrolled skeletal muscle contraction can produce severe and potentially fatal hyperthermia.[47-49] The muscle contraction is caused by an abnormal release of intracellular calcium from the sarcoplasmic reticulum through calcium release channels (see Chapter 4). The release of calcium at an abnormally high rate also leads to a sustained hypermetabolic rate and a subsequent loss of cellular integrity. The sustained hypermetabolism results in excess lactate production, high adenosine triphosphate (ATP) consumption, increased oxygen consumption and carbon dioxide production, and elevated heat production.

In affected persons, an episode of malignant hyperthermia is triggered by exposure to certain stresses or general anesthetic agents. The syndrome most frequently is associated with the halogenated anesthetic agents and the depolarizing muscle relaxant succinylcholine. There also are various nonoperative precipitating factors, including trauma, exercise, environmental heat stress, and infection. The condition is particularly dangerous in a young person who has a large muscle mass to generate heat.

During malignant hyperthermia, the body temperature can rise to as high as 43°C (109.4°F) at a rate of 1°C (2°F) every 5 minutes. In addition to a steady rise in end-tidal carbon dioxide levels, an initial sign of the disorder, when the condition occurs during anesthesia, is skeletal muscle rigidity. Cardiac arrhythmias and a hypermetabolic state follow in rapid sequence unless the triggering event is immediately discontinued. In addition to discontinuing the triggering agents, treatment includes measures to cool the body, cardiopulmonary support, and the administration of dantrolene, a muscle relaxant drug that acts by blocking the release of calcium from the sarcoplasmic reticulum.

At present, there is no accurate screening test for the condition. A family history of malignant hyperthermia should be considered when general anesthesia is needed because there are anesthetic agents available that do not trigger the hyperthermic response. A halothane–caffeine contracture test performed on muscle tissue obtained during biopsy can confirm the diagnosis; however, this test is performed only at selected centers. Molecular genetic testing for malignant hyperthermia is being developed. In the future, DNA testing may be used for determining malignant hyperthermia in some individuals.

Neuroleptic Malignant Syndrome

The neuroleptic malignant syndrome is associated with neuroleptic (psychotropic) medications and may occur in as much as 0.02% to 3.23% of persons taking such drugs.[50] Some of the most commonly implicated drugs are haloperidol, chlorpromazine, thioridazine, thiothixene, and olanzapine. All of these drugs block dopamine receptors in the basal ganglia and hypothalamus. Hyperthermia is thought to result from alterations in the function of the hypothalamic thermoregulatory center caused by decreased dopamine levels or from uncontrolled muscle contraction like that occurring with anesthetic-induced malignant hyperthermia.[50,51] Because many of the neuroleptic drugs produce an increase in muscle contraction similar to that of malignant hyperthermia, it has been suggested that the disorder may be caused by a spectrum of inherited defects in genes that are responsible for a variety of calcium regulatory mechanisms in sympathetic neurons (*e.g.,* dopaminergic neurons) or higher-order assemblies that regulate them.[52]

The syndrome usually has an explosive onset and is characterized by hyperthermia, muscle rigidity, alterations in consciousness, and autonomic nervous system dysfunction. The hyperthermia is accompanied by tachycardia (120 to 180 beats/minute), cardiac dysrhythmias, labile blood pressure (70/50 to 180/130 mm Hg), postural instability, dyspnea, and tachypnea (18 to 40 breaths/minute).[50,51]

Treatment for neuroleptic malignant syndrome includes the immediate discontinuance of the neuroleptic drug, measures to decrease body temperature, and treatment of dysrhythmias and other complications of the disorder. Bromocriptine (a dopamine agonist) and dantrolene (a muscle relaxant) may be used as part of the treatment regimen.

IN SUMMARY, fever and hyperthermia refer to an increase in body temperature outside the normal range. True fever is a disorder of thermoregulation in which there is an upward displacement of the set-point for temperature control. In hyperthermia, the set-point is unchanged, but the challenge to temperature regulation exceeds the thermoregulatory center's ability to control body temperature. Fever can be caused by a number of factors, including microorganisms, trauma, and drugs or chemicals, all of which incite the release of endogenous pyrogens. The reactions that occur during fever consist of four stages: a prodrome, a chill, a flush, and defervescence. A fever can follow an intermittent, remittent, sustained, or recurrent pattern. The manifestations of fever are largely related to dehydration and an increased metabolic rate. Even a low-grade fever in high-risk infants or in the elderly can indicate serious infection.

The treatment of fever focuses on modifying the external environment as a means of increasing heat transfer to the external environment; supporting the hypermetabolic state that accompanies fever; protecting vulnerable body tissues; and treating the infection or condition causing the fever.

Hyperthermia, which varies in severity based on the degree of core temperature elevation and the severity of cardiovascular and nervous system involvement, includes heat cramps, heat exhaustion, and heatstroke. Among the factors that contribute to the development of hyperthermia are prolonged muscular exertion in a hot environment, disorders that compromise heat dissipation, and hypersensitivity drug reactions. Malignant hyperthermia is an autosomal dominant disorder that can produce a severe and potentially fatal increase in body temperature. The condition commonly is triggered by general anesthetic agents and muscle relaxants used during surgery. The neuroleptic malignant syndrome is associated with neuroleptic drug therapy and is thought to result from alterations in the function of the thermoregulatory center or from uncontrolled muscle contraction. ■

DECREASED BODY TEMPERATURE

After completing this section of the chapter, you should be able to meet the following objectives:

- Define *hypothermia.*
- Compare the manifestations of mild, moderate, and severe hypothermia and relate them to changes in physiologic functioning that occur with decreased body temperature.
- Describe the causes of heat loss and hypothermia in the newborn infant and patient undergoing surgery.

Hypothermia

Hypothermia is defined as a core temperature (*i.e.*, rectal, esophageal, or tympanic) less than 35°C (95°F).[53,54] Core body temperatures in the range of 34°C to 35°C (93.2°F to 95°F) are considered mildly hypothermic; 30°C to 34°C (86°F to 93.2°F), moderately hypothermic; and less than 30°C (86°F), severely hypothermic.[53] In the United States, 4607 deaths from 1999 to 2002 were attributable to hypothermia.[55]

 HYPOTHERMIA

- Hypothermia is a pathologic decrease in core body temperature without a change in the hypothalamic set point.

- The compensatory physiologic responses meant to produce heat (shivering) and retain heat (vasoconstriction) are overwhelmed by unprotected exposure to cold environments.

Accidental hypothermia may be defined as a spontaneous decrease in core temperature, usually in a cold environment and associated with an acute problem but without a primary disorder of the temperature-regulating center. The term *submersion hypothermia* is used when cooling follows acute asphyxia, as occurs in drowning.[56] In children, the rapid cooling process, in addition to the diving reflex that triggers apnea and circulatory shunting to establish a heart–brain circulation, may account for the surprisingly high survival rate after submersion. The diving reflex is greatly diminished in adults. Children have been reported to survive 10 to 40 minutes of submersion asphyxia.[56,57] Controlled hypothermia may be used after brain injury and during certain types of surgery to decrease brain metabolism.

Systemic hypothermia may result from exposure to prolonged cold (atmospheric or submersion). The condition may develop in otherwise healthy persons in the course of accidental exposure. Because water conducts heat more readily than air, body temperature drops rapidly when the body is submerged in cold water or when clothing becomes wet. In persons with altered homeostasis due to debility or disease, hypothermia may follow exposure to relatively small decreases in atmospheric temperature.

Many underlying conditions can contribute to the development of hypothermia. Malnutrition decreases the fuel available for heat generation and loss of body fat decreases tissue insulation. Alcohol and sedative drugs dull mental awareness to cold and impair judgment to seek shelter or put on additional clothing. Alcohol also inhibits shivering. Persons with cardiovascular disease, cerebrovascular disease, spinal cord injury, and hypothyroidism also are predisposed to hypothermia. Elderly and inactive persons living in inadequately heated quarters are particularly vulnerable to hypothermia.[58,59]

 ## Neonatal Hypothermia

Infants are particularly at risk for hypothermia because of their high ratio of surface area to body mass. Relative to body weight, the body surface area of an infant is three times that of an adult, and in infants with low birth weight the insulating layer of subcutaneous fat is thinner. The newborn infant is particularly at risk. Under the usual delivery room conditions (20°C to 25°C), an infant's skin temperature falls approximately 0.3°C/minute and deep body temperature by approximately 0.1°C/minute.[60] The heat loss occurs by convection to the cooler surrounding air; by conduction to cooler materials on which the infant is resting; by radiation to nearby cooler solid objects; and by evaporation from the moist skin. The body temperature of a preterm infant can drop precipitously after delivery, and this hypothermia is associated with an increase in morbidity and mortality.[61,62] The use of occlusive polyethylene wrap applied immediately after birth of the preterm infant, an intervention that is easy to apply and does not interfere with resuscitation, is reported to reduce evaporative and convective heat losses.[62]

Perioperative Hypothermia

Persons who undergo surgical procedures are also at risk for hypothermia. Most open heart surgeries (adult and pediatric) involve intentionally induced hypothermia, whereas many other surgical patients undergoing general and regional anesthesia experience unintentional hypothermia.[63] Perioperative hypothermia is the result of a cold environment and impaired thermoregulatory mechanisms brought about by anesthetics and other drugs. Among the environmental factors that contribute to the loss of body heat are the cool temperature of the operating room and its equipment, air turnover rates that increase convective losses, use of cold antiseptic solutions that are allowed to evaporate from the skin, instillation of cold fluids into body cavities, and administration of cool intravenous infusions.[64] Both general and regional anesthetic agents disrupt many of the body's thermoregulatory mechanisms. General anesthetic agents lower the metabolic rate and decrease vasoconstriction and shivering thresholds, whereas epidural and spinal anesthesia decrease the vasoconstriction and shivering thresholds.[64] Postanesthetic shivering is a common complication of modern anesthesia, affecting up to 65% of patients after general anesthesia and 33% of patients during epidural anesthesia.[64] Apart from discomfort, postanesthesia shivering is associated with a number of potentially dangerous sequelae, including increased oxygen consumption and carbon dioxide production, increased cardiorespiratory effort, and effects of increased catecholamine (epinephrine and norepinephrine) release. These effects can pose a problem to recovery in vulnerable populations such as the elderly and persons with marginal cardiopulmonary reserves, impaired oxygen-carrying capacity (anemia), and other health problems.

A number of methods are used to prevent heat loss during surgery. Core temperature monitoring, accompanied by passive and active methods to maintain normal body temperature, should be part of routine inoperative monitoring. In many cases, some form of active rewarming is required. At present, forced-air warming is the most effective method available.[64] When necessary, centrally active drugs (meperidine, chlorpromazine) may be used to reduce postanesthesia shivering.

Manifestations

The signs and symptoms of hypothermia include poor coordination, stumbling, slurred speech, irrationality and poor judgment, amnesia, hallucinations, blueness and puffiness of the skin, dilation of the pupils, decreased respiratory rate, weak and irregular pulse, and stupor. With mild hypothermia, intense shivering generates heat and sympathetic nervous system activity is raised to resist lowering of temperature. Vasoconstriction can be profound, heart rate is accelerated, and stroke volume is increased. Blood pressure increases slightly, and hyperventilation is common. Exposure to cold augments urinary flow (i.e., cold diuresis) before there is any fall in temperature. Dehydration and increased hematocrit may develop within a few hours of even mild hypothermia, augmented by an extracellular-to-intracellular water shift.

With moderate hypothermia, shivering gradually decreases, and the muscles become rigid. Shivering usually ceases at 27°C (80.6°F). Heart rate and stroke volume are reduced, and blood pressure falls. The greatest effect of hypothermia is exerted through a decrease in the metabolic rate, which falls to 50% of normal at 28°C (82.4°F).[65] Associated with this decrease in metabolic rate is a decrease in oxygen consumption and carbon dioxide production. There is roughly a 6% decrease in oxygen consumption for every 1°C (2°F) decrease in temperature. A decrease in carbon dioxide production leads to a decrease in respiratory rate. Respirations decrease as temperatures drop below 32.2°C (90°F). Decreases in mentation, the cough reflex, and respiratory tract secretions may lead to difficulty in clearing secretions and aspiration. Consciousness usually is lost at 30°C (86°F).[65]

In terms of cardiovascular function, a gradual decline in heart rate and cardiac output occurs as hypothermia progresses. Blood pressure initially rises and then gradually falls. There is increased risk of dysrhythmia developing, probably from myocardial hypoxia and autonomic nervous system imbalance. Ventricular fibrillation is a major cause of death in hypothermia.

Carbohydrate metabolism and insulin activity are decreased, resulting in a hyperglycemia that is proportional to the level of cooling. A cold-induced loss of cell membrane integrity allows intravascular fluids to move into the skin, giving the skin a puffy appearance. Acid-base disorders occur with increased frequency at temperatures below 25°C (77°F) unless adequate ventilation is maintained. Extracellular sodium and potassium concentrations decrease, and chloride levels increase. There is a temporary loss of plasma from the circulation along with sludging of red blood cells and increased blood viscosity as the result of trapping in the small vessels and skin.

Diagnosis and Treatment

Oral temperatures are markedly inaccurate during hypothermia because of severe vasoconstriction and sluggish blood flow. Electronic thermometers with flexible probes are available for measuring rectal, bladder, and esophageal temperatures. However, rectal and bladder temperatures often lag behind fluctuations in core temperature, and esophageal temperatures may be elevated during inhalation of heated air.[66,67] Most clinical thermometers measure temperature only in the range of 35°C to 42°C (95°F to 107.6°F); a special thermometer that registers as low as 25°C (77°F) or an electrical thermistor probe is needed for monitoring temperatures in persons with hypothermia.

The treatment of hypothermia consists of rewarming, support of vital functions, and the prevention and treatment of complications. There are three methods of rewarming: passive external rewarming, active external rewarming, and active core rewarming.[54,67] Passive external rewarming is done by removing the person from the cold environment, covering with a blanket, supplying warm fluids (oral or intravenous), and allowing rewarming to occur at the person's own pace. Active external rewarming involves immersing the person in warm water, using forced-air warming systems, or placing heating pads or hot water bottles on the surface of the body, including the extremities. Active core rewarming can be done by instilling warmed fluids into the gastrointestinal tract; through peritoneal dialysis; by extracorporeal blood warming, in which blood is removed from the body and passed through a heat exchanger and then returned to the body; or by inhalation of an oxygen mixture warmed to 42°C to 46°C (107.6°F to 114.8°F). It places a greater emphasis on rewarming the trunk, leaving the extremities, containing the major metabolic mass, cold until the heart rewarms.

Persons with mild hypothermia usually respond well to passive rewarming in a warm bed. Persons with moderate or severe hypothermia do not have the thermoregulatory shivering mechanism and require active rewarming. During rewarming, the cold acidotic blood from the peripheral tissues is returned to the heart and central circulation. If this is done too rapidly or before cardiopulmonary function has been adequately reestablished, the hypothermic heart cannot respond to the increased metabolic demands of warm peripheral tissues.

IN SUMMARY, hypothermia is a potentially life-threatening disorder in which the body's core temperature drops below 35°C (95°F). Accidental hypothermia can develop in otherwise healthy persons in the course of accidental exposure and in elderly or disabled persons with impaired perception of or response to cold. Alcoholism, cardiovascular disease, malnutrition, and hypothyroidism contribute to the risk of hypothermia. Hypothermia is also a common occurrence in the operative patient and in newborn infants, particularly those born prematurely. The greatest effect of hypothermia is a decrease in the metabolic rate, leading to a decrease in carbon dioxide production and respiratory rate. The signs and symptoms of hypothermia include poor coordination, stumbling, slurred speech, irrationality, poor judgment, amnesia, hallucinations, blueness and puffiness of the skin, dilation of the pupils, decreased respiratory rate, weak and irregular pulse, stupor, and coma. The treatment of hypothermia includes passive or active rewarming, support of vital functions, and the prevention and treatment of complications. ■

Review Exercises

1. A 3-year-old child is seen in a pediatric clinic with a temperature of 39°C (102.2°F). Her skin is warm and flushed, her pulse is 120 beats/minute, and her respirations are shallow and rapid at 32 breaths/minute. Her mother states that her daughter has complained of a sore throat and has refused to drink or take medications to bring her temperature down.

   A. *Explain the physiologic mechanisms of fever generation.*

   B. *Are the warm and flushed skin, rapid heart rate, and respirations consistent with this level of fever?*

   C. *After receiving an appropriate dose of acetaminophen, the child begins to sweat, and the temperature drops to 37.2°C. Explain the physiologic mechanisms responsible for the drop in temperature.*

2. A 25-year-old man was brought to the emergency department after having been found unconscious in a snow bank. The outdoor temperature at the time he was discovered was −23.3°C (−10°F). His car, which was stalled a short distance away, contained liquor bottles, suggesting that he had been drinking. His temperature on admission was 29.8°C (85.6°F). His heart rate was 40 beats/minute and his respirations 18 breaths/minute and shallow. His skin was cool, his muscles rigid, and his digits blue.

   A. *What factors might have contributed to this man's state of hypothermia?*

   B. *Is this man able to engage in physiologic behaviors to control loss of body heat (refer to Fig. 10-3)?*

   C. *Given two methods that are available for taking this man's temperature (oral or rectal), which would be more accurate? Explain.*

   D. *What precautions should be considered when deciding on a method for rewarming this man?*

References

1. Guyton A. C., Hall J. E. (2006). *Textbook of medical physiology* (11th ed., pp. 822–833). Philadelphia: Elsevier Saunders.

2. Wenger C. B. (2003). The regulation of body temperature. In Rhoades R. A., Tanner G. A. (Eds.), *Medical physiology* (2nd ed., pp. 527–550). Philadelphia: Lippincott Williams & Wilkins.

3. Gisolfi C. V., Mora F. (2000). *The hot brain: Survival, temperature, and the human body.* Cambridge, MA: MIT Press.

4. Vick R. (1984). *Contemporary medical physiology* (p. 886). Menlo Park, CA: Addison Wesley.

5. Erickson R. S. (1999). The continuing question of how best to measure body temperature. *Critical Care Medicine* 27, 2307–2314.

6. Beach P. S., McCormick D. P. (1991). Clinical applications of ear thermometry [editorial]. *Clinical Pediatrics* 30(Suppl. 4), 3–4.

7. Dodd, S. R., Lancaster G. A., Craig J. V., et al. (2006). In a systematic review, infrared ear thermometry for fever diagnosis in children finds poor sensitivity. *Journal of Clinical Epidemiology* 59, 354–357.

8. Hooper V. D., Andrews J. O. (2006). Accuracy of noninvasive core temperature measurement in acutely ill adults: The state of the science. *Biological Research in Nursing* 8(1), 24–34.

9. Dhaka A., Viswanath V., Patapoutian A. (2006). TRP ion channels and temperature sensation. *Annual Review of Neuroscience* 29, 135–161.

10. Jansky L. (1998). Shivering. In Blatteis C. M. (Ed.), *Physiology and pathophysiology of temperature regulation* (pp. 48–58). River Edge, NJ: World Scientific Publishing.

11. Atkins L. (1984). Fever: The old and new. *Journal of Infectious Diseases* 149, 339–348.

12. Stein M. T. (1991). Historical perspectives in fever and thermometry. *Clinical Pediatrics* 30(Suppl. 4), 5–7.

13. Mackowiak P. A. (1998). Concepts of fever. *Archives of Internal Medicine* 158, 1870–1881.

14. Dinarello C. A., Gatti S., Bartfai T. (1999). Fever: Links with an ancient receptor. *Current Biology* 9, R147–R150.

15. Blatteis C. M., Li S., Li Z., et al. (2005). Cytokines, PGE_2, and endotoxic fever: A re-assessment. *Prostaglandins and Other Lipid Mediators* 76, 1–18.

16. Blatteis C. M. (2006). Endotoxic fever: New concepts of its regulation suggest new approaches to its management. *Pharmacology and Therapeutics* 111, 194–223.

17. Blatteis C. M. (1998). Fever. In Blatteis C. M. (Ed.), *Physiology and pathophysiology of temperature regulation* (pp. 178–192). River Edge, NJ: World Scientific Publishing.

18. Rodbard D. (1981). The role of regional temperature in the pathogenesis of disease. *New England Journal of Medicine* 305, 808–814.

19. McGee Z. A., Gorby G. L. (1987). The diagnostic value of fever patterns. *Hospital Practice* 22(10), 103–110.

20. Cunha B. A. (1984). Implications of fever in the critical care setting. *Heart and Lung* 13, 460–465.

21. Cunha B. A. (1996). The clinical significance of fever patterns. *Infectious Disease Clinics of North America* 10, 33–43.

22. Saper C. B., Breder C. D. (1994). The neurologic basis of fever. *New England Journal of Medicine* 330, 1880–1886.

23. Champi C., Gaffney-Yocum P. A. (1999). Managing febrile seizures in children. *Nurse Practitioner* 24(10), 28–30, 34–35.

24. Cunha B. A. (1996). Fever without source. *Infectious Disease Clinics of North America* 10, 111–127.

25. John C. C., Gillsdorf J. R (2002). Recurrent fever in children. *Pediatric Infectious Disease Journal* 21, 1071–1077.

26. Drenth J. P. H., van der Meer J. W. M. (2001). Hereditary periodic fever. *New England Journal of Medicine* 345, 1748–1756.

27. Plaisance K. I., Mackowiak P. A. (2000). Antipyretic therapy: Physiologic rationale, diagnostic implications, and clinical consequences. *Archives of Internal Medicine* 160, 449–456.

28. Baker M. D. (1999). Evaluation and management of infants with fever. *Pediatric Clinics of North America* 46, 1061–1072.

29. Luszczak M. (2001). Evaluation and management of infants and young children with fever. *American Family Physician* 64, 1219–1226.

30. Ishimine P. (2006). Fever without source in children 0 to 36 months of age. *Pediatric Clinics of North America* 53, 167–194.

31. ACEP Clinical Policy Committee and Clinical Policies Subcommittee on Pediatric Care. (2003). Clinical policy for children less than 3 years pre-

senting to the emergency department with fever. *Annals of Emergency Medicine* 42, 530–545.

32. Baraff, L. J. (2003). Clinical policy for children less than 3 years presenting to the emergency department with fever [editorial]. *Annals of Emergency Medicine* 42, 546–549.

33. Castle S. C., Norman D. C., Yeh M., et al. (1991). Fever response in elderly nursing home residents: Are the older truly colder? *Journal of the American Geriatrics Society* 39, 853–857.

34. Woolery W. A., Franco, F. R. (2004). Fever of unknown origin: Keys to determining the etiology in older patients. *Geriatrics* 59(10), 41–45.

35. Yoshikawa T. T., Norman, D. C. (1998). Fever in the elderly. *Infectious Medicine* 15, 704–706, 708.

36. Castle S. C., Yeh M., Toledo S., et al. (1993). Lowering the temperature criterion improves detection of infections in nursing home residents. *Aging Immunology and Infectious Disease* 4, 67–76.

37. Wexler R. K. (2002). Evaluation and treatment of heat-related illnesses. *American Family Physician* 65, 2307–2314.

38. Bouchama A., Knochel, J. P. (2002). Heat stroke. *New England Journal of Medicine* 346, 1978–1988.

39. Hamdy R. C. (2002). Heat stroke. *Southern Medical Journal* 95, 791–792.

40. Yeo T. P. (2004). Heat stroke. *AACN Critical Issues* 15, 280–293.

41. Ballester J. M., Harchelroad F. P. (1999). Hyperthermia: How to recognize and prevent heat-related illnesses. *Geriatrics* 54(7), 20–24.

42. Sharma H. S., Hoopes P. J. (2003). Hyperthermia induced pathophysiology of the central nervous system. *International Journal of Hyperthermia* 19, 325–354.

43. Cuddy M. L. S. (2004). The effects of drugs on thermoregulation. *AACN Critical Issues* 15, 238–253.

44. Mackowiak P. A., LeMaistre C. F. (1986). Drug fever: A critical appraisal of conventional concepts. *Annals of Internal Medicine* 106, 728–733.

45. Johnson D. H., Cunha B. A. (1996). Drug fever. *Infectious Disease Clinics of North America* 10, 85–99.

46. Olson K. R. (2007). Poisoning. In McPhee S. J., Papadakis M. A., Tierney L. M. (Eds.), *Current medical diagnosis and treatment* (p. 1642). New York: McGraw-Hill Medical.

47. Jurkat-Rott K., McCarthy T., Lehmann-Horn F. (2000). Genetics and pathogenesis of malignant hyperthermia. *Muscle and Nerve* 23, 4–17.

48. Denborough M. (1998). Malignant hyperthermia. *Lancet* 352, 1131–1136.

49. McCarthy E. J. (2004). Malignant hyperthermia: Pathophysiology, clinical presentation, and treatment. *AACN Critical Issues* 15, 231–237.

50. Adnet P., Lestavel P., Krivosic-Horber R. (2000). Neuroleptic malignant syndrome. *British Journal of Anaesthesia* 85, 129–135.

51. Pelonero A. L., Levenson J. L., Pandurangi A. K. (1998). Neuroleptic malignant syndrome: A review. *Psychiatric Services* 49, 1163–1172.

52. Gurrera R. J. (2002). Is neuroleptic syndrome a neurogenic form of malignant hyperthermia? *Clinical Neuropharmacology* 25, 183–193.

53. Mercer J. B. (1998). Hypothermia and cold injuries in man. In Blatteis C. M. (Ed.), *Physiology and pathophysiology of temperature regulation* (pp. 246–256). River Edge, NJ: World Scientific Publishing.

54. Kempainen R. R., Brunnette D. D. (2004). The evaluation and management of accidental hypothermia. *Respiratory Care* 49, 192–204.

55. Centers for Disease Control and Prevention. (2006). Hypothermia-related deaths—United States, 1999–2002 and 2005. *Morbidity and Mortality Weekly Reports* 55, 282–284.

56. Conn A. W. (1979). Near drowning and hypothermia. *Canadian Medical Association Journal* 120, 397–400.

57. Siebke H., Beivik H., Rod T. (1975). Survival after 40 minutes submersion with cerebral sequelae. *Lancet* 1, 1275–1277.

58. Biem J., Koehncke N., Classen D., et al. (2003). Out of the cold: Management of hypothermia and frostbite. *Canadian Medical Association Journal* 168, 305–311.

59. Ballester J. M., Harchelroad F. P. (1999). Hypothermia: An easy-to-miss, dangerous disorder in winter weather. *Geriatrics* 54(2), 51–57.

60. Stoll B. J., Kleigman R. M. (2004). The newborn infant. In Behrman R. E., Kliegman R. M., Jenson H. B. (Eds.), *Nelson textbook of pediatrics* (17th ed., p. 528). Philadelphia: Elsevier Saunders.

61. Watkinson H. (2006). Temperature control of premature infants in the delivery room. *Clinical Perinatology* 33, 43–53.

62. Bredemeyer S., Reid S., Wallace M. (2005). Thermal regulation for premature births. *Journal of Advanced Nursing* 52, 482–489.

63. Herschman Z. (2004). Hypothermia: In the operating room and beyond. *Respiratory Care* 49, 158–159.

64. Buggy D. J., Crossley A. W. A. (2000). Thermoregulation, mild perioperative hypothermia, and post-anaesthetic shivering. *British Journal of Anaesthesiology* 84, 615–628.

65. Wong K. C. (1983). Physiology and pharmacology of hypothermia. *Western Journal of Medicine* 138, 227–232.

66. Danzl D. F., Pozos R. S. (1994). Accidental hypothermia. *New England Journal of Medicine* 331, 1756–1760.

67. Hanania N. A., Zimmerman J. L. (1999). Accidental hypothermia. *Critical Care Clinics* 15, 235–249.

Visit the Point. **http://thePoint.lww.com for animations, journal articles, and more!**

Activity Tolerance and Fatigue

Chapter **11**

MARY KAY JIRICKA

EXERCISE AND ACTIVITY TOLERANCE
  Types of Exercise
    Aerobic Exercise
    Isometric Exercise
    Flexibility Exercise
  Physiologic and Psychological Responses
    Cardiopulmonary Responses
    Neuromuscular Responses
    Metabolic and Thermal Responses
    Gastrointestinal Responses
    Hemostasis and Immune Function
    Psychological Responses
  Assessment of Activity and Exercise Tolerance
    Activity Tolerance and Fatigue
    Aerobic Fitness
  Exercise and Activity Tolerance in the Elderly
ACTIVITY INTOLERANCE AND FATIGUE
  Mechanisms of Fatigue
  Acute Physical Fatigue
  Chronic Fatigue
    Chronic Fatigue Syndrome
BED REST AND IMMOBILITY
  Physiologic Effects of Bed Rest
    Cardiovascular Responses
    Pulmonary Responses
    Urinary Tract Responses
    Musculoskeletal Responses
    Metabolic, Endocrine, and Immune Responses
    Gastrointestinal Responses
    Sensory Responses
    Skin Responses
  Psychosocial Responses
  Time Course of Physiologic Responses
  Interventions

➤ Exercise, or physical activity, is a physiologic state, so common in its many forms that true physiologic rest is seldom achieved. Defined ultimately in terms of skeletal muscle contraction, exercise involves the coordinated responses of every body system to provide the energy needed for increased muscle activity. Fatigue represents the perceived lack of sufficient energy to engage fully in physical activities. Fatigue may be acute, as in that resulting from increased physical activity, or it may be chronic, as in the chronic fatigue syndrome. Conditions that restrict physical activity, such as bed rest and immobility, can impair a person's exercise reserve and ability to perform work and other activities.

This chapter focuses on activity tolerance and exercise, activity intolerance and fatigue; and the physiologic and psychosocial responses to immobility and bed rest.

 ## EXERCISE AND ACTIVITY TOLERANCE

After completing this section of the chapter, you should be able to meet the following objectives:

■ Differentiate among aerobic, isometric, and flexibility exercises.
■ Describe the physiologic and psychological responses to exercise.
■ Define the term *maximal oxygen consumption* and state how it is measured.
■ Describe methods that can be used to assess a person's activity tolerance and ability to engage in an exercise program.
■ Describe the physiologic effects of exercise in the elderly population.

Physical activity is defined as the process of energy expenditure for the purpose of accomplishing an effect. Humans interact with their environment in a cyclic pattern involving periods of activity and rest, both of which have physical and psychological elements. Physical activity and exercise denote the process of skeletal muscle movement and energy expenditure, whereas rest is characterized by inactivity and minimal energy expenditure.

🔑 ACTIVITY TOLERANCE

- Activity is the process of purposeful energy expenditure. Exercise, a form of activity that results in overall conditioning of the body, can be aerobic or isometric.

- Exercise depends on the availability of energy substrates, cardiovascular fitness, muscle strength and flexibility, and motivation.

- The cardiovascular response to exercise includes increased heart rate, stroke volume, and mean arterial pressure. An increased percentage of cardiac output is distributed to working muscle.

- Pulmonary perfusion and pulmonary ventilation increase in response to exercise.

- Psychological effects of exercise include an increase in energy and in the ability to adapt to stress.

There is increasing interest in both the preventative and therapeutic effects of physical activity and exercise. A regular program of exercise is recommended as a means of maintaining weight control and cardiovascular fitness.[1–3] Exercise partnered with diet control also is becoming recognized as an integral part of the treatment regimen for many diseases. It is recommended as a means of slowing, or even halting, the progression of atherosclerotic coronary heart disease (CHD); of lowering low-density lipoproteins (LDL) and increasing high-density lipoproteins (HDL) in persons with hyperlipidemia; of providing better regulation of blood glucose in persons with diabetes; and of improving activity tolerance in persons with cardiovascular and respiratory diseases. Regular exercise can also have psychological benefits: it can improve self-esteem, remedy depressive moods, and enhance quality of life.[1]

Although there is a growing consensus regarding the importance of physical activity and exercise, there are questions regarding the type, intensity, frequency, and duration. A single episode of acute exercise may provoke responses quite different from the adaptations seen when exercise is chronic.

Types of Exercise

There are two main types of skeletal muscle exercise: aerobic and isometric. Another type—flexibility or stretching exercise—promotes flexibility and improved range of joint motion. Most exercise programs use a combination of all three types of exercise.

Aerobic Exercise

Aerobic, or *endurance, exercise* involves the body's ability to improve its use of oxygen for energy during prolonged strenuous exercise. It involves rhythmic changes in muscle length (contraction and elongation) during activities such as walking,

running, bicycling, or swimming. During aerobic exercise that uses large muscle groups (*e.g.,* running), each person has a maximal oxygen uptake that cannot be exceeded, although it can be increased with appropriate training.[4,5] Although aerobic exercise training results in muscles that use oxygen more efficiently such that the body can do more work with less cardiac and respiratory effort, it does not promote significant increase in muscle mass, even though the exercise may go on for hours.

Whatever type of exercise a person chooses, the Centers for Disease Control and Prevention (CDC) and the American College of Sports Medicine (ACSM) recommend that adults strive for at least 30 minutes of moderate-intensity (60% to 70% of maximum heart rate) physical activity 5 or more days a week or 20 minutes or more of vigorous-intensity (70% to 85% of maximum heart rate) activity for 3 or more days a week.[6] Persons who are unfamiliar with exercise training, those who are extremely deconditioned, and elderly persons may benefit from 60 minutes of low-intensity (20% to 39% of maximum heart rate) exercise most (preferably all) days of the week. High-intensity exercise includes activities such as jogging and swimming; moderate-intensity exercise, brisk walking (15 to 20 minutes per mile) and dancing; and low-intensity exercise, light walking and gardening.

Isometric Exercise

In *isometric,* or *resistance, exercise,* sustained muscle contraction is generated against an immovable load with no change in length of the involved muscle group or joint movement.[7] It involves activities, such as weight lifting and repeated movement against low to moderate resistance, that improve overall muscle strength and tone and build muscle mass.

Although resistance training has long been accepted as a means of developing strength and muscle mass, its beneficial relationship to health factors and chronic diseases has been recognized only recently.[7] Despite the fact that the mechanisms may differ, both aerobic exercise and resistance training have similar effects on bone density, glucose tolerance, and insulin sensitivity. For weight control, aerobic exercise is considered a calorie burner; whereas resistance training assists the body in expending calories through an increase in lean body mass and basal metabolism. Many leisure and occupational tasks require isometric muscle efforts, often involving the arms rather than the legs. Because the blood pressure response to resistance exercise is proportionate to the maximal voluntary contraction as well as muscle mass involved, increased muscle strength results in an attenuated heart rate and blood pressure response to a given load.

Flexibility Exercise

In contrast to aerobic and resistance exercises, stretching as an isolated activity increases neither strength nor endurance, but should be included in an overall fitness regimen. Considerable evidence suggests that stretching exercises increase tendon flexibility, improve joint range of motion, and enhance muscular performance. When properly performed, these exercises promote a transient increase in muscle-tendon length that results from relaxation of the actin–myosin complex and a more lasting increase in length through alterations in the surrounding extracellular matrix.[7] Thus, it is recommended that aerobic and resistance training be accompanied by a stretching program that exercises the major muscle or tendon groups at least 2 to 3 days per week.[7]

Physiologic and Psychological Responses

The physiologic and psychological benefits of exercise involve four major components: cardiopulmonary fitness; increased muscle strength, flexibility, and endurance; availability of energy substrates to meet the increased energy demands imposed by increased physical activity; and motivation and mental endurance (Fig. 11-1). These benefits incorporate cardiopulmonary, neuromuscular, metabolic and thermal, and gastrointestinal responses; changes in hemostasis and immune function; and psychological behaviors that accompany physical activity and exercise.

Cardiopulmonary Responses

The cardiopulmonary responses to exercise involve the circulatory functions of the heart and blood vessels and the gas exchange functions of the respiratory system. Collectively, they function to supply oxygen and energy substrates to the working

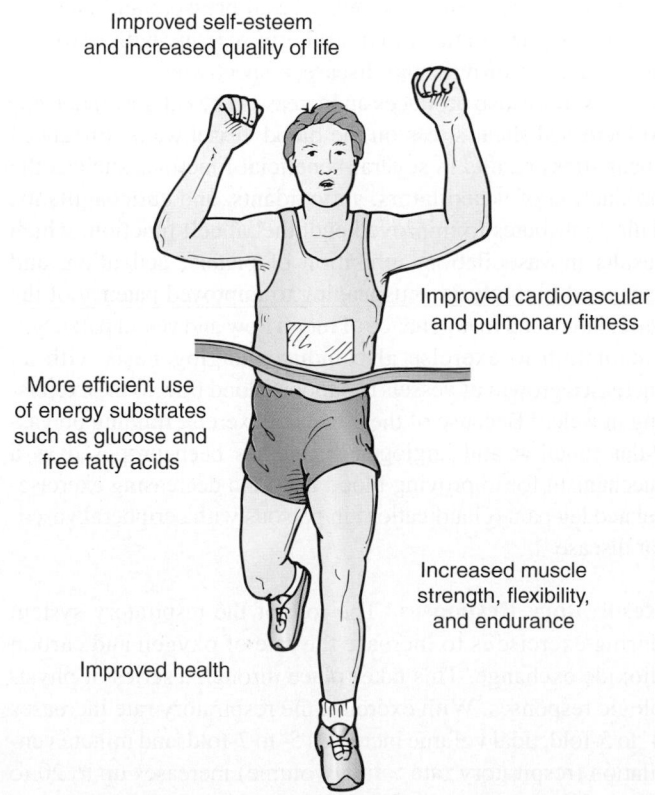

Improved self-esteem and increased quality of life

Improved cardiovascular and pulmonary fitness

More efficient use of energy substrates such as glucose and free fatty acids

Increased muscle strength, flexibility, and endurance

Improved health

FIGURE 11-1 • Beneficial effects of physical activity and exercise.

muscles and exchange oxygen and carbon dioxide with the atmosphere. Cardiopulmonary or aerobic exercise involves repetitive and rhythmic movements, uses large muscle groups, and results in the ability to perform vigorous exercise for an extended period.[1]

The principal factor that determines how long and effectively a person will be able to exercise is the capacity of the heart, lungs, and circulation to deliver oxygen to the working muscles. The term *maximal oxygen consumption* ($\dot{V}O_2max$) represents this principle. The $\dot{V}O_2max$ is determined by the rate at which oxygen is delivered to the working muscles, the oxygen-carrying capacity of blood, and the amount of oxygen extracted from the blood by the working muscles. It is measured as the volume of oxygen consumed, usually in liters or milliliters, per unit of time (*i.e.,* liters/minute). The $\dot{V}O_2max$ is an important determinant of a person's capacity to perform work and can increase up to 20-fold with strenuous exercise.[1,8,9] An exercise training program can accelerate the rate of increased $\dot{V}O_2max$ so that the trained athlete has a more rapid increase in cardiac output and skeletal muscle blood flow during the first minute of exercise.

The cardiovascular responses to exercise are regulated by output from centers in the central nervous system (CNS) and autonomic nervous system to the heart and blood vessels in tandem with local mechanisms that further regulate cardiac output and muscle blood flow.[10,11] Recent research using brain mapping demonstrates specific areas of the brain, including the insular cortex and anterior cingulate cortex, that communicate with hypothalamic centers responsible for coordinating a pattern of increased sympathetic and decreased parasympathetic (vagal) outflow to the medullary cardiovascular centers[10] (Fig. 11-2). This leads to an increase in cardiac output and baroreceptor-mediated control of arterial blood pressure. Local control is derived from the release of metabolic end products (*e.g.,* lactic acid) and local vasoactive factors that dilate blood vessels. Local factors in the coronary blood vessels mediate vasodilation, whereas increased sympathetic activity produces vasoconstriction of renal and gastrointestinal vessels, reducing blood flow to these organs.[1,10,11]

Cardiac Output. Exercise produces an increase in heart rate and stroke volume (amount of blood pumped with each heart beat), which in turn increases cardiac output. During exercise, the cardiac output may increase from a resting level of 4 to 8 L/minute to as high as 15 L/minute for women and 22 L/minute for men. The increase in heart rate is mediated through neural, hormonal, and intrinsic cardiovascular mechanisms. With anticipation of exercise, cardiovascular centers in the brain stem are stimulated to initiate an increase in sympathetic activity concomitant with an inhibition of parasympathetic mechanisms. Stimulation of the sympathetic nervous system produces an increase in heart rate and cardiac contractility. At the start of exercise, the heart rate increases immediately and continues to increase until a plateau is reached. This plateau, or steady-state heart rate, is maintained until exercise is terminated. Release of epinephrine and norepinephrine from the adrenal glands helps to sustain the increased heart rate.[1]

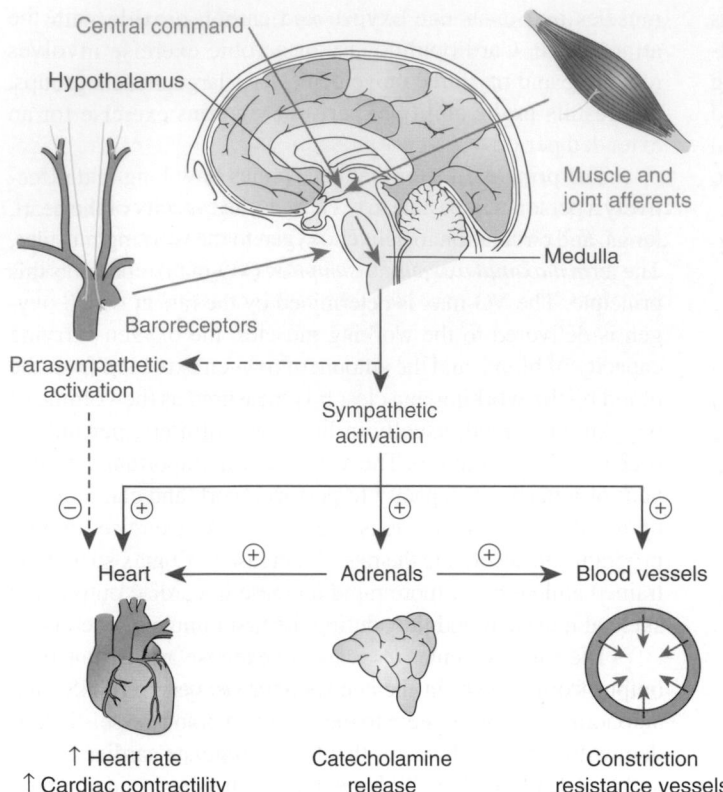

FIGURE 11-2 • Mechanisms of neural cardiovascular control during exercise.

Also contributing to the increased heart rate are mechanisms intrinsic to the heart. An increase in venous return stimulates right atrial stretch receptors that initiate an increase in heart rate, and an increase in ventricular filling stretches the myocardial fibers, resulting in a more forceful contraction and a more complete emptying of the ventricles with each beat through the *Frank-Starling mechanism* (see Chapter 21).[1,10]

Blood Pressure and Blood Flow. Blood pressure and blood flow also change with exercise. Increased sympathetic activity constricts the resistance vessels, leading to an increase in blood pressure; and it dilates the capacitance vessels in the visceral circulation, leading to an increase in venous return to the heart and maintenance of the cardiac output. It is important to note that the vasoconstriction produced by sympathetic innervation and circulating catecholamines (*i.e.,* epinephrine) does not occur in the active skeletal muscles, coronary circulation, or brain.

With the onset of aerobic exercise, the systolic blood pressure increases largely due to an increase in cardiac output, whereas the diastolic pressure remains relatively unchanged because of vasodilation and increased blood flow to the working muscles. The increased systolic pressure that occurs along with a nearly constant diastolic blood pressure produces an increase in pulse pressure and mean arterial pressure.[12] With isometric exercise, the increase in heart rate and blood pressure is proportionate to the maximal voluntary contraction (% MVC) and is most pronounced when a medium muscle mass is working, such as the arms.[1] Shoveling snow, which is a good example of an isometric-type exercise using primarily the arms, can substantially raise the systemic arterial pressure and increase the risk for heart attack and stroke in persons with coronary artery and cerebrovascular disease, respectively.

Exercise also produces an increase in blood flow that leads to increased shear stress on the blood vessel walls. Enhanced shear stress results in several beneficial functions such as the production of vasodilators, antioxidants, and anticoagulants. This contributes to improved endothelial cell function, which results in vasodilation, inhibition of platelet activation, and increased fibrinolysis, thus leading to improved patency of the vasculature and maintenance of blood flow and vessel patency.[13] Adaptation to exercise also induces angiogenesis with an increased growth of vessels to support blood flow to the exercising muscle.[14] Because of the effects of exercise training on vascular function and angiogenesis, it has been proposed as a mechanism for improving blood flow and decreasing exercise-related leg pain (claudication) in persons with peripheral vascular disease.[15]

Respiratory Responses. The role of the respiratory system during exercise is to increase the rate of oxygen and carbon dioxide exchange. This takes place through a series of physiologic responses. With exercise, the respiratory rate increases 4- to 5-fold, tidal volume increases 5- to 7-fold, and minute ventilation (respiratory rate × tidal volume) increases up to 20 to 30 times its resting value.[16] With the increase in cardiac output, a greater volume of blood under slightly increased pressure is delivered to the pulmonary vessels in the lungs. This results in the opening of more pulmonary capillary beds, producing better alveolar perfusion and more efficient exchange of oxygen and carbon dioxide. In addition to pulmonary perfusion being enhanced during exercise, pulmonary ventilation is increased, resulting in a more optimal ventilation-perfusion ratio. This response is controlled by chemoreceptors—located in the brain stem, aorta, and carotid arteries—that monitor blood gases and pH. During exercise, decreases in blood oxygen and pH and increases in carbon dioxide stimulate these receptors, producing an increase in both the rate and depth of respiration.[1,16]

Neuromuscular Responses

The integration of the neurologic and musculoskeletal systems is essential for body movement and participation in activity. To initiate and sustain increased activity, muscle strength, flexibility, and endurance are needed. *Muscle strength* is defined as the ability of muscle groups to produce force against resistance. *Flexibility* involves the range of movement of joints, and *muscle endurance* refers to the ability of the body or muscle groups to perform increased activity for an extended time.

Types of Muscle. Skeletal muscle consists of two distinct types of muscle fibers based on differences in their size, speed, contractile properties, endurance, and metabolic characteristics: red (dark) slow-twitch (type I) and white (light) fast-twitch (type II) muscle fibers.[1] Both heredity and activity influence the distribution of fast-twitch and slow-twitch fibers. Heredity appears to contribute to differences in muscle fiber composition, such that some people have considerably more fast-twitch than slow-twitch fibers, and others have more slow-twitch than fast-twitch fibers. This could determine, to some extent, the area of athletics for which a person is best suited.

The slow-twitch fibers, which are smaller than the fast-twitch fibers, tend to produce less overall force but are more energy efficient than fast-twitch fibers. They are better-suited biochemically to perform lower-intensity work for prolonged periods. These fibers have a high oxidative capacity as a result of high concentrations of mitochondria and myoglobin. Slow-twitch fibers are highly fatigue resistant and ideally suited for prolonged aerobic exercise or activity. Slow-twitch fibers predominate in the large muscle groups such as the leg muscles; therefore, they play a major role in sustaining activity during prolonged exercise or endurance activities. Periods of sustained inactivity, such as prolonged immobility or bed rest, primarily affect slow-twitch fibers, which quickly decondition.[1,15]

In contrast to slow-twitch fibers, fast-twitch fibers are larger and better suited for high-intensity work, but they fatigue more easily. These fibers have high myosin adenosine triphosphatase (ATPase) activity, few mitochondria, low myoglobin concentration, and high glycolytic capacity, resulting in dependence on anaerobic metabolism to supply adenosine triphosphate (ATP) for energy. Fast-twitch fibers predominate during activities in which short bursts of intense energy are required,

such as sprinting or weight lifting. Anabolic steroids enhance fast-twitch fiber activity.[1,15]

Persons with heart failure (HF) typically experience symptoms of breathlessness, exertional fatigue, and exercise intolerance resulting in atrophy of skeletal muscles. When these individuals engage in exercise, there is a shift toward using fast-twitch muscle fibers. This causes an early dependence on anaerobic metabolism and excessive intramuscular acidification that leads to increased fatigability.[17] The increased reliance on anaerobic metabolism and subsequent vasoconstrictor response can also lead to an increase in afterload work (see Chapter 21) for an already compromised left ventricle. Thus, it is imperative that individuals with HF have their exercise regimens monitored closely.

Muscle Blood Flow. During aerobic activity, working muscles use 10 to 20 times more oxygen than nonworking muscles. This increased oxygen demand is met by an increase in cardiac output and muscle blood flow. Skeletal muscles receive 85% to 95% of the cardiac output during aerobic activities, and only 15% to 20% of the cardiac output at rest. The increased blood flow is achieved through two mechanisms: dilation of blood vessels in the working muscles and constriction of those in organs of low priority.[18]

Increased blood flow to working muscles is achieved by relaxation of the arterioles and the precapillary sphincters. Chemical changes such as decreased oxygen and pH and increased levels of potassium, adenosine, carbon dioxide, and phosphate contribute to the vasodilation during prolonged exercise and recovery from exercise.[18] Increased venous blood flow and central venous pressure are enhanced by the alternate contraction and relaxation of working muscles.

Another mechanism that increases blood flow to the working muscles is the diversion of blood from organs such as the kidneys and gastrointestinal structures that are less active than the working muscles.[1,10,18] The amount of blood flow diverted from the visceral organs is proportional to the level of exercise, and as exercise is increased, more blood is diverted to working muscles.

Metabolic and Thermal Responses

Skeletal muscles hypertrophy and undergo other anatomic changes in response to exercise training. "Trained muscles" have an increased number of capillaries surrounding each muscle fiber that facilitates the delivery of oxygen to the working muscle cells during exercise. They are able to use oxygen more efficiently, probably because of enhanced enzymatic activity that increases oxidative capacity. The mitochondria appear to adapt by increasing the transport of oxygen and other substrates to the inner regions of the muscle fiber.[1]

Unlike other tissues in the body, skeletal muscles switch between virtual inactivity when they are relaxed and using only minimal amounts of ATP, to extremes of physical activity during which they use ATP at a rapid rate. However, they have only enough ATP to power contraction for a few seconds. If strenuous exercise is to continue beyond this time, additional sources of ATP must be generated. The ATP that is used to power muscle contraction is obtained from three sources: creatine phosphate, glycogen, and fatty acids. Much like ATP, *creatine phosphate* (also known as *phosphocreatine*) contains high-energy phosphate bonds. It is unique to muscle fibers and is 8 to 10 times as abundant as ATP. Creatine is a small, amino-acid–like molecule that is both synthesized in the body and derived from foods (Fig. 11-3). The enzyme creatine kinase (CK) catalyzes the transfer of the high-energy phosphate groups from ATP to creatine, forming creatine phosphate and adenosine diphosphate (ADP). When muscle contraction begins and ADP levels start to rise, CK catalyzes the transfer of a high-energy phosphate group back to ADP, thus forming new ATP molecules that can be used by the muscle for energy.

During exercise, particularly aerobic exercise, the body uses its energy sources in a characteristic pattern. The first sources for energy are stored ATP, creatine phosphate, and muscle glycogen. Short, intense periods of activity lasting 1 to 2 minutes exploit these energy sources through anaerobic metabolism. If the activity is to be performed for a period of 3 to 40 minutes, muscle glycogen and creatine phosphate are used to meet the energy requirements through both anaerobic and aerobic metabolism. For intense, prolonged periods of activity lasting more than 40 minutes, aerobic metabolism and the use of glucose, fatty acids, and amino acids becomes essential.[1]

Nutritional and Hydration Status. To supply the energy needed for increased activity, a person must consume a balanced diet and have adequate hydration. Although proteins are not used for energy sources during increased activity, they have an essential role in the building and rebuilding of tissues and organs. During increased activity and exercise, it is essential that an individual maintain adequate hydration. Increased activity can result in loss of fluids from the vascular compartment. If this is allowed to progress, the person may experience severe dehydration that may lead to vascular collapse. Before and during vigorous activity, a person should replenish body fluids with water and electrolyte solutions.[1]

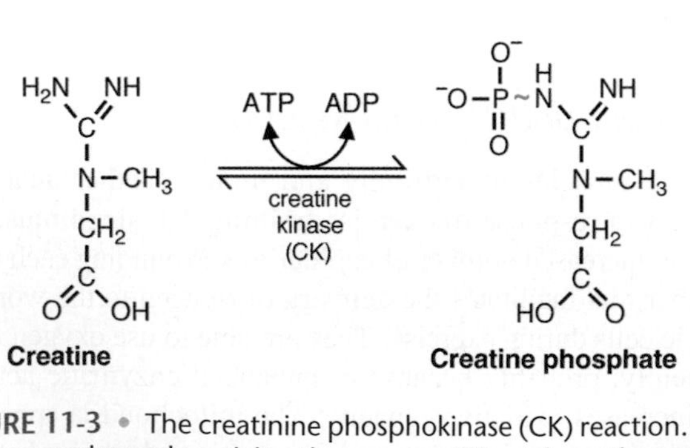

Temperature Regulation. Almost all the energy released from metabolic processes involved in muscle contraction is converted to heat. Under normal resting conditions, the body is able to maintain its temperature within a set range. It does this by two mechanisms. The first mechanism used by the body to regulate temperature is to change blood flow to the skin. When the blood vessels of the skin dilate, warm blood is shunted from the core tissues and organs to the skin surface, where heat is lost more easily to the surrounding environment (see Chapter 10). The second mechanism is through sweating, in which the evaporation of sweat from the skin surface contributes to the loss of body heat. Depending on training level and environmental conditions, the body may have difficulty regulating its temperature during vigorous exercise.[1,19] With sufficient training, the body adapts by increasing the rate of sweat production. As temperature regulation improves with training, the trained person begins to sweat sooner, often within 1 to 2 minutes of the start of exercise. Sweat production begins even before the core temperature rises, and a cooling effect is initiated soon after the start of exercise; the sweat produced is more dilute than that produced by a non-trained person. Sweat normally contains large amounts of sodium chloride; production of a dilute sweat allows evaporative cooling to take place while sodium chloride is conserved.[1]

During exercise, plasma proteins are shifted from the interstitial to the vascular compartment so that there is an increase in the amount of proteins in the blood. These proteins exert an osmotic force that draws fluid from the interstitial space into the vascular compartment. This contributes to an increase in vascular volume, which in turn is delivered to the working muscles and which also provides more efficient heat dissipation.[1]

Gastrointestinal Responses

The gastrointestinal system is affected by intense physical activity. During intense physical activity, blood flow is shunted away from the gastrointestinal tract toward the active skeletal muscles. As a result, gastrointestinal motility, secretory activity, and absorptive capacity are decreased. This can result in heartburn (reflux), vomiting, bloating, stomach pain, and gastrointestinal bleeding. It may also cause cramping, urge to defecate, and diarrhea. Although athletes may experience these symptoms, they are usually transient and do not have an effect on long-term health. Light and moderate exercise can benefit individuals with inflammatory bowel disease and liver disease. Evidence suggests that physical activity improves gastric emptying and lowers the risk of colon cancer and reduces the risks for diverticulosis, gastrointestinal hemorrhage, and inflammatory bowel disease.[1,20]

FIGURE 11-3 • The creatinine phosphokinase (CK) reaction. During increased muscle activity, the enzyme CK catalyzes the transfer of the high-energy phosphate group from creatine phosphate to adenosine diphosphate (ADP) to form adenosine triphosphate (ATP). During periods of inactivity, ATP transfers its high-energy phosphate group to creatine to form creatine phosphate. (The high-energy bond is indicated by a blue squiggle.)(From Smith C., Marks A. D., Lieberman M. [2005]. *Marks' basic medical biochemistry* (2nd ed., p. 870). Philadelphia: Lippincott Williams & Wilkins.)

Hemostasis and Immune Function

Increased physical activity affects both hemostasis and the immune system. Increased epinephrine levels stimulate increased fibrinolytic (*i.e.,* breakdown of the fibrin strands in a blood clot) activity. Thus, regular strenuous exercise can result in increased fibrinolytic activity and a slowing of coagulation activity.[1]

The response of the immune system to exercise is varied and depends on frequency, intensity, and duration of the exercise. The immune system is stimulated by regular, moderate exercise and impaired with regular, repetitive, intense exercise. A period of moderate-intensity exercise has been found to boost the immune system for several hours by producing an increase in circulating white blood cells, including neutrophils and lymphocytes. Of special note is the increased activity of natural killer cells. Chronic, intense, and exhausting exercise produces different effects on the immune system. Elevation in body temperature, cytokine release, and increased levels of various stress-related hormones (*e.g.,* epinephrine, growth hormone, cortisol) may result in a temporary depression of the body's innate immune defenses. Strenuous exercise alters mucosal immunity of the upper respiratory tract. This may explain why elite athletes are susceptible to illness, especially upper respiratory tract infections. Strenuous exercise also lowers the production of the nonessential amino acid glutamine, which serves as an energy source for lymphocytes and macrophages.[1,21,22]

Psychological Responses

There is a mental component to the performance of increased activity and exercise. The mental aspect entails the motivation to initiate an activity, or exercise program, and the dedication to incorporate the regimen into one's lifestyle. Positive effects of regularly performed exercise include increased energy and motivation, positive self-image and self-esteem, decreased anxiety, and better management of stress.

Assessment of Activity and Exercise Tolerance

A person's ability to tolerate exercise and perform work can be assessed in several ways. One way is by having the person report his or her perceived response to different types of physical activity or exercise. This method is particularly useful in assessing persons for activity intolerance and fatigue (to be discussed). Another method, exercise stress testing, is used to measure aerobic fitness.

Activity Tolerance and Fatigue

One method of assessing activity tolerance involves the administration of a paper-and-pencil test in which participants describe their normal activities, their perceived level of activity tolerance, or their level of fatigue. An example of a paper-and-pencil test is the *Human Activity Profile* (HAP).[23] The HAP originally was developed to assess the quality of life for persons participating in a rehabilitation program for chronic obstructive pulmonary disease. After investigating numerous physiologic and psychological measures, it was noted that the most important aspect of quality of life was the amount of daily activity the person was able to perform. The HAP consists of 94 items representing common activities that require known amounts of average energy expenditure. The person marks each item based on whether he or she is still able to perform the activity or has stopped performing the activity.

Another paper-and-pencil test is the *Fatigue Severity Scale.*[24] This tool consists of nine statements that describe symptoms of fatigue (*e.g.,* exercise brings on my fatigue; fatigue causes frequent problems for me; fatigue interferes with my work, family, social life). Persons are instructed to choose a number from 1 to 7 that best indicates their agreement with each statement. The tool is brief, easy to administer, and easily interpreted.

Aerobic Fitness

A number of tests are available to measure aerobic fitness, including the Rockport One Mile Test, the step test, and treadmill or bicycle ergometry.[2] Often heart rate is used to estimate $\dot{V}O_2$max without measuring oxygen consumption.

Ergometry is a procedure for determining physical performance capacity. The ergometer is a specific tool that imposes a constant level of work. A specified workload, expressed in terms of watts or joules per second, is imposed while the person performs the task. Two examples of ergometers include the bicycle ergometer and the treadmill ergometer. A bicycle ergometer is a stationary bicycle that has a friction belt attached. The front wheel of the bicycle is rotated, and the braking force of the belt can be adjusted to alter the workload. A treadmill ergometer is used more frequently to assess workload performance, especially cardiac function. During treadmill testing, the person walks or runs on a moving belt. Changing the speed and incline of the treadmill alters the workload. This change usually is done in predetermined stages. During treadmill testing, the heart rate and electrocardiogram are monitored continuously, and the blood pressure is checked intermittently. Usually, the person being tested continues to exercise, completing successive stages of the test, until exhaustion intervenes or a predetermined or maximal heart rate is reached.

Maximal heart rate is estimated by age. Tables of maximal heart rate by age are available, but as a general rule, the predicted maximal heart rate can be estimated by subtracting age from 220 (*e.g.,* the target heart rate for a 40-year-old person would be 180 beats/minute). The person may continue to exercise until the predicted maximum heart rate is achieved, or until 85% to 90% of the predicted maximal rate is reached.

Metabolic Equivalents. Metabolic equivalents (METs), which are multiples of the basal metabolic rate, are commonly used to express workload at various stages of work. The energy expended in a resting position is equivalent to 1 MET and it changes as the type of activity performed (*e.g.,* walking, running) changes. For example, walking at 4 miles per hour (mph), cycling at 11 mph, playing tennis (singles), or doing carpentry requires 5 to 6 METs. Running at 6 mph requires 10 METs, and running at 10 mph requires 17 METs. Healthy sedentary persons seldom are able to exercise beyond 10 or 11 METs, whereas highly trained persons are able to achieve workloads of 16 METs or greater. In persons with coronary heart disease, workloads of 8 METs often produce angina.

During exercise stress testing, persons are asked to rate their subjective responses to the exercise experience. A commonly used tool to measure the person's perception of the amount of work being performed is the Borg Rating of Perceived Exertion (RPE) Scale, which is based on research that correlates heart rate to feelings of perceived exertion.[25] The scale values range from 6 through 20 (e.g., 7 represents very, very light; 9, very light; 13, somewhat hard; 15, hard; and 19 very, very hard). The numeric values on the RPE Scale increase linearly with workload, and the total scale reflects a 10-fold increase in heart rate. As the person is performing the exercise stress test, he or she is asked to select a number that best corresponds to his or her feelings of exertion for the work being performed. The number chosen should be approximately 10 times the heart rate (e.g., if the person rates the exercise experience as a 7, the heart rate should be 70 beats/minute). A newer category of scale with ratio properties has been developed. The numbers used on this scale range from 0 to 10, with 0 representing nothing; 0.5, very, very weak; and 10, very, very strong. With this method, the expressions and the numbers they represent are placed in the correct position for a ratio scale. For example, because 1 represents very weak, 0.5 represents very, very weak or half that intensity.[26] When using this scale in a phase II cardiac rehabilitation program, it is often recommended that individuals not exceed 30 beats/minute above their resting heart rate.

Exercise and Activity Tolerance in the Elderly

As the population of elderly adults in Western societies increases, so does the concern over exercise and activity tolerance. It is anticipated that by 2020, persons aged 65 and older will make up approximately 30% of the population.[27] Regular exercise benefits older adults through a variety of physical and psychosocial components. These physical benefits include improved overall health and physical fitness, enhanced maximal aerobic capacity, prevention of a decline in the basal metabolic rate, gains in cerebral function, and improved balance and coordination. Psychologically, the older adult may experience a greater sense of well-being, increased opportunities for social interactions, lower rates of mortality, and fewer years of disability.

The capacity of the elderly to undertake aerobic activities such as walking and running is adversely affected by advancing age. Current evidence supports a 5% to 15% decline per decade in $\dot{V}O_2$max in men and women beginning at 25 years of age. Maximal heart rate decreases 6 to 10 beats/minute per decade, and it is this decrease in heart rate that is believed to contribute to a decreased cardiac output.[27] The decline in $\dot{V}O_2$max seems to be due to both central and peripheral adaptations. Reductions in maximal heart rate, stroke volume, and lean body mass all contribute to a reduced $\dot{V}O_2$max. Also contributing to a reduced $\dot{V}O_2$max are a decrease in plasma volume, red blood cell count, and total blood volume.[28]

In terms of skeletal muscle function, there is a decrease in muscle mass and strength, flexibility and range of joint movement, and muscle endurance. There is a decrease in size of the individual muscles that occurs with aging, particularly beyond 60 years of age. Muscle strength and mass reportedly decline 30% to 50% between 30 and 80 years of age, with loss of muscle mass accounting for most of the decrease observed in muscle strength.[28] The most important factor in muscle atrophy in elderly persons is the reduction in type II fibers and the size of the muscle fiber areas. Muscle mass loss is subordinate to an age-related denervation of type II fibers, which removes the trophic effect on the fibers, leading to atrophy. Type I fiber collaterals expand to some of the denervated type II fiber areas in an attempt to lessen muscle fiber loss. This leads to an increase in type I motor neuron units at the expense of type II fibers, resulting in a reduction in muscle mass and muscle strength. There is also a slowing of muscle contraction and rate of force development, and reduced ability to accelerate limb movement. Changes in the elastic and collagen fibers of tendons and ligaments lead to decreased flexibility and loss of mobility and stability of the joints.[29]

As with exercise programs for younger persons, exercise programs for older persons should include an emphasis on aerobic activities, resistance training, flexibility or stretching exercises, and lifestyle changes.[30] Resistance exercise, which improves muscle strength, is particularly important for the elderly. Most of the variance of walking speed in the elderly is related to leg strength, and increased strength has been shown to increase walking endurance and stair climbing. Flexibility training is also important because limited range of motion in the hip, knee, and ankle joints increases the risk of falls and contributes to age-related changes in gait. Lifestyle modification involves finding opportunities within a person's existing routines to increase physical activity (e.g., taking stairs rather than an elevator, parking farther from entrances).

IN SUMMARY, physical activity and exercise denote the process of skeletal muscle movement and energy expenditure. There are two main types of exercise: aerobic and isometric. *Aerobic,* or *endurance, exercise* involves rhythmic changes in muscle length and increases the ability of muscles to use oxygen more efficiently so that the body can do more work with less cardiac and respiratory effort. *Isometric,* or *resistance, exercise* involves the generation of force against low to moderate resistance, improves overall muscle strength and tone, and builds muscle mass. Flexibility, or stretching, exercise promotes flexibility and improves range of motion of the joints.

The body reacts to exercise by a series of physiologic responses that increase its level of performance. Heart rate, cardiac output, and stroke volume increase to deliver more blood to working muscles; minute ventilation and diffusion of oxygen and carbon dioxide increase to provide oxygen more efficiently to meet the rising metabolic demands; and local changes in the arterioles and capillaries contribute to enhanced perfusion of the working muscles. The *maximal oxygen consumption* ($\dot{V}O_2max$), which is the volume of oxygen consumed (*i.e.,* liters/minute), is an important determinant of the person's capacity to perform work. Activity and exercise tolerance can be assessed in several ways, including through the use of paper-and-pencil tests that measure subjective responses or through tests such as bicycle or treadmill ergometry that measure heart rate, $\dot{V}O_2max$, and other responses during exercise.

The capacity of the elderly to undertake aerobic activities such as walking and running is adversely affected by reductions in maximal heart rate, stroke volume, and $\dot{V}O_2max$, along with a decrease in muscle mass and strength, flexibility and range of joint movement, and muscle endurance. Exercise programs for older persons should include an emphasis on aerobic activities, resistance training, flexibility or stretching exercises, and lifestyle changes. ■

Like dyspnea and pain, fatigue is a subjective symptom. It often is described as a subjective feeling of tiredness that varies in terms of pleasantness, intensity, and duration and often is influenced by the time of day and a person's biorhythms.[31] Fatigue is different from the normal tiredness that people experience at the end of the day. Tiredness is relieved by a good night's sleep, whereas fatigue persists despite sufficient or adequate sleep. Although fatigue is one of the most common symptoms reported to health care professionals, it is one of the least understood of all health problems.

Fatigue may be described in terms of its underlying physiologic basis, by its origin or cause, or by its temporal patterns over time.[31] The physiologic basis of fatigue includes factors such as diaphragmatic, motor, and neurologic mechanisms. Diaphragmatic fatigue occurs in both acute and chronic respiratory conditions where the force and duration of muscle work exceeds muscle energy stores. Neuromuscular fatigue involves the loss of maximal capacity to generate force during exercise.

ACTIVITY INTOLERANCE AND FATIGUE

- Activity intolerance is the inability of a person to complete activities because of insufficient psychological or physiologic energy.
- Fatigue is the sensation of having exhausted one's energy reserves.
- Acute fatigue is muscle fatigue with a rapid onset and duration limited to the duration of the exercise. The time it takes to develop acute fatigue at any level of exercise depends on conditioning.
- Chronic fatigue has an insidious onset, a long duration unrelated to duration of activity, and intensity not related to the intensity of activity.
- Chronic fatigue syndrome (CFS) is characterized by disabling fatigue and many nonspecific symptoms, including cognitive impairments, sleep disturbances, and musculoskeletal pain. The etiology of CFS is unknown, but it is associated with several chronic diseases such as fibromyalgia, depression, and irritable bowel syndrome.

ACTIVITY INTOLERANCE AND FATIGUE

After completing this section of the chapter, you should be able to meet the following objectives:

- Define fatigue and describe its manifestations.
- Differentiate acute from chronic fatigue.
- List at least four health problems that are associated with chronic fatigue.
- Define *chronic fatigue syndrome* and describe assessment findings, presenting symptoms, and laboratory values associated with the disorder.
- Discuss treatment modalities for chronic fatigue syndrome.

Activity intolerance can be viewed as not having sufficient physical or psychological energy reserve to endure or complete required or desired daily activities. Fatigue is the sensation that comes with having exhausted those energy reserves. It is a state that is experienced by everyone at some time in his or her life. Fatigue can be a normal physical response, such as that following extreme exercise in healthy people, or it can be a symptom that is experienced by people with limited exercise reserve, such as people with cardiac or respiratory disease, anemia, or malnutrition, or those on certain types of drug therapy. Fatigue also may be related to lack of sleep or mental stress.

Mechanisms of Fatigue

The origin or cause of fatigue can be physiologic, psychological, pathologic, or unknown (*e.g.,* chronic fatigue syndrome). It can be caused by environmental factors (*e.g.,* excessive noise, temperature extremes, changes in weather); drug-related incidents (*e.g.,* use of tranquilizers, alcohol, toxic chemical exposure); treatment-related causes (*e.g.,* chemotherapy, radiation therapy, surgery, anesthesia, diagnostic testing); physical exertion (*e.g.,* exercise); and psychological factors (*e.g.,* stress, monotony).

Clinically, fatigue can be defined or described by its temporal patterns over time, such as acute (*e.g.,* less than 4 weeks) or chronic (*e.g.,* present for 50% of the day, or lasting 1 to 6 months or longer).[31] It is thought that both acute and chronic fatigue can exist in the same person, similar to acute and chronic pain.

Acute Physical Fatigue

Acute fatigue has a rapid onset and is often defined as muscle fatigue associated with increased activity, or exercise, that is carried out to the point of exhaustion. It is relieved shortly after the activity ceases, and serves as a protective mechanism. Physical conditioning can influence the onset of acute fatigue. People who engage in regular exercise compared with sedentary persons are able to perform an activity for longer periods before acute fatigue develops. They probably are able to do so because their muscles use oxygen and nutrients more efficiently and their circulatory and respiratory systems are better able to deliver oxygen and nutrients to the exercising muscles.

Acute physical fatigue occurs more rapidly in deconditioned muscle. For example, acute fatigue often is seen in people who have been on bed rest because of a surgical procedure or in people who have had their activity curtailed because of chronic illness, such as heart or respiratory disease. In such cases, the acute fatigue often is out of proportion to the activity that is being performed (*e.g.,* dangling at the bedside, sitting in a chair for the first time). When resuming activity for the first time after a prolonged period of bed rest or inactivity, the person may experience tachycardia and hypotension. Unless these parameters are changed by medications such as β-adrenergic blocking drugs, heart rate and blood pressure become particularly sensitive indicators of activity tolerance or intolerance.

Another example of acute fatigue is that which occurs in people who require the use of assistive devices such as wheelchairs, walkers, or crutches. The upper arm muscles are less well adapted to prolonged exercise than the leg muscles. This is because arm muscles are primarily composed of type II muscle fibers. Type II muscle fibers, which are used when the body requires short bursts of energy, fatigue quickly. As a result, people who use wheelchairs or a pair of crutches may quickly experience fatigue until their arms become conditioned to the increased activity.

Chronic Fatigue

Chronic fatigue differs from acute fatigue in terms of onset, intensity, perception, duration, and relief. In contrast to acute fatigue, chronic fatigue has an insidious onset, is typically perceived as being unusually intense relative to the amount of activity performed, lasts longer than 1 month, has a cumulative effect, and is not relieved by cessation of activity.[31] It is one of the more common problems experienced by people with chronic health problems (Table 11-1). In the primary care setting, 11% to 25%

TABLE 11-1 Chronic Illnesses and Causes of Chronic Fatigue

CHRONIC ILLNESS	CAUSE OF FATIGUE
Acquired immunodeficiency syndrome	Impaired immune function, anorexia, muscle weakness, and psychosocial factors associated with the disease
Anemia	Decreased oxygen-carrying capacity of blood
Arthritis	Pain and joint dysfunction lead to impaired mobility, loss of sleep, and emotional factors
Cancer	Presence of chemical products and catabolic processes associated with tumor growth; anorexia and difficulty eating; effects of chemotherapy and radiation therapy; and psychosocial factors such as depression, grieving, hopelessness, and fear
Cardiac disease	
Myocardial infarction	Death of myocardial tissue results in decreased cardiac output, poor tissue perfusion, and impaired delivery of oxygen and nutrients to vital organs
Congestive heart failure	Impaired pumping ability of the heart results in poor perfusion of muscle tissue and vital organs
Neurologic disorders	
Multiple sclerosis	Demyelinating disease of CNS characterized by slowing of nerve conduction, resulting in lower extremity weakness and fatigue
Myasthenia gravis	Disorder of postsynaptic acetylcholine receptors of the myoneural junction, resulting in muscle weakness and fatigue
Chronic lung disease	Increased work of breathing and impaired gas exchange
Chronic renal failure	Accumulation of metabolic wastes; fluid, electrolyte, and acid-base disorders; decreased red blood cell count and oxygen-carrying capacity due to impaired erythropoietin production
Metabolic disorders	
Hypothyroidism	Decrease in basal metabolic rate manifested by fatigue
Diabetes mellitus	Impaired cellular use of glucose by muscle cells
Obesity	Imbalance in nutritional intake and energy expenditure; increased workload due to excess weight
Steroid myopathy	Glucocorticosteroids interfere with protein and glycogen synthesis, which leads to muscle wasting

of patients present with chronic fatigue as their chief complaint. Of these, 20% to 45% will have a primary organic cause diagnosed for their fatigue, and 40% to 45% will have a primary psychiatric disorder diagnosed.[31] The remainder will either meet the criteria for diagnosis of chronic fatigue syndrome (to be discussed) or will remain undiagnosed.

Although acute fatigue often serves a protective function, chronic fatigue does not. It limits the amount of activity that a person can perform and may interfere with employment, the performance of activities of daily living, and the quality of life in general. Although fatigue often is viewed as a symptom of anxiety and depression, it is important to recognize that these psychological manifestations may be symptoms of the fatigue. For example, people with persistent fatigue due to a chronic illness may have to curtail their work schedules, decrease social activities, and limit their usual family responsibilities. These lifestyle changes may be the reasons for the depression rather than the depression being a cause of the fatigue.

Chronic fatigue occurs across a broad spectrum of disease states. It is a common complaint of persons with cancer, cardiac disease, end-stage renal disease, chronic lung disease, hepatitis C, arthritis, human immunodeficiency virus (HIV) infection and acquired immunodeficiency syndrome (AIDS), and neurologic disorders such as multiple sclerosis, postpolio syndrome, and Parkinson disease.

Chronic fatigue is almost a universal phenomenon in persons with cancer, with prevalence rates ranging from 75% to 96%, depending on the form of treatment and stage of disease.[32–34] Cancer-related fatigue may be caused by the disease itself, or it may be caused by treatment. In fact, the majority of persons undergoing cancer chemotherapy or radiation therapy have reported significant fatigue during the course of treatment.[35] Cancer-related fatigue involves a number of physiologic, sensory, affective, and cognitive dimensions. There is often a sensation of feeling unusually tired with generalized weakness and a greater need for rest. There may also be a disturbing lack of motivation, anxiety, and sadness as well as an inability to concentrate or difficulty in thinking.

There are several types of cancer-related factors that may cause fatigue, the most prominent of which are factors related to energy imbalance. They include anemia, cachexia, stress, pain, infection, medications, and metabolic disorders.[34,36] The cytokine theory of cancer-related fatigue is just emerging. This theory is based, at least in part, on the observation that patients receiving agents such as interferon-α as part of their treatment plan experienced devastating fatigue that was dose limited. Interferon-α and other agents used to treat cancer also influence the release of other cytokines that are related to fatigue. Cancer cells and the immune system appear to produce or express a number of cytokines with the potential for manufacturing many of the factors that contribute to fatigue. One of these cytokines, tumor necrosis factor-α (TNF-α), is thought to interfere with appetite, produce weight loss, and cause depletion of skeletal muscle protein stores. As a result, muscle wasting occurs, and people have to expend more energy to perform simple activities such as sitting and standing.[36]

Management. Pathologic factors associated with fatigue include insomnia, anemia, psychological stress, and wasting or weakness.[31] Many of these conditions respond to appropriate treatment measures. Anemia, which is common among persons with HIV/AIDS, patients with end-stage renal disease, and cancer patients receiving chemotherapy, causes fatigue by interfering with the oxygen-carrying capacity of the blood. It can often be treated with recombinant forms of erythropoietin (epoetin-alfa), an endogenous hormone normally produced by the kidney (see Chapter 14). Insomnia, which occurs for a number of reasons, including anxiety and depression, hot flashes, nocturia, and pain, is often amenable to nonpharmacologic and pharmacologic methods of treatment. Psychological disturbances, such as anxiety and depression, which are frequently associated with fatigue, can be treated with selected pharmacologic agents. Another cause of fatigue is loss of muscle mass, muscle strength, and endurance. This type of fatigue is common among persons with forced immobility, musculoskeletal disorders such as arthritis,[37] neuromuscular disorders such as multiple sclerosis, and wasting syndromes such as HIV/AIDS. Aerobic exercise has been shown to decrease this type of fatigue in patients with AIDS[38] and multiple sclerosis.[39]

Chronic Fatigue Syndrome

Chronic fatigue syndrome (CFS) is a condition of disabling fatigue of at least 6 months' duration that is typically accompanied by an array of self-reported, nonspecific symptoms such as cognitive impairments, sleep disturbances, and musculoskeletal pain. CFS probably is not a new disease. Indeed, in the 19th century, the diagnosis of "neurasthenia" was commonly applied to a group of symptoms that are very similar to those found in CFS.[40] In the late 20th century and now into the 21st century, the disorder continues to be a relatively common problem. Because of differences in who is included in the diagnostic category of CFS, the prevalence data vary among studies. In community surveys, 1% to 3% of the population is reported to be affected by CFS.[41–43]

Definition. Because the etiology of CFS is unknown, there are no biologic markers for the diagnosis of CFS, and there are no definitive treatments. Furthermore, the overlap of symptoms of CFS with other functional disorders such as fibromyalgia, multiple chemical sensitivities, depression, and irritable bowel syndrome, which also are characterized by fatigue, complicates the ability to define the syndrome with any degree of certainty. In fact, CFS may describe a group of similar symptoms that develop with different pathophysiologic disturbances.

Because of the need for diagnostic criteria, the case definition for CFS was established in 1988[44] by the CDC and revised through its International Chronic Fatigue Syndrome study group in 1994.[45] To be classified as CFS, the fatigue must be clinically evaluated, cause severe mental and physical exhaustion, and result in a significant reduction in the individual's premorbid activity level. In addition, there must be evidence of the concurrent occurrence of four of the following eight symptoms: sore throat, tender cervical or axillary lymph nodes, muscle pain, multijoint pain without swelling or redness, headaches, unrefreshing sleep, and postexertional malaise lasting more than 24 hours. The fatigue and concurrent symptoms must be of 6 months' duration or longer. Chart 11-1 outlines the criteria for diagnosis of CFS.[45]

Pathophysiology. Theories of the pathogenesis of CFS include infections, psychological disorders, a dysfunction in the hypothalamic-pituitary-adrenal axis, or an alteration in the autonomic nervous system.[46] Despite much research and the development of several theories, the underlying pathophysiology of CFS remains elusive. Many people with CFS attribute the onset of their disease to an influenza-like infection. Thus, the link between infectious agents such as Epstein-Barr virus, human herpesvirus 6, enterovirus, and others has been extensively studied. To date, however, none of these agents has been conclusively linked in a cause-and-effect relationship with the development of CFS.[42] Several studies have also suggested that CFS may be due to a primary alteration in immune function. A number of immunologic abnormalities have been described in persons with CFS.[41] It is hypothesized that the immune system may overreact to an environmental agent (most likely an infectious agent) or internal stimuli and be unable to self-regulate after the infectious insult is over. It has also been suggested that cytokines such as interleukin (IL)-6 might have an important role in CFS because they are also involved in the stress response and are crucial inducers of some of the manifestations of the disorder, such as sleepiness, anorexia, mild fever, and increased sensitivity to pain.[41]

Psychological disorders often are associated with CFS, especially anxiety and depression, but this is difficult to evaluate. Persons with CFS are more likely than the general population to have experienced a psychological disorder such as major depression or panic disorder before the development of CFS; however, it also is true that a significant proportion of those persons with CFS have not had such episodes, either before or after the development of CFS.[47]

Diagnostic imaging studies have provided preliminary data suggesting that the CNS may be the final common pathway in the development of this disorder.[48] In brain imaging studies using magnetic resonance imaging (MRI) and positron emission tomography (PET) scans, white matter abnormalities and hypoperfusion of the brain stem have been found in persons with CFS.[49] In other studies, abnormalities of the hypothalamic-pituitary-adrenal axis, such as attenuated activity of corticotropin-releasing hormone and changes in the circadian rhythm of cortisol secretion, have been documented. However, the findings remain unexplained.

Manifestations. One of the most important findings in persons with CFS is the complaint of fatigue. Often, the symptom of fatigue is preceded by a cold or flulike illness. Frequently, the person describes the illness as recurring, with periods of exacerbations and remissions. With each subsequent episode of the illness, the fatigue increases.

Physical findings include low-grade fever. The fever is intermittent and occurs only when the illness recurs. Other findings include nonexudative pharyngitis, palpable and tender cervical lymph nodes, a mildly enlarged thyroid gland, wheezing, splenomegaly, myalgia, arthralgia, and heme-positive stool with subsequent negative sigmoidoscopy.

Psychological problems include impaired cognition, which the person describes as an inability to concentrate and perform previously mundane tasks. There are reports of mood and sleep disturbances, balance problems, visual disturbances, and various degrees of anxiety and depression.

Diagnosis and Treatment. The diagnosis of CFS is based on integration of the entire clinical picture of the client's symptoms, physical assessment findings, and the results of diagnostic tests. Laboratory investigations are used to detect other disorders. Usually the final diagnosis is based on the definition of CFS provided by the CDC[45] (see Chart 11-1).

Because there is no known cause of CFS, current treatment tends to remain symptomatic, with a focus on management rather than cure. It centers on education, emotional support,

---

CHART 11-1   CRITERIA FOR DIAGNOSIS OF CHRONIC FATIGUE SYNDROME

Clinically evaluated fatigue
- Fatigue of ≥ 6 months' duration (new or definite onset)
- Not relieved by rest
- Significant reduction in premorbid occupational, educational, social, or personal activities

Concurrent experience of at least four of the following symptoms:
- Impaired memory or concentration
- Sore throat
- Tender cervical or axillary lymph nodes
- Muscle pain
- Multijoint pain
- New headaches
- Unrefreshing sleep
- Postexertional malaise

Exclusionary diagnoses
- Any active medical condition that could explain the chronic fatigue
- Any previously diagnosed but incompletely resolved medical condition that could explain the chronic fatigue
- Any past or current diagnosis of a major depressive disorder, schizophrenia, delusional disorder, dementia, or anorexia or bulimia nervosa
- Alcohol or other substance abuse within 2 years of onset of chronic fatigue symptoms

Developed from Fukuda K., Straus S. E., Hickie I., et al. (1994). The chronic fatigue syndrome: A comprehensive approach to its definition and study. *Annals of Internal Medicine* 121, 953–959.

treatment of symptoms, and overall management of general health. Symptom management includes development of an exercise program that helps the person regain strength. Along with a structured activity program, persons should be encouraged to be as active as possible as they resume their activities of daily living.

A holistic approach to the treatment of CFS is essential. With proper treatment and support, most persons with CFS demonstrate improvement. However, relapses can occur. Persons diagnosed with CFS must continue to receive follow-up care and treatment on a regular basis. Local and national support groups are available for persons who experience CFS.

IN SUMMARY, fatigue is a nonspecific, self-recognized state of physical and psychological exhaustion. It results in the person's not being able to perform routine activities and is not relieved with sleep or rest. Acute fatigue results from excessive use of the body or specific muscle groups and often is related to depletion of energy sources. Chronic fatigue often is associated with a specific disease or chronic illness and may be relieved when the effects of the disease are corrected. CFS is a complex illness that has physiologic and psychological manifestations. It is characterized by debilitating fatigue. Diagnosis often is made by a process of elimination, and treatment requires a holistic approach. ■

wheelchair; or involve the entire body, as in a person confined to bed rest. Bed rest and immobility are associated with various complications that include generalized weakness, orthostatic intolerance, atelectasis, pneumonia, thromboemboli, urinary retention, constipation, muscle atrophy, osteoporosis, and impaired sensory perception[50–53] (Table 11-2). This section of the chapter focuses on the physiologic changes that occur with bed rest and immobility and the interventions to counteract their effects.

Bed rest is one of the oldest and most commonly used methods of treatment for various medical conditions. Before the 1940s, bed rest was prescribed for 2 weeks after childbirth, 3 weeks after herniorrhaphy, and 4 to 6 weeks after myocardial infarction. It was believed that the complex biochemical and physical demands of physical activity diverted energy from the restorative and reparative processes of healing. Rest in bed was regarded as tantamount to optimal rest of the heart and entire body.[52,53]

During World War II, the shortage of hospital beds and medical personnel forced early mobilization of many patients. As often happens with this kind of action, it soon was discovered that early mobilization lessened complications and improved patient outcome. Studies by the National Aeronautics and Space Administration (NASA) that described the damaging effects of prolonged inactivity and weightlessness during space flight have also contributed to a further understanding of the antigravity effects of bed rest.

BED REST AND IMMOBILITY

After completing this section of the chapter, you should be able to meet the following objectives:

- Describe the effects of immobility and prolonged bed rest on cardiovascular, pulmonary, renal, metabolic, musculoskeletal, gastrointestinal, and sensory function.
- Describe the time course of the physiologic changes associated with immobility and prolonged bed rest.
- Identify physical assessment findings that are related to the effects of immobility and prolonged bed rest.
- Describe treatment interventions that counteract the negative effects of immobility and prolonged bed rest.

Bed rest and immobility are the antithesis of exercise and mobility. They defy the active use of skeletal muscles, movement against gravity, conservation of body fluids, normal distribution of blood flow, and maintenance of cardiopulmonary reserves. Immobility may be dictated by an injury that requires stabilization to facilitate the healing process, or it may result from conditions that limit physical reserve. The effects of immobility can be restricted to a single extremity that is encased in a plaster cast; involve both legs, as in a person confined to a

BED REST AND IMMOBILITY

- The cardiovascular responses to bed rest include a redistribution of blood volume from the lower body to the central circulation, a deconditioning of the heart, and a reduction in total body water. Orthostatic intolerance may develop.
- Venous stasis due to bed rest encourages the development of deep vein thrombosis.
- Pulmonary changes due to bed rest include decreased tidal volume and functional residual capacity. Alveoli tend to collapse, resulting in areas of decreased pulmonary ventilation.
- Bed rest increases the risk for development of renal calculi and urinary tract infections.
- Muscle mass is reduced owing to disuse atrophy and bone mass is reduced because of an imbalance of activity between osteoclasts (bone resorption) and osteoblasts (bone generation).
- Pressure ulcers due to tissue ischemia may develop in areas in constant contact with the bed surface.
- Psychological effects of bed rest include anxiety and depression and decreased ability to concentrate and learn.

TABLE 11-2 Complications of Bed Rest and Immobility

SYSTEM	COMPLICATION
Cardiovascular	Increased heart rate; decreased cardiac output and stroke volume contributing to decreased aerobic capacity; decreased size of the heart; decreased left ventricular end-diastolic volume; unchanged systolic-diastolic blood pressure; decreased fluid volume; orthostatic intolerance; venous thrombophlebitis
Pulmonary	Mechanical resistance to breathing; reduced cardiopulmonary functional capacity; relative hypoxemia; pneumonia
Musculoskeletal	Muscle atrophy and loss of strength and endurance; decreased strength of tendons and ligaments and their insertions on bone; decreased muscle oxidative capacity contributing to decreased aerobic capacity; osteoporosis (bone loss); contractures; immobilization hypercalcemia; osteoarthritis
Gastrointestinal	Loss of appetite; constipation
Genitourinary	Incontinence; renal calculi; urinary stasis and infection; electrolyte imbalance
Hematologic	Decreased total fluid volume; increased blood viscosity; thromboembolism
Metabolic and endocrine	Glucose intolerance; hyperglycemia; hyperinsulinemia; increased parathyroid hormone production
Skin	Pressure ulcers
Functional	Impaired ambulation and activity tolerance; impaired balance and coordination
Psychological	Sensory deprivation; altered sensory perception; confusion and disorientation; anxiety; depression; decreased intellectual capacity

Developed from information in Harper C. M., Lyles Y. M. (1988). Physiology and complications of bed rest. *Journal of the American Geriatric Society* 36, 1048.

Physiologic Effects of Bed Rest

The supine position that often accompanies immobility and bed rest interferes with the effects of gravity and exercise stimuli (Fig. 11-4). While in the upright position, the body compensates for the effects of gravity in a variety of ways. The skeletal muscles contract and exert pressure against veins and lymph vessels, counteracting the hydrostatic effects of gravity that cause blood and fluid to pool in the lower extremities. Movement against the forces of gravity maintains muscle tone and bones remain stronger because longitudinal weight bearing keeps essential minerals, such as calcium, inside the structure of the bone.

Cardiovascular Responses

After a period of bed rest and assumption of the supine position, the cardiovascular system exhibits changes that reflect the loss of gravitational and exercise stimuli. These changes include (1) a redistribution and change in blood volume, (2) increased cardiac workload, (3) orthostatic hypotension, and (4) venous stasis with the potential for development of deep vein thrombosis.

One of the most striking responses to assumption of the supine position during bed rest is the redistribution and change in blood volume. In the supine position, approximately 500 mL of blood is redistributed from the lower extremities to the central circulation. Most of this blood is diverted to the thoracic

cavity; a smaller portion is diverted to the arms and head. The increased fluid shifted to the head may result in the person experiencing headache, swelling of the nasal sinuses, nasal congestion, and puffiness of the eyelids.[53–56]

A major cardiovascular manifestation of bed rest is an increased workload on the heart. The increase in thoracic blood volume that occurs on assumption of the supine position results in an increase in central venous pressure and left ventricular end-diastolic volume, and an increase in stroke volume and cardiac output through the Frank-Starling mechanism (see Chapter 21). In the supine position, the normal cardiac output is 7 to 8 L/minute, compared with a cardiac output of 5 to 6 L/minute for a person in the standing position. Initially, the increase in cardiac output is accompanied by a slight decrease in heart rate and systemic vascular resistance and maintenance of arterial blood pressure.

With extended periods of bed rest, there is an increase in venous distention; this leads to a decrease in venous return to the heart, along with a stabilization of the stroke volume and cardiac output. The heart rate, however, continues to increase. During periods of tachycardia, the diastolic filling time is decreased; as a result, the heart has to expend more energy and use more oxygen to perfuse vital organs and meet the metabolic demands of the body. This response is exaggerated when a person has to assume the upright position and begin activity after a prolonged period of bed rest. When a person begins submaximal exercise after prolonged bed rest, heart rate increases while stroke volume and cardiac output decrease. Between 5

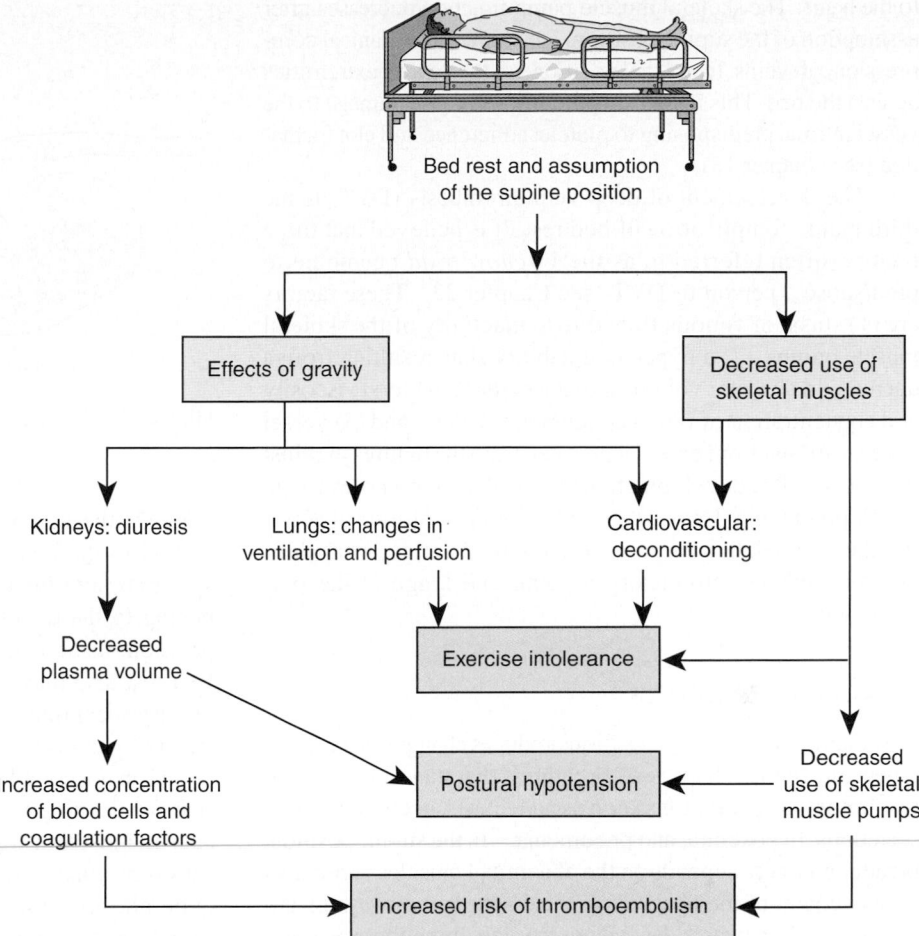

Bed rest and assumption
of the supine position

Effects of gravity

Decreased use of
skeletal muscles

Kidneys: diuresis

Lungs: changes in
ventilation and perfusion

Cardiovascular:
deconditioning

Decreased
plasma volume

Exercise intolerance

Increased concentration
of blood cells and
coagulation factors

Postural hypotension

Decreased
use of skeletal
muscle pumps

Increased risk of thromboembolism

FIGURE 11-4 • The effects of gravity and decreased use of the skeletal muscles during bed rest and assumption of the supine position on cardiovascular, respiratory, and renal function, and their impact on exercise tolerance and the risk of complications such as thromboembolism and postural hypotension.

and 10 weeks of reconditioning exercise is required for return of heart rate, stroke volume, and cardiac output parameters to their levels before bed rest.[53,56–58]

Bed rest also affects fluid balance. The increase in central blood volume results in an inhibition of antidiuretic hormone and aldosterone, with a resultant water and sodium diuresis. In the supine position, diuresis begins on the first day with the shift of blood from the lower extremities to the thoracic cavity. The loss of water and sodium results in an increase in hematocrit, hemoglobin, and red blood cell mass owing to the loss of plasma volume.[50,54,55] After approximately 4 days of bed rest, fluid losses reach an equilibrium. A possible explanation for this is that fluid is lost from the vascular compartment with a subsequent shift of fluid from the interstitial to the vascular fluid compartment. With a decrease in the interstitial fluid volume and the reestablishment of intravascular volume, the stimuli for salt and water diuresis are lost.[54,55]

Orthostatic Hypotension. During bed rest, the forces of gravity and hydrostatic pressure are removed from the cardiovascular system. After 3 to 4 days of bed rest, resumption of the upright position results in orthostatic or postural intolerance. Standing after prolonged bed rest results in a decrease in central

blood volume as blood is displaced to the lower extremities and dependent parts of the body.[59–61] Decreases in stroke volume and cardiac output occur along with increases in heart rate and systemic vascular resistance. The signs and symptoms of postural intolerance include tachycardia, nausea, diaphoresis, and sometimes syncope or fainting (discussed in Chapter 23).

The mechanism of orthostatic intolerance after bed rest involves multiple factors, including a decrease in vascular volume, a decline in skeletal muscle pump function, reduced sympathetic innervation of the resistance vessels, and resetting of the baroreceptors that control blood pressure. Because changes in plasma volume do not fully explain the orthostatic intolerance that occurs with bed rest, it would appear that at least part of the explanation rests with the functions of the baroreceptors and sympathetic nervous system control of vasomotor tone.[59,60] It has also been suggested that the decrease in stroke volume that occurs with assumption of the upright position after bed rest may be due to a reduction in left ventricular size and distensibility that occurs in response to a decrease in loading conditions of the heart.[55]

Venous Stasis. Venous stasis in the legs results from a lack of the skeletal muscle pump function that promotes venous return to the heart. The skeletal muscle pump function decreases after assumption of the supine position, and there is mechanical compression of veins from the position of the lower extremities against the bed. This increased pressure can cause damage to the vessel intima, predisposing to platelet adherence and clot formation (see Chapter 13).

The development of deep vein thrombosis (DVT) is the third major complication of bed rest. It is believed that three factors (often referred to as the *Virchow triad*) combine to predispose a person to DVT (see Chapter 22). These factors are (1) stasis of venous flow due to inactivity of the skeletal muscle pumps, (2) a hypercoagulability state resulting from a decrease in vascular volume and an increase in blood viscosity and concentration of blood coagulation factors, and (3) vessel injury resulting from external pressure from the mattress against the veins.[62] The development of DVT also predisposes to the development of pulmonary emboli. With resumption of activity, there is risk that large thrombi may dislodge, work their way through the circulatory system, and lodge in the pulmonary vessel.

Pulmonary Responses

Assumption of the supine position produces changes in lung volumes and the mechanics of breathing that can contribute to respiratory complications such as atelectasis, accumulation of secretions, hypoxemia, and pneumonia.[63] In the supine position, breathing largely depends on the abdominal muscles rather than on movement of the chest cage; the diaphragm moves upward rather than downward, decreasing the size of the thoracic compartment, and chest and lung expansion are limited because of the resistance of the bed. As a result, the tidal volume and functional residual capacity are decreased, and the efficiency and effectiveness of ventilation are hindered. Thus, persons on bed rest need to work harder to breathe, and consequently they take fewer deep breaths.

A reduction in functional residual capacity predisposes to airway collapse, ventilation-perfusion inequalities, and impaired oxygen transport. Alveoli tend to collapse, resulting in areas of atelectasis and a decrease in the surface area for gas exchange (see Chapter 29). This may result in arteriovenous shunting with a concomitant decrease in arterial oxygenation. Also, poor fluid intake and dehydration may cause secretions to become thick and tenacious. Stasis of secretions provides an ideal medium for bacterial growth and increases the risk for development of pneumonia. Reduced activity and the recumbent position inhibit coughing, foster the retention of secretions, and adversely affect secretion distribution in the airways. Coughing and deep-breathing are necessary to prevent accumulation of secretions and airway collapse.

Urinary Tract Responses

The kidneys are designed to function optimally with the body in the erect position (Fig. 11-5). The anatomy of the kidney is such that urine flows from the kidney pelvis by gravity,

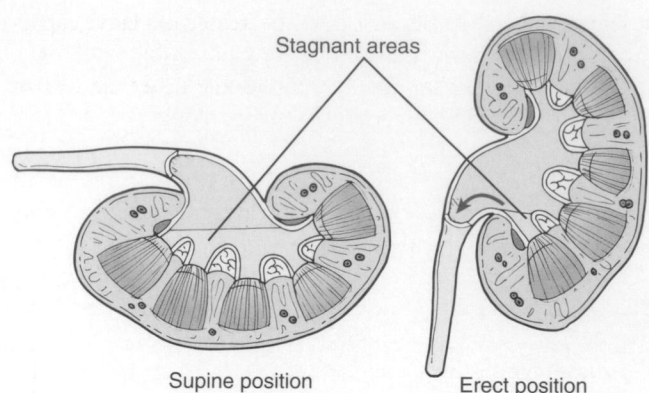

FIGURE 11-5 • Effect of body position on urine flow in the kidney.

whereas the action of peristalsis moves urine through the ureters to the bladder. Prolonged bed rest affects the renal system by altering the composition of body fluids and predisposing to the development of kidney stones. In the supine position, urine is not readily drained from the renal pelvis. Bed rest also may predispose to urinary tract infections and urinary incontinence because of positional changes and difficulty in emptying the bladder.[64]

A major complication of prolonged bed rest is the increased risk for development of kidney stones. Prolonged bed rest causes muscle atrophy, protein breakdown, and decalcification of bone with the development of hypercalcemia and hyperphosphatemia. Saturation of the urine with calcium salts (*i.e.*, calcium oxalate and calcium phosphate) coupled with urinary stasis increases the risk for the development of calcium-containing kidney stones (see Chapter 33). Also, urine levels of citrate, a prominent inhibitor of calcium stone formation, do not increase during bed rest.[64] Dehydration further increases urine concentration of stone-forming elements and risk of kidney stone formation.

Urinary tract infections and incontinence also may occur. The cause of incontinence is inadequate emptying of the bladder while the person is in the supine position. This position contributes to stagnation of urine in the bladder and may predispose the person to bladder and urinary tract infections.

Musculoskeletal Responses

Musculoskeletal responses to bed rest and immobility reflect changes associated with the loss of both gravitational and exercise stress. In addition to a loss of strength, muscles atrophy, change shape and appearance, and shorten when immobilized. Disuse atrophy can lead to loss of approximately one eighth of the muscle's strength with each week of disuse.[56,65,66] These changes affect individual muscle fibers and total muscle mass.

Immobilization also causes a reduction in force-generating capacity along with increased fatigability, primarily owing to a decrease in muscle mass and the cross-sectional area of muscle fiber.[56,67] There also is a decrease in the oxidative capacity of the muscle mitochondria. Because of the decreased oxidative capacity of the mitochondria, muscles fatigue more easily.[50,56,65,66] The larger and the better trained the muscle, the faster the loss of muscle strength and the quicker the deconditioning occurs. Leg muscles tend to lose strength more rapidly than arm muscles, but it is not clear whether it is because legs are relatively better trained than arms, have a larger muscle mass, or bed rest results in a greater decrease in activity for legs than arms.

Along with muscle, the supporting connective tissues undergo changes when subjected to immobility or bed rest. Periarticular connective tissue, ligaments, tendons, and articular cartilage require motion to maintain health. Changes in structure and function of connective tissue become apparent 4 to 6 days after immobilization and remain even after normal activity has been resumed. It is believed that changes in the structure of collagen fibers contribute to the connective tissue changes associated with immobility.[56,65]

Muscle atrophy and disuse not only contribute to wasting and weakening of muscle tissue, they play a role in the development of joint *contractures*. A contracture is the abnormal shortening of muscle tissue and connective tissue, rendering the muscle highly resistant to stretch. Contractures occur when muscles do not have the necessary strength to maintain their integrity (*i.e.,* their proper function and full range of motion). Contractures mainly develop over joints when there is an imbalance in the muscle strength of the antagonistic muscle groups. If allowed to progress, the contracture eventually involves the muscle groups, tendons, ligaments, and joint capsule. The joint becomes limited in its full use and range of motion. Proper body alignment decreases the risk for development of contractures.[50]

Another consequence of prolonged immobility and bed rest for the musculoskeletal system is the loss of bone mineralization. Bone is a dynamic tissue that undergoes continual deposition and replacement of minerals in response to the dual stimuli of weight bearing and muscle pull. According to the Wolff law, the density of bone is directly proportional to the stress placed on it.

The maintenance of normal bone function depends on two types of cells: osteoblasts and osteoclasts. Osteoblasts function in building the osseous matrix of the bone, and osteoclasts function in the breakdown of the bone matrix (see Chapter 56). Osteoblasts depend on the stress of mobility and weight bearing to perform their function. During immobility and bed rest, the building of new bone stops, but the osteoclasts continue to perform their function. When bone experiences a lack of stress, as occurs with bed rest or immobility, there is a greater amount of bone resorption than bone formation, resulting in loss of bone mineralization.[56] The degree to which bone demineralization can be reversed is not known; however, permanent loss of bone mass and osteoporosis can result from long-term immobilization.

Osteoporosis represents an increase in skeletal porosity resulting from reduced bone mass. The bones may easily compress and become deformed. Because of the lack of structural firmness, the bones may easily fracture. The best measure to prevent the occurrence of osteoporosis is to begin weight-bearing exercises as soon as possible. The type of exercise that is performed is particularly important because load magnitude influences bone density more than the number of load cycles.

Metabolic, Endocrine, and Immune Responses

Metabolic Responses. Metabolic and endocrine changes reflect the absence of both gravitational and exercise stimulation during bed rest and immobility. The basal metabolic rate drops in response to decreased energy requirements of the body. Anabolic processes are slowed, and catabolic processes become accelerated. Protein breakdown occurs and leads to a protein deficiency and a negative nitrogen balance.[51] Persons in a negative nitrogen balance experience nausea and anorexia, which contribute to the catabolic state.

Endocrine Responses. In general, bed rest results in an uncoupling of hormonal stimulation and target organ unresponsiveness. Thyroid hormone concentrations tend to fluctuate, and levels of other hormones such as insulin and cortisol tend to be reduced. A major hormonal change that occurs with prolonged periods of bed rest and immobility is an increase in the serum parathyroid hormone (PTH) and 1,25-dihydroxyvitamin D$_3$.[65] The increased level of PTH is related to the hypercalcemia that occurs secondary to immobility.

Persons who experience prolonged periods of bed rest often have changes in the circadian release of various hormones. Normally, insulin and growth hormone peak twice a day. In people who experienced 30 days of bed rest, a single daily peak of these hormones occurred. Other hormonal changes include an afternoon peak of epinephrine rather than the normal early morning peak, and an early morning peak of aldosterone rather than the usual noonday peak that is seen in normally active persons.

The person on bed rest also experiences an impaired responsiveness to the actions of insulin. After 10 days of bed rest, there is a 100% increase in basal insulin concentration to maintain normal glucose control.[67] The reason for this intolerance is not due to lack of insulin, but rather to an increased resistance to the action of insulin that then results in a hyperglycemic and hyperinsulinemic state. Possible reasons for the unresponsiveness of glucose to hyperinsulinemia include defects in suppression of hepatic glucose production, defects in insulin stimulation of glucose uptake by peripheral tissues, or both. Insulin also plays a role in regulating protein metabolism by inhibiting protein breakdown.[67–69] This induced insulin resistance may explain the negative nitrogen balance seen in patients who experience prolonged bed rest.

Immune Responses. The immune system also is subject to physiologic changes associated with bed rest or immobility. Research demonstrates that there is an increase in IL-1, IL-6, and TNF-α production (see Chapter 18). An increase in these mediators has been associated with hyperinflammatory reactions and tissue injury or wasting.[70] Increased IL-1 production contributes to the bone and mineral loss that occurs during bed rest. Also seen is decreased IL-2 secretion, which may play a part in the infectious diseases that often occur during periods of bed rest.[71]

Gastrointestinal Responses

Gastrointestinal responses to bed rest vary. Loss of appetite, slowed rate of absorption, and distaste for food combine to contribute to nutritional hypoproteinemia. Passage of food through the gastrointestinal tract is slowed when the person is placed in the supine position. In a supine position the velocity of peristalsis decreases by 60%. Also, the loss of plasma volume and dehydration can combine to exacerbate gastrointestinal problems. Thus, constipation and fecal impaction are frequent complications that occur when persons experience prolonged periods of immobility and bed rest. With inactivity, there is slowed movement of feces through the colon. The act of defecation requires the integration of the abdominal muscles, the diaphragm, and the levator ani. Muscle atrophy and loss of tone occur in the immobilized person and interfere with the normal act of defecation. Lack of privacy and the supine position may also compound problems with defecation.[51,63]

Sensory Responses

Bed rest and immobility reduces the quality and quantity of sensory information available from kinesthetic, visual, auditory, and tactile sensation. It also reduces the person's ability to interact with the environment and contributes to impaired sensory responses. Common occurrences include impaired sense of motion and limb movement, visual and auditory hallucinations, vivid dreams, inefficient thought processes, loss of contact with reality, and alteration in tactile stimulation.

In addition to sensory deprivation related to prolonged bed rest and immobility, persons may experience a sensory monotony from the hospital environment. Repetitious and meaningless sounds from cardiac monitors, respirators, and hospital personnel, along with an environment that may be void of a normal day–night cycle, also contribute to impaired sensory perception.

Skin Responses

Except for the soles of the feet, the skin is not designed for weight bearing. However, during bed rest, the large surface area of the skin bears weight and is in constant contact with the surface of the bed. Constant pressure is transmitted to the skin, subcutaneous tissue, and muscle, especially to those tissues over bony prominences. This constant contact causes increased pressure and impairs normal capillary blood flow, which interferes with the exchange of nutrients and waste products. Tissue ischemia and necrosis may result and lead to the development of pressure ulcers. Also contributing to the development of pressure ulcers is moisture from skin that is in constant contact with bed linens, along with the forces of friction and shear that occur when the person is repositioned in bed (see Chapter 61).[72]

Psychosocial Responses

Immobility often sets the stage for changes in the person's response to illness. Persons adapt to prolonged bed rest and immobility through a series of physiologic responses and through changes in affect, perception, and cognition. Affective changes include increased anxiety, fear, depression, hostility, rapid mood changes, and alterations in normal sleep patterns. These changes in mood occur with hospitalized patients who are subjected to periods of prolonged bed rest and immobility, and in persons in confinement, such as astronauts and prisoners. Research on immobilized or isolated persons has demonstrated that the motivation to learn decreases with periods of prolonged immobility, as does the ability to learn and retain new material and transfer newly learned material to a different situation. Persons are less able and less motivated to perform problem-solving activities; they are less able to concentrate on and discriminate among information.[73] These studies present major implications for the timing of patient education and the preparation of education materials.

Prolonged bed rest and immobility also contribute to the social isolation of the hospitalized person. Confined to a hospital bed, the person is unable to assume certain societal roles. The roles of spouse, parent, sibling, worker, and friend are altered either temporarily or permanently while the person is hospitalized. People may respond to this isolation by exhibiting various effective and ineffective coping behaviors, including increased anxiety, depression, restlessness, fear, and rapid mood changes.[73]

Time Course of Physiologic Responses

The deconditioning responses to the inactivity of immobility and bed rest affect all body systems. One of the important factors to keep in mind is the rapidity with which the changes occur and the length of time required to overcome these effects. The body responds in a characteristic pattern to the effects of the supine position and bed rest (Table 11-3). During the first 3 days of bed rest, one of the first changes to occur is a massive diuresis. Accompanying the diuresis are increases in serum osmolality, hematocrit, venous compliance, and urinary sodium and chloride excretion. Fluid losses stabilize by approximately the fourth day. By days 4 to 7, there are changes in the hemolytic system. Fibrinogen and fibrinolytic activity increase, and clotting time is prolonged. The cardiovascular system responds with a decrease in cardiac output and stroke volume. The basal metabolic rate decreases and glucose intolerance and a negative nitrogen balance begin to develop.[74]

Additional effects on the hemolytic system are observed on days 8 to 14. Red blood cell number is decreased and the phagocytic ability of leukocytes is reduced. There is a decrease in lean body mass and, after 15 days of bed rest, osteoporosis and hypercalciuria occur. Aerobic power decreases, the cyclic excretion of some hormones is changed, and the person's thought patterns and sensory perception are altered.[74]

TABLE 11-3 **Physiologic Changes During Bed Rest**			
0–3 DAYS	**4–7 DAYS**	**8–14 DAYS**	**OVER 15 DAYS**
Increases in Urine volume Urine Na, Cl, Ca, and osmol excretion Plasma osmolality Hematocrit Venous compliance	**Increases in** Urine creatinine, hydroxyproline, PO_4, N, and K excretion Plasma globulin, phosphate, and glucose levels Blood fibrinogen Fibrinolytic activity and clotting time Visual focal point Hyperthermia of eye conjunctiva, dilation of retinal arteries and veins Auditory threshold	**Increases in** Urine pyrophosphate Sweating sensitivity Exercise hyperthermia Exercise maximal heart rate	**Increases in** Peak hypercalciuria Sensitivity to thermal threshold Auditory threshold (secondary)
Decreases in Total fluid intake Extracellular and intracellular fluid Calf blood flow Resting heart rate Secretion of gastric acid Glucose tolerance	**Decreases in** Near point of visual acuity Orthostatic tolerance Nitrogen balance	**Decreases in** Red blood cell mass Leukocyte phagocytosis Tissue heat conductance Lean body mass	**Decreases in** Bone density

Greenleaf J.E. (1984). Physiological responses to prolonged bed rest and fluid immersion in humans. *Journal of Applied Physiology: Respiratory, Environmental and Exercise Physiology* 57, 619–633.

Interventions

A holistic approach should be taken when caring for persons who are immobile or require prolonged periods of bed rest. Interventions and treatment should include actions that address the person's physical and psychosocial needs. The goals of care for the immobilized person include structuring a safe environment in which the person is not at risk for complications; providing diversional activities to offset problems with sensory deprivation; and preventing complications of bed rest by implementing an interdisciplinary plan of care that includes repositioning schedules, prophylactic interventions to prevent DVT, and consultation with various disciplines to provide a comprehensive approach to care and treatment.

IN SUMMARY, during the last 75 years, the use of bed rest has undergone a complete reversal as a standard of treatment for a variety of medical conditions. Over time, research findings have described the deleterious consequences of inactivity. All body systems are affected by complications of immobility and prolonged bed rest.

The responses to bed rest and immobility affect all body systems. One of the important factors is the rapidity with which the changes occur and the long time required to overcome the effects of prolonged bed rest and immobility. Adverse effects of prolonged immobility and bed rest include a decreased cardiac output, orthostatic intolerance, dehydration, and sensory deprivation, as well as the potential for development of thrombophlebitis, pneumonia, kidney stones, and pressure ulcers. ■

Review Exercises

1. A 60-year-old man sustains an acute myocardial infarction (heart attack). He has been discharged from the hospital and is about to enter a phase II cardiac rehabilitation program. On his first day of the program he is being examined for his tolerance to the exercise program.

   A. *One of the tests that he is scheduled to undergo is the treadmill stress test. How will this test contribute to the evaluation of his ability to engage in exercise?*

   B. *What other subjective tests might be used to determine his exercise tolerance?*

2. A 40-year-old woman who is being treated with chemotherapy for breast cancer complains of excessive fatigue and activity intolerance. She claims she has so little energy she can hardly get up in the morning and has difficulty concentrating and doing such simple activities as shopping.

   A. *What are some of the possible explanations for this woman's excessive fatigue?*

   B. *What types of medical tests might be done to identify possible causes of fatigue?*

   C. *What types of treatment might be used to alleviate some of her symptoms?*

3. A 23-year-old man, who has sustained multiple fractures and contusions in a motorcycle accident, is confined to bed rest in the supine position. He has been on bed rest for 2 days and has lost about 500 mL of extracellular fluid volume because of diuresis.

   A. *Explain the physiologic rationale for the excessive diuresis.*

   B. *Identify two complications of bed rest that might occur as the result of this loss of extracellular fluid volume.*

   C. *Upon getting out of bed on the fourth day he suddenly turns pale, has an increase in heart rate, and complains of dizziness. What has happened to this man?*

References

1. Brooks G. A., Fahey T. D., Baldwin K. M. (2004). *Exercise physiology: Human bioenergetics and its applications* (4th ed.). Boston: McGraw-Hill.

2. Warburton D. E. R., Nicol C. W., Bredin S. S. D. (2006). Prescribing exercise as preventative therapy. *Canadian Medical Association Journal* 174, 961–974.

3. Fletcher G., Trejo J. E. (2005). Why and how to prescribe exercise: Overcoming the barriers. *Cleveland Clinic Journal of Medicine* 72, 645–656.

4. Hughson R. L., Tschakovsky M. E., Houston M. E. (2001). Regulation of oxygen consumption at the onset of exercise. *Exercise and Sport Sciences Reviews* 729, 129–133.

5. Pollock M. L., Gaesser G. A., Butcher J. D., et al. (1998). ACSM position stand: The recommended quantity and quality of exercise for developing and maintaining cardiorespiratory and muscular fitness, and flexibility in healthy adults. *Medicine & Science in Sports & Exercise* 30, 975–991.

6. Pate R. R., Pratt M., Blair S. N., et al. (1995). Physical activity and public health: A recommendation from the Centers for Disease Control and Prevention and the American College of Sports Medicine. *Journal of the American Medical Association* 273, 402–407.

7. Pollock M. L., Franklin B., Balady G. J., et al. (Committee on Exercise, Rehabilitation, and Prevention, Council Clinical Cardiology, American Heart Association). (2000). Resistance exercise for persons with and without cardiovascular disease. *Circulation* 101, 828–833.

8. Rowland T. W. (2005). Circulatory responses to exercise: Are we misreading Fick? *Chest* 127, 1023–1030.

9. Schnermann J. (2002). Exercise. *American Journal of Physiology: Regulatory, Integrative and Comparative Physiology* 283, R2–R6.

10. Klabunde R. E. (2005). *Cardiovascular physiology concepts.* Philadelphia: Lippincott Williams & Wilkins.

11. Williamson J. W., Fadel P. J., Mitchell J. H. (2006). New insights into central cardiovascular control during exercise in humans: A central command update. *Experimental Physiology* 91, 51–58.

12. Thompson P. D., Crouse S. F., Goodpaster B., et al. (2001). The acute versus the chronic response to exercise. *Medicine & Science in Sports & Exercise* 33(6 Suppl.), S438–S445.

13. Sherman D. L. (2000). Exercise and endothelial function. *Coronary Artery Disease* 11, 117–122.

14. Smith J. K. (2001). Exercise and atherogenesis. *Exercise and Sport Sciences Reviews* 29(2), 49–53.

15. Tonkonogi M., Sahlin K. (2002). Physical exercise and mitochondrial function in human skeletal muscle. *Exercise and Sport Sciences Reviews* 30(3), 129–137.

16. Booher M. A., Smith B. W. (2003). Physiological effects of exercise on the cardiopulmonary system. *Clinics in Sports Medicine* 22, 1–21.

17. Fischer J. P., White M. J. (2004). Muscle afferent contributions to the cardiovascular response to isometric exercise. *Experimental Physiology* 89, 639–646.

18. Buckwalter J. B., Clifford P. S. (2001). The paradox of sympathetic vasoconstriction in exercising skeletal muscle. *Exercise and Sport Sciences Reviews* 29(4), 159–163.

19. Casa D. J. (1999). Exercise in the heat: I. Fundamentals of thermal physiology, performance implications, and dehydration. *Journal of Athletic Training* 34, 246–252.

20. Bi L., Triadafilopoulos G. (2003). Exercise and gastrointestinal function and disease: An evidence-based review of risks and benefits. *Clinical Gastroenterology and Hepatology* 1, 345–355.

21. MacKinnon L. T. (2000). Chronic exercise effects on immune function. *Medicine & Science in Sports & Exercise* 32(7 Suppl.), S369–S376.

22. Rowbottom D. G., Green K. J. (2000). Acute exercise effects on the immune system. *Medicine & Science in Sports & Exercise* 32(7 Suppl.), S396–S405.

23. Fix A. J., Daughton D. (1986). *Human activity profile (HAP) manual.* Lutz, FL: Psychological Assessment Resources.

24. Krupp L. B., LaRocca N. G., Muir-Nash J., et al. (1989). The Fatigue Severity Scale: Application to patients with multiple sclerosis and systemic lupus erythematosus. *Archives of Neurology* 46, 1121–1123.

25. Borg G. A. V. (1973). Perceived exertion: A note on "history" and methods. *Medicine and Science in Sports* 5, 90–93.

26. Borg G. A. V. (1982). Psychophysical bases of perceived exertion. *Medicine and Science in Sports* 14, 377–381.

27. Daley M. J., Spinks W. L. (2000). Exercise, mobility, and aging. *Sports Medicine* 29, 1–12.

28. Mazzeo R. S., Cavanagh P., Evans W. J., et al. (1999). Exercise and physical activity for older adults: American College of Sports Medicine Position Stand. *The Physician and Sports Medicine* 27(11), 115–142.

29. Close G. L., Kayani A., Vasilaski A., et al. (2005). Skeletal muscle damage with exercise and aging. *Sports Medicine* 35, 413–427.

30. McDermott A. Y., Mernitz H. (2006). Exercise and older patients: Prescribing guidelines. *American Family Physician* 74, 437–744.

31. Piper B. F. (2003). Fatigue. In Carrieri-Kohlman V., Lindsey A. M., West C. W. (Eds.), *Pathophysiological phenomena in nursing: Human responses to illness* (pp. 209–234). Philadelphia: Elsevier Saunders.

32. Curt C. A. (2000). The impact of fatigue on patients with cancer: Overview of fatigue 1 and 2. *The Oncologist* 5(Suppl. 2), 9–12.

33. Berger A. (2003). Treating fatigue in cancer patients. *The Oncologist* 8(Suppl. 1), 10–14.

34. Gutstein H. B. (2001). The biologic basis of fatigue. *Cancer* 92(6 Suppl.), 1678–1683.

35. Prue G., Rankin J., Allen J., et al. (2006). Cancer-related fatigue: A critical appraisal. *European Journal of Cancer* 42, 846–863.

36. Kurzock R. (2001). The role of cytokines in cancer-related fatigue. *Cancer* 92 (6 Suppl.), 1684–1688.

37. Belza B. (1994). The impact of fatigue on exercise performance. *Arthritis Care and Research* 7, 176–180.

38. Smith B. A., Neidig J. L., Mitchell G. L., et al. (2001). Aerobic exercise: Effects on parameters related to fatigue, dyspnea, weight, and body composition in HIV-infected adults. *AIDS* 15, 693–701.

39. MacAllister W. S., Krupp L. B. (2005). Multiple sclerosis-related fatigue. *Physical Medicine and Rehabilitation Clinics of North America* 16, 483–502.

40. Straus S. E. (1991). History of chronic fatigue syndrome. *Reviews of Infectious Diseases* 13(Suppl. 1), S2–S7.

41. Evengaard E., Klimas N. (2002). Chronic fatigue syndrome: Probable pathogenesis and possible treatments. *Drugs* 62, 2433–2446.

42. Prins J. B., van der Meer J. W. M., Bleijenber G. (2006). Chronic fatigue syndrome. *Lancet* 367, 346–355.

43. Afari N., Buchwald D. (2003). Chronic fatigue syndrome: A review. *American Journal of Psychiatry* 160, 221–236.

44. Holmes G. P., Kaplan J. E., Gantz N. M., et al. (1988). Chronic fatigue syndrome: A working definition. *Annals of Internal Medicine* 108, 387–389.

45. Fukuda K., Straus S. E., Hickie I., et al. (1994). The chronic fatigue syndrome: A comprehensive approach to its definition and study. *Annals of Internal Medicine* 121, 953–959.

46. Cleare A. J. (2003). The neuroendocrinology of the chronic fatigue syndrome. *Endocrine Reviews* 24, 236–252.

47. Evengard B., Schacterle R. S., Komaroff L. (1999). Chronic fatigue syndrome: New insights and old ignorance. *Journal of Internal Medicine* 256, 455–469.

48. Craig T., Kakumanu S. (2002). Chronic fatigue syndrome: Evaluation and treatment. *American Family Physician* 65, 1083–1090.

49. Lange G., Wang S., DeLuca J., et al. (1998). Neuroimaging in chronic fatigue syndrome. *American Journal of Medicine* 105(3A), 50S–53S.

50. Harper C. M., Lyles Y. M. (1988). Physiology and complications of bed rest. *Journal of the American Geriatrics Society* 36, 1047–1054.

51. Dittmer D. K., Teasel R. (1993). Complications of immobilization and bed rest: Part 1 and Part 2. *Canadian Family Physician* 39, 1428–1437, 1440–1446.

52. Convertino V. A., Bloomfield S. A., Greenleaf J. E. (1997). An overview of the issues: Physiological effects of bed rest and restricted physical activity. *Medicine & Science in Sports & Exercise* 29, 187–190.

53. Allen C., Glasziou P., Del Mar C. (1999). Bed rest: A potentially harmful treatment needing more careful evaluation. *Lancet* 354, 1229–1233.

54. Taylor H. L., Henschel A., Broek J., et al. (1949). Effects of bed rest on cardiovascular function and work performance. *Journal of Applied Physiology* 11, 223–239.

55. Convertino V. A. (1997). Cardiovascular consequences of bed rest: Effect on maximal oxygen uptake. *Medicine & Science in Sports & Exercise* 29, 191–197.

56. Topp R., Ditmyer M., King K., et al. (2002). The effect of bed rest and potential of prehabilitation on patients in the intensive care unit. *AACN Clinical Issues* 13, 263–276.

57. Fortrat J. O., Sigaudo D., Hughson R. L., et al. (2001). Effect of prolonged head-down bed rest on complex cardiovascular dynamics. *Autonomic Neuroscience* 86, 192–201.

58. Saltin B., Blomquist G., Mitchell J. H., et al. (1968). Response to exercise after bed rest and after training: A longitudinal study of adaptive changes in oxygen transport and body composition. *Circulation* 38(Suppl. 7), 1–65.

59. Kamiya A., Michikami D., Fu Q., et al. (2003). Pathophysiology of orthostatic hypotension after bed rest: Paradoxical sympathetic withdrawal. *American Journal of Physiology: Heart and Circulatory Physiology* 285, H1158–H1167.

60. Hirayanagi K., Kamiya A., Iwase S., et al. (2004). Autonomic cardiovascular changes during and after 14 days of head-down bed rest. *Autonomic Neuroscience* 110, 121–128.

61. Kamiya A., Iwase S., Sugiyama Y., et al. (2000). Vasomotor sympathetic nerve activity in men during bed rest and on orthostasis after bed rest. *Aviation, Space, and Environmental Medicine* 71, 142–149.

62. Slipman C. W., Lipetz J. S., Jackson H. B., et al. (2000). Deep venous thrombosis and pulmonary embolism as a complication of bed rest and low back pain. *Archives of Physical Medicine and Rehabilitation* 81, 127–129.

63. Gunji A. (1997). Short review of human prolonged horizontal bed rest studies in Japan. *Journal of Gravitational Physiology* 4(1), S1–S9.

64. Krasnoff J., Painter P. (1999). The physiological consequences of bed rest and inactivity. *Advances in Renal Replacement Therapy* 6, 124–132.

65. Mobily P. R., Kelley L. S. (1991). Iatrogenesis in the elderly: Factors of immobility. *Journal of Gerontological Nursing* 17(9), 5–10.

66. Uebelhart D., Bernard J., Hartmann D. J., et al. (2000). Modifications of bone and connective tissue after orthostatic bedrest. *Osteoporosis International* 11, 59–67.

67. Ibebunjo C., Martyn J. A. J. (1999). Fiber atrophy, but not changes in acetylcholine receptor expression, contributes to the muscle dysfunction after immobilization. *Critical Care Medicine* 27, 275–285.

68. Dolkas C. B., Greenleaf J. E. (1977). Insulin and glucose responses during bed rest with isotonic and isometric exercise. *Journal of Applied Physiology* 43, 1033–1038.

69. Shangraw R. E., Stuart C. A., Prince M. J., et al. (1988). Insulin responsiveness of protein metabolism in vivo following bedrest in humans. *American Journal of Physiology: Endocrinology and Metabolism* 255, E548–E558.

70. Winkleman C. (2004). Inactivity and inflammation. *AACN Clinical Issues* 15, 74–82.

71. Schmitt D. A., Schaffar L., Taylor G. R., et al. (1996). Use of bed rest and head-down tilt to simulate spaceflight-induced immune system changes. *Journal of Interferon and Cytokine Research* 16, 151–157.

72. Lindgren M., Unosson M., Fredrikson M., et al. (2004). Immobility—a major risk factor for development of pressure ulcers among adult hospitalized patients: A prospective study. *Scandinavian Journal of Caring Science* 18, 57–64.

73. Cunningham E. (2001). Coping with bed rest. *AWHONN Lifelines* 5(5), 50–55.

74. Greenleaf J. E., Kozlowski S. (1982). Physiological consequences of reduced physical activity during bed rest. *Exercise and Sport Sciences Reviews* 10, 84–119.

Visit thePoint **http://thePoint.lww.com for animations, journal articles, and more!**

Disorders of the Hematopoietic System

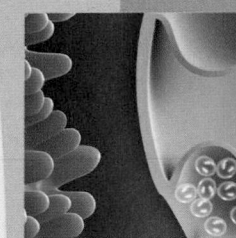

From ancient times, the importance of blood as a determinant of health was recognized. Its life-affecting powers are well described in the written treatises of Greek physician Galen (AD 130–200). Galen, who reigned as the foremost medical authority for nearly 1500 years, believed that an individual stayed healthy as long as four body fluids—blood, phlegm, yellow bile, and black bile—remained in the right proportion. He also believed that the four humors determined one's basic temperament. Whether an individual was sanguine, sluggish and dull, quick to anger, or melancholy was determined by the degree to which one or another of the humors predominated. The most desirable personality type was achieved when blood was thought to predominate, yielding a warm and cheerful person.

The workings of blood were traced by Galen from its creation, which he believed took place in the liver, throughout the body. He came to believe that disease manifested itself if any one of the fluids was in excess or deficient and was carried in the blood. The theory led to bloodletting—the drawing of blood from the vein of a sick person so the disease could flow out with the blood. For many centuries, bloodletting was the standard treatment for a myriad of ills.

Chapter 12

Blood Cells and the Hematopoietic System

KATHRYN J. GASPARD

➤ Blood is unique in that it is the only liquid tissue in the body. Blood is a specialized connective tissue that consists of blood cells (red blood cells, white blood cells, and platelets) suspended in an extracellular fluid, known as *plasma.* Blood accounts for about 7% to 8% of total body weight. The total volume of blood in the average adult is about 5 to 6 L, and it circulates throughout the body within the confines of the circulatory system. Because blood circulates throughout the body, it is an ideal vehicle for transport of materials to and from the many cells of the body.

COMPOSITION OF BLOOD AND FORMATION OF BLOOD CELLS

After completing this section of the chapter, you should be able to meet the following objectives:

- Describe the composition and functions of plasma.
- Name the formed elements of blood and cite their function and life span.
- Trace the process of hematopoiesis from stem cell to mature blood cell.

When blood is removed from the circulatory system, it clots. The clot contains the blood cells and fibrin strands formed from the conversion of the plasma protein fibrinogen. It is surrounded by a yellow liquid called *serum.* Blood that is kept from clotting by the addition of an anticoagulant (*e.g.,* heparin, citrate) and then centrifuged separates into layers (Fig. 12-1). The bottom layer (approximately 42% to 47% of the whole-blood volume) contains the erythrocytes, or red blood cells, and is referred to as the *hematocrit.* The intermediate layer (approximately 1%) containing the leukocytes, or white blood cells, is white or gray and is called the *buffy layer.* Above the leukocytes is a thin layer of thrombocytes or platelets that is not discernible to the naked eye. The translucent, yellowish fluid that forms on the top of the cells is the *plasma,* which comprises approximately 55% of the total volume.

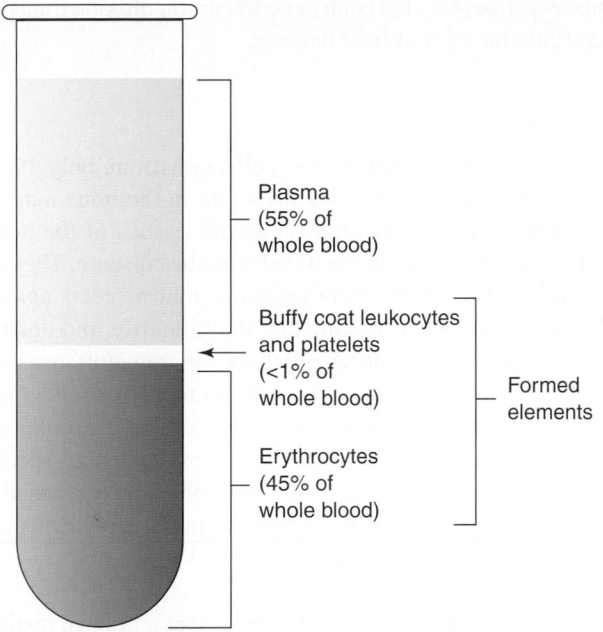

FIGURE 12-1 • Layering of blood components in an anticoagulated and centrifuged blood sample.

🔑 COMPOSITION OF THE BLOOD

- Blood is a liquid that fills the vascular compartment and serves to transport dissolved materials and blood cells throughout the body.

- The most abundant of the blood cells, the erythrocytes or red blood cells, function in oxygen and carbon dioxide transport.

- The leukocytes, or white blood cells, serve various roles in immunity and inflammation.

- Platelets are small cell fragments that are involved in blood clotting.

Plasma

Plasma, being a liquid, is 90% to 91% water by weight, 6.5% to 8% proteins by weight, and 2% other small molecular substances (Table 12-1). Plasma water serves as a transport vehicle for materials carried in the blood. As a transport medium, plasma carries nutrients from the gastrointestinal tract and oxygen from the lungs to body cells while picking up waste products from the cells for delivery to excretory organs; it transports hormones and facilitates the exchange of chemical mediators; it participates in electrolyte and acid-base balance; and it contains the plasma proteins that contribute to the osmotic regulation of body fluids. In addition, because water has a high capacity to hold heat, plasma can absorb and distribute much of the heat that is generated in the body.

Plasma Proteins

The plasma proteins are the most abundant solutes in plasma. Except for the blood-borne hormones and gamma globulins, most plasma proteins are produced by the liver. The major types of plasma proteins are albumin, globulins, and fibrinogen. Albumin is the most abundant and makes up approximately 54% of the plasma proteins. It does not pass through the pores in the capillary wall to enter the interstitial fluid and therefore contributes to the plasma osmotic pressure and maintenance of blood volume (see Chapter 31). Albumin also serves as a carrier for certain substances and acts as a blood buffer. The globulins comprise approximately 38% of plasma proteins. There are three types of globulins: the *alpha globulins* that transport bilirubin and steroids, the *beta globulins* that transport iron and copper, and the *gamma globulins* that constitute the antibodies of the immune system. Fibrinogen makes up approximately 7% of the plasma proteins and is a key factor in blood clotting. The remaining 1% of the circulating proteins is hormones, enzymes, complement, and carriers for lipids.

Blood Cells

The blood cells include the erythrocytes, leukocytes, and platelets (Fig. 12-2). The blood cells, or formed elements, are not all true cells. Erythrocytes have no nuclei or organelles and platelets are just cell fragments. Most blood cells do not divide, so they must be continually renewed by division of cells in the bone marrow, where they originate. Table 12-2 lists the normal values for the blood cells.

TABLE 12-1 **Plasma Components**		
PLASMA	**PERCENTAGE OF PLASMA VOLUME**	**DESCRIPTION**
Water	90–91	
Proteins	6.5–8	
Albumin		54% Plasma proteins
Globulins		38% Plasma proteins
Fibrinogen		7% Plasma proteins
Other substances	1–2	Hormones, enzymes, carbohydrates, fats, amino acids, gases, electrolytes, excretory products

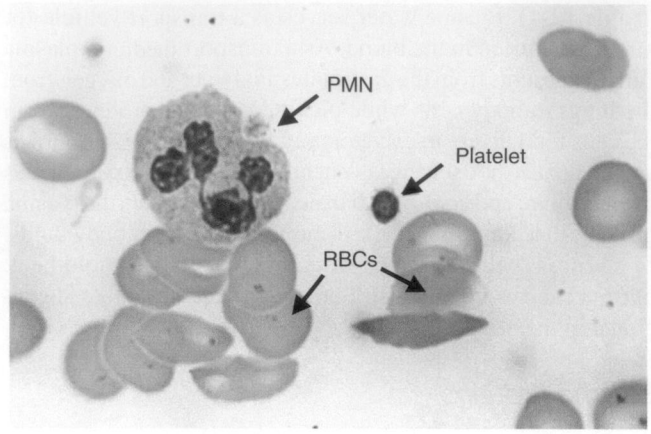

FIGURE 12-2 • Micrograph of a fixed blood smear revealing a round aggregate of platelets (*arrow*), a polymorphonuclear (PMN) leukocyte, and a number of red blood cells (RBCs). Original magnification ×1000. (Adapted from the Centers for Disease Control and Prevention Health Image Library.)

Erythrocytes

The erythrocytes, or red blood cells, are the most numerous of the formed elements. They are small, biconcave disks with a large surface area and can easily deform to move through the small capillaries of the circulatory system. They contain the oxygen-carrying protein, *hemoglobin,* that functions in the transport of oxygen. The erythrocytes, which have their origin in the bone marrow, live approximately 120 days in the circulation (see Chapter 14). Erythrocyte precursors in the bone marrow possess nuclei, but expel not only their nuclei but also all organelles before entering the circulation. Although erythrocytes have no organelles, they have soluble enzymes, including carbonic anhydrase, within their cytosol. This enzyme facilitates the formation of carbonic acid from carbon dioxide and water, which in turn dissociate into bicarbonate and hydrogen ions.

Thus, erythrocytes also contribute to carbon dioxide transport and regulation of acid-base balance.

Leukocytes

The leukocytes, or white blood cells, constitute only 1% of the total blood volume. They originate in the bone marrow and circulate throughout the lymphoid tissues of the body. Leukocytes are crucial to our defense against disease. They are responsible for the immune response that protects against disease-causing microorganisms; they identify and destroy cancer cells; and they participate in the inflammatory response and wound healing. Leukocytes are commonly classified into two groups based on presence or absence of specific prominent granules in their cytoplasm (Fig. 12-3). Those containing specific granules (neutrophils, eosinophils, basophils) are classified as *granulocytes* and those that lack granules (lymphocytes and monocytes) as *agranulocytes.*

Granulocytes. Granulocytes are spherical and have distinctive multilobar nuclei. They are all phagocytic cells that are identifiable because of their cytoplasmic granules. They have two types of granules: the *specific granules* that bind neutral, basic, or acidic dye components, and *azurophilic granules.* The azurophilic granules stain purple and are lysosomes. The granulocytes are divided into three types—neutrophils, eosinophils, and basophils—according to the staining properties of their specific granules.

Neutrophils. The neutrophils, which constitute 55% to 65% of the total white blood cells, have granules that are neutral and hence do not stain with an acidic or a basic dye. Because these white cells have nuclei that are divided into three to five lobes, they are often called *polymorphonuclear leukocytes* or *PMNs.*

The neutrophils are primarily responsible for maintaining normal host defenses against invading bacteria and fungi, cell

TABLE 12-2 **Blood Cell Counts**		
BLOOD CELLS	**NUMBER OF CELLS/μL (SI Units)**	**PERCENTAGE OF WHITE BLOOD CELLS**
Red blood cell count	Male: $4.2–5.4 \times 10^6$/μL ($4.2–5.4 \times 10^{12}$/L) Female: $3.6–5.0 \times 10^6$/μL ($3.6–5.0 \times 10^{12}$/L)	
White blood cell count Differential count Granulocytes Neutrophils	$4.8–10.8 \times 10^3$/μL ($4.8–10.8 \times 10^9$/L)	
Segs		47–63
Bands		0–4
Eosinophils		0–3
Basophils		0–2
Lymphocytes		24–40
Monocytes		4–9
Platelet count	$150–400 \times 10^3$	

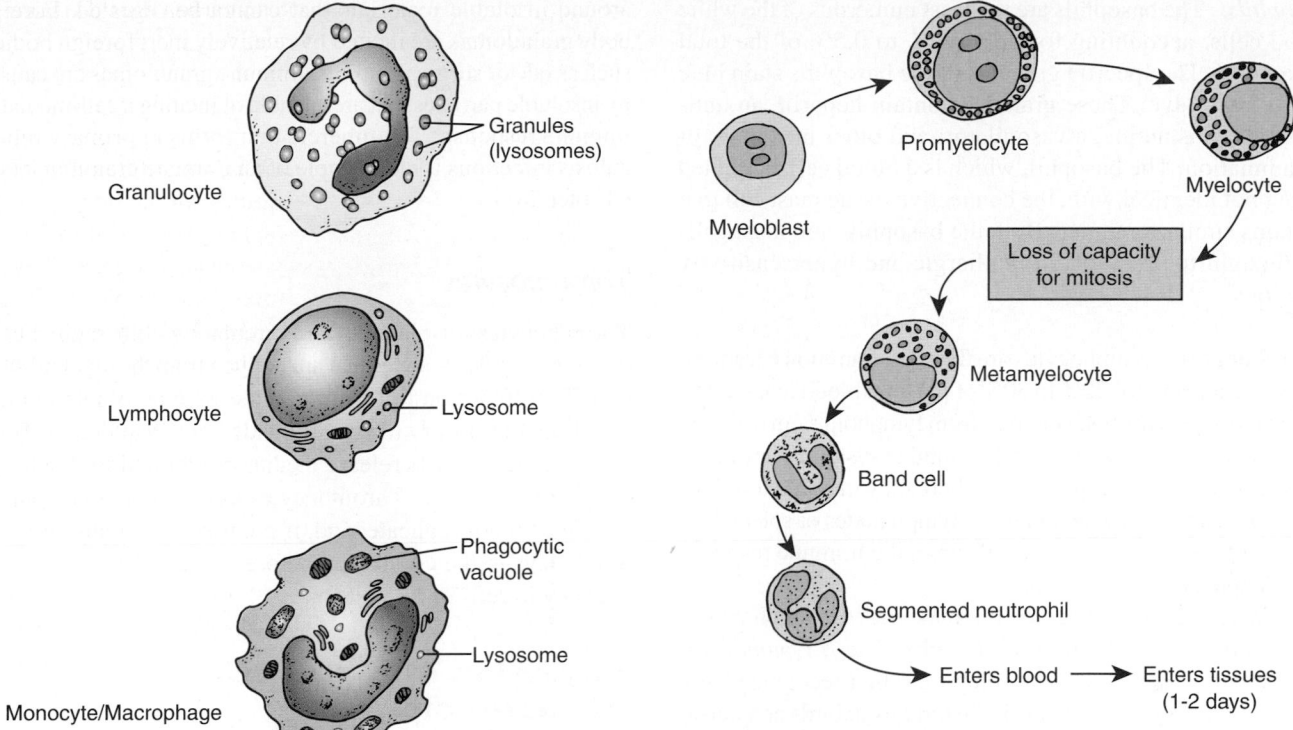

FIGURE 12-3 • White blood cells.

FIGURE 12-4 • Developmental stages of the neutrophil, which begins its development in the bone marrow as a myeloblast.

debris, and a variety of foreign substances. The cytoplasm of mature neutrophils has three types of granules: small specific granules that contain complement activators and bacteriostatic and bacteriocidal agents; larger azurophilic granules that contain peroxidases and other hydrolytic enzymes; and the newly discovered tertiary granules, which contain proteins thought to facilitate movement and migration of the neutrophil.

The neutrophils have their origin in the myeloblasts that are found in the bone marrow (Fig. 12-4). The myeloblasts are the committed precursors of the granulocyte pathway and do not normally appear in the peripheral circulation. When they are present, it suggests a disorder of blood cell proliferation and differentiation. The myeloblasts differentiate into promyelocytes and then myelocytes. Usually, a cell is not called a *myelocyte* until it has at least 12 granules. The myelocytes mature to become metamyelocytes (from the Greek *meta,* "beyond"), at which point they lose their capacity for mitosis. Subsequent development of the neutrophil involves reduction in size, with transformation from an oval to a horseshoe-shaped nucleus (*i.e.,* band cell) and then to a mature cell with a segmented nucleus. Mature neutrophils are often referred to as *segs* because of their segmented nucleus. Development from stem cell to mature neutrophil takes approximately 2 weeks. It is at this point that the neutrophil enters the bloodstream. *Neutrophilia* is an increase in immature neutrophils ("band" forms) seen in the peripheral blood. It is most commonly seen in acute infections and tissue

injuries that promote the accelerated release of neutrophils and their precursors into the circulation.

After release from the marrow, the neutrophils spend only approximately 4 to 8 hours in the circulation before moving into the tissues. They survive in the tissues for approximately 4 to 5 days. They die in the tissues by discharging their phagocytic function or from senescence. The pool of circulating neutrophils (*i.e.,* those that appear in the blood count) is in a closely maintained equilibrium with a similar-sized pool of cells marginating along the walls of small blood vessels. These are the neutrophils that respond to chemotactic factors and migrate into the tissues toward the offending agent. Epinephrine, exercise, stress, and corticosteroid drug therapy can cause rapid increases in the circulating neutrophil count by shifting cells from the marginating to the circulating pool. Endotoxins or microbes have the opposite effect, producing a transient decrease in neutrophils by attracting neutrophils into the tissues.

Eosinophils. The specific cytoplasmic granules of the eosinophils stain red with the acidic dye eosin. These leukocytes constitute 1% to 3% of the total white blood cells and increase in number during allergic reactions and parasitic infections. In allergic reactions, it is thought that they release enzymes or chemical mediators that detoxify the agents associated with allergic reactions. In parasitic infections, the eosinophils use surface markers to attach themselves to the parasite and then release hydrolytic enzymes that kill it.

Basophils. The basophils are the least numerous of the white blood cells, accounting for only 0.3% to 0.5% of the total leukocytes. The specific granules of the basophils stain blue with a basic dye. These granules contain heparin, an anticoagulant; histamine, a vasodilator; and other mediators of inflammation. The basophil, which is a blood cell, is related to, but not identical with, the connective tissue mast cell that contains similar granules. Both the basophils and mast cells are thought to be involved in allergic and hypersensitivity reactions.

Lymphocytes. Lymphocytes are the most common agranulocytes and account for 20% to 30% of the total blood leukocytes. They originate in the bone marrow from lymphoid stem cells and are the main functional cells of the immune system. They move between blood and lymph tissue, where they may be stored for hours or years. Their function in the lymph nodes or spleen is to defend against microorganisms through the immune response (see Chapter 17).

There are three types of lymphocytes: B lymphocytes, T lymphocytes, and natural killer cells. The *B lymphocytes (B cells)* are so named because they were first recognized as a separate population in the bursa of Fabricius in birds and bursa-equivalent organs (*e.g.*, bone marrow) in mammals. They differentiate to form antibody-producing plasma cells and are involved in humoral-mediated immunity. The *T lymphocytes (T cells)* differentiate in the thymus. They activate other cells of the immune system (helper T cells) and are involved in cell-mediated immunity (cytotoxic T cells). *Natural killer (NK) cells* participate in innate or natural immunity and their function is to destroy foreign cells. The lymphocytes of the three different subsets have unique surface markers that can be identified and help to define their function and diagnose disease (discussed in Chapters 17 and 18).

Monocytes and Macrophages. Monocytes are the largest of the white blood cells and constitute approximately 3% to 8% of the total leukocyte count. They are distinguished by a large amount of cytoplasm and a dark-stained nucleus in the shape of a kidney. The life span of the circulating monocyte is approximately 1 to 3 days, three to four times longer than that of the granulocytes. These cells survive for months to years in the tissues. The monocytes, which are precursors of the mononuclear phagocyte system, are often referred to as *macrophages* when they enter the tissues. The monocytes engulf larger and greater quantities of foreign material than the neutrophils. These leukocytes play an important role in chronic inflammation and are also involved in the immune response by activating lymphocytes and by presenting antigen to T cells. When the monocyte leaves the vascular system and enters the tissues, it functions as a macrophage with specific activity. The macrophages are known as *histiocytes* in loose connective tissue, *microglial cells* in the brain, and *Kupffer cells* in the liver. Other macrophages function in the alveoli, lymph nodes, and other tissues.

Granulomatous inflammation is a distinctive pattern of chronic inflammation in which the macrophages form a capsule around insoluble materials that cannot be digested. Foreign body granulomas are incited by relatively inert foreign bodies, such as talc or surgical sutures. Immune granulomas are caused by insoluble particles that are capable of inciting a cell-mediated immune response. The tubercle that forms in primary tuberculosis infections is an example of an immune granuloma (see Chapter 28).

Thrombocytes

Thrombocytes, or platelets, are circulating cell fragments of the large megakaryocytes that are derived from the myeloid stem cell. They function to form the platelet plug to help control bleeding after injury to a vessel wall (see Chapter 13). Their cytoplasmic granules release mediators required for the blood coagulation process. Thrombocytes have a membrane but no nucleus, cannot replicate, and, if not used, last approximately 8 to 9 days in the circulation before they are removed by the phagocytic cells of the spleen.

Formation of Blood Cells (Hematopoiesis)

The generation of blood cells takes place in the *hematopoietic* (from the Greek *haima*, "blood," and *poiesis*, "making") system. The hematopoietic system encompasses all of the blood cells and their precursors, the bone marrow where blood cells have their origin, and the lymphoid tissues where some blood cells circulate as they develop and mature.

Hematopoiesis begins in the endothelial cells of the developing blood vessels during the fifth week of gestation and then continues in the liver and spleen. After birth, this function is gradually taken over by the bone marrow. Some hematopoiesis may also occur in the spleen and the liver. The marrow is a network of connective tissue containing immature blood cells. At sites where the marrow is hematopoietically active, it produces so many erythrocytes that it is red, hence the name *red bone marrow*. Fat cells are also present in bone marrow, but they are inactive in terms of blood cell generation. Marrow that is made up predominantly of fat cells is called *yellow bone marrow*. During active skeletal growth, red marrow is gradually replaced by yellow marrow in most of the long bones. In adults, red marrow is largely restricted to the flat bones of the pelvis, ribs, and sternum. The cellularity of the bone marrow normally decreases as a person ages. When the demand for red cell replacement increases, as in hemolytic anemia, there can be resubstitution of red marrow for yellow marrow.

Blood Cell Precursors

The blood-forming population of bone marrow is made up of three types of cells: self-renewing stem cells, differentiated progenitor (parent) cells, and functional mature blood cells. All of the blood cell precursors of the erythrocyte (*i.e.*, red cell), myelocyte (*i.e.*, granulocyte or monocyte), lymphocyte (*i.e.*, T lymphocyte and B lymphocyte), and megakaryocyte

HEMATOPOIESIS

- White blood cells (granulocytes, monocytes, and lymphocytes) are formed in the bone marrow, circulate in the blood, and, in the case of lymphocytes, move into the peripheral lymphoid organs where they respond to antigens.

- They are formed from hematopoietic stem cells that differentiate into committed progenitor cells that in turn develop into the myelogenous and lymphocytic lineages needed for the formation of the different types of white blood cell.

- The growth and reproduction of the different stem cells is controlled by CSFs and other cytokines and chemical mediators.

- The life span of white blood cells is relatively short so that constant renewal is necessary to maintain normal blood levels. Any conditions that decrease the availability of stem cells or hematopoietic growth factors produce a decrease in white blood cells.

(*i.e.*, platelet) series are derived from a small population of primitive cells called the *pluripotent stem cells* (Fig. 12-5). Their lifelong potential for proliferation and self-renewal makes them an indispensable and lifesaving source of reserve cells for the entire hematopoietic system. Several levels of differentiation lead to the development of committed unipotential cells, which are the progenitors for each of the blood cell types. These cells are referred to as *colony-forming units* (CFUs). These progenitor cells have only limited capacity for self-renewal but retain the potential to differentiate into lineage-specific precursor cells. Precursor cells have morphologic characteristics that permit them to be recognized as the first cell of a particular cell line. They have lost their ability for self-renewal but undergo cell division and differentiation, eventually giving rise to mature lymphocytes, myelocytes, megakaryocytes, or erythrocytes.

Disorders of hematopoietic stem cells include aplastic anemia and the leukemias. Today, potential cures for these and many other disorders use hematopoietic stem cell transplantation. Stem cell transplants correct bone marrow failure, immune deficiencies, hematologic defects and malignancies, and inherited errors of metabolism. Sources of the stem cells include

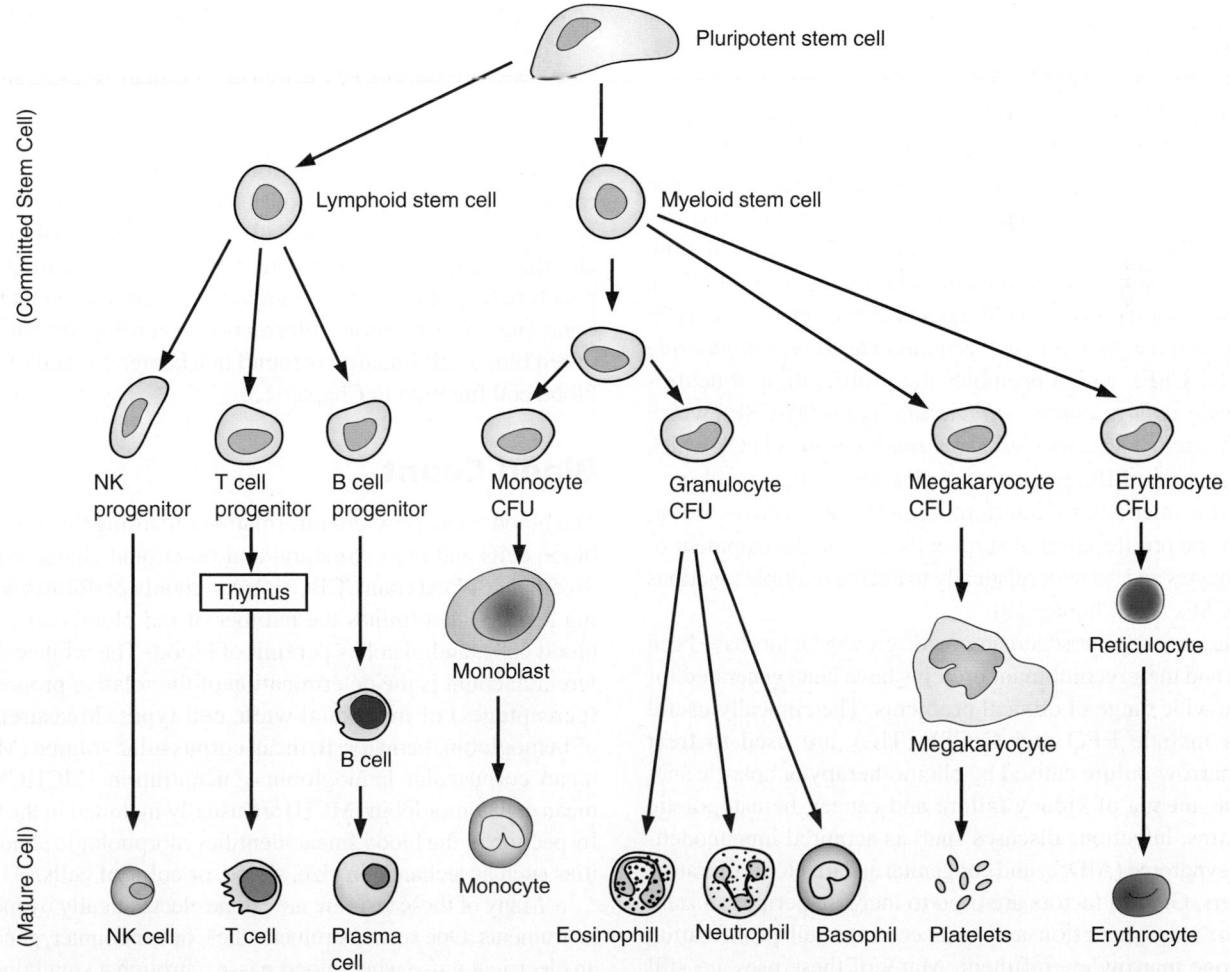

FIGURE 12-5 • Major maturational stages of blood cells. CFU, colony-forming unit; NK, natural killer cell.

bone marrow, peripheral blood, and umbilical cord blood, all of which replenish the recipient with a normal population of pluripotent stem cells. Bone marrow and peripheral blood transplants may be derived from the patient (autologous) or from a histocompatible donor (allogeneic). Autologous transplants are often used to replenish stem cells after high-dose chemotherapy or irradiation. Peripheral blood stem cells are harvested from the blood after the administration of a cytokine growth factor that increases the quantity and migration of the cells from the bone marrow. Umbilical cord blood from human leukocyte antigen (HLA)–matched donors is a transplant option for children and carries less risk of graft-versus-host disease. Methods of collecting, propagating, and preserving stem cells are still being investigated.

Regulation of Hematopoiesis

Under normal conditions, the numbers and total mass for each type of circulating blood cell remain relatively constant. The blood cells are produced in different numbers according to needs and regulatory factors. This regulation of blood cells is thought to be at least partially controlled by hormone-like growth factors called *cytokines*. The cytokines are a family of short-lived mediators that stimulate the proliferation, differentiation, and functional activation of the various blood cells.

Many cytokines derived from lymphocytes or bone marrow stromal cells stimulate the growth and production of new blood cells. Several members of this family are called *colony-stimulating factors* (CSFs) because of their ability to promote the growth of hematopoietic cell colonies in the laboratory. The CSFs that act on committed progenitor cells include *erythropoietin* (EPO), which stimulates red blood cell production; *granulocyte–monocyte colony-stimulating factor* (GM-CSF), which stimulates progenitors for granulocytes, monocytes, erythrocytes, and megakaryocytes; *granulocyte colony-stimulating factor* (G-CSF), which promotes the proliferation of neutrophils; *macrophage colony-stimulating factor* (M-CSF), which induces macrophage colonies; and *thrombopoietin* (TPO), which stimulates the differentiation of platelets. Other cytokines, such as the interleukins, interferons, and tumor necrosis factor, support the proliferation of stem cells and the development of lymphocytes and act synergistically to aid the multiple functions of the CSFs (see Chapter 18).

The genes for most hematopoietic growth factors have been cloned and their recombinant proteins have been generated for use in a wide range of clinical problems. The clinically useful factors include EPO and G-CSF. They are used to treat bone marrow failure caused by chemotherapy or aplastic anemia, the anemia of kidney failure and cancer, hematopoietic neoplasms, infectious diseases such as acquired immunodeficiency syndrome (AIDS), and congenital and myeloproliferative disorders. Growth factors are used to increase peripheral stem cells for transplantation and to accelerate cell proliferation after bone marrow engraftment. Many of these uses are still investigational.

IN SUMMARY, blood is composed of plasma, plasma proteins, fixed elements or blood cells, and substances such as hormones, enzymes, electrolytes, and byproducts of cellular waste. The blood cells consist of erythrocytes or red blood cells, leukocytes or white blood cells, and thrombocytes or platelets. Mature blood cells have a relatively short life span and must be continuously replaced. All of the different types of blood cells arise from pluripotent stem cells located in the bone marrow. The pluripotent stem cells, in turn, differentiate into unipotential colony-forming units, which are the progenitors for each of the blood cell types. Blood cell production is largely regulated by chemical messengers called *cytokines* (interleukins, interferons, and others) and growth factors (colony-stimulating factors). ■

DIAGNOSTIC TESTS

After completing this section of the chapter, you should be able to meet the following objectives:

■ Cite information gained from a complete blood count.
■ State the purpose of the erythrocyte sedimentation rate.
■ Describe the procedure used in bone marrow aspiration.

Blood tests provide information about the oxygen-carrying capacity of the blood (red blood cells), the presence of infection or tissue injury (white blood cells), and the ability of blood to clot (platelets). Blood specimens can be obtained through skin puncture (capillary blood), venipuncture, arterial puncture, or bone marrow aspiration. Information regarding specific tests of red blood cell function is found in Chapter 14, and of white blood cell function in Chapter 15.

Blood Count

The blood count provides information regarding the number of blood cells and their structural and functional characteristics. A complete blood count (CBC) is a commonly performed screening test that determines the number of red blood cells, white blood cells, and platelets per unit of blood. The white cell differential count is the determination of the relative proportions (percentages) of individual white cell types. Measurements of hemoglobin, hematocrit, mean corpuscular volume (MCV), mean corpuscular hemoglobin concentration (MCHC), and mean cell hemoglobin (MCH) are usually included in the CBC. Inspection of the blood smear identifies morphologic abnormalities such as a change in size, shape, or color of cells.

Many of these tests are now done electronically by modern instruments. One such instrument, the Coulter counter, generates an electrical pulse when blood passes through a small opening surrounded by electrodes. Each electrical pulse indicates the passage of an individual cell and the height of the pulse indicates its size. Modern electronic counters are also capable of multimodal assessment of cell size and content for the various categories of white blood cells. A spectrophotometer is used to measure the hemoglobin in the red blood cells and a microhematocrit centrifuge to measure the hematocrit.

Erythrocyte Sedimentation Rate

The erythrocyte sedimentation rate (ESR) is a screening test for monitoring the fluctuations in the clinical course of a disease. In anticoagulated blood, red blood cells aggregate and sediment to the bottom of a tube. The rate of fall of the aggregates is accelerated in the presence of fibrinogen and other plasma proteins that are often increased in inflammatory diseases. The ESR is the distance in millimeters that a red cell column travels in 1 hour. Normal values are 0 to 15 mm/hour for men and 1 to 20 mm/hour for women.

Bone Marrow Aspiration and Biopsy

Tests of bone marrow function are done on samples obtained using bone marrow aspiration or bone marrow biopsy. Bone marrow aspiration is performed with a special needle inserted into the bone marrow cavity, through which a sample of marrow is withdrawn. Usually, the posterior iliac crest is used in all persons older than 12 to 18 months of age. Other sites include the anterior iliac crest, sternum, and spinous processes T10 through L4. The sternum is not commonly used in children because the cavity is too shallow and there is danger of mediastinal and cardiac perforation. Because aspiration disturbs the marrow architecture, this technique is used primarily to determine the type of cells present and their relative numbers. Stained smears of bone marrow aspirates are usually subjected to several studies: determination of the erythroid to myeloid cell count (i.e., normal ratio is 1:3), differential cell count, search for abnormal cells, evaluation of iron stores in reticulum cells, and special stains and immunochemical studies.

Bone marrow biopsy is done with a special biopsy needle inserted into the posterior iliac crest. Biopsy removes an actual sample of bone marrow tissue and allows study of the architecture of the tissue. It is used to determine the marrow-to-fat ratio and the presence of fibrosis, plasma cells, granulomas, and cancer cells. The major hazard of these procedures is the slight risk of hemorrhage. This risk is increased in persons with a reduced platelet count.

IN SUMMARY, diagnostic tests of the blood include the complete blood count, which is used to describe the number and characteristics of the erythrocytes, leukocytes, and platelets. The erythrocyte sedimentation rate is used to detect inflammation. Bone marrow aspiration is used to determine the function of the bone marrow in generating blood cells. ∎

Review Exercises

1. A 14-year-old boy is admitted to the emergency department with severe abdominal pain and a tentative diagnosis of appendicitis. His white blood cell count shows an elevated number of white blood cells with an increased percentage of "band cells."

   A. Explain the significance of this finding.

2. Many of the primary immunodeficiency disorders, in which there is a defect in the development of immune cells of T- or B-lymphocyte origin, can be cured with allogeneic stem cell transplantation from an unaffected donor.

   A. Explain why stem cells are used rather than mature lymphocytes. You might want to refer to Figure 12-5.

   B. Describe how the stem cells would go about the process of repopulating the bone marrow.

Bibliography

Alexander W. S. (1998). Cytokines in hematopoiesis. *International Reviews of Immunology* 16, 651–682.

Guyton A. C., Hall J. E. (2006). *Textbook of medical physiology* (11th ed., pp. 419–438). Philadelphia: Elsevier Saunders.

Fischbach F. (2004). *A manual of laboratory diagnostic tests* (7th ed.). Philadelphia: Lippincott Williams & Wilkins.

Hoffman R., Benz E. J., Shattil S. J., et al. (2000). *Hematology: Basic principles and practice* (3rd ed.). New York: Churchill Livingstone.

Jansen J., Thompson J. M., Dugan M. J., et al. (2002). Peripheral blood progenitor cell transplantation. *Therapeutic Apheresis* 6(1), 5–14.

Junqueira L. C., Carneiro J. (2005). *Basic histology: Text and atlas* (11th ed., pp. 223–253). New York: McGraw-Hill.

Kaushansky K. (2006). Lineage-specific hematopoietic growth factors. *New England Journal of Medicine* 354, 2034–2045.

Lovell-Badge R. (2001). The future for stem cell research. *Nature* 414, 88–91.

Ross M. H., Kaye G. I., Pawlina W. (2003). *Histology: A text and atlas* (4th ed., pp. 214–245). Philadelphia: Lippincott Williams & Wilkins.

Schwarting R., Kocher W. D., McKenzie S., et al. (2005). Hematopathology. In Rubin E., Gorstein F., Rubin R., et al. (Eds.), *Rubin's pathology: Clinicopathologic foundations of medicine* (4th ed., pp. 1019–1070). Philadelphia: Lippincott Williams & Wilkins.

Smith C. (2003). Hematopoietic stem cells and hematopoiesis. *Cancer Control* 10, 9–16.

Stamatoyannopoulos G., Majerus P. W., Perlmutter R. M., et al. (2001). *The molecular basis of blood diseases* (3rd ed.). Philadelphia: W. B. Saunders.

Tavian M., Péault B. (2005). Embryonic development of the human hematopoietic system. *International Journal of Developmental Biology* 49, 243–250.

Tefferi A., Hanson C. A., Inwards D. J. (2005). How to interpret and pursue an abnormal complete blood count in adults. *Mayo Clinic Proceedings* 80, 923–936.

Wadlow R. C., Porter D. L. (2002). Umbilical cord blood transplant: Where do we stand? *Biology of Blood and Marrow Transplantation* 8, 637–647.

Visit thePoint http://thePoint.lww.com for animations, journal articles, and more!

Disorders of Hemostasis

KATHRYN J. GASPARD

> The term *hemostasis* refers to the stoppage of blood flow. The normal process of hemostasis is regulated by a complex array of activators and inhibitors that maintain blood fluidity and prevent blood from leaving the vascular compartment. Hemostasis is normal when it seals a blood vessel to prevent blood loss and hemorrhage. It is abnormal when it causes inappropriate blood clotting or when clotting is insufficient to stop the flow of blood from the vascular compartment. Disorders of hemostasis fall into two main categories: the inappropriate formation of clots within the vascular system (thrombosis) and the failure of blood to clot in response to an appropriate stimulus (bleeding).

MECHANISMS OF HEMOSTASIS

After completing this section of the chapter, you should be able to meet the following objectives:

- Describe the five stages of hemostasis.
- Explain the formation of the platelet plug.
- State the purpose of blood coagulation.
- State the function of clot retraction.
- Trace the process of fibrinolysis.

Hemostasis is divided into five stages: (1) vessel spasm, (2) formation of the platelet plug, (3) blood coagulation or development of an insoluble fibrin clot, (4) clot retraction, and (5) clot dissolution. During the process of hemostasis, hairlike fibrin strands glue the aggregated platelets together and intertwine to form the structural basis of the blood clot. In the presence of fibrin, plasma becomes gel-like and traps red blood cells and other formed elements in the blood (Fig. 13-1). Hemostasis is complete when fibrous tissue grows into the clot and seals the hole in the vessel.

Vessel Spasm

Vessel spasm constricts the vessel and reduces blood flow. It is a transient event that usually lasts less than 1 minute. Vessel spasm is initiated by endothelial injury and caused by local and humoral mechanisms. Neural reflexes and thromboxane A_2

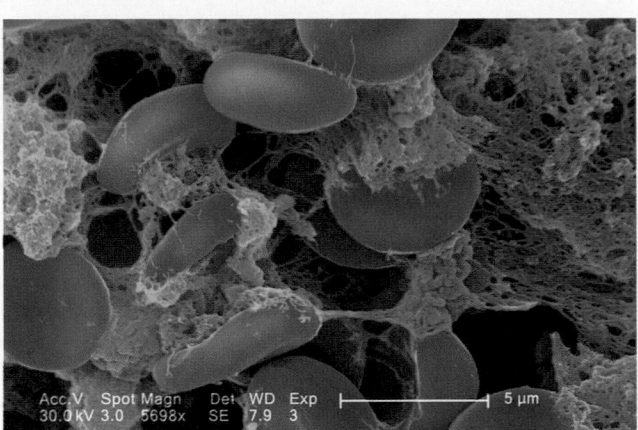

FIGURE 13-1 • A scanning electron micrograph depicting a number of red cells enmeshed in a fibrinous matrix on the luminal surface of an indwelling catheter (magnification ×5698). (From the Centers for Disease Control and Prevention Public Images Library, Courtesy Janice Carr.)

(TXA$_2$), a prostaglandin released from platelets, and other mediators contribute to vasoconstriction. Prostacyclin, another prostaglandin released from the vessel endothelium, produces vasodilation and inhibits platelet aggregation in the surrounding uninjured endothelium.

🔑 HEMOSTASIS

- Hemostasis is the orderly, stepwise process for stopping bleeding that involves vasospasm, formation of a platelet plug, and the development of a fibrin clot.

- The blood clotting process requires the presence of platelets produced in the bone marrow, von Willebrand factor generated by the vessel endothelium, and clotting factors synthesized in the liver, using vitamin K.

- The final step of the process involves fibrinolysis or clot dissolution, which prevents excess clot formation.

Formation of the Platelet Plug

The platelet plug, the second line of defense, is initiated as platelets come in contact with the vessel wall. Small breaks in the vessel wall are often sealed with the platelet plug rather than a blood clot.

Platelets, also called *thrombocytes,* are large fragments from the cytoplasm of bone marrow cells called *megakaryocytes.*[1] Each megakaryocyte releases from 1000 to 4000 platelets into the circulation. The normal serum concentration is about 150,000 to 400,000 platelets per microliter (µL) of blood.[2] The newly formed platelets that are released from the bone marrow spend up to 8 hours in the spleen before they are released into the blood, where their life span is only 8 to 9 days. Platelet pro-

duction is controlled by a protein called *thrombopoietin* that causes proliferation and maturation of megakaryocytes.[3] The sources of thrombopoietin include the liver, kidney, smooth muscle, and bone marrow.

Platelets have a cell membrane but no nucleus, and cannot reproduce. Although they lack a nucleus, they have many of the characteristics of a whole cell. The outer cell membrane is covered with a glycocalyx or coat of glycoproteins, glycosaminoglycans, and coagulation proteins (Fig. 13-2). One of the important glycoproteins is GPIIb/IIIa, which binds fibrinogen and bridges platelets to one another.[2] The platelet shape is maintained by microtubules and actin and myosin filaments that support the cell membrane. Platelets have mitochondria and enzyme systems capable of producing adenosine triphosphate (ATP) and adenosine diphosphate (ADP), and they have the enzymes needed for synthesis of the prostaglandin, TXA$_2$, required for their function in hemostasis.

Platelets contain two specific types of granules (α- and δ-granules) that release mediators for hemostasis.[2,4] The α-granules express the P-selectin, an adhesive protein, on their surface (see Chapter 4) and contain fibrinogen, von Willebrand factor, fibronectin, factors V and VIII, platelet factor 4 (a heparin-binding chemokine), platelet-derived growth factor (PDGF), and transforming growth factor-α (TGF-α). The release of growth factors results in the proliferation and growth of vascular endothelial cells, smooth muscle cells, and fibroblasts and is important in vessel repair. The δ-granules, or dense granules, contain ADP and ATP, ionized calcium, histamine, serotonin, and epinephrine, which contribute to vasoconstriction.[2]

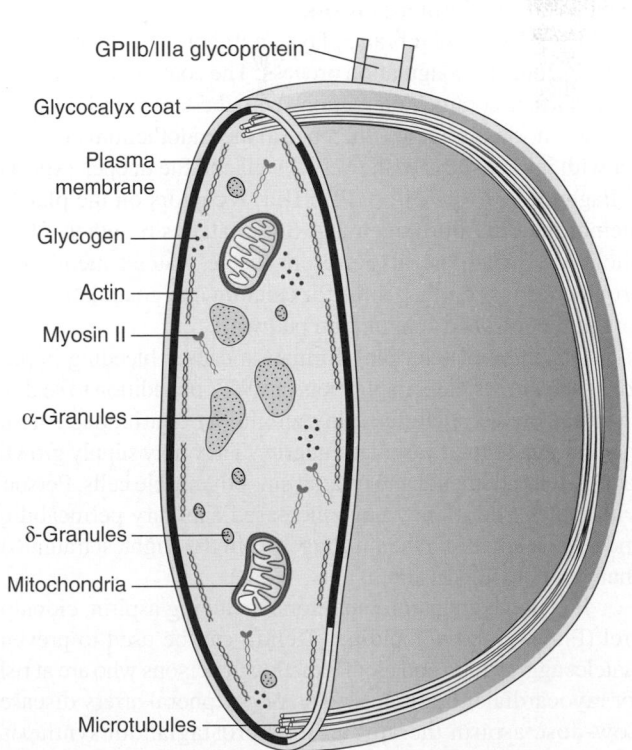

FIGURE 13-2 • Platelet structure.

Platelet plug formation involves adhesion and aggregation of platelets. Platelets are attracted to a damaged vessel wall, become activated, and change from smooth disks to spiny spheres, exposing glycoprotein receptors on their surfaces. Platelet adhesion requires a protein molecule called *von Willebrand factor* (vWF). This factor is produced by the endothelial cells of blood vessels and circulates in the blood as a carrier protein for coagulation factor VIII. Adhesion to the vessel subendothelial layer occurs when the platelet receptor binds to vWF at the injury site, linking the platelet to exposed collagen fibers.

Platelet aggregation occurs soon after adhesion. It is mediated by the secretion of the contents of the platelet granules. The release of the dense body contents is particularly important because calcium is required for the coagulation component of hemostasis, and ADP is a mediator of platelet aggregation. ADP release also facilitates the release of ADP from other platelets, leading to amplification of the aggregation process. Besides ADP, platelets secrete the prostaglandin TXA_2, which is an important stimulus for platelet aggregation. The combined actions of ADP and TXA_2 lead to the expansion of the enlarging platelet aggregate, which becomes the primary hemostatic plug. Stabilization of the platelet plug occurs as the coagulation pathway is activated on the platelet surface and fibrinogen is converted to fibrin, thereby creating a fibrin meshwork that cements the platelets and other blood components together (see Fig. 13-1). P-selectin also participates in platelet aggregation by binding leukocytes, which, with platelet substances such as PDGF, participate in healing of the vessel wall. The primary aggregation and formation of the platelet plug is reversible up to the point where the coagulation cascade has been activated and the platelets have been irreversibly fused together by the fibrin meshwork.

The platelet membrane plays an important role in platelet adhesion and the coagulation process. The coat of glycoproteins on its surface controls interactions with the vessel endothelium. Platelets normally avoid adherence to the endothelium but interact with injured areas of the vessel wall and the deeper exposed collagen.[1] Glycoprotein (GPIIb/IIIa) receptors on the platelet membrane bind fibrinogen and link platelets together. Phospholipids, which are also present in the platelet membrane, provide critical binding sites for calcium and coagulation factors in the intrinsic coagulation pathway.

Defective platelet plug formation causes bleeding in persons who are deficient in platelets or vWF. In addition to sealing vascular breaks, platelets play an almost continuous role in maintaining normal vascular integrity. They may supply growth factors for endothelial and arterial smooth muscle cells. Persons with platelet deficiency have increased capillary permeability and sustain small skin hemorrhages from the slightest trauma or change in blood pressure.

Platelet aggregation inhibitors, including aspirin, clopidogrel (Plavix), and ticlopidine (Ticlid), can be used to prevent platelet aggregation and clot formation in persons who are at risk for myocardial infarction, stroke, or peripheral artery disease. Low-dose aspirin therapy inhibits prostaglandin synthesis, including TXA_2. Clopidogrel and ticlopidine achieve their antiplatelet effects by inhibiting the ADP pathway in platelets.

Unlike aspirin, these drugs have an effect on prostaglandin synthesis. Both clopidogrel and ticlopidine prolong the bleeding time; however, the most serious side effects of ticlopidine have been neutropenia and thrombotic thrombocytopenic purpura. Studies from three large, randomized trials and numerous registry data have shown that clopidogrel in combination with aspirin is associated with a reduction in major cardiac events, similar to ticlopidine plus aspirin, and appeared safer.[5] Drugs that act as GPIIb/IIIa receptor inhibitors (tirofiban, eptifibatide, abciximab) have been developed for use in the treatment of acute myocardial infarction (see Chapter 24). However, acute and delayed thrombocytopenia has been reported after use of these agents, suggesting that further investigation is needed to understand the mechanisms leading to the thrombocytopenia and improve methods for detection.[6]

Blood Coagulation

The coagulation cascade is the third component of the hemostatic process. It is a stepwise process resulting in the conversion of the soluble plasma protein, fibrinogen, into fibrin. The insoluble fibrin strands create a meshwork that cements platelets and other blood components together to form the clot.

The coagulation process is controlled by many substances that promote clotting (procoagulation factors) or inhibit it (anticoagulation factors). Each of the procoagulation or coagulation factors, identified by Roman numerals, performs a specific step in the coagulation process. The activation of one procoagulation factor or proenzyme is designed to activate the next factor in the sequence (cascade effect). Because most of the inactive procoagulation factors are present in the blood at all times, the multistep process ensures that a massive episode of intravascular clotting does not occur by chance. It also means that abnormalities of the clotting process occur when one or more of the factors are deficient or when conditions lead to inappropriate activation of any of the steps.

Most of the coagulation factors are proteins synthesized in the liver. Vitamin K is necessary for the synthesis of factors II, VII, IX, and X, prothrombin, and protein C. Calcium (factor IV) is required in all but the first two steps of the clotting process.[1] The body usually has sufficient amounts of calcium for these reactions. Inactivation of the calcium ion prevents blood from clotting when it is removed from the body. The addition of citrate to blood stored for transfusion purposes prevents clotting by chelating ionic calcium. EDTA, another chelator, is often added to blood samples used for analysis in the clinical laboratory.

The coagulation process results from the activation of what have traditionally been designated the *intrinsic* and the *extrinsic* pathways[1] (Fig. 13-3). The intrinsic pathway, which is a relatively slow process, begins in the circulation with the activation of factor XII. The extrinsic pathway, which is a much faster process, begins with trauma to the blood vessel or surrounding tissues and the release of tissue factor, an adhesive lipoprotein, from the subendothelial cells. The terminal steps in both pathways are the same: the activation of factor X and the conversion of prothrombin to thrombin. Thrombin then acts as an enzyme

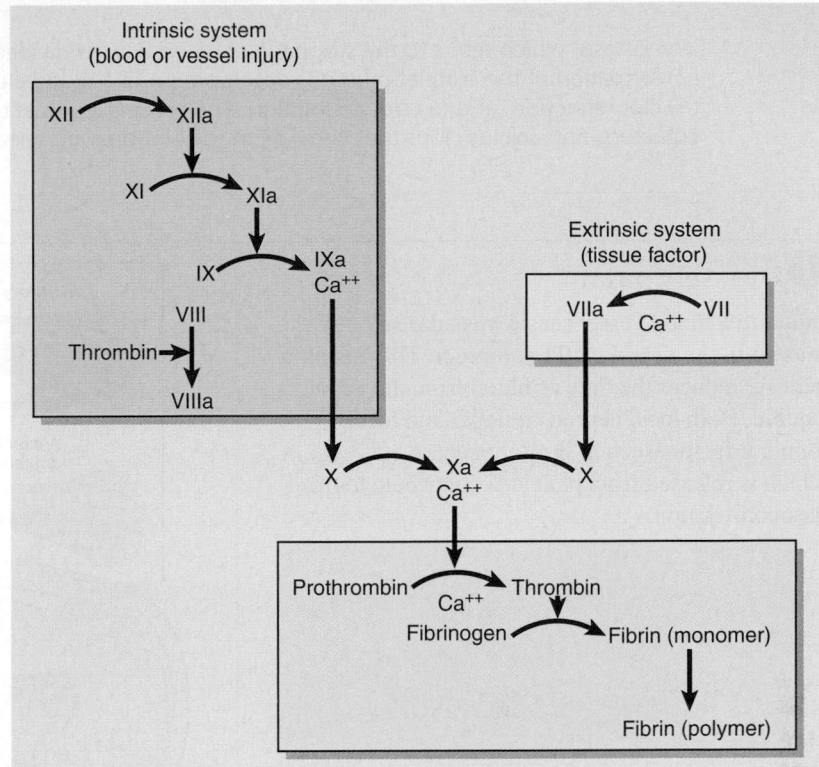

Intrinsic system
(blood or vessel injury)

Extrinsic system
(tissue factor)

FIGURE 13-3 • The intrinsic and extrinsic coagulation pathways. The terminal steps in both pathways are the same. Calcium, factors X and V, and platelet phospholipids combine to form prothrombin activator, which then converts prothrombin to thrombin. This interaction causes conversion of fibrinogen into the fibrin strands that create the insoluble blood clot.

to convert fibrinogen to fibrin, the material that stabilizes a clot. Both pathways are needed for normal hemostasis, and many interrelations exist between them. Each system is activated when blood passes out of the vascular system. The intrinsic system is activated as blood comes in contact with collagen in the injured vessel wall; the extrinsic system is activated when blood is exposed to tissue extracts. However, bleeding that occurs because of defects in the extrinsic system usually is not as severe as that resulting from defects in the intrinsic pathway.

Blood coagulation is regulated by several natural anticoagulants. Antithrombin III inactivates coagulation factors and neutralizes thrombin, the last enzyme in the pathway for the conversion of fibrinogen to fibrin. When antithrombin III is complexed with naturally occurring heparin, its action is accelerated to inactivate thrombin, factor Xa, and other coagulation factors. This complex activation provides protection against uncontrolled thrombus formation on the endothelial surface. Protein C, a plasma protein, acts as an anticoagulant by inactivating factors V and VIII. Protein S, another plasma protein, accelerates the action of protein C. Plasmin breaks down fibrin into fibrin degradation products that act as anticoagulants. It has been suggested that some of these natural anticoagulants may play a role in the bleeding that occurs with disseminated intravascular coagulation (DIC; discussed later).

The anticoagulant drugs warfarin and heparin are used to prevent thromboembolic disorders, such as deep vein thrombosis and pulmonary embolism.[7] Warfarin acts by decreasing pro-

thrombin and other procoagulation factors. It alters vitamin K in a manner that reduces its ability to participate in synthesis of the vitamin K–dependent coagulation factors in the liver. Warfarin is readily absorbed after oral administration. Its maximum effect takes 36 to 72 hours because of the varying half-lives of preformed clotting factors that remain in the circulation. Heparin is naturally formed and released in small amounts by mast cells in connective tissue surrounding capillaries. Pharmacologic preparations of heparin are extracted from animal tissues. Heparin binds to antithrombin III, causing a conformational change that increases the ability of antithrombin III to inactivate thrombin, factor Xa, and other clotting factors. By promoting the inactivation of clotting factors, heparin ultimately suppresses the formation of fibrin. Heparin is unable to cross the membranes of the gastrointestinal tract and must be given by injection, usually by intravenous infusion. Low–molecular-weight heparins have been developed that inhibit activation of factor X, but have little effect on thrombin and other coagulation factors. The low–molecular-weight-heparins are given by subcutaneous injection and require less frequent administration and monitoring compared with the standard (unfractionated) heparin.

Clot Retraction

Clot retraction normally occurs within 20 to 60 minutes after a clot has formed, contributing to hemostasis by squeezing serum from the clot and joining the edges of the broken vessel. Platelets, through the action of their actin and myosin filaments, also contribute to clot retraction. Clot retraction there-

Understanding • Hemostasis

Hemostasis, which refers to the stoppage of blood flow, is divided into five stages: (1) vessel spasm, (2) formation of the platelet plug, (3) development of a blood clot as a result of the coagulation process, (4) clot retraction, and (5) clot dissolution. The process involves the interaction of substrates, enzymes, protein cofactors, and calcium ions that circulate in the blood or are released from platelets and cells in the vessel wall.

❶ Vessel Spasm

Injury to a blood vessel causes vascular smooth muscle in the vessel wall to contract. This instantaneously reduces the flow of blood from the vessel rupture. Both local nervous reflexes and local humoral factors such as thromboxane A_2 (TXA_2), which is released from platelets, contribute to the vasoconstriction.

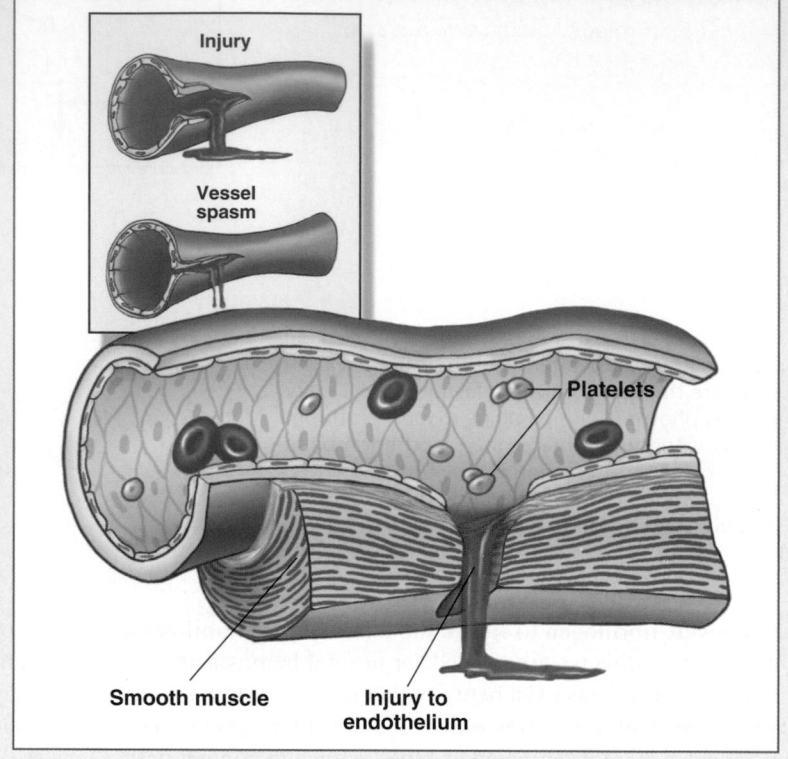

❷ Formation of the Platelet Plug

Seconds after vessel injury, von Willebrand factor, released from the endothelium, binds to platelet receptors, causing adhesion of the platelets to the exposed collagen fibers *(inset)*. As the platelets adhere to the collagen fibers on the damaged vessel wall, they become activated and release adenosine diphosphate (ADP) and TXA_2. The ADP and TXA_2 attract additional platelets, leading to platelet aggregation.

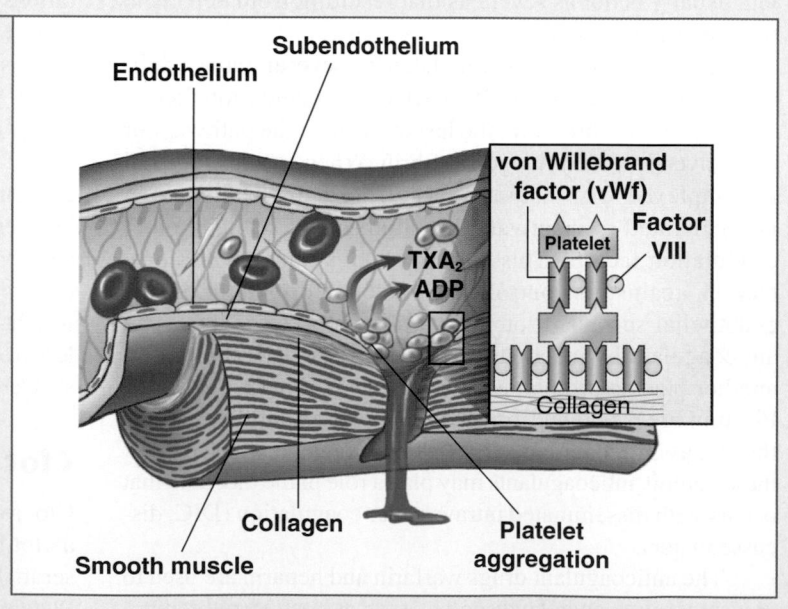

❸ Blood Coagulation

Blood coagulation is a complex process involving the sequential activation of various factors in the blood. There are two coagulation pathways: (1) the intrinsic pathway begins in the circulation and is initiated by activation of circulating factor XII; and (2) the extrinsic pathway, which is activated by a cellular lipoprotein called *tissue factor* that becomes exposed when tissues are injured. Both pathways lead to the activation of factor X, the conversion of prothrombin to thrombin, and conversion of fibrinogen to the insoluble fibrin threads that hold the clot together.

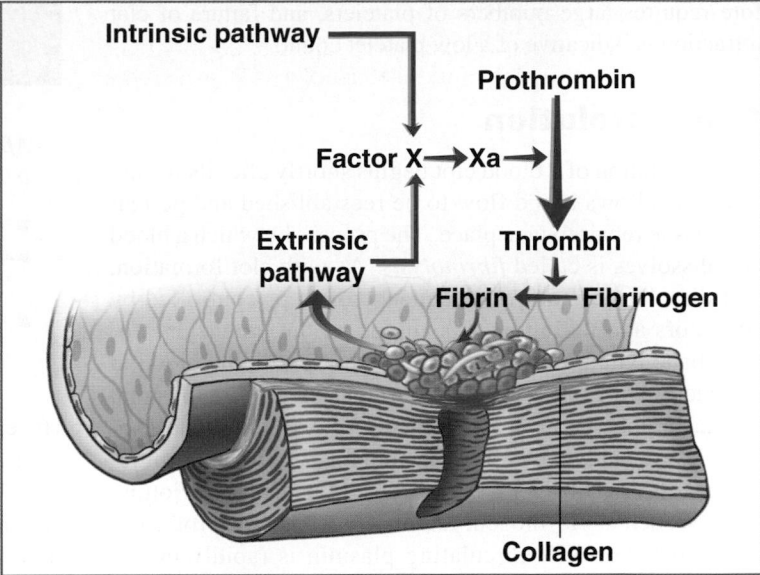

❹ Clot Retraction

Within a few minutes after a clot is formed, the actin and myosin in the platelets that are trapped in the clot begin to contract in a manner similar to that in muscles. As a result, the fibrin strands of the clot are pulled toward the platelets, thereby squeezing serum (plasma without fibrinogen) from the clot and causing it to shrink.

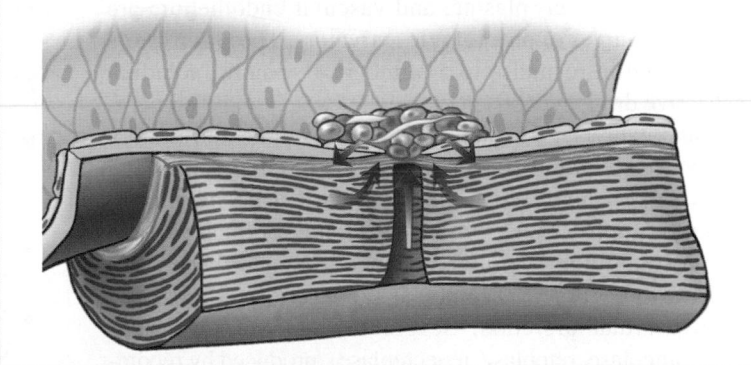

❺ Clot Dissolution or Lysis

Clot dissolution begins shortly after a clot is formed. It begins with activation of plasminogen, an inactive precursor of the proteolytic enzyme, plasmin. When a clot is formed, large amounts of plasminogen are trapped in the clot. The slow release of a very powerful activator called tissue plasminogen activator (t-PA) from injured tissues and vascular endothelium converts plasminogen to plasmin, which digests the fibrin strands, causing the clot to dissolve.

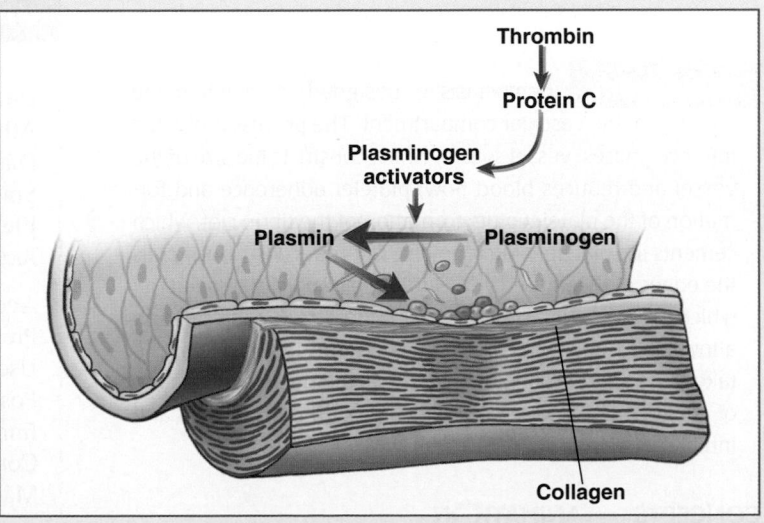

fore requires large numbers of platelets, and failure of clot retraction is indicative of a low platelet count.

Clot Dissolution

The dissolution of a blood clot begins shortly after its formation; this allows blood flow to be reestablished and permanent tissue repair to take place. The process by which a blood clot dissolves is called *fibrinolysis*. As with clot formation, clot dissolution requires a sequence of steps controlled by activators and inhibitors. Plasminogen, the proenzyme for the fibrinolytic process, normally is present in the blood in its inactive form. It is converted to its active form, plasmin, by plasminogen activators formed in the vascular endothelium, liver, and kidneys. The plasmin formed from plasminogen digests the fibrin strands of the clot and certain clotting factors, such as fibrinogen, factor V, factor VIII, prothrombin, and factor XII. Circulating plasmin is rapidly inactivated by α_2-plasmin inhibitor, which limits the fibrinolytic process to the local clot and prevents it from occurring in the entire circulation.

Two naturally occurring plasminogen activators are tissue-type plasminogen activator and urokinase-type plasminogen activator. The liver, plasma, and vascular endothelium are the major sources of physiologic activators. These activators are released in response to a number of stimuli, including vasoactive drugs, venous occlusion, elevated body temperature, and exercise. The activators are unstable and rapidly inactivated by inhibitors synthesized by the endothelium and the liver. For this reason, chronic liver disease may cause altered fibrinolytic activity. A major inhibitor, plasminogen activator inhibitor-1, in high concentrations has been associated with deep vein thrombosis, coronary artery disease, and myocardial infarction.[7] Several tissue plasminogen activators (alteplase, reteplase, tenecteplase), produced by recombinant DNA technology, are available for use in treatment of acute myocardial infarction (see Chapter 24), acute ischemic stroke (see Chapter 51), and pulmonary embolism (see Chapter 28).

IN SUMMARY, hemostasis is designed to maintain the integrity of the vascular compartment. The process is divided into five phases: vessel spasm, which constricts the size of the vessel and reduces blood flow; platelet adherence and formation of the platelet plug; formation of the fibrin clot, which cements the platelet plug together; clot retraction, which pulls the edges of the injured vessel together; and clot dissolution, which involves the action of plasmin to dissolve the clot and allow blood flow to be reestablished and tissue healing to take place. Blood coagulation requires the stepwise activation of coagulation factors, carefully controlled by activators and inhibitors. ∎

CONCEPTSin action**ANIMATION**

HYPERCOAGULABILITY STATES

After completing this section of the chapter, you should be able to meet the following objectives:

- Compare normal and abnormal clotting.
- Describe the causes and effects of increased platelet function.
- State two conditions that contribute to increased clotting activity.

Hypercoagulability represents an exaggerated form of hemostasis that predisposes to thrombosis and blood vessel occlusion. There are two general forms of hypercoagulability states: conditions that create increased platelet function and conditions that cause accelerated activity of the coagulation system. Chart 13-1 summarizes conditions commonly associated with hypercoagulability states. Arterial thrombi are usually due to turbulence and composed largely of platelet aggregates, whereas venous thrombi are usually due to stasis of flow and composed largely of platelet aggregates and fibrin complexes that result from activation of the coagulation cascade.

 HYPERCOAGULABILITY STATES

- Hypercoagulability states increase the risk of clot or thrombus formation in either the arterial or venous circulations.
- Arterial thrombi are associated with conditions that produce turbulent blood flow and platelet adherence.
- Venous thrombi are associated with conditions that cause stasis of blood flow with increased concentrations of coagulation factors.

CHART 13-1	CONDITIONS ASSOCIATED WITH HYPERCOAGULABILITY STATES

Increased Platelet Function
Atherosclerosis
Diabetes mellitus
Smoking
Elevated blood lipid and cholesterol levels
Increased platelet levels

Accelerated Activity of the Clotting System
Pregnancy and the puerperium
Use of oral contraceptives
Postsurgical state
Immobility
Congestive heart failure
Malignant diseases

Hypercoagulability Associated With Increased Platelet Function

Hypercoagulability due to increased platelet function results in platelet adhesion, formation of platelet clots, and disruption of blood flow. The causes of increased platelet function are disturbances in flow, endothelial damage, and increased sensitivity of platelets to factors that cause adhesiveness and aggregation. Atherosclerotic plaques disturb blood flow, causing endothelial damage and promoting platelet adherence. Platelets that adhere to the vessel wall release growth factors that cause proliferation of smooth muscle and thereby contribute to the development of atherosclerosis (discussed in Chapter 22). Smoking, elevated levels of blood lipids and cholesterol, hemodynamic stress, and diabetes mellitus predispose to vessel damage, platelet adherence, and eventual thrombosis.

Thrombocytosis

The term *thrombocytosis* is used to describe elevations in the platelet count above 1,000,000/μL. Thrombocytosis can occur as a reactive process (secondary thrombocytosis) or as an essential process (primary thrombocytosis).[3]

Thrombopoietin is the key hormone in the regulation of megakaryocyte differentiation and platelet formation, although various cytokines (*e.g.,* interleukin-6 and interleukin-11) may play a role.[3] Megakaryocytes and their platelet progeny have receptors for thrombopoietin. Thrombopoietin is carried in the plasma attached to receptors on the surface of circulating platelets and in an unbound form that is free to promote megakaryocyte proliferation. When the platelet count falls, more unbound thrombopoietin is available to stimulate megakaryocyte proliferation, and when the platelet count rises, less thrombopoietin is available to stimulate proliferation. Thus, megakaryocyte proliferation and platelet production are normally controlled in a negative feedback manner by the platelet count.

The most common cause of secondary thrombocytosis is a disease state that stimulates thrombopoietin production. The result is increased megakaryocyte proliferation and platelet production. However, the platelet count seldom exceeds 1,000,000/μL. The common underlying causes of secondary thrombocytosis include tissue damage due to surgery, infection, cancer, and chronic inflammatory conditions such as rheumatoid arthritis and Crohn disease. Usually the only clinically apparent signs are those of the underlying disease. Thrombocytosis may also occur in other myeloproliferative disorders such as polycythemia vera (discussed in Chapter 14) and myelogenous leukemia (discussed in Chapter 15).

Primary or essential thrombocytosis represents a myeloproliferative (bone marrow) disorder of the hematopoietic stem cells.[3] Although thrombopoietin levels are often normal in essential thrombocytosis, abnormalities in the thrombopoietin receptor and platelet binding cause higher-than-expected levels of free thrombopoietin. This leads to increased megakaryocyte proliferation and platelet production. Dysfunction of the platelets produced contributes to the major clinical features of bleeding and thrombosis.

The common clinical manifestations of essential thrombocytosis are thrombosis and hemorrhage. Thrombotic events include deep vein thrombosis and pulmonary embolism and portal and hepatic vein thrombosis. Some persons experience erythromelalgia, a painful throbbing and burning of the fingers caused by occlusion of the arterioles by platelet aggregates. Typically, the disorder is characterized by long asymptomatic periods punctuated by occasional thrombotic episodes and hemorrhagic crises, both of which occur in persons with very high platelet counts. Treatment includes the use of platelet-lowering drugs (*e.g.,* hydroxyurea) in high-risk cases.[3] Aspirin may be a highly effective adjunctive therapy in persons with recurrent thrombotic complications.

Hypercoagulability Associated With Increased Clotting Activity

Thrombus formation due to activation of the coagulation system can result from primary (genetic) or secondary (acquired) disorders affecting the coagulation components of the blood clotting process (*i.e.,* an increase in procoagulation factors or a decrease in anticoagulation factors).

Inherited Disorders

Of the inherited causes of hypercoagulability, mutations in the factor V gene and prothrombin gene are the most common.[2] Approximately 2% to 15% of whites carry a specific factor V mutation (referred to as the *Leiden mutation,* because of the Dutch city where it was first discovered).[2] In persons with inherited defects in factor V, the mutant factor Va cannot be inactivated by protein C; as a result, an important antithrombotic counter-regulatory mechanism is lost. The defect predisposes to venous thrombosis, and among persons with recurrent deep vein thrombosis, the frequency of the mutation may be as high as 60%.[2] It is one of the most common causes of primary and recurrent thromboembolism in pregnancy and is also associated with abruptio placentae (premature placental separation) and fetal growth disturbance.[8]

A single nucleotide change in the prothrombin gene, which affects 1% to 2% of the population, is associated with elevated prothrombin levels and an almost threefold increase in venous thromboses. Less common primary hypercoagulable states include inherited deficiencies of anticoagulants such as antithrombin III, protein C, and protein S.[9] Another hereditary defect results in high circulating levels of homocysteine, which predisposes to venous and arterial thrombosis by activating platelets and altering antithrombotic mechanisms.[2,9]

Acquired Disorders

Among the acquired or secondary factors that lead to increased coagulation and thrombosis are venous stasis due to prolonged bed rest and immobility, myocardial infarction, cancer, hyperestrogenic states, and oral contraceptives. Smoking and obesity promote hypercoagulability for unknown reasons.

Stasis of blood flow causes accumulation of activated clotting factors and platelets and prevents their interactions with inhibitors. Slow and disturbed flow is a common cause of venous thrombosis in the immobilized or postsurgical patient. Heart failure also contributes to venous congestion and thrombosis. Hyperviscosity syndromes (polycythemia) and deformed red blood cells in sickle cell disease increase the resistance to flow and cause small vessel stasis.

Elevated levels of estrogen increase hepatic synthesis of many coagulation factors and decrease the synthesis of antithrombin III.[10] The incidence of stroke, thromboemboli, and myocardial infarction is greater in women who use oral contraceptives, particularly those older than 35 years of age and those who are heavy smokers. Clotting factors are also increased during normal pregnancy. These changes, along with limited activity during the puerperium (immediate postpartum period), predispose to venous thrombosis.

Hypercoagulability also is common in cancer and sepsis. Many tumor cells are thought to release tissue factor molecules, which, along with the increased immobility and sepsis seen in patients with malignant disease, contribute to thrombosis in these patients.

Antiphospholipid Syndrome. Another cause of increased venous and arterial thrombosis is the *antiphospholipid syndrome*, a condition associated with autoantibodies (primarily immunoglobulin G [IgG]) directed against protein-binding phospholipids that results in increased coagulation activity.[11,12] The common features of antiphospholipid syndrome are venous and arterial thrombi, recurrent fetal loss, and thrombocytopenia. The disorder can be manifest as a primary condition occurring in isolation with signs of hypercoagulability, or as a secondary condition most often associated with connective tissue disorders, particularly systemic lupus erythematosus.

Persons with the disorder present with a variety of clinical manifestations, typically those characterized by recurrent venous and arterial thrombi. Cardiac valvular vegetations associated with adherence of thrombi and thrombocytopenia due to excessive platelet consumption may also occur. Venous thrombosis, especially in the deep leg veins, occurs in up to 50% of persons with the syndrome, half of whom develop pulmonary emboli. Arterial thrombosis involves the brain in up to 50% of cases, causing transient ischemic attacks or strokes.[9] Other sites for arterial thrombosis are the coronary arteries of the heart and the retinal, renal, and peripheral arteries. Women with the disorder commonly have a history of recurrent pregnancy losses after the 10th week of gestation because of ischemia and thrombosis of the placental vessels. These women also have increased risk of giving birth to a premature infant owing to pregnancy-associated hypertension and uteroplacental insufficiency.

Although the mechanisms for this syndrome are unknown, several potential pathways have been identified. The antibodies may interfere with the coagulation cascade, leading to a hypercoagulability state; directly bind to the endothelial cell surface, causing secretion of cytokines that result in activation and aggregation of platelets; or target a serum phospholipid binding pro-

tein that functions as an anticoagulant. In addition to the action of the antibodies, it seems likely that other factors play a role in determining whether a person develops clinical manifestations of the disorder. Although speculative, these factors may include vascular trauma or the presence of infection that leads to cytokine production and endothelial cell activation.

In most persons with antiphospholipid syndrome, the thrombotic events occur as a single episode at one anatomic site. In some persons recurrences may occur months or years later and mimic the initial event. Occasionally, someone may present with multiple vascular occlusions involving many organ systems. This rapid onset condition is termed *catastrophic antiphospholipid syndrome* and is associated with a high mortality rate.

Treatment of the syndrome focuses on removal or reduction in factors that predispose to thrombosis, including advice to stop smoking and counseling against use of estrogen-containing oral contraceptives by women. The acute thrombotic event is treated with anticoagulants (heparin and warfarin) and immune suppression in refractory cases. Aspirin and anticoagulant drugs may be used to prevent future thrombosis.[13]

IN SUMMARY, hypercoagulability causes excessive clotting and contributes to thrombus formation. It results from conditions that foster an increase in platelet numbers or function or accelerated activity of the coagulation system. Thrombocytosis, an elevation in the platelet count, can occur as a reactive process (secondary thrombocytosis) or an essential process (primary thrombocytosis). Increased platelet function usually results from disorders such as atherosclerosis that damage the vascular endothelium and disturb blood flow, or from conditions such as smoking that increase sensitivity of platelets to factors that promote adhesiveness and aggregation.

Factors that cause accelerated activity of the coagulation system include blood flow stasis, resulting in an accumulation of coagulation factors, and alterations in the components of the coagulation system (*i.e.,* an increase in procoagulation factors or a decrease in anticoagulation factors). The antiphospholipid syndrome, another cause of venous and arterial clotting, manifests as a primary disorder or a secondary disorder associated with systemic lupus erythematosus. It is associated with antiphospholipid antibodies, which promote thrombosis that can affect many organs. ■

BLEEDING DISORDERS

After completing this section of the chapter, you should be able to meet the following objectives:

- State the mechanisms of drug-induced thrombocytopenia and idiopathic thrombocytopenia, and the differing features of the disorders in terms of onset and resolution.

- Describe the manifestations of thrombocytopenia.
- Characterize the role of vitamin K in coagulation.
- State three common defects of coagulation factors and the causes of each.
- Differentiate between the mechanisms of bleeding in hemophilia A and von Willebrand disease.
- Describe the effect of vascular disorders on hemostasis.
- Explain the physiologic basis of acute disseminated intravascular coagulation.

Bleeding disorders or impairment of blood coagulation can result from defects in any of the factors that contribute to hemostasis. Bleeding can occur as a result of disorders associated with platelet number or function, coagulation factors, and blood vessel integrity.

BLEEDING DISORDERS

- Bleeding disorders are caused by defects associated with platelets, coagulation factors, and vessel integrity.
- Disorders of platelet plug formation include a decrease in platelet numbers due to inadequate platelet production (bone marrow dysfunction), excess platelet destruction (thrombocytopenia), abnormal platelet function (thrombocytopathia), or defects in von Willebrand factor.
- Impairment of the coagulation stage of hemostasis is caused by a deficiency in one or more of the clotting factors.
- Disorders of blood vessel integrity result from structurally weak vessels or vessel damage due to inflammation and immune mechanisms.

Bleeding Associated With Platelet Disorders

Bleeding due to platelet disorders reflects a decrease in platelet number due to decreased production or increased destruction or impaired function of platelets. Spontaneous bleeding from platelet disorders most often involves small vessels of the mucous membranes and skin. Common sites of bleeding are the mucous membranes of the nose, mouth, gastrointestinal tract, and uterine cavity. Cutaneous bleeding is seen as pinpoint hemorrhages (petechiae) and purple areas of bruising (purpura) in dependent areas where the capillary pressure is higher (Fig. 13-4). Petechiae are seen almost exclusively in conditions of platelet deficiency, and not platelet dysfunction. Bleeding of the intracranial vessels is a rare danger with severe platelet depletion.

Thrombocytopenia

A reduction in platelet number, also referred to as *thrombocytopenia,* is an important cause of generalized bleeding.

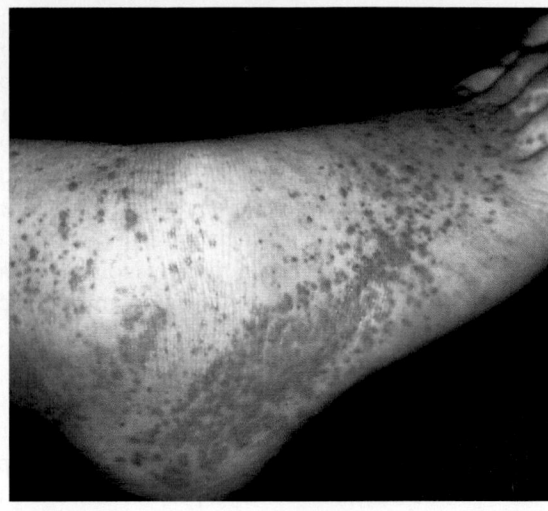

FIGURE 13-4 • Foot with acute purpura and petechiae. (From Hall J. C. [2000]. *Sauer's manual of skin diseases* [8th ed., p. 112]. Philadelphia: Lippincott Williams & Wilkins.)

Thrombocytopenia usually refers to a decrease in the number of circulating platelets to a level less than 100,000/μL.[2] The greater the decrease in the platelet count, the greater the risk of bleeding. Thrombocytopenia can result from a decrease in platelet production, increased sequestration of platelets in the spleen, or decreased platelet survival.

Decreased platelet production due to loss of bone marrow function occurs in aplastic anemia (see Chapter 14); replacement of bone marrow by malignant cells, such as occurs in leukemia, also results in decreased production of platelets. Radiation therapy and drugs such as those used in the treatment of cancer may depress bone marrow function and reduce platelet production. Infection with human immunodeficiency virus (HIV) or cytomegalovirus may suppress the production of megakaryocytes, the platelet precursors.

Production of platelets may be normal, but excessive pooling of platelets in the spleen may occur. Although the spleen normally sequesters 30% to 40% of the platelets before release into the circulation, the proportion can be as great as 90% when the spleen is enlarged in splenomegaly.[1] When necessary, hypersplenic thrombocytopenia may be treated with splenectomy.

Reduced platelet survival is caused by a variety of immune and nonimmune mechanisms. Platelet destruction may be caused by antiplatelet antibodies. The antibodies may be directed against platelet self-antigens or against antigens on the platelets from blood transfusions or pregnancy. The antibodies target the platelet membrane glycoproteins GPIIb/IIIa and GPIb/Ix. Nonimmune destruction of platelets results from mechanical injury due to prosthetic heart valves or malignant hypertension, which results in small vessel narrowing. In acute DIC or thrombotic thrombocytopenic purpura, excessive platelet consumption leads to a deficiency. Massive blood or plasma transfusions may cause a dilutional thrombocytopenia because blood stored for more than 24 hours has no viable platelets.[14]

Drug-Induced Thrombocytopenia. Some drugs, such as quinine, quinidine, and certain sulfa-containing antibiotics, may induce thrombocytopenia.[15] These drugs act as haptens to induce an antigen–antibody response and formation of immune complexes that cause platelet destruction by complement-mediated lysis (see Chapter 17). In persons with drug-associated thrombocytopenia, there is a rapid fall in the platelet count within 2 to 3 days of resuming a drug, or 7 or more days (*i.e.,* the time needed to mount an immune response) after starting a drug for the first time. The platelet count rises rapidly after the drug is discontinued.

Heparin-Induced Thrombocytopenia. Heparin-induced thrombocytopenia (HIT) is associated with the anticoagulant drug heparin. Ten percent of patients treated with heparin develop a mild, transient thrombocytopenia within 2 to 5 days of starting the drug.[16] However, approximately 1% to 5% of heparin-treated patients experience life-threatening thromboembolic events 1 to 2 weeks after the start of therapy.[16] HIT is caused by an immune reaction directed against a complex of heparin and platelet factor 4, a normal component of platelet granules that binds tightly to heparin. The binding of antibody to platelet factor 4 produces immune complexes that activate the remaining platelets, leading to thrombosis. In addition, prothrombotic platelet particles and induction of tissue factor continue to promote coagulation.

The thrombosis of HIT results in complications such as deep vein thrombosis, pulmonary embolism, myocardial infarction, and stroke, and is associated with a mortality rate of about 20% to 30%.[16] The thrombocytopenia of HIT is due to the clearance of platelets by the reticuloendothelial system and results in only a moderate reduction in the platelet count.

The treatment of HIT requires the immediate discontinuation of heparin therapy and the use of alternative anticoagulants to prevent thrombosis recurrence. The newer low–molecular-weight heparin has been shown to be effective in reducing the incidence of heparin-induced complications compared with the older, high–molecular-weight form of the drug.

Immune Thrombocytopenic Purpura. Immune thrombocytopenic purpura (ITP), an autoimmune disorder, results in platelet antibody formation and excess destruction of platelets. The disorder can occur in the absence of any known risk factors (primary or idiopathic ITP) or as a secondary disorder due to an underlying disorder, and as an acute (duration of 6 months or less) or chronic disorder. Secondary forms of ITP may be associated with acquired immunodeficiency syndrome (AIDS), systemic lupus erythematosus, antiphospholipid syndrome, chronic lymphocytic leukemia, lymphoma, hepatitis C, and drugs such as heparin and quinidine.

About half of the cases of ITP occur as an acute primary disorder in children, affecting both boys and girls.[17] The disorder occurs in young children (5 years of age) and usually follows a viral infection. It is characterized by sudden onset of petechiae and purpura and is usually a self-limited disorder requiring no treatment. Most children recover in a few weeks.

In contrast, primary ITP is often a chronic disorder in adults with an insidious onset that seldom follows an infection. It is a disease of young people, with a peak incidence between the ages of 18 and 40 years, and is seen three times as often in women as in men.

The thrombocytopenia that occurs in ITP is thought to result from multiple mechanisms, including antiplatelet antibodies against glycoproteins (IIb/IIIa and Ib/IX) in the platelet membrane. The platelets, which are made more susceptible to phagocytosis because of the antibody, are destroyed in the spleen. In addition, plasma levels of thrombopoietin, the major factor that stimulates growth and development of megakaryocytes, is not elevated in persons with ITP, as opposed to persons with thrombocytopenia from other causes such as chemotherapy or bone marrow failure.[18]

Manifestations of ITP include a history of bruising, bleeding from gums, epistaxis (*i.e.,* nosebleed), melena, and abnormal menstrual bleeding in those with moderately reduced platelet counts. Because the spleen is the site of platelet destruction, splenic enlargement may occur. The condition may be discovered incidentally or as a result of signs of bleeding, often into the skin (*i.e.,* purpura and petechiae) or oral mucosa. About half of adults with primary ITP present with a platelet count of less than 10,000/μL and are at risk for internal hemorrhage.[17]

Diagnosis of ITP usually is based on severe thrombocytopenia (platelet counts less than 20,000 to 30,000/μL), and exclusion of other causes. Tests for the platelet-bound antibodies are available but lack specificity (*e.g.,* they react with platelet antibodies from other sources). The secondary form of ITP sometimes mimics the idiopathic form of the disorder; therefore, the diagnosis is made only after excluding other known causes of thrombocytopenia.

The decision to treat ITP is based on the platelet count and the degree of bleeding. Many persons with ITP do well without treatment. Corticosteroids are usually used as initial therapy. Other effective initial treatments include intravenous immune globulin. However, this treatment is expensive and the beneficial effect lasts only 1 to 2 weeks. Because the spleen is the major site of antibody formation and platelet destruction, splenectomy is the traditional second-line treatment for persons who relapse or do not respond to drugs.[17] Immunosuppressive therapy may be used for persons who are refractory to other forms of treatment.

Thrombotic Thrombocytopenic Purpura. Thrombotic thrombocytopenic purpura (TTP) is a combination of thrombocytopenia, hemolytic anemia, renal failure, fever, and neurologic abnormalities. It is a rare disorder, occurring predominantly in adult women. The pathogenesis is elusive but likely results from introduction of platelet-aggregating substances into the circulation. The underlying cause of many cases is the deficiency of an enzyme (designated ADAMTS 13) that degrades large–molecular-weight multimers of vWF, allowing them to accumulate and cause platelet aggregation and adhesion to the endothelium.[14] The enzyme deficiency may be inherited or acquired as a result of antibody directed against the enzyme.

TTP usually occurs in previously healthy persons but may be associated with autoimmune collagen diseases, drugs, infections such as HIV, and pregnancy.[2] The disorder is similar to DIC but does not involve the clotting system. Toxins produced by some strains of *Escherichia coli* (*e.g., E. coli* O157:H7) cause endothelial injury and are responsible for a similar condition, *hemolytic uremic syndrome.*

The onset of TTP is abrupt and the outcome may be fatal. Widespread vascular occlusions result from thrombi in the arterioles and capillaries of many organs, including the heart, brain, and kidneys. Erythrocytes become fragmented as they circulate through the partly occluded vessels, causing hemolytic anemia and jaundice. The clinical manifestations include purpura, petechiae, vaginal bleeding, and neurologic symptoms ranging from headache to seizures and altered consciousness. Anemia is universal and may be marked. About half of patients have azotemia due to renal failure.[2]

Emergency treatment for TTP includes *plasmapheresis,* a procedure that involves removal of plasma from withdrawn blood and replacement with fresh-frozen plasma. Plasma infusion provides the deficient enzyme. With plasmapheresis and plasma infusion treatment, there is a complete recovery in 80% of cases.[2]

Impaired Platelet Function

Impaired platelet function (also called *thrombocytopathia*) may result from inherited disorders of adhesion (*e.g.,* von Willebrand disease) or acquired defects caused by drugs, disease, or surgery involving extracorporeal circulation (*i.e.,* cardiopulmonary bypass). Defective platelet function is also common in uremia, presumably because of unexcreted waste products.

The use of aspirin and other nonsteroidal anti-inflammatory drugs (NSAIDs) is the most common cause of impaired platelet function. Aspirin produces irreversible acetylation of platelet cyclooxygenase activity and consequently the synthesis of TXA_2, which is required for platelet aggregation. The effect of aspirin on platelet aggregation lasts for the life of the platelet—usually approximately 8 to 9 days. In contrast to the effects of aspirin, the inhibition of cyclooxygenase by other NSAIDs is reversible and lasts only for the duration of drug action. Aspirin (81 mg daily) commonly is used to prevent formation of arterial thrombi and reduce the risk for heart attack and stroke. Chart 13-2 lists other drugs that impair platelet function.

Bleeding Associated With Coagulation Factor Deficiencies

Blood coagulation defects can result from deficiencies or impaired function of one or more of the clotting factors, including vWF. Deficiencies can arise because of inherited disease, or defective synthesis or increased consumption of the clotting factors. Bleeding resulting from clotting factor deficiencies typically occurs after injury or trauma. Large bruises, hematomas, and prolonged bleeding into the gastrointestinal or urinary tracts or joints are common.

| CHART 13-2 | **DRUGS THAT MAY PREDISPOSE TO BLEEDING*** |

Interference With Platelet Production or Function
Acetazolamide
Antimetabolite and anticancer drugs
Antibiotics such as penicillin and the cephalosporins
Aspirin and salicylates
Carbamazepine
Clofibrate
Colchicine
Dipyridamole
Thiazide diuretics
Gold salts
Heparin
Nonsteroidal anti-inflammatory drugs (NSAIDs)
Quinine derivatives (quinidine and hydroxychloroquine)
Sulfonamides

Interference With Coagulation Factors
Amiodarone
Anabolic steroids
Warfarin
Heparin

Decrease in Vitamin K Levels
Antibiotics
Clofibrate

*This list is not intended to be inclusive.

Inherited Disorders

Hemophilia A and von Willebrand disease are two of the most common inherited disorders of bleeding. Hemophilia A (factor VIII deficiency) affects 1 in 5000 male live births and von Willebrand disease more than 1 in 1000 persons.[19] Hemophilia B, a deficiency of factor IX, occurs in approximately 1 in 20,000 persons, accounting for 15% of people with hemophilia.[2] It is genetically and clinically similar to hemophilia A.

Hemophilia A and von Willebrand disease are caused by defects involving the factor VIII–vWF complex. Von Willebrand factor, which is synthesized by the endothelium and megakaryocytes, is required for platelet adhesion to the subendothelial matrix of the blood vessel. It also serves as the carrier for factor VIII, and is important for the stability of factor VIII in the circulation by preventing its proteolysis. Factor VIII coagulant protein, the functional portion, is produced by the liver and endothelial cells. Thus, factor VIII and vWF, synthesized separately, come together and circulate in the plasma as a unit that serves to promote clotting and adhesion of platelets to the vessel wall.

Von Willebrand Disease. Von Willebrand disease is a relatively common hereditary bleeding disorder characterized by a deficiency or defect in vWF. It affects both men and women and is typically diagnosed in adulthood.[20,21] In most cases, it is transmitted as an autosomal dominant disorder, but several rare autosomal recessive variants have been identified.[14]

As many as 20 variants of von Willebrand disease have been described.[14] These variants can be grouped into two categories: types 1 and 3, which are associated with reduced levels of vWF; and type 2, which is characterized by defects in vWF. Type 1, an autosomal dominant disorder, accounts for approximately 70% of cases and is relatively mild. Type 2, also an autosomal dominant disorder, accounts for about 25% of cases and is associated with mild to moderate bleeding. Type 3, which is a relatively rare autosomal recessive disorder, is associated with extremely low levels of functional vWF and correspondingly severe clinical manifestations.

Persons with von Willebrand disease have a compound defect involving platelet function and the coagulation pathway. Clinical manifestations include spontaneous bleeding from the nose, mouth, and gastrointestinal tract, excessive menstrual flow, and a prolonged bleeding time in the presence of a normal platelet count. Most cases (*i.e.,* types 1 and 2) are mild and require no treatment, and many persons with the disorder are diagnosed when surgery or dental extraction results in prolonged bleeding. In severe cases (*i.e.,* type 3), life-threatening gastrointestinal bleeding and joint hemorrhage may be similar to that seen in hemophilia.

The bleeding associated with von Willebrand disease is usually mild, and no treatment is routinely administered other than avoidance of aspirin. Desmopressin acetate (DDAVP), a synthetic analog of the hormone vasopressin, is used in the treatment of type 1 von Willebrand disease and for establishing hemostasis during surgical or dental procedures.[20,22] DDAVP stimulates the endothelial cells to release stored vWF and plasminogen activator. The drug is available as an intranasal spray. In the future, recombinant vWF may be available, and clinical trials determining the efficacy of interleukin-11 in increasing vWF and factor VIII levels are in progress.[20]

Hemophilia A. Hemophilia A is an X-linked recessive disorder that primarily affects males. Although it is a hereditary disorder, there is no family history of the disorder in approximately 30% of newly diagnosed cases, suggesting that it has arisen as a new mutation in the factor VIII gene.[14] Approximately 90% of persons with hemophilia produce insufficient quantities of the factor, and 10% produce a defective form. The percentage of normal factor VIII activity in the circulation depends on the genetic defect and determines the severity of hemophilia (*i.e.,* 6% to 30% in mild hemophilia, 2% to 5% in moderate hemophilia, and 1% or less in severe forms of hemophilia). In mild or moderate forms of the disease, bleeding usually does not occur unless there is a local lesion or trauma such as surgery or a dental procedure. The mild disorder may not be detected in childhood. In severe hemophilia, bleeding usually occurs in childhood (*e.g.,* it may be noticed at the time of circumcision) and is spontaneous and severe, often occurring several times a month.

Characteristically, bleeding occurs in soft tissues, the gastrointestinal tract, and the hip, knee, elbow, and ankle joints. Spontaneous joint bleeding usually begins when a child begins to walk. Often, a target joint is prone to repeated bleeding. The bleeding causes inflammation of the synovium, with acute pain and swelling. Without proper treatment, chronic bleeding and inflammation cause joint fibrosis and contractures, resulting in major disability. Muscle hematomas may be present in 30% of episodes, and intracranial hemorrhage, although uncommon, is an important cause of death.[23]

The prevention of trauma is important in persons with hemophilia. Aspirin and other NSAIDs that affect platelet function should be avoided. Factor VIII replacement therapy (either recombinant or heat-treated concentrates from human plasma) administered at home has reduced the typical musculoskeletal damage. It is initiated when bleeding occurs or as prophylaxis with repeated bleeding episodes. The newer recombinant products and continuous-infusion pumps may allow prevention rather than therapy for hemorrhage. The development of inhibitory antibodies to recombinant factor VIII is still a major complication of treatment; 10% to 15% of treated persons produce high titers of antibodies that bind to and inhibit factor VIII. The rate of antibody production for plasma-derived products is approximately the same.

Current factor VIII products (both plasma derived and recombinant) are considered very safe as a result of technological advances of the last two decades.[24] Until the mid-1980s, before routine screening of blood for HIV antibodies was instituted, thousands of patients with hemophilia received plasma-derived factor VIII that was contaminated with HIV, and many developed AIDS.[14] Effective donor screening and development of purification and viral inactivation procedures now provide a safer product. A number of recombinant factor VIII preparations are available, the first being approved by the U.S. Food and Drug Administration (FDA) in 1992. These products were made with the use of blood-derived additives of human or animal origin, such as albumin. These additives were needed to keep the cells viable so they could produce the factor VIII protein. In 2003, the FDA approved a new recombinant factor VIII product (Advate) produced without using additives derived from human or animal blood in the manufacturing process.[24]

The cloning of the factor VIII gene and progress in gene delivery systems have led to the hope that hemophilia A may be cured by gene replacement therapy. Carrier detection and prenatal diagnosis can now be done by analysis of direct gene mutation or DNA linkage studies. Prenatal amniocentesis or chorionic villus sampling is used to predict complications and determine therapy. It may eventually be used to select patients for gene addition.

With mild hemophilia A, the person's endogenously produced factor VIII can be released by the administration of DDAVP.[14] In persons with moderate to severe factor VIII deficiency, the stored levels of factor VIII are insufficient, and DDAVP treatment is ineffective.

Acquired Disorders

Coagulation factors V, VII, IX, X, XI, and XII, prothrombin, and fibrinogen are synthesized in the liver. In liver disease, synthesis of these clotting factors is reduced, and bleeding may result. Of the coagulation factors synthesized in the liver, factors II, VII, IX, and X and prothrombin require the presence of vitamin K for normal activity. In vitamin K deficiency, the liver produces the clotting factor, but in an inactive form. Vitamin K is a fat-soluble vitamin that is continuously being synthesized by intestinal bacteria. This means that a deficiency in vitamin K is not likely to occur unless intestinal synthesis is interrupted or absorption of the vitamin is impaired. Vitamin K deficiency can occur in the newborn infant before the establishment of the intestinal flora; it can also occur as a result of treatment with broad-spectrum antibiotics that destroy intestinal flora. Because vitamin K is a fat-soluble vitamin, its absorption requires bile salts. Vitamin K deficiency may result from impaired fat absorption caused by liver or gallbladder disease.

Bleeding Associated With Vascular Disorders

Bleeding resulting from vascular disorders, sometimes called *nonthrombocytopenic purpura,* is relatively common and results in mild bleeding disorders.[14] These disorders may occur because of structurally weak vessel walls or because of damage to vessels by inflammation or immune responses. Most often they are characterized by easy bruising and the spontaneous appearance of petechiae and purpura of the skin and mucous membranes. In persons with bleeding disorders caused by vascular defects, the platelet count and results of other tests for coagulation factors are normal.

Among the vascular disorders that cause bleeding are hemorrhagic telangiectasia, an uncommon autosomal dominant disorder characterized by thin-walled, dilated capillaries and arterioles; vitamin C deficiency (*i.e.,* scurvy), resulting in poor collagen synthesis and failure of the endothelial cells to be cemented together properly, which causes a fragile vascular wall; Cushing disease, causing protein wasting and loss of vessel tissue support because of excess cortisol; and senile purpura (*i.e.,* bruising in elderly persons), caused by impaired collagen synthesis in the aging process. Vascular defects also occur in the course of DIC or as a result of microthrombi and corticosteroid therapy.

Disseminated Intravascular Coagulation

Disseminated intravascular coagulation is a paradox in the hemostatic sequence and is characterized by widespread coagulation and bleeding in the vascular compartment. It is not a primary disease but occurs as a complication of a wide variety of conditions. DIC begins with massive activation of the coagulation sequence as a result of unregulated generation of thrombin, resulting in systemic formation of fibrin. In addition, levels of all the major anticoagulants are reduced (Fig. 13-5). The microthrombi that

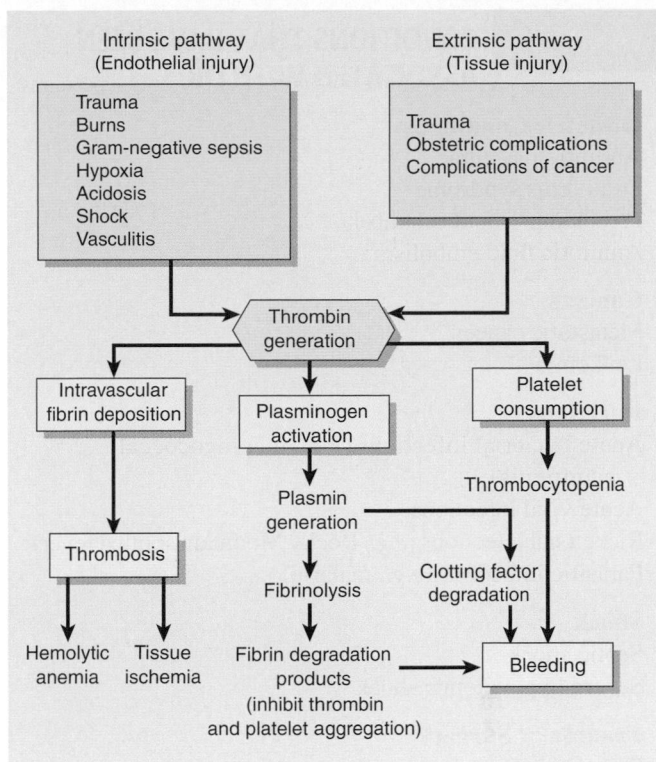

FIGURE 13-5 • Pathophysiology of disseminated intravascular coagulation.

result cause vessel occlusion and tissue ischemia. Multiple organ failure may ensue. Clot formation consumes all available coagulation proteins and platelets, and severe hemorrhage results.

The disorder can be initiated by activation of the intrinsic or extrinsic pathway, or both. Activation through the extrinsic pathway occurs with liberation of tissue factors, and is associated with obstetric complications, trauma, bacterial sepsis, and cancers. The intrinsic pathway may be activated through extensive endothelial damage, with activation of factor XII. Endothelial damage may be caused by viruses, infections, immune mechanisms, stasis of blood, or temperature extremes. Impaired anticoagulation pathways are also associated with reduced levels of antithrombin and the protein C anticoagulant system in DIC. There is increasing evidence that the underlying cause of DIC is infection or inflammation, and the cytokines (tumor necrosis factor, interleukin-1, and others) liberated in the process are the pivotal mediators.[25,26] These cytokines not only mediate inflammation, but can also increase the expression of tissue factor on endothelial cells and simultaneously decrease the expression of thrombomodulin. Thrombomodulin, a glycoprotein that is present on the cell membrane of endothelial cells, binds thrombin and acts as an additional regulatory mechanism in coagulation. The net effect is a shift in balance toward a procoagulant state.[25]

Common clinical conditions that may cause DIC include obstetric disorders, accounting for 50% of cases, massive trauma, shock, sepsis, and malignant disease.[14] Chart 13-3 summarizes the conditions associated with DIC.

| CHART 13-3 | CONDITIONS THAT HAVE BEEN ASSOCIATED WITH DIC |

Obstetric Conditions
Abruptio placentae
Dead fetus syndrome
Preeclampsia and eclampsia
Amniotic fluid embolism

Cancers
Metastatic cancer
Leukemia

Infections
Acute bacterial infections (*e.g.*, meningococcal meningitis)
Acute viral infections
Rickettsial infections (*e.g.*, Rocky Mountain spotted fever)
Parasitic infections (*e.g.*, malaria)

Shock
Septic shock
Severe hypovolemic shock

Trauma or Surgery
Burns
Massive trauma
Surgery involving extracorporeal circulation
Snake bite
Heatstroke

Hematologic Conditions
Blood transfusion reactions

The factors involved in the conditions that cause DIC are often interrelated. In obstetric complications, tissue factors released from necrotic placental or fetal tissue or amniotic fluid may enter the circulation, inciting DIC. The hypoxia, shock, and acidosis that may coexist also contribute by causing endothelial injury. Gram-negative bacterial infections result in the release of endotoxins, which activate both the extrinsic pathway by release of tissue factor and the intrinsic pathway through endothelial damage. Endotoxins also inhibit the activity of protein C. Antigen–antibody complexes associated with infection can activate platelets through complement fragments.[14]

Although coagulation and formation of microemboli characterize DIC, its acute manifestations usually are more directly related to the bleeding problems that occur. The bleeding may be present as petechiae, purpura, oozing from puncture sites, or severe hemorrhage. Uncontrolled postpartum bleeding may indicate DIC. Microemboli may obstruct blood vessels and cause tissue hypoxia and necrotic damage to organ structures, such as the kidneys, heart, lungs, and brain. As a result, common clinical signs may be due to renal, circulatory, or respiratory failure, acute bleeding ulcers, or convulsions and coma.

A form of hemolytic anemia may develop as red cells are damaged passing through vessels partially blocked by thrombus.

The treatment of DIC is directed toward managing the primary disease, replacing clotting components, and preventing further activation of clotting mechanisms. Transfusions of fresh-frozen plasma, platelets, or fibrinogen-containing cryoprecipitate may correct the clotting factor deficiency. Heparin may be given to decrease blood coagulation, thereby interrupting the clotting process. Heparin therapy is controversial, however, and the risk of hemorrhage may limit its use to severe cases. It typically is given as a continuous intravenous infusion that can be interrupted promptly if bleeding is accentuated. Tissue factor pathway inhibitors, antithrombin, protein C concentrates, and anti-inflammatory cytokines such as interleukin-10 are being evaluated in clinical trials as potential therapies.[25]

IN SUMMARY, bleeding disorders or impairment of blood coagulation can result from defects in any of the factors that contribute to hemostasis: platelets, coagulation factors, or vascular integrity. The number of circulating platelets can be decreased (*i.e.*, thrombocytopenia) because of reduced bone marrow production, excess pooling in the spleen, or immune destruction. Impaired platelet function (*i.e.*, thrombocytopathia) is caused by inherited disorders (von Willebrand disease) or results from drugs or disease. Impairment of blood coagulation can result from deficiencies of one or more of the known clotting factors. Deficiencies can arise because of acquired disorders (*i.e.*, liver disease or vitamin K deficiency) or inherited diseases (*i.e.*, hemophilia A or von Willebrand disease). Bleeding may also occur from structurally weak vessels that result from impaired synthesis of vessel wall components (*i.e.*, vitamin C deficiency, excessive cortisol levels as in Cushing disease, or the aging process) or from damage by genetic mechanisms (*i.e.*, hemorrhagic telangiectasia) or the presence of microthrombi.

Disseminated intravascular coagulation (DIC) is characterized by widespread coagulation and bleeding in the vascular compartment. It begins with massive activation of the coagulation cascade and generation of microthrombi that cause vessel occlusion and tissue ischemia. Clot formation consumes all available coagulation proteins and platelets, and severe hemorrhage results. ■

Review Exercises

1. A 55-year-old man has begun taking one 81-mg aspirin tablet daily on the recommendation of his physician. The physician had told him that this would help to prevent heart attack and stroke.

   A. *What is the action of aspirin in terms of heart attack and stroke prevention?*

B. The drug clopidogrel (Plavix) is often prescribed along with aspirin to prevent thrombosis in persons with severe atherosclerotic disease who are at risk for myocardial infarction or stroke. Explain the rationale for using the two drugs.

2. The drug desmopressin acetate (DDAVP), which is a synthetic analog of arginine vasopressin, increases the half-life of factor VIII and is sometimes used to treat bleeding in males with mild hemophilia.

   A. Explain.

3. A 29-year-old new mother, who delivered her infant 3 days ago, is admitted to the hospital with chest pain and is diagnosed as having venous thrombosis with pulmonary emboli.

   A. What factors would contribute to this woman's risk of developing thromboemboli?

4. The new mother is admitted to the intensive care unit and started on low–molecular-weight heparin and warfarin. She is told that she will be discharged in a day or two and will remain on the heparin for 5 days and the warfarin for at least 3 months.

   A. Use Figure 13-3 to explain the action of heparin and warfarin. Why is heparin administered for 5 days during the initiation of warfarin treatment?

   B. Anticoagulation with heparin and warfarin is not a definitive treatment for clot removal in pulmonary embolism, but a form of secondary prevention. Explain.

References

1. Guyton A. C., Hall J. E. (2006). *Textbook of medical physiology* (11th ed., pp. 457–468). Philadelphia: Elsevier Saunders.
2. Schwarting R., Kocher W. D., McKenzie S., et al. (2005). Hematopathology. In Rubin E., Gorstein F., Rubin R., et al. (Eds.), *Rubin's pathology: Clinicopathologic foundations of medicine* (4th ed., pp. 1048–1062). Philadelphia: Lippincott Williams & Wilkins.
3. Schafer, A. I. (2004). Thrombocytosis. *New England Journal of Medicine* 350, 1211–1219.
4. Ross M. H., Kaye G. I., Wojciech P. (2003). *Histology: A text and atlas* (4th ed., pp. 229–231). Philadelphia: Lippincott Williams & Wilkins.
5. Messmore H. L., Jeske W. P., Wehrmacher W., et al. (2005). Antiplatelet agents: Current drugs and future trends. *Hematology and Oncology Clinics of North America* 19, 87–117.
6. Aster R. H., Curtis B. R., Bougie D. W., et al. (on behalf of the Scientific and Standardization Committee of the International Society of Thrombo-sis and Hemostasis). (2006). Thrombocytopenia associated with the use of GP IIb/IIIa inhibitors: Position paper of the 15th Working Group on Thrombocytopenia and GP IIB/IIIa Inhibitors. *Journal of Thrombosis and Hemostasis* 6, 678–679.
7. Hambleton J., O'Reilly R. A. (2001). Drugs used in disorders of coagulation. In Katzung B. G. (Ed.), *Basic and clinical pharmacology* (8th ed., pp. 564–574). Norwalk, CT: Appleton & Lange.
8. Bloomenthal D., von Dadelszen P., Liston R., et al. (2002). The effect of factor V Leiden carriage on maternal and fetal health. *Canadian Medical Association Journal* 167, 48–54.
9. Mitchell R. N. (2005). Hemodynamic disorders, thrombosis, and shock. In Kumar V., Abbas A. K., Fausto N. (Eds.), *Robbins and Cotran pathologic basis of disease* (7th ed., pp. 124–135). Philadelphia: Elsevier Saunders.
10. Chrousos G. P., Zoumakis E. N., Gravania A. (2001). The gonadal hormones and inhibitors. In Katzung B. G. (Ed.), *Basic and clinical pharmacology* (8th ed., pp. 683–684). Norwalk, CT: Appleton & Lange.
11. Levine J. S., Branch D. W., Rausch J. (2002). The antiphospholipid syndrome. *New England Journal of Medicine* 346, 752–763.
12. Hanly J. C. (2003). Antiphospholipid syndrome: An overview. *Canadian Medical Association Journal* 168, 1675–1682.
13. Lim W., Crowther M. A., Eikelboom J. W. (2006). Management of antiphospholipid antibody syndrome. *Journal of the American Medical Association* 295, 1050–1057.
14. Aster J. C. (2005). Red cells and bleeding disorders. In Kumar V., Abbas K., Fausto N. (Eds.), *Robbins and Cotran pathologic basis of disease* (7th ed., pp. 649–659). Philadelphia: Elsevier Saunders.
15. van den Bemt P. M., Meyboom R. H., Egberts A. C. (2004). Drug-induced immune thrombocytopenia. *Drug Safety* 27, 1243–1252.
16. Franchini M. (2005). Heparin-induced thrombocytopenia: An update. *Thrombosis Journal* 3, 14–18.
17. Cines D. B., Blanchette V. S. (2002). Immune thrombocytopenic purpura. *New England Journal of Medicine* 346, 995–1008.
18. Bromberg M. E. (2006). Immune thrombocytopenia purpura: The changing therapeutic landscape. *New England Journal of Medicine* 355, 1643–1645.
19. Mannucci P. M., Tuddenham E. G. D. (2001). The hemophilias: From royal genes to gene therapy. *New England Journal of Medicine* 344, 1773–1779.
20. Mannucci P. M. (2004). Treatment of von Willebrand's disease. *New England Journal of Medicine* 351, 683–694.
21. Sadler J. V. (2005). New concepts in von Willebrand disease. *Annual Review of Medicine* 56, 173–180.
22. Mannucci P. M. (1997). Desmopressin (DDAVP) in the treatment of bleeding disorders: The first 20 years. *Blood* 90, 2515–2521.
23. Klinge J., Ananyeva N. M., Hauser C., et al. (2002). Hemophilia A: From basic science to clinical practice. *Seminars in Thrombosis and Hemostasis* 28, 309–322.
24. FDA Talk Paper. (2003). New recombinant antihemophilic factor licensed. [On-line.] Available: www.fda.gov/bbs/topics/ANSWERS/2003/ANSO1241.html. Accessed February 1, 2008.
25. Franchini M., Lippi G., Manzato F. (2006). Recent acquisitions in the pathophysiology, diagnosis and treatment of disseminated intravascular coagulation. *Thrombosis Journal* 4, 4–12.
26. Van der Poll T., Jonge E., Levi M. (2001). Regulatory role of cytokines in disseminated intravascular coagulation. *Seminars in Thrombosis and Hemostasis* 27, 639–651.

Visit the**Point** **http://thePoint.lww.com for animations, journal articles, and more!**

Chapter 14

Disorders of Red Blood Cells

KATHRYN J. GASPARD

> Although the lungs provide the means for gas exchange between the external and internal environments, it is the hemoglobin in the red blood cells that transports oxygen to the tissues. The red blood cells also function as carriers of carbon dioxide and participate in acid-base balance. The function of the red blood cells, in terms of oxygen transport, is discussed in Chapter 27, and acid-base balance in Chapter 32. This chapter focuses on the red blood cell, anemia, transfusion therapy, polycythemia, and age-related changes in the red blood cells.

THE RED BLOOD CELL

After completing this section of the chapter, you should be able to meet the following objectives:

- Trace the development of a red blood cell from erythroblast to erythrocyte.
- Discuss the function of iron in the formation of hemoglobin.
- Describe the formation, transport, and elimination of bilirubin.
- Explain the function of the enzyme glucose-6-phosphate dehydrogenase in the red blood cell.
- State the meaning of the red blood cell count, percentage of reticulocytes, hemoglobin, hematocrit, mean corpuscular volume, and mean corpuscular hemoglobin concentration as it relates to the diagnosis of anemia.

The erythrocytes, 500 to 1000 times more numerous than other blood cells, are the most common type of blood cell. The mature red blood cell, the erythrocyte, is a non-nucleated, biconcave disk (Fig. 14-1). This unique shape contributes in two ways to the oxygen transport function of the erythrocyte. The biconcave shape provides a larger surface area for oxygen diffusion than would a spherical cell of the same volume, and the thinness of the cell membrane enables oxygen to diffuse rapidly between the exterior and the innermost regions of the cell (Fig. 14-2A).

Another structural feature that facilitates the transport function of the red blood cell is the flexibility of its membrane.

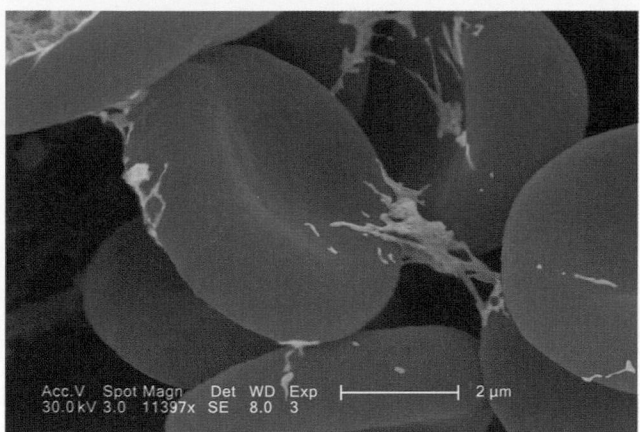

FIGURE 14-1 • A highly magnified (×11,397) scanning electron micrograph of a number of red blood cells found enmeshed in a fibrinous matrix on the luminal surface of an indwelling vascular catheter. Note the biconcave shape of each erythrocyte, which increases the surface area of these hemoglobin-filled cells, thus promoting more effective gas exchange. (Centers for Disease Control and Prevention Public Images Library, Courtesy Janice Carr.)

The biconcave shape and flexibility of the red cell membrane are maintained by a complex network of fibrous proteins, especially one called *spectrin* (Fig. 14-3). Spectrin forms an attachment with another protein, called *ankyrin,* that resides on the inner surface of the membrane and is anchored to an integral protein that spans the membrane. This unique arrangement of proteins imparts elasticity and stability to the membrane and allows it to deform easily.

The function of the red blood cell, facilitated by the hemoglobin molecule, is to transport oxygen to the tissues. Because oxygen is poorly soluble in plasma, about 95% to 98% is carried bound to hemoglobin. The hemoglobin molecule is composed of two pairs of structurally different alpha (α) and beta (β) polypeptide chains (see Fig. 14-2B). Each of the four polypeptide chains consists of a globin (protein) portion and a heme unit, which surrounds an atom of iron that binds oxygen.[1] Thus, each molecule of hemoglobin can carry four molecules of oxygen. Hemoglobin

is a natural pigment; because of its iron content, it appears reddish when oxygen is attached and has a bluish cast when deoxygenated. The production of each type of globin chain is controlled by individual structural genes with five different gene loci. Mutations, which can occur anywhere in these five loci, have resulted in over 550 types of abnormal hemoglobin molecules.[1]

RED BLOOD CELLS

- The function of red blood cells, facilitated by the iron-containing hemoglobin molecule, is to transport oxygen from the lungs to the tissues.

- The production of red blood cells, which is regulated by erythropoietin, occurs in the bone marrow and requires iron, vitamin B_{12}, and folate.

- The red blood cell, which has a life span of approximately 120 days, is broken down in the spleen; the degradation products such as iron and amino acids are recycled.

- The heme molecule, which is released from the red blood cell during the degradation process, is converted to bilirubin and transported to the liver, where it is removed and rendered water soluble for elimination in the bile.

The two major types of normal hemoglobin are adult hemoglobin (HbA) and fetal hemoglobin (HbF). HbA consists of a pair of α chains and a pair of β chains. HbF is the predominant hemoglobin in the fetus from the third through the ninth months of gestation. It has a pair of gamma (γ) chains substituted for the α chains. Because of this chain substitution, HbF has a higher affinity for oxygen than adult hemoglobin. This affinity facilitates the transfer of oxygen across the placenta from the HbA in the mother's blood to the HbF in the fetus's blood. HbF is replaced within 6 months of birth with HbA.

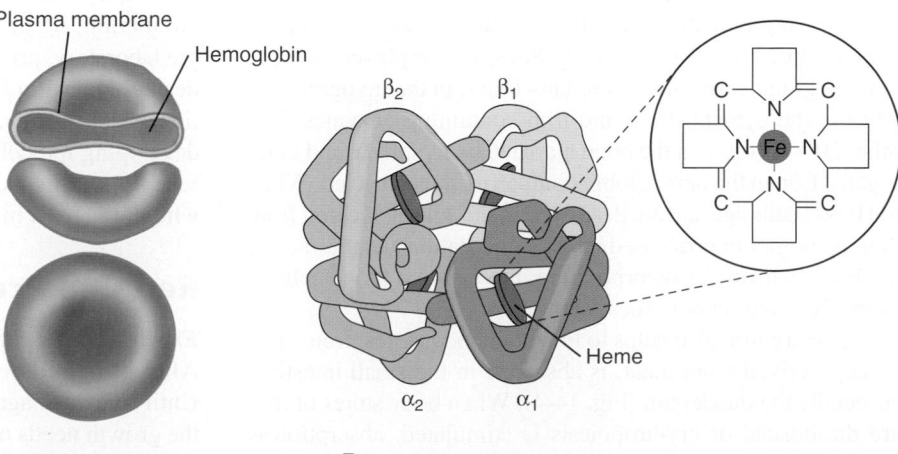

FIGURE 14-2 • (A) Biconcave structure of the red blood cell as shown in cross-section and in lateral surface view. (B) Hemoglobin molecule, showing the four iron(Fe)-containing heme subunits and their structure.

Plasma membrane
Hemoglobin

β_2 β_1

Heme

α_2 α_1

A Red blood cell

B Hemoglobin

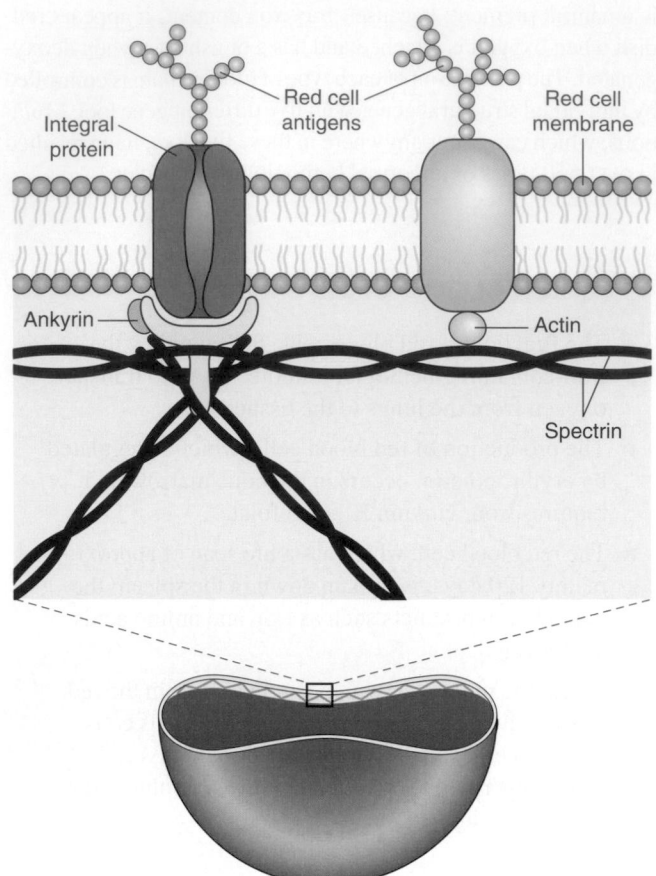

FIGURE 14-3 • Cross-sectional side view of the biconcave structure of the red blood cell and diagram showing the cytoskeleton and flexible network of spectrin proteins that attach to the ankyrin protein, a transmembrane protein that resides on the inner surface of the membrane and is anchored to an integral protein that spans the membrane.

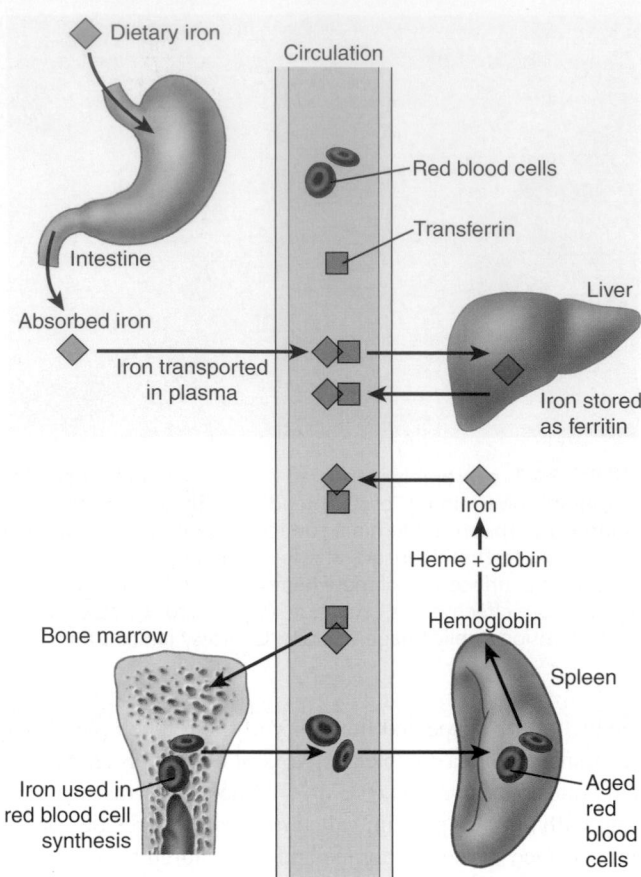

FIGURE 14-4 • Diagrammatic representation of the iron cycle, including its absorption from the gastrointestinal tract, transport in the circulation, storage in the liver, recycling from aged red cells destroyed in the spleen, and use in the bone marrow synthesis of red blood cells.

Hemoglobin Synthesis

The rate at which hemoglobin is synthesized depends on the availability of iron for heme synthesis. A lack of iron results in relatively small amounts of hemoglobin in the red blood cells. The amount of iron in the body is approximately 2 g in women and up to 6 g in men.[2] Body iron is found in several compartments. Most iron (approximately 80%) is complexed to heme in hemoglobin, with small amounts found in the myoglobin of muscle, the cytochromes, and iron-containing enzymes. The other 20% is stored in the bone marrow, liver, spleen, and other organs. Iron in the hemoglobin compartment is recycled. When red blood cells age and are destroyed in the spleen, the iron from their hemoglobin is released into the circulation and returned to the bone marrow for incorporation into new red blood cells or to the liver and other tissues for storage.

Dietary iron also helps to maintain body stores. Iron, principally derived from meat, is absorbed in the small intestine, especially the duodenum (Fig. 14-4). When body stores of iron are diminished or erythropoiesis is stimulated, absorption is increased. In iron overload, excretion of iron is accelerated. Nor-

mally, some iron is sequestered in the intestinal epithelial cells and is lost in the feces as these cells slough off. The iron that is absorbed enters the circulation, where it immediately combines with an β-globulin, *apotransferrin,* to form *transferrin,* which is then transported in the plasma. From the plasma, iron can be deposited in tissues such as the liver, where it is stored as *ferritin,* a protein–iron complex, which can easily return to the circulation. Serum ferritin levels, which can be measured in the laboratory, provide an index of body iron stores. Clinically, decreased ferritin levels usually indicate the need for prescription of iron supplements. Transferrin can also deliver iron to the developing red cell in bone marrow by binding to membrane receptors. This iron is taken up by the developing red cell, where it is used in heme synthesis.

Red Cell Production

Erythropoiesis refers to the production of red blood cells. After birth, red cells are produced in the red bone marrow. Until 5 years of age, almost all bones produce red cells to meet the growth needs of a child, after which bone marrow activity gradually declines. After 20 years of age, red cell production takes place mainly in the membranous bones of the vertebrae, sternum, ribs, and pelvis. With this reduction in activity, the red bone marrow is replaced with fatty yellow bone marrow.

The red blood cells are derived from precursor cells called *erythroblasts,* which are formed continuously from the pluripotent stem cells in the bone marrow (Fig. 14-5). The red cell precursors move through a series of divisions, each producing a smaller cell as they continue to develop into mature red blood cells. Hemoglobin synthesis begins at the early erythroblast stage and continues until the cell becomes a mature erythrocyte. During its transformation from normoblast to reticulocyte, the red blood cell accumulates hemoglobin as the nucleus condenses and is finally lost. The period from stem cell to emergence of the reticulocyte in the circulation normally takes approximately 1 week. Maturation of reticulocyte to erythrocyte takes approximately 24 to 48 hours. During this process, the red cell loses its mitochondria and ribosomes, along with its ability to produce hemoglobin and engage in oxidative metabolism. Most maturing red cells enter the blood as reticulocytes. Approximately 1% of the body's total complement of red blood cells is generated from bone marrow each day, and the reticulocyte count therefore serves as an index of the erythropoietic activity of the bone marrow.

Erythropoiesis is governed for the most part by tissue oxygen needs. Any condition that causes a decrease in the amount of oxygen that is transported in the blood produces an increase in red cell production. The oxygen content of the blood does not act directly on the bone marrow to stimulate red blood cell production. Instead, the decreased oxygen content is sensed by the peritubular cells in the kidneys, which then produce a hormone called *erythropoietin.* Normally, about 90% of all erythropoietin is produced by the kidneys, with the remaining 10% formed in the liver. Although erythropoietin is the key regulator of erythropoiesis, a number of growth factors, including granulocyte colony-stimulating factor (G-CSF), granulocyte–macrophage (GM)-CSF, and insulin-like growth factor-1 (IGF-1), are involved in the early stages of erythropoiesis.[3] Erythropoietin acts primarily in later stages of erythropoiesis to induce the erythrocyte colony-forming units to proliferate and mature through the normoblast stage into reticulocytes and mature erythrocytes. In the absence of erythropoietin, as in kidney failure, hypoxia has little or no effect on red blood cell production. Human erythropoietin can be produced by recombinant deoxyribonucleic acid (DNA) technology. It is used for the management of anemia in cases of chronic renal failure, for anemias induced by chemotherapy in persons with malignancies, and in the treatment of anemia in human immunodeficiency virus (HIV)–infected persons treated with zidovudine.[3]

Because red blood cells are released into the blood as reticulocytes, the percentage of these cells is higher when there is a marked increase in red blood cell production. In some severe forms of anemia, the reticulocytes (normally about 1%) may account for as much as 30% of the total red cell count. In some situations, red cell production is so accelerated that numerous erythroblasts appear in the blood.

Red Cell Destruction

Mature red blood cells have a life span of approximately 4 months, or 120 days. As the red blood cell ages, a number of changes occur: metabolic activity in the cell decreases, enzyme activity declines, and adenosine triphosphate (ATP) decreases.

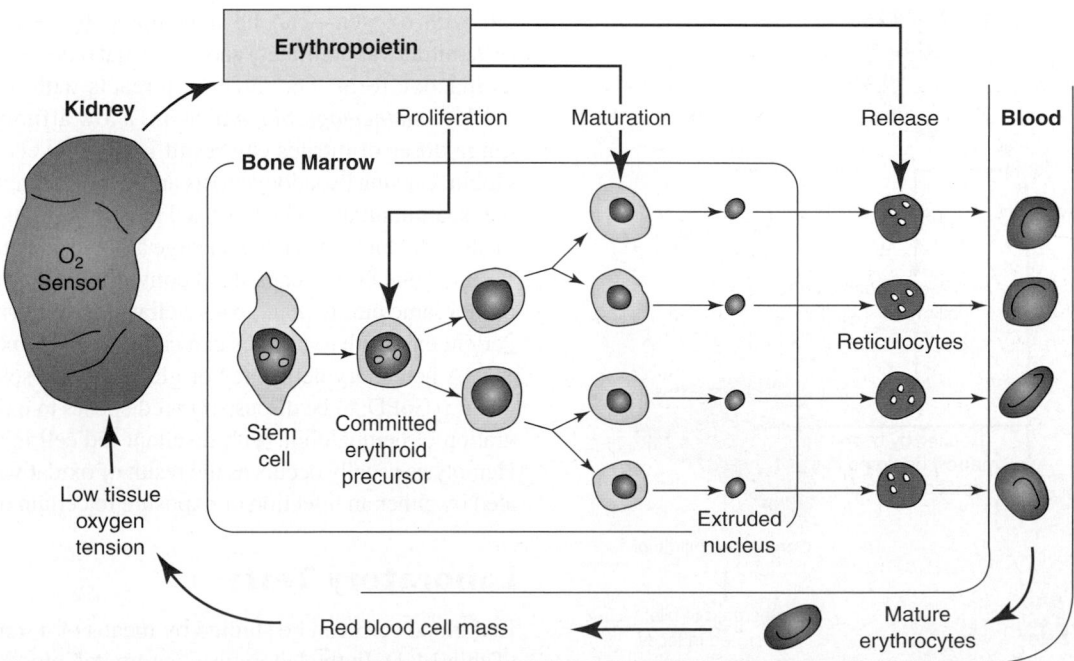

FIGURE 14-5 • Red blood cell development involves the proliferation and differentiation of committed bone marrow cells through the erythroblast and normoblast stages to reticulocytes, which are released into the bloodstream and finally become erythrocytes.

Membrane lipids become reduced and the cell membrane becomes more fragile, causing the red cell to self-destruct as it passes through narrow places in the circulation and in the small trabecular spaces in the spleen. The rate of red cell destruction (1% per day) normally is equal to the rate of red cell production, but in conditions such as hemolytic anemia, the cell's life span may be shorter.

The destruction of red blood cells is facilitated by a group of large phagocytic cells found in the spleen, liver, bone marrow, and lymph nodes. These phagocytic cells recognize old and defective red cells and then ingest and destroy them in a series of enzymatic reactions. During these reactions, the amino acids from the globulin chains and iron from the heme units are salvaged and reused (Fig. 14-6). The bulk of the heme unit is converted to bilirubin, the pigment of bile, which is insoluble in plasma and attaches to plasma proteins for transport. Bilirubin is removed from the blood by the liver and conjugated with glucuronide to render it water soluble so that it can be excreted in the bile. Excess elimination of bilirubin in the bile due to increased red cell destruction can lead to the development of bilirubin gallstones. The plasma-insoluble form of bilirubin is referred to as *unconjugated bilirubin* and the water-soluble form as *conjugated bilirubin*. Serum levels of conjugated and unconjugated bilirubin can be measured in the laboratory and are reported as direct and indirect, respectively. If red cell destruction and consequent bilirubin production are excessive, unconjugated bilirubin accumulates in the

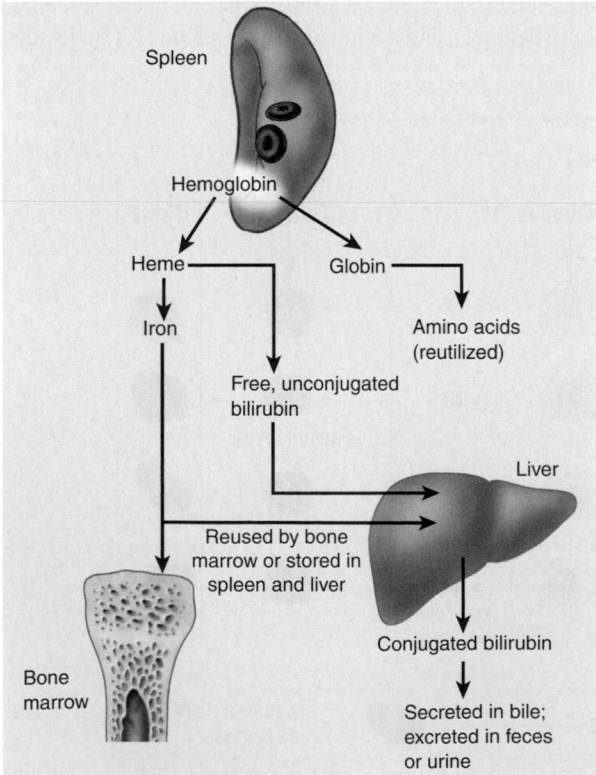

Spleen

Hemoglobin

Heme

Globin

Iron

Amino acids (reutilized)

Free, unconjugated bilirubin

Liver

Reused by bone marrow or stored in spleen and liver

Bone marrow

Conjugated bilirubin

Secreted in bile; excreted in feces or urine

FIGURE 14-6 • Destruction of red blood cells and fate of hemoglobin.

blood. This results in a yellow discoloration of the skin, called *jaundice.*

When red blood cell destruction takes place in the circulation, as in hemolytic anemia, the hemoglobin remains in the plasma. The plasma contains a hemoglobin-binding protein called *haptoglobin.* Other plasma proteins, such as albumin, can also bind hemoglobin. With extensive intravascular destruction of red blood cells, hemoglobin levels may exceed the hemoglobin-binding capacity of haptoglobin and other plasma proteins. When this happens, free hemoglobin appears in the blood (*i.e.,* hemoglobinemia) and is excreted in the urine (*i.e.,* hemoglobinuria). Because excessive red blood cell destruction can occur in hemolytic transfusion reactions, urine samples are tested for free hemoglobin after a transfusion reaction.

Red Cell Metabolism and Hemoglobin Oxidation

The red blood cell, which lacks mitochondria, relies on glucose and the glycolytic pathway for its metabolic needs (see Chapter 4). The enzyme-mediated anaerobic metabolism of glucose generates the ATP needed for normal membrane function and ion transport. The depletion of glucose or the functional deficiency of one of the glycolytic enzymes leads to the premature death of the red blood cell. An offshoot of the glycolytic pathway is the production of 2,3-diphosphoglycerate (2,3-DPG), which binds to the hemoglobin molecule and reduces the affinity of hemoglobin for oxygen. This facilitates the release of oxygen at the tissue level. An increase in the concentration of 2,3-DPG occurs in conditions of chronic hypoxia such as chronic lung disease, anemia, and residence at high altitudes.

The oxidation of hemoglobin—the combining of hemoglobin with oxygen—can be interrupted by certain chemicals (*e.g.,* nitrates and sulfates) and drugs that oxidize hemoglobin to an inactive form. The nitrite ion reacts with hemoglobin to produce *methemoglobin,* which has a low affinity for oxygen. Large doses of nitrites can result in high levels of methemoglobin, causing pseudocyanosis and tissue hypoxia. For example, sodium nitrate, which is used in curing meats, can produce methemoglobin when taken in large amounts. In nursing infants, the intestinal flora is capable of converting significant amounts of inorganic nitrate (*e.g.,* from well water) to nitrite. This inadvertent exposure to nitrates can cause serious toxic effects.

A hereditary deficiency of glucose-6-phosphate dehydrogenase (G6PD; to be discussed) predisposes to oxidative denaturation of hemoglobin, with resultant red cell injury and lysis. Hemolysis usually occurs as the result of oxidative stress generated by either an infection or exposure to certain drugs.

Laboratory Tests

Red blood cells can be studied by means of a sample of blood (Table 14-1). In the laboratory, automated blood cell counters rapidly provide accurate measurements of red cell content and cell indices. The *red blood cell count* measures the total number of red blood cells in a microliter (μL) of blood. The *percentage*

TABLE 14-1 **Standard Laboratory Values for Red Blood Cells**		
TEST	**NORMAL VALUES**	**SIGNIFICANCE**
Red blood cell count (RBC)		
Men	$4.2–5.4 \times 10^6/\mu L$	Number of red cells in the blood
Women	$3.6–5.0 \times 10^6/\mu L$	
Reticulocytes	1.0%–1.5% of total RBC	Rate of red cell production
Hemoglobin		
Men	14–16.5 g/dL	Hemoglobin content of the blood
Women	12–15 g/dL	
Hematocrit		
Men	40%–50%	Volume of cells in 100 mL of blood
Women	37%–47%	
Mean corpuscular volume	85–100 fL	Size of the red cell
Mean corpuscular hemoglobin concentration	31–35 g/dL	Concentration of hemoglobin in the red cell
Mean cell hemoglobin	27–34 pg/cell	Red cell mass

of reticulocytes (normally approximately 1%) provides an index of the rate of red cell production. The *hemoglobin* (grams per deciliter [dL] or 100 milliliters [mL] of blood) measures the hemoglobin content of the blood. The major components of blood are the red cell mass and plasma volume. The *hematocrit* measures the red cell mass in a 100-mL plasma volume. To determine the hematocrit, a sample of blood is placed in a glass tube, which is then centrifuged to separate the cells and the plasma. The hematocrit may be deceptive because it varies with the quantity of extracellular fluid, rising with dehydration and falling with overexpansion of extracellular fluid volume (Fig 14-7).

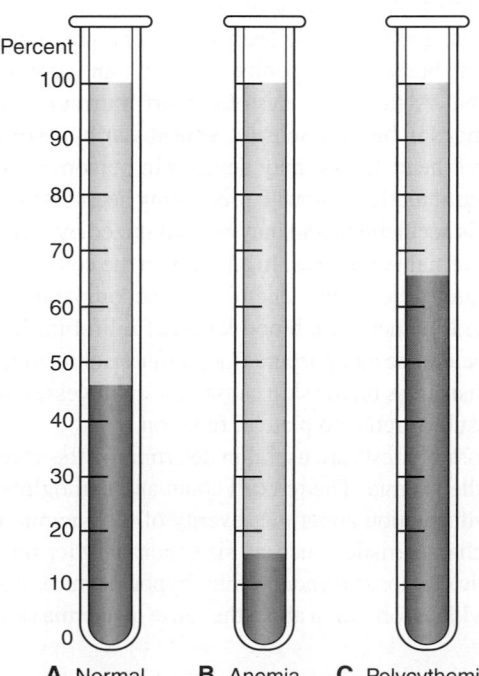

FIGURE 14-7 • Hematocrit. The hematocrit measures the percentage of cells in 100 mL of plasma: (**A**) normal, (**B**) decreased in anemia, and (**C**) increased in polycythemia.

Red cell indices are used to differentiate types of anemias by size or color of red cells. The *mean corpuscular volume* (MCV) reflects the volume or size of the red cells. The MCV falls in microcytic (small cell) anemia and rises in macrocytic (large cell) anemia. Some anemias are normocytic (*i.e.*, cells are of normal size or MCV). The *mean corpuscular hemoglobin concentration* (MCHC) is the concentration of hemoglobin in each cell. Hemoglobin accounts for the color of red blood cells. Anemias are described as *normochromic* (normal color or MCHC) or *hypochromic* (decreased color or MCHC). *Mean cell hemoglobin* (MCH) refers to the mass of the red cell and is less useful in classifying anemias.

A stained blood smear provides information about the size, color, and shape of red cells and the presence of immature or abnormal cells. If blood smear results are abnormal, examination of the bone marrow may be indicated. Bone marrow commonly is aspirated with a special needle from the posterior iliac crest or the sternum. The aspirate is stained and observed for number and maturity of cells and abnormal types.

IN SUMMARY, the red blood cell provides the means for transporting oxygen from the lungs to the tissues. The biconcave shape of the red cell increases the surface area for diffusion of oxygen across the thin cell membrane. A complex cytoskeleton of proteins attached to the interior of the membrane maintains its shape and allows the cell to be deformed while passing through the small capillaries. The red cell contains hemoglobin, a molecule composed of two polypeptide chains each consisting of a globin (protein) portion and a heme unit, which surrounds an iron atom that combines reversibly with oxygen. Red cells develop from stem cells in the bone marrow and are released as reticulocytes into the blood, where they become mature erythrocytes. Red blood cell production is regulated by the hormone erythropoietin, which is produced by the kidney in response to a decrease in oxygen levels.

The life span of a red blood cell is approximately 120 days. Red cell destruction normally occurs in the spleen, liver, bone marrow, and lymph nodes. In the process of destruction, the heme portion of the hemoglobin molecule is converted to bilirubin. Bilirubin, which is insoluble in plasma, attaches to plasma proteins for transport in the blood. It is removed from the blood by the liver and conjugated to a water-soluble form so that it can be excreted in the bile.

The red blood cell, which lacks mitochondria, relies on glucose and the glycolytic pathway for its metabolic needs. The end product of the glycolytic pathway, 2,3-DPG, increases the release of oxygen to the tissues during conditions of hypoxia by reducing hemoglobin's affinity for oxygen.

In the laboratory, automated blood cell counters rapidly provide accurate measurements of red blood cell count and cell indices. A stained blood smear provides information about the size, color, and shape of red cells, and the presence of immature or abnormal cells. If blood smear results are abnormal, examination of the bone marrow may be indicated. ■

ANEMIA

- Anemia, which is a deficiency of red cells or hemoglobin, results from excessive loss (blood loss anemia), increased destruction (hemolytic anemia), or impaired production of red blood cells (iron-deficiency, megaloblastic, and aplastic anemias).
- Blood loss anemia is characterized by loss of iron-containing red blood cells from the body; hemolytic anemia involves destruction of red blood cells in the body with iron being retained in the body.
- Manifestations of anemia are caused by the decreased presence of hemoglobin in the blood (pallor), tissue hypoxia due to deficient oxygen transport (weakness and fatigue), and recruitment of compensatory mechanisms (tachycardia and palpitations) designed to increase oxygen delivery to the tissues.

ANEMIA

After completing this section of the chapter, you should be able to meet the following objectives:

- Describe the manifestations of anemia and their mechanisms.
- Explain the difference between intravascular and extravascular hemolysis.
- Compare the hemoglobinopathies associated with sickle cell disease and thalassemia.
- Explain the cause of sickling in sickle cell disease.
- Cite common causes of iron-deficiency anemia in infancy, adolescence, and adulthood.
- Describe the relation between vitamin B$_{12}$ deficiency and megaloblastic anemia.
- List three causes of aplastic anemia.
- Compare characteristics of the red blood cells in acute blood loss, hereditary spherocytosis, sickle cell disease, iron-deficiency anemia, and aplastic anemia.

Anemia is defined as an abnormally low number of circulating red blood cells or level of hemoglobin, or both, resulting in diminished oxygen-carrying capacity. Anemia usually results from excessive loss (bleeding) or destruction (hemolysis) of red blood cells or from deficient red blood cell production because of a lack of nutritional elements or bone marrow failure.

Anemia is not a disease, but an indication of some disease process or alteration in body function. The effects of anemia can be grouped into three categories: (1) manifestations of impaired oxygen transport and the resulting compensatory mechanisms, (2) reduction in red cell indices and hemoglobin levels, and (3) signs and symptoms associated with the pathologic process that is causing the anemia. The manifestations of anemia depend on its severity, the rapidity of its development, and the person's age and health status.

In anemia, the oxygen-carrying capacity of hemoglobin is reduced, causing tissue hypoxia. Tissue hypoxia can give rise to fatigue, weakness, dyspnea, and sometimes angina. Hypoxia of brain tissue results in headache, faintness, and dim vision. The redistribution of the blood from cutaneous tissues or a lack of hemoglobin causes pallor of the skin, mucous membranes, conjunctiva, and nail beds. Tachycardia and palpitations may occur as the body tries to compensate with an increase in cardiac output. A flow-type systolic heart murmur may result from changes in blood viscosity. Ventricular hypertrophy and high-output heart failure may develop in persons with severe anemia, particularly those with preexisting heart disease. Erythropoiesis is accelerated and may be recognized by diffuse bone pain and sternal tenderness. In addition to the common anemic manifestations, hemolytic anemias are accompanied by jaundice caused by increased blood levels of bilirubin. In aplastic anemia, petechiae and purpura (*i.e.,* minute hemorrhagic spots and purplish areas on the skin caused by small vessel bleeding) are the result of reduced platelet function.

Laboratory tests are useful in determining the severity and cause of the anemia. The red cell count and hemoglobin levels provide information about the severity of the anemia, whereas red cell characteristics such as size (normocytic, microcytic, macrocytic), color (normochromic, hypochromic), and shape often provide information about the cause of anemia (Fig. 14-8).

Blood Loss Anemia

The clinical and red cell manifestations associated with blood loss anemia depend on the rate of hemorrhage and whether the

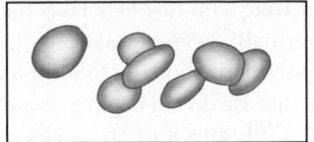
A Iron-deficiency anemia

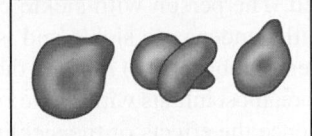
B Megaloblastic anemia

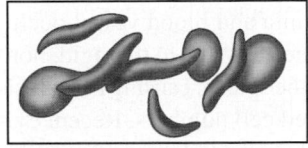
C Sickle cell disease

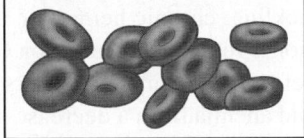
D Normal

FIGURE 14-8 • Red cell characteristics seen in different types of anemia: **(A)** microcytic and hypochromic red cells, characteristic of iron-deficiency anemia; **(B)** macrocytic and misshaped red blood cells, characteristic of megaloblastic anemia; **(C)** abnormally shaped red blood cells seen in sickle cell disease; and **(D)** normocytic and normochromic red blood cells, as a comparison.

bleeding loss is internal or external. With rapid blood loss, circulatory shock and circulatory collapse may occur. With more slowly developing anemia, the amount of red cell mass lost may reach 50% without the occurrence of signs and symptoms.[4]

The effects of acute blood loss are mainly due to loss of intravascular volume, which can lead to cardiovascular collapse and shock (see Chapter 26). A fall in the red blood cell count, hematocrit, and hemoglobin is caused by hemodilution resulting from movement of fluid into the vascular compartment. Initially, the red cells are normal in size and color (normocytic, normochromic). The hypoxia that results from blood loss stimulates proliferation of committed erythroid stem cells in the bone marrow. It takes about 5 days for the progeny of stem cells to differentiate fully, an event that is marked by increased reticulocytes in the blood. If the bleeding is controlled and sufficient iron stores are available, the red cell concentration returns to normal within 3 to 4 weeks. External bleeding leads to iron loss and possible iron deficiency, which can hamper restoration of red cell counts.

Chronic blood loss does not affect blood volume but instead leads to iron-deficiency anemia when iron stores are depleted. It is commonly caused by gastrointestinal bleeding and menstrual disorders. Because of compensatory mechanisms, patients are commonly asymptomatic until the hemoglobin level is less than 8 g/dL. The red cells that are produced have too little hemoglobin, giving rise to microcytic hypochromic anemia (see Fig. 14-8).

Hemolytic Anemias

Hemolytic anemia is characterized by the premature destruction of red cells, the retention in the body of iron and the other products of hemoglobin destruction, and an increase in erythropoiesis. Almost all types of hemolytic anemia are distinguished by normocytic and normochromic red cells. Because of the red blood cell's shortened life span, the bone marrow usually is hyperactive, resulting in an increased number of reticulocytes in the circulating blood. As with other types of anemias, the person experiences easy fatigability, dyspnea, and other signs and symptoms of impaired oxygen transport.

In hemolytic anemia, red cell breakdown can occur within or outside the vascular compartment. Intravascular hemolysis is less common and occurs as a result of complement fixation in transfusion reactions, mechanical injury, or toxic factors. It is characterized by hemoglobinemia, hemoglobinuria, jaundice, and hemosiderinuria.[2] Extravascular hemolysis occurs when red cells become less deformable, making it difficult for them to traverse the splenic sinusoids. The abnormal red cells are sequestered and phagocytized by macrophages in the spleen. The manifestations of extravascular hemolysis include anemia and jaundice.

Another classification of hemolytic anemia is based on whether the cause is intrinsic or extrinsic. Intrinsic causes include defects of the red cell membrane, the various hemoglobinopathies, and inherited enzyme defects. Two main types of hemoglobinopathies can cause red cell hemolysis: the abnormal substitution of an amino acid in the hemoglobin molecule, as in sickle cell disease, and the defective synthesis of one of the polypeptide chains that form the globin portion of hemoglobin, as in the thalassemias. Extrinsic or acquired forms of hemolytic anemia are caused by agents external to the red blood cell, such as drugs, bacterial and other toxins, antibodies, and physical trauma. Although all these factors can cause premature and accelerated destruction of red cells, they cannot all be treated in the same way. Some respond to splenectomy, others to treatment with corticosteroid hormones, and still others do not resolve until the primary disorder is corrected.

Inherited Disorders of the Red Cell Membrane

Hereditary spherocytosis, transmitted as an autosomal dominant trait in 75% of the cases, is the most common inherited disorder of the red cell membrane.[2] The disorder is caused by abnormalities of the spectrin and ankyrin membrane proteins that lead to a gradual loss of the membrane surface. The loss of membrane relative to cytoplasm causes the cell to become a tight sphere instead of a concave disk. Although the spherical cell retains its ability to transport oxygen, it is poorly deformable and susceptible to destruction as it passes through the venous sinuses of the splenic circulation. Clinical signs are variable but typically include mild hemolytic anemia, jaundice, splenomegaly, and bilirubin gallstones. A life-threatening aplastic crisis may occur when a sudden disruption of red cell production (often from a viral infection) causes a rapid drop in hematocrit and the hemoglobin level. The disorder usually is treated with splenectomy to reduce red cell destruction, and blood transfusions may be required in a crisis.

Sickle Cell Disease

Sickle cell disease is an inherited disorder in which an abnormal hemoglobin (hemoglobin S [HbS]) leads to chronic hemolytic anemia, pain, and organ failure. The HbS gene is transmitted by recessive inheritance and can manifest as sickle cell trait (*i.e.,* heterozygote with one HbS gene) or sickle cell disease (*i.e.,* homozygote with two HbS genes). Sickle cell disease affects approximately 50,000 (0.1% to 0.2%) black Americans and about 10% of black Americans carry the trait.[5] In parts of Africa, where malaria is endemic, the gene frequency approaches 30%, attributed to the slight protective effect it confers against *Plasmodium falciparum* malaria.[5]

The abnormal structure of HbS results from a point mutation in the β chain of the hemoglobin molecule, with an abnormal substitution of a single amino acid, valine, for glutamic acid (Fig. 14-9). In the heterozygote, only approximately 40% of the hemoglobin is HbS, but in the homozygote, 80% to 95% of the hemoglobin is HbS.[6] Variations in proportions exist, and the concentration of HbS correlates with the risk of sickling. In the homozygote with sickle cell disease, the HbS becomes sickled when deoxygenated or at a low oxygen tension. The deoxygenated hemoglobin aggregates and polymerizes in the cytoplasm, creating a semisolid gel that changes the shape and deformability of the cell. The sickled cell may return to normal shape with oxygenation in the lungs. However, after repeated episodes of deoxygenation, the cells remain permanently sick-

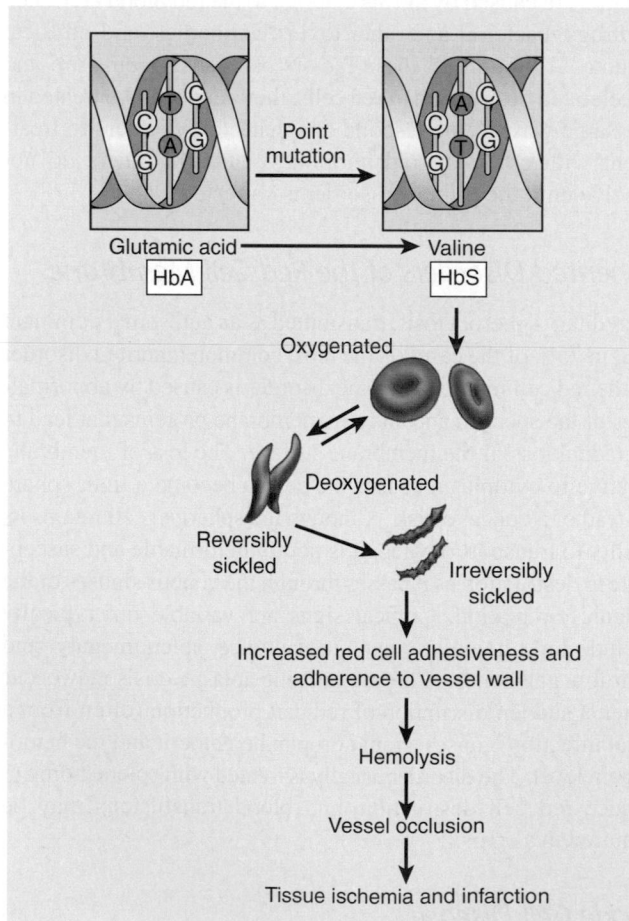

FIGURE 14-9 • Mechanism of sickling and its consequences in sickle cell disease.

led. The person with sickle cell trait who has less HbS has little tendency to sickle and is virtually asymptomatic. Fetal hemoglobin (HbF) inhibits the polymerization of HbS; therefore, most infants with sickle cell disease do not begin to experience the effects of the sickling until after 8 to 10 weeks of age, when the HbF has been replaced by HbS.[5]

There are two major consequences of red blood cell sickling: chronic hemolytic anemia and blood vessel occlusion. Premature destruction of the cells due to the rigid, nondeformable membrane occurs in the spleen, causing hemolysis and anemia from a decrease in red cell numbers. Recent evidence suggests that vessel occlusion is a complex process involving an interaction among the sickled cells, endothelial cells, leukocytes, platelets, other plasma proteins.[7] The process is initiated by the adherence of sickled cells to the vessel endothelium through adhesion molecules, causing endothelial activation with liberation of inflammatory mediators and substances that increase platelet activation and promote blood coagulation. The process also leads to the release of vasoconstrictor substances, whereas the liberation of nitric oxide, an important vasodilator, is impaired.[2,5,7]

Factors associated with sickling and vessel occlusion include cold, stress, physical exertion, infection, and illnesses that cause hypoxia, dehydration, or acidosis. The rate of HbS polymerization is affected by the concentration of hemoglobin in the cell. Dehydration increases the hemoglobin concentration and contributes to the polymerization and resulting sickling. Acidosis reduces the affinity of hemoglobin for oxygen, resulting in more deoxygenated hemoglobin and increased sickling. Even such trivial incidents as reduced oxygen tension induced by sleep may contribute to the sickling process.

Clinical Course. Persons who are homozygous for the HbS gene experience severe hemolytic anemia, chronic hyperbilirubinemia, and vaso-occlusive crises. Hemolysis produces an anemia with hematocrit values ranging from 18% to 30%.[2] The hyperbilirubinemia that results from the breakdown products of hemoglobin often leads to jaundice and the production of pigment stones in the gallbladder.

Blood vessel occlusion causes most of the severe complications. An acute pain episode results from vessel occlusion and hypoxia and can occur suddenly in almost any part of the body.[8] Common sites obstructed by sickled cells include the abdomen, chest, bones, and joints. Many areas may be affected simultaneously. Infarctions caused by sluggish blood flow may cause chronic damage to the liver, spleen, heart, kidneys, retina, and other organs (Fig. 14-10). *Acute chest syndrome* is an atypical pneumonia resulting from pulmonary infarction. It is the second leading cause of hospitalization in persons with sickle cell disease and is characterized by pulmonary infiltrates, shortness of breath, fever, chest pain, and cough.[8,9] The syndrome can cause chronic respiratory insufficiency and is a leading cause of death in sickle cell disease. Children may experience growth retardation and susceptibility to osteomyelitis. Painful bone crises may be caused by marrow infarcts of the bones of the

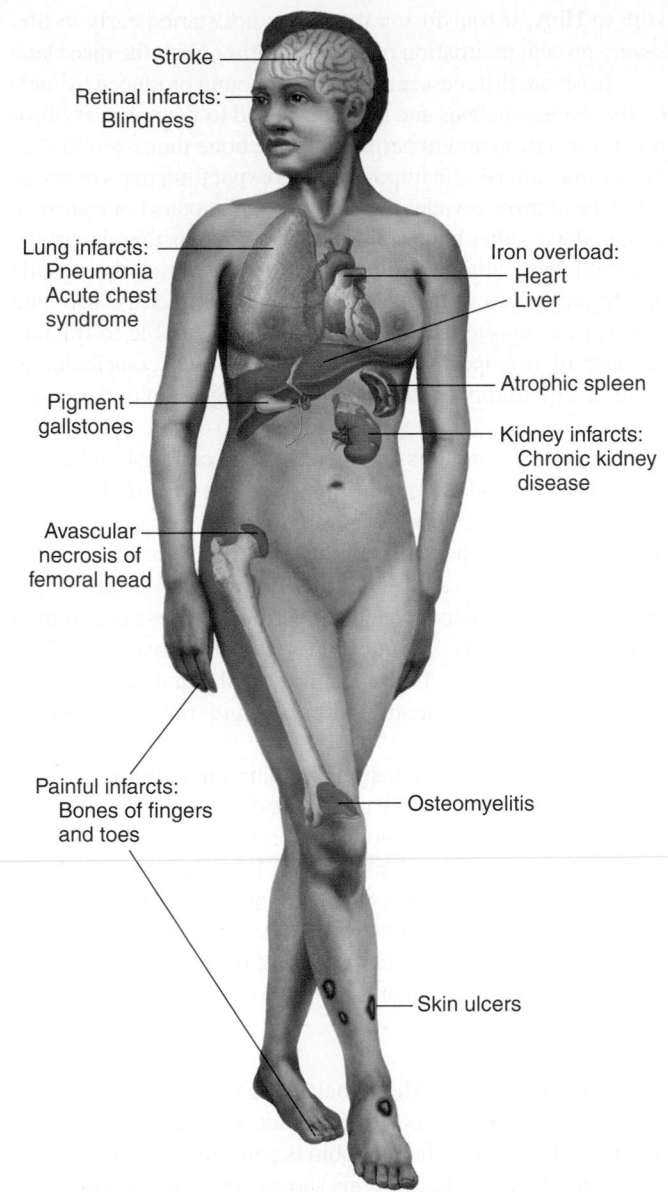

Stroke

Retinal infarcts:
Blindness

Lung infarcts:
Pneumonia
Acute chest
syndrome

Iron overload:
Heart
Liver

Pigment
gallstones

Atrophic spleen

Kidney infarcts:
Chronic kidney
disease

Avascular
necrosis of
femoral head

Painful infarcts:
Bones of fingers
and toes

Osteomyelitis

Skin ulcers

FIGURE 14-10 • Clinical manifestations of sickle cell disease.

small children have not had time to create antibodies to these organisms and rely on the spleen for their removal. In the absence of specific antibody to the polysaccharide capsular antigens of these organisms, splenic activity is essential for removing these organisms when they enter the blood.

Diagnosis and Screening. Neonatal diagnosis of sickle cell disease is made on the basis of clinical findings and hemoglobin solubility results, which are confirmed by hemoglobin electrophoresis. Prenatal diagnosis is done by the analysis of fetal DNA obtained by amniocentesis.[6]

In the United States, screening programs have been implemented to detect newborns with sickle cell disease and other hemoglobinopathies. Cord blood or heel-stick samples are subjected to electrophoresis to separate the HbF from the small amount of HbA and HbS. Other hemoglobins may be detected and quantified by further laboratory evaluation. Many states mandate screening of all newborns, regardless of ethnic origin. Ideally, the effective screening program also includes expert genetic counseling and education about pregnancy options.

Management. Currently, there is no known cure for sickle cell disease; hence, treatment strategies focus on prevention of sickling episodes, symptom management, and treatment of complications. The person is advised to avoid situations that precipitate sickling episodes, such as infections, cold exposure, severe physical exertion, acidosis, and dehydration. Infections are aggressively treated, and blood transfusions may be warranted in a crisis or given chronically in severe disease.

Most children with sickle cell disease are at risk for fulminant septicemia from encapsulated organisms during the first 3 years of life. Prophylactic penicillin should be begun as early as 2 months of age and continued until at least 5 years of age.[10] Maintaining full immunization, including *H. influenzae* vaccine and hepatitis B vaccine, is recommended. The National Institutes of Health Committee on Management of Sickle Cell Disease also recommends administration of the 7-valent pneumococcal vaccine beginning at 2 to 6 months of age.[10] The 7-valent vaccine should be followed by immunization with the 23-valent pneumococcal vaccine at 24 months of age or later.

Hydroxyurea is a cytotoxic drug used to prevent complications of sickle cell disease. The drug allows synthesis of more HbF and less HbS, thereby decreasing sickling. Hydroxyurea reduces by 50% the pain episodes and pulmonary events in about 60% of the persons treated.[11] The others do not respond. Long-term effects regarding organ damage, growth and development, and risk of malignancies are unknown. Other therapies under investigation include drugs that affect globin gene expression; prevent polymerization, membrane damage, and cell dehydration; and inhibit sickle cell adhesion to endothelial cells and promote anticoagulation.[11] Nitric oxide appears to be a promising new drug. It regulates blood vessel tone, platelet activity, and endothelial cell adhesion—all factors that contribute to vessel occlusion. It has been shown that when nitric oxide concentrations, which are low in sickle cell disease, are increased through the use of supplemental oral arginine (a precursor of nitric oxide), pulmonary complications are reduced.[11]

hands and feet, resulting in swelling of those extremities. Approximately 25% of persons with sickle cell disease have neurologic complications related to vessel occlusion.[9] Stroke occurs in children 1 to 15 years of age and may recur in two thirds of those afflicted. Transient ischemic attack or cerebral hemorrhage may precede the stroke.

The spleen is especially susceptible to damage by HbS. Because of the spleen's sluggish blood flow and low oxygen tension, hemoglobin in red cells traversing the spleen becomes deoxygenated, causing ischemia. Splenic injury begins in early childhood, characterized by intense congestion, and is usually asymptomatic. The congestion causes functional asplenia and predisposes the person to life-threatening infections by encapsulated organisms such as *Streptococcus pneumoniae, Haemophilus influenzae* type b, and *Klebsiella* species. Neonates and

Bone marrow or stem cell transplantation has the potential for cure in symptomatic children but carries the risk of graft-versus-host disease. The bone marrow transplantation survival rate for human leukocyte antigen (HLA)–identical sibling donor transplants is about 93%. For those without family donors, transplants of unrelated donor stem cells, cord blood, and mixed donor–host transplants offer possibilities of cure with about a 70% success rate.[11] Progress in gene therapy to treat sickle cell disease has been slow but promising, and may be a future option.

The Thalassemias

The thalassemias are a group of inherited disorders of hemoglobin synthesis leading to decreased synthesis of either the α- or β-globin chains of HbA. β-Thalassemias are caused by deficient synthesis of the β chain and α-thalassemias by deficient synthesis of the α chain.[2,5] The defect is inherited as a mendelian trait, and a person may be heterozygous for the trait and have a mild form of the disease or be homozygous and have the severe form of the disease. Like sickle cell disease, the thalassemias occur with high degree of frequency in certain populations. The β-thalassemias, sometimes called *Cooley anemia* or *Mediterranean anemia,* are most common in the Mediterranean populations of southern Italy and Greece, and the α-thalassemias are most common among Asians. Both α- and β-thalassemias are common in Africans and African Americans.

Two factors contribute to the anemia that occurs in thalassemia: low intracellular hemoglobin (hypochromia) due to the decreased synthesis of the affected chain, coupled with continued production and accumulation of the unaffected globin chain. The reduced hemoglobin synthesis results in a hypochromic, microcytic anemia, whereas the accumulation of the unaffected chain interferes with normal red cell maturation and contributes to membrane changes that lead to hemolysis and anemia.

The β-Thalassemias. The β-thalassemias result from 1 of nearly 200 point mutations in the β-globin gene causing a defect in β-chain synthesis.[12] In β-thalassemias, the excess α chains are denatured to form precipitates (*i.e.,* Heinz bodies) in the bone marrow red cell precursors. The Heinz bodies impair DNA synthesis and cause damage to the red cell membrane. Severely affected red cell precursors are destroyed in the bone marrow, and those that escape intramedullary death are at increased risk of destruction in the spleen. In addition to the anemia, persons with moderate to severe forms of the disease suffer from coagulation abnormalities. Thrombotic events (stroke and pulmonary embolism) appear to be related to altered platelet function, endothelial activation, and an imbalance of procoagulants and anticoagulants.[12]

The clinical manifestations of the β-thalassemias are based on the severity of the anemia. The presence of one normal gene in heterozygous persons (thalassemia minor) usually results in sufficient normal hemoglobin synthesis to prevent severe anemia. Persons who are homozygous for the trait (thalassemia major) have severe, transfusion-dependent anemia that is evident at 6 to 9 months of age when the hemoglobin switches from HbF to HbA. If transfusion therapy is not started early in life, severe growth retardation occurs in children with the disorder.

In severe β-thalassemia, marked anemia produced by ineffective hematopoiesis and hemolysis lead to increased erythropoietin secretion and hyperplasia in the bone marrow and sites of extramedullary hematopoiesis. The expanding mass of erythropoietic marrow invades the bony cortex, impairs bone growth, and produces other bone abnormalities. There is thinning of the cortical bone, with new bone formation evident on the maxilla and frontal bones of the face (*i.e., chipmunk facies*). The long bones, ribs, and vertebrae may become vulnerable to fracture because of osteoporosis or osteopenia, which contributes to increased morbidity in older patients. Enlargement of the spleen (splenomegaly) and liver (hepatomegaly) result from extramedullary hematopoiesis and increased red cell destruction.

Iron overload is a major complication of β-thalassemia. Excess iron stores, which accumulate from increased dietary absorption and repeated transfusions, are deposited in the myocardium, liver, and endocrine organs and induce organ damage. Cardiac, hepatic, and endocrine diseases are common causes of morbidity and mortality from iron overload. Disorders of the pituitary, thyroid, and adrenal glands and the pancreas result in significant morbidity and require hormone replacement therapy.[12]

Regular blood transfusions to maintain hemoglobin levels at 9 to 10 g/dL improve growth and development and prevent most of the complications, and iron chelation therapy can reduce the iron overload and extend life expectancy.[12] Stem cell transplantation is a potential cure for low-risk patients, particularly in younger persons with no complications of the disease or its treatment, and has excellent results.[12] In the future, stem cell gene replacement may provide a cure for many with the disease.

The α-Thalassemias. The α-thalassemias are caused by a gene deletion that results in defective α-chain synthesis. Synthesis of the α-globin chains of hemoglobin is controlled by two pairs or four genes; hence, α-thalassemia shows great variation in severity related to the number of gene deletions. Silent carriers who have a deletion of a single α-globin gene are asymptomatic, and those with deletion of two genes have the α-thalassemia trait and exhibit mild hemolytic anemia. Deletion of three of the four α-chain genes leads to unstable aggregates of α chains called *hemoglobin H* (HbH). This disorder is the most important clinical form and is common in Asians. The β chains are more soluble than the α chains, and their accumulation is less toxic to the red cells, so that senescent rather than precursor red cells are affected. Most persons with HbH have chronic moderate hemolytic anemia and may require transfusions in time of fever or illness or with certain medications.[13] The most severe form of α-thalassemia occurs in infants in whom all four α-globin genes are deleted. Such a defect results in a hemoglobin molecule (Hb Bart) that is formed exclusively from the chains of HbF. Hb Bart, which has an extremely high oxygen affinity, cannot release oxygen in the tissues. This disorder usually results in death *in utero* or shortly after birth. The few survivors are transfusion dependent and have other malformations.[13]

Inherited Enzyme Defects

The most common inherited enzyme defect that results in hemolytic anemia is a deficiency of G6PD. The gene that determines this enzyme is located on the X chromosome, and the defect is expressed only in males and homozygous females. There are more than 350 genetic variants of this disorder found in all populations, but particularly in African and Mediterranean groups. The African variant has been found in 10% to 15% of African Americans.[5] The disorder makes red cells more vulnerable to oxidants and causes direct oxidation of hemoglobin to methemoglobin, which cannot transport oxygen, and denaturing of the hemoglobin molecule to form Heinz bodies, which are precipitated in the red blood cell. Hemolysis usually occurs as the damaged red blood cells move through the narrow vessels of the spleen, causing hemoglobinemia, hemoglobinuria, and jaundice. The hemolysis is short-lived, occurring 2 to 3 days after the trigger event. In blacks, the defect is mildly expressed and is not associated with chronic hemolytic anemia unless triggered by oxidant drugs, acidosis, or infection.

The antimalarial drug primaquine, the sulfonamides, nitrofurantoin, aspirin, phenacetin, some chemotherapeutics, and other drugs cause hemolysis. Free radicals generated by phagocytes during infections also are possible triggers. A more severe deficiency of G6PD is found in people of Mediterranean descent (*e.g.,* Sardinians, Sephardic Jews, Arabs). In some of these persons, chronic hemolysis occurs in the absence of exposure to oxidants. The disorder can be diagnosed through the use of a G6PD assay or screening test.

Acquired Hemolytic Anemias

Several acquired factors exogenous to the red blood cell produce hemolysis by direct membrane destruction or by antibody-mediated lysis. Various drugs, chemicals, toxins, venoms, and infections such as malaria destroy red cell membranes. Hemolysis can also be caused by mechanical factors such as prosthetic heart valves, vasculitis, and severe burns. Obstructions in the microcirculation, as in disseminated intravascular coagulation, thrombotic thrombocytopenic purpura, and renal disease, may traumatize the red cells by producing turbulence and changing pressure gradients.

Many hemolytic anemias are immune mediated, caused by antibodies that destroy the red cell. Autoantibodies may be produced in response to drugs and disease. Alloantibodies come from an exogenous source and are responsible for transfusion reactions and hemolytic disease of the newborn.

The autoantibodies that cause red cell destruction are of two types: warm-reacting antibodies of the immunoglobulin G (IgG) type, which are maximally active at 37°C, and cold-reacting antibodies of the IgM type, which are optimally active at or near 4°C. The warm-reacting antibodies account for 80% of cases of hemolytic anemia.[5] They cause no morphologic or metabolic alteration in the red cell. Instead, they react with antigens on the red cell membrane, causing destructive changes that lead to spherocytosis, with subsequent phagocytic destruction in the spleen or reticuloendothelial system. They lack specificity for the ABO antigens but may react with the Rh antigens. The hemolytic reactions associated with the warm-reacting antibodies occur with an incidence of approximately 10 per 1 million and affect women more frequently than men. The reactions have a rapid onset and may be severe and life-threatening. Fatigue is a common complaint and jaundice and moderate splenomegaly are present. Angina or congestive heart failure may also occur. There are varied causes for this anemia; approximately 50% are idiopathic, and 50% are drug induced (*e.g.,* penicillin) or related to cancers of the lymphoproliferative system (*e.g.,* chronic lymphocytic leukemia, lymphoma), collagen diseases (*e.g.,* systemic lupus erythematosus), viral infections, and inflammatory disorders (*e.g.,* ulcerative colitis).[5] The antihypertensive drug alpha-methyldopa and the antiarrhythmic drug quinidine account for a small number of cases.[2] The drug-induced hemolysis is commonly benign.

The cold-reacting antibodies activate complement. Chronic hemolytic anemia caused by cold-reacting antibodies occurs with lymphoproliferative disorders and as an idiopathic disorder of unknown cause. The hemolytic process occurs in distal body parts, where the temperature may fall below 30°C. Vascular obstruction by red cells results in pallor, cyanosis of the body parts exposed to cold temperatures, and Raynaud phenomenon (see Chapter 22). Hemolytic anemia caused by cold-reacting antibodies develops in only a few persons and is rarely severe.

The Coombs test, or antiglobulin test, is used to diagnose immune hemolytic anemias. It detects the presence of antibody or complement on the surface of the red cell. The direct antiglobulin test (DAT) detects the antibody on red blood cells. In this test, red cells that have been washed free of serum are mixed with anti–human globulin reagent. The red cells agglutinate if the reagent binds to and bridges the antibody or complement on adjacent red cells. The DAT result is positive in cases of autoimmune hemolytic anemia, erythroblastosis fetalis (Rh disease of the newborn), transfusion reactions, and drug-induced hemolysis. The indirect antiglobulin test detects antibody in the serum, and the result is positive for specific antibodies. It is used for antibody detection and crossmatching before transfusion.

Anemias of Deficient Red Cell Production

Anemia may result from the decreased production of erythrocytes by the bone marrow. A deficiency of nutrients for hemoglobin synthesis (iron) or DNA synthesis (cobalamin or folic acid) may reduce red cell production by the bone marrow. A deficiency of red cells also results when the marrow itself fails or is replaced by nonfunctional tissue.

Iron-Deficiency Anemia

Iron deficiency is a common worldwide cause of anemia affecting persons of all ages. The anemia results from dietary deficiency, loss of iron through bleeding, or increased demands. Because iron is a component of heme, a deficiency leads to decreased hemoglobin synthesis and consequent impairment of oxygen delivery.

Body iron is used repeatedly. When red cells become senescent and are broken down, their iron is released and reused in the production of new red cells. Despite this efficiency, small amounts of iron are lost in the feces and need to be replaced by dietary uptake. Iron balance is maintained by the absorption of 0.5 to 1.5 mg daily to replace the 1 mg lost in the feces. The average Western diet supplies about 20 mg.[5] The absorbed iron is more than sufficient to supply the needs of most individuals, but may be barely adequate in toddlers, adolescents, and women of child-bearing age. Dietary deficiency of iron is not common in developed countries except in certain populations. Most iron is derived from meat, and when meat is not available, as for deprived populations, or is not a dietary constituent, as for vegetarians, iron deficiency may occur.

The usual reason for iron deficiency in adults in the Western world is chronic blood loss because iron cannot be recycled to the pool. In men and postmenopausal women, blood loss may occur from gastrointestinal bleeding because of peptic ulcer, intestinal polyps, hemorrhoids, or cancer. Excessive aspirin intake may cause undetected gastrointestinal bleeding. In women, menstruation may account for an average of 1.5 mg of iron lost per day, causing a deficiency.[14] Although cessation of menstruation removes a major source of iron loss in the pregnant woman, iron requirements increase at this time, and deficiency is common. The expansion of the mother's blood volume requires approximately 500 mg of additional iron, and the growing fetus requires approximately 360 mg during pregnancy. In the postnatal period, lactation requires approximately 1 mg of iron daily.[14]

A child's growth places extra demands on the body. Blood volume increases, with a greater need for iron. Iron requirements are proportionally higher in infancy (3 to 24 months) than at any other age, although they are also increased in childhood and adolescence. In infancy, the two main causes of iron-deficiency anemia are low iron levels at birth because of maternal deficiency and a diet consisting mainly of cow's milk, which is low in absorbable iron. Adolescents are also susceptible to iron deficiency because of high requirements due to growth spurts, dietary deficiencies, and menstrual loss.[15]

Iron-deficiency anemia is characterized by low hemoglobin and hematocrit, decreased iron stores, and low serum iron and ferritin. The red cells are decreased in number and are microcytic and hypochromic (see Fig. 14-8). Poikilocytosis (irregular shape) and anisocytosis (irregular size) are also present. Laboratory values indicate reduced MCHC and MCV. Membrane changes may predispose to hemolysis, causing further loss of red cells.

The manifestations of iron-deficiency anemia are related to impaired oxygen transport and lack of hemoglobin. Depending on the severity of the anemia, fatigability, palpitations, dyspnea, angina, and tachycardia may occur. Epithelial atrophy is common and results in waxy pallor, brittle hair and nails, sometimes a spoon-shaped deformity of the fingernails, smooth tongue,

sores in the corners of the mouth, and sometimes dysphagia and decreased acid secretion. A poorly understood symptom occasionally seen is pica, the bizarre, compulsive eating of ice, dirt, or other abnormal substances. Iron deficiency in infants may also result in long-term manifestations such as poor cognitive, motor, and emotional function that may be related to effects on brain development or neurotransmitter function.[16]

Prevention of iron deficiency is a primary concern in infants and children. Avoidance of cow's milk, iron supplementation at 4 to 6 months of age in breast-fed infants, and use of iron-fortified formulas and cereals are recommended for infants younger than 1 year of age.[17] In the second year, a diet rich in iron-containing foods and use of iron-fortified vitamins will help prevent iron deficiency. The treatment of iron-deficiency anemia in children and adults is directed toward controlling chronic blood loss, increasing dietary intake of iron, and administering supplemental iron. Ferrous sulfate, which is the usual oral replacement therapy, replenishes iron stores in several months. Parenteral iron (iron dextran or sodium ferric gluconate) therapy may be used when oral forms are not tolerated or are ineffective. Because of the possibility of severe hypersensitivity reactions, an initial test dose should be done before administration of the first therapeutic dose of the drug. It is recommended that the test dose be administered in an environment equipped for treatment of severe allergic or anaphylactic reactions. Parenteral iron can be given intravenously or as a deep intramuscular injection by the Z-track method, in which the skin is pulled to one side before inserting the needle to prevent leakage into the tissues, with subsequent skin discoloration. In the future, gastric delivery systems may provide good therapy without side effects.

Megaloblastic Anemias

Megaloblastic anemias are caused by impaired DNA synthesis that results in enlarged red cells (MCV >100 fL) due to impaired maturation and division.[18] Vitamin B_{12} and folic acid deficiencies are the most common conditions associated with megaloblastic anemias. Because megaloblastic anemias develop slowly, there are often few symptoms until the anemia is far advanced.

Vitamin B_{12}–Deficiency Anemia. Vitamin B_{12}, also known as *cobalamin,* serves as a cofactor for two important reactions in humans. It is essential for DNA synthesis and nuclear maturation, which in turn leads to normal red cell maturation and division.[2,19] Vitamin B_{12} is also involved in a reaction that prevents abnormal fatty acids from being incorporated into neuronal lipids. This abnormality may predispose to myelin breakdown and produce some of the neurologic complications of vitamin B_{12} deficiency.[2]

Vitamin B_{12} is found in all foods of animal origin. Dietary deficiency is rare and usually found only in strict vegetarians who avoid all dairy products as well as meat and fish. Normal body stores of 1000 to 5000 micrograms (μg) provide the daily requirement of 1 μg for a number of years.[5] Therefore, deficiency of vitamin B_{12} develops slowly. Vitamin B_{12} is absorbed by a unique process. After release from the animal protein, it is bound to intrinsic factor, a protein secreted by the gastric parietal cells (Fig. 14-11). The vitamin B_{12}–intrinsic factor complex protects vitamin B_{12} from digestion by intestinal enzymes. The complex travels to the ileum, where it binds to membrane receptors on the epithelial cells. Vitamin B_{12} is then separated from intrinsic factor and transported across the membrane into the circulation. There it is bound to its carrier protein, transcobalamin II, which transports vitamin B_{12} to its storage and tissue sites. Any defects in this pathway may cause a deficiency.

Pernicious anemia is a specific form of megaloblastic anemia caused by atrophic gastritis (see Chapter 37) and an attendant failure to produce intrinsic factor that leads to failure to absorb vitamin B_{12}. Pernicious anemia is believed to result from immunologically mediated, possibly autoimmune, destruction of the gastric mucosa. The resultant chronic atrophic gastritis is marked by loss of parietal cells and production of antibodies that interfere with binding of vitamin B_{12} to intrinsic factor. Other causes of vitamin B_{12}–deficiency anemia include gastrectomy, ileal resection, inflammation or neoplasms in the terminal ileum, and malabsorption syndromes in which vitamin B_{12} and other vitamin B compounds are poorly absorbed.

The hallmark of vitamin B_{12} deficiency is megaloblastic anemia. When vitamin B_{12} is deficient, the red cells that are produced are abnormally large because of excess cytoplasmic growth and structural proteins (see Fig. 14-8). The cells have immature nuclei and show evidence of cellular destruction. They have flimsy membranes and are oval rather than biconcave. These oddly shaped cells have a short life span that can be measured in weeks rather than months. The loss of red cells results in a moderate to severe anemia and mild jaundice. The MCV is elevated, and the MCHC is normal.

Neurologic changes that accompany the disorder are caused by deranged methylation of myelin protein. Demyelination of the dorsal and lateral columns of the spinal cord causes

symmetric paresthesias of the feet and fingers, loss of vibratory and position sense, and eventual spastic ataxia. In more advanced cases, cerebral function may be altered. In some cases, dementia and other neuropsychiatric changes may precede hematologic changes.

Diagnosis of vitamin B_{12} deficiency is made by finding an abnormally low vitamin B_{12} serum level. The Schilling test, which measures the 24-hour urinary excretion of radiolabeled vitamin B_{12} administered orally, has been commonly used in the past to document decreased absorption of vitamin B_{12}. Currently, the diagnosis of pernicious anemia is usually made by the detection of parietal cell and intrinsic factor antibodies.[18] Lifelong treatment consisting of intramuscular injections or high oral doses of vitamin B_{12} reverses the anemia and improves the neurologic changes.

Folic Acid–Deficiency Anemia. Folic acid is also required for DNA synthesis and red cell maturation, and its deficiency produces the same type of megaloblastic red cell changes that occur in vitamin B_{12}–deficiency anemia (*i.e.,* increased MCV and normal MCHC). Symptoms are also similar, but without the neurologic manifestations.

Folic acid is readily absorbed from the intestine. It is found in vegetables (particularly the green leafy types), fruits, cereals, and meats. Much of the vitamin, however, is lost in cooking. The most common causes of folic acid deficiency are malnutrition or dietary lack, especially in the elderly or in association with alcoholism. Total body stores of folic acid amount to 2000 to 5000 μg, and 50 μg is required in the daily diet.[5] A dietary deficiency may result in anemia in a few months. Malabsorption of folic acid may be due to syndromes such as sprue or other intestinal disorders. Some drugs used to treat seizure disorders (*e.g.,* primidone, phenytoin, phenobarbital) and triamterene, a diuretic, predispose to a deficiency by interfering with folic acid absorption. In neoplastic disease, tumor cells compete for folate, and deficiency is common. Methotrexate, a folic acid analog used in the treatment of cancer, impairs the action of folic acid by blocking its conversion to the active form.

Because pregnancy increases the need for folic acid 5- to 10-fold, a deficiency commonly occurs. Poor dietary habits, anorexia, and nausea are other reasons for folic acid deficiency during pregnancy. Studies also show an association between folate deficiency and neural tube defects.[18] The U.S. Public Health Service recommends that all women of childbearing age should take 400 μg of folic acid daily. It is estimated that 50% of neural tube defects could thus be prevented.[20] The Institute of Medicine Panel on Folate and Other B Vitamins has revised the recommended daily allowance for pregnant women to 600 μg/day.[21] To ensure adequate folate consumption, the U.S. Food and Drug Administration mandated the addition of folate to cereal grain products, effective January 1, 1998.

Aplastic Anemia

Aplastic anemia describes a disorder of pluripotential bone marrow stem cells that results in a reduction of all three hemato-

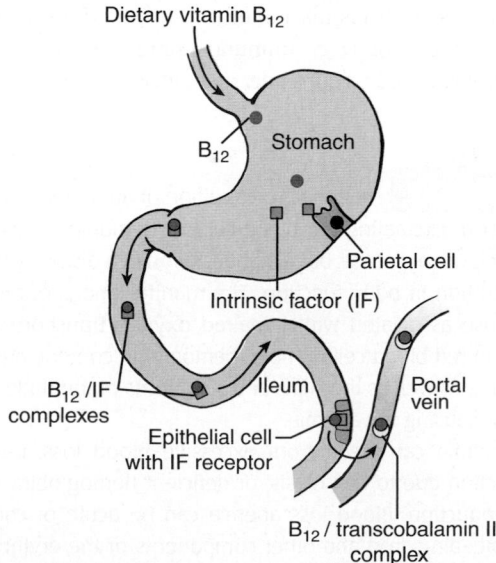

FIGURE 14-11 • Absorption of vitamin B_{12}.

poietic cell lines—red blood cells, white blood cells, and platelets.[22,23] Pure red cell aplasia, in which only the red cells are affected, rarely occurs. Anemia results from the failure of the marrow to replace senescent red cells that are destroyed and leave the circulation, although the cells that remain are of normal size and color. At the same time, because the leukocytes, particularly the neutrophils, and the thrombocytes have a short life span, a deficiency of these cells usually is apparent before the anemia becomes severe.

The onset of aplastic anemia may be insidious, or it may strike with suddenness and great severity. It can occur at any age. The initial presenting symptoms include weakness, fatigability, and pallor caused by anemia. Petechiae (*i.e.*, small, punctate skin hemorrhages) and ecchymoses (*i.e.*, bruises) often occur on the skin, and bleeding from the nose, gums, vagina, or gastrointestinal tract may occur because of decreased platelet levels. The decrease in the number of neutrophils increases susceptibility to infection.

Among the causes of aplastic anemia are exposure to high doses of radiation, chemicals, and toxins that suppress hematopoiesis directly or through immune mechanisms. Chemotherapy and irradiation commonly result in bone marrow depression, which causes anemia, thrombocytopenia, and neutropenia. Identified toxic agents include benzene, the antibiotic chloramphenicol, and the alkylating agents and antimetabolites used in the treatment of cancer (see Chapter 8). Aplastic anemia caused by exposure to chemical agents may be an idiosyncratic reaction because it affects only certain susceptible persons. It typically occurs weeks after a drug is initiated. Such reactions often are severe and sometimes irreversible and fatal. Aplastic anemia can develop in the course of many infections and has been reported most often as a complication of viral hepatitis, mononucleosis, and other viral illnesses, including acquired immunodeficiency syndrome (AIDS). In two thirds of cases, the cause is unknown, and these are called *idiopathic aplastic anemia*. The mechanisms underlying the pathogenesis of aplastic anemia are unknown. It is suggested that exposure to the chemicals, infectious agents, and other insults generates a cellular immune response resulting in production of cytokines by activated T cells. These cytokines (*e.g.*, interferon, tumor necrosis factor [TNF]) then suppress normal stem cell growth and development.[2]

Therapy for aplastic anemia in the young and severely affected includes stem cell replacement by bone marrow or peripheral blood transplantation. Histocompatible donors supply the stem cells to replace the patient's destroyed marrow cells. Graft-versus-host disease, rejection, and infection are major risks of the procedure, yet 75% or more survive.[23] For those who are not transplantation candidates, immunosuppressive therapy with lymphocyte immune globulin (*i.e.*, antithymocyte globulin) prevents suppression of proliferating stem cells, producing remission in up to 50% of patients.[22,23] Persons with aplastic anemia should avoid the offending agents and be treated with antibiotics for infection. Red cell transfusions to correct the anemia and platelets and corticosteroid therapy to minimize bleeding may also be required.

Chronic Disease Anemias

Anemia often occurs as a complication of chronic infections, inflammation, and cancer. The most common causes of chronic disease anemias are acute and chronic infections, including AIDS and osteomyelitis; cancers; autoimmune disorders such as rheumatoid arthritis, systemic lupus erythematosus, and inflammatory bowel disease; and chronic kidney disease.[24] It is theorized that the short red cell life span, deficient red cell production, a blunted response to erythropoietin, and low serum iron are caused by actions of cytokines and cells of the reticuloendothelial system (RES). Microorganisms, tumor cells, and autoimmune dysregulation lead to T-cell activation and production of cytokines (*e.g.*, interleukin-1, interferon, and TNF) that suppress the erythropoietin response, inhibit erythroid precursors, and cause changes in iron homeostasis.[24] In addition, macrophages take up iron and store it, thus reducing its availability for erythropoiesis. The mild anemia is normocytic and normochromic with low reticulocyte counts.

Chronic renal failure almost always results in anemia, primarily because of a deficiency of erythropoietin. Unidentified uremic toxins and retained nitrogen also interfere with the actions of erythropoietin and with red cell production and survival. Hemolysis and blood loss associated with hemodialysis and bleeding tendencies also contribute to the anemia of renal failure. Therapy for these anemias includes treatment for the underlying disease, short-term erythropoietin therapy, iron supplementation, and blood transfusions. Future treatments may include iron-chelating drugs, agents that lower iron retention in RES cells, and cytokines to stimulate erythropoietin production.[24]

"Anemia of critical illness" is common in the intensive care unit, with more than 90% of patients having subnormal hemoglobin levels by the third day.[25] In critically ill persons, low erythropoietin concentrations and anemia also appear to be caused by inflammatory cytokines. In this population, it is suggested that red blood cell transfusions be restricted to reduce the risk of transmission of newer infectious agents and immune modulation (*e.g.*, immunosuppression) predisposing to infections, cancer recurrence, and autoimmune disease.[25]

IN SUMMARY, anemia is a condition of an abnormally low number of circulating red blood cells or hemoglobin level, or both. It is not a disease, but a manifestation of a disease process or alteration in body function. The manifestations of anemia are those associated with impaired oxygen transport; alterations in red blood cell number, hemoglobin content, and cell structure, as well as the signs and symptoms of the underlying process causing the anemia.

Anemia can result from excessive blood loss, red cell destruction due to hemolysis, or deficient hemoglobin or red cell production. Blood loss anemia can be acute or chronic. With bleeding, iron and other components of the erythrocyte are lost from the body. Hemolytic anemia is characterized by the premature destruction of red cells, with retention in the body of iron and the other products of red cell destruction. Hemolytic anemia can be caused by defects in the red cell membrane, hemoglobinopathies (sickle cell disease or thalassemia), or inherited enzyme defects (G6PD deficiency). Acquired forms of hemolytic anemia are caused by agents extrinsic to the red blood cell, such as drugs, bacterial and other toxins, antibodies, and physical trauma. Iron-deficiency anemia, which is characterized by decreased hemoglobin synthesis, can result from dietary deficiency, loss of iron through bleeding, or increased demands for red cell production. Vitamin B_{12} and folic acid deficiencies impair red cell production by interfering with DNA synthesis. Aplastic anemia is caused by bone marrow suppression and usually results in a reduction of white blood cells and platelets, as well as red blood cells. Chronic diseases such as inflammatory disorders (rheumatoid arthritis), cancers, and renal failure cause anemia through the production of inflammatory cytokines that interfere with erythropoietin production or response. ■

TRANSFUSION THERAPY

After completing this section of the chapter, you should be able to meet the following objectives:

- Differentiate red cell antigens from antibodies in persons with type A, B, AB, or O blood.
- Explain the determination of the Rh factor.
- List the signs and symptoms of a blood transfusion reaction.

Anemias of various causes are treated with transfusions of whole blood or red blood cells only when oxygen delivery to the tissues is compromised, as evidenced by measures of oxygen transport and use, hemoglobin, and hematocrit. Current recommendations suggest transfusion for patients with hemoglobin levels less than 7 g/dL, depending on age, illness, risk factors, and surgical procedures.[25] Acute massive blood loss usually is replaced with whole-blood transfusion. Most anemias, however, are treated with transfusions of red cell concentrates, which supply only the blood component that is deficient. Since the 1960s, devices that mechanically separate a unit of blood into its constituents provide red cell components, platelets, fresh-frozen plasma, cryoprecipitate, and clotting factor concentrates. In this way, a unit of blood can be used efficiently for several recipients to correct specific deficiencies.

Several red cell components that are used for transfusion are prepared and stored under specific conditions and have unique uses, as described in Table 14-2. These red cell components are derived principally from voluntary blood donors. In the future, red cell substitutes, such as hemoglobin solutions,

may be used, particularly in the trauma setting.[26] The potential advantages are better storage, longer shelf life, and no risk of transfusion reaction.

The use of autologous donation and transfusion has been advocated since the early 1980s. Autologous transfusion refers to the procedure of receiving one's own blood—usually to replenish a surgical loss—thereby eliminating the risk of blood-borne disease or transfusion reaction. In 1992, a reported 8.5% of transfusions were autologous.[27] Autologous blood can be provided by several means: predeposit, hemodilution, and intraoperative salvage. A patient who is anticipating elective orthopedic, vascular, or open heart surgery may predeposit blood (*i.e.*, have the blood collected up to 6 weeks in advance and stored) for later transfusion during the surgery. Hemodilution involves phlebotomy before surgery with transfusion of the patient's blood at the completion of surgery. The procedure requires the use of fluid infusions to maintain blood volume and is commonly used in open heart surgery. Intraoperative blood salvage is the collection of blood shed from the operative site for reinfusion into the patient. Semiautomated devices are used to collect, anticoagulate, wash, and resuspend red cells for reinfusion during many procedures, including vascular, cardiac, and orthopedic surgery. Potential risks of autologous transfusion may include bacterial and other contamination, volume overload, and administrative errors.[27]

Before a red cell or whole-blood transfusion from a volunteer donor source can occur, a series of procedures is required to ensure a successful transfusion. Donor samples are first tested for blood-borne diseases, such as hepatitis B and C viruses, HIV types 1 and 2, human T-cell lymphotropic viruses (HTLV-I and -II), and syphilis. Donor and recipient samples are typed to determine ABO and Rh groups and screened for unexpected red cell antibodies. The cross-match is performed by incubating the donor cells with the recipient's serum and observing for agglutination. If none appears, the donor and recipient blood types are compatible.

ABO Blood Groups

ABO compatibility is essential for effective transfusion therapy and requires knowledge of ABO antigens and antibodies. There are four major ABO blood groups determined by the presence or absence of two red cell antigens (A and B). Persons who have neither A nor B antigens are classified as having type O blood; those with A antigens are classified as having type A blood; those with B antigens, as having type B blood; and those with A and B antigens, as having type AB blood (Table 14-3). The ABO blood groups are genetically determined. The type O gene is apparently functionless in production of a red cell antigen. Each of the other genes is expressed by the presence of a strong antigen on the surface of the red cell. Six genotypes, or gene combinations, result in four phenotypes, or blood type expressions. In the United States the frequencies of ABO blood groups among whites are approximately 46% for type O, 41% for type A, 9% for type B, and 4% for type AB. Although the distribution varies

TABLE 14-2 Red Blood Cell Components Used in Transfusion Therapy

COMPONENT	PREPARATION	USE	LIMITATIONS
Whole blood	Drawn from donor Anticoagulant–preservative solutions added, usually citrate-phosphate-dextrose (CPDA-1) adenine; stored at 1°–6°C until expiration, up to 35 days	Replacement of blood volume and oxygen-carrying capacity lost in massive bleeding	Contains few viable platelets or granulocytes and is deficient in coagulation factors V and VIII; may cause hypervolemia, febrile and allergic reactions, and infectious disease (i.e., hepatitis and AIDS)
Red blood cells	Removal of two thirds of plasma by centrifugation; additive solution contains adenine and dextrose to extend shelf life up to 42 days and maintain ATP levels	Standard transfusion to increase oxygen-carrying capacity in chronic anemia and slow hemorrhage; reduce danger of hypervolemia	Contains no viable platelets or granulocytes; risk of reactions and infectious disease
Leukocyte-reduced red blood cells	Removal of 99% of leukocytes, platelets, and debris by centrifugation or filtration	Reduces risk of nonhemolytic febrile reactions in susceptible persons	Preparation may reduce red cell mass to 80%; 24-hr outdate and infectious disease risk
Washed red blood cells	Red cells washed in normal saline solution and centrifuged several times to remove plasma and constituents	Reduces risk of febrile and allergic reactions	Loss of red cell mass, 24-hr outdate, costly preparation, and infectious disease risk
Frozen red blood cells	Red cells mixed with glycerol to prevent ice crystals from forming and rupturing the cell membrane; cells must be thawed, deglycerolized, and washed before transfusing	Reduces risk of severe febrile reactions; preserves rare and autologous (self-donated) units for transfusion up to 10 yr	Costly and lengthy preparation; loss of red cell mass, 24-hr outdate, and infectious disease risk

ATP, adenosine triphosphate.

Data from Vengelen-Tyler V. (Ed.) (1996). *Technical manual* (12th ed., pp. 135–142). Bethesda, MD: American Association of Blood Banks.

somewhat among other racial groups, types O and A are always the most common.

ABO antibodies predictably develop in the serum of persons whose red cells lack the corresponding antigen. Persons with type A antigens on their red cells develop type B antibodies; persons with type B antigens develop type A antibodies in their serum; persons with type O blood develop type A and type B antibodies; and persons with type AB blood develop neither A nor B antibodies. The ABO antibodies usually are

TABLE 14-3 ABO System for Blood Typing

GENOTYPE	RED CELL ANTIGENS	BLOOD TYPE	SERUM ANTIBODIES
OO	None	O	AB
AO	A	A	B
AA	A	A	B
BO	B	B	A
BB	B	B	A
AB	AB	AB	None

not present at birth but begin to develop at 3 to 6 months of age and reach maximum levels between the ages of 5 and 10 years.

Rh Types

The D antigen of the Rh system is also important in transfusion compatibility and is routinely tested. The Rh type is coded by three gene pairs: C, c; D, d; and E, e. Each allele, with the exception of d, codes for a specific antigen. The D antigen is the most immunogenic. Persons who express the D antigen are designated Rh positive, and those who do not express the D antigen are Rh negative. Unlike serum antibodies for the ABO blood types, which develop spontaneously after birth, Rh antibodies develop after exposure to one or more of the Rh antigens, usually through pregnancy or transfusions, and persist for many years. More than 80% of Rh-negative persons develop the antibody to D antigen if they are exposed to Rh-positive blood.[28] Because it takes several weeks to produce antibodies, a reaction may be delayed and usually is mild. If subsequent transfusions of Rh-positive blood are given to a person who has become sensitized, the person may have a severe, immediate reaction.

Blood Transfusion Reactions

The seriousness of blood transfusion reactions prompts the need for extreme caution when blood is administered. Because most transfusion reactions result from administrative errors or misidentification, care should be taken correctly to identify the recipient and the transfusion source. The recipient's vital signs should be monitored before and during the transfusion, and careful observation for signs of transfusion reaction is imperative. The most feared and lethal transfusion reaction is the destruction of donor red cells by reaction with antibody in the recipient's serum. This immediate hemolytic reaction usually is caused by ABO incompatibility. The signs and symptoms of such a reaction include sensation of heat along the vein where the blood is being infused, flushing of the face, urticaria, headache, pain in the lumbar area, chills, fever, constricting pain in the chest, cramping pain in the abdomen, nausea, vomiting, tachycardia, hypotension, and dyspnea. If any of these adverse effects occur, the transfusion should be stopped immediately. Access to a vein should be maintained because it may be necessary to infuse intravenous solutions to ensure diuresis, administer medications, and take blood samples. The blood must be saved for studies to determine the cause of the reaction.

Hemoglobin that is released from the hemolyzed donor cells is filtered in the glomeruli of the kidneys. Two possible complications of a blood transfusion reaction are oliguria and renal shutdown because of the adverse effects of the filtered hemoglobin on renal tubular flow. The urine should be examined for the presence of hemoglobin, urobilinogen, and red blood cells. Delayed hemolytic reactions may occur more than 10 days after transfusion and are caused by undetected antibodies in the recipient's serum. The reaction is accompanied by a fall in hematocrit and jaundice, but most recipients are asymptomatic.

A febrile reaction, the most common transfusion reaction, occurs in approximately 2% of transfusions. Recipient antibodies directed against the donor's white cells or platelets cause chills and fever. Antipyretics are used to treat this reaction. Future febrile reactions may be avoided by the use of leukocyte-reduced blood.

Allergic reactions are caused by patient antibodies against donor proteins, particularly IgG. Urticaria and itching occur and can be relieved with antihistamines. Susceptible persons may be transfused with washed red cells to prevent reactions.

IN SUMMARY, transfusion therapy provides the means for replacement of red blood cells and other blood components. Red blood cells contain surface antigens, and reciprocal antibodies are found in the serum. Four major ABO blood types are determined by the presence or absence of two red cell antigens: A and B. The D antigen determines the Rh-positive type; absence of the D antigen determines the Rh-negative type. ABO and Rh types must be determined in recipient and donor blood before transfusion to ensure compatibility. ∎

POLYCYTHEMIA

After completing this section of the chapter, you should be able to meet the following objectives:

- Define the term *polycythemia*.
- Compare causes of polycythemia vera and secondary polycythemia.
- Describe the manifestations of polycythemia.

Polycythemia is an abnormally high total red blood cell mass with a hematocrit greater than 50%. It is categorized as *relative* or *absolute*. In *relative* polycythemia, the hematocrit rises because of a loss of plasma volume without a corresponding decrease in red cells. This may occur with water deprivation, excess use of diuretics, or gastrointestinal losses. Relative polycythemia is corrected by increasing the vascular fluid volume.

Absolute polycythemia is a rise in hematocrit due to an increase in total red cell mass and is classified as primary or secondary. Primary polycythemia, or *polycythemia vera,* is a neoplastic disease of the pluripotent cells of the bone marrow characterized by an absolute increase in total red blood cell mass accompanied by elevated white cell and platelet counts. It most commonly is seen in men with a median age of 62 years, but may occur at any age.[29] In polycythemia vera, the manifestations are variable and are related to an increase in the red cell count, hemoglobin level, and hematocrit with increased blood volume and viscosity. Additional early findings include splenomegaly and depletion of iron stores.[29] Viscosity rises exponentially with the hematocrit and interferes with cardiac output and blood flow. Hypertension is common and there may be complaints of headache, dizziness, inability to concentrate, and some difficulty with hearing and vision because of decreased cerebral blood flow. Venous stasis gives rise to a plethoric appearance or dusky redness, even cyanosis, particularly of the lips, fingernails, and mucous membranes. Because of the increased concentration of blood cells, the person may experience itching and pain in the fingers or toes, and the hypermetabolism may induce night sweats and weight loss. Thromboembolism and hemorrhage, due to platelet abnormalities, are common complications that can be prevented by phlebotomy to reduce the hematocrit to less than 42% in women and less than 45% in men.[29] The goal of treatment in primary polycythemia is to reduce blood viscosity. This can be done by withdrawing blood by periodic phlebotomy to reduce red cell volume. Low-dose aspirin may control the high platelet counts, and suppression of bone marrow function with chemotherapy (hydroxyurea) controls the elevated white cell count.[29]

Secondary polycythemia results from a physiologic increase in the level of erythropoietin, commonly as a compensatory response to hypoxia. Conditions causing hypoxia include living at high altitudes, chronic heart and lung disease, and smoking. The resultant release of erythropoietin by the kidney causes the increased formation of red blood cells in the bone marrow. Neoplasms that secrete erythropoietin may also cause a secondary polycythemia. Kidney disease such as hydronephrosis or renal cysts may obstruct blood flow, cause hypoxia, and lead to an increase in erythropoietin. Treatment of secondary polycythemia focuses on relieving hypoxia. For example, continuous low-flow oxygen therapy can be used to correct the severe hypoxia that occurs in some persons with chronic obstructive pulmonary disease. This form of treatment is thought to relieve the pulmonary hypertension and polycythemia and to delay the onset of cor pulmonale.

IN SUMMARY, polycythemia describes a condition in which the red blood cell mass is increased. It can present as a relative, primary, or secondary disorder. Relative polycythemia results from a loss of vascular fluid and is corrected by replacing the fluid. Primary polycythemia, or polycythemia vera, is a proliferative disease of the bone marrow with an absolute increase in total red blood cell mass accompanied by elevated white cell and platelet counts. Secondary polycythemia results from increased erythropoietin levels caused by hypoxic conditions such as chronic heart and lung disease. Many of the manifestations of polycythemia are related to increased blood volume and viscosity that lead to hypertension and stagnation of blood flow. ■

AGE-RELATED CHANGES IN RED BLOOD CELLS

After completing this section of the chapter, you should be able to meet the following objectives:

■ Cite the function of hemoglobin F in the neonate and describe the red blood cell changes that occur during the early neonatal period.

■ Cite the factors that predispose to hyperbilirubinemia in the infant.
■ Describe the pathogenesis of hemolytic disease of the newborn.
■ Compare conjugated and unconjugated bilirubin in terms of production of encephalopathy in the neonate.
■ Explain the action of phototherapy in the treatment of hyperbilirubinemia in the neonate.
■ State the changes in the red blood cells that occur with aging.

Red Cell Changes in the Neonate

At birth, changes in the red blood cell indices reflect the transition to extrauterine life and the need to transport oxygen from the lungs (Table 14-4). Hemoglobin concentrations at birth are high, reflecting the high synthetic activity in utero to provide adequate oxygen delivery. Toward the end of the first postnatal week, hemoglobin concentration begins to decline, gradually falling to a minimum value at approximately age 2 months. The red cell count, hematocrit, and MCV likewise fall. The factors responsible for the decline include reduced red cell production and plasma dilution caused by increased blood volume with growth. Neonatal red cells also have a shorter life span of 50 to 70 days, and are thought to be more fragile than those of older persons. During the early neonatal period, there is also a switch from HbF to HbA. The amount of HbF in term infants averages about 70% of the total hemoglobin and declines to trace amounts by 6 to 12 months of age.[30] The switch to HbA provides greater unloading of oxygen to the tissues because HbA has a lower affinity for oxygen compared with HbF. Infants who are small for gestational age or born to diabetic or smoking mothers or who experienced hypoxia in utero have higher total hemoglobin levels, higher HbF levels, and a delayed switch to HbA.

TABLE 14-4 **Red Cell Values for Term Infants**				
AGE	**RBC × 10⁶/μL** **MEAN ± SD**	**Hb (g/dL)** **MEAN ± SD**	**Hct (%)** **MEAN ± SD**	**MCV (fL)** **MEAN ± SD**
Days				
1	5.14 ± 0.7	19.3 ± 2.2	61 ± 7.4	119 ± 9.4
4	5.00 ± 0.6	18.6 ± 2.1	57 ± 8.1	114 ± 7.5
7	4.86 ± 0.6	17.9 ± 2.5	56 ± 9.4	118 ± 11.2
Weeks				
1–2	4.80 ± 0.8	17.3 ± 2.3	54 ± 8.3	112 ± 19.0
3–4	4.00 ± 0.6	14.2 ± 2.1	43 ± 5.7	105 ± 7.5
8–9	3.40 ± 0.5	10.7 ± 0.9	31 ± 2.5	93 ± 12.0
11–12	3.70 ± 0.3	11.3 ± 0.9	33 ± 3.3	88 ± 7.9

Hb, hemoglobin; Hct, hematocrit; MCV, mean corpuscular volume; RBC, red blood cell count.
Adapted from Matoth Y., Zaizor R., Varsano I. (1971). Postnatal changes in some red cell parameters. *Acta Paediatrica Scandinavica* 60, 317.

A physiologic anemia of the newborn develops at approximately 2 months of age. It seldom produces symptoms and cannot be altered by nutritional supplements. Anemia of prematurity, an exaggerated physiologic response in infants with low birth weight, is thought to result from a poor erythropoietin response. A contributing factor is the frequent blood sampling often required in these infants. The hemoglobin level rapidly declines after birth to a low of 7 to 10 g/dL at approximately 6 weeks of age. Signs and symptoms include apnea, poor weight gain, pallor, decreased activity, and tachycardia. In infants born before 33 weeks' gestation or those with hematocrits below 33%, the clinical features are more evident.

Anemia at birth, characterized by pallor, congestive heart failure, or shock, usually is caused by hemolytic disease of the newborn. Bleeding from the umbilical cord, internal hemorrhage, congenital hemolytic disease, or frequent blood sampling are other possible causes of anemia. The severity of symptoms and presence of coexisting disease may warrant red cell transfusion.

Hyperbilirubinemia in the Neonate

Hyperbilirubinemia, an increased level of serum bilirubin, is a common cause of jaundice in the neonate. A benign, self-limited condition, it most often is related to the developmental state of the neonate. Rarely, cases of hyperbilirubinemia are pathologic and may lead to kernicterus and serious brain damage.

In the first week of life, approximately 60% of term and 80% of preterm neonates are jaundiced.[30] This physiologic jaundice appears in term infants on the second or third day of life. Ordinarily, the indirect bilirubin in umbilical cord blood is 1 to 3 mg/dL and increases by no more than 5 mg/dL in 24 hours, giving rise to jaundice. The levels peak at 5 to 6 mg/dL between days 2 and 4 and decrease to less than 2 mg/dL by days 5 to 7.[30] The increase in bilirubin is related to the increased red cell breakdown and the inability of the immature liver to conjugate bilirubin. Premature infants exhibit a slower rise and longer duration of serum bilirubin levels, perhaps because of poor hepatic uptake and reduced albumin binding of bilirubin. Peak bilirubin levels of 8 to 12 mg/dL appear on days 5 to 7. Most neonatal jaundice resolves within 1 week and is untreated.

The cause of jaundice is made on the basis of history and clinical and laboratory findings. Generally, a search for the cause should be made when (1) the jaundice appears in the first 24 to 36 hours after birth and lasts more than 10 to 14 days, (2) serum bilirubin rises at a rate greater than 5 mg/dL per 24 hours, (3) serum bilirubin is greater than 12 mg/dL in a full-term infant or 10 to 14 mg/dL in a preterm infant, (4) or the direct-reacting bilirubin is greater than 2 mg/dL at any time.[31] Many factors cause elevated bilirubin levels in the neonate, including breast-feeding, hemolytic disease of the newborn, hypoxia, infections, and acidosis. Bowel or biliary obstruction and liver disease are less common causes. Associated risk factors include prematurity, Asian ancestry, and maternal diabetes. Breast milk jaundice occurs in approximately 2% of breast-fed infants.[31] These neonates accumulate significant levels of uncon-

jugated bilirubin 7 days after birth, with maximum levels of 10 to 30 mg/dL reached in the third week of life. It is thought that the breast milk contains fatty acids that inhibit bilirubin conjugation in the neonatal liver. A factor in breast milk is also thought to increase the absorption of bilirubin in the duodenum. This type of jaundice disappears if breast-feeding is discontinued. Nursing can be resumed in 3 to 4 days without any hyperbilirubinemia ensuing.

Hyperbilirubinemia places the neonate at risk for the development of a neurologic syndrome called *kernicterus*. This condition is caused by the accumulation of unconjugated bilirubin in brain cells. Unconjugated bilirubin is lipid soluble, crosses the permeable blood-brain barrier of the neonate, and is deposited in cells of the basal ganglia, causing brain damage. Asphyxia and hyperosmolality may also contribute by damaging the blood-brain barrier and allowing bilirubin to cross and enter the cells. The level of unconjugated bilirubin and the duration of exposure that will be toxic to the infant are unknown. The less mature infant, however, is at greater risk for kernicterus.[31]

Symptoms may appear 2 to 5 days after birth in term infants or by day 7 in premature infants. Lethargy, poor feeding, and short-term behavioral changes may be evident in mildly affected infants. Severe manifestations include rigidity, tremors, ataxia, and hearing loss. Extreme cases cause seizures and death. Most survivors are seriously damaged and by 3 years of age exhibit involuntary muscle spasm, seizures, mental retardation, and deafness.

Hyperbilirubinemia in the neonate is treated with phototherapy or exchange transfusion. Phototherapy is more commonly used to treat jaundiced infants and reduce the risk of kernicterus. Exposure to fluorescent light in the blue range of the visible spectrum (420- to 470-nm wavelength) reduces bilirubin levels. Bilirubin in the skin absorbs the light energy and is converted to a structural isomer that is more water soluble and can be excreted in the stool and urine. Effective treatment depends on the area of skin exposed and the infant's ability to metabolize and excrete bilirubin. Frequent monitoring of bilirubin levels, body temperature, and hydration is critical to the infant's care. Exchange transfusion is considered when signs of kernicterus are evident or hyperbilirubinemia is sustained or rising and unresponsive to phototherapy.

 ## Hemolytic Disease of the Newborn

Erythroblastosis fetalis, or hemolytic disease of the newborn, occurs in Rh-positive infants of Rh-negative mothers who have been sensitized. The mother can produce anti-Rh antibodies from pregnancies in which the infants are Rh positive or by blood transfusions of Rh-positive blood. The Rh-negative mother usually becomes sensitized during the first few days after delivery, when fetal Rh-positive red cells from the placental site are released into the maternal circulation. Because the antibodies take several weeks to develop, the first Rh-positive infant of an Rh-negative mother usually is not affected. Infants with Rh-negative blood have no antigens on their red cells to react with the maternal antibodies and are not affected.

After an Rh-negative mother has been sensitized, the Rh antibodies from her blood are transferred to subsequent infants through the placental circulation. These antibodies react with the red cell antigens of the Rh-positive infant, causing agglutination and hemolysis. This leads to severe anemia with compensatory hyperplasia and enlargement of the blood-forming organs, including the spleen and liver, in the fetus. Liver function may be impaired, with decreased production of albumin causing massive edema, called *hydrops fetalis.* If blood levels of unconjugated bilirubin are abnormally high because of red cell hemolysis, there is a danger of kernicterus developing in the infant, resulting in severe brain damage or death.

Several advances have served significantly to decrease the threat to infants born to Rh-negative mothers: prevention of sensitization, antenatal identification of the at-risk fetus, and intrauterine transfusion to the affected fetus. The injection of Rh immune globulin (*i.e.,* gamma-globulin containing Rh antibody) prevents sensitization in Rh-negative mothers who have given birth to Rh-positive infants if administered at 28 weeks' gestation and within 72 hours of delivery, abortion, genetic amniocentesis, or fetal-maternal bleeding. After sensitization has developed, the immune globulin is of no value. Since 1968, the year Rh immune globulin was introduced, the incidence of sensitization of Rh-negative women has dropped dramatically. Early prenatal care and screening of maternal blood continue to be important in reducing immunization. Efforts to improve therapy are aimed at production of monoclonal anti-D, the Rh antibody.

In the past, approximately 20% of erythroblastotic fetuses died in utero. Fetal Rh phenotyping can now be performed to identify at-risk fetuses in the first trimester using fetal blood or amniotic cells.[32] Hemolysis in these fetuses can be treated by intrauterine transfusions of red cells through the umbilical cord. Exchange transfusions are administered after birth by removing and replacing the infant's blood volume with type O Rh-negative blood. The exchange transfusion removes most of the hemolyzed red cells and some of the total bilirubin, treating the anemia and hyperbilirubinemia.

Red Cell Changes With Aging

Anemia is an increasingly common health problem in the elderly, affecting approximately one fourth of 80-year-olds in the community and half of the chronically ill elderly.[33] Its prevalence is known to increase with age, with the highest prevalence in men aged 85 years and older. Undiagnosed and untreated anemia can have severe complications and is associated with increased risk of mortality, cardiovascular disease, lower functional ability, self-care deficits, cognitive disorders, and reduced bone density that increases the risk for fractures with falls.[33]

Hemoglobin levels decline after middle age. In studies of men older than 60 years of age, mean hemoglobin levels ranged

from 15.3 to 12.4 g/dL, with the lowest levels found in the oldest persons. The decline is less in women, with mean levels ranging from 13.8 to 11.7 mg/dL.[34] In most asymptomatic elderly persons, lower hemoglobin levels result from iron deficiency and anemia of chronic disease.

As with other body systems, the capacity for red cell production changes with aging. The location of bone cells involved in red cell production shifts toward the axial skeleton, and the number of progenitor cells declines from approximately 50% of younger adult numbers at age 65, to approximately 30% at age 75 years.[34] Despite these changes, the elderly are able to maintain hemoglobin and hematocrit levels within a range similar to that of younger adults.[35] However, during a stress situation such as bleeding, the red blood cells of the elderly are not replaced as promptly as those of their younger counterparts. This inability to replace red blood cells closely correlates with the increased prevalence of anemia in the elderly.

Although the age-associated decline in the hematopoietic reserve in the elderly is not completely understood, several factors seem to play a role, including a reduction in hematopoietic progenitors, reduced production of hematopoietic growth factors, and inhibition of erythropoietin or its interaction with its receptors.[33,36] Inflammatory cytokines, which have been found to increase with age, may mediate this reduced sensitivity to erythropoietin.

The diagnosis of anemia in the elderly requires a complete physical examination, a complete blood count, and studies to rule out comorbid conditions such as malignancy, gastrointestinal conditions that cause bleeding, and pernicious anemia. The complete blood count should include a peripheral blood smear and a reticulocyte count and index. If the reticulocyte index is appropriately increased for the level of anemia, then blood loss or red cell destruction should be suspected. If the reticulocyte index is inappropriately low, then decreased red cell production is indicated.[36]

The treatment of anemia in the elderly should focus on the underlying cause and correction of the red cell deficit. An important aspect of anemia of chronic disease is the inability to use and mobilize iron effectively.[33] Orally administered iron is poorly used in older adults, despite normal iron absorption.[34] Although erythropoietin remains the treatment of choice for anemias associated with cancer and renal disease, its potential use in treating anemias associated with aging remains to be established.

IN SUMMARY, hemoglobin concentrations at birth are high, reflecting the in utero need for oxygen delivery; toward the end of the first postnatal week, these levels begin to decline, gradually falling to a minimum value at approximately 2 months of age. During the early neonatal period, there is a shift from fetal to adult hemoglobin. Many infants have physiologic jaundice because of hyperbilirubinemia during the first week of life, probably related to increased red cell breakdown and the inability of the infant's liver to conjugate bilirubin. The term *kernicterus* describes elevated levels of lipid-soluble, unconjugated bilirubin, which can be toxic to brain cells. Depending on severity, it is treated with phototherapy or exchange transfusions (or both). Hemolytic disease of the newborn occurs in Rh-positive infants of Rh-negative mothers who have been sensitized. It involves hemolysis of infant red cells in response to maternal Rh antibodies that have crossed the placenta. Administration of Rh immune globulin to the mother within 72 hours of delivery of an Rh-positive infant, abortion, or amniocentesis prevents sensitization.

Anemia is an increasingly common health problem in the elderly, affecting approximately 25% of persons aged 80 years and older. As with many other tissue cells, the capacity for red cell replacement decreases with aging. Although most elderly persons are able to maintain their hemoglobin and hematocrit levels within a normal range, they are unable to replace their red cells as promptly as their younger counterparts during a stress situation such as bleeding. This inability to replace red blood cells closely correlates with the increased prevalence of anemia in the elderly, which is usually the result of bleeding, infection, malignancy, or chronic disease. ■

Review Exercises

1. A 29-year-old woman complains of generalized fatigue. Her physical examination reveals a heart rate of 115 beats/minute, blood pressure 115/75, respiratory rate 28 breaths/minute Her skin and nail beds are pale. Her laboratory results include red blood cell count $3.0 \times 10^6/\mu L$, hematocrit 30%, hemoglobin 9 g/dL, and a decrease in serum ferritin levels.

   A. *What disorder do you suspect this woman has?*

   B. *What additional data would be helpful in determining the etiology of her condition?*

   C. *Which of her signs reflect the body's attempt to compensate for the disorder?*

   D. *What is the significance of the low ferritin level, and how could it be used to make decisions related to her treatment?*

2. A 65-year-old woman is being seen in the clinic because of numbness in her lower legs and feet and difficulty walking. She has no other complaints. She takes a blood pressure pill, two calcium pills, and a multivitamin pill daily. Her laboratory results include red blood cell count $3.0 \times 10^6/\mu L$, hematocrit 20%, hemoglobin 9 g/dL, and a markedly elevated MVC.

   A. *What type of anemia does she have?*

   B. *What is the reason for her neurologic symptoms?*

   C. *What type of treatment would be appropriate?*

3. A 12-year-old boy with sickle cell disease presents in the emergency department with severe chest pain. His mother reports that he was doing well until he came down with a respiratory tract infection. She also states he insisted on playing basketball with the other boys in the neighborhood even though he wasn't feeling well.

   A. *What is the most likely cause of pain in this boy?*

   B. *Infections and aerobic-type exercise that increase the levels of deoxygenated hemoglobin produce sickling in persons who are homozygous for the sickle cell gene and have sickle cell disease, but not in persons who are heterozygous and have sickle cell trait. Explain.*

   C. *People with sickle disease experience anemia but not iron deficiency. Explain.*

4. Forty students in a hematology class conducted a laboratory exercise that involved determining their blood type. In a subsequent laboratory discussion, they discovered that 16 fellow students had type A blood, 20 had type O blood, 3 had type B blood, and only 1 had type AB blood.

   A. *What types of blood antigens and antibodies would students with type A, type O, and type AB blood have?*

   B. *What could be the possible blood types of the parents of students with type B blood, type O blood, and type AB blood?*

   C. *If these students required a blood transfusion, what type of blood could those with type A, type O, and type AB receive? (Assume the blood is of the same Rh type.)*

References

1. English E. (2003). Blood components, immunity, and hemostasis. In Rhoades R. A., Tanner R. A. (Eds.), *Medical physiology* (2nd ed., pp. 191–197). Philadelphia: Lippincott Williams & Wilkins.

2. Aster J. C. (2005). Red blood cell and bleeding disorders. In Kumar V., Abbas A. K., Fausto N. (Eds.), *Robbins and Cotran pathophysiologic basis of disease* (7th ed., pp. 619–649). Philadelphia: Elsevier Saunders.

3. Fisher J. W. (2003). Erythropoietin: Physiology and pharmacology update. *Experimental Biology and Medicine* 228, 1–14.

4. Guyton A. C., Hall J. E. (2006). *Textbook of medical physiology* (11th ed., pp. 419–438). Philadelphia: W. B. Saunders.

5. Schwarting R., Kocher W. D., McKenzie S., et al. (2005). Hematopathology. In Rubin E., Gorstein F., Rubin R., et al. (Eds.), *Rubin's pathology: Clinicopathologic foundations of medicine* (4th ed., pp. 1026–1051). Philadelphia: Lippincott Williams & Wilkins.

6. Steinberg M. H., Rodgers G. P. (2001). Pathophysiology of sickle cell disease: Role of cellular and genetic modifiers. *Seminars in Hematology* 38, 299–306.

7. Chiang E. Y., Frenette P. S. (2005). Sickle cell vaso-occlusion. *Hematology and Oncology Clinics of North America* 19, 771–784.

8. Ballas S. K. (2001). Sickle cell disease. *Seminars in Hematology* 38, 307–314.

9. Stuart M. J., Nagel R. L. (2004). Sickle-cell disease. *Lancet* 364, 1343–1360.

10. National Institutes of Health. (2002). The management of sickle cell disease. NIH publication no. 02-2117. [On-line.] Available: www.nhlbi.nih.gov/health/prof/blood/sickle/index.htm. Accessed January 10, 2007.

11. Vichinsky E. (2002). New therapies in sickle cell disease. *Lancet* 360, 629–631

12. Rund D., Rachmilewitz E. (2005). β-Thalassemia. *New England Journal of Medicine* 353, 1135–1146.

13. Lo L., Singer S. T. (2002). Thalassemia: Current approach to an old disease. *Pediatric Clinics of North America* 49, 1165–1191.

14. Brittenham G. M. (2000). Disorders of iron metabolism: Iron deficiency and overload. In Hoffman R., Benz E. J., Shattil S. J., et al. (Eds.), *Hematology: Basic principles and practice* (3rd ed., pp. 405, 413). New York: Churchill Livingstone.

15. Glader B. (2004). Anemia of inadequate production. In Behrman R. E., Kliegman R. M., Jenson H. B. (Eds.), *Nelson textbook of pediatrics* (17th ed., pp. 1606–1607), Philadelphia: Elsevier Saunders.

16. Lozoff B., Beard J., Connor J., et al. (2006). Long-lasting neural and behavioral effects of iron deficiency in infancy. *Nutritional Reviews* 64, S34–43.

17. Kazal L. A. (2002). Prevention of iron deficiency in infants and toddlers. *American Family Physician* 66, 1217–1224.

18. Aslinia F., Mazza J. J., Yale S. H. (2006). Megaloblastic anemia and other causes of macrocytosis. *Clinical Medicine and Research* 3, 236–241.

19. Oh R., Brown D. L. (2003). Vitamin B_{12} deficiency. *American Family Physician* 67, 979–986.

20. Johnston M. V., Kinsman S. (2004). Congenital anomalies of the central nervous system. In Behrman R. E., Kliegman R. M., Jenson H. B. (Eds.), *Nelson textbook of pediatrics* (17th ed., pp. 1983–1984), Philadelphia: Elsevier Saunders.

21. Bailey L. B. (2000). New standard for folate intake in pregnant women. *American Journal of Clinical Nutrition* 71(5 Suppl.), 1304S–1307S.

22. Young N. S. (2002). Acquired aplastic anemia. *Annals of Internal Medicine* 136, 534–546.

23. Young N. S., Calada R. T., Scheinberg P. (2006). Current concepts in the pathophysiology and treatment of aplastic anemia. *Blood* 108, 2509–2519.

24. Weiss G., Goodnough L. T. (2005). Anemia of chronic disease. *New England Journal of Medicine* 352, 1011–1023.

25. Raghavan M., Marik P. E. (2005). Anemia, allogenic blood transfusion, and immunomodulation in the critically ill. *Chest* 127, 295–307.

26. Goodnough L. T., Brecher M. E., Kanter M. H., et al. (1999). Blood conservation. *New England Journal of Medicine* 340, 525–533.

27. Goodnough L. T., Brecher M. E., Kanter M. H., et al. (1999). Blood transfusion. *New England Journal of Medicine* 340, 438–447.

28. Brecher M. E. (Ed.). (2005). *Technical manual* (15th ed., pp. 175–176, 485–486). Bethesda, MD: American Association of Blood Banks.

29. Tefferi A., Spivak J. L. (2005). Polycythemia vera: Scientific advances and current practice. *Seminars in Hematology* 42, 206–220.

30. Ohls R. K., Christensen R. D. (2004). Development of the hematopoietic system. In Behrman R. E., Kliegman R. M., Jenson H. B. (Eds.), *Nelson textbook of pediatrics* (17th ed., pp. 1599–1604). Philadelphia: Elsevier Saunders.

31. Stoll B. J., Kliegman R. M. (2004). Jaundice and hyperbilirubinemia in the newborn. In Behrman R. E., Kliegman R. M., Jenson H. B. (Eds.), *Nelson textbook of pediatrics* (17th ed., pp. 592–599). Philadelphia: Elsevier Saunders.

32. Kramer K., Cohen H. J. (2000). Antenatal diagnosis of hematologic disorders. In Hoffman R., Benz E. J., Shattil S. J., et al. (Eds.), *Hematology: Basic principles and practice* (3rd ed., p. 2495). New York: Churchill Livingstone.

33. Eisenstaedt R., Pennix B. W., Woodman R. C. (2006). Anemia in the elderly: Current understanding and emerging concepts. *Blood Review* 20, 213–226.

34. Balducci L. (2003). Epidemiology of anemia in the elderly: Information on diagnostic evaluation. *Journal of the American Geriatrics Society* 51(Suppl. 3), S2–S9.

35. Rothstein G. (2003). Disordered hematopoiesis and myelodysplasia in the elderly. *Journal of the American Geriatrics Society* 51(Suppl. 3), S22–S26.

36. Lipschitz D. (2003). Medical and functional consequences of anemia in the elderly. *Journal of the American Geriatrics Society* 51(Suppl. 3), S10–S13.

Visit the**Point** http://thePoint.lww.com for animations, journal articles, and more!

Disorders of White Blood Cells and Lymphoid Tissues

CAROL M. PORTH

➤ The white blood cells and lymphoid tissues where these cells originate and mature function to protect the body against invasion by foreign agents. Disorders of the white blood cells include leukopenia, in which there is a deficiency in leukocytes, and proliferative disorders, in which there is an expansion of leukocytes. The proliferative disorders may be reactive, as occurs with infection, or neoplastic, as occurs with malignant lymphomas and leukemia. This chapter focuses on leukopenia, infectious mononucleosis, malignant lymphomas, leukemias, and plasma cell dyscrasias (multiple myeloma).

HEMATOPOIETIC AND LYMPHOID TISSUES

After completing this section of the chapter, you should be able to meet the following objectives:

- Describe the different types of white blood cells and structures of the lymphoid system where they circulate and mature.
- Trace the development of the different white blood cells from their origin in the pluripotent bone marrow stem cell to their circulation in the bloodstream.

The hematopoietic system encompasses all the blood cells and their precursors. It includes the myeloid or bone marrow tissue in which the blood cells are formed, and the lymphoid tissues of the lymph nodes, thymus, and spleen, in which the white blood cells circulate, mature, and function. The development of the different blood cells involves interactions among precursor bone marrow cells and a variety of growth factors, cytokines (chemical messengers), and gene products such as transcription factors.

Leukocytes (White Blood Cells)

The white blood cells include the granulocytes (*i.e.,* neutrophils, eosinophils, and basophils), monocytes/macrophages, and lymphocytes. The granulocytes and the agranular monocytes/macrophages are derived from the myeloid stem cell in the bone

HEMATOPOIESIS

- The white blood cells are formed from hematopoietic stem cells that differentiate into committed progenitor cells that in turn develop into the myelocytic and lymphocytic lineages needed for the formation of the different types of white blood cell.

- The growth and reproduction of the different stem cells is controlled by colony-stimulating factors, other growth factors, and chemical mediators.

- The life span of white blood cells is relatively short so that constant renewal is necessary to maintain normal blood levels. Any conditions that decrease the availability of stem cells or hematopoietic growth factors produce a decrease in white blood cells.

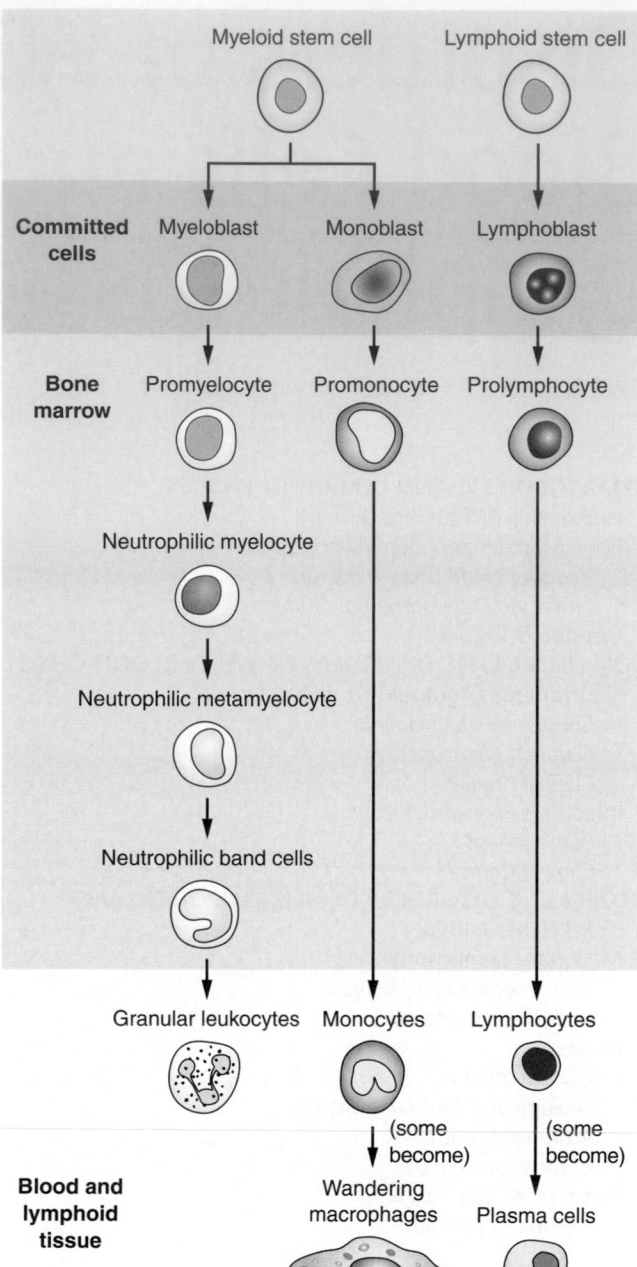

FIGURE 15-1 • Leukocytes originate from multipotential stem cells in the bone marrow. Granular leukocytes (neutrophils, eosinophils, basophils) have their origin in the myeloid stem cells and develop through a sequence involving myeloblasts. Monocytes, like granulocytes, are progeny of the myeloid stem cell line, but develop along a pathway involving monoblasts. Only lymphocytes originate from the lymphoid stem cell line. They develop through a sequence involving lymphoblasts and are released from the bone marrow as prolymphocytes, which undergo further differentiation in the lymphoid organs.

marrow and circulate in the blood (Fig. 15-1). The T lymphocytes (T cells) and B lymphocytes (B cells) originate from lymphoid stem cells in the bone marrow and migrate between the blood and the lymphatic system (see Chapter 12). T lymphocytes mature in the thymus, and B lymphocytes in the bone marrow—the mammalian equivalent of the avian bursa of Fabricius. The T lymphocytes differentiate to form CD4+ helper T cells, which serve to orchestrate the immune response, and CD8+ cytotoxic T cells, which provide for cell-mediated immune responses (see Chapter 17). The B lymphocytes differentiate to form immunoglobulin-producing plasma cells. Another population of lymphocytes includes the large granular lymphocytes, or natural killer (NK) cells, which do not share the specificity or characteristics of the T or the B lymphocytes, but have the ability to lyse target cells.[1]

Bone Marrow and Hematopoiesis

The entire hematopoietic system, with all its complexity, arises from a small number of stem cells that differentiate to form blood cells and replenish the bone marrow by a process of self-renewal. All the hematopoietic precursors, including the erythroid (red blood cell), myelocyte (granulocyte and monocyte), lymphocyte (T cell and B cell), and megakaryocyte (platelet) series, are derived from a small population of cells called *pluripotent stem cells*. These cells are capable of providing *progenitor cells* (*i.e.*, parent cells) for myelopoiesis and lymphopoiesis, processes by which myeloid and lymphoid blood cells are made. Several levels of differentiation lead to the development of committed *unipotent cells*, which are the progenitors for each of the different blood cell types.

Hematopoietic Growth Factors

Like erythropoiesis, which is described in Chapter 14, leukopoiesis or production of white blood cells is controlled by hematopoietic growth factors. The *hematopoietic growth factors* are a family of glycoproteins that support hematopoietic colony formation (see Chapter 12). These growth factors can be categorized into three functional groups: those that are involved in the development of a specific cell lineage, those that affect the early multipotential progenitor cells, and those that indirectly regulate hematopoiesis by inducing the expression of growth factor genes in other cells.[2] Cytokines or chemical messengers, such as interleukin (IL)-1, IL-4, IL-6, and interferon, act synergistically to support the functions of the growth factors.

There are several lineage-specific growth factors: erythropoietin, granulocyte-macrophage colony–stimulating factor (GM-CSF), and monocyte-macrophage colony–stimulating factor (M-CSF). Although the hematopoietic growth factors act at different points in the proliferation and differentiation pathway, their functions overlap. For example, GM-CSF stimulates the growth and function of granulocyte, macrophage, and eosinophil progenitor cells and induces IL-1 gene expression in neutrophils and peripheral mononuclear leukocytes. Cytokines, such as IL-3, act on the most immature bone marrow progenitor cells, thereby promoting the development of cells that can differentiate into a number of cell types. The identification and characterization of the various growth factors and cytokines has led to their use in treating a wide range of diseases, including bone marrow failure, hematopoietic neoplasms, infectious diseases, and congenital and myeloproliferative disorders.

Leukocyte Developmental Stages

Leukocyte development begins with the myeloid and lymphoid stem cells in the bone marrow. The granulocyte and monocyte cell lines derive from the myeloid stem cells and the lymphocytes from the lymphoid stem cells (see Fig. 15-1). The immature precursor cells for each of the cell lines are called *blast cells. Myeloblasts,* which are the granulocytic precursor cells, have round to oval nuclei, with delicate chromatin and a blue to gray cytoplasm. During the next stage of development, the myeloblasts are transformed into *promyelocytes* with similar nuclei, but with a cytoplasm containing many primary granules. In the subsequent *metamyelocyte* stage, the nuclei distort and become arclike, producing the band developmental stage. Maturation from metamyelocyte to mature neutrophil involves progressive condensation of nuclear chromatin, increasing nuclear lobulation, and the appearance of secondary (specific) granules. Eosinophils and basophils undergo similar developmental stages, but develop different secondary granules. Like granulocytes, monocytes develop from the granulocyte-monocyte progenitor cell and progress through a monoblast and promonocyte stage. By contrast, lymphocytes derive from lymphoid stem cells and progress through the lymphoblast and prolymphocyte stages. The prolymphocytes leave the bone marrow and travel to the lymphoid tissues, where further differentiation into T and B lymphocytes occurs. The names of the various leukocyte developmental stages are often used in describing blood cell changes that occur in hematopoietic disorders (*e.g.,* acute lymphoblastic leukemia, acute promyelocytic leukemia).

Lymphoid Tissues

The body's lymphatic system consists of the lymphatic vessels, lymphoid tissue and lymph nodes, thymus, and spleen (see Chapter 17). Although both precursor B and T lymphocytes begin their development in the bone marrow, they migrate to peripheral lymphoid structures to complete the differentiation process. B lymphocytes leave the bone marrow, differentiate into plasma cells, and then move to the lymph nodes, where they continue to proliferate and produce antibodies. T lymphocytes leave the bone marrow as precursor T lymphocytes travel to the thymus, where they differentiate into CD4+ helper T cells and CD8+ cytotoxic T cells, after which many of them move to lymph nodes, where they undergo further proliferation.

Lymph nodes, which are the site where many lymphomas originate, consist of organized collections of lymphoid tissue located along the lymphatic vessels.[3–5] Typically grayish-white and ovoid or bean-shaped, they range in size from 1 mm to about 1 to 2 cm in diameter. A fibrous capsule and radiating trabeculae provide a supporting structure, and a delicate reticular network contributes to internal support (Fig. 15-2). The parenchyma of the lymph node is divided into an outer or superficial cortex and an inner medulla. The superficial cortex contains well-defined B-cell and T-cell domains. The B-cell–dependent cortex consists of two types of follicles: immunologically inactive follicles, called *primary follicles,* and active follicles that contain germinal centers, called *secondary follicles.* Germinal centers contain large lymphocytes (centroblasts) and small lymphocytes with cleaved nuclei (centrocytes). The mantle zone is the small layer of B cells surrounding the germinal centers. The portion of the cortex between the medullary and superficial cortex is called the *paracortex.* This region contains most of the T cells in the lymph nodes.

Although some lymphocytes enter the lymph nodes through the afferent lymphatic channels, most enter through the wall of postcapillary venules located in the deep cortex. These vessels, which are lined with specialized endothelial cells that possess receptors for antigen-primed lymphocytes, signal lymphocytes

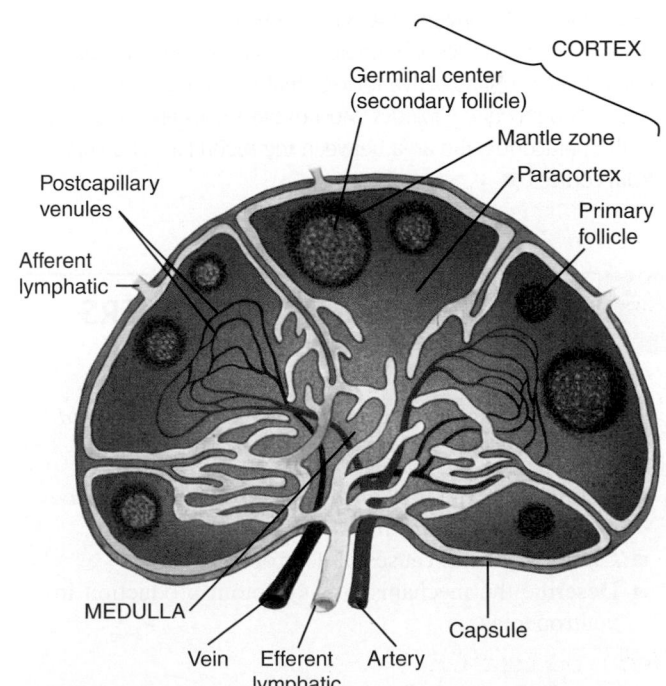

FIGURE 15-2 • Structures of normal lymph node. (From Schwarting R., McKenzie S., Rubin R. [2008]. Hematopathology. In Rubin R., Strayer D. E. [Eds.], *Rubin's pathology: Clinicopathologic foundations of medicine* [5th ed., p. 905]. Philadelphia: Lippincott Williams & Wilkins.)

to leave the circulation and migrate through the lymph nodes. Both B and T cells leave the bloodstream through these channels.[3] The T cells remain in the paracortex and the B cells migrate to the follicular area of the cortex. Most lymphocytes leave the lymph node by entering the lymphatic sinuses, from which they enter the efferent lymphatic vessel.

The alimentary canal, respiratory passages, and genitourinary systems are guarded by accumulations of lymphoid tissue that are not enclosed in a capsule. This form of lymphoid tissue is called *diffuse lymphoid tissue* or *mucosa-associated lymphoid tissue* (MALT) because of its association with mucous membranes. Lymphocytes are found in the subepithelium of these tissues. Lymphomas can arise from MALT as well as lymph node tissue.

IN SUMMARY, leukocyte or white blood cell development begins with the myeloid and lymphoid stem cells in the bone marrow. The granulocyte and monocyte cell lines derive from the myeloid stem cells, and lymphocytes from the lymphoid stem cells. The immature precursor cells for each of the cell lines are called *blast cells.* The blast cells progress through subsequent maturational stages before becoming mature granulocytes, monocytes, or lymphocytes. The names of these developmental stages are often used in describing blood cell changes that occur in hematopoietic disorders.

The lymphatic system consists of a network of lymphatic vessels, nodes, and tissues where B and T lymphocytes complete their differentiation. Lymph nodes, which are the site where many lymphomas originate, exhibit an outer or superficial cortex and an inner medulla. The cortex contains well-defined B-cell and T-cell domains. The B-cell–dependent cortex consists of two types of follicles: immunologically inactive follicles, called *primary follicles,* and active follicles that contain germinal centers, called *secondary follicles.* Most of the T cells are contained in the paracortex, the area between the medullary and superficial cortices. ■

NON-NEOPLASTIC DISORDERS OF WHITE BLOOD CELLS

After completing this section of the chapter, you should be able to meet the following objectives:

■ Define the terms *leukopenia, neutropenia, granulocytopenia,* and *aplastic anemia.*
■ Cite two general causes of neutropenia.
■ Describe the mechanism of symptom production in neutropenia.

The number of leukocytes, or white blood cells, in the peripheral circulation normally ranges from 5000 to 10,000 cells/μL (also expressed as 5 to 10×10^3 cells/μL, or 5000 to 10,000 cells/mm³ of blood). The non-neoplastic disorders of white blood cells

include a deficiency of leukocytes (leukopenia) and proliferative disorders in which there are increased numbers of leukocytes.

Neutropenia (Agranulocytosis)

The term *leukopenia* describes a decrease in the absolute number of leukocytes in the blood. Although leukopenia may affect any of the specific types of white blood cells, it most often affects the neutrophil. Neutrophils constitute the majority of blood leukocytes and play a critical role in host defense mechanisms against infection. They migrate to sites of infection and engulf, digest, and destroy microorganisms. Thus a decrease in the number of neutrophils (neutropenia) places a person at risk for infection. The risk for and severity of neutropenia-associated infection are directly proportional to the absolute neutrophil count and duration of the neutropenia.

Neutropenia refers specifically to an abnormally low number of neutrophils, and is commonly defined as a circulating neutrophil count of less than 1500/μL.[4–6] It can be further graded as mild (1000/μL), moderate (500 to 1000/μL), or severe (<500/μL) based on an absolute number of neutrophils circulating in the blood. *Agranulocytosis* denotes a virtual absence of neutrophils. In *aplastic anemia,* all of the myeloid stem cells are affected, resulting in anemia, thrombocytopenia, and agranulocytosis.

Neutropenia can result from decreased neutrophil production, accelerated utilization or destruction, or a shift from the blood to the tissue compartments. It can be present at birth (congenital) or arise from a number of factors that occur later in life and do not have a hereditary component (acquired).

Congenital Neutropenia

Inherited disorders of proliferation and maturation of myeloid stem cell lines are relatively rare. Two of the more severe inherited types of congenital neutropenia are cyclic neutropenia and severe congenital neutropenia.[6,7] There are also several congenital immunodeficiency disorders that are accompanied by severe neutropenia, including the severe combined immunodeficiencies and common variable immunodeficiency (discussed in Chapter 19). In addition to the inherited forms of neutropenia that present in infancy, an alloimmune neonatal neutropenia can occur because of the transplacental transfer of maternal antibodies.

Alloimmune neonatal neutropenia is neutropenia that occurs after transplacental transfer of maternal alloantibodies directed at an infant's neutrophils, analogous to Rh hemolytic disease discussed in Chapter 14. The disorder usually involves phagocytic destruction of antibody-coated neutrophils by splenic macrophages. Affected infants may present with delayed separation of the umbilical cord, mild skin infection, fever, and pneumonia within the first 2 weeks of life. These manifestations resolve with antimicrobial therapy.[7]

Periodic or *cyclic neutropenia* is a rare autosomal dominant disorder with variable expression that begins in infancy and persists for decades. The disorder arises from a regulatory abnormality involving early hematopoietic precursors and is associated with the neutrophil elastase (a protease that degrades virulent factors in bacteria) gene.[6,7] It is characterized by regular, periodic oscillations of peripheral neutrophils from normal to neutropenic values every 18 to 24 days.[7] During the neutropenic periods, most persons suffer from fever, stomatitis, and pharyngitis, occasionally associated with lymph node enlargement. Serious infections may occur occasionally. The cycles often become less noticeable in older persons, and the disorder then begins to resemble that of chronic neutropenia.

Severe congenital neutropenia, or *Kostmann syndrome,* is characterized by an arrest in myeloid maturation at the promyelocyte stage of development resulting in an absolute neutrophil count of less than 200 cells/μL.[7] It can be inherited as either an autosomal dominant or autosomal recessive trait. The disease is usually associated with mutations in the neutrophil elastase gene, which in turn leads to apoptosis of bone marrow myeloid cells. The disorder is characterized by severe bacterial infections. Before the GM-CSFs became available for clinical use, two thirds of children died of fatal infections before reaching adolescence. Approximately 5% to 10% of persons with the disorder develop myelogenous leukemia.[6,7]

Acquired Neutropenia

Acquired neutropenia encompasses a broad spectrum of causative processes and includes primary and secondary autoimmune neutropenia, infection-related neutropenia, and drug-induced neutropenia (Chart 15-1). It also may be caused by a number of bone marrow disorders, hematopoietic malignancies, and radiation therapy.

Autoimmune Neutropenia. Autoimmune neutropenia results from antibodies directed against neutrophil cell membrane antigens or bone marrow progenitors. The autoimmune forms of neutropenia may be classified as primary (*i.e.,* those not associated with other detectable pathologic processes) or secondary (*i.e.,* those associated with another disease condition).[6,8]

Primary autoimmune neutropenia is a rare disorder of early childhood, during which a moderate to severe neutropenia is observed. The condition is usually benign, with mild to moderate infections. Spontaneous remission occurs in 95% of children by 2 to 3 years of age.[6] The disorder is rare in adults. Because primary autoimmune neutropenia is self-limiting, treatment is usually restricted to the use of antimicrobial agents for persons who experience recurrent infections.

Secondary immune-associated neutropenia is often associated with systemic autoimmune disorders, mainly rheumatoid arthritis (RA) and systemic lupus erythematosus (SLE).[6,8] Felty syndrome, a variant of RA, is a triad of splenomegaly, deforming RA, and neutropenia. The neutropenia is the result of antineutrophil antibodies and high levels of circulating immune complexes, which induce neutrophil apoptosis. Coupled with the end-organ manifestations of RA (discussed in Chapter 59), the majority of persons with Felty syndrome are susceptible to serious bacterial infection that sometimes leads to sepsis and poor clinical outcome.

<table>
<tr><td colspan="2">CHART 15-1   PRINCIPAL CAUSES OF NEUTROPENIA</td></tr>
</table>

Congenital
- Alloimmune neonatal neutropenia (transfer of maternal antibodies)
- Cyclic neutropenia
- Kostmann syndrome (severe congenital neutropenia)

Acquired
Autoimmune
- Primary (rare, usually occurs in children and runs a benign course)
- Secondary
  - Systemic lupus erythematous
  - Felty syndrome in persons with rheumatoid arthritis

Infection related
- Many types of infections agents, but most commonly viruses
- Mechanisms include increased consumption of neutrophils, production of autoantibodies, direct infiltration of hematopoietic cells, bone marrow suppression

Drug related
- Immune-mediated reactions in which drugs act as haptens (*e.g.,* penicillin, propylthiouracil, aminopyrine)
- Accelerated apoptosis (clozapine [antipsychotic agent])
- Cancer chemotherapeutic drugs (bone marrow depression)

Radiation therapy to bone marrow
Hematologic malignancies

Several antibody-mediated mechanisms are believed to be responsible for the neutropenia seen in persons with SLE. These include the development of antineutrophil antibodies, along with increased neutrophil apoptosis, and decreased neutrophil production by the bone marrow. Similar to Felty syndrome, continued treatment of SLE to control symptoms is the preferred method of treatment.

Infection-Related Neutropenia. Many different types of infectious diseases, including viral, bacterial, rickettsial, and parasitic, may cause neutropenia, the most common being viral. Infections may produce neutropenia by a variety of mechanisms, including production of autoantibodies that cause increased and premature destruction of neutrophils; direct infiltration of developing hematopoietic cell lines; elaboration of toxins that suppress bone marrow function; and production of splenomegaly with increased neutrophil sequestration and destruction.[6] Neutropenia is a common manifestation of acquired immunodeficiency syndrome (AIDS), in which a virus-induced suppression of marrow cell proliferation is often aggravated by infectious consumption of neutrophils and the action of antiviral drugs (*e.g.,* zidovudine).[4]

Drug-Related Neutropenia. The incidence of drug-induced neutropenia has increased significantly over the last several decades and is attributed primarily to a wider use of drugs in general and more specifically to the use of chemotherapeutic drugs in the treatment of cancer. Persons with almost any malignancy who receive chemotherapy with or without radiation therapy are at risk for development of chemotherapy-induced neutropenia.[6] The risk for development of chemotherapy-induced neutropenia is influenced by patient-, disease-, and treatment-related factors. One of the most important patient-related factors is age. Elderly patients are at greater risk than younger persons because of age-related cellular changes in neutrophils.[6] Other patient-related factors include poor nutritional status and comorbid conditions such as kidney disease.[6] Disease-related factors include neoplastic bone involvement, type of cancer, and history of anemia or neutropenia with prior chemotherapy regimens. Treatment-related factors include radiation therapy to the bone marrow, extensive prior chemotherapy, and treatment regimen. Treatment regimens for hematologic malignancies are more likely to generate chemotherapy-induced neutropenia than some other treatment regimens.

The term *idiosyncratic* is used to describe drug reactions that are different from the effect obtained in most persons and that cannot be explained in terms of allergy. A number of idiosyncratic cases of drug-induced neutropenia are thought to be caused by immunologic mechanisms, with the drug or its metabolites acting as antigens (*i.e.,* haptens) to incite the production of antibodies reactive against neutrophils.[6] In the case of hapten formation, discontinuation of the drug usually results in resolution of neutropenia within a week or two. Some drugs, such as the antipsychotic drug clozapine, have been shown to cause accelerated apoptosis of neutrophils. Clozapine has been shown to cause agranulocytosis in a small but significant number of persons. This serious, potentially fatal effect can develop rapidly, usually within the 6th to 18th weeks of therapy.[9] The reaction is reversible on discontinuation of the drug. Because of the risk of agranulocytosis, persons receiving clozapine must have weekly blood counts done for the first 6 months of therapy.

Other drugs, such as the β-lactam antibiotics (*e.g.,* cephalosporins), particularly when given in high doses, and some anticonvulsant drugs (*e.g.,* carbamazepine) may inhibit the colony-forming units of granulocytes and monocytes-macrophages in bone marrow. Suppression of myeloid precursors in the bone marrow also has been noted with administration of ticlopidine (an antiplatelet drug), sulfasalazine, and chlorpromazine (an antipsychotic drug).[6]

Clinical Course

The clinical features of neutropenia usually depend on the severity of neutropenia and the cause of the disorder.[10] Neutropenia from any cause increases the risk for infection by gram-positive and gram-negative bacteria and fungi.

Neutrophils provide the first line of defense against organisms that inhabit the skin and gastrointestinal tract. Thus early signs of infection due to neutropenia, particularly those asso-

ciated with a mild to moderate decrease in neutrophils, include mild skin lesions, stomatitis, pharyngitis, and diarrhea. Signs and symptoms of more severe neutropenia include malaise, chills, and fever, followed in sequence by marked weakness and fatigability. Untreated infections can be rapidly fatal, particularly if the absolute neutrophil count drops below 250/μL. With severe neutropenia, the usual signs of infection may not be present because of a lack of a sufficient number of neutrophils to produce an inflammatory response.

Antimicrobial agents are used to treat infections in situations in which neutrophil destruction cannot be controlled or the neutropoietic function of the bone marrow cannot be recovered. Hematopoietic growth factors such as recombinant human granulocyte CSF (filgrastim, pegfilgrastim) may be used to stimulate the maturation and differentiation of the granulocyte cell lineage.[11] In patients receiving chemotherapy for solid tumors, lymphoma, and acute myelogenous leukemia, these agents reduce the duration of severe neutropenia, decrease the incidence of febrile neutropenia, and facilitate on-time delivery of scheduled doses of chemotherapy.

Infectious Mononucleosis

Infectious mononucleosis is a self-limiting lymphoproliferative disorder caused by the Epstein-Barr virus (EBV), a member of the herpesvirus family.[12-16] The term *EBV-associated infectious mononucleosis* is often used to designate infectious mononucleosis caused by EBV as opposed to non–EBV-associated clinical syndromes of infectious mononucleosis caused by other agents. Infectious mononucleosis may occur at any age, but occurs principally in adolescents and young adults in developed countries. In areas of the world where children often live in crowded conditions, asymptomatic infection with EBV occurs in childhood and infectious mononucleosis is not encountered. Two thirds of persons newly infected with EBV after childhood develop clinically evident infectious mononucleosis.[16]

EBV spreads from person to person primarily through contact with infected oral secretions. Transmission requires close contact with infected persons. Thus, the virus spreads readily among young children in crowded conditions, where there is considerable sharing of oral secretions. Kissing is also an effective mode of transmission, hence the term "kissing disease" among adolescents.[14]

Pathogenesis

Epstein-Barr virus initially penetrates the nasopharyngeal, oropharyngeal, and salivary epithelial cells. It then spreads to the underlying oropharyngeal lymphoid tissue and, more specifically, to B lymphocytes, all of which have receptors for EBV. Infection of the B cells may take one of two forms—it may kill the infected B cell, or the virus may incorporate itself into the cell's genome. The B cells that harbor the EBV genome proliferate in the circulation and produce the well-known *heterophil* antibodies that are used for the diagnosis of infectious mononucleosis.[12-14] A heterophil antibody is an immunoglobulin that reacts with antigens from another species—in this case, sheep red blood cells.

The normal immune response is important in controlling the proliferation of the EBV-infected B cells and cell-free virus. Most important in controlling the proliferation of EBV-infected B cells are the CD8⁺ cytotoxic T cells and NK cells. These virus-specific T cells appear as large, atypical lymphocytes that are characteristic of the infection (Fig. 15-3). In otherwise healthy persons, the humoral and cellular immune responses serve to control viral shedding by limiting the number of infected B cells rather than eliminating them.

Although infected B cells and free virions disappear from the blood after recovery from the disease, the virus remains in a few transformed B cells in the oropharyngeal region and is shed in the saliva. Once infected with the virus, persons remain asymptomatically infected for life, and a few such persons intermittently shed EBV. Immunosuppressed persons shed the virus more frequently. Asymptomatic shedding of EBV by healthy persons is thought to account for most of the spread of infectious mononucleosis, despite the fact that it is not a highly contagious disease.

Clinical Course

The onset of infectious mononucleosis usually is insidious. The incubation period lasts 4 to 8 weeks.[15,16] A prodromal period, which lasts for several days, follows and is characterized by malaise, anorexia, and chills. The prodromal period precedes the onset of fever, pharyngitis, and lymphadenopathy. Occasionally, the disorder comes on abruptly with a high fever. Most persons seek medical attention for severe pharyngitis, which usually is most severe on days 5 to 7 and persists for 7 to 14 days. The lymph nodes are typically enlarged throughout the body, particularly in the cervical, axillary, and groin areas. Hepatitis and splenomegaly are common manifestations of the disease

and are thought to be immune mediated. Hepatitis is characterized by hepatomegaly, nausea, anorexia, and jaundice. Although discomforting, it usually is a benign condition that resolves without causing permanent liver damage. The spleen may be enlarged two to three times its normal size, and rupture of the spleen is an infrequent complication. In less than 1% of cases, mostly in the adult age group, complications of the central nervous system (CNS) develop. These complications include cranial nerve palsies, encephalitis, meningitis, transverse myelitis, and Guillain-Barré syndrome.

The peripheral blood usually shows an increase in the number of leukocytes, with a white blood cell count between 12,000 and 18,000 cells/μL, 60% of which are lymphocytes.[14] The rise in white blood cells begins during the first week, continues during the second week of the infection, and then returns to normal around the fourth week. Although leukocytosis is common, leukopenia may be seen in some persons during the first 3 days of illness. Atypical lymphocytes are common, constituting more than 20% of the total lymphocyte count. Heterophil antibodies usually appear during the second or third week and decline after the acute illness has subsided. They may, however, be detectable for up to 9 months after onset of the disease.

Most persons with infectious mononucleosis recover without incident. The acute phase of the illness usually lasts for 2 to 3 weeks, after which recovery occurs rapidly. Some degree of debility and lethargy may persist for 2 to 3 months. Treatment is primarily symptomatic and supportive. It includes bed rest and analgesics such as aspirin to relieve the fever, headache, and sore throat.[15]

In persons with immunodeficiency disorders that lead to defects in cellular immunity (e.g., human immunodeficiency virus [HIV] infection, immunosuppressant-treated recipients of organ or bone marrow transplants), EBV infection may contribute to the development of lymphoproliferative disorders (e.g., non-Hodgkin lymphoma).[12,13] These persons have impaired T-cell immunity and are unable to control the proliferation of EBV-infected B cells.

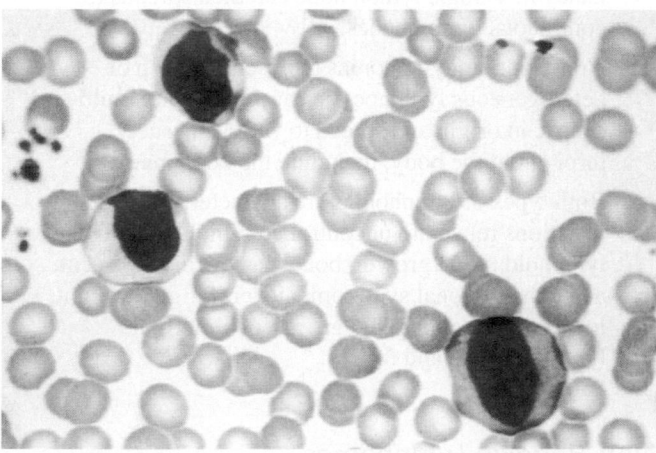

FIGURE 15-3 • Infectious mononucleosis. Atypical lymphocytes are characteristic. (From Schwarting R., McKenzie S., Rubin R. [2008]. Hematopathology. In Rubin R., Strayer D. E. [Eds.], *Rubin's pathology: Clinicopathologic foundations of medicine* [5th ed., p. 908]. Philadelphia: Lippincott Williams & Wilkins.)

IN SUMMARY, neutropenia, which represents a marked reduction in the absolute number of neutrophils, is one of the major disorders of the white blood cells. It can occur as a congenital or acquired disorder. Congenital neutropenia consists primarily of cyclic neutropenia, which is characterized by cyclic (18- to 24-day) oscillations of peripheral neutrophils, and severe congenital neutropenia or Kostmann syndrome, which is associated with severe bacterial infections. The acquired neutropenias encompass a wide spectrum of causative processes, including immunologically mediated bone marrow suppression or neutrophil injury and destruction; infection-mediated mechanisms, including increased peripheral utilization; and drug-mediated mechanisms, particularly those related to the use of cancer chemotherapeutic agents. Neutropenia may also be caused by a number of bone marrow conditions, hematopoietic malignancies, and radiation therapy. Because the neutrophil is essential to host defenses against bacterial and fungal infections, severe and often life-threatening infections are common in persons with neutropenia.

Infectious mononucleosis is a self-limited lymphoproliferative disorder caused by the B-lymphotropic EBV, a member of the herpesvirus family. The highest incidence of infectious mononucleosis is found in adolescents and young adults, and it is seen more frequently in the upper socioeconomic classes of developed countries. The virus is usually transmitted in the saliva. The disease is characterized by fever, generalized lymphadenopathy, sore throat, and the appearance in the blood of atypical lymphocytes and several antibodies, including the well-known heterophil antibodies that are used in the diagnosis of infectious mononucleosis. Most persons with infectious mononucleosis recover without incident. Treatment is largely symptomatic and supportive. ■

NEOPLASTIC DISORDERS OF HEMATOPOIETIC AND LYMPHOID ORIGIN

After completing this section of the chapter, you should be able to meet the following objectives:

- Use the concepts regarding the central and peripheral lymphoid tissues to describe the site of origin of the malignant lymphomas, leukemias, and plasma cell dyscrasias.
- Explain how changes in chromosomal structure and gene function can contribute to the development of malignant lymphomas, leukemias, and plasma cell dyscrasias.
- Contrast and compare the signs and symptoms of non-Hodgkin and Hodgkin lymphomas.
- Describe the measures used in treatment of non-Hodgkin and Hodgkin lymphomas.
- Use the predominant white blood cell type and classification of acute or chronic to describe the four general types of leukemia.
- Explain the manifestations of leukemia in terms of altered cell differentiation.
- Describe the following complications of acute leukemia and its treatment: leukostasis, tumor lysis syndrome, hyperuricemia, and blast crisis.
- Relate the clonal expansion of immunoglobulin-producing plasma cells and accompanying destructive skeletal changes that occur with multiple myeloma in terms of manifestations and clinical course of the disorder.

The neoplastic disorders of hematopoietic and lymphoid origin represent the most important of the white blood cell disorders. They include the somewhat overlapping categories of the lym-

phomas (non-Hodgkin and Hodgkin lymphomas), acute and chronic leukemias, and plasma cell dyscrasias (multiple myeloma). The clinical features of these neoplasms are largely determined by their site of origin, the progenitor cell from which they originated, and the molecular events involved in their transformation into a malignant neoplasm (Fig. 15-4). The leukemias, which arise from hematopoietic precursors in the bone marrow, can involve the T and B lymphocytes, granulocytes, and other blood cells (see Fig. 15-4). The lymphomas originate in peripheral lymphoid structures such as the lymph nodes, where B and T lymphocytes undergo differentiation and proliferation as they interact with antigens. The plasma cell dyscrasias originate in the lymph nodes, where B cells differentiate into plasma cells. Because blood cells circulate throughout the body, these neoplasms are often disseminated from the onset.

Malignant Lymphomas

The lymphomas are a diverse group of solid tumors composed of neoplastic lymphoid cells that vary with respect to molecular features, genetics, clinical presentation, and treatment. An estimated 74,340 new cases of lymphomas were diagnosed in the United States in 2008, of which 66,120 cases were non-Hodgkins lymphomas (NHLs) and 8,220 were Hodgkin lymphoma (HL).[18] Since the early 1970s the incidence rates for NHL have nearly doubled. Although some of this increase was due to AIDS-related NHL, for the most part the increase is unexplained.[18,19] During the same period, the incidence rates for HL have decreased in men, while they slightly increased for women.

🔑 MALIGNANT LYMPHOMAS

- The lymphomas represent malignancies that arise in the peripheral lymphoid tissues.
- Hodgkin lymphoma is a group of cancers characterized by Reed-Sternberg cells that begins as a malignancy in a single lymph node and then spreads to contiguous lymph nodes.
- Non-Hodgkin lymphomas represent a group of heterogeneous lymphocytic cancers that are multicentric in origin and spread to various tissues throughout the body, including the bone marrow.
- Both types of lymphomas are characterized by manifestations related to uncontrolled lymph node and lymphoid tissue growth, bone marrow involvement, and constitutional symptoms (fever, fatigue, weight loss) related to the rapid growth of abnormal lymphoid cells and tissues.

Non-Hodgkin Lymphomas

The NHLs represent a clinically diverse group of either B-cell or T-cell neoplasms, the etiology of which is largely unknown. They represent about 4% of all new cases of cancer diagnosed in the United States each year, making them the fifth most common cause of cancer death in the United States.[17]

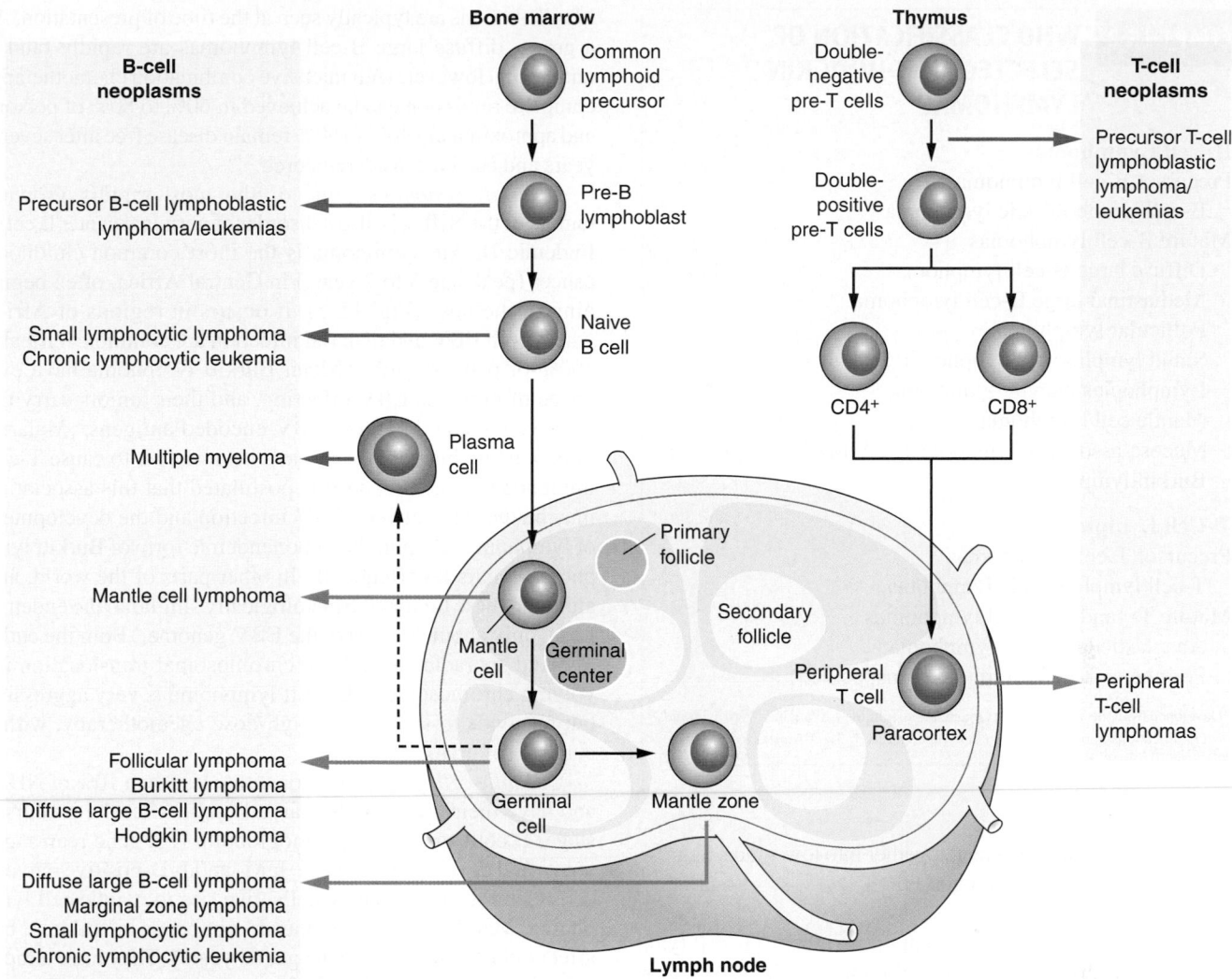

FIGURE 15-4 • Origin of lymphoid neoplasms, showing the stages of B- and T-cell differentiation from which specific lymphoid tumors emerge. (Double-negative pre-T cells express neither CD4 nor CD8; double-positive T cells express both CD4 and CD8.) (Modified from Kumar V., Abbas A. K., Fausto N. [Eds]. [2005]. *Robbins and Cotran pathologic basis of disease* [7th ed., p. 669]. Philadelphia: Elsevier Saunders.)

As with most other malignancies, the cause of NHL is largely unknown. However, impairment of the immune system and infectious agents may play a role. There is evidence of EBV infection in essentially all people with Burkitt lymphoma, which is endemic to some parts of Africa.[4,5,20] A second virus, the human T-cell lymphotropic virus (HTLV-1), which is endemic in the southwestern islands of Japan, has been associated with adult T-cell leukemia/lymphoma. The NHLs are also seen with increased frequency in persons infected with HIV, in those who have received chronic immunosuppressive therapy after organ transplantation, and in individuals with acquired or congenital immunodeficiencies.[20–22] There is also a reported association between chronic *Helicobacter pylori* infection and low-grade MALT lymphoma of the stomach.[22]

Although the NHLs can originate in any of the lymphoid tissues, they most commonly originate in the lymph nodes. Like normal lymphocytes, transformed B and T cells tend to home in to particular lymph node sites, leading to characteristic pat-

terns of involvement. For example, B-cell lymphomas tend to proliferate in the B-cell areas of the lymph node, whereas T-cell lymphomas typically grow in the paracortical T-cell areas[4,5] (see Fig. 15-4). All have the potential to spread to various lymphoid tissues throughout the body, especially the liver, spleen, and bone marrow.

The classification of NHLs remains controversial and is still evolving. A commonly used classification is the World Health Organization (WHO) system[4,5,17,19,20] (Chart 15-2). The WHO system classifies lymphomas in terms of cell type (B or T cell); level of maturation (*e.g.,* immature or mature), and anatomic sites (*e.g.,* MALT lymphoma of the stomach).[4] The NHLs are actually a complex group of almost 40 distinct entities, based on the appearance of the lymphoma cells, the presence of surface markers (*e.g.,* antigens, CD markers), and genetic features.[4,5,19] Neoplasms of immature B cells include lymphoblastic leukemia/lymphoma (*i.e.,* acute lymphocytic leukemia, to be discussed). In addition, the specific types of lymphomas are sometimes grouped together into low-grade, aggressive, and very aggressive categories.

Mature B-Cell Lymphomas. Mature (peripheral) B-cell lymphomas are the most common type of lymphoma in the Western world. The most common of the mature B-cell lymphomas are the follicular lymphomas (22%) and diffuse large B-cell lymphomas (31%). Small lymphocytic lymphoma, mantle cell lymphoma, peripheral T-cell lymphoma, and MALT lymphoma together account for 28% of NHLs.[4]

Follicular lymphomas are derived from germinal center B cells and consist of a mixture of centroblasts and centrocytes. Follicular lymphomas are a particularly common neoplasm in the United States, where they constitute about one third of all adult NHLs, with a peak incidence at 60 years of age. The lymphoma predominantly affects lymph nodes. Other sites of involvement include the spleen, bone marrow, peripheral blood, head and neck region, gastrointestinal tract, and skin. Most persons have advanced disease at presentation and an indolent clinical course, with a median survival of 6 to 10 years.[5,19] Over time, approximately one of three follicular lymphomas transforms into a fast-growing diffuse large B-cell lymphoma.[20]

Diffuse large B-cell lymphomas are a heterogeneous group of aggressive germinal or postgerminal center neoplasms. The disease occurs in all age groups but is most prevalent between 60 and 70 years of age. The cause of diffuse large B-cell lymphoma is unknown, but may involve EBV or HIV infections. It is a rapidly evolving, multifocal, nodal and extranodal tumor.

Manifestations are typically seen at the time of presentation. As a group, diffuse large B-cell lymphomas are rapidly fatal if untreated. However, with intensive combination chemotherapy, complete remission can be achieved in 60% to 80% of persons and approximately 40% to 50% remain disease free after several years and can be considered cured.[5,19]

Burkitt lymphoma, one of the most rapidly growing tumors of the NHLs, is also a disorder of germinal center B cells. Endemic Burkitt lymphoma is the most common childhood cancer (peak age 3 to 7 years) in Central Africa, often beginning in the jaw[4] (Fig. 15-5). It occurs in regions of Africa where both EBV and malarial infection are common. Virtually 100% of patients with African Burkitt lymphoma have evidence of previous EBV infection, and their tumors carry the EBV genome and express EBV-encoded antigens.[3] Malarial infections in this population have been shown to cause T-cell immunodeficiencies, and it is postulated that this association may be the link between EBV infection and the development of lymphoma.[3] A sporadic or nonendemic form of Burkitt lymphoma occurs less frequently in other parts of the world, and although these tumors are histologically similar to the endemic form, only about 20% carry the EBV genome.[3] Both the endemic and sporadic forms have chromosomal translocation involving chromosome 8. Burkitt lymphoma is very aggressive but responds to short-term, high-dose chemotherapy, with a cure rate of up to 50%.[21]

Mantle cell lymphomas constitute less than 10% of NHLs and have their origin in the naive B cell. After the precursor stage, B cells undergo immunoglobulin (Ig) gene rearrangements and develop into surface IgM- and IgD-positive naive B cells (see Fig. 15-4). These cells give rise to mantle cell lymphoma. Mantle cell lymphomas do not occur in children, but affect older persons (median age, 60 years). They have a rapid rate of progression, and half of persons do not survive 3 years.

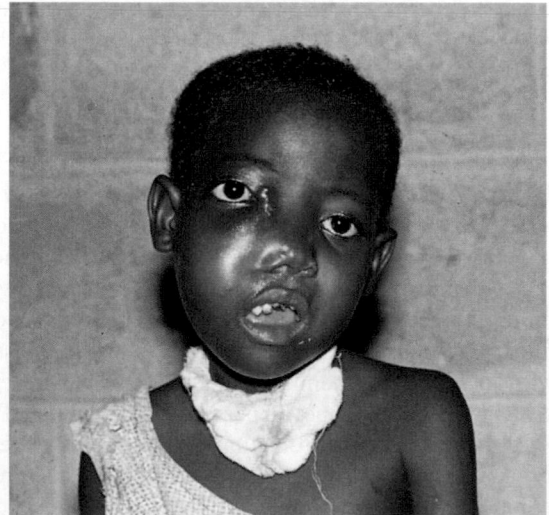

FIGURE 15-5 • African Burkitt lymphoma. A tumor of the jaw distorts the child's face. (From Schwarting R., McKenzie S., Rubin R. [2008]. Hematopathology. In Rubin R., Strayer D. E. [Eds.], *Rubin's pathology: Clinicopathologic foundations of medicine* [5th ed., p. 915]. Philadelphia: Lippincott Williams & Wilkins.)

Marginal zone lymphomas involve late-stage memory B cells that reside in the marginal zone or outermost compartment of the lymph node follicle. Variants of marginal node lymphoma include splenic marginal zone lymphoma and MALT lymphomas of the stomach and other mucosal surfaces. *MALT lymphomas* constitute 5% to 10% of all B-cell NHLs. Most MALT lymphomas involve the stomach or other mucosal sites, including the respiratory system. MALT lymphomas tend to remain localized for prolonged periods and to follow an indolent course. Extranodal marginal B cell lymphomas of the MALT type are curable by radiation or surgery when localized. MALT lymphomas that occur in the stomach secondary to *H. pylori* infection often respond to treatment with appropriate antimicrobial agents.

Clinical Manifestations. The manifestations of NHL depend on lymphoma type (*i.e.,* indolent or aggressive) and the stage of the disease. Persons with indolent or slow-growing lymphomas usually present with painless lymphadenopathy, which may be isolated or widespread. Involved lymph nodes may be present in the retroperitoneum, mesentery, and pelvis. The indolent lymphomas are usually disseminated at the time of diagnosis, and bone marrow involvement is frequent. With or without treatment, the natural course of the disease may fluctuate over 5 to 10 or more years. Many low-grade lymphomas eventually transform into more aggressive forms of lymphoma/leukemia.

Persons with intermediate or more aggressive forms of lymphoma usually present with accompanying constitutional symptoms such as fever, drenching night sweats, or weight loss. Frequently, there is increased susceptibility to bacterial, viral, and fungal infections associated with hypogammaglobulinemia and a poor humoral antibody response, rather than the impaired cellular immunity seen with Hodgkin lymphoma. Because of their high growth fraction, these lymphomas tend to be sensitive to radiation and chemotherapy. Hence, with intensive combination chemotherapy, complete remission can be achieved in 60% to 80% of cases.[23]

Diagnosis and Treatment. A lymph node biopsy is used to confirm the diagnosis of NHL and immunophenotyping to determine the lineage and clonality. Lymphomas can be grouped according to surface markers or phenotypic markers (*e.g.,* CD20).[23] Staging of the disease is important in selecting a treatment for persons with NHL. Bone marrow biopsy, blood studies, chest and abdominal computed tomography (CT) scans, magnetic resonance imaging (MRI), positron emission tomography (PET), gallium scans, and bone scans may be used to determine the stage of the disease.[21] Newer technologies, such as deoxyribonucleic acid (DNA) microarray analysis, which identifies genes that are either overexpressed or underexpressed by tumor cells, may be used to distinguish persons further into distinct risk groups.[17]

Treatment of NHL depends on the histologic type, stage of the disease, and clinical status of the person. For early-stage disease involving a single or limited node involvement, localized radiation may be used as a single treatment modality. However, because most people who present with indolent lymphoma have disseminated disease at the time of diagnosis, combination chemotherapy, combined adjuvant radiation therapy, or both are recommended. Persons with lymphomas that carry a risk of CNS involvement usually receive CNS prophylaxis with high doses of chemotherapeutic agents or cranial irradiation.

Several monoclonal antibodies (MOAs) have recently become available for use in the targeted treatment of NHL. Rituximab (Rituxan), which was the first to be approved by the U.S. Food and Drug Administration (FDA), recognizes and attaches to the CD20 antigen found on most B-cell lymphomas.[17,21,24] This MOA has been widely accepted because of its activity and favorable toxicity profile. Most adverse effects occur during infusion and consist mainly of chills, with occasional hypotension. For aggressive lymphomas, the combination of chemotherapy and rituximab has shown dramatic response rates, indicating a synergistic effect.[17] Because lymphoma cells tend to be very sensitive to radiation, newer forms of MOAs have been developed that are similar to rituximab, but with a radioactive isotope such as radioactive iodine (Bexxar) or radioactive yttrium (Zevalin) attached.[17] Another MOA (alemtuzumab) is directed at the CD52 antigen.[17] It is useful in some types of peripheral T-cell lymphomas. Bone marrow and peripheral stem cell transplantation are potentially curative treatments for people with highly resistant forms of the disease.

Hodgkin Lymphoma

Hodgkin lymphoma (HL), previously known as *Hodgkin disease,* is a specialized form of lymphoma that features the presence of an abnormal cell called a *Reed-Sternberg cell.*[4,5] Because of improved treatment methods, death rates have decreased by more than 60% since the early 1970s. Distribution of the disease is bimodal; it occurs more frequently in two separate groups, the first in early adulthood (15 to 40 years) and the second in older adulthood (55 years of age or older).[19]

HL differs from NHL in several respects. First, it usually arises in a single node or chain of nodes, whereas NHL frequently originates at extranodal sites and spreads to anatomically contiguous nodes.[25] Second, HL is characterized by the presence of large, atypical, mononuclear tumor cells, called *Reed-Sternberg cells* (Fig. 15-6). These cells, which frequently constitute less than 1% of the total cell population, are a diagnostic hallmark of the disease.

Etiology and Pathogenesis. As with NHLs, the cause of HL is largely unknown. Although exposure to carcinogens and viruses as well as genetic and immune mechanisms have been proposed as causes, none has been proved to be involved in the pathogenesis of the disease. It appears that people with a history of infectious mononucleosis are at increased risk for development of HL.[4,5,19]

The origin of the neoplastic Reed-Sternberg cell of HL has been difficult to study, in large part because these cells do

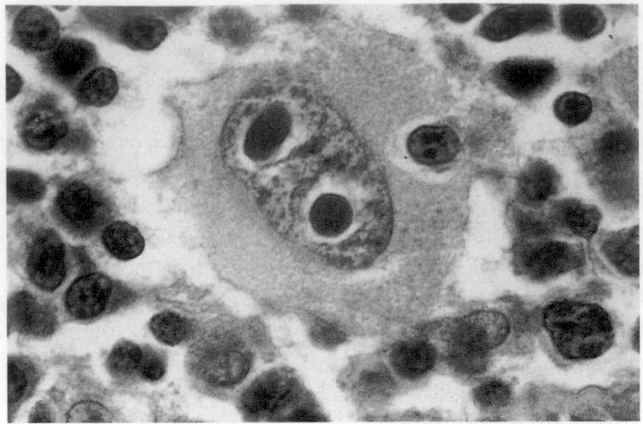

FIGURE 15-6 • Classic Reed-Sternberg cell. Mirror-image nuclei contain large eosinophilic nucleoli. (From Schwarting R., McKenzie S., Rubin R. [2008]. Hematopathology. In Rubin R., Strayer D. E. [Eds.], *Rubin's pathology: Clinicopathologic foundations of medicine* [5th ed., p. 922]. Philadelphia: Lippincott Williams & Wilkins.)

not express many of the markers found on lymphocytes. It is only recently that methods have been developed that allow for the microanalysis of these cells and their variants. These studies have shown that the Reed-Sternberg cells of most individual cases harbor identical immunoglobulin genes that show evidence of mutation, establishing the cell of origin as a germinal center or postgerminal center B cell.

Classification. The WHO classification proposed classifying HL into two major categories: nodular lymphocyte-predominant HL and classic HL.[4,25–28] Nodular lymphocyte-predominant HL represents only a small portion of all cases of HL and is a unique form that generally exhibits a nodular growth pattern, with or without diffuse areas and with rare Reed-Sternberg cells called "popcorn" or "L&H" (lymphohistiocytic) cells. It is often localized rather than disseminated at the time of diagnosis, exhibits a slowly progressive course, and has an overall survival rate greater than 80%.[4]

Classic HL is characterized by clonal proliferation of typical mononuclear Hodgkin cells and multinucleated Reed-Sternberg cells with invariable expression of CD30. Four variants of classic HL have been described: nodular sclerosis, mixed cellularity, lymphocyte-rich, and lymphocyte-depleted. The nodular sclerotic type is the most common and is often found in adolescent and young adult women, 15 to 35 years of age.[4] Lymphocyte-rich HL is a newly defined entity, and lymphocyte-depleted HL is rarely diagnosed. At present, all subtypes of classic HL are treated in the same manner.[28]

Manifestations. Most persons with HL present with painless enlargement of a single node or group of nodes. The initial lymph node involvement typically is above the level of the diaphragm (*i.e.,* in the neck, supraclavicular area, or axilla). Mediastinal masses are frequent and are sometimes discovered on routine chest radiography. There may be complaints of chest discomfort with cough or dyspnea. Involvement of subdiaphrag-

matic lymph nodes at the time of presentation is unusual and more common in elderly men. Additional symptoms that suggest HL include fevers, chills, night sweats, and weight loss. Pruritus and intermittent fevers associated with night sweats are classic symptoms of HL.

Other symptoms such as fatigue and anemia are indicative of disease spread. In the advanced stages of HL, the liver, spleen, lungs, digestive tract, and, occasionally, the CNS may be involved (Fig. 15-7). As the disease progresses, the rapid proliferation of abnormal lymphocytes leads to an immunologic defect, particularly in cell-mediated responses, rendering the person more susceptible to viral, fungal, and protozoal infections. Anergy, or the failure to develop a positive response to skin tests such as the tuberculin test, is common early in the course of the disease.

Diagnosis and Treatment. A definitive diagnosis of HL requires that the Reed-Sternberg cell be present in a biopsy specimen of lymph node tissue. CT scans of the chest and abdomen commonly are used to assess for involvement of mediastinal, abdominal, and pelvic lymph nodes.[25] A bipedal lymphangiogram may detect structural changes in the lymph nodes too small to visualize on CT scan. If with initial screening the extent of lymph node involvement cannot be determined, PET imaging may be helpful.[25] A bilateral bone marrow biopsy is usually performed on patients who are suspected of having disseminated disease.

Persons with HL are staged according to the number of lymph nodes involved, whether the lymph nodes are on one or both sides of the diaphragm, and whether there is disseminated disease involving the bone marrow, liver, lung, or skin. The staging of HL is of great clinical importance because the choice of treatment and the prognosis ultimately are related to the distribution of the disease.

Irradiation and chemotherapy are used in treating the disease. Most people with localized disease are treated with

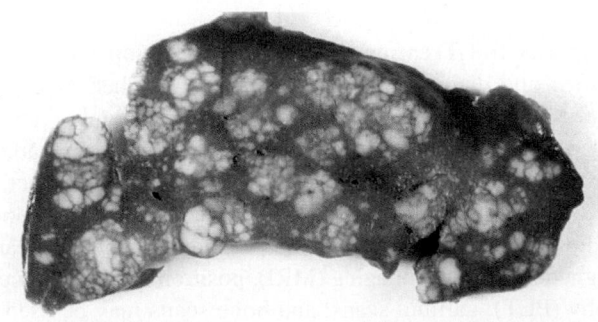

FIGURE 15-7 • Hodgkin lymphoma involving the spleen. Multinodular tumor masses replace the normal splenic tissue. (From Schwarting R., McKenzie S., Rubin R. [2008]. Hematopathology. In Rubin R., Strayer D. E. [Eds.], *Rubin's pathology: Clinicopathologic foundations of medicine* [5th ed., p. 924]. Philadelphia: Lippincott Williams & Wilkins.)

radiation therapy. A combined approach using radiation and chemotherapy is used in persons with advanced disease. As the accuracy of staging techniques, delivery of radiation, and curative efficacy of combination chemotherapy regimens have improved, the survival of people with HL also has improved. With modern treatment methods, a 5-year cure rate of 85% can be achieved.[18] As the cure rate for HL has risen and longer-term follow-up data have become available, the importance of the late effects of treatment, including secondary malignancies, has become more apparent.[17,28] Because these malignancies have mainly been attributed to radiation therapy, studies are being conducted to determine the lowest effective radiation dose. Current trials are also seeking to determine whether chemotherapy can replace radiation therapy altogether.[17]

Leukemias

The leukemias are malignant neoplasms of cells originally derived from hematopoietic precursor cells (see Fig. 15-4). They are characterized by diffuse replacement of bone marrow with unregulated, proliferating, immature neoplastic cells. In most cases, the leukemic cells spill out into the blood, where they are seen in large numbers. The term *leukemia* (i.e., "white blood") was first used by Virchow to describe a reversal of the usual ratio of red blood cells to white blood cells. The leukemic cells may also infiltrate the liver, spleen, lymph nodes, and other tissues throughout the body, causing enlargement of these organs.

🔑 LEUKEMIAS

- Leukemias are malignant neoplasms arising from the transformation of a single blood cell line derived from hematopoietic stem cells.

- The leukemias are classified as acute and chronic lymphocytic (lymphocytes) or myelocytic (granulocytes, monocytes) leukemias according to their cell lineage.

- Because leukemic cells are immature and poorly differentiated, they proliferate rapidly and have a long life span, they do not function normally, they interfere with the maturation of normal blood cells, and they circulate in the bloodstream, cross the blood-brain barrier, and infiltrate many body organs.

An estimated 44,270 new cases of leukemia were diagnosed in the U.S. in 2008, and approximately 21,710 persons died of the disease.[18] Leukemia is the most common cause of cancer in children and adolescents. It accounts for about one of three cancers in children. Although it commonly is thought of as a childhood disease, leukemia is diagnosed 10 times more frequently in adults than children.

Classification

The leukemias commonly are classified according to their predominant cell type (i.e., lymphocytic or myelocytic) and whether the condition is acute or chronic. Biphenotypic leukemias demonstrate characteristics of both lymphoid and myeloid lineages. A rudimentary classification system divides leukemia into four types: acute lymphocytic (lymphoblastic) leukemia (ALL), chronic lymphocytic leukemia (CLL), acute myelogenous (myeloblastic) leukemia (AML), and chronic myelogenous leukemia (CML).[29] The *lymphocytic leukemias* involve immature lymphocytes and their progenitors that originate in the bone marrow but infiltrate the spleen, lymph nodes, CNS, and other tissues. The *myelogenous leukemias,* which involve the pluripotent myeloid stem cells in bone marrow, interfere with the maturation of all blood cells, including the granulocytes, erythrocytes, and thrombocytes.

Etiology and Molecular Biology

The causes of leukemia are largely unknown. The incidence of leukemia among persons who have been exposed to high levels of radiation is unusually high. An increased incidence of leukemia also is associated with exposure to benzene and the use of antitumor drugs (i.e., mechlorethamine, procarbazine, cyclophosphamide, chloramphenicol, and the epipodophyllotoxins).[30] Leukemia may occur as a second cancer after aggressive chemotherapy for other cancers, such as HL. The existence of a genetic predisposition to development of acute leukemia is suggested by the increased leukemia incidence among a number of congenital disorders, including Down syndrome, neurofibromatosis, and Fanconi anemia. In individuals with Down syndrome, the incidence of acute leukemia is 10 times that of the general population.[31] There also are numerous reports of multiple cases of acute leukemia occurring within the same family.

The molecular biology of leukemia suggests that the event or events causing the disorders exert their effects through disruption or dysregulation of genes that normally regulate blood cell development, blood cell homeostasis, or both.[32] Cytogenetic studies have shown that recurrent chromosomal changes occur in over one half of all cases of leukemia.[33] Most commonly, these are structural changes classified as translocations, written t(8;21), in which a part of one (e.g., 8) chromosome becomes located on another chromosome (e.g., 21) and vice versa; inversions, written inv(16), in which part of a chromosome (e.g., 16) is upside down and now in reverse order, but still attached to the original chromosome; and deletions, written del(7) or −7, in which part of a chromosome (e.g., 7) has been lost. It is the disruption or dysregulation of specific genes and gene products occurring at the site of these chromosome aberrations that contributes to the development of leukemia.[32] In many instances, these genes and their products have been shown to be directly or indirectly involved in the normal development or maintenance of the hematopoietic system. Thus, it would appear that leukemia results, at least in part, from disruption in the activity of genes that normally regulate blood cell development. Currently, more than 500 recurring translocations have been described in hematologic malignancies.[33] Advances in the understanding of the molecular biology of leukemia are beginning to provide a more complete understanding of the molecular complexity of leukemia for the purposes of diagnosis, classification, treatment, and monitoring of clinical outcomes.

One of the more studied translocations is the Philadelphia chromosome, which was the first chromosomal abnormality identified in cancer. The Philadelphia chromosome translocation, t(9;22), represents a reciprocal translocation between the long arm of chromosome 22 and the long arm of chromosome 9.[4,5] During the translocation, a large portion of 22q is translocated to 9q, and a smaller piece of 9q is moved to 22q (Fig. 15-8). The portion of 9q that is translocated contains *ABL*, a proto-oncogene that is the cellular homolog of the Abelson murine leukemic virus. The *ABL* gene is received at a specific site on 22q called the *breakpoint cluster* (BCR). The resulting *BCR-ABL* fusion gene codes for a novel protein that differs from that of the normal *ABL* gene in that it possesses tyrosine kinase activity (a characteristic activity of transforming genes).[4,34,35] The presence of the tyrosine kinase generated by the fusion gene allows affected cells to bypass the regulated signals that control normal cell growth and differentia-

tion and instead undergo malignant transformation to become leukemic cells. The Philadelphia chromosome translocation is found in more than 90% of persons with CML and in some persons with acute leukemia. The recent development of tyrosine kinase inhibitors (*e.g.*, imatinib mesylate) has contributed to the targeted approach for treatment of leukemias that display the Philadelphia chromosome translocation.[35]

Acute Leukemias

The acute leukemias are cancers of the hematopoietic progenitor cells.[36–38] They usually have a sudden and stormy onset with signs and symptoms related to depressed bone marrow function (Table 15-1). There are two types of acute leukemia: ALL and AML. ALL is the most common cancer in children and adults. It accounts for three of four cases of childhood cancer, with AML accounting for most of the remaining cases.[36] AML is mainly a disease of older adults, but is also seen in children and young adults.[39]

ALL encompasses a group of neoplasms composed of precursor B (pre-B) or T (pre-T) lymphocytes referred to as *lymphoblasts* (see Fig. 15-4). Most cases (about 85%) of ALL are of pre–B-cell origin.[5] Approximately 90% of persons with ALL have numeric and structural changes in the chromosomes of their leukemic cells. They include hyperploidy (*i.e.,* more than 50 chromosomes), polyploidy (*i.e.,* 3 or more sets of chromosomes), and chromosomal translocations and deletions. Many of these chromosomal aberrations serve to dysregulate the expression and function of transcription factors required for normal hematopoietic cell development.

The AMLs are a diverse group of neoplasms affecting myeloid precursor cells in the bone marrow.[4,5,40,41] Most are associated with acquired genetic alterations that inhibit terminal myeloid differentiation. As a result, normal marrow elements are replaced by an accumulation of relatively undifferentiated blast cells with a resultant suppression of the remaining progenitor cells that leads to anemia, neutropenia, and thrombocytopenia. Specific chromosomal abnormalities, including translocations, are seen in a large number of AMLs. One subtype of AML, acute promyelocytic leukemia, which represents 10% of adult cases of AML, is associated with a t(15;17) chromosomal translocation.[42] This translocation produces a fusion gene that encodes a portion of the transcription factor, retinoic acid receptor-a (RARa), fused to a portion of another protein, PML. This change in the retinoic acid receptor produces a block in differentiation that can be overcome with pharmacologic doses of retinoic acid (to be discussed).

Manifestations. Although ALL and AML are distinct disorders, they typically present with similar clinical features. Both are characterized by an abrupt onset of symptoms, including fatigue resulting from anemia; low-grade fever, night sweats, and weight loss due to the rapid proliferation and hypermetabolism of the leukemic cells; bleeding due to a decreased platelet count; and bone pain and tenderness due to bone marrow expansion.[39] Infection results from neutropenia, with the risk

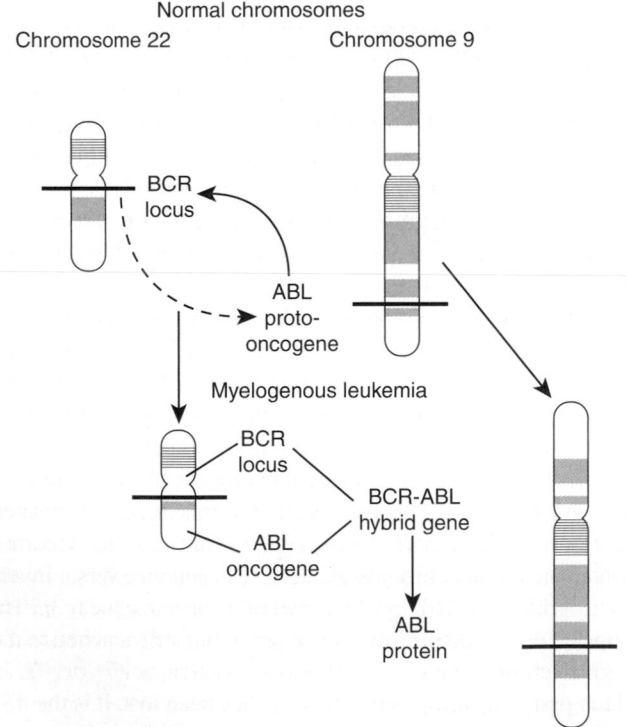

FIGURE 15-8 • The Philadelphia (Ph) chromosome is formed by breaks at the ends of the long arms of chromosomes 9 and 22, allowing the *ABL* proto-oncogene on chromosome 9 to be translocated to the breakpoint cluster region (*BCR*) on chromosome 22. The result is a new fusion gene coding for the BCR-ABL protein, which is presumably involved in the pathogenesis of chronic myelogenous leukemia.

TABLE 15-1 Clinical Manifestations of Leukemia and Their Pathologic Basis*

CLINICAL MANIFESTATIONS	PATHOLOGIC BASIS
Bone marrow depression	
Malaise, easy fatigability	Anemia
Fever	Infection or increased metabolism by neoplastic cells
Bleeding	Decreased thrombocytes
Petechiae	
Ecchymosis	
Gingival bleeding	
Epistaxis	
Bone pain and tenderness upon palpation	Subperiosteal bone infiltration, bone marrow expansion, and bone resorption
Headache, nausea, vomiting, papilledema, cranial nerve palsies, seizures, coma	Leukemic infiltration of the central nervous system
Abdominal discomfort	Generalized lymphadenopathy, hepatomegaly, splenomegaly due to leukemic cell infiltration
Increased vulnerability to infections	Immaturity of the white cells and ineffective immune function
Hematologic abnormalities	Physical and metabolic encroachment of leukemia cells on red blood cells
Anemia	and thrombocyte precursors
Thrombocytopenia	
Hyperuricemia and other metabolic disorders	Abnormal proliferation and metabolism of leukemia cells

*Manifestations vary with the type of leukemia.

of infection rising steeply as the neutrophil count falls below 500 cells/µL. Generalized lymphadenopathy, splenomegaly, and hepatomegaly caused by infiltration of leukemic cells occur in all acute leukemias but are more common in ALL.

In addition to the common manifestations of acute leukemia (*i.e.,* fatigue, weight loss, fever, easy bruising), infiltration of malignant cells in the skin, gums, and other soft tissues is particularly common in the monocytic form of AML. The leukemic cells may also cross the blood-brain barrier and establish sanctuary in the CNS. CNS involvement is more common in ALL than AML, and is more common in children than adults. Signs and symptoms of CNS involvement include cranial nerve palsies, headache, nausea, vomiting, papilledema, and occasionally seizures and coma.

Leukostasis is a condition in which the circulating blast count is markedly elevated (usually 100,000 cells/µL). The high number of circulating leukemic blasts increases blood viscosity and predisposes to the development of leukoblastic emboli with obstruction of small blood vessels in the pulmonary and cerebral circulations. Occlusion of the pulmonary vessels leads to vessel rupture and infiltration of lung tissue, resulting in sudden shortness of breath and progressive dyspnea. Cerebral leukostasis leads to diffuse headache and lethargy, which can progress to confusion and coma. Once identified, leukostasis requires immediate and effective treatment to lower the blast count rapidly. Initial treatment uses apheresis to remove excess blast cells, followed by chemotherapy to stop leukemic cell production in the bone marrow.[39]

Hyperuricemia occurs as the result of increased proliferation or increased breakdown of purine nucleotides (*i.e.,* one of the components of nucleic acids) secondary to the leukemic cell death that results from chemotherapy. It may increase before and during treatment. Prophylactic therapy with allopurinol, a

drug that inhibits uric acid synthesis, is routinely administered to prevent renal complications secondary to uric acid crystallization in the urine filtrate.

Diagnosis. A definitive diagnosis of acute leukemia is based on blood and bone marrow studies; it requires the demonstration of leukemic cells in the peripheral blood, bone marrow, or extramedullary tissue. Laboratory findings reveal the presence of immature white blood cells (blasts) in the circulation and bone marrow, where they may constitute 60% to 100% of the cells. As these cells proliferate and begin to crowd the bone marrow, the development of other blood cell lines in the marrow is suppressed. Consequently, there is a loss of mature myeloid cells, such as erythrocytes, granulocytes, and platelets. Anemia is almost always present, and the platelet count is decreased. Immunophenotyping is performed to determine the lineage subtype of the leukemia.[39]

Bone marrow biopsy may be used to determine the molecular characteristics of the leukemia, the degree of bone marrow involvement, and the morphology and histology of the disease. Cytogenetic studies, which are used to determine chromosomal abnormalities, are one of the most powerful prognostic indicators in acute leukemia. Certain chromosomal abnormalities respond more favorably to certain types of treatment and have a better prognosis than other abnormalities.

In ALL, the staging includes a lumbar puncture to assess CNS involvement. Imaging studies that include CT scans of the chest, abdomen, and pelvis may also be obtained to identify additional sites of disease.

Treatment. Treatment of ALL and AML consists of several phases and includes *induction therapy,* which is designed to elicit a remission; *intensification therapy,* which is used to produce a further reduction in leukemic cells after a remission is achieved; and *maintenance therapy,* which serves to maintain the remission. The goal of induction therapy is the production of a severe bone marrow response with destruction of leukemic progenitor cells followed by normal bone marrow recovery. The likelihood of achieving a remission depends on a number of factors, including age, type of leukemia, and stage of the disease at time of presentation. Of these factors, age is probably the most significant prognostic variable.

Treatment of ALL usually consists of four phases: induction therapy, CNS prophylaxis, consolidation or intensification therapy, and maintenance therapy.[43,44] Induction therapy incorporates a number of chemotherapeutic agents designed to achieve remission. CNS prophylaxis may be accomplished through the administration of intrathecal chemotherapy by lumbar puncture or by cranial irradiation concurrent with systemic chemotherapy.[39] Because of its side effects, CNS irradiation is being used less frequently than in the past. The use of high-dose chemotherapy that crosses the blood-brain barrier may make separate CNS treatment unnecessary in the future. Although CNS involvement is a major problem in children, the incidence in adults at the time of diagnosis is less than 10%. Consolidation therapy consists of high doses of chemotherapy given to patients who have achieved remission with their induction therapy. Maintenance therapy usually is accomplished with lower doses of chemotherapy given over a long period (*e.g.,* 2 years) to patients after consolidation therapy. Although almost 80% of children are cured of ALL, only about 30% to 40% of adults achieve long-term disease-free survival.[45]

Massive necrosis of malignant cells can occur during the initial phase of treatment. This phenomenon, known as *tumor lysis syndrome,* can lead to life-threatening metabolic disorders, including hyperkalemia, hyperphosphatemia, hyperuricemia, hypomagnesemia, hypocalcemia, and acidosis, with the potential for causing acute renal failure. Aggressive prophylactic hydration with alkaline solutions and administration of allopurinol to reduce uric acid levels are used to counteract these effects.

As with ALL, treatment of AML consists of a number of phases. Treatment usually consists of induction therapy followed by intensive consolidation therapy. Induction therapy consists of intensive chemotherapy to effect aplasia of the bone marrow. During this period, supportive transfusion and treatment with antimicrobial agents often are needed. An MOA conjugated with a chemotherapeutic agent (gemtuzumab ozogamicin) that targets the CD33 antigen found on 90% of AML blast cells is another treatment option for patients older than 60 years of age who are not candidates for intensive chemotherapy.[45] Acute promyelocytic leukemia is treated differently from other forms of AML.[46] Induction therapy includes an anthracycline (*e.g.,* idarubicin) plus all-*trans*-retinoic acid (ATRA). This agent is an analog of vitamin A that leads to terminal differentiation of acute promyelocytic cells through an interaction with the abnormal retinoic acid receptor created by the specific chromosomal translocation that is a hallmark of this subtype of leukemia.

Bone marrow or stem cell transplantation may be considered for persons with ALL and AML who have failed to respond to other forms of therapy.[39] Because of the risk of complications, bone marrow transplantation is not usually recommended for patients older than 50 to 55 years of age.[30]

Chronic Leukemias

In contrast to acute leukemias, chronic leukemias are malignancies involving proliferation of more fully differentiated myeloid and lymphoid cells. As with acute leukemia, there are two major types of chronic leukemia: CLL and CML.[47,48] CLL accounts for about one third of all leukemias.[47] It is mainly a disorder of older persons. The average age at time of diagnosis is approximately 72 years. It is rarely seen in people younger than 40 years of age, and is extremely rare in children.[47] CML accounts for 10% to 15% of all leukemias. As with CLL, it is predominantly a disorder of older adults, with an average age of approximately 67 years at time of diagnosis.[48]

Chronic Lymphocytic Leukemia. CLL, a clonal malignancy of B lymphocytes, is the most common form of leukemia in adults in the Western world. In the past, CLL was viewed as a homogeneous disease of immature, immune-incompetent, minimally self-renewing B cells, which accumulated because of faulty apoptotic mechanisms. CLL is now becoming viewed as two related entities based on aggressiveness of the disease.[49] Some persons with CLL survive for many years without therapy and eventually succumb to unrelated diseases, whereas others have a rapidly fatal disease despite aggressive therapy. Its heterogeneity is thought to reflect differences in immunoglobulin V-gene mutations, expression of cell surface CD markers (*e.g.,* CD38), and presence of the zeta-associated protein (ZAP-70). ZAP-70 is an intracellular protein that promulgates activation signals delivered to T cells and NK cells by their surface receptors for antigens. It is rarely present in normal B cells but is found in persons with CLL. Persons with leukemic cells having few or no V-gene mutations or with many CD38+ or ZAP-70+ B cells often have an aggressive course, whereas those with V-gene mutations but few CD38+ or ZAP-70+ B cells usually have a more indolent course. The analysis of DNA sequences to determine the status of immunoglobulin V-gene mutations is laborious and not performed routinely in clinical laboratories, whereas testing for ZAP-10, when appropriately standardized, can more readily serve as a diagnostic test.[49]

The clinical signs and symptoms of CLL are largely related to the progressive infiltration of the bone marrow and lymphoid tissues by neoplastic lymphocytes and to secondary immunologic defects. Persons with the indolent form of CLL are often asymptomatic at the time of diagnosis, and lymphocytosis is noted on a complete blood count obtained for another, unrelated disorder. As the disease progresses, lymph nodes gradually increase in size and new nodes are involved, sometimes in unusual areas such as the scalp, orbit, pharynx, pleura, gastrointestinal tract, liver, prostate, and gonads. Persons with the aggressive form of CLL experience a more rapid sequence of clinical detcrioration characterized by increasing lymphadenopathy, hepatosplenomegaly, fever, abdominal pain, weight loss, progressive anemia, and thrombocytopenia, with a rapid rise in lymphocyte count.

Hypogammaglobulinemia is common in CLL, especially in persons with advanced disease. An increased susceptibility to infection reflects an inability to produce specific antibodies and abnormal activation of complement. The most common infectious organisms are those that require opsonization for bacterial killing, such as *Streptococcus pneumoniae, Staphylococcus aureus,* and *Haemophilus influenzae.*

The diagnostic hallmark of CLL is isolated lymphocytosis. The white blood cell count is usually greater than 20,000/µL and may be elevated to several hundred thousand. Usually, 75% to 98% are lymphocytes. The hematocrit and platelet counts are usually normal at presentation. Tests to determine the presence of mutated forms of the immunoglobulin gene (which currently can be detected only in research laboratories) and expression of the C38 surface antigen and the ZAP-70 protein may be used to determine whether the leukemia is the indolent or aggressive type. Cytogenetic studies may also provide prognostic information. The finding of deletion of chromosome 17p or 11q is a poor prognostic indicator.

Treatment of CLL usually depends on the presence of prognostic indicators.[47] Persons with the low-risk or indolent form of CLL usually do not require specific treatment for many years after diagnosis and eventually die of apparently unrelated causes. Reassurance that persons with the disorder can live a normal life for many years is important. Many persons with intermediate-risk disease may remain stable for many years as well, whereas others may develop complications and need treatment within a few months. Most persons with high-risk CLL require treatment at diagnosis.

The current treatment of choice is combination chemotherapy plus the MOA rituximab that targets CD20⁺ B lymphocytes. Alemtuzumab, an MOA directed against the CD52 antigen, may be used to treat persons who have not responded to chemotherapy.[47,50,51] Complications such as autoimmune hemolytic anemia or thrombocytopenia may require treatment with corticosteroids or splenectomy.

In younger patients with aggressive disease, an allogeneic ablative (destruction of bone marrow cells by irradiation or chemotherapy) or nonmyeloablative stem cell transplant is a treatment option. In a nonmyeloablative type of transplant, the goal is marrow suppression, destruction of leukemia cells by the donor's lymphocytes, known as "graft-versus-leukemia" effect, and marrow recovery with donor cells.

Chronic Myelogenous Leukemia. CML is a disorder of the pluripotent hematopoietic progenitor cell. It is characterized by excessive proliferation of marrow granulocytes, erythroid precursors, and megakaryocytes. The CML cells harbor a distinctive cytogenic abnormality, the previously described *Philadelphia chromosome.*[4,5] It is generally believed that CML develops when a single, pluripotent hematopoietic stem cell acquires a Philadelphia chromosome. Although CML originates in the pluripotent

stem cells, granulocyte precursors remain the dominant leukemic cell type.

The clinical course of CML is commonly divided into three phases: (1) a chronic phase of variable length, (2) a short accelerated phase, and (3) a terminal blast crisis phase. The onset of the chronic phase is usually slow, with nonspecific symptoms such as weakness and weight loss. The most characteristic laboratory finding at the time of presentation is leukocytosis with immature granulocyte cell types in the peripheral blood. Anemia and, eventually, thrombocytopenia develop. Anemia causes weakness, easy fatigability, and exertional dyspnea. Splenomegaly is often present at the time of diagnosis; hepatomegaly is less common; and lymphadenopathy is relatively uncommon. Persons in the early chronic phase of CML generally are asymptomatic, but without effective treatment most will enter the accelerated phase within 4 years.[51]

The accelerated phase of CML is characterized by enlargement of the spleen and progressive symptoms. Splenomegaly often causes a feeling of abdominal fullness and discomfort. An increase in basophil count and more immature cells in the blood or bone marrow confirm transformation to the accelerated phase. During this phase, constitutional symptoms such as low-grade fever, night sweats, bone pain, and weight loss develop because of rapid proliferation and hypermetabolism of the leukemic cells. Bleeding and easy bruising may arise from dysfunctional platelets. Generally, the accelerated phase is short (6 to 12 months).

The terminal blast crisis phase of CML represents evolution to acute leukemia and is characterized by an increasing number of myeloid precursors, especially blast cells, in the blood (Fig. 15-9). Constitutional symptoms become more pronounced during this period, and splenomegaly may increase significantly. Isolated infiltrates of leukemic cells can involve the skin, lymph nodes, bones, and CNS. With very high blast counts (>100,000 cells/µL), symptoms of leukostasis may occur. The prognosis for patients who are in the blast crisis phase is poor, with a median survival of 3 months.[51]

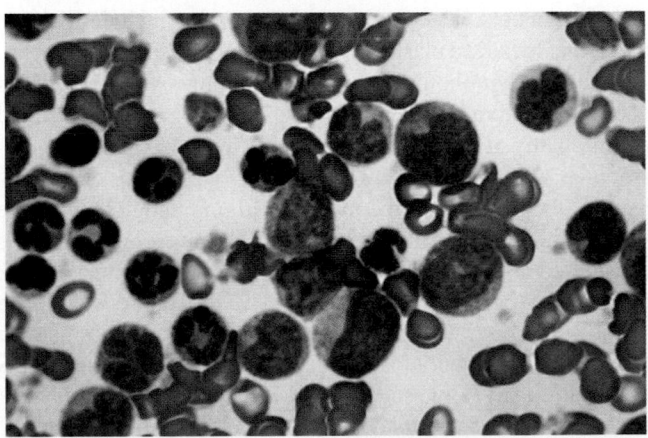

FIGURE 15-9 • Peripheral blood showing blast crisis in chronic myelogenous leukemia. (From Centers for Disease Control and Prevention. [2008]. Public Health Image Library. [Online.] Available: http://phil.cdc.gov/phil/home.asp.)

A diagnostic feature of CML is an elevated white blood count, with a median count of 150,000/μL at the time of diagnosis, although is some cases it is only modestly increased. The hallmark of the disease is the presence of the BCR-ABL gene product, which can be detected in the peripheral blood. This is best done using the polymerase chain reaction (PCR), which has supplanted cytogenetics in identifying the Philadelphia chromosome. Bone marrow examination is not usually necessary for diagnosis, but is useful for prognosis and detecting additional chromosomal abnormalities.

The goals of treatment for CML include a hematologic response characterized by normalized blood counts; a cytogenetic response demonstrated by the reduction or elimination of the Philadelphia chromosome from the bone marrow; and a molecular response confirmed by the elimination of the BCR-ABL fusion protein.[51] In the past, standard treatment included the use of single-agent chemotherapy (hydroxyurea) as well as alpha-interferon. In patients in the chronic phase, both agents normalized blood counts and reduced symptoms, but cytogenetic and molecular responses were rare. With its FDA approval in 2001, imatinib mesylate, a specifically designed inhibitor of the tyrosine kinase activity of the BCR-ABL oncogene product, has largely replaced hydroxyurea and interferon as standard therapy for CML.[52,53] Its side effect profile and ease of administration (oral route) have dramatically changed the treatment of CML.

The only available curative treatment for CML is allogeneic bone marrow or stem cell transplantation. In most transplantation centers, full myoablative transplants are available to children and adults younger than 60 years of age who have an HLA-matched sibling donor or an unrelated molecular-matched donor. Nonmyeloablative or "mini-transplants" are available to patients younger than 70 years of age who have sibling HLA-matched or unrelated HLA-matched donors.

Plasma Cell Dyscrasias

Plasma cell dyscrasias are characterized by expansion of a single clone of immunoglobulin-producing plasma cells and a resultant increase in serum levels of a single monoclonal immunoglobulin or its fragments. The plasma cell dyscrasias include multiple myeloma; localized plasmacytoma (solitary myeloma); lymphoplasmacytic lymphoma; primary or immunocyte amyloidosis due to excessive production of light chains; and monoclonal gammopathy of undetermined significance. *Monoclonal gammopathy of undetermined significance* (MGUS) is characterized by the presence of the monoclonal immunoglobulin in the serum without other findings of multiple myeloma. MGUS is considered a premalignant condition.[4,5,54,55] Approximately 2% per year of persons with MGUS will go on to develop a plasma cell dyscrasia (multiple myeloma, lymphoplasmacytic lymphoma, or amyloidosis). The strong link between MGUS and multiple myeloma suggests that a first oncogenic event produces MGUS and a second event results in multiple myeloma.[4]

Multiple Myeloma

Multiple myeloma is a B-cell malignancy of terminally differentiated plasma cells. It accounts for 1% of all cancers and 10% of all hematologic malignancies in whites and 20% in African Americans.[56] It occurs most frequently in persons older than 60 years of age, with the median age of patients with multiple myeloma being 71 years.

The cause of multiple myeloma is unknown. Risk factors are thought to include chronic immune stimulation, autoimmune disorders, exposure to ionizing radiation, and occupational exposure to pesticides or herbicides (*e.g.,* dioxin). Myeloma has been associated with exposure to Agent Orange during the Vietnam War. A number of viruses have been associated with the pathogenesis of myeloma. There is a 4.5-fold increase in the likelihood of development of multiple myeloma for persons with HIV infection.[57]

Pathogenesis. Multiple myeloma is characterized by proliferation of malignant plasma cells in the bone marrow and osteolytic bone lesions throughout the skeletal system. As with other hematopoietic malignancies, it is now recognized that multiple myeloma is associated with chromosomal abnormalities, including deletions of 13q and translocations involving the IgG locus on chromosome 14.[5] One fusion partner is a fibroblast growth factor receptor gene on chromosome 4, which is truncated to produce a constitutively active receptor. Changes also occur in the bone marrow microenvironment, including the induction of angiogenesis, the suppression of cell-mediated immunity, and the development of paracrine signaling loops involving cytokines such as IL-6 and vascular endothelial growth factor. Other growth factors that are implicated in multiple myeloma include granulocyte CSF, interferon-α, and IL-10. The development of bone lesions in multiple myeloma is thought to be related to an increase in expression by osteoblasts of the receptor activator of the nuclear factor-κB (NF-κB) ligand (RANKL) and the reduction of the level of its decoy receptor, osteoprotegerin[54] (see Chapter 58).

One of the characteristic features resulting from the proliferating osteoclasts in multiple myeloma is the unregulated production of a monoclonal antibody referred to as the *M protein* because it is detected as an M spike on protein electrophoresis. In most cases the M protein is either IgG (60%) or IgA (20% to 25%).[54] In the remaining 15% to 20% of cases, the plasma cells produce only abnormal proteins, termed *Bence Jones proteins,* that consist of light chains of the immunoglobulin molecule. Because of their low molecular weight, the Bence Jones proteins are readily excreted in the urine. Persons with this form of the disease (light-chain disease) have Bence Jones proteins in their serum, but lack the M component. However, up to 80% of myeloma cells produce both complete immunoglobulins as well as excess light chains; therefore, both M proteins and Bence Jones proteins are present. Many of the light-chain proteins are directly toxic to renal tubular structures, which may lead to tubular destruction and, eventually, to renal failure.

Manifestations. The main sites involved in multiple myeloma are the bones and bone marrow. In addition to the abnormal proliferation of marrow plasma cells, there is proliferation and activation of osteoclasts, which leads to bone resorption and destruction (Fig. 15-10). This increased bone resorption pre-

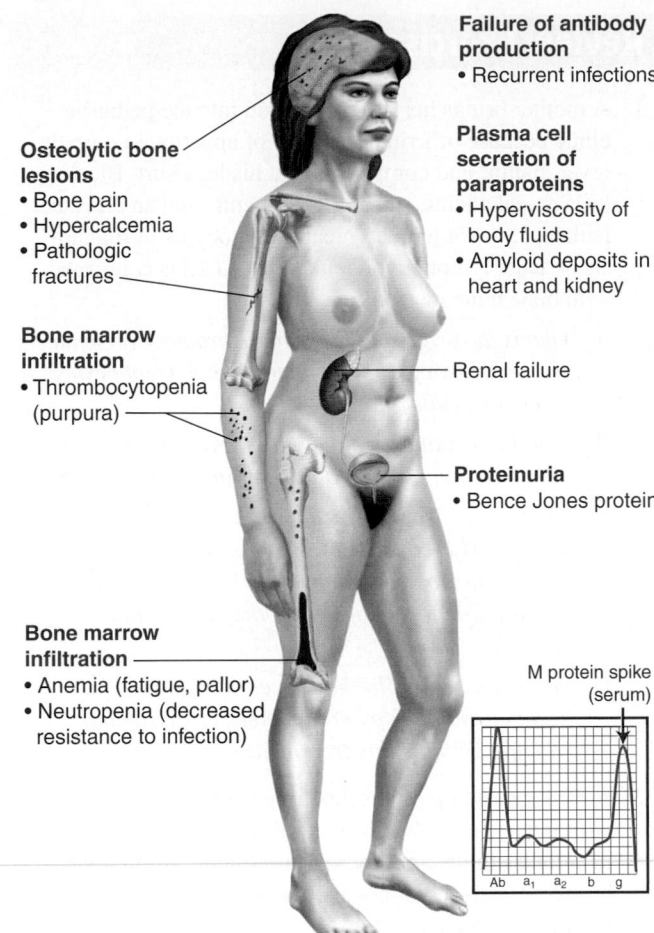

Failure of antibody production
- Recurrent infections

Plasma cell secretion of paraproteins
- Hyperviscosity of body fluids
- Amyloid deposits in heart and kidney

Renal failure

Proteinuria
- Bence Jones protein

Osteolytic bone lesions
- Bone pain
- Hypercalcemia
- Pathologic fractures

Bone marrow infiltration
- Thrombocytopenia (purpura)

Bone marrow infiltration
- Anemia (fatigue, pallor)
- Neutropenia (decreased resistance to infection)

M protein spike (serum)

Ab a₁ a₂ b g

FIGURE 15-10 • Clinical features of multiple myeloma.

disposes the individual to pathologic fractures and hypercalcemia. Paraproteins secreted by the plasma cells may cause a hyperviscosity of body fluids and may break down into amyloid, a proteinaceous substance deposited between cells, causing heart failure and nephropathy. Although multiple myeloma is characterized by excessive production of monoclonal immunoglobulin, levels of normal immunoglobulins are usually depressed. This contributes to a general susceptibility to recurrent bacterial infections.

The malignant plasma cells also can form plasmacytomas (plasma cell tumors) in bone and soft tissue sites. The most common site of soft tissue plasmacytomas is the gastrointestinal tract. The development of plasmacytomas in bone tissue is associated with bone destruction and localized pain. Osteolytic lesions and compression fractures may be seen in the axial skeleton and proximal long bones. Occasionally, the lesions may affect the spinal column, causing vertebral collapse and spinal cord compression.

Bone pain is one of the first symptoms to occur in approximately three fourths of all individuals diagnosed with multiple myeloma. Bone destruction also impairs the production of erythrocytes and leukocytes and predisposes the patient to anemia and recurrent infections. Many patients experience weight loss and weakness. Renal insufficiency occurs in 50% of patients.

Neurologic manifestations caused by neuropathy or spinal cord compression also may be present.

Diagnosis and Treatment. Diagnosis of multiple myeloma is based on clinical manifestations, blood tests, and bone marrow examination.[58] The classic triad of bone marrow plasmacytosis (more than 10% plasma cells), lytic bone lesions, and either the serum M-protein spike or the presence of Bence Jones proteins in the urine is definitive for a diagnosis of multiple myeloma. Bone radiographs are important in establishing the presence of bone lesions. Anemia is almost universal. Other laboratory features include hypercalcemia, an elevated erythrocyte sedimentation rate, and signs of kidney failure. The strongest predictors of outcome are low serum beta-2 microglobulin (a small subunit of the major histocompatibility complex I molecule) and C-reactive protein levels.[58]

The treatment of multiple myeloma is changing rapidly.[55,58] For several decades, melphalan (an alkylating agent) and prednisone have remained the cornerstone for treatment of multiple myeloma. Cumulative exposure to melphalan, however, is associated with increased risk of marrow toxicity, including myelodysplasia, acute leukemia, and impaired stem cell production. This is an important consideration in persons who are candidates for autologous stem cell transplants. The addition of anthracyclines, alternative alkylating agents, and interferon has yielded minimal improvement in treatment outcomes (see Chapter 8). Although the incorporation of new classes of medications in the treatment of multiple myeloma has seen a shift in the older treatment regimens, the conventional approaches have not been excluded.

Recently, thalidomide combined with dexamethasone (a corticosteroid) has emerged as an active agent for use in the initial treatment of multiple myeloma.[54] The combination is given orally and has shown promising results in newly diagnosed patients. The exact mechanism of action of thalidomide is unknown. Proposed mechanisms include angiogenesis inhibition; immune modulation by increasing NK cell activity, IL-2, and interferon-γ; and increasing apoptosis. Thalidomide is reasonably well tolerated; the toxicities include increased risk of venous thromboembolism (*i.e.,* deep vein thrombosis). Its efficacy as a front-line therapy has been supported by clinical trials. Because of its teratogenicity, the use of thalidomide in pregnant women is absolutely contraindicated. Lenalidomide, an oral agent, is an analog of thalidomide with both improved efficacy and reduced toxicity.

Another agent, a reversible 26S proteosome inhibitor (bortezomib), was recently approved for treatment of multiple myeloma. Proteosomes are intracellular enzymes that degrade many proteins regulating the cell cycle, ribonucleic acid (RNA) transcription, apoptosis, cell adhesion, angiogenesis, and antigen presentation.[54] Proteolysis by the 26S proteosome is fundamental to multiple signaling pathways within the cell, and disruption of this homeostatic pathway by bortezomib can lead to cell death and a delay in tumor growth.

High-dose chemotherapy with autologous stem cell transplantation is now considered appropriate front-line therapy for patients younger than 70 years of age newly diagnosed with multiple myeloma. Allogeneic transplantation offers prolonged disease-free outcomes and potential cure, but at a high cost of treatment-related mortality. Because of this, "mini-transplants" using non–marrow-ablative chemotherapy may be used to provide sufficient immune suppression to allow donor engraftment and subsequent graft-versus-tumor effect.

IN SUMMARY, the lymphomas (NHL and HL) represent malignant neoplasms of cells native to lymphoid tissue that have their origin in the secondary lymphoid structures such as the lymph nodes and mucosa-associated lymphoid tissues. The NHLs are a group of neoplastic disorders that originate in the lymphoid tissues, usually the lymph nodes. The NHLs are multicentric in origin and spread early to various lymphoid tissues throughout the body, especially the liver, spleen, and bone marrow. HL is characterized by painless and progressive enlargement of a single node or group of nodes. It is believed to originate in one area of the lymphatic system and, if unchecked, spreads throughout the lymphatic network.

The leukemias are malignant neoplasms of the hematopoietic precursor cells that originate in the bone marrow. They are classified according to cell type (i.e., lymphocytic or myelocytic) and whether the disease is acute or chronic. The lymphocytic leukemias involve immature lymphocytes and their progenitors that originate in the bone marrow but infiltrate the spleen, lymph nodes, CNS, and other tissues. The myelogenous leukemias involve the pluripotent myeloid stem cells in bone marrow and interfere with the maturation of all blood cells, including the granulocytes, erythrocytes, and thrombocytes.

The acute leukemias (i.e., ALL, which primarily affects children, and AML, which primarily affects adults) have a sudden and stormy onset with symptoms of depressed bone marrow function (anemia, fatigue, bleeding, and infections); bone pain; and generalized lymphadenopathy, splenomegaly, and hepatomegaly. The chronic leukemias, which largely affect adults, have a more insidious onset. CLL often has the most favorable clinical course, with many persons living long enough to die of other, unrelated causes. The course of CML is slow and progressive, with transformation to a course resembling that of AML.

Multiple myeloma is a plasma cell dyscrasia characterized by expansion of a single clone of immunoglobulin-producing plasma cells and a resultant increase in serum levels of a single monoclonal immunoglobulin or its fragments. The main sites involved in multiple myeloma are the bones and bone marrow. In addition to the abnormal proliferation of marrow plasma cells, there is proliferation and activation of osteoclasts that leads to bone resorption and destruction, and predisposes to increased risk for pathologic fractures and development of hypercalcemia. Paraproteins secreted by the plasma cells may cause hyperviscosity of body fluids and may break down into amyloid, a proteinaceous substance deposited between cells that can cause heart failure and neuropathy. Bone marrow involvement leads to increased risk of infection due to suppressed humoral and cell-mediated immunity and anemia due to impaired red cell production. ∎

Review Exercises

1. A mother brings her 4-year-old son into the pediatric clinic because of irritability, loss of appetite, low-grade fever, pallor, and complaints that his legs hurt. Blood tests reveal anemia, thrombocytopenia, and an elevated leukocyte count with atypical lymphocytes. A diagnosis of acute lymphocytic leukemia (ALL) is confirmed with bone marrow studies.

   A. *What is the origin of the anemia, thrombocytopenia, elevated leukocyte count, and atypical lymphocytes seen in this child?*

   B. *Explain the cause of the child's fever, pallor, increased bleeding, and bone pain.*

   C. *The parents are informed that the preferred treatment for ALL consists of aggressive chemotherapy with the purpose of achieving a remission. Explain the rationale for using chemotherapy to treat leukemia.*

   D. *The parents are told that the child will need intrathecal chemotherapy administered by a lumbar puncture. Why is this treatment necessary?*

2. A 36-year-old man presents to his health care clinic with fever, night sweats, weight loss, and a feeling of fullness in his abdomen. Subsequent lymph node biopsy reveals a diagnosis of non-Hodgkin lymphoma (NHL).

   A. *Although lymphomas can originate in any of the lymphoid tissues of the body, most originate in the lymph nodes, and most (80% to 85%) are of B-cell origin. Hypothesize as to why B cells are more commonly affected than T cells.*

   B. *A newly developed monoclonal antibody, rituximab, is being used in the treatment of NHL. Explain how this agent exerts its effect and why it is specific for B-cell lymphomas.*

References

1. Guyton A. C., Hall J. E. (2006). *Textbook of medical physiology* (11th ed., pp. 429–456). Philadelphia: Elsevier Saunders.
2. Abbas A. K., Lichtman A. H. (2003). *Cellular and molecular immunology* (5th ed., pp. 3–39, 273). Philadelphia: W. B. Saunders.
3. Ross M. H., Kaye G. I., Pawline W. (2003). *Histology: A text and atlas* (4th ed., pp. 371–378, 398–399). Philadelphia: Lippincott Williams & Wilkins.
4. Schwarting R., McKenzie S., Rubin R. (2008). Hematopathology. In Rubin R., Strayer D. E. [Eds.], *Rubin's pathology: Clinicopathologic foundations of medicine* (5th ed. pp. 893–927). Philadelphia: Lippincott Williams & Wilkins.
5. Aster J. (2005). Diseases of the white blood cells, lymph nodes, spleen, and thymus. In Kumar V., Abbas A. K., Fausto N. [Eds.], *Robbins and Cotran pathologic basis of disease* (7th ed., pp. 661–695). Philadelphia: Elsevier Saunders.

6. Schwartzberg L. S. (2006). Neutropenia: Etiology and pathogenesis. *Clinical Cornerstone* 8(Suppl. 5), S5–S11.

7. Boxer L. A. (2004). Disorders of phagocyte function and leukopenia. In Behrman R. E., Kliegman R. M., Jenson H. B. [Eds.], *Nelson textbook of pediatrics* (17th ed., pp. 710–723). Philadelphia: Elsevier Saunders.

8. Capsoni F., Sarzi-Puttini P., Zanella A. (2005). Primary and secondary autoimmune neutropenia. *Arthritis Research and Therapy* 7, 208–214.

9. Katzung B. G. (2007). *Basic and clinical pharmacology* (10th ed., p. 467). New York: McGraw-Hill Medical.

10. Schouten H. C. (2006). Neutropenia management. *Annals of Oncology* 17(Suppl. 10), x85–x89.

11. Gabrilove J. L. (2006). An analysis of current neutropenia therapies, including pegfilgrastim. *Clinical Cornerstone* 8(Suppl. 5), S19–S28.

12. Cohen J. I. (2000). Epstein-Barr virus infection. *New England Journal of Medicine* 343, 481–492.

13. McAdam A. J., Sharpe A. H. (2005). Infectious diseases. In Kumar V., Abbas A. K., Fausto N. [Eds.], *Robbins and Cotran pathologic basis of disease* (7th ed., pp. 369–371). Philadelphia: Elsevier Saunders.

14. Schwartz D. A., Genta R. M., Bennett D. P., et al. (2008). Infectious and parasitic diseases. In Rubin R., Strayer D. S. [Eds.], *Rubin's pathology: Clinicopathologic foundations of medicine* (5th ed., pp. 285–386). Philadelphia: Lippincott Williams & Wilkins.

15. Godshall S. E., Kirscher J. T. (2000). Infectious mononucleosis: Complexities of a common syndrome. *Postgraduate Medicine* 107, 175–186.

16. Ebell M. H. (2004). Epstein-Barr virus infectious mononucleosis. *American Family Physician* 70, 1279–1287, 1289–1290.

17. Cheson B. D. (2004). What is new in lymphoma? *CA: A Cancer Journal for Clinicians* 54, 260–272.

18. American Cancer Society. (2008). *Cancer facts and figures 2007.* [Online.] Available: http://www.cancer.org/downloads/STT/2008CAFFfinalsecured.pdf. Accessed April 12, 2008.

19. Rademaker J. (2007). Hodgkin's and non-Hodgkin's lymphoma. *Radiologic Clinics of North America* 45, 69–83.

20. Armitage J. O. (2005). Staging of non-Hodgkin lymphoma. *CA: A Cancer Journal for Clinicians* 55, 368–376.

21. American Cancer Society. (2007). *Non-Hodgkin lymphoma.* Atlanta: Author.

22. Cheson B. D. (2001). Hodgkin's and non-Hodgkin's lymphomas. In Lenbard R. E. Jr., Osteen R. T., Gansler T. [Eds.], *The American Cancer Society's clinical oncology* (pp. 497–516). Atlanta: American Cancer Society.

23. Reiser M., Diehl V. (2002). Current treatment of follicular non-Hodgkin's lymphoma. *European Journal of Cancer* 38, 1167–1172.

24. Vose J. M. (2002). Immunotherapy for non-Hodgkin's lymphoma. *Clinical Oncology Updates* 5(4), 1–15.

25. National Comprehensive Cancer Network. (2008). *NCCN clinical practice guidelines in oncology: Hodgkin lymphoma.* [Online.] Available: http://www.nccn.org/professionals/physician_gls/PDF/hodgkins.pdf. Accessed April 12, 2008.

26. Re D., Thomas R. K., Behringer K., et al. (2005). From Hodgkin disease to Hodgkin lymphoma: Biologic insights and therapeutic potential. *Blood* 105, 4553–4560.

27. Armitage J. O. (2005). Staging of non-Hodgkin lymphoma. *CA: A Cancer Journal for Clinicians* 55, 368–376.

28. Yung L., Linch D. (2003). Hodgkin's lymphoma. *Lancet* 361, 943–951.

29. American Cancer Society. (2007). *Leukemia—acute lymphocytic.* Atlanta: Author.

30. Scheinberg D. A., Maslak P., Weiss M. (2001). Acute leukemias. In DeVita V. T. Jr., Hellman S., Rosenberg S. A. (Eds.), *Cancer: Principles and practice of oncology* (6th ed., pp. 2404–2433). Philadelphia: Lippincott Williams & Wilkins.

31. Miller K. B., Grodman H. M. (2001). Leukemia. In Lenbard R. E. Jr., Osteen R. T., Gansler T. [Eds.], *The American Cancer Society's clinical oncology* (pp. 527–551). Atlanta: Author.

32. Bloomfield C. D., Caligiuri M. A. (2001). Biology of leukemias. In DeVita V. T. Jr., Hellman S., Rosenberg S. A. (Eds.), *Cancer: Principles and practice of oncology* (6th ed., pp. 2390–2402). Philadelphia: Lippincott Williams & Wilkins.

33. Wujcik D. (2003). Molecular biology of leukemia. *Seminars in Oncology Nursing* 19(2), 83–89.

34. Sherbenou D. W., Druker B. J. (2007). Applying the discovery of the Philadelphia chromosome. *Journal of Clinical Investigation* 117, 2067–2074.

35. Kurzrock R., Kantarjian H. M., Druker B. J., et al. (2003). Philadelphia chromosome–positive leukemias: From basic mechanisms to molecular therapeutics. *Annals of Internal Medicine* 138, 819–830.

36. Faderi S., Jeha S., Kantajian H. M. (2003). The biology and therapy of adult acute lymphoblastic leukemia. *Cancer* 98, 1337–1354.

37. Jabbour E. J., Faderl S., Kantarjian H. M. (2005). Adult acute lymphoblastic leukemia. *Mayo Clinic Proceedings* 80, 1517–1527.

38. Pui C., Reiling M. V., Downin J. R. (2004). Acute lymphoblastic leukemia. *New England Journal of Medicine* 350, 1535–1548.

39. Viele C. S. (2003). Diagnosis, treatment, and nursing care of acute leukemia. *Seminars in Oncology Nursing* 19(2), 98–108.

40. American Cancer Society. (2007). *Leukemia—acute myeioid (myelogenous).* Atlanta: Author.

41. Stone R. M., O'Donnell R. R., Sekeres M. A. (2004). Acute myeloid leukemia. *Hematology (American Society of Hematology Education Program) 2004,* 98–117.

42. Lo-Coco F., Ammatuna E. (2006). The biology of acute promyelocytic leukemia and its on diagnosis and treatment. *Hematology (American Society of Hematology Education Program) 2006,* 156–160.

43. Pui C.-H., Evans W. E. (2006). Treatment of acute lymphoblastic leukemia. *New England Journal of Medicine* 354, 166–178.

44. Gökbuget N., Hoelzer D. (2006). Treatment of adult acute lymphoblastic leukemia. *Hematology (American Society of Hematology Education Program) 2006,* 133–141.

45. Stull D. M. (2003). Targeted therapies for the treatment of leukemia. *Seminars in Oncology Nursing* 19(2), 90–97.

46. Sanz M. A. (2006). Treatment of acute promyelocytic leukemia. *Hematology (American Society of Hematology Education Program) 2006,* 147–155.

47. American Cancer Society. (2007). *Leukemia—chronic lymphocytic.* Atlanta: Author.

48. American Cancer Society. (2007). *Leukemia—chronic myeloid (myelogenous).* Atlanta: Author.

49. Chiorazzi N., Rai K. R., Farrarini M. (2005). Chronic lymphocytic leukemia. *New England Journal of Medicine* 352, 804–815.

50. Shanafelt T. D., Byrd J. C., Call T. G., et al. (2006). Narrative review: Initial management of newly diagnosed, early-stage chronic lymphocytic leukemia. *Annals of Internal Medicine* 145, 435–447.

51. Breed C. D. (2003). Diagnosis, treatment, and nursing care of patients with chronic leukemia. *Seminars in Oncology Nursing* 19(2), 109–117.

52. Vlahorvic G., Crawford J. (2003). Activation of tyrosine kinases in cancer. *Oncologist* 8, 531–538.

53. Goldman J. M., Melo J. V. (2003). Chronic myeloid leukemia: Advances in biology and new approaches to treatment. *New England Journal of Medicine* 349, 1451–1464.

54. Kyle R. A., Rajkumar S. V. (2004). Multiple myeloma. *New England Journal of Medicine* 351, 1860–1873.

55. Rajkumar S., Kyle R. A. (2005). Multiple myeloma: Diagnosis and treatment. *Mayo Clinic Proceedings* 80, 1371–1382.

56. Katzel J. A. (2007). Multiple myeloma: Charging toward a bright future. *CA: A Cancer Journal for Clinicians* 57, 301–318.

57. Zaidi A. A., Vesole D. H. (2001). Multiple myeloma: An old disease with a new hope for the future. *CA: A Cancer Journal for Clinicians* 51, 273–285.

58. National Comprehensive Cancer Network. (2007). *NCCN clinical practice guidelines in oncology: Multiple myeloma.* V.1.2008. [Online.] Available: www.nccn.org/professionals/physician_gls/f_guidelines.asp. Accessed April 12, 2008.

Visit thePoint **http://thePoint.lww.com for animations, journal articles, and more!**

Infection, Inflammation, and Immunity

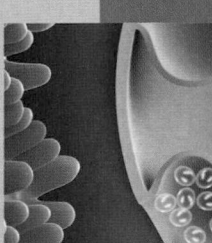

The quest to understand the mechanism of disease and ways to prevent it permeates humankind's history. Many civilizations contributed to the storehouse of knowledge. Among the early accomplishments of the Chinese are a number of practices they developed to prevent disease, one of which took the form of inoculation.

The deadly smallpox had been one of the world's most dreaded diseases. During the Middle Ages, epidemics were frequent; they swept across Asia and other parts of the world, leaving widespread death in their wake. In the 1400s, the Chinese created a technique to protect themselves during an epidemic. They collected the crusts of smallpox sores and allowed them to dry. The dried material was ground into powder and inhaled. The procedure was found to be hazardous, but it remains one of the first attempts at vaccination.

Chapter 16

Mechanisms of Infectious Disease

W. MICHAEL DUNNE, JR. AND NATHAN A. LEDEBOER

➤ All living creatures share two basic objectives in life: survival and reproduction. This doctrine applies equally to all members of the living world, including bacteria, viruses, fungi, and protozoa. To satisfy these goals, organisms must extract from the environment essential nutrients for growth and proliferation; for countless microscopic organisms, that environment includes the human body. Normally, the contact between humans and microorganisms is incidental and, in certain situations, may actually benefit both organisms. Under extraordinary circumstances, however, the invasion of the human body by microorganisms can produce harmful and potentially lethal consequences. The consequences of these invasions are collectively called *infectious diseases.*

 **INFECTIOUS DISEASES**

After completing this section of the chapter, you should be able to meet the following objectives:

■ Define the terms *host, infectious disease, colonization, microflora, virulence, pathogen,* and *saprophyte.*
■ Describe the concept of host–microorganism interaction using the concepts of commensalism, mutualism, and parasitic relationships.
■ Describe the structural characteristics and mechanisms of reproduction for prions, viruses, bacteria, fungi, and parasites.
■ Use the concepts of incidence, portal of entry, source of infection, symptomatology, disease course, site of infection, agent, and host characteristics to explain the mechanisms of infectious diseases.

Terminology

All scientific disciplines evolve with a distinct vocabulary, and the study of infectious diseases is no exception. The most appropriate way to approach this subject is with a brief discussion of the terminology used to characterize interactions between humans and microbes.

Any organism capable of supporting the nutritional and physical growth requirements of another is called a *host*. Throughout this chapter, the term *host* most often refers to humans supporting the growth of microorganisms. Occasionally, *infection* and *colonization* are used interchangeably. However, the term *infection* describes the presence and multiplication within a host of another living organism, with subsequent injury to the host, whereas *colonization* describes the act of establishing a presence, a step required in the multifaceted process of infection.

One common misconception should be dispelled from the start: not all interactions between microorganisms and humans are detrimental. The internal and external exposed surfaces of the human body are normally and harmlessly inhabited by a multitude of bacteria, collectively referred to as the normal *microflora.* Although the colonizing bacteria acquire nutritional needs and shelter, the host is not adversely affected by the relationship. An interaction such as this is called *commensalism,* and the colonizing microorganisms are sometimes referred to as *commensal flora.* The term *mutualism* is applied to an interaction in which the microorganism and the host both derive benefits from the interaction. For example, certain inhabitants of the human intestinal tract extract nutrients from the host and secrete essential vitamin byproducts of metabolism (*e.g.,* vitamin K) that are absorbed and used by the host. A *parasitic relationship* is one in which only the infecting organism benefits from the relationship and the host either gains nothing from the relationship or sustains injury from the interaction. If the host sustains injury or pathologic damage in response to a parasitic infection, the process is called an *infectious disease.*

The severity of an infectious disease can range from mild to life-threatening, depending on many variables, including the health of the host at the time of infection and the *virulence* (disease-producing potential) of the microorganism. A select group of microorganisms called *pathogens* are so virulent that they are rarely found in the absence of disease. Fortunately, there are few human pathogens in the microbial world. Most microorganisms are harmless *saprophytes,* free-living organisms obtaining their growth from dead or decaying organic material in the environment. All microorganisms, even saprophytes and members of the normal flora, can be *opportunistic pathogens,* capable of producing an infectious disease when the health and immunity of the host have been severely weakened by illness, malnutrition, or medical therapy.

Agents of Infectious Disease

The agents of infectious disease include prions, viruses, bacteria, *Rickettsiaceae* and *Chlamydiaceae,* fungi, and parasites. A summary of the salient characteristics of these human microbial pathogens is presented in Table 16-1.

Prions

Can a protein alone cause a transmissible infectious disease? Until recently, microbiologists assumed that all infectious agents must possess a genetic master plan (a genome of either ribonucleic acid [RNA] or deoxyribonucleic acid [DNA]) that codes for the production of the essential proteins and enzymes necessary for survival and reproduction. Prions, protein particles that lack any kind of a demonstrable genome, appear to be an exception to this rule. A number of prion-associated diseases have been identified, including Creutzfeldt-Jakob disease and kuru in humans, scrapie in sheep, chronic wasting disease in deer and elk, and bovine spongiform encephalopathy (BSE or mad cow disease) in cattle. The various prion-associated diseases produce very similar pathologic processes and symptoms in the hosts and are collectively called *transmissible neurodegenerative diseases.* All are characterized by a slowly progressive, noninflammatory neuronal degeneration, leading to loss of coordination (ataxia), dementia, and death over a period ranging from months to years. In fact, recent studies indicate that prion proteins (called PrP^SC) are actually altered or mutated

TABLE 16-1 **Comparison of Characteristics of Human Microbial Pathogens**

ORGANISM	DEFINED NUCLEUS	GENOMIC MATERIAL	SIZE*	INTRACELLULAR OR EXTRACELLULAR	MOTILITY
Prions	No	Unknown	55 kDa	E	–
Viruses	No	DNA or RNA	0.02–0.3	I	–
Bacteria	No	DNA	0.5–15	I/E	±
Mycoplasmas	No	DNA	0.2–0.3	E	–
Spirochetes	No	DNA	6–15	E	+
Rickettsiaceae	No	DNA	0.2–2	I	–
Chlamydiaceae	No	DNA	0.3–1	I	–
Yeasts	Yes	DNA	2–60	I/E	–
Molds	Yes	DNA	2–15 (hyphal width)	E	–
Protozoans	Yes	DNA	1–60	I/E	+
Helminths	Yes	DNA	2 mm to >1 m	E	+

*Micrometers unless indicated.

forms of a normal host protein called PrP^C. Differences in the post-translational structure cause the two proteins to behave differently. The PrP^SC is resistant to the action of proteases (enzymes that degrade excess or deformed proteins) and aggregates in the cytoplasm of affected neurons as amyloid fibrils. The normal PrP^C is protease sensitive and appears on the cell surface.

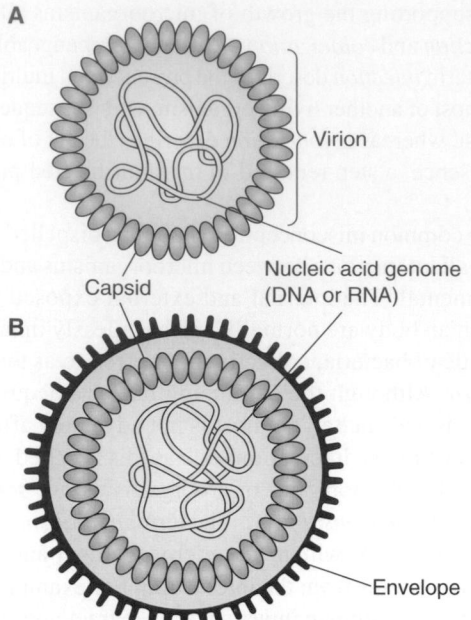

FIGURE 16-1 • **(A)** The basic structure of a virus includes a protein coat surrounding an inner core of nucleic acid (DNA or RNA). **(B)** Some viruses may also be enclosed in a lipoprotein outer envelope.

AGENTS OF INFECTIOUS DISEASE

- The agents of infectious disease represent a diversity of microorganisms that are usually not visible to the human eye.
- Microorganisms can be separated into eukaryotes (fungi and parasites), organisms containing a membrane-bound nucleus, and prokaryotes (bacteria), organisms in which the nucleus is not separated.
- Eukaryotes and prokaryotes are organisms because they contain all the enzymes and biologic equipment necessary for replication and exploiting metabolic energy.
- Viruses, which are the smallest pathogens, have no organized cellular structure, but consist of a protein coat surrounding a nucleic acid core of DNA or RNA. Unlike eukaryotes and prokaryotes, viruses are incapable of replication outside of a living cell.
- Parasites (protozoa, helminths, and arthropods) are members of the animal kingdom that infect or colonize other animals, which then transmit them to humans or in some cases directly infect the human host.

Prion diseases present significant problems to the medical community because their method of replication is not clearly understood. Studies investigating transmission of prion diseases in animals clearly demonstrate that prions replicate, leading researchers to investigate how proteins can reproduce in the absence of genetic material. Based on current models, it is believed that PrP^SC binds to the normal PrP^C on the cell surface, causing it to be processed into PrP^SC, which is released from the cell and then aggregates into amyloid-like plaques in the brain. The cell then replenishes the PrP^C and the cycle continues. As PrP^SC accumulates, it spreads within the axons of the nerve cells, causing progressively greater damage of host neurons and the eventual incapacitation of the host. In addition, because prions lack reproductive and metabolic functions, the currently available antimicrobial agents are useless against them.

Viruses

Viruses are the smallest obligate intracellular pathogens. They have no organized cellular structures but instead consist of a protein coat, or capsid, surrounding a nucleic acid core, or genome, of RNA or DNA—never both (Fig. 16-1). Some viruses are enclosed within a lipoprotein envelope derived from the cytoplasmic membrane of the parasitized host cell. Enveloped viruses include members of the herpesvirus group and paramyxoviruses, such as influenza and poxviruses. Certain enveloped viruses are continuously shed from the infected cell surface enveloped in buds pinched from the cell membrane.

The viruses of humans and animals have been categorized somewhat arbitrarily according to various characteristics. These include the type of viral genome (single-stranded or double-stranded DNA or RNA), physical characteristics (*e.g.*, size, presence or absence of a membrane envelope), the mechanism of replication (*e.g.*, retroviruses), the mode of transmission (*e.g.*, arthropod-borne viruses, enteroviruses), target tissue, and the type of disease produced (*e.g.*, hepatitis A, B, C, D, and E viruses), to name just a few.

Viruses are incapable of replication outside of a living cell. They must penetrate a susceptible living cell and use the biosynthetic machinery of the cell to produce viral progeny. The process of viral replication is shown in Figure 16-2. Not every viral agent causes lysis and death of the host cell during the course of replication. Some viruses enter the host cell and insert their genome into the host cell chromosome, where it remains in a latent, nonreplicating state for long periods without causing disease. Under the appropriate stimulation, the virus undergoes active replication and produces symptoms of disease months to years later. Members of the herpesvirus group and adenovirus are the best examples of latent viruses. Herpesviruses include the viral agents of chickenpox and zoster (varicella-zoster), cold sores (herpes simplex virus [HSV] type 1), genital herpes (HSV type 2), cytomegalovirus infec-

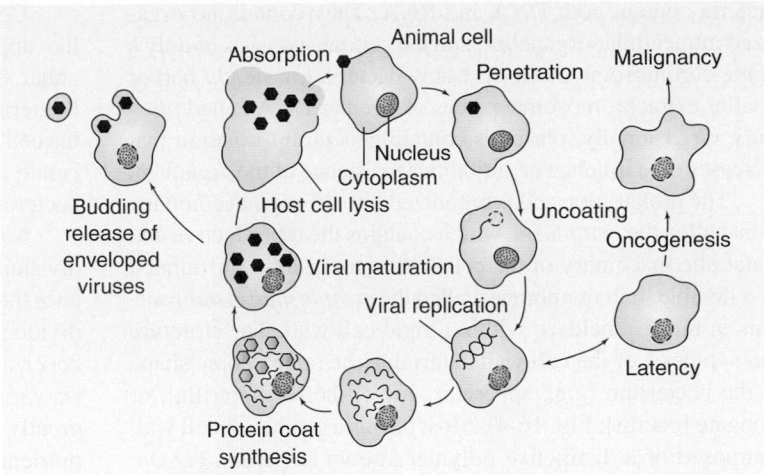

FIGURE 16-2 • Schematic representation of the many possible consequences of viral infection of host cells, including cell lysis (poliovirus), continuous release of budding viral particles, or latency (herpesviruses) and oncogenesis (papovaviruses).

tions, roseola (human herpesvirus 6), infectious mononucleosis (Epstein-Barr virus), and Kaposi sarcoma (herpesvirus 8). The resumption of the latent viral replication may produce symptoms of primary disease (*e.g.*, genital herpes) or cause an entirely different symptomatology (*e.g.*, shingles instead of chickenpox).

A family of viruses that has gained a great deal of attention in the media recently are the Orthomyxoviridae or flu viruses. Most of the recent attention has been focused on the H5N1 variant, commonly known as the *avian influenza virus*. The avian influenza viruses differ from the usual human influenza viruses by the hosts they normally infect. Avian influenza viruses typically infect wild birds; however, on occasion a new virus may result from genetic rearrangements that make it better fit to infect humans. When this occurs, the human population is more susceptible because the virus is unfamiliar to most of our immune systems.

Since the early 1980s, members of the retrovirus group have received considerable attention after identification of the human immunodeficiency viruses (HIV) as the causative agent of acquired immunodeficiency syndrome (AIDS). The retroviruses have a unique mechanism of replication. After entry into the host cell, the viral RNA genome is first translated into DNA by a viral enzyme called *reverse transcriptase* (see Chapter 20). The viral DNA copy is then integrated into the host chromosome where it exists in a latent state, similar to the herpesviruses. Reactivation and replication require a reversal of the entire process. Some retroviruses lyse the host cell during the process of replication. In the case of HIV, the infected cells regulate the immunologic defense system of the host and their lysis leads to a permanent suppression of the immune response.

In addition to causing infectious diseases, certain viruses also have the ability to transform normal host cells into malignant cells during the replication cycle. This group of viruses is referred to as *oncogenic* and includes certain retroviruses and DNA viruses, such as the herpesviruses, adenoviruses, and papovaviruses. Human papillomaviruses (HPVs), members of the papovavirus family, cause cutaneous and genital warts, and several genotypes are associated with cervical cancer (see Chapter 47). In June 2006, the U.S. Food and Drug Administration and Health Canada approved the first vaccine (Gardasil) to prevent cervical cancer, precancerous genital lesions, and genital warts due to HPV types 6, 11, 16, and 18.

Bacteria

Bacteria are autonomously replicating unicellular organisms known as *prokaryotes* because they lack an organized nucleus. Compared with nucleated eukaryotic cells (see Chapter 4), the bacterial cell is small and structurally relatively primitive (Fig. 16-3). Similar to eukaryotic cells, but unlike viruses,

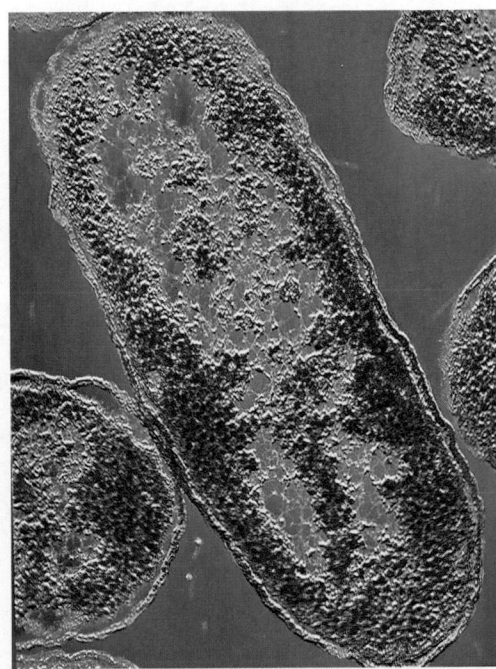

FIGURE 16-3 • False-color transmission electron micrograph of the rod-shaped, gram-negative bacterium *Escherichia coli*, showing the simple prokaryotic cell structure including the cytoplasm, the cytoplasmic membrane, and the rigid cell wall. (© Science Source/Photo Researchers.)

bacteria contain both DNA and RNA. They contain no organized intracellular organelles, and the genome consists of only a single chromosome of DNA. Many bacteria transiently harbor smaller extrachromosomal pieces of circular DNA called *plasmids*. Occasionally, plasmids contain genetic information that increases the virulence or antibiotics resistance of the organism.

The prokaryotic cell is organized into an internal compartment called the *cytoplasm,* which contains the reproductive and metabolic machinery of the cell. The cytoplasm is surrounded by a flexible lipid membrane, called the *cytoplasmic membrane.* This in turn is enclosed within a rigid cell wall. The structure and synthesis of the cell wall determine the microscopic shape of the bacterium (*e.g.,* spherical [cocci], helical [spirilla], or elongate [bacilli]; Fig. 16-4). Most bacteria produce a cell wall composed of a distinctive polymer known as *peptidoglycan*. This polymer is produced only by prokaryotes and is therefore an attractive target for antibacterial therapy. Several bacteria synthesize an extracellular capsule composed of protein or carbohydrate. The capsule protects the organism from environmental hazards such as the immunologic defenses of the host.

Certain bacteria are motile as the result of external whip-like appendages called *flagella*. The flagella rotate like a propeller, transporting the organism through a liquid environment. Bacteria can also produce hairlike structures projecting from the cell surface called *pili* or *fimbriae,* which enable the organism to adhere to surfaces such as mucous membranes or other bacteria.

Most prokaryotes reproduce asexually by simple cellular division. The manner in which an organism divides can influence the microscopic morphology. For instance, when the cocci divide in chains, they are called *streptococci;* in pairs, *diplococci*; and in clusters, *staphylococci*. The growth rate of bacteria varies significantly among different species and depends greatly on physical growth conditions and the availability of nutrients. In the laboratory, a single bacterium placed in a suitable growth environment, such as an agar plate, reproduces to the extent that it forms a visible colony composed of millions of bacteria within a few hours.

In nature, however, bacteria rarely exist as single cells floating in an aqueous environment. Rather, bacteria prefer

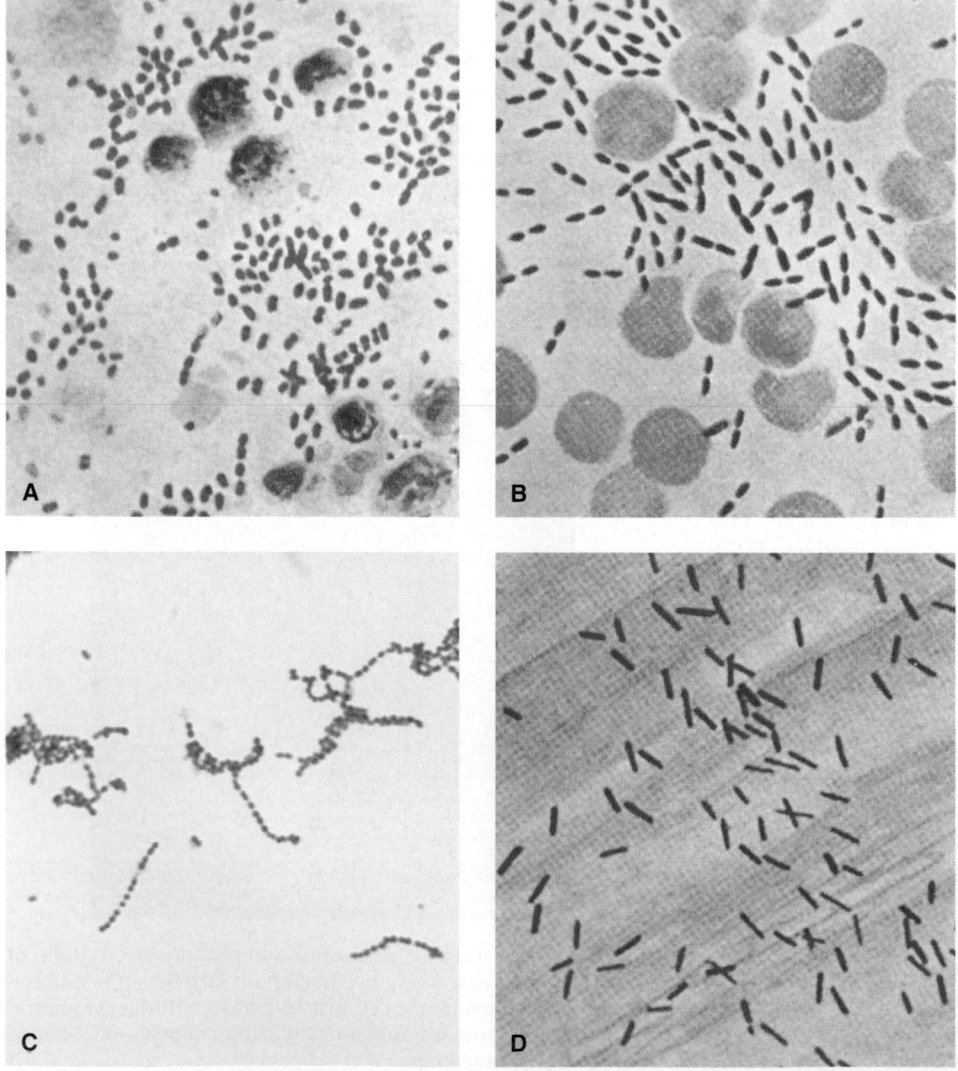

FIGURE 16-4 • A sampling of microscopic morphology of bacteria demonstrating their variability in size and shape: (**A**) *Yersinia pestis;* (**B**) gram-positive diplococci typical of *Streptococcus pneumoniae;* (**C**) *Streptococcus species* (Gram stain); (**D**) *Escherichia coli* (Gram stain). (Public Images Library, Centers for Disease Control and Prevention. Available at http://phil.cdc.gov/phil/detail.asp.)

to stick to and colonize environmental surfaces, producing structured communities called *biofilms.* The organization and structure of biofilms permit access to available nutrients and elimination of metabolic waste. Within the biofilm, individual organisms use chemical signaling as a form of primitive intercellular communication to represent the state of the environment. These signals inform members of the community when sufficient nutrients are available for proliferation or when environmental conditions warrant dormancy or evacuation. Examples of biofilms abound in nature and are found on surfaces of aquatic environments and on humans. One has only to disassemble a clogged sink drain to see a perfect example of a bacterial biofilm.

The physical appearance of a colony of bacteria grown on an agar plate can be quite distinctive for different species. Some produce pigments that give colonies a unique color. Some bacteria produce highly resistant spores when faced with an unfavorable environment. The spores can exist in a quiescent state almost indefinitely until suitable growth conditions are encountered, at which time the spores germinate and the organism resumes normal metabolism and replication.

Bacteria are extremely adaptable life forms. They are found not just in humans and other hosts, but in almost every environmental extreme on earth. However, each individual bacterial species has a well-defined set of growth parameters, including nutrition, temperature, light, humidity, and atmosphere. Bacteria with extremely strict growth requirements are called *fastidious.* For example, *Neisseria gonorrhoeae,* the bacterium that causes gonorrhea, cannot live for extended periods outside the human body. Some bacteria require oxygen for growth and metabolism and are called *aerobes;* others cannot survive in an oxygen-containing environment and are called *anaerobes.* An organism capable of adapting its metabolism to aerobic or anaerobic conditions is called *facultatively anaerobic.*

In the laboratory, bacteria are generally classified according to the microscopic appearance and staining properties of the cell. The Gram stain, originally developed in 1884 by the Danish bacteriologist Christian Gram, is still the most widely used staining procedure. Bacteria are designated as *gram-positive* organisms if they are stained purple by a primary basic dye (usually crystal violet); those that are not stained by the crystal violet but are counterstained red by a second dye (safranin) are called *gram-negative* organisms. Staining characteristics and microscopic morphology are used in combination to describe bacteria. For example, *Streptococcus pyogenes,* the agent of scarlet fever and rheumatic fever, is a gram-positive streptococcal organism that is spherical, grows in chains, and stains purple by Gram stain. *Legionella pneumophila,* the bacterium responsible for Legionnaire disease, is a gram-negative rod.

Another means of classifying bacteria according to microscopic staining properties is the *acid-fast stain.* Because of their unique cell membrane fatty acid content and composition, certain bacteria are resistant to the decolorization of a primary stain (either carbol fuchsin or a combination of auramine and rhodamine) when treated with a solution of acid alcohol. These organisms are termed *acid-fast* and include a number of signif-

icant human pathogens, most notably *Mycobacterium tuberculosis* (the cause of tuberculosis) and other mycobacteria.

For purposes of taxonomy (*i.e.,* identification and classification), each member of the bacterial kingdom is categorized into a small group of biochemically and genetically related organisms called the *genus,* and further subdivided into distinct individuals within the genus called *species.* The genus and species assignment of the organism is reflected in its name (*e.g., Staphylococcus* [genus] *aureus* [species]).

Spirochetes. The spirochetes are an eccentric category of bacteria that are mentioned separately because of their unusual cellular morphology and distinctive mechanism of motility. Technically, the spirochetes are gram-negative rods but are unique in that the cell's shape is helical and the length of the organism is many times its width. A series of filaments are wound about the cell wall and extend the entire length of the cell. These filaments propel the organism through an aqueous environment in a corkscrew motion.

Spirochetes are anaerobic organisms and comprise three genera: *Leptospira, Borrelia,* and *Treponema.* Each genus has saprophytic and pathogenic strains. The pathogenic leptospires infect a wide variety of wild and domestic animals. Infected animals shed the organisms into the environment through the urinary tract. Transmission to humans occurs by contact with infected animals or urine-contaminated surroundings. Leptospires gain access to the host directly through mucous membranes or breaks in the skin and can produce a severe and potentially fatal illness called *Weil syndrome.* In contrast, the borreliae are transmitted from infected animals to humans through the bite of an arthropod vector such as lice or ticks. Included in the genus *Borrelia* are the agents of relapsing fever (*Borrelia recurrentis*) and Lyme disease (*Borrelia burgdorferi*). Pathogenic *Treponema* species require no intermediates and are spread from person to person by direct contact. The most important member of the genus is *Treponema pallidum,* the causative agent of syphilis.

Mycoplasmas. The mycoplasmas are unicellular prokaryotes capable of independent replication. These organisms are less than one third the size of bacteria and contain a small DNA genome approximately one half the size of the bacterial chromosome. The cell is composed of cytoplasm surrounded by a membrane but, unlike bacteria, the mycoplasmas do not produce a rigid peptidoglycan cell wall. As a consequence, the microscopic appearance of the cell is highly variable, ranging from coccoid forms to filaments, and the mycoplasmas are resistant to cell-wall–inhibiting antibiotics such as penicillins and cephalosporins.

The mycoplasmas affecting humans are divided into three genera: *Mycoplasma, Ureaplasma,* and *Acholeplasma.* The first two require cholesterol from the environment to produce the cell membrane; the acholeplasmas do not. In the human host, mycoplasmas are commensals. However, a number of species are capable of producing serious diseases, including pneumonia (*Mycoplasma pneumoniae*), genital infections (*Mycoplasma hominis* and *Ureaplasma urealyticum*), and maternally transmitted respiratory infections to infants with low birth weight (*U. urealyticum*).

Rickettsiaceae, Anaplasmataceae, Chlamydiaceae, and Coxiellai

This interesting group of organisms combines the characteristics of viral and bacterial agents to produce disease in humans. All are obligate intracellular pathogens, like the viruses, but produce a rigid peptidoglycan cell wall, reproduce asexually by cellular division, and contain RNA and DNA, similar to the bacteria.

The *Rickettsiaceae* depend on the host cell for essential vitamins and nutrients, but the *Chlamydiaceae* appear to scavenge intermediates of energy metabolism such as adenosine triphosphate (ATP). The *Rickettsiaceae* infect but do not produce disease in the cells of certain arthropods such as fleas, ticks, and lice. The organisms are accidentally transmitted to humans through the bite of the arthropod (*i.e.*, the vector) and produce a number of potentially lethal diseases, including Rocky Mountain spotted fever and epidemic typhus.

The *Chlamydiaceae* are slightly smaller than the *Rickettsiaceae* but are structurally similar and are transmitted directly between susceptible vertebrates without an intermediate arthropod host. Transmission and replication of *Chlamydiaceae* occur through a defined life cycle. The infectious form, called an *elementary body,* attaches to and enters the host cell, where it transforms into a larger *reticulate body.* This undergoes active replication into multiple elementary bodies, which are then shed into the extracellular environment to initiate another infectious cycle. Chlamydial diseases of humans include sexually transmitted genital infections (*Chlamydophila trachomatis;* see Chapter 47); ocular infections and pneumonia of newborns (*C. trachomatis*); upper and lower respiratory tract infections in children, adolescents, and young adults (*Chlamydophila pneumoniae*); and respiratory disease acquired from infected birds (*Chlamydia psittaci*).

Organisms within the family *Anaplasmataceae* (including the reorganized genera *Ehrlichia, Anaplasma, Neorickettsia,* and *Wolbachia*) are also obligate intracellular organisms that resemble the *Rickettsiaceae* in structure and produce a variety of veterinary and human diseases, some of which have a tick vector. These organisms target host mononuclear and polymorphonuclear white blood cells for infection and, similar to the *Chlamydiaceae*, multiply in the cytoplasm of infected leukocytes within vacuoles called *morulae.* Unlike the *Chlamydiaceae*, however, the *Anaplasmataceae* do not have a defined life cycle and are independent of the host cell for energy production. *Ehrlichia sennetsu,* which is primarily restricted to Japan, produces a disease called *sennetsu fever* that resembles infectious mononucleosis. Disease caused by this organism differs from other *Anaplasmataceae* because it is associated with eating raw fish infested with *E. sennetsu*-infected parasites. The most common infections caused by *Anaplasmataceae* are human monocytic and granulocytic ehrlichiosis. Human monocytic ehrlichiosis is a disease caused by *Ehrlichia chaffeensis* and *E. canis* that can easily be confused with Rocky Mountain

spotted fever. Clinical disease severity ranges from mild to life-threatening. Manifestations include generalized malaise, anorexia and nausea, fever, and headache. Decreases in white blood cells (leukopenia) and platelets (thrombocytopenia) often occur. Severe sequelae include severe respiratory failure, encephalopathy, and acute renal failure. The disease is usually more severe in the elderly and persons with compromised immune function (*e.g.*, HIV/AIDS). Human granulocytic ehrlichiosis, which is caused by two species (*Anaplasma phagocytophilium,* and *Ehrlichia ewingii*), is also transmitted by ticks. The symptoms are similar to those seen with human monocytotropic ehrlichiosis.

The genus *Coxiella* contains only one species, *C. burnetii.* Like its rickettsial counterparts, it is a gram-negative intracellular organism that infects a variety of animals, including cattle, sheep, and goats. In humans, *Coxiellai* infection produces a disease called *Q fever,* characterized by a nonspecific febrile illness often accompanied by headache, chills, arthralgias, and mild pneumonia. The organism produces a highly resistant spore-like stage that is transmitted to humans when contaminated animal tissue is aerosolized (*e.g.*, during meat processing) or by ingestion of contaminated milk.

Fungi

The fungi are free-living, eukaryotic saprophytes found in every habitat on earth. Some are members of the normal human microflora. Fortunately, few fungi are capable of causing diseases in humans, and most of these are incidental, self-limited infections of skin and subcutaneous tissue. Serious fungal infections are rare and usually initiated through puncture wounds or inhalation. Despite their normally harmless nature, fungi can cause life-threatening opportunistic diseases when host defense capabilities have been disabled.

The fungi can be separated into two groups, yeasts and molds, based on rudimentary differences in their morphology (Fig. 16-5). The yeasts are single-celled organisms, approximately the size of red blood cells, that reproduce by a budding process. The buds separate from the parent cell and mature into identical daughter cells. Molds produce long, hollow, branching filaments called *hyphae.* Some molds produce cross walls, which segregate the hyphae into compartments, and others do not. A limited number of fungi are capable of growing as yeasts at one temperature and as molds at another. These organisms are called *dimorphic fungi* and include a number of human pathogens such as the agents of blastomycosis (*Blastomyces dermatitidis*), histoplasmosis (*Histoplasma capsulatum*), and coccidioidomycosis (*Coccidioides immitis*).

The appearance of a fungal colony tends to reflect its cellular composition. Colonies of yeast are generally smooth with a waxy or creamy texture. Molds tend to produce cottony or powdery colonies composed of mats of hyphae collectively called a *mycelium.* The mycelium can penetrate the growth surface or project above the colony like the roots and branches of a tree. Yeasts and molds produce a rigid cell wall layer that is chemically unrelated to the peptidoglycan of bacteria and is therefore not susceptible to the effects of penicillin-like antibiotics.

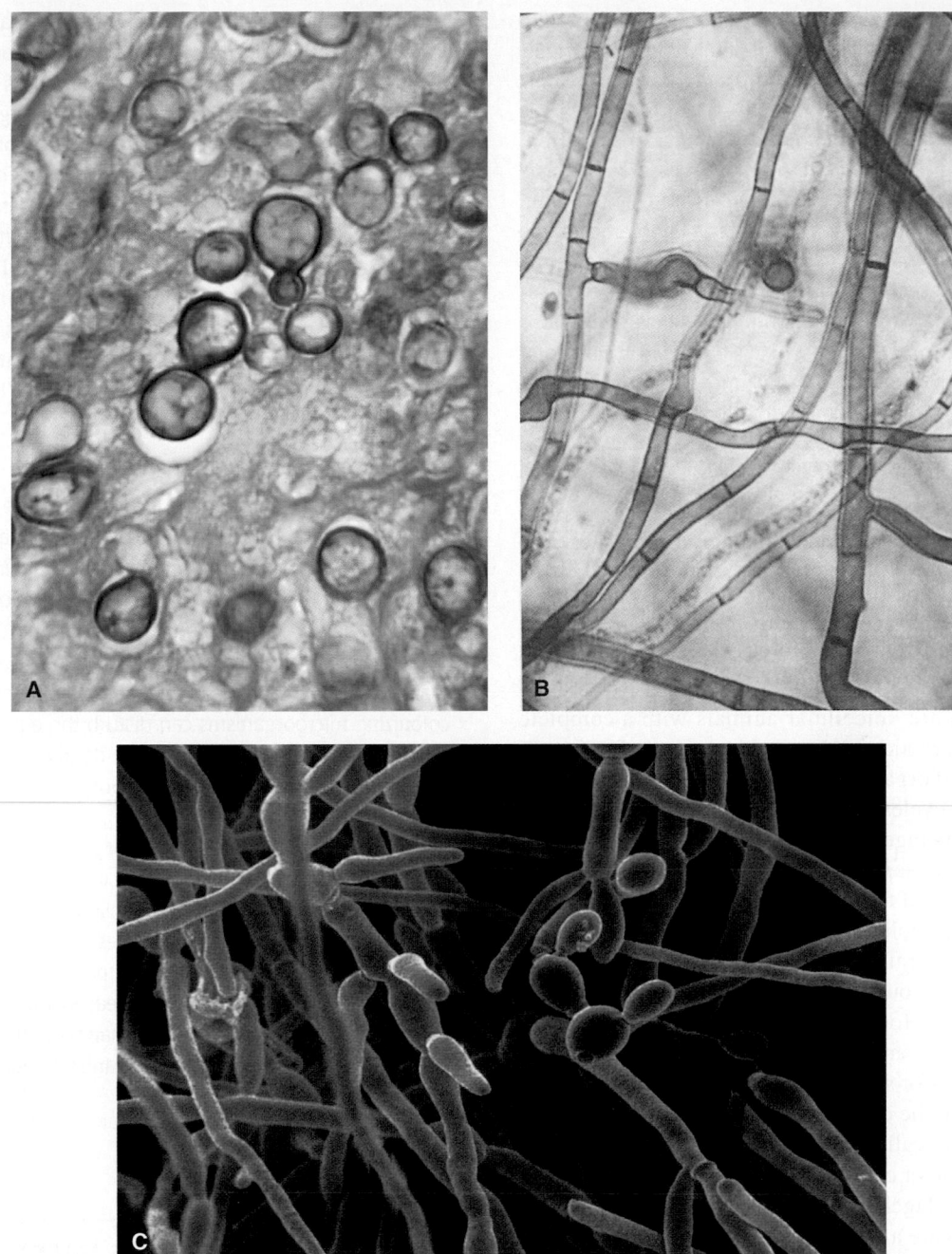

FIGURE 16-5 • The microscopic morphology of fungal pathogens in humans. (A) Histopathologic changes seen in histoplasmosis due to *Histoplasma capsulatum var. duboisii.* Note the presence of typical yeast cells, some of which are undergoing replication by budding. (B) The molds produce long branched and unbranched filaments called *hyphae.* (C) *Candida albicans* is a budding yeast that produces pseudohyphae both in culture and in tissues and exudate. (A, Public Images Library, Centers for Disease Control and Prevention. Available at http://phil.cdc.gov/phil/detail.asp; C, © Science Source/Photo Researchers.)

Most fungi are capable of sexual or asexual reproduction. The former process involves the fusion of zygotes with the production of a recombinant zygospore. Asexual reproduction involves the formation of highly resistant spores called *conidia* or *sporangiospores,* which are borne by specialized structures that arise from the hyphae. Molds are identified in the

laboratory by the characteristic microscopic appearance of the asexual fruiting structures and spores.

Like the bacterial pathogens of humans, fungi can produce disease in the human host only if they can grow at the temperature of the infected body site. For example, a number of fungal pathogens called *dermatophytes* are incapable of growing at core body temperature (37°C), and the infection is limited to the cooler cutaneous surfaces. Diseases caused by these organisms, including ringworm, athlete's foot, and jock itch, are collectively called *superficial mycoses*. Systemic mycoses are serious fungal infections of deep tissues and, by definition, are caused by organisms capable of growth at 37°C. Yeasts such as *Candida albicans* are commensal flora of the skin, mucous membranes, and gastrointestinal tract and are capable of growth at a wider range of temperatures. Intact immune mechanisms and competition for nutrients provided by the bacterial flora normally keep colonizing fungi in check. Alterations in either of these components by disease states or antibiotic therapy can upset the balance, permitting fungal overgrowth and setting the stage for opportunistic infections.

Parasites

In a strict sense, any organism that derives benefits from its biologic relationship with another organism is a parasite. In the study of clinical microbiology, however, the term *parasite* has evolved to designate members of the animal kingdom that infect and cause disease in other animals, and includes protozoa, helminths, and arthropods.

The protozoa are unicellular animals with a complete complement of eukaryotic cellular machinery, including a well-defined nucleus and organelles. Reproduction may be sexual or asexual, and life cycles may be simple or complicated, with several maturation stages requiring more than one host for completion. Most are saprophytes, but a few have adapted to the accommodations of the human environment and produce a variety of diseases, including malaria, amebic dysentery, and giardiasis. Protozoan infections can be passed directly from host to host such as through sexual contact, indirectly through contaminated water or food, or by way of an arthropod vector. Direct or indirect transmission results from the ingestion of highly resistant cysts or spores that are shed in the feces of an infected host. When the cysts reach the intestine, they mature into vegetative forms called *trophozoites,* which are capable of asexual reproduction or cyst formation. Most trophozoites are motile by means of flagella, cilia, or ameboid motion.

The helminths are a collection of wormlike parasites that include the nematodes or roundworms, cestodes or tapeworms, and trematodes or flukes. The helminths reproduce sexually within the definitive host, and some require an intermediate host for the development and maturation of offspring. Humans can serve as the definitive or intermediate host and, in certain diseases such as trichinosis, as both. Transmission of helminth diseases occurs primarily through the ingestion of fertilized eggs (ova) or the penetration of infectious larval stages through the skin—directly or with the aid of an arthropod vector. Helminth infections can involve many organ systems and sites, including the liver and lung, urinary and intestinal tracts, circulatory and central nervous systems, and muscle. Although most helminth diseases have been eradicated from the United States, they are still a major health concern of developing nations.

The parasitic arthropods of humans and animals include the vectors of infectious diseases (*e.g.*, ticks, mosquitoes, biting flies) and the ectoparasites. The ectoparasites infest external body surfaces and cause localized tissue damage or inflammation secondary to the bite or burrowing action of the arthropod. The most prominent human ectoparasites are mites (scabies), chiggers, lice (head, body, and pubic), and fleas. Transmission of ectoparasites occurs directly by contact with immature or mature forms of the arthropod or its eggs found on the infested host or the host's clothing, bedding, or grooming articles such as combs and brushes. Many of the ectoparasites are vectors of other infectious diseases, including endemic typhus and bubonic plague (fleas) and epidemic typhus (lice).

IN SUMMARY, throughout life, humans are continuously and harmlessly exposed to and colonized by a multitude of microscopic organisms. This relationship is kept in check by the intact defense mechanisms of the host (*e.g.*, mucosal and cutaneous barriers, normal immune function) and the innocuous nature of most environmental microorganisms. Those factors that weaken the host's resistance or increase the virulence of colonizing microorganisms can disturb the equilibrium of the relationship and cause disease. The degree to which the balance is shifted in favor of the microorganism determines the severity of illness.

There is an extreme diversity of prokaryotic and eukaryotic microorganisms capable of causing infectious diseases in humans. With the advent of immunosuppressive medical therapy and immunosuppressive diseases such as AIDS, the number and type of potential microbic pathogens, the so-called opportunistic pathogens, have increased dramatically. However, most infectious illnesses in humans continue to be caused by only a small fraction of the organisms that comprise the microscopic world. ■

MECHANISMS OF INFECTION

After completing this section of the chapter, you should be able to meet the following objectives:

- Differentiate between incidence and prevalence and among endemic, epidemic, and pandemic.
- Describe the stages of an infectious disease after the potential pathogen has entered the body.
- List the systemic manifestations of infectious disease.
- Describe mechanisms and significance of antimicrobial and antiviral drug resistance.
- Explain the actions of intravenous immunoglobulin and cytokines in the treatment of infectious illnesses.

Epidemiology of Infectious Diseases

Epidemiology, in the context of this chapter, is the study of factors, events, and circumstances that influence the transmission of infectious diseases among humans. The ultimate goal of the epidemiologist is to devise strategies that interrupt or eliminate the spread of an infectious agent. To accomplish this, infectious diseases must be classified according to incidence, portal of entry, source, symptoms, disease course, site of infection, and virulence factors so that potential outbreaks may be predicted and averted or appropriately treated.

 EPIDEMIOLOGY OF INFECTIOUS DISEASES

- Epidemiology is the study of factors, events, and circumstances that influence the transmission of infectious diseases in human populations.

- Epidemiology focuses on the incidence (number of new cases) and prevalence (number of active cases at any given time) of an infectious disease; the source of infection and its portal of entry, site of infection, and virulence factors of the infecting organism; and the signs and symptoms of the infection and its course.

- The ultimate goals of epidemiologic studies are the interruption of the spread of infectious diseases and their eradication.

Epidemiology is a science of rates and statistics. The expected frequency of any infectious disease must be calculated so that gradual or abrupt changes in frequency can be observed. The term *incidence* is used to describe the number of new cases of an infectious disease that occur within a defined population (*e.g.,* per 100,000 persons) over an established period of time (*e.g.,* monthly, quarterly, yearly). Disease *prevalence* indicates the number of active cases at any given time. A disease is considered *endemic* in a particular geographic region if the incidence and prevalence are expected and relatively stable. An *epidemic* describes an abrupt and unexpected increase in the incidence of disease over endemic rates. A *pandemic* refers to the spread of disease beyond continental boundaries. The advent of rapid worldwide travel increased the likelihood of pandemic transmission of pathogenic microorganisms.

As an illustration of these principles, an outbreak of a suspected respiratory viral illness—subsequently identified as severe acute respiratory syndrome (SARS)—was recognized in the Guangdong province in southern China beginning in November 2002. The illness was highly transmissible, as evidenced by the first recognized occurrence in Taiwan. Four days after returning to Taiwan from work in the Guangdong province, a businessman developed a febrile illness and was admitted to a local hospital. Within 1 month, a large nosocomial outbreak of SARS was documented to have affected approximately 3000 people in Taipei City, Taiwan. Once the SARS outbreak had crossed continental borders for the first time, its classification was changed from an epidemic to a pandemic.

Portal of Entry

The portal of entry refers to the process by which a pathogen enters the body, gains access to susceptible tissues, and causes disease. Among the potential modes of transmission are penetration, direct contact, ingestion, and inhalation. The portal of entry does not dictate the site of infection. Ingested pathogens may penetrate the intestinal mucosa, disseminate through the circulatory system, and cause diseases in other organs such as the lung or liver. Whatever the mechanisms of entry, the transmission of infectious agents is directly related to the number of infectious agents absorbed by the host.

Penetration

Any disruption in the integrity of the body's surface barrier—skin or mucous membranes—is a potential site for invasion of microorganisms. The break may be the result of an accidental injury causing abrasions, burns, or penetrating wounds; medical procedures such as surgery or catheterization; or a primary infectious process that produces surface lesions such as chickenpox or impetigo. Direct inoculation from intravenous drug use or an animal or arthropod bite also can occur.

Direct Contact

Some pathogens are transmitted directly from infected tissue or secretions to exposed, intact mucous membranes. This is especially true of certain sexually transmitted infections (STIs) such as gonorrhea, syphilis, chlamydia, and genital herpes, for which exposure of uninfected membranes to pathogens occurs during intimate contact (see Chapter 47).

The transmission of STIs is not limited to sexual contact. *Vertical transmission* of these agents, from mother to child, can occur across the placenta or during birth when the mucous membranes of the child come in contact with infected vaginal secretions of the mother. When an infectious disease is transmitted from mother to child during gestation or birth, it is classified as a *congenital infection*. The most frequently observed congenital infections include toxoplasmosis (caused by the parasite *Toxoplasma gondii*), syphilis, rubella, cytomegalovirus infection, and herpes simplex virus infections (the so-called TORCH infections, discussed in Chapter 7); varicella-zoster (chickenpox); parvovirus B19; group B streptococci (*Streptococcus agalactiae*); and HIV. Of these, cytomegalovirus is by far the most common cause of congenital infection in the United States, affecting nearly 1% of all newborns. However, with more than 6000 HIV-infected women giving birth each year in the United States and Canada, and with a 13% to 30% chance of vertical transmission, HIV is rapidly gaining in stature as a congenitally transmitted infection (see Chapter 20).

The severity of congenital defects associated with these infections depends greatly on the gestational age of the fetus when transmission occurs, but most of these agents can cause profound mental retardation and neurosensory deficits, including blindness and hearing loss. HIV rarely produces overt signs and symptoms in the infected newborn, and it sometimes takes years for the effects of the illness to manifest.

Ingestion

The entry of pathogenic microorganisms or their toxic products through the oral cavity and gastrointestinal tract represents one of the more efficient means of disease transmission in humans. Many bacterial, viral, and parasitic infections, including cholera, typhoid fever, dysentery (amebic and bacillary), food poisoning, traveler's diarrhea, cryptosporidiosis, and hepatitis A, are initiated through the ingestion of contaminated food and water. This mechanism of transmission necessitates that an infectious agent survive the low pH and enzyme activity of gastric secretions and the peristaltic action of the intestines in numbers sufficient to establish infection, deemed an *infectious dose*. Ingested pathogens also must compete successfully with the normal bacterial flora of the bowel for nutritional needs. Persons with reduced gastric acidity because of disease or medication are more susceptible to infection by this route because the number of ingested microorganisms surviving the gastric environment is greater. Ingestion has also been postulated as a means of transmission of HIV infection from mother to child through breast-feeding.

Inhalation

The respiratory tract of healthy persons is equipped with a multitiered defense system to prevent potential pathogens from entering the lungs. The surface of the respiratory tree is lined with a layer of mucus that is continuously swept up and away from the lungs and toward the mouth by the beating motion of ciliated epithelial cells. Humidification of inspired air increases the size of aerosolized particles, which are effectively filtered by the mucous membranes of the upper respiratory tract. Coughing also aids in the removal of particulate matter from the lower respiratory tract. Respiratory secretions contain antibodies and enzymes capable of inactivating infectious agents. Particulate matter and microorganisms that ultimately reach the lung are cleared by phagocytic cells.

Despite this impressive array of protective mechanisms, a number of pathogens can invade the human body through the respiratory tract, including agents of bacterial pneumonia (*S. pneumoniae, L. pneumophila*), meningitis (*Neisseria meningitidis, Haemophilus influenzae*), and tuberculosis, as well as the viruses responsible for measles, mumps, chickenpox, influenza, and the common cold. Defective pulmonary function or mucociliary clearance caused by noninfectious processes such as cystic fibrosis, emphysema, or smoking can increase the risk of inhalation-acquired diseases.

Source

The source of an infectious disease refers to the location, host, object, or substance from which the infectious agent was acquired: essentially the "who, what, where, and when" of disease transmission. The source may be endogenous (acquired from the host's own microbial flora, as would be the case in an opportunistic infection) or exogenous (acquired from sources in the external environment, such as the water, food, soil, or air). The source of the infectious agent can also be another human being, as from mother to child during gestation (congenital infections); an inanimate object; an animal; or a biting arthropod. Inanimate objects that carry an infectious agent are known as *fomites*. For example, rhinoviruses and many other non-enveloped viruses can be spread by contact with contaminated fomites such as handkerchiefs and toys. Zoonoses are a category of infectious diseases passed from other animal species to humans. Examples of zoonoses include cat-scratch disease, rabies, and visceral or cutaneous larval migrans. The spread of infectious diseases such as Lyme disease through biting arthropod vectors has already been mentioned.

Source can denote a place. For instance, infections that develop in patients while they are hospitalized are called *nosocomial,* and those that are acquired outside of health care facilities are called *community acquired.* The source may also pertain to the body substance that is the most likely vehicle for transmission, such as feces, blood, body fluids, respiratory secretions, and urine. Infections can be transmitted from person to person through shared inanimate objects (fomites) contaminated with infected body fluids. An example of this mechanism of transmission would include the spread of the HIV and hepatitis B virus through the use of shared syringes by intravenous drug users. Infection can also be spread through a complex combination of source, portal of entry, and vector. The well-publicized 1993 outbreak of hantavirus pulmonary syndrome in the southwestern United States is a prime example. This viral illness was transmitted to humans by inhalation of dust contaminated with saliva, feces, and urine of infected rodents.

Symptomatology

The term *symptomatology* refers to the collection of signs and symptoms expressed by the host during the disease course. This is also known as the *clinical picture* or *disease presentation,* and can be characteristic of any given infectious agent. In terms of pathophysiology, symptoms are the outward expression of the struggle between invading organisms and the retaliatory inflammatory and immune responses of the host. The symptoms of an infectious disease may be specific and reflect the site of infection (*e.g.,* diarrhea, rash, convulsions, hemorrhage, and pneumonia). Conversely, symptoms such as fever, myalgia, headache, and lethargy are relatively nonspecific and can be shared by a number of diverse infectious diseases. The symptoms of a diseased host can be obvious, as in the case of chickenpox or measles. Other, covert symptoms, such as an increased white blood cell count, may require laboratory testing to detect. Accurate recognition and documentation of symptomatology can aid in the diagnosis of an infectious disease.

Disease Course

The course of any infectious disease can be divided into several distinguishable stages after the point when the potential pathogen enters the host. These stages are the incubation period, the prodromal stage, the acute stage, the convalescent stage, and the resolution stage (Fig. 16-6). The stages are based on the progression and intensity of the host's symptoms over time. The duration of each phase and the pattern of the overall illness can be specific for different pathogens, thereby aiding in the diagnosis of an infectious disease.

The incubation period is the phase during which the pathogen begins active replication without producing recognizable symptoms in the host. The incubation period may be short, as in the case of salmonellosis (6 to 24 hours), or prolonged, such as that of hepatitis B (50 to 180 days) or HIV (months to years). The duration of the incubation period can be influenced by additional factors, including the general health of the host, the portal of entry, and the infectious dose of the pathogen.

The hallmark of the *prodromal stage* is the initial appearance of symptoms in the host, although the clinical presentation during this time may be only a vague sense of malaise. The host may experience mild fever, myalgia, headache, and fatigue. These are constitutional changes shared by a great number of disease processes. The duration of the prodromal stage can vary considerably from host to host.

The *acute stage* is the period during which the host experiences the maximum impact of the infectious process corresponding to rapid proliferation and dissemination of the pathogen. During this phase, toxic byproducts of microbial metabolism, cell lysis, and the immune response mounted by the host combine to produce tissue damage and inflammation. The symptoms of the host are pronounced and more specific than in the prodromal stage, usually typifying the pathogen and sites of involvement.

The *convalescent period* is characterized by the containment of infection, progressive elimination of the pathogen, repair of damaged tissue, and resolution of associated symptoms. Similar to the incubation period, the time required for complete convalescence may be days, weeks, or months, depending on the type of pathogen and the voracity of the host's immune response. The *resolution* is the total elimination of a pathogen from the body without residual signs or symptoms of disease.

Several notable exceptions to the classic presentation of an infectious process have been recognized. Chronic infectious diseases have a markedly protracted and sometimes irregular course. The host may experience symptoms of the infectious process continuously or sporadically for months or years without a convalescent phase. In contrast, *subclinical* or *subacute illness* progresses from infection to resolution without clinically apparent symptoms. A disease is called *insidious* if the prodromal phase is protracted; a fulminant illness is characterized by abrupt onset of symptoms with little or no prodrome. Fatal infections are variants of the typical disease course.

Site of Infection

Inflammation of an anatomic location is usually designated by adding the suffix *-itis* to the name of the involved tissue (*e.g.,* bronchitis, infection of the bronchi and bronchioles; encephalitis, brain infection; carditis, infection of the heart). These are general terms, however, and they apply equally to inflammation from infectious and noninfectious causes. The suffix *-emia* is used to designate the presence of a substance in the blood (*e.g., bacteremia, viremia,* and *fungemia* describe the presence of these infectious agents in the bloodstream). The term *sepsis,* or *septicemia,* refers to the presence of microbial toxins in the blood.

The site of an infectious disease is determined ultimately by the type of pathogen, the portal of entry, and the competence of the host's immunologic defense system. Many pathogenic microorganisms are restricted in their capacity to invade the human body. *M. pneumoniae,* influenza viruses, and *L. pneumophila* rarely cause disease outside the respiratory tract; infections caused by *N. gonorrhoeae* are generally confined to the genitourinary tract; and shigellosis and giardiasis seldom extend beyond the gastrointestinal tract. These are considered localized infectious diseases. The bacterium *Helicobacter pylori* is an extreme example of a site-specific pathogen. *H. pylori* is a significant cause of gastric ulcers but has not been implicated in disease processes elsewhere in the human body. Bacteria such as *N. meningitidis,* a prominent pathogen of children and

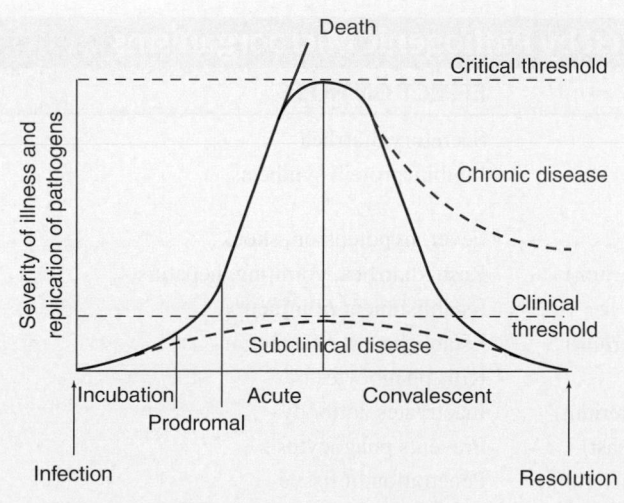

FIGURE 16-6 • Stages of a primary infectious disease as they appear in relation to the severity of symptoms and numbers of infectious agents. The clinical threshold corresponds with the initial expression of recognizable symptoms, whereas the critical threshold represents the peak of disease intensity.

young adults; *Salmonella typhi,* the cause of typhoid fever; and *B. burgdorferi,* the agent of Lyme disease, tend to disseminate from the primary site of infection to involve other locations and organ systems. These are examples of systemic pathogens disseminated throughout the body by the circulatory system.

An *abscess* is a localized pocket of infection composed of devitalized tissue, microorganisms, and the host's phagocytic white blood cells: in essence, a stalemate in the infectious process. In this case, the dissemination of the pathogen has been contained by the host, but white cell function within the toxic environment of the abscess is hampered, and the elimination of microorganisms is retarded. Abscesses usually must be surgically drained to effect a complete cure. Similarly, infections of biomedical implants such as catheters, artificial heart valves, and prosthetic bone implants are seldom cured by the host's immune response and antimicrobial therapy. The infecting organism colonizes the surface of the implant, producing a dense matrix of cells, host proteins, and capsular material—a biofilm—necessitating the removal of the device.

Virulence Factors

Virulence factors are substances or products generated by infectious agents that enhance their ability to cause disease. Although a large number of microbial products fit this description, they can be grouped generally into four categories: toxins, adhesion factors, evasive factors, and invasive factors (Table 16-2).

Toxins

Toxins are substances that alter or destroy the normal function of the host or host's cells. Toxin production is a trait chiefly monopolized by bacterial pathogens, although certain fungal and protozoan pathogens also elaborate substances toxic to humans. Bacterial toxins have a diverse spectrum of activity and exert their effects on a wide variety of host target cells. For classification purposes, however, the bacterial toxins can be divided into two main types: *exotoxins* and *endotoxins.*

Exotoxins. Exotoxins are proteins released from the bacterial cell during growth. Bacterial exotoxins enzymatically inactivate or modify key cellular constituents, leading to cell death or dysfunction. Diphtheria toxin, for example, inhibits cellular protein synthesis; botulism toxin decreases the release of neurotransmitter from cholinergic neurons, causing flaccid paralysis; tetanus toxin decreases the release of neurotransmitter from inhibitory neurons, producing spastic paralysis; and cholera toxin induces fluid secretion into the lumen of the intestine, causing diarrhea. Other examples of exotoxin-induced diseases include pertussis (whooping cough), anthrax, traveler's diarrhea, toxic shock syndrome, and a host of food-borne illnesses (*i.e.,* food poisoning).

Bacterial exotoxins that produce vomiting and diarrhea are sometimes referred to as *enterotoxins.* There has been resurgent interest in streptococcal pyrogenic exotoxin A (SPEA), an exotoxin produced by certain strains of group A, beta-hemolytic streptococci (*S. pyogenes*) that causes a life-threatening toxic shock–like syndrome similar to the disease associated with tampon use produced by *S. aureus.* The streptococcal form of intoxication is sometimes called *Henson disease* because it was this infection that caused the death of the famous puppeteer Jim Henson. Other exotoxins that have gained notoriety include the Shiga toxins produced by *Escherichia coli* O157:H7 and other select strains. The ingestion of undercooked hamburger meat or unpasteurized fruit juices contaminated with this organism

TABLE 16-2 Examples of Virulence Factors Produced by Pathogenic Microorganisms

FACTOR	CATEGORY	ORGANISM	EFFECT ON HOST
Cholera toxin	Exotoxin	*Vibrio cholerae* (bacterium)	Secretory diarrhea
Diphtheria toxin	Exotoxin	*Corynebacterium diphtheriae* (bacterium)	Inhibits protein synthesis
Lipopolysaccharide	Endotoxin	Many gram-negative bacteria	Fever, hypotension, shock
Toxic shock toxin	Enterotoxin	*Staphylococcus aureus* (bacterium)	Rash, diarrhea, vomiting, hepatitis
Hemagglutinin	Adherence	Influenza virus	Establishment of infection
Pili	Adherence	*Neisseria gonorrhoeae* (bacterium)	Establishment of infection
Leukocidin	Evasive	*S. aureus*	Kills phagocytes
IgA protease	Evasive	*Haemophilus influenzae* (bacterium)	Inactivates antibody
Capsule	Evasive	*Cryptococcus neoformans* (yeast)	Prevents phagocytosis
Collagenase	Invasive	*Pseudomonas aeruginosa* (bacterium)	Penetration of tissue
Protease	Invasive	*Aspergillus* (mold)	Penetration of tissue
Phospholipase	Invasive	*Clostridium perfringens* (bacterium)	Penetration of tissue
Botulinum toxin	Exotoxin	*Clostridium botulinum* (bacterium)	Neuroparalysis, inhibits acetylcholine release
Pneumolysin	Exotoxin	*Streptococcus pneumoniae* (bacterium)	Inhibition of respiratory ciliated and phagocytic cell function

produces hemorrhagic colitis and a sometimes fatal illness called *hemolytic uremic syndrome* (HUS), characterized by vascular endothelial damage, acute renal failure, and thrombocytopenia. HUS occurs primarily in infants and young children who have not developed antibodies to the Shiga toxins. Over time, the incidence of disease caused by food-borne exotoxins has grown. One such event occurred in the late summer of 2006. Small clusters of infections appeared in sporadic locations throughout the United States. Epidemiologists interviewed affected individuals and identified fresh spinach as the suspected source of infection. Tracking the outbreaks led investigators from the Centers for Disease Control and Prevention (CDC) to a California produce company bagging fresh spinach.

Endotoxins. In contrast to exotoxins, endotoxins do not contain protein, are not actively released from the bacterium during growth, and have no enzymatic activity. Rather, endotoxins are complex molecules composed of lipid and polysaccharides found in the cell wall of gram-negative bacteria. Studies of different endotoxins have indicated that the lipid portion of the endotoxin confers the toxic properties to the molecule. Endotoxins are potent activators of a number of regulatory systems in humans. A small amount of endotoxin in the circulatory system (endotoxemia) can induce clotting, bleeding, inflammation, hypotension, and fever. The sum of the physiologic reactions to endotoxins is sometimes called *endotoxic shock.*

Adhesion Factors

No interaction between microorganisms and humans can progress to infection or disease if the pathogen is unable to attach to and colonize the host. The process of microbial attachment may be site specific (*e.g.,* mucous membranes, skin surfaces), cell specific (*e.g.,* T lymphocytes, respiratory epithelium, intestinal epithelium), or nonspecific (*e.g.,* moist areas, charged surfaces). In any of these cases, adhesion requires a positive interaction between the surfaces of host cells and the infectious agent.

The site to which microorganisms adhere is called a *receptor,* and the reciprocal molecule or substance that binds to the receptor is called a *ligand* or *adhesin.* Receptors may be proteins, carbohydrates, lipids, or complex molecules composed of all three. Similarly, ligands may be simple or complex molecules and, in some cases, highly specific structures. Ligands that bind to specific carbohydrates are called *lectins.* After initial attachment, a number of bacterial agents become embedded in a gelatinous matrix of polysaccharides called a *slime* or *mucous layer.* The slime layer serves two purposes: it anchors the agent firmly to host tissue surfaces and it protects the agent from the immunologic defenses of the host.

Many viral agents, including influenza, mumps, measles, and adenovirus, produce filamentous appendages or spikes called *hemagglutinins* that recognize carbohydrate receptors on the surfaces of specific cells in the upper respiratory tract of the host.

Evasive Factors

A number of factors produced by microorganisms enhance virulence by evading various components of the host's immune system. Extracellular polysaccharides, including capsules, slime, and mucous layers, discourage engulfment and killing of pathogens by the host's phagocytic white blood cells (*i.e.,* neutrophils and macrophages). Encapsulated organisms such as *S. agalactiae, S. pneumoniae, N. meningitidis,* and *H. influenzae* type b (before the vaccine) are a cause of significant morbidity and mortality in neonates and children who lack protective anticapsular antibodies. Certain bacterial, fungal, and parasitic pathogens avoid phagocytosis by excreting leukocidin C toxins, which cause specific and lethal damage to the cell membrane of host neutrophils and macrophages. Other pathogens, such as the bacterial agents of salmonellosis, listeriosis, and Legionnaire disease, are adapted to survive and reproduce within phagocytic white blood cells after ingestion, avoiding or neutralizing the usually lethal products contained within the lysosomes of the cell. *H. pylori,* the infectious cause of gastritis and gastric ulcers, produces a urease enzyme on its outer cell wall. The urease converts gastric urea into ammonia, thus neutralizing the acidic environment of the stomach and allowing the organism to survive in this hostile environment.

Other unique strategies used by pathogenic microbes to evade immunologic surveillance have evolved solely to avoid recognition by host antibodies. Strains of *S. aureus* produce a surface protein (protein A) that immobilizes immunoglobulin G (IgG), holding the antigen-binding region harmlessly away from the organisms. This pathogen also secretes a unique enzyme called *coagulase.* Coagulase converts soluble human coagulation factors into a solid clot, which envelops and protects the organism from phagocytic host cells and antibodies. *H. influenzae* and *N. gonorrhoeae* secrete enzymes that cleave and inactivate secretory IgA, neutralizing the primary defense of the respiratory and genital tracts at the site of infection. *Borrelia* species, including the agents of Lyme disease and relapsing fever, alter surface antigens during the disease course to avoid immunologic detection. It appears that the capability to devise strategic defense systems and stealth technologies is not limited to humans.

Some viruses, such as HIV, impair the function of immunoregulatory cells. Although this property increases the virulence of these agents, it is not considered a virulence factor in the true sense of the definition.

Invasive Factors

Invasive factors are products produced by infectious agents that facilitate the penetration of anatomic barriers and host tissue. Most invasive factors are enzymes capable of destroying cellular membranes (*e.g.,* phospholipases), connective tissue (*e.g.,* elastases, collagenases), intercellular matrices (*e.g.,* hyaluronidase), and structural protein complexes (*e.g.,* proteases). It is the combined effects of invasive factors, toxins, and antimicrobial and inflammatory substances released by host cells to counter infection that mediate the tissue damage and pathophysiology of infectious diseases.

IN SUMMARY, epidemiology is the study of factors, events, and circumstances that influence the transmission of disease. *Incidence* refers to the number of new cases of an infectious disease that occur in a defined population, and *prevalence* to the number of active cases that are present at any given time. Infectious diseases are considered endemic in a geographic area if the incidence and prevalence are expected and relatively stable. An epidemic refers to an abrupt and unexpected increase in the incidence of a disease over endemic rates, and a pandemic to the spread of disease beyond continental boundaries.

The ultimate goal of epidemiology and epidemiologic studies is to devise strategies to interrupt or eliminate the spread of infectious disease. To accomplish this, infectious diseases are classified according to incidence, portal of entry, source, symptoms, disease course, site of infection, and virulence factors. ■

DIAGNOSIS AND TREATMENT OF INFECTIOUS DISEASES

After completing this section of the chapter, you should be able to meet the following objectives:

- State the two criteria used in the diagnosis of an infectious disease.
- Explain the differences among culture, serology, and antigen, metabolite, or molecular detection methods for diagnosis of infectious disease.
- Cite three general intervention methods that can be used in treatment of infectious illnesses.
- State four basic mechanisms by which antibiotics exert their action.
- Differentiate *bactericidal* from *bacteriostatic*.

Diagnosis

The diagnosis of an infectious disease requires two criteria: the recovery of a probable pathogen or evidence of its presence from the infected sites of a diseased host, and accurate documentation of clinical signs and symptoms (symptomatology) compatible with an infectious process. In the laboratory, the diagnosis of an infectious agent is accomplished using three basic techniques: culture, serology, or the detection of characteristic antigens, genomic sequences, or metabolites produced by the pathogen.

Culture

Culture refers to the propagation of a microorganism outside of the body, usually on or in artificial growth media such as agar plates or broth (Fig. 16-7). The specimen from the host is inoculated into broth or onto the surface of an agar plate, and the culture is placed in a controlled environment such as an incubator until the growth of microorganisms becomes detectable. In the case of a bacterial pathogen, identification is based on microscopic appearance and Gram stain reaction, shape, texture, and color (*i.e.,* morphology) of the colonies, and by a panel of biochemical reactions that fingerprint salient biochemical characteristics of the organism. Certain bacteria such as *Mycobacterium leprae,* the agent of leprosy, and *T. pallidum,* the syphilis spirochete, do not grow on artificial media and require additional methods of identification. Fungi and mycoplasmas are cultured in much the same way as bacteria, but with more reliance on microscopic and colonial morphology for identification.

DIAGNOSIS AND TREATMENT OF INFECTIOUS DISEASES

- The definitive diagnosis of an infectious disease requires recovery and identification of the infecting organism by microscopic identification of the agent in stains of specimens or sections of tissue, culture isolation and identification of the agents, demonstration of antibody- or cell-mediated immune responses to an infectious agent, or DNA or RNA identification of infectious agents.

- Treatment of infectious disease is aimed at eliminating the infectious organism and promoting recovery of the infected person. Treatment is provided through the use of antimicrobial agents, immunotherapy, and, when necessary, surgical interventions.

- Prevention of infectious disease is accomplished through the use of immunization methods.

Chlamydiaceae, Rickettsiaceae, and all human viruses are obligate intracellular pathogens. As a result, the propagation of these agents in the laboratory requires the inoculation of eukaryotic cells grown in culture (cell cultures). A cell culture consists of a flask containing a single layer, or monolayer, of eukaryotic cells covering the bottom and overlaid with broth containing essential nutrients and growth factors. When a virus infects and replicates within cultured eukaryotic cells, it produces pathologic changes in the appearance of the cell called the *cytopathic effect* (CPE; Fig. 16-8). The CPE can be detected microscopically, and the pattern and extent of cellular destruction is often characteristic of a particular virus.

Although culture media have been developed for the growth of certain human-infecting protozoa and helminths in the laboratory, the diagnosis of parasitic infectious diseases has traditionally relied on microscopic or, in the case of worms, visible identification of organisms, cysts, or ova directly from infected patient specimens.

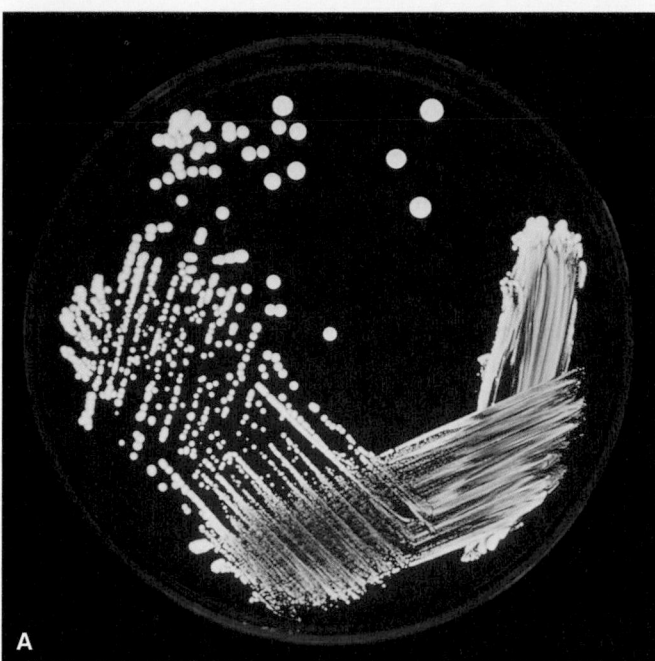
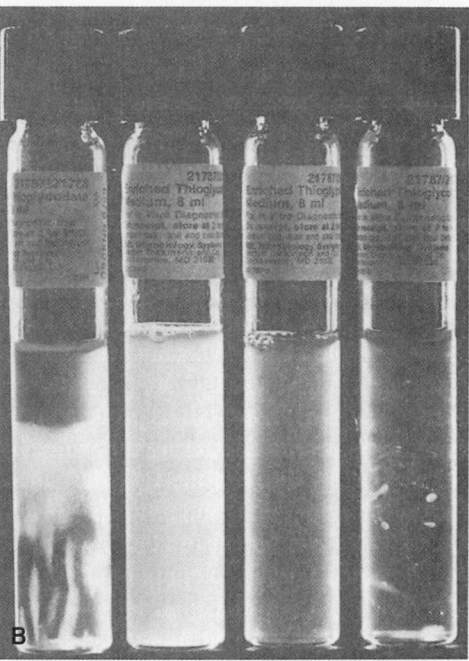

FIGURE 16-7 • Variability of the macroscopic appearance of bacteria cultured on solid, agar-containing medium and liquid broth medium. (**A**) Photograph showing numerous *Legionella* species colonies that have been cultivated on an agar culture plate and illuminated using ultraviolet light. (**B**) Bacteria cultured in broth form a variety of growth patterns, ranging from particulate to homogeneous, turbid suspensions. Anaerobic bacteria cultured in liquid medium tend to grow best at the bottom of the tube, where the concentration of molecular oxygen is lowest. (Public Images Library, Centers for Disease Control and Prevention. Available at http://phil.cdc.gov/phil/detail.asp.)

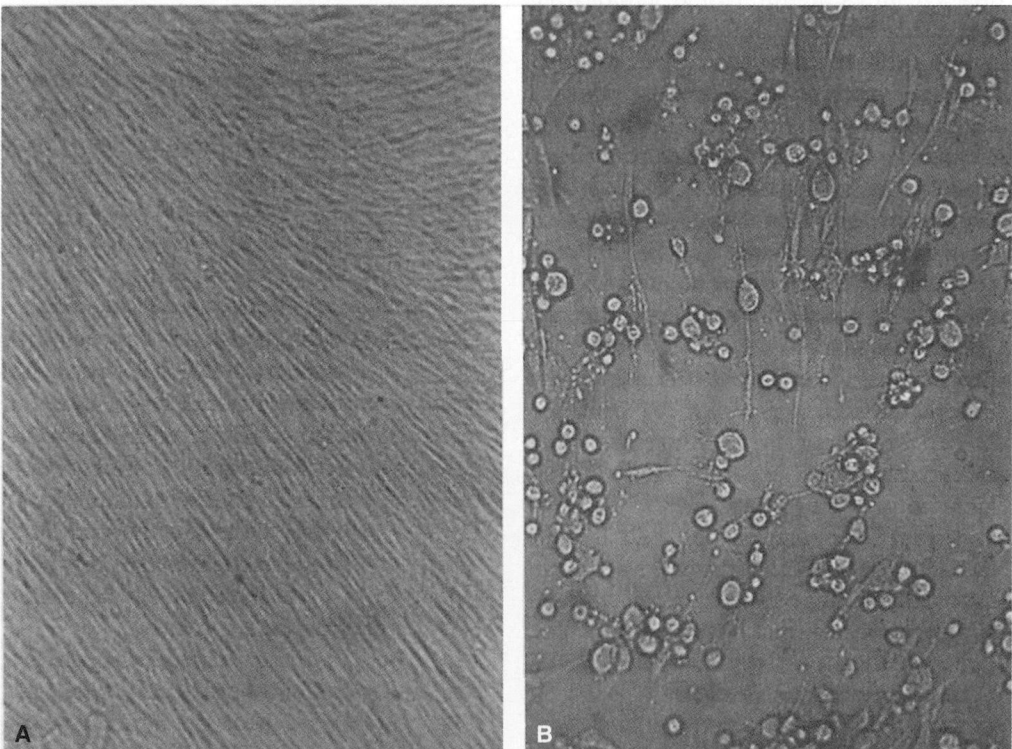

FIGURE 16-8 • The microscopic appearance of a monolayer of uninfected human fibroblasts grown in cell culture (**A**), and the same cells after infection with herpes simplex virus (**B**), demonstrating the cytopathic effect caused by viral replication and concomitant cell lysis.

Serology

Serology—literally, "the study of serum "—is an indirect means of identifying infectious agents by measuring serum antibodies in the diseased host. A tentative diagnosis can be made if the antibody level, also called *antibody titer,* against a specific pathogen rises during the acute phase of the disease and falls during convalescence. Serologic identification of an infectious agent is not as accurate as culture, but it may be a useful adjunct, especially for the diagnosis of diseases caused by pathogens such as the hepatitis B virus that cannot be cultured. The measurement of antibody titers has another advantage in that specific antibody types such as IgM and IgG are produced by the host during different phases of an infectious process. IgM-specific antibodies generally rise and fall during the acute phase of the disease, whereas the synthesis of the IgG class of antibodies increases during the acute phase and remains elevated until or beyond resolution. Measurements of class-specific antibodies are also useful in the diagnosis of congenital infections. IgM antibodies do not cross the placenta, but certain IgG antibodies are transferred passively from mother to child during the final trimester of gestation. Consequently, an elevated level of pathogen-specific IgM antibodies in the serum of a neonate must have originated from the child and therefore indicates congenital infection. A similarly increased IgG titer in the neonate does not differentiate congenital from maternal infection.

The technology of *direct antigen detection* has evolved rapidly over the past decade and in the process has revolutionized the diagnosis of certain infectious diseases. Antigen detection incorporates features of culture and serology but reduces to a fraction the time required for diagnosis. In principle, this method relies on purified antibodies to detect antigens of infectious agents in specimens obtained from the diseased host. The source of antibodies used for antigen detection can be animals immunized against a particular pathogen or *hybridomas.* Hybridomas are created by fusing normal antibody-producing spleen cells from an immunized animal with malignant myeloma cells; the resulting hybrid synthesizes large quantities of antibody. An antibody produced by a hybridoma is called a *monoclonal antibody,* and is highly specific for a single antigen and a single pathogen. Regardless of the source, the antibodies are labeled with a substance that allows microscopic or overt detection when bound to the pathogen or its products. In general, the three types of labels used for this purpose are fluorescent dyes, enzymes, and particles such as latex beads. Fluorescent antibodies allow visualization of an infectious agent with the aid of fluorescence microscopy. Depending on the type of fluorescent dye used, the organism may appear bright green or orange against a black background, making detection extremely easy. Enzyme-labeled antibodies function in a similar manner. The enzyme is capable of converting a colorless compound into a colored substance, thereby permitting detection of antibody bound to an infectious agent without the use of a fluorescent microscope. Particles coated with antibodies clump together, or agglutinate, when the appropriate antigen is present in a specimen. Particle agglutination is especially useful when examining infected body fluids such as urine, serum, or spinal fluid.

DNA and RNA Sequencing

Methods for identifying infectious agents through the detection of DNA or RNA sequences unique to a single agent have recently seen rapid development and increased use. Several techniques have been devised to accomplish this goal, each having different degrees of sensitivity regarding the number of organisms that need to be present in a specimen for detection. The first of these methods is called *DNA probe hybridization.* Small fragments of DNA are cut from the genome of a specific pathogen and labeled with compounds (photoemitting chemicals or antigens) that allow detection. The labeled DNA probes are added to specimens from an infected host. If the pathogen is present, the probe attaches to the complementary strand of DNA on the genome of the infectious agent, permitting rapid diagnosis. The use of labeled probes has allowed visualization of particular agents within and around individual cells in histologic sections of tissue.

A second and more sensitive method of DNA detection is called the *polymerase chain reaction* (PCR; Fig. 16-9). This method incorporates two unique reagents: a specific pair of oligonucleotides (usually less than 25 nucleotides long) called *primers* and a heat-stable DNA polymerase. To perform the assay, the primers are added to the specimen containing the suspect pathogen, and the sample is heated to melt the DNA in the specimen and then allowed to cool. The primers locate and bind only to the complementary target DNA of the pathogen in question. The heat-stable polymerase begins to replicate the DNA from the point at which the primers attached, similar to two trains approaching one another on separate but converging tracks. After the initial cycle, DNA polymerization ceases at the point where the primers were located, producing a strand of DNA with a distinct size, depending on the distance separating the two primers. The specimen is heated again, and the process starts anew. After many cycles of heating, cooling, and polymerization, a large number of uniformly sized DNA fragments are produced only if the specific pathogen (or its DNA) is present in the specimen. The polymerized DNA fragments are separated by electrophoresis and visualized with a dye or identified by hybridization with a specific probe.

A modification of PCR, known as real-time PCR, continues to revolutionize medical diagnostics. Real-time PCR uses the same principles as PCR, but includes a fluorescence-labeled probe that specifically binds a target DNA sequence between the oligonucleotide primers. As the DNA is replicated by the DNA polymerase, the level of fluorescence in the reaction is measured. If fluorescence increases beyond a minimum threshold, the PCR is considered positive and indicates the presence of the target DNA in a specimen.

Several variations of molecular gene detection techniques in addition to PCR have been developed and incorporated into diagnostic kits for use in the clinical laboratory, including ligase chain reaction (LCR), transcription-mediated amplification (TMA), strand displacement amplification, branched-chain DNA signal amplification (bDNA), hybrid capture assays, and DNA sequencing.

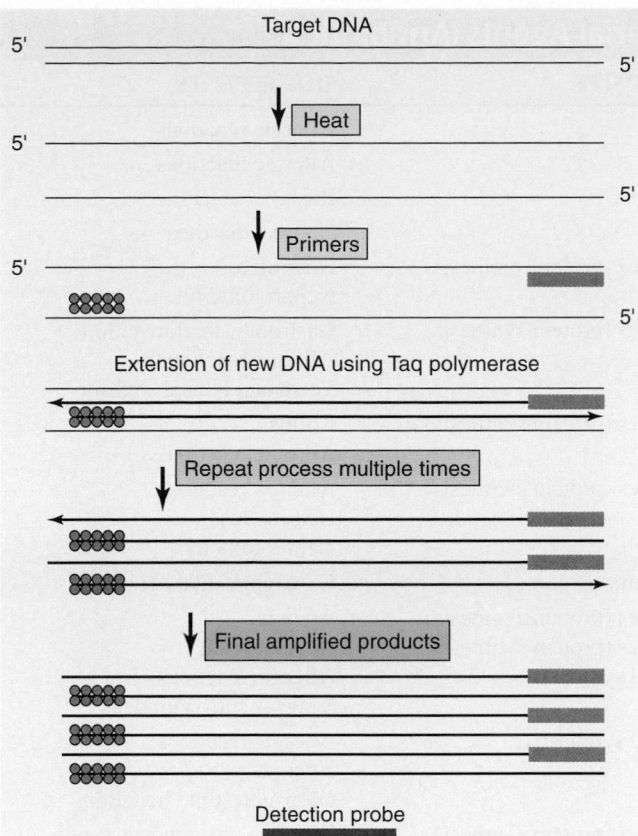

FIGURE 16-9 • Polymerase chain reaction. The target DNA is first melted using heat (generally around 94°C) to separate the strands of DNA. Primers that recognize specific sequences in the target DNA are allowed to bind as the reaction cools. Using a unique, thermostable DNA polymerase called Taq and an abundance of deoxynucleoside triphosphates, new DNA strands are amplified from the point of the primer attachment. The process is repeated many times (called *cycles*) until millions of copies of DNA are produced, all of which have the same length defined by the distance (in base pairs) between the primer binding sites. These copies are then detected by electrophoresis and staining or through the use of labeled DNA probes that, similar to the primers, recognize a specific sequence located in the amplified section of DNA.

Many of the newer gene detection technologies have been adapted for quantitation of the target DNA or RNA in serum specimens of patients infected with viruses such as HIV and hepatitis C. If the therapy is effective, viral replication is suppressed and the viral load (level of viral genome) in the peripheral blood is reduced. Conversely, if mutations in the viral genome lead to resistant strains or if the antiviral therapy is ineffective, viral replication continues and the patient's viral load rises, indicating a need to change the therapeutic approach.

Molecular biology has revolutionized medical diagnostics. Using techniques such as PCR, laboratories now can detect as little as one virus or bacterium in a single specimen, allowing for the diagnosis of infections caused by microorganisms that are impossible or difficult to grow in culture. These methods have increased sensitivity while decreasing the time required to identify the etiologic agent of infectious disease. For example, using standard viral culture, it can take days to weeks to grow a virus and correlate the CPE with the virus. Using molecular biologic techniques, laboratories are able to complete the same work in a few hours.

Treatment

The goal of treatment for an infectious disease is complete removal of the pathogen from the host and the restoration of normal physiologic function to damaged tissues. Most infectious diseases of humans are self-limiting in that they require little or no medical therapy for a complete cure. When an infectious process gains the upper hand and therapeutic intervention is essential, the choice of treatment may be medicinal through the use of antimicrobial agents; immunologic with antibody preparations, vaccines, or substances that stimulate and improve the host's immune function; or surgical by removing infected tissues. The decision about which therapeutic modality or combination of therapies to use is based on the extent, urgency, and location of the disease process, the pathogen, and the availability of effective antimicrobial agents.

Antimicrobial Agents

The use of chemicals, potions, and elixirs in the treatment of infectious diseases dates back to the earliest records of medicine. More than 2000 years ago, Greek and Chinese physicians recognized that certain substances were useful for preventing or curing wound infections. Although the biologic activity of these compounds was not understood, some may have inadvertently contained byproducts of molds that resemble modern antibiotics. From that time until the late 1800s, when the relation between infection and microorganisms was finally accepted, the evolution of anti-infective therapy was less than explosive. It was not until the advent of World War II, after the introduction of sulfonamides and penicillin, that the development of antimicrobial compounds matured into a science of great consequence. Today, the comprehensive list of effective anti-infective agents is burgeoning. Most antimicrobial compounds can be categorized roughly according to mechanism of anti-infective activity, chemical structure, and target pathogen (*e.g.,* antibacterial, antiviral, antifungal, or antiparasitic agents).

Antibacterial Agents. Antibacterial agents are generally called *antibiotics.* Most antibiotics are actually produced by other microorganisms, primarily bacteria and fungi, as byproducts of metabolism, and usually are effective only against other prokaryotic organisms. An antibiotic is considered *bactericidal* if it causes irreversible and lethal damage to the bacterial pathogen, and *bacteriostatic* if its inhibitory effects on bacterial growth are reversed when the agent is eliminated. Antibiotics can be classified into families of compounds with related chemical structure and activity (Table 16-3).

Not all antibiotics are effective against all pathogenic bacteria. Some agents are effective only against gram-negative

TABLE 16-3 Classification and Activity of Antibacterial Agents (Antibiotics)

FAMILY	EXAMPLE	TARGET SITE	SIDE EFFECTS
Penicillins	Ampicillin	Cell wall	Allergic reactions
Cephalosporins	Cephalexin	Cell wall	Allergic reactions
Monobactams	Aztreonam	Cell wall	Rash
Carbapenem	Imipenem	Cell wall	Nausea, diarrhea
Aminoglycosides	Tobramycin	Ribosomes (protein synthesis)	Hearing loss / Nephrotoxicity
Tetracyclines	Doxycycline	Ribosomes (protein synthesis)	Gastrointestinal irritation / Allergic reactions / Teeth and bone dysplasia
Macrolides	Clarithromycin	Ribosomes (protein synthesis)	Colitis / Allergic reactions
Glycopeptides	Vancomycin	Ribosomes (protein synthesis)	Allergic reactions / Hearing loss / Nephrotoxicity
Quinolones	Ciprofloxacin	DNA synthesis	Gastrointestinal irritation
Miscellaneous	Chloramphenicol	Ribosomes (protein synthesis)	Anemia
	Rifampin	Ribosomes (protein synthesis)	Hepatotoxicity
	Trimethoprim	Folic acid synthesis	Allergic reactions / Same as sulfonamides
Sulfonamides	Sulfadiazine	Folic acid synthesis	Allergic reactions / Anemia / Gastrointestinal irritation
Oxazolidinone	Linezolid	Ribosomes (protein synthesis)	Diarrhea, thrombocytopenia
Streptogramin	Quinupristin/dalfopristin	Ribosomes (protein synthesis)	Muscle and joint aches
Glycylcycline	Tigecycline	Ribosomes	Nausea, vomiting, diarrhea
Polymyxins	Colistin	Membrane	Confusion, visual disturbances, vertigo, kidney damage
Lipopeptide	Daptomycin	Membrane depolarization	Nausea, vomiting, constipation, diarrhea, headache

bacteria, and others are specific for gram-positive organisms (e.g., vancomycin). The so-called broad-spectrum antibiotics, such as the newest class of cephalosporins, are active against a wide variety of gram-positive and gram-negative bacteria. Members of the *Mycobacterium* genus, including *M. tuberculosis,* are extremely resistant to the effects of the major classes of antibiotics and require an entirely different spectrum of agents for therapy. The four basic mechanisms of the antibiotic action are interference with a specific step in bacterial cell wall synthesis (e.g., penicillins, cephalosporins, glycopeptides, monobactams, carbapenems); inhibition of bacterial protein synthesis (e.g., aminoglycosides, macrolides, ketolides, tetracyclines, chloramphenicol, oxazolidinones, streptogramins, and rifampin); interruption of nucleic acid synthesis (e.g., fluoroquinolones, nalidixic acid); and interference with normal metabolism (e.g., sulfonamides, trimethoprim).

Despite lack of antibiotic activity against eukaryotic cells, many agents cause unwanted or toxic side effects in humans, including allergic responses (penicillins, cephalosporins, sulfonamides, glycopeptides), hearing and kidney impairment (aminoglycosides), and liver or bone marrow toxicity (chloramphenicol, fluoroquinolones, vancomycin). Of greater concern is the increasing prevalence of bacteria resistant to the effects of antibiotics. The ways in which bacteria acquire resistance to antibiotics are becoming as numerous as the types of antibiotics. Bacterial resistance mechanisms include the production of enzymes that inactivate antibiotics, such as β-lactamases; genetic mutations that alter antibiotic binding sites; alternative metabolic pathways that bypass antibiotic activity; and changes in the filtration qualities of the bacterial cell wall that prevent access of antibiotics to the target site in the organism. It is the continuous search for a "better mousetrap" that makes anti-infective therapy such a fascinating aspect of infectious diseases.

Antiviral Agents. Until recently, few effective antiviral agents were available for treating human infections. The reason for this is host toxicity; viral replication requires the use of eukaryotic host cell enzymes, and the drugs that effectively interrupt viral replication are likely to interfere with host cell reproduction as well. However, in response to the AIDS epidemic, there has been massive, albeit delayed, development of antiretroviral agents. Almost all antiviral compounds are synthetic and, with few exceptions, the primary target of antiviral compounds is viral RNA or DNA synthesis. Agents such as acyclovir, ganciclovir, vidarabine, and ribavirin mimic the nucleoside building blocks of RNA and DNA. During active viral replication, the nucleoside analogs inhibit the viral DNA polymerase, preventing duplication of the viral genome and spread of infectious viral progeny to other susceptible host cells. Similar to the specificity of antibiotics, antiviral agents may be active against RNA viruses only, DNA viruses only, or occasionally both. Other nucleoside analogs such as zidovudine, lamivudine, didanosine, stavudine, and zalcitabine, and non-nucleoside inhibitors, including nevirapine, efavirenz, and delavirdine, were developed specifically for the treatment of AIDS by targeting the HIV-specific enzyme, reverse transcriptase, for inhibition. This key enzyme is essential for viral replication and has no counterpart in the infected eukaryotic host cells.

Another class of antiviral agents developed solely for the treatment of HIV infections are the *protease inhibitors* (e.g., indinavir, ritonavir, saquinavir, tipranavir, atazanvir, nelfinavir). These drugs inhibit an HIV-specific enzyme that is necessary for late maturation events in the virus life cycle.

Experimental approaches to antiviral therapy include compounds that inhibit viral attachment to susceptible host cells, drugs that prevent uncoating of the viral genome once inside the host cell, and agents that directly inhibit viral DNA polymerase, such as foscarnet. An example of drugs that prevent attachment is enfuvirtide, a peptide that binds to the docking glycopeptide (gp41) of HIV-1 and prevents its binding and fusion to the target CD4+ lymphocytes (see Chapter 20). Recently, a new class of antiviral agents has been developed and released that specifically inhibits influenza virus neuraminidase B, which is an essential enzyme for viral replication. Two agents in this class, zanamivir and oseltamivir, have been approved for treatment of both influenza A and B.

Although the treatment of viral infections with antimicrobial agents is a relatively recent endeavor, reports of viral mutations resulting in resistant strains are very common. This is especially troubling in the case of HIV, in which resistance to relatively new antiviral agents, including nucleoside analogs and protease inhibitors, has already been described, prompting the need for combination or alternating therapy with multiple antiretroviral agents.

Antifungal Agents. The target site of the two most important families of antifungal agents is the cytoplasmic membranes of yeasts or molds. Fungal membranes differ from human cell membranes in that they contain the sterol ergosterol instead of cholesterol. The polyene family of antifungal compounds (*e.g.,* amphotericin B, nystatin) preferentially binds to ergosterol and forms holes in the cytoplasmic membrane, causing leakage of the fungal cell contents and, eventually, lysis of the cell. The imidazole class of drugs (*e.g.,* fluconazole, itraconazole, voriconazole, posaconazole) inhibits the synthesis of ergosterol, thereby damaging the integrity of the fungal cytoplasmic membrane. Both types of drugs bind to a certain extent to the cholesterol component of host cell membranes and elicit a variety of toxic side effects in treated patients. The nucleoside analog 5-fluorocytosine (5-FC) disrupts fungal

RNA and DNA synthesis but without the toxicity associated with the polyene and imidazole drugs. Unfortunately, 5-FC demonstrates little or no antifungal activity against molds or dimorphic fungi and is primarily reserved for infections caused by yeasts.

A novel class of antifungal compounds called *echinocandins* has received considerable attention because these drugs inhibit the synthesis of β-1,3-glucan, a major cell wall polysaccharide found in many fungi, including *C. albicans, Aspergillus* species, and *Pneumocystis carinii.* The drugs included in this class are caspofungin, micafungin, and anidulafungin. These inhibitors are available for treatment of patients with fungal infections, such as candidiasis or invasive aspergillosis, that are refractory to treatment with other antifungal agents.

Antiparasitic Agents. Because of the extreme diversity of human parasites and their growth cycles, a review of antiparasitic therapies and agents would be highly impractical and lengthy. Similar to other infectious diseases caused by eukaryotic microorganisms, treatment of parasitic illnesses is based on exploiting essential components of the parasite's metabolism or cellular anatomy that are not shared by the host. Any relatedness between the target site of the parasite and the cells of the host increases the likelihood of toxic reactions in the host.

Continued development of improved antiparasitic agents suffers greatly from economic considerations. Parasitic diseases of humans are primarily the scourge of the world's poor, developing nations. As a result, financial incentives to produce more effective therapies are nonexistent. Resistance among human parasites to standard, effective therapy is also a major concern. In Africa, Asia, and South America, the incidence of chloroquine-resistant malaria (*Plasmodium falciparum*) is on the rise. Resistant strains require more complicated, expensive, and potentially toxic therapy with a combination of agents.

Immunotherapy

An exciting approach to the treatment of infectious diseases is immunotherapy. This strategy involves supplementing or stimulating the host's immune response so that the spread of a pathogen is limited or reversed. Several products are available for this purpose, including intravenous immune globulin (IVIG) and cytokines. IVIG is a pooled preparation of antibodies obtained from normal, healthy immune human donors that is infused as an intravenous solution. In theory, pathogen-specific antibodies present in the infusion facilitate neutralization, phagocytosis, and clearance of infectious agents above and beyond the capabilities of the diseased host. Hyperimmune immune globulin preparations, which are also commercially available, contain high titers of antibodies against specific pathogens, including hepatitis B virus, cytomegalovirus, rabies, and varicella-zoster virus.

Cytokines are substances produced by various cells that, in small quantities, stimulate white cell replication, phagocytosis, antibody production, and the induction of fever, inflammation, and tissue repair—all of which counteract infectious agents and hasten recovery (see Chapter 17). With the advent of genetic engineering and cloning, many cytokines, including interferons and interleukins, have been produced in the laboratory and are being evaluated experimentally as anti-infective agents. As we learn more about the action of cytokines, we are beginning to appreciate that some of the adverse reactions associated with infectious processes result from the body's own inflammatory response. Interventional therapies designed to inactivate certain cytokines such as tumor necrosis factor have proven to be helpful in animal models of infection. It is not unlikely that therapies based on the regulation of the inflammatory response will become widely used in human medicine over the next few years.

One of the most efficient but often overlooked means of preventing infectious diseases is immunization. Proper and timely adherence to recommended vaccination schedules in children and booster immunizations in adults effectively reduces the senseless spread of vaccine-preventable illnesses such as measles, mumps, pertussis, and rubella, which still occur with alarming frequency. The potential benefits of the new HPV vaccine, Gardasil, have been reviewed earlier in this chapter. New strategies for the development of vaccines carried by harmless viral vectors are currently being developed that someday might lead to inexpensive and effective oral immunization against HIV, hepatitis C, malaria, and other potentially lethal infectious diseases.

Surgical Intervention

Before the discovery of antimicrobial agents, surgical removal of infected tissues, organs, or limbs was occasionally the only option available to prevent the demise of the infected host. Today, medicinal therapy with antibiotics and other anti-infective agents is an effective solution for most infectious diseases. However, surgical intervention is still an important option for cases in which the pathogen is resistant to available treatments. Surgical interventions may be used to hasten the recovery process by providing access to an infected site by antimicrobial agents (drainage of an abscess), cleaning the site (debridement), or removing infected organs or tissue (*e.g.*, appendectomy). In some situations, surgery may be the only means of affecting a complete cure, as in the case of endocarditis resulting in an infected heart valve, in which the diseased valve must be replaced with a mechanical or biologic valve to restore normal function. In other situations, surgical containment of a rapidly progressing infectious process such as gas gangrene may be the only means of saving a person's life.

IN SUMMARY, the ultimate outcome of any interaction between microorganisms and the human host is decided by a complex and ever-changing set of variables that take into account the overall health and physiologic function of the host and the virulence and infectious dose of the microbe. In many instances, disease is an inevitable consequence, but with continuing advances in science and technology, the majority of

cases can now be eliminated or rapidly cured with appropriate therapy. It is the intent of those who study infectious diseases to understand thoroughly the pathogen, the disease course, the mechanisms of transmission, and the host response to infection. This knowledge will lead to development of improved diagnostic techniques, revolutionary approaches to anti-infective therapy, and eradication or control of microscopic agents that cause frightening devastation and loss of life throughout the world. ■

 # BIOTERRORISM AND EMERGING GLOBAL INFECTIOUS DISEASES

After completing this section of the chapter, you should be able to meet the following objectives:

- List the infectious agents considered to pose the highest level of bioterrorism threat.
- Describe the effect of international travel on the spread of infection.
- State an important concept in containment of infections due to bioterrorism and global travel.

Bioterrorism

In October of 2001, less than 1 month after the tragedy of September 11, the world became instantly acquainted with the term *bioterrorism*. By the end of November of that year, 22 cases of human anthrax (11 cutaneous and 11 inhalation) had been identified, resulting in five deaths, and all cases were associated with exposure to four intentionally contaminated envelopes delivered through the U.S. Postal Service. Although the possibility of such an attack had been discussed in a workshop hosted by the CDC 3 years earlier, the reality of the 2001 outbreak brought a new sense of awareness concerning the use of microorganisms as weapons.

Anthrax is an ancient disease caused by the cutaneous inoculation, inhalation, or ingestion of the spores of *Bacillus anthracis*, a gram-positive bacillus. Anthrax is more commonly known as a disease of herbivores that can be transmitted to humans through contact with infected secretions, soil, or animal products. It is a rare disease in the United States, and so the sudden increase in cases over a short time was a chilling indication that the spread of the organism had been intentional. Fortunately, the number of deaths was limited thanks to prompt recognition of cases by physicians and public health personnel and rapid institution of antimicrobial prophylaxis to exposed individuals.

To prepare for the possibility of bioterrorist attacks, the CDC along with other federal, state, and local agencies has created the laboratory response network (LRN). The LRN is a four-tiered structure consisting of laboratories with ever-increasing expertise, responsibility, and biocontainment facilities that allow for the rapid and coordinated detection and identification of bioterrorism events under safe working conditions.

Potential agents of bioterrorism have been categorized into three levels (A, B, C) based on risk of use, transmissibility, invasiveness, and mortality rate. The agents placed in the highest bioterrorism threat level include *B. anthracis, Yersinia pestis* (the cause of bubonic plague), *Francisella tularensis* (the cause of tularemia), variola major virus (the cause of smallpox), and several hemorrhagic fever viruses (Ebola, Marburg, Lassa, and Junin). The toxin of the anaerobic gram-positive organism *Clostridium botulinum,* which causes the neuromuscular paralysis termed *botulism,* is also listed as a category A agent. Interestingly, purified *C. botulinum* toxins A and B are finding increasing use under the trade names Botox, Myobloc, and Neurobloc for various medicinal and cosmetic purposes. The category B agents include agents of food-borne and water-borne diseases (*Salmonella, Shigella, Vibrio cholerae, E. coli* O157:H7), agents of zoonotic infections (*Brucella* species, *C. burnetii, Burkholderia mallei*), viral encephalitides (Venezuelan, Western, and Eastern equine encephalitis viruses), as well as toxins from *S. aureus, Clostridium perfringens,* and *Ricinus communis* (the castor bean). Category C agents are defined as emerging pathogens and potential risks for the future, even though many of these organisms are causes of ancient diseases. Category C agents include *M. tuberculosis,* Nipah virus, hantavirus, tickborne and yellow fever viruses, and the only protozoan of the group, *Cryptosporidium parvum.* An excellent website available through the CDC is the "CDC Public Health Emergency Preparedness & Response Site," which provides detailed information on agents of bioterrorism, emergency contacts, and contingency plans in the event of an outbreak (www.bt.cdc.gov).

Global Infectious Diseases

Aided by a global market and the ease of international travel, the first years of the 21st century have witnessed the importation or emergence of a host of novel infectious diseases. During the late summer and early fall of 1999, West Nile virus (WNV an arthropod-borne flavivirus) was identified as the cause of an epidemic involving 56 patients in the New York City area. This outbreak, which led to seven deaths (primarily in the elderly), marked the first time that WNV had been recognized in the Western Hemisphere since its discovery in Uganda nearly 60 years earlier. Because WNV is a mosquito-borne disease and is transmitted to a number of susceptible avian (*e.g.,* blue jays, crows, and hawks) and equine hosts, the potential for rapid and sustained spread of the disease across the United States was appreciated early. By the fall of 2002, a national surveillance network had detected WNV activity in 2289 counties from 44 states, including Los Angeles County, and had identified more than 3000 human cases. The disease ranges in intensity from a nonspecific febrile illness to fulminant meningoencephalitis. In 2002 alone, 3389 cases of WNV-associated illness were identified in the United States with 201 deaths, making this the largest arboviral meningoencephalitis outbreak ever described in the Western Hemisphere. Efforts to prevent further spread of the disease are currently centered on surveillance of WNV-associated illness in birds, humans, and other mammals, as well as mosquito control.

In the winter of 2002, SARS emerged as a global threat. The first inkling of the impending threat was when the Chinese Ministry of Health reported 305 cases of a mysterious and virulent respiratory tract illness that had appeared in Guangdong province in southern China in a 4-month period of time. The spread of the disease to household contacts of sick individuals and medical personnel caring for patients with the disease identified it as highly transmissible. In a very short time, patients with compatible symptoms were recognized in Hong Kong and Vietnam. The World Health Organization (WHO) promptly issued a global alert and started international surveillance for patients with typical symptomatology who had a history of travel to the endemic region. As of June, 2003, more than 8000 cases of SARS from 29 countries and 809 deaths were reported to the WHO. In a remarkable feat of molecular technology, the etiology of SARS was quickly determined to be a novel coronavirus, possibly of mammalian or avian origin, and its entire genome was sequenced by the end of May 2003.

In May of 2003, a child was seen in central Wisconsin for fever, lymphadenopathy, and a papular rash. Electron microscopic examination of tissue from one of the patient's skin lesions revealed a virus that morphologically resembled poxvirus, obviously generating some concern because of the awareness of the potential for bioterrorism using smallpox virus. However, the same virus was identified from a lymph node biopsy of the patient's ill pet prairie dog. Additional testing of the patient and the prairie dog specimens indicated that the virus was a monkeypox virus, one of the orthopoxvirus family of viruses. By the beginning of June, 53 possible cases of monkeypox infection were being followed in Wisconsin, Illinois, and Indiana. Epidemiologic investigations conducted by state and federal health care agencies identified the potential source of the virus as nine different species of small mammals, including Gambian giant rats that had been imported from Ghana in April and were housed in common facilities with prairie dogs. A number of these animals were then shipped to a pet distributor in Illinois and subsequently sold to the public.

These three scenarios highlight the rapidity with which novel or exotic diseases can be introduced into nonindigenous regions of the world and to a susceptible population. Although great strides in molecular microbiology have allowed for the rapid identification of new or rare microorganisms, the potential devastation in terms of human life and economic loss is great, underscoring the need to maintain resources for public health surveillance and intervention. For more detail on these and other intriguing cases of infectious disease detective work, refer to these excellent websites: www.who.int/en/ and www.cdc.gov.

IN SUMMARY, the challenges associated with maintaining health throughout a global community are becoming increasingly apparent. Aided by a global market and the ease of international travel, the past decade has witnessed the importation and emergence of a host of novel infectious diseases. There is also the potential threat of the deliberate use of microorganisms as weapons of bioterrorism. ∎

Review Exercises

1. Newborn infants who have not yet developed an intestinal flora are routinely given an intramuscular injection of vitamin K to prevent bleeding due a deficiency in vitamin K–dependent coagulation factors.

   A. *Use the concept of mutualism to explain why this is done.*

2. Persons with human granulocytic ehrlichiosis may be co-infected with Lyme disease.

   A. *Explain.*

3. Persons with chronic lung disease are often taught to contact their health care provider when they notice a change in the color of their sputum (*i.e.*, from white or clear to yellow- or green-tinged) because it might be a sign of a bacterial infection.

   A. *Explain.*

4. Microorganisms are capable of causing infection only if they can grow at the temperature of the infected body site.

   A. *Using this concept, explain the different sites of fungal infections due to the dermatophyte fungal species that cause tinea pedis (athlete's foot), and* Candida albicans, *which causes infections of the mouth (thrush) and female genitalia (vulvovaginitis).*

5. The threat of global infections, such as severe acute respiratory syndrome (SARS), continues to grow.

   A. *What would you propose to be one of the most important functions of health care professionals in terms of controlling the spread of such infections?*

Bibliography

Buller R. S., Arens M., Hmiel S. P., et al. (1999). *Ehrlichia ewingii,* a newly recognized agent of human ehrlichiosis. *New England Journal of Medicine* 341, 148–155.

Bush K., Jacoby G. A., Medeiros A. A. (1995). A functional classification scheme for β-lactamases and its correlation with molecular structure. *Antimicrobial Agents and Chemotherapy* 39, 1211–1233.

Butler J. C., Peters C. J. (1994). Hantaviruses and hantavirus pulmonary syndrome. *Clinical Infectious Diseases* 19, 387–395.

Centers for Disease Control and Prevention. (1999). Outbreak of West Nile-like viral encephalitis—New York, 1999. *Morbidity and Mortality Weekly Report* 48, 845–849.

Centers for Disease Control and Prevention. (2002). Provisional surveillance summary of the West Nile virus epidemic—United States, January–November 2002. *Morbidity and Mortality Weekly Report* 51, 1129–1133.

Centers for Disease Control and Prevention. (2003). Update: Severe acute respiratory syndrome—worldwide and United States, 2003. *Morbidity and Mortality Weekly Report* 52, 664–665.

Centers for Disease Control and Prevention. (2003). Multistate outbreak of monkeypox—Illinois, Indiana, and Wisconsin, 2003. *Morbidity and Mortality Weekly Report* 52, 537–540.

Centers for Disease Control and Prevention. (2006). Ongoing multistate outbreak of *Escherichia coli* serotype O157:H7 infections associated with consumption of fresh spinach—United States, September 2006. *Morbidity and Mortality Weekly Report* 55(Dispatch), 1–2.

Drusano G. L. (2004). Antimicrobial pharmacodynamics: Critical interactions of "bug and drug." *Nature Reviews Microbiology* 2, 289–300.

Dumler J. S., Bakken J. S. (1995). Ehrlichial diseases in humans: Emerging tick-borne infections. *Clinical Infectious Diseases* 20, 1102–1110.

Dunne W. M., Jr. (2002). Bacterial adhesion: Seen any good biofilms lately? *Clinical Microbiology Review* 15, 155–166.

Hsueh P. R., Yang P. C. (2005). Severe acute respiratory syndrome epidemic in Taiwan, 2003. *Journal of Microbiology, Immunology and Infection* 38, 82–88.

Jernigan D. M., Raghunathan P. L., Bell B. P., et al. (2002). Investigation of bioterrorism-related anthrax, United States, 2001: Epidemiologic findings. *Emerging Infectious Diseases* 8, 1019–1028.

Lampiris H. W., Maddix D. S. (2004). Clinical use of antimicrobial agents. In Katzung B. G. (Ed.), *Basic and clinical pharmacology* (9th ed.). New York: McGraw-Hill.

Medical Letter. (2006). The human papillomavirus vaccine. *The Medical Letter* 1241, 65.

O'Brien K. K., Higdon M. L., Halverson J. J. (2003). Recognition and management of bioterrorism infections. *American Family Physician* 67, 1927–1934.

Peiris J. S. M., Lai S. T., Poon L. L. M., et al. (2003). Coronavirus as a possible cause of severe acute respiratory syndrome. *Lancet* 361, 1319–1325.

Prince A. S. (2002). Biofilms, antimicrobial resistance, and airway infection. *New England Journal of Medicine* 347, 1110–1111.

Roden R., Wu T. C. (2006). How will HPV vaccines affect cervical cancer? *National Review of Cancer* 6, 753–763.

Ruan Y. J., Wei C. L., Ling A. E., et al. (2003). Comparative full-length genome sequence analysis of 14 SARS coronavirus isolates and common mutations associated with putative origins of infection. *Lancet* 361, 1779–1785.

Ryan E. T., Wilson M. E., Kain K. C. (2002). Illness after international travel. *New England Journal of Medicine* 347, 505–516.

Stone J. H., Dierberg K., Aram G., et al. (2004). Human monocytic ehrlichiosis. *Journal of the American Medical Association* 292, 2263–2270.

Suebaum S., Michetti P. (2002). *Helicobacter pylori* infection. *New England Journal of Medicine* 347, 1175–1186.

Tang Y.-W., Persing D. H. (2003). Molecular detection and identification of microorganisms. In Murray P. R., Baron E. J., Pfaller M. A., et al. (Eds.), *Manual of clinical microbiology* (7th ed., pp. 215–244). Washington, DC: American Society for Microbiology.

Tyler K. L. (2000). Prions and prion diseases of the central nervous system (neurodegenerative diseases). In Mandell G. L., Bennett J. E., Dolin R. (Eds.), *Mandell, Douglas, and Bennett's principles and practice of infectious diseases* (5th ed., pp. 1971–1985). Philadelphia: Churchill Livingstone.

U.S. Food and Drug Administration. (2006). FDA licenses new vaccine for prevention of cervical cancer and other diseases in females caused by human papillomavirus. FDA News. [On-line.] Available: www.Fda.gov/bbs/topics/NEWS/2006/NEW01385.html. Accessed June 8, 2007.

Writing Committee of the World Health Organization (WHO) Consultation on Human Influenza A/H5. (2005). Avian influenza A (H5N1) infection in humans. *New England Journal of Medicine* 353, 1374–1385.

Visit thePoint **http://thePoint.lww.com for animations, journal articles, and more!**

Innate and Adaptive Immunity

Chapter 17

CYNTHIA SOMMER

> The immune system has evolved in multicellular organisms to defend against bacteria, viruses, and other foreign substances. Through recognition of molecular patterns, the immune system can distinguish itself from foreign substances and can discriminate potentially harmful from nonharmful agents. It also defends against abnormal cells and molecules that periodically develop. Although the immune response normally is protective, it also can produce undesirable effects such as when the response is excessive, as in allergies, or when it recognizes self-tissue as foreign, as in autoimmune disease.

   This chapter is divided into three parts: (1) immunity and the immune system, (2) innate immunity, and (3) adaptive immunity. The key cells, molecules, recognition systems, and effector responses integral to immunity are discussed.

IMMUNITY AND THE IMMUNE SYSTEM

After completing this section of the chapter, you should be able to meet the following objectives:

- Discuss the function of the immune system.
- Contrast and compare the general properties of innate and adaptive immunity.
- Describe the cells of the immune system.
- Characterize the chemical mediators that orchestrate the immune response.

The term *immunity* has come to mean the protection from disease and, more specifically, infectious disease. The collective, coordinated response of the cells and molecules of the immune system is called the *immune response*. Although the relationship between microbes and infectious diseases dates far back in history, it has only been within the last 50 to 60 years that an understanding of the cellular and biochemical mechanisms involved in the immune response has begun to emerge. Advances in cell culture techniques, immunochemistry, recombinant deoxyribonucleic acid (DNA) technology, and the creation of genetically altered animals, such as "transgenic" and "knockout" mice, have transformed immunology from a largely descriptive science to one of immune phenomena that can be explained in structural and biochemical terms.

Innate and Adaptive Immunity

There are two host defenses that cooperate to protect the body—the early, rapid responses of innate immunity and the very effective, but later responses of adaptive immunity (Table 17-1). As the first line of defense, *innate immunity* (also called *natural* or *native immunity*) consists of the physical, chemical, molecular, and cellular defenses that are in place before infection and can function immediately as an effective barrier to microbes. *Adaptive* (also called *specific* or *acquired*) *immunity* is the second major immune defense, responding less rapidly than innate immunity but more effectively. Adaptive immunity uses focused recognition of each unique type of foreign agent followed in days by an amplified and effective response.

The major components of innate immunity are the skin and mucous membranes; phagocytic cells (mainly neutrophils and macrophages); specialized lymphocytes called *natural killer (NK) cells;* and several plasma proteins, including the proteins of the complement system. The innate immune system is able to distinguish self from nonself and is able to recognize and react against classes of microbial agents. The response of the innate immune system is rapid, usually within minutes to hours, and prevents the establishment of infection and deeper tissue penetration of microorganisms. The effector responses used by the innate immune system to eliminate the microbes are very similar for different classes of microorganisms. Although most innate responses are very effective in controlling and destroying the invader, pathogenic microbes have evolved several approaches to evade innate defenses. The microorganisms not controlled by innate immunity are usually controlled by the more specific approaches of adaptive immunity.

The adaptive immune system consists of lymphocytes and their products, including antibodies. Whereas the cells of the innate immune system recognize structures shared by classes of microorganisms, the cells of the adaptive immune system (*i.e.,* lymphocytes) are capable of recognizing a vast array of substances produced by microorganisms as well as noninfectious substances and developing a specific immune response that differs with each substance. Substances that elicit adaptive immune responses are called *antigens.* A memory of the substance is also developed so that a repeat exposure to the same microbe or agent produces a quicker and more vigorous response. The practical aspect of immunization is based on this ability to generate an adaptive memory response. There are two types of adaptive immune responses: humoral and cell-mediated immunity. *Humoral immunity,* generated by *B lymphocytes,* is mediated by molecules called *antibodies* and is the principal defense against extracellular microbes and toxins. *Cell-mediated immunity,* or *cellular immunity,* is mediated by specific *T lymphocytes* (T-helper and T-cytotoxic lymphocytes) and defends against intracellular microbes such as viruses.

Recent studies have shown that essential, cooperative interactions exist between innate and adaptive immunity. Innate immunity communicates to lymphocytes involved in adaptive immunity the characteristics of the pathogen and information about its intracellular or extracellular location. The innate immune response also stimulates and influences the nature of adaptive immune responses. At the effector stage of immunity, the adaptive immune response amplifies and increases its efficiency by recruitment and activation of additional phagocytes and molecules of the innate immune system. Both innate and adaptive immunity destroy the invading agent by using the effector responses of phagocytosis and the complement system. Thus, immunity is truly an interactive, cooperative effort.

Cells of the Immune System

The cells of the immune system consist of phagocytic leukocytes, lymphocytes, and antigen-presenting cells. The key cells of innate immunity include phagocytic leukocytes (neutrophils and macrophages) and NK cells. Adaptive immune responses depend on lymphocytes, which provide lifelong immunity after exposure to disease-producing microbes or environmental agents. Dendritic cells and macrophages function as antigen-presenting cells for adaptive immunity. The general properties of these cells are presented in this section, whereas their specific functions in relation to innate or adaptive immunity are discussed in those sections of the chapter.

TABLE 17-1 Features of Innate and Adaptive Immunity

FEATURE	INNATE	ADAPTIVE
Time of response	Rapid (minutes/hours)	Slower (days/weeks)
Diversity	Limited to classes or groups of microbes	Very large; specific for each unique antigen
Microbe recognition	General patterns on microbes; nonspecific	Specific to microbes and antigens
Nonself recognition	Yes	Yes
Response to repeated infection	Similar with each exposure	Immunologic memory; more rapid and efficient with subsequent exposure
Defense	Barriers (skin, mucous membranes), phagocytes, inflammation, fever	Cell killing; tagging of antigen by antibody for removal
Cells	Phagocytes (macrophages, neutrophils), natural killer cells, dendritic cells	T and B lymphocytes
Molecules	Cytokines, complement proteins, acute-phase proteins, soluble mediators	Antibodies, cytokines

Phagocytic Leukocytes

Leukocytes are subclassified into two general groups based on the presence or absence of specific staining granules in their cytoplasm. Cells containing granules are classified as granulocytes (neutrophils, eosinophils, and basophils) and cells that lack granules are classified as agranulocytes (lymphocytes, monocytes, and macrophages). Neutrophils, which are named for their neutral-staining granules, are the early responding cells of innate immunity. Macrophages are part of the monocytic phagocyte system. During an inflammation response, the monocyte leaves the blood vessel, transforms into a tissue macrophage, and phagocytizes bacteria, damaged cells, and tissue debris (discussed in Chapter 18). Both neutrophils and macrophages are equipped with recognition receptors, phagocytic potential, antimicrobial molecules, and metabolic systems for producing toxic oxygen and nitrogen intermediates for killing infectious agents.

In addition to phagocytosis, macrophages function early in the immune response to amplify the inflammatory response and initiate adaptive immunity. Macrophages direct these processes through the secretion of cell communication molecules that initiate and coordinate the inflammatory response or activate lymphocytes. Macrophages also function at the end of an immune response as effector cells in both humoral and cell-mediated immune responses. Macrophages can remove antigen–antibody aggregates or, under the influence of T cells, they can destroy virus-infected cells or tumor cells.

Lymphocytes

There are three distinct subtypes of lymphocytes: B lymphocytes, T lymphocytes, and NK cells. These subtypes are different in their functions and protein products but are morphologically similar.

T and B Lymphocytes. T and B lymphocytes represent 25% to 35% of blood leukocytes. They are the only cells in the body capable of specifically recognizing different antigenic determinants of microbial agents and other pathogens and therefore are responsible for two defining characteristics of adaptive immunity, specificity and memory.

Like other blood cells, T and B lymphocytes are generated from hematopoietic stem cells in the bone marrow. Undifferentiated immature lymphocytes congregate in the central lymphoid tissues, where they develop into distinct types of mature lymphocytes. One class of lymphocyte, the *B lymphocytes* (B cells), is essential for humoral immunity. The other class of lymphocyte, the *T lymphocytes,* is responsible for cell-mediated immunity, as well as aiding in antibody production. The various types of lymphocytes are distinguished by their function and response to antigen, cell membrane molecules and receptors, types of secreted proteins, and tissue location.

Lymphocyte Markers and the CD Nomenclature System. From the time that functionally distinct types of lymphocytes were first recognized, immunologists have worked to develop methods for distinguishing them. The development of laboratory reagents such as monoclonal antibodies allowed the recognition of distinct classes of lymphocytes based on their unique pattern of cell surface proteins. These identified proteins were then correlated with cell functions. The standard nomenclature for these proteins is the "CD" (clusters of differentiation) numeric designation (CD1, CD2), which is used to delineate surface proteins that define a particular cell type or stage of cell differentiation and are recognized by a cluster or group of antibodies. Although this nomenclature was originally developed for lymphocytes, it is now common practice to refer to homologous markers on cells other than lymphocytes by the same CD designation.

The classification of lymphocytes and other immune cells by CD antigen expression is now widely used in clinical medicine and experimental immunology. For example, the declining number of blood CD4+ T cells is often used to follow the disease progression and response to treatment of persons with human immunodeficiency virus (HIV) infection. Further investigation of the CD molecules has shown that they are not merely phenotypic markers of cell type but are themselves involved in a variety of lymphocyte functions, including promotion of cell-to-cell adhesion and transduction of signals that lead to lymphocyte activation.

Natural Killer Cells. Natural killer cells comprise approximately 10% to 15% of peripheral blood lymphocytes and do not bear T-cell receptors or cell surface immunoglobulins. Morphologically, they are somewhat larger than the smaller T and B lymphocytes and contain abundant cytoplasmic granules. NK cells are part of the innate immune system, and may be the first line of defense against viral infections. They also have the ability to recognize and kill tumor cells, abnormal body cells, and cells infected with *intracellular pathogens,* such as viruses and intracellular bacteria. Two cell surface molecules, CD16 and CD56, are widely used to identify NK cells. CD16 serves as a receptor for the immunoglobulin (Ig) G molecule, which provides NK cells with the ability to lyse IgG-coated target cells.

Dendritic Cells

Dendritic cells are specialized, bone marrow–derived leukocytes found in lymphoid tissue that are important intermediaries between the innate and adaptive immune systems. Most dendritic cells are found as immature cells under epithelial tissue and in most organs, where they are poised to capture foreign agents and transport them to peripheral lymphoid organs. Once activated, they undergo a complex maturation process as they migrate to the first regional lymph node. These cells function as key antigen-presenting cells that are needed to initiate adaptive immunity, by processing and presenting molecules of the foreign antigen to the lymphocytes. Thus, the dendritic cell functions as an important intermediary between innate and adaptive immunity. Dendritic cells, like macrophages, also release several communication molecules that direct the nature of adaptive immune responses.

Understanding • Innate and Adaptive Immunity

The body's defense against microbes is mediated by two types of immunity: (1) innate immunity and (2) adaptive immunity. Both types of immunity are members of an integrated system in which numerous cells and molecules function cooperatively to protect the body against foreign invaders. The innate immune system stimulates adaptive immunity and influences the nature of the adaptive immune responses to make them more effective. Although they use different mechanisms of pathogen recognition, both types of immunity use many of the same effector mechanisms, including destruction of the pathogen by phagocytosis and the complement system.

❶ Innate Immunity

Innate immunity (also called *natural immunity*) consists of the cellular and biochemical defenses that are in place before an encounter with an infectious agent and provide rapid protection against infection. The major effector components of innate immunity include epithelial cells, which block the entry of infectious agents and secrete antimicrobial enzymes, proteins, and peptides; phagocytic neutrophils and macrophages, which engulf and digest microbes; natural killer (NK) cells, which kill intracellular microbes and foreign agents; and the complement system, which amplifies the inflammatory response and uses the membrane attack response to lyse microbes. The cells of the innate immune system also produce chemical messengers that stimulate and influence the adaptive immune response.

The innate immune system uses pattern recognition receptors that recognize microbial structures (*e.g.,* sugars, lipid molecules, proteins) that are shared by microbes and are often necessary for their survival, but are not present on human cells. Thus, the innate immune system is able to distinguish between self and nonself, but is unable to distinguish between agents.

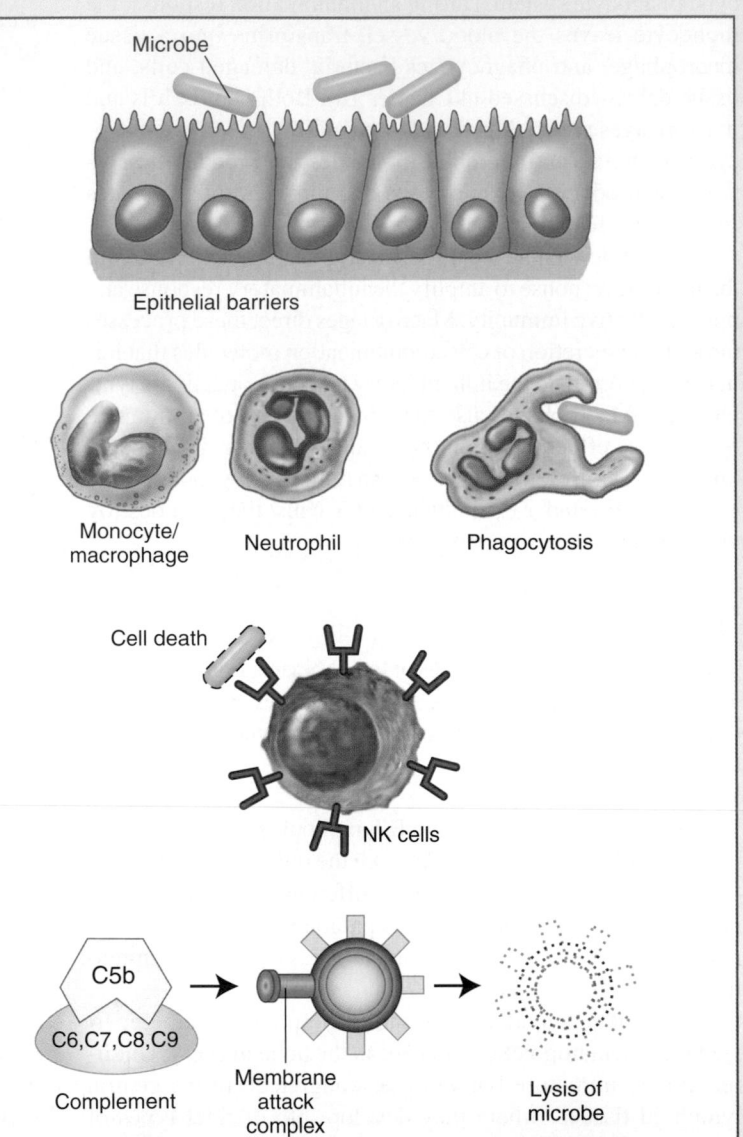

Microbe

Epithelial barriers

Monocyte/macrophage   Neutrophil   Phagocytosis

Cell death

NK cells

C5b

C6,C7,C8,C9

Complement   Membrane attack complex   Lysis of microbe

❷ Adaptive Immunity

Adaptive immunity (also called *acquired immunity*) refers to immunity that is acquired through previous exposure to infectious and other foreign agents. A defining characteristic of adaptive immunity is the ability not only to distinguish self from nonself, but to recognize and destroy specific foreign agents based on their distinct antigenic properties. The components of the adaptive immune system are the T and B lymphocytes and their products. There are two types of adaptive immune responses, humoral and cell-mediated immunity, that function to eliminate different types of microbes.

Humoral immunity is mediated by the B lymphocytes (B cells) and is the principal defense against extracellular microbes and their toxins. The B cells differentiate into antibody-secreting plasma cells. The circulating antibodies then interact with and destroy the microbes that are present in the blood or mucosal surfaces.

Cell-mediated, or cellular, immunity is mediated by the cytotoxic T lymphocytes (T cells) and functions in the elimination of intracellular pathogens (*e.g.,* viruses). T cells develop receptors that recognize the viral peptides displayed on the surface of infected cells and then signal destruction of the infected cells.

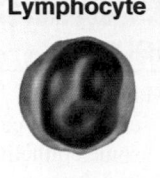

Lymphocyte

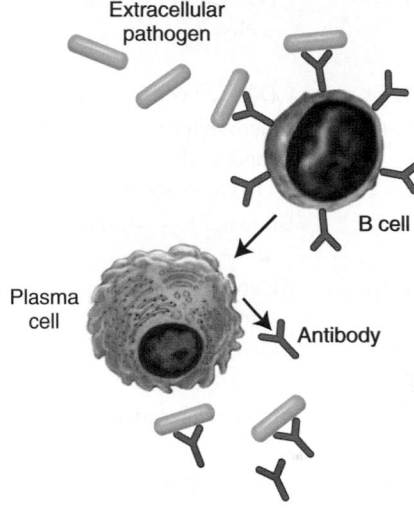

Humoral immunity (B lymphocytes)

Extracellular pathogen / B cell / Plasma cell / Antibody

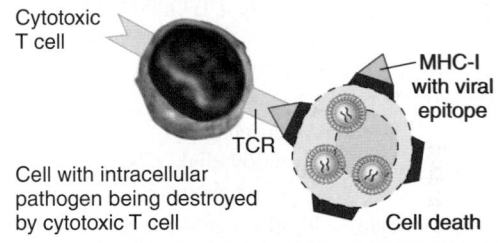

Cell-mediated immunity (T lymphocytes)

Cytotoxic T cell / MHC-I with viral epitope / TCR / Cell with intracellular pathogen being destroyed by cytotoxic T cell / Cell death

Cytokines That Mediate and Regulate Immunity

Although cells of both the innate and adaptive immune systems communicate critical information by cell-to-cell contact, many interactions and effector responses depend on the secretion of short-acting soluble molecules called *cytokines*. Chemokines are a family of cytokines that direct leukocyte movement and migration, and colony-stimulating factors are cytokines that promote the proliferation and differentiation of bone marrow progenitor cells. The sources and properties of the main cytokines that participate in innate and adaptive immunity are summarized in Table 17-2.

General Properties of Cytokines

Cytokines are low–molecular-weight regulatory proteins that are produced by cells of the innate and adaptive immune systems

and that mediate many of the actions of these cells. Cytokines were originally named for the general cell type that produced them (*e.g.,* monokines for those produced by monocytes and lymphokines for those produced by lymphocytes). With the development of advanced technology, however, it became clear that the same protein can be produced by monocytes, lymphocytes, and a variety of tissue cells, including endothelial cells. Therefore, the generic term *cytokine* has become the preferred name for this class of mediators. Cytokines are also named for the biologic property that was first ascribed to them. For example *interleukins* (ILs) are synthesized by leukocytes and act on other leukocytes, and *interferons* (IFNs) interfere with virus multiplication.

Although cytokines have many diverse actions, all share several important properties. All cytokines are secreted in a brief, self-limited manner. They are not usually stored as preformed molecules and their synthesis is limited to new gene transcription resulting from cellular activation. The actions of cytokines

TABLE 17-2 Cytokines of Innate and Adaptive Immunity

CYTOKINES	SOURCE	BIOLOGIC ACTIVITY
Interleukin-1 (IL-1)	Macrophages, endothelial cells, some epithelial cells	Wide variety of biologic effects; activates endothelium in inflammation; induces fever and acute-phase response; stimulates neutrophil production
Interleukin-2 (IL-2)	CD4$^+$, CD8$^+$ T cells	Growth factor for activated T cells; induces synthesis of other cytokines; activates cytotoxic T lymphocytes and NK cells
Interleukin-3 (IL-3)	CD4$^+$ T cells	Growth factor for progenitor hematopoietic cells
Interleukin-4 (IL-4)	CD4$^+$ T$_H$2 cells, mast cells	Promotes growth and survival of T, B, and mast cells; causes T$_H$2 cell differentiation; activates B cells and eosinophils and induces IgE-type responses
Interleukin-5 (IL-5)	CD4$^+$ T$_H$2 cells,	Induces eosinophil growth and development
Interleukin-6 (IL-6)	Macrophages, endothelial cells, T lymphocytes	Stimulates the liver to produce mediators of acute-phase inflammatory response; also induces proliferation of antibody-producing cells by the adaptive immune system
Interleukin-7 (IL-7)	Bone marrow stromal cells	Primary function in adaptive immunity; stimulates pre-B cells and thymocyte development and proliferation
Interleukin-8 (IL-8)	Macrophages, endothelial cells	Primary function in adaptive immunity; chemoattracts neutrophils and T lymphocytes; regulates lymphocyte homing and neutrophil infiltration
Interleukin-10 (IL-10)	Macrophages, some T-helper cells	Inhibitor of activated macrophages and dendritic cells; decreases inflammation by inhibiting T$_H$1 cells and release of IL-12 from macrophages
Interleukin-12 (IL-12)	Macrophages, dendritic cells	Enhances NK cell cytotoxicity in innate immunity; induces T$_H$1 cell differentiation in adaptive immunity
Type I interferons (IFN-α, IFN-β)	Macrophages, fibroblasts	Inhibit viral replication, activate NK cells, and increase expression of MHC-I molecules on virus-infected cells
Interferon-γ (IFN-γ)	NK cells, CD4$^+$ and CD8$^+$ T lymphocytes	Activates macrophages in both innate immune responses and adaptive cell-mediated immune responses; increases expression of MHC-I and -II and antigen processing and presentation
Tumor necrosis factor-α (TNF-α)	Macrophages, T cells	Induces inflammation, fever, and acute-phase response; activates neutrophils and endothelial cells; kills cells through apoptosis
Chemokines	Macrophages, endothelial cells, T lymphocytes	Large family of structurally similar cytokines that stimulate leukocyte movement and regulate the migration of leukocytes from the blood to the tissues
Granulocyte-monocyte CSF (GM-CSF)	T cells, macrophages, endothelial cells, fibroblasts	Promotes neutrophil, eosinophil, and monocyte maturation and growth; activates mature granulocytes
Granulocyte CSF (G-CSF)	Macrophages, fibroblasts, endothelial cells	Promotes growth and maturation of neutrophils consumed in inflammatory reactions
Monocyte CSF (M-CSF)	Macrophages, activated T cells, endothelial cells	Promotes growth and maturation of mononuclear phagocytes

CSF, colony-stimulating factor; NK, natural killer; T$_H$1, T-helper type 1; T$_H$2, T-helper type 2; MHC, major histocompatibility complex.

are often pleiotropic and redundant. Pleiotropism refers to the ability of a cytokine to act on different cell types. For example IL-2, initially discovered as a T-cell growth factor, is also known to affect the growth of B cells and NK cells. Interferon-γ is the key macrophage-activating cytokine that functions in both innate and adaptive immune responses. Although pleiotropism allows cytokines to mediate diverse effects, it greatly limits their use for therapeutic purposes because of numerous unwanted side effects. Redundancy refers to the ability of different cytokines to stimulate the same or overlapping biologic functions. Because of this redundancy, antagonists against a single cytokine may not

have functional consequences because other cytokines may compensate.

Not only are the actions of cytokines pleiotropic and redundant, but cytokines are produced by several different cell types. For example, IL-1 can be produced by virtually all leukocytes, endothelial cells, and fibroblasts. Cytokines often influence the synthesis and actions of other cytokines. The ability of one cytokine to stimulate the production of others often leads to cascades in which the second and third cytokines may mediate the biologic effects of the first. Cytokines may also serve as antagonists to inhibit the action of another cytokine or, in some cases, they may produce additive or greater-than-anticipated effects.

Cytokine actions may be local or systemic. Most cytokines act close to where they are produced, acting on the same cell that secreted the cytokine (autocrine mechanism), or they may influence the activity of nearby cells in a paracrine fashion. When produced in large amounts, cytokines may enter the bloodstream and exert their action on distant cells in an endocrine manner, the best examples being IL-1 and tumor necrosis factor-α (TNF-α), which produce the systemic acute-phase response during inflammation.

Cytokines generate their responses by binding to specific receptors on their target cells. Many cytokine receptors share a common structural shape and a cytoplasmic tail that interacts with a family of signaling proteins (Janus kinases [JAKs]). These signaling molecules then interact with cytoplasmic intermediary molecules (signal transducers and activators of transcription [STATs]) that are responsible for the induction of the genes for cell responses.

Chemokines

Chemokines are cytokines that stimulate the migration and activation of immune and inflammatory cells. Chemokines are synthesized as secretory proteins consisting of approximately 70 to 130 amino acids, with 4 conserved cysteine amino acids linked with disulfide bonds. Two major subclasses, termed *CC chemokines* or *CXC chemokines,* are distinguished by the position of the first two cysteines being located adjacent to each other (CC) or separated by an amino acid (CXC). The largest family, the CC chemokines attract mononuclear leukocytes to sites of chronic inflammation. The CXC chemokines attract neutrophils to sites of acute inflammation.

Chemokines are named according to structure, followed by "L" and the number of their gene (*e.g.,* CCL1, CXCL1). Likewise, chemokine receptors are named according to the structure, followed by an "R" and a number (*e.g.,* CCR1, CXCR1). Six receptors for CXC (CXCRs) and 10 for CC (CCRs) chemokines have been characterized in terms of their structure and function. Most receptors recognize more than one chemokine, and most chemokines recognize more than one receptor. Binding of a chemokine to a receptor can result in agonist or antagonist activity, with the same chemokine acting as an agonist at one type of receptor and as an antagonist at another.

Chemokines are implicated in a number of acute and chronic diseases, including atherosclerosis, rheumatoid arthritis, inflammatory bowel disease (Crohn disease, ulcerative colitis), allergic asthma and chronic bronchitis, multiple sclerosis, systemic lupus erythematosus, and HIV infection. To enter target cells, HIV type 1 requires two distinct elements: the CD4 recognition molecule of the helper T cell and either the CXCR4 or CCR5 chemokine. The targeting of T cells and monocytes allows HIV-1 access to sanctuary sites throughout the body and also cripples the CD4+ T-helper cells that orchestrate antiviral immunity (discussed in Chapter 20). Genetic evidence of the central role of CCR5 in the pathogenesis of HIV-1 came from the identification of multiply exposed noninfected persons, who proved to be homozygous for a nonfunctional variant of CCR5.

Drugs that target these chemokine receptors for HIV are currently in advanced clinical trials.

Colony-Stimulating Factors

Colony-stimulating factors (CSFs) are cytokines that stimulate bone marrow pluripotent stem and progenitor or precursor cells to produce large numbers of platelets, erythrocytes, lymphocytes, neutrophils, monocytes, eosinophils, basophils, and dendritic cells. The CSFs were named according to the type of target cell on which they act (see Table 17-2). GM-CSF acts on the granulocyte–monocyte progenitor cells to produce monocytes, neutrophils, and dendritic cells; G-CSF specifically induces neutrophil proliferation; and M-CSF directs the mononuclear phagocyte progenitor. Other cytokines, including IL-3, IL-7, and IL-11, also influence hematopoiesis (see Chapter 12). Recombinant CSF molecules are being used to increase the success rates of bone marrow transplantations. The availability of recombinant CSFs and cytokines offers the possibility of several clinical therapies where stimulation or inhibition of the immune response or cell production is desirable.

IN SUMMARY, immunity is the resistance to a disease that is provided by the immune system. Immune mechanisms can be divided into two types: innate and adaptive immunity. Innate immunity is the first line of defense against microbial agents. It can distinguish between self and nonself through recognition of conserved broad patterns on microbes. Adaptive immunity involves humoral and cellular mechanisms that respond to a unique antigen, can amplify and sustain its responses, distinguish self from nonself, and remember the antigen to quickly produce a heightened response on subsequent encounters with the same agent. There is a dynamic interplay between innate and adaptive immunity both in the early initiation stages and the final response to the foreign invader.

The cellular components of the innate and adaptive immunity include the T and B lymphocytes, NK cells, dendritic cells, and phagocytic leukocytes (neutrophils and macrophages). The phagocytic leukocytes, NK cells, and dendritic cells participate in innate immunity. The T and B lymphocytes are the only cells in the body capable of specifically recognizing different antigenic determinants of microbial agents and other pathogens and therefore are responsible for two defining characteristics of adaptive immunity, specificity and memory.

Although cells of both the innate and adaptive immune systems communicate critical information about the invading microbe or pathogen by cell-to-cell contact, many interactions and effector responses depend on the secretion of chemical mediators (cytokines, chemokines, and colony-stimulating factors). Cytokines are soluble proteins secreted by cells of both the innate and adaptive immune systems that mediate many of the functions of these cells. Chemokines are cytokines that stimulate the migration and activation of immune and inflammatory cells. Colony-stimulating factors stimulate the growth and differentiation of bone marrow progenitors of immune cells. ∎

CONCEPTS in action **ANIMATION**

INNATE IMMUNITY

The innate immune system consists of the epithelial barriers, phagocytic cells (mainly neutrophils and macrophages), NK cells, and several plasma proteins, including those of the complement system. These mechanisms are present in the body before an encounter with an infectious agent and are rapidly activated by microbes before the development of adaptive immunity. The innate immune system also interacts with and directs adaptive immune responses.

INNATE IMMUNITY

- Innate immunity consists of physical, chemical, cellular, and molecular defenses that are ready for activation and mediate rapid, initial protection against infection.

- Skin and mucous membranes are highly effective physical barriers against microorganisms. Antimicrobial molecules can effectively kill a wide variety of microbes.

- The cells of innate immunity express pattern recognition receptors (PRRs) that bind with broad patterns shared by groups of microbes but not present on mammalian cells. Toll-like receptors, a major type of PRR, are expressed on phagocytes and are potent activators of innate immune system cells and molecules.

- The effector responses of innate immunity involve the inflammatory response, the complement system, natural killer cells, and phagocytosis by neutrophils and monocyte/macrophages.

- Cytokines released from activated leukocytes regulate the activity of other cells, amplify inflammation, stimulate the production of acute-phase proteins, and aid in the initiation of an adaptive immune response.

With the ever-expanding wealth of information on immune system function, it is becoming clear that the innate immune system not only protects against microbial agents, but may play a role in the pathogenesis of disease. Among the functions of the innate immune system is induction of a complex cascade of events known as the *inflammatory response* (discussed in Chapter 18). Recent evidence suggests that inflammation plays a key role in the pathogenesis of a number of disorders such as atherosclerosis and coronary artery disease, bronchial asthma, type 2 diabetes mellitus, rheumatoid arthritis, multiple sclerosis, and systemic lupus erythematosus.

Epithelial Barriers

Physical and chemical barriers against infection are found in all common portals of entry of microbes, namely, the skin and respiratory, gastrointestinal, and urogenital tracts. The intact skin is a formidable physical barrier because of its closely packed cells, multiple layering, continuous shedding of cells, and presence of the protective protein keratin. In addition to its barrier function, the skin has simple chemicals that create a nonspecific, salty, acidic environment and antibacterial proteins, such as the enzyme lysozyme, that inhibit the colonization of microorganisms and aid in their destruction.

The mucous membrane linings of the gastrointestinal, respiratory, and urogenital tracts are protected by sheets of tightly packed epithelial cells that block the entry of microbes and destroy them by secreting antimicrobial enzymes, proteins, and peptides. Specialized cells in these linings secrete a viscous material called *mucus.* Mucus traps and washes away potential invaders, especially with the help of additional secretions such as saliva and excess mucus. Also in the lower respiratory tract, hairlike structures called *cilia* protrude through the epithelial cells. The synchronous action of the cilia moves many microbes trapped in the mucus toward the throat. The physiologic responses of coughing and sneezing further aid in their removal from the body.

Once microbes are trapped, various chemical defenses come into play. These include lysozyme, a hydrolytic enzyme capable of cleaving the walls of bacterial cells; complement, which binds and aggregates bacteria to increase their susceptibility to phagocytosis or disrupt their lipid membrane; and members of the *collectin* family of surfactant proteins (*e.g.,* surfactants [SP]-A and SP-D) in the respiratory tract (see Chapter 27). Both SP-A and SP-D bind a variety of pathogens and are important defense molecules in the lung. The best-defined function of the collectins is their ability to opsonize pathogens, including bacteria and viruses, and to facilitate phagocytosis by innate immune cells such as macrophages. SP-A and SP-D also regulate production of inflammatory mediators. In the stomach and intestines, death of microbes results from the action of digestive enzymes, acidic conditions, and secretions of *defensins,* small cationic peptides that kill within minutes both gram-positive and -negative microorganisms by disrupting the microbial membrane.

Some pathogens can penetrate the anatomic layers of the host and cause physiologic changes that result in infectious disease. The subsequent innate immune response to the penetration of these invaders is initiated by various leukocytes through their recognition of common molecular motifs on microbes.

Cells of Innate Immunity

Several types of innate immune cells with receptors for recognition of general groups of microbes can provide an array of responses to the invader. The key cells of innate immunity include neutrophils, macrophages, dendritic cells, NK cells, and intraepithelial lymphocytes.

Neutrophils and Macrophages

Several phagocytic cells recruited during an inflammatory response are innate immune cells that recognize and kill infectious invaders. The early-responding innate immune cell is the neutrophil, followed shortly by the more efficient, multifunctional macrophage. Phagocytes are activated to engulf and digest microbes that attach to their cell membrane. The initial attachment of the microbe to the phagocyte can be aided by pathogen-associated molecular pattern receptors (*i.e.,* Toll-like receptors), receptors for opsonins (*e.g.,* complement or antibodies), and receptors for lectins. Once the cell is activated and the microbe is ingested, the cell generates digestive enzymes and toxic oxygen and nitrogen intermediates (*i.e.,* hydrogen peroxide or nitric oxide) through metabolic pathways. The phagocytic killing of microorganisms helps to contain infectious agents until adaptive immunity can be marshaled.

Natural Killer Cells and Intraepithelial Lymphocytes

Other cells involved in innate immunity include NK cells and intraepithelial lymphocytes (IELs). Neither IELs nor NK cells express the specific, highly diverse receptors or antibodies associated with adaptive immunity. Like other cells in the innate immune system, they can recognize only broad patterns associated with classes of microbes.

NK cells control their responses by using both activating and inhibitory receptors (Fig. 17-1). Their activating receptors (*i.e.,* killer cell receptors) recognize altered host molecules expressed on stressed tissue cells that may be infected with intracellular microbes. The inhibitory receptors on NK cells recognize molecules (major histocompatibility complex [MHC]-I, lectins) on normal host cells and function to stop the killing response of NK cells. This control ensures that normal body cells are not inappropriately destroyed. In contrast to the cytotoxic T lymphocyte, which needs to undergo amplification and maturation to become cytotoxic, the NK cell is programmed directly to kill foreign cells. Depending on the type or combination of NK cell receptors that are activated, the effect is cell death or no response. If an abnormal cell is correctly recognized, the NK cells will cause the death of the altered target cell by producing pore-forming proteins (*i.e.,* NK perforins), enzymes, and toxic cytokines.

The IELs, which express a receptor similar in general structure to the T-cell receptor, often recognize microbial lipids and other structures that are shared by microbes of the same type. Although they appear to function as early sentinels against infec-

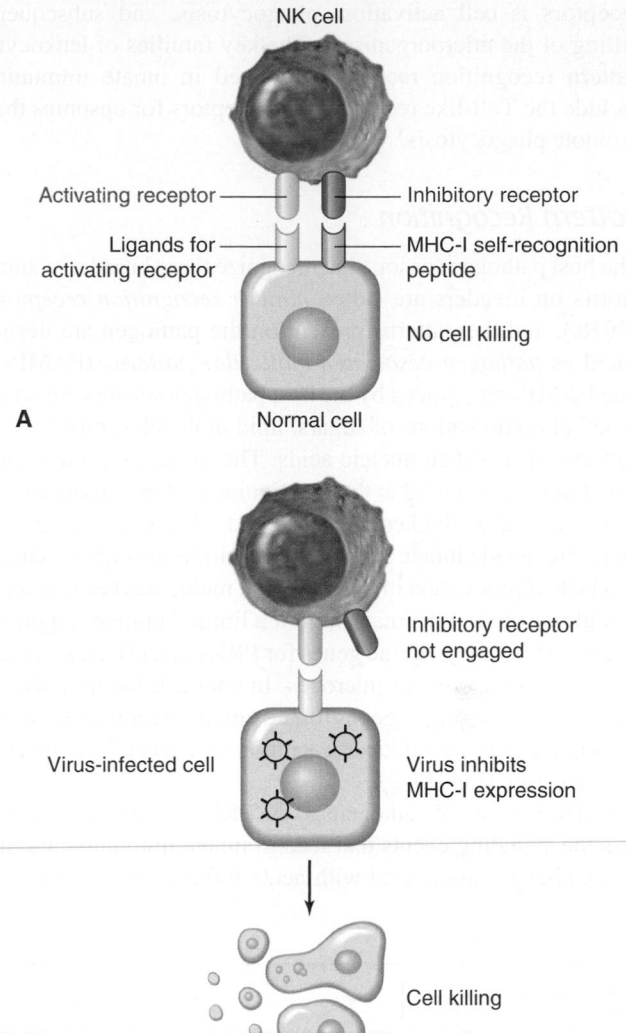

FIGURE 17-1 • Natural killer (NK) cell receptors. **(A)** NK cells express activating receptors that respond to ligands from virus-infected or injured cells, and inhibiting receptors that bind to the class I major histocompatibility complex (MHC-I) self-recognition molecules expressed by normal cells. Normal cells are not killed because inhibitory signals from normal MHC-I molecules override activating signals. **(B)** In virus-infected or tumor cells, increased expression of ligands for activating receptors and reduced expression or alteration of MHC molecules interrupts the inhibitory signals, allowing activation of NK cells and lysis of target cells.

tious microbes at the epithelial layers, our knowledge of how they function is limited.

Pathogen Recognition

The ability of any of the leukocytes to participate in innate immunity depends on first recognizing the invader. The leukocyte receptors that bind these microbial molecules may be membrane-associated receptors or soluble pattern recognition molecules that first tag the microbes and subsequently bind to their complementary membrane receptors on the phagocytes. The impact of microbial binding to the leukocyte membrane receptors is cell activation, phagocytosis, and subsequent killing of the microorganisms. The key families of leukocyte pattern recognition receptors involved in innate immunity include the Toll-like receptors and receptors for opsonins that promote phagocytosis.

Pattern Recognition

The host pathogen sensors that recognize these broad structural motifs on invaders are called *pattern recognition receptors* (PRRs), and the patterns present on the pathogen are designated as *pathogen-associated molecular patterns* (PAMPs). The PAMPs recognized by the host pathogen sensors are composed of combinations of sugars, lipid molecules, proteins, or patterns of modified nucleic acids. The recognized microbial structures are essential to the functioning and infectivity of the pathogen and are defined as "conserved." The microbe cannot, therefore, evade innate immune recognition through mutation or a lack of production of the microbial molecules because they would not survive. Humans inherit a limited number (approximately 1000) of germline genes for PRRs that effectively recognize major groups of microbes. In contrast, the millions of somatically rearranged genes for the unique receptors involved in adaptive immunity allow recognition of fine details of molecular structure (Fig. 17-2).

The binding of pathogens to the PRRs on leukocytes initiates the signaling events that lead to innate immunity and the tissue changes associated with acute inflammation. After the inflammatory changes in the blood vessels near the site of infection, white blood cells, neutrophils, and monocytes are directed in their migration from the blood to the tissues, along with body fluids. The blood monocytes mature into macrophages as they traverse the tissues. Resident tissue macrophages and immature dendritic cells add to the responding cellular recruits. Triggering of PRRs on these new recruits amplifies the initial inflammatory response by inducing antimicrobial genes and secreting inflammatory cytokines. These cytokines amplify the production of soluble mediators of inflammation, including soluble PRRs and complement. The soluble pathogen sensors also tag pathogens to allow for activation of the complement system. In addition to these inflammatory and killing responses, activation of PRRs on macrophages and dendritic cells can lead to their maturation, secretion of cytokines, and expression of costimulatory molecules needed for activation of adaptive immunity.

Toll-like Receptors

The main pathogen sensors important in innate immunity include the family of PRRs called *Toll-like receptors* (TLRs). Interestingly, the first protein to be identified in this family was the *Drosophila* Toll protein, which was found on the fruit fly *Drosophila,* where it functions in embryonic development as well as in protecting the fly from lethal fungal infections. The importance of this innate immune pathway is evident because it was maintained through evolution and expanded in its antimicrobial potential between the fly and humans. Eleven differ-

Characteristics	Innate immunity	Adaptive immunity
Recognition	Molecular patterns common to microbes 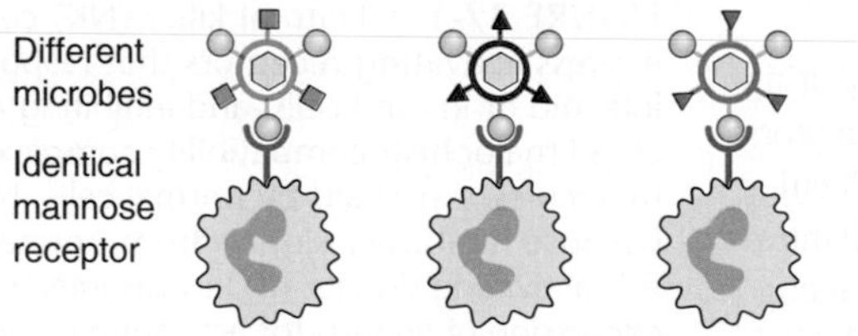 Different microbes Identical mannose receptor	Specific microbial molecules 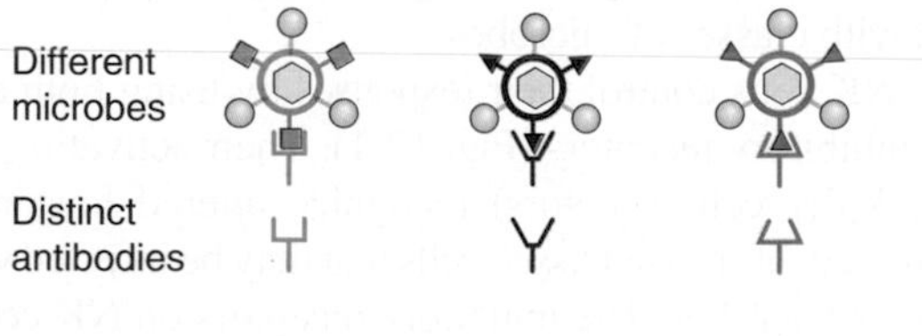 Different microbes Distinct antibodies
Receptors	Limited diversity expressed by germline genes 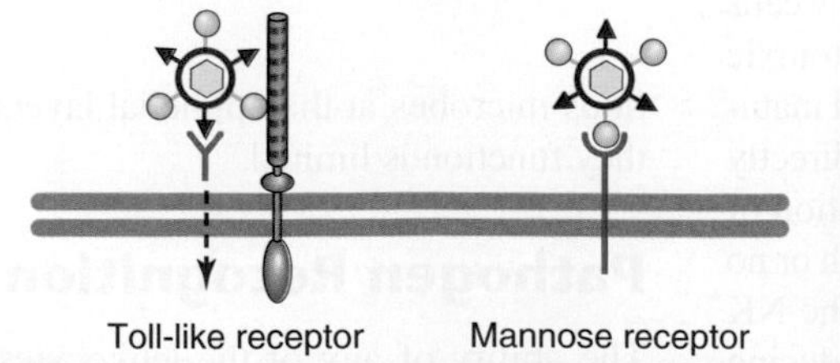 Toll-like receptor Mannose receptor	Great diversity expressed through recombination of somatic genes 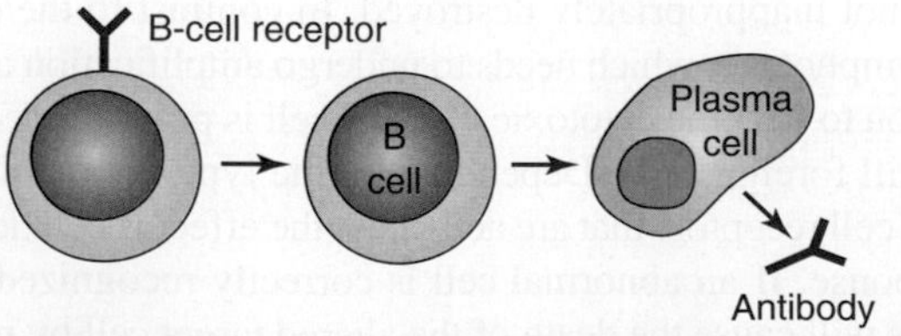 B-cell receptor B cell → Plasma cell Antibody
Cellular expression	Effector cell types express identical receptors (*e.g.,* neutrophils express Toll-like receptors).	Each clone of lymphocytes expresses unique receptors.
Self–nonself discrimination	Yes, by recognizing molecules unique to pathogen, NK cells recognize MHC-I self-recognizing molecules.	Yes, lymphocytes use MHC-I and -II and foreign peptides (*e.g.,* microbial peptides in recognition).

FIGURE 17-2 • Recognition systems of innate and adaptive immunity.

ent mammalian TLRs, TLR1 through TLR11, have so far been identified based on sequence homology to *Drosophila* Toll (Fig. 17-3A). All of these receptors are membrane-spanning proteins that contain an external horseshoe-shaped PAMP binding structure and an internal signaling domain essential for activating the leukocyte (see Fig. 17-3B). The TLRs are expressed on many different cell types that participate in innate immunity, including endothelial cells, neutrophils, macrophages, dendritic cells, and NK cells.

Human TLRs are involved in responses to widely divergent types of molecules that are commonly expressed by microbial but not mammalian cell types. For example, TLR4 is essential for phagocytic recognition and response to lipopolysaccharides (LPS or endotoxin) present in gram-negative bacteria; TLR2 binds to peptidoglycan, an essential component of the cell wall of gram-positive bacteria; and TLR5 can recognize the protein flagellin found in flagellated bacteria. Although most TLRs that recognize extracellular ligands on microbes are found on the surface of the leukocytes, a few are located on the membranes of intracellular compartments of the leukocyte, where they recognize viruses and intracellular pathogens such as *Mycobacterium*. Single-stranded ribonucleic acid (RNA), expressed during intracellular virus infections, is recognized by TLR7 and TLR8.

Ligand binding to the TLR at the cell surface leads to recruitment of cytoplasmic signaling molecules and eventual activation of transcription factors, notably nuclear factor κβ (NF-κβ). NF-κβ regulates the production of a number of proteins that are important components of innate immunity. These include inflammatory cytokines, endothelial adhesion molecules, and proteins involved in the antimicrobial activities of phagocytic leukocytes. Some TLRs function individually, whereas some dimerize to themselves (*e.g.*, TLR4–TLR4) or pair with other TLRs (*e.g.*, TLR2–TLR6) to expand their recognition of PAMPs. Recent research suggests that most TLRs need a coreceptor (*e.g.*, CD14 for TLR4) to serve as an accessory molecule, and some may recognize endogenous host molecules (*e.g.*, heat-shock proteins) for tissue regeneration and repair. Alterations in the structure of TLRs or mutations in the signaling system associated with TLRs have been suggested to play a pathologic role in disorders such as atherosclerosis, allergies, and certain autoimmune diseases.

Soluble Mediators of Innate Immunity

Although cells of the innate immune system can communicate critical information about the invader and self–nonself recognition through cell-to-cell contact, soluble mediators are essential for many other aspects of the innate immune response. Development of innate immunity and regulation of the behavior of effector cells all depend on the secretion of soluble molecules such as opsonins, cytokines, and acute-phase proteins.

Opsonins

Various soluble molecules can tag microorganisms for more efficient recognition by phagocytes. The coating of particles, such as microbes, is called *opsonization*, and the coating materials are called *opsonins*. The opsonin bound to the microbe

TRLs	Ligands	Type of microorganisms
TRL1	Lipopeptides	Mycobacteria
TRL2	Peptidoglycan Lipoprotein Zymosan	Gram-positive bacteria Mycobacteria Yeast and other fungi
TRL3	Double-stranded RNA	Viruses
TRL4	Lipopolysaccharide	Gram-negative bacteria
TRL5	Flagellin	Flagellated bacteria
TRL6	Lipopolypeptide Zymosan	Mycobacteria Yeast and fungi
TRL7	Single-stranded RNA (ssRNA)	Viruses
TRL8	Single-stranded RNA (ssRNA)	Viruses
TRL9	CpG unmethylated dinucleotides	Bacterial DNA
TRLs10,11	Unknown	

A

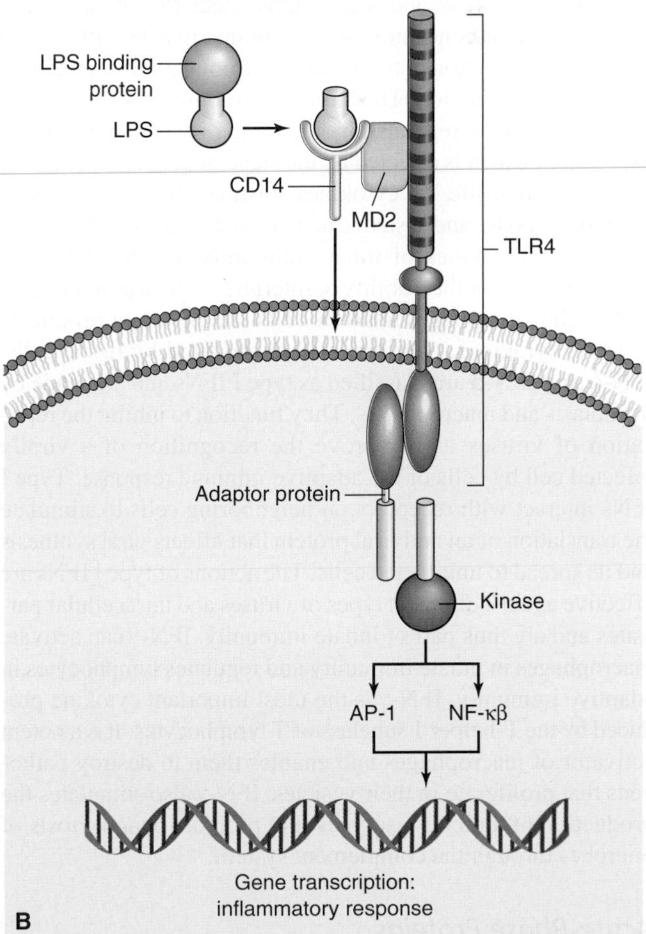

B

FIGURE 17-3 • **(A)** Different Toll-like receptors (TLRs) are involved in responses to different organisms. **(B)** Signaling by a prototypic TLR, TLR4, in response to bacterial lipopolysaccharide (LPS). An adaptor protein links the TLR to a kinase, which activates transcription factors such as NF-κβ. (Modified from Kumar V., Abbas A. K., Fausto N. [2005]. *Robbins and Cotran pathologic basis of disease* [7th ed., p. 195]. Philadelphia: Elsevier Saunders.)

then activates the phagocyte after attachment to a complementary receptor on the phagocyte. Opsonins important in innate immunity and acute inflammation include acute-phase proteins, lectins, and complement. With the activation of adaptive humoral immunity, IgG and IgM antibodies can coat microbes and act as an opsonin by binding to Fc receptors on neutrophils and macrophages. The adaptive immune response can thus enhance the phagocytic function of innate cells.

Inflammatory Cytokines

The cytokines involved in innate immunity include TNF-α, the interleukins IL-1, IL-6, and IL-12, interferons (IFN-γ, IFN-α, IFN-β), and chemokines (see Table 17-2). These cytokines serve various functions. They influence the events of inflammation and innate immunity by producing chemotaxis of leukocytes, stimulating acute-phase protein production, inhibiting virus replication, and affecting the development of cells of the innate and adaptive immune systems. A leukocyte exposed to an external stimulus (*i.e.,* bacteria) can be activated through appropriately triggered receptors (*e.g.,* TLRs) and respond by secreting small amounts of cytokines and other soluble mediators. If many cells are activated, the concentration of cytokines may be sufficient to influence the function of tissues distant from the site of infection, a true endocrine action. The biologic responses associated with cytokines are also regulated by the timing of cytokine receptor expression, which is affected by the stage of activation of a cell. The short half-life of cytokines ensures that an excessive immune response and systemic activation does not usually occur.

Other cytokines of innate immunity are the IFNs, so-named because of their ability to interfere with virus infections. Although macrophages and NK cells are the major producers of these cytokines, they can also be secreted by tissue cells. IFN-α and IFN-β are classified as type I IFNs and are made by fibroblasts and macrophages. They function to inhibit the replication of viruses and improve the recognition of a virally infected cell by cells of the adaptive immune response. Type I IFNs interact with receptors on neighboring cells to stimulate the translation of an antiviral protein that affects viral synthesis and its spread to uninfected cells. The actions of type I IFNs are effective against different types of viruses and intracellular parasites and are thus part of innate immunity. IFN-γ can activate macrophages in innate immunity and regulates lymphocytes in adaptive immunity. IFN-γ is the most important cytokine produced by the T-helper 1 subclass of T lymphocytes. It is a potent activator of macrophages and enables them to destroy pathogens that proliferate in their vesicles. IFN-γ also stimulates the production of antibody isotypes that promote phagocytosis of microbes through the complement system.

Acute-Phase Proteins

Two acute-phase proteins that are involved in the defense against infections are the mannose-binding ligand (MBL) and C-reactive protein (CRP). MBL and CRP are produced in the liver after cytokine activation and function as opsonins as well as activators of the alternative complement pathway. The binding of MBL to mannose residues and CRP to phospholipids and sugars on microbes and their subsequent binding to their complementary receptors on leukocytes leads to phagocytosis and immune cell activation.

The Complement System

The complement system is an important effector of both innate and humoral immunity that enables the body to localize and destroy infective agents. The complement system, like the blood coagulation system, consists of a group of proteins that are present in the circulation as functionally inactive precursors. These proteins, mainly proteolytic enzymes, make up 10% to 15% of the plasma proteins. For a complement reaction to occur, the complement components must be activated in the proper sequence. Uncontrolled activation of the complement system is prevented by inhibitor proteins and the instability of the activated complement proteins at each step of the process.

There are three parallel but independent pathways for recognizing microorganisms that result in activation of the complement system: the classical, the lectin, and the alternative pathways. The reactions of the complement systems can be divided into three phases: (1) initiation or activation, (2) amplification of inflammation, and (3) membrane attack response. The pathways differ slightly in the proteins used in the early stage of activation, but all converge in the process by acting on the key complement protein C3, essential for the amplification stage. Activated C3 then affects all subsequent complement molecules (C5 through C9). Inactive circulating complement proteins can be activated by microbial surface polysaccharides, MBL, and other soluble mediators in the lectin or alternative complement pathways that are integral to innate immunity, or by complement-fixing antibodies (IgG, IgM) of adaptive immunity that bind to microbial surfaces or other substances in the classical complement pathway. All activating pathways generate a series of enzymatic reactions that proteolytically cleave successive complement proteins in the pathway. New complement fragments (*e.g.,* C3a, C3b) are regularly generated in this manner.

During the activation process, the enzymatic cleavage of C3 produces C3b, a key opsonin that coats microbes and allows them to be phagocytized after binding to the type 1 complement receptor on leukocytes. The small C3 complement fragment (C3a) can trigger an influx of neutrophils to enhance the inflammatory response. Production of C3a and C5a also leads to activation of basophils and mast cells and release of inflammatory mediators that produce smooth muscle contraction, increased vascular permeability, and changes in endothelial cells to enhance migration of phagocytes. The late phase of the complement cascade triggers the assembly of a membrane attack complex (MAC; C5 to C9) that leads to the lytic destruction of many kinds of cells, including bacteria and altered blood cells. The multiple functions of the complement system, including enhanced inflammatory responses, increased phagocytosis, and destruction and clearance of the pathogen from the body, make it an integral component of innate immunity and inflammation. Clinical changes associated with inherited deficiencies of complement range from increased susceptibility to infection to inflammatory tissue damage caused by complement-activated immune complexes not properly cleared by macrophages.

IN SUMMARY, the innate immune system consists of the epithelial cells of the skin and mucous membranes, phagocytic cells (neutrophils and macrophages), NK cells, and several plasma proteins, including those of the complement system. These defenses are in place before an encounter with a microbial agent and are rapidly activated by microbes before the development of adaptive immunity. The epithelial cells of the skin and mucous membranes, which are the first line of defense, block the entry of infectious agents and secrete antimicrobial enzymes, proteins, and peptides.

The cells of the innate immunity include the phagocytic leukocytes (neutrophils and macrophages), which engulf and digest infectious agents, and NK cells, which kill microbes and foreign agents. These cells express pattern recognition receptors (PRRs) on their membranes that bind broad patterns of molecules shared by microbes and that are essential for their survival. Toll-like receptors (TLRs), a major group of PRRs, are expressed on many cell types (neutrophils, macrophages, NK cells) and are potent activators of innate immune cells and molecules. TLRs are involved in responses to widely divergent types of molecules that are commonly expressed by microbial but not mammalian cell types.

Development of innate immunity and regulation of the behavior of effector cells all depend on the secretion of soluble molecules, such as opsonins, cytokines, acute-phase proteins, and complement. Opsonins bind to and tag microorganisms for more efficient recognition by phagocytes. Activated leukocytes release cytokines that regulate innate immunity and inflammation by directing the migration of leukocytes, stimulating production of acute-phase proteins, and enhancing phagocytosis.

The complement system is a primary effector system for both the innate and adaptive immune systems and consists of a group of proteins that are activated by microbes and promote inflammation and destruction of the microbes. Recognition of microbes by complement occurs in three ways: by the classical pathway, which recognizes antibody bound to the surface of a microbe or other structure; by the alternative pathway, which recognizes certain microbial molecules; and by the lectin pathway, which uses a plasma protein called the *mannose-binding protein* to bind mannose residues on microbial glycoproteins or glycolipids. ■

ADAPTIVE IMMUNITY

After completing this section of the chapter, you should be able to meet the following objectives:

- State the properties associated with adaptive immunity.
- Define and describe the characteristics of an antigen.

- Characterize the significance and function of major histocompatibility complex molecules.
- Describe the antigen-presenting functions of macrophages and dendritic cells.
- Contrast and compare the development and function of the T and B lymphocytes.
- State the function of the five classes of immunoglobulins.
- Differentiate between the central and peripheral lymphoid structures.
- Describe the function of cytokines involved in the adaptive immune response.
- Compare passive and active immunity.

The adaptive immune system is able to recognize and react to a large number of microbes and nonmicrobial substances. Integral to the system is the ability to distinguish among different, even closely related, microbes and molecules and to "remember" the pathogen by quickly producing a heightened immune response on subsequent encounters with the same agent. The components of the adaptive immune system are lymphocytes and their products. Foreign substances that elicit specific responses are called *antigens*. There are two types of adaptive immune responses: humoral and cell-mediated immunity. *Humoral immunity* is mediated by secreted molecules and is the principal defense against extracellular microbes and toxins. *Cell-mediated immunity*, or *cellular immunity*, is mediated by specific T lymphocytes and defends against intracellular microbes such as viruses. By convention, the terms *immune response* and *immune system* usually refer to adaptive immunity.

ADAPTIVE IMMUNITY

- The adaptive immune response involves a complex series of interactions between components of the immune system and the antigens of a foreign pathogen. It is able to distinguish between self and nonself, recognize and specifically react to large numbers of different microbes and pathogens, and remember the specific agents.

- Humoral immunity consists of protection provided by the B lymphocyte–derived plasma cells, which produce antibodies that travel in the blood and interact with circulating and cell surface antigens.

- Cell-mediated immunity consists of protection provided by cytotoxic T lymphocytes, which protect against virus-infected or cancer cells.

- Passive immunity represents a temporary type of immunity that is transferred from another source (e.g., in utero transfer of antibodies from mother to infant), and active immunity is the response by the person's immune system that is acquired through immunization or actually having a disease.

Understanding • The Complement System

The complement system provides one of the major effector mechanisms of both humoral and innate immunity. The system consists of a group of proteins (complement proteins C1 through C9) that are normally present in the plasma in an inactive form. Activation of the complement system is a highly regulated process, involving the sequential breakdown of the complement proteins to generate a cascade of cleavage products capable of proteolytic enzyme activity. This allows for tremendous amplification because each enzyme molecule activated by one step can generate multiple activated enzyme molecules at the next step. Complement activation is inhibited by proteins that are present on normal host cells; thus, its actions are limited to microbes and other antigens that lack these inhibitory proteins.

The reactions of the complement system can be divided into three phases: (1) the initial activation phase, (2) the early-step inflammatory responses, and (3) the late-step membrane attack responses.

❶ Initial Activation Phase

There are three pathways for recognizing microbes and activating the complement system: (1) the alternative pathway, which is activated on microbial cell surfaces in the absence of antibody and is a component of innate immunity; (2) the classical pathway, which is activated by certain types of antibodies bound to antigen and is part of humoral immunity; and (3) the lectin pathway, which is activated by a plasma lectin that binds to mannose on microbes and activates the classical system pathway in the absence of antibody.

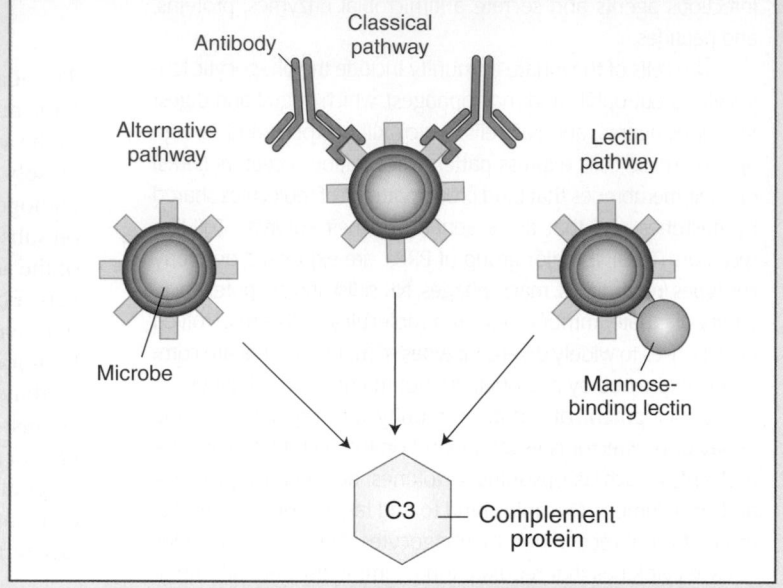

❷ Early-Step Inflammatory Responses

The central component of complement for all three pathways is the activation of the complement protein C3 and its enzymatic cleavage into a larger C3b fragment and a smaller C3a fragment. The smaller 3a fragment stimulates inflammation by acting as a chemoattractant for neutrophils. The larger 3b fragment becomes attached to the microbe and acts as an opsonin for phagocytosis. It also acts as an enzyme to cleave C5 into two components: a C5a fragment, which produces vasodilation and increases vascular permeability; and a C5b fragment, which leads to the late-step membrane attack responses.

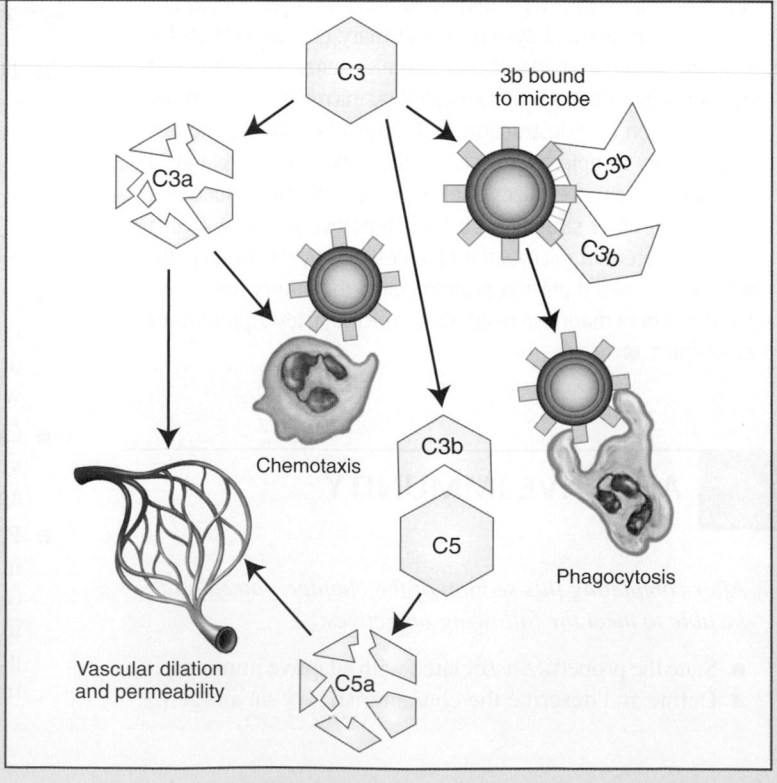

❸ Late-Step Membrane Attack

In the late-step responses, C3b binds to other complement proteins to form an enzyme that cleaves C5, generating C5a and C5b fragments. C5a stimulates the influx of neutrophils and the vascular phase of acute inflammation. The C5b fragment, which remains attached to the microbe, initiates the formation of a complex of complement proteins C6, C7, C8, and C9 into a membrane attack complex protein, or pore, that allows fluids and ions to enter and cause cell lysis.

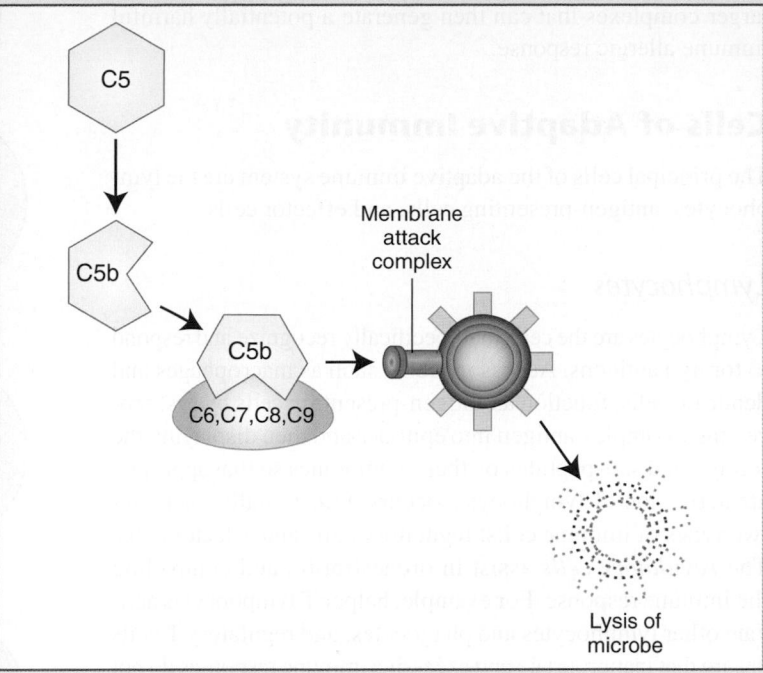

Antigens

Before discussing the cells and responses inherent to adaptive immunity, it is important to understand the substances that elicit a response from the host. *Antigens,* or *immunogens,* are substances foreign to the host that can stimulate an immune response. These foreign molecules are recognized by receptors on immune cells and by secreted proteins, called *antibodies* or *immunoglobulins,* made in response to the antigen. Antigens include bacteria, fungi, viruses, protozoa, and parasites. Nonmicrobial agents such as plant pollens, poison ivy resin, insect venom, and transplanted organs can also act as antigens. Most antigens are macromolecules, such as proteins and polysaccharides, although lipids and nucleic acids occasionally can serve as antigens.

Antigens, which in general are large and chemically complex, are biologically degraded into smaller chemical units or peptides. These discrete, immunologically active sites on antigens are called *antigenic determinants,* or *epitopes.* It is the unique molecular shape of an epitope that is recognized by a specific immunoglobulin receptor found on the surface of the lymphocyte or by an antigen-binding site of a secreted antibody (Fig. 17-4). A single antigen may contain multiple antigenic determinants, each stimulating a distinct clone of T and B lymphocytes. For example, different proteins that comprise the influenza virus may function as unique antigens (A, B, C, H, and N antigens), each of which contains several antigenic determinants. Hundreds of antigenic determinants are found on structures such as the bacterial cell wall.

Smaller substances (molecular masses <10,000 daltons) usually are unable to stimulate an adequate immune response by themselves. When these low–molecular-weight compounds,

known as *haptens,* combine with larger protein molecules, they function as antigens. The proteins act as carrier molecules for the haptens to form antigenic hapten–carrier complexes. An allergic response to the antibiotic penicillin is an example of a medically important reaction due to hapten–carrier complexes. Penicillin (molecular mass of approximately 350 daltons) is normally a nonantigenic molecule. However, in some individuals, it can chemically combine with body proteins to form

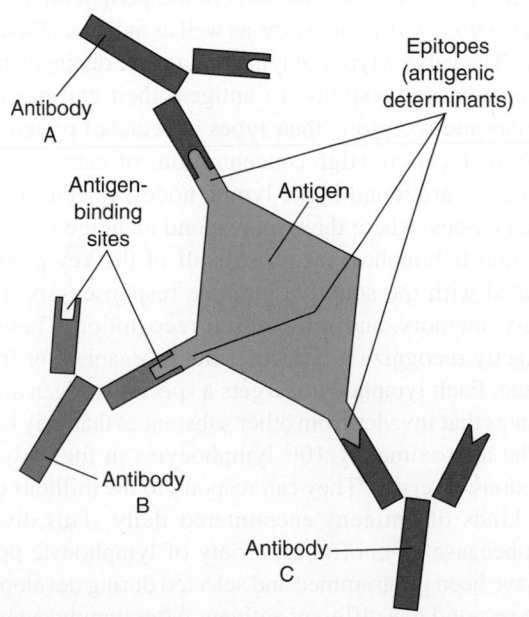

FIGURE 17-4 • Multiple epitopes on a complex antigen being recognized by their respective (A, B, C) antibodies.

larger complexes that can then generate a potentially harmful immune allergic response.

Cells of Adaptive Immunity

The principal cells of the adaptive immune system are the lymphocytes, antigen-presenting cells, and effector cells.

Lymphocytes

Lymphocytes are the cells that specifically recognize and respond to foreign antigens. Accessory cells, such as macrophages and dendritic cells, function as antigen-presenting cells by first processing a complex antigen into epitopes and then displaying the foreign and self-peptides on their membranes so that appropriate activation of lymphocytes occurs. Functionally, there are two types of immune cells: regulatory cells and effector cells. The *regulatory cells* assist in orchestrating and controlling the immune response. For example, helper T lymphocytes activate other lymphocytes and phagocytes, and regulatory T cells ensure that inappropriate and excessive immune responses do not occur. The final stages of the immune response are accomplished with the elimination of the antigen by *effector cells.* Cytotoxic T lymphocytes, macrophages, and other leukocytes function as effector cells in different immune responses.

Like other blood cells, T and B lymphocytes are generated from stem cells in the bone marrow. Undifferentiated, immature lymphocytes congregate in the central lymphoid tissues, where they develop into distinct types of mature lymphocytes (Fig. 17-5). One class of lymphocyte, the *B lymphocytes* (B cells), matures in the bone marrow and is essential for *humoral,* or *antibody-mediated, immunity.* The other class of lymphocyte, the *T lymphocytes* (T cells), completes its maturation in the thymus and functions in the peripheral tissues to produce *cell-mediated immunity,* as well as aiding antibody production. The various types of lymphocytes are distinguished by their function and response to antigen, their cell membrane molecules and receptors, their types of secreted proteins, and their tissue location. High concentrations of mature T and B lymphocytes are found in the lymph nodes, spleen, skin, and mucosal tissues, where they can respond to antigen.

T and B lymphocytes possess all of the key properties associated with the adaptive immune response—specificity, diversity, memory, and self–nonself recognition. These cells can exactly recognize a particular microorganism or foreign molecule. Each lymphocyte targets a specific antigen and differentiates that invader from other substances that may be similar. The approximately 10^{12} lymphocytes in the body have tremendous diversity. They can respond to the millions of different kinds of antigens encountered daily. This diversity occurs because an enormous variety of lymphocyte populations have been programmed and selected during development, each to respond to a different antigen. After lymphocytes have been stimulated by their antigen, they can acquire a memory response. The memory T and B lymphocytes that are generated

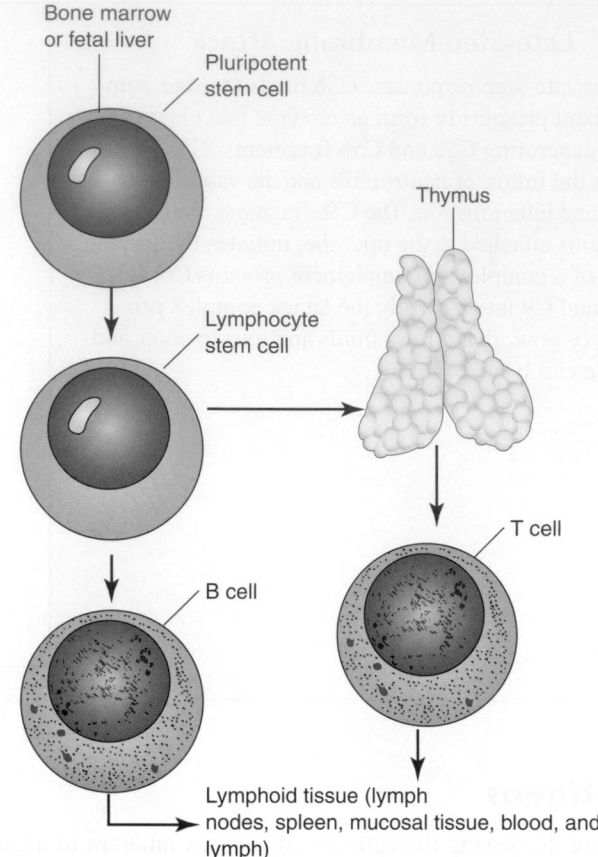

FIGURE 17-5 • Pathway for T- and B-cell differentiation.

remain in the body for a longer time and can respond more rapidly on repeat exposure than naive cells. Because of this heightened state of immune reactivity, the immune system usually can respond to commonly encountered microorganisms so efficiently that we are unaware of the response.

The key trigger for the activation of B and T cells is the recognition of the antigen by unique surface receptors. The B-cell antigen receptor consists of membrane-bound immunoglobulin molecules that can bind a specific epitope. The T-cell receptor recognizes a processed antigen peptide in association with a self-recognition protein, called a *major histocompatibility complex* (MHC) molecule (to be discussed). The appropriate recognition of MHC and self-peptides or MHC associated with foreign peptides is essential for lymphocytes to differentiate "self" from "foreign."

Activation of the lymphocytes depends on appropriate processing and presentation of antigen to T lymphocytes by antigen-presenting cells such as macrophages (Fig. 17-6). On recognition of antigen and after additional stimulation by cytokines, the B and T lymphocytes divide several times to form populations or clones of cells that continue to differentiate into several types of effector and memory cells. In an immune response, the effector cells destroy the antigens and the memory cells retain the potential needed for future encounters with the antigen.

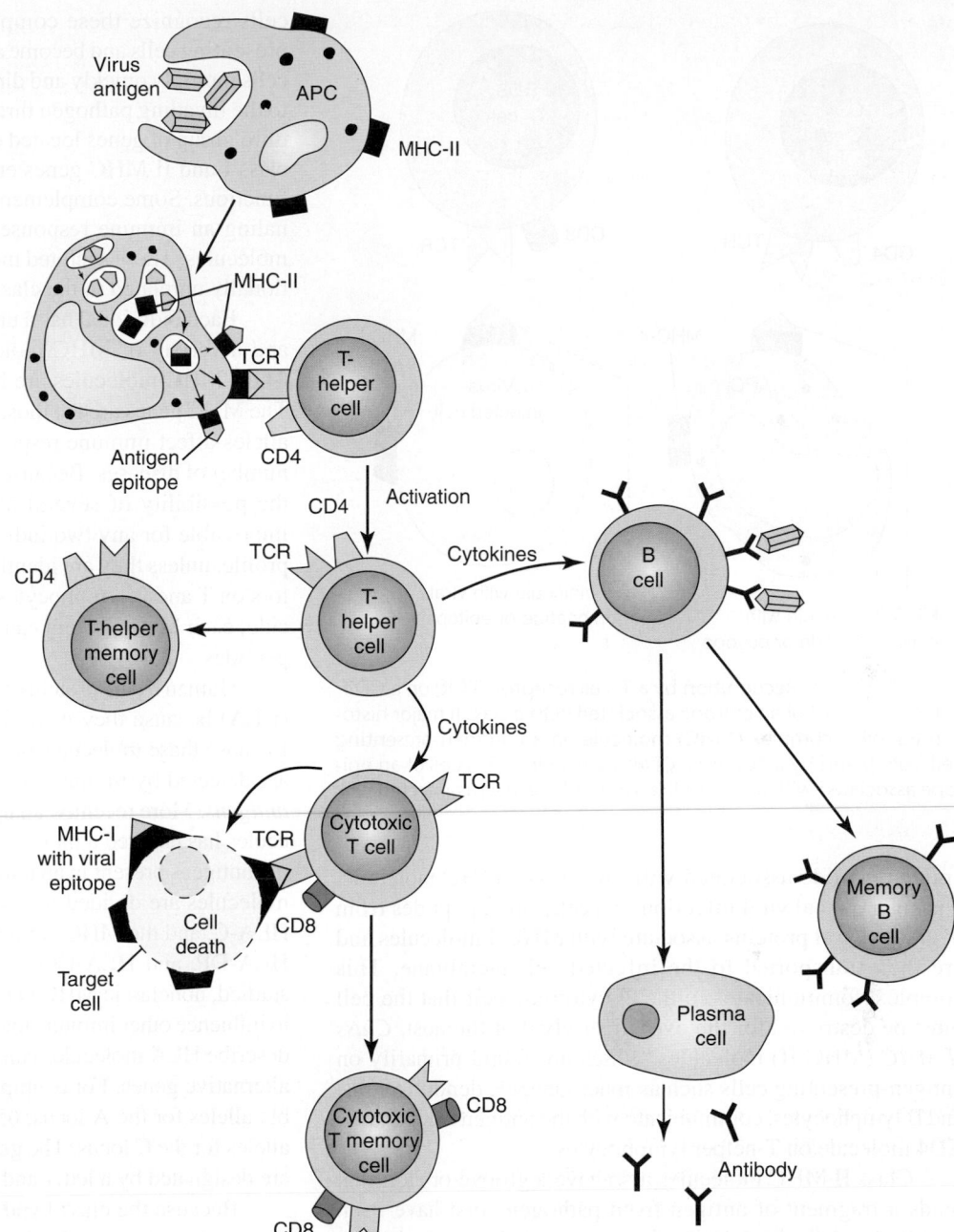

FIGURE 17-6 • Pathway for immune cell participation in an immune response. APC, antigen-presenting cell; MHC, major histocompatibility complex; TCR, T-cell receptor.

Major Histocompatibility Complex Molecules

An essential feature of adaptive or specific immunity is the ability to discriminate between the body's own molecules and foreign antigens. Key recognition molecules essential for distinguishing self from nonself are the cell surface MHC molecules. These proteins, which in humans are coded by closely linked genes on chromosome 6, were first identified because of their role in organ and tissue transplantation. When cells are transplanted between individuals who are not identical for their MHC molecules, the immune system produces a vigorous response leading to rejection of the transferred cells or organs. MHC molecules did not evolve to reject transplanted tissues, a situation not encountered in nature. Rather, these molecules are essential for correct cell-to-cell interactions among immune and body cells.

The MHC molecules involved in self-recognition and cell-to-cell communication fall into two classes, class I and class II (Fig. 17-7). *Class I MHC* (MHC-I) molecules are cell surface glycoproteins that interact with the antigen receptor–foreign peptide complex and the CD8 molecule on T-cytotoxic lymphocytes. MHC-I molecules are found on nearly all nucleated cells in the body and hence are capable of alerting the immune system to any cellular changes due to viruses, intracellular bacteria, or cancer.

The MHC-I molecule contains a groove that accommodates a peptide fragment of antigen. T-cytotoxic cells can become activated only when they are presented with the foreign

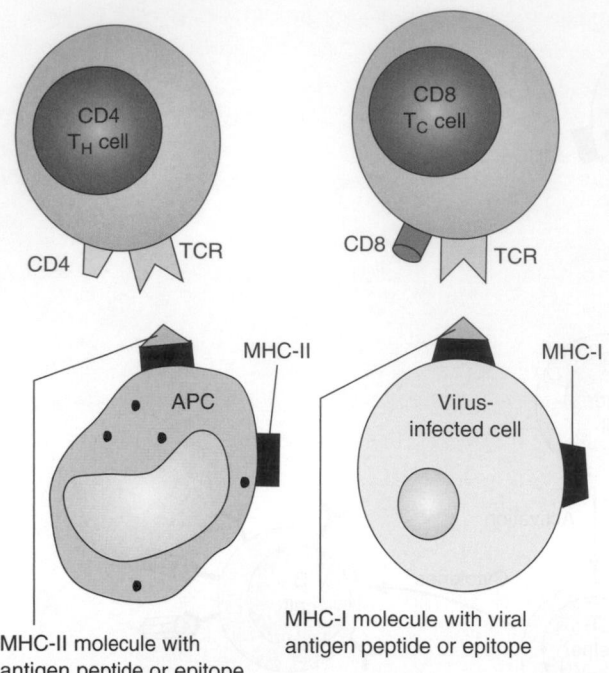

FIGURE 17-7 • Recognition by a T-cell receptor (TCR) on a CD4+ helper T (T$_H$) cell of an epitope associated with a class II major histocompatibility complex (MHC) molecule on an antigen-presenting cell (APC); and by a TCR on a CD8+ cytotoxic T (T$_C$) cell of an epitope associated with a class I MHC molecule on a virus-infected cell.

antigen peptide associated with the class I MHC molecule. During a typical viral infection of a cell, small peptides from degraded viral proteins associate with MHC-I molecules and are then transported to the infected cell membrane. This complex communicates to the T-cytotoxic cell that the cell must be destroyed for the overall survival of the host. *Class II MHC* (MHC-II) molecules, which are found primarily on antigen-presenting cells such as macrophages, dendritic cells, and B lymphocytes, communicate with the antigen receptor and CD4 molecule on T-helper lymphocytes.

Class II MHC molecules also have a groove or cleft that binds a fragment of antigen from pathogens that have been engulfed and digested during the process of phagocytosis. The engulfed pathogen is degraded into peptide in cytoplasmic vesicles and then complexed with MHC-II molecules. T-helper cells recognize these complexes on the surface of antigen-presenting cells and become activated. These triggered T-helper cells multiply quickly and direct other immune cells to respond to the invading pathogen through the secretion of cytokines. A third group of genes located on the same chromosome near the class I and II MHC genes encode other proteins with diverse functions. Some complement and cytokines important for signaling an immune response are examples of class III MHC molecules. These secreted molecules are structurally and functionally unrelated to the class I and II MHC molecules.

Each individual has a unique collection of MHC proteins, and a variety of MHC molecules can exist in a population. Thus, MHC molecules are both polygenic and polymorphic. The MHC genes are the most polymorphic genes known. MHC alleles affect immune responses as well as susceptibility to a number of diseases. Because of the number of MHC genes and the possibility of several alleles for each gene, it is almost impossible for any two individuals to have an identical MHC profile, unless they are identical twins. In contrast to the receptors on T and B lymphocytes that bind a unique antigen molecule, each MHC protein can bind a broad spectrum of antigen peptides.

Human MHC proteins are called *human leukocyte antigens* (HLA) because they were first detected on white blood cells. Because these molecules play a role in transplant rejection and are detected by immunologic tests, they are commonly called *antigens*. More recently, analysis of the genes for the HLA molecules has ensured a more complete identification of the potential antigens present in an individual. The classic human MHC-I molecules are divided into types called HLA-A, HLA-B, and HLA-C, and the MHC-II molecules are identified as HLA-DR, HLA-DP, and HLA-DQ (Table 17-3). Additional, less well-studied, nonclassic MHC genes have been described and shown to influence other immune interactions. Each of the gene loci that describe HLA molecules can be occupied by multiple alleles or alternative genes. For example, there are more than 350 possible alleles for the A locus, 650 alleles for the B locus, and 180 alleles for the C locus. The genes and their expressed molecules are designated by a letter and numbers (*i.e.*, HLA-B27).

Because the class I and II MHC genes are closely linked on one chromosome, the combination of HLA genes usually is inherited as a unit, called a *haplotype*. Each person inherits a chromosome from each parent and therefore has two HLA

TABLE 17-3 **Properties of Class I and II MHC Molecules**			
PROPERTIES	**HLA ANTIGENS**	**DISTRIBUTION**	**FUNCTIONS**
Class I MHC	HLA-A, HLA-B, HLA-C	Virtually all nucleated cells	Present processed antigen to cytotoxic CD8+ T cells; restrict cytolysis to virus-infected cells, tumor cells, and transplanted cells
Class II MHC	HLA-DR, HLA-DP, HLA-DQ	Immune cells, antigen-presenting cells, B cells, and macrophages	Present processed antigenic fragments to CD4+ T cells; necessary for effective interaction among immune cells

HLA, human leukocyte antigen; MHC, major histocompatibility complex.

haplotypes. The identification or typing of HLA molecules is important in tissue or organ transplantation, forensics, and paternity evaluations. In organ or tissue transplantation, the closer the matching of HLA types, the greater is the probability of identical antigens and the lower the chance of rejection.

Antigen-Presenting Cells

To be activated, a T lymphocyte must recognize a foreign peptide bound to a self-MHC molecule. That requires simultaneous delivery of costimulatory signals by a specialized antigen-presenting cell (APC). APCs acquire the capacity to present antigens to T lymphocytes in the context of histocompatibility after cytokine-driven up-regulation of MHC-II molecules. Only cells that can express both classes of MHC molecules, such as dendritic cells, monocytes, macrophages, and B lymphocytes residing in lymphoid follicles and, under certain conditions, endothelial cells, are able to function as APCs.

Macrophages are key members of the mononuclear phagocytic system that engulf and digest microbes and other foreign substances. The monocytes migrate from the blood to various tissues, where they mature into the major tissue phagocyte, the macrophages. As the general scavenger cells of the body, the macrophage can be fixed in a tissue or free to migrate from an organ to lymphoid tissues. The tissue macrophages are scattered in connective tissue or clustered in organs such as the lung (*i.e.,* alveolar macrophages), liver (*i.e.,* Kupffer cells), spleen, lymph nodes, peritoneum, central nervous system (*i.e.,* microglial cells), and other areas. Macrophages are activated to engulf and break down complex antigens into peptide fragments for association with MHC-II molecules. Macrophages then present these complexes to the helper T cell so that self–nonself recognition and activation of the immune response can occur.

Dendritic cells share with the macrophage the important task of presenting processed antigen to T lymphocytes. These distinctive, star-shaped cells with long extensions of their cytoplasmic membrane provide an extensive surface rich in MHC-II molecules and other membrane molecules important for initiation of adaptive immunity. Dendritic cells are found in most tissues where antigen enters the body and in the peripheral lymphoid tissues, where they function as potent APCs. In these different environments, dendritic cells can acquire specialized functions and appearances, as do macrophages. Langerhans cells are specialized dendritic cells in the skin, whereas follicular dendritic cells are found in the lymph nodes. Langerhans cells are constantly surveying the skin for antigen and can transport foreign material to a nearby lymph node. Skin dendritic cells and macrophages also are involved in cell-mediated immune reactions of the skin such as allergic contact dermatitis.

B Lymphocytes and Humoral Immunity

Humoral immunity is mediated by antibodies, which are produced by B lymphocytes and their progeny. It is the arm of the adaptive immune response that functions to eliminate extra-cellular microbes and microbial toxins. Humoral immunity is more important than cellular immunity in defending against microbes with capsules rich in polysaccharides and lipid toxins. The reason for this is that B cells respond to and produce antibodies specific for many types of molecules, whereas T cells, the mediators of cellular immunity, respond primarily to protein antigens.

B lymphocytes can be identified by the presence of membrane immunoglobulin that functions as the antigen receptor, class II MHC proteins, complement receptors, and specific CD molecules. During the maturation process in the bone marrow, B-cell progenitors (pro-B and pre-B cells) develop into mature or naive B cells. Naive B cells express membrane-bound IgD and IgM that function as receptors for antibody but do not secrete antibody. The mature B cell leaves the bone marrow, enters the circulation, and migrates to the various peripheral lymphoid tissues, where it is stimulated to respond to a specific antigen. Each of the stages of B cell development are characterized by a specific pattern of Ig gene expression and the expression of other cell surface proteins that serve as phenotypic markers of these maturational stages.

The commitment of a B-cell line to a specific antigen is evidenced by the expression of the membrane-bound Ig receptors that recognize antigen. B cells that encounter antigen complementary to their surface immunoglobulin receptor and receive T-cell help undergo a series of changes that transform them into antibody-secreting plasma cells or into memory B cells (Fig. 17-8). The antibodies produced by the plasma cells are released into the lymph and blood, where they bind and remove their unique antigen with the help of other immune effector cells and molecules. The longer-lived memory B cells are distributed to the peripheral tissues in preparation for subsequent antigen exposure.

Immunoglobulins

Antibodies comprise a class of proteins called *immunoglobulins.* The immunoglobulins have been divided into five classes, IgG, IgA, IgM, IgD, and IgE, each with a different role in the immune defense strategy (Table 17-4). Immunoglobulins have a characteristic four-polypeptide structure consisting of at least two identical antigen-binding sites (Fig. 17-9). Each immunoglobulin is composed of two identical light (L) chains and two identical heavy (H) chains to form a "Y"-shaped molecule. The two forked ends of the immunoglobulin molecule bind antigen and are called *Fab* (*i.e.,* antigen-binding) fragments, and the tail of the molecule, which is called the *Fc* fragment, determines the biologic properties that are characteristic of a particular class of immunoglobulins.

The amino acid sequence of the heavy and light chains shows constant (C) regions and variable (V) regions. The *constant regions* have sequences of amino acids that vary little among the antibodies of a particular class of immunoglobulin. The constant regions are the basis for the separation of immunoglobulins into classes (*e.g.,* IgM, IgG), and allow each class of

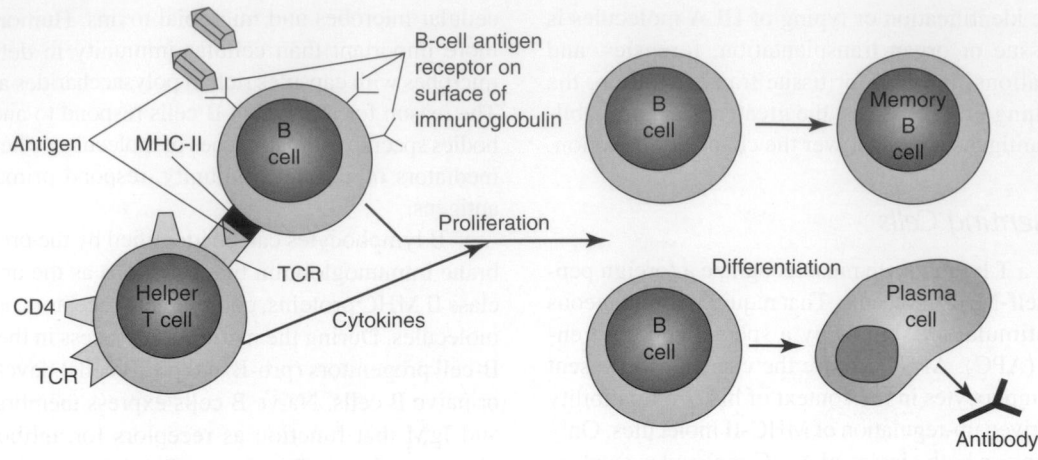

FIGURE 17-8 • Pathway for B-cell differentiation.

TABLE 17-4 **Classes and Characteristics of Immunoglobulins**

FIGURE	CLASS	PERCENTAGE OF TOTAL	CHARACTERISTICS
	IgG	75.0	Displays antiviral, antitoxin, and antibacterial properties; only Ig that crosses the placenta; responsible for protection of newborn; activates complement and binds to macrophages
	IgA	15.0	Predominant Ig in body secretions, such as saliva, nasal and respiratory secretions, and breast milk; protects mucous membranes
	IgM	10.0	Forms the natural antibodies such as those for ABO blood antigens; prominent in early immune responses; activates complement
	IgD	0.2	Found on B lymphocytes; needed for maturation of B cells
	IgE	0.004	Binds to mast cells and basophils; involved in parasitic infections, allergic and hypersensitivity reactions

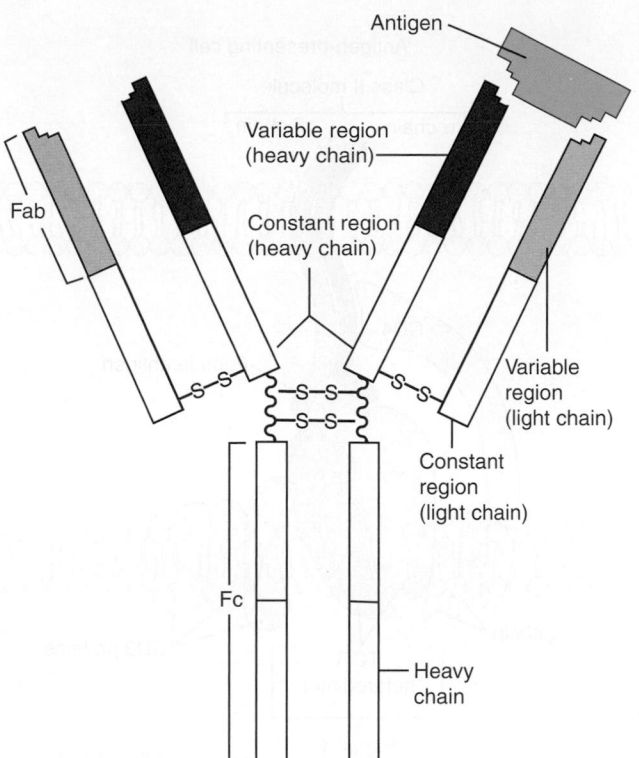

FIGURE 17-9 • Schematic model of an immunoglobulin G (IgG) molecule showing the constant and variable regions of the light and heavy chains.

antibody to interact with certain effector cells and molecules. For example, IgG can tag an antigen for recognition and destruction by phagocytes. The *variable regions* contain the antigen-binding sites of the molecule. The wide variation in the amino acid sequence of the variable regions seen from antibody to antibody allows this region to recognize its complementary epitope. A unique amino acid sequence in this region determines a distinctive three-dimensional pocket that is complementary to the antigen, allowing recognition and binding. Each B-cell clone produces antibody with one specific antigen-binding variable region or domain. During the course of the immune response, class switching (*e.g.,* from IgM to IgG) can occur, causing the B-cell clone to produce one of the different immunoglobulin types.

IgG (gamma globulin) is the most abundant of the circulating immunoglobulins. It is present in body fluids and readily enters the tissues. IgG is the only immunoglobulin that crosses the placenta and can transfer immunity from the mother to the fetus. This class of immunoglobulin protects against bacteria, toxins, and viruses in body fluids and activates the complement system. This antibody can also bind to target cells and Fc receptors on NK cells and macrophages, leading to lysis of the target cell. There are four subclasses of IgG (*i.e.,* IgG1, IgG2, IgG3, and IgG4), each of which has some restrictions in its response to certain types of antigens. For example, IgG2 appears to be responsive to bacteria that are encapsulated with a polysaccharide layer, such as *Streptococcus pneumoniae, Haemophilus influenzae,* and *Neisseria meningitidis.*

IgA, a secretory immunoglobulin, is found in saliva, tears, colostrum (*i.e.,* first milk of a nursing mother), and bronchial, gastrointestinal, prostatic, and vaginal secretions. This dimeric secretory immunoglobulin is considered a primary defense against local infections in mucosal tissues. IgA prevents the attachment of viruses and bacteria to epithelial cells.

IgM is a macromolecule that forms a polymer of five basic immunoglobulin units. It cannot cross the placenta and does not transfer maternal immunity. It is the first circulating immunoglobulin to appear in response to an antigen and is the first antibody type made by a newborn. This is diagnostically useful because the presence of IgM suggests a current infection in the infant by a specific pathogen. The identification of newborn IgM rather than maternally transferred IgG to the specific pathogen is indicative of an in utero or newborn infection.

IgD is found primarily on the cell membranes of B lymphocytes. It serves as an antigen receptor for initiating the differentiation of B cells.

IgE is involved in inflammation, allergic responses, and combating parasitic infections. It binds to mast cells and basophils. The binding of antigen to mast cell– or basophil-bound IgE triggers these cells to release histamine and other mediators important in inflammation and allergies.

Humoral Immunity

Humoral immunity depends on maturation of B lymphocytes into plasma cells, which produce and secrete antibodies. The combination of antigen with antibody can result in several effector responses, such as precipitation of antigen–antibody complexes, agglutination or clumping of cells, neutralization of bacterial toxins and viruses, lysis and destruction of pathogens or cells, adherence of antigen to immune cells, facilitation of phagocytosis, and complement activation. For example, antibodies can neutralize a virus by blocking the sites on the virus that it uses to bind to the host cell, thereby negating its ability to infect the cell.

Two types of responses occur in the development of humoral immunity: a primary and a secondary response (Fig. 17-10). A *primary immune response* occurs when the antigen is first introduced into the body. During the primary response, there is a latent period or lag before the antibody can be detected in the serum. This latent period involves the processing of antigen by the APCs and its recognition by CD4+ helper T cells. After the antigen receptors on CD4+ helper T cells recognize the antigenic peptide–class II MHC complex, the T cells become activated and produce cytokines to further stimulate and direct the immune system. In humoral immunity, activated CD4+ helper T cells trigger B cells to proliferate and differentiate into a clone of plasma cells that produce antibody. This activation process takes 1 to 2 weeks, but once generated, detectable antibody continues to rise for several weeks. Recovery from many infectious diseases occurs during the primary response when the antibody concentration is reaching its peak. The *secondary* or *memory response* occurs on second or subsequent exposures to the antigen. During the secondary response,

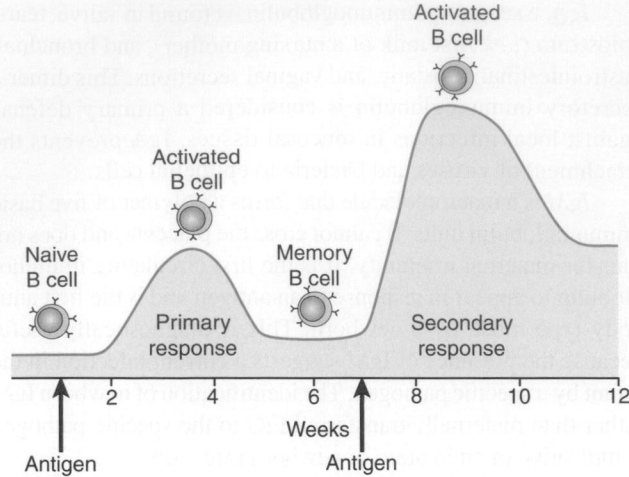

FIGURE 17-10 • Primary and secondary or memory phases of the humoral immune response to the same antigen.

the rise in antibody occurs sooner and reaches a higher level because of available memory cells.

During the primary response, B cells are activated to proliferate and differentiate into antibody-secreting plasma cells. A fraction of activated B cells does not differentiate into plasma cells but forms a pool of memory B cells. During the secondary response, the memory cells recognize the antigen and respond more efficiently to produce the specific antibody. The booster immunization given for some diseases, such as tetanus, makes use of the memory response. For a person who has been previously immunized, administration of a booster shot causes an almost immediate rise in antibody to a level sufficient to prevent development of the disease. Activated T cells can also generate primary and secondary cell-mediated immune responses and the concurrent development of T memory cells.

T Lymphocytes and Cellular Immunity

T lymphocytes function in the activation of other T cells and B cells, in the control of intracellular viral infections, in the rejection of foreign tissue grafts, and in delayed hypersensitivity reactions (see Chapter 19). Collectively, these immune responses are referred to as *cell-mediated* or *cellular immunity*. The effector phase of cell-mediated immunity is carried out by T lymphocytes and macrophages.

T lymphocytes arise from bone marrow stem cells, but unlike B cells, pre-T cells migrate to the thymus for their maturation. There, the immature T lymphocytes undergo rearrangement of the genes needed for expression of a unique T-cell antigen receptor similar to but distinct from the B-cell receptor. The T-cell receptor (TCR) is composed of two polypeptides that fold to form a groove that recognizes processed antigen peptide–MHC complexes (Fig. 17-11). The TCR–antigen–MHC complex is further stabilized during cell activation by the CD4 molecule on the helper T cell or the CD8 molecule on the cytotoxic

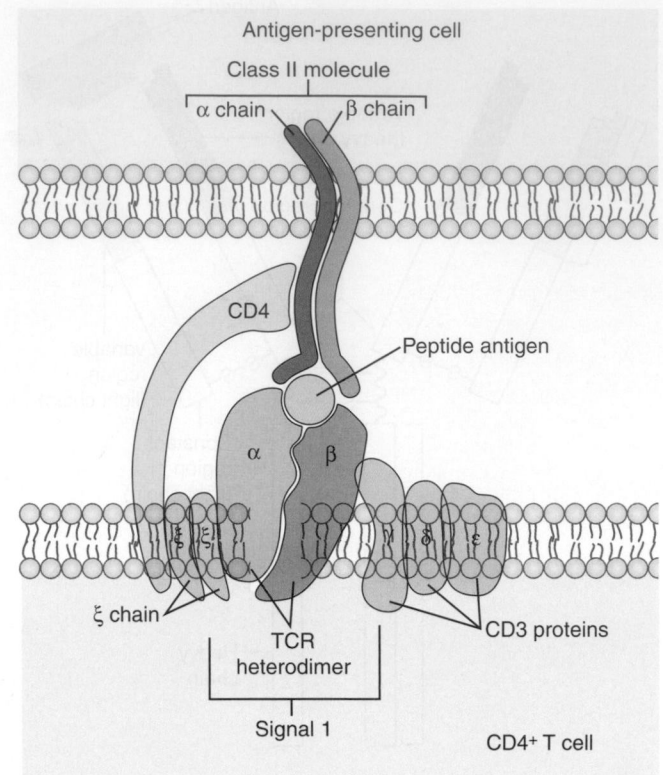

FIGURE 17-11 • The T-cell receptor (TCR) on a CD4+ T cell and its interaction with the class II major histocompatibility complex (MHC) molecule on the antigen-presenting cell. Notice that the αβ TCR heterodimer recognizes a peptide fragment of antigen bound to the MHC class II molecule. The CD4 molecule binds to the nonpolymorphic portion of the class II MHC molecule, stabilizing the interaction. The CD3 proteins associated with the TCR aid in cell signaling. (Adapted from Kumar V., Cotran R. S., Robbins S. L [2003]. *Robbins basic pathology* [7th ed., p. 106]. Philadelphia: WB Saunders.)

T cell. The TCR is associated with other surface molecules known as the *CD3 complex* that aid cell signaling. Maturation of subpopulations of T cells (*i.e.,* CD4+ and CD8+) also occurs in the thymus. Mature T cells migrate to the peripheral lymphoid tissues and, on encountering antigen, multiply and differentiate into memory T cells and various mature T cells. The two main populations of mature T cells are CD4+ (helper) and CD8+ (cytotoxic or killer) T cells.

Helper T Cells and Cytokines in Adaptive Immunity

The CD4+ helper T cell (T_H) serves as a master regulator for the immune system. Activation of CD4+ helper T cells depends on the recognition of antigen in association with class II MHC molecules. Once activated, the cytokines they secrete influence the function of nearly all other cells of the immune system (see Table 17-1). Differences in the types of cytokines made by the CD4+ T cell produce different types of immune responses. These cytokines activate and regulate B cells, cytotoxic T lymphocytes, NK cells, macrophages, and other immune cells. The first cytokine to be produced by CD4$^+$ T cells after activation is IL-2. IL-2 is necessary for the proliferation and function of helper T cells, cytotoxic T cells, B cells, and NK cells. IL-2 interacts with T lymphocytes by binding to specific membrane receptors that are present on activated T cells but not on resting T cells. The expression of high-affinity IL-2 receptors can be triggered by specific antigen peptide–MHC II interactions and other stimulatory signals. Sustained T-cell amplification relies on the presence of both IL-2 and IL-2 receptors; if either is missing, cell proliferation ceases. Severe combined immunodeficiency diseases have been associated with mutations in IL-2 and the IL-2 receptor, thereby documenting the importance of these molecules. Cyclosporine and tacrolimus are drugs used to prevent rejection of heart, kidney, and liver transplants, and function primarily by inhibiting the synthesis of IL-2.

The activated CD4$^+$ helper T cell can differentiate into distinct subpopulations of helper T cells (*i.e.,* T$_H$1 or T$_H$2) based on the cytokines secreted by the APC at the site of activation (Table 17-5). The cytokine IL-12 produced by macrophages and dendritic cells directs the maturation of CD4$^+$ helper T cells toward T$_H$1 cells, whereas IL-4 produced by mast cells and T cells induces differentiation toward T$_H$2 cells. The distinct pattern of cytokine secreted by mature T$_H$1 and T$_H$2 cells defines these subpopulations of T$_H$ cells and determines whether a humoral or cell-mediated response will occur. Activated T$_H$1 cells characteristically produce the cytokines IL-2 and IFN-γ, whereas T$_H$2 cells produce IL-4 and IL-5. Some of the cytokines (*e.g.,* IL-10) made by T$_H$2 cells inhibit macrophage activation and suppresses T$_H$1 responses.

IL-4 is the major regulatory molecule for the development of T$_H$2 cells, which direct B cells in the class switching needed to produce IgE antibodies. IL-4 can further expand T$_H$2 cell populations in an autocrine manner and at the same time inhibit T$_H$1-directed cell-mediated immunity. The detrimental impact of increased IL-4 on excessive IgE production is evident in allergic individuals. IL-5 is an activator of eosinophils that, along with IgE, functions in the control of helminth (intestinal parasite) infections.

In most immune responses, a balanced response of T$_H$1 and T$_H$2 cells occurs, but immunization or exposure to antigen can skew the response to one or the other subset. For example, the extensive exposure to an allergen in atopic individuals has been shown to shift the naive T-helper cell toward a T$_H$2 response, with the production of the cytokines that influence IgE production and mast cell priming. An appreciation of these processes has led to clinical research that suggests redirection of an allergic T$_H$2 response to a nonallergic T$_H$1 response can occur in atopic individuals through modified immunization protocols.

Regulatory T Cells

A recently defined type of T lymphocyte is the *regulatory T cell,* which has CD4 and CD25 expressed on its cell membrane. Regulatory T cells, in contrast to CD4$^+$ helper T cells, suppress immune responses by inhibiting the proliferation of other potentially harmful self-reactive lymphocytes. The regulation by these cells is antigen specific and controlled through activation of a TCR by the antigen and subsequent secretion of the cytokines IL-10 and transforming growth factor-β (TGF-β). These cytokines inhibit the proliferation and activation of lymphocytes and macrophages. There is also recent evidence of regulatory CD8$^+$ T cells that can selectively downregulate T cells that are activated by either self or foreign antigens. These cells are thought to differentiate into effector cells during the primary immune response and function as suppressor cells during the secondary or memory phases of immunity, and are primarily involved in self–nonself discrimination. The potential clinical importance of regulatory T cells is suggested from animal studies showing inhibition of inflammatory bowel disease, experimental allergic encephalitis, and autoimmune diabetes by increased activity of regulatory T cells.

Cytotoxic T Cells

Activated CD8$^+$ cytotoxic T cells become cytotoxic T lymphocytes after recognition of class I MHC–antigen complexes on target cell surfaces, such as body cells infected by viruses or transformed by cancer (Fig. 17-12). The recognition of class I MHC–antigen complexes on infected target cells ensures that

TABLE 17-5 **Comparison of Properties of Helper T-Cell Subtypes 1 (T$_H$1) and 2 (T$_H$2)**		
	T$_H$1	**T$_H$2**
Stimulus for differentiation to T$_H$ subtype	Microbes	Allergens and parasitic worms
Cells and cytokines influencing T$_H$ subtype maturation	IL-12 produced by macrophages and dendritic cells	IL-4 produced by mast cells and T cells
Cytokines secreted by T$_H$ subtype	IFN-γ, IL-2	IL-4, IL-5
Effector functions	Phagocyte-mediated defense against infections, especially intracellular microbes; stimulates production of IgG	IgE- and eosinophil/mast cell–mediated immune reactions; stimulates production of IgE

NK, natural killer; IL, interleukin; IFN, interferon; Ig, immunoglobulin.

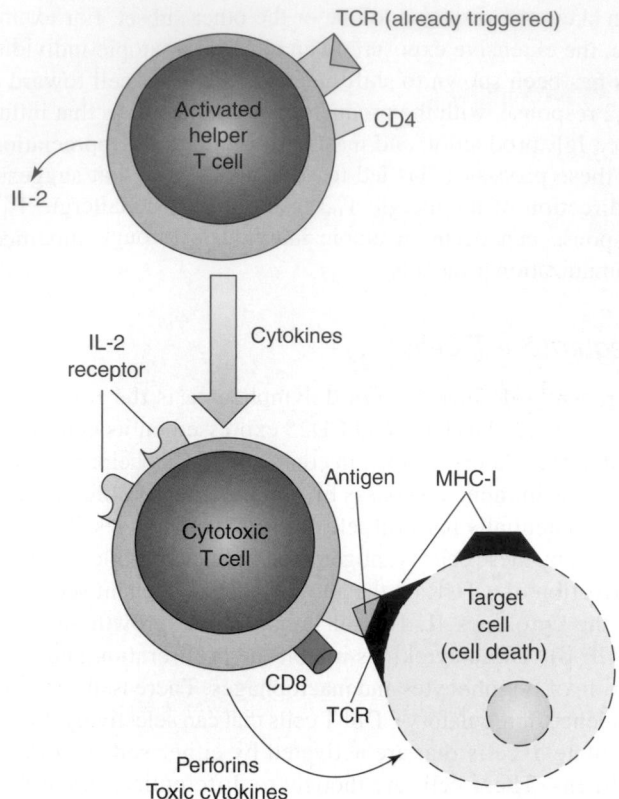

FIGURE 17-12 • Destruction of target cell by cytotoxic T cell. Cytokines released from the activated helper T cell enhance the potential of the cytotoxic T cell in destruction of the target cell.

neighboring uninfected host cells, which express class I MHC molecules alone or with self-peptide, are not indiscriminately destroyed. The CD8+ cytotoxic T lymphocytes destroy target cells by releasing cytolytic enzymes, toxic cytokines, and pore-forming molecules (*i.e.,* perforins), or through programmed cell death of the target cell by triggering membrane molecules and intracellular apoptosis. Apoptosis is a conserved cell process for the controlled elimination of excessive, dangerous, or damaged cells. In addition, the perforin proteins can produce pores in the target cell membrane, allowing entry of toxic molecules and loss of cell constituents. The CD8+ T cells are especially important in controlling replicating viruses and intracellular bacteria because antibody cannot readily penetrate the membrane of living cells.

Cell-Mediated Immunity

Cell-mediated immunity involves both CD4+ and CD8+ T lymphocytes. Activated CD4+ helper T cells release various cytokines (*i.e.,* IFN-γ) that recruit and activate other CD8+ cytotoxic T cells, macrophages, and inflammatory cells. Cytokines (*e.g.,* chemokines) can induce positive migration or chemotaxis of several types of inflammatory cells, including macrophages, neutrophils, and basophils. Activation of macrophages ensures enhanced phagocytic, metabolic, and enzymatic potential,

resulting in more efficient destruction of infected cells. This type of defense is important against intracellular pathogens such as *Mycobacterium* species and *Listeria monocytogenes*. A similar sequence of T-cell and macrophage activation, but with sustained inflammation, is elicited in delayed hypersensitivity reactions. Contact dermatitis due to a poison ivy reaction or sensitivity to dyes is an example of delayed or cell-mediated hypersensitivity caused by hapten–carrier complexes.

In cell-mediated immunity, the actions of T lymphocytes and effector macrophages predominate. The most aggressive phagocyte, the macrophage, becomes activated after exposure to T-cell cytokines, especially IFN-γ. As in humoral immunity, the initial stages of cell-mediated immunity are directed by an APC displaying the antigen peptide–class II MHC complex to the CD4+ helper T cell. CD4+ helper T cells become activated after antigen recognition and by induction with IL-12. The activated helper T cell then synthesizes IL-2, IL-4, and other cytokines. These molecules drive the multiplication of clones of CD4+ helper T cells, which amplify the response. Further differentiation of the CD4+ helper T cells leads to production of additional cytokines (*e.g.,* IFN-γ) that enhance the activity of cytotoxic T cells and effector macrophages.

Lymphoid Organs

The cells of the immune system are present in large numbers in the central and peripheral lymphoid organs. These organs and tissues are widely distributed in the body and provide different, but often overlapping, functions (Fig. 17-13). The central lymphoid organs, the bone marrow and the thymus, provide the environment for immune cell production and maturation. The structure and cells of the peripheral lymphoid organs function to concentrate antigen, aid processing of antigen, and promote cellular interactions necessary for development of adaptive immune responses. Lymph nodes, spleen, tonsils, appendix, Peyer patches in the intestine, and mucosa-associated lymphoid tissues in the respiratory, gastrointestinal, and reproductive systems comprise the peripheral lymphoid organs. The lymphoid organs are connected by networks of lymph channels, blood vessels, and capillaries. The immune cells continuously circulate through the various tissues and organs to seek out and destroy foreign material. The structure and organization of the cellular components of the peripheral lymphoid tissues ensure that the rare antigen-specific B and T cells will see each other and antigen peptide-MHC–coated antigen-presenting cells (*e.g.,* dendritic cells).

Thymus

The thymus is an elongated, bilobed structure located in the neck region above the heart. Each lobe is surrounded by a connective tissue capsule layer and is divided into lobules. Each lobule is composed of two compartments: an outer area or cortex, which is densely packed with thymocytes or immature T lymphocytes, and an inner, less dense area or medulla that contains fewer but

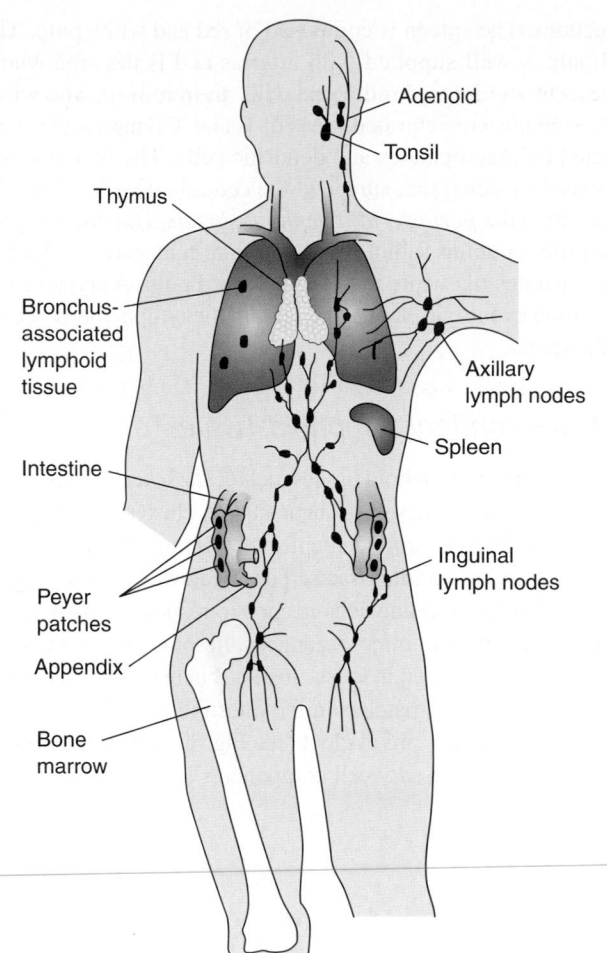

FIGURE 17-13 • Central and peripheral lymphoid organs and tissues.

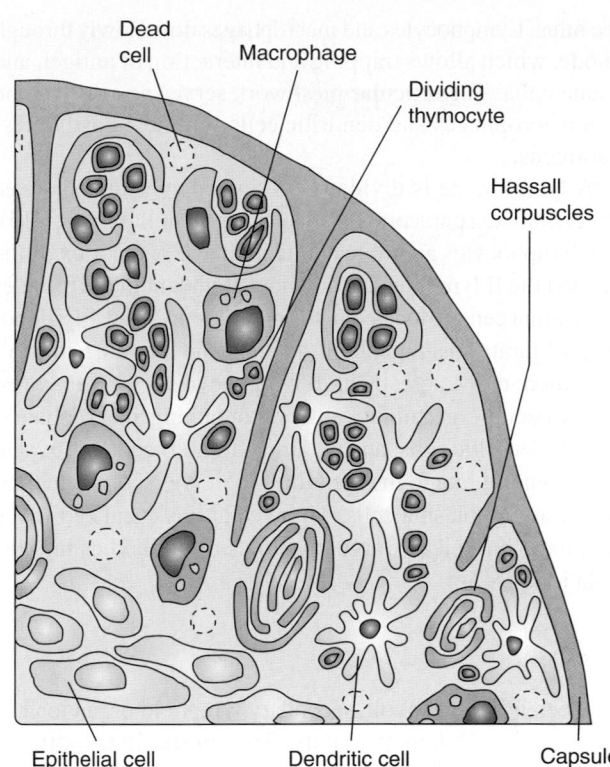

FIGURE 17-14 • Structural features of the thymus gland. The thymus gland is divided into lobules containing an outer cortex densely packed with dividing thymocytes or premature T cells and an inner medulla that contains mature T lymphocytes, macrophages, dendritic cells, and Hassall corpuscles.

more mature lymphocytes. The medulla also contains dendritic cells, macrophages, and the distinctive morphologic structure of the thymus, Hassall corpuscles (Fig. 17-14).

The function of the thymus is central to the development of the immune system because it generates mature, immunocompetent T lymphocytes expressing appropriate receptors. The thymus is a fully developed organ at birth, weighing approximately 15 to 20 g. At puberty, when the immune cells are well established in peripheral lymphoid tissues, the thymus begins slowly regressing and is replaced by adipose tissue. Nevertheless, some thymus tissue persists into old age. Precursor T (pre-T) cells enter the thymus as functionally and phenotypically immature T cells. They undergo cycles of proliferation and selection as they move from the cortical to medullary compartments of the thymus. Rapid cell multiplication, maturation, and selection occur in the cortex under the influence of the microenvironment, thymic hormones, and cytokines. As the T cells multiply and mature, they acquire TCRs, surface markers that distinguish among the different types of T cells, and antigens that distinguish them from nonself. More than 95% of the thymocytes die in the cortex and never leave the thymus because, in the random rearrangement of genes, cells are produced with inappropriate receptors. Only those T cells able to recognize foreign antigen displayed by self-MHC are allowed to mature. This process is called *thymic selection.* The thymus must be extremely thorough in eliminating self-reactive cells to ensure that autoimmune reactivity and disease do not result. Mature, immunocompetent T-helper and T-cytotoxic cells leave the thymus in 2 to 3 days and enter the peripheral lymphoid tissues through the bloodstream.

Lymph Nodes

Lymph nodes are small aggregates of lymphoid tissue located along lymphatic vessels throughout the body. Each lymph node processes lymph from a discrete, adjacent anatomic site. Many lymph nodes are in the axillae and groin, and along the great vessels of the neck, thorax, and abdomen. The lymph nodes are located along the lymph ducts, which lead from the tissues to the thoracic duct. Lymph nodes have two functions: removal of foreign material from lymph before it enters the bloodstream, and serving as centers for proliferation and response of immune cells.

A lymph node is a bean-shaped tissue surrounded by a connective tissue capsule. Lymph enters the node through afferent lymph channels that penetrate the capsule, and leaves through the efferent lymph vessels located in the deep indentation of the hilus. Lymphocytes and macrophages flow slowly through the node, which allows trapping and interaction of antigen and immune cells. The reticular meshwork serves as a surface on which macrophages and dendritic cells can more easily present antigens.

A lymph node is divided into several specialized areas, an outer cortex, a paracortex, and an inner medulla (Fig. 17-15). The T lymphocytes are more abundant in the paracortex of the node, and the B lymphocytes are more abundant in the follicles and germinal centers located in the outer cortex. The T lymphocytes proliferate on antigenic stimulation and migrate to the follicles, where they interact with B lymphocytes. These activated follicles become germinal centers, containing macrophages, follicular dendritic cells, and maturing T and B cells. Activated B cells then migrate to the medulla, where they complete their maturation into plasma cells. These cells stay localized in the lymph node but release large quantities of antibodies into the circulation.

Spleen

The spleen is a large, ovoid secondary lymphoid organ located high in the left abdominal cavity. The spleen filters antigens from the blood and is important in the response to systemic infections. The spleen is composed of red and white pulp. The red pulp is well supplied with arteries and is the area where senescent and injured red blood cells are removed. The white pulp contains concentrated areas of B and T lymphocytes permeated by macrophages and dendritic cells. The lymphocytes (primarily T cells) that surround the central arterioles form the area called the *periarterial lymphoid sheath.* The diffuse marginal zone contains follicles and germinal centers rich in B cells and separates the white pulp from the red pulp. A sequence of activation events similar to that seen in the lymph nodes occurs in the spleen.

Other Secondary Lymphoid Tissues

Other secondary lymphoid tissues include the *mucosa-associated lymphoid tissues.* These nonencapsulated clusters of lymphoid tissues are located around membranes lining the respiratory, digestive, and urogenital tracts. These gateways into the body must harbor the immune cells needed to respond to a large and diverse population of microorganisms. In some tissues, the lymphocytes are organized in loose clusters, but in other tissues such as the tonsils, Peyer patches in the intestine, and the appendix, organized structures are evident (see Fig. 17-13). These tissues contain all the necessary cell components (*i.e.,* T cells, B cells,

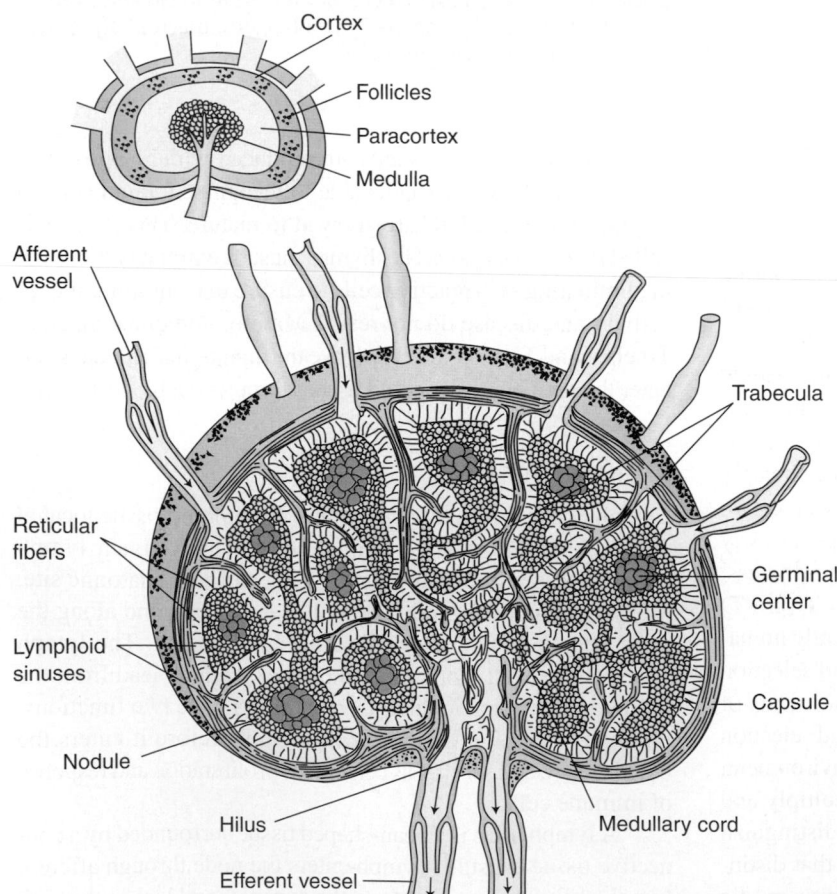

Cortex
Follicles
Paracortex
Medulla

Afferent vessel

Trabecula

Reticular fibers

Germinal center

Lymphoid sinuses

Capsule

Nodule

Hilus

Medullary cord

Efferent vessel

FIGURE 17-15 • Structural features of a lymph node. Bacteria that gain entry to the body are filtered out of the lymph as it flows through the node.

macrophages, and dendritic cells) for an immune response. Because of the continuous stimulation of the lymphocytes in these tissues by microorganisms constantly entering the body, large numbers of plasma cells are evident. Immunity at the mucosal layers helps to exclude many pathogens and thus protects the vulnerable internal organs.

Active Versus Passive Immunity

Adaptive immune responses are designed to protect the body against potentially harmful foreign substances, infections, and other sources of non–self-antigens. Protection is induced after exposure to antigens (active immunity) or through transfer of protective antibodies against an antigen (passive immunity).

Active immunity is acquired through immunization or actually having a disease. It is called *active immunity* because it depends on a response to the antigen by the person's immune system. Active immunity, although long lasting once established, requires a few days to weeks after a first exposure before the immune response is sufficiently developed to contribute to the destruction of the pathogen. However, the immune system usually is able to react within hours to subsequent exposure to the same agent because of the presence of memory B and T lymphocytes and circulating antibodies. The process of acquiring the ability to respond to an antigen after its administration by vaccine is known as *immunization*. An acquired immune response can improve on repeated exposures to an injected antigen or a natural infection.

Passive immunity is immunity transferred from another source. An infant receives passive immunity naturally from the transfer of antibodies from its mother in utero and through breast milk. Maternal IgG crosses the placenta and protects the newborn during the first few months of life. Normally, an infant has few infectious diseases during the first 3 to 6 months owing to the protection provided by the mother's antibodies. Passive immunity also can be artificially provided by the transfer of antibodies produced by other people or animals. Some protection against infectious disease can be provided by the injection of hyperimmune serum, which contains high concentrations of antibodies for a specific disease, or immune serum or gamma globulin, which contains a pool of antibodies from many individuals providing protection against many infectious agents. Passive immunity produces only short-term protection that lasts weeks to months.

Regulation of the Immune Response

Self-regulation is an essential property of the immune system. An inadequate immune response may lead to immunodeficiency, but an inappropriate or excessive response may lead to conditions varying from allergic reactions to autoimmune diseases. This regulation is not well understood and involves all aspects of the immune response—antigen, antibody, cytokines, regulatory T cells, and the neuroendocrine system.

With each exposure to antigen, the immune system must determine the branch of the immune system to be activated and the extent and duration of the immune response. After exposure to an antigen, the immune response to that antigen develops after a brief lag, reaches a peak, and then recedes. Normal immune responses are self-limited because the response eliminates the antigen, and the products of the response, such as cytokines and antibodies, have a short or limited life span and are secreted only for brief periods after antigen recognition. Evidence suggests that cytokine feedback from the helper T or regulatory T cells controls several aspects of the immune response.

Another facet of immune self-regulation is inhibition of immune responses by tolerance. The term *tolerance* is used to define the ability of the immune system to be nonreactive to self-antigens while producing immunity to foreign agents. Tolerance to self-antigens protects an individual from harmful autoimmune reactions. Exposure of an individual to foreign antigens may lead to tolerance and the inability to respond to potential pathogens that cause infection. Tolerance exists not only to self-tissues but to maternal-fetal tissues. Special regulation of the immune system is evident in defined privileged sites such as the brain, testes, ovaries, and eyes. Immune damage in these areas could result in serious consequences to the individual and the species.

IN SUMMARY, Adaptive immunity involves humoral and cellular mechanisms that respond to a unique antigen, can amplify and sustain its responses, distinguish self from nonself, and remember the antigen to produce quickly a heightened response on subsequent encounters with the same agent. Antigens are substances foreign to the host that can stimulate an immune response. They have antigenic determinant sites or epitopes, which the adaptive immune system recognizes with specific receptors that distinguish the antigens as nonself and as unique foreign molecules.

The principal cells of the adaptive immune system are the lymphocytes, antigen-presenting cells, and effector cells that eliminate the antigen. There are two types of lymphocytes: T lymphocytes and B lymphocytes. B lymphocytes differentiate into plasma cells that produce antibodies and provide for the elimination of microbes in the extracellular fluid (humoral immunity). T lymphocytes differentiate into regulatory (helper T and regulatory T cells) and effector (cytotoxic T cells) cells. Antigen-presenting cells consist of macrophages and dendritic cells that process and present antigen peptides to CD4$^+$ helper T cells.

Central to the identity of the immune cells are CD molecules that distinguish among the different immune cells and their level of differentiation. The regulatory CD4$^+$ helper T cells serve as a trigger for the immune response and are essential for the differentiation of B cells into antibody-producing plasma cells and the differentiation of T lymphocytes into effector CD8$^+$ cytotoxic T cells that eliminate intracellular microbes, such as viruses. Cytokines function as communication molecules for the cells of the adaptive immune system, activate their proliferation and differentiation, and ensure the appropriate development of T and B lymphocytes into effector and memory cells. The cell surface MHC molecules are key recognition molecules that the immune system uses in distinguishing self from non-self. Class I MHC molecules, which are present on body cells other than those of the immune system, interact with cytotoxic CD8+ T cells in the destruction of cells that have been affected by intracellular pathogens or cancer. Class II MHC molecules, found on immune cells, aid in cell-to-cell communication between different cells of the immune system.

Adaptive he cells of the immune system are present in large numbers in the central and peripheral lymphoid organs. The central lymphoid organs (bone marrow and thymus) provide the environment for immune cell production and maturation, whereas the peripheral lymphoid structures (lymph nodes, spleen, mucosa-associated lymphoid tissues in the respiratory, gastrointestinal, and reproductive systems) function to concentrate antigen, aid in the processing of antigen, and promote cellular interactions necessary for development of adaptive immune responses.

Adaptive immunity can be acquired actively through immunization or by having a disease (active immunity), or by receiving antibodies or immune cells from another source (passive immunity). An acquired immune response can improve with repeated exposure to an injected antigen or a natural infection. ■

DEVELOPMENTAL ASPECTS OF THE IMMUNE SYSTEM

After completing this section of the chapter, you should be able to meet the following objectives:

■ Explain the transfer of passive immunity from mother to fetus and from mother to infant during breast-feeding.
■ Characterize the development of active immunity in the infant and small child.
■ Describe changes in the immune response that occur with aging.

Embryologically, the immune system develops in several stages, beginning at 5 to 6 weeks as the fetal liver becomes active in hematopoiesis. Development of the primary lymphoid organs (*i.e.*, thymus and bone marrow) begins during the middle of the first trimester and proceeds rapidly. Secondary lymphoid organs (*i.e.*, spleen, lymph nodes, and mucosa-associated lymphoid tissues) develop soon after. These secondary lymphoid organs are rather small but well developed at birth and mature rapidly after exposure to microbes during the postnatal period. The thymus at birth is the largest lymphoid tissue relative to body size and normally is approximately two thirds its mature weight, which it achieves during the first year of life.

Transfer of Immunity From Mother to Infant

Protection of a newborn against antigens occurs through transfer of maternal antibodies. Maternal IgG antibodies cross the placenta during fetal development and remain functional in the newborn for the first months of life (Fig. 17-16). IgG is the only class of immunoglobulins to cross the placenta. Levels of maternal IgG decrease significantly during the first 3 to 6 months of life, while infant synthesis of immunoglobulins increases. Maternally transmitted IgG is effective against most microorganisms and viruses. The largest amount of IgG crosses the placenta during the last weeks of pregnancy and is stored in fetal tissues, and infants born prematurely may be deficient. Because of transfer of IgG antibodies to the fetus, an infant born to a mother infected with HIV has a positive HIV antibody test result, although the child may not be infected with the virus.

Cord blood does not normally contain IgM or IgA. If present, these antibodies are of fetal origin and represent exposure to intrauterine infection. The infant begins producing IgM antibodies shortly after birth, in response to the immense antigenic stimulation of his or her new environment. Premature infants appear to be able to produce IgM as well as term infants. At approximately 6 days of age the IgM rises sharply, and this rise continues until approximately 1 year of age, when the adult level is achieved.

Serum IgA normally is first detected at approximately 13 days after birth. The level increases during early childhood until adult levels are reached between the sixth and seventh year. Maternal IgA also is transferred to the infant in colostrum, or milk, by breast-feeding. These antibodies provide local immunity for the intestinal system and have been shown to decrease diarrheal infections in underdeveloped countries. These evolutionary adaptations of the immune system have increased the survival of our species and opti-

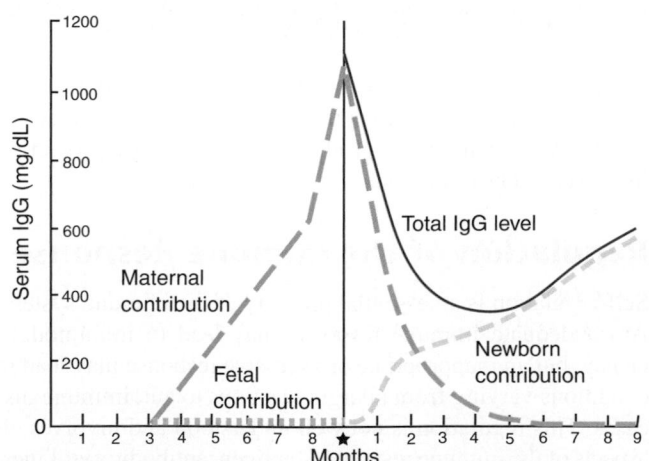

FIGURE 17-16 • Maternal/neonatal serum immunoglobulin G levels. (From Allansmith M., McClellan B. H., Butterworth M., et al. [1968]. The development of immunoglobulin levels in man. *Journal of Pediatrics* 72, 289.)

mized the development of other important organs in the early months of life.

 Immune Response in the Elderly

Aging is characterized by a declining ability to adapt to environmental stresses. One of the factors thought to contribute to this problem is a decline in immune responsiveness. This includes changes in cell-mediated and humoral immune responses. Elderly persons tend to be more susceptible to infections, have more evidence of autoimmune and immune complex disorders than younger persons, and have a higher incidence of cancer. Experimental evidence suggests that vaccination is less successful in inducing immunization in older persons than in younger adults. However, the effect of altered immune function on the health of elderly persons is clouded by the fact that age-related changes or disease may affect the immune response.

The alterations in immune function that occur with advanced age are not fully understood. There is a decrease in the size of the thymus gland, which is thought to affect T-cell function. The size of the gland begins to decline shortly after sexual maturity, and by 50 years of age, it usually has diminished to 15% or less of its maximum size. There are conflicting reports regarding age-related changes in the peripheral lymphocytes. A suggested biologic clock in T cells that determines the number of times it divides may regulate cell number with age. Some researchers have reported a decrease in the absolute number of lymphocytes, and others have found little, if any, change. The most common finding is a slight decrease in the proportion of T cells to other lymphocytes and a decrease in CD4+ and CD8+ cells.

More evident are altered responses of the immune cells to antigen stimulation; increasing proportions of lymphocytes become unresponsive, whereas the remainder continue to function relatively normally. T and B cells show deficiencies in activation. In the T-cell types, the CD4+ subset is most severely affected. Evidence indicates that aged T cells have a decreased rate of synthesis of the cytokines that drive the proliferation of lymphocytes and a diminished expression of the receptors that interact with those cytokines. For example, it has been shown that IL-2, IL-4, and IL-12 levels decrease with aging. Although B-cell function is compromised with age, the range of antigens that can be recognized is not diminished. If anything, the repertoire, including outgrowths of auto-reactive B-cell clones, is increased to the extent that B cells begin to recognize some self-antigens as foreign antigens. This may be the basis for the increased incidence of autoimmune disease in the elderly.

> **IN SUMMARY,** a newborn is protected against antigens in early life by passive transfer of maternal antibodies through the placenta (IgG) and in colostrum (IgA) through breast-feeding. Some changes are seen with aging, including an increase in autoimmune diseases. The impact of alterations in immune function that occur with aging is not fully understood. ∎

Review Exercises

1. The systemic manifestations (*e.g.,* generalized muscle aches, chills and fever, loss of appetite) that accompany a severe sore throat or acute respiratory infection are stimulated by reactions to cytokines of the innate immune system rather than by the antibodies or cell-mediated responses of the adaptive immune response.

   A. *Explain.*

2. A nursing student is working in a community clinic as a volunteer. Each time she enters the clinic, she suffers bouts of sneezing and runny nose. She has a history of mold allergy and her younger brother has asthma. Analysis at the allergy clinic indicates a strong reaction to latex. She is advised to avoid exposure to all forms of latex.

   A. *What class of immunoglobulin and what type of mediator cells are responsible for the symptoms expressed in this individual?*

   B. *What type of T-helper cell and cytokines direct the expression of this humoral immune response?*

   C. *Is this an example of active or passive immunity? Is this likely to be a primary or secondary immune response?*

3. A child of 5 months of age presents with thrush, a yeast infection of the mouth. In the last 2 months, he has had recurrent bouts of otitis media. His tonsils are very small. Laboratory analysis indicates a low lymphocyte count and no T lymphocytes. Further analysis indicates a genetic mutation in the T-cell receptor molecule complex (TCR–CD3) that affects maturation of all T cells. The final diagnosis is severe combined immunodeficiency disease. A bone marrow transplant is being pursued with cells from his HLA-matched sibling.

   A. *Why were infections not present in the first few months of this child's life?*

   B. *What would be the impact of an absence of T cells on both humoral and cell-mediated immunity?*

   C. *Why would it not be advisable to administer a live virus vaccine in this child?*

Bibliography

Abbas A. K., Litchman A. H. (2006). *Basic immunology: Functions and disorders of the immune system* (2nd ed., updated edition 2006–2007). Philadelphia: Elsevier Saunders.

Akashi-Takamura S., Miyake K. (2006). Toll-like receptors (TLRs) and immune disorders. *Journal of Infection Chemotherapy* 12, 233–240.

Akira S., Ishii K. J. (2006). Innate immune recognition of and regulation by DNA. *Trends in Immunology* 27, 525–532.

Akira S., Uematsu S., Takeuchi O. (2006). Pathogen recognition and innate immunity. *Cell* 124, 783–801.

Bluestone J. A. (2005). Regulatory T cell therapy: Is it ready for the clinic? *Nature Reviews Immunology* 5, 343–349.

Chapin D. D. (2006). Overview of the human immune response. *Journal of Clinical Immunology* 117, S430–S435.

Clark R., Kupper T. (2005). Old meets new: The interaction between innate and adaptive immunity. *Journal of Investigative Dermatology* 125, 629–637.

Deane J. A., Bolland S. (2006). Nucleic acid-sensing TLRs as modifiers of autoimmunity. *Journal of Immunology* 177, 6573–6578.

Esche C., Stellato C., Beck L. A. (2005). Chemokines: Key players in innate and adaptive immunity. *Journal of Investigative Dermatology* 125, 615–628.

Fehervari Z., Sakaguchi S. (2006). Peacekeepers of the immune system. *Scientific American* 295(4), 56–63.

Goain A., Gamelli R. L. (2005). A primer on cytokines. *Journal of Burn Care and Rehabilitation* 26, 7–12.

Hoebe K, Janssen E., Beutler B. (2004). The interface between innate and adaptive immunity. *Nature Immunology* 5, 971–974.

Horton R., Wilming L., Rand V., et al. (2004). Gene map of the extended human MHC. *Nature Reviews Genetics* 5, 889–899.

Ishii K. J., Akira S. (2006). Innate immune recognition of, and regulation by DNA. *Trends in Immunology* 27, 525–532.

Janeway C. A., Jr., Medzhitov R. (2002). Innate immune recognition. *Annual Review of Immunology* 20, 197–216.

Jiang H., Chess L. (2006). Regulation of immune responses by T cells. *New England Journal of Medicine* 354, 1166–1176.

Jones S. A. (2005). Directing transition from innate to acquired immunity. *Journal of Immunology* 175, 3463–3468.

Kindt T., Goldsby R., Osbourne B. (2007). *Kuby immunology* (6th ed.). New York: WH Freeman.

Lanier L. L. (2005). NK cell recognition. *Annual Review of Immunology* 23, 225–274.

Lasker M. V., Nair S. K. (2006). Intracellular TLR signaling: A structural perspective on human disease. *Journal of Immunology* 177, 11–16.

Lui Y. J. (2001). Dendritic cell subsets and lineages and their functions in innate and adaptive immunity. *Cell* 106, 259–262.

Nairn R., Helbert M. (2004). *Immunology for medical students.* New York: Mosby/Elsevier.

Rakoff-Nahoum S., Medzhitov R. (2006). Role of the innate immune system and host-commensal mutualism. *Current Topics in Microbiology and Immunology* 308, 1–18.

Ridker P. M., Cannon C. P., Morrow D., et al. (2005). C-reactive protein and outcomes of statin therapy. *New England Journal of Medicine* 351, 20–28.

Roozendaal R., Carroll M. C. (2006). Emerging patterns in complement-mediated pathogen recognition. *Cell* 125, 29–32.

Rossi M., Young J. W. (2005). Human dendritic cells: Potent antigen-presenting cells at the crossroads of innate and adaptive immunity. *Journal of Immunology* 175, 1373–1381.

Russell J. H., Ley T. J. (2002). Lymphocyte mediated cytotoxicity. *Annual Review of Immunology* 20, 323–370.

Staros E. B. (2005). Innate immunity: New approaches to understanding its clinical significance. *American Journal of Clinical Pathology* 123, 305–312.

Sunyer J. O., Boshra H., Lorenzo, G., et al. (2003). Evolution of complement as an effector system in innate and adaptive immunity. *Immunologic Research* 27, 549–564.

Takeda K., Kaisho T., Akira S. (2003). Toll-like receptors. *Annual Review of Immunology* 21, 335–376.

Ulevitch R. J. (2004). Therapeutics targeting the innate immune system. *Nature Reviews Immunology* 4, 512–520.

Underhill D. M., Ozinski A. (2002). Phagocytosis of microbes: Complexity in action. *Annual Review of Immunology* 20, 825–852.

Walport M. J. (2001). Complement: Parts 1 and 2. *New England Journal of Medicine* 344, 1058–1066, 1141–1144.

Wright J. (2005). Immunoregulatory functions of surfactant proteins. *Nature Reviews Immunology* 5, 58–68.

Visit the Point. **http://thePoint.lww.com for animations, journal articles, and more!**

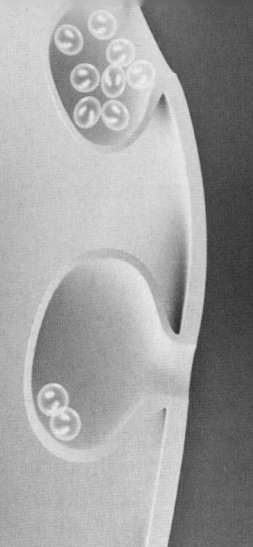

Inflammation, Tissue Repair, and Wound Healing

CAROL M. PORTH AND CYNTHIA SOMMER

➤ Inflammation is a protective response intended to eliminate the initial cause of cell injury, remove the damaged tissue, and generate new tissue. It accomplishes this by diluting, destroying, or otherwise neutralizing the harmful agents. It then sets the stage for the events that will eventually heal and reconstitute the damaged tissue. Thus, inflammation is intimately interwoven with the repair processes that replace damaged tissue or fill in the residual defects with fibrous scar tissue.

Although first described over 2000 years ago, the inflammatory response has evoked renewed interest during the past several decades. As a result, a number of diseases are now known be linked to the inflammatory response. For example, the role of the inflammatory response in producing the incapacitating effects of bronchial asthma and the crippling effects of rheumatoid arthritis has been well established. There is also increasing evidence that the inflammatory response may play a role in the pathogenesis of a number of other diseases, such as atherosclerosis, diabetes mellitus, and Alzheimer disease.

This chapter focuses on the morphologic and functional manifestations of acute and chronic inflammation, tissue repair, and wound healing. The innate and adaptive immune response, which is closely intertwined with the inflammatory response is discussed in Chapter 17.

 **THE INFLAMMATORY RESPONSE**

After completing this section of the chapter, you should be able to meet the following objectives:

■ State the five cardinal signs of acute inflammation and describe the physiologic mechanisms involved in production of these signs.
■ Describe the vascular changes in an acute inflammatory response.
■ Characterize the interaction of adhesion molecules, chemokines, and cytokines in leukocyte adhesion, migration, and phagocytosis, which are part of the cellular phase of inflammation.

(objectives continue)

Inflammation is the reaction of vascularized tissues to injury. It is characterized by the elaboration of inflammatory mediators and the movement of fluid and leukocytes from the blood into the extravascular tissues. This response localizes and eliminates microbes, foreign particles, and abnormal cells and paves the way for repair of the injured tissue. Inflammatory conditions are commonly named by adding the suffix *-itis* to the affected organ or system. For example, *appendicitis* refers to inflammation of the appendix, *pericarditis* to inflammation of the pericardium, and *neuritis* to inflammation of a nerve. More descriptive expressions of the inflammatory process might indicate whether the process was acute or chronic and what type of exudate was formed (*e.g.,* acute fibrinous pericarditis).

The classic description of inflammation has been handed down through the ages. In the first century AD, the Roman physician Celsus described the local reaction of injury in terms that are now known as the *cardinal signs* of inflammation.[1] These signs are *rubor* (redness), *tumor* (swelling), *calor* (heat), and *dolor* (pain). In the second century AD, the Greek physician Galen added a fifth cardinal sign, *functio laesa* (loss of function). In addition to the cardinal signs that appear at the site of injury, systemic manifestations (*e.g.,* fever) may occur as chemical mediators (*e.g.,* cytokines) produced at the site of inflammation gain entrance to the circulatory system. The constellation of systemic manifestations that may occur during acute inflammation is known as the *acute-phase response* (to be discussed).

Inflammation can be divided into two types: acute and chronic.[1,2] *Acute inflammation* is of relatively short duration, lasting from a few minutes to several days, and is characterized by the exudation of fluid and plasma components and emigration of leukocytes, predominantly neutrophils, into the extravascular tissues. *Chronic inflammation* is of a longer duration, lasting for days to years, and is associated with the presence of lymphocytes and macrophages, proliferation of blood vessels, fibrosis, and tissue necrosis. These basic forms of inflammation often overlap, and many factors may influence their course.

Acute Inflammation

Acute inflammation is the early (almost immediate) reaction of local tissues and their blood vessels to injury. It typically occurs before adaptive immunity becomes established and is aimed primarily at removing the injurious agent and limiting the extent of tissue damage. Acute inflammation can be triggered by a variety of stimuli, including infections, immune reactions, blunt and penetrating trauma, physical or chemical agents (*e.g.,* burns, frostbite, irradiation, caustic chemicals), and tissue necrosis from any cause.

Cells of Inflammation

Acute inflammation involves two major components: the vascular and cellular stages.[1,2,3] Many tissues and cells are involved in these reactions, including the endothelial cells that line blood vessels, circulating white blood cells, connective tissue cells (mast cells, fibroblasts, tissue macrophages, and lymphocytes), and components of the extracellular matrix (Fig. 18-1). The extracellular matrix consists of fibrous proteins (collagen and elastin), adhesive glycoproteins, and proteoglycans. At the biochemical level, the inflammatory mediators, acting together or in sequence, amplify the initial response and influence its evolution by regulating the subsequent vascular and cellular responses.

Endothelial Cells. Endothelial cells comprise the single cell–thick epithelial lining of blood vessels.[1,4,5] They produce antiplatelet and antithrombotic agents that maintain vessel patency and vasodilators and vasoconstrictors that regulate blood flow. Endothelial cells are also key players in the inflammatory response. As such, they provide a selective permeability barrier to exogenous (microbial) and endogenous inflammatory stimuli; regulate leukocyte extravasation by expression of cell adhesion molecules and receptors; contribute to the regulation and modulation of immune responses through synthesis and release of inflammatory mediators; and regulate immune cell proliferation through secretion of hematopoietic colony-stimulating factors (CSFs). Endothelial cells also participate in the repair process that accompanies inflammation through the production of growth factors that stimulate angiogenesis (formation of new blood vessels) and extracellular matrix synthesis.

Platelets. Platelets or thrombocytes are the cell fragments circulating in the blood that are involved in the cellular mechanisms of primary hemostasis (see Chapter 13). Activated platelets also release a number of potent inflammatory mediators, thereby increasing vascular permeability and altering the chemotactic, adhesive, and proteolytic properties of the

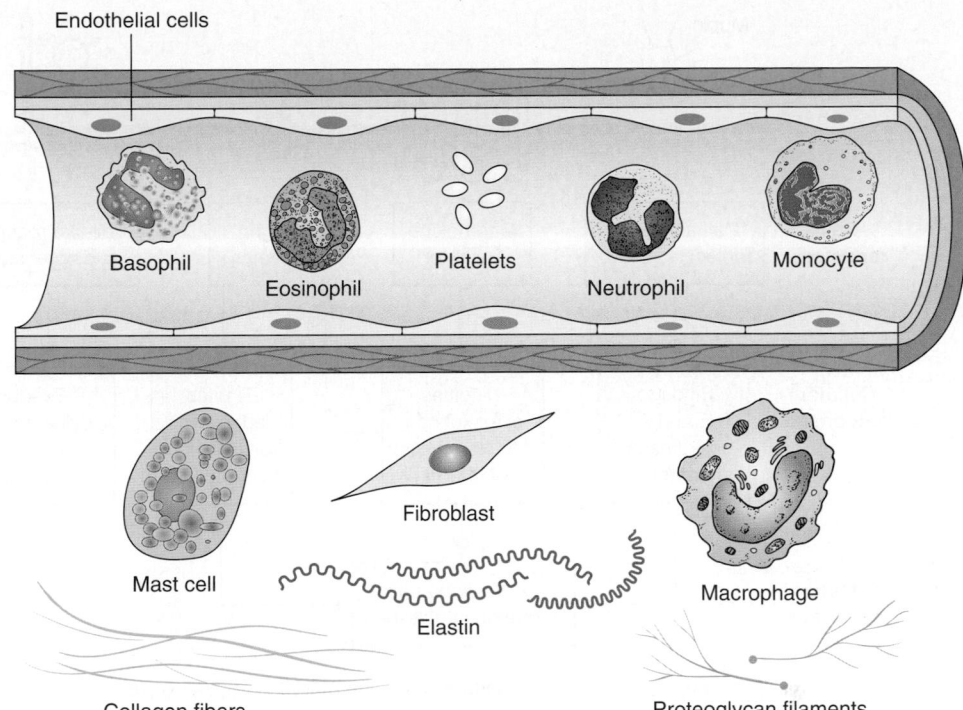

Endothelial cells

Basophil

Eosinophil

Platelets

Neutrophil

Monocyte

Mast cell

Fibroblast

Elastin

Macrophage

Collagen fibers

Proteoglycan filaments

FIGURE 18-1 • Cells of acute inflammation.

endothelial cells.[6,7] When a platelet undergoes activation, over 300 proteins are released. Although only a relatively small proportion of these have been identified, it appears that a significant number are inflammatory mediators.[6] The association between the platelet and inflammatory diseases is highlighted by the number of inflammatory disease processes (*e.g.*, atherosclerosis, migraine headache, systemic lupus erythematosus) shown to be associated with platelet activation.[6]

Neutrophils and Monocytes/Macrophages. The neutrophils and macrophages are phagocytic leukocytes that are present in large numbers and are evident within hours at the site of inflammation. Both types of leukocytes express a number of surface receptors and molecules that are involved in their activation. They include mannose receptors that bind glycoproteins of bacteria; Toll-like receptors that respond to different types and components of microbes; cell communication receptors that recognize specific cytokines and chemokines produced in response to infections and tissue injury; cell adhesion molecules that affect leukocyte adhesion; and complement receptors that recognize degraded fragments of complement deposited on the microbial surface (Fig. 18-2).

The *neutrophil* is the primary phagocyte that arrives early at the site of inflammation, usually within 90 minutes of injury. These leukocytes have nuclei that are divided into three to five lobes; therefore, they often are referred to *polymorphonuclear neutrophils (PMNs)* or *segmented neutrophils (segs)*. The neutrophil is a type of granulocyte, a white blood cell identified by distinctive cytoplasmic granules. Their cytoplasmic granules, which resist staining and remain a neutral color, contain enzymes and other antibacterial substances that are used in destroying and degrading engulfed microbes and dead tissue. Neutrophils also have oxygen-dependent metabolic pathways that generate toxic oxygen (*e.g.*, hydrogen peroxide) and nitrogen (*e.g.*, nitric oxide) products that aid in the destruction of engulfed pathogens.[3,8–10]

The neutrophil count in the blood often increases greatly during an inflammatory process, especially with bacterial infections. After being released from the bone marrow, circulating neutrophils have a life span of only approximately 10 hours and therefore must be constantly replaced if their numbers are to remain adequate. This requires an increase in circulating white blood cells, a condition called *leukocytosis*. With excessive demand for phagocytes, immature forms of neutrophils are released from the bone marrow. These immature cells often are called *bands* because of the horseshoe shape of their nuclei.

Circulating monocytes, which have a single kidney-shaped nucleus and are the largest of the circulating leukocytes, constitute 3% to 8% of the white blood cell count. They are derived from the bone marrow and can exit the circulation in response to inflammatory stimuli and become tissue macrophages.[9–11] Within 24 hours, mononuclear cells arrive at the inflammatory site, and by 48 hours, monocytes and macrophages are the predominant cell types.

Monocytes and macrophages produce potent vasoactive mediators, including prostaglandins and leukotrienes, platelet-activating factor (PAF), inflammatory cytokines, and growth factors that promote regeneration of tissues. The macrophages engulf larger and greater quantities of foreign material than the neutrophils. The circulating life span of the monocyte is three to four times longer than that of the granulocytes. These longer-lived phagocytes help to destroy the causative agent, aid in the signaling processes of immunity, serve to resolve the inflammatory process, and contribute to initiation of the healing processes. They also play an important role in chronic inflammation, where they can surround and wall off foreign material that cannot be digested.

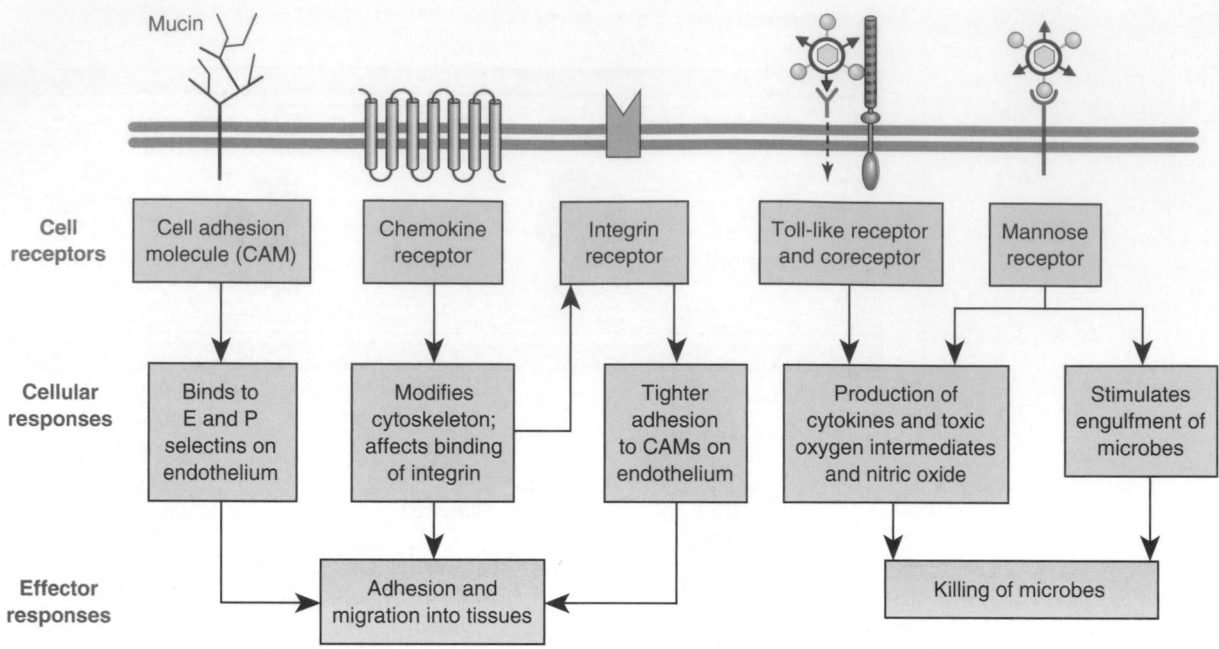

FIGURE 18-2 • Leukocyte activation. Different classes of leukocyte cell surface receptors recognize different stimuli. The receptors initiate responses that mediate the functions of the leukocytes.

Eosinophils, Basophils, and Mast Cells. Eosinophils, basophils, and mast cells produce lipid mediators and cytokines that induce inflammation. Although all three cell types have unique characteristics, they all contain cytoplasmic granules that induce inflammation. They are particularly important in inflammation associated with immediate hypersensitivity reactions and allergic disorders (discussed in Chapter 19).

Eosinophils circulate in the blood and are recruited to tissues, similar to neutrophils. These granulocytes increase in the blood during allergic reactions and parasitic infections. The granules of eosinophils, which stain red with the acid dye eosin, contain a protein that is highly toxic to large parasitic worms that cannot be phagocytized. They also play an important role in allergic reactions by controlling the release of specific chemical mediators.

Basophils are blood granulocytes with structural and functional similarities to mast cells of the connective tissue. They are derived from bone marrow progenitors and circulate in blood. The granules of the *basophils,* which stain blue with a basic dye, contain histamine and other bioactive mediators of inflammation. Both basophils and mast cells bind an antibody, immunoglobulin E (IgE), secreted by plasma cells through receptors on their cell surface. Binding of IgE triggers release of histamine and vasoactive agents from the basophil granules.

Mast cells derive from the same hematopoietic stem cells as basophils, but do not develop until they leave the circulation and lodge in tissue sites. They are particularly prevalent along mucosal surfaces of the lung and gastrointestinal tract and the dermis of the skin.[2,12] This distribution places the mast cell in a sentinel position between environmental antigens and the host for a variety of acute and chronic inflammatory conditions.[2]

Activation of mast cells results in release of preformed contents of their granules (histamine, proteoglycans, proteases, and cytokines such as tumor necrosis factor-α [TNF-α] and interleukin [IL]-16), synthesis of lipid mediators derived from cell membrane precursors (arachidonic acid metabolites, such as prostaglandins, and platelet-activating factor), and stimulation of cytokine and chemokine synthesis by other inflammatory cells such as monocytes and macrophages.

Vascular Stage

The vascular changes that occur with inflammation involve the arterioles, capillaries, and venules of the microcirculation. These changes begin almost immediately after injury and are characterized by vasodilation and changes in blood flow followed by increased vascular permeability and leakage of protein-rich fluid into the extravascular tissues.[1,2]

Vasodilation, which is one of the earliest manifestations of inflammation, follows a transient constriction of the arterioles, lasting a few seconds. Vasodilation first involves the arterioles and then results in opening of capillary beds in the area. As a result, the area becomes congested, causing the redness (erythema) and warmth associated with acute inflammation. Vasodilation is induced by the action of several mediators, most notably histamine and nitric oxide.

Vasodilation is quickly followed by increased permeability of the microvasculature, with the outpouring of a protein-rich fluid (exudate) into the extravascular spaces. The loss of fluid results in an increased concentration of blood constituents (red cells, leukocytes, platelets, and clotting factors), stagnation of flow, and clotting of blood at the site of injury. This aids in localizing the spread of infectious microorganisms. The loss of plasma proteins reduces the intracapillary osmotic pressure and increases the osmotic pressure of the interstitial fluid, causing fluid to move into the tissues and produce the swelling (*i.e.,* edema), pain, and impaired function that are the cardinal signs of acute inflammation. The exudation of fluid into the tissue spaces also serves to dilute the offending agent.

The increased permeability characteristic of acute inflammation results from formation of endothelial gaps in the venules of the microcirculation. Binding of the chemical mediators to endothelial receptors causes contraction of endothelial cells and separation of intercellular junctions. This is the most common mechanism of vascular leakage and is elicited by histamine, bradykinin, leukotrienes, and many other classes of chemical mediators.

Vascular Response Patterns. Depending on the severity of injury, the vascular changes that occur with inflammation follow one of three patterns of responses.[2] The first pattern is an *immediate transient response,* which occurs with minor injury. It develops rapidly after injury and is usually reversible and of short duration (15 to 30 minutes). Typically, this type of leakage affects venules 20 to 60 μm in diameter, leaving capillaries and arterioles unaffected.[2] Although the precise mechanism for restriction of this effect to the venules is unknown, it may reflect the greater density of receptors in the endothelium of the venules. It has also been suggested that the later leukocyte events of inflammation (*i.e.,* adhesion and emigration) also occur predominantly in the venules of most organs.

The second pattern is *an immediate sustained response,* which occurs with more serious types of injury and continues for several days. It affects all levels of the microcirculation (arterioles, capillaries, and venules) and is usually due to direct damage of the endothelium by injurious stimuli, such as burns or the products of bacterial infections.[2] Neutrophils that adhere to the endothelium may also injure endothelial cells.

The third pattern is a *delayed hemodynamic response,* in which the increased permeability begins after a delay of 2 to 12 hours, lasts for several hours or even days, and involves venules as well as capillaries.[2] A delayed response often accompanies injuries due to radiation, such as sunburn. The mechanism of the leakage is unknown, but it may result from the direct effect of the injurious agent, leading to delayed endothelial cell damage.

Cellular Stage

The cellular stage of acute inflammation is marked by changes in the endothelial cells lining the vasculature and movement of phagocytic leukocytes into the area of injury or infection. Although attention has been focused on the recruitment of leukocytes from the blood, a rapid response also requires the release of chemical mediators from tissue cells (mast cells and macrophages) that are prepositioned in the tissues. The sequence of events in the cellular response to inflammation includes leukocyte (1) margination and adhesion to the endothelium, (2) transmigration across the endothelium, (3) chemotaxis, and (4) activation and phagocytosis.[1,2,3]

Margination, Adhesion, and Transmigration. During the early stages of the inflammatory response, cross-talk between the blood leukocytes and the vascular endothelium defines a definite inflammatory event and ensures secure adhesion and arrest of the leukocytes along the endothelium.[9] As a consequence, the leukocytes slow their migration, adhere tightly to the endothelium, and begin to move along the periphery of the blood vessels. This process of leukocyte accumulation is called *margination.* The subsequent release of cell communication molecules called *cytokines* causes the endothelial cells lining the vessels to express cell adhesion molecules, such as *selectins,* that bind to carbohydrates on the leukocytes. This interaction, which is called *tethering,* slows their flow and causes the leukocytes to move along the endothelial cell surface with a rolling movement, finally coming to rest and adhering strongly to intercellular adhesion molecules (ICAMs) on the endothelium.[1-3] The adhesion causes the endothelial cells to separate, allowing the leukocytes to extend pseudopodia and *transmigrate* through the vessel wall and then, under the influence of chemotactic factors, migrate into the tissue spaces.

Several families of adhesion molecules, including selectins, integrins, and the immunoglobulin superfamily, are involved in leukocyte recruitment.[9,13,14] The selectins are a family of three closely related proteins (P-selectin, E-selectin, and L-selectin) that differ in their cellular distribution but all function in adhesion of leukocytes to endothelial cells. The integrin superfamily consists of 30 structurally similar proteins that promote cell-to-cell and cell-to-extracellular matrix interactions. The name *integrin* derives from the hypothesis that they coordinate (integrate) signals of extracellular ligands with cytoskeleton-dependent motility, shape change, and phagocytic responses of immune cells. Adhesion molecules of the immunoglobulin superfamily include ICAM-1, ICAM-2, and vascular adhesion molecule (VCAM)-1, all of which interact with integrins on leukocytes to mediate their recruitment.

Chemotaxis. Chemotaxis is the dynamic and energy-directed process of directed cell migration.[1] Once leukocytes exit the capillary, they wander through the tissue guided by a gradient of secreted chemoattractants, such as chemokines, bacterial and cellular debris, and protein fragments generated from activation of the complement system (*e.g.,* C3a, C5a). Chemokines, an important subgroup of chemotactic cytokines, are small proteins that direct the trafficking of leukocytes during the early stages of inflammation or injury.[15] Several immune (*e.g.,* macrophages) and nonimmune cells secrete these chemoattractants to ensure the directed movement of leukocytes to the site of infection.

Leukocyte Activation and Phagocytosis. During the next and final stage of the cellular response, monocytes, neutrophils, and tissue macrophages are activated to engulf and

Understanding • Acute Inflammation

Acute inflammation is the immediate and early response to an injurious agent. The response, which serves to control and eliminate altered cells, microorganisms, and antigens, occurs in two phases: (1) the vascular phase, which leads to an increase in blood flow and changes in the small blood vessels of the microcirculation; and (2) the cellular phase, which leads to the migration of leukocytes from the circulation and their activation to eliminate the injurious agent. The primary function of inflammatory response is to limit the injurious effect of the pathologic agent and remove the injured tissue components, thereby allowing tissue repair to take place.

❶ Vascular Phase

The vascular phase of acute inflammation is characterized by changes in the small blood vessels at the site of injury. It begins with momentary vasoconstriction followed rapidly by vasodilation. Vasodilation involves the arterioles and venules with a resultant increase in capillary blood flow, causing heat and redness, which are two of the cardinal signs of inflammation. This is accompanied by an increase in vascular permeability with outpouring of protein-rich fluid (exudate) into the extravascular spaces. The loss of proteins reduces the capillary osmotic pressure and increases the interstitial osmotic pressure. This, coupled with an increase in capillary pressure, causes a marked outflow of fluid and its accumulation in the tissue spaces, producing the swelling, pain, and impaired function that represent the other cardinal signs of acute inflammation. As fluid moves out of the vessels, stagnation of flow and clotting of blood occur. This aids in localizing the spread of infectious microorganisms.

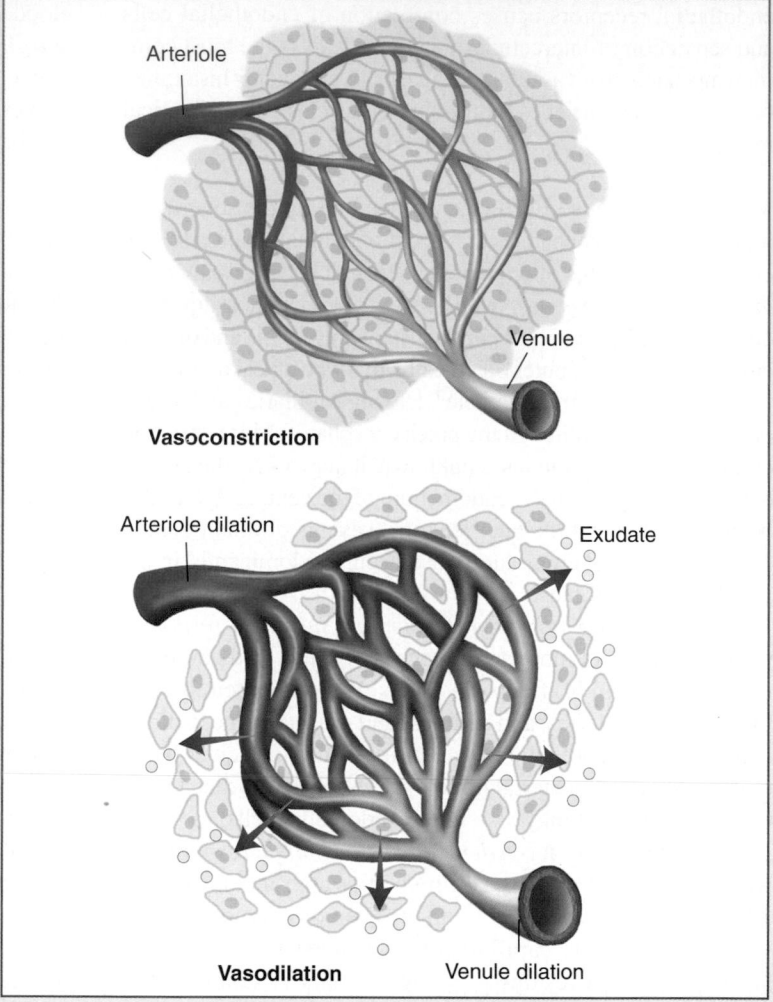

Arteriole

Venule

Vasoconstriction

Arteriole dilation

Exudate

Vasodilation   Venule dilation

Cellular Phase: Leukocyte Margination, Adhesion, and Transmigration

The cellular phase of acute inflammation involves the delivery of leukocytes, mainly neutrophils, to the site of injury so they can perform their normal functions of host defense. The delivery and activation of leukocytes can be divided into the following steps: adhesion and margination, transmigration, and chemotaxis. The recruitment of leukocytes to the precapillary venules, where they exit the circulation, is facilitated by the slowing of blood flow and margination along the vessel surface. Leukocyte adhesion and transmigration from the vascular space into the extravascular tissue is facilitated by complementary adhesion molecules (*e.g.*, selectins, integrins) on the leukocyte and endothelial surfaces. After extravasation, leukocytes migrate in the tissues toward the site of injury by chemotaxis, or locomotion oriented along a chemical gradient.

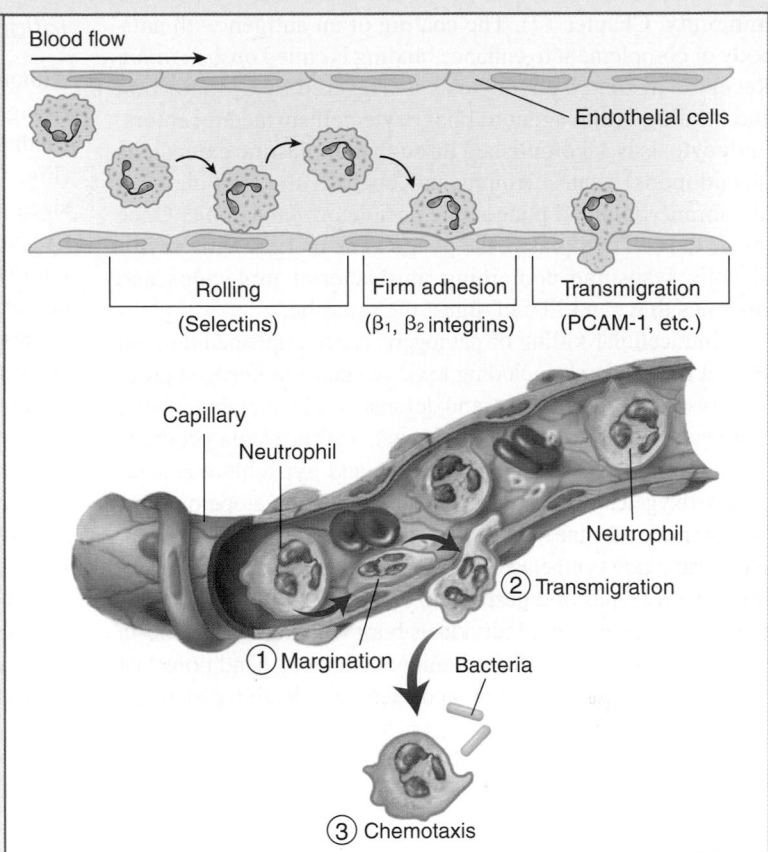

 Leukocyte Activation and Phagocytosis

Once at the sight of injury, the products generated by tissue injury trigger a number of leukocyte responses, including phagocytosis and cell killing. Opsonization of microbes (1) by complement factor C3b and antibody facilitates recognition by neutrophil C3b and the antibody Fc receptor. Receptor activation (2) triggers intracellular signaling and actin assembly in the neutrophil, leading to formation of pseudopods that enclose the microbe within a phagosome. The phagosome (3) then fuses with an intracellular lysosome to form a phagolysosome into which lysosomal enzymes and oxygen radicals (4) are released to kill and degrade the microbe.

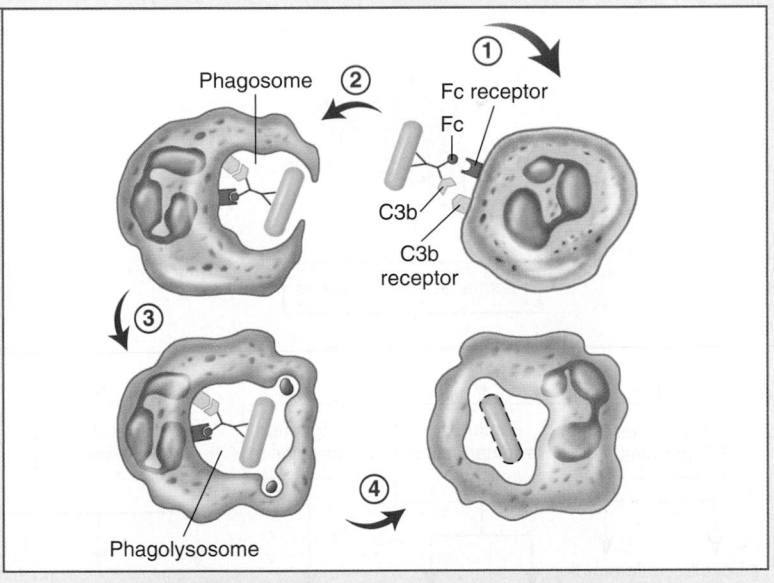

degrade the bacteria and cellular debris in a process called *phagocytosis*.[1,2,16] Phagocytosis involves three distinct steps: (1) recognition and adherence, (2) engulfment, and (3) intracellular killing. Phagocytosis is initiated by the recognition and binding of particles by specific receptors on the surface of phagocytic cells. This binding is essential for trapping the agent, which triggers engulfment and activates the killing potential of the cell. Microbes can be bound directly to the membrane of phagocytic cells by several types of pattern recognition receptors (*e.g.*, Toll-like and mannose receptors) or indirectly by receptors that recognize microbes coated with carbohydrate-binding lectins, antibody, or complement (see section on Innate

Immunity, Chapter 17). The coating of an antigen with antibody or complement to enhance binding is called *opsonization*. Receptor-mediated endocytosis is triggered by opsonization and binding of the agent to phagocyte cell surface receptors. Endocytosis is accomplished through cytoplasmic extensions (pseudopods) that surround and enclose the particle in a membrane-bounded phagocytic vesicle or *phagosome*. Once inside the cell cytoplasm, the phagosome merges with a cytoplasmic lysosome containing antibacterial molecules and enzymes that can kill and digest the microbe.

Intracellular killing of pathogens is accomplished through several mechanisms, including toxic oxygen and nitrogen products, lysozymes, proteases, and defensins. The metabolic burst pathways that generate toxic oxygen and nitrogen products (*i.e.,* nitric oxide, hydrogen peroxide, and hypochlorous acid) require oxygen and metabolic enzymes such as myeloperoxidase, nicotinamide adenine dinucleotide phosphate (NADPH) oxidase, and nitric oxide synthetase. Oxygen-independent pathways generate several types of digestive enzymes and antimicrobial molecules (*e.g.,* defensins). Individuals born with genetic defects in some of these enzymes have immunodeficiency conditions that make them susceptible to repeated bacterial infection (discussed in Chapter 19).

Inflammatory Mediators

Although inflammation is precipitated by infection and injury, its signs and symptoms are produced by chemical mediators. Mediators can originate either from the plasma or from cells (Fig. 18-3). The plasma-derived mediators, which are synthesized in the liver, include the coagulation factors (discussed in Chapter 13) and the complement proteins (discussed in Chapter 17). These mediators are present in the plasma in a precursor form that must be activated by a series of proteolytic processes to acquire their biologic properties. Cell-derived mediators are normally sequestered in intracellular granules that need to be secreted (*e.g.,* histamine from mast cells), or are newly synthesized (*e.g.,* cytokines) in response to a stimulus. Although the major sources of these mediators are platelets, neutrophils, monocytes/macrophages, and mast cells, endothelial cells, smooth muscle, fibroblasts, and most epithelial cells can be induced to produce some of the mediators.

The production of active mediators is triggered by microbes or host proteins, such as those of the complement, kinin, or coagulation systems, that are themselves activated by microbes or damaged tissues. Mediators can act on one or a few target cells, have diverse targets, or have differing effects on

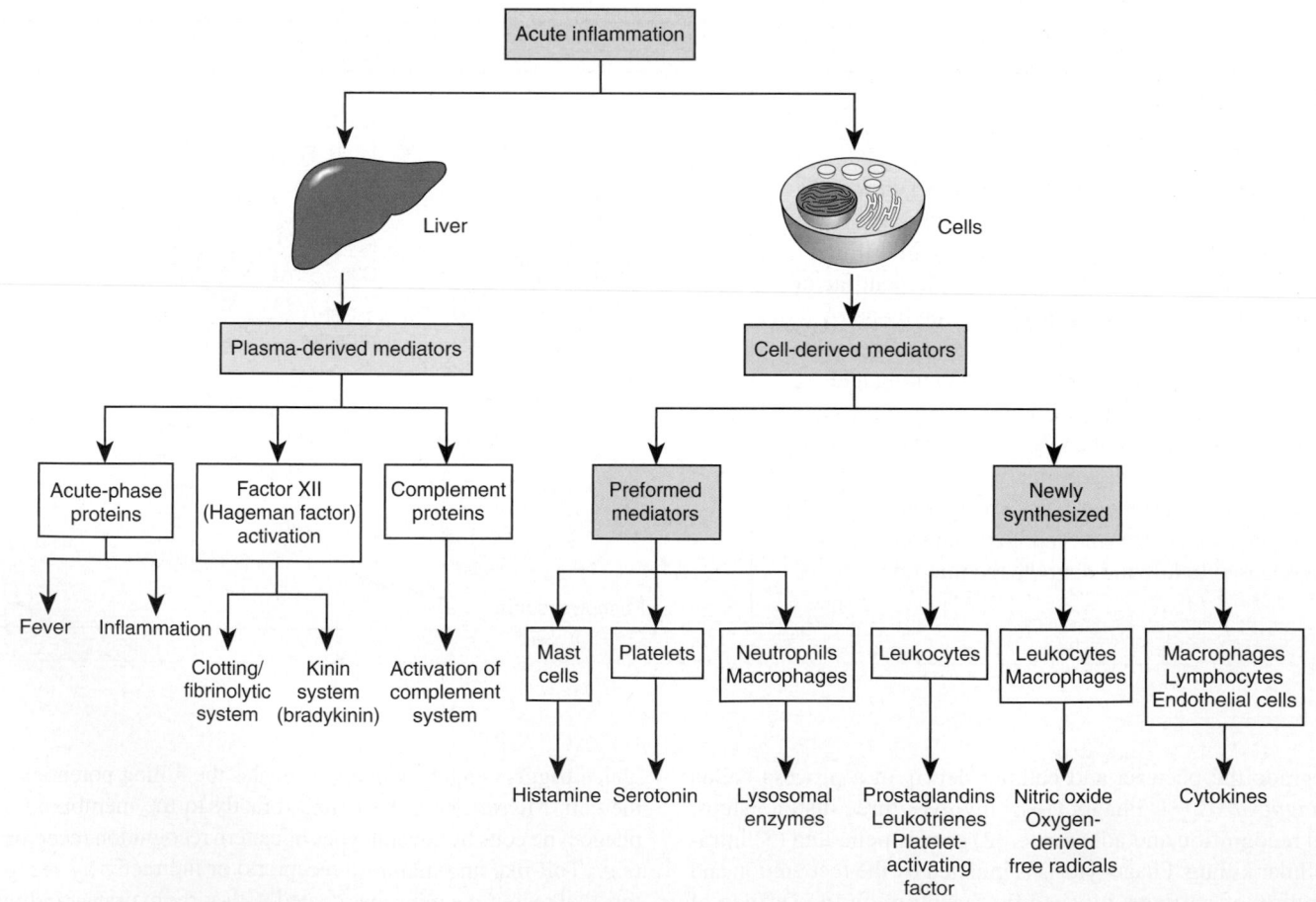

FIGURE 18-3 • Plasma- and cell-derived mediators of acute inflammation.

different types of cells. Once activated and released from the cell, most mediators are short-lived. They may be transformed into inactive metabolites, inactivated by enzymes, or otherwise scavenged or degraded.

Inflammatory mediators can be classified by function: (1) those with vasoactive and smooth muscle–constricting properties such as histamine, arachidonic acid metabolites (prostaglandins and leukotrienes), and platelet-activating factor; (2) plasma proteases that activate members of the complement system, coagulation factors of the clotting cascade, and vasoactive peptides of the kinin system; (3) chemotactic factors such as complement fragments and chemokines; and (4) reactive molecules and cytokines liberated from leukocytes, which when released into the extracellular environment can affect the surrounding tissue and cells.

Histamine. Histamine is present in preformed stores in cells and is therefore among the first mediators to be released during an acute inflammatory reaction. Preformed histamine is widely distributed in tissues, the highest concentrations being found in the connective tissues adjacent to blood vessels. It is also found in circulating blood platelets and basophils. Preformed histamine is found in mast cell granules and is released in response to a variety of stimuli, including trauma and immune reactions involving binding of IgE antibodies. Histamine causes dilation of arterioles and increases the permeability of venules. It acts at the level of the microcirculation by binding to histamine type 1 (H_1) receptors on endothelial cells, and is considered the principal mediator of the immediate transient phase of increased vascular permeability in the acute inflammatory response. Antihistamine drugs (H_1 receptor antagonists), which bind to the H_1 receptors, act competitively to antagonize many of the effects of the immediate inflammatory response.

Arachidonic Acid Metabolites. Arachidonic acid is a 20-carbon unsaturated fatty acid found in phospholipids of cell membranes. Release of arachidonic acid by phospholipases initiates a series of complex reactions that lead to the production of the *eicosanoid* family inflammatory mediators (prostaglandins, leukotrienes, and related metabolites). Eicosanoid synthesis follows one of two pathways: the cyclooxygenase pathway, which culminates in the synthesis of prostaglandins, and the lipoxygenase pathway, which culminates in the synthesis of the leukotrienes (Fig. 18-4).

Several prostaglandins are synthesized from arachidonic acid through the cyclooxygenase metabolic pathway.[17] The prostaglandins (*e.g.*, PGD_2, PGE_2, $PGF_{2\alpha}$, and PGI_2) induce inflammation and potentiate the effects of histamine and other inflammatory mediators. The prostaglandin thromboxane A_2 promotes platelet aggregation and vasoconstriction. Aspirin and the nonsteroidal anti-inflammatory drugs (NSAIDs) reduce inflammation by inactivating the first enzyme in the cyclooxygenase pathway for prostaglandin synthesis.

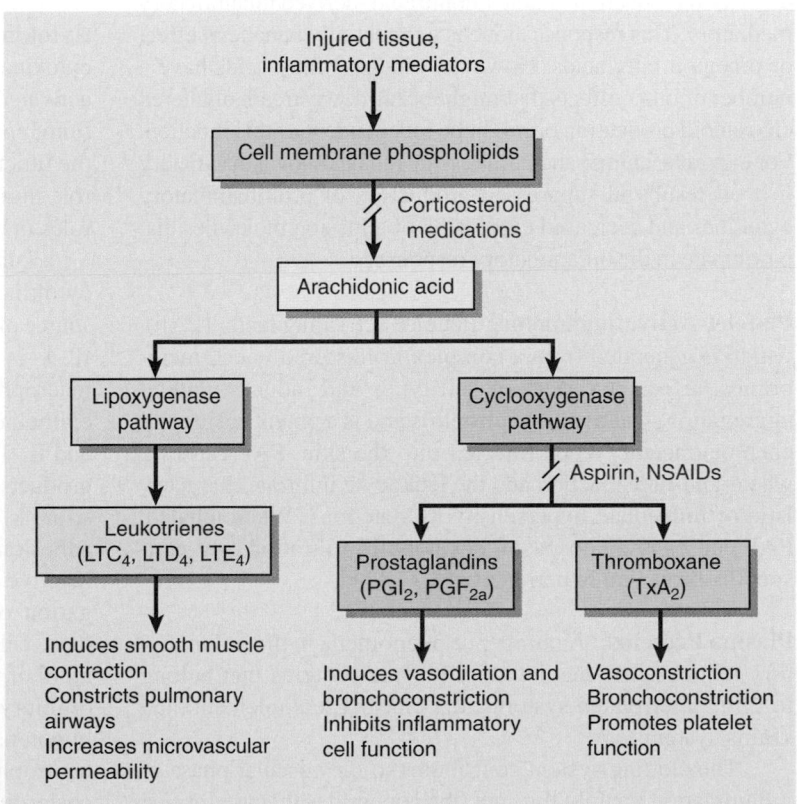

FIGURE 18-4 • The cyclooxygenase and lipoxygenase pathways and sites where the corticosteroids and nonsteroidal anti-inflammatory drugs (NSAIDs) exert their action.

Like the prostaglandins, the leukotrienes are formed from arachidonic acid, but through the lipoxygenase pathway. Histamine and leukotrienes are complementary in action in that they have similar functions. Histamine is produced rapidly and transiently while the more potent leukotrienes are being synthesized. The leukotrienes also have been reported to affect the permeability of the postcapillary venules, the adhesion properties of endothelial cells, and the extravasation and chemotaxis of neutrophils, eosinophils, and monocytes. Leukotrienes (LT) C_4, LTD_4, and LTE_4, collectively known as the *slow-reacting substance of anaphylaxis* (SRS-A), cause slow and sustained constriction of the bronchioles and are important inflammatory mediators in bronchial asthma and anaphylaxis.

There has been recent interest in dietary modification of the inflammatory response through the use of omega-3 polyunsaturated fatty acids, specifically eicosapentaenoic acid and docosahexaenoic acid, which are present in oily fish and fish oil.[18-20] Alpha-linolenic acid, which is present in flaxseed, canola oil, green leafy vegetables, walnuts, and soybeans, is another source of omega-3 fatty acid. The omega-3 polyunsaturated fatty acids, which are considered antithrombotic and anti-inflammatory, are structurally different from the prothrombotic and proinflammatory omega-6 polyunsaturated fatty acids, which are present in most seeds, vegetable oils, and meats. Typically, the cell membranes of inflammatory cells contain high proportions of omega-6 arachidonic acid, which is the source of prostaglandin and leukotriene inflammatory mediators. Eating oily fish and other foods that are high in omega-3 fatty acids results in partial replacement of arachidonic acid in inflammatory cell membranes by eicosapentaenoic acid, a change that leads to decreased production of arachidonic acid–derived inflammatory mediators. This response alone is a potentially beneficial effect of omega-3 fatty acids. However, omega-3 fatty acids have a number of other effects that might occur downstream of altered eicosanoid production or might be independent of this function. For example, animal and human research has shown that dietary fish oil results in suppressed production of proinflammatory cytokines and decreased expression of adhesion molecules that participate in the inflammatory response.

Platelet-Activating Factor.   Platelet-activating factor (PAF), which is generated from a complex lipid stored in cell membranes, affects a variety of cell types and induces platelet aggregation. It activates neutrophils and is a potent eosinophil chemoattractant. When injected into the skin, PAF causes a wheal-and-flare reaction and the leukocyte infiltrate characteristic of immediate hypersensitivity reactions. When inhaled, PAF causes bronchospasm, eosinophil infiltration, and nonspecific bronchial hyperreactivity.

Plasma Proteins.   A number of phenomena in the inflammatory response are mediated by plasma proteins that belong to three interrelated systems, the clotting, complement, and kinins systems.

The clotting system contributes to the vascular phase of inflammation, mainly through fibrinopeptides that are formed during the final steps of the clotting process (discussed in Chapter 13). The protease thrombin, which binds to receptors called *protease-activated receptors* (PARs), provides the final link between the coagulation system and inflammation. Engagement of the so-called type-1 receptor (PAR-1) by proteases, particularly thrombin, triggers several responses that induce inflammation, including production of chemokines, expression of endothelial adhesion molecules, induction of prostaglandin synthesis, and production of PAF.

The complement system consists of 20 component proteins (and their cleavage products) that are found in greatest concentration in the plasma (see Chapter 17). The complement proteins are present in inactive forms in the plasma. Many of them are activated to become proteolytic enzymes that degrade other complement proteins, thus forming a cascade that plays an important role in both immunity and inflammation. Complement fragments contribute to the inflammatory response by causing vasodilation, increasing vascular permeability, and enhancing the activity of phagocytes.[2]

The kinin system generates vasoactive peptides from plasma proteins called *kininogens,* by the action of proteases called *kallikreins.*[2] Activation of the kinin system results in release of bradykinin, which increases vascular permeability and causes contraction of smooth muscle, dilation of blood vessels, and pain when injected into the skin. These effects are similar to those of histamine. The action of bradykinin is short lived because it is quickly inactivated by an enzyme called *kininase.* Any bradykinin that escapes inactivation by the kininase enzyme is degraded by the angiotensin-converting enzyme in the lung.

Cytokines and Chemokines.   As discussed in Chapter 17, cytokines are proteins produced by many cell types (principally activated macrophages and lymphocytes, but also endothelium, epithelium, and connective tissue types) that modulate the function of other cells.[1,2,9,21] Although well known for their role in immune responses, these products also play important roles in both acute and chronic inflammation.

Tumor necrosis factor-α and IL-1 are two of the major cytokines that mediate inflammation. The major cellular source of TNF-α and IL-1 is activated macrophages (Fig. 18-5). IL-1 is also produced by many cell types other than macrophages, including neutrophils, endothelial cells, and epithelial cells (*e.g.,* keratinocytes). The secretion of TNF-α and IL-1 can be stimulated by endotoxin and other microbial products, immune cells, injury, and a variety of inflammatory stimuli. TNF-α and IL-1 induce endothelial cells to express adhesion molecules and release cytokines, chemokines, and reactive oxygen species. TNF-α induces priming and aggregation of neutrophils, leading to augmented responses of these cells to other mediators. IL-1 and TNF-α are also mediators of the acute-phase responses associated with infection or injury. Features of these systemic responses include fever, hypotension and increased heart rate, anorexia, release of neutrophils into the circulation, and increased levels of corticosteroid hormones.

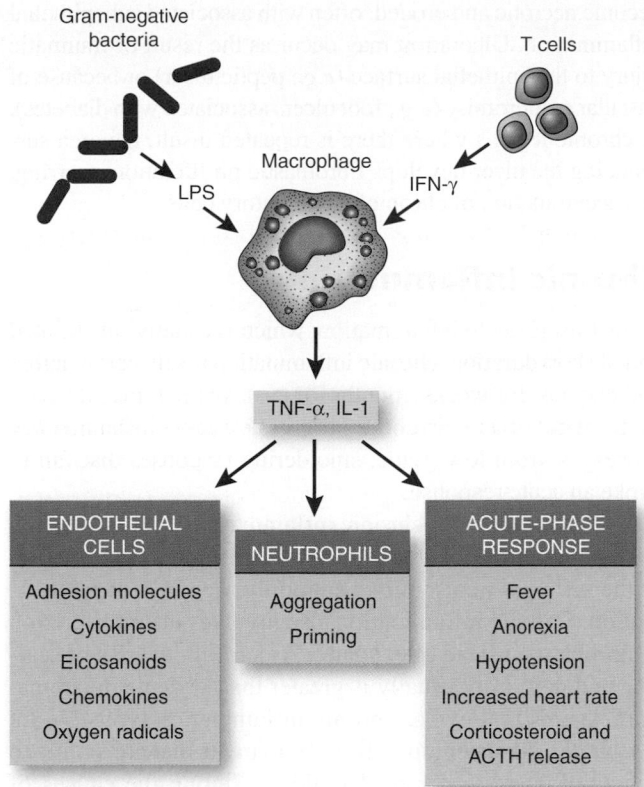

FIGURE 18-5 • Central role of interleukin (IL)-1 and tumor necrosis factor (TNF)-α in the acute inflammatory response. Lipopolysaccharide (LPS) and interferon (IFN)-γ activate macrophages to release inflammatory cytokines, principally IL-1 and TNF-α, responsible for directing both local and systemic inflammatory responses. ACTH, adrenocorticotropic hormone. (From Murphy H. S. [2007]. Inflammation. In Rubin R., Strayer D. E. [Eds.], *Rubin's pathology: Clinicopathologic foundations of medicine* [5th ed., p. 50]. Philadelphia: Lippincott Williams & Wilkins.)

Chemotactic cytokines, or *chemokines,* are a family of small proteins that act primarily as chemoattractants to recruit and direct the migration of immune and inflammatory cells[22] (discussed in Chapter 17). Chemokines generate a chemotactic gradient by binding to proteoglycans on the surface of endothelial cells or in the extracellular matrix. As a result, high concentrations of chemokines persist at sites of tissue injury or infection. Two classes of chemokines have been identified: inflammatory chemokines and homing chemokines. Inflammatory chemokines are produced in response to bacterial toxins and inflammatory cytokines (*i.e.,* IL-1, TNF-α). These chemokines recruit leukocytes during an inflammatory response. Homing chemokines are constitutively expressed and are up-regulated during inflammatory reactions and immune responses.

Nitric Oxide and Oxygen-Derived Free Radicals. Nitric oxide (NO) and oxygen-derived free radicals play an important role in the inflammatory response. NO, which is produced by a variety of cells, plays multiple roles in inflammation,

including smooth muscle relaxation and antagonism of platelet adhesion, aggregation, and degranulation; and it serves as an endogenous regulator of leukocyte recruitment. Blocking of NO production under normal conditions promotes leukocyte rolling and adhesion to postcapillary venules, and delivery of exogenous NO reduces leukocyte recruitment.[2] Thus, production of NO appears to be a compensatory mechanism that reduces the cellular phase of inflammation. Impaired production of NO by vascular endothelial cells is implicated in the inflammatory changes that occur with atherosclerosis (see Chapter 22). NO and its derivatives also have antimicrobial actions and thus NO is also a host mediator against infection.

Oxygen free radicals may be released extracellularly from leukocytes after exposure to microbes, cytokines, and immune complexes, or during the phagocytic process that occurs during the cellular phase of the inflammatory process. The superoxide radical, hydrogen peroxide, and the hydroxyl radical (discussed in Chapter 5) are the major species produced in the cell. These species can combine with NO to form other reactive nitrogen intermediates. Extracellular release of low levels of these potent mediators can increase the expression of cytokines and endothelial adhesion molecules, amplifying the cascade that elicits the inflammatory process.[2] At higher levels, these potent mediators can produce endothelial cell damage, with a resultant increase in vascular permeability; inactivate antiproteases, such as α_1-antitrypsin, which protects against lung damage in smokers; and produce injury to other cell types, including red blood cells.[2]

Local Manifestations

Although all acute inflammatory reactions are characterized by vascular changes and leukocyte infiltration, the severity of the reaction, its specific cause, and the site of involvement introduce variations in its manifestations and clinical correlates. These manifestations can range from swelling and the formation of exudates to abscess formation or ulceration.

Characteristically, the acute inflammatory response involves the production of exudates. These exudates vary in terms of fluid type, plasma protein content, and the presence or absence of cells. They can be serous, hemorrhagic, fibrinous, membranous, or purulent. Often the exudate is composed of a combination of these types. *Serous exudates* are watery fluids low in protein content that result from plasma entering the inflammatory site. *Hemorrhagic exudates* occur when there is severe tissue injury that damages blood vessels or when there is significant leakage of red cells from the capillaries. *Fibrinous exudates* contain large amounts of fibrinogen and form a thick and sticky meshwork, much like the fibers of a blood clot. *Membranous* or *pseudomembranous exudates* develop on mucous membrane surfaces and are composed of necrotic cells enmeshed in a fibropurulent exudate.

A *purulent* or *suppurative exudate* contains pus, which is composed of degraded white blood cells, proteins, and tissue debris. Certain microorganisms, such as *Staphylococcus,* are more likely to induce localized suppurative inflammation than others. An abscess is a localized area of inflammation containing a purulent exudate (Fig. 18-6). Abscesses typically have a central necrotic core containing purulent exudates surrounded by a layer of neutrophils.[2] Fibroblasts may eventually enter the area and wall off the abscess. Because antimicrobial agents cannot penetrate the abscess wall, surgical incision and drainage may be required to effect a cure.

An *ulceration* refers to a site of inflammation where an epithelial surface (*e.g.*, skin or gastrointestinal epithelium) has

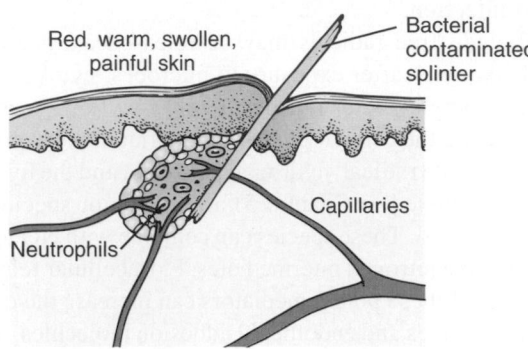

A Inflammation
Capillary dilation, fluid exudation, neutrophil migration

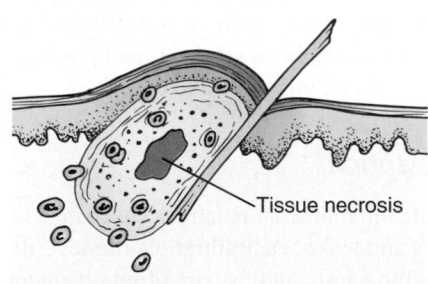

B Suppuration
Development of suppurative or purulent exudate containing degraded neutrophils and tissue debris

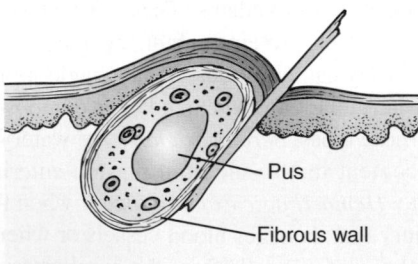

C Abscess formation
Walling off of the area of purulent (pus) exudate to form an abscess

FIGURE 18-6 • Abscess formation. **(A)** Bacterial invasion and development of inflammation. **(B)** Continued bacterial growth, neutrophil migration, liquefaction tissue necrosis, and development of a purulent exudate. **(C)** Walling off of the inflamed area and its purulent exudate to form an abscess.

become necrotic and eroded, often with associated subepithelial inflammation. Ulceration may occur as the result of traumatic injury to the epithelial surface (*e.g.*, peptic ulcer) or because of vascular compromise (*e.g.*, foot ulcers associated with diabetes). In chronic lesions where there is repeated insult, the area surrounding the ulcer develops fibroblastic proliferation, scarring, and accumulation of chronic inflammatory cells.[2]

Chronic Inflammation

In contrast to acute inflammation, which is usually self-limited and of short duration, chronic inflammation is self-perpetuating and may last for weeks, months, or even years. It may develop as the result of a recurrent or progressive acute inflammatory process or from low-grade, smoldering responses that fail to evoke an acute response.

Characteristic of chronic inflammation is an infiltration by mononuclear cells (macrophages) and lymphocytes instead of the influx of neutrophils commonly seen in acute inflammation. Chronic inflammation also involves the proliferation of fibroblasts instead of exudates. As a result, the risk of scarring and deformity usually is greater than in acute inflammation. Agents that evoke chronic inflammation typically are low-grade, persistent infections or irritants that are unable to penetrate deeply or spread rapidly. Among the causes of chronic inflammation are foreign bodies such as talc, silica, asbestos, and surgical suture materials. Many viruses provoke chronic inflammatory responses, as do certain bacteria, fungi, and larger parasites of moderate to low virulence. Examples are the tubercle bacillus, the treponeme of syphilis, and the *Actinomyces* species. The presence of injured tissue such as that surrounding a healing fracture also may incite chronic inflammation. Immunologic mechanisms are thought to play an important role in chronic inflammation. The two patterns of chronic inflammation are a nonspecific chronic inflammation and granulomatous inflammation.

Nonspecific Chronic Inflammation

Nonspecific chronic inflammation involves a diffuse accumulation of macrophages and lymphocytes at the site of injury. Ongoing chemotaxis causes macrophages to infiltrate the inflamed site, where they accumulate owing to prolonged survival and immobilization. These mechanisms lead to fibroblast proliferation, with subsequent scar formation that in many cases replaces the normal connective tissue or the functional parenchymal tissues of the involved structures. For example, scar tissue resulting from chronic inflammation of the bowel causes narrowing of the bowel lumen.

Granulomatous Inflammation

A granulomatous lesion is a distinctive form of chronic inflammation. A *granuloma* typically is a small, 1- to 2-mm lesion in which there is a massing of macrophages surrounded by lymphocytes. These modified macrophages resemble epithelial cells and sometimes are called *epithelioid cells*.[1,2] Like other macrophages, the epithelioid cells are derived originally from blood monocytes. Granulomatous inflammation is associated with foreign bodies such as splinters, sutures, silica, and asbestos and with microorganisms that cause tuberculosis, syphilis, sarcoidosis, deep fungal infections, and brucellosis. These types of agents have one thing in common: they are poorly digested and usually are not easily controlled by other inflammatory mechanisms. The epithelioid cells in granulomatous inflammation may clump in a mass or coalesce, forming a multinucleated giant cell that attempts to surround the foreign agent (Fig. 18-7). A dense membrane of connective tissue eventually encapsulates the lesion and isolates it. These cells are often referred to as *foreign body giant cells*.

Systemic Manifestations of Inflammation

Under optimal conditions, the inflammatory response remains confined to a localized area. In some cases, however, local injury can result in prominent systemic manifestations as inflammatory mediators are released into the circulation. The most prominent systemic manifestations of inflammation include the acute-phase response, alterations in white blood cell count (leukocytosis or leukopenia), and fever. Localized acute and chronic inflammation may extend to the lymphatic system and lead to a reaction in the lymph nodes that drain the affected area.

Acute-Phase Response

Along with the cellular responses that occur during the inflammatory response, a constellation of systemic effects called the *acute-phase response* occurs. The acute-phase response, which usually begins within hours or days of the onset of inflammation or infection, includes changes in the concentrations of plasma proteins (*i.e.,* acute-phase proteins),

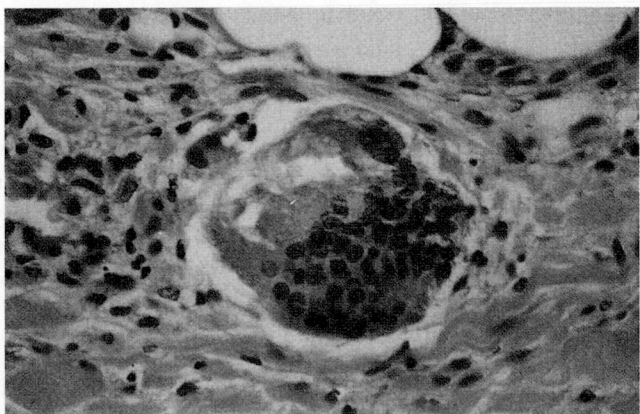

FIGURE 18-7 • Foreign body giant cell. The numerous nuclei are randomly arranged in the cytoplasm. (From Rubin E., Farber J. L. [Eds.]. [1999]. *Pathology* [3rd ed., p. 40]. Philadelphia: Lippincott-Raven.)

skeletal muscle catabolism, negative nitrogen balance, elevated erythrocyte sedimentation rate, and increased numbers of leukocytes. These responses are generated by the release of cytokines, particularly IL-1, IL-6, and TNF-α. These cytokines affect the thermoregulatory center in the hypothalamus to produce fever, the most obvious sign of the acute-phase response. IL-1 and other cytokines induce an increase in the number and immaturity of circulating neutrophils by stimulating their production in the bone marrow. Other manifestations of the acute-phase response include anorexia, somnolence, and malaise, probably because of the actions of IL-1 and TNF-α on the central nervous system. The metabolic changes, including skeletal muscle catabolism, provide amino acids that can be used in the immune response and for tissue repair. In general, the acute-phase response serves to coordinate the various changes in body function to enable an optimal host response.

In severe bacterial infections (sepsis), the large quantities of microorganisms in the blood result in an uncontrolled inflammatory response with the production and release of enormous quantities of inflammatory cytokines (most notably IL-1 and TNF-α) and development of what is referred to as the *systemic inflammatory response syndrome*[23] (see Chapter 26). These cytokines cause generalized vasodilation, increased vascular permeability, intravascular fluid loss, myocardial depression, and circulatory shock.

Acute-Phase Proteins. During the acute-phase response, the liver dramatically increases the synthesis of acute-phase proteins such as fibrinogen, C-reactive protein (CRP), serum amyloid A protein (SAA), which serve several different defense functions.[1,2] The synthesis of these proteins is up-regulated by cytokines, especially TNF-α, IL-1 (for SAA), and IL-6 (for fibrinogen and CRP).

CRP was named because it precipitated with the C fraction (C-polypeptide) of pneumococci. The function of CRP is thought to be protective, in that it binds to the surface of invading microorganisms and targets them for destruction by complement and phagocytosis. Although everyone maintains a low level of CRP, this level rises when there is an acute inflammatory response.[24,25] Recent interest has focused on the use of high-sensitivity CRP (hsCRP) as a marker for increased risk of myocardial infarction in persons with coronary heart disease.[26,27] It is believed that inflammation involving atherosclerotic plaques in coronary arteries may predispose to thrombosis and myocardial infarction (see Chapter 22).

During the acute-phase response, SAA protein replaces apolipoprotein A, a component of high-density lipoprotein (HDL) particles; this presumably increases the transfer of HDL from liver cells to macrophages, which can then use these particles for energy. The rise in fibrinogen causes red cells to form stacks (rouleaux) that sediment more rapidly than do individual erythrocytes. This is the basis for the accelerated erythrocyte sedimentation rate (ESR) that occurs in disease conditions characterized by a systemic inflammatory response.

White Blood Cell Response

Leukocytosis, or increased white blood cells, is a frequent sign of an inflammatory response, especially one caused by bacterial infection. The white blood cell count commonly increases from a normal value of 4000 to 10,000 cells/μL to 15,000 to 20,000 cells/μL in acute inflammatory conditions. After being released from the bone marrow, circulating neutrophils have a life span of only about 10 hours and therefore must be constantly replaced if their numbers are to be adequate. With excessive demand for phagocytes, immature forms of neutrophils (bands) are released from the bone marrow.

Bacterial infections produce a relatively selective increase in neutrophils (neutrophilia), whereas parasitic and allergic responses induce eosinophilia. Viral infections tend to produce a decrease in neutrophils (neutropenia) and an increase in lymphocytes (lymphocytosis).[3] A decrease in white blood cells (leukopenia) may occur with overwhelming infections or an impaired ability to produce white blood cells.

Lymphadenitis

Localized acute and chronic inflammation may lead to a reaction in the lymph nodes that drain the affected area. This response represents a nonspecific response to mediators released from the injured tissue or an immunologic response to a specific antigen. Painful palpable nodes are more commonly associated with inflammatory processes, whereas nonpainful lymph nodes are more characteristic of neoplasms.

IN SUMMARY, inflammation describes a local response to tissue injury and can present as an acute or chronic condition. The classic signs of an acute inflammatory response are redness, swelling, local heat, pain, and loss of function. Acute inflammation is orchestrated by the endothelial cells that line blood vessels, phagocytic leukocytes (mainly neutrophils and monocytes) that circulate in the blood, and tissue cells (macrophages, mast cells) that direct the tissues responses. Acute inflammation involves a hemodynamic phase during which blood flow and capillary permeability are increased, and a cellular phase during which phagocytic white blood cells move into the area to engulf and degrade the inciting agent. The inflammatory response is orchestrated by chemical mediators such as cytokines and chemokines, histamine, prostaglandins, PAF, complement fragments, and reactive molecules liberated by leukocytes. Acute inflammation may involve the production of exudates containing serous fluid (serous exudate), red blood cells (hemorrhagic exudate), fibrinogen (fibrinous exudate), or tissue debris and white blood cell breakdown products (purulent exudate).

In contrast to acute inflammation, which is self-limiting, chronic inflammation is prolonged and usually is caused by persistent irritants, most of which are insoluble and resistant to phagocytosis and other inflammatory mechanisms. Chronic inflammation involves the presence of mononuclear cells (lymphocytes and macrophages) rather than granulocytes.

The systemic manifestations of inflammation include the systemic effects of the acute-phase response, such as fever and lethargy; increased ESR and levels of CRP and other acute-phase proteins; leukocytosis or, in some cases, leukopenia; and enlargement of the lymph nodes that drain the affected area. ■

CONCEPTS in action **ANIMATION**

TISSUE REPAIR AND WOUND HEALING

After completing this section of the chapter, you should be able to meet the following objectives:

- Define the terms *parenchymal* and *stromal* as they relate to the tissues of an organ.
- Compare labile, stable, and permanent cell types in terms of their capacity for regeneration.
- Describe healing by primary and secondary intention.
- Explain the effects of soluble mediators and the extracellular matrix on tissue repair and wound healing.
- Trace the wound-healing process through the inflammatory, proliferative, and remodeling phases.
- Explain the effects of malnutrition; ischemia and oxygen deprivation; impaired immune and inflammatory responses; and infection, wound separation, and foreign bodies on wound healing.
- Discuss the effect of age on wound healing.

Tissue Repair

Tissue repair, which overlaps the inflammatory process, is a response to tissue injury and represents an attempt to maintain normal body structure and function. It can take the form of regeneration in which the injured cells are replaced with cells of the same type, sometimes leaving no residual trace of previous injury, or it can take the form of replacement by connective tissue, which leaves a permanent scar. Both regeneration and repair by connective tissue replacement are determined by similar mechanisms involving cell migration, proliferation, and differentiation, as well as interaction with the extracellular matrix.

Tissue Regeneration

Body organs and tissues are composed of two types of structures: parenchymal and stromal. The parenchymal (from the Greek for "anything poured in") tissues contain the functioning cells of an organ or body part (*e.g.*, hepatocytes, renal tubu-

TISSUE REPAIR AND WOUND HEALING

- Injured tissues can be repaired by regeneration of the injured tissue cells with cells of the same tissue or parenchymal type, or by connective repair processes in which scar tissue is used to effect healing.

- Regeneration is limited to tissues with cells that are able to undergo mitosis.

- Connective tissue repair occurs by primary or secondary intention and involves the inflammatory phase, the proliferative phase, and remodeling phase of the wound healing process.

- Wound healing is impaired by conditions that diminish blood flow and oxygen delivery, restrict nutrients and other materials needed for healing, and depress the inflammatory and immune responses; and by infection, wound separation, and the presence of foreign bodies.

lar cells). The stromal tissues (from the Greek for "something laid out to lie on") consist of the supporting connective tissues, blood vessels, extracellular matrix, and nerve fibers.

Tissue regeneration involves replacement of the injured tissue with cells of the same type, leaving little or no evidence of the previous injury. The capacity for regeneration varies with the tissue and cell type. Body cells are divided into three types according to their ability to undergo regeneration: labile, stable, or permanent cells.[28,29] *Labile cells* are those that continue to divide and replicate throughout life, replacing cells that are continually being destroyed. They include the surface epithelial cells of the skin, oral cavity, vagina, and cervix; the columnar epithelium of the gastrointestinal tract, uterus, and fallopian tubes; the transitional epithelium of the urinary tract; and bone marrow cells. *Stable cells* are those that normally stop dividing when growth ceases. However, these cells are capable of undergoing regeneration when confronted with an appropriate stimulus and are thus capable of reconstituting the tissue of origin. This category includes the parenchymal cells of the liver and kidney, smooth muscle cells, and vascular endothelial cells. *Permanent* or *fixed cells* cannot undergo mitotic division. The fixed cells include nerve cells, skeletal muscle cells, and cardiac muscle cells. These cells do not normally regenerate; once destroyed, they are replaced with fibrous scar tissue that lacks the functional characteristics of the destroyed tissue.

Fibrous Tissue Repair

Severe or persistent injury with damage to both the parenchymal cells and extracellular matrix leads to a situation in which the repair cannot be accomplished with regeneration alone. Under these conditions, repair occurs by replacement with connective tissue, a process that involves generation of granulation tissue and formation of scar tissue.

Granulation tissue is a glistening red, moist connective tissue that contains newly formed capillaries, proliferating fibroblasts, and residual inflammatory cells. The development of granulation tissue involves the growth of new capillaries (angiogenesis), fibrogenesis, and involution to the formation of scar tissue. Angiogenesis involves the generation and sprouting of new blood vessels from preexisting vessels. These sprouting capillaries tend to protrude from the surface of the wound as minute red granules, imparting the name *granulation tissue*. Eventually, portions of the new capillary bed differentiate into arterioles and venules.

Fibrogenesis involves the influx of activated fibroblasts. Activated fibroblasts secrete extracellular matrix (ECM) components, including fibronectin, hyaluronic acid, proteoglycans, and collagen (to be discussed). Fibronectin and hyaluronic acid are the first to be deposited in the healing wound, and proteoglycans appear later. Because the proteoglycans are hydrophilic, their accumulation contributes to the edematous appearance of the wound. The initiation of collagen synthesis contributes to the subsequent formation of scar tissue.

Scar formation builds on the granulation tissue framework of new vessels and loose ECM. The process occurs in two phases: (1) emigration and proliferation of fibroblasts into the site of injury, and (2) deposition of extracellular matrix by these cells. As healing progresses, the number of proliferating fibroblasts and new vessels decreases and there is increased synthesis and deposition of collagen. Collagen synthesis is important to the development of strength in the healing wound site. Ultimately, the granulation tissue scaffolding evolves into a scar composed of largely inactive spindle-shaped fibroblasts, dense collagen fibers, fragments of elastic tissue, and other ECM components. As the scar matures, vascular degeneration eventually transforms the highly vascular granulation tissue into a pale, largely avascular scar.

Regulation of the Healing Process

Tissue healing is regulated by the actions of chemical mediators and growth factors that mediate the healing process as well as orchestrate the interactions between the extracellular and cell matrix.[28–36]

Chemical Mediators and Growth Factors. Considerable research has contributed to the understanding of chemical mediators and growth factors that orchestrate the healing process. These chemical mediators and growth factors are released in an orderly manner from many of the cells that participate in tissue regeneration and the healing process. The chemical mediators include the interleukins, interferons, TNF-α, and arachidonic acid derivatives (prostaglandins and leukotrienes) that participate in the inflammatory response. The growth factors are hormone-like molecules that interact with specific cell surface receptors to control processes involved in tissue repair and wound healing.[37–40] They may act on adjacent cells or on the cell producing the growth factor. The growth factors are named for their tissue of origin (*e.g.,* platelet-derived growth factor

[PDGF], fibroblast growth factor [FGF]), their biologic activity (*e.g.,* transforming growth factor [TGF]), or the cells on which they act (*e.g.,* epithelial growth factor [EGF]). The growth factors control the proliferation, differentiation, and metabolism of cells during wound healing. They assist in regulating the inflammatory process; serve as chemoattractants for neutrophils, monocytes (macrophages), fibroblasts, and epithelial cells; stimulate angiogenesis; and contribute to the generation of the ECM.

Extracellular Matrix. The understanding of tissue regeneration and repair has expanded over the past several decades to encompass the complex environment of the ECM. The ECM is secreted locally and assembles into a network of spaces surrounding tissue cells. There are three basic components of the ECM: fibrous structural proteins (*e.g.,* collagen and elastin fibers), water-hydrated gels (*e.g.,* proteoglycans and hyaluronic acid) that permit resilience and lubrication, and adhesive glycoproteins (*e.g.,* fibronectin and laminin) that connect the matrix elements to each other and to cells (see Chapter 4). The ECM occurs in two basic forms: (1) the *basement membrane* that surrounds epithelial, endothelial, and smooth muscle cells; and (2) the *interstitial matrix,* which is present in the spaces between cells in connective tissue and between the epithelium and supporting cells of blood vessels.

The ECM provides turgor to soft tissue and rigidity to bone; it supplies the substratum for cell adhesion; it is involved in the regulation of growth, movement, and differentiation of the cells surrounding it; and it provides for the storage and presentation of regulatory molecules that control the repair process. The ECM also provides the scaffolding for tissue renewal. Although the cells in many tissues are capable of regeneration, injury does not always result in restoration of normal structure unless the ECM is intact. The integrity of the underlying basement membrane, in particular, is critical to the regeneration of tissue. When the basement membrane is disrupted, cells proliferate in a haphazard way, resulting in disorganized and nonfunctional tissues.

Critical to the process of wound healing is the transition from granulation tissue to scar tissue, which involves shifts in the composition of the ECM. In the transitional process, the ECM components are degraded by proteases (enzymes) that are secreted locally by a variety of cells (fibroblasts, macrophages, neutrophils, synovial cells, and epithelial cells). Some of the proteases, such as the collagenases, are highly specific, cleaving particular proteins at a small number of sites.[41] This allows for the structural integrity of the ECM to be retained while cell migration occurs. Because of their potential to produce havoc in tissues, the actions of the proteases are tightly controlled. They are typically elaborated in an inactive form that must be activated by chemical mediators that are present at the site of injury, and they are rapidly inactivated by tissue inhibitors. Recent research has focused on the unregulated action of the proteases in disorders such as cartilage matrix breakdown in arthritis and neuroinflammation in multiple sclerosis.[41]

Wound Healing

Injured tissues are repaired by regeneration of parenchymal cells or by connective tissue repair in which scar tissue is substituted for the parenchymal cells of the injured tissue. The primary objective of the healing process is to fill the gap created by tissue destruction and to restore the structural continuity of the injured part. When regeneration cannot occur, healing by replacement with a connective tissue scar provides the means for maintaining this continuity. Although scar tissue fills the gap created by tissue death, it does not repair the structure with functioning parenchymal cells. Because the regenerative capabilities of most tissues are limited, wound healing usually involves some connective tissue repair. The following discussion particularly addresses skin wounds.

Healing by Primary and Secondary Intention

Depending on the extent of tissue loss, wound closure and healing occur by *primary* or *secondary intention* (Fig. 18-8). A sutured surgical incision is an example of healing by primary intention. Larger wounds (*e.g.,* burns and large surface wounds) that have a greater loss of tissue and contamination heal by secondary intention. Healing by secondary intention is slower than healing by primary intention and results in the formation of larger amounts of scar tissue. A wound that might otherwise have healed by primary intention may become infected and heal by secondary intention.

Phases of Wound Healing

Wound healing is commonly divided into three phases: (1) the inflammatory phase, (2) the proliferative phase, and (3) the mat-

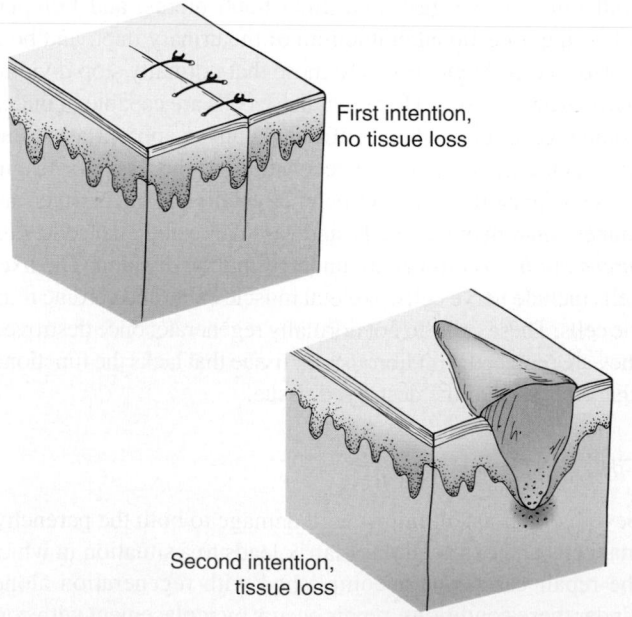

First intention,
no tissue loss

Second intention,
tissue loss

FIGURE 18-8 • Healing of a skin wound by first and second intention.

urational or remodeling phase.[28,29,33–37] The duration of the phases is fairly predictable in wounds healing by primary intention. In wounds healing by secondary intention, the process depends on the extent of injury and the healing environment.

Inflammatory Phase. The inflammatory phase of wound healing begins at the time of injury and is a critical period because it prepares the wound environment for healing. It includes hemostasis (see Chapter 13) and the vascular and cellular phases of inflammation. Hemostatic processes are activated immediately at the time of injury. There is constriction of injured blood vessels and initiation of blood clotting through platelet activation and aggregation. After a brief period of constriction, the same vessels dilate and capillaries increase their permeability, allowing plasma and blood components to leak into the injured area. In small surface wounds, the clot loses fluid and becomes a hard, desiccated scab that protects the area.

The cellular phase of inflammation follows and is evidenced by the migration of phagocytic white blood cells that digest and remove invading organisms, fibrin, extracellular debris, and other foreign matter. The neutrophils are the first cells to arrive and are usually gone by day 3 or 4. They ingest bacteria and cellular debris. After approximately 24 hours, macrophages, which are larger phagocytic cells, enter the wound area and remain for an extended period. These cells, arising from blood monocytes, are essential to the healing process. Their functions include phagocytosis and release of growth factors that stimulate epithelial cell growth and angiogenesis, and attract fibroblasts. When a large defect occurs in deeper tissues, neutrophils and macrophages are required to remove the debris and facilitate wound closure. Although a wound may heal in the absence of neutrophils, it cannot heal in the absence of macrophages.

Proliferative Phase. The proliferative phase of healing usually begins within 2 to 3 days of injury and may last as long as 3 weeks in wounds healing by primary intention. The primary processes during this time focus on the building of new tissue to fill the wound space. The key cell during this phase is the *fibroblast*. The fibroblast is a connective tissue cell that synthesizes and secretes collagen and other intercellular elements needed for wound healing. Fibroblasts also produce a family of growth factors that induce angiogenesis and endothelial cell proliferation and migration.

As early as 24 to 48 hours after injury, fibroblasts and vascular endothelial cells begin proliferating to form the granulation tissue that serves as the foundation for scar tissue development. This tissue is fragile and bleeds easily because of the numerous, newly developed capillary buds. Wounds that heal by secondary intention have more necrotic debris and exudate that must be removed, and they involve larger amounts of granulation tissue. The newly formed blood vessels are semipermeable and allow plasma proteins and white blood cells to leak into the tissues.

The final component of the proliferative phase is epithelialization, which is the migration, proliferation, and differentiation of the epithelial cells at the wound edges to form a new surface layer that is similar to the one destroyed by the injury. In wounds that heal by primary intention, these epidermal cells proliferate and seal the wound within 24 to 48 hours.[29] Because epithelial cell migration requires a moist vascular wound surface and is impeded by a dry or necrotic wound surface, epithelialization is delayed in open wounds until a bed of granulation tissue has formed. When a scab has formed on the wound, the epithelial cells migrate between it and the underlying viable tissue; when a significant portion of the wound has been covered with epithelial tissue, the scab lifts off.

At times, excessive granulation tissue, sometimes referred to as *proud flesh,* may form and extend above the edges of the wound, preventing reepithelialization from taking place. Surgical removal or chemical cauterization of the defect allows healing to proceed.

As the proliferative phase progresses, there is continued accumulation of collagen and proliferation of fibroblasts. Collagen synthesis reaches a peak within 5 to 7 days and continues for several weeks, depending on wound size. By the second week, the white blood cells have largely left the area, the edema has diminished, and the wound begins to blanch as the small blood vessels become thrombosed and degenerate.

Remodeling Phase. The third phase of wound healing, the remodeling process, begins approximately 3 weeks after injury and can continue for 6 months or longer, depending on the extent of the wound. As the term implies, there is continued remodeling of scar tissue by simultaneous synthesis of collagen by fibroblasts and lysis by collagenase enzymes. As a result of these two processes, the architecture of the scar becomes reoriented to increase the tensile strength of the wound.

Most wounds do not regain the full tensile strength of unwounded skin after healing is completed. Carefully sutured wounds immediately after surgery have approximately 70% of the strength of unwounded skin, largely because of the placement of the sutures. This allows persons to move about freely after surgery without fear of wound separation. When the sutures are removed, usually at the end of the first week, wound strength is approximately 10%. It increases rapidly over the next 4 weeks and then slows, reaching a plateau of approximately 70% to 80% of the tensile strength of unwounded skin at the end of 3 months.[29] An injury that heals by secondary intention undergoes wound contraction during the proliferative and remodeling phases. As a result, the scar that forms is considerably smaller than the original wound. Cosmetically, this may be desirable because it reduces the size of the visible defect. However, contraction of scar tissue over joints and other body structures tends to limit movement and cause deformities. As a result of loss of elasticity, scar tissue that is stretched fails to return to its original length.

An abnormality in healing by scar tissue repair is *keloid* formation. Keloids are tumor-like masses caused by excess production of scar tissue (Fig. 18-9). The tendency toward development of keloids is more common in African Americans and seems to have a genetic basis.

Understanding • Wound Healing

Wound healing involves the restoration of the integrity of injured tissue. The healing of skin wounds, which are commonly used to illustrate the general principles of wound healing, is generally divided into three phases: (1) the inflammatory phase, (2) the proliferative phase, and (3) the wound contraction and remodeling phase. Each of these phases is mediated through cytokines and growth factors.

❶ Inflammatory Phase

The inflammatory phase begins at the time of injury with the formation of a blood clot and the migration of phagocytic white blood cells into the wound site. The first cells to arrive, the neutrophils, ingest and remove bacteria and cellular debris. After 24 hours, the neutrophils are joined by macrophages, which continue to ingest cellular debris and play an essential role in the production of growth factors for the proliferative phase.

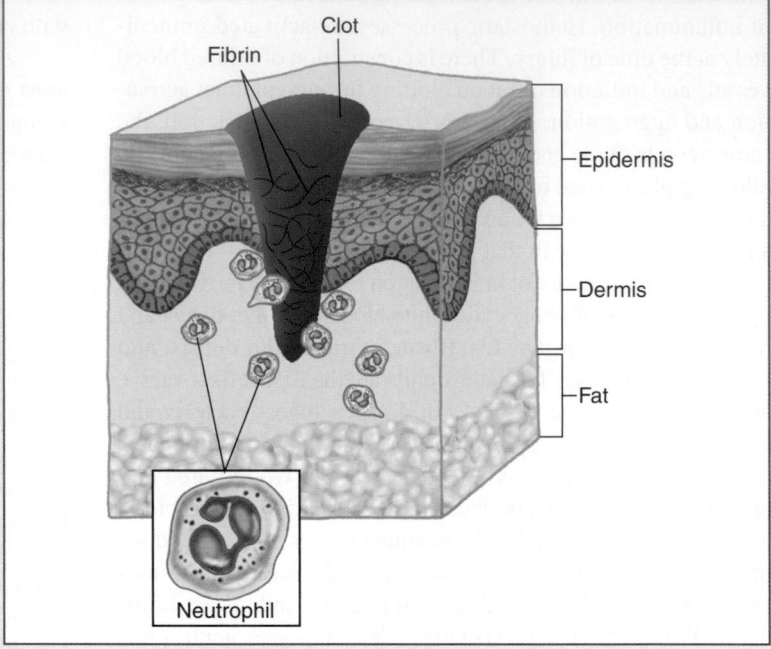

❷ Proliferative Phase

The primary processes during this phase focus on the building of new tissue to fill the wound space. The key cell during this phase is the *fibroblast,* a connective tissue cell that synthesizes and secretes the collagen, proteoglycans, and glycoproteins needed for wound healing. Fibroblasts also produce a family of growth factors that induce angiogenesis (growth of new blood vessels) and endothelial cell proliferation and migration. The final component of the proliferative phase is epithelialization, during which epithelial cells at the wound edges proliferate to form a new surface layer that is similar to that which was destroyed by the injury.

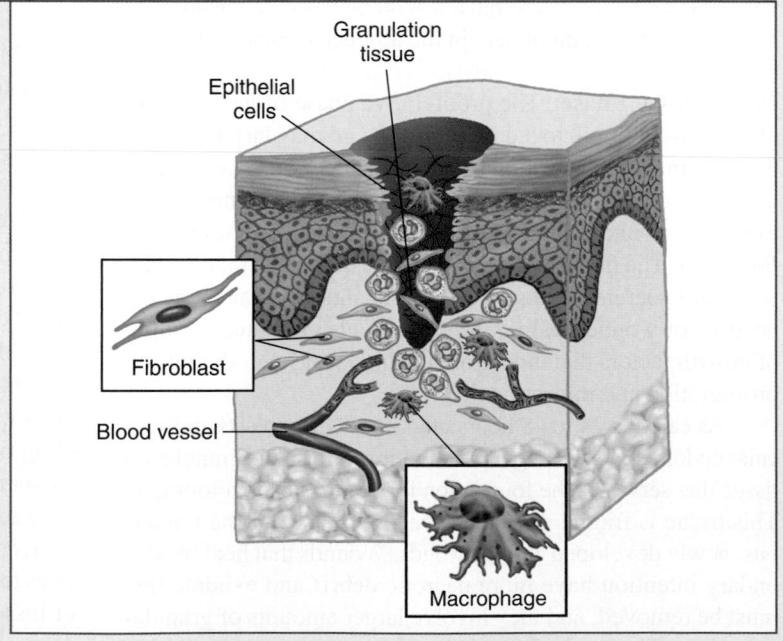

❸ Wound Contraction and Remodeling Phase

This phase begins approximately 3 weeks after injury with the development of the fibrous scar, and can continue for 6 months or longer, depending on the extent of the wound. During this phase, there is a decrease in vascularity and continued remodeling of scar tissue by simultaneous synthesis of collagen by fibroblasts and lysis by collagenase enzymes. As a result of these two processes, the architecture of the scar becomes reoriented to increase its tensile strength, and the scar shrinks so it is less visible.

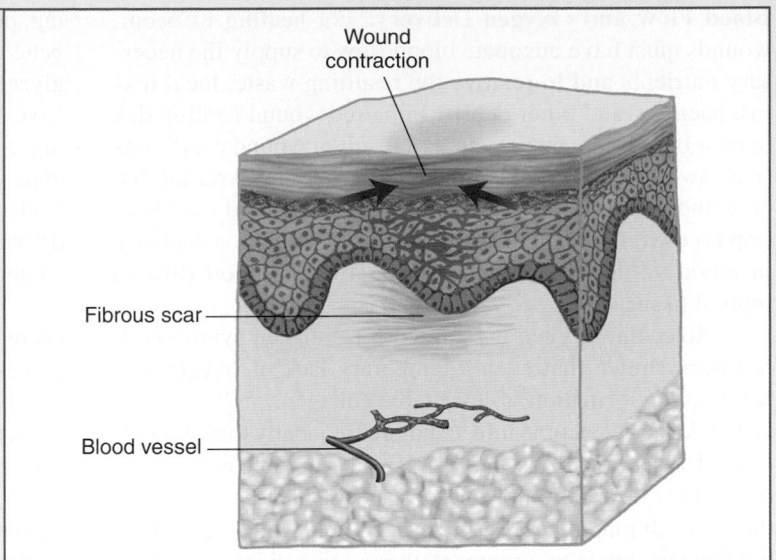

Factors That Affect Wound Healing

Many local and systemic factors influence wound healing. Although there are many factors that impair healing, science has found few ways to hasten the normal process of wound repair. Among the causes of impaired wound healing are malnutrition; impaired blood flow and oxygen delivery; impaired inflammatory and immune responses; infection, wound separation, and foreign bodies; and age effects.[42]

Malnutrition. Successful wound healing depends in part on adequate stores of proteins, carbohydrates, fats, vitamins, and minerals. It is well recognized that malnutrition slows the healing process, causing wounds to heal inadequately or incompletely.[36,43,44] Protein deficiencies prolong the inflammatory phase of healing and impair fibroblast proliferation, collagen and protein matrix synthesis, angiogenesis, and wound remodeling. Carbohydrates are needed as an energy source for white blood cells. Carbohydrates also have a protein-sparing effect and help to prevent the use of amino acids for fuel when they are needed for the healing process. Fats are essential constituents of cell membranes and are needed for the synthesis of new cells.

Although most vitamins are essential cofactors for the daily functions of the body, vitamins A and C play an essential role in the healing process. Vitamin C is needed for collagen synthesis. In vitamin C deficiency, improper sequencing of amino acids occurs, proper linking of amino acids does not take place, the byproducts of collagen synthesis are not removed from the cell, new wounds do not heal properly, and old wounds may fall apart. Administration of vitamin C rapidly restores the healing process to normal. Vitamin A functions in stimulating and supporting epithelialization, capillary formation, and collagen synthesis. Vitamin A also has been shown to counteract the anti-inflammatory effects of corticosteroid drugs and can be used to reverse these effects in persons who are on chronic steroid therapy. The B vitamins are important cofactors in enzymatic reactions that contribute to the wound-healing process. All are water soluble and, with the exception of vitamin B_{12}, which is stored in the liver, almost all must be replaced daily. Vitamin K plays an indirect role in wound healing by preventing bleeding disorders that contribute to hematoma formation and subsequent infection.

The role of minerals in wound healing is less clearly defined. The macrominerals, including sodium, potassium, calcium, and phosphorus, as well as the microminerals such as copper and zinc, must be present for normal cell function. Zinc is a cofactor in a variety of enzyme systems responsible for cell proliferation. In animal studies, zinc has been found to aid in reepithelialization.

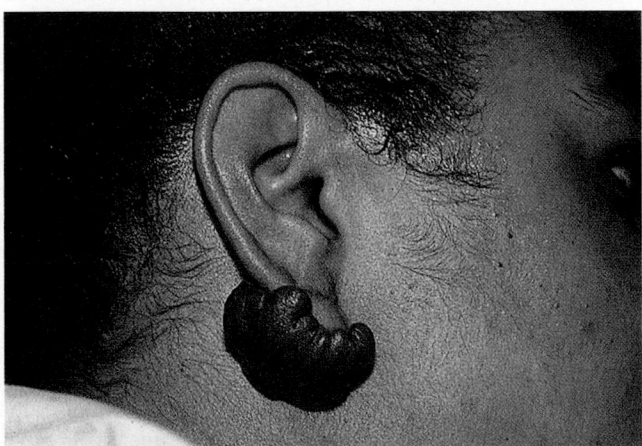

FIGURE 18-9 • Keloid. A light-skinned black woman with keloid that developed after ear piercing. (From Sephel G. C., Woodward S. C. [2007]. Repair, regeneration, and fibrosis. In Rubin R., Strayer D. E. [Eds.], *Rubin's pathology: Clinicopathologic foundations of medicine* [5th ed., p. 97]. Philadelphia: Lippincott Williams & Wilkins.)

Blood Flow and Oxygen Delivery. For healing to occur, wounds must have adequate blood flow to supply the necessary nutrients and to remove the resulting waste, local toxins, bacteria, and other debris. Impaired wound healing due to poor blood flow may occur as a result of wound conditions (*e.g.,* swelling) or preexisting health problems. Arterial disease and venous pathology are well-documented causes of impaired wound healing. In situations of trauma, a decrease in blood volume may cause a reduction in blood flow to injured tissues.

Molecular oxygen is required for collagen synthesis. It has been shown that even a temporary lack of oxygen can result in the formation of less stable collagen.[45,46] Wounds in ischemic tissue become infected more frequently than wounds in well vascularized tissue. PMNs and macrophages require oxygen for destruction of microorganisms that have invaded the area. Although these cells can accomplish phagocytosis in a relatively anoxic environment, they cannot digest bacteria.

Hyperbaric oxygen is a treatment in which 100% oxygen is delivered at greater than twice the normal atmospheric pressure at sea level.[47] The goal is to increase oxygen delivery to tissues by increasing the partial pressure of oxygen dissolved in the plasma. An increase in tissue oxygen tension by hyperbaric oxygen enhances wound healing by a number of mechanisms, including the increased killing of bacteria by neutrophils, impaired growth of anaerobic bacteria, and the promotion of angiogenesis and fibroblast activity. Hyperbaric oxygen is currently reserved for the treatment of problem wounds in which hypoxia and infection interfere with healing.

Impaired Inflammatory and Immune Responses. Inflammatory and immune mechanisms function in wound healing. Inflammation is essential to the first phase of wound healing, and immune mechanisms prevent infections that impair wound healing. Among the conditions that impair inflammation and immune function are disorders of phagocytic function, diabetes mellitus, and therapeutic administration of corticosteroid drugs.

Phagocytic disorders may be divided into extrinsic and intrinsic defects. Extrinsic disorders are those that reduce the total number of phagocytic cells (*e.g.,* immunosuppressive agents), impair the attraction of phagocytic cells to the wound site, interfere with the engulfment of bacteria and foreign agents by the phagocytic cells (*i.e.,* opsonization), or suppress the total number of phagocytic cells (*e.g.,* immunosuppressive agents). Intrinsic phagocytic disorders are the result of enzymatic deficiencies in the metabolic pathway for destroying the ingested bacteria by the phagocytic cell. The intrinsic phagocytic disorders include chronic granulomatous disease (see Chapter 19), an X-linked inherited disease in which there is a deficiency of the myeloperoxidase or NADPH oxidase enzymes. Deficiencies of these compounds prevent generation of superoxide and hydrogen peroxide needed for killing bacteria.

Wound healing is a problem in persons with diabetes mellitus, particularly those who have poorly controlled blood glucose levels.[48,49] Studies have shown delayed wound healing, poor collagen formation, and poor tensile strength in diabetic animals. Of particular importance is the effect of hyperglycemia on phagocytic function. Neutrophils, for example, have diminished chemotactic and phagocytic function, including engulfment and intracellular killing of bacteria, when exposed to altered glucose levels. Small blood vessel disease is also common among persons with diabetes, impairing the delivery of inflammatory cells, oxygen, and nutrients to the wound site.

The therapeutic administration of corticosteroid drugs decreases the inflammatory process and may delay the healing process. These hormones decrease capillary permeability during the early stages of inflammation, impair the phagocytic property of the leukocytes, and inhibit fibroblast proliferation and function.

Infection, Wound Separation, and Foreign Bodies. Wound contamination, wound separation, and foreign bodies delay wound healing. Infection impairs all dimensions of wound healing.[50] It prolongs the inflammatory phase, impairs the formation of granulation tissue, and inhibits proliferation of fibroblasts and deposition of collagen fibers. All wounds are contaminated at the time of injury. Although body defenses can handle the invasion of microorganisms at the time of wounding, badly contaminated wounds can overwhelm host defenses. Trauma and existing impairment of host defenses also can contribute to the development of wound infections.

Approximation of the wound edges (*i.e.,* suturing of an incision type of wound) greatly enhances healing and prevents infection. Epithelialization of a wound with closely approximated edges occurs within 1 to 2 days. Large, gaping wounds tend to heal more slowly because it is often impossible to effect wound closure with this type of wound. Mechanical factors such as increased local pressure or torsion can cause wounds to pull apart, or *dehisce.* Foreign bodies tend to invite bacterial contamination and delay healing. Fragments of wood, steel, glass, and other compounds may have entered the wound at the site of injury and can be difficult to locate when the wound is treated. Sutures are also foreign bodies, and although needed for the closure of surgical wounds, they are an impediment to healing. This is why sutures are removed as soon as possible after surgery. Wound infections are of special concern in persons with implantation of foreign bodies such as orthopedic devices (*e.g.,* pins, stabilization devices), cardiac pacemakers, and shunt catheters. These infections are difficult to treat and may require removal of the device.

Bite Wounds. Animal and human bites are particularly troublesome in terms of infection.[51,52] The animal inflicting the bite, the location of the bite, and the type of injury are all important determinants of whether the wound becomes infected. Approximately 28% to 80% of all cat bites become infected. Dog bites, for unclear reasons, become infected only approximately 3% to 18% of the time. Bites inflicted by children are usually superficial and seldom become infected, whereas bites inflicted by adults have a much higher rate of infection.

Puncture wounds are more likely to become infected than lacerations, probably because lacerations are easier to irrigate and debride.

Treatment of bite wounds involves vigorous irrigation and cleansing as well as debridement or removal of necrotic tissue. Whether bite wounds are closed with sutures to promote healing by primary intention depends on the location of the bite and whether the wound is already infected. Wounds that are not infected and require closure for mechanical or cosmetic reasons may be sutured. Wounds of the hand are not usually sutured because closed-space infection of the hand can produce loss of function. Antibiotics are usually administered prophylactically to persons with high-risk bites (*e.g.*, cat bites in any location and human or animal bites to the hand). All persons with bites should be evaluated to determine if tetanus or rabies prophylaxis is needed.

The Effect of Age on Wound Healing

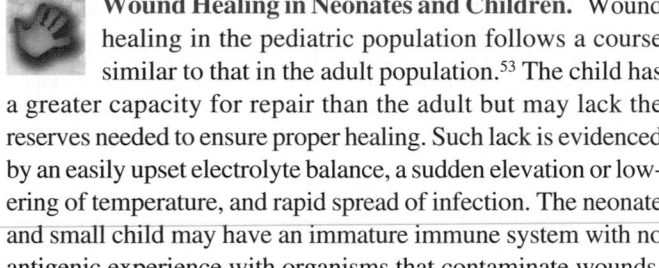

Wound Healing in Neonates and Children. Wound healing in the pediatric population follows a course similar to that in the adult population.[53] The child has a greater capacity for repair than the adult but may lack the reserves needed to ensure proper healing. Such lack is evidenced by an easily upset electrolyte balance, a sudden elevation or lowering of temperature, and rapid spread of infection. The neonate and small child may have an immature immune system with no antigenic experience with organisms that contaminate wounds. The younger the child, the more likely that the immune system is not fully developed.

Successful wound healing also depends on adequate nutrition. Children need sufficient calories to maintain growth and wound healing. The premature infant is often born with immature organ systems and minimal energy stores but high metabolic requirements—a condition that predisposes to impaired wound healing.

Wound Healing in Aged Persons. A number of structural and functional changes occur in aging skin, including a decrease in dermal thickness, a decline in collagen content, and a loss of elasticity.[54] The observed changes in skin that occur with aging are complicated by the effects of sun exposure. Since the effects of sun exposure are cumulative, older persons show more changes in skin structure.

Wound healing is thought to be progressively impaired with aging. The elderly have reduced collagen and fibroblast synthesis, impaired wound contraction, and slower reepithelialization of open wounds.[55] Although wound healing may be delayed, most wounds heal, even in the debilitated elderly undergoing major surgical procedures.

The elderly are more vulnerable to chronic wounds, chiefly pressure, diabetic, and ischemic ulcers, than younger persons, and these wounds heal more slowly. However, these wounds are more likely due to other disorders such as immobility, diabetes mellitus, or vascular disease, rather than aging.

IN SUMMARY, the ability of tissues to repair damage due to injury depends on the body's ability to replace the parenchymal cells and to organize them as they were originally. Regeneration describes the process by which tissue is replaced with cells of a similar type and function. Healing by regeneration is limited to tissue with cells that are able to divide and replace the injured cells. Body cells are divided into types according to their ability to regenerate: labile cells, such as the epithelial cells of the skin and gastrointestinal tract, which continue to regenerate throughout life; stable cells, such as those in the liver, which normally do not divide but are capable of regeneration when confronted with an appropriate stimulus; and permanent or fixed cells, such as nerve cells, which are unable to regenerate. Scar tissue repair involves the substitution of fibrous connective tissue for injured tissue that cannot be repaired by regeneration.

Wound healing occurs by primary and secondary intention and is commonly divided into three phases: the inflammatory phase, the proliferative phase, and the maturational or remodeling phase. In wounds healing by primary intention, the duration of the phases is fairly predictable. In wounds healing by secondary intention, the process depends on the extent of injury and the healing environment. Wound healing can be impaired or complicated by factors such as malnutrition; restricted blood flow and oxygen delivery; diminished inflammatory and immune responses; and infection, wound separation, and the presence of foreign bodies. ■

CONCEPTS in action **ANIMATION**

Review Exercises

1. A 15-year-old boy presents with abdominal pain, a temperature of 38°C (100.5°F), and an elevated white blood cell count of 13,000/μL, with an increase in neutrophils. A tentative diagnosis of appendicitis is made.

   A. *Explain the significance of pain as it relates to the inflammatory response.*

   B. *What is the cause of the fever and elevated white blood cell count?*

   C. *What would be the preferred treatment for this boy?*

2. Aspirin and other NSAIDs are used to control the manifestations of chronic inflammatory disorders such as arthritis.

   A. *Explain their mechanism of action in terms of controlling the inflammatory response.*

3. After a heart attack, the area of heart muscle that has undergone necrosis because of a lack of blood supply undergoes healing by replacement with scar tissue.

   A. *Compare the functioning of the heart muscle that has been replaced by scar tissue with that of the normal surrounding heart muscle.*

4. A 35-year-old man presents with a large abscess on his leg. He tells you he injured his leg while doing repair work on his house and he thinks there might be a wood sliver in the infected area.

   A. *Explain the events that participate in formation of an abscess.*

   B. *He is told that incision and drainage of the lesion will be needed so healing can take place. Explain.*

   C. *He is reluctant to have the procedure done and asks whether an antibiotic would work as well. Explain why antibiotics alone are usually not effective in eliminating the microorganisms contained in an abscess.*

References

1. Murphy H. S. (2008). Inflammation. In Rubin E., Strayer D. S. (Eds.), *Rubin's pathology: Clinicopathologic foundations of medicine* (5th ed., pp. 37–70). Philadelphia: Lippincott Williams & Wilkins.

2. Kumar V., Abbas A. K., Fausto N. (2005). Acute and chronic inflammation. In Kumar V., Abbas A. K., Fausto N. (Eds.), *Robbins and Cotran pathologic basis of disease* (7th ed., pp. 47–86). Philadelphia: Elsevier Saunders.

3. Schmid-Schonbein G. W. (2006). Analysis of inflammation. *Annual Review of Biochemistry* 8, 93–131.

4. Szekanecz Z., Koch A. E. (2004). Vascular endothelium and immune responses: Implications for inflammation and angiogenesis. *Rheumatology Clinics of North America* 30, 97–114.

5. Wiel E., Vallet B., ten Cate H. (2005). The endothelium in intensive care. *Critical Care Clinics* 21, 403–416.

6. Steinhubl S. R. (2007). Platelets as mediators of inflammation. *Hematology/Oncology Clinics of North America* 21, 115–121.

7. Gawaz, M., Langer H., May A. E. (2005). Platelets in inflammation and atherogenesis. *Journal of Clinical Investigation* 115, 3378–3384.

8. Abbas A. K., Lichtman A. H. (2006). Basic immunology: Functions and disorders of the immune system (2nd ed., pp. 34–35). Philadelphia: Elsevier Saunders.

9. Kindt T. J., Osborne B. A., Goldsby R. A. (2007). *Kuby immunology* (6th ed., pp. 327–349). New York: WH Freeman.

10. Nathan C. (2002). Points of control in inflammation. *Nature* 420, 848–852.

11. Luster A. D., Alon R., von Andrian U. H. (2005). Immune cell migration in inflammation: Present and future therapeutic targets. *Nature Immunology* 6, 1182–1190

12. Bachelet I., Levi-Schaffer F., Mekori Y. A. (2006). Mast cells: Not only in allergy. *Immunology and Allergy Clinics of North America* 26, 407–425.

13. Frenette P. S., Wagner D. D. (1996). Adhesion molecules: Parts I and II. *New England Journal of Medicine* 334, 1526–1529; 335, 43–45.

14. Bochner B. S. (2004). Adhesion molecules as therapeutic targets. *Immunology Clinics of North America* 24, 615–630.

15. Stein D. M., Nombela-Arrieta C. (2005). Chemokine control of lymphocyte trafficking: A general review. *Immunology* 116, 1–12.

16. Underhill D. M., Ozinsky A. (2002). Phagocytosis of microbes. *Annual Review of Microbiology* 20, 825–852.

17. Simmons D. L., Botting R. M., Hla T. (2004). Cyclooxygenase isoenzymes: The biology of prostaglandin synthesis and inhibition. *Pharmacological Reviews* 56, 387–437.

18. Covington M. B. (2004). Omega-3 fatty acids. *American Family Physician* 70, 133–140.

19. Harper C. R., Jacobson T. A. (2005). Usefulness of omega-3 fatty acids and prevention of coronary heart disease. *American Journal of Cardiology* 96, 1521–1529.

20. Calder P. C. (2002). Dietary modification of inflammation with lipids. *Proceedings of the Nutrition Society* 61, 345–358.

21. Gossain A., Gamelli R. L (2005). A primer on cytokines. *Journal of Burn Care and Rehabilitation* 26, 7–12.

22. Charo I., Ransohoff R. M. (2006). The many roles of chemokines and chemokine receptors in inflammation. *New England Journal of Medicine* 354, 610–621.

23. Hotchiss R. S., Karl I. E. (2003). The pathophysiology and treatment of sepsis. *New England Journal of Medicine* 348, 138–150.

24. Ridker P. M. (1999). Novel inflammatory markers of coronary risk. *Circulation* 100, 1148–1150.

25. Ridker P. M. (2005). C-reactive protein, inflammation, and cardiovascular disease. *Current Issues in Cardiology* 32, 384–386.

26. Ridker P. M. (2001). High-sensitivity C-reactive protein: Potential adjunct for global risk assessment in primary prevention of cardiovascular disease. *Circulation* 103, 1813–1818.

27. Pearson T. A., Mensah G. A. (Co-chairs), Alexander R. W., et al. (2003). Markers of inflammation and cardiovascular disease: Application to clinical and public health practice: A statement for healthcare professionals from the Centers for Disease Control and Prevention and the American Heart Association. *Circulation* 107, 499–511.

28. Sephel G. C., Woodward S. C. (2008). Repair, regeneration, and fibrosis. In Rubin R., Strayer D. S. (Eds.), *Rubin's pathology: Clinicopathologic foundations of medicine* (5th ed., pp. 71–93). Philadelphia: Lippincott Williams & Wilkins.

29. Kumar V., Abbas A. K., Fausto N. (2005). Tissue repair: Cellular growth, fibrosis, and wound healing. In Kumar V., Abbas A. K., Fausto N. (Eds.), *Robbins and Cotran pathologic basis of disease* (7th ed., pp. 87–118). Philadelphia: Elsevier Saunders.

30. Whitney J. D. (2005). Overview: Acute and chronic wounds. *Nursing Clinics of North America* 40, 191–205.

31. Wei L., Dasgeb B., Phillips T., et al. (2005). Wound-healing perspectives. *Dermatology Clinics* 23, 181–192.

32. Strecker-McGraw M. K., Jones T. R., Baer D. G. (2007). Soft tissue wounds and principles of healing. *Emergency Medical Clinics of North America* 25, 1–22.

33. Singer A. J., Clark R. A. F. (1999). Cutaneous wound healing. *New England Journal of Medicine* 341, 738–746.

34. Monaco J. L., Lawrence W. T. (2003). Acute wound healing: An overview. *Clinical Plastic Surgery* 30, 1–12.

35. Waldrop J., Doughty D. (2000). Wound-healing physiology. In Bryant R. A. (Ed.), *Acute and chronic wounds* (2nd ed., pp. 17–35). St. Louis: Mosby.

36. Harding K. G., Morris H. L., Patel K. G. (2002). Healing chronic wounds. *British Medical Journal* 324, 160–163.

37. Steed D. L. (1997). The role of growth factors in wound healing. *Surgical Clinics of North America* 77, 575–585.

38. Werner S., Grose R. (2003). Regulation of wound healing by growth factors and cytokines. *Physiological Reviews* 83, 835–870.

39. Cross K. J., Mustoe T. A. (2003). Growth factors in wound healing. *Surgical Clinics of North America* 83, 531–545.

40. Robson M. C. (2003). Cytokine manipulation of the wound. *Clinical Plastic Surgery* 30, 57–65.

41. Parks W. C. (1999). Matrix metalloproteinases in repair. *Wound Repair and Regeneration* 7, 423–432.

42. Burns J. L., Mancoll J. S., Phillips L. G. (2003). Impairments of wound healing. *Clinical Plastic Surgery* 30, 47–56.

43. Albina J. E. (1995). Nutrition and wound healing. *Journal of Parenteral and Enteral Nutrition* 18, 367–376.

44. Mechanick J. I. (2004). Practical aspects of nutrition support for wound-healing patients. *American Journal of Surgery* 188(Suppl.), 52S–56S.

45. Whitney J. D. (1990). The influence of tissue oxygenation and perfusion on wound healing. *Clinical Issues in Critical Care Nursing* 1, 578–584.

46. Whitney J. D. (1989). Physiologic effects of tissue oxygenation on wound healing. *Heart and Lung* 18, 466–474.

47. Zamboni W. A., Browder L. K., Martinez J. (2003). Hyperbaric oxygen and wound healing. *Clinics in Plastic Surgery* 30, 67–75.

48. King L. (2000). Impaired wound healing in patients with diabetes. *Nursing Standards* 15(38), 39–45.

49. Greenhalgh D. G. (2003). Wound healing and diabetes mellitus. *Clinics in Plastic Surgery* 30, 37–45.

50. Hunt T. K., Hopf H. W. (1977). Wound healing and wound infection. *Surgical Clinics of North America* 77, 587–605.

51. Fleisher G. R. (1999). The management of bite wounds. *New England Journal of Medicine* 340, 138–140.

52. Talan D. A., Citron D. M., Abrahamian F. M., et al. (1999). Bacteriologic analysis of infected dog and cat bites. *New England Journal of Medicine* 340, 85–92.

53. Garvin G. (1990). Wound healing in pediatrics. *Nursing Clinics of North America* 25, 181–191.

54. Boynton P. R., Jaworski D., Paustian C. (1999). Meeting the challenges of healing chronic wounds in older adults. *Nursing Clinics of North America* 34, 921–932.

55. Thomas D. R. (2001). Age-related changes in wound healing. *Drugs & Aging* 18, 607–620.

Visit thePoint **http://thePoint.lww.com for animations, journal articles, and more!**

Disorders of the Immune Response

CAROL M. PORTH

IMMUNODEFICIENCY DISORDERS
Humoral (B-Cell) Immunodeficiencies
Transient Hypogammaglobulinemia of Infancy
Primary Humoral Immunodeficiency Disorders
Secondary Humoral Immunodeficiency Disorders
Cell-Mediated (T-Cell) Immunodeficiencies
Primary Cell-Mediated Immunodeficiency Disorders
Secondary Cell-Mediated Immunodeficiency Disorders
Combined T-Cell and B-Cell Immunodeficiencies
Severe Combined Immunodeficiency Disorders
Combined Immunodeficiency Disorders
Disorders of the Complement System
Primary Disorders of the Complement System
Secondary Disorders of the Complement System
Disorders of Phagocytosis
Primary Disorders of Phagocytosis
Secondary Disorders of Phagocytosis
Stem Cell Transplantation
HYPERSENSITIVITY DISORDERS
Type I, Immediate Hypersensitivity Disorders
Anaphylactic (Systemic) Reactions
Type II, Antibody-Mediated Disorders
Complement- and Antibody-Mediated Cell Destruction
Complement- and Antibody-Mediated Inflammation
Antibody-Mediated Cellular Dysfunction
Type III, Immune Complex–Mediated Disorders
Systemic Immune Complex Disorders
Localized Immune Complex Reactions
Type IV, Cell-Mediated Hypersensitivity Disorders
Direct Cell-Mediated Cytotoxicity
Delayed-Type Hypersensitivity Disorders
TRANSPLANTATION IMMUNOPATHOLOGY
Mechanisms Involved in Transplant Rejection
Graft-Versus-Host Disease
Mechanisms of Autoimmune Disease
Diagnosis and Treatment of Autoimmune Disease

▶ The immune system is a multifaceted defense network that has evolved to protect against invading microorganisms, prevent the proliferation of cancer cells, and mediate the healing of damaged tissue. Under normal conditions, the immune response deters or prevents disease. Occasionally, however, the inadequate, inappropriate, or misdirected activation of the immune system can lead to debilitating or life-threatening illnesses, typified by immunodeficiency states, allergic or hypersensitivity reactions, transplantation rejection, and autoimmune disorders.

 **IMMUNODEFICIENCY DISORDERS**

After completing this section of the chapter, you should be able to meet the following objectives:

■ State the difference in causes of primary and secondary immunodeficiency disorders.
■ Compare and contrast pathology and manifestations of humoral (B-cell), cellular (T-cell), and combined T- and B-cell immunodeficiency disorders.
■ State the function of the complement system and relate it to the manifestations of complement deficiencies and hereditary angioneurotic edema.
■ State the proposed mechanisms of dysfunction and manifestations of phagocytosis disorders.

Immunodeficiency can be defined as an abnormality in the immune system that renders a person susceptible to diseases normally prevented by an intact immune system. Immunodeficiency states can be classified as primary (*i.e.,* congenital or inherited) or secondary (acquired later in life).[1] Secondary immunodeficiency can be the result of malnutrition; disseminated cancers; infection of the cells of the immune system, most notably with human immunodeficiency virus (HIV), the etiologic agent of acquired immunodeficiency syndrome (AIDS); and treatment with immunosuppressive drugs (*e.g.,* corticosteroids or transplant rejection medications). The severity and symptomatology of the various immunodeficiencies depend on the disorder and extent of immune system involvement. The various categories of immunodeficiency disorders are summarized in Chart 19-1. HIV infection/AIDS is discussed in Chapter 20.

The immune system is historically divided into two basic arms: the innate and adaptive immune systems (see Chapter 17). The innate immune system uses the defenses of the phagocytic leukocytes (*i.e.,* neutrophils, macrophages), natural killer (NK) cells, and complement proteins. This arm responds rapidly to infections in a relatively nonspecific manner. The adaptive immune response is composed mainly of T and B cells and responds to infections more slowly, but more specifically than the innate immune system. The specificity of the adaptive immune response has evolved primarily through the ability of T and B cells to rearrange their receptors (T cells) and immunoglobulins (B cells) into billions of different combinations. This diversification, in turn, allows the adaptive immune system to recognize billions of different epitopes on infectious organisms.

The adaptive immune system is further divided into the humoral and cellular immune systems. The humoral immune system classically has been limited to B cells and their production of immunoglobulins or antibodies, whereas the cellular immune system has been restricted to T cells and their ability to produce various cytokines and, in the case of cytotoxic T cells, to kill cells infected with intracellular organisms. What has become clear in recent years is that the humoral and cellular immune systems are functionally dependent on each other for mounting an immune response.[2] B cells, for example, depend on certain cytokines produced by helper T cells to produce different classes of immunoglobulin (*i.e.,* IgG versus IgA). Likewise, cytotoxic T cells depend on specific immunoglobulins produced by B cells to clear viral infections effectively by destroying cell-free virus particles and preventing their spread to other cellular targets.

Although primary immunodeficiencies are thought to be rare, it has been estimated that there are over 500,000 cases in the United States, with 50,000 new cases being diagnosed each year.[2] Until recently, little was known about the causes of primary immunodeficiency diseases. However, this has changed with recent advances in genetic technology.[1–5] To date, more than 100 primary immunodeficiency syndromes have been identified, and specific molecular defects have been identified in more than one third of these diseases.[2,5] Most are transmitted as recessive traits, several of which are caused by mutations in genes on the X chromosome and others by mutations on autosomal chromosomes. Many of these disorders have been traced to mutations affecting signaling pathways (*e.g.,* cytokines and cytokine signaling, receptor subunits, and metabolic pathways) that dictate immune cell development and function. Furthermore, it has been shown that the immune system is a carefully balanced system that is designed to distinguish between self and nonself; therefore, symptoms of autoimmunity often are observed with primary immunodeficiency disease.[2]

Early detection is possible for most primary immunodeficiency diseases, is critical for the success of some treat-

---

CHART 19-1   IMMUNODEFICIENCY STATES

Humoral (B-Cell) Immunodeficiency
Primary
 X-linked hypogammaglobulinemia
 Common variable immunodeficiency
 Selective deficiency of IgG, IgA, IgM
Secondary
 Increased loss of immunoglobulin (nephrotic syndrome)

Cellular (T-Cell) Immunodeficiency
Primary
 Congenital thymic aplasia (DiGeorge syndrome)
 Hyper-IgM syndrome
Secondary
 Malignant disease (Hodgkin disease and others)
 Transient suppression of T-cell production and function
  due to acute viral infection
 HIV-AIDS

Combined B-Cell and T-Cell Immunodeficiency
Primary
 Severe combined immunodeficiency syndrome (SCID)
  X-linked
  Autosomal recessive (ADA deficiency, Jak3 deficiency)
 Wiskott-Aldrich syndrome
 Ataxia-telangiectasia
 Combined immunodeficiency syndrome (CID)
Secondary
 Irradiation
 Immune suppression and cytotoxic drugs

Complement System Disorders
Primary
 Hereditary deficiency of complement proteins
 Hereditary deficiency of C1 inhibitor (angioneurotic edema)
Secondary
 Acquired disorders that consume complement factors

Disorders of Phagocytosis
Primary
 Chronic granulomatous disease
 Chédiak-Higashi syndrome
Secondary
 Drug induced (corticosteroid and immunosuppressive
  therapy)
 Diabetes mellitus

---

ments, and can be lifesaving. For infants with severe combined T- and B-cell immunodeficiency, early diagnosis is essential not only in terms of preventing life-threatening infections, but in preventing administration of live attenuated virus vaccines (*e.g.,* measles, mumps, rubella, varicella, bacillus Calmette-Guérin), which could prove fatal.[2] The first clinical clue for diagnosis of primary immunodeficiency disease is usually a history of infections that are per-

> **CHART 19-2   TEN WARNING SIGNS OF PRIMARY IMMUNODEFICIENCY**
>
> - Eight or more new ear infections within 1 year
> - Two or more serious sinus infections within 1 year
> - Two or more months on antibiotics with little effect
> - Two or more pneumonias within 1 year
> - Failure of an infant to gain weight or grow normally
> - Recurrent, deep skin or organ abscesses
> - Persistent thrush in mouth or elsewhere on skin, after 1 year of age
> - Need for intravenous antibiotics to clear infections
> - Two or more deep-seated infections
> - A family history of primary immunodeficiency
>
> From the Jeffrey Modell Foundation. (n.d.) [Online]. Available: www.info4pi.org.

sistent, difficult to treat, or caused by unusual microbes. The Jeffrey Modell Foundation/Immune Deficiency Foundation has developed a set of warning signs that serve as an excellent tool for determining what should be considered abnormal[6] (Chart 19-2). Because these disorders are frequently inherited, a positive family history is also a key diagnostic tool. The type of infection can provide information regarding the type of defect that is present. Infections with bacterial organisms are frequently observed in cases of antibody deficiency, whereas severe viral, fungal, and opportunistic infections characterize T-cell deficiencies. Recurrent *Strep-* *tococcus pneumoniae* or *Neisseria* infections characterize persons with complement deficiencies, and recurrent infections with staphylococcal and other catalase-positive organisms indicate disorders of phagocytosis. Table 19-1 summarizes types of infections that occur with the different types of primary immunodeficiency disorders.

Humoral (B-Cell) Immunodeficiencies

Humoral immunodeficiencies involve B-cell function and immunoglobulin (*i.e.,* antibody) production. Defects in humoral immunity increase the risk of recurrent pyogenic infections, including those caused by *S. pneumoniae, Haemophilus influenzae, Staphylococcus aureus,* and gram-negative organisms such as *Pseudomonas* species. Humoral immunity usually is not as important in defending against intracellular bacteria (mycobacteria), fungi, and protozoa. Viruses usually are handled normally, except for the enteroviruses that cause gastrointestinal infections.

 Transient Hypogammaglobulinemia of Infancy

During the first few months of life, infants are protected from infection by IgG antibodies that have been transferred from the maternal circulation during fetal life. IgA, IgM, IgD, and IgE do not normally cross the placenta. The presence of elevated levels of IgA or IgM in the infant cord blood suggests prema-

TABLE 19-1 Infectious Organisms Frequently Associated With Major Categories of Immunodeficiency Disorders

IMMUNODEFICIENCY DISORDER	VIRUSES	BACTERIA	FUNGI	PROTOZOA
B-cell (humoral) immunodeficiency	Enteroviruses	*Streptococcus pneumoniae, Staphylococcus aureus, Haemophilus influenzae*	No	*Giardia lamblia*
T-cell (cell-mediated) immunodeficiency	Herpesvirus	*Salmonella typhi,* all mycobacteria	*Candida albicans, Coccidioides immitis, Histoplasma capsulatum, Aspergillus fumigatus*	
Combined T-cell and B-cell immunodeficiency	All	*S. pneumoniae, S. aureus, H. influenzae, Pseudomonas aeruginosa, Neisseria meningitidis, Mycoplasma hominis,* enteric flora	*C. albicans, Pneumocystis jiroveci* (formerly *carinii*)	*Toxoplasma gondii*
Complement system disorders		*S. pneumoniae, S. aureus, H. influenzae*		
Phagocytosis (neutrophils and monocytes) disorders		*S. aureus,* enteric flora, *P. aeruginosa,* all mycobacteria	*A. fumigatus, C. albicans, Nocardia asteroides*	

Information from Abbas A. K. (2005). Diseases of immunity. In Kumar V., Abbas A. K., Fausto N. (Eds.), *Pathologic basis of disease* (7th ed., p. 240). Philadelphia: Elsevier Saunders; Verbsky J. W., Grossman W. J. (2006). Cellular and genetic basis of primary immune deficiencies. *Pediatric Clinics of North America* 53, 649–684; and Bonilla F. A., Geha R. S. (2006). Update on primary immunodeficiency diseases. *Journal of Allergy and Clinical Immunology* 117, S435–S441.

PRIMARY IMMUNODEFICIENCY DISORDERS

- Primary immunodeficiency disorders are congenital or inherited abnormalities of immune function that render a person susceptible to diseases normally prevented by an intact immune system.

- Disorders of B-cell function impair the ability to produce antibodies and defend against microorganisms and toxins that circulate in body fluids (IgM and IgG) or enter the body through the mucosal surface of the respiratory or gastrointestinal tract (IgA). Persons with primary B-cell immunodeficiency are particularly prone to pyogenic infections due to encapsulated organisms.

- Disorders of T-cell function impair the ability to orchestrate the immune response (CD4+ helper T cells) and to protect against fungal, protozoan, viral, and intracellular bacterial infections (CD8+ cytotoxic T cells). T cells also play an important role in surveillance against oncogenic viruses and tumors; hence, persons with impaired T-cell function are at increased risk for certain types of cancers.

- Combined T-cell and B-cell immunodeficiency states affect all aspects of immune function. Severe combined immunodeficiency represents a life-threatening absence of immune function that requires bone marrow or stem cell transplantation for survival.

ture antibody production in response to an intrauterine infection. An infant's level of maternal IgG gradually declines over a period of approximately 6 months (see Chapter 17, Fig. 17-17). Concomitant with the loss of maternal antibody, the infant's immature humoral immune system begins to function, and between the ages of 1 and 2 years, the child's antibody production reaches adult levels.

Any abnormality that interferes with the production of immunoglobulin-producing plasma cells can produce a state of immunodeficiency. For example, certain infants may experience a delay in IgG production (IgM and IgA levels are normal) beyond 6 months of age. The total number and antigenic response of circulating B cells are normal, but the chemical communication between B and T cells that leads to clonal proliferation of antibody-producing plasma cells seems to be reduced.[5] This condition is referred to as *transient hypogammaglobulinemia of infancy*. The result of this condition usually is limited to repeated bouts of upper respiratory and middle ear infections. This condition usually resolves by the time the child is 2 to 4 years of age.

Primary Humoral Immunodeficiency Disorders

Of all the primary immunodeficiency diseases, those affecting antibody production are the most common.[5] Antibody production depends on the differentiation of hematopoietic stem cells into mature B lymphocytes and the antigen-dependent generation of immunoglobulin-producing plasma cells (Fig. 19-1). This maturation cycle initially involves the production of surface IgM, migration from the bone marrow to the peripheral lymphoid tissue, and switching to the production of specialized

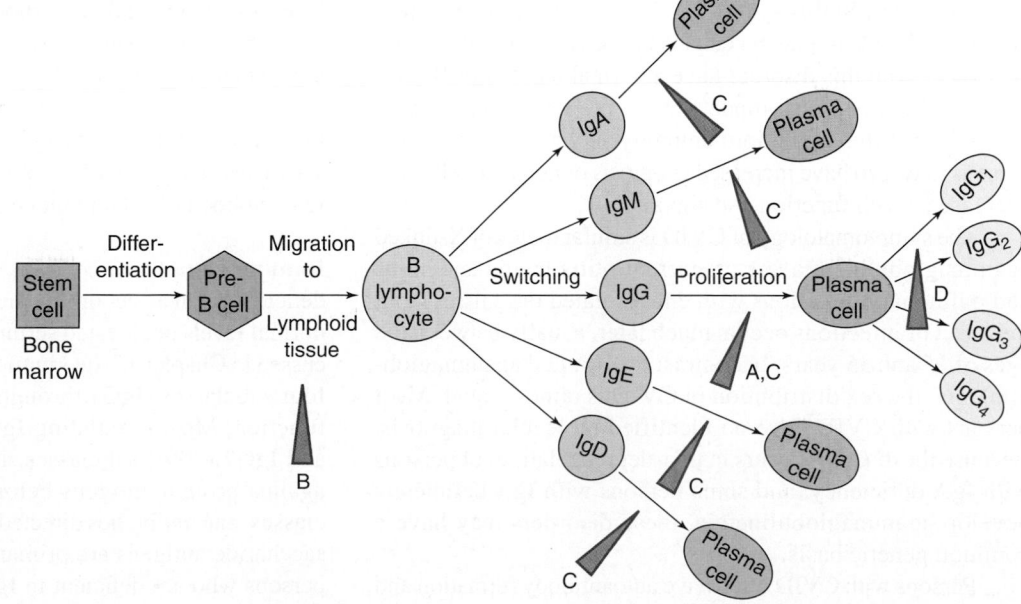

FIGURE 19-1 • Stem cells to mature immunoglobulin-secreting plasma cells. *Arrows* indicate the stage of the maturation process that is interrupted in (**A**) transient hypogammaglobulinemia, (**B**) X-linked agammaglobulinemia, (**C**) common variable immunodeficiency, and (**D**) IgG subclass deficiency.

IgM-, IgA-, IgD-, IgE-, or IgG-secreting plasma cells after antigenic stimulation. Primary humoral immunodeficiency disorders can interrupt the production of one or all of the immunoglobulins.

X-Linked Agammaglobulinemia. X-linked (Bruton) agammaglobulinemia is a recessive trait that affects only boys.[2–5,7–10] As the name implies, persons with this disorder have essentially undetectable levels of all serum immunoglobulins. Therefore, they are susceptible to meningitis and recurrent otitis media and to sinus and pulmonary infections with encapsulated organisms such as *S. pneumoniae, H. influenzae* type b, *S. aureus,* and *Neisseria meningitidis.*[3]

The abnormal gene in X-linked agammaglobulinemia maps to the long arm of the X chromosome and encodes the B-cell protein tyrosine kinase (Bruton tyrosine kinase [*Btk*]). *Btk* appears to be necessary for pre–B-cell expansion and maturation into surface immunoglobulin-expressing B cells, but probably has a role in all stages of B-cell development. Mutation in the *Btk* gene results in an absence of mature circulating B cells and plasma cells. T lymphocytes, however, are normal in number and function.

Most boys with the disorder remain asymptomatic until 6 to 9 months of life because of the presence of maternal antibodies. A clue to the presence of the disorder is the failure of an infection to respond completely and promptly to antibiotic therapy. Diagnosis is based on demonstration of low or absent serum immunoglobulins. Therapy consists of prophylaxis with intravenous immunoglobulin (IVIG) and prompt antimicrobial therapy for suspected infections. The prognosis of this condition depends on the prompt recognition and treatment of infections. Chronic pulmonary disease is an ever-present danger.

Common Variable Immunodeficiency. Another disorder of B-cell maturation, which is similar to X-linked agammaglobulinemia, is a condition called *common variable immunodeficiency* (CVID). In this syndrome, the terminal differentiation of mature B cells to plasma cells is blocked.[7,8] More than 80% of persons with this disorder have a normal number of B lymphocytes, but when the lymphocytes are presented with antigen, they fail to differentiate into antibody-secreting cells.[9] Some persons may also have increased apoptosis of helper T cells, and decreased T-cell function and signaling.

The symptomatology of CVID is similar to that of X-linked agammaglobulinemia (*i.e.,* recurrent otitis media and sinus and pulmonary infections with encapsulated organisms), but the onset of infections occurs much later, usually between the ages of 15 and 35 years. In contrast to X-linked agammaglobulinemia, the sex distribution in CVID is almost equal. Most persons with CVID have no identified molecular diagnosis. Because the disorder occurs in first-degree relatives of persons with IgA deficiency, and some persons with IgA deficiency develop agammaglobulinemia, these disorders may have a common genetic basis.

Persons with CVID often have autoantibody formation and normal-sized or enlarged tonsils and lymph nodes, and approx-imately 25% have splenomegaly.[5] They have an increased tendency toward development of interstitial lung disease, autoimmune disorders, hepatitis, and chronic diarrhea with associated intestinal malabsorption. There is also an increased risk of gastric cancer and non-Hodgkin B-cell lymphoma.

Treatment methods for CVID are similar to those used for X-linked agammaglobulinemia, with IVIG being the cornerstone of therapy. Anaphylaxis to IgA in the IVIG can occur in persons with CVID who are IgA deficient. The use of IgA-depleted IVIG has greatly reduced this risk.

Selective Immunoglobulin A Deficiency. Selective IgA deficiency is the most common type of immunoglobulin deficiency, affecting 1 in 400 to 1 in 1000 persons.[4] The syndrome is characterized by moderate to marked reduction in levels of serum and secretory IgA. It is likely that the cause of this deficiency is a block in the pathway that promotes terminal differentiation of mature B cells to IgA-secreting plasma cells. The occurrence of IgA deficiency in both men and women and in members of successive generations within families suggests autosomal inheritance with variable expressivity. The disorder has also been noted in persons treated with certain drugs (*e.g.,* phenytoin, sulfasalazine), suggesting that environmental factors may trigger the disorder.[5]

Approximately two thirds of persons with selective IgA deficiency have no overt symptoms, presumably because IgG and IgM levels are normal and compensate for the defect. At least 50% of affected children overcome the deficiency by the age of 14 years. Persons with markedly reduced levels of IgA often experience repeated upper respiratory and gastrointestinal infections and have an increased incidence of allergic manifestations, such as asthma, and autoimmune disorders. Persons with IgA deficiency also can develop antibodies against IgA, which can lead to severe anaphylactic reactions when blood components containing IgA are given.[5] Therefore, only specially washed erythrocytes from normal donors or erythrocytes from IgA-deficient donors should be used.

There is no treatment available for selective IgA deficiency unless there is a concomitant reduction in IgG levels. Administration of IgA immune globulin is of little benefit because IgA has a short half-life and is not secreted across the mucosa. There also is the risk of anaphylactic reactions associated with IgA antibodies in the immune globulin.

Immunoglobulin G Subclass Deficiency. An IgG subclass deficiency can affect one or more of the IgG subtypes, despite normal levels or elevated serum concentrations of IgG. As discussed in Chapter 17, IgG immunoglobulins can be divided into four subclasses (IgG1 through IgG4) based on structure and function. Most circulating IgG belongs to the IgG1 (70%) and IgG2 (20%) subclasses. In general, antibodies directed against protein antigens belong to the IgG1 and IgG3 subclasses, and antibodies directed against carbohydrate and polysaccharide antigens are primarily IgG2 subclass. As a result, persons who are deficient in IgG2 subclass antibodies can be at greater risk for development of sinusitis, otitis media, and pneumonia caused by polysaccharide-encapsulated micro-organisms such as *S. pneumoniae, H. influenzae* type b, and *N. meningitidis*.

Children with mild forms of the deficiency can be treated with prophylactic antibiotics to prevent repeated infections. IGIV can be given to children with severe manifestations of this deficiency. The use of polysaccharide vaccines conjugated to protein carriers can provide protection against some of these infections, rather than the protein conjugated to protein carriers that would stimulate an IgG1 response.

Secondary Humoral Immunodeficiency Disorders

Secondary deficiencies in humoral immunity can develop as a consequence of conditions that increase immunoglobulin loss, diseases that decrease immunoglobulin production, or drug-induced states that cause a decrease in immunoglobulin levels.

Abnormal immunoglobulin loss can occur with chronic kidney disease and protein-losing enteropathies. Such is the case in persons with nephrotic syndrome who, because of abnormal glomerular filtration, lose serum IgA and IgG in their urine. Because of its larger molecular size, IgM is not filtered into the urine, and serum levels remain normal. Protein-losing enteropathies that commonly present with decreased immuno-globulin levels include autoimmune enteropathy and intestinal lymphangiectasis (blocked interstitial lymphatics with loss of lymph fluid and immunoglobulins in the gastrointestinal tract).

Secondary humoral immunodeficiencies can also result from a number of malignancies, including chronic lymphocytic leukemia, lymphoma, and multiple myeloma, that interfere with normal immunoglobulin production. Medications that cause reversible secondary hypogammaglobulinemia include the disease-modifying antirheumatic drugs, corticosteroid agents, and the antiepileptic drugs phenytoin and carbamazepine.[11]

Cell-Mediated (T-Cell) Immunodeficiencies

Unlike B cells, in which a well-defined series of differentiation steps ultimately leads to the production of immunoglobulins, mature T lymphocytes consist of distinct subpopulations whose immunologic assignments are diverse. T cells can be function-ally divided into two subtypes (CD4+ helper and CD8+ cytotoxic T cells). Collectively, T lymphocytes protect against fungal, pro-tozoan, viral, and intracellular bacterial infections; control malig-nant cell proliferation; and are responsible for coordinating the overall immune response.

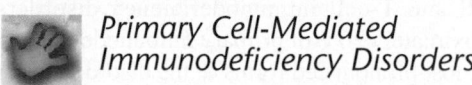

Primary Cell-Mediated Immunodeficiency Disorders

In general, persons with cell-mediated immunodeficiency dis-orders have infections or other clinical problems that are more severe than those seen with antibody disorders. Children with defects in this branch of the immune response rarely survive beyond infancy or childhood unless immunologic reconstitu-

tion is achieved through bone marrow transplantation.[5] How-ever, exceptions are being recognized as newer T-cell defects, such as the X-linked hyper-IgM syndrome, are identified. Other recently identified primary T-cell immunodeficiency disorders result from defective expression of the T-cell receptor (TCR) complex, defective cytokine production, and defects in T-cell activation.

For children with fatal forms of T-cell defects, transplan-tation of thymic tissue or major histocompatibility complex (MHC)–compatible bone marrow is currently the treatment of choice.[4] Stem cell transplantation (to be discussed), an alterna-tive to bone marrow transplantation, has also proved useful in treating some disorders. The major risk to recipients of bone marrow transplantation is that of graft-versus-host disease. Gene replacement therapy remains a distant goal for most immuno-deficiencies at present. The main obstacles to this type of ther-apy are purifying self-renewing stem cells, which are the ideal target for introduction of the replacement gene, and lack of methods for introducing the genes into the stem cell.

DiGeorge Syndrome. DiGeorge syndrome stems from an embryonic developmental defect. The defect is thought to occur before the 12th week of gestation, when the thymus gland, parathyroid gland, and parts of the head, neck, and heart are developing. The disorder affects both sexes. Because familial occurrence is rare, it seems unlikely that the disorder is inherited. Formerly thought to be caused by a variety of factors, including extrinsic teratogens, this defect has been traced to microdeletion of specific deoxyribonucleic acid (DNA) sequences from chro-mosome 22 (22q11).[5,8,11]

Infants born with this defect have partial or complete fail-ure of development of the thymus and parathyroid glands and have congenital defects of the head, neck, and heart. The extent of immune and parathyroid abnormalities is highly variable, as are the other defects. Occasionally, a child has no heart defect. In some children, the thymus is not absent but is in an abnor-mal location and is extremely small. These infants can have partial DiGeorge syndrome, in which hypertrophy of the thy-mus occurs with development of normal immune function. The facial disorders can include hypertelorism (*i.e.,* increased dis-tance between the eyes); micrognathia (*i.e.,* abnormally small jaw); low-set, posteriorly angulated ears; split uvula; and high-arched palate (Fig. 19-2). Urinary tract abnormalities also are common. The most frequent presenting sign is hypocalcemia and tetany that develop in the first 24 hours of life. It is caused by the absence of the parathyroid gland and is resistant to stan-dard therapy.

Children who survive the immediate neonatal period may have recurrent or chronic infections because of impaired T-cell immunity. Children also may have an absence of immunoglob-ulin production, caused by a lack of helper T-cell function. For children who do require treatment, thymus transplantation can be performed to reconstitute T-cell immunity. Bone marrow transplantation also has been successfully used to restore nor-mal T-cell populations. If blood transfusions are needed, as during corrective heart surgery, special processing is required to prevent graft-versus-host disease.

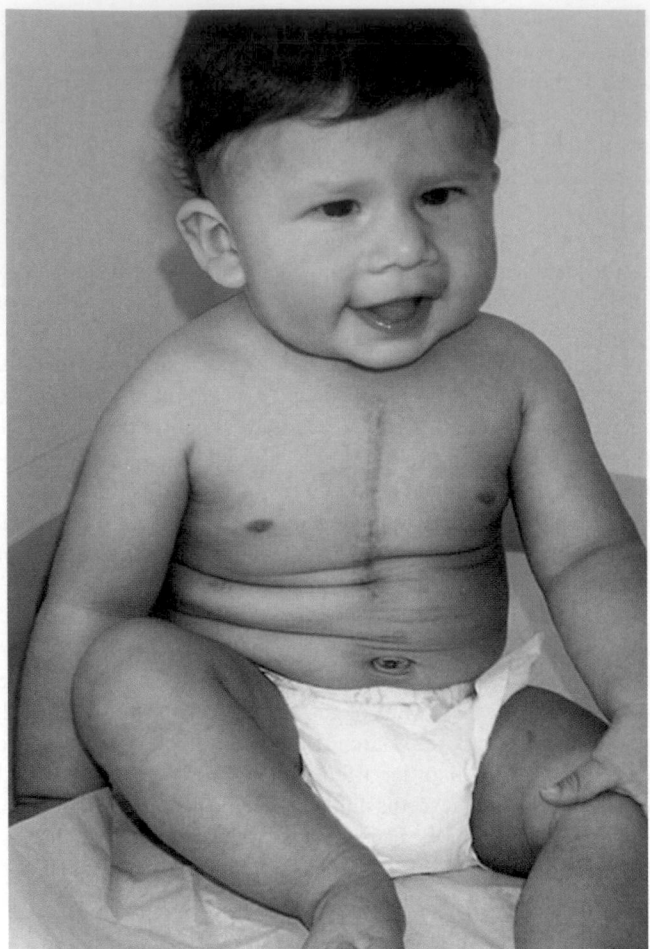

FIGURE 19-2 • An infant with DiGeorge syndrome. The surgical scar on the chest indicates repair of heart disease caused by truncus arteriosus or interrupted aortic arch, which is common in this syndrome. The infant also has the facial features of a child with DiGeorge syndrome, as illustrated by hypertelorism, low-set ears, hypoplastic mandible, and bowing upward of the upper lip. (From Roberts R. *Atlas of infectious diseases.* Edited by Gerald Mandell (series editor), Catherine M. Wilfert. © 1998 Current Medicine, Inc.)

X-Linked Immunodeficiency With Hyper-IgM. The X-linked immunodeficiency of hyper-IgM, also known as the *hyper-IgM syndrome,* is characterized by low IgG and IgA levels with normal or, more frequently, high IgM concentrations. Being X-linked, the disorder is confined to boys. Formerly classified as a B-cell defect, it now has been traced to a T-cell defect.[8] The disorder results from the inability of T cells to signal B cells to undergo isotype switching to IgG and IgA; thus, they produce only IgM.[11] Although the disorder was identified on the basis of an antibody defect, its primary cause is a defect in cell-mediated immunity.

Like boys with X-linked agammaglobulinemia, affected boys become symptomatic during the first and second years of life. They have recurrent pyogenic infections, including otitis media, sinusitis, tonsillitis, and pneumonia. They are also susceptible to opportunistic infections, especially *Pneumocystis jiroveci* (formerly *Pneumocystis carinii*), because of the defect

in cell-mediated immunity. Persons with the syndrome are also at increased risk for development of autoimmune diseases of the formed elements of the blood, including hemolytic anemia, thrombocytopenia, and recurrent severe neutropenia.[11]

Secondary Cell-Mediated Immunodeficiency Disorders

Secondary deficiencies of T-cell function are more common than primary deficiencies and have been described in conjunction with acute viral infections (*e.g.,* measles virus, cytomegalovirus) and with certain malignancies such as Hodgkin disease and other lymphomas. In the case of viruses, direct infection of specific T-lymphocyte subpopulations (*e.g.,* helper cells) by lymphotropic viruses such as HIV and human herpesvirus type 6 can lead to loss of cellular function and selective subtype depletion with a concomitant loss of immunologic function associated with that subtype. Persons with neoplastic disorders can have impaired T-cell function based on unregulated multiplication or dysfunction of one particular subclone of T cells. The outward expression of this may be an increased susceptibility to infections caused by normally harmless pathogens (*i.e.,* opportunistic infections) or failure to generate delayed-type hypersensitivity reactions (*i.e.,* anergy). Persons with anergy have a diminished or absent reaction to a battery of skin test antigens, including *Candida* and the tuberculin test, even when infected with *Mycobacterium tuberculosis* (see Chapter 28).

 Combined T-Cell and B-Cell Immunodeficiencies

Disorders that affect both B and T lymphocytes, with resultant defects in both humoral and cell-mediated immunity, fall under the broad classification of combined immunodeficiency syndrome (CIDS). A single mutation in any one of the many genes that influence lymphocyte development or response, including lymphocyte receptors, cytokines, or MHC antigens, could lead to combined immunodeficiency. Regardless of the affected gene, the net result is a disruption in the normal communication system between B and T lymphocytes and deregulation of the immune response. The spectrum of disease resulting from combined immunodeficiency disorders ranges from mild to severe to ultimately fatal forms.

Severe Combined Immunodeficiency Disorders

Combined B-cell and T-cell immunodeficiency disorders account for approximately 20% of primary immunodeficiency disorders. In the most pronounced forms of the disorder, often referred to as *severe combined immunodeficiency* (SCID), genetic mutations lead to absence of all T- and B-cell function and, in some cases, a lack of NK cells.[5,7,10-12] Affected infants have a disease course that resembles AIDS, with failure to thrive, chronic diarrhea, and opportunistic infections. Survival beyond the first year of life is rare without prompt immune reconstitution through bone marrow or hematopoietic stem cell transplantation. Early diagnosis is critical because the chances of successful treatment are highest in infants who have not experienced severe opportunistic infections. There is also hope that gene therapy will someday be available for some, if not all, forms of SCID.

The first discovered cause of SCID, adenosine deaminase (ADA) deficiency, was reported in 1972. It was not until 21 years later, however, that a second cause, the molecular basis of X-linked SCID, was found. Since then, remarkable progress has been made in elucidating several other causes of SCID. It is now known that SCID can be caused by mutations in at least nine different genes.[13,14] The products of three of the mutated genes that cause SCID are components of cytokine receptors that control T-cell differentiation; the products of three others are essential for rearrangement of antigen receptor genes; and the product of another is a component of the T-cell antigen receptor that appears essential for T-cell development. The product of yet another gene codes for ADA, an enzyme that prevents the accumulation of toxic metabolites that cause T-cell destruction. The product of the remaining mutated gene is the common leukocyte antigen, CD45, a phosphatase critical for regulating signaling thresholds in immune cells.

The most common form of SCID, accounting for half of all cases, is X-linked, and hence SCID is more common in boys than girls. It is caused by a genetic defect in the common gamma-chain subunit (γc) of cytokine receptors. This transmembrane receptor is a component of multiple interleukin (IL) receptors, including the IL-7 receptor, which is responsible for proliferation of T-lymphocyte precursors.[13] As a result of defective IL-7 signaling, there is a profound defect in the earliest stages of lymphocyte development with a greatly reduced number of T cells. Although the B cells are normal in number, antibody production is impaired because of a lack of T-cell help.

The remaining cases of SCID show an autosomal recessive pattern of inheritance. The most common cause of autosomal recessive SCID is an ADA deficiency.[13,14] Absence of this enzyme leads to the accumulation of toxic metabolites that kill dividing and resting T cells. Infants with ADA-deficiency SCID usually have a much more profound lymphopenia than do infants with other forms of SCID, often manifesting as absolute lymphocyte counts of less than 500/mm³. The absolute numbers of both T and B cells are very low. Although the number of NK cells is low, their function is normal. Other distinguishing features of ADA deficiency include the presence of rib cage deformity and numerous skeletal deformities. Bone marrow transplantation has been successful in treating children with ADA-deficiency SCID.[5,10,11] Enzyme replacement therapy also may be used in the management of persons with this form of SCID. However, it should not be used if bone marrow transplantation is anticipated because it can predispose to graft rejection.[5,11]

Several other, less common causes of SCID are recombinase-activating gene (RAG) deficiencies, Janus kinase 3 (Jak3) deficiency, and mutations that impair the expression of class II MHC molecules.[5,11] Defects in RAG activity prevent the somatic gene rearrangements necessary for the assembly of the T-cell receptor and block the development of T and B cells. Jak3 is essential for signal transduction through the common γc, which is mutated in X-linked SCID. Therefore, mutations in Jak3 have the same effect as X-linked SCID. Mutations that impair expression of MHC II prevent the development of CD4+ helper T cells.

Combined Immunodeficiency Disorders

Combined immunodeficiency (CID) is distinguished from SCID by the presence of low, but not absent, T-cell function. Although antibody-forming capacity is impaired in most cases, it is not absent. Like SCID, however, CID is a syndrome of diverse genetic causes and is often associated with other disorders such as ataxia-telangiectasia and Wiskott-Aldrich syndrome. An autosomal pattern of inheritance is common.

Children with CID are prone to development of recurrent pulmonary infections, failure to thrive, oral and cutaneous candidiasis, chronic diarrhea, recurrent skin infections, gram-negative sepsis, and urinary tract infections. Although they usually survive longer than children with SCID, they fail to thrive and often die early in life.

Ataxia-Telangiectasia. Ataxia-telangiectasia is a complex syndrome of neurologic, immunologic, endocrinologic, hepatic, and cutaneous abnormalities. It is an autosomal recessive disorder that is thought to result from the mutation of a single gene located on the long arm of chromosome 11.[11,13,15] As the name implies, this syndrome is characterized by worsening cerebellar *ataxia (i.e.,* poor muscle coordination) and the appearance of *telangiectases (i.e.,* lesions consisting of dilated capillaries and arterioles) on the skin and conjunctival surfaces of the eye. The ataxia usually goes unnoticed until the child begins to walk and the telangiectases begin to develop shortly thereafter, especially on skin surfaces exposed to the sun. The ataxia progresses slowly and relentlessly to severe disability. Intellectual development is normal at first but seems to stop at the 10-year level in many of these children.

Children with ataxia-telangiectasia have deficiencies in both cellular and humoral immunity, including absolute lymphopenia and a decrease in the ratio of CD4+ helper T cells to CD8+ suppressor T cells. Approximately 70% have an IgA deficiency, and approximately half also have an IgG subclass deficiency. There is increased susceptibility to recurrent upper and lower respiratory tract infections (particularly those caused by encapsulated bacteria) and an increased risk for the development of malignancies. Death from malignant lymphoma is common.

Wiskott-Aldrich Syndrome. The Wiskott-Aldrich syndrome is an X-linked recessive disorder that becomes symptomatic during the first year of life.[11,12,16] Infants with this syndrome are plagued by eczema, low platelet counts, and susceptibility to bacterial infections. Bleeding episodes or symptoms due to infection usually begin within the first 6 months of life. Abnormalities of humoral immunity include decreased serum levels of IgM and markedly elevated serum IgA and IgE concentrations. T-cell dysfunction initially is mild but progressively deteriorates, and persons with the disorder become increasingly susceptible to development of malignancies of the mononuclear phagocytic system, including Hodgkin lymphoma and leukemia. Children with Wiskott-Aldrich syndrome typically are unable to produce antibody to polysaccharide antigens and therefore are susceptible to infections caused by encapsulated microorganisms. They also are prone to septicemia and meningitis caused by these organisms. Varicella infection can be lethal to children with this condition.

Management of persons with Wiskott-Aldrich syndrome focuses on treatment of eczema, control of infections, and management of bleeding episodes. If an infection is suspected, careful evaluation for bacterial, viral, and fungal causes followed by administration of appropriate antimicrobial therapy is required. Bone marrow transplantation has been successful in children with Wiskott-Aldrich syndrome. Splenectomy, sometimes recommended for persons with thrombocytopenia, effectively stops the bleeding episodes, but increases the risk of septicemia.[16]

Disorders of the Complement System

The complement system is an integral part of the innate or nonspecific immune response (see Chapter 17). The activation of the complement network through the classic, lectin-mediated, or alternative pathways promotes chemotaxis, opsonization, and phagocytosis of invasive pathogens, bacteriolysis, and anaphylactic reactions. Thus, alterations in normal levels of complement or the absence of a particular complement component can lead to enhanced susceptibility to infectious diseases and also to autoimmune diseases, particularly systemic lupus erythematosus (SLE).[2]

Primary Disorders of the Complement System

Most primary disorders of the complement system are transmitted as autosomal recessive traits and can involve one or more complement components (the complement components are designated by "C" and enzyme subcomponents by "q," "r," and "s"). Deficiencies of C1r, C1rs, C2, C3, C4, C5, C6, C7, C8, and C9 are transmitted as autosomal codominant traits, in which each parent transmits a gene that codes for half the serum level of the component.[10,11] Because 50% activity is sufficient to prevent disease, persons who are heterozygous and have one normally functioning gene seldom have problems.

In general, persons with deficiencies in factors C1 (C1q, r, and s) and C4 are not necessarily at increased risk for recurrent infections because the lectin-mediated and alternative pathways can be activated normally through C3 (see Chapter 17). However, many of them acquire autoimmune diseases, particularly lupus-like syndromes.[2] Persons with primary deficiency of C1q have a high incidence of SLE, an SLE-like syndrome without typical SLE serology, a chronic rash with underlying vasculitis on biopsy, or membranoproliferative glomerulonephritis.[17,18] Like persons with C1q deficiency, persons with C1r, C1r/C1s, C4, C2, and C3 deficiencies have a high incidence of vasculitis syndromes, especially SLE or SLE-like syndrome.

A C2 deficiency causes a susceptibility to multiple and potentially life-threatening infections caused by encapsulated bacteria, especially S. pneumoniae. Similarly, persons with C3 deficiency are predisposed to infections that trigger the lectin-mediated or alternative pathway (e.g., those caused by encapsulated bacteria and S. aureus) because of their inability to opsonize and lyse bacteria. Although persons with deficiencies in the terminal components of complement (C5 through C9) are susceptible to repeated episodes of meningitis and sepsis caused by N. meningitidis or systemic gonococcal disease, they are less likely to have autoimmune disorders than persons with other complement deficiencies.[18]

Only supportive measures are available for treatment of primary disorders of the complement system. Measures to prevent bacterial infections are important. The affected person and close contacts should be immunized with vaccines for S. pneumoniae, H. influenzae, and N. meningitidis.

Hereditary Angioneurotic Edema. Hereditary angioneurotic edema is a particularly interesting form of complement deficiency. Persons with this disorder do not produce a functional C1 inhibitor.[17–20] Activation of the classic complement pathway is uncontrolled, leading to increased breakdown of C4 and C2 with concomitant generation of bradykinin, a vasodilator. This causes episodic attacks of localized edema involving the face, neck, joints, abdomen, and sites of trauma. Swelling of the subcutaneous tissues, especially of the face, can be disfiguring, and swelling of the gastric mucosa causes nausea, vomiting, and diarrhea. If the trachea or larynx is involved, the episode can prove fatal. The attacks associated with this inherited disease can begin before the age of 2 years but usually are not severe until late childhood or adolescence. Symptoms can last from 1 to 4 days, and most persons with the disorder have more than one attack a month. Adults with hereditary angioneurotic edema can be treated with danazol, a synthetic androgen with weak virilizing and mild anabolic potential. The drug, given orally, increases C1 inhibitor levels and prevents attacks. Two new groups of drugs, plasma-derived and recombinant human C1 inhibitors and agents that inhibit the bradykinin-mediated increase in vascular permeability, are currently in the clinical trial stage.

Secondary Disorders of the Complement System

Secondary complement deficiencies also can occur in persons with functionally normal complement systems because of rapid activation and turnover of complement components (as is seen in immune complex disease) or reduced synthesis of components, as would be the case in chronic cirrhosis of the liver or malnutrition.

Disorders of Phagocytosis

The phagocytic system is composed primarily of polymorphonuclear leukocytes (i.e., neutrophils and eosinophils) and mononuclear phagocytes (i.e., circulating monocytes and tissue and fixed [spleen] macrophages). The primary purpose of phagocytic cells is to migrate to the site of infection (*i.e.,* chemotaxis), aggregate around the affected tissue (*i.e.,* adherence), envelope invading microorganisms or foreign substances (*i.e.,* phagocytosis), and generate microbicidal substances (*e.g.,* enzymes or byproducts of metabolism) to kill the ingested pathogens. A defect in any of these functions or a reduction in the absolute number of available cells can disrupt the phagocytic system. Patients with phagocytic disorders are particularly prone to infections by bacteria and often by *Candida* species and filamentous fungi, although the types of pathogens vary with different disorders.[21] As with other alterations in immune function, defects in phagocytosis can be primary or secondary disorders.

Primary Disorders of Phagocytosis

Primary disorders of phagocytosis include leukocyte adhesion deficiency disorders, defects in microbicidal activity (*e.g.,* chronic granulomatous disease), and degranulation abnormalities (*e.g.,* Chédiak-Higashi syndrome).

Perhaps the best known of the primary disorders of phagocytosis is *chronic granulomatous disease* (CGD). CGD represents a group of inherited disorders that greatly reduce or inactivate the ability of phagocytic cells to produce the so-called *respiratory burst* that results in the generation of toxic derivatives of oxygen (superoxide anion and hydrogen peroxide).[22,23] These oxygen species participate in creating an intracellular environment that kills ingested microorganisms. Recurrent infections, along with granulomatous lesions, in persons with CGD are thought to be due to persistence of viable microorganisms in impaired phagocytic cells. Other aspects of phagocyte function, such as engulfment of microorganisms, are normal. About two thirds of persons with CGD are males who inherit their disorder as a result of mutations in the X chromosome; about one third inherit CGD as a result of mutations on chromosome 7; and a small number (about 5%) result from mutations on chromosome 1.

Children with CGD are subject to chronic and acute infections of the skin, liver, lung, and other soft tissues despite aggressive antibiotic therapy. Severe facial acne and painful inflammation of the nares is common. Organisms responsible for the infections include *S. aureus, Serratia marcescens, Pseudomonas cepacia, Escherichia coli, Candida albicans,* and *Aspergillus* species.[22,23] These infections usually begin during the first 2 years of life. The disorder is diagnosed by examining the ability of a person's phagocytes to reduce a yellow dye (*i.e.,* nitroblue tetrazolium) to a blue compound during active respiration. Bone marrow transplantation is the only known cure for CGD. Supportive care includes the use of recombinant interferon-gamma and prophylactic antibiotic therapy.

Chédiak-Higashi syndrome is a rare autosomal recessive disorder characterized by increased susceptibility to infection owing to defective degranulation of neutrophils, a mild bleeding disorder, partial oculocutaneous albinism, progressive peripheral neuropathy, and a tendency to develop a life-threatening lymphoma-like syndrome. The neutrophils (and other leukocytes) of persons with the disorder have giant granules, which can be seen on peripheral blood smears and which are thought to result from aberrant organelle fusion. In this syndrome, there is reduced transfer of lysosomal enzymes to phagocytic vacuoles in phagocytes (causing susceptibility to infections) and abnormalities in melanocytes (leading to albinism), cells in the nervous system (associated with nerve disorders), and platelets (generating bleeding disorders). Bone marrow transplantation reconstitutes normal hematopoietic and immunologic function, but does not correct or prevent peripheral neuropathy.

Secondary Disorders of Phagocytosis

Secondary deficiencies of the phagocytic system can be caused by a number of conditions such as leukemia, malnutrition, viral infections, or diabetes mellitus. Persons with diabetes mellitus may demonstrate poor phagocytic function, primarily because of altered chemotaxis. The reason for this dysfunction is not understood, but it is unrelated to the person's age or the severity of the metabolic disorder. Apparently, this is a separate genetic disorder that is coinherited at a higher frequency among persons with diabetes and among family members. Drugs that impair or prevent inflammation and T-cell function, such as corticosteroids or cyclosporine, also alter phagocytic response through modulation of cytokines.

HIV infection and AIDS represent another form of acquired or secondary deficiency of phagocytic function. However, in this case, the deficiency is due to direct infection and destruction of helper T cells and monocytes–macrophages by the virus (see Chapter 20).

Stem Cell Transplantation

Many of the primary immunodeficiency disorders in which the defect has been traced to the stem cell can be cured with allogeneic stem cell transplantation from an unaffected donor.[24] These include disorders such as SCID, Wiskott-Aldrich syndrome, and CGD.

It has been shown that stem cells can repopulate the bone marrow and reestablish hematopoiesis. For the procedure to be effective, the bone marrow cells of the host are destroyed by myeloablative doses of chemotherapy. The exception is children with SCID. Because of the profound cellular immune defect that is present in children with SCID, pretransplantation myeloablation may not be necessary.[24] After transplantation, a lineage-specific chimeric state usually develops in these children, in which the T-cell component is of donor origin and the B-cell component, although variable, remains largely of host origin.[24] Chronic immunoglobulin therapy may be necessary for transplant recipients who primarily retain B cells of host origin.

Stem cells can be collected from the bone marrow or peripheral blood. Donors with identical human leukocyte antigen (HLA) types (*i.e.,* matched for at least three of the six HLA loci) are associated with the least risk of graft-versus-host disease or graft rejection. HLA-matched siblings usually produce the best results. Stem cell aspiration from the bone marrow is the most common form of allograft collection. Only a few (less than 1 in 100,000) nucleated bone marrow cells are true hematopoietic stem cells. These stem cells are separated from other bone marrow cells before transplantation. Peripheral blood offers a less invasive method for obtaining stem cells. Hematopoietic growth factors, such as granulocyte colony-stimulating factor, often are used to induce stem cells to move out of the bone marrow into the blood. Many of these stem cells can be collected from the blood using leukapheresis, a process that separates the stem cells from other blood cells. A third potential source of stem cells is umbilical cord blood. Umbilical cord blood is a rich source of primitive hematopoietic blood. Up to 250 mL of umbilical cord blood can be collected at the time of delivery without producing detrimental effects to the mother and newborn. Although reliable engraftment of bone marrow can be achieved in children, it is uncertain whether cord blood contains enough stem cells to engraft adult recipients.[24]

IN SUMMARY, an immunodeficiency is defined as an absolute or partial loss of the normal immune response, which places a person in a state of compromise and increases the risk for development of infections or malignant complications. Immunodeficiency states can affect components of the innate or adaptive immune systems. The variety of defects known to involve the immune response can be classified as primary (*i.e.,* congenital or inherited) or secondary (*i.e.,* due another disease or condition). The extent to which any or all of these components are compromised dictates the severity of the immunodeficiency.

Immunodeficiency can affect the humoral or cellular components of the adaptive immune system. B-cell or humoral immunodeficiency disorders can selectively involve a single immunoglobulin (*e.g.,* IgA immunodeficiency) or all of the immunoglobulins (agammaglobulinemia). Defects in humoral immunity increase the risk of recurrent pyogenic infections but have less effect on the defense against intracellular bacteria (mycobacteria), fungi, protozoa, and viruses (except for the enteroviruses that cause gastrointestinal infections). T lymphocytes protect against fungal, protozoan, viral, and intracellular bacterial infections; control malignant cell proliferation; and are responsible for coordinating the overall immune response. T-cell or cellular immune disorders can present as selective T-cell immunodeficiency states or as combined T- and B-cell immunodeficiency disorders. Infants with severe combined immunodeficiency have a disease course that resembles AIDS, with failure to thrive, chronic diarrhea, and opportunistic infections. Survival beyond the first year of life is rare without prompt immune reconstitution through bone marrow or hematopoietic stem cell transplantation.

The complement system and phagocytosis are integral components of innate immunity. Activation of the complement system promotes chemotaxis, opsonization, and phagocytosis and destruction of invasive pathogens. Thus, deficiencies in normal levels of complement or the absence of a particular

complement component can lead to enhanced susceptibility to infectious diseases and also to autoimmune diseases, particularly SLE. Persons with phagocytic disorders are particularly prone to infections by bacteria and often by *Candida* species and filamentous fungi, although the types of pathogens vary with different disorders. Primary disorders of phagocytosis include leukocyte adhesion deficiency disorders, degranulation abnormalities, and defects in microbicidal activity. ■

HYPERSENSITIVITY DISORDERS

After completing this section of the chapter, you should be able to meet the following objectives:

■ Differentiate between adaptive immune responses that protect against microbial agents and hypersensitivity responses.

■ Describe the immune mechanisms involved in a type I, type II, type III, and type IV hypersensitivity reaction.

■ Describe the pathogenesis of allergic rhinitis, food allergy, serum sickness, Arthus reaction, contact dermatitis, and hypersensitivity pneumonitis.

■ Characterize the differences in latex allergy caused by a type I, IgE-mediated hypersensitivity response and that caused by a type IV, cell-mediated response.

Hypersensitivity disorders refer to excessive or inappropriate activation of the immune system. Although activation of the immune system normally leads to production of antibodies and T-cell responses that protect the body against attack by microorganisms, it is also capable of causing tissue injury and disease. Disorders caused by immune responses are collectively referred to as *hypersensitivity reactions.*

Historically, hypersensitivity disorders have been subdivided into four types: type I, IgE-mediated disorders; type II, antibody-mediated disorders; type III, complement-mediated immune disorders; and type IV, T-cell–mediated disorders[1,7,10] (Table 19-2). These categories differ in terms of the type of immune response causing the injury and the nature and location of the antigen that is the target of the response. Latex allergy can result from an IgE-mediated or T-cell–mediated hypersensitivity response. It is discussed separately at the end of this section. Transplant rejections and autoimmune disorders (discussed separately) may also be regarded as hypersensitivity responses.

Type I, Immediate Hypersensitivity Disorders

Type I hypersensitivity reactions are IgE-mediated reactions that begin rapidly, often within minutes of an antigen challenge.

TABLE 19-2 Classification of Hypersensitivity Responses

TYPE OF HYPERSENSITIVITY	IMMUNE MECHANISM	MECHANISM OF INJURY
Type I, immediate hypersensitivity	IgE antibody	Release of mast cell mediators
Type II, antibody mediated	IgM, IgG antibodies against cell surface or extracellular matrix	Phagocytosis and opsonization of cells; complement- and receptor-mediated recruitment and activation of inflammatory cells (neutrophils, macrophages); abnormalities in cellular functioning (e.g., hormone receptor signaling)
Type III, immune complex mediated	Formation of immune complexes involving circulating antigens and IgM or IgG antibodies	Complement-mediated recruitment and activation of inflammatory cells
Type IV, T-cell mediated	CD4$^+$ T cells (delayed-type hypersensitivity, or CD8$^+$ cytotoxic T-cell–mediated cytolysis)	Macrophage activation of cytokine-mediated inflammation; direct target cell killing, cytokine-mediated inflammation

ALLERGIC AND HYPERSENSITIVITY DISORDERS

- Hypersensitivity disorders result from immune responses to exogenous and endogenous antigens that produce inflammation and cause tissue damage.

- Type I hypersensitivity is an IgE-mediated immune response that leads to the release of inflammatory mediators for sensitized mast cells.

- Type II disorders involve humoral antibodies against cell surface or extracellular matrix antigens that result in complement-mediated phagocytosis or inflammation and cell injury, or, in some cases, abnormal physiologic responses without cell injury.

- Type III disorders result in generation of circulating immune complexes in which humoral antibodies bind antigen and activate complement. The fractions of complement attract inflammatory cells that release tissue-damaging products.

- Type IV disorders involve tissue damage in which cell-mediated immune responses with sensitized T lymphocytes cause cell and tissue injury.

These types of reactions to antigens are often referred to as *allergic reactions*. In the context of an allergic response, the antigens usually are referred to as *allergens*. Typical allergens include the protein in pollen, house dust mites, animal dander, foods, and chemicals like the antibiotic penicillin. Exposure to the allergen can be through inhalation, ingestion, injection, or skin contact. Depending on the portal of entry, type I reactions may occur as a local or atopic reaction that is merely annoying (*e.g.*, seasonal rhinitis) or severely debilitating (asthma), or as a systemic and potentially life-threatening reaction (anaphylaxis).

Two types of cells are central to a type I hypersensitivity reaction: type 2 helper T (T$_H$2) cells and mast cells or basophils.[1,7,25] There are two subsets of helper T cells (T$_H$1 and T$_H$2) that develop from the same precursor CD4$^+$ T lymphocyte (see Chapter 17). T$_H$1 cells differentiate in response to microbes and stimulate the differentiation of B cells into IgM- and IgG-producing plasma cells. T$_H$2 cell differentiation occurs in response to allergens and helminths (intestinal parasites).[1] Cytokines (*i.e.*, IL-4, IL-5, IL-13) secreted by T$_H$2 cells stimulate differentiation of B cells into IgE-producing plasma cells, act as growth factors for mast cells, and recruit and activate eosinophils.

Mast cells, which are tissue cells, and basophils, which are blood cells, are derived from hematopoietic precursor cells. Mast cells and basophils have granules that contain mediators that are released to initiate the early events in type I hypersensitivity reactions. These mediators are preformed in the cell or activated through enzymatic processing. Mast cells normally are distributed throughout connective tissue, especially in areas beneath the skin and mucous membranes of the respiratory, gastrointestinal, and genitourinary tracts, and adjacent to blood and lymph vessels.[26,27] This location places them near surfaces that are exposed to environmental antigens and parasites. Mast cells in different parts of the body and even in a single site can have significant differences in mediator content and sensitivity to agents that produce mast cell degranulation.

Type I hypersensitivity reactions begin with mast cell or basophil sensitization. During the sensitization or priming stage, allergen-specific IgE antibodies attach to receptors on the surface of mast cells and basophils. With subsequent exposure, the sensitizing allergen binds to the cell-associated IgE and triggers a series of events that ultimately lead to degranulation of the sensitized mast cells or basophils, causing release of their preformed mediators (Fig. 19-3). Mast cells are also the source of lipid-derived membrane products (*e.g.*, prostaglandins and leukotrienes) and cytokines that participate in the continued response to the allergen.

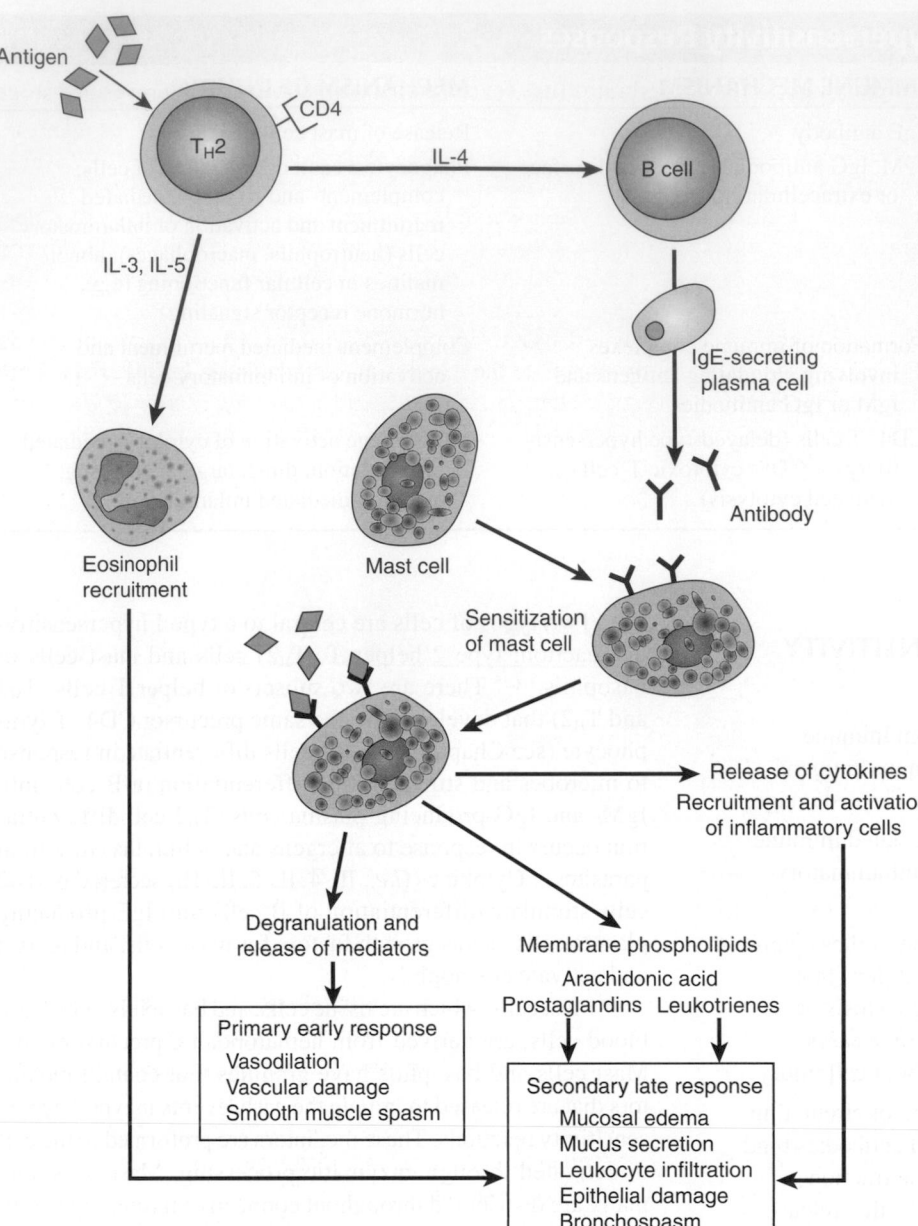

FIGURE 19-3 • Type I, IgE-mediated hypersensitivity reaction. The stimulation of B-cell differentiation by an antigen-stimulated type 2 helper (T$_H$2) T cell leads to plasma cell production of IgE and mast cell sensitization. Subsequent binding of the antigen produces degranulation of the sensitized mast cell with release of preformed mediators that leads to a primary, or early-phase response. T$_H$2 T-cell recruitment of eosinophils, along with the release of cytokines and membrane phospholipids from the mast cell, leads to a secondary, or late-phase response.

Many type I hypersensitivity reactions such as bronchial asthma have two well-defined phases: (1) a primary or initial-phase response characterized by vasodilation, vascular leakage, and smooth muscle contraction; and (2) a secondary or late-phase response characterized by more intense infiltration of tissues with eosinophils and other acute and chronic inflammatory cells, as well as tissue destruction in the form of epithelial cell damage.

The primary or initial-phase response usually occurs within 5 to 30 minutes of exposure to antigen and subsides within 60 minutes. It is mediated by mast cell degranulation and the release of preformed mediators. These mediators include histamine, acetylcholine, adenosine, chemotactic mediators, and enzymes such as chymase and trypsin that

lead to generation of kinins. Histamine is a potent vasodilator that increases the permeability of capillaries and venules and causes smooth muscle contraction and bronchial constriction. Acetylcholine produces bronchial smooth muscle contraction and dilation of small blood vessels. The kinins, which are a group of potent inflammatory peptides, require activation through enzymatic modification. Once activated, these peptide mediators produce vasodilation and smooth muscle contraction.

The secondary or late-phase response occurs about 2 to 8 hours later and lasts for several days. It results from the action of lipid mediators and cytokines involved in the inflammatory response. The lipid mediators are derived from mast cell membrane phospholipids, which are broken down to form arachidonic acid. Arachidonic acid, in turn, is the parent compound from which the leukotrienes and prostaglandins are synthesized (see Chapter 18). The leukotrienes and prostaglandins produce responses similar to histamine and acetylcholine, although their effects are delayed and prolonged by comparison. Mast cells also produce cytokines and chemotactic factors that prompt the influx of eosinophils and leukocytes to the site of allergen contact, contributing to the inflammatory response.

At this point, it is important to note that not all IgE-mediated responses produce discomfort and disease. Type I hypersensitivity, particularly the late-phase response, plays a protective role in the control of parasitic infections. IgE antibodies directly damage the larvae of these parasites by recruiting inflammatory cells and causing antibody-dependent cell-mediated cytotoxicity. This type of type I hypersensitivity reaction is particularly important in developing countries where much of the population is infected with intestinal parasites.

Anaphylactic (Systemic) Reactions

Anaphylaxis is a systemic life-threatening hypersensitivity reaction characterized by widespread edema, vascular shock secondary to vasodilation, and difficulty breathing[7,28–30] (see section on Anaphylactic Shock, Chapter 26). It results from the presence of antigen introduced by injection, insect sting, or absorption across the epithelial surface of the skin or gastrointestinal mucosa. The level of severity depends on the level of sensitization. Even small amounts of antigen, such as the presence of residual amounts of peanut that remain on equipment used for preparing foods containing peanuts, can be sufficient to cause anaphylaxis in an extremely sensitive person. Within minutes after exposure, itching, hives, and skin erythema develop, followed shortly by bronchospasm and respiratory distress. Vomiting, abdominal cramps, diarrhea, and laryngeal edema and obstruction follow, and the person may go into shock and die within the hour.

The initial management of anaphylaxis focuses on establishment of a stable airway and intravenous access, and administration of epinephrine.[28,30] Persons with a history of anaphylaxis should be provided with preloaded epinephrine syringes and instructed in their use. They should also be instructed to seek immediate professional help regardless of the initial response to self-treatment. Family members and caregivers of young children should be trained to inject epinephrine. Prevention of exposure to potential triggers that cause anaphylaxis is particularly important. Finally, all persons with potential for anaphylaxis should be advised to wear or carry a medical alert bracelet, necklace, or other identification to inform emergency personnel of the possibility of anaphylaxis.

Atopic (Local) Reactions

Local or atopic reactions usually occur when the antigen is confined to a particular site by virtue of exposure. The term *atopic* refers to a genetically determined hypersensitivity to common environmental allergens mediated by an IgE–mast cell reaction. Persons with atopic disorders commonly are allergic to more than one, and often many, environmental allergens. The most common atopic disorders are urticaria (hives), allergic rhinitis (hay fever), atopic dermatitis, food allergies, and some forms of asthma. The discussion in this section focuses on allergic rhinitis and food allergy. Allergic asthma is discussed in Chapter 29 and atopic dermatitis in Chapter 61.

The susceptibility to immediate hypersensitivity disorders tends to be genetically determined, and a positive family history of allergy is found in about 50% of atopic individuals.[7] The genetic basis of atopy is unclear; however, linkage studies suggest an association with cytokine genes on chromosome 5q that regulate the expression of circulating IgE.[7] Persons with atopic allergic conditions tend to have high serum levels of IgE and increased numbers of basophils and mast cells. Although the IgE-triggered response is likely a key factor in the pathophysiology of atopic allergic disorders, it is not the only factor and may not be responsible for conditions such as atopic dermatitis and certain forms of asthma.

Allergic Rhinitis. Allergic rhinitis is characterized by symptoms of sneezing, itching, and watery discharge from the nose and eyes (rhinoconjunctivitis). Allergic rhinitis not only produces nasal symptoms but frequently is associated with other chronic airway disorders, such as sinusitis and bronchial asthma.[31–33] Severe attacks may be accompanied by systemic malaise, fatigue, and muscle soreness from sneezing. Fever is absent. Sinus obstruction may cause headache. Typical allergens include pollens from ragweed, grasses, trees, and weeds; fungal spores; house dust mites; animal dander; and feathers. Allergic rhinitis can be divided into perennial and seasonal allergic rhinitis depending on the chronology of symptoms. Persons with the perennial type of allergic rhinitis experience symptoms throughout the year, but those with seasonal allergic rhinitis (*i.e.,* hay fever) are plagued with intense symptoms in conjunction with periods of high allergen (*e.g.,* pollens, fungal spores) exposure. Symptoms that become worse at night suggest a household allergen, and symptoms that disappear on weekends suggest occupational exposure.

Diagnosis depends on a careful history and physical examination, microscopic identification of an increased number of eosinophils on a nasal smear, and skin testing to identify the offending allergens.[31] When possible, avoidance of the offending allergen is recommended. Treatment is symptomatic in most cases and includes the use of oral antihistamines and oral or topical decongestants.[32] Tolerance and rebound congestion may occur when topical decongestants are used for longer than 1 week. Intranasal corticosteroids often are effective when used appropriately. Intranasal cromolyn, a drug that stabilizes mast cells and prevents their degranulation, may be useful, especially when administered before expected contact with an offending allergen. A program of specific immunotherapy ("allergy shots") may be used when symptoms are particularly bothersome.[30,32] Desensitization involves frequent (usually weekly) injections of the offending antigens. The antigens, which are given in increasing doses, stimulate production of high levels of IgG, which acts as a blocking antibody by combining with the antigen before it can combine with the cell-bound IgE antibodies.

Food Allergies. Virtually any food can produce atopic or nonatopic allergies. The primary target of food allergy may be the skin, the gastrointestinal tract, and the respiratory system. The foods most commonly causing these reactions in children are milk, eggs, peanuts, soy, tree nuts, fish, and shellfish (*i.e.*, crustaceans and mollusks).[34,35] In adults, they are peanuts,[36] shellfish, and fish.[34] The allergenicity of a food may be changed by heating or cooking. A person may be allergic to drinking milk but may not have symptoms when milk is included in cooked foods. Both acute reactions (hives and anaphylaxis) and chronic reactions (asthma, atopic dermatitis, and gastrointestinal disorders) can occur. Anaphylaxis occurs as a multiorgan response associated with IgE-mediated hypersensitivity. The foods most responsible for anaphylaxis are peanuts, tree nuts (*e.g.*, walnuts, almonds, pecans, cashews, hazelnuts), and shellfish.[34,37,38] One form of food-associated anaphylaxis occurs with exercise.[34,37,38] Food-associated, exercise-induced anaphylaxis may occur when exercise follows ingestion of a particular food to which IgE sensitivity has been demonstrated, or it may occur after ingestion of any food. Exercise without ingestion of the incriminated food does not produce symptoms.

Food allergies can occur at any age but, similar to atopic dermatitis and rhinitis, they tend to manifest during childhood. The allergic response is thought to occur after contact between specific food allergens and sensitizing IgE in the intestinal mucosa causes local and systemic release of histamine and other mediators of the allergic response. In this disorder, allergens usually are food proteins and partially digested food products. Carbohydrates, lipids, or food additives, such as preservatives, colorings, or flavorings, also are potential allergens. Closely related food groups can contain common cross-reacting allergens. For example, some persons are allergic to all legumes (*i.e.*, beans, peas, and peanuts).

Diagnosis of food allergies usually is based on careful food history and provocative diet testing. Provocative testing involves careful elimination of a suspected allergen from the diet for a time to see if the symptoms disappear and reintroducing the food to see if the symptoms reappear. Only one food should be tested at a time. Treatment focuses on avoidance of the food or foods responsible for the allergy. However, avoidance may be difficult for persons who are exquisitely sensitive to a particular food protein because foods may be contaminated with the protein during processing or handling of the food. For example, contamination may occur when chocolate candies without peanuts are processed with the same equipment used for making candies with peanuts. Even using the same spatula to serve cookies with and without peanuts can cause enough contamination to produce a severe reaction.

Type II, Antibody-Mediated Disorders

Type II (antibody-mediated) hypersensitivity reactions are mediated by IgG or IgM antibodies directed against target antigens on cell surfaces or in connective tissues.[7,10] The antigens may be endogenous antigens that are present on the membranes of body cells or exogenous antigens that are adsorbed on the membrane surface. There are three different types of antibody-mediated mechanisms involved in type II reactions: opsonization and complement- and antibody receptor–mediated phagocytosis, complement- and antibody receptor–mediated inflammation, and antibody-mediated cellular dysfunction[7] (Fig. 19-4).

Complement- and Antibody-Mediated Cell Destruction

The deletion of cells targeted by antibody can occur by way of either the complement system or by antibody-dependent cell-mediated cytotoxicity (ADCC), which does not require complement. Complement-mediated cell destruction can occur because the cells are coated (opsonized) with molecules that make them attractive to phagocytes or because of the formation of membrane attack proteins that disrupt the integrity of the cell membrane and cause cell lysis (see Chapter 17, Understanding the Complement System). With ADCC destruction, cells that are coated with low levels of IgG antibody are killed by a variety of effector cells that bind to their target by their receptors for IgG, and cell lysis occurs without phagocytosis.

Examples of antibody-mediated cell destruction include mismatched blood transfusion reactions, hemolytic disease of the newborn due to ABO or Rh incompatibility (see Chapter 14), and certain drug reactions. In the latter, the binding of certain drugs or drug metabolites to the surface of red or white blood cells elicits an antibody response that lyses the drug-coated cell. Lytic drug reactions can produce transient anemia, leukopenia, or thrombocytopenia, which are corrected by the removal of the offending drug.

Complement- and Antibody-Mediated Inflammation

When antibodies are deposited in the extracellular tissues, such as basement membranes and matrix, the injury is the result of inflammation rather than phagocytosis or cell lysis.[7,10] In this case, the deposited antibodies activate complement, generating chemotactic byproducts that recruit and activate neutrophils and monocytes. The activated leukocytes release injurious substances, such as enzymes and reactive oxygen intermediates, that result in inflammation and tissue damage. Antibody-mediated inflammation is responsible for the tissue injury seen in some forms of glomerulonephritis, vascular rejection in organ grafts, and other diseases. In Goodpasture syndrome, for example, antibody binds to a major structural component of pulmonary and glomerular basement membranes, causing pulmonary hemorrhage and glomerulonephritis[10] (see Chapter 33).

Antibody-Mediated Cellular Dysfunction

In some type II reactions, antibody binding to specific target cell receptors does not lead to cell death, but to a change in cell function. In Graves disease, for example, autoantibody directed against thyroid-stimulating hormone (TSH) receptors on thyroid cells stimulates thyroxine production, leading to hyperthyroidism[7,10] (discussed in Chapter 41). In contrast, in

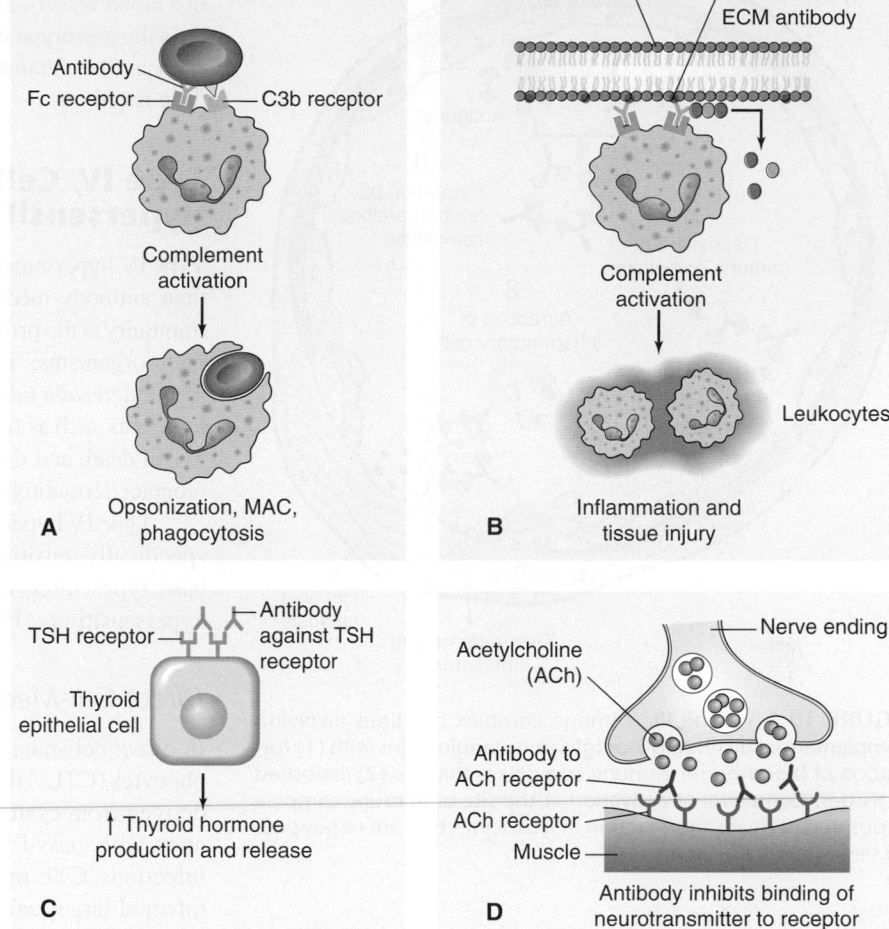

FIGURE 19-4 • Type II, hypersensitivity reactions result from binding of antibodies to normal or altered surface antigens. **(A)** Opsonization and complement- or antibody receptor–mediated phagocytosis or cell lysis through membrane attack complex (MAC). **(B)** Complement- and antibody receptor–mediated inflammation resulting from recruitment and activation of inflammation-producing leukocytes (neutrophils and monocytes). **(C)** Antibody-mediated cellular dysfunction, in which antibody against the thyroid-stimulating hormone (TSH) receptor increases thyroid hormone production, and **(D)** antibody to acetylcholine receptor inhibits receptor binding of the neurotransmitter in myasthenia gravis.

myasthenia gravis, autoantibodies to acetylcholine receptors on the neuromuscular endplates either block the action of acetylcholine or mediate internalization or destruction of receptors, leading to decreased neuromuscular function.

Type III, Immune Complex–Mediated Disorders

Immune complex allergic disorders are mediated by the formation of insoluble antigen–antibody complexes, complement fixation, and localized inflammation[7,10] (Fig. 19-5). Immune complexes formed in the circulation produce damage when they come in contact with the vessel lining or are deposited in tissues, including the renal glomerulus, skin venules, lung, and joint synovium. Once deposited, the immune complexes elicit an inflammatory response by activating complement, thereby leading to chemotactic recruitment of neutrophils and other inflammatory cells. The activation of these inflammatory cells by immune complexes and complement, accompanied by the release of potent inflammatory mediators, is directly responsible for the injury.

Type III reactions are responsible for the vasculitis seen in certain autoimmune diseases such as SLE or the kidney damage seen with acute glomerulonephritis. Type III immune complex disorders can be generalized if the immune complexes are formed in the circulation and deposited in many organs, or localized to a particular organ, such as the kidney, joints, or small blood vessels of the skin.

Systemic Immune Complex Disorders

Serum sickness is a systemic immune complex disorder that is triggered by the deposition of insoluble antigen–antibody (IgM, IgG, and occasionally IgA) complexes in blood vessels, joints, and heart and kidney tissue.[7,10] The deposited complexes activate complement, increase vascular permeability, and recruit phagocytic cells, all of which can promote focal tissue damage and edema. The term *serum sickness* was originally coined to describe a syndrome consisting of rash, lymphadenopathy, arthralgias, and occasionally neurologic disorders that appeared 7 or more days after injections of horse antiserum (tetanus). Although this therapy is not used today, the name remains. Currently, the most common causes of this allergic disorder include antibiotics (especially penicillin) and other drugs, various foods, and insect venoms.

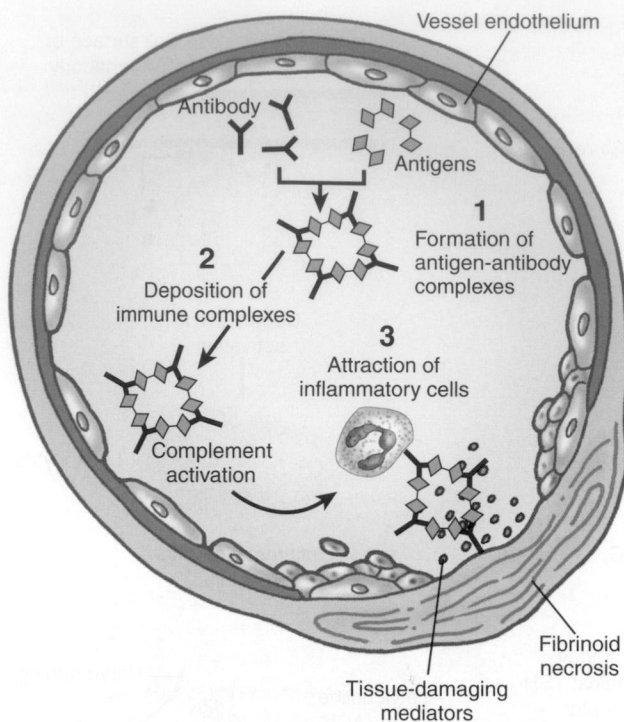

FIGURE 19-5 • Type III, immune complex reactions involving complement-activating IgG or IgM immunoglobulins with (1) formation of blood-borne immune complexes that are (2) deposited in tissues. Complement activation at the site of immune complex deposition (3) leads to attraction of leukocytes that are responsible for vessel and tissue injury.

The signs and symptoms include urticaria, patchy or generalized rash, extensive edema (usually of the face, neck, and joints), and fever. In most cases, the damage is temporary, and symptoms resolve within a few days. However, a prolonged and continuous exposure to the sensitizing antigen can lead to irreversible damage. In previously sensitized persons, severe and even fatal forms of serum sickness may occur immediately or within several days after the sensitizing drug or serum is administered.

Treatment of serum sickness usually is directed toward removal of the sensitizing antigen and providing symptom relief. This may include aspirin for joint pain and antihistamines for pruritus. Epinephrine or systemic corticosteroids may be used for severe reactions.

Localized Immune Complex Reactions

The *Arthus reaction* is a term used by pathologists and immunologists to describe localized tissue necrosis (usually in the skin) caused by immune complexes. In the laboratory, an Arthus reaction can be produced by injecting an antigen preparation into the skin of an immune animal with high levels of circulating antibody. Within 4 to 10 hours, a red, raised lesion appears on the skin at the site of the injection.[7] An ulcer often forms in the center of the lesion. It is thought that the injected antigen diffuses into local blood vessels, where it comes in contact with specific antibody (IgG) to incite a localized vasculitis (*i.e.,* inflammation of a blood vessel). This experimental model of localized vasculitis is the prototype of many forms of vasculitis seen in humans, such as the cutaneous vasculitides that characterize certain drug reactions.

Type IV, Cell-Mediated Hypersensitivity Disorders

Type IV hypersensitivity reactions involve cell-mediated rather than antibody-mediated immune responses.[7,10] Cell-mediated immunity is the principal mechanism of response to a variety of microorganisms, including intracellular pathogens such as *Mycobacterium tuberculosis* and viruses, as well as extracellular agents such as fungi, protozoa, and parasites. It can also lead to cell death and tissue injury in response to chemical antigens (contact dermatitis) or self-antigens (autoimmunity).

Type IV hypersensitivity reactions, which are mediated by specifically sensitized T lymphocytes, can be divided into two basic types: direct cell-mediated cytotoxicity and delayed-type hypersensitivity (Fig. 19-6).

Direct Cell-Mediated Cytotoxicity

In direct cell-mediated cytotoxicity, CD8+ cytotoxic T lymphocytes (CTLs) directly kill target cells that express peptides derived from cystosolic antigens that are presented in association with class I MHC molecules (see Chapter 17). In viral infections, CTL responses can lead to tissue injury by killing infected target cells even if the virus itself has no cytotoxic effects.[7] Some viruses directly injure infected cells and are said to be cytopathic, whereas other, noncytopathic viruses do not. Because CTLs cannot distinguish between cytopathic and noncytopathic viruses, they kill virtually all infected cells regardless of whether the infection is harmful. In certain forms of hepatitis, for example, the destruction of liver cells is due to the host CTL response and not the virus.

Delayed-Type Hypersensitivity Disorders

Delayed-type hypersensitivity (DTH) reactions occur in response to soluble protein antigens and primarily involve antigen-presenting cells such as macrophages and CD4+ helper T cells of the T_H1 type. During the reaction T_H1 cells are activated and secrete an array of cytokines that recruit and activate monocytes, lymphocytes, fibroblasts, and other inflammatory cells.[7] These T-cell–mediated responses require the synthesis of effector molecules and take 24 to 72 hours to develop, which is why they are called "delayed-type" hypersensitivity disorders.

The best-known DTH response is the reaction to the tuberculin test, in which inactivated tuberculin or purified protein derivative is injected under the skin. In a person who has been sensitized by previous infection, a local area of redness and induration develops within 8 to 12 hours, reaching a peak in 24 to 72 hours. The tuberculin reaction is characterized by

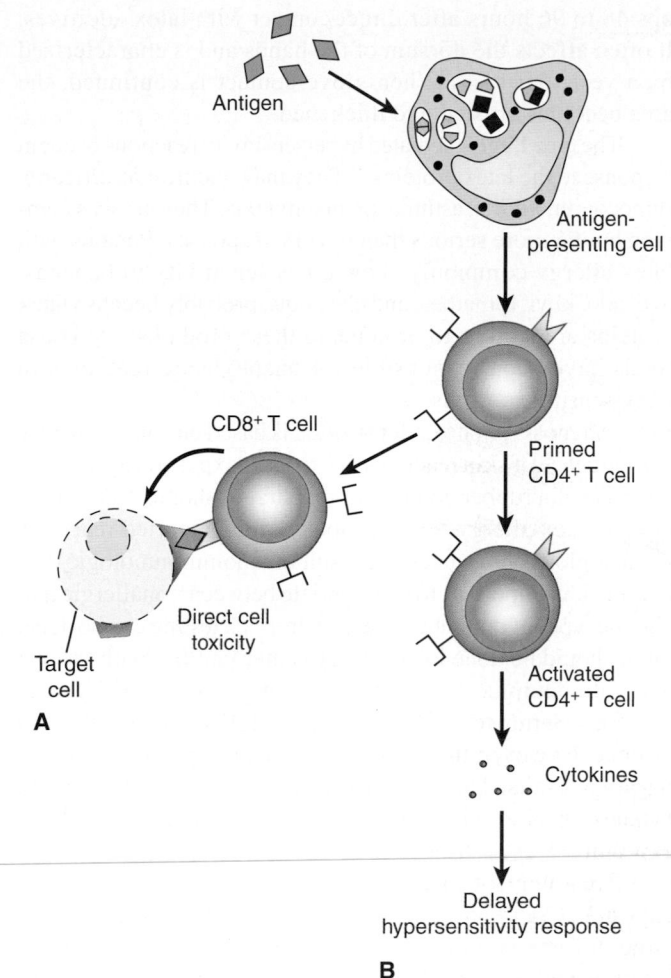

Allergic Contact Dermatitis. Allergic contact dermatitis denotes an inflammatory response confined to the skin that is initiated by reexposure to an allergen to which a person had previously become sensitized (*e.g.,* cosmetics, hair dyes, metals, topical drugs).[39] The most common form of this condition is the dermatitis that follows an intimate encounter with poison ivy or poison oak antigens, although many other substances can trigger a reaction.

Contact dermatitis is characterized by erythematous, papular, and vesicular lesions associated with intense pruritus and weeping. The affected area often becomes swollen and warm, with exudation, crusting, and development of a secondary infection. The location of the lesions often provides a clue about the antigen causing the disorder. The severity of the reaction associated with contact dermatitis ranges from mild to intense, depending on the person and the allergen. Because this condition follows the mechanism of a DTH response, the reaction does not become apparent for at least 12 hours and usually more than 24 hours after exposure. Depending on the antigen and the duration of exposure, the reaction may last from days to weeks.

Diagnosis of contact dermatitis is made by observing the distribution of lesions on the skin surface and associating a particular pattern with exposure to possible allergens. If a particular allergen is suspected, a patch test can be used to confirm the suspicion. Treatment usually is limited to removal of the irritant and application of topical preparations (*e.g.,* ointments, corticosteroid creams) to relieve symptomatic skin lesions and prevent secondary bacterial infections. Severe reactions may require systemic corticosteroid therapy.

FIGURE 19-6 • Type IV, cell-mediated hypersensitivity reactions, which include (**A**) direct cell-mediated cytotoxicity in which CD8⁺ T cells kill the antigen-bearing target cells, and (**B**) delayed-type hypersensitivity reactions in which presensitized CD4⁺ cells release cell-damaging cytokines.

Hypersensitivity Pneumonitis. Hypersensitivity pneumonitis, which is associated with exposure to inhaled organic dusts or related occupational antigens, is another example of a DTH reaction.[40] The disorder is thought to involve a susceptible host and activation of pulmonary T cells, followed by the release of cytokine mediators of inflammation. The inflammatory response that ensues (usually several hours after exposure) produces labored breathing, dry cough, chills and fever, headache, and malaise. The symptoms usually subside within hours after the sensitizing antigens are removed. A primary example of hypersensitivity pneumonitis is "farmer's lung," a condition resulting from exposure to moldy hay. Other sensitizing antigens include tree bark, sawdust, animal dander, and *Actinomycetes* bacteria that are occasionally found in humidifiers, hot tubs, and swimming pools. Exposure to small amounts of antigen for a long period may lead to chronic lung disease with minimal reversibility. This can happen to persons exposed to avian or animal antigens or a contaminated home air humidifier.

The most important element in the diagnosis of hypersensitivity pneumonitis is to obtain a good history (occupational and otherwise) of exposure to possible antigens. Treatment consists of identifying and avoiding the offending antigens. Severe forms of the disorder may be treated with systemic corticosteroid therapy.

perivascular accumulation of T$_H$1 cells and, to a lesser extent, macrophages. Local secretion of cytokines by these mononuclear inflammatory cells leads to increased microvascular permeability with local redness and swelling. The sequence of events in DTH, as demonstrated by the tuberculin reaction, begins with the first exposure to the tubercle bacilli (see Chapter 28). The T$_H$1 cells recognize the peptide antigens of the tubercle bacilli in association with class II MHC antigens on the surface of monocytes and antigen-presenting cells that have processed the mycobacterial antigens. This process leads to formation of sensitized T$_H$1 memory cells that remain in the circulation for years. Subsequent injection of tuberculin into such an individual results in the secretion of T$_H$1 cell cytokines that are ultimately responsible for the DTH response.

In addition to its beneficial protective role, DTH can also be the cause of disease, including allergic contact dermatitis and hypersensitivity pneumonitis. It also can be involved in transplant rejection and autoimmune disorders.

Latex Allergy

With the advent of HIV and other blood-borne diseases, the use of natural latex gloves has spiraled. Between 1988 and 1992, an estimated 11.8 billion examining gloves and 1.8 billion surgical gloves were used in the United States.[41] Along with the expanded use of latex gloves have come increased reports of latex allergy among health care workers. It has been estimated that 1% to 6% of the general population has some sensitivity or allergy to latex, and 8% to 12% of health care workers regularly exposed to latex develop sensitivity.[42] Other persons at high risk of sensitization are those with prolonged exposure to latex, including persons who have undergone repeated surgeries.

Exposure to latex may occur by cutaneous, mucous membrane, inhalation, internal tissue, or intravascular routes. Most severe reactions have resulted from latex proteins coming in contact with the mucous membranes of the mouth, vagina, urethra, or rectum. Although their allergen content is not very high, condoms can cause severe reactions because they come in contact with the mucous membranes.[43] Children with meningomyelocele (spina bifida) who undergo frequent examinations and treatments involving the mucosal surface of the bladder or rectum are at particular risk for development of latex allergy.[41,44,45] A large number of latex products are used in dentistry, and oral mucosal contact is common during dental procedures. Anaphylactic reactions have been caused by exposure of the internal organs to the surgeon's gloves during surgery.

Natural rubber latex, derived from the milky sap of the *Heva brasiliensis* plant or rubber tree, is a milky mixture of proteins, phospholipids, and polyisoprene. Various accelerants, curing agents, antioxidants, and stabilizers are added to the liquid latex during the manufacturing process. Allergic reactions to latex products can be triggered by the latex proteins or by the additives used in the manufacturing process.[42] Cornstarch powder is applied to the gloves during the manufacturing process to prevent stickiness and give the gloves a smooth feel. The cornstarch glove powder has an important role in the allergic response. Latex proteins are readily absorbed by glove powder and become airborne during removal of the gloves.[42] High-exposure areas such as operating rooms where powdered gloves are used contain sufficiently high levels of aerosolized latex to produce symptoms in sensitized persons.

The allergy to latex products can involve a type I, IgE-mediated hypersensitivity reaction or a type IV, T-cell–mediated response. Irritant dermatitis, which can result from glove use, is an entirely nonimmunologic response and should not be regarded as an allergy.[43] The distinction between type I and type IV reactions to latex products is not always clear. Affected individuals may experience both types of reactions. The most common type of reaction to latex gloves is contact dermatitis caused by a type IV, DTH response to the chemical additives used to process most gloves. It presents as a contact dermatitis that usually develops 48 to 96 hours after direct contact with latex additives. It often affects the dorsum of the hands and is characterized by a vesicular rash. When glove contact is continued, the area becomes crusted and thickened.

The type I, IgE-mediated hypersensitivity reactions occur in response to the latex proteins.[42] They may manifest as urticaria, rhinoconjunctivitis, asthma, or anaphylaxis. They are less common but far more serious than type IV responses. Persons with latex allergy commonly show cross-sensitivity to bananas, avocado, kiwi, tomatoes, and chestnuts, probably because latex proteins are similar to proteins in these products.[41,44] These foods have been responsible for anaphylactic reactions in latex-sensitive persons.

Diagnosis of latex allergy often is based on careful history and evidence of skin reactions due to latex exposure. Symptoms after use of a rubber condom or diaphragm should raise suspicion of latex allergy. Because many of the reported reactions to latex gloves have been the result of a nonimmunologic dermatitis, it is important to differentiate between nonallergic and allergic types of dermatitis. Latex skin-prick testing can be done, but it should be done in an allergy center familiar with the test and with equipment available to treat possible anaphylactic reactions. Serum tests for latex-specific IgE antibodies also can be done. However, these tests may give false-positive or false-negative results. Thus, at this time, diagnosis usually is based on latex-specific symptoms of IgE-mediated reactions to latex exposure.[44]

Treatment of latex allergy consists of avoiding latex exposure. Use of powder-free gloves can reduce the amount of airborne latex particles. Health care workers with severe and life-threatening allergy may be forced to change employment. Patients at high risk for latex allergy (*e.g.,* children with spina bifida, health care workers with atopy) should be offered clinical testing for latex allergy before undergoing procedures that expose them to natural rubber latex. All surgical or other procedures on persons with latex allergy should be done in a latex-free environment in which no latex gloves are used in the room or surgical suite and no latex accessories (*e.g.,* catheters, adhesives, tourniquets, and anesthesia equipment) come in contact with the patient.[43] In health care settings, general use of latex gloves with negligible allergen content, powder-free latex gloves, and nonlatex gloves and medical articles should be considered to minimize latex exposure.[43]

IN SUMMARY, hypersensitivity and allergic disorders are responses to environmental, food, or drug antigens that would not affect most of the population. There are four basic categories of hypersensitivity responses: (1) type I responses, which are mediated by the IgE-class immunoglobulins and include anaphylactic shock, hay fever, and bronchial asthma; (2) type II responses, which involve an antibody-mediated cell destruction (*e.g.,* transfusion reactions and hemolytic anemia), complement- and antibody-mediated inflammation (*e.g.,* some forms of glomerulonephritis), and antibody-mediated cell dysfunction (*e.g.,* Graves disease and myasthenia gravis); (3) type III hypersensitivity reactions, which involve the formation and deposition of insoluble antigen–antibody complexes, and are responsible for the vasculitis (seen in SLE or acute glomerulonephritis), systemic immune complex disease (serum sickness), and local immune complex disease (Arthus reaction); and (4) type IV cell-mediated hypersensitivity reactions, which include direct cell cytotoxicity, in which sensitized CD8+ T cells kill antigen-bearing target cells; and delayed-type hypersensitivity reactions, in which presensitized CD4+ T cells release cytokines that damage and kill antigen-containing cells.

Latex allergy can involve a type I, IgE-mediated reaction or a type IV, cell-mediated response. The most common type of allergic reaction to latex gloves is a contact dermatitis caused by a type IV, delayed-type hypersensitivity reaction to rubber additives. The type I, IgE-mediated response to the latex protein is less common but can cause far more serious anaphylactic reactions. ∎

TRANSPLANTATION IMMUNOPATHOLOGY

After completing this section of the chapter, you should be able to meet the following objectives:

- Discuss the rationale for matching of human leukocyte antigen or major histocompatibility complex types in organ transplantation.
- Compare the immune mechanisms involved in allogeneic transplant rejection.
- Describe the mechanisms and manifestations of graft-versus-host disease.

Transplantation is the process of taking cells, tissues, or organs, called a *graft,* from one individual, and placing them into another individual. Sometimes grafts are transplanted from another site in the same person. The individual who provided the tissue is called the *donor,* and the individual who receives the graft is called either the *recipient* or the *host.* Transplantation rejection is discussed here because it involves several of the previously discussed immunologic reactions. A major barrier to transplantation is the process of rejection, in which the recipient's immune system recognizes the graft as foreign and attacks it.

The cell surface antigens that determine whether the tissue of transplanted organs is recognized as foreign are the MHC or *human leukocyte antigens* (HLA; see Chapter 17). Transplanted tissue can be categorized as an *autologous* graft if donor and recipient are the same person, *syngeneic* graft if the donor and recipient are identical twins, and *allogeneic* (or allograft) if the donor and recipient are related or unrelated but share similar HLA types. The molecules that are recognized as foreign on

allografts are called *alloantigens.* Donors of solid organ transplants can be living or dead (cadaver) and related or nonrelated (heterologous). The likelihood of rejection varies indirectly with the degree of MHC or HLA relatedness between donor and recipient.

Mechanisms Involved in Transplant Rejection

Rejection is a complex process that involves cell-mediated immunity and circulating antibodies. Although many cells may participate in the process of acute transplant rejection, only the T lymphocytes seem to be absolutely required.[1,7] The critical role of T cells has been documented in both humans and experimental animals. T-cell–mediated graft rejection is called *cellular rejection* and is induced by two mechanisms: destruction of graft cells by CD8+ cytotoxic T cells and delayed hypersensitivity reactions triggered by CD4+ helper T cells.[7] The recipient's T cells recognize allogeneic antigens in the graft by two pathways: the direct and indirect pathways. It has been suggested that the direct pathway is the major pathway in acute rejection and the indirect pathway is more important in chronic rejection.[7]

In the *direct pathway,* T cells of the recipient recognize allogeneic MHC molecules on the surface of antigen-presenting cells on the graft. Both the CD4+ and CD8+ cells of the transplant recipient are involved in the reaction. CD8+ cells recognize class I MHC molecules and differentiate into mature CTLs. Once mature CTLs are generated, they kill the grafted tissue by mechanisms already discussed. The CD4+ helper T-cell subset is triggered into proliferation and differentiation into T_h1 effector cells by recognition of allogeneic class II MHC molecules. As in delayed hypersensitivity reactions, cytokines secreted by activated CD4+ cells cause increased vascular permeability and local accumulation and activation of macrophages, resulting in graft injury.

In the *indirect pathway,* recipient T lymphocytes recognize antigens of the graft donor after they have been presented by the recipient's own antigen-presenting cells. This process involves the uptake and processing of MHC molecules from the grafted organ by the host antigen-presenting cells. Thus, the indirect pathway is similar to the physiologic processing and presentation of other foreign (*i.e.,* microbial) antigens. It results in T cells that react with graft cells through cytokine production and delayed hypersensitivity responses.

Although there is little doubt that T cells are essential to the rejection process, antibodies evoked against alloantigens can also mediate rejection.[7] The process, which is called *humoral rejection,* can take one of two forms. *Hyperacute rejection* occurs when preformed antidonor antibodies are present in the circulation of the recipient. Such antibodies may be present if the recipient has already rejected a kidney transplant or received blood products with nonidentical HLA antigens. When preformed antidonor antibodies are present, rejection occurs immediately after transplantation. The second form of antigen–antibody rejection occurs in recipients who were not previously sensitized, but who develop antibodies to graft alloantigens. The antibodies formed by the recipient may cause injury by several mechanisms, including complement-dependent cytotoxicity, inflammation, and antibody-dependent cell-mediated cytotoxicity. The initial target of these antibodies in rejection appears to be the graft vasculature.

Patterns of Rejection

The basic patterns of transplant rejection have historically been classified as hyperacute, acute, and chronic, based on the clinical tempo of the response and the pathologic mechanisms involved.[1,7,10] In actual practice, however, there is often an overlap in features. The diagnosis is further complicated by the effects of immunosuppressant drugs or recurrence of the original disease. The following section characterizes the rejection patterns in the context of renal transplantation. Similar responses occur with other types of organ transplants.

A *hyperacute reaction* occurs almost immediately after transplantation. In kidney transplants, it can often be seen at the time of surgery. As soon as blood flow from the recipient to the donor kidney begins, it takes on a cyanotic, mottled appearance. At other times, the reaction may take hours or days to develop. The hyperacute response is produced by existing recipient antibodies to graft antigens that initiate a type III, Arthus-type hypersensitivity reaction in the blood vessels of the graft. These antibodies usually have developed in response to previous blood transfusions, pregnancies in which the mother makes antibodies to fetal antigens, or infections with bacteria or viruses possessing antigens that mimic MHC antigens.

Acute rejection usually occurs within the first few months after transplantation and is evidenced by signs of organ failure. It also may occur suddenly months or even years later, after immunosuppression has been used and terminated. T lymphocytes play a central role in acute rejection, responding to antigens in the graft tissue. The activated T cells cause direct lysis of graft cells and recruit and activate inflammatory cells that injure the graft. In vascularized grafts such as kidney grafts, the endothelial cells of blood vessels are the earliest targets of acute rejection.

Chronic rejection occurs over a prolonged period. It manifests with dense intimal fibrosis of blood vessels of the transplanted organ. In renal transplantation, it is characterized by a gradual rise in serum creatinine over a period of 4 to 6 months. The actual mechanism of this type of response is unclear but may include release of cytokines that stimulate fibrosis.

Graft-Versus-Host Disease

Graft-versus-host disease (GVHD) occurs when immuno-logically competent cells or precursors are transplanted into recipients who are immunologically compromised. Although GVHD occurs most often in persons who have undergone allogeneic bone marrow transplantation, it may also follow transplantation of organs rich in lymphoid tissue (*e.g.*, the liver) or follow transfusions with nonirradiated blood.[7]

Three basic requirements are necessary for GVHD to develop: (1) the transplant must have a functional cellular immune component; (2) the recipient tissue must bear antigens foreign to the donor tissue; and (3) recipient immunity must be compromised to the point that it cannot destroy the transplanted cells.[1,46,47] The primary agents of GVHD are the donor immunocompetent T cells derived from the donor marrow and the recipient tissue that they recognize as foreign and react against.[7] GVHD results in activation of both CD4+ and CD8+ T cells with ultimate generation of a type IV, cell-mediated DTH and CTL reactions. The greater the difference in tissue antigens between the donor and recipient, the greater is the likelihood of GVHD.

GVHD can occur as an acute or chronic reaction. Acute GVHD, which develops within days to weeks after transplantation, involves the epithelial cells of the skin, liver, and gastrointestinal tract.[7] The organ most commonly affected in acute GVHD is the skin. There is development of a pruritic, maculopapular rash, which begins on the palms and soles and frequently extends over the entire body, with subsequent desquamation. Involvement of the gastrointestinal tract usually parallels the development of skin and liver involvement. Gastrointestinal symptoms include nausea, bloody diarrhea, and abdominal pain. GVHD of the liver is heralded by painless jaundice, hyperbilirubinemia, and abnormal liver function test results. Liver involvement can progress to development of veno-occlusive disease, drug toxicity, viral infection, iron overload, extrahepatic biliary obstruction, sepsis, and coma. *Veno-occlusive disease* is characterized by obliteration of the small hepatic veins and venules.[48] In acute veno-occlusive disease there is striking centrilobular congestion and hepatocellular necrosis. As the disease progresses, connective tissue is deposited in the lumen of venules and the centrilobular congestion becomes less evident.

GVHD is considered chronic if symptoms persist or begin 100 days or more after transplantation.[7] Chronic GVHD may follow acute GVHD or it may develop insidiously. While persons in whom chronic GVHD develops are profoundly immunocompromised, they develop skin lesions resembling systemic sclerosis (discussed in Chapter 59) and manifestations mimicking other autoimmune diseases.

A second type of GVHD can follow the transplantation of genetically identical tissue (*i.e.*, syngeneic or autologous). This type of GVHD stems from the use of pretreatment conditioning regimens (*e.g.*, total-body irradiation or treatment with cytotoxic drugs). The conditioning therapy disrupts the normal immune surveillance system and allows "rogue" autoreactive T cells to proliferate and attack native tissue. This type of GVHD usually is self-limited and not severe.

GVHD can be prevented by blocking any of the three steps of pathogenesis. For example, donor T cells can be selectively removed from the transplanted tissue or destroyed using various treatments such as monoclonal antibodies with attached toxins, equivalent to heat-seeking missiles. Alternatively, immunosuppressive or anti-inflammatory drugs such as cyclosporine and tacrolimus or glucocorticoids can be used to block T-cell activation and the action of cytokines.

IN SUMMARY, transplantation is the process of taking cells, tissues, or organs, called a *graft*, from one individual (a donor), and placing them into another individual (recipient). A major barrier to transplantation is the process of rejection in which the recipient's immune system recognizes the graft as foreign and attacks it. Destruction of the cells or tissues of the graft can result from direct action of the recipient's cytotoxic T cells; from T-cell–generated cytokines and a delayed hypersensitivity reaction; or from antibodies generated against antigens in the graft. Hyperacute rejection occurs almost immediately after transplantation and is caused by existing recipient antibodies to graft antigens that initiate a type III, Arthus-type hypersensitivity reaction in the blood vessels of the graft. Acute rejection occurs within the first few months after transplantation and occurs when cytotoxic T cells cause direct lysis of graft cells and recruit and activate inflammatory cells that injure the graft. Chronic rejection occurs over a prolonged period and is caused by T-cell–generated cytokines that stimulate fibrosis of graft tissue.

Graft-versus-host disease occurs when immunologically competent cells or precursors are transplanted into recipients who are immunologically compromised. Three basic requirements are necessary for GVHD to develop: (1) the transplant must have a functional cellular immune component; (2) the recipient tissue must bear antigens foreign to the donor tissue; and (3) recipient immunity must be compromised to the point that it cannot destroy the transplanted cells. ■

CHART 19-3 PROBABLE AUTOIMMUNE DISEASE*

Systemic
Mixed connective tissue disease
Polymyositis-dermatomyositis
Rheumatoid arthritis
Scleroderma
Sjögren syndrome
Systemic lupus erythematosus

Blood
Autoimmune hemolytic anemia
Autoimmune neutropenia and lymphopenia
Idiopathic thrombocytopenic purpura

Other Organs
Acute idiopathic polyneuritis
Atrophic gastritis and pernicious anemia
Autoimmune adrenalitis
Goodpasture syndrome
Hashimoto thyroiditis
Type 1 diabetes mellitus
Myasthenia gravis
Premature gonadal (ovarian) failure
Primary biliary cirrhosis
Sympathetic ophthalmia
Temporal arteritis
Thyrotoxicosis (Graves disease)
Crohn disease, ulcerative colitis

*Examples are not inclusive.

AUTOIMMUNE DISEASE

After completing this section of the chapter, you should be able to meet the following objectives:

- Relate the mechanisms of self-tolerance to the possible explanations for development of autoimmune disease.
- Name four or more diseases attributed to autoimmunity.
- Describe three or more postulated mechanisms underlying autoimmune disease.
- State the criteria for establishing an autoimmune basis for a disease.

Autoimmune diseases represent a group of disorders that are caused by a breakdown in the ability of the immune system to differentiate between self- and nonself-antigens. Autoimmune diseases can affect almost any cell or tissue in the body. Some autoimmune disorders, such as Hashimoto thyroiditis, are tissue specific; others, such as SLE, affect multiple organs and systems. Chart 19-3 lists some of the probable autoimmune diseases. Many of these disorders are discussed elsewhere in this book.

Immunologic Tolerance

To function properly, the immune system must be able to differentiate foreign antigens from self-antigens. The ability of the immune system to differentiate self from nonself is called *self-tolerance*. It is the HLA antigens encoded by MHC genes that serve as recognition markers of self and nonself for the immune system (see Chapter 17). To elicit an immune response, an antigen must first be processed by an antigen-presenting cell (APC), such as a macrophage, which then presents the antigenic determinants along with an MHC II molecule to a CD4+ helper T cell. The dual recognition of the MHC–antigen complex by the T-cell receptor (TCR) of the CD4+ helper T cell acts like a security check. Similar recognition checks occur between CD8+ cytotoxic T cells and the MHC I–antigen complex of tissue cells that have been targeted for elimination. A number of chemical messengers (*e.g.*, interleukins) and costimulatory signals are essential to the activation of immune responses and the preservation of self-tolerance.

Several mechanisms have been postulated to explain the tolerant state, including central tolerance and peripheral tolerance.[7,49–52] *Central tolerance* refers to the elimination of self-reactive T cells and B cells in the central lymphoid organs (*i.e.*, the thymus for T cells and the bone marrow for B cells). *Peripheral tolerance* derives from the deletion or inactivation of autoreactive T cells or B cells that escaped elimination in the

IMMUNOLOGIC TOLERANCE

■ Immunologic tolerance is the ability of the immune system to differentiate self from nonself. It results from central and peripheral mechanisms that delete self-reactive immune cells that cause autoimmunity or render their response ineffective in destroying self-cells and self-tissue.

■ Central tolerance involves the elimination of self-reactive T and B cells in the central lymphoid organs. Self-reactive T cells are deleted in the thymus and self-reactive B cells in the bone marrow.

■ Peripheral tolerance derives from the deletion or inactivation of self-reactive T and B cells that escaped deletion in the central lymphoid organs. It involves mechanisms such as receptor editing, absence of necessary costimulatory signals, production of immunologic ignorance by separating self-reactive immune cells from target tissues, and the presence of suppressor immune cells.

central lymphoid organs. *Anergy* represents the state of immunologic tolerance to specific antigens. It may take the form of diminished immediate hypersensitivity or delayed-type hypersensitivity, or both.

B-Cell Tolerance

Loss of self-tolerance with development of autoantibodies is characteristic of a number of autoimmune disorders. For example, hyperthyroidism in Graves disease is due to autoantibodies to the TSH receptor (see Fig. 19-4 and Chapter 41). Several mechanisms are available to filter autoreactive B cells out of the B-cell population: clonal deletion of immature B cells in the bone marrow; deletion of autoreactive B cells in the spleen or lymph nodes; functional inactivation or anergy; and receptor editing, a process that changes the specificity of a B-cell receptor when autoantigen is encountered.[49] There is increasing evidence that B-cell tolerance is predominantly due to help from T cells.[49]

T-Cell Tolerance

The central mechanisms of T-cell tolerance involve the deletion of self-reactive T cells in the thymus (Fig. 19-7). T cells develop from bone marrow–derived progenitor cells that migrate to the thymus, where they encounter self-peptides bound to MHC molecules. T cells that display the host's MHC antigens and T-cell receptors for a nonself-antigen are allowed to mature in the thymus (*i.e.,* positive selection). T cells that have a high affinity for host cells are sorted out and undergo apoptosis or cell death (*i.e.,* negative selection). The deletion of self-reactive T cells in the thymus requires the presence of autoantigens. Because many autoantigens are

not present in the thymus, self-reactive T cells may escape the thymus, so peripheral mechanisms that participate in T-cell tolerance are required.

Several peripheral mechanisms are available to control the responsiveness of self-reactive T cells in the periphery. Sometimes the host antigens are not available in the appropriate immunologic form or are separated from the T cells (*e.g.,* by the blood-brain barrier) so that corresponding T cells remain *immunologically ignorant* of their presence.[49] In other cases, the autoreactive T cell encounters its corresponding antigen in the absence of the costimulatory signals that are necessary for its activation. The peripheral activation of T cells requires two signals: recognition of the peptide antigen in association with the MHC molecules on the APCs and a set of secondary costimulatory signals. Because costimulatory signals are not strongly expressed on most normal tissues, the encounter of the autoreactive T cells and their specific target antigens frequently results in anergy.[7]

Another mechanism involves the apoptotic death of autoreactive T cells.[49,50,53] This type of apoptosis is mediated by an apoptotic cell surface receptor (called FAS) that is present on the T cell and a soluble membrane messenger molecule (FAS ligand) that binds to the apoptotic receptor and activates the death program (see Chapter 5). The expression of the apoptotic FAS receptor is markedly increased in activated T cells; thus, coexpression of the FAS messenger molecule by the same cohort of activated autoreactive T cells may serve to induce their death.

Suppressor T cells with the ability to down-regulate the function of autoreactive T cells are also thought to play an essential role in peripheral T-cell tolerance. These cells are believed to be a distinct subset of CD4+ and CD8+ T cells.[54–56] The mechanism by which these T cells exert their suppressor function is unclear. They may secrete cytokines that suppress the activity of self-reactive immune cells, or they may delete the self-reactive T-cell clones.

Mechanisms of Autoimmune Disease

It is obvious that autoimmunity results from loss of self-tolerance. Just how this happens is largely unknown, but both inheritance of susceptibility genes that contribute to the maintenance of self-tolerance and environmental factors, such as infections that promote the activation of self-reactive lymphocytes, are clearly important. Gender may also play a role in the development of autoimmune disorders. A number of autoimmune disorders such as SLE occur more commonly in women than men, suggesting that estrogens may play a role in the development of autoimmune disease. Evidence suggests that estrogens stimulate and androgens suppress the immune response.[57,58] For example, estrogen stimulates a DNA sequence that promotes the production of interferon-γ, which is thought to assist in the induction of an autoimmune response. Because of the complexity of the immune system, it seems unlikely that autoimmune disorders arise from a single defect.

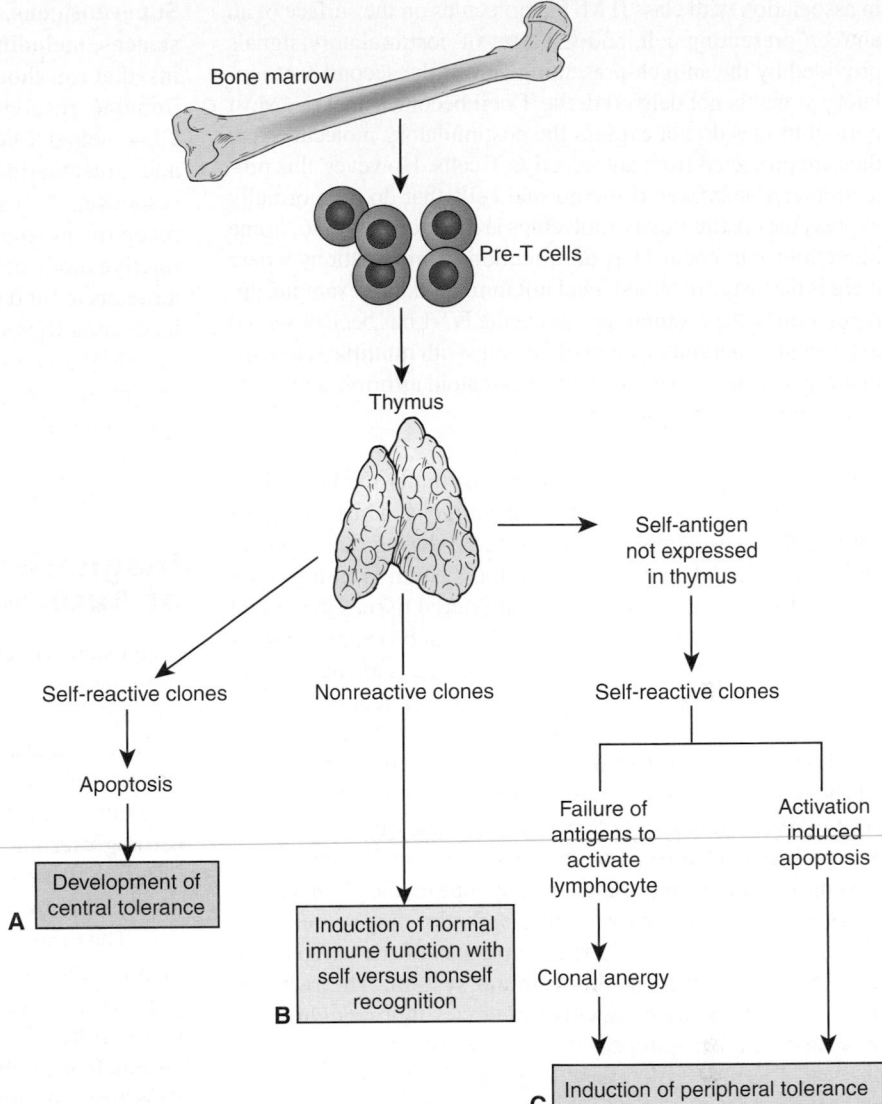

Bone marrow

Pre-T cells

Thymus

Self-antigen not expressed in thymus

Self-reactive clones   Nonreactive clones   Self-reactive clones

Apoptosis

Failure of antigens to activate lymphocyte   Activation induced apoptosis

A Development of central tolerance

B Induction of normal immune function with self versus nonself recognition

Clonal anergy

C Induction of peripheral tolerance

FIGURE 19-7 • Development of immunologic tolerance. **(A)** Development of central tolerance with deletion of self-reactive T lymphocytes in the thymus. **(B)** Nonreactive lymphocytes with development of normal immune function. **(C)** Induction of peripheral tolerance in self-reactive cells that are not eliminated in the thymus.

Heredity

Genetic factors can increase the incidence and severity of autoimmune diseases, as shown by the familial clustering of several autoimmune diseases and the observation that certain inherited HLA types occur more frequently in persons with a variety of immunologic and lymphoproliferative disorders.[7,51,52] For example, 90% of persons with ankylosing spondylitis carry the HLA-B27 antigen, compared with 7% of persons without the disease.[7] Other HLA-associated diseases are Reiter syndrome and HLA-B27, rheumatoid arthritis and HLA-DR4, and SLE and HLA-DR3 (see Chapter 59). The molecular basis for these associations is unknown. Because autoimmunity does not develop in all persons with genetic predisposition, it appears that other factors such as a "trigger event" interact to precipitate the altered immune state. The event or events that trigger the development of an autoimmune response are unknown. It has been suggested that the "trigger" may be a virus or other

microorganism, a chemical substance, or a self-antigen from a body tissue that has been hidden from the immune system during development.

Environmental Factors

Although environmental factors, such as infectious agents, appear to be involved in the pathogenesis of autoimmune disorders, their precise role in initiating or perpetuating the autoreactive response is largely unknown. Among the proposed mechanisms involved in loss of self-tolerance are breakdown of T-cell anergy, release of sequestered antigens, molecular mimicry, and superantigens.

Breakdown in T-Cell Anergy. *Anergy* is a state of unresponsiveness to antigen. It involves the prolonged or irreversible inactivation of lymphocytes, such as that induced by an encounter with self-antigens. Activation of antigen-specific CD4+ T cells requires two signals: (1) recognition of the antigen in association with class II MHC molecules on the surface of an antigen-presenting cell, and (2) a set of costimulatory signals provided by the antigen-presenting cell. If the second costimulatory signal is not delivered, the T cell becomes anergic. Most normal tissues do not express the costimulatory molecules and thus are protected from autoreactive T cells. However, this protection can be broken if the normal cells that do not normally express the costimulatory molecules are induced to do so. Some inductions can occur after an infection or in situations where there is tissue necrosis and local inflammation. For example, up-regulation of the costimulator molecule B7-1 has been observed in the central nervous system of persons with multiple sclerosis, in the synovium of persons with rheumatoid arthritis, and in the skin of persons with psoriasis.[1]

Release of Sequestered Antigens. Normally the body does not produce antibodies against self-antigens. Thus, any self-antigen that was completely sequestered during development and then reintroduced to the immune system is likely to be regarded as foreign. Among the sequestered tissues that could be regarded as foreign are spermatozoa and ocular antigens such as those found in uveal tissue. Post-traumatic uveitis and orchiditis after vasectomy may fall into this category.

Changes in antigen structure or release of hidden antigens may also account for the persistence of autoimmune disorders. Once an autoimmune disorder has been induced, it tends to be progressive, sometimes with sporadic relapses and remissions. A possible mechanism for the persistence and evolution of autoimmunity is the phenomenon of epitope reading.[2] Infections, and even the initial autoimmune episode, may release and damage self-antigens and expose epitopes of the antigen that have been hidden from the immune system. The result is continued activation of new lymphocytes that recognize the previously hidden epitopes.

Molecular Mimicry. Many autoimmune diseases are associated with infections, and clinical flare-ups are often preceded by infectious processes. One proposed link between infections and autoimmunity is *molecular mimicry,* in which a microbe shares an immunologic epitope with the host.[59–61] In rheumatic fever and acute glomerulonephritis, for example, a protein in the cell wall of group A, beta-hemolytic streptococci has considerable similarity with antigens in heart and kidney tissue, respectively. After infection, antibodies directed against the microorganism cause a classic case of mistaken identity, which leads to inflammation of the heart or kidney. Not everyone exposed to group A, beta-hemolytic streptococci has an autoimmune reaction. The reason that only certain persons are targeted for autoimmune reactions to a particular self-mimicry molecule may be determined by differences in HLA types. The HLA type determines exactly which fragments of a pathogen are displayed on the cell surface for presentation to T cells. One individual's HLA may bind self-mimicry molecules for presentation to T cells, and another's HLA type may not. In the spondyloarthropathies, particularly Reiter syndrome and reactive arthritis, there is a clear relationship between arthritis and a prior bacterial infection, combined with the inherited HLA-B27 antigens.[59]

Superantigens. Superantigens are a family of related substances, including staphylococcal and streptococcal exotoxins, that can short-circuit the normal sequence of events in an immune response, leading to inappropriate activation of CD4+ helper T cells. Superantigens do not require processing and presentation of antigen by APCs to induce a T-cell response.[62,63] Instead, they are able to interact with a T-cell receptor outside the normal antigen-binding site. This distinctive mode of activation, together with the ability of superantigens to bind to a wide variety of MHC class II molecules, leads to activation of large numbers of T cells regardless of their MHC/peptide specificity. Superantigens are involved in several diseases, including food poisoning and toxic shock syndrome. Recently, a bacterial superantigen was isolated that may be important in the pathogenesis of Crohn disease[62] (see Chapter 37).

Diagnosis and Treatment of Autoimmune Disease

Suggested criteria for determining that a disorder is an autoimmune disorder are evidence of an autoimmune reaction, determination that the immunologic findings are not secondary to another condition, and the lack of other identified causes for the disorder. Currently, the diagnosis of autoimmune disease is based primarily on clinical findings and serologic testing. In the future, it is likely that autoimmune disorders will be diagnosed by directly identifying the genes responsible for the condition.

The basis for most serologic assays is the demonstration of antibodies directed against tissue antigens or cellular components. For example, a child with chronic or acute history of fever, arthritis, and a macular rash along with high levels of antinuclear antibody has a probable diagnosis of SLE. The detection of autoantibodies in the laboratory usually is accomplished by one of three methods: indirect fluorescent antibody assays (IFA), enzyme-linked immunosorbent assay (ELISA), or particle agglutination of some kind. The rationale behind each of these methods is similar: the patient's serum is diluted and allowed to react with an antigen-coated surface (*i.e.,* whole, fixed cells for the detection of antinuclear antibodies). In the case of IFA and ELISA, a second "labeled" antibody is added, which binds to the patient's antibody and forms a visible reaction. Particle agglutination assays are much simpler—the binding of the patient's antibody to antigen-coated particles causes a visible agglutination reaction. For most serologic assays, the patient's serum is serially diluted until it no longer produces a visible reaction (e.g., 1:100 dilution). This is called a *positive titer.* Healthy persons sometimes have low titers of antibody against cellular and tissue antigens, but their titers usually are far lower than in patients with autoimmune disease.

Treatment of autoimmune disease is based on the tissue or organ that is involved, the effector mechanism involved, and the magnitude and chronicity of the effector processes. Ideally, treatment should focus on the mechanism underlying the autoimmune disorder. Corticosteroids and immunosuppressive drugs may be used to arrest or reverse the downhill course of some autoimmune disorders. Purging autoreactive cells from the immune repertoire, through the use of plasmapheresis, is also an option in some severe cases of autoimmunity.[56]

Recent research has focused on the cytokines involved in the inflammatory response that accompanies many of the autoimmune disorders. Notably, interferon beta for multiple sclerosis and tumor necrosis factor-α antibodies (*e.g.,* infliximab) for rheumatoid arthritis and Crohn disease are the first new treatments for autoimmunity approved by the U.S. Food and Drug Administration in the past 20 years.[56] Finally, research into the development of vaccines that target critical pathways in the emergence of autoimmune responses is ongoing.

IN SUMMARY, autoimmune diseases represent a disruption in self-tolerance that results in damage to body tissues by the immune system. Autoimmune diseases can affect almost any cell or tissue of the body. The ability of the immune system to differentiate self from nonself is called *self-tolerance.* Normally, self-tolerance is maintained through central and peripheral mechanisms that delete autoreactive B or T cells or otherwise suppress or inactivate immune responses that would be destructive to host tissues. Defects in any of these mechanisms could impair self-tolerance and predispose to development of autoimmune disease.

The ability of the immune system to differentiate foreign from self-antigens is the responsibility of HLA encoded by MHC genes. Antigen is presented to receptors of T cells in combination with MHC molecules. Among the possible mechanisms responsible for development of autoimmune disease are failure of T-cell–mediated immune suppression; aberrations in MHC–antigen–TCR interactions; molecular mimicry; and superantigens. The suggested criteria for determining that a disorder results from an autoimmune disorder are evidence of an autoimmune reaction, determination that the immunologic findings are not secondary to another condition, and the lack of other identifiable causes for the disorder. ■

Review Exercises

1. A 20-year-old woman has been diagnosed with IgA deficiency. She has been plagued with frequent bouts of bronchitis and sinus infections.

   A. *Why are these types of infections particularly prominent in persons with an IgA deficiency?*

   B. *She has been told that she needs to be aware that she could have a severe reaction when given unwashed blood transfusions. Explain.*

2. Persons with impaired cellular immunity may not respond to the tuberculin test, even when infected with *Mycobacterium tuberculosis.*

   A. *Explain.*

3. A 32-year-old man presents in the allergy clinic with complaints of allergic rhinitis or hay fever. His major complaints are those of nasal pruritus (itching), nasal congestion with profuse watery drainage, sneezing, and eye irritation. The physical examination reveals edematous and inflamed nasal mucosa and redness of the ocular conjunctiva. He relates that this happens every fall during "ragweed season."

   A. *Explain the immunologic mechanisms that are responsible for this man's symptoms.*

   B. *What type of diagnostic test might be used?*

   C. *What type of treatment(s) might be used to relieve his symptoms?*

4. Persons with intestinal parasites and those with allergies may both have elevated levels of eosinophils in their blood.

   A. *Explain.*

References

1. Abbas A. K., Lichtman A. H. (2003). *Cellular and molecular immunology* (5th ed., pp. 453–464, 369–390). Philadelphia: W. B. Saunders.
2. Verbsky J. W., Grossman W. J. (2006). Cellular and genetic basis of primary immune deficiencies. *Pediatric Clinics of North America* 53, 649–684.
3. Bonilla F. A., Geha R. S. (2006). Update on primary immunodeficiency diseases. *Journal of Allergy and Clinical Immunology* 117(2 Suppl.), S435–S441.
4. Buckley R. H. (2000). Primary immunodeficiency diseases due to defects in lymphocytes. *New England Journal of Medicine* 343, 1313–1324.
5. Buckley R. (2004). T-, B-, and NK-cell systems. In Behrman R. E., Kliegman R. M., Jenson H. B. (Eds.), *Nelson textbook of pediatrics* (17th ed., pp. 683–700). Philadelphia: Elsevier Saunders.
6. The Jeffrey Modell Foundation Medical Advisory Board. (2008). Ten warning signs of primary immunodeficiency. [Online.] Available: www.info4pi.org/index.cfm?CFID=11982666&CFTOKEN=43062451. Accessed March 5, 2008.
7. Abbas A. K. (2005). Diseases of immunity. In Kumar V., Abbas A. K., Fausto N. (Eds.), *Robbins and Cotran pathologic basis of disease* (7th ed., pp. 205–227, 240–245). Philadelphia: Elsevier Saunders.
8. Sorensen R. U., Moore C. (2000). Antibody deficiency syndromes. *Pediatric Clinics of North America* 47, 1225–1252.
9. Rose M. E., Lang D. M. (2006). Evaluating and managing hypogammaglobulinemia. *Cleveland Clinic Journal of Medicine* 73, 133–144.
10. Warren J. S., Bennett D. P., Pomerantz R. J. (2008). Immunopathology. In Rubin R., Strayer D. S. (Eds.), *Rubin's pathology: Clinicopathologic foundations of medicine* (5th ed., pp. 99–131). Philadelphia: Lippincott Williams & Wilkins.
11. Elder M. E. (2000). T-cell immunodeficiencies. *Pediatric Clinics of North America* 47, 1253–1274.
12. Buckley R. H. (2002). Primary cellular immunodeficiency. *Journal of Allergy and Clinical Immunology* 109, 747–757.

13. Buckley R. H. (2004). Molecular defects in human severe combined immunodeficiency and approaches to immune reconstitution. *Annual Review of Immunology* 22, 625–655.

14. Rudd C. E. (2006). Disabled receptor signaling and new primary immunodeficiency disorders. *New England Journal of Medicine* 354, 1874–1877.

15. McKinnon P. J. (2004). ATM and ataxia telangiectasia. *EMBO Reports* 5, 772–776.

16. Ochs H. D., Thrasher A. J. (2006). The Wiskott-Aldrich syndrome. *Journal of Allergy and Clinical Immunology* 117, 725–738.

17. Johnston R. B. Jr. (2004). The complement system. In Behrman R. E., Kliegman R. M., Jenson H. B. (Eds.), *Nelson textbook of pediatrics* (17th ed., pp. 725–731). Philadelphia: Elsevier Saunders.

18. Frank M. M. (2000). Complement deficiencies. *Pediatric Clinics of North America* 47, 1339–1353.

19. Davis A. E. (2006). Mechanism of angioedema in first complement component inhibitor deficiency. *Immunology and Allergy Clinics of North America* 26, 633–651.

20. Zuraw B. L. (2006). Novel therapies for hereditary angioedema. *Immunology and Allergy Clinics of North America* 26, 691–708.

21. Rosenzweig S. D., Holland S. M. (2004). Phagocyte immunodeficiencies and their infections. *Journal of Allergy and Clinical Immunology* 113, 620–626.

22. Boxer L. A. (2004). Disorders of phagocyte function. In Behrman R. E., Kliegman R. M., Jenson H. B. (Eds.), *Nelson textbook of pediatrics* (17th ed., pp. 701–717). Philadelphia: Elsevier Saunders.

23. Lekstrom-Himes J. A., Gallin J. I. (2000). Immunodeficiency diseases caused by defects in phagocytes. *New England Journal of Medicine* 343, 1703–1714.

24. Horwitz M. E. (2000). Stem-cell transplantation for inherited immunodeficiency disorders. *Pediatric Clinics of North America* 47, 1371–1384.

25. Kay A. B. (2001). Allergy and allergic disease (parts 1 and 2). *New England Journal of Medicine* 344, 30–37, 109–113.

26. Galli S. J. (1993). New concepts about the mast cell. *New England Journal of Medicine* 328, 257–265.

27. Benoist C., Mathias D. (2003). Mast cells in autoimmune disease. *Nature* 420, 875–878.

28. Tang A. W. (2003). A practical guide to anaphylaxis. *American Family Physician* 68, 1325–1340.

29. Lieberman P. (2006). Anaphylaxis. *Medical Clinics of North America* 90, 77–95.

30. Lieberman P. Kemp S. F., Oppenheimer J., et al. (Chief Editors, Joint Task Force on Practice Parameters, Joint Counsel of Allergy, Asthma and Immunology). (2005). The diagnosis and management of anaphylaxis: An updated practice parameter. *Journal of Allergy and Clinical Immunology* 115(3 Suppl.), S483–S523.

31. Rachelefsky G. S. (1999). National guidelines need to manage rhinitis and prevent complications. *Annals of Allergy, Asthma, and Immunology* 82, 296–305.

32. Quillen D. M., Feller D. B. (2006). Diagnosis of rhinitis: Allergic vs. nonallergic. *American Family Physician* 73, 1583–1590.

33. Greiner A. N. (2006). Allergic rhinitis: Impact of the disease and consideration for management. *Medical Clinics of North America* 90, 17–38.

34. Sampson H. A. (2004). Update on food allergy. *Journal of Allergy and Clinical Immunology* 113, 805–819.

35. Sicherer S. H. (1999). Manifestations of food allergy: Evaluation and management. *American Family Physician* 57, 93–102.

36. Sampson H. A. (2002). Peanut allergy. *New England Journal of Medicine* 346, 1294–1299.

37. Keet C. A., Wood R. A. (2007). Food allergy and anaphylaxis. *Immunology and Allergy Clinics of North America* 27, 193–212.

38. Sampson H. A. (1998). Fatal food-induced anaphylaxis. *Allergy* 53(Suppl. 46), 125–130.

39. Mark B. J., Slavin R. G. (2006). Allergic contact dermatitis. *Medical Clinics of North America* 90, 169–185.

40. Selman M. (2004). Hypersensitivity pneumonitis: A multifaceted deceiving disorder. *Clinical Chest Medicine* 25, 531–547.

41. Sussman G. L. (1995). Allergy to latex rubber. *Annals of Internal Medicine* 122, 43–46.

42. Reines H. D., Seifert P. C. (2005). Patient safety: Latex allergy. *Surgical Clinics of North America* 85, 13–40.

43. Zucker-Pinchoff B., Stadtmauer G. J. (2002). Latex allergy. *Mount Sinai Journal of Medicine* 69, 88–95.

44. Reddy S. (1998). Latex allergy. *American Family Physician* 57, 93–102.

45. Poley G. E., Slater J. E. (2000). Latex allergy. *Journal of Allergy and Clinical Immunology* 105, 1054–1062.

46. Gilliam A. C. (2004). Update on graft versus host disease. *Journal of Investigative Dermatology* 123, 251–257.

47. Couriel D., Caldera H., Champlin R. E., et al. (2004). Acute graft-versus-host disease: Pathophysiology, clinical manifestations, and management. *Cancer* 101, 1936–1946.

48. Crawford J. M. (2005). The liver and biliary tract. In Kumar V., Abbas A. K., Fausto N. (Eds.), *Robbins and Cotran pathologic basis of disease* (7th ed., pp. 919–920). Philadelphia: Elsevier Saunders.

49. Kamradt T., Mitchison N. A. (2001). Advances in immunology: Tolerance and autoimmunity. *New England Journal of Medicine* 344, 655–664.

50. Davidson A., Diamond B. (2001). Autoimmune disease. *New England Journal of Medicine* 345, 340–350.

51. Rioux J. D., Abbas A. K. (2005). Paths to understanding the genetic basis of autoimmune disease. *Nature* 435, 584–589.

52. Goodnow C. C., Sprent J., de St Groth B. F., et al. (2005). Cellular and genetic mechanisms of self tolerance and autoimmunity. *Nature* 435, 590–597.

53. Navratil J. S., Sabatine J. M., Ahearn J. M. (2004). Apoptosis and immune responses to self. *Rheumatic Disease Clinics of North America* 30, 193–212.

54. Jiang H., Chess L. (2006). Regulation of immune responses by T cells. *New England Journal of Medicine* 354, 166–176.

55. Kronberg M., Rudensky A. (2005). Regulation of immunity by self-reactive T cells. *Nature* 435, 598–604.

56. Chatenoud L., Salomon B., Bluestone J. A. (2001). Suppressor T cells—they're back and critical to the regulation of autoimmunity. *Immunological Reviews* 182, 149–163.

57. Zandman-Goddard G., Peeva E., Shoenfeld Y. (2007). Gender and autoimmunity. *Autoimmunity Review* 6, 366–372.

58. Cutolo M., Sulli A., Seriolo S., et al. (1995). Estrogens, the immune response and autoimmunity. *Clinical and Experimental Rheumatology* 13, 217–226.

59. Albert L. J., Inman R. D. (1999). Molecular mimicry and autoimmunity. *New England Journal of Medicine* 341, 2068–2074.

60. Fujinami R. S., von Herrath M. G., Christen U., et al. (2006). Molecular mimicry, bystander activation, or viral persistence: Infections and autoimmune disease. *Clinical Microbiology Reviews* 19, 80–94.

61. Anders H.-J., Zecher D., Pawar R. D., et al. (2005). Molecular mechanisms of autoimmunity triggered by microbial infection. *Arthritis Research & Therapy* 7, 215–224.

62. Wucherfennig K. W. (2001). Mechanisms of induction of disease by infectious agents. *Journal of Clinical Investigation* 108, 1097–1104.

63. Llewelyn M., Cohen J. (2001). Superantigen antagonist peptides. *Critical Care* 5, 53–55.

Visit the Point **http://thePoint.lww.com for animations, journal articles, and more!**

Acquired Immunodeficiency Syndrome

Chapter **20**

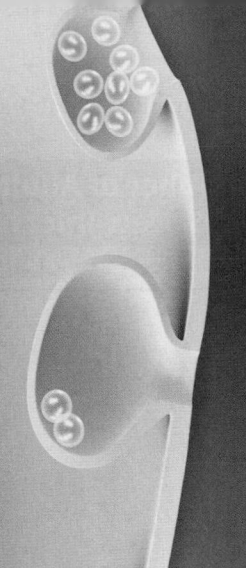

JASON FAULHABER AND JUDITH A. ABERG

➤ The acquired immunodeficiency syndrome (AIDS) is a disease caused by infection with the human immunodeficiency virus (HIV) and is characterized by profound immunosuppression with associated opportunistic infections, malignancies, wasting, and central nervous system degeneration. Because the disease affects an exceptionally high proportion of the population throughout the world, it is often referred to as a *pandemic.*[1]

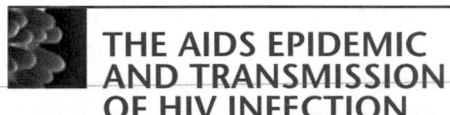

THE AIDS EPIDEMIC AND TRANSMISSION OF HIV INFECTION

After completing this section of the chapter, you should be able to meet the following objectives:

- Briefly trace the history of the AIDS epidemic.
- State the virus responsible for AIDS and explain how it differs from most other viruses.
- Describe the mechanisms of HIV transmission and relate them to the need for public awareness and concern regarding the spread of AIDS.

As a national and global epidemic, the degree of morbidity and mortality caused by HIV, as well as its impact on health care resources and the economy, is tremendous and unrelenting. At the end of 2006, it was estimated that there were nearly 40 million people worldwide living with HIV/AIDS and that over 25 million had died of the infection[2] (Table 20-1). During the same year, 4.3 million people were newly infected with HIV, with women and young people (*i.e.,* those 15 to 24 years of age) accounting for nearly 50% of the infections. Because the reporting of cases is not uniform throughout the world, many countries may not be accurately represented in this number. Projections for the next 10 years suggest that there will be 100 million people infected with HIV.

Most of the new infections worldwide are in people younger than 25 years of age who live in developing countries. Sub-Saharan Africa has been hardest hit by HIV. There are 24.7 million people living with HIV in Africa, with a reported

TABLE 20-1 Estimated Number of Adults and Children Living With HIV Infection/AIDS, New Infections, and Deaths at the End of 2006

	LIVING WITH	NEW INFECTIONS	DEATHS
North America	1,400,000	43,000	18,000
Sub-Saharan Africa	24,700,000	2,800,000	2,100,000
Eastern Europe and Central Asia	1,700,000	270,000	84,000
East Asia and Pacific	750,000	100,000	43,000
South and Southeast Asia	7,800,000	860,000	590,000
Western Europe	740,000	22,000	12,000
Caribbean	250,000	27,000	19,000
Latin America	1,700,000	140,000	65,000
Australia and New Zealand	81,000	7100	4000
Total	39.5 million	4.3 million	2.9 million

Data from UNAIDS. (2006). AIDS epidemic update—December 2006. [Online.] Available: www.unaids.org/en/HIV_data/epi2006/default.asp.

2.8 million new infections in 2006. Almost two thirds (63%) of all persons infected with HIV are living in sub-Saharan Africa. There are countries in Africa where more than 30% of the adults are infected with HIV. Because of the large number of infected people in Africa, the average life expectancy is expected to drop from 59 years to 45 years by 2005.[2] The death toll in sub-Saharan Africa represents 72% of global AIDS deaths.

Eastern Europe and central Asia have the world's fastest-growing HIV populations. Almost one third of all newly diagnosed HIV infections in Eastern Europe and central Asia are in people aged 15 to 24 years, with the Russian Federation and Ukraine accounting for 90% of all people living with HIV in this region.[2]

In the United States, 1.2 million people were living with HIV by the end of 2005, the most ever. The number of deaths in 2006 approximated 30,000, with racial and ethnic minorities being disproportionately affected.[2] Although blacks and Hispanics represent a minority of the population in the United States, they account for 55% of HIV infections.[3]

Emergence of the AIDS Epidemic

Compared with other human pathogens, HIV evolved very recently. In 1981, clinicians in New York, San Francisco, and Los Angeles recognized a new immunodeficiency syndrome in homosexual men. Initially, the syndrome was called GRIDS, for "gay-related immunodeficiency syndrome." By the end of 1981, there had been several hundred cases reported, and the name was changed to *acquired immunodeficiency syndrome,* or AIDS.[4] It soon became apparent that this disease was not confined to one segment of the population, but was also occurring in intravenous drug users, people with hemophilia, blood transfusion recipients, infants born to infected mothers, and high-risk heterosexuals. Studies of these diverse groups led to the conclusion that AIDS was an infectious disease spread by blood, sexual contact, and perinatally from mother to child.

An understanding of the virology of AIDS progressed with amazing efficiency; within 3 years of the first cases being recognized, the virus that causes AIDS had been identified. The virus was initially known by various names, including human T-cell lymphotropic virus type 3 (HTLV-III), lymphadenopathy-associated virus (LAV), and AIDS-associated retrovirus (ARV).[5] In 1986, the name *human immunodeficiency virus* became internationally accepted.[6]

Transmission of HIV Infection

HIV is a retrovirus that selectively attacks the CD4+ T lymphocytes, the immune cells responsible for orchestrating and coordinating the immune response to infection. As a consequence, persons with HIV infection have a deteriorating immune system, and thus are more susceptible to severe infections with ordinarily harmless organisms. The virus responsible for most HIV infection worldwide is called *HIV type 1* (HIV-1). A second type, *HIV type 2* (HIV-2), is endemic in many countries in West Africa but is rarely seen in other parts of the world.[7]

HIV is transmitted from one person to another through sexual contact, blood-to-blood contact, or perinatally. It is not transmitted through casual contact. Several studies involving more than 1000 uninfected, nonsexual household contacts with persons with HIV infection (including siblings, parents, and children) have shown no evidence of casual transmission.[8] HIV is not spread by mosquitoes or other insect vectors.[8] Transmission can occur when infected blood, semen, or vaginal secretions from one person are deposited onto a mucous membrane or into the bloodstream of another person.

Sexual contact is the most frequent mode of HIV transmission. Worldwide, 75% to 85% of HIV infections are transmitted through unprotected sex.[9] HIV is present in semen and vaginal fluids. There is a risk of transmitting HIV when these fluids come in contact with a part of the body that lets them enter the bloodstream. This can include the vaginal mucosa, anal mucosa,

PATHOPHYSIOLOGY OF HIV/AIDS

- The HIV is a retrovirus that destroys the body's immune system by taking over and destroying CD4+ T cells.

- In the process of taking over the CD4+ T cell, the virus attaches to receptors on the CD4+ cell, fuses to and enters the cell, incorporates its RNA into the cell's DNA, and then uses the CD4+ cell's DNA to reproduce large amounts of HIV, which are released into the blood.

- The three phases of HIV are primary HIV acute infection; latency, during which there are no signs or symptoms of disease; and overt AIDS, during which the CD4+ cell count falls to low levels and signs of opportunistic infections and other disease manifestations develop.

- As the CD4+ T-cell count decreases, the body becomes susceptible to opportunistic infections.

and wounds or sores on the skin.[9] Contact with semen occurs during vaginal and anal sexual intercourse, oral sex (*i.e.,* fellatio), and donor insemination. Exposure to vaginal or cervical secretions occurs during vaginal intercourse and oral sex (*i.e.,* cunnilingus). Condoms are highly effective in preventing the transmission of HIV. In most cities in the United States, sexual transmission of HIV is primarily related to vaginal or anal intercourse. In the United States, about 45% of HIV infections are among men who have sex with men, and 11% are from heterosexual contact.[2] In the developing world, heterosexual transmission is the major route of HIV infection.[6]

Because HIV is found in blood, the use of needles, syringes, and other drug injection paraphernalia is a direct route of transmission. Of the reported cases of AIDS in the United States, almost 25% occurred among persons who injected drugs.[2] HIV-infected injecting drug users can pass the virus to their needle-sharing and sex partners and, in the case of pregnant women, to their offspring.[6] Although alcohol, cocaine, and other noninjected drugs do not directly transmit infection, their use alters perception of risk and reduces inhibitions about engaging in behaviors that pose a high risk of transmitting HIV infection.

Transfusions of whole blood, plasma, platelets, or blood cells before 1985 resulted in the transmission of HIV. Since 1985, all blood donations in the United States have been screened for HIV, so this is no longer a transmission risk. The clotting factor used by persons with hemophilia is derived from the pooled plasma of hundreds of donors. Before HIV testing of plasma donors was implemented in 1985, the virus was transmitted to persons with hemophilia through infusions of these clotting factors.[6] Seventy percent to 80% of people with hemophilia who were treated with factor before 1985 became infected. Other blood products, such as gamma globulin or hepatitis B immune globulin, have not been implicated in the transmission of HIV.

Transmission from mother to infant is the most common way that children become infected with HIV. HIV may be transmitted from infected women to their offspring in utero, during labor and delivery, or through breast-feeding.[10] Ninety percent of infected children acquired the virus from their mother. In the 33 most affected countries, 26% of children born to HIV-infected mothers were estimated to be infected in 2005. Although this represents a 10% decrease from the estimated transmission rate in 2001, it is significantly higher than in developed countries, where transmission rates are less than 2%.[11]

Occupational HIV infection among health care workers is uncommon. Through December 2001, the Centers for Disease Control and Prevention (CDC) had received only 57 documented occupational HIV infections in the United States.[12] Fewer than 20 additional cases of occupational infections have been reported from outside the United States through the 1990s.[13] Universal Blood and Body Fluid Precautions should be used in encounters with all patients in the health care setting because HIV status is not always known. Occupational risk of infection for health care workers most often is associated with percutaneous inoculation (*i.e.,* needle stick) of blood from a patient with HIV infection. Transmission is associated with the size of the needle, amount of blood present, depth of the injury, type of fluid contamination, stage of illness of the patient, and viral load of the patient. The average risk for HIV infection from percutaneous exposure to HIV-infected blood is about 0.3%, and about 0.9% after a mucous membrane exposure.[12]

People with other sexually transmitted diseases (STDs) are at increased risk for HIV infection. The risk of HIV transmission is increased in the presence of genital ulcerative STDs (*i.e.,* syphilis, herpes simplex virus infection, and chancroid) and nonulcerative STDs (*i.e.,* gonorrhea, chlamydial infection, and trichomoniasis). HIV increases the duration and recurrence of STD lesions, treatment failures, and atypical presentation of genital ulcerative diseases because of the suppression of the immune system.

The HIV-infected person is infectious even when no symptoms are present. The point at which an infected person converts from being negative for the presence of HIV antibodies in the blood to being positive is called *seroconversion*. Seroconversion typically occurs within 1 to 3 months after exposure to HIV, but can take up to 6 months. Recent data suggest that 50% of transmissions occur during primary HIV infection (PHI) and early HIV infection.[14] The time after infection and before seroconversion is known as the *window period*. During the window period, a person's HIV antibody test result will be negative. Rarely, infection can occur from transfused blood that was screened for HIV antibody and found negative because the donor was recently infected and still in the window period. Consequently, the U.S. Food and Drug Administration (FDA) requires blood collection centers to screen potential donors through interviews designed to identify behaviors known to present a risk for HIV infection. In addition, nucleic acid amplification testing (NAAT) of blood donors has reduced the risk of transfusion transmission of HIV and hepatitis C virus to approximately 1 in 2 million blood units.[15]

IN SUMMARY, AIDS is an infectious disease of the immune system caused by HIV, a retrovirus that causes profound immunosuppression. First described in June 1981, the disease is one of the leading causes of morbidity and mortality worldwide. The severity of the clinical disease and the absence of a cure or preventive vaccine have increased public awareness and concern. Most recently, the greatest increase in incidence of the disease has been in women and young people 15 to 24 years of age.

HIV is transmitted from one person to another through sexual contact, blood-to-blood contact, or perinatally. Transmission occurs when the infected blood, semen, or vaginal secretions from one person are deposited onto a mucous membrane or into the bloodstream of another person. The primary routes of transmission are through sexual intercourse, intravenous drug use, and from mother to infant. Blood transfusions and other blood products continue to be routes of transmission in some underdeveloped countries. Occupational exposure in health care settings accounts for only a tiny percentage of HIV transmission. HIV infection is not transmitted through casual contact or by insect vectors. There is growing evidence of an association between HIV infection and other STDs. Infected individuals can transmit the virus to others before their own infections can be detected by antibody tests. ■

PATHOPHYSIOLOGY AND CLINICAL COURSE

After completing this section of the chapter, you should be able to meet the following objectives:

- Describe the structure of HIV and trace its entry and steps in replication within the CD4+ T lymphocyte.
- Describe the alterations in immune function that occur in persons with AIDS.
- Describe the CDC HIV/AIDS classification system.
- Relate the altered immune function in persons with HIV infection and AIDS to the development of opportunistic infections, malignant tumors, nervous system manifestations, the wasting syndrome, and metabolic disorders.

Molecular and Biologic Features of HIV

HIV is a member of the lentivirus family of animal retroviruses.[16,17] Lentiviruses, including feline immunodeficiency virus, simian immunodeficiency virus, and the visna virus of

sheep, are capable of long-term latency and short-term cytopathic effects. They can all produce slowly progressive fatal diseases that include wasting syndromes and central nervous system (CNS) degeneration. Two genetically different but antigenically related forms of HIV, HIV-1 and HIV-2, have been isolated in people with AIDS. HIV-1 is the type most associated with AIDS in the United States, Europe, and Central Africa, whereas HIV-2 causes a similar disease principally in West Africa. HIV-2 appears to be transmitted in the same manner as HIV-1; it can also cause immunodeficiency as evidenced by a reduction in the number of CD4+ T cells and the development of AIDS. Although the spectrum of disease for HIV-2 is similar to that of HIV-1, it spreads more slowly and causes disease more slowly than HIV-1. Specific tests are now available for HIV-2, and blood collected for transfusion is routinely screened for HIV-2. The ensuing discussion focuses on HIV-1.

HIV infects a limited number of cell types in the body, including a subset of lymphocytes called CD4+ T lymphocytes (also known as *T-helper cells* or *CD4+ T cells*), macrophages, and dendritic cells[6] (see Chapter 17). The CD4+ T cells are necessary for normal immune function. Among other functions, the CD4+ T cell recognizes foreign antigens and helps activate antibody-producing B lymphocytes.[6] The CD4+ T cells also orchestrate cell-mediated immunity, in which cytotoxic CD8+ T cells and natural killer (NK) cells directly destroy virus-infected cells, tubercle bacilli, and foreign antigens. The phagocytic function of monocytes and macrophages is also influenced by CD4+ T cells.

Like other retroviruses, HIV carries its genetic information in ribonucleic acid (RNA) rather than deoxyribonucleic acid (DNA). The HIV virion is spherical and contains an electron-dense core surrounded by a lipid envelope (Fig. 20-1). The virus core contains the major capsid protein p24, two copies of the genomic RNA, and three viral enzymes (protease, reverse transcriptase, and integrase). Because p24 is the most readily detected antigen, it is the target for the antibodies used in screening for HIV infection. The viral core is surrounded by a matrix protein called p17, which lies beneath the viral envelope. The viral envelope is studded with two viral glycoproteins, gp120 and gp41, which are critical for the infection of cells.

THE AIDS EPIDEMIC AND TRANSMISSION OF HIV

- Acquired immunodeficiency syndrome (AIDS) is caused by the human immunodeficiency virus (HIV).
- HIV is transmitted through blood, semen, vaginal fluids, and breast milk.
- Persons with HIV infection are infectious even when asymptomatic.

Replication of HIV occurs in eight steps[16,17] (see Fig. 20-1). Each of these steps provides insights into the development of methods used for preventing or treating the infection. The *first*

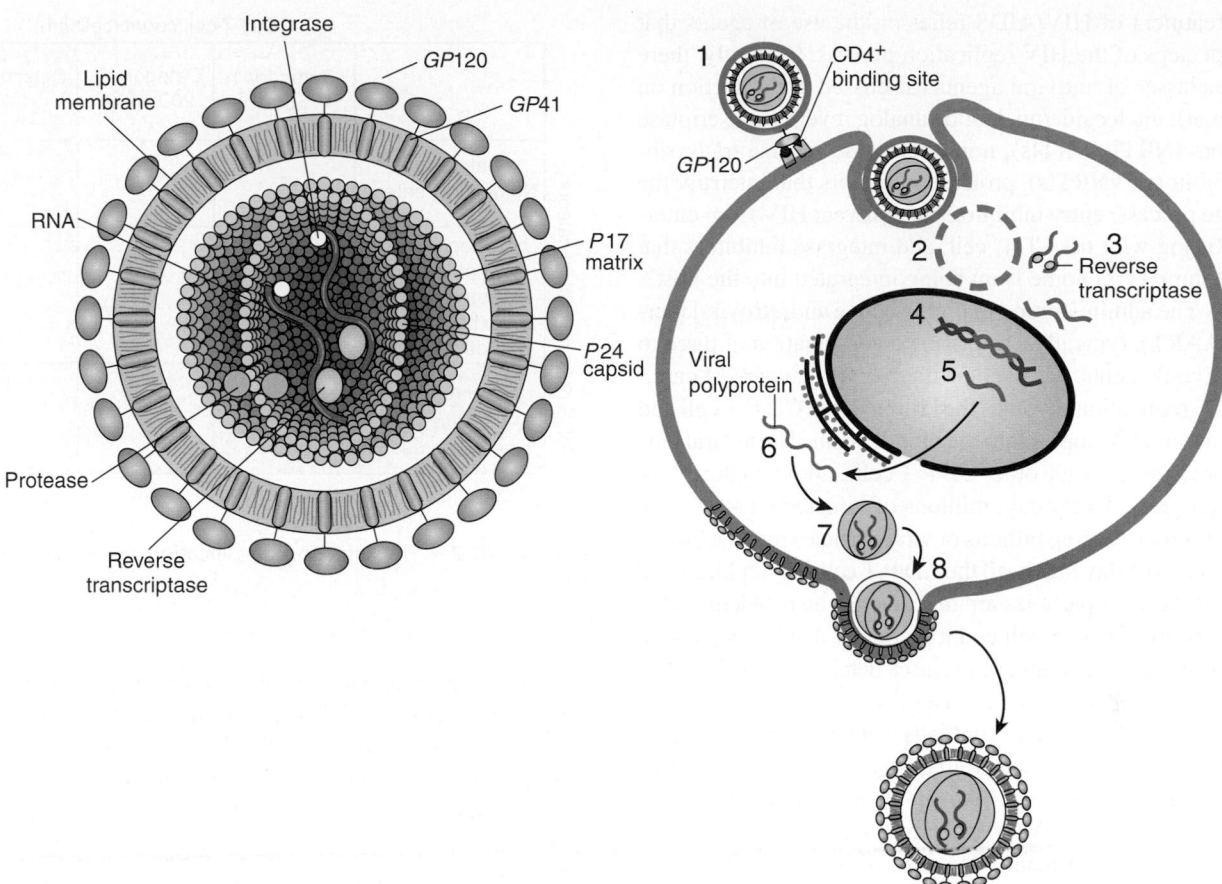

FIGURE 20-1 • Life cycle of the type 1 human immunodeficiency virus (HIV-1). **(1)** Attachment of the HIV virus to CD4+ T-cell receptor; **(2)** internalization and uncoating of the virus with viral RNA and reverse transcriptase; **(3)** reverse transcription, which produces a mirror image of the viral RNA and double-stranded DNA molecule; **(4)** integration of viral DNA into host DNA using the integrase enzyme; **(5)** transcription of the inserted viral DNA to produce viral messenger RNA; **(6)** translation of viral messenger RNA to create viral polyprotein; **(7)** cleavage of viral polyprotein into individual viral proteins that make up the new virus; and **(8)** assembly and release of the new virus from the host cell.

step involves the binding of the virus to the CD4+ T cell. Once HIV has entered the bloodstream, it attaches to the surface of a CD4+ T cell by binding to a CD4 receptor that has a high affinity for HIV. However, binding to the CD4 receptor is not sufficient for infection; the virus must also bind with other surface molecules (chemokine coreceptors, such as CCR5 and CXCR4) that bind the gp120 and gp41 envelope glycoproteins. This process is known as *attachment*. The *second step* allows for the internalization of the virus. After attachment, the viral envelope peptides fuse to the CD4+ T-cell membrane. Fusion results in an *uncoating* of the virus, allowing the contents of the viral core (the two single strands of viral RNA and the reverse transcriptase, integrase, and protease enzymes) to enter the host cell. The chemokine coreceptors are critical components of the HIV infection process. It has been reported that people with defective coreceptors are more resistant to development of HIV infection, despite repeated exposure.[18]

The *third step* consists of DNA synthesis. In order for HIV to reproduce, it must change its RNA into DNA. It does this by using the *reverse transcriptase* enzyme. Reverse transcriptase

makes a copy of the viral RNA, and then in reverse makes another mirror-image copy. The result is double-stranded DNA that carries instructions for viral replication. The *fourth step* is called *integration*. During integration, the new DNA enters the nucleus of the CD4+ T cell and, with the help of the enzyme integrase, is inserted into the cell's original DNA. The *fifth step* involves *transcription* of the double-stranded viral DNA to form a single-stranded messenger RNA (mRNA) with the instructions for building new viruses. Transcription involves activation of the T cell and induction of host cell transcription factors. The *sixth step* includes translation of mRNA. During *translation*, ribosomal RNA (rRNA) uses the instructions in the mRNA to create a chain of proteins and enzymes called a *polyprotein*. These polyproteins contain the components needed for the next stages in the construction of new viruses. The *seventh step* is called *cleavage*. During cleavage, the protease enzyme cuts the polyprotein chain into the individual proteins that will make up the new viruses. Finally, during the *eighth step,* the proteins and viral RNA are assembled into new HIV viruses and released from the CD4+ T cell.

Treatment of HIV/AIDS relies on the use of agents that interrupt steps of the HIV replication process. Currently, there are five classes of antiviral agents (discussed in the section on Treatment): nucleoside/nucleotide analog reverse transcriptase inhibitors (NRTIs/NRTIs), non-nucleoside reverse transcriptase inhibitors (NNRTIs), protease inhibitors that interrupt the cleavage process, entry inhibitors that prevent HIV from entering or fusing with the CD4+ cell, and integrase inhibitors that prevent the HIV genome from being integrated into the host's genome. The administration of highly active antiretroviral therapy (HAART), typically comprising a combination of three to four antiviral agents, has become the current standard of care.

HIV replication involves the killing of the CD4+ T cell and the release of HIV copies into the bloodstream. These viral particles, or *virions,* invade other CD4+ T cells, allowing the infection to progress. Every day, millions of infected CD4+ T cells are destroyed, releasing billions of viral particles into the bloodstream, but each day nearly all the CD4+ T cells are replaced and nearly all the viral particles are destroyed. The problem is that over years, the CD4+ T-cell count gradually decreases through this process, and the number of viruses detected in the blood of persons infected with HIV increases.[17]

Until the CD4+ T-cell count falls to a very low level, a person infected with HIV can remain asymptomatic, although active viral replication is still taking place and serologic tests can identify antibodies to HIV.[19] These antibodies, unfortunately, do not convey protection against the virus. Although symptoms are not evident, the infection proceeds on a microbiologic level, including the invasion and selective destruction of CD4+ T cells. The continual decline of CD4+ T cells, which are pivotal cells in the immune response, strips the person with HIV of protection against common organisms and cancerous cells.[20]

Classification and Phases of HIV Infection

HIV Infection and AIDS Case Definition Classification

Effective January 1, 1993, the CDC implemented a classification system for HIV infection and an AIDS case definition for adolescents and adults that emphasizes the clinical importance of the CD4+ cell count in the categorization of HIV-related clinical conditions.[21] The classification system defines three categories that correspond to CD4+ cell counts per microliter (μL) of blood: *category 1:* >500 cells/μL, *category 2:* 200 to 499 cells/μL, and *category 3:* < 200 cells/μL (Fig. 20-2).

There also are three clinical categories. *Clinical category A* includes persons who are asymptomatic or have persistent generalized lymphadenopathy or symptoms of primary HIV infection (*i.e.,* acute seroconversion illness). *Clinical category B* includes persons with symptoms of immune deficiency not serious enough to be AIDS defining. *Clinical category C* includes AIDS-defining illnesses that are listed in the AIDS surveillance case definition shown in Chart 20-1. Each HIV-infected person has a CD4+ T-cell count category and a clinical

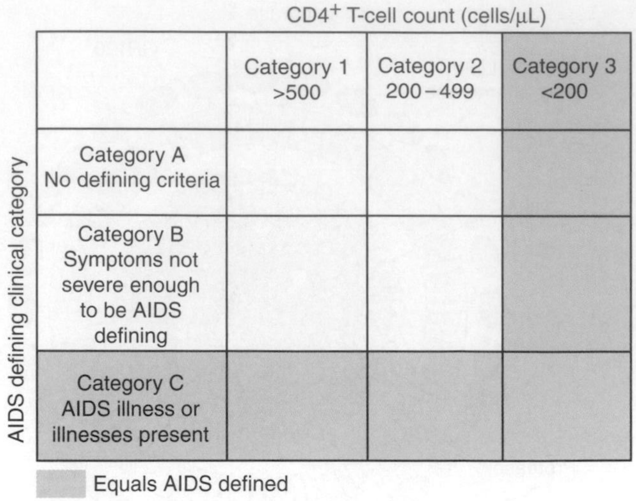

	CD4+ T-cell count (cells/μL)		
AIDS defining clinical category	Category 1 >500	Category 2 200–499	Category 3 <200
Category A No defining criteria			
Category B Symptoms not severe enough to be AIDS defining			
Category C AIDS illness or illnesses present			

☐ Equals AIDS defined

FIGURE 20-2 • HIV infection classification for adolescents and adults.

category. The combination of these two categorizations, CD4+ cell count categories 1, 2, and 3 and clinical categories A, B, and C, was initially created to guide clinical and therapeutic decisions in the management of HIV infection (see Fig. 20-2). This classification scheme is rarely used in clinical practice today, but remains a tool for epidemiologic reporting. According to the 1993 case definition, persons in category 3 or category C are considered to have AIDS.

Phases of HIV Infection

The typical course of HIV infection is defined by three phases, which usually occur over a period of 8 to 12 years. The three phases are the primary infection phase, chronic asymptomatic or latency phase, and overt AIDS phase[22] (Fig. 20-3).

Many persons, when they are initially infected with HIV, have an acute mononucleosis-like syndrome known as *primary infection.* This acute phase may include fever, fatigue, myalgias, sore throat, night sweats, gastrointestinal problems, lymphadenopathy, maculopapular rash, and headache (Chart 20-2). Fever and malaise are the symptoms most commonly associated with primary infection.[23] During primary infection, there is an increase in viral replication, which leads to very high viral loads, sometimes greater than 1,000,000 copies/mL, and a decrease in the CD4+ T-cell count. The signs and symptoms of primary HIV infection usually appear 1 to 4 weeks after exposure to HIV, and have an average duration of 7 to 10 days.[23] After several weeks, the immune system acts to control viral replication and reduces the viral load to a lower level, where it often remains for several years.

People who are diagnosed with HIV infection while they are in the primary infection phase may have a unique opportunity for treatment. Some experts hypothesize that if started early, treatment may reduce the number of long-living HIV-infected cells (*e.g.,* CD4+ memory cells).[24] Early therapy may also pro-

CHART 20-1	CONDITIONS INCLUDED IN THE 1993 AIDS SURVEILLANCE CASE DEFINITION

Candidiasis of bronchi, trachea, or lungs
Candidiasis, esophageal
Cervical cancer, invasive*
Coccidioidomycosis, disseminated or extrapulmonary
Cryptococcosis, extrapulmonary
Cryptosporidiosis, chronic intestinal (>1 month's duration)
Cytomegalovirus disease (other than liver, spleen, or nodes)
Cytomegalovirus retinitis (with loss of vision)
Encephalopathy, HIV-related
Herpes simplex: chronic ulcer(s) (>1 month's duration) or bronchitis, pneumonitis, or esophagitis
Histoplasmosis, disseminated or extrapulmonary
Isosporiasis, chronic intestinal (>1 month's duration)
Kaposi sarcoma
Lymphoma, Burkitt (or equivalent term)
Lymphoma, immunoblastic (or equivalent term)
Lymphoma, primary, of brain
Mycobacterium avium-intracellulare complex or *M. kansasii*, disseminated or extrapulmonary
Mycobacterium tuberculosis, any site (pulmonary* or extrapulmonary)
Mycobacterium, other species or unidentified species, disseminated or extrapulmonary
Pneumocystis jiroveci pneumonia
Pneumonia, recurrent*
Progressive multifocal leukoencephalopathy
Salmonella septicemia, recurrent
Toxoplasmosis of the brain
Wasting syndrome due to HIV

*Added to the 1993 expansion of the AIDS surveillance case definition.
(Centers for Disease Control and Prevention. [1992]. 1993 Revised classification system for HIV infection and expanded surveillance case definition for AIDS among adolescents and adults. *Morbidity and Mortality Weekly Report* 41 [RR-17], 19.)

during this phase.[26] Persistent generalized lymphadenopathy usually is defined as lymph nodes that are chronically swollen for more than 3 months in at least two locations, not including the groin. The lymph nodes may be sore or visible externally.

The third phase, overt AIDS, occurs when a person has a CD4+ cell count of less than 200 cells/μL or an AIDS-defining illness.[22] Without antiretroviral therapy, this phase can lead to death within 2 to 3 years. The risk of opportunistic infections and death increases significantly when the CD4+ cell count falls below 200 cells/μL.

Clinical Course

The clinical course of HIV varies from person to person. Most—60% to 70%—of those infected with HIV develop AIDS 10 to 11 years after infection. These people are the *typical progressors*.[22] Another 10% to 20% of those infected progress rapidly, with development of AIDS in less than 5 years, and are called *rapid progressors*. The final 5% to 15% are *slow progressors*, who do not progress to AIDS for more than 15 years. There is a subset of slow progressors, called *long-term nonprogressors*, who account for 1% of all HIV infections. These people have been infected for at least 8 years, are antiretroviral naive, have high CD4+ cell counts, and usually have very low viral loads. Among this group, the *elite controllers* consist of individuals who have spontaneous and sustained virologic suppression without the use of antiretroviral medications. This group of HIV-infected individuals is currently being investigated to assist in determining the immunologic and virologic interactions that allow those individuals to maintain virologic suppression of HIV.[27]

Opportunistic Infections

Opportunistic infections begin to occur as the immune system becomes severely compromised. The number of CD4+ T cells directly correlates with the risk of development of opportunistic infections. In addition, the baseline HIV RNA level contributes and serves as an independent risk factor.[28] Opportunistic infections involve common organisms that do not produce infection unless there is impaired immune function. Although a person with AIDS may live for many years after the first serious illness, as the immune system fails, these opportunistic illnesses become progressively more severe and difficult to treat.

Opportunistic infections are most often categorized by the type of organism (*e.g.,* fungal, protozoal, bacterial and mycobacterial, viral). Bacterial and mycobacterial opportunistic infections include bacterial pneumonia, salmonellosis, bartonellosis, *Mycobacterium tuberculosis* (TB), and *Mycobacterium avium-intracellulare* complex (MAC). Fungal opportunistic infections include candidiasis, coccidioidomycosis, cryptococcosis, histoplasmosis, penicilliosis, and pneumocystosis. Protozoal opportunistic infections include cryptosporidiosis, microsporidiosis, isosporiasis, and toxoplasmosis. Viral infections include those caused by cytomegalovirus (CMV), herpes simplex and zoster viruses, human papillomavirus,

tect the functioning of HIV-infected CD4+ T cells and cytotoxic T cells. Finally, early treatment could potentially help maintain a homogeneous viral population that will be better controlled by antiretroviral therapy and the immune system.

The primary phase is followed by a latent period during which the person has no signs or symptoms of illness. The median time of the latent period is about 10 years. During this time, the CD4+ T-cell count falls gradually from the normal range of 800 to 1000 cells/μL to 200 cells/μL or lower. More recent data suggest that the CD4+ T-cell decline may not fall in an even slope based on level of HIV RNA levels, and the factors related to variability in the decline in CD4+ cells are under investigation.[25] Lymphadenopathy develops in some persons with HIV infection

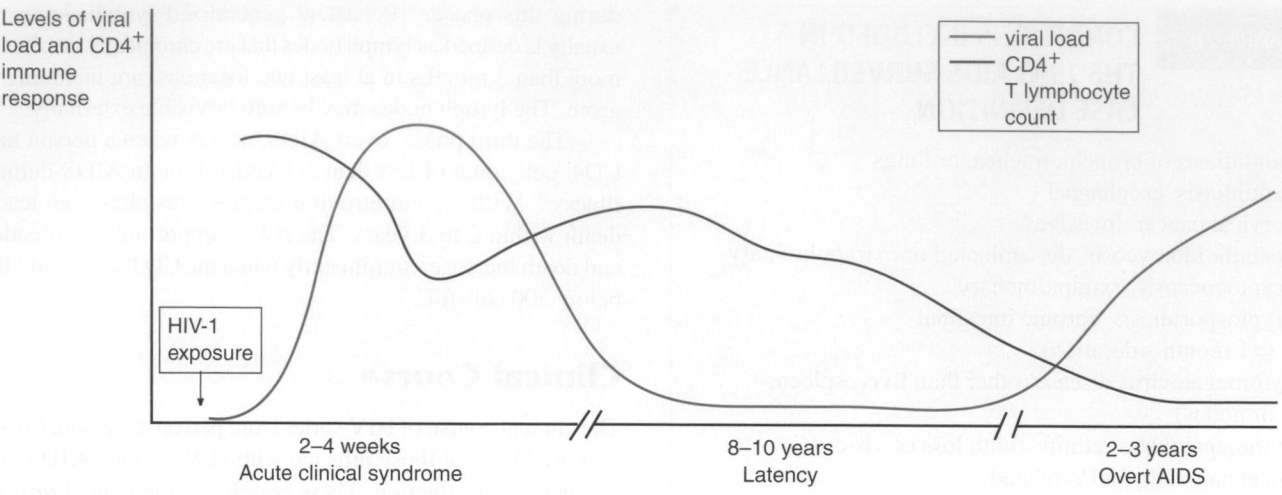

FIGURE 20-3 • Viral load and CD4+ cell count during the phases of HIV infection.

and JC virus, the causative agent of progressive multifocal leukoencephalopathy (PML).

In the United States, the most common opportunistic infections are bacterial pneumonia, *Pneumocystis jiroveci* pneumonia, oropharyngeal (thrush) or esophageal candidiasis, CMV retinitis, and infections caused by MAC.[29]

Respiratory Manifestations

The most common causes of respiratory disease in persons with HIV infection are bacterial pneumonia, *P. jiroveci* pneumonia, and pulmonary TB. Other organisms that cause opportunistic pulmonary infections in persons with AIDS include CMV, MAC, *Toxoplasma gondii,* and *Cryptococcus neoformans.* Pneumonia also may occur because of more common bacterial pulmonary pathogens, including *Streptococcus pneumoniae, Pseudomonas aeruginosa,* and *Haemophilus influenzae.*[30] Some persons may become infected with multiple organisms, and it is not uncommon to find more than one pathogen present. Kaposi sarcoma (to be discussed) also can occur in the lungs.

***P. jiroveci* Pneumonia.** *P. jiroveci* (formerly known as *Pneumocystis carinii*) pneumonia (PCP) was the most common presenting manifestation of AIDS during the first decade of the epidemic. PCP is caused by *P. jiroveci,* an organism that is common in soil, houses, and many other places in the environment. In persons with healthy immune systems, *P. jiroveci* does not cause infection or disease. In persons with HIV infection, *P. jiroveci* can multiply quickly in the lungs and cause pneumonia. As the disease progresses, the alveoli become filled with a foamy, protein-rich fluid that impairs gas exchange (Fig. 20-4). Since HAART and prophylaxis for PCP were instituted, the incidence has decreased.[29] PCP still is common in people unaware of their HIV-positive status, in those who choose not to treat their HIV infection or take prophylaxis, and in those with poor access to health care. The best predictor of PCP is a CD4+ cell count below 200 cells/μL,[29] and it is at this point that prophylaxis with trimethoprim-sulfamethoxazole (or an alternative agent in the case of adverse reactions to sulfa compounds) is strongly recommended.[27]

The symptoms of PCP may be acute or gradually progressive. Patients may present with complaints of a mild cough, fever, shortness of breath, and weight loss. Physical examination may demonstrate only fever and tachypnea, and breath sounds may be normal. The chest x-ray film may show interstitial infiltrates, but may be reported negative in up to 30% of cases.[31] Diagnosis of PCP is made on recognition of the organism in pulmonary secretions. This can be done through examination of induced sputum, bronchoalveolar lavage, transbronchial biopsy, and, rarely, open lung biopsy.

Mycobacterium Tuberculosis. Tuberculosis is the leading cause of death for people with HIV infection worldwide, and is often the first manifestation of HIV infection. At least one third of the 40 million people estimated to be living with HIV are likely to be infected with TB (UNAIDS press release, March 20, 2007). TB cases in the United States decreased from the 1950s to 1985; then, in 1986, the number of TB cases began to increase (see Chapter 28).[32] A number of factors contributed to this increase, including changes in immigration patterns and increased numbers of people living in group settings like prisons,

CHART 20-2	SIGNS AND SYMPTOMS OF ACUTE HIV INFECTION

- Fever
- Fatigue
- Rash
- Headache
- Lymphadenopathy
- Pharyngitis
- Arthralgia
- Myalgia
- Night sweats
- Gastrointestinal problems
- Aseptic meningitis
- Oral or genital ulcers

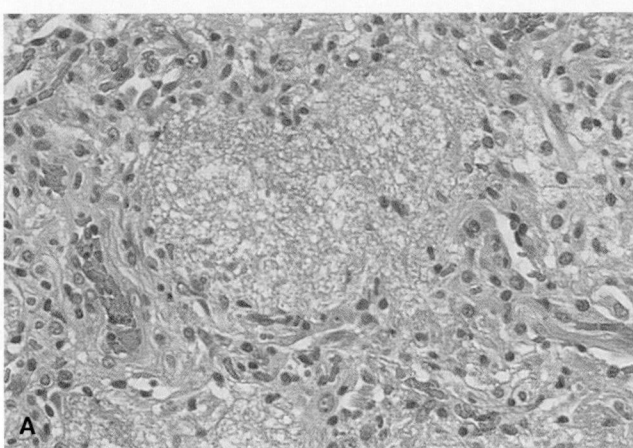 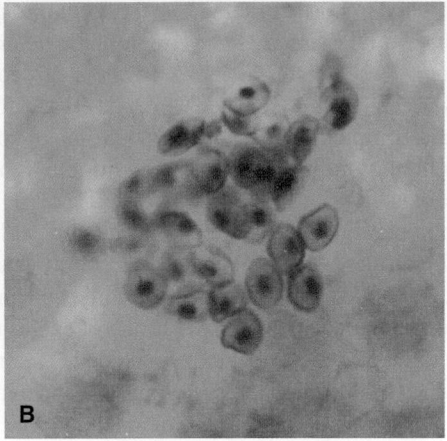

FIGURE 20-4 • *Pneumocystis jiroveci* pneumonia. (**A**) The alveoli are filled with a foamy exudate, and the interstitium is thickened and contains a chronic inflammatory infiltrate. (**B**) A centrifuged bronchoalveolar lavage specimen impregnated with silver shows a cluster of *P. jiroveci* cysts. (From Rubin E., Farber J. L. [Eds.]. [1994]. *Pathology* [2nd ed.]. Philadelphia: Lippincott Williams & Wilkins.)

shelters, and nursing homes, but the most profound factor was HIV infection.

The lungs are the most common site of *M. tuberculosis* infection, but extrapulmonary infection of the kidney, bone marrow, and other organs also occurs in people with HIV infection. Whether a person has pulmonary or extrapulmonary TB, most persons present with fever, night sweats, cough, and weight loss. Persons infected with *M. tuberculosis* (*i.e.*, those with positive tuberculin skin test results) are more likely to develop reactivated TB if they become infected with HIV. Coinfected individuals (*i.e.*, those with both HIV and TB infection) are also more likely to have a rapidly progressive form of TB. Equally important, HIV-infected persons with TB coinfection usually have an increase in viral load, which decreases the success of TB therapy. They also have an increased number of other opportunistic infections and an increased mortality rate.

Since the late 1960s, most persons with TB have responded well to therapy. However, in 1991, there were outbreaks of multidrug-resistant (MDR) TB. To be classified as MDR TB, the tubercle bacilli must be resistant to at least isoniazid and rifampin. The tubercle bacilli have recently developed more extensive resistance to include fluoroquinolones and other second-line agents, including capreomycin and kanamycin. These tuberculous strains are called extensively drug-resistant (XDR) TB.[33] Since the original outbreak of MDR TB in the early 1990s, new cases of MDR TB have declined, largely because of improved infection control practices and the expansion of directly observed therapy programs.

Gastrointestinal Manifestations

Diseases of the gastrointestinal tract are some of the most frequent complications of HIV infection and AIDS. Esophageal candidiasis, CMV infection, and herpes simplex virus infection are common opportunistic infections that cause esophagitis in people with HIV infection.[34] Aphthous ulcers presumed secondary to HIV are also common. Persons experiencing these infections usually complain of painful swallowing or retrosternal pain. The clinical presentation can range from asymptomatic to a complete inability to swallow and resulting dehydration. Endoscopy or barium esophagography is required for definitive diagnosis.

Diarrhea or gastroenteritis is a common complaint in persons with HIV infection. Patients should be evaluated for the same common causes of diarrhea as in the general population. The most common protozoal opportunistic infection that causes diarrhea is due to *Cryptosporidium parvum*. The clinical features of cryptosporidiosis can range from mild diarrhea to severe, watery diarrhea with a loss of up to several liters of water per day. The most severe form usually occurs in persons with a CD4$^+$ cell count of less than 50 cells/µL, and also can include malabsorption, electrolyte disturbances, dehydration, and weight loss.[20] Other organisms that cause gastroenteritis and diarrhea are *Salmonella*, CMV, *Clostridium difficile*, *Escherichia coli*, *Shigella*, *Giardia*, and microsporidia.[31] These organisms are identified by examination of stool cultures or endoscopy.

Nervous System Manifestations

HIV infection, particularly in its late stages of severe immunocompromise, leaves the nervous system vulnerable to an array of neurologic disorders, including HIV-associated neurocognitive disorders (HAND), toxoplasmosis, and PML. These disorders can affect the peripheral nervous system or CNS and contribute to the morbidity and mortality of persons with HIV infection.

HIV-Associated Neurocognitive Disorders. In 2007, the National Institute of Mental Health and National Institute of Neurologic Diseases and Stroke developed a new classification with standardized diagnostic criteria. The three conditions comprising HAND are HIV-associated asymptomatic neurocognitive impairment (ANI); HIV-associated mild neurocognitive disorder (MND); and HIV-associated dementia (HAD, formerly AIDS dementia complex).[35] HAND is a syndrome of cognitive impairment with motor dysfunction or behavioral/psychosocial symptoms associated with HIV infection itself.[35] HAD is usually a late complication of HIV infection. The clinical features of HAD are impairment of attention and concentration, slowing of mental speed and agility, slowing of motor speed, and apathetic behavior. The diagnosis of HAD is one of exclusion, and all other potential etiologies need to be excluded. Treatment of HAD consists of HAART to decrease symptoms and may result in significant improvement of both motor and cognitive skills.

Toxoplasmosis. Toxoplasmosis is a common opportunistic infection in persons with AIDS. The organism responsible, *T. gondii,* is a parasite that most often affects the CNS.[36] Toxoplasmosis usually is a reactivation of a latent *T. gondii* infection that has been dormant in the CNS. The typical presentation includes fever, headaches, and neurologic dysfunction, including confusion and lethargy, visual disturbances, and seizures. Computed tomography scans or, preferably, magnetic resonance imaging (MRI) should be performed immediately to detect the presence of neurologic lesions. Prophylactic treatment with trimethoprim-sulfamethoxazole, dapsone-pyrimethamine, or atovaquone is effective against *T. gondii* when the CD4+ cell count falls below 100 cells/μL. Given that these medications are also used for prevention of PCP, almost all persons under care with a CD4+ count lower than 200 cells/μL will be receiving effective toxoplasmosis prophylaxis. Since the use of trimethoprim-sulfamethoxazole and HAART began, the incidence of toxoplasmosis has decreased.[36]

Progressive Multifocal Leukoencephalopathy. Progressive multifocal leukoencephalopathy is a demyelinating disease of the white matter of the brain caused by the JC virus, a DNA papovavirus that attacks the oligodendrocytes.[37] PML advances slowly, and it can be weeks to months before the patient seeks medical care. PML is characterized by progressive limb weakness, sensory loss, difficulty controlling the digits, visual disturbances, subtle alterations in mental status, hemiparesis, ataxia, diplopia, and seizures.[37] The mortality rate is high, and the average survival time is 2 to 4 months. Diagnosis is based on clinical findings and an MRI, and confirmed by the presence of the JC virus.[37] There is no proven cure for PML, but improvement can occur after starting effective HAART. In patients who develop PML while on HAART, however, the outcome may be worse secondary to immune reconstitution syndrome.[38]

Cancers and Malignancies

Persons with AIDS have a high incidence of certain malignancies, especially Kaposi sarcoma (KS), non-Hodgkin lymphoma, and noninvasive cervical carcinoma. The increased incidence of

malignancies probably is a function of impaired cell-mediated immunity. As persons with HIV infection are living longer, there have been reports of the increasing incidence of age- and gender-specific malignancies.[39] Persons with HIV infection appear to have an increased risk of lung cancer even after adjusting for tobacco history. Non–AIDS-defining malignancies account for more morbidity and mortality than AIDS-defining malignancies in the antiretroviral therapy era. Traditional risk factors play a significant role in the increased risk of non–AIDS-defining malignancies for HIV-infected individuals, but do not entirely explain the excess cancer risk.[39] Increased incidences of lip cancer, penile cancer, and breast cancer have also been demonstrated in the post-HAART era.[40]

Kaposi Sarcoma. Kaposi sarcoma is a malignancy of the endothelial cells that line small blood vessels.[41] An opportunistic cancer, KS occurs in immunosuppressed persons (*e.g.,* transplant recipients or persons with AIDS). KS was one of the first opportunistic cancers associated with AIDS, and still is the most frequent malignancy related to HIV infection. It is 2000 times more common in people infected with HIV than in the rest of the population.[41] Before 1981, most cases of KS were found in North America among elderly men of Mediterranean or Eastern European Jewish descent and in Africa among young black adults and children.[41]

There is evidence linking KS to a herpesvirus (herpesvirus 8, also called KS-associated herpes virus [KSHV]).[41] Over 95% of KS lesions, regardless of the source or clinical subtype, have reportedly been found to be infected with KSHV. The virus is readily transmitted through homosexual and heterosexual activities; however, there is a disproportionately higher incidence of KS in men who have sex with men compared with women and other men. Maternal–infant transmission also can occur. The virus has been detected in saliva from infected persons, and other modes of transmission are suspected.

The lesions of KS can be found on the skin and in the oral cavity, gastrointestinal tract, and the lungs. More than 50% of people with skin lesions also have gastrointestinal lesions. The disease usually begins as one or more macules, papules, or violet skin lesions that enlarge and become darker (Fig. 20-5). They may enlarge to form raised plaques or tumors. These irregularly shaped tumors can range from 0.8 to 1.5 inches in size. Tumor nodules frequently are located on the trunk, neck, and head, especially the tip of the nose. They usually are painless in the early stages, but discomfort may develop as the tumor develops. Invasion of internal organs, including the lungs, gastrointestinal tract, and lymphatic system, commonly occurs. Gastrointestinal tract KS is often asymptomatic, but can cause pain, bleeding, or obstruction.[41] Pulmonary KS usually is a late development of the disease and causes dyspnea, cough, and hemoptysis.[41] The tumors may obstruct organ function or rupture and cause internal bleeding. The progression of KS may be slow or rapid.

A presumptive diagnosis of KS usually is made based on visual identification of red or violet skin or oral lesions.[41] Biopsy of at least one lesion should be done to establish the diagnosis

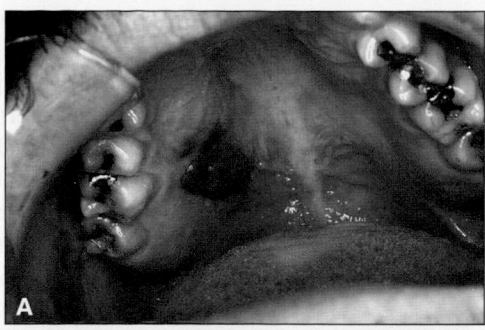

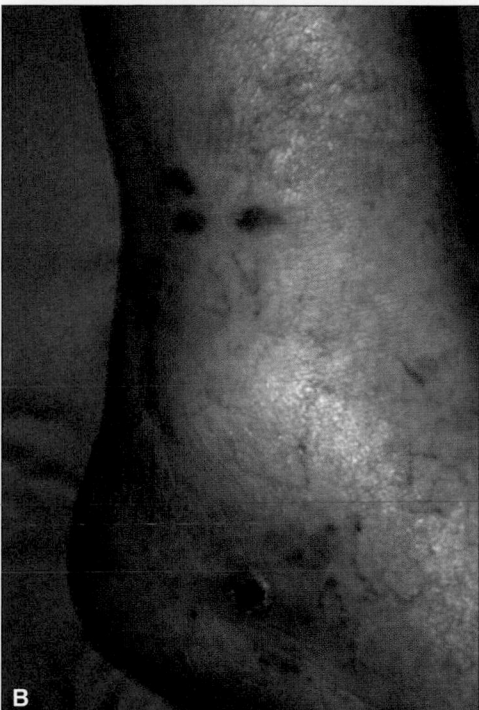

FIGURE 20-5 • Kaposi sarcoma. **(A)** Intraoral Kaposi sarcoma of the hard palate secondary to HIV infection. **(B)** Cutaneous brown Kaposi sarcoma lesions located over the maximal left ankle and foot. (From Centers for Disease Control and Prevention Public Image Library. [Online.] Available: http://phil.cdc.gov/phil/details.asp.)

and to distinguish KS from other skin lesions that may resemble it. Diagnosis of solitary gastrointestinal or pulmonary KS is more difficult because endoscopy and bronchoscopy are needed for diagnosis and biopsy of such lesions is contraindicated because of the risk of severe bleeding. Effective HAART is the treatment of choice for localized KS. Local therapy with liquid nitrogen or vinblastine, chemotherapy, radiation, and interferon injections are the most common therapies for those with extensive or systemic disease.[41]

Non-Hodgkin Lymphoma. Non-Hodgkin lymphoma (see Chapter 15) develops in 3% to 4% of people with HIV infection. The clinical features are fever, night sweats, and weight loss.

Because the manifestations of non-Hodgkin lymphoma are similar to those of other opportunistic infections, diagnosis often is difficult. Diagnosis can be made by biopsy of the affected tissue. Treatment consists of aggressive combination chemotherapy that may include intrathecal chemotherapy. In the post-HAART era, outcomes of patients with non-Hodgkin lymphoma have significantly improved, with a 57% complete remission rate and median survival rates of 50% to 64% at 3 years, depending on the lymphoma subtype and tumor burden.[42,43]

Noninvasive Cervical and Anal Carcinoma. The human papillomavirus (HPV) has been linked to the development of cervical carcinoma and anal carcinoma in both HIV-positive men and women.[44] Women with HIV infection experience a higher incidence of cervical intraepithelial neoplasia (CIN) than non–HIV-infected women.[45] HIV-infected women often experience persistent and recurrent HPV-associated anogenital disease but may not be at a higher risk for development of invasive cervical cancer.[45] Occurrence of cervical dysplasia is detected by Papanicolaou smear and cervical colposcopy. Routine screening for anal intraepithelial neoplasia should be encouraged in all HIV-positive patients regardless of history of receptive anal intercourse.[46] In 2007, a quadrivalent vaccine to prevent HPV infection was FDA approved.[47] The safety and immunogenicity of this vaccine among HIV-infected men and women are being studied.

Wasting Syndrome

In 1997, wasting became an AIDS-defining illness. The syndrome is common in persons with HIV infection or AIDS. Wasting is characterized by involuntary weight loss of at least 10% of baseline body weight in the presence of diarrhea, more than two stools per day, or chronic weakness and a fever.[48] This diagnosis is made when no other opportunistic infections or neoplasms can be identified as causing these symptoms. Factors that contribute to wasting are anorexia, metabolic abnormalities, endocrine dysfunction, malabsorption, and cytokine dysregulation. Treatment for wasting includes nutritional interventions like oral supplements or enteral or parenteral nutrition. There also are numerous pharmacologic agents used to treat wasting, including appetite stimulants, cannabinoids, and megestrol acetate.

Metabolic and Morphologic Disorders

A wide range of metabolic and morphologic disorders is associated with HIV infection, including lipoatrophy and mitochondrial disorders, lipohypertrophy, hypercholesterolemia, hypertriglyceridemia, insulin resistance, and impaired glucose tolerance. The term *lipodystrophy* is frequently used to describe the body composition changes with or without the other metabolic derangements. Metabolic complications among people with HIV infection on HAART have been increasing since the introduction of potent HAART.[49] Insulin resistance and diabetes appear to be higher among those with HIV infection compared with the general population, although traditional risk factors contribute significantly.[50,51] Insulin resistance and diabetes also appear to be more associated with the use of specific nucleosides in combination with protease inhibitors rather than just the protease inhibitors, as initially thought. The one protease inhibitor exception is indinavir, which does alter the GLUT-4 transport system.[52,53] It is still not known why insulin resistance occurs in people with HIV infection, and most experts believe it is secondary to dysregulation of metabolic pathways or to indirect effects through mitochondrial toxicity linked to adipocyte toxicity. Treatment of insulin resistance is the same as for people without HIV infection—a healthy, balanced diet; exercise; and weight loss, if needed (see Chapter 42).

HIV and its therapies have been associated with dyslipidemia independent of HAART.[54] The severity of the dyslipidemia and the typical pattern of the lipid profile differ among the classes and within the classes of antiretroviral agents.[55] The class of protease inhibitors is generally associated with elevated total cholesterol and triglyceride levels. The antiretroviral class of NNRTIs has been associated with elevated high-density lipoprotein (HDL) cholesterol and total cholesterol levels. NRTIs are a heterogeneous class in regard to lipids. Stavudine is more commonly associated with dyslipidemia with elevated total cholesterol, low-density lipoprotein (LDL) cholesterol, and triglyceride levels.

Before beginning antiretroviral therapy, a fasting lipid panel should be drawn, repeated in 3 to 6 months, and then repeated yearly. Currently, treatment of these lipid abnormalities is based on a modified version of the National Cholesterol Education Program (NCEP) endorsed by the HIV Medicine Association.[56] One strategy in attempting to correct or reverse these abnormalities is to switch the HAART regimen to an equally suppressive one that contains medications less likely to cause dyslipidemia. It is important to carefully weigh the risks of potential loss of virologic suppression when alterations in HAART are made. One study compared the benefits of switching from a protease inhibitor to an NNRTI (efavirenz or nevirapine) with those of adding a lipid-lowering drug (pravastatin or bezafibrate), and found that lipid-lowering therapy was more effective than switching.[57] The statins (*e.g.*, atorvastatin, fluvastatin, pravastatin, simvastatin; discussed in Chapter 22) are the recommended medications to manage elevated LDL cholesterol. However, caution must be used because there can be serious drug-metabolizing interactions between the protease inhibitors, NNRTIs, and statins. Because increased triglycerides can lead to pancreatitis and may be an independent risk factor for coronary heart disease, the fibric acid derivatives (*e.g.*, fenofibrate), niacin, or fish oil may be prescribed as a means of decreasing triglyceride levels.[56]

Lipodystrophy. Lipodystrophy related to HIV infection includes symptoms that fall into two categories: changes in body composition and metabolic changes.[58] The alterations in body appearance are an increase in abdominal girth, buffalo hump

development (abnormal distribution of fat in the supraclavicular area), wasting of fat from the face and extremities, and breast enlargement in men and women. Most individuals experience either lipohypertrophy or lipoatrophy. Mixed patterns of fat changes are less common.[59] The metabolic changes include elevated serum cholesterol, low HDL cholesterol, elevated triglyceride levels, and insulin resistance. Originally attributed to the use of protease inhibitors, the pathogenesis of these metabolic derangements is complex and there may be multiple confounding factors.[60]

Diagnosis of lipodystrophy is difficult because it may depend on subjective measures of reports of alteration in body shape and also because the term has not been standardized. The Lipodystrophy Case Definition Study Group developed a definition that incorporated 10 clinical, metabolic, and body composition variables that can diagnose lipodystrophy with 80% accuracy.[61] The Study of Fat Redistribution and Metabolic Change in HIV Infection (FRAM) also developed a model to define lipodystrophy.[62] However, neither study's definitions have gained wide acceptance, and most clinicians prefer to describe the spectrum of signs and symptoms their patients experience. Therefore, it is critical when interpreting the vast number of clinical trials that one note the definition used for that particular study. There is no consensus on the best treatment for lipohypertrophy or lipoatrophy.[63] Some preliminary data are available on the use of recombinant human growth hormone to decrease visceral adipose tissue and subcutaneous adipose tissue. Metformin and thiazolidinedione, oral antidiabetic drugs, have also been studied; results have been inconsistent. Some experts recommend switching to a non–protease inhibitor-based HAART regimen for treatment of lipohypertrophy, although this has not resulted in consistent results either. There is some evidence that switching from a thymidine analog to a nonthymidine analog may improve lipoatrophy. Surgical intervention (*e.g.*, liposuction, implantation or injection of synthetic substances) has been used with some success.

Mitochondrial Disorders. The mitochondria control many of the oxidative chemical reactions that release energy from glucose and other organic molecules. The mitochondria transform this newly released energy into adenosine triphosphate (ATP), which cells use as an energy source. In the absence of normal mitochondrial function, cells revert to anaerobic metabolism with generation of lactic acid. The mitochondrial disorders seen in persons with HIV infection are attributed to NRTIs, particularly the thymidine analogs.[64] The most common presentations are lipoatrophy and peripheral neuropathy, although patients may not experience both. Patients may also present with nonspecific gastrointestinal symptoms, including nausea, vomiting, and abdominal pain. They may develop altered liver function and lactic acidosis. Since the recognition of the ascending polyneuropathy syndrome and reports of hepatic failure due to combination therapy with stavudine and didanosine, reports of life-threatening events due to mitochondrial toxicities have dramatically decreased.

IN SUMMARY, HIV is a retrovirus that infects the body's CD4⁺ T cells and macrophages. HIV genetic material becomes integrated into the host cell DNA, so new HIV can be made.

Manifestations of infection, such as acute mononucleosis-like symptoms, may occur shortly after infection, and this is followed by a latent phase that may last for many years. The end of the latent period is marked by the onset of opportunistic infections and cancers as the person is diagnosed with AIDS. The complications of these infections can manifest throughout the respiratory, gastrointestinal, and nervous systems, and can include pneumonia, esophagitis, diarrhea, gastroenteritis, tumors, wasting syndrome, altered mental status, seizures, motor deficits, and metabolic disorders. ∎

PREVENTION, DIAGNOSIS, AND TREATMENT

After completing this section of the chapter, you should be able to meet the following objectives:

- Discuss the transmission of HIV.
- Describe preventive strategies to decrease the transmission of HIV.
- Explain the possible significance of a positive antibody test for HIV infection.
- Differentiate between the enzyme immunoassay (enzyme-linked immunosorbent assay) and Western blot antibody detection tests for HIV infection.
- Describe the methods used in the early management of HIV infection.
- Compare the actions of the reverse transcriptase inhibitors (*e.g.*, nucleoside/nucleotide analog reverse transcriptase inhibitors, non-nucleoside reverse transcriptase inhibitors), protease inhibitors, and fusion inhibitors in terms of controlling HIV replication.
- Enumerate some of the psychosocial issues associated with HIV infection/AIDS.

Since the first description of AIDS, considerable strides have been made in understanding the pathophysiology of the disease. The virus and its mechanism of action, HIV antibody screening tests, and some treatment methods were discovered within a few years after the recognition of the first cases. Further progress in understanding the pathophysiology of AIDS and the development of more powerful treatments continues to be made.

Prevention

Because there is no cure for HIV infection or AIDS, adopting risk-free or low-risk behavior is the best protection against the disease. Abstinence or long-term, mutually monogamous sexual relationships between two uninfected partners are the best ways to avoid HIV infection and other STDs. Correct and consistent use of latex condoms can provide protection from HIV by not allowing contact with semen or vaginal secretions during intercourse.[10] Natural or lambskin condoms do not provide the same protection from HIV as latex because of the larger pores in the material. Only water-based lubricants should be used with condoms; petroleum (oil-based) products weaken the structure of the latex.

Injection of drugs provides another opportunity for HIV transmission. Avoiding recreational drug use and particularly avoiding the practice of using syringes that may have been used by another person are important to HIV prevention. Medical and public health authorities recommend that persons who inject drugs use a new sterile syringe for each injection, or if this is not possible, clean their syringes thoroughly with a household bleach mixture. Other substances that alter inhibitions can lead to risky sexual behavior and increase the risk of exposure to HIV. For example, smoking cocaine (*i.e.*, "crack") heightens the perception of sexual arousal, and this can influence the user to practice unsafe sexual behavior.[65] The addictive nature of many recreational drugs can lead to an increase in the frequency of unsafe sexual behavior and the number of partners as the user engages in sex in exchange for money or drugs. Persons concerned about their risk should be encouraged to get information and counseling and be tested to find out their infection status.

Public health programs in the United States have been profoundly affected by the HIV epidemic. Although standard methods for disease intervention and statistical analysis are applied to HIV infection, public health programs have become more responsive to community concerns, confidentiality, and long-term follow-up of clients as a direct result of the HIV epidemic. In 2006, the CDC issued an update on the recommendations for testing for HIV.[66] The CDC now recommends that all individuals 13 to 64 years of age should be routinely screened for HIV. Anyone who is at continued risk for HIV infection should be tested at least annually; those who are at high risk—injection drug users and their partners, persons who exchange sex for money or drugs, anyone who has had more than one sex partner since the last HIV test—should be tested more frequently. Whenever HIV testing is performed, pretest and post-test counseling should be offered. HIV prevention counseling should be culturally competent, sensitive to issues of sexual identity, developmentally appropriate, and linguistically relevant.[12]

The essential elements of any HIV prevention/counseling interaction include a personalized risk assessment and prevention plan.[66] Education and behavioral intervention continue to be the mainstays of HIV prevention programs. Individual risk assessment and education regarding HIV transmission and possible prevention techniques or skills are delivered to persons in clinical settings and to those at high risk of infection in community settings. Community-wide education is provided in schools, the workplace, and the media. Training for professionals can have an impact on the spread of HIV and is an important element of prevention. The constant addition of new information on HIV makes prevention an ever-changing and challenging endeavor.

Diagnostic Methods

The diagnostic methods used for HIV infection include laboratory methods to determine infection and clinical methods to evaluate the progression of the disease. The most accurate and inexpensive method for identifying HIV infection is the HIV antibody test. The first commercial assays for HIV were introduced in 1985 to screen donated blood. Since then, use of antibody detection tests has been expanded to include evaluating persons at increased risk for HIV infection. The HIV antibody test procedure consists of screening with an *enzyme immunoassay* (EIA), also known as *enzyme-linked immunosorbent assay* (ELISA), followed by a confirmatory test, the *Western blot* assay, which is performed if the EIA is positive.[67] In light of the psychosocial issues related to HIV infection and AIDS, sensitivity and confidentiality must be maintained whenever testing is implemented. Counseling before and after testing to allay fears, provide accurate information, ensure appropriate follow-up testing, and provide referral to needed medical and psychosocial services is essential.

The EIA detects antibodies produced in response to HIV infection.[21] In an EIA, when blood is added, antibodies to HIV bind to HIV antigens. The antigen–antibody complex is then detected using an anti–human immunoglobulin G (IgG) antibody conjugated to an enzyme such as alkaline phosphatase. A substrate is then added from which the enzyme produces a color reaction. Color development, indicating the amount of HIV antibodies found, is measured. The test is considered reactive, or positive, if color is produced, and negative, or nonreactive, if there is no color. EIA tests have high false-positive rates, so samples that are repeatedly reactive are tested by a confirmatory test such as the Western blot.

The Western blot test is more specific than the EIA, and in the case of a false-positive EIA result, the Western blot test can identify the person as uninfected. The Western blot is a more sensitive assay that looks for the presence of antibodies to specific viral antigens.[21] For the test, HIV antigens are separated by electrophoresis based on their weight, and then transferred to nitrocellulose paper and arranged in strips, with larger proteins at the top and smaller proteins at the bottom. The serum sample is then added. If HIV antibodies are present, they bind with the specific viral antigen on the paper. An enzyme and substrate then are added to produce a color reaction as in the EIA. If there are no colored bands present, the test is negative. A test is positive when certain combinations of bands are present. A test can be indeterminate if there are bands present but they do not meet the criteria for a positive test result. An indeterminate or false-positive test result can occur during the window period before seroconversion. When a serum antibody test result is reactive or borderline by EIA and positive by Western blot, the person is considered to be infected with HIV. When an EIA is reactive and the Western blot is negative, the person in not infected with HIV. Both tests are important because, in some situations, misinformation can be generated by EIA testing alone because there are many situations that can produce a false-positive (Chart 20-3) or a false-negative EIA result. The Western blot test therefore is essential to determine which persons with positive EIA results are truly infected.

CHART 20-3 **CAUSES OF FALSE-POSITIVE OR FALSE-NEGATIVE HIV ELISA TEST RESULTS**

False-Positive Results
- Hematologic malignant disorders (*e.g.,* malignant melanoma)
- DNA viral infections (*e.g.,* infectious mononucleosis [Epstein-Barr virus])
- Autoimmune disorders
- Primary biliary cirrhosis
- Immunizations (*e.g.,* influenza, hepatitis)
- Passive transfer of HIV antibodies (mother to infant)
- Antibodies to class II leukocytes
- Chronic renal failure/renal transplant
- Stevens-Johnson syndrome
- Positive rapid plasma reagin test

False-Negative Results
- "Window" period after infection
- Immunosuppression therapy
- Replacement transfusion
- B-cell dysfunction
- Bone marrow transplant
- Contamination of specimen with starch powder from gloves
- Use of kits that detect primary antibody to the p24 viral core protein

---

Millions of HIV antibody tests are performed in the United States each year. New technology has led to new forms of testing, like the oral test, home testing kits, and the new rapid blood test. Oral fluids contain antibodies to HIV. In the late 1990s, the FDA approved the OraSure test.[20] The OraSure uses a cotton swab, which is inserted into the mouth for 2 minutes, placed in a transport container with preservative, and then sent to a laboratory for EIA and Western blot testing. Home HIV testing kits can be bought over the counter. The kits, approved by the FDA, allow persons to collect their own blood sample through a finger-stick process, mail the specimen to a laboratory for EIA and confirmatory Western blot tests, and receive results by telephone in 3 to 7 days. In November 2002, the FDA approved the Ora Quick Rapid HIV-1 Antibody Test.[68] The Ora Quick uses a whole-blood specimen from a finger stick and can provide results in about 20 minutes. Reactive, or positive, test results require confirmation using Western blot testing. A person with a reactive result needs to be told that the preliminary test was positive, but he or she needs a confirmatory test. The use of a rapid test should facilitate people receiving the results of their HIV test more regularly because they do not need to return for their test results 2 weeks later unless it is positive or there is concern that the person may be in the window period before seroconversion.

Polymerase chain reaction (PCR) is a technique for detecting HIV DNA (see Chapter 16). PCR detects the presence of the virus rather than the antibody to the virus, which the EIA and

Western blot tests detect. PCR is useful in diagnosing HIV infection in infants born to infected mothers because these infants have their mothers' HIV antibody regardless of whether the children are infected. Because the amount of viral DNA in the HIV-infected cell is small compared with the amount of human DNA, direct detection of viral genetic material is difficult. PCR is a method for amplifying the viral DNA up to 1 million times or more to increase the probability of detection.

Early Management

The management of HIV infection has changed dramatically since the mid-1990s. This change is due to a better understanding of the pathogenesis of HIV, the emergence of viral load testing, and the increased number of medications available to fight the virus. After HIV infection is confirmed, a baseline evaluation should be done.[67] This evaluation should include a complete history and physical examination and baseline laboratory tests. Routine follow-up care of a stable, asymptomatic HIV-infected patient should include a history and physical examination along with CD4+ cell count and viral load testing every 3 to 4 months. Persons who are symptomatic may need to be seen more frequently.

Therapeutic interventions are determined by the level of disease activity based on the viral load, the degree of immunodeficiency based on the CD4+ cell count, and the appearance of specific opportunistic infections. The U.S. Department of Health and Human Services (DHHS) guidelines released in October 2006 recommend the initiation of antiretroviral therapy based on symptomatic disease and CD4+ cell counts.[69] According to these guidelines, all symptomatic patients should be treated with antiretroviral therapy. If the individual is asymptomatic, therapy is recommended when the person's CD4+ cell counts are 200/μL or less. For those who have a CD4+ cell count greater than 350/μL, antiretroviral therapy is generally not recommended. For those whose CD4+ cell count is 200 to 350/μL, antiretroviral therapy should be considered and a decision individualized to the patient should be made.[69] Because recent studies suggest that non–HIV-related conditions such as renal, liver, and heart disease may occur more frequently among those not on HAART, some experts are reverting back to previous recommendations to start therapy when the CD4+ count is higher.[70,71] In addition, patients are more likely to experience toxicities due to HAART at lower CD4+ counts compared with those who begin HAART at higher CD4+ counts.[72] As HIV infection progresses, prophylaxis and treatment of opportunistic infections are critical.[73,74] Prophylaxis may differ based on geographic and environmental exposures and tolerability of medications, as well as the person's CD4+ cell count. Early recognition of HIV infection is becoming more common, and medical intervention in the early stages may delay life-threatening symptoms and slow the progression of the disease.

Because of frequent advances in the management of HIV infection, primary care providers must be prepared to update their knowledge of diagnosis, testing, evaluation, and medical intervention. The Infectious Diseases Society of America/HIV Medicine Association, the CDC, the DHHS, and the U.S. Public Health Service regularly issue guidelines to assist clinicians in caring for persons with HIV infection.

Treatment

There is no cure for HIV infection. The medications that are currently available to treat HIV infection decrease the amount of virus in the body, but they do not eradicate HIV. The treatment of HIV infection is one of the most rapidly evolving fields in medicine. Because different drugs act on different stages of the replication cycle, optimal treatment includes a combination of at least two to three drugs, often referred to as HAART.[69] The goal of HAART is sustained suppression of HIV replication, resulting in an undetectable viral load and an increasing CD4+ cell count. In general, antiretroviral therapies are prescribed to slow the progression to AIDS and improve the overall survival time of persons with HIV infection.

The first drug that was approved by the FDA for the treatment of HIV was zidovudine in 1987. Since then, an increasing number of therapeutics has been approved by the FDA for treatment of HIV infection. There currently are five classes of HIV antiretroviral medications: nucleoside and nucleotide analog reverse transcriptase inhibitors; non-nucleoside reverse transcriptase inhibitors; protease inhibitors; entry inhibitors; and the newest class, integrase inhibitors (Table 20-2). Each type of agent attempts to interrupt viral replication at a different point.

Reverse transcriptase inhibitors inhibit HIV replication by acting on the enzyme reverse transcriptase. There are three types of HIV medications that work on this enzyme, nucleoside analog reverse transcriptase inhibitors (NRTIs), nucleotide reverse transcriptase inhibitors (NRTIs), and non-nucleoside reverse transcriptase inhibitors (NNRTIs). *Nucleoside analog reverse transcriptase inhibitors* and *nucleotide reverse transcriptase inhibitors* act by blocking the elongation of the DNA chain by stopping more nucleosides from being added. *Non-nucleoside reverse transcriptase inhibitors* work by binding to the reverse transcriptase enzyme so it cannot copy the virus's RNA into DNA (see Fig. 20-1).

Protease inhibitors bind to the protease enzyme and inhibit its action. This inhibition prevents the cleavage of the polyprotein chain into individual proteins, which would be used to construct the new virus. Because the information inside the nucleus is not put together properly, the new viruses that are released into the body are immature and noninfectious (see Fig. 20-1).

The two newest classes of antiretroviral therapy are the *entry inhibitors* and *integrase inhibitors*. The entry inhibitors prevent HIV from entering or fusing with the CD4+ cell, thus blocking the virus from inserting its genetic information into the CD4+ T cell[75] (see Fig. 20-1). There are two types of entry inhibitors: *fusion inhibitors* and *CCR5 antagonists*. The FDA approved the first fusion inhibitor, enfuvirtide, in March 2003. It is a subcutaneous injection given twice daily. In September 2007, the FDA approved the first CCR5 antagonist, maraviroc. *Integrase inhibitors* block the integration step of the viral cycle, thus preventing the HIV genome from integrating into the host's genome.[76] This is the newest class of inhibitors; the FDA approved the first drug in this class, raltegravir, in October 2007.

Preventive and therapeutic vaccines for HIV are also being investigated.[77] The preventive vaccine would be given to someone who is HIV negative, with the goal of preventing infection if exposed to HIV. These vaccines have focused mainly on

TABLE 20-2 Antiviral Medications Used in Treatment of HIV Infection

MEDICATION (GENERIC NAME AND INITIALS) BY CLASSIFICATION	MEDICATION TRADE NAME	DOSING SCHEDULE
Nucleoside Reverse Transcriptase Inhibitors (NRTIs)		
Zidovudine (AZT)	Retrovir	Twice daily
Didanosine (ddl)	Videx	Twice daily
Didanosine (ddl) enteric coated	Videx EC	Once daily
Lamivudine (3TC)	Epivir	Once or twice daily
Stavudine (d4T)	Zerit	Twice daily
Abacavir (ABC)	Ziagen	Once or twice daily
Zalcitabine (ddC)	Hivid	Every 8 hours
Emtricitabine (FTC)	Emtriva	Once daily
Nucleotide Reverse Transcriptase Inhibitor (NRTI)		
Tenofovir (TDFNV)	Viread	Once daily
Non-nucleoside Reverse Transcriptase Inhibitors (NNRTIs)		
Nevirapine (NVP)	Viramune	Once or twice daily
Efavirenz (EFV)	Sustiva	Once daily
Delavirdine (DLV)	Rescriptor	Three times daily
Etravirine	Intelence	Twice daily
Protease Inhibitors (PIs)		
Ritonavir (RTV)	Norvir	Varies
Saquinavir (SQV)*	Invirase	Every 12 or 24 hours
Indinavir (IDV)*	Crixivan	Every 8 or 12 hours
Nelfinavir (NLF)	Viracept	Every 12 hours
Fosamprenavir (fAPV)*	Lexiva	Every 12 or 24 hours
Lopinavir/ritonavir (LPV/r)	Kaletra	Every 12 or 24 hours
Atazanavir (ATV)*	Reyataz	Every 24 hours
Tipranavir (TPV)*	Aptivus	Every 12 hours
Darunavir (DRV)*	Prezista	Every 12 hours
Entry Inhibitors		
Enfuvirtide (T-20)	Fuzeon	Every 12 hours
Maraviroc	Selzentry	Every 12 hours
Integrase Inhibitor		
Raltegravir	Isentress	Every 12 hours
Combination Medications		
AZT + 3TC	Combivir	Twice daily
ABC + 3TC	Epzicom	Once daily
AZT + 3TC + ABC	Trizivir	Twice daily
TDFNV + FTC	Truvada	Once daily
TDFNV + FTC + EFV	Atripla	Once daily

*Recommended to be boosted with ritonavir.

inducing neutralizing antibodies to prevent infections. The second type of vaccine would be used in people who are already infected with HIV as a therapeutic strategy to control HIV replication. The goal of these vaccines would be to better control the HIV viremia by lowering the viral load set point, changing the viral load trajectories, and preserving immune function for longer periods of time. These vaccines have focused on bringing about cellular immune responses and preparing the immune system for the lysis of infected cells. To date, these strategies have proved disappointing.

Opportunistic infections occur as a consequence of immunodeficiency, which is caused by the progressive loss of CD4+ T cells. Drugs and vaccines commonly are used for the prevention and treatment of opportunistic infections and conditions, including PCP, toxoplasmosis, MAC infection, candidiasis, CMV infection, influenza, hepatitis B, and *S. pneumoniae* infection.[73,74] Prophylactic medications are used once an individual's CD4+ cell count has dropped below a certain level that indicates his or her immune system is no longer able to fight off opportunistic infections.[73,74]

Persons with HIV infection should be advised to avoid infections as much as possible and seek evaluation promptly when they occur. Immunization is important because persons infected with HIV are at risk for contracting other infectious diseases. Some of these diseases can be avoided by vaccination while the immune system's responsiveness is relatively intact. Persons with asymptomatic HIV infection and CD4+ cell counts greater than 200 cells/µL should be vaccinated against measles, mumps, and rubella. Pneumococcal vaccine should be given once, as soon as possible after HIV infection is diagnosed, and then every 10 years, and influenza vaccine should be given yearly.[67] Hepatitis A and B vaccines appear to be more immunogenic when the HIV viral load is suppressed.[78,79] Live-virus vaccines should not be given to persons with HIV infection; however, there is much interest in the possibility of vaccinating those HIV-infected persons with varicella-zoster virus (VZV) vaccine to decrease the risk of VZV disease recurrences, or shingles. A study conducted among children with HIV infection demonstrated virus-specific lymphocyte proliferative responses in all subjects by 4 weeks and in 90% by 1 year after VZV vaccination.[80] All subjects tolerated the vaccination without adverse reactions or rises in HIV viral load.

Psychosocial Issues

HIV infection and AIDS affect all spheres of life.[81] The psychological effects of HIV infection or AIDS may be just as significant as the physical effects. The dramatic impact of this illness is compounded by complex reactions on the part of the person with HIV or AIDS; his or her partner, friends, and family; members of the health care team; and the community. These reactions may be influenced by inadequate information, fear of contagion, shame, prejudices, and condemnation of risk behaviors.[82] Acknowledging a diagnosis of HIV infection or AIDS may be the first indication to family and colleagues of an otherwise hidden lifestyle (*i.e.*, homosexuality or drug use). This increases the strain on relationships with important support persons. Shock is a common reaction people have when they are diagnosed with HIV infection, often followed by anger at themselves or others and denial or guilt. In addition to the fear and grief associated with death, the person with HIV infection or AIDS also may experience uncertainty and may feel helpless, hopeless, stigmatized, and out of control.[81]

Many people with HIV infection have preexisting mental health conditions such as depression or anxiety disorders as well as alcohol and other drug abuse (AODA). Appropriate diagnosis and treatment should be made available when mental health problems or AODA are evident. Diagnosis and treatment of cognitive and affective disorders are essential parts of ongoing care for the HIV-infected person.[81] The emotional stress, feelings of isolation, and sadness experienced by the person with HIV infection or AIDS can be overwhelming. Most persons, however, manage to learn to cope and live with their HIV infection. Persons with the disease must have as much information and control as possible. They should be encouraged to direct their energies in a positive manner and continue with their social and group activities as long as such activities are helpful. Appropri-

ate social support systems (*e.g.*, AIDS service organizations, community groups, religious organizations) should be called on to assist whenever possible. When they learn they can live with HIV infection, many persons acquire a positive outlook based on living their lives to the fullest.

To deal with these complex issues, the health care team must recognize and accept their own fears, prejudices, and emotions concerning those with HIV infection or AIDS. Personal feelings must not prevent caregivers from acknowledging the intrinsic human worth of all persons and their right to be treated with dignity and respect. Members of the health care team should have adequate support for their own emotional needs generated from working with persons with HIV infection. Grief, anxiety, and concern over stigmatization are normal feelings and should be acknowledged and dealt with through peer support or professional counseling to reduce burnout and emotional strain among members of the health care provider team.

IN SUMMARY, because there is no cure for HIV infection, risk-free or low-risk behavior is the best protection against it. Abstinence or long-term, mutually monogamous sexual relationships between two uninfected partners, use of condoms, avoiding drug use, and the use of sterile syringes if drug use cannot be avoided are essential to halting the transmission of HIV.

HIV infection is diagnosed using the EIA or rapid test together with the Western blot assay, both of which are antibody detection tests. The emotional stress, feelings of isolation, and sadness experienced by the person with HIV infection or AIDS can be overwhelming, but most persons adjust to living with HIV infection. Diagnosis and treatment of cognitive and affective disorders are an essential part of ongoing care for the HIV-infected person. Appropriate treatment should be made available when alcohol or other drug dependence is noted.

The management of HIV infection/AIDS incorporates the use of HAART; early recognition and treatment of opportunistic infections and other clinical disorders; as well as acknowledgment and support of the psychosocial issues that are an ongoing concern for those who are infected with the virus. ■

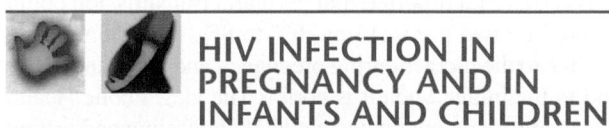

HIV INFECTION IN PREGNANCY AND IN INFANTS AND CHILDREN

After completing this section of the chapter, you should be able to meet the following objectives:

- Discuss the vertical transmission of HIV from mother to child and recommended prevention measures.
- Cite problems with the diagnosis of HIV infection in the infant.
- Compare the progress of HIV infection in infants and children with HIV infection in adults.

Early in the epidemic, children who acquired HIV could have become infected through blood products or perinatally. Now, almost all of the children who become infected with HIV at a young age in the United States get the infection perinatally. Fortunately, the incidence of perinatally infected children in the United States has markedly decreased and, as of 2006, only about 300 infants have been infected.[83] Infected women may transmit the virus to their offspring in utero, during labor and delivery, or through breast milk.[84] The risk of transmission is increased if the mother has advanced HIV disease as evidenced by low CD4+ cell counts or high levels of HIV in the blood (high viral load); if there was prolonged time from rupture of membranes to delivery; if the mother breast-feeds the child; or if there is increased exposure of the fetus to maternal blood.[84]

HIV INFECTION IN PREGNANCY AND IN INFANTS AND CHILDREN

- HIV can be passed from mother to infant during labor and delivery or through breast-feeding.
- The course of HIV infection is different for children than adults.

Diagnosis of HIV infection in children born to HIV-infected mothers is complicated by the presence of maternal anti-HIV IgG antibody, which crosses the placenta to the fetus.[11] Consequently, infants born to HIV-infected women can be HIV antibody positive by ELISA for up to 18 months of age even though they are not infected with HIV. PCR testing for HIV DNA is used most often to diagnose HIV infection in infants younger than 18 months of age. Two positive PCR tests for HIV DNA are needed to diagnose a child with HIV infection. Children born to mothers with HIV infection are considered uninfected if they become HIV antibody negative after 6 months of age, have no other laboratory evidence of HIV infection, and have not met the surveillance case definition criteria for AIDS in children.

The landmark Pediatric AIDS Clinical Trials Group (PACTG) 076 trial reported that perinatal transmission could be lowered by two thirds, from 26% to 8%, by administering zidovudine to the mother during pregnancy and labor and delivery and to the infant when it is born.[10] The U.S. Public Health Service therefore recommends that HIV counseling and testing should be offered to all pregnant women.[66] The recommendations also stress that women who test positive for HIV antibodies should be informed of the perinatal prevention benefits of zidovudine therapy and offered HAART, which often includes zidovudine. This is done because it has now been found that women receiving antiretroviral therapy who also have a viral load less than 1000 copies/mL have very low rates of perinatal transmission. One caveat to antiretroviral therapy in pregnancy is that efavirenz cannot be used during the first trimester because it is a teratogen, causing neural tube defects. Benefits of volun-

tary testing for mothers and newborns include reduced morbidity because of intensive treatment and supportive health care, the opportunity for early antiretroviral therapy for mother and child, and information regarding the risk of transmission from breast milk.

Because pregnant women in less developed countries do not always have access to zidovudine, studies are being conducted in Africa to determine if other, simpler and less expensive antiretroviral regimens can be used to decrease transmission from mother to infant. One such study, HIVNET 012, evaluated single-dose nevirapine compared with zidovudine and found that nevirapine lowered the risk of HIV transmission by almost 50%.[85] However, this strategy could lead to nevirapine resistance, and other studies evaluating drug combinations and strategies are being conducted.

Children may have a different clinical presentation of HIV infection than adults. Failure to thrive, CNS abnormalities, and developmental delays are the most prominent primary manifestations of HIV infection in children.[10] Children born with HIV infection usually weigh less and are shorter than noninfected infants. A major cause of early mortality for HIV-infected children is PCP, which may also be transmitted vertically. As opposed to adults, in whom PCP occurs in the late stages, PCP occurs early in children, with the peak age of onset at 3 to 6 months. For this reason, prophylaxis with trimethoprim-sulfamethoxazole is started by 4 to 6 weeks for all infants born to HIV-infected mothers, regardless of their CD4+ cell count or infection status.

IN SUMMARY, infected women may transmit the virus to their offspring in utero, during labor and delivery, or through breast milk. It is recommended that all pregnant women be tested for HIV at the time of diagnosis of pregnancy and again at the time of labor and delivery. Diagnosis of HIV infection in children born to HIV-infected mothers is complicated by the presence of maternal HIV antibody, which crosses the placenta to the fetus. This antibody usually disappears within 18 months in uninfected children. Administration of antiretroviral therapy to the mother during pregnancy and labor and delivery and to the infant when it is born decreases perinatal transmission. ∎

Review Exercises

1. A 29-year-old woman presents to the clinic for her initial obstetrics visit, about 10 weeks into her pregnancy.

   A. *This woman is in a monogamous relationship. Should an HIV test be a part of her initial blood work? Why?*

   B. *The woman's HIV test comes back positive. What should be done to decrease the risk of her passing on HIV to her infant?*

C. *The infant is born, and its initial antibody test is positive. Does this mean the infant is infected? How is the diagnosis of HIV infection in an infant younger than 18 months made, and why is this different than the diagnosis for adults?*

2. A 40-year-old man presents to the clinic very short of breath, and based on radiography and examination, he is diagnosed with *Pneumocystis jiroveci* pneumonia (PCP). His provider does an HIV test, which is positive. On further testing, the man's CD4$^+$ count is found to be 100 cells/μL and his viral load is 250,000 copies/mL.

A. *Why did the provider do an HIV test after the man was diagnosed with PCP?*

B. *Is there a way to prevent PCP?*

C. *What CDC classification does this man fall into based on his CD4$^+$ count and symptomatology? Why?*

References

1. Quinn T. C. (2003). World AIDS Day: Reflections on the pandemic. *The Hopkins HIV Report* 15(1), 12–14.
2. UNAIDS. (2007). AIDS epidemic update, December 2006. [Online.] Available: http://www.unaids.org/en/KnowledgeCentre/HIVData/Epi Update/EpiUpdArchive/2006/default.asp. Accessed March 20, 2008.
3. Wisconsin Department of Health and Family Services. (2000). *Wisconsin AIDS/HIV update.* Madison, WI: Author.
4. Quinn T. C. (2001). The global HIV pandemic: Lessons from the past and glimpses into the future. *The Hopkins HIV Report* 13(1), 4–5, 16.
5. Montagnier L., Alizon M. (1986). The human immune deficiency virus (HIV): An update. In Gluckman J. C., Vilmer E. (Eds.), *Proceedings of the Second International Conference on AIDS* (p. 13). Paris: Elsevier.
6. Friedland G. H., Klein R. S. (1987). Transmission of the human immunodeficiency virus. *New England Journal of Medicine* 317, 1125–1135.
7. O'Brien T. R., George J. R., Holmberg S. D. (1992). Human immunodeficiency virus type-2 infection in the United States: Epidemiology, diagnosis, and public health implications. *Journal of the American Medical Association* 267, 2775–2779.
8. Gershon R. R. M., Vlahov D., Nelson K. E. (1990). The risk of transmission of HIV-1 through non-percutaneous, non-sexual modes: A review. *AIDS* 4, 645–650.
9. Colpin H. (1999). Prevention of HIV transmission through behavioral changes and sexual means. In Armstrong D., Cohen J. (Eds.), *Infectious diseases* (Section 5, Chapter 2, pp. 1–4). London: Harcourt.
10. Connor E. M., Sperling R. S., Gelber R., et al. (1994). Reduction of maternal-infant transmission of human immunodeficiency virus type 1 with zidovudine treatment. *New England Journal of Medicine* 331, 1173–1180.
11. Havens P. L. (1999). Pediatric AIDS. In Armstrong D., Cohen J. (Eds.), *Infectious diseases* (Section 5, Chapter 20). London: Harcourt.
12. Centers for Disease Control and Prevention. (2002). Preventing occupational HIV transmission to healthcare personnel. [Online.] Available: www.cdc.gov/hiv/resources/factsheets/hcwprev.htm. Accessed March 30, 2008.
13. McIntyre, J. (2008). Managing pregnant patients. In Doiln R., Masur H., Saag M. (Eds.), *AIDS therapy* (3rd ed., pp. 595–597). London: Churchill Livingstone.
14. Brenner B. G., Roger M., Routy J. P., et al. (2007). Amplified transmission in early HIV infection. *Journal of Infectious Disease* 195, 951–959.
15. Stramer S. L., Glynn S. A., Kleinman S. H., et al. (2004). Detection of HIV-1 and HCV infections among antibody-negative blood donors by nucleic acid-amplification testing. *New England Journal of Medicine* 351, 760–768.
16. Abbas A. K. (2005). Diseases of immunity. In Kumar V., Abbas A. K., Fausto N. (Eds.), *Robbins and Cotran pathologic basis of disease* (7th ed., pp. 245–258). Philadelphia: Elsevier Saunders.
17. Warren J. S., Bennett D. P., Pomerantz R. J. (2008). Immunopathology. In Rubin R., Strayer D. E. (Eds.), *Rubin's pathology: Clinicopathologic foundations of medicine* (5th ed., pp. 131–136). Philadelphia: Lippincott Williams & Wilkins.
18. Trecarichi E. M., Tumbarello M., de Gaetano Donati K., et al. (2006). Partial protective effect of CCR5-delta 32 heterozygosity in a cohort of heterosexual Italian HIV-1 exposed uninfected individuals. *AIDS Research and Therapy* 3, 22.
19. Fauci A. S. (1988). The human immunodeficiency virus: Infectivity and mechanisms of pathogenesis. *Science* 239, 617–622.
20. Holodniy M. (1999). Establishing the diagnosis of HIV infection. In Dolin R., Masur H., Saag M. S. (Eds.), *AIDS therapy* (pp. 3–14). Philadelphia: Churchill Livingstone.
21. Centers for Disease Control and Prevention. (1992). 1993 Revised classification system for HIV infection and expanded surveillance case definition for AIDS among adolescents and adults. *Morbidity and Mortality Weekly Report* 41(RR-17), 1–23.
22. Rizzardi G. P., Pantaleo G. (1999). The immunopathogenesis of HIV-1 infection. In Armstrong D., Cohen J. (Eds.), *Infectious diseases* (Section 5, Chapter 6, pp. 1–12). London: Harcourt.
23. Hecht F. M., Busch M. P., Rawal B., et al. (2002). Use of laboratory tests and clinical symptoms for identification of primary HIV infections *AIDS* 16, 1119–1129.
24. Hecht F. M., Wang L., Collier A. (2006). A multicenter observational study of potential benefits of initiating combination antiretroviral therapy during acute infection. *Journal of Infectious Disease* 194, 725–733.
25. Rodriguez B., Sethi A. K., Cheruvu V. K. (2006). Predictive value of plasma HIV RNA level on rate of CD4 T-cell decline in untreated HIV infection. *Journal of the American Medical Association* 296, 1498–1506.
26. Pantaleo G., Graziosi C., Fauci A. S. (1993). The immunopathogenesis of human immunodeficiency virus infection. *New England Journal of Medicine* 328, 327–335.
27. Walker B. (2007). Elite control of HIV infection: Implications for vaccine and treatment. *Top HIV MED* 15(4), 134–136. Review.
28. Kaplan J. E., Hanson D. L., Jones J. L., et al. (2001).Viral load as an independent risk factor for opportunistic infections in HIV-infected adults and adolescents. *AIDS* 15, 1831–1836.
29. Kaplan J. E., Hanson D., Dworkin M. S., et al. (2000). Epidemiology of HIV associated opportunistic infections in the United States in the era of highly active antiretroviral therapy. *Clinical Infectious Diseases* 30(Suppl. 1), S5–S14.
30. Afessa B., Green B. (2000). Bacterial pneumonia in hospitalized patients with HIV. *Chest* 117, 1017–1022.
31. Huang L., Stansell J., Osmond D. (1999). Performance of an algorithm to detect *Pneumocystis carinii* pneumonia in symptomatic HIV-infected persons. *Chest* 115, 1025–1032.
32. UNAIDS. (2006). Frequently asked questions about tuberculosis. [Online.] Avaliable: http://data.unaids.org/pub/factsheet/2006/tb_hiv_qa.pdf. Accessed March 28, 2008.
33. Shah N. S., Wright A., Bai G. H., et al. (2007). Worldwide emergence of extensively drug-resistant tuberculosis. *Emerging Infectious Diseases* 13(3), 380–387.
34. Wilcox C. M. (2004). Gastrointestinal manifestations of AIDS. *Nutrition in Clinical Practice* 19, 356–364.
35. Antinori A., Arendt G., Becker J. T. (2007). Updated research nosology for HIV-associated neurocognitive disorders. *Neurology* 69, 1789–1799.
36. Dedicoat M., Livesley N. (2006). Management of toxoplasmic encephalitis in HIV-infected adults (with an emphasis on resource-poor settings). *Cochrane Database of Systematic Reviews*, July 19, 3, CD005420.
37. Berger J. R., Houff S. (2006). Progressive multifocal leukoencephalopathy: Lessons from AIDS and natalizumab. *Neurological Research* 28, 299–305.

38. Roberts M. T. (2005). AIDS-associated progressive multifocal leuko-encephalopathy: Current management strategies. *CNS Drugs* 19, 671–682.

39. Silverberg M. J., Abrams D. I. (2007). AIDS-defining and non-AIDS-defining malignancies: Cancer occurrence in the antiretroviral therapy era. *Current Opinion in Oncology* 19, 446–451.

40. Frisch M., Biggar R. J., Engels E. A. (2001). Association of cancer with AIDS-related immunosuppression in adults. *Journal of the American Medical Association* 285, 1736–1745.

41. Antman K., Chang Y. (2000). Kaposi's sarcoma. *New England Journal of Medicine* 342, 1027–1038.

42. Lim S. T., Karim R., Nathwani B. N., et al. (2005). AIDS-related Burkitt's lymphoma versus diffuse large-cell lymphoma in the pre-highly active antiretroviral therapy (HAART) and HAART eras: Significant differences in survival with standard chemotherapy. *Journal of Clinical Oncology* 23, 4430–4438.

43. Mounier N., Spina M., Gisselbrecht C. (2007). Modern management of non-Hodgkin lymphoma in HIV-infected patients. *British Journal of Haematology* 136, 685–698.

44. Einstein M. H., Kadish A. S. (2004). Anogenital neoplasia in AIDS. *Current Opinion in Oncology* 16, 455–462.

45. Massad L. S., Fazzari M. J., Anastos K., et al. (2007). Outcomes after treatment of cervical intraepithelial neoplasia among women with HIV. *Journal of Lower Genital Tract Disease* 11, 90–97.

46. Abramowitz L., Benabderrahmane D., Ravaud P., et al. (2007). Anal squamous intraepithelial lesions and condyloma in HIV-infected heterosexual men, homosexual men and women: Prevalence and associated factors. *AIDS* 21, 1457–1465.

47. De Vuyst H., Franceschi S. (2007). Human papillomavirus vaccines in HIV-positive men and women. *Current Opinion in Oncology* 19, 470–475.

48. Polsky B., Kotler D., Steinhart C. (2004). Treatment guidelines for HIV-associated wasting. *HIV Clinical Trials* 5, 50–61.

49. Umeh O. C., Currier J. S. (2005). Lipids, metabolic syndrome, and risk factors for future cardiovascular disease among HIV-infected patients. *Current HIV/AIDS Reports* 2, 132–139.

50. Brown T. T., Cole S. R., Li X., et al. (2005). Antiretroviral therapy and the prevalence and incidence of diabetes mellitus in the multicenter AIDS cohort study. *Archives of Internal Medicine* 165, 1179–1184.

51. Howard A. A., Floris-Moore M., Arnsten J. H., et al. (2005). Disorders of glucose metabolism among HIV-infected women. *Clinical Infectious Diseases* 40, 1492–1499.

52. Hertel J., Struthers H., Horj C. B., et al. (2004). A structural basis for the acute effects of HIV protease inhibitors on GLUT4 intrinsic activity. *Journal of Biological Chemistry* 279, 55147–55152.

53. Koster J. C., Remedi M. S., Qiu H., et al. (2003). HIV protease inhibitors acutely impair glucose-stimulated insulin release. *Diabetes* 52, 1695–1700.

54. Riddler S. A., Smit E., Cole S. R., et al. (2003). Impact of HIV infection and HAART on serum lipids in men. *Journal of the American Medical Association* 289, 2978–2982.

55. Tungsiripat M., Aberg J. A. (2005). Dyslipidemia in HIV-infected individuals [invited review]. *Cleveland Clinic Journal of Medicine* 72, 1113–1120.

56. Dubé M. P., Stein J. H., Aberg J. A., et al. (2003). Guidelines for the evaluation and management of dyslipidemia in human immunodeficiency virus (HIV) infected adults receiving antiretroviral therapy: Recommendations of the HIV Medical Association of the Infectious Disease Society of America and the Adult AIDS Clinical Trials Group. *Clinical Infectious Diseases* 37, 613–627.

57. Calza L., Manfredi R., Colangeli V., et al. (2005). Substitution of nevirapine or efavirenz for protease inhibitor versus lipid-lowering therapy for the management of dyslipidaemia. *AIDS* 19, 1051–1058.

58. Tershakovec A. M., Frank I., Rader D. (2004). HIV-related lipodystrophy and related factors. *Atherosclerosis* 174, 1–10.

59. Mulligan K., Parker R. A., Komarow L., et al. (2006). Mixed patterns of changes in central and peripheral fat following initiation of antiretroviral therapy in a randomized trial. *Journal of Acquired Immune Deficiency Syndromes* 41, 590–597.

60. Grinspoon S., Carr A. (2005). Cardiovascular risk and body-fat abnormalities in HIV-infected adults. *New England Journal of Medicine* 352, 48–62.

61. Carr A., Law M. (2003). HIV Lipodystrophy Case Definition Study Group: An objective lipodystrophy severity grading scale derived from the lipodystrophy case definition score. *Journal of Acquired Immune Deficiency Syndromes* 33, 571–576.

62. Tien P. C., Benson C., Zolopa A. R., et al. (2006). The Study of Fat Redistribution and Metabolic Change in HIV Infection (FRAM): Methods, design, and sample characteristics. *American Journal of Epidemiology* 163, 860–869.

63. Wohl D. A. (2004). Diagnosis and management of body morphology changes and lipid abnormalities associated with HIV Infection and its therapies. *Topics in HIV Medicine* 12(3), 89–93.

64. McComsey G., Lonergan J. T. (2004). Mitochondrial dysfunction: Patient monitoring and toxicity management. *Journal of Acquired Immune Deficiency Syndromes* 37(Suppl. 1), S30–S35.

65. Edlin B. R., Irwin K. L., Faruque S., et al., and the Multicenter Crack Cocaine and HIV Infection Study Team. (1994). Intersecting epidemics: Crack cocaine use and HIV infection among inner-city young adults. *New England Journal of Medicine* 331, 1422–1427.

66. Centers for Disease Control and Prevention. (2006). Revised recommendations for HIV testing of adults, adolescents, and pregnant women in health-care settings. *Morbidity and Mortality Weekly Report* 55(RR14), 1–17.

67. Aberg J. A., Gallant J. E., Anderson J., et al. (2004). Primary care guidelines for the management of persons infected with human immunodeficiency virus: Recommendations of the HIV Medicine Association of the Infectious Disease Society of America. *Clinical Infectious Diseases* 39, 609–629.

68. Centers for Disease Control and Prevention. (2002). Notice to readers: Approval of a new rapid test for HIV antibody. *Morbidity and Mortality Weekly Report* 51(46), 1051–1052.

69. Panel on Antiretroviral Guidelines for Adult and Adolescents. (2008). Guidelines for the use of antiretroviral agents in HIV-infected adults and adolescents. Department of Health and Human Services. [Online.] Available: www.aidsinfo.nih.gov/ContentFiles/AdultandAdolescentGL.pdf. Accessed March 30, 2008.

70. El-Sadr W. M., Lundgren J. D., Neaton J. D., et al. (2006). Strategies for Management of Antiretroviral Therapy (SMART) Study Group: CD4+ count-guided interruption of antiretroviral treatment. *New England Journal of Medicine* 355, 2283–2296.

71. Palella F. J. Jr., Deloria-Knoll M., Chmiel J. S., et al., HIV Outpatient Study (HOPS) Investigators. (2003). Survival benefit of initiating antiretroviral therapy in HIV-infected persons in different CD4+ cell strata. *Annals of Internal Medicine* 138, 620–626.

72. Lichtenstein K., Armon C., Moorman A., et al. (2007). Initiation of antiretroviral therapy at higher CD4+ T cell counts $\geq$ 350 cells/mm^3 does not increase incidence or risk of peripheral neuropathy, anemia, or renal insufficiency. *Journal of Acquired Immune Deficiency Syndromes* 247(1), 27–35.

73. Masur H., Kaplan J. E., Holmes K. K., U.S. Public Health Service; Infectious Diseases Society of America. (2002). Guidelines for preventing opportunistic infections among HIV-infected persons—2002: Recommendations of the U.S. Public Health Service and the Infectious Diseases Society of America. *Annals of Internal Medicine* 137, 435–478.

74. Benson C. A., Kaplan J. E., Masur H., et al. (2004). Treating opportunistic infections among HIV-infected adults and adolescents: Recommendations from CDC, the National Institutes of Health, and the HIV Medicine Association/Infectious Diseases Society of America. *Morbidity and Mortality Weekly Report Recommended Reports* 53(RR-15), 1–112 [erratum in *Morbidity and Mortality Weekly Report* 2005, 54(12), 311].

75. Rusconi S., Scozzafava A., Mastrolorenzo A., et al. (2007). An update in the development of HIV entry inhibitors. *Current Topics in Medical Chemistry* 7, 1273–1289.

76. Gardelli C., Nizi E., Muraglia E., et al. (2007). Discovery and synthesis of HIV integrase inhibitors: Development of potent and orally bio-available N-methyl pyrimidones. *Journal of Medical Chemistry* 50, 4953–4975.

77. Maplanka C. (2007). AIDS: Is there an answer to the global pandemic? The immune system in HIV infection and control. *Viral Immunology* 20, 331–342.

78. Overton E. T., Sungkanuparph S., Powderly W. G., et al. (2005). Un-detectable plasma HIV RNA load predicts success after hepatitis B vaccination in HIV-infected persons. *Clinical Infectious Diseases* 41, 1045–1048.

79. Overton E. T., Nurutdinova D., Sungkanuparph S., et al. (2007). Predic-tors of immunity after hepatitis A vaccination in HIV-infected persons. *Journal of Viral Hepatitis* 14, 189–193.

80. Armenian S. H., Han J. Y., Dunaway T. M., et al. (2006). Safety and immunogenicity of live varicella virus vaccine in children with human immunodeficiency virus type 1. *Pediatric Infectious Diseases Journal* 25, 368–370.

81. O'Brien A. M., Oerlemans-Bunn M., Blachfield J. C. (1987). Nursing the AIDS patient at home. *AIDS Patient Care* 1, 21.

82. Lippman S. W., James W. A., Frierson R. L. (1993). AIDS and the family: Implications for counseling. *AIDS Care* 5, 71–78.

83. AIDSinfo. (2006). Perinatal guidelines from the AETC National Resource Center. [Online.] Available: www.aidsinfo.nih.gov/Guidelines/Guideline Detail.aspx?MenuItem=Guidelines&Search=Off&GuidelineID=9.

84. Boyer P., Dillon M., Navaie M., et al. (1994). Factors predictive of maternal-fetal transmission of HIV-1. *Journal of the American Medical Association* 271, 1925–1930.

85. Guay L., Muskoe P., Fleming T., et. al. (1999). Intrapartum and neonatal single-dose nevirapine compared with zidovudine for prevention of mother-to-child transmission of HIV-1 in Kampala, Uganda: HIVNET 012 randomised trial. *Lancet* 354, 795–802.

Visit thePoint **http://thePoint.lww.com for animations, journal articles, and more**

Disorders of Cardiovascular Function

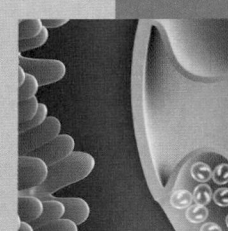

Of all body systems, the heart and circulation presented the most difficult puzzle to solve. From the fifth century BC, theories about blood and its movement were linked to the concept of the four elements (fire, earth, air, and water) and the *pneuma,* or life force. According to the Greek physician Galen (AD 130–200), the starting point of the circulatory system was the gut, where food was made into "chyle" and then carried to the liver where it was converted into blood. From the liver, which was believed to be the center of the circulation, a small amount of blood was sent to the heart and lungs where heat from the heart and pneuma from the air were added, producing an ultimate concoction of "vital spirits" that was carried in the arteries to all parts of the body.

It was not until the work of the English physician William Harvey (1578–1657) that answers to the mysteries of the circulation began to emerge. It was he who first proposed that blood traveled in a circuitous route through the body, being pumped by the active phase of the heart's contraction, not relaxation as had previously been believed. In his studies, Harvey showed that a cut artery in an animal spurts during the heart's contraction. He also demonstrated that the atria of the heart had the same relationship to the ventricles as the ventricles do to the arteries and that blood from the heart was circulated through the lungs, where it was oxygenated. As strange as it may seem today, these concepts were so revolutionary to Harvey's contemporaries that the world's basic understanding of how the body functions was thrown into turmoil.

Chapter 21

Structure and Function of the Cardiovascular System

CAROL M. PORTH AND GLENN MATFIN

➤ The main function of the circulatory system, which consists of the heart and blood vessels, is that of transport. The circulatory system delivers oxygen and nutrients needed for metabolic processes to the tissues; carries waste products from the tissues to the kidneys and other excretory organs for elimination; and circulates electrolytes and hormones needed to regulate body function. It also plays an important role in body temperature regulation, which relies on the circulatory system for transport of core heat to the periphery, where it can be dissipated into the external environment.

ORGANIZATION OF THE CIRCULATORY SYSTEM

After completing this section of the chapter, you should be able to meet the following objectives:

■ Compare the function and distribution of blood flow and blood pressure in the systemic and pulmonary circulations.
■ State the relation between blood volume and blood pressure in arteries, veins, and capillaries of the circulatory system.

Pulmonary and Systemic Circulations

The circulatory system can be divided into two parts: the *pulmonary circulation,* which moves blood through the lungs and creates a link with the gas-exchange function of the respiratory system, and the *systemic circulation,* which supplies all the other tissues of the body (Fig. 21-1). The blood that is in the heart and pulmonary circulation is sometimes referred to as the *central circulation* and that outside the central circulation as the *peripheral circulation.*

The pulmonary circulation consists of the right heart, the pulmonary artery, the pulmonary capillaries, and the pulmonary veins. The large pulmonary vessels are unique in that the pulmonary artery is the only artery that carries venous blood and the pulmonary veins, the only veins that carry arterial blood. The systemic circulation consists of the left heart, the aorta and its branches, the capillaries that supply the brain and peripheral tissues, and the systemic venous system and the vena cava. The veins from the lower portion of the body merge to form the inferior vena cava and those from the head and upper extremities merge to form the superior vena cava, both of which empty into the right heart.

FUNCTIONAL ORGANIZATION OF THE CIRCULATORY SYSTEM

■ The circulatory system consists of the heart, which pumps blood; the arterial system, which distributes oxygenated blood to the tissues; the venous system, which collects deoxygenated blood from the tissues and returns it to the heart; and the capillaries, where exchange of gases, nutrients, and wastes takes place.

■ The circulatory system is divided into two parts: the low-pressure pulmonary circulation, linking circulation and gas exchange in the lungs, and the high-pressure systemic circulation, providing oxygen and nutrients to the tissues.

■ Blood flows down a pressure gradient from the high-pressure arterial circulation to the low-pressure venous circulation.

■ The circulation is a closed system, so the output of the right and left heart must be equal over time for effective functioning of the circulation.

Although the pulmonary and systemic circulations function similarly, they have some important differences. The pulmonary circulation, which is located in the chest and near the heart, is the smaller of the two circulations and functions as a low-pressure system with a mean arterial pressure of approximately 12 mm Hg. The low pressure of the pulmonary circulation allows blood to move through the lungs more slowly, which is important for gas exchange. In contrast, the systemic circulation, which must transport blood to distant parts of the body, often against the effects of gravity, functions as a high-pressure system, with a mean arterial pressure of 90 to 100 mm Hg.

The heart, which propels blood through the circulatory system, consists of two pumps in series—the right heart, which propels blood through the gas-exchange vessels in the lungs, and the left heart, which propels blood through the vessels that supply all the other tissues in the body. Both sides of the heart are further divided into two chambers, an *atrium* and a *ventricle.* The atria function as collection chambers for blood returning to the heart and as auxiliary pumps that assist in filling the ventricles. The ventricles are the main pumping chambers of the heart. The right ventricle pumps blood through the pulmonary artery to the lungs and the left ventricle pumps blood through the aorta into the systemic circulation. The ventricular chambers of the right and left heart have inlet valves and outlet valves that act reciprocally (*i.e.,* one set of valves is open while the other is closed) to control the direction of blood flow through the cardiac chambers.

Because it is a closed system, the effective function of the circulatory system requires that the outputs of both sides of the

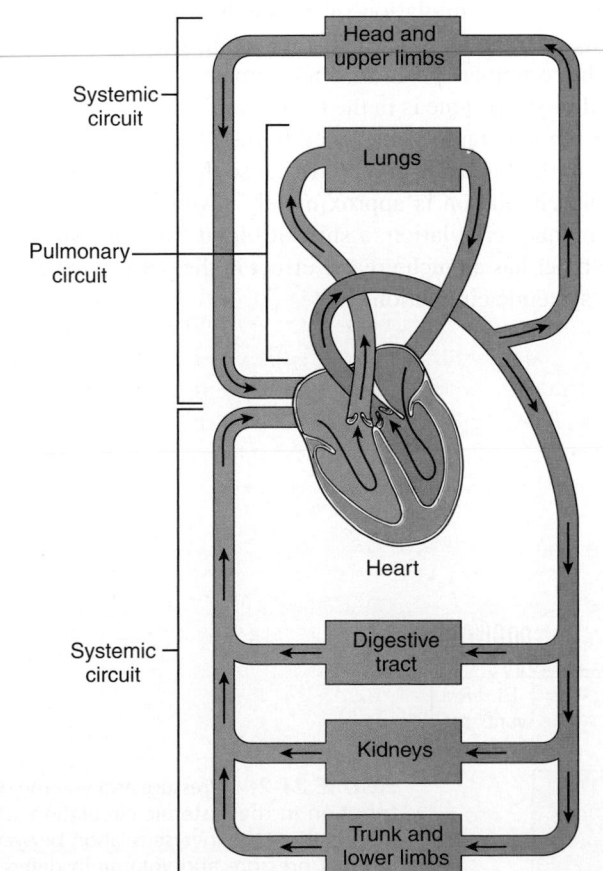

FIGURE 21-1 • Systemic and pulmonary circulations. The right side of the heart pumps blood to the lungs, and the left side of the heart pumps blood to the systemic circulation.

heart must pump the same amount of blood over time. If the output of the left heart were to fall below that of the right heart, blood would accumulate in the pulmonary circulation. Likewise, if the right heart were to pump less effectively than the left heart, blood would accumulate in the systemic circulation. However, the left and right heart seldom ejects exactly the same amount of blood with each beat. This is because blood return to the heart is affected by activities of daily living such as taking a deep breath or moving from the seated to standing position. These beat-by-beat variations in cardiac output are accommodated by the large storage capabilities of the venous system that allow for temporary changes in blood volume. The accumulation of blood occurs only when the storage capacity of the venous system has been exceeded.

Volume and Pressure Distribution

Blood flow in the circulatory system depends on a blood volume that is sufficient to fill the blood vessels and a pressure difference across the system that provides the force to move blood forward. The total blood volume is a function of age and body weight, ranging from 85 to 90 mL/kg in the neonate and from 70 to 75 mL/kg in the adult. As shown in Figure 21-2, approximately 4% of the blood at any given time is in the left heart, 16% is in the arteries and arterioles, 4% is in the capillaries, 64% is in the venules and veins, and 4% is in the right heart. The arteries and arterioles, which have thick, elastic walls and function as a distribution system, have the highest pressure. The capillaries are small, thin-walled vessels that link the arterial and venous sides of the circulation. Because of their small size and large surface area, the capillaries contain the smallest amount of blood. The venules and veins, which contain the largest amount of blood, are thin-walled, distensible vessels that function as a reservoir to collect blood from the capillaries and return it to the right heart.

Blood moves from the arterial to the venous side of the circulation along a pressure gradient, moving from an area of higher pressure to one of lower pressure. The pressure distribution in the different parts of the circulation is almost an inverse of the volume distribution (see Fig. 21-2). Thus, the pressure in the arterial side of the systemic circulation, which contains only approximately one sixth of the blood volume, is much greater than the pressure on the venous side of the circulation, which contains approximately two thirds of the blood. This pressure and volume distribution is due in large part to the structure and relative elasticity of the arteries and veins. It is the pressure difference between the arterial and venous sides of the circulation (approximately 84 mm Hg) that provides the driving force for flow of blood in the systemic circulation. The pulmonary circulation has a similar arterial–venous pressure difference, albeit of a lesser magnitude, that facilitates blood flow.

Because the pulmonary and systemic circulations are connected and function as a closed system, blood can be shifted from one circulation to the other. In the pulmonary circulation, the blood volume, which approximates 450 mL in the average-size adult, can vary from as low as 50% of normal to as high as 200% of normal. An increase in intrathoracic pressure, which impedes venous return to the right heart, can produce a transient shift from the pulmonary to the systemic circulation of as much as 250 mL of blood. Body position also affects the distribution of blood volume. In the recumbent position, approximately 25% to 30% of the total blood volume is in the central circulation. On standing, this blood is rapidly displaced to the lower part of the body due to the forces of gravity. Because the volume of the systemic circulation is approximately seven times that of the pulmonary circulation, a shift of blood from one system to the other has a much greater effect in the pulmonary than in the systemic circulation.

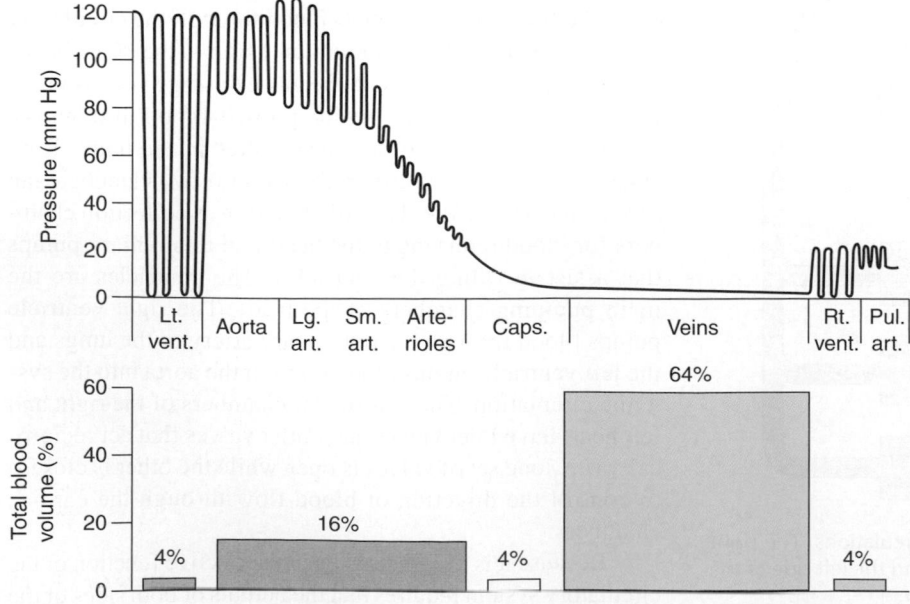

FIGURE 21-2 • Pressure and volume distribution in the systemic circulation. The graphs show the inverse relation between internal pressure and volume in different portions of the circulatory system. (From Smith J. J., Kampine J. P. [1990]. *Circulatory physiology: The essentials* [3rd ed.]. Baltimore: Williams & Wilkins.)

IN SUMMARY, the circulatory system functions as a transport system that circulates nutrients and other materials to the tissues and removes waste products. The circulatory system can be divided into two parts: the pulmonary circulation and the systemic circulation. The heart pumps blood throughout the system, and the blood vessels serve as tubes through which blood flows. The arterial system carries blood from the heart to the tissues and the veins carry it back to the heart. The cardiovascular system is a closed system with a right and left heart connected in series. The systemic circulation, which is served by the left heart, provides blood flow for all the tissues except the lungs, which are served by the right heart and the pulmonary circulation. Blood moves throughout the circulation along a pressure gradient, moving from the high-pressure arterial system to the low-pressure venous system. In the circulatory system, pressure is inversely related to volume. The pressure on the arterial side of the circulation, which contains only approximately one sixth of the blood volume, is much greater than the pressure on the venous side of the circulation, which contains approximately two thirds of the blood. ■

PRINCIPLES OF BLOOD FLOW

After completing this section of the chapter, you should be able to meet the following objectives:

- Define the term *hemodynamics* and describe the effects of blood pressure, vessel radius, vessel length, vessel cross-sectional area, and blood viscosity on blood flow.
- Use the law of Laplace to explain the effect of radius size on the pressure and wall tension in a vessel.
- Use the term *compliance* to describe the characteristics of arterial and venous blood vessels.

The term *hemodynamics* refers to the principles that govern blood flow in the circulatory system. These basic principles of physics are the same as those applied to the movement of fluid in general. The concepts of flow, pressure, resistance, and capacitance as applied to blood flow in the cardiovascular system will be used in subsequent chapters to describe the hemodynamic changes that occur with disorders of the cardiovascular system.

Relationships Between Blood Flow, Pressure, and Resistance

The most important factors governing the flow of blood in the cardiovascular system are *pressure, resistance,* and *flow*. Blood flow (F) through a vessel or series of blood vessels is determined by the pressure difference (ΔP) between the two ends of a vessel (the inlet and the outlet) and the resistance (R) that

blood must overcome as it moves through the vessel (F = ΔP/R). In the cardiovascular system, blood flow is represented by the cardiac output. Resistance is the opposition to flow caused by friction between the moving blood and the stationary vessel wall. In the peripheral circulation, the collective resistance of all the vessels in that part of the circulation is referred to as the *peripheral vascular resistance* (PVR) or, sometimes, as the *systemic vascular resistance*. The flow, pressure, and resistance relationships also can be applied on a smaller scale to determine the blood flow and resistance to flow of a single organ.

Resistance to Flow

The blood vessels and the blood itself constitute resistance to flow. A helpful equation for understanding the relationship between resistance, blood vessel diameter (radius), and blood viscosity factors that affect blood flow was derived by the French physician Poiseuille more than a century ago. The equation F = ΔP (pressure) × π × r (radius)^4/8 × L (length) × η (viscosity) expands on the previous equation, F = ΔP/R, by relating flow to several determinants of resistance—vessel radius and blood viscosity. The length of vessels does not usually change and 8 is a constant that does not change. Because flow is directly related to the fourth power of the radius, small changes in vessel radius can produce large changes in flow to an organ or tissue. For example, if the pressure remains constant, the rate of flow is 16 times greater in a vessel with a radius of 2 mm (2 × 2 × 2 × 2) than in a vessel with a radius of 1 mm. The total resistance offered by a set of blood vessels also depends on whether the vessels are arranged in series, in which blood flows sequentially from one vessel to another, or arranged in parallel, in which the total blood flow is distributed simultaneously among parallel vessels.

Viscosity is the resistance to flow caused by the friction of molecules in a fluid. The viscosity of a fluid is largely related to its thickness. The more particles that are present in a solution, the greater the frictional forces that develop between the molecules. Unlike water that flows through plumbing pipes, blood is a nonhomogeneous liquid. It contains blood cells, platelets, fat globules, and plasma proteins that increase its viscosity. The red blood cells, which constitute 40% to 45% of the formed elements of the blood, largely determine the viscosity of the blood. Under special conditions, temperature may affect viscosity. There is a 2% rise in viscosity for each 1°C decrease in body temperature, a fact that helps explain the sluggish blood flow seen in persons with hypothermia.

Velocity and Cross-Sectional Area

Velocity is a distance measurement; it refers to the rate of displacement of a particle of fluid with respect to time (centimeters per second). *Flow* is a volume measurement. It refers to the displacement of a volume of fluid with respect to time (mL/second); it is determined by the cross-sectional area of a vessel and the velocity of flow. When the flow through a given segment of the circulatory system is constant—as it must be for continuous flow—the velocity is inversely proportional to the cross-sectional area of the vessel (*i.e.,* the smaller the cross-sectional area, the

Understanding • The Hemodynamics of Blood Flow

The term *hemodynamics* is used to describe factors such as (1) pressure and resistance, (2) vessel radius, (3) cross-sectional area and velocity of flow, and (4) laminar versus turbulent flow that affect blood flow through the blood vessels in the body.

❶ Pressure, Resistance, and Flow

The flow (F) of fluid through a tube, such as blood through a blood vessel, is directly related to a pressure difference $(P_1 - P_2)$ between the two ends of the tube and inversely proportional to the resistance (R) that the fluid encounters as it moves through the tube.

The resistance to flow, in peripheral resistance units (PRU), is determined by the blood viscosity, vessel radius, and whether the vessels are aligned in series or in parallel. In vessels aligned in series, blood travels sequentially from one vessel to another such that the resistance becomes additive (*e.g.*, $2 + 2 + 2 = 6$ PRU). In vessels aligned in parallel, such as capillaries, the blood is not confined to a single channel but can travel through each of several parallel channels such that the resistance becomes the reciprocal of the total resistance (*i.e.*, 1/R). As a result, there is no loss of pressure, and the total resistance (*e.g.*, $1/2 + 1/2 + 1/2 = 3/2$ PRU) is less than the resistance of any of the channels (*i.e.*, 2) taken separately.

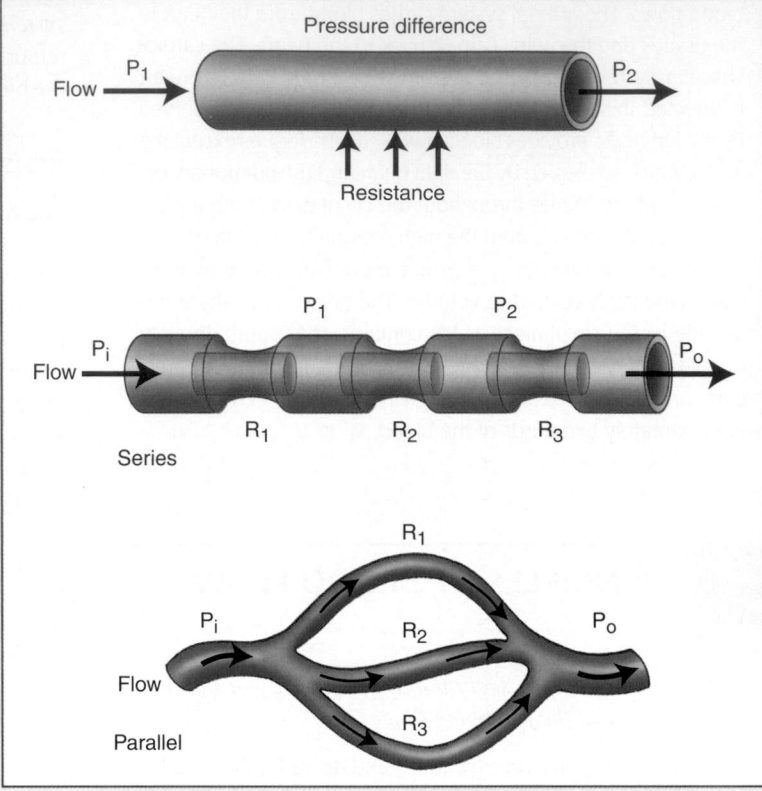

P_i, pressure in; P_o, pressure out.

❷ Vessel Radius

In addition to pressure and resistance, the rate of blood flow through a vessel is affected by the fourth power of its radius (the radius multiplied by itself four times). Thus, blood flow in vessel B with a radius of 2 mm will be 16 times greater than in vessel A with a radius of 1 mm.

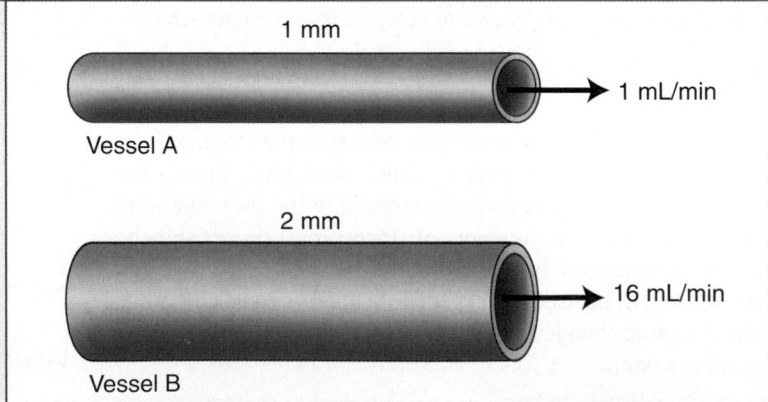

❸ Cross-sectional Area and Velocity of Flow

The velocity or rate of forward movement of the blood is affected by the cross-sectional area of a blood vessel. As the cross-sectional area of a vessel increases (sections 1 and 3), blood must flow laterally as well as forward to fill the increased area. As a result, the mean forward velocity decreases. In contrast, when the cross-sectional area is decreased (section 2), the lateral flow decreases and the mean forward velocity is increased.

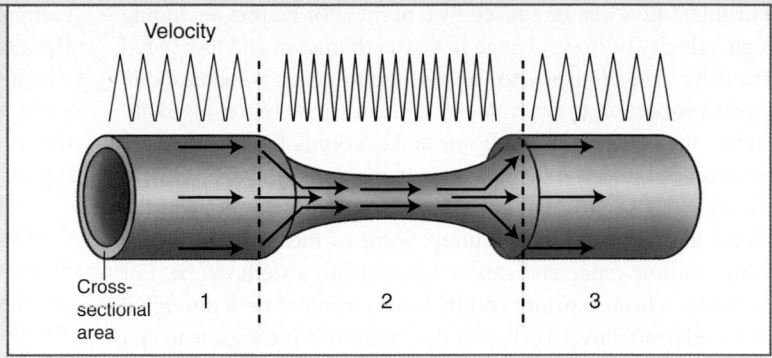

❹ Laminar and Turbulent Flow

Blood flow is normally laminar, with platelets and blood cells remaining in the center or axis of the bloodstream. Laminar blood flow can be described as layered flow in which a thin layer of plasma adheres to the vessel wall, while the inner layers of blood cells and platelets shear against this motionless layer. This allows each layer to move at a slightly faster velocity, with the greatest velocity occurring in the central part of the bloodstream.

Turbulent blood flow is flow in which the blood elements do not remain confined to a definite lamina or layer, but develop vortices (*i.e.*, a whirlpool effect) that push blood cells and platelets against the wall of the vessel. More pressure is required to force a given flow of blood through the same vessel (or heart valve) when the flow is turbulent rather than laminar. Turbulence can result from an increase in velocity of flow, a decrease in vessel diameter, or low blood viscosity. Turbulence is usually accompanied by vibrations of the fluid and surrounding structures. Some of these vibrations in the cardiovascular system are in the audible frequency range and may be detected as murmurs or bruits.

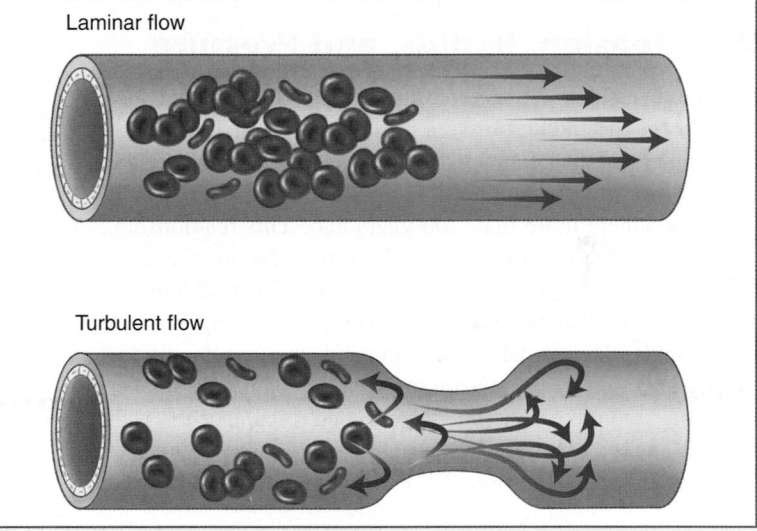

greater the velocity of flow). This phenomenon can be compared with cars moving from a two-lane to a single-lane section of a highway. To keep traffic moving at its original pace, cars would have to double their speed in the single-lane section of the highway. So it is with blood flow in the circulatory system.

The linear velocity of blood flow in the circulatory system varies widely from 30 to 35 cm/second in the aorta to 0.2 to 0.3 mm/second in the capillaries. This is because even though each individual capillary is very small, the total cross-sectional area of all the systemic capillaries greatly exceeds the cross-sectional area of other parts of the circulation. As a result of this large surface area, the slower movement of blood allows ample time for exchange of nutrients, gases, and metabolites between the tissues and the blood.

Laminar Versus Turbulent Flow

Ideally, blood flow is *laminar* or *streamlined,* with the blood components arranged in layers so that the plasma is adjacent to the smooth, slippery endothelial surface of the blood vessel, and the blood elements, including the platelets, are in the center or *axis* of the bloodstream. This arrangement reduces friction by allowing the blood layers to slide smoothly over one another, with the axial layer having the most rapid rate of flow.

Under certain conditions, blood flow switches from laminar to turbulent flow. In turbulent flow, the laminar stream is disrupted and the fluid particles become mixed radially (crosswise) and axially (lengthwise). Because energy is wasted in propelling blood both radially and axially, more energy (pressure) is required to drive turbulent flow than laminar flow.

Turbulent flow can be caused by a number of factors, including high velocity of flow, change in vessel diameter, and low blood viscosity. The tendency for turbulence to occur is increased in direct proportion to the velocity of flow. Low blood viscosity allows the blood to move faster and accounts for the transient occurrence of heart murmurs in some persons who are severely anemic. Turbulence is often accompanied by vibrations of the blood and surrounding structures. Some of these vibrations are in the audible range and can be heard using a stethoscope. For example, a heart murmur results from turbulent flow through a diseased heart valve. Turbulent flow may also predispose to clot formation as platelets and other coagulation factors come in contact with the endothelial lining of the vessel.

Wall Tension, Radius, and Pressure

In a blood vessel, *wall tension* is the force in the vessel wall that opposes the distending pressure inside the vessel. The French astronomer and mathematician Pierre de Laplace described the relationship between wall tension, pressure, and the radius of a vessel or sphere more than 200 years ago. This relationship, which has come to be known as the *law of Laplace,* can be expressed by the equation, $P = T/r$, in which T is wall tension, P is the intraluminal pressure, and r is vessel radius (Fig. 21-3A). Accordingly, the internal pressure expands the vessel until it is exactly balanced by the tension in the vessel wall. The smaller the radius, the greater the pressure needed to balance the wall tension. The law of Laplace can also be used to express the effect of the radius on wall tension ($T = P \times r$). This correlation can be

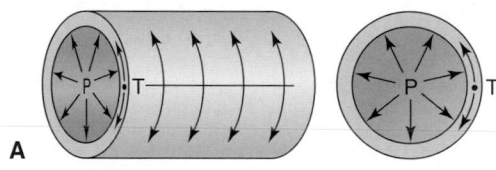

A

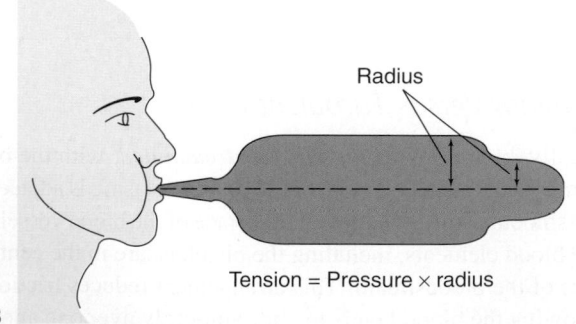

Radius

Tension = Pressure × radius

B

FIGURE 21-3 • The law of Laplace relates pressure (P), tension (T), and radius in a cylindrical blood vessel. (**A**) The pressure expanding the vessel is equal to the wall tension divided by the vessel radius. (**B**) Effect of the radius of a cylindrical balloon on tension. In a balloon, the tension in the wall is proportional to the radius because the pressure is the same everywhere inside the balloon. The tension is lower in the portion of the balloon with the smaller radius. (From Rhoades R. A., Tanner G. A. [1996]. *Medical physiology* [p. 627]. Boston: Little, Brown.)

compared with a partially inflated balloon (see Fig. 21-3B). Because the pressure in the balloon is equal throughout, the tension in the section with the smaller radius is less than the tension in the section with the larger radius. The same principle holds true for an arterial aneurysm, in which the tension and risk of rupture increase as the aneurysm grows (see Chapter 22).

The law of Laplace was later expanded to include wall thickness ($T = P \times r$/wall thickness). Thus, wall tension is inversely related to wall thickness, such that the thicker the vessel wall, the lower the tension, and vice versa. In hypertension, arterial vessel walls hypertrophy and become thicker, thereby reducing the tension and minimizing wall stress. The law of Laplace can also be applied to the pressure required to maintain the patency of small blood vessels. Providing that the thickness of a vessel wall remains constant, it takes more pressure to overcome wall tension and keep a vessel open as its radius decreases in size. The *critical closing pressure* refers to the point at which blood vessels collapse so that blood can no longer flow through them. For example, in circulatory shock there is a decrease in blood volume and vessel radii, along with a drop in blood pressure. As a result, many of the small blood vessels collapse as blood pressure drops to the point where it can no longer overcome the wall tension. The collapse of peripheral veins often makes it difficult to insert venous lines that are needed for fluid and blood replacement.

Distention and Compliance

Compliance refers to the total quantity of blood that can be stored in a given portion of the circulation for each millimeter of mercury (mm Hg) rise in pressure. Compliance reflects the *distensibility* of the blood vessel. The distensibility of the aorta and large arteries allows them to accommodate the pulsatile output of the heart. The most distensible of all vessels are the veins, which can increase their volume with only slight changes in pressure, allowing them to function as a reservoir for storing large quantities of blood that can be returned to the circulation when it is needed. The compliance of a vein is approximately 24 times that of its corresponding artery because it is 8 times as distensible and has a volume 3 times as great.

IN SUMMARY, blood flow is influenced by the pressure difference between the two ends of the vessel, the vessel length, its radius and cross-sectional area, the viscosity of the blood, and tension of the vessel wall. The rate of flow is directly related to the pressure difference between the two ends of the vessel and the vessel radius and inversely related to vessel length and blood viscosity. The cross-sectional area of a vessel influences the velocity of flow; as the cross-sectional area decreases, the velocity is increased, and vice versa. Laminar blood flow is flow in which there is layering of blood components in the center of the bloodstream. This reduces frictional forces and prevents clotting factors from coming in contact with the vessel wall. In contrast to laminar flow, turbulent flow is disordered flow, in which the blood moves crosswise and lengthwise in blood vessels. The relation between wall tension, transmural pressure, and radius is described by the law of Laplace, which states that the pressure needed to overcome wall tension becomes greater as the radius decreases. Wall tension is also affected by wall thickness; it increases as the wall becomes thinner and decreases as the wall becomes thicker. Compliance, which reflects the distensibility of blood vessels, refers to the total quantity of blood that can be stored in a given part of the circulatory system for each mm Hg rise in pressure. ■

THE HEART AS A PUMP

After completing this section of the chapter, you should be able to meet the following objectives:

- Describe the structural components and function of the pericardium, myocardium, endocardium, and the heart valves and fibrous skeleton.
- Draw a figure of the cardiac cycle, incorporating the volume, pressure, phonocardiographic, and electrocardiographic changes that occur during atrial and ventricular systole and diastole.
- Define the terms *preload* and *afterload*.
- State the formula for calculating the cardiac output and explain the effects that venous return, cardiac contractility, and heart rate have on cardiac output.
- Describe the cardiac reserve and relate it to the Frank-Starling mechanism.

The heart is a four-chambered muscular pump approximately the size of a man's fist that beats an average of 70 times each minute, 24 hours each day, 365 days each year for a lifetime. In 1 day, this pump moves more than 1800 gallons of blood throughout the body, and the work performed by the heart over a lifetime would lift 30 tons to a height of 30,000 feet.

Functional Anatomy of the Heart

The heart is located between the lungs in the mediastinal space of the intrathoracic cavity in a loose-fitting sac called the *pericardium*. It is suspended by the great vessels, with its broader side (*i.e.*, base) facing upward and its tip (*i.e.*, apex) pointing downward, forward, and to the left. The heart is positioned obliquely, so that the right side of the heart is almost fully in front of the left side of the heart, with only a small portion of the lateral left ventricle on the frontal plane of the heart (Fig. 21-4). When the hand is placed on the thorax, the main impact of the heart's contraction is felt against the chest wall at a point between the fifth and sixth ribs, a little below the nipple and approximately 3 inches to the left of the midline. This is called the *point of maximum impulse*.

The wall of the heart is composed of an outer epicardium, which lines the pericardial cavity; the myocardium or muscle

THE HEART

- The heart is a four-chambered pump consisting of two atria (the right atrium, which receives blood returning to the heart from the systemic circulation, and the left atrium, which receives oxygenated blood from the lungs) and two ventricles (a right ventricle, which pumps blood to the lungs, and a left ventricle, which pumps blood into the systemic circulation).
- Heart valves control the direction of blood flow from the atria to the ventricles (the atrioventricular valves), from the right side of the heart to the lungs (pulmonic valve), and from the left side of the heart to the systemic circulation (aortic valve).
- The myocardium, or muscle layer of the atria and ventricles, produces the pumping action of the heart. Intercalated disks between cardiac muscle cells contain gap junctions that allow for immediate communication of electrical signals from one cell to another so the cardiac muscle acts as a single unit, or syncytium.
- The cardiac cycle is divided into two major periods: systole, when the ventricles are contracting, and diastole, when the ventricles are relaxed and filling.
- The cardiac output or amount of blood that the heart pumps each minute is determined by the amount of blood pumped with each beat (stroke volume) and the number of times the heart beats each minute (heart rate). Cardiac reserve refers to the maximum percentage of increase in cardiac output that can be achieved above the normal resting level.
- The work of the heart is determined by the volume of blood it pumps out (preload) and the pressure that it must generate to pump the blood out of the heart (afterload).

layer; and the smooth endocardium, which lines the chambers of the heart (Fig. 21-5). A fibrous skeleton supports the valvular structures of the heart. The interatrial and interventricular septa divide the heart into a right and a left pump, each composed of two muscular chambers: a thin-walled atrium, which serves as a reservoir for blood coming into the heart, and a thick-walled ventricle, which pumps blood out of the heart. The increased thickness of the left ventricular wall results from the additional work this ventricle is required to perform.

Pericardium

The pericardium forms a fibrous covering around the heart, holding it in a fixed position in the thorax and providing physical protection and a barrier to infection. The pericardium consists of a tough, outer fibrous layer and a thin, inner serous layer. The outer fibrous layer is attached to the great vessels

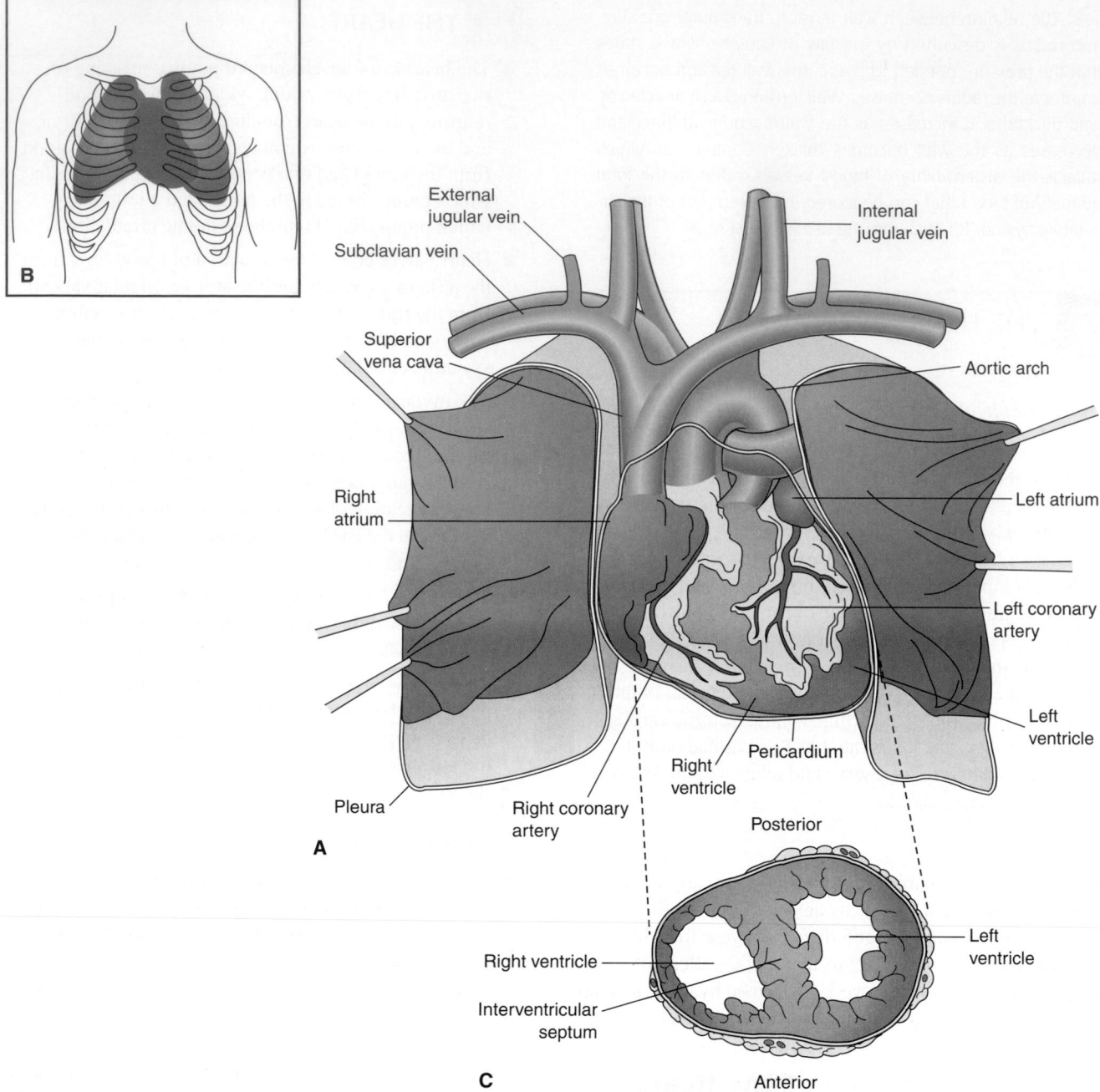

FIGURE 21-4 • **(A)** Anterior view of the heart, lungs, and great vessels (note that the lungs, which normally fold over part of the heart's anterior, have been pulled back). **(B)** The heart in relation to the sternum, ribs, and lungs. **(C)** Cross-section of the heart showing the increased thickness of the left ventricle compared with the right.

that enter and leave the heart, the sternum, and the diaphragm. The fibrous pericardium is highly resistant to distention; it prevents acute dilation of the heart chambers and exerts a restraining effect on the left ventricle. The inner serous layer consists of a visceral layer and a parietal layer. The visceral layer, also known as the *epicardium,* covers the entire heart and great vessels and then folds over to form the parietal layer that lines the fibrous pericardium (see Fig. 21-5). Between the visceral and parietal layers is the *pericardial cavity,* a potential space that

contains 30 to 50 mL of serous fluid. This fluid acts as a lubricant to minimize friction as the heart contracts and relaxes.

Myocardium

The myocardium, or muscular portion of the heart, forms the wall of the atria and ventricles. Cardiac muscle cells, like skeletal muscle, are striated and composed of *sarcomeres* that contain actin and myosin filaments (see Chapter 4). They are smaller and

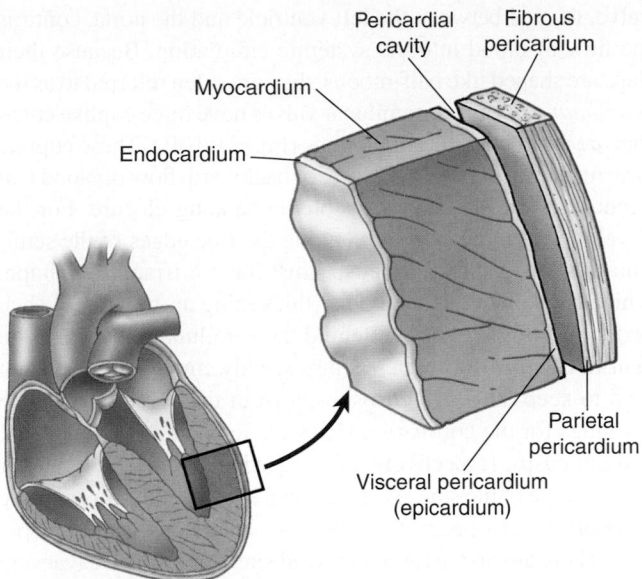

FIGURE 21-5 • Layers of the heart, showing the visceral pericardium, pericardial cavity, parietal pericardium, fibrous pericardium, myocardium, and endocardium.

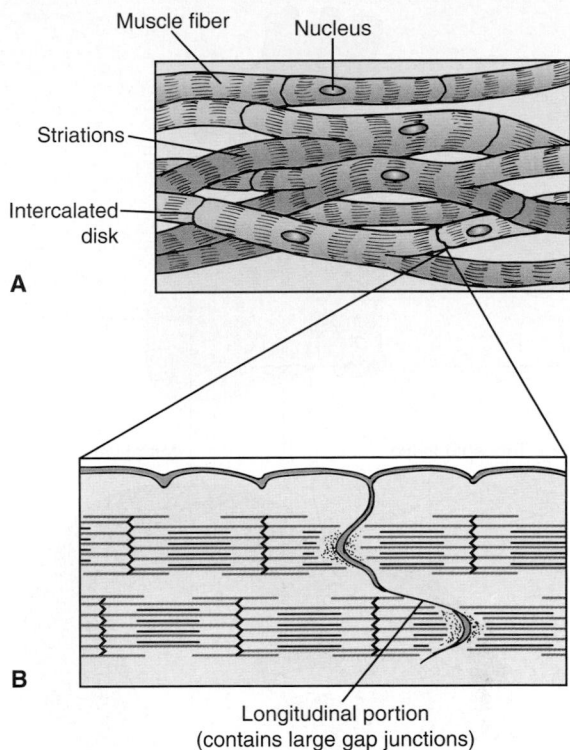

FIGURE 21-6 • **(A)** Cardiac muscle fibers, showing their branching structure. **(B)** Area indicated where cell junctions lie in the intercalated disks.

more compact than skeletal muscle cells and contain many large mitochondria, reflecting their continuous energy needs.

The contractile properties of cardiac muscle are similar to those of skeletal muscle, except the contractions are involuntary and the duration of contraction is much longer. Unlike the orderly longitudinal arrangement of skeletal muscle fibers, cardiac muscle cells are arranged as an interconnecting latticework, with their fibers dividing, recombining, and then dividing again (Fig. 21-6A). The fibers are separated from neighboring cardiac muscle cells by dense structures called *intercalated disks*. The intercalated disks, which are unique to cardiac muscle, contain gap junctions that serve as low-resistance pathways for passage of ions and electrical impulses from one cardiac cell to another (see Fig. 21-6B). Thus, the myocardium behaves as a single unit, or *syncytium*, rather than as a group of isolated units, as does skeletal muscle. When one myocardial cell becomes excited, the impulse travels rapidly so the heart can beat as a unit.

As in skeletal muscle, cardiac muscle contraction involves actin and myosin filaments, which interact and slide along one another during muscle contraction. A number of important proteins regulate actin–myosin binding. These include tropomyosin and the troponin complex (see Chapter 4, Fig. 4-22). The troponin complex consists of three subunits (troponin T, troponin I, and troponin C) that regulate calcium-mediated contraction in striated muscle. In clinical practice, the measurement of serum levels of the cardiac forms of troponin T and troponin I are used in the diagnosis of myocardial infarction (see Chapter 24).

Although cardiac muscle cells require calcium for contraction, they have a less well-defined sarcoplasmic reticulum for storing calcium than skeletal muscle cells. Thus, cardiac muscle relies more heavily than skeletal muscle on an influx of extracellular calcium ions for contraction. The cardiac glycosides (*e.g.*, digoxin) are inotropic drugs that increase cardiac contractility by increasing the free calcium concentration in the vicinity of the actin and myosin filaments.

Endocardium

The endocardium is a thin, three-layered membrane that lines the heart. The innermost layer consists of smooth endothelial cells supported by a thin layer of connective tissue. The endothelial lining of the endocardium is continuous with the lining of the blood vessels that enter and leave the heart. The middle layer consists of dense connective tissue with elastic fibers. The outer layer, composed of irregularly arranged connective tissue cells, contains blood vessels and branches of the conduction system and is continuous with the myocardium.

Heart Valves and Fibrous Skeleton

An important structural feature of the heart is its fibrous skeleton, which consists of four interconnecting valve rings and surrounding connective tissue. It separates the atria and ventricles and forms a rigid support for attachment of the valves and insertion of the cardiac muscle (Fig. 21-7). The tops of the valve rings are attached to the muscle tissue of the atria, pulmonary trunks, and aorta. The bottoms are attached to the ventricular walls. For the heart to function effectively, blood flow must occur in a one-way direction, moving in a forward (antegrade) manner through the chambers of the right heart to the lungs and then through the chambers of the left heart to the systemic

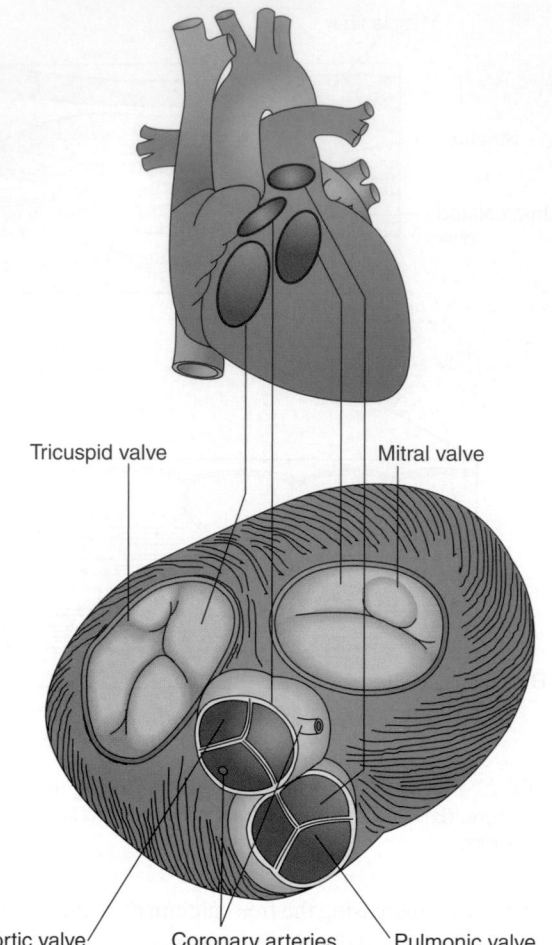

Tricuspid valve

Mitral valve

Aortic valve

Coronary arteries

Pulmonic valve

FIGURE 21-7 • Fibrous skeleton of the heart, which forms the four interconnecting valve rings and support for attachment of the valves and insertion of cardiac muscle.

circulation (Fig. 21-8). This unidirectional flow is provided by the heart's two atrioventricular (*i.e.,* tricuspid and mitral) valves and two semilunar (*i.e.,* pulmonary and aortic) valves.

The atrioventricular (AV) valves control the flow of blood between the atria and the ventricles. The thin edges of the AV valves form cusps, two on the left side of the heart (*i.e., bicuspid valve*) and three on the right side (*i.e., tricuspid valve*). The bicuspid valve is also known as the *mitral valve.* The AV valves are supported by the *papillary muscles,* which project from the wall of the ventricles, and the *chordae tendineae,* which attach to the valve (Fig. 21-9). Contraction of the papillary muscles at the onset of systole ensures closure by producing tension on the leaflets of the AV valves before the full force of ventricular contraction pushes against them. The chordae tendineae are cord-like structures that support the AV valves and prevent them from everting into the atria during systole.

The *aortic* and *pulmonic valves* control the movement of blood out of the ventricles. The pulmonic valve, which is located between the right ventricle and the pulmonary artery, controls the flow of blood into the pulmonary circulation, and the aortic

valve, located between the left ventricle and the aorta, controls the flow of blood into the systemic circulation. Because their flaps are shaped like half-moons, they are often referred to as the *semilunar valves.* The semilunar valves have three cuplike cusps that are attached to the valve rings (Fig. 21-10B). These cuplike structures collect the *retrograde,* or backward, flow of blood that occurs toward the end of systole, enhancing closure. For the development of a perfect seal along the free edges of the semi-lunar valves, each valve cusp must have a triangular shape, which is facilitated by a nodular thickening at the apex of each leaflet (see Fig. 21-10A). Behind the semilunar valves are the *sinuses of Valsalva.* In these sinuses, eddy currents develop that tend to keep the valve cusps away from the vessel walls. The openings for the coronary arteries are located behind the right and left cusps, respectively, of the aortic valve. Were it not for the presence of the sinuses of Valsalva and the eddy currents, the coronary artery openings would be blocked by the valve cusps.

There are no valves at the atrial sites (*i.e.,* venae cavae and pulmonary veins) where blood enters the heart. This means that excess blood is pushed back into the veins when the atria become distended. For example, the jugular veins typically become prominent in severe right-sided heart failure when they normally should be flat or collapsed. Likewise, the pulmonary venous system becomes congested when outflow from the left atrium is impeded.

Cardiac Cycle

The term *cardiac cycle* is used to describe the rhythmic pumping action of the heart. The cardiac cycle is divided into two parts: *systole,* the period during which the ventricles are contracting, and *diastole,* the period during which the ventricles are relaxed and filling with blood. Simultaneous changes occur in left atrial pressure, left ventricular pressure, aortic pressure, ventricular volume, the electrocardiogram (ECG), and heart sounds during the cardiac cycle (Fig. 21-11).

The electrical activity, recorded on the ECG, precedes the mechanical events of the cardiac cycle. The small, rounded P wave of the ECG represents depolarization of the sinoatrial node (*i.e.,* pacemaker of the heart), the atrial conduction tissue, and the atrial muscle mass. The QRS complex registers the depolarization of the ventricular conduction system and the ventricular muscle mass. The T wave on the ECG occurs during the last half of systole and represents repolarization of the ventricles. The cardiac conduction system and the ECG are discussed in detail in Chapter 25.

Ventricular Systole and Diastole

Ventricular systole is divided into two periods: the isovolumetric contraction period and the ejection period. The *isovolumetric contraction period,* which begins with closure of the AV valves and occurrence of the first heart sound, heralds the onset of systole. Immediately after closure of the AV valves, there is an additional 0.02 to 0.03 second during which the semilunar (pulmonary and aortic) valves remain closed. During

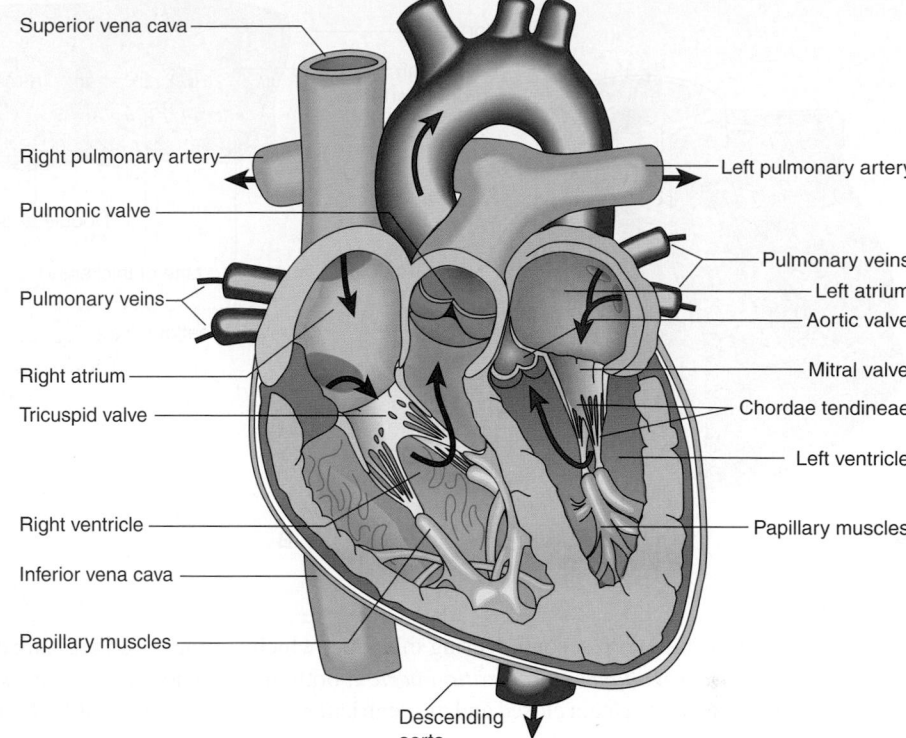

Superior vena cava

Right pulmonary artery

Pulmonic valve

Pulmonary veins

Right atrium

Tricuspid valve

Right ventricle

Inferior vena cava

Papillary muscles

Left pulmonary artery

Pulmonary veins

Left atrium

Aortic valve

Mitral valve

Chordae tendineae

Left ventricle

Papillary muscles

Descending aorta

FIGURE 21-8 • Valvular structures of the heart. *Arrows* show the course of blood flow through the heart chambers. The atrioventricular valves are in an open position, and the semilunar valves are closed. There are no valves to control the flow of blood at the inflow channels (*i.e.,* vena cava and pulmonary veins) to the heart. (Modified from Smeltzer S. C., Bare B. G. [2004]. *Brunner and Suddarth's textbook of medical-surgical nursing* [10th ed., p. 648]. Philadelphia: Lippincott Williams & Wilkins.)

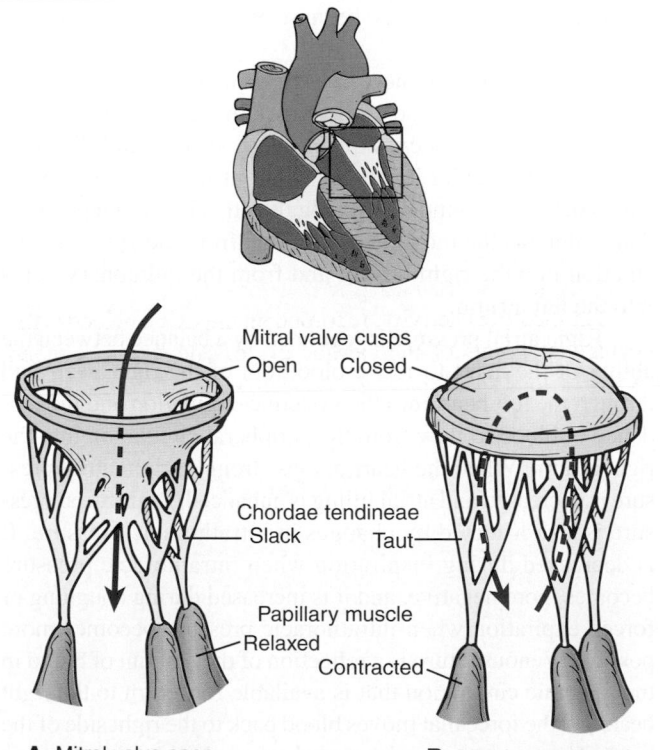

Mitral valve cusps
Open   Closed

Chordae tendineae
Slack   Taut

Papillary muscle
Relaxed
Contracted

A Mitral valve open

B Mitral valve closed

FIGURE 21-9 • The mitral (atrioventricular) valve showing the papillary muscles and chordae tendineae. (**A**) The open mitral valve with relaxed papillary muscles and slack chordae tendineae. (**B**) The closed mitral valve with contracted papillary muscles and taut chordae tendineae that prevent the valve cusps from everting into the atria.

this period (see Fig. 21-11), the ventricular pressures rise abruptly because both the AV and semilunar valves are closed and no blood is leaving the ventricles. The ventricles continue to contract until left ventricular pressure is slightly higher than aortic pressure and right ventricular pressure is higher than pulmonary artery pressure. At this point, the semilunar valves open, signaling the onset of the *ejection period.* Approximately 60% of the stroke volume is ejected during the first quarter of systole, and the remaining 40% is ejected during the next two quarters of systole. Little blood is ejected from the heart during the last quarter of systole, although the ventricle remains contracted. At the end of systole, the ventricles relax, causing a precipitous fall in intraventricular pressures. As this occurs, blood from the large arteries flows back toward the ventricles, causing the aortic and pulmonic valves to snap shut—an event that is marked by the second heart sound.

The aortic pressure reflects changes in the ejection of blood from the left ventricle. There is a rise in pressure and stretching of the elastic fibers in the aorta as blood is ejected into the aorta at the onset of systole. The aortic pressure continues to rise and then begins to fall during the last quarter of systole as blood flows out of the aorta into the peripheral vessels. The *incisura,* or notch, in the aortic pressure tracing represents closure of the aortic valve. The aorta is highly elastic and as such stretches during systole to accommodate the blood that is being ejected from the left heart. During diastole, recoil of the elastic fibers in the aorta serves to maintain the aortic pressure.

Diastole is marked by ventricular relaxation and filling. After closure of the semilunar valves, the ventricles continue to

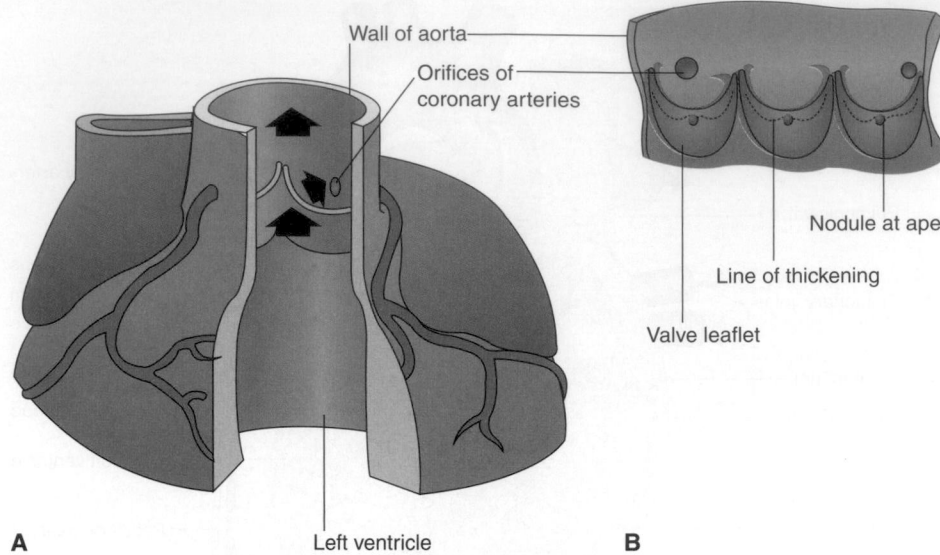

Wall of aorta

Orifices of coronary arteries

Nodule at apex

Line of thickening

Valve leaflet

A Left ventricle

B

FIGURE 21-10 • Diagram of the aortic valve. **(A)** The position of the aortic valve at the base of the ascending aorta is indicated. **(B)** The appearance of the three leaflets of the aortic valve when the aorta is cut open and spread out, flat. (From Cormack D. H. [1987]. *Ham's histology* [9th ed.]. Philadelphia: J. B. Lippincott.)

relax for another 0.03 to 0.06 second. During this time, which is referred to as the *isovolumetric relaxation period,* both the semilunar and AV valves remain closed and the ventricular volume remains the same, as the ventricular pressure drops until it becomes less than the atrial pressure (see Fig. 21-11). As this occurs, the AV valves open and blood that has been accumulating in the atria during systole moves into the ventricles. Most of ventricular filling occurs during the first third of diastole, which is called the *rapid filling period.* During the middle third of diastole, inflow into the ventricles is almost at a standstill. The last third of diastole is marked by atrial contraction, which gives an additional thrust to ventricular filling. When audible, the third heart sound is heard during the rapid filling period of diastole as blood flows into a distended or noncompliant ventricle. The fourth heart sound occurs during the last third of diastole as the atria contract.

During diastole, the ventricles increase their volume to approximately 120 mL (*i.e.,* the *end-diastolic volume*), and at the end of systole, approximately 50 mL of blood (*i.e.,* the *end-systolic volume*) remains in the ventricles (see Fig. 21-11). The difference between the end-diastolic and end-systolic volumes (approximately 70 mL) is called the *stroke volume.* The *ejection fraction,* which is the stroke volume divided by the end-diastolic volume, represents the fraction or percentage of the end-diastolic volume that is ejected from the heart during systole. The left ventricular ejection fraction (normally about 55% to 75% when determined by echocardiography or angiocardiography) is frequently used to evaluate the prognosis of persons with a variety of heart diseases.

Atrial Filling and Contraction

There are three main atrial pressure waves that occur during the cardiac cycle—the a, c, and v waves. The *a wave* occurs during the last part of diastole and is caused by atrial contraction. The *c wave* occurs as the ventricles begin to contract and their

increased pressure causes the AV valves to bulge into the atria. The *v wave* occurs toward the end of systole when the AV valves are still closed and results from a slow buildup of blood in the atria. The right atrial pressure waves are transmitted to the internal jugular veins as pulsations. These pulsations can be observed visually and may be used to assess cardiac function. For example, exaggerated a waves occur when the volume of the right atrium is increased because of impaired emptying into the right ventricle.

Because there are no valves between the junctions of the central veins (*i.e.,* venae cavae and pulmonary veins) and the atria, atrial filling occurs during both systole and diastole. During normal quiet breathing, right atrial pressure usually varies between −2 and +2 mm Hg. It is this low atrial pressure that maintains the movement of blood from the systemic circulation into the right atrium and from the pulmonary veins into the left atrium.

Right atrial pressure is regulated by a balance between the ability of the heart to move blood out of the right heart and through the left heart into the systemic circulation and the tendency of blood to flow from the peripheral circulation into the right atrium. When the heart pumps strongly, right atrial pressure is decreased and atrial filling is enhanced. Right atrial pressure is also affected by changes in intrathoracic pressure. It is decreased during inspiration when intrathoracic pressure becomes more negative, and it is increased during coughing or forced expiration when intrathoracic pressure becomes more positive. Venous return is a reflection of the amount of blood in the systemic circulation that is available for return to the right heart and the force that moves blood back to the right side of the heart. Venous return is increased when the blood volume is expanded or when right atrial pressure falls, and it is decreased in hypovolemic shock or when right atrial pressure rises.

Although the main function of the atria is to store blood as it enters the heart, these chambers also act as pumps that aid in ventricular filling. This function becomes more important

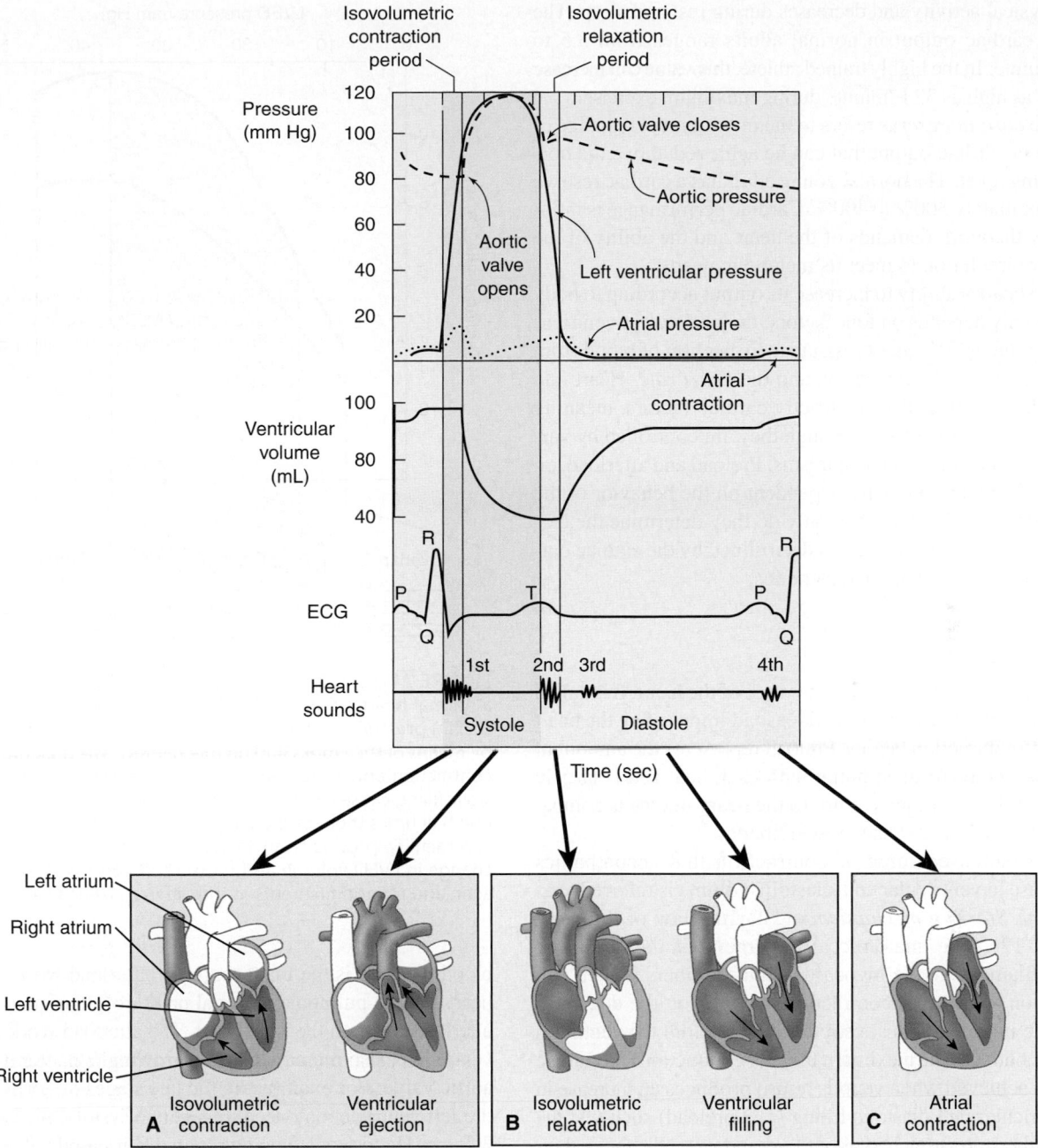

FIGURE 21-11 • **(Top)** Events in the left side of the heart, showing changes in aortic pressure, left ventricular pressure, atrial pressure, left ventricular volume, the electrocardiogram (ECG), and heart sounds during the cardiac cycle. **(Bottom)** Position of the atrioventricular and semilunar valves during **(A)** isovolumetric contraction and ventricular ejection, **(B)** isovolumetric relaxation and ventricular filling, and **(C)** atrial contraction.

during periods of increased activity when the diastolic filling time is decreased because of an increase in heart rate or when heart disease impairs ventricular filling. In these two situations, the cardiac output would fall drastically were it not for the action of the atria. It has been estimated that atrial contraction can contribute as much as 30% to cardiac reserve during periods of increased need, while having little or no effect on cardiac output during rest.

Regulation of Cardiac Performance

The efficiency of the heart as a pump often is measured in terms of *cardiac output* or the amount of blood the heart pumps each minute. The cardiac output (CO) is the product of the *stroke volume* (SV) and the *heart rate* (HR) and can be expressed by the equation: $CO = SV \times HR$. The cardiac output varies with body size and the metabolic needs of the tissues. It increases with physical activity and decreases during rest and sleep. The average cardiac output in normal adults ranges from 3.5 to 8.0 L/minute. In the highly trained athlete, this value can increase to levels as high as 32 L/minute during maximum exercise.

The *cardiac reserve* refers to the maximum percentage of increase in cardiac output that can be achieved above the normal resting level. The normal young adult has a cardiac reserve of approximately 300% to 400%. Cardiac performance is influenced by the work demands of the heart and the ability of the coronary circulation to meet its metabolic needs.

The heart's ability to increase its output according to body needs mainly depends on four factors: the *preload,* or ventricular filling; the *afterload,* or resistance to ejection of blood from the heart; *cardiac contractility;* and the *heart rate.* Heart rate and cardiac contractility are strictly cardiac factors, meaning they originate in the heart, although they are controlled by various neural and humoral mechanisms. Preload and afterload, on the other hand, are mutually dependent on the behavior of the heart and the vasculature. Not only do they determine the cardiac output, they are themselves determined by the cardiac output and certain vascular characteristics.

Preload

The preload represents the volume work of the heart. It is called the *preload* because it is the work or load imposed on the heart before the contraction begins. Preload represents the amount of blood that the heart must pump with each beat and is largely determined by the venous return to the heart and the accompanying stretch of the cardiac muscle fibers.

The increased force of contraction that accompanies an increase in ventricular end-diastolic volume is referred to as the *Frank-Starling mechanism* or Starling law of the heart (Fig. 21-12). The anatomic arrangement of the actin and myosin filaments in the myocardial muscle fibers is such that the tension or force of contraction depends on the degree to which the muscle fibers are stretched just before the ventricles begin to contract. The maximum force of contraction and cardiac output is achieved when venous return produces an increase in left ventricular end-diastolic filling (*i.e.,* preload) such that the muscle fibers are stretched about two and one-half times their normal resting length. When the muscle fibers are stretched to this degree, there is optimal overlap of the actin and myosin filaments needed for maximal contraction.

The Frank-Starling mechanism allows the heart to adjust its pumping ability to accommodate various levels of venous return. Cardiac output is less when decreased filling causes excessive overlap of the actin and myosin filaments or when excessive filling causes the filaments to be pulled too far apart.

Afterload

The afterload is the pressure or tension work of the heart. It is the pressure that the heart must generate to move blood into the aorta. It is called the *afterload* because it is the work presented to the heart after the contraction has commenced. The systemic arterial

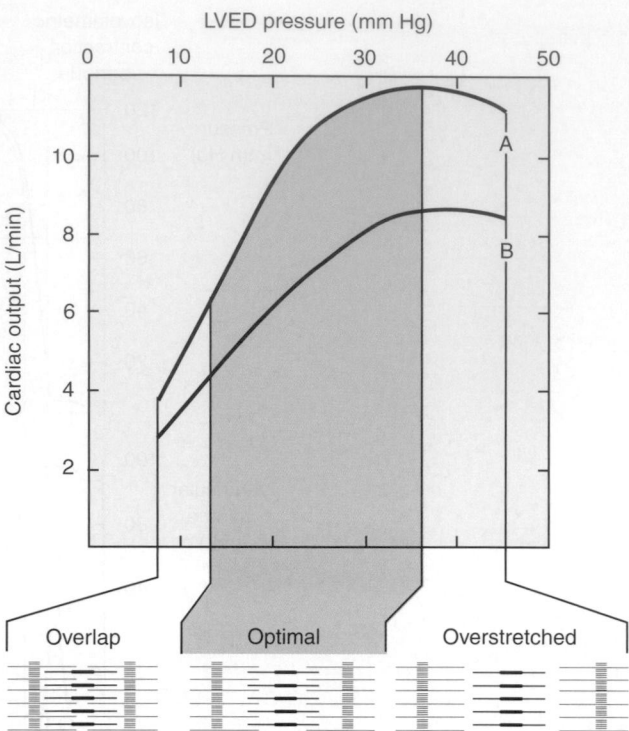

FIGURE 21-12 • The Frank-Starling ventricular function curve in a normal heart. (**Top**) An increase in left ventricular end-diastolic (LVED) pressure produces an increase in cardiac output (*curve B*) by means of the Frank-Starling mechanism. The maximum force of contraction and increased stroke volume are achieved when diastolic filling causes the muscle fibers to be stretched about two and one-half times their resting length. In *curve A,* an increase in cardiac contractility produces an increase in cardiac output without a change in LVED volume and pressure. (**Bottom**) Stretching of the actin and myosin filaments at the different LVED filling pressures.

blood pressure is the main source of afterload work on the left heart and the pulmonary arterial pressure is the main source of afterload work on the right heart. The afterload work of the left ventricle is also increased with narrowing (*i.e.,* stenosis) of the aortic valve. For example, in the late stages of aortic stenosis, the left ventricle may need to generate systolic pressures up to 300 mm Hg to move blood through the diseased valve.

Cardiac Contractility

Cardiac contractility refers to the ability of the heart to change its force of contraction without changing its resting (*i.e.,* diastolic) length. The contractile state of the myocardial muscle is determined by biochemical and biophysical properties that govern the actin and myosin interactions in the myocardial cells. It is strongly influenced by the number of calcium ions that are available to participate in the contractile process.

An *inotropic* influence is one that modifies the contractile state of the myocardium independent of the Frank-Starling mechanism (see Fig. 21-12, top curve). For example, sympathetic stimulation produces a positive inotropic effect by increasing the calcium that is available for interaction between the actin and myosin filaments. Hypoxia exerts a negative inotropic effect by interfering with the generation of adenosine triphosphate (ATP), which is needed for muscle contraction.

Heart Rate

The heart rate determines the frequency with which blood is ejected from the heart. Therefore, as the heart rate increases, cardiac output tends to increase. As the heart rate increases, the time spent in diastole is reduced, and there is less time for the ventricles to fill. At a heart rate of 75 beats per minute, one cardiac cycle lasts 0.8 second, of which approximately 0.3 second is spent in systole and approximately 0.5 second in diastole. As the heart rate increases, the time spent in systole remains approximately the same, whereas that spent in diastole decreases. This leads to a decrease in stroke volume and, at high heart rates, a decrease in cardiac output. One of the dangers of ventricular tachycardia is a reduction in cardiac output because the heart does not have time to fill adequately.

IN SUMMARY, the heart is a four-chambered muscular pump that lies in the pericardial sac within the mediastinal space of the intrathoracic cavity. The wall of the heart is composed of an outer epicardium, which lines the pericardial cavity; a fibrous skeleton; the myocardium, or muscle layer; and the smooth endocardium, which lines the chambers of the heart. The four heart valves control the direction of blood flow.

The cardiac cycle describes the pumping action of the heart. It is divided into two parts: systole, during which the ventricles contract and blood is ejected from the heart, and diastole, during which the ventricles are relaxed and blood is filling the heart. The stroke volume (approximately 70 mL) represents the difference between the end-diastolic volume (approximately 120 mL) and the end-systolic volume (approximately 50 mL). The electrical activity of the heart, as represented on the ECG, precedes the mechanical events of the cardiac cycle. The heart sounds signal the closing of the heart valves during the cardiac cycle. Atrial contraction occurs during the last third of diastole. Although the main function of the atria is to store blood as it enters the heart, atrial contraction acts to increase cardiac output during periods of increased activity when the filling time is reduced or in disease conditions in which ventricular filling is impaired.

The heart's ability to increase its output according to body needs depends on the preload, or filling of the ventricles (i.e., end-diastolic volume); the afterload, or resistance to ejection of blood from the heart; cardiac contractility, which determines the force of contraction; and the heart rate, which determines the frequency with which blood is ejected from the heart. The maximum force of cardiac contraction occurs when an increase in preload stretches muscle fibers of the heart to approximately two and one-half times their resting length (i.e., Frank-Starling mechanism). A rapid heart rate decreases the time spent in diastolic filling of the ventricles, with a resultant decrease in stroke volume. ■

CONCEPTSin action**ANIMATI:·N**

THE SYSTEMIC CIRCULATION AND CONTROL OF BLOOD FLOW

After completing this section of the chapter, you should be able to meet the following objectives:

- Compare the structure and function of arteries and veins.
- Describe the structure and function of vascular smooth muscle.
- Use the equation blood pressure = cardiac output × peripheral vascular resistance to explain the regulation of arterial blood pressure.
- Define autoregulation and characterize mechanisms responsible for short-term and long-term regulation of blood flow.
- Describe mechanisms involved in the humoral control of blood flow.

The vascular system functions in the delivery of oxygen and nutrients and removal of waste products from the tissues. It consists of the arteries and arterioles, the capillaries, and the venules and veins. Although blood vessels of the vascular system are often compared with a system of rigid pipes and tubes, this analogy serves only as a starting point. Blood vessels are dynamic structures that constrict and relax to adjust blood pressure and flow to meet the varying needs of the many different tissue types and organ systems. Structures such as the heart, brain, liver, and kidneys require a large and continuous flow to carry out their vital functions. In other tissues such as the skin and skeletal muscle, the need for blood flow varies with the level of function. For example, there is a need for increased blood flow to the skin during fever and for increased skeletal muscle blood flow during exercise.

Blood Vessels

All blood vessels, except the capillaries, have walls composed of three layers, or coats, called *tunicae* (Fig. 21-13). The outermost layer of a vessel, called the *tunica externa* or *tunica adventitia*, is composed primarily of loosely woven collagen fibers that protect the blood vessel and anchor it to the surrounding structures. The middle layer, the *tunica media*, is largely a smooth muscle layer that constricts to regulate and control the diameter of the vessel. Larger arteries have an external elastic lamina that separates the tunica media from the tunica externa. The innermost layer, the *tunica intima*, consists of a single layer of flattened endothelial cells with minimal underlying subendothelial connective tissue. The endothelial layer provides a smooth and slippery inner surface for the vessel. This smooth inner lining, as long as it remains intact, prevents platelet adherence and blood clotting.

The layers of the different types of blood vessels vary with vessel function. The walls of the arterioles, which control blood pressure, have large amounts of smooth muscle. Veins

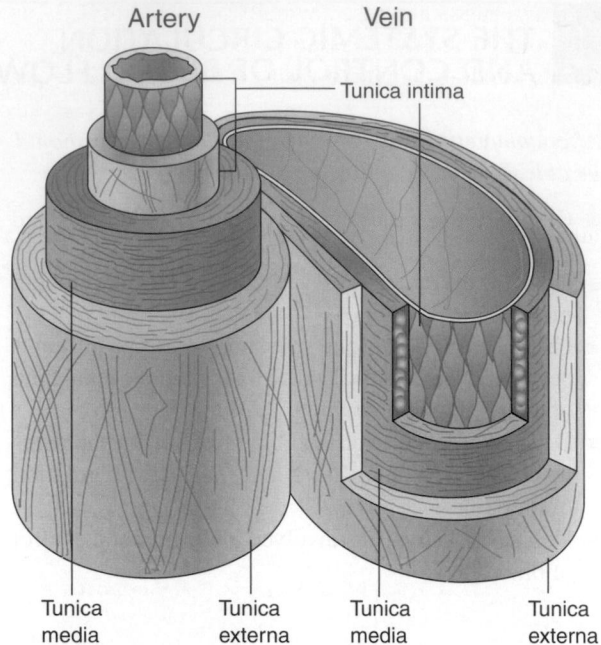

Artery   Vein

Tunica intima

Tunica   Tunica   Tunica   Tunica
media   externa   media   externa

FIGURE 21-13 • Medium-sized artery and vein, showing the relative thicknesses of the three layers.

are thin-walled, distensible, and collapsible vessels. Capillaries are single-cell–thick vessels designed for the exchange of gases, nutrients, and waste materials.

Vascular Smooth Muscle

Vascular smooth muscle cells, which form the predominant cellular layer in the tunica media, produce vasoconstriction or dilation of blood vessels. Smooth muscle contracts slowly and generates high forces for long periods with low energy requirements; it uses only 1/10 to 1/300 the energy of skeletal muscle. These characteristics are important in structures, such as blood vessels, that must maintain their tone day in and day out.

Compared with skeletal and cardiac muscles, smooth muscle has less well-developed sarcoplasmic reticulum for storing intracellular calcium, and it has very few fast sodium channels. Depolarization of smooth muscle instead relies largely on extracellular calcium, which enters through calcium channels in the muscle membrane. Sympathetic nervous system control of vascular smooth muscle tone occurs through receptor-activated opening and closing of the calcium channels. In general, α-adrenergic receptors are excitatory in that they cause the channels to open and produce vasoconstriction, and β-adrenergic receptors are inhibitory in that they cause the channels to close and produce vasodilation. Calcium channel blocking drugs cause vasodilation by blocking calcium entry through the calcium channels.

Smooth muscle contraction and relaxation also occur in response to local tissue factors such as lack of oxygen, increased hydrogen ion concentrations, and excess carbon dioxide. Nitric

oxide (formerly known as the *endothelial relaxing factor*) acts locally to produce smooth muscle relaxation and regulate blood flow. These factors are discussed more fully in the section on Local and Humoral Control of Blood Flow.

🔑 THE VASCULAR SYSTEM AND CONTROL OF BLOOD FLOW

■ The vascular system, which consists of the arterial system, the venous system, and the capillaries, functions in the delivery of oxygen and nutrients and in the removal of wastes from the tissues.

■ The arterial system is a high-pressure system that delivers blood to the tissues. It relies on the intermittent ejection of blood from the left ventricle and the generation of arterial pressure pulsations or waves that move blood toward the capillaries where the exchange of gases, nutrients, and wastes occur.

■ The venous system is a low-pressure system that collects blood from the capillaries. It relies on the presence of valves in the veins of the extremities to prevent retrograde flow and on the milking action of the skeletal muscles that surround the veins to return blood to the right heart.

■ Local control of blood flow is regulated by mechanisms that match blood flow to the metabolic needs of the tissue. Over the short term, the tissues auto-regulate flow through the synthesis of vasodilators and vasoconstrictors derived from the tissue, smooth muscle, or endothelial cells; over the long term, blood flow is regulated by creation of a collateral circulation.

■ Neural control of circulatory function occurs through the sympathetic and parasympathetic divisions of the autonomic nervous system. Sympathetic stimulation increases heart rate, cardiac contractility, and vessel tone (vascular resistance), whereas parasympathetic stimulation decreases heart rate.

Arterial System

The arterial system consists of the large and medium-sized arteries and the arterioles. Arteries are thick-walled vessels with large amounts of elastic fibers. The elasticity of these vessels allows them to stretch during systole, when the heart contracts and blood enters the circulation, and to recoil during diastole, when the heart relaxes. The arterioles, which are predominantly smooth muscle, serve as resistance vessels for the circulatory system. They act as control valves through which blood is released as it moves into the capillaries. Changes in the activity of sympathetic fibers that innervate these vessels cause them to constrict or to relax as needed to maintain blood pressure.

Arterial Pressure Pulsations

The delivery of blood to the tissues of the body depends on pressure pulsations or waves of pressure that are generated by the intermittent ejection of blood from the left ventricle into the distensible aorta and large arteries of the arterial system. The arterial pressure pulse represents the energy that is transmitted from molecule to molecule along the length of the vessel (Fig. 21-14). In the aorta, this pressure pulse is transmitted at a velocity of 4 to 6 m/second, which is approximately 20 times faster than the flow of blood. Therefore, the pressure pulse has no direct relation to blood flow and could occur if there was no flow at all. When taking a pulse, it is the pressure pulses that are felt, and it is the pressure pulses that produce the Korotkoff sounds heard during blood pressure measurement. The tip or maximum deflection of the pressure pulsation coincides with the systolic blood pressure, and the minimum point of deflection coincides with the diastolic pressure. The pulse pressure is the difference between systolic and diastolic pressure. If all other factors are equal, the magnitude of the pulse pressure reflects the volume of blood ejected from the left ventricle in a single beat.

Both the pressure values and the conformation of the pressure wave change as it moves though the peripheral arteries, such that pulsations in the large arteries are even greater than those in the aorta (see Fig. 21-14). In other words, systolic pressure and pulse pressure are higher in large arteries than in the aorta. The increase in pulse pressure in the "downstream" arteries is due to the fact that immediately after ejection from the left ventricle, the pressure wave travels at a higher velocity than the blood itself, augmenting the downhill pressure. Furthermore, at branch points of arteries, pressure points are reflected backward, which also tends to augment pressure at those sites. With peripheral arterial disease, there is a delay in the transmission of the reflected wave so that the pulse decreases rather than increases in amplitude.

After its initial amplification, the pressure pulse becomes smaller and smaller as it moves through the smaller arteries and arterioles, until it disappears almost entirely in the capillaries. This damping of the pressure pulse is caused by the resistance and distensibility characteristics of these vessels. The increased resistance of these small vessels impedes the transmission of the pressure waves, whereas their distensibility is great enough that any small change in flow does not cause a pressure change. Although the pressure pulses usually are not transmitted to the capillaries, there are situations in which this does occur. For example, injury to a finger or other area of the body often results in a throbbing sensation. In this case, extreme dilation of the small vessels in the injured area produces a reduction in the dampening of the pressure pulse. Capillary pulsations also occur in conditions that cause exaggeration of aortic pressure pulses, such as aortic regurgitation or patent ductus arteriosus (see Chapter 24).

Venous System

The venous system is a low-pressure system that returns blood to the heart. The venules collect blood from the capillaries, and the veins transport blood back to the right heart. Blood from the systemic veins flows into the right atrium of the heart; therefore, the pressure in the right atrium is called the *central venous pressure*. Right atrial pressure is regulated by the ability of the right ventricle to pump blood into the lungs and the tendency of blood to flow from the peripheral veins into the right atrium. The normal right atrial pressure is about 0 mm Hg, which is equal to atmospheric pressure. It can increase to 20 to 30 mm Hg in conditions such as right heart failure and the rapid transfusion of blood at a rate that greatly increases total blood volume and causes excessive quantities of blood to attempt to flow into the heart from the systemic veins.

The veins and venules are thin-walled, distensible, and collapsible vessels. The veins are capable of enlarging and storing large quantities of blood, which can be made available to the circulation as needed. Even though the veins are thin walled, they are muscular. This allows them to contract or expand to accommodate varying amounts of blood. Veins are innervated by the sympathetic nervous system. When blood is lost from the circulation, the veins constrict as a means of maintaining intravascular volume.

Valves in the veins of extremities prevent retrograde flow (Fig. 21-15) and with the help of skeletal muscles that surround and intermittently compress the leg veins in a milking manner, blood is moved forward to the heart. This pumping action is known as the *venous* or *muscle pump*. There are no valves in the abdominal or thoracic veins, and blood flow in these veins is heavily influenced by the pressure in the abdominal and thoracic cavities, respectively.

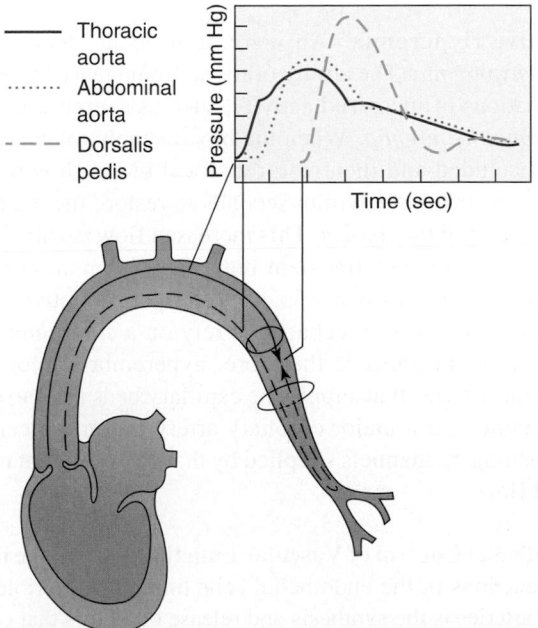

FIGURE 21-14 • Amplification of the arterial pressure wave as it moves forward in the peripheral arteries. This amplification occurs as a forward-moving pressure wave merges with a backward-moving reflected pressure wave. (**Inset**) The amplitude of the pressure pulse increases in the thoracic aorta, abdominal aorta, and dorsalis pedis.

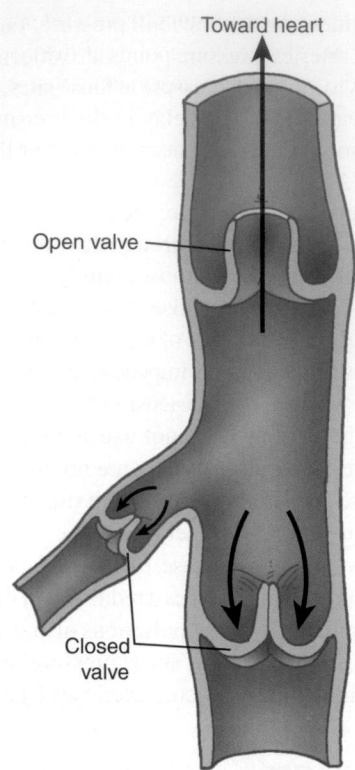

FIGURE 21-15 • Portion of a femoral vein opened, to show the valves. The direction of flow is upward. Backward flow closes the valve.

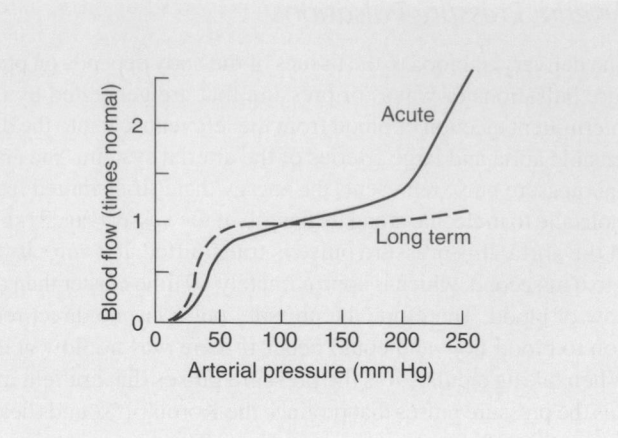

FIGURE 21-16 • Effect of increasing arterial pressure on blood flow through a muscle. The *solid curve* shows the effect if pressure is raised over a few minutes. The *dashed curve* shows the effect if the arterial pressure is raised slowly over many weeks. (From Guyton A. C., Hall J. E. [1996]. *Textbook of medical physiology* [9th ed., p. 203]. Philadelphia: W. B. Saunders.)

Because the venous system is a low-pressure system, blood flow must oppose the effects of gravity. In a person in the standing position, the weight of the blood in the vascular column causes an increase of 1 mm Hg in pressure for every 13.6 mm of distance below the level of the heart. Were it not for the valves in the veins and the action of the skeletal muscles, the venous pressure in the feet would be about +90 mm Hg in the standing adult. Gravity has no effect on the venous pressure in a person in the recumbent position because the blood in the veins is then at the level of the heart.

Local and Humoral Control of Blood Flow

Tissue blood flow is regulated on a minute-to-minute basis in relation to tissue needs and on a longer-term basis through the development of collateral circulation. Neural mechanisms regulate the cardiac output and blood pressure needed to support these local mechanisms.

Short-Term Autoregulation

Local control of blood flow is governed largely by the nutritional needs of the tissue. For example, blood flow to organs such as the heart, brain, and kidneys remains relatively constant, although blood pressure may vary over a range of 60 to 180 mm Hg (Fig. 21-16). The ability of the tissues to regulate their own blood flow over a wide range of pressures is called *autoregulation*. Autoregulation of blood flow is mediated by changes in blood vessel tone due to changes in flow through the vessel or by local tissue factors, such as lack of oxygen or accumulation of tissue metabolites (*i.e.,* potassium, lactic acid, or adenosine, which is a breakdown product of ATP). Local control is particularly important in tissues such as skeletal muscle, which has blood flow requirements that vary according to the level of activity.

Reactive Hyperemia. An increase in local blood flow is called *hyperemia*. The ability of tissues to increase blood flow in situations of increased activity, such as exercise, is called *functional hyperemia*. When the blood supply to an area has been occluded and then restored, local blood flow through the tissues increases within seconds to restore the metabolic equilibrium of the tissues. This increased flow is called *reactive hyperemia*. The transient redness seen on an arm after leaning on a hard surface is an example of reactive hyperemia. Local control mechanisms rely on a continuous flow from the main arteries; therefore, hyperemia cannot occur when the arteries that supply the capillary beds are narrowed. For example, if a major coronary artery becomes occluded, the opening of channels supplied by that vessel cannot restore blood flow.

Endothelial Control of Vascular Function. One of the important functions of the endothelial cells lining the arterioles and small arteries is the synthesis and release of factors that control vessel dilation. Of particular importance was the discovery, first reported in the early 1980s, that the intact endothelium was able to produce a factor that caused relaxation of vascular smooth muscle. This factor was originally named *endothelium-derived relaxing factor* and is now known to be *nitric oxide*. The normal endothelium maintains a continuous release of nitric oxide, which is formed from L-arginine through the action of an enzyme called *nitric oxide synthase* (Fig. 21-17). The production of nitric oxide can be stimulated by a variety of endothelial *agonists,* including acetylcholine, bradykinin, histamine, and thrombin. *Shear stress* on the endothelium resulting from an increase in blood flow or blood pressure also stimulates nitric oxide production and vessel relaxation. Nitric oxide also inhibits platelet aggregation and secretion of platelet contents, many of which cause vasoconstriction. The fact that nitric oxide is released into the vessel lumen (to inactivate platelets) and away from the lumen (to relax smooth muscle) suggests that it protects against both thrombosis and vasoconstriction. Nitroglycerin, which is used in the treatment of angina, produces its effects by causing the release of nitric oxide in vascular smooth muscle of the target tissues.

The endothelium also produces a number of vasoconstrictor substances, including *angiotensin II,* vasoconstrictor prostaglandins, and a family of peptides called *endothelins.* There are at least three endothelins. Endothelin-1, made by human endothelial cells, is the most potent endogenous vasoconstrictor known. Receptors for endothelins also have been identified.

Long-Term Regulation of Blood Flow

Collateral circulation is a mechanism for the long-term regulation of local blood flow. In the heart and other vital structures, anastomotic channels exist between some of the smaller arteries. These channels permit perfusion of an area by more than one artery. When one artery becomes occluded, these anastomotic channels increase in size, allowing blood from a patent artery to perfuse the area supplied by the occluded vessel. For example,

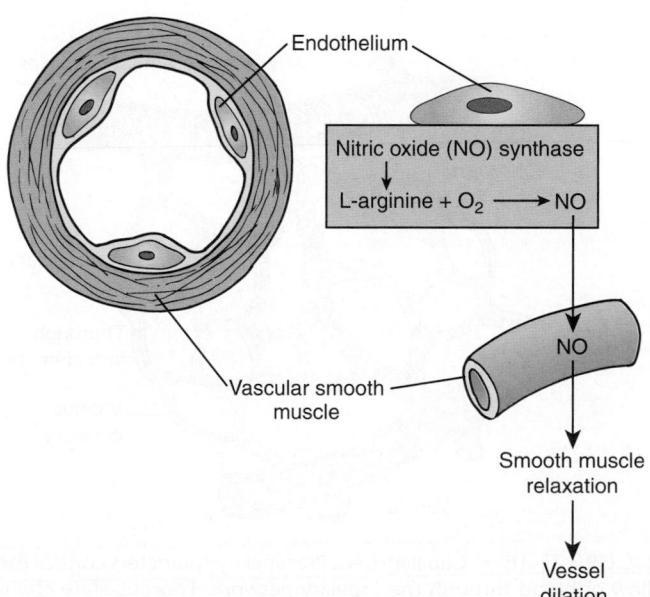

FIGURE 21-17 • Function of nitric oxide in smooth muscle relaxation.

persons with extensive obstruction of a coronary blood vessel may rely on collateral circulation to meet the oxygen needs of the myocardial tissue normally supplied by that vessel. As with other long-term compensatory mechanisms, the recruitment of collateral circulation is most efficient when obstruction to flow is gradual rather than sudden.

Humoral Control of Vascular Function

Humoral control of blood flow involves the effect of vasodilator and vasoconstrictor substances in the blood. Some of these substances are formed by special glands and transported in the blood throughout the entire circulation. Others are formed in local tissues and aid in the local control of blood flow. Among the most important of the humoral factors are norepinephrine and epinephrine, angiotensin II, histamine, serotonin, bradykinin, and the prostaglandins.

Norepinephrine and Epinephrine. Norepinephrine is an especially powerful vasoconstrictor hormone; epinephrine is less so and in some tissues (*e.g.,* skeletal muscle) even causes mild vasodilation. Stimulation of the sympathetic nervous system during stress or exercise causes local constriction of veins and arterioles because of the release of norepinephrine from sympathetic nerve endings. In addition, sympathetic stimulation causes the adrenal medullae to secrete both norepinephrine and epinephrine into the blood. These hormones then circulate in the blood, causing direct sympathetic stimulation of blood vessels in all parts of the body.

Angiotensin II. Angiotensin II is another powerful vasoconstrictor substance. Angiotensin II is produced as a part of the renin-angiotensin-aldosterone system and normally acts on many arterioles simultaneously to increase the peripheral vascular resistance, thereby increasing the arterial blood pressure (discussed in Chapter 23).

Histamine. Histamine has a powerful vasodilator effect on arterioles and has the ability to increase capillary permeability, allowing leakage of both fluid and plasma proteins into the tissues. Histamine is largely derived from mast cells in injured tissues and basophils in the blood. In certain tissues, such as skeletal muscle, the activity of the mast cells is mediated by the sympathetic nervous system; when sympathetic control is withdrawn, the mast cells release histamine.

Serotonin. Serotonin is liberated from aggregating platelets during the clotting process; it causes vasoconstriction and plays a major role in control of bleeding. Serotonin is found in brain and lung tissues, and there is some speculation that it may be involved in the vascular spasm associated with some allergic pulmonary reactions and migraine headaches.

Bradykinin. The kinins (*i.e.,* kallidins and bradykinin) are liberated from the globulin kininogen, which is present in body fluids. Bradykinin causes intense dilation of arterioles, increased capillary permeability, and constriction of venules. It is thought that the kinins play special roles in regulating blood flow and capillary leakage in inflamed tissues. It is also believed that bradykinin helps to regulate blood flow in the skin as well in the salivary and gastrointestinal glands.

Prostaglandins. Prostaglandins are synthesized from constituents of the cell membrane (*i.e.*, the long-chain fatty acid *arachidonic acid*). Tissue injury incites the release of arachidonic acid from the cell membrane, which initiates prostaglandin synthesis. There are several prostaglandins (*e.g.*, E_2, F_2, D_2), which are subgrouped according to their solubility; some produce vasoconstriction and some produce vasodilation. As a rule of thumb, those in the E group are vasodilators, and those in the F group are vasoconstrictors. The corticosteroid hormones produce an anti-inflammatory response by blocking the release of arachidonic acid, preventing prostaglandin synthesis.

IN SUMMARY, the walls of all blood vessels, except the capillaries, are composed of three layers: the tunica externa, tunica media, and tunica intima. The layers of the vessel vary with its function. Arteries are thick-walled vessels with large amounts of elastic fibers. The walls of the arterioles, which control blood pressure, have large amounts of smooth muscle. Veins are thin-walled, distensible, and collapsible vessels. Venous flow is designed to return blood to the heart. It is a low-pressure system and relies on venous valves and the action of muscle pumps to offset the effects of gravity.

The delivery of blood to the tissues of the body depends on pressure pulses that are generated by the intermittent ejection of blood from the left ventricle into the distensible aorta and large arteries of the arterial system. The combination of distensibility of the arteries and their resistance to flow reduces the pressure pulsations so that constant blood flow occurs by the time blood reaches the capillaries.

The mechanisms that control local blood flow are designed to ensure adequate delivery of blood to the capillaries in the microcirculation, where the exchange of cellular nutrients and wastes occurs. Local control is governed largely by the needs of the tissues and is regulated by local tissue factors such as lack of oxygen and the accumulation of metabolites. Hyperemia is a local increase in blood flow that occurs after a temporary occlusion of blood flow. It is a compensatory mechanism that decreases the oxygen debt of the deprived tissues. Collateral circulation is a mechanism for long-term regulation of local blood flow that involves the development of collateral vessels. The endothelial relaxing factor (mainly nitric oxide) and humoral factors, such as norepinephrine and epinephrine, angiotensin II, histamine, serotonin, bradykinin, and the prostaglandins, contribute to the regulation of blood flow. ∎

THE MICROCIRCULATION AND LYMPHATIC SYSTEM

After completing this section of the chapter, you should be able to meet the following objectives:

- Define the term *microcirculation*.
- Describe the structure and function of the capillaries.
- Explain the forces that control the fluid exchange between the capillaries and the interstitial spaces.
- Describe the structures of the lymphatic system and relate them to the role of the lymphatics in controlling interstitial fluid volume.

The term *microcirculation* refers to the functions of the smallest blood vessels, the capillaries and the neighboring lymphatic vessels. The microcirculation is the site of exchange of gases, nutrients, and waste products in the tissues, as well as the site of vascular and interstitial fluid exchange.

Structure and Function of the Microcirculation

The structures of the microcirculation include the arterioles, capillaries, and venules. Blood enters the microcirculation through an arteriole, passes through the capillaries, and leaves through a small venule. The metarterioles serve as thoroughfare channels that link arterioles and capillaries (Fig. 21-18). Small cuffs of smooth muscle, the precapillary sphincters, are positioned at the arterial end of the capillary. The smooth muscle tone of the arterioles, venules, and precapillary sphincters

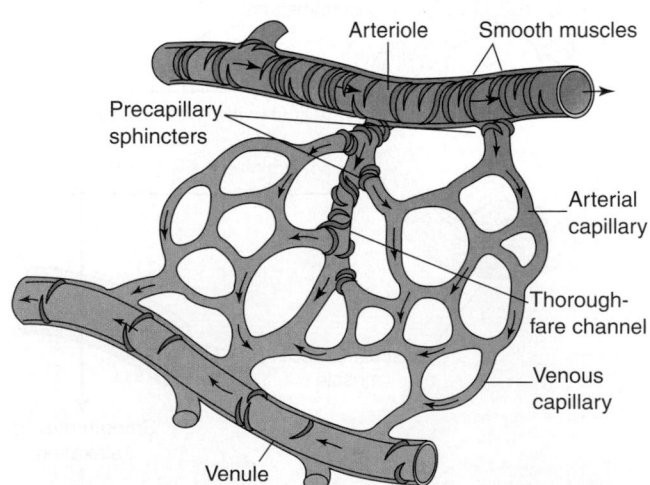

FIGURE 21-18 • Capillary bed. Precapillary sphincters control the flow of blood through the capillary network. Thoroughfare channels (*i.e.*, arteriovenous shunts) allow blood to move directly from the arteriole into the venule without moving through nutrient channels of the capillary.

serves to control blood flow through the capillary bed. Depending on venous pressure, blood flows through the capillary channels when the precapillary sphincters are open.

Capillary Structure and Function

Capillaries are microscopic vessels that connect the arterial and venous segments of the circulation. In each person, there are approximately 10 billion capillaries, with a total surface area of 500 to 700 m^2. The capillary wall is composed of a single layer of endothelial cells and their basement membrane (Fig. 21-19). The endothelial cells form a tube just large enough to allow the passage of red blood cells, one at a time.

Water-filled junctions, called the *capillary pores,* join the capillary endothelial cells and provide a pathway for passage of substances through the capillary wall. The size of the capillary pores varies with capillary function. In the brain, the endothelial cells are joined by tight junctions that form the blood-brain barrier. This prevents substances that would alter neural excitability from leaving the capillary. In organs that process blood contents, such as the liver, capillaries have large pores so that substances can pass easily through the capillary wall. The glomerular capillaries in the kidney have small openings called *fenestrations* that pass directly through the middle of the endothelial cells, a property that is consistent with the filtration function of the glomerulus.

Because of their thin walls and close proximity to the cells of metabolically active tissues, capillaries are particularly well suited for the exchange of gases and metabolites between cells and the bloodstream. This exchange of substances occurs through spaces between tissue cells called the *interstitium* (Fig. 21-20). The interstitium is supported by *collagen* and *elastin* fibers and filled with *proteoglycan* (sugar–protein) molecules that combine with water to form a tissue gel. The tissue gel acts like a sponge to entrap the interstitial fluid and provide for distribution of the fluid, even to those cells that are most distant from the capillary.

Fluids, electrolytes, gases, and substances of small and large molecular weights move across the capillary endothelium by diffusion, filtration, and pinocytosis. The exchange of gases and fluids across the capillary wall occurs by simple diffusion. Lipid-soluble substances such as oxygen and carbon dioxide readily exchange across the endothelial cells by diffusion. Water flows through the capillary endothelial cell membranes through water-selective channels called *aquaporins.* Water and water-soluble substances such as electrolytes, glucose, and amino acids also diffuse between the endothelial cells in the capillary pores. Pinocytosis (discussed in Chapter 4) is responsible for the movement of white blood cells and large protein molecules.

Control of Blood Flow in the Microcirculation

Blood flow through capillary channels, designed for exchange of nutrients and metabolites, is called *nutrient flow.* In some parts of the microcirculation, blood flow bypasses the capillary bed, moving through a connection called an *arteriovenous shunt,* which directly connects an arteriole and a venule. This type of blood flow is called *non-nutrient flow* because it does not allow for nutrient exchange. Non-nutrient channels are common in the

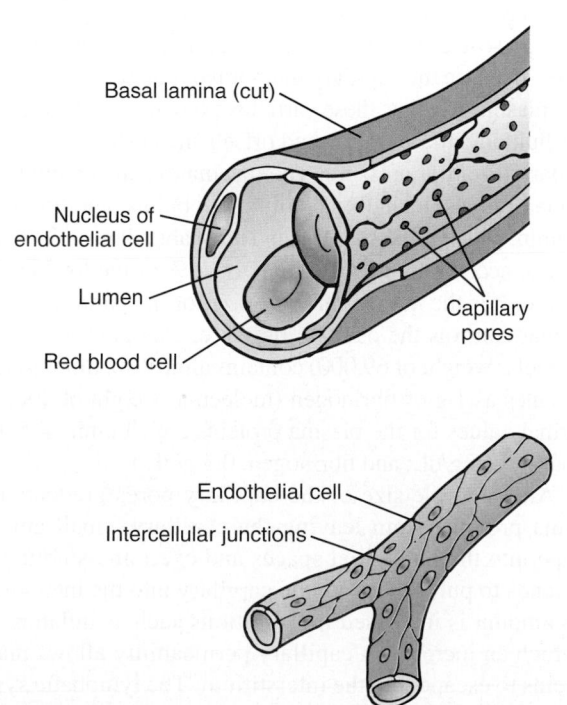

FIGURE 21-19 • Endothelial cells and intercellular junctions in a section of capillary.

Basal lamina (cut)

Nucleus of endothelial cell

Lumen

Red blood cell

Capillary pores

Endothelial cell

Intercellular junctions

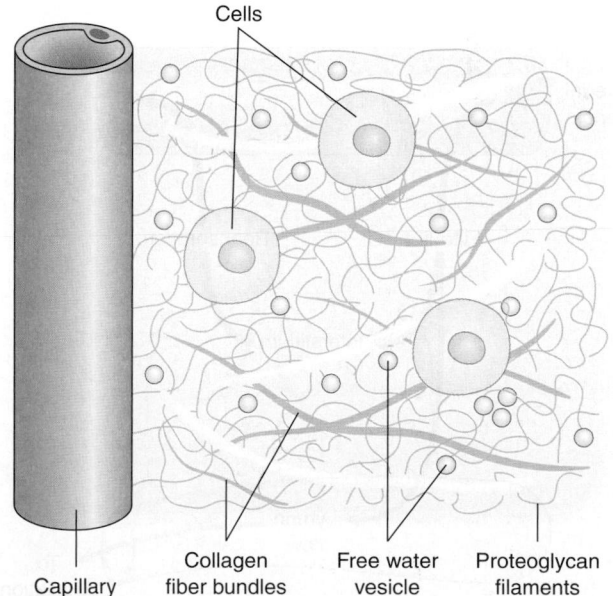

Cells

Capillary

Collagen fiber bundles

Free water vesicle

Proteoglycan filaments

FIGURE 21-20 • Structure of the interstitium. Proteoglycan filaments are everywhere in the spaces between the collagen fiber bundles. Free water vesicles and small amounts of free fluid in the form of rivulets occasionally may occur. (Adapted from Guyton A. C., Hall J. E. [2006]. *Textbook of medical physiology* [11th ed., p. 184]. Philadelphia: Elsevier Saunders.)

skin and are important in terms of heat exchange and temperature regulation (discussed in Chapter 10).

Capillary–Interstitial Fluid Exchange

The direction and magnitude of fluid movement across the capillary wall are largely controlled by the hydrostatic and osmotic pressures of the capillary and interstitial fluids, as well as the permeability of the capillary wall. The direction of fluid movement can either be into or out of the capillary. When net fluid movement is out of the capillary into the interstitial spaces, it is called *filtration,* and when net movement is from the interstitium into the capillary, it is called *absorption* (Fig. 21-21).

The capillary hydrostatic pressure represents the fluid pressure that tends to push water and its dissolved substances through the capillary pores into the interstitium. The osmotic pressure caused by the plasma proteins in the blood tends to pull fluid from the interstitial spaces back into the capillary. This pressure is termed *colloidal osmotic pressure* to differentiate the osmotic effects of the plasma proteins, which are suspended colloids, from the osmotic effects of substances such as sodium and glucose, which are dissolved crystalloids. Capillary permeability controls the movement of water and substances, such as the plasma proteins that influence osmotic pressure, into the interstitial spaces. Also important to this exchange mechanism is the lymphatic system, which removes excess fluid and osmotically active proteins and large particles from the interstitial spaces and returns them to the circulation.

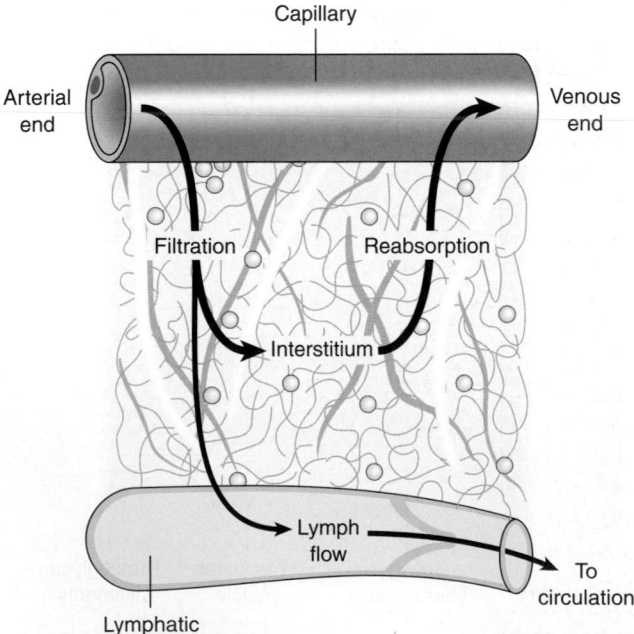

FIGURE 21-21 • Capillary filtration and lymph flow. Fluid is filtered out of the capillary and into the interstitium at the arterial end of the capillary. Most of the fluid is reabsorbed at the venous end of the capillary, with the rest of the fluid entering the terminal lymphatics for return to the circulation.

Hydrostatic Forces

The capillary hydrostatic pressure is the principal force in capillary filtration. The hydrostatic pressure (blood pressure) within the capillaries is determined by both the arterial and venous pressures (the capillaries being interspersed between the arteries and veins). An increase in small artery and arterial pressure elevates capillary hydrostatic pressure, whereas a reduction in each of these pressures has the opposite effect. A change in venous pressure has a greater effect on the capillary hydrostatic pressure than does the same change in arterial pressure. About 80% of increased venous pressure, such as that caused by venous thrombosis or congestive heart failure, is transmitted back to the capillary. Capillary hydrostatic pressure is also affected by the previously discussed effects of gravity on venous pressure. When a person stands, the hydrostatic pressure is greater in the legs and lower in the head.

The interstitial hydrostatic pressure is the pressure exerted by the interstitial fluids outside the capillary. It can be positive or negative. A positive interstitial fluid pressure opposes capillary filtration and a negative interstitial fluid pressure increases the movement of fluid out of the capillary into the interstitium. In the normal nonedematous state, the interstitial hydrostatic pressure is close to zero or slightly negative (−1 to −4 mm Hg) and has very little effect on capillary filtration or outward movement of fluid.

Osmotic Forces

The key factor that restrains fluid loss from the capillaries is the colloidal osmotic pressure (approximately 28 mm Hg) generated by the plasma proteins. The plasma proteins are large molecules that disperse in the blood and occasionally escape into the tissue spaces. Because the capillary membrane is almost impermeable to the plasma proteins, these particles exert an osmotic force that pulls fluid into the capillary and offsets the pushing force of the capillary filtration pressure. The plasma contains a mixture of plasma proteins, including albumin, globulins, and fibrinogen. Albumin, which is the smallest and most abundant of the plasma proteins, accounts for approximately 70% of the total osmotic pressure. It is the number, not the size, of the particles in solution that controls the osmotic pressure. One gram of albumin (molecular weight of 69,000) contains almost six times as many molecules as 1 g of fibrinogen (molecular weight of 400,000). (Normal values for the plasma proteins are albumin, 4.5 g/dL; globulins, 2.5 g/dL; and fibrinogen, 0.3 g/dL.)

Although the size of the capillary pores prevents most plasma proteins from leaving the capillary, small amounts escape into the interstitial spaces and exert an osmotic force that tends to pull fluid from the capillary into the interstitium. This amount is increased in conditions such as inflammation in which an increase in capillary permeability allows plasma proteins to escape into the interstitium. The lymphatic system is responsible for removing proteins from the interstitium. In the absence of a functioning lymphatic system, interstitial colloidal osmotic pressure increases, causing fluid to accumulate.

Normally, a few white blood cells, plasma proteins, and other large molecules enter the interstitial spaces; these cells and molecules, which are too large to reenter the capillary, rely on the loosely structured wall of the lymphatic vessels for return to the vascular compartment.

Balance of Hydrostatic and Osmotic Forces

Normally, the movement of fluid between the capillary bed and the interstitial spaces is continuous. As E. H. Starling pointed out more than a century ago, a state of equilibrium exists as long as equal amounts of fluid enter and leave the interstitial spaces. The forces that contribute to the Starling equilibrium are illustrated in Figure 21-22. In the diagram, the hydrostatic pressure at the arterial end of the capillary is higher than at the venous end. The pushing force of the capillary hydrostatic pressure on the arterial end of the capillary, along with the pulling effects of the interstitial colloidal osmotic pressure, contribute to the net outward movement of fluid. The capillary colloidal osmotic pressure and opposing interstitial osmotic pressure determine the reabsorption of fluid at the venous end of the capillary. A slight imbalance in forces causes slightly more filtration of fluid into interstitial spaces than absorption back into the capillary; it is this fluid that is returned to the circulation by the lymphatic system. Disorders of capillary fluid exchange are discussed in Chapter 31.

The Lymphatic System

The lymphatic system, commonly called the *lymphatics,* serves almost all body tissues, except cartilage, bone, epithelial tissue, and tissues of the central nervous system (CNS). Most of these tissues, however, have prelymphatic channels that eventually flow into areas supplied by the lymphatics. Lymph is derived from interstitial fluids that flow through the lymph channels. It contains plasma proteins and other osmotically active particles that rely on the lymphatics for movement back into the circulatory system. The lymphatic system is also the main route for absorption of nutrients, particularly fats, from the gastrointestinal tract. The lymphatic system also filters the fluid at the lymph nodes and removes foreign particles such as bacteria. When lymph flow is obstructed, a condition called *lymphedema* occurs. Involvement of lymphatic structures by malignant tumors and removal of lymph nodes at the time of cancer surgery are common causes of lymphedema.

The lymphatic system is made up of vessels similar to those of the circulatory system. These vessels commonly travel along with an arteriole or venule or with its companion artery and vein. The terminal lymphatic vessels are made up of a single layer of connective tissue with an endothelial lining and resemble blood capillaries. The lymphatic vessels lack tight junctions and are loosely anchored to the surrounding tissues by fine filaments (Fig. 21-23). The loose junctions permit the entry of large particles, and the filaments hold the vessels open under conditions of edema, when the pressure of the surrounding tissues would otherwise cause them to collapse. The lymph capillaries drain into larger lymph vessels that ultimately empty into the right and left thoracic ducts (Fig. 21-24). The thoracic ducts empty into the circulation at the junctions of the subclavian and internal jugular veins.

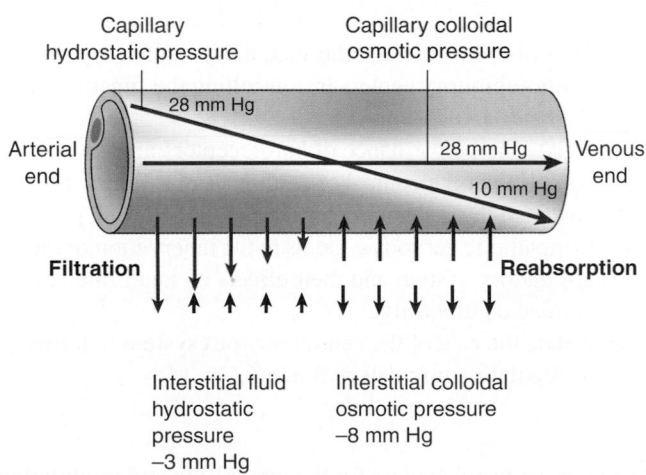

FIGURE 21-22 • Capillary–interstitial fluid exchange equilibrium. Normally, the forces (capillary hydrostatic pressure, interstitial colloidal osmotic pressure, and the opposing interstitial fluid pressure) that control the outward movement of fluid from the capillary (filtration) are almost balanced by the forces (capillary colloidal osmotic pressure and interstitial colloidal osmotic pressure) that pull fluid back into the capillary (reabsorption).

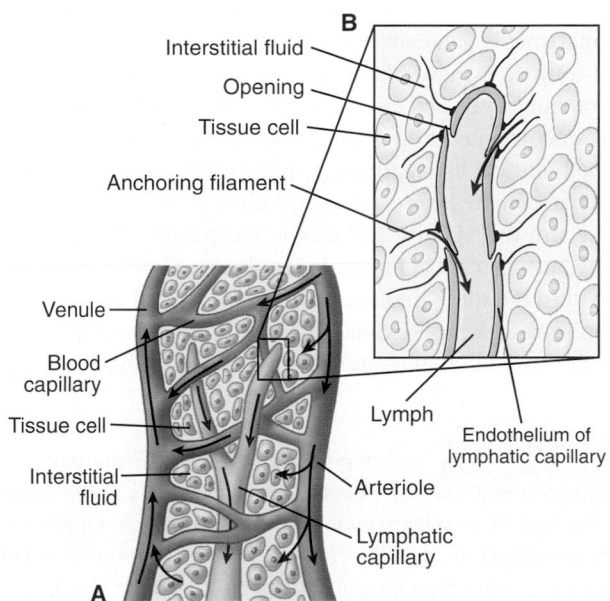

FIGURE 21-23 • (A) Location of the lymphatic capillary. Fluid from the arterial side of the capillary bed moves into the interstitial spaces and is reabsorbed in the venous side of the capillary bed. (B) Details of the lymphatic capillary with its anchoring filaments and overlapping edges that serve as valves and can be pushed open, allowing the inflow of interstitial fluid and its suspended particles.

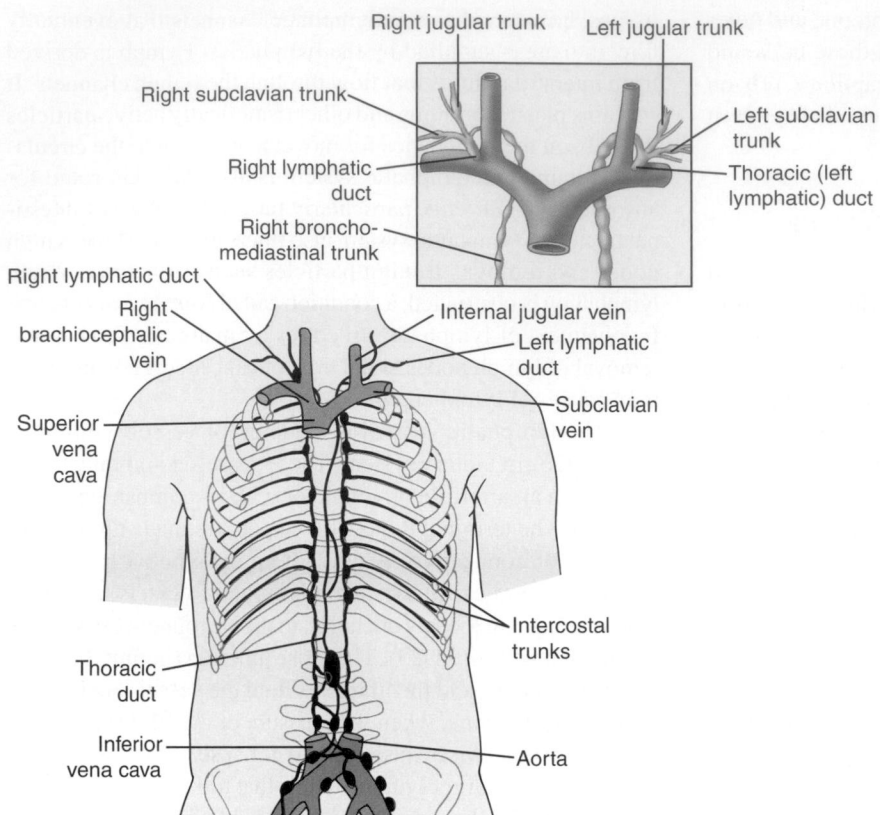

FIGURE 21-24 • Lymphatic system, showing the thoracic duct and position of the left and right lymphatic ducts (**inset**).

Although the divisions are not as distinct as in the circulatory system, the larger lymph vessels show evidence of having intimal, medial, and adventitial layers similar to blood vessels. The intima of these channels contains elastic tissue and an endothelial layer, and the larger collecting lymph channels contain smooth muscle in their medial layer. Contraction of this smooth muscle assists in propelling lymph toward the thorax. External compression of the lymph channels by pulsating blood vessels in the vicinity and active and passive movements of body parts also aid in forward propulsion of lymph. The rate of flow through the lymphatic system through all of the various lymph channels, approximately 120 mL/hour, is determined by the interstitial fluid pressure and the activity of lymph pumps.

IN SUMMARY, exchange of fluids between the vascular compartment and the interstitial spaces occurs at the capillary level. The capillary hydrostatic pressure pushes fluids out of the capillaries, and the colloidal osmotic pressure exerted by the plasma proteins pulls fluids back into the capillaries. Albumin, which is the smallest and most abundant of the plasma proteins, provides the major osmotic force for return of fluid to the vascular compartment. Normally, slightly more fluid leaves the capillary bed than can be reabsorbed. This excess fluid is returned to the circulation by way of the lymphatic channels. ∎

NEURAL CONTROL OF CIRCULATORY FUNCTION

After completing this section of the chapter, you should be able to meet the following objectives:

- Describe the roles of the medullary vasomotor and cardioinhibitory centers in controlling the function of the heart and blood vessels.
- Relate the performance of baroreceptors and chemoreceptors in the control of cardiovascular function.
- Describe the distribution of the sympathetic and parasympathetic nervous systems in the innervation of the circulatory system and their effects on heart rate and cardiac contractility.
- Relate the role of the central nervous system in terms of regulating circulatory function.

The neural control centers for the integration and modulation of cardiac function and blood pressure are located bilaterally in the medulla oblongata. The medullary cardiovascular neurons are grouped into three distinct pools that lead to sympathetic innervation of the heart and blood vessels and parasympathetic innervation of the heart. The first two, which control sympathetic-mediated acceleration of heart rate and blood vessel tone, are called the *vasomotor center*. The third, which controls parasympathetic-mediated slowing of heart rate, is called the *cardioinhibitory center*. These brain stem centers receive information from many areas of the nervous system, including the hypothalamus. The arterial baroreceptors and chemoreceptors provide the medullary cardiovascular center with continuous information regarding changes in blood pressure (see Chapter 23).

Autonomic Nervous System Regulation

The neural control of the circulatory system occurs primarily through the *sympathetic* and *parasympathetic* divisions of the autonomic nervous system (ANS). The ANS contributes to the control of cardiovascular function through modulation of cardiac (*i.e.,* heart rate and cardiac contractility) and vascular (*i.e.,* peripheral vascular resistance) functions.

Autonomic Regulation of Cardiac Function

The heart is innervated by the parasympathetic and sympathetic nervous systems. Parasympathetic innervation of the heart is achieved by means of the *vagus nerve*. The parasympathetic outflow to the heart originates from the vagal nucleus in the medulla. The axons of these neurons pass to the heart in the cardiac branches of the vagus nerve. The effect of vagal stimulation on heart function is largely limited to heart rate, with increased vagal activity producing a slowing of the pulse. Sympathetic outflow to the heart and blood vessels arises from neurons located in the reticular formation of the brain stem. The axons of these neurons exit the thoracic segments of the spinal cord to synapse with the postganglionic neurons that innervate the heart. Cardiac sympathetic fibers are widely distributed to the sinoatrial and AV nodes and the myocardium. Increased sympathetic activity produces an increase in the heart rate and the velocity and force of cardiac contraction.

Autonomic Regulation of Vascular Function

The sympathetic nervous system serves as the final common pathway for controlling the smooth muscle tone of the blood vessels. Most of the sympathetic preganglionic fibers that control vessel function originate in the vasomotor center of the brain stem, travel down the spinal cord, and exit in the thoracic and lumbar (T1–L2) segments. The sympathetic neurons that supply the blood vessels maintain them in a state of tonic activity, so that even under resting conditions, the blood vessels are partially constricted. Vessel constriction and relaxation are accomplished by altering this basal input. Increasing sympathetic activity causes constriction of some vessels, such as those of the skin, the gastrointestinal tract, and the kidneys. Blood vessels in skeletal muscle are supplied by both vasoconstrictor and vasodilator fibers. Activation of sympathetic vasodilator fibers causes vessel relaxation and provides the muscles with increased blood flow during exercise. Although the parasympathetic nervous

system contributes to the regulation of heart function, it has little or no control over blood vessels.

Autonomic Neurotransmitters

The actions of the ANS are mediated by chemical neurotransmitters. *Acetylcholine* is the postganglionic neurotransmitter for parasympathetic neurons and *norepinephrine* is the main neurotransmitter for postganglionic sympathetic neurons. Sympathetic neurons also respond to epinephrine, which is released into the bloodstream by the adrenal medulla. The neurotransmitter *dopamine* can also act as a neurotransmitter for some sympathetic neurons. The synthesis, release, and inactivation of the autonomic neurotransmitters are discussed in Chapter 48.

Central Nervous System Responses

It is not surprising that the CNS, which plays an essential role in regulating vasomotor tone and blood pressure, would have a mechanism for controlling the blood flow to the cardiovascular centers that control circulatory function. When the blood flow to the brain has been sufficiently interrupted to cause ischemia of the vasomotor center, these vasomotor neurons become strongly excited, causing massive vasoconstriction as a means of raising the blood pressure to levels as high as the heart can pump against. This response is called the *CNS ischemic response,* and it can raise the blood pressure to levels as high as 270 mm Hg for as long as 10 minutes. The CNS ischemic response is a last-ditch stand to preserve the blood flow to vital brain centers; it does not become activated until blood pressure has fallen to at least 60 mm Hg, and it is most effective in the range of 15 to 20 mm Hg. If the cerebral circulation is not reestablished within 3 to 10 minutes, the neurons of the vasomotor center cease to function, so that the tonic impulses to the blood vessels stop and the blood pressure falls precipitously.

The *Cushing reflex* is a special type of CNS reflex resulting from an increase in intracranial pressure. When the intracranial pressure rises to levels that equal intra-arterial pressure, blood vessels to the vasomotor center become compressed, initiating the CNS ischemic response. The purpose of this reflex is to produce a rise in arterial pressure to levels above intracranial pressure so that the blood flow to the vasomotor center can be reestablished. Should the intracranial pressure rise to the point that the blood supply to the vasomotor center becomes inadequate, vasoconstrictor tone is lost, and the blood pressure begins to fall. The elevation in blood pressure associated with the Cushing reflex is usually of short duration and should be considered a protective homeostatic mechanism. The brain and other cerebral structures are located within the rigid confines of the skull, with no room for expansion, and any increase in intracranial pressure tends to compress the blood vessels that supply the brain.

IN SUMMARY, the neural control centers for the regulation of cardiac function and blood pressure are located in the reticular formation of the lower pons and medulla of the brain stem, where the integration and modulation of ANS responses occur.

These brain stem centers receive information from many areas of the nervous system, including the hypothalamus. Both the parasympathetic and sympathetic nervous systems innervate the heart. The parasympathetic nervous system functions in regulating heart rate through the vagus nerve, with increased vagal activity producing a slowing of heart rate. The sympathetic nervous system has an excitatory influence on heart rate and contractility, and it serves as the final common pathway for controlling the smooth muscle tone of the blood vessels. ■

Review Exercises

1. In persons with atherosclerosis of the coronary arteries, symptoms of myocardial ischemia do not usually occur until the vessel has been 75% occluded.

   A. *Use the Poiseuille law to explain.*

2. Once an arterial aneurysm has begun to form, it continues to enlarge as the result of the increased tension in its wall.

   A. *Explain the continued increase in size using the law of Laplace.*

   B. *Using information related to cross-sectional area and velocity of flow, explain why there is stasis of blood flow with the tendency to form clots in aneurysms with a large cross-sectional area.*

3. Use events in the cardiac cycle depicted in Figure 21-11 to explain:

   A. *The effect of hypertension on the isovolumetric contraction period.*

   B. *The effect of an increase in heart rate on the time spent in diastole.*

   C. *The effect of an increase in the isovolumetric relaxation period on the diastolic filling of the ventricle*

4. Use the Frank-Starling ventricular function curve depicted in Figure 21-12 to explain the changes in cardiac output that occur with changes in respiratory effort.

   A. *What happens to cardiac output during increased inspiratory effort in which a marked decrease in intrathoracic pressure produces an increase in venous return to the right heart?*

   B. *What happens to cardiac output during increased expiratory effort in which a marked increase in intrathoracic pressure produces a decrease in venous return to the right heart?*

   C. *Given these changes in cardiac output that occur during increased respiratory effort, what would you propose as one of the functions of the Frank-Starling curve?*

Bibliography

Aukland K., Reed R. K. (1993). Interstitial-lymphatic mechanisms in the control of extracellular fluid volume. *Physiological Reviews* 73, 1–78.

Costano L. S. (2002). *Physiology* (2nd ed., pp. 101–166). Philadelphia: W. B. Saunders.

Davis M. J., Hill M. A. (1999). Signaling mechanisms underlying the vascular myogenic response. *Physiological Reviews* 79, 387–423.

Ellis C. G., Jagger J., Sharpe M. (2005). The microcirculation as a functional system. *Critical Care* 9(Suppl. 4), S3–S8.

Feletou M., Vanhoutte P. M. (1999). The alternative: EDHF. *Journal of Molecular and Cellular Cardiology* 31, 15–22.

Ganong W. F. (2005). *Review of medical physiology* (22nd ed., pp. 515–630). New York: Lange Medical Books/McGraw-Hill.

Guyton A. C., Hall J. E. (2006). *Medical physiology* (11th ed., pp. 161–277). Philadelphia: Elsevier Saunders.

Klabunde R. E. (2005). *Cardiovascular physiology concepts.* Philadelphia: Lippincott Williams & Wilkins.

Levy M. N., Pappano A. J. (2007). *Cardiovascular physiology* (9th ed.). Philadelphia: Mosby Elsevier.

Mifflin S. W. (2001). What does the brain know about blood pressure? *News in Physiological Science* 16, 266.

Norton J. M. (2001). Toward consistent definitions for preload and afterload. *Advances in Physiological Education* 25(1), 53–61.

Rhoades R. S., Tanner G. A. (2003). *Medical physiology* (2nd ed., pp. 191–308). Boston: Little, Brown.

Ross M. H., Kaye G. L., Pawlina W. (2003). *Histology: A text and atlas* (4th ed., pp. 326–354). Philadelphia: Lippincott Williams & Wilkins.

Segal S. S. (2005). Regulation of blood flow in the microcirculation. *Microcirculation* 12, 33–45.

Smith J. J., Kampine J. P. (1989). *Circulatory physiology: The essentials* (3rd ed.). Baltimore: Williams & Wilkins.

Toda N., Okamura T. (2003). The pharmacology of nitric oxide in the peripheral nervous system of blood vessels. *Pharmacological Reviews* 55, 271–324.

Vanhoutte P. M. (1999). How to assess endothelial function in human blood vessels. *Journal of Hypertension* 17, 1047–1058.

Visit thePoint **http://thePoint.lww.com for animations, journal articles, and more!**

Disorders of Blood Flow in the Systemic Circulation

GLENN MATFIN

Chapter **22**

➤ Blood flow in the arterial and venous systems depends on a system of patent blood vessels and adequate perfusion pressure. Unlike disorders of the respiratory system or central circulation that cause hypoxia and impair oxygenation of tissues throughout the body, the effects of blood vessel disease usually are limited to local tissues supplied by a particular vessel or group of vessels. With arterial disorders, there is decreased blood flow to the tissues along with impaired delivery of oxygen and nutrients, and with venous disorders there is interference with the outflow of blood and removal of waste products.

Disturbances in blood flow can result from pathologic changes in the vessel wall (*i.e.,* atherosclerosis and vasculitis), acute vessel obstruction due to thrombus or embolus, vasospasm (*i.e.,* Raynaud phenomenon), or abnormal vessel dilation (*i.e.,* arterial aneurysms or varicose veins).

BLOOD VESSEL STRUCTURE AND FUNCTION

After completing this section of the chapter, you should be able to meet the following objectives:

- Describe the functions of the endothelial cells and define the term *endothelial dysfunction.*
- Describe the function of vascular smooth muscle and its role in vascular repair.

Although the heart is at the center of the cardiovascular system, it is the blood vessels that transport blood throughout the body. The walls of all blood vessels, except the very smallest, are composed of three distinct layers: an outer layer of loosely woven collagen tissue, the *tunica externa,* which is composed of loose connective tissue; a middle layer, the *tunica media,* which consists primarily of circumferentially arranged layers of smooth muscle cells; and an inner layer, the *tunica intima,* which consists of a single layer of endothelial cells that line the lumen of the vessel, and the underlying subendothelial connective tissue (Fig. 22-1). As the main cellular components of the blood vessel wall, the

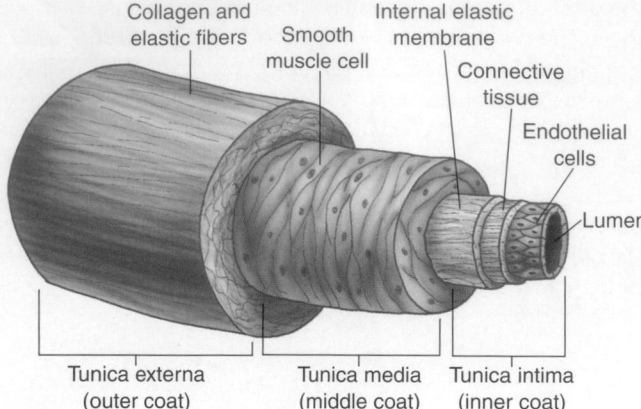

FIGURE 22-1 • Diagram of a typical artery showing the tunica externa, tunica media, and tunica intima.

endothelial and smooth muscle cells play an important role in the pathogenesis of many disorders of the arterial circulation.

Endothelial Cells

Endothelial cells form a continuous lining for the entire vascular system called the *endothelium*. Once thought to be nothing more than a lining for blood vessels, it is now known that the endothelium is a versatile, multifunctional tissue that plays an active role in controlling vascular function[1,2] (Table 22-1). As a semipermeable membrane, the endothelium controls the transfer of molecules across the vascular wall. The endothelium also plays a role in the control of platelet adhesion and blood clotting; modulation of blood flow and vascular resistance; metabolism of hormones; regulation of immune and inflammatory reactions; and elaboration of factors that influence the growth of other cell types, particularly vascular smooth muscle cells.

Endothelial Dysfunction

Structurally intact endothelial cells respond to various abnormal stimuli by adjusting their usual functions and by expressing newly acquired functions.[1] The term *endothelial dysfunction* describes several types of potentially reversible changes in endothelial function that occur in response to environmental stimuli. Inducers of endothelial dysfunction include cytokines and bacterial and viral products that cause inflammation; hemodynamic stresses and lipid products that are critical to the pathogenesis of atherosclerosis; and hypoxia. Dysfunctional endothelial cells, in turn, produce other cytokines, growth factors, procoagulant or anticoagulant substances, and a variety of other biologically active products. They also influence the reactivity of underlying smooth muscle cells through production of both relaxing factors (*e.g.*, nitric oxide) and contracting factors (*e.g.*, endothelins; see Chapter 21).

Vascular Smooth Muscle Cells

Vascular smooth muscle cells, which form the predominant cellular layer in the tunica media, produce vasoconstriction or dilation of blood vessels. A network of vasomotor nerves of the sympathetic component of the autonomic nervous system supplies the smooth muscle in the blood vessels. These nerves are responsible for vasoconstriction of the vessel walls. Because they do not enter the tunica media of the blood vessel, the nerves do not synapse directly on the smooth muscle cells. Instead, they release the neurotransmitter norepinephrine, which diffuses into the media and acts on the nearby smooth muscle cells. The resulting impulses are propagated along the smooth muscle cells through their gap junctions, causing contraction of the entire muscle cell layer and thus reducing the radius of the vessel lumen.

Vascular smooth muscle cells also synthesize collagen, elastin, and other components of the extracellular matrix; elaborate growth factors and cytokines; and after vascular injury mi-

TABLE 22-1 **Endothelial Cell Properties and Functions**

MAJOR PROPERTIES	ASSOCIATED FUNCTIONS/FACTORS
Maintenance of a selective permeability barrier	Controls the transfer of small and large molecules across the vessel wall
Regulation of thrombosis	Elaboration of prothrombogenic molecules (von Willebrand factor, plasminogen activator) and antithrombotic molecules (prostacyclin, heparin-like molecules, plasminogen activator)
Modulation of blood flow and vascular reactivity	Elaboration of vasodilators (nitric oxide, prostacyclin) and vasoconstrictors (endothelins, angiotensin-converting enzyme)
Regulation of cell growth, particularly smooth muscle cells	Production of growth-stimulating factors (platelet-derived growth factor, hematopoietic colony-stimulating factor) and growth-inhibiting factors (heparin, transforming growth factor-β)
Regulation of inflammatory/immune responses	Expression of adhesion molecules that regulate leukocyte migration and release of inflammatory and immune system mediators (*e.g.*, interleukins, interferons)
Maintenance of the extracellular matrix	Synthesis of collagen, laminin, proteoglycans
Involvement in lipoprotein metabolism	Oxidation of VLDL, LDL, cholesterol

Data from Schoen F. J. (2005). Blood vessels. In Kumar V., Abbas A. K., Fausto N. (Eds.), *Robbins and Cotran pathologic basis of disease* (7th ed., p. 514). Philadelphia: Elsevier Saunders; and Ross M. H., Kaye G. L., Pawlina W. (2003). *Histology: A text and atlas* (4th ed., p. 332). Philadelphia: Lippincott Williams & Wilkins.

grate into the intima and proliferate.[1] Thus, smooth muscle cells are important in both normal vascular repair as well as pathologic processes such as atherosclerosis. The migratory and proliferative activities of vascular smooth muscle cells are stimulated by growth promoters and inhibitors. Promoters include platelet-derived growth factor, thrombin, fibroblast growth factor, and cytokines such as interferon gamma and interleukin-1. Growth inhibitors include nitric oxide. Other regulators include the renin-angiotensin system (angiotensin II) and the catecholamines.

IN SUMMARY, the walls of blood vessels are composed of three layers: an outer layer of loosely woven collagen tissue, a middle layer of vascular smooth muscle, and an inner layer of endothelial cells. The endothelium controls the transfer of molecules across the vascular wall, plays a role in the control of platelet adhesion and blood clotting, modulation of blood flow and vascular resistance, metabolism of hormones, regulation of immune and inflammatory reactions, and elaboration of factors that influence the growth of other cell types, particularly the smooth muscle cells. The term *endothelial dysfunction* describes several types of potentially reversible changes in endothelial function that occur in response to environmental stimuli. Vascular smooth muscle cells not only control dilation and vasoconstriction of blood vessels, but elaborate growth factors and synthesize collagen, elastin, and other components of the extracellular matrix that are important in both normal vascular repair as well as pathologic processes such as atherosclerosis. ■

DISORDERS OF THE ARTERIAL CIRCULATION

After completing this section of the chapter, you should be able to meet the following objectives:

- List the five types of lipoproteins and state their function in terms of lipid transport and development of atherosclerosis.
- Describe the role of lipoprotein receptors in removal of cholesterol from the blood.
- Cite the criteria for diagnosis of hypercholesterolemia.
- Describe possible mechanisms involved in the development of atherosclerosis.
- List risk factors in atherosclerosis.
- List the vessels most commonly affected by atherosclerosis and describe the vessel changes that occur.
- State the signs and symptoms of acute arterial occlusion.
- Describe the pathology associated with the vasculitides and relate it to four disease conditions associated with vasculitis.
- Compare the mechanisms and manifestations of ischemia associated with atherosclerotic peripheral vascular disease, Raynaud phenomenon, and thromboangiitis obliterans (*i.e.,* Buerger disease).
- Distinguish between the pathology and manifestations of aortic aneurysms and dissection of the aorta.

The arterial system distributes blood to all the tissues in the body. There are three types of arteries: large elastic arteries, including the aorta and its distal branches; medium-sized arteries, such as the coronary and renal arteries; and small arteries and arterioles that pass through the tissues. The large arteries function mainly in transport of blood. The medium-sized arteries are composed predominantly of circular and spirally arranged smooth muscle cells. Distribution of blood flow to the various organs and tissues of the body is controlled by contraction and relaxation of the smooth muscle of these vessels. The small arteries and arterioles regulate capillary blood flow. Each of these different types of arteries tends to be affected by different disease processes.

Disease of the arterial system affects body function by impairing blood flow. The effect of impaired blood flow on the body depends on the structures involved and the extent of altered flow. The term *ischemia* (*i.e.,* "holding back of blood") denotes a reduction in arterial flow to a level that is insufficient to meet the oxygen demands of the tissues. *Infarction* refers to an area of ischemic necrosis in an organ produced by occlusion of its arterial blood supply or its venous drainage. The discussion in this section focuses on blood lipids and hypercholesterolemia, atherosclerosis, vasculitis, arterial disease of the extremities, and arterial aneurysms.

DISORDERS OF THE ARTERIAL CIRCULATION

- The arterial system delivers oxygen and nutrients to the tissues.
- Disorders of the arterial circulation produce ischemia owing to narrowing of blood vessels, thrombus formation associated with platelet adhesion, and weakening of the vessel wall.
- Atherosclerosis is a progressive disease characterized by the formation of fibrofatty plaques in the intima of large and medium-sized vessels, including the aorta, coronary arteries, and cerebral vessels. The major risk factors for atherosclerosis are hypercholesterolemia and inflammation.
- Vasculitis is an inflammation of the blood vessel wall resulting in vascular tissue injury and necrosis. Arteries, capillaries, and veins may be affected. The inflammatory process may be initiated by direct injury, infectious agents, or immune processes.
- Aneurysms represent an abnormal localized dilatation of an artery due to a weakness in the vessel wall. As the aneurysm increases in size, the tension in the wall of the vessel increases and it may rupture. The increased size of the vessel also may exert pressure on adjacent structures.

Hyperlipidemia

Triglycerides, phospholipids, and cholesterol, which are classified as lipids, are a diverse group of compounds that have many key biological functions. Triglycerides, which are used in energy metabolism, are combinations of three fatty acids condensed with a single glycerol molecule. Phospholipids, which contain a phosphate group, are important structural constituents of lipoproteins, blood clotting components, the myelin sheath, and cell membranes. Although cholesterol is not composed of fatty acids, its steroid nucleus is synthesized from fatty acids and thus its chemical activity is similar to that of other lipid substances.[3]

Elevated levels of blood cholesterol (*hypercholesterolemia*) are implicated in the development of atherosclerosis with its attendant risk of heart attack and stroke. This is a major public health issue that is underscored by striking statistics released by the American Heart Association (AHA). An estimated 37.2 million Americans have high-risk serum cholesterol levels (240 mg/dL or greater) that could contribute to a heart attack, stroke, or other cardiovascular event associated with atherosclerosis.[4]

Lipoproteins

Because cholesterol and triglyceride are insoluble in plasma, they are encapsulated by a stabilizing coat of water-soluble phospholipids and proteins (called *apoproteins*). These particles, which are called *lipoproteins,* transport cholesterol and triglyceride to various tissues for energy utilization, lipid deposition, steroid hormone production, and bile acid formation. There are five types of lipoproteins, classified according to their densities as measured by ultracentrifugation: chylomicrons, very–low-density lipoprotein (VLDL), intermediate-density lipoprotein (IDL), low-density lipoprotein (LDL), and high-density lipoprotein (HDL). VLDL carries large amounts of triglycerides that have a lower density than cholesterol. LDL is the main carrier of cholesterol, whereas HDL actually is 50% protein (Fig. 22-2).

Each type of lipoprotein consists of a large molecular complex of lipids combined with apoproteins.[5,6] The major lipid constituents are cholesterol esters, triglycerides, nonesterified (or free) cholesterol, and phospholipids. The insoluble cholesterol esters and triglycerides are located in the hydrophobic core of the lipoprotein macromolecule, surrounded by the soluble phospholipids, nonesterified cholesterol, and apoproteins (Fig. 22-3). Nonesterified cholesterol and phospholipids provide a negative charge that allows the lipoprotein to be soluble in plasma.

There are four major classes of apoproteins: A (*i.e.,* apoA-I, apoA-II, and apoA-IV), B (*i.e.,* apoB-48, apoB-100), C (*i.e.,* apoC-I, apoC-II, and apoC-III), and apoE.[4,5] The apoproteins control the interactions and ultimate metabolic fate of the lipoproteins. Some of the apoproteins activate the lipolytic enzymes that facilitate the removal of lipids from the lipoproteins; others serve as a reactive site that cellular receptors can recognize and use in the endocytosis and metabolism of the lipoproteins. The major apoprotein in LDL is apoB-100, whereas in HDL it is apoA-I. Research findings suggest that genetic defects in the apoproteins may be involved in hyperlipidemia and accelerated atherosclerosis.[5–8]

There are two sites of lipoprotein synthesis: the small intestine and the liver. The chylomicrons, which are the largest

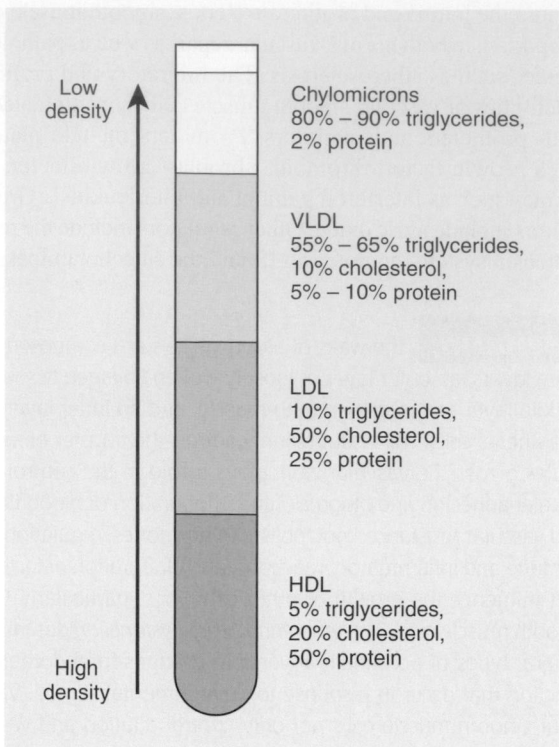

FIGURE 22-2 • Lipoproteins are named based on their protein content, which is measured in density. Because fats are less dense than proteins, as the proportion of triglycerides decreases, the density increases.

of the lipoprotein molecules, are synthesized in the wall of the small intestine. They are involved in the transport of dietary (exogenous pathway) triglycerides and cholesterol that have been absorbed from the gastrointestinal tract. Chylomicrons transfer their triglycerides to the cells of adipose and skeletal muscle tissue. The remnant chylomicron particles, which contain cholesterol, are then taken up by the liver and the cholesterol used in the synthesis of VLDL or excreted in the bile.

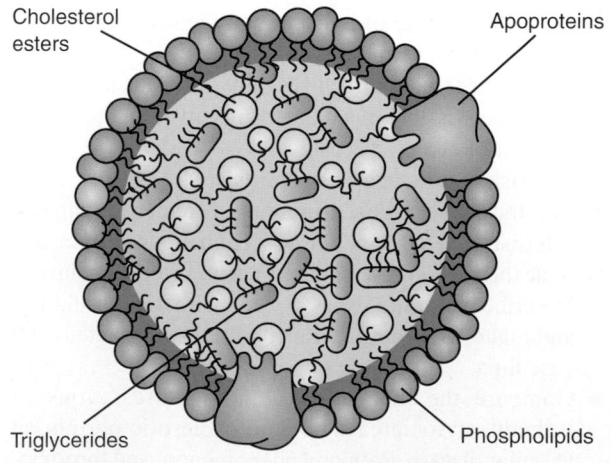

FIGURE 22-3 • General structure of a lipoprotein. The cholesterol esters and triglycerides are located in the hydrophobic core of the macromolecule, surrounded by phospholipids and apoproteins.

The liver synthesizes and releases VLDL and HDL. The VLDLs contain large amounts of triglycerides and lesser amounts of cholesterol esters.[1] They provide the primary pathway for transport of the endogenous triglycerides produced in the liver, as opposed to those obtained from the diet. They are also the body's main source of energy during prolonged fasting. Like chylomicrons, VLDLs carry their triglycerides to fat and muscle cells, where the triglycerides are removed. The resulting IDL fragments are reduced in triglyceride content and enriched in cholesterol. They are taken to the liver and recycled to form VLDL, or converted to LDL in the vascular compartment. IDLs are the main source of LDL. The exogenous and endogenous pathways for triglyceride and cholesterol transport are shown in Figure 22-4.

LDL, sometimes called the *bad cholesterol*, is the main carrier of cholesterol. LDL is removed from the circulation by either LDL receptors or by scavenger cells such as monocytes or macrophages. Approximately 70% of LDL is removed through the LDL receptor-dependent pathway, and the rest is removed by the scavenger pathway.[1] Although LDL receptors are widely distributed, approximately 75% are located on hepatocytes; thus,

the liver plays an extremely important role in LDL metabolism. LDL receptor-mediated removal involves binding of LDL to cell surface receptors, followed by *endocytosis,* a phagocytic process in which LDL is engulfed and moved into the cell in the form of a membrane-covered endocytic vesicle. Within the cell, the endocytic vesicles fuse with lysosomes, and the LDL molecule is enzymatically degraded, causing free cholesterol to be released into the cytoplasm.

Other, nonhepatic tissues (*i.e.,* adrenal glands, smooth muscle cells, endothelial cells, and lymphoid cells) also use the LDL receptor-dependent pathway to obtain cholesterol needed for membrane and hormone synthesis. These tissues can control their cholesterol intake by adding or removing LDL receptors. The scavenger pathway involves ingestion by phagocytic monocytes and macrophages. These scavenger cells have receptors that bind LDL that has been oxidized or chemically modified. The amount of LDL that is removed by the scavenger pathway is directly related to the plasma cholesterol level. When there is a decrease in LDL receptors or when LDL levels exceed receptor availability, the amount of LDL that is removed by scavenger cells is greatly increased. The uptake of

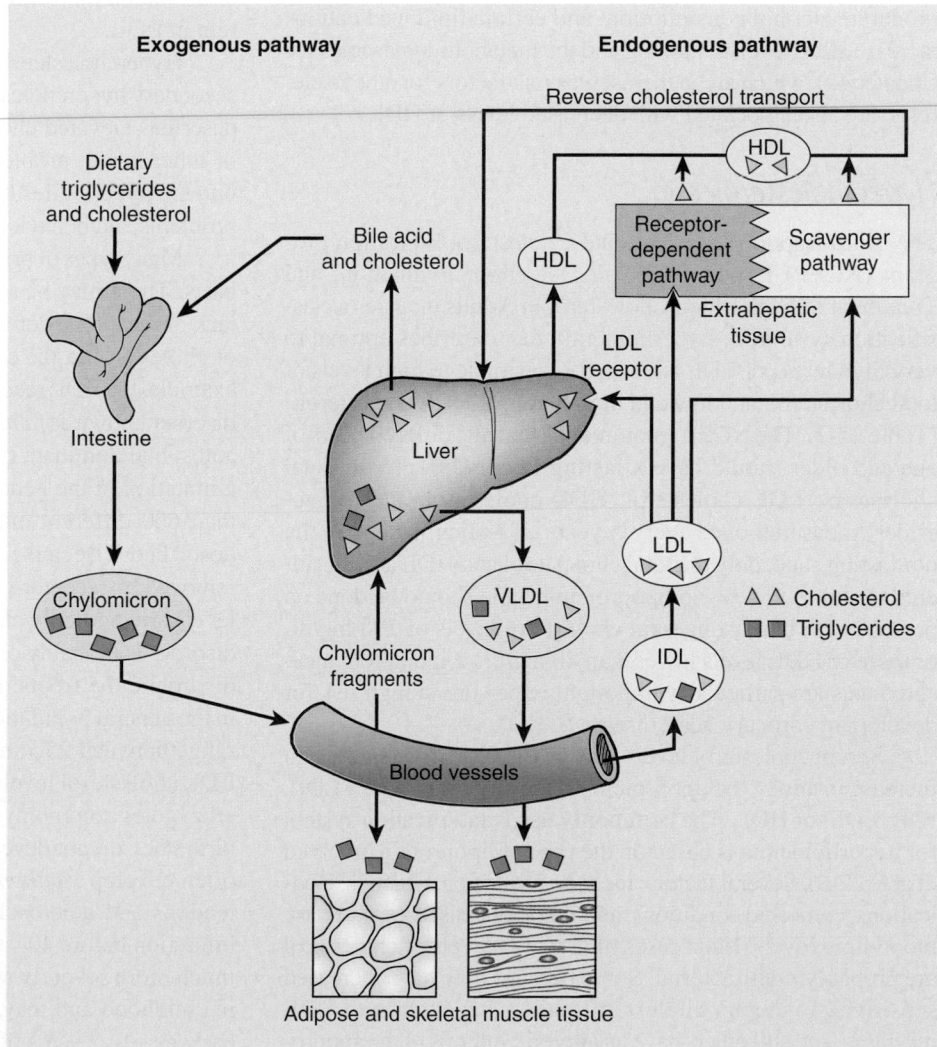

FIGURE 22-4 • Schematic representation of the exogenous and endogenous pathways for triglyceride and cholesterol transport.

LDL by macrophages in the arterial wall can result in the accumulation of insoluble cholesterol esters, the formation of foam cells, and the development of atherosclerosis.

HDL is synthesized in the liver and often is referred to as the *good cholesterol*. HDL participates in the reverse transport of cholesterol by carrying cholesterol from the peripheral tissues back to the liver. Epidemiologic studies have shown an inverse relation between HDL levels and the development of atherosclerosis.[9,10] It is thought that HDL, which is low in cholesterol and rich in surface phospholipids, facilitates the clearance of cholesterol from the periphery (including atheromatous plaques) and transports it to the liver, where it may be excreted rather than reused in the formation of VLDL (reverse cholesterol transport). The mechanism whereby HDL promotes the movement of cholesterol from peripheral cells to lipid-poor HDL, involves a specialized lipid transporter called the *ATP-binding cassette transporter A class 1* (ABCA1).[11] Defects in this system (resulting from mutations in the ABCA1 transporter) are responsible for Tangier disease, which is characterized by accelerated atherosclerosis and little or no HDL. HDL is also believed to inhibit cellular uptake of LDL by reducing oxidation, thereby preventing uptake of oxidized LDL by the scavenger receptors on macrophages. It has been observed that regular exercise, moderate alcohol consumption, and certain lipid medications increase HDL levels. Smoking and the metabolic syndrome (see Chapter 42), which are in themselves risk factors for atherosclerosis, are also associated with decreased levels of HDL.[1,10]

Hypercholesterolemia

The Third Report of the National Cholesterol Education Program (NCEP) Expert Panel on Detection, Evaluation, and Treatment of High Blood Cholesterol in Adults includes a classification system for hyperlipidemia that describes optimal to very high levels of LDL cholesterol, desirable to high levels of total cholesterol, and low and high levels of HDL cholesterol[12] (Table 22-2). The NCEP recommends that all adults 20 years of age and older should have a fasting lipoprotein profile (total cholesterol, LDL cholesterol, HDL cholesterol, and triglycerides) measured once every 5 years. If testing is done in the nonfasting state, only the total cholesterol and HDL are considered useful. A follow-up lipoprotein profile should be done on persons with nonfasting total cholesterol levels of 200 mg/dL or more or HDL levels lower than 40 mg/dL. Lipoprotein measurements are particularly important in persons at high risk for developing coronary heart disease (CHD).

Serum cholesterol levels may be elevated as a result of an increase in any of the lipoproteins—the chylomicrons, VLDL, IDL, LDL, or HDL. The commonly used classification system for hyperlipidemia is based on the type of lipoprotein involved (Table 22-3). Several factors, including nutrition, genetics, medications, comorbid conditions, and metabolic diseases, can raise blood lipid levels. Most cases of elevated levels of cholesterol are probably multifactorial. Some persons may have increased sensitivity to dietary cholesterol, others have a lack of LDL receptors, and still others have an altered synthesis of the apoproteins, including oversynthesis of apoB-100, the major apoprotein in LDL.

Hypercholesterolemia can be classified as either primary or secondary hypercholesterolemia. Primary hypercholesterolemia describes elevated cholesterol levels that develop independent of other health problems or lifestyle behaviors, whereas secondary hypercholesterolemia is associated with other health problems and behaviors.

Many types of primary hypercholesterolemia have a genetic basis. There may be a defective synthesis of the apoproteins, a lack of receptors, defective receptors, or defects in the handling of cholesterol in the cell that are genetically determined.[5,6] For example, the LDL receptor is deficient or defective in the genetic disorder known as *familial hypercholesterolemia (type 2A)*. This autosomal dominant type of hyperlipoproteinemia results from a mutation in the gene specifying the receptor for LDL. More than 600 different mutations in the LDL receptor have been described.[6] Because most of the circulating cholesterol is removed by receptor-dependent mechanisms, blood cholesterol levels are markedly elevated in persons with this disorder. The disorder is probably one of the most common of all mendelian disorders; the frequency of heterozygotes is 1 in 500 persons in the general population.[6] Plasma LDL levels in heterozygotes range between 250 and 500 mg/dL, whereas in homozygotes LDL cholesterol levels may rise to 1000 mg/dL. Although heterozygotes commonly have an elevated cholesterol level from birth, they do not develop symptoms until adult life, when they often develop *xanthomas* (i.e., cholesterol deposits) along the tendons and atherosclerosis appears (Fig. 22-5). Myocardial infarction before 40 years of age is common. Homozygotes are much more severely affected; they have cutaneous xanthomas in childhood and may experience myocardial infarction by as early as 1 to 2 years of age.

TABLE 22-2 NCEP Adult Treatment Panel III Classification of LDL, Total, and HDL Cholesterol (mg/dL)

LDL Cholesterol	
<100	Optimal
100–129	Near optimal/above optimal
130–159	Borderline high
160–189	High
≥ 190	Very high
Total Cholesterol	
<200	Desirable
200–239	Borderline high
≥ 240	High
HDL Cholesterol	
<40	Low
≥ 60	High

(National Institutes of Health Expert Panel [2001]. *Third report of the National Cholesterol Education Program [NCEP] Expert Panel on Detection, Evaluation, and Treatment of High Blood Cholesterol in Adults [Adult Treatment Panel III]*. [NIH Publication No. 01–3670]. Bethesda, MD: National Institutes of Health.)

TABLE 22-3 **Classification of Hyperlipoproteinemias and Their Genetic Basis**

TYPE	FAMILIAR NAME	LIPOPROTEIN ABNORMALITY	KNOWN UNDERLYING GENETIC DEFECTS
1	Exogenous dietary hypertriglyceridemia	Elevated chylomicrons and triglycerides	Mutation in lipoprotein lipase gene
2a	Familial hypercholesterolemia	Elevated LDL cholesterol	Mutation in LDL receptor gene or in apoprotein B gene
2b	Combined hyperlipidemia	Elevated LDL, VLDL, and triglycerides	Mutation in LDL receptor gene or apoprotein B gene
3	Remnant hyperlipidemia	Increased remnants (chylomicrons), IDL triglycerides, and cholesterol	Mutation in apolipoprotein E gene
4	Endogenous hypertriglyceridemia	Elevated VLDL and triglycerides	Unknown
5	Mixed hypertriglyceridemia	Elevated VLDL, chylomicrons, and cholesterol; triglycerides greatly elevated	Mutation in apolipoprotein C-II gene

IDL, intermediate-density lipoprotein; LDL, low-density lipoprotein; VLDL, very–low-density lipoprotein.
(Data developed from Cotran R.S., Kumar V., Robbins S.L. [1994]. *Robbins pathologic basis of disease* [5th ed., pp. 481–482].
  Philadelphia: W.B. Saunders; and Gotto A.M. [1988]. Lipoprotein metabolism and etiology of hyperlipidemia. *Hospital Practice*, 23[Suppl. 1], 4)

Causes of secondary hyperlipoproteinemia include obesity with high-calorie intake and diabetes mellitus. High-calorie diets increase the production of VLDL, with triglyceride elevation and high conversion of VLDL to LDL. Excess ingestion of cholesterol may reduce the formation of LDL receptors and thereby decrease LDL removal. Diets that are high in triglycerides and saturated fats increase cholesterol synthesis and suppress LDL receptor activity. In diabetes mellitus and the metabolic syndrome, typical dyslipidemia is seen with elevation of triglycerides, low HDL, and minimal or modest elevation of LDL.[10,12] Other systemic disorders that can elevate lipids include hypothyroidism, nephrotic syndrome, and obstructive liver disease. Medications such as beta blockers, estrogens, and protease inhibitors (used in the treatment of human immunodeficiency virus [HIV] infection) can also increase lipid levels.

Management of Hyperlipidemia. The NCEP continues to identify reduction in LDL cholesterol as the primary target for cholesterol-lowering therapy, particularly in people at risk for CHD. The major risk factors for CHD, exclusive of LDL cholesterol levels, that modify LDL cholesterol goals include cigarette smoking, hypertension, family history of premature CHD in a first-degree relative, age (men ≥45 years; women ≥55 years), and an HDL cholesterol level less than 40 mg/dL (Chart 22-1). Accordingly, the NCEP has updated the 2001 guidelines for management of LDL cholesterol based on risk factors.[13] The updated guidelines recommend that persons with zero or no major risk factors should have an LDL cholesterol goal of 160 mg/dL or less; those with two or more of the major risk factors should have an LDL cholesterol goal of less than 130 mg/dL; persons with *high-risk* factors (*i.e.,* those with

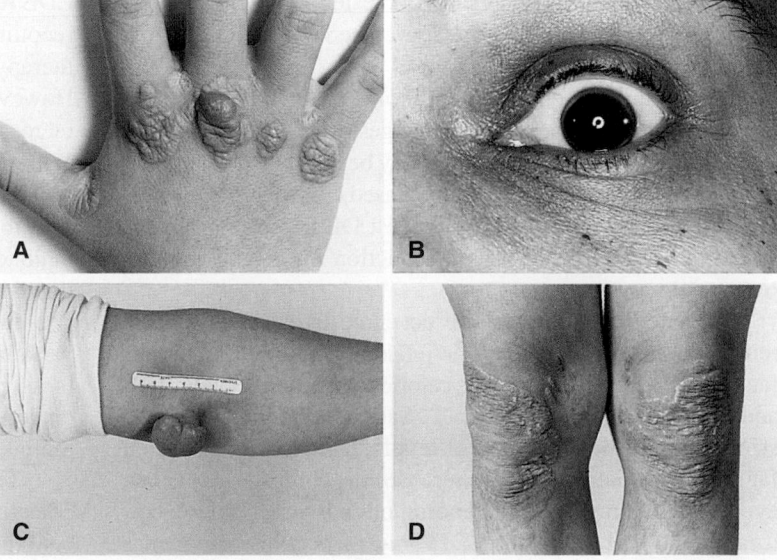

FIGURE 22-5 • Xanthomas in the skin and tendons (**A, C, D**). Arcus lipoides represents the deposition of lipids in the peripheral cornea (**B**). (From Gotlieb A. I. [2005]. Blood vessels. In Rubin E., Gorstein F., Rubin R., et al. [Eds.], *Pathology: Clinicopathologic foundations of medicine* [4th ed., p. 499]. Philadelphia: Lippincott Williams & Wilkins.)

RISK FACTORS IN CORONARY HEART DISEASE OTHER THAN LOW-DENSITY LIPOPROTEINS

Positive Risk Factors

Age

Men: ≥45 years

Women: ≥55 years or premature menopause without estrogen replacement therapy

Family history of premature coronary heart disease (definite myocardial infarction or sudden death before 55 years of age in father or other male first-degree relative, or before 65 years of age in mother or other female first-degree relative)

Current cigarette smoking

Hypertension (≥140/90 mm Hg* or on antihypertensive medication)

Low HDL cholesterol (<40 mg/dL*)

Diabetes mellitus

Negative Risk Factor

High HDL cholesterol (≥60 mg/dL)

HDL, high-density lipoprotein.
*Confirmed by measurements on several occasions.
(Modified from National Institutes of Health Expert Panel [2001]. *Third report of the National Cholesterol Education Program [NCEP] Expert Panel on Detection, Evaluation, and Treatment of High Blood Cholesterol in Adults [Adult Treatment Panel III]*. [NIH Publication No. 01-3670]. Bethesda, MD: National Institutes of Health.)

factured from vegetable oils and are used to enhance the taste and extend the shelf-life of fast foods, are more atherogenic than saturated fats. Dietary cholesterol tends to increase LDL cholesterol. On average, each 100 mg of ingested cholesterol raises the serum cholesterol 8 to 10 mg/dL.[14]

The aim of dietary therapy is to reduce total and LDL cholesterol levels and increase HDL cholesterol by reduction in total calories, and to reduce the percentage of total calories from saturated fat and cholesterol. The AHA has issued new dietary guidelines that focus on an overall plan of healthy food choices and increased physical activity to decrease the risk for development of cardiovascular disease.[15] The specific guidelines are intended to assist the general public in the maintenance of a body mass index lower than 25 (weight in kilograms divided by body surface area in square meters), to achieve and maintain a low total cholesterol and LDL and a high HDL, and to maintain a blood pressure within normal limits. In general, the dietary guidelines emphasize an increased intake of fruits, vegetables, and fish, and decreased intake of fat, cholesterol, sugars, alcohol, and salt. For persons who already have an elevated LDL, the AHA recommends that saturated fat be restricted to less than 7% of the total daily intake, trans fat to less than 1% of the total daily intake, and cholesterol to less than 300 mg/day. However, even with strict adherence to the diet, drug therapy is usually necessary. Clinical data suggest that drug therapy may be efficacious even for those with normal LDL cholesterol.[15] The Heart Protection Study showed cardiovascular benefit from statin therapy (to be discussed) in patients who had a baseline LDL less than 100 mg/dL.[16] This also suggests that some of the cardioprotective effects of the statin drugs are not just related to LDL lowering, but to their anti-inflammatory effects.[17]

Lipid-lowering drugs work in several ways, including decreasing cholesterol production, decreasing cholesterol absorption from the intestine, and removing cholesterol from the bloodstream. Drugs that act directly to decrease cholesterol levels also have the beneficial effect of further lowering cholesterol levels by stimulating the production of additional LDL receptors. Unless lipid levels are severely elevated, it is recommended that a minimum of 3 months of intensive diet therapy be undertaken before drug therapy is considered.[12,13] However, certain high-risk groups (*e.g.,* diabetic patients with increased cardiovascular risk) are now started on statin therapy at the same time as therapeutic lifestyle changes are initiated.

There currently are five major types of medications available for treating hypercholesterolemia: HMG-CoA reductase inhibitors (statins), bile acid–binding resins, cholesterol absorption inhibitor agents, niacin and its congeners, and the fibrates.[9]

Inhibitors of HMG-CoA reductase (*e.g.,* atorvastatin, rosuvastatin, simvastatin), a key enzyme in the cholesterol biosynthetic pathway, can reduce or block the hepatic synthesis of cholesterol and are the cornerstone of LDL-reducing therapy. Statins also reduce triglyceride levels.

The bile acid–binding resins (*e.g.,* cholestyramine, colestipol, colesevelam) bind and sequester cholesterol-containing bile acids in the intestine. This leads to increased

CHD, other forms of atherosclerotic disease, or diabetes) should have a LDL cholesterol goal of less than 100 mg/dL; and persons with *very–high-risk* factors (*i.e.,* acute coronary syndromes or CHD with other risk factors), an LDL cholesterol of less than 70 mg/dL.[12,13] The guidelines also recommend that persons with a greater than 20% 10-year risk of experiencing myocardial infarction or coronary death, as determined by the risk assessment tool developed from Framingham Heart Study data, should have an LDL cholesterol goal of less than 100 mg/dL. (To calculate a risk score, see www.nhlbi.nih.gov/guidelines/cholesterol.)

The management of hypercholesterolemia focuses on dietary and therapeutic lifestyle changes; when these are unsuccessful, pharmacologic treatment may be necessary. Therapeutic lifestyle changes include an increased emphasis on physical activity, dietary measures to reduce LDL cholesterol levels, smoking cessation, and weight reduction for people who are overweight.

Several dietary elements affect cholesterol and its lipoprotein fractions: (1) excess calorie intake, (2) saturated and trans fats, and (3) cholesterol. Excess calories consistently lower HDL and less consistently elevate LDL. Saturated fats in the diet can strongly influence cholesterol levels. Each 1% of saturated fat relative to caloric intake increases the cholesterol level an average of 2.8 mg/dL.[13] Depending on individual differences, it raises the VLDL and the LDL. Trans fats, which are manu-

production of LDL receptors by the liver, with resulting increased removal of cholesterol from the blood for synthesis of new bile acids. The cholesterol absorption inhibitor (ezetimibe) interferes with the absorption of cholesterol.[10] Both of these agents are typically used as adjuncts to statin therapy for patients requiring further reductions in LDL.

Nicotinic acid, a niacin congener, blocks the synthesis and release of VLDL by the liver, thereby lowering not only VLDL levels but IDL and LDL levels. Nicotinic acid also increases HDL concentrations up to 30%. The fibrates (*e.g.,* fenofibrate and gemfibrozil) also decrease the synthesis of VLDL by the liver, but also enhance the clearance of triglycerides from the circulation. The resulting decrease in triglycerides and increase in HDL with these agents are especially important in treatment of the metabolic syndrome.[10]

Atherosclerosis

Atherosclerosis is a type of arteriosclerosis or hardening of the arteries. The term *atherosclerosis,* which comes from the Greek words *atheros* ("gruel" or "paste") and *sclerosis* ("hardness"), denotes the formation of fibrofatty lesions in the intimal lining of the large and medium-sized arteries such as the aorta and its branches, the coronary arteries, and the large vessels that supply the brain (Fig. 22-6).

Although there has been a gradual decline in deaths from atherosclerosis over the past several decades, CHD remains the leading cause of death among men and women in the United States.[3] The reported decline in death rate probably reflects new and improved methods of medical treatment and improved health care practices resulting from an increased public awareness of the factors that predispose to the development of this disorder. In 2004, the major complications of atherosclerosis, including ischemic heart disease, stroke, and peripheral vascular disease, accounted for approximately 36.3% of the deaths in the United States.[18]

Atherosclerosis begins as an insidious process, and clinical manifestations of the disease typically do not become evident for 20 to 40 years or longer. Fibrous plaques commonly begin to appear in the arteries of Americans in their third decade. Necropsy findings from 300 American soldiers (average age of 22 years) killed during the Korean War indicated that 77% had gross evidence of atherosclerosis.[19]

Risk Factors

The cause or causes of atherosclerosis have not been determined with certainty. Epidemiologic studies have, however, identified predisposing risk factors, which are listed in Chart 22-1.[5,10,12,13,16,20,21] In terms of health care behaviors, some of these risk factors can be affected by a change in behavior, and others cannot.

The major risk factor for atherosclerosis is hypercholesterolemia. Nonlipid risk factors such as increasing age, family history of premature coronary heart disease, and male sex cannot be changed. The tendency toward the development of ath-

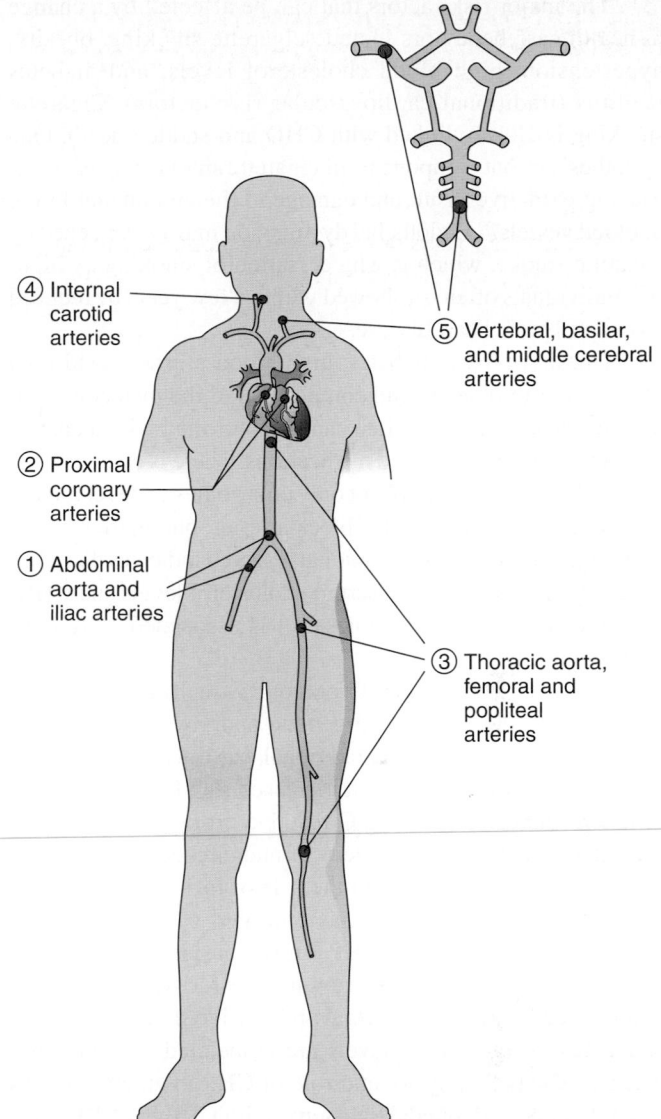

FIGURE 22-6 • Sites of severe atherosclerosis in order of frequency. (From Gotlieb A. I. [2005]. Blood vessels. In Rubin E., Gorstein F., Rubin R., et al. [Eds.], *Pathology: Clinicopathologic foundations of medicine* [4th ed., p. 491]. Philadelphia: Lippincott Williams & Wilkins.)

erosclerosis appears to run in families. Persons who come from families with a strong history of heart disease or stroke due to atherosclerosis are at greater risk for developing atherosclerosis than those with a negative family history. Several genetically determined alterations in lipoprotein and cholesterol metabolism have been identified, and it seems likely that others will be identified in the future.[5] The incidence of atherosclerosis increases with age. Other factors being equal, men are at greater risk for development of CHD than are premenopausal women, probably because of the protective effects of natural estrogens. After menopause, the incidence of atherosclerosis-related diseases in women increases, and by the seventh to eighth decade of life, the frequency of myocardial infarction in the two sexes tends to equalize.[1]

The major risk factors that can be affected by a change in health care behaviors include cigarette smoking, obesity, hypertension, high blood cholesterol levels, and diabetes mellitus (traditional cardiovascular risk factors). Cigarette smoking is closely linked with CHD and sudden death. One hypothesis is that components of cigarette smoke may be toxic, causing oxidative insult and damage to the endothelial lining of blood vessels.[22] Endothelial dysfunction may be worsened by cigarette smoke, which is why cessation of smoking by high-risk individuals often is followed within a few years by reduced risk of ischemic heart disease.

Obesity, type 2 diabetes, high blood pressure, and high blood cholesterol levels (all components of the metabolic syndrome; see Chapter 42) often can be controlled with a change in health care behaviors and medications. There is evidence that elevated serum cholesterol not only contributes to development of atherosclerotic lesions that block arteries, but interferes with vessel relaxation.[23,24] Observational research indicates that a linear relation exists between serum cholesterol levels and CHD; a 1% decrease in serum cholesterol is associated with a 2% decrease in CHD.[24]

However, not all atherothrombotic vascular disease can be explained by the established genetic and environmental risk factors. Other, so-called nontraditional, cardiovascular risk factors can be associated with an increased risk for development of atherosclerosis, including C-reactive protein (CRP), serum homocysteine, serum lipoprotein(a), and infectious agents.[5,20,21]

Considerable interest in the role of inflammation in the etiology of atherosclerosis has emerged over the last few years.[10,17,20,21] In particular, CRP is now considered a major risk factor marker.[25,26] CRP is a serum marker for systemic inflammation (see Chapter 18). Several prospective studies have indicated that elevated CRP levels are associated with vascular disease. The pathophysiologic role of CRP in atherosclerosis has not yet been defined. High-sensitivity CRP (hs-CRP) may be a better predictor of cardiovascular risk than lipid measurement alone.[26] Indeed, approximately 50% of patients with myocardial infarction have a normal LDL.[16] In the Heart Protection Study, statin therapy decreased cardiovascular complications even in patients with a normal LDL. This was thought to be due to the anti-inflammatory effects of these agents. Inflammation (as assessed by a decrease in hs-CRP) can be reduced by using certain lifestyle changes and by drugs (including statins, fibrates, and thiazolidinediones). Serum hs-CRP levels of less than 1, 1 to 3, and over 3 mg/L correspond, respectively, to low-, moderate-, and high-risk groups for future cardiovascular events.[26] In most clinical settings, a single hs-CRP assessment is likely to be adequate as long as levels less than 10 mg/L are observed. Because CRP is an acute inflammatory phase reactant, major infections, trauma, or acute hospitalization can elevate CRP levels (usually 100-fold or more). Thus, CRP levels to determine cardiovascular risk should be performed when the person is clinically stable. If the level remains markedly elevated, an alternative source of systemic inflammation should be considered.[26]

Homocysteine is derived from the metabolism of dietary methionine, an amino acid that is abundant in animal protein. The normal metabolism of homocysteine requires adequate levels of folate, vitamin B_6, vitamin B_{12}, and riboflavin. Homocysteine inhibits elements of the anticoagulant cascade and is associated with endothelial damage, which is thought to be an important first step in the development of atherosclerosis.[5,21,27] However, supplementation with folic acid, vitamin B_6, and vitamin B_{12} to decrease plasma homocysteine levels is not generally recommended for either primary or secondary prevention of cardiovascular disease based on recent clinical evidence.

Lipoprotein(a) is similar to LDL in composition and is an independent risk factor for the development of premature coronary heart disease in men. Lipoprotein(a) can cause atherosclerosis by binding to macrophages through a high-affinity receptor that promotes foam cell formation and the deposition of cholesterol in atherosclerotic plaques. Lipoprotein(a) levels should be determined in persons who have premature coronary artery disease or a positive family history.[21] There also has been increased interest in the possible connection between infectious agents (*e.g., Chlamydia pneumoniae,* herpesvirus, cytomegalovirus) and the development of vascular disease. The presence of these organisms in atheromatous lesions has been demonstrated by immunocytochemistry, but no cause-and-effect relationship has been established. The organisms may play a role in atherosclerotic development by initiating and enhancing the inflammatory response.[28]

Mechanisms of Development

The lesions associated with atherosclerosis are of three types: the fatty streak, the fibrous atheromatous plaque, and the complicated lesion. The latter two are responsible for the clinically significant manifestations of the disease.

Fatty streaks are thin, flat, yellow intimal discolorations that progressively enlarge by becoming thicker and slightly elevated as they grow in length. Histologically, they consist of macrophages and smooth muscle cells that have become distended with lipid to form foam cells. Fatty streaks are present in children, often in the first year of life.[1,5] This occurs regardless of geographic setting, sex, or race. They increase in number until about 20 years of age, and then they remain static or regress. There is controversy about whether fatty streaks, in and of themselves, are precursors of atherosclerotic lesions.

The *fibrous atheromatous plaque* is the basic lesion of clinical atherosclerosis. It is characterized by the accumulation of intracellular and extracellular lipids, proliferation of vascular smooth muscle cells, formation of scar tissue, and calcification. The lesions begin as a gray to pearly white, elevated thickening of the vessel intima with a core of extracellular lipid (mainly cholesterol, which usually is complexed to proteins) covered by a fibrous cap of connective tissue and smooth muscle (Fig. 22-7). As the lesions increase in size, they encroach on the lumen of the artery and eventually may occlude the vessel or predispose to thrombus formation, causing a reduction of blood flow. Because blood flow is related to the fourth power

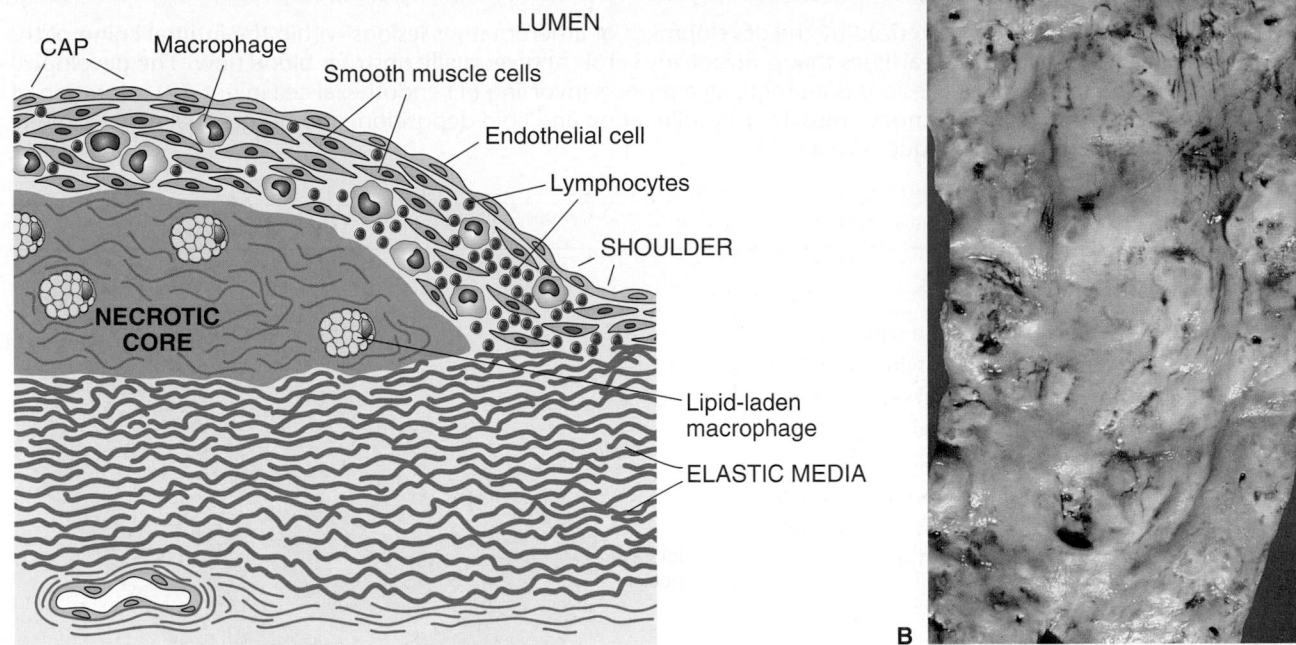

LUMEN
CAP Macrophage
Smooth muscle cells
Endothelial cell
Lymphocytes
SHOULDER
NECROTIC CORE
Lipid-laden macrophage
ELASTIC MEDIA

A B

FIGURE 22-7 • Fibrofatty plaque of atherosclerosis. **(A)** In this fully developed fibrous plaque, the core contains lipid-filled macrophages and necrotic smooth muscle cell debris. The "fibrous" cap is composed largely of smooth muscle cells, which produce collagen, small amounts of elastin, and glycosaminoglycans. Also shown are infiltrating macrophages and lymphocytes. Note that the endothelium over the surface of the fibrous cap frequently appears intact. **(B)** The aorta shows discrete raised, tan plaques. Focal plaque ulcerations are also evident. (From Gotlieb A. I. [2005]. Blood vessels. In Rubin E., Gorstein F., Rubin R., et al. [Eds.], *Pathology: Clinicopathologic foundations of medicine* [4th ed., p. 487]. Philadelphia: Lippincott Williams & Wilkins.)

of the vessel radius (see Chapter 21), the reduction in blood flow becomes increasingly greater as the disease progresses.

The more advanced complicated lesions contain hemorrhage, ulceration, and scar tissue deposits. Thrombosis is the most important complication of atherosclerosis. It is caused by slowing and turbulence of blood flow in the region of the plaque and ulceration of the plaque. The thrombus may cause occlusion of small vessels in the heart and brain. Aneurysms may develop in arteries weakened by extensive plaque formation.

Although the risk factors associated with atherosclerosis have been identified through epidemiologic studies, many unanswered questions remain regarding the mechanisms by which these risk factors contribute to the development of atherosclerosis. The vascular endothelial layer, which consists of a single layer of cells with cell-to-cell attachments, normally serves as a selective barrier that protects the subendothelial layers by interacting with blood cells and other blood components. One hypothesis of plaque formation suggests that injury to the endothelial vessel layer is the initiating factor in the development of atherosclerosis.[1,5] A number of factors are regarded as possible injurious agents, including products associated with smoking, immune mechanisms, and mechanical stress such as that associated with hypertension. The fact that atherosclerotic lesions tend to form where vessels branch or where there is turbulent flow suggests that hemodynamic factors also play a role.

Hyperlipidemia, particularly LDL with its high cholesterol content, is also believed to play an active role in the pathogenesis of the atherosclerotic lesion. Interactions between the endothelial layer of the vessel wall and white blood cells, particularly the monocytes (blood macrophages), normally occur throughout life; these interactions increase when blood cholesterol levels are elevated. One of the earliest responses to elevated cholesterol levels is the attachment of monocytes to the endothelium.[25] The monocytes have been observed to emigrate through the cell-to-cell attachments of the endothelial layer into the subendothelial spaces, where they are transformed into macrophages.

Activated macrophages release free radicals that oxidize LDL. Oxidized LDL is toxic to the endothelium, causing endothelial loss and exposure of the subendothelial tissue to blood components. This leads to platelet adhesion and aggregation and fibrin deposition. Platelets and activated macrophages release various factors that are thought to promote growth factors that modulate the proliferation of smooth muscle cells and deposition of extracellular matrix in the lesions.[1,5] Activated macrophages also ingest oxidized LDL (by uptake through the scavenger receptor) to become foam cells, which are present in all stages of atherosclerotic plaque formation. Lipids released from necrotic foam cells accumulate to form the lipid core of unstable plaques. Unstable plaques typically

Understanding • The Development of Atherosclerosis

Atherosclerosis is characterized by the development of atheromatous lesions within the intimal lining of the large and medium-sized arteries that protrude into and can eventually obstruct blood flow. The development of atherosclerotic lesions is a progressive process involving (1) endothelial cell injury, (2) migration of inflammatory cells, (3) smooth muscle cell proliferation and lipid deposition, and (4) gradual development of the atheromatous plaque with a lipid core.

❶ Endothelial Cell Injury

The vascular endothelium consists of a single layer of cells with cell-to-cell attachments, which normally protects the subendothelial layers from interacting with blood cells and other blood components. Agents such as smoking, elevated low-density lipoprotein (LDL) levels, immune mechanisms, and mechanical stress associated with hypertension share the potential for causing endothelial injury with adhesion of monocytes and platelets.

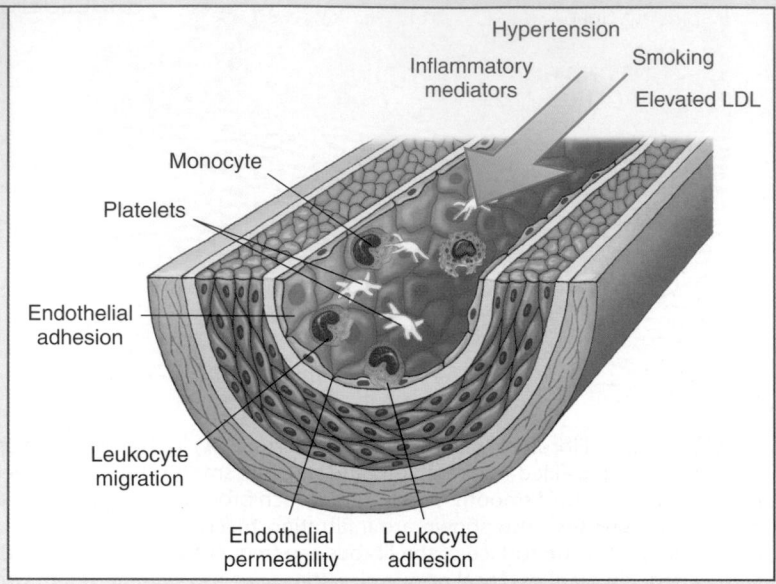

❷ Migration of Inflammatory Cells

Early in the development of atherosclerotic lesions, endothelial cells begin to express selective adhesion molecules that bind monocytes and other inflammatory cells that initiate the atherosclerotic lesions. After monocytes adhere to the endothelium, they migrate between the endothelial cells to localize in the intima, transform into macrophages, and engulf lipoproteins, largely LDL.

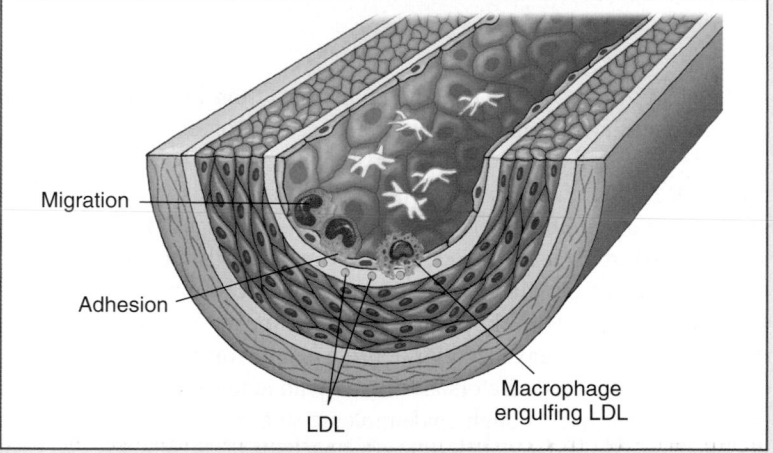

❸ Lipid Accumulation and Smooth Muscle Cell Proliferation

Although the recruitment of monocytes, their differentiation into macrophages and subsequent ingestion of lipids, and their ultimate transformation into foam cells is protective in that it removes excess lipids from the circulation, progressive accumulation eventually leads to lesion progression. Activated macrophages release toxic oxygen species that oxidize LDL; they then ingest the oxidized LDL to become foam cells. They also produce growth factors that contribute to the migration and proliferation of smooth muscle cells (SMCs) and the elaboration of extracellular matrix (ECM).

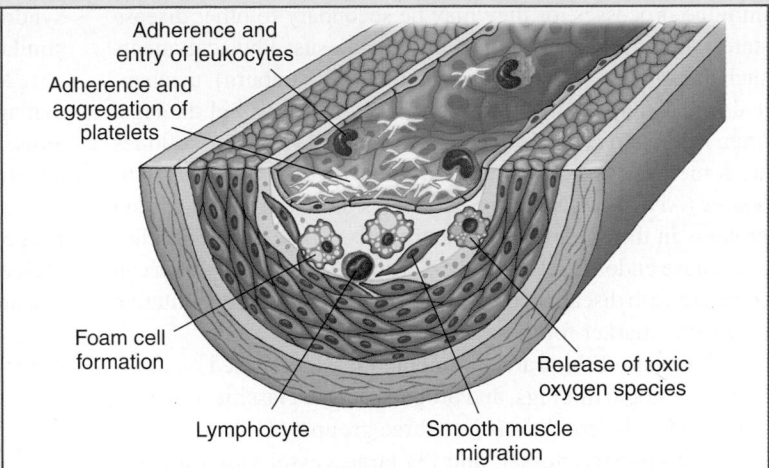

❹ Plaque Structure

Atherosclerotic plaques consist of an aggregation of SMCs, macrophages, and other leukocytes; ECM, including collagen and elastic fibers; and intracellular and extracellular lipids. Typically, the superficial fibrous cap is composed of SMCs and dense ECM. Immediately beneath and to the side of the fibrous cap is a cellular area (the shoulder) consisting of macrophages, SMCs, and lymphocytes. Below the fibrous cap is a central core of lipid-laden foam cells and fatty debris. Rupture, ulceration, or erosion of an unstable or vulnerable fibrous cap may lead to hemorrhage into the plaque or thrombotic occlusion of the vessel lumen.

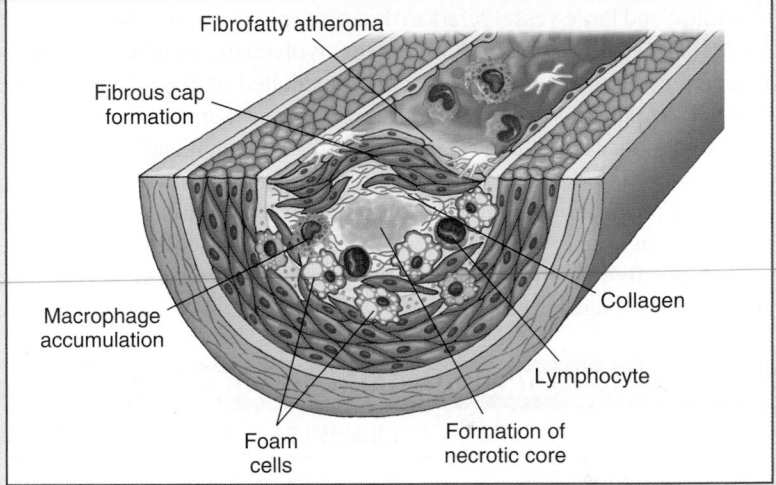

are characterized histologically by a large central lipid core, inflammatory infiltrate, and a thin fibrous cap.[29] These "vulnerable plaques" are at risk of rupture (plaque rupture), often at the shoulder of the plaque (see Fig. 22-7A) where the fibrous cap is thinnest (because of the presence of local inflammatory cells and mediators that degrade the cap) and the mechanical stresses highest.[25] Thus, "active" atherosclerosis is associated with evidence of inflammation both systemically (which can be assessed using hs-CRP) and at the level of the arterial wall.

Clinical Manifestations

The clinical manifestations of atherosclerosis depend on the vessels involved and the extent of vessel obstruction. Atherosclerotic lesions produce their effects through narrowing of the vessel and production of ischemia; sudden vessel obstruction due to plaque hemorrhage or rupture; thrombosis and formation of emboli resulting from damage to the vessel endothelium; and aneurysm formation due to weakening of the vessel wall.[1] In larger vessels, such as the aorta, the impor-

tant complications are those of thrombus formation and weakening of the vessel wall. In medium-sized arteries, such as the coronary and cerebral arteries, ischemia and infarction due to vessel occlusion are more common. Although atherosclerosis can affect any organ or tissue, the arteries supplying the heart, brain, kidneys, lower extremities, and small intestine are most frequently involved.

Vasculitis

The vasculitides are a group of vascular disorders that cause inflammatory injury and necrosis of the blood vessel wall (i.e., vasculitis). The vasculitides, which are a common pathway for tissue and organ involvement in many different disease conditions, involve the endothelial cells and smooth muscle cells of the vessel wall.[30,31] Vessels of any type (arteries, veins, and capillaries) in virtually any organ can be affected. Because they may affect veins and capillaries, the terms *vasculitis, angiitis,* and *arteritis* often are used interchangeably. Clinical manifestations often include fever, myalgia, arthralgia, and malaise. Vasculitis may result from direct injury to the vessel, infectious agents, or immune processes, or they may be secondary to other disease states such as systemic lupus erythematosus. Physical agents such as cold (*i.e.,* frostbite), irradiation (*i.e.,* sunburn), mechanical injury, and toxins may secondarily cause vessel damage, often leading to necrosis of the vessels. Small vessel vasculitides are sometimes associated with *anti-neutrophil cytoplasmic antibodies* (ANCA). ANCA are antibodies directed against certain proteins in the cytoplasm of neutrophils. These autoantibodies may cause endothelial damage.[5] Serum ANCA titers, which can correlate with disease activity, may serve as a useful quantitative diagnostic marker for these disorders.

The vasculitides are commonly classified based on etiology, pathologic findings, and prognosis. One classification system divides the conditions into three groups: (1) small vessel, (2) medium-sized vessel, and (3) large vessel vasculitides[1,5] (Table 22-4). Small vessel refers to small arteries (ANCA-associated disease only), arterioles, venules, and capillaries; medium vessels refer to medium- and small-sized arteries and arterioles; and large vessel refers to the aorta and its major tributaries. The small vessel vasculitides are involved in a number of different diseases, most of which are mediated by type III immune complex hypersensitivity reaction (see Chapter 19). They commonly involve the skin and are often a complication of an underlying disease (*i.e.,* vasculitis associated with neoplasms or connective tissue disease) and exposure to environmental agents (*i.e.,* serum sickness and urticarial vasculitis). ANCA-positive small vessel vasculitis include microscopic polyangiitis, Wegener granulomatosis, and the Churg-Strauss syndrome. These ANCA-positive vasculitides are treated by similar regimens.[32]

Medium-sized vessel vasculitides produce necrotizing damage to medium-sized muscular arteries of major organ systems. This group includes polyarteritis nodosa, Kawasaki disease (discussed in Chapter 24), and thromboangiitis obliterans (discussed in the section on Arterial Disease of the Extremities). Large vessel vasculitides involve large elastic arteries. They include giant cell (temporal) arteritis, polymyalgia rheumatica, and Takayasu arteritis. The following discussion focuses on two of the vasculitides: polyarteritis nodosa and giant cell (temporal) arteritis.

Polyarteritis Nodosa

Polyarteritis nodosa, so named because of the numerous nodules found along the course of muscular arteries, is a primary multisystem inflammatory disease of smaller and medium-sized blood vessels, especially those of the kidney, liver, intestine, peripheral nerve, skin, and muscle. The disease is seen more commonly in men than women.

The cause of polyarteritis nodosa remains unknown. It can occur in drug abusers and may be associated with the use of certain drugs such as allopurinol and the sulfonamides. There is an association between polyarteritis nodosa and hepatitis B and C infection, with 10% to 30% of persons with the disease having antibodies to hepatitis B or C in their serum. Other associations include serous otitis media, hairy cell leukemia, and

TABLE 22-4 **Classification of the Vasculitides**

GROUP	EXAMPLES	CHARACTERISTICS
Small vessel vasculitis	Microscopic polyangiitis	Necrotizing vasculitis with few or no immune deposits affecting medium and small blood vessels, including capillaries, venules, arterioles; necrotizing glomerulonephritis and involvement of the pulmonary capillaries is common
	Wegener granulomatosis	Granulomatous inflammation involving the respiratory tract and necrotizing vasculitis affecting capillaries, venules, arterioles, and arteries; necrotizing glomerulonephritis is common
Medium-sized vessel vasculitis	Polyarteritis nodosa	Necrotizing inflammation of medium-sized or small arteries without vasculitis in arteries, capillaries, or venules; usually associated with underlying disease or environmental agents
	Kawasaki disease	Involves large, medium-sized, and small arteries (frequently the coronaries) and is associated with mucocutaneous lymph node syndrome; usually occurs in small children
	Thromboangiitis obliterans	Segmental, thrombosing, acute and chronic inflammation of the medium-sized and small arteries, principally the tibial and radial arteries but sometimes extending to the veins and nerves of the extremities; occurs almost exclusively in men who are heavy smokers
Large vessel vasculitis	Giant cell (temporal) arteritis	Granulomatous inflammation of the aorta and its major branches with predilection for extracranial vessels of the carotid artery; infiltration of vessel wall with giant cells and mononuclear cells; usually occurs in people older than 50 years of age and is often associated with polymyalgia rheumatica
	Takayasu arteritis	Granulomatous inflammation of the aorta and its branches; usually occurs in people younger than 50 years of age

hyposensitization therapy for allergies. Persons with connective tissue diseases such as systemic lupus erythematosus, rheumatoid arthritis, and primary Sjögren syndrome may have manifestations similar to those of primary polyarteritis nodosa.

The onset of polyarteritis nodosa usually is abrupt, with complaints of anorexia, weight loss, fever, and fatigue often accompanied by signs of organ involvement. The kidney is the most frequently affected organ, and hypertension is a common manifestation of the disorder. Gastrointestinal involvement may manifest as abdominal pain, nausea, vomiting, or diarrhea. Myalgia, arthralgia, and arthritis are common, as are peripheral neuropathies such as paresthesias, pain, and weakness. Central nervous system complications include thrombotic and hemorrhagic stroke. Cardiac manifestations result from involvement of the coronary arteries. Skin lesions also may occur and are highly variable. They include reddish blue, mottled areas of discoloration of the skin of the extremities called *livedo reticularis*, purpura (*i.e.*, black and blue discoloration from bleeding into the skin), urticaria (*i.e.*, hives), and ulcers.

Laboratory findings, although variable, include an elevated erythrocyte sedimentation rate, leukocytosis, anemia, and signs of organ involvement such as hematuria and abnormal liver function test results. The diagnosis is confirmed through biopsy specimens demonstrating necrotizing vasculitis of the small and large arteries. Treatment involves use of high-dose corticosteroid therapy and often cytotoxic immunosuppressant agents (*e.g.*, azathioprine, cyclophosphamide). Before the availability of corticosteroids and immunosuppressive agents, the disease commonly was fatal. With the use of these agents, the 5-year survival rate is greater than 50%.[33] After the disease is under control, treatment usually is continued for 18 to 24 months and then gradually tapered.[30] For persons with polyarteritis nodosa associated with hepatitis B or C, aggressive simultaneous treatment of the hepatitis is indicated.

Giant Cell Temporal Arteritis

Temporal arteritis (*i.e.*, giant cell arteritis), the most common of the vasculitides, is a focal inflammatory condition of medium-sized and large arteries. It predominantly affects branches of arteries originating from the aortic arch, including the superficial temporal, vertebral, ophthalmic, and posterior ciliary arteries. The disorder progresses to involve the entire artery wall with focal necrosis and granulomatous inflammation involving multinucleated giant cells (Fig. 22-8). It is more common in elderly persons, with a 2:1 female-to-male ratio. The cause is unknown, although an autoimmune origin has been suggested.[34]

The disorder often is insidious in onset and may be heralded by the sudden onset of headache, tenderness over the artery, swelling and redness of the overlying skin, blurred vision or diplopia, and facial pain. Almost one half of affected persons have systemic involvement in the form of polymyalgia rheumatica (see Chapter 59). Up to 10% of patients with giant cell arteritis go on to develop aortic aneurysm (especially thoracic).

Diagnosis is based on the clinical manifestations, a characteristically elevated erythrocyte sedimentation rate and CRP,

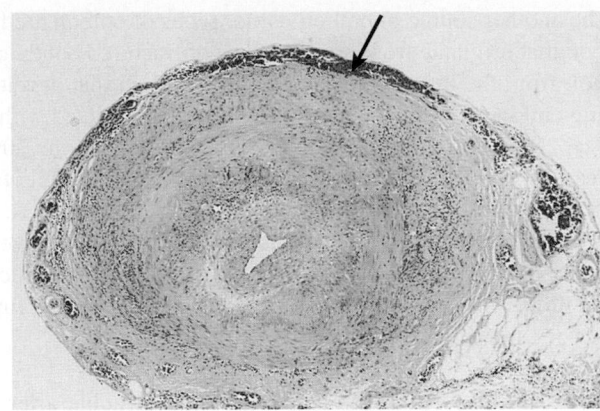

FIGURE 22-8 • Temporal arteritis. A cross-sectional photograph of a temporal artery shows inflammation throughout the wall, giant cells (*arrow*), and a lumen severely narrowed by intimal thickening. (From Gotlieb A. I. [2005]. Blood vessels. In Rubin E., Gorstein F., Rubin R, et al. [Eds.], *Pathology: Clinicopathologic foundations of medicine* [4th ed., p. 507]. Philadelphia: Lippincott Williams & Wilkins.)

and temporal artery biopsy. Treatment includes use of high-dose corticosteroids. Before persons with the disorder were treated with corticosteroids, blindness developed in almost 80% of cases due to involvement of the posterior ciliary artery.

Arterial Disease of the Extremities

Disorders of the circulation in the extremities often are referred to as *peripheral vascular disorders*. In many respects, the disorders that affect arteries in the extremities are the same as those affecting the coronary and cerebral arteries in that they produce ischemia, pain, impaired function, and in some cases infarction and tissue necrosis. Not only are the effects similar, but the pathologic conditions that impair circulation in the extremities are identical. This section focuses on acute arterial occlusion of the extremities, atherosclerotic occlusive disease, thromboangiitis obliterans, and Raynaud disease and phenomenon.

Acute Arterial Occlusion

Acute arterial occlusion is a sudden event that interrupts arterial flow to the affected tissues or organ. Most acute arterial occlusions are the result of an embolus or a thrombus. Rarely, the tips of catheters that have been inserted into a vessel can break off and become emboli. Although much less common than emboli and thrombus, trauma or arterial spasm caused by arterial cannulation can be another cause of acute arterial occlusion.

An embolus is a freely moving particle such as a blood clot that breaks loose and travels in the larger vessels of the circulation until lodging in a smaller vessel and occluding blood flow. Most emboli arise in the heart and are caused by conditions that cause blood clots to develop on the wall of a heart chamber or valve surface. Emboli usually are a complication of heart disease: ischemic heart disease with or without infarction, atrial fibrillation, or rheumatic heart disease. Prosthetic heart valves can be another source of emboli. Other types of emboli are fat emboli that originate from bone marrow of fractured bones, air emboli from the lung, and amniotic fluid emboli that develop during childbirth. Acute arterial embolism is associated with a 5% to 25% risk of affected limb loss, and a 25% to 30% increase in hospital mortality. Heart disease is responsible for over half these deaths.

A thrombus is a blood clot that forms on the wall of a vessel and continues to grow until reaching a size that obstructs blood flow. Thrombi often arise as the result of erosion or rupture of the fibrous cap of an arteriosclerotic plaque.

Manifestations. The signs and symptoms of acute arterial occlusion depend on the artery involved and the adequacy of the collateral circulation. Emboli tend to lodge in bifurcations of the major arteries, including the aorta and iliac, femoral, and popliteal arteries. The presentation of acute arterial embolism is often described as that of the seven "P's": (1) pistolshot (acute onset); (2) pallor; (3) polar (cold); (4) pulselessness; (5) pain; (6) paresthesia; and (7) paralysis. Occlusion in an extremity causes sudden onset of acute pain with numbness, tingling, weakness, pallor, and coldness. There often is a sharp line of demarcation between the oxygenated tissue above the line of obstruction and the ischemic tissue below the line of obstruction. Pulses are absent below the level of the occlusion. These changes are followed rapidly by cyanosis, mottling, and loss of sensory, reflex, and motor function. Tissue death occurs unless blood flow is restored.

Diagnosis and Treatment. Diagnosis of acute arterial occlusion is based on signs of impaired blood flow. It uses visual assessment, palpation of pulses, and methods to assess blood flow. Treatment of acute arterial occlusion is aimed at restoring blood flow. An embolectomy—surgical removal of the embolus—is the optimal therapy when a large artery is occluded.

Thrombolytic therapy (*i.e.,* streptokinase or tissue plasminogen activator) may be used in an attempt to dissolve the clot. Anticoagulant therapy (*i.e.,* heparin) usually is given to prevent extension of the embolus and to prevent progression of the original thrombus. Application of cold should be avoided, and the extremity should be protected from injury resulting from hard surfaces and overlying bedclothes.

Atherosclerotic Occlusive Disease

Atherosclerosis is an important cause of peripheral artery disease (PAD) and is seen most commonly in the vessels of the lower extremities. The condition is sometimes referred to as *arteriosclerosis obliterans*. The superficial femoral and popliteal arteries are the most commonly affected vessels. When lesions develop in the lower leg and foot, the tibial, common peroneal, or pedal vessels are the arteries most commonly affected. The disease is seen most commonly in men in their sixties and seventies.[35–37] At least one in five of the population older than 65 years of age has PAD.[37] The risk factors for this

disorder are similar to those for atherosclerosis. Cigarette smoking contributes to the progress of the atherosclerosis of the lower extremities and to the development of symptoms of ischemia. Persons with diabetes mellitus develop more extensive and rapidly progressive vascular disease than do nondiabetic individuals.

Manifestations. As with atherosclerosis in other locations, the signs and symptoms of vessel occlusion are gradual. Usually, there is at least a 50% narrowing of the vessel before symptoms of ischemia arise. The primary symptom of chronic obstructive arterial disease is *intermittent claudication* or pain with walking.[35,37] Typically, persons with the disorder complain of calf pain because the gastrocnemius muscle has the highest oxygen consumption of any muscle group in the leg during walking. Some persons may complain of a vague aching feeling or numbness, rather than pain. Other activities such as swimming, bicycling, and climbing stairs use other muscle groups and may not incite the same degree of discomfort as walking. Intermittent claudication affects at least 1 in 20 people older than 65 years of age.[37] Other signs of ischemia include atrophic changes and thinning of the skin and subcutaneous tissues of the lower leg and diminution in the size of the leg muscles. The foot often is cool, and the popliteal and pedal pulses are weak or absent. Limb color blanches with elevation of the leg because of the effects of gravity on perfusion pressure and becomes deep red when the leg is in the dependent position because of an autoregulatory increase in blood flow and a gravitational increase in perfusion pressure.

When blood flow is reduced to the extent that it no longer meets the minimal needs of resting muscle and nerves, ischemic pain at rest, ulceration, and gangrene develop. As tissue necrosis develops there typically is severe pain in the region of skin breakdown, which is worse at night with limb elevation and is improved with standing.[35]

Diagnosis and Treatment. Diagnostic methods include inspection of the limbs for signs of chronic low-grade ischemia such as subcutaneous atrophy, brittle toenails, hair loss, pallor, coolness, or dependent rubor. Palpation of the femoral, popliteal, posterior tibial, and dorsalis pedis pulses allows for an estimation of the level and degree of obstruction. The ratio of ankle to arm (*i.e.,* tibial and brachial arteries) systolic blood pressure is used to detect significant obstruction, with a ratio of less than 0.9 indicating occlusion. Normally, systolic pressure in the ankle exceeds that in the brachial artery because systolic pressure and pulse pressure tend to increase as the pressure wave moves away from the heart (see Chapter 21). Blood pressures may be taken at various levels on the leg to determine the level of obstruction. A Doppler ultrasound stethoscope may be used for detecting pulses and measuring blood pressure. Ultrasound imaging, magnetic resonance imaging (MRI) arteriography, spiral computed tomographic (CT) arteriography, and invasive contrast angiography may also be used as diagnostic methods.[35–37]

The two goals of treatment in persons with PAD are (1) to decrease their considerable cardiovascular risk, and (2) to reduce symptoms. Patients should be evaluated for coexisting coronary and cerebrovascular atherosclerosis. The risk of death, mainly from coronary and cerebrovascular events, is high (5% to 10% per year).[37] The other cardiovascular risk factors that should be addressed include smoking cessation, hypertension, lipid lowering, and diabetes. Antiplatelet agents (aspirin or clopidogrel) reduce the vascular death rate in patients with PAD by about 25%.[37] Other medications that are useful include statins, cilostazol (a phosphodiesterase inhibitor), and pentoxifylline (an adenosine diphosphate [ADP] receptor antagonist that decreases blood viscosity and improves erythrocyte flexibility). The tissues of extremities affected by atherosclerosis are easily injured and slow to heal. Treatment includes measures directed at protection of the affected tissues and preservation of functional capacity. Walking (slowly) to the point of claudication usually is encouraged because it increases collateral circulation.

Percutaneous or surgical intervention is typically reserved for the patient with disabling claudication or limb-threatening ischemia. Surgery (*i.e.,* femoropopliteal bypass grafting using a section of saphenous vein) may be indicated in severe cases. In persons with diabetes, the peroneal arteries between the knees and ankles commonly are involved, making revascularization difficult. Thromboendarterectomy with removal of the occluding core of atherosclerotic tissue may be done if the section of diseased vessel is short. Percutaneous transluminal angioplasty and stent placement, in which a balloon catheter is inserted into the area of stenosis and the balloon inflated to increase vessel diameter, is another form of treatment.[35–37]

Thromboangiitis Obliterans

Thromboangiitis obliterans, or Buerger disease, is an inflammatory (*i.e.,* vasculitis) arterial disorder that causes thrombus formation. The disorder affects the medium-sized arteries, usually the plantar and digital vessels in the foot and lower leg. Arteries in the arm and hand also may be affected. Although primarily an arterial disorder, the inflammatory process often extends to involve adjacent veins and nerves. Usually it is a disease of men between the ages of 25 and 40 years who are heavy cigarette smokers, but it is now also being reported with increasing frequency in young female smokers. The pathogenesis of Buerger disease remains speculative, although cigarette smoking and in some instances tobacco chewing seem to be involved. It has been suggested that the tobacco may trigger an immune response in susceptible persons or it may unmask a clotting defect, either of which could incite an inflammatory reaction of the vessel wall.[38]

Manifestations. Pain is the predominant symptom of the disorder. It usually is related to distal arterial ischemia. During the early stages of the disease, there is intermittent claudication in the arch of the foot and the digits. In severe cases, pain is present even when the person is at rest. The impaired circulation increases sensitivity to cold. The peripheral pulses are diminished or absent, and there are changes in the color of the extremity. In moderately advanced cases, the extremity becomes cyanotic when the person assumes a dependent position, and the digits may turn reddish blue even when in a nondependent position. With lack of blood flow, the skin assumes a thin, shiny look and hair growth and skin nutrition suffer. Chronic ischemia causes thick, malformed nails. If the disease continues to progress, tissues eventually ulcerate and gangrenous changes arise that may necessitate amputation.

Diagnosis and Treatment. Diagnostic methods are similar to those for atherosclerotic disease of the lower extremities. As part of the treatment program for thromboangiitis obliterans, it is mandatory that the person stop smoking cigarettes or using tobacco. Even passive smoking and nicotine replacement therapy should be eliminated. Other treatment measures are of secondary importance and focus on methods for producing vasodilation and preventing tissue injury. Sympathectomy may be done to alleviate the vasospastic manifestations of the disease.

Raynaud Disease and Phenomenon

Raynaud disease or phenomenon is a functional disorder caused by intense vasospasm of the arteries and arterioles in the fingers and, less often, the toes. This is a common disorder affecting 10% of the population. The disorder is divided into two types: the primary type, called *Raynaud disease,* occurs without demonstrable cause, and the secondary type, called *Raynaud phenomenon,* is associated with other disease states or known causes of vasospasm.[39–41]

Vasospasm implies an excessive vasoconstrictor response to stimuli that normally produce only moderate vasoconstriction. In contrast to other regional circulations that are supplied by vasodilator and vasoconstrictor fibers, the cutaneous vessels of the fingers and toes are innervated only by sympathetic vasoconstrictor fibers. In these vessels, vasodilation occurs by withdrawal of sympathetic stimulation. Cooling of specific body parts such as the head, neck, and trunk produces a sympathetic-mediated reduction in digital blood flow, as does emotional stress.

Raynaud disease is seen in otherwise healthy young women, and it often is precipitated by exposure to cold or by strong emotions and usually is limited to the fingers. It also follows a more benign course than Raynaud phenomenon, seldom causing tissue necrosis. The cause of vasospasm in primary Raynaud disease is unknown. Hyperreactivity of the sympathetic nervous system has been suggested as a contributing cause.[39] Raynaud phenomenon is associated with previous vessel injury, such as frostbite, occupational trauma associated with the use of heavy vibrating tools, collagen diseases, neurologic disorders, and chronic arterial occlusive disorders. Another occupation-related cause is the exposure to alternating hot and cold temperatures such as that experienced by butchers and food preparers.[39] Raynaud phenomenon often is the first symptom of collagen diseases. It occurs in almost 100% of scleroderma cases, and can precede the diagnosis of scleroderma by many years.[41]

Manifestations. In Raynaud disease and Raynaud phenomenon, ischemia due to vasospasm causes changes in skin color that progress from pallor to cyanosis, a sensation of cold, and changes in sensory perception, such as numbness and tingling. The color changes usually are first noticed in the tips of the fingers, later moving into one or more of the distal phalanges (Fig. 22-9). After the ischemic episode, there is a period of hyperemia with intense redness, throbbing, and paresthesias. The period of hyperemia is followed by a return to normal color. Although all of the fingers usually are affected symmetrically, in some cases only one or two digits are involved, or only a portion of the digit is affected.

In severe, progressive cases usually associated with Raynaud phenomenon, trophic changes may develop. The nails may become brittle, and the skin over the tips of the affected fingers may thicken. Nutritional impairment of these structures may give rise to arthritis. Ulceration and superficial gangrene of the fingers, although infrequent, may occur.

Diagnosis and Treatment. The initial diagnosis is based on history of vasospastic attacks supported by other evidence of the disorder. Immersion of the hand in cold water may be used to initiate an attack as an aid to diagnosis. Laser Doppler flow velocimetry may be used to quantify digital blood flow during changes in temperature. Raynaud disease is differentiated from Raynaud phenomenon by excluding secondary disorders known to cause vasospasm.[41]

Treatment measures are directed toward eliminating factors that cause vasospasm and protecting the digits from trauma during an ischemic episode. Abstinence from smoking and protection from cold are priorities. The entire body must be protected from cold, not just the extremities. Avoidance of emotional stress is another important factor in controlling the disorder because anxiety and stress may precipitate a vascular spasm in predisposed persons. Vasoconstrictor medications, such as the decongestants contained in allergy and cold preparations, should be avoided. Treatment with vasodilator drugs may be indicated, particularly if episodes are frequent, because frequency encourages the potential for development of thrombosis and gangrene. The calcium channel blocking drugs (*e.g.,* nifedipine, diltiazem) decrease the severity and frequency of attacks. Prazosin, an α-adrenergic receptor blocking drug, also may be used. Surgical interruption of sympathetic nerve pathways (sympathectomy) may be used for persons with severe symptoms.[41]

Aneurysms and Dissection

An *aneurysm* is an abnormal localized dilation of a blood vessel. Aneurysms can occur in arteries and veins, but they are most common in the aorta. There are two types of aneurysms: true aneurysms and false aneurysms. A *true aneurysm* is one in which the aneurysm is bounded by a complete vessel wall.[42] The blood in a true aneurysm remains within the vascular compartment. A *false aneurysm* or *pseudoaneurysm* represents a localized dissection or tear in the inner wall of the artery with formation of an extravascular hematoma that causes vessel enlargement. Unlike true aneurysms, false aneurysms are bounded only by the outer layers of the vessel wall or supporting tissues.

Aneurysms can assume several forms and may be classified according to their cause, location, and anatomic features (Fig. 22-10). A *berry aneurysm* consists of a small, spherical dilation of the vessel at a bifurcation.[1,5] This type of aneurysm usually is found in the circle of Willis in the cerebral circulation. A *fusiform aneurysm* involves the entire circumference of the vessel and is characterized by a gradual and progressive dilation of the vessel. These aneurysms, which vary in diameter (up to 20 cm) and length, may involve the entire ascending and transverse portions of the thoracic aorta or may extend over large segments of the abdominal aorta. A *saccular aneurysm* extends over part of the circumference of the vessel and appears saclike. A *dissecting aneurysm* is a false aneurysm resulting from a tear in the intimal layer of the vessel that allows blood to enter the vessel wall, dissecting its layers to create a blood-filled cavity.

The weakness that leads to aneurysm formation may be caused by several factors, including congenital defects, trauma, infections, and atherosclerosis. Once initiated, the aneurysm grows larger as the tension in the vessel increases. This is because the tension in the wall of a vessel is equal to the pressure multiplied by the radius (*i.e.,* tension = pressure × radius; see Chapter 21). In this case, the pressure in the segment of the vessel affected by the aneurysm does not change but remains the same as that of adjacent portions of the vessel. As an aneurysm increases in diameter, the tension in the wall of the vessel increases in direct proportion to its increased size. If untreated, the aneurysm may rupture because of the increased tension. Even an unruptured aneurysm can cause damage by exerting pressure on adjacent structures and interrupting blood flow.

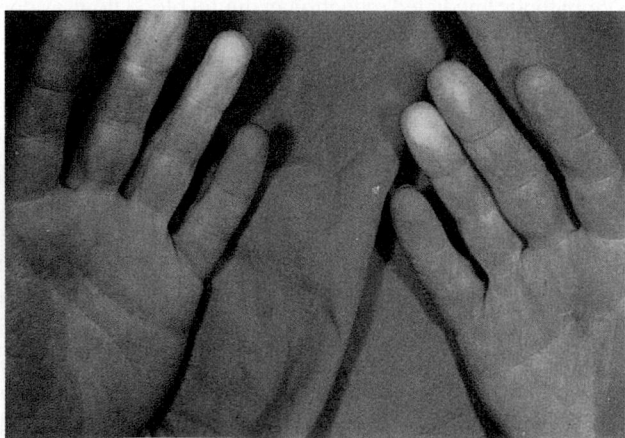

FIGURE 22-9 • Raynaud phenomenon. The tips of the fingers show marked pallor. (From Gotlieb A. I. [2005]. Blood vessels. In Rubin E., Gorstein F., Rubin R., et al. [Eds.], *Pathology: Clinicopathologic foundations of medicine* [4th ed., p. 504]. Philadelphia: Lippincott Williams & Wilkins.)

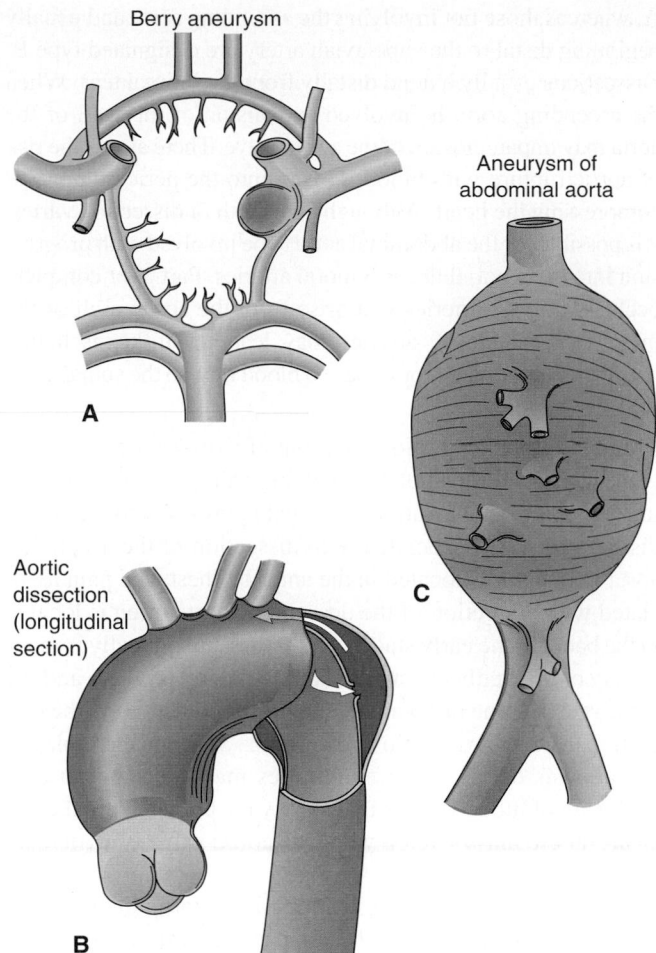

Berry aneurysm

A

Aneurysm of abdominal aorta

C

Aortic dissection (longitudinal section)

B

FIGURE 22-10 • Three forms of aneurysms: (**A**) berry aneurysm in the circle of Willis, (**B**) aortic dissection, and (**C**) fusiform-type aneurysm of the abdominal aorta.

Aortic Aneurysms

Aortic aneurysms may involve any part of the aorta: the ascending aorta, aortic arch, descending aorta, thoracoabdominal aorta, or abdominal aorta. Multiple aneurysms may be present. The two most common causes of aortic aneurysms are atherosclerosis and degeneration of the vessel media. Half of the people with aortic aneurysms have hypertension.[5] Population-based studies suggest that up to 9% of persons older than 65 years of age have unsuspected and asymptomatic abdominal aortic aneurysms, and that ruptured abdominal aortic aneurysms cause at least 15,000 deaths each year in the United States.[43]

Manifestations. The signs and symptoms of aortic aneurysms depend on the size and location. An aneurysm also may be asymptomatic, with the first evidence of its presence being associated with vessel rupture. Aneurysms of the thoracic aorta are less common than abdominal aortic aneurysms. They account for less than 10% of aortic aneurysms and may present with substernal, back, and neck pain. There also may be dyspnea, stridor,

or a brassy cough caused by pressure on the trachea. Hoarseness may result from pressure on the recurrent laryngeal nerve, and there may be difficulty swallowing because of pressure on the esophagus.[44] The aneurysm also may compress the superior vena cava, causing distention of neck veins and edema of the face and neck.

Abdominal aortic aneurysms are located most commonly below the level of the renal artery (>90%) and involve the bifurcation of the aorta and proximal end of the common iliac arteries.[1,5] The infrarenal aorta is normally 2 cm in diameter; an aneurysm is defined as an aortic diameter greater than 3 cm. They can involve any part of the vessel circumference (saccular) or extend to involve the entire circumference (fusiform). Most abdominal aneurysms are asymptomatic. Because an aneurysm is of arterial origin, a pulsating mass may provide the first evidence of the disorder. Typically, aneurysms larger than 4 cm are palpable. The mass may be discovered during a routine physical examination or the affected person may complain of its presence. Calcification, which frequently exists on the wall of the aneurysm, may be detected during abdominal radiologic examination. Pain may be present and varies from mild mid-abdominal or lumbar discomfort to severe abdominal and back pain. As the aneurysm expands, it may compress the lumbar nerve roots, causing lower back pain that radiates to the posterior aspects of the legs. The aneurysm may extend to and impinge on the renal, iliac, or mesenteric arteries, or to the vertebral arteries that supply the spinal cord. An abdominal aneurysm also may cause erosion of vertebrae. Stasis of blood favors thrombus formation along the wall of the vessel (Fig. 22-11), and peripheral emboli may develop, causing symptomatic arterial insufficiency.

With thoracic and abdominal aneurysms, the most dreaded complication is rupture. The likelihood of rupture correlates with increasing aneurysm size. The risk of rupture rises from less than 2% for small abdominal aneurysms (<4 cm in diameter) to 5% to 10% per year for aneurysms larger than 5 cm in diameter.[1]

Diagnosis and Treatment. Diagnostic methods include use of ultrasonography, echocardiography, CT scans, and MRI. Surgical repair, in which the involved section of the aorta is replaced with a synthetic graft of woven Dacron, frequently is the treatment of choice.[42,44]

Aortic Dissection

Aortic dissection (dissecting aneurysm) is an acute, life-threatening condition. It involves hemorrhage into the vessel wall with longitudinal tearing of the vessel wall to form a blood-filled channel (see Fig. 22-10B). Unlike atherosclerotic aneurysms, aortic dissection often occurs without evidence of previous vessel dilation. The dissection can originate anywhere along the length of the aorta. Two thirds of dissections involve the ascending aorta.[45] The second most common site is the thoracic aorta just distal to the origin of the subclavian artery.

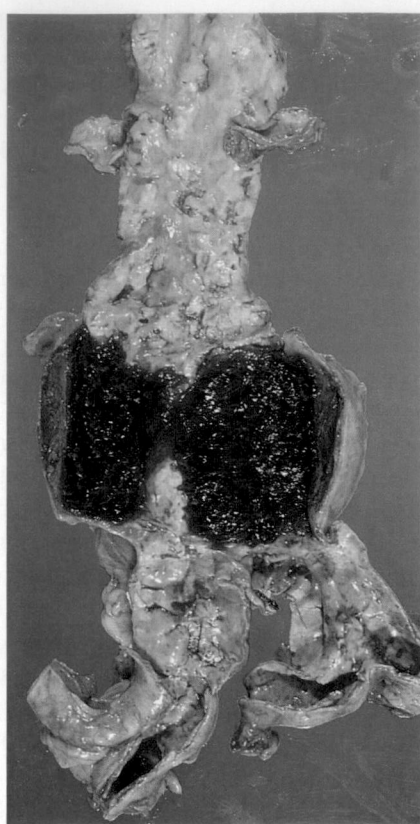

FIGURE 22-11 • Atherosclerotic aneurysm of the abdominal aorta. The aneurysm has been opened longitudinally to reveal a large thrombus in the lumen. The aorta and common iliac arteries display complicated lesions of atherosclerosis. (From Gotlieb A. I. [2005]. Blood vessels. In Rubin E., Gorstein F., Rubin R., et al. [Eds.], *Pathology: Clinicopathologic foundations of medicine* [4th ed., p. 511]. Philadelphia: Lippincott Williams & Wilkins.)

Aortic dissection is caused by conditions that weaken or cause degenerative changes in the elastic and smooth muscle of the layers of the aorta. It is most common in the 40- to 60-year-old age group and more prevalent in men than in women.[1] There are two risk factors that predispose to dissection: hypertension and degeneration of the medial layer of the vessel wall. There is a history of hypertension in most cases.[1] Aortic dissection also is associated with connective tissue diseases, such as Marfan syndrome. It also may occur during pregnancy because of changes in the aorta that occur during this time. Other factors that predispose to dissection are congenital defects of the aortic valve (*i.e.*, bicuspid or unicuspid valve structures) and aortic coarctation. Aortic dissection is a potential complication of cardiac surgery or catheterization. Surgically related dissection may occur at the points where the aorta has been incised or cross-clamped; it also has been reported at the site where the saphenous vein was sutured to the aorta during coronary artery bypass surgery.

Aortic aneurysms are commonly classified into two types, type A and type B, as determined by the level of dissection. The more common (and potentially serious in terms of complications) proximal lesions, involving the ascending aorta only or both the ascending and the descending aorta, are designated type A; whereas those not involving the ascending aorta and usually beginning distal to the subclavian artery are designated type B. Dissections usually extend distally from the intimal tear. When the ascending aorta is involved, expansion of the wall of the aorta may impair closure of the aortic valve. There also is the risk of aortic rupture with blood moving into the pericardium and compressing the heart. Although the length of dissection varies, it is possible for the abdominal aorta to be involved with progression into the renal, iliac, or femoral arteries. Partial or complete occlusion of the arteries that arise from the aortic arch or the intercostal or lumbar arteries may lead to stroke, ischemic peripheral neuropathy, or impaired blood flow to the spinal cord.

Manifestations. A major symptom of a dissecting aneurysm is the abrupt presence of excruciating pain, described as tearing or ripping. The location of the pain may point to the site of dissection.[1] Pain associated with dissection of the ascending aorta frequently is located in the anterior chest, and pain associated with dissection of the descending aorta often is located in the back. In the early stages, blood pressure typically is moderately or markedly elevated. Later, the blood pressure and the pulse rate become unobtainable in one or both arms as the dissection disrupts arterial flow to the arms. Syncope, hemiplegia, or paralysis of the lower extremities may occur because of occlusion of blood vessels that supply the brain or spinal cord. Heart failure may develop when the aortic valve is involved.

Diagnosis and Treatment. Diagnosis of aortic dissection is based on history and physical examination. Aortic angiography, transesophageal echocardiography, CT scans, and MRI studies aid in the diagnosis.

The treatment of dissecting aortic aneurysm may be medical or surgical. Aortic dissection is a life-threatening emergency; persons with a probable diagnosis are stabilized medically even before the diagnosis is confirmed. Two important factors that participate in propagating the dissection are high blood pressure and the steepness of the pulse wave. Without intervention, these forces continue to cause extension of the dissection. Medical treatment therefore focuses on control of hypertension and the use of drugs that lessen the force of systolic blood ejection from the heart. Two commonly used drugs, given in combination, are intravenous sodium nitroprusside and a β-adrenergic blocking drug. Surgical treatment consists of resection of the involved segment of the aorta and replacement with a prosthetic graft. The mortality rate due to untreated dissecting aneurysm is high, exceeding 50% within the first 48 hours, and 80% within 6 weeks.[46]

IN SUMMARY, the arterial system distributes blood to all the tissues of the body, and lesions of the arterial system exert their effects through ischemia or impaired blood flow. There are two types of arterial disorders: diseases such as atherosclerosis, vasculitis, and peripheral arterial diseases that obstruct blood flow, and disorders such as aneurysms that weaken the vessel wall.

Cholesterol relies on lipoproteins (LDLs and HDLs) for transport in the blood. The LDLs, which are atherogenic, carry cholesterol to the peripheral tissues. The HDLs, which are protective, remove cholesterol from the tissues and carry it back to the liver for disposal (reverse cholesterol transport). LDL receptors play a major role in removing cholesterol from the blood; persons with reduced numbers of receptors are at particularly high risk for development of atherosclerosis.

Atherosclerosis, a leading cause of death in the United States, affects large and medium-sized arteries, such as the coronary and cerebral arteries. It has an insidious onset, and its lesions usually are far advanced before symptoms appear. Although the mechanisms of atherosclerosis are uncertain, risk factors associated with its development have been identified. These include factors such as heredity, sex, and age, which cannot be controlled; and factors such as smoking, high blood pressure, high serum cholesterol levels, diabetes, obesity, and inflammation, which can be controlled or modified.

The vasculitides are a group of vascular disorders characterized by vasculitis or inflammation and necrosis of the blood vessels in various tissues and organs of the body. They can be caused by injury to the vessel, infectious agents, or immune processes, or can occur secondary to other disease states such as systemic lupus erythematosus.

Occlusive disorders interrupt arterial flow of blood and interfere with the delivery of oxygen and nutrients to the tissues. Occlusion of flow can result from a thrombus, emboli, vessel compression, vasospasm, or structural changes in the vessel. Peripheral arterial diseases affect blood vessels outside the heart and thorax. They include Raynaud disease or phenomenon, caused by vessel spasm, and thromboangiitis obliterans (Buerger disease), characterized by an inflammatory process that involves medium-sized arteries.

Aneurysms are localized areas of vessel dilation caused by weakness of the arterial wall. A berry aneurysm, most often found in the circle of Willis in the brain circulation, consists of a small, spherical vessel dilation. Fusiform and saccular aneurysms, most often found in the thoracic and abdominal aorta, are characterized by gradual and progressive enlargement of the aorta. They can involve part of the vessel circumference (saccular) or extend to involve the entire circumference of the vessel (fusiform). A dissecting aneurysm is an acute, life-threatening condition. It involves hemorrhage into the vessel wall with longitudinal tearing (dissection) of the vessel wall to form a blood-filled channel. The most serious consequence of aneurysms is rupture. ■

DISORDERS OF THE VENOUS CIRCULATION

After completing this section of the chapter, you should be able to meet the following objectives:

- Describe venous return of blood from the lower extremities, including the function of the muscle pumps and the effects of gravity, and relate to the development of varicose veins.
- Differentiate primary from secondary varicose veins.
- Characterize the pathology of venous insufficiency and relate to the development of stasis dermatitis and venous ulcers.
- List the four most common causes of lower leg ulcer.
- Cite risk factors associated with venous thrombosis and describe the manifestation of the disorder and its treatment.

Veins are low-pressure, thin-walled vessels that rely on the ancillary action of skeletal muscle pumps and changes in abdominal and intrathoracic pressure to return blood to the heart. Unlike the arterial system, the venous system is equipped with valves that prevent retrograde flow of blood. Although its structure enables the venous system to serve as a storage area for blood, it also renders the system susceptible to problems related to stasis and venous insufficiency. This section focuses on three common problems of the venous system: varicose veins, venous insufficiency, and venous thrombosis.

Venous Circulation of the Lower Extremities

The venous system in the legs consists of two components: the superficial veins (*i.e.*, saphenous vein and its tributaries) and the deep venous channels (Fig. 22-12A). Perforating or communicating veins connect these two systems. Blood from the skin and subcutaneous tissues in the leg collects in the superficial veins and is then transported across the communicating veins into the deeper venous channels for return to the heart. Venous valves prevent the retrograde flow of blood and play an important role in the function of the venous system. Although these valves are irregularly located along the length of the veins, they almost always are found at junctions where the communicating veins merge with the larger deep veins and where two veins meet. The number of venous valves differs somewhat from one person to another, as does their structural competence, factors that may help explain the familial predisposition to development of varicose veins.

The action of the leg muscles assists in moving venous blood from the lower extremities back to the heart. When a person walks, the action of the leg muscles serves to increase flow in the deep venous channels and return venous blood to the heart (Fig. 22-13). The function of the so-called *muscle pump*, located in the gastrocnemius and soleus muscles of the lower extremities, can be compared with the pumping action of the heart.[47] During muscle contraction, which is similar to systole, valves in the communicating channels close to prevent backward flow of blood into the superficial system, as blood in the deep veins is moved forward by the action of the contracting

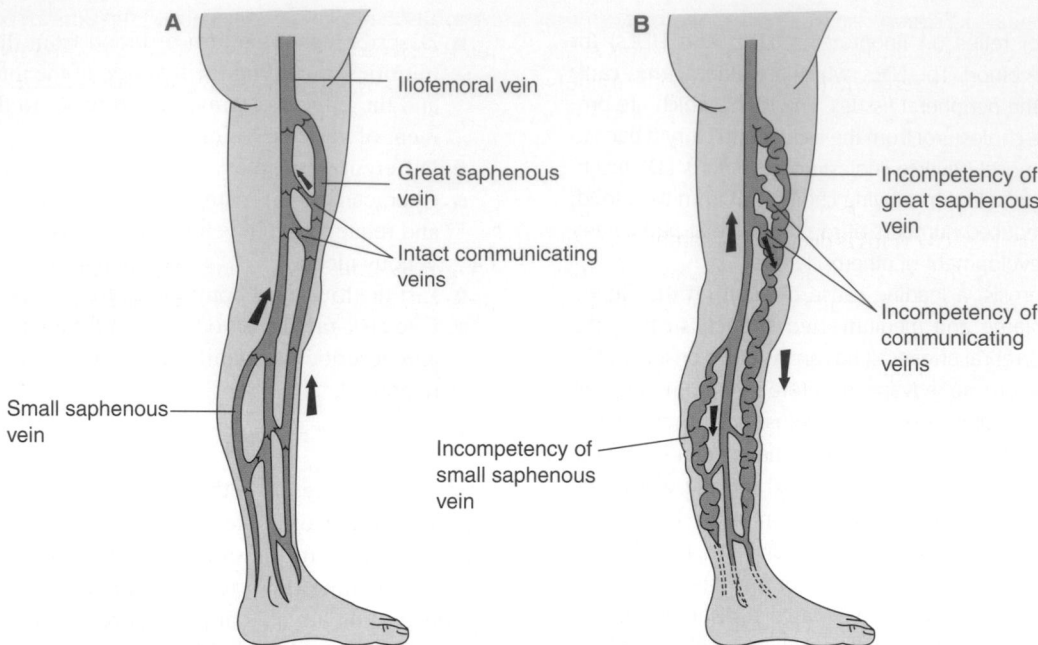

FIGURE 22-12 • Superficial and deep venous channels of the leg. **(A)** Normal venous structures and flow patterns. **(B)** Varicosities in the superficial venous system are the result of incompetent valves in the communicating veins. The *arrows* in both views indicate the direction of blood flow. (Modified from Abramson D. I. [1974]. *Vascular disorders of the extremities* [2nd ed.]. New York: Harper & Row.)

muscles. During muscle relaxation, which is similar to diastole, the communicating valves open, allowing blood from the superficial veins to move into the deep veins.

DISORDERS OF THE VENOUS CIRCULATION

- Veins are thin-walled, distensible vessels that collect blood from the tissues and return it to the heart. The venous system is a low-pressure system that relies on the pumping action of the skeletal muscles to move blood forward and the presence of venous valves to prevent retrograde flow.

- Disorders of the venous system produce congestion of the affected tissues and predispose to clot formation because of stagnation of flow and activation of the clotting system.

- Varicose veins are dilated and tortuous veins that result from a sustained increase in pressure that causes the venous valves to become incompetent, allowing for reflux of blood and vein engorgement.

- Thrombophlebitis refers to thrombus formation in a vein and the accompanying inflammatory response in the vessel wall as a result of conditions that obstruct or slow blood flow, increase the activity of the coagulation system, or cause vessel injury. Deep vein thrombosis may be a precursor to pulmonary embolism.

Disorders of the Venous Circulation of the Lower Extremities

Varicose Veins

Varicose, or dilated, tortuous veins of the lower extremities are common and often lead to secondary problems of venous insufficiency (see Fig. 22-12B). Varicose veins are described as being

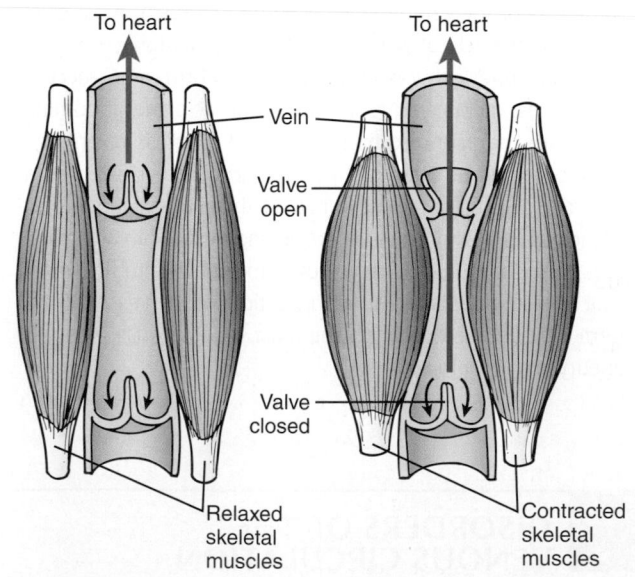

FIGURE 22-13 • The skeletal muscle pumps and their function in promoting blood flow in the deep and superficial calf vessels of the leg.

primary or secondary. Primary varicose veins originate in the superficial saphenous veins, and secondary varicose veins result from impaired flow in the deep venous channels. Approximately 80% to 90% of venous blood from the lower extremities is transported through the deep channels. The development of secondary varicose veins becomes inevitable when flow in these deep channels is impaired or blocked. The most common cause of secondary varicose veins is deep vein thrombosis. Other causes include congenital or acquired arteriovenous fistulas, congenital venous malformations, and pressure on the abdominal veins caused by pregnancy or a tumor.

The prevalence of varicose veins in Western populations is about 25% to 30% in women and 10% to 20% in men. The condition is more common after 50 years of age and in obese persons, and it occurs more often in women, probably because of venous stasis caused by pregnancy.[5] More than 50% of persons with primary varicose veins have a family history of the disorder, suggesting that heredity may play a role.

Mechanisms of Development. Prolonged standing and increased intra-abdominal pressure are important contributing factors in the development of primary varicose veins. Prolonged standing increases venous pressure and causes dilation and stretching of the vessel wall. One of the most important factors in the elevation of venous pressure is the hydrostatic effect associated with the standing position. When a person is in the erect position, the full weight of the venous columns of blood is transmitted to the leg veins. The effects of gravity are compounded in persons who stand for long periods without using their leg muscles to assist in pumping blood back to the heart.

Because there are no valves in the inferior vena cava or common iliac veins, blood in the abdominal veins must be supported by the valves located in the external iliac or femoral veins. When intra-abdominal pressure increases, as it does during pregnancy, or when the valves in these two veins are absent or defective, the stress on the saphenofemoral junction is increased. The high incidence of varicose veins in women who have been pregnant also suggests a hormonal effect on venous smooth muscle contributing to venous dilation and valvular incompetence. Lifting also increases intra-abdominal pressure and decreases flow of blood through the abdominal veins. Occupations that require repeated heavy lifting also predispose to development of varicose veins.

Prolonged exposure to increased pressure causes the venous valves to become incompetent so they no longer close properly. When this happens, the reflux of blood causes further venous enlargement, pulling the valve leaflet apart and causing more valvular incompetence in sections of adjacent distal veins. Another consideration in the development of varicose veins is the fact that the superficial veins have only subcutaneous fat and superficial fascia for support, but the deep venous channels are supported by muscle, bone, and connective tissue. Obesity reduces the support provided by the superficial fascia and tissues, increasing the risk for development of varicose veins.

Manifestations. The signs and symptoms associated with primary varicose veins vary. Most women with superficial varicose veins complain of their unsightly appearance. In many cases, aching in the lower extremities and edema, especially after long periods of standing, may occur. The edema usually subsides at night when the legs are elevated. When the communicating veins are incompetent, symptoms are more common.

Diagnosis and Treatment. The diagnosis of varicose veins often can be made after physical inspection. Several procedures are used to assess the extent of venous involvement associated with varicose veins. In one of these, the Trendelenburg test, a tourniquet is applied to the affected leg while it is elevated and the veins are empty. The person then assumes the standing position, and the tourniquet is removed. If the superficial veins are involved, the veins distend quickly. To assess the deep channels, the tourniquet is applied while the person is standing and the veins are filled. The person then lies down and the affected leg is elevated. Emptying of the superficial veins indicates that the deep channels are patent. The Doppler ultrasonic flow probe also may be used to assess flow in the large vessels. Angiographic studies using a radiopaque contrast medium also are used to assess venous function.

After the venous channels have been repeatedly stretched and the valves rendered incompetent, little can be done to restore normal venous tone and function. Ideally, measures should be taken to prevent the development and progression of varicose veins. These measures center on avoiding activities such as continued standing that produce prolonged elevation of venous pressure. Treatment measures for varicose veins focus on improving venous flow and preventing tissue injury. When correctly fitted, elastic support stockings or leggings compress the superficial veins and prevent distention. The most precise control is afforded by prescription stockings, measured to fit properly. These stockings should be applied before the standing position is assumed, when the leg veins are empty.

Sclerotherapy, which often is used in the treatment of small residual varicosities, involves the injection of a sclerosing agent into the collapsed superficial veins to produce fibrosis of the vessel lumen. Surgical treatment consists of removing the varicosities and the incompetent perforating veins, but it is limited to persons with patent deep venous channels.

Chronic Venous Insufficiency

The term *venous insufficiency* refers to the physiologic consequences of deep vein thrombosis (DVT), valvular incompetence, or a combination of both conditions. The most common cause is DVT, which causes deformity of the valve leaflets, rendering them incapable of closure. In the presence of valvular incompetence, effective unidirectional flow of blood and emptying of the deep veins cannot occur. The muscle pumps also are ineffective, often driving blood in retrograde directions. Secondary failure of the communicating and superficial veins subjects the subcutaneous tissues to high pressures.

With venous insufficiency, there are signs and symptoms associated with impaired blood flow. In contrast to the ischemia caused by arterial insufficiency, venous insufficiency leads to tissue congestion, edema, and eventual impairment of tissue nutrition.[48] The edema is exacerbated by long periods of standing. Necrosis of subcutaneous fat deposits occurs, followed by skin atrophy. Brown pigmentation of the skin caused by hemosiderin deposits resulting from the breakdown of red blood cells is common. Secondary lymphatic insufficiency occurs, with progressive sclerosis of the lymph channels in the face of increased demand for clearance of interstitial fluid.

In advanced venous insufficiency, impaired tissue nutrition causes stasis dermatitis and the development of stasis or venous ulcers (Fig. 22-14). Stasis dermatitis is characterized by the presence of thin, shiny, bluish brown, irregularly pigmented desquamative skin that lacks the support of the underlying subcutaneous tissues. Minor injury leads to relatively painless ulcerations that are difficult to heal. The lower part of the leg is particularly prone to development of stasis dermatitis and venous ulcers. Most lesions are located medially over the ankle and lower leg, with the highest frequency just above the medial malleolus. Venous insufficiency is the most common cause of lower leg ulcers, accounting for nearly 80% of all cases.[49] The other common causes of lower extremity ulcers are arterial insufficiency, neuropathy (often due to diabetes), and pressure ulcers.

Treatment of venous ulcers includes compression therapy with dressings and inelastic or elastic bandages. Medications that help include aspirin and pentoxifylline. Occasionally skin grafting is required for large or slow-healing venous ulcers. Growth factors (which are administered topically or by perilesional injection) may also be warranted.[49] Persons with long-standing venous insufficiency may also experience stiffening of the ankle joint and loss of muscle mass and strength.

Venous Thrombosis

The term *venous thrombosis,* or *thrombophlebitis,* describes the presence of thrombus in a vein and the accompanying inflammatory response in the vessel wall. Thrombi can develop in the superficial or the deep veins. DVT most commonly occurs in the lower extremities. DVT of the lower extremity is a serious disorder, complicated by pulmonary embolism (see Chapter 29), recurrent episodes of DVT, and development of chronic venous insufficiency. Most postoperative thrombi arise in the soleal sinuses or the large veins draining the gastrocnemius muscles.[50] Isolated calf thrombi often are asymptomatic. If left untreated, they may extend to the larger, more proximal veins, with an increased risk of pulmonary emboli (up to 50% risk from proximal DVTs).

In 1846, Virchow described the triad that has come to be associated with venous thrombosis: stasis of blood, increased blood coagulability, and vessel wall injury.[51] Risk factors for venous thrombosis are summarized in Chart 22-2. Stasis of blood occurs with immobility of an extremity or the entire body. Bed rest and immobilization are associated with decreased blood flow, venous pooling in the lower extremities, and increased risk of DVT. Persons who are immobilized by a hip fracture, joint replacement, or spinal cord injury are particularly vulnerable to DVT. The risk of DVT is increased in situations of impaired cardiac function. This may account for the relatively high incidence in persons with acute myocardial infarction and congestive heart failure. Elderly persons are more susceptible than younger persons, probably because disorders that produce venous stasis occur more frequently in older persons. Long airplane travel poses a particular threat in persons predisposed to DVT because of prolonged sitting and increased blood viscosity due to dehydration.[52]

Hypercoagulability is a homeostatic mechanism designed to increase clot formation, and conditions that increase the concentration or activation of clotting factors predispose to DVT. Thrombosis also can be caused by inherited or acquired deficiencies in certain plasma proteins that normally inhibit thrombus formation, such as antithrombin III, protein C, and protein S.[53] However, the most common inherited risk factors are the factor V Leiden and prothrombin gene mutations.[7] The postpartum state is associated with increased levels of fibrinogen, prothrombin, and other coagulation factors. The use of oral

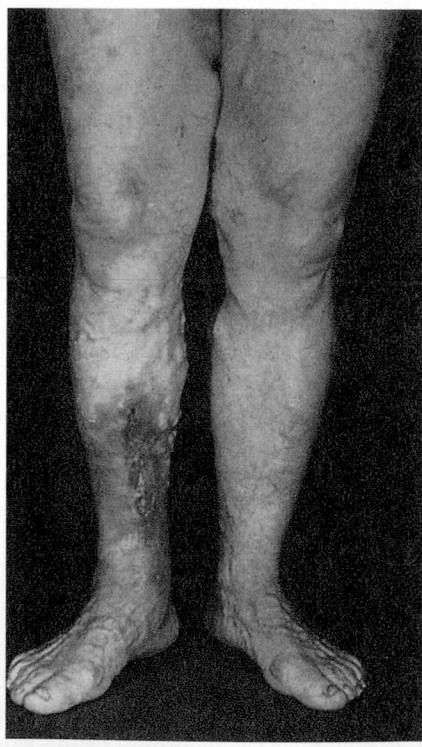

FIGURE 22-14 • Varicose veins of the legs. Severe varicosities of the superficial leg veins have led to stasis dermatitis and secondary ulcerations. (From Gotlieb A. I. [2005]. Blood vessels. In Rubin E., Gorstein F., Rubin R., et al. [Eds.], *Pathology: Clinicopathologic foundations of medicine* [4th ed., p. 514]. Philadelphia: Lippincott Williams & Wilkins.)

CHART 22-2	**RISK FACTORS ASSOCIATED WITH VENOUS THROMBOSIS***

Venous Stasis
Bed rest
Immobility
Spinal cord injury
Acute myocardial infarction
Congestive heart failure
Shock
Venous obstruction

Hyperreactivity of Blood Coagulation
Genetic factors
Stress and trauma
Pregnancy
Childbirth
Oral contraceptive and hormone replacement use
Dehydration
Cancer
Antiphospholipid syndrome
Hyperhomocysteinemia

Vascular Trauma
Indwelling venous catheters
Surgery
Massive trauma or infection
Fractured hip
Orthopedic surgery

*Many of these disorders involve more than one mechanism.

contraceptives and hormone replacement therapy appears to increase coagulability and predispose to venous thrombosis, a risk that is further increased in women who smoke. Certain cancers are associated with increased clotting tendencies, and although the reason for this is largely unknown, substances that promote blood coagulation may be produced by the tumor cells or released from the surrounding tissues in response to the cancerous growth. Immune interactions with cancer cells can result in the release of cytokines that can cause endothelial damage and predispose to thrombosis.[54] Aggressive antitumor therapy can also cause vascular damage. When body fluid is lost because of injury or disease, the resulting hemoconcentration causes clotting factors to become more concentrated. Other important risk factors include the antiphospholipid syndrome and hyperhomocysteinemia.[55]

Vessel injury can result from a trauma situation or from surgical intervention. It also may occur secondary to infection or inflammation of the vessel wall. Persons undergoing hip surgery and total hip replacement are at particular risk because of trauma to the femoral and iliac veins, and in the case of hip replacement, thermal damage from heat generated by the polymerization of the acrylic cement that is used in the procedure.[50] Venous catheters are another source of vascular injury.

Manifestations. Many persons with venous thrombosis are asymptomatic, probably because the vein is not totally occluded or because of collateral circulation.[56] When present, the most common signs and symptoms of venous thrombosis are those related to the inflammatory process: pain, swelling, and deep muscle tenderness. Fever, general malaise, and an elevated white blood cell count and erythrocyte sedimentation rate are accompanying indications of inflammation. There may be tenderness and pain along the vein. Swelling may vary from minimal to maximal. As much as 50% of persons with DVT are asymptomatic.

The site of thrombus formation determines the location of the physical findings. The most common site is in the venous sinuses in the soleus muscle and posterior tibial and peroneal veins (Fig. 22-15). Swelling in these cases involves the foot and ankle, although it may be slight or absent. Calf pain and tenderness are common. Femoral vein thrombosis produces pain and tenderness in the distal thigh and popliteal area. Thrombi in ileofemoral veins produce the most profound manifestations, with swelling, pain, and tenderness of the entire extremity. With DVT in the calf veins, active dorsiflexion produces calf pain (*i.e.,* Homans sign).

Diagnosis and Treatment. The risk of pulmonary embolism emphasizes the need for early detection and treatment of DVT. Several tests are useful for this purpose: ascending venography, ultrasonography (*e.g.,* real-time, B-mode, duplex), and plasma D-dimer assessment[56,57] (see Chapter 29).

Whenever possible, venous thrombosis should be prevented in preference to being treated. Early ambulation after childbirth and surgery is one measure that decreases the risk of thrombus formation. Exercising the legs and wearing support stockings improve venous flow. A further precautionary measure is to avoid assuming body positions that favor venous pooling. Antiembolism stockings of the proper fit and length should be used routinely in persons at risk for DVT. Another strategy used for immobile persons at risk for development of DVT is a sequential pneumatic compression device. This consists of a plastic sleeve that encircles the legs and provides alternating periods of compression on the lower extremity. When properly used, these devices enhance venous emptying to augment flow and reduce stasis. Prophylactic anticoagulation often is used in persons who are at high risk for development of venous thrombi.

The objectives of treatment of venous thrombosis are to prevent the formation of additional thrombi, prevent extension and embolization of existing thrombi, and minimize venous valve damage. A 15- to 20-degree elevation of the legs prevents stasis. It is important that the entire lower extremity or extremities be carefully extended to avoid acute flexion of the knee or hip. Heat often is applied to the leg to relieve venospasm and to aid in the resolution of the inflammatory process. Bed rest usually is maintained until local tenderness and swelling have subsided. Gradual ambulation with elastic support is then permitted. Standing and sitting increase venous pressure and are to be avoided. Elastic support is needed for 3 to 6 months to

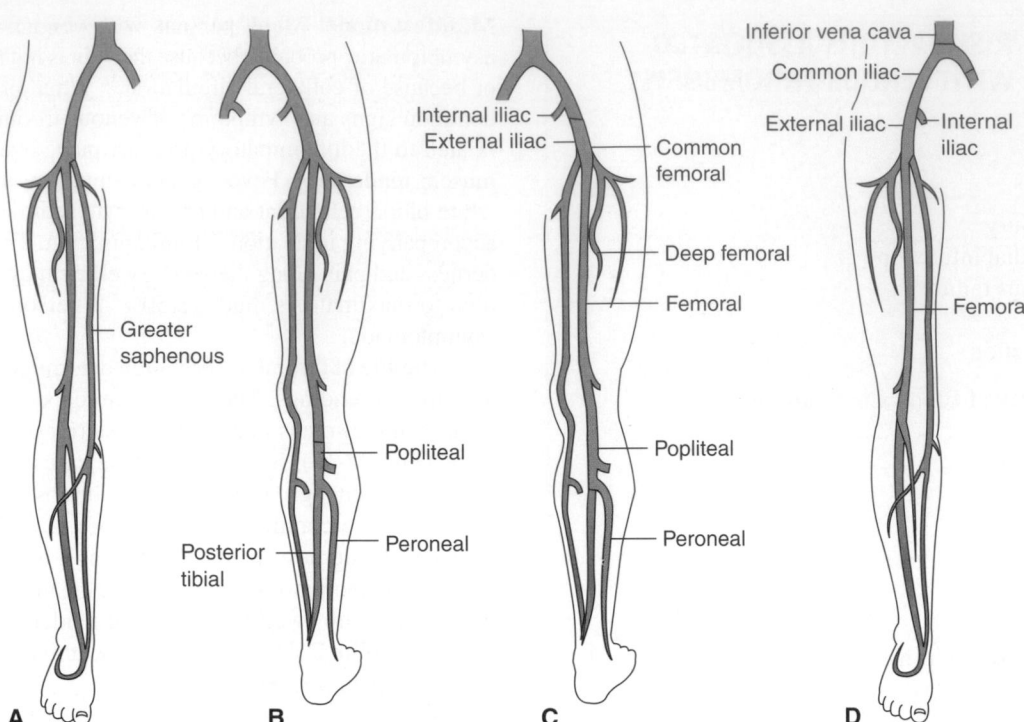

FIGURE 22-15 • Common sites of venous thrombosis. **(A)** Superficial thrombophlebitis. **(B)** Most common form of deep thrombophlebitis. **(C, D)** Deep thrombophlebitis from the calf to iliac veins. (From Haller J. A. Jr. [1967]. *Deep thrombophlebitis: Pathophysiology and treatment.* Philadelphia: W. B. Saunders.)

permit recanalization and collateralization and to prevent venous insufficiency.

Anticoagulation therapy (*i.e.*, heparin and warfarin) is used to treat and prevent venous thrombosis. Treatment typically is initiated with either continuous intravenous infusion of heparin followed by prophylactic therapy with oral anticoagulants to prevent further thrombus formation, or with subcutaneous injections of low–molecular-weight heparin (LMWH). LMWH may also be given on an outpatient basis.[58] The mechanisms of action of the anticoagulant drugs are discussed in Chapter 13. Thrombolytic therapy (*i.e.*, streptokinase, urokinase, or tissue plasminogen activator) may be used in an attempt to dissolve the clot.

Surgical removal of the thrombus may be undertaken in selected cases. Percutaneous (through the skin) insertion of intracaval filters may be done in persons at high risk for development of pulmonary emboli. This procedure prevents large clots from moving through the vessel. However, although filters prevent the development of pulmonary emboli, an increase in thrombosis occurs at the site of the filter itself in the absence of anticoagulation.

IN SUMMARY,   the storage function of the venous system renders it susceptible to venous insufficiency, stasis, and thrombus formation. Varicose veins occur with prolonged distention and stretching of the superficial veins owing to venous insuffi-

ciency. Varicosities can arise because of defects in the superficial veins (*i.e.*, primary varicose veins) or because of impaired blood flow in the deep venous channels (*i.e.*, secondary varicose veins). Venous insufficiency reflects chronic venous stasis resulting from valvular incompetence. It is associated with stasis dermatitis and stasis or venous ulcers. Venous thrombosis describes the presence of thrombus in a vein and the accompanying inflammatory response in the vessel wall. It is associated with vessel injury, stasis of venous flow, and hypercoagulability states. Thrombi can develop in the superficial or the deep veins (*i.e.*, DVT). Thrombus formation in deep veins is a precursor to venous insufficiency and embolus formation. ■

Review Exercises

1. The Third Report of the NCEP Expert Panel on Detection, Evaluation, and Treatment of High Cholesterol in Adults recommends that a person's HDL should be above 40 mg/dL.

   A. *Explain the role of HDL in prevention of atherosclerosis.*

2. A 55-year-old male executive presents at the clinic for his regular check-up. He was diagnosed with

hypertension 5 years ago and has been taking a diuretic and a β-adrenergic blocker to control his blood pressure. His blood pressure is currently being maintained at about 135/70 mm Hg. His total cholesterol level is 180 mg/dL and his HDL cholesterol is 30 mg/dL. He is otherwise well. He is a nonsmoker. He has recently read in the media about "inflammation" and the heart and expresses concern about his risk of coronary heart disease.

A. *Use the risk assessment tool based on the Framingham Heart Study to calculate this man's 10-year risk of developing myocardial infarction and coronary death (available at www.nhlbi.nih.gov/ guidelines/cholesterol/).*

3. A 55-year-old man presents at the emergency department of his local hospital with complaints of excruciating, "ripping" pain in his upper back. He has a history of poorly controlled hypertension. His radial pulse and blood pressure, which on admission were 92 and 140/80 mm Hg, respectively, become unobtainable in both arms. A transesophageal echocardiogram reveals a dissection of the descending aorta. Aggressive blood pressure control is initiated with the goal of reducing the systolic pressure and pulsatile blood flow (pulse pressure).

A. *Explain how aortic dissection differs from a thoracic aorta aneurysm.*

B. *Explain the role of poorly controlled hypertension as an etiologic factor in dissecting aneurysms.*

C. *Why did his radial pulse and blood pressure become unobtainable?*

D. *Explain the need for aggressive control of aortic pressure and pulsatile blood flow.*

4. A 34-year-old, otherwise healthy woman complains of episodes lasting several hours in which her fingers become pale and numb. This is followed by a period during which the fingers become red, throbbing, and painful.

A. *What do you think is causing this woman's problem?*

B. *She relates that the episodes often occur when her fingers become cold or when she becomes upset. Explain the possible underlying mechanisms.*

C. *What types of measures could be used to treat this woman?*

References

1. Schoen F. J., Cotran R. S. (2005). Blood vessels. In Kumar V., Abbas A. K., Fausto N. (Eds.), *Pathologic basis of disease* (8th ed., pp. 511–541). Philadelphia: Elsevier Saunders.
2. Ross M. H., Kaye G. L., Pawlina W. (2005). *Histology: A text and atlas* (4th ed., pp. 326–342). Philadelphia: Lippincott Williams & Wilkins.
3. Guyton A., Hall J. E. (2006). *Textbook of medical physiology* (11th ed., pp. 840–851). Philadelphia: W. B. Saunders.
4. American Heart Association. (2008). Cholesterol statistics. [Online.] Available: www.americanheart.org/presenter.jhtml?identifier=4506. Accessed March 12, 2008.
5. Gottlieb A. I. (2005). Blood vessels. In Rubin E., Gorstein F., Rubin R., et al. (Eds.), *Pathology: Clinicopathologic foundations of medicine* (4th ed., pp. 473–519). Philadelphia: Lippincott Williams & Wilkins.
6. Beisiegel U. (1998). Lipoprotein metabolism. *European Heart Journal* 19(Suppl. A), A20–A23.
7. Nabel E. G. (2003). Genomic medicine—cardiovascular disease. *New England Journal of Medicine* 349, 60–72.
8. Lusis A. J. (2000). Atherosclerosis. *Nature* 407, 233–241.
9. Harper C. R., Jacobson T. A. (1999). New perspectives on the management of low levels of high-density lipoprotein cholesterol. *Archives of Internal Medicine* 159, 1049–1057.
10. Kreisberg R. A., Oberman A. (2003). Medical management of hyperlipidemia/dyslipidemia. *Journal of Clinical Endocrinology and Metabolism* 88, 2445–2461.
11. Oram J. F. (2002). ATP-binding cassette transporter A1 and cholesterol trafficking. *Current Opinions in Lipidology* 13, 373–381.
12. National Institute of Health Expert Panel. (2001). *Third Report of the National Cholesterol Education Program (NCEP) Expert Panel on Detection, Evaluation, and Treatment of High Blood Cholesterol in Adults (Adult Treatment Panel III).* NIH publication no. 01-3670. Bethesda, MD: National Institutes of Health.
13. Grundy S. M., Cleeman J. I., Merz C. N., et al. (2004). Implications of recent clinical trials for the National Cholesterol Education Program (NCEP) Adult Treatment Panel III guidelines. *Journal of the American College of Cardiology* 44, 720–732.
14. Goldberg R. B. (1988). Dietary modification of cholesterol levels. *Consultant* 28(Suppl. 6), 35–41.
15. American Heart Association Dietary Guidelines Revision. (2006). A statement for healthcare professionals from the Nutrition Committee of the American Heart Association. *Circulation* 114, 82–96.
16. Heart Protection Study Collaborative Group. (2002). MRC/BHF Heart Protection Study of cholesterol lowering with simvastatin in 20,536 high-risk individuals: A randomised placebo-controlled trial. *Lancet* 360, 7–22.
17. Sinatra S. T. (2003). Is cholesterol lowering with statins the gold standard for treating patients with cardiovascular risk and disease? *Southern Medical Journal* 96, 220–223.
18. American Heart Association. (2008). Heart disease and stroke statistics. [Online.] Available: www.americanheart.org/downloadable/heart/1200082005246GHS_Stats%202008.final.pdf. Accessed March 12, 2008.
19. Enos W. F., Beyer J. C., Holmes R. F. (1955). Pathogenesis of coronary artery disease in American soldiers killed in Korea. *Journal of the American Medical Association* 158, 912.
20. Ross R. (1999). Mechanisms of disease: Atherosclerosis—an inflammatory disease. *New England Journal of Medicine* 340, 115–126.
21. Kullo I. J., Gau G. T., Tajik A. J. (2000). Novel risk factors for atherosclerosis. *Mayo Clinic Proceedings* 75, 369–380.
22. Glasser S. P., Selwyn A. P., Ganz P. (1996). Atherosclerosis: Risk factors and the vascular endothelium. *American Heart Journal* 31, 379–384.
23. Levine G. N., Keaney J. F., Vita J. A. (1995). Cholesterol reduction in cardiovascular disease. *New England Journal of Medicine* 332, 512–521.
24. Gaziano J. M., Hebert P. R., Hennekens C. H. (1996). Cholesterol reduction: Weighing the benefits and risks. *Annals of Internal Medicine* 124, 914–918.
25. Libby P., Ridker P. M., Maseri A. (2003). Inflammation and atherosclerosis. *Circulation* 105, 1135–1143.
26. Lloyd Jones D. M. (2006). Assessment of C-reactive protein for risk prediction for cardiovascular. *Annals of Internal Medicine* 145, 5–42.
27. Lonn E., Yusuf S., Arnold M. J., et al. (2006). Homocysteine lowering with folic acid and B vitamins in vascular disease. *New England Journal of Medicine* 354, 1567–1577.
28. Fong I. W. (2000). Emerging relations between infectious diseases and coronary artery disease and atherosclerosis. *Canadian Medical Association Journal* 163, 49–56.

29. Fuster V., Moreno P. R., Fayad Z. A., et al. (2005). Atherothrombosis and high-risk plaque: Part I. Evolving concepts. *Journal of the American College of Cardiology* 46, 937–954.

30. Savage C. O. S., Harper L., Cockwell P., et al. (2000). Vasculitis. Clinical review: ABC of arterial and vascular disease. *British Medical Journal* 320, 1325–1328.

31. Gross W. L., Trabandt A., Reinhold-Keller E. (2000). Diagnosis and evaluation of vasculitis. *Rheumatology* 39, 245–252.

32. Longford C. A. (2003) Treatment of ANCA-associated vasculitis. *New England Journal of Medicine* 349, 3–5.

33. Jayne D. (2000). Evidence-based treatment of systemic vasculitis. *Rheumatology* 39, 585–595.

34. Weyand C. M., Goronzy J. J. (2003). Medium- and large-vessel vasculitis. *New England Journal of Medicine* 349, 160–169.

35. Bartholomew J. R., Gray B. H. (1999). Large artery occlusive disease. *Rheumatic Disease Clinics of North America* 25, 669–686.

36. Cassar K., Bachoo P. (2006). Peripheral arterial disease. *Clinical Evidence Concise* 15, 35–37.

37. Burns P., Gough S., Bradbury A. W. (2003). The management of peripheral artery disease in primary care. *British Medical Journal* 326, 584–588.

38. Olin J. W. (2000). Thromboangiitis obliterans (Buerger's disease). *New England Journal of Medicine* 343, 864–869.

39. Belch J. (1997). Raynaud's phenomenon. *Cardiovascular Research* 33, 25–30.

40. Pope J. (2006). Raynaud's phenomenon. *Clinical Evidence Concise* 15, 436–437.

41. Block J. A., Sequeira W. (2001). Raynaud's phenomenon. *Lancet* 357, 2042–2048.

42. Sakalihasen N. (2005). Abdominal aortic aneurysms. *Lancet* 365, 1577–1589.

43. Thompson R. W. (2002). Detection and management of small aortic aneurysms. *New England Journal of Medicine* 346, 1484–1486.

44. Isselbacher E. M. (2005). Thoracic and abdominal aortic aneurysm. *Circulation* 111, 816–828.

45. Coady M. A., Rizzo J. A., Goldstein L. J., et al. (1999). Natural history, pathogenesis, and etiology of thoracic aortic aneurysms and dissections. *Cardiology Clinics of North America* 17, 615–635.

46. House-Fancher M. A. (1996). Aortic dissection: Pathophysiology, diagnosis, and acute care management. *AACN Clinical Issues* 6, 602–614.

47. Alguire P. C., Mathes B. M. (1999). Chronic venous insufficiency and venous ulceration. *Journal of General Internal Medicine* 12, 374–334.

48. Tisi P. (2006). Varicose veins. *Clinical Evidence Concise* 15, 61–63.

49. Nelson E. A., Cullun N., Jones J. (2006). Venous leg ulcers. *Clinical Evidence Concise* 15, 657–660.

50. McManus R. (2006). Thromboembolism. *Clinical Evidence Concise* 15, 56–60.

51. Virchow R. (1846). Weinere Untersuchungen uber die Verstropfung der Lungenrarterie und ihre Folgen. *Beitrage zur Experimentelle Pathologie und Physiologie* 2, 21.

52. Schurr J. H., Machin S. J., Bailey-King S., et al. (2001). Frequency and prevention of symptomless deep-vein thrombosis in long-haul flights. *Lancet* 357, 1485–1489.

53. Sheppard D. R. (2000). Activated protein C resistance: The most common risk factor for venous thromboembolism. *Journal of the American Board of Family Practice* 13, 111–115.

54. Bick R. L. (2003). Cancer-associated thrombosis. *New England Journal of Medicine* 349, 109–111.

55. Levine J. S., Branch D. W., Rauch J. (2002). The antiphospholipid syndrome. *New England Journal of Medicine* 346, 752–763.

56. Wells P. S., Owen C., Doucette S., et al. (2006). Does this patient have deep vein thrombosis? *Journal of the American Medical Association* 295, 199–207.

57. Kelly J., Hunt B. J. (2002). Role of D-dimers in diagnosis of venous thromboembolism. *Lancet* 359, 456–458.

58. Blann A. D., Lip G. Y. (2006). Venous thromboembolism. *British Medical Journal* 332, 215–219.

Visit the Point. **http://thePoint.lww.com for animations, journal articles, and more!**

Disorders of Blood Pressure Regulation

CAROL M. PORTH

➤ Blood pressure is probably one of the most variable but best-regulated functions of the body. The purpose of the control of blood pressure is to keep blood flow constant to vital organs such as the heart, brain, and kidneys. Without constant blood flow to these organs, death ensues within seconds, minutes, or days. Although a decrease in flow produces an immediate threat to life, the continuous elevation of blood pressure that occurs with hypertension is a contributor to premature death and disability because of its effects on the heart, blood vessels, and kidneys.

The discussion in this chapter focuses on determinants of blood pressure and conditions of altered arterial pressure—hypertension and orthostatic hypotension.

THE ARTERIAL BLOOD PRESSURE

After completing this section of the chapter, you should be able to meet the following objectives:

■ Define the terms *systolic blood pressure, diastolic blood pressure, pulse pressure,* and *mean arterial blood pressure.*

■ Explain how cardiac output and peripheral vascular resistance interact in determining systolic and diastolic blood pressure.

■ Describe the mechanisms for short-term and long-term regulation of blood pressure.

■ Describe the requirements for accurate and reliable blood pressure measurement in terms of cuff size, determining the maximum inflation pressure, and deflation rate.

The arterial blood pressure reflects the rhythmic ejection of blood from the left ventricle into the aorta.[1-3] It rises during systole as the left ventricle contracts and falls as the heart relaxes during diastole. The contour of the arterial pressure tracing shown in Figure 23-1 is typical of the pressure changes that occur in the large arteries of the systemic circulation. There is a rapid rise in the pulse contour during left ventricular contraction, followed by a slower rise to peak pressure. Approximately 70% of the blood that leaves the left ventricle is ejected during the first one third of systole, accounting for the rapid rise in the pressure contour. The end of systole is marked by a brief down-

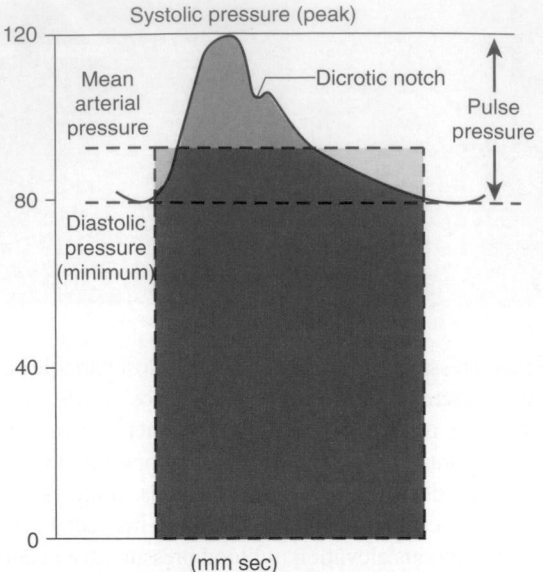

FIGURE 23-1 • Intra-arterial pressure tracing made from the brachial artery. Pulse pressure is the difference between systolic and diastolic pressures. The darker area represents the mean arterial pressure, which can be calculated by using the formula of mean arterial pressure = diastolic pressure + pulse pressure/3.

ward deflection and formation of the dicrotic notch, which occurs when ventricular pressure falls below that in the aorta. The sudden closure of the aortic valve is associated with a small rise in pressure caused by continued contraction of the aorta and other large vessels against the closed valve. As the ventricles relax and blood flows into the peripheral vessels during diastole, the arterial pressure falls rapidly at first and then declines slowly as the driving force decreases.

The pressure at the height of the pressure pulse, called the *systolic pressure,* ideally is less than 120 mm Hg, and the lowest pressure, called the *diastolic pressure,* is less than 80 mm Hg (Fig. 23-2). The difference between the systolic and diastolic pressure (approximately 40 mm Hg in healthy adults) is called the *pulse pressure.* The magnitude of the pulse pressure reflects the volume of blood ejected from the left ventricle during a single beat (stroke volume) and the total distensibility of the atrial tree. The *mean arterial pressure* (approximately 90 to 100 mm Hg), represents the average pressure in the arterial system during ventricular contraction and relaxation and is a good indicator of tissue perfusion. Notice that the mean arterial pressure is not a simple mathematical average of systolic and diastolic pressures. This is because a greater fraction of each cardiac cycle is spent in diastole rather than in systole.

The mean arterial blood pressure is determined mainly by the cardiac output (stroke volume × heart rate) and the peripheral vascular resistance, and can be expressed as the product of the two (mean arterial blood pressure = cardiac output × peripheral vascular resistance). The peripheral vascular resistance reflects changes in the radius of the arterioles as well as the viscosity or thickness of the blood (see Chapter 21 for a discussion of cardiac output and peripheral vascular resistance). The arterioles often

are referred to as the resistance vessels because they can selectively constrict or relax to control the resistance to outflow of blood into the capillaries. The body maintains its blood pressure by adjusting the cardiac output to compensate for changes in peripheral vascular resistance and changes the peripheral vascular resistance to compensate for changes in cardiac output.

In hypertension and disease conditions that affect blood pressure, changes in blood pressure usually are described in terms of the systolic and diastolic pressures, pulse pressure, and mean arterial pressure. These pressures are influenced by the stroke volume, the rapidity with which blood is ejected from the heart, the elastic properties of the aorta and large arteries and their ability to accept various amounts of blood as it is ejected from the heart, and the properties of the resistance blood vessels that control the runoff of blood into the smaller vessels and capillaries that connect the arterial and venous circulations.

Mechanisms of Blood Pressure Regulation

Although different tissues in the body are able to regulate their own blood flow, it is necessary for the arterial pressure to remain relatively constant as blood shifts from one area of the body to another. The mechanisms used to regulate the arterial pressure depend on whether short-term or long-term adaptation is needed[2] (Fig. 23-2).

Short-Term Regulation

The mechanisms for short-term regulation of blood pressure, those acting over minutes or hours, are intended to correct temporary imbalances in blood pressure, such as occur during physical exercise and changes in body position. These mechanisms also are responsible for maintenance of blood pressure at survival levels during life-threatening situations such as during an acute hemorrhagic incident. The short-term regulation of blood pressure relies mainly on neural and humoral mechanisms, the most rapid of which are the neural mechanisms.

Neural Mechanisms. The neural control centers for the regulation of blood pressure are located in the reticular formation of the medulla and lower third of the pons, where integration and modulation of autonomic nervous system (ANS) responses occur.[2] This area of the brain contains the vasomotor and cardiac control centers and is often collectively referred to as the *cardiovascular center.* The cardiovascular center transmits parasympathetic impulses to the heart through the vagus nerve and sympathetic impulses to the heart and blood vessels through the spinal cord and peripheral sympathetic nerves. Vagal stimulation of the heart produces a slowing of heart rate, whereas sympathetic stimulation produces an increase in heart rate and cardiac contractility. Blood vessels are selectively innervated by the sympathetic nervous system. Increased sympathetic activity produces constriction of the small arteries and arterioles with a resultant increase in peripheral vascular resistance.

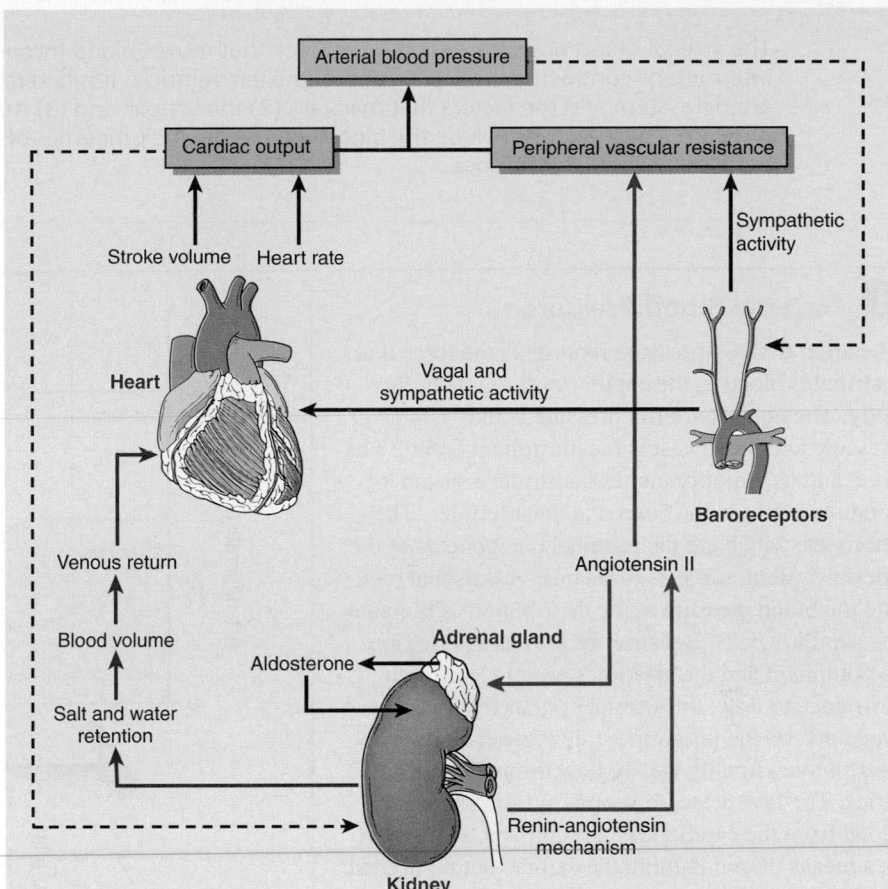

FIGURE 23-2 • Mechanisms of blood pressure regulation. The *solid lines* represent the mechanisms for renal and baroreceptor control of blood pressure through changes in cardiac output and peripheral vascular resistance. The *dashed lines* represent the stimulus for regulation of blood pressure by the baroreceptors and the kidneys.

The ANS control of blood pressure is mediated through intrinsic circulatory reflexes, extrinsic reflexes, and higher neural control centers. The *intrinsic reflexes,* including the *baroreceptor* and *chemoreceptor reflexes,* are located in the circulatory system and are essential for rapid and short-term regulation of blood pressure. The sensors for *extrinsic reflexes* are found outside the circulation. They include blood pressure responses associated with factors such as pain and cold. The neural pathways for these reactions are more diffuse, and their responses are less consistent than those of the intrinsic reflexes. Many of these responses are channeled through the hypothalamus, which plays an essential role in the control of sympathetic nervous system responses. Among higher-center responses are those caused by changes in mood and emotion.

The *baroreceptors* are pressure-sensitive receptors located in the walls of blood vessels and the heart. The carotid and aortic baroreceptors are located in strategic positions between the heart and the brain (Fig. 23-3). They respond to changes in the stretch of the vessel wall by sending impulses to cardiovascular centers in the brain stem to effect appropriate changes in heart rate and vascular smooth muscle tone. For example, the fall in blood pressure that occurs on moving from the lying to the standing position produces a decrease in the stretch of the baroreceptors with a resultant increase in heart rate and sympathetically induced

vasoconstriction that causes an increase in peripheral vascular resistance.

The *arterial chemoreceptors* are chemosensitive cells that monitor the oxygen, carbon dioxide, and hydrogen ion content of the blood. They are located in the carotid bodies, which lie in the bifurcation of the two common carotids, and in the aortic bodies of the aorta (see Fig. 23-3). Because of their location, these chemoreceptors are always in close contact with the arterial blood. Although the main function of the chemoreceptors is to regulate ventilation, they also communicate with cardiovascular centers in the brain stem and can induce widespread vasoconstriction. Whenever the arterial pressure drops below a critical level, the chemoreceptors are stimulated because of diminished oxygen supply and a buildup of carbon dioxide and hydrogen ions. In persons with chronic lung disease, systemic and pulmonary hypertension may develop because of hypoxemia (see Chapter 29). Persons with sleep apnea also may experience an increase in blood pressure because of the hypoxemia that occurs during the apneic periods.

Humoral Mechanisms. A number of humoral mechanisms contribute to blood pressure regulation, including the *renin-angiotensin-aldosterone system* and *vasopressin.* Other humoral substances, such as epinephrine, a sympathetic neurotransmitter

Understanding • Determinants of Blood Pressure

The arterial blood pressure, which is the force that moves blood through the arterial system, reflects the intermittent contraction and relaxation of the left ventricle. It is determined by (1) the properties of the arterial system and the factors that maintain (2) the systolic and (3) the diastolic components of the blood pressure. These factors include the blood volume, elastic properties of the blood vessels, cardiac output, and peripheral vascular resistance.

❶ Arterial Blood Pressure

The arterial blood pressure represents the force that distributes blood to the capillaries throughout the body. The highest arterial pressure is the systolic pressure and the lowest is the diastolic pressure. The aorta and its major branches constitute a system of conduits between the heart and the arterioles. The arterioles, which are the terminal components of the arterial system, serve as resistance vessels that regulate the blood pressure at the distribution of blood to the capillary beds. Because the normal arteries are so compliant and the arterioles present such high resistance to flow, the arterial system acts as a filter that converts the intermittent flow generated by the heart into a virtually steady flow through the capillaries. The low-pressure venous system collects blood from the capillaries and returns it to the heart as a means of maintaining the cardiac output needed to sustain arterial pressure.

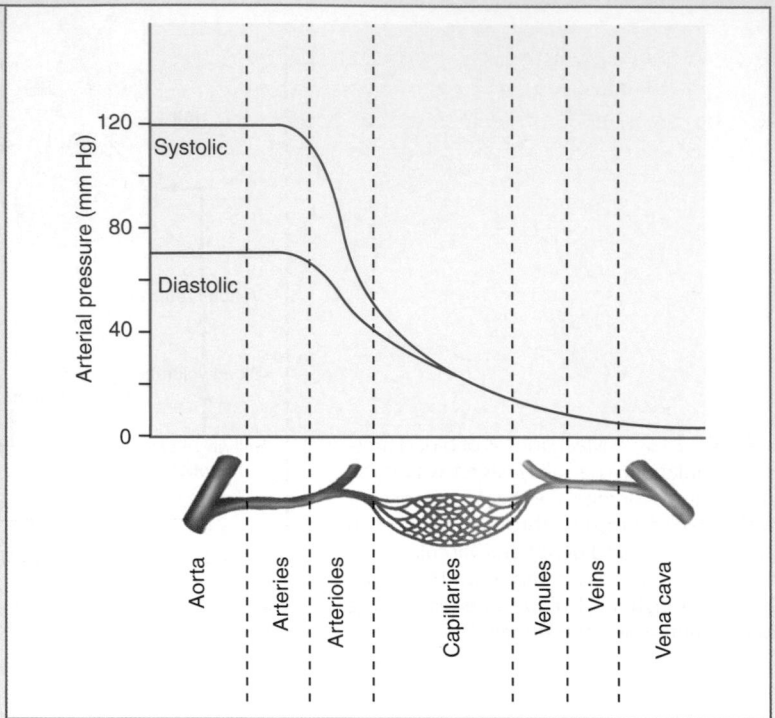

❷ Systolic Pressure

The systolic blood pressure reflects the amount of blood (stroke volume) that is ejected from the heart with each beat, the rate and force with which it is ejected, and the elasticity or compliance of the aorta and large arteries. The blood that is ejected from the heart during systole does not move directly through the circulation. Instead, a substantial fraction of the stroke volume is stored in large arteries. Because the walls of these vessels are elastic, they can be stretched to accommodate a large volume of blood without an appreciable change in pressure. The systolic pressure often increases with aging as the aorta and large arteries lose their elasticity and become more rigid.

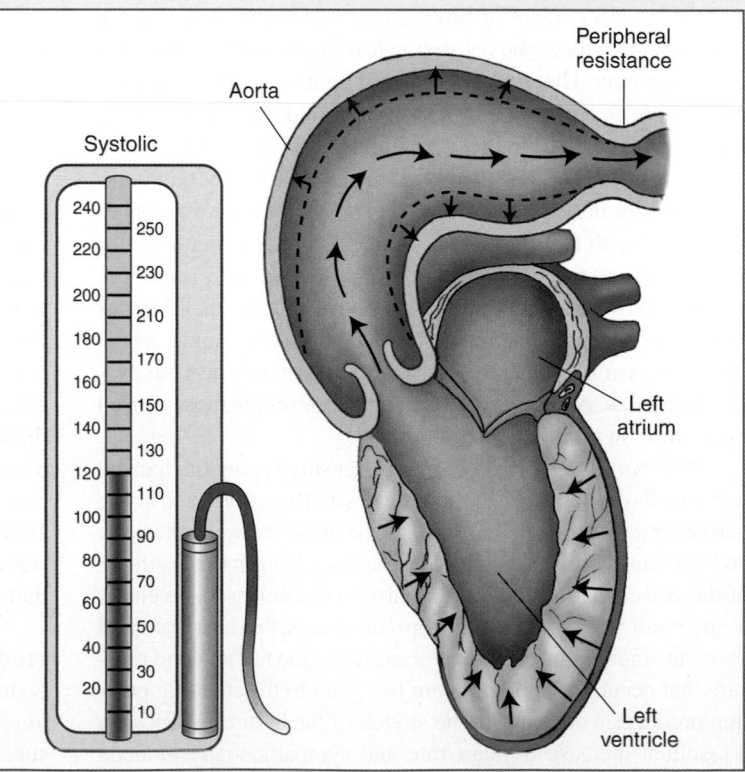

❸ Diastolic Pressure

The diastolic blood pressure reflects the closure of the aortic valve, the energy that has been stored in the elastic fibers of the large arteries during systole, and the resistance to flow through arterioles into the capillaries. Closure of the aortic valve at the onset of diastole and recoil of the elastic fibers in the aorta and large arteries continue to drive the blood forward, even though the heart is not pumping. These effects, largely restricted to the elastic vessels, convert the discontinuous systolic flow in the ascending aorta into a continuous flow in the peripheral arteries.

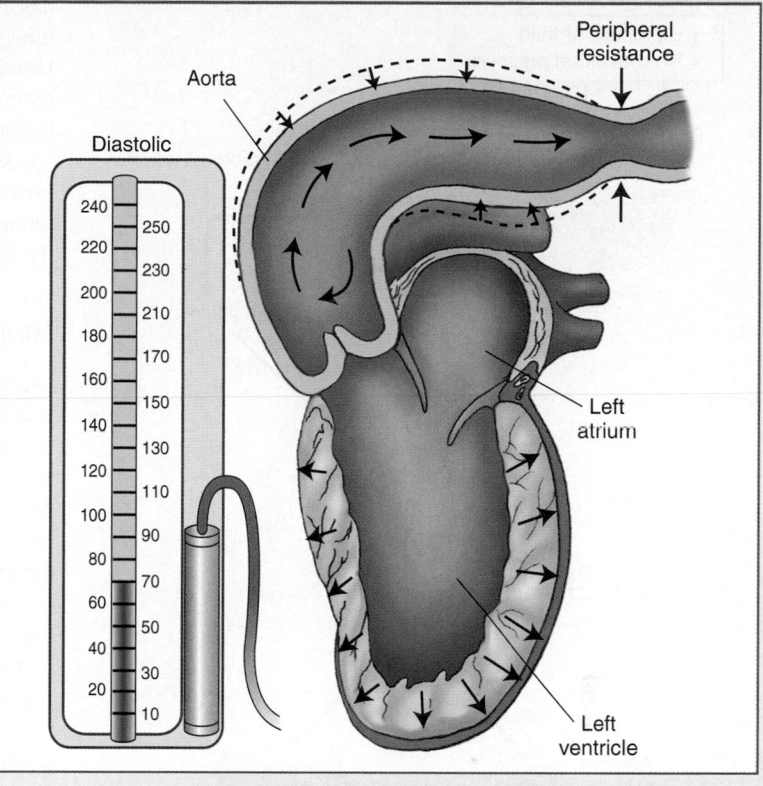

released from the adrenal gland, have the effect of directly stimulating an increase in heart rate, cardiac contractility, and vascular tone.

The *renin-angiotensin-aldosterone system* plays a central role in blood pressure regulation. Renin is an enzyme that is synthesized, stored, and released by the juxtaglomerular cells of the kidneys in response to an increase in sympathetic nervous system activity or a decrease in blood pressure, extracellular fluid volume, or extracellular sodium concentration. Most of the renin that is released leaves the kidney and enters the bloodstream, where it acts enzymatically to convert an inactive circulating plasma protein called *angiotensinogen* to angiotensin I (Fig. 23-4). Angiotensin I is then converted to angiotensin II. This conversion occurs almost entirely in the lungs, while blood flows through the small vessels of the lung, catalyzed by an enzyme called the *angiotensin-converting enzyme* that is present in the endothelium of the lung vessels. Although angiotensin II has a half-life of only several minutes, renin persists in the circulation for 30 minutes to 1 hour and continues to cause production of angiotensin II during this time.

Angiotensin II functions in both the short- and long-term regulation of blood pressure. It is a strong vasoconstrictor, particularly of arterioles and, to a lesser extent, of veins. Constriction of the arterioles increases the peripheral vascular resistance, thereby contributing to the short-term regulation of blood pressure. Angiotensin II also reduces sodium excretion by increasing sodium reabsorption by the proximal tubules of the kidney. A second major function of angiotensin II, stimulation of aldo-

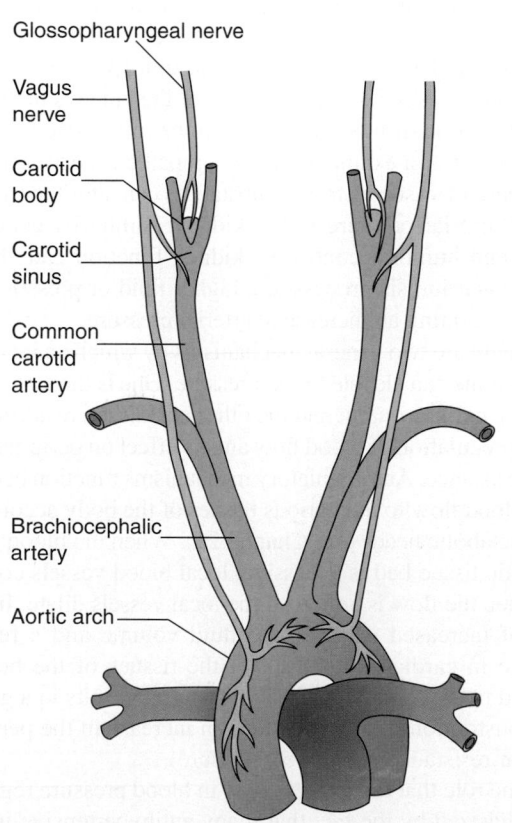

FIGURE 23-3 • Location and innervation of the aortic arch and carotid sinus baroreceptors and carotid body chemoreceptors.

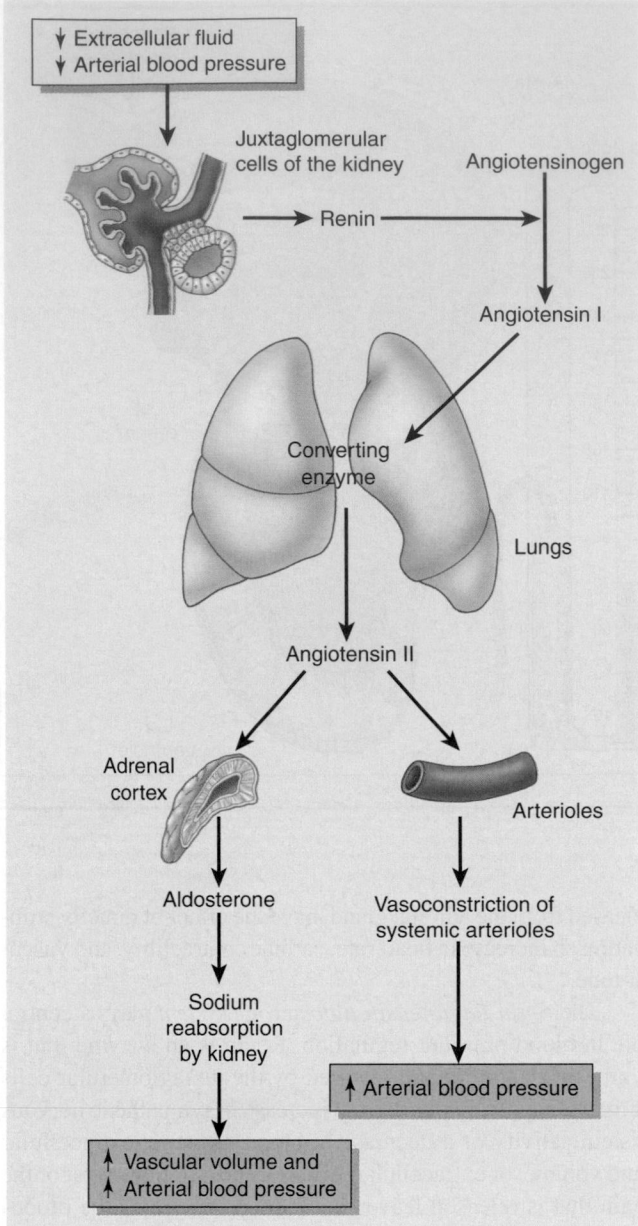

FIGURE 23-4 • Control of blood pressure by the renin-angiotensin-aldosterone system. Renin enzymatically converts the plasma protein angiotensinogen to angiotensin I; angiotensin-converting enzyme in the lung converts angiotensin I to angiotensin II; and angiotensin II produces vasoconstriction and increases salt and water retention through direct action on the kidney and through increased aldosterone secretion by the adrenal cortex.

sterone secretion from the adrenal gland, contributes to the long-term regulation of blood pressure by increasing salt and water retention by the kidney.

Vasopressin, also known as antidiuretic hormone (ADH), is released from the posterior pituitary gland in response to decreases in blood volume and blood pressure, an increase in the osmolality of body fluids, and other stimuli. The antidiuretic actions of vasopressin are discussed in Chapter 31. Vasopressin

has a direct vasoconstrictor effect, particularly on the vessels of the splanchnic circulation that supplies the abdominal viscera. However, long-term increases in vasopressin cannot maintain an increase in blood pressure, and vasopressin does not enhance hypertension produced by sodium-retaining hormones or other vasoconstricting substances. It has been suggested that vasopressin plays a permissive role in hypertension through its water-retaining properties or as a neurotransmitter that serves to modify ANS function.

Long-Term Regulation

Long-term mechanisms control the daily, weekly, and monthly regulation of blood pressure. Although the neural and hormonal mechanisms involved in the short-term regulation of blood pressure act rapidly, they are unable to maintain their effectiveness over time. Instead, the long-term regulation of blood pressure is largely vested in the kidneys and their role in the regulation of the extracellular fluid volume.[2]

According to the late Arthur Guyton, a noted physiologist, the extracellular fluid volume and arterial blood pressure are regulated around an equilibrium point, which represents the normal pressure for a given individual[2] (Fig. 23-5). When the body contains excess extracellular fluids because of increased water and salt intake, the arterial pressure rises, and the rate at which water (*i.e., pressure diuresis*) and salt (*i.e., pressure natriuresis*) are excreted by the kidney is increased. Accordingly, there are two ways that arterial pressure can be increased using this model: one is by shifting the elimination of salt and water to a higher pressure level (see Fig. 23-5A), and the second is by changing the extracellular fluid level at which diuresis and natriuresis occur (see Fig. 23-5B). The function of the kidneys in the long-term regulation of blood pressure can be influenced by a number of factors. For example, excess sympathetic nerve activity or the release of vasoconstrictor substances can alter the transmission of arterial pressure to the kidney. Similarly, changes in neural and humoral control of kidney function can shift the diuresis–natriuresis process to a higher fluid or pressure level, thereby initiating an increase in arterial pressure.

There are two general mechanisms by which an increase in fluid volume can elevate blood pressure. One is through a direct effect on cardiac output and the other is indirect, resulting from the autoregulation of blood flow and its effect on peripheral vascular resistance. Autoregulatory mechanisms function in distributing blood flow to the various tissues of the body according to their metabolic needs (see Chapter 21). When the blood flow to a specific tissue bed is excessive, local blood vessels constrict, and when the flow is deficient, the local vessels dilate. In situations of increased extracellular fluid volume and a resultant increase in cardiac output, all of the tissues of the body are exposed to the same increase in flow. This results in a generalized constriction of arterioles and an increase in the peripheral vascular resistance (and blood pressure).

The role that the kidneys play in blood pressure regulation is emphasized by the fact that many antihypertensive medications produce their blood pressure–lowering effects by increasing sodium and water elimination.

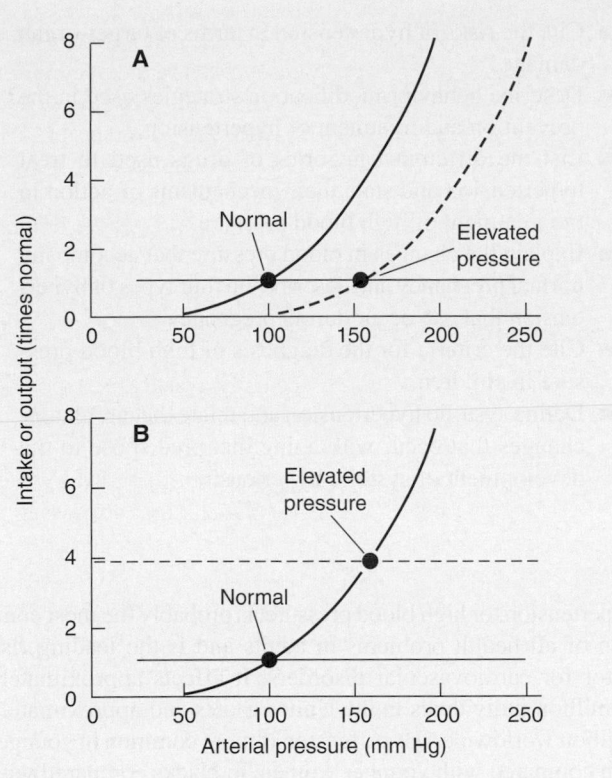

FIGURE 23-5 • Two ways in which the arterial pressure can be increased: **(A)** by shifting the renal output curve in the right-hand direction toward a higher pressure level, and **(B)** by increasing the intake of salt and water. (From Guyton A. C., Hall J. E. [2006]. *Textbook of medical physiology* [11th ed., p. 218]. Philadelphia: Elsevier Saunders.)

Blood Pressure Measurement

Arterial blood pressure measurements usually are obtained by the *indirect auscultatory method,* which uses a stethoscope and a well-calibrated sphygmomanometer. In the measurement of blood pressure, a cuff that contains an inflatable rubber bladder is placed around the upper arm. The bladder of the cuff is inflated to a point at which its pressure exceeds that of the artery, occluding the blood flow. This should be done by palpation before the actual pressure is measured to get the palpated systolic pressure. By inflating the pressure in the cuff to a level of 30 mm Hg above the palpated pressure, the observer can be certain that the cuff pressure is high enough to avoid missing the auscultatory gap. This pressure (palpated pressure + 30 mm Hg) is called the *maximum inflation level.*[4] The cuff is then slowly deflated at 2 mm Hg per second. At the point where the pressure in the vessel again exceeds the pressure in the cuff, a small amount of blood squirts through the partially obstructed artery. The sounds generated by the turbulent flow are called the *Korotkoff (K) sounds.* These low-pitched sounds are best heard with the bell of the stethoscope. Blood pressure is recorded in terms of systolic and diastolic pressures (*e.g.,* 120/70 mm Hg) unless sounds are heard to zero, in which case

three readings are required (122/64/0 or K1/K4/K5). Systolic pressure is defined as the first of two or more Korotkoff sounds heard (K1). Diastolic pressure is recorded as the last sound heard (K5) unless sounds are heard to zero, in which case the muffling sound of K4 is used.

It is important that the bladder of the cuff be appropriate for the arm size. The width of the bladder should be at least 40% of arm circumference and the length at least 80% of arm circumference.[4] Undercuffing (using a cuff with a bladder that is too small) can cause blood pressure to be overestimated.[5] This is because a cuff that is too small results in an uneven distribution of pressure across the arm, such that a greater cuff pressure is needed to occlude blood flow. Likewise, overcuffing (using a cuff with a bladder that is too large) can cause an underestimation of blood pressure.

Automated or *semiautomated methods* of blood pressure measurement use a microphone, arterial pressure pulse sensor (oscillometric method), or Doppler equipment for detecting the equivalent of the Korotkoff sounds. Oscillometric measurement, the most commonly used method, depends on the detection of the pulsatile oscillations of the brachial artery in the blood pressure cuff.[6] In contrast to the auscultatory method, this method determines the mean arterial pressure based on the amplitude of the arterial pulsations and then uses an algorithm to calculate the systolic and diastolic pressures. Blood pressures obtained by automated devices are usually less accurate than those obtained by trained observers using the auscultatory method, and it is recommended that their use be limited to situations in which frequent and less accurate measures of blood pressure trends are needed. They should not be used for the diagnosis and management of hypertension.[4]

Automated devices are useful for the self-monitoring of blood pressure and for 24-hour ambulatory monitoring of blood pressure.[7] Ambulatory blood monitors are fully automatic and can record blood pressure for 24 hours or longer while persons go about their normal activities. The monitors are typically programmed to take readings every 15 to 30 minutes throughout the day and night. The readings are stored and downloaded into a computer for analysis. Automated equipment for self-monitoring of blood pressure is sold in pharmacies and medical supply stores throughout the country and is available in many styles and price ranges. It is important that the equipment be certified as accurate and reliable. The equipment should be a validated aneroid or electronic monitor, should use an appropriate-size cuff, and be checked at least once a year for accuracy. The accuracy of an electronic device can be checked by comparing its readings with simultaneously obtained auscultatory measurements.

Intra-arterial methods provide for direct measurement of blood pressure. Intra-arterial measurement requires the insertion of a catheter into a peripheral artery. The arterial catheter is connected to a pressure transducer, which converts pressure into a digital signal that can be measured, displayed, and recorded.[1] The use of this type of blood pressure monitoring usually is restricted to intensive care units.

IN SUMMARY, the alternating contraction and relaxation of the heart produces a pressure pulse that moves blood through the circulatory system. The elastic walls of the aorta stretch during systole and relax during diastole to maintain the diastolic pressure. The systolic blood pressure denotes the highest point of the pressure pulse and the diastolic pressure the lowest point. The pulse pressure, which reflects the pulsatile nature of arterial blood flow, is the difference between the systolic and diastolic pressures, and the mean arterial pressure, the average blood pressure in the systemic circulation. Systolic pressure is determined primarily by the characteristics of the stroke volume, whereas diastolic pressure is determined largely by the conditions of the arteries and arterioles and their abilities to accept the runoff of blood from the aorta.

The regulation of blood pressure involves both short- and long-term mechanisms. The short-term mechanisms are responsible for regulating blood pressure on a minute-by-minute or hour-by-hour basis during activities such as physical exercise and changes in body position. The short-term regulation of blood pressure relies mainly on neural and humoral mechanisms, the most rapid of which are the neural mechanisms. The long-term mechanisms, those maintaining blood pressure over days, weeks, and even years, are largely vested in the kidney and the regulation of extracellular fluid volume.

Arterial blood pressure measurements usually are obtained by the indirect auscultatory method, which uses a sphygmomanometer and a stethoscope. Automated or semiautomated methods of blood pressure measurement use a microphone, arterial pressure pulse sensor (oscillometric method), or Doppler equipment for detecting the equivalent of the Korotkoff sounds. Ambulatory and self-measurement of blood pressure may provide valuable information outside the clinician's office regarding a person's blood pressure and response to treatment. Accurate blood pressure measurement, whether by auscultatory or automated methods, requires the use of accurately calibrated equipment, a properly fitted cuff, and the proper level of cuff inflation and timing for cuff deflation. ∎

HYPERTENSION

After completing this section of the chapter, you should be able to meet the following objectives:

- Cite the definition of hypertension put forth by the seventh report of the Joint National Committee on Detection, Evaluation, and Treatment of Hypertension.
- Differentiate essential, systolic, secondary, and malignant forms of hypertension.
- Describe the possible influence of genetics, age, race, obesity, diet and sodium intake, and alcohol consumption on the development of essential hypertension.

- Cite the risks of hypertension in terms of target-organ damage.
- Describe behavior modification strategies used in the prevention and treatment of hypertension.
- List the different categories of drugs used to treat hypertension and state their mechanisms of action in the treatment of high blood pressure.
- Explain the changes in blood pressure that accompany normal pregnancy and describe the four types of hypertension that can occur during pregnancy.
- Cite the criteria for the diagnosis of high blood pressure in children.
- Define systolic hypertension and relate the circulatory changes that occur with aging that predispose to the development of systolic hypertension.

Hypertension, or high blood pressure, is probably the most common of all health problems in adults and is the leading risk factor for cardiovascular disorders. It affects approximately 50 million individuals in the United States and approximately 1 billion worldwide.[8] Hypertension is more common in younger men compared with younger women, in blacks compared with whites, in persons from lower socioeconomic groups, and in older persons. Men have higher blood pressures than women up until the time of menopause, at which point women quickly lose their protection. The prevalence of hypertension increases with age. Recent data from the Framingham Study suggest that persons who are normotensive at 55 years of age have a 90% lifetime risk for development of hypertension.[9] Thus, the problem of hypertension can be expected to become even greater with the aging of the "baby-boomer" population.

Hypertension is commonly divided into the categories of primary and secondary hypertension. Primary (essential) hypertension is the term applied to 95% of cases in which no cause for hypertension can be identified. In secondary hypertension, the elevation of blood pressure results from some other disorder, such as kidney disease.

Essential Hypertension

The seventh report of the Joint National Committee on Detection, Evaluation, and Treatment of High Blood Pressure (JNC 7) of the National Institutes of Health was published in 2003.[8] According to the JNC 7 recommendations, a systolic pressure of less than 120 mm Hg and a diastolic pressure of less than 80 mm Hg are normal, and systolic pressures between 120 and 139 mm Hg and diastolic pressures between 80 and 89 mm Hg are considered prehypertensive (Table 23-1). A diagnosis of hypertension is made if the systolic blood pressure is 140 mm Hg or higher and the diastolic blood pressure is 90 mm Hg or higher. For adults with diabetes mellitus, the blood pressure goal has been lowered to less than 130/80 mm Hg.[10] Hypertension is further divided into stages 1 and 2 based on systolic and diastolic blood pressure measurements. Systolic hypertension

🔑 HYPERTENSION

- Hypertension represents an elevation in systolic and/or diastolic blood pressure.

- Essential hypertension is characterized by a chronic elevation in blood pressure that occurs without evidence of other disease, and secondary hypertension by an elevation of blood pressure that results from some other disorder, such as kidney disease.

- The pathogenesis of essential hypertension is thought to include constitutional and environmental factors involving the kidney and its role in regulating extracellular fluid volume through salt and water elimination, sympathetic nervous system hyperreactivity, renin-angiotensin system activity, or intracellular sodium and calcium levels. The medications that are used in the treatment of hypertension exert their effect through one or more of these mechanisms.

- Uncontrolled hypertension produces increased demands on the heart, resulting in left ventricular hypertrophy and heart failure, and on the vessels of the arterial system, leading to atherosclerosis, kidney disease, retinopathy, and stroke.

(to be discussed) is defined as a systolic pressure of 140 mm Hg or greater and a diastolic pressure of less than 90 mm Hg.[8]

Constitutional Risk Factors

Although the cause or causes of essential hypertension are largely unknown, both constitutional and lifestyle factors have been implicated, either singly or collectively, as contributing factors. The constitutional risk factors include a family history of hypertension, race, and age-related increases in blood pressure.[11,12] Another factor that is thought to contribute to hypertension is insulin resistance and the resultant hyperinsulinemia that occurs in metabolic abnormalities such as type 2 diabetes.

Family History. The inclusion of heredity as a contributing factor in the development of hypertension is supported by the fact that hypertension is seen most frequently among persons with a family history of hypertension. The strength of the prediction depends on the definition of positive family history and the age of the person at risk.[13] In studies of twins and family members in which the degree of familial aggregation is compared with the closeness of genetic sharing, the genetic contribution ranges from 30% to 60%.[14] Until now, however, geneticists have failed to identify common genes with large effects on hypertension. It is possible that blood pressure is determined by multiple genes at many loci, each with a small influence or with a contribution differing according to sex, race, age, and lifestyle.[11]

Age-Related Changes in Blood Pressure. Maturation and growth are known to cause predictable increases in blood pressure. For example, the arterial blood pressure in the newborn is approximately 50 mm Hg systolic and 40 mm Hg diastolic.[15] Sequentially, blood pressure increases with physical growth from a value of 78 mm Hg systolic at 10 days of age to 120 mm Hg at the end of adolescence. Diastolic pressure increases until 50 years of age and then declines from the sixth decade onward, whereas systolic blood pressure continues to rise with age.[15]

Race. Hypertension not only is more prevalent in African Americans than other ethnic groups in the United States, it is more severe.[16] The Third National Health and Nutrition Survey (NHANES) III, from 1988 to 1991, reported that diastolic blood pressures were significantly greater for African Americans than for white men and women 35 years of age and older,

TABLE 23-1 **Classification of Blood Pressure for Adults and Recommendations for Follow-up**			
BLOOD PRESSURE CLASSIFICATION	**SYSTOLIC BLOOD PRESSURE (mm Hg)**	**DIASTOLIC BLOOD PRESSURE (mm Hg)**	**FOLLOW-UP RECOMMENDATIONS FOR INITIAL BLOOD PRESSURE*†**
Normal	<120	And <80	Recheck in 2 years
Prehypertensive	120–139	or 80–89	Recheck in 1 year‡
Stage 1 hypertension	140–159	or 90–99	Confirm within 2 months‡
Stage 2 hypertension	≥160	or ≥100	Evaluate or refer to source of care within 1 month. For those with higher pressure (*e.g.,* >180/110 mm Hg), evaluate and treat immediately or within 1 week, depending on clinical situation and complications.

*Initial blood pressure: If systolic and diastolic categories are different, follow recommendations for shorter follow-up (*e.g.,* 160/86 mm Hg should be evaluated or referred to source of care with 1 month).
†Follow-up blood pressure: Modify the scheduling of follow-up according to reliable information about past blood pressure measurements, other cardiovascular risk factors, or target-organ disease.
‡Provide advice about lifestyle modification.
Modified from the National Heart, Lung, and Blood Institute. [2003]. *The seventh report of the National Committee on Detection, Evaluation, and Treatment of High Blood Pressure.* NIH publication no. 03-5233. Bethesda, MD: National Institutes of Health.

and that systolic pressures of African American women at every age were greater than those of white women.[17] Hypertension also tends to occur at an earlier age in African Americans than in whites and often is not treated early enough or aggressively enough. Blacks also tend to experience greater cardiovascular and renal damage at any level of pressure.[18]

The reasons for the increased incidence of hypertension among African Americans are largely unknown. Studies have shown that many African American persons with hypertension have lower renin levels than white persons with hypertension.[12,16] The suppression of renin has been considered a secondary response to sodium retention and volume excess. Salt sensitivity, defined as an increase in blood pressure in response to a high-salt diet, is commonly described in both normotensive and hypertensive African Americans. Recent research has focused on potential defects in renal sodium transport to explain this observation. Other factors, such as increased vasomotor function (e.g., sympathetic nervous system overactivity) or abnormalities in endothelium-dependent vasodilation have also been suggested as possible contributing factors.[16]

Evidence suggests that African Americans, when provided equal access to diagnosis and treatment, can achieve overall reductions in blood pressure and experience fewer cardiovascular complications, similar to whites.[16,18] Barriers that limit access to the health care system include inadequate financial support, inconveniently located health care facilities, long waiting times, and lack of access to culturally relevant health education about hypertension. With the high prevalence of salt sensitivity, obesity, and smoking among blacks, health education and lifestyle modifications are particularly important.

Insulin Resistance and Metabolic Abnormalities. Insulin resistance and an accompanying compensatory hyperinsulinemia have been suggested as possible etiologic links to the development of hypertension and associated metabolic disturbances such as impaired glucose tolerance, type 2 diabetes, hyperlipidemias, and obesity.[19-21] This clustering of cardiovascular risk factors has been named the *insulin resistance syndrome, cardiometabolic syndrome,* or *metabolic syndrome* (see Chapter 42).

Insulin resistance may be a genetic or acquired trait. For example, it has been shown that insulin-mediated glucose disposal declines by 30% to 40% in persons who are 40% over ideal weight.[12] Nonpharmacologic interventions, such as caloric restriction, weight loss, and exercise, tend to decrease insulin resistance, sympathetic nervous system activity, and blood pressure.

Lifestyle Risk Factors

Lifestyle factors can contribute to the development of hypertension by interacting with other risk factors. These lifestyle factors include high salt intake, excessive calorie intake and obesity, excessive alcohol consumption, and low intake of potassium. Although stress can raise blood pressure acutely, there is less evidence linking it to chronic elevations in blood pressure. Smoking and a diet high in saturated fats and cholesterol, although not identified as primary risk factors for hypertension, are independent risk factors for coronary heart disease and should be avoided.

High Salt Intake. Increased salt intake has long been suspected as an etiologic factor in the development of hypertension.[22,23] Just how increased salt intake contributes to the development of hypertension is still unclear. It may be that salt causes an elevation in blood volume, increases the sensitivity of cardiovascular or renal mechanisms to sympathetic nervous system influences, or exerts its effects through some other mechanism such as the renin-angiotensin-aldosterone system. It has also been suggested that it may be the chloride rather than the sodium in salt that is responsible for the rise in blood pressure. This is difficult to study, however, because 95% of sodium in the diet is in the form of sodium chloride.[24]

Regardless of the mechanism, numerous studies have shown that a reduction in salt intake can lower blood pressure. The strongest data come from the INTERSALT study, which measured 24-hour urine sodium excretion (an indirect measure of salt intake) in 10,079 men and women 20 to 59 years of age in 52 locations around the world.[25] In all 52 sites, there was a positive correlation between sodium excretion and both systolic and diastolic blood pressures. Furthermore, the association of sodium and blood pressure was greatest for older (40 to 59 years) subjects compared with younger (20 to 39 years) subjects in the study.

At present, salt intake among adults in the United States and United Kingdom averages at least 9 g/day, with large numbers of people consuming 12 g/day or more.[25] This is far in excess of the maximal intake of 6 g/day for adults recommended by the American Heart Association.[26] Approximately 75% of salt intake comes from salt added in the processing and manufacturing of food; 15% from the discretionary addition in cooking and at the table; and 10% from the natural sodium content of food.[22,25] The Dietary Approaches to Stop Hypertension (DASH) diet is a nutritional plan that emphasizes fruits, vegetables, low-fat dairy products, whole grains, poultry, fish, and nuts, and is reduced in fat, red meat, sweets, and sugar-containing beverages. Results from studies using the low-sodium DASH diet have shown significant reductions in both systolic and diastolic blood pressures.[27]

Obesity. Excessive weight commonly is associated with hypertension. Weight reduction of as little as 4.5 kg (10 lb) can produce a decrease in blood pressure in a large proportion of overweight people with hypertension.[8] It has been suggested that fat distribution might be a more critical indicator of hypertension risk than actual overweight. The waist-to-hip ratio commonly is used to differentiate central or upper body obesity, with fat cells located in the abdomen and viscera, from peripheral or lower body obesity, with fat cell deposits in the buttocks and legs (see Chapter 39). Studies have found an association between hypertension and increased waist-to-hip ratio (i.e., central obesity), even when body mass index and skinfold thickness are taken into account.[28,29] Abdominal or visceral fat seems to be more insulin resistant than fat deposited over the buttocks and legs. There is also an evolving understanding of the neuroendocrine effects of excess adipose tissue on blood pressure.[30] Recent evidence indicates that leptin, an adipocyte-derived hormone, may represent a link between adiposity and increased cardiovascular sympathetic activity. Besides its effect on appetite and metabolism, leptin acts on the hypothalamus to increase blood pressure through activation of the sympathetic nervous system[30] High levels of circulating free fatty acids in obese people also appear to participate in activation of the sympathetic nervous system. There is also research supporting activation of the renin-angiotensin-aldosterone system by adipocyte-derived angiotensinogen and the ability of adipose tissue to increase aldosterone levels through the production of factors that induce aldosterone production.[30]

Excess Alcohol Consumption. Regular alcohol drinking plays a role in the development of hypertension.[31–33] The effect is seen with different types of alcoholic drinks, in men and women, and in a variety of ethnic groups. One of the first reports of a link between alcohol consumption and hypertension came from the Oakland–San Francisco Kaiser Permanente Medical Care Program study that correlated known drinking patterns and blood pressure levels of 84,000 persons.[33] This study revealed that the regular consumption of three or more drinks per day increases the risk for hypertension. Systolic pressures were more markedly affected than diastolic pressures. Blood pressure may improve or return to normal when alcohol consumption is decreased or eliminated. The mechanism whereby alcohol exerts its effect on blood pressure is unclear. It has been suggested that lifestyle factors such as obesity and lack of exercise may be accompanying factors.

Dietary Intake of Potassium, Calcium, and Magnesium. Low levels of dietary potassium have also been linked to increased blood pressure. The strongest evidence comes from the previously described INTERSALT study. In this study, a 60 mmol/day or greater urinary excretion of potassium (an indirect measure of potassium intake) was associated with a reduction in systolic pressure of 3.4 mm Hg or more and a decrease in diastolic pressure of 1.9 mm Hg or more.[34] Various mechanisms have been proposed to explain the influence of potassium on blood pressure, including a purported change in the ratio of sodium to potassium in the diet, a direct natriuretic effect, and suppression of the renin-angiotensin system.[35] In terms of food intake, a diet high in potassium usually is low in sodium. One of the major benefits of increased potassium intake is increased elimination of sodium (natriuretic effect) through the renin-angiotensin-aldosterone mechanism.

The associations between high blood pressure and calcium and magnesium levels also have been investigated. Although there have been reports of high blood pressure in persons with low calcium intake or lowering of blood pressure with increased calcium intake, the link between low calcium and magnesium intake and hypertension is inconclusive.[35]

Target-Organ Damage

Essential hypertension is typically an asymptomatic disorder. When symptoms do occur, they are usually related to the long-term effects of hypertension on other organ systems such as the kidneys, heart, eyes, and blood vessels. The JNC 7 report uses the term *target-organ damage* to describe the heart, brain, peripheral vascular, kidney, and retinal complications associated with hypertension[8] (Chart 23-1). The excess morbidity and mortality related to hypertension is progressive over the whole range of systolic and diastolic pressures, with target-organ damage varying markedly among persons with similar levels of hypertension.

Hypertension is a major risk factor for atherosclerosis; it predisposes to all major atherosclerotic cardiovascular disorders, including coronary heart disease, heart failure, stroke, and peripheral artery disease. The risk for coronary artery disease and stroke depends to a great extent on other risk factors, such as obesity, smoking, and elevated cholesterol levels. In clinical trials, antihypertensive therapy has been associated with reductions in stroke incidence averaging 30% to 40%, myocardial infarction, 20% to 25%, and heart failure, more than 50%.[8,36]

An elevation in blood pressure increases the workload of the left ventricle by increasing the pressure against which the heart must pump as it ejects blood into the systemic circulation.[12] As the workload of the heart increases, the left ventricular wall hypertrophies to compensate for the increased pressure work. Despite its adaptive advantage, left ventricular hypertrophy is a major risk factor for coronary heart disease, cardiac dysrhythmias, sudden death, and congestive heart failure. Hypertensive left ventricular hypertrophy regresses with therapy. Regression is most closely related to systolic pressure reduction and does not appear to reflect the particular type of medication used.

Chronic hypertension leads to nephrosclerosis, a common cause of chronic kidney disease (see Chapter 33). Hypertensive kidney disease is more common in blacks than whites. Hypertension also plays an important role in accelerating the

---

CHART 23-1 | TARGET ORGAN DAMAGE

Heart
- Left ventricular hypertrophy
- Angina or prior myocardial infarction
- Prior coronary revascularization
- Heart failure

Brain
- Stroke or transient ischemic attack

Chronic kidney disease

Peripheral vascular disease

Retinopathy

From the National Heart, Lung, and Blood Institute. (2003). *The seventh report of the National Committee on Detection, Evaluation, and Treatment of High Blood Pressure.* Publication no. 03–5233. Bethesda, MD: National Institutes of Health.

course of other types of kidney disease, particularly diabetic nephropathy. Because of the risk for diabetic nephropathy, the American Diabetes Association recommends that persons with diabetes maintain their blood pressure at levels less than 130/80 mm Hg (see Chapter 42).

Dementia and cognitive impairment occur more commonly in persons with hypertension.[8] Hypertension, particularly systolic hypertension, is a major risk factor for ischemic stroke and intracerebral hemorrhage[12] (see Chapter 51). Narrowing and sclerosis of small penetrating arteries in the subcortical regions of the brain are common findings on autopsy in person with chronic hypertension.[8] These changes are thought to contribute to hypoperfusion, loss of autoregulation of blood flow, and impairment of the blood-brain barrier, ultimately leading to subcortical white matter demyelination. Magnetic resonance imaging (MRI) studies have revealed more extensive white matter lesions and brain atrophy in hypertensive versus normotensive persons.[37] Effective antihypertensive therapy strongly reduces the risk of development of significant white matter changes; however, existing white matter changes, once established, do not appear to be reversible.[8]

Diagnosis

Unlike disorders of other body systems that are diagnosed by methods such as radiography and tissue examination, hypertension and other blood pressure disorders are determined by repeated blood pressure measurement. Laboratory tests, x-ray films, and other diagnostic tests usually are done to exclude secondary hypertension and determine the presence or extent of target-organ damage.

Blood pressure measurements should be taken when the person is relaxed and has rested for at least 5 minutes and has not smoked or ingested caffeine within 30 minutes. At least two measurements should be made at each visit in the same arm while the person is seated in a chair (rather than on the examination table) with the feet on the floor and arm supported at heart level.[8] If the first two readings differ by more than 5 mm Hg, additional readings should be taken. Both the systolic and diastolic pressures should be recorded. The increased availability of hypertensive screening clinics provides one of the best means for early detection. Because blood pressure in many individuals is highly variable, blood pressure should be measured on different occasions over a period of several months before a diagnosis of hypertension is made unless the pressure is extremely elevated or associated with symptoms. The JNC 7 recommendations for follow-up of persons with various stages of hypertension are included in Table 23-1.

Ambulatory Blood Pressure Measurement. As previously discussed, ambulatory and self/home measurement of blood pressure may provide valuable information outside the clinician's office regarding the person's blood pressure and response to treatment. Self/home measurement can help detect "white coat hypertension," a condition in which the blood pressure is consistently elevated in the health care provider's office but normal at other times; it can be used to assess the response to treatment methods for hypertension; it can motivate adherence to treatment regimens; and it can potentially reduce health care costs.[8]

The guidelines for the 2005 Canadian Hypertension Education Program recommend short intervals between the initial and subsequent office visits (e.g., up to three visits over 6 months for a blood pressure of >140/90 mm Hg) to confirm the blood pressure elevation before pharmacologic intervention.[38] In addition, the Canadian guidelines stipulate the use of ambulatory and self/home blood pressure measurements as complements to office-based evaluations. According to these guidelines, an ambulatory or self/home awake systolic pressure of 135 mm Hg or more or a diastolic pressure of 85 mm Hg or more, or a 24-hour ambulatory systolic pressure of 130 mm Hg or more or a diastolic pressure of 80 mm Hg or more, is diagnosed as hypertension.[38]

Circadian Variations in Blood Pressure. Blood pressure normally varies in a characteristic circadian pattern. It tends to be highest in the early morning, shortly after arising from sleep, and then decreases gradually throughout the day, reaching its lowest point at approximately 2:00 to 5:00 AM.[11,39,40] The term *dippers* is used to refer to persons with a normal circadian blood pressure profile in which blood pressure falls during the night, and *nondippers* for persons whose 24-hour blood pressure profile is flattened.[39] Ambulatory blood pressure monitoring can be used to determine alterations in a person's circadian blood pressure profile.[7] Changes in the normal circadian blood pressure profile may occur in a number of conditions, including malignant hypertension, Cushing syndrome, preeclampsia, orthostatic hypotension, congestive heart failure, and sleep apnea.[11] There is increasing evidence that persons with a nondipping pattern of hypertension are at higher risk for development of target-organ damage than those with a dipping pattern; in addition, persons with an excessive morning surge in blood pressure may also be at increased risk.

Treatment

The main objective for treatment of essential hypertension is to achieve and maintain arterial blood pressure below 140/90 mm Hg, with the goal of preventing morbidity and mortality. In persons with hypertension and diabetes or renal disease, the goal is below 130/80 mm Hg. The JNC 7 report contains a treatment algorithm for hypertension that includes lifestyle modification and, when necessary, guidelines for the use of pharmacologic agents to achieve and maintain blood pressure within an optimal range[8] (Fig. 23-6).

For persons with secondary hypertension, efforts are made to correct or control the disease condition causing the hypertension. Antihypertensive medications and other measures supplement the treatment of the underlying disease.

Lifestyle Modification. Lifestyle modification has been shown to reduce blood pressure, enhance the effects of antihypertensive drug therapy, and prevent cardiovascular risk. Major life-

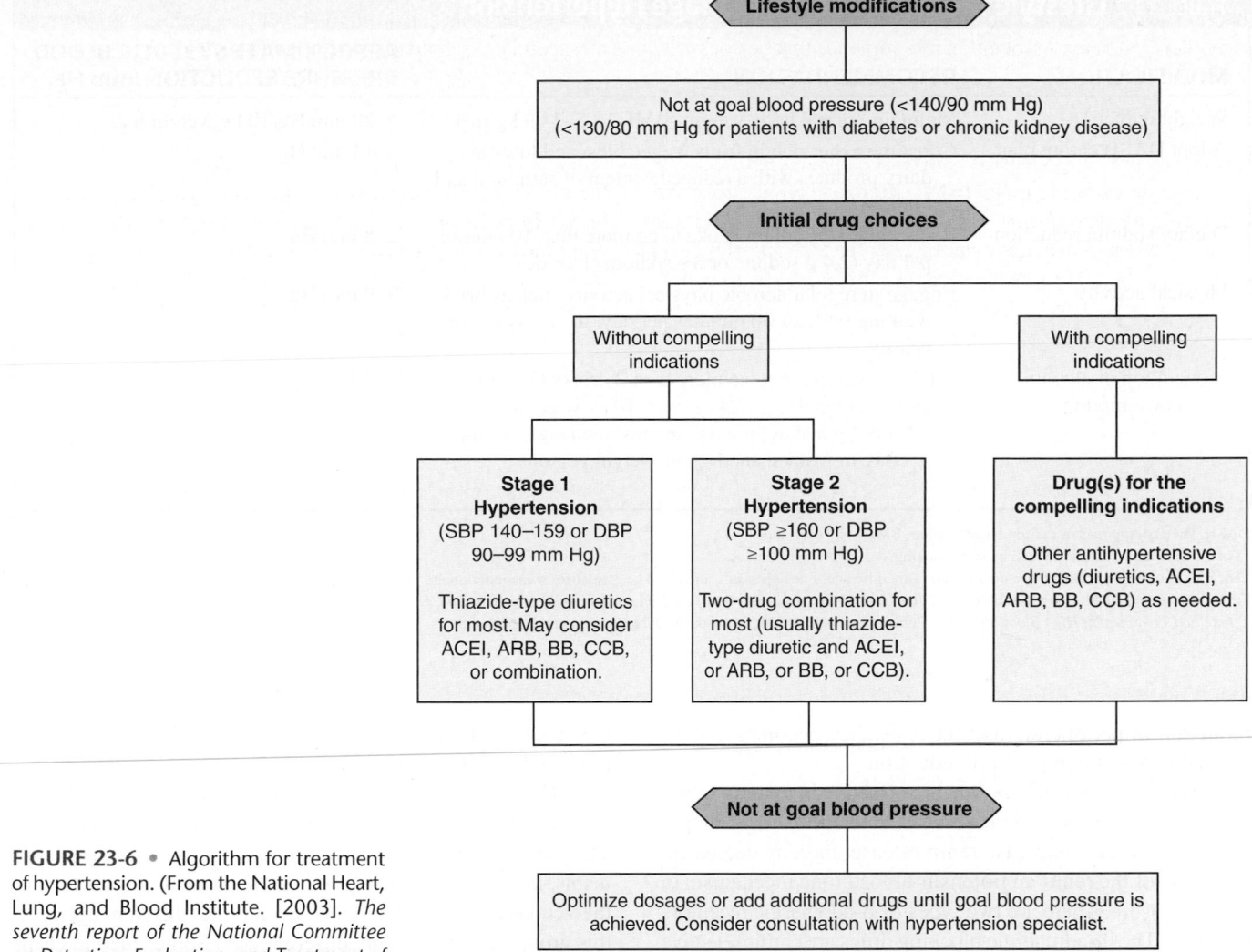

FIGURE 23-6 • Algorithm for treatment of hypertension. (From the National Heart, Lung, and Blood Institute. [2003]. *The seventh report of the National Committee on Detection, Evaluation, and Treatment of High Blood Pressure.* NIH publication no. 03-5233. Bethesda, MD: National Institutes of Health.)

DBP, diastolic blood pressure; SBP, systolic blood pressure.
Drug abbreviations: ACEI, angiotensin-converting enzyme inhibitor; ARB, angiotensin receptor blocker; BB, beta blocker; CCB, calcium channel blocker.

style modifications shown to lower blood pressure include weight reduction in persons who are overweight or obese, regular physical activity, adoption of the DASH eating plan, reduction of dietary salt intake, and limitation of alcohol intake to no more than two drinks per day for most men and one drink for women and persons of lighter weight[8] (Table 23-2). Although nicotine has not been associated with long-term elevations in blood pressure as in essential hypertension, it has been shown to increase the risk for heart disease. The fact that smoking and hypertension are major cardiovascular risk factors should be reason enough to encourage the hypertensive smoker to quit. There is conflicting evidence about the direct effects of dietary fats on blood pressure. As with smoking, the interactive effects of saturated fats and high blood pressure as cardiovascular risk factors would seem to warrant dietary modification to reduce the intake of foods high in cholesterol and saturated fats.

Pharmacologic Treatment. The decision to initiate pharmacologic treatment is based on the stage and severity of the hypertension, the presence of target-organ disease, and the existence of other disease conditions and risk factors. The JNC 7 has developed a pharmacologic treatment algorithm for use in the pharmacologic treatment of hypertension[8] (see Fig. 23-6). Among the drugs used in the treatment of hypertension are diuretics, β-adrenergic blocking agents, angiotensin-converting enzyme (ACE) inhibitors or angiotensin II receptor blockers, calcium channel blocking agents, α_1-adrenoreceptor antagonists, α_2-adrenergic agonists that act at the level of the central nervous system (CNS), and vasodilators.

Diuretics, such as the thiazides, loop diuretics, and the aldosterone antagonist (potassium-sparing) diuretics, lower blood pressure initially by decreasing vascular volume (by suppressing renal reabsorption of sodium and increasing salt and water excretion) and cardiac output. With continued therapy, a

TABLE 23-2 Lifestyle Modifications to Manage Hypertension*†

MODIFICATION	RECOMMENDATION	APPROXIMATE SYSTOLIC BLOOD PRESSURE REDUCTION (mm Hg)
Weight reduction	Maintain normal body weight (BMI, 18.5–24.9 kg/m²)	5–20 mm Hg/10 kg weight loss
Adopt DASH eating plan	Consume a diet rich in fruits, vegetables, and low-fat dairy products with a reduced content of saturated and total fat	8–14 mm Hg
Dietary sodium reduction	Reduce dietary sodium intake to no more than 100 mmol per day (2.4 g sodium or 6 g sodium chloride)	2–8 mm Hg
Physical activity	Engage in regular aerobic physical activity such as brisk walking (at least 30 minutes per day, most days of the week)	4–9 mm Hg
Moderation of alcohol consumption	Limit consumption to no more than 2 drinks (1 oz or 30 mL ethanol; *e.g.,* 24 oz beer, 10 oz wine, or 3 oz 80-proof whiskey) per day in most men and 1 drink per day in women and lighter-weight persons	2–4 mm Hg

DASH, Dietary Approaches to Stop Hypertension; BMI, body mass index.
*For overall cardiovascular reduction, stop smoking.
†The effects of implementing these modifications are dose and time dependent, and could be greater for some individuals.
From the National Heart, Lung, and Blood Institute. (2003). *The seventh report of the National Committee on Detection, Evaluation, and Treatment of High Blood Pressure.* Publication no. 03–5233. Bethesda, MD: National Institutes of Health.

reduction in peripheral vascular resistance becomes a major mechanism of blood pressure reduction.

The β-*adrenergic blockers* are effective in treating hypertension because they decrease heart rate and cardiac output. These agents also decrease renin release, thereby decreasing the effect of the renin-angiotensin-aldosterone mechanism on blood pressure. There are two types of β-adrenergic receptors: β_1 and β_2. The β_1-adrenergic blocking drugs are cardioselective, exerting their effects on the heart, whereas the β_2-adrenergic receptor blockers affect bronchodilation, relaxation of skeletal blood vessels, and other β-mediated functions. Both cardioselective (targeting β_1 receptors) and nonselective (targeting β_1 and β_2 receptors) β-adrenergic blockers are used in the treatment of hypertension.

The *ACE inhibitors* act by inhibiting the conversion of angiotensin I to angiotensin II, thus decreasing angiotensin II levels and reducing its effect on vasoconstriction, aldosterone levels, intrarenal blood flow, and the glomerular filtration rate. They also inhibit the degradation of bradykinin and stimulate the synthesis of vasodilating prostaglandins. The ACE inhibitors are increasingly used as the initial medication in mild to moderate hypertension. Because of their effect on the renin-angiotensin system, these drugs are contraindicated in persons with renal artery stenosis, in which the renin-angiotensin mechanism functions as a compensatory mechanism to maintain adequate renal perfusion. Because they inhibit aldosterone secretion, these agents also can increase serum potassium levels and cause hyperkalemia. A relative newcomer to the field of antihypertensive medications is the *angiotensin II receptor blocking* agents. Because they do not inhibit bradykinin degradation in the lungs,

they are less likely to produce a cough, which is a common side effect of ACE inhibitors.

The *calcium channel receptor blocking drugs* inhibit the movement of calcium into cardiac and vascular smooth muscle. They are thought to reduce blood pressure by several mechanisms, including a reduction of vascular smooth muscle tone in the venous and arterial systems. Each of the different agents in this group acts in a slightly different way. Some calcium channel blockers have a direct myocardial effect that reduces the cardiac output through a decrease in cardiac contractility and heart rate; others influence venous vasomotor tone and reduce the cardiac output through a decrease in venous return; still others influence arterial vascular smooth muscle tone by inhibiting calcium transport across the cell membrane channels or the vascular response to norepinephrine or angiotensin.

The α_1-*adrenergic receptor antagonists* block postsynaptic α_1 receptors and reduce the effect of the sympathetic nervous system on the vascular smooth muscle tone of the blood vessels that regulate the peripheral vascular resistance. These drugs produce a pronounced decrease in blood pressure after the first dose; therefore, treatment is initiated with a smaller dose given at bedtime. Postdosing palpitations, headache, and nervousness may continue with chronic treatment. These agents usually are more effective when used in combination with other agents.

The *centrally acting adrenergic agonists* block sympathetic outflow from the CNS. These agents are α_2-adrenergic agonists that act in a negative-feedback manner to decrease sympathetic outflow from presynaptic sympathetic neurons in the CNS. The α_2-adrenergic agonists are effective as a single therapy for some persons, but often are used as second- or third-line agents because of the high incidence of side effects associated with their use. One of the agents, clonidine, is available as a transdermal patch that is replaced weekly.

The *direct-acting smooth muscle vasodilators* promote a decrease in peripheral vascular resistance by producing relaxation of vascular smooth muscle, particularly of the arterioles. These drugs often produce tachycardia because of an initial stimulation of the sympathetic nervous system, and salt and water retention owing to decreased filling of the vascular compartment. Vasodilators are most effective when used in combination with other antihypertensive drugs that oppose the compensatory cardiovascular responses.

Treatment Strategies. Factors to be considered when hypertensive drugs are prescribed are the person's lifestyle (*i.e.,* someone with a busy schedule may have problems with medications that must be taken two or three times each day); demographics (*e.g.,* some drugs are more effective in elderly or African American persons); motivation for adhering to the drug regimen (*e.g.,* some drugs can produce undesirable and even life-threatening consequences if discontinued abruptly); other disease conditions and therapies; and potential for side effects (*e.g.,* some drugs may impair sexual functioning or mental acuity; others have not been proved safe for women of childbearing age). Particular caution should be used in persons who are at risk for orthostatic hypotension (*e.g.,* those with diabetes, ANS dysfunction, and some older individuals). Another factor to be considered is the cost of the drug in relation to financial resources. There is wide variation in the prices of antihypertensive medications, and this factor should be considered when medications are prescribed. This is particularly important for low-income persons with moderate to severe hypertension because keeping costs at an affordable level may be the key to compliance.[8]

Systolic Hypertension

The JNC 7 report defined systolic hypertension as a systolic pressure of 140 mm Hg or greater and a diastolic pressure of less than 90 mm Hg, indicating a need for increased recognition and control of isolated systolic hypertension.[8] Historically, diastolic hypertension was thought to confer a greater risk for cardiovascular events than systolic hypertension.[8] However, there is mounting evidence that elevated systolic blood pressure is at least as important, if not more so, than diastolic hypertension.[41,42]

There are two aspects of systolic hypertension that confer increased risk for cardiovascular events—one is the actual elevation in systolic pressure and the other is the disproportionate rise in pulse pressure. Elevated pressures during systole favor the development of left ventricular hypertrophy, increased myocardial oxygen demands, and eventual left heart failure. At the same time, the absolute or relative lowering of diastolic pressure is a limiting factor in coronary perfusion because coronary perfusion is greatest during diastole. Elevated pulse pressures produce greater stretch of arteries, causing damage to the elastic elements of the vessel and thus predisposing to

aneurysms and development of the intimal damage that leads to atherosclerosis and thrombosis.[42]

Secondary Hypertension

Secondary hypertension, which describes an elevation in blood pressure due to another disease condition, accounts for 5% to 10% of hypertension cases.[43] Unlike essential hypertension, many of the conditions causing secondary hypertension can be corrected or cured by surgery or specific medical treatment. Secondary hypertension tends to be seen in persons younger than 30 and older than 50 years of age. Cocaine, amphetamines, and other illicit drugs can cause significant hypertension, as can sympathomimetic agents (decongestants, anorectics), erythropoietin, and licorice (including some chewing tobaccos with licorice as an ingredient). Obstructive sleep apnea (see Chapter 52) is an independent risk factor for secondary hypertension.

Among the most common causes of secondary hypertension are kidney disease (*i.e.,* renovascular hypertension), adrenal cortical disorders, pheochromocytoma, and coarctation of the aorta. To avoid duplication in descriptions, the mechanisms associated with elevations of blood pressure in these disorders are discussed briefly, and a more detailed discussion of specific disease disorders is reserved for other sections of this book. Oral contraceptive agents are also implicated as a cause of secondary hypertension.

Renal Hypertension

With the dominant role that the kidney assumes in blood pressure regulation, it is not surprising that the largest single cause of secondary hypertension is renal disease. Most acute kidney disorders result in decreased urine formation, retention of salt and water, and hypertension. This includes acute glomerulonephritis, acute renal failure, and acute urinary tract obstruction. Hypertension also is common among persons with chronic pyelonephritis, polycystic kidney disease, diabetic nephropathy, and end-stage renal disease, regardless of cause. In older persons, the sudden onset of secondary hypertension often is associated with atherosclerotic disease of the renal blood vessels.

Renovascular hypertension refers to hypertension caused by reduced renal blood flow and activation of the renin-angiotensin-aldosterone mechanism. It is the most common cause of secondary hypertension, accounting for 1% to 2% of all cases of hypertension.[44] The reduced renal blood flow that occurs with renovascular disease causes the affected kidney to release excessive amounts of renin, increasing circulating levels of angiotensin II. Angiotensin II, in turn, acts as a vasoconstrictor to increase peripheral vascular resistance and as a stimulus for increased aldosterone levels and sodium retention by the kidney. One or both of the kidneys may be affected. When the renal artery of only one kidney is involved, the unaffected kidney is subjected to the detrimental effects of the elevated blood pressure.

There are two major types of renovascular disease: atherosclerosis of the proximal renal artery and fibromuscular dysplasia, a noninflammatory vascular disease that affects the renal arteries and branch vessels.[12,44] Atherosclerotic stenosis of the renal artery accounts for 70% to 90% of cases and is seen most often in older persons, particularly those with diabetes, aortoiliac occlusive disease, coronary artery disease, or hypertension. Fibromuscular dysplasia is more common in women and tends to occur in younger age groups, often persons in their third decade.[45] Genetic factors may be involved, and the incidence tends to increase with risk factors such as smoking and hyperlipidemia.

Renal artery stenosis should be suspected when hypertension develops in a previously normotensive person older than 50 (*i.e.,* atherosclerotic form) or younger than 30 (*i.e.,* fibromuscular dysplasia) years of age, or when accelerated hypertension occurs in a person with previously controlled hypertension. Hypokalemia (due to increased aldosterone levels), the presence of an abdominal bruit, the absence of a family history of hypertension, and a duration of hypertension of less than 1 year help to distinguish renovascular hypertension from essential hypertension. Because renal blood flow depends on the increased blood pressure generated by the renin-angiotensin system, administration of ACE inhibitors can cause a rapid decline in renal function.

Diagnostic tests for renovascular hypertension may include studies to assess overall renal function, physiologic studies to assess the renin-angiotensin system, perfusion studies to evaluate renal blood flow, and imaging studies to identify renal artery stenosis.[12] Renal arteriography remains the definitive test for identifying renal artery disease. Duplex ultrasonographic scanning, contrast-enhanced computed tomography (CT), and magnetic resonance angiography (MRA) are other tests that can be used to screen for renovascular hypertension.[12]

The goal of treatment of renal hypertension is to control the blood pressure and stabilize renal function. Angioplasty or revascularization has been shown to be an effective long-term treatment for the disorder. ACE inhibitors may be used in medical management of renal stenosis. However, these agents must be used with caution because of their ability to produce marked hypotension and renal dysfunction.

Disorders of Adrenocortical Hormones

Increased levels of adrenocortical hormones also can give rise to hypertension. Primary hyperaldosteronism (excess production of aldosterone due to adrenocortical hyperplasia or adenoma) and excess levels of glucocorticoid (Cushing disease or syndrome) tend to raise the blood pressure[12,46] (see Chapter 41). These hormones facilitate salt and water retention by the kidney; the hypertension that accompanies excessive levels of either hormone probably is related to this factor. For patients with primary hyperaldosteronism, a salt-restricted diet often produces a reduction in blood pressure. Because aldosterone acts on the distal renal tubule to increase sodium absorption in exchange for potassium elimination in the urine, persons with hyperaldosteronism usually have decreased potassium levels. Screening tests for primary hyperaldosteronism involve the determination of plasma aldosterone concentration and plasma

renin activity. CT and MRI scans are used to localize the lesion. Persons with solitary adenomas are usually treated surgically.[12] Potassium-sparing diuretics, such as spironolactone, which is an aldosterone antagonist, often are used in the medical management of persons with bilateral hyperplasia.[12]

Licorice is an extract from the roots of the *Glycyrrhiza glabra* plant that has been used in medicine since ancient times. European licorice (not licorice flavoring) is associated with sodium retention, edema, hypertension, and hypokalemia. Licorice, which is an effective analog of the steroid 11 β-dehydrogenase enzyme that modulates access to the aldosterone receptor in the kidney, produces a syndrome similar to primary hyperaldosteronism.

Pheochromocytoma

A pheochromocytoma is a tumor of chromaffin tissue, which contains sympathetic nerve cells that stain with chromium salts. The tumor is most commonly located in the adrenal medulla but can arise in other sites, such as the sympathetic ganglia, where there is chromaffin tissue.[12,47] Although only 0.1% to 0.5% of persons with hypertension have an underlying pheochromocytoma, the disorder can cause serious hypertensive crises. The tumors are malignant 8% to 10% of the time.

Like adrenal medullary cells, the tumor cells of a pheochromocytoma produce and secrete the catecholamines epinephrine and norepinephrine. The hypertension that develops is a result of the massive release of these catecholamines. Their release may be paroxysmal rather than continuous, causing periodic episodes of headache, excessive sweating, and palpitations. Headache is the most common symptom and can be quite severe. Nervousness, tremor, facial pallor, weakness, fatigue, and weight loss occur less frequently. Marked variability in blood pressure between episodes is typical. Approximately 50% of persons with pheochromocytoma have paroxysmal episodes of hypertension, sometimes to dangerously high levels. The other 50% have sustained hypertension, and some even may be normotensive.[47]

Several tests are available to differentiate hypertension due to pheochromocytoma from other forms of hypertension. The most commonly used diagnostic measure is the determination of urinary catecholamines and their metabolites. Although measurement of plasma catecholamines also may be used, other conditions can cause catecholamines to be elevated. After the presence of a pheochromocytoma has been established, the tumor needs to be located. CT and MRI scans may be used for this purpose. Radioisotopes that localize the chromaffin tissue are available. Surgical removal of operable tumors is usually curative.[12,47] If the tumor is not resectable, treatment with drugs that block the action or synthesis of catecholamines can be used.

Coarctation of the Aorta

Coarctation represents a narrowing of the aorta. In the adult form of aortic coarctation, the narrowing most commonly occurs just distal to the origin of the subclavian arteries[48] (see Chapter 24). Because of the narrowing, blood flow to the lower parts of the body and kidneys is reduced. In the infantile form of coarctation, the narrowing occurs proximal to the ductus arteriosus, in which case heart failure and other problems may occur. Many affected infants die within their first year of life.

In the adult form of aortic coarctation, the ejection of an increased stroke volume into a narrowed aorta causes an increase in systolic blood pressure and blood flow to the upper part of the body. Blood pressure in the lower extremities may be normal, although it frequently is low. It has been suggested that the increase in stroke volume and maintenance of the pressure to the lower part of the body is achieved through the renin-angiotensin-aldosterone mechanism in response to a decrease in renal blood flow. Pulse pressure in the legs almost always is narrowed, and the femoral pulses are weak. Because the aortic capacity is diminished, there usually is a marked increase in pressure (measured in the arms) during exercise, when the stroke volume and heart rate are increased. For this reason, blood pressures in both arms and one leg should be determined; a pressure that is 20 mm Hg more in the arms than in the legs suggests coarctation of the aorta. Involvement of the left subclavian artery or an anomalous origin of the right subclavian may produce decreased or absent left or right brachial pulses, respectively. Palpation of both brachial pulses and measurement of blood pressure in both arms are important.

Treatment consists of surgical repair or balloon angioplasty. Although balloon angioplasty is a relatively recent form of treatment, it has been used in children and adults with good results. However, there are few data on long-term follow-up.

Oral Contraceptive Drugs

The use of oral contraceptive pills is probably the most common cause of secondary hypertension in young women. Women taking oral contraceptive should have their blood pressure taken regularly.[8] The Nurses Health Study (a prospective cohort study of over 70,000 nurses over 4 years between 1989 and 1993) found that current users of oral contraceptives had a significant, moderately increased risk of hypertension.[49] However, among this group, only 41.5 cases per 10,000 person-years could be attributed to oral contraceptive use.

The cause of the increased blood pressure is largely unknown, although it has been suggested that the probable cause is volume expansion because both estrogens and synthetic progesterones used in oral contraceptive pills cause sodium retention. Various contraceptive drugs contain different amounts and combinations of estrogen and progestational agents, and these differences may contribute to the occurrence of hypertension in some women but not others. Fortunately, the hypertension associated with oral contraceptives usually disappears after the drug has been discontinued, although it may take as long as 3 months for this to happen.[12] However, in some women, the blood pressure may not return to normal, and they may be at risk for development of hypertension. The risk for hypertension-associated cardiovascular complications is found primarily in women older than 35 years of age and in those who smoke.

Malignant Hypertension

A small number of persons with hypertension develop an accelerated and potentially fatal form of the disease termed *malignant hypertension*.[12,50] This usually is a disease of younger persons, particularly young African American men, women with toxemia of pregnancy, and persons with renal and collagen diseases.

Malignant hypertension is characterized by sudden, marked elevations in blood pressure, with diastolic values above 120 mm Hg complicated by evidence of acute or rapidly progressive life-threatening organ dysfunction.[50] There may be intense arterial spasm of the cerebral arteries with hypertensive encephalopathy. Cerebral vasoconstriction probably is an exaggerated homeostatic response designed to protect the brain from excesses of blood pressure and flow. The regulatory mechanisms often are insufficient to protect the capillaries, and cerebral edema frequently develops. As it advances, papilledema (*i.e.*, swelling of the optic nerve at its point of entrance into the eye) ensues, giving evidence of the effects of pressure on the optic nerve and retinal vessels. The patient may have headache, restlessness, confusion, stupor, motor and sensory deficits, and visual disturbances. In severe cases, convulsions and coma follow.

Prolonged and severe exposure to exaggerated levels of blood pressure in malignant hypertension injures the walls of the arterioles, and intravascular coagulation and fragmentation of red blood cells may occur. The renal blood vessels are particularly vulnerable to hypertensive damage. Renal damage due to vascular changes probably is the most important prognostic determinant in malignant hypertension. Elevated levels of blood urea nitrogen and serum creatinine, metabolic acidosis, hypocalcemia, and proteinuria provide evidence of renal impairment.

The complications associated with a hypertensive crisis demand immediate and rigorous medical treatment in an intensive care unit with continuous monitoring of arterial blood pressure. With proper therapy, the death rate from this cause can be markedly reduced, as can complications and additional episodes. Because chronic hypertension is associated with autoregulatory changes in coronary artery, cerebral artery, and kidney blood flow, care should be taken to avoid excessively rapid decreases in blood pressure, which can lead to hypoperfusion and ischemic injury. Therefore, the goal of initial treatment measures should be to obtain a partial reduction in blood pressure to a safer, less critical level, rather than to normotensive levels.[50]

 ## High Blood Pressure in Pregnancy

Hypertensive disorders of pregnancy complicate 5% to 10% of pregnancies and remain a major cause of maternal and neonatal mortality and morbidity in the United States and worldwide.[51–54] Most adverse events are attributable directly to the preeclampsia syndrome, characterized by new-onset hypertension with proteinuria that develops in the last half of pregnancy. Women with chronic hypertension can also manifest adverse events.

Classification

In 2000, the National Institutes of Health Working Group on High Blood Pressure in Pregnancy published a revised classification system for high blood pressure in pregnancy that included preeclampsia–eclampsia, gestational hypertension, chronic hypertension, and preeclampsia superimposed on chronic hypertension[51] (Table 23-3).

Defining the cause or causes of hypertension that occurs during pregnancy is difficult because of the normal circulatory changes that occur. Blood pressure normally decreases during the first trimester, reaches its lowest point during the second trimester, and gradually rises during the third trimester. The fact that there is a large increase in cardiac output during early pregnancy suggests the decrease in blood pressure that occurs during the first part of pregnancy results from a decrease in peripheral vascular resistance. Because the cardiac output remains high throughout pregnancy, the gradual rise in blood pressure that begins during the second trimester probably represents a return of the peripheral vascular resistance to normal. Pregnancy normally is accompanied by increased levels of renin, angiotensin I and II, estrogen, progesterone, prolactin, and aldosterone, all of which may alter vascular reactivity. Women who experience preeclampsia are thought to be particularly sensitive to the vasoconstrictor activity of the renin-angiotensin-aldosterone system. They also are particularly responsive to other vasoconstrictors, including the catecholamines and vasopressin. It has been proposed that some of the sensitivity may be caused by a prostacyclin–thromboxane imbalance. Thromboxane is a prostaglandin with vasoconstrictor properties, and prostacyclin is a prostaglandin with vasodilator properties. Emerging evidence suggests that insulin resistance, including that which occurs with diabetes, obesity, and the metabolic syndrome, may predispose to the hypertensive disorders of pregnancy.

Preeclampsia–Eclampsia. Preeclampsia–eclampsia is a pregnancy-specific syndrome with both maternal and fetal manifestations.[51–54] It is defined as an elevation in blood pressure (systolic blood pressure >140 mm Hg or diastolic pressure >90 mm Hg) and proteinuria (≥300 mg in 24 hours) developing after 20 weeks of gestation. The Working Group recommends that K5 be used for determining diastolic pressure. Edema, which previously was included in definitions of preeclampsia, was excluded from this most recent definition. The presence of a systolic blood pressure of 160 mm Hg or higher or a diastolic pressure of 110 mm Hg or higher; proteinuria greater than 2 g in 24 hours; serum creatinine greater than 1.2 mg/dL; platelet counts less than 100,000 cells/mm³; elevated liver enzymes (alanine aminotransferase [ALT] or aspartate aminotransferase [AST]); persistent headache or cerebral or visual disturbances; and persistent epigastric pain serve to reinforce the diagnosis.[53] Eclampsia is the occurrence, in a woman with preeclampsia, of seizures that cannot be attributed to other causes.[53]

Preeclampsia occurs primarily during first pregnancies and during subsequent pregnancies in women with multiple fetuses, diabetes mellitus, collagen vascular disease, or underlying kidney disease.[51] It is also associated with a condition called a *hydatidiform mole* (*i.e.,* abnormal pregnancy caused by a pathologic ovum, resulting in a mass of cysts). Women with chronic hypertension who become pregnant have an increased risk for preeclampsia and adverse neonatal outcomes, particularly when associated with proteinuria early in pregnancy.

The cause of pregnancy-induced hypertension is largely unknown. Considerable evidence suggests that the placenta is the key factor in all the manifestations because delivery is the only definitive cure for this disease. Pregnancy-induced hypertension is thought to involve a decrease in placental blood flow leading to the release of toxic mediators that alter the function of endothelial cells in blood vessels throughout the body, including those of the kidney, brain, liver, and heart.[51,55] The endothelial changes result in signs and symptoms of preeclampsia and, in more severe cases, of intravascular clotting and hypoperfusion of vital organs. There is risk for development of disseminated intravascular coagulation (DIC; see Chapter 13), cerebral hemorrhage, hepatic failure, and acute renal failure. Thrombocytopenia is the most common

---

TABLE 23-3 Classification of High Blood Pressure in Pregnancy

CLASSIFICATION	DESCRIPTION
Preeclampsia–eclampsia	Pregnancy-specific syndrome of blood pressure elevation (blood pressure >140 mm Hg systolic or >90 mm Hg diastolic) that occurs after the first 20 weeks of pregnancy and is accompanied by proteinuria (urinary excretion of 0.3 g protein in a 24-hour specimen).
Gestational hypertension	Blood pressure elevation, without proteinuria, that is detected for the first time during mid-pregnancy and returns to normal by 12 weeks postpartum.
Chronic hypertension	Blood pressure ≥140 mm Hg systolic or ≥90 mm Hg diastolic that is present and observable before the 20th week of pregnancy. Hypertension that is diagnosed for the first time during pregnancy and does not resolve after pregnancy also is classified as chronic hypertension.
Preeclampsia superimposed on chronic hypertension	Chronic hypertension (blood pressure ≥140 mm Hg systolic or ≥90 mm Hg diastolic before the 20th week of pregnancy) with superimposed proteinuria and with or without signs of the preeclampsia syndrome.

Developed using information from the National Institutes of Health. (2000). *Working group report on high blood pressure in pregnancy.* NIH publication no. 00-3029. Bethesda, MD: Author. Available: www.nhlbi.gov/health/prof/heart/hbp/hbp_preg.htm.

hematologic complication of preeclampsia. Platelet counts of less than 100,000/mm³ signal serious disease. The cause of thrombocytopenia has been ascribed to platelet deposition at the site of endothelial injury. The renal changes that occur with preeclampsia include a decrease in glomerular filtration rate and renal blood flow. Sodium excretion may be impaired, although this is variable. Edema may or may not be present. Some of the severest forms of preeclampsia occur in the absence of edema. Even when there is extensive edema, the plasma volume usually is lower than that of a normal pregnancy. Liver damage, when it occurs, may range from mild hepatocellular necrosis with elevation of liver enzymes to the more ominous *h*emolysis, elevated *l*iver function test results, and *l*ow *p*latelet count (HELLP) syndrome that is associated with significant maternal mortality. Eclampsia, the convulsive stage of preeclampsia, is a significant cause of maternal mortality. The pathogenesis of eclampsia remains unclear but has been attributed to both increased blood coagulability and fibrin deposition in the cerebral vessels.

The decreased placental blood flow that occurs with preeclampsia also affects the fetus. It frequently results in intrauterine growth restriction and infants who are small for gestational age. Preeclampsia is one of the leading causes of prematurity because of frequent need for early delivery in affected women.

Gestational Hypertension. Gestational hypertension represents a blood pressure elevation without proteinuria that is detected for the first time after mid-pregnancy.[51] It includes women with preeclampsia syndrome who have not yet manifested proteinuria as well as women who do not have the syndrome. The hypertension may be accompanied by other signs of the syndrome. The final determination that a woman does not have the preeclampsia syndrome is made only postpartum. If preeclampsia has not developed and blood pressure has returned to normal by 12 weeks postpartum, the condition is considered to be gestational hypertension. If blood pressure elevation persists, a diagnosis of chronic hypertension is made.

Chronic Hypertension. Chronic hypertension is considered to be hypertension that is unrelated to the pregnancy. It is defined as a history of high blood pressure before pregnancy, identification of hypertension before 20 weeks of pregnancy, and hypertension that persists after pregnancy.[51] Hypertension that is diagnosed for the first time during pregnancy and does not resolve after pregnancy also is classified as chronic hypertension. In women with chronic hypertension, blood pressure often decreases in early pregnancy and increases during the last trimester (3 months) of pregnancy, resembling preeclampsia. Consequently, women with undiagnosed chronic hypertension who do not present for medical care until the later months of pregnancy may be incorrectly diagnosed as having preeclampsia.

Preeclampsia Superimposed on Chronic Hypertension. Women with chronic hypertension are at increased risk for the

development of preeclampsia, in which case the prognosis for the mother and fetus tends to be worse than for either condition alone. Superimposed preeclampsia should be considered in women with hypertension before 20 weeks of gestation who develop new-onset proteinuria; women with hypertension and proteinuria before 20 weeks of gestation; women with previously well-controlled hypertension who experience a sudden increase in blood pressure; and women with chronic hypertension who develop thrombocytopenia or an increase in serum ALT or AST to abnormal levels.[51]

Diagnosis and Treatment

Early prenatal care is important in the detection of high blood pressure during pregnancy. It is recommended that all pregnant women, including those with hypertension, refrain from alcohol and tobacco use. Salt restriction usually is not recommended during pregnancy because pregnant women with hypertension tend to have lower plasma volumes than normotensive pregnant women and because the severity of hypertension may reflect the degree of volume contraction. The exception is women with preexisting hypertension who have been following a salt-restricted diet.

In women with preeclampsia, delivery of the fetus is curative. The timing of delivery becomes a difficult decision in preterm pregnancies because the welfare of both the mother and the infant must be taken into account. Bed rest is a traditional therapy. Antihypertensive medications, when required, must be carefully chosen because of their potential effects on uteroplacental blood flow and on the fetus. For example, the ACE inhibitors can cause injury and even death of the fetus when given during the second and third trimesters of pregnancy.

 High Blood Pressure in Children and Adolescents

Until recently, the incidence of hypertension among children has been low, with a range of 1% to 3%.[56] Recent data, however, indicate that the prevalence and rate of diagnosis of hypertension in children and adolescents appear to be increasing.[56,57] This may be due in part to increasing prevalence of obesity and other lifestyle factors, such as decreased physical activity and increased intake of high-calorie, high-salt foods.

Blood pressure is known to increase from infancy to late adolescence. The average systolic pressure at 1 day of age is approximately 70 mm Hg and increases to approximately 85 mm Hg at 1 month of age.[58] Systolic blood pressure continues to increase with physical growth to about 120 mm Hg at the end of adolescence. During the preschool years, blood pressure begins to follow a pattern that tends to be maintained as the child grows older. This pattern continues into adolescence and adulthood, suggesting that the roots of essential hypertension have their origin early in life. A familial influence on blood pressure often can be identified early in life. Children of parents with high blood pressure tend to have higher blood pressures than do children with normotensive parents.

Blood pressure norms for children are based on age-, height-, and sex-specific percentiles[59] (Table 23-4). The National High Blood Pressure Education Program (NHBPEP) first published its recommendations in 1977. The fourth Task Force report (published in 2004) recommended classification of blood pressure (systolic or diastolic) for age, height, and gender into four categories: normal (less than the 90th percentile), high normal (between the 90th and 95th percentiles), stage 1 hypertension (between the 95th and 99th percentiles plus 5 mm Hg), and stage 2 hypertension (greater than the 99th percentile plus 5 mm Hg).[59] The height percentile is determined by using the revised Centers for Disease Control and Prevention (CDC) growth charts.[60] As with the JNC 7 report, high normal is now considered to be "prehypertensive" and is an indication for lifestyle modification. Children and adolescents with hypertension should be evaluated for target-organ damage.[59]

Secondary hypertension is the most common form of high blood pressure in infants and children. In later childhood and adolescence, essential hypertension is more common. Approximately 75% to 80% of secondary hypertension in children is caused by kidney abnormalities.[61] Coarctation of the aorta is another cause of hypertension in children and adolescents. Endocrine causes of hypertension, such as pheochromocytoma and adrenal cortical disorders, are rare. Hypertension in infants is associated most commonly with high umbilical catheterization and renal artery obstruction caused by thrombosis.[61] Most cases of essential hypertension are associated with obesity or a family history of hypertension.

A number of drugs of abuse, therapeutic agents, and toxins also may increase blood pressure. Alcohol should be considered as a risk factor in adolescents. Oral contraceptives may be a cause of hypertension in adolescent girls. The nephrotoxicity of the drug cyclosporine, an immunosuppressant used in transplant therapy, may cause hypertension in children (and adults) after

TABLE 23-4 The 90th and 95th Percentiles of Systolic and Diastolic Blood Pressure for Boys and Girls 1 to 16 Years of Age by Percentiles for Height

BLOOD PRESSURE PERCENTILE	AGE (YRS)	HEIGHT PERCENTILE FOR BOYS				HEIGHT PERCENTILE FOR GIRLS			
		5th	25th	75th	95th	5th	25th	75th	95th
Systolic Pressure									
90th	1	94	97	100	103	97	98	101	103
95th		98	101	104	106	100	102	105	107
90th	3	100	103	107	109	100	102	104	106
95th		104	107	110	113	104	105	108	110
90th	6	105	108	111	113	104	106	109	111
95th		109	112	115	117	108	110	113	115
90th	10	111	114	117	119	112	114	116	118
95th		115	117	121	123	116	117	120	122
90th	13	117	120	124	126	117	119	122	124
95th		121	124	128	130	121	123	126	128
90th	16	125	128	131	134	121	123	126	128
95th		129	132	135	137	125	127	130	132
Diastolic Pressure									
90th	1	49	51	53	54	52	53	55	56
95th		54	55	58	58	56	57	59	60
90th	3	59	60	62	63	61	62	64	65
95th		63	64	66	67	65	66	68	69
90th	6	68	69	71	72	68	69	70	72
95th		72	73	75	76	72	73	74	76
90th	10	73	74	76	78	73	73	75	76
95th		77	79	81	82	77	77	79	80
90th	13	75	76	78	79	76	76	78	79
95th		79	80	82	83	80	80	82	83
90th	16	78	79	81	82	78	79	81	82
95th		82	83	85	87	82	83	85	86

The height percentile is determined by using the newly revised CDC growth charts. Blood pressure levels are based on new data from the 1999–2000 National Health and Nutritional Examination Survey (NHANES) that have been added to the childhood BP database.

From the National High Blood Pressure Education Program Working Group on High Blood Pressure in Children and Adults. (2004). Fourth report on the diagnosis, evaluation, and treatment of high blood pressure in children and adolescents. *Pediatrics* 114, 555–576. [On-line]. Available:www.pediatrics.org/cgi/content/full/114/S2/555.

bone marrow, heart, kidney, or liver transplantation. The coadministration of corticosteroid drugs appears to increase the incidence of hypertension.

Diagnosis and Treatment

The Task Force recommended that children 3 years of age through adolescence should have their blood pressure taken once each year. The auscultatory method using a cuff of an appropriate size for the child's upper arm is recommended.[59] Repeated measurements over time, rather than a single isolated determination, are required to establish consistent and significant observations. Children with high blood pressure should be referred for medical evaluation and treatment as indicated. Treatment includes nonpharmacologic methods and, if necessary, pharmacologic therapy.

High Blood Pressure in the Elderly

The prevalence of hypertension increases with advancing age to the extent that half of people aged 60 to 69 years and approximately three fourths of people 70 years and older are affected.[8] The age-related rise in systolic blood pressure is primarily responsible for the increase in hypertension that occurs with increasing age.

Among the aging processes that contribute to an increase in blood pressure are a stiffening of the large arteries, particularly the aorta; decreased baroreceptor sensitivity; increased peripheral vascular resistance; and decreased renal blood flow.[62] Systolic blood pressure rises almost linearly between 30 and 84 years of age, whereas diastolic pressure rises until 50 years of age and then levels off or decreases.[63] This rise in systolic pressure is thought to be related to increased stiffness of the large arteries. With aging, the elastin fibers in the walls of the arteries are gradually replaced by collagen fibers that render the vessels stiffer and less compliant.[62] Differences in the central and peripheral arteries relate to the fact that the larger vessels contain more elastin, whereas the peripheral resistance vessels have more smooth muscle and less elastin. Because of increased wall stiffness, the aorta and large arteries are less able to buffer the increase in systolic pressure that occurs as blood is ejected from the left heart, and they are less able to store the energy needed to maintain the diastolic pressure. As a result, the systolic pressure increases, the diastolic pressure remains unchanged or actually decreases, and the pulse pressure or difference between the systolic pressure and diastolic pressure widens.

Isolated systolic hypertension (systolic pressure ≥140 mm Hg and diastolic pressure <90 mm Hg) is recognized as an important risk factor for cardiovascular morbidity and mortality in older persons.[8] The treatment of hypertension in the elderly has beneficial effects in terms of reducing the incidence of cardiovascular events such as stroke. Studies have shown a reduction in stroke, coronary heart disease, and congestive heart failure in persons who were treated for hypertension compared with those who were not.[62,64]

Diagnosis and Treatment

The recommendations for measurement of blood pressure in the elderly are similar to those for the rest of the population.[65] Blood pressure variability is particularly prevalent among older persons, so it is especially important to obtain multiple measurements on different occasions to establish a diagnosis of hypertension. The effects of food, position, and other environmental factors also are exaggerated in older persons. Although sitting has been the standard position for blood pressure measurement, it is recommended that blood pressure also be taken in the supine and standing positions in the elderly. In some elderly persons with hypertension, a silent interval, called the *auscultatory gap,* may occur between the end of the first and beginning of the third phases of the Korotkoff sounds, providing the potential for underestimating the systolic pressure, sometimes by as much as 50 mm Hg. Because the gap occurs only with auscultation, it is recommended that a preliminary determination of systolic blood pressure be made by palpation and the cuff be inflated 30 mm Hg above this value for auscultatory measurement of blood pressure. In some older persons, the indirect measurement using a blood pressure cuff and the Korotkoff sounds has been shown to give falsely elevated readings compared with the direct intra-arterial method. This is because excessive cuff pressure is needed to compress the rigid vessels of some older persons. Pseudohypertension should be suspected in older persons with hypertension in whom the radial or brachial artery remains palpable but pulseless at higher cuff pressures.

The JNC 7 recommendations for treating hypertension in the elderly are similar to those for the general population.[8] However, blood pressure should be reduced slowly and cautiously. When possible, appropriate lifestyle modification measures should be tried first. Antihypertensive medications should be prescribed carefully because the older person may have impaired baroreflex sensitivity and renal function. Usually, medications are initiated at smaller doses, and doses are increased more gradually. There is also the danger of adverse drug interactions in older persons, who may be taking multiple medications, including over-the-counter drugs.

IN SUMMARY, hypertension (systolic pressure ≥140 mm Hg and/or diastolic pressure ≥90 mm Hg) is one of the most common cardiovascular disorders. It may occur as a primary disorder (*i.e.,* essential hypertension) or as a symptom of some other disease (*i.e.,* secondary hypertension). The incidence of essential hypertension increases with age; the condition is seen more frequently among African Americans, and it may be associated with a family history of high blood pressure, metabolic syndrome, obesity, and increased sodium intake. Causes of secondary hypertension include kidney disease and adrenal cortical disorders (hyperaldosteronism and Cushing disease), which increase sodium and water retention; pheochromocy-tomas, which increase catecholamine levels; and coarctation of the aorta, which produces an increase in blood flow and systolic blood pressure in the arms and a decrease in blood flow and systolic pressure in the legs.

Unlike disorders of other body systems that are diagnosed by methods such as radiography and tissue examination, hypertension and other blood pressure disorders are determined by repeated blood pressure measurements. Uncontrolled hypertension increases the risk of heart disease, renal complications, retinopathy, and stroke. Treatment of essential hypertension focuses on nonpharmacologic methods such as weight reduction, reduction of sodium intake, regular physical activity, and modification of alcohol intake. Among the drugs used in the treatment of hypertension are diuretics, β-adrenergic blocking agents, ACE inhibitors, calcium channel blocking agents, α_1-adrenergic blocking agents, centrally acting α_2 agonists, and vasodilating drugs.

Hypertension that occurs during pregnancy can be divided into four categories: preeclampsia–eclampsia, gestational hypertension, chronic hypertension, and preeclampsia superimposed on chronic hypertension. Preeclampsia–eclampsia is hypertension that develops after 20 weeks' gestation and is accompanied by proteinuria. This form of hypertension, which is thought to result from impaired placental perfusion along with the release of toxic vasoactive substances that alter blood vessel tone and blood clotting mechanisms, poses a particular threat to the mother and the fetus. Gestational hypertension represents a blood pressure elevation without proteinuria that is detected for the first time after mid-pregnancy and returns to normal by 12 weeks postpartum. Chronic hypertension is hypertension that is unrelated to the pregnancy. It is characterized by hypertension that was present before pregnancy or identified before the 20th week of pregnancy and persists after pregnancy.

The prevalence of hypertension in children and adolescents appear to be increasing, partly as a result of an increase in childhood obesity, and lifestyle factors such as physical inactivity and increased intake of high-calorie and high-salt foods. During childhood, blood pressure is influenced by growth and maturation; therefore, blood pressure norms have been established using percentiles specific to age, height, and sex to identify children for further follow-up and treatment. Although hypertension occurs infrequently in children, it is recommended that children 3 years of age through adolescence should have their blood pressure taken once each year.

The most common type of hypertension in elderly persons is isolated systolic hypertension (systolic pressure ≥140 mm Hg and diastolic pressure <90 mm Hg). Its pathogenesis is related to the loss of elastin fibers in the aorta and the inability of the aorta to stretch during systole. Untreated systolic hypertension is recognized as an important risk factor for stroke and other cardiovascular morbidity and mortality in older persons. ■

CONCEPTSin action **ANIMATI**◯**N**

ORTHOSTATIC HYPOTENSION

After completing this section of the chapter, you should be able to meet the following objectives:

■ Define the term *orthostatic hypotension.*
■ Describe the cardiovascular, neurohumoral, and muscular responses that serve to maintain blood pressure when moving from the supine to standing position.
■ Explain how fluid deficit, medications, aging, disorders of the ANS, and bed rest contribute to the development of orthostatic hypotension.

Orthostatic or postural hypotension, which is a physical finding and not a disease, is an abnormal drop in blood pressure on assumption of the standing position.[66-68] In 1995, the Joint Consensus Committee of the American Autonomic Society and the American Academy of Neurology defined orthostatic hypotension as a drop in systolic pressure of 20 mm Hg or more or a drop in diastolic blood pressure of 10 mm Hg or more within 3 minutes of standing.[69] Although this is now the accepted definition, it does not take into account the possibility that different blood pressure declines may be symptomatic or asymptomatic, depending on the resting supine pressure. It also does not account for blood pressure changes that occur after 3 minutes of standing. Therefore, some authorities regard the presence of orthostatic symptoms (*e.g.*, dizziness, syncope) as being more relevant than the numeric decrease in blood pressure.[70]

⚷ ORTHOSTATIC HYPOTENSION

■ Orthostatic or postural hypotension represents an abnormal drop in blood pressure on assumption of the upright position due to pooling of blood in the lower part of the body.

■ Orthostatic hypotension may be accompanied by a decrease in cerebral perfusion that causes a feeling of lightheadedness, dizziness, and, in some cases, fainting. It poses a particular threat for falls in the elderly.

■ The fall in blood pressure is caused by conditions that decrease vascular volume (dehydration), impair muscle pump function (bed rest and spinal cord injury), or interfere with the cardiovascular reflexes (medications that decrease heart rate or cause vasodilation, disorders of the ANS, effects of aging on baroreflex function).

Pathophysiology and Causative Factors

After the assumption of the upright posture from the supine position, approximately 500 to 700 mL of blood is momentarily shifted to the lower part of the body, with an accompanying decrease in central blood volume and arterial pressure.[66] Maintenance of blood pressure during position change is quite complex, involving the rapid initiation of cardiovascular, neurohumoral, and muscular responses. When the standing position is assumed in the absence of normal circulatory reflexes or blood volume, blood pools in the lower part of the body, cardiac output falls, blood pressure drops, and blood flow to the brain is inadequate. As a result, symptoms of decreased blood flow to the CNS may occur, including feelings of weakness, nausea, lightheadedness, dizziness, blurred vision, palpitations, and syncope (*i.e.,* fainting).

The decrease in blood pressure that occurs on standing is usually transient, lasting through several cardiac cycles. Normally, the barorceptors located in the thorax and carotid sinus area sense the decreased pressure and initiate reflex constriction of the veins and arterioles and an increase in heart rate, which brings blood pressure back to normal (Fig. 23-7). The initial adjustment to orthostatic stress is mediated exclusively by the ANS.[71] Within a few minutes of standing, blood levels of antidiuretic hormone and sympathetic neuromediators increase as a secondary means of ensuring maintenance of normal blood pressure in the standing position. Under normal conditions, the renin-angiotensin-aldosterone system is also activated when the standing position is assumed, and even more so in situations of hypotensive orthostatic stress.

Muscle movement in the lower extremities also aids venous return to the heart by pumping blood out of the legs. The unconscious slight body and leg movement during standing (postural sway) is recognized as an important factor in moving venous blood back to the heart.[72] Crossing the legs, which involves contraction of the agonist and antagonist muscles, has been shown to be a simple and effective way of increasing cardiac output and, therefore, blood pressure. When leg crossing is practiced routinely by persons with autonomic failure, standing systolic and diastolic pressures can be increased by approximately 20/10 mm Hg.[72]

Causes

A wide variety of conditions, acute and chronic, are associated with orthostatic hypotension. Although orthostatic hypotension can occur in all age groups, it is seen more frequently in the elderly, especially in persons who are sick and frail. Any disease condition that reduces blood volume, impairs mobility, results in prolonged inactivity, or impairs ANS function may also predispose to orthostatic hypotension. Adverse effects of medications are also commonly encountered causes of orthostatic hypotension.

Aging. Weakness and dizziness on standing are common complaints of elderly persons. Although orthostatic tolerance is well maintained in the healthy elderly, after 70 years of age there is an increasing tendency toward arterial pressure instability and postural hypotension. Although orthostatic hypotension may be either systolic or diastolic, that associated with aging seems

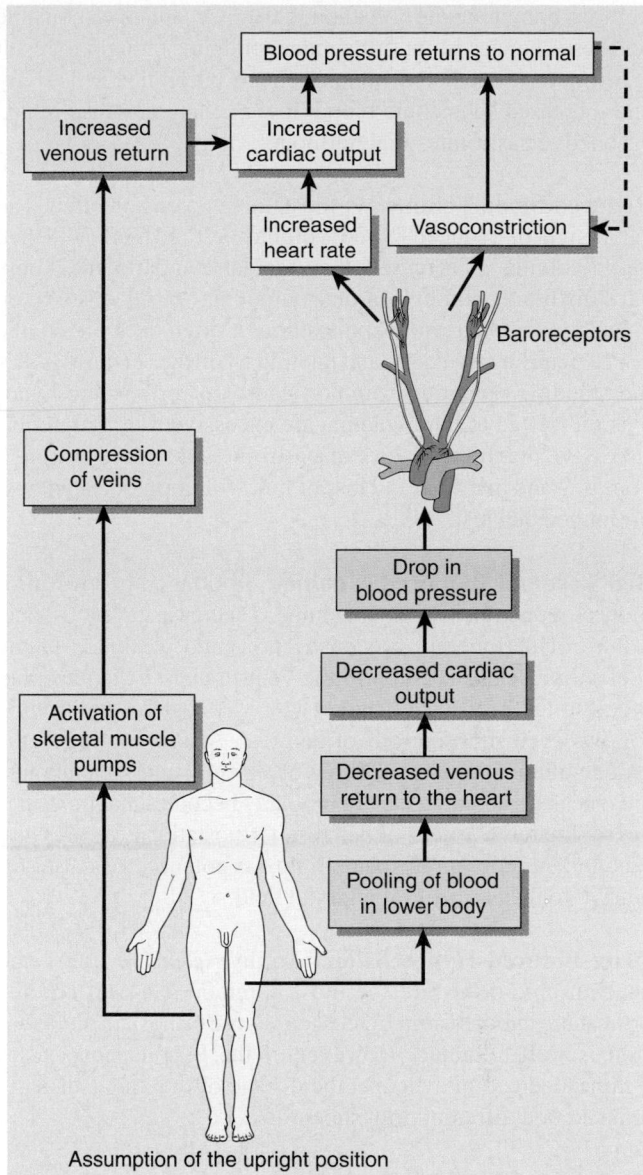

FIGURE 23-7 • Mechanisms of blood control on immediate assumption of the upright position.

more often to be systolic.[67] Several deficiencies in the circulatory response may predispose to this problem in the elderly, including diminished ability to produce an adequate increase in the heart rate, ventricular stroke volume, or peripheral vascular resistance; decreased function of the skeletal muscle pumps; and decreased blood volume. Because cerebral blood flow primarily depends on systolic pressure, patients with impaired cerebral circulation may experience symptoms of weakness, ataxia, dizziness, and syncope when their arterial pressure falls even slightly. This may happen in older persons who are immobilized for even brief periods or whose blood volume is decreased owing to inadequate fluid intake or overzealous use of diuretics.

Postprandial blood pressure often decreases in elderly persons.[73] The greatest postprandial changes occur after a high-carbohydrate meal. Although the mechanism responsible for these changes is not fully understood, it is thought to result from glucose-mediated impairment of baroreflex sensitivity and increased splanchnic blood flow mediated by insulin and vasoactive gastrointestinal hormones.

Reduced Blood Volume. Orthostatic hypotension often is an early sign of reduced blood volume or fluid deficit. When blood volume is decreased, the vascular compartment is only partially filled; although cardiac output may be adequate when a person is in the recumbent position, it often decreases to the point of causing weakness and fainting when the person assumes the standing position. Common causes of orthostatic hypotension related to hypovolemia are excessive use of diuretics, excessive diaphoresis, loss of gastrointestinal fluids through vomiting and diarrhea, and loss of fluid volume associated with prolonged bed rest.

Bed Rest and Impaired Mobility. Prolonged bed rest promotes a reduction in plasma volume, a decrease in venous tone, failure of peripheral vasoconstriction, and weakness of the skeletal muscles that support the veins and assist in returning blood to the heart (see Chapter 11). Physical deconditioning follows even short periods of bed rest. After 3 to 4 days, the blood volume is decreased. Loss of vascular and skeletal muscle tone is less predictable but probably becomes maximal after approximately 2 weeks of bed rest. Orthostatic intolerance is a recognized problem of space flight—a potential risk after re-entry into the earth's gravitational field.

Drug-Induced Hypotension. Antihypertensive drugs and psychotropic drugs are the most common cause of chronic orthostatic hypotension. In most cases, the orthostatic hypotension is well tolerated. However, if the hypotension causes lightheadedness or syncope, the dosage of the drug is usually reduced or a different drug substituted.

Disorders of the Autonomic Nervous System. The sympathetic nervous system plays an essential role in adjustment to the upright position. Sympathetic stimulation increases heart rate and cardiac contractility and causes constriction of peripheral veins and arterioles. Orthostatic hypotension caused by altered ANS function is common in peripheral neuropathies associated with diabetes mellitus, after injury or disease of the spinal cord, or as the result of a cerebral vascular accident in which sympathetic outflow from the brain stem is disrupted. The American Autonomic Society and the American Academy of Neurology have distinguished three forms of primary ANS dysfunction: (1) pure autonomic failure, which is defined as a sporadic, idiopathic cause of persistent orthostatic hypotension and other manifestations of autonomic failure such as urinary retention, impotence, or decreased sweating; (2) Parkinson disease with autonomic failure; and (3) multiple-system atrophy (Shy-Drager syndrome).[69] The Shy-Drager syndrome usually develops in middle to late life as orthostatic hypotension associated with uncoordinated movements, urinary incontinence, constipation, and other signs of neurologic deficits referable to the corticospinal, extrapyramidal, corticobulbar, and cerebellar systems.

Diagnosis and Treatment

Orthostatic hypotension can be assessed with the auscultatory method of blood pressure measurement. Measurements should be made when the person is supine, after standing for 1 minute, and again after standing for 3 minutes.[67] Because it takes approximately 5 to 10 minutes for the blood pressure to stabilize after lying down, it is recommended that the patient be supine for this period before standing. It is strongly recommended that a second person be available when blood pressure is measured in the standing position to prevent injury should the person become faint. The seated position may be used in persons who are unable to stand; however, the postural blood pressure changes may be missed.

The detection of orthostatic hypotension may require numerous blood pressure measurements under different conditions.[67] The time of day is important because postural hypotension is often worse in the morning when the person rises from bed. Food and alcohol can also exacerbate orthostatic hypotension, as can activities that raise intrathoracic pressure (urination, defecation, coughing). An orthostatic hypotensive response may be immediate or delayed. Prolonged standing or a tilt table test may be needed to detect a delayed response. With a tilt table, the recumbent person can be moved to a head-up position without voluntary movement when the table is tilted. The tilt table also has the advantage of rapidly and safely returning persons with a profound postural drop in blood pressure to the horizontal position.

The heart rate response to postural change may provide valuable information about the cause of orthostatic hypotension.[67] A minimal increase in heart rate (<10 beats/minute) in the face of hypotension suggests impairment of baroreflex function, whereas tachycardia (>100 beats/minute) is suggestive of volume depletion or orthostatic intolerance. Because of the age-related decrease in baroreflex function, the absence of an increase in heart rate does not rule out volume depletion in the elderly person.[67]

Persons with a position-related drop in blood pressure sufficient to qualify as orthostatic hypotension should be evaluated to determine the cause and seriousness of the condition. A history should be taken to elicit information about symptoms, particularly dizziness and history of syncope and falls; medical conditions, particularly those such as diabetes mellitus that predispose to orthostatic hypotension; use of prescription and over-the-counter drugs; and symptoms of ANS dysfunction, such as erectile or bladder dysfunction. A physical examination should document blood pressure in both arms and the heart rate while in the supine, sitting, and standing positions and should note the occurrence of symptoms. Noninvasive, 24-hour ambulatory blood pressure monitoring may be used to determine blood pressure responses to other stimuli of daily life, such as food ingestion and exertion.

Treatment of orthostatic hypotension usually is directed toward alleviating the cause or, if this is not possible, toward helping people learn ways to cope with the disorder and prevent falls and injuries. Medications that predispose to postural hypotension should be avoided. Correcting the fluid deficit and trying a different antihypertensive medication are examples of measures designed to correct the cause. Measures designed to help persons prevent symptomatic orthostatic drops in blood pressure include gradual ambulation to allow the circulatory system to adjust (*i.e.*, sitting on the edge of the bed for several minutes and moving the legs to initiate skeletal muscle pump function before standing); avoidance of situations that encourage excessive vasodilation (*e.g.*, drinking alcohol, exercising vigorously in a warm environment); and avoidance of excess diuresis (*e.g.*, use of diuretics), diaphoresis, or loss of body fluids. Tight-fitting elastic support hose or an abdominal support garment may help prevent pooling of blood in the lower extremities and abdomen.

Pharmacologic treatment may be used when nonpharmacologic methods are unsuccessful. A number of types of drugs can be used for this purpose.[67,69] Mineralocorticoids (*e.g.*, fludrocortisone) can be used to reduce salt and water loss and probably increase α-adrenergic sensitivity. Vasopressin-2 receptor agonists (desmopressin as a nasal spray) may be used to reduce nocturnal polyuria. Sympathomimetic drugs that act directly on the resistance vessels (*e.g.*, phenylephrine, noradrenaline, clonidine) or on the capacitance vessels (*e.g.*, dihydroergotamine) may be used. Many of these agents have undesirable side effects. Octreotide, a somatostatin analog that inhibits the release of vasodilatory gastrointestinal peptides, may prove useful in persons with postprandial hypotension.

IN SUMMARY, orthostatic hypotension refers to an abnormal decrease in systolic and diastolic blood pressures that occurs on assumption of the upright position. An important consideration in orthostatic hypotension is the occurrence of dizziness and syncope. Among the factors that contribute to its occurrence are decreased fluid volume, medications, aging, defective function of the ANS, and the effects of immobility. Diagnosis of orthostatic hypotension relies on blood pressure measurements in the supine and upright positions, and a history of symptomatology, medication use, and disease conditions that contribute to a postural drop in blood pressure. Treatment includes correcting the reversible causes and assisting the person to compensate for the disorder and prevent falls and injuries. ■

Review Exercises

1. A 47-year-old African American man who is an executive in a law firm has his blood pressure taken at a screening program and is told that his pressure is 142/90 mm Hg. His father and older brother have hypertension, and his paternal grandparents had a history of stroke and myocardial infarction. The patient enjoys salty foods and routinely uses a salt shaker to add salt to meals his wife prepares, drinks about four beers while watching television in the evening, and gained 15 pounds in the past year. Although his family has encouraged him to engage in physical activities with them, he states he is either too busy or too tired.

   A. *According to the JNC 7 guidelines, into what category does the patient's blood pressure fall?*

   B. *What are his risk factors for hypertension?*

   C. *Explain how an increased salt intake might contribute to his increase in blood pressure.*

   D. *What lifestyle changes would you suggest to the patient? Explain the rationale for your suggestions.*

2. A 36-year-old woman enters the clinic complaining of headache and not feeling well. Her blood pressure is 175/90 mm Hg. Her renal test results are abnormal, and follow-up tests confirm that she has a stricture of the left renal artery.

   A. *Would this woman's hypertension be classified as primary or secondary?*

   B. *Explain the physiologic mechanisms underlying her blood pressure elevation.*

3. A 75-year-old woman residing in an extended care facility has multiple health problems, including diabetes, hypertension, and heart failure. Lately, she has been feeling dizzy when she stands up, and she has almost fallen on several occasions. Her family is concerned and wants to know why this is happening and what they can do to prevent her from falling and breaking her hip.

   A. *How would you go about assessing this woman for orthostatic hypotension?*

   B. *What are the causes of orthostatic hypotension in elderly persons?*

   C. *How might this woman's medical conditions and their treatment contribute to her orthostatic hypotension?*

   D. *The woman tells you that she feels particularly dizzy after she has eaten, yet staff members insist that she sit up and socialize with the other residents even though she would rather lie down and rest until the dizziness goes away. Explain the possible reason for her dizziness and what measures might be used to counteract the dizziness.*

   E. *The woman recently had an episode of vomiting and diarrhea on an extremely hot day. She told her family that she was so dizzy that she was sure she would fall. Explain why her dizziness was more severe under these conditions and what might be done to alleviate the situation.*

References

1. Smith J. J., Kampine J. P. (1990). *Circulatory physiology* (3rd ed., pp. 89–109). Baltimore: Williams & Wilkins.

2. Guyton A. C., Hall J. E. (2006). *Textbook of medical physiology* (11th ed., pp. 204–231). Philadelphia: Elsevier Saunders.

3. Verdecchia P., Schillaci G., Porcella C. (1991). Dippers versus non-dippers. *Hypertension* 9(Suppl. 8), S42–S44.

4. Grim C. E., Grim C. M. (2001). Accurate and reliable blood pressure measurement in the clinic and home: The key to hypertension control. In Hollenberg N. (Ed.), *Hypertension: Mechanisms and management* (3rd ed., pp. 315–324). Philadelphia: Current Medicine.

5. O'Brien E. (1996). Review: A century of confusion; which bladder for accurate blood pressure measurement? *Journal of Human Hypertension* 10, 565–572.

6. Pickering T. (1995). American Society for Blood Pressure Ad Hoc Panel: Recommendations for use of home (self) and ambulatory blood pressure monitoring. *Journal of Hypertension* 9, 1–11.

7. Pickering T. G., Shimbo D., Haas D. (2006). Ambulatory blood-pressure monitoring. *New England Journal of Medicine* 354, 2368–2374.

8. National Heart, Lung, and Blood Institute. (2003). The seventh report of the Joint National Committee on Detection, Evaluation, and Treatment of High Blood Pressure. U.S. Department of Health and Human Services (NIH publication 03-5233). [On-line.] Available: www.nhlbi.nih.gov/guidelines/hypertension/jnc7full.pdf. Accessed April 1, 2007.

9. Vassan R. S., Larson M. G., Leip E. P., et al. (2001). Assessment of frequency of progression to hypertension in non-hypertensive participants in the Framingham Heart Study: A cohort study. *Lancet* 358, 1682–1686.

10. American Diabetes Association. (2001). Summary of revisions for the 2001 clinical practice recommendations. *Diabetes Care* 24(Suppl. 1), 1.

11. Staesen J. A., Wang J., Bianchi G., et al. (2003). Essential hypertension. *Lancet* 361, 1629–1641.

12. Kaplan N. M. (2005). Systemic hypertension. In Zipes D. P., Libby L., Bonow R. O., et al. (Eds.), *Braunwald's heart disease* (7th ed., pp. 959–985). Philadelphia: Elsevier Saunders.

13. Hunt S. C. (2003). Genetics and family history of hypertension. In Izzo J. L., Black H. R. (Eds.), *Hypertension primer* (3rd ed., pp. 218–221). Dallas: American Heart Association.

14. Iliadou A., Lichtenstein P., Morgenstern R., et al. (2002). Repeated blood pressure measurements in a sample of Swedish twins: Heritabilities and association with polymorphisms of the renin-angiotensin system. *Journal of Hypertension* 20, 1543–1550.

15. Burt V. L., Whelton P., Rocella E. J., et al. (1995). Prevalence of hypertension in the US population: Results from the Third National Health and Nutrition Examination Survey, 1988–91. *Hypertension* 25, 305–313.

16. Gadegbeku C. A., Lea J. P. (2005). Update on disparities in the pathophysiology and management of hypertension: Focus on African Americans. *Medical Clinics of North America* 89, 921–933.

17. Gillum R. F. (1996). Epidemiology of hypertension in African American women. *American Heart Journal* 131, 385–395.

18. Blaustein M. P., Grim C. E. (1991). The pathogenesis of hypertension: Black-white differences. *Cardiovascular Clinics* 21(3), 97–114.

19. Ward K. D., Sparrow D., Landsberg L. (1996). Influence of insulin, sympathetic nervous system activity, and obesity on blood pressure: The Normative Aging Study. *Journal of Hypertension* 14, 301–306.

20. Sowers J. R., Frohlich E. D. (2004). Insulin and insulin resistance: Impact on blood pressure and cardiovascular disease. *Medical Clinics of North America* 88, 63–82.

21. Natali A., Ferrannini E. (2004). Hypertension, insulin resistance, and the metabolic syndrome. *Endocrine and Metabolic Clinics of North America* 33, 417–429.

22. Wilson T. W., Grim C. E. (2000). Sodium and hypertension. In Kiple K. (Ed.), *The Cambridge world history of food and nutrition* (pp. 848–856). Cambridge: Cambridge University Press.

23. Katori M., Majima M. (2006). A missing link between high salt intake and blood pressure increase. *Journal of Pharmacological Sciences* 100, 370–390.

24. Kotchen T. A. (2005). Contributions of sodium and chloride to NaCl-induced hypertension. *Hypertension* 45, 849–850.

25. Elliott P., Stamler S., Nichols R., et al. (1996). INTERSALT revisited: Further analyses of 24 hour sodium excretion and blood pressure within and across populations. *British Medical Journal* 312, 1249–1253.

26. Kotchen T. A., McCarron D. A. (1998). Dietary electrolytes and blood pressure: A statement for healthcare professionals from the American Heart Association Nutrition Committee. *Circulation* 98, 613–617.

27. Sacks F. M., Svetkey L. P., Vollmer W. M., et al. (2001). Effects on blood pressure of reduced sodium and the Dietary Approaches to Stop Hypertension (DASH) diet. *New England Journal of Medicine* 344, 3–10.

28. Cassano P. A., Segal M. R., Vokonas P. S., et al. (1990). Body fat distribution, blood pressure, and hypertension: A prospective study of men in the normative aging study. *Annals of Epidemiology* 1, 33–48.

29. Peiris A. N., Sothmann M. S., Hoffmann R. G., et al. (1989). Obesity, fat distribution, and cardiovascular risk. *Annals of Internal Medicine* 110, 867–872.

30. Rahmouni K., Correla M. L. G., Haynes W. G., et al. (2005). Obesity-associated hypertension: New insights into mechanisms. *Hypertension* 45, 9–14.

31. Beilin L. J., Puddey I. B. (2006). Alcohol and hypertension: An update. *Hypertension* 47, 1035–1038.

32. Fuchs F. D., Chambless L. E., Whelton P. K., et al. (2001). Alcohol consumption and the incidence of hypertension. *Hypertension* 37, 1242–1250.

33. Klatsky A. L., Freidman G. D., Siegelaub A. B. (1977). Alcohol consumption and blood pressure. *New England Journal of Medicine* 296, 1194–1200.

34. INTERSALT Cooperative Research Group. (1988). INTERSALT: An international study of electrolyte excretion and blood pressure. Results of 24 hour urinary sodium and potassium excretion. *British Medical Journal* 297, 319–328.

35. Sacks F. M., Willett W. C., Smith A., et al. (1998). Effect on blood pressure of potassium, calcium, and magnesium in women with low habitual intake. *Hypertension* 31, 131–138.

36. Neal B., MacMahon S., Chapman N. (2000). Effects of ACE inhibitors, calcium antagonists, and other blood-lowering drugs: Results of prospectively designed overviews of randomized trials. Blood Pressure Treatment Trialists' Collaboration. *Lancet* 356, 1955–1964.

37. Goldstein I. B., Bartzokis G., Guthrie D., et al. (2002). Ambulatory blood pressure and brain atrophy in the healthy elderly. *Neurology* 59, 713–719.

38. McAlister F. A., Wooltorton E., Campbell N. R. C., for the Canadian Hypertension Education Program. (2005). The Canadian Hypertension Education Program (CHEP) recommendations: Launching a new series. *CMAJ* 173, 480–483.

39. Alagiakrishnan K., Masaki K., Schatz I., et al. (2001). Blood pressure dysregulation syndrome: The case for control throughout the circadian cycle. *Geriatrics* 56(3), 50–60.

40. Verdecchia P., Schillaci G., Porcella C. (1991). Dippers versus non-dippers. *Hypertension* 9(Suppl. 8), S42–S44.

41. Griffith T. F., Klassen P. S., Franklin S. S. (2005). Systolic hypertension: An overview. *American Heart Journal* 149, 769–775.

42. Lloyd-Jones D. M., Evans J. C., Larson M. G., et al. (1999). Differential impact of systolic and diastolic blood pressure level on JNC-VI staging. *Hypertension* 34, 381–385.

43. Onusko E. (2003). Diagnosing secondary hypertension. *American Family Physician* 67, 67–74.

44. Safian R. D., Textor S. C. (2001). Renal-artery stenosis. *New England Journal of Medicine* 344, 431–444.

45. Prisant L. M., Szerlip H. M., Mulloy L. L. (2006). Fibromuscular dysplasia: An uncommon cause of secondary hypertension. *Journal of Clinical Hypertension* 81, 894–898.

46. Stern N., Tuck M. (2003). Pathology of adrenal cortical hypertension. In Izzo J. L., Black H. R. (Eds.), *Hypertension primer* (3rd ed., pp. 144–148). Dallas: American Heart Association.

47. Venkata C., Ram S., Fierro-Carrion G. A. (1995). Pheochromocytoma. *Seminars in Nephrology* 15, 126–137.

48. Roa P. S. (1995). Coarctation of the aorta. *Seminars in Nephrology* 15, 87–105.

49. Chasan-Taber L., Willet W. C., Manson J. E. (1996). Prospective study of oral contraceptives and hypertension among women in the United States. *Circulation* 94, 483–489.

50. Vidt D. G. (2003). Treatment of hypertensive emergencies and urgencies. In Izzo J. L., Black H. R. (Eds.), *Hypertension primer* (3rd ed., pp. 462–455). Dallas: American Heart Association.

51. Gifford R. W., Jr. (Chair). (2000). *National High Blood Pressure Working Group report on high blood pressure in pregnancy.* NIH publication no. 00-3029. Bethesda, MD: National Institutes of Health.

52. Roberts J. M., Pearson G., Cutler J., et al. (2003). Summary of NHLBI working group on research on hypertension during pregnancy. *Hypertension* 41, 437–445.

53. Sibai B., Dekker G., Kupfemic M. (2005). Pre-eclampsia. *Lancet* 365, 785–799.

54. Solomon C. G., Seely E. W. (2006). Hypertension in pregnancy. *Endocrinology and Metabolism Clinics* 35, 157–171.

55. Sibai B. M., Lindheimer M., Hauth J., et al. (1998). Risk factors for preeclampsia, abruptio placentae, and adverse neonatal outcomes among women with chronic hypertension. *New England Journal of Medicine* 339, 667–671.

56. Luma G. B., Spiotta R. T. (2006). Hypertension in children and adolescents. *American Family Physician* 73, 1158–1168.

57. Mitsnefes M. M. (2006). Hypertension in children and adolescents. *Pediatric Clinics of North America* 53, 493–512.

58. Bartosh S. M., Aronson A. J. (1999). Childhood hypertension. *Pediatric Clinics of North America* 46, 235–251.

59. National High Blood Pressure Education Program Working Group on High Blood Pressure in Children and Adolescents. (2004). The fourth report on the diagnosis, evaluation, and treatment of high blood pressure in children and adolescents. *Pediatrics* 114, 555–576.

60. National Center for Health Statistics. (2000). 2000 CDC growth charts: United States. [On-line.] Available: www.cdc.gov/growthcharts. Accessed January 30, 2008.

61. Behrman R. E., Kliegman R. M., Arvin A. M. (2004). Systemic hypertension. In Behrman R. E., Kliegman R. M., Jenson H. B. (Eds.), *Nelson textbook of pediatrics* (17th ed., pp. 1592–1598). Philadelphia: Elsevier Saunders.

62. Maddens M., Imam K., Ashkar A. (2005). Hypertension in the elderly. *Primary Care Clinics in Office Practice* 32, 723–753.

63. Franklin S. S., Larson M. G., Khan S. A., et al. (2001). Does the relation of blood pressure to coronary heart disease risk change with aging? *Circulation* 103, 1245–1250.

64. Basile J. N. (2003). Treatment of elderly hypertensive: Systolic hypertension. In Izzo J. L., Black H. R. (Eds.), *Hypertension primer* (3rd ed., pp. 446–449). Dallas: American Heart Association.

65. Dickerson L. M., Gibson M. V. (2005). Management of hypertension in older persons. *American Family Physician* 71, 469–476.

66. Smith J. J., Porth C. J. M. (1990). Age and the response to orthostatic stress. In Smith J. J. (Ed.), *Circulatory response to the upright posture* (pp. 121–138). Boca Raton, FL: CRC Press.

67. Mukai S., Lipsitz L. A. (2002). Orthostatic hypotension. *Clinics in Geriatric Medicine* 19, 253–268.

68. Bradley J. G., Davis K. A. (2003). Orthostatic hypotension. *American Family Physician* 68, 2393–2398.

69. American Autonomic Society and American Academy of Neurologists. (1996). Consensus statement of the definition of orthostatic hypotension, pure autonomic failure, and multiple system atrophy. *Neurology* 46, 1470.

70. Kochar M. S. (1990). Orthostatic hypotension. In Smith J. J. (Ed.), *Circulatory response to the upright posture* (pp. 170–179). Boca Raton, FL: CRC Press.

71. Goldstein D. S. (Moderator), Robertson D., Murray E., Straus S. E., et al., (Discussants). (2002). NIH Conference. Dysautonomias: Clinical disorders of the autonomic nervous system. *Annals of Internal Medicine* 137, 753–763.

72. Van Lieshout J. J., Ten Harkel A. D. J., Weiling W. (1992). Physical maneuvers for combating orthostatic dizziness in autonomic failure. *Lancet* 339, 897–898.

73. Jansen R. W. M. M., Lipsitz L. A. (1995). Postprandial hypotension: Epidemiology, pathophysiology, and clinical management. *Annals of Internal Medicine* 122, 286–295.

Visit thePoint **http://thePoint.lww.com for animations, journal articles, and more!**

Chapter 24

Disorders of Cardiac Function

TONI BALISTRIERI AND KATHY MUSSATTO

➤ Cardiovascular disease (CVD) is the leading cause of death in men and women in the United States. Because of economic advances, social structures, and demographics, it is predicted that CVD will become the leading cause of death worldwide by 2020, surpassing infectious diseases.[1] It is estimated that the direct and indirect costs of CVD in the United States alone were $448.5 billion for 2008.[2] To reduce this increase in morbidity, mortality, and cost, strategies such as population-based public health measures, preventative programs for high-risk subgroups, and the allocation of resources for treatments for CVD can be useful.[1]

In an attempt to focus on common heart problems that affect persons in all age groups, this chapter is organized into six sections: disorders of the pericardium, coronary artery disease, cardiomyopathies, infectious and immunologic disorders of the heart, valvular heart disease, and heart disease in infants and children.

DISORDERS OF THE PERICARDIUM

After completing this section of the chapter, you should be able to meet the following objectives:

- Characterize the function of the pericardium.
- Compare the clinical manifestations of acute pericarditis and chronic pericarditis.
- Describe the physiologic impact of pleural effusion on cardiac function and relate it to the life-threatening nature of cardiac tamponade.
- Relate the pathophysiology of constrictive pericarditis to its clinical manifestations.

The pericardium, sometimes referred to as the *pericardial sac,* is a double-layered serous membrane that isolates the heart from other thoracic structures, maintains its position in the thorax, prevents it from overfilling, and serves as a barrier to infection. The pericardium consists of two layers: a thin inner layer, called the *visceral pericardium,* that adheres to the epicardium; and an outer fibrous layer, called the *parietal pericardium,* that is attached to the great vessels that enter and leave the heart, the sternum, and diaphragm (see Chapter 21, Fig. 21-8). These two layers of the pericardium are separated by a potential space, the *pericardial cavity,* that contains about 50 mL of serous fluid. This fluid acts as a lubricant that prevents frictional forces from developing as the heart contracts and relaxes. Although there is little blood supply to the pericardium, it is well innervated and inflammation can cause severe pain.[3]

🔑 DISORDERS OF THE PERICARDIUM

- The pericardium isolates the heart from other thoracic structures, maintains its position in the thorax, and prevents it from overfilling.

- The two layers of the pericardium are separated by a thin layer of serous fluid, which prevents frictional forces from developing between the visceral and parietal layers of the pericardium.

- Disorders that produce inflammation of the pericardium interfere with the friction-reducing properties of the pericardial fluid and produce pain.

- Disorders that increase the fluid volume of the pericardial sac interfere with cardiac filling and produce a subsequent reduction in cardiac output.

The pericardium is subject to many of the same pathologic processes (*e.g.,* congenital disorders, infections, trauma, immune mechanisms, and neoplastic disease) that affect other structures of the body. Pericardial disorders frequently are associated with or result from another disease in the heart or the surrounding structures (Chart 24-1).

Acute Pericarditis

Pericarditis represents an inflammatory process of the pericardium. *Acute pericarditis,* defined as signs and symptoms resulting from a pericardial inflammation of less than 2 weeks, may occur as an isolated disease or as the result of systemic disease. Viral infections (especially infections with coxsackieviruses and echoviruses) are the most common cause of pericarditis and probably are responsible for many cases classified as idiopathic. Other causes of acute pericarditis include bacterial or mycobacterial infections, connective tissue diseases (*e.g.,* systemic lupus erythematosus, rheumatoid arthritis), uremia, postcardiac surgery, neoplastic invasion of the peri-

---

CHART 24-1 CLASSIFICATION OF DISORDERS OF THE PERICARDIUM

Inflammation
Acute inflammatory pericarditis
1. Infectious
   Viral (echovirus, coxsackievirus, and others)
   Bacterial (*e.g.,* tuberculosis, *Staphylococcus, Streptococcus*)
   Fungal
2. Immune and collagen disorders
   Rheumatic fever
   Rheumatoid arthritis
   Systemic lupus erythematosus
3. Metabolic disorders
   Uremia and dialysis
   Myxedema
4. Ischemia and tissue injury
   Myocardial infarction
   Cardiac surgery
   Chest trauma
5. Physical and chemical agents
   Radiation therapy
   Untoward reactions to drugs, such as hydralazine, procainamide, and anticoagulants
Chronic inflammatory pericarditis
   Can be associated with most of the agents causing an acute inflammatory response

Neoplastic Disease
1. Primary
2. Secondary (*e.g.,* carcinoma of the lung or breast, lymphoma)

Congenital Disorders
1. Complete or partial absence of the pericardium
2. Congenital pericardial cysts

---

cardium, radiation, trauma, drug toxicity, and contiguous inflammatory processes of the myocardium or lung.[3,4]

Like other inflammatory conditions, acute pericarditis often is associated with increased capillary permeability. The capillaries that supply the serous pericardium become permeable, allowing plasma proteins, including fibrinogen, to leave the capillaries and enter the pericardial space. This results in an exudate that varies in type and amount according to the causative agent. Acute pericarditis frequently is associated with a fibrinous (fibrin-containing) exudate (Fig. 24-1), which heals by resolution or progresses to deposition of scar tissue and formation of adhesions between the layers of the serous pericardium. Inflammation also may involve the superficial myocardium and the adjacent pleura.

The manifestations of acute pericarditis include a triad of chest pain, pericardial friction rub, and electrocardiographic (ECG) changes. The clinical findings may vary according to

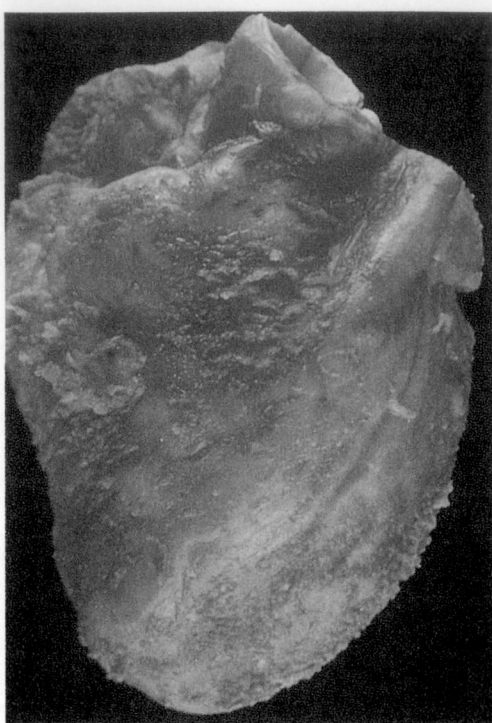

FIGURE 24-1 • Fibrinous pericarditis. The heart of a patient who died in uremia displays a shaggy, fibrinous exudate covering the visceral pericardium. (From Saffitz J. E. [2008]. The heart. In Rubin E., Strayer D. E. [Eds.], *Rubin's pathology: Clinicopathologic foundations of medicine* [5th ed., p. 479]. Philadelphia: Lippincott Williams & Wilkins.)

the causative agent. Nearly all persons with acute pericarditis have chest pain. The pain usually is abrupt in onset and sharp, occurring in the precordial area, and may radiate to the neck, back, abdomen, or side. Pain in the scapular ridge may be due to irritation of the phrenic nerve. The pain typically is worse with deep breathing, coughing, swallowing, and positional changes because of changes in venous return and cardiac filling. Many persons seek relief by sitting up and leaning forward. It is important that chest pain from pericarditis be differentiated from acute myocardial infarction or pulmonary embolism.

Diagnosis of acute pericarditis is based on clinical manifestations, ECG, chest radiography, and echocardiography. A pericardial friction rub, often described as high-pitched or scratchy, results from the rubbing and friction between the inflamed pericardial surfaces. The friction rub is typically described as having three components, which correspond to atrial systole, ventricular systole, and rapid filling of the ventricle. Because it results from the rubbing together of the inflamed pericardial surfaces, large effusions are unlikely to produce a friction rub. Except in uremic pericarditis, the ECG changes in pericarditis typically evolve through four progressive stages: diffuse ST-segment elevations and PR-segment depression; normalization of the ST and PR segments; widespread T-wave inversions; and normalization of T waves. Laboratory markers of systemic inflammation may also be present, including an elevated white blood cell count, elevated erythrocyte sedimentation rate (ESR), and increased C-reactive protein (CRP).[5]

Acute idiopathic pericarditis is frequently self-limiting. Symptoms are usually successfully treated with nonsteroidal anti-inflammatory drugs (NSAIDs).[3,4] Colchicine has also been shown to be of benefit in combination with aspirin and prednisone in initial treatment of acute pericarditis and for prevention of recurrences. Colchicine produces its anti-inflammatory effects by preventing the polymerization of microtubules, which leads to the inhibition of leukocyte migration and phagocytosis. When infection is present, antibiotics specific for the causative agent usually are prescribed. Corticosteroids may be used for treatment of persons with connective tissue disease or severely symptomatic pericarditis that is not responsive to NSAIDs and colchicine.

Relapsing pericarditis can occur in up to 30% of persons with acute pericarditis who respond satisfactorily to treatment.[3] A minority of these develop recurrent bouts of pericardial pain, which can sometimes be chronic and debilitating. The process commonly is associated with autoimmune disorders, such as lupus erythematosus, rheumatoid arthritis, scleroderma, and myxedema, but may also occur following viral pericarditis. Treatment includes the use of anti-inflammatory medications such as NSAIDs, corticosteroids, or colchicine.

Pericardial Effusion and Cardiac Tamponade

Pericardial effusion refers to the accumulation of fluid in the pericardial cavity, usually as a result of an inflammatory or infectious process. It may also develop as the result of neoplasms, cardiac surgery, trauma, cardiac rupture due to myocardial infarction, and dissecting aortic aneurysm. The pericardial cavity has little reserve volume. The pressure–volume relationship between the normal pericardial and cardiac volumes can be dramatically affected by only small amounts of fluid once critical levels of effusion are present. Because right heart filling pressures are lower than that of the left heart, increases in pressure are usually reflected in signs and symptoms of right-sided heart failure before equalization is achieved.

The amount of fluid, the rapidity with which it accumulates, and the elasticity of the pericardium determine the effect the effusion has on cardiac function. Small pericardial effusions may produce no symptoms or abnormal clinical findings. Even a large effusion that develops slowly may cause few or no symptoms, provided the pericardium is able to stretch and avoid compressing the heart. However, a sudden accumulation of even 200 mL may raise intracardiac pressure to levels that seriously limit the venous return to the heart. Symptoms of cardiac compression also may occur with relatively small accumulations of fluid if the pericardium has become thickened by scar tissue or neoplastic infiltrations.

Pericardial effusion can lead to a condition called *cardiac tamponade,* in which there is compression of the heart due to the accumulation of fluid, pus, or blood in the pericardial sac. This life-threatening condition can be caused by infections, neoplasms, and bleeding.[3,4] Cardiac tamponade results in increased intracardiac pressure, progressive limitation of ventricular diastolic filling, and reductions in stroke volume and cardiac output. The severity of the condition depends on the amount of fluid present and the rate at which it accumulates.

A significant accumulation of fluid in the pericardium results in increased adrenergic stimulation, which leads to tachycardia and increased cardiac contractility. There is elevation of central venous pressure, jugular vein distention, a fall in systolic blood pressure, narrowed pulse pressure, and signs of circulatory shock. The heart sounds may become difficult to hear because of the insulating effects of the pericardial fluid and reduced cardiac function. Persons with slowly developing cardiac tamponade usually appear acutely ill, but not to the extreme seen in those with rapidly developing tamponade.

A key diagnostic finding is *pulsus paradoxus,* or an exaggeration of the normal variation in the systemic arterial pulse volume with respiration.[3,4] Normally, the decrease in intrathoracic pressure that occurs during inspiration accelerates venous flow, increasing right atrial and right ventricular filling. This causes the interventricular septum to bulge to the left, producing a slight decrease in left ventricular filling, stroke volume output, and systolic blood pressure. In cardiac tamponade, the left ventricle is compressed from within by movement of the interventricular septum and from without by fluid in the pericardium (Fig. 24-2). This produces a marked decrease in left ventricular filling and left ventricular stroke volume output, often within a beat of the beginning of inspiration. Pulsus paradoxus can be determined by palpation, cuff sphygmomanometry, or arterial pressure monitoring. With pulsus paradoxus, the arterial pulse as palpated at the carotid or femoral artery becomes weakened or absent during inspiration and stronger during expiration. Palpation provides only a gross estimate of the degree of pulsus paradoxus. It is more sensitively estimated when the blood pressure cuff is used to compare the Korotkoff sounds during inspiration and expiration—a decline in systolic pressure greater than 10 mm Hg during inspiration is suggestive of tamponade. Arterial pressure monitoring allows visualization of the arterial pressure waveform and measurement of the blood pressure drop during inspiration.

The echocardiogram is a rapid, accurate, and widely used method of evaluating pericardial effusion. The ECG often reveals nonspecific T-wave changes and low QRS voltage. Usually only moderate to large effusions can be detected by chest radiography.

Treatment of pericardial effusions depends on the progression to cardiac tamponade. In small pericardial effusions or mild cardiac tamponade, NSAIDs, colchicine, or corticosteroids may minimize fluid accumulation. Pericardiocentesis, or removal of fluid from the pericardial sac, often with the aid of echocardiography, is the initial treatment of choice. Closed pericardiocentesis, which is performed with a needle inserted through the chest wall, may be an emergency lifesaving measure in severe cardiac tamponade. Open pericardiocentesis may be used for recurrent or loculated effusions (*i.e.,* those confined to one or more pockets in the pleural space), during which biopsies can be obtained and pericardial windows created. Aspiration and laboratory evaluation of the pericardial fluid may be used to identify the causative agent.

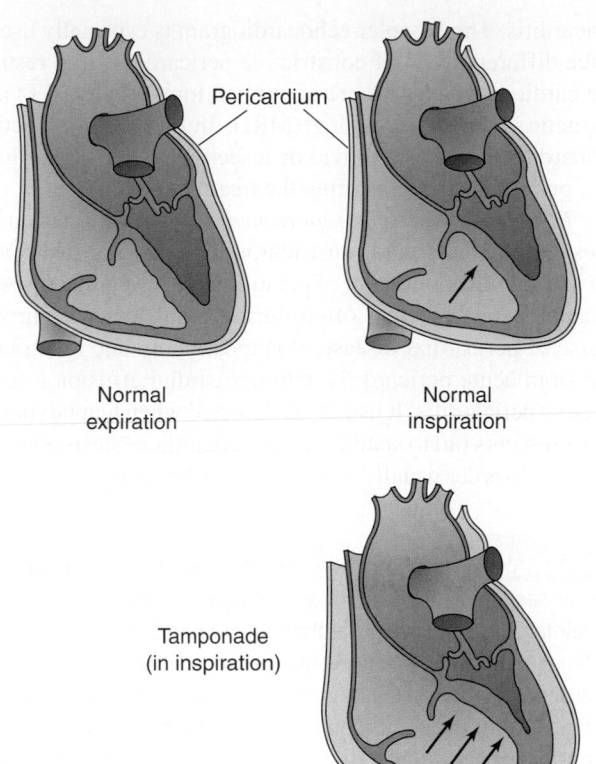

Pericardium

Normal expiration

Normal inspiration

Tamponade (in inspiration)

FIGURE 24-2 • Effects of respiration and cardiac tamponade on ventricular filling and cardiac output. During inspiration, venous flow into the right heart increases, causing the interventricular septum to bulge into the left ventricle. This produces a decrease in left ventricular volume, with a subsequent decrease in stroke volume output. In cardiac tamponade, the fluid in the pericardial sac produces further compression of the left ventricle, causing an exaggeration of the normal inspiratory decrease in stroke volume and systolic blood pressure.

Constrictive Pericarditis

In constrictive pericarditis, fibrous, calcified scar tissue develops between the visceral and parietal layers of the serous pericardium. In time, the scar tissue contracts and interferes with diastolic filling of the heart, at which point cardiac output and cardiac reserve become fixed. The equalization of end-diastolic pressures in all four cardiac chambers is the pathophysiologic hallmark of constrictive pericarditis.[5]

Long-standing inflammation from mediastinal radiation, cardiac surgery, or infection is usually the cause of constrictive pericarditis. Ascites is a prominent early finding and may be accompanied by pedal edema, dyspnea on exertion, and fatigue. The jugular veins also are distended. The Kussmaul sign is an inspiratory distention of the jugular veins caused by the inability of the right atrium, encased in its rigid pericardium, to accommodate the increase in venous return that occurs with inspiration. Exercise intolerance, muscle wasting, and weight loss develop in end-stage constrictive pericarditis.

Chest radiography and Doppler and transesophageal echocardiography are helpful in the diagnosis of constrictive pericarditis. The Doppler echocardiogram is especially useful in the differentiation of constrictive pericarditis from restrictive cardiomyopathy, as are computed tomography (CT) and magnetic resonance imaging (MRI). In chronic constrictive pericarditis, surgical removal or resection of the pericardium (*i.e.*, pericardiectomy) is often the treatment of choice.

Effusive–constrictive pericarditis, a combination of effusion-tamponade and constriction, is a syndrome that develops in a significant number of persons with pericardial disease. Because it occurs most often during a subacute or chronic course of pericardial disease, it is most likely due to a transition from acute pericarditis with pericardial effusion to constrictive pericarditis. It usually is detected when hemodynamic measurements fail to stabilize after pericardiocentesis. Persons with the disorder usually require pericardiectomy.[3,5]

IN SUMMARY, the pericardium is a two-layered membranous sac that isolates the heart from other thoracic structures, maintains its position in the thorax, and prevents it from overfilling; it also may help prevent infection. Disorders of the pericardium include acute and chronic pericarditis, pericardial effusion and cardiac tamponade, and constrictive and effusive–constrictive pericarditis. The major threat of pericardial disease is compression of the heart chambers.

Acute pericarditis may be infectious in origin or it may be due to systemic diseases. It is characterized by chest pain, ECG changes, and pericardial friction rub. Recurrent pericarditis is usually associated with autoimmune disorders, and symptoms may be minimal. Pericardial effusion, either acute or chronic, refers to the presence of an exudate in the pericardial cavity. It can increase intracardiac pressure, compress the heart, and interfere with venous return to the heart. The amount of exudate, the rapidity with which it accumulates, and the elasticity of the pericardium determine the effect the effusion has on cardiac function. Cardiac tamponade represents a life-threatening compression of the heart resulting from excess fluid in the pericardial sac. In constrictive pericarditis, scar tissue develops between the visceral and parietal layers of the serous pericardium. In time, the scar tissue contracts and interferes with cardiac filling. ■

CORONARY ARTERY DISEASE

After completing this section of the chapter, you should be able to meet the following objectives:

- Describe blood flow in the coronary circulation and relate it to the determinants of myocardial oxygen supply and demand.
- Define the term *acute coronary syndrome* and distinguish among chronic stable angina, unstable angina, non–ST-segment elevation myocardial infarction, and ST-segment elevation myocardial infarction in terms

of pathology, symptomatology, ECG changes, and serum cardiac markers.
- Compare the treatment goals for stable angina and the acute coronary syndromes.

The term *coronary artery disease* (CAD) describes heart disease caused by impaired coronary blood flow. In most cases, CAD is caused by atherosclerosis, which affects not only the coronary arteries but arteries in other areas of the body. Diseases of the coronary arteries can cause myocardial ischemia and angina, myocardial infarction or heart attack, cardiac arrhythmias, conduction defects, heart failure, and sudden death. Heart attack is the single largest killer of men and women in the United States, Canada, and other industrialized countries. Each year, more than 1.6 million Americans have new or recurrent myocardial infarctions; one third of those die within the first 24 hours, and many of those who survive suffer significant morbidity. In spite of these numbers, the overall death rate from CAD has declined over the past several decades.[2,6]

Major risk factors for CAD include cigarette smoking, elevated blood pressure, elevated serum total and low-density lipoprotein (LDL) cholesterol, low serum high-density lipoprotein (HDL) cholesterol, diabetes, advancing age, abdominal obesity, and physical inactivity.[2] Individuals with diabetes and the metabolic syndrome (discussed in Chapter 42) are at particularly increased risk for development of cardiovascular disease.[2] Risk factors for atherosclerosis and risk factor assessment are discussed in Chapter 22.

Coronary Circulation

The Coronary Arteries

The two main coronary arteries, the left and the right, arise from the coronary sinus just above the aortic valve[7–9] (Fig. 24-3). The left coronary artery extends for approximately 3.5 cm as the *left main coronary artery* and then divides into the left anterior descending and circumflex branches. The *left anterior descending artery* passes down through the groove between the two ventricles, giving off diagonal branches, which supply the left ventricle, and perforating branches, which supply the anterior portion of the interventricular septum and the anterior papillary muscle of the left ventricle. The *circumflex branch* of the left coronary artery passes to the left and moves posteriorly in the groove that separates the left atrium and ventricle, giving off branches that supply the left lateral wall of the left ventricle. The *right coronary artery* lies in the right atrioventricular groove, and its branches supply the right ventricle. The right coronary artery usually moves to the back of the heart, where it forms the *posterior descending artery,* which normally supplies the posterior portion of the heart, interventricular septum, sinoatrial (SA) and atrioventricular (AV) nodes, and posterior papillary muscle. By convention, the coronary artery that supplies the posterior third of the septum (either the right coronary artery or the left circumflex) is called *dominant.* In a right dominant circulation, present in approximately four fifths of people, the

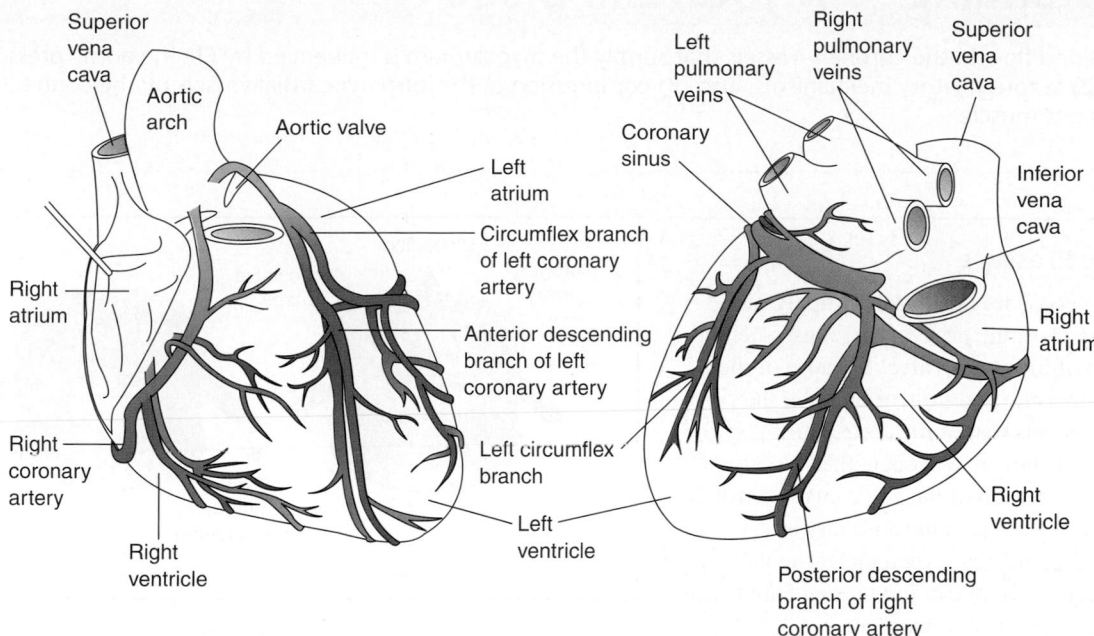

FIGURE 24-3 • Coronary arteries and some of the coronary sinus veins.

left circumflex perfuses the lateral wall of the left ventricle, and the right coronary artery supplies the entire right ventricular free wall and the posterior third of the septum.[9] Thus, occlusion of the right as well as the left coronary artery can cause left ventricular damage.

The large epicardial coronary arteries lie on the surface of the heart, with smaller intramyocardial arteries branching and penetrating the myocardium before merging with a network or plexus of subendocardial vessels. Although there are no connections between the large coronary arteries, there are anastomotic channels that join the small arteries. With gradual occlusion of the larger vessels, the smaller collateral vessels increase in size and provide alternative channels for blood flow. One of the reasons CAD does not produce symptoms until it is far advanced is that the collateral channels develop at the same time the atherosclerotic changes are occurring.

Blood flow in the coronary arteries is controlled largely by physical, neural, and metabolic factors. The openings for the coronary arteries originate in the root of the aorta just outside the aortic valve. Thus, the main factor responsible for perfusion of the coronary arteries is the aortic blood pressure, which is generated by the heart itself. Myocardial blood flow, in turn, is largely regulated by the metabolic activity of the myocardium and autoregulatory mechanisms that control vessel dilation. In addition to generating the aortic pressure that moves blood through the coronary vessels, the contracting heart muscle influences its own blood supply by compressing the intramyocardial and subendocardial blood vessels during systole. The autonomic nervous system exerts its effects on coronary blood flow through changes in heart rate, cardiac contractility, and blood pressure.

Coronary blood flow is largely regulated by the need of the cardiac muscle for oxygen. Even under normal resting condi-

tions, the heart extracts and uses 60% to 80% of oxygen in blood flowing through the coronary arteries, compared with the 25% to 30% extracted by skeletal muscle. Because there is little oxygen reserve in the blood, the coronary arteries must increase their flow to meet the metabolic needs of the myocardium during periods of increased activity. The normal resting blood flow through the coronary arteries averages approximately 225 mL/minute.[7] During strenuous exercise, coronary flow may increase four- to fivefold to meet the energy requirements of the heart.

One of the major determinants of coronary blood flow is the metabolic activity of the heart. Numerous agents, referred to as *metabolites,* are thought to act as mediators for the vasodilation that accompanies increased cardiac work. These substances, which include potassium ions, lactic acid, carbon dioxide, and adenosine, are released from working myocardial cells. Of these substances, adenosine appears to have the greatest vasodilator effect and is perhaps the critical mediator of local blood flow.[7]

The endothelial cells that line blood vessels, including the coronaries, normally form a barrier between the blood and the arterial wall. They also synthesize several substances that, when released, can affect relaxation or constriction of the smooth muscle in the arterial wall. Potent vasodilators produced by the endothelium include nitric oxide, prostacyclin, and endothelium-derived hyperpolarizing factor (EDHF). The most important of these is nitric oxide (see Chapter 21). Most vasodilators and vasodilating stimuli exert their effects through nitric oxide. Products from aggregating platelets, thrombin, the products of mast cells, and increased shear force, which is responsible for so-called flow-mediated vasodilation, stimulate the synthesis and release of nitric oxide.[8] The endothelium also is the source of vasoconstricting factors, the best known of which are the endothelins.

Understanding • Myocardial Blood Flow

Blood flow in the coronary vessels that supply the myocardium is influenced by (1) the aortic pressure, (2) autoregulatory mechanisms, and (3) compression of the intramyocardial vessels by the contracting heart muscle.

❶ Aortic Pressure

The two main coronary arteries that supply blood flow to the myocardium arise in the sinuses behind the two cusps of the aortic valve. Because of their location, the pressure and flow of blood in the coronary arteries reflects that of the aorta. During systole, when the aortic valve is open, the velocity of blood flow and position of the valve cusps cause the blood to move rapidly past the coronary artery inlets, and during diastole, when the aortic valve is closed, blood flow and the aortic pressure are transmitted directly into the coronary arteries.

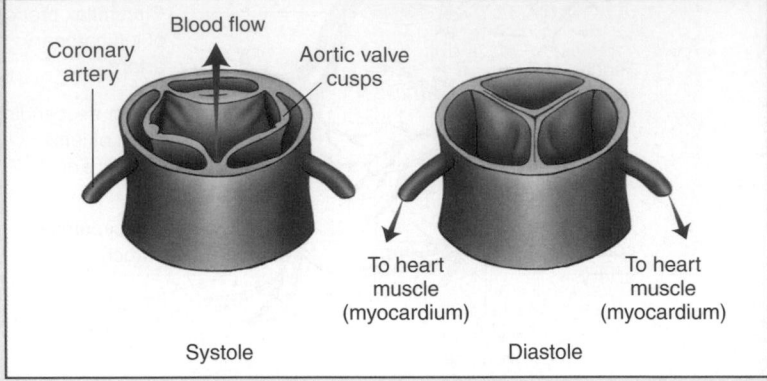

❷ Autoregulatory Mechanisms

The heart normally extracts 60% to 80% of the oxygen in the blood delivered to it, leaving little in reserve. Accordingly, oxygen delivery during periods of increased metabolic demand depends on autoregulatory mechanisms that regulate blood flow through a change in vessel tone and diameter. During increased metabolic demand, vasodilation produces an increase in blood flow; during decreased demand, vasoconstriction or return of vessel tone to normal produces a reduction in flow. The mechanisms that link the metabolic activity of the heart to changes in vessel tone result from vasoactive mediators released from myocardial cells and the vascular endothelium.

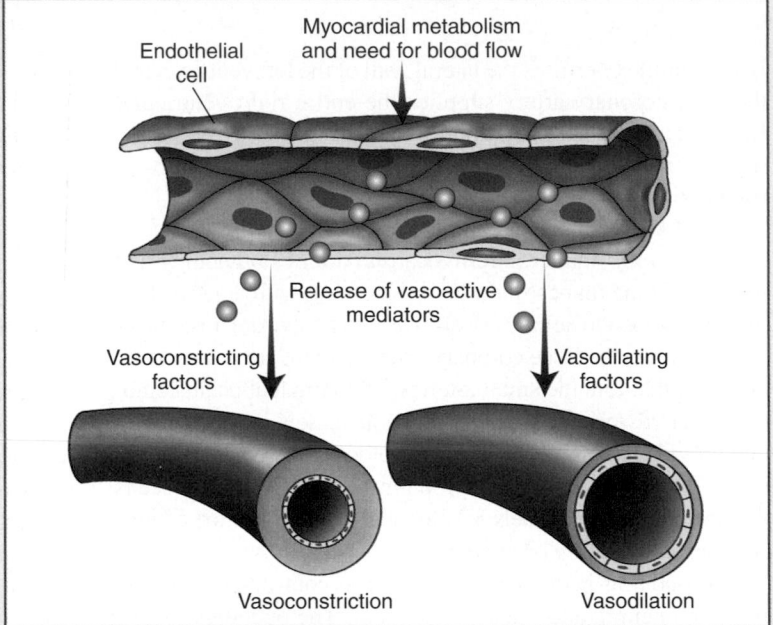

❸ Vessel Compression

The large coronary arteries lie on the epicardial surface of the heart, with smaller intramyocardial vessels branching off and moving through the myocardium before merging with a plexus of vessels that supply the subendocardial muscle with blood. During systole, the contracting cardiac muscle has a squeezing effect on the intramyocardial vessels, while at the same time producing an increase in intraventricular pressure that pushes against and compresses the subendocardial vessels. As a result, blood flow to the subendocardial muscle is greatest during diastole. Because the time spent in diastole becomes shortened as the heart rate increases, myocardial blood flow can be greatly reduced during sustained periods of tachycardia.

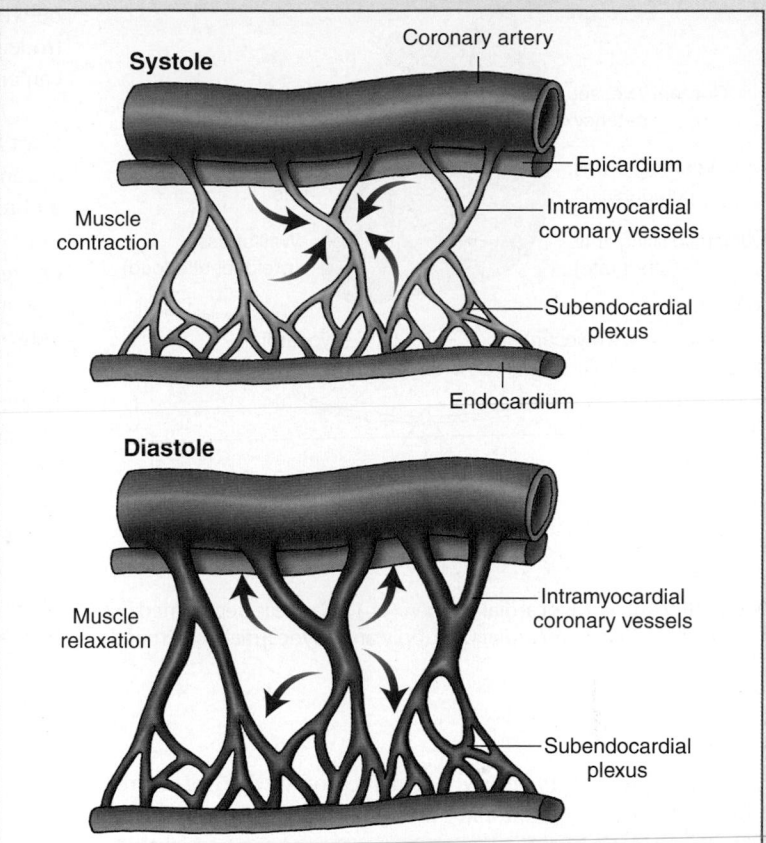

Myocardial Oxygen Supply and Demand

The coronary circulation supplies the heart muscle with the oxygen and nutrients it needs to pump blood out to the rest of the body. As the metabolic needs of the body change, cardiac function and coronary blood flow must adapt to meet these needs. If there is an imbalance in the myocardial oxygen supply and demand, myocardial ischemia and angina, myocardial infarction, or even sudden death can occur. Angina pectoris, often referred to simply as *angina,* is the severe, often constricting, chest pain associated with transient myocardial ischemia.

Myocardial Oxygen Supply. Myocardial oxygen supply is determined by the coronary arteries and capillary inflow, and the ability of hemoglobin to transport and deliver oxygen to the heart muscle. Important factors in the transport and delivery of oxygen include the fraction of inspired oxygen in the blood and the number of red blood cells with normally functioning hemoglobin. Even with adequate coronary blood flow, myocardial ischemia can occur in situations of hypoxia, anemia, or carbon monoxide poisoning.[8]

Myocardial Oxygen Demand. There are three major determinants of myocardial oxygen demand (MVO_2): the heart rate, myocardial contractility, and myocardial wall stress or tension[8] (Fig. 24-4). The heart rate is the most important factor in myocardial oxygen demand, for two reasons: (1) as the heart rate increases, myocardial oxygen consumption or demand also increases; and (2) as noted previously, subendocardial coronary blood flow is reduced because of the decreased diastolic filling time with increased heart rates.[7,8]

Myocardial contractility is the intrinsic ability of the heart muscle to shorten and generate force. It reflects the interaction between calcium ions and the contractile proteins (actin and myosin) of the muscle fibers[8] (see Chapter 4). It is normally determined by the rate of pressure development and muscle shortening. With increased myocardial contractility, the rate of change in wall stress is increased, which in turn increases myocardial oxygen uptake. Factors that increase contractility, such as exercise, sympathetic nervous system stimulation, and inotropic agents, all increase MVO_2.[8]

Wall stress develops when tension is applied to a given area. Left ventricular wall stress can be thought of as the average tension that individual muscle fibers must generate to shorten against a developed intraventricular pressure. It is proportional to the product of the intraventricular pressure and ventricle radius, divided by the thickness of the ventricle wall. Thus, at a given pressure, wall stress is increased by an increase in radius (ventricular dilation) and it is increased by a decrease in wall thickness. The term *preload* is used to describe the distending force of the ventricular wall, which is highest at the end of diastole, just before contraction.[10] Changes in preload are assessed by using the left ventricular end-diastolic pressure. This can be measured indirectly by

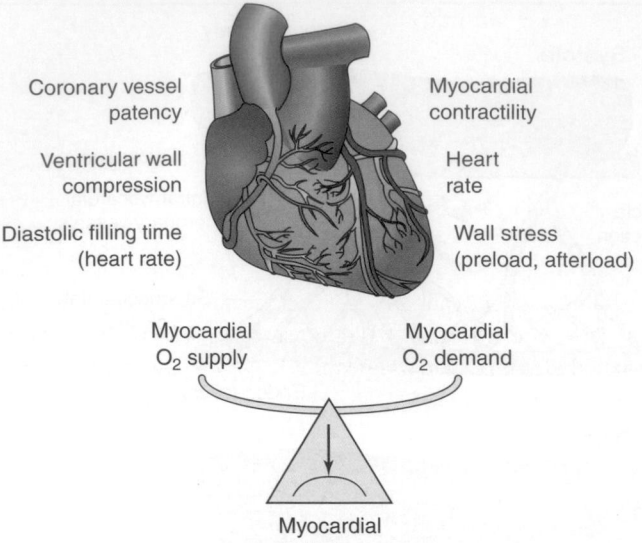

FIGURE 24-4 • Myocardial oxygen (O_2) balance is determined by factors that affect myocardial O_2 supply and myocardial O_2 demand (MVO_2).

using the pulmonary artery occlusive (or wedge) pressure, obtained through a pulmonary artery catheter. *Afterload* is the "load" against which the heart must contract to eject blood. A major component of the left ventricular afterload is the aortic pressure, or pressure that the ventricle must generate to eject blood.[10] An increase in wall stress, whether caused by an increase in preload or afterload, increases MVO_2 because as cardiac muscle fibers develop more tension, they require a greater rate of adenosine triphosphate (ATP) use. Because wall stress is inversely related to wall thickness, ventricular hypertrophy serves as an adaptive mechanism by which the ventricle is able to offset the increase in wall stress that accompanies increased aortic pressure or aortic valve stenosis.

Assessment of Coronary Blood Flow and Myocardial Perfusion

Among the methods used in the evaluation of coronary blood flow and myocardial perfusion are electrocardiography, exercise stress testing, echocardiography, and Doppler ultrasonographic imaging; cardiac MRI and CT; and cardiac catheterization and angiography. These assessment modalities vary widely and are undergoing constant technological advances.

Electrocardiography. The 12-lead ECG is the most frequently used cardiovascular diagnostic procedure. It is indispensable not only for the diagnosis and treatment of CAD, but also for the identification of ventricular conduction defects, arrhythmias, electrolyte imbalances, drug effects, and genetically mediated electrical or structural abnormalities. The standard 12-lead ECG uses electrodes to record electrical potential differences, generated by ion currents (action potentials) during the cardiac cycle,

between prescribed sites on the body (see Chapter 25). Electrode placement and patient position are important because they can change the recorded amplitudes and axes of the ECG.

Ambulatory ECG monitoring often is done to detect transient ST-segment and T-wave changes that occur and are not accompanied by symptoms (*i.e.,* silent ischemia). Continuous ambulatory ECG monitoring can be done using a Holter monitor (see Chapter 25). Another method, called *signal-averaged* or *high-resolution ECG,* accentuates the QRS complex so that low-amplitude afterpotentials that correlate with high risk of ventricular arrhythmias and sudden death can be detected.

Exercise Stress Testing. Exercise stress testing is a means of observing cardiac function under stress and is typically performed in adults with symptoms of known or suspected ischemic heart disease. It is not, however, currently recommended as a routine screening modality in asymptomatic adults.[11]

Treadmill exercise, which is the most commonly used method of cardiovascular stress testing, requires higher levels of myocardial performance than other forms of exercise. Blood pressure is monitored during exercise testing, and the ECG pattern is recorded for the purposes of determining heart rate and detecting myocardial ischemic changes. Chest pain, severe shortness of breath, arrhythmias, ST-segment changes on the ECG, or a decrease in blood pressure suggests CAD, and if one or more of these signs or symptoms is present, the test is usually terminated.

Pharmacologic stress testing may be used to simulate the stress of exercise in persons who cannot participate in active forms of exercise because of orthopedic, neurologic, peripheral vascular disorders, or other conditions. The intravenous infusion of dipyridamole, adenosine, or dobutamine can be used. Dipyridamole blocks the cellular reabsorption of adenosine, an endogenous vasodilator, and increases coronary blood flow three to five times above baseline levels. In persons with significant CAD, the resistance vessels distal to the stenosis already are maximally dilated to maintain normal resting flow. In these persons, further vasodilation does not produce an increase in blood flow. Intravenous injection of adenosine has comparable effects. Dobutamine, a sympathomimetic agent, increases myocardial contractility and stroke volume. During stress echocardiography, low-dose dobutamine identifies myocardial viability and high-dose dobutamine identifies myocardial ischemia.[11]

Echocardiography. Echocardiography uses ultrasound signals that are inaudible to the human ear.[12] The ultrasound signal is reflected (*i.e.,* echoes) whenever there is a change in the resistance to transmission of the sound beam. Thus, it is possible to create a moving image of the internal structures of the heart because the chest wall, blood, and different heart structures all reflect ultrasound differently. The echocardiogram is useful for determining ventricular dimensions and valve movements, obtaining data on the movement of the left ventricular wall and septum, estimating diastolic and systolic volumes, and viewing the motion of individual segments of the left ventricular wall during systole and diastole.

There are several different forms of echocardiography, including two-dimensional imaging, M-mode, Doppler, and contrast echocardiography. M-mode echocardiography, which was the earliest form of cardiac ultrasonography, uses a stationary ultrasound beam to produce a one-dimensional or "ice-pick" view of the heart. *Two-dimensional (2-D) echocardiography* uses a moving ultrasound beam to produce an integrated view of the heart comprising multiple pie-shaped images. *Doppler echocardiography* uses ultrasound to record blood flow within the heart. *Transesophageal echocardiography* uses a 2-D echocardiography transducer placed at the end of a flexible endoscope to obtain echocardiographic images from the esophagus. Placement of the transducer in the esophagus allows echocardiographic images of cardiac structures to be obtained from different viewpoints, rather than only from the surface of the chest. Transesophageal echocardiography is particularly useful in assessing valve function. Stress echocardiography, with or without the use of pharmacologic agents, is used in conjunction with dynamic exercise. Rest and stress images are recorded, stored, and then analyzed for global and regional left ventricular size, shape, and function. Reduced systolic wall thickening seen on stress echocardiography identifies myocardial ischemia.

Nuclear Cardiac Imaging. Nuclear cardiac imaging techniques involve the use of radionuclides (*i.e.,* radioactive substances) and are essentially noninvasive. Four types of nuclear cardiology tests are commonly used: myocardial perfusion imaging, infarct imaging, positron emission tomography, and radionuclide angiocardiography. With all four of these tests, a scintillation (gamma) camera is used to record the radiation emitted from the radionuclide. Single-photon emission computed tomography(SPECT), which uses a multiple-head camera to obtain a series of planar images over a 180- to 360-degree arc around the thorax, is the most widely used imaging technique at present.[13]

Myocardial perfusion imaging is used to visualize the regional distribution of blood flow. *Myocardial perfusion scintigraphy* uses thallium-201 or one of the newer technetium-based agents that are extracted from the blood and taken up by functioning myocardial cells. Thallium-201, an analog of potassium, is distributed to the myocardium in proportion to the magnitude of blood flow. After injection, an external detection device registers the distribution of the radioactive material. An ischemic area appears as a "cold spot" that lacks radioactive uptake. The most important application of this technique has been its use during stress testing for evaluation of ischemic heart disease.

Acute infarct imaging uses a radionuclide that is taken up by the cells in an infarcted zone. With this method, the damaged myocardium is visualized as a "hot spot," or positive area, of increased radionuclide uptake. Its usefulness usually is limited by an 18- to 26-hour lag after acute infarction before the test becomes positive, and it has limited sensitivity for small, non-transmural infarcts.

Positron emission tomography (PET) uses positron-emitting agents to demonstrate either the perfusion or metabolic status of the myocardium. The radioisotopes used as positron emitters are the naturally occurring, small atomic weight atoms

(*e.g.,* carbon, nitrogen, oxygen) that are the predominant constituents of organic compounds such as glucose.[14] During ischemia, cardiac muscle shifts from fatty acid to glucose metabolism. Thus, a radioactive tracer such as fluorodeoxyglucose can be used to distinguish a transiently dysfunctional ("stunned") myocardium from scar tissue by showing persistent glucose metabolism in areas of reduced blood flow.

Radionuclide angiocardiography provides actual visualization of the ventricular structures during systole and diastole and a means for evaluating ventricular function during rest and exercise stress testing. A radioisotope such as technetium-labeled albumin, which does not leave the capillaries but remains in the blood and is not bound to the myocardium, is used for this type of imaging. This type of nuclear imaging can be used to determine right and left ventricular volumes, ejection fractions, regional wall motion, and cardiac contractility. This method also is useful in the diagnosis of intracardiac shunts.

Cardiac Magnetic Resonance Imaging and Computed Tomography. The cardiac MRI creates a spatially resolved map of radio signals and, compared with x-ray–based techniques, is much safer. Cardiac MRI uses gadolinium as a contrast agent and ECG gating to prevent artifacts and blurring from periodic cardiac cycles.[14] In nearly all current scanners, this is achieved by gating (triggering) the acquisition of MRI data to the R wave of the ECG. Cardiac MRI is used for quantifying the volume, mass, and function of the ventricles. However, it cannot be used in persons with implanted metal pacemakers, defibrillators, or other devices.[14]

CT is an x-ray–based technique that obtains cross-sectional views of the body through rotation of the x-ray scanner around the patient. Several generations of CT technology have been developed, including conventional CT, contrast-enhanced CT, and electron-beam CT. CT cardiac imaging can be performed with or without injection of a contrast agent. Noncontrast CT studies are used primarily to assess coronary artery calcification. Contrast-enhanced studies can be used to assess cardiac chambers, great cardiac vessels, and sometimes the coronary artery lumen.[15] The electron-beam CT, developed specifically for cardiac imaging, is a useful technique for identifying persons with or at risk for CAD. Unlike conventional CT, in which the scanner moves around the patient, in electron-beam CT only the electron beam moves.

Cardiac Catheterization and Arteriography. Cardiac catheterization is one of the most widely used invasive procedures in the assessment of CAD. Cardiac catheterization involves the passage of flexible catheters into the great vessels and chambers of the heart. In right heart catheterization, the catheter is inserted into a peripheral vein (usually the femoral) and then advanced into the right heart. The left heart catheter is inserted retrograde through a peripheral artery (usually the brachial or femoral) into the aorta and left heart. The cardiac catheterization laboratory, where the procedure is done, is equipped for viewing and recording fluoroscopic images of the heart and vessels in the chest and for measuring pressures in the heart and great vessels. It also has equipment for cardiac output studies and for obtaining samples of blood for blood gas analysis. Angiographic studies are done by injecting a radiographic contrast medium into the heart so that an outline of the moving structures can be visualized and filmed.

Coronary arteriography involves the injection of a radiographic contrast medium into the coronary arteries, permitting visualization of lesions in these vessels. It is used to identify and establish the extent of coronary artery narrowing, perform percutaneous coronary intervention and placement of coronary artery stents, and determine appropriateness for coronary artery bypass graft surgery.[16] Intracoronary physiologic measurements (Doppler ultrasonography, fractional flow reserve) can also be obtained with new sensor guide wire technology.

Coronary Atherosclerosis and the Pathogenesis of Coronary Artery Disease

Atherosclerosis is by far the most common cause of CAD, and begins at a very young age in the United States and other developed countries of the world (see Chapter 22). Atherosclerosis can affect one or all three of the major epicardial coronary arteries and their branches. Clinically significant lesions may be located anywhere in these vessels, but tend to predominate in the first several centimeters of the left anterior descending and left circumflex or the entire length of the right coronary artery.[16] Sometimes the major secondary branches also are involved.

Coronary artery disease is commonly divided into two types of disorders: the acute coronary syndrome and chronic ischemic heart disease. The *acute coronary syndrome* (ACS) represents a spectrum of acute ischemic heart diseases ranging from unstable angina to myocardial infarction resulting from disruption of an atherosclerotic plaque that did not significantly compromise the coronary lumen before the event. *Chronic ischemic heart disease* is characterized by recurrent and transient episodes of myocardial ischemia and stable angina that result from narrowing of a coronary artery lumen due to atherosclerosis and/or vasospasm.

Stable Versus Unstable Plaque. There are two types of atherosclerotic lesions: the fixed or stable plaque, which obstructs blood flow, and the unstable or vulnerable plaque, which can rupture and cause platelet adhesion and thrombus formation. The fixed or stable plaque is commonly implicated in stable angina and the unstable plaque in unstable angina and myocardial infarction. In most cases the myocardial ischemia underlying unstable angina, acute myocardial infarction, and, in many cases, sudden cardiac death, is precipitated by abrupt plaque changes, followed by thrombosis. The major determinants of plaque vulnerability to disruption include the size of the lipid-rich core, the stability and thickness of its fibrous cap, the presence of inflammation, and lack of smooth muscle cells[9] (Fig. 24-5). Plaques with a thin fibrous cap overlaying a large lipid core are at high risk for rupture.

Although plaque disruption may occur spontaneously, it is often triggered by hemodynamic factors such as blood flow characteristics and vessel tension. For example, a sudden surge of sympathetic activity with an increase in blood pressure, heart rate, force of cardiac contraction, and coronary blood flow is thought to increase the risk of plaque disruption. Indeed, many

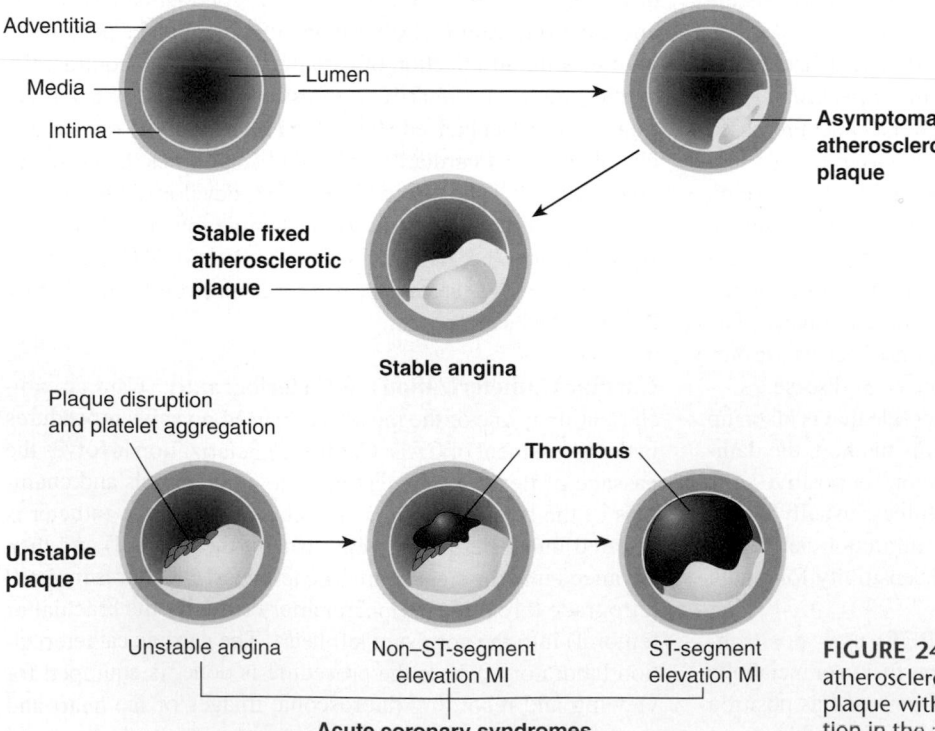

FIGURE 24-5 • Atherosclerotic plaque: stable fixed atherosclerotic plaque in stable angina and unstable plaque with plaque disruption and platelet aggregation in the acute coronary syndromes.

people with myocardial infarction report a trigger event, most often emotional stress or physical activity.[9] Plaque disruption also has a diurnal variation, occurring most frequently during the first hour after arising, suggesting that physiologic factors such as surges in coronary artery tone and blood pressure may promote atherosclerotic plaque disruption and subsequent platelet deposition.[9] It has been suggested that the sympathetic nervous system is activated on arising, resulting in changes in platelet aggregation and fibrinolytic activity that tend to favor thrombosis.

Thrombosis and Vessel Occlusion. Local thrombosis occurring after plaque disruption results from a complex interaction among its lipid core, smooth muscle cells, macrophages, and collagen. The lipid core provides a stimulus for platelet aggregation and thrombus formation.[9] Both smooth muscle and foam cells in the lipid core contribute to the expression of tissue factor in unstable plaques. Once exposed to blood, tissue factor initiates the extrinsic coagulation pathway, resulting in the local generation of thrombin and deposition of fibrin (see Chapter 13).

Platelets play an important role in linking plaque disruption to acute CAD. As a part of the response to plaque disruption, platelets adhere to the endothelium and release substances (*i.e.,* adenosine diphosphate [ADP], thromboxane A_2, and thrombin) that promote further aggregation of platelets and thrombus formation. The platelet membrane, which contains glycoprotein receptors that bind fibrinogen and link platelets together, contributes to thrombus formation. Platelet adhesion and aggregation occurs in several steps. First, release of ADP, thromboxane A_2, and thrombin initiates the aggregation process. Second, glycoprotein IIb/IIIa receptors on the platelet surface are activated. Third, fibrinogen binds to the activated glycoprotein receptors, forming bridges between adjacent platelets.

There are two types of thrombi formed as a result of plaque disruption—white platelet-containing thrombi and red fibrin-containing thrombi. The thrombi in unstable angina have been characterized as grayish-white and presumably platelet rich.[17] Red thrombi, which develop with vessel occlusion in myocardial infarction, are rich in fibrin and red blood cells superimposed on the platelet component and are extended by the stasis of blood flow.

Acute Coronary Syndrome

Acute coronary syndrome includes unstable angina, non–ST-segment elevation (non–Q-wave) myocardial infarction, and ST-segment elevation (Q-wave) myocardial infarction. Persons without ST-segment elevation on ECG are those in whom thrombotic coronary occlusion is subtotal or intermittent; whereas those with ST-segment elevation are usually found to have complete coronary occlusion on angiography, and many ultimately have Q-wave myocardial infarction. Persons with an ACS are routinely classified as low risk, intermediate risk, or high risk based on history and physical examination, the ECG, and serum cardiac markers, with primary emphasis on the ECG.

> ### 🔑 CORONARY ARTERY DISEASE
>
> - The term *coronary artery disease* refers to disorders of myocardial blood flow due to stable or unstable coronary atherosclerotic plaques.
> - Unstable atherosclerotic plaques tend to fissure or rupture, causing platelet aggregation and potential for thrombus formation with production of a spectrum of acute coronary syndromes of increasing severity, ranging from unstable angina, to non–ST-segment elevation myocardial infarction, to ST-segment elevation myocardial infarction.
> - Stable atherosclerotic plaques produce fixed obstruction of coronary blood flow with myocardial ischemia occurring during periods of increased metabolic need, such as in stable angina.

Electrocardiographic Changes. The classic ECG changes that occur with ACS involve T-wave inversion, ST-segment elevation, and development of an abnormal Q wave[18] (Fig. 24-6). The changes that occur may not be present immediately after the onset of symptoms, and vary considerably depending on the duration of the ischemic event (acute versus evolving), its extent (subendocardial versus transmural), and its location (anterior versus inferior posterior). Because these changes usually occur over time and are seen on the ECG leads that view the involved area of the myocardium, provision for continuous and serial 12-lead ECG monitoring is indicated (see Chapter 25 for a more complete discussion of the ECG).

The repolarization phase of the action potential (T wave and ST segment on the ECG) is usually the first to be involved during myocardial ischemia and injury. As the involved area becomes ischemic, myocardial repolarization is altered, causing changes in the T wave. This is usually represented by T-wave inversion, although a hyperacute T-wave elevation may occur as the earliest sign of infarction. ST-segment changes occur with ischemic myocardial injury. Normally, the ST segment of the ECG is nearly isoelectric (*e.g.,* flat along the baseline) because all healthy myocardial cells attain the same potential during early repolarization. Acute severe ischemia reduces the resting membrane potential and shortens the duration of the action potential in the ischemic area. These changes create a voltage difference between the normal and ischemic areas of the myocardium that leads to a so-called current of injury between these regions. It is these currents of injury that are represented on the surface ECG as a deviation of the ST segment. When the acute injury is transmural, the overall ST vector is shifted in the direction of the outer epicardium, resulting in ST-segment elevation[18] (see Fig. 24-6). When the injury is confined primarily to the subendocardium, the overall ST segment is shifted toward the inner ventricular layer, resulting in an overall depression of the ST segment.

With actual infarction, depolarization (QRS) changes often follow the T-wave and ST-segment abnormalities. With Q-wave

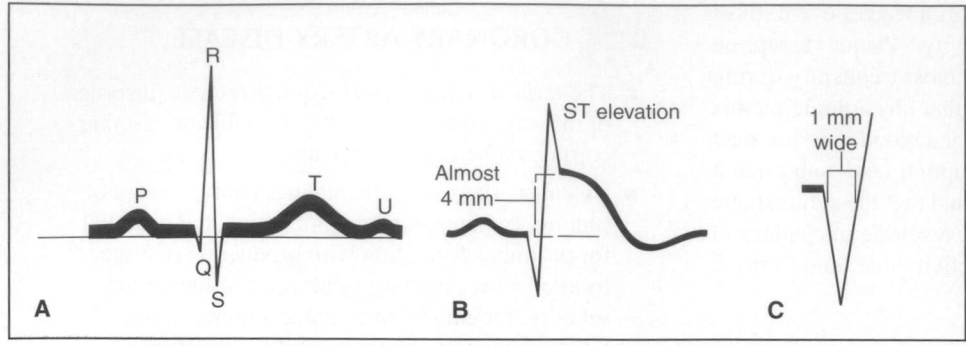

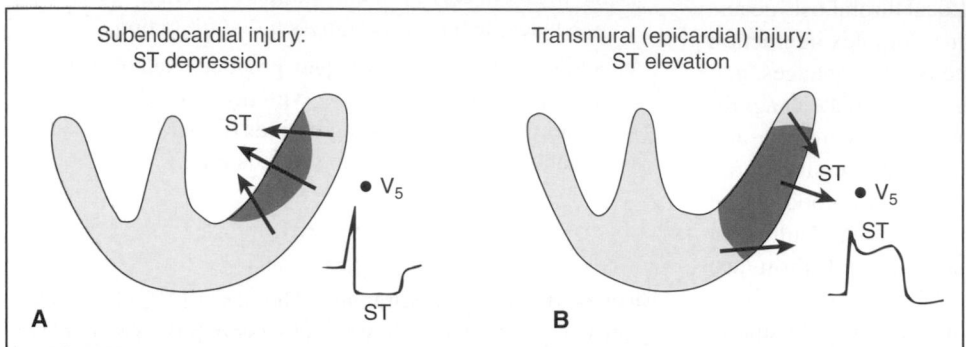

FIGURE 24-6 • (Top) (A) ECG tracing showing normal P, Q, R, S, and T waves. (B) ST-segment elevation with acute ischemia. (C) Q wave with acute myocardial infarction. (Bottom) Current-of-injury patterns with acute ischemia. (A) With predominant subendocardial ischemia, the resultant ST segment is directed toward the inner layer of the affected ventricle and the ventricular cavity. Overlying leads therefore record ST-segment depression. (B) With ischemia involving the outer ventricular layer (transmural or epicardial injury), the ST vector is directed outward. Overlying leads record ST-segment elevation. (Bottom from Braunwald E., Zipes D. P., Libby P. [Eds.]. [2002]. Heart disease: A textbook of cardiovascular medicine [6th ed., p. 108]. Philadelphia: W. B. Saunders.)

infarction, abnormal Q waves develop because there is no depolarizing current conduction from the necrotic tissue.

Serum Biomarkers. Serum biomarkers for ACS include cardiac-specific troponin I (TnI) and troponin T (TnT), myoglobin, and creatine kinase MB (CK-MB). As the myocardial cells become necrotic, their intracellular contents begin to diffuse into the surrounding interstitium and then into the blood. The rate at which the enzymes appear in the blood depends on their intracellular location, their molecular weight, and local blood flow. For example, they may appear at an earlier-than-predicted time in patients who have undergone successful reperfusion therapy.

The *troponin assays* have high specificity for myocardial tissue and have become the primary biomarker tests for the diagnosis of myocardial infarction. The troponin complex, which is part of the actin filament, consists of three subunits (*i.e.,* TnC, TnT, and TnI) that regulate calcium-mediated actin–myosin contractile process in striated muscle (see Chapter 4, Fig. 4-22). TnI and TnT, which are present in cardiac muscle, begin to rise within 3 hours after the onset of myocardial infarction and may remain elevated for 7 to 10 days after the event. This is especially advantageous in the late diagnosis of myocardial infarction.[19]

Creatine kinase is an intracellular enzyme found in muscle cells. There are three isoenzymes of CK, with the MB isoenzyme being highly specific for injury to myocardial tissue. Serum levels of CK-MB exceed normal ranges within 4 to 8 hours of myocardial injury and decline to normal within 2 to 3 days.[19]

Myoglobin is an oxygen-carrying protein, similar to hemoglobin, that is normally present in cardiac and skeletal muscle. It is a small molecule that is released quickly from infarcted myocardial tissue and becomes elevated within 1 hour after

myocardial cell death, with peak levels reached within 4 to 8 hours.[19] Because myoglobin is present in both cardiac and skeletal muscle, it is not cardiac specific.

Unstable Angina/Non–ST-Segment Elevation Myocardial Infarction

Unstable angina (UA)/non–ST-segment elevation myocardial infarction (NSTEMI) is considered to be a clinical syndrome of myocardial ischemia ranging from stable angina to myocardial infarction.[17] Typically, UA and NSTEMI differ in whether the ischemia is severe enough to cause sufficient myocardial damage to release detectable quantities of serum cardiac markers. Persons who have no evidence of serum markers for myocardial damage are considered to have UA, whereas a diagnosis of NSTEMI is indicated if a serum marker of myocardial injury is present.

The pathophysiologic process of UA/NSTEMI can be divided into three phases: the development of the unstable plaque that ruptures, the acute ischemic event, and the long-term risk of recurrent events that remains after the acute event.[20] Inflammation can play a prominent role in plaque instability, with inflammatory cells releasing cytokines that cause the fibrous cap to become thinner and more vulnerable to rupture or erosion (see Chapter 22). The acute ischemic event can be caused by an increase in myocardial oxygen demand precipitated by tachycardia or hypertension, or more commonly by a decrease in oxygen supply related to a reduction in coronary lumen diameter due to platelet-rich thrombi or vessel spasm.[20]

The pain associated with UA/NSTEMI has a persistent and severe course and is characterized by at least one of three features: (1) it occurs at rest (or with minimal exertion), usually lasting more than 20 minutes (if not interrupted by nitroglycerin); (2) it is severe and described as frank pain and of new onset (*i.e.,* within 1 month); and (3) it is more severe, prolonged, or frequent than previously experienced.[20]

Risk stratification of persons presenting with UA/NSTEMI is important because the outcome can range from excellent, with little change in treatment, to NSTEMI or death, requiring aggressive treatment. UA/NSTEMI is classified as either low, intermediate or high risk for acute myocardial infarction, based on the clinical history, ECG pattern, and serum biomarkers. The ECG pattern in UA/NSTEMI demonstrates ST-segment depression (or transient ST-segment elevation) and T-wave changes. The degree of ST-segment deviation has been shown to be an important measure of ischemia and prognosis.

ST-Segment Elevation Myocardial Infarction

Acute ST-segment elevation myocardial infarction (STEMI), also known as *heart attack,* is characterized by the ischemic death of myocardial tissue associated with atherosclerotic disease of the coronary arteries. The area of infarction is determined by the coronary artery that is affected and by its distribution of blood flow (Fig. 24-7). Approximately 30% to 40% of infarcts affect the right coronary artery, 40% to 50% affect the left anterior descending artery, and the remaining 15% to 20% affect the left circumflex artery.[9]

Pathologic Changes.   The extent of the infarct depends on the location and extent of occlusion, amount of heart tissue sup-

plied by the vessel, duration of the occlusion, metabolic needs of the affected tissue, extent of collateral circulation, and other factors such as heart rate, blood pressure, and cardiac rhythm. An infarct may involve the endocardium, myocardium, epicardium, or a combination of these. Transmural infarcts involve the full thickness of the ventricular wall and most commonly occur when there is obstruction of a single artery (Fig. 24-8). Subendocardial infarcts involve the inner one third to one half of the ventricular wall and occur more frequently in the presence of severely narrowed but still patent arteries. Most infarcts are transmural, involving the free wall of the left ventricle and the interventricular septum.

The principal biochemical consequence of myocardial infarction is the conversion from aerobic to anaerobic metabolism with inadequate production of energy to sustain normal myocardial function. As a result, a striking loss of contractile function occurs within 60 seconds of onset.[9] Changes in cell structure (*i.e.,* glycogen depletion and mitochondrial swelling) develop within several minutes. These early changes are reversible if blood flow is restored. Although gross tissue changes are not apparent for hours after onset of myocardial infarction, the ischemic area ceases to function within a matter of minutes, and irreversible damage to cells occurs in approximately 40 minutes. Irreversible myocardial cell death (necrosis) occurs after 20 to 40 minutes of severe ischemia.[9] Microvascular injury occurs in approximately 1 hour and follows irreversible cell injury. If the infarct is large enough, it depresses overall left ventricular function and pump failure ensues.

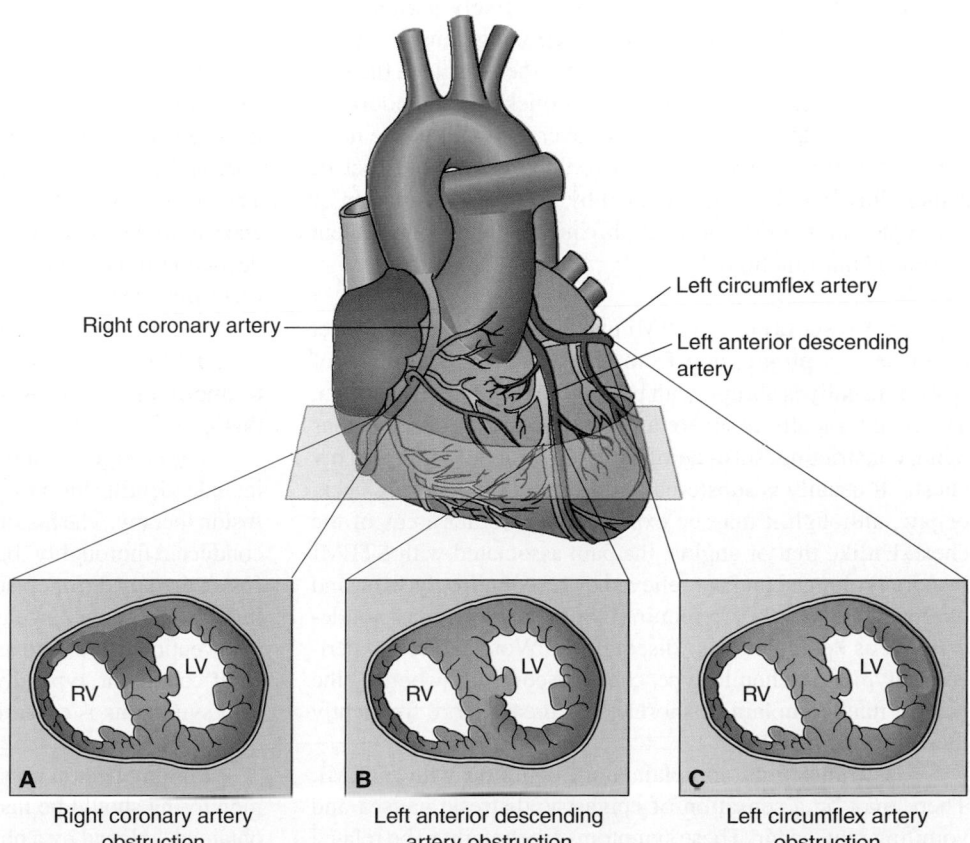

FIGURE 24-7 • Areas of the heart affected by occlusion of the **(A)** right coronary artery, **(B)** left anterior descending coronary artery, and **(C)** left circumflex coronary artery. RV, right ventricle; LV, left ventricle.

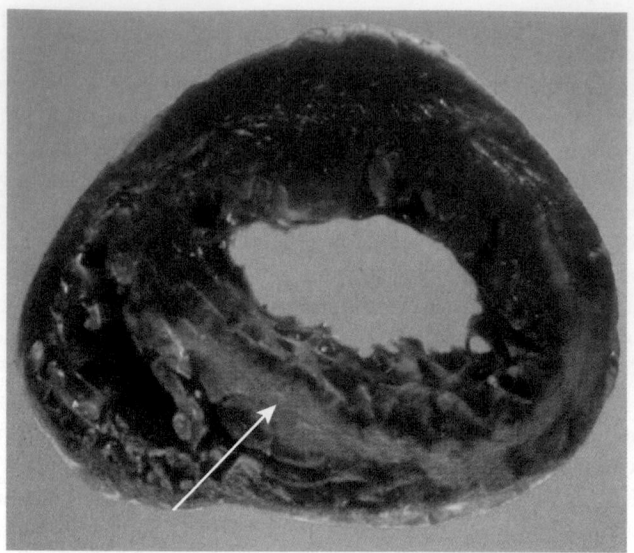

FIGURE 24-8 • Acute myocardial infarct. A cross-section of the ventricles of a man who died a few days after the onset of severe chest pain shows a transmural infarct in the posterior and septal regions of the left ventricle. The necrotic myocardium is soft, yellowish, and sharply demarcated. (From Rubin E., Farber J. L. [1999]. *Pathology* [3rd ed., p. 558]. Philadelphia: Lippincott Williams & Wilkins.)

Multiple dynamic structural changes maintain cardiac function in persons with STEMI. Both the infarcted and non-infarcted areas of the ventricle undergo progressive changes in size, shape, and thickness, comprising early wall thinning, healing, hypertrophy, and dilation, collectively termed *ventricular remodeling*. As the nonfunctioning muscle in the infarcted area becomes thin and dilated, the muscle in the surrounding, noninfarcted area becomes thicker as it undergoes adaptive hypertrophy so it can take over the work of the muscle in the infarcted zone. However, the adaptive effect of remodeling may be overwhelmed by aneurysm formation or depression of myocardial function, causing further impairment of ventricular function.[9,19]

Clinical Presentation. STEMI may occur as an abrupt-onset event or as a progression from UA/NSTEMI. The onset of STEMI usually is abrupt, with pain as the significant symptom. The pain typically is severe and crushing, often described as being constricting, suffocating, or like "someone sitting on my chest." It usually is substernal, radiating to the left arm, neck, or jaw, although it may be experienced in other areas of the chest. Unlike that of angina, the pain associated with STEMI is more prolonged and not relieved by rest or nitroglycerin, and narcotics frequently are required. Some persons may not describe it as "pain," but as "discomfort." Women often experience atypical ischemic-type chest discomfort, whereas the elderly may complain of shortness of breath more frequently than chest pain.[6]

Gastrointestinal complaints are common with STEMI. There may be a sensation of epigastric distress; nausea and vomiting may occur. These symptoms are thought to be related to the severity of the pain and vagal stimulation. The epigastric distress may be mistaken for indigestion, and the person may seek relief with antacids or other home remedies, which only delays getting medical attention. Complaints of fatigue and weakness, especially of the arms and legs, are common. Pain and sympathetic stimulation combine to give rise to tachycardia, anxiety, restlessness, and feelings of impending doom. The skin often is pale, cool, and moist. Impairment of myocardial function may lead to hypotension and shock.

Sudden death from STEMI is death that occurs within 1 hour of symptom onset.[19] It usually is attributed to fatal arrhythmias, which may occur without evidence of infarction. Early hospitalization after onset of symptoms greatly improves the chances of averting sudden death because appropriate resuscitation facilities are immediately available when the ventricular arrhythmia occurs. The recent distribution of automatic external defibrillators in multiple public arenas highlights the importance of early defibrillation in the survival of patients with STEMI.

Management of Acute Coronary Syndrome

Because the specific diagnosis of STEMI often is difficult to make at the time of entry into the health care system, the immediate management of UA/NSTEMI and STEMI is generally the same. The prognosis in STEMI is largely related to the occurrences of two general complications—arrhythmias and mechanical complications (pump failure). The majority of deaths from STEMI are due to the sudden development of ventricular fibrillation. Therefore, the major elements in management of persons with STEMI are recognition of symptoms and prompt seeking of medical care; the prompt deployment of an emergency medical team capable of resuscitation procedures, including defibrillation; expeditious transport to a hospital equipped for managing arrhythmias and providing advanced cardiac life support; and expeditious implementation of reperfusion therapy.[19] The greatest delay usually results because persons who experience signs and symptoms of STEMI delay seeking treatment, despite current public information regarding the benefits of early treatment. The development of "Systems of Care" for ACS is currently being pursued by the American Heart Association (AHA) and other national organizations with the goal of improving timely access and adherence to evidence-based therapies.[21]

The emergency department goals for management of ACS include identification of persons who are candidates for reperfusion therapy. The history and physical examination should be conducted thoroughly, but efficiently, so as not to delay reperfusion therapy. Prior episodes of cardiovascular disease, including ACS, coronary bypass surgery, or percutaneous coronary intervention, should be ascertained. Evaluation of the person's chief complaint, typically chest pain, along with other associated symptoms is essential in differentiating ACS from other diagnoses.

For any person presenting with symptoms of ACS, ECG monitoring should be instituted, and a 12-lead ECG should be obtained and read by a physician within 10 minutes of arrival at the emergency department. The typical ECG changes may not be present immediately after the onset of symptoms, except as arrhythmias. Diagnostic ECG tracings (*i.e.,* ST-segment elevation, prolongation of the Q wave, and inversion of the T wave) are absent in as much as half of persons with STEMI who present with chest pain. Premature ventricular contractions are common arrhythmias after myocardial infarction. The occurrence of other arrhythmias and conduction defects depends on the areas of the heart and conduction pathways that are included in the infarct. A new bundle branch block, particularly left bundle branch block, also serves as a criterion for STEMI and indicates a need for rapid reperfusion.

Commonly indicated treatment regimens include administration of oxygen, aspirin, nitrates, pain medications, antiplatelet and anticoagulant therapy, β-adrenergic blocking agents (beta blockers), and an angiotensin-converting enzyme (ACE) inhibitor.[19] Persons with ECG evidence of infarction should receive immediate reperfusion therapy with a thrombolytic agent or percutaneous coronary intervention (PCI).[6] The importance of intensive insulin control to maintain normal blood glucose (80 to 110 mg/dL) in critically ill patients has been supported by multiple studies. Current American College of Cardiology (ACC)/AHA guidelines recommend the maintenance of strict glucose control during STEMI.[6]

The severe pain of STEMI gives rise to anxiety and recruitment of autonomic nervous system responses, both of which increase the work demands on the heart. Sudden increases in catecholamines may also play a role in plaque fissuring and thrombus propagation, as well as lowering the threshold for ventricular fibrillation.[9] Therefore, pain relief is a major objective in the treatment of STEMI. Control of pain in STEMI is accomplished through a combination of nitrates, analgesics (*e.g.,* morphine), oxygen, and β-adrenergic blocking agents.

Nitroglycerin is given because of its vasodilating effect and ability to relieve coronary pain. The vasodilating effects of the drug decrease venous return (*i.e.,* reduce preload) and arterial blood pressure (*i.e.,* reduce afterload), thereby reducing oxygen consumption. Nitroglycerin may also limit infarction size and is most effective if given within 4 hours of symptom onset. Nitroglycerin usually is administered sublingually initially, after which the need for intravenous infusion is assessed. The use of intravenous nitroglycerin may be indicated for treatment of ongoing ischemic pain, control of hypertension, or management of pulmonary congestion. Nitroglycerin should not be administered to patients with severe hypotension or to patients who have received a phosphodiesterase inhibitor for erectile dysfunction within the previous 24 hours.

Although a number of analgesic agents have been used to treat the pain of STEMI, morphine is usually the drug of choice.[19] It usually is indicated if chest pain is unrelieved with oxygen and nitrates. The reduction in anxiety that accompanies the administration of morphine contributes to a decrease in restlessness and autonomic nervous system activity, with a subsequent decrease in the metabolic demands of the heart. It is commonly given intravenously because of the rapid onset of action and because the intravenous route does not elevate enzyme levels. The intravenous route also bypasses the variable rate of absorption of subcutaneous or intramuscular sites, which often are underperfused because of the decrease in cardiac output that occurs after infarction.

The administration of oxygen augments the oxygen content of inspired air and increases the oxygen saturation of hemoglobin. Arterial oxygen levels may fall precipitously after STEMI, and oxygen administration helps to maintain the oxygen content of the blood perfusing the coronary circulation. In patients with severe heart failure from STEMI, continuous positive-pressure ventilation or endotracheal intubation and support with mechanical ventilation may be necessary.

β-Adrenergic blocking drugs act as antagonists that block β-receptor–mediated functions of the sympathetic nervous system and thus decrease myocardial oxygen demand by reducing heart rate and cardiac contractility, and systemic arterial blood pressure. The lengthening of diastole caused by the slower heart rate may enhance myocardial perfusion, especially to the subendocardium. Beta blockers also alter resting myocardial membrane potentials and may decrease life-threatening ventricular arrhythmias. Because sympathetic nervous system activity increases the metabolic demands of the myocardium, oral or intravenous beta blockers are usually administered within the first few hours after the onset of STEMI. Beta blockers are also recommended for patients with UA/NSTEMI who do not have contraindications. They should not be given in STEMI caused by cocaine use because it could accentuate coronary spasm. Other relative contraindications to beta blockers include symptomatic bradycardia, hypotension, moderate-to-severe left ventricular failure, shock, or second- or third-degree heart block.

Platelets play a major role in the thrombotic response to atherosclerotic plaque disruption; therefore, inhibition of platelet aggregation is an important aspect in the early treatment of both UA/NSTEMI and STEMI. Aspirin (*i.e.,* acetylsalicylic acid) is the preferred antiplatelet agent for preventing platelet aggregation in persons with ACS. Aspirin, which acts by inhibiting synthesis of the prostaglandin thromboxane A_2, is thought to promote reperfusion and reduce the likelihood of rethrombosis. The actions of aspirin are related to the presence of the acetyl group, which irreversibly acetylates the critical platelet enzyme, cyclooxygenase, which is required for thromboxane A_2 synthesis. Because the action is irreversible, the effect of aspirin on platelet function lasts for the lifetime of the platelet—approximately 8 to 10 days. For patients who are unable to take aspirin because of hypersensitivity or gastrointestinal intolerance, clopidogrel may be prescribed. Clopidogrel is a thienopyridine derivative that reduces platelet aggregation by inhibiting the ADP pathway in platelets. Unlike aspirin, it has no effect on prostaglandin synthesis. Results of several studies have resulted in recommendations by the AHA for the use of clopidogrel along with aspirin for persons with UA/NSTEMI, and for pre-procedural loading and long-term therapy for persons undergoing PCI. Clopidogrel should be withheld for 5 to 7 days before coronary artery bypass graft surgery.[20]

Another class of antiplatelet agents is the platelet receptor antagonists. In contrast to aspirin and clopidogrel, which target a single step in the aggregation process, the platelet glycoprotein IIb/IIIa (GP IIb/IIIa) receptor inhibitors (*e.g.*, tirofiban, eptifibatide, abciximab) block the receptor involved in the final common pathway for platelet adhesion, activation, and aggregation. The GP IIb/IIIa receptor inhibitors are now recommended in the treatment of patients undergoing early invasive therapy (*e.g.*, PCI) based on a number of different trials.

Antithrombin agents are also used in the treatment of patients with ACS. Anticoagulation therapy, which targets the coagulation pathway and formation of the fibrin clot, involves the use of unfractionated and low–molecular-weight heparin (see Chapter 13). The rationale for the use of antithrombin therapy in patients with STEMI is the prevention of deep vein thrombosis, pulmonary emboli, and cerebral embolization.

ACE inhibitors are often used during the early and convalescent phases of STEMI, demonstrating a benefit in terms of decreased mortality rate. The greatest benefit is in those patients with previous infarctions, heart failure, and tachycardia. ACE inhibitors usually are started within the first 24 hours, after fibrinolytic therapy has been completed. Therapy with ACE inhibitors is usually begun with low-dose oral administration and increased steadily to full dose.[6] Although the use of ACE inhibitors in short-term therapy for patients with UA/NSTEMI does not appear to have benefits, long-term use is helpful in preventing recurrent ischemic episodes.[19]

Reperfusion Strategies. The term *reperfusion* refers to reestablishment of blood flow through use of pharmacologic agents (fibrinolytic therapy), PCI, or coronary artery bypass grafting. All patients presenting with STEMI should be assessed for reperfusion therapy as soon as possible on entry into the health care system. Time since onset of symptoms, risk of STEMI, possible risks associated with fibrinolytic therapy, and time required for transport to a skilled PCI laboratory should all be considered.

Early reperfusion (within 15 to 20 minutes) after onset of occlusion can prevent necrosis and improve myocardial perfusion in the infarct zone. Reperfusion after a longer interval can salvage some of the myocardial cells that would have died owing to longer periods of ischemia. It also may prevent the microvascular injury that occurs over a longer period. Even though much of the viable myocardium existing at the time of reflow, or reperfusion, ultimately recovers, critical abnormalities in biochemical function may persist, causing impaired ventricular function. The recovering area of the heart is often referred to as a *stunned myocardium.* Because myocardial function is lost before cell death occurs, a stunned myocardium may not be capable of sustaining life, and persons with large areas of dysfunctional myocardium may require life support until the stunned regions regain their function.[9]

Fibrinolytic Therapy. Fibrinolytic drugs dissolve blood and platelet clots and are used to reduce mortality, limit infarct size, encourage infarct healing and myocardial remodeling, and reduce the potential for life-threatening arrhythmias. These agents interact with plasminogen to generate plasmin, which lyses

fibrin clots and digests clotting factors V and VIII, prothrombin, and fibrinogen (see Chapter 15). The fibrinolytic agents include streptokinase, alteplase, reteplase, and tenecteplase-tPA. The best results occur if treatment is initiated within 60 to 90 minutes of symptom onset. The magnitude of the benefit declines after this period, but it is possible that some benefit can be achieved for up to 12 hours after the onset of pain. The person must be a low-risk candidate for complications caused by bleeding, with no intracranial hemorrhage or significant trauma within the last 3 months. The primary complication of fibrinolytic therapy is intracranial hemorrhage, which usually occurs within the first 24 hours of treatment.[20]

Percutaneous Coronary Intervention. PCI is indicated as an early invasive procedure for patients with UA/NSTEMI who have no serious comorbidity and who have lesions amenable to PCI.[22] PCI includes percutaneous transluminal coronary angioplasty (PTCA), stent implantation, atherectomy, and thrombectomy. Stent implantation, in conjunction with the platelet GP IIb/IIIa antagonist abciximab, is now the most frequently used procedure. The goal in PCI is to perform the procedure within 90 minutes of the patient's first medical contact (the "door-to-balloon interval").[22]

Balloon PTCA involves dilation of a stenotic atherosclerotic plaque with an inflatable balloon (Fig. 24-9). The procedure is similar to cardiac catheterization for coronary angiography, in that the double-lumen balloon dilation catheter is introduced percutaneously into the femoral or brachial artery and advanced under fluoroscopic view into the stenotic area of the affected coronary vessel. There it is used to expand the coronary arterial

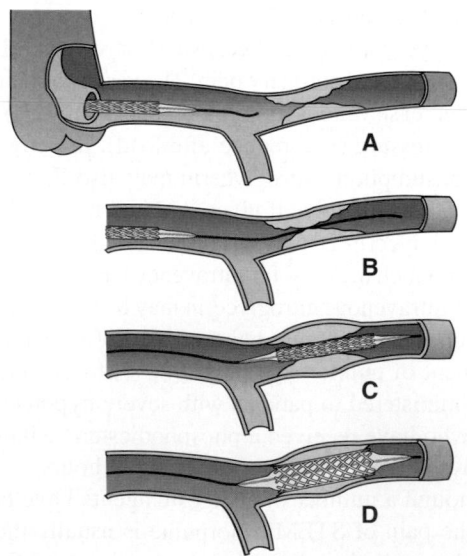

FIGURE 24-9 • Balloon-expandable stent insertion. (**A**) Insertion of a guide catheter with a collapsed balloon-expandable stent mounted over a guide wire into a coronary artery. (**B**) Advancement of guide wire across the coronary lesion. (**C**) Positioning of the balloon-expandable stent across the lesion. (**D**) Balloon inflation with expansion of the stent. Once the stent is expanded, the balloon system is removed.

lumen by stretching and tearing the atherosclerotic plaque and, to a lesser extent, by distributing the plaque along its longitudinal axis. This procedure is often used in conjunction with the placement of stents, but now rarely used alone. Acute complications of PTCA include thrombosis and vessel dissection; longer-term complications involve restenosis of the dilated vessel.

The use of *coronary stenting* has been shown to improve short- and long-term outcomes compared with PTCA alone. Persons undergoing stent procedures are treated with antiplatelet and anticoagulant drugs to prevent thrombosis, which is a major risk of the procedure.[23] The self-expanding wire mesh stents that were used initially had high thrombosis rates and have largely been replaced by balloon-expandable stents. Drug-eluting stents (with sirolimus, paclitaxel, and everolimus) are now being used to suppress local neointimal proliferation that causes restenosis of the coronary artery.[24] Radiation brachytherapy involves the use of localized intra-coronary artery radiation for reduction of in-stent restenosis. The procedure is credited with inhibiting cell proliferation and vascular lesion formation and preventing constrictive arterial remodeling.[23]

Atherectomy (i.e., cutting of the atherosclerotic plaque with a high-speed circular blade from within the vessel) is a mechanical technique to remove atherosclerotic tissue during angioplasty. Laser angioplasty devices are also used. However, with the availability of stents, these procedures are used less frequently than in the past. Thrombectomy (removal of the thrombus) involves the use of a special catheter device to fracture the thrombus into small pieces and then pull the fracture fragments into the catheter tip so they can be propelled proximally and removed.

Coronary Artery Bypass Grafting. Coronary artery bypass grafting (CABG) is one of the most common surgeries performed in the world, providing relief of angina, improvement in exercise tolerance, and prolongation of life. The procedure involves revascularization of the affected myocardium by placing a saphenous vein graft between the aorta and the affected coronary artery distal to the site of occlusion, or by using the internal mammary artery as a means of revascularizing the left anterior descending artery or its branches (Fig. 24-10). One to five distal anastomoses commonly are done.

Emergent or urgent CABG, as a reperfusion strategy, is indicated in situations such as failed PCI with persistent pain or hemodynamic instability, or for patients who are not candidates for PCI or fibrinolytic therapy.[6,25] In considering CABG as a treatment option, the risk for hospital mortality and other complications must be taken into account. Advanced age, poor left ventricular function, and the urgency with which surgery is performed increase the risk of early mortality. Serious complications, such as stroke, mediastinitis, and renal dysfunction, also increase the mortality and morbidity associated with CABG. The use of preoperative antibiotics and preoperative and postoperative administration of beta blockers help in reducing the incidence of postoperative infection and atrial fibrillation.

CABG does not alter the progress of the CAD, and although the rate of return of angina is low for the first 5 years,

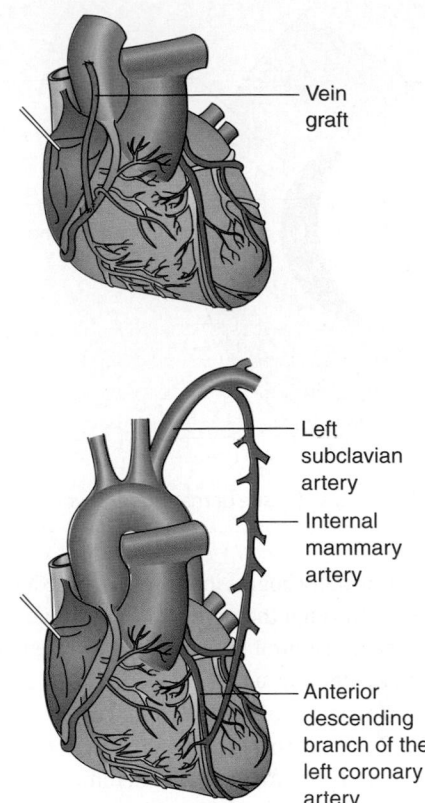

FIGURE 24-10 • Coronary artery revascularization. **(Top)** Saphenous vein bypass graft. The vein segment is sutured to the ascending aorta and the right coronary artery at a point distal to the occluding lesion. **(Bottom)** Mammary artery bypass graft. The mammary artery is anastomosed to the anterior descending left coronary artery, bypassing the obstructing lesion.

about 50% of vein grafts are closed 10 years after CABG. The use of internal mammary artery grafts, however, has shown excellent late patency. Aspirin is the drug of choice for prophylaxis against early saphenous vein graft closure and is continued indefinitely.[25] New surgical techniques in the treatment of CAD continue to evolve in an effort to reduce adverse effects of the midline sternotomy incision, cardiopulmonary bypass, and global cardioplegic arrest. Some of these include "off-pump" CABG, the development of robotic coronary bypass, and transmyocardial laser revascularization.[25]

Postinfarction Recovery Period

After a myocardial infarction, there usually are three zones of tissue damage: a zone of myocardial tissue that becomes necrotic because of an absolute lack of blood flow; a surrounding zone of injured cells, some of which will recover; and an outer zone in which cells are ischemic and can be salvaged if blood flow can be reestablished (Fig. 24-11). The boundaries of these zones may change with time after the infarction and with the success of treatment measures to reestablish blood flow. If blood flow can be restored within the 20- to 40-minute time frame, loss of cell viability does not occur or is minimal. The progression of

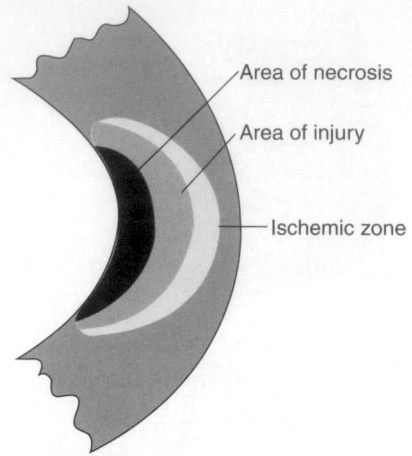

FIGURE 24-11 • Areas of tissue damage after myocardial infarction.

ischemic necrosis usually begins in the subendocardial area of the heart and extends through the myocardium to involve progressively more of the transmural thickness of the ischemic zone.

Myocardial cells that undergo necrosis are gradually replaced with scar tissue. An acute inflammatory response develops in the area of necrosis approximately 2 to 3 days after infarction. Thereafter, macrophages begin removing the necrotic tissue; the damaged area is gradually replaced with an ingrowth of highly vascularized granulation tissue, which gradually becomes less vascular and more fibrous.[9] At approximately 4 to 7 days, the center of the infarcted area is soft and yellow; if rupture of the ventricle, interventricular septum, or valve structures occurs, it usually happens at this time. Replacement of the necrotic myocardial tissue usually is complete by the seventh week. Areas of the myocardium that have been replaced with scar tissue lack the ability to contract and initiate or conduct action potentials.

Complications. The stages of recovery from STEMI are closely related to the size of the infarct and the changes that have taken place in the infarcted area. Fibrous scar tissue lacks

the contractile, elastic, and conductive properties of normal myocardial cells; the residual effects and the complications are determined essentially by the extent and location of the injury. Among the complications of STEMI are sudden death, pericarditis, stroke, thromboemboli, and mechanical defects (*e.g.*, mitral valve regurgitation, ventricular septal rupture, left ventricular wall rupture, and left ventricular aneurysm). Depending on its severity, myocardial infarction has the potential for compromising the pumping action of the heart. Heart failure and cardiogenic shock are dreaded complications of STEMI (see Chapter 26).

Life-threatening arrhythmias can be the first symptom of an ACS, differing in mechanism from chronic stable angina. With ACS, mechanisms may be related to reentry, abnormal automaticity, and electrolyte imbalances, particularly potassium and magnesium (see Chapter 25). Symptomatic bradycardia and heart block are also complications of ACS and are treated according to the guidelines for implantation of cardiac pacemakers and antiarrhythmia devices.[26]

Pericarditis tends to occur in patients with large infarcts, a lower ejection fraction, and a higher occurrence of heart failure. It may appear as early as the second or third day postinfarction or up to several weeks later. This late complication, called *Dressler syndrome,* occurs weeks to months after STEMI, and is thought to be an autoimmune response. In contrast to the pain associated with STEMI, the pain with pericarditis is sharp and stabbing and aggravated by deep inspiration and positional changes. Because of reperfusion therapy, this complication has been greatly reduced.

Acute stroke is another complication of STEMI. Risk factors for stroke after a STEMI include hypertension, older age, history of previous stroke, decreased ejection fraction, and atrial fibrillation. Thromboemboli, presenting as deep vein thrombosis or pulmonary emboli, do not present as frequently as in the past because of the use of anticoagulant therapy.

Mechanical defects result from changes that occur in the necrotic and subsequently inflamed myocardium and include rupture of the ventricular septum, papillary muscle, or free ventricular wall[9] (Fig. 24-12). Partial or complete rupture of a pap-

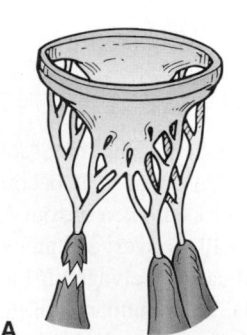
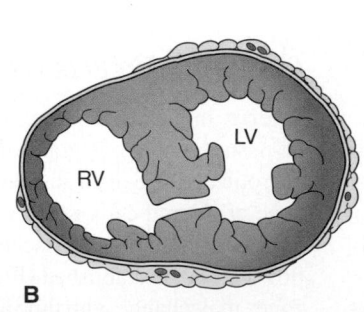
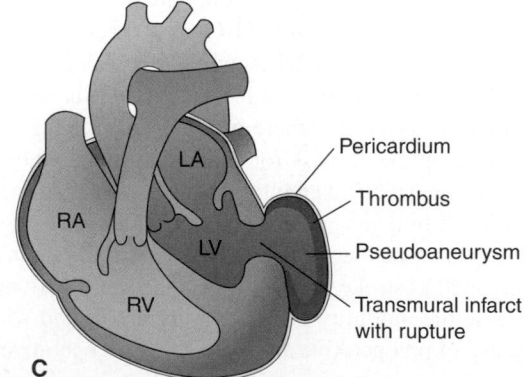

FIGURE 24-12 • Acute mechanical complications of myocardial infarction. (**A**) Papillary muscle rupture. (**B**) Interventricular septum rupture. (**C**) Rupture of the free wall of the left ventricle with pseudoaneurysm formation. RA, right atrium; LA, left atrium; RV, right ventricle; LV, left ventricle.

illary muscle is a rare but often fatal complication of transmural myocardial infarction.[19] It is detected by the presence of a new systolic murmur and clinical deterioration, often with pulmonary edema. More frequently, postinfarction mitral valve regurgitation results from early ischemic dysfunction of the papillary muscle and underlying myocardium. Ventricular septal rupture occurs less frequently than in the past because of the use of reperfusion therapy.[19] Previously thought to require surgical intervention only in symptomatic patients, surgical repair is now recommended for all patients with ventricular septal rupture. Complete rupture of the free wall of the infarcted ventricle occurs in 1% to 6% of patients and usually results in immediate death.[9] It usually occurs 3 to 7 days postinfarction, usually involves the anterior wall, and is more frequent in older women. Incomplete or gradual rupture may be sealed off by the pericardium, creating a pseudoaneurysm. It requires early surgical intervention because delayed complete rupture is common.

A left ventricular aneurysm, a sharply delineated area of scar tissue that bulges paradoxically during systole (Fig. 24-13), develops in 10% of persons dying in the hospital of STEMI.[23] They usually present on the anterior portion of the left ventricle after occlusion of the left anterior descending coronary artery and become evident 4 to 8 weeks after infarct. They rarely rupture but may be associated with arterial emboli, ventricular arrhythmias, and heart failure. Surgical resection may be performed for these indications when other treatment measures fail.[23]

Cardiac Rehabilitation

Cardiac rehabilitation programs are recommended for patients after ACS and incorporate strategies to improve adherence to medical therapies and lifestyle changes. Components of cardiac rehabilitation include exercise, nutrition, smoking cessation, psychosocial management, and education. Education is an essential component of cardiac rehabilitation programs, and is often incorporated with other aspects of the program. This includes education related to exercise, nutrition, smoking cessation, and medications. Adherence to a cardiac rehabilitation program, or to any of its components, can be extremely difficult. Among the factors that influence participation and adherence are physician referral, reimbursement issues, distance and transportation, and social support.[27]

An exercise program is an integral part of a cardiac rehabilitation program. It includes activities such as walking, swimming, and bicycling. These exercises involve changes in muscle length and rhythmic contractions of muscle groups. Most exercise programs are individually designed to meet each person's physical and psychological needs. The goal of the exercise program is to increase the maximal oxygen consumption by the muscle tissues, so that these persons are able to perform more work at a lower heart rate and blood pressure.[27]

In addition to exercise, cardiac risk factor modification incorporates strategies for smoking cessation, weight loss, stress reduction, and control of hypertension and diabetes (when present). Nutrition counseling has direct effects on weight, serum lipids, blood pressure, diabetes, and other factors. The choice of diet is based on beneficial effect, as well as the social and cultural needs of the patient. Dietary patterns are assessed and specific goals determined and communicated with the patient.[27] Cardiac rehabilitation programs should include an assessment of psychosocial problems, such as depression, anxiety, and social isolation. Behavioral therapy, such as stress management skills, and individual or group counseling can be provided, or referrals made to other experts.

Chronic Ischemic Heart Disease

Myocardial ischemia occurs when the ability of the coronary arteries to supply blood is inadequate to meet the metabolic demands of the heart. Limitations in coronary blood flow most commonly are the result of atherosclerosis, but vasospasm may serve as an initiating or contributing factor.[28] There are three types of chronic ischemic coronary artery disease: chronic stable angina, silent myocardial ischemia, and variant or vasospastic angina.

Stable Angina

Chronic stable angina is associated with a fixed coronary obstruction that produces a disparity between coronary blood flow and metabolic demands of the myocardium. Stable angina is the initial manifestation of ischemic heart disease in approximately half of persons with CAD.[29] Although most persons with stable angina have atherosclerotic heart disease, angina does not develop in a considerable number of persons with advanced coronary atherosclerosis. This probably is because of their sedentary lifestyle, the development of adequate collateral circulation, or the inability of these persons to perceive pain. In

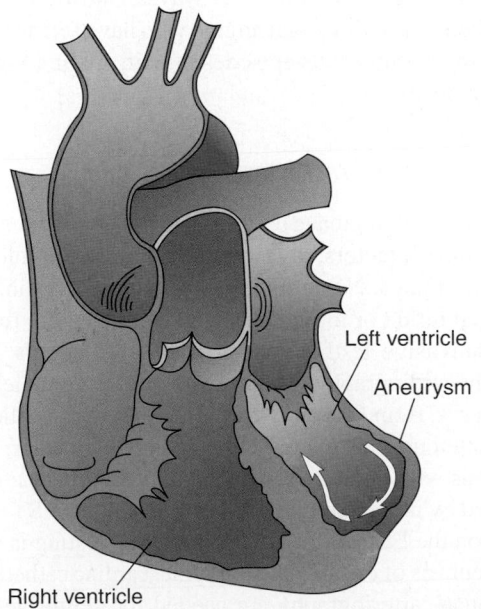

FIGURE 24-13 • Paradoxical movement of a left ventricular aneurysm during systole.

many instances, myocardial infarction occurs without a history of angina.

Angina pectoris usually is precipitated by situations that increase the work demands of the heart, such as physical exertion, exposure to cold, and emotional stress. The pain typically is described as a constricting, squeezing, or suffocating sensation. It usually is steady, increasing in intensity only at the onset and end of the attack. The pain of angina commonly is located in the precordial or substernal area of the chest; it is similar to myocardial infarction in that it may radiate to the left shoulder, jaw, arm, or other areas of the chest (Fig. 24-14). In some persons, the arm or shoulder pain may be confused with arthritis; in others, epigastric pain is confused with indigestion. Angina commonly is categorized according to whether it occurs with exercise, occurs during rest, is of new onset, or is of increasing severity.

Typically, chronic stable angina is provoked by exertion or emotional stress and relieved within minutes by rest or the use of nitroglycerin. A delay of more than 5 to 10 minutes before relief is obtained suggests that the symptoms are not due to ischemia or that they are due to severe ischemia. Angina that occurs at rest, is of new onset, or is increasing in intensity or duration denotes an increased risk for myocardial infarction and should be evaluated using the criteria for ACS.

Silent Myocardial Ischemia

Silent myocardial ischemia occurs in the absence of anginal pain. The factors that cause silent myocardial ischemia appear to be the same as those responsible for angina: impaired blood flow from the effects of coronary atherosclerosis or vasospasm. Silent myocardial ischemia affects three populations—persons who are asymptomatic without other evidence of CAD, persons who have had a myocardial infarct and continue to have episodes of silent ischemia, and persons with angina who also have episodes of silent ischemia.[28] The reason for the painless episodes of ischemia is unclear. The episodes may be shorter and involve less myocardial tissue than those producing pain. Another explanation is that persons with silent angina have defects in pain threshold or pain transmission, or autonomic neuropathy with sensory denervation. There is evidence of an increased incidence of silent myocardial ischemia in persons with diabetes mellitus, probably the result of autonomic neuropathy, which is a common complication of diabetes.[28] Silent STEMI comprises a significant proportion of all STEMIs in the elderly.

Variant (Vasospastic) Angina

Variant angina is also known as *vasospastic* or *Prinzmetal angina.* The causes of variant angina are not completely understood, but a combination of pathologic processes may be responsible. It has been suggested that it may result from endothelial dysfunction, hyperactive sympathetic nervous system responses, defects in the handling of calcium by vascular smooth muscle, or from an alteration in nitric oxide production.[28] In some persons it is associated with hypercontractility of vascular smooth muscle and is associated with migraine headaches or Raynaud phenomenon.

Unlike stable angina that occurs with exertion or stress, variant angina usually occurs during rest or with minimal exercise and frequently occurs nocturnally (between midnight and 8 AM). Arrhythmias often occur when the pain is severe, and most persons are aware of their presence during an attack. ECG changes are significant if recorded during an attack. These abnormalities include ST-segment elevation or depression, T-wave peaking, inversion of U waves, and rhythm disturbances. Persons with variant angina who have serious arrhythmias during spontaneous episodes of pain are at a higher risk of sudden death.

Diagnosis and Treatment

The diagnosis of angina is based on a detailed pain history, the presence of risk factors, invasive and noninvasive studies, and laboratory studies. Noncoronary causes of chest pain, such as esophageal reflux or musculoskeletal disorders, are ruled out.

Noninvasive testing for chronic stable angina includes ECG, echocardiography, exercise stress testing, nuclear imaging studies, CT, and possibly cardiac MRI. Because the resting ECG is often normal, exercise testing is often used in evaluating persons with angina. Ischemia that is asymptomatic at rest is detected by precipitation of typical chest pain or ST-segment changes on the ECG. Although noninvasive testing is valuable in the diagnosis of chronic stable angina, cardiac catheterization and coronary arteriography are needed for definitive diagnosis.[28] Serum biochemical markers for myocardial infarction are normal in patients with chronic stable angina. Metabolic abnor-

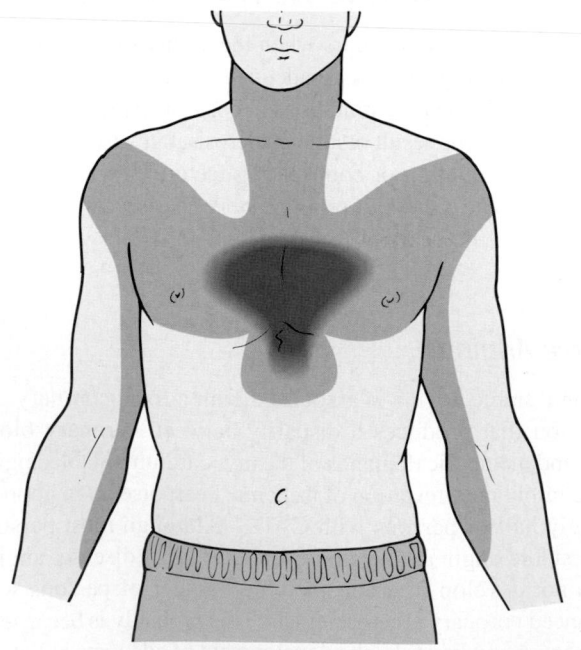

FIGURE 24-14 • Areas of pain due to angina.

malities are frequently detected, such as hypercholesterolemia and other dyslipidemias, carbohydrate intolerance, and insulin resistance.

Comprehensive and individualized assessment, lifestyle changes, and treatments are needed for patients with chronic stable angina. The treatment goals for stable angina are directed toward symptom reduction and prevention of myocardial infarction through nonpharmacologic strategies, pharmacologic therapy, and coronary interventions. PCI relieves symptoms for patients with chronic stable angina, but does not extend the life span. CABG is usually indicated in patients with double- or triple-vessel disease.[29]

Nonpharmacologic methods are aimed at symptom control and lifestyle modifications to reduce risk factors for coronary disease. They include smoking cessation in persons who smoke, stress reduction, a regular exercise program, limiting dietary intake of cholesterol and saturated fats, weight reduction if obesity is present, and avoidance of cold or other stresses that produce vasoconstriction. Immediate cessation of activity often is sufficient to abort an angina attack. Sitting down or standing quietly may be preferable to lying down because these positions decrease preload by producing pooling of blood in the lower extremities.

The goal of pharmacologic treatment of angina is to relieve ischemia and alleviate symptoms, prevent myocardial infarction and death, and improve the quality of life. Pharmacologic agents used in chronic stable angina include aspirin or clopidogrel, beta blockers in persons without contraindications or calcium antagonists when beta blockers are contraindicated, and ACE inhibitors in patients who also have diabetes or left ventricular systolic dysfunction (see previous discussion in section on Acute Coronary Syndrome). In patients with established CAD, including chronic stable angina, the use of lipid-lowering agents or statins is recommended, even in the presence of mild to moderate elevations of LDL cholesterol (see Chapter 22).

Nitrates, both short acting and long acting, are vasodilators used in the treatment of chronic stable angina and in silent myocardial ischemia.[28] Nitrates exert their effect mainly through a decrease in venous return to the heart with a resultant decrease in intraventricular volume. Arterial pressure also decreases. Decreased intraventricular pressure and volume are associated with decreased wall tension and myocardial oxygen requirement. Although they are not vasodilators, beta blocking drugs are extremely useful in management of angina associated with effort. The benefits of beta blocking agents are due primarily to their hemodynamic effects—decreased heart rate, blood pressure, and myocardial contractility—which decrease myocardial oxygen requirements at rest and during exercise. The calcium channel blocking drugs, also called *calcium antagonists,* block activated and inactivated L-type calcium channels in cardiac and smooth muscle. The therapeutic effects of the calcium channel blocking agents result from coronary and peripheral artery dilation and from decreased myocardial metabolism associated with the decrease in myocardial contractility. Persons with variant angina usually respond to treatment with calcium antagonists.

IN SUMMARY, CAD is a disorder of impaired coronary blood flow, usually caused by atherosclerosis. Myocardial ischemia occurs when there is a disparity between myocardial oxygen supply and demand and can present as chronic ischemic heart disease or ACS. Diagnostic methods for CAD include ECG, exercise stress testing, nuclear imaging studies, CT, MRI, and angiographic studies in the cardiac catheterization laboratory.

The ACS, which includes UA/NSTEMI and STEMI, results from multiple pathophysiologic processes, including unstable atherosclerotic plaques, platelet aggregation, and thrombus formation. Unstable angina is an accelerated form of angina in which the pain occurs more frequently, is more severe, and lasts longer than in chronic stable angina. Myocardial infarction refers to the ischemic death of myocardial tissue associated with obstructed blood flow in the coronary arteries due to plaque disruption and occlusion of blood flow. NSTEMI and STEMI differ in terms of extent of myocardial damage. The complications of STEMI include potentially fatal arrhythmias, heart failure and cardiogenic shock, pericarditis, thromboemboli, rupture of cardiac structures, and ventricular aneurysms. Diagnostic methods include the use of ECG monitoring and serum biomarkers. Treatment goals focus on reestablishment of myocardial blood flow through rapid reperfusion of the occluded coronary artery, prevention of clot extension through use of aspirin and other antiplatelet and antithrombotic agents, alleviation of pain, administration of oxygen, and the use of vasodilators (nitroglycerin) and β-adrenergic blocking agents to reduce the work demands on the heart.

The chronic ischemic heart diseases include chronic stable angina, silent myocardial ischemia, and variant (vasospastic) angina. Chronic stable angina is associated with a fixed atherosclerotic obstruction and pain that is precipitated by increased work demands on the heart and relieved by rest. Variant angina can result from spasms of the coronary arteries or other dysfunctions. Silent myocardial ischemia occurs without symptoms. ■

CONCEPTSin action**ANIMATI**  **N**

CARDIOMYOPATHIES

After completing this section of the chapter, you should be able to meet the following objectives:

- Define the term *cardiomyopathy* as it relates to both the mechanical and electrical function of the myocardium.
- Describe the role of genetics in the etiology of the primary cardiomyopathies.
- Differentiate among the pathophysiologic changes that occur with hypertrophic cardiomyopathy, arrhythmogenic right ventricular cardiomyopathy, dilated cardiomyopathies, and myocarditis.

(objectives continue)

- List four causes of secondary cardiomyopathy.
- Describe the treatment strategies of both primary and secondary cardiomyopathy.

The definition and classification of the cardiomyopathies have evolved tremendously with the advance of molecular genetics. In 2006, the definition and classification of cardiomyopathies were updated in an AHA scientific statement incorporating not only the advances of cardiac molecular genetics, but other newly diagnosed diseases, as well as ion channelopathies.[30] This scientific statement defines cardiomyopathies as

> a heterogeneous group of diseases of the myocardium associated with mechanical and/or electrical dysfunction that usually (but not invariably) exhibit inappropriate ventricular hypertrophy or dilatation and are due to a variety of causes that frequently are genetic. Cardiomyopathies either are confined to the heart or are part of generalized systemic disorders, often leading to cardiovascular death or progressive heart failure–related disability.[30]

Based on this definition, the classification of cardiomyopathies is divided into two major groups: *primary* and *secondary*. The primary cardiomyopathies represent heart disorders that are confined to the myocardium, whereas the secondary cardiomyopathies represent myocardial changes that occur with a variety of systemic (multiorgan) disorders. Cardiomyopathies are usually associated with disorders of myocardial performance, which may be mechanical (*e.g.,* heart failure) or electrical (*e.g.,* life-threatening arrhythmias).

Primary Cardiomyopathies

The primary cardiomyopathies are classified as genetic, mixed, or acquired, based on their etiology.[30] The genetic cardiomyopathies include hypertrophic cardiomyopathy, arrhythmogenic right ventricular cardiomyopathy, left ventricular noncompaction cardiomyopathy, inherited conduction system disorders, and ion channelopathies. The mixed cardiomyopathies, which include dilated cardiomyopathy, are of both genetic and nongenetic origin. Acquired cardiomyopathies include those that have their origin in the inflammatory process (*e.g.,* myocarditis), stress ("tako-tsubo" pericarditis), or pregnancy (peripartum cardiomyopathy). In many cases the cause is unknown, in which case it is referred to as an *idiopathic cardiomyopathy.*

Genetic Cardiomyopathies

Hypertrophic Cardiomyopathy. Hypertrophic cardiomyopathy (HCM) is characterized by unexplained left ventricular hypertrophy with disproportionate thickening of the ventricular septum, abnormal diastolic filling, cardiac arrhythmias, and, in some cases, intermittent left ventricular outflow obstruction[31] (Fig. 24-15). It is one of the most common types of cardiomyopathy, occurring in approximately 1 person in 500 of the general population.[31] HCM is the most common cause of sudden cardiac death (SCD) in young athletes. The propensity to sud-

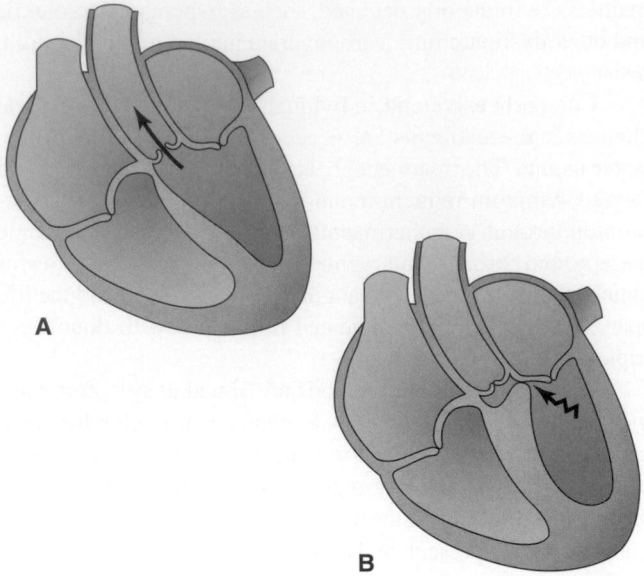

FIGURE 24-15 • Vertical section of the heart showing (**A**) normal heart and (**B**) a heart with hypertrophic cardiomyopathy in which disproportionate thickening of intraventricular septum causes intermittent left ventricular outflow obstruction.

den death seems to be genetic. Other complications that occur include atrial fibrillation, stroke, and heart failure.

HCM is an autosomal dominant heart disease caused by mutations in the genes encoding proteins of the cardiac sarcomere (*i.e.,* muscle fibers). Histologically, HCM appears as myocyte hypertrophy with myofibril disarray and increased cardiac fibrosis. At least 10 different genes are associated with HCM, with the β-myosin heavy chain and the myosin-binding protein C genes being the most common. More than 400 individual mutations have been identified and are unique from family to family. Some phenotypic correlates can be made from specific mutations; however, there are many exceptions, indicating that genetic modifiers and environmental factors are also important.[31,32] Although HCM is inherited, it may present anywhere from early childhood to late adulthood with a broad category of manifestations and variable clinical course. Up to 25% of persons with the disorder remain stable and achieve normal longevity, with mild or no disability, thereby requiring minimal or no therapeutic intervention.[9]

The basic physiologic abnormalities in HCM are reduced left ventricular chamber size; poor compliance with reduced stroke volume that results from impaired diastolic filling; and, in about 25% of cases, dynamic obstruction of left ventricular outflow.[9] Clinical manifestations may include dyspnea, chest pain during exertion, or exercise intolerance. Owing to massive hypertrophy, high left ventricular chamber pressure, and potentially abnormal intramural arteries, focal myocardial ischemia often develops even in the absence of CAD; thus, anginal pain is common. HCM is frequently associated with the development of left ventricular outflow obstruction during rest or exertion that is caused by systolic anterior motion of the mitral valve and contact of the mitral valve with the ventricular septum. SCD and atrial fibrillation are also complications of HCM. Clinical manifestations are highly variable and may progress to end-stage heart failure with left ventricular remodeling and systolic dysfunction.

Diagnosis of HCM is frequently established with 2-D echocardiography, demonstrating nondilated left ventricular hypertrophy, in the absence of other cardiac or systemic diseases. ECG, continuous ambulatory monitoring, and cardiac MRI can also be helpful. The value of electrophysiologic testing remains controversial. Genetic testing, through bidirectional deoxyribonucleic acid (DNA) sequence analysis, provides accurate diagnosis and precise identification of gene mutations, although with some limitations.[33]

Medical management of HCM is primarily focused on symptom management. The first-line approach to relief of symptoms is pharmacologic therapy designed to block the effects of catecholamines that exacerbate outflow obstruction and to slow the heart rate to enhance diastolic filling. β-Adrenergic blockers are generally the initial choice for persons with symptomatic HCM. The calcium channel blocker verapamil can also be used. It can, however, exacerbate left ventricular outflow obstruction and is not recommended for persons with severe outflow obstruction and pronounced symptoms.

In obstructive HCM that is refractory to drug therapy, septal myectomy, alcohol ablation of the interventricular septum, and dual-chamber and biventricular pacing are alternative treatment options. Atrial fibrillation is treated with pharmacologic rate control, cardioversion, and coagulation. An implantable cardioverter–defibrillator (ICD) should be used for persons with HCM who have sustained ventricular tachycardia or ventricular fibrillation and are receiving optimal medical therapy.[31] About 5% of patients develop end-stage HCM and require standard therapy for advanced heart failure, including consideration for heart transplantation.

Arrhythmogenic Right Ventricular Cardiomyopathy/Dysplasia. Arrhythmogenic right ventricular cardiomyopathy/dysplasia (ARVC/D) is a heart muscle disease that affects primarily the right ventricle, causing right-sided heart failure and various rhythm disturbances, particularly ventricular tachycardia.[34,35] It ranks second, after HCM, as the leading cause of SCD in young athletes. The incidence of ARVC/D varies from about 1 in 2000 to 1 in 5000, affecting men more frequently than women. It is inherited as an autosomal dominant trait in greater than 50% of cases, although often with incomplete penetrance and variable expression.[34] Although a gene defect was recently located on chromosome 14, the pathogenesis of the disorder remains unclear.

The disorder is characterized by progressive loss of myocytes, with partial or complete replacement of the right ventricular muscle with fatty or fibrofatty tissue. The disorder is associated with reentrant ventricular tachyarrhythmias of right ventricular origin that are often precipitated by exercise-induced discharge of catecholamines. Clinical manifestations include palpitations, syncope, or cardiac arrest, usually in young or middle-aged men. Other symptoms may include abdominal pain and mental confusion.

Diagnosis of ARVC/D is based on clinical, ECG, echocardiographic, and histologic findings. Personal and family history, including first- and second-degree relatives, is important.

Characteristic findings on 12-lead ECG include ventricular tachycardia with left bundle branch block pattern, T-wave inversion in the right precordial leads, and epsilon waves (small deflections just beyond the QRS complex). Right ventricular bundle branch block may also be present. Other diagnostic studies that may be used in assessing ARVC/D include signal-averaged ECG, MRI, electrophysiologic studies, and right ventricular angiography.

Treatment for ARVC/D is aimed at prevention of SCD. Although ARVC/D cannot be cured, the goal of treatment is to control the arrhythmias with antiarrhythmic agents.[35] Combinations of various antiarrhythmic agents are often used. Radiofrequency ablation is used in drug-refractory cases, although it is completely successful in only 30% to 65% of cases, with multiple ablations sometimes needed. ICD placement is also indicated for drug-refractory cases and for those who have survived a SCD episode. ICD placement for others is debatable because no risk stratification system exists. Final options for treatment include ventriculotomy and heart transplantation.[35]

Left Ventricular Noncompaction. Left ventricular noncompaction is a primary congenital cardiomyopathy that is thought to develop because of abnormal embryogenesis in which there is failure of trabecular compaction in the developing myocardium. The disorder may be isolated or associated with other congenital heart diseases.[30] Both familial and nonfamilial cases of left ventricular noncompaction have been identified, and mutations of several genes have been reported.[30]

Signs and symptoms are primarily related to arrhythmias, embolic events, and heart failure. Diagnosis is made primarily with 2-D and color echocardiography, but cardiac MRI or left ventricular angiography may also be helpful.[30] Treatment focuses on preventing symptoms of heart failure, arrhythmias, and systemic embolic events.

Ion Channelopathies. Ion channels are pore-forming proteins that provide pathways for movement of ions across cell membranes (see Chapter 4). Diseases caused by mutations in genes encoding ion channel subunits or proteins are called *ion channelopathies*.[30] In the heart, these ion channel disorders include the long QT syndrome (LQTS), short QT syndrome (SQTS), Brugada syndrome, and catecholaminergic polymorphic ventricular tachycardia.

LQTS and SQTS are caused by sodium or potassium ion channel gene mutations. LQTS, which is probably the most common of the ion channelopathies, is identified on 12-lead ECG by a prolonged QT interval. It causes a polymorphic ventricular tachycardia known as *torsade de pointes* (discussed in Chapter 25). First described in 2000, the short QT syndrome is characterized by short QT interval (<330 milliseconds) on the ECG, which can lead to ventricular tachycardia or fibrillation and SCD.[30]

Brugada syndrome is a relatively newly described clinical entity related to a sodium channel gene mutation. It is associated with SCD in young people, particularly young Southeast Asian men who experience SCD during sleep. The disorder is characterized on ECG by right bundle branch block and ST-segment elevation in the anterior pericardial leads.[30] Catecholaminergic polymorphic ventricular tachycardia is caused by an abnormal receptor that regulates calcium release from the sarcoplasmic reticulum. It is triggered by vigorous physical activity or acute emotion, and leads to syncope, polymorphic ventricular tachycardia, and SCD. The resting ECG is usually normal.[30]

Mixed (Genetic and Nongenetic) Cardiomyopathies

Dilated Cardiomyopathy. Dilated cardiomyopathy (DCM) is a common cause of heart failure and the leading indication for heart transplantation. Up to 35% of cases of dilated cardiomyopathy are reported as familial; that proportion may be even higher because incomplete penetrance often makes it difficult to identify early or latent disease in family members.[9,36] Most familial cases appear to be transmitted as an autosomal dominant trait, but autosomal recessive, X-linked recessive, and mitochondrial inheritance patterns have been identified. Other causes include infections (i.e, viral, bacterial, fungal, mycobacterial, parasitic), toxins, alcoholism, chemotherapeutic agents, metals, and multiple other disorders. Often no cause is found, in which case it is often referred to as *idiopathic DCM.*

DCM is characterized by ventricular enlargement, a reduction in ventricular wall thickness, and impaired systolic function of one or both ventricles (Fig. 24-16). Histologically, DCM is characterized by atrophic and hypertrophic myocardial fibers and interstitial fibrosis. Cardiac myocytes, particularly those in the subendocardium, often show advanced degenerative changes.

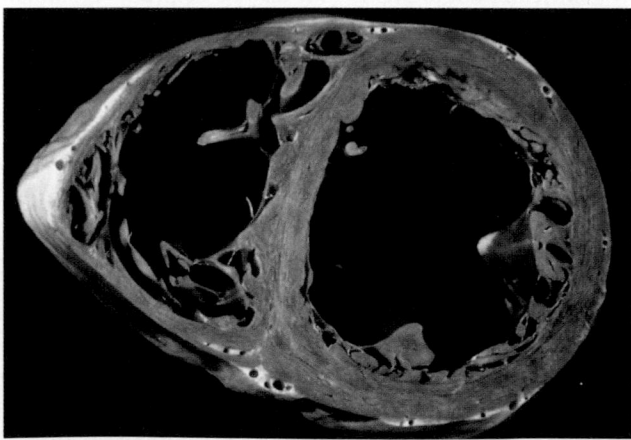

FIGURE 24-16 • Idiopathic dilated cardiomyopathy. A transverse section of the enlarged heart reveals conspicuous dilation of both ventricles. Although the ventricular wall appears thinned, the increased mass of the heart indicates considerable hypertrophy. (From Saffitz J. E. [2008]. The heart. In Rubin E., Strayer D. E. [Eds.], *Rubin's pathology: Clinicopathologic foundations of medicine* [5th ed., p. 470]. Philadelphia: Lippincott Williams & Wilkins.)

Interstitial fibrosis is present, also most prominently in the subendocardial zone. Scattered inflammatory cells may be present.

The most common clinical manifestations of dilated cardiomyopathy are those related to heart failure, such as dyspnea, orthopnea, and reduced exercise capacity. In the end stages, persons with DCM often have ejection fractions of less than 25% (normal is approximately 50% to 60%).[9] As the disease progresses, stasis of blood in the walls of the heart chambers can lead to thrombus formation and systemic emboli. Secondary mitral valve regurgitation and abnormal cardiac rhythms are common. Death is usually due to heart failure or arrhythmias, and can occur suddenly.

The treatment of DCM is directed toward relieving the symptoms of heart failure and reducing the work of the heart. Pharmacologic agents include diuretics to reduce preload, beta blockers to reduce heart rate and myocardial oxygen demand, afterload-reducing agents to improve contractility and decrease left ventricular filling pressures, and ACE inhibitors to prevent vasoconstriction. Anticoagulants and antiarrhythmics may also be used. Other treatments may include a biventricular pacemaker, an ICD, and in cases that are refractory to treatment, cardiac transplantation. Removing or avoiding causative agents (if identified); avoiding myocardial depressants, including alcohol; and pacing rest with asymptomatic levels of exercise or activity are also important.

Primary Restrictive Cardiomyopathy. Restrictive cardiomyopathy is a rare form of heart muscle disease in which ventricular filling is restricted because of excessive rigidity of the ventricular walls, although the contractile properties of the heart remain relatively normal.[9] Restrictive cardiomyopathy can be idiopathic or associated with distinct diseases that affect the myocardium, principally radiation fibrosis, amyloidosis, sarcoidosis, or metastatic tumors. Genetics may also play a role because familial forms of restrictive cardiomyopathy have been reported.[30]

Symptoms of restrictive cardiomyopathy include dyspnea, paroxysmal nocturnal dyspnea, orthopnea, peripheral edema, ascites, fatigue, and weakness. The manifestations of restrictive cardiomyopathy resemble those of constrictive pericarditis. In the advanced form of the disease, all the signs of heart failure are present except cardiomegaly.

Acquired Cardiomyopathies

Myocarditis (Inflammatory Cardiomyopathy). Myocarditis can be defined simply as "an inflammation of the heart," but the classification, diagnosis, and treatment are complex.[9,36] Clinical findings can vary greatly, from nonspecific symptoms, such as fever, myalgias, or exertional dyspnea, to hemodynamic collapse and sudden death. The incidence and prevalence of myocarditis have been difficult to ascertain because of the wide variation in clinical presentation.

Although there are a number of etiologies associated with myocarditis, it is usually caused by a viral infection, most commonly an enterovirus (coxsackievirus group B).[9,36–38] Adenovirus and parvovirus in young children have also been identified as causative agents. Other etiologies include bacterial or fungal infections, hypersensitivity to certain drugs, and autoimmune diseases, such as systemic lupus erythematosus. Myocarditis is a frequent pathologic cardiac finding in persons with acquired immunodeficiency syndrome (AIDS), although it is unclear whether it is due to the human immunodeficiency virus infection itself or to a secondary infection.

Acute viral myocarditis appears to progress through three phases: the acute viral infection, autoimmune activation, and ongoing myocardial injury, resulting in dilated cardiomyopathy.[37] The three phases present with varying clinical manifestations and varying indications for treatment. Phases 1 and 2 produce inflammatory responses to the initial viral infection. However, activation of the immune system in response to virus-specific antigens can also illicit inflammatory responses by the host, independent of the initial viral infection, which can lead to tissue damage in the host organism. As leukocytes, lymphocytes, and macrophages penetrate the myocardium, interstitial edema and focal myocyte necrosis lead to replacement fibrosis.[9] It has been suggested that autoreactive T cells and host-generated cytokines, including tumor necrosis factor-α, interleukin-1, and interleukin-6, may play prominent roles in the myocardial changes that occur with mycocarditis.[37] Some cases of myocarditis progress to phase 3, which is characterized by ongoing myocardial injury that ultimately results in acute or chronic dilated cardiomyopathy, severe left ventricular failure, or life-threatening arrhythmias.

The signs and symptoms of myocarditis vary from person to person.[38] Some persons may present with fever, chills, nausea, vomiting, arthralgia, and myalgia, occurring up to 6 weeks before the diagnosis of myocarditis. Other persons may present with heart failure without antecedent symptoms. The onset of heart failure may be gradual or abrupt and fulminant. Emboli may occur because of the procoagulant effect of cytokines combined with decreased myocardial contractility. At times, the presentation may mimic ACS, with ST-segment and T-wave changes, positive cardiac markers, and regional wall motion abnormalities despite normal coronary arteries. Viral myocarditis in children or young adults is often nonspecific, with symptoms such as fever and poor eating.

No clinical practice guidelines exist, and although standardized diagnostic guidelines have been proposed (i.e., Dallas criteria), several factors suggest they are no longer adequate.[39]

Endomyocardial biopsy findings, obtained through cardiac catheterization, remain the gold standard for establishing the diagnosis of acute myocarditis, despite limited accuracy.[38–40] Other diagnostic methods include the use of serum cardiac biomarkers (i.e., CK, TnI, TnT), and immunohistochemical staining. Echocardiography is usually performed in the initial evaluation of suspected myocarditis, although the findings can be nonspecific. Other myocardial imaging techniques that are being evaluated include nuclear imaging with gallium- or indium-labeled antimyosin antibodies, and MRI.

Many cases of myocarditis are mild and self-limiting, so first-line treatment remains largely supportive.[37–40] Initial treatments include supplemental oxygen, bed rest, and antibiotics, if needed. In persons with more severe myocarditis, hemodynamic support with vasopressors and positive inotropic agents may be needed. ACE inhibitors, beta blockers, and spironolactone (an aldosterone antagonist) may be used to prevent further clinical deterioration in persons with dilated cardiomyopathy due to myocarditis.[37] An ICD should be considered for those with documented life-threatening arrhythmias. Some persons with severe fulminant myocarditis who develop severe hemodynamic compromise may have a better prognosis than those with acute or chronic forms of myocarditis. Because there is a high likelihood of recovery, they require aggressive support with left ventricular assist devices if necessary.[37] Immunosuppressive therapy continues to be investigated as a treatment for myocarditis.

 Peripartum Cardiomyopathy. Peripartum cardiomyopathy is a rare heart muscle disorder that occurs during the last trimester of pregnancy or the first 6 months after delivery. The disorder is relatively rare in the United States, but in some regions of Africa it is encountered in as much as 1% of pregnant women. The incidence is greater in African American, multiparous, or older women, and in women with twin fetuses, preeclampsia, or use of tocolytic therapy to prevent premature labor and delivery.[41,42]

Although the etiology of peripartum cardiomyopathy is unknown, several causes have been proposed, including infectious, immunologic, nutritional, drug-induced, and genetic factors. Some women exhibit inflammatory cells in heart biopsies taken during the symptomatic phase of the disorder, suggesting a disordered immune response.

Diagnosis of peripartum cardiomyopathy can be challenging because symptoms that can occur normally in late pregnancy are similar to the early signs of heart failure. A joint workshop of the National Heart, Lung, and Blood Institute and the Office of Rare Diseases of the National Institutes of Health, in 1997, identified four criteria for the definition of peripartum cardiomyopathy: (1) heart failure in the last month of pregnancy or within 5 months after delivery; (2) no identifiable cause of heart failure; (3) no identifiable cause of heart failure before the last month of pregnancy; and (4) evidence of systolic dysfunction.[42]

Management of peripartum cardiomyopathy includes standard therapy for heart failure. However, potential teratogenic effects and excretion of drugs during breast-feeding need to be considered. Prognosis depends on resolution of the heart failure. About half of women with peripartum cardiomyopathy spontaneously recover normal cardiac function; the other half are left with persistent left ventricular dysfunction or progress to overt heart failure and early death.[42]

Stress or "Tako-Tsubo" Cardiomyopathy. Stress cardiomyopathy was first described in Japan, where most cases have occurred, although cases have been described in the United States.[30] In Japan, it was called *tako-tsubo* after the fishing pot with a narrow neck and wide base used to trap octopus. The term *transient left ventricular apical ballooning* has also been used to describe this syndrome.

Stress or tako-tsubo cardiomyopathy has been identified in the clinical setting as a transient, reversible left ventricular dysfunction in response to profound psychological or emotional stress. The syndrome occurs primarily in middle-aged women who present with acute STEMI, but who, on cardiac catheterization, have no evidence of CAD. There is, however, impaired myocardial contractility characterized by apical ballooning of the left ventricle with hypercontractility of the basal left ventricle.[43]

The mechanism for myocardial stunning in stress cardiomyopathy is unclear, although some theories suggest ischemia from coronary artery spasm, microvascular spasm, or direct myocyte injury. When catecholamine levels return to normal, the interventricular gradient resolves and left ventricular function recovers.[44] Treatment is the same as that for heart failure, and most patients demonstrate rapid improvement and an excellent prognosis.

Secondary Cardiomyopathies

Secondary cardiomyopathy is a heart muscle disease in the presence of a multisystem disorder (Chart 24-2). There are numerous conditions reported to involve the myocardium. Some of these disorders produce accumulation of abnormal substances between myocytes (extracellular), whereas others produce accumulation of abnormal substances within myocytes (intracellular).

Almost 100 distinct myocardial diseases can result in the clinical features of DCM. They include cardiomyopathies associated with drugs, diabetes mellitus, muscular dystrophy, autoimmune disorders, and cancer treatment agents (radiation and cancer drugs).[30] Alcoholic cardiomyopathy is the single most common identifiable cause of DCM in the United States and Europe. Doxorubicin (Adriamycin) and other anthracycline drugs, used in the treatment of cancer, are potent agents whose usefulness is limited by cumulative dose-dependent cardiac toxicity. Another cancer chemotherapeutic agent with cardiotoxic potential is cyclophosphamide (Cytoxan). Unlike the primary myocyte injury that occurs with doxorubicin, the principal insult with cyclophosphamide appears to be vascular, leading to myocardial hemorrhage.

CHART 24-2　CONDITIONS ASSOCIATED WITH SECONDARY CARDIOMYOPATHIES*

Autoimmune Disorders
Systemic lupus erythematosus
Rheumatoid arthritis
Scleroderma
Polyarteritis nodosa

Endocrine Disorders
Acromegaly
Diabetes mellitus
Hypothyroidism and hyperthyroidism
Hyperparathyroidism

Familial Storage Diseases
Glycogen storage disease
Mucopolysaccharidoses
Hemochromatosis

Infiltrative Disorders
Amyloidosis
Sarcoidosis
Radiation-induced fibrosis

Neuromuscular/Neurologic Disorders
Friedreich ataxia
Muscular dystrophy
Neurofibromatosis

Nutritional Deficiencies
Thiamine (beriberi)
Protein (kwashiorkor)

Toxins
Alcohol and its metabolites
Arsenic
Cancer chemotherapeutic agents (anthracyclines [doxorubicin, daunorubicin], cyclophosphamide)
Catecholamines
Hydrocarbons

*Not intended to be inclusive.

IN SUMMARY, the cardiomyopathies involve both mechanical and electrical etiologies of myocardial dysfunction. They are currently identified as either primary or secondary cardiomyopathies, based on genetic or other organ system involvement. Symptoms related to most cardiomyopathies, whether primary or secondary, are those associated with heart failure and SCD. Treatments are related to symptom management and prevention of lethal arrhythmias.

The primary cardiomyopathies include genetic, mixed, or acquired types. The genetic cardiomyopathies include hypertrophic cardiomyopathy, arrhythmogenic right ventricular cardiomyopathy, left ventricular noncompaction cardiomyopathy, inherited conduction system disorders, and ion channelopathies.

The mixed cardiomyopathies, which include dilated cardiomyopathy, are of both genetic and acquired origin. Acquired cardiomyopathies include those that have their origin in the inflammatory process (*e.g.,* myocarditis), stress (tako-tsubo pericarditis), or pregnancy (peripartum cardiomyopathy). In many cases the cause is unknown, in which case it is referred to as an *idiopathic cardiomyopathy*.

The secondary cardiomyopathies are heart diseases in which myocardial involvement occurs as part of a generalized systemic (multiorgan) disorder. They include cardiomyopathies associated with drugs, diabetes mellitus, muscular dystrophy, autoimmune disorders, and cancer treatment agents (radiation and chemotherapeutic drugs). ∎

INFECTIOUS AND IMMUNOLOGIC DISORDERS

After completing this section of the chapter, you should be able to meet the following objectives:

■ Distinguish between the roles of infectious organisms and the immune system in infective endocarditis and rheumatic fever.

■ Describe the relation between the infective vegetations associated with infective endocarditis and the extracardiac manifestations of the disease.

■ Describe the long-term effects of rheumatic fever and primary and secondary prevention strategies for rheumatic fever and rheumatic heart disease.

Infective Endocarditis

Infective endocarditis (IE) is a serious and potentially life-threatening infection of the inner surface of the heart. It is characterized by colonization or invasion of the heart valves and the mural endocardium by a microbial agent, leading to the formation of bulky, friable vegetations and destruction of underlying cardiac tissues.[9]

The incidence, demographics, and characteristics of IE have changed over the past decade.[45] The classic picture of a person with preexisting rheumatic heart disease and community-associated bacteremia no longer represents the majority of cases of IE. More common causes now are mitral valve prolapse, congenital heart disease, and prosthetic heart valves. Host factors such as neutropenia, immunodeficiency, malignancy, therapeutic immunosuppression, diabetes, and alcohol or intravenous drug use are predisposing factors.[9] A more recently identified cause of IE is infection involving a variety of cardiovascular prostheses and devices, such as pacemakers, defibrillators, and left ventricular assist devices. Infections of these intracardiac, arterial, and venous devices are nosocomially acquired in medical centers throughout the developed world.[46]

Traditionally, IE has been classified on clinical grounds into acute or subacute–chronic forms, depending on the onset, etiology, and severity of the disease.[45] Usually, the onset of acute cases is rapid and involves patients with normal cardiac valves who are either healthy and perhaps have a history of intravenous drug use, or are debilitated. Subacute–chronic cases evolve over months; these patients usually have valve abnormalities. The development of drug-resistant strains of microorganisms due to the indiscriminate use of antibiotics and an increase in the number of immunocompromised persons has made classification of acute and subacute–chronic cases more difficult.[47]

Etiology and Pathogenesis

Staphylococcal infections have now emerged as the leading cause of IE, with streptococci and enterococci as the other two

most common causes. Other causative agents include the so called HACEK group (*Haemophilus* species, *Actinobacillus actinomycetemcomitans, Cardiobacterium hominis, Eikenella corrodens,* and *Kingella kingae*), gram-negative bacilli, and fungi.[9,45] The causative agents differ somewhat in the major high-risk groups. For example, *Staphylococcus aureus* is the major offender in intravenous drug abusers, whereas prosthetic heart valve IE tends to be caused by coagulase-negative staphylococci (*e.g., Staphylococcus epidermidis*).[9] Foremost among the factors leading to the development of IE is seeding of the blood with microbes. The portal of entry into the bloodstream may be an obvious infection, a dental or surgical procedure that causes transient bacteremia, injection of a contaminated substance directly into the blood by intravenous drug users, or an occult source in the oral cavity, gut, or a trivial injury.[9] Endothelial injury, bacteremia, and altered hemodynamics can all incite the formation of a fibrin–platelet thrombus along the endothelial lining. The thrombus is susceptible to bacterial seeding from transient bacteremia, causing continued monocyte activation and cytokine and tissue factor production. This results in progressive enlargement of infected valvular vegetations.

In both acute and subacute–chronic forms of IE, friable, bulky, and potentially destructive vegetative lesions form on the heart valves (Fig. 24-17). The aortic and mitral valves are the most common sites of infection, although the right heart may also be involved, particularly in intravenous drug abusers. These vegetative lesions consist of a collection of infectious organisms and cellular debris enmeshed in the fibrin strands of clotted blood. The lesions may be singular or multiple, may grow as large as several centimeters, and usually are found loosely attached to the free edges of the valve surface.[9] The infectious loci continuously release bacteria into the bloodstream and are a source of persistent bacteremia. As the lesions grow, they cause valve destruction, leading to valvular regurgitation, ring abscesses with heart block, pericarditis, aneurysm, and valve perforation.

The intracardiac vegetative lesions also have local and distant systemic effects.[9,45] The loose organization of these lesions

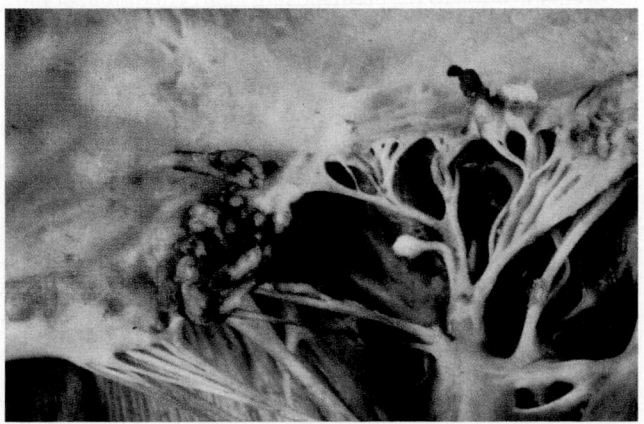

FIGURE 24-17 • Bacterial endocarditis. The mitral valve shows destructive vegetations, which have eroded through the free margin of the valve leaflet. (From Rubin E., Farber J. I. [1999]. *Pathology* [3rd ed., p. 572]. Philadelphia: Lippincott-Raven.)

permits the organisms and fragments of the lesions to form emboli and travel in the bloodstream, causing cerebral, systemic, or pulmonary emboli. The fragments may lodge in small blood vessels, causing small hemorrhages, abscesses, and infarction of tissue. The bacteremia also can initiate immune responses thought to be responsible for skin manifestations, polyarthritis, glomerulonephritis, and other immune disorders. Other complications from IE include heart failure, periannular extension of the infection, and mycotic aneurysms.

Clinical Features

Signs and symptoms of IE can include fever and signs of systemic infection, change in the character of an existing heart murmur, and evidence of embolic distribution of the vegetative lesions.[45] In the acute form, the fever usually is spiking and accompanied by chills. In the subacute form, the fever usually is low grade, of gradual onset, and frequently accompanied by other systemic signs of inflammation, such as anorexia, malaise, and lethargy. Small petechial hemorrhages frequently result when emboli lodge in the small vessels of the skin, nail beds, and mucous membranes. Splinter hemorrhages (*i.e.,* dark red lines) under the nails of the fingers and toes are common.[45] Cough, dyspnea, arthralgia or arthritis, diarrhea, and abdominal or flank pain may occur as the result of systemic emboli.

Diagnosis. Infective endocarditis continues to pose major challenges in diagnosis and treatment, despite advances in its epidemiology and microbiology. The diagnosis of IE cannot be made through any single test, but rather includes the use of clinical, laboratory, and echocardiographic features.[45,47–50] The Duke criteria, which were modified by a committee of the AHA in 2005, provide health care professionals with a standardized assessment of persons with suspected IE that integrates blood culture evidence of infection, echocardiographic findings, clinical findings, and laboratory information.[48] The modified Duke criteria are classified into major criteria (positive blood culture for IE, evidence of endocardial involvement) and minor criteria (predisposition to IE, predisposing heart condition, or intravenous drug use; fever with a temperature >38°C; vascular phenomenon such as evidence of arterial emboli; immunologic phenomenon such as glomerulonephritis; microbiologic evidence such as blood culture that does not meet major criteria). Cases are classified as "definite" if they fulfill two major criteria, one major criterion plus two minor criteria, or five minor criteria. Cases are defined as "possible" if they fulfill one major criterion and one minor criterion, or three minor criteria. Diagnosis of IE is rejected if an alternative diagnosis is made, the infection resolves with antibiotic treatment for 4 days or less, or there is no histologic evidence of infection.

The blood culture remains the most definitive diagnostic procedure and is essential to guide treatment. However, the indiscriminate use of antibiotics has made identifying the causative organism much more difficult. The modified Duke criteria recommend the inclusion of *S. aureus* as a major criterion, whether it is a nosocomial or a community-acquired infection. Positive serologic results for *Coxiella burnetii, Chlamydia psittaci,* and *Bartonella* species are also considered major criteria. Negative blood cultures can occur in up to 30% of cases of IE, delaying diagnosis and treatment and having a profound effect on outcome.[48] This can occur because of prior antibiotic administration, or because the causative organisms are slow growing, require special culture media, or are not readily cultured.

Echocardiography is the primary technique for detection of vegetations and cardiac complications resulting from IE, and is an important tool in the diagnosis and management of disease. Echocardiographic evidence of endocardial involvement is now the major criterion in the modified Duke criteria. It is recommended that echocardiography be performed in all suspected cases of IE.[45]

Treatment. Treatment of IE focuses on identifying and eliminating the causative microorganism, minimizing the residual cardiac effects, and treating the pathologic effect of emboli. The choice of antimicrobial therapy depends on the organism cultured and whether it occurs in a native or prosthetic valve. *S. aureus,* the most common cause of IE, is primarily the result of nosocomial infections from intravascular catheters, surgical wounds, and indwelling prosthetic devices. Guidelines for the prevention and management of nonvalvular cardiovascular device–related infections are presented in the literature.[47,51] The widespread emergence of multidrug-resistant organisms, including *S. aureus,* poses a serious challenge in the treatment of IE. In addition to antibiotic therapy, surgery may be needed for unresolved infection, severe heart failure, and significant emboli.

The majority of persons with IE are cured with medical or surgical treatment. Persons who have had infectious endocarditis should be educated about its signs and symptoms and informed of the possibility of relapse or recurrence. Immediate medical attention should be sought if signs or symptoms recur. Prevention of IE through the use of prophylactic antibiotics is controversial. The current recommendations conclude that only a very small number of IE cases might be prevented by antibiotic prophylaxis for dental procedures. Therefore, prophylaxis is recommended only for patients with underlying cardiac conditions and the highest risk for adverse outcomes from IE. It is not recommended based solely on an increased lifetime risk of acquiring IE.[50,51]

Rheumatic Heart Disease

Rheumatic fever (RF) and rheumatic heart disease (RHD) are complications of the immune-mediated response to group A (beta-hemolytic) streptococcal (GAS) throat infection.[9] The most serious aspect of RF is the development of chronic valvular disorders that produce permanent cardiac dysfunction and sometimes cause fatal heart failure years later. Although RF and RHD are rare in developed countries, they continue to be major health problems in underdeveloped countries, where inadequate health care, poor nutrition, and crowded living conditions still prevail.[52]

Pathogenesis

Beta-hemolytic streptococci are divided into several serologic groups based on their cell wall polysaccharide antigen. Group A is further subdivided into more than 130 distinct M types, which are responsible for the vast majority of infections. The M protein best defines the virulence of the bacterium, and has been studied most intensively with regard to cross-reactivity with heart tissue.[9] Although GAS causes both pharyngitis and skin (impetigo) infections, only the pharyngitis has been linked with RF and RHD.

The pathogenesis of RF is unclear. The time frame for development of symptoms in relation to the sore throat and the presence of antibodies to GAS strongly suggests an immunologic origin.[9,52–54] It is thought that antibodies directed against the M protein of certain strains of streptococci cross-react with glycoprotein antigens in the heart, joints, and other tissues to produce an autoimmune response through a phenomenon called *molecular mimicry*[52] (see Chapter 19). The onset of symptoms 2 to 3 weeks after infection and the absence of streptococci in the lesion support this belief. Although only a small percentage of persons with untreated GAS pharyngitis develop RF, the incidence of recurrence with a subsequent untreated infection is substantially greater. These observations and more recent studies suggest a genetic predisposition to development of the disease.[9]

Clinical Features

Rheumatic fever can manifest as an acute, recurrent, or chronic disorder. The *acute stage* of RF includes a history of an initiating streptococcal infection and subsequent involvement of the connective tissue elements of the heart, blood vessels, joints, and subcutaneous tissues. Common to all is a lesion called the *Aschoff body*,[9] which is a localized area of tissue necrosis surrounded by immune cells. The *recurrent phase* usually involves extension of the cardiac effects of the disease. The *chronic phase* of RF is characterized by permanent deformity of the heart valves and is a common cause of mitral valve stenosis. Chronic RHD usually does not appear until at least 10 years after the initial attack, sometimes decades later.

Most persons with RF have a history of sore throat, headache, fever, abdominal pain, nausea, vomiting, swollen glands (usually at the angle of the jaw), and other signs and symptoms of streptococcal infection. Other clinical features associated with an acute episode of RF are related to the acute inflammatory process and the structures involved in the disease process. The course of the disease is characterized by a constellation of findings that includes migratory polyarthritis of the large joints, carditis, erythema marginatum, subcutaneous nodules, and Sydenham chorea.[9] Laboratory markers of acute inflammation include an elevated white blood cell count, ESR, and CRP. These elevated levels of acute-phase reactants are not specific for RF but provide evidence of an acute inflammatory response.

Polyarthritis. Polyarthritis is the most common, and frequently the first, manifestation of RF. It may be the only major criterion in adolescents and adults. The arthritis, which may range from arthralgia to disabling arthritis, most often involves the larger joints, particularly the knees and ankles, and occurs less frequently in the wrists, elbows, shoulders, and hips. It is almost always migratory, affecting one joint and then moving to another. Untreated, the arthritis lasts approximately 4 weeks. A striking feature of rheumatic arthritis is the dramatic response (usually within 48 hours) to salicylates. Arthritis usually heals completely and leaves no functional residua.

Carditis. Acute rheumatic carditis, which complicates the acute phase of RF, can affect the endocardium, myocardium, or pericardium. Usually all three layers are involved. Both the pericarditis and myocarditis usually are self-limited manifestations of the acute stage of RF. The involvement of the endocardium and valvular structures produces the permanent and disabling effects of RF. Although any of the four valves can be involved, the mitral and aortic valves are affected most often. During the acute inflammatory stage of the disease, the valvular structures become red and swollen, and small vegetative lesions develop on the valve leaflets. The acute inflammatory changes gradually proceed to development of fibrous scar tissue, which tends to contract and cause deformity of the valve leaflets and shortening of the chordae tendineae. In some cases, the edges or commissures of the valve leaflets fuse together as healing occurs.

Clinical features of endocarditis/valvulitis, without a history of RHD, include the presence of an apical holosystolic murmur of mitral regurgitation or a basal early diastolic murmur of aortic regurgitation. In someone with a history of RHD, a change in the character of these murmurs or a new murmur would indicate acute rheumatic carditis. In patients with recurrent carditis and a history of RHD, the condition is sometimes difficult to distinguish from acute endocarditis.[54]

Subcutaneous Nodules, Erythema Marginatum, and Sydenham Chorea. *Subcutaneous nodules* are hard, painless, and freely movable and usually occur over the extensor muscles of the wrist, elbow, ankle, and knee joints, ranging in size from 0.5 to 2 cm. Subcutaneous nodules rarely occur alone in RF and occur most often in association with carditis.

Erythema marginatum lesions are maplike, macular areas most commonly seen on the trunk or inner aspects of the upper arm and thigh, but never on the face. They occur early in the course of a rheumatic attack and tend to occur with subcutaneous nodules. They are transitory and disappear during the course of the disease.

Sydenham chorea is the major central nervous system manifestation of RF. It is seen most frequently in young girls and rarely occurs after 20 years of age. There typically is an insidious onset of irritability and other behavior problems. The child often is fidgety, cries easily, begins to walk clumsily, and drops things. The choreiform movements are spontaneous, rapid, purposeless, jerking movements that interfere with voluntary activities. Facial grimaces are common, and even speech may be affected. The chorea is self-limited, usually running its course within a matter of weeks or months, but recurrences are not uncommon. A previous streptococcal infection can be detected only in about two thirds of cases, making differential diagnosis more difficult.

Diagnosis. There are no specific laboratory tests that can establish a diagnosis of RF. Because of the variety of signs and symptoms, the Jones criteria for the diagnosis of RF, which were first proposed in 1944 and have undergone multiple reviews by the AHA and the World Health Organization (WHO), are designed to assist in standardizing the diagnosis of RF.[53,55] The Jones criteria divide the clinical features of RF into major and minor categories, based on prevalence and specificity. The presence of two major signs (*i.e.,* carditis, polyarthritis, chorea, erythema marginatum, and subcutaneous nodules) or one major and two minor signs (*i.e.,* arthralgia, fever, and elevated ESR, CRP, or leukocyte count), accompanied by evidence of a preceding GAS infection, indicates a high probability of RF. The latest review, in 2004 by the WHO, proposes the diagnosis of a primary episode of RF, recurrent attacks of RF with or without RHD, rheumatic chorea, insidious onset of rheumatic carditis, and chronic RHD.[53] The epidemiologic setting in which the diagnosis of RF is made is also considered important.

The use of echocardiography has enhanced the understanding of both acute and chronic RHD. It is useful in assessing the severity of valvular stenosis and regurgitation, chamber size and ventricular function, and the presence and size of pleural effusions. Doppler ultrasonography may be useful in identifying cardiac lesions in persons who do not show typical signs of cardiac involvement during an attack of RF, but is not considered either a major or minor Jones criterion at this time.[55]

Treatment and Prevention. It is important that streptococcal infections be promptly diagnosed and treated to prevent RF. The gold standard for detecting a streptococcal infection is throat culture. However, it takes 24 to 48 hours to produce a result, delaying treatment. The development of rapid tests for direct detection of GAS antigens has provided at least a partial solution for this problem. Both the throat culture and the rapid antigen tests are highly specific for GAS infection but are limited in terms of their sensitivity (*e.g.,* the person may have a negative test result but have a streptococcal infection). A negative antigen test result should be confirmed with a throat culture when a streptococcal infection is suspected.[55] The presence of GAS in the upper respiratory tract can indicate either a carrier or infectious state, the latter of which can be defined by a rising antibody response. Serologic examinations for streptococcal antibodies (antistreptolysin O and antideoxyribonuclease B) are measured for retrospective confirmation of recent streptococcal infections in persons thought to have acute RF. There is, however, no single specific laboratory test result that is pathognomonic for acute or recurrent RF.

Treatment of acute RF is designed to control the acute inflammatory response and prevent cardiac complications and recurrence of the disease. During the acute phase, antibiotics, anti-inflammatory drugs, and selective restriction of activities are prescribed. No clinical isolate of GAS is resistant to penicillin; therefore, penicillin, or another antibiotic in penicillin-

sensitive patients, is the treatment of choice for GAS infection.[55] First-generation cephalosporins have also been given successfully. Salicylates and corticosteroids can be used to suppress the inflammatory response, but should not be given until the diagnosis of RF is confirmed. Surgery is indicated for chronic rheumatic valve disease, and is determined by the severity of the symptom or the evidence that cardiac function is significantly impaired. Procedures used include closed mitral commissurotomy, valve repair, and valve replacement.

The person who has had an attack of RF is at high risk for recurrence after subsequent GAS throat infections. Penicillin is the treatment of choice for secondary prophylaxis, but sulfadiazine or erythromycin may be used in penicillin-allergic individuals. The duration of prophylaxis depends on whether residual valvular disease is present or absent. It is recommended that persons with persistent valvular disease receive prophylaxis for at least 5 years after the last episode of acute RF or age 21 years.[54] Compliance with a plan for prophylactic administration of penicillin requires that the person and his or her family understand the rationale for such measures. They also need to be instructed to report possible streptococcal infections to their physicians and to inform their dentists about the disease so that they can be adequately protected during dental procedures that may traumatize the oral mucosa.

> **IN SUMMARY,** infective endocarditis involves the invasion of the endocardium by pathogens that produce vegetative lesions on the endocardial surface. The loose organization of these lesions permits the organisms and fragments of the lesions to be disseminated throughout the systemic circulation. Although several organisms can cause the condition, staphylococci have now become the leading cause of IE. Treatment of IE focuses on identifying and eliminating the causative microorganism, minimizing the residual cardiac effects, and treating the pathologic effect of emboli.
>
> Rheumatic fever, which is associated with an antecedent GAS throat infection, is an important cause of heart disease. Its most serious and disabling effects result from involvement of the heart valves. Because there is no single laboratory test result, sign, or symptom that is pathognomonic for acute rheumatic fever, the Jones criteria are used to establish the diagnosis during the acute stage of the disease. Primary and secondary prevention strategies focus on appropriate antibiotic therapy. ∎

VALVULAR HEART DISEASE

After completing this section of the chapter, you should be able to meet the following objectives:

- State the function of the heart valves and relate alterations in hemodynamic function of the heart that occur with valvular disease.

- Compare the effects of stenotic and regurgitant mitral and aortic valvular heart disease on cardiovascular function.
- Compare the methods of and diagnostic information obtained from cardiac auscultation and echocardiography as they relate to valvular heart disease.

The past several decades have brought remarkable advances in the treatment and outlook for people with valvular heart disease. This is undoubtedly due to improved methods for non-invasive monitoring of ventricular function, improvement in prosthetic valves, advances in valve reconstruction procedures, and the development of useful guidelines to improve the timing of surgical interventions.[56] Nonetheless, valvular heart disease continues to produce considerable mortality and morbidity.

Hemodynamic Derangements

The function of the heart valves is to promote unidirectional flow of blood through the chambers of the heart. Dysfunction of the heart valves can result from a number of disorders, including congenital defects, trauma, ischemic damage, degenerative changes, and inflammation. Although any of the four heart valves can become diseased, the most commonly affected are the mitral and aortic valves. Disorders of the pulmonary and tricuspid valves are uncommon, probably because of the low pressure in the right side of the heart.

The heart valves consist of thin leaflets of tough, flexible, endothelium-covered fibrous tissue firmly attached at the base to the fibrous valve rings (see Chapter 21). Capillaries and smooth muscle are present at the base of the leaflet but do not extend up into the valve. The leaflets of the heart valves may be injured or become the site of an inflammatory process that can deform their line of closure. Healing of the valve leaflets often is associated with increased collagen content and scarring, causing the leaflets to shorten and become stiffer. The edges of the healing valve leaflets can fuse together so that the valve does not open or close properly.

Two types of mechanical disruptions occur with valvular heart disease: narrowing of the valve opening so it does not open properly, and distortion of the valve so it does not close properly (Fig. 24-18). *Stenosis* refers to a narrowing of the valve orifice and failure of the valve leaflets to open normally. Blood flow through a normal valve can increase by five to seven times the resting volume; consequently, valvular stenosis must be severe before it causes problems. Significant narrowing of the valve orifice increases the resistance to blood flow through the valve, converting the normally smooth laminar flow to a less efficient turbulent flow (see Chapter 21). This increases the volume and work of the chamber emptying through the narrowed valve—the left atrium in the case of mitral stenosis and the left ventricle in aortic stenosis. Symptoms usually are noticed first during situations of increased flow, such as exercise. An incompetent or regurgitant valve permits backward flow to occur when the valve should be closed—flowing back into the left ventricle during

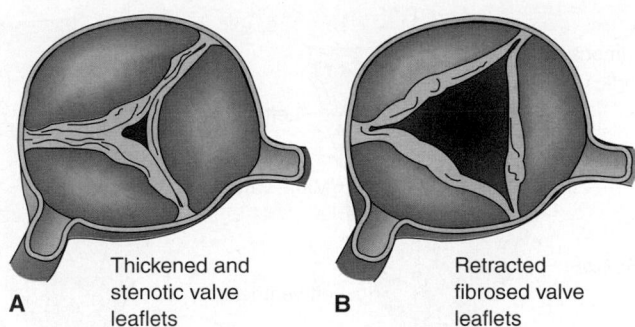

FIGURE 24-18 • Disease of the aortic valve as viewed from the aorta. **(A)** Stenosis of the valve opening. **(B)** An incompetent or regurgitant valve that is unable to close completely.

diastole when the aortic valve is affected and back into the left atrium during systole when the mitral valve is diseased.

The effects of valvular heart disease on cardiac function are related to alterations in blood flow across the valve and to the resultant increase in work demands on the heart the disorder generates. Many valvular heart defects are characterized by heart murmurs resulting from turbulent blood flow through a diseased valve. Disorders in valve flow and heart chamber size for mitral and aortic valve disorders are illustrated in Figure 24-19.

Echocardiography, described earlier in the chapter, provides a means of visualizing valvular motion, patterns of flow, and closure patterns. Pulsed Doppler ultrasonography provides a semiquantitative or qualitative estimation of the severity of transvalvular gradients, right ventricular systolic pressure, and valvular regurgitation. Color flow Doppler provides a visual pattern of flow velocities over the anatomic 2-D echocardiographic image. This allows for demonstration of turbulence from stenotic and regurgitant valves.

Transesophageal echocardiography with Doppler ultrasonography is used to obtain echocardiographic data when surface sound transmission is poor, particularly of the AV valves and prosthetic heart valves.

VALVULAR HEART DISEASE

- The heart valves determine the direction of blood flow through the heart chambers.
- Valvular heart defects exert their effects by obstructing flow of blood (stenotic valve disorders) or allowing backward flow of blood (regurgitant valve disorders).
- Stenotic valvular defects produce distention of the heart chamber that empties blood through the diseased valve and impaired filling of the chamber that receives blood that moves through the valve.
- Regurgitant valves allow blood to move back through the valve when it should be closed. This produces distention and places increased work demands on the chamber ejecting blood through the diseased valve.

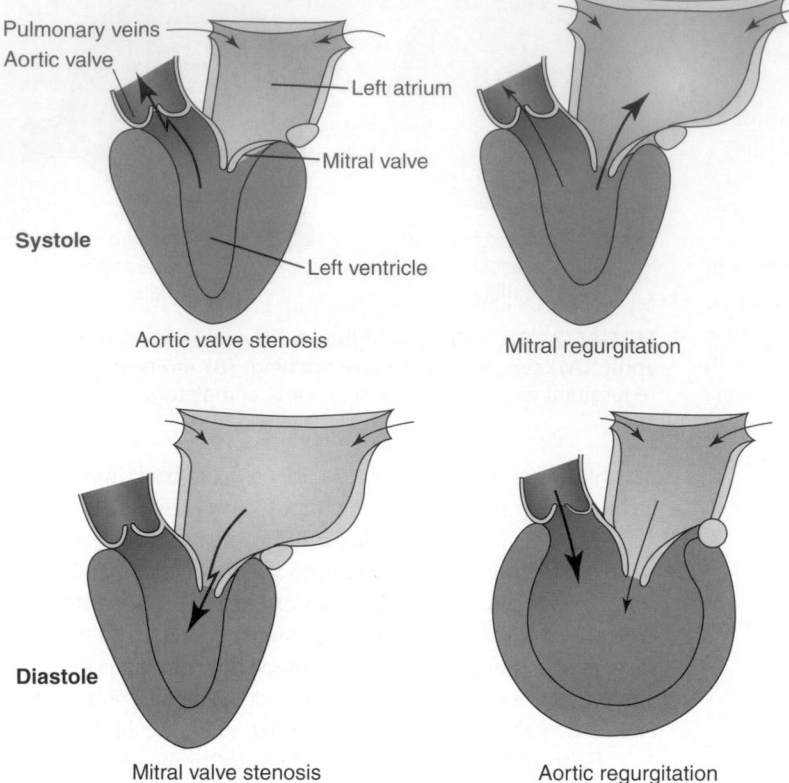

Systole

Pulmonary veins
Aortic valve
Left atrium
Mitral valve
Left ventricle
Aortic valve stenosis
Mitral regurgitation

Diastole

Mitral valve stenosis
Aortic regurgitation

FIGURE 24-19 • Alterations in hemodynamic function that accompany aortic valve stenosis, mitral valve regurgitation, mitral valve stenosis, and aortic valve regurgitation. The *thin arrows* indicate direction of normal flow, and *thick arrows* the direction of abnormal flow.

Mitral Valve Disorders

The mitral valve controls the directional flow of blood between the left atrium and the left ventricle. The edges or cusps of the AV valves are thinner than those of the semilunar valves; they are anchored to the papillary muscles by the chordae tendineae. During much of systole, the mitral valve is subjected to the high pressure generated by the left ventricle as it pumps blood into the systemic circulation. During this period of increased pressure, the chordae tendineae prevent the eversion of the valve leaflets into the left atrium.

Mitral Valve Stenosis

Mitral valve stenosis represents the incomplete opening of the mitral valve during diastole, with left atrial distention and impaired filling of the left ventricle. Mitral valve stenosis most commonly is the result of RF.[56,57] Less frequently, the defect is congenital and manifests during infancy or early childhood. Mitral valve stenosis is a continuous, progressive, lifelong disorder consisting of a slow, stable course in the early years and progressive acceleration in later years.

Mitral valve stenosis is characterized by fibrous replacement of valvular tissue, along with stiffness and fusion of the valve apparatus (Fig. 24-20). Typically, the mitral cusps fuse at the edges and involvement of the chordae tendineae causes shortening, which pulls the valvular structures more deeply into the ventricles. As the resistance to flow through the valve increases, the left atrium becomes dilated and left atrial pres-

sure rises. The increased left atrial pressure eventually is transmitted to the pulmonary venous system, causing pulmonary congestion.

The rate of flow across the valve depends on the size of the valve orifice, the driving pressure (*i.e.,* atrial minus ventricular pressure), and the time available for flow during diastole. The normal mitral valve area is 4 to 6 cm². Narrowing of the valve area to less than 2 cm² must occur before mild symptoms begin to develop.[56] As the condition progresses, symptoms of

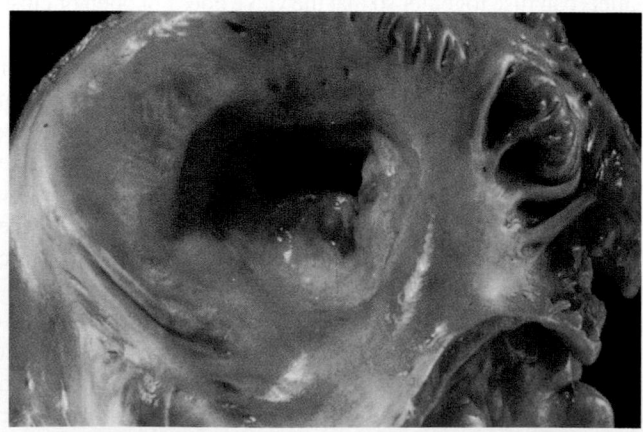

FIGURE 24-20 • Chronic rheumatic valvulitis. A view of the mitral valve from the left atrium shows rigid, thickened, and fused leaflets with a narrow orifice, creating the characteristic "fish mouth" appearance of rheumatic mitral stenosis. (From Rubin E., Farber J. L. [1999]. *Pathology* [3rd ed., p. 570]. Philadelphia: Lippincott-Raven.)

decreased cardiac output occur during extreme exertion or other situations that cause tachycardia and thereby reduce diastolic filling time. In the late stages of the disease, pulmonary vascular resistance increases with the development of pulmonary hypertension; this increases the pressure against which the right heart must pump and eventually leads to right-sided heart failure.

The signs and symptoms of mitral valve stenosis depend on the severity of the obstruction and are related to the elevation in left atrial pressure and pulmonary congestion, decreased cardiac output owing to impaired left ventricular filling, and left atrial enlargement with development of atrial arrhythmias and mural thrombi. The symptoms are those of pulmonary congestion, including nocturnal paroxysmal dyspnea and orthopnea. Palpitations, chest pain, weakness, and fatigue are common complaints.

Premature atrial beats, paroxysmal atrial tachycardia, and atrial fibrillation may occur as a result of distention of the left atrium. Fibrosis of the internodal and interatrial tracts, along with damage to the sinoatrial node, may occur from the rheumatic process itself. Atrial fibrillation develops in 30% to 40% of persons with symptomatic mitral stenosis.[57] Together, the fibrillation and distention predispose to mural thrombus formation. The risk of arterial embolization, particularly stroke, is significantly increased in persons with atrial fibrillation.

The murmur of mitral valve stenosis is heard during diastole when blood is flowing through the constricted valve orifice; it is characteristically a low-pitched, rumbling murmur, best heard at the apex of the heart. The first heart sound often is accentuated and somewhat delayed because of the increased left atrial pressure; an opening snap may precede the diastolic murmur as a result of the elevation in left atrial pressure. The 2-D and Doppler echocardiograms are most commonly used to diagnose mitral stenosis. These echocardiograms confirm the diagnosis of mitral stenosis, evaluate mitral valve morphology and hemodynamics, and measure pulmonary artery pressures. They also rule out other causes of mitral stenosis and assist in identifying the most appropriate treatment.

Medical treatment of mitral valve stenosis is aimed at relieving signs of decreased cardiac output and pulmonary congestion. In atrial fibrillation, the goals are to control ventricular rate and prevent systemic embolization with anticoagulation therapy. Antibiotic prophylaxis against recurrent RF is recommended. Surgical interventions, including commissurotomy, balloon valvotomy, and valve repair or replacement, may be used to treat degenerative and functional mitral valve disease and, in some cases, IE.[57–59]

Mitral valve commissurotomy can be performed percutaneously with a balloon catheter or surgically through a left thoracotomy. These procedures open the commissures that were fused by scar tissue, decreasing the gradient and increasing the valve area, and, as a result, improve clinical symptoms.[57] Mechanical or biologic prostheses can be used for mitral valve replacement. Because of the risk of thromboembolism, persons with mechanical prostheses usually require indefinite anticoagulation therapy.[57]

Mitral Valve Regurgitation

Mitral valve regurgitation is characterized by incomplete closure of the mitral valve, with the left ventricular stroke volume being divided between the forward stroke volume that moves into the aorta and the regurgitant stroke volume that moves back into the left atrium during systole (see Fig. 24-19). Mitral valve regurgitation can result from many processes. RHD is associated with a rigid and thickened valve that does not open or close completely. In addition to RHD, mitral regurgitation can result from rupture of the chordae tendineae or papillary muscles, papillary muscle dysfunction, or stretching of the valve structures due to dilation of the left ventricle or valve orifice. Mitral valve prolapse is a common cause of mitral valve regurgitation.

Acute mitral valve regurgitation may occur abruptly, such as with papillary muscle dysfunction after myocardial infarction, valve perforation in IE, or ruptured chordae tendineae in mitral valve prolapse. In acute severe mitral regurgitation, acute volume overload increases left ventricular preload, allowing a modest increase in left ventricular stroke volume. However, the forward stroke volume (that moving through the aorta into the systemic circulation) is reduced and the regurgitant stroke volume leads to a rapid rise in left atrial pressure and pulmonary edema. Acute mitral valve regurgitation almost always is symptomatic; if severe, mitral valve replacement often is indicated.

The hemodynamic changes associated with chronic mitral valve regurgitation occur more slowly, allowing for recruitment of compensatory mechanisms. An increase in left ventricular end-diastolic volume permits an increase in total stroke volume, with restoration of forward flow into the aorta. Augmented preload and reduced or normal afterload (provided by unloading the left ventricle into the left atrium) facilitates left ventricular ejection. At the same time, a gradual increase in left atrial size allows for accommodation of the regurgitant volume at a lower filling pressure.

The increased volume work associated with mitral regurgitation is relatively well tolerated, and many persons with the disorder remain asymptomatic for many years, developing symptoms between 6 and 10 years after diagnosis. The degree of left ventricular enlargement reflects the severity of regurgitation. As the disorder progresses, left ventricular function becomes impaired, the forward (aortic) stroke volume decreases, and the left atrial pressure increases, with the subsequent development of pulmonary congestion. Surgery should be performed before the onset of these symptoms.

A characteristic feature of mitral valve regurgitation is an enlarged left ventricle, a hyperdynamic left ventricular impulse, and a pansystolic (throughout systole) murmur. Mitral regurgitation, like mitral stenosis, predisposes to atrial fibrillation.

The 2-D Doppler echocardiogram is useful in mitral regurgitation to evaluate left ventricular and atrial size, measure the ejection fraction, and assist in decision making regarding surgery through assessment of the severity of the regurgitation. In some patients with mitral regurgitation, preload reduction can be beneficial and may be treated with ACE inhibitors and biventricular pacing. Surgeries used in the treatment of mitral regurgitation include mitral valve repair and valve replacement with or without removal of the mitral apparatus. Mitral valve repair avoids the use of anticoagulation needed with artificial valves.[59] Conservation of the mitral apparatus is always the goal in mitral valve replacement because it ensures competence of the mitral valve and preserves left ventricular function.

Mitral Valve Prolapse

Sometimes referred to as the *floppy mitral valve syndrome,* mitral valve prolapse occurs in 1% to 2.5% of the general population.[57] The disorder is seen more frequently in women than in men and may have a familial basis. Familial mitral valve prolapse is transmitted as an autosomal trait, and several chromosomal loci have been identified. Although the exact cause of the disorder usually is unknown, it has been associated with Marfan syndrome, osteogenesis imperfecta, and other connective tissue disorders, and with cardiac, hematologic, neuroendocrine, metabolic, and psychological disorders.

Pathologic findings in persons with mitral valve prolapse include a myxedematous (mucinous) degeneration of mitral valve leaflets that causes them to become enlarged and floppy so that they prolapse or balloon back into the left atrium during systole[56] (Fig. 24-21). Secondary fibrotic changes reflect the stresses and injury that the ballooning movements impose on the valve. Certain forms of mitral valve prolapse may arise from disorders of the myocardium that place undue stress on the mitral valve because of abnormal movement of the ventricular wall or papillary muscle. Mitral valve prolapse may or may not cause mitral regurgitation.

Most persons with mitral valve prolapse are asymptomatic and the disorder is discovered during a routine physical examination. A minority of people have chest pain mimicking angina, dyspnea, fatigue, anxiety, palpitations, and lightheadedness. Unlike angina, the chest pain often is prolonged, ill defined, and not associated with exercise or exertion. The pain has been attributed to ischemia resulting from traction of the prolapsing valve leaflets. The anxiety, palpitations, and arrhythmias may result from abnormal autonomic nervous system function that commonly accompanies the disorder. Rare cases of sudden death have been reported for persons with mitral valve prolapse, mainly those with a family history of similar occurrences.

The disorder is characterized by a spectrum of auscultatory findings, ranging from a silent form to one or more mid-systolic clicks followed by a late systolic or holosystolic murmur. The clicks are caused by the sudden tensing of the mitral valve apparatus as the leaflets prolapse. Two-dimensional and Doppler echocardiography are valuable noninvasive studies used to diagnose mitral valve prolapse.

The treatment of mitral valve prolapse focuses on the relief of symptoms and the prevention of complications.[57] Persons with palpitations and mild tachyarrhythmias or increased adrenergic symptoms, and those with chest discomfort, anxiety, and fatigue often respond to therapy with the β-adrenergic blocking drugs. In many cases, the cessation of stimulants such as caffeine, alcohol, and cigarettes may be sufficient to control symptoms. IE is an uncommon complication in persons with a murmur; antibiotic prophylaxis usually is recommended before dental or surgical procedures associated with bacteremia. Transient ischemic attacks occur more frequently in persons with mitral valve prolapse. Therefore, in persons with documented events who are in sinus rhythm with no atrial thrombi, daily aspirin therapy is recommended. Most persons with mitral valve prolapse are encouraged to participate in regular exercise and lead a normal life. Persons with severe valve dysfunction may require valve surgery.

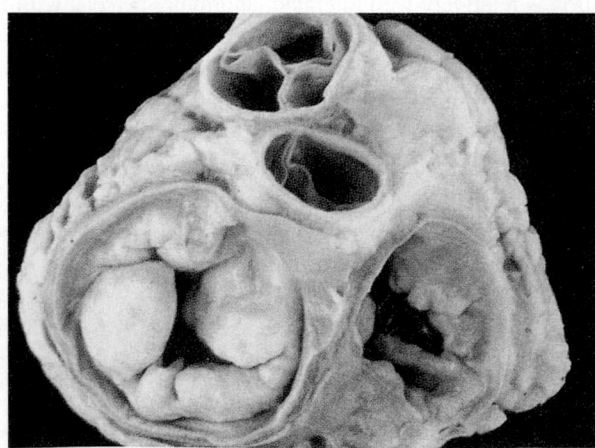

FIGURE 24-21 • Mitral valve prolapse. A view of the mitral valve from the left atrium shows redundant and deformed leaflets that billow into the left atrial cavity. (From Saffitz J. E. [2008]. The heart. In Rubin E., Strayer D. E. [Eds.], *Rubin's pathology: Clinicopathologic foundations of medicine* [5th ed., p. 464]. Philadelphia: Lippincott Williams & Wilkins.)

Aortic Valve Disorders

The aortic valve is located between the left ventricle and the aorta. The aortic valve has three cusps and sometimes is referred to as the *aortic semilunar valve* because its leaflets are crescent or moon shaped (see Chapter 21, Fig. 21-9). The aortic valve has no chordae tendineae. Although their structures are similar, the cusps of the aortic valve are thicker than those of the mitral valve. The middle layer of the aortic valve is thickened near the middle, where the three leaflets meet, ensuring a tight seal. Between the thickened tissue and their free margins, the leaflets are more thin and flimsy.

An important aspect of the aortic valve is the location of the orifices for the two main coronary arteries, which are located behind the valve and at right angles to the direction of blood flow. It is the lateral pressure in the aorta that propels blood into the coronary arteries. During the ejection phase of the cardiac cycle, the lateral pressure is diminished by conversion of potential energy to kinetic energy as blood moves forward into the aorta. This process is grossly exaggerated in aortic valve stenosis because of the high flow velocities.

Aortic Valve Stenosis

Aortic valve stenosis, often referred to simply as *aortic stenosis,* is characterized by increased resistance to ejection of blood from the left ventricle into the aorta (see Fig. 24-19). The most common causes of aortic valve stenosis are congenital valve malformations and acquired calcification of a normal tricuspid valve. Congenital malformations may result in unicuspid, bicuspid, or misshaped valve leaflets. Acquired aortic stenosis is usually the consequence of calcification associated with the normal "wear and tear" of either a previously normal aortic valve or congenitally bicuspid valves (with which approximately 1% of the population are born).[9] The incidence of acquired aortic valve stenosis is increasing with the rising average age of the population.[9,60]

The progression of calcific aortic stenosis is usually slow and varies widely among individuals. It usually becomes clinically evident in the sixth and seventh decades in persons with bicuspid aortic valves, and not until the eight and ninth decades in those with previously normal valves. Valve changes range from mild thickening without obstruction to severe calcification with impaired leaflet motion and obstructed left ventricular outflow.[61] Processes in the development of calcific aortic valve disease have been shown to be similar to those in CAD. Both conditions are more common in men, older persons, and persons with hypercholesteremia and both derive in part from an active inflammatory process.[60] Early lesions of aortic sclerosis show focal subendothelial plaquelike lesions, similar to the initial phases of an atherosclerotic lesion. Aortic sclerosis is distinguished from aortic stenosis by the degree of valve impairment. In aortic sclerosis the valve leaflets are abnormally thickened, but the obstruction to outflow is minimal, whereas in aortic stenosis the functional area of the valve has decreased enough to cause measurable obstruction to outflow. Calcification of the aortic valve progresses from the base of the cusps to the leaflets. This reduces leaflet motion and effective valve area, but without commissural fusion. As calcification progresses, the leaflets become more rigid, there is worsening obstruction to left ventricular outflow, and fusion of the commissures leads to aortic stenosis.

Because aortic stenosis develops gradually, the left ventricle has time to adapt. With increased systolic pressure from obstruction, the left ventricular wall becomes thicker, or hypertrophies, but a normal chamber volume is maintained. This increase in wall thickness can maintain a normal ejection fraction. Little hemodynamic disturbance occurs as the valve area is reduced by half its normal area (from a normal 3 to 4 cm² to 1.5 to 2 cm²). However, an additional reduction in valve area from one half to one fourth of its normal size produces severe obstruction to flow and a progressive pressure overload on the left ventricle. At this point, the increased work of the heart begins to exceed the coronary blood flow reserve, causing both systolic and diastolic dysfunction and signs of heart failure.[57,60,61]

Aortic stenosis is usually first diagnosed with auscultation of a loud systolic ejection murmur or a single or paradoxically split second heart sound. Eventually, the classic symptoms of angina, syncope, and heart failure develop, although more subtle signs of a decrease in exercise tolerance or exertional dyspnea should be monitored closely. Angina occurs in approximately two thirds of persons with advanced aortic stenosis and is similar to that observed in CAD. Dyspnea, marked fatigability, peripheral cyanosis, and other signs of low-output heart failure usually are not prominent until late in the course of the disease. Syncope (fainting) is most commonly due to the reduced cerebral circulation that occurs during exertion when the arterial pressure declines consequent to vasodilation in the presence of a fixed cardiac output.

Echocardiography can be used to evaluate the severity of calcified aortic lesions, left ventricular size and function, degree of ventricular hypertrophy, and presence of associated valve disorders, and plays a major part in decision making for aortic valve replacement.

There is no effective medical therapy for severe aortic stenosis. In children with congenital aortic stenosis, the valve leaflets are merely fused and balloon valvulotomy may provide substantial benefit; valve replacement is the most effective treatment. Medical interventions are prescribed to relieve symptoms of heart failure for those patients who are ineligible for surgical intervention. For prevention of IE and recurrent RF, antibiotics are prescribed. Two pharmacologic agents currently being evaluated as treatment options for delaying disease progression are the statins and ACE inhibitors.[61]

Aortic Valve Regurgitation

Aortic valve regurgitation (or aortic regurgitation) is the result of an incompetent aortic valve that allows blood to flow back to the left ventricle during diastole (see Fig. 24-19). As a result, the left ventricle must increase its stroke volume to include blood entering from the lungs as well as that leaking back through the regurgitant valve. This defect may result from conditions that cause scarring of the valve leaflets or from enlargement of the valve orifice to the extent that the valve leaflets no longer meet. There are various causes of aortic regurgitation, including RF, idiopathic dilation of the aorta, congenital abnormalities, IE, and Marfan syndrome. Other causes include hypertension, trauma, and failure of a prosthetic valve.

Acute aortic regurgitation is characterized by the presentation of a sudden, large regurgitant volume to a left ventricle of normal size that has not had time to adapt to the volume overload. It is caused most commonly by disorders such as IE, trauma, or aortic dissection. Although the heart responds with use of the Frank-Starling mechanisms and an increase in heart rate, these compensatory mechanisms fail to maintain the cardiac output. As a result, there is severe elevation in left ventricular end-diastolic pressure, which is transmitted to the left atrium and pulmonary veins, culminating in pulmonary edema. A decrease in cardiac output leads to sympathetic stimulation and a resultant increase in heart rate and peripheral vascular resistance that cause the regurgitation to worsen. Death from pulmonary edema, ventricular arrhythmias, or circulatory collapse is common in severe acute aortic regurgitation.

Chronic aortic regurgitation, which usually has a gradual onset, represents a condition of combined left ventricular volume and pressure overload. As the valve deformity increases, regurgitant flow into the left ventricle increases, diastolic blood pressure falls, and the left ventricle progressively enlarges. Hemodynamically, the increase in left ventricular volume results in the ejection of a large stroke volume that usually is adequate to maintain the forward cardiac output until late in the course of the disease. Most persons remain asymptomatic during this compensated phase, which may last decades. The only sign for many years may be a soft systolic aortic murmur.

As the disease progresses, signs and symptoms of left ventricular failure begin to appear. These include exertional dyspnea, orthopnea, and paroxysmal nocturnal dyspnea. In aortic regurgitation, failure of aortic valve closure during diastole causes an abnormal drop in diastolic pressure. Because coronary blood flow is greatest during diastole, the drop in diastolic pressure produces a decrease in coronary perfusion. Although angina is rare, it may occur when the heart rate and diastolic pressure fall to low levels. Persons with severe aortic regurgitation often complain of an uncomfortable awareness of heartbeat, particularly when lying down, and chest discomfort due to pounding of the heart against the chest wall. Tachycardia, occurring with emotional stress or exertion, may produce palpitations, head pounding, and premature ventricular contractions.

The major physical findings relate to the widening of the arterial pulse pressure. The pulse has a rapid rise and fall (Corrigan pulse), with an elevated systolic pressure and low diastolic pressure owing to the large stroke volume and rapid diastolic runoff of blood back into the left ventricle. Korotkoff sounds may persist to zero, even though intra-arterial pressure rarely falls below 30 mm Hg.[56] The large stroke volume and wide pulse pressure may result in prominent carotid pulsations in the neck, throbbing peripheral pulses, and a left ventricular impulse that causes the chest to move with each beat. The hyperkinetic pulse of more severe aortic regurgitation, called a *water-hammer pulse,* is characterized by distention and quick collapse of the artery. The turbulence of flow across the aortic valve during diastole produces a high-pitched or blowing sound.

The treatment for acute or severe chronic aortic regurgitation is aortic valve replacement. Surgery is recommended whenever patients are symptomatic, regardless of left ventricular function. In asymptomatic patients, valve replacement is controversial. However, in patients with left ventricular systolic dysfunction or with severe left ventricular dilation, valve replacement is also recommended, even if patients are asymptomatic.[57]

The goal of medical therapy is to improve forward stroke volume and reduce regurgitant volume, usually through the use of vasodilator therapy. This is indicated in symptomatic patients with severe aortic regurgitation when surgery is not recommended, or for short-term therapy to improve hemodynamics of a patient preparing for valve replacement.[57]

IN SUMMARY, dysfunction of the heart valves can result from a number of disorders, including congenital defects, trauma, ischemic heart disease, degenerative changes, and inflammation. Rheumatic endocarditis is a common cause. Valvular heart disease produces its effects through disturbances of blood flow. A stenotic valvular defect is one that causes a decrease in blood flow through a valve, resulting in impaired emptying and increased work demands on the heart chamber that empties blood across the diseased valve. A regurgitant valvular defect permits the blood flow to continue when the valve is closed. Valvular heart disorders produce blood flow turbulence and often are detected through cardiac auscultation. ∎

HEART DISEASE IN INFANTS AND CHILDREN

After completing this section of the chapter, you should be able to meet the following objectives:

- Trace the flow of blood in the fetal circulation, state the function of the foramen ovale and ductus arteriosus, and describe the changes in circulatory function that occur at birth.
- Compare the effects of left-to-right and right-to-left shunts on the pulmonary circulation and production of cyanosis.
- Describe the anatomic defects and altered patterns of blood flow in children with atrial septal defects, ventricular septal defects, endocardial cushion defects, pulmonary stenosis, tetralogy of Fallot, patent ductus arteriosus, transposition of the great vessels, coarctation of the aorta, and single-ventricle anatomy.
- Describe the prevalence of the condition and issues of concern for adults with congenital heart disease.
- Describe the manifestations related to the acute, subacute, and convalescent phases of Kawasaki disease.

Approximately 1 of every 125 infants born has a congenital heart defect, making this the most common form of structural birth defect.[1,62] Advances in diagnostic methods and surgical treatment have greatly increased the long-term survival and outcomes for children born with congenital heart defects. Surgical correction of most defects is now possible, often within the first weeks of life, and the majority of affected children are expected to survive into adulthood.

Although thousands of infants born each year will have a congenital heart disease, other children will develop an acquired heart disease, including Kawasaki disease. Two other acquired disorders that affect children, the cardiomyopathies and RF, were discussed earlier in the chapter.

Embryonic Development of the Heart

The heart is the first functioning organ in the embryo; its first pulsatile movements begin during the third week after conception. This early development of the heart is essential to the rapidly growing embryo as a means of circulating nutrients and removing waste products. Most of the development of the heart and blood vessels occurs between the third and eighth weeks of embryonic life.[63]

The developing heart begins as two endothelial tubes that fuse into a single tubular structure.[63] The early heart structures develop as the tubular heart elongates and forms alternating dilations and constrictions. A single atrium and ventricle along with the bulbus cordis develop first (Fig. 24-22). This is followed by formation of the truncus arteriosus and the sinus venosus, a large venous sinus that receives blood from the embryo and developing placenta. The early pulsatile movements of the heart begin in the sinus venosus and move blood out of the heart by way of the bulbus cordis, truncus arteriosus, and aortic arches.

A differential growth rate in the early cardiac structures, along with fixation of the heart at the venous and arterial ends, causes the tubular heart to bend over on itself. As the heart bends, the atrium and the sinus venosus come to lie behind the bulbus cordis, truncus arteriosus, and ventricle. This looping of the primitive heart results in the heart's alignment in the left side of the chest with the atrium located behind the ventricle. Malrotation during formation of the ventricular loop can cause various malpositions, such as dextroposition of the heart.

The embryonic heart undergoes further development as partitioning of the chambers occurs. Partitioning of the AV canal, atrium, and ventricle begins in the fourth week and essentially is complete by the fifth week. Septation of the heart begins as tissue bundles called the *endocardial cushions* form in the mid-portion of the dorsal and ventral walls of the heart in the region of the AV canal and begin to grow inward. Until septation begins, a single AV canal exists between the atria and the ventricles. As the endocardial cushions enlarge, they meet and fuse to form separate right and left AV canals (Fig. 24-23). The mitral and tricuspid valves develop in these canals. The

FIGURE 24-23 • Development of the endocardial cushions, right and left atrioventricular canals, interventricular septum, and septum primum and septum secundum of the foramen ovale. Note that blood from the right atrium flows through the foramen ovale to the left atrium.

endocardial cushions also contribute to formation of parts of the atrial and ventricular septa. Defects in endocardial cushion formation can result in atrial and ventricular septal defects, complete AV canal defects, and anomalies of the mitral and tricuspid valves.

Compartmentalization of the ventricles begins with the growth of the interventricular septum from the floor of the ventricle moving upward toward the endocardial cushions. Fusion of the endocardial cushions with the interventricular septum usually is completed by the end of the seventh week.

Partitioning of the atrial septum is more complex and occurs in two stages, beginning with the formation of a thin, crescent-shaped membrane called the *septum primum* that emerges from the anterosuperior portion of the heart and grows toward the endocardial cushions, leaving an opening called the *foramen*

FIGURE 24-22 • Ventral view of the developing heart. **(A)** Fusion of the heart tubes to form a single tube, it is at this stage that the heart begins to beat. **(B)** Cardiac looping, in which the heart begins to bend ventrally and to the right, bringing the primitive ventricle leftward and in continuity with the sinus venosus (future left and right atria), with the future right ventricle being shifted rightward and in continuity with the bulbus cordis (future aorta and pulmonary artery), and **(C)** folding is complete.

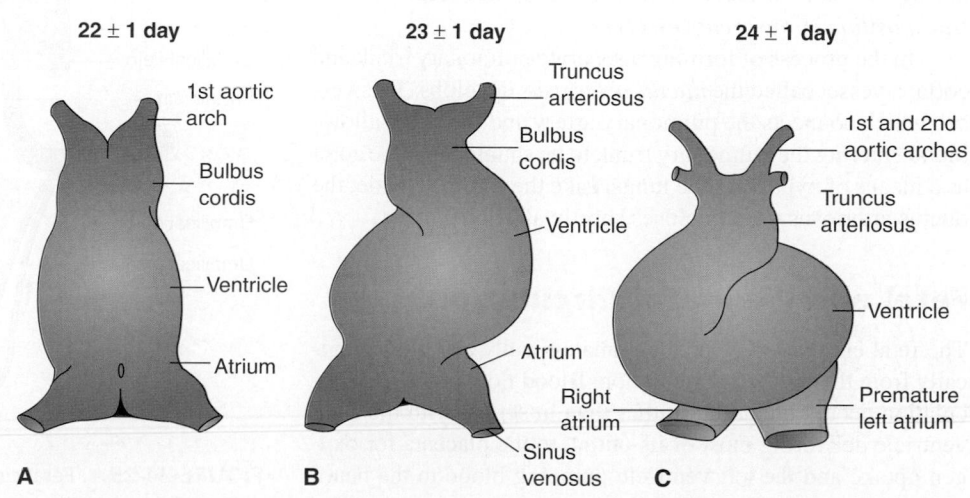

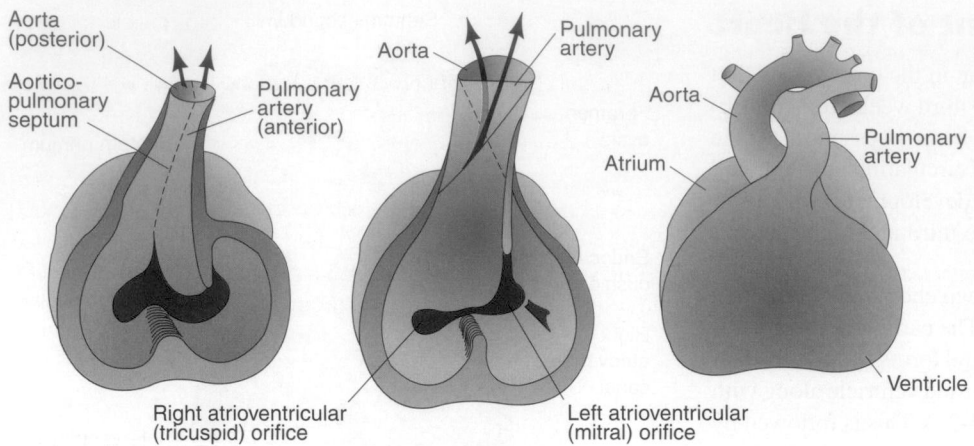

FIGURE 24-24 • Separation and twisting of the truncus arteriosus to form the pulmonary artery and aorta.

primum between its lower edge and the endocardial cushions. A second membrane, called *septum secundum,* also begins to grow from the upper wall of the atrium on the right side of the septum primum. As this membrane grows toward the endocardial cushions, it gradually overlaps an opening in the upper part of the septum primum, forming an oval opening with a flap-type valve called the *foramen ovale* (see Fig. 24-23). The upper part of the septum primum gradually disappears, with the remaining part becoming the valve of the foramen ovale. The foramen ovale forms a communicating channel between the two upper chambers of the heart. This opening, which typically closes shortly after birth, allows blood from the umbilical vein to pass directly into the left heart, bypassing the lungs.

To complete the transformation into a four-chambered heart, provision must be made for separating the blood pumped from the right side of the heart, which is to be diverted into the pulmonary circulation, from the blood pumped from the left side of the heart, which is to be pumped to the systemic circulation. This separation of blood flow is accomplished by developmental changes in the outflow channels of the tubular heart, the *bulbus cordis* and the *truncus arteriosus,* which undergo spiral twisting and vertical partitioning (Fig. 24-24). As these vessels spiral and divide, the aorta takes up position posterior to and to the right of the pulmonary artery. Impaired spiraling during this stage of development can lead to defects such as *transposition of the great vessels.*

In the process of forming a separate pulmonary trunk and aorta, a vessel called the *ductus arteriosus* develops. This vessel, which connects the pulmonary artery and the aorta, allows blood entering the pulmonary trunk to be shunted into the aorta as a means of bypassing the lungs. Like the foramen ovale, the ductus arteriosus usually closes shortly after birth.[63]

Fetal and Perinatal Circulation

The fetal circulation is different anatomically and physiologically from the postnatal circulation. Blood flow in the fetal circulation occurs in parallel rather than in series, with the right ventricle delivering most of its output to the placenta for oxygen uptake and the left ventricle pumping blood to the heart,

brain, and primarily upper body of the fetus.[64] Before birth, oxygenation of blood occurs through the placenta, and after birth, it occurs through the lungs. The fetus is maintained in a low-oxygen state (PO_2 30 to 35 mm Hg; hemoglobin O_2 saturation 60% to 70%). To compensate, fetal cardiac output is higher than at any other time in life (400 to 500 mL/kg/minute) and fetal hemoglobin has a higher affinity for oxygen.[64] Also, the pulmonary vessels in the fetus are markedly constricted because of the fluid-filled lungs and the heightened hypoxic stimulus for vasoconstriction that is present in the fetus. As a result, blood flow through the lungs is less than at any other time in life.

In the fetus, blood enters the circulation through the umbilical vein and returns to the placenta through the two umbilical arteries (Fig. 24-25). A vessel called the *ductus venosum* allows

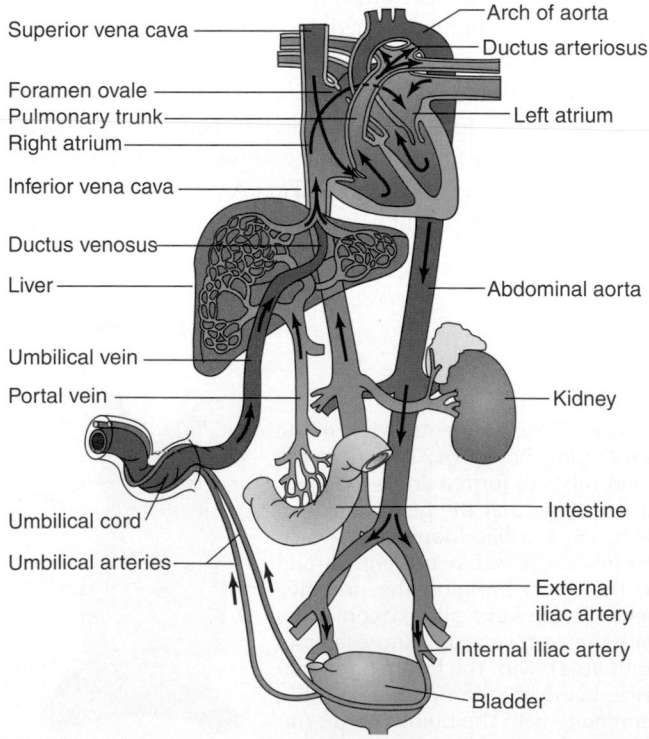

FIGURE 24-25 • Fetal circulation.

the majority of blood from the umbilical vein to bypass the hepatic circulation and pass directly into the inferior vena cava. From the inferior vena cava, blood flows into the right atrium, where approximately 40% of the blood volume moves through the foramen ovale into the left atrium. It then passes into the left ventricle and is ejected into the ascending aorta to perfuse the head and upper extremities. In this way, the best-oxygenated blood from the placenta is used to perfuse the brain. At the same time, venous blood from the head and upper extremities returns to the right side of the heart through the superior vena cava, moves into the right ventricle, and is ejected into the pulmonary artery. Because of the very high pulmonary vascular resistance that is present, almost 90% of blood ejected into the pulmonary artery gets diverted through the ductus arteriosus into the descending aorta. This blood perfuses the lower extremities and is returned to the placenta by the umbilical arteries.

At birth, the infant takes its first breath and switches from placental to pulmonary oxygenation of the blood. The most dramatic alterations in the circulation after birth are the elimination of the low-resistance placental vascular bed and the marked pulmonary vasodilation that is produced by initiation of ventilation. Within minutes of birth, pulmonary blood flow increases from 35 mL/kg/minute to 160 to 200 mL/kg/minute.[64] The pressure in the pulmonary circulation and the right side of the heart falls as fetal lung fluid is replaced by air and as lung expansion decreases the pressure transmitted to the pulmonary blood vessels. With lung inflation, the alveolar oxygen tension increases, causing reversal of the hypoxemia-induced pulmonary vasoconstriction of the fetal circulation. Cord clamping and removal of the low-resistance placental circulation produce an increase in systemic vascular resistance and a resultant increase in left ventricular pressure. The resultant decrease in right atrial pressure and increase in left atrial pressure produce closure of the foramen ovale flap valve. Reversal of the fetal hypoxemic state also produces constriction of ductal smooth muscle, contributing to closure of the ductus arteriosus. The foramen ovale and the ductus arteriosus normally close within the first day of life, effectively separating the pulmonary and systemic circulations.

After the initial precipitous fall in pulmonary vascular resistance, a more gradual decrease in pulmonary vascular resistance is related to regression of the medial smooth muscle layer in the pulmonary arteries. During the first 2 to 9 weeks of life, gradual thinning of the smooth muscle layer results in further decreases in pulmonary vascular resistance. By the time a healthy, term infant is several weeks old, the pulmonary vascular resistance has fallen to adult levels.

Several factors, including alveolar hypoxia, prematurity, lung disease, and congenital heart defects, may affect postnatal pulmonary vascular development. Alveolar hypoxia is one of the most potent stimuli of pulmonary vasoconstriction and pulmonary hypertension in the neonate. During this period, the pulmonary arteries remain highly reactive and can constrict in response to hypoxia, acidosis, hyperinflation of the alveoli, and hypothermia. Thus, hypoxia during the first days of life may delay or prevent the normal decrease in pulmonary vascular resistance.

Much of the development of the smooth muscle layer in the pulmonary arterioles occurs during late gestation; as a result, infants born prematurely have less medial smooth muscle. These infants follow the same pattern of smooth muscle regression, but because less muscle exists, the muscle layer may regress in a shorter time. The pulmonary vascular smooth muscle in premature infants also may be less responsive to hypoxia. For these reasons, a premature infant may demonstrate a larger decrease in pulmonary vascular resistance and a resultant shunting of blood from the aorta through the ductus arteriosus to the pulmonary artery within hours of birth.

Congenital Heart Defects

The major development of the fetal heart occurs between the fourth and seventh weeks of gestation, and most congenital heart defects arise during this time. Most congenital heart defects are thought to be multifactorial in origin, resulting from an interaction between a genetic predisposition toward development of a heart defect and environmental influences.

Knowledge about the genetic basis of congenital heart defects has grown dramatically in recent years. This area of research is particularly important as more individuals with congenital heart disease survive into adulthood and consider having children of their own. Recent knowledge suggests that the genetic contribution to congenital heart disease has been underestimated in the past.[65,66] Some heart defects, such as aortic stenosis, atrial septal defect of the secundum type, pulmonary valve stenosis, tetralogy of Fallot, and certain ventricular septal defects, have a stronger familial predisposition than others.

Chromosomal abnormalities are also associated with congenital heart defects, as evidenced by the observation that as much as 30% of children with congenital heart disease have an associated chromosomal abnormality. Heart disease is found in nearly 100% of children with trisomy 18; 50% of those with trisomy 21; and 35% of those with Turner syndrome.[66] Other syndromes that commonly include cardiac malformations are DiGeorge syndrome (22q11 deletion), which is frequently associated with conotruncal defects such as interrupted aortic arch, truncus arteriosus, and tetralogy of Fallot; and Williams syndrome (7q11.23 microdeletion), which is associated with supravalvar aortic and pulmonary stenoses.[65,66]

As much as 30% of congenital cardiac defects may be attributable to identifiable and potentially modifiable risk factors, including teratogenic influences, and adverse maternal conditions such as febrile illnesses, systemic lupus erythematosus, diabetes mellitus, maternal alcohol ingestion, and treatment with anticonvulsant drugs, retinoids, lithium, and other prescription or nonprescription drugs. Periconceptive multivitamin intake with folic acid may reduce the risk of cardiac disease in the fetus.[67]

Pathophysiology

Congenital heart defects produce their effects mainly through abnormal shunting of blood, production of cyanosis, and disruption of pulmonary blood flow.

Abnormal Shunting of Blood. Shunting of blood refers to the diversion of blood flow from one system to the other— from the arterial to the venous system (*i.e.,* left-to-right shunt) or from the venous to the arterial system (*i.e.,* right-to-left shunt). The shunting of blood in congenital heart defects is determined by the presence, position, and size of an abnormal opening between the right and left circulations and the degree of resistance to flow through the opening.

The vascular resistance of the systemic and pulmonary circulations influences the direction of shunting. Because of the high pulmonary vascular resistance in the neonate, atrial and ventricular septal defects usually do not produce significant shunt or symptoms during the first weeks of life.

As the pulmonary vascular smooth muscle regresses in the neonate, the resistance in the pulmonary circulation falls below that of the systemic circulation; in uncomplicated atrial or ventricular septal defects, blood shunts from the left side of the heart to the right. In more complicated ventricular septal defects, increased resistance to outflow may affect the pattern of shunting. For example, defects that increase resistance to aortic outflow (*e.g.,* aortic valve stenosis, coarctation of the aorta, hypoplastic left heart syndrome) increase left-to-right shunting, and defects that obstruct pulmonary outflow (*e.g.,* pulmonary valve stenosis, tetralogy of Fallot) increase right-to-left shunting. Crying, defecating, or even the stress of feeding may increase pulmonary vascular resistance and cause an increase in right-to-left shunting and cyanosis in infants with septal defects.

Cyanotic Versus Acyanotic Disorders. Congenital heart diseases are commonly divided into two categories: acyanotic and cyanotic. Defects that result in a left-to-right shunt are usually categorized as acyanotic disorders because they do not compromise oxygenation of blood in the pulmonary circulation.

Defects that produce shunting of blood from the right to the left side of the heart or result in obstruction of pulmonary blood flow are categorized as cyanotic disorders.[68] Cyanosis, a bluish color of the skin, most notable in the nail beds and mucous membranes, develops when sufficient deoxygenated blood from the right side of the heart mixes with oxygenated blood in the left side of the heart. Abnormal color becomes obvious when the oxygen saturation falls below 80% in the capillaries (equal to 5 g of deoxygenated hemoglobin).

A right-to-left shunt results in deoxygenated blood moving from the right side of the heart to the left side and then being ejected into the systemic circulation. With a left-to-right shunt, oxygenated blood intended for ejection into the systemic circulation is recirculated through the right side of the heart and back through the lungs. This increased volume distends the right side of the heart and pulmonary circulation and increases the workload placed on the right ventricle. A child with a defect that causes left-to-right shunting usually has an enlarged right side of the heart and pulmonary blood vessels. Of the congenital defects discussed in this chapter, patent ductus arteriosus, atrial and ventricular septal defects, endocardial cushion defects, pulmonary valve stenosis, and coarctation of the aorta

are considered defects with little or no cyanosis; tetralogy of Fallot, transposition of the great vessels, and single-ventricle anatomy are considered defects with cyanosis.

Disruption of Pulmonary Blood Flow. Many of the complications of congenital heart disorders result from a decrease or an increase in pulmonary blood flow. Defects that reduce pulmonary blood flow (*e.g.,* pulmonary stenosis) typically cause symptoms of fatigue, dyspnea, and failure to thrive. In contrast to the arterioles in the systemic circulation, the arterioles in the pulmonary circulation are normally thin-walled vessels that can accommodate the various levels of stroke volume that are ejected from the right heart. The thinning of the pulmonary vessels occurs during the first weeks after birth, during which the vessel media thin and pulmonary vascular resistance decreases. In a term infant who has a congenital heart defect that produces markedly increased pulmonary blood flow (*e.g.,* ventricular septal defect), the increased flow stimulates pulmonary vasoconstriction and delays or reduces the normal involutional thinning of the small pulmonary arterioles. In most cases during early infancy, pulmonary vascular resistance is only slightly elevated, and the major contribution to pulmonary hypertension is the increased blood flow. However, in some infants with a large right-to-left shunt, the pulmonary vascular resistance never decreases.

Congenital heart defects that persistently increase pulmonary blood flow or pulmonary vascular resistance have the potential of causing pulmonary hypertension and producing irreversible pathologic changes in the pulmonary vasculature. When shunting of systemic blood flow into the pulmonary circulation threatens permanent injury to the pulmonary vessels, a surgical procedure should be done to reduce the flow temporarily or permanently. Pulmonary artery banding consists of placing a constrictive band around the main pulmonary artery, thereby increasing resistance to outflow from the right ventricle. The banding technique is a temporary measure to alleviate symptoms and protect the pulmonary vasculature in anticipation of later surgical repair of the defect.

Manifestations and Treatment

It is increasingly common for heart defects to be diagnosed prenatally. In this case, the infant can be evaluated shortly after birth to confirm the diagnosis and develop a treatment plan. Reliable diagnostic images of the fetal heart can be obtained as early as 16 weeks of gestation and research using transvaginal ultrasonography is underway to view the heart even earlier. Among the disorders that can be diagnosed with certainty by fetal echocardiography are AV septal defects, hypoplastic left heart syndrome, aortic valve stenosis, hypertrophic cardiomyopathy, pulmonic valve stenosis, and transposition of the great arteries. Disorders that result in an abnormal four-chamber view, an image typically obtained during routine prenatal ultrasonography, are the most likely to be detected.[69]

In the postnatal period, congenital heart defects may present with numerous signs and symptoms. Over 40 different types of congenital heart defects have been described, and even individual lesions can vary along a spectrum of severity; therefore, there is no standard presentation for infants and children with congenital heart disease. Some defects, such as patent ductus arteriosus and small ventricular septal defects, close spontaneously. In other, less severe defects, there may be no obvious signs and symptoms and the disorder may be discovered during a routine health examination. Cyanosis, pulmonary congestion, cardiac failure, and decreased peripheral perfusion are the chief concerns in children with more severe defects. Such defects often cause problems immediately after birth or early in infancy. The child may exhibit cyanosis, respiratory difficulty, and fatigability, and is likely to have difficulty with feeding and failure to thrive. A generalized cyanosis that persists longer than 3 hours after birth suggests congenital heart disease.

An oxygen challenge (administration of 100% oxygen for 5 to 10 minutes) can help to determine whether congenital heart disease is present in a cyanotic newborn. An arterial blood sample is taken during this time. If the partial pressure of oxygen (PO_2) is greater than 250 mm Hg, cyanotic heart disease can be ruled out; if the PO_2 is 160 to 250 mm Hg, heart disease is unlikely; failure of the PO_2 to rise to these levels is strongly suggestive of cyanotic heart disease.[70] Because infant cyanosis may appear as duskiness, it is important to assess the color of the mucous membranes, fingernails, toenails, tongue, and lips. Pulmonary congestion in the infant causes an increase in respiratory rate, orthopnea, grunting, wheezing, coughing, and crackles. A chest radiograph can quickly differentiate infants who have reduced pulmonary vascular markings (densities) from those who have normal or increased markings. The infant whose peripheral perfusion is markedly decreased may be in a shocklike state.

Heart failure manifests itself as tachypnea or dyspnea at rest or on exertion. For the infant, this most commonly occurs during feeding. Recurrent respiratory infections and excessive sweating may also be reported. Growth failure results from unresolved heart failure.[70] The treatment plan usually includes supportive therapy (e.g., digoxin, diuretics, and feeding supplementation) designed to help the infant compensate for the limitations in cardiac reserve and to prevent complications. Surgical intervention often is required for severe defects. It may be done in the early weeks of life or, conditions permitting, delayed until the child is older. A discussion of congestive heart failure in children is presented in Chapter 26.

Children with structural congenital heart disease and those who have had corrective surgery may have a higher-than-expected risk for development of IE. Prophylactic antibiotic therapy before dental procedures or other periods of increased risk for bacteremia is suggested for children with (1) unrepaired cyanotic heart disease, including those with palliative shunts and conduits; (2) completely repaired congenital heart disease with prosthetic material or device, whether placed by surgery or catheter intervention, during the first 6 months after the procedure; and (3) repaired congenital heart disease with residual defects at the site or adjacent to the site of a prosthetic patch or prosthetic device (which inhibit endothelialization).[71]

Types of Defects

Congenital heart defects can affect almost any of the cardiac structures or central blood vessels. Defects include communication between heart chambers, interrupted development of the heart chambers or valve structures, malposition of heart chambers and great vessels, and altered closure of fetal communication channels. The particular defect reflects the embryo's stage of development at the time it occurred. It is common for multiple defects to be present in one child and for some congenital heart disorders, such as tetralogy of Fallot, to involve several defects.

The development of the heart is simultaneous and sequential; a heart defect may reflect the multiple developmental events that were occurring simultaneously or sequentially. Over 40 types of defects have been identified, the most common being patent ductus arteriosus (6% to 8%), atrial septal defects (6% to 8%), and ventricular septal defects (27% to 42%).[72]

Patent Ductus Arteriosus. The ductus arteriosus plays a vital role in diverting blood from the right side of the heart and away from the lungs to the systemic circulation during fetal life (Fig. 24-26G). With the onset of spontaneous respiration after birth, muscular constriction of the ductal tissue typically closes this vessel. The initiating step of ductal closure in the healthy infant is believed to be the sharp increase in arterial oxygen saturation and subsequent fall in pulmonary vascular resistance after birth. Additional factors that are thought to contribute to ductal closure are a fall in endogenous levels of prostaglandins and adenosine and the release of vasoactive substances. After constriction, the lumen of the ductus becomes permanently sealed with fibrous tissue within 2 to 3 weeks.

For 90% of full-term infants, the ductus is functionally closed by 48 hours of age.[73] Full-term infants with abnormalities of circulation or ventilation and premature infants are those most likely to exhibit persistent patency of the ductus arteriosus. Arterial oxygenation, circulating prostaglandins, genetic predetermination, and other, unknown factors interact to determine the mechanism of ductal closure.[73] Circulating prostaglandin levels are directly related to gestational age, and the incidence of patent ductus arteriosus in infants with birth weights less than 1000 g may be as high as 50%.[73]

Persistent patency of the ductus arteriosus is defined as a duct that remains open beyond 3 months in the full-term infant. The incidence of this lesion is estimated at 80 per 100,000 live births, and female infants with the disorder outnumber males by a ratio of 2:1.[74] The size of the persistent ductus and the difference between the systemic and pulmonary vascular resistance determine its clinical manifestations. Blood typically shunts across the ductus from the higher-pressure left side (systemic circulation) to the lower-pressure right side (pulmonary circulation). A murmur is typically detected within days or weeks of birth. The murmur is loudest at the second left intercostal space, is continuous through systole and diastole, and has a characteristic "machinery" sound.[73] A widened pulse pressure is common due to the continuous runoff of aortic blood into the pulmonary artery. Diagnostic methods include chest radiography and

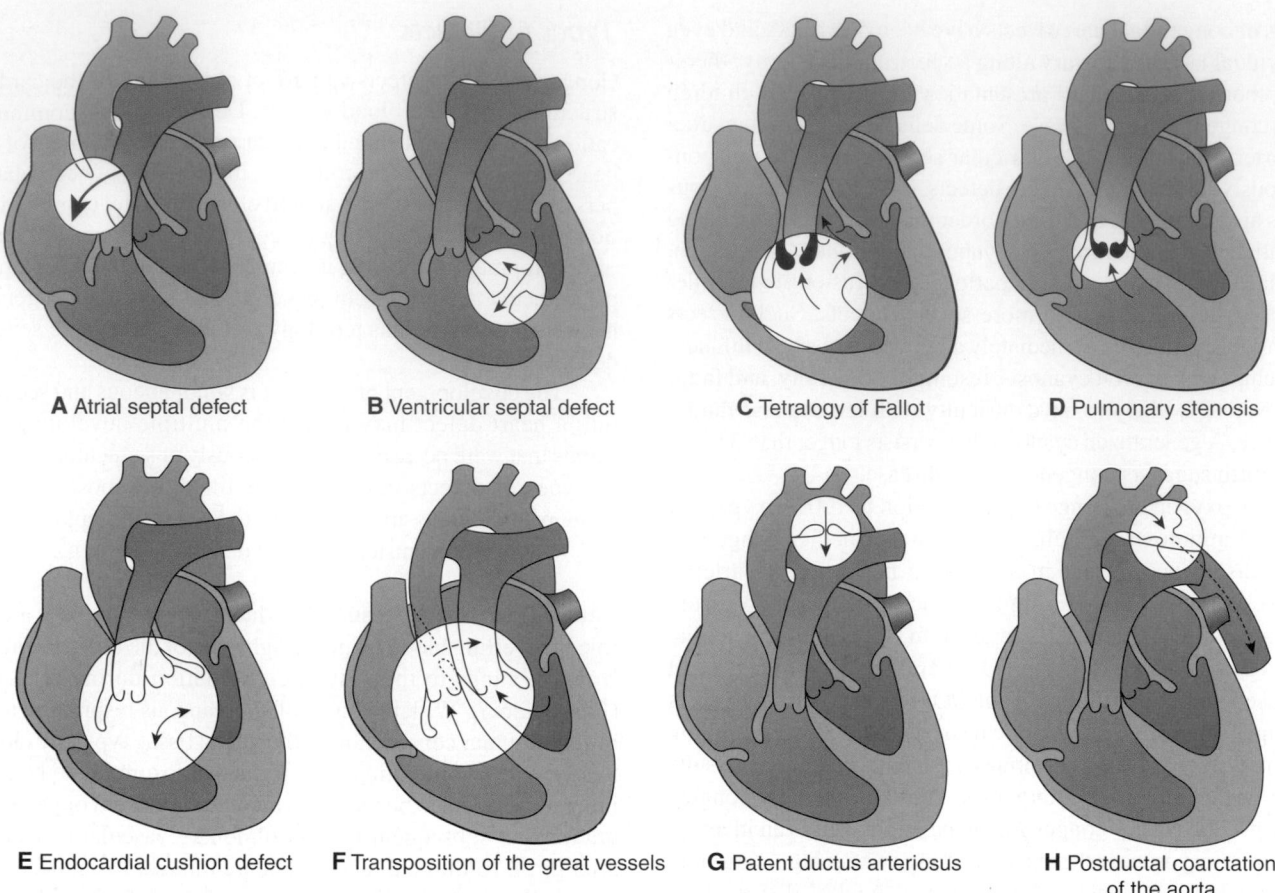

A Atrial septal defect   **B** Ventricular septal defect   **C** Tetralogy of Fallot   **D** Pulmonary stenosis

E Endocardial cushion defect   **F** Transposition of the great vessels   **G** Patent ductus arteriosus   **H** Postductal coarctation of the aorta

FIGURE 24-26 • Congenital heart defects. (**A**) Atrial septal defect. Blood is shunted from left to right. (**B**) Ventricular septal defect. Blood is usually shunted from left to right. (**C**) Tetralogy of Fallot. This involves a ventricular septal defect, dextroposition of the aorta, right ventricular outflow obstruction, and right ventricular hypertrophy. Blood is shunted from right to left. (**D**) Pulmonary stenosis, with decreased pulmonary blood flow and right ventricular hypertrophy. (**E**) Endocardial cushion defects. Blood flows between the chambers of the heart. (**F**) Transposition of the great vessels. The pulmonary artery is attached to the left side of the heart and the aorta to the right side. (**G**) Patent ductus arteriosus. The high-pressure blood of the aorta is shunted back to the pulmonary artery. (**H**) Postductal coarctation of the aorta.

echocardiography. There are increased pulmonary markings on chest radiography and enlargement of the left heart from the increased pulmonary venous return.[75] Echocardiography is used to determine the presence, size, direction (*i.e.*, left to right or right to left), and physical consequences of the shunt.

An untreated patent ductus can result in important long-term complications that may include congestive heart failure, IE, pulmonary vascular disease, aneurysm formation, thromboembolism, and calcification.[75] The potential risk of complications and the extremely low procedural morbidity and mortality justify closure of a patent arterial ductus even when the shunt is small. In the full-term infant or older child, closure can be achieved with either surgical ligation or device occlusion. Surgery typically involves a small left thoracotomy or thoracoscopic approach that allows ligation of the vessel. Implantable devices, most commonly coils, have allowed successful ductus closure to be done in the catheterization laboratory on an outpatient basis. The anatomy of the ductus and the size of the

patient are key determinants of the applicability of this technique. In the premature infant, a patent ductus can produce respiratory distress and impede weaning from mechanical ventilation. Indomethacin, an inhibitor of prostaglandin synthesis, has proven effective in up to 79% of premature infants.[76] When this medical management fails, surgical intervention is recommended.

Although closure of a patent ductus is uniformly recommended when it is present as an isolated lesion, deliberate maintenance of ductal patency can be a lifesaving therapy for children with complex forms of congenital heart disease who have ductal-dependent pulmonary or systemic blood flow, or those with obligatory mixing of the arterial and venous circulations (*i.e.*, transposition of the great arteries). Intravenous infusion of prostaglandin E_1 has proved extremely effective in maintaining ductal patency or reopening the ductus in newborns. Today, this therapy is routinely administered to newborns with suspected congenital heart defects until they can be transported to a specialized center where a diagnosis can be confirmed.[74] The ductus has also been successfully stented to maintain patency in hypoplastic left heart syndrome,[77] and implantation of a synthetic aortopulmonary shunt has been used to mimic the function of a patent ductus in other defects.

Atrial Septal Defects. Any persistent opening that allows shunting of blood across the atrial septum is considered an atrial septal defect. The defect may be single or multiple and vary from a small, asymptomatic opening to a large, symptomatic opening. The typology of the defect is determined by its position and may include a secundum atrial defect (the most common form), an ostium primum defect, a sinus venosus defect, or a patent foramen ovale (see Fig. 24-26A). The incidence of the defect is estimated at 1 per 1000 live births, and it occurs more frequently in girls (63%) than boys.[74] As much as 50% of children with congenital heart disorders have an atrial septal defect as a part of their diagnosis.

Many atrial septal defects are asymptomatic and discovered inadvertently during a routine physical examination at a few years of age.[73] Intracardiac shunting is usually from left to right and may increase with age as the right ventricle becomes more compliant. In most cases there is a moderate shunt resulting in dilation of the right heart chambers and overperfusion of the pulmonary circulation. The increased volume of blood that must be ejected from the right heart prolongs closure of the pulmonary valve and produces a separation (fixed splitting) of the aortic and pulmonary components of the second heart sound. Children with undiagnosed atrial defects are at risk for pulmonary vascular disease, although this is a rare occurrence before 20 years of age. Rarely, infants with a large shunt may develop congestive heart failure and failure to thrive, prompting early closure of the defect.[73]

Atrial septal defects that measure 8 mm or more are unlikely to undergo spontaneous closure. Smaller defects may be observed for spontaneous closure in the young child. However, surgical or transcatheter closure is recommended in children with persistent defects to reduce the long-term risk of pulmonary vascular disease and atrial arrhythmias.[73] Both transcatheter device and surgical closure are effective and of low risk. Use of the transcatheter approach is determined by the position and size of the defect. Transcatheter device closure has been particularly effective for small to medium-sized secundum septal defects and patent foramen ovale. Sinus venosus defects, which are frequently associated with partial anomalous pulmonary venous return and ostium primum defects, require surgical closure. Surgery requires the use of cardiopulmonary bypass and mild hypothermia. Most defects are effectively closed using the patient's native septal tissue or a pericardial or synthetic patch. There is a very low incidence of residual sequelae or need for reintervention.

Ventricular Septal Defects. A ventricular septal defect is an opening in the ventricular septum that results from an incomplete separation of the ventricles during early fetal development (see Fig. 24-26B). These defects may be single or multiple and may occur in any position along the ventricular septum. Ventricular septal defects are the most common form of congenital heart defect, accounting for 27% to 42% of congenital heart disorders[72] and a reported prevalence of 2.5 per 1000 live births.[73] Distribution between boys and girls is relatively even. Ventricular septal defect may be the only cardiac defect, or it may occur in association with multiple cardiac anomalies.

The ventricular septum originates from two sources: the interventricular groove of the folded tubular heart that gives rise to the muscular part of the septum, and the endocardial cushions that extend to form the membranous portion of the septum. The upper membranous portion of the septum is the last area to close, typically by the seventh week of gestation, and it is here that most defects occur. Depending on the size of the opening and the pulmonary vascular resistance, the signs and symptoms of a ventricular septal defect may range from an asymptomatic murmur to congestive heart failure.[70]

The physical size of the ventricular septal defect is a major, but not the only, determinant of left-to-right shunt. The pulmonary vascular resistance in relation to systemic vascular resistance also determines the shunt's magnitude. In a small communicating defect (<5 cm^2), the higher pressure in the left ventricle drives the shunt to the left and the size of the defect limits the magnitude of the shunt. Most children with such defects are asymptomatic and have a low risk for development of pulmonary vascular disease.

In a larger, nonrestrictive shunt (usually >1 cm^2), right and left ventricular pressure is equalized and the degree of shunting is determined by the ratio of pulmonary to systemic vascular resistance. After birth in infants with large ventricular septal defects, pulmonary vascular resistance may remain higher than normal, and the size of the left-to-right shunt may initially be limited. As the pulmonary vascular resistance continues to fall in the first few weeks after birth because of normal involution of the media of the small pulmonary arterioles, the magnitude of the left-to-right shunt increases. Eventually, a large left-to-right shunt develops, and clinical symptoms (*e.g.,* tachypnea, diaphoresis, especially with feeding, and failure to thrive) become apparent. In most cases during infancy, pulmonary vascular pressure is only slightly elevated, and the major contributor to pulmonary hypertension is an increase in pulmonary blood flow. In some infants with a large septal defect, pulmonary arteriolar thickness never decreases. With continued exposure to high pulmonary blood flow, pulmonary vascular obstructive disease develops. In untreated patients, the pulmonary vascular resistance can eventually exceed the systemic resistance. In this case, a reversal of shunt flow occurs and the child demonstrates progressive cyanosis as deoxygenated blood moves from the right to the left side of the heart. These symptoms, coupled with irreversible changes in the pulmonary vasculature, represent an end-stage form of congenital heart disease called *Eisenmenger syndrome.*

The treatment of a ventricular septal defect depends on the size of the defect, accompanying hemodynamic derangements, and symptomatology. Children with small or medium-sized defects may be followed without intervention if they remain free from signs of congestive heart failure or pulmonary hypertension. Ventricular defects do not increase in size, and some spontaneously close over time.[73] Detailed 2-D echocardiography is usually adequate to diagnosis the size and position of a defect as well as to estimate pulmonary pressures. Cardiac catheterization is usually reserved for cases where it is necessary to confirm the degree and reversibility of pulmonary vascular resistance.[70]

Congestive heart failure is treated medically. Symptomatic infants may require feeding supplements or tube feeding to promote growth and development. In the symptomatic infant in whom complete repair cannot be achieved because of size or other complicating lesions, a palliative procedure may be performed to reduce symptoms. Placement of a synthetic band around the main pulmonary artery (pulmonary artery banding) can reduce pulmonary blood flow until complete repair can be accomplished. Surgical closure of the defect is completed by placement of a synthetic or autologous patch effectively to close the shunt across the ventricular septum. These procedures are typically done electively in the infant or young child, and are associated with low morbidity and mortality rates. Transcatheter device closure of ventricular septal defects remains an area of interest; however, difficulty with successful positioning of the devices has limited its applicability.

Endocardial Cushion Defects. The AV canal connects the atria to the ventricles during early cardiac development. The endocardial cushions surround this canal and contribute tissue to the lower part of the atrial septum, the upper part of the ventricular septum, the septal leaflet of the tricuspid valve, and the anterior leaflet of the mitral valve.[78] Any flaw in the development of these tissues results in an endocardial cushion defect. Approximately 3% of all congenital heart defects are endocardial cushion defects, with a nearly equal incidence in boys and girls. Endocardial cushion defects have a strong association with Down syndrome, and are seen in as much as 50% of children with Down syndrome.[79]

Several variations of endocardial cushion defects are possible. The defect may be described as *partial* or *complete*. The anatomy of the AV valve determines the classification. In partial AV canal defects, the two AV valve rings are complete and separate. The most common type of partial AV canal defect is an ostium primum defect, often associated with a cleft in the mitral valve. In a complete canal defect, there is a common AV valve orifice along with defects in both the atrial and ventricular septal tissue (see Fig. 24-26E). Other cardiac defects may be associated with endocardial cushion defects and most commonly include cardiac malposition defects and tetralogy of Fallot.[78]

Physiologically, endocardial cushion defects result in abnormalities similar to those described for atrial or ventricular septal defects. The direction and magnitude of a shunt in a child with an endocardial cushion defect are determined by the combination of defects and the child's pulmonary and systemic vascular resistance. The hemodynamic effects of an isolated ostium primum defect are those of the previously described atrial septal defect. These children are largely asymptomatic

during childhood. With a complete AV canal defect, pulmonary blood flow is increased after pulmonary vascular resistance falls because of left-to-right shunting across both the ventricular and atrial septal defects. Children with complete defects often have effort intolerance, easy fatigability, failure to thrive, recurrent infections, and other signs of congestive heart failure, particularly when the shunt is large. Pulmonary hypertension and increased pulmonary vascular resistance result if the lesion is left untreated.

The timing of treatment for endocardial cushion defects is determined by the severity of the defect and symptoms. With an ostium primum defect, surgical repair usually is planned on an elective basis before the child reaches school age. The defect in the atrial septum is closed with a patch and mitral valvuloplasty is performed if the valve is regurgitant. Corrective surgery is required for all complete AV canal defects. This is typically performed in infants at 3 to 6 months of age and requires patching of both the atrial and ventricular septal defects and separation of the AV valve apparatus to create competent mitral and tricuspid valves. Infants with severe symptoms may require a palliative procedure where the main pulmonary artery is banded to reduce pulmonary blood flow. This typically improves the infant's ability to grow and develop until a complete repair can be performed. Total surgical repair of complete AV canal defects can be accomplished with low operative risk. Reoperation may be required in 6% to 13% of children. Late sequelae include AV valve regurgitation, subaortic stenosis, and arrhythmias.[70,73]

Pulmonary Stenosis. Obstruction of blood flow from the right ventricle to the pulmonary circulation is termed *pulmonary stenosis*. The obstruction can occur as an isolated valvular lesion, within the right ventricular chamber, in the pulmonary arteries, or as a combination of stenoses in multiple areas. It is a relatively common defect, estimated to account for approximately 10% of all congenital cardiac disease, and is often associated with other abnormalities.[70,73]

Pulmonary valvular defects, the most common type of obstruction, usually produce some impairment of pulmonary blood flow and increase the workload imposed on the right side of the heart (see Fig. 24-26D). Most children with pulmonic valve stenosis have mild stenosis that does not increase in severity. These children are largely asymptomatic and are diagnosed by the presence of a systolic murmur. Moderate or greater stenosis has been shown to progress over time, particularly before 12 years of age, so these children require careful follow-up. Critical pulmonary stenosis in the neonate is evidenced by cyanosis due to right-to-left atrial-level shunting and right ventricular hypertension. These infants require prostaglandin E_1 to maintain circulation to the lungs through the ductus arteriosus.[70,73]

Pulmonary valvotomy is the treatment of choice for all valvular defects with pressure gradients from the right ventricle to the pulmonary circulation greater than 30 mm Hg. Transcatheter balloon valvuloplasty has been quite successful in this lesion. Stenosis in the peripheral pulmonary arteries can also be effectively treated with balloon angioplasty, with or without stent placement.[70,73]

Tetralogy of Fallot. Tetralogy of Fallot is the most common cyanotic congenital heart defect, accounting for approximately 5% to 7% of all congenital heart defects.[80] As the name implies, tetralogy of Fallot consists of four associated defects: (1) a ventricular septal defect involving the membranous septum and the anterior portion of the muscular septum; (2) dextroposition or shifting to the right of the aorta, so that it overrides the right ventricle and is in communication with the septal defect; (3) obstruction or narrowing of the pulmonary outflow channel, including pulmonic valve stenosis, a decrease in the size of the pulmonary trunk, or both; and (4) hypertrophy of the right ventricle because of the increased work required to pump blood through the obstructed pulmonary channels[80,81] (see Fig. 24-26C). Variations of the defect can include complete atresia of the pulmonary valve or absence of pulmonary valve tissue altogether.

Cyanosis is caused by a right-to-left shunt across the ventricular septal defect. The degree of cyanosis is determined by the restriction of blood flow into the pulmonary bed. Right ventricular outflow obstruction causes deoxygenated blood from the right ventricle to shunt across the ventricular septal defect and be ejected into the systemic circulation. The degree of obstruction may be dynamic and can increase during periods of stress, causing hypercyanotic attacks ("tet spells"). These spells typically occur in the morning during crying, feeding, or defecating. These activities increase the infant's oxygen requirements. Crying and defecating may further increase pulmonary vascular resistance, thereby increasing right-to-left shunting and decreasing pulmonary blood flow. With the hypercyanotic spell, the infant becomes acutely cyanotic, hyperpneic, irritable, and diaphoretic. Later in the spell, the infant becomes limp and may lose consciousness. Placing the infant in the knee–chest position increases systemic vascular resistance, which increases pulmonary blood flow and decreases right-to-left shunting. During a hypercyanotic spell, toddlers and older children may spontaneously assume the squatting position, which functions like the knee–chest position to relieve the spell. Turbulent flow across the narrow right ventricular outflow track produces a characteristic harsh systolic ejection murmur. Auscultation during a hypercyanotic spell reveals a diminished or absent murmur due to the dramatic reduction in pulmonary blood flow.[81]

Total surgical correction is required for all children with tetralogy of Fallot. Early definitive repair in infancy is currently advocated in most centers experienced in intracardiac surgery in infants. When extreme cyanosis is present in a small infant or when there is associated marked hypoplasia of the pulmonary arteries, a palliative procedure to facilitate pulmonary blood flow may be necessary. This is accomplished by placing a prosthetic shunt between a systemic artery and the pulmonary artery (modified Blalock-Taussig shunt). Balloon dilation of the pulmonary valve may also afford palliation in some infants. Total correction is then carried out later in infancy or early childhood. Complete repair includes patch closure of the ventricular septal defect and relief of any right ventricular outflow tract obstruction. Repair is associated with a mortality rate of less than 3%; however, patients need long-term follow-up to monitor for residual lesions, right ventricular dilation or dysfunction, and arrhythmias.[80,81]

Transposition of the Great Arteries. In complete transposition of the great arteries, the aorta arises from the right ventricle, and the pulmonary artery arises from the left ventricle (see Fig. 24-26F). Complete transposition occurs in 24 per 100,000 live births and is the most common reason for pediatric cardiology referral in the first 2 weeks of life. The defect is more common in infants whose mothers have diabetes, and is two to three times more common in boys.[82]

Cyanosis is the most common presenting symptom resulting from an anomaly that allows the systemic venous return to be circulated through the right heart and ejected into the aorta, and the pulmonary venous return to be recirculated to the lungs through the left ventricle and main pulmonary artery.[70] In infants born with this defect, survival depends on communication between the right and left sides of the heart in the form of a patent ductus arteriosus or septal defect. Ventricular septal defects are present in 50% of infants with transposition of the great arteries at birth and may allow effective mixing of blood. Prostaglandin E_1 should be administered to neonates when this lesion is suspected in an effort to maintain the patency of the ductus arteriosus. Balloon atrial septostomy may be done to increase the blood flow between the two sides of the heart. In this procedure, a balloon-tipped catheter is inserted into the heart through the vena cava and then passed through the foramen ovale into the left atrium. The balloon is then inflated and pulled back through the foramen ovale, enlarging the opening as it goes.

Corrective surgery is essential for long-term survival. An arterial switch procedure, the current operation of choice, has survival rates greater than 90%.[70] This procedure, which corrects the relation of the systemic and pulmonary blood flows, is preferably performed in the first 2 to 3 weeks of life, before the postnatal reduction in pulmonary vascular resistance occurs. The coronary arteries are moved to the left-sided great artery and any ventricular septal defects are closed during the same operation. Complications of the arterial switch procedure may include coronary insufficiency, supravalvar pulmonary stenosis, neoaortic regurgitation, and rhythm abnormalities.[82]

Coarctation of the Aorta. Coarctation of the aorta is a localized narrowing of the aorta, proximal to (preductal), distal to (postductal), or opposite the entry of the ductus arteriosus (juxtaductal; see Fig. 24-26H). Approximately 98% of coarctations are juxtaductal. Constriction of aberrant ductal tissue extending into the aortic wall is believed to be the cause of obstruction.[73] The anomaly occurs in approximately 1 in 12,000 live births.[82] It is frequently associated with other congenital cardiac lesions, most commonly bicuspid aortic valve, and occurs in approximately 10% of subjects with Turner syndrome, suggesting a genetic linkage[73,83] (see Chapter 7).

The classic sign of coarctation of the aorta is a disparity in pulsations and blood pressures in the arms and legs. The femoral, popliteal, and dorsalis pedis pulsations are weak or delayed compared with the bounding pulses of the arms and carotid vessels. Normally, the systolic blood pressure in the legs obtained by the cuff method is 10 to 20 mm Hg higher than in the arms. In coarctation, the pressure in the legs is lower and may be difficult to obtain. Patients with coarctation are often identified during a diagnostic work-up for hypertension. Most patients with moderate coarctation remain otherwise asymptomatic owing to collateral vessels that form around the area of narrowing. Left untreated, however, coarctation will result in left ventricular hypertension and hypertrophy and significant systemic hypertension (see Chapter 23). Infants with severe coarctation demonstrate early symptoms of heart failure and may present in critical condition upon ductal closure. Reopening of the duct with prostaglandin E_1, if possible, and emergent surgery are needed in this subgroup.[70,73]

Children with coarctation causing a blood pressure gradient between the arms and legs of 20 mm Hg or greater should be treated ideally by 2 years of age to reduce the likelihood of persistent hypertension.[70,73] A surgical approach typically involves resection of the narrowed segment of the aorta and end-to-end anastomosis of healthy tissue. This can usually be accomplished without cardiopulmonary bypass, with a mortality rate near zero. Balloon angioplasty with or without stent placement has also been used, although the presence of residual gradients and the reliability of the surgical approach have limited this technique.[70,73] The most common complications after repair of coarctation are persistent hypertension and recoarctation.

Functional Single-Ventricle Anatomy. Several forms of complex congenital heart disease result in only one functional ventricle. There may be a single right or a single left ventricle, or a ventricle of indeterminate morphology. Functional single-ventricle anatomy is the most common form of congenital heart disease diagnosed during fetal life because of the inability to obtain a four-chamber cardiac view on routine prenatal ultrasonography. Hypoplastic left heart syndrome is the most common form of single right ventricular anatomy. Tricuspid valve atresia is the most common cause of a single left ventricle. Several other forms of double-inlet ventricle have been described; however, all forms of this disease result in similar pathologic effects and follow a common pathway of intervention.[84-86]

All forms of single-ventricle anatomy result in a common mixing chamber of pulmonary and systemic venous return and cause varying degrees of cyanosis. The single ventricle must supply both the pulmonary and systemic circulations.[85,86] The amount of blood flow to each circulation is determined by the resistance in each system. As pulmonary vascular resistance falls, flow to the pulmonary circulation will be preferential and systemic circulation will be compromised. In some defects, such as hypoplastic left heart syndrome, systemic flow depends on a patent ductus arteriosus. Neonates with this lesion typically present with extreme cyanosis and symptoms of heart failure as the duct begins to close.[73,87]

Although functional single-ventricle anatomy cannot be completely repaired, the surgical palliation of these defects has been one of the most innovative accomplishments in intervention for congenital heart disease. The goal of surgical palliation is to redirect systemic venous return directly to the pulmonary arteries and allow the single ventricle to deliver oxygenated blood to the systemic circulation. This is accomplished in a series of two to three staged surgical interventions during the child's first years of life. Stage one palliation is designed to ensure unobstructed systemic blood flow and adequate flow to the pulmonary circulation. Stage two palliation, the bidirectional cavopulmonary shunt, redirects systemic venous return from the superior vena cava directly to the pulmonary arteries. Finally, the completion Fontan procedure connects flow from the inferior vena cava directly into the pulmonary arteries, and the pulmonary and systemic circulations are effectively separated[84-87] (Fig. 24-27). Cardiac transplantation is also used as an intervention for the most complex forms of single-ventricle congenital heart disease.

Survival rates for children with complex forms of single-ventricle heart disease have improved markedly, but long-term outcomes remain uncertain. Ventricular dysfunction, arrhythmias, and thromboses plague this population of patients. Defining the optimal medical and surgical management strategies for these patients remains an active area of research in pediatric cardiology and cardiac surgery.[84-87]

Adults With Congenital Heart Disease

Successful treatment of congenital heart disease in the pediatric population has resulted in a growing number of adult survivors with a variety of repaired, unrepaired, and palliated congenital

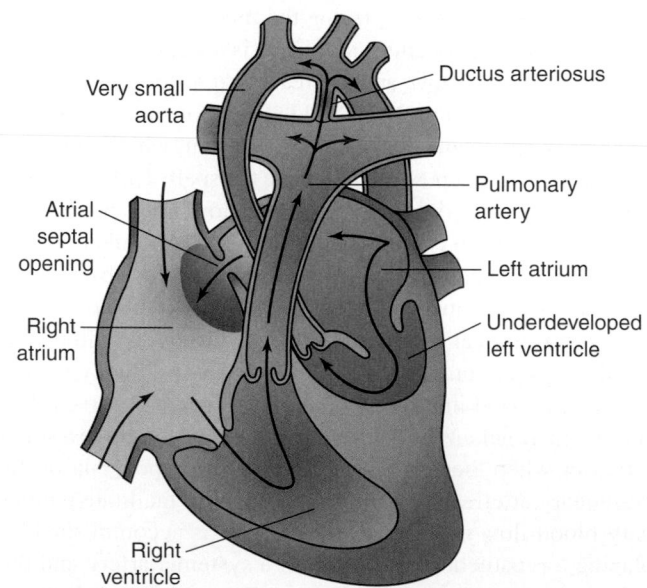

FIGURE 24-27 • Functional single-ventricle anatomy with an underdeveloped left ventricle and small ascending aorta. Because of the markedly decreased left ventricular compliance, most of the pulmonary venous blood returning to the left atrium shunts left to right at the atrial level. Pulmonary arterial blood flows into the pulmonary arteries as well as right to left across a patent ductus arteriosus into the aorta.

cardiac lesions. Since 1985, there have been more adults living with congenital heart disease than children.[88-90] An epidemiologic study on the prevalence and age distribution of congenital heart disease identified a prevalence of 4.09 per 1000 adults.[88] Extrapolating these data to the U.S. population would predict nearly 1 million adults living with congenital heart disease, and growth of this population of approximately 5% per year.[88]

Although the majority of adults with congenital heart disease will have undergone treatment and perhaps surgery as children, most congenital heart defects must be considered chronic conditions requiring long-term surveillance and care. Only the simplest lesions, such as patent ductus arteriosus and uncomplicated secundum atrial septal defect, can be considered completely repaired.[89] Chronic physiologic concerns include arrhythmias, hemodynamic problems, complications of prolonged cyanosis, endocarditis, residual lesions, and the need for reoperation. The underlying heart defect can also have significant implications for other aspects of health, such as exercise tolerance, noncardiac surgery, and pregnancy. Several important psychosocial issues also require consideration, including neurocognitive achievement, employment, insurability, family planning, treatment adherence, and understanding of the underlying condition and risks. Life expectancy for some of the most complex lesions (*e.g.*, hypoplastic left heart syndrome) is unknown because the oldest survivors to date were born in the 1980s. A growing medical specialty has emerged designed specifically to provide adults with congenital heart disease the specialized services they need from practitioners who understand both the complexities of their cardiac problems and other issues of adult health care.

Kawasaki Disease

Kawasaki disease, also known as *mucocutaneous lymph node syndrome,* is an acute febrile disease of young children. First described in Japan in 1967 by Dr. Tomisaku Kawasaki, the disease affects the skin, brain, eyes, joints, liver, lymph nodes, and heart. The disease is the most common cause of acquired heart disease in young children, with 15% to 25% of cases resulting in coronary artery aneurysms or ectasias that may lead to myocardial infarction, sudden death, or chronic coronary insufficiency.[91] More than 4000 children with Kawasaki disease are hospitalized annually in the United States.[91] Over 80% of patients with Kawasaki disease are 4 years of age or younger, with a male-to-female ratio of 1.4:1. Although most common in Japan, the disease affects children of many races, occurs worldwide, and is increasing in frequency.

The disease is characterized by a vasculitis (*i.e.*, inflammation of the blood vessels) that begins in the small vessels (*i.e.*, arterioles, venules, and capillaries) and progresses to involve some of the larger arteries, such as the coronaries. The exact etiology and pathogenesis of the disease remain unknown, but it is thought to be of immunologic origin.[92] Immunologic abnormalities, including increased activation of helper T cells and increased levels of immune mediators and antibodies that destroy endothelial cells, have been detected during the acute phase of the disease. It has been hypothesized that some unknown antigen, possibly a common infectious agent, triggers the immune response in a genetically predisposed child.

Manifestations and Clinical Course

The clinical course of the disease has been described in three phases: the acute, subacute, and convalescent phases.[91,92] The *acute phase* begins with an abrupt onset of fever, followed by conjunctivitis, rash, involvement of the oral mucosa, redness and swelling of the hands and feet, and enlarged cervical lymph nodes (Fig. 24-28). The fever typically is high, reaching 40°C (104°F) or more, has an erratic spiking pattern, is unresponsive to antibiotics, and persists for 5 or more days. The conjunctivitis, which is bilateral, begins shortly after the onset of fever, persists throughout the febrile course of the disease, and may last as long as 3 to 5 weeks. There is no exudate, discharge, or

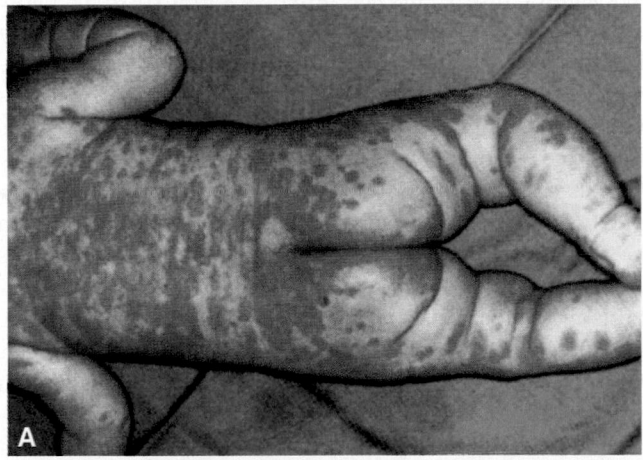
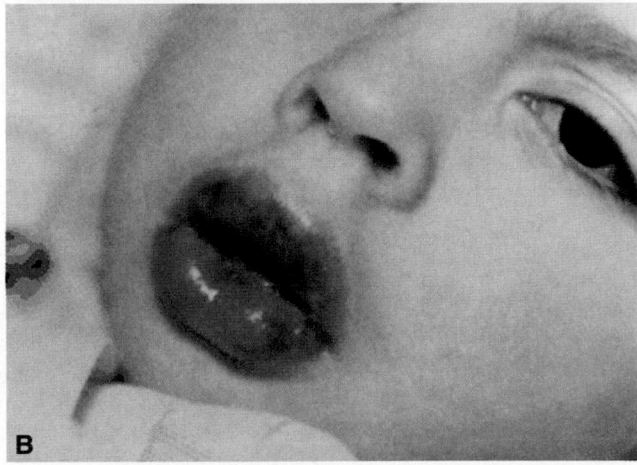

FIGURE 24-28 • Kawasaki disease. (**A**) Rash of Kawasaki disease in a 7-month-old child on the 4th day of illness. (**B**) Conjunctival infection, lip edema in a 2-year-old boy on the 6th day of illness. (From The Council on Cardiovascular Disease in Young, Committee on Rheumatic Fever, Endocarditis, and Kawasaki Disease. [2001]. Diagnostic guidelines for Kawasaki disease. *Circulation* 103, 335–336.)

conjunctival ulceration, differentiating it from many other types of conjunctivitis. The rash usually is deeply erythematous and may take several forms, the most common of which is a nonpruritic urticarial rash with large erythematous plaques, or a measles-type rash. Although the rash usually is generalized, it may be accentuated centrally or peripherally. Some children have a perianal rash with a diaper-like distribution. Oropharyngeal manifestations include fissuring of the lips, diffuse erythema of the oropharynx, and hypertrophic papillae of the tongue, creating a "strawberry" appearance. The hands and feet become swollen and painful, and have reddened palms and soles. The rash, oropharyngeal manifestations, and changes in hands and feet appear within 1 to 3 days of fever onset and usually disappear as the fever subsides. Lymph node involvement is the least constant feature of the disease. It is cervical and unilateral, with a single, firm, enlarged lymph node mass that usually is larger than 1.5 cm in diameter.

The *subacute phase* begins with defervescence and lasts until all signs of the disease have disappeared. During the subacute phase, desquamation (*i.e.*, peeling) of the skin of the fingers and toe tips begins and progresses to involve the entire surface of the palms and soles. Patchy peeling of skin areas other than the hands and feet may occur in some children. The convalescent stage persists from the complete resolution of symptoms until all signs of inflammation have disappeared. This usually takes approximately 8 weeks, although inflammatory changes in the coronary arteries may persist as long as 4 years.

In addition to the major manifestations that occur during the acute stage of the illness, there are several associated, less specific characteristics of the disease, including arthritis, urethritis and pyuria, gastrointestinal manifestations (*e.g.*, diarrhea, abdominal pain), hepatitis, and hydrops of the gallbladder. Arthritis or arthralgia occurs in approximately 30% of children with the disease, characterized by symmetric joint swelling involving large and small joints. Central nervous system involvement occurs in almost all children and is characterized by pronounced irritability and lability of mood.

Cardiac involvement is the most important manifestation of Kawasaki disease. Coronary artery abnormalities develop in approximately 15% to 25% of children, manifested by coronary artery dilation and aneurysm formation as seen on 2-D echocardiography. The manifestations of coronary artery involvement include signs and symptoms of myocardial ischemia or, rarely, overt myocardial infarction or rupture of the aneurysm. Pericarditis, myocarditis, endocarditis, heart failure, and arrhythmias also may develop. Death from Kawasaki disease is estimated to occur in 0.4% of patients and is almost always cardiac in nature, most often occurring during the convalescent phase of the illness, usually from thromboses or coronary arterial aneurysms.[92]

Diagnosis and Treatment

No specific diagnostic test for Kawasaki disease is available; therefore, the diagnosis is made on clinical grounds following published guidelines.[93] The guidelines specify fever persisting at least 5 days or more without another source in association with at least four principal features, including oral changes that may include erythema or cracking of the lips, strawberry tongue, erythema of the oral mucosa; bilateral, nonexudative conjunctivitis; polymorphous rash, generally truncal involvement, nonvesicular; changes of extremities that may include erythema and edema of the hands or feet, desquamation of fingers and toes 1 to 3 weeks after onset of illness; and cervical lymphadenopathy, often unilateral, with at least one node that is 1.5 cm in size.[93] Chest radiographs, ECG tests, and 2-D echocardiography are used to detect coronary artery involvement and follow its progress. Coronary angiography may be used to determine the extent of coronary artery involvement.

Intravenous gamma globulin and aspirin are considered the best therapies for prevention of coronary artery abnormalities in children with Kawasaki disease. During the acute phase of the illness, aspirin usually is given in larger doses (80 to 100 mg/kg/day divided in four doses) for its anti-inflammatory and antipyretic effects. After the fever is controlled, the aspirin dose is lowered (3 to 5 mg/kg/day, single dose), and the drug is given for its anti–platelet-aggregating effects for 6 to 8 weeks.[91]

Recommendations for cardiac follow-up evaluation (*i.e.*, stress testing and sometimes coronary angiography) are based on the level of coronary artery changes. Anticoagulant therapy may be recommended for children with multiple or large coronary aneurysms. Some restrictions in activities such as competitive sports may be advised for children with significant coronary artery abnormalities.[9]

IN SUMMARY, congenital heart defects arise during fetal heart development, which occurs during weeks 3 through 8 after conception, and reflect the stage of development at the time the causative event occurred. Several factors contribute to the development of congenital heart defects, including genetic and chromosomal influences, viruses, and environmental agents such as drugs and radiation. The exact cause of the defect often is unknown. These defects are relatively common, occurring in 1 of every 125 births, and are the most common cause of death related to a birth defect.

Congenital heart defects may produce no effects, or they may markedly affect cardiac function. The defects may produce shunting of blood from the right to the left side of the heart or from the left to the right side of the heart. Left-to-right shunts typically increase the volume of the right side of the heart and pulmonary circulation, and right-to-left shunts transfer deoxygenated blood from the right side of the heart to the left side, diluting the oxygen content of blood that is being ejected into the systemic circulation and causing cyanosis. The direction and degree of shunt depend on the size and position of the defect that connects the two sides of the heart and the difference in resistance between the two sides of the circulation. Congenital heart defects often are classified as defects that produce cyanosis and those that produce little or no cyanosis. Depending on the severity of the defect, congenital heart defects may be treated medically or surgically. Medical and surgical treatment often is indicated in children with severe defects.

Kawasaki disease is an acute febrile disease of young children that affects the skin, brain, eyes, joints, liver, lymph nodes, and heart. The disease can produce aneurysmal disease of the coronary arteries and is the most common cause of acquired heart disease in young children. ■

Review Exercises

1. A 40-year-old man presents in the emergency department complaining of substernal chest pain that is also felt in his left shoulder. He is short of breath and nauseated. His blood pressure is 148/90 mm Hg and his heart rate is 110 beats/minute. His ECG shows an ST-segment elevation with T-wave inversion. He is given aspirin, morphine, and oxygen. Blood tests reveal elevated CK-MB and troponin I.

   A. *What is the probable cause of the man's symptoms?*

   B. *Explain the origin of the left arm pain, nausea, and increased heart rate.*

   C. *What is the significance of the ST-segment changes and elevation in CK-MB and troponin I?*

   D. *Relate the actions of aspirin, morphine, and oxygen to the treatment of this man's condition.*

2. A 50-year-old woman presents with complaints of nocturnal paroxysmal dyspnea and orthopnea, palpitations, and fatigue. An echocardiogram demonstrates a thickened, immobile mitral valve with anterior and posterior leaflets moving together; slow early diastolic filling of the ventricle; and left atrial enlargement.

   A. *What is the probable cause of this woman's symptoms?*

   B. *Explain the pathologic significance of the slow early diastolic filling, distended left atrium, and palpitations.*

   C. *Given the echocardiographic data, what type of cardiac murmur would you expect to find in this woman?*

   D. *Which circulation (systemic or pulmonary) would you expect to be affected as this woman's mitral valve disorder progresses?*

3. A 4-month-old male infant is brought into the pediatric clinic by his mother. She reports that she noted over the past several weeks that her baby's lips and mouth and his fingernails and toenails have become a bluish-gray color. She also states that he seems to tire easily and that even nursing seems to wear him out. Lately, he has had several spells where he has sud-

denly turned blue, has had difficulty breathing, and been very irritable. During one of these spells he turned limp and seemed to have passed out for a short time. An echocardiogram reveals a thickening of the right ventricular wall with overriding of the aorta, a large subaortic ventricular septal defect, and narrowing of the pulmonary outflow with stenosis of the pulmonary valve.

   A. *What is this infant's probable diagnosis?*

   B. *Describe the shunting of blood that occurs with this disorder and its relationship to the development of cyanosis.*

   C. *The mother is instructed to place the infant in the knee–chest position when he has one of the spells in which he becomes blue and irritable. How does this position help to relieve the cyanosis and impaired oxygenation of tissues?*

   D. *The surgical creation of a shunt between the aorta and pulmonary artery may be performed as a palliative procedure for infants with marked hypoplasia of the pulmonary artery, with corrective surgery performed later in childhood. Explain how this procedure increases blood flow to the lungs.*

References

1. Gaziano J. M. (2005). Global burden of cardiovascular disease. In Zipes D. P., Libby P., Bonow R. O., et al. (Eds.), *Braunwald's heart disease: A textbook of cardiovascular medicine* (7th ed., pp. 1–19). Philadelphia: Elsevier Saunders.
2. American Heart Association. (2008). Heart disease and stroke statistics: 2008 at a glance. [Online.] Available: http://www.americanheart.org/downloadable/heart/1200082005246HS–Stats%202008.final.pdf. Accessed April 20, 2008.
3. LeWinter M. M., Kabban S. (2005). Pericardial diseases. In Zipes D. P., Libby P., Bonow R. O., et al. (Eds.), *Braunwald's heart disease: A textbook of cardiovascular medicine* (7th ed., pp. 1757–1780). Philadelphia: Elsevier Saunders.
4. Lange R. A., Hillis L. (2004). Acute pericarditis. *New England Journal of Medicine* 351, 2195–2202.
5. Little W. C., Freeman G. L. (2006). Pericardial disease. *Circulation* 113, 1622–1632.
6. Antman E. M., Anbe D. T., Armstrong P. W., et al. (2004). ACC/AHA guidelines for the management of patients with ST-elevation myocardial infarction. *Circulation* 110, e82–e293.
7. Guyton A., Hall J. E. (2006). *Textbook of medical physiology* (11th ed., pp. 249–253). Philadelphia: Elsevier Saunders.
8. Kern M. J. (2005). Coronary blood flow and myocardial ischemia. In Zipes D. P., Libby P., Bonow R. O., et al. (Eds.), *Braunwald's heart disease: A textbook of cardiovascular medicine* (7th ed., pp. 1103–1127). Philadelphia: Elsevier Saunders.
9. Schoen F. J. (2005). The heart. In Kumar V., Abbas A. K., Fausto N. (Eds.), *Robbins and Cotran pathologic basis of disease* (7th ed., pp. 555–617). Philadelphia: Elsevier Saunders.
10. Carroll J. D., Hess O. M. (2005). Assessment of normal and abnormal cardiac function. In Zipes D. P, Libby P., Bonow R. O., et al. (Eds.), *Braunwald's heart disease: A textbook of cardiovascular medicine* (7th ed., pp. 491–507). Philadelphia: Elsevier Saunders.

11. Lauer M., Froelicher E. S., Williams M., et al. (2005). Exercise testing in asymptomatic adults. *Circulation* 112, 771–776.

12. Armstrong W. F. (2005). Echocardiography. In Zipes D. P, Libby P., Bonow R. O., et al. (Eds.), *Braunwald's heart disease: A textbook of cardiovascular medicine* (7th ed., pp. 187–270). Philadelphia: Elsevier Saunders.

13. Udelson J. E., Dilsizian V., Bonow R. O. (2005). Nuclear cardiology. In Zipes D. P, Libby P., Bonow R. O., et al. (Eds.), *Braunwald's heart disease: A textbook of cardiovascular medicine* (7th ed., pp. 287–333). Philadelphia: Elsevier Saunders.

14. Pennell D. (2005). Cardiovascular magnetic resonance. In Zipes D. P., Libby P., Bonow R. O., et al. (Eds.), *Braunwald's heart disease: A textbook of cardiovascular medicine* (7th ed., pp. 335–353). Philadelphia: Elsevier Saunders.

15. Achenback S., Daniel W. G. (2005). Computed tomography of the heart. In Zipes D. P, Libby P., Bonow R. O., et al. (Eds.), *Braunwald's heart disease: A textbook of cardiovascular medicine* (7th ed., pp. 355–371). Philadelphia: Elsevier Saunders.

16. Davidson C. J., Bonow R. O. (2005). Cardiac catheterization. In Zipes D. P, Libby P., Bonow R. O., et al. (Eds.), *Braunwald's heart disease: A textbook of cardiovascular medicine* (7th ed., pp. 355–371). Philadelphia: Elsevier Saunders.

17. Yeghiazarians Y., Braunstein J. B., Askari A., et al. (2000). Unstable angina pectoris. *New England Journal of Medicine* 342, 101–114.

18. Mirvis D. M., Goldberger A. L. (2005). Electrocardiography. In Zipes D. P, Libby P., Bonow R. O., et al. (Eds.), *Braunwald's heart disease: A textbook of cardiovascular medicine* (7th ed., pp. 107–151). Philadelphia: Elsevier Saunders.

19. Antman E. M., Braunwald E. (2005). ST-elevation myocardial infarction: Pathology, pathophysiology, and clinical features; and ST-elevation myocardial infarction: Management. In Zipes D. P, Libby P., Bonow R. O., et al. (Eds.), *Braunwald's heart disease: A textbook of cardiovascular medicine* (7th ed., pp. 1141–1165, 1167–1226). Philadelphia: Elsevier Saunders.

20. Cannon C. P., Braunwald E. (2005). Unstable angina and non-ST elevation myocardial infarction. In Zipes D. P, Libby P., Bonow R. O., et al. (Eds.), *Braunwald's heart disease: A textbook of cardiovascular medicine* (7th ed., pp. 1243–1279). Philadelphia: Elsevier Saunders.

21. Jacobs A. K., Antman E. M., Faxon D. P., et al. (2007). Development of systems of care for ST-elevation myocardial infarction patients. *Circulation* 116, 217–230.

22. Smith S. C. Jr., Feldman T. E., Hirshfeld J. W. Jr., et al. (2006). ACC/AHA/SCAI 2005 guideline update for percutaneous coronary intervention. *Circulation* 113, 156–175.

23. Popma J. J., Kuntz R. E., Baim D. S. (2005). Percutaneous coronary and valvular interventions. In Zipes D. P, Libby P., Bonow R. O., et al. (Eds.), *Braunwald's heart disease: A textbook of cardiovascular medicine* (7th ed., pp. 1367–1393). Philadelphia: Elsevier Saunders.

24. Levine G. N., Berer P. B., Cohen D. J., et al. (2006). Newer pharmacotherapy in patients undergoing percutaneous coronary interventions: A guide for pharmacists and other health care professionals. *Pharmacotherapy* 26, 1537–1556.

25. Eagle K. A., Guyton R. A., Davidoff R., et al. (2004). ACC/AHA 2004 guideline update for coronary artery bypass graft surgery. *Circulation* 110, 1168–1176.

26. Gregoratos G., Abrams J., Epstein A. E., et al. (2002). ACC/AHA/NASPE 2002 guideline update for implantation of cardiac pacemakers and antiarrhythmia devices. *Journal of the American College of Cardiology* 40, 1703–1719.

27. Pasternak R. C. (2000). Comprehensive rehabilitation of patients with cardiovascular disease. In Zipes D. P, Libby P., Bonow R. O., et al. (Eds.), *Braunwald's heart disease: A textbook of cardiovascular medicine* (7th ed., pp. 1085–1102). Philadelphia: Elsevier Saunders.

28. Morrow D. A., Gersh B. J., Braunwald E. (2005). Chronic coronary artery disease. In Zipes D. P., Libby P, Bonow R. O., et al. (Eds.), *Braunwald's heart disease: A textbook of cardiovascular medicine* (7th ed., pp. 1281–1354). Philadelphia: Elsevier Saunders.

29. Gibbons R. J., Abrams J., Chatterjee K., et al. (2003). ACC/AHA 2002 guideline update for the management of patients with chronic stable angina. *Circulation* 107, 149–158.

30. Maron B. J., Towbin J. A., Thiene G., et al. (2006). Contemporary definitions and classification of the cardiomyopathies. *Circulation* 113, 1807–1816.

31. Nishimura R. A., Holmes D. R. (2004). Hypertrophic obstructive cardiomyopathy. *New England Journal of Medicine* 350, 1320–1327.

32. Moran B. J., McKenna W. J., Danielson G. K., et al. (2003). ACC/ESC clinical expert consensus document on hypertrophic cardiomyopathy. *European Heart Journal* 24, 1965–1991.

33. Ho C. Y., Seidman C. E. (2006). A contemporary approach to hypertrophic cardiomyopathy. *Circulation* 113, 858–862.

34. Corrado D., Thiene G. (2005). Arrhythmogenic right ventricular cardiomyopathy/dysplasia: Clinical impact of molecular genetic studies. *Circulation* 113, 1634–1637.

35. Anderson E. L. (2006). Arrhythmic right ventricular dysplasia. *American Family Physician* 73, 1391–1398.

36. Saffitz J. E. (2008). The heart. In Rubin E., Strayer D. E. (Eds.), *Rubin's pathology: Clinicopathologic foundations of medicine* (5th ed., pp. 465–474). Philadelphia: Lippincott Williams & Wilkins.

37. Liu P. P., Mason J. W. (2001). Advances in the understanding of myocarditis. *Circulation* 104, 1076–1082.

38. Feldman A. M., McNammara D. (2000). Myocarditis. *New England Journal of Medicine* 343, 1387–1398.

39. Baughman K. L. (2006). Diagnosis of myocarditis: Death of Dallas criteria. *Circulation* 113, 593–595.

40. Magnani J. W., Dec G. W. (2006). Myocarditis: Current trends in diagnosis and treatment. *Circulation* 113, 876–890.

41. Ro A., Frishman W. H. (2006). Peripartum cardiomyopathy. *Cardiology in Review* 14(1), 35–42.

42. Pearson G. D., Veille J. C., Rahimtoola S., et al. (2000). Peripartum cardiomyopathy: National Heart, Lung, and Blood Institute and Office of Rare Diseases (National Institutes of Health) Workshop Recommendations and Review. *Journal of the American Medical Association* 283, 1183–1188.

43. Wittstein I. S., Thiemann D. R., Lima J. A. C, et al. (2005). Neurohumoral features of myocardial stunning due to sudden emotional stress. *New England Journal of Medicine* 352, 539–548.

44. Merli E., Sutcliffe S., Gori M., et al. (2006). Tako-tsubo cardiomyopathy: New insights into the possible underlying pathophysiology. *European Journal of Echocardiography* 7, 53–61.

45. Mylonakis E., Calderwood S. B. (2001). Infective endocarditis in adults. *New England Journal of Medicine* 345, 1318–1330.

46. Baddour L. M., Bettman M. A., Bolger A. F. (2003). Nonvalvular cardiovascular device-related infections. *Circulation* 108, 2015–2031.

47. Holcomb S. (2005). Infective endocarditis guidelines assist in early identification. *Nurse Practitioner* 30(11), 7–17.

48. Baddour L. M., Wilson W. R., Bayer A. S., et al. (2005). Infective endocarditis: Diagnosis, antimicrobial therapy, and management of complications. *Circulation* 111, 394–434.

49. Devlin R. K., Andrews M. M., von Reyn C. F. (2004). Recent trends in infective endocarditis: Influence of case definitions. *Current Opinion in Cardiology* 19, 134–139.

50. Prendergast B. D. (2006). The changing face of infective endocarditis. *Heart* 92, 879–885.

51. Wilson W., Taubert K. A., Gewitz M., et al. (2007). Prevention of infective endocarditis: Guidelines from the American Heart Association. *Circulation* 115, 1656–1658.

52. Guilherme L., Cury P., Demarchi L. M. F., et al. (2004). Rheumatic heart disease. *American Journal of Pathology* 165, 1583–1591.

53. World Health Organization. (2004). *Rheumatic fever and rheumatic heart disease: Report of WHO expert consultation.* [Online.] Available: www.who.int/cardiovascular_diseases/resources/en/cvd_trs923.pdf. Accessed April 22, 2008.

54. Dajani A. S. (2005). Rheumatic fever. In Zipes D. P., Libby P., Bonow R. O., et al. (Eds.). *Braunwald's heart disease: A textbook of cardiovascular medicine* (7th ed., pp. 2093–2099). Philadelphia: Elsevier Saunders.

55. Ferrieri P., for the Jones Criteria Working Group. (2002). Proceedings of the Jones criteria workshop. *Circulation* 106, 2521–2527.

56. Bonow R. O., Braunwald E. (2005). Valvular heart disease. In Zipes D. P, Libby P., Bonow R. O., et al. (Eds.), *Braunwald's heart disease: A textbook of cardiovascular medicine* (7th ed., pp. 1553–1632). Philadelphia: Elsevier Saunders.

57. Bonow R. O., Carabello B. A., Chatterjee K., et al. (2006). ACC/AHA 2006 guidelines for the management of patients with valvular heart disease. *Circulation* 114, e84–e231.

58. Sfeir P. M., Febara V. A., Ayoub C. M. (2006). Mitral valve repair or replacement in elderly people. *Current Opinion in Anaesthesiology* 19, 82–87.

59. Walkes J.-C. M., Reardon M. J. (2004). Status of mitral valve surgery. *Current Opinion in Cardiology* 19, 117–122.

60. Carabello B. A. (2004). Aortic stenosis. *New England Journal of Medicine* 346, 677–682.

61. Freeman R. V., Otto C. M. (2005). Spectrum of calcific aortic valve disease: Pathogenesis, disease progression, and treatment strategies. *Circulation* 111, 3316–3326.

62. March of Dimes. (2007). Congenital heart defects. [Online.] Available: http://search.marchofdimes.com. Accessed August 13, 2007.

63. Van Praagh R. (2006). Embryology. In Keane J. F., Lock J. E., Fyler D. C. (Eds.), *Nadas' pediatric cardiology* (2nd ed., pp. 13–25). Philadelphia: Elsevier Saunders.

64. Freed M. D. (2006). Fetal and transitional circulation. In Keane J. F., Lock J. E., Fyler D. C. (Eds.), *Nadas' pediatric cardiology* (2nd ed., pp. 75–79). Philadelphia: Elsevier Saunders.

65. Sander T. L., Klinkner D. B., Tomita-Mitchell A., et al. (2006). Molecular and cellular basis of congenital heart disease. *Pediatric Clinics of North America* 53, 989–1009.

66. Pierpont M. E., Basson C. T., Benson D. W., et al. (2007). Genetic basis for congenital heart defects: Current knowledge. *Circulation* 115, 1–24.

67. Jenkins K. J., Correa A., Feinstein J. A., et al. (2007). Noninherited risk factors and congenital cardiovascular defects: Current knowledge. *Circulation* 115, 2995–3014.

68. Nadas A. S., Fyler D. C. (2006). Hypoxemia. In Keane J. F., Lock J. E., Fyler D. C. (Eds.), *Nadas' pediatric cardiology* (2nd ed., pp. 97–101). Philadelphia: Elsevier Saunders.

69. Allan L. D. (2002). Prenatal detection of congenital heart disease. In Anderson R. H., Baker E. J., Macartney F. J., et al. (Eds.), *Paediatric cardiology* (2nd ed., pp. 687–699). London: Churchill Livingstone.

70. Tynan M., Anderson R. H. (2002). Clinical presentation of heart disease in infants and children, ventricular septal defect, complete transposition, pulmonary stenosis. In Anderson R. H., Baker E. J., Macartney F. J., et al. (Eds.), *Paediatric cardiology* (2nd ed., pp. 275–283, 983–1014, 1281–1320, 1461–1479). London: Churchill Livingstone.

71. Wilson W., Taubert K. A., Gewitz M., et al. (2007). Prevention of infective endocarditis. *Circulation* 106, 1–20.

72. Hoffman J. I. E. (2002). Incidence, mortality and natural history. In Anderson R. H., Baker E. J., Macartney F. J., et al. (Eds.), *Paediatric cardiology* (2nd ed., pp. 111–139). London: Churchill Livingstone.

73. Keane J. F., Geva T., Fyler D. C. (2006). Atrial septal defect, ventricular septal defect, coarctation of the aorta, single ventricle, pulmonary stenosis. In Keane J. F., Lock J. E., Fyler D. C. (Eds.), *Nadas' pediatric cardiology* (2nd ed., pp. 527–558, 603–616, 627–644, 743–752). Philadelphia: Elsevier Saunders.

74. Botto L. D., Correa A., Erickson J. D. (2001). Racial and temporal variation in the prevalence of heart defects. *Pediatrics* 107, E32.

75. Benson L. N., Cowan K. N. (2002). Persistent patency of the arterial duct. In Anderson R. H., Baker E. J., Macartney F. J., et al. (Eds.), *Paediatric cardiology* (2nd ed., pp. 1405–1460).

76. Gersony W. M., Peckham G. J., Ellison R. C., et al. (1983). Effects of indomethacin in premature infants with patent ductus arteriosus: Results of a national collaborative study. *Journal of Pediatrics* 102, 895–906.

77. Bacha E. A., Daves S., Hardin J., et al. (2006). Single-ventricle palliation for high-risk neonates: The emergence of an alternative hybrid stage I strategy. *Journal of Thoracic and Cardiovascular Surgery* 131, 163–171.

78. Marx G. R., Fyler D. C. (2006). Endocardial cushion defects. In Keane J. F., Lock J. E., Fyler D. C. (Eds.), *Nadas' pediatric cardiology* (2nd ed., pp. 663–674). Philadelphia: Elsevier Saunders.

79. Ebels T., Anderson R. H. (2002). Atrioventricular septal defect. In Anderson R. H., Baker E. J., Macartney F. J., et al. (Eds.), *Paediatric cardiology* (2nd ed., pp. 939–982). London: Churchill Livingstone.

80. Shinebourne E. A., Anderson R. H. (2002). Fallot's tetralogy. In Anderson R. H., Baker E. J., Macartney F. J., et al. (Eds.), *Paediatric cardiology* (2nd ed., pp. 1213–1250). London: Churchill Livingstone.

81. LoBreitbart R. E., Fyler D. C. (2006). Tetralogy of Fallot. In Keane J. F., Lock J. E., Fyler D. C. (Eds.), *Nadas' pediatric cardiology* (2nd ed., pp. 559–580). Philadelphia: Elsevier Saunders.

82. Fulton D. R., Fyler D. C. (2006). D-Transposition of the great arteries. In Keane J. F., Lock J. E., Fyler D. C. (Eds.), *Nadas' pediatric cardiology* (2nd ed., pp. 645–662). Philadelphia: Elsevier Saunders.

83. Brierley J., Redington A. N. (2002). Aorta coarctation and interrupted aortic arch. In Anderson R. H., Baker E. J., Macartney F. J., et al. (Eds.), *Paediatric cardiology* (2nd ed., pp. 1523–1558). London: Churchill Livingstone.

84. O'Brien P., Boisvert J. T. (2001). Current management of infants and children with single ventricle anatomy. *Journal of Pediatric Nursing* 16, 338–350.

85. Khairy P., Poirier N., Mercier L. A. (2007). Univentricular heart. *Circulation* 115, 800–812.

86. Tweddell J. S., Litwin S. B., Thomas J. P., Mussatto K. A. (1999). Recent advances in the surgical management of the single ventricle pediatric patient. *Pediatric Clinics of North America* 46, 465–480.

87. Alsoufi B., Bennetts J., Verma S., et al. (2007). New developments in the treatment of hypoplastic left heart syndrome. *Pediatrics* 119, 109–117.

88. Marelli A. J., Mackie A. S., Ionescu-Ittu R., et al. (2007). Congenital heart disease in the general population: Changing prevalence and age distribution. *Circulation* 115, 163–172.

89. Deanfield J. E., Cullen S., Celermajer D. S. (2002). Congenital heart disease in adolescents and adults. In Anderson R. H., Baker E. J., Macartney F. J., et al. (Eds.), *Paediatric cardiology* (2nd ed., pp. 1893–1930). London: Churchill.

90. Landzberg M. (2006). Adult congenital heart disease. In Keane J. F., Lock J. E., Fyler D. C. (Eds.), *Nadas' pediatric cardiology* (2nd ed., pp. 833–841). Philadelphia: Elsevier Saunders.

91. Fulton D. R., Newburger J. W. (2006). Kawasaki disease. In Keane J. F., Lock J. E., Fyler D. C. (Eds.), *Nadas' pediatric cardiology* (2nd ed., pp. 401–413). Philadelphia: Elsevier Saunders.

92. Neches W. H. (2002). Kawasaki disease. In Anderson R. H., Baker E. J., Macartney F. J., et al. (Eds.), *Paediatric cardiology* (2nd ed., pp. 1683–1696). London: Churchill Livingstone.

93. American Heart Association, Committee on Rheumatic Fever, Endocarditis, and Kawasaki Disease. (2004). Diagnostic guidelines for Kawasaki disease. *Circulation* 110, 2747–2711.

Visit thePoint. **http://thePoint.lww.com for animations, journal articles, and more!**

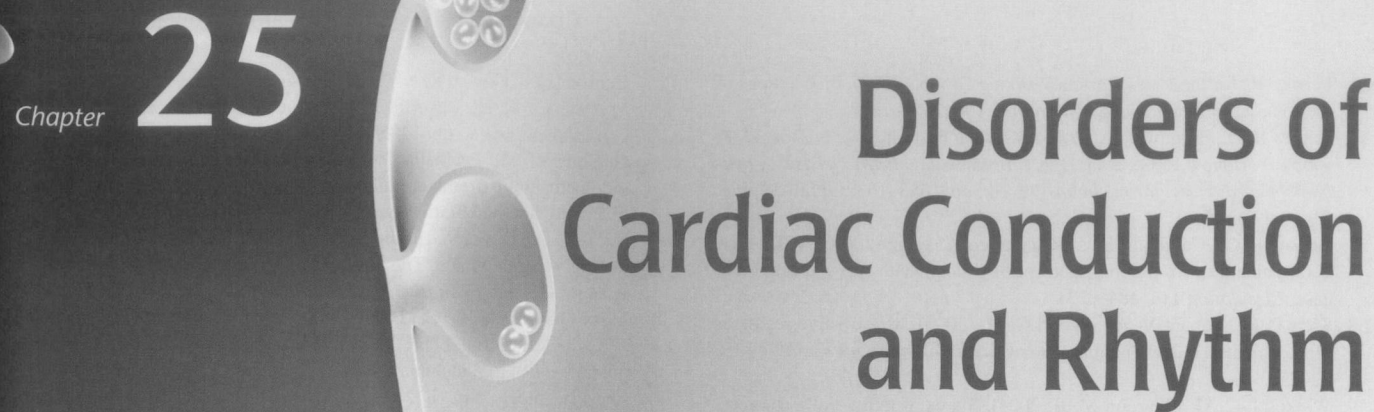

Chapter 25

Disorders of Cardiac Conduction and Rhythm

JILL WINTERS

➤ Heart muscle is unique in that it is capable of generating and rapidly conducting its own electrical impulses or action potentials. These action potentials result in excitation of muscle fibers throughout the myocardium. Impulse formation and conduction result in weak electrical currents that spread through the entire body. It is these impulses that are recorded on an electrocardiogram. Disorders of cardiac impulse generation and conduction range from benign arrhythmias that are merely annoying to those causing serious disruption of heart function and sudden cardiac death.

CARDIAC CONDUCTION SYSTEM

After completing this section of the chapter, you should be able to meet the following objectives:

■ Describe the cardiac conduction system and relate it to the mechanical functioning of the heart.
■ Characterize the four phases of a cardiac action potential and differentiate between the fast and slow responses.
■ Draw an ECG tracing and state the origin of the component parts of the tracing.
■ Provide a rationale for the importance of careful lead placement and monitoring of ischemic events.

In certain areas of the heart, the myocardial cells have been modified to form the specialized cells of the conduction system. Although most myocardial cells are capable of initiating and conducting impulses, it is the conduction system that maintains the pumping efficiency of the heart. Specialized pacemaker cells generate impulses at a faster rate than other types of heart tissue, and the conduction tissue transmits these impulses more rapidly than other cardiac cell types. Because of these properties, the conduction system usually controls the rhythm of the heart. Blood reaches the conduction tissues by way of the coronary blood vessels. Coronary heart disease that interrupts blood flow through the vessels supplying tissues of the conduction system can induce serious and sometimes fatal disturbances in cardiac rhythm.

The specialized excitatory and conduction system of the heart consists of the sinoatrial (SA) node, in which the normal rhythmic impulse is generated; the internodal pathways between the atria and the ventricles; the atrioventricular (AV) node and bundle of His, which conduct the impulse from the atria to the ventricles; and the Purkinje fibers, which conduct the impulses to all parts of the ventricle (Fig. 25-1).

The SA node, which has the fastest intrinsic rate of firing (60 to 100 beats per minute), normally serves as the pacemaker of the heart. It is a spindle-shaped strip of specialized muscle tissue, about 10 to 20 mm in length and 2 to 3 mm wide; located in the posterior wall of the right atrium just below the opening of the superior vena cava and less than 1 mm from the epicardial surface.[1] It has been suggested that no single cell in the SA node serves as the pacemaker, but rather that sinus nodal cells discharge synchronously because of mutual entrainment.[2] As a result, the firing of faster-discharging cells is slowed down by slower-discharging cells and the firing rate of slower-discharging cells is sped up by faster-discharging cells, resulting in a synchronization of their firing rates.

Impulses originating in the SA node travel through the atria to the AV node. Because of the anatomic location of the SA node, the progression of atrial depolarization occurs in an inferior, leftward, and somewhat posterior direction, and the right atrium is depolarized slightly before the left atrium.[2] There are three internodal pathways between the SA node and the AV node, including the anterior (Bachmann), middle (Wenckebach), and posterior (Thorel) internodal tracts. These three tracts anastomose with each other proximally to the AV node. Interatrial conduction appears to be accomplished through the Bachmann bundle. This large muscle bundle originates along the anterior border of the SA node and travels posteriorly around the aorta to the left atrium.[3]

CARDIAC CONDUCTION SYSTEM

- The cardiac conduction system controls the rate and direction of electrical impulse conduction in the heart.

- Normally, impulses are generated in the SA node, which has the fastest rate of firing, and travel through the AV node to the Purkinje system in the ventricles.

- Cardiac action potentials are divided into five phases: phase 0, or the rapid upstroke of the action potential; phase 1, or early repolarization; phase 2, or the plateau; phase 3, or final repolarization period; and phase 4, or diastolic repolarization period.

- Cardiac muscle has two types of ion channels that function in producing the voltage changes that occur during the depolarization phase of the action potential: the fast sodium channels and the slow calcium channels.

- There are two types of cardiac action potentials: the fast response, which occurs in atrial and ventricular muscle cells and the Purkinje conduction system and uses the fast sodium channels; and the slow response of the SA and AV nodes, which uses the slow calcium channels.

The heart essentially has two conduction systems: one that controls atrial activity and one that controls ventricular activity. The AV junction connects the two conduction systems and provides for one-way conduction between the atria and ventricles. The AV node is a compact, ovoid structure measuring approximately $1 \times 3 \times 5$ mm and located slightly beneath the right atrial endocardium, anterior to the opening of the coronary sinus, and immediately above the insertion of the sep-

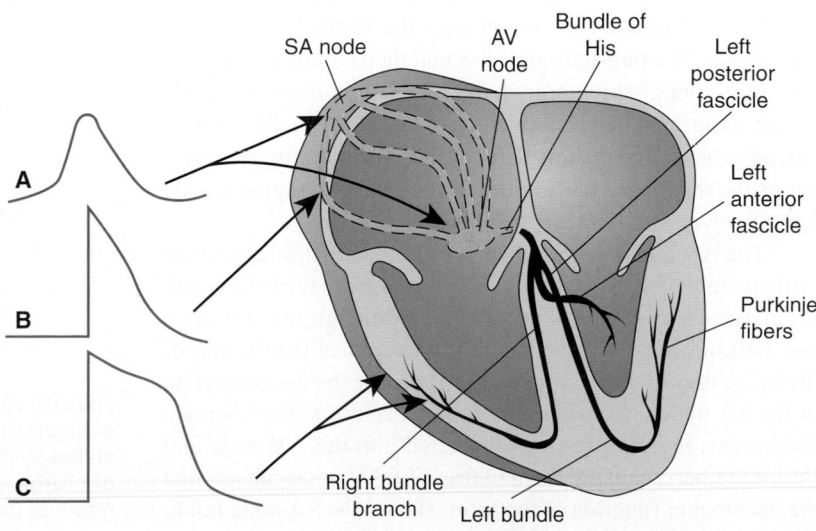

FIGURE 25-1 • Conduction system of the heart and action potentials. **(A)** Action potential of sinoatrial (SA) and atrioventricular (AV) nodes; **(B)** atrial muscle action potential; **(C)** action potential of ventricular muscle and Purkinje fibers.

tal leaflet of the tricuspid valve.[1,3] The AV node is divided into three functional regions: the AN or transitional region, located between the atria and the rest of the node; the N or middle region (*i.e.*, the node proper); and the NH region, in which nodal fibers merge with the bundle of His, which is the upper portion of the specialized conduction system.[1,4] In the AN portion of the node, atrial fibers connect with very small junctional fibers of the node itself. The velocity of conduction through the AN and N fibers is very slow (approximately one half that of normal cardiac muscle), which greatly delays transmission of the impulse.[4,5] A further delay occurs as the impulse travels through the N region into the NH region, which connects with the *bundle of His* (also called the *AV bundle*). This delay provides a mechanical advantage whereby the atria complete their ejection of blood before ventricular contraction begins. Under normal circumstances, the AV node provides the only connection between the atrial and ventricular conduction systems. The atria and ventricles would beat independently of each other if the transmission of impulses through the AV node were blocked.

The *Purkinje system,* which supplies the ventricles, has large fibers that allow for rapid conduction and almost simultaneous excitation of the entire right and left ventricles (0.06 second).[5] This rapid rate of conduction throughout the Purkinje system is necessary for the swift and efficient ejection of blood from the heart. The fibers of the Purkinje system originate in the AV node and proceed to form the bundle of His, which extends through the fibrous tissue between the valves of the heart and into the ventricular system. Because of its proximity to the aortic valve and the mitral valve ring, the bundle of His is predisposed to inflammation and deposits of calcified debris that can interfere with impulse conduction.[5] The bundle of His penetrates into the ventricles and almost immediately divides into *right* and *left bundle branches* that straddle the interventricular septum. Branches from the anterior and posterior descending coronary arteries provide the blood supply for the His bundle, making this conduction site less susceptible to ischemic damage, unless the damage is extensive.[1] The bundle branches move through the subendocardial tissues toward the papillary muscles and then subdivide into the Purkinje fibers, which branch out and supply the outer walls of the ventricles. The main trunk of the left bundle branch extends for approximately 1 to 2 cm before fanning out as it enters the septal area and divides further into two segments: the *left posterior* and *anterior fascicles.*

The AV nodal fibers, when not stimulated, discharge at an intrinsic rate of 40 to 60 times a minute, and the Purkinje fibers discharge 15 to 40 times per minute. Although the AV node and Purkinje system have the ability to control the rhythm of the heart, they do not normally do so because the discharge rate of the SA node is considerably faster. Each time the SA node discharges, its impulses are conducted into the AV node and Purkinje fibers, causing them to fire. The AV node can assume the pacemaker function of the heart, should the SA node fail to discharge, and the Purkinje system can assume the pacemaker function of the ventricles should the AV node fail to conduct impulses from the atria to the ventricles. Under these circumstances, the heart rate reflects the intrinsic firing rate of the prevailing structures.

Action Potentials

An action potential represents the sequential change in electrical potential that occurs across a cell membrane when excitation occurs (see Chapter 4, Understanding Membrane Potentials). These potential or voltage differences, often referred to as membrane potentials, represent the flow of current associated with the passage of ions through ion channels in the cell membrane. The sodium (Na^+), potassium (K^+), and calcium (Ca^{++}) ions are the major charge carriers in cardiac muscle cells. Disorders of the ion channels along with disruption in the flow of these current-carrying ions are increasingly being linked to the generation of cardiac arrhythmias and conduction disorders.

Action potentials can be divided into three phases: the resting or unexcited state, depolarization, and repolarization. During the resting phase, cardiac cells exhibit a resting membrane potential that typically ranges from −60 to −90 millivolts (mV). The negative sign before the voltage indicates that the inside of the membrane is negatively charged in relation to the outside (Fig. 25-2A). Although different kinds of ions are found both inside and outside of the membrane, the membrane potential is determined largely by Na^+ and K^+ and the membrane permeability for these two ions. During the resting phase of the membrane potential, the membrane is selectively permeable to K^+ and nearly impermeable to Na^+. As a result, K^+ diffuses out of the cell along its concentration gradient, causing a relative loss of positive ions from inside the membrane. The result is an uneven distribution of charge with negativity on the inside and positivity on the outside.

Depolarization represents the period of time (measured in milliseconds [msec]) during which the polarity of the membrane potential is reversed. It occurs when the cell mem-

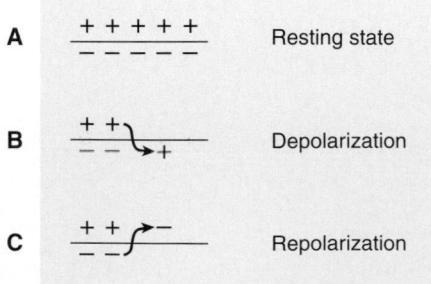

FIGURE 25-2 • The flow of charge during impulse generation in excitable tissue. During the resting state, opposite charges are separated by the cell membrane. Depolarization represents the flow of charge across the membrane, and repolarization denotes the return of the membrane potential to its resting state.

brane suddenly becomes selectively permeable to a current-carrying ion such as Na$^+$, allowing it move into a cell and change the membrane potential so it becomes positive on the inside and negative on the outside (Fig. 25-2B).

Repolarization involves reestablishment of the resting membrane potential. It is a complex and somewhat slower process, involving the outward flow of electrical charges and the return of the membrane potential to its resting state.[6] During repolarization, membrane permeability for K$^+$ again increases, allowing the positively charged K$^+$ to move outward across the membrane. This outward movement removes positive charges from inside the cell; thus, the voltage across the membrane again becomes negative on the inside and positive on the outside (Fig. 25-2C). The adenosine triphosphatase (ATPase)-dependent sodium–potassium pump assists in repolarization by pumping positively charged Na$^+$ out across the cell membrane and returning K$^+$ to the inside of the membrane.[7]

Action Potential Phases

The action potentials in cardiac muscle are typically divided into five phases: *phase 0*—upstroke or rapid depolarization; *phase 1*—early repolarization period; *phase 2*—plateau; *phase 3*—final, rapid repolarization period; and *phase 4*—

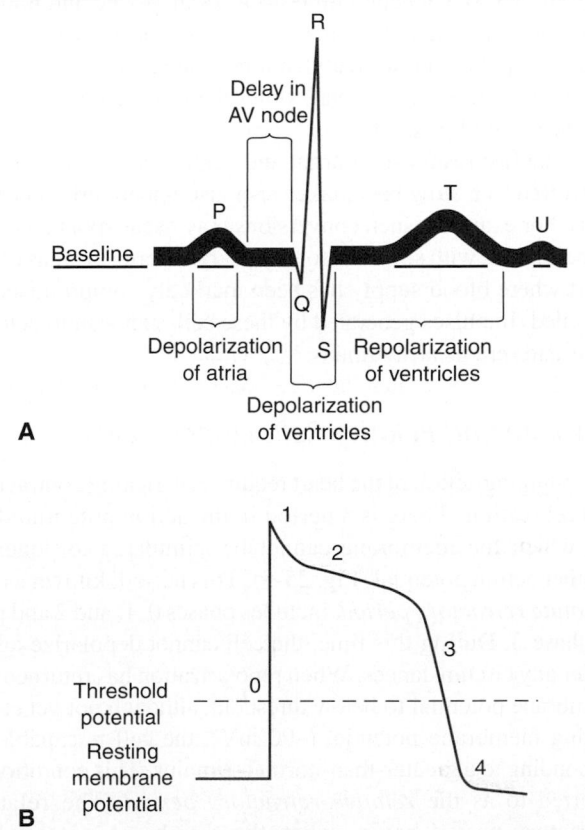

A

B

FIGURE 25-3 • Relation between **(A)** the electrocardiogram and **(B)** phases of the ventricular action potential.

diastolic depolarization (Fig. 25-3B). Cardiac muscle has three types of membrane ion channels that contribute to the voltage changes that occur during the different phases of the cardiac action potential. They are the fast Na$^+$ channels, slow calcium (Ca^{++}) channels, and K$^+$ channels.

During *phase 0,* in atrial and ventricular muscle and in the Purkinje system, the fast Na$^+$ channels in the cell membrane are stimulated to open, resulting in the rapid influx of Na$^+$. The point at which the Na$^+$ channels open is called the *depolarization threshold.* When the cell has reached this threshold, a rapid influx of Na$^+$ occurs. The exterior of the cell now is negatively charged in relation to the highly positive interior of the cell. This influx of Na$^+$ produces a rapid, positively directed change in the membrane potential, resulting in the electrical spike and overshoot during phase 0 of the action potential.[6] The membrane potential shifts from a resting membrane potential of approximately −90 to +20 mV. The rapid depolarization that comprises phase 0 is responsible for the QRS complex on the electrocardiogram (ECG; see Fig. 25-3A). Depolarization of a cardiac cell tends to cause adjacent cells to depolarize because the voltage spike of the cell's depolarization stimulates the Na$^+$ channels in nearby cells to open. Therefore, when a cardiac cell is stimulated to depolarize, a wave of depolarization is propagated across the heart, cell by cell.

Phase 1 occurs at the peak of the action potential and signifies inactivation of the fast Na$^+$ channels with an abrupt decrease in sodium permeability. The slight downward slope is thought to be caused by the influx of a small amount of negatively charged chloride ions and efflux of potassium.[1] The decrease in intracellular positivity reduces the membrane potential to a level near 0 mV, from which the plateau, or phase 2, arises.

Phase 2 represents the plateau of the action potential. If K$^+$ permeability increased to its resting level at this time, as it does in nerve fibers or skeletal muscle, the cell would repolarize rapidly. Instead, K$^+$ permeability is low, allowing the membrane to remain depolarized throughout the phase 2 plateau. A concomitant influx of Ca^{++} into the cell through the slow Ca^{++} channels contributes to the phase 2 plateau.[6] Calcium ions entering the muscle during this phase also play a key role in the contractile process.[1] These unique features of the phase 2 plateau cause the action potential of cardiac muscle (several hundred msec) to last 3 to 15 times longer than that of skeletal muscle and produce a corresponding increased period of contraction.[5] The phase 2 plateau coincides with the ST segment of the ECG.

Phase 3 reflects rapid repolarization and begins with the downslope of the action potential. During the phase 3 repolarization period, the slow Ca^{++} channels close and the influx of Ca^{++} and Na$^+$ ceases. There is a sharp rise in K$^+$ permeability, contributing to the rapid outward movement of K$^+$ and reestablishment of the resting membrane potential (−90 mV). At the conclusion of phase 3, the distribution of K$^+$ and Na$^+$ returns the membrane to the normal resting state. The T wave on the ECG corresponds with phase 3 of the action potential.

Phase 4 represents the resting membrane potential. During phase 4, the activity of the Na$^+$/K$^+$-ATPase pump contributes to maintaining the resting membrane potential by transporting Na$^+$ out of the cell and moving K$^+$ back in. Phase 4 corresponds to diastole.

Fast and Slow Responses

There are two main types of action potentials in the heart—the fast response and the slow response. The *fast response* occurs in the normal myocardial cells of the atria, the ventricles, and the Purkinje fibers (Fig. 25-4A). It is characterized by the opening of voltage-dependent Na$^+$ channels called the *fast sodium channels.* The fast-response cardiac cells do not normally initiate cardiac action potentials. Instead, impulses

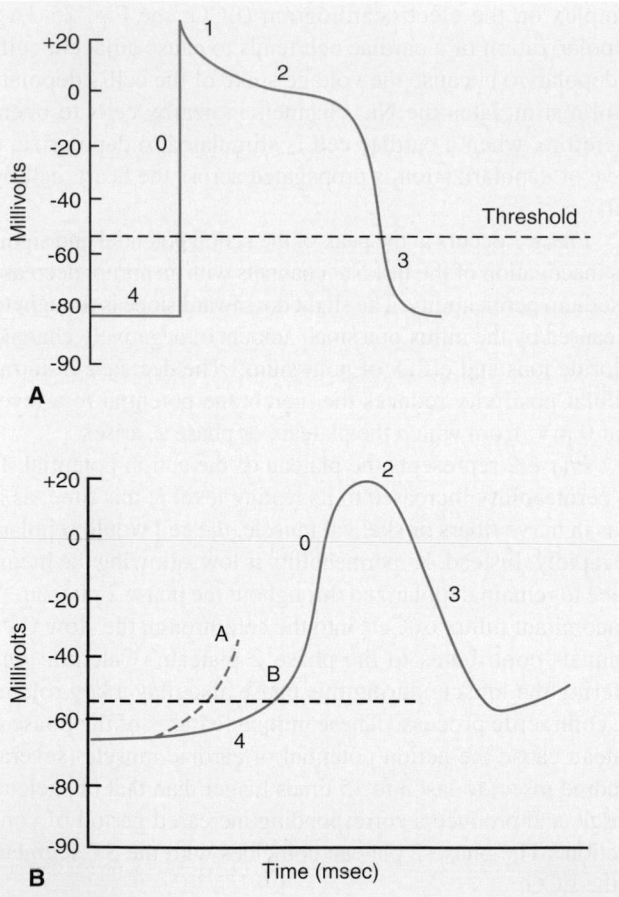

A

B

FIGURE 25-4 • Changes in action potential recorded from a fast response in cardiac muscle cell (**A**) and from a slow response recorded in the sinoatrial and atrioventricular nodes (**B**). The phases of the action potential are identified by numbers: phase 4, resting membrane potential; phase 0, depolarization; phase 1, brief period of repolarization; phase 2, plateau; phase 3, repolarization. The slow response is characterized by a slow, spontaneous rise in the phase 4 membrane potential to threshold levels; it has a lesser amplitude and shorter duration than the fast response. Increased automaticity (A) occurs when the rate of phase 4 depolarization is increased.

originating in the specialized cells of the SA node are conducted to the fast-response myocardial cells, where they effect a change in the membrane potential to the threshold level. On reaching threshold, the voltage-dependent Na$^+$ channels open to initiate the rapid upstroke of the phase 1 action potential. The amplitude and the rate of rise of phase 1 are important to the conduction velocity of the fast response. Myocardial fibers with a fast response are capable of conducting electrical activity at relatively rapid rates (0.5 to 5.0 m/second), thereby providing a high safety factor for conduction.[8]

The *slow response* occurs in the SA node, which is the natural pacemaker of the heart, and the conduction fibers of the AV node (see Fig. 25-4B). The hallmark of these pacemaker cells is a spontaneous phase 4 depolarization. The membrane permeability of these cells allows a slow inward leak of current to occur through the slow channels during phase 4. This leak continues until the threshold for firing is reached, at which point the cell spontaneously depolarizes. Under normal conditions, the slow response, sometimes referred to as the *calcium current,* does not contribute significantly to depolarization of the atria and ventricles. Its primary role in normal atrial and ventricular cells is to provide for the entrance of calcium for the excitation–contraction mechanism that couples the electrical activity with muscle contraction.

The rate of pacemaker cell discharge varies with the resting membrane potential and the slope of phase 4 depolarization (see Fig. 25-3). Catecholamines (*i.e.,* epinephrine and norepinephrine) increase heart rate by increasing the slope or rate of phase 4 depolarization. Acetylcholine, which is released during vagal stimulation of the heart, slows the heart rate by decreasing the slope of phase 4.

The fast response of atrial and ventricular muscle can be converted to a slow pacemaker response under certain conditions. For example, such conversions may occur spontaneously in individuals with severe coronary artery disease, in areas of the heart where blood supply has been markedly compromised or curtailed. Impulses generated by these cells can lead to ectopic beats and serious arrhythmias.

Absolute and Relative Refractory Periods

The pumping action of the heart requires alternating contraction and relaxation. There is a period in the action potential during which the membrane cannot be stimulated to generate another action potential (Fig. 25-5). This period, known as the *absolute refractory period,* includes phases 0, 1, and 2 and part of phase 3. During this time, the cell cannot depolarize again under any circumstances. When repolarization has returned the membrane potential to below threshold, although not yet at the resting membrane potential (–90 mV), the cell is capable of responding to a greater-than-normal stimulus. This condition is referred to as the *relative refractory period.* The relative refractory period begins when the membrane potential in phase 3 reaches threshold level and ends just before the end of phase 3. After the relative refractory period is a short period called the *supernormal excitatory period,* during which a weak

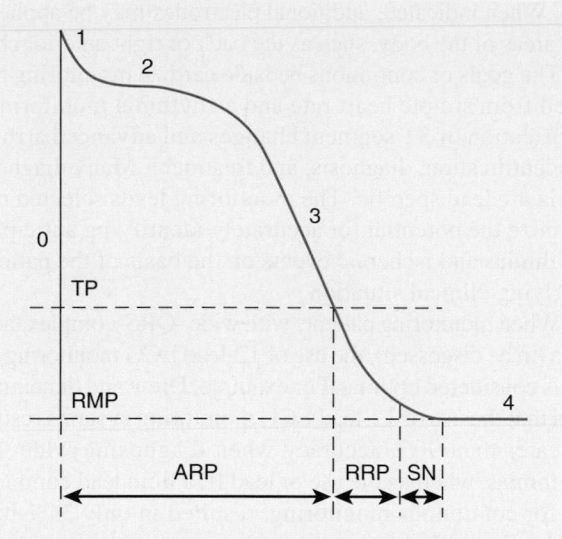

FIGURE 25-5 • Diagram of an action potential of a ventricular muscle cell, showing the threshold potential (TP), resting membrane potential (RMP), absolute refractory period (ARP), relative refractory period (RRP), and supernormal (SN) period.

stimulus can evoke a response. The supernormal excitatory period extends from the terminal portion of phase 3 until the beginning of phase 4. It is during this period that cardiac arrhythmias develop.

In skeletal muscle, the refractory period is very short compared with the duration of contraction such that a second contraction cannot be initiated before the first is over, resulting in a

summated tetanized contraction. In cardiac muscle, the absolute refractory period is almost as long as the contraction itself, ensuring that a second contraction cannot be stimulated until the first one is complete. The longer length of the absolute refractory period of cardiac muscle is important in maintaining the alternating contraction and relaxation that is essential to the pumping action of the heart and for the prevention of fatal arrhythmias.

Electrocardiography

The electrocardiogram (ECG) is a graphic recording of the electrical activity of the heart. The electrical currents generated by the heart spread through the body to the skin, where they can be sensed by appropriately placed electrodes, amplified, and viewed on an oscilloscope or chart recorder.

The deflection points of an ECG are designated by the letters P, Q, R, S, and T. Figure 25-6 depicts the electrical activity of the conduction system on an ECG tracing. The P wave represents the SA node and atrial depolarization; the QRS complex (i.e., beginning of the Q wave to the end of the S wave) depicts ventricular depolarization; and the T wave portrays ventricular repolarization. The isoelectric line between the P wave and the Q wave represents depolarization of the AV node, bundle branches, and Purkinje system (Fig. 25-7). Atrial repolarization occurs during ventricular depolarization and is hidden in the QRS complex.

The ECG records the potential difference in charge between two electrodes as the depolarization and repolarization waves move through the heart and are conducted to the skin surface. The shape of the recorder tracing is determined by the direction in

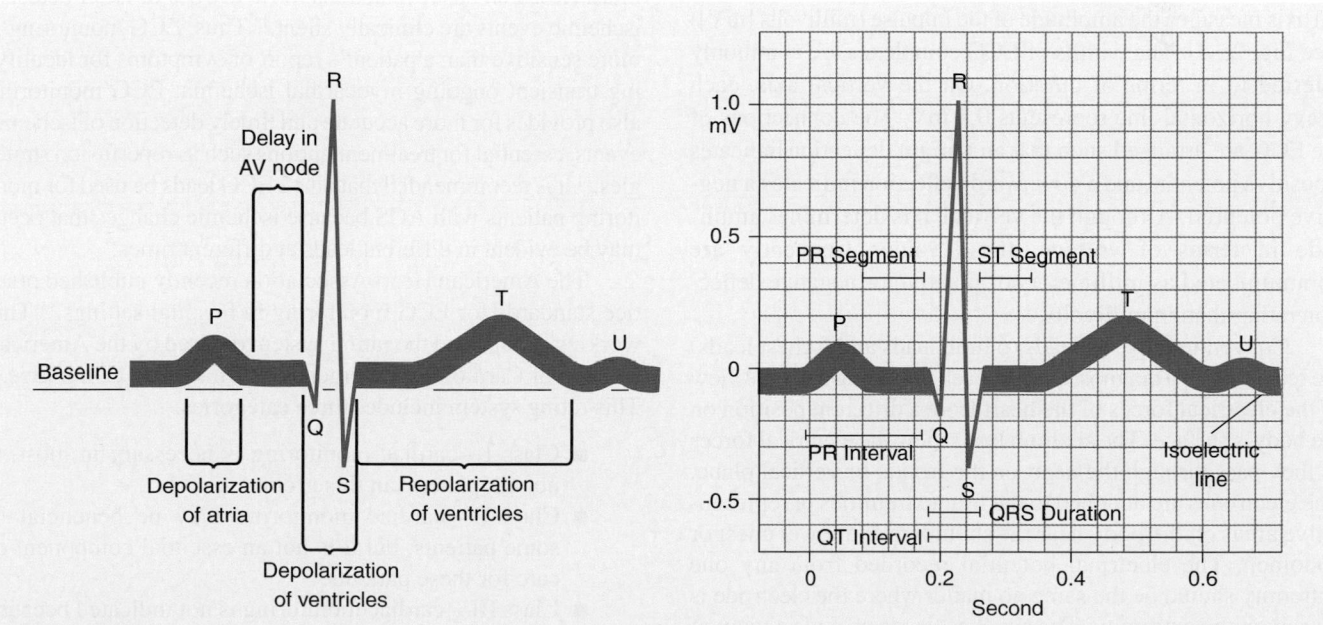

FIGURE 25-6 • Diagram of the electrocardiogram (lead II) and representative depolarization and repolarization of the atria and ventricles. The P wave represents atrial depolarization, the QRS complex ventricular depolarization, and the T wave ventricular repolarization. Atrial repolarization occurs during ventricular depolarization and is hidden under the QRS complex.

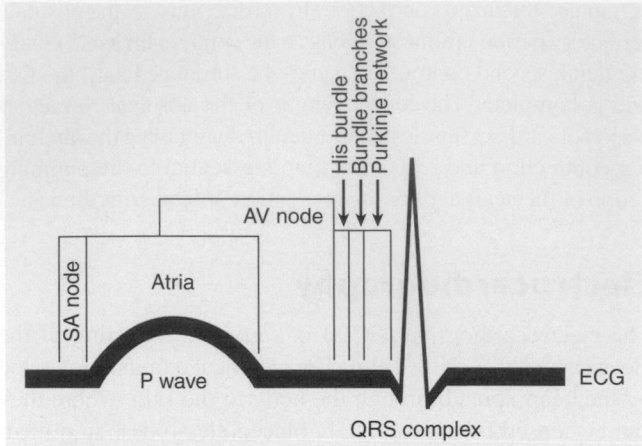

FIGURE 25-7 • Tissues depolarized by a wave of activation commencing in the sinoatrial (SA) node are shown in a series of blocks superimposed on the deflections of the electrocardiogram (ECG). (From Katz A. M. [1992]. *Physiology of the heart* [p. 483]. New York: Raven Press.)

which the impulse spreads through the heart muscle in relation to electrode placement. A depolarization wave that moves toward the recording electrode registers as a positive, or upward, deflection. Conversely, if the impulse moves away from the recording electrode, the deflection is downward, or negative. When there is no flow of charge between electrodes, the potential is zero, and a straight line is recorded at the baseline of the chart.

The ECG recorder is much like a camera in that it can record different views of the electrical activity of the heart, depending on where the recording electrode is placed. The horizontal axis of the ECG measures time (seconds), and the vertical axis measures the amplitude of the impulse (millivolts [mV]) (see Fig. 25-6). The widths of ECG complexes are commonly referred to in terms of duration. On the vertical axis, each heavy horizontal line represents 0.5 mV. The connections of the ECG are arranged such that an upright deflection indicates a positive potential and a downward deflection indicates a negative potential. Although the vertical axis determines amplitude in terms of voltage, these values frequently are communicated as millimeters of positive or negative deflection rather than in millivolts.

Conventionally, 12 leads (6 limb leads and 6 chest leads) are recorded for a diagnostic ECG, each providing a unique view of the electrical forces of the heart from a different position on the body's surface. The six limb leads view the electrical forces as they pass through the heart on the frontal or vertical plane. The electrodes are attached to the four extremities or representative areas on the body near the shoulders and lower chest or abdomen. The electrical potential recorded from any one extremity should be the same no matter where the electrode is placed on the extremity. The six chest leads provide a view of the electrical forces as they pass through the heart on the horizontal plane. They are moved to different positions on the chest, including the right and left sternal borders and the left anterior surface. The right lower extremity lead is used as a ground elec-

trode. When indicated, additional electrodes may be applied to other areas of the body, such as the back or right anterior chest.

The goals of continuous bedside cardiac monitoring have shifted from simple heart rate and arrhythmia monitoring to identification of ST segment changes and advanced arrhythmia identification, diagnosis, and treatment. Many diagnostic criteria are lead specific. The monitoring leads selected must maximize the potential for accurately identifying anticipated arrhythmias and ischemic events on the basis of the patient's underlying clinical situation.

When monitoring patients with wide–QRS-complex tachycardia (to be discussed), the use of 12-lead ECG monitoring systems is considered optimal. For example, Drew and Scheinman[9] found that the use of 12-lead ECG monitoring systems resulted in greater than 90% accuracy when diagnosing wide-QRS arrhythmias, whereas the use of lead II, a limb lead commonly used for continuous monitoring, resulted in only 34% being correctly identified.

Although accurate ECG placement and lead selection are important aspects of ECG monitoring, two national surveys conducted in 1991 and 1995, respectively,[10,11] identified two common errors: inaccurate electrode placement and inappropriate lead selection for individual clinical situations. Improper lead placement can significantly change QRS morphology, resulting in misdiagnosis of cardiac arrhythmias or failure to detect existing conduction defects.

In persons with acute coronary syndromes (ACS), including unstable angina and ST-segment elevation and non–ST-segment elevation myocardial infarction, careful cardiac ECG monitoring is imperative[12] (see Chapter 24). Persons with ACS are at risk for development of extension of an infarcted area, ongoing myocardial ischemia, and life-threatening arrhythmias. Research has revealed that 80% to 90% of ECG-detected ischemic events are clinically silent.[13] Thus, ECG monitoring is more sensitive than a patient's report of symptoms for identifying transient ongoing myocardial ischemia. ECG monitoring also provides for more accurate and timely detection of ischemic events, essential for treatment options such as reperfusion strategies.[14] It is recommended that all 12 ECG leads be used for monitoring patients with ACS because ischemic changes that occur may be evident in different leads at different times.

The American Heart Association recently published practice standards for ECG monitoring in hospital settings.[15] This working group used the rating system devised by the American College of Cardiology Emergency Cardiac Care Committee.[16] This rating system includes three categories:

- Class I—cardiac monitoring is necessary in most, if not all, patients in this group.
- Class II—cardiac monitoring may be beneficial in some patients, but it is not an essential component of care for these patients.
- Class III—cardiac monitoring is not indicated because the risk of a serious event for these patients is so low that monitoring is not viewed as therapeutic.

Examples of patients categorized as class I are those who have been resuscitated from a cardiac arrest, are in the early phase of ACS, have unstable coronary syndromes or newly diagnosed high-risk coronary lesions, or have undergone cardiac surgery within the past 48 to 72 hours. In addition, recommendations for staffing, training, documentation, and approaches for improving quality of ECG monitoring were presented. It is recommended that these practice standards be adhered to when making determinations about ECG monitoring.

IN SUMMARY, the rhythmic contraction and relaxation of the heart rely on the specialized cells of the heart's conduction system. Specialized cells in the SA node have the fastest inherent rate of impulse generation and act as the pacemaker of the heart. Impulses from the SA node travel through the atria to the AV node and then to the AV bundle and the ventricular Purkinje system. The AV node provides the only connection between the atrial and ventricular conduction systems. The atria and the ventricles function independently of each other when AV node conduction is blocked.

Action potentials represent the sequential changes in electrical potentials that are associated with the movement of current-carrying ions through ion channels in the cell membrane. The action potentials of cardiac muscle are divided into five phases: phase 0 represents depolarization and is characterized by the rapid upstroke of the action potential; phase 1 is characterized by a brief period of repolarization; phase 2 consists of a plateau, which prolongs the duration of the action potential; phase 3 represents repolarization; and phase 4 is the resting membrane potential. After an action potential, there is a refractory period during which the membrane is resistant to a second stimulus. During the absolute refractory period, the membrane is insensitive to stimulation. This period is followed by the relative refractory period, during which a more intense stimulus is needed to initiate an action potential. The relative refractory period is followed by a supernormal excitatory period, during which a weak stimulus can evoke a response.

The ECG provides a means for monitoring the electrical activity of the heart. Conventionally, 12 leads (6 limb leads and 6 chest leads) are recorded for a diagnostic ECG, each providing a unique view of the electrical forces of the heart from a different position on the body's surface. This procedure allows for advanced arrhythmia detection, detection of wide–QRS-complex tachycardia, and early identification of ischemia- and infarction-related changes in persons with ACS. ∎

DISORDERS OF CARDIAC RHYTHM AND CONDUCTION

After completing this section of the chapter, you should be able to meet the following objectives:

- Describe the possible mechanisms for arrhythmia generation.
- Compare sinus arrhythmias with atrial arrhythmias.

- Characterize the effects of atrial flutter and atrial fibrillation on heart rhythm.
- Describe the significance of long QT syndrome.
- Describe the characteristics of first-, second-, and third-degree heart block.
- Compare the effects of premature ventricular contractions, ventricular tachycardia, and ventricular fibrillation on cardiac function.
- Cite the types of cardiac conditions that can be diagnosed using the ECG.
- Describe the methods used in diagnosis of cardiac arrhythmias.
- Explain the mechanisms, criteria for use, and benefits of antiarrhythmic drugs, internal cardioverter-defibrillator therapy, ablation therapy, and surgical procedures in the treatment of persons with recurrent, symptomatic arrhythmias.

There are two types of disorders of the cardiac conduction system: disorders of rhythm and disorders of impulse conduction. The terms *dysrhythmia* and *arrhythmia* have sometimes been used interchangeably to describe disorders of cardiac rhythm. Marriott[17] has pointed out that the term *arrhythmia* was originally based on the inaccurate usage of the alpha privative (the prefix *a-*) to imply "imperfection in" as opposed to "absence of" cardiac rhythms. However, Marriott[17] further pointed out that the term *dysrhythmia* has not been generally accepted and conventional use of the term *arrhythmia* continues. Therefore, the term *arrhythmia* is used throughout this chapter.

There are many causes of cardiac arrhythmias and conduction disorders, including congenital defects or degenerative changes in the conduction system, myocardial ischemia and infarction, fluid and electrolyte imbalances, and the effects of pharmacologic agents. Arrhythmias are not necessarily pathologic; they can occur in both healthy and diseased hearts. Disturbances in cardiac rhythms exert their harmful effects by interfering with the heart's pumping ability. Excessively rapid heart rates (tachyarrhythmias) reduce the diastolic filling time, causing a subsequent decrease in the stroke volume output and in coronary perfusion while increasing the myocardial oxygen needs. Abnormally slow heart rates (bradyarrhythmias) may impair blood flow to vital organs such as the brain.

Mechanisms of Arrhythmias and Conduction Disorders

The specialized cells in the conduction system manifest four inherent properties that contribute to the genesis of all cardiac rhythms, both normal and abnormal. They are automaticity, excitability, conductivity, and refractoriness. An alteration in any of these four properties may produce arrhythmias or conduction defects.

The ability of certain cells in the conduction system spontaneously to initiate an impulse or action potential is referred

PHYSIOLOGIC BASIS OF ARRHYTHMIA GENERATION

- Cardiac arrhythmias represent disorders of cardiac rhythm related to alterations in automaticity, excitability, conductivity, or refractoriness of specialized cells in the conduction system of the heart.

- Automaticity refers to the ability of pacemaker cells in the heart to spontaneously generate an action potential. Normally, the SA node is the pacemaker of the heart because of its intrinsic automaticity.

- Excitability is the ability of cardiac tissue to respond to an impulse and generate an action potential.

- Conductivity and refractoriness represent the ability of cardiac tissue to conduct action potentials.

- Whereas conductivity relates to the ability of cardiac tissue to conduct impulses, refractoriness represents temporary interruptions in conductivity related to the repolarization phase of the action potential.

to as *automaticity*. The SA node has an inherent discharge rate of 60 to 100 times per minute. It normally acts as the pacemaker of the heart because it reaches the threshold for excitation before other parts of the conduction system have recovered sufficiently to be depolarized. If the SA node fires more slowly or SA node conduction is blocked, another site that is capable of automaticity takes over as pacemaker. Other regions that are capable of automaticity include the atrial fibers that have plateau-type action potentials, the AV node, the bundle of His, and the bundle branch Purkinje fibers. These pacemakers have a slower rate of discharge than the SA node. The AV node has an inherent firing rate of 40 to 60 times per minute, and the Purkinje system fires at a rate of 15 to 40 times per minute. The SA node may be functioning properly, but because of additional precipitating factors, other cardiac cells can assume accelerated properties of automaticity and begin to initiate impulses. These additional factors might include injury, hypoxia, electrolyte disturbances, enlargement or hypertrophy of the atria or ventricles, and exposure to certain chemicals or drugs.

An *ectopic pacemaker* is an excitable focus outside the normally functioning SA node. These pacemakers can reside in other parts of the conduction system or in muscle cells of the atria or ventricles. A premature contraction occurs when an ectopic pacemaker initiates a beat. Premature contractions do not follow the normal conduction pathways, they are not coupled with normal mechanical events, and they often render the heart refractory or incapable of responding to the next normal impulse arising in the SA node. They occur without incident in persons with healthy hearts in response to sympathetic nervous system stimulation or other stimulants, such as caffeine. In the diseased heart, premature contractions may lead to more serious arrhythmias.

Excitability describes the ability of a cell to respond to an impulse and generate an action potential. Myocardial cells that have been injured or replaced by scar tissue do not possess normal excitability. For example, during the acute phase of an ischemic event, involved cells become depolarized. These ischemic cells remain electrically coupled to the adjacent nonischemic area; current from the ischemic zone can induce reexcitation of cells in the nonischemic zone.

Conductivity is the ability to conduct impulses, and *refractoriness* refers to the extent to which the cell is able to respond to an incoming stimulus. The refractory period of cardiac muscle is the interval in the repolarization period during which an excitable cell has not recovered sufficiently to be reexcited. Disturbances in conductivity or refractoriness predispose to arrhythmias.

Almost all tachyarrhythmias are the result of a phenomenon known as *reentry*.[4,7,18] Under normal conditions, an electrical impulse is conducted through the heart in an orderly, sequential manner. The electrical impulse then dies out and does not reenter adjacent tissue because that tissue has already been depolarized and is refractory to immediate stimulation. However, fibers that were not activated during the initial wave of depolarization can recover excitability before the initial impulse dies out, and they may serve as a link to reexcite areas of the heart that were just discharged and have recovered from the initial depolarization.[1] This activity disrupts the normal conduction sequence. For reentry to occur, there must be areas of slow conduction and a unidirectional conduction block (Fig. 25-8). For previously depolarized areas to repolarize adequately to conduct an impulse again, slow conduction is necessary. Uni-

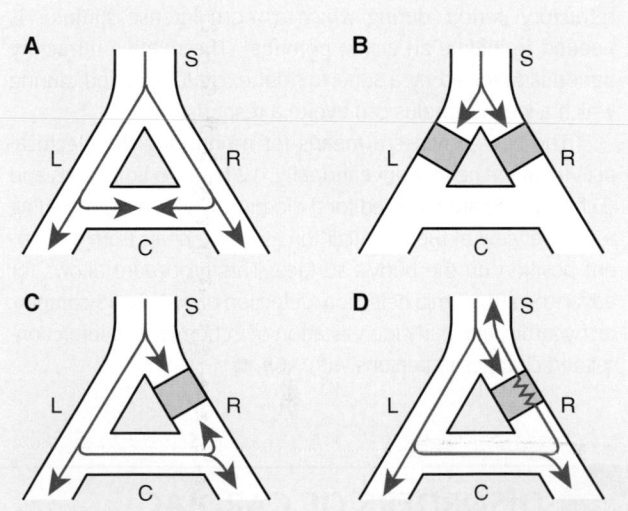

FIGURE 25-8 • The role of unidirectional block in reentry. **(A)** An excitation wave traveling down a single bundle (S) of fibers continues down the left (L) and right (R) branches. The depolarization wave enters the connecting branch (C) from both ends and is extinguished at the zone of collision. **(B)** The wave is blocked in the L and R branches. **(C)** Bidirectional block exists in the R branch. **(D)** The antegrade impulse is blocked, but the retrograde impulse is conducted through and reenters bundle S. (From Berne R. M., Levy M. N. [1988]. *Physiology* [2nd ed., p. 417]. St. Louis: C.V. Mosby.)

directional block is necessary to provide a one-way route for the original impulse to reenter, thereby blocking other impulses entering from the opposite direction from extinguishing the reentrant circuit.[4] Reentry requires a triggering stimulus such as an extrasystole. If sufficient time has elapsed for the refractory period in the reentered area to end, a self-perpetuating, circuitous movement can be initiated.[1]

Reentry may occur anywhere in the conduction system. The functional components of a reentry circuit can be large and include an entire specialized conduction system, or the circuit can be microscopic. It can include myocardial tissue, AV nodal cells, junctional tissue, or the ventricles. Factors contributing to the development of a reentrant circuit include ischemia, infarction, and elevated serum potassium levels.[19] Scar tissue interrupts the normally low-resistance paths between viable myocardial cells, slowing conduction, promoting asynchronous myocardial activation, and predisposing to unidirectional conduction block. Specially filtered signal-averaged electrocardiography can be used to detect the resultant late potentials. Effects of drugs such as epinephrine can produce a shortened refractory period, thereby increasing the likelihood of reentrant arrhythmias.

There are several forms of reentry. The first is anatomic reentry. It involves an anatomic obstacle around which the circulating current must pass and results in an excitation wave that travels in a set pathway.[1,20] Arrhythmias that arise as a result of anatomic reentry are paroxysmal supraventricular tachycardias, as seen in Wolff-Parkinson-White syndrome, atrial fibrillation, atrial flutter, AV nodal reentry, and some ventricular tachycardias. Functional reentry does not rely on an anatomic structure to circle, but instead depends on the local differences in conduction velocity and refractoriness among neighboring fibers that allow an impulse to circulate repeatedly around an area.[1,21,22] Spiral reentry is the most common form of this type of reentry.[21,22] It is initiated by a wave of current that does not propagate normally after meeting refractory tissue. The broken end of the wave curls, forms a vortex, and permanently rotates. This phenomenon suppresses normal pacemaker activity and can result in atrial fibrillation.[22,23] Arrhythmias observed with functional reentry are likely to be polymorphic because of changing circuits.[1] Reflection is sometimes considered another form of reentry that can occur in parallel pathways of myocardial tissue or the Purkinje network. With reflection, the cardiac impulse reaches an area of depressed conduction, triggers the surrounding tissue, and then returns in a retrograde direction through the severely depressed region. Reflection differs from true reentry in that the impulse travels along the same pathway in both directions and does not require a circuit.[1]

Types of Arrhythmias and Conduction Disorders

Sinus Node Arrhythmias

In a healthy heart driven by sinus node discharge, the rate ranges between 60 and 100 beats per minute. On the ECG, a P wave may be observed to precede every QRS complex. Historically,

normal sinus rhythm has been considered the "normal" rhythm of a healthy heart. In normal sinus rhythm, a P wave precedes each QRS complex and the RR intervals remain relatively constant over time (Fig. 25-9). Alterations in the function of the SA node lead to changes in rate or rhythm of the heartbeat.

Years ago, it was believed that sinus rhythm should be regular—that is, all RR intervals should be equal. Today, it is accepted that a more optimal rhythm is respiratory sinus arrhythmia. Respiratory sinus arrhythmia is a cardiac rhythm characterized by gradual lengthening and shortening of RR intervals (see Fig. 25-9). This variation in cardiac cycles is related to intrathoracic pressure changes that occur with respiration and resultant alterations in autonomic control of the SA node. Inspiration causes acceleration of the heart rate, and expiration causes slowing. Respiratory sinus arrhythmia accounts for most heart rate variability in healthy individuals. Decreased heart rate variability has been associated with altered health states, including myocardial infarction, congestive heart failure, hypertension, diabetes mellitus, and prematurity in infants.

Sinus Bradycardia. Sinus bradycardia describes a slow (<60 beats per minute) heart rate (see Fig. 25-9). In sinus bradycardia, a P wave precedes each QRS. A normal P wave and PR interval (0.12 to 0.20 second) indicates that the impulse

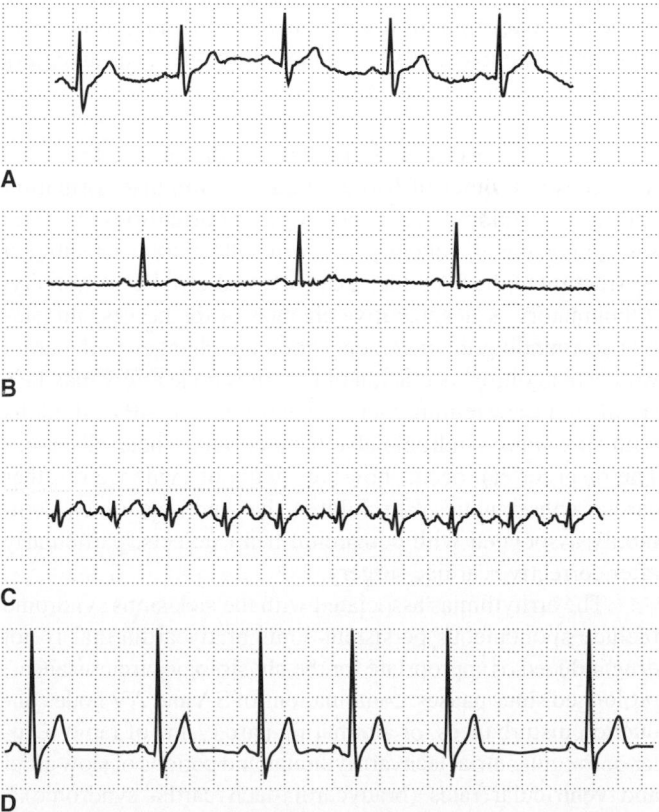

FIGURE 25-9 • Electrocardiographic tracings of rhythms originating in the sinus node. **(A)** Normal sinus rhythm (60 to 100 beats/minute). **(B)** Sinus bradycardia (<60 beats/minute). **(C)** Sinus tachycardia (>100 beats/minute). **(D)** Respiratory sinus arrhythmia, characterized by gradual lengthening and shortening of RR intervals.

originated in the SA node rather than in another area of the conduction system that has a slower inherent rate. Vagal stimulation decreases the firing rate of the SA node and conduction through the AV node to cause a decrease in heart rate. This rhythm may be normal in trained athletes, who maintain a large stroke volume, and during sleep. Sinus bradycardia may be an indicator of poor prognosis when it occurs in conjunction with acute myocardial infarction, particularly if associated with hypotension.

Sinus Tachycardia. Sinus tachycardia refers to a rapid heart rate (>100 beats per minute) that has its origin in the SA node (see Fig. 25-9). A normal P wave and PR interval should precede each QRS complex. The mechanism of sinus tachycardia is enhanced automaticity related to sympathetic stimulation or withdrawal of vagal tone. Sinus tachycardia is a normal response during fever and exercise, and in situations that incite sympathetic stimulation. It may be associated with congestive heart failure, myocardial infarction, and hyperthyroidism. Pharmacologic agents such as atropine, isoproterenol, epinephrine, and quinidine also can cause sinus tachycardia.

Sinus Arrest. Sinus arrest refers to failure of the SA node to discharge and results in an irregular pulse. An escape rhythm develops as another pacemaker takes over. Sinus arrest may result in prolonged periods of asystole and often predisposes to other arrhythmias. Causes of sinus arrest include disease of the SA node, digitalis toxicity, myocardial infarction, acute myocarditis, excessive vagal tone, quinidine, lidocaine, and hyperkalemia or hypokalemia.[24–27]

Sick Sinus Syndrome. Sick sinus syndrome is a term that describes a number of forms of cardiac impulse formation and intra-atrial and AV conduction abnormalities.[28–31] The syndrome most frequently is the result of total or subtotal destruction of the SA node, areas of nodal-atrial discontinuity, inflammatory or degenerative changes of the nerves and ganglia surrounding the node, or pathologic changes in the atrial wall.[30] In addition, occlusion of the sinus node artery may be a significant contributing factor. Approximately 40% of adults with sick sinus syndrome also have coronary heart disease.[32] The disorder can occur, however, without evidence of other cardiac abnormalities.[30] In children, the syndrome is most commonly associated with congenital heart defects, particularly after corrective cardiac surgery.[30]

The arrhythmias associated with the sick sinus syndrome include spontaneous persistent sinus bradycardia that is not drug induced or appropriate for the physiologic circumstances, prolonged sinus pauses, combinations of SA and AV node conduction disturbances, or alternating paroxysms of rapid regular or irregular atrial tachyarrhythmias and periods of slow atrial and ventricular rates (bradycardia-tachycardia syndrome).[33] Most commonly, the term *sick sinus syndrome* is used to refer to the bradycardia-tachycardia syndrome. The bradycardia is caused by disease of the sinus node (or other intra-atrial conduction pathways), and the tachycardia is caused by paroxysmal

atrial or junctional arrhythmias. Individuals with this syndrome often are asymptomatic. Ironically, the development of atrial fibrillation may alleviate symptoms in persons who are symptomatic because heart rate can be controlled more consistently under these circumstances.[29]

The most common manifestations of sick sinus syndrome are lightheadedness, dizziness, and syncope, and these symptoms are related to the bradyarrhythmias.[32,34] When persons with sick sinus syndrome experience palpitations, they are generally the result of tachyarrhythmias and are suggestive of the presence of bradycardia-tachycardia syndrome.[32]

Treatment depends on the rhythm problem and frequently involves the implantation of a permanent pacemaker. Pacing for the bradycardia, combined with drug therapy to treat the tachycardia, often is required in the bradycardia-tachycardia syndrome.[30] Medications that affect SA node discharge must be used cautiously.

⚡ SUPRAVENTRICULAR AND VENTRICULAR ARRHYTHMIAS

- Supraventricular arrhythmias represent disorders of atrial rhythm or conduction.

- Atrioventricular nodal and junctional arrhythmias result from disruption in conduction of impulses from the atria to the ventricles.

- Ventricular arrhythmias represent disorders of ventricular rhythm or conduction.

- Because the ventricles are pumping chambers of the heart, arrhythmias that produce an abnormally slow (*e.g.,* heart block) or rapid ventricular rate (*e.g.,* ventricular tachycardia or fibrillation) are potentially life threatening.

Arrhythmias of Atrial Origin

Impulses from the SA node pass through the conductive pathways in the atria to the AV node. Arrhythmias of atrial origin include premature atrial contractions, paroxysmal supraventricular tachycardia, atrial flutter, and atrial fibrillation (Fig. 25-10).

Premature Atrial Contractions. Premature atrial contractions (PACs) are contractions that originate in the atrial conduction pathways or atrial muscle cells and occur before the next expected SA node impulse. This impulse to contract usually is transmitted to the ventricle and back to the SA node. The location of the ectopic focus determines the configuration of the P wave. In general, the closer the ectopic focus is to the SA node, the more the ectopic complex resembles a normal sinus complex. The retrograde transmission to the SA node often interrupts the timing of the next sinus beat, such that a pause occurs between the two normally conducted beats. In

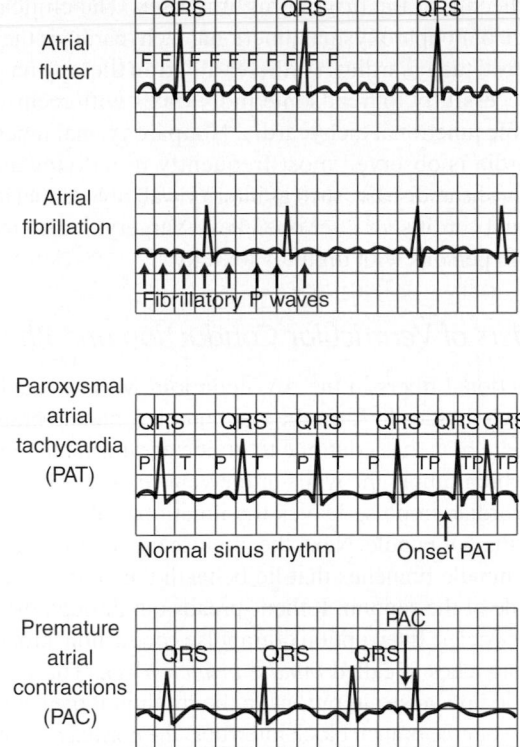

FIGURE 25-10 • Electrocardiographic tracings of atrial arrhythmias. Atrial flutter (*first tracing*) is characterized by the atrial flutter (F) waves occurring at a rate of 240 to 450 beats per minute. The ventricular rate remains regular because of the conduction of every sixth atrial contraction. Atrial fibrillation (*second tracing*) has grossly disorganized atrial electrical activity that is irregular with respect to rate and rhythm. The ventricular response is irregular, and no distinct P waves are visible. The *third tracing* illustrates paroxysmal atrial tachycardia (PAT), preceded by a normal sinus rhythm. The *fourth tracing* illustrates premature atrial complexes (PACs).

healthy individuals, PACs may be the result of stress, tobacco, or caffeine. They also have been associated with myocardial infarction, digitalis toxicity, low serum potassium or magnesium levels, and hypoxia.

Paroxysmal Supraventricular Tachycardia. Paroxysmal supraventricular tachycardia refers to tachyarrhythmias that originate above the bifurcation of the bundle of His and have a sudden onset and termination. The heart rate may be 140 to 240 beats per minute and be perfectly regular despite exercise or change in position. Most persons remain asymptomatic except for an awareness of the rapid heartbeat, but some may experience shortness of breath, especially if the episodes are prolonged. The most common mechanism for paroxysmal supraventricular tachycardia is reentry. It may be the result of AV nodal reentry, Wolff-Parkinson-White syndrome (caused by an accessory conduction pathway between the atria and ventricles), or intra-atrial or sinus node reentry.

Atrial Flutter. Atrial flutter is a rapid atrial ectopic tachycardia, with a rate that ranges from 240 to 450 beats per minute. There are two types of atrial flutter.[29,30] Typical atrial flutter

(sometimes called type I) is the result of a reentry rhythm in the right atrium that can be entrained and interrupted with atrial pacing techniques. The atrial rate in typical type I flutter usually is in the vicinity of 300 beats per minute, but it can range from 240 to 340 beats per minute. Other forms of atrial flutter (*i.e.,* the so-called atypical or type II flutters) are now recognized as distinct types and include atrial macro-reentry caused by surgical scars, idiopathic fibrosis in areas of the atrium, or other anatomic or functional barriers in the atria.[30] Because the barriers that constrain these flutters are variable, the ECG pattern of the atypical flutters can vary. Often, the flutter wave changes morphologically during the same episode of flutter, indicating multiple circuits or nonfixed conduction barriers.[30]

In typical atrial flutter, the ECG reveals a defined sawtooth pattern in leads aVF, V_1, and V_5.[35] The ventricular response rate and regularity are variable and depend on the AV conduction sequence. When regular, the ventricular response rate usually is a defined fraction of the atrial rate (*i.e.,* when conduction from the atria to the ventricles is 2:1, an atrial flutter rate of 300 would result in a ventricular response rate of 150 beats per minute). The QRS complex may be normal or abnormal, depending on the presence or absence of preexisting intraventricular conduction defects or aberrant ventricular conduction.

Atrial flutter rarely is seen in normal, healthy individuals. It may be seen in persons of any age in the presence of underlying atrial abnormalities. Subgroups that are at particularly high risk for development of atrial flutter include children, adolescents, and young adults who have undergone corrective surgery for complex congenital heart diseases.[29]

Atrial Fibrillation. Atrial fibrillation is characterized by chaotic impulses propagating in different directions and causing disorganized atrial depolarizations without effective atrial contraction.[36] In most cases multiple, small reentrant circuits are constantly arising in the atria, colliding, being extinguished, and arising again. Fibrillation occurs when the atrial cells cannot repolarize in time for the next incoming stimulus. Atrial fibrillation is characterized on the ECG by a grossly disorganized pattern of atrial electrical activity that is irregular with respect to rate and rhythm and the absence of discernible P waves. Atrial activity is depicted by fibrillatory (f) waves of varying amplitude, duration, and morphology. These f waves appear as random oscillation of the baseline. Because of the random conduction through the AV node, QRS complexes appear in an irregular pattern.

Atrial fibrillation is the "only common arrhythmia in which the ventricular rate is rapid and the rhythm irregular."[37] The atrial rate typically ranges from 400 to 600 beats/minute, with many impulses blocked at the AV node. The ventricular response is completely irregular ranging from 80 to 180 beats/minute in the untreated state. Because of changes in stroke volumes resulting from varying periods of diastolic filling, not all ventricular beats produce a palpable pulse. The difference between the apical rate and the palpable peripheral pulses is called the *pulse deficit.* The pulse deficit increases when the ventricular rate is high.

Atrial fibrillation may appear paroxysmally or as a chronic phenomenon. It can be seen in persons without any apparent disease, or it may occur in individuals with coronary artery disease, mitral valve disease, ischemic heart disease, hypertension, myocardial infarction, pericarditis, congestive heart failure, digitalis toxicity, and hyperthyroidism. Spontaneous conversion to sinus rhythm within 24 hours of atrial fibrillation is common, occurring in up to two thirds of persons with the disorder.[36] If the duration of atrial fibrillation exceeds 24 hours, the likelihood of conversion decreases, and after 1 week of persistent arrhythmia, spontaneous conversion is rare.[36]

Atrial fibrillation is the most common chronic arrhythmia, with an incidence and prevalence that increase with age. Atrial fibrillation often is considered a benign arrhythmia, but it has been associated with increased mortality after adjustment for other risk factors in both community[38] and patient studies.[39,40] The incidence of chronic atrial fibrillation doubles with each decade of life and ranges from 2 or 3 new cases per year per 1000 persons between 55 and 64 years of age, to 35 new cases per year per 1000 persons between 85 and 95 years of age.[39]

The symptoms of chronic atrial fibrillation vary. Some people have minimal symptoms, and others have severe symptoms, particularly at the onset of the arrhythmia. The symptoms may range from palpitations to acute pulmonary edema. Fatigue and other nonspecific symptoms are common in the elderly. The condition predisposes individuals to thrombus formation in the atria, with subsequent risk of embolic stroke.

The treatment of atrial fibrillation depends on its cause, recency of onset, and persistence. Anticoagulant medications may be used to prevent embolic stroke, and medications (*e.g.,* digitalis, beta blockers) may be used to control the ventricular rate in persons with persistent atrial fibrillation.[39,40] Cardioversion may be considered in some persons, particularly when pulmonary edema or unstable cardiac status is present. Because conversion to sinus rhythm is associated with increased risk of thromboembolism, anticoagulation therapy is usually administered for at least 3 weeks before cardioversion is attempted in persons in whom the duration of atrial fibrillation is unknown or exceeds 2 to 3 days.[39] Transesophageal echocardiography can be used to detect atrial thrombus, and transesophageal echo-guided cardioversion provides a means of ensuring that atrial thrombi are not present when cardioversion is attempted. Anticoagulant medication usually is continued after cardioversion.

Junctional Arrhythmias

The AV node can act as a pacemaker in the event the SA node fails to initiate an impulse. Junctional rhythms can be transient or permanent, and they usually have a rate of 40 to 60 beats per minute. Junctional fibers in the AV node or bundle of His also can serve as ectopic pacemakers, producing premature junctional complexes. Another rhythm originating in the junctional tissues is nonparoxysmal junctional tachycardia. This rhythm usually is of gradual onset and termination. However, it may occur abruptly if the dominant pacemaker slows sufficiently. The rate associated with junctional tachycardia ranges from 70 to 130 beats per minute, but it may be faster.[1] The P waves may precede, be buried in, or follow the QRS complexes, depend-

ing on the site of the originating impulses. The clinical significance of nonparoxysmal junctional tachycardia is the same as for atrial tachycardias. Catheter ablation therapy has been used successfully to treat some individuals with recurrent or intractable junctional tachycardia. Nonparoxysmal junctional tachycardia is observed most frequently in individuals with underlying heart disease, such as inferior wall myocardial infarction or myocarditis, or after open heart surgery. It also may be present in persons with digitalis toxicity.

Disorders of Ventricular Conduction and Rhythm

The junctional fibers in the AV node join with the bundle of His, which divides to form the right and left bundle branches. The bundle branches continue to divide and form the Purkinje fibers, which supply the walls of the ventricles (see Fig. 25-1). As the cardiac impulse leaves the junctional fibers, it travels through the AV bundle. Next, the impulse moves down the right and left bundle branches that lie beneath the endocardium on either side of the septum. It then spreads out through the walls of the ventricles. Interruption of impulse conduction through the bundle branches is called *bundle branch block*. These blocks usually do not cause alterations in the rhythm of the heartbeat. Instead, a bundle branch block interrupts the normal progression of depolarization, causing the ventricles to depolarize one after the other because the impulses must travel through muscle tissue rather than through the specialized conduction tissue. This prolonged conduction causes the QRS complex to be wider than the normal 0.08 to 0.12 second. The left bundle branch bifurcates into the left anterior and posterior fascicles. An interruption of one of these fascicles is referred to as a *hemiblock*.

Long QT Syndrome and Torsades de Pointes

The *long QT syndrome* (LQTS) is characterized by a prolongation of the QT interval that may result in a characteristic type of polymorphic ventricular tachycardia called *torsades de pointes* and sudden cardiac death.[30,41,42] *Torsades de pointes* (*i.e.,* "twisting or rotating around a point") is a specific type of ventricular tachycardia (Fig. 25-11). The term refers to the polarity of the QRS complex, which swings from positive to negative and vice versa. The QRS abnormality is characterized by large, bizarre, polymorphic QRS complexes that vary, often from beat to beat, in amplitude and direction, as well as in rotation of the complexes around the isoelectric line. The rate of tachycardia is 100 to 180, but it can be as fast as 200 to 300 per minute. The rhythm is highly unstable and may terminate in ventricular fibrillation or revert to sinus rhythm.

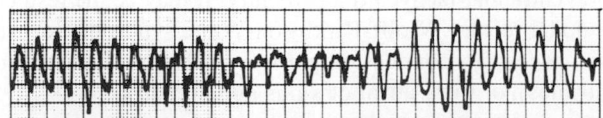

FIGURE 25-11 • Torsades de pointes. (From Hudak C. M., Gallo B. M., Morton P. G. [1998]. *Critical care nursing: A holistic approach* [7th ed., p. 216]. Philadelphia: Lippincott-Raven.)

LQTS can be caused by various agents and conditions that reduce the magnitude of outward repolarizing potassium currents, enhance the magnitude of the inward depolarizing sodium and calcium currents, or both. Thus, there is delayed repolarization of the ventricles with development of early depolarizing afterpotentials that initiate the arrhythmia. Typically, the QT interval is measured in a lead in which the T wave is prominent and its end is easily distinguished, such as V_2 or V_3. Because the QT interval shortens with tachycardia and lengthens with bradycardia, it is typically corrected for heart rate and is noted as QT_c.[43,44] Nonetheless, a QT_c greater than 440 msec in men and greater than 460 msec in women has been linked with episodes of sudden arrhythmia death syndromes. In addition, T-wave morphology frequently is abnormal in patients with LQTS.[1]

LQTSs have been classified into inherited and acquired forms, both of which are associated with the development of torsades de pointes and sudden cardiac death. The hereditary forms of LQTS are caused by disorders of membrane ion channel proteins, with either potassium channel defects or sodium channel defects (to be discussed).[1]

Acquired LQTS has been linked to a variety of conditions, including cocaine use, exposure to organophosphorus compounds, electrolyte imbalances, marked bradycardia, myocardial infarction, subarachnoid hemorrhage, autonomic neuropathy, human immunodeficiency virus infection, and protein-sparing fasting.[41,42,45] Medications linked to LQTS include digitalis, antiarrhythmic agents (*e.g.*, amiodarone, procainamide, and quinidine), verapamil (calcium channel blocker), haloperidol (antipsychotic agent), and erythromycin (antibiotic).[42] The acquired forms of LQTS often are classified as pause-dependent because the torsades de pointes associated with them generally occurs at slow heart rates or in response to short–long–short RR interval sequences. Treatment of acquired forms of LQTS is directed primarily at identifying and withdrawing the offending agent, although emergency measures that modulate the function of transmembrane ion currents can be lifesaving.

Ventricular Arrhythmias

Arrhythmias that arise in the ventricles generally are considered more serious than those that arise in the atria because they afford the potential for interfering with the pumping action of the heart.

Premature Ventricular Contractions. A premature ventricular contraction (PVC) is caused by a ventricular ectopic pacemaker. After a PVC occurs, the ventricle usually is unable to repolarize sufficiently to respond to the next impulse that arises in the SA node. This delay, commonly referred to as a *compensatory pause,* occurs while the ventricle waits to reestablish its previous rhythm (Fig. 25-12). When a PVC occurs, the diastolic volume usually is insufficient for ejection of blood into the arterial system. As a result, PVCs usually do not produce a palpable pulse, or the pulse amplitude is significantly diminished. In the absence of heart disease, PVCs typically are not clinically significant. The incidence of PVCs is greatest with

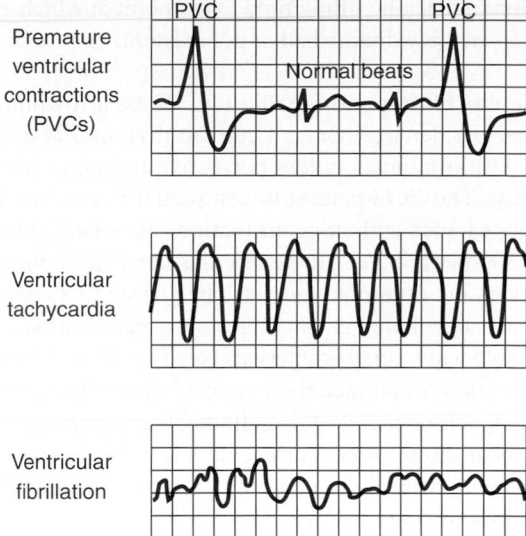

FIGURE 25-12 • Electrocardiographic (ECG) tracings of ventricular arrhythmias. Premature ventricular contractions (PVCs) *(top tracing)* originate from an ectopic focus in the ventricles, causing a distortion of the QRS complex. Because the ventricle usually cannot repolarize sufficiently to respond to the next impulse that arises in the sinoatrial node, a PVC frequently is followed by a compensatory pause. Ventricular tachycardia *(middle tracing)* is characterized by a rapid ventricular rate of 70 to 250 beats per minute and the absence of P waves. In ventricular fibrillation *(bottom tracing)*, there are no regular or effective ventricular contractions, and the ECG tracing is totally disorganized.

ischemia, acute myocardial infarction, history of myocardial infarction, ventricular hypertrophy, infection, increased sympathetic nervous system activity, or increased heart rate.[46] PVCs also can be the result of electrolyte disturbances or medications.

A special pattern of PVC called *ventricular bigeminy* is a condition in which each normal beat is followed by or paired with a PVC. This pattern often is an indication of digitalis toxicity or heart disease. The occurrence of frequent PVCs in the diseased heart predisposes to the development of other, more serious arrhythmias, including ventricular tachycardia and ventricular fibrillation.

Ventricular Tachycardia. Ventricular tachycardia describes a cardiac rhythm originating distal to the bifurcation of the bundle of His, in the specialized conduction system in ventricular muscle, or both.[1] It is characterized by a ventricular rate of 70 to 250 beats per minute, and the onset can be sudden or insidious. Usually, ventricular tachycardia is exhibited electrocardiographically by wide, tall, bizarre-looking QRS complexes that persist longer than 0.12 second (see Fig. 25-12). QRS complexes can be uniform in appearance, or they can vary randomly, in a repetitive manner (*e.g.*, torsades de pointes), in an alternating pattern (*e.g.*, bidirectional), or in a stable but changing fashion. Ventricular tachycardia can be sustained, lasting more than 30 seconds and requiring intervention, or it can be nonsustained and stop spontaneously. This rhythm is dangerous because it eliminates atrial kick and can cause a reduction in diastolic filling time to the point at which cardiac output is severely diminished or nonexistent.

Ventricular Flutter and Fibrillation. These arrhythmias represent severe derangements of cardiac rhythm that terminate fatally within minutes unless corrective measures are taken promptly. The ECG pattern in ventricular flutter has a sine-wave appearance with large oscillations occurring at a rate of 150 to 300 per minute.[30] In ventricular fibrillation, the ventricle quivers but does not contract. The classic ECG pattern of ventricular fibrillation is that of gross disorganization without identifiable waveforms or intervals (see Fig. 25-12). When the ventricles do not contract, there is no cardiac output, and there are no palpable or audible pulses. Immediate defibrillation using a nonsynchronized, direct-current electrical shock is mandatory for ventricular fibrillation and for ventricular flutter that has caused loss of consciousness.[30]

Disorders of Atrioventricular Conduction

Under normal conditions, the AV junction, which consists of the AV node with its connections to the entering atrial internodal pathways, the AV bundle, and the nonbranching portion of the bundle of His, provides the only connection for transmission of impulses between the atrial and ventricular conduction systems. Junctional fibers in the AV node have high-resistance characteristics that cause a delay in the transmission of impulses from the atria to the ventricles. This delay provides optimal timing for the atrial contribution to ventricular filling and protects the ventricles from abnormally rapid rates that arise in the atria. Conduction defects of the AV node are most commonly associated with fibrosis or scar tissue in fibers of the conduction system. Conduction defects also may result from medications, including digoxin, β-adrenergic blocking agents, calcium channel blocking agents, and class 1A antiarrhythmic agents.[47] Additional contributing factors include electrolyte imbalances, inflammatory disease, or cardiac surgery.

Heart block refers to abnormalities of impulse conduction. It may be normal, physiologic (*e.g.,* vagal tone), or pathologic. It may occur in the AV nodal fibers or in the AV bundle (*i.e.,* bundle of His), which is continuous with the Purkinje conduction system that supplies the ventricles. The PR interval on the ECG corresponds with the time it takes for the cardiac impulse to travel from the SA node to the ventricular pathways. Normally, the PR interval ranges from 0.12 to 0.20 second.

First-Degree AV Block. First-degree AV block is characterized by a prolonged PR interval (>0.20 second; Fig. 25-13). The prolonged PR interval indicates delayed AV conduction, but all atrial impulses are conducted to the ventricles. This condition usually produces a regular atrial and ventricular rhythm. Clinically significant PR interval prolongation can result from conduction delays in the AV node itself, the His-Purkinje system, or both.[1] When the QRS complex is normal in contour and duration, the AV delay almost always occurs in the AV node and rarely in the bundle of His. In contrast, when the QRS

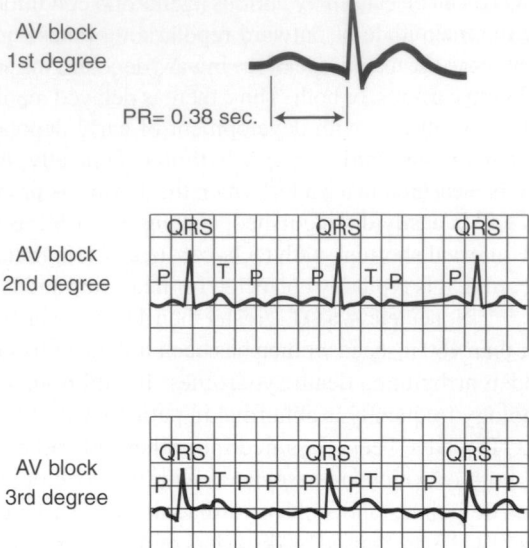

FIGURE 25-13 • Electrocardiographic changes that occur with alterations in atrioventricular (AV) node conduction. The *top tracing* shows the prolongation of the PR interval, which is characteristic of first-degree AV block. The *middle tracing* illustrates Mobitz-type II second-degree AV block, in which the conduction of one or more P waves is blocked. In third-degree AV block *(bottom tracing),* impulses conducted through the AV node are completely blocked, and the atria and ventricles develop their own rates of impulse generation.

complex is prolonged, showing a bundle branch block pattern, conduction delays may be in the AV node or the His-Purkinje system. First-degree block may be the result of disease in the AV node, such as ischemia or infarction, or of infections such as rheumatic fever or myocarditis.[48,49] Isolated first-degree heart block usually is not symptomatic, and temporary or permanent cardiac pacing is not indicated.

Second-Degree AV Block. Second-degree AV block is characterized by intermittent failure of conduction of one or more impulses from the atria to the ventricles. The nonconducted P wave can appear intermittently or frequently. A distinguishing feature of second-degree AV block is that conducted P waves relate to QRS complexes with recurring PR intervals; that is, the association of P waves with QRS complexes is not random.[1] Second-degree AV block has been divided into two types: type I (*i.e.,* Mobitz type I or Wenckebach phenomenon) and type II (*i.e.,* Mobitz type II). A *Mobitz type I* AV block is characterized by progressive lengthening of the PR interval until an impulse is blocked and the sequence begins again. It frequently occurs in persons with inferior wall myocardial infarction, particularly with concomitant right ventricular infarction.[1] The condition usually is associated with an adequate ventricular rate and rarely is symptomatic. It usually is transient and does not require temporary pacing.[29] In the *Mobitz type II* AV block, an intermittent block of atrial impulses occurs, with a constant PR interval (see Fig. 25-13). It frequently accompanies anterior wall myocardial infarction and can require temporary or permanent pacing. This condition is associated with a high mortality rate. In addition, Mobitz type II AV block is associated with other types of organic heart disease and often progresses to complete heart block.

Third-Degree AV Block. Third-degree, or complete AV block, occurs when the conduction link between the atria and ventricles is lost, resulting in atrial and ventricular depolarization being controlled by separate pacemakers (see Fig. 25-13). The atrial pacemaker can be sinus or ectopic in origin. The ventricular pacemaker usually is located just below the region of the block. The atria usually continue to beat at a normal rate and the ventricles develop their own rate, which normally is slow (30 to 40 beats per minute). The atrial and ventricular rates are regular but dissociated. Third-degree AV block can result from an interruption at the level of the AV node, in the bundle of His, or in the Purkinje system. Third-degree blocks at the level of the AV node usually are congenital, whereas blocks in the Purkinje system usually are acquired. Normal QRS complexes, with rates ranging from 40 to 60 complexes per minute, usually are displayed on the ECG when the block occurs proximal to the bundle of His.

Complete heart block causes a decrease in cardiac output with possible periods of syncope (fainting), known as a *Stokes-Adams attack.*[1] Other symptoms include dizziness, fatigue, exercise intolerance, or episodes of acute heart failure.[30] Most persons with complete heart block require a permanent cardiac pacemaker.

Inherited Types of Arrhythmias

Cardiac arrhythmias most commonly occur in the presence of cardiac disease, electrolyte disorders, or other demonstrable abnormalities. Ischemic heart disease is the primary cause for the development of ventricular fibrillation, and structural heart defects such as hypertrophic and dilated cardiomyopathies account for most of the remaining cases. However, in victims of what for many years was referred to as *idiopathic ventricular fibrillation,* structural abnormalities were present at autopsy in only 5% to 10% of cases.[50] Over the past several decades, considerable evidence has been collected indicating that these cases are genetically determined abnormalities of proteins in the ion channels that control the electrical activity of the heart. At least nine genes have been associated with inherited arrhythmogenic cardiomyopathies (see Chapter 24), and it is expected that more will be identified and linked to sudden death in persons with apparently healthy hearts.[50] Among the inherited arrhythmogenic disorders are congenital LQTS, Brugada syndrome, and catecholamine polymorphic ventricular tachycardia.

Congenital Long QT Syndrome. Congenital LQTS is an inherited arrhythmogenic disease characterized by life-threatening ventricular arrhythmias. Two major forms of LQTS have been identified, one transmitted as an autosomal dominant trait (Romano-Ward syndrome) and the second as an autosomal recessive trait in which the cardiac phenotype is accompanied by neurosensory deafness (Jervell and Lange-Neilsen syndrome).[50,51]

The ECG marker for LQTS consists of a prolonged QT interval, abnormal morphology of the T wave, and a characteristic polymorphic ventricular tachycardia (torsades de pointes). Onset of symptoms is typically in the first two decades of life, including the neonatal period, where it can be misdiagnosed as sudden infant death.[50] The severity of the clinical manifestations in LQTS varies, ranging from full-blown disease with marked prolongation of the QT interval and recurrent syncope to subclinical forms with borderline QT interval prolongation and no arrhythmias or syncopal episodes.

The hereditary forms of LQTS are typically considered adrenergic dependent because they are generally triggered by increased activity of the sympathetic nervous system.[41,50] Long-term treatment with β-adrenergic receptor blockers, permanent pacing, or left cardiac sympathetic denervation is frequently effective.[50] Placement of an implantable cardioverter-defibrillator is recommended for persons in whom recurrent syncope, sustained ventricular arrhythmias, or sudden cardiac arrest occurs despite drug treatment.

Brugada Syndrome. First described in 1992, Brugada syndrome is an autosomal dominant disorder characterized by ST segment elevation in precordial leads V_1 to V_3, right bundle branch block, and susceptibility to ventricular tachycardia.[50] It has so far been associated with a single gene encoding for the cardiac sodium channel. The disorder typically manifests in adulthood with very incomplete penetrance, and a high percentage of mutation carriers are asymptomatic.[51] Cardiac events typically occur during sleep or rest. Even though the disorder is inherited as an autosomal trait, a male-to-female ratio of 8:1 is observed in clinical manifestations.[50]

Catecholaminergic Polymorphic Ventricular Tachycardia. Catecholaminergic polymorphic ventricular tachycardia (CPVT) was first described in 1978.[50] It was reported that the disorder was characterized by ventricular tachycardia, syncope, and sudden death occurring in familial or sporadic cases in the absence of cardiac disease or ECG abnormalities.

The ECG of persons with CPVT is usually remarkably normal with the exception of sinus bradycardia reported in some persons. Physical activity and acute emotions are the specific triggers for arrhythmias in persons with CPVT. The complexity of the arrhythmias progressively increases with an increase in workload, from isolated premature beats to bigeminy to runs of ventricular tachycardia. Although clinical diagnosis of CPVT is rather elusive because of the absence of abnormal ECG findings, genetic analysis can identify the mutations in approximately 70% of persons with the disorder.[50] This is particularly important because if left untreated, the disorder is highly malignant, but the prognosis improves considerably once the disorder is correctly identified and treatment is implemented.[51]

Antiadrenergic treatment with beta blockers is the cornerstone of therapy for CPVT. The use of an implantable cardioverter-defibrillator may be necessary when exercise stress testing and Holter monitoring indicate that beta blockers do not provide complete arrhythmia protection.[50]

Diagnostic Methods

The diagnosis of disorders of cardiac rhythm and conduction usually is made on the basis of the surface ECG. Further clarification of conduction defects and cardiac arrhythmias can be obtained using electrophysiologic studies.

A resting surface ECG records the impulses originating in the heart as they are recorded at the body surface. These impulses are recorded for a limited time and during periods of inactivity. Although there are no complications related to the procedure, errors related to misdiagnosis may result in iatrogenic heart disease.[2] The resting ECG is the first approach to the clinical diagnosis of disorders of cardiac rhythm and conduction, but it is limited to events that occur during the period the ECG is being monitored.

Signal-Averaged Electrocardiogram

Signal-averaged ECG is a special type of ECG that is used to detect ventricular late action potentials that are thought to originate from slow-conducting areas of the myocardium.[52] Ventricular late action potentials are low-amplitude, high-frequency waveforms in the terminal QRS complex, and they persist for tens of milliseconds into the ST segment. The presence of late potentials indicates high risk for development of ventricular tachycardia and sudden cardiac death. These late potentials are detectable from leads of the surface ECG when signal averaging is performed.

The intent of signal averaging is reduction of noise that makes surface ECG analysis more difficult to interpret. This technique averages multiple samples of QRS waveforms and creates a tracing that is an average of all the repetitive signals. Signal averaging can be carried out by using either temporal or spatial averaging. Both approaches are based on the assumption that the noise is random and that the signal of interest is coherent and repetitive.[20] As a result, when several inputs that represent the same event are combined, the coherent signal will be reinforced and the noise will cancel itself.

Temporal averaging frequently is referred to as signal averaging. Most studies use temporal averaging as opposed to spatial averaging because it affords greater noise reduction. Six standard bipolar orthogonal leads and one ground are typically used over a large number of beats (generally 100 or more). Theoretically, this method allows for noise reduction by a factor of 10 or more.[20] The implicit assumption underlying signal averaging is that the waveform is repetitive and can be captured without loss of beat-to-beat synchronization.

Spatial averaging uses anywhere from 4 to 16 electrodes,[53] and inputs are averaged to provide noise reduction. The degree of noise reduction is limited by the number of electrodes that can be placed, the potential that closely spaced electrodes will respond to a common noise source and not cancel effectively,

and the theoretical limit of a two- to fourfold reduction in noise.[20] The advantage of using spatial averaging is that it enhances the ability to obtain a signal-averaged ECG from a single beat, thereby permitting beat-to-beat analysis of transient events and complex arrhythmias.

Signal averaging is a computer-based process. Each electrode input is amplified, its voltage is sampled or measured at intervals of 1 msec or less, and each sample is converted into a digital number with at least 12-bit precision.[54] The ECG waveform is converted from an analog waveform to digital numbers that become a computer-readable ECG.

Holter Monitoring

Holter monitoring is one form of long-term monitoring during which a person wears a device that digitally records two or three ECG leads for up to 48 hours. During this time, the person keeps a diary of his or her activities or symptoms, which later are correlated with the ECG recording. Most recording devices also have an event marker button that can be pressed when the individual experiences symptoms, which assists the technician or physician in correlating the diary, symptoms, and ECG changes during analysis. Newer Holter recorders are capable of providing a derived 12-lead ECG. Holter monitoring is useful for documenting arrhythmias, conduction abnormalities, and ST segment changes. The interpretative accuracy of long-term Holter recordings varies with the system used and clinician expertise. Most computer software packages used to scan Holter recordings are sufficiently accurate to meet clinical demand. The majority of patients who have ischemic heart disease exhibit PVCs, particularly those who have recently experienced myocardial infarction.[55] The frequency of PVCs increases progressively over the first several weeks, and decreases approximately 6 months postinfarction. Holter recordings also are used to determine antiarrhythmic drug efficacy, episodes of myocardial ischemia, QT prolongation, and heart rate variability.

Intermittent ECG recorders also are used in the diagnosis of arrhythmias and conduction defects. There are two basic types of recorders that perform this type of monitoring.[55] The first continuously monitors rhythm and is programmed to recognize abnormalities. In the second variety, the unit does not continuously monitor the ECG and therefore cannot automatically recognize abnormalities. The latter form relies on the person to activate the unit when he or she is symptomatic. The data are stored in memory or transmitted telephonically to an ECG receiver, where they are recorded. These types of ECG recordings are useful in persons who have transient symptoms.

Exercise Stress Testing

The exercise stress test elicits the body's response to measured increases in acute exercise (see Chapter 24). This technique provides information about changes in heart rate, blood pressure, respiration, and perceived level of exercise. It is useful in determining exercise-induced alterations in hemodynamic response and ECG ischemic-type ST segment changes, and can detect and classify disturbances in cardiac rhythm and conduction associated with exercise. These changes are indicative of a poorer prognosis in persons with known coronary disease and recent myocardial infarction.

Electrophysiologic Studies

Electrophysiologic testing is used for the diagnosis and management of complex arrhythmias. It involves the passage of two or more electrode catheters into the right side of the heart. These catheters are inserted into the femoral, subclavian, internal jugular, or antecubital veins and positioned with fluoroscopy into the high right atrium near the sinus node, the area of the His bundle, the coronary sinus that lies in the posterior AV groove, and into the right ventricle.[6] The electrode catheters are used to stimulate the heart and record intracardiac ECGs. During the study, overdrive pacing, cardioversion, or defibrillation may be necessary to terminate tachycardia induced during the stimulation procedures.

The primary indications for electrophysiologic testing are to determine a person's potential for arrhythmia formation; evaluate recurrent syncope of cardiac origin, when ambulatory ECG has not provided the diagnosis; differentiate supraventricular from ventricular arrhythmias; and locate arrhythmogenic foci for therapeutic interventions such as catheter ablation procedures or antitachycardia devices.[37] Testing can also define reproducible arrhythmia induction characteristics and hence can be used to evaluate the therapeutic efficacy of a particular treatment modality.

Electrophysiologic methods can also be used as interventions. These interventions may include pacing a person out of tachycardia or ablation therapy. Ablation therapy involves the destruction of myocardial tissue by delivering electrical energy over electrodes on a catheter placed next to an area related to the onset or maintenance of arrhythmias.

Risks associated with electrophysiologic testing are small.[56] Most electrophysiologic studies do not involve left-sided heart access, and therefore the risk of myocardial infarction, stroke, or systemic embolism is less than observed with coronary arteriography. The addition of therapeutic maneuvers, such as ablation therapy, to the procedure increases the risk of complications.[56] Predictors of major complications include an ejection fraction of less than 35% and multiple ablation targets.[57]

QT Dispersion

A hallmark of reentrant arrhythmias is heterogeneity in refractoriness and conduction velocity. An index of the heterogeneity of ventricular refractoriness is found by examining the differences in the length of QT intervals using the surface ECG. The most common index used to examine QT dispersion is the difference between the longest and shortest QT_c intervals on the 12-lead ECG. Unusually high QT dispersion has been associated with the risk of life-threatening arrhythmias in a variety of disorders,[58] but these results have been inconsistent.[59] Many

different techniques exist for determining QT dispersion, often making it difficult to compare results of various studies.

Treatment

The treatment of cardiac rhythm or conduction disorders is directed toward controlling the arrhythmia, correcting the cause, and preventing more serious or fatal arrhythmias. Correction may involve simply adjusting an electrolyte disturbance or withholding a medication such as digitalis. Preventing more serious arrhythmias often involves drug therapy, electrical stimulation, or surgical intervention.

Pharmacologic Treatment

Antiarrhythmic drugs act by modifying the disordered formation and conduction of impulses that induce cardiac muscle contraction. These drugs are classified into four major groups according to the drug's effect on the action potential of the cardiac cells.[7,37,60] Although drugs in one category have similar effects on conduction, they may vary significantly in their hemodynamic effects.

Class I drugs act by blocking the fast sodium channels. These drugs affect impulse conduction, excitability, and automaticity to various degrees and therefore have been divided further into three groups: IA, IB, and IC. Class IA drugs (e.g., quinidine, procainamide, disopyramide) decrease automaticity by depressing phase 4 of the action potential, decrease conductivity by moderately prolonging phase 0, and prolong repolarization by extending phase 3 of the action potential.[7] Because these drugs are effective in suppressing ectopic foci and treating reentrant arrhythmias, they are used for supraventricular and ventricular arrhythmias. Class IB drugs (e.g., lidocaine, mexiletine) decrease automaticity by depressing phase 4 of the action potential, have little effect on conductivity, decrease refractoriness by decreasing phase 2, and shorten repolarization by decreasing phase 3. These drugs have little or no effect on sodium channels in resting cells. However, they shorten the action potential and are powerful inhibitors of sodium-dependent conduction in depolarized cells, making them effective in depressing conduction in ischemic areas of the heart.[7] Drugs in this group are used for treating ventricular arrhythmias only and have little or no effect on myocardial contractility. Class IC drugs (e.g., propafenone, moricizine, flecainide) decrease conductivity by markedly depressing phase 0 of the action potential but have little effect on refractoriness or repolarization. Their primary action is inhibition of sodium channel opening.[7] Drugs in this class are used for life-threatening ventricular arrhythmias and supraventricular tachycardias.

Class II agents (e.g., propranolol, metoprolol, atenolol, timolol, sotalol) are β-adrenergic blocking drugs that act by blunting the effect of sympathetic nervous system stimulation on the heart, thereby inhibiting calcium channel opening. These drugs decrease automaticity by depressing phase 4 of the action potential; they also decrease heart rate and cardiac contractility. These medications are effective for treatment of supraventricular arrhythmias and tachyarrhythmias secondary to excessive sympathetic activity, but they are not very effective in treating severe arrhythmias such as recurrent ventricular tachycardia.[60]

Class III drugs (*e.g.,* amiodarone, bretylium, ibutilide, dofetilide, sotalol) act by inhibiting the potassium current and repolarization, thereby extending the action potential and refractoriness. They have little inhibiting effect on depolarizing currents. Sotalol has both β-adrenergic receptor blocking (class II) and action potential prolonging (class III) actions. These agents are used in the treatment of serious ventricular arrhythmias.

Class IV drugs (*e.g.,* verapamil, diltiazem, mibefradil) act by blocking the slow calcium channels, thereby depressing phase 4 and lengthening phases 1 and 2 of the action potential. By blocking the release of intracellular calcium ions, these agents reduce the force of myocardial contractility, thereby decreasing myocardial oxygen demand. These drugs are used to slow the SA node pacemaker and inhibit conduction in the AV node, slowing the ventricular response in atrial tachycardias, and to terminate reentrant paroxysmal supraventricular tachycardias when the AV node functions as a reentrant pathway.[37]

Two other types of antiarrhythmic drugs, the cardiac glycosides and adenosine, are not included in this classification schema. The cardiac glycosides (*i.e.,* digitalis drugs) slow the heart rate and are used in the management of arrhythmias such as atrial tachycardia, atrial flutter, and atrial fibrillation. Adenosine, an endogenous nucleoside that is present in every cell, is used for emergency intravenous treatment of paroxysmal supraventricular tachycardia involving the AV node. It interrupts AV node conduction and slows SA node firing.

Electrical Interventions

The correction of conduction defects, bradycardias, and tachycardias can involve the use of an electronic pacemaker, cardioversion, or defibrillation. Electrical interventions can be used in emergency and elective situations.

Efforts directed at cardiac electrostimulation date back more than a century. During this time, tremendous strides have been made in the effectiveness of cardiac pacing. A cardiac pacemaker is an electronic device that delivers an electrical stimulus to the heart. It is used to initiate heartbeats in situations when the normal pacemaker of the heart is defective, with certain types of AV heart block, with symptomatic bradycardia in which the rate of cardiac contraction and consequent cardiac output are inadequate to perfuse vital tissues, as well as in other cardiac arrhythmias. A pacemaker may be used as a temporary or a permanent measure. Pacemakers can pace the atria, the ventricles, or the atria and ventricles sequentially, or overdrive pacing can be used. Overdrive pacing is used to treat recurrent ventricular tachycardia and reentrant atrial or ventricular tachyarrhythmias, and to terminate atrial flutter.

Temporary pacemakers are useful for treatment of symptomatic bradycardias and to perform overdrive pacing. They can be placed transcutaneously, transvenously, or epicardially. External temporary pacing, also known as *transcuta-*

neous pacing, involves the placement of large patch electrodes on the anterior and posterior chest wall, which then are connected by a cable to an external pulse generator. Many defibrillators today have transcutaneous pacing capabilities. Internal temporary pacing, also known as *transvenous pacing,* involves the passage of a venous catheter with electrodes on its tip into the right atrium or ventricle, where it is wedged against the endocardium. The electrode then is attached to an external pulse generator. This procedure is performed under fluoroscopic or electrocardiographic direction. During open thoracotomy procedures, epicardial pacing wires sometimes are placed. These wires are brought out directly through the chest wall and also can be attached to an external pulse generator, if necessary.

Permanent cardiac pacemakers may become necessary for a variety of reasons. Permanent pacemakers require a pulse generator and implantation of pacing wires into the epicardium. The pulse generator typically weighs approximately 25 to 40 g.[61] Ongoing evaluation of the pacemaker's sensing and firing capabilities is necessary.

Defibrillation and synchronized cardioversion are two reliable methods for treating ventricular tachycardia, and defibrillation is the definitive treatment for atrial fibrillation. The discharge of electrical energy that is synchronized with the R wave of the ECG is referred to as *synchronized cardioversion,* and unsynchronized discharge is known as *defibrillation.* The goal of both of these techniques is to provide an electrical pulse to the heart in such a way as to depolarize the heart completely during passage of the current. This electrical current interrupts the disorganized impulses, allowing the SA node to regain control of the heart. Defibrillation and synchronized cardioversion can be delivered externally through large patch electrodes on the chest or internally through small paddle electrodes placed directly on the myocardium, patch electrodes sewn into the epicardium, or transvenous wires placed in the right ventricle. Electrical devices that combine antitachycardia pacing, cardioversion, defibrillation, and bradycardial pacing are under investigation.

Automatic implantable cardioverter-defibrillators (AICDs) are being used successfully to treat individuals with life-threatening ventricular tachyarrhythmias by the use of intrathoracic electrical countershock.[62] Reliable sensing and detection of ventricular tachyarrhythmias are essential for proper functioning of the AICD. Sensing and detection are accomplished through endocardial leads. The AICD responds to ventricular tachyarrhythmia by delivering an electrical shock between intrathoracic electrodes within 10 to 20 seconds of its onset. This time frame provides nearly a 100% likelihood of reversal of the arrhythmia, supporting the utility of this device as a reliable and effective means of preventing sudden cardiac death in survivors of out-of-hospital cardiac arrest.

Ablation and Surgical Interventions

Ablation therapy is used for treating recurrent, life-threatening supraventricular and ventricular tachyarrhythmias. Ablative therapy may be performed by catheter or surgical techniques.

It involves localized destruction, isolation, or excision of cardiac tissue that is considered to be arrhythmogenic.[6,63,64]

The first catheter ablation procedures were performed using direct-current shocks, but this energy source has largely been replaced by radiofrequency (RF) energy, which is delivered by an external generator and destroys tissue by heat production.[64] Radiofrequency ablation uses radiofrequency waves to destroy defective or aberrant electrical conduction pathways. Cryoablation involves the direct application of an extremely cold probe to arrhythmogenic cardiac tissue. Catheter-delivered cryoablation causes damage by freezing cellular structures of defective or aberrant electrical conduction pathways.[63–66]

Additional surgical interventions such as coronary artery bypass surgery, ventriculotomy, and endocardial resection may be used to improve myocardial oxygenation, remove arrhythmogenic foci, or alter electrical conduction pathways. Coronary artery bypass surgery improves myocardial oxygenation by increasing blood supply to the myocardium. Ventriculotomy involves the removal of aneurysm tissue and the resuturing of the myocardial walls to eliminate the paradoxical ventricular movement and the foci of arrhythmias. In endocardial resection, endocardial tissue that has been identified as arrhythmogenic through the use of electrophysiologic testing or intraoperative mapping is surgically removed. Ventriculotomy and endocardial resection have been performed with cryoablation or laser ablation as an adjunctive therapy.

IN SUMMARY, disorders of cardiac rhythm arise as the result of disturbances in impulse generation or conduction in the heart. Normal sinus rhythm and respiratory sinus arrhythmia (*i.e.,* heart rate speeds up and slows down in concert with respiratory cycle) are considered normal cardiac rhythms. Cardiac arrhythmias are not necessarily pathologic; they occur in healthy and diseased hearts. Sinus arrhythmias originate in the SA node. They include sinus bradycardia (heart rate <60 beats per minute); sinus tachycardia (heart rate >100 beats per minute); sinus arrest, in which there are prolonged periods of asystole; and sick sinus syndrome, a condition characterized by periods of bradycardia alternating with tachycardia.

Atrial arrhythmias arise from alterations in impulse generation that occur in the conduction pathways or muscle of the atria. They include premature atrial contractions, atrial flutter (*i.e.,* atrial depolarization rate of 240 to 450 beats per minute), and atrial fibrillation (*i.e.,* grossly disorganized atrial depolarization that is irregular with regard to rate and rhythm). Atrial arrhythmias often go unnoticed unless they are transmitted to the ventricles.

Arrhythmias that arise in the ventricles commonly are considered more serious than those that arise in the atria because they afford the potential for interfering with the pumping action of the heart. The long QT syndrome represents a prolongation of the QT interval that may result in torsades de pointes and sudden cardiac death. A premature ventricular contraction is caused by a ventricular ectopic pacemaker. Ventricular tachycardia is characterized by a ventricular rate of 70 to 250 beats per minute. Ventricular fibrillation (*e.g.,* ventricular rate >350 beats per minute) is a fatal arrhythmia unless it is successfully treated with defibrillation. Arrhythmogenic cardiomyopathies are inherited disorders of the ion channels that control the electrical activity of the heart. Among the inherited arrhythmogenic disorders are congenital Long QT syndrome, Brugada syndrome, and catecholamine polymorphic ventricular tachycardia.

Alterations in the conduction of impulses through the AV node lead to disturbances in the transmission of impulses from the atria to the ventricles. There can be a delay in transmission (*i.e.,* first-degree heart block), failure to conduct one or more impulses (*i.e.,* second-degree heart block), or complete failure to conduct impulses between the atria and the ventricles (*i.e.,* third-degree heart block). Conduction disorders of the bundle of His and Purkinje system, called *bundle branch blocks,* cause a widening of and changes in the configuration of the QRS complex of the ECG.

The diagnosis of disorders of cardiac rhythm and conduction typically is accomplished using surface ECG recordings or electrophysiologic studies. Surface electrodes can be used to obtain a 12-lead ECG; signal-averaged electrocardiographic studies in which multiple samples of QRS waves are averaged to detect ventricular late action potentials; and Holter monitoring, which provides continuous ECG recordings for up to 48 hours. Electrophysiologic studies use electrode catheters inserted into the right heart through a peripheral vein as a means of directly stimulating the heart while obtaining an intracardiac ECG recording.

Both medications and electrical devices are used in the treatment of arrhythmias and conduction disorders. Antiarrhythmic drugs act by modifying disordered formation and conduction of impulses that induce cardiac muscle contraction. They include drugs that act by blocking the fast sodium channels, β-adrenergic blocking drugs that decrease sympathetic outflow to the heart, drugs that act by inhibiting the potassium current and repolarization, calcium-channel blocking agents, cardiac glycosides (*i.e.,* digitalis drugs), and adenosine, which is used for emergency intravenous treatment of paroxysmal supraventricular tachycardia involving the AV mode. Electrical devices include temporary and permanent cardiac pacemakers that are used to treat symptomatic bradycardias or to provide overdrive pacing procedures; defibrillators that are used to treat atrial and ventricular fibrillation; external or internally implanted cardioversion devices, which can be used to treat ventricular tachycardia; and radiofrequency ablation and cryoablation therapy, which are used to destroy specific irritable foci in the heart. Surgical procedures can be performed to excise irritable or dysfunctional tissue, replace cardiac valves, or to provide better blood supply to the myocardial muscle wall. ■

Review Exercises

1. A 63-year-old woman with a history of congestive heart failure comes to the clinic complaining of feeling tired. Her heart rate is 97 beats per minute and the rhythm is irregular.

   A. *What type of arrhythmia do you think she might be having? What would it look like if you were to obtain an ECG?*

   B. *What causes this irregularity?*

   C. *Why do you think she is feeling tired?*

   D. *What are some of the concerns with this type of arrhythmia?*

2. A 42-year-old man appears at the urgent care center with complaints of chest discomfort, shortness of breath, and generally not feeling well. You assess vital signs and find that his temperature is 99.2°F, blood pressure 166/90, pulse 87 and slightly irregular, and respiratory rate 26. You do an ECG, and the readings from the anterior leads indicate that he is experiencing an ischemic episode.

   A. *You attach him to a cardiac monitor and see that his underlying rhythm is normal sinus rhythm, but he is having frequent premature contractions that are more than 0.10 sec in duration. What type of premature contractions do you suspect?*

   B. *What would you expect his pulse to feel like?*

   C. *What leads would you want to monitor?*

   D. *What do you think the etiology of this arrhythmia might be? How might it be treated?*

References

1. Rubart M., Zipes D. P. (2005). Genesis of cardiac arrhythmias: Electrophysiologic considerations. In Zipes D. P., Libby P., Bonow R. O., et al. (Eds.), *Braunwald's heart disease: A textbook of cardiovascular medicine* (7th ed., pp. 653–687). Philadelphia: Elsevier Saunders.
2. Castellanos A., Iterian A., Myerburg R. J. (2001). The resting electrocardiogram. In Fuster V., Alexander R. W., King S. B., et al. (Eds.), *Hurst's the heart* (10th ed., pp. 281–314). New York: McGraw-Hill.
3. Malouf J. F., Edwards W. D., Tajik A. J. (2001). Functional anatomy of the heart. In Fuster V., Alexander R. W., King S. B., et al. (Eds.), *Hurst's the heart* (10th ed., pp. 19–62). New York: McGraw-Hill.
4. Levy M. N., Pappano A. J. (2007). *Cardiovascular physiology* (9th ed., pp. 13–54). Philadelphia: Mosby Elsevier.
5. Guyton A. C., Hall J. E. (2006). *Textbook of medical physiology* (11th ed., pp. 116–122, 157). Philadelphia: Elsevier Saunders.
6. Fogoros R. N. (2006). *Electrophysiologic testing.* Malden, MA: Blackwell Science.
7. Katz A. M. (2006). *Physiology of the heart* (4th ed.). Philadelphia: Lippincott Williams & Wilkins.
8. Wit A. L., Friedman P. L. (1975). Basis for ventricular arrhythmias accompanying myocardial infarction: Alterations in electrical activity of ventricular muscle and Purkinje fibers after coronary artery occlusion. *Archives of Internal Medicine* 135, 459–472.
9. Drew B. J., Scheinman M. M. (1995). ECG criteria to distinguish between aberrantly conducted supraventricular tachycardia and ventricular tachycardia: Practical aspects for the immediate care setting. *Pacing and Clinical Electrophysiology* 18, 2194–2208.
10. Drew B. J., Ide B., Sparacino P. S. (1991). Accuracy of bedside electrocardiographic monitoring: A report on current practices of critical care nurses. *Heart and Lung* 20, 597–607.
11. Thomason T. R., Riegel B., Carlson B., et al. (1995). Monitoring electrocardiographic changes: Results of a national survey. *Journal of Cardiovascular Nursing* 9, 1–9.
12. Mirvis D. M., Goldberger A. L. (2005). Electrocardiography. In Zipes D. P., Libby P., Bonow R. O., et al. (Eds.), *Braunwald's heart disease: A textbook of cardiovascular medicine* (7th ed., pp. 107–151). Philadelphia: Elsevier Saunders.
13. Adams M. G., Pelter M. M., Wung S. F., et al. (1999). Frequency of silent myocardial ischemia with 12-lead ST segment monitoring in the coronary care unit: Are there sex-related differences? *Heart and Lung* 28, 81–86.
14. Drew B. J., Krucoff M. W. (1999). Multilead ST-segment monitoring in patients with acute coronary syndromes: A consensus statement for healthcare professionals. ST-Segment Monitoring Practice Guideline International Working Group. *American Journal of Critical Care* 8, 372–386.
15. Drew B. J., Califf R. M., Funk M., et al. (2005). AHA scientific statement: Practice standards for electrocardiographic monitoring in hospital settings: An American Heart Association Scientific Statement from the Councils on Cardiovascular Nursing, Clinical Cardiology, and Cardiovascular Disease in the Young: Endorsed by the International Society of Computerized Electrocardiology and the American Association of Critical-Care Nurses. *Journal of Cardiovascular Nursing* 20, 76–106.
16. American College of Cardiology Emergency Cardiac Care Committee. (1991). Recommended guidelines for in-hospital cardiac monitoring of adults for detection of arrhythmia. *Journal of the American College of Cardiology* 18, 1431–1433.
17. Marriott H. J. (1984). Arrhythmia versus dysrhythmia. *American Journal of Cardiology* 53, 628.
18. Waldo A. L., Wit A. L. (2001). Mechanisms of cardiac arrhythmias and conduction disturbances. In Fuster V., Alexander R. W., King S. B., et al. (Eds.), *Hurst's the heart* (10th ed., pp. 751–796). New York: McGraw-Hill.
19. Kay G. N., Bubien R. S. (1992). *Clinical management of cardiac arrhythmias.* Gaithersburg, MD: Aspen.
20. Conover M. (2003). Mechanisms of arrhythmias. In Conover M. (Ed.), *Understanding electrocardiography* (pp. 25–31). St. Louis: Mosby.
21. Yang M. J., Tran D. X., Weiss J. N., et al. (2007). The pinwheel experiment revisited: Effects of cellular electrophysiological properties on vulnerability to cardiac reentry. *American Journal of Physiology: Heart and Circulatory Physiology* 293, H1781–H1790.
22. Luqman N., Sung R. J., Wang C. L., et al. (2007). Myocardial ischemia and ventricular fibrillation: Pathophysiology and clinical implications. *International Journal of Cardiology* 119, 283–290.
23. Kuo S. R., Trayanova N. A. (2006). Action potential morphology heterogeneity in the atrium and its effect on atrial reentry: A two-dimensional and quasi-three-dimensional study. *Philosophical Transactions of the Royal Society, Series A: Mathematical, Physical and Engineering Sciences* 364, 1349–1366.
24. Nakagawa M., Takahashi N., Yufu K., et al. (2000). Malignant neurocardiogenic vasovagal syncope associated with chronic exaggerated vagal tone. *Pacing and Clinical Electrophysiology* 23, 1695–1697.
25. Kyriakidis M., Barbetseas J., Antonopoulos A., et al. (1992). Early atrial arrhythmias in acute myocardial infarction: Role of the sinus node artery. *Chest* 101, 944–947.
26. Bonvini R. F., Hendiri T., Anwar A. (2006). Sinus arrest and moderate hyperkalemia, *Annales de Cardiologie et d'Angeiologie (Paris)* 55, 161–163.
27. Applebaum D., Halperin E. (1986). Asystole following a conventional therapeutic dose of lidocaine. *American Journal of Emergency Medicine* 4, 143–145.
28. Kastor J. A. (2000). Sick sinus syndrome. In J. A. Kastor (Ed.), *Arrhythmias* (pp. 566–591). Philadelphia: W.B. Saunders.

29. Myerburg R. J., Kloosterman E. M., Castellanos A. (2001). Recognition, clinical assessment, and management of arrhythmias and conduction disturbances. In Fuster V., Alexander R. W., King S. B., et al. (Eds.), *Hurst's the heart* (10th ed., pp. 797–874). New York: McGraw-Hill.

30. Olgin J. L., Zipes D. P. (2005). Specific arrhythmias: Diagnosis and treatment. In Zipes D. P., Libby P., Bonow R. O., et al. (Eds.), *Braunwald's heart disease: A textbook of cardiovascular medicine* (7th ed., pp. 803–863). Philadelphia: Elsevier Saunders.

31. Keller K. B., Lemberg L. (2007). Iatrogenic sick sinus syndrome. *American Journal of Critical Care* 16, 294–297.

32. Rubenstein J. J., Schulman C. L., Yurchak P. M., et al. (1972). Clinical spectrum of the sick sinus syndrome. *Circulation* 46, 5–13.

33. Marriott H. J. L., Conover M. (1998). *Advanced concepts in arrhythmias.* St. Louis: Mosby.

34. Brignole M., Menozzi C., Bottoni N., et al. (1995). Mechanisms of syncope caused by transient bradycardia and the diagnostic value of electrophysiologic testing and cardiovascular reflexivity maneuvers. *American Journal of Cardiology* 76, 273–278.

35. Kahn A. M., Krummen D. E., Feld G. K., et al. (2007). Localizing circuits of atrial macroreentry using electrocardiographic planes of coherent atrial activation. *Heart Rhythm* 4, 445–451.

36. Falk R. H. (2001). Atrial fibrillation. *New England Journal of Medicine* 344, 1067–1078.

37. Bashore T. M., Granger C. B. (2007). The heart. In Tierney L. M, McPhee S. J., Papadakis M. A. (Eds.), *Current medical diagnosis and treatment* (46th ed., pp. 376–386). New York: McGraw-Hill.

38. Benjamin E. J., Wolf P. A., D'Agostino R. B., et al. (1998). Impact of atrial fibrillation on the risk of death: The Framingham Heart Study. *Circulation* 98, 946–952.

39. Dries D. L., Exner D. V., Gersh B. J., et al. (1998). Atrial fibrillation is associated with an increased risk for mortality and heart failure progression in patients with asymptomatic and symptomatic left ventricular systolic dysfunction: A retrospective analysis of the SOLVD trials. Studies of Left Ventricular Dysfunction. *Journal of the American College of Cardiology* 32, 695–703.

40. Wyse D. G., Love J. C., Yao Q., et al. (2001). Atrial fibrillation: A risk factor for increased mortality—an AVID registry analysis. *Journal of Interventional Cardiac Electrophysiology* 5, 267–273.

41. Khan I. A. (2002). Long QT syndrome: Diagnosis and management. *American Heart Journal* 143, 7–14.

42. Tan H. L., Hou C. J., Lauer M. R., et al. (1995). Electrophysiologic mechanisms of the long QT interval syndromes and torsade de pointes. *Annals of Internal Medicine* 122, 701–714.

43. Sagie A., Larson M. G., Goldberg R. J., et al. (1992). An improved method for adjusting the QT interval for heart rate (the Framingham Heart Study). *American Journal of Cardiology* 70, 797–801.

44. Smetana P., Batchvarov V., Hnatkova K., et al. (2003). Circadian rhythm of the corrected QT interval: Impact of different heart rate correction models. *Pacing and Clinical Electrophysiology* 26, 383–386.

45. Vincent G. M. (2000). Long QT syndrome. *Cardiology Clinics* 18, 309–325.

46. Bigger T. J., Jr. (2000). Ventricular premature complexes. In J. A. Kastor (Ed.), *Arrhythmias* (pp. 310–325). Philadelphia: W.B. Saunders.

47. Moungey S. J. (1994). Patients with sinus node dysfunction or atrioventricular blocks. *Critical Care Nursing Clinics of North America* 6, 55–68.

48. Rosenfeld L. E. (1988). Bradyarrhythmias, abnormalities of conduction, and indications for pacing in acute myocardial infarction. *Cardiology Clinics* 6, 49–61.

49. Wellens H. J. (1993). Right ventricular infarction. *New England Journal of Medicine* 328, 1036–1038.

50. Priori S. G., Napolitano C., Schwartz P. J. (2005). Genetics of cardiac arrhythmias. In Zipes D. P., Libby P., Bonow R. O., et al. (Eds.), *Braunwald's heart disease: A textbook of cardiovascular medicine* (7th ed., pp. 689–695). Philadelphia: Elsevier Saunders.

51. Priori S. G., Napolitano C. (2006). Role of genetic analysis in cardiology: Part I. Mendelian diseases: Cardiac channelopathies. *Circulation* 113, 1130–1135.

52. Miller J. M., Zipes D. P. (2005). Diagnosis of cardiac arrhythmias. In Zipes D. P., Libby P., Bonow R. O., et al. (Eds.), *Braunwald's heart disease: A textbook of cardiovascular medicine* (7th ed., pp. 697–712). Philadelphia: Elsevier Saunders.

53. Flowers N. C., Shvartsman V., Kennelly B. M., et al. (1981). Surface recording of His-Purkinje activity on an every-beat basis without digital averaging. *Circulation* 63, 948–952.

54. Gomes J. A., Cain M. E., Buxton A. E., et al. (2001). Prediction of long-term outcomes by signal-averaged electrocardiography in patients with unsustained ventricular tachycardia, coronary artery disease, and left ventricular dysfunction. *Circulation* 104, 436–441.

55. Manolio T. A., Furberg C. D., Rautaharju P. M., et al. (1994). Cardiac arrhythmias on 24-h ambulatory electrocardiography in older women and men: The Cardiovascular Health Study. *Journal of the American College of Cardiology* 23, 916–925.

56. Horowitz L. N., Kay H. R., Kutalek S. P., et al. (1987). Risks and complications of clinical cardiac electrophysiologic studies: A prospective analysis of 1,000 consecutive patients. *Journal of the American College of Cardiology* 9, 1261–1268.

57. Calkins H., Epstein A., Packer D., et al. (2000). Catheter ablation of ventricular tachycardia in patients with structural heart disease using cooled radiofrequency energy: Results of a prospective multicenter study. Cooled RF Multi Center Investigators Group. *Journal of the American College of Cardiology* 35, 1905–1914.

58. Spargias K. S., Lindsay S. J., Kawar G. I., et al. (1999). QT dispersion as a predictor of long-term mortality in patients with acute myocardial infarction and clinical evidence of heart failure. *European Heart Journal* 20, 1158–1165.

59. Gang Y., Ono T., Hnatkova K., et al. (2003). QT dispersion has no prognostic value in patients with symptomatic heart failure: An ELITE II substudy. *Pacing and Clinical Electrophysiology* 26, 394–400.

60. Woosley R. L. (2001). Antiarrhythmic drugs. In Fuster V., Alexander R. W., King S. B., et al. (Eds.), *Hurst's the heart* (10th ed., pp. 899–924). New York: McGraw-Hill.

61. Mitrani R. D., Myerburg R. J., Castellanos A. (2001). Cardiac pacemakers. In Fuster V., Alexander R. W., King S. B., et al. (Eds.), *Hurst's the heart* (10th ed., pp. 963–994). New York: McGraw-Hill.

62. O'Callaghan P. A., Ruskin J. N. (2001). The implantable cardioverter defibrillator. In Fuster V., Alexander R. W., King S. B., et al. (Eds.), *Hurst's the heart* (10th ed., pp. 945–962). New York: McGraw-Hill.

63. O'Neill M. D., Jais P., Hocini M., et al. (2007). Catheter ablation for atrial fibrillation. *Circulation* 116, 1515–1523.

64. Miller J. M., Zipes D. P. (2005). Therapy for cardiac arrhythmias. In Zipes D. P., Libby P., Bonow R. O., et al. (Eds.), *Braunwald's heart disease: A textbook of cardiovascular medicine* (7th ed., pp. 739–753). Philadelphia: Elsevier Saunders.

65. Lukac P., Hjortdal V. E., Pedersen A. K., et al. (2007). Prevention of atrial flutter with cryoablation may be proarrhythmogenic. *Annals of Thoracic Surgery* 83, 1717–1723.

66. Collins K. K., Rhee E. K., Kirsh J. A., et al. (2007). Cryoablation of accessory pathways in the coronary sinus in young patients: A multicenter study from the Pediatric and Congenital Electrophysiology Society's Working Group on Cryoablation. *Journal of Cardiovascular Electrophysiology* 18, 592–597.

Visit thePoint http://thePoint.lww.com for animations, journal articles, and more!

Chapter 26

Heart Failure and Circulatory Shock

ANNA BARKMAN AND CHARLOTTE POOLER

➤ Adequate perfusion of body tissues depends on the pumping ability of the heart, a vascular system that transports blood to the cells and back to the heart, sufficient blood to fill the circulatory system, and tissues that are able to extract and use oxygen and nutrients from the blood. Heart failure and circulatory shock are separate conditions that reflect failure of the circulatory system. Both conditions exhibit common compensatory mechanisms even though they differ in terms of pathogenesis and causes.

HEART FAILURE

After completing this section of the chapter, you should be able to meet the following objectives:

- Define heart failure.
- Describe the contractile properties of the myocardium.
- Explain how the Frank-Starling mechanism, sympathetic nervous system, renin-angiotensin-aldosterone mechanism, natriuretic peptides, endothelins, and myocardial hypertrophy and remodeling function as adaptive and maladaptive mechanisms in heart failure.
- Differentiate high-output versus low-output heart failure, systolic versus diastolic heart failure, and right-sided versus left-sided heart failure in terms of causes, impact on cardiac function, and major manifestations.
- Differentiate chronic heart failure from acute heart failure syndromes.
- Describe the manifestations of heart failure and relate to the function of the heart.
- Describe the methods used in diagnosis and assessment of cardiac function in persons with heart failure.
- Relate the pharmacologic actions of angiotensin-converting enzyme inhibitors and receptor blockers, β-adrenergic blockers, diuretics, digoxin, and vasodilatory agents to the treatment of heart failure.
- Relate the use of cardiac resynchronization, implantable cardioverter–defibrillators, left ventricular assist devices, heart transplantation, and other surgical alternatives to the treatment of selected types of heart failure.

Heart failure has been defined as a complex syndrome resulting from any functional or structural disorder of the heart that results in or increases the risk of developing manifestations of low cardiac output and/or pulmonary or systemic congestion.[1,2] In the United States, heart failure affected an estimated 5,200,000 persons in 2004,[3] and in Canada, it affected an estimated 400,000 persons.[4] Heart failure can occur in any age group but primarily affects the elderly. Although morbidity and mortality rates from other cardiovascular diseases have decreased over the past several decades, the incidence of heart failure is increasing at an alarming rate. In the United States alone, the number of hospital discharges of patients with heart failure has increased by 175% from 1979 to 2004.[3] This change undoubtedly reflects improved treatment methods and increased survival from other forms of heart disease.

HEART FAILURE

- The function of the heart is to move deoxygenated blood from the venous system through the right heart into the pulmonary circulation, and oxygenated blood from the pulmonary circulation through the left heart and into the arterial circulation.

- Systolic dysfunction represents a decrease in cardiac myocardial contractility and an impaired ability to eject blood from the left ventricle, whereas diastolic dysfunction represents an abnormality in ventricular relaxation and filling.

- Right-sided heart failure represents failure of the right ventricle to move unoxygenated blood from the venous system into the pulmonary circulation, with an eventual backup in the systemic venous circulation, whereas left-sided heart failure represents failure of the left ventricle to move oxygenated blood from the pulmonary circulation into the arterial circulation with eventual backup of blood in the lungs. Both types result in decreased forward flow, resulting in poor circulation of oxygenated blood in the body.

The syndrome of heart failure can be produced by any heart condition that reduces the pumping ability of the heart. Among the most common causes of heart failure are coronary artery disease, hypertension, dilated cardiomyopathy, and valvular heart disease.[1] Because many of the processes leading to heart failure are long standing and progress gradually, heart failure can often be prevented or its progression slowed by early detection and intervention. The importance of these approaches is emphasized by the American College of Cardiology (ACC)/ American Heart Association (AHA) guidelines that have incorporated a classification system of heart failure that includes four stages (Table 26-1).[1] This staging system recognizes that there are established risk factors and structural abnormalities that are characteristic of the four stages of heart failure, and that patients normally progress from one stage to another unless disease progression is slowed or stopped by treatment.

Pathophysiology of Heart Failure

Cardiac output is the amount of blood that the ventricles eject each minute. The heart has the amazing capacity to adjust its cardiac output to meet the varying needs of the body. During sleep, the cardiac output declines, and during exercise, it increases markedly. The ability to increase cardiac output during increased activity is called the *cardiac reserve*. For example, competitive swimmers and long-distance runners have large cardiac reserves. During exercise, the cardiac output of these athletes rapidly increases to as much as five to six times their resting level.[5] In sharp contrast with healthy athletes, persons with heart failure often use their cardiac reserve at rest. For them, just climbing a flight of stairs may cause shortness of breath because they have exceeded their cardiac reserve.

Control of Cardiac Performance and Output

Cardiac output, which is the major determinant of cardiac performance, reflects how often the heart beats each minute (heart rate) and how much blood it pumps with each beat (stroke volume) and can be expressed as the product of the heart rate and stroke volume (*i.e.*, cardiac output = heart rate × stroke volume). The heart rate is regulated by a balance between the activity of the sympathetic nervous system, which produces an increase in heart rate, and the parasympathetic nervous system, which slows it down, whereas the stroke volume is a function of preload, afterload, and myocardial contractility.[5–7]

Preload and Afterload. The work that the heart performs consists mainly of ejecting blood that has returned to the ventricles during diastole into the pulmonary or systemic circulation. It is determined largely by the loading conditions, or what are called the *preload* and *afterload*.

Preload reflects the volume or loading conditions of the ventricle at the end of diastole, just before the onset of systole. It is the volume of blood stretching the heart muscle at the end of diastole and is normally determined by the venous return to the heart. During any given cardiac cycle, the maximum volume of blood filling the ventricle is present at the end of diastole. Known as the *end-diastolic volume,* this volume causes an increase in the length of the myocardial muscle fibers. Within limits, as end-diastolic volume or preload increases, the stroke volume increases in accord with the Frank-Starling mechanism.

Afterload represents the force that the contracting heart muscle must generate to eject blood from the filled heart. The main components of afterload are the systemic (peripheral) vascular resistance and ventricular wall tension. When the systemic vascular resistance is elevated, as with arterial hypertension, an increased left intraventricular pressure must be generated to first open the aortic valve and then move blood out of the ventricle and into the systemic circulation. This increased pressure

TABLE 26-1 ACC/AHA Stages of Heart Failure

STAGE	DESCRIPTION	EXAMPLES
A	High risk for developing heart failure because of conditions that are strongly associated with heart failure No identified structural or functional abnormalities of pericardium, myocardium, or heart valves No history of signs or symptoms of heart failure	Systemic hypertension Coronary heart disease Diabetes mellitus History of cardiotoxic drug therapy History of alcohol abuse Family history of cardiomyopathy
B	Presence of structural heart disease that is strongly associated with heart failure No history of signs or symptoms of heart failure	Left ventricular hypertrophy or fibrosis Left ventricular dilation or dysfunction Asymptomatic valvular heart disease Previous myocardial infarction
C	Current or prior symptoms of heart failure with underlying structural heart disease	Dyspnea or fatigue due to left ventricular systolic dysfunction Asymptomatic patients receiving treatment for prior symptoms of heart failure
D	Advanced structural heart disease and marked symptoms of heart failure at rest despite maximal medical therapy Require specialized interventions	Frequent heart failure hospitalizations and cannot be discharged In the hospital awaiting heart transplantation At home with continuous inotropic or mechanical support In hospice setting for management of heart failure

From Hunt S. A., Chair. (2001). ACC/AHA guidelines for evaluation and management of chronic heart failure in the adult. *Circulation* 104, 2997.

equates to an increase in ventricular wall stress or tension. As a result, excessive afterload may impair ventricular ejection and increase wall tension.

Myocardial Contractility. Myocardial contractility, also known as *inotropy,* refers to the contractile performance of the heart. It represents the ability of the contractile elements (actin and myosin filaments) of the heart muscle to interact and shorten against a load[5–7] (see Chapter 4, Fig. 4-22). Contractility increases cardiac output independent of preload and afterload.

The interaction between the actin and myosin filaments during cardiac muscle contraction (*i.e.,* cross-bridge attachment and detachment) requires the use of energy supplied by the breakdown of adenosine triphosphate (ATP) and the presence of calcium ions (Ca^{++}). ATP provides the energy needed for cross-bridge formation during cardiac muscle contraction and for cross-bridge detachment during muscle relaxation.

As with skeletal muscle, when an action potential passes over the cardiac muscle fiber, the impulse spreads to the interior of the muscle fiber along the membranes of the transverse (T) tubules. The T tubule action potentials in turn act to cause release of Ca^{++} from the sarcoplasmic reticulum (Fig. 26-1). These Ca^{++} ions diffuse into the myofibrils and catalyze the chemical reactions that promote sliding of the actin and myosin filaments along one another to produce muscle shortening. In addition to the Ca^{++} ions released from the sarcoplasmic reticulum, a large quantity of extracellular Ca^{++} also diffuses into sarcoplasm through voltage-dependent L-type Ca^{++} channels in T tubules at the time of the action potential. Without the extra Ca^{++} that enters through the L-type Ca^{++} channels, the strength of the cardiac contraction would be considerably weaker. Opening of the L-type Ca^{++} channels is facilitated by the second messenger cyclic adenosine monophosphate (cAMP), the formation of which is coupled to β-adrenergic receptors. The catecholamines (norepinephrine and epinephrine) exert their inotropic effects by binding to these receptors. The L-type calcium channel also contains several other types of drug receptors. The dihydropyridine Ca^{++} channel blocking drugs (*e.g.,* nifedipine) exert their effects by binding to one site, while diltiazem and verapamil appear to bind to closely related but not identical receptors in another region. Blockade of the Ca^{++} channels in cardiac muscle by these drugs results in a reduction in contractility throughout the heart and a decrease in sinus node pacemaker rate and in atrioventricular node conduction velocity.

Another mechanism that can modulate inotropy is the sodium ion (Na^+)/Ca^{++} exchange pump and the ATPase-dependent Ca^{++} pump on the myocardial cell membrane (see Fig. 26-1). These pumps transport Ca^{++} out of the cell, thereby preventing the cell from becoming overloaded with Ca^{++}. If Ca^{++} extrusion is inhibited, the rise in intracellular Ca^{++} can increase inotropy. Digitalis and related cardiac glycosides are inotropic agents that exert their effects by inhibiting the Na^+/potassium ion (K^+)-ATPase pump, which increases intracellular Na^+; this in turn leads to an increase in intracellular Ca^{++} through the Na^+/Ca^{++} exchange pump.

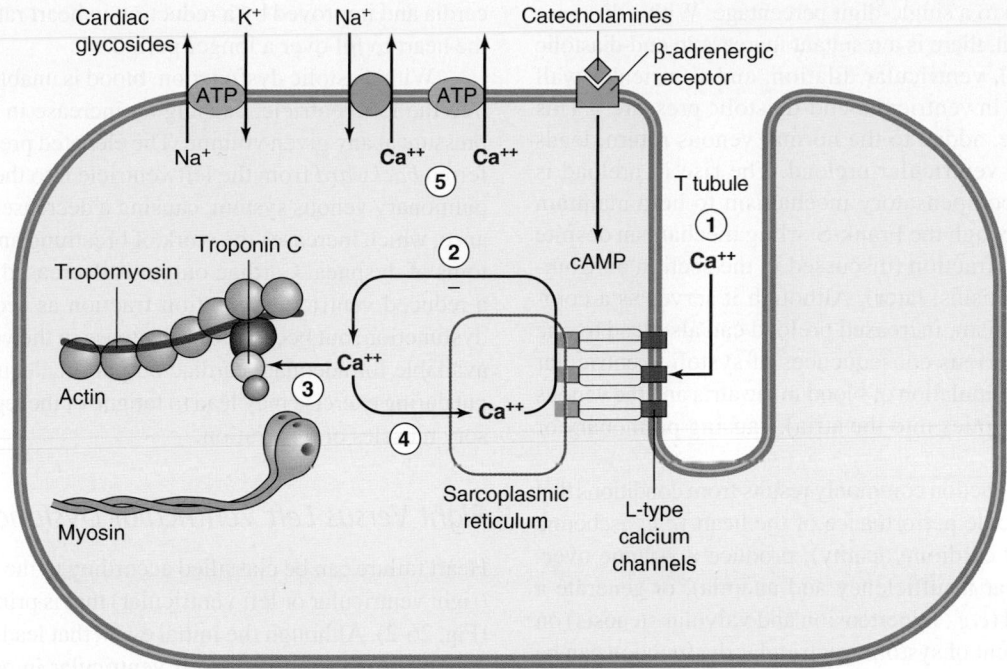

FIGURE 26-1 • Schematic representation of the role of calcium ions (Ca⁺⁺) in cardiac excitation–contraction coupling. The influx (site 1) of extracellular Ca⁺⁺ through the L-type Ca⁺⁺ channels in the T tubules during excitation triggers (site 2) release of Ca⁺⁺ by the sarcoplasmic reticulum. This Ca⁺⁺ binds to troponin C (site 3). The Ca⁺⁺–troponin complex interacts with tropomyosin to unblock active sites on the actin and myosin filaments, allowing cross-bridge attachment and contraction of the myofibrils (systole). Relaxation (diastole) occurs as a result of calcium reuptake by the sarcoplasmic reticulum (site 4) and extrusion of intracellular Ca⁺⁺ by the sodium Na⁺/Ca⁺⁺ exchange transporter or, to a lesser extent, by the Ca⁺⁺ ATPase pump (site 5). Mechanisms that raise systolic Ca⁺⁺ increase the level of developed force (inotropy). Binding of catecholamines to β-adrenergic receptors increases Ca⁺⁺ entry by phosphorylation of the Ca⁺⁺ channels through a cyclic adenosine monophosphate (cAMP)–dependent second messenger mechanism. The cardiac glycosides increase intracellular Ca⁺⁺ by inhibiting the Na⁺/K⁺-ATPase pump. The elevated intracellular Na⁺ reverses the Na⁺/Ca⁺⁺ exchange transporter (site 5), so less Ca⁺⁺ is removed from the cell. (Modified from Klabunde R. E. [2005]. *Cardiovascular physiology concepts* [p. 46]. Philadelphia: Lippincott Williams & Wilkins.)

Systolic Versus Diastolic Dysfunction

Until recently, heart failure was viewed mainly in terms of backward and forward failure. *Backward failure* represented failure of one of the ventricles to effectively eject blood during systole, such that blood backs up in the venous system, causing congestion. *Forward failure* was characterized by impaired forward movement of blood into the arterial system emerging from the heart, resulting in reduced cardiac output.

A more recent classification separates the pathophysiology of heart failure into systolic and diastolic failure or dysfunction based on the ventricular ejection fraction.[8] *Ejection fraction* is the percentage of blood pumped out of the ventricles with each contraction. In systolic ventricular dysfunction, myocardial contractility is impaired, leading to a decrease in the ejection fraction and cardiac output. Diastolic ventricular dysfunction is characterized by a normal ejection fraction but impaired diastolic ventricular relaxation, leading to a decrease in ventricular filling that ultimately causes a decrease in preload, stroke volume, and cardiac output. Many persons with

heart failure have combined elements of both systolic and diastolic ventricular dysfunction, and the division between systolic and diastolic dysfunction may be somewhat artificial, particularly as it relates to manifestations and treatment.[9] It is important to note that ventricular dysfunction is not synonymous with heart failure. It can, however, lead to heart failure.

With both systolic and diastolic ventricular dysfunction, compensatory mechanisms are usually able to maintain adequate resting cardiac function until the later stages of heart failure. Therefore, cardiac function measured at rest is a poor clinical indicator of the extent of cardiac impairment because cardiac output may be relatively normal at rest.[5]

Systolic Dysfunction. Systolic dysfunction is primarily defined as a decrease in myocardial contractility, characterized by an ejection fraction of less than 40%.[10] A normal heart ejects approximately 65% of the blood that is present in the ventricle at the end of diastole. In systolic heart failure, the ejection fraction declines progressively with increasing degrees of myocardial dysfunction. In very severe forms of heart failure, the ejection fraction may drop to a single-digit percentage. With a decrease in ejection fraction, there is a resultant increase in end-diastolic volume (preload), ventricular dilation, and ventricular wall tension and a rise in ventricular end-diastolic pressure.[11] This increased volume, added to the normal venous return, leads to an increase in ventricular preload. The rise in preload is thought to be a compensatory mechanism to help maintain stroke volume through the Frank-Starling mechanism despite a drop in ejection fraction (discussed in the section on Compensatory Mechanisms, later). Although it serves as a compensatory mechanism, increased preload can also lead to one of the most deleterious consequences of systolic ventricular dysfunction—accumulation of blood in the atria and the venous system (which empties into the atria), causing pulmonary or peripheral edema.

Systolic dysfunction commonly results from conditions that impair the contractile performance of the heart (*e.g.,* ischemic heart disease and cardiomyopathy), produce a volume overload (*e.g.,* valvular insufficiency and anemia), or generate a pressure overload (*e.g.,* hypertension and valvular stenosis) on the heart. The extent of systolic ventricular dysfunction can be estimated by measuring the cardiac output and ejection fraction and by assessment for manifestations of left-sided heart failure, particularly pulmonary congestion.

Diastolic Dysfunction. Although heart failure is commonly associated with impaired systolic function, in approximately 35% to 55% of cases systolic function has been preserved and heart failure occurs exclusively on the basis of left ventricular diastolic dysfunction.[12,13] Although such hearts contract normally, relaxation is abnormal. Cardiac output, especially during exercise, is compromised by the abnormal filling of the ventricle. For any given ventricular volume, ventricular pressures are elevated, leading to signs of pulmonary and systemic venous congestion identical to those seen in persons with a dilated, poorly contracting heart. The prevalence of diastolic failure increases with age and is higher in women than men, and in persons with obesity, hypertension, and diabetes.[12,13]

Among the conditions that cause diastolic dysfunction are those that impede expansion of the ventricle (*e.g.,* pericardial effusion, constrictive pericarditis), those that increase wall thickness and reduce chamber size (*e.g.,* myocardial hypertrophy, hypertrophic cardiomyopathy), and those that delay diastolic relaxation (*e.g.,* aging, ischemic heart disease).[13] Aging is often accompanied by a delay in relaxation of the heart during diastole such that diastolic filling begins while the ventricle is still stiff and resistant to stretching to accept an increase in volume. A similar delay occurs in myocardial ischemia, resulting from a lack of energy to break the rigor bonds that forms between the actin and myosin filaments and to move Ca^{++} out of the cytosol and back into the sarcoplasmic reticulum.[13]

Diastolic function is further influenced by the heart rate, which determines how much time is available for ventricular filling. An increase in heart rate shortens the diastolic filling [14] Thus, diastolic dysfunction can be aggravated by tachy-cardia and improved by a reduction in heart rate, which allows the heart to fill over a longer period.

With diastolic dysfunction, blood is unable to move freely into the left ventricle, causing an increase in intraventricular pressure at any given volume. The elevated pressures are transferred *backward* from the left ventricle into the left atrium and pulmonary venous system, causing a decrease in lung compliance, which increases the work of breathing and evokes symptoms of dyspnea. Cardiac output is decreased, not because of a reduced ventricular ejection fraction as seen with systolic dysfunction, but because of a decrease in the volume (preload) available for adequate cardiac output. Inadequate cardiac output during exercise may lead to fatigue of the legs and the accessory muscles of respiration.

Right Versus Left Ventricular Dysfunction

Heart failure can be classified according to the side of the heart (right ventricular or left ventricular) that is primarily affected[10] (Fig. 26-2). Although the initial event that leads to heart failure may be primarily right or left ventricular in origin, long-term heart failure usually involves both sides. The pathophysiologic changes that occur in the myocardium itself, including the compensatory responses in conditions like myocardial infarction, are not significantly different between right and left ventricular dysfunction and are not addressed in detail in this section.

Right Ventricular Dysfunction. Right-sided heart failure impairs the ability to move deoxygenated blood from the systemic circulation into the pulmonary circulation. Consequently, when the right ventricle fails, there is a reduction in the amount of blood moved forward into the pulmonary circulation and then into the left side of the heart, ultimately causing a reduction of left ventricular cardiac output. Also, if the blood is not moved forward by the right ventricle, there is accumulation or congestion of blood into the systemic venous system. This causes an increase in right ventricular end-diastolic, right atrial, and systemic venous pressures. A major effect of right-sided heart failure is the development of peripheral edema (see Fig. 26-2). Because of the effects of gravity, the edema is most pronounced in the dependent parts of the body—in the lower extremities when the person is in the upright position and in the area over the sacrum when the person is supine. The accumulation of edema fluid is evidenced by a gain in weight (*i.e.,* 1 pint [568 mL] of accumulated fluid results in a 1 lb [0.45 kg] weight gain). Daily measurement of weight can be used as a means of assessing fluid accumulation in a patient with chronic heart failure. As a rule, a weight gain of more than 2 lb (0.90 kg) in 24 hours or 5 lb (2.27 kg) in 1 week is considered a sign of worsening failure.

Right-sided heart failure also produces congestion of the viscera. As venous distention progresses, blood backs up in the hepatic veins that drain into the inferior vena cava, and the liver becomes engorged. This may cause hepatomegaly and right upper quadrant pain. In severe and prolonged right-sided failure,

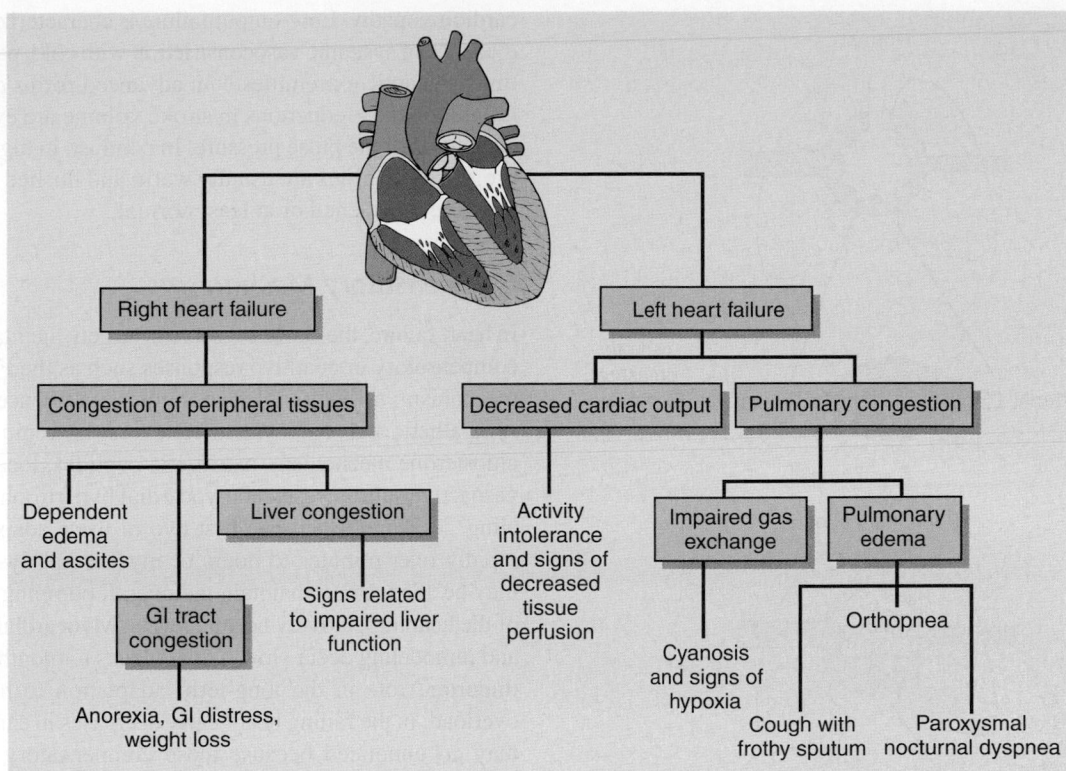

FIGURE 26-2 • Manifestations of left- and right-sided heart failure. GI, gastrointestinal.

liver function is impaired and hepatic cells may die. Congestion of the portal circulation also may lead to engorgement of the spleen and the development of ascites. Congestion of the gastrointestinal tract may interfere with digestion and absorption of nutrients, causing anorexia and abdominal discomfort. The jugular veins, which are above the level of the heart, are normally not visible in the standing position or when sitting with the head at higher than a 30-degree angle. In severe right-sided failure, the external jugular veins become distended and can be visualized when the person is sitting up or standing.

The causes of right ventricular dysfunction include conditions that impede blood flow into the lungs or compromise the pumping effectiveness of the right ventricle. Left ventricular failure is the most common cause of right ventricular failure. Sustained pulmonary hypertension also causes right ventricular dysfunction and failure. Pulmonary hypertension occurs in persons with chronic pulmonary disease, severe pneumonia, pulmonary embolus, or aortic or mitral stenosis. When the right heart failure occurs in response to chronic pulmonary disease, it is referred to as *cor pulmonale*[15] (see Chapter 29). Other common causes include stenosis or regurgitation of the tricuspid or pulmonic valves, right ventricular infarction, and cardiomyopathy. Right ventricular dysfunction with heart failure is also caused by congenital heart defects such as tetralogy of Fallot and ventricular septal defect (see Chapter 24).

Left Ventricular Dysfunction. Left-sided heart failure impairs the movement of blood from the low-pressure pulmonary circu-

lation into the high-pressure arterial side of the systemic circulation. With impairment of left heart function, there is a decrease in cardiac output to the systemic circulation; blood accumulates in the left ventricle, left atrium, and pulmonary circulation, which causes an elevation in pulmonary venous pressure (see Fig. 26-2). When the pressure in the pulmonary capillaries (normally approximately 10 mm Hg) exceeds the capillary osmotic pressure (normally approximately 25 mm Hg), there is a shift of intravascular fluid into the interstitium of the lung and development of pulmonary edema (Fig. 26-3). An episode of pulmonary edema often occurs at night, after the person has been reclining for some time and the gravitational forces have been removed from the circulatory system. It is then that the edema fluid that had been sequestered in the lower extremities during the day is returned to the vascular compartment and redistributed to the pulmonary circulation.

The most common causes of left ventricular dysfunction are hypertension and acute myocardial infarction. Left ventricular heart failure and pulmonary congestion can develop very rapidly in persons with acute myocardial infarction. Even when the infarcted area is small, there may be a surrounding area of ischemic tissue. This may result in large areas of ventricular wall hypokinesis or akinesis and rapid onset of pulmonary congestion and edema. Stenosis or regurgitation of the aortic or mitral valves also creates the level of left-sided backflow that results in pulmonary congestion. As pulmonary pressure rises as a result of congestion it may progress to produce right-sided heart failure. Pulmonary edema also may develop

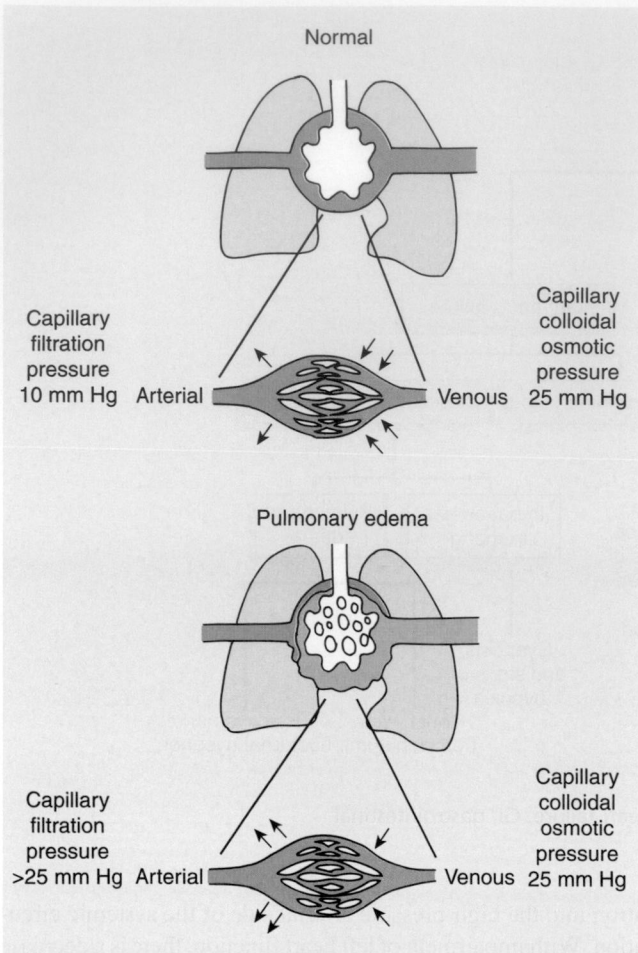

FIGURE 26-3 • Mechanism of respiratory symptoms in left-sided heart failure. In the normal exchange of fluid in the pulmonary capillaries **(top)**, the capillary filtration pressure that moves fluid out of the capillary into the lung is less than the capillary colloidal osmotic pressure that pulls fluid back into the capillary. Development of pulmonary edema **(bottom)** occurs when the capillary filtration pressure exceeds the capillary colloidal osmotic pressure that pulls fluid back into the capillary.

during rapid infusion of intravenous fluids or blood transfusions in an elderly person or in a person with limited cardiac reserve.

High-Output Versus Low-Output Failure

High- and low-output heart failure are described in terms of cardiac output. *High-output failure* is an uncommon type of heart failure that is caused by an excessive need for cardiac output. With high-output failure, the function of the heart may be supranormal but inadequate owing to excessive metabolic needs. Causes of high-output failure include severe anemia, thyrotoxicosis, conditions that cause arteriovenous shunting, and Paget disease.

Low-output failure is caused by disorders that impair the pumping ability of the heart, such as ischemic heart disease and

cardiomyopathy. Low-output failure is characterized by clinical evidence of systemic vasoconstriction with cold, pale, and sometimes cyanotic extremities.[10] In advanced forms of low-output failure, marked reductions in stroke volume are evidenced by a narrowing of the pulse pressure. In contrast, in high-output failure, the extremities are usually warm and flushed and the pulse pressure is widened or at least normal.

Compensatory Mechanisms

In heart failure, the cardiac reserve is largely maintained through compensatory or adaptive responses such as the Frank-Starling mechanism; activation of neurohumoral influences such as the sympathetic nervous system reflexes, the renin-angiotensin-aldosterone mechanism, natriuretic peptides, locally produced vasoactive substances, and myocardial hypertrophy and remodeling[5–7,14] (Fig. 26-4). The first two of these adaptations occur rapidly over minutes to hours of myocardial dysfunction and may be adequate to maintain the overall pumping performance of the heart at relatively normal levels. Myocardial hypertrophy and remodeling occur slowly over weeks to months and play an important role in the long-term adaptation to hemodynamic overload. In the failing heart, early decreases in cardiac function may go unnoticed because these compensatory mechanisms maintain the cardiac output. However, these mechanisms contribute not only to the adaptation of the failing heart but also to the pathophysiology of heart failure.[14]

Length Tension/Frank-Starling Mechanism. The Frank-Starling mechanism operates through an increase in preload (Fig. 26-5). With increased diastolic filling, there is increased stretching of the myocardial fibers and more optimal approximation of the heads on the thick myosin filaments to the troponin binding sites on the thin actin filaments, with a resultant increase in the force of the next contraction (see Chapter 21). In the normally functioning heart, the Frank-Starling mechanism serves to match the outputs of the two ventricles. As illustrated in Figure 26-5, there is no one single Frank-Starling curve.[6] An increase in contractility, or inotropy, will increase cardiac output at any end-diastolic volume, causing the curve to move up and to the left, whereas a decrease in inotropy will cause the curve to move down and to the right. In heart failure, inotropy is decreased compared with normal; thus, the stroke volume will not be as high as with normal inotropy, regardless of the increase in preload.

In heart failure, a decrease in cardiac output and renal blood flow leads to increased sodium and water retention, a resultant increase in vascular volume and venous return to the heart, and an increase in ventricular end-diastolic volume. Within limits, as preload and ventricular end-diastolic volume increase, there is a resultant increase in cardiac output. Although this may preserve the resting cardiac output, the resulting chronic elevation of left ventricular end-diastolic pressure is transmitted to the atria and the pulmonary circulation, causing pulmonary congestion.

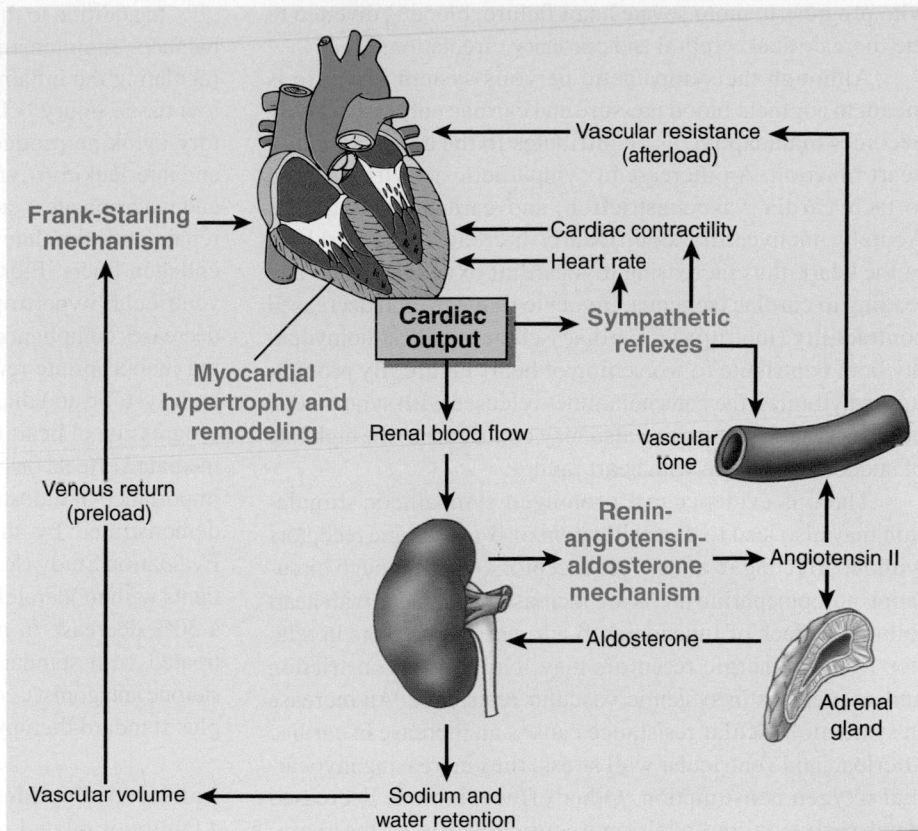

FIGURE 26-4 • Compensatory mechanisms in heart failure. The Frank-Starling mechanism, sympathetic reflexes, renin-angiotensin-aldosterone mechanism, and myocardial hypertrophy function in maintaining cardiac output for the failing heart.

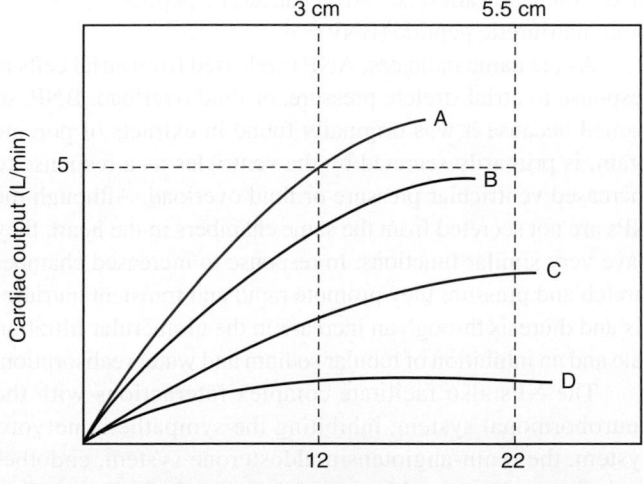

FIGURE 26-5 • Left ventricular function curves. *Curve A:* Normal function curve, with a normal cardiac output and optimal left ventricular end-diastolic (LVED) filling pressure. *Curve B:* Compensated heart failure with normal cardiac output at higher LVED pressures. *Curve C:* Decompensated heart failure with a decrease in cardiac output and elevated LVED, with eventual elevation of pulmonary capillary pressure and development of pulmonary congestion. *Curve D:* Cardiogenic shock, with an extreme decrease in cardiac output and marked increase in LVED pressures.

An increase in muscle stretch, as occurs with the Frank-Starling mechanism, also causes an increase in ventricular wall tension with a resultant increase in myocardial oxygen consumption. Because increased wall tension increases myocardial oxygen requirements, it can produce ischemia and contribute to further impairment of inotropy, moving the Frank-Starling curve farther down and to the right (see Fig. 26-5). In this situation, the increase in preload is no longer contributing to compensation but rather causing heart failure to worsen. The use of diuretics in persons with heart failure helps to reduce vascular volume and ventricular filling, thereby unloading the heart and reducing ventricular wall tension.

Sympathetic Nervous System Activity. Stimulation of the sympathetic nervous system plays an important role in the compensatory response to decreased cardiac output and in the pathogenesis of acute heart failure.[14,16] Both cardiac sympathetic tone and catecholamine (epinephrine and norepinephrine) levels are elevated during the late stages of most forms of heart failure. By direct stimulation of heart rate and cardiac contractility, regulation of vascular tone, and enhancement of renal sodium and water retention, the sympathetic nervous system initially helps to maintain perfusion of the various body organs. In persons who progress to more severe heart failure, blood is diverted to the more critical cerebral and coronary circulations.

Although the sympathetic nervous system response is meant to augment blood pressure and cardiac output, it quickly becomes maladaptive and contributes to the deterioration of heart function. An increase in sympathetic activity can lead to tachycardia, vasoconstriction, and cardiac arrhythmias. Acutely, tachycardia significantly increases the workload of the heart, thus increasing myocardial oxygen demand and leading to cardiac ischemia, myocyte damage, and decreased contractility (inotropy).[17] Cardiac ischemia and cardiomyopathy both contribute to worsening of heart failure. By promoting arrhythmias, the catecholamines released with sympathetic nervous system stimulation also may contribute to the high rate of sudden death seen with heart failure.

There is evidence that prolonged sympathetic stimulation may also lead to desensitization of β-adrenergic receptors without affecting α-adrenergic receptors.[7] Even though circulating norepinephrine levels are increased in persons with heart failure, the lack of functioning β-adrenergic receptors in relation to α-adrenergic receptors may lead to vasoconstriction and an increase in systemic vascular resistance. An increase in systemic vascular resistance causes an increase in cardiac afterload and ventricular wall stress, thus increasing myocardial oxygen consumption. Other effects include decreased renal perfusion and additional augmentation of the renin-angiotensin-aldosterone system, as well as decreased blood flow to skin, muscle, and abdominal organs.[17]

Renin-Angiotensin-Aldosterone Mechanism. One of the most important effects of lowered cardiac output in heart failure is a reduction in renal blood flow and glomerular filtration rate, which leads to sodium and water retention. With decreased renal blood flow, there is a progressive increase in renin secretion by the kidneys with parallel increases in circulating levels of angiotensin II. The increased concentration of angiotensin II contributes directly to a generalized and excessive vasoconstriction, as well as facilitating norepinephrine release and inhibiting reuptake of norepinephrine by the sympathetic nervous system.[6]

Angiotensin II also provides a powerful stimulus for aldosterone production by the adrenal cortex (see Chapter 23). Aldosterone increases tubular reabsorption of sodium, with an accompanying increase in water retention. Because aldosterone is metabolized in the liver, its levels are further increased when heart failure causes liver congestion. Angiotensin II also increases the level of antidiuretic hormone (ADH), which serves as a vasoconstrictor and inhibitor of water excretion (see Chapter 31). In heart failure, the progressive accumulation of fluid leads to ventricular dilation and increased wall tension. As described earlier, the increased oxygen demand that accompanies increased wall tension eventually outweighs the compensatory Frank-Starling mechanism, reducing inotropy and exacerbating heart failure.

In addition to their individual effects on sodium and water balance, angiotensin II and aldosterone are also involved in regulating the inflammatory and reparative processes that follow tissue injury.[18] In this capacity, they stimulate inflammatory cytokine production (e.g., tumor necrosis factor [TNF] and interleukin-6), attract inflammatory cells (e.g., neutrophils and macrophages), activate macrophages at sites of injury and repair, and stimulate the growth of fibroblasts and synthesis of collagen fibers. Fibroblast and collagen deposition results in ventricular hypertrophy and myocardial wall fibrosis, which decreases compliance (i.e., increases stiffness), ultimately causing inappropriate remodeling of the heart and progression of both systolic and diastolic ventricular dysfunction.[19] Thus, the progression of heart failure may be augmented by aldosterone-mediated effects on both the vasculature and myocardium. The importance of aldosterone, independent of angiotensin II, was demonstrated by the International Randomized Aldactone Evaluation Study (RALES) trial involving more than 1600 patients with moderately severe to severe heart failure: there was a 30% decrease in mortality from any cause among patients treated with standard therapy plus spironolactone (an aldosterone antagonist), compared with those who received a placebo plus standard therapy.[20]

Natriuretic Peptides. The heart muscle produces and secretes a family of related peptide hormones, the cardiac natriuretic hormones or natriuretic peptides (NPs), that have potent diuretic, natriuretic, and vascular smooth muscle effects and also interact with other neurohumoral mechanisms that affect cardiovascular function. Two of the four known NPs most commonly associated with heart failure are atrial natriuretic peptide (ANP) and brain natriuretic peptide (BNP).[21,22]

As the name indicates, ANP is released from atrial cells in response to atrial stretch, pressure, or fluid overload. BNP, so named because it was originally found in extracts of porcine brain, is primarily secreted by the ventricles as a response to increased ventricular pressure or fluid overload. Although the NPs are not secreted from the same chambers in the heart, they have very similar functions. In response to increased chamber stretch and pressure they promote rapid and transient natriuresis and diuresis through an increase in the glomerular filtration rate and an inhibition of tubular sodium and water reabsorption.

The NPs also facilitate complex interactions with the neurohormonal system, inhibiting the sympathetic nervous system, the renin-angiotensin-aldosterone system, endothelin inflammatory cytokines, and vasopressin.[23] Suppression of the sympathetic nervous system causes both venous and arterial dilation with consequent reduction in venous return to the heart (decreased preload) and cardiac filling pressures, and a decrease in afterload (arterial vasodilation). Inhibition of angiotensin II and vasopressin by the NPs reduces renal fluid retention. In addition, the NPs directly affect the central nervous system and the brain, inhibiting the secretion of vasopressin and the function of the salt appetite and thirst center.[23]

Circulating levels of both ANP and BNP are reportedly elevated in persons with heart failure. The concentrations are well correlated with the extent of ventricular dysfunction, increasing up to 30-fold in persons with advanced heart disease.[21] Assays of BNP are used clinically in the diagnosis of heart failure and to predict the severity of the condition. Many of the medications used to treat heart failure (*e.g.,* diuretics such as spironolactone, and the angiotensin-converting enzyme inhibitors) reduce BNP concentrations. Therefore, many persons with chronic stable heart failure have BNP levels in the normal diagnostic range. However, digoxin and beta blockers appear to increase BNP levels. Human BNP, synthesized by recombinant DNA technology, is now available for treatment of persons with acutely decompensated heart failure (discussed later).

Endothelins. The endothelins, released from the endothelial cells throughout the circulation, are potent vasoconstrictors. Like angiotensin II, endothelin can also be synthesized and released by a variety of cell types, such as cardiac myocytes. Four endothelin peptides (endothelin-1 [ET-1], ET-2, ET-3, and ET-4) have been identified.[24] In addition to vasoconstrictor actions, the endothelins induce vascular smooth muscle cell proliferation and cardiac myocyte hypertrophy; increase the release of ANP, aldosterone, and catecholamines; and exert antinatriuretic effects on the kidneys. They also have been shown to have a negative inotropic action in patients with heart failure.[25] Production of ET-1 is regulated by many factors that are significant for cardiovascular function and have implications for heart failure; for example, it is enhanced by angiotensin-II, vasopressin, and norepinephrine and by factors such as shear stress and endothelial stretching.[25] Plasma ET-1 levels also correlate directly with pulmonary vascular resistance, and it is thought that the peptide may play a role in mediating pulmonary hypertension in persons with heart failure. There are at least two types of endothelin receptors—type A and type B.[24] An endothelin receptor antagonist is now available for use in persons with pulmonary arterial hypertension due to severe heart failure.

Inflammatory Mediators. There is ongoing research examining the relationship between inflammatory markers, especially C-reactive protein (CRP), and heart failure. Elevated CRP levels have been associated with adverse consequences in persons with heart failure, and have been shown to be predictive of the development of heart failure in high-risk groups. Of particular interest are the interactions between CRP and mediators, such as angiotensin II and norepinephrine. As previously mentioned, these associations relate to left ventricular dysfunction, ventricular hypertrophy and remodeling, progressive loss of myocardial cells through apoptosis (programmed cell death), and endothelial dysfunction. It has been suggested that many of the conventional treatments for heart failure (*e.g.,* angiotensin-converting enzyme inhibitors and beta blockers) may work, at least in part, through modulation of the proinflammatory cytokines.[26]

Myocardial Hypertrophy and Remodeling. The development of myocardial hypertrophy constitutes one of the principal mechanisms by which the heart compensates for an increase in workload.[14,16] Although ventricular hypertrophy improves the work performance of the heart, it is also an important risk factor for subsequent cardiac morbidity and mortality. Inappropriate hypertrophy and remodeling can result in changes in structure (*i.e.,* muscle mass, chamber dilation) and function (*i.e.,* impaired systolic or diastolic function) that often lead to further pump dysfunction and hemodynamic overload.

Myocardial hypertrophy and remodeling involve a series of complex events at both the molecular and cellular levels. The myocardium is composed of myocytes, or muscle cells, and nonmyocytes. The myocytes are the functional units of cardiac muscle. Their growth is limited by an increment in cell size, as opposed to an increase in cell number. The nonmyocytes include cardiac macrophages, fibroblasts, vascular smooth muscle, and endothelial cells. These cells, which are present in the interstitial space, remain capable of an increase in cell number, and provide support for the myocytes. The nonmyocytes also determine many of the inappropriate changes that occur during myocardial hypertrophy. For example, uncontrolled cardiac fibroblast growth is associated with increased synthesis of collagen fibers, myocardial fibrosis, and ventricular wall stiffness. Not only does ventricular wall stiffness increase the workload of the heart, but the fibrosis and remodeling that occur may lead to electrical conduction abnormalities in which the heart contracts in an uncoordinated manner, known as *cardiac dyssynchrony,* causing reduced systolic heart function.[27]

Recent research has focused on the type of hypertrophy that develops in persons with heart failure. At the cellular level, cardiac muscle cells respond to stimuli from stress placed on the ventricular wall by pressure and volume overload by initiating several different processes that lead to hypertrophy. These include stimuli that produce a *symmetric hypertrophy* with a proportionate increase in muscle length and width, as occurs in athletes; *concentric hypertrophy* with an increase in wall thickness, as occurs in hypertension; and *eccentric hypertrophy* with a disproportionate increase in muscle length, as occurs in dilated cardiomyopathy[28] (Fig. 26-6). When the primary stimulus for hypertrophy is *pressure overload,* the increase in wall stress leads to parallel replication of myofibrils, thickening of the individual myocytes, and concentric hypertrophy. Concentric hypertrophy may preserve systolic function for a time, but eventually the work performed by the ventricle exceeds the vascular reserve, predisposing to ischemia. When the primary stimulus is *ventricular volume overload,* the increase in wall stress leads to replication of myofibrils in series, elongation of the cardiac muscle cells, and eccentric hypertrophy. Eccentric hypertrophy leads to a decrease in ventricular wall thickness with an increase in diastolic volume and wall tension.

The stimuli for hypertrophy and remodeling are thought to reflect not only the mechanical stress placed on the myocytes, but growth signals provided by the release of substances such as angiotensin II, ANP, and ET-1. It is hoped that further research into the signals that cause specific features of inappropriate

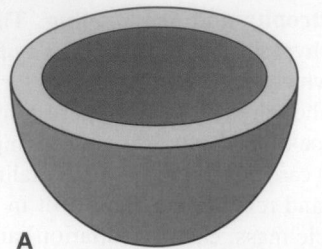 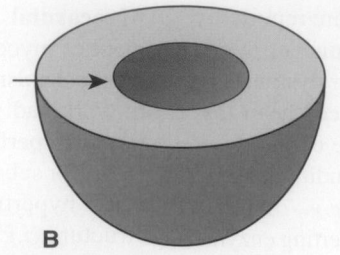 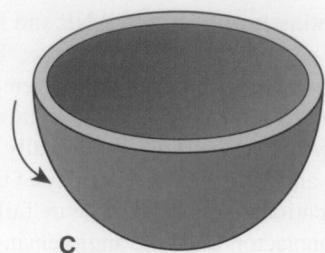

FIGURE 26-6 • Different types of myocardial hypertrophy. **(A)** Normal symmetric hypertrophy with proportionate increases in myocardial wall thickness and length. **(B)** Concentric hypertrophy with a disproportionate increase in wall thickness. **(C)** Eccentric hypertrophy with a disproportionate decrease in wall thickness and ventricular dilation.

myocardial hypertrophy and remodeling will lead to the identification of targets whose actions can be interrupted or modified.

Acute Heart Failure Syndromes

The acute heart failure syndromes (AHFS) are "defined as gradual or rapid change in heart failure signs and symptoms resulting in a need for urgent therapy."[29] These symptoms are primarily the result of severe pulmonary edema due to elevated left ventricular filling pressures, with or without a low cardiac output.[29] The syndromes are among the most common disorders seen in emergency departments, and chronic heart failure, often complicated by episodes of acute worsening, is the most common cause of the syndrome. Until recently, the underlying cause of heart failure hospitalization was viewed as merely a problem with volume overload or low cardiac output precipitated by dietary indiscretions or medication nonadherence. Hospitalization therefore was considered to be an expected part of the chronic heart failure trajectory.

AHFS are thought to encompass three different types of conditions: (1) worsening of chronic systolic or diastolic dysfunction that appears to respond to treatment; (2) new-onset acute heart failure that occurs secondary to a precipitating event such as a large myocardial infarction or a sudden increase in blood pressure superimposed on a noncompliant left ventricle; and (3) worsening of end-stage/advanced heart failure that is refractory to treatment, with predominantly left ventricular systolic dysfunction associated with a low-output state.[29–31] The difference between new-onset AHFS and AHFS caused by chronic heart failure is in the degree of physiologic response, which is more pronounced in the new-onset AHFS and more subtle in chronic heart failure because of the compensatory pathophysiology. For example, with new-onset AHFS, the person will have a stronger sympathetic response with enhanced pulmonary vascular permeability causing rapid and dramatic symptoms of pulmonary edema. Because many compensatory mechanisms operate in persons with chronic heart failure, they tolerate higher pulmonary vascular pressures. Chronic changes in neurohormonal regulation lead to stronger activation of the angiotensin-aldosterone system with a resultant volume overload, and venous congestion is more prominent in both the systemic and pulmonary circulations.[30]

Manifestations of Heart Failure

The manifestations of heart failure depend on the extent and type of cardiac dysfunction that is present and the rapidity with which it develops. A person with previously stable compensated heart failure may develop signs of heart failure for the first time when the condition has advanced to a critical point, such as with a progressive increase in pulmonary hypertension in a person with mitral valve regurgitation. Overt heart failure also may be precipitated by conditions such as infection, emotional stress, uncontrolled hypertension, or fluid overload.[11] Many persons with serious underlying heart disease, regardless of whether they have previously experienced heart failure, may be relatively asymptomatic as long they carefully adhere to their treatment regimen. A dietary excess of sodium is a frequent cause of sudden cardiac decompensation.

The manifestations of heart failure reflect the physiologic effects of the impaired pumping ability of the heart, decreased renal blood flow, and activation of the sympathetic compensatory mechanisms. The severity and progression of symptoms depend on the extent and type of dysfunction that is present (systolic versus diastolic, right- versus left-sided). The signs and symptoms include shortness of breath and other respiratory manifestations, fatigue and limited exercise tolerance, fluid retention and edema, cachexia and malnutrition, and cyanosis. Persons with severe heart failure may exhibit diaphoresis and tachycardia.

Respiratory Manifestations

Shortness of breath due to congestion of the pulmonary circulation is one of the major manifestations of left-sided heart failure. Perceived shortness of breath (*i.e.,* breathlessness) is called *dyspnea.* Dyspnea related to an increase in activity is called *exertional dyspnea. Orthopnea* is shortness of breath that occurs when a person is supine. Gravitational forces cause fluid to become sequestered in the lower legs and feet when the person is standing or sitting. When the person assumes the recumbent position, fluid from the legs and dependent parts of the body is mobilized and redistributed to an already distended pulmonary circulation. *Paroxysmal nocturnal dyspnea* is a sudden attack of dyspnea that occurs during sleep. It disrupts sleep, and the person awakens with a feeling of extreme suffocation that resolves when he or she sits up. Initially, the experience may be interpreted as awakening from a bad dream.

A subtle and often overlooked symptom of heart failure is a chronic dry, nonproductive cough that becomes worse when the person is lying down. Bronchospasm due to congestion of the bronchial mucosa may cause wheezing and difficulty in breathing. This condition is sometimes referred to as *cardiac asthma*.[11]

Cheyne-Stokes Respiration. Cheyne-Stokes respiration is a pattern of periodic breathing characterized by gradual increase in depth (and sometimes rate) of breathing to a maximum, followed by a decrease resulting in apnea (see Chapter 27). Although no longer associated solely with heart failure, it is recognized as an independent risk factor for worsening of heart failure. It has been suggested that Cheyne-Stokes respirations may not be just a marker for increasing severity of heart failure, but may also aggravate it.[32] During sleep, Cheyne-Stokes breathing causes recurrent awakening and thereby reduces slow-wave and rapid eye movement (REM) sleep. The recurrent cycling of hypoventilation/apnea and hyperventilation may also increase sympathetic activity and predispose to arrhythmias.

Acute Pulmonary Edema. Acute pulmonary edema is the most dramatic symptom of AHFS. It is a life-threatening condition in which capillary fluid moves into the alveoli.[11] The accumulated fluid in the alveoli and airways causes lung stiffness, makes lung expansion more difficult, and impairs the gas exchange function of the lung. With the decreased ability of the lungs to oxygenate the blood, the hemoglobin leaves the pulmonary circulation without being fully oxygenated, resulting in shortness of breath and cyanosis.

The person with severe pulmonary edema is usually seen sitting and gasping for air. The pulse is rapid, the skin is moist and cool, and the lips and nail beds are cyanotic. As the pulmonary edema worsens and oxygen supply to the brain drops, confusion and stupor appear. Dyspnea and air hunger are accompanied by a productive cough with frothy (resembling beaten egg whites) and often blood-tinged sputum—the effect of air mixing with the serum albumin and red blood cells that have moved into the alveoli. The movement of air through the alveolar fluid produces fine crepitant sounds called *crackles,* which can be heard with chest auscultation. As fluid moves into the larger airways, the crackles become louder and coarser.

Fatigue, Weakness, and Mental Confusion

Fatigue and weakness often accompany diminished output from the left ventricle. Cardiac fatigue is different from general fatigue in that it usually is not present in the morning but appears and progresses as activity increases during the day.

In acute or severe left-sided failure, cardiac output may fall to levels that are insufficient for providing the brain with adequate oxygen, and there are indications of mental confusion and disturbed behavior. Confusion, impairment of memory,

anxiety, restlessness, and insomnia are common in elderly persons with advanced heart failure, particularly in those with cerebral atherosclerosis. These symptoms may confuse the diagnosis of heart failure in the elderly because of their myriad other causes associated with aging.

Fluid Retention and Edema

Many of the manifestations of heart failure result from the increased capillary pressures (increased hydrostatic pressures) that develop in the peripheral circulation in persons with right-sided heart failure and in the pulmonary circulation in persons with left-sided heart failure. The increased capillary pressure reflects an overfilling of the vascular system because of increased sodium and water retention and venous congestion, referred to earlier as *backward* failure, resulting from impaired cardiac output.[11]

Nocturia is a nightly increase in urine output that occurs relatively early in the course of heart failure. It occurs because of the increased cardiac output, renal blood flow, and glomerular filtration rate that follow the increased blood return to the heart when the person is in a supine position. *Oliguria,* which is a decrease in urine output, is a late sign related to a severely reduced cardiac output and resultant renal failure.

Transudation of fluid into the pleural cavity (hydrothorax) or the peritoneal cavity (ascites) may occur in persons with advanced heart failure. Because the pleural veins drain into both the systemic and pulmonary venous beds, hydrothorax is observed more commonly in persons with hypertension involving both venous systems.[11] Pleural effusion occurs as the excess fluid in the lung interstitial spaces crosses the visceral pleura, which in turn overwhelms the capacity of the pulmonary lymphatic system. Ascites occurs in persons with increased pressure in the hepatic veins and veins draining the peritoneum. It usually reflects right ventricular failure and long-standing elevation of systemic venous pressure.[11]

Cachexia and Malnutrition

Cardiac cachexia is a condition of malnutrition and tissue wasting that occurs in persons with end-stage heart failure. A number of factors probably contribute to its development, including the fatigue and depression that interfere with food intake, congestion of the liver and gastrointestinal structures that impairs digestion and absorption and produces feelings of fullness, and the circulating toxins and mediators released from poorly perfused tissues that impair appetite and contribute to tissue wasting.

Cyanosis

Cyanosis is the bluish discoloration of the skin and mucous membranes caused by excess desaturated hemoglobin in the blood; it often is a late sign of heart failure. Cyanosis may be central, caused by arterial desaturation resulting from impaired pulmonary gas exchange, or peripheral, caused by venous desaturation resulting from extensive extraction of oxygen at the capillary level. Central cyanosis is caused by conditions that impair oxygenation of the arterial blood, such as pulmonary edema, left heart failure, or right-to-left cardiac shunting. Peripheral cyanosis is caused by conditions such as low-output failure that result in delivery of poorly oxygenated blood to the peripheral tissues, or by conditions such as peripheral vasoconstriction that cause excessive removal of oxygen from the blood. Central cyanosis is best monitored in the lips and mucous membranes because these areas are not subject to conditions, such as a cold environment, that cause peripheral cyanosis. Persons with right-sided or left-sided heart failure may develop cyanosis especially around the lips and in the peripheral parts of the extremities.

Arrhythmias and Sudden Cardiac Death

Both atrial and ventricular arrhythmias occur in persons with heart failure. Atrial fibrillation is the most common arrhythmia (see Chapter 25). Manifestations associated with atrial fibrillation are related to loss of atrial contraction, tachycardia, irregular heart rate, and symptoms related to a drop in blood pressure.[33] There is also strong evidence that persons with heart failure are at increased risk for sudden cardiac arrest; that is, unwitnessed death or death that occurs within 1 hour of the symptom onset.[27] In persons with ventricular dysfunction, sudden death is caused most commonly by ventricular tachycardia or ventricular fibrillation.[27]

Diagnosis and Treatment

Diagnostic Methods

Diagnostic methods in heart failure are directed toward establishing the cause of the disorder and determining the extent of the dysfunction. Medical guidelines for diagnosis and treatment are clearly described in the Canadian Heart Association and AHA guidelines for heart failure management.[1,2,34] Because heart failure represents the failure of the heart as a pump and can occur in the course of a number of heart diseases or other systemic disorders, the diagnosis of heart failure often is based on signs and symptoms related to the failing heart itself, such as shortness of breath and fatigue. The functional classification of the New York Heart Association (NYHA) is one guide to classifying the extent of dysfunction (Table 26-2).

The methods used in the diagnosis of heart failure include risk factor assessment, history and physical examination, laboratory studies, electrocardiography, chest radiography, and echocardiography. The history should include information related to dyspnea, cough, nocturia, generalized fatigue, and other signs and symptoms of heart failure. A complete physical examination includes assessment of heart rate, heart sounds, blood pressure, jugular veins for venous congestion, lungs for signs of pulmonary congestion, and lower extremities for edema. Laboratory tests are used in the diagnosis of anemia and electrolyte imbalances, and to detect signs of chronic liver congestion. Measurements of BNP are recommended to con-

TABLE 26-2 New York Heart Association Functional Classification of Patients With Heart Disease

CLASSIFICATION	CHARACTERISTICS
Class I	Patients with cardiac disease but without the resulting limitations in physical activity. Ordinary activity does not cause undue fatigue, palpitation, dyspnea, or anginal pain.
Class II	Patients with heart disease resulting in slight limitations of physical activity. They are comfortable at rest. Ordinary physical activity results in fatigue, palpitation, dyspnea, or anginal pain.
Class III	Patients with cardiac disease resulting in marked limitation of physical activity. They are comfortable at rest. Less than ordinary physical activity causes fatigue, palpitation, dyspnea, or anginal pain.
Class IV	Patients with cardiac disease resulting in inability to carry on any physical activity without discomfort. The symptoms of cardiac insufficiency or of the anginal syndrome may be present even at rest. If any physical activity is undertaken, discomfort increases.

From Criteria Committee of the New York Heart Association. (1964). *Diseases of the heart and blood vessels: Nomenclature and criteria for diagnosis* (6th ed., pp. 112–113). Boston: Little, Brown.

firm the diagnosis of heart failure; to evaluate the severity of left ventricular compromise, estimate the prognosis, and predict future cardiac events such as sudden death; and to evaluate the effectiveness of treatment.[2,34]

Echocardiography plays a key role in assessing right and left ventricular wall motion (normal, akinesis, or hypokinesis), wall thickness, ventricular chamber size, valve function, heart defects, ejection fraction, and pericardial disease.[2,34] Electrocardiographic findings may indicate atrial or ventricular hypertrophy, underlying disorders of cardiac rhythm, or conduction abnormalities such as right or left bundle branch block. Radionuclide ventriculography and cardiac angiography are recommended if there is reason to suspect coronary artery disease as the underlying cause for heart failure. Chest x-rays provide information about the size and shape of the heart and pulmonary vasculature. The cardiac silhouette can be used to detect cardiac hypertrophy and dilatation. Chest x-rays can indicate the relative severity of the failure by revealing if pulmonary edema is predominantly vascular or interstitial, or has advanced to the alveolar and bronchial stages. Cardiac magnetic resonance imaging (CMRI) and cardiac computed tomography (CCT) are used to document ejection fraction, ventricular preload, and regional wall motion.

Invasive hemodynamic monitoring may be used for assessment in acute, life-threatening episodes of heart failure. These monitoring methods include central venous pressure (CVP), pulmonary artery pressure monitoring, thermodilution measurements of cardiac output, and intra-arterial measurements of blood pressure. CVP reflects the amount of blood returning to the heart. Measurements of CVP are best obtained by a catheter inserted into the right atrium through a peripheral vein, or by the right atrial port (opening) in a pulmonary artery catheter. This pressure is decreased in hypovolemia and increased in right heart failure. The changes that occur in CVP over time usually are more significant than the absolute numeric values obtained during a single reading.

Ventricular volume pressures are obtained by means of a flow-directed, balloon-tipped pulmonary artery catheter. This catheter is introduced through a peripheral or central vein and then advanced into the right atrium. The balloon is then inflated with air, enabling the catheter to float through the right ventricle into the pulmonary artery until it becomes wedged in a small pulmonary vessel (Fig. 26-7). With the balloon inflated, the catheter monitors pulmonary capillary pressures (also called *pulmonary capillary wedge pressure* [PCWP]), which is in direct communication with pressures from the left heart. The pulmonary capillary pressures provide a means of assessing the pumping ability of the left heart.

One type of pulmonary artery catheter is equipped with a thermistor probe to obtain *thermodilution measurements* of cardiac output. A known amount of solution of a known temperature (iced or room temperature) is injected into the right atrium through an opening in the catheter, and the temperature of the blood is measured downstream in the pulmonary artery by the thermistor probe located at the end of that catheter. A microcomputer calculates the cardiac output from changes in the temperature of the blood as it flows past the thermistor. Catheters with oximeters built into their tips that permit continuous monitoring of oxygen saturation (SvO_2) also are available.

Intra-arterial blood pressure monitoring provides a means for continuous monitoring of blood pressure. It is used in persons with acute heart failure when aggressive intravenous medication therapy or a mechanical assist device is required. Measurements are obtained through a small catheter inserted into a peripheral artery, usually the radial artery. The catheter is connected to a pressure transducer, and beat-by-beat measurements of blood pressure are recorded. The monitoring system displays the contour of the pressure waveform, the systolic, diastolic, and mean arterial pressures, along with the heart rate and rhythm.

Treatment

The goals of treatment are determined by the rapidity of onset and severity of the heart failure. Persons with acute heart failure syndromes require urgent therapy directed at stabilizing and correcting the cause of the cardiac dysfunction. For persons with chronic heart failure, the goals of treatment are directed toward relieving the symptoms, improving the quality of life, and reducing or eliminating risk factors (*e.g.,* hypertension, diabetes, obesity) with a long-term goal of slowing, halting, or reversing the cardiac dysfunction.[1,2,34,35]

Treatment measures for both acute and chronic heart failure include nonpharmacologic and pharmacologic approaches. Mechanical support devices, including the intra-aortic balloon pump (for acute failure) and the ventricular assist device (VAD), sustain life in persons with severe heart failure. Heart transplantation remains the treatment of choice for many persons with end-stage heart failure.

Nonpharmacologic Methods. Exercise intolerance is typical in individuals with chronic heart failure.[36] Consequently, individualized exercise training is important to maximize muscle conditioning; persons who are not accustomed to exercise and those with more severe heart failure are started at a lower intensity and shorter sessions than those who are mostly asymptomatic. Sodium and fluid restriction and weight management are important for all individuals with heart failure; the degree of sodium and fluid restriction is individualized to the severity of heart failure. Counseling, health teaching, and ongoing evaluation programs help persons with heart failure to manage and cope with their treatment regimen.

Pharmacologic Treatment. Once heart failure is moderate to severe, pharmacologic in conjunction with nonpharma-

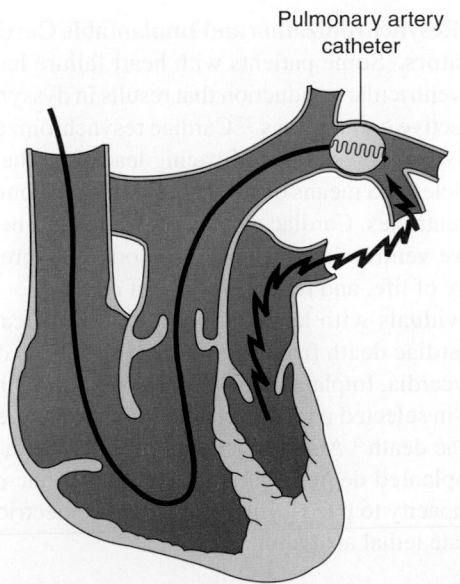

Pulmonary artery catheter

FIGURE 26-7 • Balloon-tipped pulmonary artery catheter positioned in a small pulmonary vessel. The pulmonary capillary wedge pressure, which reflects the left ventricular diastolic pressure, is measured with the balloon inflated.

cologic management is important to prevent and treat acute heart failure and manage chronic heart failure. Evidence-based agents recommended for treatment and management include diuretics, angiotensin-converting enzyme (ACE) inhibitors or angiotensin II receptor blockers, β-adrenergic blockers, and digoxin.[1,2,34,35,37] The choice of pharmacologic agents is based on symptomatology of the person.

Diuretics are among the most frequently prescribed medications for moderate to severe heart failure.[1,2,34] They promote the excretion of fluid and help to sustain cardiac output and tissue perfusion by reducing preload and allowing the heart to operate at a more optimal part of the Frank-Starling curve. Thiazide and loop diuretics are used. In emergencies, such as acute pulmonary edema, loop diuretics such as furosemide can be administered intravenously. When given as a bolus infusion, intravenous furosemide acts within minutes to increase venous capacitance so that right ventricular output and pulmonary capillary pressures are decreased.

The *ACE inhibitors,* which prevent the conversion of angiotensin I to angiotensin II, have been used effectively in the treatment of chronic heart failure. The renin-angiotensin-aldosterone system is activated early in the course of heart failure and plays an important role in its progression. It results in an increase in angiotensin II, which causes vasoconstriction, unregulated ventricular remodeling, and increased aldosterone production with a subsequent increase in sodium and water retention by the kidneys. ACE inhibitors have been shown to limit these harmful complications. The *angiotensin II receptor blockers* appear to have similar but more limited beneficial effects. They have the advantage of not causing a cough, which is a troublesome side effect of the ACE inhibitors for many persons. Aldosterone has a number of deleterious effects in individuals with heart failure. *Aldosterone receptor antagonists* may be used in combination with other agents for persons with moderately severe to severe heart failure.

β-*Adrenergic receptor blocking drugs* are used to decrease left ventricular dysfunction associated with activation of the sympathetic nervous system. Large clinical trials have shown that long-term therapy with β-adrenergic receptor blocking agents reduces morbidity and mortality in persons with chronic heart failure. The mechanism of this benefit remains unclear, but it is likely that chronic elevations of catecholamines and sympathetic nervous system activity cause progressive myocardial damage, leading to a worsening of left ventricular function and a poorer prognosis in persons with heart failure. Large, landmark clinical trials of persons with stable NYHA class II and III heart failure have demonstrated significant reductions in the overall mortality rate with treatment with various β-adrenergic receptor blocking agents.[37,38]

Digitalis has been a recognized treatment for heart failure for over 200 years. The various forms of digitalis are called *cardiac glycosides.* They improve cardiac function by increasing the force and strength of ventricular contractions. By decreasing sinoatrial node activity and decreasing conduction through the atrioventricular node, they also slow the heart rate

and increase diastolic filling time. Although not a diuretic, digitalis promotes urine output by improving cardiac output and renal blood flow. The role of digitalis in the treatment of heart failure has been studied in clinical trials over the past several decades. Although the results of these studies remain controversial, there seems to be a growing consensus that although it does not necessarily reduce mortality rates, digitalis prevents clinical deterioration and hospitalization, and improves exercise tolerance.[39]

Vasodilator drugs are included as recommended agents by the Canadian Heart Failure Guidelines in combination therapy for heart failure.[34] Agents such as isosorbide dinitrate and hydralazine may be added to other standard medications for patients with chronic heart failure.[39] Vasodilators such as nitroglycerin, nitroprusside, and nesiritide (B-type natriuretic peptide) are used in AHFS to improve left heart performance by decreasing the preload (through vasodilation) or reducing the afterload (through arteriolar dilation), or both.[34,40]

Oxygen Therapy. Oxygen therapy increases the oxygen content of the blood and is most often used in patients with acute episodes of heart failure. Continuous positive airway pressure (CPAP) is recommended to reduce the need for endotracheal intubation in patients with AHFS.[41] Because CPAP increases intrathoracic pressure, it also has the potential for decreasing venous return and left ventricular preload, thereby improving the cardiac ejection fraction and stabilizing the hemodynamic status in persons with severe heart failure.[42] Bilevel positive airway pressure (BiPAP), which is like CPAP but also delivers higher pressures during inspiration, is argued by some to be superior to CPAP in that it decreases the respiratory rate and heart rate and improves oxygenation more quickly or more substantially than CPAP.[41]

Cardiac Resynchronization and Implantable Cardioverter–Defibrillators. Some patients with heart failure have abnormal intraventricular conduction that results in dyssynchronous and ineffective contractions.[27] Cardiac resynchronization therapy involves the placement of pacing leads into the right and left ventricles as a means of resynchronizing the contraction of the two ventricles. Cardiac resynchronization has been shown to improve ventricular function and blood pressure, increase the quality of life, and reduce the risk of death.[43]

Individuals with heart failure are at significant risk of sudden cardiac death from ventricular fibrillation or ventricular tachycardia. Implantation of a cardioverter–defibrillator is indicated in selected patients with heart failure to prevent sudden cardiac death.[2] A cardioverter–defibrillator is a programmable implanted device that monitors the cardiac rhythm. It has the capacity to pace the heart and deliver electrical shocks to terminate lethal arrhythmias.

Mechanical Support and Heart Transplantation. Refractory heart failure reflects deterioration in cardiac function that is unresponsive to medical or surgical interventions. With improved methods of treatment, more people are reaching a point where a cure is unachievable and death is imminent without mechanical support or heart transplantation.

Since the early 1960s, significant progress has been made in improving the efficacy of *ventricular assist devices* (VADs), which are mechanical pumps used to support ventricular function. VADs are used to decrease the workload of the myocardium while maintaining cardiac output and systemic arterial pressure. This decreases the workload on the ventricle and allows it to rest and recover. Most VADs require an invasive open chest procedure for implantation. They may be used in patients who fail or have difficulty being weaned from cardiopulmonary bypass after cardiac surgery; those who develop cardiogenic shock after myocardial infarction; those with end-stage cardiomyopathy; and those who are awaiting cardiac transplantation. Earlier and more aggressive use of VADs as a bridge to transplantation and destination therapy (permanent support) has been shown to increase survival.[44] VADs that allow the patient to be mobile and managed at home are sometimes used for long-term or permanent support for treatment of end-stage heart failure, rather than simply as a bridge to transplantation. VADs can be used to support the function of the left ventricle, right ventricle, or both.[44]

Heart transplantation is the preferred treatment for patients with end-stage cardiac failure and otherwise good life expectancy.[2,45] In the United States, 5-year survival rates of persons with heart transplants are approximately 71.2% for males and 66.9% for females.[3] Despite the overall success of heart transplantation, donor availability remains a key problem, and thousands are denied transplantation each year.

Other novel surgical therapies that are being explored include left ventricular remodeling and isolated cell transplantation[46] or gene therapy.[47] Left ventricular remodeling is a surgical procedure designed to restore the size and shape of the ventricle, and is thought to be a viable surgical alternative to cardiac transplantation for persons with severe left ventricular dysfunction.[48]

IN SUMMARY, heart failure occurs when the heart fails to pump sufficient blood to meet the metabolic needs of body tissues. The physiology of heart failure reflects the interplay between a decrease in cardiac output that accompanies impaired function of the failing heart and the compensatory mechanisms that preserve the cardiac reserve. Compensatory mechanisms include the Frank-Starling mechanism, sympathetic nervous system activation, the renin-angiotensin-aldosterone mechanism, natriuretic peptides, the endothelins, and myocardial hypertrophy and remodeling. In the failing heart, early decreases in cardiac function may go unnoticed because these compensatory mechanisms maintain the cardiac output. Unfortunately, the mechanisms were not intended for long-term use, and in severe and prolonged heart failure the compensatory mechanisms no longer are effective, and instead contribute to the progression of heart failure.

Heart failure may be described in terms of systolic versus diastolic dysfunction and right ventricular versus left ventricular dysfunction. With systolic dysfunction, there is impaired ejection of blood from the heart during systole; with diastolic dysfunction, there is impaired filling of the heart during diastole. Right ventricular dysfunction is characterized by congestion in the peripheral circulation, and left ventricular dysfunction by congestion in the pulmonary circulation. Heart failure can present as a chronic condition characterized by decreased cardiac function or as an acute heart failure syndrome. The acute heart failure syndromes represent a gradual or rapid change in heart failure signs and symptoms, indicating need for urgent therapy. These symptoms are primarily the result of pulmonary congestion due to elevated left ventricular filling pressures with or without a low cardiac output.

The manifestations of heart failure include edema, nocturia, fatigue and impaired exercise tolerance, cyanosis, signs of increased sympathetic nervous system activity, and impaired gastrointestinal function and malnutrition. In right-sided failure, there is dependent edema of the lower parts of the body, engorgement of the liver, and ascites. In left-sided failure, pulmonary congestion with shortness of breath and chronic, nonproductive cough are common.

The diagnostic methods in heart failure are directed toward establishing the cause and extent of the disorder. Treatment is directed toward correcting the cause whenever possible, improving cardiac function, maintaining the fluid volume within a compensatory range, and developing an activity pattern consistent with individual limitations in cardiac reserve. Among the medications used in the treatment of heart failure are diuretics, ACE inhibitors and angiotensin receptor blocking agents, β-adrenergic receptor blockers, digoxin, and vasodilators. Mechanical support devices, including the VAD, sustain life in persons with severe heart failure. Heart transplantation remains the treatment of choice for many persons with end-stage heart failure. ■

CONCEPTS in action ANIMATIN

CIRCULATORY FAILURE (SHOCK)

After completing this section of the chapter, you should be able to meet the following objectives:

- State a clinical definition of shock.
- Compare the causes, pathophysiology, and chief characteristics of cardiogenic, hypovolemic, obstructive, and distributive shock.
- Describe the complications of shock as they relate to the lungs, kidneys, gastrointestinal tract, and blood clotting.
- State the rationale for treatment measures to correct and reverse shock.
- Define multiple organ dysfunction syndrome and cite its significance in shock.

Circulatory shock can be described as an acute failure of the circulatory system to supply the peripheral tissues and organs of the body with an adequate blood supply, resulting in cellular hypoxia.[5,49] Most often hypotension and hypoperfusion are present, but shock may occur in the presence of normal vital signs. Shock is not a specific disease but a syndrome that can occur in the course of many life-threatening traumatic conditions or disease states. It can be caused by an alteration in cardiac function (cardiogenic shock), a decrease in blood volume (hypovolemic shock), excessive vasodilation with maldistribution of blood flow (distributive shock), or obstruction of blood flow through the circulatory system (obstructive shock). The main types of shock are summarized in Chart 26-1 and depicted in Figure 26-8.

Pathophysiology of Circulatory Shock

Circulatory failure results in hypoperfusion of organs and tissues, which in turn results in insufficient supply of oxygen and nutrients for cellular function. There are compensatory physiologic responses that eventually decompensate into various shock states if the condition is not properly treated in a timely manner. The most immediate of the compensatory mechanisms are the sympathetic and renin systems, which are designed to maintain cardiac output and blood pressure.

There are two types of adrenergic receptors for the sympathetic nervous system: α and β. The β receptors are further subdivided into β_1 and β_2 receptors. Stimulation of the α receptors causes vasoconstriction; stimulation of β_1 receptors, an increase

---

CHART 26-1   CLASSIFICATION OF CIRCULATORY SHOCK

Cardiogenic
Myocardial damage (myocardial infarction, contusion)
Sustained arrhythmias
Acute valve damage, ventricular septal defect
Cardiac surgery

Hypovolemic
Loss of whole blood
Loss of plasma
Loss of extracellular fluid

Obstructive
Inability of the heart to fill properly (cardiac tamponade)
Obstruction to outflow from the heart (pulmonary embolus, cardiac myxoma, pneumothorax, or dissecting aneurysm)

Distributive
Loss of sympathetic vasomotor tone (neurogenic shock)
Presence of vasodilating substances in the blood (anaphylactic shock)
Presence of inflammatory mediators (septic shock)

⚷ CIRCULATORY SHOCK

- Circulatory shock represents the inability of the circulation to adequately perfuse the tissues of the body.

- It can result from failure of the heart as a pump, a loss of fluid from the vascular compartment (hypovolemic shock), obstruction of flow through the vascular compartment (obstructive shock), or an increase in the size of the vascular compartment that interferes with the distribution of blood (distributive shock).

- The manifestations of shock reflect both the impaired perfusion of body tissues and the body's attempt to maintain tissue perfusion through conservation of water by the kidney, translocation of fluid from extracellular to the intravascular compartment, and activation of sympathetic nervous system mechanisms that increase heart rate and divert blood from less to more essential body tissues.

---

in heart rate and force of myocardial contraction; and of β_2 receptors, vasodilation of the skeletal muscle beds and relaxation of the bronchioles. In shock, there is an increase in sympathetic outflow that results in increased epinephrine and norepinephrine release, and activation of both α and β receptors. Thus, increases in heart rate and vasoconstriction occur in most types of shock. There also is an increase in renin release, leading to an increase in angiotensin II, which augments vasoconstriction and leads to an aldosterone-mediated increase in sodium and water retention by the kidneys. In addition, there is local release of vasoconstrictors, including norepinephrine, angiotensin II, vasopressin, and endothelin, which contribute to arterial and venous vasoconstriction.

The compensatory mechanisms that the body recruits are not effective over the long term and become detrimental when the shock state is prolonged. The intense vasoconstriction causes a decrease in tissue perfusion and insufficient supply of oxygen. Cellular metabolism is impaired, vasoactive inflammatory mediators such as histamine are released, production of oxygen free radicals is increased, and excessive lactic acid and hydrogen ions result in intracellular acidity.[5] Each of these factors promotes cellular dysfunction or death. If circulatory function is reestablished, whether the shock is irreversible or the patient will survive is determined largely at the cellular level.

Shock ultimately exerts its effect at the cellular level, with failure of the circulation to supply the cell with the oxygen and nutrients needed for production of ATP. The cell uses ATP for a number of purposes, including operation of the sodium-potassium membrane pump that moves sodium out of the cell and potassium back into the cell. The cell uses two pathways to convert nutrients to energy (see Chapter 4). The first is the anaerobic (non–oxygen-dependent) glycolytic pathway, which is located in the cytoplasm. Glycolysis converts glucose to ATP and pyruvate. The second pathway is the aerobic (oxygen-

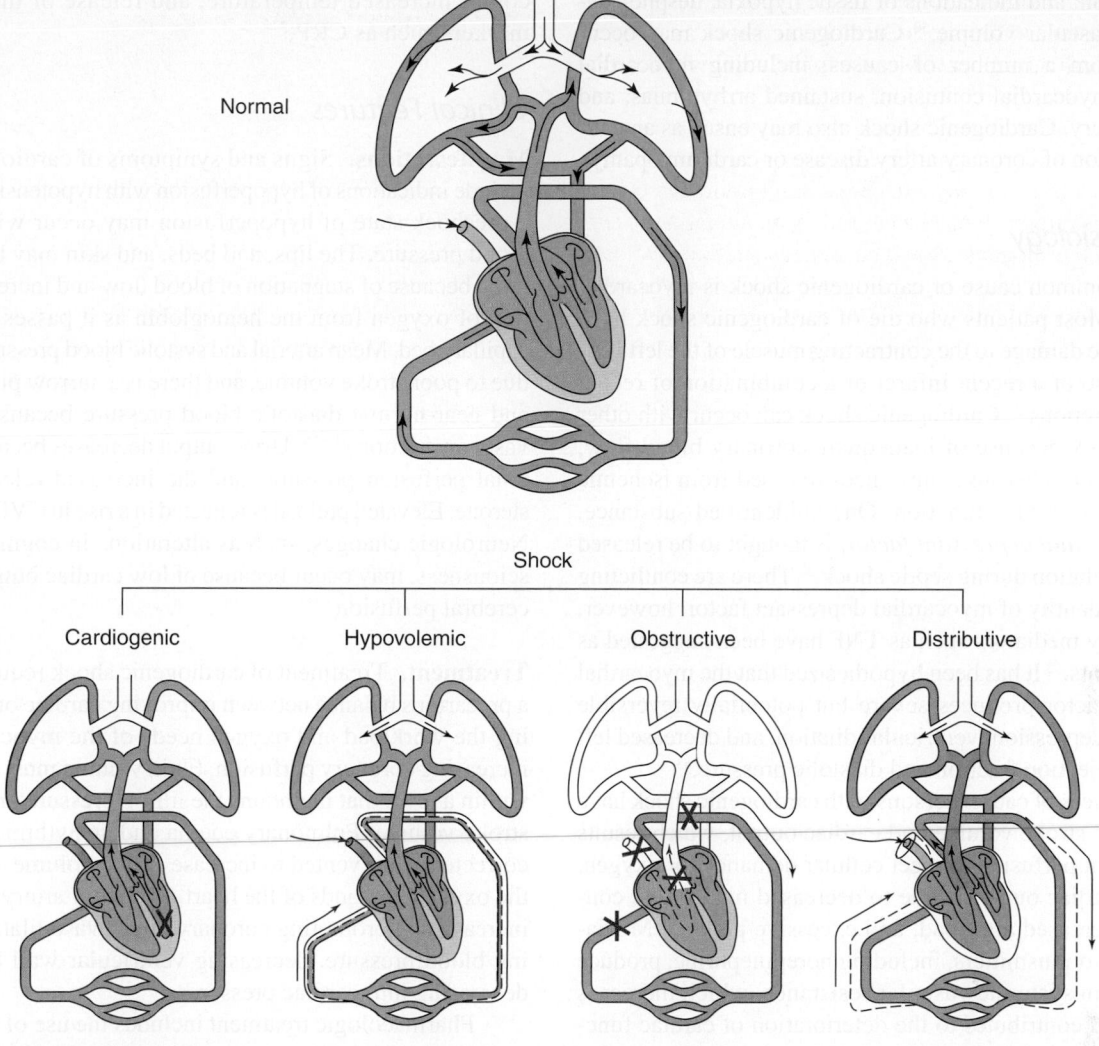

FIGURE 26-8 • Types of shock.

dependent) pathway, called the *citric acid cycle,* which is located in the mitochondria. When oxygen is available, pyruvate from the glycolytic pathway moves into the mitochondria and enters the citric acid cycle, where it is transformed into ATP and the metabolic byproducts carbon dioxide and water. When oxygen is lacking, pyruvate does not enter the citric acid cycle; instead, it is converted to lactic acid. The anaerobic pathway, although allowing energy production to continue in the absence of oxygen, is relatively inefficient and produces significantly less ATP than the aerobic pathway.

In severe shock, cellular metabolic processes are essentially anaerobic owing to the decreased availability of oxygen. Excess amounts of lactic acid accumulate in the cellular and the extracellular compartments, and limited amounts of ATP are produced. Without sufficient energy production, normal cell function cannot be maintained. The sodium-potassium membrane pump is impaired, resulting in excess sodium inside the cells and potassium loss from cells. The increase in intracellular sodium results in cellular edema and

increased cell membrane permeability. Mitochondrial activity becomes severely depressed and lysosomal membranes may rupture, resulting in the release of enzymes that cause further intracellular destruction. This is followed by cell death and the release of intracellular contents into the extracellular space. The destruction of the cell membrane activates the arachidonic acid cascade, release of inflammatory mediators, and production of oxygen free radicals that extend cellular damage.

The extent of the microvascular injury and organ dysfunction is primarily determined by the extent of the shock state and whether it is prolonged. Interventions are targeted at both prevention and early intervention, when possible.

Cardiogenic Shock

Cardiogenic shock occurs when the heart fails to pump blood sufficiently to meet the body's demands (see Fig. 26-8). Clinically, it is defined as decreased cardiac output, hypotension, hypoperfusion, and indications of tissue hypoxia, despite adequate intravascular volume.[50] Cardiogenic shock may occur suddenly from a number of causes, including myocardial infarction, myocardial contusion, sustained arrhythmias, and cardiac surgery. Cardiogenic shock also may ensue as an end-stage condition of coronary artery disease or cardiomyopathy.

Pathophysiology

The most common cause of cardiogenic shock is myocardial infarction. Most patients who die of cardiogenic shock have had extensive damage to the contracting muscle of the left ventricle because of a recent infarct or a combination of recent and old infarctions.[51] Cardiogenic shock can occur with other types of shock because of inadequate coronary blood flow, or it can develop because substances released from ischemic tissues impair cardiac function. One unidentified substance, called *myocardial depressant factor,* is thought to be released into the circulation during septic shock.[52] There are conflicting data on the identity of myocardial depressant factor; however, inflammatory mediators such as TNF have been suggested as possible agents.[52] It has been hypothesized that the myocardial depressant factor produces severe but potentially reversible myocardial depression, ventricular dilation, and decreased left ventricular ejection fraction and diastolic pressure.[53]

Regardless of cause, persons with cardiogenic shock have a decrease in stroke volume and cardiac output, which results in insufficient perfusion to meet cellular demands for oxygen. The poor cardiac output is due to decreased myocardial contractility, increased afterload, and excessive preload. Mediators and neurotransmitters, including norepinephrine, produce an increase in systemic vascular resistance, which increases afterload and contributes to the deterioration of cardiac function. Preload, or the filling pressure of the heart, is increased as blood returning to the heart is added to blood that previously was not pumped forward, resulting in an increase in left ventricular end-systolic volume. Activation of the renin-angiotensin-aldosterone mechanism worsens both preload and afterload by producing an aldosterone-mediated increase in fluid retention and an angiotensin-II–mediated increase in vasoconstriction. The increased resistance (*i.e.,* afterload) to ejection of blood from the left ventricle, in combination with a decrease in myocardial contractility, results in an increase in end-systolic ventricular volume and preload, which further impairs the heart's ability to pump effectively.

Eventually, coronary artery perfusion is impaired because of the increased preload and afterload, and cardiac function decreases because of poor myocardial oxygen supply. There is an increase in intracardiac pressures due to volume overload and ventricular wall tension in both diastole and systole. Excessive pressures decrease coronary artery perfusion during diastole, and increased wall tension decreases coronary artery perfusion during systole. If treatment is unsuccessful, cardiogenic shock may result in a systemic inflammatory response syndrome (discussed in the section on Sepsis and Septic Shock, later), evidenced by increased white blood cell count, increased temperature, and release of inflammatory markers such as CRP.[54]

Clinical Features

Manifestations. Signs and symptoms of cardiogenic shock include indications of hypoperfusion with hypotension, although a preshock state of hypoperfusion may occur with a normal blood pressure. The lips, nail beds, and skin may become cyanotic because of stagnation of blood flow and increased extraction of oxygen from the hemoglobin as it passes through the capillary bed. Mean arterial and systolic blood pressures decrease due to poor stroke volume, and there is a narrow pulse pressure and near-normal diastolic blood pressure because of arterial vasoconstriction.[51,53,54] Urine output decreases because of lower renal perfusion pressures and the increased release of aldosterone. Elevated preload is reflected in a rise in CVP and PCWP. Neurologic changes, such as alterations in cognition or consciousness, may occur because of low cardiac output and poor cerebral perfusion.

Treatment. Treatment of cardiogenic shock requires striking a precarious balance between improving cardiac output, reducing the workload and oxygen needs of the myocardium, and increasing coronary perfusion. Fluid volume must be regulated within a level that maintains the filling pressure and optimizes stroke volume. Pulmonary edema and arrhythmias should be corrected or prevented to increase stroke volume and decrease the oxygen demands of the heart. Coronary artery perfusion is increased by promoting coronary artery vasodilation, increasing blood pressure, decreasing ventricular wall tension, and decreasing intracardiac pressures.

Pharmacologic treatment includes the use of vasodilators such as nitroprusside and nitroglycerin. Both nitroprusside and nitroglycerin cause coronary artery dilation, which increases myocardial oxygen delivery. Nitroprusside causes arterial and venous dilation, producing a decrease in venous return to the heart and a reduction in arterial resistance against which the left heart must pump.[37] At lower doses, the main effects of nitroglycerin are on the venous vascular beds and coronary arteries; at high doses, it also dilates the arterial beds. Both medications may result in a decrease in diastolic arterial pressure that results in a lower systemic vascular resistance (afterload). The systolic arterial pressure is maintained by an increase in ventricular stroke volume, which is ejected against the lowered systemic vascular resistance. The improvement in heart function increases stroke volume and enables blood to be redistributed from the pulmonary vascular bed to the systemic circulation.

Positive inotropic agents are used to improve cardiac contractility. Both dobutamine and milrinone are effective medications in that they result in increased contractility and arterial vasodilation. Dobutamine is a synthetic agent consisting of two isomers, one of which is a potent β_1-adrenergic receptor agonist and α_1-adrenergic receptor antagonist and the other that is a mild β_2-adrenergic receptor agonist and α_1-adrenergic receptor agonist. The combination tends to produce vasodilation and a positive inotropic action. Milrinone increases myocardial contractility by increasing the movement of Ca⁺⁺ into myocardial cells during an action potential (see Fig. 26-1). The increase in stroke volume results in a decrease in end-systolic volume and a reduction in preload. With a decrease in preload pressures, coronary artery perfusion is improved during diastole. Thus, stroke volume and myocardial oxygen supply are improved with a minimal increase in myocardial oxygen demand. Catecholamines increase cardiac contractility but must be used with extreme caution because they also result in arterial constriction and increased heart rates, which worsens the imbalance between myocardial oxygen supply and demand.

The intra-aortic balloon pump, also referred to as *counterpulsation,* enhances coronary and systemic perfusion, yet decreases afterload and myocardial oxygen demands.[55] The device, which pumps in synchrony with the heart, consists of a 10-inch-long balloon that is inserted through a catheter into the descending aorta (Fig. 26-9). The balloon is timed to inflate during ventricular diastole and deflate just before ventricular systole. Diastolic inflation creates a pressure wave in the ascending aorta that increases coronary artery blood flow and a less intense wave in the lower aorta that enhances organ perfusion. The abrupt balloon deflation at the onset of systole results in a displacement of blood volume that lowers the resistance to ejection of blood from the left ventricle. Thus, the heart's pumping efficiency is increased, myocardial oxygen supply is increased, and myocardial oxygen consumption is decreased.

When cardiogenic shock is caused by myocardial infarction, several aggressive interventions can be used successfully.

Either fibrinolytic therapy or percutaneous coronary intervention (see Chapter 24) may be used to prevent or treat cardiogenic shock.[56] Reperfusion of the coronary arteries is expected to improve myocardial function.

Hypovolemic Shock

Hypovolemic shock is characterized by diminished blood volume such that there is inadequate filling of the vascular compartment[5,57,58] (see Fig. 26-8). It occurs when there is an acute loss of 15% to 20% of the circulating blood volume. The decrease may be caused by an external loss of whole blood (*e.g.,* hemorrhage), plasma (*e.g.,* severe burns), or extracellular fluid (*e.g.,* severe dehydration or loss of gastrointestinal fluids with vomiting or diarrhea). Hypovolemic shock also can result from an internal hemorrhage or from third-space losses, when extracellular fluid is shifted from the vascular compartment to the interstitial space or compartment.

Pathophysiology

Hypovolemic shock, which has been the most widely studied type of shock, is often used as a prototype in discussions of the manifestations of shock. Figure 26-10 shows the effect of removing blood from the circulatory system during approximately 30 minutes.[5] Approximately 10% of the total blood volume can be removed without changing cardiac output or arterial pressure. The average blood donor loses approximately 500 mL or 10% of their blood without experiencing adverse effects. As increasing amounts of blood (10% to 25%) are removed, the stroke volume falls but arterial pressure is maintained because of sympathetic-mediated increases in heart rate and vasoconstriction. Vasoconstriction results in an increased diastolic pressure and narrow pulse pressure. Blood pressure is the product of cardiac output and systemic vascular resistance

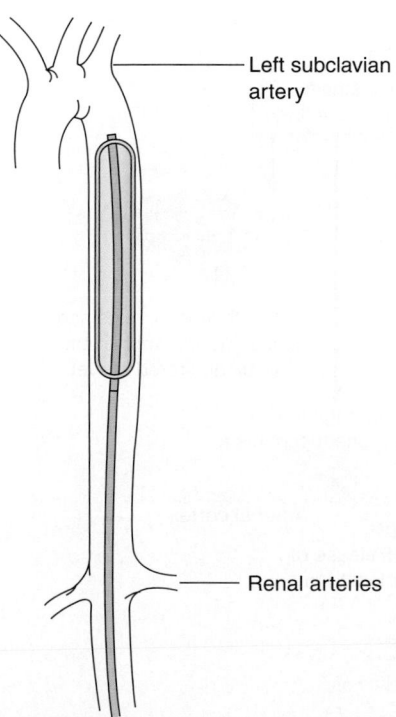

FIGURE 26-9 • Aortic balloon pump. (From Hudak C. M., Gallo B. M. [1994]. *Critical care nursing* [6th ed.]. Philadelphia: J. B. Lippincott.)

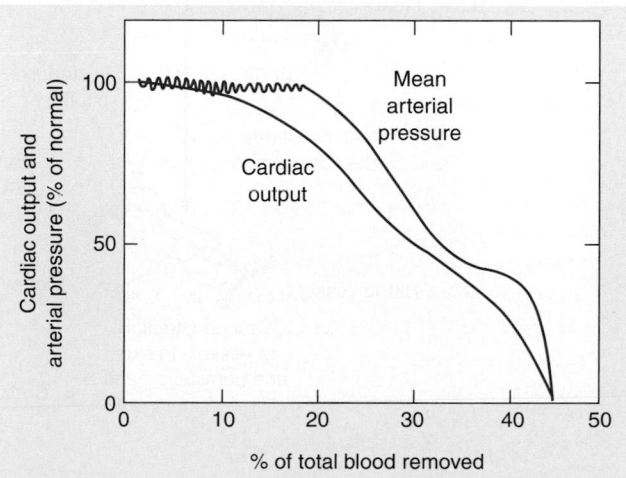

FIGURE 26-10 • Effect of hemorrhage on cardiac output and arterial pressure. (From Guyton A. C., Hall J. E. [2006]. *Textbook of medical physiology* [11th ed., p. 279]. Philadelphia: Elsevier Saunders.)

(blood pressure = cardiac output × systemic vascular resistance). An increase in systemic vascular resistance maintains mean arterial pressure for a short time despite decreased cardiac output. Cardiac output and tissue perfusion decrease before signs of hypotension appear. Cardiac output and arterial pressure fall to zero when approximately 35% to 45% of the total blood volume has been removed.[5]

Compensatory Mechanisms. Without compensatory mechanisms to maintain cardiac output and blood pressure, the loss of vascular volume would result in a rapid progression from the initial to the progressive and irreversible stages of shock. The most immediate of the compensatory mechanisms are the sympathetic-mediated responses designed to maintain cardiac output and blood pressure (Fig. 26-11). Within seconds after the onset of hemorrhage or the loss of blood volume, tachycardia, increased cardiac contractility, vasoconstriction, and other signs of sympathetic and adrenal medullary activity appear. The sympathetic vasoconstrictor response also mobilizes blood that has been stored in the venous side of the circulation as a means of increasing venous return to the heart. There is considerable capacity for blood storage in the large veins of the abdomen,

and approximately 350 mL of blood that can be mobilized in shock is stored in the liver.[5] Sympathetic stimulation does not initially cause constriction of the cerebral and coronary vessels, and blood flow to the heart and brain is maintained at essentially normal levels as long as the mean arterial pressure remains above 70 mm Hg.[5]

Compensatory mechanisms designed to restore blood volume include absorption of fluid from the interstitial spaces, conservation of sodium and water by the kidneys, and thirst. Extracellular fluid is distributed between the interstitial spaces and the vascular compartment. When there is a loss of vascular volume, capillary pressures decrease and water is drawn into the vascular compartment from the interstitial spaces. The maintenance of vascular volume is further enhanced by renal mechanisms that conserve fluid. A decrease in renal blood flow and glomerular filtration rate results in activation of the renin-angiotensin-aldosterone mechanism, which produces an increase in sodium reabsorption by the kidneys. The decrease in blood volume also stimulates centers in the hypothalamus that regulate ADH release and thirst. ADH, also known as *vasopressin*, constricts the peripheral arteries and veins and greatly increases water retention by the kidneys. Although the mechanism of

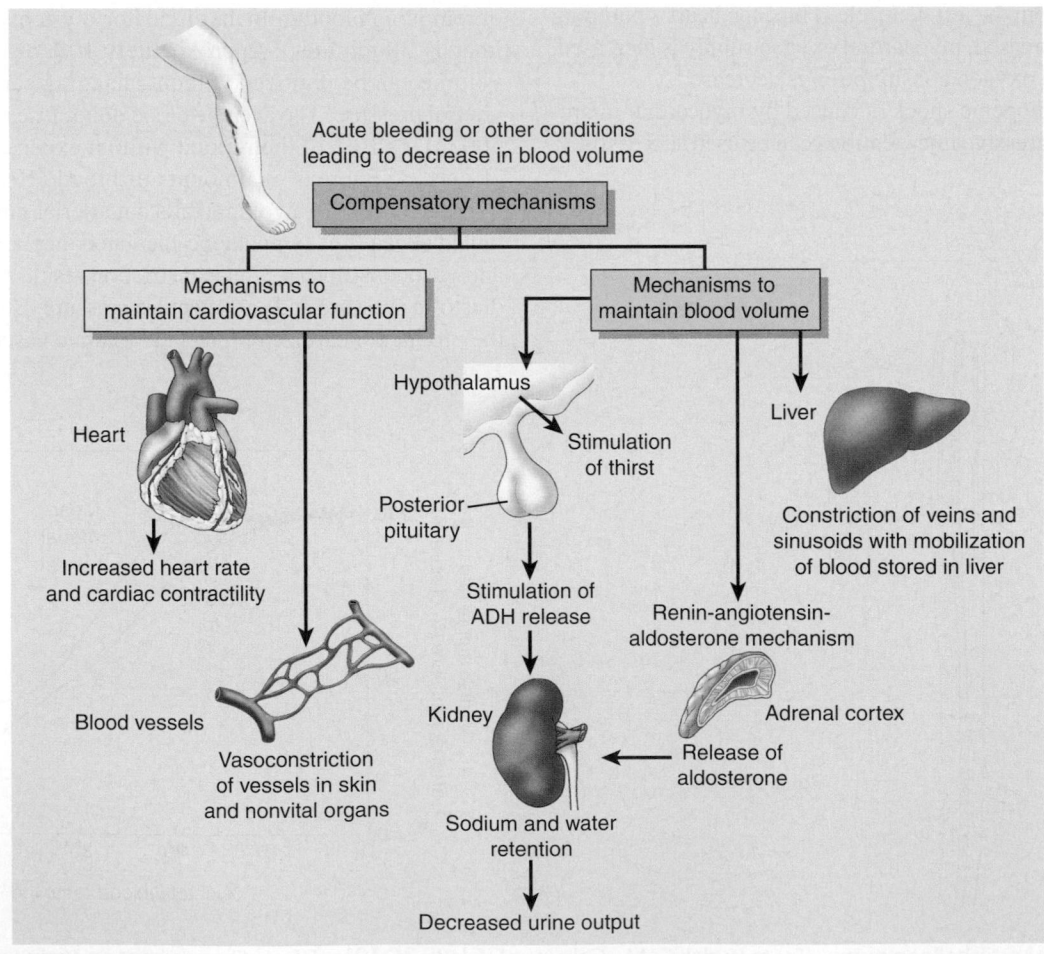

FIGURE 26-11 • Compensatory mechanisms used to maintain circulatory function and blood volume in hypovolemic shock. ADH, antidiuretic hormone.

ADH is more sensitive to changes in serum osmolality, a decrease of 10% to 15% in blood volume serves as a strong stimulus for thirst.[5]

During the early stages of hypovolemic shock, vasoconstriction decreases the size of the vascular compartment and increases systemic vascular resistance. This response usually is all that is needed when the injury is slight and blood loss is minimal. As hypovolemic shock progresses, vasoconstriction of the blood vessels that supply the skin, skeletal muscles, kidneys, and abdominal organs becomes more severe, with a further decrease in blood flow and conversion to anaerobic metabolism resulting in cellular injury.

Clinical Features

The signs and symptoms of hypovolemic shock depend on its severity and are closely related to low peripheral blood flow and excessive sympathetic stimulation. They include thirst, increased heart rate, cool and clammy skin, decreased arterial blood pressure, decreased urine output, and changes in mentation. Laboratory tests of hemoglobin and hematocrit provide information regarding the severity of blood loss or hemoconcentration due to dehydration. Serum lactate and arterial pH provide information about the severity of acidosis due to anaerobic metabolism. Metabolic acidosis revealed by arterial blood gas measurement is the gold standard diagnostic test.[58] Acute, fatal hemorrhagic shock is characterized by metabolic acidosis, coagulopathy, and hypothermia, followed by circulatory failure.[58]

An increase in heart rate is an early sign of hypovolemic shock, as the body tries to maintain cardiac output despite the decrease in stroke volume. As shock progresses, the pulse becomes weak and thready, indicating vasoconstriction and reduced filling of the vascular compartment. Thirst is an early symptom in hypovolemic shock. Although the underlying cause is not fully understood, it probably is related to decreased blood volume and increased serum osmolality (see Chapter 31).

Arterial blood pressure is decreased in moderate to severe shock. However, controversy exists over the value of blood pressure measurements in the early diagnosis and management of shock. This is because compensatory mechanisms tend to preserve blood pressure until shock is relatively far advanced. Furthermore, a normal arterial pressure does not ensure adequate perfusion and oxygenation of vital organs at the cellular level. This does not imply that blood pressure should not be closely monitored in patients at risk for development of shock, but it does indicate the need for other assessment measures.

As shock progresses, the respirations become rapid and deep, to compensate for the increased production of acid and decreased availability of oxygen. Decreased intravascular volume results in decreased venous return to the heart and a decreased CVP. When shock becomes severe, the peripheral veins may collapse. Sympathetic stimulation leads to intense vasoconstriction of the skin vessels, which results in cool and mottled skin. In hemorrhagic shock, the loss of red blood cells results in pallor of the skin and mucous membranes.

Urine output decreases very quickly in hypovolemic shock. Compensatory mechanisms decrease renal blood flow as a means of diverting blood flow to the heart and brain. Oliguria of 20 mL/hour or less indicates inadequate renal perfusion. Continuous measurement of urine output is essential for assessing the circulatory and volume status of the person in shock.

Restlessness, agitation, and apprehension are common in early shock because of increased sympathetic outflow and increased levels of epinephrine. As the shock progresses and blood flow to the brain decreases, restlessness is replaced by altered arousal and mentation. Loss of consciousness and coma may occur if the person does not receive or respond to treatment.

Treatment. The treatment of hypovolemic shock is directed toward correcting or controlling the underlying cause and improving tissue perfusion. Ongoing loss of blood must be corrected, such as in surgery. Oxygen is administered to increase oxygen delivery to the tissues. Medications usually are administered intravenously. Frequent measurements of heart rate and cardiac rhythm, blood pressure, and urine output are used to assess the severity of circulatory compromise and to monitor treatment.

In hypovolemic shock, the goal of treatment is to restore vascular volume.[57,58] This can be accomplished through intravenous administration of fluids and blood. The crystalloids (*e.g.,* isotonic saline and Ringer's lactate) are readily available and effective, at least temporarily. Plasma volume expanders (*e.g.,* pentastarch and colloidal albumin) have a high molecular weight, do not necessitate blood typing, and remain in the vascular space for longer periods than crystalloids such as dextrose and saline. Blood or blood products (packed or frozen red cells) are administered based on hematocrit and hemodynamic findings. Fluids and blood are best administered based on volume indicators such as CVP and urine output.

Vasoactive medications are agents capable of constricting or dilating blood vessels. Considerable controversy exists about the advantages or disadvantages related to the use of these drugs. As a general rule, vasoconstrictor agents are not used as a primary form of therapy in hypovolemic shock, and may be detrimental. These agents are given only when volume deficits have been corrected yet hypotension persists.

Distributive Shock

Distributive or vasodilatory shock is characterized by loss of blood vessel tone, enlargement of the vascular compartment, and displacement of the vascular volume away from the heart and central circulation.[59] In distributive shock, the capacity of the vascular compartment expands to the extent that a normal volume of blood does not fill the circulatory system (see Fig. 26-8). Therefore, this type of shock is also referred to as *normovolemic shock.* Two main causes result in the loss of vascular tone: a decrease in the sympathetic control of vasomotor tone or the release of excessive vasodilator substances. It can also occur as a complication of vessel damage resulting from prolonged and severe hypotension due to hemorrhage, known as *irreversible* or *late-phase hemorrhagic shock*.[59] There are three shock states that share the basic circulatory pattern of distributive shock: neurogenic shock, anaphylactic shock, and septic shock.

Neurogenic Shock

Neurogenic shock is caused by decreased sympathetic control of blood vessel tone due to a defect in the vasomotor center in the brain stem or the sympathetic outflow to the blood vessels.[5] The term *spinal shock* describes the neurogenic shock that occurs in persons with spinal cord injury (see Chapter 50). Output from the vasomotor center can be interrupted by brain injury, the depressant action of drugs, general anesthesia, hypoxia, or lack of glucose (*e.g.,* insulin reaction). Fainting due to emotional causes is a transient form of impaired sympathetic outflow. Many general anesthetic agents can cause a neurogenic shock–like reaction, especially during induction, because of interference with sympathetic nervous system function. Spinal anesthesia or spinal cord injury above the mid-thoracic region can interrupt the transmission of outflow from the vasomotor center. In contrast to other shock states due to the loss of blood volume or impaired cardiac function, the heart rate in neurogenic shock often is slower than normal, and the skin is dry and warm. This type of distributive shock is rare and usually transitory.

Anaphylactic Shock

Anaphylaxis is a clinical syndrome that represents the most severe systemic allergic reaction.[60–62] Anaphylactic shock results from an immunologically mediated reaction in which vasodilator substances such as histamine are released into the blood (see Chapter 19). These substances cause vasodilation of arterioles and venules along with a marked increase in capillary permeability. The vascular response in anaphylaxis is often accompanied by life-threatening laryngeal edema and bronchospasm, circulatory collapse, contraction of gastrointestinal and uterine smooth muscle, and urticaria (hives) or angioedema.

Among the most frequent causes of anaphylactic shock are reactions to medications, such as penicillin; foods, such as nuts and shellfish; and insect venoms. The most common cause is stings from insects of the order Hymenoptera (*i.e.,* bees, wasps, and fire ants). Latex allergy causes life-threatening anaphylaxis in a growing segment of the population (see Chapter 19). Health care workers and others who are exposed to latex are developing latex sensitivities that range from mild urticaria, contact dermatitis, and mild respiratory distress to anaphylactic shock.[63] Children with spina bifida also are at extreme risk for this serious and increasingly common allergy.

The onset and severity of anaphylaxis depend on the sensitivity of the person and the rate and quantity of antigen exposure. Signs and symptoms associated with impending anaphylactic shock include abdominal cramps; apprehension; warm or burning sensation of the skin, itching, and urticaria (*i.e.,* hives); and coughing, choking, wheezing, chest tightness, and difficulty in

breathing. After blood begins to pool peripherally, there is a precipitous drop in blood pressure and the pulse becomes so weak that it is difficult to detect. Life-threatening airway obstruction may ensue as a result of laryngeal angioedema or bronchial spasm. Anaphylactic shock often develops suddenly; death can occur within minutes unless appropriate medical intervention is promptly instituted.

Treatment includes immediate discontinuation of the inciting agent or institution of measures to decrease its absorption (*e.g.,* application of ice to the site of an insect bite); close monitoring of cardiovascular and respiratory function; and maintenance of respiratory gas exchange, cardiac output, and tissue perfusion. Epinephrine is given in an anaphylactic reaction because it constricts blood vessels and relaxes the smooth muscle in the bronchioles, thus restoring cardiac and respiratory function.[61] Other treatment measures include the administration of oxygen, antihistamine drugs, and corticosteroids. The person should be placed in a supine position. This is extremely important because venous return can be severely compromised in the sitting position. This in turn produces a pulseless mechanical contraction of the heart and predisposes to arrhythmias. In several cases, death has occurred immediately after assuming the sitting position.[61]

The prevention of anaphylactic shock is preferable to treatment. Once a person has been sensitized to an antigen, the risk of repeated anaphylactic reactions with subsequent exposure is high. All health care providers should question patients regarding previous drug reactions and inform patients as to the name of the medication they are to receive before it is administered or prescribed. Persons with known hypersensitivities should wear Medic Alert jewelry and carry an identification card to alert medical personnel if they become unconscious or unable to relate this information. Persons who are at risk for anaphylaxis should be provided with emergency medications (*e.g.,* epinephrine autoinjector) and instructed in procedures to follow in case they are inadvertently exposed to the offending antigen.[61]

Sepsis and Septic Shock

Septic shock, which is the most common type of vasodilatory shock, is associated with severe infection and the systemic response to infection (Fig. 26-12).[64–71] The nomenclature related to sepsis and septic shock has been evolving.[65,66] *Sepsis* is currently defined as suspected or proven infection, plus a systemic inflammatory response (*e.g.,* fever, tachycardia, tachypnea, and elevated white blood cell count, altered mental state, and hyperglycemia in the absence of diabetes).[70] *Severe sepsis* is defined as sepsis with organ dysfunction (*e.g.,* hypotension, hypoxemia, oliguria, metabolic acidosis, thrombocytopenia, or obtundation).[65] *Septic shock* is defined as severe sepsis with hypotension, despite fluid resuscitation.[64–66]

It is estimated that more than 750,000 cases of sepsis occur each year in the United States, leading to approximately 225,000 deaths.[66,67] The growing incidence has been attributed to enhanced awareness of the diagnosis, increased number of resistant organisms, growing number of immunocompromised and elderly persons, and greater use of invasive procedures. With early intervention and advances in treatment methods, the mortality rate has decreased; however, the number of deaths has increased because of the increased prevalence.[68]

Mechanisms. The pathogenesis of sepsis involves a complex process of cellular activation resulting in the release of proinflammatory mediators such as cytokines; recruitment of neutrophils and monocytes; involvement of neuroendocrine reflexes; and activation of complement, coagulation, and fibrinolytic systems. Initiation of the response begins with activation of the innate immune system by pattern-recognition receptors (e.g., Toll-like receptors [TLRs]) that interact with specific molecules present on microorganisms[65] (see Chapter 17). Binding of TLRs to epitopes on microorganisms stimulates transcription and release of a number of proinflammatory and anti-inflammatory mediators. Two of these mediators, TNF-α and interleukin-1, are involved in leukocyte adhesion, local inflammation, neutrophil activation, suppression of erythropoiesis, generation of fever, tachycardia, lactic acidosis, ventilation-perfusion abnormalities, and other signs of sepsis (see section on The Inflammatory Response, Chapter 18). Although activated neutrophils kill microorganisms, they also injure the endothelium by releasing mediators that increase vascular permeability. In addition, activated endothelial cells release nitric oxide, a potent vasodilator that acts as a key mediator of septic shock.

Another important aspect of sepsis is an alteration of the procoagulation–anticoagulation balance with an increase in procoagulation factors and a decrease in anticoagulation factors. Lipopolysaccharide on the surface of microorganisms stimulates endothelial cells lining blood vessels to increase their production of tissue factor, thus activating coagulation[66] (see Chapter 13). Fibrinogen is then converted to fibrin, leading to the formation of microvascular thrombi that further amplify tissue injury. In addition, sepsis lowers levels of protein C, protein S, antithrombin III, and tissue factor pathway inhibitor, substances that modulate and inhibit coagulation. Lipopolysaccharide and TNF-α also decrease the synthesis of thrombomodulin and endothelial protein C receptor, impairing activation of protein C, and they increase the synthesis of plasminogen activator inhibitor-1, impairing fibrinolysis.[66]

Manifestations. Sepsis and septic shock typically manifests with hypotension and warm, flushed skin. Whereas other forms of shock (i.e., cardiogenic, hypovolemic, and obstructive) are characterized by a compensatory increase in systemic vascular resistance, septic shock often presents with a decrease in systemic vascular resistance. There is hypovolemia due to arterial and venous dilatation, plus leakage of plasma into the interstitial spaces. Abrupt changes in cognition or behavior are due to reduced cerebral blood flow, and may be early indications of septic shock. Regardless of the underlying cause, fever and increased leukocytes are present. An elevated serum lactate or metabolic acidosis indicates anaerobic metabolism due to tissue hypoxia or cellular dysfunction and altered cellular metabolism.[68] Tissue hypoxia produces continued production and activation of inflammatory mediators, resulting in further increases in vascular permeability, impaired vascular regulation, and altered hemostasis.

Treatment. The treatment of sepsis and septic shock focuses on control of the causative agent and support of the circulation. Early use of antibiotics is essential, followed by antibiotic therapy specific to the infectious agent.[70] However, antibiotics do not treat the inflammatory response to the infection; thus, the cardiovascular status of the patient must be supported to increase

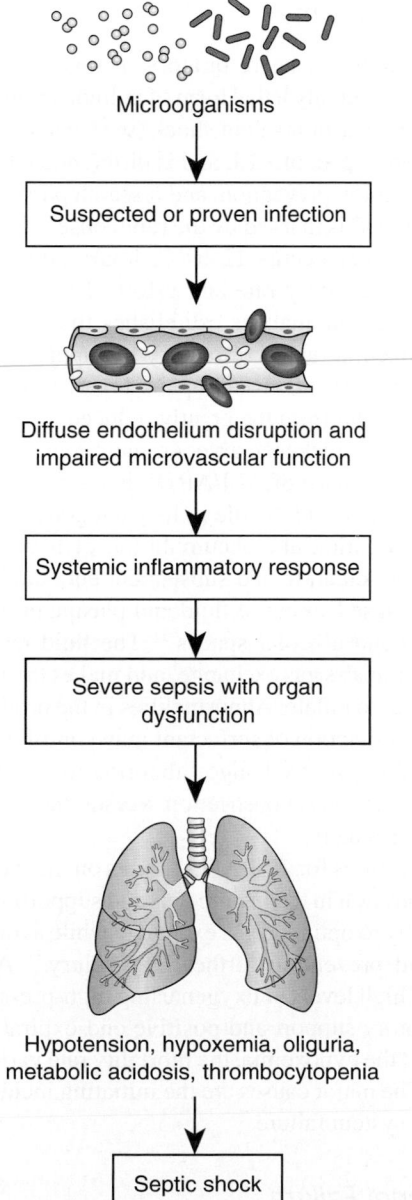

FIGURE 26-12 • Pathogenic mechanisms leading from infection to septic shock.

The flow diagram shows:

Microorganisms → Suspected or proven infection → Diffuse endothelium disruption and impaired microvascular function → Systemic inflammatory response → Severe sepsis with organ dysfunction → Hypotension, hypoxemia, oliguria, metabolic acidosis, thrombocytopenia → Septic shock

oxygen delivery to the cells and prevent further cellular injury. Swift and aggressive fluid administration is needed to compensate for third spacing. Equally aggressive use of vasoconstrictive agents, such as vasopressin, norepinephrine, and phenylephrine, is needed to counteract the vasodilation caused by inflammatory mediators. A positive inotrope, such as dobutamine or milrinone, may be used to augment cardiac output. Ongoing assessment of CVP, central or mixed venous oxygen saturation, mean arterial pressure, urinary output, and laboratory measurements of serum lactate, base deficit, and pH are used to evaluate the progression of sepsis and adequacy of treatment.[65–67,70]

Among the more recent advances in the treatment of sepsis are the use of intensive insulin therapy for hyperglycemia and the administration of recombinant human activated protein C.[67,71] It has been demonstrated that intensive insulin therapy that maintained blood glucose levels at 80 to 110 mg/dL (4.4 to 6.1 mmol/L) resulted in lower mortality and morbidity than did conventional therapy that maintained blood glucose levels at 180 to 200 mg/dL (10 to 11 mmol/L).[72] Hyperglycemia is potentially harmful because it acts as a procoagulant, induces apoptosis, impairs neutrophil function, increases the risk of infection, and impairs wound healing.[66] Recombinant human activated protein C (drotrecogin alfa), a naturally occurring anticoagulant factor that acts by inactivating coagulation factors Va and VIII (see Chapter 13), is the first agent that has demonstrated effectiveness in the treatment of sepsis.[66–68] In addition to its anticoagulant actions, activated protein C has direct anti-inflammatory properties, including blocking the production of cytokines by monocytes and blocking cell adhesion. Activated protein C also has antiapoptotic actions that may contribute to its effectiveness. The use of corticosteroids, once considered a mainstay in the treatment of sepsis, remains controversial. Use of high-dose corticosteroids, in particular, has not been shown to improve survival and may worsen outcomes by increasing the risk of secondary infections.

Obstructive Shock

The term *obstructive shock* describes circulatory shock that results from mechanical obstruction of the flow of blood through the central circulation (great veins, heart, or lungs; see Fig. 26-8). Obstructive shock may be caused by a number of conditions, including dissecting aortic aneurysm, cardiac tamponade, pneumothorax, atrial myxoma, and evisceration of abdominal contents into the thoracic cavity because of a ruptured hemidiaphragm. The most frequent cause of obstructive shock is pulmonary embolism.

The primary physiologic result of obstructive shock is elevated right heart pressure due to impaired right ventricular function. Pressures are increased despite impaired venous return to the heart. Signs of right heart failure occur, including elevation of CVP and jugular venous distention. Treatment modalities focus on correcting the cause of the disorder, frequently with surgical interventions such as pulmonary embolectomy, pericardiocentesis (*i.e.,* removal of fluid from the pericardial sac) for cardiac tamponade, or the insertion of a chest tube for cor-

rection of a tension pneumothorax or hemothorax. In severe or massive pulmonary embolus, fibrinolytic drugs may be used to break down the clots causing the obstruction.

Complications of Shock

Carl Wiggers, a noted circulatory physiologist, stated, "Shock not only stops the machine, but it wrecks the machinery."[73] Many body systems are wrecked by severe shock. Five major complications of severe shock are pulmonary injury, acute renal failure, gastrointestinal ulceration, disseminated intravascular coagulation, and multiple organ dysfunction syndrome. These complications of shock are serious and often fatal.

Acute Lung Injury/Acute Respiratory Distress Syndrome

Acute lung injury/acute respiratory distress syndrome (ALI/ARDS) is a potentially lethal form of pulmonary injury that may be either the cause or result of shock (see Chapter 29). ARDS is a more severe aspect of ALI, and is differentiated primarily for early intervention, prevention, and research purposes.

ALI/ARDS is marked by the rapid onset of profound dyspnea that usually occurs 12 to 48 hours after the initiating event. The respiratory rate and effort of breathing increase. Arterial blood gas analysis establishes the presence of profound hypoxemia that is refractory to supplemental oxygen. The hypoxemia results from impaired matching of ventilation and perfusion and from the greatly reduced diffusion of blood gases across the thickened alveolar membranes.

The exact cause of ALI/ARDS is unknown. Neutrophils are thought to play a key role in its pathogenesis. A cytokine-mediated activation and accumulation of neutrophils in the pulmonary vasculature and subsequent endothelial injury are thought to cause leaking of fluid and plasma proteins into the interstitium and alveolar spaces.[74] The fluid leakage causes atelectasis, impairs gas exchange, and makes the lung stiff and more difficult to inflate. Abnormalities in the production, composition, and function of surfactant may contribute to alveolar collapse and gas exchange abnormalities. Inappropriate vasodilation and vasoconstriction worsen the ventilation and perfusion mismatch.

Interventions for ALI/ARDS focus on increasing the oxygen concentration in the inspired air and supporting ventilation mechanically to optimize gas exchange while avoiding oxygen toxicity and preventing further lung injury.[75] Although the delivery of high levels of oxygen using high-pressure mechanical ventilatory support and positive end-expiratory pressure may correct the hypoxemia, the mortality rate varies from 35% to 40%.[76] The major causes are the initiating incident and multiple organ system failure.

Acute Renal Failure

The renal tubules are particularly vulnerable to ischemia, and acute renal failure is an important factor in mortality due to severe shock. Most cases of acute renal failure are due to impaired renal perfusion or direct injury to the kidneys. The degree of renal damage is related to the severity and duration of shock. The normal kidney is able to tolerate severe ischemia for 15 to 20 minutes. The renal dysfunction most frequently seen after severe shock is acute tubular necrosis. Acute tubular necrosis usually is reversible, although return to normal renal function may require weeks or months (see Chapter 33). Continuous monitoring of urinary output during shock provides a means of assessing renal blood flow. Frequent monitoring of serum creatinine and blood urea nitrogen levels also provides valuable information regarding renal status.

Mediators implicated in septic shock are powerful vasoconstrictors capable of activating the sympathetic nervous system and causing intravascular clotting. They have been shown to trigger all the separate physiologic mechanisms that contribute to the onset of acute renal failure.

Gastrointestinal Complications

The gastrointestinal tract is particularly vulnerable to ischemia because of the changes in distribution of blood flow to its mucosal surface. In shock, there is widespread constriction of blood vessels that supply the gastrointestinal tract, causing a redistribution of blood flow and a severe decrease in mucosal perfusion. Patients may experience loss of appetite, nausea, or vomiting. Superficial mucosal lesions of the stomach and duodenum can develop within hours of severe trauma, sepsis, or burns. Bowel obstruction or bleeding may occur after the decrease in perfusion in shock. Hemorrhage usually has its onset within 2 to 10 days after the original insult and often begins without warning. Poor perfusion in the gastrointestinal tract has been credited with allowing intestinal bacteria to enter the bloodstream, thereby contributing to the development of sepsis and shock.[77]

Histamine type 2 receptor antagonists, proton pump inhibitors, or sucralfate may be given prophylactically to prevent gastrointestinal ulcerations caused by shock.[77] Nasogastric tubes, when attached to intermittent suction, also help to diminish the accumulation of hydrogen ions in the stomach.

Disseminated Intravascular Coagulation

Disseminated intravascular coagulation (DIC) is characterized by widespread activation of the coagulation system with resultant formation of fibrin clots and thrombotic occlusion of small and midsized vessels (see Chapter 13). The systemic formation of fibrin results from increased generation of thrombin, the simultaneous suppression of physiologic anticoagulation mechanisms, and the delayed removal of fibrin as a consequence of impaired fibrinolysis. Clinically overt DIC is reported to occur in as much as 30% to 50% of persons with sepsis and septic shock.[78] As with other systemic inflammatory responses, the derangement of coagulation and fibrinolysis is thought to be mediated by inflammatory mediators and cytokines.

The contribution of DIC to morbidity and mortality in sepsis depends on the underlying clinical condition and the intensity of the coagulation disorder. Depletion of the platelets and coagulation factors increases the risk of bleeding. Deposition of fibrin in the vasculature of organs contributes to ischemic damage and organ failure. In a large number of clinical trials, the occurrence of DIC appeared to be associated with an unfavorable outcome and was an independent predictor of mortality.[78] However, it remains uncertain whether DIC was a predictor of unfavorable outcome, or merely a marker of the seriousness of the underlying condition causing the DIC.

The management of sepsis-induced DIC focuses on treatment of the underlying disorder and measures to interrupt the coagulation process. Anticoagulation therapy and administration of platelets and plasma may be used. Clinical trials have shown modest to marked reductions in mortality based on the dose of antithrombin III used.[78] Other therapeutic options, aimed at interrupting the intrinsic coagulation pathway at the point where tissue factor complexes with factor VIIa, also are being investigated.[78]

Multiple Organ Dysfunction Syndrome

Multiple organ dysfunction syndrome (MODS) represents the presence of altered organ function in an acutely ill patient such that homeostasis cannot be maintained without intervention. As the name implies, MODS commonly affects multiple organ systems, including the kidneys, lungs, liver, brain, and heart. MODS is a particularly life-threatening complication of shock, especially septic shock. It has been reported as the most frequent cause of death in the noncoronary intensive care unit. Mortality rates vary from 30% to 100%, depending on the number of organs involved.[79] Mortality rates increase with an increased number of organs failing. A high mortality rate is associated with failure of the brain, liver, kidneys, and lungs. The pathogenesis of MODS is not clearly understood, and current management therefore is primarily supportive. Major risk factors for the development of MODS are severe trauma, sepsis, prolonged periods of hypotension, hepatic dysfunction, infarcted bowel, advanced age, and alcohol abuse.[79] Interventions for multiple organ failure are focused on support of the affected organs.

IN SUMMARY, circulatory shock is an acute emergency in which body tissues are deprived of oxygen and cellular nutrients or are unable to use these materials in their metabolic processes. Circulatory shock may develop because the heart is unable to adequately pump blood through the circulatory system (cardiogenic shock), there is insufficient blood in the circulatory system (i.e., hypovolemic shock), there is a maldistribution of blood due to abnormalities in the vascular resistance (i.e., distributive shock), or blood flow or venous return is obstructed (i.e., obstructive shock). Three types of shock share the basic circulatory pattern of distributive shock: neurogenic shock, anaphylactic shock, and septic shock. Sepsis and septic shock, which is the most common of the three types, is associated with a severe, overwhelming inflammatory response and has a high mortality rate.

The manifestations of hypovolemic shock, which serves as a prototype for circulatory shock, are related to low peripheral blood flow and excessive sympathetic stimulation. The low peripheral blood flow produces thirst, changes in skin temperature, decreased blood pressure, increased heart rate, decreased venous pressure, decreased urine output, and changes in the sensorium. The intense vasoconstriction that serves to maintain blood flow to the heart and brain causes a decrease in tissue perfusion, impaired cellular metabolism, liberation of lactic acid, and, eventually, cell death. Whether the shock is irreversible or the patient will survive is determined largely by changes that occur at the cellular level.

The complications of shock result from the deprivation of blood flow to vital organs or systems, such as the lungs, kidneys, gastrointestinal tract, and blood coagulation system. Shock can cause or be accompanied by ALI/ARDS, which is characterized by changes in the permeability of the alveolar-capillary membrane with development of interstitial edema and severe hypoxemia that does not respond to oxygen therapy. The renal tubules are particularly vulnerable to ischemia, and acute renal failure is an important complication of shock. Gastrointestinal ischemia may lead to gastrointestinal bleeding and increased vascular permeability to intestinal bacteria, which can cause further sepsis and shock. DIC is characterized by formation of small clots in the circulation. It is thought to be caused by inappropriate activation of the coagulation cascade because of toxins or other products released as a result of the shock state. Multiple organ failure, perhaps the most ominous complication of shock, rapidly depletes the body's ability to compensate and recover from a shock state. ■

HEART FAILURE IN CHILDREN AND THE ELDERLY

After completing this section of the chapter, you should be able to meet the following objectives:

■ Describe the causes of heart failure in infants and children.

■ Cite how the aging process affects cardiac function and predisposes to ventricular dysfunction.

■ State how the signs and symptoms of heart failure may differ between younger and older adults.

Heart Failure in Infants and Children

As in adults, heart failure in infants and children results from the inability of the heart to maintain the cardiac output required to sustain metabolic demands.[80–82] The etiology of heart failure, however, is very different between children and adults. Structural (congenital) heart defects are the most common cause of heart failure in children. Surgical correction of congenital heart defects may cause heart failure as a result of intraoperative

manipulation of the heart and resection of heart tissue, with subsequent alterations in pressure, flow, and resistance relations. Usually, the heart failure that results is acute and resolves after the effects of the surgical procedure have subsided. Another cause of heart failure in children is cardiomyopathy related to a genetic or inherited disorder, infectious disease, drugs, toxins, and Kawasaki disease.[81] Chart 26-2 lists some of the more common causes of heart failure in children. Inflammatory heart disorders (*e.g.,* myocarditis, rheumatic fever, bacterial endocarditis, Kawasaki disease), cardiomyopathy, and congenital heart disorders are discussed in Chapter 24.

CHART 26-2   CAUSES OF HEART FAILURE IN CHILDREN

Newborn Period
Congenital heart defects
    Severe left ventricular outflow disorders
        Hypoplastic left heart
        Critical aortic stenosis or coarctation of the aorta
    Large arteriovenous shunts
        Ventricular septal defects
        Patent ductus arteriosus
    Transposition of the great vessels
Heart muscle dysfunction (secondary)
    Asphyxia
    Sepsis
    Hypoglycemia
Hematologic disorders (*e.g.,* anemia)

Infants 1 to 6 Months
Congenital heart disease
    Large arteriovenous shunts (ventricular septal defect)
Heart muscle dysfunction
    Myocarditis
    Cardiomyopathy
Pulmonary abnormalities
    Bronchopulmonary dysplasia
    Persistent pulmonary hypertension

Toddlers, Children, and Adolescents
Acquired heart disease
    Cardiomyopathy
    Viral myocarditis
    Rheumatic fever
    Endocarditis
    Systemic disease
        Sepsis
        Kawasaki disease
        Renal disease
        Sickle cell disease
Congenital heart defects
    Nonsurgically treated disorders
    Surgically treated disorders

Clinical Features

Manifestations. Many of the signs and symptoms of heart failure in infants and children are similar to those in adults. In children, overt symptoms of heart failure occur late in the disease process.[83] Breathlessness, tachypnea, and tachycardia felt as palpitations are the most common symptoms.[80] Other symptoms include fatigue, effort intolerance, cough, anorexia, and abdominal pain. A subtle sign of cardiorespiratory distress in infants and children is a change in disposition or responsiveness, including irritability or lethargy. Sympathetic stimulation produces peripheral vasoconstriction and diaphoresis. Decreased renal blood flow often results in a decrease in urine output despite adequate fluid intake.

When right ventricular function is impaired, systemic venous congestion develops. Hepatomegaly due to liver congestion often is one of the first signs of systemic venous congestion in infants and children. However, dependent edema or ascites rarely is seen unless the CVP is extremely high. Because of their short, fat necks, jugular venous distention is difficult to detect in infants; it is not a reliable sign until the child is of school age or older. A third heart sound, or gallop rhythm, is a common finding in infants and children with heart failure. It results from rapid filling of a noncompliant ventricle. However, it is difficult to distinguish at high heart rates.

Most commonly, children develop interstitial pulmonary edema rather than alveolar pulmonary edema. This reduces lung compliance and increases the work of breathing, causing tachypnea and increased respiratory effort. Older children display use of accessory muscles (*i.e.,* scapular and sternocleidomastoid). Head bobbing and nasal flaring may be observed in infants. Signs of respiratory distress often are the first and most noticeable indication of heart failure in infants and young children. Pulmonary congestion may be mistaken for bronchiolitis or lower respiratory tract infection. The infant or young child with respiratory distress often grunts with expiration. This grunting effort (essentially, exhaling against a closed glottis) is an instinctive effort to increase end-expiratory pressures and prevent collapse of small airways and the development of atelectasis. Respiratory crackles are uncommon in infants and usually suggest development of a respiratory tract infection. Wheezes may be heard, particularly if there is a large left-to-right shunt.

Infants with heart failure often show increased tachypnea, fatigue, and diaphoresis during feeding.[80,83] Weight gain is slow owing to high energy requirements and low calorie intake. Diaphoresis occurs (because of increased sympathetic tone) particularly over the head and neck. They may have repeated lower respiratory tract infections. Peripheral perfusion usually is poor, with cool extremities; tachycardia is common (resting heart rate >150 beats per minute); and the respiratory rate is increased (resting rate >50 breaths per minute).[80]

Diagnosis and Treatment. Diagnosis of heart failure in infants and children is based on symptomatology, chest radiographic films, electrocardiographic findings, echocardiographic techniques to assess cardiac structures and ventricular function

(*i.e.,* end-systolic and end-diastolic diameters), arterial blood gases to determine intracardiac shunting and ventilation-perfusion inequalities, and other laboratory studies to determine anemia and electrolyte imbalances.

Treatment of heart failure in infants and children includes measures aimed at improving cardiac function and eliminating excess intravascular fluid. Oxygen delivery must be supported and oxygen demands controlled or minimized. Whenever possible, the cause of the disorder is corrected (*e.g.,* medical treatment of sepsis and anemia, surgical correction of congenital heart defects). With congenital anomalies that are amenable to surgery, medical treatment often is needed for a time before surgery and usually is continued in the immediate postoperative period. For some children, only medical management can be provided.

Medical management of heart failure in infants and children is similar to that in the adult, although it is tailored to the special developmental needs of the child. Inotropic agents such as digitalis often are used to increase cardiac contractility. Diuretics may be given to reduce preload and vasodilating medications used to manipulate the afterload. Medication doses must be carefully tailored to control for the child's weight and conditions such as reduced renal function. Daily weighing and accurate measurement of intake and output are imperative during acute episodes of failure. Most children feel better in the semi-upright position. An infant seat is useful for infants with chronic heart failure. Activity restrictions usually are designed to allow children to be as active as possible within the limitations of their heart disease. Infants with heart failure often have problems feeding. Small, frequent feedings usually are more successful than larger, less frequent feedings. Severely ill infants may lack sufficient strength to suck and may need to be tube fed.

The treatment of heart failure in children should be designed to allow optimal physical and psychosocial development. It requires the full involvement of the parents, who often are the primary care providers; therefore, parent education and support are essential.

Heart Failure in the Elderly

Heart failure is one of the most common causes of disability in the elderly and is the most frequent hospital discharge diagnosis for the elderly in the United States and Canada. An estimated 90% of people with heart failure are older than 60 years of age.[3] Among the factors that have contributed to the increased numbers of older people with heart failure are the improved therapies for ischemic and hypertensive heart disease.[84] Thus, persons who would have died from acute myocardial disease 20 years ago are now surviving, but with residual left ventricular dysfunction. Advances in treatment of other diseases have also contributed indirectly to the rising prevalence of heart failure in the older population.

Coronary heart disease, hypertension, and valvular heart disease (particularly aortic stenosis and mitral regurgitation) are common causes of heart failure in older adults.[85,86] In contrast to the etiology in middle-aged persons with heart failure, factors other than systolic failure contribute to heart failure in the elderly. Preserved left ventricular function may be seen in 40% to 80% of older persons with heart failure.[86] Aging is associated with impaired left ventricular filling due to changes in myocardial relaxation and compliance. These alterations lead to a shift in the left ventricular pressure–volume relationship, such that small increases in left ventricular volume lead to greater increases in left ventricular diastolic pressure. This increase in diastolic pressure further compromises left ventricular filling and leads to increases in left atrial, pulmonary venous, and pulmonary capillary pressures, and thus predisposes to pulmonary congestion and heart failure.[85] Although diastolic heart failure accounts for less than 10% of heart failure cases in persons younger than 60 years of age, it accounts for greater than 50% of cases after age 75 years.[85]

There are a number of changes associated with aging that contribute to the development of heart failure in the elderly.[84–86] First, reduced responsiveness to β-adrenergic stimulation limits the heart's capacity to maximally increase heart rate and contractility. A second major effect of aging is increased vascular stiffness, which leads to a progressive increase in systolic blood pressure with advancing age, which in turn contributes to the development of left ventricular hypertrophy and altered diastolic filling. Third, in addition to increased vascular stiffness, the heart itself becomes stiffer and less compliant with age. The changes in diastolic stiffness result in important alterations in diastolic filling and atrial function. A reduction in ventricular filling not only affects cardiac output, but produces an elevation in diastolic pressure that is transmitted back to the left atrium, where it stretches the muscle wall and predisposes to atrial ectopic beats and atrial fibrillation. The fourth major effect of cardiovascular aging is altered myocardial metabolism at the level of the mitochondria. Although older mitochondria may be able to generate sufficient ATP to meet the normal energy needs of the heart, they may not be able to respond under stress.

Clinical Features

Manifestations. The manifestations of heart failure in the elderly often are masked by other disease conditions.[2] Nocturia and nocturnal incontinence is an early symptom but may be caused by other conditions such as prostatic hypertrophy. Lower extremity edema may reflect venous insufficiency. Impaired perfusion of the gastrointestinal tract is a common cause of anorexia and profound loss of lean body mass. Loss of lean body mass may be masked by edema. Exertional dyspnea, orthopnea, and impaired exercise tolerance are cardinal symptoms of heart failure in both younger and older persons with heart failure. However, with increasing age, which is often accompanied by a more sedentary lifestyle, exertional dyspnea becomes less prominent. Instead of dyspnea, the prominent sign may be restlessness. Chart 26-3 summarizes the manifestations of heart failure in the elderly.

Physical signs of heart failure, such as elevated jugular venous pressure, hepatic congestion, S_3 gallop, and pulmonary

---

CHART 26-3   MANIFESTATIONS OF HEART FAILURE IN THE ELDERLY

Symptoms
Nocturia or nocturnal incontinence
Fatigue
Cognitive impairment (*e.g.,* problem solving, decision making)
Depression
Restlessness/acute delirium
Sleep disturbance
History of falls
Loss of appetite

Signs
Dependent edema (ankles when sitting up and sacral edema when supine)
Pulmonary crackles (usually late sign)

---

crackles, occur less commonly in the elderly, in part because of the increased incidence of diastolic failure, in which signs of right-sided heart failure are late manifestations and a third heart sound is typically absent.[86] Instead, behavioral changes and altered cognition such as short-term memory loss and impaired problem solving are more common.[2] With exacerbation of heart failure, the elderly often present with acute delirium and dementia.[34] Depression is common in the elderly with heart failure and shares the symptoms of sleep disturbances, cognitive changes, and fatigue.[2]

The elderly also maintain a precarious balance between the managed symptom state and acute symptom exacerbation. During the managed symptom state, they are relatively symptom free while adhering to their treatment regimen. Acute symptom exacerbation, often requiring emergency medical treatment, can be precipitated by seemingly minor conditions such as poor adherence to sodium restriction, infection, or stress. Failure to promptly seek medical care is a common cause of progressive acceleration of symptoms.

Diagnosis and Treatment. The diagnosis of heart failure in the elderly is based on the history, physical examination, chest radiograph, and electrocardiographic findings.[87] However, the presenting symptoms of heart failure often are difficult to evaluate. Symptoms of dyspnea on exertion are often interpreted as a sign of "getting older" or attributed to deconditioning from other diseases. Ankle edema is not unusual in the elderly because of decreased skin turgor and the tendency of the elderly to be more sedentary with the legs in a dependent position.

Treatment of heart failure in the elderly involves many of the same methods as in younger persons, with medication dose adaptations to reduce age-related adverse and toxic events.[2] ACE inhibitors may be particularly beneficial to preserve cognitive and functional capacities.[2] Activities are restricted to a level that is commensurate with the cardiac reserve. Seldom is bed rest recommended or advised. Bed rest causes rapid deconditioning of skeletal muscles and increases the risk of complications such as orthostatic hypotension and thromboemboli. Instead, carefully prescribed exercise programs can help to maintain activity tolerance. Even walking around a room usually is preferable to continuous bed rest. Sodium restriction usually is indicated.

IN SUMMARY, the mechanisms of heart failure in children and the elderly are similar to those in adults. However, the causes and manifestations may differ because of age. In children, heart failure is seen most commonly during infancy and immediately after heart surgery. It can be caused by congenital and acquired heart defects and is characterized by fatigue, effort intolerance, cough, anorexia, abdominal pain, and impaired growth. Treatment of heart failure in children includes correction of the underlying cause whenever possible. For congenital anomalies that are amenable to surgery, medical treatment often is needed for a time before surgery and usually is continued in the immediate postoperative period. For many children, only medical management can be provided.

In the elderly, age-related changes in cardiovascular functioning contribute to heart failure but are not in themselves sufficient to cause heart failure. The manifestations of heart failure often are different and superimposed on other disease conditions; therefore, heart failure often is more difficult to diagnose in the elderly than in younger persons. Because the elderly are more susceptible to adverse and toxic medication reactions, medication doses need to be adapted and more closely monitored. ■

Review Exercises

1. A 75-year-old woman with long-standing hypertension and angina due to coronary heart disease presents with ankle edema, nocturia, increased shortness of breath with activity, and a chronic nonproductive cough. Her blood pressure is 170/80 and her heart rate 92. Electrocardiography and chest radiography indicate the presence of left ventricular hypertrophy.

   A. *Relate the presence of uncontrolled hypertension and coronary artery disease to the development of heart failure in this woman.*

   B. *Explain the significance of left ventricular hypertrophy in terms of both a compensatory mechanism and as a pathologic mechanism in the progression of heart failure.*

   C. *Use Figure 26-2 to explain this woman's symptoms, including shortness of breath and nonproductive cough.*

2. A 26-year-old man is admitted to the emergency department after an automobile injury with excessive blood loss. He is alert and anxious, his skin is cool and moist, his heart rate is 135, and his blood pressure is 100/85. He is receiving intravenous fluids, which were started at the scene of the accident by an emergency medical technician. He has been typed and cross-matched for blood transfusions and a urinary catheter has been inserted to monitor his urinary output. His urinary output has been less than 10 mL since admission and his blood pressure has dropped to 85/70. Efforts to control his bleeding have been unsuccessful and he is being prepared for emergency surgery.

   A. *Use information regarding the compensatory mechanisms in circulatory shock to explain this man's presenting symptoms, including urinary output.*

   B. *Use Figure 26-11 to hypothesize about this man's blood loss and maintenance of blood pressure.*

   C. *The treatment of hypovolemic shock is usually directed at maintaining the circulatory volume through fluid resuscitation rather than maintaining the blood pressure through the use of vasoactive medications. Explain.*

References

1. Hunt S. A., Abraham W. T., Chin M. H., et al. (2005). ACC/AHA 2005 guidelines for diagnosis and management of chronic heart failure in the adult. *Circulation* 112, e154–e235.
2. Arnold J. M. O., Liu P., Demers C., et al. (2006). Canadian Cardiovascular Society consensus conference recommendations on heart failure 2006: Diagnosis and management. *Canadian Journal of Cardiology* 22, 23–45.
3. American Heart Association. (2007). Heart disease and stroke statistics: 2007 update at a glance. [Online.] Available: www.americanheart.org/downloadable/heart/1166711577754HS_StatsInsideText.pdf. Accessed March 4, 2007.
4. Chow C. M., Donovan L., Manuel D., et al. (2005) Regional variation in self-reported heart disease prevalence in Canada [abstract]. *Canadian Journal of Cardiology* 21, 1265–1271.
5. Guyton A. C., Hall J. E. (2006). *Textbook of medical physiology* (11th ed., pp. 103–115, 264, 278–288). Philadelphia: Elsevier Saunders.
6. Klabunde R. E. (2005). *Cardiovascular physiology concepts.* Philadelphia: Lippincott Williams & Wilkins.
7. Opie L. H. (2005). Mechanisms of cardiac contraction and relaxation. In Zipes D. P., Libbey P., Bonow R. O., et al. (Eds.), *Braunwald's heart disease: A textbook of cardiovascular medicine* (7th ed., pp. 457–489). Philadelphia: Elsevier Saunders.
8. Carroll J. D., Hess O. M. (2005). Assessment of normal and abnormal cardiac function. In Zipes D. P., Libbey P., Bonow R. O., et al. (Eds.), *Braunwald's heart disease: A textbook of cardiovascular medicine* (7th ed., pp. 491–507). Philadelphia: Elsevier Saunders.
9. Wu E. B., Yu C. M. (2005). Management of diastolic heart failure: A practical review of pathophysiology and treatment trial data. *International Journal of Clinical Practice* 59, 1239–1246.
10. Fletcher L., Thomas D. (2001). Congestive heart failure: Understanding the pathophysiology and management. *Journal of the American Academy of Nurse Practitioners* 13, 249–257.
11. Givertz M. M., Colucci W. S., Braunwald E. (2005). Clinical aspects of heart failure: Pulmonary edema, high-output failure. In Zipes D. P., Libbey P., Bonow R. O., et al. (Eds.), *Braunwald's heart disease: A textbook of cardiovascular medicine* (7th ed., pp. 539–568). Philadelphia: Elsevier Saunders.

12. Aurigemma G. P., Gaasch W. H. (2004). Diastolic heart failure. *New England Journal of Medicine* 351, 1095–1105.

13. Haney S., Sur D., Xu Z. (2005). Diastolic heart failure: A review and primary care perspective. *Journal of the American Board of Family Practice* 18, 189–195.

14. Colucci W. C. (2005). Pathophysiology of heart failure. In Zipes D. P., Libbey P., Bonow R. O., et al. (Eds.), *Braunwald's heart disease: A textbook of cardiovascular medicine* (7th ed., pp. 509–568). Philadelphia: Elsevier Saunders.

15. Budev M. M., Arroliga A. C., Wiedemann H. P., et al. (2003). Cor pulmonale: An overview. *Seminars in Respiratory Critical Care Medicine* 23, 233–243.

16. Francis G. S., Tang W. H. W. (2003). Pathophysiology of congestive heart failure. *Reviews in Cardiovascular Medicine* 4(Suppl. 2), S14–S20.

17. Adams K. F. (2004). Pathophysiologic role of the renin-angiotensin-aldosterone and sympathetic nervous system in HF. *American Journal of Health-System Pharmacy* 61(Suppl. 2), S4–S13.

18. Weber K. T. (2001). Aldosterone in congestive heart failure. *New England Journal of Medicine* 345, 1689–1697.

19. Struthers A. D. (2005). Pathophysiology of heart failure following myocardial infarction. *Heart* 91, 14–16.

20. Pitt B., Zannad F., Remme W. J., et al. (1999). The effect of spironolactone on morbidity and mortality in patients with severe heart failure. *New England Journal of Medicine* 341, 709–717.

21. Levin E. R., Gardner D. G., Samson W. K. (1998). Natriuretic peptides. *New England Journal of Medicine* 339, 321–328.

22. Baughman K. L. (2002). B-type natriuretic peptide: A window to the heart. *New England Journal of Medicine* 347, 158–159.

23. Nathisuwan S., Talbert R. L. (2002). A review of vasopeptidase inhibitors: A new modality in the treatment of hypertension and chronic heart failure. *Pharmacotherapy* 22, 27–42.

24. Spieker L. E., Lüscher T. F. (2003). Will endothelin receptor antagonists have a role in heart failure? *Medical Clinics of North America* 87, 459–474.

25. Ergul A. (2002). Endothelin-1 and endothelin receptor antagonists as potential cardiovascular therapeutic agents. *Pharmacotherapy* 22, 54–65.

26. Kardys I., Knetsch A. M., Bleumink G. S., et al. (2006). C-reactive protein and risk of heart failure: The Rotterdam Study. *American Heart Journal* 152, 514–520.

27. Estes N. A. M. III. (2006). Implantable cardioverter defibrillator and cardiac resynchronization therapy in patients with left ventricular dysfunction: Evidence based medicine, economics, and guidelines: CME. [Online.] Available:www.medscape.com/viewprogram/5242. Accessed February 24, 2007.

28. Hunter J. J., Chien K. R. (1999). Signaling pathways for cardiac hypertrophy and failure. *New England Journal of Medicine* 341, 1276–1284.

29. Gheorghiade M., Zannad F., Sopko G., et al. (2005). Acute heart failure syndrome: Current state and framework for future research. *Circulation* 112, 3958–3968.

30. Nieminen M. S., Harjola V.-P. (2005). Definition and epidemiology of acute heart failure syndrome. *American Journal of Cardiology* 95 (Suppl. G), 5G–10G.

31. Filippatos G., Zannad F. (2007). An introduction to acute heart failure syndromes: Definition and classification. *Heart Failure Review* 12, 87–90.

32. Brack T. (2003). Cheyne-Stokes respiration in patients with congestive heart failure. *Swiss Medical Weekly* 133, 605–610.

33. Crijns H. J., Tjeerdsma G., De Kam P. J., et al. (2000). Prognostic value of the presence and development of atrial fibrillation in patients with advanced chronic HF. *European Heart Journal* 21, 1238–1245.

34. Arnold J. M. O., Howlett J. G., Dorian P., et al. (2007). Canadian Cardiovascular Society consensus conference recommendations on heart failure update 2007: Prevention, management during intercurrent illness or acute decompensation, and use of biomarkers. *Canadian Journal of Cardiology*, 23, 21–45. [Online.] Available: www.ccs.ca/consensus_conferences/cc_library_e.aspx. Accessed March 4, 2007.

35. Nolan P. E. (2004). Integrating traditional and emerging treatment options in heart failure. *American Journal of Health-System Pharmacy* 61(Suppl. 2), S14–S22.

36. Piña H. L. (Chair, Writing Group). (2003). Exercise and heart failure: A statement from the American Heart Association Committee on Exercise, Rehabilitation, and Prevention. *Circulation* 107, 1210–1225.

37. Bristow M. R., Linas S., Port J. D. (2005). Drugs in treatment of heart failure. In Zipes D. P., Libbey P., Bonow R. O., et al. (Eds.), *Braunwald's heart disease: A textbook of cardiovascular medicine* (7th ed., pp. 569–601). Philadelphia: Elsevier Saunders.

38. MERIT-HF Study Group. (1999). Effect of metoprolol CR/XL in chronic heart failure: Metoprolol CR/XL Randomised Intervention Trial in Congestive Heart Failure (MERIT-HF). *Lancet* 353, 2001–2007.

39. Dee W. J. (2003). Digoxin remains useful in the management of chronic heart failure. *Medical Clinics of North America* 87, 317–337.

40. Hachey D. M., Smith T. (2003). Use of nesiritide to treat acute decompensated HF. *Critical Care Nurse* 23, 53–55.

41. Stoltzfus S. (2006). The role of noninvasive ventilation: CPAP and BiPAP in the treatment of congestive HF. *Dimensions of Critical Care Nursing* 25(2), 66–70.

42. Bendjelid K., Schutz N., Suter P. M., et al. (2005). Does continuous positive airway pressure by face mask improve patients with acute cardiogenic pulmonary edema due to left ventricular diastolic dysfunction? *Chest* 127, 1053–1056.

43. Albert N. M. (2003). Cardiac resynchronization therapy through biventricular pacing in patients with HF and ventricular dyssynchrony. *Critical Care Nurse* 23(June Suppl.), 2–13.

44. Wheeldon D. R. (2003). Mechanical circulatory support: State of the art and future perspectives. *Perfusion* 8, 233–243.

45. Hunt S. A., Kouretas P. C., Balsam L. B., et al. (2005). Heart transplantation. In Zipes D. P., Libbey P., Bonow R. W., et al. (Eds.), *Braunwald's heart disease: A textbook of cardiovascular medicine* (7th ed., pp. 641–651). Philadelphia: Elsevier Saunders.

46. Vilquin J. T., Marolleau J. P. (2004). Cell transplantation in heart failure management [abstract]. *Médecine Sciences* 20(6–7), 651–662.

47. Giordano A., Galderisi U., Marino I. R. (2007). From the laboratory bench to the patient's bedside: An update on clinical trials with mesenchymal stem cells [abstract]. *Journal of Cell Physiology* 211, 27–35.

48. Patel N. D., Barreiro C. J., Williams J. A., et al. (2005). Surgical ventricular remodeling for patients with clinically advanced congestive HF and severe left ventricular dysfunction. *Journal of Heart and Lung Transplantation* 24, 2202–2210.

49. Holmes C. L., Walley K. R. (2003). The evaluation and management of shock. *Clinical Chest Medicine* 24, 775–789.

50. Aymong E. D., Ramanathan K., Buller C. E. (2007). Pathophysiology of cardiogenic shock complicating acute myocardial infarction. *Medical Clinics of North America* 91, 701–712.

51. Antman E. M. (2005). Cardiogenic shock. In Zipes D. P., Libbey P., Bonow R. O., et al. (Eds.), *Braunwald's heart disease: A textbook of cardiovascular medicine* (7th ed., pp. 1200–1202). Philadelphia: Elsevier Saunders.

52. Parrillo J. E. (1995). Pathogenic mechanisms of septic shock. *New England Journal of Medicine* 328, 1471–1477.

53. Hollenberg S. M., Kavinsky C. J., Parrillo J. E. (1999). Cardiogenic shock. *Annals of Internal Medicine* 131, 47–59.

54. Hochmann J. S. (2003). Cardiogenic shock complicating acute myocardial infarction: Expanding the paradigm. *Circulation* 107, 2998–3002.

55. Naka Y., Chen J. M., Rose E. A. (2005). Assisted circulation in the treatment of heart failure. In Zipes D. P., Libbey P., Bonow R. O., et al. (Eds.), *Braunwald's heart disease: A textbook of cardiovascular medicine* (7th ed., pp. 625–640). Philadelphia: Elsevier Saunders.

56. Antman E. M., Anbe D. T., Armstrong P. W., et al. (2004). ACC/AHA guidelines for the management of patients with ST-elevation myocardial infarction: Executive summary: A report of the ACC/AHA Task Force on Practice Guidelines (Committee to Revise the 1999 Guidelines on the Management of Patients with Acute Myocardial Infarction). *Journal of the American College of Cardiology* 44, 671–719.

57. Kelley D. M. (2005). Hypovolemic shock. *Critical Care Nursing Quarterly* 28(1), 2–19.

58. Dutton R. P. (2007). Current concepts in hemorrhagic shock. *Anesthesiology Clinics* 25, 23–34.
59. Landry D. W., Oliver J. A. (2001). The pathogenesis of vasodilatory shock. *New England Journal of Medicine* 345, 588–595.
60. Lieberman P. (2006). Anaphylaxis. *Medical Clinics of North America* 90, 77–95.
61. Brown S. G. A. (2007). The pathophysiology of shock in anaphylaxis. *Immunology and Allergy Clinics of North America* 27, 165–175.
62. Ellis A. K., Day J. H. (2003). Diagnosis and management of anaphylaxis. *Canadian Medical Association Journal* 169, 307–312.
63. Stankiewicz J., Ruta W., Gorski P. (1995). Latex allergy. *International Journal of Occupational Medicine and Environmental Health* 8, 139–148.
64. Levy M. M., Fink M. P., Marshall J. C., et al. (2003). SCCM/ESICM/ACCP/ATS/SIS International sepsis definitions conference. *Critical Care Medicine* 31, 1250–1256.
65. Nguyen H. B., Rivers E. P., Abrahamian F. M. (2006). Severe sepsis and septic shock: Review of the literature and emergency department management guidelines. *Annals of Emergency Medicine* 48, 28–54.
66. Russell J. A. (2006). Management of sepsis. *New England Journal of Medicine* 355, 1699–1711.
67. Howell G., Tisherman S. A. (2006). Management of sepsis. *Surgical Clinics of North America* 86, 1523–1539.
68. Vincent J. L., Taccone F., Schmit X. (2007). Classification, incidence, and outcomes of sepsis and multiple organ failure. *Contributions to Nephrology* 156, 64–74.
69. Annane D., Bellissant I., Cavaillon J.-M. (2005). Septic shock. *Lancet* 365, 63–78.
70. Rivers E. P., McIntyre L., Morro D. C., et al. (2005). Early and innovative interventions for severe sepsis and septic shock: Taking advantage of the window of opportunity. *Canadian Medical Association Journal* 173, 1054–1065.
71. Gullo A., Bianco N., Berlot G. (2006). Management of severe sepsis and septic shock: Challenges and recommendations. *Critical Care Clinics* 22, 489–501.
72. Van den Berghe G., Woulters P., Weekers F., et al. (2001). Intensive insulin therapy in critically ill patients. *New England Journal of Medicine* 345, 1359–1367.
73. Smith J. J., Kampine J. P. (1980). *Circulatory physiology* (p. 298). Baltimore: Williams & Wilkins.
74. Abraham, E. (2003). Neutrophils and acute lung injury. *Critical Care Medicine* 31, S195–S199.
75. Ausiello D. A., Benos D. J., Aboud F., et al. (2004). The acute respiratory distress syndrome. *Annals of Internal Medicine* 141, 460–470.
76. Rubenfeld, G. D., Herridge M. S. (2007). Epidemiology and outcomes of acute lung injury. *Chest* 131, 554–562.
77. Fink M. (1991). Gastrointestinal mucosal injury in experimental models of shock, trauma and sepsis. *Critical Care Medicine* 19, 627–641.
78. Levi M., Ten Cate H. T. (1999). Disseminated intravascular coagulation. *New England Journal of Medicine* 341, 586–592.
79. Balk R. A. (2000). Pathogenesis and management of multiple organ dysfunction or failure in acute sepsis and septic shock. *Critical Care Clinics* 16, 337–352.
80. Bernstein D. (2004). Heart failure. In Behrman R. E., Kliegman R. M., Nelson W., Jenson H. B. (Eds.), *Nelson textbook of pediatrics* (17th ed., pp. 1582–1587). Philadelphia: Elsevier Saunders.
81. Kay J. D., Colan S. D., Graham T. P. (2001). Congestive heart failure in pediatric patients. *American Heart Journal* 142, 923–928.
82. O'Laughlin M. P. (1999). Congestive heart failure in children. *Pediatric Clinics of North America* 46, 263–273.
83. Rosenthal D., Chrisant M., Edens E., et al. (2004). International Society for Heart and Lung Transplantation: Practice guidelines for management of heart failure in children. *Journal of Heart and Lung Transplantation* 23, 1313–1333.
84. Thomas S., Rich M. W. (2007). Epidemiology, pathophysiology, and prognosis of heart failure in the elderly. *Clinics in Geriatric Medicine* 23, 1–10.
85. Schwartz J. B., Zipes D. P. (2005). Cardiovascular disease in the elderly. In Zipes D. P., Libbey P., Bonow R. O., et al. (Eds.), *Braunwald's heart disease: A textbook of cardiovascular medicine* (7th ed., pp. 1925–1949). Philadelphia: Elsevier Saunders.
86. Rich M. W. (2006). Heart failure in older adults. *Medical Clinics of North America* 90, 863 885.
87. Abdelhafiz A. H. (2002). Heart failure in older people: Causes, diagnosis, and treatment. *Age and Aging* 31, 29–36.

Visit the Point. **http://thePoint.lww.com for animations, journal articles, and more!**

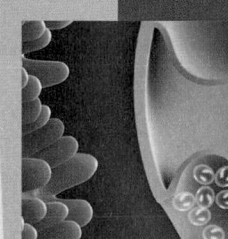

Disorders of Respiratory Function

In the early studies of the body, there is almost no mention of the lungs or respiratory passages. Although the pneuma, or "vital spirits," of the body were closely related to the air and vapors of the universe, the lungs and air passages were almost disregarded. It was not until the circulation of blood had been charted that real progress in understanding the respiratory system took place.

A major step in the understanding of respiration began with the work of Robert Boyle (1627–1691), an Irish scholar. Using an air pump, Boyle proved that a candle would not burn and a small bird or mouse could not live inside a jar from which the air had been removed. Scientists at this time believed that when something burned, air lost a mysterious substance called *phlogiston*. It was the British clergyman Joseph Priestley (1733–1804) who discovered that a gas made by heating oxide of mercury supported combustion. He called this gas, which later became known as oxygen, *dephlogisticated* air. Priestley showed that a mouse lived longer in a given volume of dephlogisticated air than it did in ordinary air. Antoine Lavoisier (1743–1794), a French chemist, confirmed that oxygen was present in inspired air and carbon dioxide in expired air and gave oxygen its name. In 1791, just 16 years after Priestley's discovery of oxygen, it was shown that blood contained both oxygen and carbon dioxide. From this point on, a detailed understanding of the respiratory system and its function proceeded rapidly.

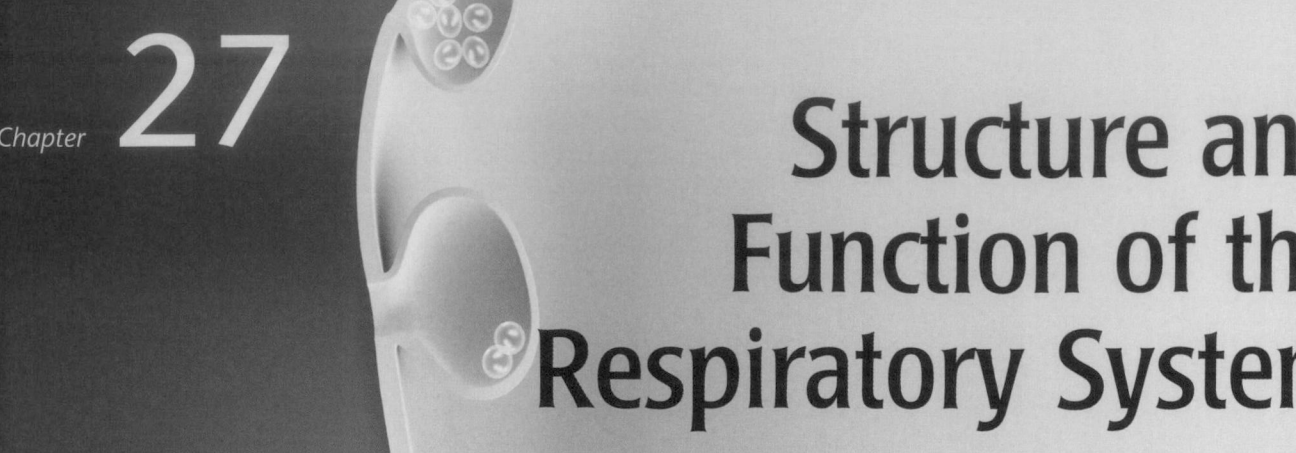

Chapter 27

Structure and Function of the Respiratory System

CAROL M. PORTH AND KIM LITWACK

The primary function of the respiratory system, which consists of the airways and lungs, is gas exchange. Oxygen from the air is transferred to the blood and carbon dioxide from the blood is eliminated into the atmosphere. In addition to gas exchange, the lungs serve as a host defense by providing a barrier between the external environment and the inside of the body. Finally, the lung is also a metabolic organ that synthesizes and metabolizes different compounds.

This chapter focuses on the structural organization of the respiratory system; exchange of gases between the atmosphere and the lungs; exchange of gases in the lungs and its transport in the blood; and control of breathing. The function of the red blood cell in the transport of oxygen is discussed in Chapter 14.

STRUCTURAL ORGANIZATION OF THE RESPIRATORY SYSTEM

After completing this section of the chapter, you should be able to meet the following objectives:

- State the difference between the conducting and the respiratory airways.
- Trace the movement of air through the airways, beginning in the nose and oropharynx and moving into the respiratory tissues of the lung.
- Describe the function of the mucociliary blanket.
- Compare the supporting structures of the large and small airways in terms of cartilaginous and smooth muscle support.
- State the function of the two types of alveolar cells.
- Differentiate the function of the bronchial and pulmonary circulations that supply the lungs.

The respiratory system consists of the air passages, the two lungs and the blood vessels that supply them, and the structures that provide a ventilator mechanism, that is, the rib cage and the respiratory muscles, which includes the diaphragm—the principal respiratory muscle. Functionally, the respiratory system can be divided into two parts: the *conducting airways,* through which air moves as it passes between the atmosphere and the lungs, and the *respiratory tissues* of the lungs, where gas exchange takes place.

The lungs are soft, spongy, cone-shaped organs located side by side in the chest cavity (Fig. 27-1). They are separated from each other by the *mediastinum (i.e.,* the space between the lungs) and its contents—the heart, blood vessels, lymph nodes, nerve fibers, thymus gland, and esophagus. The upper part of the lung, which lies against the top of the thoracic cavity, is called the *apex,* and the lower part, which lies against the diaphragm, is called the *base.* The lungs are divided into lobes: three in the right lung and two in the left.

CONDUCTING AND RESPIRATORY AIRWAYS

- Respiration requires ventilation, or movement of gases into and out of the lungs; perfusion, or movement of blood through the lungs; and diffusion of gases between the lungs and the blood.

- Ventilation depends on the conducting airways, including the nasopharynx and oropharynx, larynx, and tracheobronchial tree, which move air into and out of the lungs but do not participate in gas exchange.

- Gas exchange takes place in the respiratory airways of the lungs, where gases diffuse across the alveolar-capillary membrane as they are exchanged between the air in the lungs and the blood that flows through the pulmonary capillaries.

Conducting Airways

The conducting airways consist of the nasal passages, mouth and pharynx, larynx, trachea, bronchi, and bronchioles (see Fig. 27-1). Besides functioning as a conduit for airflow, the conducting airways serve to "condition" the inspired air. The air we breathe is warmed, filtered, and moistened as it moves through these structures. Heat is transferred to the air from the blood flowing through the walls of the respiratory passages; the mucociliary blanket removes foreign materials; and water from the mucous membranes is used to moisten the air.

A combination of cartilage, elastic and collagen fibers, and smooth muscle provides the airways with the rigidity and flexibility needed to maintain airway patency and ensure an uninterrupted supply of air. Most of the conducting airways are lined with ciliated pseudostratified columnar epithelium, containing a mosaic of mucus-secreting glands, ciliated cells with hairlike projections, and serous glands that secrete a watery fluid containing antibacterial enzymes (Fig. 27-2). The epithelial layer gradually becomes thinner as it moves from the pseudostratified epithelium of the bronchi to cuboidal epithelium of the bronchioles and then to squamous epithelium of the alveoli.

The mucus produced by the epithelial cells in the conducting airways forms a layer, called the *mucociliary blanket,* that protects the respiratory system by entrapping dust, bacteria, and other foreign particles that enter the airways. The cilia, which are in constant motion, move the mucociliary blanket with its entrapped particles in an escalator-like fashion toward the oropharynx, from which it is expectorated or swallowed. The function of cilia in clearing the lower airways is optimal at normal oxygen levels and is impaired when oxygen levels are higher or lower than normal. It is also impaired by drying conditions, such as breathing heated but unhumidified indoor air during the winter months. Cigarette smoking slows down or paralyzes the motility of the cilia. This slowing allows the

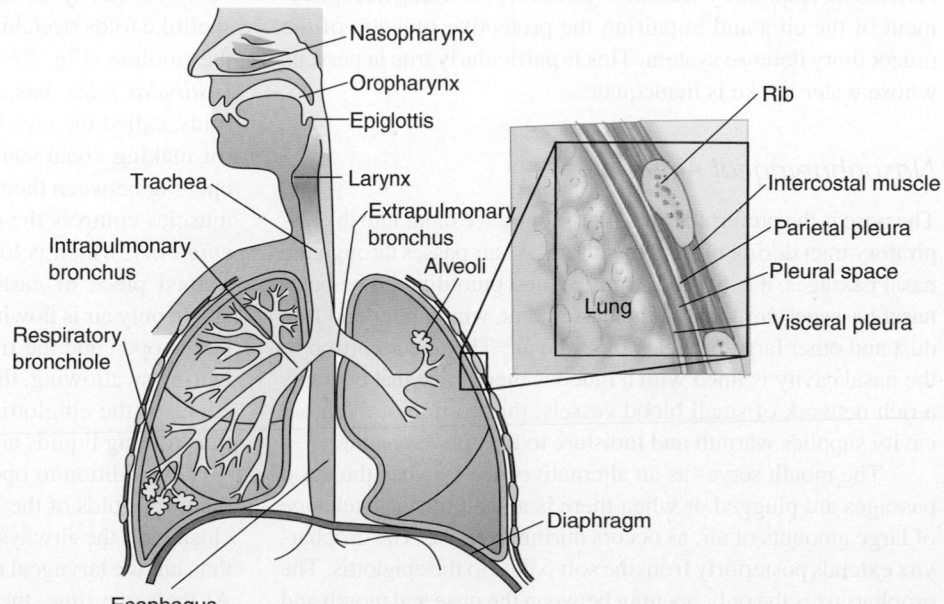

FIGURE 27-1 • Structures of the respiratory system. The structures of the pleura are shown in the inset.

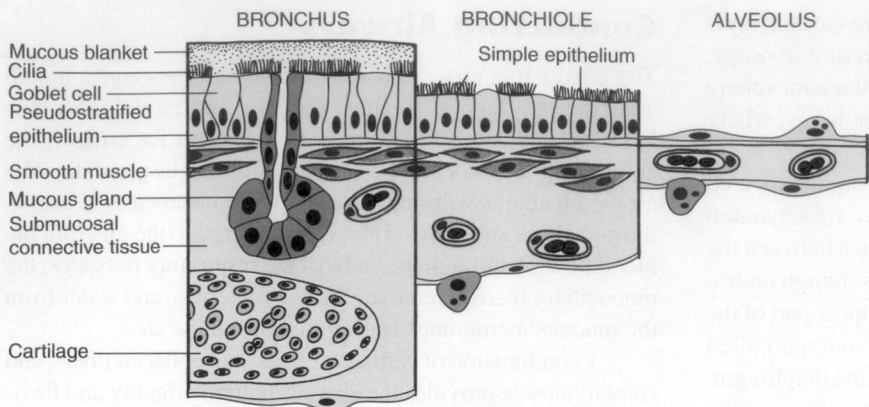

FIGURE 27-2 • Airway wall structure: bronchus, bronchiole, and alveolus. The bronchial wall contains pseudostratified epithelium, smooth muscle cells, mucous glands, connective tissue, and cartilage. In smaller bronchioles, a simple epithelium is found, cartilage is absent, and the wall is thinner. The alveolar wall is designed for gas exchange, rather than structural support. (From Weibel E. R., Taylor R. C. [1988]. Design and structure of the human lung. In Fishman A. P. [Ed.], *Pulmonary diseases and disorders* [Vol. 1., p. 14]. New York: McGraw-Hill.)

residue from tobacco smoke, dust, and other particles to accumulate in the lungs, decreasing the efficiency of this pulmonary defense system. As discussed in Chapter 29, these changes are thought to contribute to the development of chronic bronchitis and emphysema.

The conducting airways are kept moist by water contained in the mucous membranes of the upper airways and the tracheobronchial tree. The capacity of the air to contain moisture without condensation increases as the temperature rises. Thus, the air in the alveoli, which is maintained at body temperature, usually contains considerably more moisture than the atmosphere-temperature air that we breathe. The difference between the moisture contained in the air we breathe and that found in the alveoli is drawn from the moist surface of the mucous membranes that line the conducting airways and is a source of insensible water loss. Under normal conditions, approximately 1 pint of water per day is lost in humidifying the air breathed. During fever, the water vapor in the lungs increases, causing more water to be lost from the respiratory mucosa. Also, fever usually is accompanied by an increase in respiratory rate so that more air needing to be moisturized passes through the airways. As a result, respiratory secretions thicken, preventing free movement of the cilia and impairing the protective function of the mucociliary defense system. This is particularly true in persons whose water intake is inadequate.

Nasopharyngeal Airways

The nose is the preferred route for the entrance of air into the respiratory tract during normal breathing. As air passes through the nasal passages, it is filtered, warmed, and humidified. The outer nasal passages are lined with coarse hairs, which filter and trap dust and other large particles from the air. The upper portion of the nasal cavity is lined with a mucous membrane that contains a rich network of small blood vessels; this portion of the nasal cavity supplies warmth and moisture to the air we breathe.

The mouth serves as an alternative airway when the nasal passages are plugged or when there is a need for the exchange of large amounts of air, as occurs during exercise. The oropharynx extends posteriorly from the soft palate to the epiglottis. The oropharynx is the only opening between the nose and mouth and

the lungs. Both swallowed food on its way to the esophagus and air on its way to the larynx pass through it. Obstruction of the oropharynx leads to immediate cessation of ventilation. Neural control of the tongue and pharyngeal muscles may be impaired in coma and other neurologic disorders. In these conditions, the tongue falls back into the pharynx and obstructs the airway, particularly if the person is lying on his or her back. Swelling of the pharyngeal structures caused by injury, infection, or severe allergic reaction also predisposes a person to airway obstruction, as does the presence of a foreign body.

Larynx

The larynx connects the oropharynx with the trachea. The walls of the larynx are supported by firm cartilaginous structures that prevent collapse during inspiration. The functions of the larynx can be divided into two categories: those associated with speech and those associated with protecting the lungs from substances other than air. The larynx is located in a strategic position between the upper airways and the lungs and sometimes is referred to as the "watchdog of the lungs."

The cavity of the larynx is divided into two pairs of shelflike folds stretching from front to back with an opening in the midline (Fig. 27-3). The upper pair of folds, called the *vestibular folds,* has a protective function. The lower pair of folds, called the *vocal folds,* produces the vibrations required for making vocal sounds. The vocal folds and the elongated opening between them are called the *glottis.* A complex set of muscles controls the opening and closing of the glottis. The *epiglottis,* which is located above the larynx, is a large, leaf-shaped piece of cartilage that is covered with epithelium. When only air is flowing through the larynx, the inlet of the larynx is open and the free edges of the epiglottis point upward. During swallowing, the larynx is pulled superiorly and the free edges of the epiglottis move downward to cover the larynx, thus routing liquids and foods into the esophagus.

In addition to opening and closing the glottis for speech, the vocal folds of the larynx can perform a sphincter function, closing off the airways. When confronted with substances other than air, the laryngeal muscles contract and close off the airway. At the same time, the cough reflex is initiated as a means of

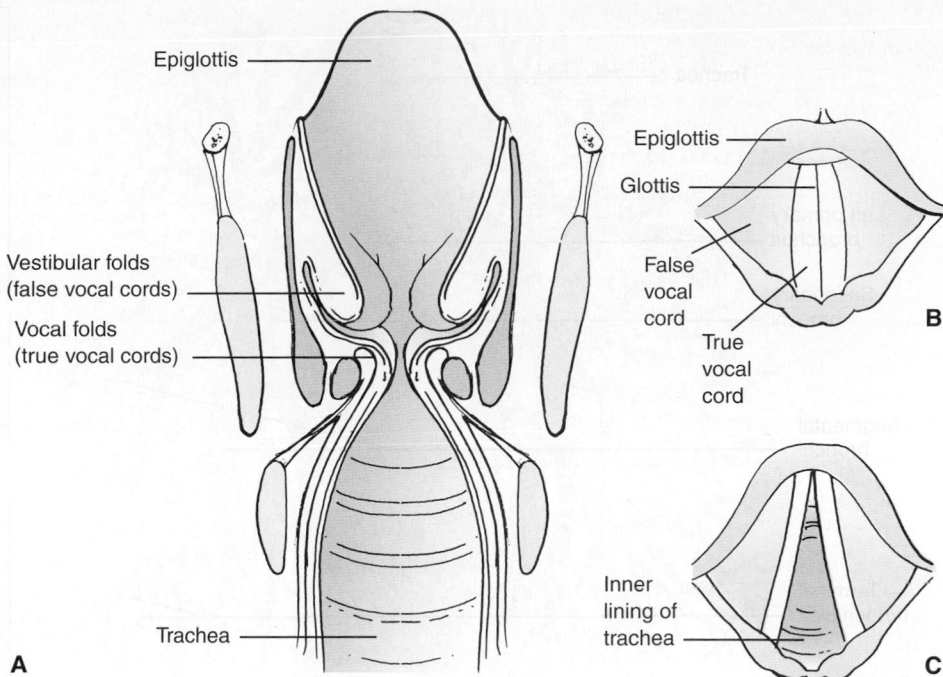

Epiglottis

Vestibular folds
(false vocal cords)

Vocal folds
(true vocal cords)

Trachea

Epiglottis

Glottis

False
vocal
cord

True
vocal
cord

B

Inner
lining of
trachea

C

FIGURE 27-3 • (**A**) Coronal section showing the position of the epiglottis, the vestibular folds (true vocal cords), and vocal folds (false vocal cords), and glottis. (**B**) Vocal cords viewed from above with glottis closed and (**C**) with glottis open.

A

removing a foreign substance from the airway. If the swallowing mechanism is partially or totally paralyzed, food and fluids can enter the airways instead of the esophagus when a person attempts to swallow. These substances are not easily removed; and when they are pulled into the lungs, they can cause a serious inflammatory condition called *aspiration pneumonia.*

Tracheobronchial Tree

The tracheobronchial tree, which consists of the trachea, bronchi, and bronchioles, can be viewed as a system of branching tubes. It is similar to a tree whose branches become smaller and more numerous as they divide (Fig. 27-4A). There are approximately 23 levels of branching, beginning with the conducting airways and ending with the respiratory airways, where gas exchange takes place (see Fig. 27-4B).

The trachea, or windpipe, is a continuous tube that connects the larynx and the major bronchi of the lungs. The walls of the trachea are supported by horseshoe- or C-shaped rings of hyaline cartilage, which prevent it from collapsing when the pressure in the thorax becomes negative (Fig. 27-5). The open part of the C ring, which abuts the esophagus, is connected by smooth muscle. Since this portion of the trachea is not rigid, the esophagus can expand anteriorly as swallowed food passes through it.

The trachea extends to the superior border of the fifth thoracic vertebra, where it divides to form the right and left main or primary bronchi. Between the main bronchi is a keel-like ridge, called the *carina* (Fig. 27-6). The mucosa of the carina is highly sensitive; violent coughing is initiated when a foreign object (*e.g.,* suction catheter) makes contact with it. The structure of the primary bronchi is similar to that of the trachea in

that these airways are lined with a mucosal surface and supported by cartilaginous rings. Each primary bronchus, accompanied by the pulmonary arteries, veins, and lymph vessels, enters the lung through a slit called the *hilum.*

On entering the lungs, each primary bronchus divides into secondary or lobular bronchi that supply each of the lobes of the lung—three in the right lung and two in the left (see Fig. 27-6). The right middle lobe bronchus is of relatively small diameter and length and sometimes bends sharply near its bifurcation. It is surrounded by a collar of lymph nodes that drain the middle and the lower lobe and is particularly subject to obstruction. The secondary bronchi, in turn, divide to form the segmental bronchi, which supply the bronchopulmonary segments of the lung. There are 10 segments on the right lung and 9 on the left (Fig. 27-7). These segments are identified according to their location in the lung (*e.g.,* the apical segment of the right upper lobe) and are the smallest named units in the lung. Lung disorders such as atelectasis and pneumonia often are localized to a particular bronchopulmonary segment. The structure of the secondary and segmental bronchi is similar, for the most part, to that of the primary bronchi; however, the C-shaped cartilage rings are replaced by irregular plates of hyaline cartilage that completely surround the lumina of the bronchi, and there are two layers of smooth muscle spiraling in opposite directions (Fig. 27-8).

The segmental bronchi continue to branch, forming smaller bronchi, until they become the terminal bronchioles, the smallest of the conducting airways. As these bronchi branch and become smaller, their wall structure changes. The cartilage gradually decreases and there is an increase in smooth muscle and elastic tissue (with respect to the thickness of the wall). By the time the bronchioles are reached, there is no cartilage present and their walls are composed mainly of smooth muscle and

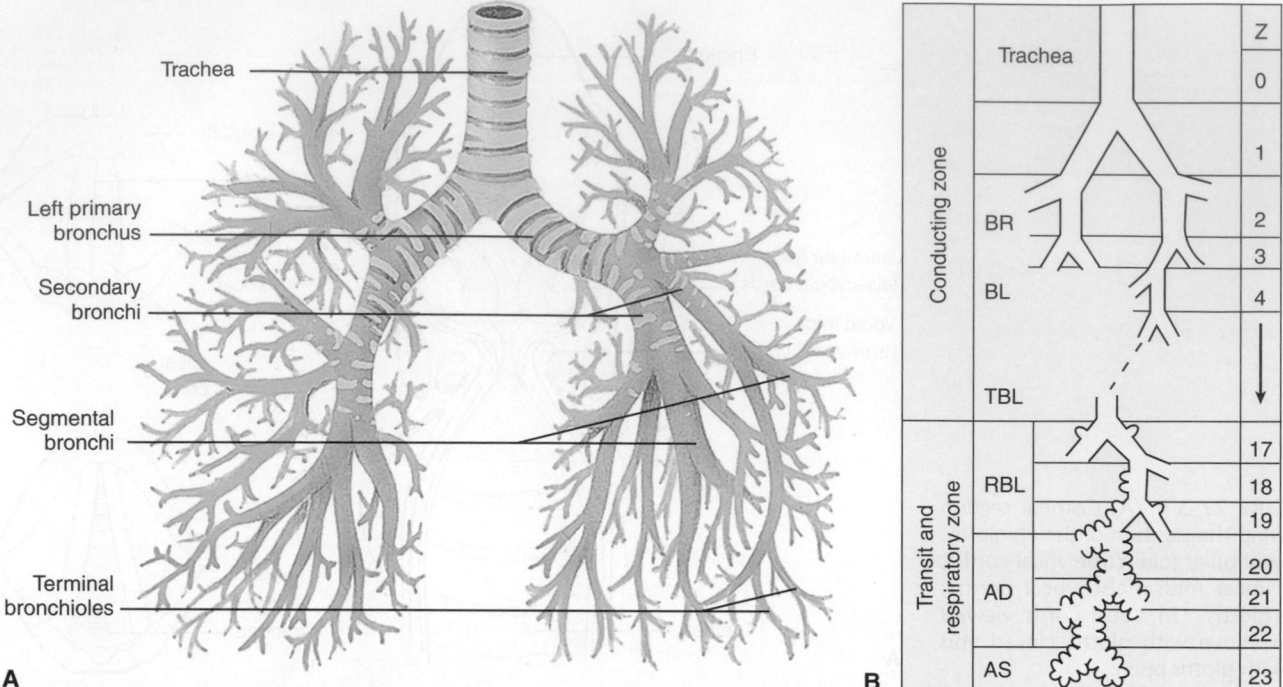

FIGURE 27-4 • **(A)** Conducting and respiratory air pathways inferior to the larynx. (From Anatomic Chart Company. *Atlas of human anatomy* [p. 175]. Springhouse, PA: Springhouse.) **(B)** Idealization of the human airways. The first 16 generations of branching (Z) make up the conducting airways, and the last 7 constitute the respiratory zone (or transitional and respiratory zone). BR, bronchus; BL, bronchiole; TBL, terminal bronchiole; RBL, respiratory bronchiole; AD, alveolar ducts; AS, alveolar sacs. (From Weibel E. R. [1962]. *Morphometry of the human lung* [p. 111]. Berlin: Springer-Verlag.)

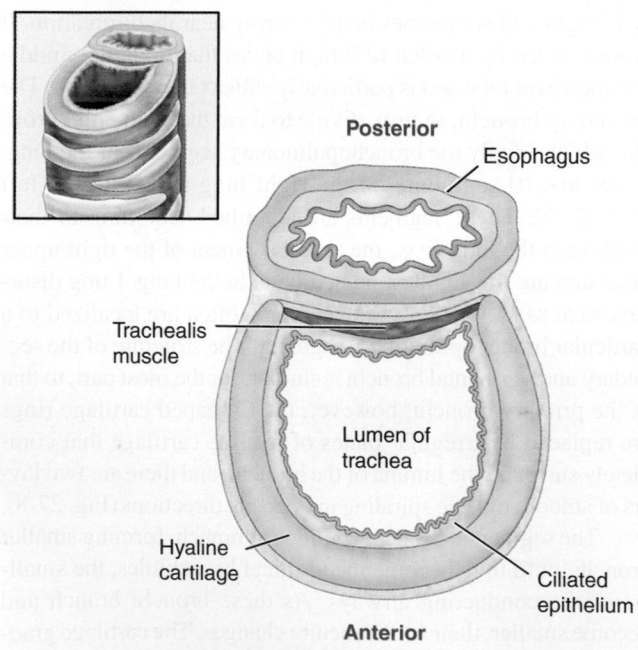

FIGURE 27-5 • Cross-section of the trachea, illustrating its relationship to the esophagus, the position of the supporting hyaline cartilage rings in its wall, and the trachealis muscle connecting the free ends of the cartilage rings.

elastic fibers. Bronchospasm, or contraction of these muscles, causes narrowing of the bronchioles and impairs air flow. The elastic fibers, which radiate from the outer layer of the bronchial wall and connect with elastic fibers arising from other parts of the bronchial tree, exert tension on the bronchial walls; by pulling uniformly in all directions, they help maintain airway patency.

Lungs and Respiratory Airways

The lungs are the functional structures of the respiratory system. In addition to their gas exchange function, they inactivate vasoactive substances such as bradykinin; they convert angiotensin I to angiotensin II; and they serve as a reservoir for blood storage. Heparin-producing cells are particularly abundant in the capillaries of the lung, where small clots may be trapped.

The gas exchange function of the lung takes place in the lobules of the lungs. Each lobule, which is the smallest functional unit of the lung, is supplied by a branch of a terminal bronchiole, an arteriole, the pulmonary capillaries, and a venule (see Fig. 27-8). Gas exchange takes place in the terminal respiratory bronchioles and the alveolar ducts and sacs. Blood enters the lobules through a pulmonary artery and exits through a pulmonary vein. Lymphatic structures surround the lobule and aid in the removal of plasma proteins and other particles from the interstitial spaces.

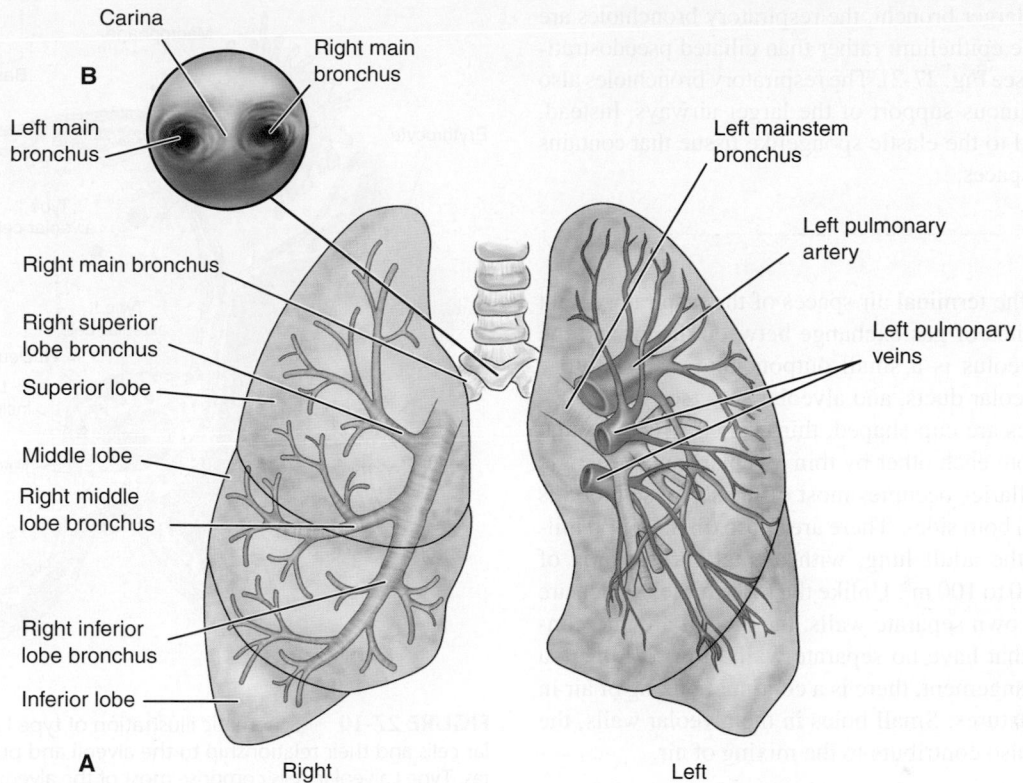

FIGURE 27-6 • **(A)** Anterior view of respiratory structures, including the lobes of the lung, the larynx, trachea, and the main bronchi on the left and the main pulmonary artery and vein on the right. **(B)** The carina is located at the bifurcation of the right and left mainstem bronchi.

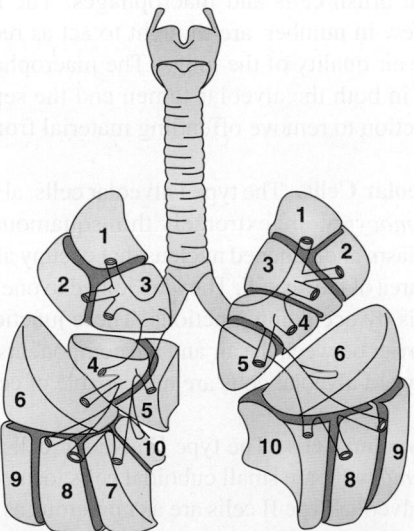

FIGURE 27-7 • Bronchopulmonary segments of the human lung. Left and right upper lobes: (1) apical, (2) posterior, (3) anterior, (4) superior lingular, and (5) inferior lingular segments. Right middle lobe: (4) lateral and (5) medial segments. Lower lobes: (6) superior (apical), (7) medial-basal, (8) anterior-basal, (9) lateral-basal, and (10) posterior-basal segments. The medial-basal segment (7) is absent in the left lung. (From Fishman A. P. [1980]. *Assessment of pulmonary function* [p. 19]. New York: McGraw-Hill.)

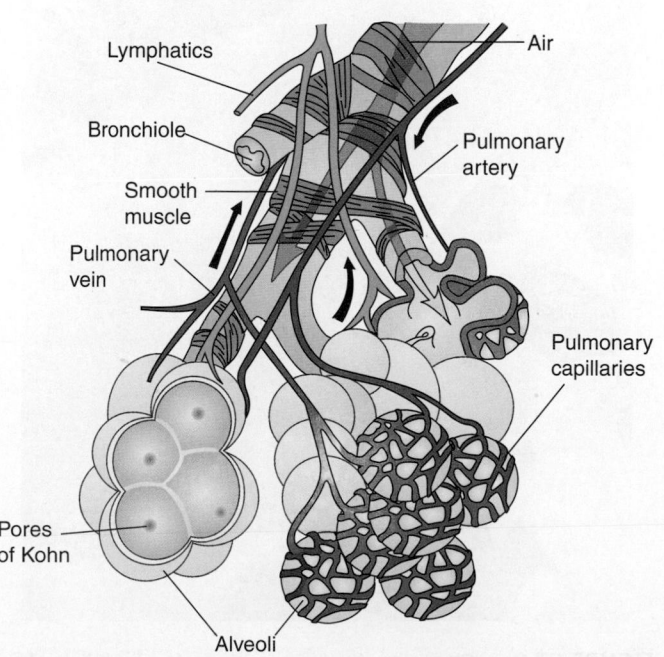

FIGURE 27-8 • Lobule of the lung, showing the bronchial smooth muscle fibers, pulmonary blood vessels, and lymphatics.

Unlike the larger bronchi, the respiratory bronchioles are lined with simple epithelium rather than ciliated pseudostratified epithelium (see Fig. 27-2). The respiratory bronchioles also lack the cartilaginous support of the larger airways. Instead, they are attached to the elastic spongelike tissue that contains the alveolar air spaces.

Alveoli

The alveoli are the terminal air spaces of the respiratory tract and the actual sites of gas exchange between the air and the blood. Each alveolus is a small outpouching of respiratory bronchioles, alveolar ducts, and alveolar sacs (see Fig. 27-8). The alveolar sacs are cup-shaped, thin-walled structures that are separated from each other by thin alveolar septa. A single network of capillaries occupies most of the septa, so blood is exposed to air on both sides. There are approximately 300 million alveoli in the adult lung, with a total surface area of approximately 50 to 100 m². Unlike the bronchioles, which are tubes with their own separate walls, the alveoli are interconnecting spaces that have no separate walls (Fig. 27-9). As a result of this arrangement, there is a continual mixing of air in the alveolar structures. Small holes in the alveolar walls, the pores of Kohn, also contribute to the mixing of air.

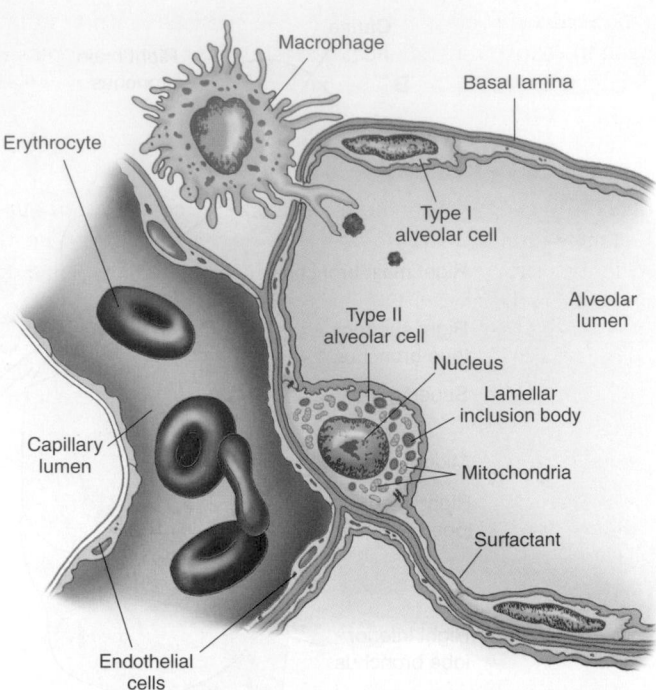

FIGURE 27-10 • Schematic illustration of type I and type II alveolar cells and their relationship to the alveoli and pulmonary capillaries. Type I alveolar cells comprise most of the alveolar surface. Type II alveolar cells, which produce surfactant, are located at the corners between adjacent alveoli. Also shown are the endothelial cells, which line the pulmonary capillaries, and an alveolar macrophage.

The alveolar epithelium is composed of two types of cells: type I and type II alveolar cells (Fig. 27-10). The alveoli also contain brush cells and macrophages. The brush cells, which are few in number, are thought to act as receptors that monitor the air quality of the lungs. The macrophages, which are present in both the alveolar lumen and the septum of the alveoli, function to remove offending material from the lung.

Type I Alveolar Cells. The type I alveolar cells, also known as *type I pneumocytes,* are extremely thin squamous cells with a thin cytoplasm and flattened nucleus that occupy about 95% of the surface area of the alveoli. They are joined to one another and to other cells by occluding junctions. These junctions form an effective barrier between the air and the components of the alveolar wall. Type I alveolar cells are not capable of cell division.

Type II Alveolar Cells. The type II alveolar cells, also called *type II pneumocytes,* are small cuboidal cells located at the corners of the alveoli. Type II cells are as numerous as type I cells, but because of their different shape, they cover only about 5% of the alveolar surface area. The type II cells synthesize pulmonary surfactant, a substance that decreases the surface tension in the alveoli and allows for greater ease of lung inflation. They are also the progenitor cells for type I cells. After lung injury, they proliferate and restore both type I and type II alveolar cells.

Pulmonary surfactant is a complex mixture of phospholipids, neutral lipids, and proteins that is synthesized in the

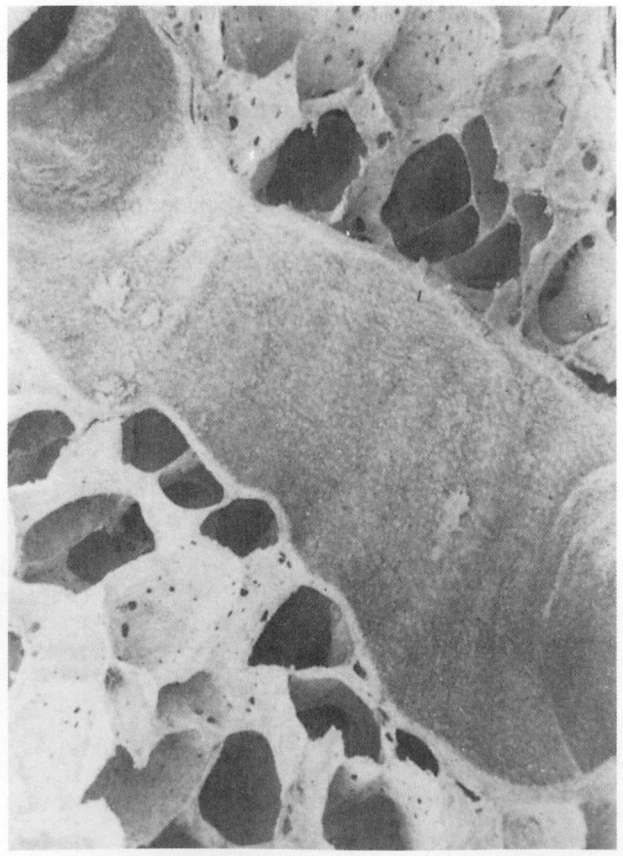

FIGURE 27-9 • Close-up of a cross-section of a small bronchus and surrounding alveoli. (Courtesy of Janice A. Nowell, University of California, Santa Cruz.)

type II alveolar cells. Type II alveolar cells are rich in mitochondria and are metabolically active. Their apical cytoplasm contains stacks of parallel membrane sheets or lamellae, called the lamellar bodies. All of the components of surfactant are synthesized by the alveolar type II cells and stored as preformed units in the lamellar bodies. Secretion of surfactant occurs by exocytosis. The major route of clearance of surfactant within the lung is through reuptake by the type II cells. After reuptake, the phospholipids are either recycled or degraded and reused in the synthesis of new phospholipids.

The surfactant molecules produced by the type II alveolar cells reduce the surface tension at the air–epithelium interface and modulate the immune functions of the lung. Recent research has revealed four types of surfactant, each with a different molecular structure: surfactant proteins A (SP-A), B (SP-B), C (SP-C), and D (SP-D). SP-B and SP-C reduce the surface tension at the air–epithelium interface and increase lung compliance and ease of lung inflation. SP-B is particularly important to the generation of the surface-reducing film that makes lung expansion possible (to be discussed). SP-A and SP-D do not reduce surface tension, but contribute to host defenses that protect against pathogens that have entered the lung. They are members of the collectin protein family that function as a part of the innate immune system (see Chapter 17). Collectively, they opsonize pathogens, including bacteria and viruses, to facilitate phagocytosis by macrophages. They also regulate the production of inflammatory mediators. Evidence also suggests that SP-A and SP-D are directly bactericidal, meaning they can kill bacteria in the absence of immune system effector cells.

Alveolar Macrophages. The macrophages, which are present in both the connective tissue of the septum and in the air spaces of the alveolus, are responsible for the removal of offending substances from the alveoli. In the air spaces, they scavenge the surface to remove inhaled particulate matter, such as dust and pollen. Some macrophages pass up the bronchial tree in the mucus and are disposed of by swallowing or coughing when they reach the pharynx. Others enter the septal connective tissue, where, filled with phagocytosed materials, they remain for life. Thus, at autopsy, urban dwellers, as well as smokers, usually show many alveolar macrophages filled with carbon and other polluting particles from the environment. The alveolar macrophages also phagocytose insoluble infectious agents such as *Mycobacterium tuberculosis.* The activated macrophages then aggregate to form a fibrin-encapsulated granuloma, called a *tubercle,* to contain the infection. The tubercle bacillus can remain dormant in this stage or be reactivated years later, when the person's immunologic tolerance wanes as the result of old age or immunosuppressive disease or therapy (see Chapter 28).

Pulmonary Vasculature and Lymphatic Supply

Pulmonary and Bronchial Circulations

The lungs are provided with a dual blood supply, the pulmonary and bronchial circulations. The pulmonary circulation arises from the pulmonary artery and provides for the gas exchange function of the lungs (see Fig. 27-8). Deoxygenated blood leaves the right heart through the pulmonary artery, which divides into a left pulmonary artery that enters the left lung and a right pulmonary artery that enters the right lung. Return of oxygenated blood to the heart occurs by way of the pulmonary veins, which empty into the left atrium. This is the only part of the circulation where arteries carry deoxygenated blood and veins carry oxygenated blood.

The bronchial circulation distributes blood to the conducting airways and the supporting structures of the lung. The bronchial circulation has a secondary function of warming and humidifying incoming air as it moves through the conducting airways. The bronchial arteries arise from the thoracic aorta and enter the lungs with the major bronchi, dividing and subdividing along with the bronchi as they move out into the lung, supplying them and other lung structures with oxygen. The blood from the capillaries in the bronchial circulation drains into the bronchial veins, with the blood from the larger bronchial veins emptying into the vena cava. Blood from the smaller bronchial veins empties into the pulmonary veins. Because the bronchial circulation does not participate in gas exchange, this blood is deoxygenated. As a result, it dilutes the oxygenated blood returning to the left side of the heart through the pulmonary veins.

The bronchial blood vessels are the only ones that can undergo angiogenesis (formation of new vessels) and develop collateral circulation when vessels in the pulmonary circulation are obstructed, as in pulmonary embolism. The development of new blood vessels helps to keep lung tissue alive until the pulmonary circulation can be restored.

Lymphatic Circulation

The lungs are also supplied with lymphatic drainage that parallels that of their dual blood supply. One set of lymph vessels, the superficial vessels, drains the surface of the lung and travels in the connective tissue of the visceral pleura. A second set of the vessels, the deep lymphatic vessels, follows the pulmonary arteries, pulmonary veins, and bronchial tree down to the level of the respiratory bronchioles (see Fig. 27-8). Both of these systems have numerous interconnections and both form networks that drain into the hilar lymph nodes at the base of each lung. Particulate matter entering the lung is partly removed through these channels, as are the plasma proteins that have escaped from the pulmonary capillaries. The latter function is particularly important in keeping the lungs dry and in preventing the accumulation of fluid in the pleural cavity.

Innervation

The lung is innervated by the sympathetic and parasympathetic divisions of the autonomic nervous system. It is parasympathetic stimulation, through the vagus nerve, that is responsible for the slightly constricted smooth muscle tone in the normal resting lung. There is no voluntary motor innervation of the lung, nor are there pain fibers. Pain fibers are found only in the pleura.

Stimulation of the parasympathetic nervous system leads to airway constriction and increased glandular secretion. Parasympathetic innervation of the lung arises from the vagal nuclei in the medulla. Preganglionic fibers from the vagal nuclei descend in the vagus nerve to ganglia adjacent to the airways and blood vessels of the lung. Postganglionic fibers from the ganglia then complete the network that innervates smooth muscle, blood vessels, and epithelial cells, including the goblet and submucosal glands. Both the preganglionic and postganglionic fibers contain excitatory (cholinergic) motor neurons that respond to acetylcholine. Parasympathetic innervation is greater in the large airways and diminishes toward the smaller airways.

Stimulation of the sympathetic nervous system causes airway relaxation, blood vessel constriction, and inhibition of glandular secretion. Sympathetic innervation arises from the cell bodies in paravertebral sympathetic ganglia. Neurotransmitters of the sympathetic nervous system include the catecholamines norepinephrine and epinephrine.

Pleura

A thin, transparent, double-layered serous membrane, called the *pleura*, lines the thoracic cavity and encases the lungs (see Fig. 27-1). The outer parietal layer lines the pulmonary cavities and adheres to the thoracic wall, the mediastinum, and the diaphragm. The inner visceral pleura closely covers the lung and is adherent to all its surfaces. It is continuous with the parietal pleura at the hilum of the lung, where the major bronchus and pulmonary vessels enter and leave the lung. A thin film of serous fluid separates the two pleural layers, allowing the two layers to glide over each other and yet hold together, so there is no separation between the lungs and the chest wall. The pleural cavity is a potential space in which serous fluid or inflammatory exudate can accumulate. The term *pleural effusion* is used to describe an abnormal collection of fluid or exudate in the pleural cavity.

IN SUMMARY, the respiratory system consists of the air passages and the lungs, where gas exchange takes place. Functionally, the air passages of the respiratory system can be divided into two parts: the conducting airways, through which air moves as it passes into and out of the lungs, and the respiratory tissues, where gas exchange actually takes place. The conducting airways include the nasal passages, mouth and nasopharynx, larynx, and tracheobronchial tree. Air is warmed, filtered, and humidified as it passes through these structures.

The lungs are the functional structures of the respiratory system. In addition to their gas exchange function, they inactivate vasoactive substances such as bradykinin; they convert angiotensin I to angiotensin II; and they serve as a reservoir for blood. The lobules, which are the functional units of the lung, consist of the respiratory bronchioles, alveoli, and pulmonary capillaries. It is here that gas exchange takes place. Oxygen from the alveoli diffuses across the alveolar capillary membrane into the blood, and carbon dioxide from the blood diffuses into the alveoli. There are two types of alveolar cells: type I and type II. Type I cells, which provide the gas exchange function of the lung, are extremely thin squamous cells lining most of the surface of the alveoli. Type II cells, which produce surfactant and serve as progenitor cells for type I cells, are small cuboidal cells. There are four types of surfactant protein (SP): SP-A, SP-B, SP-C, and SP-D. SP-B and SP-C provide the critical surface tension–lowering properties necessary for ease of lung inflation. SP-A and SP-D modulate the immune response to foreign pathogens and participate in local inflammatory responses.

The lungs are provided with a dual blood supply: the pulmonary circulation provides for the gas exchange function of the lungs and the bronchial circulation distributes blood to the conducting airways and supporting structures of the lung. The lungs are also supplied by a dual system of lymphatic vessels: a superficial system in the visceral pleura and a deep system that supplies deeper pulmonary structures, including the respiratory bronchioles.

The respiratory system is innervated by the sympathetic and parasympathetic divisions of the autonomic nervous system. Parasympathetic innervation causes airway constriction and an increase in respiratory secretions, whereas sympathetic innervation causes bronchial dilation and a decrease in respiratory tract secretions. There is no voluntary motor innervation of the lung, nor are there pain fibers. Pain fibers are found only in the pleura.

The lungs are encased in a thin, transparent, double-layered serous membrane called the *pleura*. A thin film of serous fluid separates the outer parietal and inner visceral pleural layers, allowing the two layers to glide over each other and yet hold together, so there is no separation between the lungs and the chest wall. The pleural cavity is a potential space in which serous fluid or inflammatory exudate can accumulate. ■

CONCEPTS in action **ANIMATI☆N**

EXCHANGE OF GASES BETWEEN THE ATMOSPHERE AND THE LUNGS

After completing this section of the chapter, you should be able to meet the following objectives:

- Describe the basic properties of gases in relation to their partial pressures and their pressures in relation to volume and temperature.
- State the definition of intrathoracic, intrapleural, and intra-alveolar pressures, and state how each of these pressures changes in relation to atmospheric pressure during inspiration and expiration.
- Use the law of Laplace to explain the need for surfactant in maintaining the inflation of small alveoli.

■ Differentiate between the determinants of airway resistance and lung compliance and their effect on the work of breathing.

■ Define inspiratory reserve, expiratory reserve, vital capacity, residual lung volume, and $FEV_{1.0}$.

Basic Properties of Gases

The air we breathe is made up of a mixture of gases, mainly nitrogen and oxygen. These gases exert a combined pressure called the *atmospheric* or *barometric pressure*. The pressure at sea level, which is defined as 1 atmosphere, is 760 millimeters of mercury (mm Hg, or torr) or 14.7 pounds per square inch (PSI). When measuring respiratory pressures, atmospheric pressure is assigned a value of zero. A respiratory pressure of +15 mm Hg means that the pressure is 15 mm Hg above atmospheric pressure, and a respiratory pressure of −15 mm Hg is 15 mm Hg less than atmospheric pressure. Respiratory pressures often are expressed in centimeters of water (cm H_2O) because of the small pressures involved (1 mm Hg = 1.35 cm H_2O pressure).

The pressure exerted by a single gas in a mixture is called the *partial pressure*. The capital letter "P" followed by the chemical symbol of the gas (PO_2) is used to denote its partial pressure. The law of partial pressures states that the total pressure of a mixture of gases, as in the atmosphere, is equal to the sum of the partial pressures of the different gases in the mixture. If the concentration of oxygen at 760 mm Hg (1 atmosphere) is 20%, its partial pressure is 152 mm Hg (760×0.20).

Water vapor is different from other types of gases in that its partial pressure is affected by temperature but not atmospheric pressure. The relative humidity refers to the percentage of moisture in the air compared with the amount that the air can hold without causing condensation (100% saturation). Warm air holds more moisture than cold air. This is the reason that precipitation in the form of rain or snow commonly occurs when the relative humidity is high and there is a sudden drop in atmospheric temperature. The air in the alveoli, which is 100% saturated at normal body temperature, has a water vapor pressure of 47 mm Hg. The water vapor pressure must be included in the sum of the total pressure of the gases in the alveoli (*i.e.,* the total pressure of the other gases in the alveoli is $760 - 47 = 713$ mm Hg).

Air moves between the atmosphere and the lungs because of a pressure difference. According to the laws of physics, the pressure of a gas varies inversely with the volume of its container, provided the temperature remains constant. If equal amounts of a gas were placed in two different-sized containers, the pressure of the gas in the smaller container would be greater than the pressure in the larger container. The movement of gases is always from the container with the greater pressure to the one with the lesser pressure. The chest cavity can be viewed as a volume container. During inspiration, the size of the chest cavity increases and air moves into the lungs; during expiration, air moves out of the lungs as the size of the chest cavity decreases.

Ventilation and the Mechanics of Breathing

Ventilation is concerned with the movement of gases into and out of the lungs. There is nothing complicated about ventilation. It is purely a mechanical event that obeys the laws of physics as they relate to the behavior of gases. It relies on a system of open airways and the respiratory pressures created as the movements of the respiratory muscles change the size of the chest cage. The degree to which the lungs inflate and deflate depends on the respiratory pressures inflating the lung, compliance of the lungs, and airway resistance.

VENTILATION AND GAS EXCHANGE

■ Ventilation refers to the movement of gases into and out of the lungs through a system of open airways and along a pressure gradient resulting from a change in chest volume.

■ During inspiration, air is drawn into the lungs as the respiratory muscles expand the chest cavity; during expiration, air moves out of the lungs as the chest muscles recoil and the chest cavity becomes smaller.

■ The ease with which air is moved into and out of the lung depends on the resistance of the airways, which is inversely related to the fourth power of the airway radius, and lung compliance, or the ease with which the lungs can be inflated.

■ The minute volume, which is determined by the metabolic needs of the body, is the amount of air that is exchanged each minute. It is the product of the tidal volume or amount of air exchanged with each breath multiplied by the respiratory rate.

Respiratory Pressures

The pressure inside the airways and alveoli of the lungs is called the *intrapulmonary pressure* or *alveolar pressure*. The gases in this area of the lungs are in communication with atmospheric pressure (Fig. 27-11). When the glottis is open and air is not moving into or out of the lungs, as occurs just before inspiration or expiration, the intrapulmonary pressure is zero or equal to atmospheric pressure.

The pressure in the pleural cavity is called the *intrapleural pressure*. The intrapleural pressure of a normal inflated lung is always negative in relation to alveolar pressure, approximately −4 mm Hg between breaths when the glottis is open and the alveolar spaces are open to the atmosphere. The lungs and the chest wall have elastic properties, each pulling in the opposite direction. If removed from the chest, the lungs would contract to a smaller size, and the chest wall, if freed from the lungs, would expand. The opposing forces of the chest wall and lungs create a pull against the visceral and parietal layers of the

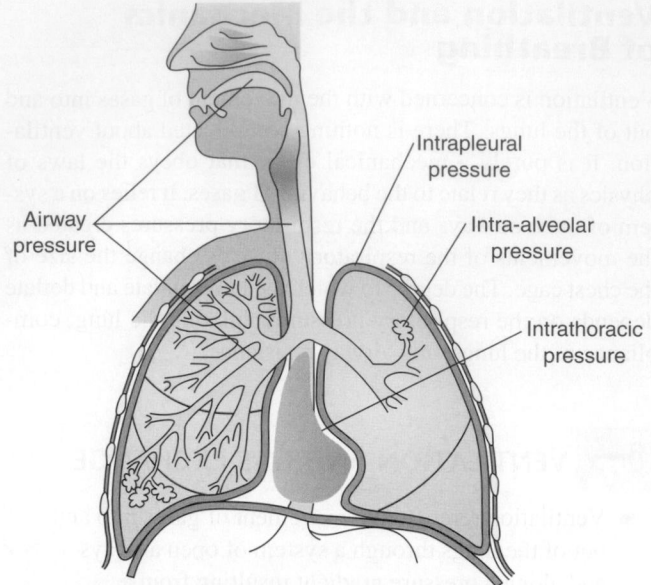

FIGURE 27-11 • Partitioning of respiratory pressures.

pleura, causing the pressure in the pleural cavity to become negative. During inspiration, the elastic recoil of the lungs increases, causing intrapleural pressure to become more negative than during expiration. Without the negative intrapleural pressure holding the lungs against the chest wall, their elastic recoil properties would cause them to collapse. Although intrapleural pressure is negative in relation to alveolar pressure, it may become positive in relation to atmospheric pressure (*e.g.*, during forced expiration and coughing). The *transpulmonary* (*trans* = "across") *pressure* is the difference between the alveolar and intrapleural pressures. As will be explained later, it is used in determining pulmonary compliance.

The *intrathoracic pressure* is the pressure in the thoracic cavity. It is essentially equal to the intrapleural pressure and is the pressure to which the lungs, heart, and great vessels are exposed. Forced expiration against a closed glottis, such as occurs during defecation and the Valsalva maneuver, produces marked increases in intrathoracic pressure and impedes venous

return to the right atrium. The Valsalva maneuver is used to study the cardiovascular effects of increased intrathoracic pressure on peripheral venous pressures, cardiac filling, and cardiac output, as well as post-strain heart rate and blood pressure responses.

Chest Cage and Respiratory Muscles

The lungs and major airways share the chest cavity with the heart, great vessels, and esophagus. The chest cavity is a closed compartment bounded on the top by the neck muscles and at the bottom by the diaphragm. The outer walls of the chest cavity are formed by 12 pairs of ribs, the sternum, the thoracic vertebrae, and the intercostal muscles that lie between the ribs. Mechanically, the act of breathing depends on the fact that the chest cavity is a closed compartment whose only opening to the external atmosphere is through the trachea.

Ventilation consists of inspiration and expiration. During *inspiration,* the size of the chest cavity increases, the intrathoracic pressure becomes more negative, and air is drawn into the lungs. *Expiration* occurs as the elastic components of the chest wall and lung structures that were stretched during inspiration recoil, causing the size of the chest cavity to decrease and the pressure in the chest cavity to increase.

The diaphragm is the principal muscle of inspiration. When the diaphragm contracts, the abdominal contents are forced downward and the chest expands from top to bottom (Fig. 27-12). During normal levels of inspiration, the diaphragm moves approximately 1 cm, but this can be increased to 10 cm on forced inspiration. The diaphragm is innervated by the phrenic nerve roots, which arise from the cervical level of the spinal cord, mainly from C4 but also from C3 and C5. Persons who sustain spinal cord injury above C3 lose the function of the diaphragm and require mechanical ventilation (see Chapter 50). Paralysis of one side of the diaphragm causes the chest to move up on that side rather than down during inspiration because of the negative pressure in the chest. This is called *paradoxical movement.*

The external intercostal muscles, which also aid in inspiration, connect to the adjacent ribs and slope downward and for-

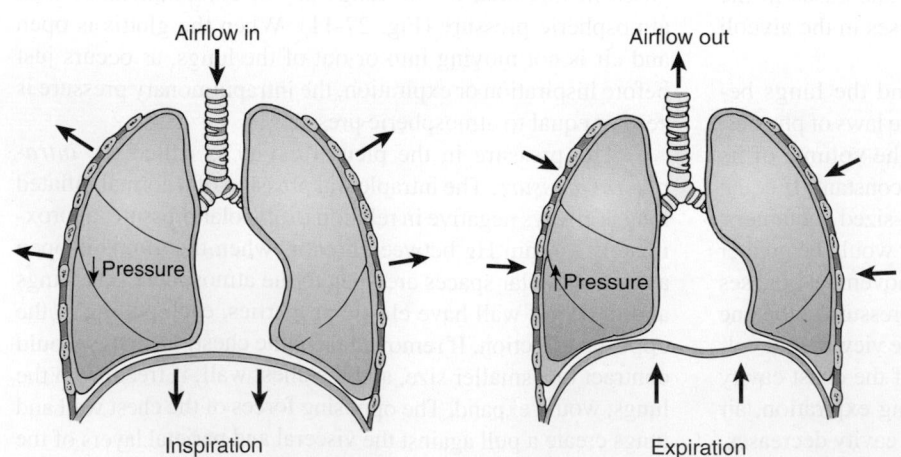

FIGURE 27-12 • Movement of the diaphragm and changes in chest volume and pressure during inspiration and expiration. During inspiration, contraction of the diaphragm and expansion of the chest cavity produce a decrease in intrathoracic pressure, causing air to move into the lungs. During expiration, relaxation of the diaphragm and chest cavity produces an increase in intrathoracic pressure, causing air to move out of the lungs.

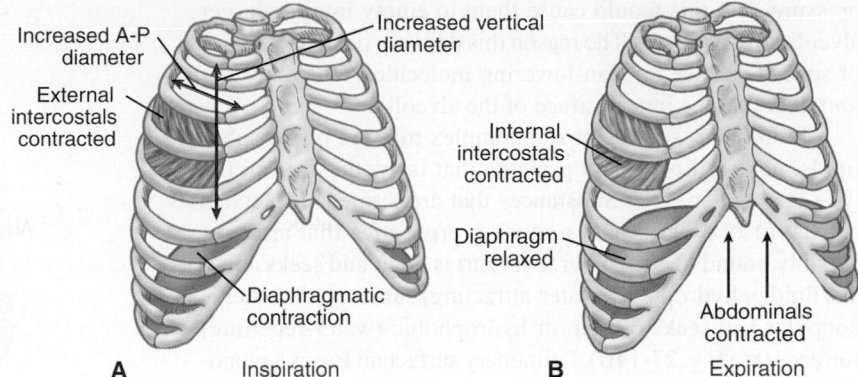

FIGURE 27-13 • Expansion and contraction of the chest cage during expiration and inspiration, demonstrating especially diaphragmatic contraction, elevation of the rib cage, and function of the (**A**) external and (**B**) internal intercostals.

ward (Fig. 27-13). When they contract, they raise the ribs and rotate them slightly so that the sternum is pushed forward; this enlarges the chest from side to side and from front to back. The intercostal muscles receive their innervation from nerves that exit the central nervous system at the thoracic level of the spinal cord. Paralysis of these muscles usually does not have a serious effect on respiration because of the effectiveness of the diaphragm.

The accessory muscles of inspiration include the scalene muscles and the sternocleidomastoid muscles. The scalene muscles elevate the first two ribs, and the sternocleidomastoid muscles raise the sternum to increase the size of the chest cavity. These muscles contribute little to quiet breathing but contract vigorously during exercise. For the accessory muscles to assist in ventilation, they must be stabilized in some way. For example, persons with bronchial asthma often brace their arms against a firm object during an attack as a means of stabilizing their shoulders so that the attached accessory muscles can exert their full effect on ventilation. The head commonly is bent backward so that the scalene and sternocleidomastoid muscles can elevate the ribs more effectively. Other muscles that play a minor role in inspiration are the alae nasi, which produce flaring of the nostrils during obstructed breathing.

Expiration is largely passive. It occurs as the elastic components of the chest wall and lung structures that were stretched during inspiration recoil, causing air to leave the lungs as the intrathoracic pressure increases. When needed, the abdominal and the internal intercostal muscles can be used to increase expiratory effort (see Fig. 27-13B). The increase in intra-abdominal pressure that accompanies the forceful contraction of the abdominal muscles pushes the diaphragm upward and results in an increase in intrathoracic pressure. The internal intercostal muscles move inward, which pulls the chest downward, increasing expiratory effort.

Lung Compliance

Lung compliance refers to the ease with which the lungs can be inflated. Compliance can be appreciated by comparing the ease of blowing up a noncompliant new balloon that is stiff and resistant with a compliant one that has been previously blown up and is easy to inflate. Specifically, lung compliance (C) de-

scribes the change in lung volume (ΔV) that can be accomplished with a given change in respiratory pressure (ΔP); thus, $C = \Delta V / \Delta P$. It takes more pressure to move the same amount of air into a noncompliant lung than it does into a compliant one.

Lung compliance is determined by the elastin and collagen fibers of the lung, its water content, and surface tension. It also depends on the compliance of the thoracic or chest cage. It is diminished by conditions that reduce the natural elasticity of the lung, block the bronchi or smaller airways, increase the surface tension in the alveoli, or impair the flexibility of the thoracic cage.

Lung tissue is made up of elastin and collagen fibers. The elastin fibers are easily stretched and increase the ease of lung inflation, whereas the collagen fibers resist stretching and make lung inflation more difficult. In lung diseases such as interstitial lung disease and pulmonary fibrosis, the lungs become stiff and noncompliant as the elastin fibers are replaced with scar tissue. Pulmonary congestion and edema produce a reversible decrease in pulmonary compliance.

Elastic recoil describes the ability of the elastic components of the lung to recoil to their original position after having been stretched. Overstretching lung tissues, as occurs with emphysema, causes the elastic components of the lung to lose their recoil, making the lung easier to inflate but more difficult to deflate because of its inability to recoil.

Surface Tension. An important factor in lung compliance is the *surface tension* or attraction forces of the surface molecules in the alveoli. The alveoli are lined with a thin film of liquid, and it is at the interface between this liquid film and the alveolar air that surface tension develops. This is because the forces that hold the water molecules of the liquid film together are stronger than those that hold the air molecules in the alveoli together. In the alveoli, excess surface tension causes water molecules in the liquid film to contract, making lung inflation difficult.

The units of surface tension are those of force per unit length. The relationship between the pressure within a sphere such as an alveolus and the tension in the wall can be described using the law of Laplace (pressure = 2 × surface tension/radius). If the surface tension were equal throughout the lungs, the alveoli with the smallest radii would have the greatest pressure, and this would cause them to empty into the larger alveoli (Fig. 27-14A). The reason this does not occur is because of special surface tension-lowering molecules, called *surfactant*, that line the inner surface of the alveoli.

Pulmonary surfactant is a complex mixture of phospholipids, neutral lipids, and proteins that is synthesized in the type II alveolar cells. Substances that are termed surfactants consist of two parts with opposing properties that are irreversibly bound to each other. One part is polar and seeks aqueous fluid or hydrophilic (water-attracting) surfaces; the other is nonpolar and seeks oil, air, or hydrophobic (water-repelling) surfaces (see Fig. 27-14B). Pulmonary surfactant forms a monolayer, with its hydrophilic surface binding to liquid film on the surface of the alveoli and its hydrophobic surface facing outward toward the gases in the alveolar air. It is this monolayer that interrupts the surface tension that develops at the air–liquid interface in the alveoli.

Pulmonary surfactant, particularly SP-B, exerts several important effects on lung inflation: it lowers the surface tension and it increases lung compliance and ease of lung inflation. Without surfactant, lung inflation would be extremely difficult. In addition, it helps to keep the alveoli dry and prevent pulmonary edema. This is because water is pulled out of the pulmonary capillaries into the alveoli when increased surface tension causes the alveoli to contract. Surfactant also provides for stability and more even inflation of the alveoli. Alveoli, except those at the pleural surface, are surrounded by other alveoli. Thus, the tendency of one alveolus to collapse is opposed by the traction exerted by the surrounding alveolus. The surfactant molecules are also more densely packed in small alveoli than in large alveoli (see Fig. 27-14C). In surgical and bedridden patients, shallow and quiet breathing often impairs the spreading of surfactant. Encouraging these patients to cough and deep breathe enhances the spreading of surfactant. This allows for a more even distribution of ventilation and prevention of atelectasis.

The type II alveolar cells that produce surfactant do not begin to mature until the 26th to 27th week of gestation; consequently, many premature infants have difficulty producing sufficient amounts of surfactant. This can lead to alveolar collapse and severe respiratory distress. This condition, called *infant respiratory distress syndrome,* is the single most common cause of respiratory disease in premature infants. Surfactant dysfunction also is possible in the adult. This usually occurs as the result of severe injury or infection and can contribute to the development of a condition called *acute respiratory distress syndrome* (see Chapter 29).

Airway Airflow

The volume of air that moves into and out of the air exchange portion of the lungs is directly related to the pressure difference between the lungs and the atmosphere and inversely related to the resistance that the air encounters as it moves through the airways. Depending on the velocity and pattern of flow, airflow can be laminar or turbulent.

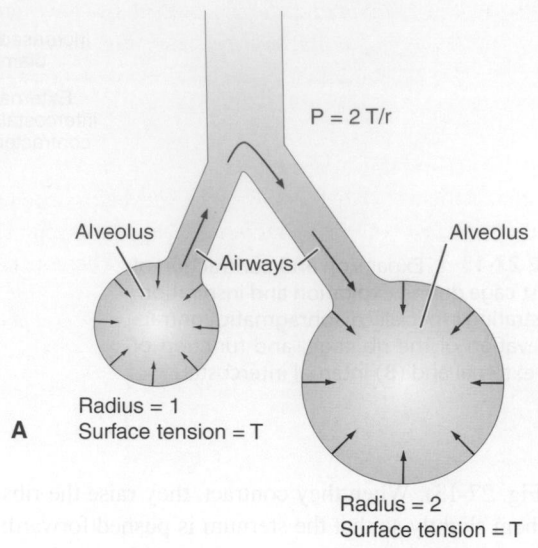

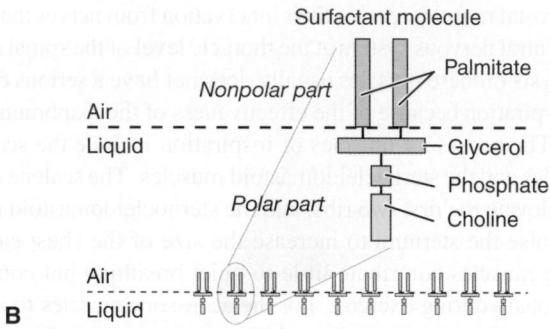

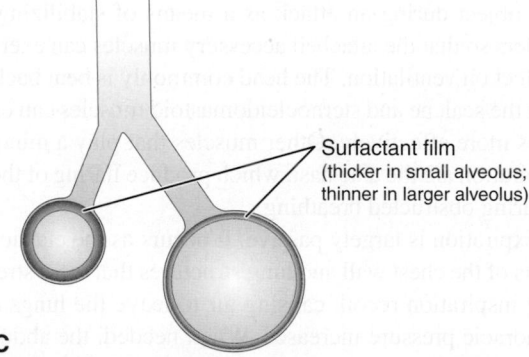

FIGURE 27-14 • **(A)** The effect of the surface tension (forces generated at the fluid–air interface) and radius on the pressure and movement of gases in the alveolar structures. According to the law of Laplace ($P = 2T/r$, P = pressure, T = tension, r = radius), the pressure generated within the sphere is inversely proportional to the radius. Air moves from the alveolus with a small radius and higher pressure to the alveolus with the larger radius and lower pressure. **(B)** Surfactant molecules, showing their hydrophilic heads attached to the fluid lining of the alveolus and their hydrophobic tails oriented toward the air interface. **(C)** The surfactant molecules form a monolayer (*shaded in blue*) that disrupts the intermolecular forces and lowers the surface tension more in the smaller alveolus with its higher concentration of surfactant than in the larger alveolus with the lower concentration.

Laminar or *streamlined airflow* occurs at low flow rates in which the air stream is parallel to the sides of the airway. With laminar flow, the air at the periphery must overcome the resistance to flow, and as a result, the air in the center of the airway moves faster. *Turbulent airflow* is disorganized flow in which the molecules of the gas move laterally, collide with one another, and change their velocities. Whether turbulence develops depends on the radius of the airways, the interaction of the gas molecules, and the velocity of airflow. It is most likely to occur when the radius of the airways is large and the velocity of flow is high. Turbulent flow occurs regularly in the trachea. Turbulence of airflow accounts for the respiratory sounds that are heard during chest auscultation (*i.e.,* listening to chest sounds using a stethoscope).

In the bronchial tree with its many branches, laminar airflow probably occurs only in the very small airways, where the velocity of flow is low. Because the small airways contribute little resistance to airflow, they constitute a silent zone (to be discussed).

Airway Resistance. Airway resistance is the ratio of the pressure driving inspiration or expiration to airflow. The French physician Jean Léonard Marie Poiseuille first described the pressure–flow characteristics of laminar flow in a straight circular tube, a correlation that has become known as the *Poiseuille law.* According to the Poiseuille law, the resistance to flow is inversely related to the fourth power of the radius ($R = 1/r^4$). If the radius is reduced by one half, the resistance increases 16-fold ($2 \times 2 \times 2 \times 2 = 16$).

Airway resistance differs in large (*e.g.,* trachea and bronchi), medium-sized (*e.g.,* segmental), and small (*e.g.,* bronchioles) airways. Therefore, the total airway resistance is equal to the sum of the resistances in these three types of airways. The site of most of the resistance along the bronchial tree is the large bronchi, with the smallest airways contributing very little to the total airway resistance. This is because most of these airways are arranged in parallel and their resistances are added as reciprocals (*i.e.,* total combined resistance = 1/R + 1/R, etc.). Although the resistance of each individual bronchiole may be relatively high, their great number results in a large total cross-sectional area, causing their total resistance to be low. Many airway diseases, such as emphysema and chronic bronchitis, begin in the small airways. Early detection of these diseases is often difficult because a considerable amount of damage must be present before the usual measurements of airway resistance can detect them.

Airway resistance is greatly affected by lung volumes, being less during inspiration than expiration. This is because elastic fibers connect the outside of the airways to the surrounding lung tissues. As a result, these airways are pulled open as the lungs expand during inspiration, and they become narrower as the lungs deflate during expiration (Fig. 27-15). This is one of the reasons why persons with conditions that increase airway resistance, such as bronchial asthma, usually have less difficulty during inspiration than during expiration.

Airway resistance is also affected by the bronchial smooth tone that controls airway diameter. The smooth muscles in the

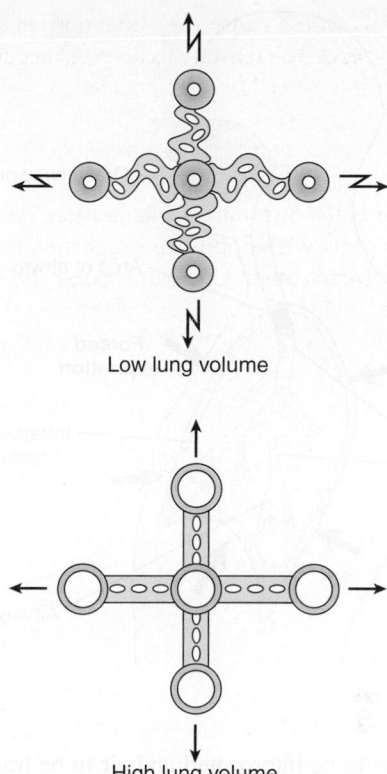

FIGURE 27-15 • Interaction of tissue forces on airways during low and high lung volumes. At low lung volumes, the tissue forces tend to fold and place less tension on the airways and they become smaller; during high lung volumes, the tissue forces are stretched and pull the airways open.

airway, from the trachea down to the terminal bronchioles, are under autonomic nervous system control. Stimulation of the parasympathetic nervous system causes bronchial constriction as well as increased mucus secretion, whereas sympathetic stimulation has the opposite effect.

Airway Compression During Forced Expiration. Airway resistance does not change much during normal quiet breathing; however, it is significantly increased during forced expiration, such as in vigorous exercise. Airflow through the collapsible airways in the lungs depends on the distending airway (intrapulmonary) pressures that hold the airways open and the external (intrapleural or intrathoracic) pressures that surround and compress the airways. The difference between these two pressures (intrathoracic pressure minus airway pressure) is called the *transpulmonary pressure.* For airflow to occur, the distending pressure inside the airways must be greater than the compressing pressure outside the airways. During forced expiration, the transpulmonary pressure is decreased because of a disproportionate increase in the intrathoracic pressure compared with airway pressure. The resistance that air encounters as it moves out of the lungs causes a further drop in airway pressure. If this drop in airway pressure is sufficiently great, the surrounding intrathoracic pressure will compress the collapsible airways (*i.e.,* those that lack cartilaginous support),

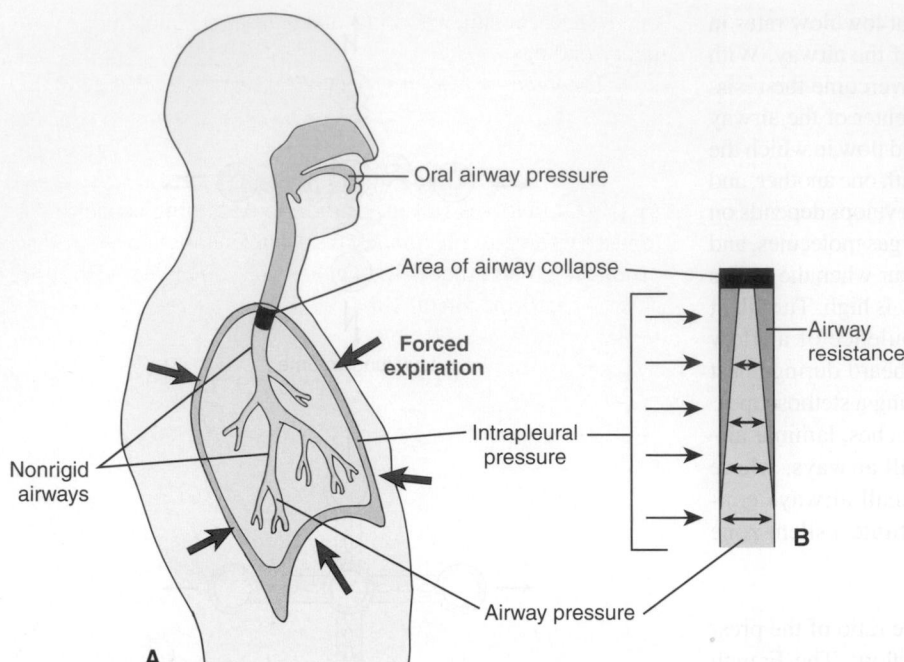

FIGURE 27-16 • Mechanism that limits maximal expiratory flow rate. **(A)** Airway patency and airflow in the nonrigid airways of the lungs rely on a transpulmonary pressure gradient in which airway pressure is greater than intrapleural pressure. **(B)** Airway resistance normally produces a drop in airway pressure as air moves out of the lungs. The increased intrapleural pressure that occurs with forced expiration produces airway collapse in the nonrigid airways at the point where intrapleural pressure exceeds airway pressure.

causing airflow to be interrupted and air to be trapped in the terminal airways (Fig. 27-16).

Although this type of airway compression usually is seen only during forced expiration in persons with normal respiratory function, it may occur during normal breathing in persons with lung diseases. For example, in conditions that increase airway resistance, such as emphysema, the pressure drop along the smaller airways is magnified, and an increase in intra-airway pressure is needed to maintain airway patency. Measures such as pursed-lip breathing increase airway pressure and improve expiratory flow rates in persons with chronic obstructive pulmonary disease (discussed in Chapter 29). This is also the basis for using positive end-expiratory pressure in persons who are being mechanically ventilated. Infants who are having trouble breathing often grunt to increase their expiratory airway pressures and keep their airways open.

Lung Volumes

Lung volumes, or the amount of air exchanged during ventilation, can be subdivided into three components: (1) the tidal volume, (2) the inspiratory reserve volume, and (3) the expiratory reserve volume (Fig. 27-17). The *tidal volume* (TV) is the volume of air inspired (or exhaled) with each breath. It varies with age, gender, body position, and metabolic activity. It usually is about 500 mL in the average-sized adult and about 3 to 5 mL/kg in children. The maximum amount of air that can be inspired in excess of the normal TV is called the *inspiratory reserve volume* (IRV), and the maximum amount that can be exhaled in excess of the normal TV is the *expiratory reserve volume* (ERV). Approximately 1200 mL of air always remains in the lungs after forced expiration; this air is the *residual volume* (RV). The RV increases with age because there is more trapping of air in the

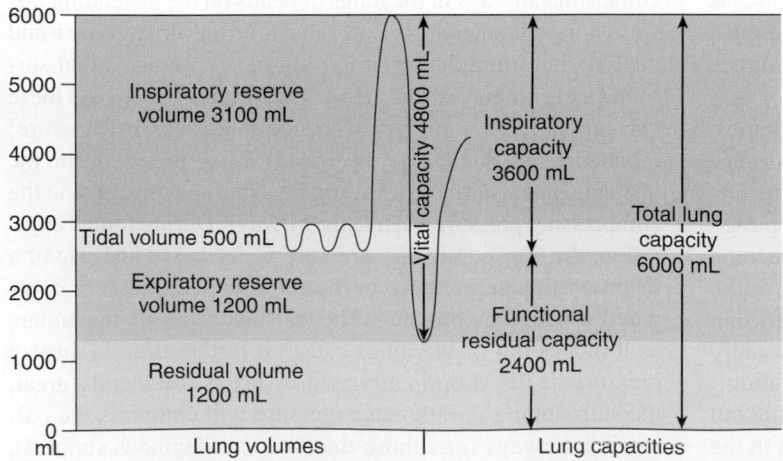

FIGURE 27-17 • Tracings of respiratory volumes (*left*) and lung capacities (*right*) as they would appear if made using a spirometer. The tidal volume (*yellow*) represents the amount of air inhaled and exhaled during normal breathing; the inspiratory reserve volume (*pink*), the maximal amount of air in excess of the tidal volume that can be forcefully inhaled; the maximal expiratory reserve (*blue*), the maximal amount of air that can be exhaled in excess of the tidal volume; and the residual volume (*green*), the air that continues to remain in the lung after maximal expiratory effort. The inspiratory capacity represents the sum of the inspiratory reserve volume and the tidal volume; the functional residual capacity, the sum of the maximal expiratory reserve and residual volumes; and the total lung capacity, the sum of all the volumes.

lungs at the end of expiration. These volumes can be measured using an instrument called a *spirometer*.

Lung capacities include two or more lung volumes. The *vital capacity* equals the IRV plus the TV plus the ERV and is the amount of air that can be exhaled from the point of maximal inspiration. The *inspiratory capacity* equals the TV plus the IRV. It is the amount of air a person can breathe in beginning at the normal expiratory level and distending the lungs to the maximal amount. The *functional residual capacity* is the sum of the RV and ERV; it is the volume of air that remains in the lungs at the end of normal expiration. The *total lung capacity* is the sum of all the volumes in the lungs. The RV cannot be measured with the spirometer because this air cannot be expressed from the lungs. It is measured by indirect methods, such as the helium dilution method, nitrogen washout method, or body plethysmography. Lung volumes and capacities are summarized in Table 27-1.

Pulmonary Function Studies

The previously described lung volumes and capacities are anatomic or static measures determined by lung volumes and measured without relation to time. The spirometer also is used to measure dynamic lung function (*i.e.,* ventilation with respect to time); these tests often are used in assessing pulmonary function. Pulmonary function measures include maximum voluntary ventilation, forced vital capacity, forced expiratory volumes and flow rates, and forced inspiratory flow rates (Table 27-2). Pulmonary function is measured for various clinical purposes, including diagnosis of respiratory disease, preoperative surgical and anesthetic risk evaluation, and symptom and disability evaluation for legal or insurance purposes. The tests also are used for evaluating dyspnea, cough, wheezing, and abnormal radiologic or laboratory findings.

The *maximum voluntary ventilation* measures the volume of air that a person can move into and out of the lungs during maximum effort lasting for 12 to 15 seconds. This measurement usually is converted to liters per minute. The *forced vital capacity* (FVC) involves full inspiration to total lung capacity followed by forceful maximal expiration. Obstruction of airways produces a FVC that is lower than that observed with more slowly performed vital capacity measurements. The *forced expiratory volume* (FEV) is the expiratory volume achieved in a given time period. The $FEV_{1.0}$ is the FEV that can be exhaled in 1 second. The $FEV_{1.0}$ frequently is expressed as a percentage of the FVC. The $FEV_{1.0}$ and FVC are used in the diagnosis of obstructive lung disorders.

The *forced inspiratory vital flow* (FIF) measures the respiratory response during rapid maximal inspiration. Calculation of airflow during the middle half of inspiration ($FIF_{25\%-75\%}$) relative to the forced mid-expiratory flow rate ($FEF_{25\%-75\%}$) is used as a measure of respiratory muscle dysfunction because inspiratory flow depends more on effort than does expiration.

Efficiency and the Work of Breathing

The *minute volume,* or total ventilation, is the amount of air that is exchanged in 1 minute. It is determined by the metabolic needs of the body. The minute volume is equal to the TV multiplied by the respiratory rate, which is normally about 6000 mL (500 mL TV × respiratory rate of 12 breaths per minute) in the average-sized adult during normal activity. The efficiency of breathing is determined by matching the TV and respiratory

TABLE 27-1 **Lung Volumes and Capacities**		
VOLUME	**SYMBOL**	**MEASUREMENT**
Tidal volume (about 500 mL at rest)	TV	Amount of air that moves into and out of the lungs with each breath
Inspiratory reserve volume (about 3000 mL)	IRV	Maximum amount of air that can be inhaled from the point of maximal expiration
Expiratory reserve volume (about 1100 mL)	ERV	Maximum volume of air that can be exhaled from the resting end-expiratory level
Residual volume (about 1200 mL)	RV	Volume of air remaining in the lungs after maximal expiration. This volume cannot be measured with the spirometer; it is measured indirectly using methods such as the helium dilution method, the nitrogen washout technique, or body plethysmography.
Functional residual capacity (about 2300 mL)	FRC	Volume of air remaining in the lungs at end-expiration (sum of RV and ERV)
Inspiratory capacity (about 3500 mL)	IC	Sum of IRV and TV
Vital capacity (about 4600 mL)	VC	Maximal amount of air that can be forcibly exhaled from the point of maximal inspiration
Total lung capacity (about 5800 mL)	TLC	Total amount of air that the lungs can hold; it is the sum of all the volume components after maximal inspiration. This value is about 20% to 25% less in females than in males.

TABLE 27-2 Pulmonary Function Tests

TEST	SYMBOL	MEASUREMENT*
Maximal voluntary ventilation	MVV	Maximum amount of air that can be breathed in a given time
Forced vital capacity	FVC	Maximum amount of air that can be rapidly and forcefully exhaled from the lungs after full inspiration. The expired volume is plotted against time.
Forced expiratory volume achieved in 1 second	$FEV_{1.0}$	Volume of air expired in the first second of FVC
Percentage of forced vital capacity	$FEV_{1.0}/FVC\%$	Volume of air expired in the first second, expressed as a percentage of FVC
Forced midexpiratory flow rate	$FEF_{25\%-75\%}$	The forced midexpiratory flow rate determined by locating the points on the volume-time curve recording obtained during FVC corresponding to 25% and 75% of FVC and drawing a straight line through these points. The slope of this line represents the average midexpiratory flow rate.
Forced inspiratory flow rate	$FIF_{25\%-75\%}$	FIF is the volume inspired from RV at the point of measurement. $FIF_{25\%-75\%}$ is the slope of a line between the points on the volume pressure tracing corresponding to 25% and 75% of the inspired volume.

*By convention, all the lung volumes and rates of flow are expressed in terms of body temperature and pressure and saturated with water vapor (BTPS), which allows for a comparison of the pulmonary function data from laboratories with different ambient temperatures and altitudes.

rate in a manner that provides an optimal minute volume while minimizing the work of breathing.

The work of breathing is determined by the amount of effort required to move air through the conducting airways and by the ease of lung expansion, or compliance. Expansion of the lungs is difficult for persons with stiff and noncompliant lungs; they usually find it easier to breathe if they keep their TV low and breathe at a more rapid rate (*e.g.*, $300 \times 20 = 6000$ mL) to achieve their minute volume and meet their oxygen needs. In contrast, persons with obstructive airway disease usually find it less difficult to inflate their lungs but expend more energy in moving air through the airways. As a result, these persons take deeper breaths and breathe at a slower rate (*e.g.*, $600 \times 10 = 6000$ mL) to achieve their oxygen needs.

IN SUMMARY, the movement of air between the atmosphere and the lungs follows the laws of physics as they relate to gases. The air in the alveoli contains a mixture of gases, including nitrogen, oxygen, carbon dioxide, and water vapor. With the exception of water vapor, each gas exerts a pressure that is determined by the atmospheric pressure and the concentration of the gas in the mixture. Water vapor pressure is affected by temperature but not atmospheric pressure. Air moves into the lungs along a pressure gradient. The pressure inside the airways and alveoli of the lungs is called *intrapulmonary* (or *alveolar*) *pressure;* the pressure in the pleural cavity is called *pleural pressure;* and the pressure in the thoracic cavity is called *intrathoracic pressure.*

Breathing is the movement of gases between the atmosphere and the lungs. It requires a system of open airways and pressure changes resulting from the action of the respiratory mus-

cles in changing the volume of the chest cage. The diaphragm is the principal muscle of inspiration, assisted by the external intercostal muscles. The scalene and sternocleidomastoid muscles elevate the ribs and act as accessory muscles for inspiration. Expiration is largely passive, aided by the elastic recoil of the respiratory muscles that were stretched during inspiration. When needed, the abdominal and internal intercostal muscles can be used to increase expiratory effort.

Lung compliance describes the ease with which the lungs can be inflated. It is determined by the elastic and collagen fibers of the lung, the water content, the surface tension of the alveoli, and the compliance of the chest cage. It also reflects the surface tension at the air–epithelium interface of the alveoli. Surfactant molecules, produced by type II alveolar cells, reduce the surface tension in the lungs and thereby increase lung compliance.

The volume of air that moves into and out of the air exchange portion of the lungs is directly related to the pressure difference between the lungs and the atmosphere and inversely related to the resistance that the air encounters as it moves through the airways. Depending on the velocity and pattern of flow, airflow can be laminar or turbulent. Airway resistance refers to the impediment to flow that the air encounters as it moves through the airways. It differs with airway size, being greatest in the medium-sized bronchi and lowest in the smaller bronchioles.

Lung volumes and lung capacities reflect the amount of air that is exchanged during normal and forced breathing. The tidal volume (TV) is the amount of air that moves into and out of the lungs during normal breathing; the inspiratory reserve volume (IRV) is the maximum amount of air that can be inspired in excess of the normal TV; and the expiratory reserve volume (ERV) is the maximum amount that can be exhaled in excess of the normal TV. The residual volume (RV) is the amount of air that remains in the lungs after forced expiration. Lung capacities include two or more lung volumes. The vital capacity equals the IRV plus the TV plus the ERV and is the amount of air that can be exhaled from the point of maximal inspiration. The minute volume, which is determined by the metabolic needs of the body, is the amount of air that is exchanged in 1 minute (*i.e.,* respiratory rate and TV). ■

CONCEPTSin action **ANIMATION**

EXCHANGE AND TRANSPORT OF GASES

After completing this section of the chapter, you should be able to meet the following objectives:

- Trace the exchange of gases between the air in the alveoli and the blood in the pulmonary capillaries.
- Differentiate between pulmonary and alveolar ventilation.
- Explain why ventilation and perfusion must be matched.
- Cite the difference between dead air space and shunt.
- List four factors that affect the diffusion of gases in the alveoli.
- Explain the difference between PO$_2$ and hemoglobin-bound oxygen and O$_2$ saturation, and oxygen content.
- Explain the significance of a shift to the right and a shift to the left in the oxygen–hemoglobin dissociation curve.

The primary functions of the lungs are oxygenation of the blood and removal of carbon dioxide. Pulmonary gas exchange is conventionally divided into three processes: ventilation, or the flow of gases into and out of the alveoli of the lungs; perfusion, or flow of blood in the adjacent pulmonary capillaries; and diffusion, or transfer of gases between the alveoli and the pulmonary capillaries. The efficiency of gas exchange requires that alveolar ventilation occur adjacent to perfused pulmonary capillaries.

Ventilation

Ventilation refers to the exchange of gases in the respiratory system. There are two types of ventilation: pulmonary and alveolar. *Pulmonary ventilation* refers to the total exchange of gases between the atmosphere and the lungs. *Alveolar ventilation* is the exchange of gases within the gas exchange portion of the lungs. Ventilation requires a system of open airways and a pressure difference that moves air into and out of the lungs. It is affected by body position and lung volume as well as by disease conditions that affect the heart and respiratory system.

Distribution of Ventilation

The distribution of ventilation between the apex and base of the lung varies with body position and the effects of gravity on intrapleural pressure (Fig. 27-18). In the seated or standing position, gravity exerts a downward pull on the lung, causing intrapleural pressure at the apex of the lung to become more negative than that at the base of the lung. As a result, the alveoli at the apex of the lung are more fully expanded than those at the base of the lung. The same holds true for dependent portions of the lung in the supine or lateral position. In the supine position, ventilation in the lowermost (posterior) parts of the lung exceeds that in the uppermost (anterior) parts. In the lateral position (*i.e.,* lying on the side), the dependent lung is better ventilated.

The distribution of ventilation also is affected by lung volumes. Compliance reflects the change in volume that occurs with a change in pressure. It is less in fully expanded alveoli, which have difficulty accommodating more air, and greater in alveoli that are less inflated. During full inspiration in the seated or standing position, the airways are pulled open and air moves into the more compliant portions of the lower lung. At low lung volumes, the opposite occurs. In this case, the pleural pressure at the base of the lung exceeds airway pressure compressing the airways so that ventilation is greatly reduced, while the airways in the upper part of the lung

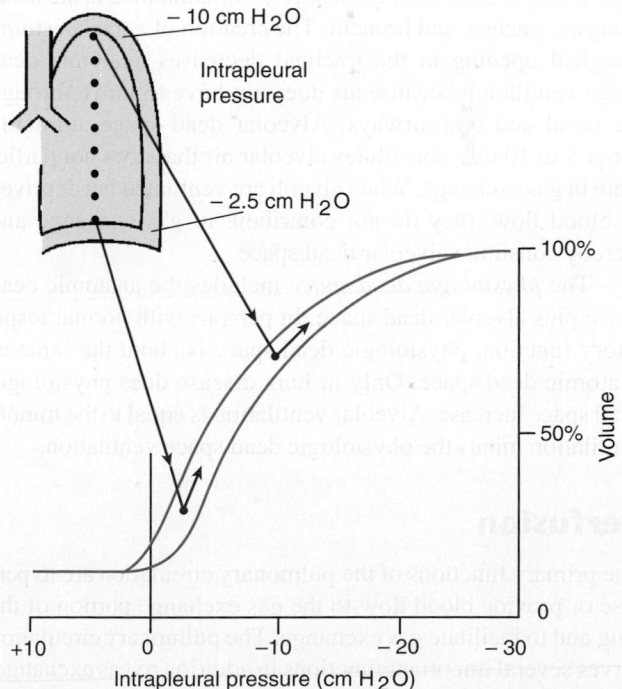

FIGURE 27-18 • Explanation of the regional differences in ventilation down the lung; the intrapleural pressure is less negative at the base than at the apex. As a consequence, the basal lung is relatively compressed in its resting state but expands more on inspiration than the apex. (From West J. B. [2001]. *Pulmonary physiology and pathophysiology* [p. 99]. Philadelphia: Lippincott Williams & Wilkins.)

remain open so that the top of the lung is better ventilated than the bottom.

Even at low lung volumes, some air remains in the alveoli of the lower portion of the lungs, preventing their collapse. According to the law of Laplace (discussed previously), the pressure needed to overcome the tension in the wall of a sphere or an elastic tube is inversely related to its radius; therefore, the small airways close first, trapping some gas in the alveoli. There may be increased trapping of air in the alveoli of the lower part of the lungs in older persons and in those with lung disease (*e.g.,* emphysema). This condition is thought to result from a loss in the elastic recoil properties of the lungs, so that the intrapleural pressure, created by the elastic recoil of the lung and chest wall, becomes less negative. In these persons, airway closure occurs at the end of normal instead of low lung volumes, trapping larger amounts of air with a resultant increase in the residual lung volume.

Dead Air Space

Dead space refers to the air that must be moved with each breath but does not participate in gas exchange. The movement of air through dead space contributes to the work of breathing but not to gas exchange. There are two types of dead space: that contained in the conducting airways, called the *anatomic dead space,* and that contained in the respiratory portion of the lung, called the *alveolar dead space.* The volume of anatomic airway dead space is fixed at approximately 150 to 200 mL, depending on body size. It constitutes air contained in the nose, pharynx, trachea, and bronchi. The creation of a tracheostomy (surgical opening in the trachea) decreases anatomic dead space ventilation because air does not have to move through the nasal and oral airways. Alveolar dead space, normally about 5 to 10 mL, constitutes alveolar air that does not participate in gas exchange. When alveoli are ventilated but deprived of blood flow, they do not contribute to gas exchange and thereby constitute alveolar dead space.

The *physiologic dead space* includes the anatomic dead space plus alveolar dead space. In persons with normal respiratory function, physiologic dead space is about the same as anatomic dead space. Only in lung disease does physiologic dead space increase. Alveolar ventilation is equal to the minute ventilation minus the physiologic dead space ventilation.

Perfusion

The primary functions of the pulmonary circulation are to perfuse or provide blood flow to the gas exchange portion of the lung and to facilitate gas exchange. The pulmonary circulation serves several important functions in addition to gas exchange. It filters all the blood that moves from the right to the left side of the circulation; it removes most of the thromboemboli that might form; and it serves as a reservoir of blood for the left side of the heart.

The gas exchange function of the lungs requires a continuous flow of blood through the respiratory portion of the lungs. Deoxygenated blood enters the lung through the pulmonary artery, which has its origin in the right side of the heart and enters the lung at the hilus, along with the primary bronchus. The pulmonary arteries branch in a manner similar to that of the airways. The small pulmonary arteries accompany the bronchi as they move down the lobules and branch to supply the capillary network that surrounds the alveoli (see Fig. 27-8). The oxygenated capillary blood is collected in the small pulmonary veins of the lobules, and then it moves to the larger veins to be collected in the four large pulmonary veins that empty into the left atrium.

The pulmonary blood vessels are thinner, more compliant, and offer less resistance to flow than those in the systemic circulation, and the pressures in the pulmonary system are much lower (*e.g.,* 22/8 mm Hg versus 120/70 mm Hg). The low pressure and low resistance of the pulmonary circulation accommodate the delivery of varying amounts of blood from the systemic circulation without producing signs and symptoms of congestion. The volume in the pulmonary circulation is approximately 500 mL, with approximately 100 mL of this volume located in the pulmonary capillary bed. When the input of blood from the right heart and output of blood to the left heart are equal, pulmonary blood flow remains constant. Small differences between input and output can result in large changes in pulmonary volume if the differences continue for many heart beats. The movement of blood through the pulmonary capillary bed requires that the mean pulmonary arterial pressure be greater than the mean pulmonary venous pressure. Pulmonary venous pressure increases in left-sided heart failure, allowing blood to accumulate in the pulmonary capillary bed and cause pulmonary edema (see Chapter 26).

Distribution of Blood Flow

As with ventilation, the distribution of pulmonary blood flow is affected by body position and gravity. In the upright position, the distance of the upper apices of the lung above the level of the heart may exceed the perfusion capabilities of the mean pulmonary arterial pressure (approximately 12 mm Hg); therefore, blood flow in the upper part of the lungs is less than that in the base or bottom part of the lungs (Fig. 27-19). In the supine position, the lungs and the heart are at the same level, and blood flow to the apices and base of the lungs becomes more uniform. In this position, blood flow to the posterior or dependent portions (*e.g.,* bottom of the lung when lying on the side) exceeds flow in the anterior or nondependent portions of the lungs.

Hypoxia-Induced Vasoconstriction

The blood vessels in the pulmonary circulation are highly sensitive to alveolar oxygen levels and undergo marked vasoconstriction when exposed to hypoxia. The precise mechanism for this response is unclear. When alveolar oxygen levels drop below 60 mm Hg, marked vasoconstriction may occur, and at very low oxygen levels, the local flow may be almost abolished. In regional hypoxia, as occurs with atelectasis, vasoconstriction is localized to a specific region of the lung. In this case, vasoconstriction has the effect of directing blood flow

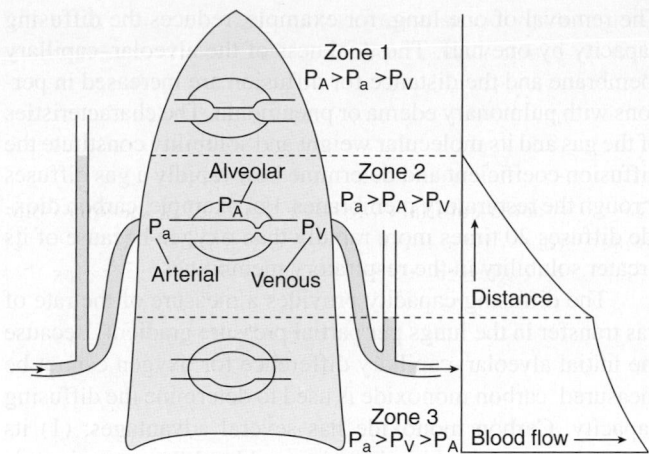

FIGURE 27-19 • The uneven distribution of blood flow in the lung results from different pressures affecting the capillaries, which are affected by body position and gravity. (From West J. B. [2000]. *Respiratory physiology: The essentials* [p. 41]. Philadelphia: Lippincott Williams & Wilkins.)

away from the hypoxic regions of the lungs. When alveolar hypoxia no longer exists, blood flow is restored.

Generalized hypoxia, such as occurs at high altitudes and in persons with chronic hypoxia due to lung disease, causes vasoconstriction throughout the lung. Prolonged hypoxia can lead to pulmonary hypertension and increased workload on the right heart (discussed in Chapter 29). A low blood pH produces a similar effect, particularly when alveolar hypoxia is present (*e.g.,* during circulatory shock).

Shunt

Shunt refers to blood that moves from the right to the left side of the circulation without being oxygenated. As with dead air space, there are two types of shunts: physiologic and anatomic. In an *anatomic shunt,* blood moves from the venous to the arterial side of the circulation without moving through the lungs. Anatomic intracardiac shunting of blood due to congenital heart defects is discussed in Chapter 24. In a *physiologic shunt,* there is mismatching of ventilation and perfusion within the lung, resulting in insufficient ventilation to provide the oxygen needed to oxygenate the blood flowing through the alveolar capillaries. Physiologic shunting of blood usually results from destructive lung disease that impairs ventilation or from heart failure that interferes with movement of blood through sections of the lungs.

Mismatching of Ventilation and Perfusion

The gas exchange properties of the lung depend on matching ventilation and perfusion, ensuring that equal amounts of air and blood are entering the respiratory portion of the lungs. Both dead air space and shunt produce a mismatching of ventilation and perfusion, as depicted in Figure 27-20. With shunt (depicted on the left), there is perfusion without ventilation,

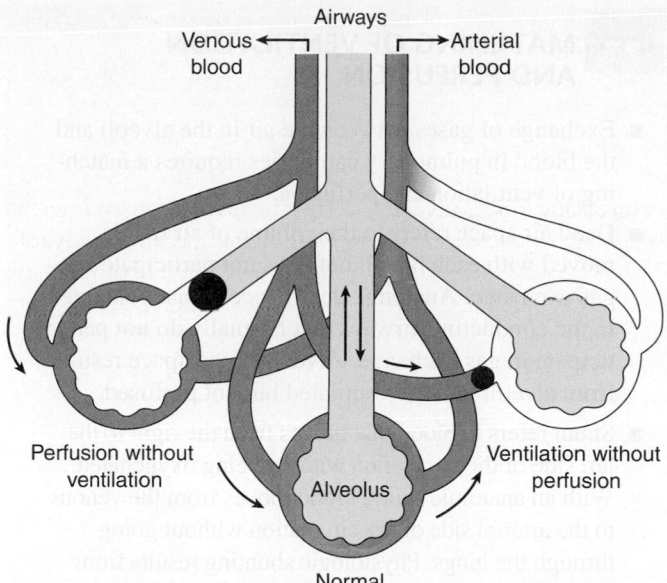

FIGURE 27-20 • Matching of ventilation and perfusion. (*Center*) Normal matching of ventilation and perfusion; (*left*) perfusion without ventilation (*i.e.,* shunt); (*right*) ventilation without perfusion (*i.e.,* dead air space).

resulting in a low ventilation–perfusion ratio. It occurs in conditions such as atelectasis in which there is airway obstruction (see Chapter 29). With dead air space (depicted on the right), there is ventilation without perfusion, resulting in a high ventilation–perfusion ratio. It occurs in conditions such as pulmonary embolism, which impairs blood flow to a part of the lung. The arterial blood leaving the pulmonary circulation reflects mixing of blood from normally ventilated and perfused areas of the lung as well as areas that are not ventilated (dead air space) or perfused (shunt). Many of the conditions that cause mismatching of ventilation and perfusion involve both dead air space and shunt. In chronic obstructive lung disease, for example, there may be impaired ventilation in one area of the lung and impaired perfusion in another area.

Diffusion

Diffusion occurs in the respiratory portions of the lung and refers to the movement of gases across the alveolar–capillary membrane. Gas diffusion in the lung can be described by the *Fick law of diffusion.* The Fick law states that the volume of a gas ($\dot{V}gas$) diffusing across the membrane per unit time is directly proportional to the partial pressure difference of the gas ($P_1 - P_2$), the surface area (SA) of the membrane, and the diffusion coefficient (D), and is inversely proportional to the thickness (T) of the membrane (Fig. 27-21).

Several factors influence the diffusion of gases in the lung. The administration of high concentrations of oxygen increases the difference in partial pressure between the two sides of the membrane and increases the diffusion of the gas. Diseases that destroy lung tissue (*i.e.,* surface area for diffusion) or increase the thickness of the alveolar–capillary membrane adversely influence the diffusing capacity of the lungs.

MATCHING OF VENTILATION AND PERFUSION

- Exchange of gases between the air in the alveoli and the blood in pulmonary capillaries requires a matching of ventilation and perfusion.

- Dead air space refers to the volume of air that is moved with each breath but does not participate in gas exchange. Anatomic dead space is that contained in the conducting airways that normally do not participate in gas exchange. Alveolar dead space results from alveoli that are ventilated but not perfused.

- Shunt refers to blood that moves from the right to the left side of the circulation without being oxygenated. With an anatomic shunt, blood moves from the venous to the arterial side of the circulation without going through the lungs. Physiologic shunting results from blood moving through unventilated parts of the lung.

- The blood oxygen level reflects the mixing of blood from alveolar dead space and physiologic shunting areas as it moves into the pulmonary veins.

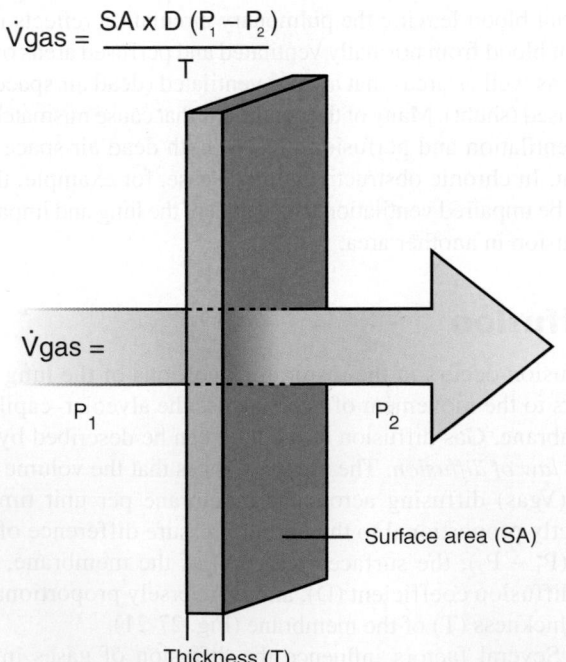

$$\dot{V}gas = \frac{SA \times D\,(P_1 - P_2)}{T}$$

FIGURE 27-21 • The Fick law of diffusion states that the diffusion of a gas ($\dot{V}gas$) across a sheet of tissue is related to the surface area (SA) of the tissue, the diffusion constant (D) for the gas, and the partial pressure difference ($P_1 - P_2$) on either side of the tissue, and is inversely proportional to the thickness (T) of the tissue.

The removal of one lung, for example, reduces the diffusing capacity by one half. The thickness of the alveolar–capillary membrane and the distance for diffusion are increased in persons with pulmonary edema or pneumonia. The characteristics of the gas and its molecular weight and solubility constitute the diffusion coefficient and determine how rapidly a gas diffuses through the respiratory membranes. For example, carbon dioxide diffuses 20 times more rapidly than oxygen because of its greater solubility in the respiratory membranes.

The diffusing capacity provides a measure of the rate of gas transfer in the lungs per partial pressure gradient. Because the initial alveolar–capillary difference for oxygen cannot be measured, carbon monoxide is used to determine the diffusing capacity. Carbon monoxide has several advantages: (1) its uptake is not limited by diffusion or blood flow; (2) there is essentially no carbon monoxide in venous blood; and (3) its affinity for hemoglobin is 210 times that of oxygen, ensuring that its partial pressure will remain essentially zero in the pulmonary capillary. The most common technique for making this measurement is the *single-breath test*. This test involves the inhalation of a single breath of dilute carbon monoxide (CO), followed by a breath-hold of 10 seconds. The diffusing capacity can be calculated using the lung volume and the percentage of CO in the alveoli at the beginning and end of the 10-second breath-hold.

Oxygen and Carbon Dioxide Transport

Although the lungs are responsible for the exchange of gases with the external environment, it is the blood that transports these gases between the lungs and body tissues. The blood carries oxygen and carbon dioxide in the physically dissolved state and in combination with hemoglobin. Carbon dioxide also is converted to bicarbonate and transported in that form.

Dissolved oxygen and carbon dioxide exert a partial pressure that is designated in the same manner as the partial pressures in the gas state. In the clinical setting, blood gas measurements are used to determine the partial pressure of oxygen (PO_2) and carbon dioxide (PCO_2) in the blood. Arterial blood commonly is used for measuring blood gases. Venous blood is not used because venous levels of oxygen and carbon dioxide reflect the metabolic demands of the tissues rather than the gas exchange function of the lungs. The PO_2 of arterial blood normally is above 80 mm Hg, and the PCO_2 is in the range of 35 to 45 mm Hg. Normally, the arterial blood gases are the same or nearly the same as the partial pressure of the gases in the alveoli. The arterial PO_2 often is written PaO_2, and the alveolar PO_2 as PAO_2, with the same types of designations being used for PCO_2. This text uses PO_2 and PCO_2 to designate both arterial and alveolar levels of the gases.

Oxygen Transport

Oxygen is transported in two forms: (1) in chemical combination with hemoglobin, and (2) in the dissolved state. Hemoglobin carries about 98% to 99% of oxygen in the blood and is the main transporter of oxygen. The remaining 1% to 2% of the oxygen is carried in the dissolved state. Only the dissolved form of oxygen passes through the capillary wall, diffuses through the cell membrane, and makes itself available for use in cell metabolism. The oxygen content (measured in mL/100 mL) of the blood includes the oxygen carried by hemoglobin and in the dissolved state.

Hemoglobin Transport. Hemoglobin is a highly efficient carrier of oxygen. Hemoglobin with bound oxygen is called *oxyhemoglobin,* and when oxygen is removed, it is called *deoxygenated* or *reduced hemoglobin.* Each gram of hemoglobin carries approximately 1.34 mL of oxygen when it is fully saturated. This means that a person with a hemoglobin level of 14 g/100 mL carries 18.8 mL of oxygen per 100 mL of blood.

In the lungs, oxygen moves across the alveolar–capillary membrane, through the plasma, and into the red blood cell, where it forms a loose and reversible bond with the hemoglobin molecule. In normal lungs, this process is rapid, so that even with a fast heart rate the hemoglobin is almost completely saturated with oxygen during the short time it spends in the pulmonary capillaries. As the oxygen moves out of the capillaries in response to the needs of the tissues, the hemoglobin saturation, which usually is approximately 95% to 97% as the blood leaves the left side of the heart, drops to approximately 75% as the mixed venous blood returns to the right side of the heart.

Dissolved Oxygen. The partial pressure of oxygen represents the level of dissolved oxygen in plasma. The amount of dissolved oxygen depends on its partial pressure and its solubility in the plasma. In the normal lung at 760 mm Hg atmospheric pressure, the PO_2 of arterial blood is approximately 100 mm Hg. The solubility of oxygen in plasma is fixed and very small. For every 1 mm Hg of PO_2 present, 0.003 mL of oxygen becomes dissolved in 100 mL of plasma. This means that at a normal arterial PO_2 of 100 mm Hg, the blood carries only 0.3 mL of dissolved oxygen in each 100 mL of plasma. This amount (approximately 1%) is very small compared with the amount that can be carried in an equal amount of blood when oxygen is attached to hemoglobin.

Although the amount of oxygen carried in plasma under normal conditions is small, it can become a lifesaving mode of transport in cases of carbon monoxide poisoning, when most of the hemoglobin sites are occupied by carbon monoxide and are unavailable for transport of oxygen. The use of a hyperbaric chamber, in which 100% oxygen can be administered at high atmospheric pressures, increases the amount of oxygen that can be carried in the dissolved state.

Binding Affinity of Hemoglobin for Oxygen. The efficiency of the hemoglobin transport system depends on the ability of the hemoglobin molecule to bind oxygen in the lungs and release it as it is needed in the tissues. Oxygen that remains bound to hemoglobin cannot participate in tissue metabolism. The term *affinity* refers to hemoglobin's ability to bind oxygen. Hemoglobin binds oxygen more readily when its affinity is increased and releases it more readily when its affinity is decreased.

As described in Chapter 14, the hemoglobin molecule is composed of four polypeptide chains with an iron-containing heme group. Because oxygen binds to the iron atom, each hemoglobin molecule can bind four molecules of oxygen when it is fully saturated. Oxygen binds cooperatively with the heme groups on the hemoglobin molecule. After the first molecule of oxygen binds to hemoglobin, the molecule undergoes a change in shape. As a result, the second and third molecules bind more readily, and binding of the fourth molecule is even easier. In a like manner, the unloading of the first molecule of oxygen enhances the unloading of the next molecule and so on. Thus, the affinity of hemoglobin for oxygen changes with hemoglobin saturation.

Hemoglobin's affinity for oxygen is also influenced by pH, carbon dioxide concentration, and body temperature. It binds oxygen more readily under conditions of increased pH (alkalosis), decreased carbon dioxide concentration, and decreased body temperature and it releases it more readily under conditions of decreased pH (acidosis), increased carbon dioxide concentration, and fever. For example, increased tissue metabolism generates carbon dioxide and metabolic acids and thereby decreases the affinity of hemoglobin for oxygen. Heat also is a byproduct of tissue metabolism, explaining the effect of fever on oxygen binding.

Red blood cells contain a metabolic intermediate called *2,3-diphosphoglycerate (2,3-DPG)* that also affects the affinity of hemoglobin for oxygen. An increase in 2,3-DPG enhances unloading of oxygen from hemoglobin at the tissue level. Conditions that increase 2,3-DPG include exercise, hypoxia that occurs at high altitude, and chronic lung disease.

The Oxygen Dissociation Curve. The relation between the oxygen carried in combination with hemoglobin and the PO_2 of the blood is described by the *oxygen–hemoglobin dissociation curve,* which is shown in Figure 27-22. The x axis of the graph depicts the PO_2 or dissolved oxygen. It reflects the partial pressure of the oxygen in the lungs (*i.e.,* the PO_2 is approximately 100 mm Hg when room air is being breathed, but can rise to 200 mm Hg or higher when oxygen-enriched air is breathed). The left y axis depicts hemoglobin saturation or the amount of oxygen that is carried by the hemoglobin. The right y axis depicts oxygen content or total amount of the oxygen content being carried in the blood.

The S-shaped oxygen dissociation curve has a flat top portion representing binding of oxygen to hemoglobin in the lungs and a steep portion representing its release into the tissue capillaries (see Fig. 27-22A). The S shape of the curve reflects the effect that oxygen saturation has on the conformation of the hemoglobin molecule and its affinity for oxygen. At approximately 100 mm Hg PO_2, a plateau occurs, at which point the hemoglobin is approximately 98% saturated. Increasing the alveolar PO_2 above this level does not increase the hemoglobin saturation. Even at high altitudes, when the partial pressure of oxygen is considerably decreased, the hemoglobin remains

Understanding • Oxygen Transport

All body tissues rely on oxygen (O_2) that is transported in the blood to meet their metabolic needs. Oxygen is carried in two forms: dissolved and bound to hemoglobin. About 98% of O_2 is carried by hemoglobin and the remaining 2% is carried in the dissolved state. Dissolved oxygen is the only form that diffuses across cell membranes and produces a partial pressure (PO_2), which, in turn, drives diffusion. The transport of O_2 involves (1) transfer from the alveoli to the pulmonary capillaries in the lung; (2) hemoglobin binding and transport; and (3) the dissociation from hemoglobin in the tissue capillaries.

❶ Alveoli-to-Capillary Transfer

In the lung, O_2 moves from the alveoli to the pulmonary capillaries as a dissolved gas. Its movement occurs along a concentration gradient, moving from the alveoli, where the partial pressure of PO_2 is about 100 mm Hg, to the venous end of the pulmonary capillaries with their lesser O_2 concentration and lower PO_2. The dissolved O_2 moves rapidly between the alveoli and the pulmonary capillaries, such that the PO_2 at the arterial end of the capillary is almost if not the same as that in the alveoli.

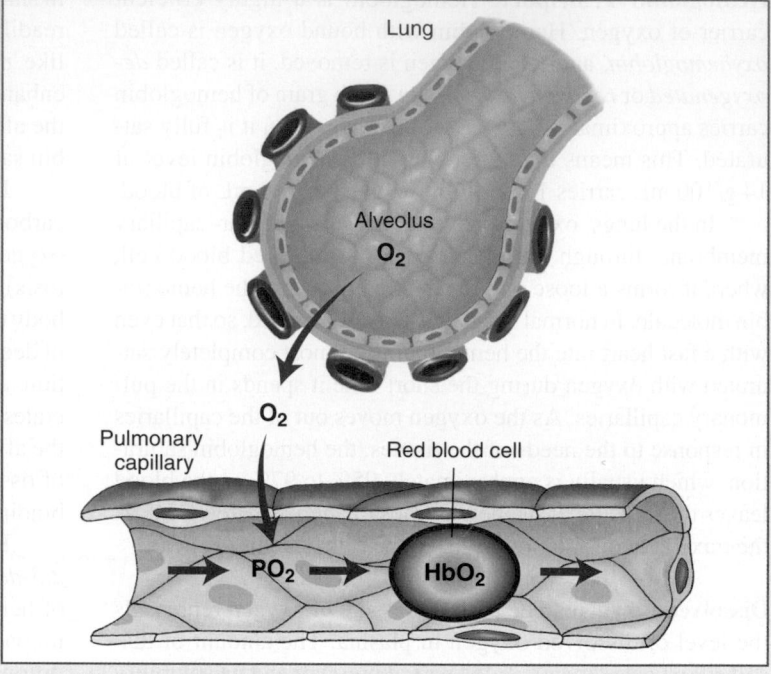

relatively well saturated. At 60 mm Hg PO_2, for example, the hemoglobin is still approximately 89% saturated.

The steep portion of the dissociation curve—between 60 and 40 mm Hg—represents the removal of oxygen from the hemoglobin as it moves through the tissue capillaries. This portion of the curve reflects the fact that there is considerable transfer of oxygen from hemoglobin to the tissues with only a small drop in PO_2, thereby ensuring a gradient for oxygen to move into body cells. The tissues normally remove approximately 5 mL of oxygen per 100 mL of blood, and the hemoglobin of mixed venous blood is approximately 75% saturated as it returns to the right side of the heart. In this portion of the dissociation curve (saturation <75%), the rate at which oxygen is released from hemoglobin is determined largely by tissue uptake. During strenuous exercise, for example, the muscle

cells may remove as much as 15 mL of oxygen per 100 mL of blood from hemoglobin.

Hemoglobin can be regarded as a buffer system that regulates the delivery of oxygen to the tissues. In order to function as a buffer system, the affinity of hemoglobin for oxygen must change with the metabolic needs of the tissues. This change is represented by a shift to the right or left in the dissociation curve (see Fig. 27-22B). A shift to the right indicates that the tissue PO_2 is greater for any given level of hemoglobin saturation and represents reduced affinity of the hemoglobin for oxygen at any given PO_2. It usually is caused by conditions that reflect increased tissue metabolism, such as fever or acidosis, or by an increase in PCO_2. High altitude and conditions such as pulmonary insufficiency, heart failure, and severe anemia also cause the oxygen dissociation curve to shift to the right. A shift to the left in the

② Hemoglobin Binding and Transport

Oxygen, which is relatively insoluble in plasma, relies on hemoglobin for transport in the blood. Once oxygen has diffused into the pulmonary capillary, it moves rapidly into the red blood cells and reversibly binds to hemoglobin to form HbO_2. The hemoglobin molecule contains four heme units, each capable of attaching an oxygen molecule. Hemoglobin is 100% saturated when all four units are occupied and is usually about 97% saturated in the systemic arterial blood. The capacity of the blood to carry O_2 is dependent both on hemoglobin levels and the ability of the lungs to oxygenate the hemoglobin.

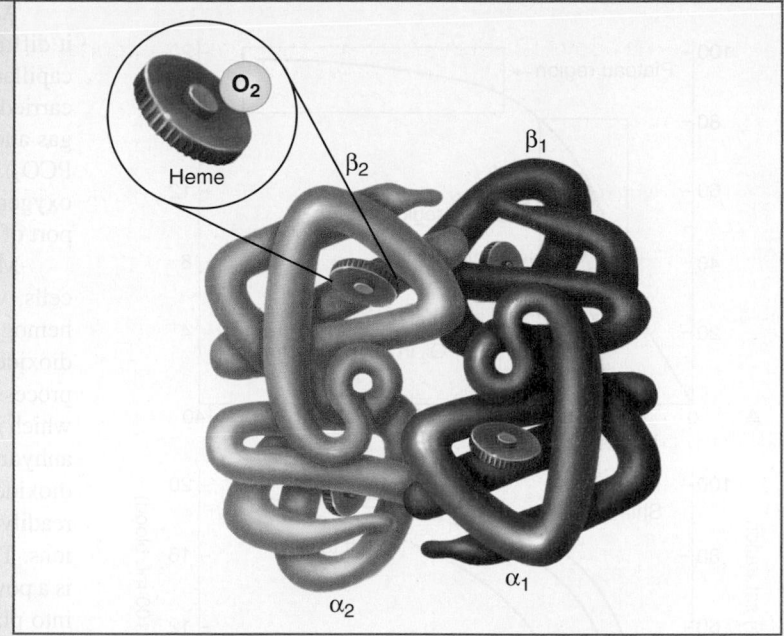

③ Oxygen Dissociation in the Tissues

The dissociation or release of O_2 from hemoglobin occurs in the tissue capillaries where the PO_2 is less than that of the arterial blood. As oxygen dissociates from hemoglobin, it dissolves in the plasma and then moves into the tissues where the PO_2 is less than that in the capillaries. The affinity of hemoglobin for O_2 is influenced by the carbon dioxide (PCO_2) content of the blood and its pH temperature, and 2,3-diphosphoglycerate (2,3-DPG), a byproduct of glycolysis in red blood cells. Under conditions of high metabolic demand, in which the PCO_2 is increased and the pH is decreased, the binding affinity of hemoglobin is decreased, and during decreased metabolic demand, when the PCO_2 is decreased and the pH is increased, the affinity is increased.

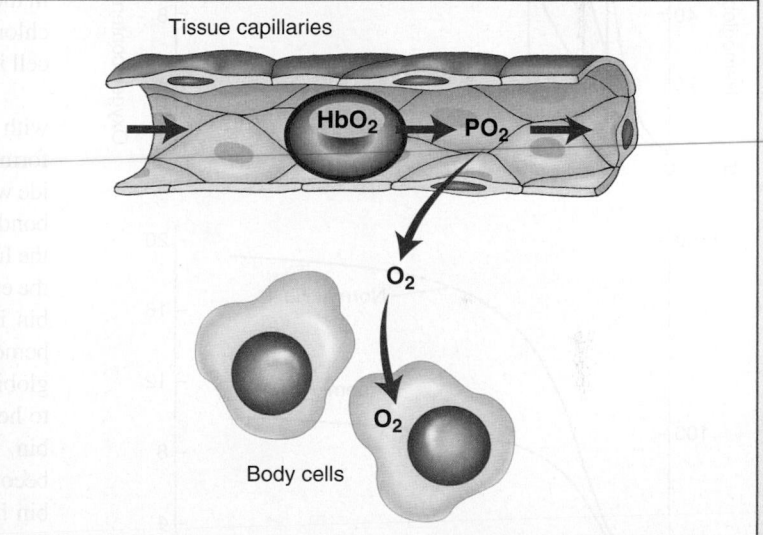

oxygen dissociation curve represents an increased affinity of hemoglobin for oxygen and occurs in situations associated with a decrease in tissue metabolism, such as alkalosis, decreased body temperature, and decreased PCO_2 levels. The degree of shift can be determined by the P_{50}, or the partial pressure of oxygen that is needed to achieve a 50% saturation of hemoglobin. Returning to Figure 27-23B, the dissociation curve on the left has a P_{50} of approximately 20 mm Hg; the normal curve, a P_{50} of 26; and the curve on the right, a P_{50} of 39 mm Hg.

The oxygen content (measured in mL/dL blood) represents the total amount of oxygen carried in the blood, including the dissolved oxygen and that carried by the hemoglobin (see Fig. 27-22C). The amount of hemoglobin-bound oxygen is determined by the concentration of hemoglobin (in g/dL), the oxygen-binding capacity of hemoglobin (1.34 mL O_2/g hemo-

globin), and the percentage saturation of the hemoglobin. The dissolved oxygen content is the product of the oxygen solubility (0.0003 mL O_2/dL) times the PO_2. Thus, an anemic person may have a normal PO_2 and hemoglobin saturation level but decreased oxygen content because of the lower amount of hemoglobin for binding oxygen.

Carbon Dioxide Transport

Carbon dioxide is transported in the blood in three forms (see Understanding Carbon Dioxide Transport, Chapter 32): as dissolved carbon dioxide (10%), attached to hemoglobin (30%), and as bicarbonate (60%). Acid-base balance is influenced by the amount of dissolved carbon dioxide and the bicarbonate level in the blood.

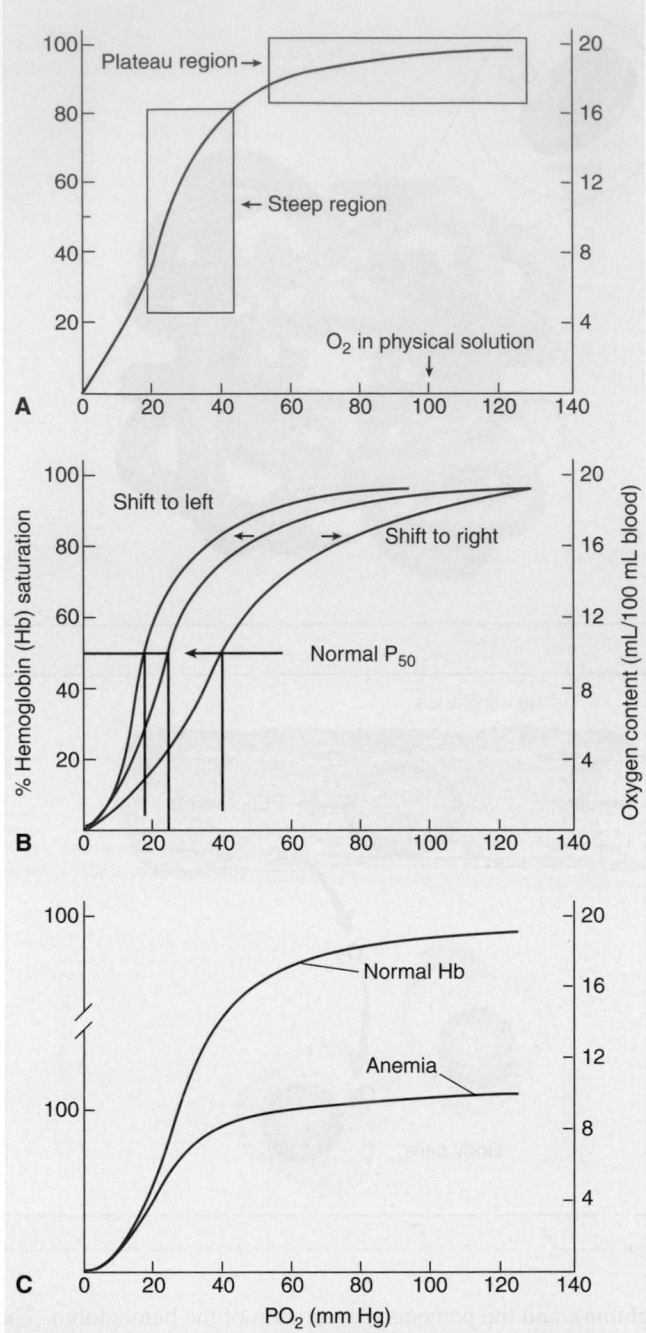

As carbon dioxide is formed during the metabolic process, it diffuses out of cells into the tissue spaces and then into the capillaries. The amount of dissolved carbon dioxide that can be carried in plasma is determined by the partial pressure of the gas and its solubility coefficient (0.03 mL/100 mL/1 mm Hg PCO_2). Carbon dioxide is 20 times more soluble in plasma than oxygen. Thus, the dissolved state plays a greater role in transport of carbon dioxide compared with oxygen.

Most of the carbon dioxide diffuses into the red blood cells, where it either forms carbonic acid or combines with hemoglobin. *Carbonic acid* (H_2CO_3) is formed when carbon dioxide combines with water ($CO_2 + H_2O = H^+ + HCO_3^-$). The process is catalyzed by an enzyme called *carbonic anhydrase*, which is present in large quantities in red blood cells. Carbonic anhydrase increases the rate of the reaction between carbon dioxide and water approximately 5000-fold. Carbonic acid readily ionizes to form bicarbonate (HCO_3^-) and hydrogen (H^+) ions. The hydrogen ion combines with the hemoglobin, which is a powerful acid-base buffer, and the bicarbonate ion diffuses into plasma in exchange for a chloride ion. This exchange is made possible by a special bicarbonate–chloride carrier protein in the red blood cell membrane. As a result of the bicarbonate–chloride shift, the chloride and water content of the red blood cell is greater in venous blood than in arterial blood.

In addition to the carbonic anhydrase–mediated reaction with water, carbon dioxide reacts directly with hemoglobin to form *carbaminohemoglobin*. The combination of carbon dioxide with hemoglobin is a reversible reaction that involves a loose bond, which allows transport of carbon dioxide from tissues to the lungs, where it is released into the alveoli for exchange with the external environment. The release of oxygen from hemoglobin in the tissues enhances the binding of carbon dioxide to hemoglobin; in the lungs, the combining of oxygen with hemoglobin displaces carbon dioxide. The binding of carbon dioxide to hemoglobin is determined by the acidic nature of hemoglobin. Binding with carbon dioxide causes the hemoglobin to become a stronger acid. In the lungs, the highly acidic hemoglobin has a lesser tendency to form carbaminohemoglobin, and carbon dioxide is released from hemoglobin into the alveoli. In the tissues, the release of oxygen from hemoglobin causes hemoglobin to become less acid, thereby increasing its ability to combine with carbon dioxide and form carbaminohemoglobin.

FIGURE 27-22 • Oxygen–hemoglobin dissociation curve. **(A)** Left boxed area represents the steep portion of the curve where oxygen is released from hemoglobin (Hb) to the tissues, and the top boxed area the plateau of the curve where oxygen is loaded onto hemoglobin in the lung. **(B)** The effect of body temperature, arterial PCO_2, and pH on hemoglobin affinity for oxygen as indicated by a shift in the curve and position of the P_{50}. A shift of the curve to the right due to an increase in temperature, PCO_2 or decreased pH favors release of oxygen to the tissues. A decrease in temperature, PCO_2 or increase in pH shifts the curve to the left and has the opposite effect. The P_{50} is the partial pressure of oxygen required to saturate 50% of hemoglobin with oxygen. **(C)** Effect of anemia on the oxygen-carrying capacity of blood. The hemoglobin can be completely saturated, but the oxygen content of the blood is reduced.

IN SUMMARY, the primary functions of the lungs are oxygenation of the blood and removal of carbon dioxide. Pulmonary gas exchange is conventionally divided into three processes: ventilation, or the flow of gases into the alveoli of the lungs; perfusion, or movement of blood through the adjacent pulmonary capillaries; and diffusion, or transfer of gases between the alveoli and the pulmonary capillaries.

Ventilation is the movement of air between the atmosphere and the lungs and perfusion is the flow of blood into and out of the gas exchange portions of the lung. Pulmonary ventilation refers to the total exchange of gases between the atmosphere and the lungs, and alveolar ventilation to ventilation in the gas exchange portion of the lungs. The distribution of alveolar ventilation and pulmonary capillary blood flow varies with lung volume and body position. In the upright position and at high lung volumes, ventilation is greatest in the lower parts of the lungs. The upright position also produces a decrease in blood flow to the upper parts of the lung, resulting from the distance above the level of the heart and the low mean arterial pressure in the pulmonary circulation. The efficiency of gas exchange requires matching of ventilation and perfusion, so that equal amounts of air and blood enter the respiratory portion of the lungs. Two conditions interfere with matching of ventilation and perfusion: dead air space, in which areas of the lungs are ventilated but not perfused, and shunt, in which areas of the lungs are perfused but not ventilated.

The diffusion of gases in the lungs is influenced by four factors: the surface area available for diffusion; the thickness of the alveolar–capillary membrane, through which the gases diffuse; the differences in the partial pressure of the gas on either side of the membrane; and the diffusion characteristics of the gas.

The blood transports oxygen to the cells and returns carbon dioxide to the lungs. Oxygen is transported in two forms: in chemical combination with hemoglobin and physically dissolved in plasma (PO_2). Hemoglobin is an efficient carrier of oxygen, and approximately 98% to 99% of oxygen is transported in this manner. The relationship between the oxygen carried in combination with hemoglobin and the PO_2 of the blood is described by the oxygen–hemoglobin dissociation curve. Carbon dioxide is carried in three forms: attached to hemoglobin (30%), dissolved carbon dioxide (10%), and bicarbonate (60%). ■

CONCEPTSin action**ANIMATI◌N**

CONTROL OF BREATHING

After completing this section of the chapter, you should be able to meet the following objectives:

- Compare the neural control of the respiratory muscles, which control breathing, with that of cardiac muscle, which controls the pumping action of the heart.
- Describe the function of the chemoreceptors and lung receptors in the regulation of ventilation.
- Trace the integration of the cough reflex from stimulus to explosive expulsion of air that constitutes the cough.
- Describe the type of periodic breathing known as Cheyne-Stokes breathing.
- Define dyspnea and list three types of conditions in which dyspnea occurs.

Unlike the heart, which has inherent rhythmic properties and can beat independently of the nervous system, the muscles that control respiration require continuous input from the nervous system. Movement of the diaphragm, intercostal muscles, sternocleidomastoid, and other accessory muscles that control ventilation is integrated by neurons located in the pons and medulla. These neurons are collectively referred to as the *respiratory center* (Fig. 27-23).

Respiratory Center

The respiratory center consists of two dense, bilateral aggregates of respiratory neurons involved in initiating inspiration and expiration and incorporating afferent impulses into motor responses of the respiratory muscles. The first, or dorsal, group of neurons in the respiratory center is concerned primarily with inspiration. These neurons control the activity of the phrenic nerves that innervate the diaphragm and drive the second, or ventral, group of respiratory neurons. They are thought to integrate sensory input from the lungs and airways into the ventilatory response. The second group of neurons, which contains inspiratory and expiratory neurons, controls the spinal motor neurons of the intercostal and abdominal muscles.

The pacemaker properties of the respiratory center result from the cycling of the two groups of respiratory neurons: the *pneumotaxic center* in the upper pons and the *apneustic center* in the lower pons (see Fig. 27-23). These two groups of neurons contribute to the function of the respiratory center in the medulla. The apneustic center has an excitatory effect on inspiration, tending to prolong inspiration. The pneumotaxic center switches inspiration off, assisting in the control of respiratory rate and inspiratory volume. Brain injuries that damage the connection between the pneumotaxic and apneustic centers result in an irregular breathing pattern that consists of prolonged inspiratory gasps interrupted by expiratory efforts.

Axons from the neurons in the respiratory center cross in the midline and descend in the ventrolateral columns of the spinal cord. The tracts that control expiration and inspiration are spatially separated in the cord, as are the tracts that transmit specialized reflexes (*i.e.*, coughing and hiccupping) and voluntary control of ventilation. Only at the level of the spinal cord are the respiratory impulses integrated to produce a reflex response.

Regulation of Breathing

The control of breathing has automatic and voluntary components. The automatic regulation of ventilation is controlled by input from two types of sensors or receptors: chemoreceptors and lung receptors. Chemoreceptors monitor blood levels of oxygen, carbon dioxide, and pH and adjust ventilation to meet the changing metabolic needs of the body. Lung receptors monitor breathing patterns and lung function.

Voluntary regulation of ventilation integrates breathing with voluntary acts such as speaking, blowing, and singing.

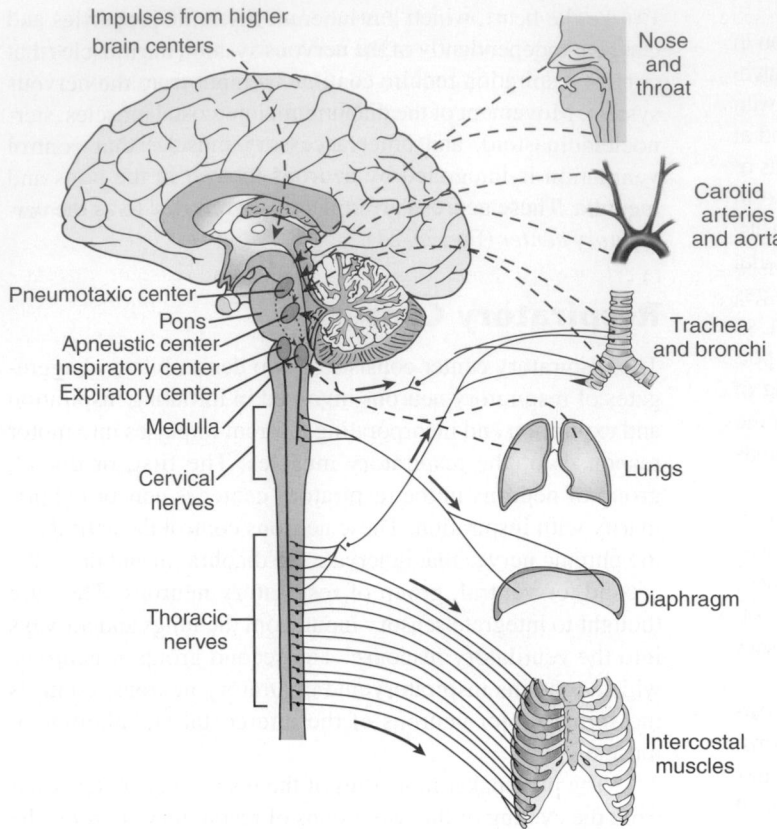

FIGURE 27-23 • Schematic representation of activity in the respiratory center. Impulses traveling over afferent neurons (*dashed lines*) communicate with central neurons, which activate efferent neurons that supply the muscles of respiration. Respiratory movements can be altered by a variety of stimuli.

These acts, which are initiated by the motor and premotor cortex, cause a temporary suspension of automatic breathing. The automatic and voluntary components of respiration are regulated by afferent impulses that are transmitted to the respiratory center from a number of sources. Afferent input from higher brain centers is evidenced by the fact that a person can consciously alter the depth and rate of respiration. Fever, pain, and emotion exert their influence through lower brain centers. Vagal afferents from sensory receptors in the lungs and airways are integrated in the dorsal area of the respiratory center.

Chemoreceptors

Tissue needs for oxygen and the removal of carbon dioxide are regulated by chemoreceptors that monitor blood levels of these gases. Input from these sensors is transmitted to the respiratory center, and ventilation is adjusted to maintain the arterial blood gases within a normal range.

There are two types of chemoreceptors: central and peripheral. The most important chemoreceptors for sensing changes in the PCO_2 of the blood are the *central chemoreceptors,* which are located in chemosensitive regions near the respiratory center in the medulla. The central chemoreceptors are surrounded by brain extracellular fluid and respond to changes in its hydrogen ion (H^+) concentration. The composi-

tion of the extracellular fluid surrounding the chemoreceptors is governed by the cerebral spinal fluid (CSF), local blood flow, and tissue metabolism. Of these, the CSF is apparently the most important. The CSF is separated from the blood by the blood-brain barrier, which permits free diffusion of carbon dioxide but not bicarbonate (HCO_3^-) or H^+. The carbon dioxide combines rapidly with water to form carbonic acid (H_2CO_3), which dissociates into H^+ and HCO_3^-. When the PCO_2 rises, carbon dioxide from the blood diffuses into the CSF, liberating H^+, which then stimulates the chemoreceptors. The central chemoreceptors are extremely sensitive to short-term changes in PCO_2. An increase in PCO_2 levels produces an increase in ventilation that reaches its peak within a minute or so and then declines if the PCO_2 level remains elevated. Thus, persons with chronically elevated levels of PCO_2 no longer have a response to this stimulus for increased ventilation but rely on the stimulus provided by a decrease in blood PO_2 levels.

The *peripheral chemoreceptors* are located in the carotid and aortic bodies, which are found at the bifurcation of the common carotid arteries and in the arch of the aorta, respectively (see Fig. 27-23). These chemoreceptors monitor arterial blood oxygen levels. Although the peripheral chemoreceptors also monitor carbon dioxide, they play a much more important role in monitoring oxygen levels. These receptors exert little control over ventilation until the PO_2 has dropped below 60 mm Hg. Thus, hypoxia is the main stimulus for ventilation in persons with chronically elevated levels of carbon dioxide. If these patients are given oxygen therapy at a level sufficient to increase the PO_2 above that needed to stimulate the peripheral chemoreceptors, their ventilation may be seriously depressed.

Lung Receptors

Lung and chest wall receptors monitor the status of breathing in terms of airway resistance and lung expansion. There are three types of lung receptors: stretch, irritant, and juxtacapillary receptors.

Stretch receptors are located in the smooth muscle layers of the conducting airways. They respond to changes in pressure in the walls of the airways. When the lungs are inflated, these receptors inhibit inspiration and promote expiration. They are important in establishing breathing patterns and minimizing the work of breathing by adjusting respiratory rate and TV to accommodate changes in lung compliance and airway resistance.

The *irritant receptors* are located between the airway epithelial cells. They are stimulated by noxious gases, cigarette smoke, inhaled dust, and cold air. Stimulation of the irritant receptors leads to airway constriction and a pattern of rapid, shallow breathing. This pattern of breathing probably protects respiratory tissues from the damaging effects of toxic inhalants. It also is thought that the mechanical stimulation of these receptors may ensure more uniform lung expansion by initiating periodic sighing and yawning. It is also possible that these receptors are involved in the bronchoconstriction response that occurs in some persons with bronchial asthma.

The *juxtacapillary* or *J receptors* are located in the alveolar wall, close to the pulmonary capillaries. It is thought that these receptors sense lung congestion. These receptors may be responsible for the rapid, shallow breathing that occurs with pulmonary edema, pulmonary embolism, and pneumonia.

Cough Reflex

Coughing is a neurally mediated reflex that protects the lungs from accumulation of secretions and from entry of irritating and destructive substances. It is one of the primary defense mechanisms of the respiratory tract. The cough reflex is initiated by receptors located in the tracheobronchial wall; these receptors are extremely sensitive to irritating substances and to the presence of excess secretions. Afferent impulses from these receptors are transmitted through the vagus to the medullary center, which integrates the cough response.

Coughing itself requires the rapid inspiration of a large volume of air (usually about 2.5 L), followed by rapid closure of the glottis and forceful contraction of the abdominal and expiratory muscles. As these muscles contract, intrathoracic pressures are elevated to levels of 100 mm Hg or more. The rapid opening of the glottis at this point leads to an explosive expulsion of air.

Many conditions can interfere with the cough reflex and its protective function. The reflex is impaired in persons whose abdominal or respiratory muscles are weak. This problem can be caused by disease conditions that lead to muscle weakness or paralysis, and by prolonged inactivity, or can arise as an outcome of surgery involving these muscles. Bed rest interferes with expansion of the chest and limits the amount of air that can be taken into the lungs in preparation for coughing, making the cough weak and ineffective. Disease conditions that prevent effective closure of the glottis and laryngeal muscles interfere with production of the marked increase in intrathoracic pressure that is needed for effective coughing. The presence of a nasogastric tube, for example, may prevent closure of the upper airway structures and may fatigue the receptors for the cough reflex that are located in the area. The cough reflex also is impaired when there is depressed function of the medullary centers in the brain that integrate the cough reflex. Interruption of the central integration aspect of the cough reflex can arise as the result of disease of this part of the brain or the action of drugs that depress the cough center.

Although the cough reflex is a protective mechanism, frequent and prolonged coughing can be exhausting and painful and can exert undesirable effects on the cardiovascular and respiratory systems and on the elastic tissues of the lungs. This is particularly true in young children and elderly persons.

Dyspnea

Dyspnea is a subjective sensation or a person's perception of difficulty in breathing that includes the perception of labored breathing and the reaction to that sensation. The terms *dyspnea, breathlessness,* and *shortness of breath* often are used interchangeably. Dyspnea is observed in at least three major cardiopulmonary disease states: primary lung diseases such as pneumonia, asthma, and emphysema; heart disease that is characterized by pulmonary congestion; and neuromuscular disorders such as myasthenia gravis and muscular dystrophy that affect the respiratory muscles. Although dyspnea commonly is associated with respiratory disease, it also occurs during exercise, particularly in untrained persons.

The cause of dyspnea is unknown. Four types of mechanisms have been proposed to explain the sensation: stimulation of lung receptors; increased sensitivity to changes in ventilation perceived through central nervous system mechanisms; reduced ventilatory capacity or breathing reserve; and stimulation of neural receptors in the muscle fibers of the intercostals and diaphragm and of receptors in the skeletal joints. The first of the suggested mechanisms is stimulation of lung receptors. These receptors are stimulated by the contraction of bronchial smooth muscle, the stretch of the bronchial wall, pulmonary congestion, and conditions that decrease lung compliance. The second category of proposed mechanisms focuses on central nervous system mechanisms that transmit information to the cortex regarding respiratory muscle weakness or a discrepancy between the increased effort of breathing and inadequate respiratory muscle contraction. The third type of mechanism focuses on a reduction in ventilatory capacity or breathing reserve. A reduction in breathing reserve (*i.e.*, maximum voluntary ventilation not being used during a given activity) to less than 65% to 75% usually correlates well with dyspnea. The fourth possible mechanism is stimulation of muscle and joint receptors in the respiratory musculature because of a discrepancy in the tension generated by these muscles and the TV that results. These receptors, once stimulated, transmit signals that bring about an awareness of the breathing discrepancy. Like other subjective symptoms, such as fatigue and pain, dyspnea is difficult to quantify because it relies on a person's perception of the problem.

The most common method for measuring dyspnea is a retrospective determination of the level of daily activity at which a person experiences dyspnea. Several scales are available for this use. One of these uses four grades of dyspnea to evaluate disability. The visual analog scale may be used to assess breathing difficulty that occurs with a given activity, such as walking a certain distance. The visual analog scale consists of a line (often 10 cm in length) with descriptors such as "easy to breathe" on one end and "very difficult to breathe" on the other. The person being assessed selects a point on the scale that describes his or her perceived dyspnea. It also can be used to assess dyspnea over time.

The treatment of dyspnea depends on the cause. For example, persons with impaired respiratory function may require oxygen therapy, and those with pulmonary edema may require measures to improve heart function. Methods to decrease anxiety, breathing retraining, and energy conservation measures may be used to decrease the subjective sensation of dyspnea.

IN SUMMARY, the respiratory system requires continuous input from the nervous system. Movement of the diaphragm, intercostal muscles, and other respiratory muscles is controlled by neurons of the respiratory center located in the pons and medulla. The control of breathing has automatic and voluntary components. The automatic regulation of ventilation is controlled by two types of receptors: lung receptors, which protect respiratory structures, and chemoreceptors, which monitor the gas exchange function of the lungs by sensing changes in blood levels of carbon dioxide, oxygen, and pH. There are three types of lung receptors: stretch receptors, which monitor lung inflation; irritant receptors, which protect against the damaging effects of toxic inhalants; and J receptors, which are thought to sense lung congestion. There are two groups of chemoreceptors: central and peripheral. The central chemoreceptors are the most important in sensing changes in carbon dioxide levels, and the peripheral chemoreceptors function in sensing arterial blood oxygen levels.

Voluntary respiratory control is needed for integrating breathing and actions such as speaking, blowing, and singing.

These acts, which are initiated by the motor and premotor cortex, cause temporary suspension of automatic breathing. The cough reflex protects the lungs from the accumulation of secretions and from the entry of irritating and destructive substances; it is one of the primary defense mechanisms of the respiratory tract. Dyspnea is a subjective sensation of difficulty in breathing that is seen in cardiac, pulmonary, and neuromuscular disorders that affect the respiratory muscles. It can also occur during strenuous work and exercise in healthy persons. ■

Review Exercises

1. Calculate the *partial pressure* of oxygen (PO_2) in the alveoli at an atmospheric pressure at sea level (760 mm Hg); Denver, Colorado, at 5431 feet (621 mm Hg); and Berthoud Pass, Colorado at 12,490 feet (477 mm Hg). Consider that the oxygen concentration is 21% and the water vapor pressure in the lungs is 47 mm Hg.

2. Use the solubility coefficient for oxygen and the oxygen dissociation curve depicted in Figure 27-22 to answer the following questions:

   A. *What is the hemoglobin saturation at a high altitude in which the barometric pressure is 500 mm Hg (consider oxygen to represent 21% of the total gases)?*

   B. *It is usually recommended that the hemoglobin saturation of persons with chronic lung disease be maintained at about 89% to 90% when they are receiving supplemental low-flow oxygen. What would their PO_2 be at this level of hemoglobin saturation and what is the rationale for keeping the PO_2 at this level?*

   C. *What is the oxygen content of a person with a hemoglobin level of 6 gm/dL who is breathing room air?*

   D. *What is the oxygen content of a person with carbon monoxide poisoning who is receiving 100% oxygen at 3 atmospheres' pressure in a hyperbaric chamber? Consider that most of the person's hemoglobin is saturated with carbon monoxide.*

Bibliography

Berne R. M., Levy M. N., Koeppen B. M., et al. (2004). *Physiology* (5th ed., pp. 443–520). Philadelphia: Elsevier Saunders.

Cole F. S. (2003). Surfactant protein B: Unambiguously necessary for adult pulmonary function. *American Journal of Physiology: Lung and Cell Molecular Physiology* 285, L540–L545.

Costanzo L. S. (2002). *Physiology* (2nd ed., pp. 167–214). Philadelphia: WB Saunders.

Crapo R. O. (1994). Pulmonary function testing. *New England Journal of Medicine* 331, 25–30.

DeTroyer A., Kirkwood P. A., Wilson T. A. (2005). Respiratory action of inspiratory muscles. *Physiology Reviews* 85, 717–756.

Ganong W. F. (2005). *Review of medical physiology* (22nd ed., pp. 647–697). New York: Lange Medical Books/McGraw-Hill.

Gartner L. P., Hiatt J. L. (2001). *Color textbook of histology* (2nd ed., pp. 343–364). Philadelphia: WB Saunders.

Guyton A., Hall J. E. (2006). *Textbook of medical physiology* (11th ed., pp. 471–522). Philadelphia: Elsevier Saunders.

Hills B. A. (1999). An alternative view of the role(s) of surfactant and the alveolar model. *Journal of Applied Physiology* 87, 1567–1583.

Junqueira L. C., Carneiro J., Kelly R. O. (2005). *Basic histology* (11th ed.). Stamford, CT: Appleton & Lange.

Moore K. L., Dalley A. F. (2003). *Clinically oriented anatomy* (5th ed., pp. 241–252). Philadelphia: Lippincott Williams & Wilkins.

Porth C. J., Bamrah V. S., Tristani F. E., et al. (1984). The Valsalva maneuver: Mechanisms and clinical implications. *Heart & Lung* 13, 507–518.

Prabhakar N. R., Peng Y.-J. (2004). Peripheral chemoreceptors in health and disease. *Journal of Applied Physiology* 96, 359–366.

Rhoades R. A., Tanner G. A. (2003). *Medical physiology* (2nd ed., pp. 309–375). Philadelphia: Lippincott Williams & Wilkins.

Ross M. H. (2003). *Histology: A text and atlas* (4th ed., pp. 568–590). Philadelphia: Lippincott Williams & Wilkins.

West J. B. (2004). *Respiratory physiology: The essentials* (7th ed.). Philadelphia: Lippincott Williams & Wilkins.

Whitsett J. A., Weaver T. E. (2002). Hydrophobic surfactant proteins in lung function and disease. *New England Journal of Medicine* 347, 2141–2148.

Wright J. R. (2005). Immunoregulatory functions of surfactant proteins. *Nature Reviews Immunology* 5, 58–68.

Visit thePoint. **http://thePoint.lww.com for animations, journal articles, and more!**

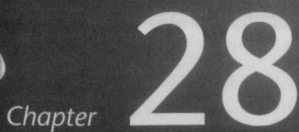

Chapter 28

Respiratory Tract Infections, Neoplasms, and Childhood Disorders

CAROL M. PORTH

➤ Respiratory illnesses represent one of the more common reasons for visits to the physician, admission to the hospital, and forced inactivity among all age groups. The common cold, although not usually serious, is a common cause of missed work and school days. Pneumonia is the sixth leading cause of death in the United States, particularly among the elderly and those with compromised immune function. Tuberculosis remains one of the deadliest diseases in the world. It has been estimated that between 19% and 43% of the world's population is infected with tuberculosis.[1] Although the rate of tuberculosis infection has declined slightly since its resurgence in the early 1990s, there remains a large number of people who are infected; without effective treatment for latent infection, new cases can be expected to emerge from within this group. Lung cancer remains the leading cause of cancer death worldwide.

RESPIRATORY TRACT INFECTIONS

After completing this section of the chapter, you should be able to meet the following objectives:

- Describe the transmission of the common cold from one person to another.
- Describe the causes, manifestations, and treatment of acute and chronic sinusitis.

- Relate the characteristics of the influenza virus to its contagious properties and the need for a yearly "flu shot."
- Characterize community-acquired pneumonia, hospital-acquired pneumonia, and pneumonia in immuno-compromised persons in terms of pathogens, manifestations, and prognosis.
- Describe the immunologic properties of the tubercle bacillus, and differentiate between primary tuberculosis and reactivated tuberculosis on the basis of their pathophysiology.
- State the mechanism for the transmission of fungal infections of the lung.

The respiratory tract is susceptible to infectious processes caused by many different types of microorganisms. Infections can involve the upper respiratory tract (*i.e.,* nose, oropharynx, and larynx), the lower respiratory tract (*i.e.,* lower airways and lungs), or the upper and lower airways. For the most part, the signs and symptoms of respiratory tract infections depend on the function of the structure involved, the severity of the infectious process, and the person's age and general health status. The discussion in this section of the chapter focuses on the common cold, rhinosinusitis, influenza, pneumonia, tuberculosis, and fungal infections of the lung. Acute respiratory infections in children are discussed in the last section of the chapter.

Viruses are the most frequent cause of respiratory tract infections. They can cause infections ranging from a self-limited cold to life-threatening pneumonia. Moreover, viral infections can damage bronchial epithelium, obstruct airways, and lead to secondary bacterial infections. Each viral species has its own pattern of respiratory tract involvement. The rhinoviruses grow best at 33°C to 35°C and remain strictly confined to the upper respiratory tract.[2] Other microorganisms, such as bacteria (*e.g.,* pneumococci, staphylococci), mycobacteria (*e.g., Mycobacterium tuberculosis*), fungi (*e.g., Histoplasma capsulatum* [histoplasmosis], *Coccidioides immitis* [coccidioidomycosis], and *Blastomyces dermatitidis* [blastomycosis]), and opportunistic organisms (*e.g., Pneumocystis jiroveci* [formerly *Pneumocystis carinii*]), also produce infections of the lung, many of which produce significant morbidity and mortality.

The Common Cold

The common cold is a viral infection of the upper respiratory tract. It occurs more frequently than any other respiratory tract infection. Most adults have two to three colds per year, whereas the average school child may have up to 12 per year.[3] The condition usually begins with a feeling of dryness and stuffiness affecting mainly the nasopharynx, followed by excessive production of nasal secretions and tearing of the eyes. Usually, the secretions remain clear and watery. The mucous membranes of the upper respiratory tract become reddened, swollen, and bathed in secretions. Involvement of the pharynx and larynx causes sore throat and hoarseness. The affected person may

experience headache and generalized malaise. In severe cases, there may be chills, fever, and exhaustion. The disease process is usually self-limited, lasting approximately 7 days.

Initially thought to be caused by either a single "cold virus" or a group of them, the common cold is now recognized to be associated with a number of viruses.[3,4] The most common of these are the rhinoviruses, parainfluenza viruses, respiratory syncytial virus, coronaviruses, and adenoviruses. The season of the year and the person's age and prior exposure are important factors in the type of virus causing the infection and the type of symptoms that occur. For example, outbreaks of colds due to rhinoviruses are most common in early fall and late spring; those due to respiratory syncytial virus peak in the winter and spring months; and infections due to the adenoviruses and coronaviruses are more frequent during the winter and spring months. Infections resulting from the respiratory syncytial virus and parainfluenza viruses are most common and severe in children younger than 3 years of age. Infections occur less frequently and with milder symptoms with increasing age. Parainfluenza viruses often produce lower respiratory symptoms with first infections, but less severe upper respiratory symptoms with reinfections. The rhinoviruses are the most common cause of colds in persons between 5 and 40 years of age. There are more than 100 serotypes of rhinoviruses.[4,5] Although people acquire lifetime immunity to an individual serotype, it would take a long time to become immune to all serotypes.

The "cold viruses" are rapidly spread from person to person. Children are the major reservoir of cold viruses, often acquiring a new virus from another child in school or day care. The fingers are the greatest source of spread, and the nasal mucosa and conjunctival surface of the eyes are the most common portals for entry of the virus. The most highly contagious period is during the first 3 days after the onset of symptoms, and the incubation period is approximately 5 days. Cold viruses have been found to survive for more than 5 hours on the skin and hard surfaces, such as plastic countertops.[4,5] Aerosol spread of colds through coughing and sneezing is much less important than the spread by fingers picking up the virus from contaminated surfaces and carrying it to the nasal membranes and eyes.[6] This suggests that careful attention to hand washing is one of the most important preventive measures for avoiding the common cold.

Because the common cold is an acute and self-limited illness in persons who are otherwise healthy, symptomatic treatment with rest and antipyretic drugs is usually all that is needed. Antibiotics are ineffective against viral infections and are not recommended. Many over-the-counter (OTC) remedies are available for treating the common cold. Antihistamines are popular OTC drugs because of their action in drying nasal secretions. However, they may dry up bronchial secretions and worsen the cough, and they may cause dizziness, drowsiness, and impaired judgment. There is no evidence that they shorten the duration of the cold. Decongestant drugs (*i.e.,* sympathomimetic agents) are available in OTC nasal sprays, drops, and oral cold medications. These drugs constrict the blood vessels in the swollen nasal mucosa and reduce nasal swelling. Rebound nasal swelling can occur with indiscriminate use of nasal drops and sprays. Oral preparations containing decongestants may cause systemic vasoconstriction and elevation of blood pressure when given in doses large enough to relieve nasal congestion, and they should be avoided by persons with hypertension, heart disease, hyperthyroidism, diabetes mellitus, or other health problems.[3]

There is controversy regarding the use of vitamin C to reduce the incidence and severity of colds and influenza. Some studies have found vitamin C intake to be beneficial, and others have found it to be of questionable value.[3,4,7] Zinc lozenges are also marketed as an OTC remedy for colds. As with vitamin C, some studies have shown the lozenges to be beneficial, and others have not.[7]

Rhinosinusitis

Rhinitis refers to inflammation of the nasal passages and sinusitis as inflammation of the paranasal sinuses. Although it has not been universally accepted, the suggestion has been made that the term *rhinosinusitis* is a more accurate term for what is commonly referred to as *sinusitis,* because the mucosa of the nasal cavities and paranasal sinuses are lined with a continuous mucous membrane layer and viral upper respiratory tract infections frequently precede or occur along with sinus infections.[8–10]

The paranasal sinuses are air sacs that develop during embryogenesis from a series of ridges and furrows within the cartilaginous capsule surrounding the developing nasal cavity. As development progresses, outpouchings from these furrows become lined with ciliated respiratory epithelium and invade the surrounding facial bones to become the major sinuses. Each sinus remains in constant communication with the nasal cavity through narrow openings or *ostia.* The sinuses are named for the bone in which in which they are located—frontal, ethmoid, maxillary, and sphenoidal (Fig. 28-1A). The *maxillary sinuses* are located inferior to the bony orbit and superior to the hard palate and their openings are located superiorly and medially in the sinus, a location that impedes drainage. The *frontal sinuses* open into the middle meatus of the nasal cavity. The *ethmoid sinuses* consist of 3 to 15 air cells on each side of the ethmoid, with each maintaining a separate path to the nasal chamber. The anterior ethmoid, frontal, and maxillary sinuses all drain into the nasal cavity through a relatively convoluted and narrow passage called the *ostiomeatal complex* (see Fig. 28-1B). Because of this anatomic configuration, any defects in the anterior ethmoid sinus can obstruct the ostiomeatal complex and cause secondary disease of the frontal or maxillary sinuses.[9,10] The *sphenoidal sinuses* are located just anterior to the pituitary fossa behind the posterior ethmoid sinuses, with their openings draining into the sphenoethmoid recess at the top of the nasal cavity (see Fig. 28-1C).

Each sinus is lined with a mucosal surface that is continuous with that of the nasal passages. An active mucociliary clearance mechanism helps move fluid and microorganisms out of the sinuses and into the nasal cavity. Mucociliary clearance, along with innate and adaptive immune mechanisms, helps to keep the sinuses sterile. The lower oxygen content in the sinuses facilitates the growth of organisms, impairs local defenses, and alters the function of immune cells.

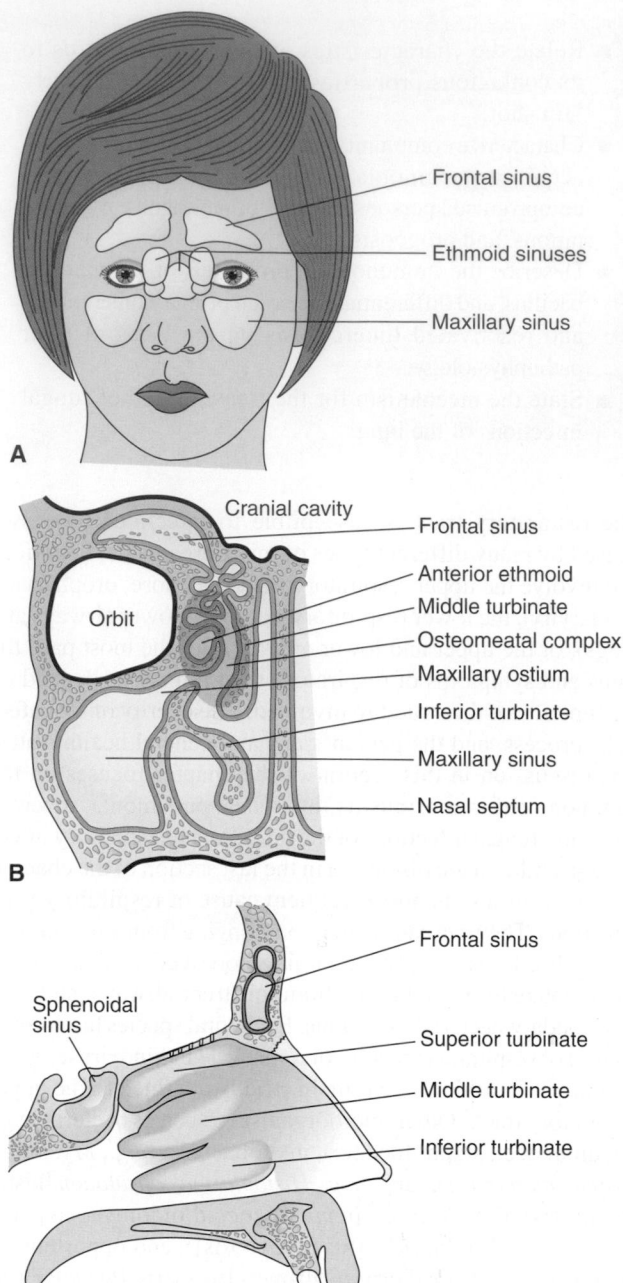

FIGURE 28-1 • Paranasal sinuses. (**A**) Frontal view showing the frontal, ethmoid, and maxillary sinuses. (**B**) Cross-section of nasal cavity (anterior view). The shaded area is the osteomeatal complex, which is the final common pathway for drainage of the anterior ethmoid, frontal, and maxillary sinuses. (**C**) Lateral wall, left nasal cavity showing the frontal sphenoidal sinuses and the superior, middle, and inferior turbinates.

Etiology

The most common causes of rhinosinusitis are conditions that obstruct the narrow ostia that drain the sinuses.[9,10] Most commonly, rhinosinusitis develops when a viral upper respiratory tract infection or allergic rhinitis obstructs the ostia and impairs the mucociliary clearance mechanism. Nasal polyps also can obstruct the sinus openings and facilitate sinus infection. Infections associated with nasal polyps can be self-perpetuating because constant irritation from the infection can facilitate polyp growth. Barotrauma caused by changes in barometric pressure, as occurs in airline pilots and flight attendants, may lead to impaired sinus ventilation and clearance of secretions. Swimming, diving, and abuse of nasal decongestants are other causes of sinus irritation and impaired drainage.

Clinical Features

Rhinosinusitis can be classified as acute, subacute, or chronic.[9] Acute rhinosinusitis may be of viral, bacterial, or mixed viral-bacterial origin and may last from 5 to 7 days in the case of acute viral rhinosinusitis and up to 4 weeks in the case of acute bacterial rhinosinusitis. Recurrent acute rhinosinusitis is defined as four or more episodes of acute disease within a 12-month period. Subacute rhinosinusitis lasts from 4 weeks to less than 12 weeks, whereas chronic rhinosinusitis lasts beyond 12 weeks.

Acute bacterial rhinosinusitis most commonly results from infection with *Haemophilus influenzae* or *Streptococcus pneumoniae*.[8-11] In chronic rhinosinusitis, anaerobic organisms, including species of *Peptostreptococcus, Fusobacterium,* and *Prevotella,* tend to predominate, alone or in combination with aerobes such as the *Streptococcus* species or *Staphylococcus aureus*. In immunocompromised persons, such as those with human immunodeficiency virus (HIV) infection, the sinuses may become infected with gram-negative species and opportunistic fungi. In this group, particularly those with leukopenia, the disease may have a fulminant and even fatal course.

Manifestations. The symptoms of acute viral rhinosinusitis often are difficult to differentiate from those of the common cold and allergic rhinitis (discussed in Chapter 19). They include facial pain, headache, purulent nasal discharge, decreased sense of smell, and fever. A history of a preceding common cold and the presence of purulent nasal drainage, pain on bending, unilateral maxillary pain, and pain in the teeth are common findings with involvement of the maxillary sinuses. The symptoms of acute viral rhinosinusitis usually resolve within 5 to 7 days without medical treatment. Acute bacterial rhinosinusitis is suggested by symptoms that worsen after 5 to 7 days or persist beyond 10 days, or symptoms that are out of proportion to those usually associated with a viral upper respiratory tract infection.[10,11] Persons who are immunocompromised, such as those with leukemia, aplastic anemia, a bone marrow transplant, or HIV infection, often present with fever of unknown origin, rhinorrhea, or facial edema. Often, other signs of inflammation such as purulent drainage are absent.

In persons with chronic rhinosinusitis, the only symptoms may be those such as nasal obstruction, a sense of fullness in the ears, postnasal drip, hoarseness, chronic cough, loss of taste and smell, or unpleasant breath.[12] Sinus pain often is absent; instead, the person may complain of a headache that is dull and constant. Persons with chronic rhinosinusitis may have super-imposed bouts of acute rhinosinusitis. The epithelial changes that occur during acute and subacute forms of rhinosinusitis usually are reversible, but the mucosal changes that occur with chronic rhinosinusitis often are irreversible.

Diagnosis and Treatment. The diagnosis of rhinosinusitis usually is based on symptom history and a physical examination that includes inspection of the nose and throat.[8-11] Headache due to sinusitis needs to be differentiated from other types of headache. Sinusitis headache usually is exaggerated by bending forward, coughing, or sneezing. Physical examination findings in acute bacterial sinusitis include turbinate edema, nasal crusts, purulence of the nasal cavity, and failure of transillumination of the maxillary sinuses.[11] Transillumination is done in a completely darkened room by placing a flashlight against the skin overlying the infraorbital rim, directing the light inferiorly, having the person open his or her mouth, and observing the hard palate for light transmission. Sinus radiographs and computed tomography (CT) scans may be used. CT scans usually are reserved for diagnosis of chronic rhinosinusitis or to exclude complications. Magnetic resonance imaging (MRI) is expensive and usually reserved for cases of suspected neoplasms or fungal sinusitis.[9]

Treatment of rhinosinusitis depends on cause and includes appropriate use of antibiotics, mucolytic agents, and symptom relief measures. About two thirds of persons with acute bacterial rhinosinusitis improve without antibiotic treatment, and most persons with viral upper respiratory infections improve within 7 days. Therefore, treatment with antibiotics is usually reserved for persons who have had symptoms for more than 7 days and who present with two or more manifestations of acute bacterial rhinosinusitis (*i.e.,* purulent nasal drainage; maxillary, tooth, or facial pain [especially if it is unilateral]; unilateral maxillary tenderness; or worsening of symptoms after initial improvement), or for those with severe symptoms.[11] In addition to antibiotic therapy, the treatment of acute rhinosinusitis includes measures to promote adequate drainage by reducing nasal congestion. Oral and topical decongestants may be used for this purpose. The use of intranasal decongestants should be limited to 3 to 5 days to prevent rebound vasodilation.[8] Antihistamines tend to dry up secretions and are not recommended as adjunctive treatment in acute viral or bacterial rhinosinusitis. Mucolytic agents such as guaifenesin may be used to thin secretions. Topical corticosteroids may be used to decrease inflammation in persons with allergic rhinitis or rhinosinusitis. Nonpharmacologic measures include saline nasal sprays, nasal irrigation, and mist humidification.

Surgical intervention directed at correcting obstruction of the ostiomeatal openings may be indicated in persons with chronic rhinosinusitis that is resistant to other forms of therapy. Indications for surgical intervention include obstructive nasal polyps and obstructive nasal deformities.

Complications. Because of the sinuses' proximity to the brain and orbital wall, sinusitis can lead to intracranial and orbital wall complications. Intracranial complications are seen most commonly with infection of the frontal and ethmoid sinuses because of their proximity to the dura and drainage of the veins from the frontal sinus into the dural sinus. Orbital complications can range from edema of the eyelids to orbital cellulitis and subperiosteal abscess formation. Facial swelling over the involved sinus, abnormal extraocular movements, protrusion of the eyeball, periorbital edema, or changes in mental status may indicate intracranial complications and require immediate medical attention.[8]

Influenza

Influenza is one of the most important causes of acute upper respiratory tract infection in humans. Until the advent of acquired immunodeficiency syndrome (AIDS), it was the last uncontrolled pandemic killer of humans. In the United States, approximately 36,000 persons die each year of influenza-related illness during nonpandemic years.[13] Rates of infection are highest among children, but rates of serious illness and death are highest among persons who are 65 years of age or older.[14]

The viruses that cause influenza belong to the Orthomyxoviridae family, whose members are characterized by a segmented, single-stranded ribonucleic acid (RNA) genome[15]

(Fig. 28-2). There are three types of influenza viruses that cause epidemics in humans: types A, B, and C. Influenza A differs in its ability to infect multiple species, including avian and mammalian species. The influenza A virus is further divided into subtypes based on two surface glycoproteins: hemagglutinin (HA) and neuraminidase (NA).[15,16] HA is an attachment protein that allows the virus to enter epithelial cells in the respiratory tract, and NA facilitates viral replication and release from the cell. Host antibodies to HA and NA prevent or ameliorate infection by the influenza virus. There are 16 known HA subtypes (*i.e.,* H1 to H16) and 9 known subtypes for NA (*i.e.,* N1 to N9). Contagion results from the ability of the influenza A virus to develop new HA and NA subtypes against which the population is not protected. An antigenic shift, which involves a major genetic rearrangement in either antigen, may lead to epidemic or pandemic infection. Lesser changes, called *antigenic drift,* find the population partially protected by cross-reacting antibodies. Influenza B and C undergo less frequent antigenic shifts than influenza A, probably because few related viruses exist in mammalian or avian species.[15–17]

As with many viral respiratory tract infections, influenza is more contagious than bacterial respiratory tract infections. In contrast to the rhinoviruses, transmission occurs by inhalation of droplet nuclei rather than touching contaminated objects. Most

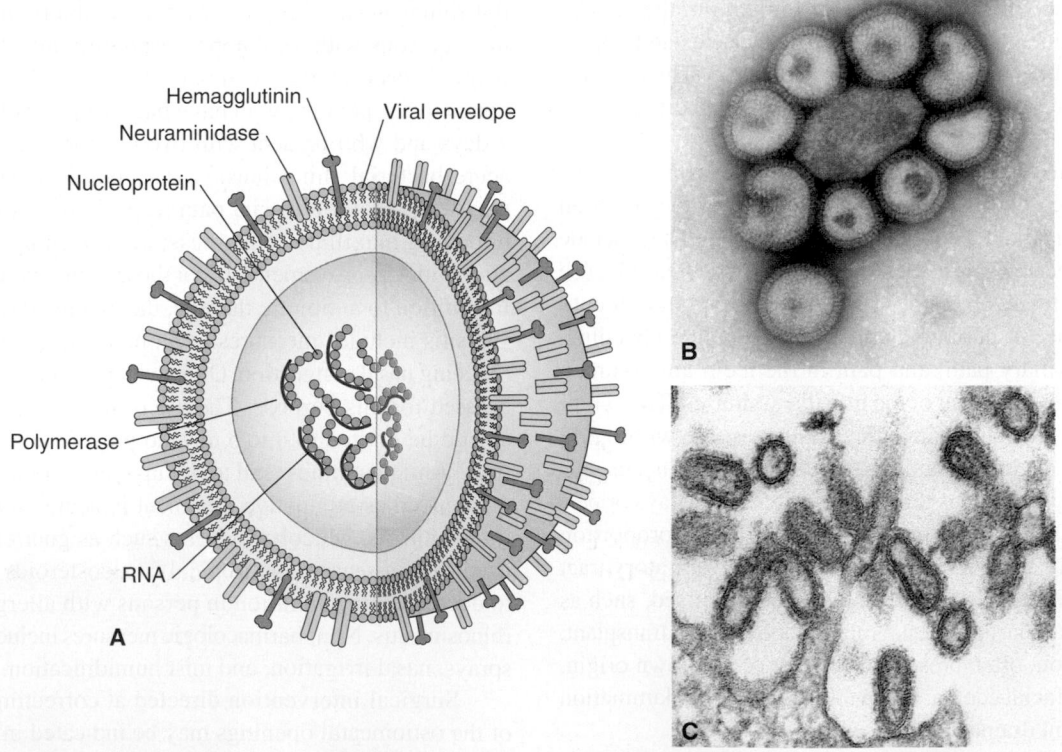

FIGURE 28-2 • Influenza type A virus. (**A**) Model of the RNA influenza A virus, showing the hemagglutinin and neuraminidase envelope glycoproteins that provide access to host cells. (**B**) Negative-stained transmission electron micrograph (TEM) depicting the ultrastructural details of a number of influenza viral particles, or "virions." (**C**) TEM revealing ultrastructural features of the 1918 influenza pandemic virus virions. (**B** and **C** Courtesy Public Image Library, Centers for Disease Control and Prevention. [Online.] Available: http://phil.cdc.gov/phil/home.asp.)

infected people develop symptoms of the disease, increasing the likelihood of contagion through spread of infectious droplets. Young children are most likely to become infected and also to spread the infection. The incubation period for influenza is 1 to 4 days, with 2 days being the average. Persons become infectious starting 1 day before their symptoms begin and remain infectious through approximately 5 days after illness onset.[13] Children can be infectious for greater than 10 days, and young children can shed virus for up to 6 days before their illness onset. Severely immunocompromised persons can shed virus for weeks or months.

Pathogenesis

The influenza viruses can cause three types of infections: an uncomplicated upper respiratory infection (rhinotracheitis), viral pneumonia, and a respiratory viral infection followed by a bacterial infection. Influenza initially establishes upper airway infection. In doing this, the virus first targets and kills mucous-secreting, ciliated, and other epithelial cells, leaving gaping holes between the underlying basal cells and allowing extracellular fluid to escape. This is the reason for the "runny nose" that is characteristic of this phase of the infection. If the virus spreads to the lower respiratory tract, the infection can cause severe shedding of bronchial and alveolar cells down to a single-cell–thick basal layer. In addition to compromising the natural defenses of the respiratory tract, influenza infection promotes bacterial adhesion to epithelial cells. Pneumonia may result from a viral pathogenesis or from a secondary bacterial infection.

Clinical Features

In the early stages, the symptoms of influenza often are indistinguishable from other viral infections. There is an abrupt onset of fever and chills, malaise, muscle aching, headache, profuse, watery nasal discharge, nonproductive cough, and sore throat.[18,19] One distinguishing feature of an influenza viral infection is the rapid onset, sometimes in as little as 1 to 2 minutes, of profound malaise. The symptoms of uncomplicated rhinotracheitis usually peak by days 3 to 5 and disappear by days 7 to 10. The aforementioned symptoms can be caused by any of the influenza A or B viruses. Influenza C virus infection causes symptoms similar to the common cold.

Viral pneumonia occurs as a complication of influenza, most frequently in the elderly or in persons with cardiopulmonary disease, but has been reported in pregnant women and in healthy, immunocompetent people. It typically develops within 1 day after onset of influenza and is characterized by rapid progression of fever, tachypnea, tachycardia, cyanosis, and hypotension.[20] The clinical course of influenza pneumonia progresses rapidly. It can cause hypoxemia and death within a few days of onset. Survivors often develop diffuse pulmonary fibrosis.

Secondary complications typically include sinusitis, otitis media, bronchitis, and bacterial pneumonia.[20] Persons in whom secondary bacterial pneumonia develops usually report that they were beginning to feel better when they experienced a return of fever, shaking chills, pleuritic chest pain, and productive cough. The most common causes of secondary bacterial pneumonia are *S. pneumoniae, S. aureus, H. influenzae,* and *Moraxella catarrhalis.* This form of pneumonia commonly produces less cyanosis and tachypnea and is usually milder than primary influenza pneumonia. Influenza-related deaths can result from pneumonia as well as exacerbations of cardiopulmonary conditions and other disease. Reye syndrome (fatty liver with encephalitis) is a rare complication of influenza, particularly in young children who have been given aspirin as an antipyretic agent.

Diagnosis and Treatment. The appropriate treatment of people with influenza depends on accurate and timely diagnosis. The early diagnosis can reduce the inappropriate use of antibiotics and provide the opportunity for use of an antiviral drug. Rapid diagnostic tests, which are available for use in outpatient settings, allow health care providers to diagnose influenza more accurately, consider treatment options more carefully, and monitor the influenza type and its prevalence in their community.[21]

The goals of treatment for influenza are designed to limit the infection to the upper respiratory tract. The symptomatic approach for treatment of uncomplicated influenza rhinotracheitis focuses on rest, keeping warm, and drinking large amounts of liquids. Analgesics and cough medications can also be used. Rest decreases the oxygen requirements of the body and reduces the respiratory rate and the chance of spreading the virus from the upper to lower respiratory tract. Keeping warm helps maintain the respiratory epithelium at a core body temperature of 37°C (or higher if fever is present), thereby inhibiting viral replication, which is optimal at 35°C. Drinking large amounts of liquids ensures that the function of the epithelial lining of the respiratory tract is not further compromised by dehydration. Antiviral medications may be indicated in some persons. Antibacterial antibiotics should be reserved for bacterial complications. The use of aspirin to treat fever should be avoided in children because of the risk of Reye syndrome.

Four antiviral drugs are available for treatment of influenza: amantadine, rimantadine, zanamivir, and oseltamivir.[21,22] The first-generation antiviral drugs amantadine and rimantadine are similarly effective against influenza A but not influenza B. These agents inhibit the uncoating of viral RNA in the host cells and prevent its replication. Both drugs are effective in prevention of influenza A in high-risk groups and in treatment of persons who acquire the disease. Unfortunately, resistance to the drugs develops rapidly and strains that are resistant to amantadine also are resistant to rimantadine. Amantadine stimulates release of catecholamines, which can produce central nervous system side effects such as anxiety, depression, and insomnia.

The second-generation antiviral drugs zanamivir and oseltamivir are inhibitors of NA, a viral glycoprotein that is necessary for viral replication and release. These drugs, which have been approved for treatment of acute uncomplicated influenza infection, are effective against both influenza A and

B viruses. Zanamivir and oseltamivir result in less resistance than amantadine and rimantadine. Zanamivir is administered intranasally and oseltamivir is administered orally. Zanamivir can cause bronchospasm and is not recommended for persons with asthma or chronic obstructive lung disease. To be effective, the antiviral drugs should be initiated within 30 hours after onset of symptoms.

Influenza Immunization

Because influenza is so highly contagious, prevention relies primarily on vaccination. Currently, there are two types of influenza vaccines available: the trivalent inactivated influenza vaccine (TIIV), which was developed in the 1940s, and the live, attenuated influenza vaccine (LAIV).[13] The formulation of the vaccines must be changed yearly in response to antigenic changes in the influenza virus. The Centers for Disease Control and Prevention (CDC) Advisory Committee on Immunization Practices (ACIP) annually updates its recommendations for the composition of the vaccine. The influenza vaccines are contraindicated in persons with anaphylactic hypersensitivity to eggs or to other components of the vaccine, persons with a history Guillain-Barré syndrome, and persons with acute febrile illness.[13]

The TIIV, which is administered by injection, has become the mainstay for prevention of influenza. It has proved to be inexpensive and effective in reducing illness caused by influenza. Immunization is recommended for high-risk groups who, because of their age or underlying health problems, are unable to cope well with the infection and often require medical attention, including hospitalization. The effectiveness of the influenza vaccine in preventing and lessening the effects of influenza infection depend primarily on the age and immunocompetence of the recipient and the match between the virus strains included in the vaccine and those that circulate during the influenza season.[13] When there is a good match, the vaccine is effective in preventing the illness in approximately 70% to 90% of healthy persons younger than 65 years of age.[13]

The LAIVs are cold-adapted viruses that replicate efficiently in the 25°C temperatures of the nasopharynx, inducing protective immunity against viruses included in the vaccine, but replicate inefficiently at the 38°C to 39°C temperature of the lower airways. LAIV is an option for vaccination of healthy, nonpregnant persons, 2 to 49 years of age.[13]

Avian Influenza (Bird Flu)

Avian influenza, or "bird flu," is an infection caused by avian influenza viruses. The normal hosts for avian influenza viruses are birds and occasionally pigs. These influenza viruses occur naturally among birds.[23–25] Wild birds carry the viruses in their intestines, but usually are not affected by them. However, the virus is highly contagious among avian species and can infect and kill domestic poultry, such as chickens, ducks, and turkeys. Infected birds shed the virus in their saliva, nasal secretions, and

feces. Susceptible birds become infected when they have contact with contaminated secretions or feces. Avian strains of the influenza virus do not usually cause outbreaks of disease in humans unless a reassortment of the virus genome has occurred within an intermediate mammalian host such as a pig.[23] In this setting, a virus is produced that contains mammalian characteristics as well as avian characteristics to which humans may not be immune. It is noteworthy that many of the pandemics of the past were thought to arise in Asia, where large human populations live in close proximity to ducks, chickens, and pigs, thus facilitating the phenomenon of viral reassortment.[24]

Recently, a highly pathogenic influenza A subtype, H5N1, was found in poultry in East and Southeast Asian countries.[25] Although the H5N1 strain is highly contagious from one bird to another, its transmission from human to human is relatively inefficient and not sustained. The result is only rare cases of person-to-person transmission. Most cases occur after exposure to infected poultry or surfaces contaminated with poultry droppings. Because infection in humans is associated with a high mortality rate, there is considerable concern that the H5N1 strain might mutate and initiate a pandemic.

There currently is no commercially available vaccine to protect humans against the bird flu. Current commercial rapid diagnostic tests are not optimally sensitive or specific for detection of the virus. Most Asian H5N1 influenza strains are resistant to amantadine and rimantadine. The NA inhibitors, oseltamivir and zanamivir, would probably be effective if administered within 48 hours, but additional studies are needed to demonstrate their effectiveness.

Pneumonias

The term *pneumonia* describes inflammation of parenchymal structures of the lung, such as the alveoli and the bronchioles. An estimated 4 to 5 million cases occur annually in the United States each year.[26] Pneumonia is the sixth leading cause of death in the United States and the most common cause of death from infectious disease.[27–29] Etiologic agents include infectious and noninfectious agents. Inhalation of irritating fumes or aspiration of gastric contents, although much less common than infectious causes, can result in severe pneumonia.

Although antibiotics have significantly reduced the mortality rate from pneumonias, these diseases remain an important immediate cause of death of the elderly and persons with debilitating diseases. There have been subtle changes in the spectrum of microorganisms that cause infectious pneumonias, including a decrease in pneumonias caused by *S. pneumoniae* and an increase in pneumonias caused by other microorganisms such as *Pseudomonas, Candida* and other fungi, and nonspecific viruses. Many of these pneumonias occur in persons with impaired immune defenses, including persons who are on immunosuppressant drugs to prevent rejection of a bone marrow or organ transplant.

Pneumonias can be commonly classified according to the type of agent (typical or atypical) causing the infection, distribution of the infection (lobar pneumonia or bronchopneumonia),

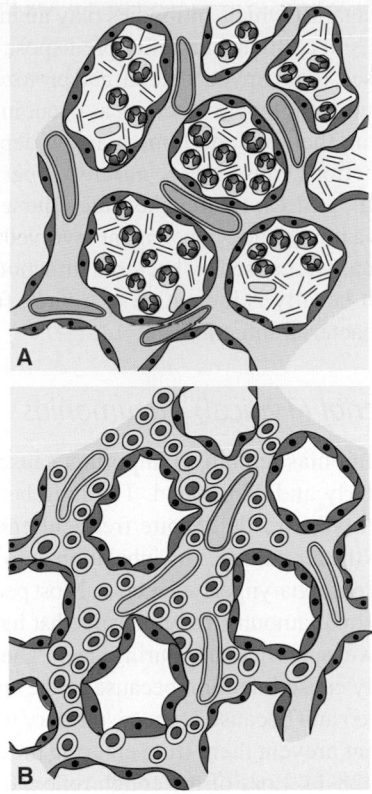

FIGURE 28-3 • Location of inflammatory processes in (A) typical and (B) atypical forms of pneumonia.

and setting (community or hospital) in which it occurs. *Typical pneumonias* result from infection by bacteria that multiply extracellularly in the alveoli and cause inflammation and exudation of fluid into the air-filled spaces of the alveoli (Fig. 28-3). *Atypical pneumonias* are caused by viral and mycoplasma infections that involve the alveolar septum and the interstitium of the lung. They produce less striking symptoms and physical findings than bacterial pneumonia; there is a lack of alveolar infiltration and purulent sputum, leukocytosis, and lobar consolidation on the radiograph. Acute bacterial pneumonias can be classified as lobar pneumonia or bronchopneumonia, based on their anatomic pattern of distribution (Fig. 28-4). In general, *lobar pneumonia* refers to consolidation of a part or all of a lung lobe, and *bronchopneumonia* signifies a patchy consolidation involving more than one lobe (see Fig. 28-4).

Because of the overlap in symptomatology and changing spectrum of infectious organisms involved, pneumonias are increasingly being classified as community-acquired and hospital-acquired (nosocomial) pneumonias.[27,29,30] Persons with compromised immune function constitute a special concern in both categories.

Community-Acquired Pneumonia

The term *community-acquired pneumonia* is used to describe infections from organisms found in the community rather than in the hospital or nursing home. It is defined as an infection that

begins outside the hospital or is diagnosed within 48 hours after admission to the hospital in a person who has not resided in a long-term care facility for 14 days or more before admission.[31] Community-acquired pneumonia may be further categorized according to risk of mortality and need for hospitalization based on age, presence of coexisting disease, and severity of illness, using physical examination, laboratory, and radiologic findings.[32]

Community-acquired pneumonia may be either bacterial or viral. The most common cause of infection in all categories is *S. pneumoniae*.[33–35] Other common pathogens include *H. influenzae*, *S. aureus*, and gram-negative bacilli. Less common agents are *Mycoplasma pneumoniae*, *Chlamydia* species, and viruses, sometimes called *atypical agents*. Common viral causes of

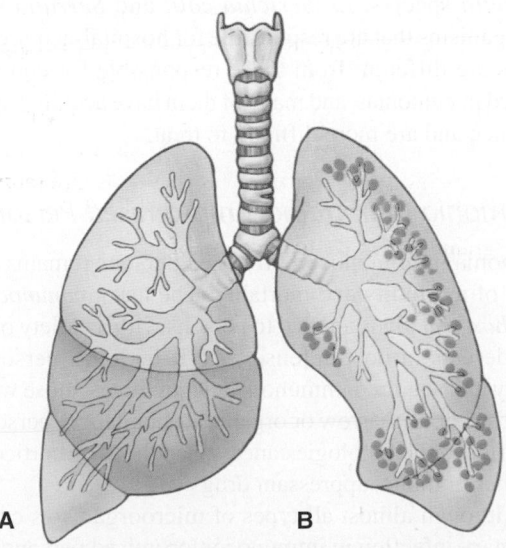

FIGURE 28-4 • Distribution of lung involvement in (A) lobar pneumonia and (B) bronchopneumonia.

community-acquired pneumonia include the influenza virus, respiratory syncytial virus, adenovirus, and parainfluenza virus.

The methods used in the diagnosis of community-acquired pneumonia depend on age, coexisting health problems, and the severity of illness. In persons younger than 65 years of age and without coexisting disease, the diagnosis usually is based on history and physical examination, chest radiographs, and knowledge of the microorganisms currently causing infections in the community. Sputum specimens may be obtained for staining procedures and culture. Blood cultures may be done for persons requiring hospitalization.

Treatment involves the use of appropriate antibiotic therapy.[35] Empiric antibiotic therapy, based on knowledge regarding an antibiotic's spectrum of action and ability to penetrate bronchopulmonary secretions, often is used for persons with community-acquired pneumonia who do not require hospitalization. Hospitalization and more intensive care may be required depending on the person's age, preexisting health status, and severity of the infection.

Hospital-Acquired Pneumonia

Hospital-acquired, or nosocomial, pneumonia is defined as a lower respiratory tract infection that was not present or incubating on admission to the hospital. Usually, infections occurring 48 hours or more after admission are considered hospital acquired.[30] Hospital-acquired pneumonia is the second most common cause of hospital-acquired infection and has a mortality rate of 20% to 50%.[30] Persons requiring intubation and mechanical ventilation are particularly at risk, as are those with compromised immune function, chronic lung disease, and airway instrumentation, such as endotracheal intubation or tracheotomy.

Most hospital-acquired infections are bacterial. The organisms are those present in the hospital environment and include *Pseudomonas aeruginosa, S. aureus, Enterobacter* species, *Klebsiella* species, *Escherichia coli,* and *Serratia* species. The organisms that are responsible for hospital-acquired pneumonias are different from those responsible for community-acquired pneumonias, and many of them have acquired antibiotic resistance and are more difficult to treat.

Pneumonia in Immunocompromised Persons

Pneumonia in immunocompromised persons remains a major source of morbidity and mortality. The term *immunocompromised host* usually is applied to persons with a variety of underlying defects in host defenses.[15,30] It includes persons with primary and acquired immunodeficiency states, those who have undergone bone marrow or organ transplantation, persons with solid organ or hematologic cancers, and those on corticosteroid and other immunosuppressant drugs.

Although almost all types of microorganisms can cause pulmonary infection in immunocompromised persons, certain types of immunologic defects tend to favor certain types of infections.[15] Defects in humoral immunity predispose to bacte-

rial infections against which antibodies play an important role, whereas defects in cellular immunity predispose to infections caused by viruses, fungi, mycobacteria, and protozoa. Neutropenia and impaired granulocyte function, as occur in persons with leukemia, chemotherapy, and bone marrow depression, predispose to infections caused by *S. aureus, Aspergillus,* gram-negative bacilli, and *Candida.* The time course of infection often provides a hint to the type of agent involved. A fulminant pneumonia usually is caused by bacterial infection, whereas an insidious onset usually is indicative of a viral, fungal, protozoal, or mycobacterial infection.

Acute Bacterial (Typical) Pneumonias

Bacterial pneumonias remain an important cause of mortality among the elderly and debilitated. The lung below the main bronchi is normally sterile despite frequent entry of microorganisms into the air passages by inhalation during ventilation or aspiration of nasopharyngeal secretions. Most people unknowingly aspirate small amounts of organisms that have colonized their upper airways, particularly during sleep. These organisms do not normally cause infection because of the small numbers that are aspirated and because of the respiratory tract's defense mechanisms that prevent them from entering the distal air passages[15] (Table 28-1). Loss of the cough reflex, damage to the ciliated endothelium that lines the respiratory tract, or impaired immune defenses predispose to colonization and infection of the lower respiratory system. Bacterial adherence also plays a role in colonization of the lower airways. The epithelial cells of critically and chronically ill persons are more receptive to binding microorganisms that cause pneumonia. Other clinical risk factors favoring colonization of the tracheobronchial tree include antibiotic therapy that alters the normal bacterial flora, diabetes, smoking, chronic bronchitis, and viral infection.

Bacterial pneumonias are commonly classified according to etiologic agent. This is because the clinical and morphologic features, and thus the therapeutic implications, often vary with the causative agent. The discussion in this section focuses on two types of bacterial pneumonia: pneumococcal pneumonia and Legionnaire disease.

Pneumococcal Pneumonia. *S. pneumoniae* (pneumococcus) remains the most common cause of bacterial pneumonia.[30,36] *S. pneumoniae* is a gram-positive diplococcus, possessing a capsule of polysaccharide. The virulence of the pneumococcus is a function of its capsule, which prevents or delays digestion by phagocytes. The polysaccharide is an antigen that primarily elicits a B-cell response with antibody production. In the absence of antibody, clearance of the pneumococci from the body relies on the reticuloendothelial system, with the macrophages in the spleen playing a major role in elimination of the organism.[36] This, along with the spleen's role in antibody production, increases the risk for pneumococcal bacteremia in persons who are anatomically or functionally asplenic, such as children with sickle cell disease. The initial step in the pathogenesis of pneumococcal infection is the attachment and colonization of the

TABLE 28-1 Respiratory Defense Mechanisms and Conditions That Impair Their Effectiveness

DEFENSE MECHANISM	FUNCTION	FACTORS THAT IMPAIR EFFECTIVENESS
Glottic and cough reflexes	Protect against aspiration into tracheo-bronchial tree	Loss of cough reflex due to stroke or neural lesion, neuromuscular disease, abdominal or chest surgery, depression of the cough reflex due to sedation or anesthesia, presence of a nasogastric tube (tends to cause adaptation of afferent receptors)
Mucociliary blanket	Removes secretions, microorganisms, and particles from the respiratory tract	Smoking, viral diseases, chilling, inhalation of irritating gases
Phagocytic and bactericidal action of alveolar macrophages	Removes microorganisms and foreign particles from the lung	Tobacco smoke, chilling, alcohol, oxygen intoxication
Immune defenses (IgA and IgG and cell-mediated immunity)	Destroy microorganisms	Congenital and acquired immunodeficiency states

organism to the mucus and cells of the nasopharynx. Colonization does not equate with signs of infection. Perfectly healthy people can be colonized and carry the organism without evidence of infection. The spread of particular strains of pneumococci, particularly antibiotic-resistant strains, is largely by healthy colonized individuals.

The pathologic process of pneumococcal pneumonia can be divided into the four stages—edema, red hepatization, gray hepatization, and resolution.[29] During the first stage of pneumococcal pneumonia, the alveoli become filled with a protein-rich edema fluid containing numerous organisms (Fig. 28-5). Marked capillary congestion follows, leading to massive outpouring of polymorphonuclear leukocytes and red blood cells. Because the first consistency of the affected lung resembles that of the liver, this stage is referred to as the *red hepatization* stage. The next stage, occurring after 2 or more days, depending on the success of treatment, involves the arrival of macrophages that phagocytose the fragmented polymorphonuclear cells, red blood cells, and other cellular debris. During this stage, which is termed the *gray hepatization* stage, the congestion has diminished but the lung is still firm. The alveolar exudate is then removed and the lung gradually returns to normal.

The signs and symptoms of pneumococcal pneumonia vary widely, depending on the age and health status of the infected person.[36] In previously healthy persons, the onset usually is sudden and is characterized by malaise, severe, shaking chills, and fever. The temperature may go as high as 106°F. During the initial or congestive stage, coughing brings up watery sputum and breath sounds are limited, with fine crackles. As the disease progresses, the character of the sputum changes; it may be blood tinged or rust colored to purulent. Pleuritic pain, a sharp pain that is more severe with respiratory movements, is common. With antibiotic therapy, fever usually subsides in approximately 48 to 72 hours, and recovery is uneventful. Elderly persons are less likely to experience marked elevations in temperature; in these persons, the only

sign of pneumonia may be a loss of appetite and deterioration in mental status.

Treatment includes the use of antibiotics that are effective against *S. pneumoniae*. In the past, *S. pneumoniae* was uniformly susceptible to penicillin. However, penicillin-resistant and multidrug-resistant strains have been emerging in the United States and other countries.[36]

Pneumococcal pneumonia can be prevented through immunization. A 23-valent pneumococcal vaccine, composed of antigens from 23 types of *S. pneumoniae* capsular polysaccharides, is used. The capsular polysaccharides induce antibodies primarily by T-cell–independent mechanisms. The vaccine is recommended for persons 65 years of age or older and persons aged 2 to 65 years with chronic illnesses, particularly cardiovascular and pulmonary diseases, diabetes mellitus, and alcoholism, who sustain increased morbidity with respiratory infections. Immunization also is recommended for immunocompromised persons 2 years of age or older, including those with sickle cell disease, splenectomy, Hodgkin disease, multiple myeloma, renal failure, nephrotic syndrome, organ transplantation, and HIV infection.[37] Immunization is also recommended for residents in special environments or social settings in which the risk for invasive pneumococcal disease is increased (*e.g.*, Alaskan Natives, certain Native American populations), and for residents of nursing homes and long-term care facilities.

A single dose of pneumococcal vaccine usually confers some lifetime immunity. Serotype antibody levels decline after 5 to 10 years and decrease more rapidly in some groups than others.[37] Although not currently recommended for immunocompetent people who received the 23-valent vaccine, a second dose of vaccine is recommended for immunocompromised persons and persons older than 65 years of age if 5 years or more have elapsed since the previous vaccine was given. A second dose is also recommended for persons with hematologic cancer, nephrotic syndrome and chronic kidney diseases, and those with selected immunodeficiency states.[37]

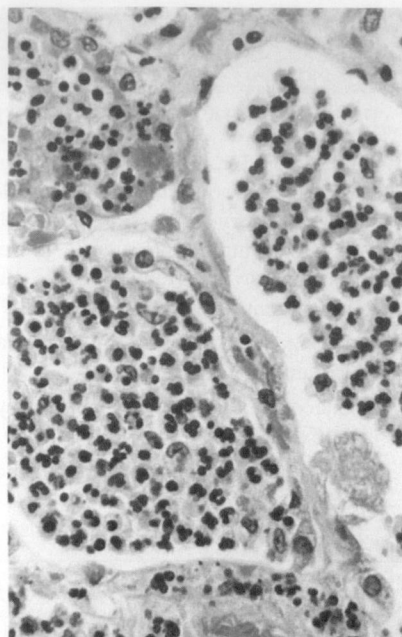

FIGURE 28-5 • Pneumococcal pneumonia. The alveoli are packed with an exudate composed of polymorphonuclear leukocytes and occasional macrophages. (From Beasley M. B., Travis W. D., Rubin E. [2008]. The respiratory system. In Rubin R., Strayer D. S. [Eds.], *Rubin's pathology: Clinicopathologic foundations of medicine* [5th ed., p. 493]. Philadelphia: Lippincott Williams & Wilkins.)

Because their immune system is immature, the antibody response to most pneumococcal capsular polysaccharides usually is poor or inconsistent in children younger than 2 years of age. A 7-valent pneumococcal polysaccharide-protein conjugate vaccine is now available for use among infants and children.[38] With the success of *H. influenzae* type B vaccine, *S. pneumoniae* has become the leading cause of bacterial meningitis in the United States. *S. pneumoniae* also contributes substantially to noninvasive respiratory infections and is the most common cause of community-acquired pneumonia, acute otitis media, and sinusitis among young children. The ACIP recommends that conjugate vaccine be used for all children aged 2 to 23 months and for children aged 24 to 49 months who are at increased risk for pneumococcal disease (*e.g.,* children with sickle cell disease, HIV infection, and other immunocompromising or chronic medical conditions).[38]

Legionnaire Disease. Legionnaire disease is a form of bronchopneumonia caused by a gram-negative rod, *Legionella pneumophila.*[15,39] Transmission from person to person has not been documented, and infection normally occurs by acquiring the organism from the environment. Infection typically occurs when water that contains the pathogen is aerosolized into appropriately sized droplets and is inhaled or aspirated by a susceptible host.[39] The disease was first recognized and received its name after an epidemic of severe and, for some, fatal pneumonia that developed among delegates to the 1976 American

Legion convention held in a Philadelphia hotel. The spread of infection was traced to a water-cooled air-conditioning system. Although healthy persons can contract the infection, the risk is greatest among smokers, persons with chronic diseases, and those with impaired cell-mediated immunity.[15,39]

Symptoms of the disease typically begin approximately 2 to 10 days after infection. Onset is usually abrupt, with malaise, weakness, lethargy, fever, and dry cough. Other manifestations include disturbances of central nervous system function, gastrointestinal tract involvement, arthralgias, and elevation in body temperature, sometimes to more than 104°F.[39] The presence of pneumonia along with diarrhea, hyponatremia, and confusion is characteristic of *Legionella* pneumonia. The disease causes consolidation of lung tissues and impairs gas exchange.

Diagnosis is based on clinical manifestations, radiologic studies, and specialized laboratory tests to detect the presence of the organism. Of these, the *Legionella* urinary antigen test is a relatively inexpensive, rapid test that detects antigens of *L. pneumophila* in the urine.[39] The urine test usually is easier to obtain because people with legionellosis often have a nonproductive cough and the test results remain positive for weeks despite antibiotic therapy. The test is available as both a radioimmunoassay and an enzyme immunoassay.

Treatment consists of administration of antibiotics that are known to be effective against *L. pneumophila.* Delay in instituting antibiotic therapy significantly increases mortality rates; therefore, antibiotics known to be effective against *L. pneumophila* should be included in the treatment regimen for severe community-acquired pneumonia.[39]

Primary Atypical Pneumonia

The primary atypical pneumonias are caused by a variety of agents, the most common being *Mycoplasma pneumoniae.* Mycoplasma infections are particularly common among children and young adults. Other etiologic agents include viruses (*e.g.,* influenza virus, respiratory syncytial viruses, adenoviruses, rhinoviruses, and the rubeola [measles] and varicella [chickenpox] viruses), and *Chlamydia pneumoniae.*[15,30] In some cases, the cause is unknown.

The atypical pneumonias are characterized by patchy involvement of the lung, largely confined to the alveolar septum and pulmonary interstitium. The term *atypical* denotes a lack of lung consolidation, production of moderate amounts of sputum, moderate elevation of white blood cell count, and lack of alveolar exudate.[15,30] The agents that cause atypical pneumonias damage the respiratory tract epithelium and impair respiratory tract defenses, thereby predisposing to secondary bacterial infections. The sporadic form of atypical pneumonia is usually mild with a low mortality rate. It may, however, assume epidemic proportions with intensified severity and greater mortality, as in the influenza pandemics of 1915 and 1918.

The clinical course among persons with mycoplasmal and viral pneumonias varies widely from a mild infection (*e.g.,* influenza types A and B, adenovirus) that masquerades as a chest cold to a more serious and even fatal outcome (*e.g.,* chickenpox pneumonia). The symptoms may remain confined to fever, headache, and muscle aches and pains. Cough, when present, is characteristically dry, hacking, and nonproductive. The diagnosis is usually made based on history, physical findings, and chest radiographs.

Tuberculosis

Tuberculosis is the world's foremost cause of death from a single infectious agent. It is estimated that each year more than 8 million new cases of tuberculosis occur worldwide and approximately 2 million persons die of the disease.[40–43] In the United States, there were approximately 15,000 new cases and 750 deaths attributed to tuberculosis in 2003.[40] With the introduction of antibiotics in the 1950s, the United States and other Western countries enjoyed a long decline in the number of infections until the mid-1980s. Since that time, the rate of infection has increased, particularly among HIV-infected people. In the United States, the biggest increase in new cases was from 1985 to 1993, after which the rate of cases reported yearly has again declined. In part, this decline reflects the impact of resources committed to assist state and local control efforts, wider screening and prevention programs, and increased support for prevention programs among HIV-infected persons. Tuberculosis is more common among foreign-born persons from countries with a high incidence of tuberculosis and among residents of high-risk congregate settings such as correctional facilities, drug treatment facilities, and homeless shelters. Outbreaks of a drug-resistant form of tuberculosis have emerged, complicating the selection of drugs and affecting the duration of treatment.

Tuberculosis is an infectious disease caused by the mycobacterium, *M. tuberculosis.* The mycobacteria are slender, rod-shaped, aerobic bacteria that do not form spores (Fig. 28-6). They are similar to other bacterial organisms except for an outer

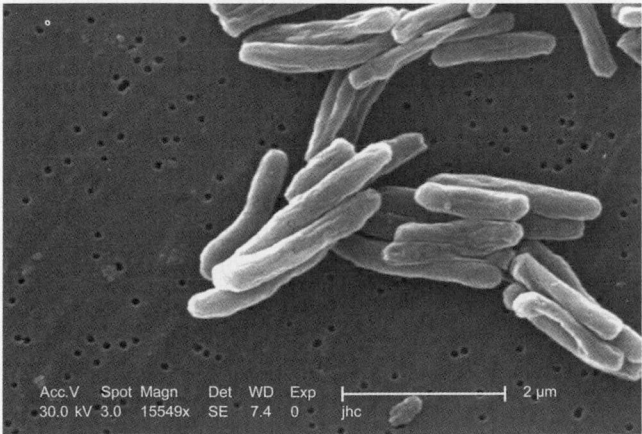

FIGURE 28-6 • Scanning electron micrograph (SEM) depicting some of the ultrastructural details seen in the cell wall configuration of a number of gram-positive *Mycobacterium tuberculosis* bacteria. (Courtesy Public Image Library, Centers for Disease Control and Prevention. [Online.] Available: http://phil.cdc.gov/phil/home.asp.)

waxy capsule that makes them more resistant to destruction; the organism can persist in old necrotic and calcified lesions and remain capable of reinitiating growth. The waxy coat also causes the organism to retain red dye when treated with acid in acid-fast staining.[15,44] Thus, the mycobacteria are often referred to as *acid-fast bacilli.* Although *M. tuberculosis* can infect practically any organ of the body, the lungs are most frequently involved. The tubercle bacilli are strict aerobes that thrive in an oxygen-rich environment. This explains their tendency to cause disease in the upper lobe or upper parts of the lower lobe of the lung, where the ventilation and oxygen content are greatest.

Two forms of tuberculosis pose a particular threat to humans: those caused by *M. tuberculosis hominis* (human tuberculosis) and *M. tuberculosis bovis* (bovine tuberculosis). Bovine tuberculosis is acquired by drinking milk from infected cows, and it initially affects the gastrointestinal tract. This form of tuberculosis has been virtually eradicated in North America and other developed countries as a result of rigorous controls on dairy herds and the pasteurization of milk.[15] Other mycobacteria, including *Mycobacterium avium-intracellulare* complex, are much less virulent than *M. tuberculosis hominis* and *M. tuberculosis bovis* and rarely cause disease except in severely immunosuppressed persons, such as those with HIV infection.[15]

M. tuberculosis hominis is an airborne infection spread by minute, invisible particles, called *droplet nuclei,* that are harbored in the respiratory secretions of persons with active tuberculosis. Coughing, sneezing, and talking all create respiratory droplets; these droplets evaporate, leaving the organisms (droplet nuclei), which remain suspended in the air and are circulated by air currents. Thus, living under crowded and confined conditions increases the risk for spread of the disease.

Pathogenesis

The pathogenesis of tuberculosis in a previously unexposed immunocompetent person is centered on the development of a cell-mediated immune response that confers resistance to the organism and development of tissue hypersensitivity to the tubercular antigens.[15,44] The destructive features of the disease, such as caseating necrosis and cavitation, result from the hypersensitivity immune response rather than the destructive capabilities of the tubercle bacillus.

Macrophages are the primary cell infected with *M. tuberculosis.* Inhaled droplet nuclei pass down the bronchial tree without settling on the epithelium and are deposited in the alveoli. Soon after entering the lung, the bacilli are phagocytosed by alveolar macrophages but resist killing, apparently because cell wall lipids of *M. tuberculosis* block fusion of phagosomes and lysosomes (see Chapter 18, Fig. 18-3). Although the macrophages that first ingest *M. tuberculosis* cannot kill the organisms, they initiate a cell-mediated immune response that eventually contains the infection. As the tubercle bacilli multiply, the infected macrophages degrade the mycobacteria and present their antigens to T lymphocytes. The sensitized T lymphocytes, in turn, stimulate the macrophages to increase their concentration of lytic enzymes and ability to kill the mycobac-

TUBERCULOSIS

- Tuberculosis is an infectious disease caused by *Mycobacterium tuberculosis,* a rod-shaped, aerobic bacterium that is resistant to destruction and can persist in necrotic and calcified lesions for prolonged periods and remain capable of reinstating growth.

- The organism is spread by inhaling the mycobacterium-containing droplet nuclei that circulate in the air. Overcrowded living conditions increase the risk of tuberculosis spread.

- The tubercle bacillus has no known antigens to stimulate an early immunoglobulin response; instead, the host mounts a delayed-type cell-mediated immune response.

- The cell-mediated response plays a dominant role in walling off the tubercle bacilli and preventing the development of active tuberculosis. People with impaired cell-mediated immunity are more likely to develop active tuberculosis when infected.

- A positive tuberculin skin test results from a cell-mediated immune response and implies that a person has been infected with *M. tuberculosis* and has mounted a cell-mediated immune response. It does not mean that the person has active tuberculosis.

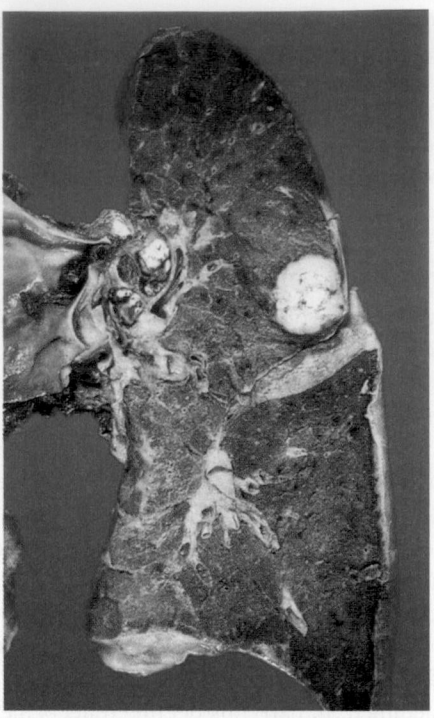

FIGURE 28-7 • Primary tuberculosis. A healed Ghon complex is represented by a subpleural nodule and involved hilar lymph nodes. (From Beasley M. B., Travis W. D., Rubin E. [2008]. The respiratory system. In Rubin R., Strayer D. S. [Eds.], *Rubin's pathology: Clinicopathologic foundations of medicine* [5th ed., p. 496]. Philadelphia: Lippincott Williams & Wilkins.)

teria. When released, these lytic enzymes also damage lung tissue. The development of a population of activated T lymphocytes and related development of activated macrophages capable of ingesting and destroying the bacilli constitutes the cell-mediated immune response, a process that takes about 3 to 6 weeks to become effective.

In persons with intact cell-mediated immunity, the cell-mediated immune response results in the development of a gray-white, circumscribed granulomatous lesion, called a *Ghon focus,* that contains the tubercle bacilli, modified macrophages, and other immune cells.[15,44] It is usually located in the subpleural area of the upper segments of the lower lobes or in the lower segments of the upper lobe. When the number of organisms is high, the hypersensitivity reaction produces significant tissue necrosis, causing the central portion of the Ghon focus to undergo soft, caseous (cheeselike) necrosis. During this same period, tubercle bacilli, free or inside macrophages, drain along the lymph channels to the tracheobronchial lymph nodes of the affected lung and there evoke the formation of caseous granulomas. The combination of the primary lung lesion and lymph node granulomas is called a *Ghon complex* (Fig. 28-7). The Ghon complex eventually heals, undergoing shrinkage, fibrous scarring, and calcification, the latter visible radiographically. However, small numbers of organisms may remain viable for years. Later, if immune mechanisms decline or fail, latent tuberculosis infection has the potential to develop into secondary tuberculosis.

Primary Tuberculosis

Primary tuberculosis is a form of the disease that develops in previously unexposed, and therefore unsensitized persons. It typically is initiated as a result of inhaling droplet nuclei that contain the tubercle bacillus (Fig. 28-8). Most people with primary tuberculosis go on to develop *latent infection* in which T lymphocytes and macrophages surround the organism in granulomas that limit their spread.[15,44] Individuals with latent tuberculosis do not have active disease and cannot transmit the organism to others.

In approximately 5% of newly infected people, the immune response is inadequate; these people go on to develop progressive primary tuberculosis with continued destruction of lung tissue and spread to multiple sites within the lung.[15] People with HIV infection and others with disorders of cell-mediated immunity are more likely to develop progressive tuberculosis if they become infected. In those who develop progressive disease, the symptoms are usually insidious and nonspecific, with fever, weight loss, fatigue, and night sweats.[42,44] Sometimes the onset of symptoms is abrupt, with high fever, pleuritis, and lymphadenitis. As the disease spreads, the organism gains access to the sputum, allowing the person to infect others.

In rare instances, tuberculosis may erode into a blood vessel, giving rise to hematogenic dissemination. *Miliary tuberculosis* describes minute lesions, resembling millet seeds, resulting

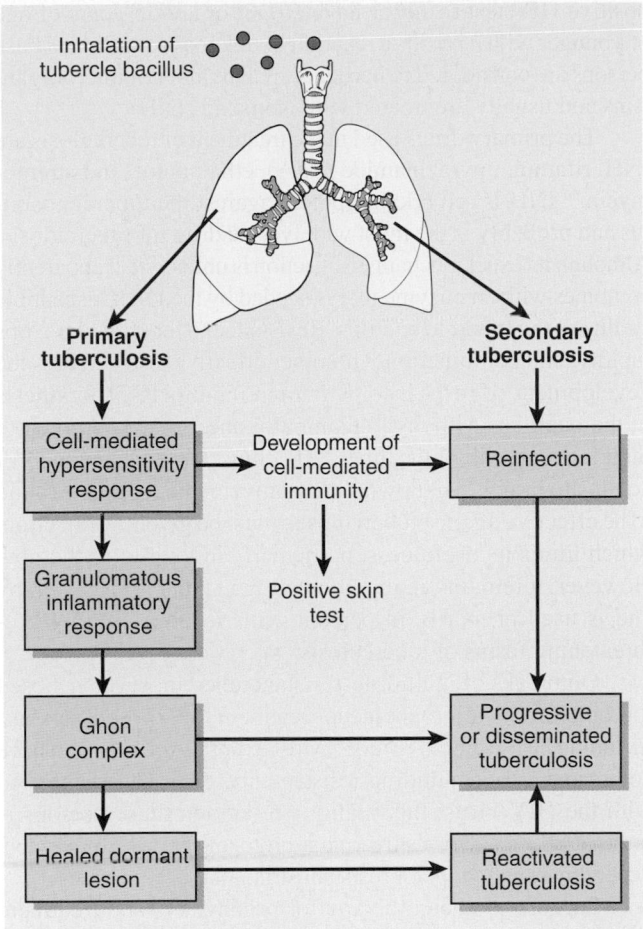

FIGURE 28-8 • Pathogenesis of tuberculosis infection.

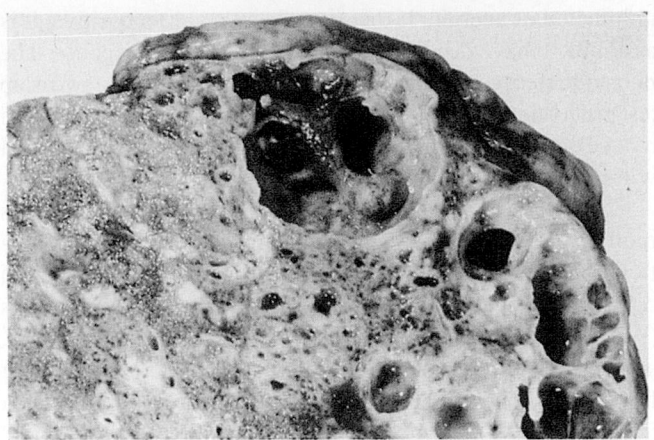

FIGURE 28-9 • Cavitary tuberculosis in the apex of the left upper lobe of the lung. (From Beasley M. B., Travis W. D., Rubin E. [2008]. The respiratory system. In Rubin R., Strayer D. S. [Eds.], *Rubin's pathology: Clinicopathologic foundations of medicine* [5th ed., p. 496]. Philadelphia: Lippincott Williams & Wilkins.)

Diagnosis

The most frequently used screening methods for pulmonary tuberculosis are the tuberculin skin tests and chest radiographic studies. The tuberculin skin test measures the delayed hypersensitivity (*i.e.,* cell-mediated, type IV) that follows exposure to the tubercle bacillus. Persons who become tuberculin positive usually remain so for the remainder of their lives. A positive reaction to the skin test does not mean that a person has active tuberculosis, only that there has been exposure to the bacillus and that cell-mediated immunity to the organism has developed. False-positive and false-negative skin test reactions can occur. False-positive reactions often result from cross-reactions with nontuberculosis mycobacteria, such as *M. avium-intracellulare* complex.[45] Because the hypersensitivity response to the tuberculin test depends on cell-mediated immunity, a false-negative test result can occur because of immunodeficiency states that result from HIV infection, immunosuppressive therapy, lymphoreticular malignancies, or aging. This is called *anergy.* In the immunocompromised person, a negative tuberculin test result can mean that the person has a true lack of exposure to tuberculosis or is unable to mount an immune response to the test. Because of the problem with anergy in persons with HIV infection and other immunocompromised states, the use of control tests is recommended. Three antigens that can be used for control testing are *Candida,* mumps virus, and tetanus toxoid. Most people have been exposed to the antigens used in these control tests; therefore, persons with a healthy immune system will respond with a positive test result and those with anergy will be unable to respond.[45]

A two-step testing procedure, which uses a "boosting" phenomenon, may be used to increase the reaction to a subsequent tuberculin test in persons who have been infected with tuberculosis.[40,45] If the first test result of the two-step procedure is negative, a second test is administered 1 week later. If the second test result is negative, the person is considered to be

from this type of dissemination that can involve almost any organ, particularly the brain, meninges, liver, kidney, and bone marrow.

Secondary Tuberculosis

Secondary tuberculosis represents either reinfection from inhaled droplet nuclei or reactivation of a previously healed primary lesion[15,44] (see Fig. 28-8). It often occurs in situations of impaired body defense mechanisms. The partial immunity that follows primary tuberculosis affords protection against reinfection and to some extent aids in localizing the disease should reactivation occur. In secondary tuberculosis, the cell-mediated hypersensitivity reaction can be an aggravating factor, as evidenced by the frequency of cavitation and bronchial dissemination. The cavities may coalesce to a size of up to 10 to 15 cm in diameter[15,44] (Fig. 28-9). Pleural effusion and tuberculous empyema are common as the disease progresses.

Persons with secondary tuberculosis commonly present with low-grade fevers, night sweats, easy fatigability, anorexia, and weight loss.[44] A cough initially is dry but later becomes productive with purulent and sometimes blood-tinged sputum. Dyspnea and orthopnea develop as the disease advances.

uninfected or anergic. If the second test result is positive, it is assumed to have occurred because of a boosted response. The boosted effect can last for 1 year or longer. Use of the two-step test procedure for employee health or institutional screening can reduce the likelihood that a boosted response in a subsequent test will not be interpreted as a recent infection.

Definitive diagnosis of active pulmonary tuberculosis requires identification of the organism from cultures or identification of the organism from deoxyribonucleic acid (DNA) or RNA amplification techniques.[46–48] Bacteriologic studies (*i.e.,* acid-fast stain and cultures) of early sputum specimens, gastric aspirations, or bronchial washings obtained during fiberoptic bronchoscopy may be used. Cultures of solid media to identify *M. tuberculosis* may take up to 12 weeks. Liquid medium culture systems allow for detection of mycobacterial growth in several days. Once mycobacteria have been grown in culture, nucleic acid probes or high-performance liquid chromatography can be used to identify the species within hours. Genotyping can be done to identify different strains of *M. tuberculosis*. It can be used to evaluate second episodes of tuberculosis to determine whether the second episode was due to relapse or reinfection. Genotyping also permits the evaluation of isolates with different patterns of drug susceptibility.[46] In addition, genotyping is useful in investigating outbreaks of infection and determining sites and patterns of *M. tuberculosis* transmission in communities.

Treatment

The goals of treatment are to eliminate all tubercle bacilli from an infected person while avoiding emergence of significant drug resistance. Treatment of active tuberculosis requires the use of multiple drugs.[49,50] Tuberculosis is an unusual disease in that chemotherapy is required for a relatively long period. The tubercle bacillus is an aerobic organism that multiplies slowly and remains relatively dormant in oxygen-poor caseous material. It undergoes a high rate of mutation and tends to acquire resistance to any one drug. For this reason, multidrug regimens are used for treating persons with active tuberculosis. Drug susceptibility tests are used to guide treatment in drug-resistant forms of the disease.

Two groups meet the criteria established for the use of antimycobacterial therapy for tuberculosis: persons with active tuberculosis and those who have had contact with cases of active tuberculosis and who are at risk for development of an active form of the disease. Prophylactic treatment is used for persons who are infected with *M. tuberculosis* but do not have active disease.[50] This group includes persons with a positive skin test result who have had close contact with active cases of tuberculosis; have converted from a negative to positive skin test result within 2 years; have a history of untreated or inadequately treated tuberculosis; have chest radiographs with evidence of tuberculosis but no bacteriologic evidence of the active disease; have special risk factors such as silicosis, diabetes mellitus, prolonged corticosteroid therapy, immunosuppression therapy, end-stage renal disease, chronic malnutrition from any cause, or hematologic or reticuloendothelial cancers; have a

positive HIV test result or have AIDS; or are 35 years of age or younger with a positive reaction of unknown duration. These persons are considered to harbor a small number of microorganisms and usually are treated with isoniazid (INH).

The primary drugs used in the treatment of tuberculosis are INH, rifampin, pyrazinamide (PZA), ethambutol, and streptomycin.[50] INH is remarkably potent against the tubercle bacillus and probably is the most widely used drug for tuberculosis. Although its exact mechanism of action is unknown, it apparently combines with an enzyme that is needed by the INH-susceptible strains of the tubercle bacillus. Resistance to the drug develops rapidly, and combination with other effective drugs delays the development of resistance. Rifampin inhibits RNA synthesis in the bacillus. Although ethambutol and PZA are known to inhibit the growth of the tubercle bacillus, their mechanisms of action are largely unknown. Streptomycin, the first drug found to be effective against tuberculosis, must be given by injection, which limits its usefulness, particularly in long-term therapy. However, it remains an important drug in tuberculosis therapy and is used primarily in persons with severe, possibly life-threatening forms of tuberculosis.

Outbreaks of multidrug-resistant tuberculosis have posed a problem for the prophylactic treatment of exposed persons, including health care workers.[51] Most exposed persons who have contracted active multidrug-resistant tuberculosis were infected with the HIV virus; the fatality rate among these persons is high, at 80%.[52] Various treatment protocols are recommended, depending on the type of resistant strain that is identified.

Success of chemotherapy for prophylaxis and treatment of tuberculosis depends on strict adherence to a lengthy drug regimen. This often is a problem, particularly for persons with asymptomatic tuberculosis infections and for poorly motivated groups such as intravenous drug users. Directly observed therapy, which requires that a health care worker observe while the person takes the antituberculosis drug, is recommended for some persons and for some types of treatment protocols.[51]

First administered to humans in 1921, the bacillus Calmette-Guérin (BCG) vaccine is used to prevent the development of tuberculosis in persons who are at high risk for infection. BCG is an attenuated strain of *M. tuberculosis bovis*.[53] It is administered only to persons who have a negative tuberculin skin test result. The vaccine, which is given intradermally, produces a local reaction that can last as long as 3 months and may result in scarring at the injection site. Persons who have been vaccinated with BCG usually have a positive tuberculin skin test result that wanes with time and is unlikely to persist beyond 10 years.

Today, more than 70 years after its development, BCG remains the only tuberculosis vaccine available. Currently, several candidate vaccines are being prepared or are already in the early stages of human testing. Worldwide, BCG is currently used as a major method of prevention for tuberculosis. However, it is not generally recommended in the United States because of the low prevalence of tuberculosis infection, the vaccine's interference with the ability to determine latent tuberculosis with skin tests, and variable effectiveness against pulmonary tuberculosis.[54] Vaccination of health care workers may be considered on an individual basis in settings where patients are infected with drug-resistant strains of tuberculosis.

Fungal Infections

Fungi are classified as yeasts and molds. Yeasts are round and grow by budding. Molds form tubular structures called *hyphae* and grow by branching and forming spores (see Chapter 16). Some fungi are *dimorphic,* meaning that they grow as yeasts at body temperatures and as molds at room temperatures. A simple classification of mycoses or diseases caused by fungi divides them into superficial, cutaneous, subcutaneous, or deep (systemic) mycoses. The superficial, cutaneous, or subcutaneous mycoses cause disease of the skin, hair, and nails (discussed in Chapter 61). Deep fungal infections may produce pulmonary and systemic infections and are sometimes fatal. They are caused by virulent fungi that live free in nature or soil or in decaying organic matter and are frequently limited to certain geographic regions. The most common of these are the dimorphic fungi, which include *Histoplasma capsulatum* (histoplasmosis), *Coccidioides immitis* (coccidioidomycosis), and *Blastomyces dermatitidis* (blastomycosis). These fungi form infectious spores, which enter the body through the respiratory system. Most people who become infected with these fungi develop only minor symptoms or none at all; only a small minority develops serious disease.

The host's cell-mediated immune response is paramount in controlling such infections. Pathologic fungi generally produce no toxins. In the host, they induce a delayed cell-mediated hypersensitivity response to their chemical constituents (see Chapter 19). Cellular immunity is mediated by antigen-specific T lymphocytes and cytokine-activated macrophages that assume fungicidal properties. The primary pulmonary lesions consist of aggregates of macrophages stuffed with organisms, with similar lesions developing in the lymph nodes that drain the area. These lesions develop into granulomas complete with giant cells and may develop central necrosis and calcification resembling that of primary tuberculosis.

Although most fungal infections are asymptomatic, they can be severe or even fatal in persons who have experienced a heavy exposure, have underlying immune deficiencies, or develop progressive disease that is not recognized or treated. Immunocompromised persons, particularly those with HIV infection, are particularly prone to development of disseminated infection.

Histoplasmosis

Histoplasmosis is caused by the dimorphic fungus *H. capsulatum* and is one of the most common fungal infections in the United States. Most cases occur along the major river valleys of the Midwest—the Ohio, the Mississippi, and the Missouri.[55,56] The organism grows in soil and other areas that have been enriched with bird excreta: old chicken houses, pigeon lofts, barns, and trees where birds roost. Many caves also contain enormous numbers of *H. capsulatum* growing in bat guano.[56] The infection is acquired by inhaling the fungal spores that are released when the dirt or dust from the infected areas is disturbed. The spores convert to the parasitic yeast phase when exposed to body temperature in the alveoli. They are then carried to the regional lymphatics and from there are disseminated throughout the body in the bloodstream. Dissemination occurs during the first several weeks of infection before specific immunity has developed. After 2 to 3 weeks, cellular immunity develops, establishing the body's ability to control the infection.

Depending on the host's resistance and immunocompetence, the disease usually takes one of four forms: (1) latent asymptomatic disease, (2) self-limited primary disease, (3) chronic pulmonary disease, or (4) disseminated infection. The average incubation period for the infection is approximately 14 days. Most persons with *H. capsulatum* infection remain asymptomatic or have mild respiratory illness that is not diagnosed as histoplasmosis. Latent asymptomatic histoplasmosis is characterized by evidence of healed lesions in the lungs or hilar lymph nodes. Primary pulmonary histoplasmosis occurs in otherwise healthy persons as a mild, self-limited, febrile respiratory infection. Its symptoms include muscle and joint pains and a nonproductive cough. Erythema nodosum (*i.e.,* subcutaneous nodules) or erythema multiforme (*i.e.,* hivelike lesions) sometimes appears. During this stage of the disease, chest radiographs usually show single or multiple infiltrates.

Chronic histoplasmosis resembles reactivation tuberculosis. Infiltration of the upper lobes of one or both lungs occurs with cavitation. This form of the disease is more common in middle-aged men who smoke and in persons with chronic lung disease. The most common manifestations are a productive cough, fever, night sweats, and weight loss. In many persons, the disease is self-limited. In others, there is progressive destruction of lung tissue and dissemination of the disease.

Disseminated histoplasmosis can follow primary or chronic histoplasmosis but most often develops as an acute and fulminating infection in the very old or the very young or in persons who are immunocompromised, including persons who have undergone transplantations, those with hematologic malignancies, and persons with AIDS. Although the macrophages of the reticuloendothelial system can remove the fungi from the bloodstream, they are unable to destroy them. Characteristically, this form of the disease produces a high fever, generalized lymph node enlargement, hepatosplenomegaly, muscle wasting, anemia, leukopenia, and thrombocytopenia. There may be hoarseness, ulcerations of the mouth and tongue, nausea, vomiting, diarrhea, and abdominal pain. Often, meningitis becomes a dominant feature of the disease.

A number of laboratory tests, including cultures, fungal stain, antigen detection, and serologic tests for antibodies, are used in the diagnosis of histoplasmosis. The type of test that is used depends on the type of involvement that is present. In pulmonary disease, sputum culture is rarely positive, whereas blood or bone marrow cultures from immunocompromised people with acute disseminated disease are positive in 80% to 90% of cases. Antigen tests can be performed on blood, urine, cerebrospinal fluid, or bronchoalveolar lavage fluid. A urine antigen assay is particularly useful in detecting disseminated histoplasmosis.

The antifungal drug, itraconazole, usually is the drug of choice for treatment of persons with disease severe enough to require treatment or those with compromised immune function who are at risk for the development of disseminated disease.[55,56] Amphotericin B, which is administered intravenously, usually is the drug of choice in severe disease. Persons with HIV-related histoplasmosis usually require lifelong suppression therapy with itraconazole.

Coccidioidomycosis

Coccidioidomycosis is a common fungal infection caused by inhaling the spores of *C. immitis*.[57–59] The disease resembles tuberculosis, and its mechanisms of infection are similar to those of histoplasmosis. It is most prevalent in the southwestern United States, principally in parts of California, Arizona, Nevada, New Mexico, and Texas. Because of its prevalence in the San Joaquin Valley, the disease is sometimes referred to as *San Joaquin fever* or *valley fever*. The *C. immitis* organism lives in soil and can establish new sites in the soil. Events such as dust storms and digging for construction have been associated with increased incidence of the disease.

The disease most commonly occurs as an acute, primary, self-limited pulmonary infection with or without systemic involvement, but in some cases it progresses to a disseminated disease. The incubation period is 10 to 30 days. About 40% of infected persons develop symptoms of primary coccidioidomycosis. The symptoms are usually those of a respiratory tract infection with fever, cough, and pleuritic pain. Erythema nodosum may occur 2 to 20 days after onset of symptoms. The skin lesions usually are accompanied by arthralgias or arthritis without effusion, particularly of the ankles and knees. The terms *desert bumps* and *desert arthritis* are used to describe these manifestations. The presence of skin and joint manifestations indicates strong host defenses because persons who have had such manifestations seldom acquire disseminated disease.

Disseminated disease occurs in approximately 0.5% to 1% of infected persons. Commonly affected structures in disseminated disease are the lymph nodes, meninges, spleen, liver, kidney, skin, and adrenal glands. Meningitis is the most common cause of death. Persons with diabetes or compromised immune function, infants, and members of dark-skinned races tend to localize the disease poorly and are at higher risk for disseminated disease. In HIV-infected persons in endemic areas, coccidioidomycosis is now a common opportunistic infection.

Radiologic studies, including chest radiographic studies and bone scans, are useful in determining disease but cannot distinguish coccidioidomycosis from other pulmonary diseases. A definitive diagnosis requires microscopic or serologic evidence that *C. immitis* is present in body tissues or fluids. *C. immitis* spherules can be visualized in specially stained biopsy specimens. Serologic tests can be done for immunoglobulin M (IgM) and IgG antibody detection.

Treatment depends on the severity of infection. Persons without associated risk factors such as HIV infection or without specific evidence of progressive disease usually can be managed without antifungal therapy. The oral antifungal drugs itraconazole and fluconazole are used for treatment of less severe forms of infection. Intravenous amphotericin B is used in the treatment of persons with progressive disease. Long-term treatment is often required.

Blastomycosis

Blastomycosis is a fungal infection caused by inhaling the spores of *B. dermatitidis*. The disease is most commonly found in the southern and north central United States, especially in areas bordering the Mississippi and Ohio River basins and the Great Lakes.[55,60] *B. dermatitidis* is most commonly found in soil containing decayed vegetation or decomposed wood. The disease occurs most often in men infected during occupational or recreational outdoor activities.

The infection is characterized by local suppurative (pus-forming) and granulomatous lesions of the lungs and skin. The symptoms of acute infection, which are similar to those of acute histoplasmosis, include fever, cough, aching joints and muscles, and, uncommonly, pleuritic pain. In contrast to histoplasmosis, the cough in blastomycosis often is productive, and the sputum is purulent. Acute pulmonary infections may be self-limited or progressive. In persons with overwhelming pulmonary disease, diffuse interalveolar infiltrates and evidence of acute respiratory distress syndrome may develop (see Chapter 29). Extrapulmonary spread most commonly involves the skin, bones, or prostate. These lesions may provide the first evidence of the disease.

The definitive diagnostic test for *B. dermatitidis* infection is growth of the organism from sputum, tissue biopsy, or body fluid. It generally takes several weeks to grow in mold phase at room temperature. Once growth has occurred, laboratories that use the highly specific and sensitive DNA probe for *B. dermatitidis* can rapidly identify the organism.

Treatment of the progressive or disseminated form of the disease includes the use of itraconazole or amphotericin B.[55,60] Most persons with blastomycosis are identified and treated before the development of overwhelming or fatal disease.

> **IN SUMMARY,** respiratory infections are the most common cause of respiratory illness. They include the common cold, influenza, pneumonias, tuberculosis, and fungal infections. The common cold occurs more frequently than any other respiratory infection. The fingers are the usual source of transmission, and the most common portals of entry are the nasal mucosa and the conjunctiva of the eye. The influenza virus causes three syndromes: an uncomplicated rhinotracheitis, a respiratory viral infection followed by a bacterial infection, and viral pneumonia. The contagiousness of influenza results from the ability of the virus to mutate and form subtypes against which the population is unprotected.
>
> Pneumonia describes an infection of the parenchymal tissues of the lung. Loss of the cough reflex, damage to the

ciliated endothelium that lines the respiratory tract, or impaired immune defenses predispose to pneumonia. Pneumonia can be classified according to the type of organism causing the infection (typical or atypical), location of the infection (lobar pneumonia or bronchopneumonia), and setting in which it occurs (community- or hospital-acquired). Persons with compromised immune function constitute a special concern in both categories. Community-acquired pneumonia involves infections from organisms that are present more often in the community than in the hospital or nursing home. The most common cause of community-acquired pneumonia is *S. pneumoniae.* Hospital-acquired (nosocomial) pneumonia is defined as a lower respiratory tract infection occurring 48 hours or more after admission. Hospital-acquired pneumonia is the second most common cause of hospital-acquired infection. Acute typical pneumonias, including *S. pneumoniae* and *L. pneumophila* pneumonia, are caused by organisms that multiply extracellularly in the alveoli and cause inflammation and transudation of fluid into the air-filled spaces of the alveoli. Atypical pneumonias are caused by a variety of agents, including *M. pneumoniae* and viruses that invade the alveolar septum and interstitium of the lung.

Tuberculosis is a chronic respiratory infection caused by *M. tuberculosis,* which is spread by minute, invisible particles called *droplet nuclei.* Tuberculosis is a particular threat among HIV-infected persons, foreign-born persons from countries with a high incidence of tuberculosis, and residents of high-risk congregate settings such as correctional facilities, drug treatment facilities, and homeless shelters. The tubercle bacillus incites a distinctive chronic inflammatory response referred to as *granulomatous inflammation.* The destructiveness of the disease results from the cell-mediated hypersensitivity response that the bacillus evokes rather than its inherent destructive capabilities. Cell-mediated immunity and hypersensitivity reactions contribute to the evolution of the disease. The treatment of tuberculosis has been complicated by outbreaks of drug-resistant forms of the disease.

Infections caused by the fungi *H. capsulatum* (histoplasmosis), *C. immitis* (coccidioidomycosis), and *B. dermatitidis* (blastomycosis) produce pulmonary manifestations that resemble tuberculosis. These infections are common but seldom serious unless they produce progressive destruction of lung tissue or the infection disseminates to organs and tissues outside the lungs. ■

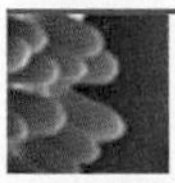

CANCER OF THE LUNG

After completing this section of the chapter, you should be able to meet the following objectives:

- Cite risk factors associated with lung cancer.
- Compare small cell lung cancer and non–small cell lung cancer in terms of histopathology, prognosis, and treatment methods.
- Describe the manifestations of lung cancer and list two symptoms of lung cancer that are related to the invasion of the mediastinum.
- Define the term *paraneoplastic* and cite three paraneoplastic manifestations of lung cancer.
- Characterize the effect of age on treatment of lung cancer.

Lung cancer is the leading cause of cancer death among men and women in the United States.[61–63] The American Cancer Society estimates there were 213,380 new diagnoses and 160,390 deaths from lung cancer in the United States in 2007, accounting for approximately 15% of cancer diagnoses and 29% of all cancer deaths.[61] Because smoking tobacco accounts for the majority of cases of lung cancer, this cancer is largely preventable.[61] The number of Americans who develop lung cancer is decreasing, primarily because of a decrease in smoking over the past 30 years.[61] However, smoking among teens and preteens has increased in recent years, raising the potential for increased rates of lung cancer in the future. Because lung cancer usually is far advanced before it is discovered, the prognosis in general is poor. The overall 5-year survival rate for all stages combined is 16%, a dismal statistic that has not changed since the late 1960s.[61]

Cigarette smoking causes more that 80% of cases of lung cancer. The risk for lung cancer among cigarette smokers increases with duration of smoking and the number of cigarettes smoked per day. Cigarette smokers can benefit at any age from smoking cessation. However, even for periods of abstinence greater than 40 years, the risk for lung cancer among former smokers remains elevated compared with that of nonsmokers.[63,64] Industrial hazards also contribute to the incidence of lung cancer. A commonly recognized hazard is exposure to asbestos, with the mean risk for lung cancer being significantly greater in asbestos workers than in the general population. Tobacco smoke contributes heavily to the development of lung cancer in persons exposed to asbestos; the risk in this population group is estimated to be 60 to 90 times greater than that for nonsmokers.[63] There is also evidence to suggest a familial predisposition to lung cancer. This occurrence may be due to a genetic predisposition, with the trait being expressed only in the presence of its major predisposing factor—cigarette smoking.[63]

Histologic Subtypes and Pathogenesis

Most (about 95%) primary lung tumors are carcinomas that arise from the lung tissue.[15] The remaining 5% are a miscellaneous group that includes bronchial carcinoid tumors (neuroendocrine tumors), bronchial gland tumors, fibrosarcomas, and lymphomas. The lung is also a frequent site of metastasis from cancers in other parts of the body.

Lung cancers are aggressive, locally invasive, and widely metastatic tumors that arise from the epithelial lining of major bronchi. These tumors begin as small mucosal lesions that may follow one of several patterns of growth. They may form intra-luminal masses that invade the bronchial mucosa and infiltrate the peribronchial connective tissue, or they may form large, bulky masses that extend into the adjacent lung tissue. Some large tumors undergo central necrosis and acquire local areas of hemorrhage, and some invade the pleural cavity and chest wall and spread to adjacent intrathoracic structures.[15] All types of lung cancer, especially small cell lung carcinoma, have the capacity to synthesize bioactive products and produce para-neoplastic syndromes.

Lung cancer is commonly subdivided into four major cat-egories: squamous cell lung carcinoma (25% to 40%), adeno-carcinoma (20% to 40%), small cell carcinoma (20% to 25%), and large cell carcinoma (10% to 15%).[15] For purposes of staging and treatment, lung cancers are commonly identified as small cell lung cancer (SCLC) or non–small cell lung cancer (NSCLC).[15] The key reason for this classification is that most SCLCs have metastasized by the time of diagnosis and hence are not amenable to cancer surgery. They are usually best treated with chemotherapy, with or without radiation.

Small Cell Lung Cancers

The SCLCs are characterized by a distinctive cell type—small round to oval cells that are approximately the size of a lym-phocyte.[15,65] The cells grow in clusters that exhibit neither glan-dular nor squamous organization. Electron microscopic studies demonstrate the presence of neurosecretory granules in some of the tumor cells similar to those found in the bronchial epithe-lium of the fetus or neonate.[15] The presence of these granules suggests the ability of some of these tumors to secrete polypep-tide hormones, and the presence of neuroendocrine markers such as neuron-specific enolase and parathormone-like and other hormonally active products suggest that these tumors may arise from the neuroendocrine cells of the bronchial epithelium. This cell type has the strongest association with cigarette smoking and is rarely observed in someone who has not smoked.[65–67]

The SCLCs are highly malignant, tend to infiltrate widely, disseminate early in their course, and rarely are resectable. About 70% have detectable metastases at the time of diagnosis[66]; the rest are assumed to have micrometastases. Brain metastases are particularly common with SCLC and may provide the first evidence of the tumor. Without treatment, one half of persons with SCLC die within 12 to 15 weeks.

This type of lung cancer is associated with several types of paraneoplastic syndrome, including the syndrome of inappro-priate antidiuretic hormone secretion (SIADH; see Chapter 31), Cushing syndrome associated with ectopic production of adreno-corticotropic hormone (ACTH; see Chapter 41), and the Eaton-Lambert syndrome of neuromuscular disorder (see Chapter 8).

Non–Small Cell Lung Cancers

The NSCLCs include squamous cell carcinomas, adenocarci-nomas, and large cell carcinomas. Like the SCLCs, these cancers

have the capacity to synthesize bioactive products and produce paraneoplastic syndromes.

Squamous Cell Carcinoma. Squamous cell carcinoma is found most commonly in men and is closely correlated with a smoking history. Squamous cell carcinoma tends to originate in the cen-tral bronchi as an intraluminal growth and is thus more amenable to early detection through cytologic examination of the sputum than other forms of lung cancer. It tends to spread centrally into major bronchi and hilar lymph nodes and disseminates outside the thorax later than other types of bronchogenic cancers. Squamous cell carcinoma is associated with the paraneoplastic syndromes that produce hypercalcemia.

Adenocarcinoma. Currently, adenocarcinoma is the most com-mon type of lung cancer in North America. Its association with cigarette smoking is weaker than for squamous cell carcinoma. It is the most common type of lung cancer in women and non-smokers. Adenocarcinomas can have their origin in either the bronchiolar or alveolar tissues of the lung. These tumors tend to be located more peripherally than squamous cell sarcomas and sometimes are associated with areas of scarring (Fig. 28-10). The scars may be due to old infarcts, metallic foreign bodies, wounds, and granulomatous infections such as tuberculosis. In general, adenocarcinomas have a poorer stage-for-stage prog-nosis than squamous cell carcinomas.

Large Cell Carcinoma. Large cell carcinomas have large, polygonal cells. They constitute a group of neoplasms that are highly anaplastic and difficult to categorize as squamous cell carcinoma or adenocarcinoma. They tend to occur in the periph-ery of the lung, invading subsegmental bronchi and larger air-

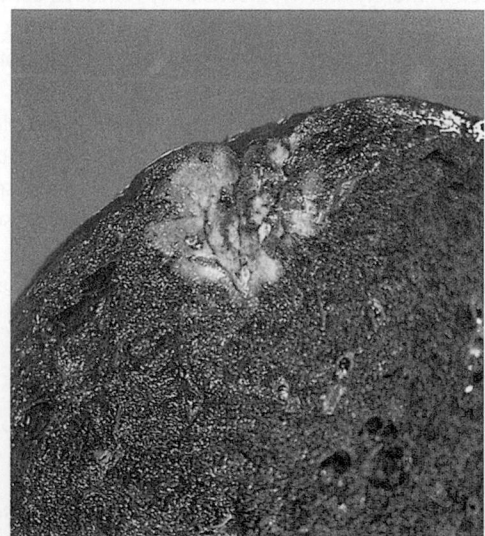

FIGURE 28-10 • Adenocarcinoma of the lung. A peripheral tumor is located in the upper right lobe of the lung. (From Beasley M. B., Travis W. D., Rubin E. [2008]. The respiratory system. In Rubin R., Strayer D. S. [Eds.], *Rubin's pathology: Clinicopathologic foundations of medicine* [5th ed., p. 541]. Philadelphia: Lippincott Williams & Wilkins.)

ways. They have a poor prognosis because of their tendency to spread to distant sites early in their course.

Clinical Features

Manifestations

The manifestations of lung cancer can be divided into three categories: (1) those due to involvement of the lung and adjacent structures; (2) the effects of local spread and metastasis; and (3) nonmetastatic paraneoplastic manifestations involving endocrine, neurologic, and connective tissue function. As with other cancers, lung cancer also causes nonspecific symptoms such as anorexia and weight loss. Because its symptoms are similar to those associated with smoking and chronic bronchitis, they often are disregarded. Metastases already exist in many patients presenting with evidence of lung cancer. The most common sites of these metastases are the brain, bone, and liver.

Many of the manifestations of lung cancers result from local irritation and obstruction of the airways and from invasion of the mediastinum and pleural space. The earliest symptoms usually are chronic cough, shortness of breath, and wheezing because of airway irritation and obstruction. Hemoptysis (*i.e.,* blood in the sputum) occurs when the lesion erodes blood vessels. Pain receptors in the chest are limited to the parietal pleura, mediastinum, larger blood vessels, and peribronchial afferent vagal fibers. Dull, intermittent, poorly localized retrosternal pain is common in tumors that involve the mediastinum. Pain becomes persistent, localized, and more severe when the disease invades the pleura.

Tumors that invade the mediastinum may cause hoarseness because of the involvement of the recurrent laryngeal nerve and cause difficulty in swallowing because of compression of the esophagus. An uncommon complication called the *superior vena cava syndrome* occurs in some persons with mediastinal involvement. Interruption of blood flow in this vessel usually results from compression by the tumor or involved lymph nodes. The disorder can interfere with venous drainage from the head, neck, and chest wall. The outcome is determined by the speed with which the disorder develops and the adequacy of the collateral circulation. Tumors adjacent to the visceral pleura often insidiously produce pleural effusion. This effusion can compress the lung and cause atelectasis and dyspnea. It is less likely to cause fever, pleural friction rub, or pain than pleural effusion resulting from other causes.

Paraneoplastic disorders are those that are unrelated to metastasis (see Chapter 8). These include hypercalcemia from secretion of parathyroid-like peptide, Cushing syndrome from ACTH secretion, SIADH, neuromuscular syndromes (*e.g.,* Eaton-Lambert syndrome), and hematologic disorders (*e.g.,* migratory thrombophlebitis, nonbacterial endocarditis, disseminated intravascular coagulation). Neurologic or muscular symptoms can develop 6 months to 4 years before the lung tumor is detected. One of the more common of these problems is weakness and wasting of the proximal muscles of the pelvic and shoulder girdles, with decreased deep tendon reflexes

but without sensory changes. Hypercalcemia is seen most often in persons with squamous cell carcinoma, hematologic syndromes in persons with adenocarcinomas, and the remaining syndromes in persons with small cell neoplasms. Manifestations of the paraneoplastic syndrome may precede the onset of other signs of lung cancer and may lead to discovery of an occult tumor.

Diagnosis and Treatment

The diagnosis of lung cancer is based on a careful history and physical examination and on other tests such as chest radiography, bronchoscopy, cytologic studies (Papanicolaou [Pap] test) of the sputum or bronchial washings, percutaneous needle biopsy of lung tissue, and scalene lymph node biopsy.[64] CT scans, MRI studies, and ultrasonography are used to locate lesions and evaluate the extent of the disease. Positron emission tomography (PET) is a noninvasive alternative for identifying metastatic lesions in the mediastinum or distant sites. Persons with SCLC should also have a CT scan or MRI of the brain for detection of metastasis.

Like other cancers, lung cancer is classified according to extent of disease. NSCLCs are usually classified according to cell type (*i.e.,* squamous cell carcinoma, adenocarcinoma, and large cell carcinoma) and staged according to the TNM international staging system[15] (see Chapter 8). SCLCs are not staged using the TNM system because micrometastases are assumed to be present at the time of diagnosis. Instead, they are usually classified as limited disease, when the tumor is limited to the unilateral hemithorax, or extensive disease, when it extends beyond these boundaries.[15]

Treatment methods for NSCLC include surgery, radiation therapy, and chemotherapy.[64,68] These treatments may be used singly or in combination. Surgery is used for the removal of small, localized NSCLC tumors. It can involve a lobectomy, pneumonectomy, or segmental resection of the lung. Radiation therapy can be used as a definitive or main treatment modality, as part of a combined treatment plan, or for palliation of symptoms. Because of the frequency of metastases, chemotherapy often is used in treating lung cancer. Combination chemotherapy, which uses a regimen of several drugs, usually is used. New targeted treatments are under development with the goal of increasing survival and ultimately providing a cure for this type of cancer.

Therapy for SCLC is based on chemotherapy and radiation therapy.[64,68] Advances in the use of combination chemotherapy, along with thoracic irradiation, have improved the outlook for persons with SCLC. Because SCLC may metastasize to the brain, prophylactic cranial irradiation is often indicated. In most persons who achieve a complete remission from SCLC, the brain is the most frequent site of relapse. About half of such persons develop clinical metastasis within 3 years. Newer combination chemotherapy regimens and targeted therapies are being developed in hopes of providing treatment alternatives that increase survival and produce fewer treatment liabilities.

Management of Lung Cancer in Older Adults

At the time of diagnosis, most people with lung cancer are older than 65 years of age and have stage III or IV disease.[69] Knowledge about the optimal treatment for older persons is limited because of underrepresentation in clinical trials and failure to evaluate younger versus older persons in randomized clinical trials. At present, it is recommended that the elderly should be treated based on their general physiologic rather than chronologic age. This includes an evaluation of functional status (ability to be independent in daily tasks at home and in the community), coexisting medical conditions, nutritional status, cognition, psychological functioning, social support, and medication review. Those with good performance status and normal renal and hematologic parameters may be treated surgically or receive standard chemoradiation for limited-stage disease and combination chemotherapy for extensive-stage disease.

Surgery remains the mainstay for older persons with stages I to III NSCLC. Curative resection is feasible in older persons. The challenge for surgical treatment for older persons is age-related physiologic changes in cardiovascular and respiratory systems that may affect tolerance of surgery.

Radiation can be given with curative intent for older persons who are not surgical candidates. It may also be used for palliation of cancer-related symptoms. Evidence suggests that treatment tolerance and efficacy of thoracic radiation are similar in younger and older patients. Age is reported to have no effect on acute or late radiation toxicity, including nausea, dyspnea, esophagitis, or weakness. Older patients are more likely, however, to experience weight loss than younger patients.[69]

Chemotherapy is the mainstay of treatment of SCLC. Older persons with good performance status may receive standard chemotherapy for limited disease and combination chemotherapy for extensive-stage disease. Some older persons may require dose reductions or be unable to complete the full chemotherapy course.

IN SUMMARY, cancer of the lung is a leading cause of death worldwide. Cigarette smoking is implicated in the majority of cases of lung cancer. The risk for lung cancer among cigarette smokers increases with duration of smoking and the number of cigarettes smoked per day. Industrial hazards, such as exposure to asbestos, increase the risk for development of lung cancer. Because lung cancer develops insidiously, it often is far advanced before it is diagnosed, a fact that is used to explain the poor 5-year survival rate. Carcinoma, which accounts for 95% of all primary lung cancers, can be subdivided into four major categories: squamous cell carcinoma, adenocarcinoma, large cell carcinoma, and small cell carcinoma. For purposes of staging and treatment, lung cancer is divided into small cell lung cancer and non–small cell lung cancer. The main reason for this is that almost all small cell lung

cancers have metastasized at the time of diagnosis and are not amenable to surgical resection.

The manifestations of lung cancer can be attributed to the involvement of the lung and adjacent structures, the effects of local spread and metastasis, and paraneoplastic syndromes involving endocrine, neurologic, and hematologic dysfunction. As with other cancers, lung cancer causes nonspecific symptoms such as anorexia and weight loss. Treatment methods for lung cancer include surgery, irradiation, and chemotherapy. The current increase in lung cancer among persons 65 years of age and older has required a rethinking of the treatment strategies for this age group, with the trend being to base treatment on physiologic rather than chronologic age. ∎

RESPIRATORY DISORDERS IN CHILDREN

After completing this section of the chapter, you should be able to meet the following objectives:

- Trace the development of the respiratory tract through the five stages of embryonic and fetal development.
- Cite the role of surfactant in lung function in the neonate.
- Cite the possible cause and manifestations of respiratory distress syndrome and bronchopulmonary dysplasia.
- Describe the physiologic basis for sternal and chest wall retractions and grunting, stridor, and wheezing as signs of respiratory distress in infants and small children.
- Compare croup, epiglottitis, and bronchiolitis in terms of incidence by age, site of infection, and signs and symptoms.
- List the signs of impending respiratory failure in small children.

Acute respiratory diseases are the most common cause of illness in infancy and childhood. This section focuses on (1) lung development, with an emphasis on the developmental basis for lung disorders in children; (2) respiratory disorders in the neonate; and (3) respiratory infections in children. A discussion of bronchial asthma in children and cystic fibrosis is included in Chapter 29.

Lung Development

Although other body systems are physiologically ready for extrauterine life as early as 25 weeks of gestation, the lungs require much longer. Immaturity of the respiratory system is a major cause of morbidity and mortality in infants born prematurely. Even at birth, the lungs are not fully mature, and additional growth and maturation continue well into childhood.

Lung development may be divided into five stages: embryonic period, pseudoglandular period, canalicular period, saccular period, and alveolar period[70,71] (Fig. 28-11). The development of the respiratory system begins with the *embryonic period* (weeks 4 to 6 of gestation), during which a rudimentary bronchial bud branches from the esophagus to begin formation of the airways and alveolar spaces. The bronchial bud divides into two lung buds that grow laterally; the right bud gives rise to two secondary bronchial buds and the left bud to one secondary bronchial bud. Consequently, at maturity, there are three main (primary) bronchi and three lung lobes on the right and only two main bronchi and two lung lobes on the left. Each secondary bronchial bud subsequently undergoes continuous branching. The tertiary (segmental) bronchi (10 in the right lung and 8 or 9 in the left lung) begin to form during the seventh week. The pulmonary vasculature is a mesenchymal derivative. Soon after their appearance, the bronchial buds are surrounded by a vascular plexus, which originates from the aorta and drains into the major somatic veins. This vascular plexus connects with the pulmonary artery and veins at the seventh week of gestation.

During the *pseudoglandular period* (weeks 5 to 16), the lungs resemble a gland. During this period, the conducting airways are formed. At 17 weeks, all of the major elements of the lung have formed except the gas exchange structures. Respiration is not possible because the airways end in blind tubes. The *canalicular period* (weeks 17 to 27) marks the formation of the primitive alveoli. The lumina of the bronchi and bronchioles become much larger, and the lung tissue becomes more highly vascularized. By the 24th week, each bronchiole has given rise to two or more respiratory bronchioles. Respiration is possible at this time because some primitive alveoli have developed at the ends of the bronchioles.[71]

The *saccular period* (weeks 27 to 35) is devoted to the development of the terminal alveolar sacs, which facilitate gas exchange. During this period, the terminal sacs thin out, and capillaries begin to bulge into the terminal sacs. These thin cells are known as type I alveolar cells. By the 25th to 28th weeks, sufficient terminal sacs are present to permit survival. Before this time, the premature lungs are incapable of adequate gas exchange. It is not so much the presence of the thin alveolar epithelium as it is the adequate matching of pulmonary vasculature to it that is critical to survival.[71] Type II alveolar cells begin to develop at approximately 24 weeks. These cells produce surfactant, a substance capable of lowering the surface tension of the air–alveoli interface (see Chapter 27). By the 28th to 30th weeks, sufficient amounts of surfactant are available to prevent alveolar collapse when breathing begins.

The *alveolar period* (late fetal to early childhood) marks the maturation and expansion of the alveoli. Starting as early as 30 weeks and usually by 36 weeks of gestation, the saccular structures become alveoli.[70,71] Alveolar development is characterized by thinning of the pulmonary interstitium and the appearance of a single-capillary network, in which one capillary bulges into each terminal alveolar sac. By the late fetal period, the lungs are capable of respiration because the alveolar–capillary membrane is sufficiently thin to allow for gas exchange.

Although transformation of the lungs from glandlike structures to highly vascular, alveoli-like organs occurs during the late fetal period, mature alveoli do not form for some time after birth. The growth of the lung during infancy and early childhood involves an increase in the number rather than the size of the alveoli. Only one eighth to one sixth of the adult number of alveoli is present at birth. There is a relative slowing of alveolar growth during the first 3 months after birth, and this is followed by a rapid increase in alveolar number during the rest of the first year of life, reaching approximately the adult number of 300 million alveoli by 8 years of age.[71]

Development of Breathing in the Fetus and Neonate

The fetal lung is a secretory organ, and fluids and electrolytes are secreted into the potential air spaces. This fluid appears to be important in stimulating alveolar development. For the fetus to complete the transition from intrauterine to extrauterine life, this fluid must be cleared from the lung soon after birth. Presumably with the onset of labor, the secretion of fluid ceases. During the birth process, pressure on the fetal thorax causes the fluid to be expelled from the mouth and nose. When the lungs expand after birth, the fluid moves into the tissues surrounding the alveoli and is then absorbed into the pulmonary capillaries or removed by the lymphatic system.

Fetal breathing movements occur in utero. These movements are irregular in rate and amplitude, ranging from 30 to 70 breaths per minute, and become more rapid as gestation advances. Because they are rapid and shallow, these movements do not result in movement of fluid into or out of the fetal lung. Instead, they are thought to condition the respiratory mus-

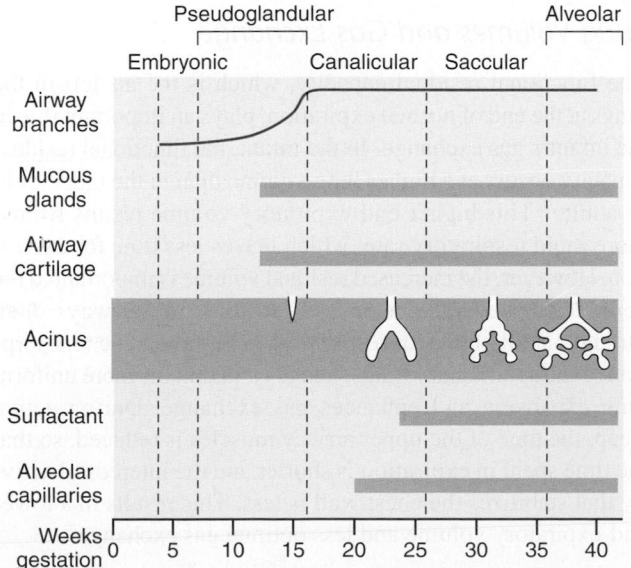

FIGURE 28-11 • Development of various respiratory structures during the five stages of lung development. (From Behrman R. E., Kliegman R. M., Jenson H. B. [Eds.]. (2004). *Nelson textbook of pediatrics* [17th ed., p. 1358]. Philadelphia: Elsevier Saunders.)

cles and stimulate lung development. The breathing movements in the fetus become more rapid in response to an increase in carbon dioxide levels and become slower in response to hypoxia.

The major difference between respiration in the fetus and the neonate is that there is complete separation between gas exchange and breathing movements in the fetus. The gas supply and exchange depend entirely on maternal mechanisms controlling placental circulation. At birth, dependence on the placental circulation is terminated, and the infant must integrate the two previously separate functions of gas exchange and respiratory movements. Within seconds of clamping the umbilical cord, the infant takes its first breath, and rhythmic breathing begins and persists for life.

Effective ventilation requires coordinated interaction between the muscles of the upper airways, including those of the pharynx and larynx, the diaphragm, and the intercostal muscles of the chest wall. In infants, a specific sequence of upper airway nerve and muscle activity occurs before and early in inspiration: the tongue moves forward to prevent airway obstruction, and the vocal cord abducts, reducing laryngeal resistance. By moving downward, the action of the diaphragm increases chest volume in both the longitudinal and transverse directions. In the infant, the diaphragm inserts more horizontally than in the adult. As a result, contraction of the diaphragm tends to draw the lower ribs inward, especially if the infant is placed in the horizontal position. The function of the intercostal muscles is to lift the ribs during inspiration. In the infant, however, the intercostal muscles are not fully developed, so they function largely to stabilize the chest rather than lift the chest wall.

The chest wall of the neonate is highly compliant; although this is advantageous during the birth process in that it allows for marked distortion to occur without damaging chest structures, it has implications for ventilation during the postnatal period. A striking characteristic of neonatal breathing is the paradoxical inward movement of the upper chest during inspiration, especially during active sleep. This occurs because of decreased activity of the intercostal muscles during active sleep, which allows the contracting diaphragm to pull the highly compliant chest wall inward. Under circumstances such as crying, the intercostal muscles of the neonate function together with the diaphragm to splint the chest wall and prevent its collapse.

Normally, the infant's lungs also are compliant; this is advantageous to the infant with a compliant chest cage because it takes only small changes in inspiratory pressure to inflate a compliant lung. When respiratory disease develops, lung compliance is reduced, and it takes more effort to inflate the lungs. The diaphragm must generate more negative pressure, causing the compliant chest wall structures to be sucked inward. *Retractions* are abnormal inward movements of the chest wall during inspiration; they may occur intercostally (between the ribs), in the substernal or epigastric area, and in the supraclavicular spaces. Because the chest wall of the infant is compliant, substernal retractions become more obvious with small changes in lung function. Retractions can indicate airway obstruction or atelectasis.

Airway Resistance

Normal lung inflation requires uninterrupted movement of air through the extrathoracic airways (*i.e.,* nose, pharynx, larynx, and upper trachea) and intrathoracic airways (*i.e.,* bronchi and bronchioles). The neonate (0 to 4 weeks of age) breathes predominantly through the nose and does not adapt well to mouth breathing. Any obstruction of the nose or nasopharynx may increase upper airway resistance and increase the work of breathing.

The airways of the infant and small child are much smaller than those of the adult.[72] Because the resistance to airflow is inversely related to the fourth power of the radius (resistance = $1/r^4$), relatively small amounts of mucus secretion, edema, or airway constriction can produce marked changes in airway resistance and airflow. Nasal flaring is a method that infants use to take in more air. This method of breathing increases the size of the nares and decreases the resistance of the small airways.

Normally, the extrathoracic airways in the infant narrow during inspiration and widen during expiration, and the intrathoracic airways widen during inspiration and narrow during expiration.[73] This occurs because the pressure inside the extrathoracic airways reflects the intrapleural pressures that are generated during breathing, whereas the pressure outside the airways is similar to atmospheric pressure. Thus, during inspiration, the pressure inside becomes more negative, causing the airways to narrow, and during expiration it becomes more positive, causing them to widen. In contrast to the extrathoracic airways, the pressure outside the intrathoracic airways is equal to the intrapleural pressure. These airways widen during inspiration as the surrounding intrapleural pressure becomes more negative and pulls them open, and they narrow during expiration as the surrounding pressure becomes more positive.

Lung Volumes and Gas Exchange

The functional residual capacity, which is the air left in the lungs at the end of normal expiration, plays an important role in the infant's gas exchange. In the infant, the functional residual capacity occurs at a higher lung volume than in the older child or adult.[74] This higher end-expiratory volume results from a more rapid respiratory rate, which leaves less time for expiration. However, the increased residual volume is important to the neonate for several reasons: (1) it holds the airways open throughout all phases of respiration, (2) it favors the reabsorption of intrapulmonary fluids, and (3) it maintains more uniform lung expansion and enhances gas exchange. During active sleep, the tone of the upper airway muscles is reduced, so that the time spent in expiration is shorter and the intercostal activity that stabilizes the chest wall is less. This results in a lower end-expiratory volume and less optimal gas exchange.

Control of Ventilation

Fetal arterial oxygen pressures (PO_2) normally range from 25 to 30 mm Hg, and carbon dioxide pressures (PCO_2) range from

45 to 50 mm Hg, independent of any respiratory movements. Any decrease in oxygen levels induces quiet sleep in the fetus with subsequent cessation of breathing movements, both of which lead to a decrease in oxygen consumption. Switching to oxygen derived from the aerated lung at birth causes an immediate increase in arterial PO_2 to approximately 50 mm Hg; within a few hours, it increases to approximately 70 mm Hg.[73] These levels, which greatly exceed fetal levels, cause the chemoreceptors that sense arterial PO_2 levels to become silent for several days. Although the infant's arterial PO_2 may fluctuate during this critical time, the chemoreceptors do not respond appropriately. It is not until several days after birth that the chemoreceptors "reset" their PO_2 threshold; only then do they become the major controller of breathing. However, the response seems to be biphasic, with an initial hyperventilation followed by a decreased respiratory rate and even apnea. In normal infants, especially those that are born prematurely, breathing patterns and respiratory reflexes depend on the arousal state.[74] Periodic breathing and apnea are characteristic of premature infants and reflect patterns of fetal breathing. The fact that they occur with sleep and disappear during wakefulness underscores the importance of arousal.

Alterations in Breathing

Most respiratory disorders in the infant or small child produce a decrease in lung compliance or an increase in airway resistance manifested by changes in breathing patterns, rib cage distortion (retractions), audible sounds, and use of accessory muscles.[73]

Children with restrictive lung disorders, such as pulmonary edema or respiratory distress syndrome, breathe at faster rates, and their respiratory excursions are shallow. *Grunting* is an audible noise emitted during expiration. An expiratory grunt is common as the child tries to raise the end-expiratory pressure and thus prolong the period of oxygen and carbon dioxide exchange across the alveolar–capillary membrane.

Increased airway resistance can occur in either the extrathoracic or intrathoracic airways. When the obstruction is in the extrathoracic airways, inspiration is more prolonged than expiration. *Nasal flaring* (enlargement of the nares) helps reduce the nasal resistance and maintain airway patency. It can be a sign of increased work of breathing and is a significant finding in an infant. *Inspiratory retractions,* or pulling in of the soft tissue surrounding the cartilaginous and bony thorax, is often observed with airway obstruction in infants and small children (Fig. 28-12). In conditions such as croup, the pressures distal to the point of obstruction must become more negative to overcome the resistance; this causes collapse of the distal airways, and the increased turbulence of air moving through the obstructed airways produces an audible crowing sound called a *stridor* during inspiration.

When the obstruction is in the intrathoracic airways, as occurs with bronchiolitis and bronchial asthma, expiration is prolonged and the child makes use of the accessory expiratory muscles (abdominals). Rib cage retractions may also be present. Intrapleural pressure becomes more positive during expiration

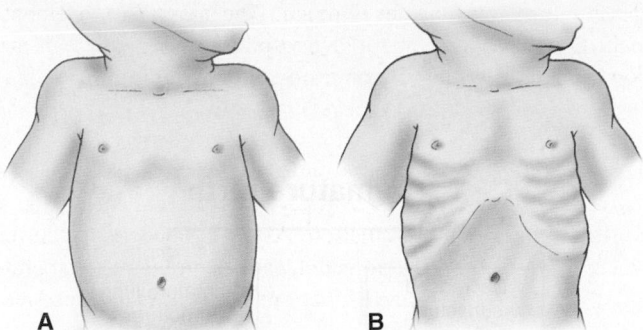

FIGURE 28-12 • **(A)** Normal inspiratory appearance of the chest during unobstructed breathing in the neonate. **(B)** Sternal and intercostal retractions during obstructed breathing in the neonate.

because of air trapping; this causes collapse of intrathoracic airways and produces an audible wheezing or whistling sound during expiration.

Respiratory Disorders in the Neonate

The neonatal period is one of transition from placental dependency to air breathing. This transition requires functioning of the surfactant system, conditioning of the respiratory muscles, and establishment of parallel pulmonary and systemic circulations. Respiratory disorders develop in infants who are born prematurely or who have other problems that impair this transition. Among the respiratory disorders of the neonate are the respiratory distress syndrome, bronchopulmonary dysplasia, and persistent fetal circulation (*i.e.,* delayed closure of the ductus arteriosus and foramen ovale; see Chapter 24).

Respiratory Distress Syndrome

Respiratory distress syndrome (RDS), also known as *hyaline membrane disease,* is one of the most common causes of respiratory disease in premature infants.[75,76] In these infants, pulmonary immaturity, together with surfactant deficiency, leads to alveolar collapse (Fig. 28-13). The type II alveolar cells that produce surfactant do not begin to mature until approximately the 25th to 28th weeks of gestation; consequently, many premature infants are born with poorly functioning type II alveolar cells and have difficulty producing sufficient amounts of surfactant. The incidence of RDS is higher among preterm male infants, white infants, infants of diabetic mothers, and those subjected to asphyxia, cold stress, precipitous deliveries, and delivery by cesarean section (when performed before the 38th week of gestation).

Surfactant synthesis is influenced by several hormones, including insulin and cortisol. Insulin tends to inhibit surfactant production; this explains why infants of insulin-dependent diabetic mothers are at increased risk for development of RDS. Cortisol can accelerate maturation of type II cells and formation of surfactant. The reason that premature infants born by

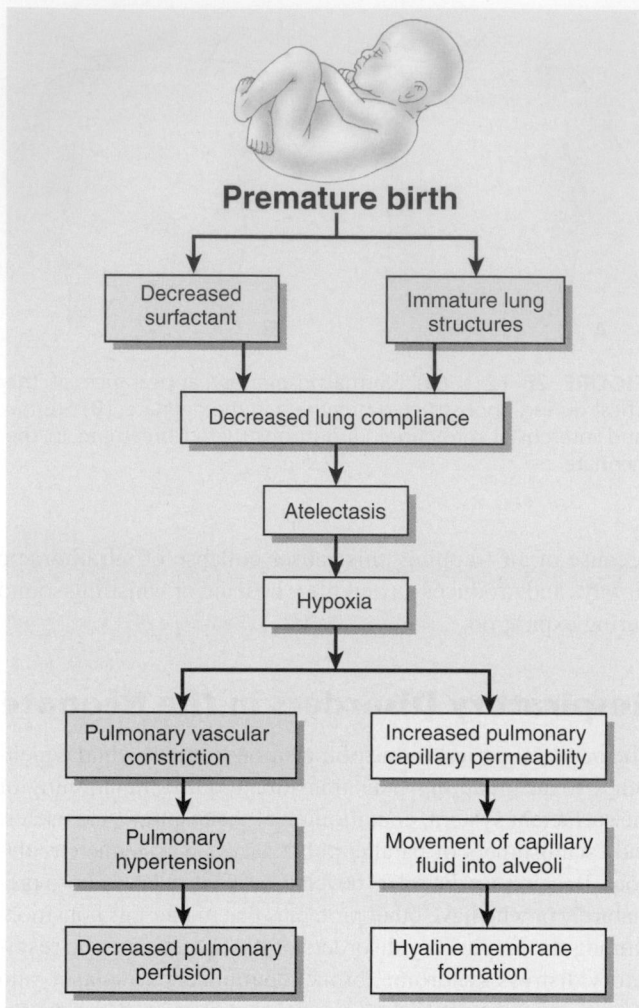

Premature birth

Decreased surfactant → Decreased lung compliance ← Immature lung structures

Decreased lung compliance → Atelectasis → Hypoxia

Hypoxia →

Pulmonary vascular constriction → Pulmonary hypertension → Decreased pulmonary perfusion

Increased pulmonary capillary permeability → Movement of capillary fluid into alveoli → Hyaline membrane formation

FIGURE 28-13 • Pathogenesis of respiratory distress syndrome (RDS) in the infant.

cesarean section presumably are at greater risk for development of RDS is that they are not subjected to the stress of vaginal delivery, which is thought to increase the infants' cortisol levels. These observations have led to administration of corticosteroid drugs before delivery to mothers with infants at high risk for development of RDS.[75]

Surfactant reduces the surface tension in the alveoli, thereby equalizing the retractive forces in the large and small alveoli and reducing the amount of pressure needed to inflate and hold the alveoli open (see Chapter 27). Without surfactant, the large alveoli remain inflated, whereas the small alveoli become difficult to inflate. At birth, the first breath requires high inspiratory pressures to expand the lungs. With normal levels of surfactant, the lungs retain up to 40% of the residual volume after the first breath, and subsequent breaths require far lower inspiratory pressures. With a surfactant deficiency, the lungs collapse between breaths, making the infant work as hard with each successive breath as with the first breath. The airless portions of the lungs become stiff and noncompliant. A hyaline membrane forms inside the alveoli as protein- and fibrin-rich fluids are pulled into the alveolar spaces. The fibrin–hyaline membrane constitutes a barrier to gas exchange, leading to hypoxemia and carbon dioxide retention, a condition that further impairs surfactant production.

Infants with RDS present with multiple signs of respiratory distress, usually within the first 24 hours of birth. Central cyanosis is a prominent sign. Breathing becomes more difficult, and retractions occur as the infant's soft chest wall is pulled in as the diaphragm descends. Grunting sounds accompany expiration. As the tidal volume drops because of atelectasis, the respiration rate increases (usually to 60 to 120 breaths/minute) in an effort to maintain normal minute ventilation. Fatigue may develop rapidly because of the increased work of breathing. The stiff lungs of infants with RDS also increase the resistance to blood flow in the pulmonary circulation. As a result, a hemodynamically significant patent ductus arteriosus may develop in infants with RDS (see Chapter 24).

The basic principles of treatment for infants with suspected RDS focus on the provision of supportive care, including gentle handling and minimal disturbance.[75] An incubator or radiant warmer is used to prevent hypothermia and increased oxygen consumption. Continuous cardiorespiratory monitoring is needed. Monitoring of blood glucose and prevention of hypoglycemia are also recommended. Oxygen levels can be assessed through an arterial (umbilical) line or by a transcutaneous oxygen sensor. Treatment includes administration of supplemental oxygen, continuous positive airway pressure through nasal prongs, and often assisted mechanical ventilation.

Exogenous surfactant therapy is used to prevent and treat RDS.[75,76] There are two types of surfactants: natural surfactants prepared from animal sources and synthetic surfactants. Currently, only the natural surfactants are approved for clinical use in the United States.[76] The surfactants are suspended in saline and administered into the airways, usually through an endotracheal tube. The treatment often is initiated soon after birth in infants who are at high risk for RDS.

Bronchopulmonary Dysplasia

Bronchopulmonary dysplasia (BPD) is a chronic lung disease that develops in premature infants who were treated with mechanical ventilation, mainly for RDS.[77] The condition is considered to be present if the neonate is oxygen dependent at 36 weeks after gestation. The disorder is thought to be a response of the premature lung to early injury. High inspired oxygen concentration and injury from positive-pressure ventilation (*i.e.,* barotrauma) have been implicated.

BPD is characterized by chronic respiratory distress, persistent hypoxemia when breathing room air, reduced lung compliance, increased airway resistance, and severe expiratory flow limitation. There is a mismatching of ventilation and perfusion with development of hypoxemia and hypercapnia. Pulmonary vascular resistance may be increased and pulmonary hypertension and cor pulmonale (*i.e.,* right heart failure associated with lung disease) may develop. The infant with BPD often demonstrates a barrel chest, tachycardia, rapid and shallow breathing, chest retractions, cough, and poor weight gain.[75,77]

Clubbing of the fingers occurs in children with severe disease. Hepatomegaly and periorbital edema may develop in infants with right heart failure.

The treatment of BPD includes mechanical ventilation and administration of supplemental oxygen. Weaning from ventilation is accomplished gradually, and some infants may require ventilation at home. Rapid lung growth occurs during the first year of life, and lung function usually improves.

Adequate nutrition is essential for recovery of infants with BPD. There has been an interest in the protective effect of polyunsaturated fatty acids, vitamin A, and other nutrients such as inositol (a sulfur-containing amino acid) and selenium in preventing lung injury in high-risk premature infants.[77] Research into the effects of some of these dietary substances is ongoing. Other areas of investigation include developmental influences such as glucocorticoid hormones, which accelerate the maturation of lung tissue, increase surfactant production and lung compliance, reduce vascular permeability, and increase lung water clearance.

Most adolescents and young adults who had severe BPD during infancy have some degree of pulmonary dysfunction, consisting of airway obstruction, airway hyperreactivity, or hyperinflation.

Respiratory Infections in Children

In children, respiratory tract infections are common, and although they are troublesome, they usually are not serious. Frequent infections occur because the immune system of infants and small children has not been exposed to many common pathogens; consequently, they tend to contract infections with each new exposure. Although most of these infections are not serious, the small size of an infant or child's airways tends to foster impaired airflow and obstruction. For example, an infection that causes only sore throat and hoarseness in an adult may result in serious airway obstruction in a small child.

Upper Airway Infections

Acute upper airway infections are important in infants and small children. They include croup (laryngotracheobronchitis) and epiglottitis.[78-80] Croup is the more common and usually is benign and self-limited. Epiglottitis is a rapidly progressive and life-threatening condition. The site of involvement is illustrated in Figure 28-14, and the characteristics of both infections are described in Table 28-2.

Obstruction of the upper airways because of infection tends to exert its greatest effect during the inspiratory phase of respiration. Movement of air through an obstructed upper airway, particularly the vocal cords in the larynx, causes stridor.[78] Impairment of the expiratory phase of respiration also can occur, causing wheezing. With mild to moderate obstruction, inspiratory stridor is more prominent than expiratory wheezing because the airways tend to dilate with expiration. When the swelling and obstruction become severe, the airways no longer can dilate during expiration, and both stridor and wheezing occur.

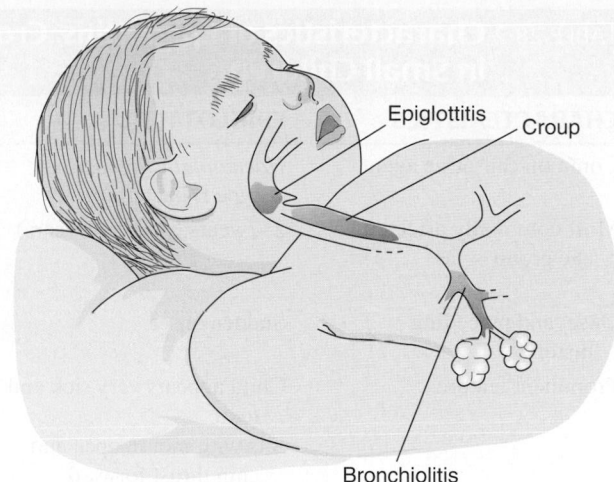

FIGURE 28-14 • Location of airway obstruction in epiglottitis, acute laryngotracheobronchitis (croup), and bronchiolitis. (Courtesy of Carole Russell Hilmer, C.M.I.)

Cartilaginous support of the trachea and the larynx is poorly developed in infants and small children. These structures are soft and tend to collapse when the airway is obstructed and the child cries, causing the inspiratory pressures to become more negative. When this happens, the stridor and inspiratory effort are increased. The phenomenon of airway collapse in the small child is analogous to what happens when a thick beverage, such as a milkshake, is drunk through a soft paper or plastic straw. The straw collapses when the negative pressure produced by the sucking effort exceeds the flow of liquid through the straw.

Viral Croup. Croup is characterized by inspiratory stridor, hoarseness, and a barking cough. The British use the term *croup* to describe the cry of the crow or raven, and this is undoubtedly how the term originated.

Viral croup, more appropriately called *acute laryngotracheobronchitis*, is a viral infection that affects the larynx, trachea, and bronchi. The parainfluenza viruses account for approximately 75% all cases; the remaining 25% are caused by adenoviruses, respiratory syncytial virus, influenza A and B viruses, and measles virus.[81,82] Viral croup usually is seen in children 3 months to 5 years of age. The condition may affect the entire laryngotracheal tree, but because the subglottic area is the narrowest part of the respiratory tree in this age group, the obstruction usually is greatest in this area. For example, the subglottic airway in the 1- to 2-year-old child is approximately 6.5 mm in diameter, and 1 mm of edema can reduce the cross-sectional area by 50%.[83]

Although the respiratory manifestations of croup often appear suddenly, they usually are preceded by upper respiratory infections that cause rhinorrhea (*i.e.*, runny nose), coryza (*i.e.*, common cold), hoarseness, and a low-grade fever. In most children, the manifestation of croup advances only to stridor and slight dyspnea before they begin to recover. The symptoms usually subside when the child is exposed to moist air.

TABLE 28-2 Characteristics of Epiglottitis, Croup, and Bronchiolitis in Small Children

CHARACTERISTICS	EPIGLOTTITIS	CROUP	BRONCHIOLITIS
Common causative agent	*Haemophilus influenzae* type B bacterium	Mainly parainfluenza virus	Respiratory syncytial virus
Most commonly affected age group	2–7 years (peak 3–5 years)	3 months to 5 years	Less than 2 years (most severe in infants younger than 6 months)
Onset and preceding history	Sudden onset	Usually follows symptoms of a cold	Preceded by stuffy nose and other signs
Prominent features	Child appears very sick and toxic	Stridor and a wet, barking cough	Breathlessness, rapid, shallow breathing, wheezing, cough, and retractions of lower ribs and sternum during inspiration
	Sits with mouth open and chin thrust forward	Usually occurs at night	
	Low-pitched stridor, difficulty swallowing, fever, drooling, anxiety	Relieved by exposure to cold or moist air	
	Danger of airway obstruction and asphyxia		
Usual treatment	Hospitalization	Mist tent or vaporizer	Supportive treatment, administration of oxygen and hydration
	Intubation or tracheotomy	Administration of oxygen	
	Treatment with appropriate antibiotic		

For example, letting the bathroom shower run and then taking the child into the bathroom often brings prompt and dramatic relief of symptoms. Exposure to cold air also seems to relieve the airway spasm; often, the severe symptoms are relieved simply because the child is exposed to cold air on the way to the hospital emergency department. Viral croup does not respond to antibiotics; expectorants, bronchodilating agents, and antihistamines are not helpful. The child should be disturbed as little as possible and carefully monitored for signs of respiratory distress.

Airway obstruction may progress in some children. As obstruction increases, the stridor becomes continuous and is associated with nasal flaring with substernal and intercostal retractions. Agitation and crying aggravate the signs and symptoms, and the child prefers to sit up or be held upright. In the cyanotic, pale, or obstructed child, any manipulation of the pharynx, including use of a tongue depressor, can cause cardiorespiratory arrest and should be done only in a medical setting that has the facilities for emergency airway management. Other treatments may be required when a humidifier or mist tent is ineffective. One method is to administer a racemic mixture of epinephrine (L-epinephrine and D-epinephrine) by positive-pressure breathing through a face mask.[78] Establishment of an artificial airway may become necessary in severe airway obstruction.

Spasmodic Croup. Spasmodic croup manifests with symptoms similar to those of acute viral croup. Because the child is afebrile and lacks other manifestations of the viral prodrome, it is thought that it may have an allergic origin. Spasmodic croup characteristically occurs at night and tends to recur with respiratory tract

infections. The episode usually lasts several hours and may recur several nights in a row.

Most children with spasmodic croup can be effectively managed at home. An environment of high humidification (*i.e.,* cold-water room humidifier or taking the child into a bathroom with a warm, running shower) lessens irritation and prevents drying of secretions.

Epiglottitis. Acute epiglottitis is a dramatic, potentially fatal condition characterized by inflammatory edema of the supraglottic area, including the epiglottis and pharyngeal structures (see Fig. 28-14), that comes on suddenly, bringing danger of airway obstruction and asphyxia.[78–80] In the past, the *H. influenzae* type B bacterium was the most commonly identified etiologic agent. It is seen less commonly since the widespread use of immunization against *H. influenzae* type B. Therefore, other agents such as *Streptococcus pyogenes, S. pneumoniae,* and *S. aureus* now represent the larger cause of pediatric epiglottitis.

The child appears pale, toxic, and lethargic and assumes a distinctive position—sitting up with the mouth open and the chin thrust forward. The child has difficulty in swallowing, a muffled voice, drooling, fever, and extreme anxiety. Moderate to severe respiratory distress is evident. There is inspiratory and sometimes expiratory stridor, flaring of the nares, and inspiratory retractions of the suprasternal notch and supraclavicular and intercostal spaces. Within a matter of hours, epiglottitis may progress to complete obstruction of the airway and death unless adequate treatment is instituted. Epiglottitis is a medical emergency and immediate establishment of an airway by endotracheal tube or tracheotomy usually is needed. If epiglottitis is suspected, the child should never be forced to lie down because this causes the epiglottis to fall backward and may lead to complete airway obstruction. Examination of the throat with a tongue blade or other instrument may cause cardiopulmonary arrest and should be done only by medical personnel experienced in intubation of small children. It also is unwise to attempt any procedure, such as drawing blood, that would heighten the child's anxiety because this also could precipitate airway spasm and cause death. Recovery from epiglottitis usually is rapid and uneventful after an adequate airway has been established and appropriate antibiotic therapy initiated.

Lower Airway Infections

Lower airway infections produce air trapping with prolonged expiration. Wheezing results from bronchospasm, mucosal inflammation, and edema. The child presents with increased expiratory effort, increased respiratory rate, and wheezing. If the infection is severe, there also are marked intercostal retractions and signs of impending respiratory failure.

Acute bronchiolitis is a viral infection of the lower airways, most commonly caused by the respiratory syncytial virus.[84–86] Other viruses, such as parainfluenza-3 virus and some adenoviruses, as well as mycoplasmas, also are causative. The infection produces inflammatory obstruction of the small airways and necrosis of the cells lining the lower airways. It usually occurs during the first 2 years of life, with a peak incidence between 3 and 6 months of age. The source of infection usually is a family member with a minor respiratory illness. Older children and adults tolerate bronchiolar edema much better than infants and do not manifest the clinical picture of bronchiolitis. Because the resistance to airflow in a tube is inversely related to the fourth power of the radius, even minor swelling of bronchioles in an infant can produce profound changes in airflow.

Most affected infants in whom bronchiolitis develops have a history of a mild upper respiratory tract infection. These symptoms usually last several days and may be accompanied by fever and diminished appetite. There is then a gradual development of respiratory distress, characterized by a wheezy cough, dyspnea, and irritability. The infant usually is able to take in sufficient air but has trouble exhaling it. Air becomes trapped in the lung distal to the site of obstruction and interferes with gas exchange. Hypoxemia and, in severe cases, hypercapnia may develop. Airway obstruction may produce air trapping and hyperinflation of the lungs or collapse of the alveoli. Infants with acute bronchiolitis have a typical appearance, marked by breathlessness with rapid respirations, a distressing cough, and retractions of the lower ribs and sternum. Crying and feeding exaggerate these signs. Wheezing and crackles may or may not be present, depending on the degree of airway obstruction. In infants with severe airway obstruction, wheezing decreases as the airflow diminishes. Usually, the most critical phase of the disease is the first 48 to 72 hours. Cyanosis, pallor, listlessness, and sudden diminution or absence of breath sounds indicate impending respiratory failure. The characteristics of bronchiolitis are described in Table 28-2.

Infants with respiratory distress usually are hospitalized. Treatment is supportive and includes administration of supplemental oxygen if the oxygen saturation consistently falls below 90%.[85] Elevation of the head facilitates respiratory movements and avoids airway compression. Handling is kept at a minimum to avoid tiring. Because the infection is viral, antibiotics are not effective and are given only for a secondary bacterial infection. Dehydration may occur as the result of increased insensible water losses because of the rapid respiratory rate and feeding difficulties, and measures to ensure adequate hydration are needed. If the child is in respiratory distress and adequate hydration cannot be achieved, the child should receive intravenous fluids.[85] Recovery usually begins after the first 48 to 72 hours and usually is rapid and complete. Adequate hand washing is essential to prevent the nosocomial spread of respiratory syncytial virus.

Signs of Impending Respiratory Failure

Respiratory problems of infants and small children often originate suddenly, and recovery usually is rapid and complete. Children are at risk for the development of airway obstruction and respiratory failure resulting from obstructive disorders or lung infection. The child with epiglottitis is at risk for airway obstruction. The child with bronchiolitis is at risk for respiratory failure resulting from impaired gas exchange. Children with impending respiratory failure due to airway or lung disease have rapid breathing; exaggerated use of the accessory muscles; retractions, which are more pronounced in the child than in the adult because of more compliant chest; nasal flaring; and grunting during expiration.[87] The signs and symptoms of impending respiratory failure are listed in Chart 28-1.

CHART 28-1   SIGNS OF RESPIRATORY DISTRESS AND IMPENDING RESPIRATORY FAILURE IN THE INFANT AND SMALL CHILD

Severe increase in respiratory effort, including severe retractions or grunting, decreased chest movement
Cyanosis that is not relieved by administration of oxygen (40%)
Heart rate of 150 per minute or greater and increasing bradycardia
Very rapid breathing (rate 60 per minute in the newborn to 6 months or above 30 per minute in children 6 months to 2 years)
Very depressed breathing (rate 20 per minute or below)
Retractions of the supraclavicular area, sternum, epigastrium, and intercostal spaces
Extreme anxiety and agitation
Fatigue
Decreased level of consciousness

IN SUMMARY, acute respiratory disease is the most common cause of illness in infancy and childhood, accounting for 50% of illnesses in children younger than 5 years of age and 30% of illnesses in children between 5 and 12 years of age. Although other body systems are physiologically ready for extrauterine life as early as 25 weeks of gestation, the lungs take longer. Immaturity of the respiratory system is a major cause of morbidity and mortality in premature infants.

Lung development may be divided into five stages: embryonic period, pseudoglandular period, canalicular period, saccular period, and alveolar period. The first three phases are devoted to development of the conducting airways, and the last two phases are devoted to development of the gas exchange portion of the lung. By the 25th to 28th weeks of gestation, sufficient terminal air sacs are present to permit survival. It is also during this period that type II alveolar cells, which produce surfactant, begin to function. Lung development is incomplete at birth; an infant is born with only one-eighth to one-sixth the adult number of alveoli. Alveoli continue to be formed during early childhood, reaching the adult number of 300 million alveoli by 8 years of age.

Children with restrictive lung disease breathe at faster rates, and their respiratory excursions are shallow. An expiratory grunt is common as the child tries to raise the functional residual capacity by closing the glottis at the end of expiration. Obstruction of the extrathoracic airways often produces turbulence of airflow and an audible inspiratory crowing sound called *stridor,* and obstruction of the intrathoracic airways produces an audible expiratory wheezing or whistling sound. RDS is one of the most common causes of respiratory disease in premature infants. In these infants, pulmonary immaturity, together with surfactant deficiency, leads to alveolar collapse. BPD is a chronic pulmonary disease that develops in premature infants who were treated with mechanical ventilation.

Because of the small size of the airway of infants and children, respiratory tract infections in these groups often are more serious. Infections that may cause only a sore throat and hoarseness in the adult may produce serious obstruction in the child. Among the respiratory tract infections that affect small children are croup, epiglottitis, and bronchiolitis. Epiglottitis is a life-threatening supraglottic infection that may cause airway obstruction and asphyxia. ■

Review Exercises

1. It is flu season, and although you had a flu shot last year, you have not had one this year. Imagine yourself experiencing an abrupt onset of fever, chills, malaise, muscle aching, and nasal stuffiness.

   A. *Which of these symptoms would lead you to believe you are coming down with the flu?*

   B. *Because you hate to miss classes, you decide to go to the student health center to get an antibiotic. After being seen by a health professional, you are told that antibiotics are ineffective against the flu virus, and you are instructed not to attend classes but instead to go home, take acetaminophen for your fever, go to bed and stay warm, and drink a lot of fluids. Explain the rationale for each of these recommendations.*

   C. *Explain why last year's flu shot did not protect you during this year's flu season.*

   D. *There is current concern about the possibility of an influenza pandemic such as the one that occurred during the 1917–1918 season. What is the rationale for this concern?*

2. Bacterial (*e.g., S. pneumoniae*) pneumonia is commonly manifested by a cough productive of sputum, whereas with atypical (*e.g., Mycoplasma pneumoniae*) pneumonia, the cough is usually nonproductive or absent.

   A. *Explain.*

3. A 4-month-old infant is admitted to the pediatric intensive care unit with a diagnosis of bronchiolitis. The infant is tachypneic, with wheezing, nasal flaring, and retractions of the lower sternum and intercostal spaces during inspiration.

   A. *What is the usual pathogen in bronchiolitis? Would this infection be treated with an antibiotic?*

   B. *Explain the physiologic mechanism involved in the retraction of the lower sternum and intercostal spaces during inspiration.*

   C. *What would be the signs of impending respiratory failure in this infant?*

References

1. Maher D., Raviglione M. (2005). Global epidemiology of tuberculosis. *Clinics in Chest Medicine* 26, 167–182.
2. McAdam A. J., Sharpe A. H. (2005). Infectious diseases. In Kumar V., Abbas A. K., Fausto N. (Eds.), *Robbins and Cotran pathologic basis of disease* (7th ed., p. 353). Philadelphia: Elsevier Saunders.
3. Covington T. R., Henkin R., Miller S., et al. (2004). Treating the common cold. *American Journal of Nurse Practitioners* 8(11), 77–88.
4. Heikkinen T., Järvinsen A. (2003). The common cold. *Lancet* 361, 51–59.
5. Greenberg S. B. (2003). Respiratory consequences of rhinovirus infection. *Archives of Internal Medicine* 163, 278–284.
6. Goldman D. A. (2000). Transmission of viral respiratory tract infections in the home. *Pediatric Infectious Disease Journal* 19, S97–S107.
7. Simasek M., Blandino D. A. (2007). Treatment of the common cold. *American Family Physician* 75, 512–522.
8. Dykewicz M. S. (2003). Rhinitis and sinusitis. *Journal of Allergy and Clinical Immunology* 111, S520–S539.
9. Slavin R. G. Spector S. L., Bernstein I. L., Chief editors, American Academy of Allergy, Asthma and Immunology; American College of Allergy,

Asthma and Immunology; Joint Council of Allergy, Asthma and Immunology. (2005). The diagnosis and management of sinusitis: A practice parameter update. *Journal of Allergy and Clinical Immunology* 116(Suppl. 6), S13–S17.

10. Scheid D. C., Hamm R. M. (2004). Acute bacterial rhinosinusitis in adults: Part I. Evaluation; Part II. Treatment. *American Family Physician* 70, 1685–1692, 1697–1704.

11. Piccirillo J. F. (2004). Acute bacterial sinusitis. *New England Journal of Medicine* 351, 902–910.

12. Lockey R. F. (1996). Management of chronic sinusitis. *Hospital Practice* 31, 141–151.

13. Advisory Committee on Immunization Practices. (2007). Prevention and control of influenza: Recommendations of the Advisory Committee on Immunization Practices (ACIP). *Morbidity and Mortality Weekly Report* 56(RR-06), 1–54.

14. Cunha B. A. (2004). Influenza: Historical aspects of epidemics and panepidemics. *Infectious Disease Clinics of North America* 18, 141–155.

15. Hussain A. N., Kumar V. (2005). The lung. In Kumar V., Abbas A. K., Fausto N. (Eds.), *Robbins and Cotran pathologic basis of disease* (7th ed., 747–756). Philadelphia: Elsevier Saunders.

16. Moorman J. P. (2003). Viral characteristics of influenza. *Southern Medical Journal* 96, 758–761.

17. Shorman M., Moorman J. P. (2003). Clinical manifestations and diagnosis of influenza. *Southern Medical Journal* 96, 737–739.

18. Olshaker J. S. (2003). Influenza. *Emergency Medicine Clinics of North America* 21, 353–361.

19. Khater F., Moorman J. P. (2003). Complications of influenza. *Southern Medical Journal* 96, 740–743.

20. Montal N. J. (2003). An office-based approach to influenza: Clinical diagnosis and laboratory testing. *American Family Physician* 67, 111–118.

21. Stiver G. (2003). The treatment of influenza with antiviral drugs. *Canadian Medical Association Journal* 168, 49–57.

22. Palese P., Garcia-Sastre A. (2002). Influenza vaccines: Present and future. *Journal of Clinical Investigation* 110, 9–13.

23. Liptov A., Govorkova E. A., Webby R. J., et al. (2004). Influenza: Emergence and control. *Journal of Virology* 78, 8951–8959.

24. Webby R. J., Webster R. G. (2003). Are we ready for pandemic influenza? *Science* 302, 1519–1522.

25. Beigel J. H., Farrar J., Han A. M., et al., Writing Committee of the World Health Organization (WHO) Consultation on Human Influenza A/H5. (2005). Avian influenza A (H5N1) infections in humans. *New England Journal of Medicine* 353, 1374–1385.

26. Apisarnthanarak A., Mundy L. M. (2005). Etiology of community-acquired pneumonia. *Clinics in Chest Medicine* 26, 47–55.

27. Alcón A., Fabregas N., Torres A. (2005). Pathophysiology of pneumonia. *Clinics in Chest Medicine* 26, 39–46.

28. Waite S., Jeudy J., White C. S. (2006). Acute lung infections in normal and immunocompromised hosts. *Radiologic Clinics of North America* 44, 295–316.

29. Beasley M. B., Travis W. D., Rubin E. (2008). The respiratory system. In Rubin R., Strayer D. (Eds.), *Rubin's pathology: Clinicopathologic foundations of medicine* (5th ed., pp. 491–503). Philadelphia: Lippincott Williams & Wilkins.

30. Chestnut M. S., Prendergast T. J. (2007). The lung. In Tierney L. M., McPhee S. J., Papadakis M. A. (Eds.), *Current medical diagnosis and treatment* (46th ed., pp. 251–260, 261–268). New York: Lange Medical Books/McGraw-Hill.

31. Halm E. A., Teirstein A. S. (2002). Management of community-acquired pneumonia. *New England Journal of Medicine* 347, 2039–2045.

32. Neiderman M. S., Mandell L. A., Anzueto A., et al., American Thoracic Society. (2001). Guidelines for the initial management of adults with community-acquired pneumonia: Diagnosis, assessment of severity, antimicrobial therapy, and prevention. *American Journal of Respiratory Critical Care Medicine* 163, 1730–1754.

33. Mandell L. A. (2004). Epidemiology and etiology of community-acquired pneumonia. *Infectious Disease Clinics of North America* 18, 761–776.

34. Ramirez J. A. (2003). Community-acquired pneumonia in adults. *Primary Care Clinics and Office Practice* 30, 155–171.

35. Lutfiyya N. N., Henley E., Chang L. F. (2006). Diagnosis and treatment of community-acquired pneumonia. *American Family Physician* 73, 442–450.

36. Catterall J. R. (1999). *Streptococcus pneumoniae. Thorax* 54, 929–937.

37. Centers for Disease Control and Prevention. (1996). Prevention of pneumococcal disease: Recommendations of the Advisory Committee on Immunization Practices (ACIP). *Morbidity and Mortality Weekly Report* 46(RR-8), 1–24.

38. Centers for Disease Control and Prevention. (2000). Preventing pneumococcal disease among infants and small children: Recommendations of the Advisory Committee on Immunization Practices (ACIP). *Morbidity and Mortality Weekly Report* 46(RR-9), 1–38.

39. Stout J. E., Yu V. C. (1997). Legionellosis. *New England Journal of Medicine* 337, 682–688.

40. American Lung Association. (2003). Search Lung USA: Tuberculosis. [Online.] Available: www.lungusa.org. Accessed May, 1, 2007.

41. Jasmer R. M., Nahid P., Hopewell P. C. (2002). Latent tuberculosis infection. *New England Journal of Medicine* 347, 1860–1866.

42. Goldberg S. (2004). Tuberculosis. *Clinics in Family Practice* 6, 175–197.

43. American Thoracic Society/Centers for Disease Control and Prevention/Infectious Diseases Society of America. (2005). Controlling tuberculosis in the United States. *American Journal of Respiratory Critical Care Medicine* 172, 1169–1227.

44. Schwartz D. A., Genta R. M., Bennett D. P., et al. (2008). Infectious and parasitic diseases. In Rubin R., Strayer D. (Eds.), *Rubin's pathology: Clinicopathologic foundations of medicine* (5th ed., pp. 341–344). Philadelphia: Lippincott Williams & Wilkins.

45. American Thoracic Society and Centers for Disease Control and Prevention. (2000). Diagnostic standards and classification of tuberculosis in adults and children. *American Review of Respiratory Disease* 161, 1376–1395.

46. Barnes P. F., Cave M. D. (2003). Molecular epidemiology of tuberculosis. *New England Journal of Medicine* 349, 1149–1156.

47. Nahid P., Pal M., Hopewell P. C. (2006). Advances in the diagnosis and treatment of tuberculosis. *Proceedings of the American Thoracic Society* 3, 103–110.

48. Brodie D., Schluger N. W. (2005). The diagnosis of tuberculosis. *Clinics in Chest Medicine* 26, 247–271.

49. Potter B., Rindfleisch K. (2005). Management of active tuberculosis. *American Family Physician* 72, 2225–2232.

50. American Thoracic Society, Centers for Disease Control and Prevention, and Infectious Diseases Society of America. (2003). Treatment of tuberculosis. *Morbidity and Mortality Weekly Report* 52(RR-11), 1–14.

51. Spiegler P., Ilowitz J. (1999). Multiple-drug-resistant tuberculosis: Parts 1 and 2. *Emergency Medicine* 31(6,7), 10–23.

52. Havlir D. V., Barnes P. F. (1999). Tuberculosis in patients with human immunodeficiency virus infection. *New England Journal of Medicine* 380, 367–372.

53. Centers for Disease Control and Prevention. (1996). The role of BCG vaccine in the prevention and control of tuberculosis in the United States. *Morbidity and Mortality Weekly Report* 45(RR-4), 1–19.

54. Centers for Disease Control and Prevention. (2006). Fact sheets: BCG vaccine. [Online.] Available www.cdc.gov/tb/tbfactsheets/BCG.htm. Accessed March 6, 2008.

55. Kauffman C. A. (2006). Endemic mycoses: Blastomycosis, histoplasmosis, and sporotrichosis. *Infectious Disease Clinics of North America* 20, 645–662.

56. Wheat L. J., Kauffman C. A. (2003). Histoplasmosis. *Infectious Disease Clinics of North America* 17, 1–19.

57. Galgiani J. N. (1999). Coccidioidomycosis: A regional disease of national importance. *Annals of Internal Medicine* 130, 293–300.

58. Anstead G. M., Grayhill J. R. (2006). Coccidioidomycosis. *Infectious Disease Clinics of North America* 20, 621–643.

59. Chiller T. M., Galgiani J. N., Stevens D. A. (2003). Coccidioidomycosis. *Infectious Disease Clinics of North America* 17, 41–57.

60. Bradsher R. W., Chapman S. W., Pappas P. G. (2003). Blastocytosis. *Infectious Disease Clinics of North America* 17, 21–40.

61. American Cancer Society. (2007). Lung cancer. [Online]. Available: www.cancer.org. Accessed March 6, 2008.

62. Ginsberg M. S., Grewal R. K., Heelan R. T. (2007). Lung cancer. *Radiological Clinics of North America 45*, 21–43.

63. Alberg A. J., Samet J. M. (2003). Epidemiology of lung cancer. *Chest* 123(Suppl. 1), 21S–44S.

64. Thomas C. R., Williams T. E., Cobos E., et al. (2001). Lung cancer. In Lenhard R. E., Osteen R. T., Gansler T. (Eds.), *The American Cancer Society: Clinical oncology* (pp. 269–295). Atlanta, GA: American Cancer Society.

65. Oklund S. H., Jett J. R. (2002). Small cell lung cancer: Current therapy and promising new regimens. *Oncologist 7*, 563–568.

66. Walker S. (2003). Updates in small cell lung cancer treatment. *Clinical Journal of Oncology Nursing 7*, 563–568.

67. Simson G. R. (2003). Small cell lung cancer. *Chest* 123(Suppl.), 259S–268S.

68. Spira A., Ettinger D. S. (2004). Multidisciplinary management of lung cancer. *New England Journal of Medicine 350*, 379–392.

69. Hurria A. (2003). Management of lung cancer in older adults. *CA: A Cancer Journal for Clinicians 53*, 325–341.

70. Haddad G. G., Fontán J. J. P. (2004). Development of the respiratory system. In Behrman R. E., Kliegman R. M., Jenson H. L. (Eds.), *Nelson textbook of pediatrics* (17th ed., pp. 1362–1370). Philadelphia: W. B. Saunders.

71. Moore K., Persaud T. V. N. (2003). *The developing human* (6th ed., pp. 242–253). Philadelphia: W. B. Saunders.

72. Hazinski F. (1999). *Manual of pediatric critical care* (pp. 289–356). St. Louis: Mosby.

73. Fontán J. J. P., Haddad G. G. (2004). Respiratory pathophysiology. In Behrman R. E., Kliegman R. M., Jensen H. L. (Eds.), *Nelson textbook of pediatrics* (17th ed., pp. 1362–1367). Philadelphia: Elsevier Saunders.

74. Crocetti M., Barone M. A. (Eds.). (2004). *Oski's essential pediatrics* (2nd ed., pp. 44–52, 374–388). Philadelphia: Lippincott Williams & Wilkins.

75. Stoll B. J., Kliegman R. M. (2004). The fetus and neonatal infant. In Behrman R. E., Kliegman R. M., Jenson H. L. (Eds.), *Nelson textbook of pediatrics* (17th ed., pp. 573–583). Philadelphia: Elsevier Saunders.

76. Rodriguez R. J. (2003). Management of respiratory distress syndrome. *Respiratory Care 48*, 279–286.

77. Jobe A. H., Bancalari E. (2001). Bronchopulmonary dysplasia. *American Journal of Respiratory Critical Care 163*, 1723–1729.

78. Roosevelt G. E. (2004). Acute inflammatory upper airway obstruction. In Behrman R. E., Kliegman R. M., Jenson H. L. (Eds.), *Nelson textbook of pediatrics* (17th ed., pp. 1405–1409). Philadelphia: Elsevier Saunders.

79. Rafei K., Lichenstein R. (2006). Airway infectious disease emergencies. *Pediatric Clinics of North America 53*, 215–242.

80. Rotta A. T., Wiryawan B. (2003). Respiratory emergencies in children. *Respiratory Care 43*, 248–258.

81. Klassen T. P. (1999). Croup: A current perspective. *Pediatric Clinics of North America 46*, 1167–1177.

82. Knutson D., Arling A. (2004). Viral croup. *American Family Physician 69*, 535–542.

83. Wright R. B., Pomerantz W. J., Luria J. W. (2002). New approaches to respiratory infections in children. *Emergency Medicine Clinics of North America 20*, 93–111.

84. Smyth R. L., Openshaw P. J. M. (2006). Bronchiolitis. *Lancet 368*, 312–322.

85. American Academy of Pediatrics Subcommittee on Diagnosis and Management of Bronchiolitis. (2006). Diagnosis and management of bronchiolitis. *Pediatrics 118*, 1774–1793.

86. Coffin S. E. (2005). Bronchiolitis: In-patient focus. *Pediatrics 52*, 1047–1057.

87. Frankel L. R. (2004). Respiratory distress and failure. In Behrman R. E., Kliegman R. M., Jenson H. L. (Eds.), *Nelson textbook of pediatrics* (17th ed., pp. 301–306). Philadelphia: Elsevier Saunders.

Visit the Point http://thePoint.lww.com for animations, journal articles, and more!

Disorders of Ventilation and Gas Exchange

CHARLOTTE POOLER

Chapter 29

➤ The major function of the lungs is to exchange oxygen and carbon dioxide to support the metabolic functions of the body's tissues. The gas exchange function of the lungs depends on a system of open airways, expansion of the lungs, an adequate surface area for gas diffusion, and blood flow through the pulmonary capillary bed. Many types of disease are capable of disrupting the normal gas-exchanging function of the lungs. In some cases the disruption is temporary and in other cases it is marked and disabling. This chapter focuses on disorders that disrupt ventilation and pulmonary gas exchange. It is divided into six sections: the physiologic effects of altered ventilation and gas exchange, disorders of lung inflation, obstructive airway disorders, chronic interstitial lung disorders, disorders of the pulmonary circulation, and acute respiratory disorders.

PHYSIOLOGIC EFFECTS OF VENTILATION AND DIFFUSION DISORDERS

After completing this section of the chapter, you should be able to meet the following objectives:

- Define the terms *hypoxemia* and *hypercapnia*.
- Characterize the mechanisms whereby disorders of ventilation and diffusion cause hypoxemia and hypercapnia.
- Compare the manifestations of hypoxemia and hypercapnia.

The primary function of the respiratory system is to remove appropriate amounts of carbon dioxide (CO_2) from the blood entering the pulmonary circulation and to add adequate amounts of oxygen (O_2) to the blood leaving the pulmonary circulation[1,2] (discussed in Chapter 27). This section of the chapter provides a brief overview of the causes and manifestations of the hypoxemia and hypercapnia that develop as the result of the impaired ventilation and gas exchange that occurs with many of the disorders discussed in the chapter.

Ventilation involves the movement of fresh atmospheric air to the alveoli for provision of O_2 and removal of CO_2. Minute ventilation is the volume of air exchanged per minute and is determined by both the amount of air exchanged with each breath (tidal volume) and the respiratory rate (breaths per minute). *Gas exchange* takes place within the lungs and involves the exchange of O_2 and CO_2 between air in the alveoli and the blood in the pulmonary capillaries. The process involves the diffusion or movement of O_2 from the air in the alveoli (which is rich in O_2 and low in CO_2) to the blood in the pulmonary capillaries and the transfer of CO_2 from the blood in the pulmonary capillaries (which has low amounts of O_2 and high amounts of CO_2) to the alveoli. Adequate oxygenation of the blood and removal of CO_2 also depend on adequate circulation of blood through the pulmonary blood vessels (perfusion) and appropriate contact between ventilated alveoli and perfused capillaries of the pulmonary circulation (ventilation and perfusion matching).

As a general rule, oxygenation of the blood depends primarily on factors that promote diffusion of O_2 from the alveoli into the pulmonary capillaries, whereas removal of CO_2 depends primarily on the minute ventilation and elimination of CO_2 from the alveoli.

Hypoxemia

Hypoxemia refers to a reduction in blood O_2 levels (designated as the partial pressure of oxygen [PO_2]). Hypoxemia can result from an inadequate amount of O_2 in the air, disease of the respiratory system, dysfunction of the neurologic system, or alterations in circulatory function. The mechanisms whereby respiratory disorders lead to a significant reduction in PO_2 are hypoventilation, impaired diffusion of gases, inadequate circulation of blood through the pulmonary capillaries, and mismatching of ventilation and perfusion[2] (see Chapter 27). Often, more than one mechanism contributes to hypoxemia in a person with respiratory or cardiac disease.

Clinical Manifestations and Treatment

Hypoxemia produces its effects through tissue hypoxia and the compensatory mechanisms that the body uses to adapt to the lowered oxygen level. Body tissues vary considerably in their vulnerability to hypoxia; those with the greatest need are the brain and heart. If the PO_2 of the tissues falls below a critical level, aerobic metabolism ceases and anaerobic metabolism takes over, with formation and release of lactic acid. This results in increased serum lactate levels and metabolic acidosis (see Chapter 32).

Mild hypoxemia produces few manifestations. Recruitment of sympathetic nervous system compensatory mechanisms produces an increase in heart rate, peripheral vasoconstriction, diaphoresis, and a mild increase in blood pressure. There may be slight impairment of mental performance and visual acuity and sometimes hyperventilation. This is because hemoglobin saturation still is approximately 90% when the PO_2 is only 60 mm Hg (see Chapter 27, Fig. 27-22). More pronounced hypoxemia may produce personality changes, restlessness, agitated or combative behavior, uncoordinated muscle movements, euphoria, impaired judgment, delirium, and, eventually, stupor and coma.

The manifestations of chronic hypoxemia may be insidious in onset and attributed to other causes, particularly in persons with chronic lung disease. The body compensates for chronic hypoxemia by increased ventilation, pulmonary vasoconstriction, and increased production of red blood cells. Pulmonary vasoconstriction occurs as a local response to alveolar hypoxia; it increases pulmonary arterial pressure and improves the matching of ventilation and blood flow. Increased production of red blood cells results from the release of erythropoietin from the kidneys in response to hypoxia (see Chapter 14). Polycythemia increases the red blood cell concentration and the oxygen-carrying capacity of the blood. Other adaptive mechanisms include a shift to the right in the oxygen dissociation curve, which increases O_2 release to the tissues (see Chapter 27).

Cyanosis refers to the bluish discoloration of the skin and mucous membranes that results from an excessive concentration of reduced or deoxygenated hemoglobin in the small blood vessels. It usually is most marked in the lips, nail beds, ears, and cheeks. The degree of cyanosis is modified by the amount of cutaneous pigment, skin thickness, and the state of the cutaneous capillaries. Cyanosis is more difficult to distinguish in persons with dark skin and in areas of the body with increased skin thickness. Although cyanosis may be evident in persons with respiratory failure, it often is a late sign. A concentration of approximately 5 g/dL of deoxygenated hemoglobin is required in the circulating blood for cyanosis to occur.[1] The absolute quantity of reduced hemoglobin, rather than the relative quantity, is important in producing cyanosis. Persons with anemia and low hemoglobin levels are less likely to exhibit cyanosis (because they have less hemoglobin to deoxygenate), even though they may be relatively hypoxic because of their decreased ability to transport oxygen, than persons who have high hemoglobin concentrations. A person with a high hemoglobin level because of polycythemia may be cyanotic without being hypoxic.

Cyanosis can be divided into two types: central and peripheral. *Central cyanosis* is evident in the tongue and lips. It is caused by an increased amount of deoxygenated hemoglobin or an abnormal hemoglobin derivative in the arterial blood. Abnormal hemoglobin derivatives include *methemoglobin*, in which the nitrite ion reacts with hemoglobin. Because methemoglobin has a low affinity for O_2, large doses of nitrites can result in cyanosis and tissue hypoxia. Although nitrites are used in treating angina, the therapeutic dose is too small to cause cyanosis. *Peripheral cyanosis* occurs in the extremities and on the tip of the nose or ears. It is caused by slowing of blood flow to an area of the body, with increased extraction of oxygen from the blood. It results from vasoconstriction and diminished peripheral blood flow, as occurs with cold exposure, shock, heart failure, or peripheral vascular disease.

Diagnosis. Diagnosis of hypoxemia is based on clinical observation and diagnostic measures of PO_2 levels. The analysis of arterial blood gases provides a direct measure of the O_2 content of the blood and is the best indicator of the ability of the lungs to oxygenate the blood. Venous oxygen saturation (SvO_2) reflects the body's extraction and utilization of O_2 at the tissue levels. Venous blood samples can be obtained either through a pulmonary artery catheter or a central line. The latter is less invasive but slightly less accurate because the blood has not yet been mixed in the right ventricle.

Noninvasive measurements of arterial O_2 saturation of hemoglobin can be obtained using an instrument called the *pulse oximeter.* The pulse oximeter uses light-emitting diodes and combines plethysmography (*i.e.,* changes in light absorbance and vasodilation) with spectrophotometry.[3,4] Spectrophotometry uses a red-wavelength light that passes through oxygenated hemoglobin and is absorbed by deoxygenated hemoglobin, and an infrared-wavelength light that is absorbed by oxygenated hemoglobin and passes through deoxygenated hemoglobin. Sensors that can be placed on the ear, finger, toe, or forehead are available. The pulse oximeter cannot distinguish between oxygen-carrying hemoglobin and carbon monoxide–carrying hemoglobin. In addition, the pulse oximeter cannot detect elevated levels of methemoglobin. Although pulse oximetry is not as accurate as arterial blood gas measurements, it provides the means for noninvasive and continuous monitoring of O_2 saturation, which is a useful indicator of respiratory and circulatory status.

The ratio between the arterial PO_2 and the fraction of inspired oxygen (FiO_2), termed the *PF ratio,* is an additional indicator of alterations in diffusion of O_2 at the lung level. In determining this ratio, the PO_2 is divided by the FiO_2. For example, the FiO_2 of a person breathing room air is 0.21 because 21% of atmospheric air is O_2, whereas for the person receiving 40% O_2, the FiO_2 is 0.40. The normal value of the PF ratio is greater than 300.[5] The PF ratio is useful for evaluating improvements or deteriorations in oxygen diffusion regardless of the percentage of supplemental oxygen that is being administered. In addition, the PF ratio is a diagnostic indicator of acute lung injury and acute respiratory distress syndrome (discussed later in the chapter).

Treatment. Treatment of hypoxemia is directed toward correcting the cause of the disorder and increasing the gradient for diffusion through the administration of supplemental oxygen. Oxygen may be delivered by nasal cannula or mask, or administered directly into an endotracheal or tracheostomy tube in persons who are mechanically ventilated. A high-flow administration system is one in which the flow rate and reserve capacity are sufficient to provide all the inspired air.[6] A low-flow administration system delivers less than the total inspired air.[6] The concentration of O_2 being administered (usually determined by the flow rate) is based on the PO_2. A high flow rate must be carefully monitored in persons with chronic lung disease because increases in PO_2 above 60 mm Hg may depress the ventilatory drive. There also is the danger of oxygen toxicity with high concentrations of oxygen. Continuous breathing of oxygen at high concentrations can lead to diffuse parenchymal lung injury. Persons with healthy lungs begin to experience respiratory symptoms such as cough, sore throat, substernal distress, nasal congestion, and painful inspiration after breathing pure oxygen for 24 hours.[2]

Hypercapnia

Hypercapnia refers to an increase in the carbon dioxide content of the arterial blood.[7] The carbon dioxide level in the arterial blood, or PCO_2, is proportional to carbon dioxide production and inversely related to alveolar ventilation. The diagnosis of hypercapnia is based on physiologic manifestations, arterial pH, and arterial blood gas levels.

Hypercapnia can occur in a number of disorders that cause hypoventilation or mismatching of ventilation and perfusion.[7] The diffusing capacity of carbon dioxide is 20 times that of oxygen; therefore, hypercapnia without hypoxemia is usually observed only in situations of hypoventilation.[2] In cases of ventilation–perfusion mismatching, hypercapnia is usually accompanied by a decrease in arterial PO_2 levels.

Conditions that increase carbon dioxide production, such as an increase in metabolic rate or a high-carbohydrate diet, can contribute to the degree of hypercapnia that occurs in persons with impaired respiratory function. Changes in the metabolic rate resulting from an increase in activity, fever, or disease can have profound effects on carbon dioxide production. Alveolar ventilation usually rises proportionally with these changes, and hypercapnia occurs only when this increase is inappropriate.

The respiratory quotient (RQ), which is the ratio of carbon dioxide production to oxygen consumption (RQ = CO_2 production/O_2 consumption), varies with the type of food metabolized.[1] A characteristic of carbohydrate metabolism is an RQ of 1.0, with equal amounts of carbon dioxide being produced and oxygen being consumed. Because fats contain less oxygen than carbohydrates, their oxidation produces less carbon dioxide (RQ = 0.7). The metabolism of pure proteins (RQ = 0.81) results in the production of more carbon dioxide than the metabolism of fat, but less than the metabolism of carbohydrates. The type of food that is eaten or the types of nutrients that are delivered through enteral feedings (*i.e.,* through a tube placed in the small intestine) or parenteral nutrition (*i.e.,* through a venous catheter placed in the central vena cava) may influence PCO_2 levels.

Clinical Manifestations and Treatment

Hypercapnia affects a number of body functions, including acid-base balance and kidney, nervous system, and cardiovascular function. Elevated levels of PCO_2 produce a decrease in pH and respiratory acidosis (see Chapter 32). The body normally compensates for an increase in PCO_2 by increasing renal bicarbonate (HCO_3^-) retention, which results in an increase in serum HCO_3^- and pH levels. As long as the pH is within normal range, the main complications of hypercapnia are those resulting from the accompanying hypoxia. Because the body adapts to chronic increases in blood levels of carbon dioxide, persons with chronic hypercapnia may not have symptoms until the PCO_2 becomes markedly elevated.

Treatment. The treatment of hypercapnia is directed at decreasing the work of breathing and improving the ventilation–perfusion balance. The use of intermittent rest therapy, such as nocturnal negative-pressure ventilation, in persons with chronic obstructive disease or chest wall disease may be effective in increasing the strength and endurance of the respiratory muscles and improving the PCO_2. Respiratory muscle retraining aimed at improving the respiratory muscles, their endurance, or both has been used to improve exercise tolerance and diminish the likelihood of respiratory fatigue. Mechanical ventilation (discussed in the section on Acute Respiratory Failure) may become necessary in situations of acute hypercapnia.

IN SUMMARY, the primary function of the respiratory system is to remove appropriate amounts of CO_2 from the blood entering the pulmonary circulation and provide adequate O_2 to blood leaving the pulmonary circulation. This is accomplished through the process of ventilation, in which air moves into and out of the lungs, and diffusion, in which gases move between the alveoli and the pulmonary capillaries. Although both diffusion and ventilation affect gas exchange, oxygenation of the blood largely depends on diffusion, and removal of carbon dioxide on ventilation.

Hypoxemia refers to a decrease in arterial blood oxygen levels that results in a decrease in tissue oxygenation. Hypoxemia can occur as the result of hypoventilation, diffusion impairment, shunt, and ventilation–perfusion impairment. Acute hypoxemia is manifested by increased respiratory effort (increased respiratory and heart rates), cyanosis, and impaired sensory and neurologic function. The body compensates for chronic hypoxemia by increased ventilation, pulmonary vasoconstriction, and increased production of red blood cells.

Hypercapnia refers to an increase in carbon dioxide levels. In the clinical setting, four factors contribute to hypercapnia: alterations in carbon dioxide production, disturbance in the gas exchange function of the lungs, abnormalities in function of the chest wall and respiratory muscles, and changes in neural control of respiration. Alterations in respiratory function or rate decrease minute volume, which is the most common cause of hypercapnia. The manifestations of hypercapnia consist of those associated with a decrease in pH (respiratory acidosis); vasodilation of blood vessels, including those in the brain; and depression of central nervous system function. ∎

 DISORDERS OF LUNG INFLATION

After completing this section of the chapter, you should be able to meet the following objectives:

- Characterize the pathogenesis and manifestations of transudative and exudative pleural effusion, chylothorax, and hemothorax.
- Differentiate among the causes and manifestations of spontaneous pneumothorax, secondary pneumothorax, and tension pneumothorax.
- Describe the causes of pleurisy and differentiate the characteristics of pleural pain from other types of chest pain.
- Describe the causes and manifestations of atelectasis.

Air entering through the airways inflates the lung, and the negative pressure in the pleural cavity keeps the lung from collapsing. Disorders of lung inflation are caused by conditions that obstruct the airways, cause lung compression, or produce lung collapse. There can be compression of the lung by an accumulation of fluid in the intrapleural space, complete collapse of an entire lung, as in pneumothorax, or collapse of a segment of the lung due to airway obstruction, as in atelectasis.

Disorders of the Pleura

The pleura is a thin, double-layered serous membrane that encases the lungs (Fig. 29-1). The outer *parietal layer* lines the thoracic wall and superior aspect of the diaphragm. It continues around the heart and between the lungs, forming the lateral walls of the mediastinum. The inner *visceral layer* covers the

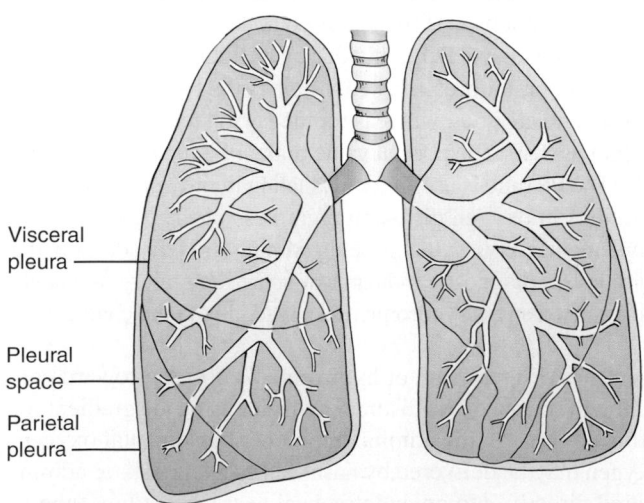

FIGURE 29-1 • The relationship between the parietal and visceral pleurae and the pleural space, which is the site of fluid accumulation in pleural effusions.

Visceral pleura — Pleural space — Parietal pleura —

lung and is adherent to all its surfaces. The pleural cavity or space between the two layers contains a thin layer of serous fluid that lubricates the pleural surfaces and allows the parietal and visceral pleurae to slide smoothly over each other during breathing movements. The pressure in the pleural cavity, which is negative in relation to atmospheric pressure, holds the lungs against the chest wall and keeps them from collapsing (see Chapter 27). Disorders of the pleura include pleural effusion, hemothorax, pneumothorax, and pleural inflammation.

Pleural Effusion

Pleural effusion refers to an abnormal collection of fluid in the pleural cavity.[8,9] Like fluid developing in other transcellular spaces in the body, pleural effusion occurs when the rate of fluid formation exceeds the rate of its removal (see Chapter 31). Normally, fluid enters the pleural space from capillaries in the parietal pleura and is removed by the lymphatics situated in the parietal pleura. Fluid can also enter from the interstitial spaces of the lung through the visceral pleura or from small holes in the diaphragm. The lymphatics have the capacity to reabsorb about 20 times the fluid that is formed.[9] Accordingly, fluid may accumulate when there is excess fluid formation (from the interstitium of the lung, the parietal pleura, or peritoneal cavity) or when there is decreased removal by the lymphatics.

The fluid that accumulates in a pleural effusion may be a transudate or exudate, purulent (containing pus), chyle, or sanguineous (bloody). The accumulation of a serous transudate (clear fluid) in the pleural cavity often is referred to as *hydrothorax*. The condition may be unilateral or bilateral. The most common cause of hydrothorax is congestive heart failure.[9] Other causes are renal failure, nephrosis, liver failure, and malignancy. An *exudate* is a pleural fluid that has a specific gravity greater than 1.020 and often contains inflammatory cells.

Transudative and exudative pleural effusions are distinguished by measuring the lactate dehydrogenase (LDH) and protein levels in the pleural fluid.[9] Exudative pleural effusion meets at least one of the following criteria: (1) a pleural fluid protein/serum protein ratio greater than 0.5; (2) a pleural fluid LDH/serum LDH ratio greater than 0.6; and (3) a pleural fluid LDH greater than two thirds the upper limit of normal serum LDH.[9] LDH is an enzyme that is released from inflamed and injured pleural tissue. Because measurements of LDH are easily obtained from a sample of pleural fluid, it is a useful marker for diagnosis of exudative pleural disorders. Conditions that produce exudative pleural effusions are bacterial pneumonia, viral infection, pulmonary infarction, and malignancies.

Empyema refers to an infection in the pleural cavity that results in exudate containing glucose, proteins, leukocytes, and debris from dead cells and tissue.[9] It is caused by an adjacent bacterial pneumonia, rupture of a lung abscess into the pleural space, invasion from a subdiaphragmatic infection, or infection associated with trauma.

Chylothorax is the effusion of lymph in the thoracic cavity.[10] Chyle, a milky fluid containing chylomicrons, is found in the lymph fluid originating in the gastrointestinal tract. The thoracic duct transports chyle to the central circulation. Chylothorax also results from trauma, inflammation, or malignant infiltration obstructing chyle transport from the thoracic duct into the central circulation. It is the most common cause of pleural effusion in the fetus and neonate, resulting from congenital malformation of the thoracic duct or lymph channels. Chylothorax also can occur as a complication of intrathoracic surgical procedures and use of the great veins for total parenteral nutrition and hemodynamic monitoring.

Manifestations. The manifestations of pleural effusion vary with the cause. Empyema may be accompanied by fever, increased white blood cell count, and other signs of inflammation. Fluid in the pleural cavity acts as a space-occupying mass; it causes a decrease in lung expansion on the affected side that is proportional to the amount of fluid collected. Characteristic signs of pleural effusion are dullness or flatness to percussion and diminished breath sounds. Hypoxemia may occur due to the decreased surface area and usually is corrected with supplemental oxygen. Dyspnea, the most common symptom, occurs when fluid compresses the lung, resulting in increased effort or rate of breathing. Pleuritic pain usually occurs only when inflammation is present, although constant discomfort may be felt with large effusions.

Diagnosis and Treatment. Diagnosis of pleural effusion is based on chest radiographs, chest ultrasonography, and computed tomography (CT). Thoracentesis (aspiration of fluid from the pleural space) can be used to obtain a sample of pleural fluid for diagnosis. The treatment of pleural effusion is directed at the cause of the disorder. With large effusions, thoracentesis may be used to remove fluid from the intrapleural space and allow for reexpansion of the lung. A palliative method used for treatment of pleural effusions caused by a malignancy is the injection of a sclerosing agent into the pleural cavity. This method of treatment causes obliteration of the pleural space and prevents the reaccumulation of fluid. Chest tube drainage may be necessary in cases of continued effusion.

Hemothorax

Hemothorax is a specific type of pleural effusion in which there is blood in the pleural cavity. Bleeding may be the result of chest injury, a complication of chest surgery, malignancies, or rupture of a great vessel such as an aortic aneurysm. Hemothorax may be classified as minimal, moderate, or large.[11] A minimal hemothorax involves the presence of 300 to 500 mL of blood in the pleural space. Small amounts of blood usually are absorbed from the pleural space, and the hemothorax usually clears in 10 to 14 days without complication. A moderate hemothorax (500 to 1000 mL of blood) fills approximately one third of the pleural space and may produce signs of lung compression and loss of intravascular volume. It requires immediate drainage and replacement of intravascular fluids. A large hemothorax fills one half or more of one side of the chest; it indicates the presence of 1000 mL or more of blood in the thorax and usually is caused by bleeding from a high-pressure vessel such as an intercostal or mammary artery. It requires immediate drainage and, if the bleeding continues, surgery to control the bleeding.

In addition to alterations in oxygenation, ventilation, respiration effort, and breath sounds, hemothorax may be accompanied by signs of blood loss, including increased heart rate. Because hemothorax is abrupt in onset, the manifestations are usually sudden and distressing. One of the complications of untreated moderate or large hemothorax is fibrothorax—the fusion of the pleural surfaces by fibrin, hyalin, and connective tissue—and in some cases, calcification of the fibrous tissue, which restricts lung expansion.

Diagnosis of hemothorax is based on chest radiographs and decreased arterial saturation, which is indicative of decreased oxygen exchange. If the person is symptomatic or oxygen exchange is compromised, chest tube drainage is indicated.

Pneumothorax

Pneumothorax refers to the presence of air in the pleural space. Pneumothorax causes partial or complete collapse of the affected lung. Pneumothorax can occur without an obvious cause or injury (*i.e.,* spontaneous pneumothorax) or as a result of direct injury to the chest or major airways (*i.e.,* traumatic pneumothorax). Tension pneumothorax describes a life-threatening condition in which increased pressure within the pleural cavity impairs both respiratory and cardiac function.

Spontaneous Pneumothorax. Spontaneous pneumothorax is hypothesized to occur due to the rupture of an air-filled bleb, or blister, on the surface of the lung. Rupture of these blebs allows atmospheric air from the airways to enter the pleural cavity (Fig. 29-2). Because alveolar pressure normally is greater than pleural pressure, air flows from the alveoli into the pleural space,

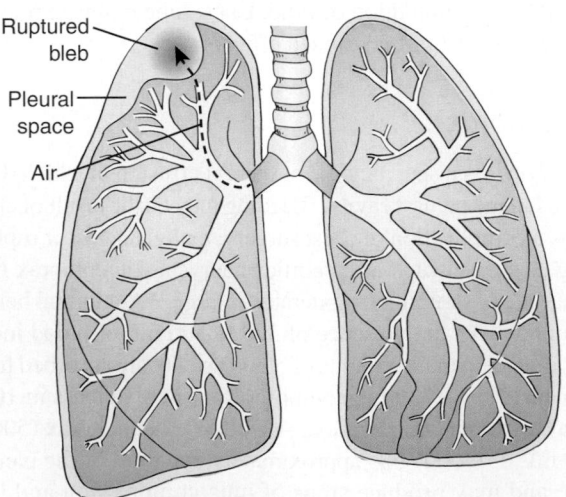

FIGURE 29-2 • Mechanism for development of spontaneous pneumothorax, in which an air-filled bleb on the surface of the lung ruptures, allowing atmospheric air from the airways to enter the pleural space.

causing the involved portion of the lung to collapse as a result of its own recoil. Air continues to flow into the pleural space until a pressure gradient no longer exists or until the decline in lung size causes the leak to seal. Spontaneous pneumothoraces can be divided into primary and secondary pneumothoraces. Primary pneumothorax occurs in otherwise healthy persons, whereas secondary pneumothorax occurs in persons with underlying lung disease.

In primary spontaneous pneumothorax, the blebs usually are located at the top of the lungs.[12] The condition is seen most often in tall boys and young men between 10 and 30 years of age.[13] It has been suggested that the difference in pleural pressure from the top to the bottom of the lung is greater in tall persons and that this difference in pressure may contribute to the development of blebs. Smoking is another factor that has been associated with primary spontaneous pneumothorax. Inflammation of the small airways related to smoking probably contributes to the condition, and cessation of smoking may reduce the recurrence.[14] Persons with *talc lung* are also highly susceptible to the occurrence of pneumothorax. Talc lung may result from inhalation of talc particles from household or industrial sources, but is more commonly associated with injected or inhaled talc powder used as a filler with heroin, methamphetamine, or cocaine.[15]

Secondary spontaneous pneumothoraces usually are more serious because they occur in persons with lung disease. They are associated with many different types of lung conditions that cause trapping of gases and destruction of lung tissue, including asthma, tuberculosis, cystic fibrosis, sarcoidosis, bronchogenic carcinoma, and metastatic pleural diseases. The most common cause of secondary spontaneous pneumothorax is emphysema. Secondary spontaneous pneumothorax may be life-threatening because of the underlying lung injury and poor compensatory reserves.

Catamenial pneumothorax occurs in relation to the menstrual cycle and usually is recurrent.[16] It typically occurs in women who are 30 to 40 years of age and have a history of endometriosis. It usually affects the right lung and develops within 72 hours of onset of menses. Although the cause of catamenial pneumothorax is unknown, it has been suggested that air may gain access to the peritoneal cavity during menstruation and then enter the pleural cavity through a diaphragmatic defect.[16] Pleural and diaphragmatic endometriosis also have been implicated as causes of the condition.

Traumatic Pneumothorax. Traumatic pneumothorax may be caused by penetrating or nonpenetrating injuries. Fractured or dislocated ribs that penetrate the pleura are the most common cause of pneumothorax from nonpenetrating chest injuries. Hemothorax may accompany these injuries. Pneumothorax also may accompany fracture of the trachea or major bronchus or rupture of the esophagus. Persons with pneumothorax due to chest trauma frequently have other complications and may require chest surgery. Medical procedures such as transthoracic needle aspirations, central line insertion, intubation, and positive-pressure ventilation occasionally may cause pneumothorax. Traumatic pneumothorax also can occur as a complication of cardiopulmonary resuscitation.

Tension Pneumothorax.

Tension pneumothorax occurs when the intrapleural pressure exceeds atmospheric pressure. It is a life-threatening condition and occurs when injury to the chest or respiratory structures permits air to enter but not leave the pleural space (Fig. 29-3). This results in a rapid increase in pressure within the chest that causes compression atelectasis of the unaffected lung, a shift in the mediastinum to the opposite side of the chest, and compression of the vena cava, which results in a decrease in venous return to the heart and reduced cardiac output.[9] Although tension pneumothorax can develop in persons with spontaneous pneumothoraces, it is seen most often in persons with traumatic pneumothoraces. It also may result from mechanical ventilation.

Manifestations.

The manifestations of pneumothorax depend on its size and the integrity of the underlying lung. In spontaneous pneumothorax, manifestations of the disorder include development of ipsilateral chest pain. There is an almost immediate increase in respiratory rate, often accompanied by dyspnea that occurs as a result of the activation of receptors that monitor lung volume. Asymmetry of the chest may occur because of the air trapped in the pleural cavity on the affected side. This asymmetry may be evidenced during inspiration as a lag in the movement of the affected side, with inspiration delayed until the unaffected lung reaches the same level of pressure as the lung with the air trapped in the pleural space. Percussion of the chest produces a more hyperresonant sound, and breath sounds are decreased or absent over the area of the pneumothorax.

With tension pneumothorax, the structures in the mediastinal space shift toward the opposite side of the chest (see Fig. 29-3). When this occurs, the position of the trachea, normally located in the midline of the neck, deviates with the mediastinum. The position of the trachea can be used as a means of assessing for a mediastinal shift. Because of the increase in intrathoracic pressure, stroke volume is impaired to such an extent that cardiac output is decreased despite an increase in heart rate. There may be distention of the neck veins, subcutaneous emphysema (*i.e.,* presence of air in the subcutaneous tissues of the chest and neck), and clinical signs of shock due to impaired cardiac function.

Hypoxemia usually develops immediately after a large pneumothorax, followed by vasoconstriction of the blood vessels in the affected lung, causing the blood flow to shift to the unaffected lung. In persons with primary spontaneous pneumothorax, this mechanism usually returns oxygen saturation to normal within 24 hours. Hypoxemia usually is more serious in persons with underlying lung disease in whom secondary spontaneous pneumothorax develops or in persons with underlying heart disease who are unable to compensate with an increase in heart rate and stroke volumes. Regardless of etiology, the hypoxemia caused by the partial or total loss of lung function can be life-threatening. Without immediate intervention, the increased thoracic pressure will further impair both cardiac and pulmonary function, resulting in severe hypoxemia and hypotension.

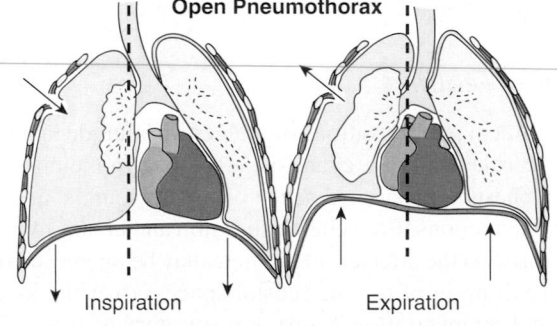

Open Pneumothorax

Inspiration   Expiration

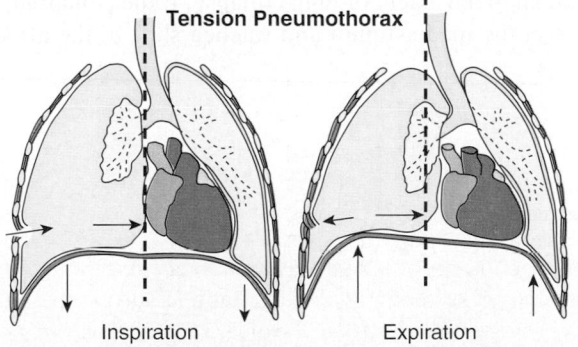

Tension Pneumothorax

Inspiration   Expiration

FIGURE 29-3 • Open or communicating pneumothorax (**top**) and tension pneumothorax (**bottom**). In an open pneumothorax, air enters the chest during inspiration and exits during expiration. There may be slight inflation of the affected lung because of a decrease in pressure as air moves out of the chest. In tension pneumothorax, air can enter but not leave the chest. As the pressure in the chest increases, the heart and great vessels are compressed and the mediastinal structures are shifted toward the opposite side of the chest. The trachea is pushed from its normal midline position toward the opposite side of the chest, and the unaffected lung is compressed.

Diagnosis and Treatment.

Diagnosis of pneumothorax can be confirmed by chest radiograph or CT scan. Pulse oximetry and blood gas analysis may be done to determine the effect on blood oxygen levels.

Treatment of pneumothorax varies with the cause and extent of the disorder. In small spontaneous pneumothoraces, the air usually reabsorbs spontaneously, and only observation and follow-up chest radiographs are required. Supplemental oxygen may be used to correct the hypoxemia until the air is reabsorbed. In larger pneumothoraces, the air is removed by needle aspiration or a closed drainage system used with or without suction. This type of drainage system uses a one-way valve or a water-seal chamber to allow air to exit the pleural space and prevent it from reentering the chest.

Emergency treatment of tension pneumothorax involves the prompt insertion of a large-bore needle or chest tube into the affected side of the chest along with one-way valve drainage or continuous chest suction to aid in lung reexpansion. Sucking chest wounds, which allow air to pass in and out of the chest cavity, should be treated by promptly covering the area with an airtight covering (*e.g.,* Vaseline gauze, firm piece of plastic). Chest tubes are inserted as soon as possible.

Because of the risk for recurrence, persons with primary spontaneous pneumothorax should be advised against cigarette smoking, exposure to high altitudes, flying in nonpressurized aircraft, and scuba diving.

Pleuritis

Pleuritis (also called *pleurisy*) refers to inflammation of the pleura. Pleuritis is common in infectious processes such as respiratory infections that extend to involve the pleura. Pain is a frequent symptom, and most commonly is unilateral and abrupt in onset. When the central part of the diaphragm is irritated, the pain may be referred to the shoulder. The pain is usually made worse by chest movements such as deep breathing and coughing that exaggerate pressure changes in the pleural cavity and increase movement of the inflamed or injured pleural surfaces. Because deep breathing is painful, tidal volumes usually are kept small, and breathing becomes more rapid to maintain minute volume. Reflex splinting of the chest muscles may occur, causing a lesser respiratory expansion on the affected side.

It is important to differentiate pleural pain from pain produced by other conditions, such as musculoskeletal strain of chest muscles, bronchial irritation, and myocardial disease. Musculoskeletal pain may occur as the result of frequent, forceful coughing. This type of pain usually is bilateral and located in the inferior portions of the rib cage, where the abdominal muscles insert into the anterior rib cage. It is made worse by movements associated with contraction of the abdominal muscles. The pain associated with irritation of the bronchi usually is substernal and dull in character rather than sharp. It is made worse with coughing but is not affected by deep breathing. Myocardial pain, which is discussed in Chapter 24, usually is located in the substernal area and is not affected by respiratory movements.

Treatment of pleuritis consists of treating the underlying disease and inflammation. Analgesics and nonsteroidal anti-inflammatory drugs (NSAIDs; *e.g.,* indomethacin) may be used for pleural pain. Although these agents reduce inflammation, they may not entirely relieve the discomfort associated with deep breathing and coughing.

Atelectasis

Atelectasis refers to an incomplete expansion of a lung or portion of a lung. It can be caused by airway obstruction, lung compression such as occurs in pneumothorax or pleural effusion, or increased recoil of the lung due to loss of pulmonary surfactant (see Chapter 27). The disorder may be present at birth (*i.e.,* primary atelectasis) or develop during the neonatal period or later in life (*i.e.,* acquired or secondary atelectasis).

Primary atelectasis of the newborn implies that the lung has never been inflated. It is seen most frequently in premature and high-risk infants. A secondary form of atelectasis can occur in infants who established respiration and subsequently experienced impairment of lung expansion. Among the causes of secondary atelectasis in the newborn is the respiratory dis-

tress syndrome associated with lack of surfactant and airway obstruction due to aspiration of amniotic fluid or blood.

Acquired atelectasis occurs mainly in adults. It is caused most commonly by airway obstruction and lung compression (Fig. 29-4). Obstruction can be caused by a mucus plug in the airway or by external compression by fluid, tumor mass, exudate, or other matter in the area surrounding the airway. Portions of alveoli, a small segment of lung, or an entire lung lobe may be involved in obstructive atelectasis. Complete obstruction of an airway is followed by the absorption of air from the dependent alveoli and collapse of that portion of the lung. Breathing high concentrations of oxygen increases the rate at which gases are absorbed from the alveoli and predisposes to atelectasis. The danger of obstructive atelectasis increases after surgery. Anesthesia, pain, administration of narcotics, and immobility tend to promote retention of viscid bronchial secretions and hence airway obstruction. The encouragement of coughing and deep breathing, frequent change of position, adequate hydration, and early ambulation decrease the likelihood of atelectasis developing.

Another cause of atelectasis is compression of lung tissue. It occurs when the pleural cavity is partially or completely filled with fluid, exudate, blood, a tumor mass, or air. It is observed most commonly in persons with pleural effusion from congestive heart failure or cancer.

Clinical Features

The clinical manifestations of atelectasis include tachypnea, tachycardia, dyspnea, cyanosis, signs of hypoxemia, diminished chest expansion, absence of breath sounds, and intercostal retractions. Both chest expansion and breath sounds are decreased on the affected area. There may be intercostal retraction (pulling in of the intercostal spaces) over the involved area during inspiration. Signs of respiratory distress are proportional to the extent of lung collapse. If the collapsed area is large, the mediastinum and trachea shift to the affected

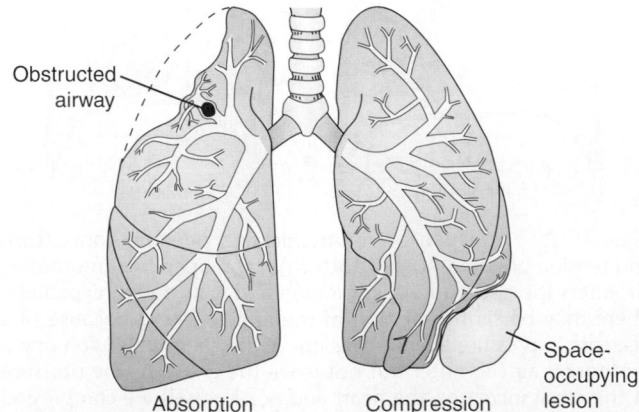

Obstructed airway

Absorption   Compression

Space-occupying lesion

FIGURE 29-4 • Atelectasis caused by airway obstruction and absorption of air from the involved lung area (**left**) and by compression of lung tissue (**right**).

side. In compression atelectasis, the mediastinum shifts away from the affected lung.

The diagnosis of atelectasis is based on signs and symptoms. Chest radiographs are used to confirm the diagnosis. CT scans may be used to show the exact location of the obstruction.

Treatment depends on the cause and extent of lung involvement. It is directed at reducing the airway obstruction or lung compression and at reinflating the collapsed area of the lung. Ambulation, deep breathing, and body positions that favor increased lung expansion are used when appropriate. Administration of oxygen may be needed to correct the hypoxemia. Bronchoscopy may be used as both a diagnostic and treatment method.

IN SUMMARY, disorders of the pleura include pleural effusion, hemothorax, pneumothorax, and pleuritis. Pleural effusion refers to the abnormal accumulation of fluid in the pleural cavity. The fluid may be a transudate (*i.e.,* hydrothorax), exudate (*i.e.,* empyema), or chyle (*i.e.,* chylothorax). Hemothorax refers to the presence of blood in the pleural cavity. Pain is a common symptom of conditions that produce pleuritis or inflammation of the pleura. Characteristically, the pain is unilateral, abrupt in onset, and exaggerated by respiratory movements. Pneumothorax refers to an accumulation of air in the pleural cavity that causes partial or complete collapse of the lung. Pneumothorax can result from rupture of an air-filled bleb on the lung surface or from penetrating or nonpenetrating injuries. A tension pneumothorax is a life-threatening event in which air progressively accumulates in the thorax, collapsing the lung on the injured side and progressively shifting the mediastinum to the opposite side of the thorax, producing severe cardiac and respiratory impairment.

Atelectasis refers to an incomplete expansion of the lung. Primary atelectasis occurs most often in premature and high-risk infants. Acquired atelectasis occurs mainly in adults and is caused most commonly by a mucus plug in the airway or by external compression by fluid, tumor mass, exudate, or other matter in the area surrounding the airway. ■

OBSTRUCTIVE AIRWAY DISORDERS

After completing this section of the chapter, you should be able to meet the following objectives:

- Describe the physiology of bronchial smooth muscle as it relates to airway disease.
- Describe the interaction between heredity, alterations in the immune response, and environmental agents in the pathogenesis of bronchial asthma.

- Characterize the acute- or early-phase and late-phase responses in the pathogenesis of bronchial asthma and relate them to current methods for treatment of the disorder.
- Explain the changes in pulmonary function studies that occur with chronic airway disease.
- Explain the distinction between chronic bronchitis and emphysema in terms of pathology and clinical manifestations.
- State the chief manifestations of bronchiectasis.
- Describe the genetic abnormality responsible for cystic fibrosis and relate it to the manifestations of the disorder.

Obstructive airway disorders are caused by disorders that limit expiratory airflow. Bronchial asthma represents an acute and reversible form of airway disease caused by narrowing of airways due to bronchospasm, inflammation, and increased airway secretions. Chronic obstructive disorders include a variety of airway diseases, such as chronic bronchitis, emphysema, bronchiectasis, and cystic fibrosis.

Physiology of Airway Disease

Air moves through the upper airways (*i.e.,* trachea and major bronchi) into the lower or pulmonary airways (*i.e.,* bronchi and alveoli), which are located in the lung. In the pulmonary airways, the cartilaginous layer that provides support for the trachea and major bronchi gradually disappears and is replaced with crisscrossing strips of smooth muscle (see Chapter 27). The contraction and relaxation of the smooth muscle layer, which is innervated by the autonomic nervous system, controls the diameter of the bronchial airways and consequent resistance to airflow. Parasympathetic stimulation, through the vagus nerve and cholinergic receptors, produces bronchial constriction, whereas sympathetic stimulation, through β_2-adrenergic receptors, increases bronchial dilation. At rest, a slight vagal-mediated bronchoconstrictor tone predominates. When there is need for increased airflow, as during exercise, the bronchodilator effects of the sympathetic nervous system are stimulated and the bronchoconstrictor effects of the parasympathetic nervous system are inhibited. Bronchial smooth muscle also responds to inflammatory mediators, such as histamine, that act directly on bronchial smooth muscle cells to produce constriction.

Bronchial Asthma

Bronchial asthma is a chronic disorder of the airways that causes episodes of airway obstruction, bronchial hyperresponsiveness, and airway inflammation that are usually reversible.[17,18] According to 2005 data, an estimated 22.2 million Americans (3.8 million children younger than 18 years of age) had an asthma attack.[19] Although the prevalence rates for asthma have increased over

⚷— AIRWAY DISORDERS

■ Airway disorders affect airway patency and movement of atmospheric air into and out of the gas exchange portion of the lung.

■ Changes in airway patency involve changes in airway diameter due to bronchial smooth muscle hyperreactivity or changes in bronchial wall structure, injury to the mucosal lining of the airways, or excess respiratory tract secretions.

■ Bronchial asthma is a chronic disorder of the airways that causes episodes of airway obstruction due to bronchial smooth muscle hyperreactivity and airway inflammation. The episodes usually are reversible.

■ Chronic obstructive pulmonary disease represents a group of disorders that cause chronic and recurrent obstruction of the pulmonary airways. These disorders can affect patency of the bronchial structures (chronic bronchitis), the gas-diffusing airspaces distal to the terminal bronchioles (emphysema), or a combination of both.

the past several decades, the mortality rate and hospitalizations due to asthma have stabilized, indicating a higher level of disease management.[19]

The National Heart, Lung, and Blood Institute's Second Expert Panel on the Management of Asthma defined bronchial asthma as "a chronic inflammatory disorder of the airways in which many cells and cellular elements play a role, in particular, mast cells, eosinophils, T lymphocytes, and epithelial cells."[17,18] This inflammatory process produces recurrent episodes of airway obstruction, characterized by wheezing, breathlessness, chest tightness, and a cough that often is worse at night and in the early morning. These episodes, which usually are reversible either spontaneously or with treatment, also cause an associated increase in bronchial responsiveness to a variety of stimuli.[17]

In susceptible persons, an asthma attack can be triggered by a variety of stimuli that do not normally cause symptoms. Typically, asthma has been categorized into extrinsic (initiated by a type I hypersensitivity [atopic] response to an extrinsic antigen) and intrinsic (initiated by diverse nonimmune mechanisms, including respiratory tract infections, exercise, ingestion of aspirin, emotional upset, and exposure to bronchial irritants such as cigarette smoke.).[18] Although this distinction is useful from the perspective of pathophysiology, it is less useful clinically because many persons with asthma manifest overlapping characteristics of both extrinsic and intrinsic asthma.

Etiology and Pathogenesis

The common denominator underlying all forms of asthma is an exaggerated hypersensitivity response to a variety of stimuli.

Most current information suggests that airway inflammation manifested by the presence of inflammatory cells (particularly eosinophils, lymphocytes, and mast cells) and by damage to the bronchial epithelium contributes to the pathogenesis of the disease.

Recent research has focused on the role of T lymphocytes in the pathogenesis of bronchial asthma. It is now known that there are two subsets of T-helper cells (T_H1 and T_H2) that develop from the same precursor CD4$^+$ T lymphocyte (see Chapter 17).[20,21] T_H1 cells differentiate in response to microbes and stimulate the differentiation of B cells into immunoglobulin (Ig)M– and IgG-producing plasma cells. T_H2 cells, on the other hand, respond to allergens and helminths (intestinal parasites) by stimulating B cells to differentiate into IgE-producing plasma cells, produce growth factors for mast cells, and recruit and activate eosinophils (see Chapter 19, Fig. 19-3). In persons with allergic asthma, T-cell differentiation appears to be skewed toward T_H2 cells. Although the molecular basis for this preferential differentiation is unclear, it seems likely that both genetic and environmental factors play a role.[21]

Cytokines also have an apparent role in the chronic inflammatory response and complications of asthma. Tumor necrosis factor (TNF)-α and interleukins 4 and 5 (IL-4, IL-5) participate in the pathogenesis of bronchial asthma through their effects on the bronchial epithelial and smooth muscle cells.[21,22] Recent studies suggest that TNF-α, an inflammatory cytokine that is stored and released from mast cells, plays a critical role in the initiation and amplification of airway inflammation in persons with asthma. TNF-α is credited with increasing the migration and activation of inflammatory cells (*i.e.,* eosinophils and neutrophils) and contributing to all aspects of airway remodeling, including proliferation and activation of fibroblasts, increased production of extracellular matrix glycoproteins, and mucous cell hyperplasia.[22]

Extrinsic (Atopic) Asthma. Extrinsic or atopic asthma is typically initiated by a type I hypersensitivity reaction induced by exposure to an extrinsic antigen or allergen.[23,24] It usually has its onset in childhood or adolescence and is seen in persons with a family history of atopic allergy (see Chapter 19). Candidate genes for predisposition to atopy and airway hyperresponsiveness are currently subjects for intensive research and include genes involved in antigen presentation, T-cell activation, regulation of cytokine production or function, and receptors for bronchodilating substances.[21]

Persons with atopic asthma often have other allergic disorders, such as hay fever, urticaria, and eczema. Attacks are related to exposure to specific allergens. Among airborne allergens implicated in perennial (year-round) asthma are house dust mite allergens, cockroach allergens, animal danders, and *Alternaria* (a fungus).

The mechanisms of response to antigens in atopic asthma can be described in terms of the early- or acute-phase response and the late-phase response[20,21] (Fig. 29-5). Recall that IgE-mediated hypersensitivity responses (discussed in Chapter 19) involve an initial antigen (allergen) sensitization, which leads

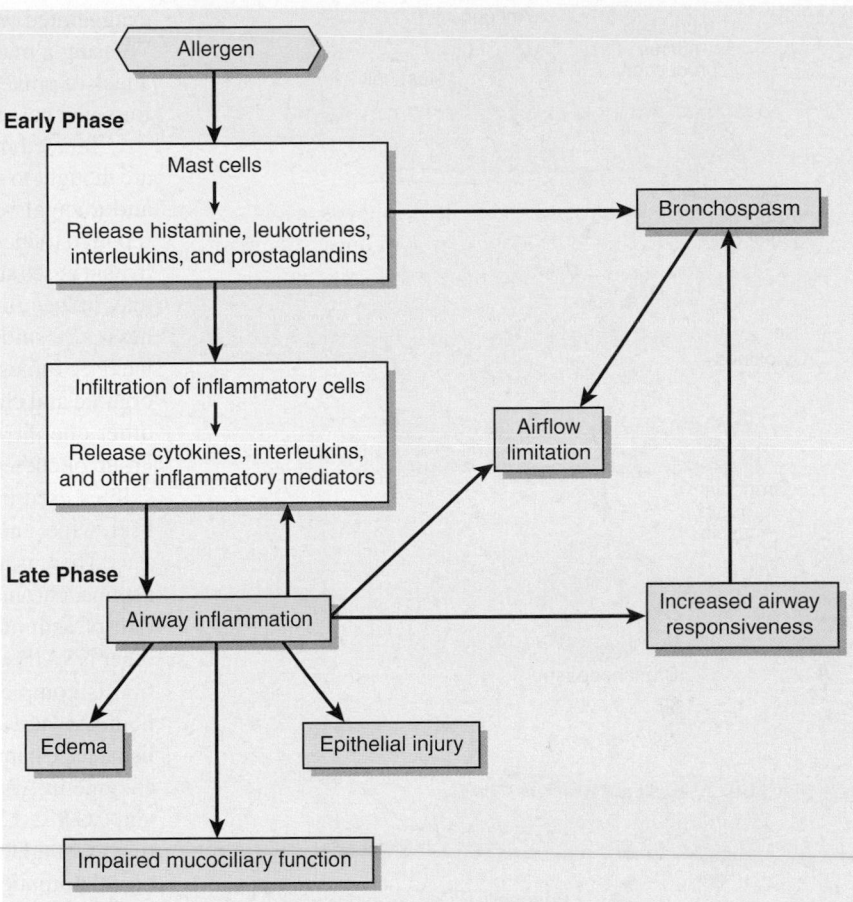

FIGURE 29-5 • Mechanisms of early- and late-phase IgE-mediated bronchospasm.

to the production of presensitized IgE-coated mast cells. The symptoms of the *acute-phase response,* which usually develop within 10 to 20 minutes, are caused by the release of chemical mediators from the presensitized mast cells. In the case of airborne antigens, the reaction occurs when antigen binds to previously sensitized mast cells on the mucosal surface of the airways (Fig. 29-6). Mediator release results in the infiltration of inflammatory cells, opening of the mucosal intercellular junctions, and increased access of antigen to the more prevalent submucosal mast cells. In addition, there is bronchospasm caused by direct stimulation of parasympathetic receptors, mucosal edema caused by increased vascular permeability, and increased mucus secretions. The acute response usually can be inhibited or reversed by bronchodilators, such as β_2-adrenergic agonists, but not by the anti-inflammatory actions of the corticosteroids.

The *late-phase response,* which develops 4 to 8 hours after exposure to an asthmatic trigger, involves inflammation and increased airway responsiveness that prolong the asthma attack and set into motion a vicious cycle of exacerbations.[23] Typically, the response reaches a maximum within a few hours and may last for days or even weeks. An initial trigger in the late-phase response causes the release of inflammatory mediators from mast cells, macrophages, and epithelial cells. These substances induce the migration and activation of other inflammatory cells

(*e.g.,* basophils, eosinophils, neutrophils), which then produce epithelial injury and edema, changes in mucociliary function and reduced clearance of respiratory tract secretions, and increased airway responsiveness (see Fig. 29-6). Responsiveness to cholinergic mediators often is heightened, suggesting changes in parasympathetic control of airway function. Chronic inflammation can lead to airway remodeling, in which case airflow limitations may be only partially reversible.[20]

Intrinsic (Nonatopic) Asthma. Intrinsic or nonatopic asthma triggers include respiratory tract infections, exercise, hyperventilation, cold air, exercise, drugs and chemicals, hormonal changes and emotional upsets, airborne pollutants, and gastroesophageal reflux. Respiratory tract infections, especially those caused by viruses, may produce their effects by causing epithelial damage and stimulating the production of IgE antibodies directed toward the viral antigens. In addition to precipitating an asthmatic attack, viral respiratory infections increase airway responsiveness to other asthma triggers that may persist for weeks beyond the original infection.

Exercise-induced asthma occurs in 40% to 90% of persons with bronchial asthma.[25] The cause of exercise-induced asthma is unclear. One possible cause is the loss of heat and water from the tracheobronchial tree because of the need for warming and humidifying large volumes of air.[26] The response commonly is

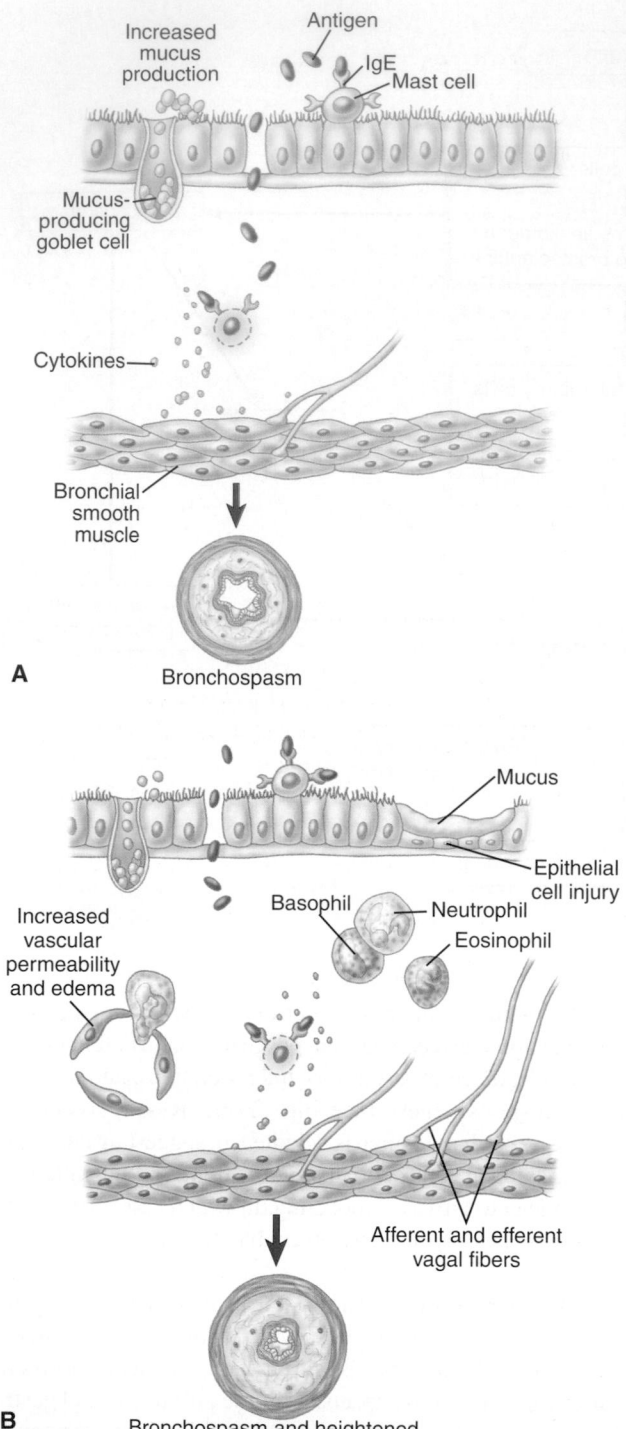

A   Bronchospasm

B   Bronchospasm and heightened airway responsiveness

FIGURE 29-6 • Pathogenesis of bronchial asthma. **(A)** The immediate or early-phase response triggered by an IgE-mediated release of mediators from sensitized mast cells. The release of chemical mediators results in increased mucus production, opening of mucosal intercellular junctions with exposure of submucosal mast cells to antigen, and bronchospasm. **(B)** The late-phase response involves epithelial cell injury with decreased mucociliary function and accumulation of mucus; release of inflammatory mediators with recruitment of neutrophils, eosinophils, and basophils; increased vascular permeability and edema; and increased airway responsiveness and bronchospasm.

exaggerated when the person exercises in a cold environment. Wearing a mask over the nose and mouth often minimizes the attack or prevents it. A warm-up period alleviates the symptoms for some persons.

Inhaled irritants, such as tobacco smoke and strong odors, are thought to induce bronchospasm by way of irritant receptors and a vagal reflex. Exposure to parental smoking has been reported to increase asthma severity in children.[27] High doses of irritant gases such as sulfur dioxide, nitrogen dioxide, and ozone may induce inflammatory exacerbations of airway responsiveness (*e.g.*, smog-related asthma). Occupational asthma is stimulated by fumes and gases (*e.g.*, epoxy resins, plastics, toluene), organic and chemical dusts (*e.g.*, wood, cotton, platinum), and other chemicals (*e.g.*, formaldehyde) in the workplace.[28] A group of chemicals that can provoke an asthmatic attack are the sulfites used in food processing and as preservatives added to beer, wine, and fresh vegetables.

There is a small group of persons with the clinical triad of asthma, chronic rhinosinusitis with nasal polyps, and precipitation of asthma and rhinitis attacks in response to aspirin and other NSAIDs.[29,30] The mechanism of the hypersensitivity reaction is complex and not fully understood, but most evidence points toward an abnormality in arachidonic acid (AA) metabolism (see Chapter 18). Cyclooxygenase (COX), the rate-limiting enzyme in AA metabolism, exists in two main forms: COX-1 and COX-2. COX-1 is responsible for the synthesis of protective prostaglandins and COX-2 for the synthesis of mediators of inflammation and bronchoconstriction. It has been hypothesized that in persons with aspirin-induced asthma, the inhibition of COX-1 shunts the metabolism of AA away from the production of protective prostaglandins and toward the generation of COX-2 and other mediators of inflammation and bronchoconstriction.[30] Avoidance of aspirin and all NSAIDs is a necessary part of the treatment program.

Both emotional factors and changes in hormone levels are thought to contribute to an increase in asthma symptoms. Emotional factors produce bronchospasm by way of vagal pathways. They can act as a bronchospastic trigger, or they can increase airway responsiveness to other triggers through noninflammatory mechanisms. The role of sex hormones in asthma is unclear, although there is much circumstantial evidence to suggest that they may be important. Up to 40% of women with asthma report a premenstrual increase in asthma symptoms.[31] Female sex hormones have a regulatory role on β_2-adrenergic function, and it has been suggested that abnormal regulation may be a possible mechanism for premenstrual asthma.[31]

Symptoms of gastroesophageal reflux are common in both adults and children with asthma, suggesting that reflux of gastric secretions may act as a bronchospastic trigger. Reflux during sleep can contribute to nocturnal asthma.[18]

Clinical Features

Manifestations. Persons with asthma exhibit a wide range of signs and symptoms, from episodic wheezing and feelings of chest tightness to an acute, immobilizing attack. The attacks differ from person to person, and between attacks, many persons are symptom free. Attacks may occur spontaneously or in response to various triggers, respiratory infections, emotional stress, or weather changes. Asthma is often worse at night, referred to as *nocturnal asthma*. Studies of nocturnal asthma suggest that there is a circadian and sleep-related variation in hormones and respiratory function.[32] The greatest decrease in respiratory function occurs at about 4:00 AM, at which time cortisol levels are low, melatonin levels high, and eosinophil activity increased.[33]

During an asthmatic attack, the airways narrow because of bronchospasm, edema of the bronchial mucosa, and mucus plugging. Expiration becomes prolonged because of progressive airway obstruction. The amount of air that can be forcibly expired in 1 second (forced expiratory volume in 1 second [$FEV_{1.0}$]) and the peak expiratory flow rate (PEF), measured in liters per second, are decreased. A fall in the PEF to levels below 50% of the predicted value during an acute asthmatic attack indicates a severe exacerbation and the need for emergency department treatment.[18]

During a prolonged attack, air becomes trapped behind the occluded and narrowed airways, causing hyperinflation of the lungs. This produces an increase in the residual volume (RV) along with a decrease in the inspiratory reserve capacity (tidal volume + inspiratory reserve volume [IRC]) and forced vital capacity (FVC), such that the person breathes close to his or her functional residual capacity (residual volume + expiratory reserve volume; see Chapter 27, Fig. 27-17). As a result, more energy is needed to overcome the tension already present in the lungs, and the accessory muscles (*e.g.*, sternocleidomastoid muscles) are required to maintain ventilation and gas exchange. This increased work of breathing further increases oxygen demands and causes dyspnea and fatigue. Because air is trapped in the alveoli and inspiration is occurring at higher residual lung volumes, the cough becomes less effective. As the condition progresses, the effectiveness of alveolar ventilation declines, and mismatching of ventilation and perfusion occurs, causing hypoxemia and hypercapnia. Pulmonary vascular resistance may increase as a result of the hypoxemia and hyperinflation, leading to a rise in pulmonary arterial pressure and increased work demands on the right heart.

The physical signs of bronchial asthma vary with the severity of the attack. A mild attack may produce a feeling of chest tightness, a slight increase in respiratory rate with prolonged expiration, and mild wheezing. A cough may accompany the wheezing. More severe attacks are accompanied by use of the accessory muscles, distant breath sounds due to air trapping, and loud wheezing. As the condition progresses, fatigue develops, the skin becomes moist, and anxiety and apprehension are obvious. Sensations of shortness of breath may be severe, and often the person is able to speak only one or two words before taking a breath. At the point at which airflow is markedly decreased, breath sounds become inaudible with diminished wheezing, and the cough becomes ineffective despite being repetitive and hacking.[18] This point often marks the onset of respiratory failure.

Diagnosis. The diagnosis of asthma is based on a careful history and physical examination, laboratory findings, and pulmonary function studies (see Chapter 27). Spirometry provides a means for measuring FVC, $FEV_{1.0}$, PEF, tidal volume, expiratory reserve capacity, and inspiratory reserve capacity. The $FEV_{1.0}$/FVC ratio can then be calculated. The level of airway responsiveness can be measured by inhalation challenge tests using methacholine (a cholinergic agonist), histamine, or exposure to a nonpharmacologic agent such as cold air.

Small, inexpensive, portable meters that measure PEF are available. Although not intended for use in the diagnosis of asthma, they can be used in clinics and physicians' offices and in the home to provide frequent measures of flow rates. Day–night (circadian) variations in asthma symptoms and PEF variability can be used to indicate the severity of bronchial hyperresponsiveness. The person's best performance is established from readings taken over several weeks. This often is referred to as the individual's *personal best* and is used as a reference to indicate changes in respiratory function.[17]

Treatment. The Expert Panel of the National Asthma Education and Prevention Program (NAEPP) has developed classification systems intended for use in directing asthma treatment and identifying persons at high risk for development of life-threatening asthma attacks[17,18] (Table 29-1). Based on these classifications systems, the panel recommends two categories for management and treatment of asthma: control of factors contributing to asthma severity and pharmacologic treatment.[17,18]

Measures to control factors contributing to asthma severity are aimed at prevention of exposure to irritants and factors that increase asthma symptoms and precipitate asthma exacerbations. They include education of the patient and family regarding measures used in avoiding exposure to irritants and allergens that are known to induce or trigger an attack. A careful history often is needed to identify all the contributory factors. Factors such as nasal polyps, a history of aspirin sensitivity, and gastroesophageal reflux should be considered. Annual influenza vaccination is recommended for persons with persistent asthma.

Relaxation techniques and controlled breathing often help to allay the panic and anxiety that aggravate breathing difficulties. The hyperventilation that often accompanies anxiety and panic is known to act as an asthmatic trigger. In a child, measures to encourage independence as it relates to symptom control, along with those directed at helping to develop a positive self-concept, are essential.

A program of desensitization may be undertaken in persons with persistent asthma who react to allergens, such as house dust mites, that cannot be avoided. This involves the injection of selected antigens (based on skin tests) to stimulate the production of IgG antibodies that block the IgE response. A course of allergen immunotherapy is typically of 3 to 5 years' duration.[17]

Pharmacologic treatment is used to prevent or treat reversible airway obstruction and airway hyperresponsiveness caused by the inflammatory process. The Expert Panel recommends a stepwise approach to pharmacologic therapy based on

TABLE 29-1 Classification of Asthma Severity

	SYMPTOMS	NIGHTTIME SYMPTOMS	LUNG FUNCTION
Mild intermittent	Symptoms ≤2 times a week Asymptomatic and normal PEF between exacerbations Exacerbations brief (from a few hours to a few days); intensity may vary	≤2 times a month	$FEV_{1.0}$ or PEF ≥80% predicted PEF variability <20%
Mild persistent	Symptoms >2 times a week but <1 time a day Exacerbations may affect activity	>2 times a month	$FEV_{1.0}$ or PEF ≥80% predicted PEF variability 20%–30%
Moderate persistent	Daily symptoms Daily use of inhaled short-acting β_2-adrenergic agonist Exacerbations affect activity Exacerbations ≥2 times a week; may last days	>1 time a week	$FEV_{1.0}$ or PEF >60%–<80% predicted PEF variability >30%
Severe persistent	Continual symptoms Limited physical activity Frequent exacerbations	Frequent	$FEV_{1.0}$ or PEF ≤60% predicted PEF variability >30%

$FEV_{1.0}$, forced expiratory volume in 1 second; PEF, peak expiratory flow rate.

Adapted from National Asthma Education and Prevention Program. (2003). *Expert Panel report 2: Guidelines for the diagnosis and management of asthma: Update of selected topics—2002.* National Institutes of Health publication no. 02-5074. Bethesda, MD: National Institutes of Health.

frequency and severity of disease symptoms.[18] The medications used in the treatment of asthma include those with bronchodilator and anti-inflammatory actions. They are categorized into two general categories: quick-relief medications and long-term control medications.

The *quick-relief medications* include the short-acting β_2-adrenergic agonists, anticholinergic agents, and systemic corticosteroids. The short-acting β_2-adrenergic agonists (*e.g.,* albuterol, bitolterol, pirbuterol, terbutaline) relax bronchial smooth muscle and provide prompt relief of symptoms, usually within 30 minutes. They are administered by inhalation (*i.e.,* metered-dose inhaler [MDI] or nebulizer), and their recommended use is in alleviating acute attacks of asthma because regular use does not produce beneficial effects.[18] An increase in the use of short-acting β_2-adrenergic agonists or use of more than one canisters in a month indicates progression or inadequate control of the disease. The anticholinergic medications (*e.g.,* ipratropium) block the postganglionic efferent vagal pathways that cause bronchoconstriction. These medications, which are administered by inhalation, produce bronchodilation by direct action on the large airways and do not change the composition or viscosity of the bronchial mucus. It is thought that they may provide some additive benefit for treatment of asthma exacerbations when administered with inhaled β_2-adrenergic agonists.[17] A short course of systemic corticosteroids, administered orally or parenterally, may be used for treating the inflammatory reaction associated with the late-phase response. Although their onset of action is slow (>4 hours), systemic corticosteroids may be used in the treatment of moderate to severe exacerba-

tions because of their action in preventing the progression of the exacerbation, speeding recovery, and preventing early relapses.[17]

The *long-term medications* are taken on a daily basis to achieve and maintain control of persistent asthma symptoms. They include anti-inflammatory agents, long-acting bronchodilators, and leukotriene modifiers. The Expert Panel defines anti-inflammatory medications as "those that cause a reduction in markers of airway inflammation in airway tissues and airway secretions (*e.g.,* eosinophils, mast cells, activated lymphocytes, macrophages, cytokines, or inflammatory mediators) and thus decrease the intensity of airway hyperresponsiveness."[18] The corticosteroids are considered the most effective anti-inflammatory agents for use in long-term treatment of asthma. Inhaled corticosteroids administered by MDI usually are preferred because of minimal systemic absorption and degree of disruption in hypothalamic-pituitary-adrenal function. In severe cases, oral or parenterally administered corticosteroids may be necessary.

The anti-inflammatory agents sodium cromolyn and nedocromil are also used to prevent an asthmatic attack. These agents act by stabilizing mast cells, thereby preventing release of the inflammatory mediators that cause an asthmatic attack. They are used prophylactically to prevent early and late responses but are of no benefit when taken during an attack.

The long-acting β_2-adrenergic agonists, which are available for administration in inhaled (*e.g.,* salmeterol, formoterol) or oral (*e.g.,* albuterol sustained release) routes, act by relaxing bronchial smooth muscle. They are used as an adjunct to anti-inflammatory medications for providing long-term control of symptoms, especially nocturnal symptoms, and for preventing exercise-induced bronchospasm. The long-acting β_2-adrenergic agonists have durations of action of at least 12 hours and should not be used to treat acute symptoms or exacerbations.[18]

Theophylline, a methylxanthine, is a bronchodilator that acts by relaxing bronchial smooth muscle. The sustained-release form of the drug is used as an adjuvant therapy and is particularly useful in relieving nighttime symptoms. It may be used as an alternative, but not preferred, medication in long-term preventative therapy when there are issues concerning adherence with regimens using inhaled medications or when cost is a factor. Because elimination of the drug varies widely among persons, blood levels are required to ensure that the therapeutic, but not toxic, dose is achieved.[18]

A group of medications called the *leukotriene modifiers* or *anti-leukotrienes* are available for use in the treatment of asthma.[34] Leukotrienes are potent biochemical mediators released from mast cells that cause bronchoconstriction, increased mucus secretion, and attraction and activation of inflammatory cells in the airways. There are two types of leukotriene modifiers: (1) those that act by inhibiting 5-lipoxygenase (*e.g.,* zileuton), an enzyme required for leukotriene synthesis; and (2) those that act by inhibiting the binding of leukotrienes to their receptor in the target tissues (*e.g.,* zafirlukast and montelukast). A particular advantage of the leukotriene modifiers is that they are taken orally.

Severe Asthma

Severe or refractory asthma represents a subgroup (probably <5%) of persons with asthma who have more troublesome disease as evidenced by high medication requirements to maintain good symptom control or those who continue to have persistent symptoms despite high medication use.[35,36] Severe or refractory asthma has been defined as persistent asthma that requires continuous high-dose inhaled or oral corticosteroids for more than 50% of the previous year, obstructive lung function and evidence of disease exacerbations or instability, and need for additional medications.[35,36] In the population of persons with refractory asthma, approximately 10% have been hospitalized, 20% have been seen in the emergency department, and 40% have required an increase in corticosteroid dose.[37] These persons are at increased risk for fatal or near-fatal asthma.

Little is known about the causes of severe asthma. Among the proposed risk factors are genetic predisposition, continued allergen or tobacco exposure, infection, intercurrent sinusitis or gastroesophageal reflux disease, and lack of compliance or adherence with treatment measures.[36] It has been proposed that because asthma is a disease involving multiple genes, mutations in genes regulating cytokines (*e.g.,* IL-4), growth factors, or receptors for medications used in treatment of asthma (β_2-adrenergic agonist or glucocorticoid) could be involved. Environmental factors include both allergen and tobacco exposure, with the strongest response occurring in response to house dust, cockroach allergen, and *Alternaria* exposure. Infections may also play a role. Respiratory syncytial virus infections are implicated in children, and pathogens such as mycoplasma and chlamydiae may play a role in adults. Gastroesophageal reflux and chronic sinusitis may also play a role.

Fatal and near-fatal asthma attacks, although uncommon, have increased during the past several decades.[37] Although the cause of death during an acute asthmatic attack is largely unknown, both cardiac arrhythmias and asphyxia due to severe airway obstruction have been implicated. It has been suggested that an underestimation of the severity of the attack may be a contributing factor. Deterioration often occurs rapidly during an acute attack, and underestimation of its severity may lead to a life-threatening delay in seeking medical attention. Frequent and repetitive use of β_2-adrenergic agonist inhalers far in excess of the recommended doses may temporarily blunt symptoms and mask the severity of the condition. It has been suggested that persons who have a fatal or near-fatal asthmatic attack may not perceive its severity.[38] That is, they may not perceive the severity of their condition and consequently not take appropriate measures in terms of seeking medical or emergency treatment.

 ## Bronchial Asthma in Children

Asthma is a leading cause of chronic illness in children and is responsible for a significant number of lost school days. It is the most frequent admitting diagnosis in children's hospitals. Based on information collected by the National Center for Health Statistics, as many as 8.65 million children (12.1%) were reported to have had a physician or health care professional diagnosis of asthma at some time during their life.[39] Asthma may have its onset at any age; 80% of children are symptomatic by 6 years of age.[39,40] Asthma is more prevalent in black than white children and results in more frequent disability and more frequent hospitalizations in black children.[40]

As with adults, asthma in children commonly is associated with an IgE-related reaction. It has been suggested that IgE directed against respiratory viruses in particular may be important in the pathogenesis of wheezing illnesses in infants (*i.e.,* bronchiolitis), which often precede the onset of asthma. The respiratory syncytial virus and parainfluenza viruses are the most commonly involved.[39,41] Other contributing factors include exposure to environmental allergens such as pet dander, dust mite antigens, and cockroach allergens. Exposure to environmental tobacco smoke also contributes to asthma in children. Of particular concern is the effect of in utero exposure to maternal smoking on lung function in infants and children.[42,43]

The signs and symptoms of asthma in infants and small children vary with the stage and severity of an attack. Because airway patency decreases at night, many children have acute signs of asthma at this time. Often, previously well infants and children develop what may seem to be a cold with rhinorrhea, rapidly followed by irritability, a tight and nonproductive cough, wheezing, tachypnea, dyspnea with prolonged expiration, and use of accessory muscles of respiration. Cyanosis, hyperinflation of the chest, and tachycardia indicate increasing severity of the attack. Wheezing may be absent in children with extreme respiratory distress. The symptoms may progress rapidly and require a trip to the emergency department or hospitalization.

The Expert Panel of the NAEPP has developed guidelines for management of asthma in infants and children younger than 5 years of age and for adults and children older than 5 years of age.[18,44] As with adults and older children, the Expert Panel recommends a stepwise approach to diagnosing and managing asthma in infants and children younger than 5 years of age. The anti-inflammatory agents cromolyn and nedocromil are recommended as an initial therapy for mild to moderate persistent asthma in infants and children. Inhaled short-acting β_2-adrenergic agonists may be used for mild intermittent symptoms or exacerbations. More severe symptoms may require the use of inhaled corticosteroids. Systemic corticosteroids may be required during an episode of severe disease. Growth velocity should be monitored in children and adolescents receiving long-term corticosteroid therapy by any route because these drugs may suppress growth.[18]

Special delivery systems for administration of inhalation medications are available for infants and small children, including nebulizers with face masks and spacers and holding chambers for use with an MDI. For children younger than 2 years of age, nebulizer therapy usually is preferred. Children between 3 and 5 years of age may begin using an MDI with a spacer and holding chamber. The child's caregiver should be carefully instructed in the appropriate use of these devices. The Expert Panel recommends that adolescents (and younger children when appropriate) be directly involved in developing their asthma management plans.[18] Active participation in physical activities, exercise, and sports should be encouraged.

Chronic Obstructive Pulmonary Disease

Chronic obstructive pulmonary disease (COPD) is characterized by chronic and recurrent obstruction of airflow in the pulmonary airways.[45] Airflow obstruction usually is progressive and is accompanied by inflammatory responses to noxious particles or gases.[45–47] COPD is a leading cause of morbidity and mortality worldwide. It has been estimated that approximately 9 million Americans[48] and 1.9 million Canadians have COPD. COPD is the fourth leading cause of death in both the United States and Canada.[48,50] In 2004, COPD claimed the lives of more than 118,000 people in the United States, with the number of women dying from the disease surpassing that of men.[48]

The risk factors for COPD include both host and environmental factors. The most common cause of COPD is smoking, as evidenced by the fact that 80% to 85% of persons with COPD have a history of smoking.[45,46,51] A second, less common host factor is a hereditary deficiency in α_1-antitrypsin. Other predisposing factors are asthma and airway hyperresponsiveness. Unfortunately, clinical findings are almost always absent during the early stages of COPD, and as many as 50% of smokers may have undiagnosed COPD.[49,52] By the time symptoms appear or are recognized, the disease is usually far advanced. For smokers with early signs of airway disease, there is hope that early recognition, combined with appropriate treatment and smoking cessation, may prevent or delay the usually relentless progression of the disease.

Etiology and Pathogenesis

The mechanisms involved in the pathogenesis of COPD usually are multiple and include inflammation and fibrosis of the bronchial wall, hypertrophy of the submucosal glands and hypersecretion of mucus, and loss of elastic lung fibers and alveolar tissue[52] (Fig. 29-7). Inflammation and fibrosis of the bronchial wall, along with excess mucus secretion, obstruct airflow and cause mismatching of ventilation and perfusion. Destruction of alveolar tissue decreases the surface area for gas exchange, and loss of elastic fibers impairs the expiratory flow rate, increases air trapping, and predisposes to airway collapse.

The term *chronic obstructive pulmonary disease* encompasses two types of obstructive airway disease: *emphysema,* with enlargement of airspaces and destruction of lung tissue; and *chronic obstructive bronchitis,* with increased mucus production, obstruction of small airways, and a chronic productive cough. Persons with COPD often have overlapping features of both disorders.

Emphysema. Emphysema is characterized by a loss of lung elasticity and abnormal enlargement of the airspaces distal to the terminal bronchioles, with destruction of the alveolar walls and capillary beds (Fig. 29-8). Enlargement of the airspaces leads to hyperinflation of the lungs and produces an increase in total lung capacity (TLC). Two of the recognized causes of emphysema are smoking, which incites lung injury, and an inherited deficiency of α_1-antitrypsin, an antiprotease enzyme

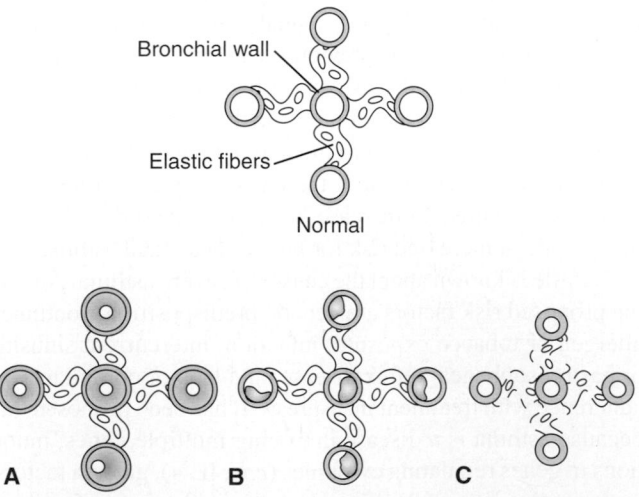

FIGURE 29-7 • Mechanisms of airflow obstruction in chronic obstructive lung disease. **(Top)** Normal bronchial airway with elastic fibers that provide traction and hold the airway open. **(Bottom)** Obstruction of the airway caused by **(A)** hypertrophy of the bronchial wall, **(B)** inflammation and hypersecretion of mucus, and **(C)** loss of elastic fibers that hold the airway open.

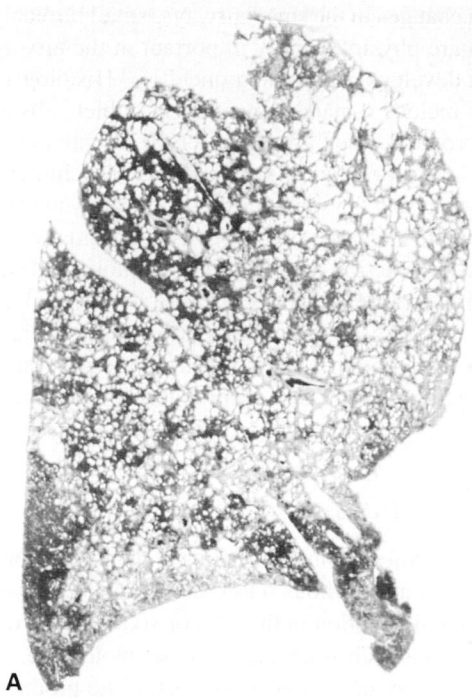

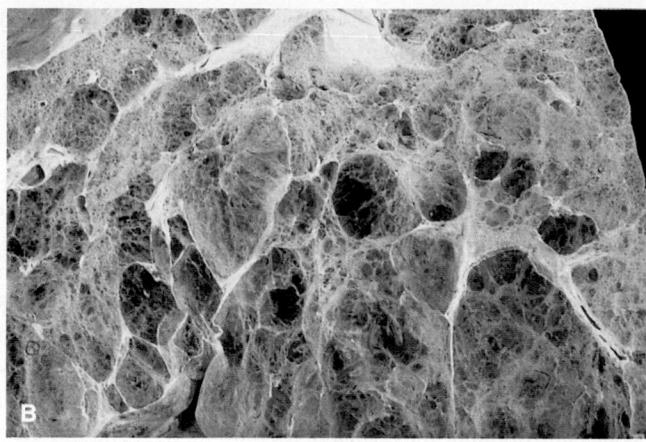

FIGURE 29-8 • Panacinar emphysema. **(A)** A whole mount of the left lung from a patient with severe emphysema reveals widespread destruction of pulmonary parenchyma that in some areas leaves behind a lacy network of supporting tissue. **(B)** The lung from a patient with α_1-antitrypsin deficiency shows a panacinar pattern of emphysema. The loss of alveolar walls has resulted in markedly enlarged airspaces. (From Bearsley M. B., Travis W. D., Rubin E. [2008]. The respiratory system. In Rubin R., Strayer D. S. [Eds.], *Rubin's pathology: Clinicopathologic foundations of medicine* [5th ed., p. 515]. Philadelphia: Lippincott Williams & Wilkins.)

that protects the lung from injury. Genetic factors other than an inherited α_1-antitrypsin deficiency also may play a role in smokers who develop COPD at an early age.[52]

Emphysema is thought to result from the breakdown of elastin and other alveolar wall components by enzymes, called *proteases,* that digest proteins. The proteases, particularly elastase, which is an enzyme that digests elastin, are released from polymorphonuclear leukocytes (*i.e.,* neutrophils), alveolar macrophages, and other inflammatory cells.[45] Normally, the lung is protected by antiprotease enzymes including α_1-antitrypsin. Cigarette smoke and other irritants stimulate the movement of inflammatory cells into the lungs, resulting in increased release of elastase and other proteases. In smokers in whom COPD develops, antiprotease production and release may be inadequate to neutralize the excess protease production such that the process of elastic tissue destruction goes unchecked (Fig. 29-9).

A hereditary deficiency in α_1-antitrypsin accounts for approximately 1% of all cases of COPD and is more common in young persons with emphysema.[45] The type and amount of α_1-antitrypsin that a person has is determined by a pair of codominant genes referred to as *PI* (protein inhibitor) genes. An α_1-antitrypsin deficiency is inherited as an autosomal recessive disorder. There are more than 75 mutations of the gene. One of these, the *PIZ* variant, which occurs in 5% of the population, causes the most serious deficiency in α_1-antitrypsin. It

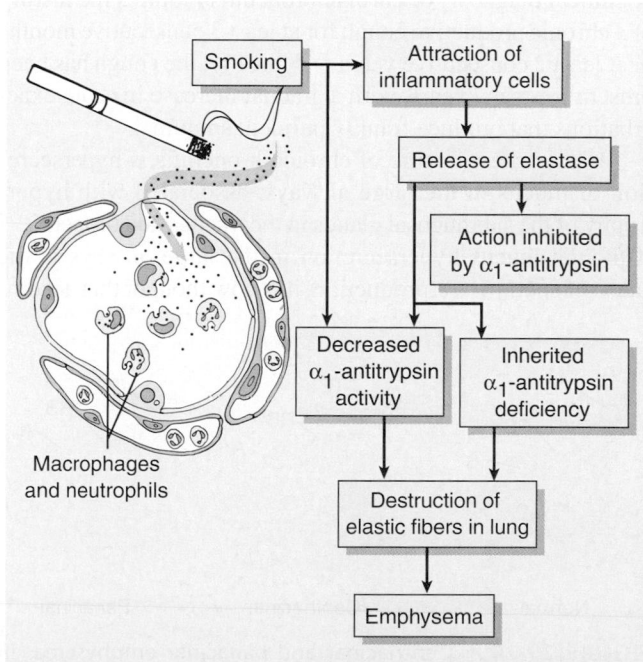

FIGURE 29-9 • Protease (elastase)–antiprotease (antitrypsin) mechanisms of emphysema. The effects of smoking and an inherited α_1-antitrypsin deficiency on the destruction of elastic fibers in the lung and development of emphysema are shown.

is most common in persons of Scandinavian descent and is rare in Jews, blacks, and the Japanese.[52] Homozygotes who carry two defective *PIZ* genes have only about 15% to 20% of the normal plasma concentration of α_1-antitrypsin.[52] Most persons with clinically diagnosed emphysema before the age of 40 years have an α_1-antitrypsin deficiency. Smoking and repeated respiratory tract infections, which also decrease α_1-antitrypsin levels, contribute to the risk for emphysema in persons with α_1-antitrypsin deficiency. Laboratory methods are available for measuring α_1-antitrypsin levels. Human α_1-antitrypsin is available for replacement therapy in persons with a hereditary deficiency of the enzyme.

There are two commonly recognized types of emphysema: centriacinar or centrilobular, and panacinar (Fig. 29-10). The centriacinar type affects the bronchioles in the central part of the respiratory lobule, with initial preservation of the alveolar ducts and sacs.[52] It is the most common type of emphysema and is seen predominantly in male smokers. The panacinar type produces initial involvement of the peripheral alveoli and later extends to involve the more central bronchioles. This type of emphysema is more common in persons with α_1-antitrypsin deficiency. It also is found in smokers in association with centriacinar emphysema. In such cases, the panacinar pattern tends to occur in the lower parts of the lung and centriacinar emphysema is seen in the upper parts of the lung.

Chronic Bronchitis. Chronic bronchitis represents airway obstruction of the major and small airways.[21,52] The condition is seen most commonly in middle-aged men and is associated with chronic irritation from smoking and recurrent infections. A clinical diagnosis of chronic bronchitis requires the history of a chronic productive cough for at least 3 consecutive months in at least 2 consecutive years.[47] Typically, the cough has been present for many years, with a gradual increase in acute exacerbations that produce frankly purulent sputum.

The earliest feature of chronic bronchitis is hypersecretion of mucus in the large airways, associated with hypertrophy of the submucosal glands in the trachea and bronchi.[21,52] Although mucus hypersecretion in the large airways is the cause of sputum overproduction, it is now thought that accompanying changes in the small airways (small bronchi and bronchioles) are physiologically important in the airway obstruction that develops in chronic bronchitis.[21] Histologically, these changes include a marked increase in goblet cells and excess mucus production with plugging of the airway lumen, inflammatory infiltration, and fibrosis of the bronchiolar wall. It is thought that both the submucosal hypertrophy in the larger airways and the increase in goblet cells in the smaller airways are a protective reaction against tobacco smoke and other pollutants. Viral and bacterial infections are common in persons with chronic bronchitis and are thought to be a result rather than a cause of the problem. While infections are not responsible for initiating the problem, they are probably important in maintaining it and may be critical in producing acute exacerbations.[21]

Clinical Features

Clinical Manifestations. The clinical manifestations of COPD usually have an insidious onset and patients characteristically seek medical attention in the fifth or sixth decade of life, with manifestations such as fatigue, exercise intolerance, cough, sputum production, or shortness of breath. The productive cough usually occurs in the morning and the dyspnea becomes more severe as the disease progresses. Frequent exacerbations of infection and respiratory insufficiency are common, causing absence from work and eventual disability. The late stages of COPD are characterized by recurrent respiratory infections and chronic respiratory failure. Death usually occurs during an exacerbation of illness associated with infection and respiratory failure.

The mnemonics "pink puffer" and "blue bloater" have been used to differentiate the clinical manifestations of emphysema and chronic obstructive bronchitis.[21,53] Persons with predominant emphysema are classically referred to as *pink puffers,* a reference to the lack of cyanosis, the use of accessory muscles, and pursed-lip ("puffer") breathing. With loss of lung elasticity and hyperinflation of the lungs, the airways often collapse during expiration because pressure in surrounding lung tissues exceeds airway pressure. Air becomes trapped in the alveoli and lungs, producing an increase in the anteroposterior dimensions of the chest, the so-called *barrel chest* that is typical of persons with emphysema (Fig. 29-11). Such persons have a dramatic decrease in breath sounds throughout the chest. Because the diaphragm may be functioning near its maximum ability, the person is vulnerable to diaphragmatic fatigue and acute respiratory failure. Persons with a clinical syndrome of chronic bronchitis are classically labeled *blue bloaters,* a reference to cyanosis and fluid retention associated with right-sided heart failure. In practice, differentiation between the two types of COPD is often difficult. This is because persons with COPD often have some degree of both emphysema and chronic bronchitis.

The manifestations of COPD represent a progressive change in respiratory function. There is moderate to severe respiratory impairment due to obstruction of airflow, which is greater on expiration than inspiration, resulting in increased work of breathing but decreased effectiveness. The development of exertional dyspnea, often described as increased effort

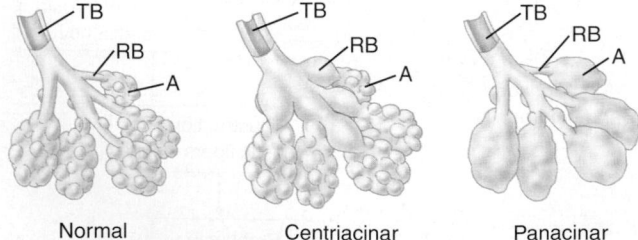

Normal   Centriacinar   Panacinar

FIGURE 29-10 • Centriacinar and panacinar emphysema. In centriacinar emphysema, the destruction is confined to the terminal (TB) and respiratory bronchioles (RB). In panacinar emphysema, the peripheral alveoli (A) are also involved. (Adapted from West J. B. [1997]. *Pulmonary pathophysiology* [5th ed., p. 53]. Philadelphia: Lippincott-Raven.)

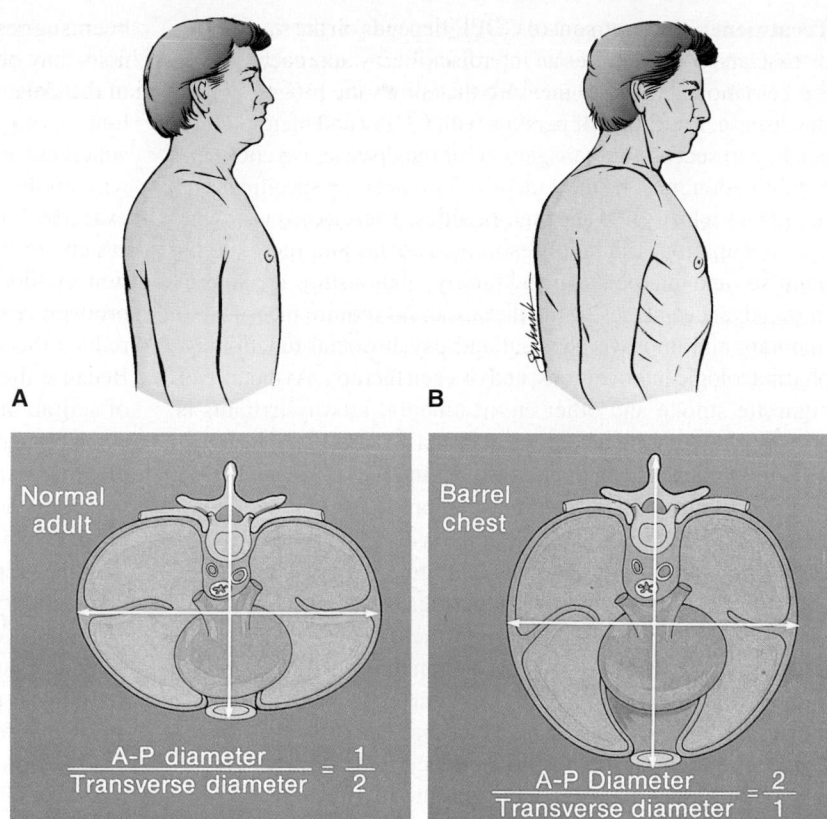

FIGURE 29-11 • Characteristics of normal chest wall and chest wall in emphysema. The normal chest wall and its cross-section are illustrated on the left (**A**). The barrel-shaped chest of emphysema and its cross-section are illustrated on the right (**B**). (From Smeltzer S. C., Bare B. G. [2004]. *Medical-surgical nursing.* [10th ed., p. 572]. Philadelphia: Lippincott Williams & Wilkins.)

to breathe, heaviness, air hunger, or gasping, can be insidious. Activities involving significant arm work, particularly above the shoulders, are particularly difficult for persons with COPD. Activities that allow the person to brace the arms and use the accessory muscles are better tolerated. As the disease progresses, breathing becomes increasingly more labored, even at rest. The expiratory phase of respiration is prolonged, and expiratory wheezes and crackles can be heard on auscultation. Persons with severe airflow obstruction may also exhibit use of the accessory muscles, sitting in the characteristic "tripod" position to facilitate use of the sternocleidomastoid, scalene, and intercostal muscles.[53] Pursed-lip breathing enhances airflow because it increases the resistance to the outflow of air and helps to prevent airway collapse by increasing airway pressure. Eventually, persons with COPD are unable to maintain normal blood gases by increasing their breathing effort. Hypoxemia, hypercapnia, and cyanosis develop, reflecting an imbalance between ventilation and perfusion.

Severe hypoxemia, in which arterial PO_2 levels fall below 55 mm Hg, causes reflex vasoconstriction of the pulmonary vessels and further impairment of gas exchange in the lung. It is more common in persons with the chronic bronchitis form of COPD. Hypoxemia also stimulates red blood cell production, causing polycythemia. The increase in pulmonary vasoconstriction and subsequent elevation in pulmonary artery pressure further increase the work of the right ventricle. As a result, persons with COPD may develop right-sided heart failure with peripheral edema (*i.e.,* cor pulmonale). However,

signs of overt right-sided heart failure are seen less frequently since the advent of supplemental oxygen therapy.

Diagnosis. The diagnosis of COPD is based on a careful history and physical examination, pulmonary function studies, chest radiographs, and laboratory tests.[52] Airway obstruction prolongs the expiratory phase of respiration and affords the potential for impaired gas exchange because of mismatching of ventilation and perfusion. The FVC is the amount of air that can be forcibly exhaled after maximal inspiration. In an adult with normal respiratory function, this should be achieved in 4 to 6 seconds. In patients with chronic lung disease, the time required for FVC is increased, the $FEV_{1.0}$ is decreased, and the ratio of $FEV_{1.0}$ to FVC is decreased. In severe disease, the FVC is markedly reduced. Lung volume measurements reveal a marked increase in RV, an increase in TLC, and elevation of the RV-to-TLC ratio. These and other measurements of expiratory flow are determined by spirometry and are used in the diagnosis of COPD (see Chapter 27, Fig. 27-17). Spirometry measurements can be used in staging disease severity. For example, an $FEV_{1.0}$-to-FVC ratio of less than 70% with an $FEV_{1.0}$ of 80% or more, with or without symptoms, indicates mild disease; and an $FEV_{1.0}$-to-FVC ratio of less than 70% with an $FEV_{1.0}$ of less than 50%, with or without symptoms, indicates severe disease.[46] Other diagnostic measures become important as the disease advances. Measures of exercise tolerance, nutritional status, hemoglobin saturation, and arterial blood gases can be used to assess the overall impact of COPD on health status and to direct treatment.

Treatment. The treatment of COPD depends on the stage of the disease and often requires an interdisciplinary approach. Smoking cessation is the only measure that slows the progression of the disease. Education of persons with COPD and their families is a key to successful management of the disease. Psychosocial rehabilitation must be individualized to meet the specific needs of persons with COPD and their families. These needs vary with age, occupation, financial resources, social and recreational interests, and interpersonal and family relationships. Persons in more advanced stages of the disease often require measures to maintain and improve physical and psychosocial functioning, pharmacologic interventions, and oxygen therapy. Avoidance of cigarette smoke and other environmental airway irritants is imperative. Wearing a cold-weather mask often prevents dyspnea and bronchospasm due to cold air and wind exposure.

Respiratory tract infections can prove life-threatening to persons with severe COPD. A person with COPD should avoid exposure to others with known respiratory tract infections and should avoid attending large gatherings during periods of the year when influenza or respiratory tract infections are prevalent. Immunization for influenza and pneumococcal infections decreases the likelihood of their occurrence. Although antibiotics are used to treat acute exacerbations of COPD due to bacterial infection, there is no evidence that the prophylactic use of antibiotics prevents acute exacerbations.[47]

Undernutrition (body weight <90% of ideal weight) affects approximately 25% of persons with COPD.[54] Many persons with COPD find it difficult to manage the effort needed to consume a large meal. This situation, combined with impaired diaphragm descent, air swallowing, and medications that cause anorexia and nausea, impairs nutrition and promotes weight loss. Specifically, nutrition depletion is associated with decreased exercise capacity, dyspnea, fatigue, and increased susceptibility to respiratory infections. Small, frequent, nutritious, and easily swallowed feedings aid in maintaining good nutrition and preventing weight loss. Excess carbohydrates in the diet can increase carbon dioxide production and arterial carbon dioxide levels. However, this usually is not a problem unless a high-carbohydrate diet is followed.

Maintaining and improving physical and psychosocial functioning is an important part of the treatment program for persons with COPD. A long-term pulmonary rehabilitation program can significantly reduce episodes of hospitalization and add measurably to a person's ability to manage and cope with his or her impairment in a positive way. This program includes breathing exercises that focus on restoring the function of the diaphragm, reducing the work of breathing, and improving gas exchange. Physical conditioning with appropriate exercise training increases maximal oxygen consumption and reduces ventilatory effort and heart rate for a given workload. Work simplification and energy conservation strategies may be needed when impairment is severe.

The pharmacologic treatment of COPD includes the use of bronchodilators, including inhaled adrenergic and anticholinergic agents.[45–47,53] Inhaled β_2-adrenergic agonists have been the mainstay of treatment of COPD for many years. It has

been suggested that long-acting inhaled β_2-adrenergic agonists may be even more effective than the short-acting forms of the drug. In addition to their action as bronchodilators, the long-acting β_2-adrenergic agonists are thought to reduce the adherence of bacteria such as *Haemophilus influenzae* to airway epithelial cells, thereby reducing the risk for infective exacerbations.[45] The anticholinergic drugs (*e.g.,* ipratropium), which are administered by inhalation, produce bronchodilation by blocking parasympathetic cholinergic receptors that produce contraction of bronchial smooth muscle. They also reduce the volume of sputum without altering its viscosity. Because these drugs have a slower onset and longer duration of action, they usually are used on a regular basis rather than on an as-needed basis. Inhalers that combine an anticholinergic drug with a β_2-adrenergic agonist are available.

Oral theophylline may be used in treatment of persons who fail to respond to inhaled bronchodilators. The long-acting theophylline preparations may be used to reduce overnight declines in respiratory function. There also is evidence that theophylline may improve respiratory muscle function, increase mucociliary clearance, and improve central respiratory drive.[45] When theophylline is prescribed, blood levels are used as a guide in arriving at an effective dose schedule.

Although inhaled corticosteroids often are used in treatment of COPD, there is controversy regarding their usefulness. There is evidence that inflammation in COPD is not suppressed by inhaled or oral corticosteroids.[45] An explanation for this lack of effect may be related to the fact that corticosteroids prolong the action of neutrophils and hence do not suppress the neutrophilic inflammation seen in COPD. Because corticosteroids are useful in relieving asthma symptoms, they may benefit persons with asthma concomitant with COPD. Inhaled corticosteroids also may be beneficial in treating acute exacerbations of COPD, minimizing the undesirable effects that often accompany systemic use.

Oxygen therapy is prescribed for selected persons with significant hypoxemia (arterial PO_2 <55 mm Hg). Administration of continuous low-flow (1 to 2 L/minute) oxygen to maintain arterial PO_2 levels between 55 and 65 mm Hg decreases dyspnea and pulmonary hypertension and improves neuropsychological function and activity tolerance. The overall goal of oxygen therapy is to maintain a hemoglobin oxygen saturation of at least 90%.[45] Oxygen usually is administered using a nasal cannula. Portable oxygen administration units, which allow mobility and the performance of activities of daily living, usually are used. Transtracheal oxygen, delivered by a small-diameter percutaneous catheter placed in the trachea, can be used to increase oxygen delivery and decrease ventilatory effort. It is particularly useful in persons with high oxygen requirements.[45] It also can be used to increase ambulation by eliminating the need to wear a nasal cannula. Because the ventilatory drive associated with hypoxic stimulation of the peripheral chemoreceptors does not occur until the arterial PO_2 has been reduced to about 60 mm Hg or less, increasing the arterial PO_2 above 60 mm Hg tends to depress the hypoxic stimulus for ventilation and often leads to hypoventilation and carbon dioxide retention.

Lung reduction surgery or bullectomy may prove useful for a limited number of persons. Lung volume reduction surgery involves the resection of the most distended areas of the lung as a means of improving respiratory function.[53] Bullectomy is a surgical procedure that involves the removal of large emphysematous bullae that compress adjacent lung tissue and cause dyspnea. Lung transplantation is becoming an alternative treatment for persons with severe lung disease, limited life expectancy without transplantation, adequate functioning of other organ systems, and a good social support system.

Bronchiectasis

Bronchiectasis is an uncommon type of COPD characterized by a permanent dilation of the bronchi and bronchioles caused by destruction of the muscle and elastic supporting tissue as the result of a vicious cycle of infection and inflammation[55] (Fig. 29-12). It is not a primary disease but secondary to persisting infection or obstruction.[21] In the past, bronchiectasis

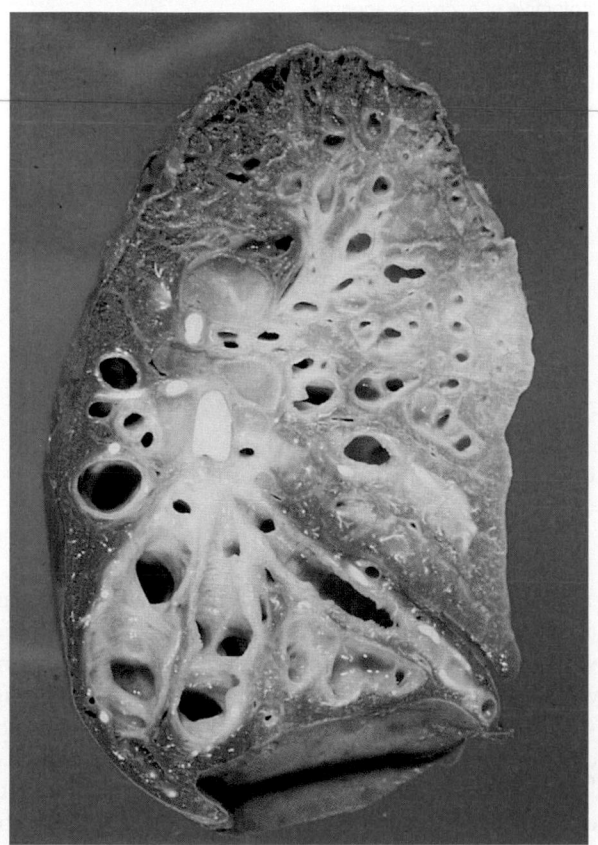

FIGURE 29-12 • Bronchiectasis. The resected upper lobe shows widely dilated bronchi, with thickening of the bronchial walls and collapse and fibrosis of the pulmonary parenchyma. (From Bearsley M. B., Travis W. D., Rubin E. [2008]. The respiratory system. In Rubin R., Strayer D. S. [Eds.], *Rubin's pathology: Clinicopathologic foundations of medicine* [5th ed., p. 490]. Philadelphia: Lippincott Williams & Wilkins.)

often followed a necrotizing bacterial pneumonia that frequently complicated measles, pertussis, or influenza. Tuberculosis was also commonly associated with bronchiectasis. Thus, with the advent of antibiotics that more effectively treat respiratory infections such as tuberculosis, and with immunization against pertussis and measles, there has been a marked decrease in the prevalence of bronchiectasis.

Etiology and Pathogenesis

Two processes are critical to the pathogenesis of bronchiectasis: obstruction and chronic persistent infection.[21] Regardless of which may come first, both cause damage to the bronchial walls, leading to weakening and dilation. On gross examination, bronchial dilation is classified as saccular, cylindrical, or varicose. Saccular bronchiectasis involves the proximal third to fourth generation of bronchi[21,52] (see Chapter 27, Fig. 27-4). These bronchi become severely dilated and end blindly in dilated sacs, with collapse and fibrosis of more distal lung tissue. Cylindrical bronchiectasis involves uniform and moderate dilation of the sixth to eighth generations of airways. It is a milder form of disease than saccular bronchiectasis and leads to fewer symptoms. Varicose bronchiectasis involves the second through eighth branchings of bronchi and results in bronchi that resemble varicose veins. Bronchiolar obliteration is not as severe and symptoms are variable.

Bronchiectasis can present in either of two forms: a local obstructive process involving a lobe or segment of a lung or a diffuse process involving much of both lungs.[52] *Localized bronchiectasis* is most commonly caused by conditions such as tumors, foreign bodies, and mucus plugs that produce atelectasis and infection due to obstructed drainage of bronchial secretions. It can affect any area of the lung, the area being determined by the site of obstruction or infection. *Generalized bronchiectasis* usually is bilateral and most commonly affects the lower lobes. It is due largely to inherited impairments of host mechanisms or acquired disorders that permit introduction of infectious organisms into the airways. They include inherited conditions such as cystic fibrosis, in which airway obstruction is caused by impairment of normal mucociliary function; congenital and acquired immunodeficiency states, which predispose to respiratory tract infections; lung infection (*e.g.,* tuberculosis, fungal infections, lung abscess); and exposure to toxic gases that cause airway obstruction.

Clinical Features

Clinical Manifestations. Bronchiectasis is associated with a number of abnormalities that profoundly affect respiratory function, including atelectasis, obstruction of the smaller airways, and diffuse bronchitis. Affected persons have recurrent bronchopulmonary infection; coughing; production of copious amounts of foul-smelling, purulent sputum; and hemoptysis. Weight loss and anemia are common.

The manifestations of bronchiectasis are similar to those seen in chronic bronchitis and emphysema. As in the latter two conditions, chronic bronchial obstruction leads to marked dyspnea and cyanosis. Clubbing of the fingers, which is not usually seen in other types of obstructive lung diseases, is more common in moderate to advanced bronchiectasis.

Diagnosis and Treatment. Diagnosis is based on history and imaging studies. The condition often is evident on chest radiographs. High-resolution CT scanning of the chest allows for definitive diagnosis. Accuracy of diagnosis is important because interventional bronchoscopy or surgery may be palliative or curative in some types of obstructive disease.

Treatment consists of early recognition and treatment of infection along with regular postural drainage and chest physical therapy. Persons with this disorder benefit from many of the rehabilitation and treatment measures used for chronic bronchitis and emphysema.

 **Cystic Fibrosis**

Cystic fibrosis (CF), which is the major cause of severe chronic respiratory disease in children, is an autosomal recessive disorder involving fluid secretion in the exocrine glands in the epithelial lining of the respiratory, gastrointestinal, and reproductive tracts.[56–59] In addition to chronic respiratory disease, CF is manifested by pancreatic exocrine deficiency and elevation of sodium chloride in the sweat. Nasal polyps, sinus infections, pancreatitis, and cholelithiasis also are common. Excessive loss of sodium in the sweat predisposes young children to salt depletion episodes. Most boys with CF have congenital bilateral absence of the vas deferens with azoospermia.

The disease affects approximately 30,000 children and adults in the United States (70,000 worldwide), and more than 10 million persons are asymptomatic carriers of the defective gene.[60] The gene is rare in African blacks and Asians. Homozygotes (*i.e.*, persons with two defective genes) have all or substantially all of the clinical symptoms of the disease, compared with heterozygotes, who are carriers of the disease but have no recognizable symptoms.

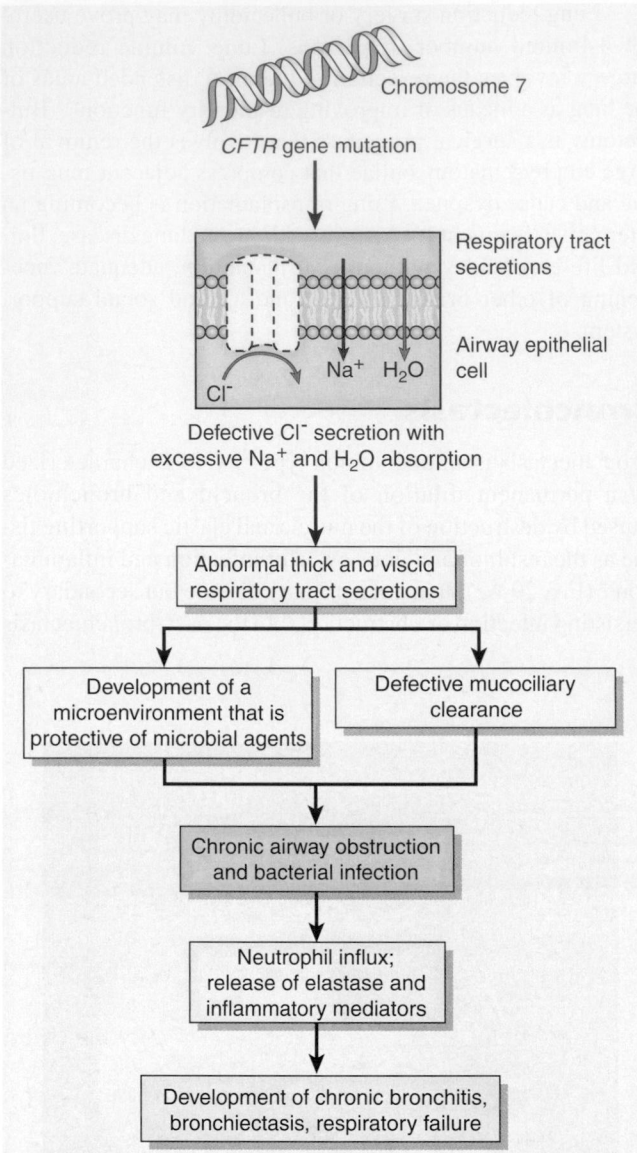

FIGURE 29-13 • Pathogenesis of cystic fibrosis.

Etiology and Pathogenesis

Cystic fibrosis is caused by mutations in a single gene on the long arm of chromosome 7 that encodes for the cystic fibrosis transmembrane regulator (CFTR), which functions as a chloride (Cl^-) channel in epithelial cell membranes. Mutations in the *CFTR* gene render the epithelial membrane relatively impermeable to the chloride ion (Fig. 29-13). Although a large number of mutations in the *CFTR* gene have been identified, the most common mutation, which involves a three–base-pair deletion that codes for phenylalanine, accounts for 90% of persons with CF in the United States.[57]

The impact on impaired Cl^- transport is relatively tissue specific. In the sweat glands, the concentration of sodium (Na^+) and Cl^- secreted into the lumen of the gland remains unaffected, whereas the reabsorption of Cl^- through the CFTR

and accompanying reabsorption of Na^+ in the ducts of the gland fail to occur. This defect accounts for the high concentration of NaCl in the sweat of persons with CF.[56–59] In the normal airway epithelium, Cl^- is secreted into airway lumen through the CFTR. The impaired transport of Cl^- ultimately leads to a series of secondary events, including increased absorption of Na^+ and water from the airways into the blood. This lowers the water content of the mucociliary blanket coating the respiratory epithelium, causing it to become more viscid. The resulting dehydration of the mucous layer leads to defective mucociliary function and accumulation of viscid secretions that obstruct the airways and predispose to recurrent pulmonary infections. Similar transport abnormalities and pathophysiologic events take place in the pancreatic and biliary ducts and in the vas deferens in boys.

Clinical Features

Respiratory manifestations of CF are caused by an accumulation of viscid mucus in the bronchi, impaired mucociliary clearance, and lung infections. Chronic bronchiolitis and bronchitis are the initial lung manifestations, but after months and years, structural changes in the bronchial wall lead to bronchiectasis. In addition to airway obstruction, the basic genetic defect that occurs with CF predisposes to chronic infection with a surprisingly limited number of organisms, the most common being *Pseudomonas aeruginosa, Burkholderia cepacia, Staphylococcus aureus,* and *Haemophilus influenzae.*[57] Soon after birth, initial infection with bacterial pathogens occurs and is associated with an excessive neutrophilic inflammatory response that appears to be independent of the infection itself. There is evidence that the CF airway epithelial cells or surface liquids provide a favorable environment for harboring these organisms. *P. aeruginosa,* in particular, has a propensity to undergo mucoid transformation in this environment.[57] The complex polysaccharide produced by these organisms provides a hypoxic environment and generates a biofilm that protects *Pseudomonas* against antimicrobial agents. Pulmonary inflammation is another cause of decline in respiratory function in persons with CF and may precede the onset of chronic infection. Elevated levels of inflammatory mediators (*e.g.,* IL-1, IL-6, TNF-α), along with reduced levels of anti-inflammatory cytokines have been found in the airways of persons with CF.[57]

Pancreatic function is abnormal in approximately 80% to 90% of affected persons.[59] Steatorrhea, diarrhea, and abdominal pain and discomfort are common. In the newborn, meconium ileus may cause intestinal obstruction, a fatal condition if left untreated. The degree of pancreatic involvement is highly variable. In some children, the defect is relatively mild, and in others, the involvement is severe and impairs intestinal absorption. In addition to exocrine pancreatic insufficiency, hyperglycemia may occur, especially after 10 years of age, when approximately 8% of persons with CF develop diabetes mellitus.[59]

Diagnosis and Treatment. Early diagnosis and treatment are important in delaying the onset and severity of chronic illness in children with CF. Diagnosis is based on the presence of respiratory and gastrointestinal manifestations typical of CF, a history of CF in a sibling, or a positive newborn screening test result. Confirmatory laboratory tests include the sweat test, assessment of bioelectrical properties of respiratory epithelia by measurement of transepithelial potential differences in the nasal membrane, and genetic tests for *CFTR* gene mutations.[59] The *sweat test,* using pilocarpine iontophoresis to collect the sweat followed by chemical analysis of its chloride content, remains the standard approach to diagnosis. Newborns with CF have elevated blood levels of immunoreactive trypsinogen, presumably because of secretory obstruction in the pancreas. *Newborn screening* consists of a test for determination of immunoreactive trypsinogen. The test can be done on blood spots collected for routine newborn screening tests.

At present, there are no approved treatments for correcting the genetic defects in CF or to reverse the ion transport abnormalities associated with the dysfunctional CFTR. Thus, treatment measures are directed toward slowing the progression of secondary organ dysfunction and sequelae such as chronic lung infection and pancreatic insufficiency.[59] They include the use of antibiotics to prevent and manage infections; the use of chest physical therapy (chest percussion and postural drainage) and mucolytic agents to prevent airway obstruction; and pancreatic enzyme replacement and nutritional therapy. Routine laboratory evaluations are key to assessing pulmonary function and response to therapeutic interventions. These studies include radiologic examinations, pulmonary function testing, and microbiologic cultures of respiratory secretions.

Appropriate antibiotic therapy directed against bacterial pathogens isolated from the respiratory tract is an essential component in the management of CF lung disease. Antibiotics are initially used to prevent colonization with *P. aeruginosa;* they are used as maintenance therapy once the airways are colonized with *P. aeruginosa* and other organisms such as *S. aureus;* and they are administered as aggressive treatment during acute exacerbations of pulmonary symptoms caused by infections.[58,61] To avoid adverse effects and to obtain high airway concentrations, the inhalation route is often used. Indications for oral antibiotics include the presence of respiratory tract symptoms and identification of pathogenic organisms in respiratory tract cultures. Intravenous antibiotics are used for progressive and unrelenting symptoms.

The abnormal viscosity of airway secretions is attributed largely to the presence of polymorphonuclear white blood cells and their degradation products. A purified recombinant human deoxyribonuclease (rhDNase), an enzyme that breaks down these products, has been developed.[56,59] Clinical trials have shown that the drug, which is administered by inhalation, can improve pulmonary symptoms and reduce the frequency of respiratory exacerbations. Although many persons benefit from the therapy, the drug is costly, and recommendations for its use are evolving.

Up to 90% of patients with CF have complete loss of exocrine pancreas function and inadequate digestion of fats and proteins. They require diet adjustment, pancreatic enzyme replacement, and supplemental vitamins and minerals. Many individuals with CF have a higher-than-normal caloric need because of the increased work of breathing and perhaps because of the increased metabolic activity related to the basic defect. Pancreatic enzyme dosage and product type are individualized for each patient. Enteric-coated, pH-sensitive enzyme microspheres are available.[59] A low-fat, high-protein, high-calorie diet was generally recommended in the past. With the advent of improved pancreatic enzyme products, however, normal amounts of fat in the diet are usually tolerated and preferred.

Progress of the disease is variable. Improved medical management has led to longer survival. Today, many people with the disease can expect to live into their 30s, 40s, and beyond.[60] Lung transplantation is being used as a treatment for persons with end-stage lung disease. Current hopes reside in research that would make gene therapy a feasible alternative for persons with the disease.

IN SUMMARY, obstructive ventilatory disorders are characterized by airway obstruction and limitation in expiratory airflow. Bronchial asthma is a chronic inflammatory disorder of the airways characterized by airway hyperreactivity and episodic attacks of airway narrowing. An asthmatic attack can be triggered by a variety of stimuli. Based on their mechanism of response, these triggers can be divided into two types: extrinsic (atopic) and intrinsic (nonatopic). Atopic asthma is typically initiated by a type I hypersensitivity reaction triggered by an extrinsic antigen or allergen; whereas intrinsic asthma has triggers such as respiratory tract infections, exercise, drugs and chemicals, airborne pollutants, and gastroesophageal reflux. There are two types of responses in persons with asthma: the acute- or early-phase response and the late-phase response. The acute-phase response results in immediate bronchoconstriction on exposure to an inhaled antigen and usually subsides within 90 minutes. The late-phase response usually develops 3 to 5 hours after exposure to an asthmatic trigger; it involves inflammation and increased airway responsiveness that prolong the attack and cause a vicious cycle of exacerbations.

Chronic obstructive pulmonary disease describes a group of conditions characterized by obstruction to airflow in the lungs. Among the conditions associated with COPD are emphysema, chronic bronchitis, and bronchiectasis. Emphysema is characterized by a loss of lung elasticity, abnormal, permanent enlargement of the airspaces distal to the terminal bronchioles, and hyperinflation of the lungs. Chronic bronchitis is caused by inflammation of major and small airways and is characterized by edema and hyperplasia of submucosal glands and excess mucus secretion into the bronchial tree. A history of a chronic productive cough that has persisted for at least 3 months and for at least 2 consecutive years in the absence of other disease is necessary for the diagnosis of chronic bronchitis. Emphysema and chronic bronchitis are manifested by eventual mismatching of ventilation and perfusion. As the condition advances, signs of respiratory distress and impaired gas exchange become evident, with development of hypercapnia and hypoxemia. Bronchiectasis is a less common form of COPD that is characterized by an abnormal dilation of the large bronchi associated with infection and destruction of the bronchial walls.

Cystic fibrosis is an autosomal recessive genetic disorder manifested by chronic lung disease, pancreatic exocrine deficiency, and elevation of sodium chloride in the sweat. The disorder is caused by a mutation of a single gene on the long arm of chromosome 7 that codes for the cystic fibrosis transmembrane regulator (CFTR), which functions in the transepithelial transport of the chloride ion. The defect causes exocrine gland secretions to become exceedingly viscid, and it promotes colonization of the respiratory tract with *P. aeruginosa* and other organisms such as *S. aureus*. Accumulation of viscid mucus in the bronchi, impaired mucociliary function, and infection contribute to the development of chronic lung disease and a decreased life expectancy. ■

CONCEPTS in action **ANIMATION**

CHRONIC INTERSTITIAL (RESTRICTIVE) LUNG DISEASES

After completing this section of the chapter, you should be able to meet the following objectives:

- State the difference between chronic obstructive pulmonary diseases and chronic restrictive lung diseases in terms of their pathology and manifestations.
- Cite the characteristics of occupational dusts that determine their pathogenicity in terms of the production of pneumoconiosis.
- Describe the causes of hypersensitivity pneumonitis.
- Characterize the organ involvement in sarcoidosis.

The diffuse interstitial diseases are a diverse group of lung disorders that produce similar inflammatory and fibrotic changes in the interstitium or interalveolar septa of the lung. Because the interstitial lung diseases result in a stiff and noncompliant lung, they are commonly classified as restrictive lung disorders. In contrast to obstructive lung diseases, the lungs are stiff and difficult to expand, despite normally functioning airways.

INTERSTITIAL OR RESTRICTIVE LUNG DISEASES

- Interstitial lung diseases result from inflammatory conditions that affect the interalveolar structures of the lung and produce lung fibrosis and a stiff lung.
- A stiff and noncompliant lung is difficult to inflate, increasing the work of breathing and causing decreased exercise tolerance due to hypoxemia.
- Because of the increased effort needed for lung expansion, persons with interstitial lung disease tend to take small but more frequent breaths.

Etiology and Pathogenesis of Interstitial Lung Diseases

The interstitial lung diseases may be acute or insidious in onset; they may be rapidly progressive, slowly progressive, or static in their course. They include occupational lung diseases such as the pneumoconioses, which are caused by the inhalation of inorganic dusts such as silica, coal dust, and asbestos; hypersensitivity pneumonitis[21,52,62] (see Chapter 19); lung diseases caused by exposure to toxic drugs (*e.g.*, the cancer drug, bleomycin; the antiarrhythmic drug, amiodarone) and radiation; and sarcoidosis. Some of the most common interstitial lung diseases are caused by exposure to inhaled dust and particles. In many cases, no specific cause can be found.[37–39]

CHART 29-1 CAUSES OF INTERSTITIAL LUNG DISEASE*

Occupational and Environmental Inhalants
Pneumoconioses
    Coal miner's pneumoconiosis
    Silicosis
    Asbestosis
Hypersensitivity pneumonitis
    Farmer's lung
    Pigeon breeder's lung

Drugs and Therapeutic Agents
Cancer drugs
    Bleomycin
    Busulfan
    Cyclophosphamide
    Methotrexate
Amiodarone
Ionizing radiation (radiation therapy)

Immunologic Lung Disease
Sarcoidosis
Collagen vascular disease
    Systemic lupus erythematosus
    Rheumatoid arthritis
    Scleroderma

*This list is not intended to be inclusive.

Examples of interstitial lung diseases and their causes are listed in Chart 29-1.

In contrast to the obstructive lung diseases, which primarily involve the airways of the lung, the interstitial lung disorders exert their effects on the collagen and elastic connective tissue found in the delicate interstitium of the alveolar walls. Many of these diseases also involve the airways, arteries, and veins. In general, these lung diseases share a pattern of lung dysfunction that includes diminished lung volumes, reduced diffusing capacity of the lung, and varying degrees of hypoxemia.

Current theory suggests that most interstitial lung diseases, regardless of their causes, have a common pathogenesis.[21,63] It is thought that these disorders are initiated by some type of injury to the alveolar epithelium, followed by an inflammatory process that involves the alveoli and interstitium of the lung. An accumulation of inflammatory and immune cells causes continued damage to lung tissue and replacement of normally functioning lung tissue with fibrous scar tissue.

In general, the interstitial lung diseases are characterized by clinical changes consistent with restrictive rather than obstructive changes in the lung. Persons with interstitial lung diseases have dyspnea, tachypnea, and eventual cyanosis, without evidence of wheezing or signs of airway obstruction. Usually, there is an insidious onset of breathlessness that initially occurs during exercise and may progress to the point at which the person is totally incapacitated. Typically, a person with a restrictive lung disease breathes with a tachypneic pattern of breathing, in which the respiratory rate is increased and the tidal volume is decreased. This pattern of breathing serves to maintain minute volume yet reduces the work of breathing because it takes less work to move air through the airways at an increased rate than it does to stretch a stiff lung to accommodate a larger tidal volume. A nonproductive cough may develop, particularly with continued exposure to the inhaled irritant. Clubbing of the fingers and toes may develop.

Lung volumes, including vital capacity and TLC, are reduced in interstitial lung disease. In contrast to COPD, in which expiratory flow rates are reduced, the $FEV_{1.0}$ usually is preserved, even though the ratio of $FEV_{1.0}$ to FVC may increase. Although resting arterial blood gases usually are normal early in the course of the disease, arterial PO_2 levels may fall during exercise. In persons with advanced disease, hypoxemia often is present, even at rest. In the late stages of the disease, hypercapnia and respiratory acidosis develop. The impaired diffusion of gases in persons with interstitial lung disease is thought to be caused by alterations in the alveolar–capillary membrane as well as an increase in shunt resulting from unventilated regions of the lung.

The diagnosis of interstitial lung disease requires a careful personal and family history, with particular emphasis on exposure to environmental, occupational, and other injurious agents. Chest radiographs may be used as an initial diagnostic method, and serial chest films often are used to follow the progress of the disease. A biopsy specimen for histologic study and culture may be obtained by surgical incision or bronchoscopy using a fiberoptic bronchoscope. In bronchoalveolar lavage, fluid is instilled into the alveoli through a bronchoscope and then removed by suction to obtain inflammatory and immune cells for laboratory study. Gallium lung scans often are used to detect and quantify the chronic alveolitis that occurs in interstitial lung disease. Gallium does not localize in normal lung tissue, but uptake of the radionuclide is increased in interstitial lung disease and other diffuse lung diseases.

The treatment goals for persons with interstitial lung disease focus on identifying and removing the injurious agent, suppressing the inflammatory response, preventing progression of the disease, and providing supportive therapy for persons with advanced disease. In general, the treatment measures vary with the type of lung disease. Corticosteroid drugs frequently are used to suppress the inflammatory response. Many of the supportive treatment measures used in the late stages of the disease, such as oxygen therapy and measures to prevent infection, are similar to those discussed for persons with COPD.

Occupational Lung Disease

The occupational lung diseases can be divided into two major groups: the pneumoconioses and the hypersensitivity diseases.[64] The *pneumoconioses* are caused by the inhalation of inorganic dusts and particulate matter. The *hypersensitivity diseases* result from the inhalation of organic dusts and related occupational antigens. A third type of occupational lung disease, byssinosis, a disease that affects cotton workers, has characteristics of the pneumoconioses and hypersensitivity lung diseases.

Among the pneumoconioses are silicosis, found in hard-rock miners, foundry workers, sandblasters, pottery makers, and workers in the slate industry; coal miner's pneumoconiosis; asbestosis, found in asbestos miners, manufacturers of asbestos products, and installers and removers of asbestos insulation; talcosis, found in talc miners, millers, or drug abusers, and in infants or small children who accidentally inhale powder containing talc; and berylliosis, found in ore extraction workers and alloy production workers. The danger of exposure to asbestos dust is not confined to the workplace. The dust pervades the general environment because it was used in the construction of buildings and in other applications before its health hazards were realized. It has been mixed into paints and plaster, wrapped around water and heating pipes, used to insulate hair dryers, and woven into theater curtains, hot pads, and ironing board covers.

Important etiologic determinants in the development of the pneumoconioses are the size of the dust particle, its chemical nature and ability to incite lung destruction, and the concentration of dust and the length of exposure to it. The most dangerous particles are those in the range of 1 to 5 μm.[21] These small particles are carried through the inspired air into the alveolar structures, whereas larger particles are trapped in the nose or mucous linings of the airways and removed by the mucociliary blanket. Exceptions are asbestos and talc particles, which range in size from 30 to 60 μm but find their way into the alveoli because of their density.

All particles in the alveoli must be cleared by the lung macrophages. Macrophages are thought to transport engulfed particles from the small bronchioles and the alveoli, which have neither cilia nor mucus-secreting cells, to the mucociliary escalator or to the lymphatic channels for removal from the lung. This clearing function is hampered when the function of the macrophage is impaired by factors such as cigarette smoking, consumption of alcohol, and hypersensitivity reactions. This helps to explain the increased incidence of lung disease among smokers exposed to asbestos. In silicosis, the ingestion of silica particles leads to the destruction of the lung macrophages and the release of substances resulting in inflammation and fibrosis.[21] Tuberculosis and other diseases caused by mycobacteria are common in persons with silicosis. Because the macrophages are responsible for protecting the lungs from tuberculosis, the destruction of macrophages accounts for an increased susceptibility to tuberculosis in persons with silicosis.

The concentration of some dusts in the environment strongly influences their effects on the lung. For example, acute silicosis is seen only in persons whose occupations entail intense exposure to silica dust over a short period. It is seen in sandblasters, who use a high-speed jet of sand to clean and polish bricks and the insides of corroded tanks; in tunnelers; and in rock drillers, particularly if they drill through sandstone. Acute silicosis is a rapidly progressive disease, usually leading to severe disability and death within 5 years of diagnosis. In contrast to acute silicosis, which is caused by exposure to extremely high concentrations of silica dust, the symptoms related to chronic, low-level exposure to silica dust usually do not begin to develop until after many years of exposure, and then the symptoms often are insidious in onset and slow to progress.

The hypersensitivity occupational lung disorders (*e.g.,* hypersensitivity pneumonitis) are caused by intense and often prolonged exposure to inhaled organic dusts and related occupational antigens. Affected persons have a heightened sensitivity to the antigen. The most common forms of hypersensitivity pneumonitis are farmer's lung, which results from exposure to moldy hay; pigeon breeder's lung, provoked by exposure to the serum, excreta, or feathers of birds; bagassosis, from contaminated sugar cane; and humidifier or air conditioner lung, caused by mold in the water reservoirs of these appliances. Unlike bronchial asthma, this type of hypersensitivity reaction involves primarily the alveoli. These disorders cause progressive fibrotic lung disease, which can be prevented by the removal of the environmental agent.

Drug- and Radiation-Induced Lung Diseases

Drugs can cause a variety of both acute and chronic alterations in lung function. For example, some of the cytotoxic drugs (*e.g.,* bleomycin, busulfan, methotrexate, cyclophosphamide) used in treatment of cancer cause pulmonary damage as a result of direct toxicity of the drug and by stimulating the influx of inflammatory cells into the alveoli.[21,52] Amiodarone, a drug used to treat resistant cardiac arrhythmias, is preferentially sequestered in the lung and causes significant pneumonitis in 5% to 15% of persons receiving it.[21]

Radiation pneumonitis is a well-known complication of therapeutic radiation for pulmonary and other thoracic malignancies (esophageal, breast, mediastinal). It most often involves the lung in the radiation field but may extend to involve adjacent lung tissue or even the contralateral lung. Two phases of the pulmonary response to radiation occur: an acute phase (radiation pneumonitis) and a chronic phase (radiation fibrosis).[52] Acute radiation pneumonitis occurs 2 to 3 months after completion of radiation and is characterized by insidious onset of dyspnea, dry cough, chest pain, weakness, and fever. Although the pathogenesis of acute radiation pneumonitis is unclear, there is speculation that hypersensitivity mechanisms are involved. Chronic radiation fibrosis develops after a period of 6 to 12 months. Most person are asymptomatic, but slowly progressive dyspnea may occur.

Sarcoidosis

Sarcoidosis is a systemic disorder in which granulomas are found in affected tissues and organ systems, particularly the lung and lymphatic system.[65-68] An important qualification is that these granulomas occur in the absence of exogenous (infection or environmental) agents known to cause granulomatous inflammation. The disorder predominantly affects adults younger than 40 years of age, although it can occur in older persons. The incidence of sarcoidosis in the United States is approximately 5.9 of

100,000 persons per year for men and 6.3 of 100,000 persons per year for women.[65] The incidence is highest among North American blacks and northern European whites; among blacks, women are affected more frequently than men.

Etiology and Pathogenesis

The characteristic lesion of sarcoidosis is the noncaseating granuloma. Unlike the granulomatous lesions that develop in tuberculosis and histoplasmosis, the collection of tissue macrophages composing the granulomas in sarcoidosis do not show evidence of necrosis or caseation. In addition to granulomas, in which multinuclear giant cells are frequently seen (see Chapter 5), there is often alveolitis or inflammation of the alveoli. The inflammation is composed largely of macrophages and lymphocytes, with the latter thought to be of particular importance in the pathogenesis of the disease.[66]

The cause of sarcoidosis remains obscure. It is thought that the disorder may result from exposure of genetically predisposed persons to specific environmental agents.[66,67] Support for a genetic influence comes from epidemiologic studies that have demonstrated the higher incidence in American blacks and Scandinavian populations. Additional evidence comes from familial clustering of the disease. Analysis of human leukocyte antigen (HLA) genes located in the major histocompatibility complex also suggests that unique HLA genes can be linked to disease susceptibility and prognosis. Despite advances, including the identification of sarcoidosis genetic factors, a specific etiologic agent has yet to be identified. Multiple lines of evidence suggest that the inciting agent triggers an immune response that depends on host susceptibility and is characterized by chronic inflammation, monocyte recruitment, and granuloma formation.

Clinical Features

Sarcoidosis has variable manifestations and an unpredictable course of progression in which any organ system can be affected. The three systems that most commonly manifest symptoms are the lungs, skin, and eyes. Persons with sarcoidosis frequently seek health care either as a result of abnormalities detected on an incidental chest film or because of insidious onset of respiratory symptoms (shortness of breath, nonproductive cough, chest pain) or constitutional signs and symptoms (*e.g.,* fever, sweating, anorexia, weight loss, fatigue, myalgia).[21,66] Eye involvement (anterior uveitis) and skin involvement (skin papules and plaques) are particularly common extrathoracic manifestations, but there may be cardiac, neuromuscular, hematologic, hepatic, endocrine, and lymph node findings.[66-68]

Sarcoidosis follows an unpredictable course characterized by either progressive chronicity or periods of activity interspersed with remissions, sometimes permanent, that may be spontaneous or induced by corticosteroid therapy. Approximately 65% to 75% of persons recover with minimal clinical and radiographic abnormalities.[21] Other persons have persistent radiographic abnormalities and progression of their respiratory symptoms, with or without additional extrathoracic disease.[66,67]

The diagnosis of sarcoidosis is based on history and physical examination, tests to exclude other diseases, chest radiography, and biopsy to obtain confirmation of noncaseating granulomas.[66-68] The use of CT scans and magnetic resonance imaging (MRI) as routine methods for diagnosis of sarcoidosis remains controversial. A thorough ophthalmologic evaluation is recommended for most persons, even those without ocular symptoms.[67]

Treatment is directed at interrupting the granulomatous inflammatory process that is characteristic of the disease and managing the associated complications. When treatment is indicated, corticosteroid drugs are used. These agents produce clearing of the lung, as seen on the chest radiograph, and improve pulmonary function, but it is not known whether they affect the long-term outcome of the disease.

IN SUMMARY, the interstitial lung diseases are characterized by fibrosis and decreased compliance of the lung. They include the occupational lung diseases, lung diseases caused by toxic drugs and radiation, and lung diseases of unknown origin, such as idiopathic pulmonary fibrosis and sarcoidosis. These disorders are thought to result from an inflammatory process that begins in the alveoli and extends to involve the interstitial tissues of the lung. Unlike COPD, which affects the airways, interstitial lung diseases affect the supporting collagen and elastic tissues that lie between the airways and blood vessels. These lung diseases decrease lung volumes, reduce the diffusing capacity of the lung, and cause various degrees of hypoxemia. Because lung compliance is reduced, persons with this form of lung disease maintain their minute volume by a rapid, shallow breathing pattern. ■

DISORDERS OF THE PULMONARY CIRCULATION

After completing this section of the chapter, you should be able to meet the following objectives:

- State the most common cause of pulmonary embolism and the clinical manifestations of the disorder.
- Describe the pathophysiology of pulmonary arterial hypertension and state three causes of secondary pulmonary hypertension.
- Describe the alterations in cardiovascular function that are characteristic of cor pulmonale.

As blood moves through the pulmonary capillaries, oxygen content increases and carbon dioxide decreases. These processes depend on the matching of ventilation (*i.e.,* gas exchange) and perfusion (*i.e.,* blood flow). This section discusses two major problems of the pulmonary circulation: pulmonary embolism and pulmonary hypertension. Pulmonary edema, another major problem of the pulmonary circulation, is discussed in Chapter 26.

🔑 DISORDERS OF THE PULMONARY CIRCULATION

■ The pulmonary circulation is a low-pressure system that links the right heart and systemic venous system with the left heart and the systemic arterial system and functions as a conduit for exchange between the dissolved gases in the blood and the ventilated air in the alveoli.

■ Pulmonary thromboemboli are blood clots that originate in the systemic venous system and become lodged in a pulmonary blood vessel as they move from the right heart into and through the pulmonary circulation.

■ Pulmonary hypertension is an elevated pulmonary arterial pressure. It may arise as a primary disorder of the pulmonary arteries in which an abnormal thickening of the vessel wall increases the resistance to blood flow, or as a secondary disorder due to chronic lung disorders or environmental conditions that produce hypoxemia and a resultant constriction of small pulmonary arteries, cardiac disorders that increase pulmonary venous pressure, or thromboembolic disorders that occlude pulmonary blood vessels.

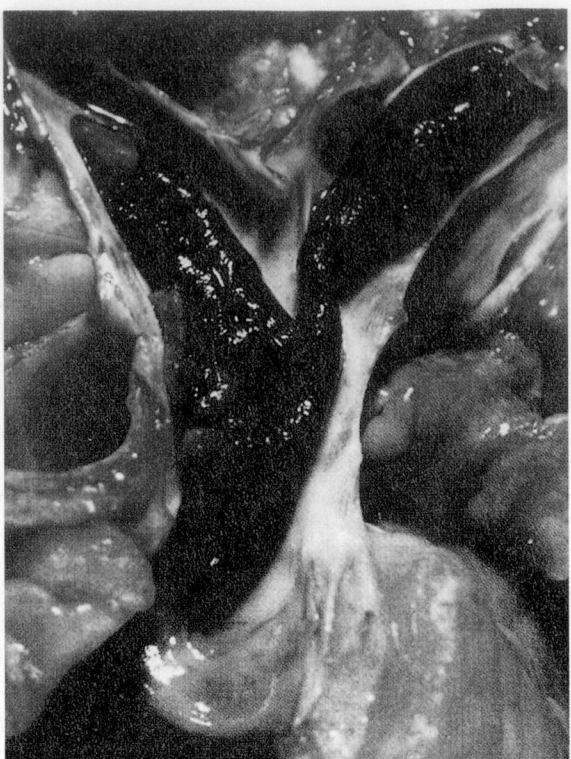

FIGURE 29-14 • Pulmonary embolism. The main pulmonary artery and its bifurcation have been opened to reveal a large saddle embolus. (From McManus B. M., Allard M. F., Yanagawa R. [2008]. Hemodynamic disorders. In Rubin R., Strayer D. S. [Eds.]. *Rubin's pathology: Clinicopathologic foundations of medicine* [5th ed., p. 236]. Philadelphia: Lippincott Williams & Wilkins.)

Pulmonary Embolism

Pulmonary embolism develops when a blood-borne substance lodges in a branch of the pulmonary artery and obstructs blood flow.[69,70] The embolism may consist of a thrombus (Fig. 29-14), air that has accidentally been injected during intravenous infusion, fat that has been mobilized from the bone marrow after a fracture or from a traumatized fat depot (see Chapter 58), or amniotic fluid that has entered the maternal circulation after rupture of the membranes at the time of delivery. The overall mortality rate of major pulmonary embolism is 30% or more.[70]

Etiology and Pathogenesis

Almost all pulmonary emboli are thrombi that arise from deep vein thrombosis (DVT) in the lower extremities[69,70] (see Chapter 22). The presence of thrombosis in the deep veins of the legs or pelvis often is unsuspected until embolism occurs. The effects of emboli on the pulmonary circulation are related to mechanical obstruction of the pulmonary circulation and neurohumoral reflexes causing vasoconstriction. Obstruction of pulmonary blood flow causes reflex bronchoconstriction in the affected area of the lung, wasted ventilation and impaired gas exchange, and loss of alveolar surfactant. Pulmonary hypertension and right heart failure may develop when there is massive vasoconstriction because of a large embolus. Although small areas of infarction may occur, frank pulmonary infarction is uncommon.

Among the physiologic factors that contribute to venous thrombosis are venous stasis, venous endothelial injury, and hypercoagulability states. The thrombophilias (*e.g.,* antithrombin III deficiency, protein C and S deficiencies, factor V Leiden mutation) are a group of inherited disorders affecting coagulation that make an individual prone to development of venous thromboemboli.[69,70] Venous stasis and venous endothelial injury can result from prolonged bed rest, trauma, surgery, childbirth, fractures of the hip and femur, myocardial infarction and congestive heart failure, and spinal cord injury. Persons undergoing orthopedic surgery and gynecologic cancer surgery are at particular risk, as are immobilized persons. Hypercoagulability is related to various factors. Cancer cells can produce thrombin and synthesize procoagulation factors, increasing the risk for thromboembolism. Use of oral contraceptives, pregnancy, and hormone replacement therapy are thought to increase the resistance to endogenous anticoagulants. The risk for pulmonary embolism among users of oral contraceptives is approximately two to four times that of nonusers.[70] Women who smoke are at particular risk.

Clinical Features

Manifestations. The manifestations of pulmonary embolism depend on the size and location of the obstruction. Chest pain, dyspnea, and increased respiratory rate are the most frequent signs and symptoms of pulmonary embolism. Pulmonary infarction often causes pleuritic pain that changes with respiration; it is more severe on inspiration and less severe on expiration. Moderate hypoxemia without carbon dioxide retention occurs as a result of impaired gas exchange. Small emboli that become lodged in the peripheral branches of the pulmonary artery may go unrecognized unless the person is compromised, such as occurs in the elderly or acutely ill. Repeated small emboli gradually reduce the size of the pulmonary capillary bed, resulting in pulmonary hypertension. Persons with moderate-sized emboli often present with breathlessness accompanied by pleuritic pain, apprehension, slight fever, and cough productive of blood-streaked sputum. Tachycardia often occurs to compensate for decreased oxygenation, and the breathing pattern is rapid and shallow. Patients with massive emboli usually present with sudden collapse, crushing substernal chest pain, shock, and sometimes loss of consciousness. The pulse is rapid and weak, the blood pressure is low, the neck veins are distended, and the skin is cyanotic and diaphoretic. Massive pulmonary emboli often are fatal.

Diagnosis and Treatment. The diagnosis of pulmonary embolism is based on clinical signs and symptoms, blood gas determinations, venous thrombosis studies, D-dimer testing, lung scans, helical CT scans of the chest, and, in selected cases, pulmonary angiography.[69–71] Laboratory studies and radiologic films are useful in ruling out other conditions that might give rise to similar symptoms. Because emboli can cause an increase in pulmonary vascular resistance, the electrocardiogram (ECG) may be used to detect signs of right heart strain. There has been recent interest in combining several noninvasive methods (lower limb compression ultrasonography, D-dimer measurements, and clinical assessment measures) as a means of establishing a diagnosis of pulmonary embolism.

Because most pulmonary emboli originate from DVT, venous studies such as *lower limb compression ultrasonography, impedance plethysmography,* and *contrast venography* are often used as initial diagnostic procedures. Of these, lower limb compression ultrasonography has become an important noninvasive means for detecting DVT. *D-dimer testing* involves the measurement of plasma D-dimer, a degradation product of coagulation factors that have been activated as the result of a thromboembolic event. The *ventilation–perfusion scan* uses radiolabeled albumin, which is injected intravenously, and a radiolabeled gas, which is inhaled. A scintillation (gamma) camera is used to scan the various lung segments for blood flow and distribution of the radiolabeled gas. Ventilation–perfusion scans are useful only when their results are either normal or indicate a high probability of pulmonary embolism. *Helical (spiral) CT angiography* requires administration of an intravenous radiocontrast medium. It is sensitive for the detection of emboli in the proximal pulmonary arteries and provides another method of diagnosis. *Pulmonary angiography* involves the passage of a venous catheter through the right heart and into the pulmonary artery under fluoroscopy. Although it remains the most accurate method of diagnosis, it is an invasive procedure; therefore, its use is reserved for selected cases. An embolectomy sometimes is performed during this procedure.

The treatment goals for pulmonary emboli focus on preventing DVT and the development of thromboemboli, protecting the lungs from exposure to thromboemboli when they occur, and in the case of large and life-threatening pulmonary emboli, sustaining life and restoring pulmonary blood flow.[69,70,72] Fibrinolytic therapy using streptokinase, urokinase, or recombinant tissue plasminogen activator may be indicated in persons with multiple or large emboli. Fibrinolytic therapy is followed by administration of heparin and then warfarin, to prevent clot reoccurrence.

Prevention. Prevention focuses on identification of persons at risk, avoidance of venous stasis and hypercoagulability states, and early detection of venous thrombosis.[72] Patients require mobilization as soon as possible after surgery or illness. For persons at risk, graded compression elastic stockings and intermittent pneumatic compression (IPC) boots can be used to prevent venous stasis. Both of these devices are safe and practical ways to prevent venous thrombosis. IPC boots provide intermittent inflation of air-filled sleeves that prevent venous stasis. Some devices produce sequential gradient compression that moves blood upward in the leg.

Pharmacologic prophylaxis involves the use of anticoagulant drugs (see Chapter 13). Anticoagulant therapy may be used to decrease the likelihood of deep vein thrombosis, thromboembolism, and fatal pulmonary embolism after major surgical procedures. Low–molecular-weight heparin, which can be administered subcutaneously on an outpatient basis, often is used. Warfarin, an oral anticoagulation drug, may be used for persons with a long-term risk for development of thromboemboli.

Surgical interruption of the vena cava may be indicated when pulmonary embolism poses a life-threatening risk.[69] There are two surgical procedures for protecting the lung from thromboemboli: venous ligation to prevent the embolus from traveling to the lung and vena caval plication. The plication procedure, which is done with a suture or by insertion of a clip, filter, or sieve, permits blood to flow while trapping the embolus. Percutaneous transjugular placement of a filter has become the preferred mode of inferior vena cava interruption.

Pulmonary Hypertension

The pulmonary circulation is a low-pressure system designed to accommodate varying amounts of blood delivered from the right heart and to facilitate gas exchange. The main pulmonary artery and major branches are relatively thin-walled, compliant vessels. The distal pulmonary arterioles also are thin walled and have the capacity to dilate, collapse, or constrict depending on the presence of vasoactive substances released from the endothelial cells of the vessel, neurohumoral influences, flow velocity, oxygen tension, and alveolar ventilation.

Pulmonary hypertension is a disorder characterized by an elevation of pressure within the pulmonary circulation, namely the pulmonary arterial system. The elevation in pressure may be acute or chronic, depending on the causative factors. A number of factors can contribute to the pathogenesis of pulmonary arterial hypertension, including a decrease in the cross-sectional area of the pulmonary arteries, a loss of blood vessels from either scarring or destructive processes affecting the alveolar walls, vasoconstriction in response to hypoxia, the need to accommodate excessive inflow of blood flow without any anatomic changes in the pulmonary arteries or arterioles, or the occlusion of outflow from the pulmonary circulation due to elevated pressures within the left atrium or ventricle. The disorder may be due to changes in the arterial wall, often referred to as *pulmonary arterial hypertension,* or it may occur as a secondary condition related to the occlusion of the pulmonary circulation by pulmonary emboli or to disruption of the pulmonary circulation due to heart or lung disease.

Pulmonary Arterial Hypertension

The term *pulmonary arterial hypertension* (PAH) is used to describe a type of pulmonary hypertension that has its origin in the pulmonary arteries. It includes primary (idiopathic or familial) pulmonary hypertension, as well as pulmonary hypertension associated with disease entities that clinically appear similar to primary pulmonary hypertension in presentation and response to treatment.[73] PAH is a rare and debilitating disorder characterized by abnormal proliferation and contraction of vascular smooth muscle, coagulation abnormalities, and marked intimal fibrosis leading to obliteration or obstruction of the pulmonary arteries and arterioles (Fig. 29-15). The resulting increase in pressure results in progressive right heart failure, low cardiac output, and death if left untreated. The incidence of idiopathic or primary pulmonary hypertension, which is the best-studied entity in this group, ranges from 1 to 2 cases per million people in the general population.[74] The past decade has witnessed dramatic advances in the treatment of PAH, with medical therapies targeting specific pathways that are believed to play pathogenetic roles in development of the disorder. Despite these achievements, PAH remains a serious, life-threatening condition.

The familial form of PAH appears to be inherited as an autosomal dominant trait with a variable but low penetrance, with some individuals inheriting the trait without exhibiting the disease. In 2000, the bone morphogenetic protein receptor type II gene (*BMPR2*), which codes for a member of the transforming growth factor-β (TGF-β) superfamily of receptors, was identified as causative of familial PAH. Mutations in these receptors are thought to prevent TGF-β and related molecules from exerting an inhibitory effect on smooth muscle and endothelial cell proliferation.[74,75] Other conditions associated with PAH include collagen vascular disorders (*e.g.,* scleroderma), drugs and toxins, human immunodeficiency virus (HIV) infection, portal hypertension, and persistent pulmonary hypertension in the newborn.[73–76] A causal relationship has been established between several appetite suppressant drugs, including

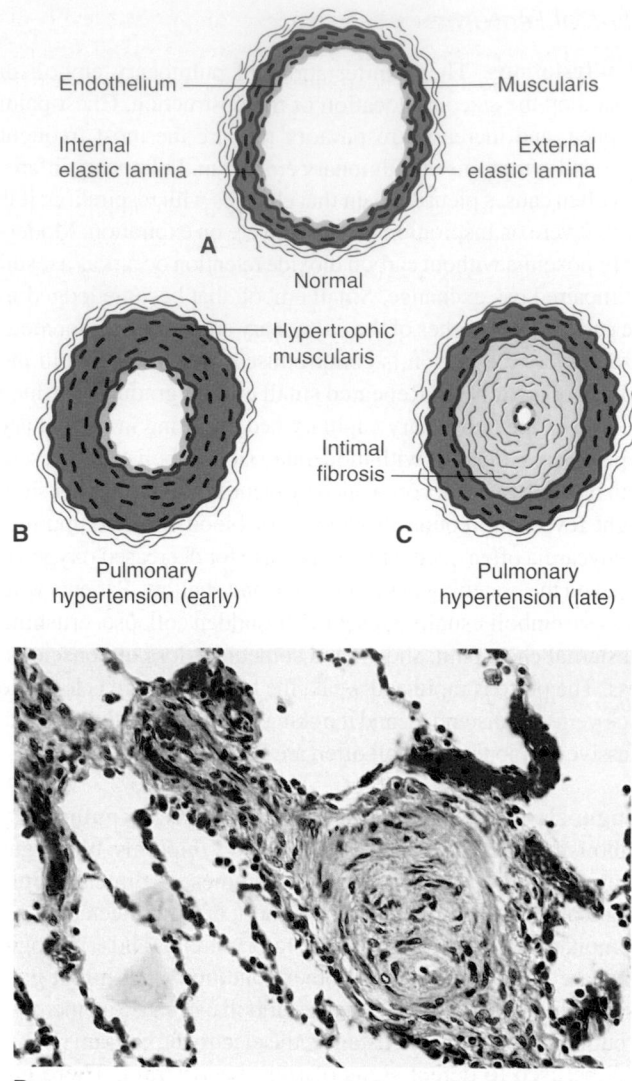

FIGURE 29-15 • (**A**) Normal pulmonary artery. (**B**) Mild pulmonary hypertension with thickening of the media of the pulmonary artery. (**C**) Pulmonary artery with extensive intimal fibrosis and thickening of vascular smooth muscle. (**D**) Micrograph of a small pulmonary artery that is virtually occluded by concentrically thickened intimal fibrosis and thickening of the media due to pulmonary arterial hypertension. (From Bearsley M. B., Travis W. D., Rubin E. [2008]. The respiratory system. In Rubin R., Strayer D. S. [Eds.], *Rubin's pathology: Clinicopathologic foundations of medicine* [5th ed., p. 537]. Philadelphia: Lippincott Williams & Wilkins.)

fenfluramine, and the development of PAH. Although the drug has been removed from the world market, there are still persons who were exposed to the drug before that time. The mechanism by which HIV infection produces PAH remains unknown, but treatment of HIV infection does not appear to affect the severity or natural history of the underlying pulmonary hypertension.

Although the specific mechanisms responsible for the vascular changes that occur in PAH remain unknown, a number of mechanisms have been proposed. These include enhanced expression of the serotonin transporter, diminished levels of nitric oxide and prostacyclin, and increased levels of several growth factors, including endothelin, vascular endothelial growth factor, and platelet-derived growth factor. The endothelium relaxing factor, nitric oxide, is a potent pulmonary vasodilator that is produced locally in the lung and has profound effects on smooth muscle relaxation and proliferation. Endothelin-1 is a peptide produced by the vascular endothelium that has potent vasoconstrictor and paracrine effects on vascular smooth muscle. The endothelium also produces prostacyclin (PGI2), an inhibitor of platelet aggregation and potent vasodilator. Results of studies relating these mechanisms to the structure and function of the pulmonary arterial circulation have already been translated into targeted therapies for PAH, with the probability that more will be investigated in the future.

PAH is defined by persistent elevation in pulmonary artery pressure with normal left-ventricular pressures, differentiating it from left-sided heart failure. Symptoms typically progress from shortness of breath and decreasing exercise tolerance to right heart failure, with marked peripheral edema and functional limitations. Other common symptoms include fatigue, angina, and syncope (fainting) or near-syncope. The diagnosis of primary pulmonary hypertension is based on an absence of disorders that cause secondary hypertension and mean pulmonary artery pressures greater than 25 mm Hg at rest or 30 mm Hg with exercise.

Treatment consists of measures to improve right heart function as a means of reducing fatigue and peripheral edema. Supplemental oxygen may be used to increase exercise tolerance. The calcium channel blockers (nifedipine, diltiazem) may be effective early in the course of the disease but offer little in advanced stages. More advanced disease has been managed with epoprostenol, a prostacyclin that has potent pulmonary vasodilator effects.[75,76] Because of its short half-life (3 to 5 minutes), the drug must be administered by continuous infusion through an indwelling catheter with an automatic ambulatory pump. Properties of the drug other than its vasodilating effects include inhibition of platelet aggregation and beneficial vascular remodeling effects. This agent often improves symptoms, sometimes dramatically, in persons who have not responded to other vasodilators. Bosentan, an oral endothelin antagonist, has proved to be effective in treating moderate to severe primary pulmonary hypertension and may become the treatment of choice for all stages of the disease.[77] Sildenafil (*e.g.,* Viagra) a highly selective phosphodiesterase-5 inhibitor, which acts in a manner similar to nitric oxide to produce vasodilation, has recently been approved in the United States for treatment of pulmonary hypertension. Lung transplantation may be an alternative for persons who do not respond to other forms of treatment.

Secondary Pulmonary Hypertension

Although pulmonary hypertension can develop as a primary disorder, most cases develop secondary to conditions such as chronic hypoxemia due to COPD, interstitial lung disease, or sleep-disordered breathing; increased resistance to pulmonary venous drainage due to conditions such as diastolic dysfunc-

tion of the left heart or disorders of mitral or aortic valves; or chronic thromboembolic disorders.

Continued exposure of the pulmonary vessels to hypoxemia is a common cause of pulmonary hypertension. Unlike blood vessels in the systemic circulation, most of which dilate in response to hypoxemia and hypercapnia, the pulmonary vessels constrict. The stimulus for constriction seems to originate in the airspaces near the smaller branches of the pulmonary arteries. In regions of the lung that are poorly ventilated, the response is adaptive in that it diverts blood flow away from the poorly ventilated areas to those areas that are more adequately ventilated. This effect, however, becomes less beneficial as more and more areas of the lung become poorly ventilated. Pulmonary hypertension is a common problem in persons with advanced COPD or interstitial lung disease. It also may develop at high altitudes in persons with normal lungs. Persons who experience marked hypoxemia during sleep (such as those with sleep apnea) often experience marked elevations in pulmonary arterial pressure.

Elevation of pulmonary venous pressure is common in conditions such as mitral valve disorders or left ventricular diastolic dysfunction. In each of these alterations, the elevated left atrial pressure is transmitted to the pulmonary circulation. Continued increases in left atrial pressure can lead to medial hypertrophy and intimal thickening of the small pulmonary arteries, causing sustained hypertension. Another cause of secondary pulmonary hypertension is obstruction of pulmonary blood flow due to pulmonary thromboemboli. Persons who are promptly treated for acute pulmonary thromboembolism with anticoagulants rarely develop pulmonary hypertension. However, in some persons chronic obstruction of the pulmonary vascular bed develops because of impaired resolution of the thromboemboli.

The signs and symptoms of secondary pulmonary hypertension reflect both the elevated pulmonary arterial pressure and the underlying heart or lung disease. As with primary pulmonary hypertension, diagnosis is based on radiographic findings, echocardiography, and Doppler ultrasonography. Treatment measures are directed toward the underlying disorder. Vasodilator therapy may be indicated for some persons.

Cor Pulmonale

The term *cor pulmonale* refers to right heart failure resulting from primary lung disease or pulmonary hypertension. The increased pressures and work result in hypertrophy and eventual failure of the right ventricle. The manifestations of cor pulmonale include the signs and symptoms of the primary lung disease and the signs of right-sided heart failure (see Chapter 26). Signs of right-sided heart failure include venous congestion, peripheral edema, shortness of breath, and a productive cough, which becomes worse during periods of heart failure. Plethora (*i.e.,* redness), cyanosis, and warm, moist skin may result from the compensatory polycythemia and desaturation of arterial blood that accompany chronic lung disease. Drowsiness and altered consciousness may occur as the result of carbon dioxide retention. Management of cor pulmonale focuses on the treatment of the lung disease and heart failure. Low-flow oxygen therapy may be used to reduce the pulmonary hypertension and polycythemia associated with severe hypoxemia caused by chronic lung disease.

IN SUMMARY, pulmonary vascular disorders include pulmonary embolism and pulmonary hypertension. Pulmonary embolism develops when a blood-borne substance lodges in a branch of the pulmonary artery and obstructs blood flow. The embolus can consist of a thrombus, air, fat, or amniotic fluid. The most common form is thromboemboli arising from the deep venous channels of the lower extremities. Pulmonary hypertension is the elevation of pulmonary arterial pressure. It can be divided into two types: (1) pulmonary arterial hypertension, which has its origin in the pulmonary arteries and includes both primary (idiopathic or familial) pulmonary hypertension and pulmonary hypertension associated with disease entities that produce a similar pathologic process; and (2) pulmonary hypertension that develops secondary to lung disease and hypoxemia (*e.g.,* chronic lung diseases, sleep-disordered breathing, or chronic exposure to high altitude), conditions that elevate pulmonary venous pressures (left ventricular dysfunction, mitral valve disease), or chronic obstruction of the pulmonary vasculature due to thromboemboli. *Cor pulmonale* describes right heart failure caused by primary pulmonary disease and long-standing pulmonary hypertension. ■

ACUTE RESPIRATORY DISORDERS

After completing this section of the chapter, you should be able to meet the following objectives:

- Describe the pathologic lung changes that occur in acute respiratory distress syndrome and relate them to the clinical manifestations of a general definition of respiratory failure.
- Differentiate between the causes and manifestations of hypoxemic and hypercapnic/hypoxemic respiratory failure.
- Describe the treatment of respiratory failure.

The function of the respiratory system is to add oxygen to the blood and remove carbon dioxide. Disruptions in this function occur with acute lung injury/respiratory distress syndrome and acute respiratory failure. Although the mechanisms that disrupt gas exchange may vary, both conditions represent a life-threatening situation with high risks of morbidity and mortality.

Acute Lung Injury/Acute Respiratory Distress Syndrome

Acute respiratory distress syndrome (ARDS) was first described in 1967 in adults, and initially called *adult respiratory distress syndrome.*[78] It later was renamed *acute respiratory distress syndrome* because it also affects children. After a consensus conference, acute lung injury (ALI) and ARDS were differentiated by the extent of hypoxemia, as evaluated by the PF (PO_2 to FiO_2) ratio.[79] ARDS is a more severe aspect of ALI, and is differentiated primarily for early intervention, prevention, and research purposes. The incidence of ALI/ARDS is not consistently reported, although it is estimated to occur in approximately 150,000 to 200,000 persons each year in North America. Despite the most sophisticated interventions, the mortality rate varies from 35% to 60% and morbidity is extensive, including physical, cognitive, and emotional sequelae.[80,81]

ARDS may result from a number of conditions, including aspiration of gastric contents, major trauma (with or without fat emboli), sepsis secondary to pulmonary or nonpulmonary infections, acute pancreatitis, hematologic disorders, metabolic events, and reactions to drugs and toxins (Chart 29-2). Chronic alcohol abuse increases both the risk for and severity of ALI/ARDS.[82] In the United States, there is a risk of transfusion-related acute lung injury (TRALI),[83] which is rare in Europe, Canada, Australia, and the United Kingdom owing to their practice of washing of packed cells. It is hypothesized that levels of mediators and cytokines are higher in unwashed packed cells.

CHART 29-2	CONDITIONS IN WHICH ARDS CAN DEVELOP*

Aspiration
Near drowning
Aspiration gastric contents

Drugs, Toxins, Therapeutic Agents
Free-base cocaine smoking
Heroin
Inhaled gases (*e.g.*, smoke, ammonia)
Breathing high concentrations of oxygen
Radiation

Infections
Septicemia

Trauma and Shock
Burns
Fat embolism
Chest trauma

Disseminated Intravascular Coagulation

Multiple Blood Transfusions

*This list is not intended to be inclusive.

Etiology and Pathogenesis

Although a number of conditions may lead to ALI/ARDS, they all produce similar pathologic lung changes that include diffuse epithelial cell injury with increased permeability of the alveolar–capillary membrane (Fig. 29-16). The increased permeability permits fluid, plasma proteins, and blood cells to move out of the vascular compartment into the interstitium and alveoli of the lung.[84,85] Diffuse alveolar cell damage leads to accumulation of fluid, surfactant inactivation, and formation of a hyaline membrane that is impervious to gas exchange. As the disease progresses, the work of breathing becomes greatly increased as the lung stiffens and becomes more difficult to inflate. There is increased intrapulmonary shunting of blood, impaired gas exchange, and hypoxemia despite high supplemental oxygen therapy. Gas exchange is further compromised by alveolar collapse resulting from abnormalities in surfactant production. When injury to the alveolar epithelium is severe, disorganized epithelial repair may lead to fibrosis.

The pathogenesis of ALI/ARDS is unclear, although both local and systemic inflammatory responses occur. Neutrophils accumulate early in the course of the disorder and are considered to play a role in the pathogenesis of ALI/ARDS.[86] Activated neutrophils synthesize and release a variety of products, including proteolytic enzymes, toxic oxygen species, and phospholipid products that increase the inflammatory response and cause further injury to the capillary endothelium and alveolar epithelium.

Clinical Features

Clinically, ALI/ARDS is marked by a rapid onset, usually within 12 to 18 hours of the initiating event, of respiratory distress, an increase in respiratory rate, and signs of respiratory failure. Chest radiography shows diffuse bilateral infiltrates of the lung tissue in the absence of cardiac dysfunction. Marked hypoxemia occurs that is refractory to treatment with supplemental oxygen therapy, which results in a decrease in the PF ratio. Many persons with ARDS have a systemic response that results in multiple organ failure, particularly of the renal, gastrointestinal, cardiovascular, and central nervous systems.

Treatment. The treatment goals in ARDS are to supply oxygen to vital organs and provide supportive care until the condition causing the pathologic process has been reversed and the lungs have had a chance to heal. Assisted ventilation using high concentrations of oxygen may be required to correct the hypoxemia (to be discussed). Positive end-expiratory pressure breathing, which increases the pressure in the airways during expiration, may be used to assist in reinflating the collapsed areas of the lung and to improve the matching of ventilation and perfusion. Extensive research has been done to determine optimal pressures and volumes to correct the hypoxemia yet prevent further lung injury due to the mechanics of ventilation.[87]

Acute Respiratory Failure

Respiratory failure can be viewed as a failure in gas exchange due to either pump (heart) or lung failure, or both. It is not a specific disease, but can occur in the course of a number of conditions that impair ventilation, compromise the matching of ventilation and perfusion, or impair gas diffusion. Acute respiratory failure may occur in previously healthy persons as the result of acute disease or trauma involving the respiratory system, or it may develop in the course of a chronic neuromuscular or lung disease.

Respiratory failure is a condition in which the respiratory system fails in one or both of its gas exchange functions—

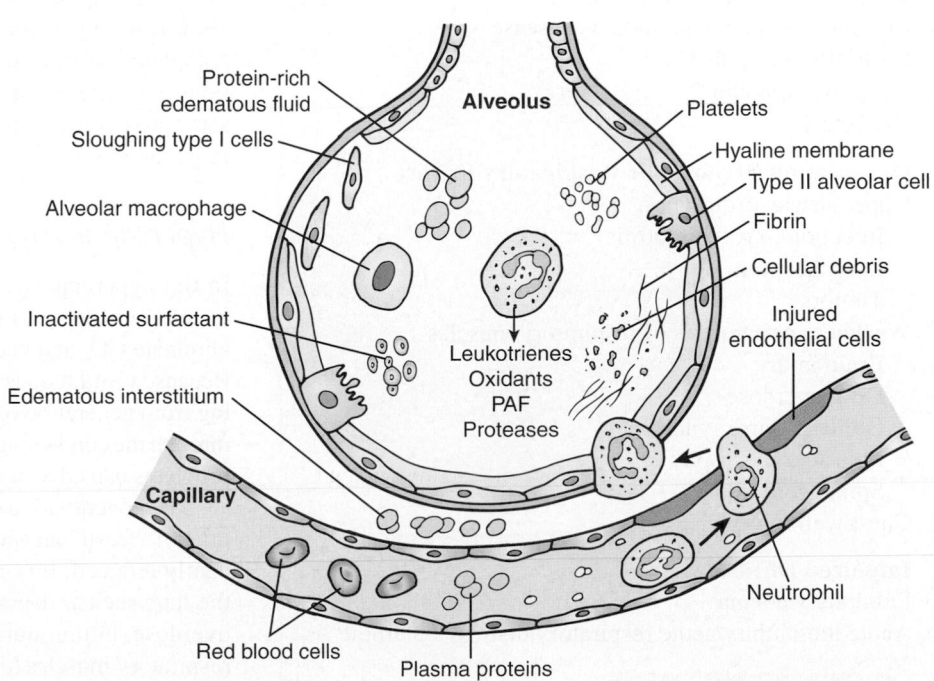

FIGURE 29-16 • The mechanism of lung changes in ARDS. Injury and increased permeability of the alveolar capillary membrane allow fluid, protein, cellular debris, platelets, and blood cells to move out of the vascular compartment and enter the interstitium and alveoli. Activated neutrophils release a variety of products that damage the alveolar cells and lead to edema, sur-factant inactivation, and formation of a hyaline membrane. PAF, platelet-activating factor.

oxygenation of mixed venous blood and elimination of carbon dioxide. The function of the respiratory system can be said to consist of two aspects: gas exchange (movement of gases across the alveolar-capillary membrane) and ventilation (movement of gases into and out of the alveoli due to the action of the respiratory muscles, respiratory center in the central nervous system [CNS], and the pathways that connect the centers in the CNS with the respiratory muscles). Thus respiratory failure is commonly divided into two types: (1) hypoxemic respiratory failure due to failure of the gas-exchange function of the lung and (2) hypercapnic/hypoxemic respiratory failure due to ventilatory failure.[88,89] The classification should not be viewed as rigid since lung disorders that cause impaired gas exchange can be complicated by ventilatory failure and ventilatory failure can be accompanied by lung disorders that impair gas diffusion. Causes of the two types of respiratory failure are summarized in Chart 29-3.

Hypoxemic Respiratory Failure

In persons with hypoxemic respiratory failure, two major pathophysiologic factors contribute to the lowering of arterial PO_2–ventilation–perfusion mismatching or impaired diffusion.

Mismatching of Ventilation and Perfusion. The mismatching of ventilation and perfusion occurs when areas of the lung are ventilated but not perfused or when areas are perfused but not ventilated. Usually the hypoxemia seen in situations of ventilation–perfusion mismatching is more severe in relation

---

CHART 29-3   **CAUSES OF RESPIRATORY FAILURE***

Hypoxemic Respiratory Failure
Chronic obstructive pulmonary disease
Restrictive lung disease
Severe pneumonia
Atelectasis

Hypercapnic/Hypoxemic Respiratory Failure
Upper airway obstruction
　Infection (*e.g.*, epiglottitis)
　Laryngospasm
　Tumors
Weakness or paralysis of respiratory muscles
　Brain injury
　Drug overdose
　Guillain-Barré syndrome
　Muscular dystrophy
　Spinal cord injury
Chest wall injury

Impaired Diffusion
Pulmonary edema
Acute lung injury/acute respiratory distress syndrome

*This list is not intended to be inclusive.

---

to hypercapnia than that seen in hypoventilation. Severe mismatching of ventilation and perfusion often is seen in persons with advanced COPD. These disorders contribute to the retention of carbon dioxide by reducing the effective alveolar ventilation, even when total ventilation is maintained. This occurs because a region of the lung is not perfused and gas exchange cannot take place or because an area of the lung is not being ventilated. Maintaining a high ventilation rate effectively prevents hypercapnia but also increases the work of breathing.

The hypoxemia associated with ventilation–perfusion disorders often is exaggerated by conditions such as hypoventilation and decreased cardiac output. For example, sedation can cause hypoventilation in persons with severe COPD, resulting in further impairment of ventilation. Likewise, a decrease in cardiac output because of myocardial infarction can exaggerate the ventilation–perfusion impairment in a person with mild pulmonary edema or COPD.

The beneficial effect of oxygen administration on PO_2 levels in ventilation–perfusion disorders depends on the degree of mismatching that is present. Because oxygen administration increases the diffusion gradient in ventilated portions of the lung, it usually is effective in raising arterial PO_2 levels. However, high-flow oxygen may decrease the respiratory drive and produce an increase in PCO_2.

Impaired Diffusion. Impaired diffusion describes a condition in which gas exchange between the alveolar air and pulmonary blood is impeded because of an increase in the distance for diffusion or a decrease in the permeability or surface area of the respiratory membranes to the movement of gases. It most commonly occurs in conditions such as interstitial lung disease, ALI/ARDS, pulmonary edema, and pneumonia.

Conditions that impair diffusion may produce severe hypoxemia but no hypercapnia because of the increase in ventilation and greater diffusion rate of carbon dioxide. Hypoxemia resulting from impaired diffusion can be partially or completely corrected by the administration of high concentrations of oxygen. In this case, the high concentration of oxygen serves to overcome the decrease in diffusion by establishing a larger alveolar-to-capillary diffusion gradient.

Hypercapnic/Hypoxemic Respiratory Failure

In the hypercapnic form of respiratory failure, patients are unable to maintain a level of alveolar ventilation sufficient to eliminate CO_2 and keep arterial O_2 levels within normal range. Because ventilation is determined by a sequence of events ranging from generation of impulses in the CNS to movement of air through the conducting airways, there are several stages at which problems can adversely affect the total minute ventilation.

Hypoventilation or ventilatory failure occurs when the volume of "fresh" air moving into and out of the lung is significantly reduced. It is commonly caused by conditions outside the lung such as depression of the respiratory center (*e.g.*, drug overdose, brain injury), diseases of the nerves supplying the respiratory muscles (*e.g.*, Guillain-Barré syndrome, spinal cord injury), disorders of the respiratory muscles (*e.g.*, muscular dystrophy), exacerbation of chronic lung disease (*e.g.*, COPD), or thoracic cage disorders (*e.g.*, severe scoliosis or crushed chest).

Hypoventilation has two important effects on arterial blood gases. First, it almost always causes an increase in PCO_2. The rise in PCO_2 is directly related to the level of ventilation; reducing the ventilation by one half causes a doubling of the PCO_2. Thus, the PCO_2 level is a good diagnostic measure for hypoventilation. Second, it may cause hypoxemia, although the hypoxemia that is caused by hypoventilation can be readily abolished by the administration of supplemental oxygen.

Clinical Features

Acute respiratory failure is usually manifested by varying degrees of hypoxemia and hypercapnia. There is no absolute definition of the levels of PO_2 and PCO_2 that indicate respiratory failure. Respiratory failure is conventionally defined by an arterial PO_2 of less than 60 mm Hg, an arterial PCO_2 of more than 45 mm Hg, or both when prior blood values have been normal.[88,89] It is important to emphasize that these cut-off values are not rigid, but simply serve as a general guide in combination with history and physical assessment information. The signs and symptoms of acute respiratory failure are those of the underlying disease combined with signs of hypoxemia and hypercapnia/hypoxemia. Respiratory acidosis is usually present because the retention of CO_2 results in increased production of acids.

Hypoxemia is accompanied by increased respiratory drive and increased sympathetic tone. Potential signs of hypoxemia include cyanosis, restlessness, confusion, anxiety, delirium, fatigue, tachypnea, hypertension, cardiac arrhythmias, and tremor. The initial cardiovascular effects are tachycardia with increased cardiac output and increased blood pressure. Serious arrhythmias may be triggered. The pulmonary vasculature constricts in response to low alveolar PO_2. If severe, the pulmonary vasoconstriction may result in acute right ventricular failure with manifestations such as jugular vein distention and dependent edema. Profound acute hypoxemia can cause convulsions, retinal hemorrhages, and permanent brain damage. Hypotension and bradycardia often are preterminal events in persons with hypoxemic respiratory failure, indicating the failure of compensatory mechanisms.

Many of the adverse consequences of hypercapnia are the result of respiratory acidosis. Direct effects of acidosis include depression of cardiac contractility, decreased respiratory muscle contractility, and arterial vasodilation (see Chapter 32). Raised levels of PCO_2 greatly increase cerebral blood flow, which may result in headache, increased cerebrospinal fluid pressure, and sometimes papilledema (see Chapter 54, Fig. 54-14). The headache is due to dilation of the cerebral vessels. Additional indicators of hypercapnia are warm and flushed skin and hyperemic conjunctivae. Hypercapnia has nervous system effects similar to those of an anesthetic—hence the term *carbon dioxide narcosis*. There is progressive somnolence, disorientation, and, if the condition is untreated, coma. Mild to moderate increases in blood pressure are common. Air hunger and rapid breathing occur when alveolar PCO_2 levels rise to approximately

60 to 75 mm Hg; as PCO_2 levels reach 80 to 100 mm Hg, the person becomes lethargic and sometimes semicomatose.

Treatment. The treatment of the person with acute respiratory failure consists of specific therapy directed toward the underlying disease, respiratory supportive care directed toward maintenance of adequate gas exchange, and general supportive care. A number of treatment modalities are available, including the establishment of an airway, use of bronchodilating drugs, and antibiotics for respiratory infections. The main therapeutic goal in acute hypoxemic respiratory failure is to ensure adequate oxygenation of vital organs. This is accomplished through administration of supplemental oxygen.

Mechanical Ventilation. When alveolar ventilation is inadequate to maintain PO_2 or PCO_2 levels because of impaired respiratory function or neurologic failure, mechanical ventilation may be necessary.[90,91] There are noninvasive forms of mechanical ventilation that use a face mask to deliver positive-pressure ventilation.[92,93] Bilevel positive airway pressure (BiPAP) ventilation mode senses inspiratory effort and delivers a higher pressure during inspiration, which decreases work and increases effectiveness of breathing.[94] The external mode of mechanical ventilation has been demonstrated to be effective in patients who are conscious, have minimal airway secretions, and a normal blood pressure. It is recommended for first consideration for the person with acute respiratory failure and underlying COPD.[95]

Usually an endotracheal tube is inserted to provide the patient with the airway needed for mechanical ventilation. There are two basic types of positive-pressure mechanical ventilators: pressure-cycled units and volume-cycled units.[91] In each type, the inspiratory pressure or tidal volume and respiratory rate are adjusted to maintain ventilation at a given minute volume. The patient does less or no work of breathing. In either type, positive pressure may also be added at the end of expiration (PEEP) to optimize the alveolar surface area for diffusion. The pressure-cycled unit delivers a preset pressure, whereas the tidal volume is determined by the airway pressure with a controlled flow rate. The volume-cycled ventilator delivers a preset tidal volume, but the pressure may vary. Thus, either pressure or volume is controlled. Both of these modes of ventilation deliver the pressure or volume at a minimum set rate per minute, and the person may initiate additional breaths at that preset volume or pressure. Thus, ventilators deliver a breath triggered by the patient or independently if such an effort does not occur.

Mandatory volume ventilation may be intermittent and synchronized to the patient, which is called *synchronized intermittent mandatory ventilation* (SIMV). In this mode, the patient receives periodic positive-pressure ventilation from the ventilator at a preset volume and rate, and pressure-support ventilation, in which the ventilator delivers a set pressure rather than volume to augment each spontaneous respiratory effort. Ventilators also can be programmed to supply positive pressure for support during inspiration (PSV) or continuous positive airway pressure (CPAP) in spontaneously breathing patients. In each of these, the work of breathing is supported by the ventilator, but the patient also provides some effort.

IN SUMMARY, the hallmark of acute lung injury and acute respiratory distress syndrome is a pronounced inflammatory response that affects the lung and may result in systemic organ failure. The acute inflammatory response results in damage and dysfunction of the alveolar–capillary membrane of the lung. Classically, there is interstitial edema of lung tissue, an increase in surface tension caused by inactivation of surfactant, collapse of the alveolar structures, a stiff and noncompliant lung that is difficult to inflate, and impaired diffusion of the respiratory gases with severe hypoxia that is resistant to oxygen therapy.

Acute respiratory failure is a condition in which the lungs fail to oxygenate the blood adequately (hypoxemic respiratory failure) or prevent undue retention of carbon dioxide (hypercapnic/hypoxemic respiratory failure). The causes of respiratory failure are many. It may arise acutely in persons with previously healthy lungs, or it may be superimposed on chronic lung disease. Treatment of acute respiratory failure is directed toward treatment of the underlying disease, maintenance of adequate gas exchange and tissue oxygenation, and general supportive care. When alveolar ventilation is inadequate to maintain PO_2 or PCO_2 levels because of impaired respiratory function or neurologic failure, mechanical ventilation may be necessary. ■

Review Exercises

1. A 30-year-old man is brought to the emergency department with a knife wound to the chest. On visual inspection, asymmetry of chest movement during inspiration, displacement of the trachea, and absence of breath sounds on the side of the wound are noted. His neck veins are distended, and his pulse is rapid and thready. A rapid diagnosis of tension pneumothorax is made.

    A. *Explain the observed respiratory and cardiovascular function in terms of the impaired lung expansion and the air that has entered the chest as a result of the injury.*

    B. *What type of emergent treatment is necessary to save this man's life?*

2. A 10-year-old boy who is having an acute asthmatic attack is brought to the emergency department by his parents. The boy is observed to be sitting up and struggling to breathe. His breathing is accompanied by use of the accessory muscles, a weak cough, and audible wheezing sounds. His pulse is rapid and weak and both heart and breath sounds are distant on auscultation. His parents relate that his asthma began to worsen after he developed a "cold," and now he doesn't even get relief from his "albuterol" inhaler.

    A. *Explain the changes in physiologic function underlying this boy's signs and symptoms.*

    B. *What is the most probable reason for the progression of this boy's asthma in terms of the early- and late-phase responses?*

    C. *The boy is treated with a systemic corticosteroid and inhaled anticholinergic and β_2-adrenergic agonist and then transferred to the intensive care unit. Explain the action of each of these medications in terms of relieving this boy's symptoms.*

3. A 62-year-old man with an 8-year history of chronic bronchitis reports to his health care provider with complaints of increasing shortness of breath, ankle swelling, and a feeling of fullness in his upper abdomen. The expiratory phase of his respirations is prolonged and expiratory wheezes and crackles are heard on auscultation. His blood pressure is 160/90 mm Hg, his red blood cell count is 6.0×10^6 µL (normal 4.2 to 5.4×10^6 µL), his hematocrit is 65% (normal male value 40% to 50%), his arterial PO_2 is 55 mm Hg, and his O_2 saturation, which is 85% while he is resting, drops to 55% during walking exercise.

    A. *Explain the physiologic mechanisms responsible for his edema, hypertension, and elevated red blood cell count.*

    B. *His arterial PO_2 and O_2 saturation indicate that he is a candidate for continuous low-flow oxygen. Explain the benefits of this treatment in terms of his activity tolerance, blood pressure, and red blood cell count.*

    C. *Explain why the oxygen flow rate for persons with COPD is normally titrated to maintain the arterial PO_2 between 60 and 65 mm Hg.*

4. An 18-year-old woman is admitted to the emergency department with a suspected drug overdose. Her respiratory rate is slow (4 to 6 breaths/minute) and shallow. Arterial blood gases reveal a PCO_2 of 80 mm Hg and a PO_2 of 60 mm Hg.

    A. *What is the cause of this woman's high PCO_2 and low PO_2?*

    B. *Hypoventilation almost always causes an increase in PCO_2. Explain.*

    C. *Even though her PO_2 increases to 90 mm Hg with institution of oxygen therapy, her PCO_2 remains elevated. Explain.*

References

1. Guyton A. C., Hall J. E. (2006). *Textbook of medical physiology* (11th ed., pp. 491–501, 524–533, 867). Philadelphia: W. B. Saunders.
2. West J. B. (2003). *Pulmonary pathophysiology: The essentials* (6th ed., p. 75). Philadelphia: Lippincott Williams & Wilkins.

3. St. John R. E., Thomson P. D. (1999). Noninvasive respiratory monitoring. *Critical Care Nursing Clinics of North America* 11, 423–434.

4. Grap M. J. (2002). Pulse oximetry. *Critical Care Nurse* 22(3), 69–74.

5. Bernard G. R., Artigas A., Brigham K. L., et al. (1994). The American-European Consensus Conference on ARDS: Definitions, mechanisms, relevant outcomes, and clinical trial coordination. *American Journal of Respiratory Critical Care Medicine* 149, 818–824.

6. Hudak C. M., Gallo B. M., Morton P. G. (1998). *Critical care nursing* (7th ed., pp. 449–455, 476–489). Philadelphia: Lippincott Williams & Wilkins.

7. Weinberger S. E., Schwartzstein R. M., Weiss J. W. (1989). Hypercapnia. *New England Journal of Medicine* 321, 1223–1230.

8. Yataco J. C., Dweik R. A. (2005). Pleural effusions: Evaluation and management. *Cleveland Clinic Journal* 72, 854–871.

9. Light R. W. (2005). Disorders of the pleura, mediastinum, and diaphragm. In Kasper A. S., Braunwald E., Fauci A. S., et al. (Eds.), *Harrison's principles of internal medicine* (16th ed., pp. 1565–1569). New York: McGraw-Hill.

10. Romero S. (2000). Nontraumatic chylothorax. *Current Opinion in Pulmonary Medicine* 6, 287–291.

11. Guenther C. A., Welch M. H. (1982). *Pulmonary medicine* (2nd ed., pp. 524–526). Philadelphia: J. B. Lippincott.

12. Sahn S. A., Heffner J. E. (2000). Spontaneous pneumothorax. *New England Journal of Medicine* 342, 868–874.

13. Nopeen M., Baumann M. H. (2003). Pathogenesis and treatment of primary spontaneous pneumothorax: An overview. *Respiration* 70, 431–438.

14. Baumann M. H., Nopeen M. (2004). Invited review: Pneumothorax. *Respirology* 9, 157–164.

15. Gotway M. B., Marder S. R., Hanks D. K., et al. (2002). Thoracic complications of illicit drug use: An organ system approach. *Radiographics* 22, S119–S135.

16. Alifano M., Roth T., Broet S. C., et al. (2003). Catamenial pneumothorax: A prospective study. *Chest* 124, 1004–1008.

17. National Asthma Education and Prevention Program. (1997). *Expert Panel report 2: Guidelines for the diagnosis and management of asthma.* NIH publication no. 98-4051. Bethesda, MD: National Institutes of Health, National Heart, Lung, and Blood Institute.

18. National Asthma Education and Prevention Program. (2003). Expert Panel report: Guidelines for the diagnosis and management of asthma: Update of selected topics—2002. NIH publication no. 02-5074. Bethesda, MD: National Institutes of Health, National Heart, Lung, and Blood Institute.

19. American Lung Association. (2007). Asthma in adults fact sheet. [Online.] Available http://www.lungusa.org/site/pp.asp?c=dvLUK9O0E&b=22542. Accessed April 9, 2008.

20. Elias J. A., Lee C. G., Zheng T., et al. (2003). New insights into the pathogenesis of asthma. *Journal of Clinical Investigation* 111, 291–297.

21. Husain A. N., Kumar V. (2005). The lung. In Kumar R. S., Abbas A. K., Fausto N. (Eds.), *Robbins and Cotran pathologic basis of disease* (7th ed., pp. 711–747). Philadelphia: Elsevier Saunders.

22. Berry M. A., Hargadon B., Shelley S., et al. (2006). Evidence of a role of tumor necrosis factor-α in refractory asthma. *New England Journal of Medicine* 354, 697–708.

23. Fireman P. (2003). Understanding asthma pathophysiology. *Allergy and Asthma Proceedings* 24(2), 79–83.

24. Busse W. W., Lemanske R. F. (2001). Asthma. *New England Journal of Medicine* 344, 350–362.

25. McFadden E. R., Gilbert I. A. (1994). Exercise-induced asthma. *New England Journal of Medicine* 330, 1362–1366.

26. Roberts J. A. (1988). Exercise-induced asthma in athletes. *Sports Medicine* 6, 193–195.

27. Young S., LeSouef P. N., Geelhoed G. C., et al. (1991). The influence of a family history of asthma and parental smoking on airway responsiveness in early infancy. *New England Journal of Medicine* 324, 1168–1173.

28. Chan-Yeung M., Malo J. (1995). Occupational asthma. *New England Journal of Medicine* 333, 107–112.

29. Babu K. S., Salvi S. S. (2000). Aspirin and asthma. *Chest* 118, 1470–1476.

30. Szczeklik A., Nizankowska E. (2000). Clinical features and diagnosis of aspirin induced asthma. *Thorax* 55(Suppl. 2), S42–S44.

31. Tan K. S., McFarlane L. C., Lipworth B. J. (1997). Loss of normal cyclical B2 adrenoreceptor regulation and increased premenstrual responsiveness to adenosine monophosphate in stable female asthmatic patients. *Thorax* 52, 608–611.

32. Haxhiu M. A., Rust C. F., Brooks C., et al. (2006). CNS determinants of sleep-related worsening of airway functions: Implications for nocturnal asthma. *Respiratory Physiology and Neurobiology* 151, 1–30.

33. Sutherland E. R. (2005). Nocturnal asthma. *Journal of Allergy and Clinical Immunology* 116, 1179–1186.

34. Drazen J. M., Israel E., O'Byrne P. M. (1999). Treatment of asthma with drugs modifying the leukotriene pathway. *New England Journal of Medicine* 340, 197–204.

35. Wenzel S. (Chair). (2000). Proceedings of the ATS workshop on refractory asthma. *American Journal of Respiratory Critical Care Medicine* 162, 2341–2351.

36. Wenzel S. (2003). Severe asthma. *Mount Sinai Journal of Medicine* 70, 185–190.

37. Papiris S., Kotanidou A., Malagari K., et al. (2002). Clinical review: Severe asthma. *Critical Care* 6, 30–44.

38. Magadle R., Berar-Yanay N., Weiner P. (2002). The risk of hospitalization and near-fatal and fatal asthma in relation to the perception of dyspnea. *Chest* 121, 329–333.

39. Lui A. H., Spahn J. D., Leung D. Y. M. (2004). Childhood asthma. In Behrman R. E., Kliegman R. M., Jenson H. B. (Eds.), *Nelson textbook of pediatrics* (16th ed., pp. 760–774). Philadelphia: Elsevier Saunders.

40. Kemp J. P., Kemp J. A. (2001). Management of asthma in children. *American Family Physician* 63, 1341–1348.

41. Gern J. E., Lemanske R. F. (2003). Infectious triggers of pediatric asthma. *Pediatric Clinics of North America* 50, 555–575.

42. Gilliland F. D., Berhane K., McConnell R., et al. (2000). Maternal smoking during pregnancy, environmental tobacco smoke exposure and childhood lung function. *Thorax* 55, 271–276.

43. Stein R. T., Holberg C. J., Sherrill D., et al. (1999). Influence of parental smoking on respiratory symptoms during the first decade of life: The Tucson Children's Respiratory Study. *American Journal of Epidemiology* 149, 1030–1037.

44. Szefler S. J. (2003). Identifying the child in need of asthma therapy. *Pediatric Clinics of North American* 50, 577–591.

45. Barnes P. J. (2000). Chronic obstructive pulmonary disease. *New England Journal of Medicine* 343, 269–280.

46. Pawels R. A., Buist A. S., Calverley P. M. A., et al. (2003). Global strategy for the diagnosis, management, and prevention of chronic obstructive pulmonary disease: NHLBI/WHO Global Initiative for Chronic Obstructive Lung Disease (GOLD) Workshop Update. [Online.] Available: www.goldcopd.com. Accessed July 23, 2007.

47. Calverley P. M. A., Walker P. (2003). Chronic obstructive pulmonary disease. *Lancet* 362, 1053–1061.

48. American Lung Association. (2007). Chronic obstructive pulmonary disease (COPD) fact sheet. [Online.] Available: http://www.lungusa.org/site/pp.asp?c=dvLUK9O0E&b=38502. Accessed April 9, 2008.

49. Canadian Lung Association. (2007). COPD: How many people have COPD. [Online.] Available: http://www.lung.ca/diseases-maladies/copd-mpoc/what-quoi/index_e.php?print=1. Accessed April 9, 2008.

50. O'Donnell D. E., Aaron S., Bourbeau J., et al. (2004). State of the art compendium: Canadian Thoracic Society recommendations for the management of chronic obstructive pulmonary disease. *Canadian Respiratory Journal* 11(Suppl.), 7B–59B.

51. Chapman, K. R., Bourbeau, J., Rance, L. (2003). The burden of COPD in Canada: Results from the confronting COPD survey. *Respiratory Medicine* 9(Suppl. C), S23–S31.

52. Bearsley M. B., Travis W. D., Rubin E. (2008). The respiratory system. In Rubin R., Strayer D. S. (Eds.), *Rubin's pathology: Clinicopathologic foundations of medicine* (5th ed., pp. 510–518, 525–534, 536–545). Philadelphia: Lippincott Ventiliams & Wilkins.

53. Reilly J. J., Silverman E. K., Shapiro S. D. (2005). Chronic obstructive pulmonary disease. In Kasper A. S., Braunwald E., Fauci A. S., et al. (Eds.), *Harrison's principles of internal medicine* (16th ed., pp. 1547–1554). New York: McGraw-Hill.

54. Berry J. K., Baum C. L. (2001). Malnutrition in chronic obstructive pulmonary disease. *AACN Clinical Issues* 18, 210–219.

55. Barker A. F. (2002). Bronchiectasis. *New England Journal of Medicine* 346, 1383–1393.

56. Ratjen F. (2003). Cystic fibrosis. *Lancet* 361, 681–689.

57. Rowe S. M., Miller S., Sorscher E. J. (2005). Cystic fibrosis. *New England Journal of Medicine* 352, 1992–2001.

58. Maitra A., Kumar V. (2005). Diseases of infancy and childhood. In Kumar V., Abbas A. K., Fausto N. R. (Eds.), *Robbins and Cotran pathologic basis of disease* (7th ed., pp. 489–495). Philadelphia: Elsevier Saunders.

59. Boat T. F. (2004). Cystic fibrosis. In Behrman R. E., Kliegman R. M., Jenson H. B. (Eds.), *Nelson textbook of pediatrics* (17th ed., pp. 1437–1450). Philadelphia: Elsevier Saunders.

60. Cystic Fibrosis Foundation. (2007). About cystic fibrosis. [Online.] Available: http://www.cff.org/AboutCF. Accessed April 9, 2008.

61. Gibsen R. L., Burns J. L., Ramsey B. W. (2003). Pathophysiology and management of pulmonary infections in cystic fibrosis. *American Journal Respiratory Critical Care Medicine* 168, 918–951.

62. Gross F. H. Y. (2002). Overview of pulmonary fibrosis. *Chest* 122(6 Suppl.), 334S–335S.

63. Gross T. J., Hunninghake G. W. (2001). Idiopathic pulmonary fibrosis. *New England Journal of Medicine* 345, 517–525.

64. Kushner W. G., Stark P. (2003). Occupational lung disease. *Postgraduate Medicine* 113(4), 81–88.

65. American Thoracic Society. (1999). Statement on sarcoidosis. *American Journal of Respiratory Critical Care Medicine* 160, 736–755.

66. Weinberger S. E. (2004). *Principles of pulmonary medicine* (4th ed., pp. 161–166). Philadelphia: Elsevier Saunders.

67. Thomas K. W., Hunninghake G. W. (2003). Sarcoidosis. *Journal of the American Medical Association* 289(24), 3300–3303.

68. Baughman R. P. (2003). Sarcoidosis. *Lancet* 361, 111–118.

69. Sadosty A. T., Boie E. T., Stead L. G. (2003). Pulmonary embolism. *Emergency Medicine Clinics of North America* 21, 363–384.

70. Cardin T., Marinelli A. (2004). Pulmonary embolism. *Critical Care Nursing Quarterly* 27, 310–332.

71. Kearon C. (2003). Diagnosis of pulmonary embolism. *Canadian Medical Association Journal* 168, 183–194.

72. Ramzi D. W., Leeper K. V. (2004). DVT and pulmonary embolism: Part II. Treatment and prevention. *American Family Physician* 69, 2841–2848.

73. McLaughlin V. V. (2004). Classification and epidemiology of pulmonary hypertension. *Cardiology Clinics* 22, 327–341.

74. Ghambra Z., Dweik R. A. (2003). Primary pulmonary hypertension: An overview of epidemiology and pathogenesis. *Cleveland Clinic Journal of Medicine* 70 (Suppl. 1), S2–S8.

75. Runo J. R., Loyd J. E. (2003). Primary pulmonary hypertension. *Lancet* 361, 1533–1544.

76. Farber H. W., Lascalzo J. (2004). Pulmonary arterial hypertension. *New England Journal of Medicine* 351, 1655–1365.

77. Rubin L. J., Badesch D. B. (2005). Evaluation and management of the patient with pulmonary arterial hypertension. *Annals Internal Medicine* 143, 282–292.

78. Ashbaugh D. G., Bigelow D. B., Petty T. L., et al. (1967). Acute respiratory distress in adults. *Lancet* 2(7511), 319–323.

79. Bernard G. R. A. Artigas K. L., Brigham J., et al. (Consensus Committee). (1994). The American-European Consensus Conference on ARDS: Definitions, mechanisms, relevant outcomes, and clinical trial coordination. *American Journal of Respiratory Critical Care Medicine* 149, 1807–1814.

80. Rubenfeld G. D., Caldwell E., Peabody E., et al. (2005). Incidence and outcomes of acute lung injury. *New England Journal of Medicine* 353, 1685–1693.

81. Orme J., Romney J. S., Hopkins R. O., et al. (2003). Pulmonary function and health-related quality of life in survivors of acute respiratory distress syndrome. *American Journal of Respiratory Critical Care Medicine* 167, 690–694.

82. Moss M., Burnham E. L. (2003). Chronic alcohol abuse, acute respiratory distress syndrome, and multiple organ dysfunction. *Critical Care Medicine* 31, S207–S212.

83. Moore S. B. (2006). Transfusion-related acute lung injury (TRALI): Clinical presentation, treatment, and prognosis. *Critical Care Medicine* 34, S114–S117.

84. Mendez J. L., Hubmar R. D. (2005). New insights into the pathology of acute respiratory failure. *Current Opinion in Critical Care* 11, 29–36.

85. Abraham E. (2003). Neutrophils and acute lung injury. *Critical Care Medicine* 31, S195–199.

86. Acute Respiratory Distress Syndrome Network. (2000). Ventilation with lower tidal volumes as compared with traditional tidal volumes for acute lung injury and acute respiratory distress syndrome. *New England Journal of Medicine* 342, 1301–1308.

87. Roussos C., Koutsoukou A. (2003). Respiratory failure. *European Respiratory Journal* 22(Suppl. 47), 3s–14s.

88. Markou N. K., Myrianthefs P. M., Batlopoulos G. J. (2004). Respiratory failure: An overview. *Critical Care Nursing Quarterly* 27, 353–379.

89. Slutsky A. S. (2001). Basic science in ventilator-induced lung injury: Implications for the bedside. *American Journal of Respiratory Critical Care Medicine* 163, 599–600.

90. Tobin M. J. (2001). Advances in mechanical ventilation. *New England Journal of Medicine* 344, 1986–1996.

91. American Thoracic Society. (2001). International consensus conference in intensive care medicine: Noninvasive positive pressure ventilation in acute respiratory failure. *American Journal of Respiratory and Critical Care Medicine* 163, 283–291.

92. Antonelli M., Conti G., Rocco M., et al. (1998). A comparison of noninvasive positive-pressure ventilation and conventional mechanical ventilation in patients with acute respiratory failure. *New England Journal of Medicine* 339, 429–435.

93. Poponick J., Renston J. P., Bennett R. P., et al. (1999). Use of a ventilatory support system (BIPAP) for acute respiratory failure in the emergency department. *Chest* 116, 166–171.

94. Lightowler J. V., Wedzicha J. A., Elliott M. W., et al. (2003). Non-invasive positive pressure ventilation to treat respiratory failure resulting from exacerbations of chronic obstructive pulmonary disease: Cochrane systematic review and meta-analysis. *British Medical Journal* 326, 185–189.

95. Tobin M. J. (2001). Advances in mechanical ventilation. *New England Journal of Medicine* 344, 1986–1996.

Visit the**Point** http://thePoint.lww.com for animations, journal articles, and more!

Disorders of Renal Function and Fluids and Electrolytes

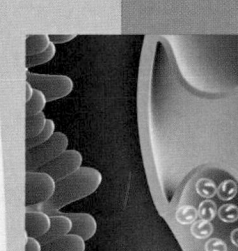

Throughout the earlier part of the Middle Ages, one of the major concerns of the physician was examination of the urine. Many physicians of this time thought that most diseases could be diagnosed by careful examination of the urine. Numerous illustrations taken from this period show early physicians holding up flasks of urine to study its color, cloudiness, and other properties. It was thought that if the cloudiness was at the top of the urine, the problem was in the head, and if it was at the bottom, the problem was in the legs.

From the 16th century on, anatomists began to acquire a fairly good understanding of the gross structure of the kidney, ureters, and bladder. The first great discovery of the minute structures of the kidney was made by Marcello Malphigi (1628–1694), one of the earliest microscopists, who described the ball-shaped structure of the glomerulus. The work of Malphigi was followed by that of Sir William Bowman (1816–1892), who described the urine collecting capsule of the nephron, Bowman's capsule. Bowman also described the relationship between the glomerulus and the tubules. German pathologist Friedrich Henle (1809–1885) described the long U-shaped loop, called the loop of Henle, that contributes to the concentrating abilities of the kidney. Once this structure of the kidney was established, other scientists began to focus on the chemical composition of urine and on the function of the kidney in the regulation of blood pressure.

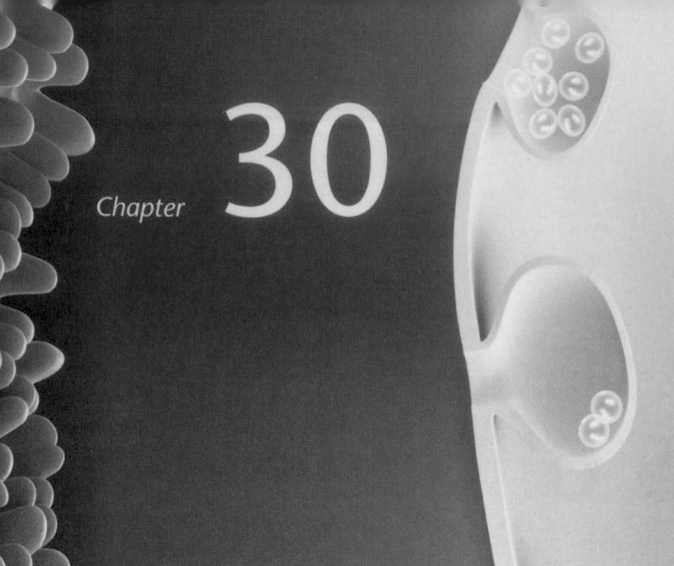

Chapter 30

Structure and Function of the Kidney

CAROL M. PORTH

It is no exaggeration to say that the composition of the blood is determined not so much by what the mouth takes in as by what the kidneys keep.

—HOMER SMITH, *FROM FISH TO PHILOSOPHER*

➤ The kidneys are remarkable organs. Each is smaller than a person's fist, but in a single day the two organs process approximately 1700 L of blood and combine its waste products into approximately 1.5 L of urine. As part of their function, the kidneys filter physiologically essential substances, such as sodium (Na^+) and potassium (K^+) ions, from the blood and selectively reabsorb those substances that are needed to maintain the normal composition of internal body fluids. Substances that are not needed or are in excess of those needed for this purpose pass into the urine. In regulating the volume and composition of body fluids, the kidneys perform excretory and endocrine functions. The renin-angiotensin mechanism participates in the regulation of blood pressure and the maintenance of circulating blood volume, and erythropoietin stimulates red blood cell production. The discussion in this chapter focuses on the structure and function of the kidneys, tests of renal function, and the physiologic action of diuretics.

 ## KIDNEY STRUCTURE AND FUNCTION

After completing this section of the chapter, you should be able to meet the following objectives:

- Describe the location and gross structure of the kidney.
- Explain why the kidney receives such a large percentage of the cardiac output and describe the mechanisms for regulating renal blood flow.
- Describe the structure and function of the glomerulus and tubular components of the nephron in terms of regulating the composition of the extracellular fluid compartment.
- Explain the function of sodium in terms of tubular transport mechanisms.
- Describe how the kidney produces a concentrated or dilute urine.

- Characterize the function of the juxtaglomerular complex.
- Relate the function of the kidney to drug elimination.
- Explain the endocrine functions of the kidney.
- Relate the sodium reabsorption function of the kidney to action of diuretics.

Gross Structure and Location

The kidneys are paired, bean-shaped organs that lie outside the peritoneal cavity in the back of the upper abdomen, one on each side of the vertebral column at the level of the 12th thoracic to 3rd lumbar vertebrae (Fig. 30-1). The right kidney normally is situated lower than the left, presumably because of the position of the liver. In the adult, each kidney is approximately 10 to 12 cm long, 5 to 6 cm wide, and 2.5 cm deep, and weighs approximately 113 to 170 g. The medial border of the kidney is indented by a deep fissure called the *hilus*. It is here that blood vessels and nerves enter and leave the kidney. The ureters, which connect the kidneys with the bladder, also enter the kidney at the hilus.

The kidney is a multilobular structure, composed of up to 18 lobes. Each lobe is composed of nephrons, which are the functional units of the kidney. Each nephron has a glomerulus that filters the blood and a system of tubular structures that

selectively reabsorb material from the filtrate back into the blood and secrete materials from the blood into the filtrate as urine is being formed.

On longitudinal section, a kidney can be divided into an outer cortex and an inner medulla (Fig. 30-2). The cortex, which is reddish-brown, contains the glomeruli and convoluted tubules of the nephron and blood vessels. The medulla consists of light-colored, cone-shaped masses—the renal pyramids—that are divided by the columns of the cortex (*i.e.,* columns of Bertin) that extend into the medulla. Each pyramid, topped by a region of cortex, forms a lobe of the kidney. The apices of the pyramids form the papillae (*i.e.,* 8 to 18 per kidney, corresponding to the number of lobes), which are perforated by the openings of the collecting ducts. The renal pelvis is a wide, funnel-shaped structure at the upper end of the ureter. It is made up of the calyces or cuplike structures that drain the upper and lower halves of the kidney.

The kidney is sheathed in a fibrous external capsule and surrounded by a mass of fatty connective tissue, especially at its ends and borders. The adipose tissue protects the kidney from mechanical blows and assists, together with the attached blood vessels and fascia, in holding the kidney in place. Although the kidneys are relatively well protected, they may be bruised by blows to the loin or by compression between the lower ribs and the ileum. Because the kidneys are located outside the peritoneal cavity, injury and rupture do not produce the same threat of peritoneal involvement as that of other organs such as the liver or spleen.

Renal Blood Supply

Each kidney is supplied by a single renal artery that arises on either side of the aorta. As the renal artery approaches the kidney, it divides into five segmental arteries that enter the hilus of the kidney. In the kidney, each segmental artery branches into several lobular arteries that supply the upper, middle, and lower parts of the kidney. The lobular arteries further subdivide to form the interlobular arteries at the level of the corticomedullary junction (Fig. 30-3). These arteries give off branches, the arcuate arteries, that arch across the top of the pyramids. Small intralobular arteries radiate from the arcuate arteries to supply the cortex of the kidney. The afferent arterioles that supply the glomeruli arise from the intralobular arteries.

Although nearly all the blood flow to the kidneys passes through the cortex, less than 10% is directed to the medulla and only approximately 1% goes to the papillae. Under conditions of decreased perfusion or increased sympathetic nervous system stimulation, blood flow is redistributed away from the cortex toward the medulla. This redistribution of blood flow decreases glomerular filtration while maintaining the urine-concentrating ability of the kidneys, a factor that is important during conditions such as shock.

The Nephron

Each kidney is composed of more than 1 million tiny, closely packed functional units called *nephrons* (Fig. 30-4A). Each

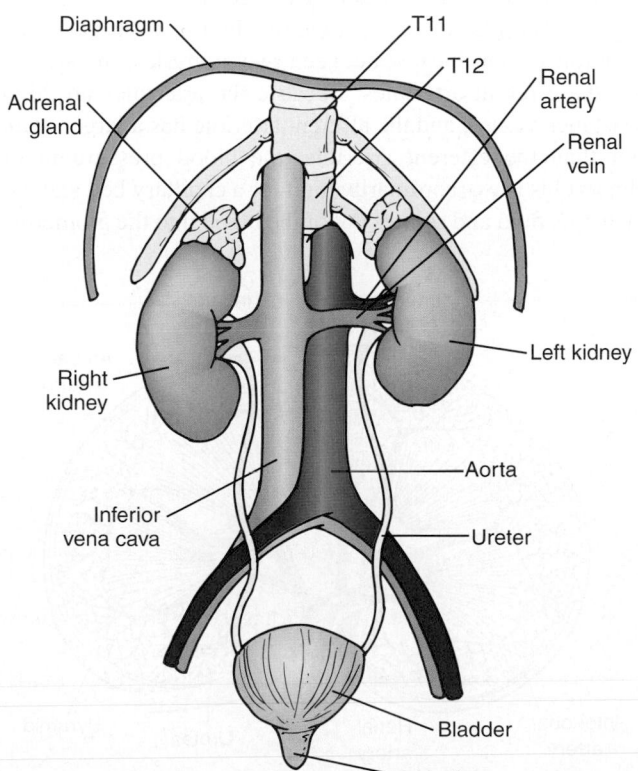

FIGURE 30-1 • Kidneys, ureters, and bladder. (The right kidney is usually lower than the left.)

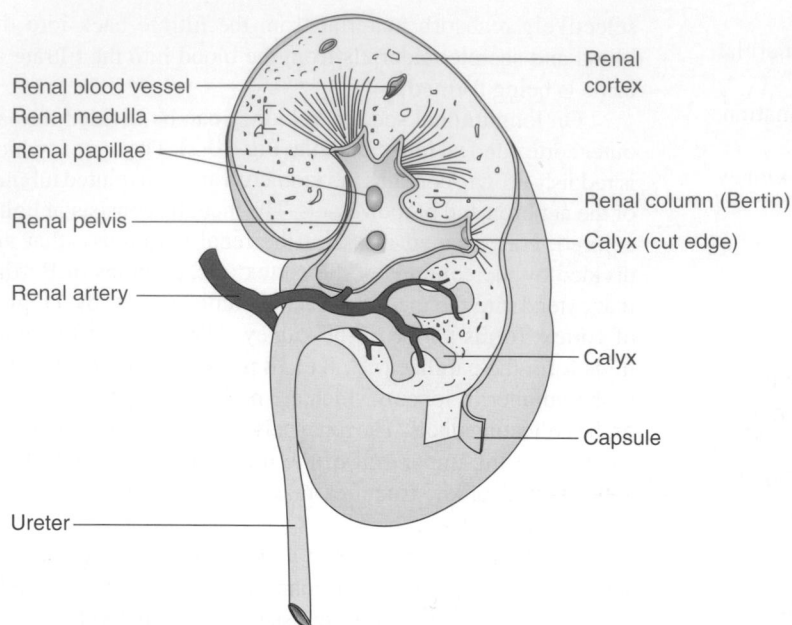

FIGURE 30-2 • Internal structure of the kidney.

nephron consists of a glomerulus, where blood is filtered, and a proximal convoluted tubule, loop of Henle, distal convoluted tubule, and collecting duct, where water, electrolytes, and other substances needed to maintain the constancy of the internal environment are reabsorbed into the bloodstream while other, unneeded materials are secreted into the tubular filtrate for elimination.

🔑 THE NEPHRON

- The nephron, which is the functional unit of the kidney, is composed of a vascular component, which connects to the circulatory system, and a tubular component, which has connections to both the circulatory system and the elimination functions of the kidney.

- The vascular component of the nephron consists of two arterioles closely associated with two capillary beds: the glomerulus (where water-soluble nutrients, wastes, and other small particles are filtered from the blood) and the peritubular capillaries (which surround the tubular structures).

- The tubular portion of the nephron processes the glomerular filtrate (urine), facilitating the reabsorption of substances from the tubular fluid into the peritubular capillaries and the secretion of substances from the peritubular capillaries into the urine filtrate.

Nephrons can be roughly grouped into two categories. Approximately 85% of the nephrons originate in the superficial part of the cortex and are called *cortical nephrons* (see Fig. 30-4B). They have short, thick loops of Henle that pene-

trate only a short distance into the medulla. The remaining 15% are called *juxtamedullary nephrons.* They originate deeper in the cortex and have longer and thinner loops of Henle that penetrate the entire length of the medulla. The juxtamedullary nephrons are largely concerned with urine concentration.

The nephrons are supplied by two capillary systems, the glomerulus and the peritubular capillary network (see Fig. 30-4A). The *glomerulus* is a unique, high-pressure capillary filtration system located between two arterioles, the afferent and the efferent arterioles. Because the arterioles are high-resistance vessels and the afferent arteriole has a larger diameter than the efferent arteriole, the blood pressure in the glomerulus is extraordinarily high for a capillary bed and easily forces fluid and solutes out of the blood into the glomerular

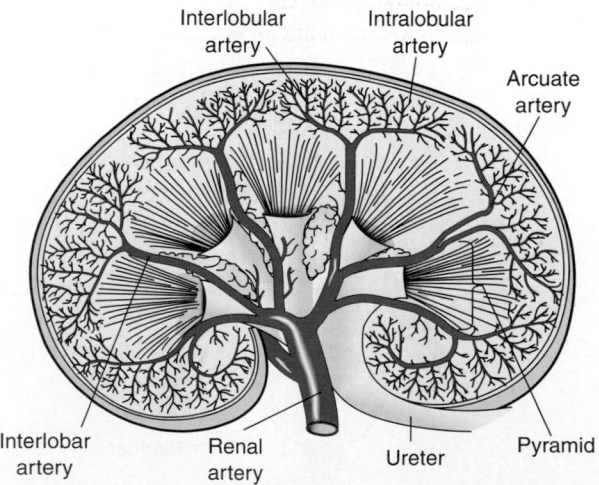

FIGURE 30-3 • Simplified illustration of the arterial supply of the kidney. (From Cormack D. H. [1987]. *Ham's histology* [9th ed.]. Philadelphia: J.B. Lippincott.)

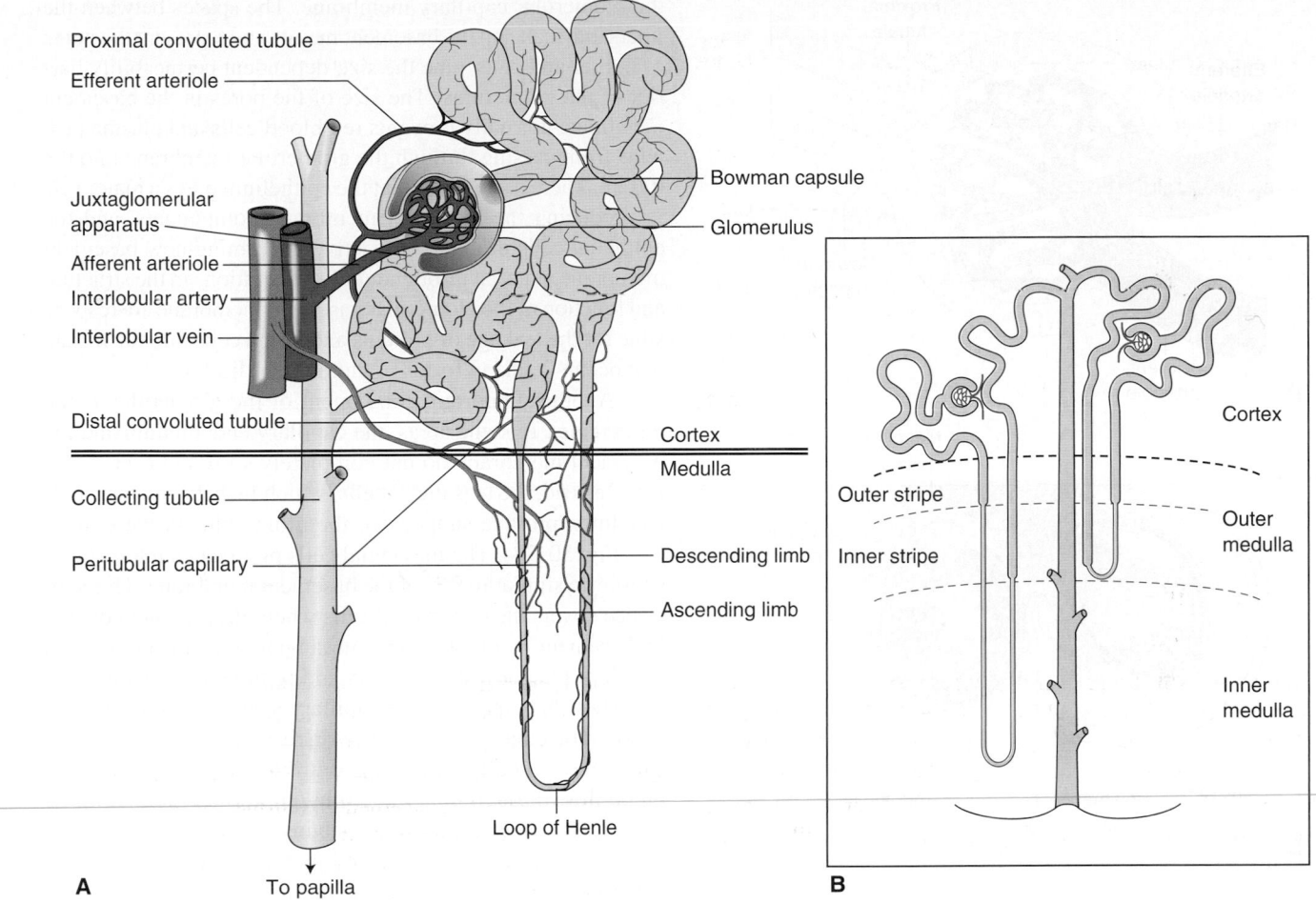

FIGURE 30-4 • **(A)** Nephron, showing the glomerular and tubular structures along with the blood supply. **(B)** Comparison of differences in location of tubular structures of the cortical and juxtamedullary nephrons.

capillary along its entire length. The *peritubular capillaries* originate from the efferent arteriole. They are low-pressure vessels that are adapted for reabsorption rather than filtration. These capillaries surround all portions of the tubules, an arrangement that permits rapid movement of solutes and water between the fluid in the tubular lumen and the blood in the capillaries. In the deepest part of the renal cortex, the efferent arterioles serving the juxtaglomerular glomeruli also continue into long, thin-walled looping vessels called the *vasa recta*. The vasa recta accompany the long loops of Henle in the medullary portion of the kidney to assist in exchange of substances flowing in and out of that portion of the kidney. The peritubular capillaries rejoin to form the venous channels by which blood leaves the kidneys and empties into the inferior vena cava.

The Glomerulus

The glomerulus consists of a compact tuft of capillaries encased in a thin, double-walled capsule called the *Bowman capsule*. Blood flows into the glomerular capillaries from the afferent arteriole and flows out of the glomerular capillaries into the efferent arteriole, which leads into the peritubular capillaries. Fluid and particles from the blood are filtered through the capillary membrane into a fluid-filled space in the Bowman capsule, called the *Bowman space*. The portion of the blood that is filtered into the capsule space is called the *filtrate*. The mass of capillaries and its surrounding epithelial capsule are collectively referred to as the *renal corpuscle* (Fig. 30-5A).

The glomerular capillary membrane is composed of three layers: the capillary endothelial layer, the basement membrane, and the single-celled capsular epithelial layer (see Fig. 30-5B). The endothelial layer lines the glomerulus and interfaces with blood as it moves through the capillary. This layer contains many small perforations, called *fenestrations*.

The epithelial layer that covers the glomerulus is continuous with the epithelium that lines the Bowman capsule. The cells of the epithelial layer have unusual octopus-like structures that possess a large number of extensions, or *foot processes* (*i.e., podocytes*), which are embedded in the basement membrane (see Fig. 30-5B). These foot processes form *slit pores* through which the glomerular filtrate passes.

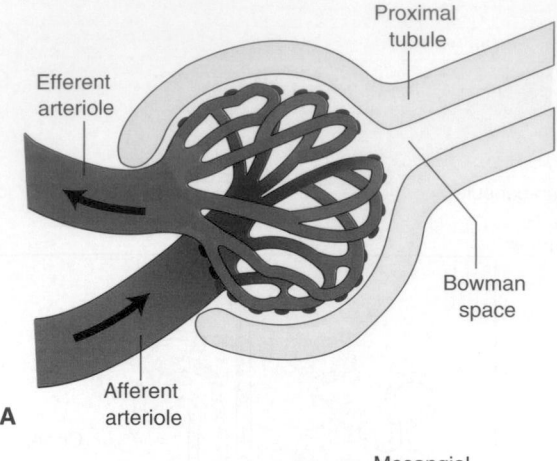

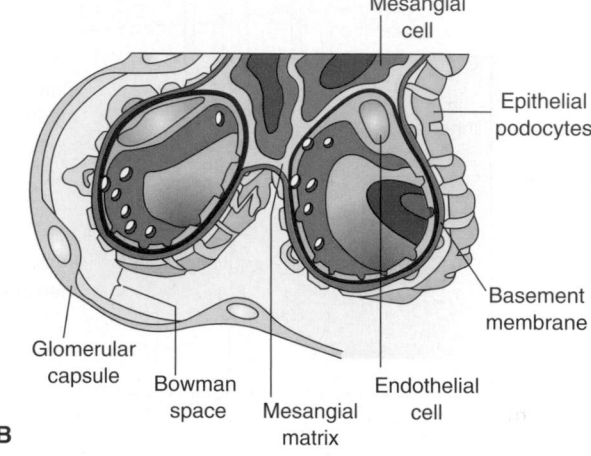

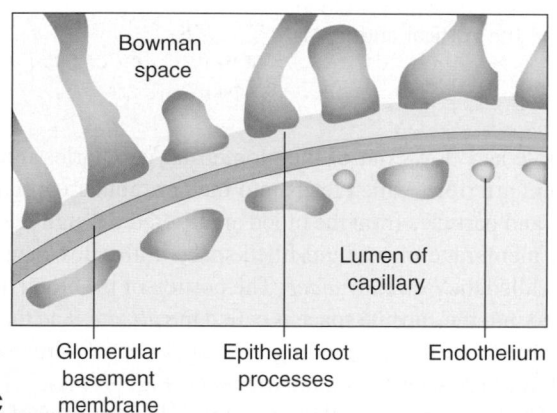

FIGURE 30-5 • Renal corpuscle. **(A)** Structures of the glomerulus. **(B)** Cross-section of the glomerular membrane, showing the position of the endothelium, basement membrane, and epithelial foot processes. **(C)** Position of the mesangial cells in relation to the capillary loops and Bowman capsule.

The basement membrane consists of a homogeneous acellular meshwork of collagen fibers, glycoproteins, and mucopolysaccharides (see Fig. 30-5C). Because the endothelial and epithelial layers of the glomerular capillary have porous structures, the basement membrane determines the permeability of

the glomerular capillary membrane. The spaces between the fibers that make up the basement membrane represent the pores of a filter and determine the size-dependent permeability barrier of the glomerulus. The size of the pores in the basement membrane normally prevents red blood cells and plasma proteins from passing through the glomerular membrane into the filtrate. There is evidence that the epithelium plays a major role in producing the basement membrane components, and the epithelial cells probably are active in forming new basement membrane material throughout life. Alterations in the structure and function of the glomerular basement membrane are responsible for the leakage of proteins and blood cells into the filtrate that occurs in many forms of glomerular disease.

Another important component of the glomerulus is the *mesangium.* In some areas, the capillary endothelium and the basement membrane do not completely surround each capillary. Instead, the mesangial cells, which lie between the capillary tufts, provide support for the glomerulus in these areas (see Fig. 30-5B). The mesangial cells produce an intercellular substance similar to that of the basement membrane. This substance covers the endothelial cells where they are not covered by basement membrane. The mesangial cells possess (or can develop) phagocytic properties and remove macromolecular materials that enter the intercapillary spaces. Mesangial cells also exhibit contractile properties in response to neurohumoral substances and are thought to contribute to the regulation of blood flow through the glomerulus. In normal glomeruli, the mesangial area is narrow and contains only a small number of cells. Mesangial hyperplasia and increased mesangial matrix occur in a number of glomerular diseases.

Tubular Components of the Nephron

The nephron tubule is divided into four segments: a highly coiled segment called the *proximal convoluted tubule,* which drains the Bowman capsule; a thin, looped structure called the *loop of Henle;* a distal coiled portion called the *distal convoluted tubule;* and the final segment, called the *collecting tubule,* which joins with several tubules to collect the filtrate. The filtrate passes through each of these segments before reaching the pelvis of the kidney.

The proximal tubule is a highly coiled structure that dips toward the renal pelvis to become the descending limb of the loop of Henle. The ascending loop of Henle returns to the region of the renal corpuscle, where it becomes the distal tubule. The distal convoluted tubule, which begins at the juxtaglomerular complex, is divided into two segments: the *diluting segment* and the *late distal tubule.* The late distal tubule fuses with the collecting tubule. Like the distal tubule, the collecting duct is divided into two segments: the *cortical collecting tubule* and the *inner medullary collecting tubule.*

Throughout its course, the tubule is composed of a single layer of epithelial cells resting on a basement membrane. The structure of the epithelial cells varies with tubular function. The cells of the proximal tubule have a fine, villous structure that increases the surface area for reabsorption; they also are rich in mitochondria, which support active transport processes. The epithelial layer of the thin segment of the loop of Henle has few mitochondria, indicating minimal metabolic activity and reabsorptive function.

Urine Formation

Urine formation involves the filtration of blood by the glomerulus to form an *ultrafiltrate of urine* and the tubular reabsorption of electrolytes and nutrients needed to maintain the constancy of the internal environment while eliminating waste materials.

Glomerular Filtration

Urine formation begins with the filtration of essentially protein-free plasma through the glomerular capillaries into the Bowman space. The movement of fluid through the glomerular capillaries is determined by the same factors (*i.e.*, capillary filtration pressure, colloidal osmotic pressure, and capillary permeability) that affect fluid movement through other capillaries in the body (see Chapter 21). The glomerular filtrate has a chemical composition similar to plasma, but it contains almost no proteins because large molecules do not readily cross the glomerular wall. Approximately 125 mL of filtrate is formed each minute. This is called the *glomerular filtration rate (GFR)*. This rate can vary from a few milliliters per minute to as high as 200 mL/minute.

The location of the glomerulus between two arterioles allows for maintenance of a high-pressure filtration system. The capillary filtration pressure (approximately 60 mm Hg) in the glomerulus is approximately two to three times higher than that of other capillary beds in the body. The filtration pressure and the GFR are regulated by the constriction and relaxation of the afferent and efferent arterioles. Constriction of the efferent arteriole increases resistance to outflow from the glomeruli and increases the glomerular pressure and the GFR. Constriction of the afferent arteriole causes a reduction in the renal blood flow, glomerular filtration pressure, and GFR. The afferent and the efferent arterioles are innervated by the sympathetic nervous system and are sensitive to vasoactive hormones, such as angiotensin II, as well. During periods of strong sympathetic stimulation, such as shock, constriction of the afferent arteriole causes a marked decrease in renal blood flow and thus glomerular filtration pressure. Consequently, urine output can fall almost to zero.

Tubular Reabsorption and Secretion

From the Bowman capsule, the glomerular filtrate moves into the tubular segments of the nephron. In its movement through the lumen of the tubular segments, the glomerular filtrate is changed considerably by the tubular transport of water and solutes. Tubular transport can result in reabsorption of substances from the tubular fluid into the peritubular capillaries or secretion of substances into the tubular fluid from the blood in the peritubular capillaries (Fig. 30-6).

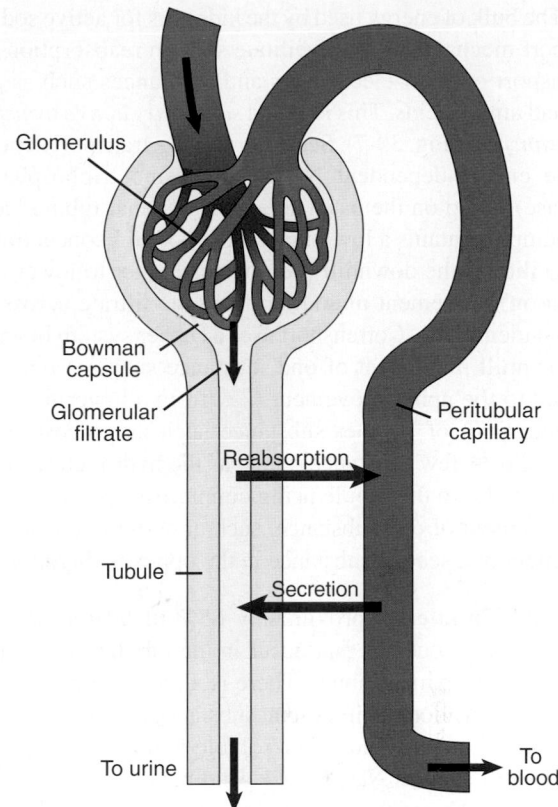

FIGURE 30-6 • Reabsorption and secretion of substances between the renal tubules and peritubular capillaries.

The basic mechanisms of transport across the tubular epithelial cell membrane are similar to those of other cell membranes in the body and include active and passive transport mechanisms. Water and urea are passively absorbed along concentration gradients. Sodium, K^+, chloride (Cl^-), calcium (Ca^{++}), and phosphate (PO_4^-) ions, as well as urate, glucose, and amino acids are reabsorbed using primary or secondary active transport mechanisms to move across the tubular membrane. Some substances, such as hydrogen, potassium, and urate ions, are secreted into the tubular fluids. Under normal conditions, only approximately 1 mL of the 125 mL of glomerular filtrate that is formed each minute is excreted in the urine. The other 124 mL is reabsorbed in the tubules. This means that the average output of urine is approximately 60 mL/hour.

Renal tubular cells have two membrane surfaces through which substances must pass as they are reabsorbed from the tubular fluid. The outside membrane that lies adjacent to the interstitial fluid is called the *basolateral membrane,* and the side that is in contact with the tubular lumen and tubular filtrate is called the *luminal membrane.* In most cases, substances move from the tubular filtrate into the tubular cell along a concentration gradient, but they require facilitated transport or carrier systems to move across the basolateral membrane into the interstitial fluid, where they are absorbed into the peritubular capillaries.

The bulk of energy used by the kidney is for active sodium transport mechanisms that facilitate sodium reabsorption and cotransport of other electrolytes and substances such as glucose and amino acids. This is called *secondary active transport* or *cotransport* (Fig. 30-7). Secondary active transport depends on the energy-dependent Na⁺/K⁺-adenosine triphosphatase (ATPase) pump on the basolateral side of renal tubular cells. The pump maintains a low intracellular sodium concentration that facilitates the downhill (*i.e.,* from a higher to lower concentration) movement of sodium from the filtrate across the luminal membrane. Cotransport uses a carrier system in which the downhill movement of one substance such as sodium is coupled to the uphill movement (*i.e.,* from a lower to higher concentration) of another substance such as glucose or an amino acid. A few substances, such as the hydrogen (H⁺) ion, are secreted into the tubule using countertransport, in which the movement of one substance, such as sodium, enables the movement of a second substance in the opposite direction.

Proximal Tubule. Approximately 65% of all reabsorptive and secretory processes that occur in the tubular system take place in the proximal tubule. There is almost complete reabsorption of nutritionally important substances, such as glucose, amino acids, lactate, and water-soluble vitamins (Fig. 30-8). Electrolytes, such as Na⁺, K⁺, Cl⁻, and bicarbonate (HCO₃⁻), are 65% to 80% reabsorbed. As these solutes move into the tubular cells, their concentration in the tubular lumen decreases, providing a concentration gradient for the osmotic reabsorption of water and urea. The proximal tubule is highly permeable to water, and the osmotic movement of water occurs so rapidly that the concentration difference of solutes on either side of the membrane seldom is more than a few milliosmoles.

Many substances, such as glucose, are freely filtered in the glomerulus and reabsorbed by energy-dependent cotransport carrier mechanisms. The maximum amount of substance that these transport systems can reabsorb per unit time is called the *transport maximum.* The transport maximum is related to the number of carrier proteins that are available for transport and usually is sufficient to ensure that all of a filtered substance such as glucose can be reabsorbed rather than being eliminated in the urine. The plasma level at which the substance appears in the urine is called the *renal threshold* (Fig. 30-9). Under some circumstances, the amount of substance filtered in the glomerulus exceeds the transport maximum. For example, when the blood glucose level is elevated in uncontrolled diabetes mellitus, the amount that is filtered in the glomerulus often exceeds the transport maximum (approximately 320 mg/minute), and glucose spills into the urine.

In addition to *reabsorbing* solutes and water, cells in the proximal tubule also *secrete* organic cations and anions into the urine filtrate (see Figs. 30-6 and 30-8). Many of these organic anions and cations are end products of metabolism (*e.g.,* urate, oxalate) that circulate in the plasma. The proximal tubule also secretes exogenous organic compounds such as penicillin, aspirin, and morphine. Many of these compounds can be bound to plasma proteins and are not freely filtered in the glomerulus. Therefore, excretion by filtration alone eliminates only a small portion of these potentially toxic substances from the body.

The Loop of Henle. The loop of Henle plays an important role in controlling the concentration of the urine. It does this by establishing a high concentration of osmotically active particles in the interstitium surrounding the medullary collecting tubules where the antidiuretic hormone exerts its effects (to be discussed).

The loop of Henle is divided into three segments: the thin descending segment, the thin ascending segment, and thick ascending segment. The loop of Henle, taken as a whole, always reabsorbs more sodium and chloride than water. This is in contrast to the proximal tubule, which reabsorbs sodium and water in equal proportions. The thin descending limb is highly permeable to water and moderately permeable to urea, sodium, and other ions. As the urine filtrate moves down the descending limb, water moves out of the filtrate into the surrounding interstitium. Thus, the osmolality of the filtrate reaches its highest point at the elbow of the loop of Henle. In contrast to the descending limb, the ascending limb of the loop of Henle is impermeable to water. In this segment, solutes are reabsorbed, but water cannot follow and remains in the filtrate; as a result, the tubular filtrate becomes more and more dilute, often reaching an osmolality of 100 mOsm/kg of H₂O as it enters the distal convoluted tubule, compared with the 285 mOsm/kg of H₂O in plasma. This allows for excretion of free water from the body. For this reason, it is often called the *diluting segment.*

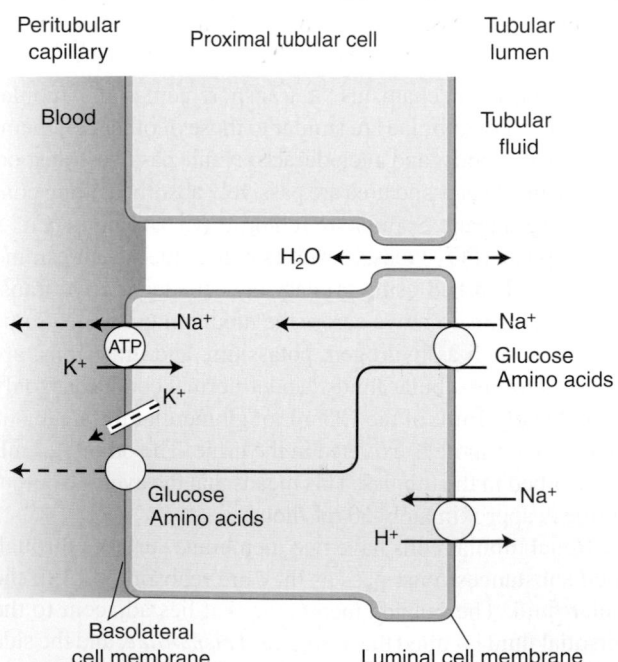

FIGURE 30-7 • Mechanism for secondary active transport or cotransport of glucose and amino acids in the proximal tubule. The energy-dependent sodium-potassium pump on the basal lateral surface of the cell maintains a low intracellular gradient that facilitates the downhill movement of sodium and glucose or amino acids (cotransport) from the tubular lumen into the tubular cell and then into the peritubular capillary.

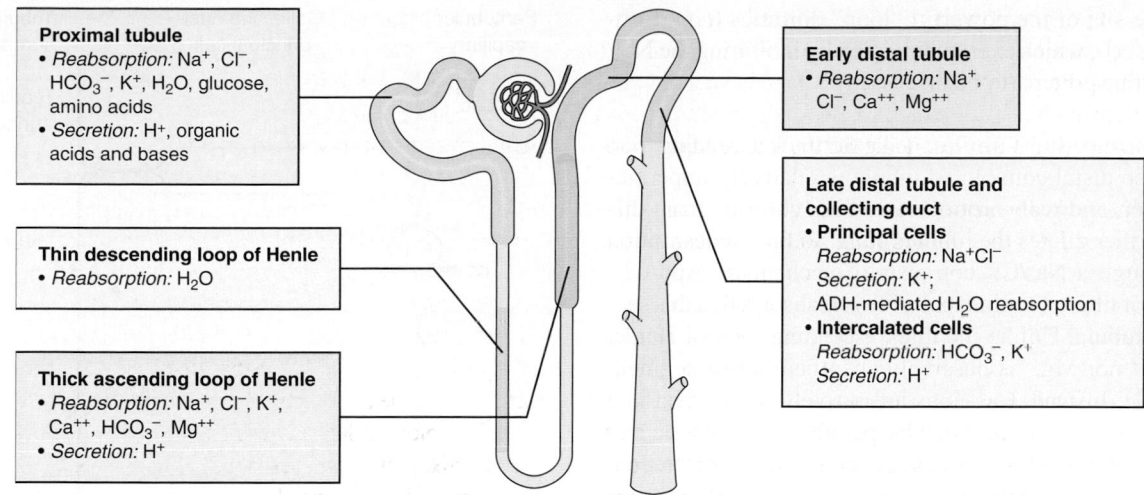

FIGURE 30-8 • Sites of tubular water (H_2O), glucose, amino acids, Na^+ (sodium), Cl^- (chloride), HCO_3^- (bicarbonate), K^+ (potassium), Ca^{++} (calcium), and Mg^{++} (magnesium) reabsorption; and organic acids and bases, H^+ (hydrogen), and K^+ secretion.

The thick segment of the loop of Henle begins in the ascending limb where the epithelial cells become thickened. As with the thin ascending limb, this segment is impermeable to water. The thick segment contains a $Na^+/K^+/2Cl^-$ cotransport system (Fig. 30-10). This system involves the cotransport of a

positively charged Na^+ and a positively charged K^+ ion accompanied by two negatively charged Cl^- ions. The gradient for the operation of this cotransport system is provided by the basolateral Na^+/K^+-ATPase pump, which maintains a low intracellular sodium concentration. Approximately 20% to 25% of the filtered load of sodium, potassium, and chloride is reabsorbed in the thick loop of Henle. Movement of these ions out of the tubule leads to the development of a transmembrane potential that favors the passive reabsorption of small divalent cations such as calcium and magnesium. The thick ascending loop of

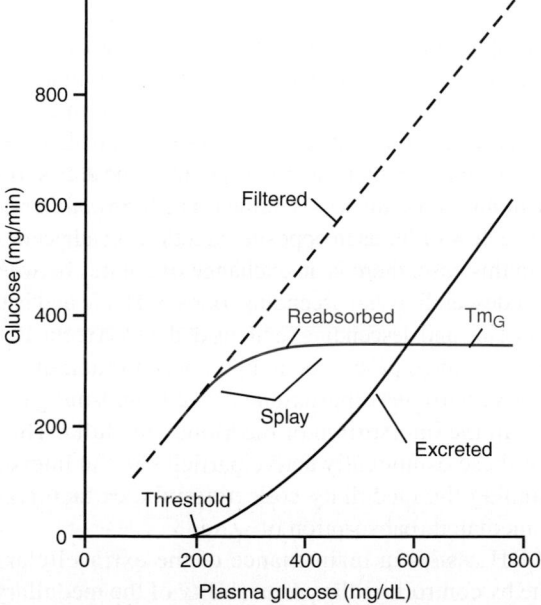

FIGURE 30-9 • Relations among the filtered load of glucose, the rate of glucose reabsorption by the renal tubules, and the rate of glucose excretion in the urine. The tubular transport maximum for glucose (Tm_G) is the maximum rate at which glucose can be reabsorbed from the tubules. The *threshold* for glucose refers to the filtered load of glucose at which glucose first begins to appear in the urine. The splay or rounding of the graph represents the fact that some nephrons reach their tubular maximum before others do. (From Rhoades R. A., Tanner G. A. [2003]. *Medical physiology* [2nd ed., p. 384]. Philadelphia: Lippincott Williams & Wilkins.)

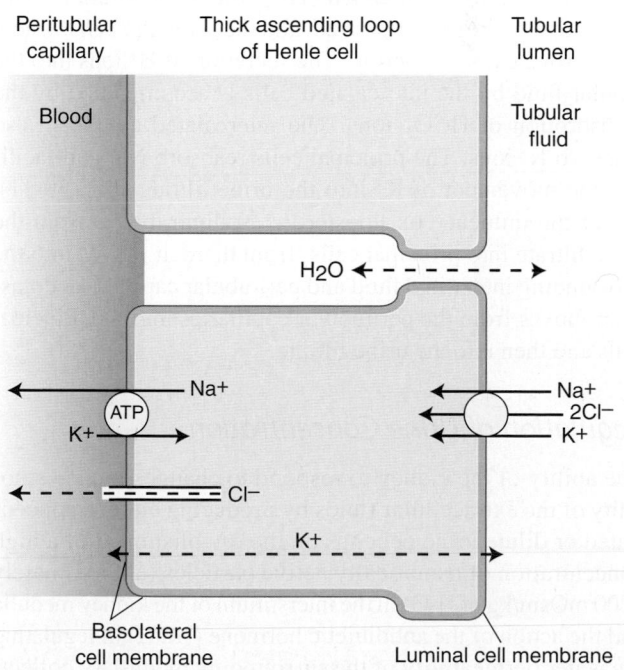

FIGURE 30-10 • Sodium, chloride, and potassium reabsorption in the thick segment of the loop of Henle.

Henle is the site of the powerful "loop" diuretics (*e.g.*, furosemide [Lasix]), which exert their action by inhibiting the $Na^+/K^+/2Cl^-$ cotransporters (to be discussed).

Distal and Collecting Tubules. Like the thick ascending loop of Henle, the distal convoluted tubule is relatively impermeable to water, and reabsorption of sodium chloride from this segment further dilutes the tubular fluid. Sodium reabsorption occurs through a Na^+/Cl^- cotransport mechanism. Approximately 5% of filtered sodium chloride is reabsorbed in this section of the tubule. Unlike the thick ascending loop of Henle, neither Ca^{++} nor Mg^{++} is passively absorbed in this segment of the tubule. Instead, Ca^{++} ions are actively reabsorbed in a process that is largely regulated by parathyroid hormone and possibly by vitamin D. The thiazide diuretics (to be discussed) exert their action by inhibiting sodium chloride reabsorption in this segment of the renal tubules.

The late distal tubule and the cortical collecting tubule constitute the site where aldosterone exerts its action on sodium reabsorption and potassium secretion and elimination. Although responsible for only 2% to 5% of sodium chloride reabsorption, this site is largely responsible for determining the final sodium concentration of the urine. The late distal tubule with the cortical collecting tubule also is the major site for regulation of potassium excretion by the kidney. When the body is confronted with a potassium excess, as occurs with a diet high in potassium content, the amount of potassium secreted at this site may exceed the amount filtered in the glomerulus.

The mechanism for sodium reabsorption and potassium secretion in this section of the nephron is distinct from other tubular segments. This tubular segment is composed of two types of cells, the *intercalated cells,* where potassium is reabsorbed and hydrogen is secreted, and the *principal cells,* where aldosterone exerts its action. The secretion of H^+ ions into the tubular fluid by the intercalated cells is accompanied by the reabsorption of HCO_3^- ions. The intercalated cells can also reabsorb K^+ ions. The principal cells reabsorb Na^+ and facilitate the movement of K^+ into the urine filtrate (Fig. 30-11). Under the influence of aldosterone, sodium moves from the urine filtrate into principal cells; from there, it moves into the surrounding interstitial fluid and peritubular capillaries. Potassium moves from the peritubular capillaries into the principal cells and then into the urine filtrate.

Regulation of Urine Concentration

The ability of the kidney to respond to changes in the osmolality of the extracellular fluids by producing either a concentrated or dilute urine depends on the establishment of a high concentration of osmotically active particles (approximately 1200 mOsm/kg of H_2O) in the interstitium of the kidney medulla and the action of the antidiuretic hormone (ADH) in regulating the water permeability of the surrounding medullary collecting tubules (see Understanding How the Kidney Concentrates Urine).

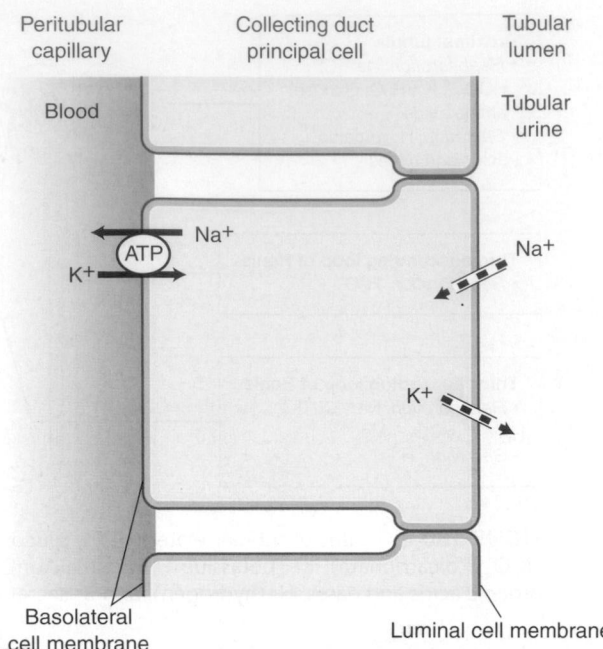

FIGURE 30-11 • Mechanism of sodium reabsorption and potassium secretion by principal cells of the late distal and collecting tubules. Aldosterone exerts its action by increasing the activity of the Na^+/K^+-ATPase pump that transports sodium outward through the basolateral membrane of the cell and into the blood at the same time it pumps potassium into the cell. Aldosterone also increases the permeability of the luminal membrane for potassium.

In approximately one fifth of the juxtamedullary nephrons, the loops of Henle and special hairpin-shaped capillaries called the *vasa recta* descend into the medullary portion of the kidney, forming a countercurrent system that controls water and solute movement so that water is kept out of the area surrounding the tubule and solutes are retained. The term *countercurrent* refers to a flow of fluids in opposite directions in adjacent structures. In this case, there is an exchange of solutes between the adjacent descending and ascending loops of Henle and between the ascending and descending sections of the vasa recta. Because of these exchange processes, a high concentration of osmotically active particles (approximately 1200 mOsm/kg of H_2O) collects in the interstitium of the kidney medulla. The presence of these osmotically active particles in the interstitium surrounding the medullary collecting tubules facilitates the ADH-mediated reabsorption of water.

ADH assists in maintenance of the extracellular fluid volume by controlling the permeability of the medullary collecting tubules. Osmoreceptors in the hypothalamus sense an increase in osmolality of extracellular fluids and stimulate the release of ADH from the posterior pituitary gland. In exerting its effect, ADH, also known as *vasopressin,* binds to receptors on the basolateral side of the tubular cells. Binding of ADH to the vasopressin receptors causes water channels, known as *aquaporin-2 channels,* to move into the luminal side of the tubular cell membrane, producing a marked increase in water permeability. At the basolateral side of the membrane, water exits the tubular cell into the hyperosmotic interstitium of the medullary area, where it enters the peritubular capillaries for return to the vascular system. The aquaporin-2 channels are thought to have a critical role in inherited and acquired disorders of water reabsorption by the kidney (*e.g.,* diabetes insipidus).

Regulation of Renal Blood Flow

In the adult, the kidneys are perfused with 1000 to 1300 mL of blood per minute, or 20% to 25% of the cardiac output. This large blood flow is mainly needed to ensure a sufficient GFR for the removal of waste products from the blood, rather than for the metabolic needs of the kidney. Feedback mechanisms, both intrinsic (*e.g.,* autoregulation, local hormones) and extrinsic (*e.g.,* sympathetic nervous system, blood-borne hormones), normally keep blood flow and GFR constant despite changes in arterial blood pressure.

Neural and Humoral Control Mechanisms

The kidney is richly innervated by the sympathetic nervous system. Increased sympathetic activity causes constriction of the afferent and efferent arterioles and thus a decrease in renal blood flow. Intense sympathetic stimulation such as occurs in shock and trauma can produce marked decreases in renal blood flow and GFR, even to the extent of causing blood flow to cease altogether.

Several humoral substances, including angiotensin II, ADH, and the endothelins, produce vasoconstriction of renal vessels. The endothelins are a group of peptides released from damaged endothelial cells in the kidney and other tissues. Although not thought to be an important regulator of renal blood flow during everyday activities, endothelin I may play a role in reduction of blood flow in conditions such as postischemic acute renal failure (see Chapter 34).

Other substances such as dopamine, nitric oxide, and prostaglandins (*i.e.,* E_2 and I_2) produce vasodilation. Nitric oxide, a vasodilator produced by the vascular endothelium, appears to be important in preventing excessive vasoconstriction of renal blood vessels and allowing normal excretion of sodium and water. Prostaglandins are a group of mediators of cell function that are produced locally and exert their effects locally. Although prostaglandins do not appear to be of major importance in regulating renal blood flow and GFR under normal conditions, they may protect the kidneys against the vasoconstricting effects of sympathetic stimulation and angiotensin II. Nonsteroidal anti-inflammatory drugs (NSAIDs) that inhibit prostaglandin synthesis may cause reduction in renal blood flow and GFR under certain conditions.

Autoregulatory Mechanisms

The constancy of renal blood flow is maintained by a process called *autoregulation* (see Chapter 21). Normally, autoregulation of blood flow is designed to maintain blood flow at a level

consistent with the metabolic needs of the tissues. In the kidney, autoregulation of blood flow also must allow for precise regulation of solute and water excretion. For autoregulation to occur, the resistance to blood flow through the kidneys must be varied in direct proportion to the arterial pressure. The exact mechanisms responsible for the intrarenal regulation of blood flow are unclear. One of the proposed mechanisms is a direct effect on vascular smooth muscle that causes the blood vessels to relax when there is an increase in blood pressure, and to constrict when there is a decrease in pressure. A second proposed mechanism is the juxtaglomerular complex.

The Juxtaglomerular Complex. The juxtaglomerular complex is thought to represent a feedback control system that links changes in the GFR with renal blood flow. The juxtaglomerular complex is located at the site where the distal tubule extends back to the glomerulus and then passes between the afferent and efferent arterioles (Fig. 30-12A). The distal tubular site that is nearest the glomerulus is characterized by densely nucleated cells called the *macula densa*. In the adjacent afferent arteriole, the smooth muscle cells of the media are modified as special secretory cells called *juxtaglomerular cells*. These cells contain granules of inactive renin, an enzyme that functions in the conversion of angiotensinogen to angiotensin. Renin functions by means of angiotensin II to produce vasoconstriction of the efferent arteriole as a means of preventing large decreases in the GFR. Angiotensin II also increases sodium reabsorption indirectly by stimulating aldosterone secretion from the adrenal gland, and directly by increasing sodium reabsorption by the proximal tubule cells.

Because of its location between the afferent and efferent arterioles, the juxtaglomerular complex is thought to play an essential feedback role in linking the level of arterial blood pressure and renal blood flow to the GFR and the composition of the distal tubular fluid (see Fig. 30-12B). It is thought to monitor the systemic arterial blood pressure by sensing the stretch of the afferent arteriole and the concentration of sodium chloride in the tubular filtrate as it passes through the macula densa. This information is then used in determining how much renin should be released to keep the arterial blood pressure within its normal range and maintain a relatively constant GFR. Studies suggest that a decrease in the GFR slows the flow rate of the urine filtrate in the ascending loop of Henle, thereby increasing sodium and chloride reabsorption. This, in turn, decreases the delivery of sodium chloride to the macula densa. The decrease in delivery of sodium chloride to the macula densa has two effects: it decreases resistance in the afferent arterioles, which raises glomerular filtration pressure, and it increases the release of renin from the juxtaglomerular cells. The renin from these cells functions as an enzyme to convert angiotensinogen to angiotensin I, which is converted to angiotensin II (see Chapter 23, Fig. 23-4). Finally, angiotensin II acts to constrict the efferent arteriole as a means of producing a further increase in the glomerular filtration pressure and thereby returning the GFR toward a more normal range.

Understanding • How the Kidney Concentrates Urine

The osmolarity of body fluids relies heavily on the ability of the kidney to produce dilute or concentrated urine. Urine concentration depends on three factors: (1) the osmolarity of interstitial fluids in the urine-concentrating part of the kidney, (2) the antidiuretic hormone (ADH), and (3) the action of ADH on the cells in the collecting tubules of the kidney.

❶ Osmolarity

In approximately one fifth of the juxtamedullary nephrons, the loops of Henle and special hairpin-shaped capillaries called the *vasa recta* descend into the medullary portion of the kidney to form a countercurrent system—a set of parallel passages in which the contents flow in opposite directions. The countercurrent design serves to increase the osmolarity in this part of the kidney by promoting the exchange of solutes between the adjacent descending and ascending loops of Henle and between the descending and ascending sections of the vasa recta. Because of these exchange processes, a high concentration of osmotically active particles (approximately 1200 mOsm/kg of H_2O) collects in the interstitium surrounding the collecting tubules where the ADH-mediated reabsorption of water takes place.

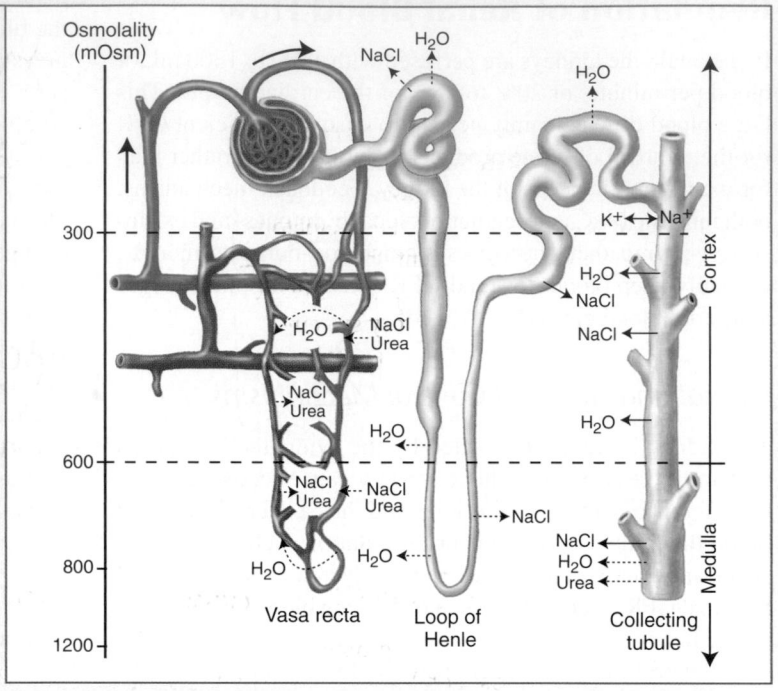

❷ Antidiuretic Hormone

ADH, which regulates the ability of the kidneys to concentrate urine, is synthesized by neurons in the hypothalamus and transported down their axons to the posterior pituitary gland and then released into the circulation. One of the main stimuli for synthesis and release of ADH is an increase in serum osmolarity. ADH release is also controlled by cardiovascular reflexes that respond to changes in blood pressure or blood volume.

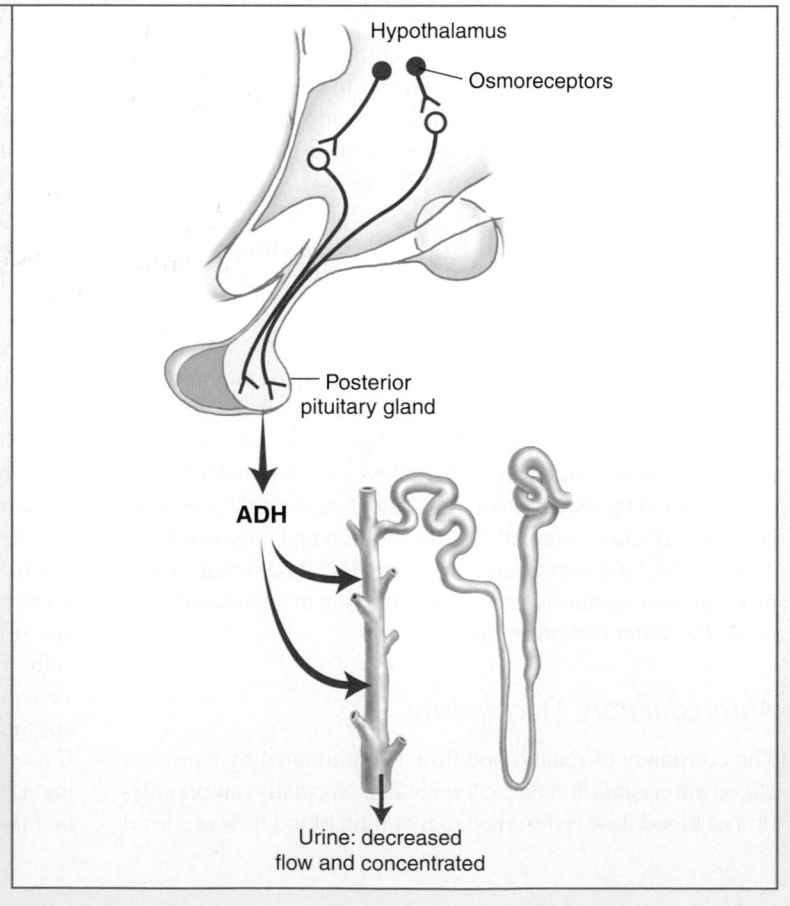

❸ Action of ADH

ADH, also known as vasopressin, acts at the level of the collecting tubule to increase water absorption. It exerts its action by binding to vasopressin receptors on the basolateral membrane of the tubular cell. Binding of ADH to the vasopressin receptors causes water channels (*aquaporin-2 channels*) to move into the luminal side of the cell membrane, which is normally impermeable to water. Insertion of the channels allows water from the tubular fluids to move into the tubular cell and then out into the surrounding hyperosmotic interstitial fluid on the basolateral side of the cell, and from there it moves into the peritubular capillaries for return to the circulatory system. Thus, when ADH is present, the water that moved from the blood into the urine filtrate in the glomeruli is returned to the circulatory system, and when ADH is absent, the water is excreted in the urine.

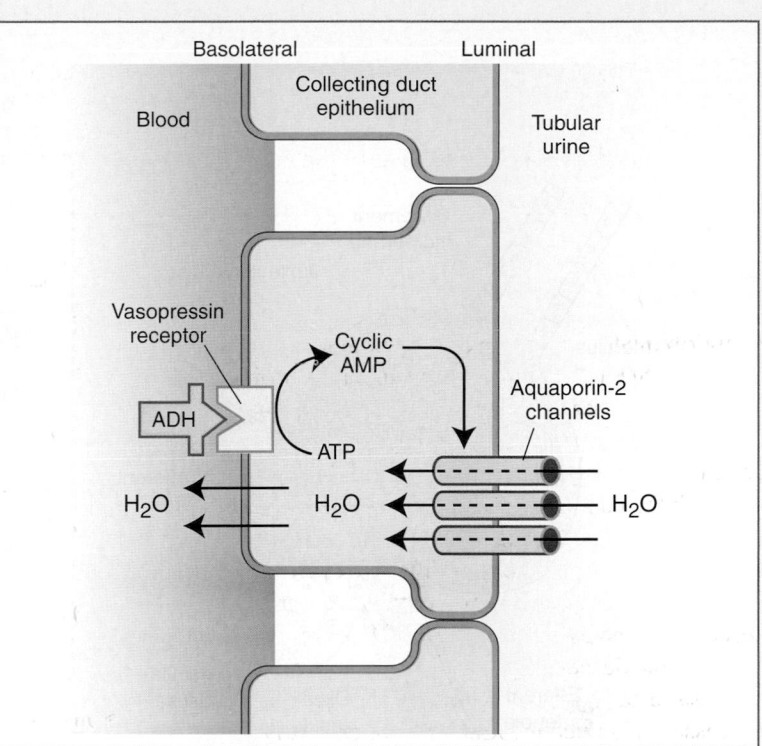

Effect of Increased Protein and Glucose Load

Even though renal blood flow and glomerular filtration are relatively stable under most conditions, two conditions can increase renal blood flow and glomerular filtration. These are an increased amount of protein in the diet and an increase in blood glucose. With ingestion of a high-protein diet, renal blood flow increases 20% to 30% within 1 to 2 hours. Although the exact mechanism for this increase is uncertain, it is thought to be related to the fact that amino acids and sodium are absorbed together in the proximal tubule (secondary active transport). As a result, delivery of sodium to the macula densa is decreased, which elicits an increase in renal blood flow through the juxtaglomerular complex feedback mechanism. The resultant increase in blood flow and GFR allows sodium excretion to be maintained at a near-normal level while increasing the excretion of the waste products of protein metabolism, such as urea. The same mechanism is thought to explain the large increases in renal blood flow and GFR that occur with high blood glucose levels in persons with uncontrolled diabetes mellitus.

Elimination Functions of the Kidney

The functions of the kidney focus on elimination of water, waste products, excess electrolytes, and unwanted substances from the blood. Blood tests can provide valuable information about the kidneys' ability to remove metabolic wastes and maintain the blood's normal electrolyte and pH composition. As renal function declines, there is an increase in serum levels of substances such urea, creatinine, phosphate, and potassium. The

effect of renal failure on the concentration of serum electrolytes and metabolic end products is discussed in Chapter 34.

Renal Clearance

Renal clearance is the volume of plasma that is completely cleared each minute of any substance that finds its way into the urine. It is determined by the ability of the substance to be filtered in the glomeruli and the capacity of the renal tubules to reabsorb or secrete the substance. Every substance has its own clearance rate, the units of which are always volume of plasma per unit time. It can be determined by measuring the amount of a substance that is excreted in the urine (*i.e.,* urine concentration × urine flow rate in milliliters per minute) and dividing by its plasma concentration. Inulin, a large polysaccharide, is freely filtered in the glomeruli and neither reabsorbed nor secreted by the tubular cells. After intravenous injection, the amount that appears in the urine is equal to the amount that is filtered in the glomeruli (*i.e.,* the clearance rate is equal to the GFR). Because of these properties, inulin can be used as a laboratory measure of the GFR. Some substances, such as urea, are freely filtered in the glomeruli, but the volume that is cleared from the plasma is less than the GFR, indicating that at least some of the substance is being reabsorbed. At normal plasma levels, glucose has a clearance of zero because it is reabsorbed in the tubules and none appears in the urine.

Regulation of Sodium and Potassium Elimination

Elimination of sodium and potassium is regulated by the GFR and by humoral agents that control their reabsorption.

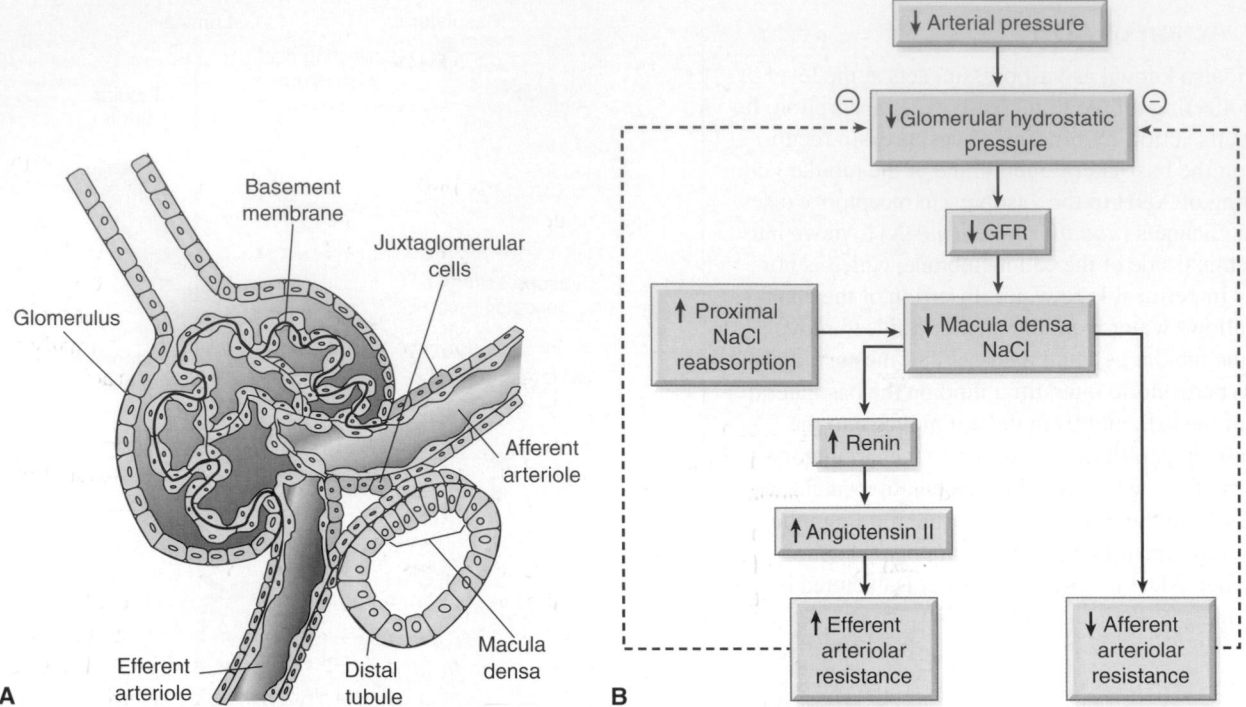

FIGURE 30-12 • **(A)** Juxtaglomerular apparatus, showing the close contact of the distal tubule with the afferent arteriole, the macula densa, and the juxtaglomerular cells. **(B)** Flow chart depicting the macula densa feedback mechanism for autoregulation of glomerular hydrostatic pressure and glomerular filtration rate (GFR) during changes in renal arterial pressure. (From Guyton A. C., Hall J. E. [2006]. *Textbook of medical physiology* [11th ed., p. 324]. Philadelphia: Elsevier Saunders.)

Aldosterone functions in the regulation of sodium and potassium elimination. Atrial natriuretic peptide (ANP) contributes to the regulation of sodium elimination. Sodium reabsorption in the distal tubule and collecting duct is highly variable and depends on the presence of aldosterone, a hormone secreted by the adrenal gland. In the presence of aldosterone, almost all the sodium in the distal tubular fluid is reabsorbed, and the urine essentially becomes sodium free. In the absence of aldosterone, virtually no sodium is reabsorbed from the distal tubule. The remarkable ability of the distal tubular and collecting duct cells to alter sodium reabsorption in relation to changes in aldosterone allows the kidneys to excrete urine with sodium levels that range from a few tenths of a gram to 40 g per day.

Like sodium, potassium is freely filtered in the glomerulus, but unlike sodium, potassium is reabsorbed from and secreted into the tubular fluid. The secretion of potassium into the tubular fluid occurs in the distal tubule and, like that of sodium, is regulated by aldosterone. Only approximately 70 mEq of potassium is delivered to the distal tubule each day, but the average person consumes this much and more potassium in the diet. Excess potassium that is not filtered in the glomerulus and delivered to the collecting tubule therefore must be secreted (*i.e.,* transported from the blood) into the tubular fluid for elimination from the body. In the absence of aldosterone (as in Addison disease; see Chapter 41), potassium secretion becomes

minimal. In these circumstances, potassium reabsorption exceeds secretion, and blood levels of potassium increase.

Atrial natriuretic peptide, discovered in 1981, is a hormone believed to have an important role in salt and water excretion by the kidney. It is synthesized in muscle cells of the atria of the heart and released when the atria are stretched. The actions of ANP include vasodilation of the afferent and efferent arterioles, which results in an increase in renal blood flow and glomerular filtration rate. ANP inhibits aldosterone secretion by the adrenal gland and sodium reabsorption from the collecting tubules through its action on aldosterone and through direct action on the tubular cells. It also inhibits ADH release from the posterior pituitary gland, thereby increasing excretion of water by the kidneys. ANP also has vasodilator properties. Whether these effects are sufficient to produce long-term changes in blood pressure is uncertain.

Regulation of pH

The kidneys regulate body pH by conserving base bicarbonate and eliminating hydrogen ions (H^+). Neither the blood buffer systems nor the respiratory control mechanisms for carbon dioxide elimination can eliminate hydrogen ions from the body. This is accomplished by the kidneys. The average North American diet results in the liberation of 40 to 80 mmol of hydrogen ions each day. Virtually all the hydrogen ions excreted

THE FUNCTIONS OF THE KIDNEY

- The kidney regulates the composition and pH of body fluids through the reabsorption and elimination or conservation of sodium, potassium, hydrogen, chloride, and bicarbonate ions.
- It functions in the elimination of metabolic wastes (urea, uric acid, creatinine) and drugs and their metabolites.
- It serves to regulate the osmolality of the extracellular fluid through the action of antidiuretic hormone (ADH).
- It plays a central role in blood pressure regulation through the renin-angiotensin-aldosterone mechanism and the regulation of salt and water elimination.
- It contributes to the metabolic functions of the skeletal system through activation of vitamin D and regulation of calcium and phosphate conservation and elimination.
- It controls the production of red blood cells in the bone marrow through the production of erythropoietin.

in the urine are secreted into the tubular fluid by means of tubular secretory mechanisms. The lowest tubular fluid pH that can be achieved is 4.4 to 4.5. The ability of the kidneys to excrete hydrogen ions depends on buffers in the urine that combine with the hydrogen ion. The three major urine buffers are bicarbonate (HCO_3^-), phosphate ($HPO_4^=$), and ammonia (NH_3). Bicarbonate ions, which are present in the urine filtrate, combine with hydrogen ions that have been secreted into the tubular fluid; this results in the formation of carbon dioxide and water. The carbon dioxide is then absorbed into the tubular cells and bicarbonate is regenerated. The phosphate ion is a metabolic end product that is filtered into the tubular fluid; it combines with a secreted hydrogen ion and is not reabsorbed. Ammonia is synthesized in tubular cells by deamination of the amino acid glutamine; it diffuses into the tubular fluid and combines with the hydrogen ion. An important aspect of this buffer system is that the deamination process increases whenever the body's hydrogen ion concentration remains elevated for 1 to 2 days. These mechanisms for pH regulation are described more fully in Chapter 32.

pH-Dependent Elimination of Organic Ions

The proximal tubule actively secretes large amounts of different organic anions. Foreign anions (*e.g.*, salicylates, penicillin) and endogenously produced anions (*e.g.*, bile acids, uric acid) are actively secreted into the tubular fluid. Most of the anions that are secreted use the same transport system, allowing the kidneys to rid the body of many different drugs and environmental agents. Because the same transport system is shared by different anions, there is competition for transport such that elevated levels of one substance tend to inhibit the secretion of other anions.

The proximal tubules also possess an active transport system for organic cations that is analogous to that for organic ions.

Uric Acid Elimination

Uric acid is a product of purine metabolism (see Chapter 59). Excessively high blood levels (*i.e.,* hyperuricemia) can cause gout, and excessive urine levels can cause kidney stones. Uric acid is freely filtered in the glomerulus and is reabsorbed and secreted into the proximal tubules. Uric acid is one of the anions that use the previously described anion transport system in the proximal tubule. Tubular reabsorption normally exceeds secretion, and the net effect is removal of uric acid from the filtrate. Although the rate of reabsorption exceeds secretion, the secretory process is homeostatically controlled to maintain a constant plasma level. Many persons with elevated uric acid levels secrete less uric acid than do persons with normal uric acid levels.

Uric acid uses the same transport systems as other anions, such as aspirin, sulfinpyrazone, and probenecid. Small doses of aspirin compete with uric acid for secretion into the tubular fluid and reduce uric acid secretion, and large doses compete with uric acid for reabsorption and increase uric acid excretion in the urine. Because of its effect on uric acid secretion, aspirin is not recommended for treatment of gouty arthritis. Thiazide and loop diuretics (*i.e.,* furosemide and ethacrynic acid) also can cause hyperuricemia and gouty arthritis, presumably through a decrease in extracellular fluid volume and enhanced uric acid reabsorption.

Urea Elimination

Urea is an end product of protein metabolism. The normal adult produces 25 to 30 g/day; the quantity rises when a high-protein diet is consumed, when there is excessive tissue breakdown, or in the presence of gastrointestinal bleeding. With gastrointestinal bleeding, the blood proteins are broken down to form ammonia in the intestine; the ammonia is then absorbed into the portal circulation and converted to urea by the liver before being released into the bloodstream. The kidneys, in their role as regulators of blood urea nitrogen (BUN) levels, filter urea in the glomeruli and then reabsorb it in the tubules. This enables maintenance of a normal BUN, which is in the range of 8 to 25 mg/dL (2.9 to 8.9 mmol/L). During periods of dehydration, the blood volume and GFR drop, and BUN levels increase. The renal tubules are permeable to urea, which means that the longer the tubular fluid remains in the kidneys, the greater is the reabsorption of urea into the blood. Only small amounts of urea are reabsorbed into the blood when the GFR is high, but relatively large amounts of urea are returned to the blood when the GFR is reduced.

Drug Elimination

Many drugs are eliminated in the urine. These drugs are selectively filtered in the glomerulus and reabsorbed or secreted into the tubular fluid. Only drugs that are not bound to plasma proteins are filtered in the glomerulus and therefore able to be eliminated by the kidneys. Many drugs are weak acids or weak bases and are present in the renal tubular fluid partly as water-soluble ions and partly as nonionized lipid-soluble molecules. The nonionized lipid-soluble form of a drug diffuses more readily through the lipid membrane of the tubule and then back into the bloodstream, whereas the water-soluble ionized form remains in the urine filtrate. The ratio of ionized to nonionized drug depends on the pH of the urine. For example, aspirin is highly ionized in alkaline urine and in this form is rapidly excreted in the urine. Aspirin is largely nonionized in acid urine and is reabsorbed rather than excreted. Alkaline or acid diuresis may be used to increase elimination of drugs in the urine, particularly in situations of drug overdose.

Endocrine Functions of the Kidney

In addition to their function in regulating body fluids and electrolytes, the kidneys function as an endocrine organ in that they produce chemical mediators that travel through the blood to distant sites where they exert their actions. The kidneys participate in control of blood pressure through the renin-angiotensin-aldosterone mechanism, in calcium metabolism by activating vitamin D, and in regulating red blood cell production through the synthesis of erythropoietin.

The Renin-Angiotensin-Aldosterone Mechanism

The renin-angiotensin-aldosterone mechanism plays an important part in short- and long-term regulation of blood pressure. Renin is an enzyme that is synthesized and stored in the juxtaglomerular cells of the kidney. This enzyme is thought to be released in response to a decrease in renal blood flow or a change in the composition of the distal tubular fluid, or as the result of sympathetic nervous system stimulation. Renin itself has no direct effect on blood pressure. Rather, it acts enzymatically to convert a circulating plasma protein called *angiotensinogen* to angiotensin I (see Chapter 23, Fig. 23-4). Angiotensin I, which has few vasoconstrictor properties, leaves the kidneys and enters the circulation; as it is circulated through the lungs, *angiotensin-converting enzyme* catalyzes the conversion of angiotensin I to angiotensin II. Angiotensin II is a potent vasoconstrictor, and it acts directly on the kidneys to decrease salt and water excretion. Both mechanisms have relatively short periods of action. Angiotensin II also stimulates aldosterone secretion by the adrenal gland. Aldosterone acts on the distal tubule to increase sodium reabsorption and exerts a longer-term effect on the maintenance of blood pressure. Renin also functions via angiotensin II to produce constriction of the efferent arteriole as a means of preventing a serious decrease in glomerular filtration pressure.

Erythropoietin

Erythropoietin is a polypeptide hormone that regulates the differentiation of red blood cells in the bone marrow (see Chapter 14). Between 89% and 95% of erythropoietin is formed in the kidneys. The synthesis of erythropoietin is stimulated by tissue hypoxia, which may be brought about by anemia, residence at high altitudes, or impaired oxygenation of tissues due to cardiac or pulmonary disease. Persons with end-stage kidney disease often are anemic because of an inability of the kidneys to produce erythropoietin. This anemia usually is managed by the administration of a recombinant erythropoietin (epoetin alfa) produced through DNA technology, to stimulate erythropoiesis.

Vitamin D

Activation of vitamin D occurs in the kidneys. Vitamin D increases calcium absorption from the gastrointestinal tract and helps to regulate calcium deposition in bone. It also has a weak stimulatory effect on renal calcium absorption. Although vitamin D is not synthesized and released from an endocrine gland, it often is considered as a hormone because of its pathway of molecular activation and mechanism of action.

Vitamin D exists in two forms: natural vitamin D (cholecalciferol), produced in the skin from ultraviolet irradiation, and synthetic vitamin D (ergocalciferol), derived from irradiation of ergosterol. The active form of vitamin D is 1,25-dihydroxycholecalciferol. Cholecalciferol and ergocalciferol must undergo chemical transformation to become active: first to 25-hydroxycholecalciferol in the liver and then to 1,25-dihydroxycholecalciferol in the kidneys. Persons with end-stage renal disease are unable to transform vitamin D to its active form and may require pharmacologic preparations of the active vitamin (calcitriol) for maintaining mineralization of their bones.

Action of Diuretics

Diuretics are drugs that increase urine volume. Many diuretic agents (loop diuretics, thiazide diuretic, and potassium-sparing diuretics) exert their effects by blocking the reabsorption of sodium in the renal tubules. Others exert osmotic effects that prevent water reabsorption in the water-permeable parts of the nephron.

Diuretics That Block Sodium Reabsorption. Most diuretics share the same mechanism of action—blockade of sodium and chloride reabsorption. By blocking the reabsorption of these solutes, diuretics create an osmotic pressure gradient within the nephron that prevents the passive reabsorption of water. Thus, diuretics cause water and sodium to be retained in the nephron, thereby promoting the excretion of both. The increase in urine flow that a diuretic produces is related to the amount of sodium and chloride reabsorption that it blocks. Because the amount of sodium becomes progressively less as the urine filtrate flows from the proximal tubule to the collecting ducts, drugs that act early in the nephron have the opportunity to block the greatest amount of sodium reabsorption. Approximately 65% of sodium that is filtered in the glomeruli of the kidney is reabsorbed in the proximal tubule, 20% is reabsorbed in the thick ascending loop of Henle, 10% in the early distal convoluted tubule, and 2% to 5% is reabsorbed in the late distal and cortical collecting tubules (Fig 30-13).

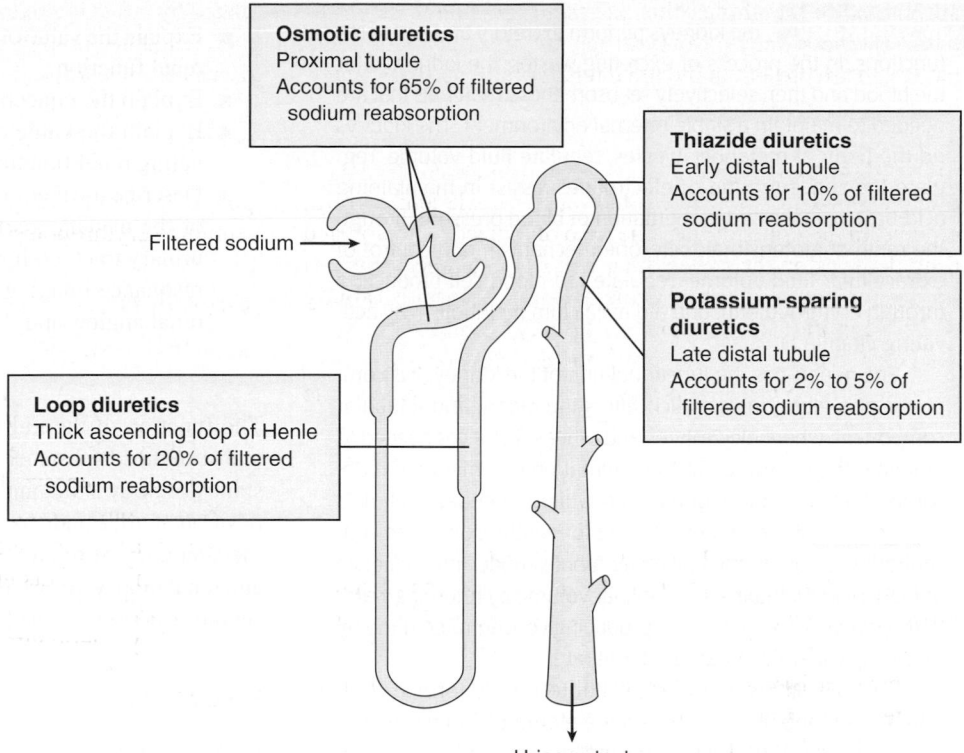

Osmotic diuretics
Proximal tubule
Accounts for 65% of filtered
    sodium reabsorption

Thiazide diuretics
Early distal tubule
Accounts for 10% of filtered
    sodium reabsorption

Filtered sodium

**Potassium-sparing
diuretics**
Late distal tubule
Accounts for 2% to 5% of
    filtered sodium reabsorption

Loop diuretics
Thick ascending loop of Henle
Accounts for 20% of filtered
    sodium reabsorption

Urine output

FIGURE 30-13 • Tubular sites of diuretic action and percentage of sodium reabsorption.

The so-called *loop diuretics* exert their effect in the thick ascending loop of Henle. Because of their site of action, these drugs are the most effective diuretic agents available. These drugs inhibit the coupled $Na^+/K^+/2Cl^-$ transport system on the luminal side of the ascending loop of Henle (see Fig. 30-10). By inhibiting this transport system, they reduce the reabsorption of sodium chloride, decrease potassium reabsorption, and increase calcium and magnesium elimination. Prolonged use can cause significant loss of magnesium in some persons. Because calcium is actively reabsorbed in the distal convoluted tubule, loop diuretics usually do not cause hypocalcemia. The loop diuretics may also increase uric acid retention and impair glucose tolerance.

The *thiazide diuretics* act by preventing the reabsorption of sodium chloride in the early distal convoluted tubule. Because of their site of action, the thiazide diuretics are less effective than loop diuretics in terms of effecting diuresis. The thiazide diuretics produce increased losses of potassium in the urine, uric acid retention, and some impairment in glucose tolerance. In contrast to the situation in the loop of Henle, where the loop diuretics inhibit calcium reabsorption, the thiazide diuretics actually enhance calcium reabsorption in the distal convoluted tubule.

The *aldosterone antagonists,* also called *potassium-sparing diuretics,* reduce sodium reabsorption and decrease potassium secretion in the late distal tubule and cortical collecting tubule site regulated by aldosterone (see Fig. 30-11). Because potassium secretion is linked to sodium reabsorption in this segment of the tubule, these agents are also effective in reducing potassium excretion and may, in some cases, cause severe hyperkalemia. These agents also tend to interfere with secretion

of hydrogen ions in the collecting duct, explaining in part the metabolic acidosis sometimes seen with the use of these agents.

There are two types of potassium-sparing diuretics: those that act as direct aldosterone antagonists and those that act independently of aldosterone. The first type (*e.g.,* spironolactone) binds to the mineralocorticoid receptor in the tubule, preventing aldosterone from entering the cell and exerting its effects. The second type (*e.g.,* triamterene, amiloride) does not bind to the receptor, but instead directly interferes with sodium entry through the sodium-selective ion channel. The potassium-sparing diuretics produce only mild diuresis because they inhibit such a small percentage of sodium reabsorption. However, as the name implies, their main use is in combination with other diuretics to inhibit K^+ secretion by the principal cells. These diuretics may also be used during states of mineralocorticoid (*i.e.,* aldosterone) excess.

Osmotic Diuretics. The osmotic diuretics act in the proximal tubule and ascending loop of Henle, both of which are highly permeable to water. In contrast to the loop, thiazide, and potassium-sparing diuretics that exert their effects by blocking specific tubular Na^+ transport mechanisms, the osmotic diuretics, which are filtered but not reabsorbed, cause water to be retained in the urine filtrate and promote water diuresis. One such agent, mannitol, is used mainly to reduce increased intracranial pressure, but is occasionally used to promote prompt removal of toxins. Because it is not absorbed, mannitol must be given parenterally to act as a diuretic. If given orally, it causes osmotic diarrhea.

IN SUMMARY, the kidneys perform excretory and endocrine functions. In the process of excreting wastes, the kidneys filter the blood and then selectively reabsorb those materials that are needed to maintain a stable internal environment. The kidneys rid the body of metabolic wastes, regulate fluid volume, regulate the concentration of electrolytes, assist in maintaining acid-base balance, aid in regulation of blood pressure through the renin-angiotensin-aldosterone mechanism and control of extracellular fluid volume, regulate red blood cell production through erythropoietin, and aid in calcium metabolism by activating vitamin D.

The nephron is the functional unit of the kidney. It is composed of a glomerulus, which filters the blood, and a tubular component, where electrolytes and other substances needed to maintain the constancy of the internal environment are reabsorbed back into the bloodstream while unneeded materials are secreted into the tubular filtrate for elimination. Urine concentration occurs in the collecting tubules under the influence of ADH. ADH maintains extracellular volume by returning water to the vascular compartment, producing concentrated urine by removing water from the tubular filtrate.

The GFR is the amount of filtrate that is formed each minute as blood moves through the glomeruli. It is regulated by the arterial blood pressure and renal blood flow in the normally functioning kidney. The juxtaglomerular complex is thought to represent a feedback control system that links changes in the GFR with renal blood flow. Renal clearance is the volume of plasma that is completely cleared each minute of any substance that finds its way into the urine. It is determined by the ability of the substance to be filtered in the glomeruli and the capacity of the renal tubules to reabsorb or secrete the substance.

Diuretics are drugs that increase urine volume. Many diuretic agents (loop diuretics, thiazide diuretics, and potassium-sparing diuretics) exert their effect by blocking the reabsorption of sodium at specific sites in the renal tubules. Others exert osmotic effects that prevent water reabsorption in the water-permeable parts of the nephron. The effectiveness of a diuretic is related to its site of action; accordingly, diuretics such as the loop diuretics that act in the thick ascending loop of Henle, where approximately 20% of sodium reabsorption takes place, produce the greatest diuresis. ■

CONCEPTSin action **ANIMATI**⚙**N**

TESTS OF RENAL FUNCTION

After completing this section of the chapter, you should be able to meet the following objectives:

- Describe the characteristics of normal urine.
- Explain the significance of casts in the urine.

- Explain the value of urine specific gravity in evaluating renal function.
- Explain the concept of the glomerular filtration rate.
- Explain the value of serum creatinine levels in evaluating renal function.
- Describe the methods used in cystoscopic examination of the urinary tract, ultrasonographic studies of the urinary tract, computed tomographic scans, magnetic resonance imaging studies, excretory urography, and renal angiography.

The function of the kidneys is to filter the blood, selectively reabsorb those substances that are needed to maintain the constancy of body fluid, and excrete metabolic wastes. The composition of urine and blood provides valuable information about the adequacy of renal function. Radiologic tests, endoscopy, and renal biopsy afford means for viewing the gross and microscopic structures of the kidneys and urinary system.

Urine Tests

Urine is a clear, amber-colored fluid that is approximately 95% water and 5% dissolved solids. The kidneys normally produce approximately 1.5 L of urine each day. Normal urine contains metabolic wastes and few or no plasma proteins, blood cells, or glucose molecules. Urine tests can be performed on a single urine specimen or on a 24-hour urine specimen. First-voided morning specimens are useful for qualitative protein and specific gravity testing. A freshly voided specimen is most reliable. Urine specimens that have been left standing may contain lysed red blood cells, disintegrating *casts,* and rapidly multiplying bacteria. Table 30-1 describes urinalysis values for normal urine.

Casts are molds of the distal nephron lumen. A gel-like substance called *Tamm-Horsfall mucoprotein,* which is formed in the tubular epithelium, is the major protein constituent of urinary casts. Casts composed of this gel but devoid of cells are called *hyaline casts.* These casts develop when the protein concentration of the urine is high (as in nephrotic syndrome), urine osmolality is high, and urine pH is low. The inclusion of granules or cells in the matrix of the protein gel leads to the formation of various other types of casts.

Proteinuria represents excessive protein excretion in the urine. Because of the glomerular capillary filtration barrier, less than 150 mg/L of protein is excreted in the urine over 24 hours in a healthy person. Urine tests for proteinuria are used to detect abnormal filtering of albumin in the glomeruli or defects in its reabsorption in the renal tubules. A protein reagent dipstick can be used as a rapid screening test for the presence of proteins in the urine. Once the presence of proteinuria has been detected, a 24-hour urine test is often used to quantify the amount of protein that is present.

Albumin, which is the smallest of the plasma proteins, is filtered more readily than globulins or other plasma proteins.

TABLE 30-1 **Normal Values for Routine Urinalysis**		
GENERAL CHARACTERISTICS AND MEASUREMENTS	**CHEMICAL DETERMINATIONS**	**MICROSCOPIC EXAMINATION OF SEDIMENT**
Color: yellow-amber—indicates a high specific gravity and small output of urine	Glucose: negative	Casts negative: occasional hyaline casts
Turbidity: clear to slightly hazy	Ketones: negative	Red blood cells: negative or rare
Specific gravity: 1.010–1.025 with a normal fluid intake	Blood: negative	Crystals: negative (none)
pH: 4.5–8.0	Protein: negative	White blood cells; negative or rare
	Bilirubin: negative	Epithelial cells: few
	Urobilinogen: 0.5–4.0 mg/d	
	Nitrate for bacteria: negative	
	Leukocyte esterase: negative	

From Fischbach F. (2004). *A manual of laboratory and diagnostic tests* (7th ed., p. 178). Philadelphia: Lippincott Williams & Wilkins.

Thus, *microalbuminuria* tends to occur long before clinical proteinuria becomes evident. A dipstick test for microalbuminuria is available for screening purposes. The microalbuminuria dipstick method, however, only indicates an increase in urinary albumin that is below the detectable range of the standard proteinuria test. It does not specify the amount of albumin that is present in the urine. Therefore, a 24-hour urine collection is the standard method for detecting microalbuminuria (an albumin excretion >30 mg/day is abnormal).

The *specific gravity* of urine varies with its concentration of solutes. Urine specific gravity provides a valuable index of the hydration status and functional ability of the kidneys. Healthy kidneys can produce a concentrated urine with a specific gravity of 1.030 to 1.040. During periods of marked hydration, the specific gravity can approach 1.000. With diminished renal function, there is a loss of renal concentrating ability, and the urine specific gravity may fall to levels of 1.006 to 1.010 (usual range is 1.010 to 1.025 with normal fluid intake). These low levels are particularly significant if they occur during periods that follow a decrease in water intake (*e.g.,* during the first urine specimen on arising in the morning).

Urine osmolality, which depends on the number of particles of solute in a unit of solution, is a more exact measurement of urine concentration than specific gravity. More information concerning renal function can be obtained if the serum and urine osmolality tests are done at the same time. The normal ratio between urine and serum osmolality is 3:1. A high urine-to-serum ratio is seen in concentrated urine. With poor concentrating ability, the ratio is low.

Glomerular Filtration Rate

The GFR provides a gauge of renal function. It can be measured clinically by collecting timed samples of blood and urine. *Creatinine,* a product of creatine metabolism by the muscle, is filtered by the kidneys but not reabsorbed in the renal tubule. Creatinine levels in the blood and urine can be used to measure GFR. The clearance rate for creatinine is the amount that is completely cleared by the kidneys in 1 minute. The formula is expressed as C = UV/P, in which C is the clearance rate (mL/minute), U is the urine concentration (mg/dL), V is the urine volume excreted (mL/minute or 24 hours), and P is plasma concentration (mg/dL).

Normal creatinine clearance is 115 to 125 mL/minute. This value is corrected for body surface area, which reflects the muscle mass where creatinine metabolism takes place. The test may be done on a 24-hour basis, with blood being drawn when the urine collection is completed. In another method, two 1-hour urine specimens are collected, and a blood sample is drawn in between.

Blood Tests

Blood tests can provide valuable information about the kidneys' ability to remove metabolic wastes from the blood and maintain normal electrolyte and pH composition of the blood. Normal blood values are listed in Table 30-2. Serum levels of potassium, phosphate, BUN, and creatinine increase in renal failure. Serum pH, calcium, and bicarbonate levels decrease in renal failure. The effect of renal failure on the concentration of serum electrolytes and metabolic end products is discussed in Chapter 34.

TABLE 30-2 **Normal Blood Chemistry Levels**	
SUBSTANCE	**NORMAL VALUE***
Blood urea nitrogen	8.0–20.0 mg/dL (2.9–7.1 mmol/L)
Creatinine	0.6–1.2 mg/dL (50–100 mmol/L)
Sodium	135–145 mEq/L (135–145 mmol/L)
Chloride	98–106 mEq/L (98–106 mmol/L)
Potassium	3.5–5 mEq/L (3.5–5 mmol/L)
Carbon dioxide (CO_2 content)	24–29 mEq/L (24–29 mmol/L)
Calcium	8.5–10.5 mg/dL (2.1–2.6 mmol/L)
Phosphate	2.5–4.5 mg/dL (0.77–1.45 mmol/L)
Uric acid	
male	2.4–7.4 mg/dL (140–440 µmol/L)
female	1.4–5.8 mg/dL (80–350 µmol/L)
pH	7.35–7.45

*Values may vary among laboratories, depending on the method of analysis used.

Serum Creatinine

Serum creatinine levels reflect the GFR. Because these measurements are easily obtained and relatively inexpensive, they often are used as a screening measure of renal function. Creatinine is a product of creatine metabolism in muscles; its formation and release are relatively constant and proportional to the amount of muscle mass present. Creatinine is freely filtered in the glomeruli, is not reabsorbed from the tubules into the blood, and is only minimally secreted into the tubules from the blood; therefore, its blood values depend closely on the GFR.

The normal creatinine value is approximately 0.7 mg/dL of blood for a woman with a small frame, approximately 1.0 mg/dL of blood for a normal adult man, and approximately 1.5 mg/dL of blood (60 to 130 mmol/L) for a muscular man. There is an age-related decline in creatinine clearance in many elderly persons because muscle mass and the GFR decline with age (see Chapter 34). A normal serum creatinine level usually indicates normal renal function. In addition to its use in calculating the GFR, the serum creatinine level is used in estimating the functional capacity of the kidneys (Fig. 30-14). If the value doubles, the GFR—and renal function—probably has fallen to one half of its normal state. A rise in the serum creatinine level to three times its normal value suggests that there is a 75% loss of renal function, and with creatinine values of 10 mg/dL or more, it can be assumed that approximately 90% of renal function has been lost.

Recently it has been proposed that another serum protein, *cystatin-C* (a cysteine protease inhibitor), could be useful as a marker of GFR because it has a stable production rate, is freely filtered at the glomerulus, and in several studies has shown a greater sensitivity in detecting a decreased GFR. Further clinical studies are needed to determine the clinical efficacy of cystatin-C as a marker and to determine whether there is an advantage to its use compared with creatinine.

Blood Urea Nitrogen

Urea is formed in the liver as a byproduct of protein metabolism and is eliminated entirely by the kidneys. BUN therefore is related to the GFR but, unlike creatinine, also is influenced by protein intake, gastrointestinal bleeding, and hydration status. In gastrointestinal bleeding, the blood is broken down by the intestinal flora, and the nitrogenous waste is absorbed into the portal vein and transported to the liver, where it is converted to urea. During dehydration, elevated BUN levels result from increased concentration. Approximately two thirds of renal function must be lost before a significant rise in the BUN level occurs.

The BUN is less specific for renal insufficiency than creatinine, but the *BUN–creatinine ratio* may provide useful diagnostic information. The ratio normally is approximately 10:1. Ratios greater than 15:1 represent prerenal conditions, such as congestive heart failure and upper gastrointestinal tract bleeding, that produce an increase in BUN but not in creatinine. A ratio of less than 10:1 occurs in persons with liver disease and in those who receive a low-protein diet or chronic dialysis, because BUN is more readily dialyzable than creatinine.

Cystoscopy

Cystoscopy provides a means for direct visualization of the urethra, bladder, and ureteral orifices. It relies on the use of a cystoscope, an instrument with a lighted lens. The cystoscope is inserted through the urethra into the bladder. Biopsy specimens, lesions, small stones, and foreign bodies can be removed from the bladder. Urethroscopy may be used to remove stones from the ureter and aid in the treatment of ureteral disorders such as ureteral strictures.

Ultrasonography

Ultrasonographic studies use the reflection of ultrasonic (high-frequency) waves to visualize the deep structures of the body. The procedure is painless and noninvasive and requires no patient preparation. Ultrasonography is used to visualize the structures of the kidneys and has proved useful in the diagnosis of many urinary tract disorders, including congenital anomalies, renal abscesses, hydronephrosis, and kidney stones. It can differentiate a renal cyst from a renal tumor. The use of ultrasonography also enables accurate placement of needles for renal biopsy and catheters for percutaneous nephrostomy.

Radiologic and Other Imaging Studies

Radiologic studies include a simple flat plate (radiograph) of the kidneys, ureters, and bladder that can be used to determine the size, shape, and position of the kidneys and observe any radiopaque stones that may be in the kidney pelvis or ureters. In excretory urography, or *intravenous pyelography,* a radiopaque dye is injected into a peripheral vein; the dye is then filtered by the glomerulus and excreted into the urine, and x-ray films are taken as it moves through the kidneys and ureters.

Urography is used to detect space-occupying lesions of the kidneys, pyelonephritis, hydronephrosis, vesicoureteral reflux, and kidney stones. Some persons are allergic to the dye

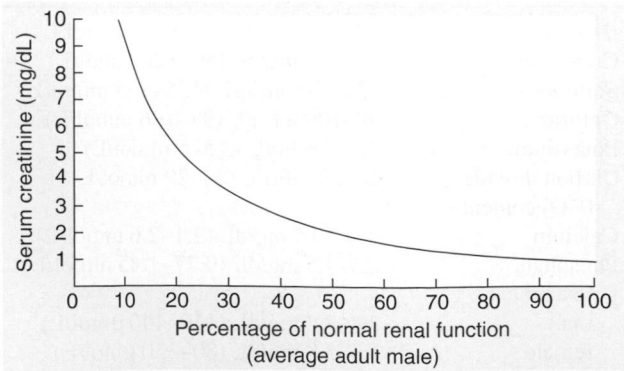

FIGURE 30-14 • Relation between the percentage of renal function and serum creatinine levels.

used for urography and may have an anaphylactic reaction after its administration. Every person undergoing urographic studies should be questioned about previous reactions to the dye or to similar dyes. If the test is considered essential in such persons, premedication with antihistamines and corticosteroids may be used. The dye also reduces renal blood flow; acute renal failure can occur, particularly in persons with vascular disease or preexisting renal insufficiency.

Other diagnostic tests include computed tomographic (CT) scans, magnetic resonance imaging (MRI), radionuclide imaging, and renal angiography. CT scans may be used to outline the kidneys and detect renal masses and tumors. MRI is becoming readily available and is used in imaging the kidneys, retroperitoneum, and urinary bladder. It is particularly useful in evaluating vascular abnormalities in and around the kidneys. Radionuclide imaging involves the injection of a radioactive material that subsequently is detected externally by a scintillation camera, which detects the radioactive emissions. Radionuclide imaging is used to evaluate renal function and structures, as well as the ureters and bladder. It is particularly useful in evaluating the function of kidney transplants. Renal angiography provides x-ray pictures of the blood vessels that supply the kidneys. It involves the injection of a radiopaque dye directly into the renal artery. A catheter usually is introduced through the femoral artery and advanced under fluoroscopic view into the abdominal aorta. The catheter tip then is maneuvered into the renal artery, and the dye is injected. This test is used to evaluate persons suspected of having renal artery stenosis, abnormalities of renal blood vessels, or vascular damage to the renal arteries after trauma.

IN SUMMARY, urinalysis and blood tests that measure serum levels of pH, electrolytes, and byproducts of metabolism provide valuable information about renal function. Urine specific gravity is used to assess the kidneys' ability to concentrate urine. Dipstick and 24-hour urine tests for proteinuria and microalbuminuria are used to detect abnormal filtering of albumin in the glomeruli or defects in its reabsorption in the renal tubules. Creatinine is a product of creatine metabolism in muscles that is freely filtered in the glomeruli and neither reabsorbed nor secreted in the tubules; therefore, serum creatinine levels are commonly used to estimate the GFR. Urea is formed in the liver as a byproduct of protein metabolism and is eliminated entirely by the kidneys. BUN is therefore related to the GFR but, unlike creatinine, also is influenced by protein intake, gastrointestinal bleeding, and hydration status.

Cystoscopic examinations can be used for direct visualization of the urethra, bladder, and ureters. Ultrasonography can be used to determine kidney size, and renal radionuclide imaging can be used to evaluate the kidney structures. Radiologic methods such as excretory urography provide a means by which kidney structures such as the renal calyces, pelvis, ureters, and bladder can be outlined. Other diagnostic tests include CT scans, MRI, radionuclide imaging, and renal angiography. ■

Review Exercises

1. A 32-year-old woman with diabetes is found to have a positive result on a urine dipstick test for microalbuminuria. A subsequent 24-hour urine specimen reveals an albumin excretion of 50 mg (an albumin excretion >30 mg/day is abnormal).

   A. *Use the structures of the glomerulus in Figure 30-5 to provide a possible explanation for this finding. Why specifically test for the albumin rather than the globulins or other plasma proteins?*

   B. *Strict control of blood sugars and treatment of hypertension have been shown to decrease the progression of kidney disease in persons with diabetes. Explain the physiologic rationale for these two types of treatments.*

2. A 10-year-old boy with bed-wetting was placed on an ADH nasal spray at bedtime as a means of treating the disorder.

   A. *Explain the rationale for using ADH to treat bed-wetting.*

3. A 54-year-old man, seen by his physician for an elevated blood pressure, was found to have a serum creatinine of 2.5. He complains that he has been urinating more frequently than usual and his first morning urine specimen reveals a dilute urine with a specific gravity of 1.010.

   A. *Explain the elevation of serum creatinine in terms of renal function.*

   B. *Explain the inability of persons with early renal failure to produce a concentrated urine as evidenced by the frequency of urination and the low specific gravity of his first morning urine specimen.*

4. A 60-year-old woman with a diagnosis of hypertension is being treated with a thiazide diuretic.

   A. *What diuretic effect would you expect the woman to have based on the percentage of sodium reaching the site where the diuretic exerted its action?*

   B. *What type of effects might be expected in terms of renal losses of potassium and calcium?*

Bibliography

Berne R. M., Levy M. N. (2004). *Physiology* (3rd ed., pp. 408–432). Philadelphia: C.V. Mosby.

Ganong W. F. (2005). *Review of medical physiology* (22nd ed., pp. 699–730). New York: Lange Medical Books/McGraw-Hill.

Gartner L. P., Hiatt J. L. (2001). *Color textbook of histology* (2nd ed., pp. 435–456). Philadelphia: W.B. Saunders.

Guyton A. C., Hall J. E. (2006). *Textbook of medical physiology* (11th ed., pp. 307–382). Philadelphia: Elsevier Saunders.

Junqueira L. C., Carneiro J. (2005). *Basic histology* (11th ed., pp. 373–391). New York: McGraw-Hill.

Koeppen B. M., Stanton B. A. (1997). *Renal physiology* (2nd ed.). St. Louis: C.V. Mosby.

Price C. P., Finney H. (2000). Developments in the assessment of glomerular filtration rate. *Clinica Chimica Acta* 297, 55–66.

Laterza O. F., Price C. P., Scott M. G. (2002). Cystatin C: An improved estimator of glomerular filtration rate. *Clinical Chemistry* 48, 699–707.

Rahn K. H., Heidenreich S., Bruckner D. (1999). How to assess glomerular function and damage in humans. *Journal of Hypertension* 17, 309–317.

Rhoades R. A., Tanner G. A. (2003). *Medical physiology* (2nd ed., pp. 377–402). Boston: Little, Brown.

Ross G. I., Pawlina W. (2003). *Histology: A text and atlas* (4th ed., pp. 604–624). Philadelphia: Lippincott Williams & Wilkins.

Schrier R. W. (2003). *Renal and electrolyte disorders* (6th ed.). Philadelphia: Lippincott Williams & Wilkins.

Smith H. (1953). *From fish to philosopher* (p. 4). Boston: Little, Brown.

Stevens L. A., Levey A. S. (2005). Measurement of kidney function. *Medical Clinics of North America* 89, 457–473.

Thomson S. C., Vallon V., Blantz R. C. (2004). Kidney function in early diabetes: The tubular hypothesis of glomerular filtration. *American Journal of Physiology: Renal Physiology* 286, F8–F15.

Vallon V. (2003). Tubuloglomerular feedback and the control of glomerular filtration rate. *News in Physiological Sciences* 18, 169–174.

Vander A. J. (1995). *Renal physiology* (5th ed.). New York: McGraw-Hill.

Visit the**Point** **http://thePoint.lww.com for animations, journal articles, and more!**

Chapter **31**

Disorders of Fluid and Electrolyte Balance

GLENN MATFIN AND CAROL M. PORTH

➤ Fluids and electrolytes are present in body cells, in the tissue spaces between the cells, and in the blood that fills the vascular compartment. Body fluids transport gases, nutrients, and wastes; help generate the electrical activity needed to power body functions; take part in the transforming of food into energy; and otherwise maintain the overall function of the body. Although fluid volume and composition remain relatively constant in the presence of a wide range of changes in intake and output, conditions such as environmental stresses and disease can impair intake, increase losses, and otherwise interfere with mechanisms that regulate fluid volume, composition, and distribution.

This chapter is divided into four sections: (1) Composition and Compartmental Distribution of Body Fluids, (2) Sodium and Water Balance, (3) Potassium Balance, and (4) Calcium, Phosphorus, and Magnesium Balance. The mechanisms of edema formation are discussed in the section on composition and compartmental distribution of body fluids.

 **COMPOSITION AND COMPARTMENTAL DISTRIBUTION OF BODY FLUIDS**

After completing this section of the chapter, you should be able to meet the following objectives:

■ Define the terms *electrolyte, ion,* and *nonelectrolytes.*
■ Differentiate the intracellular from the extracellular fluid compartments in terms of distribution and composition of water, electrolytes, and other osmotically active solutes.
■ Cite the rationale for the use of concentration rather than absolute values in describing electrolyte content of body fluids.

761

- Relate the concept of a concentration gradient to the processes of diffusion and osmosis.
- Describe the control of cell volume and the effect of isotonic, hypotonic, and hypertonic solutions on cell size.
- Describe factors that control fluid exchange between the vascular and interstitial fluid compartments and relate them to the development of edema and third spacing of extracellular fluids.
- Describe the manifestations and treatment of edema.

Body fluids are distributed between the intracellular (ICF) and extracellular fluid (ECF) compartments. The *ICF compartment* consists of fluid contained within all of the billions of cells in the body. It is the larger of the two compartments, with approximately two thirds of the body water in healthy adults. The remaining one third of body water is in the *ECF compartment,* which contains all the fluids outside the cells, including those in the interstitial or tissue spaces and blood vessels (Fig. 31-1).

The ECF, including blood plasma and interstitial fluids, contains large amounts of sodium and chloride, moderate amounts of bicarbonate, but only small quantities of potassium, magnesium, calcium, and phosphorus. In contrast to the ECF, the ICF contains almost no calcium; small amounts of sodium, chloride, bicarbonate, and phosphorus; moderate amounts of magnesium; and large amounts of potassium (Table 31-1). It is the ECF levels of electrolytes in the blood or blood plasma that are measured clinically. Although blood levels usually are representative of the total body levels of an electrolyte, this is not always the case, particularly with potassium, which is approximately 28 times more concentrated inside the cell than outside.

The cell membrane serves as the primary barrier to the movement of substances between the ECF and ICF compartments. Lipid-soluble substances (*e.g.,* oxygen [O_2] and carbon dioxide [CO_2]), which dissolve in the lipid bilayer of the cell membrane, pass directly through the membrane, whereas

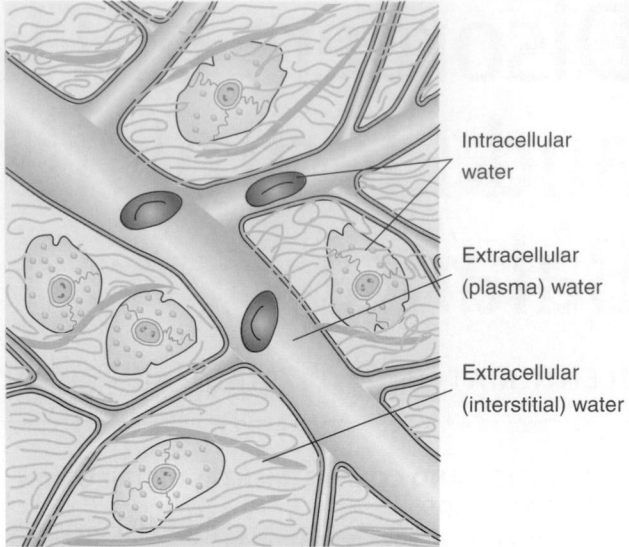

Intracellular water

Extracellular (plasma) water

Extracellular (interstitial) water

FIGURE 31-1 • Distribution of body water. The extracellular space includes the vascular compartment and the interstitial spaces.

many ions (*e.g.,* sodium [Na^+] and potassium [K^+]) rely on transport mechanisms such as the Na^+/K^+ pump located in the cell membrane for movement across the membrane. Because the Na^+/K^+ pump relies on adenosine triphosphate (ATP) and the enzyme ATPase for energy, it is often referred to as the Na^+/K^+-ATPase membrane pump. Water crosses the cell membrane by osmosis using special transmembrane protein channels called *aquaporins.*

Introductory Concepts

Dissociation of Electrolytes

Body fluids contain water and electrolytes. Electrolytes are substances that dissociate in solution to form charged particles, or *ions.* For example, a sodium chloride (NaCl) molecule dissociates to form a positively charged Na^+ and a negatively

TABLE 31-1 **Concentrations of Extracellular and Intracellular Electrolytes in Adults**				
	EXTRACELLULAR CONCENTRATION*		**INTRACELLULAR CONCENTRATION***	
ELECTROLYTE	Conventional Units	SI Units	Conventional Units	SI Units
Sodium	135–145 mEq/L	135–145 mmol/L	10–14 mEq/L	10–14 mmol/L
Potassium	3.5–5.0 mEq/L	3.5–5.0 mmol/L	140–150 mEq/L	140–150 mmol/L
Chloride	98–106 mEq/L	98–106 mmol/L	3–4 mEq/L	3–4 mmol/L
Bicarbonate	24–31 mEq/L	24–31 mmol/L	7–10 mEq/L	7–10 mmol/L
Calcium	8.5–10.5 mg/dL	2.1–2.6 mmol/L	<1 mEq/L	<0.25 mmol/L
Phosphorus	2.5–4.5 mg/dL	0.8–1.45 mmol/L	Variable	Variable
Magnesium	1.8–3.0 mg/dL	0.75–1.25 mmol/L	40 mEq/kg†	20 mmol/L

*Values may vary among laboratories, depending on the method of analysis used.
†Values vary among various tissues and with nutritional status.

charged Cl⁻ ion. Particles that do not dissociate into ions such as glucose and urea are called *nonelectrolytes*. Positively charged ions are called *cations* because they are attracted to the cathode of a wet electric cell, and negatively charged ions are called *anions* because they are attracted to the anode. The ions found in body fluids carry one charge (*i.e.*, monovalent ion) or two charges (*i.e.*, divalent ion). Because of their attraction forces, positively charged cations are always accompanied by negatively charged anions. Thus, all body fluids contain equal amounts of anions and cations. However, cations and anions may be exchanged one for another, providing they carry the same charge. For example, a positively charged H⁺ ion may be exchanged for a positively charged K⁺ ion, and a negatively charged HCO₃⁻ ion may be exchanged for a negatively charged Cl⁻ ion.

Diffusion and Osmosis

Diffusion. *Diffusion* is the movement of charged or uncharged particles along a concentration gradient. All molecules and ions, including water and dissolved molecules, are in constant random motion. It is the motion of these particles, each colliding with one another, that supplies the energy for diffusion. Because there are more molecules in constant motion in a concentrated solution, particles move from an area of higher concentration to one of lower concentration.

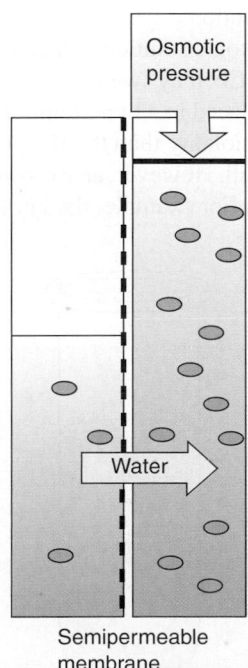

FIGURE 31-2 • Movement of water across a semipermeable membrane. Water moves from the side that has fewer nondiffusible particles to the side that has more. The osmotic pressure is equal to the hydrostatic pressure needed to oppose water movement across the membrane.

CLINICAL APPLICATION
Measurement Units

The amount of electrolytes and solutes in body fluids is expressed as a concentration or amount of solute in a given volume of fluid, such as milligrams per deciliter (mg/dL), milliequivalents per liter (mEq/L), or millimoles per liter (mmol/L). The *milligrams per deciliter* measurement unit expresses the weight of the solute in one tenth of a liter (dL) or 100 mL of solution. The concentration of electrolytes, such as calcium, phosphate, and magnesium, is often expressed in mg/dL.

The *milliequivalent* is used to express the charge equivalency for a given weight of an electrolyte. Electroneutrality requires that the total number of cations in the body equals the total number of anions. When cations and anions combine, they do so according to their ionic charge, not according to their atomic weight. Thus, 1 mEq of sodium has the same number of charges as 1 mEq of chloride, regardless of molecular weight (although sodium is positive and chloride is negative). The number of milliequivalents of an electrolyte in a liter of solution can be derived from the following equation:

$$mEq = \frac{mg/100\ mL \times 10 \times valence}{atomic\ weight}$$

The Système Internationale (SI) units express electrolyte content of body fluids in *millimoles per liter* (mmol/L). A millimole is one thousandth of a mole, or the molecular weight of a substance expressed in milligrams. The number of millimoles of an electrolyte in a liter of solution can be calculated using the following equation:

$$mmol/L = \frac{mEq/L}{valence}$$

For monovalent electrolytes such as sodium and potassium, the mmol and mEq values are identical. For example 140 mEq is equal to 140 mmol of sodium.

Osmosis. *Osmosis* is the movement of water across a semipermeable membrane (*i.e.*, one that is permeable to water but impermeable to most solutes). As with particles, water diffuses down its concentration gradient, moving from the side of the membrane with the lesser number of particles and greater concentration of water to the side with the greater number of particles and lesser concentration of water (Fig. 31-2). As water moves across the semipermeable membrane, it generates a pressure called the *osmotic pressure*. The magnitude of the osmotic pressure represents the hydrostatic pressure (measured in millimeters of mercury [mm Hg]) needed to oppose the movement of water across the membrane.

The osmotic activity that nondiffusible particles exert in pulling water from one side of the semipermeable membrane to the other is measured by a unit called an *osmole*. The osmole is derived from the gram molecular weight of a substance (*i.e.*,

1 gram molecular weight of a nondiffusible and nonionizable substance is equal to 1 osmole). In the clinical setting, osmotic activity usually is expressed in milliosmoles (one thousandth of an osmole) per liter. Each nondiffusible particle, large or small, is equally effective in its ability to pull water through a semipermeable membrane. Thus, it is the number, rather than the size, of the nondiffusible particles that determines the osmotic activity of a solution.

The osmotic activity of a solution may be expressed in terms of either its osmolarity or osmolality. *Osmolarity* refers to the osmolar concentration in 1 L of solution (mOsm/L) and *osmolality* to the osmolar concentration in 1 kg of water (mOsm/kg of H_2O). Osmolarity is usually used when referring to fluids outside the body and osmolality for describing fluids inside the body. Because 1 L of water weighs 1 kg, the terms *osmolarity* and *osmolality* are often used interchangeably.

The predominant osmotically active particles in the extracellular fluid are Na^+ and its attendant anions (Cl^- and HCO_3^-), which together account for 90% to 95% of the osmotic pressure. Blood urea nitrogen (BUN) and glucose, which also are osmotically active, account for less than 5% of the total osmotic pressure in the extracellular compartment. This can change, however, as when blood glucose levels are elevated in persons with diabetes mellitus or when BUN levels change rapidly in persons with chronic kidney disease. Serum osmolality, which normally ranges between 275 and 295 mOsm/kg, can be calculated using the following equation:

$$Osmolality\ (mOsm/kg) = 2[Na^+\ (mEg/L)]$$

$$+\frac{glucose\ (mg/dL)^*}{18} + \frac{BUN\ (mg/dL)^*}{2.8}$$

1 mOsm of glucose equals 180 mg/L,

and 1 mOsm of urea equals 28 mg/L

Ordinarily, the calculated and measured osmolality are within 10 mOsm of one another. The difference between the calculated and measured osmolality is called the *osmolar gap*. An osmolar gap larger than 10 mOsm suggests the presence of an unmeasured, osmotically active substance such as alcohol, acetone, or mannitol.

Tonicity. A change in water content causes cells to swell or shrink. The term *tonicity* refers to the tension or effect that the effective osmotic pressure of a solution with impermeable solutes exerts on cell size because of water movement across the cell membrane. An effective osmole is one that exerts an osmotic force and cannot permeate the cell membrane, whereas an ineffective osmole is one that exerts an osmotic force but crosses the cell membrane. Tonicity is determined solely by effective solutes such as glucose that cannot penetrate the cell membrane, thereby producing an osmotic force that pulls water out of the cell. In contrast, urea, which is osmotically active but lipid soluble, tends to distribute equally across the cell membrane. Therefore, when ECF levels of urea are elevated, ICF levels also are elevated. Urea is therefore considered to be an ineffective osmole. It is only when extracellular levels of urea

CLINICAL APPLICATION
Urine Osmolality

Urine osmolality reflects the kidneys' ability to produce a concentrated or diluted urine based on serum osmolality and the need for water conservation or excretion. The ratio of urine osmolality to serum osmolality in a 24-hour urine sample normally exceeds 1:1, and after a period of overnight water deprivation, it should be greater than 3:1. A dehydrated person (one who has a loss of water) may have a urine–serum ratio that approaches 4:1. In these persons, urine osmolality may exceed 1000 mOsm/kg H_2O. In those who have difficulty concentrating their urine (*e.g.*, those with diabetes insipidus or chronic renal failure), the urine–serum ratio often is less than or equal to 1:1.

Urine specific gravity compares the weight of urine with that of water, providing an index for solute concentration. Water is considered to be 1.000. A change in specific gravity of 1.010 to 1.020 is an increase of 400 mOsm/kg H_2O. In the sodium-depleted state, the kidneys usually try to conserve sodium, urine specific gravity is normal, and urine sodium and chloride concentrations are low.

change rapidly, as during hemodialysis treatment, that urea affects tonicity.

Solutions to which body cells are exposed can be classified as isotonic, hypotonic, or hypertonic depending on whether they cause cells to swell or shrink (Fig. 31-3). Cells placed in an isotonic solution, which has the same effective osmolality as the ICF (*i.e.*, 280 mOsm/L), neither shrink nor swell. An example of an isotonic solution is 0.9% sodium chloride. When cells are placed in a hypotonic solution, which has a lower effective osmolality than the ICF, they swell as water moves into the cell, and when they are placed in a hypertonic solution, which has a greater effective osmolality than the ICF, they shrink as water is pulled out of the cell. However, an iso-osmotic solution is not necessarily isotonic. For example, the intravenous administra-

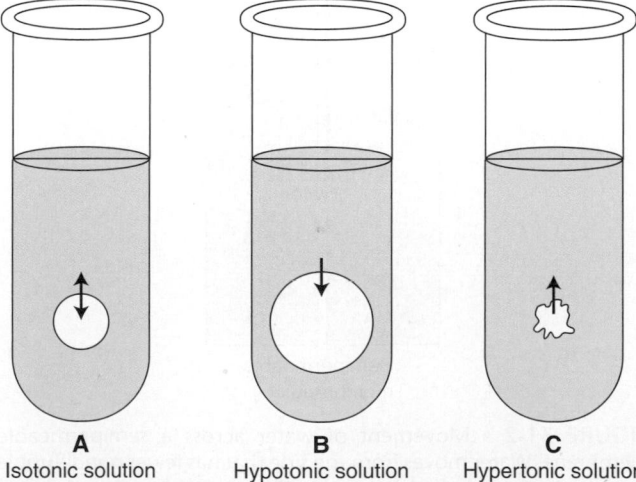

FIGURE 31-3 • Osmosis. **(A)** Red cells undergo no change in size in isotonic solutions. **(B)** They increase in size in hypotonic solutions and **(C)** decrease in size in hypertonic solutions.

tion of a solution of 5% dextrose in water, which is iso-osmotic, is equivalent to the infusion of a hypotonic solution of distilled water because the glucose is rapidly metabolized to carbon dioxide and water.

Compartmental Distribution of Body Fluids

Body water is distributed between the ICF and ECF compartments. In the adult, the fluid in the ICF compartment constitutes approximately 40% of body weight, and the ECF 20%.[1] The fluid in the ECF compartment is further divided into two major subdivisions: the plasma compartment, which constitutes approximately 5% of body weight, and the interstitial fluid compartment, which constitutes approximately 14% of body weight (Fig. 31-4).

A third, usually minor, subdivision of the ECF compartment is the transcellular compartment. It includes the cerebrospinal fluid and fluid contained in the various body spaces, such as the peritoneal, pleural, and pericardial cavities; the joint spaces; and the gastrointestinal tract. Normally, only approximately 1% of ECF is in the transcellular space. This amount can increase considerably in conditions such as ascites, in which large amounts of fluid are sequestered in the peritoneal cavity. When the transcellular fluid compartment becomes considerably enlarged, it is referred to as a *third space*, because this fluid is not readily available for exchange with the rest of the ECF.

Intracellular Fluid Volume

The ICF volume is regulated by proteins and organic compounds within the body cells and by water and solutes that move between the ECF and ICF. The membrane in most cells is freely permeable to water; therefore, water moves between the ECF and ICF as a result of osmosis. In contrast, osmotically active proteins and other organic compounds cannot pass through the membrane. Water entry into the cell is regulated by these osmotically active substances as well as by solutes such

as sodium and potassium that pass through the cell membrane. Many of the intracellular proteins are negatively charged and attract positively charged ions such as K^+, accounting for its higher concentration in the ICF. Na^+, which has a greater concentration in the ECF than the ICF, tends to enter the cell by diffusion. Na^+ is osmotically active and, if left unchecked, its entry would pull water into the cell until it ruptured. The reason this does not occur is because the Na^+/K^+-ATPase membrane pump continuously removes three Na^+ ions from the cell for every two K^+ ions that are moved back into the cell. Situations that impair the function of the Na^+/K^+-ATPase pump, such as hypoxia, cause cells to swell because of an accumulation of Na^+ ions.

The ICF volume is also affected by the concentration of osmotically active substances in the ECF that cannot cross the cell membrane. In diabetes mellitus, for example, glucose cannot enter the cell and its increased concentration in the ECF pulls water out of the cell. Some cells, such as those in the central nervous system (CNS), defend against significant shifts in fluid volume through a change in osmotically active intracellular molecules. As an initial compensatory mechanism to preserve cell volume, there is a rapid shift of sodium, potassium, chloride, and water out of brain cells in response to a decrease in ECF osmolality and into brain cells in response to an increase in ECF osmolality. After 48 to 72 hours, a slower adaptive process takes place, during which brain cells mobilize organic osmolytes, composed mainly of amino acids, in an effort to maintain a normal cellular volume.

Extracellular Fluid Volume

The ECF is divided between the vascular, interstitial, and transcellular fluid compartments. The vascular compartment contains blood, which is essential to the transport of substances such as electrolytes, gases, nutrients, and waste products throughout the body. The fluid in the interstitial spaces acts as a transport vehicle for gases, nutrients, wastes, and other materials that move between the vascular compartment and body cells. Interstitial fluid also provides a reservoir from which the vascular volume can be maintained during periods of hemorrhage or loss of vascular fluid. A tissue gel, which is a spongelike material composed of large quantities of proteoglycan filaments, fills the tissue spaces and aids in even distribution of interstitial fluid[2] (see Fig. 31-1). Normally, most of the fluid in the interstitium is in gel form. The tissue gel is supported by collagen fibers that hold the gel in place. The tissue gel, which has a firmer consistency than water, opposes the outflow of water from the capillaries and helps to prevent the accumulation of free water in the interstitial spaces.

Capillary–Interstitial Fluid Exchange

The transfer of water between the vascular and interstitial compartments occurs at the capillary level. Four forces control the movement of water between the capillary and interstitial spaces: (1) the capillary filtration pressure, which pushes water out of the capillary into the interstitial spaces; (2) the capillary colloidal osmotic pressure, which pulls water back into the capillary; (3) the interstitial hydrostatic pressure, which opposes the

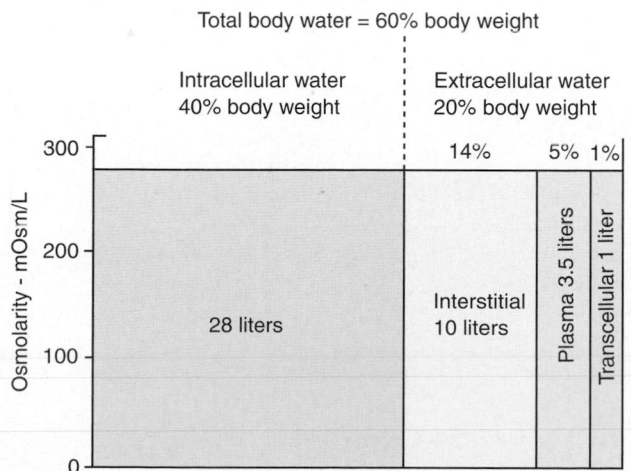

FIGURE 31-4 • Approximate sizes of body compartments in a 70-kg adult.

Understanding • Capillary Fluid Exchange

Movement of fluid between the vascular compartment and the interstitial fluid compartment surrounding the body cells occurs at the capillary level. The direction and amount of fluid that flows across the capillary wall are determined by: (1) the hydrostatic pressure of the two compartments, (2) the colloidal osmotic pressures of the two compartments, and (3) the removal of excess fluid and osmotically active particles from the interstitial spaces by the lymphatic system.

❶ Hydrostatic Pressure

The hydrostatic pressure is the pushing force exerted by a fluid. Inside the capillaries, the hydrostatic pressure is the same as the capillary filtration pressure, about 30 mm Hg at the arterial end and 10 mm Hg at the venous end. The interstitial fluid pressure is the force of fluid in the interstitial spaces pushing against the outside of the capillary wall. Evidence suggests that the interstitial pressure is slightly negative (−3 mm Hg), contributing to the outward movement of fluid from the capillary.

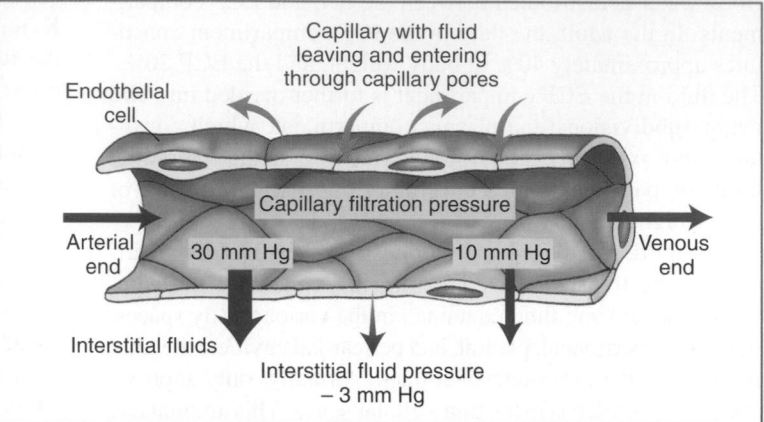

❷ Colloidal Osmotic Pressure

The colloidal osmotic pressure is the pulling force created by the presence of evenly dispersed particles, such as the plasma proteins, that cannot pass through the pores of the capillary membrane. The capillary colloidal osmotic pressure is normally about 28 mm Hg throughout the length of the capillary bed. The interstitial colloidal osmotic pressure (about 8 mm Hg) represents the pulling pressure exerted by the small amounts of plasma proteins that leak through the pores of the capillary wall into the interstitial spaces. The capillary colloidal osmotic pressure, which is greater than both the hydrostatic pressure at the venous end of the capillary and the interstitial colloidal osmotic pressure, is largely responsible for the movement of fluid back into the capillary.

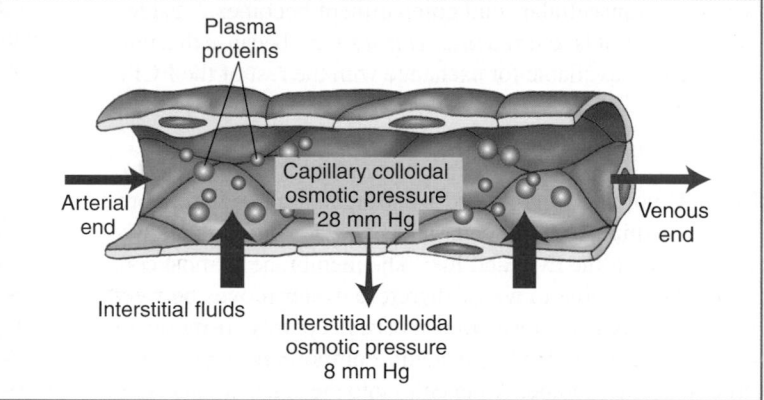

❸ Lymph Drainage

The lymphatic system represents an accessory system by which fluid can be returned to the circulatory system. Normally the forces moving fluid out of the capillary into the interstitium are greater than those returning fluid to the capillary. Any excess fluids and osmotically active plasma proteins that may have leaked into the interstitium are picked up by vessels of the lymphatic system and returned to the circulation. Without the function of the lymphatic system, excessive amounts of fluid would accumulate in the interstitial spaces.

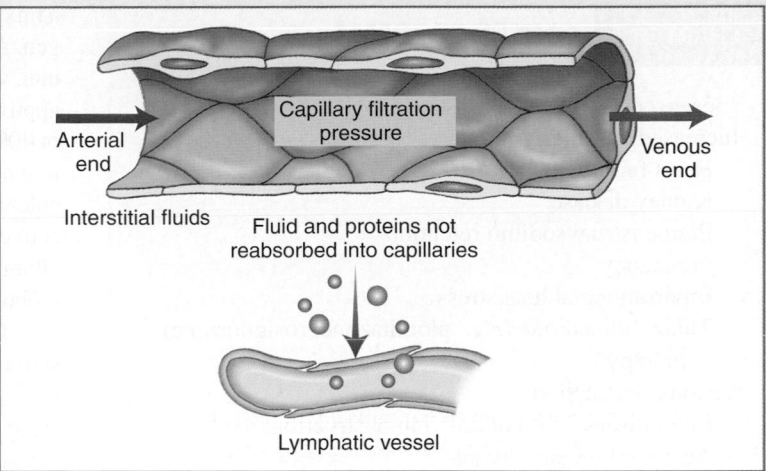

movement of water out of the capillary; and (4) the tissue colloidal osmotic pressure, which pulls water out of the capillary into the interstitial spaces. Normally, the combination of these four forces is such that only a small excess of fluid remains in the interstitial compartment. This excess fluid is removed from the interstitium by the lymphatic system and returned to the systemic circulation. The capillary–interstitial fluid exchange and lymphatic system are further discussed in Chapter 21.

Capillary filtration refers to the movement of water through capillary pores because of a mechanical, rather than an osmotic, force. The capillary filtration pressure (about 30 to 40 mm Hg at the arterial end, 10 to 15 mm Hg at the venous end, and 25 mm Hg in the middle), sometimes called the *capillary hydrostatic pressure,* is the pressure pushing water out of the capillary into the interstitial spaces. It reflects the arterial and venous pressures, the precapillary (arterioles) and postcapillary (venules) resistances, and the force of gravity.[2] A rise in arterial or venous pressure increases capillary pressure. The force of gravity increases capillary pressure in the dependent parts of the body. In a person who is standing absolutely still, the weight of blood in the vascular column causes an increase of 1 mm Hg in pressure for every 13.6 mm of distance from the heart.[2] This pressure results from the weight of water and is therefore called *hydrostatic pressure*. In the adult who is standing absolutely still, the pressure in the veins of the feet can reach 90 mm Hg. This pressure is then transmitted to the capillaries.

The *capillary colloidal osmotic pressure* (about 28 mm Hg) is the osmotic pressure generated by the plasma proteins that are too large to pass through the pores of the capillary wall.[2] The term *colloidal osmotic pressure* differentiates this type of osmotic pressure from the osmotic pressure that develops at the cell membrane from the presence of electrolytes and nonelectrolytes. Because plasma proteins do not normally penetrate the capillary pores and because their concentration is greater in the plasma than in the interstitial fluids, it is the capillary colloidal osmotic pressure that pulls fluids back into the capillary.

The interstitial fluid pressure (about −3 mm Hg) and the tissue colloidal osmotic pressure (about 8 mm Hg) contribute to movement of water into and out of the interstitial spaces.[2] The interstitial fluid pressure, which is normally negative, con-

tributes to the outward movement of water into the interstitial spaces. The tissue colloidal osmotic pressure, which reflects the small amount of plasma proteins that normally escape into the interstitial spaces from the capillary, also pulls water out of the capillary into the tissue spaces.

The lymphatic system represents an accessory route whereby fluid from the interstitial spaces can return to the circulation. More important, the lymphatic system provides a means for removing plasma proteins and osmotically active particulate matter from the tissue spaces, neither of which can be reabsorbed into the capillaries.

Edema

Edema can be defined as palpable swelling produced by expansion of the interstitial fluid volume. Edema does not become evident until the interstitial volume has been increased by 2.5 to 3 L.[3] The physiologic mechanisms that contribute to edema formation include factors that (1) increase the capillary filtration pressure, (2) decrease the capillary colloidal osmotic pressure, (3) increase capillary permeability, or (4) produce obstruction to lymph flow.[4] The causes of edema are summarized in Chart 31-1.

Increased Capillary Filtration Pressure. As the capillary filtration pressure rises, the movement of vascular fluid into the interstitial spaces increases. Among the factors that increase capillary pressure are (1) increased arterial pressure or decreased resistance to flow through the precapillary sphincters, (2) an increase in venous pressure or increased resistance to outflow at the postcapillary sphincter, and (3) capillary distention due to increased vascular volume.

Edema can be either localized or generalized. The localized edema that occurs with urticaria (*i.e.,* hives) or other allergic or inflammatory conditions results from the release of histamine and other inflammatory mediators that cause dilation of the precapillary sphincters and arterioles that supply the swollen lesions. Thrombophlebitis obstructs venous flow, producing an elevation of venous pressure and edema of the affected part, usually one of the lower extremities.

CHART 31-1   CAUSES OF EDEMA

Increased Capillary Pressure
Increased vascular volume
   Heart failure
   Kidney disease
   Premenstrual sodium retention
   Pregnancy
   Environmental heat stress
   Thiazolidinedione (*e.g.,* pioglitazone, rosiglitazone)
     therapy
Venous obstruction
   Liver disease with portal vein obstruction
   Acute pulmonary edema
   Venous thrombosis (thrombophlebitis)
Decreased arteriolar resistance
   Calcium channel–blocking drug responses

Decreased Colloidal Osmotic Pressure
Increased loss of plasma proteins
   Protein-losing kidney diseases
   Extensive burns
Decreased production of plasma proteins
   Liver disease
   Starvation, malnutrition

Increased Capillary Permeability
Inflammation
Allergic reactions (*e.g.,* hives, angioneurotic edema)
Malignancy (*e.g.,* ascites, pleural effusion)
Tissue injury and burns

Obstruction of Lymphatic Flow
Malignant obstruction of lymphatic structures
Surgical removal of lymph nodes

Generalized edema (termed *anasarca*) is generally the result of increased vascular volume. The swelling of hands and feet that occurs in healthy persons during hot weather is an example of edema that is caused by the vasodilation of superficial blood vessels along with sodium and water retention. Generalized edema is common in conditions such as congestive heart failure that produce fluid retention and venous congestion. In right-sided heart failure, blood dams up throughout the entire venous system, causing organ congestion and edema of the dependent extremities (discussed in Chapter 26).

Because of the effects of gravity, edema resulting from increased capillary pressure commonly causes fluid to accumulate in the dependent parts of the body, a condition referred to as *dependent edema.* For example, edema of the ankles and feet becomes more pronounced during prolonged periods of standing.

Decreased Capillary Colloidal Osmotic Pressure. Plasma proteins exert the osmotic force needed to pull fluid back into the capillary from the tissue spaces. The plasma proteins constitute a mixture of proteins, including albumin, globulins, and fibrinogen. Albumin, the smallest of the plasma proteins, has a molecular weight of 69,000; globulins have molecular weights of approximately 140,000; and fibrinogen has a molecular weight of 400,000.[2] Because of its lower molecular weight, 1 g of albumin has approximately twice as many osmotically active molecules as 1 g of globulin and almost six times as many osmotically active molecules as 1 g of fibrinogen. Also, the concentration of albumin (approximately 4.5 g/dL) is greater than that of the globulins (2.5 g/dL) and fibrinogen (0.3 mg/dL).

Edema due to decreased capillary colloidal osmotic pressure usually is the result of inadequate production or abnormal loss of plasma proteins, mainly albumin. The plasma proteins are synthesized in the liver. In persons with severe liver failure, the impaired synthesis of albumin results in a decrease in colloidal osmotic pressure. In starvation and malnutrition, edema develops because there is a lack of amino acids for plasma protein synthesis.

The most common site of plasma protein loss is the kidney. In kidney diseases such as glomerulonephritis, the glomerular capillaries become permeable to the plasma proteins, particularly albumin, which is the smallest of the proteins. When this happens, large amounts of albumin are filtered out of the blood and lost in the urine. An excessive loss of plasma proteins also occurs when large areas of skin are injured or destroyed. Edema is a common problem during the early stages of a burn, resulting from capillary injury and loss of plasma proteins.[5]

Because the plasma proteins are evenly distributed throughout the body and are not affected by the force of gravity, edema due to a decrease in capillary colloidal osmotic pressure tends to affect tissues in nondependent as well as dependent parts of the body. There is swelling of the face as well as the legs and feet.

Increased Capillary Permeability. When the capillary pores become enlarged or the integrity of the capillary wall is damaged, capillary permeability is increased. When this occurs, plasma proteins and other osmotically active particles leak into the interstitial spaces, increasing the tissue colloidal osmotic pressure and thereby contributing to the accumulation of interstitial fluid. Among the conditions that increase capillary permeability are burn injury, capillary congestion, inflammation, and immune responses.

Obstruction of Lymph Flow. Osmotically active plasma proteins and other large particles that cannot be reabsorbed through the pores in the capillary membrane rely on the lymphatic system for movement back into the circulatory system. Edema due to impaired lymph flow is commonly referred to as *lymphedema.*[6] Malignant involvement of lymph structures and removal of lymph nodes at the time of cancer surgery are common causes of lymphedema. Another cause of lymphedema is infection and trauma involving the lymphatic channels and lymph nodes.

Manifestations. The effects of edema are determined largely by its location. Edema of the brain, larynx, or lungs is an acute, life-threatening condition. Although not life-threatening, edema may interfere with movement, limiting joint motion. Swelling of the ankles and feet often is insidious in onset and may or may not be associated with disease. At the tissue level, edema increases the distance for diffusion of oxygen, nutrients, and wastes. Edematous tissues usually are more susceptible to injury and development of ischemic tissue damage, including pressure ulcers. Edema can also compress blood vessels. The skin of a severely swollen finger can act as a tourniquet, shutting off the blood flow to the finger. Edema can also be disfiguring, causing psychological effects and disturbances in self-concept. It can also create problems with obtaining proper-fitting clothing and shoes.

Pitting edema occurs when the accumulation of interstitial fluid exceeds the absorptive capacity of the tissue gel. In this form of edema, the tissue water becomes mobile and can be translocated with pressure exerted by a finger. *Nonpitting edema* usually reflects a condition in which plasma proteins have accumulated in the tissue spaces and coagulated. It is seen most commonly in areas of localized infection or trauma. The area often is firm and discolored. *Brawny edema* is a type of nonpitting edema in which the skin thickens and hardens.

Assessment and Treatment. Methods for assessing edema include daily weight, visual assessment, measurement of the affected part, and application of finger pressure to assess for pitting edema. Daily weight performed at the same time each day with the same amount of clothing provides a useful index of water gain (1 L of water weighs 1 kg [2.2 lb]) due to edema. Visual inspection and measurement of the circumference of an extremity can also be used to assess the degree of swelling. This is particularly useful when swelling is due to thrombophlebitis. Finger pressure can be used to assess the degree of pitting edema. If an indentation remains after the finger has been removed, pitting edema is identified. It is evaluated on a scale of +1 (minimal) to +4 (severe; Fig. 31-5).

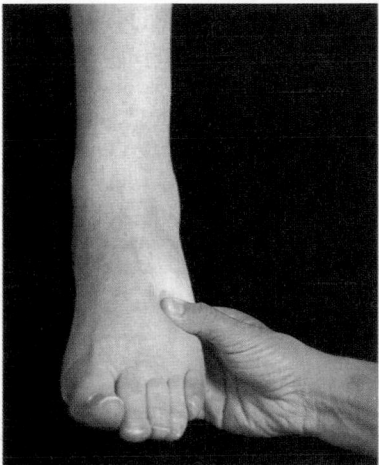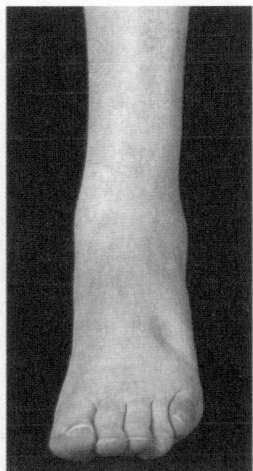

FIGURE 31-5 • 3+ pitting edema of the left foot. (Used with permission from Bates B., Bickley L. S., Hoekelman R. A. [1995]. *A guide to physical examination and history taking* [6th ed., p. 438]. Philadelphia: J. B. Lippincott.)

Distinguishing lymphedema from other forms of edema can be challenging, especially early in its course. Papillomatosis, a characteristic honeycomb appearance of the skin due to dilated lymph vessels that are enveloped in fibrotic tissue, distinguishes lymphedema from other edemas. Computed tomography (CT) or magnetic resonance imaging (MRI) may be used to confirm the diagnosis.[4,6]

Treatment of edema usually is directed toward maintaining life when the swelling involves vital structures, correcting or controlling the cause, and preventing tissue injury. Edema of the lower extremities may respond to simple measures such as elevating the feet. Diuretic therapy commonly is used to treat edema associated with an increase in ECF volume. Serum albumin levels can be measured, and albumin may be administered intravenously to raise the plasma colloidal osmotic pressure when edema is caused by hypoalbuminemia.

Elastic support stockings and sleeves increase interstitial fluid pressure and resistance to outward movement of fluid from the capillary into the tissue spaces. These support devices typically are prescribed for patients with conditions such as lymphatic or venous obstruction and are most efficient if applied before the tissue spaces have filled with fluid—in the morning, for example, before the effects of gravity have caused fluid to move into the ankles. Moderate to severe lymphedema is usually treated with light-pressure massage designed to increase lymph flow by encouraging opening and closing of lymph vessel valves; compression garments or pneumatic compression pumps; range-of-motion exercises; and scrupulous skin care to prevent infection.[4,6]

Third-Space Accumulation

Third spacing represents the loss or trapping of ECF into the transcellular space. The serous cavities are part of the transcellular compartment (*i.e.,* third space) located in strategic body areas where there is continual movement of body structures—the pericardial sac, the peritoneal cavity, and the pleural cavity. The exchange of ECF between the capillaries, the interstitial spaces, and the transcellular space of the serous cavity uses the same mechanisms as capillaries elsewhere in the body. The serous cavities are closely linked with lymphatic drainage systems. The milking action of the moving structures, such as the lungs, continually forces fluid and plasma proteins back into the circulation, keeping these cavities empty. Any obstruction to lymph flow causes fluid accumulation in the serous cavities. As with edema fluid, third-space fluids represent an accumulation or trapping of body fluids that contribute to body weight but not to fluid reserve or function.

The prefix *hydro-* may be used to indicate the presence of excessive fluid, as in *hydrothorax,* which means excessive fluid in the pleural cavity. The accumulation of fluid in the peritoneal cavity is called *ascites.* The transudation of fluid into the serous cavities is also referred to as *effusion.* Effusion can contain blood, plasma proteins, inflammatory cells (*i.e.,* pus), and ECF.

IN SUMMARY, body fluids, which contain water and electrolytes, are distributed between the ICF and ECF compartments of the body. Two thirds of body fluid is contained in the body cells of the ICF compartment and one third is contained in the vascular compartment, interstitial spaces, and third-space areas of the ECF compartment. The ICF has high concentrations of potassium, calcium, phosphorus, and magnesium, and the ECF high concentrations of sodium, chloride, and bicarbonate.

Electrolytes and nonelectrolytes move by diffusion across cell membranes that separate the ICF and ECF compartments. Water crosses the cell membrane by osmosis, using special protein channels called *aquaporins*. It moves from the side of the membrane that has the lesser number of particles and greater concentration of water to the side that has the greater number of particles and lesser concentration of water. The osmotic tension or effect that a solution exerts on cell volume in terms of causing the cell to swell or shrink is called *tonicity*.

Edema represents an increase in interstitial fluid volume. The physiologic mechanisms that contribute to the development of edema include factors that (1) increase capillary filtration pressure, (2) decrease capillary colloidal osmotic pressure, (3) increase capillary permeability, and (4) obstruct lymphatic flow. The effect that edema exerts on body function is determined by its location. Edema of the brain, larynx, or lungs is an acute, life-threatening situation, whereas swelling of the ankles and feet can be a normal discomfort that accompanies hot weather. Fluid can also accumulate in the transcellular compartment—the joint spaces, pericardial sac, the peritoneal cavity, and the pleural cavity. Because this fluid is not easily exchanged with the rest of the ECF, it is often referred to as third-space fluid. ■

CONCEPTSin action**ANIMATI⚙N**

SODIUM AND WATER BALANCE

After completing this section of the chapter, you should be able to meet the following objectives:

■ State the functions and physiologic mechanisms controlling body water levels and sodium concentration, including the effective circulating volume, sympathetic nervous system, renin-angiotensin-aldosterone system, and antidiuretic hormone.

■ Describe measures that can be used in assessing body fluid levels and sodium concentration.

■ Describe the causes, manifestations, and treatment of psychogenic polydipsia.

■ Describe the relationship between antidiuretic hormone and aquaporin-2 channels in reabsorption of water by the kidney.

■ Compare the pathology, manifestations, and treatment of diabetes insipidus and the syndrome of inappropriate antidiuretic hormone.

■ Compare and contrast the causes, manifestations, and treatment of isotonic fluid volume deficit, isotonic fluid volume excess, hyponatremia with water excess, and hypernatremia with water deficit.

The movement of body fluids between the ICF and ECF compartments occurs at the cell membrane and depends on ECF levels of water and sodium. Water provides approximately 90% to 93% of the volume of body fluids and sodium salts approximately 90% to 95% of ECF solutes. Normally, equivalent changes in sodium and water are such that the volume and osmolality of ECF are maintained within a normal range. Because it is the concentration of sodium that controls ECF osmolality, changes in sodium are usually accompanied by proportionate changes in water volume.

Body Water Balance

Total body water (TBW) varies with sex and weight. These differences can be explained by differences in body fat, which is essentially water free (*i.e.*, fat is approximately 10% water by composition, compared with 75% for skeletal muscle). In men, TBW approximates 60% of body weight during young adulthood and decreases to approximately 50% in old age; in young women it is approximately 50% and in elderly women approximately 40%.[7] Obesity produces further decreases in TBW, sometimes reducing these levels to values as low as 30% to 40% of body weight in adults (Fig. 31-6).

Infants normally have more TBW than older children or adults. TBW constitutes approximately 75% to 80% of body weight in full-term infants and an even greater proportion in premature infants. In addition to having proportionately more body water than adults, infants have relatively more water in their ECF compartment. Infants have more than half of their TBW in the ECF compartment, whereas adults have only approximately one third.[8] The greater ECF water content of an infant can be explained in terms of its higher metabolic rate, larger surface area in relation to body mass, and its inability to concentrate urine because of immature kidney structures. Because ECFs are more readily lost from the body, infants are more vulnerable to fluid deficit than older children and adults. As an infant grows older, TBW decreases, and by the second year of life, the percentages and distribution of body water approach those of an adult.[8]

Gains and Losses

Regardless of age, all healthy persons require approximately 100 mL of water per 100 calories metabolized for dissolving and eliminating metabolic wastes. This means that a person who expends 1800 calories for energy requires approximately 1800 mL of water for metabolic purposes. The metabolic rate increases with fever; it rises approximately 12% for every 1°C

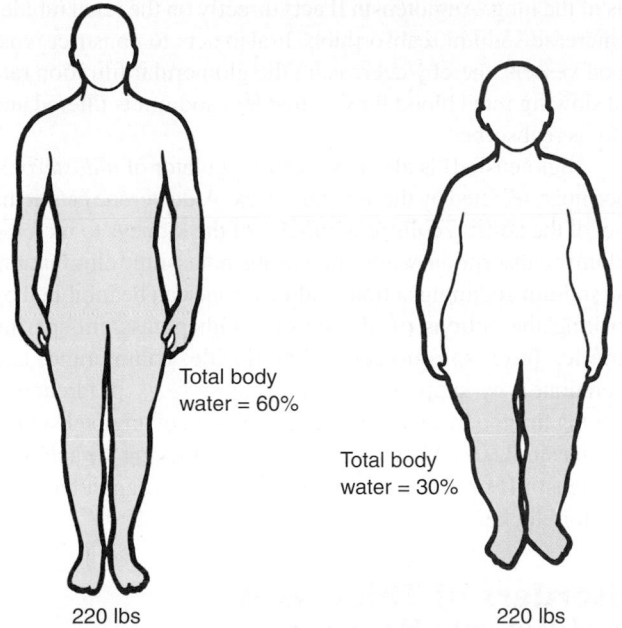

FIGURE 31-6 • Body composition of a lean and an obese individual. (Adapted with permission from Statland H. [1963]. *Fluids and electrolytes in practice* [3rd ed.]. Philadelphia: J. B. Lippincott.)

TABLE 31-2 **Sources of Body Water Gains and Losses in the Adult**			
GAINS		**LOSSES**	
Oral intake		Urine	1500 mL
As water	1000 mL	Insensible losses	
In food	1300 mL	Lungs	300 mL
Water of	200 mL	Skin	500 mL
oxidation		Feces	200 mL
Total	2500 mL	Total	2500 mL

that enters the cell is transported out of the cell against an electrochemical gradient by the Na^+/K^+-ATPase membrane pump.

Sodium functions mainly in regulating the ECF volume. As the major cation in the ECF compartment, Na^+ and its attendant anions (Cl^- and HCO_3^-) account for approximately 90% to 95% of the osmotic activity in the ECF. Because sodium is part of the sodium bicarbonate molecule, it is important in regulating acid-base balance. As a current-carrying ion, Na^+ contributes to the function of the nervous system and other excitable tissue.

Gains and Losses

Sodium normally enters the body through the gastrointestinal tract and is eliminated by the kidneys or lost from the gastrointestinal tract or skin. Sodium intake normally is derived from dietary sources. Body needs for sodium usually can be met by as little as 500 mg/day. The average salt intake is approximately 6 to 15 g/day, or 12 to 30 times the daily requirement. Dietary intake, which frequently exceeds the amount needed by the body, is often influenced by culture and food preferences rather than need. As package labels indicate, many commercially prepared foods and soft drinks contain considerable amounts of sodium. Other sources of sodium are intravenous saline infusions and medications that contain sodium.

Most sodium losses occur through the kidneys. The kidneys are extremely efficient in regulating sodium output, and when sodium intake is limited or conservation of sodium is needed, the kidneys are able to reabsorb almost all the sodium that has been filtered by the glomerulus. This results in essentially sodium-free urine. Conversely, urinary losses of sodium increase as intake increases.

Usually less than 10% of sodium intake is lost through the gastrointestinal tract and skin. Although the sodium concentration of fluids in the upper part of the gastrointestinal tract approaches that of the ECF, sodium is reabsorbed as the fluids move through the lower part of the bowel, so that the concentration of sodium in the stool is only approximately 40 mEq/L (40 mmol/L). Sodium losses increase with conditions such as vomiting, diarrhea, fistula drainage, and gastrointestinal suction that remove sodium from the gastrointestinal tract. Irrigation of gastrointestinal tubes with distilled water removes sodium from the gastrointestinal tract, as do repeated tap water enemas.

Sodium leaves the skin through the sweat glands. Sweat is a hypotonic solution containing both sodium and chloride.

(7% for every 1°F) increase in body temperature.[2] Fever also increases the respiratory rate, resulting in additional loss of water vapor through the lungs.

The main source of water gain is through oral intake and metabolism of nutrients. Water, including that obtained from liquids and solid foods, is absorbed from the gastrointestinal tract. Tube feedings and parenterally administered fluids are also sources of water gain. Metabolic processes also generate a small amount of water. The amount of water gained from these processes varies from 150 to 300 mL/day, depending on the metabolic rate.

Normally, the largest loss of water occurs through the kidneys, with lesser amounts being lost through the skin, lungs, and gastrointestinal tract. Even when oral or parenteral fluids are withheld, the kidneys continue to produce urine as a means of ridding the body of metabolic wastes. The urine output that is required to eliminate these wastes is called the *obligatory urine output*. The obligatory urine loss is approximately 300 to 500 mL/day. Water losses that occur through the skin and lungs are referred to as *insensible water losses* because they occur without a person's awareness. The gains and losses of body water are summarized in Table 31-2.

Sodium Balance

Sodium is the most abundant cation in the body, averaging approximately 60 mEq/kg of body weight.[9] Most of the body's sodium is in the ECF compartment (135 to 145 mEq/L [135 to 145 mmol/L]), with only a small amount (10 to 14 mEq/L [10 to 14 mmol/L]) located in the ICF compartment. The resting cell membrane is relatively impermeable to sodium; sodium

Although sodium losses due to sweating are usually negligible, they can increase greatly during exercise and periods of exposure to a hot environment. A person who sweats profusely can lose up to 15 to 30 g of salt each day for first few days of exposure to a hot environment. This amount usually drops to less than 3 to 5 g a day after 4 to 6 weeks of acclimatization.[2]

Mechanisms of Regulation

The major regulator of sodium and water balance is the maintenance of the *effective circulating volume* (also termed the *effective arterial blood volume*), which can be described as that portion of the ECF that fills the vascular compartment and is "effectively" perfusing the tissues.[9,10] A low effective circulating volume activates feedback mechanisms that produce an increase in renal sodium and water retention, and a high effective circulating volume triggers feedback mechanisms that decrease sodium and water retention.

The effective circulating volume is monitored by a number of sensors that are located in both the vascular system and the kidney. These sensors are commonly referred to as *baroreceptors* because they respond to pressure-induced stretch of the vessel walls in which they are located.[10] There are baroreceptors located in the low-pressure side of the circulation (walls of the cardiac atria and large pulmonary vessels) that respond primarily to fullness of the circulation. Baroreceptors are also present in the high-pressure arterial side of the circulation (aortic arch and carotid sinus) that respond primarily to changes in the arterial pressure. The activity of both types of receptors regulates renal sodium and water elimination by modulating sympathetic nervous system outflow and antidiuretic hormone (ADH) secretion.[10] The sympathetic nervous system responds to changes in arterial pressure and blood volume by adjusting the glomerular filtration rate and thus the rate at which sodium is filtered from the blood. Sympathetic activity also regulates tubular reabsorption of sodium and renin release. An additional mechanism related to renal sodium excretion is atrial natriuretic peptide (ANP), which is released from cells in the atria of the heart. ANP, which is released in response to atrial stretch and overfilling, increases sodium excretion by the kidney[3] (see Chapter 30).

Pressure-sensitive receptors in the kidney, particularly in the afferent arterioles, respond directly to changes in arterial pressure through stimulation of the sympathetic nervous system and release of renin with activation of the renin-angiotensin-aldosterone system (RAAS).[11] The RAAS exerts its action through angiotensin II and aldosterone. Renin is a small protein enzyme that is released by the kidney in response to changes in arterial pressure, the glomerular filtration rate, and the amount of sodium in the tubular fluid. Most of the renin that is released leaves the kidney and enters the bloodstream, where it interacts enzymatically to convert a circulating plasma protein called *angiotensinogen* to angiotensin I (see Chapter 23, Fig. 23-5).

Angiotensin I is rapidly converted to angiotensin II by the angiotensin-converting enzyme (ACE) in the small blood vessels of the lung. Angiotensin II acts directly on the renal tubules to increase sodium reabsorption. It also acts to constrict renal blood vessels, thereby decreasing the glomerular filtration rate and slowing renal blood flow so that less sodium is filtered and more is reabsorbed.

Angiotensin II is also a powerful regulator of *aldosterone,* a hormone secreted by the adrenal cortex. Aldosterone acts at the level of the cortical collecting tubules of the kidneys to increase sodium reabsorption while increasing potassium elimination. The sodium-retaining action of aldosterone can be inhibited by blocking the actions of aldosterone with potassium-sparing diuretics (*e.g.,* spironolactone, amiloride, triamterene, and eplerenone), by suppressing renin release (*e.g.,* β-adrenergic blocking drugs), by inhibiting the conversion of angiotensin I to angiotensin II (*i.e.,* ACE inhibitors), or by blocking the action of angiotensin II on the angiotensin receptor (*i.e.,* angiotensin II receptor blockers).[11]

Disorders of Thirst and Antidiuretic Hormone

Two other mechanisms that contribute directly to the regulation of body water and indirectly to the regulation of sodium are thirst and ADH. Thirst is primarily a regulator of water intake and ADH a regulator of water output. Both mechanisms respond to changes in extracellular osmolality and the effective circulating volume (Fig. 31-7).

Disorders of Thirst

Like appetite and eating, thirst and drinking behavior are two separate entities.[12,13] Thirst is the conscious sensation of the need to obtain and drink fluids high in water content. Drinking of water or other fluids often occurs as the result of habit or for reasons other than those related to thirst. Most people drink without being thirsty, and water is consumed before it is needed. As a result, thirst is basically an emergency response. It usually occurs only when the need for water has not been anticipated.

Thirst is controlled by the thirst center in the hypothalamus. There are two stimuli for true thirst based on water need: (1) cellular dehydration caused by an increase in ECF osmolality; and (2) a decrease in blood volume, which may or may not be associated with a decrease in serum osmolality. Sensory neurons, called *osmoreceptors,* which are located in or near the thirst center in the hypothalamus, respond to changes in ECF osmolality by swelling or shrinking (see Fig. 31-7). Thirst normally develops when there is as little as a 1% to 2% change in serum osmolality.[13] The previously described stretch receptors in the vascular system that monitor the effective circulating volume also aid in the regulation of thirst. Thirst is one of the earliest symptoms of hemorrhage and is often present before other signs of blood loss appear.

A third important stimulus for thirst is angiotensin II, levels of which increase in response to low blood volume and low blood pressure. The renin-angiotensin mechanism contributes to nonosmotic thirst. This system is considered a backup sys-

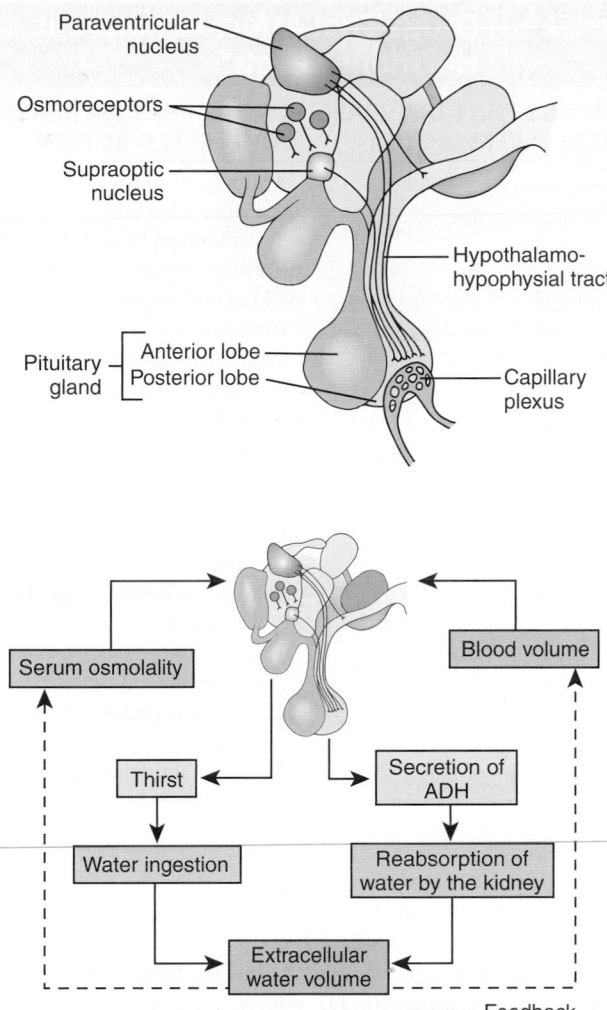

FIGURE 31-7 • **(Top)** Sagittal section through the pituitary and anterior hypothalamus. Antidiuretic hormone (ADH) is formed primarily in the supraoptic nucleus and to a lesser extent in the paraventricular nucleus of the hypothalamus. It is then transported down the hypothalamohypophysial tract and stored in secretory granules in the posterior pituitary, where it can be released into the blood. **(Bottom)** Pathways for regulation of extracellular water volume by thirst and ADH.

tem for thirst should other systems fail. Because it is a backup system, it probably does not contribute to the regulation of normal thirst. However, elevated levels of angiotensin II may lead to thirst in conditions, such as chronic kidney disease and congestive heart failure, in which renin levels may be elevated.

Dryness of the mouth, such as the thirst a lecturer experiences during speaking, produces a sensation of thirst that is not necessarily associated with the body's hydration status. Thirst sensation also occurs in those who breathe through their mouths, such as smokers and persons with chronic respiratory disease or hyperventilation syndrome.

Hypodipsia. Hypodipsia represents a decrease in the ability to sense thirst. It is commonly associated with lesions in the area of the hypothalamus (*e.g.,* head trauma, meningiomas,

occult hydrocephalus, subarachnoid hemorrhage). There is also evidence that thirst is decreased and water intake reduced in elderly persons, despite higher plasma sodium and osmolality levels.[14–16] The inability to perceive and respond to thirst is compounded in elderly persons who have had a stroke and may be further influenced by confusion, sensory deficits, and motor disturbances.

Polydipsia. Polydipsia, or excessive thirst, is normal when it accompanies conditions of water deficit. Increased thirst and drinking behavior can be classified into three categories: (1) symptomatic or true thirst, (2) inappropriate or false thirst that occurs despite normal levels of body water and serum osmolality, and (3) compulsive water drinking. *Symptomatic thirst* develops when there is a loss of body water and resolves after the loss has been replaced. Among the most common causes of symptomatic thirst are water losses associated with diarrhea, vomiting, diabetes mellitus, and diabetes insipidus. *Inappropriate or excessive thirst* may persist despite adequate hydration. It is a common complaint in persons with congestive heart failure and chronic kidney disease. Although the cause of thirst in these persons is unclear, it may result from increased angiotensin levels. Thirst is also a common complaint in persons with dry mouth caused by decreased salivary function or treatment with drugs with an anticholinergic action (*e.g.,* antihistamines, atropine) that lead to decreased salivary flow.

Psychogenic polydipsia involves compulsive water drinking and is usually seen in persons with psychiatric disorders, most commonly schizophrenia. Persons with the disorder drink large amounts of water and excrete large amounts of urine. The cause of excessive water drinking in these persons is uncertain. It has been suggested it may share the same pathologic process as the psychosis because persons with the disorder often increase their water drinking during periods of exacerbation of their psychotic symptoms.[17] The condition may be compounded by antipsychotic medications that increase ADH levels and interfere with water excretion by the kidneys. Cigarette smoking, which is common among persons with psychiatric disorders, also stimulates ADH secretion. Excessive water ingestion coupled with impaired water excretion (or rapid ingestion at a rate that exceeds renal excretion) in persons with psychogenic polydipsia can lead to water intoxication (see section on Hyponatremia). Treatment usually consists of water restriction and behavioral measures aimed at decreasing water consumption. Measurements of body weight can be used to provide an estimate of water consumption.[18]

Disorders of Antidiuretic Hormone

The reabsorption of water by the kidneys is regulated by ADH, also known as *vasopressin*. ADH is synthesized by cells in the supraoptic and paraventricular nuclei of the hypothalamus and then transported along a neural pathway (*i.e.,* hypothalamohypophysial tract) to the posterior pituitary gland, where it is stored. When the supraoptic and paraventricular nuclei in the hypothalamus are stimulated by increased serum osmolality or other factors, nerve impulses travel down the hypothalamohypo-physial tract to the posterior pituitary gland, causing the stored ADH to be released into the circulation[19,20] (see Fig. 31-7).

ADH exerts its effects through two types of vasopressin (V) receptors—V_1 and V_2. V_1 receptors, which are located in vascular smooth muscle, cause vasoconstriction—hence the name *vasopressin*. Although ADH can increase blood pressure through V_1 receptors, this response occurs only when ADH levels are very high. The V_2 receptors, which are located on the tubular cells of the cortical collecting duct, control water reabsorption by the kidney. These renal mechanisms for water reabsorption are responsible for maintaining the osmolality of body fluids.

The mechanism whereby ADH acts on the tubular cells to increase water reabsorption has recently been elucidated. Without ADH, the luminal membranes of the tubular epithelial cells of the collecting ducts are almost impermeable to water. In the presence of ADH, pores or water channels, called *aquaporins,* are inserted into the membrane of these tubular cells, making them permeable to water (see Understanding Urine Concentration, Chapter 30). The specific water channel that is controlled by ADH is aquaporin-2.[21]

As with thirst, ADH levels are controlled by ECF volume and osmolality. Osmoreceptors in the hypothalamus sense changes in ECF osmolality and stimulate the production and release of ADH. A small increase in serum osmolality of 1% is sufficient to cause ADH release.[9] Likewise, stretch receptors that are sensitive to changes in blood pressure and the effective circulating volume aid in the regulation of ADH release (*i.e.,* nonosmotic ADH secretion). A blood volume decrease of 5% to 10% produces a maximal increase in ADH levels. As with many other homeostatic mechanisms, acute conditions produce greater changes in ADH levels than do chronic conditions.

The abnormal synthesis and release of ADH occurs in a number of stress situations. Severe pain, nausea, trauma, surgery, certain anesthetic agents, and some narcotics (*e.g.,* morphine and meperidine) increase ADH levels. Among the drugs that affect ADH are nicotine, which stimulates its release, and alcohol, which inhibits it (Table 31-3). Two important conditions alter ADH levels: diabetes insipidus and inappropriate secretion of ADH.

Diabetes Insipidus. Diabetes insipidus (DI) is caused by a deficiency of or a decreased response to ADH.[22] Persons with DI are unable to concentrate their urine during periods of water restriction and they excrete large volumes of urine, usually 3 to 20 L/day, depending on the degree of ADH deficiency or renal insensitivity to ADH. This large urine output is accompanied by excessive thirst. As long as the thirst mechanism is normal and fluid is readily available, there is little or no alteration in the fluid levels of persons with DI. The danger arises when the condition develops in someone who is unable to communicate the need for water or is unable to secure the needed water. In such cases, inadequate fluid intake rapidly leads to hypertonic dehydration and increased serum osmolality.

TABLE 31-3 **Drugs That Affect Antidiuretic Hormone Levels***	
DRUGS THAT DECREASE ADH LEVELS/ACTION	**DRUGS THAT INCREASE ADH LEVELS/ACTION**
Amphotericin B Demeclocycline Ethanol Foscarnet Lithium Morphine antagonists	Anticancer drugs (vincristine and cyclophosphamide) Carbamazepine Chlorpropamide Clofibrate General anesthetics (most) Narcotics (morphine and meperidine) Nicotine Nonsteroidal anti-inflammatory drugs Phenothiazine antipsychotic drugs Selective serotonin reuptake inhibitors Thiazide diuretics (chlorothiazide) Thiothixene (antipsychotic drug) Tricyclic antidepressants

ADH, antidiuretic hormone
*List not inclusive.

There are two types of DI: neurogenic or central DI, which occurs because of a defect in the synthesis or release of ADH, and nephrogenic DI, which occurs because the kidneys do not respond to ADH.[22,23] In neurogenic DI, loss of 80% to 90% of ADH-secreting neurons is necessary before polyuria becomes evident. Most persons with neurogenic DI have an incomplete form of the disorder and retain some ability to concentrate their urine. Temporary neurogenic DI may follow head injury or surgery near the hypothalamohypophysial tract. Nephrogenic DI is characterized by impairment of urine-concentrating ability and free-water conservation. It may be due to a genetic trait that affects the V_2 receptor that binds ADH, or the aquaporin-2 protein that forms the water channels in the collecting tubules.[23] Other, acquired causes of nephrogenic DI are drugs such as lithium and electrolyte disorders such as potassium depletion or chronic hypercalcemia. Lithium and the electrolyte disorders are thought to interfere with the postreceptor actions of ADH on the permeability of the collecting ducts.

Diagnosis of DI usually starts by attempting to document the total 24-hour urine output. Also, it must be documented that an osmotic diuresis is not caused by glucose or such disorders as kidney disease. Further evaluation is based on measurement of ADH levels along with plasma and urine osmolality before and after a period of fluid deprivation or hypertonic saline infusion. Persons with neurogenic DI do not increase their ADH levels in response to increased plasma osmolality. Another diagnostic approach is to conduct a carefully monitored trial of a pharmacologic form of ADH. Persons with nephrogenic DI do not respond to pharmacologic preparations of the hormone. When central DI is suspected, diagnostic methods such as MRI studies of the pituitary-hypothalamic area are used to determine the cause of the disorder. MRI studies localize the normal posterior pituitary as a high-intensity signal on T1-weighted images. Research reports indicate the "bright spot" is related to the content of stored ADH. This high-intensity signal is present in most (but not all) normal subjects and is absent in most (but not all) patients with DI.[22]

The management of central DI depends on the cause and severity of the disorder. Many persons with incomplete neurogenic DI maintain near-normal water balance when permitted to ingest water in response to thirst. Pharmacologic preparations of ADH are available for persons who cannot be managed by conservative measures. The preferred drug for treating chronic DI is desmopressin acetate (DDAVP). It usually is given orally, but is also available in parenteral and nasal forms. The oral antidiabetic agent chlorpropamide may be used to stimulate ADH release in partial neurogenic DI. It usually is reserved for special cases because of its ability to cause hypoglycemia. Both neurogenic and nephrogenic forms of DI respond partially to the thiazide diuretics (e.g., hydrochlorothiazide). These diuretics are thought to act by increasing sodium excretion by the kidneys, leading to ECF volume contraction, a decrease in the glomerular filtration rate (along with filtered load of sodium), and an increase in sodium and water reabsorption. It also has been postulated that the thiazide diuretics increase water permeability in the collecting tubules.[23]

Syndrome of Inappropriate Antidiuretic Hormone. The syndrome of inappropriate ADH (SIADH) results from a failure of the negative feedback system that regulates the release and inhibition of ADH.[24] In persons with this syndrome, ADH secretion continues even when serum osmolality is decreased, causing marked water retention and dilutional hyponatremia.

SIADH may occur as a transient condition, as in a stress situation, or as a chronic condition, resulting from disorders such as lung tumors. Stimuli such as surgery, pain, stress, and temperature changes are capable of triggering ADH release through action of the CNS. Drugs induce SIADH in different ways; some drugs are thought to increase hypothalamic production and release of ADH, and others are believed to act directly on the renal tubules to enhance the action of ADH. More chronic forms of SIADH may result from lung tumors, chest lesions, and CNS disorders. Tumors, particularly bronchogenic carcinomas and cancers of the lymphoid tissue, prostate, and pancreas, are known to produce and release ADH independent of normal hypothalamic control mechanisms (examples of paraneoplastic conditions are described in Chapter 8). Other intrathoracic conditions, such as advanced tuberculosis, severe pneumonia, and positive-pressure breathing, also cause SIADH. The suggested mechanism for SIADH in positive-pressure ventilation is activation of baroreceptors

(e.g., aortic baroreceptors, cardiopulmonary receptors) that respond to marked changes in intrathoracic pressure. Disease and injury to the CNS can cause direct pressure on or direct involvement of the hypothalamic–posterior pituitary structures. Examples include brain tumors, hydrocephalus, head injury, meningitis, and encephalitis. Human immunodeficiency virus (HIV) infection is an established cause of SIADH (e.g., related to associated infections, tumors, drugs).

The manifestations of SIADH are those of dilutional hyponatremia (to be discussed). Urine osmolality is high and serum osmolality is low. Urine output decreases despite adequate or increased fluid intake. Hematocrit and the plasma sodium and BUN levels are all decreased because of the expansion of the ECF volume. The diagnosis of SIADH should be considered only if the five cardinal features are fulfilled: (1) hypotonic hyponatremia, (2) natriuresis (>20 mEq/L [20 mmol/L]), (3) urine osmolality in excess of plasma osmolality, (4) absence of edema and volume depletion, and (5) normal renal, thyroid, and adrenal function.[24]

The treatment of SIADH depends on its severity. In mild cases, treatment consists of fluid restriction. If fluid restriction is not sufficient, diuretics such as mannitol and furosemide (Lasix) may be given to promote diuresis and free-water clearance. Lithium and the antibiotic demeclocycline inhibit the action of ADH on the renal collecting ducts and sometimes are used in treating the disorder. In cases of severe water intoxication, a hypertonic (e.g., 3%) sodium chloride solution may be administered intravenously. The recently developed antagonists to the antidiuretic action of ADH (aquaretics) offer a new therapeutic approach to the treatment of euvolemic hyponatremia.[21] These agents (e.g., conivaptan) are specific ADH V_2 receptor antagonists and result in aquaresis (i.e., the electrolyte-sparing excretion of free water).

Disorders of Sodium and Water Balance

Disorders of sodium and water balance can be divided into two main categories: (1) isotonic contraction or expansion of ECF volume; and (2) hypotonic dilution (hyponatremia) or hypertonic concentration (hypernatremia) of extracellular sodium brought about by changes in extracellular water (Fig. 31-8). Isotonic disorders usually are confined to the ECF compartment, producing a contraction (fluid volume deficit) or expansion (fluid volume excess) of the interstitial and vascular fluids. Disorders of sodium concentration produce a change in the osmolality of the ECF, with movement of water from the ECF compartment into the ICF compartment (hyponatremia) or from the ICF compartment into the ECF compartment (hypernatremia).

Isotonic Fluid Volume Deficit

Fluid volume deficit is characterized by a decrease in the ECF, including the circulating blood volume. The term *isotonic fluid volume deficit* is used to differentiate the type of fluid deficit in

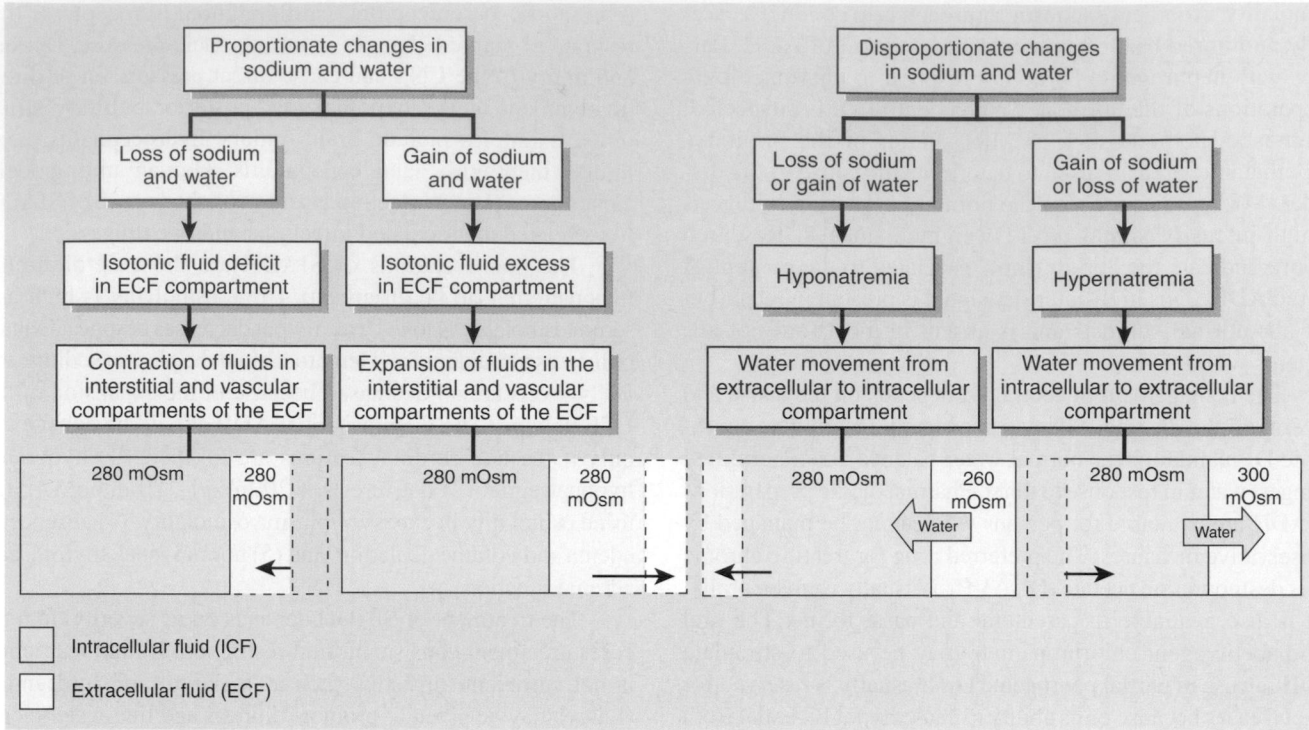

FIGURE 31-8 • Effect of isotonic fluid excess and deficit and of hyponatremia and hypernatremia on movement of water between the extracellular (ECF) and intracellular fluid (ICF) compartments.

🔑 SODIUM AND WATER BALANCE

- It is the amount of water and its effect on sodium concentration in the ECF that serves to regulate the distribution of fluid between the ICF and the ECF compartments.

- Isotonic changes in body fluids that result from proportionate gains or losses of sodium and water are largely confined to the ECF compartment. Many of the manifestations of isotonic fluid deficit or excess reflect changes in vascular and interstitial fluid volume.

- Hyponatremia or hypernatremia that is brought about by disproportionate losses or gains in sodium or water exerts its effects on the ICF compartment, causing water to move in or out of body cells. Many of the manifestations of changes in sodium concentration reflect changes in the intracellular volume of cells, particularly those in the nervous system.

which there are proportionate losses in sodium and water from water deficit and the hyperosmolar state associated with hypernatremia. Unless other fluid and electrolyte imbalances are present, the concentration of plasma electrolytes remains essentially unchanged. When the effective circulating blood volume is compromised, the condition is often referred to as *hypovolemia*.

Causes. Isotonic fluid volume deficit results when water and electrolytes are lost in isotonic proportions (Table 31-4). It is almost always caused by a loss of body fluids and is often accompanied by a decrease in fluid intake. It can occur because of a loss of gastrointestinal fluids, polyuria, or sweating due to fever and exercise. Fluid intake may be reduced because of a lack of access to fluids, impaired thirst, unconsciousness, oral trauma, impaired swallowing, or neuromuscular problems that prevent fluid access.

In a single day, 8 to 10 L of ECF is secreted into the gastrointestinal tract. Most of it is reabsorbed in the ileum and proximal colon, and only approximately 150 to 200 mL/day is eliminated in the feces. Vomiting and diarrhea interrupt the reabsorption process and, in some situations, lead to increased secretion of fluid into the intestinal tract. In Asiatic cholera, death can occur within a matter of hours as the cholera organism causes excessive amounts of fluid to be secreted into the bowel. These fluids are then lost as vomitus or excreted as diarrheal fluid. Gastrointestinal suction, fistulas, and drainage tubes can remove large amounts of fluid from the gastrointestinal tract.

Excess sodium and water losses also can occur through the kidney. Certain forms of kidney disease are characterized by salt wasting due to impaired sodium reabsorption. Fluid volume deficit also can result from osmotic diuresis or injudicious use of diuretic therapy. Glucose in the urine filtrate prevents reabsorption of water by the renal tubules, causing a loss of sodium and water. In Addison disease, a condition of chronic adrenocortical insufficiency, there is unregulated loss of sodium in the urine

TABLE 31-4 Causes and Manifestations of Isotonic Fluid Volume Deficit

CAUSES	MANIFESTATIONS
Inadequate Fluid Intake	**Acute Weight Loss (% body weight)**
Oral trauma or inability to swallow	Mild fluid volume deficit: 2%
Inability to obtain fluids	Moderate fluid volume deficit: 2%–5%
(*e.g.,* impaired mobility)	Severe fluid deficit: 8% or greater
Impaired thirst sensation	**Compensatory Increase in**
Therapeutic withholding of fluids	**Antidiuretic Hormone**
Unconsciousness or inability to	Decreased urine output
express thirst	Increased osmolality and specific gravity
Excessive Gastrointestinal Fluid Losses	**Increased Serum Osmolality**
Vomiting	Thirst
Diarrhea	Increased hematocrit and blood urea
Gastrointestinal suction	nitrogen
Draining gastrointestinal fistula	**Decreased Vascular Volume**
Excessive Renal Losses	Postural hypotension
Diuretic therapy	Tachycardia, weak and thready pulse
Osmotic diuresis (hyperglycemia)	Decreased vein filling and increased vein
Adrenal insufficiency (Addison disease)	refill time
Salt-wasting kidney disease	Hypotension and shock
Excessive Skin Losses	**Decreased Extracellular Fluid Volume**
Fever	Depressed fontanel in an infant
Exposure to hot environment	Sunken eyes and soft eyeballs
Burns and wounds that remove skin	**Impaired Temperature Regulation**
Third-Space Losses	Elevated body temperature
Intestinal obstruction	
Edema	
Ascites	
Burns (first several days)	

with a resultant loss of ECF (see Chapter 41). This is accompanied by increased potassium retention.

The skin acts as an exchange surface for heat and as a vapor barrier to prevent water from leaving the body. Body surface losses of sodium and water increase when there is excessive sweating or when large areas of skin have been damaged. Hot weather and fever increase sweating. In hot weather, water losses through sweating may be increased by as much as 1 to 3 L/hour, depending on acclimatization.[2] The respiratory rate and sweating usually are increased as body temperature rises. As much as 3 L of water may be lost in a single day as a result of fever. Burns are another cause of excess fluid loss. Evaporative losses can increase 10-fold with severe burns, up to 3 to 5 L/day.[2]

Third-space losses cause sequestering of ECF in the serous cavities, extracellular spaces in injured tissues, or lumen of the gut. Because the fluid remains in the body, fluid volume deficit caused by third spacing does not usually cause weight loss.

Manifestations. The manifestations of fluid volume deficit reflect a decrease in ECF volume. They include thirst, loss of body weight, signs of water conservation by the kidney, impaired temperature regulation, and signs of reduced interstitial and vascular volume (see Table 31-4).

A loss in fluid volume is accompanied by a decrease in body weight. One liter of water weighs 1 kg (2.2 lb). A mild ECF deficit exists when weight loss equals 2% of body weight. In a person who weighs 68 kg (150 lb), this percentage of weight loss equals 1.4 L of water. A moderate deficit equates to a 5% loss in weight and a severe deficit to an 8% or greater loss in weight.[8] To be accurate, weight must be measured at the same time each day with the person wearing the same amount of clothing. Because the ECF is trapped in the body in persons with third-space losses, their body weight may not decrease.

Thirst is a common symptom of fluid deficit, although it is not always present in the early stages of isotonic fluid deficit. It develops as the effective circulatory volume decreases to a point sufficient to stimulate the thirst mechanism. Urine output decreases and urine osmolality and specific gravity increase as ADH levels rise because of a decrease in vascular volume. Although there is an isotonic loss of fluid from the vascular compartment, the other blood components such as red blood cells and BUN become more concentrated.

The fluid content of body tissues decreases as fluid is removed from the interstitial spaces. The eyes assume a sunken appearance and feel softer than normal as the fluid content in the anterior chamber of the eye is decreased. Fluids add resiliency to the skin and underlying tissues that is referred to as *skin* or *tissue turgor*. Tissue turgor is assessed by pinching a fold of skin between the thumb and forefinger. The skin should immediately return to its original configuration when the fingers are released. A loss of 3% to 5% of body water in children causes the resiliency of the skin to be lost, and the tissue remains elevated for several seconds.[8] Decreased tissue turgor is less predictive of fluid deficit in older persons (>65 years) because of the loss of tissue elasticity. In infants, fluid deficit may be evidenced by depression of the anterior fontanel due to a decrease in cerebrospinal fluid.

Arterial and venous volumes decline during periods of fluid deficit, as does filling of the capillary circulation. As the volume in the arterial system declines, the blood pressure decreases, the heart rate increases, and the pulse becomes weak and thready. Postural hypotension (a drop in blood pressure on standing) is an early sign of fluid deficit. On the venous side of the circulation, the veins become less prominent. When volume depletion becomes severe, signs of hypovolemic shock and vascular collapse appear (see Chapter 26).

Diagnosis and Treatment. Diagnosis of fluid volume deficit is based on a history of conditions that predispose to sodium and water losses, weight loss, and observations of altered physiologic function indicative of decreased fluid volume. Intake and output measurements afford a means for assessing fluid balance. However, these measurements may not represent actual losses and gains, largely because accurate measurements of intake and output often are difficult to obtain and insensible losses are difficult to estimate.

Measurement of heart rate and blood pressure provides useful information about vascular volume. A simple test to determine venous refill time consists of compressing the distal end of a vein on the dorsal aspect of the hand when it is not in the dependent position. The vein is then emptied by "milking" the blood toward the heart. The vein should refill almost immediately when the occluding finger is removed. In the case of decreased venous volume, as occurs in fluid deficit, venous refill time increases. Capillary refill time is also increased. Capillary refill can be assessed by applying pressure to a fingernail for 5 seconds and then releasing the pressure and observing the time (normally 1 to 2 seconds) it takes for the color to return to normal.[8]

Treatment of fluid volume deficit consists of fluid replacement and measures to correct the underlying cause. Usually, isotonic electrolyte solutions are used for fluid replacement. Acute hypovolemia and hypovolemic shock can cause renal damage; therefore, prompt assessment of the degree of fluid deficit and adequate measures to resolve the deficit and treat the underlying cause are essential.

Isotonic Fluid Volume Excess

Fluid volume excess represents an isotonic expansion of the ECF compartment with increases in both interstitial and vascular volumes. Although increased fluid volume is usually the result of a disease condition, this is not always true. For example, a compensatory isotonic expansion of body fluids can occur in healthy persons during hot weather as a mechanism for increasing body heat loss.

Causes. Isotonic fluid volume excess almost always results from an increase in total body sodium that is accompanied by a proportionate increase in body water. Although it can occur as the result of excessive sodium intake, it is most commonly caused by a decrease in sodium and water elimination by the kidney.

Among the causes of decreased sodium and water elimination are disorders of renal function, heart failure, liver failure, and corticosteroid excess (Table 31-5). Heart failure (see Chapter 26) produces a decrease in the effective circulating volume and renal blood flow and a compensatory increase in sodium and water retention. Persons with severe congestive heart failure maintain a precarious balance between sodium and water intake and output. Even small increases in sodium intake can precipitate a state of fluid volume excess and a worsening of heart failure. A condition called *circulatory overload* results from an increase in blood volume; it can occur during infusion of intravenous fluids or transfusion of blood if the amount or rate of administration is excessive. Liver failure (*e.g.,* cirrhosis of the liver) impairs aldosterone metabolism and decreases effective circulating volume and renal perfusion, leading to increased salt and water retention. The corticosteroid hormones increase sodium reabsorption by the kidneys. Persons taking corticosteroid medications and those with Cushing disease (see Chapter 41) often have problems with sodium retention.

Manifestations. Isotonic fluid volume excess is manifested by an increase in interstitial and vascular fluids. It is characterized by weight gain over a short period of time. Mild fluid volume excess represents a 2% gain in weight; moderate fluid volume excess, a 5% gain in weight; and severe fluid volume excess, a gain of 8% or more in weight[8] (see Table 31-5). The presence of edema is characteristic of isotonic fluid excess. When the excess fluid accumulates gradually, as often happens in debilitating diseases and starvation, edema fluid may mask the loss of tissue mass. There may be a decrease in BUN and hematocrit as a result of dilution due to expansion of the plasma volume. An increase in vascular volume may be evidenced by distended neck veins, slow-emptying peripheral veins, a full and bounding pulse, and an increase in central venous pressure. When excess fluid accumulates in the lungs (*i.e.,* pulmonary edema), there are complaints of shortness of breath and difficult breathing, respiratory crackles, and a productive cough. Ascites and pleural effusion may occur with severe fluid volume excess.

Diagnosis and Treatment. Diagnosis of fluid volume excess is usually based on a history of factors that predispose to sodium and water retention, weight gain, and manifestations such as edema and cardiovascular symptoms indicative of an expanded ECF volume.

TABLE 31-5 Causes and Manifestations of Isotonic Fluid Volume Excess

CAUSES	MANIFESTATIONS
Inadequate Sodium and Water Elimination	**Acute Weight Gain (% body weight)**
Congestive heart failure	Mild fluid volume excess: 2%
Renal failure	Moderate fluid volume excess: 5%
Increased corticosteroid levels	Severe fluid volume excess: 8% or greater
Hyperaldosteronism	**Increased Interstitial Fluid Volume**
Cushing disease	Dependent and generalized edema
Liver failure (*e.g.,* cirrhosis)	**Increased Vascular Volume**
Excessive Sodium Intake in Relation to Output	Full and bounding pulse
Excessive dietary intake	Venous distention
Excessive ingestion of sodium-containing	Pulmonary edema
medications or home remedies	Shortness of breath
Excessive administration of sodium-	Crackles
containing parenteral fluids	Dyspnea
Excessive Fluid Intake in Relation to Output	Cough
Ingestion of fluid in excess of elimination	
Administration of parenteral fluids or	
blood at an excessive rate	

The treatment of fluid volume excess focuses on providing a more favorable balance between sodium and water intake and output. A sodium-restricted diet is often prescribed as a means of decreasing extracellular sodium and water levels. Diuretic therapy is commonly used to increase sodium elimination. When there is a need for intravenous fluid administration or transfusion of blood components, the procedure requires careful monitoring to prevent fluid overload.

Hyponatremia

The normal plasma concentration of sodium ranges from 135 to 145 mEq/L (135 to 145 mmol/L). Plasma sodium values reflect the sodium concentration expressed in milliequivalents or millimoles per liter, rather than an absolute amount. Because sodium and its attendant anions account for 90% to 95% of the osmolality of ECF, serum osmolality (normal range, 275 to 295 mOsm/kg) usually changes with changes in plasma sodium concentration.

Hyponatremia represents a plasma sodium concentration below 135 mEq/L (135 mmol/L). It is one of the most common electrolyte disorders seen in general hospital patients and is also common in the outpatient population, particularly in the elderly population. A number of age-related events make the elderly population more vulnerable to hyponatremia, including a decrease in renal function accompanied by limitations in sodium conservation. Although older people maintain body fluid homeostasis under most circumstances, the ability to withstand environmental, drug-related, and disease-associated stresses becomes progressively limited.

Types and Causes. Because of the effects of osmotically active particles such as glucose, hyponatremia can present as a hypo-

tonic or hypertonic state.[25–28] *Hypertonic (translocational) hyponatremia* results from an osmotic shift of water from the ICF to the ECF compartment, such as occurs with hyperglycemia (the correction for hyperglycemia is a 1.6 mEq/L [1.6 mmol/L] increase in plasma sodium for every 100 mg/dL rise in plasma glucose above the normal 100 mg/dL [5.5 mmol/L]). In this case, the sodium in the ECF becomes diluted as water moves out of cells in response to the osmotic effects of the elevated blood glucose level. *Hypotonic (dilutional) hyponatremia,* by far the most common type of hyponatremia, is caused by water retention. It can be classified as hypovolemic, euvolemic, or hypervolemic based on accompanying ECF fluid volumes.[19,25–28] Because of its effect on both sodium and water elimination, diuretic therapy can cause either hypovolemic or euvolemic hyponatremia.

Hypovolemic hypotonic hyponatremia occurs when water is lost along with sodium, but to a lesser extent. Among the causes of hypovolemic hyponatremia are excessive sweating in hot weather, particularly during heavy exercise, which leads to loss of salt and water. Hyponatremia develops when water, rather than electrolyte-containing liquids, is used to replace fluids lost in sweating. Another potential cause of hypovolemic hyponatremia is the loss of sodium from the gastrointestinal tract caused by frequent gastrointestinal irrigations with distilled water. Iso-osmotic fluid loss, such as occurs in vomiting or diarrhea, does not usually lower plasma sodium levels unless these losses are replaced with disproportionate amounts of orally ingested or parenterally administered water. Gastrointestinal fluid loss and ingestion of excessively diluted formula are common causes of acute hyponatremia in infants and children. Hypovolemic hyponatremia is also a common complication of adrenal insufficiency and is attributable to a decrease in aldosterone levels. A lack of aldosterone increases renal losses of sodium and a cortisol deficiency leads to increased release of ADH with water retention.

Euvolemic or *normovolemic hypotonic hyponatremia* represents retention of water with dilution of sodium while maintaining the ECF volume within a normal range. It is usually the result of SIADH. The risk of normovolemic hyponatremia is increased during the postoperative period. During this time ADH levels are often high, producing an increase in water reabsorption by the kidney (see section on SIADH). Although these elevated levels usually resolve in about 72 hours, they can persist for as long as 5 days. The hyponatremia becomes exaggerated when electrolyte-free fluids (*e.g.,* 5% glucose in water) are used for fluid replacement.

Hypervolemic hypotonic hyponatremia is seen when hyponatremia is accompanied by edema-associated disorders such as decompensated heart failure, advanced liver disease, and renal disease. Although the total body sodium is increased in heart failure, the effective circulating volume is often sensed as inadequate by the baroreceptors (*i.e.,* relative arterial underfilling), resulting in increased ADH levels (nonosmotic ADH secretion).[9]

Abuse of methylenedioxymethamphetamine (MDMA), also know as "ecstasy," can lead to severe neurologic symptoms, including seizures, brain edema, and herniation due to severe hyponatremia. MDMA and its metabolites have been shown to cause enhanced release of ADH from the hypothalamus.[27]

Manifestations. The manifestations of hypotonic hyponatremia are largely related to sodium dilution (Table 31-6). Serum osmolality is decreased and cellular swelling occurs owing to the movement of water from the ECF to the ICF compartment. The manifestations of hyponatremia depend on the rapidity of onset and the severity of the sodium dilution. The signs and symptoms may be acute (*i.e.,* onset within 48 hours), as in severe water intoxication, or more insidious in onset and less severe, as in chronic hyponatremia. Because of water movement, hyponatremia produces an increase in intracellular water, which is responsible for many of the clinical manifestations of the disorder. Fingerprint edema is a sign of excess intracellular water. This phenomenon is demonstrated by pressing the finger firmly over the bony surface of the sternum for 15 to 30 seconds. When excess intracellular water is present, a fingerprint similar to that observed when pressing on a piece of modeling clay is seen.[8]

Muscle cramps, weakness, and fatigue reflect the effects of hyponatremia on skeletal muscle function and are often early signs of hyponatremia. These effects commonly are observed in persons with hyponatremia that occurs during heavy exercise in hot weather. Gastrointestinal manifestations such as nausea and vomiting, abdominal cramps, and diarrhea may develop.

The cells of the brain and nervous system are the most seriously affected by increases in intracellular water. Symptoms include apathy, lethargy, and headache, which can progress to disorientation, confusion, gross motor weakness, and depression of deep tendon reflexes. Seizures and coma occur when plasma sodium levels reach extremely low levels. These severe effects, which are caused by brain swelling, may be irreversible. If the condition develops slowly, signs and symptoms do not develop

until plasma sodium levels approach 120 mEq/L (120 mmol/L) (*i.e.,* severe hyponatremia).[25] The term *water intoxication* is often used to describe the neurologic effects of acute hypotonic hyponatremia.

Diagnosis and Treatment. Diagnosis of hyponatremia is based on laboratory reports of a decreased plasma sodium concentration, plasma and urine osmolality, and urine sodium concentration; assessment of the person's volume status; presence of conditions that predispose to sodium loss or water retention; and signs and symptoms indicative of the disorder.

The treatment of hyponatremia with water excess focuses on the underlying cause. When hyponatremia is caused by water intoxication, limiting water intake or discontinuing medications that contribute to SIADH may be sufficient. The administration of a saline solution orally or intravenously may be needed when hyponatremia is caused by sodium deficiency. Symptomatic hyponatremia (*i.e.,* neurologic manifestations) is often treated with hypertonic saline solution and a loop diuretic, such as furosemide, to increase water elimination. This combination allows for correction of plasma sodium levels while ridding the body of excess water. New, specific ADH V_2 receptor antagonists to the antidiuretic action of ADH (aquaretics) offer a new therapeutic approach to the treatment of euvolemic hyponatremia.[21]

There is concern about the rapidity with which plasma sodium levels are corrected, particularly in persons with chronic symptomatic hyponatremia. Cells, particularly those in the brain, tend to defend against changes in cell volume caused by changes in ECF osmolality by increasing or decreasing their concentration of organic osmolytes.[29] In the case of prolonged water intoxication, brain cells reduce their concentration of osmolytes as a means of preventing an increase in cell volume. It takes several days for brain cells to restore the osmolytes lost during hyponatremia. Thus, treatment measures that produce rapid changes in serum osmolality may cause a dramatic change in brain cell volume. One of the reported effects of rapid treatment of hyponatremia is an osmotic demyelinating condition called *central pontine myelinolysis,* which produces serious neurologic sequelae and sometimes causes death.[30] This complication occurs more commonly in premenopausal women and in hypoxic patients.

Hypernatremia

Hypernatremia implies a plasma sodium level above 145 mEq/L (145 mmol/L) and a serum osmolality greater than 295 mOsm/kg. Because sodium is functionally an impermeable solute, it contributes to tonicity and induces movement of water across cell membranes. Hypernatremia is characterized by hypertonicity of ECF and almost always causes cellular dehydration.[31]

Causes. Hypernatremia represents a deficit of water in relation to the body's sodium stores. It can be caused by net loss of water or sodium gain. Net water loss can occur through the urine, gastrointestinal tract, lungs, or skin. A defect in thirst or inability to obtain or drink water can interfere with water replace-

TABLE 31-6 Causes and Manifestations of Hyponatremia

CAUSES	MANIFESTATIONS
Hypotonic Hyponatremia	**Laboratory Values**
Hypovolemic (Decreased Serum Sodium With Decreased ECF Volume)	Serum sodium levels below 135 mEq/L (135 mmol/L)
Use of excessively diluted infant formula	Hypotonic hyponatremia
Administration of sodium-free parenteral solutions	Serum osmolality <280 mOsm/kg
Gastrointestinal losses	Dilution of blood components, including hematocrit, blood urea nitrogen
Vomiting, diarrhea	Hypertonic hyponatremia
Sweating, with sodium-free fluid replacement	Serum osmolality >280 mOsm/kg
Repeated irrigation of body cavities with sodium-free solutions	**Signs Related to Hypo-osmolality of Extra-cellular Fluids and Movement of Water Into Brain Cells and Neuromuscular Tissue**
Irrigation of gastrointestinal tubes with distilled water	Muscle cramps
Tap water enemas	Weakness
Use of nonelectrolyte irrigating solutions during prostate surgery	Headache
Third-spacing (paralytic ileus, pancreatitis)	Depression
Diuretic use	Apprehension, feeling of impending doom
Mineralocorticoid deficiency (Addison disease)	Personality changes
Salt-wasting nephritis	Lethargy
Euvolemic (Decreased Serum Sodium With Normal ECF Volume)	Stupor, coma
Increased ADH levels	**Gastrointestinal Manifestations**
Trauma, stress, pain	Anorexia, nausea, vomiting
Syndrome of inappropriate ADH	Abdominal cramps, diarrhea
Use of medications that increase ADH	**Increased Intracellular Fluid**
Diuretic use	Fingerprint edema
Glucocorticoid deficiency	
Hypothyroidism	
Psychogenic polydipsia	
Endurance exercise	
Methylenedioxymethamphetamine ("ecstasy") abuse	
Hypervolemic (Decreased Serum Sodium With Increased ECF Volume)	
Decompensated heart failure	
Advanced liver disease	
Kidney failure without nephrosis	
Hypertonic Hyponatremia (Osmotic Shift of Water From the ICF to the ECF Compartment)	Manifestations largely related to hyperosmolality of extracellular fluids
Hyperglycemia	

ment. Rapid ingestion or infusion of sodium with insufficient time or opportunity for water ingestion can produce a disproportionate gain in sodium (Table 31-7).

Hypernatremia almost always follows a loss of body fluids that have a lower-than-normal concentration of sodium, so that water is lost in excess of sodium. This can result from increased losses from the respiratory tract during fever or strenuous exercise, from watery diarrhea, or when osmotically active tube feedings are given with inadequate amounts of water. With pure water loss, each body fluid compartment loses an equal percentage of its volume. Because approximately one third of the water is in the ECF compartment, compared with the two thirds in the ICF compartment, more actual water volume is lost from the ICF than the ECF compartment.[2]

Normally, water deficit stimulates thirst and increases water intake. Therefore, hypernatremia is more likely to occur in infants and in persons who cannot express their thirst or obtain water to drink. With hypodipsia, or impaired thirst, the need for fluid intake does not activate the thirst response. Hypodipsia is particularly prevalent among the elderly. In persons with DI, hyperna-

TABLE 31-7 Causes and Manifestations of Hypernatremia

CAUSES	MANIFESTATIONS
Excessive Water Losses	**Laboratory Values**
Watery diarrhea	Serum sodium level above 145 mEq/L
Excessive sweating	(145 mmol/L)
Increased respirations due to conditions such as tracheobronchitis	Increased serum osmolality
Hypertonic tube feedings	Increased hematocrit and blood urea nitrogen
Diabetes insipidus	**Thirst and Signs of Increased ADH Levels**
Decreased Water Intake	Polydipsia
Unavailability of water	Oliguria or anuria
Oral trauma or inability to swallow	High urine specific gravity
Impaired thirst sensation	**Intracellular Dehydration**
Withholding water for therapeutic reasons	Dry skin and mucous membranes
Unconsciousness or inability to express thirst	Decreased tissue turgor
	Tongue rough and fissured
Excessive Sodium Intake	Decreased salivation and lacrimation
Rapid or excessive administration of sodium-containing parenteral solutions	**Signs Related to Hyperosmolality of Extracellular Fluids and Movement of Water Out of Brain Cells**
Near-drowning in salt water	Headache
	Agitation and restlessness
	Decreased reflexes
	Seizures and coma
	Extracellular Dehydration and Decreased Vascular Volume
	Tachycardia
	Weak and thready pulse
	Decreased blood pressure
	Vascular collapse

tremia can develop when thirst is impaired or access to water is impeded.

The therapeutic administration of sodium-containing solutions may also cause hypernatremia. For example, the administration of sodium bicarbonate during cardiopulmonary resuscitation increases body sodium levels because each 50-mL ampule of 7.5% sodium bicarbonate contains 892 mEq of sodium.[8] Hypertonic saline solution intended for intra-amniotic instillation for therapeutic abortion may inadvertently be injected intravenously, causing hypernatremia. Rarely, salt intake occurs rapidly, as in taking excess salt tablets or during near-drowning in salt water.

Manifestations. The clinical manifestations of hypernatremia caused by water loss are largely those of ECF loss and cellular dehydration (see Table 31-7). The severity of signs and symptoms is greatest when the increase in plasma sodium is large and occurs rapidly. Body weight is decreased in proportion to the amount of water that has been lost. Because blood plasma is roughly 90% to 93% water, the concentrations of blood cells and other blood components increase as ECF water decreases.

Thirst is an early symptom of water deficit, occurring when water losses are equal to 0.5% of body water. Urine output is decreased and urine osmolality increased because of renal

water-conserving mechanisms. Body temperature frequently is elevated, and the skin becomes warm and flushed. The vascular volume decreases, the pulse becomes rapid and thready, and the blood pressure drops. Hypernatremia produces an increase in serum osmolality and results in water being pulled out of body cells. As a result, the skin and mucous membranes become dry, and salivation and lacrimation are decreased. The mouth becomes dry and sticky, and the tongue becomes rough and fissured. Swallowing is difficult. The subcutaneous tissues assume a firm, rubbery texture. Most significantly, water is pulled out of the cells in the CNS, causing decreased reflexes, agitation, headache, and restlessness. Coma and seizures may develop as hypernatremia progresses.

Diagnosis and Treatment. The diagnosis of hypernatremia is based on history, physical examination findings indicative of dehydration, and results of laboratory tests. The treatment of hypernatremia includes measures to treat the underlying cause of the disorder and fluid replacement therapy to treat the accompanying dehydration. Replacement fluids can be given orally or intravenously. The oral route is preferable. Oral glucose–electrolyte replacement solutions are available for the treatment of infants with diarrhea[32,33] (see Chapter 37). Until recently, these solutions were used only early in diarrheal illness or as a first step in reestablishing oral intake after parenteral replacement therapy. These solutions are now widely available in grocery stores and pharmacies for use in the treatment of diarrhea and other dehydrating disorders in infants and young children.

One of the serious aspects of fluid volume deficit is dehydration of brain and nerve cells. Serum osmolality should be corrected slowly in cases of chronic hypernatremia. As mentioned previously, brain cells mobilize organic osmolytes to protect against changes in cell volume.[29] If hypernatremia is corrected too rapidly before the osmolytes have had a chance to dissipate, the plasma may become relatively hypotonic in relation to brain cell osmolality. When this occurs, water moves into the brain cells, causing cerebral edema and potentially severe neurologic impairment.

IN SUMMARY, body fluids are distributed between the ICF and ECF compartments. Regulation of fluid volume, solute concentration, and distribution between the two compartments depends on water and sodium balance. Water provides approximately 90% to 93% of fluid volume, and sodium salts, approximately 90% to 95% of extracellular solutes. Both water and sodium are absorbed from the gastrointestinal tract and eliminated by the kidneys. The main regulator of sodium and water is the maintenance of the effective circulating blood volume, which is monitored by stretch receptors in the vascular system, which exert their effects through ADH and the sympathetic nervous system; and those in the kidney, which exert their effects through the sympathetic nervous system and the renin-angiotensin-aldosterone system. Body water and serum osmolality are also regulated by thirst, which controls water intake, and ADH, which controls urine concentration and renal output.

Isotonic fluid disorders result from contraction or expansion of ECF volume brought about by proportionate losses of sodium and water. *Isotonic fluid volume deficit* is characterized by a decrease in ECF volume. It causes thirst, decreased vascular volume and circulatory function, decreased urine output, and increased urine specific gravity. *Isotonic fluid volume excess* is characterized by an increase in ECF volume. It is manifested by signs of increased vascular volume and edema.

Alterations in extracellular sodium concentration are brought about by a disproportionate gain (hyponatremia) or loss (hypernatremia) of water. As the major cation in the ECF compartment, sodium controls the ECF osmolality and its effect on cell volume. Hyponatremia can present as a *hypertonic (translocational) hyponatremia* in which water moves out of the cell in response to elevated blood glucose levels, or as a *hypotonic (dilutional) hyponatremia* that is caused by retention of water by the body in excess of sodium. Hypotonic hyponatremia, which can present as a hypovolemic, euvolemic, or hypervolemic state, is characterized by water being pulled into the cell from the ECF compartment, causing cells to swell. It is manifested by muscle cramps and weakness; nausea, vomiting,

abdominal cramps, and diarrhea; and CNS signs such as headache, lethargy, depression of deep tendon reflexes, and in severe cases seizure and coma.

Hypernatremia represents a disproportionate loss of body water in relation to sodium. It is characterized by intracellular water being pulled into the ECF compartment, causing cells to shrink. It is manifested by thirst and decreased urine output; dry mouth and decreased tissue turgor; signs of decreased vascular volume (tachycardia, weak and thready pulse); and CNS signs, such as decreased reflexes, agitation, headache, and in severe cases seizures and coma. ■

POTASSIUM BALANCE

After completing this section of the chapter, you should be able to meet the following objectives:

- Characterize the distribution of potassium in the body and explain how extracellular potassium levels are regulated in relation to body gains and losses.
- State the causes of hypokalemia and hyperkalemia in terms of altered intake, output, and transcellular shifts.
- Relate the functions of potassium to the manifestations of hypokalemia and hyperkalemia.
- Describe methods used in diagnosis and treatment of hypokalemia and hyperkalemia.

Regulation of Potassium Balance

Potassium is the second most abundant cation in the body and the major cation in the ICF compartment. Approximately 98% of body potassium is contained within body cells, with an intracellular concentration of 140 to 150 mEq/L (140 to 150 mmol/L).[34] The potassium content of the ECF (3.5 to 5 mEq/L [3.5 to 5 mmol/L]) is considerably lower. Because potassium is an intracellular ion, total body stores of potassium are related to body size and muscle mass. In adults, total body potassium is approximately 50 mEq/kg of body weight.[35] Approximately 65% to 75% of potassium is in muscle.[36] Thus, potassium content declines with age, mainly as a result of a decrease in muscle mass.

Gains and Losses

Potassium intake is normally derived from dietary sources. In healthy persons, potassium balance usually can be maintained by a daily dietary intake of 50 to 100 mEq. Additional amounts of potassium are needed during periods of trauma and stress. The kidneys are the main source of potassium loss. Approximately 80% to 90% of potassium losses occur in the urine, with the remainder being lost in stools or sweat.

Mechanisms of Regulation

Normally, the ECF concentration of potassium is precisely regulated at about 4.2 mEq/L (4.2 mmol/L). The precise control is necessary because many cell functions are sensitive to even small changes in ECF potassium levels. An increase in potassium of as small an amount as 0.3 to 0.4 mEq/L (0.3 to 0.4 mmol/L) can cause serious cardiac dysrhythmias and even death.

Plasma potassium is largely regulated through two mechanisms: (1) renal mechanisms that conserve or eliminate potassium, and (2) a transcellular shift between the ICF and ECF compartments.

🔑 POTASSIUM BALANCE

- Potassium is mainly an intracellular ion with only a small, but vital, amount being present in the extracellular fluids.

- The distribution of potassium between the intracellular and extracellular compartments regulates electrical membrane potentials controlling the excitability of nerve and muscle cells as well as contractility of skeletal, cardiac, and smooth muscle tissue.

- Because of its vital role in regulating neuromuscular excitability, potassium regulation must be extremely efficient. Even a 1% to 2% addition of potassium to the extracellular fluid compartment can elevate serum levels to dangerously high levels.

- Two major mechanisms function in the control of serum potassium: (1) renal mechanisms that conserve or eliminate potassium, and (2) transcellular buffer systems that remove potassium from and release it into the serum as needed. Conditions that disrupt the function of either mechanism can result in a serious alteration in serum potassium levels.

Renal Regulation. The major route for potassium elimination is the kidney. Unlike other electrolytes, the regulation of potassium elimination is controlled by secretion from the blood into the tubular filtrate rather than through reabsorption from the tubular filtrate into the blood. Potassium is filtered in the glomerulus, reabsorbed along with sodium and water in the proximal tubule and with sodium and chloride in the thick ascending loop of Henle, and then secreted into the late distal and cortical collecting tubules for elimination in the urine. The latter mechanism serves to "fine-tune" the concentration of potassium in the ECF.

Aldosterone plays an essential role in regulating potassium elimination by the kidney. The effects of aldosterone on potassium elimination are mediated through an Na^+/K^+ exchange mechanism located in the late distal and cortical collecting tubules of the kidney (see Chapter 30). In the presence of aldosterone, Na^+ is transported back into the blood and K^+ is secreted in the tubular filtrate for elimination in the urine. The rate of aldosterone secretion by the adrenal gland is strongly controlled by plasma potassium levels. For example, an increase of less than 1 mEq/L (1 mmol/L) of potassium causes aldosterone levels to triple.[2] The effect of plasma potassium on aldosterone secretion is an example of the powerful feedback regulation of potassium elimination. In the absence of aldosterone, as occurs in persons with Addison disease, renal elimination of potassium is impaired, causing plasma potassium levels to rise to dangerously high levels. Aldosterone is often referred to as a *mineralocorticoid hormone* because of its effect on sodium and potassium. The term *mineralocorticoid activity* is used to describe the aldosterone-like actions of other adrenocortical hormones, such as cortisol.

There is also a K^+/H^+ exchange mechanism in the cortical collecting tubules of the kidney (see Chapter 30). When plasma potassium levels are increased, K^+ is secreted into the urine and H^+ is reabsorbed into the blood, producing a decrease in pH and metabolic acidosis. Conversely, when potassium levels are low, K^+ is reabsorbed and H^+ is secreted in the urine, leading to metabolic alkalosis.

Extracellular–Intracellular Shifts. Normally, it takes 6 to 8 hours to eliminate 50% of potassium intake.[3] To avoid an increase in extracellular potassium levels during this time, excess potassium is temporarily shifted into red blood cells and other cells such as those of muscle, liver, and bone. This movement is controlled by the function of the Na^+/K^+-ATPase membrane pump and the permeability of the ion channels in the cell membrane.

Among the factors that alter the intracellular–extracellular distribution of potassium are serum osmolality, acid-base disorders, insulin, and β-adrenergic stimulation. Acute increases in serum osmolality cause water to leave the cell. The loss of cell water produces an increase in intracellular potassium, causing it to move out of the cell into the ECF.

The H^+ and K^+ ions, which are positively charged, can be exchanged between the ICF and ECF in a cation shift (Fig. 31-9). In metabolic acidosis, for example, H^+ moves into body cells for buffering, causing K^+ to leave and move into the ECF.[8] Both insulin and the catecholamines (*e.g.,* epinephrine) increase cellular uptake of K^+ by increasing the activity of the Na^+/K^+-ATPase membrane pump.[36,37] Insulin produces an increase in cellular uptake of potassium after a meal. The catecholamines, particularly epinephrine, facilitate the movement of potassium into muscle tissue during periods of physiologic stress. β-Adrenergic agonist drugs, such as pseudoephedrine and albuterol, have a similar effect on potassium distribution.

Exercise also produces compartmental shifts in potassium. Repeated muscle contraction releases potassium into the ECF. Although the increase usually is small with modest exercise, it can be considerable during exhaustive exercise. Even the repeated clenching and unclenching of the fist during a

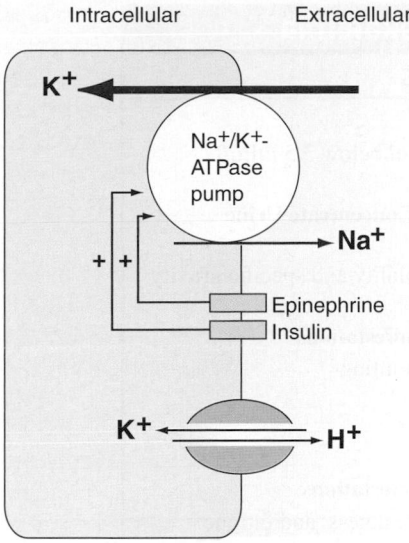

Intracellular   Extracellular

FIGURE 31-9 • Mechanisms regulating transcellular shifts in potassium.

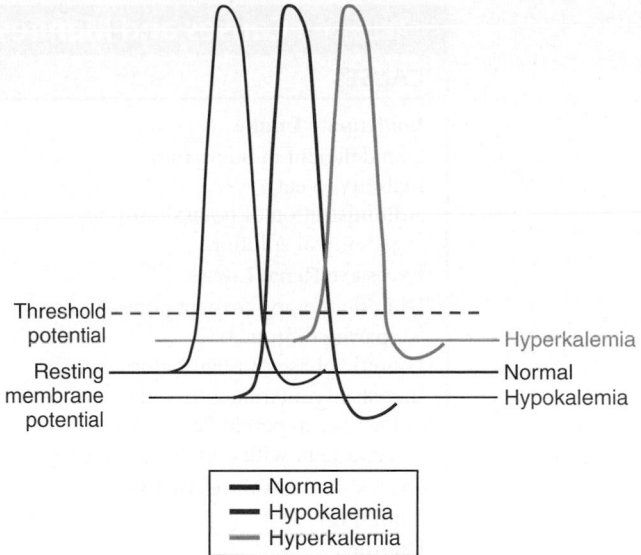

FIGURE 31-10 • Effect of changes in plasma hypokalemia (*red*) and hyperkalemia (*blue*) on the resting membrane potential, activation and opening of the sodium channels at threshold potential, and the rate of repolarization during a nerve action potential.

blood draw can cause potassium to move out of cells and artificially elevate plasma potassium levels.

Disorders of Potassium Balance

As the major intracellular cation, potassium is critical to many body functions. It is involved in a wide range of body functions, including the maintenance of the osmotic integrity of cells, acid-base balance, and the kidney's ability to concentrate urine. Potassium is necessary for growth and it contributes to the intricate chemical reactions that transform carbohydrates into energy, change glucose into glycogen, and convert amino acids to proteins. Potassium also plays a critical role in conducting nerve impulses and the excitability of skeletal, cardiac, and smooth muscle (see Chapter 4). It does this by regulating (1) the resting membrane potential, (2) the opening of the sodium channels that control the flow of current during the action potential, and (3) the rate of membrane repolarization. Changes in nerve and muscle excitability are particularly important in the heart, where alterations in plasma potassium can produce serious cardiac arrhythmias and conduction defects. Changes in plasma potassium also affect skeletal muscles and the smooth muscle in blood vessels and the gastrointestinal tract.

The *resting membrane potential* is determined by the ratio of ICF to ECF potassium concentration (Fig. 31-10). A decrease in plasma potassium causes the resting membrane potential to become more negative, moving it further from the threshold for excitation (see Chapter 4). Thus, it takes a greater stimulus to reach threshold and open the sodium channels that are responsible for the action potential. An increase in plasma potassium has the opposite effect; it causes the resting membrane potential to become more positive, moving it closer to threshold. With severe hyperkalemia, the resting membrane approaches the

threshold potential, causing sustained subthreshold depolarization with a resultant inactivation of the sodium channels and a net decrease in excitability.[3] The *rate of repolarization* also varies with plasma potassium levels. It is more rapid in hyperkalemia and delayed in hypokalemia. Both the inactivation of the sodium channels and the rate of membrane repolarization are important clinically because they predispose to cardiac arrhythmias or conduction defects (see Chapter 25).

Hypokalemia

Hypokalemia refers to a decrease in plasma potassium levels below 3.5 mEq/L (3.5 mmol/L). Because of transcellular shifts, temporary changes in plasma potassium may occur as the result of movement between the ICF and ECF compartments.

Causes. The causes of potassium deficit can be grouped into three categories: (1) inadequate intake; (2) excessive gastrointestinal, renal, and skin losses; and (3) redistribution between the ICF and ECF compartments (Table 31-8).

Inadequate Intake. Inadequate intake is a frequent cause of hypokalemia. A potassium intake of at least 40 to 50 mEq/day is needed to compensate for obligatory urine losses.[8,38] Insufficient dietary intake may result from the inability to obtain or ingest food or from a diet that is low in potassium-containing foods. Potassium intake is often inadequate in persons on fad diets and those who have eating disorders. Elderly persons are particularly likely to have potassium deficits. Many have poor eating habits as a consequence of living alone; they may have limited income, which makes

TABLE 31-8 Causes and Manifestations of Hypokalemia

CAUSES	MANIFESTATIONS
Inadequate Intake	**Laboratory Values**
Diet deficient in potassium	Serum potassium level below 3.5 mEq/L
Inability to eat	(3.5 mmol/L)
Administration of potassium-free	**Impaired Ability to Concentrate Urine**
parenteral solutions	Polyuria
Excessive Renal Losses	Urine with low osmolality and specific gravity
Diuretic therapy (except potassium-	Polydipsia
sparing diuretics)	**Gastrointestinal Manifestations**
Diuretic phase of renal failure	Anorexia, nausea, vomiting
Increased mineralocorticoid levels	Constipation
Primary hyperaldosteronism	Abdominal distention
Treatment with corticosteroid drugs	Paralytic ileus
Excessive Gastrointestinal Losses	**Neuromuscular Manifestations**
Vomiting	Muscle flabbiness, weakness, and fatigue
Diarrhea	Muscle cramps and tenderness
Gastrointestinal suction	Paresthesias
Draining gastrointestinal fistula	Paralysis
Transcompartmental Shift	**Cardiovascular Manifestations**
Administration of β-adrenergic	Postural hypotension
agonist (*e.g.*, albuterol)	Increased sensitivity to digitalis toxicity
Administration of insulin for	Changes in electrocardiogram
treatment of diabetic ketoacidosis	Cardiac dysrhythmias
Alkalosis, metabolic or respiratory	**Central Nervous System Manifestations**
	Confusion
	Depression
	Acid-Base Disorders
	Metabolic alkalosis

buying foods high in potassium difficult; they may have difficulty chewing many foods that have high potassium content because of dental problems; or they may have problems with swallowing.

Excessive Losses. The kidneys are the main source of potassium loss. Approximately 80% to 90% of potassium losses occur in the urine, with the remaining losses occurring in the stool and sweat. The kidneys do not have the homeostatic mechanisms needed to conserve potassium during periods of insufficient intake. After trauma and in stress situations, urinary losses of potassium are greatly increased, sometimes approaching levels of 150 to 200 mEq/L (150 to 200 mmol/L).[37] This means that a potassium deficit can develop rather quickly if intake is inadequate. Renal losses also can be increased by medications, metabolic alkalosis, magnesium depletion, and increased levels of aldosterone. Some antibiotics, particularly amphotericin B and gentamicin, are impermeable anions that require the presence of positively charged cations for elimination in the urine; this causes potassium wasting.

Diuretic therapy, with the exception of potassium-sparing diuretics, is the most common cause of hypokalemia. Both thiazide and loop diuretics increase the loss of potassium in the urine. The degree of hypokalemia is directly related to diuretic dose and is greater when sodium intake is higher.[36] Magnesium depletion causes renal potassium wasting. Magnesium deficiency often coexists with potassium depletion due to diuretic therapy or disease processes such as diarrhea. Importantly, the ability to correct potassium deficiency is impaired when magnesium deficiency is present.

Renal losses of potassium are accentuated by aldosterone and cortisol. Increased potassium losses occur in situations such as trauma and surgery that produce a stress-related increase in these hormones. Primary aldosteronism, caused by either a tumor or hyperplasia of the cells of the adrenal cortex that secrete aldosterone, produces severe potassium losses and a decrease in plasma potassium levels. Cortisol binds to aldosterone receptors and exerts aldosterone-like effects on potassium elimination. Licorice-induced hypokalemia results from inhibition of the enzyme that inactivates cortisol.

Other rare, genetic disorders that can also result in hypokalemia are the Bartter, Gitelman, and Liddle syndromes. *Bartter syndrome,* which involves the $Na^+/K^+/2Cl^-$ cotransporter in the thick loop of Henle, is manifested by metabolic alkalosis, hypercalciuria or excessive loss of calcium in the urine, and *normal* blood pressure. Because the loop diuretics act at the same site in the kidney, these features are identical to those seen with chronic loop diuretic ingestion. The manifestations of *Gitelman syndrome,* which involves the Na^+/Cl^- transporter in the distal tubule, are similar to those of Bartter syndrome, but with hypocalciuria and hypomagnesemia due to renal magnesium wasting. Because this is the site where the thiazide diuretics exert their action, these manifestations are identical to those seen with chronic thiazide diuretic ingestion. *Liddle syndrome* has manifestations similar to Bartter syndrome, but with *high* blood pressure due to excessive sodium reabsorption.

Although potassium losses from the skin and the gastrointestinal tract usually are minimal, these losses can become excessive under certain conditions. For example, burns increase surface losses of potassium. Losses due to sweating increase in persons who are acclimated to a hot climate, partly because increased secretion of aldosterone during heat acclimatization increases the loss of potassium in urine and sweat. Gastrointestinal losses also can become excessive; this occurs with vomiting and diarrhea and when gastrointestinal suction is being used. The potassium content of liquid stools, for example, is approximately 40 to 60 mEq/L (40 to 60 mmol/L).

Transcellular Shifts. Because of the high ratio of intracellular to extracellular potassium, conditions that produce a redistribution of potassium from the ECF to the ICF compartment can cause a marked decrease in plasma potassium levels (see Fig. 31-9). Insulin increases the movement of glucose and potassium into cells; therefore, potassium deficit often develops during treatment of diabetic ketoacidosis. A wide variety of β_2-adrenergic agonist drugs (*e.g.,* decongestants and bronchodilators) shift potassium into cells and cause transient hypokalemia. For example, a standard dose of nebulized albuterol (a bronchodilator) reduces plasma potassium by 0.2 to 0.4 mEq/L (0.2 to 0.4 mmol/L).[37]

Manifestations. The manifestations of hypokalemia include alterations in renal, gastrointestinal, cardiovascular, and neuromuscular function (see Table 31-8). These manifestations reflect both the intracellular functions of potassium as well as the body's attempt to regulate ECF potassium levels within the very narrow range needed to maintain the normal electrical activity of excitable tissues such as nerve and muscle cells. The signs and symptoms of potassium deficit seldom develop until plasma potassium levels have fallen to levels below 3 mEq/L (3 mmol/L). They are typically gradual in onset, and therefore the disorder may go undetected for some time.

The renal processes that conserve potassium during hypokalemia interfere with the kidney's ability to concentrate urine. Urine output and plasma osmolality are increased, urine specific gravity is decreased, and complaints of polyuria, nocturia, and thirst are common (an example of nephrogenic DI). Metabolic alkalosis and renal chloride wasting are signs of severe hypokalemia.

There are numerous signs and symptoms associated with gastrointestinal function, including anorexia, nausea, and vomiting. Atony of the gastrointestinal smooth muscle can cause constipation, abdominal distention, and, in severe hypokalemia, paralytic ileus. When gastrointestinal symptoms occur gradually and are not severe, they often impair potassium intake and exaggerate the condition.

The most serious effects of hypokalemia are those affecting cardiovascular function. Postural hypotension is common. Most persons with plasma potassium levels below 3 mEq/L (3 mmol/L) demonstrate electrocardiographic (ECG) changes typical of hypokalemia. These changes include prolongation of the PR interval, depression of the ST segment, flattening of the T wave, and appearance of a prominent U wave (Fig. 31-11). Normally, potassium leaves the cell during the repolarization phase of the action potential, returning the membrane potential to its normal resting value. Hypokalemia reduces the permeability of the cell membrane to potassium and thus produces a decrease in potassium efflux that prolongs the rate of repolarization and lengthens the relative refractory period. The U wave normally may be present on the ECG but should be of lower amplitude than the T wave. With hypokalemia, the amplitude of the T wave decreases as the U-wave amplitude increases. Although these changes in electrical activity of the heart usually are not serious, they may predispose to sinus bradycardia and

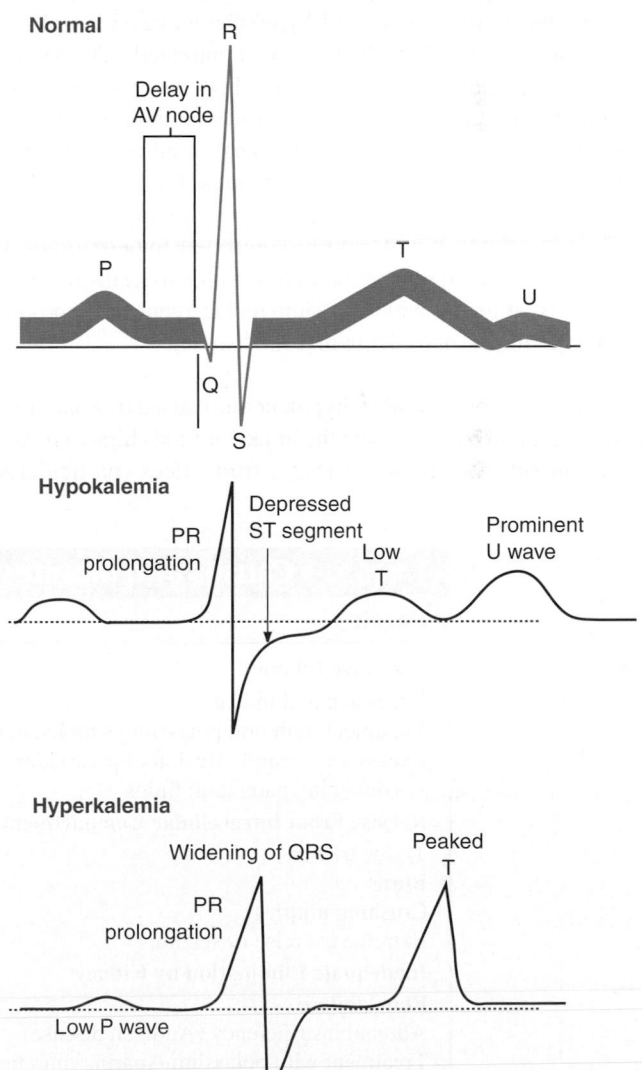

FIGURE 31-11 • Electrocardiographic changes with hypokalemia and hyperkalemia.

ectopic ventricular arrhythmias (the reader is referred to Chapter 25 for additional information on the ECG and cardiac arrhythmias). Digitalis toxicity can be provoked in persons treated with this drug and there is an increased risk of ventricular arrhythmias, particularly in persons with underlying heart disease. The dangers associated with digitalis toxicity are compounded in persons who are receiving diuretics that increase urinary losses of potassium.

Complaints of weakness, fatigue, and muscle cramps, particularly during exercise, are common in moderate hypokalemia (plasma potassium 3 to 2.5 mEq/L [3 to 2.5 mmol/L]). Muscle paralysis with life-threatening respiratory insufficiency can occur with severe hypokalemia (plasma potassium <2.5 mEq/L [2.5 mmol/L]). Leg muscles, particularly the quadriceps, are most prominently affected. Some persons complain of muscle tenderness and paresthesias rather than weakness. In chronic potassium deficiency, muscle atrophy may contribute to muscle weakness.

In a rare genetic condition called *hypokalemic familial periodic paralysis,* episodes of hypokalemia cause attacks of flaccid paralysis that last 6 to 48 hours if untreated.[3] The paralysis may be precipitated by situations that cause severe hypokalemia by producing an intracellular shift in potassium, such as ingestion of a high-carbohydrate meal or administration of insulin, epinephrine, or glucocorticoid drugs. The paralysis often can be reversed by potassium replacement therapy. A similar condition can occur with poorly controlled hyperthyroidism (thyrotoxic hypokalemic periodic paralysis), especially in Asian persons. Treatment is with potassium replacement and appropriate therapy for the underlying thyroid disorder.[39]

Treatment. When possible, hypokalemia caused by potassium deficit is treated by increasing the intake of foods high in potassium content—meats, dried fruits, fruit juices (particularly orange juice), and bananas. Oral potassium supplements are prescribed for persons whose intake of potassium is insufficient in relation to losses. This is particularly true of persons who are receiving diuretic therapy and those who are taking digitalis.

Potassium may be given intravenously when the oral route is not tolerated or when rapid replacement is needed. Magnesium deficiency may impair potassium correction; in such cases, magnesium replacement is indicated.[40] The rapid infusion of a concentrated potassium solution can cause death from cardiac arrest. Health personnel who assume responsibility for administering intravenous solutions that contain potassium should be fully aware of all the precautions pertaining to their dilution and flow rate.

Hyperkalemia

Hyperkalemia refers to an increase in plasma levels of potassium in excess of 5 mEq/L (5 mmol/L). It seldom occurs in healthy persons because the body is extremely effective in preventing excess potassium accumulation in the ECF.

Causes. The three major causes of potassium excess are (1) decreased renal elimination, (2) excessively rapid administration, and (3) movement of potassium from the ICF to ECF compartment[41] (Table 31-9). A pseudohyperkalemia can occur secondary to release of potassium from intracellular stores after a blood sample has been collected, hemolysis of red blood cells from excessive agitation of a blood sample, traumatic venipuncture, or prolonged application of a tourniquet during venipuncture.[41]

The most common cause of hyperkalemia is decreased renal function. Chronic hyperkalemia is almost always associated with renal failure. Usually, the glomerular filtration rate must decline to less than 10 mL/minute before hyperkalemia

TABLE 31-9 **Causes and Manifestations of Hyperkalemia**	
CAUSES	**MANIFESTATIONS**
Excessive Intake	**Laboratory Values**
Excessive oral intake	Serum potassium level above 5.0 mEq/L
Treatment with oral potassium supplements	(5.0 mmol/L)
Excessive or rapid infusion of potassium-containing parenteral fluids	**Gastrointestinal Manifestations**
Release From Intracellular Compartment	Nausea and vomiting
Tissue trauma	Intestinal cramps
Burns	Diarrhea
Crushing injuries	**Neuromuscular Manifestations**
Extreme exercise or seizures	Paresthesias
Inadequate Elimination by Kidneys	Weakness, dizziness
Renal failure	Muscle cramps
Adrenal insufficiency (Addison disease)	**Cardiovascular Manifestations**
Treatment with potassium-sparing diuretics	Changes in electrocardiogram
Treatment with angiotensin-converting enzyme inhibitors or angiotensin II receptor blockers	Risk of cardiac arrest with severe excess

develops. Some renal disorders, such as sickle cell nephropathy, lead nephropathy, and systemic lupus nephritis, can selectively impair tubular secretion of potassium without causing renal failure. As discussed previously, acidosis diminishes potassium elimination by the kidney. Persons with acute renal failure accompanied by lactic acidosis or ketoacidosis are at increased risk for development of hyperkalemia. Correcting the acidosis usually helps to correct the hyperkalemia.[42]

Aldosterone acts at the level of the distal tubular Na^+/K^+ exchange system to increase potassium excretion while facilitating sodium reabsorption. A decrease in aldosterone-mediated potassium elimination can result from adrenal insufficiency (*i.e.*, Addison disease), depression of aldosterone release due to a decrease in renin or angiotensin II, or impaired ability of the kidneys to respond to aldosterone. Potassium-sparing diuretics (*e.g.*, spironolactone, amiloride, triamterene, eplerenone) can produce hyperkalemia by means of the latter mechanism. Because of their ability to decrease aldosterone levels, the angiotensin-converting enzyme (ACE) inhibitors and angiotensin II receptor blockers (ARBs) can also produce an increase in plasma potassium levels.

Potassium excess can result from excessive oral ingestion or intravenous administration of potassium. It is difficult to increase potassium intake to the point of causing hyperkalemia when renal function is adequate and the aldosterone Na^+/K^+ exchange system is functioning. An exception to this rule is the intravenous route of administration. In some cases, severe and fatal incidents of hyperkalemia have occurred when intravenous potassium solutions were infused too rapidly. Because the kidneys control potassium elimination, intravenous solutions that contain potassium should never be started until urine output has been assessed and renal function has been deemed to be adequate.

The movement of potassium out of body cells into the ECF also can lead to elevated plasma potassium levels. Tissue injury causes release of intracellular potassium into the ECF compartment. For example, burns and crushing injuries cause cell death and release of potassium into the ECF. The same injuries often diminish renal function, which contributes to the development of hyperkalemia. Transient hyperkalemia may be induced during extreme exercise or seizures, when muscle cells are permeable to potassium. In a rare autosomal dominant disorder called *hyperkalemic periodic paralysis*, hyperkalemia may cause transient periods of muscle weakness and paralysis after exercise, cold exposure, or other situations that cause potassium to move out of the cells. In contrast to hypokalemic periodic paralysis, the episodes are usually mild, lasting less than 2 hours.[3]

Manifestations. The signs and symptoms of potassium excess are closely related to a decrease in neuromuscular excitability (see Table 31-9). The neuromuscular manifestations of potassium excess usually are absent until the plasma concentration exceeds 6 mEq/L (6 mmol/L). The first symptom associated with hyperkalemia typically is paresthesia. There may be complaints of generalized muscle weakness or dyspnea secondary to respiratory muscle weakness.

The most serious effect of hyperkalemia is on the heart. As potassium levels increase, disturbances in cardiac conduction occur. The earliest changes are peaked, narrow T waves and widening of the QRS complex. If plasma levels continue to rise, the PR interval becomes prolonged, followed by disappearance of P waves (see Fig. 31-11). The heart rate may be slow. Ventricular fibrillation and cardiac arrest are terminal events. Detrimental effects of hyperkalemia on the heart are most pronounced when the plasma potassium level rises rapidly.

Diagnosis and Treatment. Diagnosis of hyperkalemia is based on complete history, physical examination to detect muscle weakness and signs of volume depletion, plasma potassium levels, and ECG findings. The history should include questions about dietary intake, use of potassium-sparing diuretics, history of kidney disease, and recurrent episodes of muscle weakness.

The treatment of potassium excess varies with the degree of increase in plasma potassium and whether there are ECG and neuromuscular manifestations. Calcium antagonizes the potassium-induced decrease in membrane excitability, restoring excitability toward normal. The protective effect of calcium administration is usually short-lived (15 to 30 minutes), and it must be accompanied by other therapies to decrease the ECF potassium concentration. The administration of sodium bicarbonate, β-adrenergic agonists (*e.g.*, nebulized albuterol), or insulin distributes potassium into the ICF compartment and rapidly decreases the ECF concentration. Intravenous infusions of insulin and glucose are often used for this purpose.

Less emergent measures focus on decreasing or curtailing intake or absorption, increasing renal excretion, and increasing cellular uptake. Decreased intake can be achieved by restricting dietary sources of potassium. The major ingredient in most salt substitutes is potassium chloride, and such substitutes should not be given to patients with renal problems. Increasing potassium output often is more difficult. Patients with renal failure may require hemodialysis or peritoneal dialysis to reduce plasma potassium levels. Sodium polystyrene sulfonate, a cation exchange resin, also may be used to remove K^+ ions from the colon. The Na^+ ions in the resin are exchanged for K^+ ions, and the potassium-containing resin is eliminated in the stool.

IN SUMMARY, potassium is the major ICF cation. It contributes to the maintenance of intracellular osmolality, plays a critical role in conducting nerve impulses and in the excitability of skeletal, cardiac, and smooth muscle, and influences acid-base balance. Potassium is ingested in the diet and eliminated through the kidney. Because potassium is poorly conserved by the kidney, an adequate daily intake is needed. A transcellular shift can produce a redistribution of potassium between the ECF and ICF compartments, causing blood levels to increase or decrease.

Hypokalemia represents a decrease in plasma potassium to levels below 3.5 mEq/L (3.5 mmol/L). It can result from inadequate intake, excessive losses, or redistribution between the

ICF and ECF compartments. The manifestations of potassium deficit include alterations in renal, skeletal muscle, gastrointestinal, and cardiovascular function, reflecting the crucial role of potassium in cell metabolism and neuromuscular function.

Hyperkalemia represents an increase in plasma potassium to levels plasma greater than 5 mEq/L (5 mmol/L). It seldom occurs in healthy persons because the body is extremely effective in preventing excess potassium accumulation in the ECF. The major causes of potassium excess are decreased elimination of potassium by the kidney, excessively rapid intravenous administration of potassium, and a transcellular shift of potassium out of the cell to the ECF compartment. The most serious effect of hyperkalemia is cardiac arrest. ■

CALCIUM, PHOSPHORUS, AND MAGNESIUM BALANCE

After completing this section of the chapter, you should be able to meet the following objectives:

- Describe the associations among intestinal absorption, renal elimination, bone stores, and the functions of vitamin D and parathyroid hormone in regulating calcium, phosphorus, and magnesium levels.
- State the difference between ionized and bound or chelated forms of calcium in terms of physiologic function.
- Describe the mechanisms of calcium gain and loss and relate them to the causes of hypocalcemia and hypercalcemia.
- Relate the functions of calcium to the manifestations of hypocalcemia and hypercalcemia.
- Describe the mechanisms of phosphorus gain and loss and relate them to causes of hypophosphatemia and hyperphosphatemia.
- Relate the functions of phosphorus to the manifestations of hypophosphatemia and hyperphosphatemia.
- Describe the mechanisms of magnesium gain and loss and relate them to the causes of hypomagnesemia and hypermagnesemia.
- Relate the functions of magnesium to the manifestations of hypomagnesemia and hypermagnesemia.

Mechanisms Regulating Calcium, Phosphorus, and Magnesium Balance

Calcium, phosphorus, and magnesium are the major divalent cations in the body. They are ingested in the diet, absorbed from the intestine, filtered in the glomerulus of the kidney, reabsorbed in the renal tubules, and eliminated in the urine. Approximately 99% of calcium, 85% of phosphorus, and 50% to 60% of magnesium are found in bone. Most of the remaining calcium (approximately 1%), phosphorus (approximately 14%),

and magnesium (approximately 40% to 50%) is located inside cells. Only a small amount of these three ions is present in ECF. This small, but vital, amount of ECF calcium, phosphorus, and magnesium is directly or indirectly regulated by vitamin D and parathyroid hormone. Calcitonin, a hormone produced by C cells in the thyroid, is thought to act on the kidney and bone to remove calcium from the extracellular circulation. The roles of vitamin D, parathyroid hormone (PTH), and calcitonin in skeletal function are discussed further in Chapters 57 and 59.

Vitamin D

Although classified as a vitamin, vitamin D functions as a hormone. It acts to sustain normal plasma levels of calcium and phosphorus by increasing their absorption from the intestine, and it also is necessary for normal bone formation. Vitamin D is synthesized by ultraviolet irradiation of 7-dehydrocholesterol, which is present in the skin or obtained from foods in the diet, many of which are fortified with vitamin D. The synthesized or ingested forms of vitamin D are essentially prohormones that lack biologic activity and must undergo metabolic transformation to achieve potency. Once vitamin D enters the circulation from the skin or intestine, it is concentrated in the liver. There it is hydroxylated to form 25-hydroxyvitamin D [25-(OH)D$_3$], also called *calcidiol*. It is then transported to the kidney, where it is transformed into active 1,25-(OH)$_2$D$_3$. The major action of the activated form of vitamin D, also called *calcitriol*, is to increase the absorption of calcium from the intestine. Calcitriol also sensitizes bone to the resorptive actions of PTH. There is also recent evidence that vitamin D controls parathyroid gland growth and suppresses the synthesis and secretion of PTH.[43] The formation of 1,25-(OH)$_2$D$_3$ in the kidneys is regulated in feedback fashion by plasma calcium and phosphate levels. Low calcium levels lead to an increase in PTH, which then increases vitamin D activation. A lowering of plasma phosphate also augments vitamin D activation. Additional control of renal activation of vitamin D is exerted by a negative feedback loop that monitors 1,25-(OH)$_2$D$_3$ levels.

Parathyroid Hormone

Parathyroid hormone, a major regulator of plasma calcium and phosphorus, is secreted by the parathyroid glands. There are four parathyroid glands located on the dorsal surface of the thyroid gland. The dominant regulator of PTH is the plasma calcium concentration. A unique calcium receptor on the parathyroid cell membrane (extracellular calcium-sensing receptor) responds rapidly to changes in plasma calcium levels.[44] When the plasma calcium level is high, PTH is inhibited and the calcium is deposited in the bones. When the level is low, PTH secretion is increased and calcium is mobilized from the bones. The response to a decrease in plasma calcium is prompt, occurring within seconds. Phosphorus does not exert a direct effect on PTH secretion. Instead, it acts indirectly by forming a complex with calcium, thereby decreasing the plasma calcium concentration.

The secretion, synthesis, and action of PTH are also influenced by magnesium. Magnesium serves as a cofactor in the generation of cellular energy and is important in the function of second messenger systems. Magnesium's effects on the synthesis and release of PTH are thought to be mediated through these mechanisms. Because of its function in regulating PTH release, severe and prolonged hypomagnesemia can markedly inhibit PTH levels.

The main function of PTH is to maintain the calcium concentration of the ECF. It performs this function by promoting the release of calcium from bone, increasing the activation of vitamin D as a means of enhancing intestinal absorption of calcium, and stimulating calcium conservation by the kidney while increasing phosphate excretion (Fig. 31-12). PTH acts on bone to accelerate the mobilization and transfer of calcium to the ECF. The skeletal response to PTH is a two-step process. There is an immediate response in which calcium that is present in bone fluid is released into the ECF, and a second, more slowly developing response in which completely mineralized bone is resorbed, resulting in the release of both calcium and phosphorus. The actions of PTH in terms of bone resorption require normal levels of both vitamin D and magnesium. The activation of vitamin D by the kidney is enhanced by the pres-

ence of PTH; it is through the activation of vitamin D that PTH increases intestinal absorption of calcium and phosphorus as well as acting on the kidney to increase tubular reabsorption of calcium and magnesium while increasing phosphorus elimination. The accompanying increase in phosphorus elimination ensures that the phosphorus released from bone does not produce hyperphosphatemia and increases the risk of soft tissue deposition of calcium phosphate crystals.

Hypoparathyroidism. Hypoparathyroidism reflects deficient PTH secretion, resulting in hypocalcemia. PTH deficiency may be caused by a congenital absence of all of the parathyroid glands, as in DiGeorge syndrome (see Chapter 19). An acquired deficiency of PTH may occur after neck surgery, particularly if the surgery involves removal of a parathyroid adenoma, thyroidectomy, or bilateral neck resection for cancer. A transient form of PTH deficiency, occurring within 1 to 2 days and lasting up to 5 days, may occur after thyroid surgery owing to parathyroid gland suppression.[8] Hypoparathyroidism also may have an autoimmune origin. Antiparathyroid antibodies have been detected in some persons with hypoparathyroidism, particularly those with multiple autoimmune disorders such as type 1 diabetes, Graves disease, and vitiligo (autoimmune destruction of melanocytes resulting in the development of totally white areas of skin). Other causes of hypoparathyroidism include heavy metal damage such as occurs with Wilson disease, metastatic tumors, and surgery. Functional impairment of parathyroid function occurs with magnesium deficiency. Correction of the hypomagnesemia results in rapid disappearance of the condition.

Manifestations of acute hypoparathyroidism, which result from a decrease in plasma calcium, include tetany with muscle cramps, carpopedal spasm, and convulsions (see section on Hypocalcemia). Paresthesias, such as tingling of the circumoral area and the hands and feet, are almost always present. Low calcium levels may cause prolongation of the QT interval, resistance to digitalis, hypotension, and refractory heart failure. Symptoms of chronic PTH deficiency include lethargy, anxiety state, and personality changes. There may be blurring of vision because of cataracts, which develop over a number of years. Extrapyramidal signs, such as those seen with Parkinson disease, may occur because of calcification of the basal ganglia. Successful treatment of the hypocalcemia may improve the disorder and is sometimes associated with a decrease in basal ganglia calcification on radiography. Teeth may be defective if the disorder occurs during childhood.

Diagnosis of hypoparathyroidism is based on low plasma calcium levels, high plasma phosphate levels, and low plasma PTH levels. Plasma magnesium levels usually are measured to rule out hypomagnesemia as a cause of the disorder. Acute hypoparathyroid tetany is treated with intravenous calcium gluconate followed by oral administration of calcium salts and vitamin D. Magnesium supplementation is used when the disorder is caused by magnesium deficiency. Persons with chronic hypoparathyroidism are treated with oral calcium and vitamin D. Plasma calcium levels are monitored at regular intervals (at least every 3 months) as a means of maintaining plasma calcium

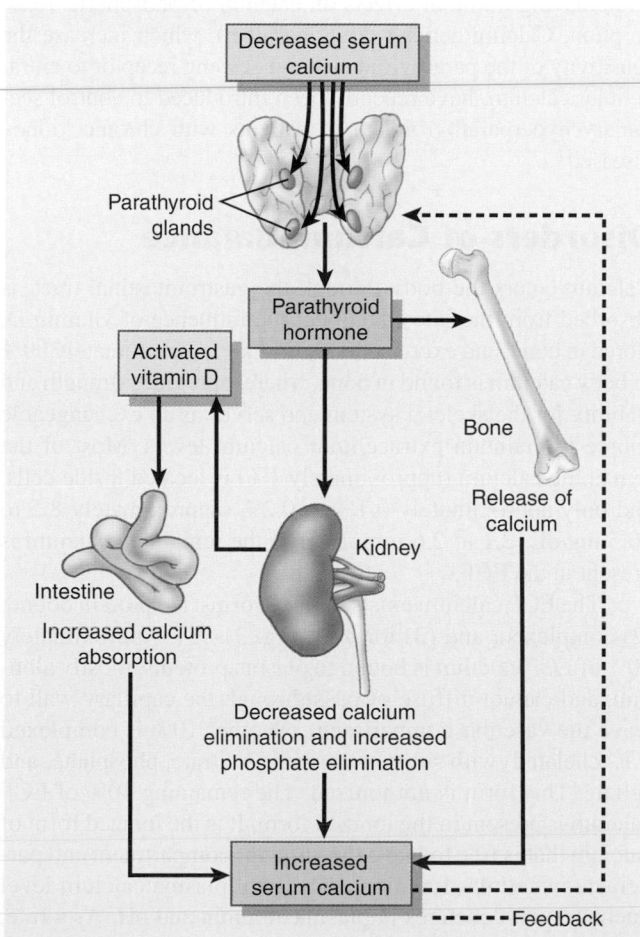

FIGURE 31-12 • Regulation of plasma calcium concentration by parathyroid hormone.

within a slightly low but asymptomatic range. Maintaining plasma calcium within this range helps to prevent hypercalciuria and kidney damage.

Pseudohypoparathyroidism is a rare familial disorder characterized by target tissue resistance to PTH. It is characterized by hypocalcemia, increased parathyroid function, and a variety of congenital defects in the growth and development of the skeleton, including short stature and short metacarpal and metatarsal bones. There are variants in the disorder, with some persons having pseudohypoparathyroidism with the congenital defects and others having the congenital defects with normal calcium and phosphate levels. The manifestations of the disorder are due primarily to chronic hypocalcemia. Treatment is similar to that for hypoparathyroidism.

Hyperparathyroidism. Hyperparathyroidism is caused by hypersecretion of PTH. Hyperparathyroidism can manifest as a primary disorder caused by hyperplasia (15%), an adenoma (85%), and rarely carcinoma of the parathyroid glands, or as a secondary disorder seen in persons with chronic renal failure or chronic malabsorption of calcium. Parathyroid adenomas and hyperplasia can occur in several distinct familial diseases (including multiple endocrine neoplasia [MEN] types 1 and 2a).

Primary hyperparathyroidism is seen more commonly after 50 years of age and is more common in women than men.[45,46] Primary hyperparathyroidism causes hypercalcemia and an increase in calcium in the urine filtrate, resulting in hypercalciuria and the potential for development of kidney stones. Chronic bone resorption may produce diffuse demineralization, pathologic fractures, and cystic bone lesions. A dual-energy x-ray absorptiometry (DEXA) bone scan may be used to assess bone mineral density (BMD). Signs and symptoms of the disorder are related to skeletal abnormalities, exposure of the kidney to high calcium levels, and elevated plasma calcium levels (see section on Hypercalcemia). At present, most patients with primary hyperparathyroidism manifest an asymptomatic disorder that is discovered in the course of routine biochemical testing.

Diagnostic procedures, which include plasma calcium levels and intact PTH levels, are used to differentiate between the two most common causes of hypercalcemia: primary hyperparathyroidism and hypercalcemia of malignancy. Assays of intact PTH use two antibodies that bind to different sites on PTH and are designed to measure the intact, biologically active hormone, specifically. In primary hyperparathyroidism the intact PTH levels are elevated in 75% to 90% of affected persons or are inappropriately "normal" in the face of hypercalcemia, when they should be suppressed. In hypercalcemia of malignancy, the intact PTH levels are suppressed. Imaging studies of the parathyroid area may be used to identify a parathyroid adenoma. However, the role of imaging studies before and during surgery is the topic of much debate.[45] Parathyroid surgery is usually the treatment of choice.

Secondary hyperparathyroidism involves hyperplasia of the parathyroid glands and occurs primarily in persons with renal failure[47,48] (see Chapter 34). In early renal failure, an increase in PTH results from decreased plasma calcium and activated vitamin D levels. As the disease progresses, there is a decrease in

vitamin D and calcium receptors, making the parathyroid glands more resistant to feedback regulation by plasma calcium and vitamin D level. At this point, elevated plasma phosphate levels induce hyperplasia of the parathyroid glands independent of calcium and activated vitamin D. The bone disease seen in persons with secondary hyperparathyroidism due to renal failure is known as *renal osteodystrophy* (see Chapter 34).

Treatment of hyperparathyroidism includes resolving the hypercalcemia with increased fluid intake. Persons with mild disease are advised to keep active and drink adequate fluids. They also are advised to avoid calcium-containing antacids, vitamin D, and thiazide diuretics, which increase reabsorption of calcium by the kidney. Parathyroidectomy may be indicated in persons with symptomatic hyperparathyroidism, kidney stones, or bone disease. Avoiding hyperphosphatemia may prevent renal osteodystrophies caused by secondary hyperparathyroidism in renal failure. Calcium acetate or a newer calcium-free agent (sevelamer HCl [Renagel]) can be given with meals to bind phosphate.[49] Calcitriol, the activated form of vitamin D, may be used to control parathyroid hyperplasia and suppress the synthesis and secretion of PTH. However, because of its potent effect on intestinal absorption and bone mobilization, calcitriol can cause hypercalcemia. Newer analogs of activated vitamin D are being developed that retain the ability to suppress parathyroid function while having minimal effects on calcium or phosphorus reabsorption. Calcimimetics (*e.g.,* cinacalcet), which increase the sensitivity of the parathyroid calcium-sensing receptor to extracellular calcium, have recently been introduced to control secondary hyperparathyroidism in patients with chronic kidney disease.[44]

Disorders of Calcium Balance

Calcium enters the body through the gastrointestinal tract, is absorbed from the intestine under the influence of vitamin D, stored in bone, and excreted by the kidney. Approximately 99% of body calcium is found in bone, where it provides strength and stability for the skeletal system and serves as an exchangeable source to maintain extracellular calcium levels. Most of the remaining calcium (approximately 1%) is located inside cells, and only approximately 0.1% to 0.2% (approximately 8.5 to 10.5 mg/dL [2.1 to 2.6 mmol/L]) of the remaining calcium is present in the ECF.

The ECF calcium exists in three forms: (1) protein bound, (2) complexed, and (3) ionized (Fig. 31-13). Approximately 40% of ECF calcium is bound to plasma proteins, mostly albumin, and cannot diffuse or pass through the capillary wall to leave the vascular compartment. Another 10% is complexed (*i.e.,* chelated) with substances such as citrate, phosphate, and sulfate. This form is not ionized. The remaining 50% of ECF calcium is present in the ionized form. It is the ionized form of calcium that is free to leave the vascular compartment and participate in cellular functions. The total plasma calcium level fluctuates with changes in plasma albumin and pH. As a rule, the total plasma calcium level is increased 0.75 to 1 mg/dL for every 1 g/dL decreased from normal in the plasma albumin level, and decreased by 0.16 mg/dL for each 0.1 unit rise in pH.[5]

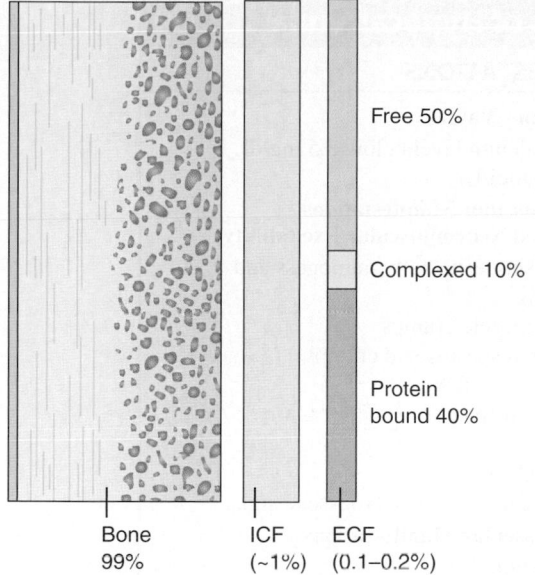

FIGURE 31-13 • Distribution of body calcium between bone and the intracellular (ICF) and extracellular fluid (ECF) compartments. The percentages of free, complexed, and protein-bound calcium in extracellular fluids are indicated.

Ionized calcium serves a number of functions. It participates in many enzyme reactions; exerts an important effect on membrane potentials and neuronal excitability; is necessary for contraction in skeletal, cardiac, and smooth muscle; participates in the release of hormones, neurotransmitters, and other chemical messengers; influences cardiac contractility and automaticity through the slow calcium channels; and is essential for blood clotting. The use of calcium channel blocking drugs in circulatory disorders demonstrates the importance of Ca^{2+} ions in the normal functioning of the heart and blood vessels. Calcium is required for all but the first two steps of the intrinsic pathway for blood coagulation. Because of its ability to bind calcium, citrate often is used to prevent clotting in blood that is to be used for transfusions.

⚷ CALCIUM BALANCE

■ About 99% of body calcium is stored in bone; 1% is located inside cells; and 0.1% is found in the extracellular fluid.

■ Extracellular fluid calcium levels are made up of free (ionized), complexed, and protein-bound fractions. Only the ionized Ca^{2+} plays an essential role in neuromuscular and cardiac excitability.

■ Serum calcium levels are regulated by parathyroid hormone and by renal mechanisms in which serum levels of calcium and phosphate are reciprocally regulated to prevent the damaging deposition of calcium phosphate crystals in the soft tissues of the body.

Gains and Losses

The major dietary sources of calcium are milk and milk products. Only 30% to 50% of dietary calcium is absorbed from the duodenum and upper jejunum; the remainder is eliminated in the stool. There is a calcium influx of approximately 150 mg/day into the intestine from the blood. Net absorption of calcium is equal to the amount that is absorbed from the intestine less the amount that moves into the intestine. Calcium balance can become negative when dietary intake (and calcium absorption) is less than intestinal secretion. A dietary intake of less than 400 mg/day can be associated with negative calcium balance.[5]

Calcium is stored in bone and excreted by the kidney. Approximately 60% to 65% of filtered calcium is passively reabsorbed in the proximal tubule, driven by the reabsorption of sodium chloride; 15% to 20% is reabsorbed in the thick ascending loop of Henle, driven by the $Na^+/K^+/2Cl^-$ cotransport system; and 5% to 10% is reabsorbed in the distal convoluted tubule (see Chapter 30). The distal convoluted tubule is an important regulatory site for controlling the amount of calcium that enters the urine. PTH and possibly vitamin D stimulate calcium reabsorption in this segment of the nephron. Thiazide diuretics, which exert their effects in the distal convoluted tubule, enhance calcium reabsorption. Other factors that may influence calcium reabsorption in the distal convoluted tubule are phosphate levels and glucose and insulin levels.

Hypocalcemia

Hypocalcemia represents a plasma calcium level of less than 8.5 mg/dL (2.1 mmol/L). Hypocalcemia occurs in many forms of critical illness and has affected as much 70% to 90% of patients in intensive care units.[50]

Causes. The causes of hypocalcemia can be divided into four categories: (1) impaired ability to mobilize calcium from bone stores, (2) abnormal losses of calcium from the kidney, (3) increased protein binding or chelation such that greater proportions of calcium are in the nonionized form, and (4) soft tissue sequestration (Table 31-10). A pseudohypocalcemia is caused by hypoalbuminemia. It results in a decrease in protein-bound, rather than ionized, calcium and usually is asymptomatic.[51]

Plasma calcium exists in a dynamic equilibrium with calcium in bone. The ability to mobilize calcium from bone depends on adequate levels of PTH. Decreased levels of PTH may result from primary or secondary forms of hypoparathyroidism. Suppression of PTH release may also occur when vitamin D levels are elevated. The activated form of vitamin D (calcitriol) can be used to suppress the secondary hyperparathyroidism that occurs in persons with chronic kidney disease. Magnesium deficiency inhibits PTH release and impairs the action of PTH on bone resorption. This form of hypocalcemia is difficult to treat with calcium supplementation alone and requires correction of the magnesium deficiency.

TABLE 31-10 Causes and Manifestations of Hypocalcemia

CAUSES	MANIFESTATIONS
Impaired Ability to Mobilize Calcium From Bone	**Laboratory Values**
Hypoparathyroidism	Serum calcium level below 8.5 mg/dL (2.1 mmol/L)
Resistance to the actions of parathyroid hormone	**Neuromuscular Manifestations (Increased Neuromuscular Excitability)**
Hypomagnesemia	Paresthesias, especially numbness and tingling
Decreased Intake or Absorption	Skeletal muscle cramps
Malabsorption	Abdominal spasms and cramps
Vitamin D deficiency	Hyperactive reflexes
Failure to activate	Carpopedal spasm
Liver disease	Tetany
Kidney disease	Laryngeal spasm
Medications that impair activation of vitamin D (*e.g.*, phenytoin)	Positive Chvostek and Trousseau signs
Abnormal Renal Losses	**Cardiovascular Manifestations**
Renal failure and hyperphosphatemia	Hypotension
Increased Protein Binding or Chelation	Signs of cardiac insufficiency
Increased pH	Failure to respond to drugs that act by calcium-mediated mechanisms
Increased fatty acids	Prolongation of QT interval predisposes to ventricular dysrhythmias
Rapid transfusion of citrated blood	**Skeletal Manifestations (Chronic Deficiency)**
Increased Sequestration	Osteomalacia
Acute pancreatitis	Bone pain, deformities, fracture

There is an inverse relation between calcium and phosphate excretion by the kidneys. Phosphate elimination is impaired in chronic kidney disease, causing plasma calcium levels to decrease. Hypocalcemia and hyperphosphatemia occur when the glomerular filtration rate falls below 59 mL/minute (normal values, which are related to age, sex, and body size, are approximately 120 mL/minute in young women and 130 mL/minute in young men; see Chapter 34).

Only the ionized form of calcium is able to leave the capillary and participate in body functions. A change in pH alters the proportion of calcium that is in the bound and ionized forms. An acid pH decreases binding of calcium to protein, causing a proportionate increase in ionized calcium, whereas total plasma calcium remains unchanged. An alkaline pH has the opposite effect. As an example, hyperventilation sufficient to cause respiratory alkalosis can produce tetany because of increased protein binding of calcium. Free fatty acids also increase binding of calcium to albumin, causing a reduction in ionized calcium. Elevations in free fatty acids sufficient to alter calcium binding may occur during stressful situations that cause elevations of epinephrine, glucagon, growth hormone, and adrenocorticotropic hormone levels. Heparin, β-adrenergic drugs (*i.e.*, epinephrine, isoproterenol, and norepinephrine), and alcohol can also produce elevations in free fatty acids levels sufficient to increase calcium binding.

Citrate, which complexes with calcium, is often used as an anticoagulant in blood transfusions. Theoretically, excess citrate in donor blood could combine with the calcium in a recipient's blood, producing a sharp drop in ionized calcium. This normally does not occur because the liver removes the citrate within a matter of minutes. When blood transfusions are administered at a slow rate, there is little danger of hypocalcemia caused by citrate binding.[2]

Hypocalcemia is a common finding in patients with acute pancreatitis. Inflammation of the pancreas causes release of proteolytic and lipolytic enzymes. It is thought that the Ca^{2+} combines with free fatty acids released by lipolysis in the pancreas, forming soaps and removing calcium from the circulation.

Calcium deficit due to dietary deficiency exerts its effects on bone stores rather than extracellular calcium levels. A dietary deficiency of vitamin D is still seen today despite many foods being fortified with vitamin D. Vitamin D deficiency is more likely to occur in malabsorption states, such as biliary obstruction, pancreatic insufficiency, and celiac disease, in which the ability to absorb fat and fat-soluble vitamins is impaired. Failure to activate vitamin D is another cause of hypocalcemia. Anticonvulsant medications, particularly phenytoin, can impair initial activation of vitamin D in the liver. The final step in activation of vitamin D is impaired in persons with chronic kidney disease (see Chapter 34). Fortunately, the activated form of vitamin D, calcitriol, has been synthesized and is available for use in the treatment of calcium deficit in persons with chronic kidney disease.

Manifestations. Hypocalcemia can manifest as an acute or chronic condition. The manifestations of acute hypocalcemia reflect the increased neuromuscular excitability and cardiovascular effects of a decrease in ionized calcium (see Table 31-10). Ionized calcium stabilizes neuromuscular excitability, thereby making nerve cells less sensitive to stimuli. Nerves exposed to low ionized calcium levels show decreased thresholds for excitation, repetitive responses to a single stimulus, and, in extreme cases, continuous activity. The severity of the manifestations depends on the underlying cause, rapidity of onset, accompanying electrolyte disorders, and extracellular pH. Increased neuromuscular excitability can manifest as paresthesias (*i.e.,* tingling around the mouth and in the hands and feet) and tetany (*i.e.,* spasms of the muscles of the face, hands, and feet).[52] Severe hypocalcemia can lead to laryngeal spasm, seizures, and even death.

Cardiovascular effects of acute hypocalcemia include hypotension, cardiac insufficiency, cardiac dysrhythmias (particularly heart block and ventricular fibrillation), and failure to respond to drugs such as digitalis, norepinephrine, and dopamine that act through calcium-mediated mechanisms.

The Chvostek and Trousseau tests can be used to assess for an increase in neuromuscular excitability and tetany[8] (Fig. 31-14). The Chvostek sign is elicited by tapping the face just below the temple at the point where the facial nerve emerges. Tapping the face over the facial nerve causes spasm of the lip, nose, or face when the test result is positive. An inflated blood pressure cuff is used to test for the Trousseau sign. The cuff is inflated 10 mm Hg above systolic blood pressure for 3 minutes. Contraction of the fingers and hands (*i.e.,* carpopedal spasm) indicates the presence of tetany.

Chronic hypocalcemia is often accompanied by skeletal manifestations and skin changes. There may be bone pain,

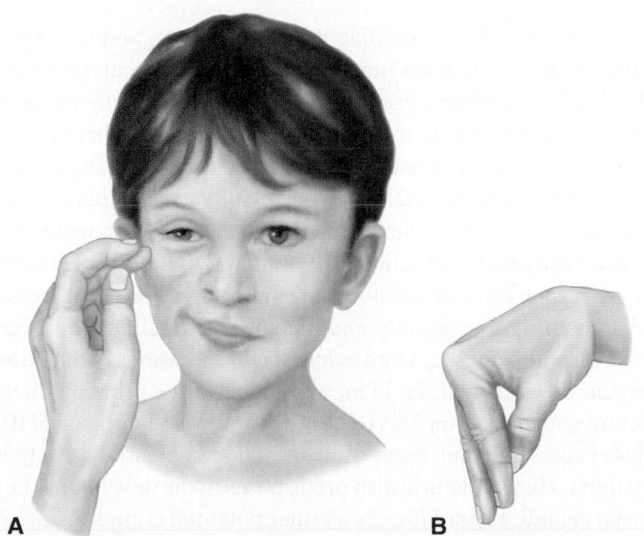

FIGURE 31-14 • **(A)** The Chvostek sign: a contraction of the facial muscles elicited in response to a light tap over the facial nerve in front of the ear. **(B)** The Trousseau sign: a carpopedal spasm induced by inflating a blood pressure cuff above systolic blood pressure. (Adapted from Bullock B. A., Henze R. J. [2000]. *Focus on pathophysiology* [p. 173]. Philadelphia: Lippincott Williams & Wilkins.)

fragility, deformities, and fractures. The skin may be dry and scaling, the nails brittle, and hair dry. Development of cataracts is common.

Treatment. Acute hypocalcemia is an emergency, requiring prompt treatment. An intravenous infusion containing calcium (*e.g.,* calcium gluconate, calcium chloride) is used when tetany or acute symptoms are present or anticipated because of a decrease in the plasma calcium level.[52]

Chronic hypocalcemia is treated with oral intake of calcium. One glass of milk contains approximately 300 mg of calcium. Oral calcium supplements of carbonate, gluconate, or lactate salts may be used. Long-term treatment may require the use of vitamin D preparations, especially in persons with hypoparathyroidism and chronic kidney disease. The active form of vitamin D is administered when the liver or kidney mechanisms needed for hormone activation are impaired. Synthetic PTH (1-34) can be administered by subcutaneous injection as replacement therapy in hypoparathyroidism.

Hypercalcemia

Hypercalcemia represents a total plasma calcium concentration greater than 10.5 mg/dL (2.6 mmol/L). Falsely elevated levels of calcium can result from prolonged drawing of blood with an excessively tight tourniquet. Increased plasma proteins (*e.g.,* hyperalbuminemia, hyperglobulinemia) may elevate the total plasma calcium but not affect the ionized calcium concentration.

Causes. A plasma calcium excess (*i.e.,* hypercalcemia) results when calcium movement into the circulation overwhelms the calcium regulatory hormones or the ability of the kidney to remove excess calcium ions (Table 31-11). The two most common causes of hypercalcemia are increased bone resorption due to neoplasms and hyperparathyroidism.[53] These two etiologies account for over 90% of all persons with hypercalcemia. Hypercalcemia is a common complication of malignancy, occurring in approximately 10% to 20% of persons with advanced disease.[53] A number of malignant tumors, including carcinoma of the lungs, have been associated with hypercalcemia. Some tumors destroy the bone, whereas others produce humoral agents that stimulate osteoclastic activity, increase bone resorption, or inhibit bone formation. Approximately 80% of patients with hypercalcemia of malignancy produce PTH-related protein (PTH-rP).[54] PTH and PTH-rP have marked homology, or structural similarity, at their amino terminal ends, with 8 of the first 13 amino acids in the same positions. This homology results in both PTH and PTH-rP binding to the same receptor (PTH/PTH-rP receptor). PTH-rP is produced by several tumors, including cancers of the lung, breast, kidney, head and neck, and ovary.[54]

Less frequent causes of hypercalcemia are prolonged immobilization, increased intestinal absorption of calcium, excessive doses of vitamin D, or the effects of drugs such as lithium and thiazide diuretics. Prolonged immobilization and

TABLE 31-11 Causes and Manifestations of Hypercalcemia

CAUSES	MANIFESTATIONS
Increased Intestinal Absorption	**Laboratory Values**
Excessive vitamin D	Serum calcium level above 10.5 mg/dL
Excessive calcium in the diet	(2.6 mmol/L)
Milk-alkali syndrome	**Impaired Ability to Concentrate Urine**
Increased Bone Resorption	**and Exposure of Kidney to Increased**
Increased levels of parathyroid hormone	**Concentration of Calcium**
Malignant neoplasms	Polyuria
Prolonged immobilization	Polydipsia
Decreased Elimination	Flank pain
Thiazide diuretics	Signs of acute and chronic renal insufficiency
Lithium therapy	Signs of kidney stones
	Gastrointestinal Manifestations
	Anorexia
	Nausea, vomiting
	Constipation
	Neuromuscular Manifestations
	(Decreased Neuromuscular Excitability)
	Muscle weakness and atrophy
	Ataxia, loss of muscle tone
	Skeletal Manifestations
	Osteopenia
	Osteoporosis
	Central Nervous System Manifestations
	Lethargy
	Personality and behavioral changes
	Stupor and coma
	Cardiovascular Manifestations
	Hypertension
	Shortening of the QT interval
	Atrioventricular block on electrocardiogram

lack of weight bearing cause demineralization of bone and release of calcium into the bloodstream. Intestinal absorption of calcium can be increased by excessive doses of vitamin D or as a result of a condition called the *milk-alkali syndrome.* The milk-alkali syndrome is caused by excessive ingestion of calcium (often in the form of milk) and absorbable antacids. Because of the availability of nonabsorbable antacids, the condition is seen less frequently than in the past, but it may occur in women who are overzealous in taking calcium preparations for osteoporosis prevention. Discontinuance of the antacid repairs the alkalosis and increases calcium elimination.

A variety of drugs elevate calcium levels. The use of lithium to treat bipolar disorders has caused hypercalcemia and hyperparathyroidism. The thiazide diuretics increase calcium reabsorption in the distal convoluted tubule of the kidney. Although the thiazide diuretics seldom cause hypercalcemia, they can unmask hypercalcemia from other causes such as underlying bone disorders and conditions that increase bone resorption.

Manifestations. The signs and symptoms associated with calcium excess reflect (1) changes in neural excitability, (2) alter-

ations in smooth and cardiac muscle function, and (3) exposure of the kidneys to high concentrations of calcium (see Table 31-11). Neural excitability is decreased in patients with hypercalcemia. There may be a dulling of consciousness, stupor, weakness, and muscle flaccidity. Behavioral changes may range from subtle alterations in personality to acute psychoses. The heart responds to elevated levels of calcium with increased contractility and ventricular arrhythmias. Digitalis accentuates these responses. Gastrointestinal symptoms reflect a decrease in smooth muscle activity and include constipation, anorexia, nausea, and vomiting. High calcium concentrations in the urine impair the ability of the kidneys to concentrate urine by interfering with the action of ADH (an example of nephrogenic DI). This causes salt and water diuresis and an increased sensation of thirst. Hypercalciuria also predisposes to the development of renal calculi. Pancreatitis is another potential complication of hypercalcemia and is probably related to stones in the pancreatic ducts.

Hypercalcemic crisis describes an acute increase in the plasma calcium level.[53] Malignant disease and hyperparathyroidism are the major causes of hypercalcemic crisis. In hypercalcemic crisis, polyuria, excessive thirst, volume depletion, fever, altered levels of consciousness, azotemia (*i.e.,* nitrogenous wastes in the blood), and a disturbed mental state accompany other signs of calcium excess. Symptomatic hypercalcemia is associated with a high mortality rate; death often is caused by cardiac arrest.

Treatment. Treatment of calcium excess usually is directed toward rehydration and use of measures to increase urinary excretion of calcium and inhibit release of calcium from bone.[53] Fluid replacement is needed in situations of volume depletion. The excretion of sodium is accompanied by calcium excretion. Diuretics and sodium chloride can be administered to increase urinary elimination of calcium after the ECF volume has been restored. Loop diuretics commonly are used rather than thiazide diuretics, which increase calcium reabsorption. Initial lowering of calcium levels is followed by measures to inhibit bone reabsorption. Drugs that are used to inhibit calcium mobilization include bisphosphonates, calcitonin, corticosteroids, mithramycin, and gallium nitrate. The bisphosphonates (*e.g.,* pamidronate, zoledronate), which act mainly by inhibiting osteoclastic activity, provide a significant reduction in calcium levels with relatively few side effects. Calcitonin inhibits osteoclastic activity, thereby decreasing resorption. The corticosteroids and mithramycin inhibit bone resorption and are used to treat hypercalcemia associated with cancer. The long-term use of mithramycin, an antineoplastic drug, is limited because of its potential for nephrotoxicity and hepatotoxicity. Gallium nitrate is highly effective in the treatment of severe hypercalcemia associated with malignancy. It is a chemical compound that inhibits bone resorption, although the precise mechanism of action is unclear. Dialysis can be used in hypercalcemic patients with renal failure and in patients with heart failure in whom fluid overload is a concern.

Disorders of Phosphorus Balance

Phosphorus is mainly an intracellular anion. Approximately 85% of phosphorus is contained in bone, and most of the remainder (14%) is located in cells. Only approximately 1% is in the ECF compartment, and of that, only a minute proportion is in the plasma. In the adult, the normal plasma phosphorus level ranges from 2.5 to 4.5 mg/dL (0.8 to 1.45 mmol/L). These values are slightly higher in infants (3.7 to 8.5 mg/dL, 01.2 to 02.7 mmol/L) and children (4 to 5.4 mg/dL, 1.3 to 1.7 mmol/L), probably because of increased growth hormone and decreased gonadal hormones.

Phosphorus exists in two forms within the body—inorganic and organic. The inorganic form (phosphate [$H_2PO_4^-$ or HPO_4^{2-}]) is the principal circulating form of phosphorus and is the form that is routinely measured (and reported as phosphorus) for laboratory purposes.[55] Most of the intracellular phosphorus (approximately 90%) is in the organic form (*e.g.,* nucleic acids, phospholipids, adenosine triphosphate [ATP]). Entry of phosphorus into cells is enhanced after glucose uptake because phosphorus is incorporated into the phosphorylated intermediates of glucose metabolism. Cell injury or atrophy leads to a loss of cell components that contain organic

> ## ⚷ PHOSPHORUS BALANCE
>
> - Approximately 85% of the phosphorus is contained in bone. Most of the remaining phosphorus is incorporated into organic compounds such as nucleic acids, high-energy compounds (*e.g.,* ATP), and coenzymes that are critically important for cell function.
>
> - Many of the manifestations of hypophosphatemia are related to a decrease in cell energy due to ATP depletion.
>
> - Serum phosphorus levels are regulated by the kidneys, which eliminate or conserve phosphate as serum levels change. Serum levels of calcium and phosphate are reciprocally regulated to prevent the damaging deposition of calcium phosphate crystals in the soft tissues of the body. Many of the manifestations of hyperphosphatemia reflect a decrease in serum calcium levels.

phosphate; regeneration of these cellular components results in withdrawal of inorganic phosphate from the ECF compartment.

Phosphorus is essential to many bodily functions. It plays a major role in bone formation; is essential to certain metabolic processes, including the formation of ATP and the enzymes needed for metabolism of glucose, fat, and protein; is a necessary component of several vital parts of the cell, being incorporated into the nucleic acids of DNA and RNA and the phospholipids of the cell membrane; and serves as an acid-base buffer in the ECF and in the renal excretion of hydrogen ions. Delivery of oxygen by the red blood cell depends on organic phosphorus in ATP and 2,3-diphosphoglycerate. Phosphorus is also needed for normal function of other blood cells, including the white blood cells and platelets.

Gains and Losses

Phosphorus is ingested in the diet and eliminated in the urine. Phosphorus is derived from many dietary sources, including milk and meats. Approximately 80% of ingested phosphorus is absorbed in the intestine, primarily in the jejunum. Absorption is diminished by concurrent ingestion of substances that bind phosphorus, including calcium, magnesium, and aluminum.

Phosphate is not bound to plasma proteins and essentially all of the phosphate that is present in the plasma is filtered in the glomerulus.[56] Renal elimination of phosphate is then regulated by an overflow mechanism in which the amount of phosphate lost in the urine is directly related to phosphate concentrations in the blood. Essentially all the filtered phosphate is reabsorbed when phosphate levels are low; when plasma phosphate levels rise above a critical level, the excess phosphate is eliminated in the urine. Phosphate is reabsorbed from the filtrate into the proximal tubular epithelial cells through the action of a sodium-phosphate cotransporter (NPT2). PTH can play a significant role in regulating phosphate reabsorption by inhibiting the synthesis and expression of the NPT2 transporter. Thus, whenever PTH is increased, tubular reabsorption of phosphate is decreased and more phosphate is lost in the urine. NPT2 is also inhibited by the recently identified hormone called *phosphatonin*.[57] When this hormone is overproduced, as in tumor-induced osteomalacia, marked hypophosphatemia occurs. In addition, increased phosphatonin causes excessive calcitriol (active vitamin D) degradation, resulting in osteomalacia or rickets[57] (see Chapter 57).

Hypophosphatemia

Hypophosphatemia is commonly defined by a plasma phosphorus level of less than 2.5 mg/dL (0.8 mmol/L) in adults; it is considered severe at concentrations of less than 1 mg/dL (0.32 mmol/L).[55] Hypophosphatemia may occur despite normal body phosphate stores as a result of movement from the ECF into the ICF compartment. Serious depletion of phosphorus may exist with low, normal, or high plasma concentrations.

Causes. The most common causes of hypophosphatemia are depletion of phosphorus because of insufficient intestinal absorption, transcompartmental shifts, and increased renal losses (Table 31-12). Often, more than one of these mechanisms is active. Unless food intake is severely restricted, dietary intake and intestinal absorption of phosphorus are usually adequate. Intestinal absorption may be inhibited by administration of glucocorticoids, high dietary levels of magnesium, and hypothyroidism. Prolonged ingestion of antacids may also interfere with intestinal absorption. Antacids that contain aluminum hydroxide, aluminum carbonate, and calcium carbonate bind with phosphate, causing increased phosphate losses in the stool. Because of their ability to bind phosphate, calcium-based antacids are sometimes used therapeutically to decrease plasma phosphate levels in persons with chronic kidney disease.

Alcoholism is a common cause of hypophosphatemia. The mechanisms underlying hypophosphatemia in the person addicted to alcohol may be related to malnutrition, increased renal excretion rates, or hypomagnesemia. Malnutrition and diabetic ketoacidosis increase phosphate excretion and phosphorus loss from the body. Refeeding of malnourished patients increases the incorporation of phosphorus into nucleic acids and phosphorylated compounds in the cell. The same thing happens when diabetic ketoacidosis is reversed with insulin therapy. Urinary losses of phosphate may be caused by drugs, such as theophylline, corticosteroids, and loop diuretics, which increase renal excretion.

Hypophosphatemia also can occur during prolonged courses of glucose administration or hyperalimentation. Glucose administration causes insulin release, with transport of glucose and phosphorus into the cell. The catabolic events that occur with diabetic ketoacidosis also deplete phosphorus stores. Usually the hypophosphatemia does not become apparent, however, until insulin and fluid replacement have reversed the dehydration and glucose has started to move back into the cell. Administration of hyperalimentation solutions without adequate phosphorus can cause a rapid influx of phosphorus into the body's muscle mass, particularly if treatment is initiated after a period of tissue catabolism. Because only a small amount of total-body phosphorus is in the ECF compartment, even a small redistribution between the ECF and ICF compartments can cause hypophosphatemia, even though total phosphorus levels have not changed.

Respiratory alkalosis due to prolonged hyperventilation can produce hypophosphatemia through decreased levels of ionized calcium from increased protein binding, increased PTH

TABLE 31-12 **Causes and Manifestations of Hypophosphatemia**	
CAUSES	**MANIFESTATIONS**
Decreased Intestinal Absorption	**Laboratory Values**
Antacids (aluminum and calcium)	Serum level below 2.5 mg/dL (0.8 mmol/L)
Severe diarrhea	in adults and 4.0 mg/dL (1.3 mmol/L) in
Lack of vitamin D	children
Increased Renal Elimination	**Neural Manifestations**
Alkalosis	Intention tremor
Hyperparathyroidism	Ataxia
Diabetic ketoacidosis	Paresthesias
Renal tubular absorption defects	Confusion, stupor, coma
Malnutrition and Intracellular Shifts	Seizures
Alcoholism	**Musculoskeletal Manifestations**
Total parenteral hyperalimentation	Muscle weakness
Recovery from malnutrition	Joint stiffness
Administration of insulin during	Bone pain
recovery from diabetic ketoacidosis	Osteomalacia
	Blood Disorders
	Hemolytic anemia
	Platelet dysfunction with bleeding disorders
	Impaired white blood cell function

release, and increased phosphate excretion. Clinical conditions associated with hyperventilation include gram-negative septicemia, alcohol withdrawal, heat stroke, and primary hyperventilation.[55,58]

Manifestations. The manifestations of phosphorus deficiency result from a decrease in cellular energy stores due to deficiency in ATP and impaired oxygen transport due to a decrease in red blood cell 2,3-diphosphoglycerate (2,3 DPG). Hypophosphatemia results in altered neural function, disturbed musculoskeletal function, and hematologic disorders (see Table 31-12).

Red blood cell metabolism is impaired by phosphorus deficiency; the cells become rigid, undergo increased hemolysis, and have diminished ATP and 2,3-DPG levels (see Chapter 14). The chemotactic and phagocytic functions of white blood cells and the hemostatic functions of the platelets are also impaired. Acute severe hypophosphatemia (0.1 to 0.2 mg/dL) can lead to acute hemolytic anemia with increased erythrocyte fragility, increased susceptibility to infection, and platelet dysfunction with petechial hemorrhages. Anorexia and dysphagia can occur. Neural manifestations (intention tremors, paresthesias, hyporeflexia, stupor, coma, and seizures) are uncommon but serious manifestations. Respiratory insufficiency resulting from impaired function of the respiratory muscles can develop in patients with severe hypophosphatemia.

Chronic phosphorus depletion interferes with mineralization of newly formed bone matrix. In growing children, this process causes abnormal endochondral growth and clinical manifestations of rickets. In adults, the condition leads to joint stiffness, bone pain, and skeletal deformities consistent with osteomalacia (see Chapter 59).

Treatment. The treatment of hypophosphatemia is usually directed toward prophylaxis. This may be accomplished with dietary sources high in phosphorus (one glass of milk contains approximately 250 mg of phosphorus) or with oral or intravenous replacement solutions. Phosphorus supplements usually are contraindicated in hyperparathyroidism, chronic kidney disease, and hypercalcemia because of the increased risk of extracellular calcifications.

Hyperphosphatemia

Hyperphosphatemia represents a plasma phosphorus concentration in excess of 4.5 mg/dL (1.45 mmol/L) in adults. Growing children normally have plasma phosphate levels higher than those of adults.

Causes. Hyperphosphatemia results from failure of the kidneys to excrete excess phosphate, rapid redistribution of intracellular phosphate to the ECF compartment, and excessive intake of phosphorus.[58] The most common cause of hyperphosphatemia is impaired renal function (Table 31-13).

Hyperphosphatemia is a common electrolyte disorder in persons with chronic kidney disease. The increase in phosphate levels in persons with chronic kidney disease occurs despite compensatory increases in PTH. Recent studies have shown an increase in soft tissue calcification (vascular and cardiac calcification especially) and mortality among patients with chronic kidney disease with hyperphosphatemia.[48,49] Release of intracellular phosphorus can result from conditions such as massive tissue injury, rhabdomyolysis, heat stroke, potassium deficiency, and seizures. Chemotherapy can raise plasma phosphate levels because of the rapid destruction of tumor cells (tumor lysis syndrome).

The administration of excess phosphate-containing antacids, laxatives, or enemas can be another cause of hyperphosphatemia, especially when there is a decrease in vascular volume and a reduced glomerular filtration rate. Phosphate-containing laxatives and enemas predispose to hypovolemia and a decreased glomerular filtration rate by inducing diarrhea, thereby increasing the risk of hypophosphatemia. Serious and even fatal hyperphosphatemia has resulted from administration of Fleet Phospho-Soda enterally[59] or as an enema.

TABLE 31-13 **Causes and Manifestations of Hyperphosphatemia**	
CAUSES	**MANIFESTATIONS**
Acute Phosphate Overload	**Laboratory Values**
Laxatives and enemas containing phosphorus	Serum level above 4.5 mg/dL (1.45 mmol/L) in adults and 5.4 mg/dL
Intravenous phosphate supplementation	(1.7 mmol/L) in children
Intracellular-to-Extracellular Shift	**Neuromuscular Manifestations (Reciprocal Decrease in Serum Calcium)**
Massive trauma	Paresthesias
Heat stroke	Tetany
Seizures	**Cardiovascular Manifestations**
Rhabdomyolysis	Hypotension
Tumor lysis syndrome	Cardiac arrhythmias
Potassium deficiency	
Impaired Elimination	
Kidney failure	
Hypoparathyroidism	

Manifestations. Hyperphosphatemia is accompanied by a decrease in plasma calcium. Many of the signs and symptoms of a phosphate excess are related to a calcium deficit (see Table 31-13). Inadequately treated hyperphosphatemia in chronic disease can lead to secondary hyperparathyroidism, renal osteodystrophies, and extraosseous calcifications in soft tissues.

Treatment. The treatment of hyperphosphatemia is directed at the cause of the disorder. Dietary restriction of foods that are high in phosphorus may be used. Calcium-based phosphate binders are useful in chronic hyperphosphatemia. Sevelamer, a recently approved calcium- and aluminum-free phosphate binder, is as effective as a calcium-based binder, but lacks its adverse manifestations such as elevation of the calcium × phosphate product, hypercalcemia, and vascular and cardiac calcifications.[49] Hemodialysis is used to reduce phosphate levels in persons with chronic kidney disease.

Disorders of Magnesium Balance

Magnesium is the fourth most abundant cation in the body and the second most abundant intracellular cation after potassium. The average adult has approximately 24 g of magnesium distributed throughout the body. Of the total magnesium content, approximately 50% to 60% is stored in bone, 39% to 49% is contained in the body cells, and the remaining 1% is dispersed in the ECF.[60–65] Approximately 20% to 30% of ECF magnesium is protein bound, and only a small fraction of ICF magnesium (15% to 30%) is exchangeable with the ECF. The normal plasma concentration of magnesium is 1.8 to 3.0 mg/dL (0.75 to 1.25 mmol/L).

Only recently has the importance of magnesium to the overall function of the body been recognized. Magnesium acts as a cofactor in many intracellular enzyme reactions, including the transfer of high-energy phosphate groups in the generation of ATP from adenosine diphosphate (ADP). It is essential to all reactions that require ATP, for every step related to replication and transcription of DNA, and for the translation of messenger RNA. It is required for cellular energy metabolism, functioning of the Na^+/K^+-ATPase membrane pump, membrane stabilization, nerve conduction, ion transport, and potassium and calcium channel activity.[61] Potassium channels, including the acetylcholine-sensitive potassium channel, depend on adequate intracellular magnesium levels. Magnesium blocks the outward movement of potassium in cardiac cells; when magnesium levels are low, the channel permits outward flow of potassium, resulting in low levels of intracellular potassium. Many calcium channels are also magnesium dependent. Higher ICF magnesium concentrations inhibit calcium transport into the cell and its release from the sarcoplasmic reticulum. Therefore, magnesium tends to act as a smooth muscle relaxant by altering calcium levels that are responsible for muscle contraction. Because of its smooth muscle relaxing effect, there has been a recent interest in the use of magnesium in the treatment of severe bronchial asthma.[64] In addition, it has been suggested that magnesium has an anticonvulsant effect. The suggested mechanism of action is cerebral vasodilation or prevention of ischemic neuronal damage by blockade of N-methyl-D-aspartate (NMDA) receptors in the brain (see Chapter 51). Magnesium is the first-line drug in the treatment of eclampsia in pregnant women.[64]

MAGNESIUM BALANCE

- Most of the body's magnesium is located within cells, where it functions in regulation of enzyme activity, generation of ATP, and calcium transport. Magnesium is necessary for parathyroid hormone function and hypomagnesemia is a common cause of hypocalcemia.

- Elimination of magnesium occurs mainly through the kidney, which adjusts urinary excretion as a means of maintaining serum magnesium levels. Diuretics tend to disrupt renal regulatory mechanisms and increase urinary losses of magnesium.

- There is an interdependency between intracellular concentrations of magnesium and potassium such that a decrease in one is accompanied by a decrease in the other. Magnesium deficiency contributes to cardiac arrhythmias that occur with hypokalemia.

Gains and Losses

Magnesium is ingested in the diet, absorbed from the intestine, and excreted by the kidneys. Intestinal absorption is not closely regulated, and approximately 25% to 65% of dietary magnesium is absorbed. Magnesium is contained in all green vegetables, grains, nuts, meats, and seafood. Magnesium is also present in much of the groundwater in North America.

The kidney is the principal organ of magnesium regulation. The kidneys filter about 70% to 80% of the plasma magnesium and excrete about 6%, although this amount can be influenced by other conditions and medications.[60] Magnesium is a unique electrolyte in that only approximately 12% to 20% of the filtered amount is reabsorbed in the proximal tubule.[62,63] The greatest quantity, approximately 70%, is passively reabsorbed in the thick ascending loop of Henle. The major driving force for magnesium absorption in the thick ascending loop of Henle is the positive voltage gradient created in the tubular lumen by the $Na^+/K^+/2Cl^-$ cotransport system (see Chapter 30). Inhibition of this transport system by loop diuretics lowers magnesium reabsorption. Active reabsorption of magnesium takes place in the distal convoluted tubule and accounts for about 10% of the filtered load. Magnesium reabsorption is stimulated by PTH and is decreased in the presence of increased plasma levels of magnesium and calcium.

Hypomagnesemia

Magnesium deficiency refers to depletion of total body stores, whereas hypomagnesemia describes a plasma magnesium concentration below 1.8 mg/dL (0.75 mmol/L).[66] It is seen in conditions that limit intake or increase intestinal or renal losses, and it is a common finding in emergency departments and intensive care units.

Causes. Magnesium deficiency can result from insufficient intake, excessive losses, or movement between the ECF and ICF compartments (Table 31-14). It can result from conditions that directly limit intake, such as malnutrition, starvation, or prolonged maintenance of magnesium-free parenteral nutrition. Other conditions, such as diarrhea, malabsorption syndromes, prolonged nasogastric suction, or laxative abuse, decrease intestinal absorption. Another common cause of magnesium deficiency is chronic alcoholism. Many factors contribute to hypomagnesemia in alcoholism, including low intake and gastrointestinal losses from diarrhea. The effects of hypomagnesemia are exaggerated by other electrolyte disorders, such as hypokalemia, hypocalcemia, and metabolic acidosis.

Although the kidneys are able to defend against hypermagnesemia, they are less able to conserve magnesium and prevent hypomagnesemia. Urine losses are increased in diabetic ketoacidosis, hyperparathyroidism, and hyperaldosteronism. Some drugs increase renal losses of magnesium, including both loop and thiazide diuretics and nephrotoxic drugs such as aminoglycoside antibiotics, cyclosporine, cisplatin, and amphotericin B. Several rare, genetic disorders can also result in hypomagnesemia (*i.e.,* Gitelman and Bartter syndromes; see discussion in section on Hypokalemia).

Relative hypomagnesemia may also develop in conditions that promote movement of magnesium between the ECF and ICF compartments, including rapid administration of glucose, insulin-containing parenteral solutions, and alkalosis. Although transient, these conditions can cause serious alterations in body function.

Manifestations. Magnesium deficiency usually occurs in conjunction with hypocalcemia and hypokalemia, producing a number of related neurologic and cardiovascular manifestations (see Table 31-14). Hypocalcemia is typical of severe hypomagnesemia. Most persons with hypomagnesemia-related hypocalcemia have decreased PTH levels, probably as a result of impaired magnesium-dependent mechanisms that control PTH release and synthesis. There is also evidence that hypomagnesemia decreases both the PTH-dependent and PTH-independent release of calcium from bone. In hypomagnesemia, magnesium ions (Mg^{2+}) are released from bone in exchange for increased uptake of calcium from the ECF.

Hypomagnesemia leads to a reduction in intracellular potassium and impairs the ability of the kidney to conserve potassium. When hypomagnesemia is present, hypokalemia is unresponsive to potassium replacement therapy.

Magnesium is vital to carbohydrate metabolism and the generation of both aerobic and anaerobic metabolisms. Many of the manifestations of magnesium deficit are due to related electrolyte disorders such as hypokalemia and hypocalcemia. Hypocalcemia may be evidenced by personality changes and neuromuscular irritability along with tremors, athetoid or choreiform movements, and positive Chvostek or Trousseau signs (see Fig. 31-14). Cardiovascular manifestations include tachycardia, hypertension, and ventricular dysrhythmias. There may be ECG changes such as widening of the QRS complex, appearance of peaked T waves, prolongation of the PR interval, T-wave inversion, and appearance of U waves. Ventricular arrhythmias, particularly in the presence of digitalis, may be difficult to treat unless magnesium levels are normalized.

Persistent magnesium deficiency has been implicated as a risk factor for osteoporosis and osteomalacia, particularly in

TABLE 31-14 **Causes and Manifestations of Hypomagnesemia**	
CAUSES	**MANIFESTATIONS**
Impaired Intake or Absorption	**Laboratory Values**
Alcoholism	Serum magnesium level below 1.8 mg/dL
Malnutrition or starvation	(0.75 mmol/L)
Malabsorption	**Neuromuscular Manifestations**
Small bowel bypass surgery	Personality change
Parenteral hyperalimentation with	Athetoid or choreiform movements
inadequate amounts of magnesium	Nystagmus
High dietary intake of calcium without	Tetany
concomitant amounts of magnesium	Positive Babinski, Chvostek,
Increased Losses	Trousseau signs
Diuretic therapy	**Cardiovascular Manifestations**
Hyperparathyroidism	Tachycardia
Hyperaldosteronism	Hypertension
Diabetic ketoacidosis	Cardiac arrhythmias
Magnesium-wasting kidney disease	

persons with chronic alcoholism, diabetes mellitus, and mal-absorption syndrome.

Treatment. Hypomagnesemia is treated with magnesium replacement. The route of administration depends on the severity of the condition. Symptomatic, moderate to severe magnesium deficiency is treated by parenteral administration. Treatment must be continued for several days to replace stored and plasma levels. In conditions of chronic intestinal or renal loss, maintenance support with oral magnesium may be required. Magnesium often is used therapeutically to treat cardiac arrhythmia, myocardial infarct, angina, bronchial asthma, and pregnancy complicated by preeclampsia or eclampsia. Caution to prevent hypermagnesemia is essential; patients with any degree of renal failure must be carefully monitored to prevent magnesium excess.

Hypermagnesemia

Hypermagnesemia represents an increase in total body magnesium and a plasma magnesium concentration in excess of 3.0 mg/dL (1.25 mmol/L). Because of the ability of the normal kidney to excrete magnesium, hypermagnesemia is rare.

Causes. When hypermagnesemia does occur, it usually is related to renal insufficiency and the injudicious use of magnesium-containing medications such as antacids, mineral supplements, or laxatives (Table 31-15). The elderly are particularly at risk because they have age-related reductions in renal function and tend to consume more magnesium-containing medications, including antacids and laxatives. Magnesium sulfate is used to treat toxemia of pregnancy and premature labor; in these cases, careful monitoring for signs of hypermagnesemia is essential.

Manifestations. Hypermagnesemia affects neuromuscular and cardiovascular function (see Table 31-15). Because magnesium tends to suppress PTH secretion, hypocalcemia may accompany hypermagnesemia. The signs and symptoms usually occur only when plasma magnesium levels exceed 4.8 mg/dL (2 mmol/L).[66]

Hypermagnesemia diminishes neuromuscular function, causing hyporeflexia, muscle weakness, and confusion. Magnesium decreases acetylcholine release at the myoneural junction and may cause neuromuscular blockade and respiratory paralysis. Cardiovascular effects are related to the calcium channel blocking effects of magnesium. Blood pressure is decreased, and the ECG shows shortening of the QT interval, T-wave abnormalities, and prolongation of the QRS and PR intervals. Severe hypermagnesemia (>12 mg/dL) is associated with muscle and respiratory paralysis, complete heart block, and cardiac arrest.

Treatment. The treatment of hypermagnesemia includes cessation of magnesium administration. Calcium is a direct antagonist of magnesium, and intravenous administration of calcium may be used. Peritoneal dialysis or hemodialysis may be required.

IN SUMMARY, calcium, phosphorus, and magnesium are major divalent ions in the body. Calcium is a major divalent cation. Approximately 99% of body calcium is found in bone; less than 1% is found in the ECF compartment. The calcium in bone is in dynamic equilibrium with ECF calcium. Of the three forms of ECF calcium (*i.e.,* protein bound, complexed, and ionized), only the ionized form can cross the cell membrane and contribute to cellular function. Ionized calcium has a number of functions. It contributes to neuromuscular function, plays a vital role in the blood clotting process, and participates in a number of enzyme reactions. Alterations in ionized calcium levels produce neural effects; neural excitability is increased in hypocalcemia and decreased in hypercalcemia.

Phosphorus is largely an ICF anion. It is incorporated into the nucleic acids and ATP. The most common causes of altered levels of ECF phosphate are alterations in intestinal absorption, transcompartmental shifts, and disorders of renal elimination. Phosphorus deficit causes signs and symptoms of neural dysfunction, disturbed musculoskeletal function, and hematologic disorders. Most of these manifestations result from a decrease in cellular energy stores due to a deficiency in ATP and oxygen

TABLE 31-15 Causes and Manifestations of Hypermagnesemia

CAUSES	MANIFESTATIONS
Excessive Intake	**Laboratory Values**
Intravenous administration of magnesium for treatment of preeclampsia	Serum magnesium level above 3.0 mg/dL (1.25 mmol/L)
Excessive use of oral magnesium-containing medications	**Neuromuscular Manifestations**
Decreased Excretion	Lethargy
Kidney disease	Hyporeflexia
Glomerulonephritis	Confusion
Tubulointerstitial kidney disease	Coma
Acute renal failure	**Cardiovascular Manifestations**
	Hypotension
	Cardiac arrhythmias
	Cardiac arrest

transport by 2,3-diphosphoglycerate in the red blood cell. Phosphorus excess occurs with renal failure and PTH deficit; it is associated with decreased plasma calcium levels.

Magnesium is the second most abundant ICF cation. It acts as a cofactor in many intracellular enzyme reactions and is required for cellular energy metabolism, functioning of the Na^+/K^+-ATPase membrane pump, nerve conduction, ion transport, and potassium and calcium channel activity. Magnesium blocks the outward movement of potassium in cardiac cells; when magnesium levels are low, the channel permits outward flow of potassium, resulting in low levels of intracellular potassium. It acts on calcium channels to inhibit the movement of calcium into cells. Magnesium deficiency can result from insufficient intake, excessive losses, or movement between the ECF and ICF compartments. Hypomagnesemia impairs PTH release and the actions of PTH; it leads to a reduction in ICF potassium and impairs the ability of the kidney to conserve potassium. Hypermagnesemia usually is related to renal insufficiency and the injudicious use of magnesium-containing medications such as antacids, mineral supplements, or laxatives. It can cause neuromuscular dysfunction with hyporeflexia, muscle weakness, and confusion. Magnesium decreases acetylcholine release at the myoneural junction and may cause neuromuscular blockade and respiratory paralysis. ∎

CONCEPTSin action **ANIMATION**

Review Exercises

1. A 40-year-old man with advanced acquired immunodeficiency syndrome (AIDS) presents with an acute chest infection. Investigations confirm a diagnosis of *Pneumocystis jiroveci* (formerly *P. carinii*) pneumonia. Although he is being treated appropriately, his plasma sodium level is 118 mEq/L (118 mmol/L). Results of adrenal function tests are normal.

    A. *What is the likely cause of his electrolyte disturbance?*

    B. *What are the five cardinal features of this condition?*

2. A 70-year-old woman who is taking furosemide (a loop diuretic) for congestive heart failure complains of weakness, fatigue, and cramping of the muscles in her legs. Her plasma potassium is 2 mEq (2 mmol/L), and her plasma sodium is 140 mEq/L (140 mmol/L). She also complains that she notices a "strange heartbeat" at times.

    A. *What is the likely cause of this woman's symptoms?*

    B. *An ECG shows depressed ST segment and low T-wave changes. Explain the physiologic mechanism underlying these changes.*

    C. *What would be the treatment for this woman?*

3. A 50-year-old woman presents with symptomatic hypercalcemia. She has a recent history of breast cancer treatment.

    A. *How do you evaluate this person with increased plasma calcium levels?*

    B. *What is the significance of the recent history of malignancy?*

    C. *What further tests may be indicated?*

References

1. Schrier R. W., Gurevich A. K., Abraham W. T. (2003). Renal sodium excretion, edematous disorders, and diuretic use. In Schrier R. W. (Ed.), *Renal and electrolyte disorders* (6th ed., pp. 64–114). Philadelphia: Lippincott Williams & Wilkins.
2. Guyton A., Hall J. E. (2006). *Textbook of medical physiology* (11th ed., pp. 177–178, 183–190, 291–306, 358–363, 383–401, 893–894). Philadelphia: Elsevier Saunders.
3. Rose B. D., Post T. W. (2001). *Clinical physiology of acid-base and electrolyte disorders* (5th ed., pp. 187–190, 478–479, 547, 823–833, 841–842, 896–897). New York: McGraw-Hill.
4. O'Brien J. G., Chennubhotla R. V. (2005). Treatment of edema. *American Family Physician* 71, 2111–2117.
5. Demling R. H. (2005). The burn edema process: Current concepts. *Journal of Burn Care and Rehabilitation* 26, 207–227.
6. Sarvis C. (2003). When lymph edema takes hold. *RN* 66(9), 32–36.
7. Stearns R. H., Spital A., Clark E. C. (1996). Disorders of water balance. In Kokko J., Tannen R. L. (Eds.), *Fluids and electrolytes* (3rd ed., pp. 65, 69, 95). Philadelphia: W. B. Saunders.
8. Metheney N. M. (2000). *Fluid and electrolyte balance* (4th ed., pp. 3, 18, 47, 56, 98, 256). Philadelphia: Lippincott Williams & Wilkins.
9. Schrier R. W. (2006). Water and sodium retention in edematous disorders: Role of vasopressin and aldosterone. *American Journal of Medicine* 119(7 Suppl. 1), S47–S53.
10. Berne R. M., Levy M. N., Koeppen B. M., et al. (Eds.). (2005). *Physiology* (5th ed. pp. 659–684). Philadelphia: Elsevier Saunders.
11. Brewster U. C., Selaro J. F., Perazella M. A. (2003). The renin-angiotensin-aldosterone system: Cardiorenal effects and implications for renal and cardiovascular disease states. *American Journal of Medical Science* 326, 15–24.
12. Porth C. J. M., Erickson M. (1992). Physiology of thirst and drinking: Implications for nursing practice. *Heart and Lung* 21, 273–284.
13. McKinley M. J., Johnson A. K. (2004). The physiological regulation of thirst and fluid intake. *News in Physiological Sciences* 19, 1–6.
14. Kenney W. L., Chiu P. (2001). Influence of age on thirst and fluid intake. *Medicine and Science in Sports and Exercise* 33, 1524–1532.
15. Ayus J. C., Arieff A. I. (1996). Abnormalities of water metabolism in the elderly. *Seminars in Nephrology* 16, 277–288.
16. Rolls B., Phillips P. A. (1990). Aging and disturbances of thirst and fluid balance. *Nutrition Reviews* 48, 137–143.
17. Illowsky B. P., Kirch D. G. (1988). Polydipsia and hyponatremia in psychiatric patients. *American Journal of Psychiatry* 145, 675–683.
18. Vieweg W. V. R. (1994). Treatment strategies for polydipsia-hyponatremia syndrome. *Journal of Clinical Psychiatry* 55(4), 154–159.
19. Lin M., Liu S. J., Lim I. T. (2005). Disorders of water imbalance. *Emergency Medicine Clinics of North America* 23, 749–770.
20. Robertson A. G., Verbalis J. G. (2003). The posterior pituitary gland. In Larsen P. R., Kronenberg H. M., Melmed S., et al. (Eds.), *Williams textbook of endocrinology* (10th ed., pp. 281–329). Philadelphia: Elsevier Saunders.
21. Palm C., Pistrosch F., Herbrig K., et al. (2006). Vasopressin antagonists as aquaretic agents for the treatment of hyponatremia. *American Journal of Medicine* 119(7 Suppl. 1), S87–S92.

22. Makaryus A. N., McFarlane S. I. (2006). Diabetes insipidus: Diagnosis and treatment of a complex disease. *Cleveland Clinic Journal of Medicine* 73, 65–71.

23. Sands J. M., Bichet D. G. (2006). Nephrogenic diabetes insipidus. *Annals of Internal Medicine* 144, 186–194.

24. Robertson G. L. (2006). Regulation of arginine vasopressin in the syndrome of inappropriate antidiuresis. *American Journal of Medicine* 119(7 Suppl. 1), S36–S42.

25. Gohl K. P. (2004). Management of hyponatremia. *American Family Physician* 69, 2387–2394.

26. Palmer B. F., Gates J. R., Lader M. (2003). Causes and management of hyponatremia. *Annals of Pharmacotherapy* 37, 1694–1702.

27. Adrogue H. J., Madias N. E. (2000). Hyponatremia. *New England Journal of Medicine* 343, 1581–1589.

28. Freda B. J., Davidson M. B., Hall P. M. (2004). Evaluation of hyponatremia: A little physiology goes a long way. *Cleveland Clinic Journal of Medicine* 71, 639–650.

29. McManus M. L., Churchwell K. B., Strange K. (1995). Regulation of cell volume in health and disease. *New England Journal of Medicine* 333, 1260–1266.

30. Murase T., Sugimura Y., Takefuji S., et al. (2006). Mechanisms and therapy of osmotic demyelination. *American Journal of Medicine* 119(7 Suppl. 1), S69–S73.

31. Adrogue H. J., Madias N. E. (2000). Hypernatremia. *New England Journal of Medicine* 342, 1493–1499.

32. Rao M. C. (2004). Oral rehydration therapy. *Annual Review of Physiology* 66, 183–417.

33. Editorial. (2002). Oral rehydration theory: Reverse transfer of technology. *Archives of Pediatric and Adolescent Medicine* 156, 1177–1179.

34. Gennari F. J. (2002). Disorders of potassium homeostasis: Hypokalemia and hyperkalemia. *Critical Care Clinics of North America* 18, 273–288.

35. Schaefer T. J., Wolford R. W. (2005). Disorders of potassium. *Medical Clinics of North America* 23, 723–747.

36. Peterson N. L., Levi M. (2003). Disorders of potassium metabolism. In Schrier R. W. (Ed.), *Renal and electrolyte disorders* (6th ed., pp. 171–215). Philadelphia: Lippincott Williams & Wilkins.

37. Gennari F. J. (1998). Hypokalemia. *New England Journal of Medicine* 339, 451–458.

38. Tannen R. L (1996). Potassium disorders. In Kokko J., Tannen R. L. (Eds.), *Fluids and electrolytes* (3rd ed., pp. 116–118). Philadelphia: W. B. Saunders.

39. Matfin G., Durand D., D'Agostino A., et al. (1998) Thyrotoxic hypokalemic periodic paralysis. *Hospital Practice* 1, 23–26.

40. Whang G., Whang G. G., Ryan M. P. (1992). Refractory potassium repletion: A consequence of magnesium deficiency. *Archives of Internal Medicine* 152, 40–45.

41. Hollander-Rodriguez J. C., Calvert J. F. (2006). Hyperkalemia. *American Family Physician* 73, 283–290.

42. Clark B. A., Brown R. S. (1995). Potassium homeostasis and hyperkalemic syndromes. *Endocrinology and Metabolism Clinics of North America* 24, 573–590.

43. Slatopolsky E., Finch J., Brown A. (2003). New vitamin D analogs. *Kidney International* 85, 83–87.

44. Quarles L. D. (2003). Extracellular calcium-sensing receptors in the parathyroid gland, kidney, and other tissues. *Current Opinion in Nephrology and Hypertension* 12, 349–355.

45. Tangiera E. D. (2004). Hyperparathyroidism. *American Family Physician* 69, 333–340.

46. Clark O. H. (2003). How should patients with primary hyperparathyroidism be treated? *Journal of Clinical Endocrinology and Metabolism* 88, 3011–3014.

47. Llach F. (1999). Hyperphosphatemia in end-stage renal disease patients: Pathological consequences. *Kidney International* 56(Suppl. 73), S31–S37.

48. Goodman W. G. (2003). Medical management of secondary hyperparathyroidism in chronic renal failure. *Nephrology, Dialysis and Transplantation* 18(Suppl. 3), S2–S8.

49. Hervas J. G., Prados D., Cerezo S. (2003). Treatment of hyperphosphatemia with sevelamer hydrochloride in hemodialysis patients. *Kidney International* 85, 69–72.

50. Zaloga G. F. (1992). Hypocalcemia in critically ill patients. *Critical Care Medicine* 20, 251–262.

51. Yucha C. B., Toto K. H. (1994). Calcium and phosphorus derangements. *Critical Care Clinics of North America* 6, 747–765.

52. Reber R. M., Heath H. (1995). Hypocalcemic emergencies. *Medical Clinics of North America* 79, 93–165.

53. Carroll M. F., Schade D. S. (2003). A practical approach to hypercalcemia. *American Family Physician* 67, 1959–1966.

54. Strewler G. J. (2000). The physiology of parathyroid hormone-related protein. *New England Journal of Medicine* 342, 177–185.

55. Dennis V. W. (1996). Phosphate disorders. In Kokko J., Tannen R. L. (Eds.), *Fluids and electrolytes* (3rd ed., pp. 359–382). Philadelphia: W. B. Saunders.

56. Yucha C., Dungan J. (2004). Renal handling of phosphorus and magnesium. *Nephrology Nursing Journal* 31(1), 33–39.

57. Schiav S. C., Kumar R. (2004). The phosphatonin pathway: New insights in phosphate homeostasis. *Kidney International* 65, 1–14.

58. Weisinger J., Bellorin-Font E. (1998). Magnesium and phosphate. *Lancet* 352, 391–396.

59. Fass R., Do S., Hixson L. J. (1993). Fatal hyperphosphatemia following Fleet Phospho-Soda in patient with colonic ileus. *American Journal of Gastroenterology* 88, 929–932.

60. Swain R., Kaplan-Machlis B. (1999). Magnesium for the next millennium. *Southern Medical Journal* 92, 1040–1046.

61. Gums J. G. (2004). Magnesium in cardiovascular and other disorders. *American Journal of Health-System Pharmacy* 61, 1569–1576.

62. Konrad M., Schlingmann K. P., Gundermann T. (2003). Insights into the molecular nature of magnesium homeostasis. *American Journal of Physiology: Renal Physiology* 286, F599–F605.

63. Konrad M., Weber S. (2003). Recent advances in molecular genetics of hereditary magnesium-losing disorders. *Journal of the American Society of Nephrology* 14, 249–260.

64. Dubé L., Granry J. (2003). The therapeutic use of magnesium in anesthesiology, intensive care, and emergency medicine: A review. *Canadian Journal of Anaesthesia* 50, 732–746.

65. Rude R. K. (1998). Magnesium deficiency: A cause for heterogenous disease in humans. *Journal of Bone and Mineral Metabolism* 13, 749–755.

66. Topf J. M., Murray P. T. (2003). Hypomagnesemia and hypermagnesemia. *Reviews in Endocrine and Metabolic Disorders* 4, 195–206.

Visit the Point.: **http://thePoint.lww.com for animations, journal articles, and more!**

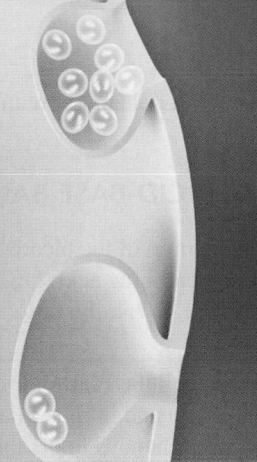

Disorders of Acid-Base Balance

CAROL M. PORTH AND KIM LITWACK

Chapter **32**

➤ The need for precise regulation of hydrogen ion (H^+) balance is similar in many ways to that of other ions in the body. Membrane excitability, enzyme systems, and chemical reactions all depend on the H^+ concentration being regulated within a narrow physiologic range to function in an optimal way. Many conditions, pathologic or otherwise, can alter H^+ concentration and acid-base balance. This chapter has been organized into two sections: Mechanisms of Acid-Base Balance and Disorders of Acid-Base Balance.

MECHANISMS OF ACID-BASE BALANCE

After completing this section of the chapter, you should be able to meet the following objectives:

- State the definition of an acid and a base.
- Cite the source of metabolic acids.
- Describe the three forms of carbon dioxide transport and their contribution to acid-base balance.
- Define pH and use the Henderson-Hasselbalch equation to calculate the pH and to compare compensatory mechanisms for regulating pH.
- Describe the intracellular and extracellular mechanisms for buffering changes in body pH.
- Compare the role of the kidneys and respiratory system in regulation of acid-base balance.
- Explain how interactions between potassium and hydrogen cations and between bicarbonate and chloride anions contribute to the regulation of pH.

Normally, the concentration of body acids and bases is regulated so that the pH of extracellular body fluids is maintained within a very narrow range of 7.35 to 7.45. This balance is maintained through mechanisms that generate, buffer, and eliminate acids and bases. This section of the chapter focuses on acid-base chemistry, the production and regulation of metabolic acids and bicarbonate, calculation of pH, and laboratory tests of acid-base balance.

🔑 MECHANISMS OF ACID-BASE BALANCE

- The pH is determined by the ratio of the bicarbonate (HCO_3^-) base to the volatile carbonic acid ($H_2CO_3 \rightleftharpoons H^+ + HCO_3^-$). At a normal pH of 7.4, the ratio is 20:1.

- The pH is regulated by extracellular (carbonic acid [H_2CO_3]/bicarbonate [HCO_3^-]) and intracellular (proteins) systems that buffer changes in pH that would otherwise occur because of the metabolic production of volatile (CO_2) and nonvolatile (*i.e.,* sulfuric and phosphoric) acids.

- The respiratory system regulates the concentration of the volatile carbonic acid ($CO_2 + H_2O \rightleftharpoons H_2CO_3 \rightleftharpoons H^+ + HCO_3^-$) by changing the rate and depth of respiration.

- The kidneys regulate the plasma concentration of HCO_3^- by two processes: reabsorption of the filtered HCO_3^- and generation of new HCO_3^- or the elimination of H^+ ions that have been buffered by tubular systems (phosphate and ammonia) to maintain a luminal pH of at least 4.5.

Acid-Base Chemistry

An *acid* is a molecule that can release an H^+ and a *base* is an ion or molecule that can accept or combine with an H^+.[1–6] For example, hydrochloric acid (HCl) dissociates in water to form H^+ and chloride (Cl^-) ions. A base, such as the bicarbonate ion (HCO_3^-), is a base because it can combine with H^+ to form carbonic acid (H_2CO_3). Most of the body's acids and bases are weak acids and bases, the most important being H_2CO_3, which is a weak acid derived from carbon dioxide (CO_2), and *bicarbonate* (HCO_3^-), which is a weak base.

Acids and bases exist as buffer pairs or systems—a mixture of a weak acid and its conjugate base or a weak base and its conjugate acid. When an acid (HA) is added to water, it dissociates reversibly to form H^+ and its conjugate anion (A^-); for example, $HA \leftrightarrow H^+ + A^-$. The degree to which an acid dissociates and acts as an H^+ donor determines whether it is a strong or weak acid. *Strong acids,* such as sulfuric acid, dissociate completely; *weak acids,* such as acetic acid, dissociate only to a limited extent. The same is true of a base and its ability to dissociate and accept an H^+.

The concentration of H^+ in body fluids is low compared with other ions. For example, the sodium ion (Na^+) is present at a concentration approximately 3.5 million times that of H^+. Because it is cumbersome to work with such a small number, the H^+ concentration is commonly expressed in terms of the *pH.* Specifically, pH represents the negative logarithm ($\log_{10}$) of the H^+ concentration expressed in milliequivalents per liter (mEq/L). Thus, a pH value of 7.0 implies an H^+ concentration of 10^{-7} (0.0000001 mEq/L). Because the pH is inversely related to the H^+ concentration, a low pH indicates a high concentration of H^+, and a high pH indicates a low concentration.

The *dissociation constant* (K_a) is used to describe the degree to which an acid or base in a buffer system dissociates. The symbol pK_a refers to the negative $\log_{10}$ of the dissociation constant for an acid and represents the pH at which an acid is 50% dissociated.[4] Use of a negative $\log_{10}$ for the dissociation constant allows pH to be expressed as a positive value. Each acid in an aqueous solution has a characteristic pK_a that varies slightly with temperature and pH. At normal body temperature, the pK_a for the HCO_3^- buffer system of the extracellular fluid compartment is 6.1.

Metabolic Acid and Bicarbonate Production

Acids are continuously generated as byproducts of metabolic processes (Fig. 32-1). Physiologically, these acids fall into two groups: the *volatile acid* H_2CO_3 and all other *nonvolatile* or *fixed acids.* The difference between the two types of acids arises because H_2CO_3 is in equilibrium with CO_2 ($H_2CO_3 \leftrightarrow CO_2 + H_2O$), which is volatile and leaves the body by way of the lungs. Therefore, the H_2CO_3 concentration is determined by the lungs and their capacity to exhale CO_2. The fixed or *nonvolatile acids* (*e.g.,* sulfuric, hydrochloric, phosphoric) are not eliminated by the lungs. Instead, they are buffered by body proteins or extracellular buffers, such as HCO_3^-, and then eliminated by the kidney.

Carbon Dioxide and Bicarbonate Production

Body metabolism results in the production of approximately 15,000 mmol of CO_2 each day.[1] Carbon dioxide is transported in the circulation in three forms: (1) as a dissolved gas, (2) as bicarbonate, and (3) as carbaminohemoglobin (see Understanding Carbon Dioxide Transport). Collectively, dissolved CO_2 and HCO_3^- account for approximately 77% of the CO_2 that is transported in the extracellular fluid; the remaining CO_2 travels as carbaminohemoglobin (CO_2 bound to amino acids in hemoglobin).[2] Although CO_2 is a gas and not an acid, a small percentage of the gas combines with water form H_2CO_3. The reaction that generates H_2CO_3 from CO_2 and water is catalyzed by an enzyme called *carbonic anhydrase,* which is present in large quantities in red blood cells, renal tubular cells, and other tissues in the body. The rate of the reaction between CO_2 and water is increased approximately 5000 times by the presence of carbonic anhydrase. Were it not for this enzyme, the reaction would occur too slowly to be of any significance.

Because it is almost impossible to measure H_2CO_3, CO_2 measurements are commonly used when calculating pH. The H_2CO_3 content of the blood can be calculated by multiplying the partial pressure of CO_2 (PCO_2) by its solubility coefficient, which is 0.03. This means that the concentration of H_2CO_3 in the arterial blood, which normally has a PCO_2 of approximately 40 mm Hg, is 1.20 mEq/L (40 × 0.03 = 1.20), and that for

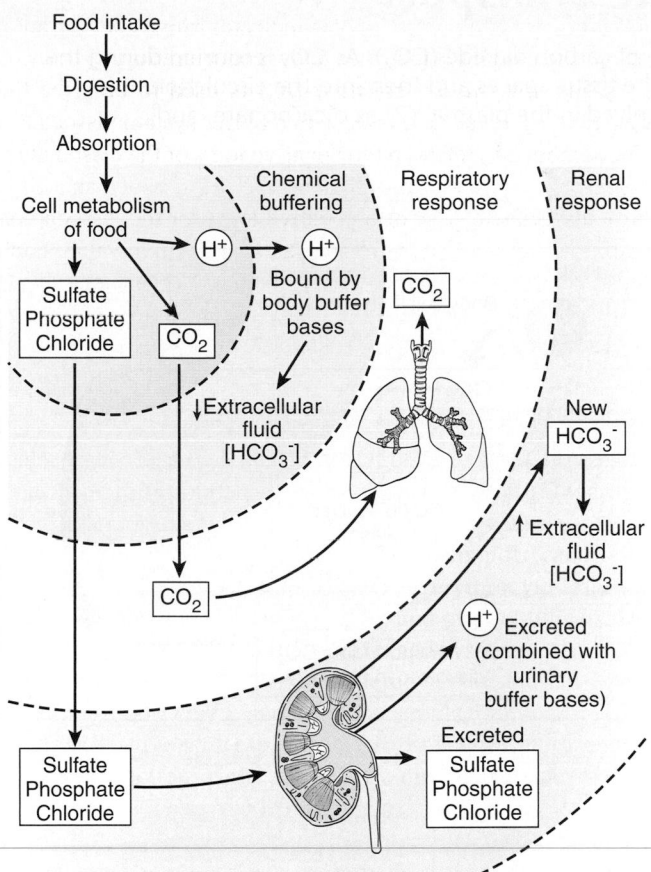

FIGURE 32-1 • The maintenance of normal blood pH by chemical buffers, the respiratory system, and the kidneys. On a mixed diet, pH is threatened by the production of strong acids (sulfuric, hydrochloric, and phosphoric) mainly as the result of protein metabolism. These strong acids are buffered in the body by chemical buffer bases, such as extracellular fluid (ECF) bicarbonate (HCO_3^-). The respiratory system disposes of carbon dioxide (CO_2). The kidneys eliminate hydrogen ions (H^+) combined with urinary buffers and anions in the urine. At the same time, they add new HCO_3^- to the ECF, to replace the HCO_3^- consumed in buffering strong acids. (From Rhoades R. A., Tanner G. A. [2003]. *Medical physiology* [2nd ed., p. 429]. Philadelphia: Lippincott Williams & Wilkins.)

venous blood, which normally has a PCO_2 of approximately 45 mm Hg, is 1.35 mEq/L.

Production of Fixed or Nonvolatile Acids and Bases

The metabolism of dietary proteins and other substances results in the generation of fixed or nonvolatile acids and bases.[1] Oxidation of the sulfur-containing amino acids (*e.g.*, methionine, cysteine) results in the production of sulfuric acid. Oxidation of arginine and lysine produces hydrochloric acid, and oxidation of phosphorus-containing nucleic acids yields phosphoric acid. Incomplete oxidation of glucose results in the formation of lactic acid and incomplete oxidation of fats, the production of ketoacids. The major source of base is the metabolism of amino

acids such as aspartate and glutamate and the metabolism of certain organic anions (*e.g.*, citrate, lactate, acetate). Acid production normally exceeds base production, with the net effect being the addition of approximately 1 mmol/kg body weight of nonvolatile or fixed acid to the body each day.[1] Consumption of a vegetarian diet, which contains large amounts of organic anions, results in the net production of base.

Calculation of pH

The plasma pH can be calculated using an equation called the *Henderson-Hasselbalch equation*. This equation uses the pK_a of the bicarbonate buffer system, which is 6.1, and $\log_{10}$ of the HCO_3^- to dissolved CO_2 (H_2CO_3) ratio:

$$pH = 6.1 + \log_{10}(HCO_3^-/PCO_2 \times 0.03)$$

It should be noted that it is the ratio rather than the absolute values for bicarbonate and dissolved CO_2 that determines pH (*e.g.*, when the ratio is 20:1, the pH = 7.4). Plasma pH decreases when the ratio is less than 20:1, and it increases when the ratio is greater than 20:1 (Fig. 32-2). Because it is the ratio rather than the absolute values of HCO_3^- or CO_2 that determines pH, the pH can remain within a relatively normal range as long as changes in HCO_3^- are accompanied by similar changes in CO_2, or vice versa. For example, the pH will remain at 7.4 when plasma HCO_3^- has increased from 24 to 48 mEq/L as long as CO_2 levels are also doubled. Likewise, the pH will remain at 7.4 when plasma HCO_3^- has decreased from 24 to 12 mEq/L as long as CO_2 levels are also reduced by one half.

Regulation of pH

The pH of body fluids is regulated by three major mechanisms: (1) chemical buffer systems of the body fluids, which immediately combine with excess acids or bases to prevent large changes in pH, (2) the lungs, which control the elimination of CO_2, and (3) the kidneys, which eliminate H^+ and both reabsorb and generate HCO_3^- (see Fig. 32-1).

Chemical Buffer Systems

The moment-by-moment regulation of pH depends on chemical buffer systems of the intracellular (ICF) and extracellular fluids (ECF). As previously discussed, a *buffer system* consists of a weak base and its conjugate acid pair or a weak acid and its conjugate base pair. In the process of preventing large changes in pH, the system trades a strong acid for a weak acid or a strong base for a weak base.

The three major buffer systems that protect the pH of body fluids are (1) the bicarbonate buffer system, (2) proteins, and (3) the transcellular H^+/K^+ exchange system.[1–6] These buffer systems are immediately available to combine with excess acids or bases and prevent large changes in pH from occurring during the time it takes for the respiratory and renal mechanisms to become effective.

Understanding • Carbon Dioxide Transport

Body metabolism results in a continuous production of carbon dioxide (CO_2). As CO_2 is formed during the metabolic process, it diffuses out of body cells into the tissue spaces and then into the circulation. It is transported in the circulation in three forms: (1) dissolved in the plasma, (2) as bicarbonate, and (3) attached to hemoglobin.

❶ Plasma

A small portion (about 10%) of the CO_2 that is produced by body cells is transported in the dissolved state to the lungs and then exhaled. The amount of dissolved CO_2 that can be carried in plasma is determined by the partial pressure of the gas (PCO_2) and its solubility coefficient (0.03 mL/100 mL plasma for each 1 mm Hg PCO_2). Thus, each 100 mL of arterial blood with a PCO_2 of 40 mm Hg would contain 1.2 mL of dissolved CO_2. It is the carbonic acid (H_2CO_3) formed from hydration of dissolved CO_2 that contributes to the pH of the blood.

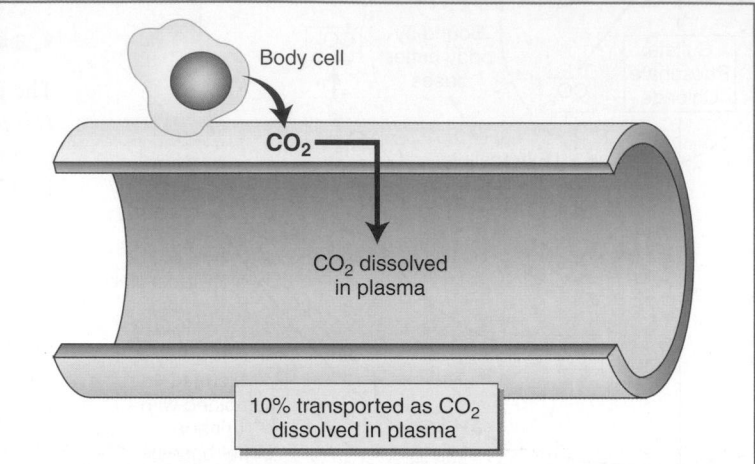

Body cell

CO_2

CO_2 dissolved in plasma

10% transported as CO_2 dissolved in plasma

Bone represents an additional source of acid-base buffering.[1] Excess H^+ ions can be exchanged for Na^+ and K^+ on the bone surface, and dissolution of bone minerals with release of compounds such as sodium bicarbonate ($NaHCO_3$) and calcium carbonate ($CaCO_3$) into the ECF can be used for buffering excess acids. It has been estimated that as much as 40% of buffering of an acute acid load takes place in bone. The role of bone buffers is even greater in the presence of chronic acidosis. The consequences of bone buffering include demineralization of bone and predisposition to development of kidney stones because of increased urinary excretion of calcium. Persons with chronic kidney disease are at particular risk for reduction in bone calcium due to acid retention.

Bicarbonate Buffer System. The HCO_3^- buffer system, which is the principal ECF buffer, uses H_2CO_3 as its weak acid and a bicarbonate salt such as sodium bicarbonate ($NaHCO_3$) as its weak base. It substitutes the weak H_2CO_3 for a strong acid such as hydrochloric acid ($HCl + NaHCO_3 \leftrightarrow H_2CO_3 + NaCl$) or the weak bicarbonate base for a strong base such as sodium hydroxide ($NaOH + H_2CO_3 \leftrightarrow NaHCO_3 + H_2O$). The bicarbonate buffer system is a particularly efficient system because its components can be readily added or removed from the body.[2,5] Metabolism provides an ample supply of CO_2, which can replace any H_2CO_3 that is lost when excess base is added, and CO_2 can be readily eliminated when excess acid is added. Likewise, the kidney can conserve or form new HCO_3^- when excess acid is added, and it can excrete HCO_3^- when excess base is added.

Protein Buffer Systems. Proteins are the largest buffer system in the body. Proteins are *amphoteric,* meaning that they can function either as acids or bases. They contain many ionizable groups that can release or bind H^+. The protein buffers are largely located in cells, and H^+ ions and CO_2 diffuse across cell membranes for buffering by intracellular proteins. Albumin and plasma globulins are the major protein buffers in the vascular compartment.

Hydrogen-Potassium Exchange. The transcompartmental exchange of H^+ and potassium ions (K^+) provides another important system for regulation of acid-base balance. Both ions are positively charged, and both ions move freely between the ICF and ECF compartments (see Chapter 31, Fig. 31-11). When excess H^+ is present in the ECF, it moves into the ICF in exchange for K^+, and when excess K^+ is present in the ECF,

❷ Bicarbonate

Carbon dioxide in excess of that which can be carried in the plasma moves into the red blood cells, where the enzyme carbonic anhydrase (CA) catalyzes its conversion to carbonic acid (H_2CO_3). The H_2CO_3, in turn, dissociates into hydrogen (H^+) and bicarbonate (HCO_3^-) ions. The H^+ combines with hemoglobin and the HCO_3^- diffuses into plasma, where it participates in acid-base regulation. The movement of HCO_3^- into the plasma is made possible by a special transport system on the red blood cell membrane in which HCO_3^- ions are exchanged for chloride ions (Cl^-).

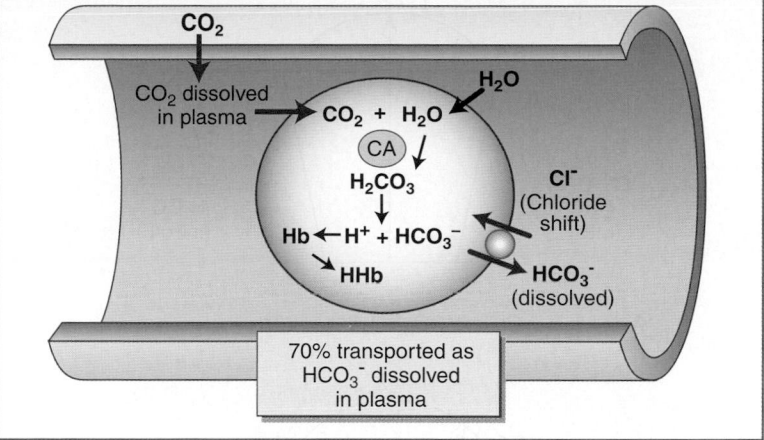

❸ Hemoglobin

The remaining CO_2 in the red blood cells combines with hemoglobin to form carbaminohemoglobin ($HbCO_2$). The combination of CO_2 with hemoglobin is a reversible reaction characterized by a loose bond, so that CO_2 can be easily released in the alveolar capillaries and exhaled from the lung.

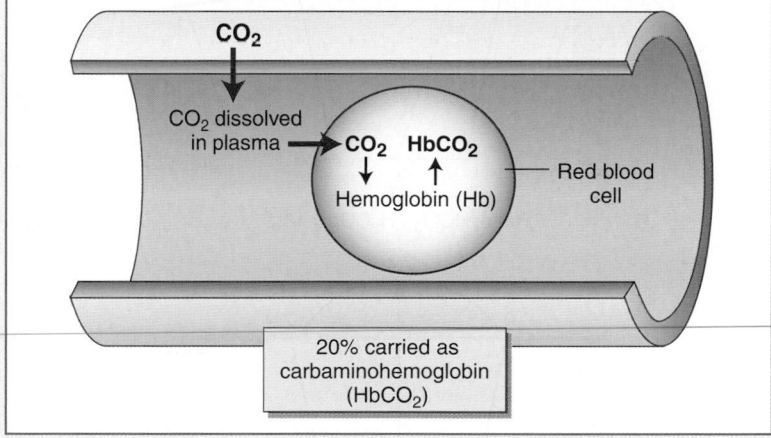

it moves into the ICF in exchange for H^+. Thus, alterations in potassium levels can affect acid-base balance, and changes in acid-base balance can influence potassium levels. Potassium shifts tend to be more pronounced in metabolic acidosis than in respiratory acidosis.[5,6] Also, metabolic acidosis caused by an accumulation of nonorganic acids (*e.g.,* hydrochloric acid that occurs in diarrhea, phosphoric acid that occurs in chronic kidney disease) produces a greater increase in extracellular K^+ levels than does acidosis caused by an accumulation of organic acids (*e.g.,* lactic acid, ketoacids).

Respiratory Control Mechanisms

The second line of defense against acid-base disturbances is the control of CO_2 by the lungs. Increased ventilation decreases PCO_2, whereas decreased ventilation increases PCO_2. The blood PCO_2 and pH are important regulators of ventilation. Chemoreceptors in the brain stem and the peripheral chemoreceptors in the carotid and aortic bodies sense changes in PCO_2 and pH and alter the ventilatory rate.

The respiratory control of pH is rapid, occurring within minutes, and is maximal within 12 to 24 hours.[1] Although the respiratory response is rapid, it does not completely return the

pH to normal. It is only about 50% to 75% effective as a buffer system.[2] This means that if the pH falls from 7.4 to 7.0, the respiratory system can return the pH to a value of about 7.2 to 7.3.[2] In acting rapidly, however, it prevents large changes in pH from occurring while waiting for the much more slowly reacting kidneys to respond.

Although CO_2 readily crosses the blood-brain barrier, there is a lag for entry of HCO_3^-. Thus, blood levels of HCO_3^- change more rapidly than cerebrospinal fluid (CSF) levels. In metabolic acidosis, for example, there is often a primary decrease in pH of the cerebral fluids and a slower decrease in HCO_3^-. When metabolic acid-base disorders are corrected rapidly, the respiratory response may persist because of a delay in adjustment of CSF HCO_3^- levels.

Renal Control Mechanisms

The kidneys play two major roles in regulating acid-base balance.[1-8] The first is accomplished through the reabsorption of the HCO_3^- that is filtered in the glomerulus so this important buffer is not lost in the urine. The second is through the excretion of H^+ from fixed acids that result from protein and lipid metabolism. The renal mechanisms for regulating acid-base

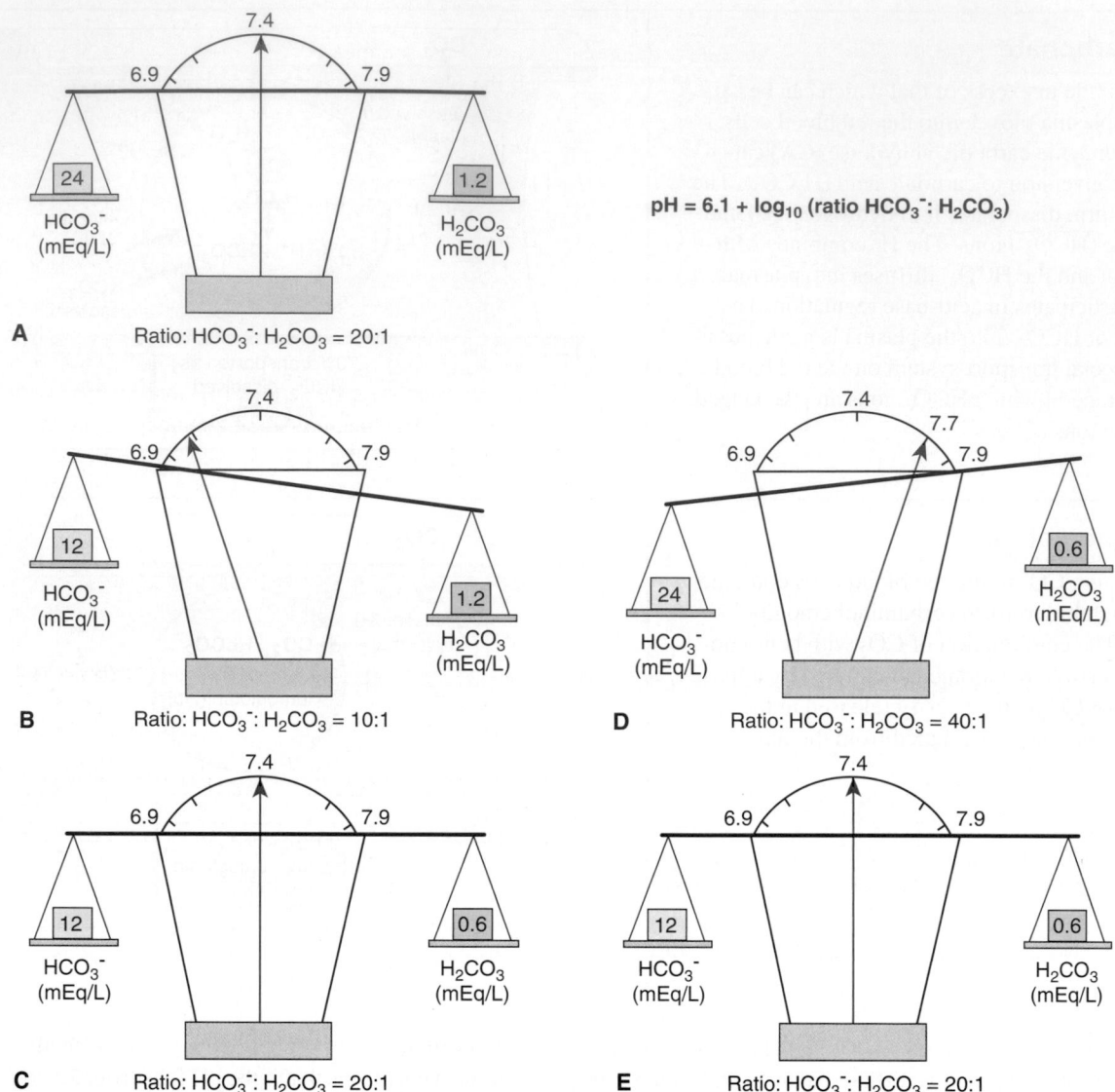

$$pH = 6.1 + \log_{10} (\text{ratio } HCO_3^-: H_2CO_3)$$

FIGURE 32-2 • Normal and compensated states of pH and acid-base balance represented as a balance scale. **(A)** When the ratio of bicarbonate (HCO_3^-) to carbonic acid (H_2CO_3, arterial $CO_2 \times 0.03$) = 20:1, the pH = 7.4. **(B)** Metabolic acidosis with a HCO_3^-:H_3CO_3 ratio of 10:1 and a pH of 7.1. **(C)** Respiratory compensation lowers the H_3CO_3 to 0.6 mEq/L and returns the HCO_3^-:H_3CO_3 ratio to 20:1 and the pH to 7.4. **(D)** Respiratory alkalosis with a HCO_3^-:H_3CO_3 ratio of 40:1 and a pH of 7.7. **(E)** Renal compensation eliminates HCO_3^-, reducing serum levels to 12 mEq/L, returning the HCO_3^-:H_3CO_3 ratio to 20:1 and the pH to 7.4. Normally, these compensatory mechanisms are capable of buffering large changes in pH, but do not return the pH completely to normal as illustrated here.

balance cannot adjust the pH within minutes, as respiratory mechanisms can, but they continue to function for days until the pH has returned to normal or near-normal range.

Hydrogen Ion Elimination and Bicarbonate Conservation. The kidney regulates pH by excreting excess H^+ and reabsorbing or regenerating HCO_3^-. Bicarbonate is freely filtered in the glomerulus (approximately 4300 mEq/day) and reabsorbed in the tubules.[2] Loss of even small amounts of HCO_3^- impairs the body's ability to buffer its daily load of metabolic acids. Because the amount of H^+ that can be filtered in the glomeruli is relatively

small compared with HCO_3^-, its elimination relies on secretion of H^+ from the blood into the urine filtrate in the tubules.

Most of the H^+ secretion and reabsorption of HCO_3^- takes place in the proximal tubule. The process begins with a coupled Na^+/H^+ transport system in which H^+ is secreted into the tubular fluid and Na^+ is reabsorbed into the tubular cell (Fig. 32-3). The secreted H^+ combines with filtered HCO_3^- to form H_2CO_3. The H_2CO_3 then decomposes into CO_2 and H_2O, catalyzed by a brush border carbonic anhydrase. The CO_2 and H_2O that are formed readily cross the luminal membrane and enter the tubular cell. Inside the cell, the reactions occur in reverse. The CO_2 and H_2O

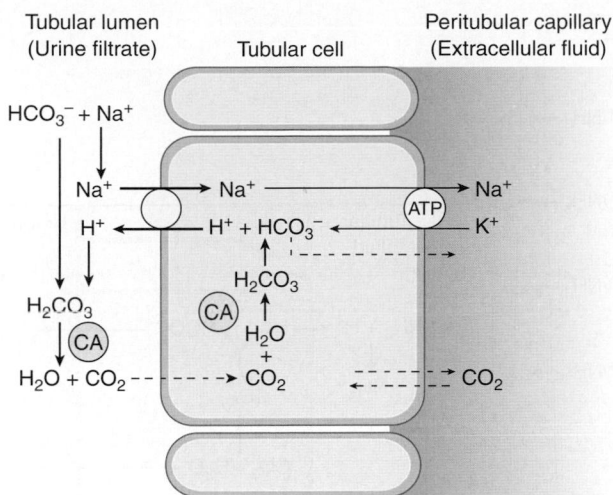

FIGURE 32-3 • Hydrogen ion (H⁺) secretion and bicarbonate ion (HCO₃⁻) reabsorption in a renal tubular cell. Carbon dioxide (CO₂) diffuses from the blood or urine filtrate into the tubular cell, where it combines with water in a carbonic anhydrase (CA)–catalyzed reaction that yields carbonic acid (H₂CO₃). The H₂CO₃ dissociates to form H⁺ and HCO₃⁻. The H⁺ is secreted into the tubular fluid in exchange for Na⁺. The Na⁺ and HCO₃⁻ enter the extracellular fluid. ATP, adenosine triphosphate.

combine to form H_2CO_3, in a carbonic anhydrase–mediated reaction. The H_2CO_3, in turn, is converted to HCO_3^- and H^+. The HCO_3^- is then reabsorbed into the blood along with Na^+, and the newly generated H^+ is secreted into the tubular fluid to begin another cycle. Normally, only a few of the secreted H^+ ions remain in the tubular fluid because the secretion of H^+ is roughly equivalent to the number of HCO_3^- ions filtered in the glomerulus.

Tubular Buffer Systems. Because an extremely acidic urine filtrate would be damaging to structures in the urinary tract, the minimum urine pH is 4.4 to 4.5. Once the urine pH reaches this level of acidity, H^+ secretion ceases. This limits the amount of unbuffered H^+ that can be eliminated by the kidney. When the amount of free H^+ secreted into the tubular fluid threatens to cause the pH of the urine to become too acidic, it must be carried in another form. This is accomplished by combining H^+ ions with intratubular buffers before they are excreted in the urine. There are two important intratubular buffer systems: the phosphate and ammonia buffer systems.[2] The HCO_3^- that is generated by these two buffer systems is new bicarbonate, demonstrating one of the ways that the kidney is able to replenish the ECF stores of HCO_3^-.

The *phosphate buffer system* uses HPO_4^{2-} and $H_2PO_4^-$ that are present in the tubular filtrate. Both forms of phosphate become concentrated in the tubular fluid because of their relatively poor absorption and because of reabsorption of water from the tubular fluid. Another factor that makes phosphate so effective as a urinary buffer is the fact that urine pH is close to the pK of the phosphate buffer system. The process of H^+ secretion in the tubules is the same as that used for reabsorption of

HCO_3^-. As long as there is excess HCO_3^- in the tubular fluid, most of the secreted H^+ combines with HCO_3^-. However, once all the HCO_3^- has been reabsorbed and is no longer available to combine with H^+, any excess H^+ combines with HPO_4^{2-} to form $H_2PO_4^-$ (Fig. 32-4). After H^+ combines with HPO_4^{2-}, it can be excreted as NaH_2PO_4, carrying the excess H^+ with it.

Another important but more complex buffer system is the *ammonia buffer system*. The excretion of H^+ and generation of HCO_3^- by the ammonia buffer system occurs in three major steps: (1) the synthesis of ammonium (NH_4^+) from the amino acid glutamine in the proximal tubule, (2) the reabsorption and recycling of NH_4^+ within the medullary portion of the kidney, and (3) the buffering of H^+ ions by NH_3 in the collecting tubules.[1-4] The metabolism of glutamate in the proximal tubule results in the formation of two NH_4^+ and two HCO_3^- ions[2] (Fig. 32-5A). The two NH_4^+ ions are secreted into the tubular fluid by a countertransport mechanism in exchange for Na^+. The two HCO_3^- ions move out of the tubular cell along with the reabsorbed Na^+ to enter the peritubular capillary system. Thus, for each molecule of glutamine metabolized in the proximal tubule, two NH_4^+ ions are secreted into the tubular filtrate, and two HCO_3^- ions are reabsorbed into the blood. The HCO_3^- generated by this process constitutes new HCO_3^-.

A significant portion of the NH_4^+ secreted by the proximal tubular cells is reabsorbed in the thick ascending loop of Henle, where the NH_4^+ substitutes for K^+ on the $Na^+/K^+/2Cl^-$ cotransporter (discussed in Chapter 30). The NH_4^+ that is reabsorbed by the thick ascending loop of Henle accumulates in the medullary interstitium of the kidney, where it exists in equilibrium with NH_3 (see Fig. 32-5B). Although both NH_4^+ and NH_3 are present in the medullary interstitial fluid, only NH_3 is

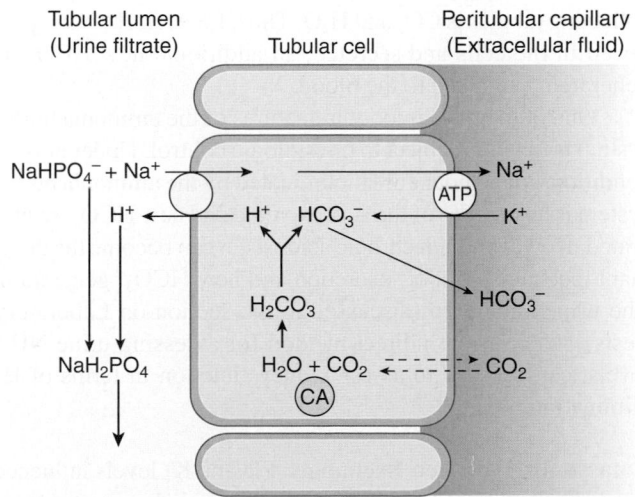

FIGURE 32-4 • The renal phosphate buffer system. The monohydrogen phosphate ion (HPO₄²⁻) enters the renal tubular fluid in the glomerulus. An H⁺ combines with the HPO₄²⁻ to form H₂PO₄⁻ and is then excreted into the urine in combination with Na⁺. The HCO₃⁻ moves into the extracellular fluid along with the Na⁺ that was exchanged during secretion of the H⁺. ATP, adenosine triphosphate; CA, carbonic anhydrase.

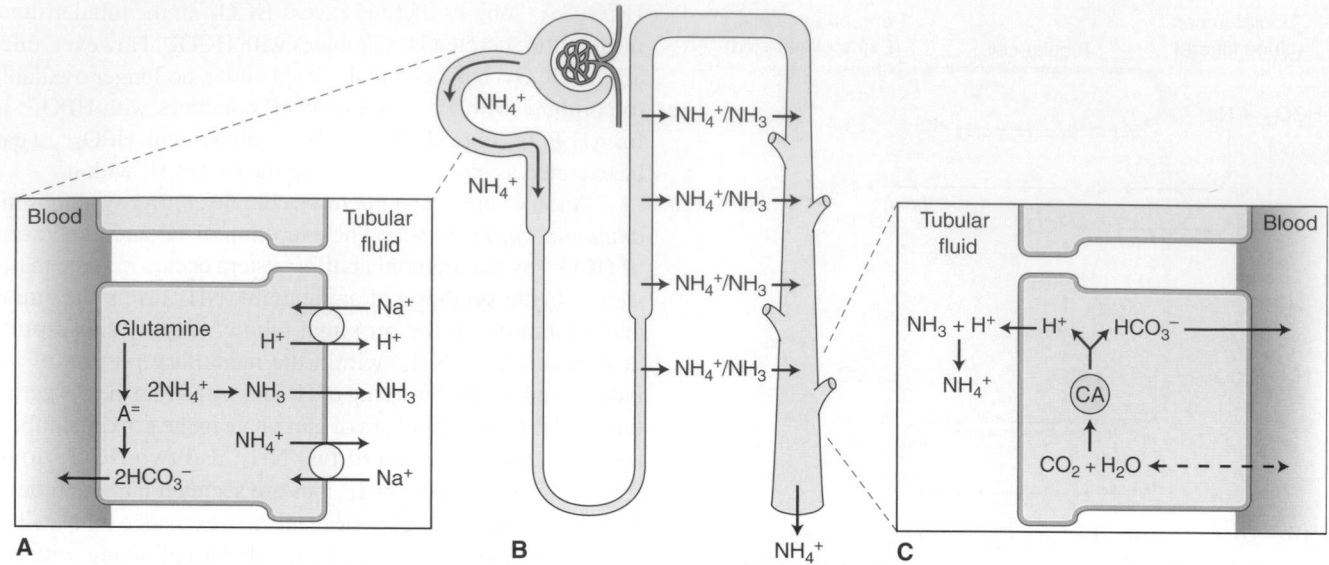

FIGURE 32-5 • Production, transport, and excretion of ammonium (NH_4^+) by the kidney. **(A)** Glutamine is metabolized in the proximal tubule to produce two NH_4^+ and two bicarbonate ions (HCO_3^-). The two NH_4^+ are secreted into the tubular fluid and the two HCO_3^- ions, which represent new HCO_3^-, are returned to the circulation. **(B)** A significant portion of the secreted NH_4^+ is reabsorbed in the medullary interstitium, where it exists as both NH_4^+ and NH_3. **(C)** The NH_3 diffuses into the tubular fluid of the collecting tubule, where it interacts with secreted hydrogen ions (H^+) to form NH_4^+, which is eliminated in the urine. For each NH_4^+ excreted in the urine, another HCO_3^- is returned to the circulation. CA, carbonic anhydrase. (From Berne R. M., Levy M. N. [2000]. *Principles of physiology* [3rd ed., p. 474]. St. Louis: Mosby.)

lipid soluble and can diffuse across the collecting duct cells into the tubular fluid. Once in the tubular fluid, NH_3 combines with secreted H^+ to form NH_4^+ (see Fig. 32-5C). NH_4^+ is not lipid soluble, and thus is trapped in the tubular fluid and excreted in urine. Note that the source of the H^+ secreted by the cells of the collecting tubules is CO_2 and H_2O. Thus, for each H^+ that is produced in the cells and secreted, an additional new HCO_3^- is generated and added to the blood.

One of the most important features of the ammonia buffer system is that it is subject to physiologic control. Under normal conditions, the amount of H^+ eliminated by the ammonia buffer system is about 50% of the acid excreted and new HCO_3^- regenerated. However, with chronic acidosis, it can become the dominant mechanism for H^+ excretion and new HCO_3^- generation. The urine anion gap (discussed in the section on Laboratory Tests), which is an indirect method for assessing urine NH_4^+ levels, can be used to assess kidney function in terms of H^+ elimination.

Potassium-Hydrogen Exchange. Plasma K^+ levels influence renal elimination of H^+ and vice versa. Hypokalemia is a potent stimulus for H^+ secretion and HCO_3^- reabsorption. When plasma K^+ levels fall, there is movement of K^+ from the ICF into the ECF compartment and a reciprocal movement of H^+ from the ECF into the ICF compartment. A similar process occurs in the distal tubules of the kidney, where the H^+/K^+-adenosine triphosphatase (ATPase) exchange pump actively reabsorbs K^+

as well as secreting H^+. An elevation in plasma K^+ levels has the opposite effect. Plasma K^+ levels are similarly altered by acid-base balance. Thus, acidosis tends to increase H^+ elimination and decrease K^+ elimination, with a resultant increase in plasma potassium levels, whereas alkalosis tends to decrease H^+ elimination and increase K^+ elimination, with a resultant decrease in plasma K^+ levels.[5,9]

Aldosterone also influences H^+ elimination by the kidney. It acts in the collecting duct to stimulate H^+ secretion indirectly, while increasing Na^+ reabsorption and K^+ secretion (see Chapter 30). Thus, hyperaldosteronism tends to lead to a decrease in plasma K^+ levels and an increase in pH because of increased H^+ secretion, whereas hypoaldosteronism has the opposite effect.

Chloride-Bicarbonate Exchange. Another mechanism that the kidney uses in regulating HCO_3^- is the chloride-bicarbonate anion exchange that occurs in association with Na^+ reabsorption. Normally, Cl^- is absorbed along with Na^+ throughout the tubules. In situations of volume depletion due to vomiting and chloride depletion, the kidney is forced to substitute HCO_3^- for the Cl^- anion, thereby increasing its absorption of HCO_3^-. *Hypochloremic alkalosis* refers to an increase in pH induced by excess HCO_3^- reabsorption due to a decrease in Cl^- levels, and *hyperchloremic acidosis* to a decrease in pH because of decreased HCO_3^- reabsorption due to an increase in Cl^- levels.

Laboratory Tests

Laboratory tests that are used in assessing acid-base balance include arterial blood gases and pH, CO_2 content and HCO_3^- levels, base excess or deficit, and blood and urine anion gaps. Although useful in determining whether acidosis or alkalosis is present, measurements of the blood pH provide little information about the cause of an acid-base disorder.

Carbon Dioxide and Bicarbonate Levels

The PCO_2 of the arterial blood gases provide a means of assessing the respiratory component of acid-base balance. Arterial blood gases are used because venous blood gases are highly variable, depending on metabolic demands of the various tissues that empty into the vein from which the sample is being drawn. The H_2CO_3 levels can be determined from arterial blood gas measurements using the PCO_2 and the solubility coefficient for CO_2 (normal arterial PCO_2 is 38 to 42 mm Hg). Arterial blood gases also provide a measure of blood oxygen (PO_2) levels. This can be important in assessing respiratory function.

The CO_2 content refers to the total CO_2 in the blood, including dissolved CO_2, that contained in HCO_3^-, and that attached to hemoglobin (carbaminohemoglobin [CO_2HHb]). The plasma HCO_3^- content normally comprises about 95% of the total CO_2 content.[10] The normal range of values for venous HCO_3^- concentration is 24 to 31 mEq/L (24 to 31 mmol/L).

Base Excess or Deficit

The total base excess or deficit, also referred to as the *whole blood buffer base,* measures the level of all the buffer systems of the blood—hemoglobin, protein, phosphate, and HCO_3^-. The base excess or deficit describes the amount of a fixed acid or base that must be added to a blood sample to achieve a pH of 7.4 (normal ± 2 mEq/L).[11] For clinical purposes, base excess or deficit can be viewed as a measurement of bicarbonate excess or deficit. A base excess indicates metabolic alkalosis, and a base deficit indicates metabolic acidosis.

Anion Gap

The anion gap describes the difference between the plasma concentration of the major measured cation (Na^+) and the sum of the measured anions (Cl^- and HCO_3^-). This difference represents the concentration of unmeasured anions, such as phosphates, sulfates, organic acids, and proteins (Fig. 32-6). Normally, the anion gap ranges between 8 and 12 mEq/L (a value of 16 mEq/L is normal if both sodium and potassium concentrations are used in the calculation). Because albumin is an anion, it is often measured and used in determining the anion gap in persons with decreased albumin levels. For every 1 g decline in plasma albumin concentration, 2.5 should be added to the gap that is calculated from the formula $Na^+ - (Cl^- + HCO_3^-)$.[12] The anion gap is increased in conditions such as lactic acidosis and ketoacidosis that result from elevated levels of metabolic acids. A low anion

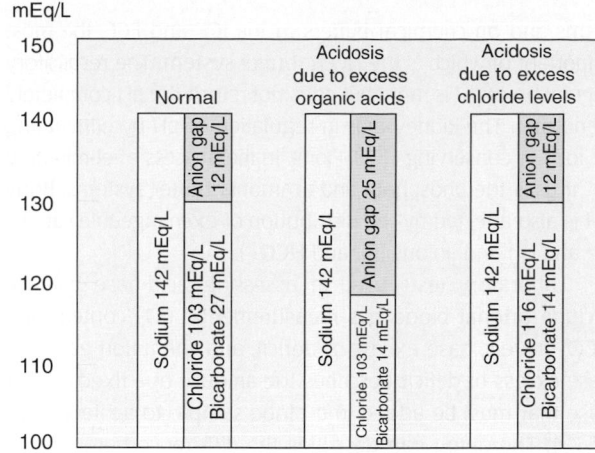

FIGURE 32-6 • The anion gap in acidosis due to excess metabolic acids and excess plasma chloride levels. Unmeasured anions such as phosphates, sulfates, and organic acids increase the anion gap because they replace bicarbonate. This assumes there is no change in sodium content.

gap is found in conditions that produce a fall in unmeasured anions (primarily albumin) or rise in unmeasured cations. The latter can occur in hyperkalemia, hypercalcemia, hypermagnesemia, lithium intoxication, or multiple myeloma, in which an abnormal immunoglobulin is produced.[1]

The anion gap of urine, also called the *delta gap,* can also be measured.[12] Urine electrolyte determinations do not include bicarbonate. Instead, the urine anion gap uses the difference between the measurable cations (Na^+ and K^+) and anions (Cl^-) to provide an estimate of ammonium (NH_4^+) excretion. Because ammonium is a cation, the value of the anion gap becomes more negative as the ammonium level increases. In normal persons secreting 20 to 40 mmol of ammonium per liter, the urine anion gap is close to zero. In metabolic acidosis, the amount of unmeasured NH_4^+ should increase if renal excretion of H^+ is intact; as a result, the urine anion gap should become more negative.

IN SUMMARY, normal body function depends on the precise regulation of acid-base balance. The pH of the extracellular fluid is normally maintained within the narrow physiologic range of 7.35 to 7.45. Metabolic processes produce volatile and fixed or nonvolatile metabolic acids that must be buffered and eliminated from the body. The volatile acid, H_2CO_3, is in equilibrium with dissolved CO_2, which is eliminated through the lungs. The nonvolatile metabolic acids, which are derived mainly from protein metabolism and incomplete carbohydrate and fat metabolism, are excreted by the kidneys. It is the ratio of the HCO_3^- concentration to dissolved CO_2 (H_2CO_3 concentration) that determines the pH of the extracellular fluids. When this ratio is 20:1, the pH is 7.4.

The ability of the body to maintain pH within the normal physiologic range depends on respiratory and renal mechanisms and on chemical buffers in the ICF and ECF, the most important of which is the HCO_3^- buffer system. The respiratory regulation of pH is rapid but does not return the pH completely to normal. The kidney aids in regulation of pH by eliminating H^+ ions or conserving HCO_3^- ions. In the process of eliminating H^+, it uses the phosphate and ammonia buffer systems. Body pH is also affected by the distribution of exchangeable cations (K^+ and H^+) and anions (Cl^- and HCO_3^-).

Laboratory tests used in assessing acid-base balance include arterial blood gas measurements, CO_2 content and HCO_3^- levels, base excess or deficit, and the anion gap. The base excess or deficit describes the amount of a fixed acid or base that must be added to a blood sample to achieve a pH of 7.4. The anion gap describes the difference between the plasma concentration of the major measured cation (Na^+) and the sum of the anions (Cl^- and HCO_3^-). This difference represents the concentration of unmeasured anions, such as phosphates, sulfates, and organic acids, that are present. The urine delta gap uses the difference between the measurable cations (Na^+ and K^+) and anions (Cl^-) to provide an estimate of ammonium (NH_4^+) excretion and the ability of the kidney to rid the body of excess H^+. ■

DISORDERS OF ACID-BASE BALANCE

After completing this section of the chapter, you should be able to meet the following objectives:

- Differentiate the terms *acidemia, alkalemia, acidosis,* and *alkalosis.*
- Describe a clinical situation involving an acid-base disorder in which both primary and compensatory mechanisms are present.
- Define metabolic acidosis, metabolic alkalosis, respiratory acidosis, and respiratory alkalosis.
- Explain the use of the plasma anion gap in differentiating types of metabolic acidosis.
- List common causes of metabolic and respiratory acidosis and metabolic and respiratory alkalosis.
- Contrast and compare the clinical manifestations and treatment of metabolic and respiratory acidosis and of metabolic and respiratory alkalosis.

The terms *acidosis* and *alkalosis* describe the clinical conditions that arise as a result of changes in dissolved CO_2 and HCO_3^- concentrations. An alkali represents a combination of one or more alkali metals such as sodium or potassium with a highly basic ion such as a hydroxyl ion (OH^-). Sodium bicarbonate is the main alkali in the extracellular fluid. Although the definitions differ somewhat, the terms *alkali* and *base* are often

used interchangeably. Hence, the term *alkalosis* has come to mean the opposite of *acidosis.*

Metabolic Versus Respiratory Acid-Base Disorders

There are two types of acid-base disorders: metabolic and respiratory (Table 32-1). *Metabolic disorders* produce an alteration in the plasma HCO_3^- concentration and result from the addition to or loss from the ECF of nonvolatile acid or alkali. A reduction in pH due to a decrease in HCO_3^- is called *metabolic acidosis,* and an elevation in pH due to increased HCO_3^- levels is called *metabolic alkalosis. Respiratory disorders* involve an alteration in the PCO_2, reflecting an increase or decrease in alveolar ventilation. *Respiratory acidosis* is characterized by a decrease in pH, reflecting a decrease in ventilation and an increase in PCO_2. *Respiratory alkalosis* involves an increase in pH, resulting from an increase in alveolar ventilation and a decrease in PCO_2.

Compensatory Mechanisms

Acidosis and alkalosis typically involve a *primary* or *initiating event* and a *compensatory* or *adaptive state* that results from homeostatic mechanisms that attempt to correct or prevent large changes in pH. For example, a person may have a primary metabolic acidosis as a result of overproduction of ketoacids and respiratory alkalosis because of a compensatory increase in ventilation (see Table 32-1).

Compensatory mechanisms provide a means to control pH when correction is impossible or cannot be immediately achieved. Often, compensatory mechanisms are interim measures that permit survival while the body attempts to correct the primary disorder. Compensation requires the use of mechanisms that are different from those that caused the primary disorder. For example, the lungs cannot compensate for respiratory acidosis that is caused by lung disease, nor can the kidneys compensate for metabolic acidosis that occurs because of chronic kidney disease. The body can, however, use renal mechanisms to compensate for respiratory-induced changes in pH, and it can use respiratory mechanisms to compensate for metabolically induced changes in acid-base balance. Because compensatory mechanisms become more effective with time, there are often differences between the level of pH change that is present in acute and chronic acid-base disorders.

Single Versus Mixed Acid-Base Disorders

Thus far we have discussed acid-base disorders as if they existed as a single primary disorder such as metabolic acidosis, accompanied by a predicted compensatory response (*i.e.,* hyperventilation and respiratory alkalosis). It is not uncommon, however, for persons to present with more than

TABLE 32-1 Summary of Single Acid-Base Disturbances and Their Compensatory Responses

ACID-BASE IMBALANCE	PRIMARY DISTURBANCE	RESPIRATORY COMPENSATION AND PREDICTED RESPONSE*	RENAL COMPENSATION AND PREDICTED RESPONSE*†
Metabolic acidosis	↓plasma pH and HCO_3^-	↑ventilation and ↓PCO_2 *1 mEq/L ↓HCO_3^- → 1 to 1.5 mm Hg ↓PCO2*	↑H^+ excretion and ↑HCO_3^- reabsorption if no renal disease
Metabolic alkalosis	↑plasma pH and HCO_3^-	↓ventilation and ↑PCO_2 *1 mEq/L ↑HCO3- → 0.25 to 1.0 ↑PCO2*	↓H^+ excretion and ↓HCO_3^- reabsorption if no renal disease
Respiratory acidosis	↓plasma pH and ↑PCO_2	None	↑H^+ excretion and ↑HCO_3^- reabsorption *Acute: 1 mm Hg ↑PCO_2 → 0.1 mEq/L ↑HCO_3^- Chronic: 1 mm Hg ↑PCO_2 → 0.4 mEq/L ↑HCO_3^-*
Respiratory alkalosis	↑plasma pH and ↓PCO_2	None	↓H^+ excretion and ↓HCO_3^- reabsorption *Acute: 1 mm Hg ↓PCO_2 → 0.2 mEq/L ↓HCO_3^- Chronic: 1 mm Hg ↓PCO_2 → 0.4 mEq/L ↓HCO_3^-*

Note: Predicted compensatory responses are in *italics*.

*If blood values are the same as predicted compensatory values, a single acid-base disorder is present; if values are different, a mixed acid-base disorder is present.[12]

†Acute renal compensation ≤48 hours, chronic renal compensation >48 hours.[12]

one primary disorder or a mixed disorder. For example, a person may present with a low plasma HCO_3^- concentration due to metabolic acidosis and a high PCO_2 due to chronic lung disease. Values for the predicted renal or respiratory compensatory responses can be used in the diagnosis of these mixed acid-base disorders[1,7,10,12] (see Table 32-1). If the values for the compensatory response fall outside the predicted plasma values, it can then be concluded that more than one disorder (*i.e.*, a mixed disorder) is present. Because the respiratory response to changes in HCO_3^- occurs almost immediately, there is only one predicted compensatory response for primary metabolic acid-base disorders. This is in contrast to the primary respiratory disorders, which have two ranges of predicted values, one for the acute and one for the chronic response. Renal compensation takes several days to become fully effective. The acute compensatory response represents the HCO_3^- levels before renal compensation has occurred, and the chronic response after it has occurred. Thus, the values for the plasma pH tend to be more normal in the chronic phase.

Metabolic Acidosis

Metabolic acidosis involves a decreased plasma HCO_3^- concentration along with a decrease in pH. In metabolic acidosis, the body compensates for the decrease in pH by increasing the respiratory rate in an effort to decrease PCO_2 and H_2CO_3 levels.

METABOLIC ACID-BASE IMBALANCE

- Metabolic acid-base disorders represent a primary change in the plasma HCO_3^- ion concentration.

- Metabolic acidosis can be defined as a decrease in plasma HCO_3^- and pH that is caused by an excess of production or accumulation of fixed acids or loss of HCO_3^- ion. Compensatory responses include an increase in ventilation and elimination of CO_2 and the reabsorption and generation of bicarbonate by the kidney.

- Metabolic alkalosis can be defined as an increase in plasma HCO_3^- and pH that is initiated by excess H^+ ion loss or HCO_3^- ion gain and maintained by conditions that impair the ability of the kidney to excrete the excess HCO_3^- ion. Compensatory responses include a decreased respiratory rate with retention of PCO_2 and increased elimination of HCO_3^- by the kidney.

The PCO_2 can be expected to fall by 1 to 1.5 mm Hg for each 1-mEq/L fall in HCO_3^-.[1,3,4,9,12]

Causes

Metabolic acidosis can be caused by one or more of the following four mechanisms: (1) increased production of fixed metabolic acids or ingestion of fixed acids such as salicylic acid, (2) inability of the kidneys to excrete the fixed acids produced from normal metabolism, (3) excessive loss of bicarbonate through the kidneys or gastrointestinal tract, or (4) increased plasma Cl^- concentration.[9,11,12] The anion gap is often useful in determining the cause of the metabolic acidosis (Chart 32-1). The presence of excess metabolic acids produces an increase in the anion gap as sodium bicarbonate is replaced by the sodium salt of the offending acid (e.g., sodium lactate). When the acidosis results from an increase in plasma Cl^- levels (e.g., hyperchloremic acidosis), the anion gap remains within normal levels. The causes of metabolic acidosis are summarized in Table 32-2.

Lactic Acidosis. Acute lactic acidosis, which is one of the most common types of metabolic acidosis, develops when there is excess production or diminished removal of lactic acid from the blood.[12–14] Lactic acid is produced by the anaerobic metabolism of glucose (see Understanding Cell Metabolism, Chapter 4). Most cases of lactic acidosis are caused by inadequate oxygen delivery, as in shock or cardiac arrest.[14] Such conditions not only increase lactic acid production, but they

---

CHART 32-1   THE ANION GAP IN DIFFERENTIAL DIAGNOSIS OF METABOLIC ACIDOSIS

Decreased Anion Gap (<8 mEq/L)
Hypoalbuminemia (decrease in unmeasured anions)
Multiple myeloma (increase in unmeasured cationic IgG paraproteins)
Increased unmeasured cations (hyperkalemia, hypercalcemia, hypermagnesemia, lithium intoxication)

Increased Anion Gap (>12 mEq/L)
Presence of unmeasured metabolic anion
    Diabetic ketoacidosis
    Alcoholic ketoacidosis
    Lactic acidosis
    Starvation
    Renal insufficiency
Presence of drug or chemical anion
    Salicylate poisoning
    Methanol poisoning
    Ethylene glycol poisoning

Normal Anion Gap (8–12 mEq/L)
Loss of bicarbonate
    Diarrhea
    Pancreatic fluid loss
    Ileostomy (unadapted)
Chloride retention
    Renal tubular acidosis
    Ileal loop bladder
    Parenteral nutrition (arginine and lysine)

---

tend to impair lactic acid clearance because of poor liver and kidney perfusion. Mortality rates are high for persons with lactic acidosis due to shock and tissue hypoxia.[13] Lactic acidosis can also occur during periods of intense exercise in which the metabolic needs of the exercising muscles outpace their aerobic capacity for production of ATP, causing them to revert to anaerobic metabolism and the production of lactic acid.[15]

Lactic acidosis is also associated with disorders in which tissue hypoxia does not appear to be present. It has been reported in patients with leukemia, lymphomas, and other cancers; those with poorly controlled diabetes; and persons with severe liver failure.[16] Mechanisms causing lactic acidosis in these conditions are poorly understood. Some conditions such as neoplasms may produce local increases in tissue metabolism and lactate production or they may interfere with blood flow to noncancerous cells.

Lactic acidosis may also occur in genetic mitochondrial disorders that impair oxidative metabolism (see Chapter 7).[17–20] One of these disorders, referred to by the acronym MELAS, involves mitochondrial encephalopathy (ME), lactic acidosis (LA), and strokelike episodes (S). Children with the disorder are normal for the first few years of life and then begin to display impaired motor and cognitive development. The mitochondrial defect also leads to short stature, seizure disorders, and multiple strokes. Lowering the plasma lactate level of children with severe lactic acidosis may result in marked clinical improvement. A variety of drugs can also produce life-threatening lactic acidosis by inhibiting mitochondrial function. These drugs include the biguanide antidiabetic drugs (metformin)[18] and the antiretroviral nucleoside analogs (e.g., zidovudine [AZT]) that are used to treat the acquired immunodeficiency syndrome (AIDS).[19]

A unique form of lactic acidosis, called D-lactic acidosis, can occur in persons with intestinal disorders that involve the generation and absorption of D-lactic acid (L-lactic acid is the usual cause of lactic acidosis). It can occur in persons with jejunoileal bypass, small bowel resection, or short bowel syndrome, in which there is impaired absorption of carbohydrate in the small intestine.[12,21] In these cases, the unabsorbed carbohydrate is delivered to the colon, where it is converted to D-lactic acid by an overgrowth of gram-positive anaerobes. Persons with D-lactic acidosis experience episodic periods of metabolic acidosis often brought on by eating a meal high in carbohydrates. Manifestations include confusion, cerebellar ataxia, slurred speech, and loss of memory. They may complain of feeling (or appear) intoxicated. Treatment includes use of antimicrobial agents to decrease the number of D-lactic acid–producing microorganisms in the bowel along with a low-carbohydrate diet.

Ketoacidosis. Ketoacids (i.e., acetoacetic and β-hydroxybutyric acid), produced in the liver from fatty acids, are the source of fuel for many body tissues. An overproduction of ketoacids occurs when carbohydrate stores are inadequate or when the body cannot use available carbohydrates as a fuel. Under these conditions, fatty acids are mobilized from adipose tissue and delivered to the liver, where they are converted to ketones. Ketoacidosis develops when ketone production by the liver exceeds tissue use.

TABLE 32-2 Causes and Manifestations of Metabolic Acidosis

CAUSES	MANIFESTATIONS
Excess Metabolic Acids (Increased Anion Gap)	**Blood pH, HCO$_3^-$, CO$_2$**
Excessive production of metabolic acids	pH decreased
Lactic acidosis	HCO$_3^-$ (primary) decreased
Diabetic ketoacidosis	PCO$_2$ (compensatory) decreased
Alcoholic ketoacidosis	**Gastrointestinal Function**
Fasting and starvation	Anorexia
Poisoning (*e.g.,* salicylate, methanol,	Nausea and vomiting
ethylene glycol)	Abdominal pain
Impaired elimination of metabolic acids	**Neural Function**
Kidney failure or dysfunction	Weakness
Excessive Bicarbonate Loss (Normal Anion Gap)	Lethargy
Loss of intestinal secretions	General malaise
Diarrhea	Confusion
Intestinal suction	Stupor
Intestinal or biliary fistula	Coma
Increased renal losses	Depression of vital functions
Renal tubular acidosis	**Cardiovascular Function**
Treatment with carbonic anhydrase	Peripheral vasodilation
inhibitors	Decreased heart rate
Hypoaldosteronism	Cardiac arrhythmias
Increased Chloride Levels (Normal Anion Gap)	**Skin**
	Warm and flushed
Excessive reabsorption of chloride by	**Skeletal System**
the kidney	Bone disease (*e.g.,* chronic acidosis)
Sodium chloride infusions	**Signs of Compensation**
Treatment with ammonium chloride	Increased rate and depth of respiration
Parenteral hyperalimentation	(*i.e.,* Kussmaul breathing)
	Hyperkalemia
	Acid urine
	Increased ammonia in urine

The most common cause of ketoacidosis is uncontrolled diabetes mellitus, in which an insulin deficiency leads to the release of fatty acids from adipose cells with subsequent production of excess ketoacids[22] (see Chapter 42). Ketoacidosis may also develop as the result of fasting or food deprivation, during which the lack of carbohydrates produces a self-limited state of ketoacidosis.[22–24]

Ketones are also formed during the oxidation of alcohol, a process that occurs in the liver. A condition called *alcoholic ketoacidosis* can develop in persons who engage in excess alcohol consumption.[25] It usually follows prolonged alcohol ingestion, particularly if accompanied by decreased food intake and vomiting—conditions that result in using fatty acids as an energy source. Ketone formation may be further enhanced by the hypoglycemia that results from alcohol-induced inhibition of glucose synthesis (*i.e.,* gluconeogenesis) by the liver and impaired ketone elimination by the kidneys because of dehydration. An ECF volume deficit caused by vomiting and decreased fluid intake often contributes to the acidosis. Numerous other factors, such as elevations in cortisol, growth hormone, glucagon, and catecholamines, mediate free fatty acid release and thereby contribute to the development of alcoholic ketoacidosis.

Salicylate Toxicity. Salicylates are another potential source of metabolic acids. Aspirin (acetylsalicylic acid) is rapidly converted to salicylic acid in the body. Although aspirin is the most common cause of salicylate toxicity, other salicylate preparations such as methyl salicylate, sodium salicylate, and salicylic acid may produce similar effects. Salicylate overdose produces serious toxic effects, including death. A fatal overdose can occur with as little as 10 to 30 g in adults and 3 g in children.[1]

A variety of acid-base disturbances occur with salicylate toxicity. The salicylates cross the blood-brain barrier and directly stimulate the respiratory center, causing hyperventilation and respiratory alkalosis. The kidneys compensate by secreting increased amounts of HCO$_3^-$, K$^+$, and Na$^+$, thereby contributing to the development of metabolic acidosis. Salicylates also interfere with carbohydrate metabolism, which results in increased production of metabolic acids.

One of the treatments for salicylate toxicity is *alkalinization* of the plasma. Salicylic acid, which is a weak acid, exists in equilibrium with the alkaline salicylate anion. It is the salicylic acid that is toxic because of its ability to cross cell membranes and enter brain cells. The salicylate anion crosses membranes poorly and is less toxic. With alkalinization of the extracellular fluids, the ratio of salicylic acid to salicylate is greatly reduced. This allows salicylic acid to move out of cells into the extracellular fluid along a concentration gradient. The renal elimination of salicylates follows a similar pattern when the urine is alkalinized.

Methanol and Ethylene Glycol Toxicity. Ingestion of methanol and ethylene glycol results in the production of metabolic acids and causes metabolic acidosis. Both produce an osmolar gap because of their small size and osmotic properties. Methanol (wood alcohol) is a component of shellac, varnish, deicing solutions, Sterno, and other commercial products. Methanol can be absorbed through the skin or gastrointestinal tract or inhaled through the lungs. A dose as small as 30 mL can be fatal.[26] In addition to metabolic acidosis, methanol produces severe optic nerve and central nervous system toxicity. Organ system damage occurs after a 24-hour period in which methanol is converted to formaldehyde and formic acid.

Ethylene glycol is a solvent found in products ranging from antifreeze and deicing solutions to carpet and fabric cleaners. It tastes sweet and is intoxicating, factors that contribute to its abuse potential. It is rapidly absorbed from the intestine, making treatment with gastric lavage and syrup of ipecac ineffective. Acidosis occurs as ethylene glycol is converted to oxalic and lactic acid. Manifestations of ethylene glycol toxicity occur in three stages: neurologic symptoms ranging from drunkenness to coma, which appear during the first 12 hours; cardiorespiratory disorders such as tachycardia and pulmonary edema; and flank pain and acute renal failure caused by plugging of the tubules with oxalate crystals (from excess oxalic acid production).[27,28]

The enzyme *alcohol dehydrogenase* metabolizes methanol and ethylene glycol into their toxic metabolites. This is the same enzyme that is used in the metabolism of ethanol. Because alcohol dehydrogenase has an affinity for ethanol 10 times its affinity for methanol or ethylene glycol, intravenous or oral ethanol is used as an antidote for methanol and ethylene glycol poisoning.[1] Extracellular volume expansion and hemodialysis are also used. Fomepizole, with specific indications for ethylene glycol poisoning, was recently approved by The U.S. Food and Drug Administration.[29] In a manner similar to ethanol, it is thought to act as an inhibitor of alcohol dehydrogenase, thereby preventing the formation of the toxic ethylene glycol metabolites.

Decreased Renal Function. Chronic kidney disease is the most common cause of chronic metabolic acidosis. The kidneys normally conserve HCO_3^- and secrete H^+ ions into the urine as a means of regulating acid-base balance. In chronic kidney disease, there is loss of both glomerular and tubular function, with retention of nitrogenous wastes and metabolic acids. In a condition called *renal tubular acidosis,* glomerular function is normal, but the tubular secretion of H^+ or reabsorption of HCO_3^- is abnormal[30] (discussed in Chapter 33).

Increased Bicarbonate Losses. Increased HCO_3^- losses occur with the loss of bicarbonate-rich body fluids or with impaired conservation of HCO_3^- by the kidney. Intestinal secretions have a high HCO_3^- concentration. Consequently, excessive loss of HCO_3^- occurs with severe diarrhea; small bowel, pancreatic, or biliary fistula drainage; ileostomy drainage; and intestinal suction. In diarrhea of microbial origin, HCO_3^- is also secreted into the bowel as a means of neutralizing the metabolic acids produced by the microorganisms causing the diarrhea. Creation of an ileal bladder, which is done for conditions such as neurogenic bladder or surgical removal of the bladder because of cancer, involves the implantation of the ureters into a short, isolated loop of ileum that serves as a conduit for urine collection. With this procedure, contact time between the urine and ileal bladder is normally too short for significant anion exchange, and HCO_3^- is lost in the urine.[1]

Hyperchloremic Acidosis. Hyperchloremic acidosis occurs when Cl^- levels are increased.[31] Because Cl^- and HCO_3^- are exchangeable anions, the plasma HCO_3^- decreases when there is an increase in Cl^-. Hyperchloremic acidosis can occur as the result of abnormal absorption of Cl^- by the kidneys or as a result of treatment with chloride-containing medications (*i.e.,* sodium chloride, amino acid–chloride hyperalimentation solutions, and ammonium chloride). Ammonium chloride is broken down into NH_4^+ and Cl^-. The ammonium ion is converted to urea in the liver, leaving the Cl^- free to react with H^+ to form HCl. The administration of intravenous sodium chloride or parenteral hyperalimentation solutions that contain an amino acid–chloride combination can cause acidosis in a similar manner.[31] With hyperchloremic acidosis, the anion gap remains within the normal range, whereas plasma Cl^- levels are increased and HCO_3^- levels are decreased.

Manifestations

Metabolic acidosis is characterized by a decrease in plasma pH (<7.35) and HCO_3^- levels (<24 mEq/L) due to a gain in H^+ or a loss of HCO_3^-. Acidosis typically produces a compensatory increase in respiratory rate with a decrease in PCO_2.

The manifestations of metabolic acidosis fall into three categories: (1) signs and symptoms of the disorder causing the acidosis; (2) changes in body function related to recruitment of compensatory mechanisms; and (3) alterations in cardiovascular, neurologic, and musculoskeletal function resulting from the decreased pH (see Table 32-2). The signs and symptoms of metabolic acidosis usually begin to appear when the plasma HCO_3^- concentration falls to 20 mEq/L or less. A fall in pH to less than 7.0 to 7.10 can reduce cardiac contractility and predispose to potentially fatal cardiac arrhythmias.[1]

Metabolic acidosis is seldom a primary disorder; it usually develops during the course of another disease. The manifestations of metabolic acidosis frequently are superimposed on the symptoms of the contributing health problem. With diabetic ketoacidosis, which is a common cause of metabolic acidosis, there is an increase in blood and urine glucose and a characteristic smell of ketones to the breath. In the metabolic acidosis that accompanies chronic kidney disease, blood urea nitrogen levels are elevated and other tests of renal function yield abnormal results.

Manifestations related to respiratory and renal compensatory mechanisms usually occur early in the course of metabolic acidosis. In situations of acute metabolic acidosis, the respiratory system compensates for a decrease in pH by increasing ventilation to reduce PCO_2; this is accomplished through deep and rapid respirations. In diabetic ketoacidosis, this breathing pattern is referred to as *Kussmaul breathing*. For descriptive purposes, it can be said that Kussmaul breathing resembles the hyperpnea of exercise—the person breathes as though he or she had been running. There may be complaints of difficult breathing or dyspnea with exertion; with severe acidosis, dyspnea may be present even at rest. Respiratory compensation for acute acidosis tends to be somewhat greater than for chronic acidosis. When kidney function is normal, H^+ excretion increases promptly in response to acidosis, and the urine becomes more acid.

Changes in pH have a direct effect on body function that can produce signs and symptoms common to most types of metabolic acidosis, regardless of cause. A person with metabolic acidosis often complains of weakness, fatigue, general malaise, and a dull headache. They also may have anorexia, nausea, vomiting, and abdominal pain. Tissue turgor is impaired, and the skin is dry when fluid deficit accompanies acidosis. In persons with undiagnosed diabetes mellitus, the nausea, vomiting, and abdominal symptoms may be misinterpreted as being caused by gastrointestinal flu or other abdominal disease, such as appendicitis. Acidosis depresses neuronal excitability and it decreases binding of calcium to plasma proteins so that more free calcium is available to decrease neural activity. As acidosis progresses, the level of consciousness declines, and stupor and coma develop. The skin is often warm and flushed because blood vessels in the skin become less responsive to sympathetic nervous system stimulation and lose their tone.

When the pH falls to 7.0 to 7.1, cardiac contractility and cardiac output decrease, the heart becomes less responsive to catecholamines (*i.e.,* epinephrine and norepinephrine), and arrhythmias, including fatal ventricular arrhythmias, can develop. A decrease in ventricular function may be particularly important in perpetuating shock-induced lactic acidosis, and partial correction of the acidemia may be necessary before tissue perfusion can be restored.[1]

Chronic acidemia, as in chronic kidney disease, can lead to a variety of musculoskeletal problems, some of which result from the release of calcium and phosphate during bone buffering of excess H^+ ions.[32] Of particular importance is impaired growth in children. In infants and children, acidemia may be associated with a variety of nonspecific symptoms such as anorexia, weight loss, muscle weakness, and listlessness.[1] Muscle weakness and listlessness may result from alterations in muscle metabolism.

Treatment

The treatment of metabolic acidosis focuses on correcting the condition that caused the disorder and restoring the fluids and electrolytes that have been lost from the body. The treatment of diabetic ketoacidosis is discussed in Chapter 42.

The use of supplemental sodium bicarbonate ($NaHCO_3$) may be indicated in the treatment of some forms of normal anion gap acidosis. However, its use in treatment of metabolic acidosis with an increased anion gap is controversial, particularly in cases of impaired tissue perfusion.[4,33] In most patients with circulatory shock, cardiac arrest, or sepsis, impaired oxygen delivery is the primary cause of lactic acidosis. In these situations, the administration of large amounts of $NaHCO_3$ does not improve oxygen delivery and may produce hypernatremia, hyperosmolality, and decreased oxygen release by hemoglobin because of a shift in the oxygen dissociation curve.[33]

Metabolic Alkalosis

Metabolic alkalosis is a systemic disorder caused by an increase in plasma pH due to a primary excess in HCO_3^-.[34,35] It is reported to be the second most common acid-base disorder in hospitalized adults, accounting for about 32% of all acid-base disorders.[35]

Causes

Metabolic alkalosis can be caused by factors that generate a loss of fixed acids or a gain of bicarbonate and those that maintain the alkalosis by interfering with excretion of the excess bicarbonate (Table 32-3). They include (1) a gain of base through the oral or intravenous route; (2) loss of fixed acids from the stomach; and (3) maintenance of the increased bicarbonate levels by contraction of the ECF volume, hypokalemia, and hypochloremia.

Excess Base Loading. Because the normal kidney is extremely efficient at excreting bicarbonate, excess base intake is rarely a cause of significant chronic metabolic alkalosis. Transient acute alkalosis, on the other hand, is a rather common occurrence during or immediately after excess oral ingestion of bicarbonate-containing antacids (*e.g.,* Alka-Seltzer) or intravenous infusion of $NaHCO_3$ or base equivalent (*e.g.,* acetate in hyperalimentation solutions, lactate in Ringer's lactate, and citrate in blood transfusions). A condition called the *milk-alkali syndrome* is a condition in which the chronic ingestion of milk or calcium carbonate antacids leads to hypercalcemia and metabolic alkalosis. In this case, the antacids raise the plasma HCO_3^- concentration, whereas the hypercalcemia prevents the urinary excretion of HCO_3^-. The most common cause at present is the administration of calcium carbonate as a phosphate binder to persons with chronic kidney disease.[1]

TABLE 32-3 Causes and Manifestations of Metabolic Alkalosis

CAUSES	MANIFESTATIONS
Excessive Gain of Bicarbonate or Alkali	**Blood pH, HCO_3^-, CO_2**
Ingestion or administration of sodium bicarbonate	pH increased
Administration of hyperalimentation solutions containing acetate	HCO_3^- (primary) increased
Administration of parenteral solutions containing lactate	PCO_2 (compensatory) increased
Administration of citrate-containing blood transfusions	**Neural Function**
	Confusion
	Hyperactive reflexes
Excessive Loss of Hydrogen Ions	Tetany
Vomiting	Convulsions
Gastric suction	**Cardiovascular Function**
Binge-purge syndrome	Hypotension
Potassium deficit	Arrhythmias
Diuretic therapy	**Respiratory Function**
Hyperaldosteronism	Respiratory acidosis due to decreased respiratory rate
Milk-alkali syndrome	**Signs of Compensation**
Increased Bicarbonate Retention	Decreased rate and depth of respiration
Loss of chloride with bicarbonate retention	Increased urine pH
Volume Contraction	
Loss of body fluids	
Diuretic therapy	

Loss of Fixed Acid. The loss of fixed acids occurs mainly through the loss of acid from the stomach and the loss of chloride in the urine. Vomiting and removal of gastric secretions by nasogastric suction are common causes of metabolic alkalosis in acutely ill or hospitalized patients. Bulimia nervosa with self-induced vomiting also is associated with metabolic alkalosis.[35] Gastric secretions contain high concentrations of HCl and lesser concentrations of potassium chloride (KCl). As Cl^- is taken from the blood and secreted into the stomach, it is replaced by HCO_3^-. Under normal conditions, each 1 mEq of H^+ that is secreted into the stomach generates 1 mEq of plasma HCO_3^-.[35] Thus, the loss of gastric secretions through vomiting or gastric suction is a common cause of metabolic alkalosis. The accompanying ECF volume depletion, hypochloremia, and hypokalemia serve to maintain the metabolic alkalosis by increasing HCO_3^- reabsorption by the kidneys (Fig. 32-7).

The loop (*e.g.,* furosemide [Lasix]) and thiazide (*e.g.,* hydrochlorothiazide) diuretics are commonly associated with metabolic alkalosis, the severity of which varies directly with the degree of diuresis. The volume contraction and loss of H^+ in the urine contribute to the problem. The latter is primarily due to the enhanced H^+ secretion in the distal tubule that results from an interplay between the diuretic-induced increase in Na^+ delivery to the distal tubule and collecting duct, where an accelerated excretion of H^+ and K^+ takes place, and an increase in aldosterone secretion resulting from the volume contraction. Although aldosterone blunts the loss of Na^+, it also accelerates the secretion of K^+ and H^+. The resulting loss of K^+ also accelerates HCO_3^- reabsorption.

Metabolic alkalosis can also occur with abrupt correction of respiratory acidosis in persons with chronic respiratory acidosis. Chronic respiratory acidosis is associated with a compensatory loss of H^+ and Cl^- in the urine along with HCO_3^- retention. When respiratory acidosis is corrected abruptly, as with mechanical ventilation, a "posthypercapneic" metabolic alkalosis may develop because although the PCO_2 drops rapidly, the plasma HCO_3^-, which must be eliminated through the kidney, remains elevated.

Maintenance of Metabolic Alkalosis. Maintenance of metabolic alkalosis resides within the kidney and its inability to rid the body of excess HCO_3^-. Many of the conditions that accompany the development of metabolic alkalosis, such as contraction of the ECF volume, hypochloremia, and hypokalemia, also increase reabsorption of HCO_3^- by the kidney, thereby contributing to its maintenance.

Depletion of the ECF causes a decline in the glomerular filtration rate with a subsequent increase in Na^+ and H_2O reabsorption. When there is Cl^- depletion from loss of HCl, the available anion for reabsorption with Na^+ is HCO_3^-. Hypokalemia, which generally accompanies metabolic alkalosis, also contributes to its maintenance. This is due partly to the direct effect of alkalosis on potassium excretion by the kidney and partly to a secondary hyperaldosteronism resulting from volume depletion. In hypokalemia, the distal tubular reabsorption of K^+ is accompanied by an increase in H^+ secretion. The secondary hyperaldosteronism, in turn, promotes extensive reabsorption of Na^+ from the distal and collecting tubules and at the same

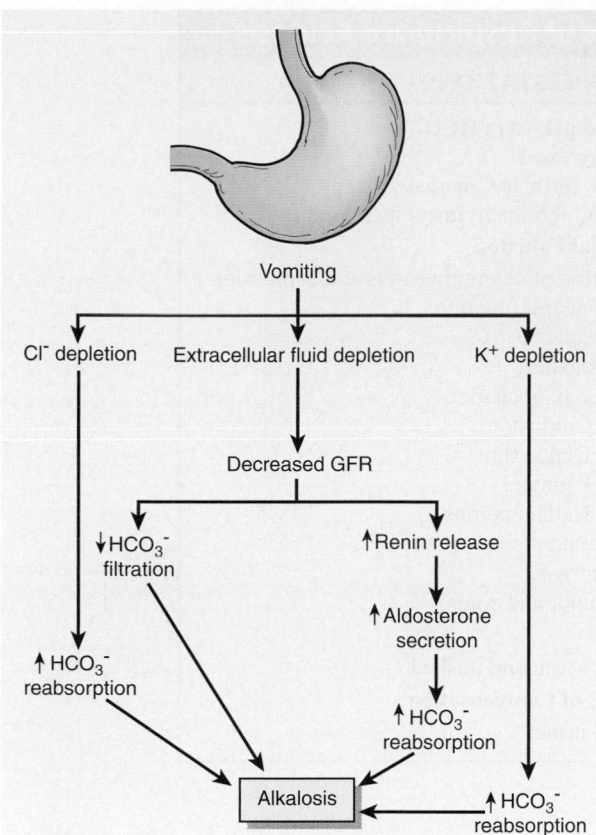

FIGURE 32-7 • Renal mechanisms for bicarbonate (HCO_3^-) reabsorption and maintenance of metabolic alkalosis after depletion of extracellular fluid volume, chloride (Cl^-), and potassium (K^+) due to vomiting. GFR, glomerular filtration rate.

time stimulates the secretion of H^+ from cells in the collecting tubules. Hypokalemia induced in this manner further worsens the metabolic alkalosis by increasing HCO_3^- reabsorption in the proximal tubule and H^+ secretion in the distal tubule.

Manifestations

Metabolic alkalosis is characterized by a plasma pH above 7.45, plasma HCO_3^- above 31 mEq/L (31 mmol/L), and base excess above 3 mEq/L (3 mmol/L; see Table 32-3). Persons with metabolic alkalosis often are asymptomatic or have signs related to ECF volume depletion or hypokalemia. Neurologic signs and symptoms (*e.g.,* hyperexcitability) occur less frequently with metabolic alkalosis than with other acid-base disorders because HCO_3^- enters the cerebrospinal fluid (CSF) more slowly than CO_2. When neurologic manifestations do occur, as in acute and severe metabolic alkalosis, they include mental confusion, hyperactive reflexes, tetany, and carpopedal spasm. Metabolic alkalosis also leads to a compensatory hypoventilation with development of various degrees of hypoxemia and respiratory acidosis. Significant morbidity occurs with severe metabolic alkalosis (pH >7.55), including respiratory failure, cardiac arrhythmias, seizures, and coma.

Treatment

The treatment of metabolic alkalosis usually is directed toward correcting the cause of the condition. A chloride deficit requires correction. Potassium chloride usually is the treatment of choice when there is an accompanying K^+ deficit. When KCl is used as a therapy, the Cl^- anion replaces the HCO_3^- anion and the K^+ corrects the potassium deficit, allowing the kidneys to retain H^+ while eliminating K^+. Fluid replacement with normal saline or one-half normal saline often is used in treatment volume contraction alkalosis.

Respiratory Acidosis

Respiratory acidosis occurs in conditions that impair alveolar ventilation and cause an increase in plasma PCO_2, also known as *hypercapnia,* along with a decrease in pH. Respiratory acidosis can occur as an acute or chronic disorder. Acute respiratory failure is associated with a rapid rise in arterial PCO_2 with a minimal increase in plasma HCO_3^- and large decrease in pH. Chronic respiratory acidosis is characterized by a sustained increase in arterial PCO_2, resulting in renal adaptation with a more marked increase in plasma HCO_3^- and a lesser decrease in pH.[36-38]

RESPIRATORY ACID-BASE IMBALANCE

- Respiratory acid-base imbalances are due to a primary disturbance in PCO_2, reflecting an increase or decrease in alveolar ventilation.

- Respiratory acidosis, or hypercapnia, represents an increase in PCO_2 and a decrease in plasma pH, resulting from a decrease in effective alveolar ventilation. Compensatory mechanisms include increased conservation and generation of HCO_3^- and elimination of H^+ by the kidney.

- Respiratory alkalosis, or hypocapnia, represents a decrease in PCO_2 and an increase in plasma pH, resulting from increased alveolar ventilation. Compensatory mechanisms include increased elimination of HCO_3^- and conservation of H^+ by the kidney.

Causes

Respiratory acidosis occurs in acute or chronic conditions that impair effective alveolar ventilation and cause an accumulation of PCO_2 (Table 32-4). Impaired ventilation can occur as the result of decreased respiratory drive, lung disease, or disorders of chest wall and respiratory muscles. Less commonly, it results from excess CO_2 production.

Acute Disorders of Ventilation. Acute respiratory acidosis can be caused by impaired function of the respiratory center in

TABLE 32-4 Causes and Manifestations of Respiratory Acidosis

CAUSES	MANIFESTATIONS
Depression of Respiratory Center	**Blood pH, CO_2, HCO_3^-**
Drug overdose	pH decreased
Head injury	PCO_2 (primary) increased
Lung Disease	HCO_3^- (compensatory) increased
Bronchial asthma	**Neural Function**
Emphysema	Dilation of cerebral vessels and depression
Chronic bronchitis	of neural function
Pneumonia	Headache
Pulmonary edema	Weakness
Respiratory distress syndrome	Behavior changes
Airway Obstruction, Disorders of Chest	Confusion
Wall and Respiratory Muscles	Depression
Paralysis of respiratory muscles	Paranoia
Chest injuries	Hallucinations
Kyphoscoliosis	Tremors
Extreme obesity	Paralysis
Treatment with paralytic drugs	Stupor and coma
Breathing Air With High CO_2 Content	**Skin**
	Skin warm and flushed
	Signs of Compensation
	Acid urine

the medulla (as in narcotic overdose), lung disease, chest injury, weakness of the respiratory muscles, or airway obstruction. Almost all persons with acute respiratory acidosis are hypoxemic if they are breathing room air. In many cases, signs of hypoxemia develop before those of respiratory acidosis because CO_2 diffuses across the alveolar capillary membrane 20 times more rapidly than oxygen.[1,2]

Chronic Disorders of Ventilation. Chronic respiratory acidosis is a relatively common disturbance in patients with chronic obstructive lung disease. In these persons, the persistent elevation of PCO_2 stimulates renal H^+ secretion and HCO_3^- reabsorption. The effectiveness of these compensatory mechanisms can often return the pH to near-normal values as long as oxygen levels are maintained within a range that does not unduly suppress chemoreceptor control of respirations.

An acute episode of respiratory acidosis can develop in persons with chronic lung disease who receive oxygen therapy at a flow rate that is sufficient to raise their PO_2 to a level that produces a decrease in ventilation (discussed in Chapter 29). In these persons, the medullary respiratory center has adapted to the elevated levels of CO_2 and no longer responds to increases in PCO_2. Instead, a decrease in the PO_2 becomes the major stimulus for respiration. If oxygen is administered at a flow rate that is sufficient to suppress this stimulus, the rate and depth of respiration decrease, and the PCO_2 increases. That being said, any person who is in need of additional oxygen should have it administered, albeit at a flow rate that does not depress the respiratory drive.

Increased Carbon Dioxide Production. Carbon dioxide is a product of the body's metabolic processes, generating a substantial amount of acid that must be excreted by the lungs or kidneys to prevent acidosis. An increase in CO_2 production can result from numerous processes, including exercise, fever, sepsis, and burns. For example, CO_2 production increases by approximately 13% for each 1°C rise in temperature above normal.[38] Nutrition also affects the production of carbon dioxide. A carbohydrate-rich diet produces larger amounts of CO_2 than one containing reasonable amounts of protein and fat. Although excess CO_2 production can lead to an increase in PCO_2, it seldom does. In healthy persons, an increase in CO_2 is usually matched by an increase in CO_2 elimination by the lungs. In contrast, persons with respiratory diseases may be unable to eliminate the excess CO_2.

Manifestations

Respiratory acidosis is associated with a plasma pH below 7.35 and an arterial PCO_2 above 50 mm Hg (see Table 32-4). The signs and symptoms of respiratory acidosis depend on the rapidity of onset and whether the condition is acute or chronic. Because respiratory acidosis often is accompanied by hypoxemia, the manifestations of respiratory acidosis often are intermixed with those of oxygen deficit. Carbon dioxide readily crosses the blood-brain barrier, exerting its effects by changing the pH of brain fluids. Elevated levels of CO_2 produce vasodilation of cerebral blood vessels, causing headache, blurred vision, irritability, muscle twitching, and psychological disturbances.

If the condition is severe and prolonged, it can cause an increase in CSF pressure and papilledema. Impaired consciousness, ranging from lethargy to coma, develops as the PCO_2 rises to extreme levels. Paralysis of the extremities may occur, and there may be respiratory depression. Less severe forms of acidosis often are accompanied by warm and flushed skin, weakness, and tachycardia.

Treatment

The treatment of acute and chronic respiratory acidosis is directed toward improving ventilation. In severe cases, mechanical ventilation may be necessary. The treatment of respiratory acidosis due to respiratory failure is discussed in Chapter 29.

Respiratory Alkalosis

Respiratory alkalosis is a systemic acid-base disorder characterized by a primary decrease in plasma PCO_2, also referred to as *hypocapnia,* which produces an elevation in pH and a subsequent decrease in HCO_3^-.[37,39,40] Because respiratory alkalosis can occur suddenly, a compensatory decrease in bicarbonate level may not occur before respiratory correction has taken place.

Causes

Respiratory alkalosis is caused by hyperventilation or a respiratory rate in excess of that needed to maintain normal plasma PCO_2 levels (Table 32-5). It may occur as the result of central stimulation of the medullary respiratory center or stimulation of peripheral (*e.g.,* carotid chemoreceptor) pathways to the medullary respiratory center.[40]

Mechanical ventilation may produce respiratory alkalosis if the rate and tidal volume are set so that CO_2 elimination exceeds CO_2 production. Carbon dioxide crosses the alveolar capillary membrane 20 times more rapidly than oxygen. Therefore, increased minute ventilation may be necessary to maintain adequate oxygen levels while producing a concomitant decrease in CO_2 levels. In some cases, respiratory alkalosis may be induced through mechanical ventilation as a means of controlling disorders such as severe intracranial hypertension.[40]

Central stimulation of the medullary respiratory center occurs with anxiety, pain, pregnancy, febrile states, sepsis, encephalitis, and salicylate toxicity. Respiratory alkalosis has long been recognized as a common acid-base disorder in critically ill patients, and is a consistent finding in both septic shock and the systemic inflammatory response syndrome[40] (see Chapter 26). Progesterone increases ventilation in women; during the progesterone phase of the menstrual cycle, normal women increase their PCO_2 values by 2 to 4 mm Hg and their pH by 0.01 to 0.02.[3] Women also develop substantial hypocapnia during pregnancy, most notably during the last trimester, with PCO_2 values of 29 to 32 mm Hg.[3]

One of the most common causes of respiratory alkalosis is hyperventilation syndrome, which is characterized by recurring episodes of overbreathing often associated with anxiety. Persons experiencing panic attacks frequently present in the emergency department with manifestations of acute respiratory alkalosis.

Hypoxemia exerts its effect on pH through the peripheral chemoreceptors in the carotid bodies. Stimulation of peripheral chemoreceptors occurs in conditions that cause hypoxemia with relatively unimpaired CO_2 transport, such as exposure to high altitudes.

Manifestations

Respiratory alkalosis manifests with a decrease in PCO_2 and a deficit in H_2CO_3 (see Table 32-5). In respiratory alkalosis, the

TABLE 32-5 **Causes and Manifestations of Respiratory Alkalosis**	
CAUSES	**MANIFESTATIONS**
Excessive Ventilation	**Blood pH, CO_2, HCO_3^-**
Anxiety and psychogenic hyperventilation	pH increased
Hypoxia and reflex stimulation of ventilation	PCO_2 (primary) decreased
Lung disease that causes a reflex stimulation of ventilation	HCO_3^- (compensatory) decreased
Stimulation of respiratory center	**Neural Function**
Elevated blood ammonia level	Constriction of cerebral vessels and increased neuronal excitability
Salicylate toxicity	Dizziness, panic, lightheadedness
Encephalitis	Tetany
Fever	Numbness and tingling of fingers and toes
Mechanical ventilation	Positive Chvostek and Trousseau signs
	Seizures
	Cardiovascular Function
	Cardiac arrhythmias

pH is above 7.45, arterial PCO_2 is below 35 mm Hg, and plasma HCO_3^- levels usually are below 24 mEq/L (24 mmol/L).

The signs and symptoms of respiratory alkalosis are associated with hyperexcitability of the nervous system and a decrease in cerebral blood flow. Alkalosis increases protein binding of extracellular calcium. This reduces ionized calcium levels, causing an increase in neuromuscular excitability. A decrease in the CO_2 content of the blood causes constriction of cerebral blood vessels. Because CO_2 crosses the blood-brain barrier rather quickly, the manifestations of acute respiratory alkalosis are usually of sudden onset. The person often experiences lightheadedness, dizziness, tingling, and numbness of the fingers and toes. These manifestations may be accompanied by sweating, palpitations, panic, air hunger, and dyspnea. Chvostek and Trousseau signs may be positive (see Chapter 31), and tetany and convulsions may occur. Because CO_2 provides the stimulus for short-term regulation of respiration, short periods of apnea may occur in persons with acute episodes of hyperventilation.

Treatment

The treatment of respiratory alkalosis focuses on measures to correct the underlying cause. Hypoxia may be corrected by administration of supplemental oxygen. Changing ventilator settings may be used to prevent or treat respiratory alkalosis in persons who are being mechanically ventilated. Persons with hyperventilation syndrome may benefit from reassurance, rebreathing from a paper bag during symptomatic attacks, and attention to the psychological stress.

IN SUMMARY, acidosis describes a decrease in pH and alkalosis a increase in pH. Acid-base disorders may be caused by alterations in the body's volatile acids (i.e., respiratory acidosis or respiratory alkalosis) or nonvolatile or fixed acids (i.e., metabolic acidosis or metabolic alkalosis). Acidosis and alkalosis typically involve a primary or initiating event and a compensatory or adaptive state that results from homeostatic mechanisms that attempt to prevent or correct large changes in pH. A mixed acid-base disorder is one in which there is both a primary and a compensatory change in acid-base balance.

Metabolic acidosis is defined as a decrease in pH due to a decrease in the HCO_3^- level, and metabolic alkalosis as an increase in pH due to an increase in the HCO_3^- level. It is caused by an increased production of nonvolatile metabolic acids such as lactic acid or ketoacids, decreased acid excretion by the kidney, excessive loss of HCO_3^- as in diarrhea, or an increase in Cl^-. Metabolic acidosis may present with an increased anion gap in which sodium bicarbonate is replaced by the sodium salt of the offending anion, or with a normal anion gap as when HCO_3^- is replaced by Cl^-. Metabolic alkalosis involves generation of the increased pH and HCO_3^- levels through a loss of H^+ or gain of HCO_3^-, and the maintenance of the alkalotic state because of the kidney's failure to eliminate the excess HCO_3^- owing to

an accompanying ECF volume contraction, increased aldosterone levels, and decreased Cl^- and K^+ levels.

Respiratory acidosis reflects an increase in PCO_2 levels and is caused by conditions that impair alveolar ventilation. It can occur as an acute disorder in which there is a rapid rise in PCO_2, a minimal increase in plasma HCO_3^-, and a large decrease in pH. Respiratory alkalosis is caused by conditions that cause hyperventilation and a reduction in PCO_2 levels. Because respiratory alkalosis often occurs suddenly, a compensatory decrease in HCO_3^- levels may not occur before corrections have been accomplished.

The signs and symptoms of acidosis and alkalosis reflect alterations in body function associated with the disorder causing the acid-base disturbance, the effect of the change of pH on body function, and the body's attempt to correct and maintain the pH within a normal physiologic range. In general, neuromuscular excitability is decreased in acidosis and increased in alkalosis. ■

Review Exercises

1. A 34-year-old woman with diabetes is admitted to the emergency department in a stuporous state. Her skin is flushed and warm, her breath has a sweet odor, her pulse is rapid and weak, and her respirations are rapid and deep. Her initial laboratory tests indicate a blood sugar of 320 mg/dL, serum HCO_3^- of 12 mEq/L (normal, 24 to 31 mEq/L), and a pH of 7.1 (normal, 7.35 to 7.45).

   A. *What is the most likely cause of her lowered pH and bicarbonate levels?*

   B. *How would you account for her rapid and deep respirations?*

   C. *Using the Henderson-Hasselbalch equation and the solubility coefficient for CO_2 given in this chapter, what would you expect her PCO_2 to be?*

   D. *How would you explain her warm, flushed skin and stuporous mental state?*

2. Explain the use of the urine anion gap to determine the kidney's ability to compensate for acid-base disorders by secreting and eliminate H^+ ions.

3. A 16-year-old girl is seen by her primary care provider because of her parents' concern over her binge eating and their recent discovery that she engages in self-induced vomiting. A tentative diagnosis of bulimia nervosa is made. Initial laboratory tests reveal a plasma K^+ of 3 mEq/L (normal, 3.5–5.0 mEq/L) and a Cl^- of 93 mEq/L (normal, 98–106 mEq/L).

   A. *Explain her low K^+ and Cl^-.*

   B. *What type of acid-base abnormality would you expect her to have?*

4. A 65-year-old man with chronic obstructive lung disease has been using low-flow oxygen therapy because of difficulty in maintaining adequate oxygenation of his blood. He has recently had a severe respiratory tract infection and has had difficulty breathing. He is admitted to the emergency department because he became increasingly lethargic and his wife has had trouble arousing him. His respirations are 12 breaths/minute. She relates that he had "turned his oxygen way up" because of difficulty breathing.

A. *What is the most likely cause of this man's problem?*

B. *How would you explain the lethargy and difficulty in arousal?*

C. *Arterial blood gases, drawn on admission to the emergency department, indicated a PO_2 of 85 mm Hg (normal, 90 to 95 mm Hg) and a PCO_2 of 90 mm Hg (normal, 40 mm Hg). His serum HCO_3^- was 34 mEq/L (normal, 24 to 31 mEq/L). What is his pH?*

D. *What would be the main goal of treatment for this man in terms of acid-base balance?*

References

1. Rose B. D. (2001). *Clinical physiology of acid-base and electrolyte disorders* (5th ed., pp. 302, 325–364, 578–647, 669). New York: McGraw-Hill.
2. Guyton A., Hall J. E. (2006). *Textbook of medical physiology* (11th ed., pp. 383–401). Philadelphia: Elsevier Saunders.
3. Adrogue H. E., Adrogue H. J. (2001). Acid-base physiology. *Respiratory Care* 46, 328–341.
4. Costanzo L. S. (2002). *Physiology* (2nd ed., pp. 275–299). Philadelphia: W. B. Saunders.
5. Tanner G. A. (2002). Acid-base balance. In Rhoades R. A., Tanner G. A. (Eds.), *Medical physiology* (2nd ed., pp. 426–447). Philadelphia: Lippincott Williams & Wilkins.
6. Berne R. M., Levy M. N., Koeppen B. M., et al. (Eds.). (2004). *Physiology* (5th ed., pp. 703–715). St. Louis: CV Mosby.
7. Yucha C. (2004). Renal regulation of acid-base disorders. *Nephrology Nursing Journal* 31, 201–208.
8. Madias N. E., Adrogue H. J. (2003). Cross-talk between two organs: How the kidney responds to disruption of acid-base balance by the lung. *Nephron Physiology* 93, 61–66.
9. Shapiro J. I., Kaehny W. D. (2003). Pathogenesis and management of metabolic acidosis and alkalosis. In Schrier R. W. (Ed.), *Renal and electrolyte disorders* (6th ed., pp. 115–153). Philadelphia: Lippincott Williams & Wilkins.
10. Kraut J. A., Madias N. E. (2001). Approach to patients with acid-base disorders. *Respiratory Care* 46, 392–402.
11. Fischbach F. (2004). *A manual of laboratory and diagnostic tests* (7th ed., p. 946). Philadelphia: Lippincott Williams & Wilkins.
12. Whittier W. L., Rutecki G. W. (2004). Primer on clinical acid-base problem solving. *Disease of the Month* 50, 117–162.
13. Adrogue H. J., Madias N. E. (1998). Management of life-threatening acid-base disorders: First of two parts. *New England Journal of Medicine* 338, 26–34.
14. Gauthier P. M., Szerlip H. M. (2002). Metabolic acidosis in the intensive care unit. *Critical Care Medicine* 18, 289–308.
15. Swenson E. R. (2001). Metabolic acidosis. *Respiratory Care* 46, 342–353.
16. Casaletto J. J. (2005). Differential diagnosis of metabolic acidosis. *Emergency Medicine Clinics of North America* 23, 771–787.
17. Rothman S. M. (1999). Mutations of the mitochondrial genome: Clinical overview and possible pathophysiology of cell damage. *Biochemical Society Symposia* 66, 111–122.
18. Miesen R. I. (2004). The phantom of lactic acidosis due to metformin in patients with diabetes. *Diabetes Care* 27, 1791–1793.
19. Claessens Y.-E., Chiche J.-D., Mira J.-P., et al. (2003). Bench-to-bedside review: Severe lactic acidosis in HIV patients treated with nucleoside analogue reverse transcription inhibitors. *Clinical Care* 7, 226–232.
20. Howell N. (1999). Human mitochondrial diseases: Answering questions and questioning answers. *International Review of Cytology* 186, 49–116.
21. Uribarri J., Oh M. S., Carroll H. J. (1998). D-Lactic acidosis: A review of clinical presentation, biochemical features and pathophysiological mechanisms. *Medicine (Baltimore)* 77, 73–82.
22. Trachtenbarg D. E. (2005). Diabetic ketoacidosis. *American Family Physician* 71, 1705–1714.
23. Chen T.-V., Smith W., Rosenstock J. L., et al. (2006). A life-threatening complication of the Atkins diet. *Lancet* 367, 958.
24. Toth H. I., Greenbaum L. A. (2003). Severe acidosis caused by starvation and stress. *American Journal of Kidney Disease* 42, E16–E19.
25. Umpierrez G. E., DiGirolamo M., Tuvlin J. A., et al. (2000). Differences in metabolic and hormonal milieu in diabetic and alcohol-induced keto-acidosis. *Journal of Critical Care* 15, 52–59.
26. Meyer R. J., Beard M. E., Ardagh M. W., et al. (2000). Methanol poisoning. *New Zealand Medical Journal* 113(1102), 3–11.
27. Scalley R. D., Smart M. L., Archie T. E. (2002). Treatment of ethylene glycol poisoning. *American Family Physician* 66, 807–812.
28. Egbert P. A., Abraham K. (1999). Ethylene glycol intoxication: Pathophysiology, diagnosis, and emergency management. *ANNA Journal* 26, 295–300.
29. Brent J., McMartin K., Phillips S. (2001). Fomepizole for treatment of methanol poisoning. *New England Journal of Medicine* 344, 424–429.
30. Soriano J. R. (2002). Renal tubular acidosis. *Journal of the American Society of Nephrology* 13, 2160–2170.
31. Powers F. (1999). The role of chloride in acid-base balance. *Journal of Intravenous Nursing* 22, 286–291.
32. Alpern R. J., Sakhaee K. (1997). The clinical spectrum of chronic metabolic acidosis: Homeostatic mechanisms produce significant morbidity. *American Journal of Kidney Diseases* 29, 291–302.
33. Forsythe S. M., Schmidt G. A. (2000). Sodium bicarbonate for the treatment of lactic acidosis. *Chest* 117, 260–267.
34. Khanna A., Kurtzman N. A. (2001). Metabolic alkalosis. *Respiratory Care* 46, 354–365.
35. Galla J. H. (2000). Metabolic alkalosis. *Journal of the American Society of Nephrology* 11, 369–375.
36. Adrogue H. J., Madias N. E. (1998). Management of life-threatening acid-base disorders. *New England Journal of Medicine* 338, 107–111.
37. Kaehny W. D. (2003). Pathogenesis and management of respiratory and mixed acid-base disorders. In Schrier R. W. (Ed.), *Renal and electrolyte disorders* (6th ed., pp. 154–170). Philadelphia: Lippincott Williams & Wilkins.
38. Epstein S. K., Singh N. (2001). Respiratory acidosis. *Respiratory Care* 46, 366–383.
39. Laffey J. H., Kavenaugh B. P. (2002). Hypocapnia. *New England Journal of Medicine* 347, 43–53.
40. Foste G. T., Vaziri N. D., Sassoon C. S. H. (2001). Respiratory alkalosis. *Respiratory Care* 46, 384–391.

Visit the**Point** **http://thePoint.lww.com for animations, journal articles, and more!**

Disorders of Renal Function

CAROL M. PORTH

> Kidney disease continues to be a major cause of work loss, physician visits, and hospitalization among both men and women. Each year, kidney stones account for 1 million physician office visits and nearly 177,500 hospitalizations, and urinary tract infections (UTIs) result in nearly 11 million office visits and 368,000 hospitalizations.[1] The kidneys filter blood from all parts of the body, and although many forms of kidney disease originate in the kidneys, others develop secondary to disorders such as hypertension, diabetes mellitus, and systemic lupus erythematosus (SLE). The content in this chapter focuses on congenital disorders of the kidneys, obstructive disorders, UTIs, disorders of glomerular function, tubulointerstitial disorders, and neoplasms of the kidneys. Acute renal failure and chronic kidney disease are discussed in Chapter 34, and disorders that predominantly affect the lower urinary tract and bladder in Chapter 35.

CONGENITAL AND INHERITED DISORDERS OF THE KIDNEYS

After completing this section of the chapter, you should be able to meet the following objectives:

■ Define the terms *agenesis, hypoplasia,* and *dysgenesis,* and discuss them as they refer to the development of the kidney.
■ Cite the effect of urinary obstruction in the fetus.
■ Describe the inheritance, pathology, and manifestations of the different types of polycystic kidney disease.

Some abnormality of the kidneys and ureters occurs in approximately 3% to 4% of newborn infants.[2] Anomalies in shape and position are the most common. Less common are disorders involving a decrease in renal mass (*e.g.,* agenesis, hypogenesis) or a change in renal structure (*e.g.,* renal dysplasia). The kidneys can be visualized as early as 12 weeks' gestation by ultrasonography, allowing many fetal urinary abnormalities to be detected before birth.

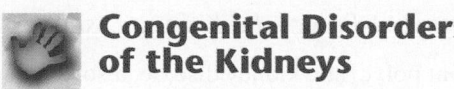
Congenital Disorders of the Kidneys

The kidneys begin to develop early in the fifth week of gestation and start to function approximately 3 weeks later. Formation of urine is thought to begin in the 9th to 12th weeks of gestation; by the 32nd week, fetal production of urine reaches approximately 28 mL/hour.[3] The urine that is produced is excreted into the amniotic cavity and is the main constituent of amniotic fluid. Thus, the relative amount of amniotic fluid can provide information about the status of fetal renal function. In pregnancies that involve infants with nonfunctional kidneys or outflow obstruction of urine from the kidneys, the amount of amniotic fluid is small—a condition called *oligohydramnios*. The condition causes compression of the developing fetus and is often associated with impaired development of lungs and other fetal structures.[2]

Agenesis and Hypoplasia

The term *dysgenesis* refers to a failure of an organ to develop normally, and *agenesis* to complete failure of an organ to develop. Unilateral renal agenesis is relatively common, being present in about 1 of 1000 newborn infants. Boys are affected more often than girls, and the left kidney is the one that is usually absent.[2] Unilateral agenesis usually does not cause symptoms and is usually not discovered during infancy because the other kidney usually undergoes compensatory hypertrophy and performs the function of the missing kidney.

Total agenesis of both kidneys is incompatible with extrauterine life. Infants are stillborn or die shortly after birth of pulmonary hypoplasia. Newborns with renal agenesis often have characteristic facial features, termed *Potter syndrome,* resulting from the effects of oligohydramnios.[4] The eyes are widely separated and have epicanthic folds, the ears are low set, the nose is broad and flat, the chin is receding, and limb defects often are present.[4,5]

In *renal hypoplasia,* the kidneys do not develop to normal size. Like agenesis, hypoplasia more commonly affects only one kidney. When both kidneys are affected, there is progressive development of renal failure. It has been suggested that true hypoplasia is extremely rare; most cases probably represent acquired scarring due to vascular, infectious, or other kidney diseases rather than an underlying developmental failure.[4,5]

Renal Dysplasia

Renal dysplasia is caused by an abnormality in the differentiation of kidney structures during embryonic development. It is characterized by undifferentiated tubular structures surrounded by primitive embryonic tissue.[5,6] The disorder may result in small, aplastic kidneys or cysts that form from the abnormal tubules. If cysts are present, the condition is referred to as *cystic dysplasia.* One or both kidneys may be involved, and the affected kidney may be abnormally large or very small. Many forms of dysplasia are accompanied by other urinary tract abnormalities, especially disorders that cause obstruction to

urine flow (*e.g.,* ureteral agenesis or atresia; ureteropelvic junction obstruction).[6]

A multicystic kidney is one in which the kidney is replaced by cysts and does not function. The kidney does not have the usual kidney shape, but is rather a mass of cysts. Unilateral multicystic renal dysplasia is the most common cause of an abdominal mass in newborns. The function of the opposite kidney is usually normal and such children have an excellent prognosis after surgical removal of the affected kidney. Bilateral renal dysplasia causes oligohydramnios and the resultant Potter facies, pulmonary hypoplasia, and renal failure.

Alterations in Kidney Position and Form

The development of the kidneys during embryonic life can result in *ectopic kidneys* that lie outside their normal position. One or both kidneys may be in an abnormal position. Most ectopic kidneys are located just above the pelvic brim or within the pelvis, but some lie in the inferior part of the abdomen. Because of the abnormal position, kinking of the ureters and obstruction of urinary flow may occur.

One of the most common alterations in kidney form is an abnormality called a *horseshoe kidney.* This abnormality occurs in approximately 1 of every 500 to 1000 persons.[4,5] In this disorder, the upper or lower poles of the two kidneys are fused, producing a horseshoe-shaped structure that is continuous along the midline of the body anterior to the great vessels. Most horseshoe kidneys are fused at the lower pole[6] (Fig. 33-1). The condition usually does not cause problems unless there is an

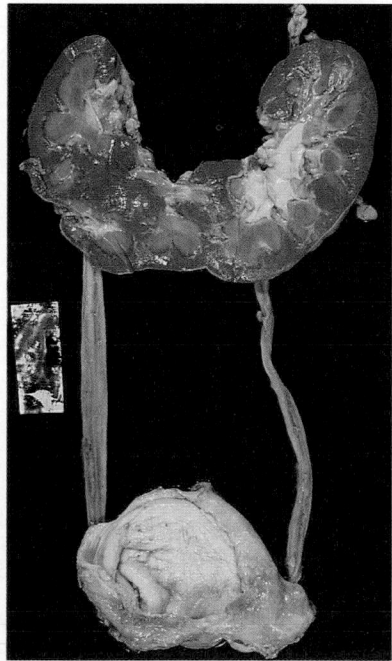

FIGURE 33-1 • Horseshoe kidney. The kidneys are fused at the lower poles. (From Jennette J. C. [2008]. The kidney. In Rubin R., Strayer D. [Eds.], *Rubin's pathology: Clinicopathologic foundations of medicine* [5th ed., p. 695]. Philadelphia: Lippincott Williams & Wilkins.)

associated defect in the renal pelvis or other urinary structures that obstructs urinary flow.

Inherited Cystic Kidney Diseases

The inherited cystic kidney diseases, which are single-gene disorders and are inherited as mendelian traits, include autosomal dominant and recessive polycystic kidney disease, and nephronophthisis–medullary cystic disease. Polycystic kidney diseases are a group of kidney disorders characterized by fluid-filled sacs or segments that have their origin in the tubular structures of the kidney. The cysts may be single or multiple and can vary in size from microscopic to several centimeters in diameter. Although they may arise as a developmental abnormality or be acquired later in life, most forms are hereditary. In the autosomal dominant form of polycystic kidney disease (ADPKD), thousands of large cysts are derived from every segment of the nephron (Fig. 33-2A). The tubule wall, which is lined by a single layer of tubular cells, expands and then rapidly closes the cyst off from the tubule of origin. In the autosomal recessive form of polycystic kidney disease (ARPKD), small, elongated cysts form in the collecting ducts and maintain contact with the nephron of origin (see Fig. 33-2B). In nephronophthisis–medullary cystic kidney disease, the cysts are restricted to the corticomedullary border. Simple cysts are acquired cysts that develop in the kidney as a consequence of aging, dialysis, or other conditions that affect tubular function.

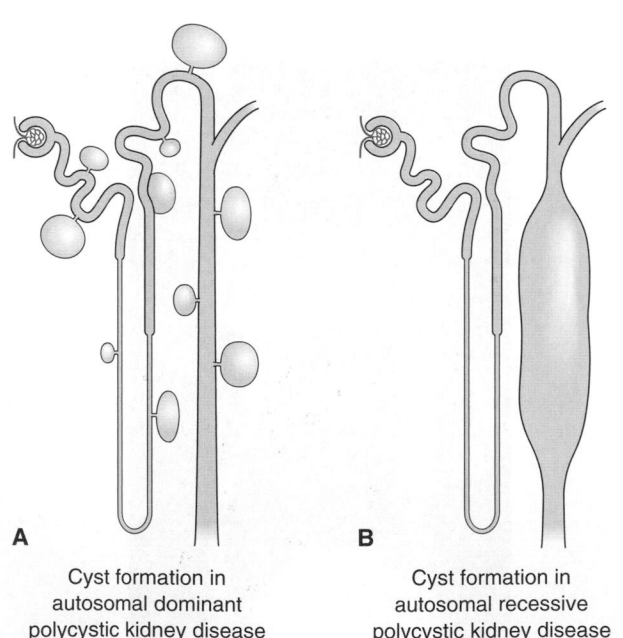

A
Cyst formation in autosomal dominant polycystic kidney disease

B
Cyst formation in autosomal recessive polycystic kidney disease

FIGURE 33-2 • Mechanism of cyst formation in polycystic kidney disease. **(A)** In autosomal dominant polycystic kidney disease, cystic outpouchings arise in every tubule segment and rapidly close off the tubule from the nephron of origin. **(B)** By contrast, in autosomal recessive polycystic kidney disease, cysts are derived from collecting tubules, which remain connected to the nephron of origin. (From Wilson P. D. [2004]. Polycystic kidney disease. *New England Journal of Medicine* 350, 155.)

Autosomal Dominant Polycystic Kidney Disease

Autosomal dominant polycystic kidney disease, also known as *adult polycystic disease,* is the most common form of renal cystic disease. The disorder, which is inherited as an autosomal trait, results in the formation of destructive fluid-filled cysts in the kidney and other organs. ADPKD affects more than 500,000 persons in the United States and 4 to 6 million worldwide.[7] The disease accounts for 10% of all cases of chronic renal disease that require dialysis or transplantation.

There are two types of ADPKD: type I, which is caused by mutations in the *PKD1* gene and accounts for 85% of cases; and type II, which is caused by mutations in the *PKD2* gene and accounts for most of the remaining 15% of cases.[5–10] Recent research has shown that the products of these genes, polycystin-1 and polycystin-2, are found in the primary cilia that line the apical surface of the tubular epithelium. These primary cilia are thought to act as sensors of urinary flow and as signal transducers for tubular cell proliferation, differentiation, and apoptosis.[6,7–10]

Although the precise pathogenesis of ADPKD remains unclear, it is thought that the cysts arise in segments of the renal tubules from a few epithelial cells that proliferate abnormally. The epithelial cells lining the cysts of ADPKD have a high proliferation rate and are relatively undifferentiated. Concomitantly, a defective basement membrane immediately underlying the abnormal epithelium allows for dilation and cyst formation. Cysts frequently detach from the tubule and grow by active fluid secretion from the epithelial lining cells. Historically, it was thought that chronic kidney disease resulted from pressure exerted by expanding cysts on the normal surrounding kidney tissue. However, it is now appreciated that cysts arise in less that 2% of nephrons, and that factors other than compression by the expanding cysts account for loss of functioning renal tissue.[6] Apoptotic loss of renal tubular cells and accumulation of inflammatory mediators are now thought to contribute to the destruction of normal kidney tissue.[6]

Mutations in the *PKD1* and *PKD2* genes produce identical renal and extrarenal disease, but disease progression is typically more rapid in people with type I disease.[5] The kidneys are usually enlarged in persons with ADPKD and may achieve enormous sizes (Fig. 33-3). The external contours of the kidneys are distorted by numerous cysts, some as large as 5 cm in diameter, which are filled with straw-colored fluid.[6] Cysts also may be found in the liver and, less commonly, the pancreas and spleen. Mitral valve prolapse and other valvular heart diseases occur in 20% to 25% of persons with ADPKD, but most are asymptomatic.[5] Many persons with polycystic disease also develop colonic diverticula. One of the most devastating extrarenal manifestations is a weakness in the walls of the cerebral arteries that can lead to aneurysm formation.

Clinical Features. The manifestations of ADPKD include pain from the enlarging cysts that may reach debilitating levels, episodes of gross hematuria from bleeding into a cyst, infected cysts from ascending UTIs, and hypertension resulting from compression of intrarenal blood vessels with activation of the

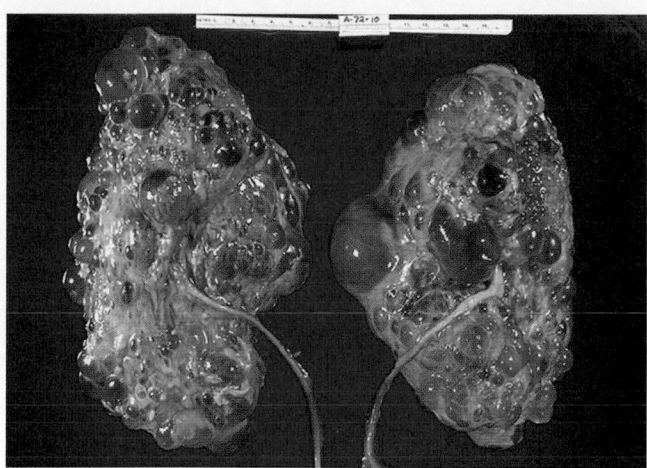

FIGURE 33-3 • Gross pathology of polycystic kidneys. (From Centers for Disease Control and Prevention Public Images Library. [Online.] Available: http://phil.cdc.gov/phil/details.asp.)

renin-angiotensin mechanism.[5,11] Nephrolithiasis occurs in 15% to 20% of patients.[11] The progress of the disease is slow, and end-stage renal disease is uncommon before 40 years of age. Extrarenal manifestations are frequent, underscoring the systemic nature of the disease. Hepatic cysts occur in 50% to 70% of persons.[11] Cysts are generally asymptomatic, and liver function is normal. Approximately 20% of persons with polycystic kidney disease have an associated aneurysm, and subarachnoid hemorrhage is a frequent cause of death.[6]

Ultrasonography usually is the preferred technique for diagnosis of ADPKD in symptomatic patients and for screening of asymptomatic family members. The ability to detect cysts increases with age; 80% to 90% of affected persons older than 20 years of age have cysts large enough to be detected by ultrasonography. Computed tomography (CT) may be used for detection of small cysts. Genetic linkage studies are now available for diagnosis of ADPKD, but are usually reserved for cases in which radiographic imaging is negative and the need for a definitive diagnosis is essential, such as when screening family members for potential kidney donation.

The treatment of ADPKD is largely supportive and aimed at delaying progression of the disease. Control of hypertension and prevention of ascending UTIs are important. Pain is a common complaint of persons with ADPKD, and a systematic approach is needed to differentiate the etiology of the pain and define an approach for management.[12] Dialysis and kidney transplantation are reserved for those who progress to kidney failure.

Autosomal Recessive Polycystic Kidney Disease

Autosomal recessive polycystic kidney disease is characterized by cystic dilation of the cortical and medullary collecting tubules[5,6] (see Fig. 33-2B). It is rare compared with ADPKD,

occurring in 1 to 10,000 to 50,000 live births. ARPKD is caused by mutations in the *PKHD1* gene. The gene product, fibrocystin, is found in the kidney, liver, and pancreas and appears to be involved in the regulation of cell proliferation and adhesion.

Clinical Features. The typical infant with ARPKD presents with bilateral flank masses, accompanied by severe renal failure, signs of impaired lung development, and variable degrees of liver fibrosis and portal hypertension.[4] Potter facies and other defects associated with oligohydramnios may be present. Hypertension is usually noted within the first few weeks of like and is often severe. Approximately 75% of infants die during the perinatal period, often of pulmonary hypoplasia.[6] Exceptional cases of ARPKD manifest in older children and adults.

The treatment of ARPKD is largely supportive. Aggressive ventilatory support is often necessary in the neonatal period because of pulmonary hypoplasia and hypoventilation. Modern neonatal respiratory techniques and renal replacement therapy have increased the 10-year survival rate of children surviving beyond the first year of life to 70% to 80%.[4] Morbidity and mortality in the older child is related to complications from chronic renal failure and liver disease.

Nephronophthisis–Medullary Cystic Disease Complex

The nephronophthisis–medullary cystic disease complex is a group of renal disorders that have their onset in childhood.[5,6] Common characteristics are small and shrunken kidneys and the presence of a variable number of cysts, usually concentrated at the corticomedullary junction. The initial insult involves the distal tubules, with tubular basement membrane disruption followed by chronic and progressive tubular atrophy involving both the medulla and cortex. Although the presence of medullary cysts is important, the cortical and tubular damage is the eventual cause of chronic kidney disease and failure.

Four variants of the disease complex are recognized: (1) sporadic, nonfamilial (20%); (2) familial juvenile nephronophthisis (40% to 50%), inherited as an autosomal recessive trait; (3) renal–retinal dysplasia (15%), also inherited as an autosomal recessive trait, in which the kidney disease is accompanied by ocular lesions; and (4) adult-onset medullary cystic disease (15%), which is inherited as an autosomal dominant trait.[5]

As a complex, the disorders account for 10% to 25% of renal failure in childhood.[6] Affected children present first with polyuria, polydipsia, and enuresis (bed-wetting), which reflect impaired ability of the kidneys to concentrate urine. Other manifestations of the disorders include salt wasting, growth retardation, anemia, and progressive renal insufficiency. Some juvenile forms of nephronophthisis have extrarenal complications, including ocular motor abnormalities, retinitis pigmentosa, liver fibrosis, and cerebellar abnormalities. Progressive azotemia and renal failure follow, usually within 5 to 10 years.[5,6]

Simple and Acquired Renal Cysts

Simple cysts are a common disorder of the kidney. The cysts may be single or multiple, unilateral or bilateral, and they usually are less than 1 cm in diameter, although they may grow larger. Most simple cysts do not produce signs or symptoms or compromise renal function. When symptomatic, they may cause flank pain, hematuria, infection, and hypertension related to ischemia-produced stimulation of the renin-angiotensin system. They are most common in older persons. Although the cysts are benign, they may be confused clinically with renal cell carcinoma.

An acquired form of renal cystic disease occurs in persons with end-stage renal failure who have undergone prolonged dialysis treatment.[6] The cysts, which measure 0.2 to 2 cm in diameter, probably develop as a result of tubular obstruction.[5] Although the condition is largely asymptomatic, the cysts may bleed, causing hematuria. Tumors, usually adenomas but occasionally adenosarcomas, may develop in the walls of these cysts.

IN SUMMARY, approximately 10% of infants are born with potentially significant malformations of the urinary system. These abnormalities can range from bilateral renal agenesis, which is incompatible with life, to hypogenesis of one kidney, which usually causes no problems unless the function of the remaining kidney is impaired. Renal dysplasia is caused by an abnormality in the differentiation of kidney structures during embryonic development. A dysplastic multicystic kidney is one in which the kidney is replaced by cysts and does not function. The horseshoe kidney is a developmental disorder in which the upper or lower poles of the two kidneys are fused, producing a horseshoe-shaped structure.

Renal cystic disease is a condition in which there is dilation of tubular structures with cyst formation. Cysts may be single or multiple. Polycystic kidney disease is an inherited form of renal cystic disease; it can be inherited as an autosomal dominant or recessive trait. The autosomal dominant form of the disease (ADPKD) results in the formation of numerous fluid-filled cysts in the tubular structures of both kidneys with the threat of progression to chronic renal failure. Other manifestations of the disease include hypertension, cardiovascular abnormalities, cerebral aneurysms, and cysts in other organs such as the liver and pancreas. The autosomal recessive form of polycystic kidney disease (ARPKD) is characterized by cystic transformation of the collecting ducts. It is rare compared with ADPKD, and usually presents as severe renal dysfunction during infancy. The nephronophthisis–medullary cystic disease complex is a group of hereditary disorders that usually have their onset during childhood and are characterized by the presence of cysts in the medullary portion of the kidney, renal atrophy, and eventual kidney failure. Single or multiple simple renal cysts most commonly occur in persons older than 50 years of age. ∎

OBSTRUCTIVE DISORDERS

After completing this section of the chapter, you should be able to meet the following objectives:

- List four common causes of urinary tract obstruction.
- Define the term *hydronephrosis* and relate it to the destructive effects of urinary tract obstruction.
- Describe the role of urine supersaturation, nucleation, and inhibitors of stone formation in the development of kidney stones.
- Explain the mechanisms of pain and infection that occur with kidney stones.
- Describe methods used in the diagnosis and treatment of kidney stones.

Urinary obstruction can occur in persons of any age and can involve any level of the urinary tract, from the urethra to the renal pelvis (Fig. 33-4). Obstruction may be sudden or insidious, partial or complete and unilateral or bilateral. The conditions that cause urinary tract obstruction include congenital anomalies, urinary calculi (*i.e.*, stones), pregnancy, benign prostatic hyperplasia, scar tissue resulting from infection and inflammation, tumors, and neurologic disorders such as spinal cord injury. The causes of urinary tract obstructions are summarized in Table 33-1.

Obstructive uropathy is usually classified according to site, degree, and duration of obstruction. Lower urinary tract

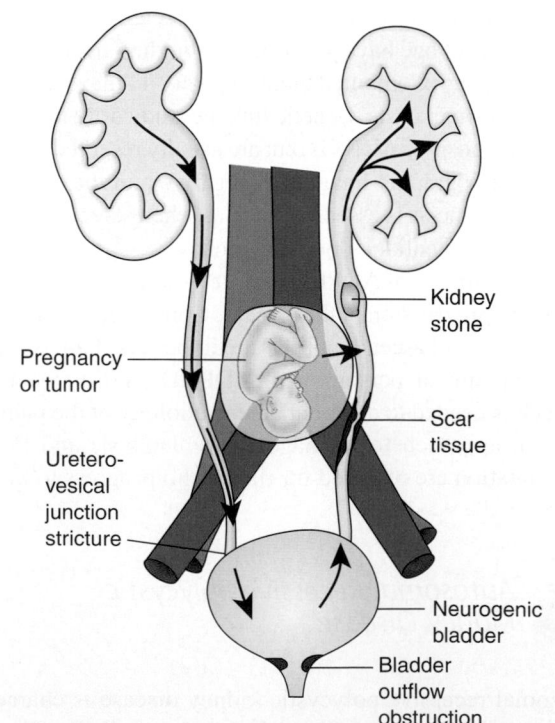

FIGURE 33-4 • Locations and causes of urinary tract obstruction.

LEVEL OF OBSTRUCTION	CAUSE
Renal pelvis	Renal calculi
	Papillary necrosis
Ureter	Renal calculi
	Pregnancy
	Tumors that compress the ureter
	Ureteral stricture
	Congenital disorders of the uretero-vesical junction and ureteropelvic junction strictures
Bladder and urethra	Bladder cancer
	Neurogenic bladder
	Bladder stones
	Prostatic hyperplasia or cancer
	Urethral strictures
	Congenital urethral defects

TABLE 33-1 Causes of Urinary Tract Obstruction

In situations of severe partial or complete obstruction, the impediment to the outflow of urine causes dilation of the renal pelvis and calices associated with progressive atrophy of the kidney. Even with complete obstruction, glomerular filtration continues for some time. Because of the continued filtration, the calices and pelvis of the affected kidney become dilated, often markedly so. The high pressure in the renal pelvis is transmitted back through the collecting ducts of the kidney, compressing renal vasculature and causing renal atrophy. Initially, the functional alterations are largely tubular, manifested primarily by impaired urine-concentrating ability. Only later does the glomerular filtration rate (GFR) begin to diminish.

Hydronephrosis

Hydronephrosis refers to urine-filled dilation of the renal pelvis and calices associated with progressive atrophy of the kidney due to obstruction of urine outflow. The degree of hydronephrosis depends on the duration, degree, and level of obstruction. In far-advanced cases, the kidney may be transformed into a thin-walled cystic structure with parenchymal atrophy, total obliteration of the pyramids, and thinning of the cortex (Fig. 33-5). The condition is usually unilateral; bilateral hydronephrosis occurs only when the obstruction is below the level of the ureterovesical junction. When the obstruction affects the outflow of urine from the distal ureter, the increased pressure dilates the ureter, a condition called *hydroureter* (Fig. 33-6). Bilateral hydroureter may develop as a complication of bladder outflow obstruction due to prostatic hyperplasia (see Chapter 44).

Clinical Features

The manifestations of urinary obstruction depend on the site of obstruction, the cause, and the rapidity with which the condi-

obstructions are located below the ureterovesical junction and are bilateral in nature. Upper urinary tract obstructions are located above the ureterovesical junction and are usually unilateral. The condition causing the obstruction can cause complete or partial occlusion of urine outflow. When the obstruction is of short duration (*i.e.*, less than a few days), it is said to be acute and is usually caused by conditions such as renal calculi. An obstruction that develops slowly and is longer lasting is said to be chronic and is usually caused by conditions such as congenital ureterovesical abnormalities. Bilateral acute urinary tract obstruction causes acute renal failure. Because many causes of acute obstruction are reversible, prompt recognition is important. When left untreated, an obstructed kidney undergoes atrophy, and in the case of bilateral obstruction, results in chronic renal failure.

Mechanisms of Renal Damage

The destructive effects of urinary obstruction on kidney structures are determined by the degree (*i.e.*, partial versus complete, unilateral versus bilateral) and the duration of the obstruction. The two most damaging effects of urinary obstruction are stasis of urine, which predisposes to infection and stone formation; and progressive dilation of the renal collecting ducts and renal tubular structures, which causes destruction and atrophy of renal tissue.

A common complication of urinary tract obstruction is infection. Stagnation of urine predisposes to infection, which may spread throughout the urinary tract. When present, urinary calculi serve as foreign bodies and contribute to the infection. Once established, the infection is difficult to treat. It often is caused by urea-splitting organisms (*e.g., Proteus,* staphylococci) that increase ammonia production and cause the urine to become alkaline.[13] Calcium salts precipitate more readily in stagnant alkaline urine; thus, urinary tract obstructions also predispose to stone formation.

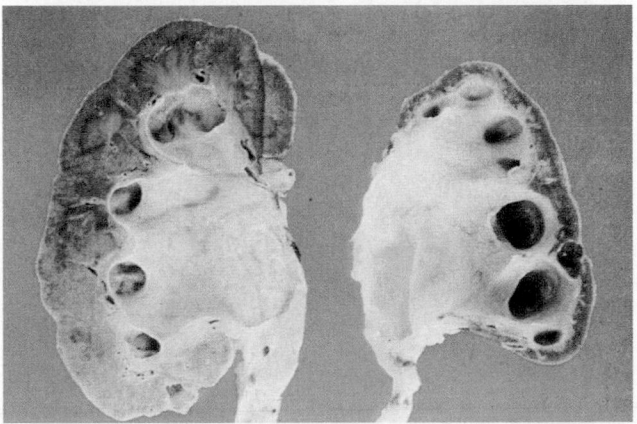

FIGURE 33-5 • Hydronephrosis. Bilateral urinary tract obstruction has led to conspicuous dilation of the ureters, pelves, and calices. The kidney on the right shows severe cortical atrophy. (From Jennette J. C. [2008]. The kidney. In Rubin R., Strayer D. [Eds.], *Rubin's pathology: Clinicopathologic foundations of medicine* [5th ed., p. 738]. Philadelphia: Lippincott Williams & Wilkins.)

tion developed. Most of the early symptoms are produced by the underlying pathologic process. Urinary tract obstruction encourages the growth of microorganisms and should be suspected in persons with recurrent UTIs.

Complete or partial unilateral hydronephrosis may remain silent for long periods because the unaffected kidney can maintain adequate kidney function. Obstruction may provoke pain due to distention of the collecting system and renal capsule. Acute supravesical obstruction, such as that due to a kidney stone lodged in the ureter, is associated with excruciatingly severe pain. By contrast, more insidious causes of obstruction, such as narrowing of the ureteropelvic junction, may produce little pain but cause total destruction of the kidney.

Complete bilateral obstruction results in oliguria and anuria and renal failure. Acute bilateral obstruction may mimic prerenal failure. With partial bilateral obstruction, the earliest manifestation is an inability to concentrate urine, reflected by polyuria and nocturia. Hypertension is an occasional complication of urinary tract obstruction. It is more common in cases of unilateral obstruction in which renin secretion is enhanced, probably secondary to impaired renal blood flow. In these circumstances, removal of the obstruction often leads to a reduction in blood pressure. When hypertension accompanies bilateral obstruction,

it is volume related. The relief of bilateral obstruction leads to a loss of volume and a decrease in blood pressure. In some cases, relieving the obstruction does not correct the hypertension.

Diagnosis and Treatment. Early diagnosis of urinary tract obstruction is important because the condition usually is treatable and a delay in therapy may result in permanent damage to the kidneys. Diagnostic methods vary with the symptoms. Ultrasonography has proved to be the single most useful noninvasive diagnostic modality for urinary obstruction. Radiologic methods, CT scans, and intravenous urography may also be used.[13] Other diagnostic methods, such as urinalysis, are used to determine the extent of renal involvement and the presence of infection.

Treatment of urinary tract obstruction depends on the cause. Urinary stone removal may be necessary, or surgical treatment of structural defects may be indicated. Treatment of complicating UTIs due to urinary stasis is also important.

Renal Calculi

The most common cause of upper urinary tract obstruction is urinary calculi. Although stones can form in any part of the urinary tract, most develop in the kidneys. Renal calculi or kidney stones are the third most common disorder of the urinary tract, exceeded only by UTIs and prostate disorders.[14]

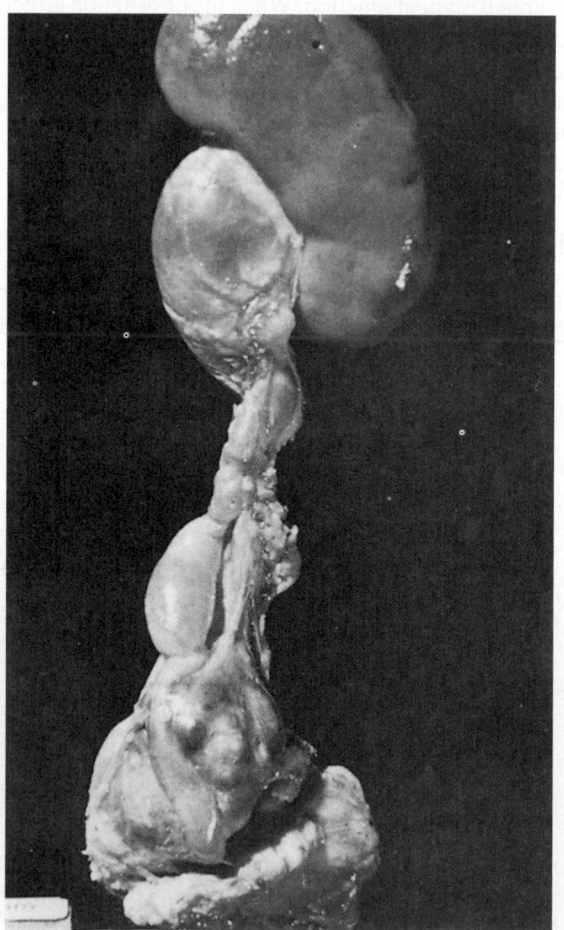

FIGURE 33-6 • Hydroureter caused by ureteral obstruction in a woman with cancer of the uterus.

KIDNEY STONES

- Kidney stones are polycrystalline structures that form from components of the urine.

- Stones require a nidus to form and a urinary environment that supports continued crystallization of stone components.

- The development of kidney stones is influenced by the concentration of stone components in the urine, the ability of the stone components to complex and form stones, and the presence of substances that inhibit stone formation.

Kidney stones are polycrystalline aggregates composed of materials that the kidneys normally excrete in the urine. The etiology of urinary stone formation is complex. It is thought to encompass a number of factors, including increases in blood and urinary levels of stone components and interactions among the components; anatomic changes in urinary tract structures; metabolic and endocrine influences; dietary and intestinal absorption factors; and UTIs. Adding to the mystery of stone formation is the fact that although both kidneys are exposed to the same urinary constituents, kidney stones tend to form in only one kidney. Several factors are used to explain stone formation, including a supersaturated urine, presence of a nucleus for crystal formation, and deficiency of inhibitors of stone formation.[14]

Kidney stone formation requires a supersaturated urine and an environment that allows the stone to grow. The risk for stone formation is increased when the urine is supersaturated with stone components (*e.g.,* calcium salts, uric acid, magnesium ammonium phosphate, cystine). Supersaturation depends on urinary pH, solute concentration, ionic strength, and complexation. The greater the concentration of two ions, the more likely they are to precipitate. Complexation influences the availability of specific ions. For example, oxalate complexes with sodium and decreases the availability of its free ionic form that participates in stone formation.

In addition to a supersaturated urine, kidney stone formation requires a nidus or nucleus that facilitates crystal aggregation. In supersaturated urine, stone formation begins with small clusters of crystals such as calcium oxalate. Most small clusters tend to disperse because the internal forces that hold them together are too weak to overcome the random tendency of ions to move apart. Larger ion clusters form nuclei and remain stable because the attraction forces balance surface losses. Once they are stable, nuclei can grow at levels of supersaturation below that needed for their creation. Organic materials, such as mucopolysaccharides derived from the epithelial cells that line the tubules, are also thought to act as nuclei for stone formation by lowering the level of supersaturation required for crystal aggregation.

The fact that many people experience supersaturation of their urine without development of kidney stones is believed to be a result of the presence of natural stone inhibitors, including magnesium, citrate, and the Tamm-Horsfall mucoprotein. To date, the measurement and manipulation of stone inhibitors has not been part of clinical practice, with the exception of citrate.[14–16] Urine citrate reduces supersaturation by binding calcium and inhibiting nucleation and growth of calcium crystals. Citrate is a normal byproduct of the citric acid cycle in renal cells. Metabolic stimuli that consume this product (as with metabolic acidosis due to fasting or hypokalemia) reduce the urinary concentration of citrate. Citrate supplementation (potassium citrate) may be used in the treatment of some forms of hypocitraturic kidney stones.[14]

Types of Stones

There are four basic types of kidney stones: calcium stones (*i.e.,* oxalate or phosphate), magnesium ammonium phosphate stones, uric acid stones, and cystine stones.[14–18] The causes and treatment measures for each of these types of renal stones are described in Table 33-2. Most kidney stones (70% to 80%) are calcium stones—calcium oxalate, calcium phosphate, or a combination of the two materials.[5,6] Calcium stones usually are associated with increased concentrations of calcium in the blood and urine. Excessive bone resorption caused by immobility, bone disease, hyperparathyroidism, and renal tubular acidosis all are contributing conditions. High oxalate concentrations in the blood and urine predispose to formation of calcium oxalate stones.

Magnesium ammonium phosphate stones, also called *struvite stones,* form only in alkaline urine and in the presence of bacteria that possess an enzyme called *urease,* which splits the urea in the urine into ammonia and carbon dioxide. The ammonia that is formed takes up a hydrogen ion to become an ammonium ion, increasing the pH of the urine so that it becomes more alkaline. Because phosphate levels are increased in alkaline urine and because magnesium always is present in the urine, struvite stones form. These stones enlarge as the bacterial count

TABLE 33-2 Composition, Contributing Factors, and Treatment of Kidney Stones

TYPE OF STONE	CONTRIBUTING FACTORS	TREATMENT
Calcium (oxalate and phosphate)	Hypercalcemia and hypercalciuria Immobilization	Treatment of underlying conditions Increased fluid intake Thiazide diuretics
	Hyperparathyroidism Vitamin D intoxication Diffuse bone disease Milk-alkali syndrome Renal tubular acidosis Hyperoxaluria Intestinal bypass surgery	Dietary restriction of foods high in oxalate
Magnesium ammonium phosphate (struvite)	Urea-splitting urinary tract infections	Treatment of urinary tract infection Acidification of the urine Increased fluid intake
Uric acid (urate)	Formed in acid urine with pH of approximately 5.5 Gout High-purine diet	Increased fluid intake Allopurinol for hyperuricosuria Alkalinization of urine
Cystine	Cystinuria (inherited disorder of amino acid metabolism)	Increased fluid intake Alkalinization of urine

grows, and they can increase in size until they fill an entire renal pelvis (Fig. 33-7). Because of their shape, they often are called *staghorn stones*. They almost always are associated with UTIs and persistently alkaline urine. Because these stones act as a foreign body, treatment of the infection often is difficult. Struvite stones usually are too large to be passed and require lithotripsy or surgical removal.

Uric acid stones develop in conditions of gout and high concentrations of uric acid in the urine. Hyperuricosuria also may contribute to calcium stone formation by acting as a nucleus for calcium oxalate stone formation. Unlike radiopaque calcium stones, uric acid stones are not visible on x-ray films. Uric acid stones form most readily in urine with a pH of 5.1 to 5.9.[16] Thus, these stones can be treated by raising the urinary pH to 6 to 6.5 with potassium alkali salts.

Cystine stones account for less than 1% of kidney stones overall but represent a significant proportion of childhood calculi.[6] They are seen in cystinuria, which results from a genetic defect in renal transport of cystine. These stones resemble struvite stones except that infection is unlikely to be present.

Clinical Features

One of the major manifestations of kidney stones is pain. Depending on location, there are two types of pain associated with kidney stones: renal colic and noncolicky renal pain.[14,17,18] *Renal colic* is the term used to describe the colicky pain that accompanies stretching of the collecting system or ureter. The symptoms of renal colic are caused by stones 1 to 5 mm in diameter that can move into the ureter and obstruct flow. Classic ureteral colic is manifested by acute, intermittent, and excruciating pain in the flank and upper outer quadrant of the abdomen on the affected side. The pain may radiate to the lower abdominal quadrant, bladder area, perineum, or scrotum in the man. The skin may be cool and clammy, and nausea and vomiting are common. Noncolicky pain is caused by stones that produce distention of the renal calyces or renal pelvis. The pain usually is a dull, deep ache in the flank or back that can vary in intensity from mild to severe. The pain is often exaggerated by drinking large amounts of fluid.

Diagnosis and Treatment. Patients with kidney stones often present with acute renal colic, and the diagnosis is based on symptomatology and diagnostic tests, which include urinalysis, plain film radiography, intravenous pyelography, and abdominal ultrasonography.[18] Urinalysis provides information related to hematuria, infection, the presence of stone-forming crystals, and urine pH. Most stones are radiopaque and readily visible on a plain radiograph of the abdomen. The noncontrast spiral CT scan is the imaging modality of choice in persons with acute renal colic.[14] Intravenous pyelography (IVP) uses an intravenously injected contrast medium that is filtered in the glomeruli to visualize the collecting system of the kidneys and ureters. Abdominal ultrasonography is highly sensitive to hydronephrosis, which may be a manifestation of ureteral obstruction. A new imaging technique called *nuclear scintigraphy* uses bisphosphonate markers as a means of imaging stones.[14] The method has been credited with identifying stones that are too small to be detected by other methods.

Treatment of acute renal colic usually is supportive. Pain relief may be needed during acute phases of obstruction, and antibiotic therapy may be necessary to treat UTIs. Most stones that are less than 5 mm in diameter pass spontaneously. All urine should be strained during an attack in the hope of retrieving the stone for chemical analysis and determination of type. This information, along with a careful history and laboratory tests, provides the basis for long-term preventive measures.

A major goal of treatment in persons who have passed kidney stones or have had them removed is to prevent their recurrence. Prevention requires investigation into the cause of stone formation using urine tests, blood chemistries, and stone analysis. Underlying disease conditions, such as hyperparathyroidism, are treated. Adequate fluid intake reduces the concentration of stone-forming crystals in the urine and needs to be encouraged. Depending on the type of stone that is formed, dietary changes, medications, or both may be used to alter the concentration of stone-forming elements in the urine. For example, persons who form calcium oxalate stones may need to decrease their intake of foods that are high in oxalate

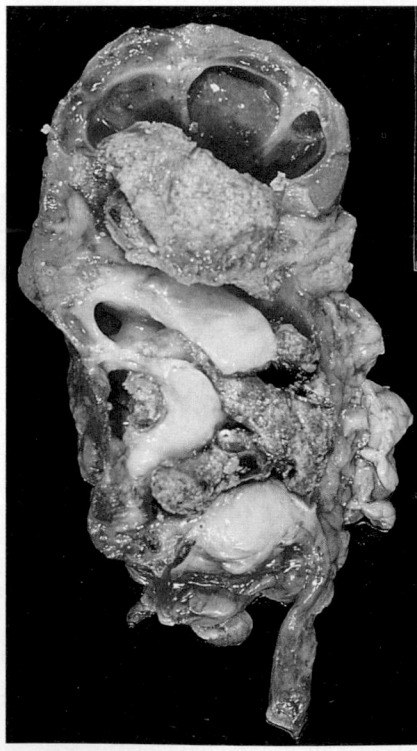

FIGURE 33-7 • Staghorn stones. The kidney shows hydronephrosis and stones that are casts of the dilated calices. (From Jennette J. C. [2008]. The kidney. In Rubin R., Strayer D. [Eds.], *Rubin's pathology: Clinicopathologic foundations of medicine* [5th ed., p. 738]. Philadelphia: Lippincott Williams & Wilkins.)

(*e.g.*, spinach, Swiss chard, cocoa, chocolate, pecans, peanuts). Calcium supplementation with calcium salts such as calcium carbonate and calcium phosphate also may be used to bind oxalate in the intestine and decrease its absorption. Thiazide diuretics lower urinary calcium by increasing tubular reabsorption so that less remains in the urine. Drugs that bind calcium in the gut (*e.g.*, cellulose phosphate) may be used to inhibit calcium absorption and urinary excretion.

Measures to change the pH of the urine also can influence kidney stone formation. In persons who lose the ability to lower the pH of (or acidify) their urine, there is an increase in the divalent and trivalent forms of urine phosphate that combine with calcium to form calcium phosphate stones. The formation of uric acid stones is increased in acid urine; stone formation can be reduced by raising the pH of urine to 6.0 to 6.5 with potassium alkali (*e.g.*, potassium citrate) salts. Table 33-2 summarizes measures for preventing the recurrence of different types of kidney stones.

In some cases, stone removal may be necessary. Several methods are available for removing kidney stones: ureteroscopic removal, percutaneous removal, and extracorporeal lithotripsy.[14] All these procedures eliminate the need for an open surgical procedure, which is another form of treatment. Open stone surgery may be required to remove large calculi or those that are resistant to other forms of removal.

Ureteroscopic removal involves the passage of an instrument through the urethra into the bladder and then into the ureter. The development of high-quality optics has improved the ease with which this procedure is performed and its outcome. The procedure, which is performed under fluoroscopic guidance, involves the use of various instruments for dilating the ureter and for grasping, fragmenting, and removing the stone. Preprocedure radiologic studies using a contrast medium (*i.e.*, excretory urography) are done to determine the position of the stone and direct the placement of the ureteroscope.

Percutaneous nephrolithotomy is the treatment of choice for removal of renal or proximal ureteral calculi.[14] It involves the insertion through the flank of a small-gauge needle into the collecting system of the kidney; the needle tract is then dilated, and an instrument called a *nephroscope* is inserted into the renal pelvis. The procedure is performed under fluoroscopic guidance. Preprocedure radiologic and ultrasonographic examinations of the kidney and ureter are used to determine the placement of the nephroscope. Stones up to 1 cm in diameter can be removed through this method. Larger stones must be broken up with an electrohydraulic or ultrasonic lithotriptor (*i.e.*, stone breaker).

A nonsurgical treatment, called *extracorporeal shock-wave lithotripsy*, uses acoustic shock waves to fragment calculi into sandlike particles that are passed in the urine over the next few days. Because of the large amount of stone particles that are generated during the procedure, a ureteral stent (*i.e.*, a tube-like device used to hold the ureter open) may be inserted to ensure adequate urine drainage.

IN SUMMARY, obstruction of urine flow can occur at any level of the urinary tract. Among the causes of urinary tract obstruction are developmental defects, pregnancy, infection and inflammation, kidney stones, neurologic defects, and prostatic hypertrophy. Obstructive disorders produce stasis of urine, increase the risk for infection and calculi formation, and produce progressive dilation of the renal collecting ducts and renal tubular structures, which causes renal atrophy.

Hydronephrosis refers to urine-filled dilation of the renal pelvis and calices associated with progressive atrophy of the kidney due to obstruction of urine outflow. Unilateral hydronephrosis may remain silent for long periods because the unaffected kidney can maintain adequate kidney function. With partial bilateral obstruction, the earliest manifestation is an inability to concentrate urine, reflected by polyuria and nocturia. Complete bilateral obstruction results in oliguria and anuria and renal failure.

Kidney stones are a major cause of upper urinary tract obstruction. There are four types of kidney stones: calcium (*i.e.*, oxalate and phosphate) stones, which are associated with increased serum calcium levels; magnesium ammonium phosphate (*i.e.*, struvite) stones, which are associated with UTIs; uric acid stones, which are related to elevated uric acid levels; and cystine stones, which are seen in cystinuria. A major goal of treatment for persons who have passed kidney stones or have had them removed is to identify stone composition and prevent their recurrence. Treatment measures depend on stone type and include adequate fluid intake to prevent urine saturation, dietary modification to decrease intake of stone-forming constituents, treatment of UTI, measures to change urine pH, and the use of diuretics that decrease the calcium concentration of urine. ■

URINARY TRACT INFECTIONS

After completing this section of the chapter, you should be able to meet the following objectives:

- Cite the organisms most responsible for UTIs and state why urinary catheters, obstruction, and reflux predispose to infections.
- List three physiologic mechanisms that protect against UTIs.
- Describe the signs and symptoms of UTIs.
- Describe factors that predispose to UTIs in children, sexually active women, pregnant women, and older adults.
- Compare the manifestations of UTIs in different age groups, including infants, toddlers, adolescents, adults, and older adults.
- Cite measures used in the diagnosis and treatment of UTIs.

Urinary tract infections are the second most common type of bacterial infection seen by health care providers, with respiratory tract infections being the first.[1] UTIs include several distinct entities, including asymptomatic bacteriuria, symptomatic infections, lower UTIs such as cystitis, and upper UTIs such as pyelonephritis. Because of their ability to cause renal damage, upper UTIs are considered more serious than lower UTIs. Acute pyelonephritis (discussed in the section on Tubulointerstitial Disorders) represents an infection of the renal parenchyma and renal pelvis. Improperly treated, it can lead to sepsis, renal abscesses, and chronic pyelonephritis.

🔑 URINARY TRACT INFECTIONS

- Urinary tract (UT) infections involve host–agent interactions that pit the defenses of the host against the virulence of the infectious agent.

- Infection is facilitated by host conditions that disrupt washout of the agent from the UT through urine flow, change the protective properties of the mucin lining of the UT, disrupt the protective function of the normal bacterial flora, or impair the function of the immune system.

- Virulence of the agent is derived from its ability to gain access to and thrive in the UT environment, adhere to the tissues of the lower or upper UT, evade the destructive effects of the host's immune system, and develop resistance to antimicrobial agents.

Etiologic Factors

Most uncomplicated lower UTIs are caused by *Escherichia coli*.[20–23] Other uropathic pathogens include *Staphylococcus saprophyticus* in uncomplicated UTIs, and both non–*E. coli* gram-negative rods (*Proteus mirabilis, Klebsiella* species, *Enterobacter* species, and *Pseudomonas aeruginosa*) and gram-positive cocci (*Staphylococcus aureus*) in complicated UTIs.[21] Most UTIs are caused by bacteria that enter through the urethra. Bacteria can also enter through the bloodstream, usually in immunocompromised persons and neonates. Although the distal portion of the urethra often contains pathogens, the urine formed in the kidneys and found in the bladder normally is sterile or free of bacteria. This is because of the *washout phenomenon,* in which urine from the bladder normally washes bacteria out of the urethra. When a UTI occurs, it is usually from bacteria that have colonized the urethra, vagina, or perianal area.

There is an increased risk for UTIs in persons with urinary obstruction and reflux, in people with neurogenic disorders that impair bladder emptying, in women who are sexually active, in postmenopausal women, in men with diseases of the prostate, and in elderly persons. Instrumentation and urinary catheterization are the most common predisposing factors for nosocomial

UTIs. UTIs occur more commonly in women with diabetes than in women without the disease. People with diabetes are also at increased risk for complications associated with UTIs, including pyelonephritis, and they are more susceptible to fungal infections (particularly *Candida* species) and infections with gram-negative pathogens other than *E. coli,* both of which are accompanied by increased severity and unusual manifestations.[22]

Host–Agent Interactions

Because certain people tend to be predisposed to development of UTIs, considerable interest has been focused on host–pathogen interactions and factors that increase the risk for UTI.[20] UTIs are more common in women than men, specifically at 16 to 35 years of age, at which time they are more than 40 times likely to develop a UTI than age-matched men.[23] In men, the longer length of the urethra and the antibacterial properties of the prostatic fluid provide some protection from ascending UTIs until approximately 50 years of age.[21] After this age, prostatic hypertrophy becomes more common, and with it may come obstruction and increased risk for UTI (see Chapter 44).

Host Defenses. In the development of a UTI, host defenses are matched against the virulence of the pathogen. The host defenses of the bladder have several components, including the washout phenomenon, in which bacteria are removed from the bladder and urethra during voiding; the protective mucin layer that lines the bladder and protects against bacterial invasion; and local immune responses.[20] In the ureters, peristaltic movements facilitate the movement of urine from the renal pelvis through the ureters and into the bladder. Immune mechanisms, particularly secretory immunoglobulin (Ig) A, appear to provide an important antibacterial defense. Phagocytic blood cells further assist in the removal of bacteria from the urinary tract.

There has been a growing appreciation of the protective function of the bladder's mucin layer.[20] It is thought that the epithelial cells that line the bladder synthesize protective substances that subsequently become incorporated into the mucin layer that adheres to the bladder wall. One theory proposes that the mucin layer acts by binding water, which then constitutes a protective barrier between the bacteria and the bladder epithelium. Elderly and postmenopausal women produce less mucin than younger women, suggesting that estrogen may play a role in mucin production in women.

Other important host factors include the normal flora of the periurethral area in women and prostate secretions in men.[20] In women, the normal flora of the periurethral area, which consists of organisms such as *Lactobacillus,* provides defense against the colonization of uropathic bacteria. Alterations in the periurethral environment, such as occurs with a decrease in estrogen levels during menopause or the use of antibiotics, can alter the protective periurethral flora, allowing uropathogens to colonize and enter the urinary tract. In men, the prostatic fluid has antimicrobial properties that protect the urethra from colonization.

Pathogen Virulence. Not all bacteria are capable of adhering and infecting the urinary tract. Of the many strains of *E. coli*, only those with increased ability to adhere to the epithelial cells of the urinary tract are able to produce UTIs. These bacteria have fine protein filaments, called *pili* or *fimbriae*, that help them adhere to receptors on the lining of urinary tract structures.[20] The two main types of pili (types 1 and P) found on *E. coli* that cause UTIs are morphologically similar but differ in their ability to mediate hemagglutination in the presence of mannose. Type P pili are mannose resistant and were named because of their high incidence in *E. coli* that cause pyelonephritis and because of their association with the P blood group system. P pili have been observed in over 90% of *E. coli* strains causing pyelonephritis but less than 20% of strains causing lower UTIs.[20]

Obstruction and Reflux

Obstruction and reflux are other contributing factors in the development of UTIs. Any microorganisms that enter the bladder normally are washed out during voiding. When outflow is obstructed, urine remains in the bladder and acts as a medium for microbial growth; the microorganisms in the contaminated urine can then ascend along the ureters to infect the kidneys. The presence of residual urine correlates closely with bacteriuria and with its recurrence after treatment. Another aspect of bladder outflow obstruction and bladder distention is increased intravesical pressure, which compresses blood vessels in the bladder wall, leading to a decrease in the mucosal defenses of the bladder.

In UTIs associated with stasis of urine flow, the obstruction may be anatomic or functional. Anatomic obstructions include urinary tract stones, prostatic hyperplasia, pregnancy, and malformations of the ureterovesical junction. Functional obstructions include neurogenic bladder, infrequent voiding, detrusor (bladder) muscle instability, and constipation.

Reflux occurs when urine from the urethra moves into the bladder (*i.e.*, urethrovesical reflux). In women, *urethrovesical reflux* can occur during activities such as coughing or squatting, in which an increase in intra-abdominal pressure causes the urine to be squeezed into the urethra and then to flow back into the bladder as the pressure decreases. This also can happen when voiding is abruptly interrupted. Because the urethral orifice frequently is contaminated with bacteria, the reflux mechanism may cause bacteria to be drawn back into the bladder.

A second type of reflux mechanism, *vesicoureteral reflux,* occurs at the level of the bladder and ureter. Normally, the distal portion of the ureter courses between the muscle layer and the mucosal surface of the bladder wall, forming a flap (Fig. 33-8). The flap is compressed against the bladder wall during micturition, preventing urine from being forced into the ureter. In persons with vesicoureteral reflux, the ureter enters the bladder at an approximate right angle such that urine is forced into the ureter during micturition. It is seen most commonly in children with UTIs and is believed to result from congenital

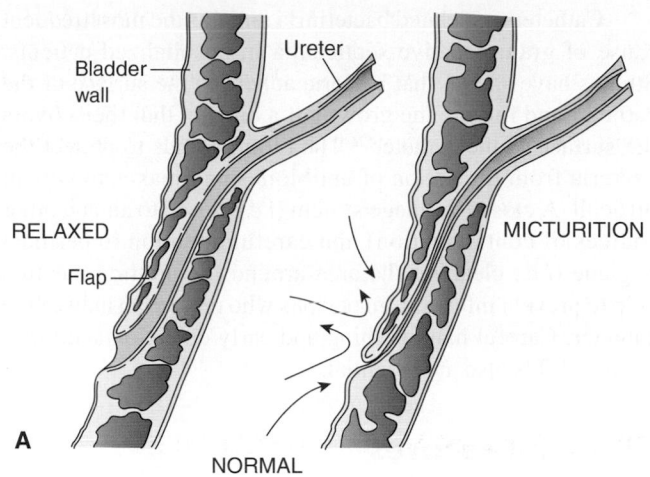

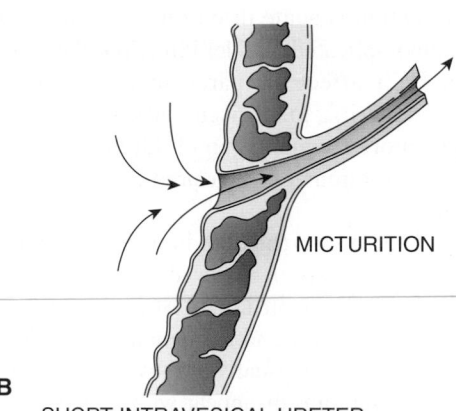

FIGURE 33-8 • Anatomic features of the ureter and bladder and their relationship to vesicoureteral reflux. **(A)** In the normal bladder, the distal portion of the intravesical ureter courses between the mucosa and the muscularis of the bladder. A mucosal flap is thus formed. On micturition, the elevated intravesicular pressure compresses the flap against the bladder wall, thereby occluding the lumen. **(B)** Persons with a congenitally short intravesical ureter have no mucosal flap because the entry of the ureter into the bladder approaches a right angle. Thus, micturition forces urine into the ureter. (Adapted from Jennette J. C. [2008]. The kidney. In Rubin R., Strayer D. [Eds.], *Rubin's pathology: Clinicopathologic foundations of medicine* [5th ed., p. 732]. Philadelphia: Lippincott Williams & Wilkins; Courtesy of Dmitri Karetnikov, artist.)

defects in length, diameter, muscle structure, or innervation of the submucosal segment of the ureter. Vesicoureteral reflux also is seen in adults with obstruction to bladder outflow, primarily due to increased bladder volume and pressure.

Catheter-Induced Infection

Urinary catheters are tubes made of latex or plastic. They are inserted through the urethra into the bladder for the purpose of draining urine. They are a source of urethral irritation and provide a means for entry of microorganisms into the urinary tract.

Catheter-associated bacteriuria remains the most frequent cause of gram-negative septicemia in hospitalized patients. Studies have shown that bacteria adhere to the surface of the catheter and initiate the growth of a biofilm that then covers the surface of the catheter.[24] The biofilm tends to protect the bacteria from the action of antibiotics and makes treatment difficult. A closed drainage system (*i.e.,* closed to air and other sources of contamination) and careful attention to perineal hygiene (*i.e.,* cleaning the area around the urethral meatus) help to prevent infections in persons who require an indwelling catheter. Careful handwashing and early detection and treatment of UTIs also are essential.

Clinical Features

The manifestations of UTI depend on whether the infection involves the lower (bladder) or upper (kidney) urinary tract and whether the infection is acute or chronic. The majority of UTIs are acute uncomplicated bladder infections that occur in women. Upper UTIs affect the parenchyma and pelvis of the kidney (pyelonephritis, to be discussed). They are less common and occur more frequently in children and adults with urinary tract obstructions or other predisposing conditions such as diabetes.

An acute episode of cystitis (bladder infection) is characterized by frequency of urination, lower abdominal or back discomfort, and burning and pain on urination (*i.e.,* dysuria).[20,23] Occasionally, the urine is cloudy and foul smelling. In adults, fever and other signs of infection usually are absent. If there are no complications, the symptoms disappear within 48 hours of treatment. The symptoms of cystitis also may represent urethritis caused by *Chlamydia trachomatis, Neisseria gonorrhoeae,* or herpes simplex virus, or vaginitis attributable to *Trichomonas vaginalis* or *Candida* species (see Chapter 47).

Diagnosis and Treatment

The diagnosis of UTI usually is based on symptoms and on examination of the urine for the presence of microorganisms. When necessary, x-ray films, ultrasonography, and CT and renal scans are used to identify contributing factors, such as obstruction.

Urine tests are used to establish the presence of bacteria in the urine and a diagnosis of UTI. A commonly accepted criterion for diagnosis of a UTI is the presence of 100,000 colony-forming units (CFU) or more bacteria per milliliter (mL) of urine.[19,20] Colonization usually is defined as the multiplication of microorganisms in or on a host without apparent evidence of invasiveness or tissue injury. Pyuria (the presence of less than five to eight leukocytes per high-power field) indicates a host response to infection rather than asymptomatic bacterial colonization. A Gram stain may be done to determine the type (gram-positive or gram-negative) of organism that is present. A urine culture may be done to confirm the presence of pathogenic bacteria in urine specimens, allow for their identification, and permit the determination of their sensitivity to specific antibiotics.

Chemical screening (urine dipstick) for markers of infection may provide useful information but is less sensitive than microscopic analysis.[19,20] These tests are relatively inexpensive, easy to perform, and can be done in the clinic setting or even in the home. Bacteria reduce nitrates in the urine to nitrites, providing a means for chemical analysis. Similarly, activated leukocytes secrete leukocyte esterase, which can be detected chemically. Leukocyte esterase is specific (94% to 98%) and reliably sensitive (75% to 96%) for detecting uropathogens equivalent to 100,000 CFU/mL urine.[19] Nitrite tests may be negative if the causative organism is not nitrate producing (*e.g.,* enterococci, *S. saprophyticus*). Therefore, the sensitivity of nitrite tests ranges from 35% to 85%, but the specificity is 95%.[20] The nitrite test can also be negative if the urine specimen is too diluted.

The treatment of UTI is based on the pathogen causing the infection, and the presence of contributing host–agent factors. Other considerations include whether the infection is acute, recurrent, or chronic. Most acute lower UTIs, which occur mainly in women and are generally caused by *E. coli,* are treated successfully with a short course of antimicrobial therapy. Forcing fluids may relieve signs and symptoms, and this approach is used as an adjunct to antimicrobial treatment. For several decades, first-line therapy for acute uncomplicated UTI has been a 3-day regimen of trimethoprim-sulfamethoxazole (TMP-SMX).[19,23,25] However, there is increasing resistance among commonly acquired *E. coli* infections to TMP-SMX in many parts of the United States, varying from 22% to 39%, depending on geographic location.[26] The resistance of *E. coli* to TMP-SMX is often accompanied by resistance to other antimicrobial drugs, including ampicillin, cephalothin, and tetracycline. Thus, selection of a therapeutic agent must now take into account the geographic location and susceptibility of the bacteria to the different antimicrobial agents.

Recurrent lower UTIs are those that recur after treatment. They are due either to bacterial persistence or reinfection. Bacterial persistence usually is curable by removal of the infectious source (*e.g.,* urinary catheter or infected bladder stones). Reinfection is managed principally through education regarding pathogen transmission and prevention measures. Cranberry juice or blueberry juice has been suggested as a preventive measure for persons with frequent UTIs. Studies suggest that these juices reduce bacterial adherence to the epithelial lining of the urinary tract.[27,28] Because of their mechanism of action, these juices are used more appropriately in prevention rather than treatment of an established UTI.

Chronic UTIs are more difficult to treat. Because they often are associated with obstructive uropathy or reflux flow of urine, diagnostic tests usually are performed to detect such abnormalities. When possible, the condition causing the reflux flow or obstruction is corrected. Most persons with recurrent UTIs are treated with antimicrobial agents for 10 to 14 days in doses sufficient to maintain high urine levels of the drug, and they are examined for obstruction or other causes of infection. Men in particular should be investigated for obstructive disorders or a prostatic focus of infection.

Infections in Special Populations

Urinary tract infections affect persons of all ages. In infants, they occur more often in boys than in girls. After the first year of life UTIs occur more often in girls. This is because of the shorter length of the female urethra and because the vaginal vestibule can be easily contaminated with fecal flora. Approximately half of all adult women have at least one UTI during their lifetime.[19,20,23] The major risk factors for women 16 to 35 years of age are related to sexual intercourse and use of spermicidal agents.[23,29] The anterior urethra usually is colonized with bacteria; urethral massage or sexual intercourse can force these bacteria back into the bladder. Using a diaphragm and spermicide enhances the susceptibility to infection. This seems to be related to the bactericidal effect on lactobacilli and normal vaginal flora.

Urinary Tract Infections in Pregnant Women

Pregnant women are at increased risk for UTIs. Normal changes in the functioning of the urinary tract that occur during pregnancy predispose to UTIs.[30,31] These changes involve the collecting system of the kidneys and include dilation of the renal calyces, pelves, and ureters that begins during the first trimester and becomes most pronounced during the third trimester. This dilation of the upper urinary system is accompanied by a reduction in the peristaltic activity of the ureters that is thought to result from the muscle-relaxing effects of progesterone-like hormones and mechanical obstruction from the enlarging uterus. In addition to the changes in the kidneys and ureters, the bladder becomes displaced from its pelvic position to a more abdominal position, producing further changes in ureteral position.

Asymptomatic UTIs are common, with a prevalence of 2% to 14% in pregnant women.[30] The complications of asymptomatic UTIs during pregnancy include persistent bacteriuria, acute and chronic pyelonephritis, and preterm delivery of infants with low birth weight. Evidence suggests that few women become bacteriuric during pregnancy. Rather, it appears that symptomatic UTIs during pregnancy reflect preexisting asymptomatic bacteriuria and that changes occurring during pregnancy simply permit the prior urinary colonization to progress to symptomatic infection and invasion of the kidneys. Incidence of pyelonephritis during pregnancy is approximately 1% to 2%. However, 20% to 40% of women with untreated bacteriuria will develop pyelonephritis during pregnancy.[30] Because bacteriuria may occur as an asymptomatic condition in pregnant women, the American College of Obstetricians and Gynecologists recommends that a urine culture be obtained at the first prenatal visit.[32] A repeat culture should be obtained during the third trimester. Women with bacteriuria should be followed closely, and infections should be properly treated to prevent complications. The choice of antimicrobial agent should address the common infecting organisms and should be safe for the mother and fetus.

Urinary Tract Infections in Children

Urinary tract infections occur in as much as 3% to 5% of female and 1% of male children.[4,33] In girls, the average age at first diagnosis is 5 years or younger, with peaks during infancy and toilet training. In boys, most UTIs occur during the first year of life; they are more common in uncircumcised than in circumcised boys.[34,35] Children who are at increased risk for bacteriuria or symptomatic UTIs are premature infants discharged from neonatal intensive care units; children with systemic or immunologic disease or urinary tract abnormalities such as neurogenic bladder or vesicoureteral reflux; those with a family history of UTI or urinary tract anomalies with reflux; and girls younger than 5 years of age with a history of UTI.[4,33]

UTIs in children frequently involve the upper urinary tract (pyelonephritis). In children in whom renal development is not complete, pyelonephritis can lead to renal scarring and permanent kidney damage. Most UTIs that lead to scarring and diminished kidney growth occur in children younger than 4 years, especially infants younger than 1 year of age. The incidence of scarring is greatest in children with gross vesicoureteral reflux or obstruction, in children with recurrent UTIs, and in those with a delay in treatment.

Unlike adults, children frequently do not present with the typical signs of a UTI.[4,34,35] Many neonates with UTIs have bacteremia and may show signs and symptoms of septicemia, including fever, hypothermia, apneic spells, poor skin perfusion, abdominal distention, diarrhea, vomiting, lethargy, and irritability. Older infants may present with feeding problems, failure to thrive, diarrhea, vomiting, fever, and foul-smelling urine. Toddlers often present with abdominal pain, vomiting, diarrhea, abnormal voiding patterns, foul-smelling urine, fever, and poor growth. In older children with lower UTIs, the classic features—enuresis, frequency, dysuria, and suprapubic discomfort—are more common. Fever is a common sign of UTI in children, and the possibility of UTI should be considered in any child with unexplained fever.

Diagnosis is based on a careful history of voiding patterns and symptomatology; physical examination to determine fever, hypertension, abdominal or suprapubic tenderness, and other manifestations of UTI; and urinalysis to determine bacteriuria, pyuria, proteinuria, and hematuria. A positive urine culture that is obtained correctly is essential for the diagnosis. Additional diagnostic methods may be needed to determine the cause of the disorder. Vesicoureteral reflux is the most commonly associated abnormality in UTIs, and reflux nephropathy is an important cause of end-stage renal disease in children and adolescents. Children with a relatively uncomplicated first UTI may turn out to have significant reflux. Therefore, even a single documented UTI in a child requires careful diagnosis. Urinary symptoms in the absence of bacteriuria suggest vaginitis, urethritis, sexual molestation, the use of irritating bubble baths, pinworms, or viral cystitis. In adolescent girls, a history of dysuria and vaginal discharge makes vaginitis or vulvitis a consideration.

The approach to treatment is based on the clinical severity of the infection, the site of infection (*i.e.*, lower versus upper urinary tract), the risk for sepsis, and the presence of structural abnormalities.[4,34–36] The immediate treatment of infants and young children is essential. Most infants with symptomatic UTIs and many children with clinical evidence of acute upper UTIs require hospitalization, rehydration, and intravenous antibiotic therapy. Follow-up is essential for children with febrile UTIs to ensure resolution of the infection. Follow-up urine cultures often are done at the end of treatment. Imaging studies often are recommended for all children after their first UTI to detect renal scarring, vesicoureteral reflux, or other abnormalities.

Urinary Tract Infections in the Elderly

Urinary tract infections are relatively common in elderly persons.[33] They are the second most common form of infection, after respiratory tract infections, among otherwise healthy community-dwelling elderly. They are particularly prevalent in elderly living in nursing homes or extended care facilities.

Most of these infections follow invasion of the urinary tract by the ascending route. Several factors predispose elderly persons to UTIs, including immobility resulting in poor bladder emptying; bladder outflow obstruction caused by prostatic hyperplasia or kidney stones; bladder ischemia caused by urine retention; constipation; senile vaginitis; and diminished bactericidal activity of urine and prostatic secretions. Added to these risks are other health problems that necessitate instrumentation of the urinary tract. UTIs develop in 1% of ambulatory patients after a single catheterization and within 3 to 4 days in essentially all patients with indwelling catheters.[37]

Elderly persons with bacteriuria have varying symptoms, ranging from the absence of symptoms to the presence of typical UTI symptoms. Even when symptoms of lower UTIs are present, they may be difficult to interpret because elderly persons without UTIs commonly experience urgency, frequency, and incontinence. Alternatively, elderly persons may have vague symptoms such as anorexia, fatigue, weakness, or change in mental status. Even with more serious upper UTIs (*e.g.*, pyelonephritis), the classic signs of infection such as fever, chills, flank pain, and tenderness may be altered or absent in elderly persons.[33] Sometimes, no symptoms occur until the infection is far advanced.

IN SUMMARY, UTI is the second most common type of bacterial infection seen by health care professionals. Infections can range from asymptomatic bacteriuria to severe kidney infections that cause irreversible kidney damage. Predisposition to infection is determined by host defenses and pathogen virulence. Host defenses include the washout phenomenon associated with voiding, the protective mucin lining of the bladder, and the local immune defenses. Pathogen virulence is enhanced by the presence of pili that facilitate adherence to structures in the urinary tract, lipopolysaccharides that bind to host cells and elicit an inflammatory reaction, and enzymes that break down red blood cells and make iron available for bacterial metabolism and multiplication.

Most UTIs ascend from the urethra and bladder. A number of factors interact in determining the predisposition to development of UTIs, including urinary tract obstruction, urine stasis and reflux, pregnancy-induced changes in urinary tract function, age-related changes in the urinary tract, changes in the protective mechanisms of the bladder and ureters, impaired immune function, and virulence of the pathogen. Urinary tract catheters and urinary instrumentation contribute to the incidence of UTIs. Early diagnosis and treatment of UTI are essential to preventing permanent kidney damage. ■

DISORDERS OF GLOMERULAR FUNCTION

After completing this section of the chapter, you should be able to meet the following objectives:

- Describe the two types of immune mechanisms involved in glomerular disorders.
- Use the terms *proliferation, sclerosis, membranous, diffuse, focal, segmental,* and *mesangial* to explain changes in glomerular structure that occur with glomerulonephritis.
- Relate the proteinuria, hematuria, pyuria, oliguria, edema, hypertension, and azotemia that occur with glomerulonephritis to changes in glomerular structure.
- Briefly describe the difference among the nephritic syndromes, rapidly progressive glomerulonephritis, nephrotic syndrome, asymptomatic glomerular disorders, and chronic glomerulonephritis.

The glomeruli are tufts of capillaries that lie between the afferent and efferent arterioles. The capillaries of the glomeruli are arranged in lobules and supported by a stalk consisting of mesangial cells and a basement membrane–like extracellular matrix (Fig. 33-9A). The glomerular capillary membrane is composed of three structural layers: an endothelial cell layer that lines the inner surface of the capillary, a basement membrane made up of a network of matrix proteins, and a layer of epithelial cells that surrounds the outer surface of the capillary and lines the inner surface of the Bowman capsule (see Chapter 30, Fig. 30-5). The epithelial cells are attached to the basement membrane by long, footlike processes (*podocytes*) that encircle the outer surface of the capillaries. The glomerular capillary membrane is selectively permeable, allowing water and small particles (*e.g.*, electrolytes, and dissolved particles, such as glucose and amino acids) to leave the blood and enter the Bowman space and preventing larger particles (*e.g.*, plasma proteins and blood cells) from leaving the blood.

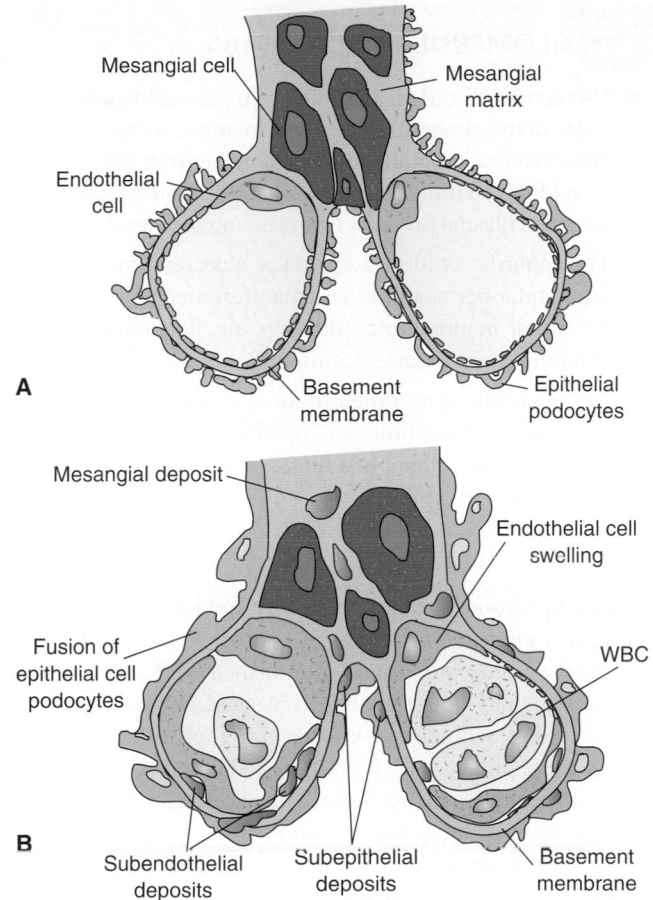

FIGURE 33-9 • Schematic representations of a glomerulus. **(A)** Normal. **(B)** Localization of immune deposits (mesangial, subendothelial, subepithelial) and changes in glomerular architecture associated with injury. WBC, white blood cell. (From Whitley K., Keane W. F., Vernier R. L. [1984]. Acute glomerulonephritis: A clinical overview. *Medical Clinics of North America* 68, 263.)

Glomerulonephritis, an inflammatory process that involves glomerular structures, is the second leading cause of kidney failure worldwide and it ranks third, after diabetes and hypertension, as a cause of chronic kidney disease in the United States.[1,38] There are many causes of glomerular disease. The

disease may occur as a primary condition in which the glomerular abnormality is the only disease present, or it may occur as a secondary condition in which the glomerular abnormality results from another disease, such as diabetes mellitus or SLE.

Etiology and Pathogenesis of Glomerular Injury

The causative agents or triggering events that produce glomerular injury include immunologic, nonimmunologic, and hereditary mechanisms. Most cases of primary and many cases of secondary glomerular disease probably have an immune origin.[5,6,38–44] Although many glomerular diseases are driven by immunologic events, a variety of nonimmunologic metabolic (*e.g.,* diabetes), hemodynamic (*e.g.,* hypertension), and toxic (*e.g.,* drugs, chemicals) stresses can induce glomerular injury, either alone or in concert with immunologic mechanisms. Hereditary glomerular diseases such as Alport syndrome, although relatively rare, are an important category of glomerular disease because of their association with progressive loss of renal function and transmission to future generations.

Two types of immune mechanisms have been implicated in the development of glomerular disease: (1) injury resulting from antibodies reacting with fixed glomerular antigens or antigens planted within the glomerulus, and (2) injury resulting from circulating antigen–antibody complexes that become trapped in the glomerular membrane (Fig. 33-10). Antigens responsible for development of the immune response may be of endogenous origin, such as autoantibodies to deoxyribonucleic acid (DNA) in SLE, or they may be of exogenous origin, such as streptococcal membrane antigens in poststreptococcal glomerulonephritis. Frequently, the source of the antigen is unknown.

The cellular changes that occur with glomerular disease include increases in glomerular or inflammatory cell number (proliferative or hypercellular), basement membrane thickening (membranous), and changes in noncellular glomerular components (sclerosis and fibrosis).[5,6,39] An increase in cell numbers is characterized by one or more of the following: proliferation of endothelial and mesangial cells, leukocyte infiltration (neutrophils, monocytes, and in some cases lymphocytes),

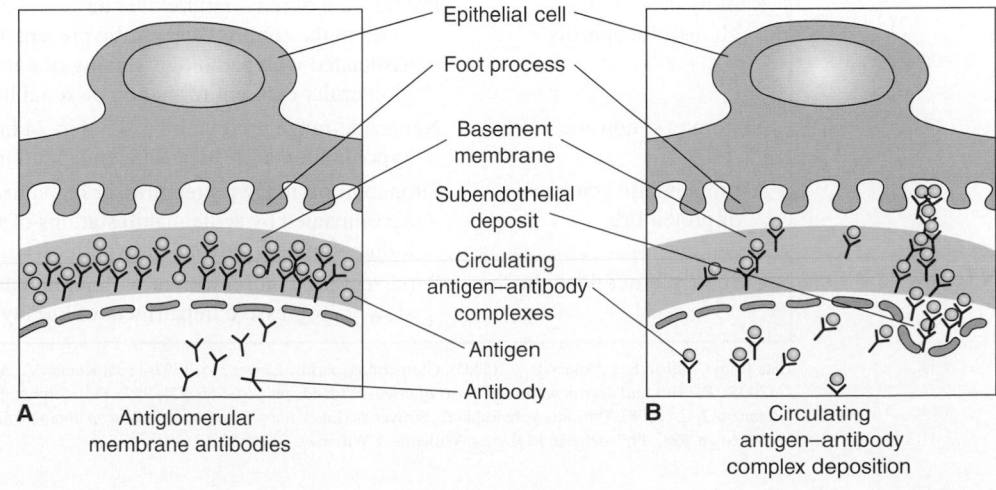

FIGURE 33-10 • Immune mechanisms of glomerular disease. **(A)** Antiglomerular membrane antibodies leave the circulation and interact with antigens that are present in the basement membrane of the glomerulus. **(B)** Antigen–antibody complexes circulating in the blood become trapped as they are filtered in the glomerulus.

and formation of crescents (half-moon–shaped collections of proliferating epithelial cells and infiltrating leukocytes) in the Bowman space.[5,6,39] *Basement membrane thickening* involves deposition of dense noncellular material on the endothelial and epithelial sides of the basement membrane or within the membrane itself. *Sclerosis* refers to an increase in the amount of extracellular material in the mesangial, subendothelial, or subepithelial tissue of the glomerulus, and *fibrosis* refers to the deposition of collagen fibers. Glomerular changes can be *diffuse,* involving all glomeruli and all parts of the glomeruli; *focal,* in which only some glomeruli are affected and others are essentially normal; *segmental,* involving only a certain segment of each glomerulus; or *mesangial,* affecting only mesangial cells.[5] Figure 33-9B illustrates the location of lesions associated with various types of glomerular disease.

Types of Glomerular Disease

The clinical manifestations of glomerular disorders generally fall into one of five categories: nephritic syndromes, rapidly progressive glomerulonephritis, the nephrotic syndrome, asymptomatic disorders of urinary sediment (*i.e.,* hematuria, proteinuria), and chronic glomerulonephritis[5,6,38,39] (Table 33-3). The nephritic syndromes produce a proliferative inflammatory response, whereas the nephrotic syndrome produces increased permeability of the glomerulus. Because most glomerular disorders can produce mixed nephritic and nephrotic syndromes, a definitive diagnosis often requires renal biopsy.

Acute Nephritic Syndrome

The acute nephritic syndrome is the clinical correlate of acute glomerular inflammation. In its most dramatic form, the acute nephritic syndrome is characterized by sudden onset of hematuria (either microscopic or grossly visible, with red cell casts), variable degrees of proteinuria, diminished GFR, oliguria, and signs of impaired renal function. It is caused by inflammatory processes that occlude the glomerular capillary lumen and damage the capillary wall, permitting red blood cells to escape into the urine and producing hemodynamic changes that decrease the GFR. Extracellular fluid accumulation, hypertension, and edema develop because of the decreased GFR and enhanced tubular reabsorption of salt and water.

The acute nephritic syndrome may occur in such systemic diseases as SLE. Typically, however, it is associated with acute proliferative glomerulonephritis such as postinfectious glomerulonephritis.

GLOMERULAR DISORDERS

- Glomerular disorders affect the semipermeable properties of the glomerular capillary membrane that allow water and small particles to move from the blood into the urine filtrate, while preventing blood cells and plasma proteins from leaving the circulation.

- The nephritic syndromes produce a decrease in glomerular permeability and manifestations related to a decrease in glomerular filtration rate, fluid retention, and nitrogenous waste accumulation.

- The nephrotic syndrome produces an increase in glomerular permeability and manifestations of altered body function related to a massive loss of plasma proteins in the urine.

TABLE 33-3 Classification and Manifestations of Glomerular Syndromes

CLASSIFICATION	MANIFESTATIONS
Acute nephritic syndrome	Recent onset of hematuria and proteinuria, impairment of kidney function (azotemia), and salt and water retention causing edema and hypertension
Rapidly progressive glomerulonephritis	Progression of renal failure over days to weeks, in most cases in the context of nephritic presentation, typically associated with pathologic finding of extensive glomerular crescent formation on renal biopsy
Nephrotic syndrome	Nephrotic-range proteinuria (>3.5 g in 24 hours), hypoalbuminemia, hyperlipidemia, and lipiduria
Asymptomatic hematuria or proteinuria	Subnephrotic-range proteinuria, or hematuria, not accompanied by acute manifestations of impaired kidney function, edema, or hypertension
Chronic glomerulonephritis	Persistent proteinuria with or without hematuria and slowly progressive impairment of kidney function

Data from Chadban S. J., Atkins R. C. (2005). Glomerulonephritis. *Lancet* 365, 1797–1806; Kumar V., Abbas A. K., Fausto N. (2005). *Robbins and Cotran pathologic basis of disease* (7th ed., pp. 961–966, 971–979). Philadelphia: Elsevier Saunders; and Jennette J. C. (2008). The kidney. In Rubin R., Strayer D. (Eds.), *Rubin's pathology: Clinicopathologic foundations of medicine* (5th ed., p. 698). Philadelphia: Lippincott Williams & Wilkins.

Acute Postinfectious Glomerulonephritis. Acute postinfectious glomerulonephritis usually occurs after infection with certain strains of group A β-hemolytic streptococci and is caused by deposition of immune complexes.[5,6,39] It also may occur after infections by other organisms, including staphylococci and a number of viral agents, such as those responsible for mumps, measles, and chickenpox. This type of glomerular disease is decreasing in frequency in the United States but continues to be a common disorder worldwide. Although the disease is seen primarily in children, persons of any age can be affected.

The acute phase of postinfectious glomerulonephritis is characterized by diffuse glomerular enlargement and hypercellularity. The hypercellularity is caused by infiltration of leukocytes, both neutrophils and monocytes; proliferation of endothelial and mesangial cells; and in severe cases, formation of crescents. There is also swelling of endothelial cells, and the combination of proliferation, swelling, and leukocyte infiltration obliterates the glomerular capillary lumens. There may be interstitial edema and inflammation, and the tubules often contain red blood cells. In the first weeks of disease, immunofluorescence microscopy typically reveals granular deposits of IgG and the complement component C3 in the mesangium and along the basement membrane (Fig. 33-11).

The classic case of poststreptococcal glomerulonephritis follows a streptococcal infection by approximately 7 to 12 days—the time needed for the development of antibodies. The primary infection usually involves the pharynx. Oliguria, which develops as the GFR decreases, is one of the first symptoms. Proteinuria and hematuria follow because of increased glomerular capillary wall permeability. The red blood cells are degraded by materials in the urine, and cola-colored urine may be the first sign of the disorder. Sodium and water retention gives rise to edema (particularly of the face and hands) and hypertension. Important laboratory findings include an elevated antistreptococcal antibody (ASO) titer, a decline in serum concentrations of C3 and other components of the complement cascade, and cryoglobulins (*i.e.*, large immune complexes) in the serum.

Treatment of acute poststreptococcal glomerulonephritis includes elimination of the streptococcal infection with antibiotics and providing supportive care. The disorder carries an excellent prognosis and rarely causes chronic kidney disease.[39] In children, spontaneous resolution of the glomerular lesion and nephritic syndrome is usually the norm and occurs within 6 to 8 weeks. Adults tend to recover more slowly, and approximately 20% have some degree of persistent proteinuria or compromise of GFR 1 year after presentation.

Rapidly Progressive Glomerulonephritis

Rapidly progressive glomerulonephritis is a clinical syndrome characterized by signs of severe glomerular injury that does not have a specific cause. As its name indicates, this type of glomerulonephritis is rapidly progressive, often within a matter of months. The disorder involves focal and segmental proliferation of glomerular cells and recruitment of monocytes and macrophages with formation of crescent-shaped structures that obliterate the Bowman space.[5] Rapidly proliferative glomerulonephritis may be caused by a number of immunologic disorders, some systemic and others restricted to the kidney. Among the diseases associated with this form of glomerulonephritis are immune complex disorders such as SLE, small vessel vasculitides (*e.g.*, microscopic polyangiitis), and an immune disorder called *Goodpasture syndrome*.

Goodpasture Syndrome. Goodpasture syndrome is an uncommon and aggressive form of glomerulonephritis that is caused by antibodies to the glomerular basement membrane (GBM). The anti-GBM antibodies cross-react with the pulmonary alveolar basement membrane to produce the syndrome of pulmonary hemorrhage associated with renal failure. The pathologic hallmark of anti-GBM glomerulonephritis is diffuse linear staining of GBMs for IgG (Fig. 33-12). The cause of the disorder is unknown, although influenza infection and exposure to hydrocarbon solvent (found in paints and dyes) have been implicated in some persons, as have various drugs and cancers. There is a high prevalence of certain human leukocyte antigen subtypes (*e.g.*, HLA-DRB1) in those affected, suggesting a genetic predisposition.[5] Treatment includes plasmapheresis to remove circulating anti-GBM antibodies and immunosuppressive therapy (*i.e.*, corticosteroids and cyclophosphamide) to inhibit antibody production.

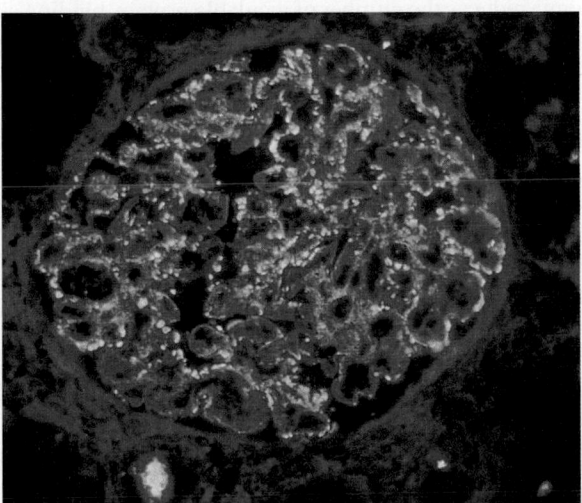

FIGURE 33-11 • Acute postinfectious glomerulonephritis. An immunofluorescence micrograph demonstrates granular staining for complement C3 in capillary walls and the mesangium. (From Jennette J. C. [2008]. The kidney. In Rubin R., Strayer D. [Eds.], *Rubin's pathology: Clinicopathologic foundations of medicine* [5th ed., p. 713]. Philadelphia: Lippincott Williams & Wilkins.)

Nephrotic Syndrome

The nephrotic syndrome is characterized by massive proteinuria (>3.5 g/day) and lipiduria (*e.g.*, free fat, oval bodies, fatty casts), along with an associated hypoalbuminemia (<3 g/dL), generalized edema, and hyperlipidemia (cholesterol >300 mg/dL).[5,6,45,46]

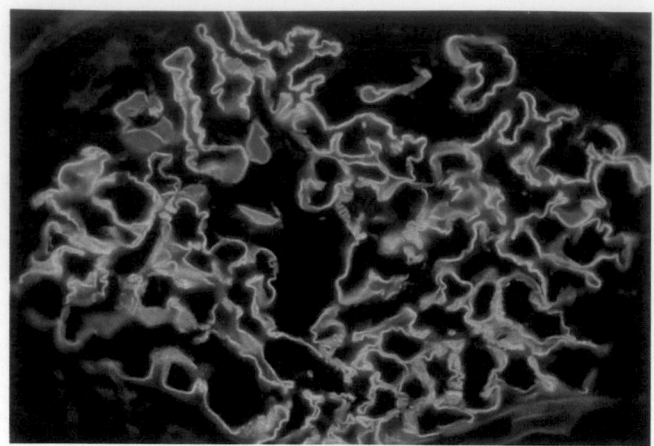

FIGURE 33-12 • Anti-glomerular basement membrane glomerulo-nephritis. Linear immunofluorescence for IgG is seen along the glomerular basement membrane. Contrast this with the granular pattern of immunofluorescence typical of most types of immune complex deposition within the capillary wall. (From Jennette J. C. [2008]. The kidney. In Rubin R., Strayer D. [Eds.], *Rubin's pathology: Clinicopathologic foundations of medicine* [5th ed., p. 720]. Philadelphia: Lippincott Williams & Wilkins.)

The nephrotic syndrome is not a specific glomerular disease, but a constellation of clinical findings that result from an increase in glomerular permeability and loss of plasma proteins in the urine[45,46] (Fig. 33-13).

The glomerular membrane acts as a size and charge barrier through which the glomerular filtrate must pass. Any increase in permeability allows proteins to escape from the plasma into the glomerular filtrate. Massive proteinuria results, leading to hypoalbuminemia. Generalized edema, which is a hallmark of the nephrotic syndrome, results from the loss of colloidal osmotic pressure of the blood with subsequent accumulation of fluid in the interstitial tissues.[5,6] There is also salt and water retention, which aggravates the edema. This appears to be due to several factors, including a compensatory increase in aldosterone, stimulation of the sympathetic nervous system, and a reduction in secretion of natriuretic factors. Initially, the edema presents in dependent parts of the body such as the lower extremities, but becomes more generalized as the disease progresses. Dyspnea due to pulmonary edema, pleural effusions, and diaphragmatic compromise due to ascites can develop in persons with nephrotic syndrome.

The hyperlipidemia that occurs in persons with nephrosis is characterized by elevated levels of triglycerides and low-density lipoproteins (LDLs). Levels of high-density lipoproteins (HDLs) usually are normal. It is thought that these abnormalities are related, at least in part, to increased synthesis of lipoproteins in the liver secondary to a compensatory increase in albumin production.[45] Because of the elevated LDL levels, persons with nephrotic syndrome are at increased risk for development of atherosclerosis.

The largest proportion of protein lost in the urine is albumin, but globulins also may be lost in some diseases. As a result, persons with nephrosis may be vulnerable to infections, particularly those caused by staphylococci and pneumococci.[5] This decreased resistance to infection probably is related to loss of both immunoglobulins and low–molecular-weight complement components in the urine. Many binding proteins also are lost in the urine. Consequently, the plasma levels of many ions (iron, copper, zinc) and hormones (thyroid and sex hormones) may be low because of decreased binding proteins. Many drugs require protein binding for transport. Hypoalbuminemia reduces the number of available protein-binding sites, thereby producing a potential increase in the amount of free (active) drug that is available.[45]

Thrombotic complications also have evolved as a risk in persons with nephrotic syndrome. These disorders reflect a disruption in the function of the coagulation system brought about by a loss of coagulation and anticoagulation factors. Renal vein thrombosis, once thought to be a cause of the disorder, is more likely a consequence of the hypercoagulable state.[45] Other thrombotic complications include deep vein thrombosis and pulmonary emboli.

Causes. The glomerular derangements that occur with nephrosis can develop as a primary disorder or secondary to changes caused by systemic diseases such as diabetes mellitus and SLE.[5,6] Among the primary glomerular lesions leading to nephrotic syndrome are minimal-change disease (lipoid nephrosis), focal segmental glomerulosclerosis, and membranous glomerulonephritis. The relative frequency of these causes varies with age. In children younger than 15 years of age, nephrotic syndrome almost always is caused by primary idiopathic glomerular disease, whereas in adults, it often is a secondary disorder.[5,46]

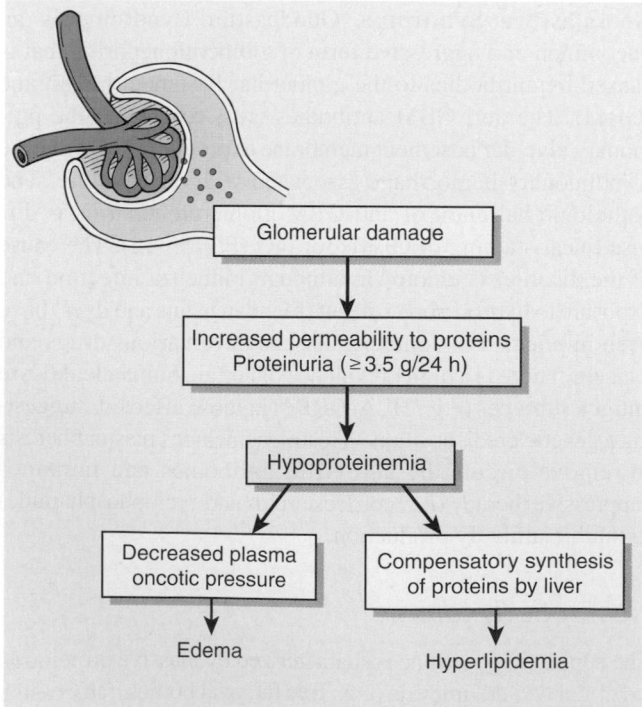

FIGURE 33-13 • Pathophysiology of the nephrotic syndrome.

Minimal-Change Disease (Lipoid Nephrosis). Minimal-change disease is characterized by diffuse loss (through fusion) of the foot processes of cells in the epithelial layer of the glomerular membrane. It is most commonly seen in children (peak incidence at 2 to 6 years of age),[5] but may occasionally occur in adults. The cause of minimal-change nephrosis is unknown; however, children in whom the disease develops often have a history of recent upper respiratory infections or of receiving routine immunizations.[5] Although minimal-change disease does not progress to renal failure, it can cause significant complications, including predisposition to infection with gram-positive organisms, a tendency toward thromboembolic events, hyperlipidemia, and protein malnutrition. There usually is a dramatic response to corticosteroid therapy.[5,45]

Membranous Glomerulonephritis. Membranous glomerulo-nephritis is the most common cause of primary nephrosis in adults, most commonly those in the fifth and sixth decades of life and almost always after 30 years of age.[5,6] The disorder is caused by diffuse thickening of the GBM due to deposition of immune complexes. The disorder may be idiopathic or associated with a number of disorders, including autoimmune diseases such as SLE, infections such as chronic hepatitis B, metabolic disorders such as diabetes mellitus and thyroiditis, and use of certain drugs such as gold compounds, penicillamine, and captopril.[5] The presence of immunoglobulins and complement in the subendothelial deposits suggests that the disease represents a chronic immune complex–mediated disorder.

The disorder usually begins with an insidious onset of the nephrotic syndrome or, in a small percentage of patients, with non-nephrotic proteinuria. Hematuria and mild hypertension may be present. The progress of the disease is variable. The nephrotic syndrome remits spontaneously in about 40% of patients, another 30% to 40% have repeated relapses and remissions, and the final 10% to 20% suffer a slow, progressive decline in GFR that terminates in kidney failure.[41] Spontaneous remissions and a relatively benign outcome occur more commonly in women and those with proteinuria in the non-nephrotic range. Treatment is controversial. Because of the variable course of the disease, the overall effectiveness of corticosteroids and other immunosuppressive therapy in controlling the progress of the disease has been difficult to evaluate.[5,39]

Focal Segmental Glomerulosclerosis. Focal segmental glomerulosclerosis is characterized by sclerosis (i.e., increased collagen deposition) of some but not all glomeruli, and in the affected glomeruli, only a portion of the glomerular tuft is involved.[5] The disorder has increased in prevalence since the late 1980s so that it now accounts for as much as one third of cases of nephrotic syndrome in adults.[39] It is a particularly common cause of nephrotic syndrome in Hispanic and African Americans.

Although focal segmental sclerosis often is an idiopathic syndrome, it may be associated with reduced oxygen in the blood (e.g., sickle cell disease and cyanotic congenital heart disease), human immunodeficiency virus (HIV) infection, or intravenous drug abuse, or it may occur as a secondary event reflecting glomerular scarring due to other forms of glomerulo-nephritis or reflux nephropathy.[5,6]

The presence of hypertension and decreased renal function distinguishes focal sclerosis from minimal-change disease. The disorder usually is treated with corticosteroids. Most persons with the disorder progress to kidney failure within 5 to 10 years.

Asymptomatic Hematuria or Proteinuria

Many cases of glomerulonephritis result in mild asymptomatic illness that is not recognized or brought to the attention of a health care professional, and therefore remains undiagnosed. Population-based screening studies have shown that kidney damage as evidenced by proteinuria, hematuria, low GFR, or a combination of these features is present in 16% of persons in Australia and a similar proportion in the United States.[47] Disorders such as Henoch-Schönlein purpura often resolve without permanent kidney damage, whereas others, such as IgA nephropathy and Alport syndrome, can progress to chronic kidney disease and renal failure.

Immunoglobulin A Nephropathy. Immunoglobulin A nephropathy (i.e., Berger disease) is a primary glomerulonephritis characterized by the presence of glomerular IgA immune complex deposits. It can occur at any age, but most commonly has its onset in the second and third decades of life.[48,49] The disease occurs more commonly in men than women and is the most common cause of glomerular nephritis in Asians.

The disorder is characterized by the deposition of IgA-containing immune complexes in the mesangium of the glomerulus. Once deposited in the kidney, the immune complexes are associated with glomerular inflammation. The cause of the disorder is unknown. Some persons with the disorder have elevated serum IgA levels. Recent studies have focused on potential abnormalities of the IgA molecule as a factor in the pathogenesis of the disorder.[48]

Early in the disease, many persons with the disorder have no obvious symptoms and are unaware of the problem. In these persons, IgA nephropathy is suspected during routine screening or examination for another condition. In other persons, the disorder presents with gross hematuria that is preceded by upper respiratory tract infection, gastrointestinal tract symptoms, or a flulike illness. The hematuria usually lasts 2 to 6 days. Approximately one half of the persons with gross hematuria have a single episode, whereas the remainder experience a gradual progression in the disease with recurrent episodes of hematuria and mild proteinuria. Progression usually is slow, extending over several decades.

Immunofluorescence microscopy is essential for diagnosis of IgA nephropathy.[6] The diagnostic finding is mesangial staining for IgA more intense than staining for IgG or IgM (Fig. 33-14). At present, there are no satisfactory treatment measures for IgA nephropathy. The role of immunosuppressive drugs such as steroids and cytotoxic drugs is not clear. There has been recent interest in the use of omega-3 fatty acids (i.e., fish

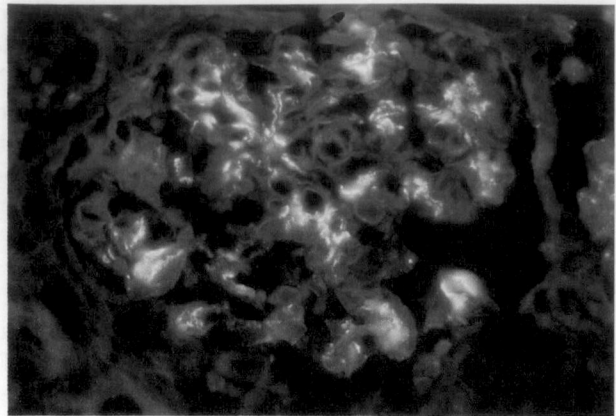

FIGURE 33-14 • IgA nephropathy. An immunofluorescence micrograph shows deposits of IgA in the mesangial areas. (From Jennette J. C. [2008]. The kidney. In Rubin R., Strayer D. [Eds.], *Rubin's pathology: Clinicopathologic foundations of medicine* [5th ed., p. 718]. Philadelphia: Lippincott Williams & Wilkins.)

oil) in delaying the progression of the disease. Randomized, clinical control studies have yielded conflicting results.

Henoch-Schönlein Purpura Nephritis. Henoch-Schönlein purpura is a small vessel vasculitis (see Chapter 22) that causes a purpuric rash largely of the lower extremities, arthritis or arthralgia, abdominal pain, and renal involvement identical to that of IgA nephropathy. The disease is seen most commonly in children (peak age 4 to 6 years) but can also occur in adults.[40,41] Renal involvement is not always present initially, but its incidence increases with time and is more common in older children who have associated abdominal pain and a persistent rash. Although hematuria and proteinuria are the most common presentation, some persons present with manifestations of acute nephritis and others may present with combined nephritis and nephrotic manifestations. Most persons recover fully over a period of several weeks.

Alport Syndrome. Alport syndrome represents a hereditary defect of the GBM that results in hematuria and may progress to chronic renal failure.[5,40] Approximately 80% of cases are inherited as an X-linked autosomal dominant trait, whereas others have autosomal dominant and recessive patterns of inheritance.[40] In X-linked pedigrees, boys are usually affected more seriously than girls. Affected boys usually progress to renal failure as adults, but progression may occur during adolescence. Although many girls never have more than mild hematuria with or without mild proteinuria, some have more significant disease and may even progress to kidney failure.

Diagnosis of Alport syndrome is often made after examination of the urine of a child from a family with multiple cases of hereditary nephritis. Children may initially present with heavy microscopic hematuria (large blood on dipstick), followed by the development of proteinuria. Many, but not all, persons with Alport syndrome have sensorineural deafness and various eye disorders, including lens dislocation, posterior

cataracts, and corneal dystrophy. The hearing loss is bilateral and often is first detected during adolescence.

Chronic Glomerulonephritis

Chronic glomerulonephritis represents the chronic phase of a number of specific types of glomerulonephritis.[5,6] Some forms of acute glomerulonephritis (*e.g.,* poststreptococcal glomerulonephritis) undergo complete resolution, whereas others progress at variable rates to chronic glomerulonephritis. Some persons who present with chronic glomerulonephritis have no history of glomerular disease. These cases may represent the end result of relatively asymptomatic forms of glomerulonephritis. Histologically, the condition is characterized by small kidneys with sclerosed glomeruli. In most cases, chronic glomerulonephritis develops insidiously and slowly progresses to chronic kidney disease over a period of years (see Chapter 34).

Glomerular Lesions Associated With Systemic Disease

Many immunologic, metabolic, or hereditary systemic diseases are associated with glomerular injury. In some diseases, such as SLE, diabetes mellitus, and hypertension, the glomerular involvement may be a major clinical manifestation.

Systemic Lupus Erythematosus Glomerulonephritis

Renal involvement is clinically evident in 40% to 85% of persons with SLE and is seen more commonly in black women.[6,39–42] The pathogenesis of SLE (discussed in Chapter 59) is uncertain, but seems to be related to dysregulated B-cell immunity with production of autoantibodies to a variety of nuclear, cytoplasmic, extracellular matrix, and cell membrane components. Most glomerular injury is triggered by the formation of immune complexes within the glomerular capillary wall.

The clinical manifestations of lupus nephritis depend on the site of immune complex–mediated injury. Immune complexes confined to the mesangium cause less inflammation than subendothelial immune complexes, which have greater exposure to inflammatory cells and mediators in the blood, and which therefore are more likely to produce inflammation.[6,50] The World Health Organization (WHO) classifies the renal glomerular lesions of SLE as class I, normal; class II, mesangial proliferation; class III, focal and segmental proliferation; class IV, diffuse proliferation; and class V, membranous proliferation.[50]

Because of the high risk for kidney disease, all persons with SLE should undergo routine urinalysis to monitor for the appearance of hematuria or proteinuria. If urinary abnormalities are noted, renal biopsy is often performed. Treatment depends on the extent of glomerular involvement. Individuals with class I or II glomerulonephritis usually require no treatment. Progression to higher classes is usually accompanied by an increase in lupus serology activity and evidence of deteriorating renal function (*i.e.,* rising serum creatinine, and a decrease in calculated GFR). Oral corticosteroids and angiotensin-converting enzyme (ACE) inhibitors are the mainstays of treatment. Persons with more advanced disease may require treatment with immunosuppressive agents (*e.g.*, intravenous cyclophosphamide or oral mycophenolate mofetil). Clinical trials using other immunosuppressant agents are ongoing.

Diabetic Glomerulosclerosis

Diabetic nephropathy is a major cause of chronic kidney disease and the most common cause of kidney failure treated by renal replacement therapy in the United States.[51–53] It occurs in both types 1 and 2 diabetes mellitus. It is more prevalent among African Americans, Asians, and Native Americans than whites. Among persons starting renal replacement therapy, the incidence of diabetic nephropathy doubled from 1991 to 2001.[51] Since that time, the rate of increase has slowed, probably because of the adoption of clinical practice guidelines that contribute to early diagnosis and prevention of the disorder.

The lesions of diabetic nephropathy most commonly involve the glomeruli and are associated with three glomerular syndromes: non-nephrotic proteinuria, nephrotic syndrome, and chronic renal failure.[5,6,51] Widespread thickening of the glomerular capillary basement membrane occurs in almost all persons with diabetes and can occur without evidence of proteinuria. This is followed by a diffuse increase in mesangial matrix, with mild proliferation of mesangial cells. As the disease progresses, the mesangial cells impinge on the capillary lumen, reducing the surface area for glomerular filtration. In nodular glomerulosclerosis, also known as *Kimmelstiel-Wilson syndrome*, there is nodular deposition of hyaline in the mesangial portion of the glomerulus. As the sclerotic process progresses in the diffuse and nodular forms of glomerulosclerosis, there is complete obliteration of the glomerulus, with impairment of renal function.

Although the mechanisms of glomerular change in diabetes are uncertain, they are thought to represent enhanced or defective synthesis of the GBM and mesangial matrix with an inappropriate incorporation of glucose into the noncellular components of these glomerular structures.[54] Alternatively, hemodynamic changes that occur secondary to elevated blood glucose levels may contribute to the initiation and progression of diabetic glomerulosclerosis.[5] It has been hypothesized that elevations in blood glucose produce an increase in GFR and glomerular pressure that leads to enlargement of glomerular capillary pores by a mechanism that is, at least partly, mediated by angiotensin II. This enlargement results in an increase in the protein content of the glomerular filtrate, which in turn requires increased endocytosis of the filtered proteins by tubular endothelial cells, a process that ultimately leads to nephron destruction and progressive deterioration of renal function.

The clinical manifestations of diabetic glomerulosclerosis are closely linked to those of diabetes. The increased GFR that occurs in persons with early alterations in renal function is associated with *microalbuminuria*, defined as urinary albumin excretion of 30 to 300 mg in 24 hours.[5] Microalbuminuria is an important predictor of future diabetic nephropathies.[5,51] In many cases, these early changes in glomerular function can be reversed by careful control of blood glucose levels (see Chapter 42). Inhibition of angiotensin by ACE inhibitors or angiotensin receptor blockers (ARBs) has been shown to have a beneficial effect, possibly by reversing increased glomerular pressure.[51] Hypertension and cigarette smoking have been implicated in the progression of diabetic nephropathy. Thus, control of blood pressure (to levels of 130/80 mm Hg or less) and smoking cessation are recommended as primary and secondary prevention strategies in persons with diabetes.

Hypertensive Glomerular Disease

Mild to moderate hypertension causes sclerotic changes in renal arterioles and small arteries, referred to as *benign nephrosclerosis*.[5,6] The condition has been identified in approximately 15% of persons with benign hypertension (hypertension is discussed in Chapter 23). It is most prevalent and most aggressive among blacks. Among African Americans, hypertension is the leading cause of end-stage renal disease.

Hypertensive nephropathy is associated with a number of changes in kidney structure and function. The kidneys are smaller than normal and are usually affected bilaterally.[5,6] On histologic examination, there is narrowing of the arterioles and small arteries, caused by thickening and hyalinization of the vessel walls. As the vascular structures thicken and perfusion diminishes, blood flow to the nephron decreases, causing patchy tubular atrophy, interstitial fibrosis, and a variety of changes in glomerular structure and function.

Although uncomplicated hypertensive nephrosclerosis is not usually associated with significant abnormalities in renal function, a few persons may progress to end-stage renal disease. Three groups of people are at particular risk for development of renal failure: blacks, persons with more severe blood pressure elevations, and persons with a second underlying disease, such as diabetes.[5]

IN SUMMARY, Glomerulonephritis, an inflammatory process that involves glomerular structures, is the second leading cause of kidney failure worldwide and ranks third, after diabetes and hypertension, as a cause of chronic kidney disease in the United States. The disease may occur as a primary condition in which the glomerular abnormality is the only disease present, or it may occur as a secondary condition in which the glomerular abnormality results from another disease, such as diabetes mellitus or SLE. Most cases of primary and many cases of secondary glomerular disease probably have an immune origin.

The clinical manifestations of glomerular disorders generally fall into one of five categories: the nephritic syndromes, rapidly progressive glomerulonephritis, nephrotic syndrome, asymptomatic disorders (*i.e.*, hematuria, proteinuria), and chronic glomerulonephritis. The nephritic syndrome evokes an inflammatory response in the glomeruli and is characterized by hematuria with red cell casts in the urine, a diminished GFR, azotemia, oliguria, and hypertension. The nephrotic syndrome affects the integrity of the glomerular capillary membrane and is characterized by massive proteinuria, hypoalbuminemia, generalized edema, lipiduria, and hyperlipidemia. Asymptomatic hematuria and proteinuria represent glomerular disorders that are not recognized or brought to the attention of a health care professional, and therefore remain undiagnosed. Chronic glomerulonephritis represents the chronic phase of a number of specific types of glomerulonephritis. Secondary causes of glomerular kidney disease include SLE, diabetes mellitus, and hypertension. ■

 ## TUBULOINTERSTITIAL DISORDERS

After completing this section of the chapter, you should be able to meet the following objectives:

- Cite a definition of tubulointerstitial kidney disease.
- Differentiate between the defects in tubular function that occur in proximal and distal tubular acidosis.
- Explain the pathogenesis of kidney damage in acute and chronic pyelonephritis.
- Explain the vulnerability of the kidneys to injury caused by drugs and toxins.

Several disorders affect renal tubular structures, including the proximal and distal tubules. Most of these disorders also affect the interstitial tissue that surrounds the tubules. These disorders, sometimes are referred to as *tubulointerstitial disorders,* include acute tubular necrosis (see Chapter 34), renal tubular acidosis, acute and chronic pyelonephritis, and the effects of drugs and toxins.

Tubulointerstitial renal diseases may be divided into acute and chronic disorders. The acute disorders are characterized by their sudden onset and by signs and symptoms of interstitial edema; they include acute pyelonephritis and acute hypersensitivity reaction to drugs. The chronic disorders produce interstitial fibrosis, atrophy, and mononuclear infiltrates; most persons are asymptomatic until late in the course of the disease. In the early stages, tubulointerstitial diseases commonly are manifested by fluid and electrolyte imbalances that reflect subtle changes in tubular function. These manifestations can include inability to concentrate urine, as evidenced by polyuria and nocturia; interference with acidification of urine, resulting in metabolic acidosis; and diminished tubular reabsorption of sodium and other substances.[5]

Renal Tubular Acidosis

Renal tubular acidosis (RTA) refers to a group of tubular defects in reabsorption of bicarbonate ions (HCO_3^-) or excretion of hydrogen ions (H^+) that result in metabolic acidosis and its

subsequent complications, including metabolic bone disease, kidney stones, and growth failure in children. There are two main types of RTA: proximal tubular disorders that affect bicarbonate reabsorption, and distal tubular defects that affect the secretion of fixed metabolic acids.[55,56] A third type of RTA results from aldosterone deficiency or resistance to its action that leads to impaired reabsorption of sodium ions (Na^+) with decreased elimination of H^+ and potassium ions (K^+). Renal acidosis also occurs in kidney failure (see Chapter 34).

Proximal Renal Tubular Acidosis

Proximal RTA involves a defect in proximal tubular reabsorption, the nephron site where 85% of filtered HCO_3^- is reabsorbed (see Chapter 32). With the onset of impaired tubular HCO_3^- reabsorption, there is a loss of HCO_3^- in the urine that reduces plasma HCO_3^- levels. The concomitant loss of Na^+ in the urine leads to contraction of the extracellular fluid volume with increased aldosterone secretion and a resultant decrease in serum K^+ levels (see Chapter 31). With proximal tubular defects in acid-base regulation, the distal tubular sites for secretion of the fixed acids into the urine continue to function, and the reabsorption of HCO_3^- eventually resumes, albeit at a lower level of serum HCO_3^-. Whenever serum levels rise above this decreased level, HCO_3^- is lost in the urine. Persons with proximal RTA generally have plasma HCO_3^- levels greater than 15 mEq/L and seldom develop severe acidosis.

Proximal RTA may occur as a hereditary or acquired disorder and may involve an isolated defect in HCO_3^- reabsorption or accompany other defects in proximal tubular function (Fanconi syndrome). Isolated defects in HCO_3^- reabsorption are relatively rare. The term *Fanconi syndrome* is used to describe a generalized proximal tubular dysfunction in which the RTA is accompanied by impaired reabsorption of glucose, amino acids, phosphate, and uric acid. Children with Fanconi syndrome are likely to have growth retardation, rickets, osteomalacia, and abnormal vitamin D metabolism in addition to mild acidosis associated with proximal RTA.

Children and infants with proximal RTA require alkali therapy because of the high incidence of growth retardation due to acidemia. Potassium supplements are also needed because of increased loss of potassium that occurs with alkali therapy. Adults may also require alkali therapy. Vitamin D and phosphate are appropriate treatments for rickets and hypophosphatemia.

Distal Renal Tubular Acidosis

Distal RTA has its origin in the distal convoluted tubule and the collecting duct, where about 15% of the filtered bicarbonate is reabsorbed. The clinical syndrome of distal RTA includes hypokalemia, hyperchloremic metabolic acidosis, inability to acidify the urine, nephrocalcinosis, and nephrolithiasis. Additional features include osteomalacia or rickets.

Distal RTA results from a distal tubular defect in H^+ secretion with failure to acidify the urine. Because the secretion of H^+ in the distal tubules is linked to sodium reabsorption, failure to secrete H⁺ results in a net loss of sodium bicarbonate in the urine. This results in contraction of fluids in the extracellular fluid compartment, a compensatory increase in aldosterone levels, and development of hypokalemia. The persistent acidosis, which requires buffering by the skeletal system, causes calcium to be released from bone. Increased losses of calcium in the urine lead to increased levels of parathyroid hormone, osteomalacia, bone pain, impaired growth in children, and development of kidney stones and nephrocalcinosis.

Long-term treatment of distal RTA requires alkali supplementation. Greater amounts are needed for children because of the need for base deposition in growing bone and because bicarbonate wastage is greater in children than in adults. Alkali therapy generally allows for correction of potassium wasting and hypokalemia. It also decreases the calcium concentration in the urine and increases citrate excretion, both of which serve to decrease the incidence of nephrocalcinosis and nephrolithiasis.[56]

Pyelonephritis

Pyelonephritis refers to infection of the kidney parenchyma and renal pelvis. There are two forms of pyelonephritis: acute and chronic.

Acute Pyelonephritis

Acute pyelonephritis represents an infection of the upper urinary tract, specifically the renal parenchyma and renal pelvis.[57] Risk factors for complicated acute pyelonephritis are those that increase the host's susceptibility or reduce the host response to infection. Persons with diabetes mellitus are at increased risk. A less frequent and more serious type of acute pyelonephritis, called *necrotizing pyelonephritis,* is characterized by necrosis of the renal papillae. It is particularly common in persons with diabetes and may also be a complication of acute pyelonephritis when there is significant urinary tract obstruction.

Gram-negative bacteria, including *E. coli* and *Proteus, Klebsiella, Enterobacter,* and *Pseudomonas* species, are the most common causative agents. The infection usually ascends from the lower urinary tract, with the exception of *S. aureus,* which is usually spread through the bloodstream. Factors that contribute to the development of acute pyelonephritis are catheterization and urinary instrumentation, vesicoureteral reflux, pregnancy, and neurogenic bladder.

Hematogenous acute pyelonephritis occurs most often in debilitated, chronically ill persons and those receiving immunosuppressive therapy. Immunosuppression favors the development of subclinical (silent) pyelonephritis and infections caused by nonenteric, aerobic, gram-negative rods, and *Candida.* Metastatic staphylococcal or fungal infections may spread to the kidney from distant foci in the skin or bone.

Clinical Features. Acute pyelonephritis tends to present with an abrupt onset of shaking chills, moderate to high fever, and a constant ache in the loin area of the back that is unilateral or bilateral.[23,57] Lower urinary tract symptoms, including dysuria,

frequency, and urgency, also are common. There may be significant malaise, and the person usually looks and feels ill. Nausea and vomiting may occur along with abdominal pain. Palpation or percussion over the costovertebral angle on the affected side usually causes pain. Pyuria occurs but is not diagnostic because it also occurs in lower UTIs. The development of necrotizing papillitis is associated with a much poorer prognosis. These persons have evidence of overwhelming sepsis with frequent development of renal failure.

Acute pyelonephritis is treated with appropriate antimicrobial drugs. Unless obstruction or other complications occur, the symptoms usually disappear within several days. Treatment with an appropriate antimicrobial agent usually is continued for 10 to 14 days. Persons with complicated acute pyelonephritis and those who do not respond to outpatient treatment may require hospitalization.[57]

Chronic Pyelonephritis

Chronic pyelonephritis represents a progressive process. There is scarring and deformation of the renal calyces and pelvis[5] (Fig. 33-15). The disorder appears to involve a bacterial infection superimposed on obstructive abnormalities or vesicoureteral reflux. Chronic obstructive pyelonephritis is associated with recurrent bouts of inflammation and scarring, which eventually lead to chronic pyelonephritis. Reflux, which is the most common cause of chronic pyelonephritis, results from superimposition of infection on congenital vesicoureteral reflux or intrarenal reflux. Reflux may be unilateral with involvement of a single kidney or bilateral, leading to scarring and atrophy of both kidneys with the eventual development of chronic renal insufficiency.

Clinical Features. Chronic pyelonephritis may cause many of the same symptoms as acute pyelonephritis, or its onset may be insidious. Often there is a history of recurrent episodes of UTI or acute pyelonephritis. Loss of tubular function and the ability to concentrate urine give rise to polyuria and nocturia, and mild proteinuria is common. Severe hypertension often is a contributing factor in the progress of the disease. Chronic pyelonephritis is a significant cause of renal failure. It is thought to be responsible for 10% to 20% of all cases of end-stage renal disease.[5]

Drug-Related Nephropathies

Drug-related nephropathies involve functional or structural changes in the kidneys that occur after exposure to a drug. Because of their large blood flow and high filtration pressure, the kidneys are exposed to any substance that is in the blood. The kidneys also are active in the metabolic transformation of drugs and therefore are exposed to a number of toxic metabolites. The tolerance to drugs varies with age and depends on renal function, state of hydration, blood pressure, and the pH of the urine. Elderly persons are particularly susceptible to kidney damage caused by drugs and toxins. The dangers of

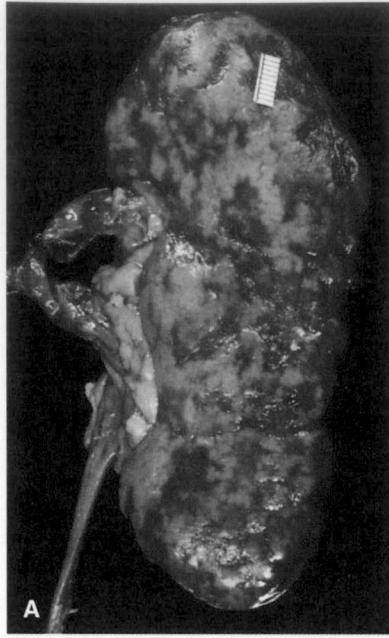
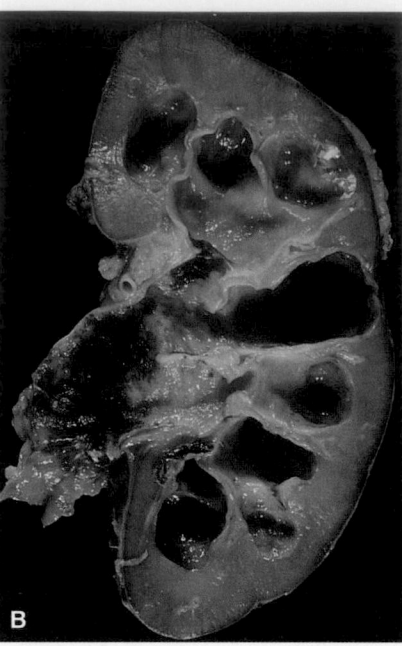

FIGURE 33-15 • Chronic pyelonephritis. **(A)** The cortical surface contains many irregular, depressed scars (reddish areas). **(B)** There is marked dilation of calyces caused by inflammatory destruction of papillae, with atrophy and scarring of the overlying cortex. (From Jennette J. C. [2008]. The kidney. In Rubin R., Strayer D. [Eds.], *Rubin's pathology: Clinicopathologic foundations of medicine* [5th ed., p. 718]. Philadelphia: Lippincott Williams & Wilkins.)

nephrotoxicity are increased when two or more drugs capable of producing kidney damage are given at the same time.

Drugs and toxic substances can damage the kidneys by causing a decrease in renal blood flow, obstructing urine flow, directly damaging tubulointerstitial structures, or producing hypersensitivity reactions.[58] Some drugs, such as diuretics, high–molecular-weight radiocontrast media, the immunosuppressive drugs cyclosporine and tacrolimus, and the nonsteroidal anti-inflammatory drugs (NSAIDs), can cause acute prerenal failure by decreasing renal blood flow (see Chapter 34). Persons at particular risk are those who already have compromised renal blood flow. Other drugs such as sulfonamides and vitamin C (due to oxalate crystals) can form crystals that cause kidney damage by obstructing urinary flow in the tubules.

Acute drug-related hypersensitivity reactions produce tubulointerstitial nephritis, with damage to the tubules and interstitium. This condition was observed initially in persons who were sensitive to the sulfonamide drugs; currently, it is observed most often with the use of methicillin and other synthetic antibiotics, and with the use of furosemide and the thiazide diuretics in persons sensitive to these drugs. The condition begins approximately 15 days (range, 2 to 40 days) after exposure to the drug.[6] At the onset, there is fever, eosinophilia, hematuria, mild proteinuria, and in approximately one fourth of cases, a rash. In approximately 50% of cases, signs and symptoms of acute renal failure develop. Withdrawal of the drug commonly is followed by complete recovery, but there may be permanent damage in some persons, usually in older persons. Drug nephritis may not be recognized in its early stage because it is relatively uncommon.

Chronic analgesic nephritis, which is associated with analgesic abuse, causes interstitial nephritis with renal papillary necrosis. When first observed, it was attributed to phenacetin, a then-common ingredient of over-the-counter medications containing aspirin, phenacetin, and caffeine. Although phenacetin is no longer contained in these preparations, it has been suggested that other ingredients, such as aspirin and acetaminophen, also may contribute to the disorder. How much analgesic it takes to produce papillary necrosis is unknown. NSAIDs also have the potential for damaging renal structures, including medullary interstitial cells. Prostaglandins (particularly PGI_2 and PGE_2) contribute to the regulation of tubular blood flow.[59] The deleterious effects of NSAIDs on the kidney are thought to result from their ability to inhibit prostaglandin synthesis. Persons particularly at risk are the elderly because of age-related changes in renal function, individuals who are dehydrated or have a decrease in blood volume, and those with preexisting kidney disease or renal insufficiency.

IN SUMMARY, tubulointerstitial diseases affect the tubules and the surrounding interstitium of the kidneys. These disorders include renal tubular acidosis, acute and chronic pyelonephritis, and the effects of drugs and toxins. Renal tubular acidosis describes a form of systemic acidosis that results from tubular defects in bicarbonate reabsorption or hydrogen ion secretion. Pyelonephritis, or infection of the kidney and kidney pelvis, can occur as an acute or a chronic condition. Acute pyelonephritis typically is caused by ascending bladder infections or infections that come from the bloodstream; it usually is successfully treated with appropriate antimicrobial drugs. Chronic pyelonephritis is a progressive disease that produces scarring and deformation of the renal calyces and pelvis. Drug-induced impairment of tubulointerstitial structure and function usually is the result of direct toxic injury, decreased blood flow, or hypersensitivity reactions. ■

MALIGNANT TUMORS OF THE KIDNEY

After completing this section of the chapter, you should be able to meet the following objectives:

- Characterize Wilms tumor in terms of age of onset, possible oncogenic origin, manifestations, and treatment.
- Cite the risk factors for renal cell carcinoma, describe its manifestations, and explain why the 5-year survival rate has been so low.

There are two major groups of malignant tumors of the kidney: embryonic kidney tumors (*i.e.,* Wilms tumor), which occur during childhood, and renal cell carcinoma, which occurs in adults.

Wilms Tumor

Wilms tumor (nephroblastoma) is one of the most common primary neoplasms of young children. It usually presents between 3 and 5 years of age and is the most common malignant abdominal tumor in children.[6] It may occur in one or both kidneys; the incidence of bilateral Wilms tumor is 6% to 7%.[6,60]

Histologically, the tumor is composed of elements that resemble normal fetal tissue: blastemic, stromal, and epithelial. An important feature of Wilms tumor is its association with other congenital anomalies, including aniridia (absence of the iris), hemihypertrophy (enlargement of one side of the face or body), and other congenital anomalies, usually of the genitourinary system. Several chromosomal abnormalities have been associated with Wilms tumor. One Wilms tumor gene, *WT1*, which is located on chromosome 11, encodes a transcription factor that is critical for normal kidney development.[60] Roughly 20% of all Wilms tumors carry *WT1* mutations.[60]

Wilms tumor usually is a solitary mass that occurs in any part of the kidney. It usually is sharply demarcated and variably encapsulated (Fig. 33-16). The tumors grow to a large size, distorting kidney structure. The tumors usually are staged using the National Wilms' Tumor Study Group classification.[60] Stage I tumors are limited to the kidney and can be excised with the capsular surface intact. Stage II tumors extend into the renal capsule but can be excised. In stage III, extension of the tumor is confined to the abdomen, and in stage IV, hematogenous metastasis most commonly involves the lung. Bilateral kidney involvement occurs in 5% to 10% of cases.

The common presenting signs are a large asymptomatic abdominal mass and hypertension.[6,60] The tumor is often discovered inadvertently, and it is not uncommon for the mother to discover it while bathing the child. Some children may present with abdominal pain, vomiting, or both. Microscopic and gross hematuria is present in 17% to 25% of children. CT scans are used to confirm the diagnosis.[60]

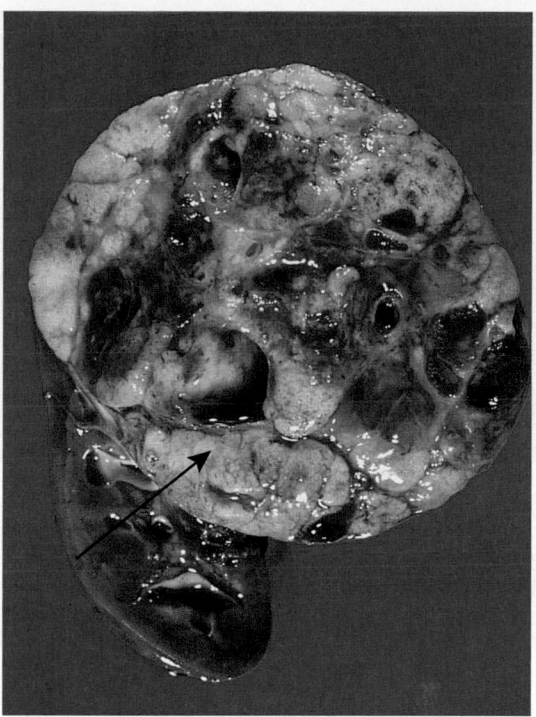

FIGURE 33-16 • Wilms tumor. A cross-section of a pale tan neoplasm (*arrow*) attached to a residual portion of the kidney. (From Jennette J. C. [2008]. The kidney. In Rubin R., Strayer D. [Eds.], *Rubin's pathology: Clinicopathologic foundations of medicine* [5th ed., p. 742]. Philadelphia: Lippincott Williams & Wilkins.)

Treatment involves surgery, chemotherapy, and sometimes radiation therapy. Long-term survival rates have increased to more than 60% for all stages and to 88% to 98% for stages I through III.[60]

Renal Cell Carcinoma

Cancer of the kidney is the 7th leading malignancy among men and the 12th among women, accounting for about 3% of all cancers.[61] Incidence peaks between 55 and 84 years of age.[62] The increased use of imaging procedures such as ultrasonography, CT scanning, and magnetic resonance imaging (MRI) has contributed significantly to earlier diagnosis and more accurate staging of kidney cancers.[61,62]

Renal cell carcinoma accounts for approximately 90% to 95% of kidney tumors.[62] The tumor may arise from any portion of the kidney, but most commonly affects the poles, most commonly the upper pole (Fig. 33-17). The cause of renal cell carcinoma remains unclear. Epidemiologic evidence suggests a correlation between heavy smoking and kidney cancer.[61,62] Obesity also is a risk factor, particularly in women. Additional risk factors include occupational exposure to petroleum products, heavy metals, and asbestos.[6] The risk for renal cell carcinoma also is increased in persons with acquired cystic kidney disease associated with chronic renal insufficiency.

There are pathologic variants of renal cell carcinoma that reflect differences in cellular pathology, genetic profile, and

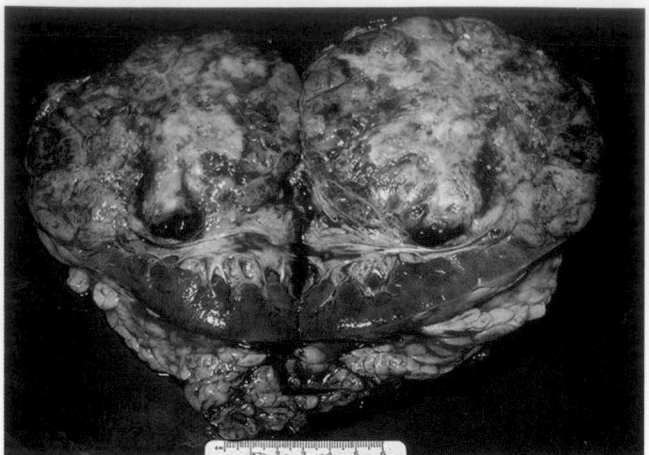

FIGURE 33-17 • Gross pathology of a bisected kidney showing large renal cell carcinoma. Much of the kidney has been replaced by gray and yellow tumor tissue. A little remaining renal cortex and pericapsular fat are visible at the bottom of this surgical specimen. (From Centers for Disease Control and Prevention Public Images Library. [Online.] Available: http://phil.cdc.gov/phil/details.asp.)

clinical features ranging from benign to highly malignant. Categories include clear cell carcinoma (60% of cases), papillary tumors (5% to 10%), chromophobic tumors (5% to 10%), oncocytomas (5% to 10%), and collecting duct tumors (<1%).[62] Clear cell tumors have a clear cytoplasm, usually show chromosome 3 deletions, and arise from proximal tubular epithelial cells. Papillary renal cell tumors tend to be bilateral and multifocal, show trisomy 7 or 17, and arise from proximal tubular cells. Chromophobic tumors are characterized by multiple chromosomal losses but do not exhibit 3 deletions or trisomy 7 or 17, have an indolent clinical course, and appear to arise from intercalated cells of the collecting tubules.[6,62] Collecting duct tumors arise from the collecting ducts within the renal medulla, are very rare, affect younger individuals, and are very aggressive. Oncocytomas do not exhibit chromosomal changes and are considered benign.

Kidney cancer is largely a silent disorder during its early stages, and symptoms usually denote advanced disease. Presenting features include hematuria, flank pain, and presence of a palpable flank mass. Gross or microscopic hematuria, which occurs in 70% to 90% of cases, is an important clinical clue. It is, however, intermittent and may be microscopic; as a result, the tumor may reach considerable size before it is detected. Because of the widespread use of ultrasonography and CT scanning for diverse indications, renal tumors are being detected incidentally in persons with no urologic symptoms.

Kidney cancer is suspected when there are findings of hematuria and a renal mass. Ultrasonography and CT scanning are used to confirm the diagnosis. MRI may be used when involvement of the inferior vena cava is suspected. Renal cancer is commonly staged using the American Joint Committee on Cancer staging system (TNM system, described in Chapter 8).

Surgery (radical nephrectomy with lymph node dissection) is the treatment of choice for all resectable tumors. Nephron-sparing surgery may be done when both kidneys are involved or when the contralateral kidney is threatened by an associated disease such as hypertension or diabetes mellitus. Single-agent and combination chemotherapic have been used with limited success. Immunotherapy involving interferon-alfa and interleukin-2 has been used with some success.[62] The 5-year survival rate is 90% if the tumor has not extended beyond the renal capsule, but drops to 30% if metastasis has occurred.[6]

IN SUMMARY,   there are two major groups of renal neoplasms: embryonic kidney tumors (*i.e.*, Wilms tumor) that occur during childhood and adult renal cell carcinomas. Wilms tumor is one of the most common malignant tumors of children. The most common presenting signs are a large abdominal mass and hypertension. Treatment is surgery, chemotherapy, and sometimes radiation therapy. The long-term survival rate for children with Wilms tumor is approximately 90%, with an aggressive plan of treatment.

Renal cancer accounts for about 3% of all cancers, with a peak incidence between 55 and 84 years of age. Renal cell carcinoma accounts for 90% to 95% of kidney tumors. These tumors are characterized by a lack of early warning signs, diverse clinical manifestations, and resistance to chemotherapy and radiation therapy. Because of the widespread use of ultrasonography and CT scanning for diverse indications, renal tumors are being detected incidentally in persons with no urologic symptoms. Diagnostic methods include ultrasonography and CT scans. The treatment of choice is surgical resection. Prognosis depends on the stage of the cancer; the 5-year survival rate is 90% if the tumor has not extended beyond the renal capsule, but drops to 30% if metastasis has occurred. ■

Review Exercises

1. A 36-year old man is admitted to the emergency department with a sudden onset of severe, intermittent, cramping pain that makes him feel nauseated. He describes the pain as originating in the left groin and radiating toward the flank. Microscopic examination of his urine reveals the presence of red blood cells. His temperature is normal, and he does not exhibit signs of sepsis.

   A. *What is the probable cause of this man's pain?*

   B. *What diagnostic measure could be used to confirm the cause of his pain?*

   C. *A plain-film radiograph reveals a 4- to 5-mm kidney stone in the left ureter. What are the chances that this man will pass the stone spontaneously?*

   D. *What type of medications and other treatments should this man receive?*

   E. *Once the stone has been passed, what type of measures can he use to prevent stone recurrence?*

2. A 6-year-old boy is diagnosed with acute glomerulo-nephritis that developed after a streptococcal throat infection. At this time, the following manifestations are noted: a decrease in urine output, increasing lethargy, hyperventilation, and generalized edema. Trace amounts of protein are detected in his urine. Blood analysis reveals the following: pH = 7.35, HCO_3 = 18 mEq/L, hematocrit = 29%, Na = 132 mEq/L, K = 5.6 mEq/L, blood urea nitrogen (BUN) = 62 mg/dL, creatinine = 4.1 mg/dL, and albumin = 2 g/dL.

   A. What is the probable cause of this boy's glomerular disease?

   B. Use the laboratory values in the Appendix to interpret his laboratory test results. Which values are significant and why?

   C. Is he progressing to uremia? How can you tell?

3. A 26-year-old woman makes an appointment with her health care provider, complaining of urinary frequency, urgency, and burning. She reports that her urine is cloudy and smells abnormal. Her urine is cultured, and she is given a prescription for antibiotics.

   A. What is the most likely cause of the woman's symptoms?

   B. What microorganism is most likely responsible for the infection?

   C. What factors may have predisposed her to this disorder?

   D. What could this woman do to prevent future infection?

References

1. National Kidney Foundation. (2006). Fact sheets: The problem of kidney and urologic diseases. [Online.] Available: www.kidney.org. Accessed May 12, 2007.
2. Moore K. L., Persaud T. V. N. (2003). *The developing human: Clinically oriented embryology* (7th ed., pp. 288–296). Philadelphia: W. B. Saunders.
3. Stewart C. L., Jose P. A. (1991). Transitional nephrology. *Urologic Clinics of North America* 18, 143–149.
4. Elder J. S. (2004). Urologic disorders in infants and children. In Behrman R. E., Kliegman R. M., Jenson H. B. (Eds.), *Nelson textbook of pediatrics* (17th ed., pp. 1783–1789). Philadelphia: Elsevier Saunders.
5. Alpers C. E. (2005). The kidney. In Kumar V., Abbas A. K., Fausto N. (Eds.), *Robbins and Cotran pathologic basis of disease* (7th ed., pp. 961–966, 971–979). Philadelphia: Elsevier Saunders.
6. Jennette J. C. (2008). The kidney. In Rubin R., Strayer D. S. (Eds.), *Rubin's pathology: Clinicopathologic foundations of medicine* (5th ed., pp. 694–698, 867–877, 881–884). Philadelphia: Lippincott Williams & Wilkins.
7. Wilson P. D. (2004). Polycystic kidney disease. *New England Journal of Medicine* 350, 151–164.
8. Sutters M., Germino G. G. (2003). Autosomal dominant polycystic kidney disease: Molecular genetics and pathophysiology. *Journal of Laboratory and Clinical Medicine* 141, 91–110.
9. Igarashi P., Somolo S. (2002). Genetics and pathogenesis of polycystic kidney disease. *Journal of the American Society of Nephrology* 13, 2384–2398.
10. Ong A. C. M., Wheatley D. N. (2003). Polycystic kidney disease: The ciliary connection. *Lancet* 361, 774–776.
11. Bajwa Z. H., Gupta S., Warfield C. A., et al. (2001). Pain management in polycystic kidney disease. *Kidney International* 60, 1631–1644.
12. Asplin J. R., Coe F. L. (2005). Tubular disorders. In Kasper D. L., Braunwald E., Fauci A. S., et al. (Eds.), *Harrison's principles of internal medicine* (16th ed., pp. 1694–1696). New York: McGraw-Hill.
13. Tanagho E. A. (2004). Urinary obstruction and stasis. In Tanagho E. A., McAninch J. W. (Eds.), *Smith's general urology* (16th ed., p. 175). New York: Lange Medical Books/McGraw-Hill.
14. Stoller M. L. (2004). Urinary stone disease. In Tanagho E. A., McAninch J. W. (Eds.), *Smith's general urology* (16th ed., pp. 256–290). New York: Lange Medical Books/McGraw-Hill.
15. Moe O. W. (2006). Kidney stones: Pathophysiology and medical management. *Lancet* 367, 333–444.
16. Coe F. L., Evan A., Worcester E. (2005). Kidney stone disease. *Journal of Clinical Investigation* 115, 2598–2608.
17. Pietrow P. E., Karellas M. E. (2006). Medical management of urinary calculi. *American Family Physician* 74, 86–94, 99–100.
18. Portis A. J., Sundram C. P. (2001). Diagnosis and initial management of kidney stones. *American Family Physician* 63, 1329–1338.
19. Menhert-Kay S. A. (2005). Diagnosis and management of uncomplicated urinary tract infections. *American Family Physician* 72, 451–456, 458.
20. Nguyen H. T. (2004). Bacterial infections of the genitourinary tract. In Tanagho E. A., McAninch J. W. (Eds.), *Smith's general urology* (16th ed., pp. 203–227). New York: Lange Medical Books/McGraw-Hill.
21. Stamm W. E. (2002). Scientific and clinical challenges in the management of urinary tract infections. *American Journal of Medicine* 113(Suppl. 1A), 1S–4S.
22. Stapleton A. (2002). Urinary tract infections in patients with diabetes. *American Journal of Medicine* 113(Suppl. 1A), 80S–84S.
23. McLaughlin S. P., Carson C. D. (2004). Urinary tract infections in women. *Medical Clinics of North America* 88, 417–429.
24. Saint S., Chenoweth C. E. (2003). Biofilms and catheter-associated urinary tract infections. *Infectious Disease Clinics of North America* 17, 411–432.
25. Nicolle L. E. (2002). Urinary tract infections: Traditional pharmacologic therapies. *American Journal of Medicine* 113(Suppl. 1A), 35S–44S.
26. Manges A. R., Johnson J. R., Foxman B., et al. (2001). Widespread distribution of urinary tract infections caused by multidrug resistant *Escherichia coli* colonial group. *New England Journal of Medicine* 345, 1007–1013.
27. Raz R., Chazan B., Dan M. (2004). Cranberry juice and urinary tract infection. *Clinical Infectious Diseases* 38, 1413–1419.
28. Lynch D. M. (2004). Cranberry for prevention of urinary tract infections. *American Family Physician* 20, 2175–2177.
29. Fihn S. D. (2003). Acute uncomplicated urinary tract infections in women. *New England Journal of Medicine* 349, 259–266.
30. Mittal P., Wing D. A. (2005). Urinary tract infections in pregnancy. *Clinics in Perinatology* 32, 749–764.
31. Macejko A. M., Schaeffer A. J. (2007). Asymptomatic bacteriuria and symptomatic urinary tract infections during pregnancy. *Urology Clinics of North America* 34, 35–42.
32. American College of Obstetricians and Gynecologists. (1998). *Antimicrobial therapy for obstetric patients* (pp. 8–10). ACOG Educational Bulletin no. 245. Washington, DC: Author.
33. Shortliffe L. M., McCue J. D. (2002). Urinary tract infections at the age extremes: Pediatrics and geriatrics. *American Journal of Medicine* 113(Suppl. 1A), 55S–66S.
34. Zorc J. L., Kiddoo D. A., Shaw K. N. (2005). Diagnosis and management of pediatric urinary tract infections. *Clinical Microbiology Reviews* 18, 417–422.
35. Chang S. L., Shortliffe L. D. (2006). Pediatric urinary tract infections. *Pediatric Clinics of North America* 53, 379–400.

36. Alper B. S., Curry S. H. (2005). Urinary tract infections in children. *American Family Physician* 72, 2483–2488.

37. Mouton C. P., Pierce B., Espino D. V. (2001). Common infections in older adults. *American Family Physician* 63, 257–268.

38. Chadban S. J., Atkins R. C. (2005). Glomerulonephritis. *Lancet* 365, 1797–1806.

39. Brady H. R., O'Meara Y. M., Brenner B. M. (2005). Glomerular diseases. In Kasper D. L., Braunwald E., Fauci A. S., et al. (Eds.), *Harrison's principles of internal medicine* (16th ed., pp. 1674–1694). New York: McGraw-Hill.

40. Lau K. K., Wyatt R. J. (2005). Glomerulonephritis. *Adolescent Medicine* 16, 67–85.

41. Vinen C. S., Oliveira D. B. G. (2003). Acute glomerulonephritis. *Postgraduate Medicine Journal* 79, 206–213.

42. Glassock R. J. (2003). The glomerulopathies. In Schrier R. W. (Ed.), *Renal and electrolyte disorders* (6th ed., pp. 623–670). Philadelphia: Lippincott Williams & Wilkins.

43. Hricik D. E., Chung-Park M., Sedor J. R. (1998). Glomerulonephritis. *New England Journal of Medicine* 339, 888–899.

44. Vincenti F. G., Amend W. J. C. (2004). Diagnosis of medical renal diseases. In Tanagho E. A., McAninch J. W. (Eds.), *Smith's general urology* (16th ed., pp. 527–537). New York: Lange Medical Books/McGraw-Hill.

45. Orth S. R., Ritz E. (1998). The nephrotic syndrome. *New England Journal of Medicine* 339, 1202–1211.

46. Eddy A. A., Symons J. M. (2003). Nephrotic syndrome in childhood. *Lancet* 362, 629–639.

47. Coresh J., Astor B. C., Greene T., et al. (2003). Prevalence of chronic kidney disease and decreased kidney function in the adult U.S. population: Third National Health and Nutrition Examination Survey. *American Journal of Kidney Disease* 42, 1–12.

48. Donadio J. V., Grande J. P. (2002). IgA nephropathy. *New England Journal of Medicine* 347, 738–748.

49. Baratt J., Feehally J. (2005). IgA nephropathy. *Journal of the American Society of Nephrology* 16, 2088–2097.

50. Weening J. J., D'Agati V. D., Schwartz M. M. (2004). The classification of glomerulonephritis in systemic lupus erythematosus. *Journal of the American Society of Nephrology* 15, 241–250.

51. Gross J. L., De Azevedo M. J., Silverdo P., et al. (2005). Diabetic nephropathy: Diagnosis, prevention, and treatment. *Diabetes Care* 28, 164–188.

52. Remuzza G., Schiepatti A., Ruggenenti P. (2002). Nephropathy in patients with type 2 diabetes. *New England Journal of Medicine* 346, 1145–1151.

53. Jawa A., Kcomt J., Fonseca V. A. (2004). Diabetic nephropathy and retinopathy. *Medical Clinics of North America* 88, 1001–1036.

54. Schena F. P., Gesualdo L. (2005). Pathogenic mechanisms of diabetic nephropathy. *Journal of the American Society of Nephrology* 16(Suppl. 1), S30–S33.

55. Soriano J. R. (2002). Renal tubular acidosis: The clinical entity. *Journal of the American Society of Nephrology* 13, 2160–2170.

56. Kurtzman N. A. (2000). Renal tubular acidosis syndromes. *Southern Medical Journal* 93, 1042–1052.

57. Ramakrishnan K., Scheid D. (2005). Diagnosis and management of acute pyelonephritis in adults. *American Family Physician* 71, 933–942.

58. Guo S., Nzerue C. (2002). How to prevent, recognize, and treat drug-induced nephrotoxicity. *Cleveland Clinic Journal of Medicine* 69, 289–297.

59. Taber S. S., Mueller B. A. (2006). Drug-associated renal dysfunction. *Critical Care Clinics* 22, 357–374.

60. Jaffe N., Huff V. (2004). Neoplasms of the kidney. In Behrman R. E., Kliegman R. M., Jenson H. B. (Eds.), *Nelson textbook of pediatrics* (17th ed., pp. 1711–1714). Philadelphia: Elsevier Saunders.

61. Cohen H. T., McGovern F. J. (2005). Renal-cell carcinoma. *New England Journal of Medicine* 353, 2477–2490.

62. Scher H. I., Motzer R. J. (2005). Bladder and renal cell carcinoma. In Kasper D. L., Braunwald E., Fauci A. S., et al. (Eds.), *Harrison's principles of internal medicine* (16th ed., pp. 541–543). New York: McGraw-Hill.

Visit the Point. **http://thePoint.lww.com for animations, journal articles, and more!**

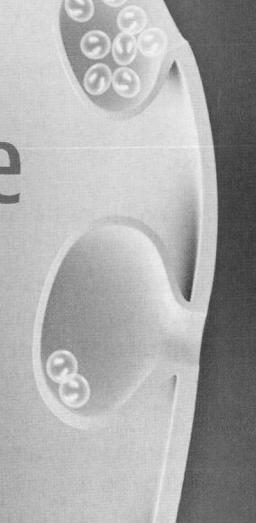

Acute Renal Failure and Chronic Kidney Disease

Chapter **34**

CAROL M. PORTH

➤ Renal failure is a condition in which the kidneys fail to remove metabolic end products from the blood and regulate the fluid, electrolyte, and pH balance of the extracellular fluids. The underlying cause may be renal disease, systemic disease, or urologic defects of nonrenal origin. Renal failure can occur as an acute or a chronic disorder. Acute renal failure is abrupt in onset and often is reversible if recognized early and treated appropriately. In contrast, chronic kidney disease is the end result of irreparable damage to the kidneys. It develops slowly, usually over the course of a number of years.

ACUTE RENAL FAILURE

After completing this section of the chapter, you should be able to meet the following objectives:

■ Describe acute renal failure in terms of its causes, treatment, and outcome.
■ Differentiate the prerenal, intrinsic, and postrenal forms of acute renal failure in terms of the mechanisms of development and manifestations.
■ Cite the two most common causes of acute tubular necrosis and describe the course of the disease in terms of the initiation, maintenance, and recovery phases.

Acute renal failure represents a rapid decline in kidney function sufficient to increase blood levels of nitrogenous wastes and impair fluid and electrolyte balance.[1-8] Unlike chronic kidney disease and failure, acute renal failure is potentially reversible if the precipitating factors can be corrected or removed before permanent kidney damage has occurred.

Acute renal failure is a common threat to seriously ill persons in intensive care units, with a mortality rate ranging from 40% to 75%.[2] Although treatment methods such as dialysis and renal replacement therapies are effective in correcting life-threatening fluid and electrolyte disorders, the mortality rate from acute renal failure has not changed substantially since the 1960s.[1] This probably is because acute renal failure is seen

🔑 ACUTE RENAL FAILURE

- Acute renal failure is caused by conditions that produce an acute shutdown in renal function.

- It can result from decreased blood flow to the kidney (prerenal failure), disorders that disrupt the structures in the kidney (intrinsic or intrarenal failure), or disorders that interfere with the elimination of urine from the kidney (postrenal failure).

- Acute renal failure, although it causes an accumulation of products normally cleared by the kidney, is a potentially reversible process if the factors causing the condition can be corrected.

more often in older persons than before, and because it frequently is superimposed on other life-threatening conditions, such as trauma, shock, and sepsis.

The most common indicator of acute renal failure is *azotemia*, an accumulation of nitrogenous wastes (urea nitrogen, uric acid, and creatinine) in the blood and a decrease in the glomerular filtration rate (GFR). As a result, excretion of nitrogenous wastes is reduced and fluid and electrolyte balance cannot be maintained.

Types of Acute Renal Failure

Acute renal failure can be caused by several types of conditions, including a decrease in blood flow without ischemic injury; ischemic, toxic, or obstructive tubular injury; and obstruction of urinary tract outflow. The causes of acute renal failure commonly are categorized as prerenal, intrinsic, and postrenal[1–8] (Fig. 34-1). Collectively, prerenal and intrinsic causes account

for 80% to 95% of acute renal failure cases.[3] Causes of renal failure within these categories are summarized in Chart 34-1.

Prerenal Failure

Prerenal failure, the most common form of acute renal failure, is characterized by a marked decrease in renal blood flow. It is reversible if the cause of the decreased renal blood flow can be identified and corrected before kidney damage occurs. Causes of prerenal failure include profound depletion of vascular volume (*e.g.,* hemorrhage, loss of extracellular fluid volume), impaired perfusion due to heart failure and cardiogenic shock, and decreased vascular filling because of increased vascular capacity (*e.g.,* anaphylaxis or sepsis). Elderly persons are particularly at risk because of their predisposition to hypovolemia and their high prevalence of renal vascular disorders.

Some vasoactive mediators, drugs, and diagnostic agents stimulate intense intrarenal vasoconstriction and can induce glomerular hypoperfusion and prerenal failure. Examples include endotoxins, radiocontrast agents such as those used for cardiac catheterization, cyclosporine (an immunosuppressant drug that is used to prevent transplant rejection), amphotericin B (an antifungal agent), epinephrine, and high doses of dopamine.[3] Many of these drugs also cause acute tubular necrosis (discussed later). In addition, several commonly used classes of drugs can impair renal adaptive mechanisms and can convert compensated renal

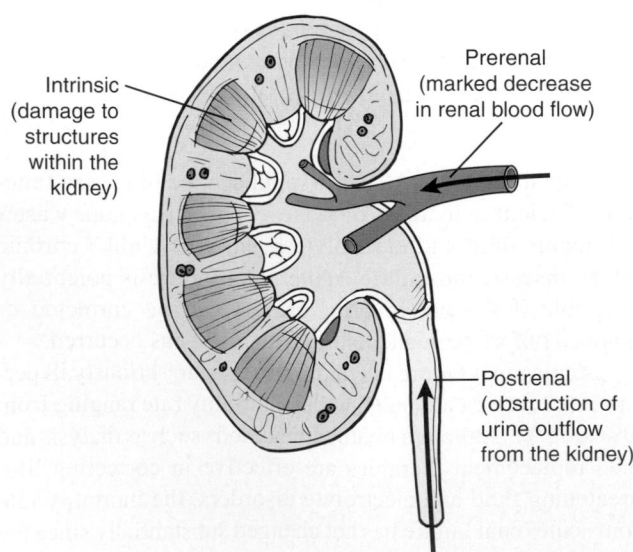

Intrinsic (damage to structures within the kidney)

Prerenal (marked decrease in renal blood flow)

Postrenal (obstruction of urine outflow from the kidney)

FIGURE 34-1 • Types of acute renal failure.

CHART 34-1	**CAUSES OF ACUTE RENAL FAILURE**

Prerenal
Hypovolemia
   Hemorrhage
   Dehydration
   Excessive loss of gastrointestinal tract fluids
   Excessive loss of fluid due to burn injury
Decreased vascular filling
   Anaphylactic shock
   Septic shock
Heart failure and cardiogenic shock
Decreased renal perfusion due to sepsis, vasoactive
   mediators, drugs, diagnostic agents

Intrinsic or intrarenal
Acute tubular necrosis
   Prolonged renal ischemia
   Exposure to nephrotoxic drugs, heavy metals, and
     organic solvents
   Intratubular obstruction resulting from hemoglobin-
     uria, myoglobinuria, myeloma light chains, or
     uric acid casts
   Acute renal disease (acute glomerulonephritis,
     pyelonephritis)

Postrenal
Bilateral ureteral obstruction
Bladder outlet obstruction

hypoperfusion into prerenal failure. Angiotensin-converting enzyme (ACE) inhibitors and angiotensin receptor blockers (ARBs) reduce the effects of renin on renal blood flow; when combined with diuretics, they may cause prerenal failure in persons with decreased blood flow due to large-vessel or small-vessel kidney disease. Prostaglandins have a vasodilatory effect on renal blood vessels. Nonsteroidal anti-inflammatory drugs (NSAIDs) can reduce renal blood flow through inhibition of prostaglandin synthesis. In some persons with diminished renal perfusion, NSAIDs can precipitate prerenal failure.

Normally, the kidneys receive 22% of the cardiac output.[9] This large blood supply is required to remove metabolic wastes and regulate body fluids and electrolytes. Fortunately, the normal kidney can tolerate relatively large reductions in blood flow before renal damage occurs. As renal blood flow is reduced, the GFR decreases, the amount of sodium and other substances that are filtered by the glomeruli is reduced, and the need for energy-dependent mechanisms to reabsorb these substance is reduced (see Chapter 30). As the GFR and urine output approach zero, oxygen consumption by the kidney approximates that required to keep renal tubular cells alive. When blood flow falls below this level, which is about 25% of normal, ischemic changes occur.[9] Because of their high metabolic rate, the tubular epithelial cells are most vulnerable to ischemic injury. Improperly treated, prolonged renal hypoperfusion can lead to ischemic tubular necrosis with significant morbidity and mortality.

Prerenal failure is manifested by a sharp decrease in urine output and a disproportionate elevation of blood urea nitrogen (BUN) in relation to serum creatinine levels. The kidney normally responds to a decrease in the GFR with a decrease in urine output. Thus, an early sign of prerenal failure is a sharp decrease in urine output. A low fractional excretion of sodium (<1%) suggests that oliguria is due to decreased renal perfusion and that the nephrons are responding appropriately by decreasing the excretion of filtered sodium in an attempt to preserve vascular volume. BUN levels also depend on the GFR. A low GFR allows more time for small particles such as urea to be reabsorbed into the blood. Creatinine, which is larger and nondiffusible, remains in the tubular fluid, and the total amount of creatinine that is filtered, although small, is excreted in the urine. Consequently, there also is a disproportionate elevation in the ratio of BUN to serum creatinine, from a normal value of 10:1 to a ratio greater than 15:1 to 20:1.[1]

Postrenal Failure

Postrenal failure results from obstruction of urine outflow from the kidneys. The obstruction can occur in the ureter (*i.e.,* calculi and strictures), bladder (*i.e.,* tumors or neurogenic bladder), or urethra (*i.e.,* prostatic hyperplasia). Prostatic hyperplasia is the most common underlying problem. Because both ureters must be occluded to produce renal failure, obstruction of the bladder rarely causes acute renal failure unless one of the kidneys already is damaged or a person has only one kidney. The treatment of acute postrenal failure consists of treating the underlying cause of obstruction so that urine flow can be reestablished before permanent nephron damage occurs.

Intrinsic Renal Failure

Intrinsic or intrarenal renal failure results from conditions that cause damage to structures within the kidney—glomerular, tubular, or interstitial. The major causes of intrarenal failure are ischemia associated with prerenal failure, toxic insult to the tubular structures of the nephron, and intratubular obstruction. Acute glomerulonephritis and acute pyelonephritis also are intrarenal causes of acute renal failure. Injury to the tubular structures of the nephron (acute tubular necrosis) is the most common cause and often is ischemic or toxic in origin.

Acute Tubular Necrosis. Acute tubular necrosis (ATN) is characterized by the destruction of tubular epithelial cells with acute suppression of renal function (Fig. 34-2). ATN can be caused by a variety of conditions, including acute tubular damage due to ischemia, sepsis, nephrotoxic effects of drugs, tubular obstruction, and toxins from a massive infection.[3–5,10] Tubular epithelial cells are particularly sensitive to ischemia and also are vulnerable to toxins. The tubular injury that occurs in ATN frequently is reversible. The process depends on recovery of the injured cells, removal of the necrotic cells and intratubular casts, and regeneration of renal cells to restore the normal continuity of the tubular epithelium.[5,11]

Ischemic ATN occurs most frequently in persons who have major surgery, severe hypovolemia, or overwhelming sepsis, trauma, or burns.[3] Sepsis produces ischemia by provoking a combination of systemic vasodilation and intrarenal hypoper-

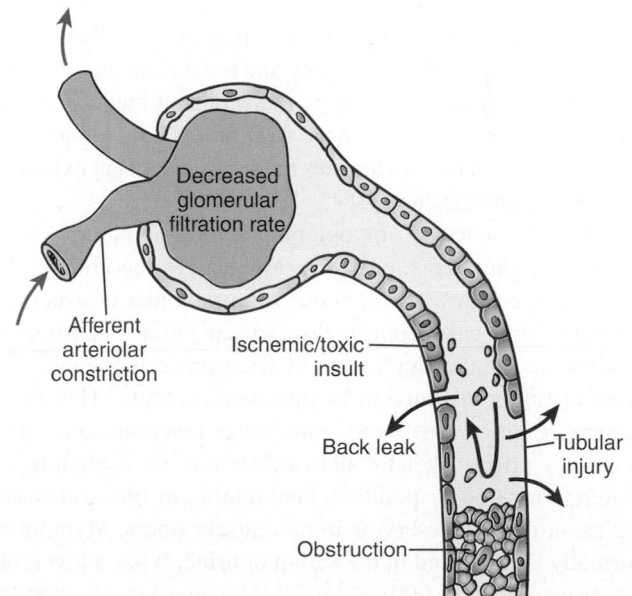

FIGURE 34-2 • Pathogenesis of acute tubular necrosis. Sloughing and necrosis of tubular epithelial cells lead to obstruction and increased intraluminal pressure, which reduce glomerular filtration. Afferent arteriolar vasoconstriction caused in part by tubuloglomerular feedback mechanisms results in decreased glomerular capillary filtration pressure. Tubular injury and increased intraluminal pressure cause fluid to move from the tubular lumen into the interstitium (back leak). (Modified from Rubin E., Farber J. L. [Eds.]. [1999]. *Pathology* [3rd ed., p. 901]. Philadelphia: Lippincott-Raven.)

fusion. In addition, sepsis results in the generation of toxins that sensitize renal tubular cells to the damaging effects of ischemia. ATN complicating trauma and burns frequently is multifactorial in origin, resulting from the combined effects of hypovolemia, myoglobinuria, and other toxins released from damaged tissue. In contrast to prerenal failure, the GFR does not improve with the restoration of renal blood flow in acute renal failure caused by ischemic ATN.

Nephrotoxic ATN complicates the administration of or exposure to many structurally diverse drugs and other nephrotoxic agents. These agents cause tubular injury by inducing varying combinations of renal vasoconstriction, direct tubular damage, or intratubular obstruction. The kidney is particularly vulnerable to nephrotoxic injury because of its rich blood supply and ability to concentrate toxins to high levels in the medullary portion of the kidney. In addition, the kidney is an important site for metabolic processes that transform relatively harmless agents into toxic metabolites. Pharmacologic agents that are directly toxic to the renal tubule include antimicrobials such as aminoglycosides (e.g., gentamicin), cancer chemotherapeutic agents such as cisplatin and ifosfamide, and radiocontrast agents.[3,5,8,10] Several factors contribute to aminoglycoside nephrotoxicity, including a decrease in the GFR, preexisting renal disease, hypovolemia, and concurrent administration of other drugs that have a nephrotoxic effect. Nonoliguric ATN occurs in 10% to 30% of courses of aminoglycoside therapy, even when the blood levels of the drug are within therapeutic ranges.[3] Cisplatin accumulates in proximal tubule cells, inducing mitochondrial injury and inhibition of adenosine triphosphatase (ATP) activity and solute transport. Radiocontrast media–induced nephrotoxicity is thought to result from direct tubular toxicity and renal ischemia.[12,13] The risk for renal damage caused by radiocontrast media is greatest in elderly persons and those with preexisting kidney disease, volume depletion, diabetes mellitus, and recent exposure to other nephrotoxic agents.

The presence of myoglobin, hemoglobin, uric acid, myeloma light chains, or excess uric acid in the urine is the most frequent cause of ATN due to intratubular obstruction. Both myeloma cast nephropathy and acute urate nephropathy usually are seen in the setting of widespread malignancy or massive tumor destruction by therapeutic agents.[3] Hemoglobinuria results from blood transfusion reactions and other hemolytic crises. Skeletal and cardiac muscles contain myoglobin, which corresponds to hemoglobin in function, serving as an oxygen reservoir in the muscle fibers. Myoglobin normally is not found in the serum or urine. It has a low molecular weight of 17,000 daltons; if it escapes into the circulation, it is rapidly filtered in the glomerulus. Myoglobinuria most commonly results from muscle trauma, but may result from extreme exertion, hyperthermia, sepsis, prolonged seizures, potassium or phosphate depletion, and alcoholism or drug abuse. Both myoglobin and hemoglobin discolor the urine, which may range from the color of tea to red, brown, or black.

The course of ATN can be divided into three phases: the onset or initiating phase, the maintenance phase, and the recovery or convalescent phase. The *onset* or *initiating phase,* which lasts hours or days, is the time from the onset of the precipitating event (*e.g.,* ischemic phase of prerenal failure or toxin exposure) until tubular injury occurs.

The *maintenance phase* of ATN is characterized by a marked decrease in the GFR, causing sudden retention of endogenous metabolites, such as urea, potassium, sulfate, and creatinine, that normally are cleared by the kidneys. The urine output usually is lowest at this point. Fluid retention gives rise to edema, water intoxication, and pulmonary congestion. If the period of oliguria is prolonged, hypertension frequently develops and with it signs of uremia. When untreated, the neurologic manifestations of uremia progress from neuromuscular irritability to seizures, somnolence, coma, and death. Hyperkalemia usually is asymptomatic until the serum potassium level rises above 6 to 6.5 mEq/L, at which point characteristic electrocardiographic changes and symptoms of muscle weakness are seen.

Formerly, most patients with ATN were oliguric. During the past several decades, a nonoliguric form of ATN has become increasingly prevalent. Persons with nonoliguric failure have higher levels of glomerular filtration and excrete more nitrogenous waste, water, and electrolytes in their urine than persons with acute oliguric renal failure. Abnormalities in blood chemistry levels usually are milder and cause fewer complications. The decrease in oliguric ATN probably reflects new approaches to the treatment of poor cardiac performance and circulatory failure that focus on vigorous plasma volume expansion and the selective use of dopamine and other drugs to improve renal blood flow (see Chapter 26). Dopamine has renal vasodilator properties and inhibits sodium reabsorption in the proximal tubule, thereby decreasing the work demands of the nephron.

The *recovery phase* is the period during which repair of renal tissue takes place. Its onset usually is heralded by a gradual increase in urine output and a fall in serum creatinine, indicating that the nephrons have recovered to the point at which urine excretion is possible. Diuresis often occurs before renal function has fully returned to normal. Consequently, BUN and serum creatinine, potassium, and phosphate levels may remain elevated or continue to rise even though urine output is increased. In some cases, the diuresis may result from impaired nephron function and may cause excessive loss of water and electrolytes. Eventually, renal tubular function is restored with improvement in concentrating ability. At about the same time, the BUN and creatinine begin to return to normal. In some cases, mild to moderate kidney damage persists.

Diagnosis and Treatment

Given the high morbidity and mortality rates associated with acute renal failure, attention should be focused on prevention and early diagnosis. This includes assessment measures to identify persons at risk for development of acute renal failure, including those with preexisting renal insufficiency and diabetes. These persons arc particularly at risk for development of acute renal failure due to nephrotoxic drugs (*e.g.*, aminoglycosides and radiocontrast agents), or drugs such as the NSAIDs that alter intrarenal hemodynamics. Elderly persons are susceptible to all forms of acute renal failure because of the effects of aging on renal reserve.

Careful observation of urine output is essential for persons at risk for development of acute renal failure. Urine tests that measure urine osmolality, urinary sodium concentration, and fractional excretion of sodium help differentiate prerenal azotemia, in which the reabsorptive capacity of the tubular cells is maintained, from tubular necrosis, in which these functions are lost. One of the earliest manifestations of tubular damage is the inability to concentrate the urine.

Further diagnostic information that can be obtained from the urinalysis includes evidence of proteinuria, hemoglobinuria, and casts or crystals in the urine. Blood tests for BUN and creatinine provide information regarding the ability to remove nitrogenous wastes from the blood. It also is important to exclude urinary obstruction.

A major concern in the treatment of acute renal failure is identifying and correcting the cause (*e.g.*, improving renal perfusion, discontinuing nephrotoxic drugs). Fluids are carefully regulated in an effort to maintain normal fluid volume and electrolyte concentrations. Adequate caloric intake is needed to prevent the breakdown of body proteins, which increases nitrogenous wastes.[5,8,10] Parenteral hyperalimentation may be used for this purpose. Because secondary infections are a major cause of death in persons with acute renal failure, constant effort is needed to prevent and treat such infections.

Hemodialysis or continuous renal replacement therapy (CRRT) may be indicated when nitrogenous wastes and the water and electrolyte balance cannot be kept under control by other means.[5,10] Venovenous or arteriovenous CRRT has emerged as a method for treating acute renal failure in patients too hemodynamically unstable to tolerate hemodialysis. An associated advantage of the CRRTs is the ability to administer nutritional support. The disadvantages are the need for prolonged anticoagulation and continuous sophisticated monitoring.

IN SUMMARY, acute renal failure is an acute, potentially reversible suppression of kidney function. It is a common threat to seriously ill persons in intensive care units, with a mortality rate of 40% to 75%. Acute renal failure is characterized by a decrease in GFR, accumulation of nitrogenous wastes in the blood (*i.e.*, azotemia), and alterations in body fluids and electrolytes. Acute renal failure is classified as prerenal, intrinsic or intrarenal, or postrenal in origin. Prerenal failure is caused by decreased blood flow to the kidneys; postrenal failure by obstruction to urine output; and intrinsic renal failure by disorders in the kidney itself. Acute tubular necrosis, due to ischemia, sepsis, or nephrotoxic agents, is a common cause of acute intrinsic renal failure. ATN typically progresses through three phases: the initiation phase, during which tubular injury is induced; the maintenance phase, during which the GFR falls, nitrogenous

wastes accumulate, and urine output decreases; and the recovery or reparative phase, during which the GFR, urine output, and blood levels of nitrogenous wastes return to normal.

Because of the high morbidity and mortality rates associated with acute renal failure, identification of persons at risk is important to clinical decision making. Acute renal failure often is reversible, making early identification and correction of the underlying cause (*e.g.*, improving renal perfusion, discontinuing nephrotoxic drugs) important. Treatment includes the judicious administration of fluids and hemodialysis or CRRT. ∎

 ## CHRONIC KIDNEY DISEASE

After completing this section of the chapter, you should be able to meet the following objectives:

- State the most common causes of chronic kidney disease.
- Describe the five stages of chronic kidney disease.
- Describe the methods used to arrive at an accurate estimation of the GFR and explain the rationale for its use in defining the stages of chronic kidney disease.
- Explain the physiologic mechanisms underlying the common problems associated with chronic kidney disease, including alterations in fluid and electrolyte balance and disorders of skeletal, hematologic, cardiovascular, immune system, neurologic, skin, and sexual function.
- State the basis for adverse drug reactions in patients with chronic kidney disease.
- Describe the scientific principles underlying dialysis treatment, and compare hemodialysis with peritoneal dialysis.
- Cite the possible complications of kidney transplantation.
- State the goals for dietary management of persons with chronic kidney disease.

Chronic kidney disease is a worldwide problem affecting people of all ages, races, and economic groups. The prevalence and incidence of the disease, which mirrors that of conditions such as diabetes, hypertension, and obesity, is rising. In the United States alone, more than 20 million people or 1 in 9 adults have chronic kidney disease, and another 20 million are at increased risk for development of the disorder.[14]

Definition and Classification

In 2002, the Kidney Disease Outcome Quality Initiative (K/DOQI) of the National Kidney Foundation (NKF) published clinical practice guidelines for chronic kidney disease.[14] The

CHRONIC KIDNEY DISEASE

- Chronic kidney disease (CKD) represents the progressive decline in kidney function due to the permanent loss of nephrons.

- CKD can result from a number of conditions, including diabetes, hypertension, glomerulonephritis, and other kidney diseases.

- The glomerular filtration rate (GFR) is considered the best measure of kidney function.

- The National Kidney Foundation (NKF) Practice Guidelines divide CKD into five stages based on GFR, beginning with minimal loss of renal function (stage 1) and progressing to kidney failure (stage 5).

- The Practice Guidelines are intended to encourage the early diagnosis of CKD so that measures to delay or prevent its progression are instituted.

goals of the Work Group that developed the guidelines were to define chronic kidney disease and classify its stages, to evaluate laboratory measures used for assessment of kidney disease, and to associate the level of kidney function with the complications of chronic kidney disease. The K/DOQI definition and classification were later accepted by participants in an International Controversies Conference on Kidney Disease: Improving Global Outcomes (KDIGO).[15] The guidelines use the GFR to classify chronic kidney disease into five stages, beginning with kidney damage with normal or elevated GFR, progressing to chronic kidney disease and, potentially, to kidney failure (Table 34-1). It is anticipated that early detection of kidney damage along with implementation of aggressive measures to decrease its progression can delay or prevent the onset of kidney failure.

According to the NKF guidelines, individuals with a GFR of 60 to 89 mL/min/1.73 m² (corrected for body surface area) without kidney damage are classified as "decreased GFR."[14] Decreased GFR without recognized markers of kidney damage can occur in infants and older adults, and is usually considered to be "normal for age." Other causes of chronically decreased GFR without kidney damage in adults include removal of one kidney, extracellular fluid volume depletion, and systemic illnesses associated with reduced kidney perfusion, such as heart failure and cir-

rhosis.[14] Even at this stage, there is often a characteristic loss of renal reserve.

Chronic kidney disease (CKD) is defined as either kidney damage or a GFR less than 60 mL/min/1.73 m² for 3 months or longer.[14–17] CKD can result from a number of conditions that cause permanent loss of nephrons, including diabetes, hypertension, glomerulonephritis, systemic lupus erythematosus, and polycystic kidney disease. Hypertension and diabetic kidney disease are the two main causes of CKD in the United States.[18]

The NKF Practice Guidelines define kidney failure "as either (1) a GFR of less than 15 mL/min/1.73 m², usually accompanied by most of the signs and symptoms of uremia, or (2) a need to start renal replacement therapy (dialysis or transplantation)."[14] These guidelines point out that kidney failure is not synonymous with end-stage renal disease (ESRD), which is an administrative term in the United States that indicates a person is being treated with dialysis and transplantation, a condition that qualifies persons to receive health care through the Medicare ESRD program.

Regardless of cause, CKD represents a loss of functioning kidney nephrons with progressive deterioration of glomerular filtration, tubular reabsorptive capacity, and endocrine functions of the kidneys (Fig. 34-3). All forms of CKD are characterized by a reduction in the GFR, reflecting a corresponding reduction in the number of functional nephrons. The rate of nephron destruction differs from case to case, ranging from several months to many years. Typically, the signs and symptoms of CKD occur gradually and do not become evident until the disease is far advanced. This is because of the amazing compensatory ability of the kidneys. As kidney structures are destroyed, the remaining nephrons undergo structural and functional hypertrophy, each increasing its function as a means of compensating for those that have been lost. In the process, each of the remaining nephrons must filter more solute particles from the blood. It is only when the few remaining nephrons are destroyed that the manifestations of kidney failure become evident.

Assessment of Glomerular Filtration Rate and Other Indicators of Renal Function

The GFR is considered the best measure of overall function of the kidney. The normal GFR, which varies with age, sex, and body

TABLE 34-1 Stages of Chronic Kidney Disease

STAGE	DESCRIPTION	GFR (mL/min/1.73 m²)
1	Kidney damage with normal or increased GFR	≥90
2	Kidney damage with mild decrease in GFR	60–89
3	Moderate decrease in GFR	30–59
4	Severe decrease in GFR	15–29
5	Kidney failure	<15 (or dialysis)

Adapted from National Kidney Foundation. (2002). K/DOQI Clinical Practice Guidelines for Chronic Kidney Disease: Evaluation, classification, and stratification. [Online.] Available: www.kidney.org/professionals/kdoqi/guidelines_ckd/toc/htm. Accessed January 19, 2007.

Chronic kidney disease is defined as either kidney damage or GFR <60 mL/min/1.73 m² for ≥3 months. Kidney damage is defined as pathologic abnormalities or markers of damage, including abnormalities in blood or urine tests or imaging studies.

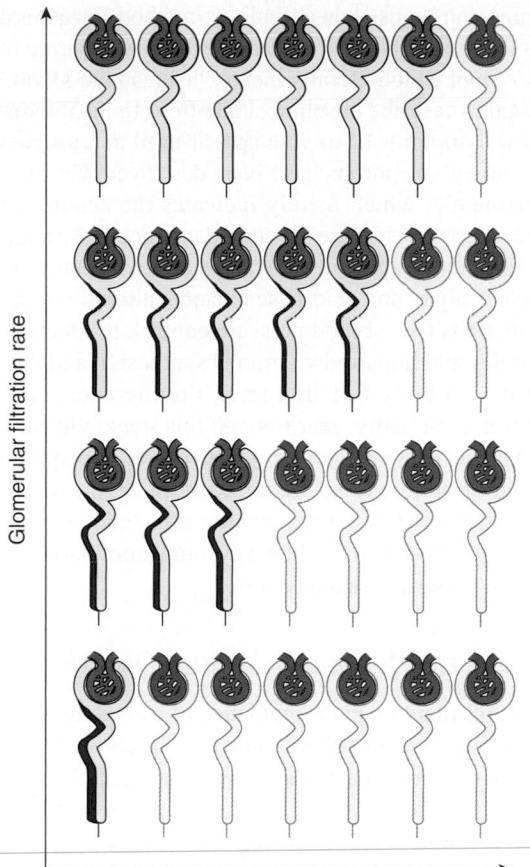

FIGURE 34-3 • Relation of renal function and nephron mass. Each kidney contains about 1 million tiny nephrons. A proportional relation exists between the number of nephrons affected by a disease process and the resulting glomerular filtration rate.

size, is approximately 120 to 130 mL/min/1.73 m² for normal young healthy adults.[14,16] A GFR below 60 mL/min/1.73 m² represents a loss of one half or more the level of normal adult kidney function.[15,16] In clinical practice, GFR is usually estimated using the serum creatinine concentration. Although the GFR can be obtained from measurements of creatinine clearance using timed (*e.g.,* 24-hour) urine collection methods, the levels gathered are reportedly no more reliable than the estimated levels obtained by using serum creatinine levels.[14] Because GFR varies with age, sex, ethnicity, and body size, the Cockroft and Gault or Modification of Diet in Renal Diseases (MDRD) equations that take these factors into account are used for estimating the GFR based on serum creatinine levels[14,16,19] (Box 34-1).

Albuminuria serves as a key adjunctive tool for measuring nephron injury and repair. Urine normally contains small amounts of protein. However, a persistent increase in protein excretion usually is a sign of kidney damage. The type of protein (*e.g.,* low–molecular-weight globulins or albumin) depends on the type of kidney disease.[20] Increased excretion of low–molecular-weight globulins is a marker of tubulointerstitial disease, and excretion of albumin a marker of CKD, resulting from hypertension or diabetes mellitus. For the diagnosis of CKD in adults and postpuberal children with diabetes, measurement of urinary albumin is preferred.[21] In most cases, urine dipstick tests are acceptable for detecting albuminuria. If the urine dipstick test is positive (1+ or greater), albuminuria is usually confirmed by quantitative measurement of the albumin-to-creatinine ratio in a spot (untimed) urine specimen.[20,21] Microalbuminuria, which is an early sign of diabetic kidney disease, refers to albumin excretion that is above the normal range, but below the range normally detected by tests of total protein excretion in the urine (see Chapter 42). Populations at risk for CKD (*i.e.,* those with diabetes mellitus, hypertension, or family history of kidney disease) should be screened for microalbuminuria, at least annually, as part of their health examination.[21]

Other markers of kidney damage include abnormalities in urine sediment (red and white blood cells) and abnormal findings on imaging studies.[20] Ultrasonography is particularly useful for detecting a number of kidney disorders, including urinary tract obstructions, infections, stones, and polycystic kidney disease.

BOX 34-1 PREDICTION OF CREATININE CLEARANCE USING SERUM CREATININE

Cockroft and Gault Equation*

$$\text{Creatinine clearance (mL/min)} = \frac{(140 - \text{age}) \times (\text{body weight in kg})}{(72 \times \text{ serum creatinine in mg/dL})}$$

The equation result should be multiplied by a factor of 0.85 for women.

Modification of Diet in Renal Diseases (MDRD)†

$$\text{GFR (mL/min/1.73m}^2) = 170 \times (\text{serum creatinine in mg/dL})^{-0.999} \times (\text{age in years})^{-0.176}$$
$$\times (\text{female})^{0.762} \times (1.18 \text{ if African American}) \times (\text{blood urea nitrogen in mg/dL})^{-0.17}$$
$$\times (\text{serum albumin in g/dL})^{+0.318}$$

*Cockroft D. W., Gault M. H. (1976). Prediction of creatinine clearance from serum creatinine. *Nephron* 16, 31.

†Levey A. S., Basch J. P., Lewis J. B., et al. (1999). A more accurate method to estimate glomerular filtration rate from serum creatinine: A new prediction equation. *Annals of Internal Medicine* 130, 461–470.

National Kidney Foundation. (2000). NFK K/DOQI Guidelines 2000: Appendix IX. [Online.] Available: www.kidney.org/professionals/kdoqi/guidelines_updates/nut_appx09a.html. Accessed March 8, 2008.

GFR calculator available online: www.kidney.org/professionals/KDOQI/gfr_calculator.cfm. Accessed January 30, 2007.

Clinical Manifestations

The manifestations of CKD include an accumulation of nitrogenous wastes; alterations in water, electrolyte, and acid-base balance; mineral and skeletal disorders; anemia and coagulation disorders; hypertension and alterations in cardiovascular function; gastrointestinal disorders; neurologic complications; disorders of skin integrity; and disorders of immunologic function [18,22] (Fig. 34-4). The point at which these disorders make their appearance and the severity of the manifestations are determined largely by the extent of renal function that is present and the coexisting disease conditions. Many of them make their appearance before the GFR has reached the kidney failure stage.

Accumulation of Nitrogenous Wastes

The accumulation of nitrogenous wastes in the blood, or azotemia, is an early sign of kidney failure, usually occurring before other symptoms become evident. Urea is one of the first nitrogenous wastes to accumulate in the blood, and the BUN level becomes increasingly elevated as CKD progresses. The normal concentration of urea in the plasma is approximately 20 mg/dL. In kidney failure, this level may rise to as high as 800 mg/dL. Creatinine, a byproduct of muscle metabolism, is freely filtered in the glomerulus and is not reabsorbed in the renal tubules. It is produced at a relatively constant rate, and essentially all the creatinine that is filtered in the glomerulus is lost in the urine rather than being reabsorbed into the blood. Thus, serum creatinine can be used as an indirect method for assessing the GFR and the extent of kidney damage that has occurred in CKD.

Uremia, which literally means "urine in the blood," is the term used to describe the clinical manifestations of kidney failure. Few symptoms of uremia appear until at least two thirds of the kidney's nephrons have been destroyed. Uremia differs from azotemia, which merely indicates the accumulation of nitrogenous wastes in the blood and can occur without symptoms. The uremic state includes signs and symptoms of altered fluid, electrolyte, and acid-base balance; alterations in regulatory functions (*e.g.,* blood pressure control, production of red blood cells, and impaired vitamin D synthesis); and the effects of uremia on body function (*e.g.,* uremic encephalopathy, peripheral neuropathy, pruritus). At this stage, virtually every organ and structure in the body is affected. The symptoms at the onset of uremia (*e.g.,* weakness, fatigue, nausea, apathy) often are subtle. More severe symptoms include extreme weakness, frequent vomiting, lethargy, and confusion. Without treatment, coma and death follow.

Fluid, Electrolyte, and Acid-Base Disorders

The kidneys function in the regulation of extracellular fluid volume. They do this by either eliminating or conserving sodium and water. Chronic renal failure can produce dehydration or fluid overload, depending on the pathologic process of the kidney disease. In addition to volume regulation, the ability of the kidneys to concentrate the urine is diminished. One of the earliest

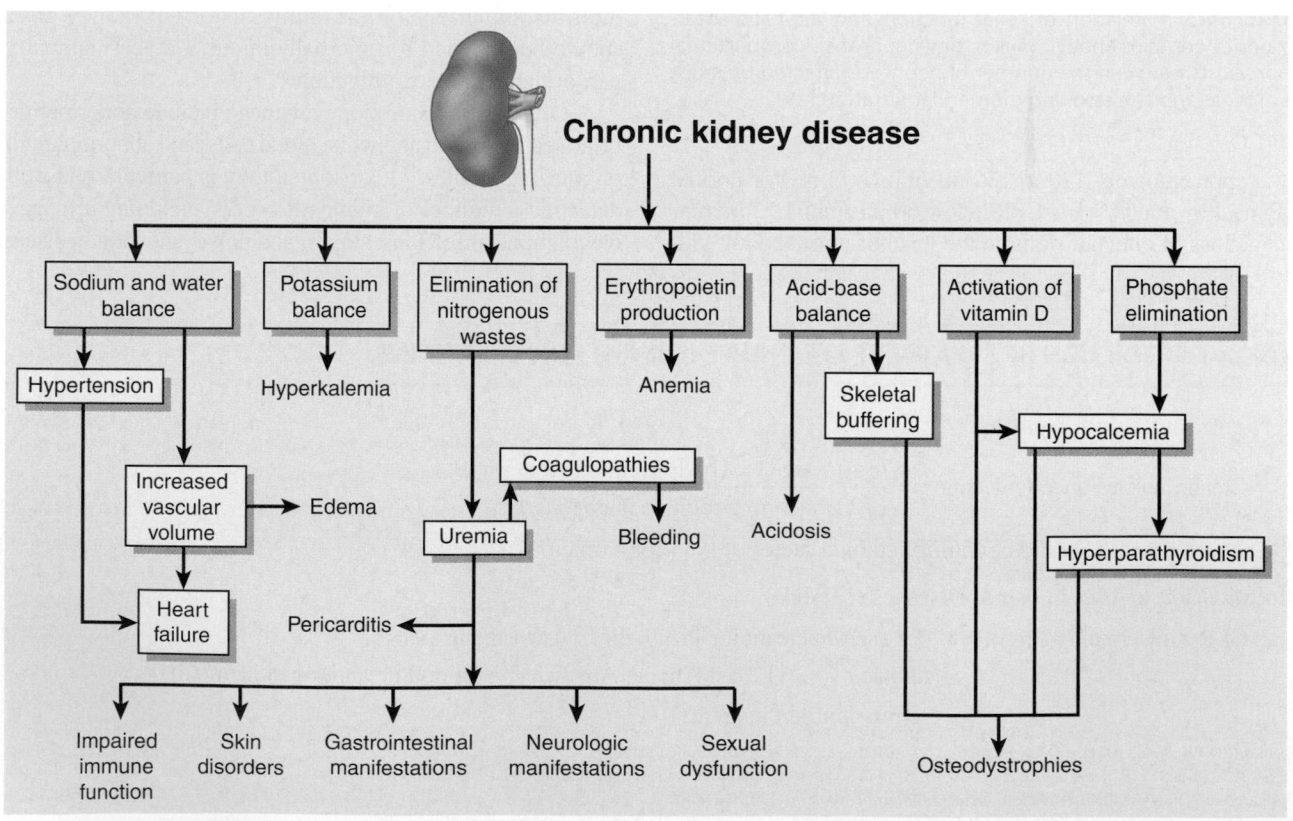

FIGURE 34-4 • Mechanisms and manifestations of chronic kidney disease.

symptoms of kidney damage is *isosthenuria,* or polyuria with urine that is almost isotonic with plasma (*i.e.,* specific gravity of 1.008 to 1.012) and varies little from voiding to voiding.

As renal function declines further, the ability to regulate sodium excretion is reduced. The kidneys normally tolerate large variations in sodium intake while maintaining normal serum sodium levels. In chronic renal failure, they lose the ability to regulate sodium excretion. There is impaired ability to adjust to a sudden reduction in sodium intake and poor tolerance of an acute sodium overload. Volume depletion with an accompanying decrease in the GFR can occur with a restricted sodium intake or excess sodium loss caused by diarrhea or vomiting. Salt wasting is a common problem in advanced kidney failure because of impaired tubular reabsorption of sodium. Increasing sodium intake in persons with kidney failure often improves the GFR and whatever renal function remains. In patients with associated hypertension, the possibility of increasing blood pressure or producing congestive heart failure often excludes supplemental sodium intake.

Approximately 90% of potassium excretion is through the kidneys. In kidney failure, potassium excretion by each nephron increases as the kidneys adapt to a decrease in the GFR. In addition, excretion in the gastrointestinal tract is increased. As a result, hyperkalemia usually does not develop until kidney function is severely compromised. Because of this adaptive mechanism, it usually is not necessary to restrict potassium intake in patients with CKD until the GFR has dropped below 5 to 10 mL/min/1.73 m^2.[21] In persons with kidney failure, hyperkalemia often results from failure to follow dietary potassium restrictions; constipation; acute acidosis that causes the release of intracellular potassium into the extracellular fluid; trauma or infection that causes release of potassium from body tissues; or exposure to medications that contain potassium, prevent its entry into cells, or block its secretion in distal nephrons.

The kidneys normally regulate blood pH by eliminating hydrogen ions produced in metabolic processes and regenerating bicarbonate. This is achieved through hydrogen ion secretion, sodium and bicarbonate reabsorption, and the production of ammonia, which acts as a buffer for titratable acids (see Chapter 32). With a decline in kidney function, these mechanisms become impaired and metabolic acidosis may occur when the person is challenged with an excessive acid load or loses excessive alkali, as in diarrhea. The acidosis that occurs in persons with kidney failure seems to stabilize as the disease progresses, probably as a result of the tremendous buffering capacity of bone. However, this buffering action is thought to increase bone resorption and contribute to the skeletal disorders that occur in persons with CKD.

Disorders of Calcium and Phosphorus Metabolism and Bone Disease

Abnormalities of calcium and phosphorus metabolism occur early in the course of CKD.[23–27] The regulation of serum phosphate levels requires a daily urinary excretion of an amount equal to that ingested in the diet. With deteriorating renal function, phosphate excretion is impaired, and as a result serum phosphate levels rise. At the same time, serum calcium levels, which are inversely regulated in relation to serum phosphate levels, fall (see Chapter 31). The drop in serum calcium, in turn, stimulates parathyroid hormone (PTH) release, with a resultant increase in calcium resorption from bone. Although serum calcium levels are maintained through increased PTH function, this adjustment is accomplished at the expense of the skeletal system and other body organs.

Vitamin D synthesis also is impaired in CKD. The kidneys regulate vitamin D activity by converting the inactive form of vitamin D (25[OH] vitamin D_3) to calcitriol (1,25[OH] vitamin D_3), the active form of vitamin D.[23,24,28] Calcitriol is known to have a direct suppressive effect on PTH production; therefore, reduced levels of calcitriol cause elevated levels of PTH. In addition, reduced calcitriol levels lead to impaired calcium absorption from the gastrointestinal tract. Vitamin D also regulates osteoblast differentiation, thereby affecting bone replacement.

Most persons with CKD develop a secondary hyperparathyroidism, the result of chronic stimulation of the parathyroid glands.[26] Over the past several decades, the principal biochemical marker for diagnosis of hyperparathyroidism in persons with CKD has been the measurement of PTH function using an immunoreactive technique called *intact PTH*[23,24] (see Chapter 31).

Skeletal Disorders. The term *renal osteodystrophy* is used to describe the skeletal complications of CKD.[23,24,27] The skeletal changes that occur with CKD have been divided into two major types of disorders: high–bone-turnover and low–bone-turnover osteodystrophy. Some persons may have predominantly one type of bone disorder, whereas others may have a mixed type of bone disease. Inherent to both of these conditions is abnormal reabsorption and defective remodeling of bone (see Chapter 58). Mild forms of defective bone metabolism may be observed in early stages of CKD (stage 2), and they become more severe as kidney function deteriorates.

High–bone-turnover osteodystrophy, sometimes referred to as *osteitis fibrosa,* is characterized by increased bone resorption and formation, with bone resorption predominating. The disorder is associated with secondary hyperparathyroidism; altered vitamin D metabolism, along with resistance to the action of vitamin D; and impaired regulation of locally produced growth factors and inhibitors. There is an increase in both osteoblast and osteoclast numbers and activity. Although the osteoblasts produce excessive amounts of bone matrix, mineralization fails to keep pace, and there is a decrease in bone density and formation of porous and coarse-fibered bone. Cortical bone is affected more severely than cancellous bone. Bone marrow fibrosis is another component of osteitis fibrosa; it occurs in areas of increased bone cell activity. In advanced stages of the disorder, cysts may develop in the bone, a condition called *osteitis fibrosa cystica.*

Low–bone-turnover osteodystrophy is characterized by decreased numbers of osteoblasts and low or reduced numbers of osteoclasts, a low rate of bone turnover, and an accumulation of unmineralized bone matrix. There are two forms of low-turnover osteodystrophy: osteomalacia and adynamic osteodystrophy. *Osteomalacia* is characterized by a slow rate of bone formation and defects in bone mineralization, which may be caused by vitamin D deficiency, excess aluminum deposition, or metabolic acidosis. Metabolic acidosis is thought to have a direct effect on both osteoblastic and osteoclastic activity, as well as on the mineralization process, by decreasing the availability of trivalent phosphate. Until the 1980s, the osteomalacia seen in CKD resulted mainly from aluminum intoxication. Aluminum intoxication causes decreased and defective mineralization of bone by existing osteoblasts and more long-term inhibition of osteoblast differentiation. During the 1970s and 1980s, it was discovered that accumulation of aluminum from water used in dialysis and aluminum salts used as phosphate binders caused osteomalacia and adynamic bone disease. This discovery led to a change in the composition of dialysis solutions and the substitution of calcium carbonate for aluminum salts as phosphate binders. As a result, the prevalence of osteomalacia in persons with CKD has declined.

The second type of low–bone-turnover osteodystrophy, *adynamic osteodystrophy,* is characterized by a low number of osteoblasts, with the osteoclast number being normal or reduced. It is now recognized as being as common as high-turnover osteodystrophy and is especially common among persons with diabetes. Adynamic bone disease is characterized by reduced bone volume and mineralization that may result, in part, from excessive suppression of PTH production with calcitriol.

Regardless of the cause of skeletal abnormalities in CKD, bone disease can lead to bone tenderness and muscle weakness. Bone fractures complicate both high- and low-turnover types of bone disease. However, it is now recognized that persons with adynamic bone disease may be more predisposed to fractures than those with osteitis fibrosa cystica. In the latter disorder, however, PTH-associated proximal muscle weakness in the lower extremities often coexists, giving rise to gait abnormalities and making it difficult to get out of a chair or climb stairs.

Early treatment of hyperphosphatemia and hypocalcemia is important to prevent or slow the development of skeletal complications. Milk products and other foods high in phosphorus content are restricted in the diet. Phosphate-binding antacids (aluminum salts, calcium carbonate, or calcium acetate) may be prescribed to decrease absorption of phosphate from the gastrointestinal tract. Calcium-containing phosphate binders can lead to hypercalcemia, thus worsening soft tissue calcification, especially in persons receiving vitamin D therapy. Aluminum-containing antacids can contribute to the development of osteodystrophy. To avoid these side effects, a new, well-tolerated aluminum- and calcium-free binder (sevelamer) has been developed. Sevelamer is a hydrogel that is resistant to digestive degradation and is not absorbed.[23,24,28]

Activated pharmacologic forms of vitamin D (*e.g.,* calcitriol) often are used to increase serum calcium levels and, at least partially, reverse the secondary hyperparathyroidism and osteitis fibrosis that occur with CKD. Although calcitriol is effective in controlling PTH overproduction, its stimulatory effects on intestinal absorption of calcium and phosphorus, along with its suppressive effects on bone turnover, predispose to hypercalcemia and hyperphosphatemia and to an increase in

the calcium–phosphate (Ca × P) product (see Chapter 31). Hypercalcemia and an elevated Ca × P product increase the risk for metastatic calcification, a complication associated with cardiac dysfunction and death; the risk is greater in patients who are also taking calcium-based phosphate binders.[23,24,28] Several vitamin D analogs (paricalcitol, doxercalciferol) have recently been approved for the treatment of secondary hyperparathyroidism due to CKD.[23,28] These analogs are cleared more rapidly from the circulation than calcitriol and are less likely to produce hypercalcemia.

Secondary hyperparathyroidism may also be treated by activating the calcium sensing receptor on the parathyroid gland (see Chapter 31). The calcimimetic agent cinacalcet, the first representative of a new class of drugs that act through the calcium sensing receptor, has been approved for treatment of secondary hyperparathyroidism in CKD.[28] However, because adynamic bone disease is often a consequence of overzealous treatment of secondary hyperthyroidism, these agents require careful use.

Hematologic Disorders

Anemia. Chronic anemia (hemoglobin levels <13.5 g/dL in adult men and <12 g/dL in adult women) is the most profound hematologic alteration that accompanies CKD.[29] In the National Health and Nutrition Examination Survey (NHANES), the prevalence of anemia in stage 3 CKD was 5.2%, rising to 44.1% in stage 4, and becoming almost universal in stage 5.[30] African Americans and persons with diabetes have even higher rates of anemia for each stage of CKD. Therefore, the NKF guidelines recommend that those persons with a GFR less than 60 mL/min per 1.73 m² should be evaluated for anemia. Assessment for anemia and its causes includes measures of hemoglobin, hematocrit, and iron stores (measured directly by bone marrow biopsy or indirectly by serum ferritin, transferrin saturation levels, and percentage of hypochromic red cells or reticulocytes; see Chapter 14). [29]

The anemia of CKD is due to several factors, including chronic blood loss, hemolysis, bone marrow suppression due to retained uremic factors, and decreased red cell production due to impaired production of erythropoietin and iron deficiency. The kidneys are the primary site for the production of the hormone *erythropoietin,* which controls red blood cell production.[29,31–33] In renal failure, erythropoietin production usually is insufficient to stimulate adequate red blood cell production by the bone marrow. Among the causes of iron deficiency in persons with CKD are anorexia and dietary restrictions that limit intake, and the blood loss that occurs during dialysis.[32]

When untreated, anemia causes or contributes to weakness, fatigue, depression, insomnia, and decreased cognitive function. There also is an increasing concern regarding the physiologic effects of anemia on cardiovascular function.[31,32] The anemia of renal failure produces a decrease in blood viscosity and a compensatory increase in heart rate. The decreased blood viscosity also exacerbates peripheral vasodilation and contributes to decreased vascular resistance. Cardiac output increases in a compensatory fashion to maintain tissue perfusion. Anemia also limits myocardial oxygen supply, particularly in persons with coronary heart disease, leading to angina pectoris and other ischemic events. It has also been suggested that anemia may contribute to the progression of CKD by subjecting the functioning nephrons that remain to increased hypoxic and oxidative stress.[33]

A remarkable advance in medical management of CKD was realized when recombinant human erythropoietin (rhEPO) became available. Since its approval by the U.S. Food and Drug Administration in June 1989, rhEPO therapy has been used to help maintain hematocrit levels in persons with kidney failure.[29,31,32] More recently, a novel erythropoiesis-stimulating protein has been introduced for treatment of anemia in CKD. This protein, darbepoetin alpha, is a hyperglycosylated analog of rhEPO that possesses great biologic activity and a prolonged half-life.[31] Secondary benefits of treating anemia with rhEPO, previously attributed to the correction of uremia, include improvement in appetite, energy level, sexual function, skin color, and hair and nail growth, and reduced cold intolerance. Because worsening of hypertension and seizures have occurred when the hematocrit was raised too suddenly, frequent measurements of hematocrit are necessary.

Because iron deficiency is common among persons with CKD, iron supplementation often is needed.[29,32] Iron can be given orally or intravenously. Intravenous iron (iron dextran and ferric sodium gluconate) is used for treatment of persons who are not able to maintain adequate iron status with oral iron. Because intravenously administered iron may cause serious immediate and delayed hypersensitivity reactions, including life-threatening anaphylactic reactions, care is required when prescribing and administering these drugs.[29]

Coagulopathies. Bleeding disorders are manifested by epistaxis, menorrhagia, gastrointestinal bleeding, and bruising of the skin and subcutaneous tissues. Although platelet production often is normal in CKD, platelet function is impaired.[22,34] Coagulative function improves with dialysis but does not completely normalize, suggesting that uremia contributes to the problem. Persons with CKD also have greater susceptibility to thrombotic disorders, particularly if their underlying disease was characterized by a nephrotic presentation.

Cardiovascular Disorders

The overall mortality rate from cardiovascular disease in people with CKD is 30 times that of the general population.[35] Even after stratification for age, the incidence of cardiovascular disease remains 10 to 20 times higher in persons with CKD than in the general population.[35]

Hypertension. Hypertension commonly is an early manifestation of CKD. The mechanisms that produce hypertension in CKD are multifactorial; they include an increased vascular volume, elevation of peripheral vascular resistance, decreased levels of renal vasodilator prostaglandins, and increased activity of the renin-angiotensin system.

Early identification and aggressive treatment of hypertension has been shown to slow the progression of renal impairment in many types of kidney disease.[18,22] Treatment involves salt and water restriction and the use of antihypertensive medications to control blood pressure. Many persons with CKD need to take several antihypertensive medications to control blood pressure (see Chapter 23).

Heart Disease. The spectrum of cardiovascular disease due to CKD includes left ventricular hypertrophy and ischemic heart disease. People with CKD tend to have an increased prevalence of left ventricular dysfunction, with both depressed left ventricular ejection fraction, as in systolic dysfunction, and impaired ventricular filling, as in diastolic failure[36–38] (see Chapter 26). Multiple factors lead to development of left ventricular dysfunction, including extracellular fluid overload, shunting of blood through an arteriovenous fistula for dialysis, and anemia. Anemia, in particular, has been correlated with the presence of left ventricular hypertrophy. These abnormalities, coupled with the hypertension that often is present, cause increased myocardial work and oxygen demand, with eventual development of heart failure.

Congestive heart failure and pulmonary edema tend to occur in the late stages of kidney failure. Coexisting conditions that have been identified as contributing to the burden of cardiovascular disease include hypertension, anemia, diabetes mellitus, dyslipidemia, and coagulopathies. PTH also may play a role in the pathogenesis of cardiomyopathy in renal failure.

Pericarditis. Pericarditis occurs in approximately 20% of persons receiving chronic dialysis.[39] It can result from metabolic toxins associated with the uremic state or from dialysis. The manifestations of uremic pericarditis resemble those of viral pericarditis, with all its potential complications, including cardiac tamponade (see Chapter 24). The presenting signs include mild to severe chest pain with respiratory accentuation and a pericardial friction rub. Fever is variable in the absence of infection and is more common in dialysis than uremic pericarditis.

Gastrointestinal Disorders

Anorexia, nausea, and vomiting are common in patients with uremia, along with a metallic taste in the mouth that further depresses the appetite.[18,22] Early-morning nausea is common. Ulceration and bleeding of the gastrointestinal mucosa may develop, and hiccups are common. A possible cause of nausea and vomiting is the decomposition of urea by intestinal flora, resulting in a high concentration of ammonia. PTH increases gastric acid secretion and contributes to gastrointestinal problems. Nausea and vomiting often improve with restriction of dietary protein and after initiation of dialysis, and disappear after kidney transplantation.

Neuromuscular Disorders

Many persons with CKD have alterations in peripheral and central nervous system function.[18,22,40] Peripheral neuropathy, or involvement of the peripheral nerves, affects the lower limbs more frequently than the upper limbs. It is symmetric and affects both sensory and motor function. Neuropathy is caused by atrophy and demyelination of nerve fibers, possibly caused by uremic toxins. Restless legs syndrome is a manifestation of peripheral nerve involvement and can be seen in as many as two thirds of patients on dialysis. This syndrome is characterized by creeping, prickling, and itching sensations that typically are more intense at rest. Temporary relief is obtained by moving the legs. A burning sensation of the feet, which may be followed by muscle weakness and atrophy, is a manifestation of uremia.

The central nervous system disturbances in uremia are similar to those caused by other metabolic and toxic disorders. Sometimes referred to as *uremic encephalopathy,* the condition is poorly understood and may result, at least in part, from an excess of toxic organic acids that alter neural function. Electrolyte abnormalities, such as sodium shifts, also may contribute. The manifestations are more closely related to the progress of the uremic disorder than to the level of the metabolic end products. Reductions in alertness and awareness are the earliest and most significant indications of uremic encephalopathy. These often are followed by an inability to fix attention, loss of recent memory, and perceptual errors in identifying persons and objects. Delirium and coma occur late in the disease course; seizures are the preterminal event.

Disorders of motor function commonly accompany the neurologic manifestations of uremic encephalopathy. During the early stages, there often is difficulty in performing fine movements of the extremities; the gait becomes unsteady and clumsy with tremulousness of movement. Asterixis (dorsiflexion movements of the hands and feet) typically occurs as the disease progresses. It can be elicited by having the person hyperextend his or her arms at the elbow and wrist with the fingers spread apart. If asterixis is present, this position causes side-to-side flapping movements of the fingers.

Altered Immune Function

Infection is a common complication and cause of hospitalization and death for persons with kidney failure. Immunologic abnormalities decrease the efficiency of the immune response to infection.[22] All aspects of inflammation and immune function may be affected adversely by the high levels of urea and metabolic wastes, including a decreased granulocyte count, impaired humoral and cell-mediated immunity, and defective phagocyte function. The acute inflammatory response and delayed-type hypersensitivity response are impaired. Although persons with CKD have normal humoral responses to vaccines, a more aggressive immunization program may be needed. Skin and mucosal barriers to infection also may be defective. In persons who are maintained on dialysis, vascular access devices are common portals of entry for pathogens. Many persons with CKD fail to mount a fever with infection, making the diagnosis more difficult.

Disorders of Skin Integrity

Skin manifestations are common in persons with CKD.[18] The skin often is pale owing to anemia and may have a sallow, yellow-brown hue. The skin and mucous membranes often are dry, and subcutaneous bruising is common. Skin dryness is caused by a reduction in perspiration owing to the decreased size of sweat glands and the diminished activity of oil glands. Pruritus is common; it results from the high serum phosphate levels and the development of phosphate crystals that occur with hyperparathyroidism. Severe scratching and repeated needle sticks, especially with hemodialysis, break the skin integrity and increase the risk for infection. In the advanced stages of untreated kidney failure, urea crystals may precipitate on the skin as a result of the high urea concentration in body fluids. The fingernails may become thin and brittle, with a dark band just behind the leading edge of the nail, followed by a white band. This appearance is known as *Terry nails.*

Sexual Dysfunction

The cause of sexual dysfunction in men and women with CKD is unclear. The cause probably is multifactorial and may result from high levels of uremic toxins, neuropathy, altered endocrine function, psychological factors, and medications (*e.g.,* antihypertensive drugs). Alterations in physiologic sexual responses, reproductive ability, and libido are common.

Impotence occurs in as much as 56% of male patients on dialysis.[41] Derangements of the pituitary and gonadal hormones, such as decreases in testosterone levels and increases in prolactin and luteinizing hormone levels, are common and cause erectile difficulties and decreased spermatocyte counts. Loss of libido may result from chronic anemia and decreased testosterone levels. Several drugs, such as exogenous testosterone and bromocriptine, have been used in an attempt to return hormone levels to normal.

Impaired sexual function in women is manifested by abnormal levels of progesterone, luteinizing hormone, and prolactin. Hypofertility, menstrual abnormalities, decreased vaginal lubrication, and various orgasmic problems have been described. Amenorrhea is common among women who are on dialysis therapy.[42]

Elimination of Drugs

The kidneys are responsible for the elimination of many drugs and their metabolites. CKD and its treatment can interfere with the absorption, distribution, and elimination of drugs.[43] The administration of large quantities of phosphate-binding antacids to control hyperphosphatemia and hypocalcemia in patients with advanced renal failure interferes with the absorption of some drugs. Many drugs are bound to plasma proteins, such as albumin, for transport in the body; the unbound portion of the drug is available to act at the various receptor sites and is free to be metabolized. A decrease in plasma proteins, particularly albumin, that occurs in many persons with CKD results in less protein-bound drug and greater amounts of free drug.

In the process of metabolism, some drugs form intermediate metabolites that are toxic if not eliminated. Some pathways of drug metabolism, such as hydrolysis, are slowed with uremia. In persons with diabetes, for example, insulin requirements may be reduced as renal function deteriorates. Decreased elimination by the kidneys allows drugs or their metabolites to accumulate in the body and requires that drug dosages be adjusted accordingly. Some drugs contain unwanted nitrogen, sodium, potassium, and magnesium and must be avoided in patients with CKD. Penicillin, for example, contains potassium. Nitrofurantoin and ammonium chloride add to the body's nitrogen pool. Many antacids contain magnesium. Because of problems with drug dosing and elimination, persons with CKD should be cautioned against the use of over-the-counter remedies.

Treatment

Chronic kidney disease is treated by conservative management to prevent or slow the rate of nephron destruction and, when necessary, by renal replacement therapy with dialysis or transplantation.

Measures to Slow Progression of the Disorder

Conservative treatment can often delay the progression of CKD.[18,44] It includes measures to retard deterioration of renal function and assist the body in managing the effects of impaired function. Urinary tract infections should be treated promptly and medication with renal damaging potential should be avoided. It should be noted that these strategies are complementary to the treatment of the original cause of the renal disorder, which is of the utmost importance and needs to be continually addressed.

Blood pressure control is important, as is control of blood sugar in persons with diabetes mellitus. Intensive glycemic control in persons with diabetes helps to prevent the development of microalbuminuria and retards the progression of diabetic nephropathy (see Chapter 42). In addition to reduction in cardiovascular risk, antihypertensive therapy in persons with CKD aims to slow the progression of nephron loss by lowering intraglomerular hypertension and hypertrophy.[18] Elevated blood pressure also increases proteinuria due to transmission of the elevated pressure to the glomeruli. This is the basis for the treatment guideline establishing 125/75 mm Hg as the target blood pressure for persons with CKD[14] (see Chapter 23). The ACE inhibitors and ARBs, which have a unique effect on the glomerular microcirculation (*i.e.,* dilation of the efferent arteriole), are increasingly being used in the treatment of hypertension and proteinuria, particularly in persons with diabetes.[18]

It has become apparent that smoking has a negative impact on kidney function, and it is one of the most remedial risk factors for CKD.[45] The mechanisms of smoking-induced renal damage appear to include both acute hemodynamic effects (*i.e.,* increase in blood pressure, intraglomerular pressure, and urinary albu-

min excretion) and chronic effects (endothelial cell dysfunction).[45] Smoking is particularly nephrotoxic in elderly persons with hypertension, and those with diabetes. Importantly, the adverse effects of smoking appear to be independent of the underlying kidney disease.

Dialysis and Transplantation

Dialysis or renal replacement therapy is indicated when advanced uremia or serious electrolyte imbalances are present. As recently as 1965, many patients with CKD progressed to the final stages of kidney failure and then died. The high mortality rate was associated with limitations in the treatment of kidney disease and with the tremendous cost of ongoing treatment. In 1972, federal support began for dialysis and transplantation through a Medicare entitlement program in the United States.[46] During the past several decades, an increasing number of persons have required renal replacement therapy with dialysis or transplantation. The number of people beginning hemodialysis has grown sevenfold since 1978, reaching 94,891 in 2004. The number of persons who received their first kidney transplant surpassed 15,000 in 2005 and is growing each year, and the total number waiting to receive a transplant has increased from 21,847 in 1995 to 57,837 in 2005.[47]

The choice between dialysis and transplantation is dictated by age, related health problems, donor availability, and personal preference. Although transplantation often is the preferred treatment, dialysis plays a critical role as a treatment method for kidney failure. It is life-sustaining for persons who are not candidates for transplantation or who are awaiting transplantation. There are two broad categories of dialysis: hemodialysis and peritoneal dialysis.

Hemodialysis. The basic principles of hemodialysis have remained unchanged over the years, although new technology has improved the efficiency and speed of dialysis.[48,49] A hemodialysis system, or artificial kidney, consists of three parts: a blood delivery system, a dialyzer, and a dialysis fluid delivery system. The dialyzer is usually a hollow cylinder composed of bundles of capillary tubes through which blood circulates, while the dialysate travels on the outside of the tubes.[48] The walls of the capillary tubes in the dialysis chamber are made up of a semipermeable membrane material that allows all molecules except blood cells and plasma proteins to move freely in both directions—from the blood into the dialyzing solution and from the dialyzing solution into the blood. The direction of flow is determined by the concentration of the substances contained in the two solutions. The waste products and excess electrolytes in the blood normally diffuse into the dialyzing solution. If there is a need to replace or add substances, such as bicarbonate, to the blood, these can be added to the dialyzing solution (Fig. 34-5).

During dialysis, blood moves from an artery through the tubing and blood chamber in the dialysis machine and then back into the body through a vein. Access to the vascular system is

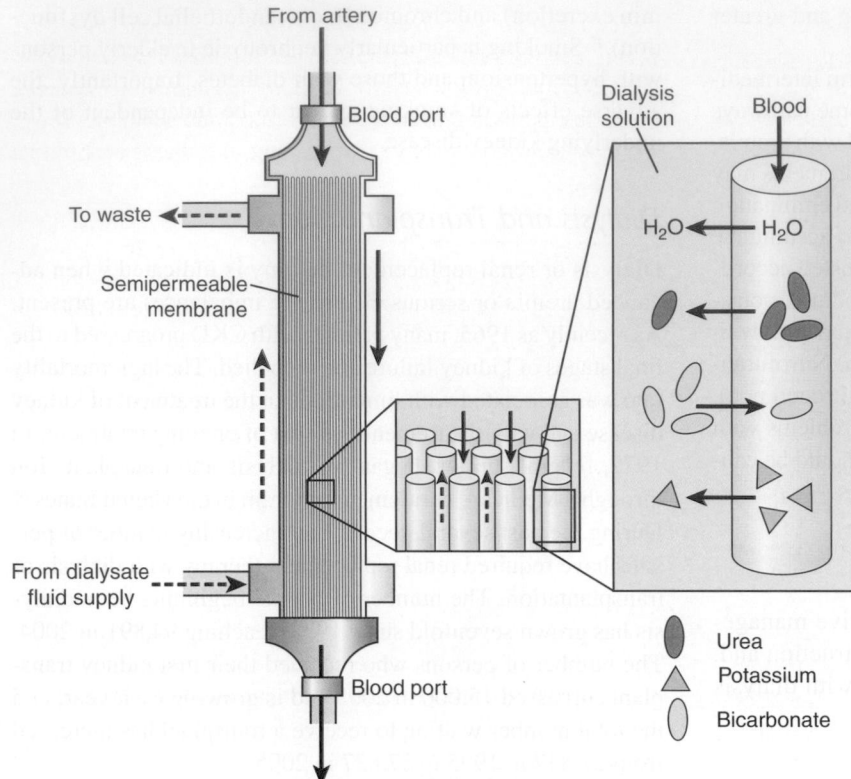

FIGURE 34-5 • Schematic diagram of a hemodialysis system. The blood compartment and dialysis solution compartment are separated by a semipermeable membrane. This membrane is porous enough to allow all the constituents, except the plasma proteins and blood cells, to diffuse between the two compartments.

accomplished through an external arteriovenous shunt (*i.e.,* tubing implanted into an artery and a vein) or, more commonly, through an internal arteriovenous fistula (*i.e.,* anastomosis of a vein to an artery, usually in the forearm). Heparin is used to prevent clotting during the dialysis treatment; it can be administered continuously or intermittently. Problems that may occur during dialysis, depending on the rates of blood flow and solute removal, include hypotension, nausea, vomiting, muscle cramps, headache, chest pain, and disequilibrium syndrome.

Most persons are dialyzed three times each week for 3 to 4 hours; treatment is determined by kinetic profiles, referred to as Kt/V values, which consider dialyzer size, dialysate, flow rate, time of dialysis, and body size. Many dialysis centers provide the option for patients to learn how to perform hemodialysis at home.

Peritoneal Dialysis. Peritoneal dialysis was introduced in the mid-1970s. Improvements in technology and the ability to deliver adequate dialysis resulted in improved outcomes and the acceptance of peritoneal dialysis as a renal replacement therapy.

The same principles of diffusion, osmosis, and ultrafiltration that apply to hemodialysis apply to peritoneal dialysis.[48] The thin serous membrane of the peritoneal cavity serves as the dialyzing membrane. A Silastic catheter is surgically implanted in the peritoneal cavity below the umbilicus to provide access. The catheter is tunneled through subcutaneous tissue and exits on the side of the abdomen (Fig. 34-6). The dialysis process involves instilling a sterile dialyzing solution (usually 1 to 3 L) through the catheter over a period of approximately 10 minutes. The solution

then is allowed to remain, or *dwell,* in the peritoneal cavity for a prescribed amount of time, during which the metabolic end products and extracellular fluid diffuse into the dialysis solution. At the end of the dwell time, the dialysis fluid is drained out of the peritoneal cavity by gravity into a sterile bag. Glucose in the dialysis solution accounts for water removal. Commercial dialysis

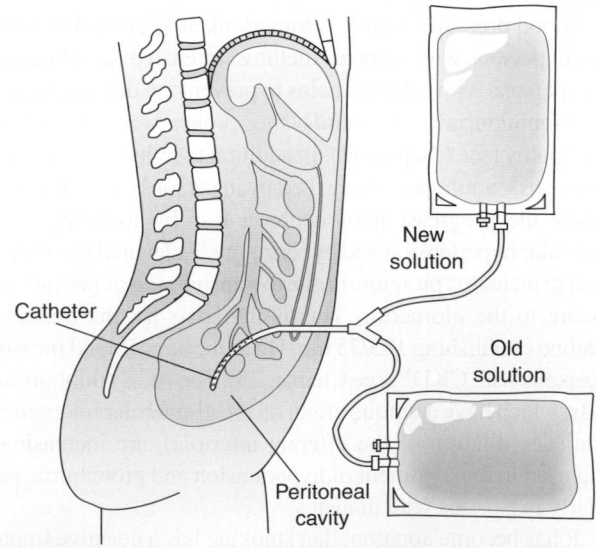

FIGURE 34-6 • Peritoneal dialysis. A semipermeable membrane, richly supplied with small blood vessels, lines the peritoneal cavity. With dialysate dwelling in the peritoneal cavity, waste products diffuse from the network of blood vessels into the dialysate.

solution is available in 1.5%, 2.5%, and 4.25% dextrose concentrations. Solutions with higher dextrose levels increase osmosis, causing more fluid to be removed. As with hemodialysis, Kt/V values are used to evaluate adequacy of peritoneal dialysis.

Peritoneal dialysis can be performed at home or in a dialysis center and can be carried out by continuous ambulatory peritoneal dialysis (CAPD), continuous cyclic peritoneal dialysis (CCPD), or nocturnal intermittent peritoneal dialysis (NIPD)—all with variations in the number of exchanges and dwell times.[48] Individual preference, manual ability, lifestyle, knowledge of the procedure, and physiologic response to treatment are used to determine the type of dialysis that is used. The most common method is CAPD, a self-care procedure in which the person manages the dialysis procedure at home. CAPD involves instilling the dialysate into the peritoneal cavity and rolling up the bag and tubing and securing them under clothing during the dwell. After the dwell time is completed (usually 4 to 6 hours during the day), the bag is unrolled and lowered, allowing the waste-containing dialysis solution to drain from the peritoneal cavity into the bag. Each exchange, which involves draining the solution and infusing a new solution, requires approximately 30 to 45 minutes. Four exchanges usually are performed each day. In CCPD, exchanges are performed in an automated manner, usually at night, with the person connected to an automatic cycler, which then performs four or five cycles, while the person sleeps. In the morning, the person, with the last exchange remaining in the abdomen, is disconnected from the cycler and goes about his or her usual activities. In NIPD, the person is given approximately 10 hours of automatic cycling each night, with the abdomen left dry during the day.

Potential problems with peritoneal dialysis include infection, catheter malfunction, dehydration caused by excessive fluid removal, hyperglycemia, and hernia. The most serious complication is infection, which can occur at the catheter exit site, in the subcutaneous tunnel, or in the peritoneal cavity (*i.e.,* peritonitis).

Transplantation. Greatly improved success rates have made kidney transplantation the treatment of choice for many patients with CKD. The availability of donor organs continues to limit the number of transplantations performed each year. Donor organs are obtained from cadavers and living related donors (*e.g.,* parent, sibling). Transplants from living unrelated donors (*e.g.,* spouse) have been used in cases of suitable ABO blood type and tissue compatibility. Of the transplantations performed in 2002, the 1-year graft survival rates for cadaver transplants were 88.8%, and for living related donors, 94.8%.[50]

The success of transplantation depends primarily on the degree of histocompatibility, adequate organ preservation, and immunologic management.[51,52] Maintenance immunosuppressive therapy typically consists of corticosteroids, azathioprine, and cyclosporine (or tacrolimus [FK506] or sirolimus). Interleukin-2, a cytokine, plays an essential role in T- and B-cell activation (see Chapter 17). Cyclosporine and tacrolimus inhibit interleukin-2 synthesis, and sirolimus inhibits the T-cell response to interleukin. Genetically engineered antibodies that selectively target interleukin receptors also are available. Mono-

clonal antibodies such as OKT-3 (directed against the CD3 T-cell receptor) and antilymphocyte antibodies may be used as induction therapy. Because of the increased number of effective immunosuppressive agents that have become available, lower corticosteroid doses are used, resulting in reduced cushingoid effects after transplantation.

Rejection, which is categorized as acute and chronic, can occur at any time (see Chapter 19). Acute rejection most commonly occurs during the first several months after transplantation and involves a cellular response with the proliferation of T lymphocytes. Chronic rejection can occur months to years after transplantation. Because chronic rejection is caused by both cellular and humoral immunity, it does not respond well to increased immunosuppressive therapy.

Maintenance immunosuppressive therapy and increased use of immunosuppression to treat rejection predispose the person to a spectrum of infectious complications. Prophylactic antimicrobials may be prescribed to decrease the incidence of common infections, such as candidiasis, herpesvirus infections, and *Pneumocystis jiroveci* (formerly *P. carinii*) pneumonia. Other infections, such as cytomegalovirus infection and aspergillosis, are seen with chronic immunosuppression.

Dietary Management

A major component in the treatment of CKD is dietary management.[53] The goal of dietary treatment is to provide optimum nutrition while maintaining tolerable levels of metabolic wastes. The specific diet prescription depends on the type and severity of renal disease and on the dialysis modality. Because of the severe restrictions placed on food and fluid intake, these diets may be complicated and unappetizing. After kidney transplantation, some dietary restrictions still may be necessary, even when renal function is normal, to control the adverse effects from immunosuppressive medication.

Protein. Restriction of dietary proteins may decrease the progress of renal impairment in persons with advanced renal disease. Proteins are broken down to form nitrogenous wastes, and reducing the amount of protein in the diet lowers the BUN and reduces symptoms. Moreover, a high-protein diet is high in phosphates and inorganic acids. The Modification of Diet in Renal Disease (MDRD) Study, which was conducted in 15 university hospital outpatient nephrology clinics and included 255 patients between the ages of 18 and 70 years, demonstrated a slower decline in GFR among patients randomized to the very–low-protein diet compared with patients on a low-protein diet.[54]

Considerable controversy exists over the degree of restriction needed. If the diet is too low in protein, protein malnutrition can occur, with a loss of strength, muscle mass, and body weight. Results of the MDRD Study indicate that protein requirements can be met by providing 0.6 g of protein per kilogram of body weight per day.[18,54] Persons on hemodialysis usually require a higher dietary protein intake to prevent protein and energy malnutrition due to anorexia from uremia itself, the dialysis procedure, intercurrent illness, and acidemia. Persons on peritoneal dialysis also have significant protein losses and require a higher dietary protein intake. At least 50% of the protein intake should consist of proteins of high biologic value, such as those in eggs, lean meat, and milk, which are rich in essential amino acids. Proteins with a high biologic value are believed to promote the reuse of endogenous nitrogen, decreasing the amount of nitrogenous wastes that are produced and ameliorating the symptoms of uremia. In reusing nitrogen, the proteins ingested in the diet are broken down into their constituent amino acids and recycled in the synthesis of protein required by the body. In contrast to proteins with a high biologic value, fewer than half of the amino acids in cereal proteins are reused. Amino acids that are not reused to build body proteins are broken down and form the end products of protein metabolism, such as urea.

Carbohydrates, Fat, and Calories. With CKD, adequate calories in the form of carbohydrates and fat are required to meet energy needs. This is particularly important when the protein content of the diet is severely restricted. If sufficient calories are not available, the limited protein in the diet goes into energy production, or body tissue itself is used for energy purposes. Caloric intake for persons on CAPD includes food intake and calories absorbed from the dialysis solution. A 2-L bag of 1.5% dialysate solution equals 105 calories, and a 4.25% solution delivers 289 calories.

Fluid and Electrolytes. The sodium and fluid restrictions depend on the kidneys' ability to excrete sodium and water and must be individually determined. Renal disease of glomerular origin is more likely to contribute to sodium retention, whereas tubular dysfunction causes salt wasting. Fluid intake in excess of what the kidneys can excrete causes circulatory overload, edema, and water intoxication. Thirst is a common problem among patients on hemodialysis, often resulting in large weight gains between treatments. Inadequate intake, on the other hand, causes volume depletion and hypotension and can cause further decreases in the already compromised GFR. It is common practice to allow a daily fluid intake of 500 to 800 mL, which is equal to insensible water loss plus a quantity equal to the 24-hour urine output.

When the GFR falls to extremely low levels in kidney failure or during hemodialysis therapy, dietary restriction of potassium becomes mandatory. Using salt substitutes that contain potassium, or ingesting fruits, fruit juice, chocolate, potatoes, or other high-potassium foods can cause hyperkalemia. Most persons on CAPD do not need to limit potassium intake and often may even need to increase intake.

Persons with CKD are usually encouraged to limit their dietary phosphorus as a means of preventing secondary hyperparathyroidism, renal osteodystrophy, and metastatic calcification. Unfortunately, many processed and convenience foods contain considerable amounts of phosphorus additives. The most notable products using phosphorus additives are restructured meats (*e.g.*, chicken nuggets, hot dogs), processed and spreadable cheeses, instant products (*e.g.*, puddings, sauces), refrigerated bakery products, and beverages.[55] These phosphorus additives are highly absorbable. In a typical diet of grains, meats, and dairy products, only about 60% of phosphorus is absorbed, whereas phosphorus additives (*e.g.*, polyphosphates, pyrophosphates) are almost 100% absorbed.[55] Identifying these newer phosphorus-containing foods is often challenging because manufacturers are no longer required to list the phosphorus content on food labels.[55]

IN SUMMARY, CKD results from the destructive effects of many forms of renal disease. Regardless of the cause, the consequences of nephron destruction in CKD are alterations in the filtration, reabsorption, and endocrine functions of the kidneys. Chronic disease is defined as either diagnosed kidney damage or GFR of less than 60 mL/min/1.73 m^2 for 3 months or more, and kidney failure as a GFR of less than 15 mL/min/1.73 m^2, usually accompanied by most of the signs and symptoms of uremia, or a need to start renal replacement therapy.

CKD affects almost every body system. It causes an accumulation of nitrogenous wastes (*i.e.,* azotemia), alters sodium and water excretion, and alters regulation of body levels of potassium, phosphate, calcium, and magnesium. It also causes skeletal disorders, anemia, cardiovascular disorders, neurologic disturbances, gastrointestinal dysfunction, and discomforting skin changes.

The treatment measures for CKD can be divided into two types: conservative treatment measures and renal replacement therapy. Conservative treatment consists of measures to prevent or retard deterioration in remaining renal function and assist the body in compensating for the existing impairment. Interventions that have been shown to retard the progression of CKD include blood pressure normalization and control of blood glucose in persons with diabetes. Activated vitamin D can be used to increase calcium absorption and control secondary hyperparathyroidism. Recombinant human erythropoietin is used to treat the profound anemia that occurs in persons with chronic kidney disease. Renal replacement therapy (dialysis or kidney transplantation) is indicated when advanced uremia and serious electrolyte problems are present. ∎

CHRONIC KIDNEY DISEASE IN CHILDREN AND ELDERLY PERSONS

After completing this section of the chapter, you should be able to meet the following objectives:

- List the causes of CKD in children and describe the special problems of children with kidney failure.
- State why CKD is more common in the elderly and describe measures to prevent or delay the onset of kidney failure in this population.
- Describe the treatment of CKD in children and the elderly.

Although the spectrum of CKD among children and elderly persons is similar to that of adults, several unique issues affecting these groups warrant further discussion.

Chronic Kidney Disease in Children

The true incidence of CKD in infants and children is unknown. Available data suggest that 1% to 2% of persons with CKD are in the pediatric age range.[56] The causes of CKD in children include congenital malformations, inherited disorders, acquired diseases, and metabolic syndromes. The underlying cause correlates closely with the age of the child.[57] In children younger than 5 years of age, CKD is commonly the result of congenital malformations such as renal dysplasia or obstructive uropathy. After 5 years of age, acquired diseases (*e.g.,* glomerulonephritis) and inherited disorders (*e.g.,* familial juvenile nephronophthisis) predominate. CKD related to metabolic disorders such as hyperoxaluria and inherited disorders such as polycystic kidney disease may present throughout childhood.

The stages for progression of CKD in children are similar to those for adults: mild reduction of GFR to 60 to 89 mL/min/1.73 m²; moderate reduction of GFR to 30 to 59 mL/min/1.73 m²; severe reduction in GFR to 15 to 29 mL/min/1.73 m²; and kidney failure with a GFR of less than 15 mL/min/1.73 m², or a need for renal replacement therapy. Because the GFR is much lower in infancy and undergoes gradual changes in relation to body size during the first 2 years of age, these values apply only to children older than 2 years of age.[58]

The manifestations of CKD in children are quite varied and depend on the underlying disease condition. Features of CKD that are marked during childhood include severe growth impairment, developmental delay, delay in sexual maturation, bone abnormalities, and development of psychosocial problems. Critical growth periods occur during the first 2 years of life and during adolescence. Physical growth and cognitive development occur at a slower rate as consequences of CKD, especially among children with congenital kidney disease.[59] Puberty usually occurs at a later age in children with CKD, partly because of endocrine abnormalities. Renal osteodystrophies are more common and extensive in children than in adults. The most common condition seen in children is high–bone-turnover bone disease caused by secondary hyperparathyroidism. Some hereditary renal diseases, such as medullary cystic disease, have patterns of skeletal involvement that further complicate the problems of renal osteodystrophy. Clinical manifestations of renal osteodystrophy include muscle weakness, bone pain, fractures with minor trauma.[57] In growing children, rachitic changes, varus and valgus deformities of long bones, and slipped capital femoral epiphysis may be seen (see Chapter 58).

Factors related to impaired growth include deficient nutrition, anemia, renal osteodystrophy, chronic acidosis, and cases of nephrotic syndrome that require high-dose corticosteroid therapy. Nutrition is believed to be the most important determinant

during infancy.[60] During childhood, growth hormone is important, and gonadotropic hormones become important during puberty.[60] Parental heights provide a means of assessing growth potential (see Chapter 41). For many children, catch-up growth is important because a growth deficit frequently is established during the first months of life. Recombinant human growth hormone therapy has been used to improve growth in children with CKD.[60,61] Success of treatment depends on the level of bone maturation at the initiation of therapy.

All forms of renal replacement therapy can be safely and reliably used for children. Age is a defining factor in dialysis modality selection; 88% of infants and children from birth to 5 years of age are treated with peritoneal dialysis, whereas 54% of children older that 12 years of age are treated with hemodialysis.[57] The majority of North American children are treated with CCPD or NIPD, which leaves the child and family free of dialysis demands during waking hours, with the exchanges being performed automatically during sleep by the machine. Renal transplantation is considered the best alternative for children.[56,62] Early transplantation in young children is regarded as the best way to promote physical growth, improve cognitive function, and foster psychosocial development. Immunosuppressive therapy in children is similar to that used in adults. All of these immunosuppressive agents have side effects, including increased risk for infection. Corticosteroids, which have been the mainstay of chronic immunosuppressive therapy for decades, carry the risk for hypertension, orthopedic complications (especially aseptic necrosis), cataracts, and growth retardation.

Chronic Kidney Disease in Elderly Persons

Since the mid-1980s, there have been increasing numbers of elderly persons accepted to renal replacement therapy programs. Data from NHANES III suggest that almost 75% of people 70 years of age or older have a GFR less than 90 mL/min/1.73 m² and almost 25% may have a GFR less than 60 mL/min/1.73 m².[63] However, the true prevalence or outcomes of CKD in the elderly have not been systematically studied. Also, the presentation and course of CKD may be altered because of age-related changes in the kidneys and concurrent medical conditions.

Normal aging is associated with a decline in the GFR and subsequently with reduced homeostatic regulation under stressful conditions.[64] This reduction in GFR makes elderly persons more susceptible to the detrimental effects of nephrotoxic drugs, such as radiographic contrast compounds. The reduction in GFR related to aging is not accompanied by a parallel rise in the serum creatinine level because the serum creatinine level, which results from muscle metabolism, is significantly reduced in elderly persons because of diminished muscle mass and other age-related changes. The NKF guidelines suggest that the same criteria for establishing the presence of CKD in younger adults (*i.e.,* GFR <60 mL/min/1.73 m²) should be used for the elderly. Evaluation of elderly persons with a GFR of 60 to

89 mL/min/1.73 m² should include age-adjusted measurements of creatinine clearance, along with assessment of CKD risks, measurement of blood pressure, albumin-to-creatinine ratio in a "spot" urine specimen, and examination of the urine sediment for red and white blood cells.[64]

The prevalence of chronic disease affecting the cerebrovascular, cardiovascular, and skeletal systems is higher in this age group.[65] Because of concurrent disease, the presenting symptoms of kidney disease in elderly persons may be less typical than those observed in younger adults. For example, congestive heart failure and hypertension may be the dominant clinical features with the onset of acute glomerulonephritis, whereas oliguria and discolored urine more often are the first signs in younger adults. The course of CKD may be more complicated in older patients with numerous chronic diseases.

The NKF guidelines indicate that clinical interventions for the elderly with CKD should be based on diagnosis, severity of kidney function impairment, and stratification of risk for progression to renal failure and cardiovascular disease.[64] Persons with low risk may require only modification of dosages of medications excreted by the kidney, monitoring of blood pressure, avoidance of drugs and procedures that increase the risk of acute renal failure, and lifestyle modification to reduce the risk of cardiovascular disease.

Elderly persons with more severe impairment of kidney function may require renal replacement therapy. Treatment options for CKD in elderly patients include hemodialysis, peritoneal dialysis, transplantation, and acceptance of death from uremia. Neither hemodialysis nor peritoneal dialysis has proved to be superior in the elderly. The mode of renal replacement therapy should be individualized, taking into account underlying medical and psychosocial factors. Age alone should not preclude renal transplantation.[65,66] With increasing experience, many transplantation centers have increased the age for acceptance on transplant waiting lists. Reluctance to provide transplantation as an alternative may have been due, at least in part, to the scarcity of available organs and the view that younger persons are more likely to benefit for a longer time. The general reduction in T-lymphocyte function that occurs with aging has been suggested as a beneficial effect that increases transplant graft survival.

IN SUMMARY, available data suggest that 1% to 2% of patients with CKD are in the pediatric age range. The causes of CKD include congenital malformations (*e.g.,* renal dysplasia and obstructive uropathy), inherited disorders (*e.g.,* polycystic kidney disease), acquired diseases (*e.g.,* glomerulonephritis), and metabolic syndromes (*e.g.,* hyperoxaluria). Problems associated with CKD in children include growth impairment, delay in sexual maturation, and more extensive bone abnormalities than in adults. Although all forms of renal replacement therapy can be safely and reliably used in children, CCPD, NIPO, or transplantation optimizes growth and development.

Since the mid-1980s, there have been increasing numbers of elderly persons accepted for renal replacement therapy programs. Normal aging is associated with a decline in the GFR, which makes elderly persons more susceptible to the detrimental effects of nephrotoxic drugs and other conditions that compromise renal function. Current guidelines for diagnosis of CKD and stratification of risk for progression to kidney failure are the same as for younger adults. Treatment options for failure in elderly patients are also similar to those for younger adults. ■

Review Exercises

1. A 55-year-old man with diabetes and coronary heart disease, who had undergone cardiac catheterization with the use of a radiocontrast agent 2 days ago, is admitted to the emergency department with a flulike syndrome including chills, nausea, vomiting, abdominal pain, fatigue, and pulmonary congestion. His serum creatinine is elevated, and he has protein in his urine. He is admitted to the intensive care unit with a tentative diagnosis of acute renal failure due to radiocontrast nephropathy.

   A. *Radiocontrast agents are thought to exert their effects through decreased renal perfusion and through direct toxic effects on renal tubular structures. Explain how each of these phenomena contributes to the development of acute renal failure.*

   B. *Explain the elevated serum creatinine, proteinuria, and presence of pulmonary congestion.*

2. A 35-year-old, 70-kg white man with diabetes mellitus is seen in the diabetic clinic for his 6-month checkup. His serum creatinine, which was slightly elevated at his last visit, is now 1.6 mg/dL. Use the following website to estimate his GFR: www.kidney.org/professionals/kdoqi/gfr_calculator.cfm.

   A. *Would he be classified as having chronic kidney disease? If so, what stage? What might be done to delay or prevent further deterioration of his kidney function?*

3. Chronic kidney disease is accompanied by hyperphosphatemia, hypocalcemia, impaired activation of vitamin D, hyperparathyroidism, and skeletal complications.

   A. *Explain the impaired activation of vitamin D and its consequences on calcium and phosphate homeostasis, parathyroid function, and mineralization of bone in persons with CKD.*

   B. *Explain the possible complications of the administration of activated forms of vitamin D on parathyroid function and calcium and phosphate homeostasis (e.g., calcium × phosphate product).*

References

1. Singri N., Ahya S. N., Levin M. L. (2003). Acute renal failure. *Journal of the American Medical Association* 289, 747–751.

2. Albright R. C. Jr. (2001). Acute renal failure: A practical update. *Mayo Clinic Proceedings* 76, 67–74.

3. Brady H. R., Clarkson M. R., Liebman W. (2004). Acute renal failure. In Brenner B. M. (Ed.), *Brenner and Rector's the kidney online* (7th ed.). Philadelphia: Elsevier Saunders.

4. Thadhani R., Pascual M., Bonventre J. V. (1996). Acute renal failure. *New England Journal of Medicine* 334, 1448–1460.

5. Lameire N., Van Biesen W., Vanholder R. (2005). Acute renal failure. *Lancet* 365, 417–430.

6. Schrier R. W., Wang W., Pooler B., et al. (2004). Acute renal failure: Definitions, diagnosis, pathogenesis, and therapy. *Journal of Clinical Investigation* 114, 5–14.

7. Mitra A., Zolty E., Wang W., et al. (2005). Clinical acute renal failure. *Comprehensive Therapy* 31, 262–269.

8. Needham E. (2005). Management of acute renal failure. *American Family Physician* 22, 1739–1746.

9. Guyton A., Hall J. E. (2006). *Textbook of medical physiology* (11th ed., pp. 309–326). Philadelphia: Elsevier Saunders.

10. Gill N., Nally J. V., Fatica R. A. (2005). Renal failure secondary to acute tubular necrosis. *Chest* 128, 2847–2863.

11. Alpers C. E. (2005). The kidney. In Kumar V., Abbas A. K., Fausto N. (Eds.), *Robbins and Cotran pathologic basis of disease* (7th ed., pp. 993–996). Philadelphia: Elsevier Saunders.

12. McCullough P. A., Soman S. S. (2005). Contrast-induced nephropathy. *Critical Care Clinics* 21, 261–280.

13. Maddox T. G. (2002). Adverse reactions to contrast material: Recognition, prevention, and treatment. *American Family Physician* 66, 1229–1234.

14. National Kidney Foundation. (2002). K/DOQI Clinical Practice Guidelines for Chronic Kidney Disease: Evaluation, classification, and stratification. [Online.] Available: www.kidney.org/professionals/kdoqi/guidelines_ckd/toc.htm. Accessed January 19, 2007.

15. Levey A. S., Eckardt K.-W., Tsukamato Y. (2005). Definition and classification of chronic kidney disease: A position statement from kidney disease: Improving global outcomes (KDIGO). *Kidney International* 67, 2089–2100.

16. Levey A. S., Coresh J., Balk E., et al. (2003). National Kidney Foundation practice guidelines for chronic kidney disease: Evaluation, classification, and stratification. *Annals of Internal Medicine* 139, 137–147.

17. Johnson C. A., Levey A. S., Coresh J., et al. (2004). Clinical practice guidelines for chronic kidney disease in adults: Part I. Definition, disease stages, evaluation, treatment, and risk factors. *American Family Physician* 70, 869–876.

18. Skorecki K., Green J., Brenner B. M. (2005). Chronic renal failure. In Kasper D. L., Braunwald E., Fauci A. S., et al. (Eds.), *Harrison's principles of internal medicine* (16th ed., pp. 1653–1663). New York: McGraw-Hill.

19. Stevens L. A., Coresh J., Greene T., et al. (2006). Assessing kidney function: Measured and estimated glomerular filtration rate. *New England Journal of Medicine* 354, 2473–2483.

20. Johnson C. A., Levey A. S., Coresh J., et al. (2004). Clinical practice guidelines for chronic kidney disease in adults: Part II. Glomerular filtration rate, proteinuria, and other markers. *American Family Physician* 70, 1091–1097.

21. Eknoyan G., Hostetter T., Barkis G. L., et al. (2003). Proteinuria and other markers of chronic kidney disease: A position statement of the National Kidney Foundation (NKF) and the National Institute of Diabetes and Digestive and Kidney Diseases (NIDDK). *American Journal of Kidney Diseases* 42, 617–622.

22. Wang W., Chan L. (2003). Chronic renal failure: Manifestations and pathogenesis. In Schrier R. W. (Ed.), *Renal and electrolyte disorders* (6th ed., pp. 456–497). Philadelphia: Lippincott Williams & Wilkins.

23. Eknoyan G., Levin N. W. (2003). Bone metabolism and disease in chronic kidney disease. *American Journal of Kidney Diseases* 42(Suppl. 3), S1–S201.

24. Goodman W. G. (2005). Calcium and phosphorous metabolism in patients who have chronic kidney disease. *Medical Clinics of North America* 89, 631–647.

25. Ritz E., Gross M.-L., Dikow R. (2005). Role of calcium-phosphorous disorders in the progression of renal failure. *Kidney International* 68(Suppl. 99), S66–S70.

26. Albaaj F., Hutchinson A. J. (2003). Hyperphosphatemia in renal failure. *Drugs* 63, 577–576.

27. Elder G. (2002). Pathophysiology and recent advances in the management of renal osteodystrophy. *Journal of Bone and Mineral Research* 17, 2094–2105.

28. Martin K. J., Olgaard K., Colburn J. W., et al. (2004). Diagnosis, assessment, and treatment of bone turnover abnormalities in renal osteodystrophy. *American Journal of Kidney Diseases* 43, 558–565.

29. National Kidney Foundation. K/DOQI Clinical Practice Guideline and Clinical Practice Recommendations for Anemia in Chronic Kidney Disease. [Online.] Available: www.kidney.org/professionals/kdoqi/guidelines_anemia/guide2.htm. Accessed February 17, 2007.

30. Hsu C. Y., McCulloch C. E., Curhan G. C. (2000). Epidemiology of anemia associated with chronic renal insufficiency among adults in the United States: Results from the Third National Health and Nutrition Examination Survey. *Journal of the American Society of Nephrology* 13, 504–510.

31. Pendse S., Singh A. K. (2005). Complications of chronic renal kidney disease: Anemia, mineral metabolism, and cardiovascular disease. *Medical Clinics of North America* 89, 549–561.

32. Nurko S. (2006). Anemia in chronic kidney disease: Causes, diagnosis, treatment. *Cleveland Clinic Journal of Medicine* 73, 289–297.

33. Rossert J., Froissart M., Jacquot C. (2005). Anemia management and renal failure progression. *Kidney International* 68(Suppl. 99), S76–S81.

34. Boccardo P., Remuzzi G., Galbusera M. (2004). Platelet dysfunction in renal failure. *Seminars in Thrombosis and Hemostasis* 30, 579–589.

35. National Kidney Foundation Task Force on Cardiovascular Disease. (1998). Controlling the epidemic of cardiovascular disease in chronic renal disease. *American Journal of Kidney Diseases* 32, 853–906.

36. Curtis B. M., Parfey P. S. (2005). Congestive heart failure in chronic kidney disease: Disease specific mechanisms of systolic and diastolic heart failure and management. *Cardiovascular Clinics* 23, 275–284.

37. Levin A., Foley R. N. (2000). Cardiovascular disease in chronic renal failure. *American Journal of Kidney Diseases* 36(6 Suppl. 3), S24–S30.

38. Al-Ahmad A., Sarnak M. J., Salem D. N., et al. (2001). Cause and management of heart failure in patients with chronic renal disease. *Seminars in Nephrology* 21, 3–12.

39. Gunukula S., Spodick D. H. (2001). Pericardial disease in renal failure. *Seminars in Nephrology* 21, 52–56.

40. Brouns R., De Deyn P. P. (2004). Neurological complications in renal failure: A review. *Clinical Neurology and Neurosurgery* 107, 1–16.

41. Foulks C. J., Cushner H. M. (1986). Sexual dysfunction in the male dialysis patient: Pathogenesis, evaluation, and therapy. *American Journal of Kidney Diseases* 8, 211–212.

42. Rickus M. A. (1987). Sexual dysfunction in the female ESRD patient. *American Nephrology Nurses' Association Journal* 14, 185–186.

43. Quan D. J., Aweeks F. T. (2005). Dosing of drugs in renal failure. In Koda-Kimble M. A., Young L. Y., Kradjan W. A., et al. (Eds.), *Applied therapeutics: The clinical use of drugs* (8th ed., pp. 34-1–34-26). Philadelphia: Lippincott Williams & Wilkins.

44. Jabor B. L., Madias N. E. (2005). Progression of chronic kidney disease: Can it be prevented or arrested? *American Journal of Medicine* 118, 1323–1330.

45. Orth S. R. (2004). Effects of smoking on systemic and intrarenal hemodynamics: Influence on renal function. *Journal of the American Society of Nephrology* 15(Suppl. 1), S58–S63.

46. Rettig R. A. (1996). The social contract and the permanent treatment of renal failure. *Journal of the American Medical Association* 274, 1123–1125.

47. United States Renal Data System. (2007). Transplant process. [Online.] Available: www.usrds.org/2007/ref/E_tx_process_07.pdf. Accessed March 8, 2007.

48. Singh A. K., Brenner B. (2005). Dialysis in treatment of renal failure. In Kasper D. L., Braunwald E., Fauci A. S., et al. (Eds.), *Harrison's principles of internal medicine* (16th ed., pp. 1663–1667). New York: McGraw-Hill.

49. Daelemans R. A., D'Haese P. C., BeBroe M. E. (2001). Dialysis. *Seminars in Nephrology* 21, 204–212.

50. National Kidney and Urologic Diseases Information Clearinghouse. (2003). Kidney and urologic diseases statistics in the United States. [Online.] Available: http://kidney.niddk.nih.gov/kudiseases/pubs/kustats/index.htm#kp. Accessed February 17, 2007.

51. Carpenter C. B., Milford E. L., Sayegh M. H. (2005). Transplantation in treatment of renal failure. In Kasper D. L., Braunwald E., Fauci A. S., et al. (Eds.), *Harrison's principles of internal medicine* (16th ed., pp. 1668–1674). New York: McGraw-Hill.

52. Ramanathan V., Goral S., Helderman J. H. (2001). Renal transplantation. *Seminars in Nephrology* 21, 213–219.

53. National Kidney Foundation. (2000). Clinical practice guidelines for nutrition in chronic renal failure. [Online.] Available: www.kidney.org/professionals/kdoqi/guidelines_updates/doqi_nut.html. Accessed January 19, 2007.

54. Levey A. S., Adler S., Caggiula A. W., et al. (1996). Effects of dietary protein restriction on the progression of advanced renal disease in the modification of diet in renal disease study. *American Journal of Kidney Diseases* 27, 652–663.

55. Karalis M. (2005). Hidden phosphorus in popular beverages: Part 1; at breakfast: Part II, and enhanced meats: Part IV. *Journal of Renal Nutrition* 15(2, 3, 4), pp. e1–e6, e1–e6, e1–e4.

56. Chan J. C. M., Williams D. M., Roth K. S. (2002). Kidney failure in infants and children. *Pediatrics in Review* 23(2), 47–60.

57. Vogt B. A., Avner E. D. (2004). Renal failure. In Behrman R. E., Kliegman R. M., Jenson H. B. (Eds.), *Nelson textbook of pediatrics* (17th ed., pp. 1767–1775). Philadelphia: Elsevier Saunders.

58. Hogg R. J., Furth S., Lemley K. V., et al. (2003). National Kidney Foundation's kidney disease outcomes quality initiative clinical practice guidelines for chronic kidney disease in children and adolescents: Evaluation, classification, and stratification. *Pediatrics* 111, 1416–1423.

59. Hanna J. D., Krieg R. J., Scheinman J. I., et al. (1996). Effects of uremia on growth in children. *Seminars in Nephrology* 16, 230–241.

60. Abitbol C., Chan J. C. M., Trachtman H., et al. (1996). Growth in children with moderate renal insufficiency: Measurement, evaluation, and treatment. *Journal of Pediatrics* 129, S3–S7.

61. Haffner D., Schaffer F., Nissel R., et al. (Study Group for Growth Hormone Treatment in Chronic Renal Failure). (2000). Effect of growth hormone treatment on the adult height of children with chronic renal failure. *New England Journal of Medicine* 343, 923–930.

62. Urizar R. E. (2004). Renal transplantation. In Behrman R. E., Kliegman R. M., Jenson H. B. (Eds.), *Nelson textbook of pediatrics* (17th ed., pp. 1775–1782). Philadelphia: Elsevier Saunders.

63. National Kidney Foundation. (2002). Decreased kidney function in the elderly. K/DOQI Guidelines. [Online.] Available: www.kidney.org. Accessed January 23, 2007.

64. Choudhury D., Raj D. S. D., Palmer B., et al. (2000). Effect of aging on renal function and disease. In Brenner B. M. (Ed.), *Brenner and Rector's the kidney* (6th ed., pp. 2187–2210). Philadelphia: W. B. Saunders.

65. Hansberry M. R., Whittier W. L., Krause M. W. (2005). The elderly patient with chronic kidney disease. *Advances in Chronic Kidney Disease* 12(1), 71–77.

66. Davison A. M. (1998). Renal disease in the elderly. *Nephron* 80, 6–16.

Visit the Point. **http://thePoint.lww.com for animations, journal articles, and more!**

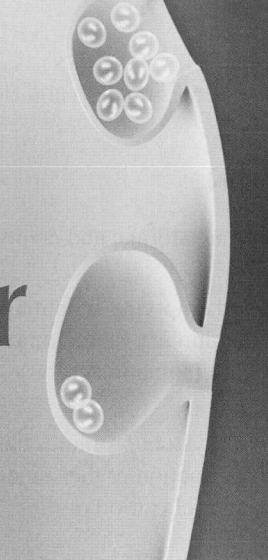

Chapter *35*

Disorders of the Bladder and Lower Urinary Tract

CAROL M. PORTH

➤ Although the kidneys control the formation of urine and regulate the composition of body fluids, it is the bladder that stores urine and controls its elimination from the body. Alterations in the storage and expulsion functions of the bladder can result in incontinence, with its accompanying social and hygienic problems, or obstruction of urinary flow, which has deleterious effects on ureteral and, ultimately, renal function. The discussion in this chapter focuses on the normal control of urine elimination, urinary obstruction and stasis, neurogenic bladder, incontinence, and bladder cancer. Urinary tract infections are discussed in Chapter 33.

CONTROL OF URINE ELIMINATION

After completing this section of the chapter, you should be able to meet the following objectives:

■ Trace the ascending sensory and descending motor impulses between the detrusor muscle and external urinary sphincter and the spinal cord, pontine micturition center, and cerebral cortex.
■ Explain the mechanism of low-pressure urine storage in the bladder.
■ List at least three classes of autonomic drugs and explain their potential effect on bladder function.
■ Describe at least three urodynamic studies that can be used to assess bladder function.

Bladder Structure

The bladder, also known as the *urinary vesicle,* is a freely movable organ located retroperitoneally on the pelvic floor, just posterior to the pubic symphysis. It consists of two main components: the body in which urine collects, and the neck, which is a funnel-shaped extension of the body that connects with the urethra.[1-5] In the male, the urethra continues anteriorly through the penis, with the prostate gland surrounding the neck of the bladder where it empties into the urethra. In the female, the bladder is located anterior to the vagina and uterus.

875

🗝 BLADDER FUNCTION

■ The functions of the bladder are storage and emptying of urine.

■ The control of the storage and emptying functions of the bladder involves both involuntary (autonomic nervous system) and voluntary (somatic nervous system) control.

■ The parasympathetic nervous system promotes bladder emptying. It produces contraction of the smooth muscle of the bladder wall and relaxation of the internal sphincter.

■ The sympathetic nervous system promotes bladder filling. It produces relaxation of the smooth muscle of the bladder wall and contraction of the internal sphincter.

■ The striated muscles in the external sphincter and pelvic floor, which are innervated by the somatic nervous system, provide for the voluntary control of urination and maintenance of continence.

Urine passes from the kidneys to the bladder through the ureters. The interior of the bladder has openings for both the ureters and the urethra. The smooth triangular area that is bounded by these three openings is called the *trigone* (Fig. 35-1). There are no valves at the ureteral openings, but as the pressure of the urine in the bladder rises, the ends of the ureters are compressed against the bladder wall to prevent the backflow of urine.

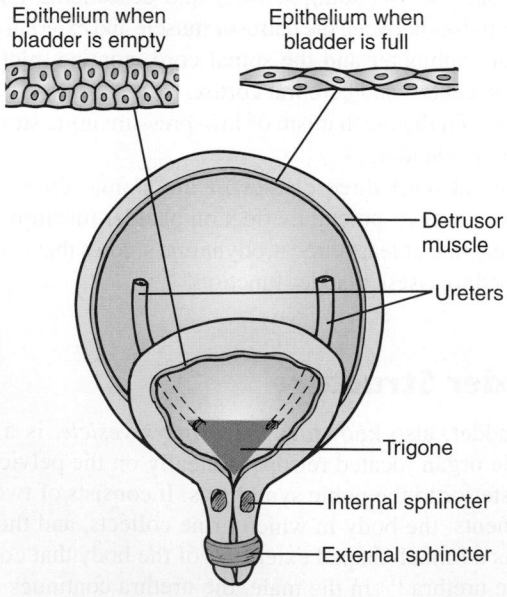

FIGURE 35-1 • Diagram of the bladder, showing the detrusor muscle, ureters, trigone area, and urethral orifice. Note the flattening of epithelial cells when the bladder is full and the wall is stretched.

The bladder is composed of four layers. The first is an outer serosal layer, which covers the upper surface and is continuous with the peritoneum. The second is a network of smooth muscle fibers called the *detrusor muscle*. The third is a submucosal layer of loose connective tissue, and the fourth is an inner mucosal lining of transitional epithelium (urothelium). This stratified epithelium is essentially impermeable to salts and water. The tonicity and composition of the urine often is quite different from that of the blood, and the epithelial lining of the bladder acts as an effective barrier to prevent the passage of water and other urine elements between the bladder and the blood. The epithelial lining of the bladder is six or more layers thick in the empty bladder. However, when the bladder is distended, as few as two or three layers are seen. This change reflects the ability of these cells to flatten and unfold to accommodate the increased surface area of a distended bladder (see Fig. 35-1).

The detrusor muscle is the muscle of micturition (passage of urine). When it contracts, urine is expelled from the bladder. Muscles in the bladder neck, sometimes referred to as the *internal urethral sphincter,* are a continuation of the detrusor muscle. They run down obliquely behind the proximal urethra, forming the posterior urethra in males and the entire urethra in females. When the bladder is relaxed, these circular muscle fibers are closed and act as a sphincter. When the detrusor muscle contracts, the sphincter is pulled open as the shape of the bladder changes. In the female, the urethra (2.5 to 3.5 cm) is shorter than in the male (16.5 to 18.5 cm), and usually affords less resistance to urine outflow.

Another muscle important to bladder function is the *external sphincter,* a circular muscle composed of striated muscle fibers that surrounds the urethra distal to the base of the bladder. The external sphincter operates as a reserve mechanism to stop micturition when it is occurring and to maintain continence in the face of unusually high bladder pressure. The skeletal muscle of the pelvic floor also contributes to the support of the bladder and the maintenance of continence.

Neural Control of Bladder Function

Normal bladder function requires the coordinated interaction between the sensory and motor components of the involuntary autonomic and voluntary somatic nervous systems. The motor component of the neural reflex that causes bladder emptying is controlled by the parasympathetic nervous system, whereas the relaxation and storage function of the bladder is controlled by the sympathetic nervous system. The somatic nervous system provides for the voluntary control of the external sphincter and pelvic floor muscles. These functions are controlled by three neurologic centers: the spinal cord reflex centers, the micturition center in the pons, and cortical and subcortical centers.

Spinal Cord Centers

The centers for reflex control of bladder function are located in the sacral (S1 through S4) and thoracolumbar (T11 through L2) segments of the spinal cord[1-6] (Fig. 35-2). The parasympathetic lower motor neurons (LMNs) for the detrusor muscle of

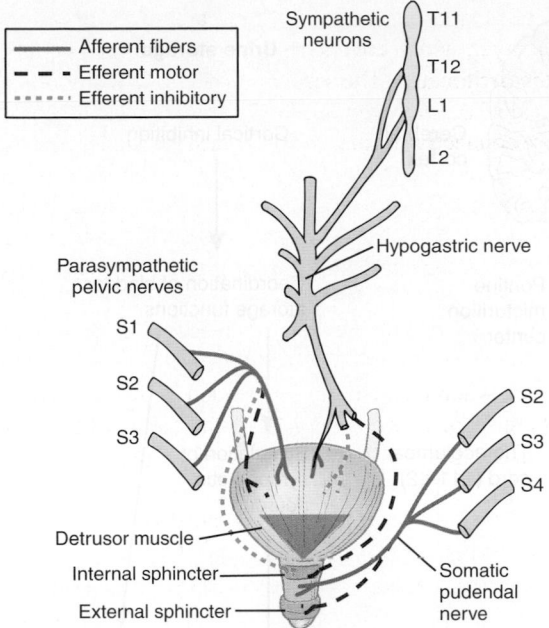

FIGURE 35-2 • Nerve supply to the bladder and the urethra.

the bladder are located in the sacral segments of the spinal cord; their axons travel to the bladder by way of the *pelvic nerve.* LMNs for the external sphincter also are located in the sacral segments of the spinal cord. These LMNs receive their control from the motor cortex through the corticospinal tract and send impulses to the external sphincter through the *pudendal nerve.* The bladder neck and trigone area of the bladder, because of their different embryonic origins, receive sympathetic outflow from the thoracolumbar (T11 to L2) segments of the spinal cord. In the male, the seminal vesicles, ampulla, and vas deferens also receive sympathetic innervation from the thoracolumbar segments of the cord.

The afferent input from the bladder and urethra is carried to the central nervous system (CNS) by fibers that travel with the parasympathetic (pelvic), somatic (pudendal), and sympathetic (hypogastric) nerves. The pelvic nerve carries sensory fibers from the stretch receptors in the bladder wall; the pudendal nerve carries sensory fibers from the external sphincter and pelvic muscles; and the hypogastric nerve carries sensory fibers from the trigone area.[3]

Pontine Micturition Center

The immediate coordination of the normal micturition reflex occurs in the micturition center in the pons, facilitated by descending input from the forebrain and ascending input from the reflex centers in the spinal cord[1,2] (Fig. 35-3). This center is thought to coordinate the activity of the detrusor muscle and the external sphincter. As bladder filling occurs, ascending spinal afferents relay this information to the micturition center, which also receives important descending information from the forebrain concerning behavioral cues for bladder emptying

and urine storage. Descending pathways from the pontine micturition center produce coordinated inhibition or relaxation of the external sphincter. Disruption of pontine control of micturition, as in spinal cord injury, results in uninhibited spinal reflex–controlled contraction of the bladder without relaxation of the external sphincter, a condition known as *detrusor–sphincter dyssynergia.*

Cortical and Subcortical Centers

Cortical brain centers enable inhibition of the micturition center in the pons and conscious control of urination. Neural influences from the subcortical centers in the basal ganglia modulate the contractile response. They modify and delay the detrusor contractile response during filling and then modulate the expulsive activity of the bladder to facilitate complete emptying.

Micturition and Maintenance of Continence

To maintain continence, or retention of urine, the bladder must function as a low-pressure storage system, with the pressure in the bladder being lower than that in the urethra. To ensure that this condition is met, the increase in intravesical pressure that accompanies bladder filling is almost imperceptible. For example, an increase in bladder volume from 10 to 400 mL may be accompanied by only a 5 cm H_2O increase in pressure.[1] Abnormal sustained elevations in intravesical pressures (>40 to 50 cm H_2O) often are associated with vesicoureteral reflux (*i.e.,* backflow of urine from the bladder into the ureter) and the development of ureteral dilation (see Chapter 33). Although the pressure in the bladder is maintained at low levels, sphincter pressure remains high (45 to 65 cm H_2O) as a means of preventing loss of urine as the bladder fills.

Micturition, or the act of bladder emptying, involves both sensory and motor functions associated with bladder emptying. When the bladder is distended to 150 to 250 mL in the adult, the sensation of fullness is transmitted to the spinal cord and then to the cerebral cortex, allowing for conscious inhibition of the micturition reflex.[4] During the act of micturition, the detrusor muscle of the bladder fundus and bladder neck contract down on the urine; the ureteral orifices are forced shut; the bladder neck is widened and shortened as it is pulled up by the globular muscles in the bladder fundus; the resistance of the internal sphincter in the bladder neck is decreased; and the external sphincter relaxes as urine moves out of the bladder.

Pharmacology of Micturition

The autonomic nervous system (ANS) and its neuromediators play a central role in micturition. Parasympathetic innervation of the bladder is mediated by the neurotransmitter acetylcholine. Two types of cholinergic receptors, nicotinic and muscarinic, affect various aspects of micturition. *Nicotinic* (N) receptors are found in the synapses between the preganglionic and postganglionic neurons of the sympathetic and the

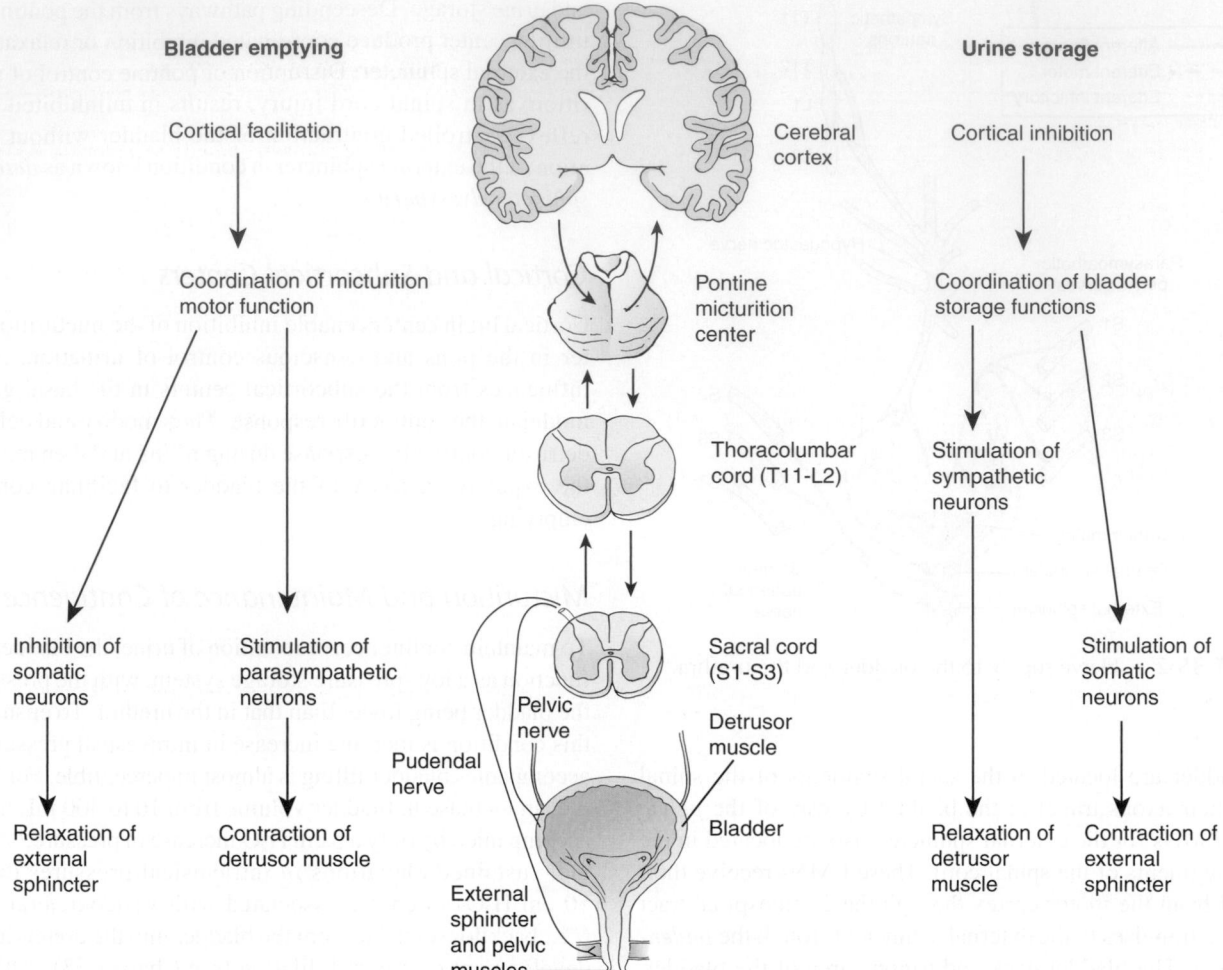

Bladder emptying

Cortical facilitation

Coordination of micturition motor function

Inhibition of somatic neurons

Stimulation of parasympathetic neurons

Relaxation of external sphincter

Contraction of detrusor muscle

Urine storage

Cortical inhibition

Coordination of bladder storage functions

Stimulation of sympathetic neurons

Stimulation of somatic neurons

Relaxation of detrusor muscle

Contraction of external sphincter

Cerebral cortex

Pontine micturition center

Thoracolumbar cord (T11-L2)

Sacral cord (S1-S3)

Pelvic nerve

Pudendal nerve

Detrusor muscle

Bladder

External sphincter and pelvic muscles

FIGURE 35-3 • Pathways and central nervous system centers involved in the control of bladder emptying (**left**) and storage (**right**) functions. Efferent pathways for micturition (**left**) and urine storage (**right**) also are shown.

parasympathetic system, as well as in the neuromuscular end-plates of the striated muscle fibers of the external sphincter and pelvic muscles. *Muscarinic* (M) receptors are found in the postganglionic parasympathetic endings of the detrusor muscle. Several subtypes of M receptors have been identified. Both M_2 and M_3 receptors appear to mediate detrusor muscle activity, with the M_3 subtype mediating direct activation of detrusor muscle contraction. The M_2 subtype appears to act indirectly by inhibiting sympathetically mediated detrusor muscle relaxation.[4,7,8] The identification of muscarinic receptor subtypes has facilitated the development of medications that selectively target bladder structures while minimizing undesired side effects.

Although sympathetic innervation is not essential to the act of micturition, it allows the bladder to store a large volume without the involuntary escape of urine—a mechanism that is consistent with the fight-or-flight function subserved by the sympathetic nervous system. The bladder is supplied with α_1- and β_2-adrenergic receptors. The β_2-adrenergic receptors are found in the detrusor muscle; they produce relaxation of the detrusor muscle, increasing the bladder volume at which the micturition reflex is triggered. The α_1-adrenergic receptors are found in the trigone area, including the intramural ureteral musculature, bladder neck, and internal sphincter. The activation of α_1-adrenergic receptors produces contraction of these muscles. Sympathetic activity ceases when the micturition reflex is activated. During male ejaculation, which is mediated by the sympathetic nervous system, the musculature of the trigone area and that of the bladder neck and prostatic urethra contract and prevent the backflow of seminal fluid into the bladder.

Because of their effects on bladder function, drugs that selectively activate or block ANS outflow or receptor activity can alter urine elimination. Table 35-1 describes the action of drug groups that can impair bladder function or can be used in the treatment of micturition disorders. Many of the nonprescription cold preparations contain α-adrenergic agonists and antihistamine agents that have anticholinergic properties. These drugs can cause urinary retention. Many of the antidepressant and antipsychotic drugs also have anticholinergic actions that influence urination.

TABLE 35-1 Action of Drug Groups on Bladder Function

FUNCTION	DRUG GROUPS	MECHANISM OF ACTION
Detrusor Muscle		
Increased tone and contraction	Cholinergic drugs	Stimulate parasympathetic receptors that cause detrusor contraction
Inhibition of detrusor muscle relaxation during filling	β_2-Adrenergic blockers	Block β_2 receptors that produce detrusor muscle relaxation
Decreased tone	Anticholinergic drugs and drugs with an anticholinergic action	Block the muscarinic receptors that cause detrusor muscle contraction
	Calcium channel blockers	May interfere with influx of calcium to support contraction of detrusor smooth muscle
Internal Bladder Sphincter		
Increased tone	α_1-Adrenergic agonists	Activate α_1 receptors that produce contraction of the smooth muscle of the internal sphincter
Decreased tone	α_1-Adrenergic blockers	Block contraction of the smooth muscle of the internal sphincter
External Sphincter		
Decreased tone	Skeletal muscle relaxants	Decrease the tone of the external sphincter by acting at the level of the spinal cord or by interfering with release of calcium in the muscle fibers

 ## Continence in Children

In infants and young children, micturition is an involuntary act that is triggered by a spinal cord reflex; when the bladder fills to a given capacity, the detrusor muscle contracts, and the external sphincter relaxes. As the child grows, the bladder gradually enlarges, with an increase in capacity, in ounces, that approximates the age of the child plus 2.[9] This formula applies up to age 12 to 14 years. As the bladder grows and increases in capacity, the tone of the external sphincter muscle increases. Toilet training begins at about 2 to 3 years of age when the child becomes conscious of the need to urinate. Conscious control of bladder function depends on (1) normal bladder growth, (2) myelination of the ascending afferents that signal awareness of bladder filling, (3) development of cortical control and descending communication with the sacral micturition center, (4) ability consciously to tighten the external sphincter to prevent incontinence, and (5) motivation of the child to stay dry. Girls typically achieve continence before boys, and bowel control is typically achieved before bladder control. By 5 years of age, 90% to 95% of children are continent during the day and 80% to 85% are continent at night.[9]

Diagnostic Methods of Evaluating Bladder Function

Bladder structure and function can be assessed by a number of methods.[10] Reports or observations of frequency, hesitancy, straining to urinate or void, and a weak or interrupted stream are suggestive of outflow obstruction. Palpation and percussion provide information about bladder distention.

Physical Examination

Postvoid residual (PVR) urine volume provides information about bladder emptying. It can be estimated by abdominal palpation and percussion. Catheterization and ultrasonography can be used to obtain specific measurements of PVR. A PVR value of less than 50 mL is considered adequate bladder emptying, and more than 200 mL indicates inadequate bladder emptying.[11]

Pelvic examination is used in women to assess perineal skin condition, perivaginal muscle tone, genital atrophy, pelvic prolapse (e.g., cystocele, rectocele, uterine prolapse), pelvic mass, or other conditions that may impair bladder function. Bimanual examination (i.e., pelvic and abdominal palpation) can be used to assess PVR volume. Rectal examination is used to test for perineal sensation, sphincter tone, fecal impaction, and rectal mass. It is also used to assess the contour of the prostate in men.

Laboratory and Radiologic Studies

Urine tests provide information about kidney function and urinary tract infections (discussed in Chapter 33). The presence of bacteriuria or pyuria suggests urinary tract infection and the possibility of urinary tract obstruction. Blood tests (i.e., blood urea nitrogen and creatinine) provide information about renal function.

Bladder structures can be visualized indirectly by taking x-ray films of the abdomen and by using excretory urography, which involves the use of a radiopaque dye, computed tomographic (CT) scanning, magnetic resonance imaging (MRI), or ultrasonography. Cystoscopy enables direct visualization of the urethra, bladder, and ureteral orifices.

Ultrasonographic Bladder Scan

The ultrasonographic bladder scan provides a noninvasive method for estimating bladder volume.[12,13] The device uses ultrasonic reflections to differentiate the urinary bladder from the surrounding tissue. A computer system calculates and displays bladder volume. The device can be used to determine the need for catheterization, for evaluation and diagnosis of urinary retention, to measure PVR volumes, and for facilitating volume-dependent or time-dependent catheterization or toileting programs.

Urodynamic Studies

Urodynamic studies are used to study bladder function and voiding problems. Three aspects of bladder function can be assessed by urodynamic studies: bladder, urethral, and intra-abdominal pressure changes; characteristics of urine flow; and the activity of the striated muscles of the external sphincter and pelvic floor. Specific urodynamic tests include uroflowmetry, cystometry, urethral pressure profile, and sphincter electromyography (EMG). It often is advantageous to evaluate several components of bladder function simultaneously.

Uroflowmetry. Uroflowmetry measures the flow rate (milliliters per minute) during urination.[10] It commonly is done using a weight-recording device located at the bottom of a commode receptacle unit. As the person being tested voids, the weight of the commode receptacle unit increases. This weight change is electronically recorded and then analyzed as volume (weight converted to milliliters) versus time.

Cystometry. Cystometry is used to measure bladder pressure during filling and voiding. It provides valuable information about total bladder capacity, intravesical pressures during bladder filling, the ability to perceive bladder fullness and the desire to urinate, the ability of the bladder to contract and sustain a contraction, uninhibited bladder contractions, and the ability to inhibit urination. Bladder pressure is measured using gas or water to transfer pressure to a transducer near a polygraph, or a pressure-tipped catheter to transfer the pressure recording directly to a polygraph.[10] The test can be done by allowing physiologic filling of the bladder with urine and recording intravesical pressure throughout a voiding cycle, or by using a catheter to fill the bladder with water and measuring intravesical pressure against the volume of water instilled into the bladder.[10]

In a normally functioning bladder, the sensation of bladder fullness is first perceived when the bladder contains 100 to 200 mL of urine while bladder pressure remains constant at approximately 8 to 15 cm H_2O. The desire to void occurs when the bladder is full (normal capacity is approximately 400 to 500 mL). At this point, a definite sensation of fullness occurs, the pressure rises sharply to 40 to 100 cm H_2O, and voiding occurs around the catheter.[10] Urinary continence requires that urethral pressure exceed bladder pressure. Bladder pressure usually rises 30 to 40 cm H_2O during voiding. If the urethral resistance is high because of obstruction, greater pressure is required, a condition that can be detected by cystometry.

Urethral Pressure Profile. The urethral pressure profile is used to evaluate the intraluminal pressure changes along the length of the urethra with the bladder at rest.[10] It provides information about smooth muscle activity along the length of the urethra. This test can be done using the infusion method (most commonly used), the membrane catheter method, or the microtip transducer. The infusion method involves the insertion of a small double-lumen urethral catheter, followed by the infusion of water into the bladder and measurement of the changes in urethral pressure as the catheter is slowly withdrawn.

Sphincter Electromyography. Sphincter EMG allows the activity of the striated (voluntary) muscles of the perineal area to be studied. Activity is recorded using an anal plug electrode, a catheter electrode, adhesive skin electrodes, or needle electrodes.[10] Electrode placement is based on the muscle groups that need to be tested. The test usually is done along with urodynamic tests such as cystometry and uroflowmetry.

IN SUMMARY, although the kidneys function in the formation of urine and the regulation of body fluids, it is the bladder that stores and controls the elimination of urine. Micturition is a function of the peripheral ANS, subject to facilitation or inhibition from higher neurologic centers. The parasympathetic nervous system controls the function of the detrusor muscle and internal sphincter; its cell bodies are located in S1 through S3 of the spinal cord and communicate with the bladder through the pelvic nerve. Efferent sympathetic control originates at the thoracolumbar level (T11 through L2) of the spinal cord and produces relaxation of the detrusor muscle and contraction of the internal sphincter. Skeletal muscle found in the external sphincter and the pelvic muscles that support the bladder are supplied by the pudendal nerve, which exits the spinal cord at the sacral level (S2 through S4) of the spinal cord. The pontine micturition center coordinates the action of the detrusor muscle and the external sphincter, whereas cortical centers permit conscious control of micturition.

Bladder function can be evaluated using urodynamic studies that measure bladder, urethral, and abdominal pressures; urine flow characteristics; and skeletal muscle activity of the external sphincter. ■

ALTERATIONS IN BLADDER FUNCTION

After completing this section of the chapter, you should be able to meet the following objectives:

■ Describe the causes of and compensatory changes that occur with urinary tract obstruction.

■ Differentiate lesions that produce storage dysfunction associated with spastic bladder from those that produce

emptying dysfunction associated with flaccid bladder in terms of the level of the lesions and their effects on bladder function.
- Describe methods used in treatment of neurogenic bladder.
- Define *incontinence* and differentiate between stress incontinence, overactive bladder/urge incontinence, and overflow incontinence.
- Describe behavioral, pharmacologic, and surgical methods used in treatment of the different types of incontinence.
- List the treatable causes of incontinence in the elderly.

Alterations in bladder function include urinary obstruction with retention or stasis of urine and urinary incontinence with involuntary loss of urine. Although the two conditions have almost opposite effects on urination, they can have similar causes. Both can result from structural changes in the bladder, urethra, or surrounding organs or from impairment of neurologic control of bladder function.

Lower Urinary Tract Obstruction and Stasis

Urinary tract obstructions are classified according to cause (congenital or acquired), degree (partial or complete), duration (acute or chronic), and level (upper or lower urinary tract).[14] In lower urinary tract obstruction and stasis, urine is produced normally by the kidneys but is retained in the bladder. Because it has the potential to produce vesicoureteral reflux and cause kidney damage, lower urinary tract obstruction and stasis is a serious disorder.

The common sites of congenital obstructions are the external meatus (*i.e.,* meatal stenosis) in boys and just inside the external urinary meatus in girls. Another congenital cause of urinary stasis is the damage to sacral nerves that is seen in spina bifida and meningomyelocele.

The acquired causes of lower urinary tract obstruction and stasis are numerous. In males, the most important cause of urinary obstruction is external compression of the urethra caused by the enlargement of the prostate gland. Gonorrhea and other sexually transmitted infections contribute to the incidence of infection-produced urethral strictures. Bladder tumors and secondary invasion of the bladder by tumors arising in structures that surround the bladder and urethra can compress the bladder neck or urethra and cause obstruction. Because of the proximity of the involved structures, constipation and fecal impaction can compress the urethra and produce urethral obstruction. This can be a particular problem in elderly persons.

Compensatory and Decompensatory Changes

The body compensates for the obstruction of urine outflow with mechanisms designed to prevent urine retention. These

NEUROGENIC BLADDER DISORDERS

- Neurogenic disorders of the bladder commonly are manifested by a spastic bladder dysfunction, in which there is failure to store urine, or as flaccid bladder dysfunction, in which bladder emptying is impaired.
- Spastic bladder dysfunction results from neurologic lesions above the level of the sacral cord that allow neurons in the micturition center to function reflexively without control from higher central nervous system centers.
- Flaccid bladder dysfunction results from neurologic disorders affecting the motor neurons in the sacral cord or peripheral nerves that control detrusor muscle contraction and bladder emptying.

mechanisms can be divided into two stages: a compensatory stage and a decompensatory stage.[14] The degree to which these changes occur and their effect on bladder structure and urinary function depend on the extent of the obstruction, the rapidity with which it occurs, and the presence of other contributing factors, such as neurologic impairment and infection.

During the early stage of obstruction, the bladder begins to hypertrophy and becomes hypersensitive to afferent stimuli arising from stretch receptors in the bladder wall. The ability to suppress urination is diminished, and bladder contraction can become so strong that it virtually produces bladder spasm. There is urgency, sometimes to the point of incontinence, and frequency during the day and at night.

With continuation and progression of the obstruction, compensatory changes begin to occur. There is further hypertrophy of the bladder muscle, the thickness of the bladder wall may double, and the pressure generated by detrusor contraction can increase from a normal 20 to 40 cm H_2O to 50 to 100 cm H_2O to overcome the resistance from the obstruction. As the force needed to expel urine from the bladder increases, compensatory mechanisms may become ineffective, causing muscle fatigue before complete emptying can be accomplished. After a few minutes, voiding can again be initiated and completed, accounting for the frequency of urination.

The inner bladder surface forms smooth folds. With continued outflow obstruction, this smooth surface is replaced with coarsely woven structures (*i.e.,* hypertrophied smooth muscle fibers) called *trabeculae*. Small pockets of mucosal tissue, called *cellules,* commonly develop between the trabecular ridges. These pockets form diverticula when they extend between the actual fibers of the bladder muscle (Fig. 35-4). Because the diverticula have no muscle, they are unable to contract and expel their urine into the bladder, and secondary infections caused by stasis are common.

Along with hypertrophy of the bladder wall, there is hypertrophy of the trigone area and the interureteric ridge, which is located between the two ureters. This causes backpressure on the ureters, the development of hydroureters (*i.e.,* dilated, urine-

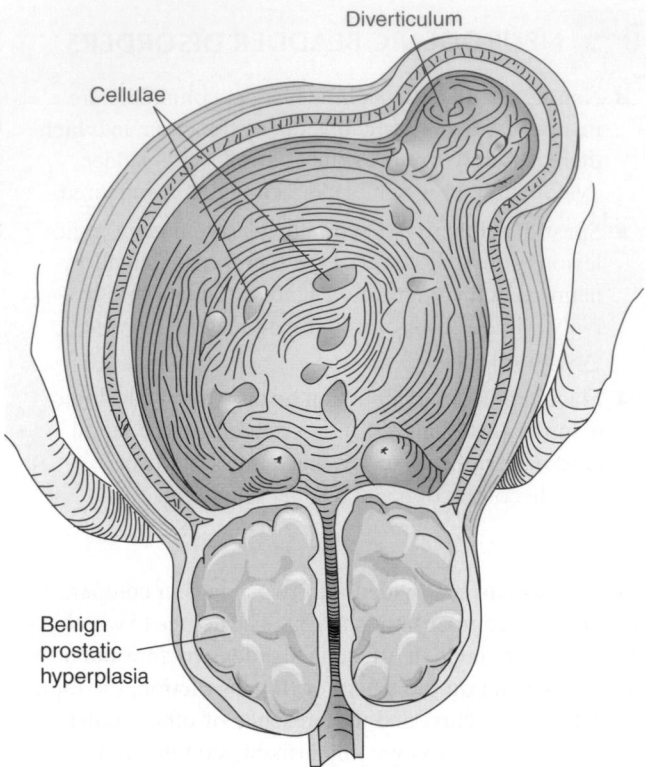

Diverticulum

Cellulae

Benign
prostatic
hyperplasia

FIGURE 35-4 • Destructive changes of the bladder wall with development of diverticulum caused by benign prostatic hypertrophy.

filled ureters), and, eventually, kidney damage (see Chapter 33, Fig. 33-5). Stasis of urine predisposes to urinary tract infections.

When compensatory mechanisms no longer are effective, signs of decompensation begin to appear. The period of detrusor muscle contraction becomes too short to expel the urine completely, and residual urine remains in the bladder. At this point, the symptoms of obstruction—frequency of urination, hesitancy, need to strain to initiate urination, a weak and small stream, and termination of the stream before the bladder is completely emptied—become pronounced. With progressive decompensation, the bladder may become severely overstretched, with a residual urine volume of 1000 to 3000 mL.[14] At this point, it loses its power of contraction and overflow incontinence occurs. The signs of outflow obstruction and urine retention are summarized in Chart 35-1.

CHART 35-1   SIGNS OF OUTFLOW OBSTRUCTION AND URINE RETENTION

Bladder distention
Hesitancy
Straining when initiating urination
Small and weak stream
Frequency
Feeling of incomplete bladder emptying
Overflow incontinence

Treatment

The immediate treatment of lower urinary tract obstruction and stasis is directed toward relief of bladder distention. This usually is accomplished through urinary catheterization (to be discussed). Constipation or fecal impaction should be corrected. Long-term treatment is directed toward correcting the problem causing the obstruction.

Neurogenic Bladder Disorders

The urinary bladder is unique in that it is probably the only autonomically innervated visceral organ that is under CNS control. The neural control of bladder function can be interrupted at any level. It can be interrupted at the level of the peripheral nerves that connect the bladder to the reflex micturition center in the sacral cord, the ascending and descending tracts in the spinal cord, the pontine micturition center, or the cortical centers that are involved in voluntary control of micturition[13,15,16] (see Fig. 35-3).

Neurogenic disorders of bladder function commonly are manifested in one of two ways: failure to store urine (spastic bladder dysfunction) or failure to empty (flaccid bladder dysfunction). Spastic bladder dysfunction usually results from neurologic lesions located above the level of the sacral micturition reflexes, whereas flaccid bladder dysfunction results from lesions at the level of the sacral micturition reflexes or the peripheral nerves that innervate the bladder. In addition to disorders of detrusor muscle function, disruption of micturition occurs when the neurologic control of external sphincter function is disrupted. Some disorders, such as stroke and Parkinson disease, may affect both the storage and emptying functions of the bladder. Table 35-2 describes the characteristics of neurogenic bladder according to the level of the lesion.

Spastic Bladder: Failure to Store Urine

Failure to store urine results from conditions that cause reflex bladder spasm and a decrease in bladder volume. It commonly is caused by conditions that produce partial or extensive neural damage above the micturition reflex center in the sacral cord (see Fig. 35-3). As a result, bladder function is regulated by segmental reflexes, without control from higher brain centers. The degree of bladder spasticity and dysfunction depends on the level and extent of neurologic dysfunction. Usually, both the ANS neurons controlling bladder function and the somatic neurons controlling the function of the striated muscles in the external sphincter are affected. In some cases, there is a detrusor–sphincter dyssynergia with uncoordinated contraction and relaxation of the detrusor and external sphincter muscles. The most common causes of spastic bladder dysfunction are spinal cord lesions such as spinal cord injury, herniated intervertebral disk, vascular lesions, tumors, and myelitis. Other neurologic conditions that affect voiding are stroke, multiple sclerosis, and brain tumors.

TABLE 35-2 Types and Characteristics of Neurogenic Bladder

LEVEL OF LESION	CHANGE IN BLADDER FUNCTION	COMMON CAUSES
Sensory cortex, motor cortex, or corticospinal tract	Loss of ability to perceive bladder filling; low-volume, physiologically normal micturition that occurs suddenly and is difficult to inhibit	Stroke and advanced age
Basal ganglia or extrapyramidal tract	Detrusor contractions are elicited suddenly without warning and are difficult to control; bladder contraction is shorter than normal and does not produce full bladder emptying	Parkinson disease
Pontine micturition center or communicating tracts in the spinal cord	Storage reflexes are provoked during filling, and external sphincter responses are heightened; uninhibited bladder contractions occur at a lower volume than normal and do not continue until the bladder is emptied; antagonistic activity occurs between the detrusor muscle and the external sphincter	Spinal cord injury
Sacral cord or nerve roots	Areflexic bladder fills but does not contract; loss of external sphincter tone occurs when the lesion affects the α-adrenergic motor neurons or pudendal nerve	Injury to sacral cord or spinal roots
Pelvic nerve	Increased filling and impaired sphincter control cause increased intravesicular pressure	Radical pelvic surgery
Autonomic peripheral sensory pathways	Bladder overfilling occurs owing to a loss of ability to perceive bladder filling	Diabetic neuropathies, multiple sclerosis

Bladder Dysfunction Caused by Spinal Cord Injury. One of the most common types of spinal cord lesions is spinal cord injury (see Chapter 50). The immediate and early effects of spinal cord injury on bladder function are quite different from those that follow recovery from the initial injury. During the period immediately after spinal cord injury, a state of spinal shock develops, during which all the reflexes, including the micturition reflex, are depressed. During this stage, the bladder becomes atonic and cannot contract. Catheterization is necessary to prevent injury to urinary structures associated with overdistention of the bladder. Aseptic intermittent catheterization is the preferred method of catheterization. Depression of reflexes lasts from a few weeks to 6 months (usually 2 to 3 months), after which the spinal reflexes return and become hyperactive.

After the acute stage of spinal cord injury, the micturition response changes from a long-tract reflex to a segmental reflex. Because the sacral reflex arc remains intact, stimuli generated by bladder stretch receptors during filling produce frequent spontaneous contractions of the detrusor muscle. This creates a small, hyperactive bladder subject to high-pressure and short-duration uninhibited bladder contractions. Voiding is interrupted, involuntary, or incomplete. Dilation of the internal sphincter and spasticity of the external sphincter and perineal muscles innervated by upper motor neurons occur, producing resistance to bladder emptying. Hypertrophy of the trigone develops, often leading to vesicoureteral reflux and risk for renal damage.

Spastic bladder due to spinal cord injuries at the cervical level is often accompanied by a condition known as *autonomic hyperreflexia* (see Chapter 50). Because the injury interrupts CNS control of sympathetic reflexes in the spinal cord, severe hypertension, bradycardia, and sweating can be triggered by insertion of a catheter or mild overdistention of the bladder.

Uninhibited Neurogenic Bladder. A mild form of reflex neurogenic bladder, sometimes called *uninhibited bladder,* can develop after a stroke, during the early stages of multiple sclerosis, or as a result of lesions located in the inhibitory centers of the cortex or the pyramidal tract. With this type of disorder, the sacral reflex arc and sensation are retained, the urine stream is normal, and there is no residual urine. Bladder capacity is diminished, however, because of increased detrusor muscle tone and spasticity.

Detrusor–Sphincter Dyssynergia. Depending on the level of the lesion, the coordinated activity of the detrusor muscle and the external sphincter may be affected. Lesions that affect the micturition center in the pons or impair communication between the micturition center and spinal cord centers interrupt the coordinated activity of the detrusor muscle and the external sphincter. This is called *detrusor–sphincter dyssynergia.* Instead of relaxing during micturition, the external sphincter becomes more constricted. This condition can lead to elevated intravesical pressures, vesicoureteral reflux, and kidney damage.

Treatment. Among the methods used to treat spastic bladder and detrusor–sphincter dyssynergia are the administration of anticholinergic medications to decrease bladder hyperactivity (to be discussed) and urinary catheterization to produce bladder emptying. A sphincterotomy (surgical resection of the external sphincter) or implantable urethral stent may be used to decrease outflow resistance in a person who cannot be managed with medications and catheterization procedures. An alternative to surgical resection of the external sphincter is the injection of botulinum toxin type A (BTX-A) to produce paralysis of the striated muscles in the external sphincter. The effects of the injection last from 3 to 9 months, after which the injection must be repeated.[15]

Flaccid Bladder: Failure to Empty Urine

Failure to empty the bladder can be due to flaccid bladder dysfunction, peripheral neuropathies that interrupt afferent or efferent communication between the bladder and the spinal cord, or conditions that prevent relaxation of the external sphincter (see Fig. 35-3).

Flaccid Bladder Dysfunction. Detrusor muscle areflexia, or flaccid neurogenic bladder, occurs when there is injury to the micturition center of the sacral cord, the cauda equina, or the sacral nerves that supply the bladder.[16] Atony of the detrusor muscle and loss of the perception of bladder fullness permit the overstretching of the detrusor muscle that contributes to weak and ineffective bladder contractions. External sphincter tone and perineal muscle tone are diminished. Voluntary urination does not occur, but fairly efficient emptying usually can be achieved by increasing the intra-abdominal pressure or applying manual suprapubic pressure. Among the causes of flaccid neurogenic bladder are trauma, tumors, and congenital anomalies (e.g., spina bifida, meningomyelocele).

Bladder Dysfunction Caused by Peripheral Neuropathies. In addition to CNS lesions and conditions that disrupt bladder function, disorders of the peripheral (pelvic, pudendal, and hypogastric) nerves that supply the muscles of micturition can occur. These neuropathies can selectively interrupt sensory or motor pathways for the bladder or involve both pathways.

Bladder atony with dysfunction is a frequent complication of diabetes mellitus.[17,18] The disorder initially affects the sensory axons of the urinary bladder without involvement of the pudendal nerve. This leads to large residual volumes after micturition, sometimes complicated by infection. There frequently is a need for straining, accompanied by hesitation, weakness of the stream, dribbling, and a sensation of incomplete bladder emptying.[18] The chief complications are vesicoureteral reflux and ascending urinary tract infection. Because persons with diabetes are already at risk for development of kidney disease, urinary stasis and reflux can have serious effects on renal function (see Chapter 33). Treatment consists of client education, including the need for frequent voiding (e.g., every 3 to 4 hours while awake), use of abdominal compression to effect more complete bladder emptying, and intermittent catheterization when necessary.[18]

Nonrelaxing External Sphincter

Another condition that affects micturition and bladder function is the nonrelaxing external sphincter. This condition usually is related to a delay in maturation, developmental regression, psychomotor disorders, or locally irritative lesions. Inadequate relaxation of the external sphincter can be the result of anxiety or depression. Any local irritation can produce spasms of the sphincter through afferent sensory input from the pudendal

nerve, including vaginitis, perineal inflammation, and inflammation or irritation of the urethra. In men, chronic prostatitis contributes to impaired relaxation of the external sphincter.

Treatment

The goals of treatment for neurogenic bladder disorders focus on preventing bladder overdistention, urinary tract infections, and potentially life-threatening kidney damage; and reducing the undesirable social and psychological effects of the disorder. The methods used in treatment of neurogenic bladder disorders are individualized based on the type of neurologic lesion that is involved; information obtained through the health history, including fluid intake; report or observation of voiding patterns; presence of other health problems; urodynamic studies when indicated; and the ability of the person to participate in the treatment. Treatment methods include catheterization, bladder training, pharmacologic manipulation of bladder function, and surgery.

Catheterization. Catheterization involves the insertion of a small-diameter latex or silicone tube into the bladder through the urethra.[19] The catheter may be inserted on a one-time basis to relieve temporary bladder distention, left indwelling (i.e., retention catheter), or inserted intermittently. With acute overdistention of the bladder, usually no more than 1000 mL of urine is removed from the bladder at one time. The theory behind this limitation is that removing more than this amount at one time releases pressure on the pelvic blood vessels and predisposes to alterations in circulatory function.

Permanent indwelling catheters sometimes are used when there is urine retention or incontinence in persons who are ill or debilitated or when conservative or surgical methods for the correction of incontinence are not feasible. The use of permanent indwelling bladder catheters in patients with spinal cord injury has been shown to produce a number of complications, including urinary tract infections, pyelonephritis, and kidney stones. Because urethral catheters often produce urethral irritation and injury, a suprapubic catheter may be inserted in persons requiring long-term catheter drainage.[13]

Intermittent catheterization is used to treat urine retention or incomplete emptying secondary to various neurologic or obstructive disorders.[19] Properly used, it prevents bladder overdistention and urethral irritation, allows more freedom of activity, and provides periodic distention of the bladder to prevent muscle atony. It often is used with pharmacologic manipulation to achieve continence; when possible, it is learned and managed as a self-care procedure (i.e., intermittent self-catheterization).[20] It may be carried out as an aseptic (sterile) or a clean procedure. Aseptic intermittent catheterization is used in persons with spinal shock and in those who need short-term catheterization.

The clean procedure typically is used for self-catheterization. It is performed at 3- to 4-hour intervals to prevent overdistention of the bladder. The best results are obtained if only 300 to 400 mL is allowed to collect in the bladder between catheterizations. The use of the clean instead of the sterile procedure has been defended on the basis that most urinary tract infections are caused by some underlying abnormality of the urinary tract that leads to impaired mucosal resistance to bacterial infection, the most common cause of which is decreased blood flow to the bladder wall because of bladder overdistention.[19]

Bladder Retraining. Bladder retraining differs with the type of disorder.[21] Methods used to supplement bladder retraining include monitoring fluid intake to prevent urinary tract infections and control urine volume and osmolality, developing scheduled times for urination, and using body positions that facilitate micturition. Adequate fluid intake also is needed to prevent urinary tract infections, the irritating effects of which increase bladder irritability and the risk for urinary incontinence and renal damage. Fluid intake must be balanced to prevent bladder overdistention from occurring during the night. Developing scheduled times for urinating prevents overdistention of the bladder.

The methods used for bladder retraining depend on the type of lesion causing the disorder. In spastic neurogenic bladder, methods designed to trigger the sacral micturition reflex are used; in flaccid neurogenic bladder, manual methods that increase intravesical pressure are used. Trigger voiding methods include manual stimulation of the afferent loop of the micturition reflex through such maneuvers as tapping the suprapubic area, pulling on the pubic hairs, stroking the glans penis, or rubbing the thighs. Credé maneuvers, which are used with the person in a sitting position, consists of applying pressure with four fingers of one hand or both hands to the suprapubic area as a means of increasing intravesical pressure. The Valsalva maneuver (*i.e.,* bearing down by exhaling against a closed glottis) increases intra-abdominal pressure and aids in bladder emptying. This maneuver is repeated until the bladder is empty. For the best results, the patient must cooperate fully with the procedures and, if possible, learn to perform them independently.

Biofeedback methods have been useful for teaching some aspects of bladder control. They involve the use of EMG or cystometry as a feedback signal for training a person to control the function of the external sphincter or raise intravesical pressure enough to overcome outflow resistance.

Pharmacologic Manipulation. Pharmacologic manipulation includes the use of drugs to alter the contractile properties of the bladder, decrease the outflow resistance of the internal sphincter, and relax the external sphincter. The usefulness of drug therapy often is evaluated during cystometric studies. Antimuscarinic drugs, such as oxybutynin, tolterodine, and propantheline, decrease detrusor muscle tone and increase bladder capacity in persons with spastic bladder dysfunction[16,22] (discussed in the section on Overactive Bladder/Urge Incontinence). Cholinergic drugs that stimulate parasympathetic receptors, such as bethanechol, provide increased bladder tonus and may prove helpful in the symptomatic treatment of milder forms of flaccid neurogenic bladder. Muscle relaxants, such as diazepam and baclofen, may be used to decrease the tone of the external sphincter. A nasal spray preparation of desmopressin (DDAVP), a synthetic antidiuretic hormone, can be used to reduce urine output in persons with nighttime frequency due to spastic bladder symptoms.

Surgical Procedures. Among the surgical procedures used in the management of neurogenic bladder are sphincterectomy, reconstruction of the sphincter, nerve resection of the sacral reflex nerves that cause spasticity or the pudendal nerve that controls the external sphincter, and urinary diversion. Urinary diversion can be done by creating an ileal or a colon loop into which the ureters are anastomosed; the distal end of the loop is brought out and attached to the abdominal wall.

Extensive research is being conducted on methods of restoring voluntary control of the storage and evacuation functions of the bladder through the use of implanted electrodes. Single and multiple electrodes can be placed on selected nerves and then coupled to a subcutaneous receiver.[13]

Urinary Incontinence

The Agency for Health Care Policy and Research Urinary Incontinence Guideline Panel[11] and the International Continence Society[23] have defined urinary incontinence as the involuntary loss or leakage of urine.[11] Urinary incontinence is a common problem, particularly in older adults, with women being affected twice as often as men.[24–28]

Incontinence can be caused by a number of conditions. It can occur without the person's knowledge; at other times, the person may be aware of the condition but be unable to prevent it. The Urinary Incontinence Guideline Panel has identified four main types of incontinence: stress incontinence, urge incontinence, overflow incontinence, and mixed incontinence, which is a combination of stress and urge incontinence.[11] Recently, the term *urge incontinence* has been expanded to include *overactive bladder* (*i.e.,* overactive bladder/urge incontinence). Table 35-3 summarizes the characteristics of stress incontinence, overactive bladder/urge incontinence, and overflow incontinence.

TABLE 35-3 Types and Characteristics of Urinary Incontinence

TYPE	CHARACTERISTICS
Stress	Involuntary loss of urine associated with activities, such as coughing, that increase intra-abdominal pressure
Overactive bladder/ urge incontinence	Urgency and frequency associated with hyperactivity of the detrusor muscle; may or may not involve involuntary loss of urine
Overflow	Involuntary loss of urine when intra-vesicular pressure exceeds maximal urethral pressure in the absence of detrusor activity

🔑 INCONTINENCE

- Incontinence represents the involuntary loss of urine due to increased bladder pressures (overactive bladder with urge incontinence or overflow incontinence) or decreased ability of the vesicourethral sphincter to prevent the escape of urine (stress incontinence).

- Stress incontinence is caused by the decreased ability of the vesicourethral sphincter to prevent the escape of urine during activities, such as lifting and coughing, that raise bladder pressure above the sphincter closing pressure.

- Overactive bladder/urge incontinence is caused by neurogenic or myogenic disorders that result in hyperactive bladder contractions.

- Overflow incontinence results from overfilling of the bladder with escape of urine.

Stress Incontinence

Stress incontinence is the involuntary loss of urine during coughing, laughing, sneezing, or lifting that increases intra-abdominal pressure.[24,29–32] With severe urinary stress incontinence, any strain or increase in bladder pressure leads to urinary leakage.

In women, the angle between the bladder and the posterior proximal urethra (*i.e.,* urethrovesical junction) is important to continence.[29] This angle normally is 90 to 100 degrees, with at least one third of the bladder base contributing to the angle when not voiding[30] (Fig. 35-5). During the first stage of voiding, this angle is lost as the bladder descends. In women, diminution of muscle tone associated with normal aging, childbirth, or surgical procedures can cause weakness of the pelvic floor muscles and result in stress incontinence by obliterating the critical posterior urethrovesical angle. In these women, loss of the posterior urethrovesical angle, descent and funneling of the bladder neck, and backward and downward rotation of the bladder occur, so that the bladder and urethra are already in an anatomic position for the first stage of voiding. Any activity that causes downward pressure on the bladder is sufficient to allow the urine to escape involuntarily.

Another cause of stress incontinence is intrinsic urethral deficiency, which may result from congenital sphincter weakness, as occurs with meningomyelocele. It also may be acquired as a result of trauma, irradiation, or sacral cord lesions. Stress incontinence in men may result from a congenital defect or from trauma or surgery to the bladder outlet, as occurs with prostatectomy. Neurologic dysfunction, as occurs with impaired sympathetic innervation of the bladder neck, impaired pelvic nerve innervation to the intrinsic sphincter, or impaired pudendal nerve innervation to the external sphincter, may also be contributing factors.

Overactive Bladder/Urge Incontinence

The Urinary Incontinence Guideline Panel has defined urge incontinence as the involuntary loss of urine associated with a strong desire to void (urgency).[11] To expand the number and types of patients eligible for clinical trials, the U.S. Food and Drug Administration adopted the term *overactive bladder* to describe the clinical syndrome that describes not only urge incontinence but frequency, dysuria, and nocturia.[33] The International Continence Society defines overactive bladder as the presence of involuntary bladder contractions during filling and while the person is trying to inhibit micturition.[34] Nocturia often occurs and is associated with sleep disruption. Although overactive bladder often is associated with urge incontinence, it can occur without incontinence. Despite recent media coverage of overactive bladder and advances in treatment, many people continue to suffer in silence, probably because they are embarrassed or think it is an inevitable consequence of aging.

The symptoms of overactive bladder, which are caused by involuntary bladder contractions during filling, may occur alone or in any combination, and they constitute overactive bladder when they occur in the absence of other pathologic processes.[35] Regardless of the primary cause of overactive bladder, two types of mechanisms are thought to contribute to its symptomatology: those involving CNS and neural control of bladder sensation and emptying (neurogenic) and those involving the smooth muscle of the bladder itself (myogenic).[8,34,35,37]

The neurogenic theory for overactive bladder postulates that the CNS functions as an on–off switching circuit for voluntary control of bladder function. Therefore, damage to the CNS inhibitory pathways may trigger bladder overactivity owing to uncontrolled voiding reflexes. Neurogenic causes of overactive bladder include stroke, Parkinson disease, and mul-

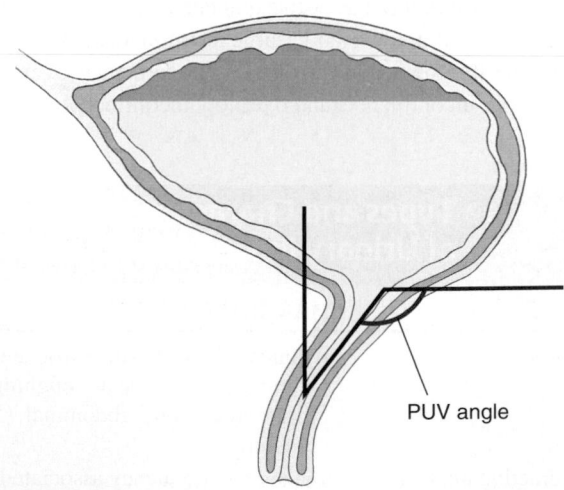

FIGURE 35-5 • Normal 90- to 100-degree posterior urethrovesical (PUV) angle. In the presence of a normal PUV angle, sudden changes in intra-abdominal pressure are transmitted optimally to all sides of the proximal urethra, ensuring that intraurethral pressure remains higher than intravesical pressure. Loss of the PUV angle results in displacement of the vesicle neck to the most dependent portion of the bladder, preventing the equal transmission of sudden increases in intra-abdominal pressure.

PUV angle

tiple sclerosis. Other neurogenic causes of overactive bladder include increased sensitization of the afferent nerves that sense bladder filling or increased sensitivity to efferent nerves that produce bladder emptying.

The myogenic causes of overactive bladder are thought to result from changes in the properties of the smooth muscle of the bladder itself. One example is overactive bladder associated with bladder outlet obstruction. It is hypothesized that the sustained increase in intravesical pressure that occurs with the outlet obstruction causes a partial destruction of the nerve endings that control bladder excitability.[8,35] This partial denervation results in increased excitability of the individual muscle cells. The result is urgency and frequency of urination due to spontaneous bladder contractions resulting from detrusor muscle hyperexcitability. Disorders of detrusor muscle structure and excitability also can occur as the result of the aging process or disease conditions such as diabetes mellitus. Overactive bladder symptoms usually are exaggerated by incomplete bladder emptying, a common accompaniment of overactive bladder.

Overflow Incontinence

Overflow incontinence is an involuntary loss of urine that occurs when intravesical pressure exceeds the maximal urethral pressure because of bladder distention in the absence of detrusor activity. It can occur with retention of urine owing to nervous system lesions or obstruction of the bladder neck. With this type of incontinence, the bladder is distended, and small amounts of urine are passed, particularly at night. In men, one of the most common causes of obstructive incontinence is enlargement of the prostate gland. Another cause that commonly is overlooked is fecal impaction (i.e., dry, hard feces in the rectum). When a large bolus of stool forms in the rectum, it can push against the urethra and block the flow of urine.

The Standardization Subcommittee of the International Continence Committee recommends that the term *overflow incontinence* should no longer be used, indicating that the term is confusing and lacking definition.[23] Instead, it suggests that more specific terms such as *reduced urethral function* or *overactivity/low bladder compliance* be used.

Other Causes of Incontinence

Other causes of incontinence include decreased bladder compliance or distensibility. This abnormal bladder condition may result from radiation therapy, radical pelvic surgery, or interstitial cystitis. Many persons with this disorder have severe urgency related to bladder hypersensitivity that results in loss of bladder elasticity, such that any small increase in bladder volume or detrusor function causes a sharp rise in bladder pressure and severe urgency.

Incontinence may occur as a transient and correctable phenomenon, or it may not be totally correctable and occur with various degrees of frequency. Among the transient causes of urinary incontinence are recurrent urinary tract infections; medications that alter bladder function or perception of blad-

der filling and the need to urinate; diuretics and conditions that increase bladder filling; stool impaction; restricted mobility; and confusional states.

Incontinence also may be caused by factors outside the lower urinary tract, such as the inability to locate, reach, or receive assistance in reaching an appropriate place to void. This may be a particular problem for elderly persons, who may have problems with mobility and manual dexterity or find themselves in unfamiliar surroundings. It occurs when a person cannot find or reach the bathroom or manipulate clothing quickly enough. Failing vision may contribute to the problem. Embarrassment in front of other persons at having to use the bathroom, particularly if the timing seems inappropriate, may cause a person to delay emptying the bladder and may lead to incontinence. Treatment with drugs such as diuretics may cause the bladder to fill more rapidly than usual, making it difficult to reach the bathroom in time if there are problems with mobility or if a bathroom is not readily available. Night sedation may cause a person to sleep through the signal that normally would waken a person so that he or she could get up and empty the bladder and avoid wetting the bed.

Diagnosis and Treatment

Urinary incontinence is not a single disease but a symptom with many possible causes. As a symptom, it requires full investigation to establish its cause.[28,32,37–39] This usually is accomplished through a careful history, physical examination, blood tests, and urinalysis. A voiding record (i.e., diary) may be used to determine the frequency, timing, and amount of voiding, as well as other factors associated with the incontinence.[32] Because many drugs affect bladder function, a full drug history is essential. Estimation of PVR volume is recommended for all persons with incontinence. Provocative stress testing is done when stress incontinence is suspected. This test is done by having the person relax and then cough vigorously while the examiner observes for urine loss. The test usually is done in the lithotomy position; if no leakage is observed, it is repeated in the standing position.[32] Urodynamic studies may be needed to provide information about urinary pressures and urine flow rates.

Treatment or management depends on the type of incontinence, accompanying health problems, and the person's age. It includes behavioral and pharmacologic measures; exercises to strengthen the pelvic muscles and surgical correction of pelvic relaxation disorders associated with stress incontinence; and, when urine flow cannot be controlled, noncatheter devices to obstruct urine flow or collect urine as it is passed.[25,37–39] Indwelling catheters (discussed earlier), although a solution to the problem of urinary incontinence, usually are considered only after all other treatment methods have failed. In some types of incontinence, such as that associated with spinal cord injury or meningomyelocele, self-catheterization may provide the best means for controlling urine elimination (see Chapter 51).

Behavioral Measures. Behavioral methods include fluid management, timed/prompted voiding, pelvic floor exercises (to be discussed), bladder retraining, and toileting assistance.[37-39] Bladder retraining and biofeedback techniques seek to reestablish cortical control over bladder function by having the person ignore urgency and respond only to cortical signals during waking hours. Toileting assistance techniques are caregiver-dependent techniques used to treat persons with cognitive and motor dysfunction.

Pharmacologic Treatment. Pharmacologic treatment is aimed at using drugs to alter the physiologic mechanisms that contribute to the neurogenic or myogenic causes of incontinence.[38-42] They include the use of drugs that increase sphincter tone in stress incontinence, decrease hyperreactivity of the detrusor muscle in overactive bladder/urge incontinence, or relieve outflow obstruction in overflow incontinence.

The α-adrenergic agonist drugs, such as pseudoephedrine, increase sympathetic relaxation of the detrusor muscle and internal sphincter tone and may be used in treating stress incontinence. The tricyclic antidepressants (particularly imipramine hydrochloride) are useful in facilitating urine storage because they decrease bladder contractility and increase outlet resistance. Although these drugs have a weak anticholinergic effect on smooth muscle, it has recently been postulated that their beneficial effects may be caused by increased serotonin activity (due to reuptake blockade) in the CNS. This may involve a direct inhibition of normal excitatory pathways or depression of afferent ascending neural activity. Duloxetine, a selective serotonin and norepinephrine reuptake inhibitor, is thought to increase external sphincter tone by stimulation of the pudendal motor α_1-adrenergic receptors and serotonin-2 receptors.[40,42] Because serious side effects (*e.g.,* CNS effects, postural hypotension, cardiac arrhythmias) can occur with imipramine and other tricyclic antidepressants, these agents need to be used with caution.

Acetylcholine is the neurotransmitter that mediates detrusor contraction in overactive bladder. Therefore, anticholinergic medications are used to suppress these contractions. Some of the newer antimuscarinic drugs (*e.g.,* oxybutynin, tolterodine, trospium, darifenacin, solifenacin) have greater selectivity for the M_3 muscarinic receptors and produce fewer side effects than some of the older agents (*e.g.,* hyoscyamine, propantheline). All anticholinergic drugs can have bothersome side effects. Although dry mouth is the most common, constipation, gastroesophageal reflux, blurred vision, urinary retention, and cognitive effects can occur. The use of controlled-release (*e.g.,* oxybutynin, atolterodine) or transdermal drug delivery (*e.g.,* oxybutynin) can reduce but not completely eliminate side effects. Botulinum toxin (BTX-A) injection into the bladder was recently introduced as an alternative treatment for persons with overactive bladder who do not respond to anticholinergic agents or cannot tolerate their side effects.[43] The duration of the injection's effect seems to be at least 6 months.

The primary treatment of overflow incontinence that results from benign prostatic hypertrophy is relief of outflow obstruction. α-Adrenergic blocker therapy is based on the hypothesis that clinical manifestations of prostatic hyperplasia are caused partly by α_1-adrenergic–mediated contraction of prostatic smooth muscle, resulting in bladder outlet obstruction. Bladder outlet obstruction contributes to overfilling of the bladder and large-volume contraction, or frequency of urination resulting from incomplete bladder emptying. α-Adrenergic antagonists such as alfuzosin, doxazosin, tamsulosin, and terazosin are treatment options for men with symptomatic prostatic hyperplasia (see Chapter 47). The primary adverse effects of α-adrenergic blocker therapy are orthostatic hypotension, dizziness, fatigue, ejaculatory problems, and nasal congestion.

Pelvic Exercises and Surgical Treatment of Stress Incontinence. Muscle-tensing exercises of the pelvic muscles may prove effective in treatment of stress incontinence.[24,25,32,44,45] These exercises were first advocated by Kegel, and they commonly are called *Kegel exercises.*[45] Two groups of muscles are strengthened: those of the back part of the pelvic floor (*i.e.,* muscles used to contract the anus and control the passing of stool) and the front muscles of the pelvic floor (*i.e.,* muscles used to stop the flow of urine during voiding). In learning the exercises, a woman concentrates on identifying the muscle groups and learning how to control contraction. After this has been accomplished, she can start an exercise program that consists of slowly contracting the muscles, beginning at the front and working to the back while counting to four and then releasing. The exercises can be done while sitting or standing and usually are performed in repetitions of 10, three times each day. A vaginal cone, a tampon-like device, may be used to enhance the benefits of the exercise. The cone is placed in the vagina, and the woman is instructed to hold it in place by contracting the proper inner muscles.

Surgical intervention may be considered when other treatment methods have proved ineffective. Three types of surgical procedures are used: procedures that increase outlet resistance, decrease detrusor muscle instability, or remove outflow obstruction to reduce overflow incontinence and detrusor muscle instability. A relatively new development for the treatment of stress incontinence is the tension-free vaginal tape procedure.[46] This procedure, which is minimally invasive and performed under local anesthesia, involves recreating suburethral support with a polypropylene mesh, without repositioning the bladder or urethra. Initial results from the procedure appear to be promising, with one study reporting a 90% cure rate.[46] Another minimally invasive procedure for the treatment of stress incontinence is the periurethral injection of a bulking agent (glutaraldehyde cross-linked bovine collagen or carbon-coated beads). Both of these agents typically require multiple treatment sessions to achieve a cure.[29,32]

Noncatheter Devices. Two types of noncatheter devices commonly are used in the management of urinary incontinence: one obstructs flow, and the other collects urine as it is passed. Obstruction of urine flow is achieved by compressing the urethra or stimulating contraction of the pelvic floor muscles. Penile clamps are available that occlude the urethra without obstructing blood circulation to the penis. Clamps must be removed at 3-hour intervals to empty the bladder. Complications such as penile and urethral erosion can occur if clamps are used incorrectly. In women, compression of the urethra usually is accomplished by intravaginal devices.

Surgically implanted artificial sphincters are available for use in men and women. These devices consist of an inflatable cuff that surrounds the proximal urethra. The cuff is connected by tubing to an implanted fluid reservoir and an inflation bulb. Pressing the bulb, which is placed in the scrotum in men, inflates the cuff. It is emptied in a similar manner.

When urinary incontinence cannot be prevented, various types of urine collection devices or protective pads are used. Men can be fitted with collection devices (*i.e.,* condom or sheath urinals) that are worn over the penis and attached to a container at the bedside or fastened to the body. There are no effective external collection devices for women. Pants and pads usually are used. Dribbling bags (men) and pads (women) in which the urine changes to a nonpourable gel are available for occasional dribbling but are unsuitable for considerable wetting.

Special Needs of Elderly Persons

Urinary incontinence is a common problem in elderly persons, both male and female.[47,48] An estimated 15% to 30% of community-dwelling elders and 50% of institutionalized elders have severe urinary incontinence.[28,47] Incontinence increases social isolation, frequently leads to institutionalization of elderly persons, and predisposes to infections and skin breakdown. The economic and social costs of incontinence are staggering. Annually, more than $3 billion is spent managing incontinence in nursing homes alone.[49]

Many factors contribute to incontinence in elderly persons, a number of which can be altered. The overall capacity of the bladder is reduced, as is the urethral closing pressure.[28] Detrusor muscle function also tends to decline with aging; thus, there is a trend toward a reduction in the strength of bladder contraction and impairment in emptying that leads to larger PVR volumes.[2,28,50] It has been proposed that many of these changes are due to degenerative detrusor muscle changes rather than neurologic changes, as was once thought. The combination of involuntary detrusor contraction (detrusor hyperactivity) leading to urge incontinence, along with impaired contractile function, leads to incomplete bladder emptying. Urge incontinence is the most frequent type of incontinence in elderly men. In about 50% of these men, detrusor overactivity is found; the urge to urinate comes on suddenly, without warning, accompanied by an uncontrolled detrusor contraction causing incontinence.[48]

Furthermore, advancing age often results in restricted mobility, an increasing number of medications being taken, comorbid illness, infection, and stool impaction, all of which can precipitate urinary incontinence.[21,50] More than half of normal elderly persons experience nocturia. Many elderly persons have difficulty getting to the toilet in time. This can be caused by arthritis that makes walking or removing clothing difficult or by failing vision that makes trips to the bathroom precarious, especially in new and unfamiliar surroundings.

Medication prescribed for other health problems may prevent a healthy bladder from functioning normally.[28,29,50] Potent, fast-acting diuretics are known for their ability to cause urge incontinence. Impaired thirst or limited access to fluids predisposes to constipation with urethral obstruction and overflow incontinence and to concentrated and infected urine, which increases bladder excitability. Drugs such as hypnotics, tranquilizers, and sedatives can interfere with the conscious inhibition of voiding, leading to urge incontinence. Diuretics, particularly in elderly persons, increase the flow of urine and may contribute to incontinence, particularly in persons with diminished bladder capacity and in those who have difficulty reaching the toilet.

Diagnosis and Treatment. According to Stanton, "there are two guiding principles in management of incontinence in the elderly. First, growing old does not imply becoming incontinent, and second, incontinence should not be left untreated just because the patient is old."[51]

As with urinary incontinence in younger persons, incontinence in elderly persons requires a thorough history and physical examination to determine the cause of the problem. A voiding history is important. A voiding diary provides a means for the person to provide objective information about the number of bathroom visits, the number of protective pads used, and even the volume of urine voided. A medication history is also important because medications can affect bladder function.[78]

There are many nonurologic conditions that predispose to urinary incontinence. The transient and often treatable causes of urinary incontinence in elderly persons may best be remembered with the acronym DIAPPERS, in which the *D* stands for dementia/dementias, *I* for infection (urinary or vaginal), *A* for atrophic vaginitis, *P* for pharmaceutical agents, *P* for psychological causes, *E* for endocrine conditions (diabetes), *R* for restricted mobility, and *S* for stool impaction.[23,38,52] These eight transient causes of incontinence should be identified and treated before other treatment options are considered.

Treatment may involve changes in the physical environment so that the older person can reach the bathroom more easily or remove clothing more quickly. Habit training with regularly scheduled toileting—usually every 2 to 4 hours—often is effective. Many elderly persons who void on a regular schedule can gradually increase the interval between toileting while improving their ability to suppress bladder instability. The treatment plan may require dietary changes to prevent constipation or a plan to promote adequate fluid intake to ensure adequate bladder filling and prevent urinary stasis and symptomatic urinary tract infections.

IN SUMMARY, alterations in bladder function include urinary obstruction with retention of urine, neurogenic bladder, and urinary incontinence with involuntary loss of urine. Urine retention occurs when the outflow of urine from the bladder is obstructed because of urethral obstruction or impaired bladder innervation. Urethral obstruction causes bladder irritability, detrusor muscle hypertrophy, formation of trabeculae and diverticula, development of hydroureters, and eventual renal failure.

Neurogenic bladder is caused by interruption in the innervation of the bladder. It can result in spastic bladder dysfunction caused by failure of the bladder to fill or flaccid bladder dysfunction caused by failure of the bladder to empty. Spastic bladder dysfunction usually results from neurologic lesions that are above the level of the sacral micturition reflex center; flaccid bladder dysfunction results from lesions at the level of the sacral micturition reflexes or peripheral innervation of the bladder. A third type of neurogenic disorder involves a nonrelaxing external sphincter.

Urinary incontinence is the involuntary loss of urine in amounts sufficient to be a problem. It may manifest as stress incontinence, in which the loss of urine occurs as a result of coughing, sneezing, laughing, or lifting; overactive bladder/urge incontinence, characterized by urgency, frequency, and nocturia associated with hyperactive bladder contractions; or overflow incontinence, which results when intravesical pressure exceeds the maximal urethral pressure because of bladder distention. Other causes of incontinence include a small, contracted bladder or external environmental conditions that make it difficult to access proper toileting facilities. Diagnosis usually is accomplished through a careful history (including a voiding record and full drug history), physical examination, blood tests and urinalysis, and in some cases urodynamic studies. Treatment methods include correction of the underlying cause, such as obstruction due to prostatic hyperplasia; pharmacologic methods to improve bladder and external sphincter tone; behavioral methods that focus on bladder and habit training; exercises to improve pelvic floor function; and the use of catheters and urine collection devices.

Urinary incontinence is a common problem in elderly persons. Many factors, including health problems, medications, and changes in bladder structure and function, contribute to incontinence in elderly persons. The acronym DIAPPERS—*D* (dementia), *I* (infection), *A* (atrophic vaginitis), *P* (pharmaceutical), *P* (psychological), *E* (endocrine), *R* (restricted mobility), and *S* (stool impaction)—emphasizes the transient and often treatable causes of incontinence in the elderly. ■

CANCER OF THE BLADDER

After completing this section of the chapter, you should be able to meet the following objectives:

■ Discuss the difference between superficial and invasive bladder cancer in terms of bladder involvement, extension of the disease, and prognosis.
■ State the most common sign of bladder cancer.

Bladder cancer is the most frequent form of urinary tract cancer in the United States, accounting for more than 68,810 new cases and 14,100 deaths each year.[53] It is the fourth most common malignancy in men and the eighth most common malignancy in women in the Western world.[54] For some as-yet unexplained reason, African Americans have only half the risk of white European Americans, but the overall survival rate among African Americans appears to be worse.[54]

Approximately 90% of bladder cancers are derived from the transitional (urothelium) cells that line the bladder.[55–58] These tumors can range from low-grade noninvasive tumors to high-grade tumors that invade the bladder wall and metastasize frequently. The low-grade tumors, which may recur after resection, have an excellent prognosis, with only a small number (<5%) progressing to higher-grade tumors, whereas 15% to 40% of persons with high-grade tumors progress.[56]

Etiology and Pathophysiology

Although the cause of bladder cancer is unknown, evidence suggests that its origin is related to local influences, such as carcinogens that are excreted in the urine and stored in the bladder. These include the breakdown products of aromatic amines used in the dye industry, and products used in the manufacture of rubber, textiles, paint, chemicals, and petroleum.[54,56–58] Smoking also deserves attention.[52,54] Thirty to 50% of all bladder cancers are associated with cigarette smoking.[54,56–58] Chronic bladder infections and bladder stones also increase the risk for bladder cancer. Bladder cancer is more frequent among persons harboring the parasite *Schistosoma haematobium* in their bladder.[57] The parasite is endemic in Egypt and Sudan. It is not known whether the parasite excretes a carcinogen or produces its effects through irritation of the bladder.

Manifestations

The most common sign of bladder cancer is painless hematuria.[53,54,56,57] Gross hematuria is a presenting sign in 75% of persons with the disease, and microscopic hematuria is present in most others. Frequency, urgency, and dysuria occasionally accompany the hematuria. Because hematuria often is intermittent, the diagnosis may be delayed. Periodic urine cytology is recommended for all persons who are at high risk for the development of bladder cancer because of exposure to urinary tract carcinogens. Ureteral invasion leading to bacterial and obstructive renal disease and dissemination of the cancer are potential complications and ultimate causes of death. The prognosis depends on the histologic grade of the cancer and the stage of the disease at the time of diagnosis.

Diagnosis and Treatment

Diagnostic methods include cytologic studies, excretory urography, cystoscopy, and biopsy. Ultrasonography, CT scans, and MRI are used as aids for staging the tumor. Cytologic studies performed on biopsy tissues or cells obtained from bladder washings may be used to detect the presence of malignant cells.[56] A technique called *flow cytometry* is helpful in screening persons at high risk for the disease and for monitoring the results of therapy. In flow cytometry, the interaction between fluorochromes or dyes with deoxyribonucleic acid (DNA) causes the emission of high-intensity light similar to that produced by a laser. Flow cytometry can be carried out on biopsy specimens, bladder washings, or cytologic preparations.

The treatment of bladder cancer depends on the extent of the lesion and the health of the patient. Endoscopic resection usually is done for diagnostic purposes and may be used as a treatment for superficial lesions. Diathermy (*i.e.,* electrocautery) may be used to remove the tumors. Segmental surgical resection may be used for removing a large single lesion. When the tumor is invasive, cystectomy with resection of the pelvic lymph nodes frequently is the treatment of choice. In men, the prostate and seminal vesicles often are removed as well. Until the 1980s, most men who underwent radical cystectomy became impotent. Newer surgical approaches designed to preserve erectile function now are being used. Cystectomy requires urinary diversion, an alternative reservoir, usually created from the ileum (*e.g.,* an ileal loop), that is designed to collect the urine. Traditionally, the ileostomy reservoir drains urine continuously into an external collecting device. External-beam radiation therapy is an alternative to radical cystectomy in some patients with deeply infiltrating bladder cancer.[56]

Although a number of chemotherapeutic drugs have been used in the treatment of bladder cancer, no chemotherapeutic regimens for the disease have been established. Perhaps of more importance is the increasing use of intravesical chemotherapy, in which the cytotoxic drug is instilled directly into the bladder; thereby avoiding the side effects of systemic therapy. These drugs can be instilled prophylactically, after surgical resection of all the demonstrable tumor tissue, or therapeutically, in the presence of residual disease. Among the chemotherapeutic drugs that have been used for this purpose are thiotepa, mitomycin C, and doxorubicin (Adriamycin).[56] The intervesicular administration of bacillus Calmette-Guérin (BCG) vaccine, made from a strain of *Mycobacterium bovis* that formerly was used to protect against tuberculosis, causes a significant reduction in the rate of relapse and prolongs relapse-free interval in persons with cancer in situ. The vaccine is thought to act as a nonspecific stimulator of cell-mediated immunity. It is not known whether the effects of BCG are immunologic or include a component of direct toxicity. Several strains of this agent exist, and it is not known which strains are the most active and least toxic.

IN SUMMARY, cancer of the bladder is the most common cause of urinary tract cancer in the United States. Bladder cancers fall into two major groups: low-grade noninvasive tumors, and high-grade invasive tumors that are associated with metastasis and a worse prognosis. Although the cause of cancer of the bladder is unknown, evidence suggests that carcinogens excreted in the urine may play a role. Microscopic and gross, painless hematuria are the most frequent presenting signs of bladder cancer. The methods used in treatment of bladder cancer depend on the cytologic grade of the tumor and the lesion's degree of invasiveness. The methods include surgical removal of the tumor, radiation therapy, and chemotherapy. In many cases, chemotherapeutic or immunotherapeutic agents can be instilled directly into the bladder, thereby avoiding the side effects of systemic therapy. ■

Review Exercises

1. A 23-year-old man is recovering after the acute phase of a cervical (C6) spinal cord injury with complete loss of motor and sensory function below the level of injury. He is now experiencing spastic bladder contractions with involuntary and incomplete urination. Urodynamic studies reveal spastic contraction of the external sphincter with urine retention and high bladder pressures.

   A. *Explain the reason for the involuntary urination and incomplete emptying of the bladder despite high bladder pressures.*

   B. *What are possible complications associated with overdistention and high pressure within the bladder?*

2. A 66-year-old woman complains of leakage of urine during coughing, sneezing, laughing, or squatting down.

   A. *Explain the source of this woman's problem.*

   B. *One of the recommended treatments for stress incontinence is the use of Kegel exercises, which focus on strengthening the muscles of the pelvic floor. Explain how these exercises contribute to the control of urine leakage in women with stress incontinence.*

References

1. Kandel E. R., Schwartz J. H., Jessel T. M. (2000). *Principles of neural science* (4th ed.). New York: McGraw-Hill.
2. Fowler C. J. (1999). Neurological disorders of micturition and their treatment. *Brain* 122, 1213–1231.
3. Guyton A. C., Hall J. E. (2006). *Textbook of medical physiology* (11th ed., pp. 311–314). Philadelphia: Elsevier Saunders.
4. Andersson K.-E., Arner A. (2004). Urinary bladder contraction and relaxation: Physiology and pathophysiology. *Physiology Review* 84, 935–986.
5. Sugaya K., Miyazato M., Ogawa Y. (2005). Central nervous control of micturition and urine storage. *Journal of Smooth Muscle Research* 41, 117–132.
6. Rhoades R. A., Tanner G. A. (2003). *Medical physiology* (2nd ed., pp. 423–424). Philadelphia: Lippincott Williams & Wilkins.

7. Dmochowski R. R., Appell R. A. (2000). Advances in pharmacologic management of overactive bladder. *Urology* 56(Suppl. 6A), 41–49.

8. Ouslander J. G. (2004). Management of overactive bladder. *New England Journal of Medicine* 350, 786–799.

9. Elder J. S. (2004). Voiding dysfunction. In Behrman R. E., Kliegman R. M., Jenson H. B. (Eds.), *Nelson textbook of pediatrics* (17th ed., pp. 1808–1809). Philadelphia: Elsevier Saunders.

10. Tanagho E. A. (2004). Urodynamic studies. In Tanagho E. A., McAninch J. W. (Eds.), *Smith's general urology* (16th ed., pp. 453–472). New York: Lange Medical Books/McGraw-Hill.

11. Fantl J. A., Newman D. K., Colling J., et al., for the Agency for Health Care Policy and Research, Public Health Service. (1996). *Urinary incontinence in adults: Acute and chronic management.* Clinical practice guideline no. 2, 1996 update. AHCPR publication no. 96-0682. Rockville, MD: U.S. Department of Health and Human Services.

12. Schott-Baer F. D., Reaume L. (2001). Accuracy of ultrasound estimates of urine volume. *Urological Nursing* 21, 193–195.

13. Fowler C. J., O'Malley K. J. (2003). Investigation and management of neurogenic bladder dysfunction. *Journal of Neurology, Neurosurgery, and Psychiatry* 74(Suppl. IV), iv27–iv31.

14. Tanagho E. A. (2004). Urinary obstruction and stasis. In Tanagho E. A., McAninch J. W. (Eds.), *Smith's general urology* (16th ed., pp. 175–187). New York: Lange Medical Books/McGraw-Hill.

15. Elliott D. S., Boone T. B. (2000). Recent advances in management of neurogenic bladder. *Urology* 56(Suppl. 6A), 76–81.

16. Tanagho E. A., Lue T. F. (2000). Neuropathic bladder disorders. In Tanagho E. A., McAninch J. W. (Eds.), *Smith's general urology* (16th ed., pp. 435–452). New York: Lange Medical Books/McGraw-Hill.

17. Sasaki K., Yoshimura N., Chancellor M. B. (2003). Implication of diabetes mellitus in urology. *Urologic Clinics of North America* 30, 1–12.

18. Vinik A. I., Maser R. E., Mitchell B. D., et al. (2003). Diabetic autonomic neuropathy. *Diabetes Care* 26, 1553–1579.

19. Cravens D. D., Zwieg S. (2000). Urinary catheter management. *American Family Physician* 61, 356–369.

20. Barton R. (2000). Intermittent self-catheterization. *Nursing Standard* 15(9), 47–52.

21. Addison R., Lopez J. (2001). Bladder retraining. *Nursing Times* 97(5), 45–46.

22. Dmochowski R. R., Appell R. A. (2000). Advancements in pharmacologic management of overactive bladder. *Urology* 56(Suppl. 6A), 41–49.

23. Abrams P., Cardozo L., Fall M., et al. (2002). The standardization of terminology in lower urinary tract function: Report from the standardization sub-committee on the international continence society. *Urology* 61, 37–49.

24. Walters M. D. (2005). Urinary incontinence in women. ACOG practice bulletin no. 63. Clinical Practice Guidelines for Obstetricians and Gynecologists. *Obstetrics and Gynecology* 105, 1533–1545.

25. Smith P. P., McCrery R. J., Appell R. A. (2006). Current trends in the evaluation and management of female urinary incontinence. *Canadian Medical Association Journal* 175, 1233–1240.

26. Sampselle C. M., Palmer M. H., Boyington A. R., et al. (2004). Prevention of urinary incontinence in adults. *Nursing Research* 53(6 Suppl.), S61–S67.

27. Wilson M.-M. G. (2006). Urinary incontinence: Selected current concepts. *Medical Clinics of North America* 90, 825–836.

28. Klausner A. P., Vapnek J. M. (2003). Urinary incontinence in the geriatric population. *Mount Sinai Journal of Medicine* 70, 54–61.

29. Tanagho E. A. (2004). Urinary incontinence. In Tanagho E. A., McAninch J. W. (Eds.), *Smith's general urology* (17th ed., pp. 473–491). New York: Lange Medical Books/McGraw-Hill.

30. Green T. H. (1975). Urinary stress incontinence: Differential diagnosis, pathophysiology, and management. *American Journal of Obstetrics and Gynecology* 122, 368–382.

31. Plzak L. III, Staskin D. (2002). Genuine stress incontinence: Theories of etiology and surgical correction. *Urologic Clinics of North America* 29, 527–535.

32. Culligan P. J., Heit M. (2000). Urinary incontinence in women: Evaluation and management. *American Family Physician* 62, 2433–2452.

33. U.S. Food and Drug Administration. (2005). Fact sheet—loss of bladder control. [Online.] Available: www.fda.gov/womens/getthefacts/bladder Control.html. Accessed February 8, 2007.

34. Hampel C., Wienhold D., Benken N., et al. (1997). Definition of overactive bladder and epidemiology of urinary incontinence. *Urology* 50(Suppl. 6A), 4–14.

35. Wein A. J. (2001). Putting overactive bladder into clinical perspective. *Patient Care for the Nurse Practitioner* (Spring Suppl.), 1–5.

36. Chu F. M., Dmochowski R. (2006). Pathology of overactive bladder. *American Journal of Medicine* 119(Suppl. 3A), 3S–8S.

37. Scientific Committee of the First International Consultation on Incontinence. (2000). Assessment and treatment of incontinence. Lancet 355, 2153–2158.

38. Lavell J. P., Karram M., Chu F. M. (2006). Management of incontinence for family practice physicians. *American Journal of Medicine* 119(Suppl. 3A), 37S–40S.

39. Erdem N., Chu F. M. (2006). Management of overactive bladder and urge incontinence in the elderly patient. *American Journal of Medicine* 119(Suppl. 3A), 29S–36S.

40. Thomas D. R. (2004). Pharmacologic management of urinary incontinence. *Clinics in Geriatric Medicine* 20, 511–523.

41. Dmochowski R. R., Appell R. A. (2000). Advancements in pharmacological management of overactive bladder. *Urology* 56(Suppl. 6A), 41–49.

42. Wein A. J., Rovner E. S. (2002). Pharmacologic management of urinary incontinence in women. *Urologic Clinics of North America* 29, 537–550.

43. Schurch B. (2006). Botulism toxin for the management of bladder dysfunction. *Drugs* 66, 1307–1318.

44. Wells T. J., Brink C. A., Kiokno A. C., et al. (1991). Pelvic muscle exercise for stress urinary incontinence in elderly women. *Journal of the American Geriatrics Society* 39, 785–791.

45. Kegel A. H. (1948). Progressive resistance exercises in the functional restoration of the perineal muscles. *American Journal of Obstetrics and Gynecology* 56, 238–248.

46. Carlin B. I., Klutke J. J., Klutke C. G. (2000). The tension-free vaginal tape procedure for treatment of stress incontinence in the female patient. *Urology* 56(Suppl. 6A), 28–31.

47. Lee S. Y., Phanumus D., Fields S. D. (2000). Urinary incontinence: A primary guide to managing acute and chronic symptoms in older adults. *Geriatrics* 55(11), 65–71.

48. Madersbacher H., Madersbacher S. (2005). Men's bladder health: Urinary incontinence in the elderly (Part I). *Journal of Men's Health & Gender* 2(1), 31–37.

49. Weiss B. D. (1998). Diagnostic evaluation of urinary incontinence in geriatric patients. *American Family Physician* 57, 2675–2684, 2688–2690.

50. Dubeau C. E. (2002). The continuum of urinary incontinence in an aging population. *Geriatrics* 57(Suppl. 1), 12–17.

51. Stanton S. L. (1984). Surgical management of female incontinence. In Brocklehurst J. C. (Ed.), *Urology in the elderly* (p. 93). New York: Churchill Livingstone.

52. Resnick N. M., Yalla S. V. (1998). Geriatric incontinence and voiding dysfunction. In Walsh P. C., Retik A. B., Vaughan E. D., et al. (Eds.), *Campbell's urology* (7th ed., p. 1045). Philadelphia: W.B. Saunders.

53. American Cancer Society. (2006). Overview of bladder cancer. [Online.] Available: http://www.cancer.org/docroot/CRI/CRI_2_1x.asp?dt=44. Accessed April 21, 2008.

54. Kirkall Z., Chan T., Manoharan M., et al. (2005). Bladder cancer: Epidemiology, staging and grading, and diagnosis. *Urology* 66(Suppl. 6A), 4–34.

55. Reuter V. E. (2006). The pathology of bladder cancer. *Urology* 67(Suppl. 3A), 11–17.

56. Grossfeld G. D., Carroll P. (2004). Urothelial carcinoma: Cancers of the bladder, ureter, and renal pelvis. In Tanagho E. A., McAninch J. W. (Eds.), *Smith's general urology* (16th ed., pp. 324–345). New York: Lange Medical Books/McGraw-Hill.

57. Epstein J. I. (2005). The lower urinary tract and male genitourinary system. In Kumar V., Abbas A. K., Fausto N. (Eds.), *Robbins and Cotran pathologic basis of disease* (7th ed., pp. 1024–1034). Philadelphia: Elsevier Saunders.

58. Damjanov I. (2005). The lower urinary tract and male reproductive system. In Rubin E., Gorstein F., Rubin R., et al. (Eds.), *Rubin's pathology: Clinicopathologic foundations of medicine* (4th ed., pp. 887–900). Philadelphia: Lippincott Williams & Wilkins.

Visit thePoint **http://thePoint.lww.com for animations, journal articles, and more!**

Disorders of Gastrointestinal Function

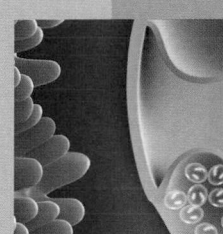

The study of the gastrointestinal system aroused none of the philosophical interest that surrounded the elements, humors, and pneuma of Galen's time. During ancient times, the gut was thought merely to provide the chyle that was turned into blood by the liver. Although the structures of the gut had been fairly well described, perhaps owing to observations made during the slaughtering of animals, it was not until the 18th and 19th centuries that the function of the gastrointestinal tract began to unfold.

One of the breakthroughs in gastrointestinal physiology came as the result of an accident. In 1822, William Beaumont (1785–1853), a self-trained surgeon in the United States Army, was called upon to render aid to Alexis St. Martin, a Canadian traveler who had suffered a large gunshot wound to the chest and abdomen. Although not expected to live, young St. Martin rallied and his wounds healed; however, he was left with a permanent fistula that opened to his stomach. Beaumont became intrigued with this patient's unique defect, using this living laboratory to study the process of digestion. He would have St. Martin swallow different types of food and then collect the stomach contents by means of a tube passed into the fistula. Beaumont described the movement of the stomach, and he confirmed the presence of hydrochloric acid and a ferment, later shown to be the result of the protein-breaking enzyme pepsin. Because of an unfortunate accident, both Beaumont and St. Martin gained a place in the history of gastrointestinal physiology.

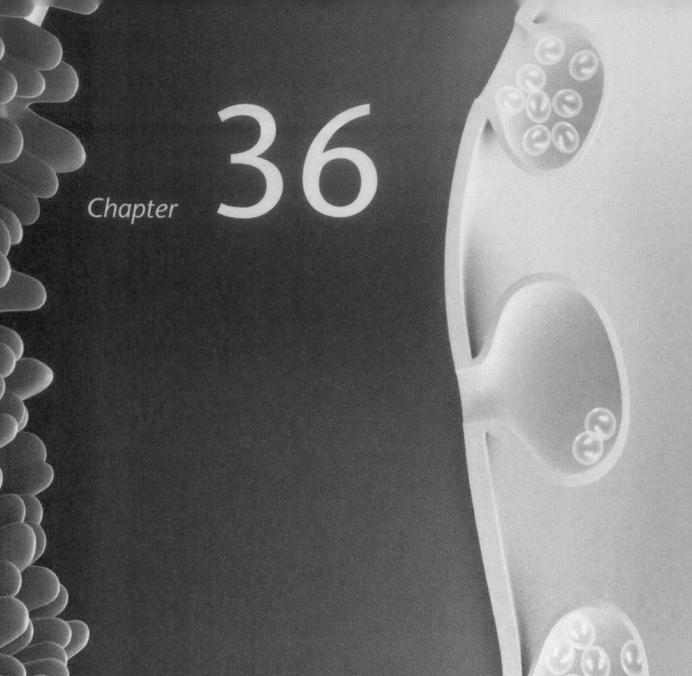

Chapter 36

Structure and Function of the Gastrointestinal System

CAROL M. PORTH

> The digestive system is an amazing structure. In this system, food is dismantled and its nutrients absorbed, wastes are collected and eliminated, vitamins are synthesized, and enzymes are produced. The gastrointestinal (GI) tract is also becoming increasingly recognized as an endocrine organ that produces and augments hormones that contribute to the regulation of appetite and nutrient intake and function in the use and storage of nutrients.

As a matter of semantics, the GI tract also is referred to as the *digestive tract,* the *alimentary canal,* and, at times, the *gut.* The intestinal portion also may be called the *bowel.* For the purposes of this text, the liver and pancreas (discussed in Chapter 38), which produce secretions that aid in digestion, are considered *accessory organs.*

STRUCTURE AND ORGANIZATION OF THE GASTROINTESTINAL TRACT

After completing this section of the chapter, you should be able to meet the following objectives:

- Describe the anatomic structures of the upper, middle, and lower gastrointestinal tract.
- List the five layers of the gastrointestinal tract wall and describe their function.
- Characterize the structure and function of the peritoneum and describe its attachment to the abdominal wall.

The major physiologic functions of the GI system are to digest food and absorb nutrients into the bloodstream. It carries out these functions by motility, secretion, digestion, and absorption. In the digestive tract, food and other materials move slowly along its length as they are systematically broken down into ions and molecules that can be absorbed into the body. In the large intestine, unabsorbed nutrients and wastes are collected for later elimination.

Structurally, the GI tract is a long, hollow tube, the lumen (*i.e.,* hollow center) of which is an extension of the external environment (Fig. 36-1). Nutrients do not become part of the internal environment until they have passed through the intestinal wall and have entered the blood or lymph channels. For simplicity and understanding, the GI tract can be divided into three parts. The upper part—the mouth, esophagus, and stomach—acts as an intake source and receptacle through which food passes and in which initial digestive processes take place. The middle portion—the duodenum, jejunum, and ileum—is where most digestive and absorptive processes occur. The lower segment—the cecum, colon, and rectum—serves as a storage channel for the efficient elimination of waste. The accessory organs, which include the salivary glands, liver, and pancreas, produce secretions that aid in digestion.

Upper Gastrointestinal Tract

The mouth forms the entryway into the GI tract for food; it contains the teeth, used in the mastication of food, and the tongue and other structures needed to direct food toward the pharyngeal structures and the esophagus. The mouth also serves as a receptacle for saliva produced by the salivary glands. Saliva moistens and lubricates food, so it is easier to swallow, and contains enzymes involved in the initial digestion of lipids and starches.

Esophagus

The esophagus is a straight, collapsible tube, about 25 cm (10 in) in length, that lies behind the trachea and connects the oropharynx with the stomach. The esophagus functions primarily as a conduit for the passage of food from the pharynx to the

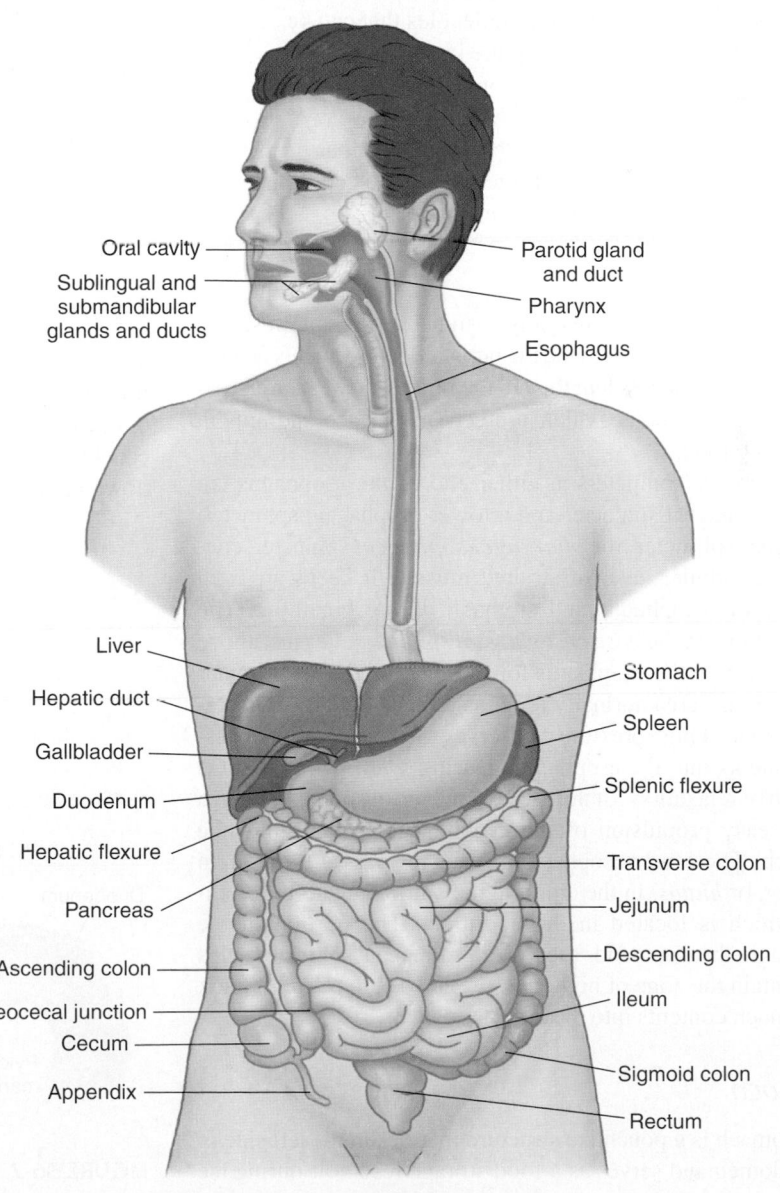

FIGURE 36-1 • The digestive system.

STRUCTURE AND FUNCTION OF THE GASTROINTESTINAL TRACT

- The gastrointestinal tract is a long, hollow tube that extends from the mouth to the anus; food and fluids that enter the gastrointestinal tract do not become part of the internal environment until they have been broken down and absorbed into the blood or lymph channels.

- The wall of the GI tract is essentially a four-layered tube: an inner mucosal layer; a supporting submucosal layer; a muscularis layer consisting of an inner circular layer and outer longitudinal layer of smooth muscle that functions propel to its contents in a proximal-to-distal direction, and an outer serosa layer that covers those parts of the GI tract that are suspended in the abdominopelvic cavity.

- The nutrients contained in ingested foods and fluids must be broken down into molecules that can be absorbed across the wall of the intestine. Gastric acids and pepsin from the stomach begin the digestive process: bile from the liver, digestive enzymes from the pancreas, and brush border enzymes break carbohydrates, fats, and proteins into molecules that can be absorbed from the intestine.

stomach. Its structure is uniquely designed for this purpose: the smooth muscle layers provide the peristaltic movements needed to move food along its length, and the mucosal and submucosal glands secrete mucus, which protects its surface and aids in lubricating food.

There are sphincters at either end of the esophagus: an upper esophageal sphincter and a lower esophageal sphincter. The upper sphincter, the *pharyngoesophageal* sphincter, consists of a circular layer of striated muscle. It keeps air from entering the esophagus and stomach during breathing. The lower sphincter, the *gastroesophageal sphincter,* lies just above the area where the esophagus joins the stomach. The circular muscle in this area normally remains tonically contracted, creating a zone of high pressure that serves to prevent reflux of gastric contents into the esophagus. During swallowing, there is "receptive relaxation" of the lower esophageal sphincter, which allows easy propulsion of the esophageal contents into the stomach. The lower esophageal sphincter passes through an opening, or *hiatus,* in the diaphragm as it joins with the stomach, which is located in the abdomen. The portion of the diaphragm that surrounds the lower esophageal sphincter helps to maintain the zone of high pressure needed to prevent reflux of stomach contents into the esophagus.

Stomach

The stomach is a pouchlike structure that lies in the left side of the abdomen and serves as a food storage reservoir during the

early stages of digestion. The esophagus opens into the stomach through an opening called the *cardiac orifice,* so named because of its proximity to the heart. The small part of the stomach that surrounds the cardiac orifice is called the *cardiac region,* the dome-shaped region that bulges above the cardiac region is called the *fundus,* the middle portion is called the *body,* and the funnel-shaped portion that connects with the small intestine is called the *pyloric region* (Fig. 36-2). The wider and more superior part of the pyloric region, the *antrum,* narrows to form the pyloric channel as it approaches the small intestine. At the end of the pyloric channel, the circular layer smooth muscle thickens to form the *pyloric sphincter.* This muscle serves as a valve that controls the rate of stomach emptying and prevents the regurgitation of intestinal contents back into the stomach.

Middle Gastrointestinal Tract

The small intestine, which forms the middle portion of the digestive tract, consists of three subdivisions: the duodenum, jejunum, and ileum (see Fig. 36-1). The duodenum, which is approximately 22 cm (10 in) long, connects the stomach to the jejunum and contains the opening for the common bile duct and the main pancreatic duct. Bile and pancreatic juices enter the intestine through these ducts. It is in the jejunum and ileum, which together are approximately 7 m (23 ft) long and must be folded onto themselves to fit into the abdominal cavity, that food is digested and absorbed.

Lower Gastrointestinal Tract

The large intestine, which forms the lower GI tract, is approximately 1.5 m (4.5 to 5 ft) long and 6 to 7 cm (2.4 to 2.7 in) in diameter. It is divided into the cecum, colon, rectum, and anal canal (see Fig. 36-1). The cecum is a blind pouch that projects down at the junction of the ileum and the colon. The ileocecal

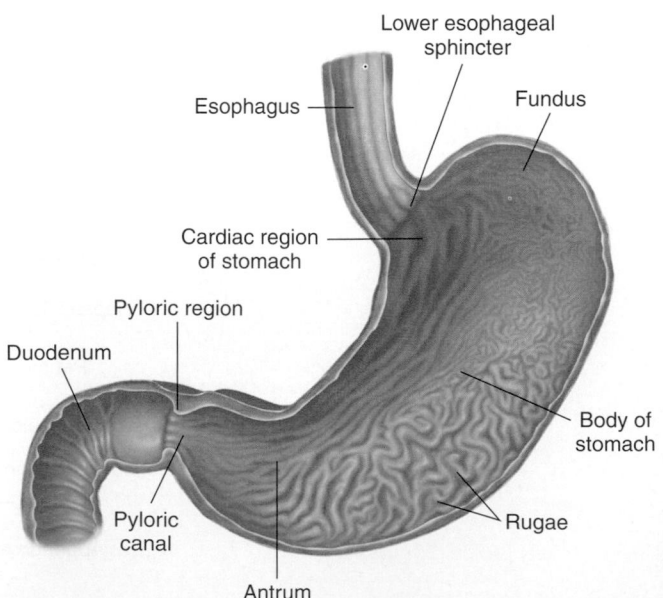

FIGURE 36-2 • Structures of the stomach.

valve lies at the upper border of the cecum and prevents the return of feces from the cecum into the small intestine. The appendix arises from the cecum approximately 2.5 cm (1 in) from the ileocecal valve. The colon is further divided into ascending, transverse, descending, and sigmoid portions. The ascending colon extends from the cecum to the undersurface of the liver, where it turns abruptly to form the right colic (hepatic) flexure. The transverse colon crosses the upper half of the abdominal cavity from right to left and then curves sharply downward beneath the lower end of the spleen, forming the left colic (splenic) flexure. The descending colon extends from the colic flexure to the rectum. The rectum extends from the sigmoid colon to the anus. The anal canal passes between the two medial borders of the levator ani muscles. Powerful sphincter muscles guard against fecal incontinence.

Gastrointestinal Wall Structure

The digestive tract, below the upper third of the esophagus, is essentially a four-layered tube (Fig. 36-3). The inner *mucosal layer* is made up of a lining epithelium, an underlying connective tissue called the *lamina propria,* and the muscularis mucosae, composed of smooth muscle cells that can contract and change the shape and surface area of the mucosal layer. The mucosal layer performs numerous functions in its role as an interface between the body and environment, including production of the mucus that lubricates and protects the inner surface of the alimentary canal, secretion of the digestive enzymes and substances that break down food, absorption of the breakdown products of digestion, and maintenance of a barrier to prevent the entry of noxious substances and pathogenic organisms; lymphatics within the mucosa serve as the

body's first line of immune defense. The epithelial cells in the mucosal layer have a rapid turnover rate and are replaced every 4 to 5 days. Because of the regenerative capabilities of the mucosal layer, injury to this layer heals rapidly without leaving scar tissue. The *submucosal* (second) *layer* consists of dense connective tissue and aggregates of adipose tissue. It contains the blood vessels, nerves, and structures responsible for secreting digestive enzymes. The submucosal glands either deliver their secretions directly to the lumen of the mucosal glands or via ducts that pass through the mucosa to the luminal surface. The third layer, the *muscularis externa,* consists of an inner layer of circularly arranged smooth muscle cells and an outer layer of longitudinally arranged smooth muscle layers, which facilitate movement of contents of the GI tract. The fourth or *serosal layer* is a serous membrane consisting of a layer of simple squamous epithelium, called the *mesothelium,* and a small amount of underlying connective tissue. It is equivalent to the visceral peritoneum and is the most superficial layer of those parts of the digestive tract that are suspended in the peritoneal cavity.

The peritoneum is the largest serous membrane in the body, having a surface area approximately equal to that of the skin. The peritoneum consists of two continuous layers: the *visceral peritoneum* and the *parietal peritoneum,* which lines the wall of the abdominopelvic cavity. Between the two layers is the *peritoneal cavity,* a potential space containing fluid secreted by the serous membranes. This serous fluid forms a moist and slippery surface that prevents friction between the continuously moving abdominal structures.

A *mesentery* is the double layer of peritoneum that encloses a portion or all of one of the abdominal viscera and attaches it to the abdominal wall (Fig. 36-4A). The mesentery contains the blood vessels, nerves, and lymphatic vessels that supply the

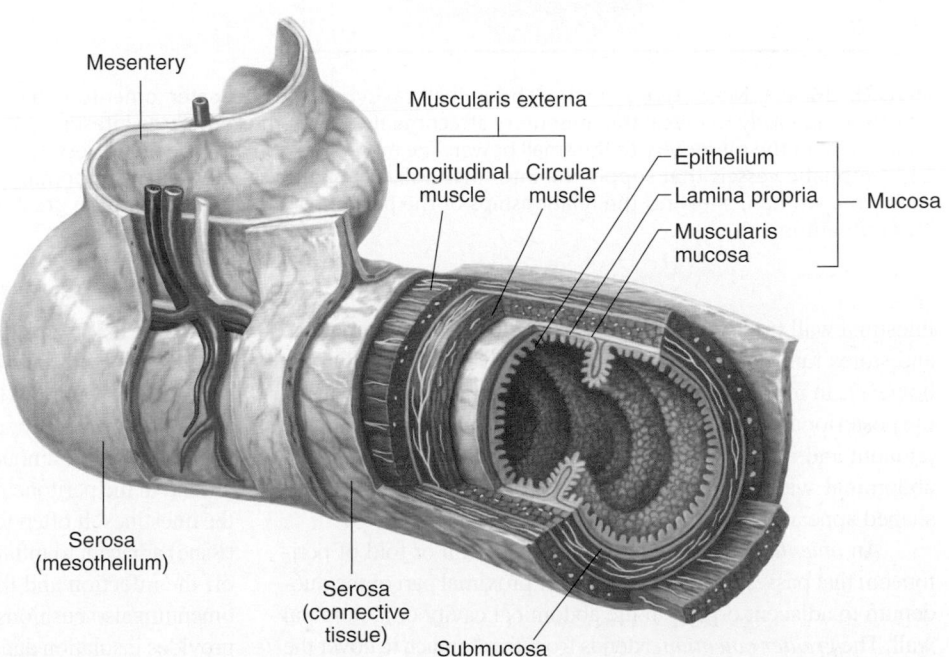

FIGURE 36-3 • Transverse section of the digestive system.

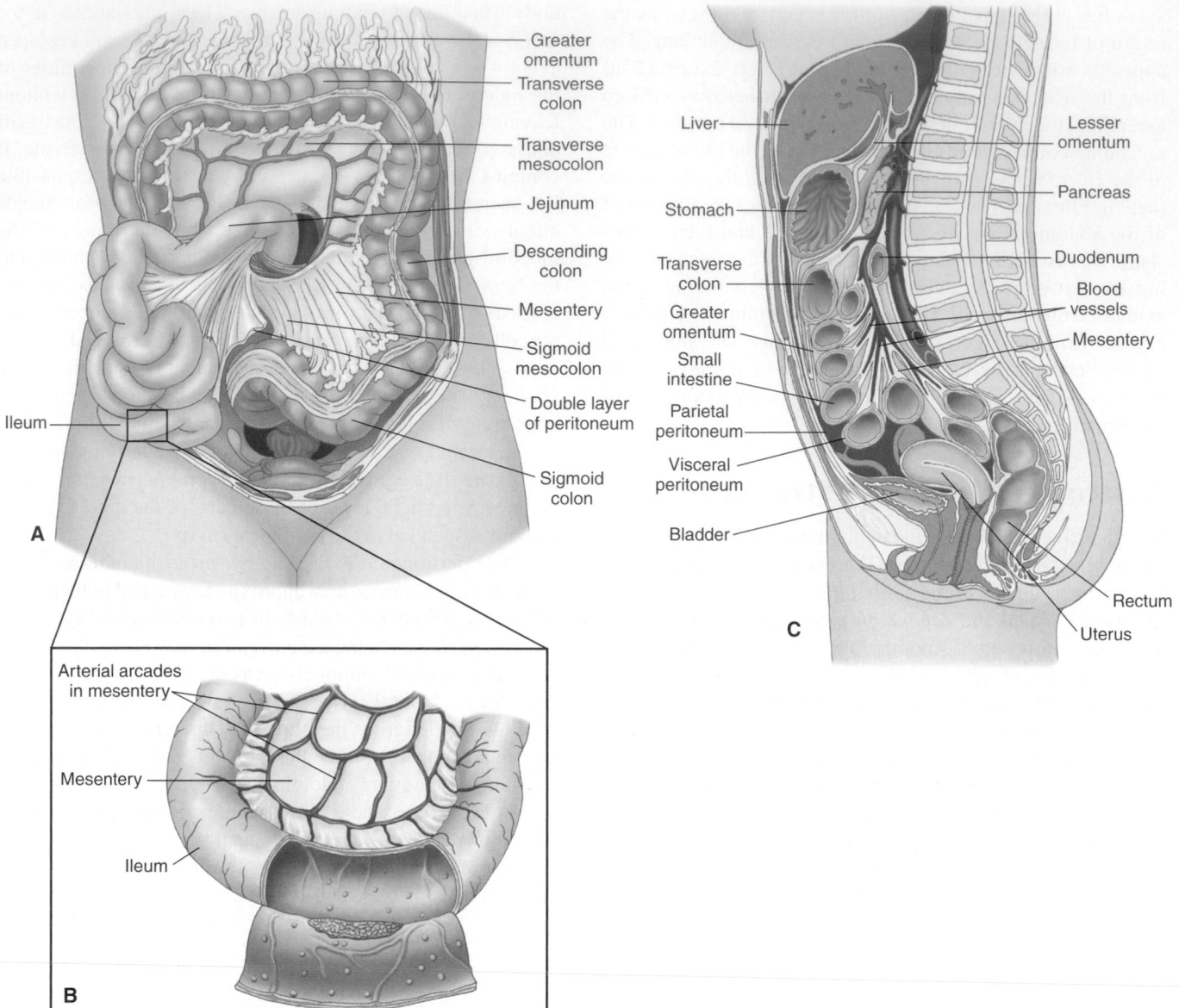

FIGURE 36-4 • Mesenteries of the abdominal cavity. (**A**) The greater omentum has been reflected superiorly to reveal the mesentery attachments to the small and large intestines. (**B**) The attachment of the mesentery to the small bowel. The mesentery contains the blood vessels, nerves, and lymphatic vessels that supply the intestinal wall. (**C**) Sagittal section of the abdominopelvic cavity in a woman, showing the relationships of the peritoneal attachments and the greater and lesser omentums.

intestinal wall (see Fig. 36-4B). It also holds the organs in place and stores fat. There are dorsal as well as ventral mesenteries; however, in most places the mesentery is dorsal and attaches to the posterior abdominal wall. The mesentery that attaches to the jejunum and ileum is gathered in folds that attach to the dorsal abdominal wall along a short line of insertion, giving a fan-shaped appearance, with the intestines at the edge.

An *omentum* is a double-layered extension or fold of peritoneum that passes from the stomach or proximal part of the duodenum to adjacent organs in the abdominal cavity or abdominal wall. The *greater omentum* extends from the stomach to cover the transverse colon and the folds of the intestine, whereas the *lesser omentum* extends between the transverse fissure of the liver and the lesser curvature of the stomach (see Fig. 36-4C). The greater omentum always contains some fat, which in obese persons can be a considerable amount. It has considerable mobility and moves around in the peritoneal cavity with the peristaltic movements of the intestines. It often forms adhesions (*i.e.,* bands of fibrous scar tissue) adjacent to inflamed organs such as the appendix, walling off the infection and thereby preventing its spread. The greater omentum also cushions the abdominal organs against injury and provides insulation against the loss of body heat.

IN SUMMARY, the GI tract is a long, hollow tube, the lumen of which is an extension of the external environment. The digestive tract can be divided into three parts: an upper part, consisting of the mouth, esophagus, and stomach; a middle part, consisting of the duodenum, jejunum, and ileum; a lower part, consisting of the cecum, colon, and rectum; and the accessory organs, consisting of the salivary glands, the liver, and the pancreas. Throughout its length, except for the mouth, throat, and upper esophagus, the GI tract is composed of five layers: an inner mucosal layer, a submucosal layer, a layer of circular smooth muscle fibers, a layer of longitudinal smooth muscle fibers, and an outer serosal layer that forms the peritoneum and is continuous with the mesentery. ■

MOTILITY

After completing this section of the chapter, you should be able to meet the following objectives:

- Characterize the properties of the interstitial smooth muscle cells that act as pacemakers for the GI tract.
- Compare the actions of the enteric and autonomic nervous systems as they relate to motility of the GI tract.
- Trace a bolus of food through the stages of swallowing.
- Differentiate tonic and peristaltic movements in the GI tract.
- Describe the action of the internal and external sphincters in the control of defecation.

Control of Gastrointestinal Motility

The motility of the GI tract propels food and fluids along its length, from mouth to anus, in a manner that facilitates digestion and absorption. The movements of the GI tract can be either rhythmic or tonic. The *rhythmic movements* consist of intermittent contractions that are responsible for mixing and moving food along the digestive tract. Rhythmic movements are found in the esophagus, antrum of the stomach, and small intestine. The *tonic movements* consist of a constant level of contraction or tone without regular periods of relaxation. They are found in the lower esophagus and the upper region of the stomach and the ileocecal valve and the internal anal sphincter.

Pacemaker-Generated Slow-Wave Activity

All of the contractile tissue in the GI tract is smooth muscle, except for that in the pharynx, the upper third of the esophagus, and the external anal sphincter. Although the smooth muscle found in each region of the GI tract exhibits structural and functional differences, certain basic properties are common to all of the muscle cells. All of the smooth muscle of the GI tract is unitary smooth muscle, in which the cells are electrically coupled by low-resistance pathways so that electrical signals initiating muscle contractions can move rapidly from one fiber to the next within each bundle.

Like the self-excitable cardiac muscle cells in the heart, some smooth muscle cells of the GI tract function as pacemaker cells. These cells display rhythmic, spontaneous oscillations in membrane potentials, called *slow waves*, ranging in frequency from about 3 per minute in the stomach to 12 per minute in the duodenum. Slow waves are generated by a thin layer of interstitial cells (*interstitial cells of Cajal*) located between the longitudinal and circular muscle layers.

The amplitude and, to a lesser extent, the frequency of the slow waves can be modulated by the enteric nervous system, which lies entirely within the wall of the GI tract, and by the parasympathetic and sympathetic divisions of the autonomic nervous system (ANS). In addition, a number of peptides, including neurotransmitters and GI hormones (to be discussed) assist in regulating GI motility. In general, the activity of the sympathetic nervous system decreases the amplitude of the slow waves or abolishes them altogether, whereas activation of the parasympathetic nervous system increases the amplitude of the slow waves.

Enteric Nervous System

The enteric nervous system consists of the myenteric and submucosal plexuses in the wall of the GI tract. These two plexuses are networks of nerve fibers and ganglion cell bodies. Interneurons in the plexuses connect afferent sensory fibers, efferent motor neurons, and secretory cells to form reflex circuits that are located entirely in the GI tract wall.

The *myenteric* (Auerbach) *plexus* consists mainly of a linear chain of interconnecting neurons that is located between the circular and longitudinal muscle layers. Because it lies between the two muscle layers and extends all the way down the intestinal wall, it is concerned mainly with motility along the length of the gut. The *submucosal* (Meissner) *plexus,* which lies between the mucosal and muscle layers of the intestinal wall, is mainly concerned with controlling the function of each segment of the intestinal tract. It integrates signals received from the mucosal layer into local control of motility, intestinal secretions, and absorption of nutrients.

The activity of the neurons in the myenteric and submucosal plexuses is regulated by local influences, input from the ANS, and by interconnecting fibers that transmit information between the two plexuses. Mechanoreceptors monitor the stretch and distention of the GI tract wall, and chemoreceptors monitor the chemical composition (*i.e.,* osmolality, pH, and digestive products of protein and fat metabolism) of its contents. These receptors can communicate directly with ganglionic cells in the intramural plexuses or with visceral afferent fibers that influence ANS control of GI function.

Autonomic Nervous System Innervation. The autonomic innervation of the GI system is mediated by both the sympa-

Understanding • Intestinal Motility

Motility of the small intestine is organized to optimize the digestion and absorption of nutrients and the propulsion of undigested material toward the colon. Peristaltic movements mix the ingested foodstuffs with digestive enzymes and secretions and circulate the intestinal contents to facilitate contact with the intestinal mucosa. The regulation of motility results from an interplay of input from the (1) enteric and (2) autonomic nervous (ANS) systems and the intrinsic pacemaker activity of the (3) intestinal smooth muscle cells.

❶ Enteric Nervous System Innervation

The gastrointestinal system has its own nervous system, called the *enteric nervous system*. The enteric nervous system is composed mainly of two plexuses: (1) the outer *myenteric (Auerbach) plexus* that is located between the longitudinal and circular layers of smooth muscle cells, and (2) an inner *submucosal (Meissner) plexus* that lies between the mucosal and circular muscle layers. The myenteric plexus controls mainly intestinal movements along the length of the gut, whereas the submucosal plexus is concerned mainly with controlling the function within each segment of the intestine. Fibers in the submucosal plexus also use signals originating from the intestinal epithelium to control intestinal secretion and local blood flow.

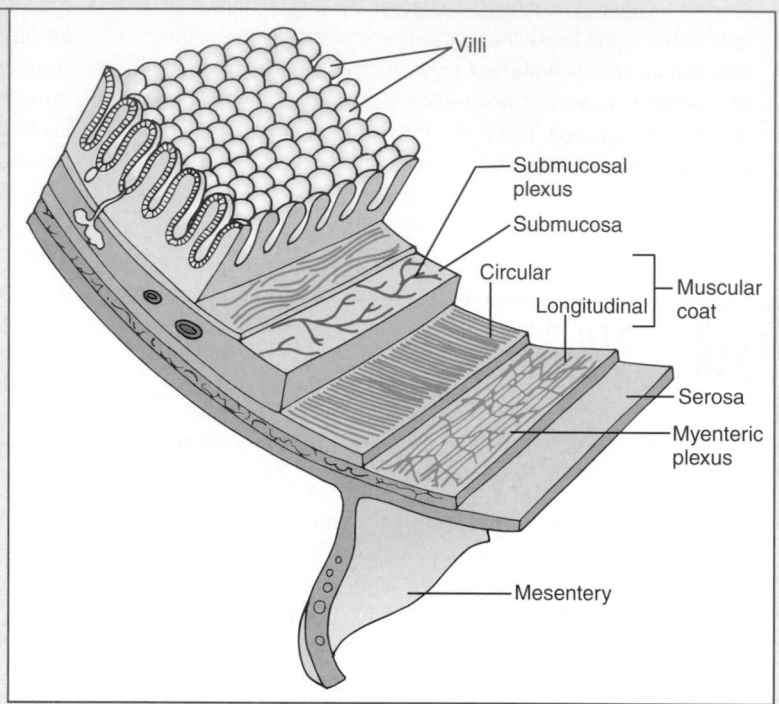

❷ ANS Innervation

The intestine is also innervated by the parasympathetic and sympathetic branches of the ANS (see Fig. 36-5). *Parasympathetic innervation* is supplied mainly by the vagus nerve with postganglionic neurons located primarily in the myenteric and submucosal plexuses. Stimulation of these parasympathetic nerves causes a general increase in both intestinal motility and secretory activity. *Sympathetic innervation* is supplied by nerves that run between the spinal cord and the prevertebral ganglia and between these ganglia and the intestine. Stimulation of the sympathetic nervous system is largely inhibitory, producing a decrease in intestinal motility and secretory activity.

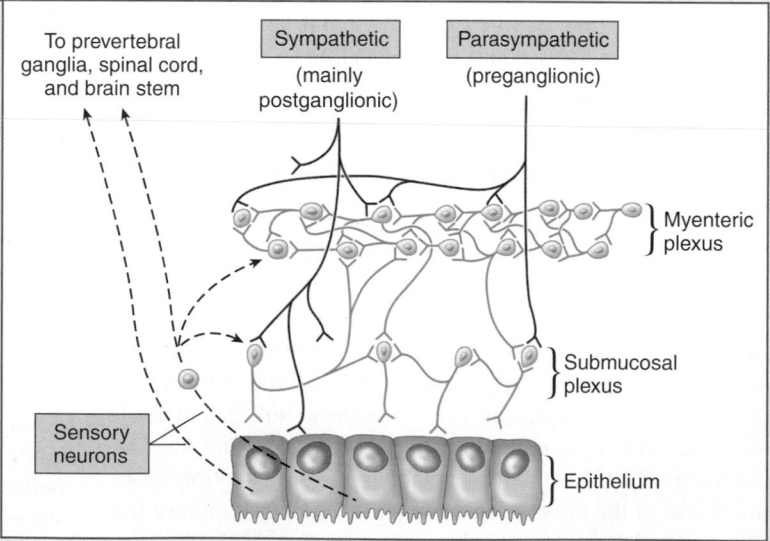

❸ Intestinal Smooth Muscle

Intestinal smooth muscle has its own intrinsic slow-wave activity, which varies from about 12 per minute in the duodenum to 8 or 9 per minute in the ileum. This slow-wave activity is thought to reside in a network of specialized pacemaker cells, the *interstitial cells of Cajal,* that are interposed between the smooth muscle cells. Slow waves are not action potentials and they do not directly induce muscle contraction; instead, they are rhythmic, wavelike fluctuations in the membrane potential that cyclically bring the membrane closer to threshold. If the peak voltage of the slow wave exceeds the cell's threshold potential, one or more action potentials may be triggered. Because action potentials occur at the peak of a smooth wave, slow-wave frequency determines the rate of smooth muscle contractions. Stretching the intestinal smooth muscle and parasympathetic nervous system stimulation increase excitability of the smooth muscle cells, whereas sympathetic stimulation decreases excitability.

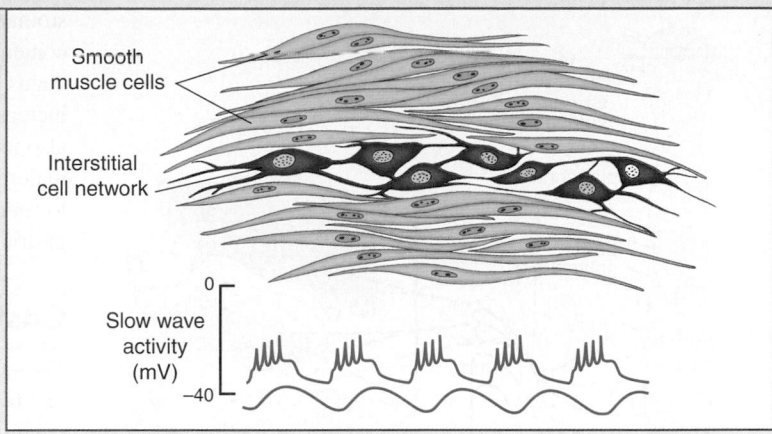

thetic and parasympathetic nervous systems (Fig. 36-5). Parasympathetic innervation to the stomach, small intestine, cecum, ascending colon, and transverse colon occurs through the vagus nerve. The remainder of the colon is innervated by parasympathetic fibers that exit the sacral segments of the spinal cord, by way of the pelvic nerves. Preganglionic parasympathetic fibers can synapse with intramural plexus neurons, or they can act directly on intestinal smooth muscle. In addition, these same nerve bundles provide many afferent nerves whose receptors lie within the various tissues of the gut. Their nerves project to the spinal cord and brain to provide sensory input for integration. Most parasympathetic innervation is excitatory. Numerous vagovagal reflexes influence motility and secretions of the digestive tract.

Sympathetic innervation occurs through the thoracic chain of sympathetic ganglia and the celiac, superior mesenteric, and inferior mesenteric ganglia. The sympathetic nervous system exerts several effects on GI function. It controls the extent of mucus secretion by the mucosal glands, reduces motility by inhibiting the activity of intramural plexus neurons, enhances sphincter function, and increases the vascular smooth muscle tone of the blood vessels that supply the GI tract. The effect of sympathetic stimulation is to block the release of the excitatory neuromediators in the intramural plexuses, inhibiting GI motility. Sympathetic control of GI function is largely mediated by activity in the intramural plexuses. For example, when gastrointestinal motility is enhanced because of increased vagal activity, stimulation of sympathetic centers in the hypothalamus promptly, and often completely, inhibits motility.

Swallowing and Esophageal Motility

Chewing begins the digestive process; it breaks the food into particles of a size that can be swallowed, lubricates it by mixing it with saliva, and mixes starch-containing food with salivary amylase. Although chewing usually is considered a voluntary act, it can be carried out involuntarily by a person who has lost the function of the cerebral cortex.

The swallowing reflex is a rigidly ordered sequence of events that results in the propulsion of food from the mouth to the stomach through the esophagus. Although swallowing is initiated as a voluntary activity, it becomes involuntary as food or fluid reaches the pharynx. Sensory impulses for the reflex begin at tactile receptors in the pharynx and esophagus and are integrated with the motor components of the response in an area of the reticular formation of the medulla and lower pons called the *swallowing center.* The motor impulses for the oral and pharyngeal phases of swallowing are carried in the trigeminal (V), glossopharyngeal (IX), vagus (X), and hypoglossal (XII) cranial nerves, and impulses for the esophageal phase are carried by the vagus nerve. Diseases that disrupt these brain centers or their cranial nerves disrupt the coordination of swallowing and predispose an individual to food and fluid lodging in the trachea and bronchi, leading to risk of asphyxiation or aspiration pneumonia.

Swallowing consists of three phases: an oral or voluntary phase; a pharyngeal phase; and an esophageal phase (Fig. 36-6). During the *oral phase,* the bolus is collected at the back of the mouth so the tongue can lift the food upward until it touches the

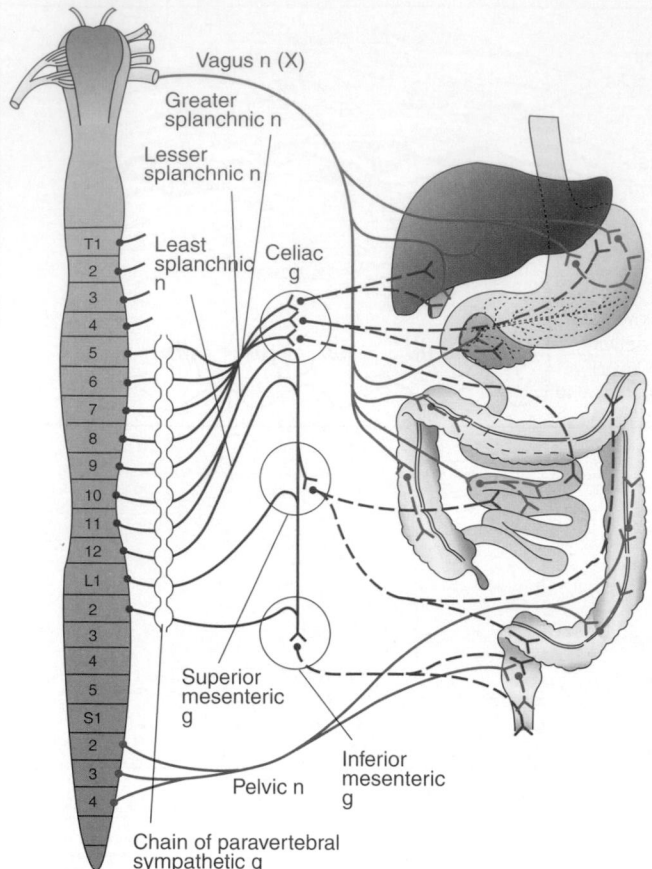

Vagus n (X)
Greater
splanchnic n
Lesser
splanchnic n
T1
2
3
4
5
6
7
8
9
10
11
12
L1
2
3
4
5
S1
2
3
4
Least
splanchnic
n
Celiac
g
Superior
mesenteric
g
Pelvic n
Inferior
mesenteric
g
Chain of paravertebral
sympathetic g

FIGURE 36-5 • Autonomic innervation of the gastrointestinal tract (g, ganglion; n, nerve). Parasympathetic innervation is indicated in *blue* and sympathetic in *red*.

stomach, an important factor in preventing the reflux of gastric contents. The lower esophageal sphincter is innervated by the vagus nerve. Increased levels of parasympathetic stimulation increase the constriction of the sphincter. The hormone gastrin also increases constriction of the sphincter. Gastrin provides the major stimulus for gastric acid production, and its action on the lower esophageal sphincter protects the esophageal mucosa when gastric acid levels are elevated.

Gastric Motility

The stomach serves as a food storage reservoir where the chemical breakdown of proteins begins and food is converted to a creamy mixture called *chyme*. Although an empty stomach has a volume of about 50 mL, it can expand to as much as 1000 mL before the intraluminal pressure begins to rise.

Motility of the stomach results in the churning and mixing of solid foods and regulates the emptying of the gastric contents, or chyme, into the duodenum. Peristaltic mixing and churning contractions begin in a pacemaker area in the middle of the stomach and move toward the antrum. They occur at a frequency of three to five contractions per minute, each lasting 2 to 20 seconds. As the peristaltic wave approaches the antrum, it speeds up, and the entire terminal 5 to 10 cm of the antrum contracts, occluding the pyloric opening. Contraction of the antrum reverses the movement of the chyme, returning the larger particles to the body of the stomach for further churning and kneading. Because the pylorus is contracted during antral contraction, the gastric contents are emptied into the duodenum between contractions.

The pyloric sphincter prevents the backflow of gastric contents and allows them to flow into the duodenum at a rate commensurate with the ability of the duodenum to accept them. This is important because the regurgitation of bile salts and duodenal contents can damage the mucosal surface of the antrum and lead to gastric ulcers. Likewise, the duodenal mucosa can be damaged by the rapid influx of highly acid gastric contents.

Like other parts of the GI tract, the stomach is richly innervated by the enteric nervous system and its connections with the sympathetic and parasympathetic nervous systems. Axons from the intramural plexuses innervate the smooth muscles and glands of the stomach. Parasympathetic innervation is provided by the vagus nerve and sympathetic innervation by the celiac ganglia. The emptying of the stomach is regulated by hormonal and neural mechanisms. The hormones cholecystokinin and glucose-dependent insulinotropic polypeptide (formerly known as *gastric inhibitory peptide*), which are thought in part to control gastric emptying, are released in response to the pH, osmolality, and fatty acid composition of the chyme. Both local and central circuitries are involved in the neural control of gastric emptying. Afferent receptor fibers synapse with the neurons in the intramural plexus or trigger intrinsic reflexes through vagal or sympathetic pathways that participate in extrinsic reflexes.

Disorders of gastric motility can occur when the rate is too slow or too fast (see Chapter 37). A rate that is too slow leads to gastric retention. It can be caused by obstruction or gastric atony. Obstruction can result from the formation of scar

posterior wall of the pharynx (Fig. 36-6A). At this point, the *pharyngeal phase* of swallowing is initiated. The soft palate is pulled upward, the palatopharyngeal folds are pulled together so that food does not enter the nasopharynx, the vocal cords are pulled together, and the epiglottis is moved so that it covers the larynx (Fig. 36-6B). Respiration is inhibited, and the bolus is moved backward into the esophagus by constrictive movements of the pharynx. Although the striated muscles of the pharynx are involved in the second stage of swallowing, it is an involuntary stage.

The third phase of swallowing is the *esophageal stage* (Fig. 36-6C). As food enters the esophagus and stretches its walls, local and central nervous system (CNS) reflexes that initiate peristalsis are triggered. There are two types of peristalsis—primary and secondary. Primary peristalsis is controlled by the swallowing center in the brain stem and begins when food enters the esophagus. Secondary peristalsis is partially mediated by smooth muscle fibers in the esophagus and occurs when primary peristalsis is inadequate to move food through the esophagus. Peristalsis begins at the site of distention and moves downward. Before the peristaltic wave reaches the stomach, the lower esophageal sphincter relaxes to allow the bolus of food to enter the stomach. The pressure in the lower esophageal sphincter normally is greater than that in the

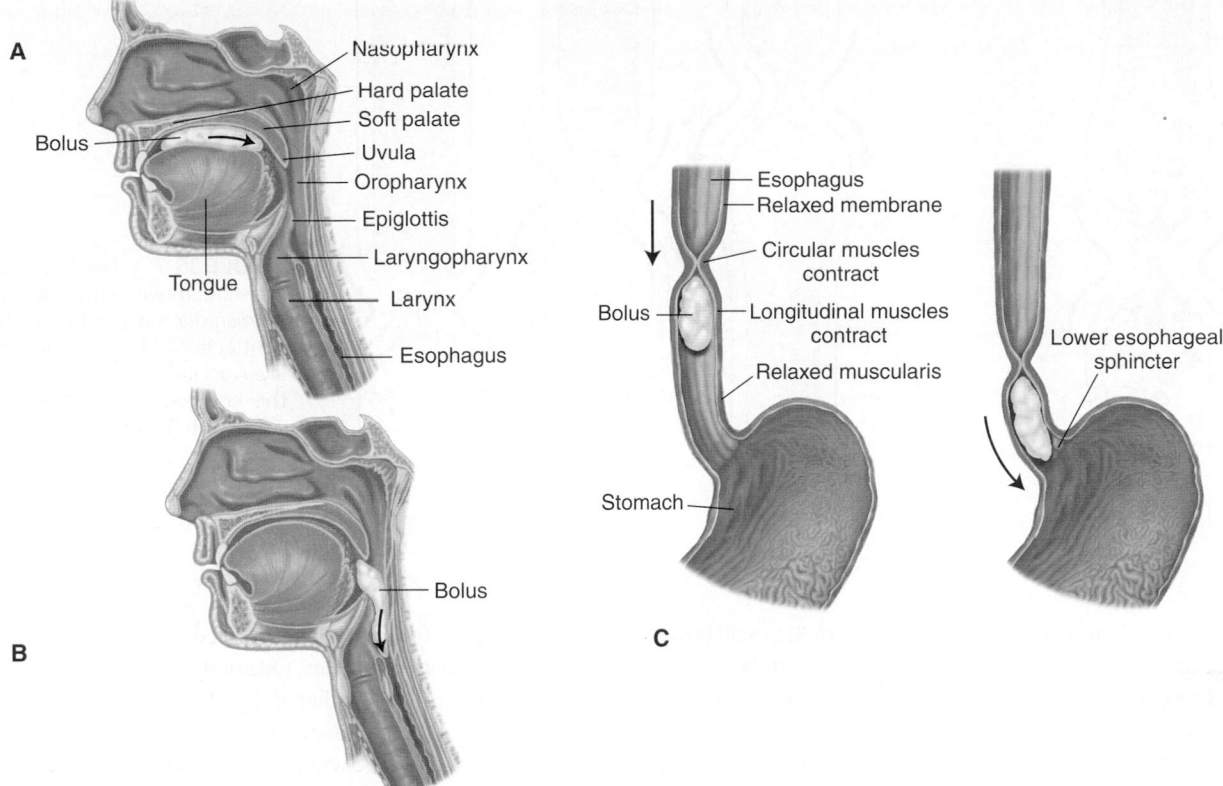

FIGURE 36-6 • Steps in the swallowing reflex. **(A)** The *oral* or *voluntary phase* during which the bolus is collected at the back of the mouth so the tongue can lift the food upward and into the pharynx; **(B)** the *pharyngeal phase* during which food movement into the respiratory passages is prevented as the tongue is elevated and pressed against the soft palate closing the epiglottis, the upper esophageal sphincter relaxes, and the superior constrictor muscle contracts forcing food into the esophagus; and **(C)** the *esophageal phase* during which peristalsis moves food through the esophagus and into the stomach.

tissue in the pyloric area after a peptic ulcer. Another example of obstruction is *hypertrophic pyloric stenosis,* which can occur in infants with an abnormally thick muscularis layer in the terminal pylorus. Myotomy, or surgical incision of the muscular ring, may be done to relieve the obstruction. Gastric atony can occur as a complication of visceral neuropathies in diabetes mellitus. Surgical procedures that disrupt vagal activity also can result in gastric atony. Abnormally fast emptying occurs in the dumping syndrome, which is a consequence of certain types of gastric operations. This condition is characterized by the rapid dumping of highly acidic and hyperosmotic gastric secretions into the duodenum and jejunum.

Small Intestinal Motility

The small intestine is the major site for the digestion and absorption of food; its movements are mixing and propulsive. There are two patterns of contractions in the small intestine: segmentation and peristaltic contractions. With *segmentation waves,* slow contractions of the circular muscle layer occlude the lumen and drive the contents forward and backward (Fig. 36-7A). Most of the contractions that produce segmentation waves are local

events involving only 1 to 4 cm of intestine at a time. They function mainly to mix the chyme with the digestive enzymes from the pancreas and to ensure adequate exposure of all parts of the chyme to the mucosal surface of the intestine, where absorption takes place. The frequency of segmenting activity increases after a meal. Presumably, it is stimulated by receptors in the stomach and intestine.

In contrast to the segmentation contractions, *peristaltic movements* are rhythmic propulsive movements designed to propel the chyme along the small intestine toward the large intestine. They occur when the smooth muscle layer constricts, forming a contractile band that forces the intraluminal contents forward. Normal peristalsis always moves in the direction from the mouth toward the anus. Regular peristaltic movements begin in the duodenum near the entry sites of the common duct and the main hepatic duct. These propulsive movements occur with synchronized activity in a section 10 to 20 cm long. They are accomplished by contraction of the proximal portion of the intestine with the sequential relaxation of its distal, or caudal, portion (see Fig. 36-7B). After material has been propelled to the ileocecal junction by peristaltic movement, stretching of the distal ileum produces a local reflex that relaxes the sphincter and allows fluid

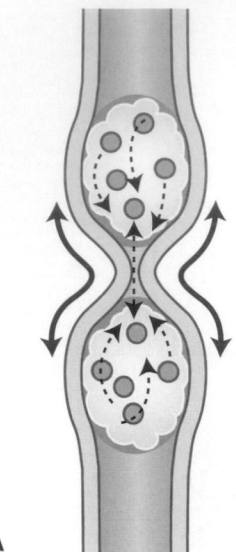

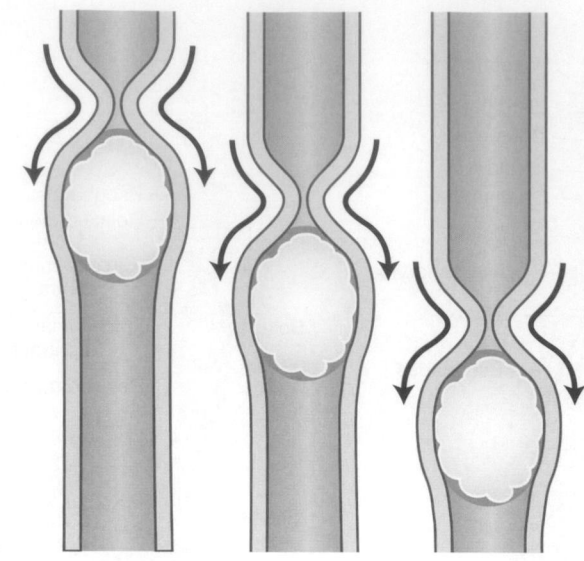

FIGURE 36-7 • Two types of small intestine movements. **(A)** Mixing *segmentation waves* in which slow contractions of the circular muscle layer occlude the lumen and drive the contents forward and backward; and **(B)** propulsive *peristaltic movements* in which segmental contractions followed by sequential relaxation moves the contents forward.

to squirt into the cecum. Motility disturbances of the small bowel are common, and auscultation of the abdomen can be used to assess bowel activity. Inflammatory changes often increase motility. In many instances, it is not certain whether changes in motility occur because of inflammation or are secondary to toxins and unabsorbed materials. Delayed passage of chyme in the small intestine also can be a problem. Transient interruption of intestinal motility often occurs after GI surgery. Intubation with suction often is required to remove the accumulating intestinal contents and gases until activity is resumed.

Colonic Motility and Defecation

The storage function of the colon dictates that movements in this section of the gut are different from those in the small intestine. Movements in the colon are of two types. First are the segmental mixing movements, called *haustrations,* so named because they occur within sacculations called *haustra.* These movements produce a local digging-type action, which ensures that all portions of the fecal mass are exposed to the intestinal surface. Second are the propulsive mass movements, in which a large segment of the colon (≥20 cm) contracts as a unit, moving the fecal contents forward as a unit. Mass movements last approximately 30 seconds, followed by a 2- to 3-minute period of relaxation, after which another contraction occurs. A series of mass movements lasts only for 10 to 30 minutes and may occur only several times a day. Defecation normally is initiated by the mass movements. The normal colonic transit time is 24 to 48 hours, with normal stool weights of up to 250 g/day.

Defecation is controlled by the action of two sphincters, the internal and external anal sphincters (Fig. 36-8). The internal sphincter is a several-centimeters-long, circular thickening of smooth muscle that lies inside the anus. The external sphincter, which is composed of striated voluntary muscle, surrounds the internal sphincter. The external sphincter is controlled by nerve fibers in the pudendal nerve, which is part of the somatic nervous

system and therefore under voluntary control. Defecation is controlled by defecation reflexes. One of these reflexes is the intrinsic myenteric reflex mediated by the local enteric nervous system. It is initiated by distention of the rectal wall, with initiation of reflex peristaltic waves that spread through the descending colon, sigmoid colon, and rectum. A second defecation reflex, the parasympathetic reflex, is integrated at the level of the sacral cord. When the nerve endings in the rectum are stimulated, signals are transmitted first to the sacral cord and then reflexly back to the descending colon, sigmoid colon, rectum, and anus by the pelvic nerves. These impulses greatly increase peristaltic movements as well as relax the internal sphincter.

To prevent involuntary defecation from occurring, the external anal sphincter is under the conscious control of the

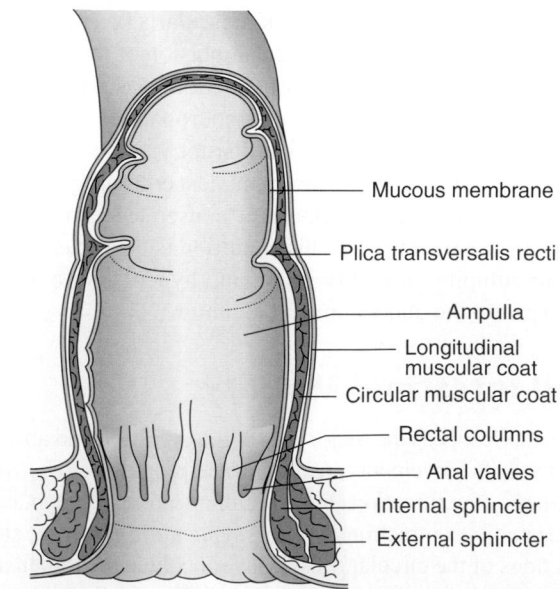

Mucous membrane

Plica transversalis recti

Ampulla

Longitudinal muscular coat

Circular muscular coat

Rectal columns

Anal valves

Internal sphincter

External sphincter

FIGURE 36-8 • Interior of the rectum and anal canal.

cortex. As afferent impulses arrive at the sacral cord, signaling the presence of a distended rectum, messages are transmitted to the cortex. If defecation is inappropriate, the cortex initiates impulses that constrict the external sphincter and inhibit efferent parasympathetic activity. Normally, the afferent impulses in this reflex loop fatigue easily, and the urge to defecate soon ceases. At a more convenient time, contraction of the abdominal muscles compresses the contents in the large bowel, reinitiating afferent impulses to the cord.

IN SUMMARY, motility of the GI tract propels food products and fluids along its length from the mouth to anus. Although the activity of GI smooth muscle is self-propagating and can continue without input from the nervous system, its rate and strength of contractions are regulated by a network of intramural neurons that receive input from the ANS and local receptors that monitor wall stretch and the chemical composition of luminal contents. Parasympathetic innervation occurs through the vagus nerve and nerve fibers from sacral segments of the spinal cord; it increases GI motility. Sympathetic activity occurs through thoracolumbar output from the spinal cord, its paravertebral ganglia, and celiac, superior mesenteric, and inferior mesenteric ganglia. Sympathetic stimulation enhances sphincter function and reduces motility by inhibiting the activity of intramural plexus neurons. ∎

HORMONAL, SECRETORY, AND DIGESTIVE FUNCTIONS

After completing this section of the chapter, you should be able to meet the following objectives:

- State the source and function of water and electrolytes that are secreted in digestive secretions.
- Explain the protective function of saliva.
- Describe the function of the gastric secretions in the process of digestion.
- List three major GI hormones and cite their function.
- Describe the site of gastric acid and pepsin production and secretion in the stomach.
- Describe the function of the gastric mucosal barrier.
- Describe the functions of the secretions of the small and the large intestines.
- Discuss the function of gut flora in terms of metabolic activities, trophic effects, and protection against invasion by pathogenic microorganisms.

Gastrointestinal Hormones

The GI tract is the largest endocrine organ in the body. It produces hormones that act locally, pass into the general circulation for distribution to more distant sites, and interact with

the CNS through the enteric and autonomic nervous systems. Among the hormones produced by the GI tract are gastrin, ghrelin, secretin, cholecystokinin, and incretin hormones (glucagon-like peptide-1 [GLP-1] and glucose-dependent insulinotropic polypeptide [GIP]). These hormones influence appetite, GI motility, enzyme activity, electrolyte levels, and the secretion and actions of hormones such as growth hormone, insulin, and glucagon. The actions of many of these hormones overlap: two or more GI hormones may affect the same process in the same direction, or they may inhibit each other. The GI tract hormones and their functions are summarized in Table 36-1.

The stomach is the source of two important GI hormones: gastrin and ghrelin. Gastrin is produced by G cells, located predominantly in the antrum of the stomach. The primary function of *gastrin* is the stimulation of gastric acid secretion. Gastrin also has a trophic, or growth-producing, effect on the mucosa of the small intestine, colon, and acid-secreting area of the stomach. Removal of the tissue that produces gastrin results in atrophy of these structures. *Ghrelin* is a newly discovered peptide hormone produced by endocrine cells in the mucosal layer of the fundus of the stomach. It displays potent growth hormone–releasing activity and has a stimulatory effect on food intake and digestive function, while reducing energy expenditure. The isolation of this hormone has led to new insights into the gut–brain regulation of growth hormone secretion and energy balance.

The intestine is the source of secretin, cholecystokinin, and incretin hormones. *Secretin*, which is secreted by S cells in the mucosa of the duodenum and jejunum, inhibits gastric acid secretion. The entry of an acid chyme into the intestine stimulates the release of secretin, which inhibits the release of gastrin. Secretin also stimulates the pancreas to secrete large quantities of fluid with a high bicarbonate concentration and low chloride concentration. The primary function of *cholecystokinin* (CCK), secreted by I cells in the intestinal mucosa, is the stimulation of pancreatic enzyme secretion. It potentiates the action of secretin, increasing the pancreatic bicarbonate response to low circulating levels of secretin, stimulates biliary secretion of fluid and bicarbonate, and regulates gallbladder contraction and gastric emptying. CCK has also been shown to inhibit food intake and to be an important mediator for appetite and the control of meal size.

Several gut-derived hormones have been identified as having what is termed an *incretin* effect, meaning that they increase insulin release after an oral glucose load. This suggests that gut-derived factors can stimulate insulin secretion after a predominantly carbohydrate meal. The two hormones that account for about 90% of the incretin effect are GLP-1, which is released from L cells in the distal small bowel, and GIP, which is released by K cells in the upper gut (mainly the jejunum). Because increased levels of GLP-1 and GIP can lower blood glucose levels by augmenting insulin release in a glucose-dependent manner (*i.e.*, at low blood glucose levels no further insulin is secreted, minimizing the risk of hypoglycemia), these hormones have been targeted as possible antidiabetic drugs. Moreover, GLP-1 can exert other metabolically beneficial effects, includ-

TABLE 36-1 Selected Gastrointestinal Hormones and Their Actions

HORMONE	SITE OF SECRETION	STIMULUS FOR SECRETION	ACTION
Cholecystokinin	Duodenum, jejunum	Products of protein digestion and long-chain fatty acids	Stimulates contraction of gallbladder and secretion of pancreatic enzymes; slows gastric emptying; inhibits food intake
Gastrin	Antrum of stomach, duodenum	Vagal stimulation; epinephrine; neutral amino acids; calcium-containing foods such as milk; alcohol Secretion inhibited by acid content of stomach antrum (pH < 2.5)	Stimulates secretion of gastric acid and pepsinogen; increases gastric blood flow; stimulates gastric smooth muscle contractions; stimulates growth of gastric and intestinal mucosal cells
Ghrelin	Fundus of stomach	Nutritional (fasting) and hormonal (decreased levels of growth hormone)	Stimulates secretion of growth hormone; acts as an appetite-stimulating signal from stomach when an increase in metabolic efficiency is necessary
Glucagon-like peptide-1 (GLP-1)	Distal small intestine	High-carbohydrate meal	Augments insulin release; suppresses glucagon release; slows gastric emptying; decreases appetite and body weight
Glucose-dependent insulinotropic polypeptide (GIP)	Small intestine, mainly jejunum	High-carbohydrate meal	Augments insulin release
Secretin	Duodenum	Acid pH or chyme entering duodenum (pH < 3.0)	Stimulates secretion of bicarbonate-containing fluids by pancreas and liver

ing suppression of glucagon release, slowing of gastric emptying, augmenting of net glucose clearance, and decreasing appetite and body weight.

Gastrointestinal Secretions

Throughout the GI tract, secretory glands serve two basic functions: (1) production of mucus to lubricate and protect the mucosal layer of the GI tract wall and (2) secretion of fluids and enzymes to aid in the digestion and absorption of nutrients. Each day, approximately 7000 mL of fluid is secreted into the GI tract (Table 36-2). Approximately 50 to 200 mL of this fluid leaves the body in the stool; the remainder is reabsorbed in the small and large intestines. These secretions are mainly water and have sodium and potassium concentrations similar to those of extracellular fluid. Because water and electrolytes for digestive tract secretions are derived from the extracellular fluid compartment, excessive secretion or impaired absorption can lead to extracellular fluid deficit.

The secretory and digestive functions of the gut are influenced by local, humoral, and neural influences. Neural control of GI secretory activity is mediated through the ANS. Secretory activity, like motility, is increased with parasympathetic stimulation and inhibited with sympathetic activity. Many of the local influences, including pH, osmolality, and chyme, consistently act as stimuli for neural and humoral mechanisms.

Salivary Secretions

Saliva is secreted by the salivary glands. The salivary glands consist of the parotid, submaxillary, sublingual, and buccal glands. Saliva has three functions. The first is protection and lubrication. Saliva is rich in mucus, which protects the oral mucosa and coats the food as it passes through the mouth, pharynx, and esophagus. The sublingual and buccal glands produce only mucus-type secretions. The second function of saliva is its protective antimicrobial action. The saliva cleans the mouth and contains the enzyme lysozyme, which has an antibacterial action. Third, saliva contains ptyalin and amylase, which initiate the digestion of dietary starches. Secretions from the salivary glands are primarily regulated by the ANS. Parasympathetic stimulation increases flow and sympathetic stimulation decreases flow. The dry mouth that accompanies anxiety attests to the effects of sympathetic activity on salivary secretions.

Mumps, or parotitis, is an infection of the parotid glands. Although most of us associate mumps with the contagious viral form of the disease, inflammation of the parotid glands can occur in the seriously ill person who does not receive adequate oral hygiene and who is unable to take fluids orally.

Gastric Secretions

In addition to mucus-secreting cells that line the entire surface of the stomach, the stomach mucosa has several other types of

TABLE 36-2 **Secretions of the Gastrointestinal Tract**	
SECRETIONS	**AMOUNT DAILY (ML)**
Salivary	1200
Gastric	2000
Pancreatic	1200
Biliary	700
Intestinal	2000
Total	7100

One of the important characteristics of the gastric mucosa is resistance to the highly acid secretions that it produces. When the gastric mucosa is damaged by aspirin, nonsteroidal anti-inflammatory drugs (NSAIDs), ethyl alcohol, or bile salts, this barrier is disrupted, and hydrogen ions move into the tissue. As the hydrogen ions accumulate in the mucosal cells, intracellular pH decreases, enzymatic reactions become impaired, and cellular structures are disrupted. The result is local ischemia, vascular stasis, hypoxia, and tissue necrosis. The mucosal surface is further protected by prostaglandins. Aspirin and NSAIDs inhibit prostaglandin synthesis by inhibition of cyclooxygenase (known as COX, hence these agents are also known as COX inhibitors), which also impairs the integrity of the mucosal surface.

cells, including the parietal (or oxyntic) cells, chief cells, and G cells. The parietal and chief cells are located in the proximal 80% (body and fundus) of the stomach. The parietal cells secrete hydrochloric acid (HCl) and intrinsic factor. The chief cells secrete pepsinogen, an enzyme that initiates proteolysis or breakdown of proteins. The antrum is located in the distal 20% of the stomach. This area contains the G cells, which secrete gastrin.

The luminal surface and gastric pits of the stomach are lined with mucus-producing epithelial cells, with the parietal and chief cells situated in the bases of the gastric pits (Fig. 36-9). There are approximately 1 billion parietal cells in the stomach; together they produce and secrete approximately 20 mEq of HCl in several hundred milliliters of gastric juice each hour. The pepsinogen that is secreted by the chief cells is rapidly converted to pepsin when exposed to the low pH of the gastric juices. Intrinsic factor, which is produced by the parietal cells, is necessary for the absorption of vitamin B_{12} (see Chapter 14).

Gastric Acid Secretion. The cellular mechanism for HCl secretion by the parietal cells in the stomach involves the hydrogen (H^+)/potassium (K^+) adenosine triphosphatase (ATPase) transporter and chloride (Cl^-) channels located on their luminal membrane (Fig. 36-10). During the process of HCl secretion, carbon dioxide (CO_2) produced by aerobic metabolism combines with water (H_2O), catalyzed by carbonic anhydrase, to form carbonic acid (H_2CO_3), which dissociates into H^+ and bicarbonate (HCO_3^-). The H^+ is secreted with Cl^- into the stomach, and the HCO_3^- moves out of the cell and into blood from the basolateral membrane. The absorbed HCO_3^- is responsible for the alkaline tide (increased pH) that occurs after a meal. At the luminal side of the membrane, H^+ is secreted into the stomach by the H^+/K^+-ATPase transporter (also known as the *proton pump*). Chloride follows H^+ into the stomach by diffusing through Cl^- channels in the luminal membrane. The proton pump

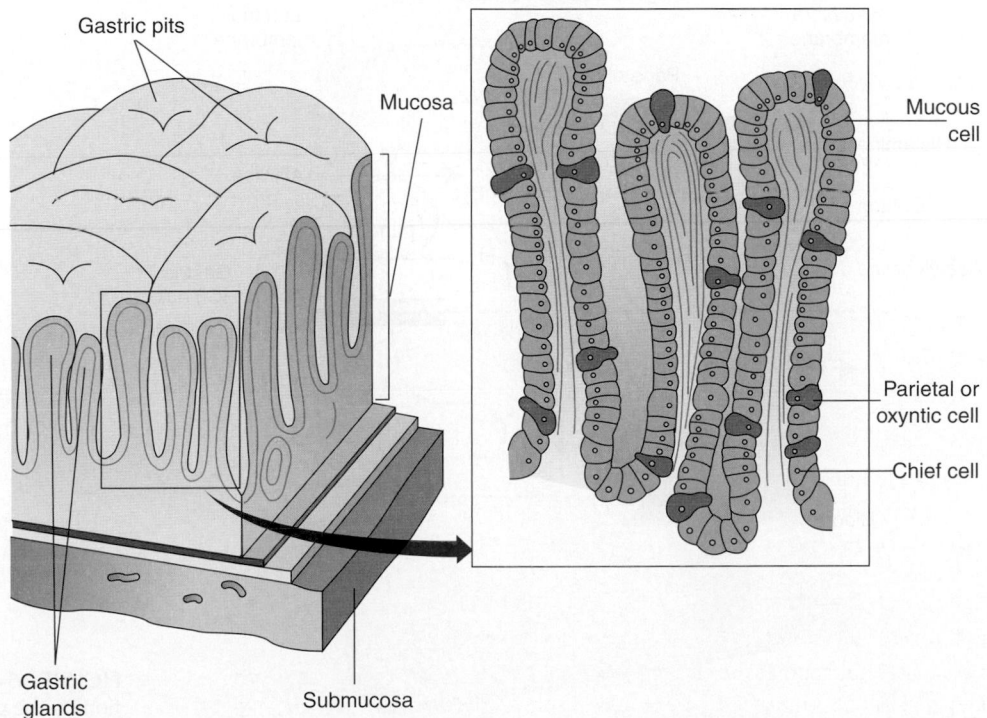

FIGURE 36-9 • Gastric pit from body of the stomach.

inhibitors (*e.g.*, omeprazole), which are used in treatment of acid reflux and peptic ulcer, inhibit gastric acid secretion by binding irreversibly to the sulfhydryl groups of the H^+/K^+-ATPase transporter.

Three substances stimulate HCl secretion by the parietal cells: acetylcholine, gastrin, and histamine. Although each substance binds to different receptors on the parietal cell and has a different mechanism of action, they all serve to stimulate an increase in H^+ secretion through the H^+/K^+-ATPase transporter. Acetylcholine is released from vagal nerves innervating the stomach and binds to acetylcholine receptors on the parietal cells. Gastrin is secreted by G cells in the antrum of the stomach and reaches the parietal cells through the circulation. It binds to as yet uncharacterized receptors on the parietal cells. Histamine is released from special endocrine cells in the gastric mucosa and diffuses to nearby parietal cells, where it binds to histamine-2 (H_2) receptors. H_2 receptor blockers (*e.g.*, cimetidine), used in treatment of peptic ulcer and gastroesophageal reflux, bind to H_2 receptors and block the action of histamine on parietal cells. In contrast to these acid-stimulatory factors, prostaglandin E_2 (after binding to its receptor) inhibits acid secretion and stimulates mucus production. Hence, it is an important factor in the maintenance of the gastric mucosal barrier. Gastric acid secretion and its relation to gastroesophageal reflux and peptic ulcer are discussed further in Chapter 37.

Intestinal Secretions

The small intestine secretes digestive juices and receives secretions from the liver and pancreas (see Chapter 38). An extensive array of mucus-producing glands, called *Brunner glands,* is concentrated at the site where the contents from the stomach and secretions from the liver and pancreas enter the duodenum. These glands secrete large amounts of alkaline mucus that protect the duodenum from the acid content in the gastric chyme and from the action of the digestive enzymes. The activity of Brunner glands is strongly influenced by ANS activity. For example, sympathetic stimulation causes a marked decrease in mucus production, leaving this area more susceptible to irritation. Between 75% and 80% of peptic ulcers occur at this site.

In addition to mucus, the intestinal mucosa produces two other types of secretions. The first is a serous fluid (pH 6.5 to 7.5) secreted by specialized cells (*i.e.,* crypts of Lieberkühn) in the intestinal mucosal layer. This fluid, which is produced at the rate of 2000 mL/day, acts as a vehicle for absorption. The second type of secretion consists of surface enzymes that aid absorption. These enzymes are the peptidases, or enzymes that separate amino acids, and the disaccharidases, or enzymes that split sugars.

The large intestine usually secretes only mucus. ANS activity strongly influences mucus production in the bowel, as in

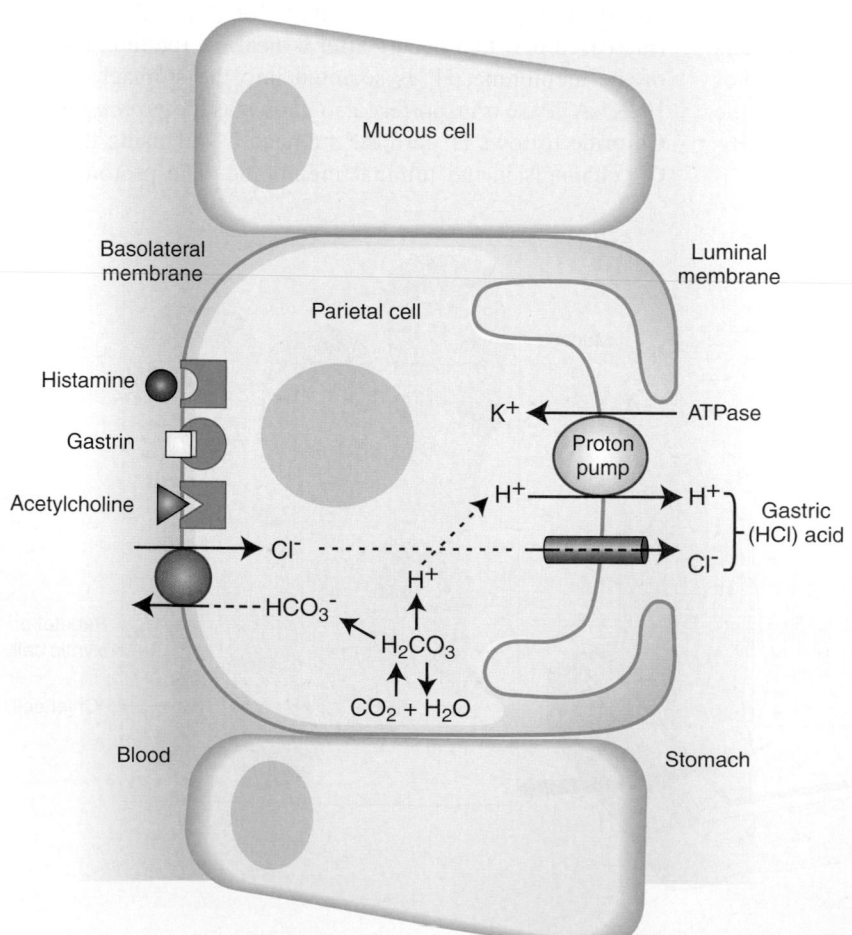

FIGURE 36-10 • Mechanism of gastric acid secretion by the parietal cells in the stomach.

other parts of the digestive tract. During intense parasympathetic stimulation, mucus secretion may increase to the point that the stool contains large amounts of obvious mucus. Although the bowel normally does not secrete water or electrolytes, these substances are lost in large quantities when the bowel becomes irritated or inflamed.

Intestinal Flora

The gut is the natural habitat of a large and diverse bacterial community. The major functions of the gut microflora include metabolic activities that salvage energy and absorbable nutrients, trophic effects on intestinal epithelial cells, and protection of the colonized host against invasion by pathogenic organisms.

The stomach and small intestine contain only a few species of bacteria, probably because of the composition of luminal contents (*i.e.*, acids, bile, pancreatic secretions), which kills most ingested microorganisms, and the propulsive movements of this area, which impedes their colonization. The large intestine, on the other hand, contains a large and complex microbial ecosystem. It has been estimated that each individual has 300 to 500 different species of intestinal bacteria, with anaerobic bacteria outnumbering aerobic bacteria by a large percentage.

Colonization of the GI tract begins shortly after birth and is influenced by passage through the birth canal and the type of diet (breast milk versus formula) the infant receives. Other environmental factors also have a role because differences exist between the intestinal flora of infants born in industrialized countries and those born in developing countries.

The major metabolic function of colonic microflora is the fermentation of undigestible dietary residue and endogenous mucus produced by the epithelial cells. The genetic diversity of the microorganisms in the gut provides various enzymes and biochemical pathways that are distinct from those of the host. Fermentation of nondigestible carbohydrates, including resistant starches, cellulose, pectins, and unabsorbed sugars, is a major source of energy in the colon. The metabolic end point is the generation of short-chain fatty acids, which play a major role in epithelial cell growth and differentiation. Colonic microorganisms also play a role in vitamin synthesis and in absorption of calcium, magnesium, and iron. Vitamin K, for example, is synthesized by the colonic flora; the newborn infant does not synthesize an adequate amount of vitamin K for the first week or so of life until the normal colonic bacterial flora becomes established. Last, the resident gut flora provides a crucial line of resistance to colonization by exogenous microbes, and therefore is highly protective against invasion of tissues by pathogens. Colonization resistance also applies to opportunistic bacteria that are present in the gut but whose growth is restricted. The administration of broad-spectrum antibiotics can disrupt the microbial balance and allow overgrowth of species with potential pathogenicity, such as *Clostridium difficile* (see Chapter 37).

The role of probiotics as a supplement to the normal diet and as a treatment for several disease states has become increasingly recognized. Probiotics are live microorganisms that, when ingested, can modify the composition of enteric microflora.

Commonly used probiotics are lactobacilli, bifidobacteria, and nonpathogenic *Escherichia coli*. Probiotics have shown value in several diseases, such as maintaining remission in ulcerative colitis.

IN SUMMARY, the secretions of the GI tract include saliva, gastric juices, bile, and pancreatic and intestinal secretions. Each day, more than 7000 mL of fluid is secreted into the digestive tract; all but 50 to 200 mL of this fluid is reabsorbed. Water, derived from the extracellular fluid compartment, is the major component of GI tract secretions. Neural, humoral, and local mechanisms contribute to the control of these secretions. The parasympathetic nervous system increases secretion, and sympathetic activity exerts an inhibitory effect. In addition to secreting fluids containing digestive enzymes, the GI tract produces and secretes hormones, such as gastrin, ghrelin, secretin, CCK, and the incretin hormones (GLP-1 and GIP) that influence appetite, GI motility, enzyme activity, and the secretions as actions of hormones such as growth hormone, insulin, and glucagon.

The gut is also the natural habitat of a large and diverse bacterial community. The major functions of the gut microflora include metabolic activities that salvage energy and absorbable nutrients, impart trophic effects on intestinal epithelial cells, and protect the colonized host against invasion by pathogenic organisms. ■

DIGESTION AND ABSORPTION

After completing this section of the chapter, you should be able to meet the following objectives:

- Differentiate digestion from absorption.
- Relate the characteristics of the small intestine to its absorptive function.
- Explain the function of intestinal brush border enzymes.
- Compare the digestion and absorption of carbohydrates, fats, and proteins.

Digestion is the process of dismantling foods into their constituent parts. Digestion requires hydrolysis, enzyme cleavage, and fat emulsification. Hydrolysis is the breakdown of a compound that involves a chemical reaction with water. The importance of hydrolysis to digestion is evidenced by the amount of water (7 to 8 L) that is secreted into the GI tract daily. The intestinal mucosa is impermeable to most large molecules: most proteins, fats, and carbohydrates must be broken down into smaller particles before they can be absorbed. Although some digestion of carbohydrates and proteins begins in the stomach, digestion takes place mainly in the small intestine. The breakdown of fats to free fatty acids and monoglycerides takes place entirely in the small intestine. The liver, with its production of bile, and the pancreas, which sup-

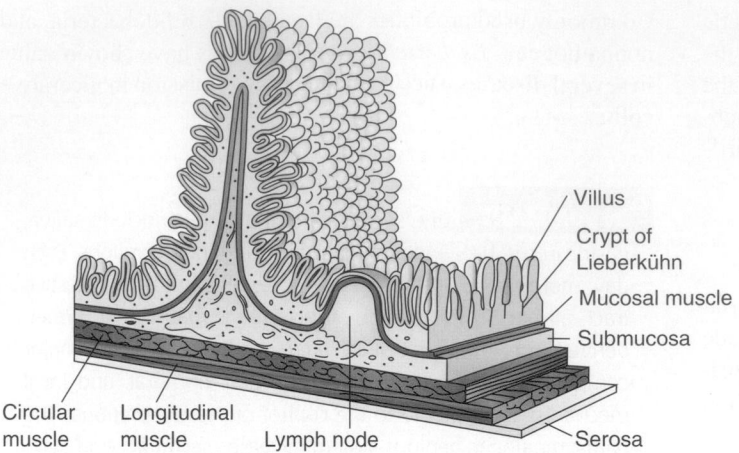

FIGURE 36-11 • The mucous membrane of the small intestine. Note the numerous villi on a circular fold.

plies a number of digestive enzymes, play important roles in digestion.

Absorption is the process of moving nutrients and other materials from the external environment in the lumen of the GI tract into the internal environment. Absorption is accomplished by active transport and diffusion. The absorptive function of the large intestine focuses mainly on water reabsorption. A number of substances require a specific carrier or transport system. For example, vitamin B$_{12}$ is not absorbed in the absence of intrinsic factor, which is secreted by the parietal cells of the stomach. Transport of amino acids and glucose occurs mainly in the presence of sodium. Water is absorbed passively along an osmotic gradient.

The distinguishing characteristic of the small intestine is its large surface area, which in the adult is estimated to be approximately 250 m^2. Anatomic features that contribute to this enlarged surface area are the circular folds that extend into the lumen of the intestine and the villi, which are finger-like projections of mucous membrane, numbering as many as 25,000, that line the entire small intestine (Fig. 36-11). Each villus is equipped with an artery, vein, and lymph vessel (*i.e.,* lacteal), which bring blood to the surface of the intestine and transport the nutrients and other materials that have passed into the blood from the lumen of the intestine (Fig. 36-12). Fats rely largely on the lymphatics for absorption.

Each villus is covered with cells called *enterocytes* that contribute to the absorptive and digestive functions of the small bowel, and goblet cells that provide mucus. The crypts of Lieberkühn are glandular structures that open into the spaces between the villi. The enterocytes have a life span of approximately 4 to 5 days, and it is believed that replacement cells differentiate from progenitor cells located in the area of the crypts. The maturing enterocytes migrate up the villus and eventually are extruded from the tip.

The enterocytes secrete enzymes that aid in the digestion of carbohydrates and proteins. These enzymes are called *brush border enzymes* because they adhere to the border of the villus structures. In this way they have access to the carbohydrates and protein molecules as they come in contact with the absorptive surface of the intestine. This mechanism of secre-

tion places the enzymes where they are needed and eliminates the need to produce enough enzymes to mix with the entire contents filling the lumen of the small bowel. The digested molecules diffuse through the membrane or are actively transported across the mucosal surface to enter the blood or, in the case of fatty acids, the lacteal. These molecules are then transported through the portal vein or lymphatics into the systemic circulation.

Carbohydrate Absorption

Carbohydrates must be broken down into monosaccharides, or single sugars, before they can be absorbed from the small intestine. The average daily intake of carbohydrate in the American diet is approximately 350 to 400 g. Starch makes up approximately 50% of this total, sucrose (*i.e.,* table sugar) approximately

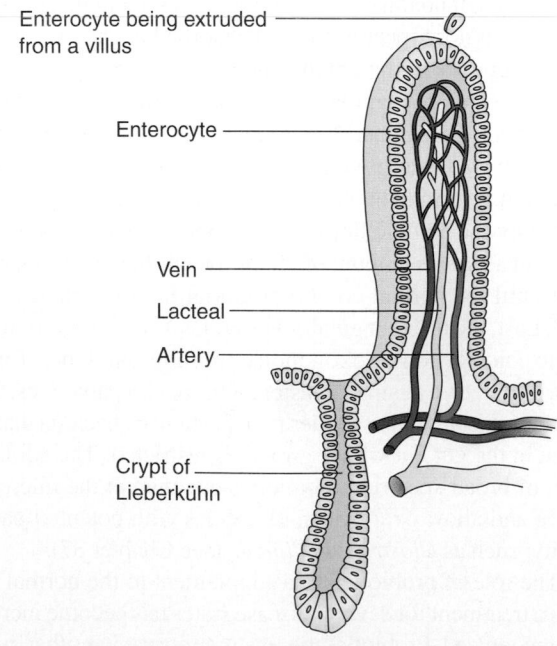

FIGURE 36-12 • A single villus from the small intestine.

TABLE 36-3 Enzymes Used in Digestion of Carbohydrates		
DIETARY CARBOHYDRATES	**ENZYME**	**MONOSACCHARIDES PRODUCED**
Lactose	Lactase	Glucose and galactose
Sucrose	Sucrase	Fructose and glucose
Starch	Amylase	Maltose, maltotriose, and α-dextrins
Maltose and maltotriose	Maltase	Glucose and glucose
α-Dextrins	α-Dextrinase	Glucose and glucose

30%, lactose (*i.e.,* milk sugar) approximately 6%, and maltose approximately 1.5%.

Digestion of starch begins in the mouth with the action of amylase. Pancreatic secretions also contain an amylase. Amylase breaks down starch into several disaccharides, including maltose, isomaltose, and α-dextrins. The brush border enzymes convert the disaccharides into monosaccharides that can be absorbed (Table 36-3). Sucrose yields glucose and fructose, lactose is converted to glucose and galactose, and maltose is converted to two glucose molecules. When the disaccharides are not broken down to monosaccharides, they cannot be absorbed but remain as osmotically active particles in the contents of the digestive system, causing diarrhea. Persons with a deficiency of lactase, the enzyme that breaks down lactose, experience diarrhea when they drink milk or eat dairy products.

Fructose is transported across the intestinal mucosa by facilitated diffusion, which does not require energy expenditure. Glucose and galactose move from the intestinal lumen into the intestinal cells by way of a sodium-glucose cotransporter (SGLT-1), against a chemical gradient. The energy for this step does not come directly from adenosine triphosphate (ATP), but from the sodium gradient created by the Na+/K+-ATPase pump located on the basolateral side of the membrane (Fig. 36-13). Glucose and galactose are transported from the cell into the blood across the basolateral membrane by facilitated diffusion using a glucose transporter-2 (GLUT-2) protein. Water absorption from the intestine is linked to absorption of osmotically active particles, such as glucose and sodium. It follows that an important consideration in facilitating the transport of water across the intestine (and decreasing diarrhea) after temporary disruption in bowel function is to include sodium and glucose in the fluids that are consumed.

Fat Absorption

The average adult eats approximately 60 to 100 g of fat daily, principally as triglycerides. The first step in digestion of lipids is to break the large globules of dietary fat into smaller sizes so that water-soluble digestive enzymes can act on the surface molecules. This process, which is called *emulsification,* begins in the stomach with agitation of the globules and continues in the duodenum under the influence of bile from the liver (Fig. 13-14). Emulsification greatly increases the number of triglyceride molecules exposed to pancreatic lipase, which splits

triglycerides into free fatty acids and monoglycerides. Bile salts play an additional role by forming micelles that transport these substances to the surface of the intestinal villi, where they are taken into the epithelial cells and used to form new triglycerides. These new triglycerides are then released into the lymphatic system as chylomicrons. Small quantities of short- and medium-chain fatty acids are absorbed directly into the portal blood rather than being converted into triglycerides and absorbed by way of the lymphatics.

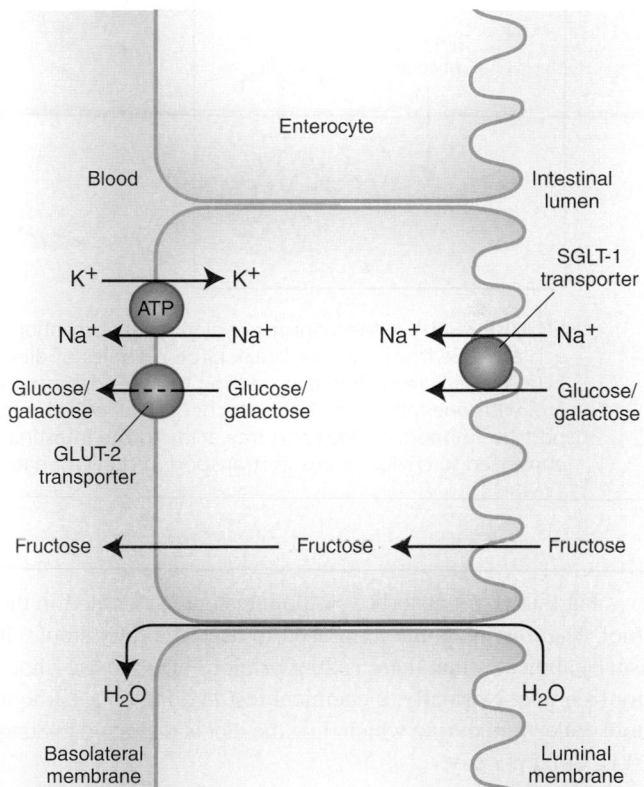

FIGURE 36-13 • Intestinal transport of glucose, galactose, and fructose. Glucose and galactose are transported across the apical membrane by the sodium-glucose cotransporter (SGLT-1). Glucose moves out of the intestinal cell and into the blood using a glucose transporter-2 (GLUT-2) protein. Sodium is transported out of the cell by the Na+/K+ ATPase sodium pump. This creates the gradient needed to operate the transport system. Fructose is passively transported across the apical and basolateral membranes of the intestinal cell.

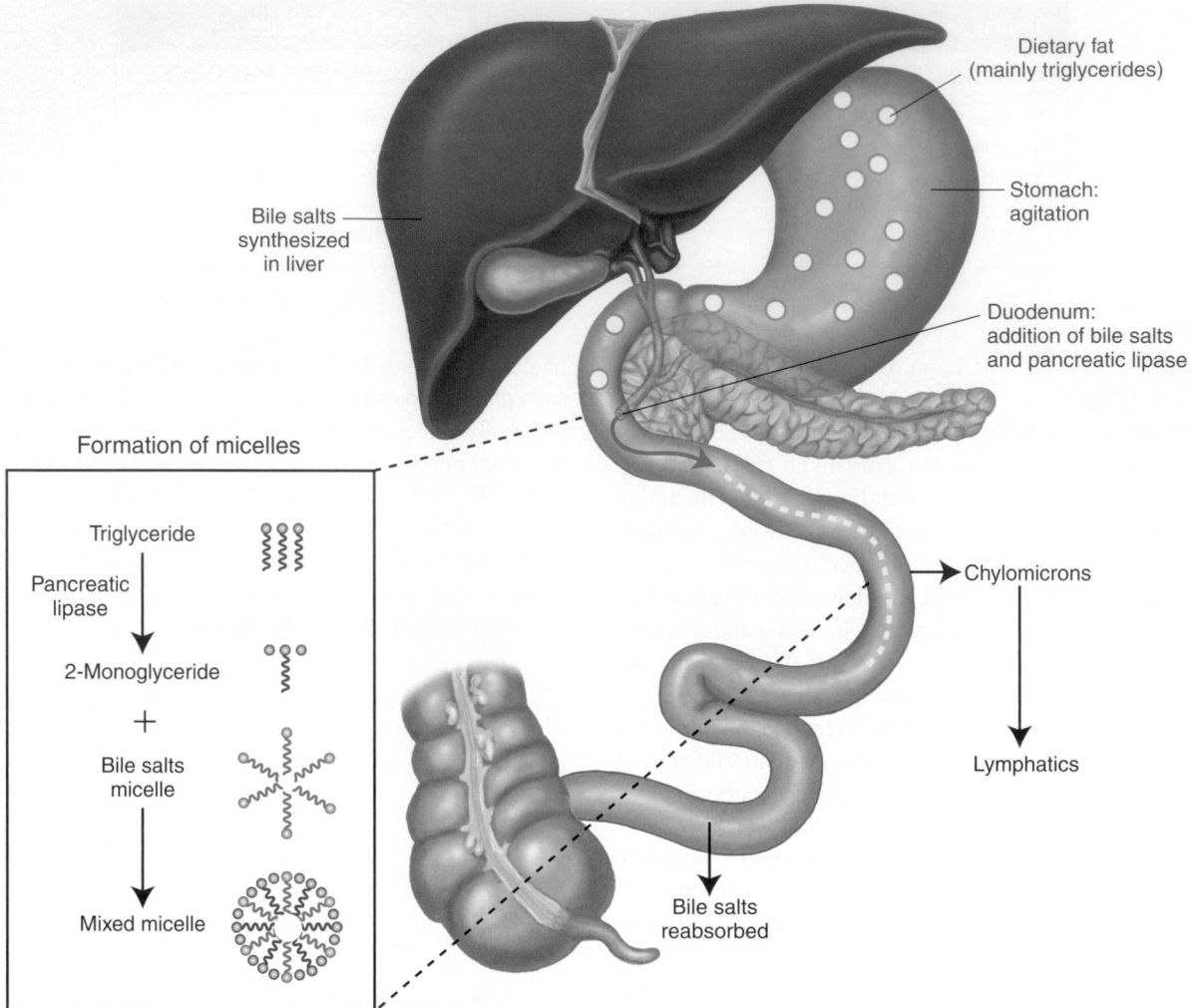

FIGURE 36-14 • Mechanisms of dietary fat absorption. During digestion, agitation in the stomach and bile from the liver break large globules of dietary fat into small sizes that facilitate the action of pancreatic lipase in splitting triglycerides into free fatty acids and monoglycerides (glycerol with one fatty acid chain attached). Bile salts also facilitate formation of micelles that transport the monoglycerides and free acids to the intestinal mucosa, where they are absorbed and converted to chylomicrons for transport in the lymphatic channels.

Fat that is not absorbed in the intestine is excreted in the stool. *Steatorrhea* is the term used to describe fatty stools. It usually indicates that there is 20 g or more of fat in a 24-hour stool sample. Normally, a chemical test is done on a 72-hour stool collection, during which time the diet is restricted to 80 to 100 g of fat per day.

Protein Absorption

Protein digestion begins in the stomach with the action of pepsin. Pepsinogen, the enzyme precursor of pepsin, is secreted by the chief cells in response to a meal and acid pH. Acid in the stomach is required for the conversion of pepsinogen to pepsin. Pepsin is inactivated when it enters the intestine by the alkaline pH.

Proteins are broken down further by pancreatic enzymes, such as trypsin, chymotrypsin, carboxypeptidase, and elastase. As with pepsin, the pancreatic enzymes are secreted as precursor molecules. Trypsinogen, which lacks enzymatic activity, is activated by an enzyme located on the brush border cells of the duodenal enterocytes. Activated trypsin activates additional trypsinogen molecules and other pancreatic precursor proteolytic enzymes. The amino acids are then liberated on the surface of the mucosal surface of the intestine by brush border enzymes that degrade proteins into peptides that are one, two, or three amino acids long. Similar to glucose, many amino acids are transported across the mucosal membrane in a sodium-linked process that uses ATP as an energy source. Some amino acids are absorbed by facilitated diffusion processes that do not require sodium.

IN SUMMARY, the digestion and absorption of foodstuffs take place mainly in the small intestine. Digestion is the process of dismantling foods into their constituent parts. Digestion requires hydrolysis, enzyme cleavage, and fat emulsification. Proteins, fats, carbohydrates, and other components of the diet are broken down into molecules that can be transported from the intestinal lumen into the body fluids. Absorption is the process of moving nutrients and other materials from the external environment of the GI tract into the internal environment. Brush border enzymes break carbohydrates into monosaccharides that can be transported across the intestine into the bloodstream. The digestion of proteins begins in the stomach with the action of pepsin and is further facilitated in the intestine by the pancreatic enzymes, such as trypsin, chymotrypsin, carboxypeptidase, and elastase. Enzymes that break down proteins are released as proenzymes that are activated in the GI tract. The absorption of glucose and amino acids is facilitated by a sodium-dependent transport system. Fat in the diet is broken down by pancreatic lipase into triglycerides containing medium- and long-chain fatty acids. Bile salts form micelles that transport these substances to the surface of intestinal villi, where they are absorbed. ■

CONCEPTSin action**ANIMATI**●**N**

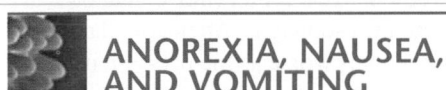

ANOREXIA, NAUSEA, AND VOMITING

After completing this section of the chapter, you should be able to meet the following objectives:

- Characterize the relationship among anorexia, nausea, retching, and vomiting.
- Describe the neural structures involved in vomiting and their mediators.

Anorexia, nausea, and vomiting are physiologic responses that are common to many GI disorders. These responses are protective to the extent that they signal the presence of disease and, in the case of vomiting, remove noxious agents from the GI tract. They also can contribute to impaired intake or loss of fluids and nutrients.

Anorexia

Anorexia represents a loss of appetite. Several factors influence appetite. One is hunger, which is stimulated by contractions of the empty stomach. Appetite or the desire for food intake is regulated by the hypothalamus and other associated centers in the brain. Smell plays an important role, as evidenced by the fact that appetite can be stimulated or suppressed by the smell of food. Loss of appetite is associated with emotional factors, such as fear, depression, frustration, and anxiety. Many drugs and disease states cause anorexia. For example, in uremia the accumulation of nitrogenous wastes in the blood contributes to the development of anorexia. Anorexia often is a forerunner of nausea, and most conditions that cause nausea and vomiting also produce anorexia.

Nausea

Nausea is an ill-defined and unpleasant subjective sensation. It is the conscious sensation resulting from stimulation of the medullary vomiting center that often precedes or accompanies vomiting. Nausea usually is preceded by anorexia, and stimuli such as foods and drugs that cause anorexia in small doses usually produce nausea when given in larger doses. A common cause of nausea is distention of the duodenum or upper small intestinal tract. Nausea frequently is accompanied by autonomic nervous system manifestations such as watery salivation and vasoconstriction with pallor, sweating, and tachycardia. Nausea may function as an early warning signal of a pathologic process.

Retching and Vomiting

Retching consists of the rhythmic spasmodic movements of the diaphragm, chest wall, and abdominal muscles. It usually precedes or alternates with periods of vomiting. Vomiting or emesis is the sudden and forceful oral expulsion of the contents of the stomach. It usually is preceded by nausea. The contents that are vomited are called *vomitus*. Vomiting, as a basic physiologic protective mechanism, limits the possibility of damage from ingested noxious agents by emptying the contents of the stomach and portions of the small intestine. Nausea and vomiting may represent a total-body response to drug therapy, including overdose, cumulative effects, toxicity, and side effects.

Vomiting involves two functionally distinct medullary centers: the *vomiting center* and the *chemoreceptor trigger zone*. The act of vomiting is thought to be a reflex that is integrated in the vomiting center, which is located in the dorsal portion of the reticular formation of the medulla near the sensory nuclei of the vagus (Fig. 36-15). The chemoreceptor trigger zone is located in a small area on the floor of the fourth ventricle, where it is exposed to both blood and cerebrospinal fluid. It is thought to mediate the emetic effects of blood-borne drugs and toxins.

The act of vomiting consists of taking a deep breath, closing the airways, and producing a strong, forceful contraction of the diaphragm and abdominal muscles along with relaxation of the gastroesophageal sphincter. Respiration ceases during the act of vomiting. Vomiting may be accompanied by dizziness, lightheadedness, a decrease in blood pressure, and bradycardia.

The vomiting center receives input from the GI tract and other organs; from the cerebral cortex; from the vestibular apparatus, which is responsible for motion sickness; and from the chemoreceptor trigger zone, which is activated by many drugs and endogenous and exogenous toxins (see Fig. 36-15). Hypoxia exerts a direct effect on the vomiting center, producing nausea and vomiting. This direct effect probably accounts for the

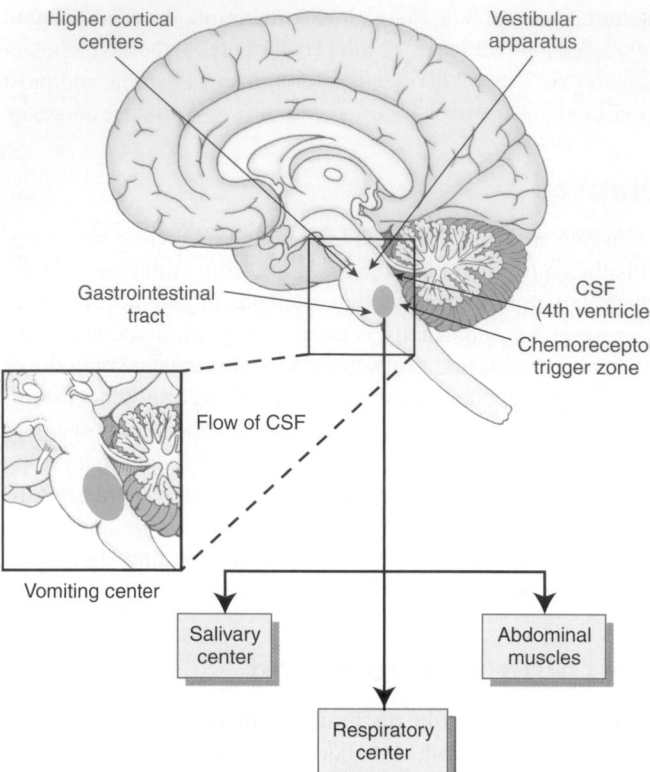

Higher cortical centers

Vestibular apparatus

Gastrointestinal tract

CSF (4th ventricle)

Chemoreceptor trigger zone

Flow of CSF

Vomiting center

Salivary center

Abdominal muscles

Respiratory center

FIGURE 36-15 • Physiologic events involved in vomiting. CSF, cerebrospinal fluid.

vomiting that occurs during periods of decreased cardiac output, shock, environmental hypoxia, and brain ischemia caused by increased intracranial pressure. Inflammation of any of the intra-abdominal organs, including the liver, gallbladder, or urinary tract, can cause vomiting because of the stimulation of the visceral afferent pathways that communicate with the vomiting center. Distention or irritation of the GI tract also causes vomiting through the stimulation of visceral afferent neurons.

Several neurotransmitters and receptor subtypes are implicated as neuromediators in nausea and vomiting. Dopamine, serotonin, and opioid receptors are found in the GI tract and in the vomiting center and chemoreceptor trigger zone. Dopamine antagonists, such as prochlorperazine, depress vomiting caused by stimulation of the chemoreceptor trigger zone. Serotonin is believed to be involved in the nausea and emesis associated with cancer chemotherapy and radiation therapy. Serotonin antagonists (e.g., granisetron, ondansetron) are effective in treating the nausea and vomiting associated with these stimuli. Motion sickness appears to be a CNS response to vestibular stimuli. Norepinephrine and acetylcholine receptors are located in the vestibular center. The acetylcholine receptors are thought to mediate the impulses responsible for exciting the vomiting center; norepinephrine receptors may have a stabilizing influence that resists motion sickness. Many of the motion sickness drugs (e.g., dimenhydrinate) have a strong CNS anticholinergic effect and act on the receptors in the vomiting center and areas related to the vestibular system.

IN SUMMARY, the signs and symptoms of many GI tract disorders are manifested by anorexia, nausea, and vomiting. Anorexia, or loss of appetite, may occur alone or may accompany nausea and vomiting. Nausea, which is an ill-defined, unpleasant sensation, signals the stimulation of the medullary vomiting center. It often precedes vomiting and frequently is accompanied by autonomic responses, such as salivation and vasoconstriction with pallor, sweating, and tachycardia. The act of vomiting, which is integrated by the vomiting center, involves the forceful oral expulsion of the gastric contents. It is a basic physiologic mechanism that rids the GI tract of noxious agents. ■

Review Exercises

1. Persons receiving chemotherapeutic agents, which interfere with mitosis of cancer cells as well as the cells of other rapidly proliferating tissues in the body, often experience disorders such as ulcerations in the mucosal tissues of the mouth and other parts of the GI tract. These disorders are resolved once the chemotherapy treatment has been completed.
   A. Explain.

2. People with gastroesophageal reflux (movement of gastric contents into the esophagus) often complain of heartburn that becomes worse as the pressure in the stomach increases.
   A. Use information on hormonal control of gastric emptying to explain why eating a meal that is high in fat content often exaggerates the problem.

3. Infections of the GI tract, such as the "GI flu," often cause profound diarrhea.
   A. Describe the neural mechanisms involved in the increase in GI motility that produces the diarrhea.
   B. Explain the rationale for using a "drink" that contains both glucose and sodium to treat the fluid deficit that often occurs with diarrhea.

4. Explain the physiologic mechanisms associated with the occurrence of diarrhea in persons with:
   A. Lactase deficiency.
   B. Obstruction of bile flow into the intestine.
   C. Disruption of the normal intestinal flora due to antibiotic therapy.

5. Anticholinergic drugs are often effective in treating the nausea and vomiting that accompany motion sickness but are relatively ineffective in treating the nausea and vomiting associated with chemotherapy agents used in the treatment of cancer.
   A. Explain.

Bibliography

Berne R. M., Levy M. N., Koeppen B. M., et al. (Eds.). (2004). *Physiology* (5th ed., pp. 539–620). St. Louis: Mosby.

Brubaker P. L., Drucker D. J. (2004). Minireview: Glucagon-like peptides regulate cell proliferation and apoptosis in the pancreas, gut, and central nervous system. *Endocrinology* 145, 2653–2659.

Costanzo L. S. (2002). *Physiology* (2nd ed., pp. 300–346). Philadelphia: W. B. Saunders.

Gershon M. D. (1999). The enteric nervous system: A second brain. *Hospital Practice* 34(7), 31–52.

Grelot L., Miller A. D. (1994). Vomiting: Its ins and outs. *News in Physiological Sciences* 9, 142–147.

Guarner F., Malagelada J.-R. (2003). Gut flora in health and disease. *Lancet* 361, 512–519.

Guyton A. C., Hall J. E. (2006). *Textbook of medical physiology* (11th ed., pp. 771–824). Philadelphia: Elsevier Saunders.

Inul A., Asakawa A., Bowers C. Y., et al. (2004). Ghrelin, appetite, and gastric motility: The emerging role of the stomach as an endocrine organ. *FASEB Journal* 18, 439–456.

Johnson L. R. (2001). *Gastrointestinal physiology* (6th ed.). St. Louis: C. V. Mosby.

Kellert G. L., Brot-Larche E. (2005). A major pathway for intestinal sugar absorption. *Diabetes* 54, 3056–3062.

Lindley C. (2005). Nausea and vomiting. In Koda-Kimble M. A., Young L. Y., Kradian W. A., et al. (Eds.), *Applied therapeutics: The clinical use of drugs* (8th ed., pp. 8-1–8-18). Philadelphia: Lippincott Williams & Wilkins.

Moore K. L., Dalley A. F. (2005). *Clinically oriented anatomy* (5th ed., pp. 231–305). Philadelphia: Lippincott Williams & Wilkins.

Moran T. H., Kinzig K. P. (2004). Gastrointestinal satiety signals: II. Cholecystokinin. *American Journal of Physiology: Gastrointestinal and Liver Physiology* 286, G183–G188.

Rhoades R. A., Tanner G. A. (2003). *Medical physiology* (2nd ed., pp. 449–511). Boston: Little, Brown.

Salehi M., D'Allessio D. (2006). New therapies for type 2 diabetes based on glucagon-like peptide 1. *Cleveland Clinic Journal of Medicine* 73, 382–389.

Sanders K. M., Koh S. D., Ward M. (2006). Interstitial cells of Cajal in the gastrointestinal tract. *Annual Review of Physiology* 68, 307–343.

Schiller L. R. (1994). Peristalsis. *Scientific American Science & Medicine* (November/December), 38–47.

Soybel D. I. (2005). Anatomy and physiology of the stomach. *Surgical Clinics of North America* 85, 875–894.

St.-Pierre D. H., Tache Y. (2003). Ghrelin: A novel player in the gut-brain regulation of growth hormone and energy balance. *News in Physiological Sciences* 18, 242–246.

Varga G., Ba'lint A., Burghardt B., et al. (2004). Involvement of endogenous CCK and CCK$_1$ receptors in colonic motor function. *British Journal of Pharmacology* 141, 1275–1284.

Ward S. M., Sanders K. M. (2001). Physiology and pathophysiology of the interstitial cells of Cajal: From bench to bedside. *American Journal of Physiology: Gastrointestinal and Liver Physiology* 281, G602–G611.

Wolfe M. M., Soll A. H. (1988). The physiology of gastric acid secretion. *New England Journal of Medicine* 319, 1707–1715.

Visit the Point. **http://thePoint.lww.com for animations, journal articles, and more!**

Chapter 37

Disorders of Gastrointestinal Function

CAROL M. PORTH

➤ Gastrointestinal disorders are not cited as the leading cause of death in the United States, nor do they receive the same publicity as heart disease and cancer. However, according to government reports, digestive diseases rank third in the total economic burden of illness, resulting in considerable human suffering, personal expenditures for treatment, and lost working hours, as well as a drain on the nation's economy. It has been estimated that 60 to 70 million people in the United States have a digestive disease and more than 6 million hospitalizations (14% of total) are for digestive disorders.[1] Even more important is the fact that proper nutrition or a change in health practices could prevent or minimize many of these disorders.

Disruption in structure and function can occur at any level of the gastrointestinal tract, from the esophagus to the colon and rectum. This chapter is divided into three sections: (1) disorders of the esophagus, (2) disorders of the stomach, and (3) disorders of the small and large intestines. Disorders of the hepatobiliary system and exocrine pancreas are discussed in Chapter 38.

DISORDERS OF THE ESOPHAGUS

After completing this section of the chapter, you should be able to meet the following objectives:

- Define and cite the causes of dysphagia, odynophagia, and achalasia.
- Relate the pathophysiology of gastroesophageal reflux to measures used in the diagnosis and treatment of the disorder in adults and children.
- State the reason for the poor prognosis associated with esophageal cancer.

The esophagus is a tube that connects the oropharynx with the stomach. It lies posterior to the trachea and larynx and extends through the mediastinum, intersecting the diaphragm at the level of the 11th thoracic vertebra.

The esophagus functions primarily as a conduit for passage of food and liquid from the pharynx to the stomach. The walls of the esophagus consist of a mucosal, submucosal, muscularis externa, and adventitial layer, reflecting the general structural organization of the gastrointestinal tract. The inner mucosal layer contains nonkeratinized stratified epithelium. At the esophageal–stomach junction, the abrasion-resistant epithelium changes abruptly to the simple columnar epithelium of the stomach. The submucosal layer contains mucus-secreting glands that provide the mucin-containing fluids that lubricate the esophageal wall and aid in the passage of food. The muscularis externa layer consists of skeletal muscle in the superior third of the esophagus, a mixture of skeletal and smooth muscle in its middle third, and entirely smooth muscle in its lower third. The outer fibrous adventitial layer of the esophagus is composed entirely of connective tissue, which blends with surrounding structures along its route.

There are sphincters at either end of the esophagus: an upper esophageal sphincter and a lower esophageal sphincter. The upper esophageal, or pharyngoesophageal, sphincter consists of a circular layer of striated muscle, the cricopharyngeal muscle. The lower esophageal, or gastroesophageal, sphincter is an area approximately 3 cm above the junction with the stomach. The gastroesophageal sphincter is a physiologic rather than a true anatomic sphincter. That is, it acts as a valve, but the only structural evidence of a sphincter is a slight thickening of the circular smooth muscle. The smooth muscle in this portion of the esophagus normally remains tonically constricted, creating an intraluminal pressure of about 30 mm Hg, in contrast to the mid-portion of the esophagus, which normally remains relaxed.[2] The lower esophageal sphincter passes through an opening, or *hiatus,* in the diaphragm as it joins with the stomach, which is located in the abdomen. The portion of the diaphragm that surrounds the lower esophageal sphincter helps to maintain the zone of high pressure needed to prevent reflux of stomach contents.

 ## Congenital Anomalies

Congenital anomalies of the esophagus require early detection and correction because they are incompatible with life. Esophageal atresia (EA) and tracheoesophageal fistula (TEF) are the two most common congenital anomalies of the esophagus.[3,4] EA, which is the most common congenital anomaly, affects about 1 in 4000 neonates.[3] Of these, more than 90% have an associated TEF. In the most common form of EA, the upper esophagus ends in a blind pouch and the TEF is connected to the trachea (Fig. 37-1). This defect now has a survival rate greater than 90% owing largely to early recognition and improved neonatal intensive care units. Infants weighing less than 1500 g have the greatest risk for mortality, as do neonates with other congenital anomalies.[3]

The newborn infant with EA/TEF typically has frothing and bubbling at the mouth and nose and episodes of coughing, cyanosis, and respiratory distress. Feeding exacerbates these manifestations, causes regurgitation, and precipitates aspiration. The inability to pass a catheter into the stomach provides

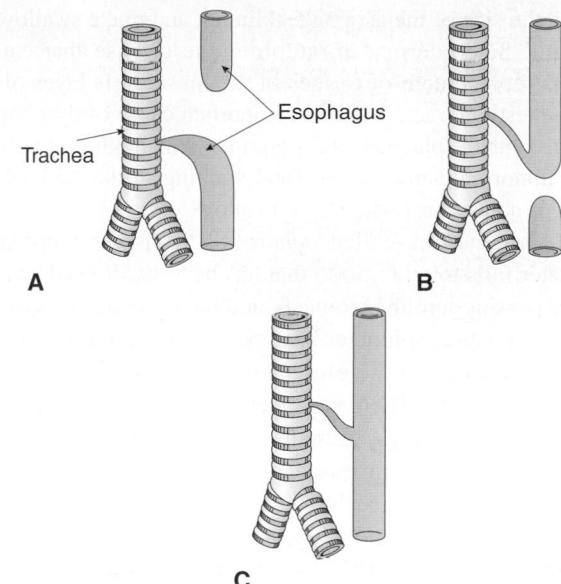

FIGURE 37-1 • Congenital tracheoesophageal fistulas. **(A)** The most common type is a communication between the trachea and the lower portion of the esophagus. The upper segment of the esophagus ends in a blind sac. **(B)** In a few cases, the proximal esophagus communicates with the trachea. **(C)** The least common anomaly, the H type, is a fistula between a continuous esophagus and the trachea. (From Mitos F. A., Rubin E. [2008]. The gastrointestinal tract. In Rubin R., Strayer D. S. [Eds.], *Rubin's pathophysiology: Clinicopathologic foundations of medicine* [5th ed., p. 551]. Philadelphia: Lippincott Williams & Wilkins.)

further evidence of the disorder. The infant with isolated TEF may develop respiratory symptoms at a later age.

Treatment of EA and TEF is surgical. Surgical ligation of the TEF and end-to-end anastomosis of the esophagus is performed when possible. Temporary ligation of the TEF and insertion of a gastrostomy tube may be used to delay the need for primary closure in preterm infants and those with more complicated lesions. The main goal of preoperative management is to maintain the airway and prevent lung damage from aspiration of gastric contents. Prone positioning minimizes movement of gastric secretions into a distal fistula and esophageal suctioning minimizes the risk of aspiration from a blind pouch.

Dysphagia

The act of swallowing depends on the coordinated action of the tongue and pharynx. These structures are innervated by cranial nerves V, IX, X, and XII. *Dysphagia* refers to difficulty in swallowing. If swallowing is painful, it is referred to as *odynophagia.* Dysphagia can result from disorders that produce narrowing of the esophagus, lack of salivary secretion, weakness of the muscular structures that propel the food bolus, or disruption of the neural networks coordinating the swallowing mechanism.[5] Lesions of the central nervous system (CNS), such as a stroke, often involve the cranial nerves that control swallowing. Cancer of the esophagus and strictures resulting from scarring can reduce the size of the esophageal lumen and make swallowing difficult. Scleroderma, an autoimmune disease that causes fibrous replacement of tissues in the muscularis layer of the gastrointestinal tract, is another important cause of dysphagia.[6] Persons with dysphagia usually complain of choking, coughing, or an abnormal sensation of food sticking in the back of the throat or upper chest when they swallow.

In a condition called *achalasia,* the lower esophageal sphincter fails to relax; food that has been swallowed has difficulty passing into the stomach, and the esophagus above the lower esophageal sphincter becomes enlarged. One or several meals may lodge in the esophagus and pass slowly into the stomach over time. There is danger of aspiration of esophageal contents into the lungs when the person lies down.

Endoscopy, barium esophagoscopy, and videoradiography may be used to determine the site and extent of a swallowing disorder. Esophageal manometry, a procedure in which a small pressure-sensing catheter is inserted into the esophagus, may be done to measure pressures in different parts of the esophagus. Treatment of swallowing disorders depends on the cause and type of altered function that is present. Treatment of dysphagia often involves a multidisciplinary team of health professionals, including a speech therapist. Mechanical dilation or surgical procedures may be done to enlarge the lower esophageal sphincter in persons with esophageal strictures.

Esophageal Diverticulum

A diverticulum of the esophagus is an outpouching of the esophageal wall caused by a weakness of the muscularis layer.[7,8] An esophageal diverticulum tends to retain food. Complaints that the food stops before it reaches the stomach are common, as are reports of gurgling, belching, coughing, and foul-smelling breath. The trapped food may cause esophagitis and ulceration. Because the condition usually is progressive, correction of the defect requires surgical intervention.

Tears (Mallory-Weiss Syndrome)

Longitudinal tears in the esophagus at the esophagogastric junction are termed *Mallory-Weiss tears.*[5,6] They are most often encountered in persons with chronic alcoholism after a bout of severe retching or vomiting, but may also occur during acute illness with severe vomiting. The presumed pathogenesis is inadequate relaxation of the esophageal sphincter during vomiting, with stretching and tearing of the esophageal junction at the moment of propulsive expulsion of gastric contents. Tears may involve only the mucosa or may penetrate the wall of the esophagus. Infection may lead to inflammatory ulcer or mediastinitis.

Esophageal lacerations account for 5% to 10% of all upper gastrointestinal bleeding episodes.[5] Most often bleeding is not severe and does require surgical intervention. Severe bleeding usually responds to vasoconstrictive medications, transfusions,

and balloon compression. Healing is usually prompt, with minimal or no residual effects.

Hiatal Hernia

Hiatal hernia is characterized by a protrusion or herniation of the stomach through the esophageal hiatus of the diaphragm. There are two anatomic patterns of hiatal herniation: axial, or sliding, and nonaxial, or paraesophageal.[7,8] The sliding hiatal hernia, which constitutes 95% of cases, is characterized by a bell-shaped protrusion of the stomach above the diaphragm[7] (Fig. 37-2). Small sliding hiatal hernias are common and considered to be of no significance in asymptomatic people. However, in cases of severe erosive esophagitis where gastroesophageal reflux and a large hiatal hernia coexist, the hernia may retard esophageal acid clearance and contribute to the more severe esophagitis, especially Barrett esophagus (to be discussed). In paraesophageal hiatal hernias, a separate portion of the stomach, usually along the greater portion of the stomach, enters the thorax through a widened opening. The hernia progressively enlarges, and increases in size. In extreme cases, most of the stomach herniates

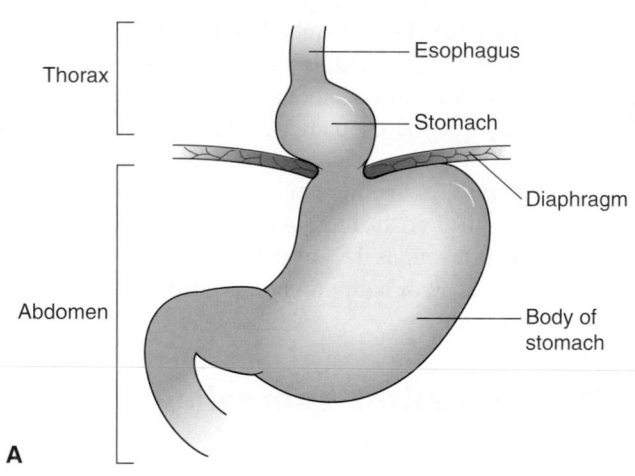

A

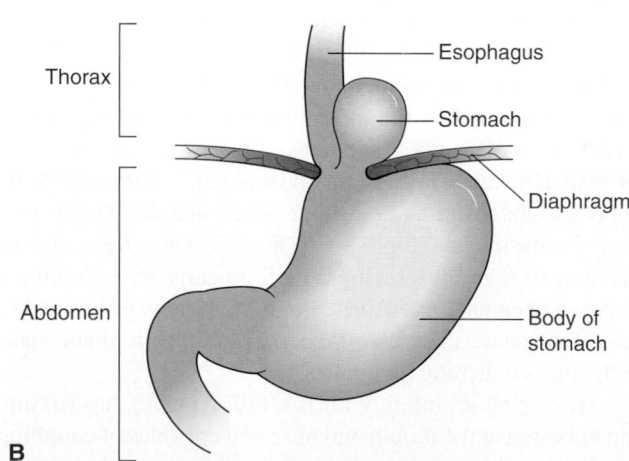

B

FIGURE 37-2 • Hiatal hernia. **(A)** Sliding hiatal hernia. **(B)** Paraesophageal hiatal hernia.

into the thorax. Large paraesophageal hiatal hernias may require surgical treatment.

Gastroesophageal Reflux

The term *reflux* refers to backward or return movement. In the context of gastroesophageal reflux, it refers to the backward movement of gastric contents into the esophagus, a condition that causes heartburn or pyrosis.[9] It probably is the most common disorder originating in the gastrointestinal tract. Most persons experience heartburn occasionally as a result of reflux. Such symptoms usually occur soon after eating, are short lived, and seldom cause more serious problems.

The lower esophageal sphincter regulates the flow of food from the esophagus into the stomach. Both internal and external mechanisms function in maintaining the antireflux function of the lower esophageal sphincter.[9,10] The circular muscles of the distal esophagus constitute the internal mechanisms, and the portion of the diaphragm that surrounds the esophagus constitutes the external mechanism. The oblique muscles of the stomach, located below the lower esophageal sphincter, form a flap that contributes to the antireflux function of the internal sphincter.[7] Relaxation of the lower esophageal sphincter is a brain stem reflex that is mediated by the vagus nerve in response to a number of afferent stimuli. Transient relaxation with reflux is common after meals. Gastric distention and meals high in fat increase the frequency of relaxation. Normally, refluxed material is returned to the stomach by secondary peristaltic waves in the esophagus and swallowed saliva neutralizes and washes away the refluxed acid.

Gastroesophageal Reflux Disease

The persistent reflux of gastric contents into the esophagus is referred to as *gastroesophageal reflux disease* (GERD). It is thought to be associated with a weak or incompetent lower esophageal sphincter that allows reflux to occur, the irritant effects of the refluxate, and decreased clearance of the refluxed acid from the esophagus after it has occurred[9,11–13] (Fig. 37-3). In most cases, reflux occurs during transient relaxation of the esophagus. Delayed gastric emptying also may contribute to reflux by increasing gastric volume and pressure with greater chance for reflux. Esophageal mucosal injury is related to the destructive nature of the refluxate and the amount of time it is in contact with mucosa. Acidic gastric fluids (pH <4.0) are particularly damaging. The gastroesophageal reflux normally is cleared and neutralized by esophageal peristalsis and salivary bicarbonate. Decreased salivation and salivary buffering capacity may contribute to impaired clearing of acid reflux from the esophagus.

Clinical Features. The most frequent symptom of GERD is heartburn. It frequently is severe, occurring 30 to 60 minutes after eating. It often is made worse by bending at the waist and recumbency and usually is relieved by sitting upright. The sever-

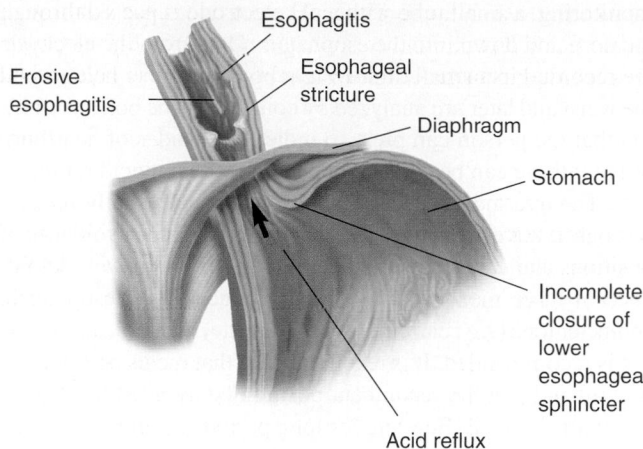

FIGURE 37-3 • Gastroesophageal junction and site of gastroesophageal reflux. (From Anatomical Chart Company. [2004]. *Atlas of pathophysiology* [p. 171]. Springhouse, PA: Springhouse.)

ity of heartburn is not indicative of the extent of mucosal injury; only a small percentage of people who complain of heartburn have mucosal injury. Often, the heartburn occurs during the night. Antacids give prompt, although transient relief. Other symptoms include belching and chest pain. The pain usually is located in the epigastric or retrosternal area and often radiates to the throat, shoulder, or back. Because of its location, the pain may be confused with angina. The reflux of gastric contents also may produce respiratory symptoms such as wheezing, chronic cough, and hoarseness.[14] There is considerable evidence linking gastroesophageal reflux with bronchial asthma.[15] The proposed mechanisms of reflux-associated asthma and chronic cough include microaspiration and macroaspiration, laryngeal injury, and vagal-mediated bronchospasm.

Reflux esophagitis involves mucosal injury to the esophagus, hyperemia, and inflammation. Complications can result from persistent reflux, which produces a cycle of mucosal damage that causes hyperemia, edema, and erosion of the luminal surface. These complications include strictures and a condition called *Barrett esophagus*.[12,16] Strictures are caused by a combination of scar tissue, spasm, and edema. They produce narrowing of the esophagus and cause dysphagia when the lumen becomes sufficiently constricted. Barrett esophagus is characterized by a reparative process in which the squamous mucosa that normally lines the esophagus gradually is replaced by columnar epithelium resembling that in the stomach or intestines.[7,8,16] It is associated with increased risk for development of esophageal cancer.

Diagnosis of gastroesophageal reflux depends on a history of reflux symptomatology and selective use of diagnostic methods, including radiographic studies using a contrast medium such as barium, esophagoscopy, and ambulatory esophageal pH monitoring.[13,17] Esophagoscopy involves the passage of a flexible fiberoptic endoscope into the esophagus for the purpose of visualizing the lumen of the upper gastrointestinal tract. It also permits performance of a biopsy, if indicated. For 24-hour pH monitoring, a small tube with a pH electrode is passed through the nose and down into the esophagus. Data from the electrode are recorded in a small, lightweight box worn on a belt around the waist and later are analyzed by computer. The box has a button that the person can press to indicate episodes of heartburn or pain; these can be correlated with episodes of acid reflux.

The treatment of gastroesophageal reflux usually focuses on conservative measures. These measures include avoidance of positions and conditions that increase gastric reflux.[13,17] Avoidance of large meals and foods that reduce lower esophageal sphincter tone (e.g., caffeine, fats, chocolate), alcohol, and smoking is recommended. It is recommended that meals be eaten sitting up and that the recumbent position be avoided for several hours after a meal. Bending for long periods should be avoided because it tends to increase intra-abdominal pressure and cause gastric reflux. Sleeping with the head elevated helps to prevent reflux during the night. This is best accomplished by placing blocks under the head of the bed or by using a wedge-shaped bolster to elevate the head and shoulders by at least 6 inches. Weight loss usually is recommended in overweight people.

Antacids or a combination of antacids and alginic acid also are recommended for mild disease. Alginic acid produces a foam when it comes in contact with gastric acid; if reflux occurs, the foam rather than acid rises into the esophagus. Histamine-2 receptor (H_2)–blocking antagonists, which inhibit gastric acid production, often are recommended when additional treatment is needed.[12] The proton pump inhibitors act by inhibiting the gastric proton pump, which regulates the final pathway for acid secretion (see Fig. 36-10, Chapter 36). These agents may be used for persons who continue to have daytime symptoms, recurrent strictures, or large esophageal ulcerations. Surgical treatment may be indicated in some people.

Gastroesophageal Reflux in Children

Gastroesophageal reflux is a common problem in infants and children. The small reservoir capacity of an infant's stomach coupled with frequent spontaneous reductions in sphincter pressure contributes to reflux. At least one episode of regurgitation a day occurs in as much as half of infants ages 0 to 3 months. By 6 months of age it becomes less frequent, and it abates by 2 years of age as the child assumes a more upright posture and eats solid foods.[3,18,19] Although many infants have minor degrees of reflux, complications can occur in children with more frequent or persistent episodes. The condition occurs more frequently in children with cerebral palsy, Down syndrome, and other neurologic disorders.

In most cases, infants with simple reflux are thriving and healthy, and symptoms resolve between 9 and 24 months of age. Pathologic reflux is classified into three categories: (1) regurgitation and malnutrition, (2) esophagitis, and (3) respiratory problems.

Clinical Features. Symptoms of reflux esophagitis include evidence of pain when swallowing, hematemesis, anemia due

to esophageal bleeding, heartburn, irritability, and sudden or inconsolable crying. Parents often report feeding problems in their infants.[18] These infants often are irritable and demonstrate early satiety. Sometimes the problems progress to actual resistance to feeding. Tilting of the head to one side and arching of the back may be noted in children with severe reflux. The head positioning is thought to represent an attempt to protect the airway or reduce the pain-associated reflux. Sometimes regurgitation is associated with dental caries and recurrent otalgia. The ear pain is thought to occur through referral from the vagus nerve in the esophagus to the ear.

A variety of respiratory symptoms are caused by damage to the respiratory mucosa when gastric reflux enters the esophagus. Reflux may cause laryngospasm, apnea, and bradycardia. A relationship between reflux and acute life-threatening events or sudden infant death syndrome has been proposed. However, the association remains controversial and the linkage may be coincidental.[3] Asthma may co-occur with GERD in about 50% of asthmatic children. Asthmatic children who are particularly likely to have GERD as a provocative factor are those with symptoms of reflux, those with refractory or steroid-dependent asthma, and those with nocturnal worsening of symptoms[3,20] (see Chapter 29 for a discussion of childhood asthma).

Diagnosis of gastroesophageal reflux in infants and children often is based on parental and clinical observations. The diagnosis may be confirmed by esophageal pH probe studies or barium fluoroscopic esophagography. In severe cases, esophagoscopy may be used to demonstrate reflux and obtain a biopsy.

Various treatment methods are available for infants and children with gastroesophageal reflux. Small, frequent feedings are recommended because of the association between gastric volume and transient relaxation of the esophagus. Thickening an infant's feedings with cereal tends to decrease the volume of reflux, decrease crying and energy expenditure, and increase the calorie density of the formula.[3,18] In infants, positioning on the left side seems to decrease reflux. In older infants and children, raising the head of the bed and keeping the child upright may help. Medications usually are not added to the treatment regimen until pathologic reflux has been documented by diagnostic testing. Antacids are the most commonly used antireflux therapy and are readily available over the counter. H_2-receptor antagonists and proton pump inhibitors may be used in children with persistent reflux. Prokinetic agents (e.g., metoclopramide, a dopamine-2 and 5-hydroxytryptamine [5-HT_3] receptor antagonist; bethanechol, a cholinergic agonist) may be used in selected cases.[3]

Cancer of the Esophagus

Carcinoma of the esophagus accounts for approximately 6% of all gastrointestinal cancers.[7] It is more common in older persons, with a mean age at diagnosis of 67 years. It occurs more frequently in men than women and is the seventh leading cause of cancer death among men, particularly black men.[21,22]

There are two types of esophageal cancer: squamous cell carcinoma and adenocarcinoma. Most squamous cell esophageal carcinomas are attributable to alcohol and tobacco use. Worldwide, squamous cell carcinomas constitute 90% of esophageal cancers, but in the United States there has been an exponential increase in adenocarcinomas associated with Barrett esophagus.[21] Molecular studies have suggested that the pathogenesis of adenocarcinoma from Barrett esophagus is a multistep process, with the development of dysplasia being a critical step in the process.[7] Thus, endoscopic surveillance of persons with Barrett esophagus provides the means for detecting adenocarcinoma at an earlier stage, when it is most amenable to curative surgical resection.[21]

Dysphagia is by far the most frequent complaint of persons with esophageal cancer. It is apparent first with ingestion of bulky food, later with soft food, and finally with liquids. Unfortunately, it is a late manifestation of the disease. Unintentional weight loss, anorexia, fatigue, and pain on swallowing also may occur.

Treatment of esophageal cancer depends on tumor stage. Surgical resection provides a means of cure when done in early disease and palliation when done in late disease. Radiation may be used as an alternative to surgery. Chemotherapy may be used before surgery to decrease the size of the tumor or it may be used along with irradiation and surgery in an effort to increase survival.[21]

The prognosis for persons with cancer of the esophagus, although poor, has improved. Even with modern forms of therapy, however, the long-term survival is limited because, in many cases, the disease has already metastasized by the time the diagnosis is made.

Gastroesophageal reflux refers to the backward movement of gastric contents into the esophagus, a condition that causes heartburn. Although most persons experience occasional gastroesophageal reflux and heartburn, persistent reflux can result in a cycle of mucosal damage that causes hyperemia, edema, erosion luminal surface, and Barrett esophagus. Reflux can cause respiratory symptoms, including chronic cough, and serve as a potential trigger for asthma. Gastroesophageal reflux is a common problem in infants and children. Reflux commonly corrects itself with age, and symptoms abate in most children by 2 years of age. Although many infants have minor degrees of reflux, some infants and small children have significant reflux that interferes with feeding, causes esophagitis, and results in respiratory symptoms and other complications.

Carcinoma of the esophagus, which accounts for 6% of all gastrointestinal cancers, is more common in older persons and occurs more frequently in men than women. There are two types of esophageal cancer: squamous cell carcinoma and adenocarcinoma. Most squamous cell carcinomas are attributable to alcohol and tobacco use, whereas adenocarcinomas are more closely linked to gastroesophageal reflux and Barrett esophagus. ■

DISORDERS OF THE STOMACH

After completing this section of the chapter, you should be able to meet the following objectives:

- Describe the anatomic and physiologic factors that contribute to the gastric mucosal barrier.
- Differentiate between the causes and manifestations of acute and chronic gastritis.
- Characterize the proposed role of *Helicobacter pylori* in the development of chronic gastritis and peptic ulcer and cite methods for diagnosis and treatment of the infection.
- Describe the predisposing factors in development of peptic ulcer and cite the three complications of peptic ulcer.
- Describe the goals for pharmacologic treatment of peptic ulcer disease.
- Cite the etiologic factors in ulcer formation related to Zollinger-Ellison syndrome and stress ulcer.
- List risk factors associated with gastric cancer.

IN SUMMARY, the esophagus is a tube that connects the oropharynx with the stomach; it functions primarily as a conduit for passage of food from the pharynx to the stomach. Although relatively uncommon, congenital anomalies (*i.e.,* esophageal atresia and tracheoesophageal fistulas) must be corrected early because they cause aspiration of gastric and oral secretions and are incompatible with life. Dysphagia refers to difficulty in swallowing; it can result from altered nerve function or from disorders that produce narrowing of the esophagus. A diverticulum of the esophagus is an outpouching of the esophageal wall caused by a weakness of the muscularis layer. Longitudinal tears (Mallory-Weiss tears) at the esophagogastric junction can occur with severe bouts of retching or vomiting. They are most often encountered in persons with chronic alcoholism, but may also occur during acute illness with severe vomiting. Hiatal hernia is characterized by a protrusion or herniation of the stomach through the esophageal hiatus of the diaphragm. There are two anatomic patterns of herniation: (1) the axial or sliding hiatal hernia, which is the most common type and is characterized by bell-shaped protrusion of the stomach above the diaphragm; and (2) the nonaxial or paraesophageal hernia, in which a portion of the stomach enters the thorax through a widened opening.

The stomach is a reservoir for contents entering the digestive tract. It lies in the upper abdomen, anterior to the pancreas, splenic vessels, and left kidney. Anteriorly, the stomach is bounded by the anterior abdominal wall and the left inferior lobe of the liver. While in the stomach, food is churned and mixed with hydrochloric acid and pepsin before being released into the small intestine. Normally, the mucosal surface of the stomach provides a barrier that protects it from the hydrochloric acid and pepsin contained in gastric secretions. Disorders of the stomach include gastritis, peptic ulcer, and gastric carcinoma.

Gastric Mucosal Barrier

The stomach lining usually is impermeable to the acid it secretes, a property that allows the stomach to contain acid and pepsin without having its walls digested. Several factors contribute to the protection of the gastric mucosa, including an impermeable epithelial cell surface covering, mechanisms for the selective transport of hydrogen and bicarbonate ions, and the characteristics of gastric mucus.[23] These mechanisms are collectively referred to as the *gastric mucosal barrier.*

DISRUPTION OF THE GASTRIC MUCOSA AND ULCER DEVELOPMENT

- The stomach is protected by a mucosal barrier that prevents gastric secretions and other destructive agents from injuring the epithelial and deeper layers of the stomach wall.

- The integrity of the mucosal layer is maintained by tight cellular junctions and the presence of a protective mucus layer.

- Prostaglandins serve as chemical messengers that protect the stomach lining by improving blood flow, increasing bicarbonate secretion, and enhancing mucus production.

- Two of the major causes of gastric irritation and ulcer formation are aspirin or nonsteroidal anti-inflammatory drugs (NSAIDs) and infection with *Helicobacter pylori.*

- Aspirin and NSAIDs exert their destructive effects by irritating the stomach and inhibiting prostaglandin synthesis.

- *H. pylori* is an infectious agent that thrives in the acid environment of the stomach and disrupts the mucosal barrier that protects the stomach from the harmful effects of its digestive enzymes.

The cells of the gastric epithelia are connected by tight junctions that prevent acid penetration, and they are covered with an impermeable hydrophobic lipid layer that prevents diffusion of ionized water-soluble molecules. Aspirin, which is nonionized and lipid soluble in acid solutions, rapidly diffuses across this lipid layer, increasing mucosal permeability and damaging epithelial cells.[23] Gastric irritation and occult bleeding due to gastric irritation occur in a significant number of persons who take aspirin on a regular basis. Alcohol, which also is lipid soluble, disrupts the mucosal barrier; when aspirin and alcohol are taken in combination, as they often are, there is increased risk of gastric irritation. Bile acids also attack the lipid components of the mucosal barrier and afford the potential for gastric irritation when there is reflux of duodenal contents into the stomach.

Normally, the secretion of hydrochloric acid by the parietal cells of the stomach is accompanied by secretion of bicarbonate ions (HCO_3^-). For every hydrogen ion (H^+) that is secreted, an HCO_3^- is produced, and as long as HCO_3^- production is equal to H^+ secretion, mucosal injury does not occur. Changes in gastric blood flow, as in shock, tend to decrease HCO_3^- production. This is particularly true in situations in which decreased blood flow is accompanied by acidosis. Aspirin and the nonsteroidal anti-inflammatory drugs (NSAIDs), such as indomethacin and ibuprofen, also impair HCO_3^- secretion.[24]

The mucus that protects the gastric mucosa is of two types: water insoluble and water soluble.[23] Water-insoluble mucus forms a thin, stable gel that adheres to the gastric mucosal surface and provides protection from the proteolytic (protein-digesting) actions of pepsin. It also forms an unstirred layer that traps bicarbonate, forming an alkaline interface between the luminal contents of the stomach and its mucosal surface. The water-soluble mucus is washed from the mucosal surface and mixes with the luminal contents; its viscid nature makes it a lubricant that prevents mechanical damage to the mucosal surface. In addition to their effects on mucosal permeability and bicarbonate production, damaging agents such as aspirin and the NSAIDs inhibit and modify the characteristics of gastric mucus.

Prostaglandins, chemical messengers derived from cell membrane lipids, play an important role in protecting the gastric mucosa from injury.[7] The prostaglandins are thought to exert their effect through improved mucosal blood flow, decreased acid secretion, increased bicarbonate ion secretion, and enhanced mucus production. The fact that drugs such as aspirin and the NSAIDs inhibit prostaglandin synthesis may contribute to their ability to produce gastric irritation.

Gastritis

Gastritis refers to inflammation of the gastric mucosa. There are many causes of gastritis, most of which can be grouped as either acute or chronic gastritis.

Acute Gastritis

Acute gastritis is characterized by an acute mucosal inflammatory process, usually transient in nature. The inflammation may be accompanied by hemorrhage into the mucosa and, in severe cases, by sloughing of the superficial mucosa. This erosive form is an important cause of acute gastrointestinal bleeding. The condition is most commonly associated with local irritants such aspirin or other NSAIDs, alcohol, or bacterial toxins.[7] Oral administration of corticosteroids may also be complicated by acute hemorrhagic gastritis. Any serious illness or trauma that is accompanied by profound physiologic stress that requires substantial medical or surgical treatment renders the gastric mucosa more vulnerable to acute hemorrhagic gastritis because of mucosal injury (discussed under stress ulcers).[8] Uremia, treatment with cancer chemotherapy drugs, and gastric radiation are other causes of acute gastritis.

The complaints of persons with acute gastritis vary. Persons with aspirin-related gastritis can be totally unaware of the condition or may complain only of heartburn or sour stomach. Gastritis associated with excessive alcohol consumption is often a different situation; it often causes transient gastric distress, which may lead to vomiting and, in more severe situations, to bleeding and hematemesis. Gastritis caused by the toxins of infectious organisms, such as the staphylococcal enterotoxins, usually has an abrupt and violent onset, with gastric distress and vomiting ensuing approximately 5 hours after the ingestion of a contaminated food source. Acute gastritis usually is a self-limiting disorder, with complete regeneration and healing occurring within several days of removal of the inciting agent.

Chronic Gastritis

Chronic gastritis is a separate entity from acute gastritis. It is characterized by the absence of grossly visible erosions and the presence of chronic inflammatory changes leading eventually to atrophy of the glandular epithelium of the stomach. There are three major types of chronic gastritis: *Helicobacter pylori* gastritis, autoimmune gastritis and multifocal atrophic gastritis, and chemical gastropathy.[8]

***Helicobacter pylori* Gastritis.** *H. pylori* infection is the most common cause of chronic gastritis. Infection occurs worldwide, but the prevalence varies greatly among countries and population groups within countries.[25] The prevalence among middle-aged adults is over 80% in many developing countries, compared with 20% to 50% in industrialized countries.[26] It has been suggested that transmission in industrialized countries is largely person-to-person by vomitus, saliva, or feces, whereas additional transmission routes such as water may be important in developing countries. In industrialized countries, the rate of infection with *H. pylori* has decreased substantially over the past several decades owing to improved sanitation. Thus, the reported increased prevalence of *H. pylori* infection in older persons (*e.g.*, over 50% in American adults older than 50 years of age) has been credited to infection that occurred at an earlier age.[26]

H. pylori gastritis is a chronic inflammatory disease of the antrum and body of the stomach. Chronic infection with *H. pylori* can lead to gastric atrophy and peptic ulcer, and is associated with increased risk of gastric adenocarcinoma and low-grade B-cell gastric lymphoma (MALToma [mucosa-associated lymphoid tissue]).[8]

H. pylori are small, curved, gram-negative rods (protobacteria) that can colonize the mucus-secreting epithelial cells of the stomach[25,26] (Fig. 37-4). *H. pylori* have multiple flagella, which allow them to move through the mucous layer of the stomach, and they secrete urease, which enables them to produce sufficient ammonia to buffer the acidity of their immediate environ-

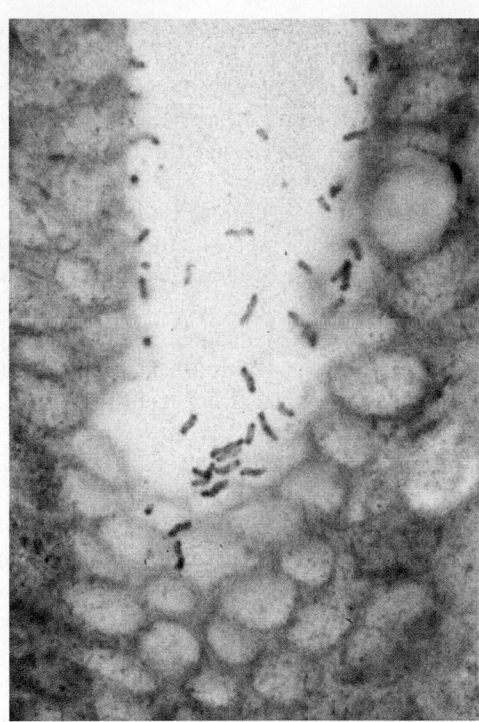

FIGURE 37-4 • Infective gastritis. *H. pylori* appear on silver staining as small, curved rods on the surface of the gastric mucosa. (From Mitos F. A., Rubin E. [2008]. The gastrointestinal tract. In Rubin R., Strayer D. S. [Eds.], *Rubin's pathophysiology: Clinicopathologic foundations of medicine* [5th ed., p. 563]. Philadelphia: Lippincott Williams & Wilkins.)

ment. These properties help to explain why the organism is able to survive in the acidic environment of the stomach. *H. pylori* produce enzymes and toxins that have the capacity to interfere with the local protection of the gastric mucosa against acid, produce intense inflammation, and elicit an immune response. There is increased production of proinflammatory cytokines that serve to recruit and activate neutrophils. Several *H. pylori* proteins are immunogenic and they evoke an intense immune response in the mucosa. Both T and B cells can be seen in the chronic gastritis caused by *H. pylori*. Although the role of T and B cells in causing epithelial injury has not been established, T-cell–driven activation of B cells may be involved in the pathogenesis of gastric lymphomas.[8]

Why some people with *H. pylori* infection develop clinical disease and others do not is unclear. Scientists are studying the different strains of the bacteria in an attempt to establish whether certain strains are more virulent than others and whether host and environmental factors contribute to the development of clinical disease.[8]

Methods for establishing the presence of *H. pylori* infection include the carbon (C) urea breath test using a radioactive carbon isotope (^{13}C or ^{14}C), the stool antigen test, and endoscopic biopsy for urease testing.[26,27] Blood tests to obtain serologic titers of *H. pylori* antibodies also can be done. The serologic test can establish that a person has been infected with *H. pylori*, but it cannot distinguish how recently the infection occurred.

Eradication of *H. pylori* has proved difficult. Treatment requires combination therapy that includes the use of two antibiotics with a proton pump inhibitor or bismuth.[13] Treatment is usually continued for 10 to 14 days. *H. pylori* mutate rapidly to develop antibiotic-resistant strains. The combination of two or more antimicrobial agents increases the rates of cure and reduces the risk of resistant strains developing. The antibiotics that have shown the greatest efficacy against *H. pylori* are clarithromycin, metronidazole, amoxicillin, and tetracycline. The proton pump inhibitors have direct antimicrobial properties against *H. pylori,* and by raising the intragastric pH they suppress bacterial growth and optimize antibiotic efficacy. Bismuth has a direct antibacterial effect against *H. pylori.*

Chronic Autoimmune and Multifocal Gastritis. *Autoimmune gastritis,* which accounts for less than 10% of cases of chronic gastritis, is a diffuse form of gastritis that is limited to the body and fundus of the stomach, with a lack or minimal involvement of the antrum. The disorder results from the presence of autoantibodies to components of gastric gland parietal cells and intrinsic factor. Gastric gland and mucosal atrophy lead to a loss of acid production. In the most severe cases, production of intrinsic factor is lost, leading to a vitamin B_{12} deficiency and pernicious anemia (see Chapter 14). This type of chronic gastritis frequently is associated with other autoimmune disorders such as Hashimoto thyroiditis and Addison disease.

Multifocal atrophic gastritis is a disorder of uncertain etiology that affects the antrum and adjacent areas of the stomach. It is more common than autoimmune gastritis, and is seen more frequently in whites than in other races. It is particularly common in Asia, Scandinavia, and parts of Europe and Latin America.[8] As with autoimmune gastritis, it is associated with reduced gastric acid secretion, but achlorhydria and pernicious anemia are uncommon.

Chronic autoimmune gastritis and multifocal atrophic gastritis usually cause few symptoms related directly to gastric changes. When severe parietal cell loss occurs in the presence of autoimmune gastritis, hypochlorhydria or achlorhydria and hypergastrinemia are characteristically present. More important is the relationship of chronic gastritis to the development of peptic ulcer and gastric carcinoma. The long-term risk of gastric cancer in persons with autoimmune gastritis is 2% to 4%, which is considerably greater than that of the general population.[7]

Chemical Gastropathy. Chemical gastropathy is a chronic gastric injury resulting from reflux of alkaline duodenal contents, pancreatic secretions, and bile into the stomach. It is most commonly seen in persons who have had gastroduodenostomy or gastrojejunostomy surgery. A milder form may occur in persons with gastric ulcer, gallbladder disease, or various motility disorders of the distal stomach.

Peptic Ulcer Disease

Peptic ulcer is a term used to describe a group of ulcerative disorders that occur in areas of the upper gastrointestinal tract that are exposed to acid–pepsin secretions.[7,8,28] The most common

forms of peptic ulcer are duodenal and gastric ulcers. Peptic ulcer disease, with its remissions and exacerbations, is a chronic health problem. Approximately 10% of the population have or will develop peptic ulcer.[8] Duodenal ulcers occur five times more commonly than gastric ulcers. The peak age for peptic ulcer has progressively increased in the last 50 years, and is now between 30 and 60 years of age for duodenal ulcers, although the disorder can occur in persons of any age. Gastric ulcers are more prevalent among middle-aged and elderly persons. For duodenal ulcers there is a male predominance, whereas the incidence of gastric ulcers is more equally distributed between men and women.[8]

Peptic Ulcers

A peptic ulcer can affect one or all layers of the stomach or duodenum (Fig. 37-5). The ulcer may penetrate only the mucosal surface, or it may extend into the smooth muscle layers. Occasionally, an ulcer penetrates the outer wall of the stomach or duodenum. Spontaneous remissions and exacerbations are common. Healing of the muscularis layer involves replacement with scar tissue; although the mucosal layers that cover the scarred muscle layer regenerate, the regeneration often is less than perfect, which contributes to repeated episodes of ulceration.

A variety of risk factors have been shown to have an association with peptic ulcer disease. The two most important are

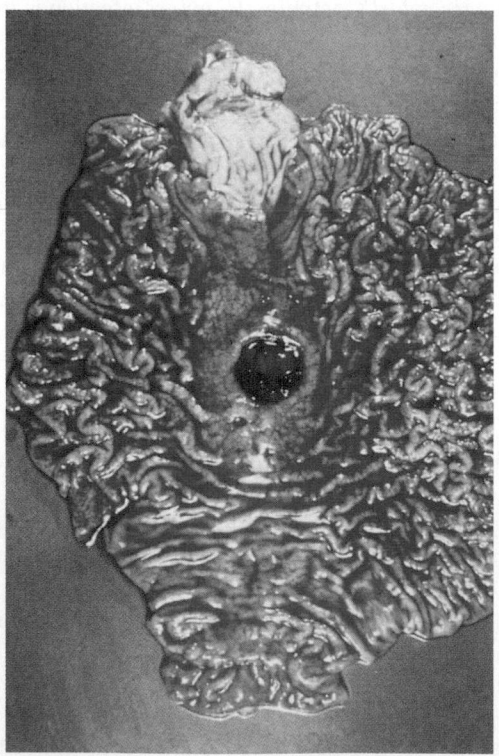

FIGURE 37-5 • Gastric ulcer. The stomach has been opened to reveal a sharply demarcated, deep peptic ulcer on the lesser curvature. (From Rubin E., Farber J. L. [Eds.]. [1999]. *Pathology* [3rd ed., p. 693]. Philadelphia: Lippincott Williams & Wilkins.)

infection with the bacteria *H. pylori* and use of aspirin and other NSAIDs.[28] Both *H. pylori* infection and exposure to NSAIDs have been shown to impair the mechanisms that protect the gastric mucosa from the destructive effects of the corrosive acid that is continually challenging the upper gastrointestinal tract mucosa, and ulceration reflects a failure of these mechanisms.

The exact mechanism by which *H. pylori* promotes the development of peptic ulcer has not been fully elucidated. *H. pylori*'s ability to induce inflammation and stimulate the release of cytokines and other mediators of inflammation contributes to mucosal damage. Infection, predominantly in the antrum of the stomach, leads to hypergastrinemia and an increased acid production. Acid injury to the duodenum is thought to promote the development of gastric metaplasia, allowing the organism to colonize these areas and promote the development of duodenal ulcers.

The pathogenesis of NSAID-induced ulcers is thought to involve mucosal injury and inhibition of prostaglandin synthesis.[28] Aspirin appears to be the most ulcerogenic of the NSAIDs. Ulcer development in NSAID users is dose dependent, but some risk occurs even with aspirin doses of 81 mg/day.[7] In contrast to peptic ulcer from other causes, NSAID-induced gastric injury often is without symptoms, and life-threatening complications can occur without warning. There is reportedly less gastric irritation with the newer class of NSAIDs that selectively inhibit cylcooxygenase-2 (COX-2–selective NSAIDs), the principal enzyme involved in prostaglandin synthesis at the site of inflammation, than with the nonselective NSAIDs that also inhibit COX-1, the enzyme involved in prostaglandin production in the gastric mucosa.

Epidemiologic studies have identified independent factors that augment the effect of *H. pylori* infection and NSAID-produced peptic ulcer disease. These factors include advancing age, a prior history of peptic ulcer, multiple NSAID use, and concurrent use of warfarin (an anticoagulant) and corticosteroid drugs. Smoking may augment the risk of peptic ulcer by impairing healing. There is no convincing evidence that dietary factors play a role in development of peptic ulcer. There is increased incidence of peptic ulcer in families. This finding is likely due to familial clustering of *H. pylori* infection, and inherited genetic factors reflecting responses to the organism likely play a secondary role.

Clinical Features. The clinical manifestations of uncomplicated peptic ulcer focus on discomfort and pain. The pain, which is described as burning, gnawing, or cramplike, usually is rhythmic and frequently occurs when the stomach is empty—between meals and at 1 or 2 o'clock in the morning. The pain usually is located over a small area near the midline in the epigastrium near the xiphoid, and may radiate below the costal margins, into the back, or, rarely, to the right shoulder. Superficial and deep epigastric tenderness and voluntary muscle guarding may occur with more extensive lesions. An additional characteristic of ulcer pain is periodicity. The pain tends to recur at intervals of weeks or months. During an exacerbation, it occurs daily for a period of several weeks and then remits until the next recurrence. Characteristically, the pain is relieved by food or antacids.

The most common complications of peptic ulcer are hemorrhage, perforation and penetration, and gastric outlet obstruction. Hemorrhage is caused by bleeding from granulation tissue or from erosion of an ulcer into an artery or vein. It occurs in up to 15% to 20% of persons with peptic ulcer.[7] Evidence of bleeding may consist of hematemesis or melena. Bleeding may be sudden, severe, and without warning, or it may be insidious, producing only occult blood in the stool. Up to 20% of persons with bleeding ulcers have no antecedent symptoms of pain; this is particularly true in persons using NSAIDs. Acute hemorrhage is evidenced by the sudden onset of weakness; dizziness; thirst; cold, moist skin; the desire to defecate; and the passage of loose, tarry, or even red stools and coffee-ground emesis. Signs of circulatory shock develop depending on the amount of blood lost.

Perforation occurs when an ulcer erodes through all the layers of the stomach or duodenum wall. Perforation develops in approximately 5% of persons with peptic ulcers, usually from ulcers on the anterior wall of the stomach or duodenum.[7] With perforation, gastrointestinal contents enter the peritoneum and cause peritonitis. Radiation of the pain into the back, severe night distress, and inadequate pain relief from eating foods or taking antacids in persons with a long history of peptic ulcer may signify perforation. Penetration is a process similar to perforation, but with penetration the ulcer crater erodes into adjacent organs, including the small bowel, pancreas, liver, or biliary tree.[28] Typically it has a subtle presentation marked by a gradual increase in severity and frequency of pain.

Outlet obstruction is caused by edema, spasm, or contraction of scar tissue and interference with the free passage of gastric contents through the pylorus or adjacent areas. The presentation of an obstruction is typically insidious, with symptoms of early satiety, feeling of epigastric fullness and heaviness after meals, gastroesophageal reflux, weight loss, and abdominal pain. With severe obstruction, there is vomiting of undigested food.

Diagnosis and Treatment. Diagnostic procedures for peptic ulcer include history taking, laboratory tests, radiologic imaging, and endoscopic examination. The history should include careful attention to aspirin and NSAID use. Peptic ulcer should be differentiated from other causes of epigastric pain. Laboratory findings of hypochromic anemia and occult blood in the stools indicate bleeding. Endoscopy (*i.e.*, gastroscopy and duodenoscopy) can be used to visualize the ulcer area and obtain biopsy specimens to test for *H. pylori* and exclude malignant disease. X-ray studies with a contrast medium such as barium are used to detect the presence of an ulcer crater and to exclude gastric carcinoma.

The treatment of peptic ulcer has changed dramatically over the past several decades and now aims to eradicate the cause and promote a permanent cure for the disease. Pharmacologic treatment focuses on eradicating *H. pylori*, relieving ulcer symptoms, and healing the ulcer crater. Acid-neutralizing, acid-inhibiting drugs and mucosa-protective agents are used to relieve symptoms and promote healing of the ulcer crater. There is no evidence that special diets are beneficial in treating peptic ulcer. Aspirin and NSAID use should be avoided when possible.

There are two pharmacologic methods for reducing gastric acid content. The first involves the neutralization of gastric acid through the use of antacids, and the second a decrease in gastric acid production through the use of H_2-receptor antagonists or proton pump inhibitors. Essentially three types of antacids are used to relieve gastric acidity: calcium carbonate, aluminum hydroxide, and magnesium hydroxide. Many antacids contain a combination of ingredients, such as magnesium aluminum hydroxide. *Calcium preparations* are constipating and may cause hypercalcemia and the milk-alkali syndrome. There also is evidence that oral calcium preparations increase gastric acid secretion after their buffering effect has been depleted. *Magnesium hydroxide* is a potent antacid that also has laxative effects. Approximately 5% to 10% of the magnesium in this preparation is absorbed from the intestine; because magnesium is excreted through the kidneys, this formulation should not be used in persons with renal failure. *Aluminum hydroxide* reacts with hydrochloric acid to form aluminum chloride. It combines with phosphate in the intestine, and prolonged use may lead to phosphate depletion and osteoporosis. Because antacids can decrease the absorption, bioavailability, and renal elimination of a number of drugs, this should be considered when antacids are administered with other medications.

Histamine is the major physiologic mediator for hydrochloric acid secretion (see Chapter 36, Fig. 36-10). The H_2-receptor antagonists block gastric acid secretion stimulated by histamine, gastrin, and acetylcholine. The volume of gastric secretion and the concentration of pepsin also are reduced. The proton pump inhibitors block the final stage of hydrogen ion secretion by blocking the action of the gastric parietal cell proton pump.

Among the agents that enhance mucosal defenses are sucralfate and prostaglandin analogs. The drug sucralfate, which is a complex salt of sucrose containing aluminum and sulfate, selectively binds to necrotic ulcer tissue and serves as a barrier to acid, pepsin, and bile. Sucralfate also can directly absorb bile salts. The drug is not absorbed systemically. The drug requires an acid pH for activation and should not be administered with antacids or an H_2 antagonist. Misoprostol, a prostaglandin E derivative, promotes ulcer healing by stimulating mucus and bicarbonate secretion and by modestly inhibiting acid secretion. It is the only drug in this class approved by the U.S. Food and Drug Administration (FDA) for clinical use in the prevention of NSAID-induced peptic ulcers. The drug causes dose-dependent diarrhea, and because of its stimulant effect on the uterus, it is contraindicated in women of childbearing age.

The current surgical management of peptic ulcer disease is largely limited to treatment of complications. When surgery is needed, it usually is performed using minimally invasive methods. With bleeding ulcers, hemostasis often can be achieved by endoscopic methods, and endoscopic balloon dilation often is effective in relieving outflow obstruction.

Zollinger-Ellison Syndrome

The Zollinger-Ellison syndrome is a rare condition caused by a gastrin-secreting tumor (gastrinoma). In persons with this disorder, gastric acid secretion reaches such levels that ulceration becomes inevitable.[29] The tumors may be single or multiple; although most tumors are located in the pancreas, a few develop in the submucosa of the stomach or duodenum. Over half of gastrin-producing tumors are malignant and have already metastasized at the time of diagnosis.[30] The increased gastric secretions cause symptoms related to peptic ulcer. Diarrhea may result from hypersecretion or from the inactivation of intestinal lipase and impaired fat digestion that occur with a decrease in intestinal pH.

Hypergastrinemia may also occur in an autosomal dominant disorder called the *multiple endocrine neoplasia type 1 (MEN 1) syndrome,* which is characterized by multiple endocrine neoplasms. The syndrome is characterized by hyperparathyroidism and multiple endocrine tumors, including gastrinomas. Approximately 25% of gastrinomas are due to MEN 1.[30]

The diagnosis of the Zollinger-Ellison syndrome is based on elevated serum gastrin and basal gastric acid levels and elimination of the MEN 1 syndrome as a cause of the disorder. Computed tomography (CT), abdominal ultrasonography, and selective angiography are used to localize the tumor and determine if metastatic disease is present.

Treatment of Zollinger-Ellison syndrome involves control of gastric acid secretion by proton pump inhibitors. Over half of gastrin-producing tumors are locally invasive or have already metastasized at the time of diagnosis.[30] Surgical removal is indicated when the tumor is malignant and has not metastasized.

Stress Ulcers

A stress ulcer, sometimes called a *Curling ulcer,* refers to gastrointestinal ulcerations that develop in relation to major physiologic stress.[8] Persons at high risk for development of stress ulcers include those with large–surface-area burns, trauma, sepsis, acute respiratory distress syndrome, severe liver failure, and major surgical procedures. These lesions occur most often in the fundus of the stomach and proximal duodenum and are thought to result from ischemia, tissue acidosis, and bile salts entering the stomach in critically ill persons with decreased gastrointestinal tract motility.[7,31,32] Another form of stress ulcer, called *Cushing ulcer,* consists of gastric, duodenal, and esophageal ulcers arising in persons with intracranial injury, operations, or tumors. They are thought to be caused by hypersecretion of gastric acid resulting from stimulation of vagal nuclei by increased intracranial pressure. These ulcers are associated with a high incidence of perforation.[31]

Persons admitted to hospital intensive care units are at particular risk for development of stress ulcers.[31] H_2-receptor antagonists and proton pump inhibitors are used in the prevention and treatment of stress ulcers.[32]

Cancer of the Stomach

Gastric carcinoma is the second most common tumor in the world. However, its incidence varies widely, being particularly high in countries such as Japan, Chile, Costa Rica, Columbia, China, Portugal, Russia, and Bulgaria. It is more common in lower socioeconomic groups and exhibits a male-to-female ratio of about 2:1. Although it is responsible for only 2.5% of all cancer deaths in the United States, it is the leading cause of cancer mortality worldwide.[7]

Factors thought to increase the risk of gastric cancer include genetic factors, carcinogenic factors in the diet (*e.g.*, *N*-nitroso compounds and benzopyrene found in smoked and preserved foods), autoimmune gastritis, and gastric adenomas or polyps. The incidence of stomach cancer in the United States has decreased fourfold since 1930, presumably because of improved storage of food with decreased consumption of salted, smoked, and preserved foods.[7] Chronic infection with *H. pylori* appears to serve as a cofactor in some types of gastric carcinomas. The bacterial infection causes gastritis, followed by atrophy, intestinal metaplasia, and carcinoma. This sequence of cellular events depends on both the presence of the bacterial proteins and the host immune response, with the latter being influenced by the host genetic background. However, the vast majority of people with *H. pylori* infection will not develop gastric cancer, and not all *H. pylori* infections increase the risk of gastric cancer, suggesting that other factors must be involved.[7] Autoimmune gastritis, like *H. pylori* infection, increases the risk of gastric cancer, presumably due to chronic inflammation and intestinal metaplasia.[7]

Between 50% and 60% of gastric cancers occur in the pyloric region or adjacent to the antrum. Compared with a benign ulcer, which has smooth margins and is concentrically shaped, gastric cancers tend to be larger, are irregularly shaped, and have irregular margins.

Clinical Features

Unfortunately, stomach cancers often are asymptomatic until late in their course. Symptoms, when they do occur, usually are vague and include indigestion, anorexia, weight loss, vague epigastric pain, vomiting, and an abdominal mass. Because these symptoms are essentially nonspecific, early detection is difficult.

Diagnosis of gastric cancer is accomplished by a variety of techniques, including barium x-ray studies, endoscopic studies with biopsy, and cytologic studies (*e.g.*, Papanicolaou smear) of gastric secretions.[33] Cytologic studies can prove particularly useful as routine screening tests for persons with atrophic gastritis or gastric polyps. CT and endoscopic ultrasonography often are used to delineate the spread of a diagnosed stomach cancer.

Depending on the location and extent of the lesion, surgery in the form of radical subtotal gastrectomy usually is the treatment of choice. Irradiation and chemotherapy have not proved particularly useful as primary treatment modalities in stomach cancer. These methods usually are used for palliative purposes or to control metastatic spread of the disease.

IN SUMMARY, disorders of the stomach include gastritis, peptic ulcer, and cancer of the stomach. Gastritis refers to inflammation of the gastric mucosa. Acute gastritis refers to a transient inflammation of the gastric mucosa; it is associated most commonly with local irritants such as bacterial endotoxins, caffeine, alcohol, and aspirin. Chronic gastritis is characterized by the absence of grossly visible erosions and the presence of chronic inflammatory changes leading eventually to atrophy of the glandular epithelium of the stomach. There are three main types of chronic gastritis: *H. pylori* gastritis, autoimmune gastritis and multifocal atrophic gastritis, and chemical gastropathy. *H. pylori* is an "S"-shaped bacterium that colonizes the mucus-secreting epithelial cells of the stomach. Infection increases the risk of chronic gastritis, peptic ulcer, gastric carcinoma, and low-grade B-cell lymphoma. Treatment of *H. pylori* infection involves the use of multidrug therapy aimed at increasing the pH of gastric secretions and antimicrobial agents designed to eradicate the organism.

Peptic ulcer is a term used to describe a group of ulcerative disorders that occur in areas of the upper gastrointestinal tract that are exposed to acid–pepsin secretions, most commonly the duodenum and stomach. There are two main causes of peptic ulcer: *H. pylori* infection and aspirin or NSAID use. The treatment of peptic ulcer focuses on eradication of *H. pylori*, avoidance of gastric irritation from NSAIDs, and conventional pharmacologic treatment directed at symptom relief and ulcer healing.

The Zollinger-Ellison syndrome is a rare condition caused by a gastrin-secreting tumor in which gastric acid secretion reaches such levels that ulceration becomes inevitable. Stress ulcers, also called *Curling ulcers*, occur in relation to major physiologic stresses such as burns and trauma and are thought to result from ischemia, tissue acidosis, and bile salts entering the stomach in critically ill persons with decreased gastrointestinal tract motility. Another form of stress ulcer, Cushing ulcer, occurs in persons with intracranial trauma or surgery and is thought to be caused by hypersecretion of gastric acid resulting from stimulation of vagal nuclei by increased intracranial pressure.

Although the incidence of cancer of the stomach has declined over the past 50 years in the United States, it remains the leading cause of death worldwide. Because there are few early symptoms with this form of cancer, the disease often is far advanced at the time of diagnosis. ■

DISORDERS OF THE SMALL AND LARGE INTESTINES

After completing this section of the chapter, you should be able to meet the following objectives:

- State the diagnostic criteria for irritable bowel syndrome.
- Compare the characteristics of Crohn disease and ulcerative colitis.

- Relate the use of a high-fiber diet in the treatment of diverticular disease to the etiologic factors for the condition.
- Describe the pathogenesis of the symptoms associated with appendicitis.
- Compare the causes and manifestations of small-volume diarrhea and large-volume diarrhea.
- Explain why a failure to respond to the defecation urge may result in constipation.
- List five causes of fecal impaction.
- Differentiate between mechanical and paralytic intestinal obstruction in terms of cause and manifestations.
- Describe the characteristics of the peritoneum that increase its vulnerability to and protect it against the effects of peritonitis.
- List three causes of intestinal malabsorption and describe their manifestations.
- List the risk factors associated with colorectal cancer and cite the screening methods for detection.

There are many similarities in conditions that disrupt the integrity and function of the small and large intestines. The walls of the small and large intestines consist of five layers (see Chapter 36, Fig. 36-3): an inner mucosal layer, which lines the lumen of the intestine; a submucosal layer; a muscularis layer, which is divided into a layer of circular and a layer of longitudinal muscle fibers; and an outer serosal layer. Among the conditions that cause altered intestinal function are irritable bowel disease, inflammatory bowel disease, diverticulitis, appendicitis, disorders of bowel motility (*i.e.,* diarrhea, constipation, and bowel obstruction), malabsorption syndrome, and cancer of the colon and rectum.

Irritable Bowel Syndrome

The term *irritable bowel syndrome* is used to describe a functional gastrointestinal disorder characterized by a variable combination of chronic and recurrent intestinal symptoms not explained by structural or biochemical abnormalities. There is evidence to suggest that 10% to 15% of the U.S. population have the disorder, although most do not seek medical attention.[34]

Irritable bowel disease is characterized by persistent or recurrent symptoms of abdominal pain, altered bowel function, and varying complaints of flatulence, bloating, nausea and anorexia, constipation or diarrhea, and anxiety or depression. A hallmark of irritable bowel syndrome is abdominal pain that is relieved by defecation and associated with a change in consistency or frequency of stools. Abdominal pain usually is intermittent, cramping, and in the lower abdomen. It does not usually occur at night or interfere with sleep. The condition is believed to result from dysregulation of intestinal motor and sensory functions modulated by the CNS.[34–36] Persons with irritable bowel syndrome tend to experience increased motility and abnormal intestinal contractions in response to psychological and physi-

ologic stresses. The role that psychological factors play in the disease is uncertain. Although changes in intestinal activity are normal responses to stress, these responses appear to be exaggerated in persons with irritable bowel syndrome. Women tend to be affected more often than men. Menarche often is associated with onset of the disorder. Women frequently notice an exacerbation of symptoms during the premenstrual period, suggesting a hormonal component.

Because irritable bowel syndrome lacks anatomic or physiologic markers, diagnosis is usually based on signs and symptoms of abdominal pain or discomfort, bloating, and constipation or diarrhea, or alternating bouts of constipation and diarrhea. A commonly used set of diagnostic criteria require continuous or recurrent symptoms of at least 12 weeks' duration (which may be nonconsecutive) of abdominal discomfort or pain in the preceding 12 months, with two of three accompanying features: relief with defecation, onset associated with a change in bowel frequency, and associated with a change in form (appearance) of stool.[37] Other symptoms that support the diagnosis of irritable bowel syndrome include abnormal stool frequency (more than 3 times per day or less than 3 times per week), abnormal stool form (lumpy/hard or loose/watery), abnormal stool passage (straining, urgency, or feeling of incomplete evacuation), passage of mucus, and bloating or feeling of abdominal distention.[37] A history of lactose intolerance should be considered because intolerance to lactose and other sugars may be a precipitating factor in some persons. The acute onset of symptoms raises the likelihood of organic disease, as does weight loss, anemia, fever, occult blood in the stool, nighttime symptoms, or signs and symptoms of malabsorption. These signs and symptoms require additional investigation.

The treatment of irritable bowel syndrome focuses on methods of stress management, particularly those related to symptom production. Reassurance is important. Usually, no special diet is indicated, although adequate fiber intake usually is recommended. Avoidance of offending dietary substances such as fatty and gas-producing foods, alcohol, and caffeine-containing beverages may be beneficial. Various pharmacologic agents, including antispasmodic and anticholinergic drugs, have been used with varying success in treatment of the disorder. Alosetron, a 5-HT$_3$ antagonist, was the first specific drug to be approved by the FDA for the treatment of irritable bowel disease. It acts by reducing intestinal secretion, decreasing visceral afferent nerve activity (thereby reducing abdominal pain), and reducing intestinal motility. The drug, which was indicated for treatment of women with the severe diarrheal form of the disease, was removed from the market in late 2000 because of serious side effects and then reintroduced in 2002 under a restricted prescribing program.[34–36]

Inflammatory Bowel Disease

The term *inflammatory bowel disease* (IBD) is used to designate two related inflammatory intestinal disorders: Crohn disease and ulcerative colitis. The annual incidence of these diseases in the United States ranges from 3 to 10 new cases per

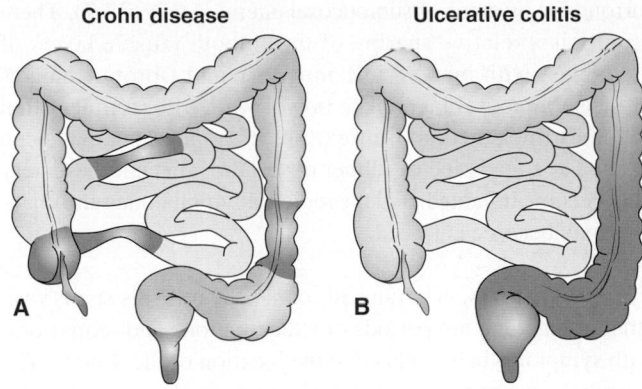

Crohn disease   **Ulcerative colitis**

A   B

FIGURE 37-6 • Distribution patterns of disease with (**A**) skip lesions in Crohn disease and (**B**) continuous involvement of the colon, beginning with the rectum, in ulcerative colitis.

100,000 people.[7] Although the two diseases differ sufficiently to be distinguishable, they have many features in common. Both diseases produce inflammation of the bowel, both lack confirming evidence of a proven causative agent, both have a pattern of familial occurrence, and both can be accompanied by systemic manifestations. Crohn disease most commonly affects the distal small intestine and proximal colon, but can affect any area of the gastrointestinal tract from the esophagus to the anus, whereas ulcerative colitis is confined to the colon and rectum (Fig. 37-6). The distinguishing characteristics of Crohn disease and ulcerative colitis are summarized in Table 37-1.

The clinical manifestations of both Crohn disease and ulcerative colitis are ultimately the result of activation of inflammatory cells with elaboration of inflammatory mediators that cause nonspecific tissue damage. Both diseases are characterized by remissions and exacerbations of diarrhea, fecal urgency, and weight loss. Acute complications, such as intestinal obstruction, may develop during periods of fulminant disease.

A number of systemic manifestations have been identified in persons with Crohn disease and ulcerative colitis. These include axial arthritis affecting the spine and sacroiliac joints and oligoarticular arthritis affecting the large joints of the arms and legs; inflammatory conditions of the eye, usually uveitis; skin lesions, especially erythema nodosum; stomatitis; and autoimmune anemia, hypercoagulability of blood, and sclerosing cholangitis. Occasionally, these systemic manifestations may herald the recurrence of intestinal disease. In children, growth retardation may occur, particularly if the symptoms are prolonged and nutrient intake has been poor.

Etiology and Pathogenesis

A remarkable feature of the gastrointestinal tract is that the mucosal immune system is always ready to respond against ingested pathogens but is unresponsive to the normal intestinal microflora. According to the currently accepted hypothesis, this normal state of homeostasis is disrupted in IBD, leading to unregulated and exaggerated immune responses against bacteria in the normal intestinal flora of genetically susceptible individuals.[38–42] Thus, as in many other autoimmune disorders, the pathogenesis of Crohn disease and ulcerative colitis involves a failure of immune regulation, genetic predisposition, and an environmental trigger, especially microbial flora.[7]

Genetic Susceptibility. The genetic basis of IBD has long been suspected. Approximately 15% of persons with IBD have affected first-degree relatives, and the lifetime risk of either a parent or sibling is 9%.[7] For Crohn disease, studies found a concordance rate of 20% to 50% in monozygotic twins and less than 10% in dizygotic twins.[7,38] With ulcerative colitis, this genetic component was found to be weaker, but still present. These associations clearly indicate that genetic susceptibility plays an important role in the development of IBD. However, classic mendelian inheritance patterns are not seen, and IBD therefore cannot be attributed to a single gene. Many candidate genes are known to be associated with, and likely to contribute to, the development of IBD. These include the human leukocyte antigen (HLA) associations. Ulcerative colitis has been associated with HLA-D2 and Crohn disease with the HLA-

CHARACTERISTIC	CROHN DISEASE	ULCERATIVE COLITIS
Types of inflammation	Granulomatous	Ulcerative and exudative
Level of involvement	Primarily submucosal	Primarily mucosal
Extent of involvement	Skip lesions	Continuous
Areas of involvement	Primarily ileum, secondarily colon	Primarily rectum and left colon
Diarrhea	Common	Common
Rectal bleeding	Rare	Common
Fistulas	Common	Rare
Strictures	Common	Rare
Perianal abscesses	Common	Rare
Development of cancer	Uncommon	Relatively common

TABLE 37-1 **Differentiating Characteristics of Crohn Disease and Ulcerative Colitis**

DR1 and HLA-DQw5 alleles, suggesting that the two diseases are genetically distinct.[7] Accumulating evidence also suggests that both Crohn disease and ulcerative colitis are associated with profound disorders of mucosal immunity. The IBD1 locus on chromosome 16 has recently been shown to contribute to Crohn disease.[7,38,39] The product of the implicated gene, NOD2 (so named because the coded protein has a nucleotide oligomerization domain) activates the nuclear kappa beta (NFκβ) transcription factor. The NOD2 protein is expressed in many types of leukocytes as well as epithelial cells and is thought to act as an intracellular receptor for lipopolysaccharides on microbes. On binding microbial products, it may trigger the NFκβ pathway, which leads to the production of cytokines and other proteins involved in the innate immune defense against microorganisms. The NOD2 mutations that are associated with Crohn disease may reduce the activity of the protein, resulting in persistence of intracellular microbes and prolonged immune responses. Another region studied extensively is IBD3 on chromosome 6. This is the area that includes the HLA complex that has been linked to Crohn disease and ulcerative colitis. Another area linked specifically to Crohn disease is on chromosome 5q (IBD5). This area is rich in genes encoding several cytokines that may contribute to the disease.

Role of Environmental Factors. Animal studies have definitively established the importance of the gut flora in IBD. The sites affected by IBD, the distal ileum and the colon, are awash with bacteria. Although it is unlikely that IBD is caused by microbes, it seems likely that microbes may provide the antigen trigger for an unregulated immune response.

Interestingly, smoking tobacco has the opposite effect on the two forms of IBD. It predisposes to development of Crohn disease, yet is associated with a reduced incidence of ulcerative colitis. Smoking also increases the likelihood of disease exaggeration and need for surgery in people with Crohn disease.[40]

Crohn Disease

Crohn disease is a recurrent, granulomatous type of inflammatory response that can affect any area of the gastrointestinal tract. In nearly 40% of persons with the disease, the lesions are restricted to the small intestine; in 30%, only the large bowel is affected; and in the remaining 30%, the large bowel and small bowel are affected.[7] It is a slowly progressive, relentless, and often disabling disease. The disease usually strikes people in their twenties or thirties, with women being affected slightly more often than men.

A characteristic feature of Crohn disease is the sharply demarcated, granulomatous lesions that are surrounded by normal-appearing mucosal tissue. When the lesions are multiple, they often are referred to as *skip lesions* because they are interspersed between what appear to be normal segments of the bowel. All the layers of the bowel are involved, with the submucosal layer affected to the greatest extent. The surface of the inflamed bowel usually has a characteristic "cobblestone" appearance resulting from the fissures and crevices that develop,

surrounded by areas of submucosal edema[7,8] (Fig. 37-7). There usually is a relative sparing of the smooth muscle layers of the bowel, with marked inflammatory and fibrotic changes of the submucosal layer. The bowel wall, after a time, often becomes thickened and inflexible; its appearance has been likened to a lead pipe or rubber hose. The adjacent mesentery may become inflamed, and the regional lymph nodes and channels may become enlarged.

Clinical Features. The clinical course of Crohn disease is variable; often, there are periods of exacerbations and remissions, with symptoms being related to the location of the lesions. The principal symptoms include intermittent diarrhea, colicky pain (usually in the lower right quadrant), weight loss, fluid and electrolyte disorders, malaise, and low-grade fever.[43,44] Because Crohn disease affects the submucosal layer to a greater extent than the mucosal layer, there is less bloody diarrhea than with ulcerative colitis. Ulceration of the perianal skin is common, largely because of the severity of the diarrhea. The absorptive surface of the intestine may be disrupted; nutritional deficiencies may occur, related to the specific segment of the intestine involved. When Crohn disease occurs in childhood, one of its major manifestations may be retardation of growth and physical development.

Complications of Crohn disease include fistula formation, abdominal abscess formation, and intestinal obstruction. Fistulas are tubelike passages that form connections between different sites in the gastrointestinal tract. They also may develop between other sites, including the bladder, vagina, urethra, and skin. Perineal fistulas that originate in the ileum are relatively common. Fistulas between segments of the gastrointestinal tract may lead to malabsorption, syndromes of bacterial overgrowth, and diarrhea. They also can become infected and cause abscess formation.

The diagnosis of Crohn disease requires a thorough history and physical examination. Sigmoidoscopy is used for direct visualization of the affected areas and to obtain biopsies. Measures are taken to exclude infectious agents as the cause of

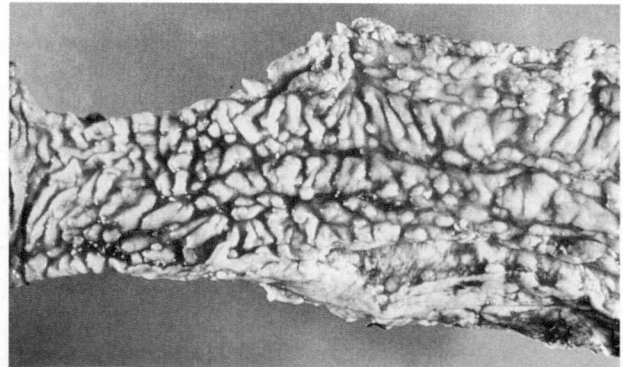

FIGURE 37-7 • Crohn disease. The mucosal surface of the colon displays a "cobblestone" appearance owing to the presence of linear ulcerations and edema and inflammation of the intervening tissue. (From Rubin E., Farber J. L. [Eds.]. [1999]. *Pathology* [3rd ed., p. 728]. Philadelphia: Lippincott Williams & Wilkins.)

the disorder. This usually is accomplished by the use of stool cultures and examination of fresh stool specimens for ova and parasites. In persons suspected of having Crohn disease, radiographic contrast studies provide a means for determining the extent of involvement of the small bowel and establishing the presence and nature of fistulas. CT scans may be used to detect an inflammatory mass or abscess.

Treatment methods focus on terminating the inflammatory response and promoting healing, maintaining adequate nutrition, and preventing and treating complications. Several medications have been successful in suppressing the inflammatory reaction, including the corticosteroids, sulfasalazine, metronidazole, azathioprine, 6-mercaptopurine, methotrexate, and infliximab. Surgical resection of damaged bowel, drainage of abscesses, or repair of fistula tracts may be necessary.

Sulfasalazine is a topically active agent that has a variety of anti-inflammatory effects. The beneficial effects of sulfasalazine are attributable to one component of the drug, 5-aminosalicylic acid (5-ASA). Agents containing 5-ASA affect multiple sites in the arachidonic acid pathway critical to the pathogenesis of inflammation. Sulfasalazine contains 5-ASA with sulfapyridine linked to an azo bond. The drug is poorly absorbed from the intestine, and the azo linkage is broken down by the bacterial flora in the ileum and colon to release 5-ASA. Metronidazole is an antibiotic used to treat bacterial overgrowth in the small intestine. Azathioprine, 6-mercaptopurine, and methotrexate are immunomodulating drugs that are used in the approximately one third of persons who do not respond to other forms of therapy.[13]

Infliximab is a monoclonal antibody that targets the destruction of tumor necrosis factor (TNF), a mediator of the inflammatory response that is known to be important in granulomatous inflammatory processes such as Crohn disease.[44] It is the first drug approved specifically for Crohn disease and is used in the treatment of persons with active moderate to severe Crohn disease who have had an inadequate response to corticosteroids or other immune modulators. Although infliximab is currently the only anti-TNF agent approved for treatment of persons with IBD, controlled studies of other anti-TNF and immunomodulating agents are ongoing.

Nutritional deficiencies are common in Crohn disease because of diarrhea, steatorrhea, and other malabsorption problems. A nutritious diet that is high in calories, vitamins, and proteins is recommended. Because fats often aggravate the diarrhea, it is recommended that they be avoided. Elemental diets, which are nutritionally balanced but residue free and bulk free, may be given during the acute phase of the illness. These diets are largely absorbed in the jejunum and allow the inflamed bowel to rest. Total parenteral nutrition (*i.e.,* parenteral hyperalimentation) consists of intravenous administration of hypertonic glucose solutions to which amino acids and fats may be added. This form of nutritional therapy may be needed when food cannot be absorbed from the intestine. Because of the hypertonicity of these solutions, they must be administered through a large-diameter central vein.

Ulcerative Colitis

Ulcerative colitis is a nonspecific inflammatory condition of the colon. The disease is more common in the United States and Western countries. The disease may arise at any age, with a peak incidence between ages 20 and 25 years.[7] Unlike Crohn disease, which can affect various sites in the gastrointestinal tract, ulcerative colitis is confined to the rectum and colon. The disease usually begins in the rectum and spreads proximally, affecting primarily the mucosal layer, although it can extend into the submucosal layer. The length of proximal extension varies. It may involve the rectum alone (ulcerative proctitis), the rectum and sigmoid colon (proctosigmoiditis), or the entire colon (pancolitis). The inflammatory process tends to be confluent and continuous instead of skipping areas, as it does in Crohn disease.

Characteristic of the disease are the lesions that form in the crypts of Lieberkühn in the base of the mucosal layer (see Chapter 36, Fig. 36-12). The inflammatory process leads to the formation of pinpoint mucosal hemorrhages, which in time suppurate and develop into *crypt abscesses*. These inflammatory lesions may become necrotic and ulcerate. Although the ulcerations usually are superficial, they often extend, causing large denuded areas (Fig. 37-8). As a result of the inflammatory process, the mucosal layer often develops tonguelike projections that resemble polyps and therefore are called *pseudopolyps*. The bowel wall thickens in response to repeated episodes of colitis.

Clinical Features. Ulcerative colitis typically presents as a relapsing disorder marked by attacks of diarrhea. The diarrhea may persist for days, weeks, or months and then subside, only to recur after an asymptomatic interval of several months to years or even decades. Because ulcerative colitis affects the mucosal layer of the bowel, the stools typically contain blood and mucus. Nocturnal diarrhea usually occurs when daytime symptoms are severe. There may be mild abdominal cramping

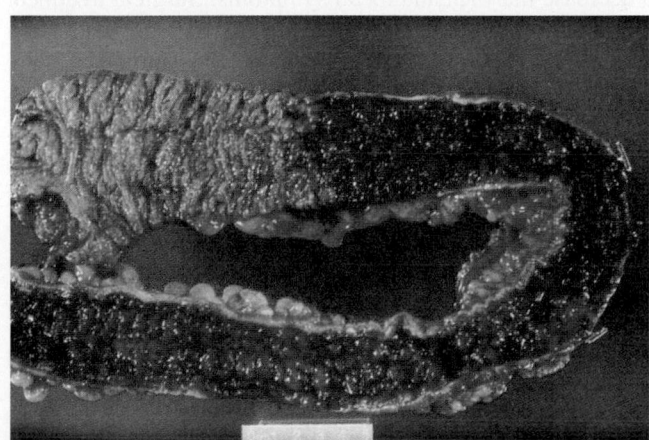

FIGURE 37-8 • Ulcerative colitis. Prominent erythema and ulceration of the colon begin in the ascending colon and are most severe in the rectosigmoid area. (From Mitos F. A., Rubin E. [2008]. The gastrointestinal tract. In Rubin R., Strayer D. S. [Eds.], *Rubin's pathophysiology: Clinicopathologic foundations of medicine* [5th ed., p. 597]. Philadelphia: Lippincott Williams & Wilkins.)

and fecal incontinence. Anorexia, weakness, and fatigability are common.

Based on clinical and endoscopic findings, the disease is characterized by its severity and extent. Severity is defined as mild, moderate, severe, or fulminant.[45] The most common form of the disease is the mild form, in which the person has less than four stools daily, with or without blood, no systemic signs of toxicity, and a normal erythrocyte sedimentation rate (ESR). Persons with moderate disease have more than four stools daily, but have minimal signs of toxicity. Severe disease is manifested by more than six bloody stools daily, and evidence of toxicity as demonstrated by fever, tachycardia, anemia, and elevated ESR. Persons with fulminant disease have features that include more than 10 bowel movements a day, continuous bleeding, fever and other signs of toxicity, abdominal tenderness and distention, need for blood transfusions, and colonic dilation on abdominal radiographs. These persons are at risk for development of toxic megacolon, which is characterized by dilation of the colon and signs of systemic toxicity. It results from extension of the inflammatory response, with involvement of neural and vascular components of the bowel.

Diagnosis of ulcerative colitis is based on history and physical examination. The diagnosis usually is confirmed by sigmoidoscopy, colonoscopy, biopsy, and by negative stool examinations for infectious or other causes. Colonoscopy should not be performed on persons with severe disease because of the danger of perforation, but may be performed after demonstrated improvement to determine the extent of disease and need for subsequent cancer surveillance.

Treatment depends on the extent of the disease and severity of symptoms. It includes measures to control the acute manifestations of the disease and prevent recurrence. Some people with mild to moderate symptoms are able to control their symptoms simply by avoiding caffeine, lactose (milk), highly spiced foods, and gas-forming foods. Fiber supplements may be used to decrease diarrhea and rectal symptoms. Surgical treatment (*i.e.,* removal of the rectum and entire colon) with the creation of an ileostomy or ileoanal anastomosis may be required for persons who do not respond to medications and conservative methods of treatment.

The medications used in treatment of ulcerative colitis are similar to those used in the treatment of Crohn disease. They include the nonabsorbable 5-ASA compounds (*e.g.,* mesalamine, olsalazine).[45] The corticosteroids are used selectively to lessen the acute inflammatory response. Many of these medications can be administered rectally by suppository or enema. Immunomodulating drugs and anti-TNF therapies may be used to treat persons with severe colitis.

Cancer of the colon is one of the feared complications of ulcerative colitis. Ulcerative colitis is characterized by deoxyribonucleic acid (DNA) damage with microsatellite instability in mucosa cells. More recently, genomic instability was detected in nondysplastic areas of persons with ulcerative colitis, suggesting that these persons have DNA repair deficiency and genomic instability throughout the intestinal tract. Historically,

the risk for development of cancer among persons who have had pancolitis for 10 years or more is 20 to 30 times that of the general population.[7] Because of this relatively high risk for development of cancer, regular annual or biannual surveillance colonoscopies with multiple biopsies are recommended for persons with extensive colitis, beginning 8 to 10 years after diagnosis.[45]

Infectious Enterocolitis

A number of microbial agents, including viruses, bacteria, and protozoa, can infect the gastrointestinal tract, causing diarrhea and sometimes ulcerative and inflammatory changes in the small or large intestine. Infectious enterocolitis is a global problem, causing more than 12,000 deaths per day among children in developing countries. Although far less common in industrialized countries, these disorders still have infection rates second only to the common cold. Most infections are spread by the oral-fecal route, often through contaminated water or food.

Viral Infection

Most viral infections affect the superficial epithelium of the small intestine, destroying these cells and disrupting their absorptive function. Repopulation of the small intestinal villi with immature enterocytes and preservation of crypt secretory cells leads to net secretion of water and electrolytes compounded by incomplete absorption of nutrients and osmotic diarrhea. Symptomatic disease is caused by several distinct viruses, including the rotavirus, which most commonly affects children 6 to 24 months of age; the Norwalk virus, which is responsible for the majority of nonbacterial food-borne epidemic gastroenteritis in all age groups: and enteric adenoviruses, which primarily affect children.[7]

Rotavirus. Worldwide, rotavirus is estimated to cause more than 125 million cases of diarrhea in children younger than 5 years of age. In the United States, the disease causes 3 million cases of diarrhea, 50,000 hospitalizations, and 20 to 40 deaths per year.[46] The disease tends to be most severe in children 3 to 24 months of age. Infants younger than 3 months of age are relatively protected by transplacental antibodies and possibly by breast-feeding. The virus is spread by a fecal-oral route and outbreaks are common in children in day care centers. The virus is shed before and for days after clinical illness. Very few infectious virions are needed to cause disease in a susceptible host.

Rotavirus infection typically begins after an incubation period of less than 24 hours, with mild to moderate fever and vomiting, followed by onset of frequent watery stools. The fever and vomiting usually disappear on about the second day, but the diarrhea continues for 5 to 7 days. Dehydration may develop rapidly, particularly in infants.

Treatment is largely supportive. Avoiding and treating dehydration are the main goals. A live oral vaccine for rotavirus

(RotaTeq) was approved by the FDA in 2006.[47] A different live vaccine was approved in 1998 but was withdrawn from the market less than a year later when several infants developed intussusception after receiving the vaccine.

Bacterial Infection

Infectious enterocolitis can be caused by a number of bacteria. There are several pathogenic mechanisms for bacterial enterocolitis: ingestion of preformed toxins that are present in contaminated food; infection by toxigenic organisms that proliferate in the gut lumen and produce an enterotoxin; and infection by enteroinvasive organisms, which proliferate in the lumen and invade and destroy mucosal epithelial cells. The pathogenic effects of bacterial infections depend on the ability of the organism to adhere to the mucosal epithelial cells, elaborate enterotoxins, then invade the mucosal epithelial cells.

In general, bacterial infections produce more severe effects than viral infections. The complications of bacterial enterocolitis result from massive fluid loss or destruction of intestinal mucosa and include dehydration, sepsis, and perforation. Among the organisms that cause bacterial enterocolitis are *Staphylococcus aureus* (toxins associated with "food poisoning"), *Escherichia coli*, *Shigella* species, *Salmonella*, and *Campylobacter*. Two particularly serious forms of bacterial enterocolitis are caused by *Clostridium difficile* and *E. coli* O157:H7.

Clostridium difficile **Colitis.** *C. difficile* colitis is associated with antibiotic therapy.[48–50] *C. difficile* is a gram-positive, spore-forming bacillus that is part of the normal flora in 1% to 3% of humans.[50] The spores are resistant to the acid environment of the stomach and convert to vegetative forms in the colon. Treatment with broad-spectrum antibiotics predisposes to disruption of the normal protective bacterial flora of the colon, leading to colonization by *C. difficile* along with the release of toxins that cause mucosal damage and inflammation. Almost any antibiotic may cause *C. difficile* colitis, but broad-spectrum antibiotics with activity against gram-negative enteric bacteria are the most frequent agents. After antibiotic therapy has made the bowel susceptible to infection, colonization by *C. difficile* occurs by the oral-fecal route. *C. difficile* infection usually is acquired in the hospital, where the organism is commonly encountered.

In general, *C. difficile* is noninvasive. Development of *C. difficile* colitis and diarrhea requires an alteration in the normal gut flora, acquisition and germination of the spores, overgrowth of *C. difficile*, and toxin production. The toxins bind to and damage the intestinal mucosa, causing hemorrhage, inflammation, and necrosis. The toxins also interfere with protein synthesis, attract inflammatory cells, increase capillary permeability, and stimulate intestinal peristalsis. The infection commonly manifests with diarrhea that is mild to moderate and sometimes is accompanied by lower abdominal cramping. Typically symptoms begin within 1 to 2 weeks after an antibiotic treatment has been started, although presentation varies from 1 day to 6 weeks.[50] In most cases, systemic manifestations are absent, and the symptoms subside after the antibiotic has been discontinued.

A more severe form of colitis, *pseudomembranous colitis*, is characterized by an adherent inflammatory membrane overlying the areas of mucosal injury. It is a life-threatening form of the disease. Persons with the disease are acutely ill, with lethargy, fever, tachycardia, abdominal pain and distention, and dehydration. The smooth muscle tone of the colon may be lost, resulting in toxic dilation of the colon. Prompt therapy is needed to prevent perforation of the bowel.

The diagnosis of *C. difficile*–associated diarrhea requires a careful history, with particular emphasis on antibiotic use. Diagnostic findings include a history of antibiotic use and laboratory tests that confirm the presence of *C. difficile* toxins in the stool. Treatment includes the immediate discontinuation of antibiotic therapy. Specific treatment aimed at eradicating *C. difficile* is used when symptoms are severe or persistent. Metronidazole is the drug of first choice, with vancomycin being reserved for persons who cannot tolerate metronidazole or do not respond to the drug. Both drugs are given orally.[48–50] Metronidazole is absorbed from the upper gastrointestinal tract and may cause side effects. Vancomycin is poorly absorbed, and its actions are limited to the gastrointestinal tract.

Escherichia coli **O157:H7 Infection.** *E. coli* O157:H7 has become recognized as an important cause of epidemic and sporadic colitis.[51] *E. coli* O157:H7 is a strain of *E. coli* found in the feces and contaminated milk of healthy dairy and beef cattle, but it also has been found in contaminated pork, poultry, and lamb. Infection usually is by food-borne transmission, often by ingesting undercooked hamburger. The organism also can be transferred to nonmeat products such as fruits and vegetables. Transmission has also been reported in persons swimming in a fecally contaminated lake as well as among visitors to farms and petting zoos, where children are in direct contact with animals. Person-to-person transmission may occur, particularly in nursing homes, day care settings, and hospitals. The very young and the very old are particularly at risk for the infection and its complications.

The infection may cause no symptoms or cause a variety of manifestations, including acute, nonbloody diarrhea; hemorrhagic colitis; hemolytic uremic syndrome; and thrombotic thrombocytopenic purpura. The infection often presents with abdominal cramping and watery diarrhea and subsequently may progress to bloody diarrhea. The diarrhea commonly lasts 3 to 7 days or longer, with 10 to 12 diarrheal episodes per day. Fever occurs in up to one third of the cases.

Most strains of *E. coli* are harmless; however, enterohemorrhagic *E. coli* can release *Shigella*-like toxins that attach to and damage the mucosal lining of the intestine, causing bloody diarrhea.[52,53] Subsequently, the *Shigella*-like toxins gain access to the circulatory system and travel in the plasma and on the surface of platelets and monocytes. The *Shigella*-like toxins bind to high-affinity galactose-containing receptors in the membranes of glomerular, cerebral, or microvascular endothelial cells; renal mesangial and tubular cells; and monocytes and platelets.[53] Two complications of the infection, hemolytic uremic syndrome and thrombotic thrombocytopenic purpura, reflect the effects of the *Shigella*-like toxins. The hemolytic uremic syndrome is characterized by hemolytic anemia, thrombocytopenia, and renal failure. It occurs predominantly in infants and young children and is the most common cause of acute renal failure in children. It has a mortality rate of 3% to 5%, and one third of the survivors are left with permanent disability.[54] Thrombotic thrombocytopenic purpura is manifested by thrombocytopenia, renal failure, fever, and neurologic manifestations. It often is regarded as the severe end of the disease that leads to hemolytic uremic syndrome plus neurologic problems.

No specific therapy is available for *E. coli* O157:H7 infection. Treatment is largely symptomatic and directed toward treating the effects of complications. The use of antibiotics or antimotility/antidiarrheal agents in the early stages of diarrhea has been shown to increase the risk of hemolytic uremic syndrome because the gut is exposed to a greater amount of toxins for a longer time.

Because of the seriousness of the infection and its complications, education of the public about techniques for decreasing primary transmission of the infection from animal sources is important. Undercooked meats and unpasteurized milk are sources of transmission. Food handlers and consumers should be aware of the proper methods for handling uncooked meat to prevent cross-contamination of other foods. Particular attention should be paid to hygiene in day care centers and nursing homes, where the spread of infection to the very young and very old may result in severe complications.

Protozoan Infection

Amebiasis refers to an infection by *Entamoeba histolytica* involving the colon and occasionally the liver.[55,56] Humans are the only known reservoir for *E. histolytica*, which reproduce in the colon and pass in the feces. Although *E. histolytica* infection occurs worldwide, it is more common and more severe in tropical and subtropical areas, where crowding and poor sanitation prevail. Intestinal amebiasis ranges from completely asymptomatic infection to serious dysenteric disease.

E. histolytica has two distinct stages: the trophozoites (ameboid form) and cysts.[55] The trophozoites thrive in the colon and feed on bacteria and human cells. They may colonize any portion of the large bowel, but the area of maximum disease is usually the cecum. Persons with symptomatic disease pass both cysts and trophozoites in their feces, but the latter survive only briefly outside the body. Only the cysts are infectious because they survive gastric acidity, which destroys the trophozoites. Once established, the trophozoites invade the crypts of colonic glands and burrow down into the submucosa; the organism then fans out to create a flask-shaped ulcer with a narrow neck and broad base. *E. histolytica* that have invaded into the submucosal veins of the colon enter the portal vein and embolize to the liver to produce solitary and, less often, multiple discrete hepatic abscesses.[56]

Some people have an acute onset of diarrhea as early as 8 days (commonly 2 to 4 weeks) after infection.[55] Others may be asymptomatic or have only mild intestinal symptoms for months or several years before either intestinal symptoms or liver abscesses appear. Manifestations include abdominal discomfort, tenderness, cramps, and fever, often accompanied by nausea, vomiting, and passage of malodorous flatus. There may be frequent passage of liquid stools containing bloody mucus, but the duration of diarrhea is not usually so prolonged as to cause dehydration. The infection often persists for months or years, causing emaciation and anemia. In severe cases, massive destruction of the colonic mucosa may lead to hemorrhage, perforation, or peritonitis. Persons with amebic liver abscesses often present with severe right upper quadrant pain, low-grade fever, and weight loss.[56]

Diagnostic methods include microscopic examination of the stool for *E. histolytica*, serum antibody tests, and colonoscopy with specimen collection or biopsy. Treatment includes use of the antimicrobial agents tinidazole and metronidazole, which act against the trophozoites, and diloxanide (not available in the United States), which is effective against the cysts.

Diverticular Disease

Diverticulosis is a condition in which the mucosal layer of the colon herniates through the muscularis layer.[57,58] There are often multiple diverticula, most of which occur in the sigmoid colon (Fig. 37-9). Diverticular disease is common in Western society, affecting approximately 5% to 10% of the population older than 45 years of age and almost 80% of those older than 85 years.[57] Although the disorder is prevalent in the developed countries of the world, it is almost nonexistent in many African nations and underdeveloped countries. This suggests that factors such as lack of fiber in the diet, a decrease in physical activity, and poor bowel habits (*e.g.,* neglecting the urge to

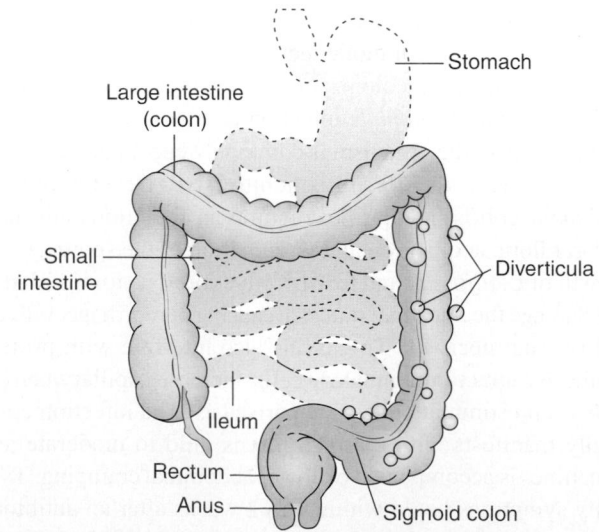

FIGURE 37-9 • Location of diverticula in the sigmoid colon.

defecate), along with the effects of aging, contribute to the development of the disease.

In the colon, the longitudinal muscle does not form a continuous layer, as it does in the small bowel. Instead, there are three separate longitudinal bands of muscle called the *teniae coli*. In a manner similar to the small intestine, bands of circular muscle constrict the large intestine. As the circular muscle contracts at each of these points (approximately every 2.5 cm), the lumen of the bowel becomes constricted, so that it is almost occluded. The combined contraction of the circular muscle and the lack of a continuous longitudinal muscle layer cause the intestine to bulge outward into pouches called *haustra*. Diverticula develop between the longitudinal muscle bands of the haustra, in the area where the blood vessels pierce the circular muscle layer to bring blood to the mucosal layer. An increase in intraluminal pressure in the haustra provides the force for creating these herniations. The increase in pressure is thought to be related to the volume of the colonic contents. The scantier the contents, the more vigorous are the contractions and the greater is the pressure in the haustra.

Most persons with diverticular disease remain asymptomatic. The disease often is found when x-ray studies are done for other purposes. When symptoms do occur, they often are attributed to irritable bowel syndrome or other causes. Ill-defined lower abdominal discomfort, a change in bowel habits (*e.g.,* diarrhea, constipation), bloating, and flatulence are common.

Diverticulitis is a complication of diverticulosis in which there is inflammation and gross or microscopic perforation of the diverticulum. One of the most common complaints of diverticulitis is pain in the lower left quadrant, accompanied by nausea and vomiting, tenderness in the lower left quadrant, a slight fever, and an elevated white blood cell count. These symptoms usually last for several days, unless complications occur, and usually are caused by localized inflammation of the diverticula with perforation and development of a small, localized abscess. Complications include perforation with peritonitis, hemorrhage, and bowel obstruction. Fistulas can form, usually involving the bladder (*i.e.,* vesicosigmoid fistula) but sometimes involving the skin, perianal area, or small bowel. Pneumaturia (*i.e.,* air in the urine) is a sign of vesicosigmoid fistula.

The diagnosis of diverticular disease is based on history and presenting clinical manifestations. The disease may be confirmed by CT scans or ultrasonographic studies. CT scans are the safest and most cost-effective method.[57] Although barium enema was used in the past, it is no longer recommended because of the risk of extravasation of contrast material if perforation has occurred.[58] Flat abdominal radiographs may be used to detect complications associated with acute diverticulitis.

The usual treatment for diverticular disease is to prevent symptoms and complications. This includes increasing the bulk in the diet and bowel retraining so that the person has at least one bowel movement each day. The increased bulk promotes regular defecation and increases colonic contents and colon diameter, thereby decreasing intraluminal pressure. Acute diverticulitis is treated by withholding solid food and administering a broad-spectrum antibiotic. Hospitalization may be required for persons who show significant inflammation, are unable to tolerate oral fluids, are older than 85 years, or have significant comorbid conditions.[58] Surgical treatment is reserved for complications.

Appendicitis

Acute appendicitis is extremely common. It is seen most frequently in the 5- to 30-year-old age group, but it can occur at any age. The appendix becomes inflamed, swollen, and gangrenous, and it eventually perforates if not treated. Although the cause of appendicitis is unknown, it is thought to be related to intraluminal obstruction with a fecalith (*i.e.,* hard piece of stool) or to twisting.

Appendicitis usually has an abrupt onset, with pain referred to the epigastric or periumbilical area. This pain is caused by stretching of the appendix during the early inflammatory process. At approximately the same time that the pain appears, there are one or two episodes of nausea. Initially, the pain is vague, but over a period of 2 to 12 hours, it gradually increases and may become colicky. When the inflammatory process has extended to involve the serosal layer of the appendix and the peritoneum, the pain becomes localized to the lower right quadrant. There usually is an elevation in temperature and a white blood cell count greater than 10,000/mm^3, with 75% or more polymorphonuclear cells. Palpation of the abdomen usually reveals a deep tenderness in the lower right quadrant, which is confined to a small area approximately the size of the fingertip. It usually is located at approximately the site of the inflamed appendix. The person with appendicitis often is able to place his or her finger directly over the tender area. Rebound tenderness, which is pain that occurs when pressure is applied to the area and then released, and spasm of the overlying abdominal muscles are common.

Diagnosis is usually based on history and findings on physical examination. Ultrasonography or CT may be used to confirm the diagnosis.[59] Treatment consists of surgical removal of the appendix. Complications include peritonitis, localized periappendiceal abscess formation, and septicemia.

Alterations in Intestinal Motility

The movement of contents through the gastrointestinal tract is controlled by neurons located in the submucosal and myenteric plexuses of the gut (see Chapter 36). The axons from the cell bodies in the myenteric plexus innervate the circular and longitudinal smooth muscle layers of the gut. These neurons receive impulses from local receptors located in the mucosal and muscle layers of the gut and extrinsic input from the parasympathetic and sympathetic nervous systems. As a general rule, the parasympathetic nervous system tends to increase the motility of the bowel, whereas sympathetic stimulation tends to slow its activity.

DISORDERS OF GASTROINTESTINAL MOTILITY

■ The luminal contents move down the gastrointestinal tract as a result of peristaltic movements regulated by a complex interaction of electrical, neural, and hormonal control mechanisms.

■ The enteric nervous system that is incorporated into the wall of the gut controls the basic movement of the gastrointestinal tract, with input from the autonomic nervous system.

■ Local irritation and the composition and constituents of gastrointestinal contents influence motility through the submucosal afferent neurons of the enteric nervous system. Gastrointestinal wall distention, chemical irritants, osmotic gradients, and bacterial toxins exert many of their effects on gastrointestinal motility through these afferent pathways.

■ Autonomic influences generated by factors such as medications, trauma, and emotional experiences interact with the enteric nervous system to alter gastrointestinal motility.

The colon has sphincters at both ends: the ileocecal sphincter, which separates it from the small intestine, and the anal sphincter, which prevents the movement of feces to the outside of the body. The colon acts as a reservoir for fecal material. Normally, approximately 400 mL of water, 55 mEq of sodium, 30 mEq of chloride, and 15 mEq of bicarbonate are absorbed each day in the colon. At the same time, approximately 5 mEq of potassium is secreted into the lumen of the colon. The amount of water and electrolytes that remains in the stool reflects the absorption or secretion that occurs in the colon. The average adult ingesting a typical American diet evacuates approximately 200 to 300 g of stool each day.

Diarrhea

The usual definition of *diarrhea* is excessively frequent passage of stools. The complaint of diarrhea is a general one and can be related to a number of pathologic and nonpathologic factors. Diarrhea can be acute or chronic and can be caused by infectious organisms, food intolerance, drugs, or intestinal disease. Acute diarrheas that last less than 4 days are predominantly caused by infectious agents and follow a self-limited course.[60]

Acute Diarrhea. Diarrhea that is acute in onset and persists for less than 2 weeks is commonly caused by infectious agents (see previous discussion of infectious enterocolitis). Acute diarrhea is commonly divided into noninflammatory (large-volume) and inflammatory (small-volume) diarrhea, based on the characteristics of the diarrheal stool. Enteric organisms cause diarrhea by several ways. Some are noninvasive and do not cause inflamma-

tion, but secrete toxins that stimulate fluid secretion.[61–63] Others invade and destroy intestinal epithelial cells, thereby altering fluid transport so that secretory activity continues while absorption activity is halted.[61]

Noninflammatory diarrhea is associated with large-volume watery and nonbloody stools, periumbilical cramps, bloating, and nausea or vomiting. It is commonly caused by toxin-producing bacteria (*e.g.,* enterotoxigenic *E. coli, S. aureus, Vibrio cholerae*) or other agents (*e.g.,* viruses, *Giardia*) that disrupt the normal absorption or secretory process in the small bowel. Prominent vomiting suggests viral enteritis or *S. aureus* food poisoning. Although typically mild, the diarrhea (which originates in the small intestine) can be voluminous and result in dehydration with hypokalemia and metabolic acidosis (*i.e.,* cholera). Because tissue invasion does not occur, leukocytes are not present in the feces.

Inflammatory diarrhea is usually characterized by the presence of fever and bloody diarrhea (dysentery). It is caused by invasion of intestinal cells (*e.g., Shigella, Salmonella, Yersinia,* and *Campylobacter*) or the toxins associated with the previously described *C. difficile* or *E. coli* O157:H7 infection. Because infections associated with these organisms predominantly affect the colon, the diarrhea is small in volume (<1 L/day) and is associated with left lower quadrant cramps, urgency, and tenesmus. Infectious dysentery must be distinguished from acute ulcerative colitis, which may present with bloody diarrhea, fever, and abdominal pain. Diarrhea that persists for 14 days is not attributable to bacterial pathogens (except for *C. difficile*), and the person should be evaluated for chronic diarrhea.

Chronic Diarrhea. Diarrhea is considered to be chronic when the symptoms persist for 3 to 4 weeks in children or adults and 4 weeks in infants. Chronic diarrhea is often associated with conditions such as IBD, IBS, malabsorption syndrome, endocrine disorders (hyperthyroidism, diabetic autonomic neuropathy), or radiation colitis. There are four major causes of chronic diarrhea: presence of hyperosmotic luminal contents, increased intestinal secretory processes, inflammatory conditions, and infectious processes[13] (Chart 37-1). Factitious diarrhea is caused by indiscriminate use of laxatives or excessive intake of laxative-type foods.

In *osmotic diarrhea,* water is pulled into the bowel by the hyperosmotic nature of its contents. It occurs when osmotically active particles are not absorbed. In persons with lactase deficiency, the lactose in milk cannot be broken down and absorbed. Magnesium salts, which are contained in milk of magnesia and many antacids, are poorly absorbed and cause diarrhea when taken in sufficient quantities. Another cause of osmotic diarrhea is decreased transit time, which interferes with absorption. Osmotic diarrhea usually disappears with fasting.

Secretory diarrhea occurs when the secretory processes of the bowel are increased. Secretory diarrhea also occurs when excess bile acids remain in the intestinal contents as they enter the colon. This often happens with disease processes of the ileum because bile salts are absorbed there. It also may occur with bacterial overgrowth in the small bowel, which interferes with bile absorption. Some tumors, such as those of the

| CHART 37-1 | **CHRONIC DIARRHEA** |

Hyperosmotic diarrhea
   Saline cathartics
   Lactase deficiency
Secretory diarrhea
   Acute infectious diarrhea
   Failure to absorb bile salts
   Fat malabsorption
   Chronic laxative abuse
   Carcinoid syndrome
   Zollinger-Ellison syndrome
   Fecal impaction
Inflammatory bowel disease
   Crohn disease
   Ulcerative colitis
Infectious disease
   Shigellosis
   Salmonellosis
Irritable colon

drugs. These drugs decrease gastrointestinal motility and stimulate water and electrolyte absorption. Adsorbents, such as kaolin and pectin, adsorb irritants and toxins from the bowel. These ingredients are included in many over-the-counter antidiarrheal preparations because they adsorb toxins responsible for certain types of diarrhea. Bismuth subsalicylate (Pepto-Bismol) can be used to reduce the frequency of unformed stools and increase stool consistency, particularly in cases of traveler's diarrhea. The drug is thought to inhibit intestinal secretion caused by enterotoxigenic *E. coli* and cholera toxins. Antidiarrheal medications should not be used in persons with bloody diarrhea, high fever, or signs of toxicity because of the risk of worsening the disease. Antibiotics should be reserved for use in persons with identified enteric pathogens.

 Acute Diarrheal Disease in Children. In developing countries, diarrhea is a common cause of mortality among children younger than 5 years of age, with an estimated 2 million deaths annually.[64] Although diarrheal diseases are less prevalent in the United States than in other countries, they place a burden on the health care system. Approximately 1.5 million children are seen in outpatient clinics, and 220,000 younger than 5 years of age are hospitalized each year for acute gastroenteritis.[64,65]

The causes of acute diarrhea in children vary with location, time of year, and population studied. There is increasing recognition of a widening array of enteric pathogens that cause acute diarrhea in children. Viruses are the most common pathogen causing diarrheal illness in the United States. Rotaviruses and noroviruses are the frequently observed pathogens. Other viruses that have been observed in the stools of children include astroviruses and enteric adenoviruses. Many of these pathogens are transmitted easily through food and water or from one person to another. Prevention remains the most vital measure in managing diarrheal disease in children. Important measures to prevent spread of pathogens include proper sanitation methods for food processing and preparation, sanitary water supplies, proper hand hygiene, exclusion of infected people from handling food or providing health care, and exclusion of people with diarrhea from using public recreational water (*i.e.*, swimming pools, ponds, and lakes).

The main objectives in the approach to a child with acute diarrhea are to assess the degree of dehydration, prevent spread of the infection, determine the nature of the etiologic agent, and provide specific therapy as needed. The hydration status of children can be assessed on the basis of easily observed signs and symptoms. Questions about oral intake, frequency and volume of stool output, general appearance and activity of the child, and frequency of urination provide essential information about hydration. Children who are not thirsty and have moist mucous membranes, wet diapers, and tears are usually not dehydrated.[65] Data should be obtained about day care attendance, recent travel to a diarrhea-endemic area, use of antimicrobial drugs, and exposure to contaminated water, unwashed fruits or vegetables, or improperly cooked meats because they may indicate the cause of the disorder. Fever is suggestive of an inflammatory process, but also occurs with dehydration.

Zollinger-Ellison syndrome and carcinoid syndrome, produce hormones that cause increased secretory activity of the bowel.

Inflammatory diarrhea commonly is associated with acute or chronic inflammation or intrinsic disease of the colon, such as ulcerative colitis or Crohn disease. Inflammatory diarrhea usually is evidenced by frequency and urgency and colicky abdominal pain. It commonly is accompanied by tenesmus (*i.e.*, painful straining at stool), fecal soiling of clothing, and awakening during the night with the urge to defecate.

Chronic parasitic infections may cause chronic diarrhea through a number of mechanisms. Pathogens most commonly associated with chronic diarrhea include the protozoans *Giardia, E. histolytica,* and *Cyclospora.* Immunocompromised persons are particularly susceptible to infectious organisms that can cause acute and chronic diarrhea (see Chapter 20), including *Cryptosporidium,* cytomegalovirus (CMV), and *Mycobacterium avium-intracellulare* complex.

Diagnosis and Treatment. The diagnosis of diarrhea is based on complaints of frequent stools and a history of accompanying factors such as concurrent illnesses, medication use, and exposure to potential intestinal pathogens. Disorders such as IBD should be considered. If the onset of diarrhea is related to travel outside the United States, the possibility of traveler's diarrhea must be considered.

Although most acute forms of diarrhea are self-limited and require no treatment, diarrhea can be particularly serious in infants and small children, persons with other illnesses, elderly persons, and even previously healthy persons if it continues for any length of time. Thus, the replacement of fluids and electrolytes is considered to be a primary therapeutic goal in the treatment of diarrhea.

Drugs used in the treatment of diarrhea include diphenoxylate (Lomotil) and loperamide (Imodium), which are opium-like

Management of dehydration remains the cornerstone of treatment of children with diarrhea. Infants in particular are more susceptible to dehydration because of their greater surface area, higher metabolic rate, and inability effectively to concentrate their urine. Oral replacement therapy (ORT) is usually the method of choice for infants and children with uncomplicated diarrhea that can be treated at home.

First applied to the treatment of diarrhea in developing countries, ORT can be regarded as a case of reverse technology, in which the protocols originally implemented in these countries have changed health care in industrialized countries as well.[64] Complete ORT solutions contain carbohydrate, sodium, potassium, chloride, and base to replace that lost in the diarrheal stool.[64-67] Commonly used beverages such as apple juice and cola drinks, which have increased osmolarity because of their high carbohydrate content and low electrolyte content, are not recommended. The effectiveness of ORT is based on the coupled transport of sodium and glucose or other actively transported small organic molecules (see Chapter 36). Bottled ORT solutions are available but can be costly, particularly in cases where large amounts of replacement fluids are needed. The cost can represent a sizable burden for socioeconomically disadvantaged families. Less expensive, premeasured packets and recipes for preparing replacement solutions are available. The use of ORT for treatment of diarrhea in infants and small children is often labor intensive, requiring frequent feeding, sometimes using a spoon.[61] More importantly, the diarrhea does not promptly cease after ORT has been instituted; this can be discouraging for parents and caregivers who desire early results from their efforts. Children who are severely dehydrated with changes in vital signs or mental status require emergency intravenous fluid resuscitation. After initial treatment with intravenous fluids, these children can be given ORT.

Evidence suggests that feeding should be continued during diarrheal illness, particularly in children.[63,64,66] It has been shown that unrestricted diets do not worsen the course or symptoms of mild diarrhea and can decrease stool output.[64,67] Starch and simple proteins are thought to provide cotransport molecules with little osmotic activity, increasing fluid and electrolyte uptake by intestinal cells. The luminal contents associated with early refeeding are also a known growth factor for enterocytes and help facilitate repair after injury. It is recommended that children who require rehydration therapy because of diarrhea be fed an age-appropriate diet. Although there is little agreement on which foods are best, fatty foods and foods high in simple sugars are best avoided. No data suggest that a diet consisting of only bananas, rice, applesauce, and toast (the BRAT diet) speeds recovery from diarrheal illnesses.[65] Almost all infants with acute gastroenteritis can tolerate breast-feeding. For formula-fed infants, diluted formula does not provide an advantage over full-strength formula.

Constipation

Constipation can be defined as the infrequent or difficult passage of stools.[68-71] The difficulty with this definition arises from the many individual variations of function that are normal. What is considered normal for one person (*e.g.*, two or three bowel movements per week) may be considered evidence of constipation by another. Constipation can occur as a primary disorder of intestinal motility, as a side effect of drugs, as a problem associated with another disease condition, or as a symptom of obstructing lesions of the gastrointestinal tract. Some common causes of constipation are failure to respond to the urge to defecate, inadequate fiber in the diet, inadequate fluid intake, weakness of the abdominal muscles, inactivity and bed rest, pregnancy, and hemorrhoids. The pathophysiology of constipation can be classified into three broad categories: normal-transit constipation, slow-transit constipation, and disorders of defecatory or rectal evacuation. Normal-transit constipation (or functional constipation) is characterized by perceived difficulty in defecation and usually responds to increased fluid and fiber intake. Slow-transit constipation, which is characterized by infrequent bowel movements, is often caused by alterations in intestinal innervation. Hirschsprung disease is an extreme form of slow-transit constipation in which the ganglion cells in the distal bowel are absent because of a defect that occurred during embryonic development; the bowel narrows at the area that lacks ganglionic cells. Although most persons with this disorder present in infancy or early childhood, some with a relatively short segment of involved colon do not have symptoms until later in life. Defecatory disorders are most commonly due to dysfunction of the pelvic floor or anal sphincter.

Diseases associated with chronic constipation include neurologic diseases such as spinal cord injury, Parkinson disease, and multiple sclerosis; endocrine disorders such as hypothyroidism; and obstructive lesions in the gastrointestinal tract. Drugs such as narcotics, anticholinergic agents, calcium channel blockers, diuretics, calcium (antacids and supplements), iron supplements, and aluminum antacids tend to cause constipation. Elderly people with long-standing constipation may develop dilation of the rectum, colon, or both. This condition allows large amounts of stool to accumulate with little or no sensation. Constipation, in the context of a change in bowel habits, may be a sign of colorectal cancer.

Diagnosis of constipation usually is based on a history of infrequent stools, straining with defecation, the passing of hard and lumpy stools, or the sense of incomplete evacuation with defecation. Rectal examination is used to determine whether fecal impaction, anal stricture, or rectal masses are present. Constipation as a sign of another disease condition should be ruled out. Tests that measure colon transit time and defecatory function are reserved for refractory cases.

The treatment of constipation usually is directed toward relieving the cause. A conscious effort should be made to respond to the defecation urge. A time should be set aside after a meal, when mass movements in the colon are most likely to occur, for a bowel movement. Adequate fluid intake and bulk in the diet should be encouraged. Moderate exercise is essential, and persons on bed rest benefit from passive and active exercises. Laxatives and enemas should be used judiciously.

They should not be used on a regular basis to treat simple constipation because they interfere with the defecation reflex and actually may damage the rectal mucosa.

Fecal Impaction

Fecal impaction is the retention of hardened or putty-like stool in the rectum and colon, which interferes with normal passage of feces. If not removed, it can cause partial or complete bowel obstruction. It may occur in any age group but is more common in incapacitated elderly persons. Fecal impaction may result from painful anorectal disease, tumors, or neurogenic disease; use of constipating antacids or bulk laxatives; a low-residue diet; drug-induced colonic stasis; or prolonged bed rest and debility. In children, a habitual neglect of the urge to defecate because it interferes with play may promote impaction.[72]

The manifestations may be those of severe constipation, but frequently there is a history of watery diarrhea, fecal soiling, and fecal incontinence.[13] This is caused by increased secretory activity of the bowel, representing the body's attempt to break up the mass so that it can be evacuated. The abdomen may be distended, and there may be blood and mucus in the stool. The fecal mass may compress the urethra, giving rise to urinary incontinence. Fecal impaction should be considered in an elderly or immobilized person who develops watery stools with fecal or urinary incontinence.

Digital examination of the rectum is done to assess for the presence of a fecal mass. The mass may need to be broken up and dislodged manually or with the use of a sigmoidoscope. Oil enemas often are used to soften the mass before removal. The best treatment is prevention.

Intestinal Obstruction

Intestinal obstruction designates an impairment of movement of intestinal contents in a cephalocaudad direction.[73] The causes can be categorized as mechanical or paralytic. Strangulation with necrosis of the bowel may occur and lead to perforation, peritonitis, and sepsis.

Mechanical obstruction can result from a number of conditions, intrinsic or extrinsic, that encroach on the patency of the bowel lumen (Fig. 37-10). Major inciting causes include external hernia (*i.e.,* inguinal, femoral, or umbilical) and postoperative adhesions. Less common causes are strictures, tumors, foreign bodies, intussusception, and volvulus.

Intussusception involves the telescoping of bowel into the adjacent segment (Fig. 37-11). It is the most common cause of intestinal obstruction in children younger than 2 years of age.[74] The most common form is intussusception of the terminal ileum into the right colon, but other areas of the bowel may be involved. In most cases, the cause of the disorder is unknown. The condition can also occur in adults when an intraluminal mass or tumor acts as a traction force and pulls the segment along as it telescopes into the distal segment. Volvulus refers to a complete twisting of the bowel on an axis formed by its mesentery (see Fig. 37-10B). It can occur in any portion of the gastrointestinal tract, but most commonly involves the cecum,

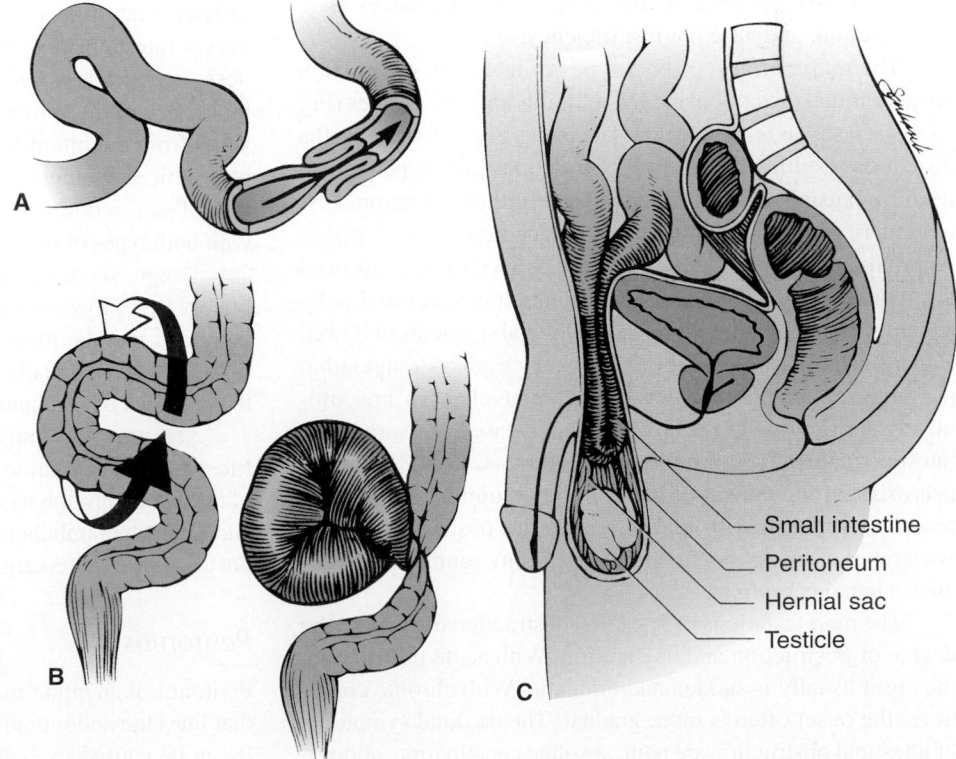

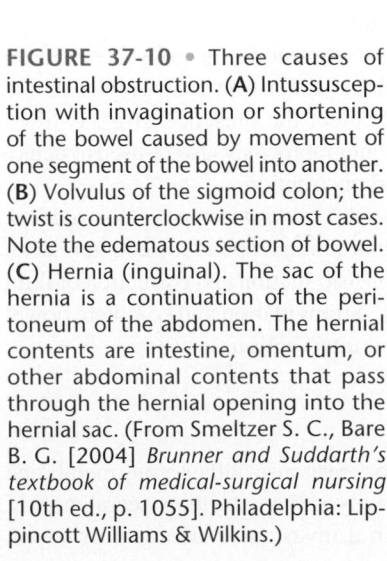

FIGURE 37-10 • Three causes of intestinal obstruction. (**A**) Intussusception with invagination or shortening of the bowel caused by movement of one segment of the bowel into another. (**B**) Volvulus of the sigmoid colon; the twist is counterclockwise in most cases. Note the edematous section of bowel. (**C**) Hernia (inguinal). The sac of the hernia is a continuation of the peritoneum of the abdomen. The hernial contents are intestine, omentum, or other abdominal contents that pass through the hernial opening into the hernial sac. (From Smeltzer S. C., Bare B. G. [2004] *Brunner and Suddarth's textbook of medical-surgical nursing* [10th ed., p. 1055]. Philadelphia: Lippincott Williams & Wilkins.)

Small intestine
Peritoneum
Hernial sac
Testicle

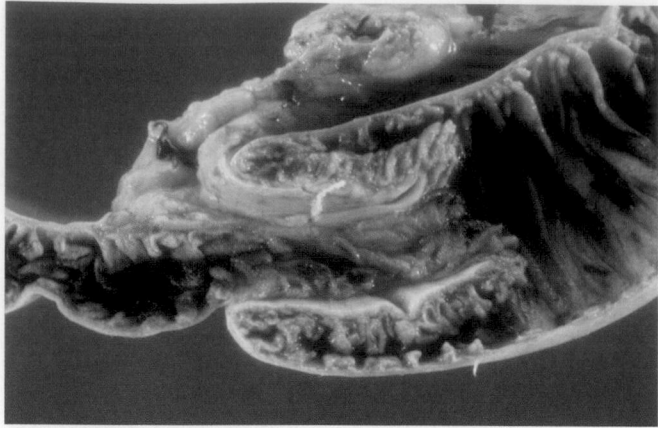

FIGURE 37-11 • Intussusception. A cross-section through the area of the obstruction shows "telescoped" small intestine surround by dilated small intestine. (From Mitos F. A., Rubin E. [2008]. The gastrointestinal tract. In Rubin R., Strayer D. S. [Eds.], *Rubin's pathophysiology: Clinicopathologic foundations of medicine* [5th ed., p. 586]. Philadelphia: Lippincott Williams & Wilkins.)

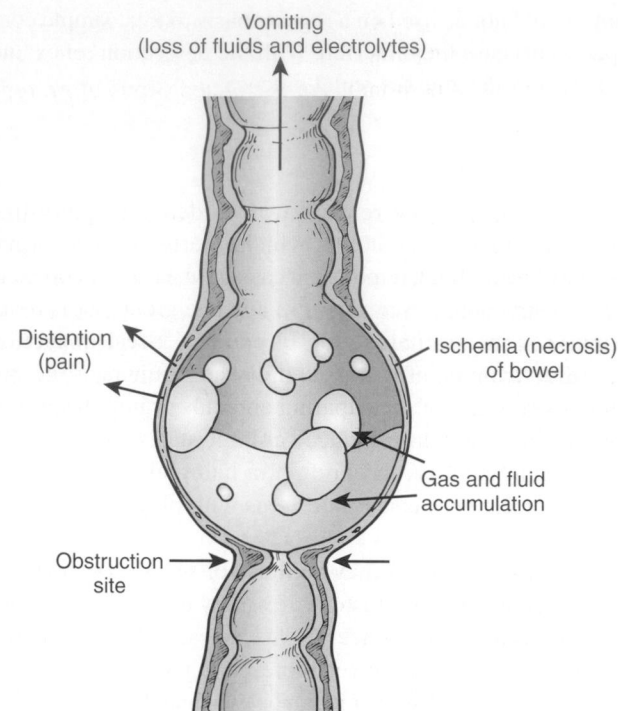

FIGURE 37-12 • Pathophysiology of intestinal obstruction.

followed by the sigmoid colon.[73] Mechanical bowel obstruction may be a simple obstruction, in which there is no alteration in blood flow, or a strangulated obstruction, in which there is impairment of blood flow and necrosis of bowel tissue.

Paralytic, or adynamic, obstruction results from neurogenic or muscular impairment of peristalsis. Paralytic ileus is seen most commonly after abdominal surgery. It also accompanies inflammatory conditions of the abdomen, intestinal ischemia, pelvic fractures, and back injuries. It occurs early in the course of peritonitis and can result from chemical irritation caused by bile, bacterial toxins, electrolyte imbalances as in hypokalemia, and vascular insufficiency.

The major effects of both types of intestinal obstruction are abdominal distention and loss of fluids and electrolytes (Fig 37-12). Gases and fluids accumulate in the area; if untreated, the distention resulting from bowel obstruction tends to perpetuate itself by causing atony of the bowel and further distention. Distention is further aggravated by the accumulation of gases. Approximately 70% of these gases are derived from swallowed air. As the process continues, the distention moves proximally (*i.e.,* toward the mouth), involving additional segments of bowel. Either form of obstruction eventually may lead to strangulation (*i.e.,* interruption of blood flow), gangrenous changes, and, ultimately, perforation of the bowel. The increased pressure in the intestine tends to compromise mucosal blood flow, leading to necrosis and movement of blood into the luminal fluids. This promotes rapid growth of bacteria in the obstructed bowel. Anaerobes grow rapidly in this favorable environment and produce a lethal endotoxin.

The manifestations of intestinal obstruction depend on the degree of obstruction and its duration. With acute obstruction, the onset usually is sudden and dramatic. With chronic conditions, the onset often is more gradual. The cardinal symptoms of intestinal obstruction are pain, absolute constipation, abdominal distention, and vomiting. With mechanical obstruction, the pain is severe and colicky, in contrast with the continuous pain and silent abdomen of paralytic ileus. There also is borborygmus (*i.e.,* rumbling sounds made by propulsion of gas in the intestine); audible, high-pitched peristalsis; and peristaltic rushes. Visible peristalsis may appear along the course of the distended intestine. Extreme restlessness and conscious awareness of intestinal movements are experienced along with weakness, perspiration, and anxiety. Should strangulation of the bowel occur, the symptoms change. The character of the pain shifts from the intermittent colicky pain caused by the hyperperistaltic movements of the intestine to a severe and steady type of pain. Vomiting and fluid and electrolyte disorders occur with both types of obstruction.

Diagnosis of intestinal obstruction usually is based on history and physical findings. Plain film radiography of the abdomen may be used to detect the presence of a gas-filled bowel. CT scans and ultrasonography may also be used to detect the presence of mechanical obstruction.

Treatment depends on the cause and type of obstruction. Most cases of adynamic obstruction respond to decompression of the bowel through nasogastric suction and correction of fluid and electrolyte imbalances. Strangulation and complete bowel obstruction require surgical intervention.

Peritonitis

Peritonitis is an inflammatory response of the serous membrane that lines the abdominal cavity and covers the visceral organs. It can be caused by bacterial invasion or chemical irritation.

Most commonly, enteric bacteria enter the peritoneum because of a defect in the wall of one of the abdominal organs. The most common causes of peritonitis are perforated peptic ulcer, ruptured appendix, perforated diverticulum, gangrenous bowel, pelvic inflammatory disease, and gangrenous gallbladder. Other causes are abdominal trauma and wounds. Generalized peritonitis, although no longer the overwhelming problem it once was, is still a leading cause of death after abdominal surgery.

The peritoneum has several characteristics that increase its vulnerability to or protect it from the effects of peritonitis. One weakness of the peritoneal cavity is that it is a large, unbroken space that favors the dissemination of contaminants. For the same reason, it has a large surface that permits rapid absorption of bacterial toxins into the blood. The peritoneum is particularly well adapted for producing an inflammatory response as a means of controlling infection. It tends, for example, to exude a thick, sticky, and fibrinous substance that adheres to other structures, such as the mesentery and omentum, and that seals off the perforated viscus and aids in localizing the process. Localization is enhanced by sympathetic stimulation that limits intestinal motility. Although the diminished or absent peristalsis that occurs tends to give rise to associated problems, it does inhibit the movement of contaminants throughout the peritoneal cavity.

One of the most important manifestations of peritonitis is the translocation of extracellular fluid into the peritoneal cavity (through weeping or serous fluid from the inflamed peritoneum) and into the bowel as a result of bowel obstruction. Nausea and vomiting cause further losses of fluid. The fluid loss may encourage development of hypovolemia and shock. The onset of peritonitis may be acute, as with a ruptured appendix, or it may have a more gradual onset, as occurs in pelvic inflammatory disease. Pain and tenderness are common symptoms. The pain usually is more intense over the inflamed area. The person with peritonitis usually lies still because any movement aggravates the pain. Breathing often is shallow to prevent movement of the abdominal muscles. The abdomen usually is rigid and sometimes described as boardlike because of reflex muscle guarding. Vomiting is common. Fever, an elevated white blood cell count, tachycardia, and hypotension are common. Hiccups may develop because of irritation of the phrenic nerve. Paralytic ileus occurs shortly after the onset of widespread peritonitis and is accompanied by abdominal distention. Peritonitis that progresses and is untreated leads to toxemia and shock.

Treatment. Treatment measures for peritonitis are directed toward preventing the extension of the inflammatory response, correcting the fluid and electrolyte imbalances that develop, and minimizing the effects of paralytic ileus and abdominal distention. Surgical intervention may be needed to remove an acutely inflamed appendix or close the opening in a perforated peptic ulcer. Oral fluids are forbidden. Nasogastric suction, which entails the insertion of a tube placed through the nose into the stomach or intestine, is used to decompress the bowel and relieve the abdominal distention. Fluid and electrolyte replacement is essential. These fluids are prescribed on the basis of frequent blood chemistry determinations. Antibiotics are given to combat infection. Narcotics often are needed for pain relief.

Alterations in Intestinal Absorption

Malabsorption is the failure to transport dietary constituents, such as fats, carbohydrates, proteins, vitamins, and minerals, from the lumen of the intestine into the extracellular fluid compartment for transport to the various parts of the body. It can selectively affect a single component, such as vitamin B_{12} or lactose, or its effects can extend to all the substances absorbed in a specific segment of the intestine. When one segment of the intestine is affected, another may compensate. For example, the ileum may compensate for malabsorption in the proximal small intestine by absorbing substantial amounts of fats, carbohydrates, and amino acids. Similarly, the colon, which normally absorbs water, sodium, chloride, and bicarbonate, can compensate for small intestine malabsorption by absorbing additional end products of bacterial carbohydrate metabolism.

The conditions that impair one or more steps involved in digestion and absorption of nutrients can be divided into three broad categories: intraluminal maldigestion, disorders of transepithelial transport, and lymphatic obstruction. Intraluminal maldigestion involves a defect in processing of nutrients in the intestinal lumen. The most common causes are pancreatic insufficiency, hepatobiliary disease, and intraluminal bacterial growth. Disorders of transepithelial transport are caused by mucosal lesions that impair uptake and transport of available intraluminal nutrients across the mucosal surface of the intestine. They include disorders such as celiac disease and Crohn disease. Lymphatic obstruction interferes with the transport of the products of fat digestion to the systemic circulation after they have been absorbed by the intestinal mucosa. The process can be interrupted by congenital defects, neoplasms, trauma, and selected infectious diseases.

Malabsorption Syndrome

Persons with intestinal malabsorption usually have symptoms directly referrable to the gastrointestinal tract that include diarrhea, steatorrhea, flatulence, bloating, abdominal pain, and cramps. Weakness, muscle wasting, weight loss, and abdominal distention often are present. Weight loss often occurs despite normal or excessive caloric intake. Steatorrheic stools contain excess fat. The fat content causes bulky, yellow-gray, malodorous stools. In a person consuming a diet containing 80 to 100 g of fat each day, excretion of 7 to 9 g of fat indicates steatorrhea.

Along with loss of fat in the stools, there is failure to absorb the fat-soluble vitamins. This can lead to easy bruising and bleeding (*i.e.,* vitamin K deficiency), bone pain, a predisposition to the development of fractures and tetany (*i.e.,* vitamin D and calcium deficiency), macrocytic anemia, and glossitis (*i.e.,* folic acid deficiency). Neuropathy, atrophy of the skin, and peripheral edema may be present. Table 37-2 describes the signs and symptoms of impaired absorption of dietary constituents.

TABLE 37-2 Sites of and Requirements for Absorption of Dietary Constituents and Manifestations of Malabsorption

DIETARY CONSTITUENT	SITE OF ABSORPTION	REQUIREMENTS	MANIFESTATIONS
Water and electrolytes	Mainly small bowel	Osmotic gradient	Diarrhea Dehydration Cramps
Fat	Upper jejunum	Pancreatic lipase Bile salts Functioning lymphatic channels	Weight loss Steatorrhea Fat-soluble vitamin deficiency
Carbohydrates			
Starch	Small intestine	Amylase Maltase Isomaltase α-dextrins	Diarrhea Flatulence Abdominal discomfort
Sucrose	Small intestine	Sucrase	
Lactose	Small intestine	Lactase	
Maltose	Small intestine	Maltase	
Fructose	Small intestine		
Protein	Small intestine	Pancreatic enzymes (*e.g.*, trypsin, chymotrypsin, elastin)	Loss of muscle mass Weakness Edema
Vitamins			
A	Upper jejunum	Bile salts	Night blindness Dry eyes Corneal irritation
Folic acid	Duodenum and jejunum	Absorptive; may be impaired by some drugs (*i.e.*, anticonvulsants)	Cheilosis Glossitis Megaloblastic anemia
B_{12}	Ileum	Intrinsic factor	Glossitis Neuropathy Megaloblastic anemia
D	Upper jejunum	Bile salts	Bone pain Fractures Tetany
E	Upper jejunum	Bile salts	Uncertain
K	Upper jejunum	Bile salts	Easy bruising and bleeding
Calcium	Duodenum	Vitamin D and parathyroid hormone	Bone pain Fractures Tetany
Iron	Duodenum and jejunum	Normal pH (hydrochloric acid secretion)	Iron-deficiency anemia Glossitis

Celiac Disease

Celiac disease, also known as *celiac sprue* and *gluten-sensitive enteropathy,* is an immune-mediated disorder triggered by ingestion of gluten-containing grains (including wheat, barley, and rye).[75–80] Until recently, celiac disease was considered to be a rare malabsorption syndrome that manifested during early childhood, but today it is known to be one of the most common genetic diseases, with a mean prevalence of 1% in the general population.[75–77] This would represent an estimated 3 million people in Europe and at least another 3 million in the United States.

The disease results from an inappropriate T-cell–mediated immune response against ingested α-gliadin (a component of gluten protein) in genetically predisposed people. Almost all persons with the disorder share the major histocompatibility complex class II allele HLA-DQ2 or HLA-DQ8. Persons with the disease have increased levels of antibodies to a variety of antigens, including transglutaminase, endomysium, and gliadin. The resultant immune response produces an intense inflammatory reaction that results in loss of absorptive villi from the small intestine (Fig. 37-13). When the resulting lesions are extensive, they may impair absorption of macronutrients (*i.e.*, proteins, carbohydrates, fats) and micronutrients (*i.e.*, vitamins and minerals). Small bowel involvement is most prominent in the proximal part of the small intestine, where the exposure to gluten is greatest.

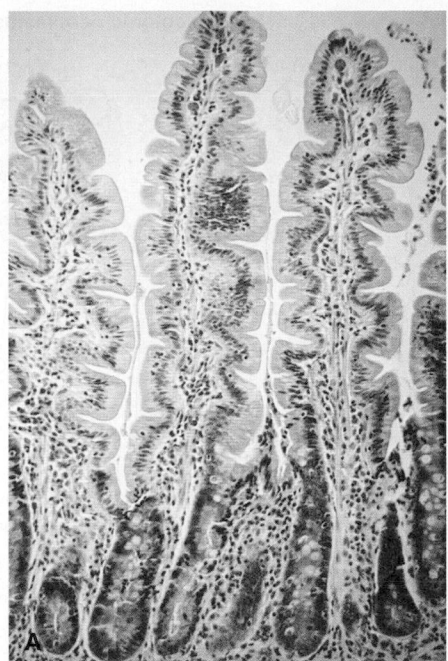

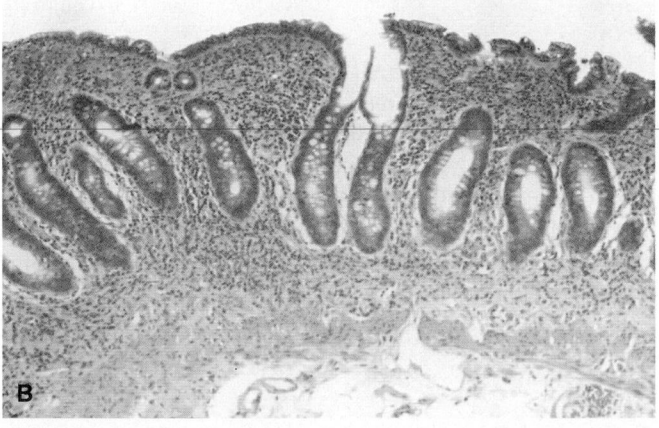

FIGURE 37-13 • Celiac disease. **(A)** Microscopic view of the normal proximal small intestine showing tall, slender villi with crypts present at the base. **(B)** A mucosal biopsy from a patient with advanced celiac disease showing complete loss of the villi with infiltration of the lamina propria by lymphocytes and plasma cells. (From Mitos F. A., Rubin E. [2008]. The gastrointestinal tract. In Rubin R., Strayer D. S. [Eds.], *Rubin's pathophysiology: Clinicopathologic foundations of medicine* [5th ed., p. 584]. Philadelphia: Lippincott Williams & Wilkins.)

There are a number of populations who are at higher risk for celiac disease. These include persons with type 1 diabetes mellitus, other autoimmune endocrinopathies, first- and second-degree relatives of persons with celiac disease, and individuals with Turner syndrome. Various malignancies also appear to be a direct result of celiac disease, in that the increased incidence seen in persons with celiac disease returns to that of the general population after several years of a gluten-free diet. These malignancies include head and neck squamous cell carcinoma, small intestinal adenocarcinoma, and non-Hodgkin lymphoma.

The classic form of celiac disease presents in infancy and manifests as failure to thrive, diarrhea, abdominal distention, and, occasionally severe malnutrition.[80] Beyond infancy, the manifestations tend to be less dramatic. Older children may present with anemia, constitutional short stature, dental enamel defects, and constipation. Women comprise about 75% of newly diagnosed adult celiac disease. In adults, gastrointestinal symptoms may manifest as diarrhea, constipation, or other symptoms of malabsorption such as bloating, flatus, or belching.

The diagnosis of celiac disease is based on clinical manifestations and confirmed by serologic tests and intestinal biopsy. Based on very high sensitivities, the best available tests are the immunoglobulin (Ig) A antihuman tissue transglutaminase (TTG) and IgA endomysial antibody immunofluorescence (EMA) tests.[78] Biopsies of the proximal small bowel are indicated in persons with a positive celiac disease antibody test.[78] Usually, additional laboratory tests are done to determine if the disorder has resulted in nutritional disorders such as iron-deficiency anemia.

The primary treatment of celiac disease consists of removal of gluten and related proteins from the diet. Gluten is the primary protein in wheat, barley, and rye. Oat products, which are nontoxic, may be contaminated with wheat during processing. Many gluten-free types of bread, cereals, cookies, and other products are available.[79] Meats, vegetables, fruits, and dairy products are free of gluten as long as they are not contaminated during processing. Complete exclusion of dietary gluten generally results in rapid and complete healing of the intestinal mucosa.

Neoplasms

Epithelial cell tumors of the intestines are a major cause of morbidity and mortality worldwide. The colon, including the rectum, is the site of more primary neoplasms than any other organ in the body.[7] Although the small intestine accounts for approximately 75% of the length of the gastrointestinal tract, it is an uncommon site of benign or malignant tumors.

Adenomatous Polyps

By far the most common types of neoplasms of the intestine are adenomatous polyps. A gastrointestinal polyp can be described as a mass that protrudes into the lumen of the gut.[7,8] Polyps can be subdivided according to their attachment to the bowel wall (sessile [raised mucosal nodules] or pedunculated [attached by a stalk]); their histopathologic appearance (hyperplastic or adenomatous); and their neoplastic potential (benign or malignant).[8]

Adenomatous polyps (adenomas) are benign neoplasms that arise from the mucosal epithelium of the intestine. They are composed of neoplastic cells that have proliferated in excess of those needed to replace the cells that normally are shed from the mucosal surface (Fig. 37-14). The pathogenesis of adenoma formation involves neoplastic alteration in the replication of the crypt epithelial cells. There may be diminished apoptosis (see Chapter 5), persistence of cell replication,

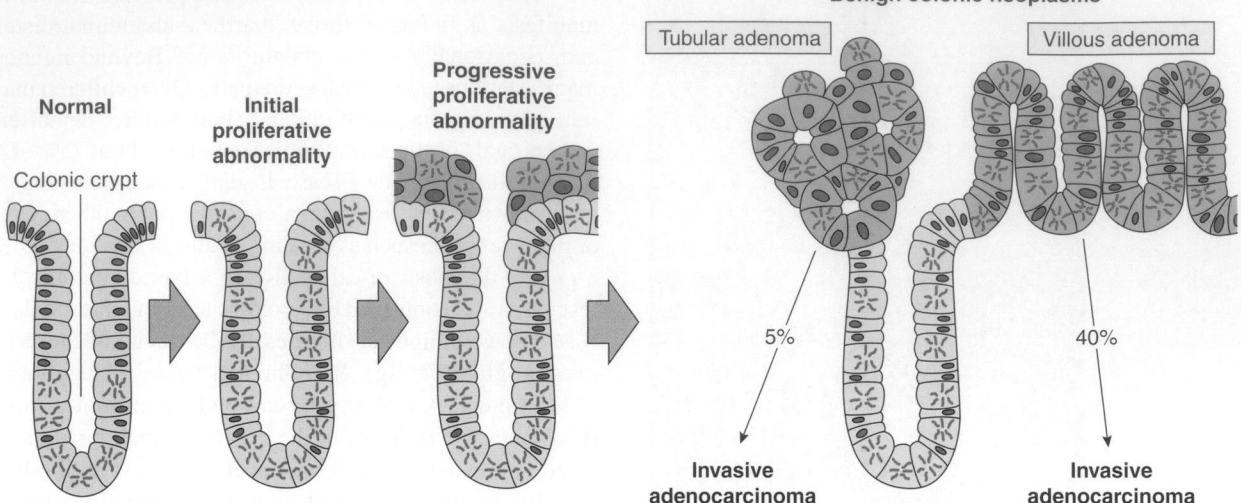

FIGURE 37-14 • The histogenesis of adenomatous polyps of the colon. The initial proliferative abnormality of the colonic mucosa, the extension of the mitotic zone in the crypts, leads to accumulation of mucosal cells. The formation of adenomas may reflect epithelial–mesenchymal interactions. (From Mitos F. A., Rubin E. [2008]. The gastrointestinal tract. In Rubin R., Strayer D. S. [Eds.], *Rubin's pathophysiology: Clinicopathologic foundations of medicine* [5th ed., p. 604]. Philadelphia: Lippincott Williams & Wilkins.)

and failure of cell maturation and differentiation of the cells that migrate to the surface of the crypts.[8] Normally, DNA synthesis ceases as the cells reach the upper two thirds of the crypts, after which they mature, migrate to the surface, and become senescent. They then become apoptotic and are shed from the surface.[8] Adenomas arise from a disruption in this sequence, such that the epithelial cells retain their proliferative ability throughout the entire length of the crypt. Alterations in cell differentiation can lead to dysplasia and progression to the development of invasive carcinoma.

More than half of all adenomatous polyps are located in the rectosigmoid colon and can be detected by rectal examination or sigmoidoscopy.[8] The remainder are evenly distributed throughout the rest of the colon. Adenomas can range in size from a barely visible nodule to a large, sessile mass. They can be classified as tubular, villous, or tubulovillous adenomas.

Tubular adenomas, which constitute approximately 65% of benign large bowel adenomas, typically are smooth-surfaced spheres, usually less than 2 cm in diameter, that are attached to the mucosal surface by a stalk.[8] Although most tubular adenomas display little epithelial dysplasia, approximately 20% show a range of dysplastic changes, from mild nuclear changes to frank invasive carcinoma. *Villous adenomas* constitute 10% of adenomas of the colon.[8] They are found predominantly in the rectosigmoid colon. They typically are broad-based, elevated lesions, with a shaggy, cauliflower-like surface. In contrast to tubular adenomas, villous adenomas are more likely to contain malignant cells. When invasive carcinoma develops, there is no stalk to isolate the tumor and invasion is directly into the wall of the colon. *Tubulovillous adenomas* manifest both tubular and villous architecture. They are intermediate between tubular and villous adenomas in terms of invasive carcinoma risk.

Most cases of colorectal cancer begin as benign adenomatous colonic polyps. The frequency of polyps increases with age, and the prevalence of adenomatous polyps, which is approximately 20% to 30% before 40 years of age, rises to 40% to 50% after 60 years of age.[22] Men and women are equally affected. The peak incidence of adenomatous polyps precedes by some years the peak for colorectal cancer. Programs that provide careful follow-up for persons with adenomatous polyps and removal of all suspect lesions have substantially reduced the incidence of colorectal cancer.[8]

Colorectal Cancer

Colorectal cancer is the third most common cancer in men and women and the second leading cause of cancer death in the United States. The annual incidence of colon and rectal cancer in the United States is approximately 148,810, with 49,960 deaths.[81] The death rate for colorectal cancer has been steadily declining since the early 1980s. This may due to a decreased number of cases, earlier diagnosis, and improved treatments.

The cause of cancer of the colon and rectum is largely unknown. Its incidence increases with age, as evidenced by the fact that approximately 90% of persons who develop this form of cancer are older than 50 years of age.[81] Its incidence is increased among persons with a family history of cancer, persons with Crohn disease or ulcerative colitis, and those with familial adenomatous polyposis of the colon. Persons with a familial risk—those who have two or more first- or second-degree relatives (or both) with colorectal cancer—make up approximately 20% of all persons with colorectal cancer.[82] Familial adenomatous polyposis is a rare autosomal dominant trait linked to a mutation in the long arm of chromosome 5.

Persons with the disorder develop multiple adenomatous polyps of the colon at an early age.[7,82] Carcinoma of the colon is inevitable, often by 40 years of age, unless a total colectomy is performed.

Diet also is thought to play a role.[81] Attention has focused on dietary fat intake, refined sugar intake, fiber intake, and the adequacy of such protective micronutrients as vitamins A, C, and E in the diet. It has been hypothesized that a high level of fat in the diet increases the synthesis of bile acids in the liver, which may be converted to potential carcinogens by the bacterial flora in the colon. Bacterial organisms in particular are suspected of converting bile acids to carcinogens; their proliferation is enhanced by a high dietary level of refined sugars. Dietary fiber is thought to increase stool bulk and thereby dilute and remove potential carcinogens. Refined diets often contain reduced amounts of vitamins A, C, and E, which may act as oxygen free radical scavengers.

Reports indicate that aspirin may protect against colorectal cancer.[83] An analysis of the incidence of colorectal cancer in the Nurses' Health Study showed a decreased incidence of colorectal cancer among women who took four to six aspirins per week.[84] Although the mechanism of aspirin's action is unknown, it may be related to its effect on the synthesis of prostaglandins, one or more of which may be involved in signal systems that influence cell proliferation or tumor growth. Aspirin inhibits cyclooxygenase, the enzyme which catalyzes the conversion of arachidonic acid in cell membranes to prostaglandins. One form of cyclooxygenase, COX-2, promotes inflammation and cell proliferation, and colorectal cancers often overexpress this enzyme. Regular use of aspirin appears to reduce the risk of colorectal cancers that overexpress COX-2 but not the risk of colorectal cancers with weak or absent expression of COX-2. Supplemental folate and calcium, selected vitamins, and postmenopausal hormone replacement therapy (estrogen) also have been proposed as potential chemoprotective agents.[85] All of these agents will require more extensive study before they can be recommended for long-term chemoprevention of colorectal cancer.

Usually, cancer of the colon and rectum is present for a long time before it produces symptoms. Bleeding is a highly significant early symptom, and usually is the one that causes persons to seek medical care. Other symptoms include a change in bowel habits, diarrhea or constipation, and sometimes a sense of urgency or incomplete emptying of the bowel. Pain usually is a late symptom.

The prognosis for persons with colorectal cancer depends largely on the extent of bowel involvement and on the presence of metastasis at the time of diagnosis. Colorectal cancer commonly is classified into four TNM (tumor, node, and metastasis) stages. In this system, a stage I tumor is limited to invasion of the mucosal and submucosal layers of the colon and has a 5-year survival rate of 90% to 100%.[13] A stage II (lymph node–negative) tumor infiltrates into, but not through the muscularis propria, and has a 5-year survival rate of 80%.[13] With a stage III (lymph node–positive) tumor, in which there is invasion of the serosal layer and regional lymph node involvement,

the 5-year survival rate is 30% to 50%.[13] Stage IV (metastatic) tumors penetrate the serosa or adjacent organs and have a much poorer prognosis.

Screening, Diagnosis, and Treatment. The single most important prognostic indicator of colorectal cancer is the extent (stage) of the tumor at time of diagnosis.[81] Therefore, the challenge is to discover the tumors at their earliest stages. Among the methods used for the detection of colorectal cancers are the digital rectal examination and the fecal occult blood test, usually done during routine physical examinations; x-ray studies using barium (*e.g.*, barium enema); and flexible sigmoidoscopy and colonoscopy.[81,86] Digital rectal examinations are most helpful in detecting neoplasms of the rectum. Rectal examination should be considered a routine part of a good physical examination. The American Cancer Society recommends that all asymptomatic men and women older than 40 years of age should have a digital rectal examination performed annually as a part of their physical examination. Beginning at 50 years of age, both men and women should follow one of these five screening options: fecal occult blood test every year; flexible sigmoidoscopy examination every 5 years; annual fecal occult blood test for blood and flexible sigmoidoscopy every 5 years; double-contrast barium enema every 5 years; or a colonoscopy every 10 years.[81] People with increased risk for colorectal cancer should be screened earlier and more often. Colonoscopy is recommended whenever a screening test is positive.

Almost all cancers of the colon and rectum bleed intermittently, although the amount of blood is small and usually not apparent in the stools. It therefore is feasible to screen for colorectal cancers using commercially prepared tests for occult blood in the stool.[13,81] Two slides must be prepared from three consecutive bowel movements. To reduce the likelihood of false-positive test results, persons are instructed to avoid NSAIDs such as ibuprofen and aspirin for 7 days before testing; to avoid vitamin C in excess of 250 mg from either supplements or citrus fruits for 3 days before testing; and to avoid red meats for 3 days before testing. The most commonly used tests are guaiac-based fecal occult blood tests, which are uncomplicated and can be processed in a health care provider's office. There are also immunochemistry-based tests that may be processed in a laboratory or in the health care provider's office, but they are less commonly used. Persons with a positive fecal occult blood test should be referred to their physician for further study. Usually, a physical examination, rectal examination, and flexible sigmoidoscopy or colonoscopy are done.

Flexible sigmoidoscopy involves examination of the rectum and sigmoid colon with a hollow, lighted tube that is inserted through the rectum. The procedure is performed without sedation and is well tolerated. Approximately 40% of cancers and polyps are out of the reach of the sigmoidoscope, emphasizing the need for fecal occult blood tests. Polyps can be removed or tissue can be obtained for biopsy during the procedure.

Colonoscopy provides a means for direct visualization of the rectum and colon. The colonoscope consists of a flexible,

4-cm–diameter glass fiber bundle that contains approximately 250,000 glass fibers and has a lens at either end to focus and magnify the image. Light from an external source is transmitted by the fiberoptic viewing bundle. Instruments are available that afford direct examination of the sigmoid colon or the entire colon. This method is used for screening persons at high risk for development of cancer of the colon (e.g., those with ulcerative colitis) and for those with symptoms. Colonoscopy also is useful for obtaining a biopsy and for removing polyps. Although this method is one of the most accurate for detecting early colorectal cancers, it is not suitable for mass screening because it is expensive and time consuming and must be done by a person who is highly trained in the use of the instrument.

The only recognized treatment for cancer of the colon and rectum is surgical removal.[86] Preoperative radiation therapy may be used and has in some cases demonstrated increased 5-year survival rates. Postoperative adjuvant chemotherapy may be used. Radiation therapy and chemotherapy are used as palliative treatment methods.

IN SUMMARY, disorders of the small and large intestines include irritable bowel syndrome, inflammatory bowel disease, diverticular disease, disorders of motility (i.e., diarrhea, constipation, fecal impaction, and intestinal obstruction), alterations in intestinal absorption, and colorectal cancer.

Irritable bowel syndrome is a functional disorder characterized by a variable combination of chronic and recurrent intestinal symptoms not explained by structural or biochemical abnormalities. The term *inflammatory bowel disease* is used to designate two inflammatory conditions: Crohn disease, which affects the small and large bowel, and ulcerative colitis, which affects the colon and rectum. Both are chronic diseases characterized by remissions and exacerbations of diarrhea, weight loss, fluid and electrolyte disorders, and systemic signs of inflammation.

Infectious forms of enterocolitis include viral (e.g., rotavirus), bacterial (e.g., C. difficile and E. coli O157:H7), and protozoal (E. histolytica) infections. Diverticular disease includes diverticulosis, which is a condition in which the mucosal layer of the colon herniates through the muscularis layer, and diverticulitis, in which there is inflammation and gross or microscopic perforation of the diverticulum.

Diarrhea and constipation represent disorders of intestinal motility. Diarrhea is characterized by excessively frequent passage of stools. It can be acute or chronic and can be caused by infectious organisms, food intolerance, drugs, or intestinal disease. Acute diarrheas that last less than 4 days are predominantly caused by infectious agents and follow a self-limited course. Chronic diarrhea persists beyond 3 to 4 weeks and is caused by the presence of hyperosmotic luminal contents, increased intestinal secretory processes, inflammatory conditions, and infectious processes. Constipation can be defined as the infrequent passage of stools; it commonly is caused by failure to respond to the urge to defecate, inadequate fiber or fluid

intake, weakness of the abdominal muscles, inactivity and bed rest, pregnancy, hemorrhoids, and gastrointestinal disease. Fecal impaction is the retention of hardened or putty-like stool in the rectum and colon, which interferes with normal passage of feces. Intestinal obstruction designates an impairment of movement of intestinal contents in a cephalocaudad direction as the result of mechanical or paralytic mechanisms. Peritonitis is an inflammatory response of the serous membrane that lines the abdominal cavity and covers the visceral organs. It can be caused by bacterial invasion or chemical irritation resulting from perforation of the viscera or abdominal organs.

Malabsorption results from the impaired absorption of nutrients and other dietary constituents from the intestine. It can involve a single dietary constituent, such as vitamin B_{12}, or extend to involve all of the substances absorbed in a particular part of the small intestine. Malabsorption can result from disease of the small bowel and disorders that impair digestion and, in some cases, obstruct the lymph flow by which fats are transported to the general circulation. Celiac disease is an immune-mediated disorder triggered by ingestion of gluten-containing grains (including wheat, barley, and rye).

Colorectal cancer, the second most common fatal cancer, is seen most commonly in persons older than 50 years of age. Most, if not all, cancers of the colon and rectum arise in pre-existing adenomatous polyps. Programs that provide careful follow-up for persons with adenomatous polyps and removal of all suspect lesions have substantially reduced the incidence of colorectal cancer. ■

Review Exercises

1. A 40-year-old man reports to his health care provider complaining of "heartburn" that occurs after eating and also wakes him up at night. He is overweight, admits to enjoying fatty foods, and usually lies down on the sofa and watches TV after dinner. He also complains that lately he has been having a cough and some wheezing. A diagnosis of gastroesophageal reflux disease (GERD) was made.

   A. *Explain the cause of heartburn and why it becomes worse after eating.*

   B. *Persons with GERD are advised to lose weight, avoid eating fatty foods, remain sitting after eating, and to sleep with their head slightly elevated. Explain the possible relationship between these situations and the occurrence of reflux.*

   C. *Explain the possible relationship between GERD and the respiratory symptoms this man is having.*

2. A 36-year-old woman who has been taking aspirin for back pain experiences a sudden episode of tachycardia and feeling faint, accompanied by the vomit-

ing of a coffee-ground emesis and the passing of a tarry stool. She relates that she has not had any signs of a "stomach ulcer" such as pain or heartburn.

A. *Relate the mucosal protective effects of prostaglandins to the development of peptic ulcer associated with aspirin or nonsteroidal anti-inflammatory drug (NSAID) use.*

B. *Explain the apparent suddenness of the bleeding and the fact that the woman did not experience pain as a warning signal.*

C. *Among the results of her initial laboratory tests is an elevated blood urea nitrogen (BUN) level. Explain the reason for the elevated BUN.*

3. A 29-year-old woman has been diagnosed with Crohn disease. Her medical history reveals that she began having symptoms of the disease at 24 years of age and that her mother died of complications of the disease at 54 years of age. She complains of diarrhea and chronic cramping abdominal pain.

A. *Define the term* inflammatory bowel disease *and compare the pathophysiologic processes and manifestations of Crohn disease and ulcerative colitis.*

B. *Describe the possible association between genetic and environmental factors in the pathogenesis of Crohn disease.*

C. *Relate the use of the monoclonal antibody infliximab to the pathogenesis of the inflammatory lesions that occur in Crohn disease.*

References

1. National Digestive Diseases Information Clearing House (NDDIC). Digestive disease statistics. [Online.] Available: http://digestive.niddk.nih.gov/statistics/statistics.htm. Accessed June 14, 2007.

2. Guyton A. C., Hall J. E. (2006). *Textbook of medical physiology* (11th ed., pp. 782–786). Philadelphia: Elsevier Saunders.

3. Orenstein S., Peters J., Khan S., et al. (2004). The esophagus. In Behrman R. E., Kliegman R. M., Jenson H. B. (Eds.), *Nelson textbook of pediatrics* (17th ed., pp. 1218–1224). Philadelphia: Elsevier Saunders.

4. Aschildi O., Grewal H. (2007). Congenital anomalies of the esophagus. *Otolaryngologic Clinics of North America* 40, 219–244.

5. Saud B. M., Szyjkowski R. (2004). A diagnostic approach to dysphagia. *Gastroenterology* 6, 525–546.

6. Spieker M. R. (2000). Evaluating dysphagia. *American Family Physician* 61, 3639–3648.

7. Liu C., Crawford J. M. (2005). The gastrointestinal tract. In Kumar V., Abbas A. K., Fausto N. (Eds.), *Robbins and Cotran pathologic basis of disease* (7th ed., pp. 797–875). Philadelphia: Elsevier Saunders.

8. Mitos F. A., Rubin E. (2008). The gastrointestinal tract. In Rubin R., Strayer D. S. (Eds.), *Rubin's pathophysiology: Clinicopathologic foundations of medicine* (5th ed., pp. 557–576, 727–746). Philadelphia: Lippincott Williams & Wilkins.

9. Orlando R. C. (2002). Pathogenesis of gastroesophageal reflux disease. *Gastroenterology Clinics of North America* 31, S35–S44.

10. Mittal R. K., Balaban D. H. (1997). The esophagogastric junction. *New England Journal of Medicine* 336, 924–931.

11. Cappell M. S. (2005). Clinical presentation, diagnosis, and management of gastroesophageal reflux disease. *Medical Clinics of North America* 84, 1137–1161.

12. Orlando R. C. (2005). Pathogenesis of reflux esophagitis and Barrett's esophagus. *Medical Clinics of North America* 89, 219–241.

13. McQuaid K. R. (2007). Alimentary tract. In Tierney L. M., McPhee S. J., Papadakis M. (Eds.), *Current medical diagnosis and treatment* (42nd ed., pp. 555, 567–585, 617–623, 652–658). New York: Lange Medical Books/McGraw-Hill.

14. Irwin R. S. (2006). Chronic cough due to gastroesophageal reflux disease. *Chest* 129, 80S–94S.

15. Harding S. M. (2005). Gastroesophageal reflux: A potential asthma trigger. *Immunology and Allergy Clinics* 25, 131–148.

16. Spechler S. J. (2002). Barrett's esophagus. *New England Journal of Medicine* 346, 836–842.

17. Heidelbaugh J. J., Nostrant T. T., Clark K. (2003). Management of gastroesophageal reflux disease. *American Family Physician* 68, 1311–1322.

18. Mason D. B. (2000). Gastroesophageal reflux in children. *Nursing Clinics of North America* 35, 15–36.

19. Hassall E. (2005). Decisions in diagnosis and managing chronic gastroesophageal reflux disease in children. *Journal of Pediatrics* 146, S3–S12.

20. Gold B. D. (2005). Asthma and gastroesophageal reflux disease in children: Exploring the relationship. *Journal of Pediatrics* 146, S13–S20.

21. Enzinger P. C., Mayer R. J. (2003). Esophageal cancer. *New England Journal of Medicine* 349, 2241–2252.

22. Layke J. C., Lopez P. P. (2006). Esophageal cancer. *American Family Physician* 73, 2187–2794.

23. Fromm D. (1987). Mechanisms involved in gastric mucosal resistance to injury. *Annual Review of Medicine* 38, 119.

24. Wolfe M. M., Lichtenstein D. R., Singh G. (1999). Gastrointestinal toxicity of nonsteroidal anti-inflammatory drugs. *New England Journal of Medicine* 340, 1888–1899.

25. Suerbaum S., Michetti P. (2002). *Helicobacter pylori* infections. *New England Journal of Medicine* 347, 1175–1186.

26. Shiotani A., Nurgalieva Z. Z., Yamaoka Y., et al. (2000). *Helicobacter pylori*. *Medical Clinics of North America* 84, 1125–1136.

27. Ables A. Z. (2007). Update on *Helicobacter pylori* treatment. *American Family Physician* 75, 351–358.

28. Saad R. J., Scheiman J. M. (2004). Diagnosis and management of peptic ulcer disease. *Clinics in Family Practice* 6, 569–587.

29. Fass R. (1995). Zollinger-Ellison syndrome: Diagnosis and management. *Hospital Practice* 30(11), 73–80.

30. Maitra A., Abbas A. K. (2005). The endocrine system. In Kumar V., Abbas A. K., Fausto N. (Eds.), *Robbins and Cotran pathologic basis of disease* (7th ed., pp. 1206–1207). Philadelphia: Elsevier Saunders.

31. Zuckerman G. R., Cort D., Schuman R. B. (1988). Stress ulcer syndrome. *Journal of Intensive Care Medicine* 3, 21.

32. Spirit M. J., Starily S. (2006). Update on stress ulcer prophylaxis in critically ill patients. *Critical Care Nurse* 26(1), 18–29.

33. Layke J. C., Lopez P. P. (2004). Gastric cancer: Diagnosis and treatment options. *American Family Physician* 69, 1133–1146.

34. Hadley S. K., Gaarder S. M. (2005). Treatment of irritable bowel syndrome. *American Family Physician* 72, 2501–2506.

35. Hassler W. L. (2002). The irritable bowel syndrome. *Medical Clinics of North America* 86, 1524–1551.

36. Olden K. W. (2003). Irritable bowel syndrome: An overview of diagnosis and pharmacologic treatment. *Cleveland Clinic Journal of Medicine* 70(Suppl. 2), S3–S17.

37. Thompson W. G., Longstreth G. E., Drossman D. A., et al. (Committee on Functional Bowel Disorders and Functional Abdominal Pain, Multinational Working Teams to Develop Diagnostic Criteria for Functional Gastrointestinal Disorders [ROME II], University Ottawa, Canada). (1999). Functional bowel disorders and functional abdominal pain. *Gut* 45(Suppl. 2), 1143–1147.

38. Thoreson R., Cullen J. J. (2007). Pathophysiology of inflammatory bowel disease: An overview. *Surgical Clinics of North America* 87, 575–585.

39. Bamias G., Nyce M. R., DeLaRue S. A., et al. (2005). New concepts of inflammatory bowel disease. *Annals of Internal Medicine* 143, 895–904.

40. Bridget S., Lee J. C., Bjarnason I., et al. (2002). In siblings with similar genetic susceptibility for inflammatory bowel disease, smokers tend to develop Crohn's disease and nonsmokers develop ulcerative colitis. *Gut* 51, 21–25.

41. Podolsky D. K. (2002). Inflammatory bowel disease. *New England Journal of Medicine* 347, 417–429.

42. Chinyu S., Lichtenstein G. R. (2002). Recent developments in inflammatory bowel disease. *Medical Clinics of North America* 86, 1497–1523.

43. Hanauer S. B., Present D. H. (2003). The state of the art in the management of inflammatory bowel disease. *Reviews in Gastroenterological Disorders* 3(2), 81–92.

44. Knutson D., Greenberg G., Cronau H. (2003). Management of Crohn's disease: A practical approach. *American Family Physician* 68, 707–714.

45. Kornbluth A., Sachar D. B. (2004). Ulcerative colitis practice guidelines in adults (update): American College of Gastroenterology, Practice Parameters Committee. *American Journal of Gastroenterology* 99, 1371–1385.

46. Bass D. M. (2004). Rotavirus and other agents of viral gastroenteritis. In Behrman R. E., Kliegman R. M., Jenson H. B. (Eds.), *Nelson textbook of pediatrics* (17th ed., pp. 1081–1083). Philadelphia: Elsevier Saunders.

47. Shatsky M. (2006). Rotavirus vaccine, live, oral, pentavalent (RotaTeq) for prevention of rotavirus gastroenteritis. *American Family Physician* 74, 1014–1016.

48. Mylonakis E., Ryan E. T., Claderswood S. B. (2001). *Clostridium difficile*–associated diarrhea: A review. *Archives of Internal Medicine* 161, 525–533.

49. Schroeder M. S. (2005). *Clostridium difficile*–associated diarrhea. *American Family Physician* 71, 921–928.

50. Yassen S. F., Young-Fadok T. M., Zein N. N., et al. (2001). *Clostridium difficile*–associated diarrhea and colitis. *Mayo Clinic Proceedings* 76, 725–730.

51. Tarr P. I., Neil M. A. (2001). *Escherichia coli* O157:H7. *Gastroenterology Clinics of North America* 30, 735–751.

52. Razzaq S. (2006). Hemolytic uremic syndrome. *American Family Physician* 74, 991–996.

53. Moake J. L. (2002). Thrombotic microangiopathies. *New England Journal of Medicine* 347, 589–600.

54. Goldman R. (2006). *Escherichia coli*. *Pediatrics in Review* 27(3), 114–115.

55. Goldsmith R. S. (2007). Infectious diseases: Protozoal and helminthic. In Tierney L. M., McPhee S. J., Papadakis M. (Eds.), *Current medical diagnosis and treatment* (46th ed., pp. 1498–1503). New York: McGraw-Hill Medical.

56. Schwartz D. A., Genta R. M., Bennett D. P., et al. (2008). Infectious and parasitic diseases. In Rubin R., Strayer D. S. (Eds.), *Rubin's pathophysiology: Clinicopathologic foundations of medicine* (5th ed., pp. 363–365). Philadelphia: Lippincott Williams & Wilkins.

57. Ferzoco L. B., Raptopoulos V., Silen W. (1998). Acute diverticulitis. *New England Journal of Medicine* 338, 1521–1526.

58. Salzman H., Lillie D. (2005). Diverticular disease: Diagnosis and treatment. *American Family Physician* 72, 1229–1234.

59. Paulson E. K., Kalady M. F., Pappas T. N. (2003). Suspected appendicitis. *New England Journal of Medicine* 348, 236–242.

60. Schiller L. R. (2000). Diarrhea. *Medical Clinics of North America* 84, 1259–1275.

61. Field M., Rao M. C., Chang E. B. (1989). Intestinal electrolyte transport and diarrheal disease (part 2). *New England Journal of Medicine* 321, 879–883.

62. Field M. (2003). Intestinal ion transport and the pathophysiology of diarrhea. *Journal of Clinical Investigation* 111, 931–943.

63. Ghishan F. K. (2004). Chronic diarrhea. In Berman R. E., Kliegman R. M., Jenson H. B. (Eds.), *Nelson textbook of pediatrics* (17th ed., pp. 1276–1281). Philadelphia: Elsevier Saunders.

64. King C. K., Glass R., Brewer J. S., et al. (2003). Managing acute gastroenteritis among children: Oral rehydration, maintenance, and nutritional therapy. *Morbidity and Mortality Weekly Report* 52(RR-16), 1–16.

65. Dennehy P. H. (2005). Acute diarrheal disease in children: Epidemiology, prevention, treatment. *Infectious Disease Clinics* 19, 585–602.

66. Limbos M. A., Lieberman J. M. (1995). Management of acute diarrhea in children. *Contemporary Pediatrics* 12(12), 68–88.

67. American Academy of Pediatrics, Subcommittee on Acute Gastroenteritis. (1996). Practice parameter: The management of acute gastroenteritis in young children. *Pediatrics* 97, 424–434.

68. Wald A. (2006). Constipation in the primary care setting. *American Journal of Medicine* 119, 736–739.

69. Wald A. (2000). Constipation. *Medical Clinics of North America* 84, 1231–1246.

70. Hsieh C. (2005). Treatment of constipation in older adults. *American Family Physician* 72, 2277–2285.

71. Lembo A., Camilleri M. (2003). Chronic constipation. *New England Journal of Medicine* 349, 1360–1368.

72. Wrenn K. (1989). Fecal impaction. *New England Journal of Medicine* 321, 658–662.

73. Kahi C. J., Rex D. K. (2003). Bowel obstruction and pseudoobstruction. *Gastroenterology Clinics of North America* 32, 1229–1247.

74. Wyllie R. (2004). Ileus, adhesions, intussusception, and closed-loop obstruction. In Berman R. E., Kliegman R. M., Jenson H. B. (Eds.), *Nelson textbook of pediatrics* (17th ed., pp. 1241–1243). Philadelphia: Elsevier Saunders.

75. Green P. H. R., Jabri B. (2006). Celiac disease. *Annual Review of Medicine* 57, 207–221.

76. Rodrigo L. (2006). Celiac disease. *World Journal of Gastroenterology* 12, 6585–6593.

77. Alaedini A., Green P. H. R. (2005). Narrative review: Celiac disease: Understanding a complex autoimmune disorder. *Annals of Internal Medicine* 142, 289–298.

78. National Institutes of Health Consensus Development Conference. (2004). NIH Consensus Statement on Celiac Disease. [Online.] Available: http://consensus.nih.gov/2004/2004CeliacDisease118PDF.pdf. Accessed March 22, 2008.

79. Celiac.com. (2008). Celiac disease and gluten-free diet information. [Online.] Available: www.celiac.com/index.html. Accessed March 22, 2008.

80. Garcia-Carega M., Kerner J. A. (2004). Malabsorption disorders. In Berman R. E., Kliegman R. M., Jenson H. B. (Eds.), *Nelson textbook of pediatrics* (16th ed., pp. 1264–1266). Philadelphia: Elsevier Saunders.

81. American Cancer Society. (2008). Colon and rectal cancer. [Online.] Available: www.cancer.org. Accessed March 22, 2008.

82. Guttmacher A. E., de la Chapelle A. (2003). Hereditary colorectal cancer. *New England Journal of Medicine* 348, 919–932.

83. Chan A. T., Ogino S., Fuchs C. S. (2007). Aspirin and the risk of colorectal cancer in relation to the expression of COX-2. *New England Journal of Medicine* 356, 2131–2142.

84. Marcus A. J. (1995). Aspirin as prophylaxis against colorectal cancer. *New England Journal of Medicine* 333, 656–657.

85. Pasi J. A., Mayer R. J. (2000). Chemoprevention of colorectal cancer. *New England Journal of Medicine* 342, 1960–1966.

86. Engstrom P. F. (2001). Colorectal cancer. In Lenhard R. E., Osteen R. T., Gansler T. (Eds.), *The American Cancer Society clinical oncology* (pp. 362–372). Atlanta: American Cancer Society.

Visit the Point. **http://thePoint.lww.com for animations, journal articles, and more!**

Disorders of Hepatobiliary and Exocrine Pancreas Function

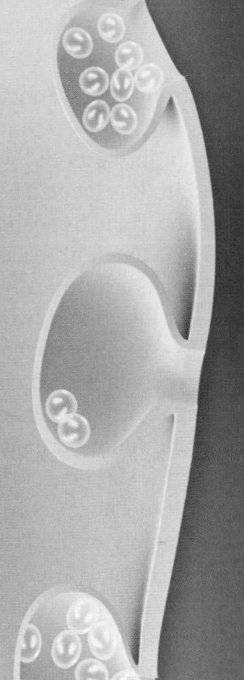

Chapter **38**

CAROL M. PORTH

➤ The liver, the gallbladder, and the exocrine pancreas are classified as accessory organs of the gastrointestinal tract. In addition to producing digestive secretions, the liver and the pancreas have other important functions. The endocrine pancreas, for example, supplies the insulin and glucagon needed in cell metabolism, whereas the liver synthesizes glucose, plasma proteins, and blood clotting factors and is responsible for the degradation and elimination of drugs and hormones, among other functions. This chapter focuses on functions and disorders of the liver, the biliary tract and gallbladder, and the exocrine pancreas.

THE LIVER AND HEPATOBILIARY SYSTEM

After completing this section of the chapter, you should be able to meet the following objectives:

- Describe the lobular structures of the liver.
- State the source and trace the movement of blood flow into, through, and out of the liver.
- Describe the function of the liver in terms of carbohydrate, protein, and fat metabolism.
- Characterize the function of the liver in terms of bilirubin elimination and describe the pathogenesis of unconjugated and conjugated hyperbilirubinemia.
- Relate the mechanism of bile formation and elimination to the development of cholestasis.
- List four laboratory tests used to assess liver function and relate them to impaired liver function.

The liver is the largest visceral organ in the body, weighing approximately 1.3 kg (3 lb) in the adult. It is located below the diaphragm and occupies much of the right hypochondrium (Fig. 38-1). The liver is surrounded by a tough fibroelastic capsule called the *Glisson capsule*. The liver is anatomically divided into two large lobes (the right and left lobes) and two smaller lobes (the caudate and quadrate lobes). Except for the portion that is in the epigastric area, the liver is contained within the rib cage, and cannot normally be palpated in healthy persons.

The liver is unique among the abdominal organs in having a dual blood supply consisting of a venous (portal) supply through the hepatic portal vein and an arterial supply through the hepatic artery. Approximately 300 mL of blood per minute enters the liver through the hepatic artery; another 1050 mL/minute enters by way of the valveless portal vein. The venous blood delivered by the hepatic portal vein comes from the digestive tract and major abdominal organs, including the pancreas and spleen (Fig. 38-2). The portal blood supply carries nutrient and toxic materials absorbed in the intestine, blood cells and their breakdown products from the spleen, and insulin and glucagon from the pancreas. Although the blood from the portal vein is incompletely saturated with oxygen, it supplies approximately 60% to 70% of the oxygen needs of the liver.

The venous outflow from the liver is carried by the valveless hepatic veins, which empty into the inferior vena cava just below the level of the diaphragm. The pressure difference between the hepatic vein and the portal vein normally is such that the liver stores approximately 450 mL of blood.[1] This blood can be shifted back into the general circulation during periods of hypovolemia and shock. In right heart failure in which the pressure in the vena cava increases, blood backs up and accumulates in the liver.

The *lobules* are the functional units of the liver. Each lobule is a cylindrical structure that measures approximately 0.8 to 2 mm in diameter and several millimeters in length. There are approximately 50,000 to 100,000 lobules in the liver.[1] Each lobule is organized around a central vein that empties into the hepatic veins and from there into the vena cava. The terminal bile ducts and small branches of the portal vein and hepatic artery are located at the periphery of the lobule. Plates of hepatic cells radiate centrifugally from the central vein like spokes on a wheel (Fig. 38-3). These hepatic plates are separated by wide, thin-walled sinusoidal capillaries, called *sinusoids,* that extend from the periphery of the lobule to its central vein. The sinusoids are supplied by blood from the portal vein and hepatic artery. The sinusoids are in intimate contact with the hepatocytes and provide for the exchange of substances between the blood and liver cells. The sinusoids are lined with two types of cells: the typical capillary endothelial cells and Kupffer cells. *Kupffer cells* are reticuloendothelial cells that are capable of removing and phagocytizing old and defective blood cells, bacteria, and other foreign material from the portal blood as it flows through the sinusoid. This phagocytic action removes enteric bacilli and other harmful substances that filter into the blood from the intestine.

A major exocrine function of the liver is bile secretion. The lobules also are supplied by small tubular channels, called *bile canaliculi,* that lie between the cell membranes of adjacent hepatocytes. The bile produced by the hepatocytes flows into the canaliculi and then to the periphery of the lobules, draining into progressively larger ducts, until it reaches the right and left hepatic ducts. The intrahepatic and extrahepatic bile ducts often are collectively referred to as the *hepatobiliary tree.* These ducts unite to form the common duct (see Fig. 38-1). The common duct, which is approximately 10 to 15 cm long,

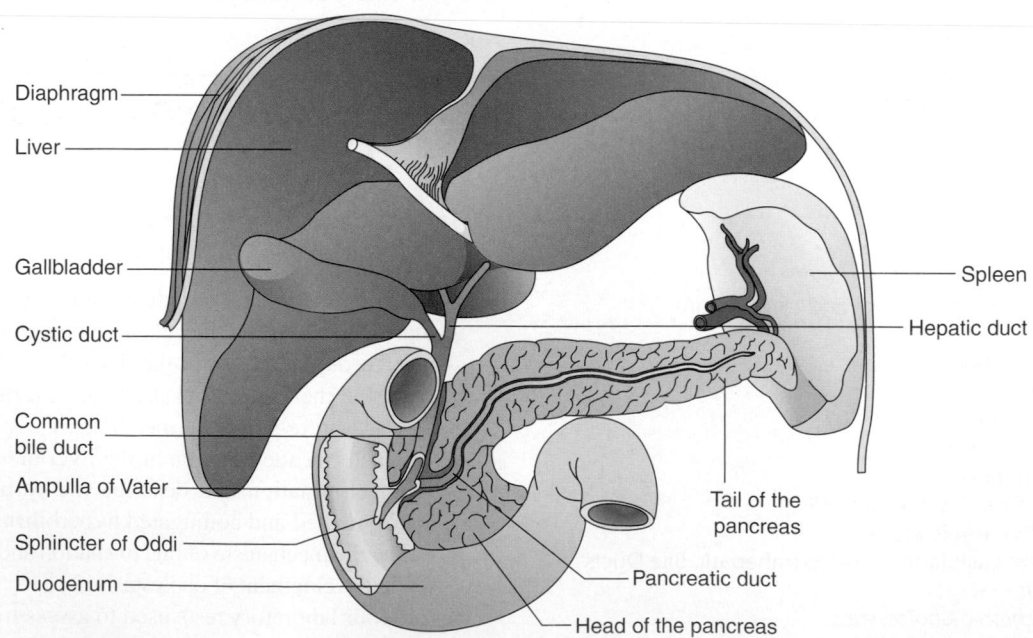

FIGURE 38-1 • The liver and biliary system, including the gallbladder and bile ducts.

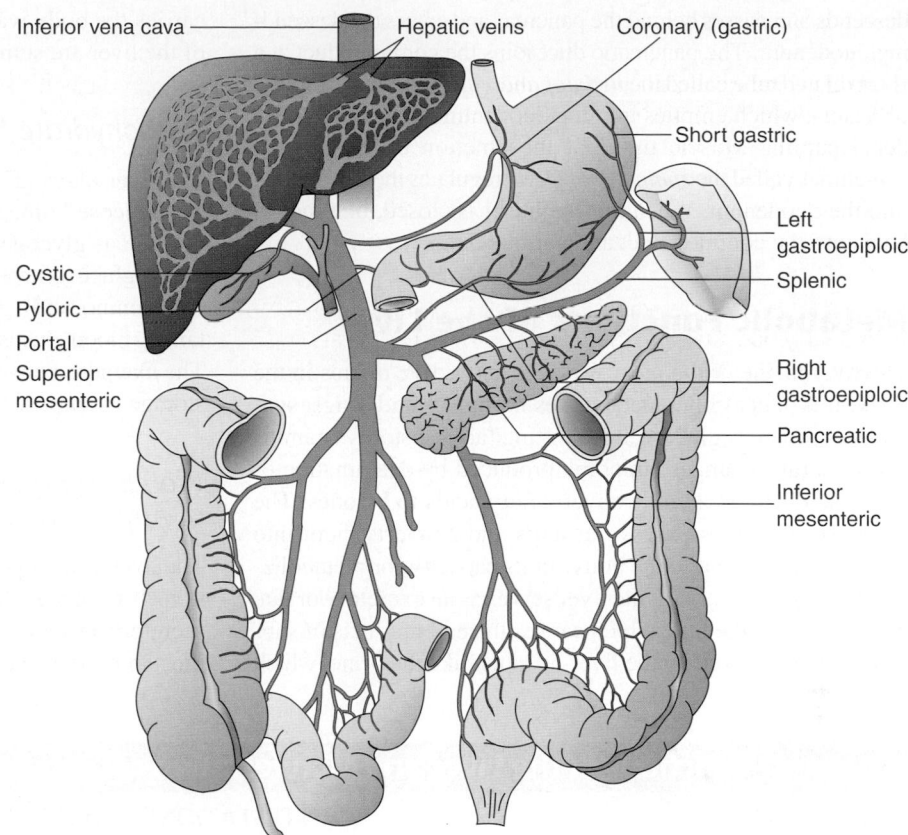

FIGURE 38-2 • The portal circulation. Blood from the gastrointestinal tract, spleen, and pancreas travels to the liver through the portal vein before moving into the vena cava for return to the heart.

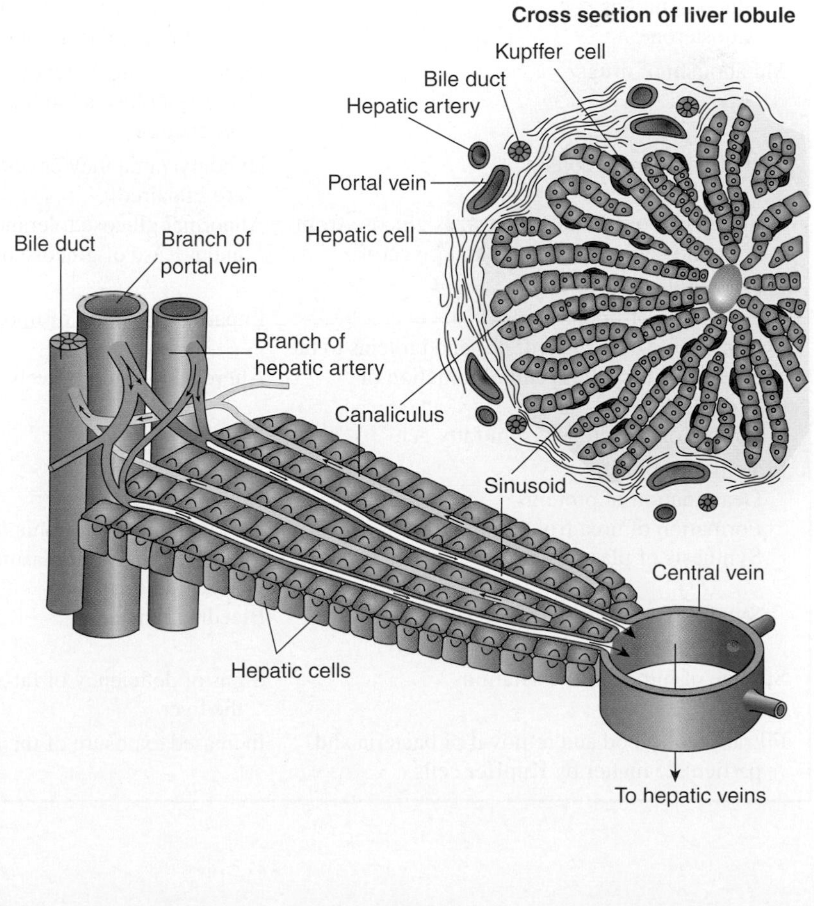

FIGURE 38-3 • A section of liver lobule showing the location of the hepatic veins, hepatic cells, liver sinusoids, and branches of the portal vein and hepatic artery.

descends and passes behind the pancreas and enters the descending duodenum. The pancreatic duct joins the common duct at a short dilated tube called the *hepatopancreatic ampulla* (ampulla of Vater), which empties into the duodenum through the duodenal papilla. Muscle tissue at the junction of the papilla, sometimes called the *sphincter of Oddi,* regulates the flow of bile into the duodenum. When this sphincter is closed, bile moves back into the common duct and gallbladder.

Metabolic Functions of the Liver

The liver is one of the most versatile and active organs in the body. It produces bile; metabolizes hormones and drugs; synthesizes proteins, glucose, and clotting factors; stores vitamins and minerals; changes ammonia produced by deamination of amino acids to urea; and converts fatty acids to ketones. The liver also degrades excess nutrients and converts them into substances essential to the body. In its capacity for metabolizing drugs and hormones, the liver serves as an excretory organ. In this respect, the bile, which carries the end products of substances metabolized by the liver, is much like the urine, which carries the body wastes filtered by the kidneys. The functions of the liver are summarized in Table 38-1.

Carbohydrate Metabolism

The liver plays an essential role in carbohydrate metabolism and glucose homeostasis (Fig. 38-4). The liver stores excess glucose as glycogen and releases it into the circulation when blood glucose levels fall. The liver also synthesizes glucose from amino acids, glycerol, and lactic acid as a means of maintaining blood glucose during periods of fasting or increased need. The liver also converts excess carbohydrates to triglycerides for storage in adipose tissue.

Protein Synthesis and Conversion of Ammonia to Urea

The liver is an important site for protein synthesis and degradation. It produces the proteins for its own cellular needs, and secretory proteins that are released into the circulation. The most important of these secretory proteins is albumin. Albumin

TABLE 38-1 Functions of the Liver and Manifestations of Altered Function

FUNCTION	MANIFESTATIONS OF ALTERED FUNCTION
Production of bile salts	Malabsorption of fat and fat-soluble vitamins
Elimination of bilirubin	Elevation in serum bilirubin and jaundice
Metabolism of steroid hormones	
Sex hormones	Disturbances in gonadal function, including gynecomastia in the male
Glucocorticoids	Signs of increased cortisol levels (*i.e.,* Cushing syndrome)
Aldosterone	Signs of hyperaldosteronism (*e.g.,* sodium retention and hypokalemia)
Metabolism of drugs	Decreased drug metabolism
	Decreased plasma binding of drugs owing to a decrease in albumin production
Carbohydrate metabolism	Hypoglycemia may develop when glycogenolysis and gluconeogenesis are impaired
Stores glycogen and synthesizes glucose from amino acids, lactic acid, and glycerol	Abnormal glucose tolerance curve may occur because of impaired uptake and release of glucose by the liver
Fat metabolism	
Formation of lipoproteins	Impaired synthesis of lipoproteins
Conversion of carbohydrates and proteins to fat	
Synthesis, recycling, and elimination of cholesterol	Altered cholesterol levels
Formation of ketones from fatty acid	
Protein metabolism	
Deamination of proteins	
Formation of urea from ammonia	Elevated blood ammonia levels
Synthesis of plasma proteins	Decreased levels of plasma proteins, particularly albumin, which contributes to edema formation
Synthesis of clotting factors (fibrinogen, prothrombin, factors V, VII, IX, X)	Bleeding tendency
Storage of minerals and vitamins	Signs of deficiency of fat-soluble and other vitamins that are stored in the liver
Filtration of blood and removal of bacteria and particulate matter by Kupffer cells	Increased exposure of the body to colonic bacteria and other foreign matter

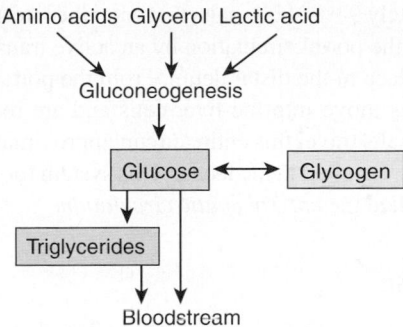

Amino acids Glycerol Lactic acid

Gluconeogenesis

Glucose ↔ Glycogen

Triglycerides

Bloodstream

FIGURE 38-4 • Hepatic pathways for storage and synthesis of glucose and conversion of glucose to fatty acids.

contributes significantly to the plasma colloidal osmotic pressure (see Chapter 31) and to the binding and transport of numerous substances, including some hormones, fatty acids, bilirubin, and other anions. The liver also produces other important proteins, such as fibrinogen and the blood clotting factors.

Through a variety of anabolic and catabolic processes, the liver is the major site of amino acid interconversion (Fig. 38-5). Hepatic catabolism and degradation involve two major reactions: transamination and deamination. In *transamination,* an amino group (NH_2) is transferred to an acceptor substance. As a result of transamination, amino acids can participate in the

intermediary metabolism of carbohydrates and lipids. During periods of fasting or starvation, amino acids are used for producing glucose (*i.e.,* gluconeogenesis). Most of the nonessential amino acids are synthesized in the liver by transamination. The process of transamination is catalyzed by *aminotransferases,* enzymes that are found in high amounts in the liver.

Oxidative *deamination* involves the removal of the amino groups from amino acids and conversion of amino acids to ketoacids and ammonia. This occurs mainly by transamination, in which the amino groups are removed and then transferred to another acceptor substance. The acceptor substance can then transfer the amino group to still another substance or release it as ammonia. Because ammonia is very toxic to body tissues, particularly neurons, the ammonia that is released during deamination is rapidly removed from the blood by the liver and converted to urea. Essentially all urea formed in the body is synthesized by the urea cycle in the liver and then excreted by the kidneys.[2] Although urea is mostly excreted by the kidneys, some diffuses into the intestine, where it is converted to ammonia by enteric bacteria. The intestinal production of ammonia also results from bacterial deamination of unabsorbed amino acids and proteins derived from the diet, exfoliated cells, or blood in the gastrointestinal tract. Ammonia produced in the intestine is absorbed into the portal circulation and transported to the liver, where it is converted to urea before being released into the systemic circulation. Intestinal production of ammonia is increased after ingestion of high-protein foods and gastrointestinal bleeding. In advanced liver disease, urea synthesis often is impaired, leading to an accumulation of blood ammonia.

Pathways of Lipid Metabolism

Although most cells of the body metabolize fat, certain aspects of lipid metabolism occur mainly in the liver, including the oxidation of free fatty acids to ketoacids that supply energy for other body functions; synthesis of cholesterol, phospholipids, and lipoproteins; and formation of triglycerides from carbohydrates and proteins (Fig. 38-6). To derive energy from triglycerides, the molecule must first be split into glycerol and fatty acids, and then the fatty acids split into two-carbon acetyl-coenzyme A (acetyl-CoA) units by a process called *beta oxidation.* Acetyl-CoA is readily channeled into the citric acid cycle to produce adenosine triphosphate (ATP). Because the liver cannot use all the acetyl-CoA that is formed, it converts the excess into acetoacetic acid, a highly soluble ketoacid that is released into the bloodstream and transported to other tissues, where it is used for energy. During periods of starvation, ketones become a major source of energy as fatty acids released from adipose tissue are converted to ketones by the liver.

Acetyl-CoA units from fat metabolism also are used to synthesize cholesterol and bile acids in the liver. Cholesterol has several fates in the liver. It can be esterified and stored; it can be exported bound to lipoproteins; or it can be converted to bile acids. The rate-limiting step in cholesterol synthesis is that which is catalyzed by 3-hydroxy-3-methylglutaryl-coenzyme A reductase (HMG-CoA reductase). The HMG-CoA

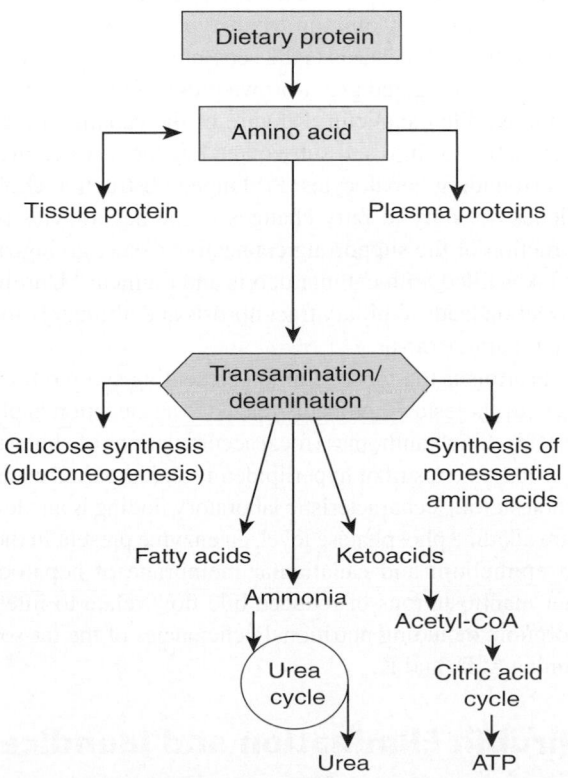

Dietary protein

Amino acid

Tissue protein

Plasma proteins

Transamination/ deamination

Glucose synthesis (gluconeogenesis)

Synthesis of nonessential amino acids

Fatty acids   Ketoacids

Ammonia

Acetyl-CoA

Urea cycle

Citric acid cycle

Urea

ATP

FIGURE 38-5 • Hepatic pathways for conversion of amino acids to proteins, nucleic acids, ketoacids, and glucose. The urea cycle converts ammonia generated by the deamination of amino acids to urea. Acetyl CoA, acetyl-coenzyme A; ATP, adenosine triphosphate.

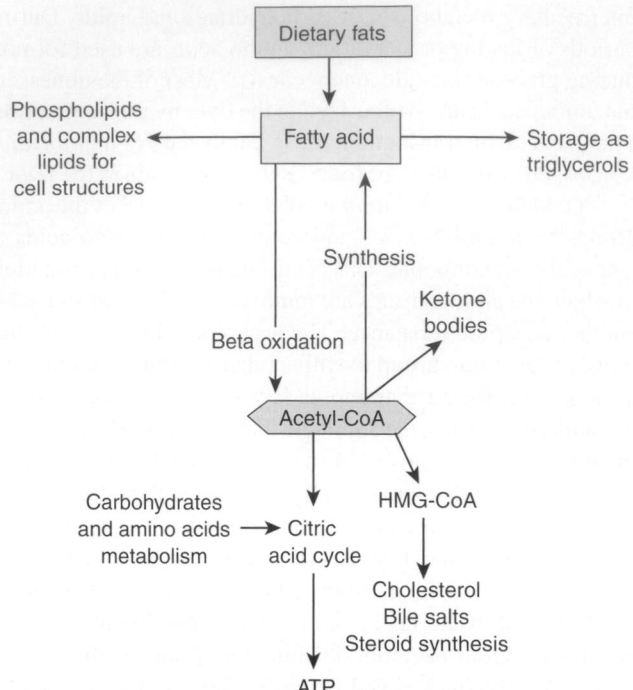

FIGURE 38-6 • Hepatic pathways for fat metabolism. Beta oxidation breaks fatty acids into two-carbon acetyl-coenzyme A (acetyl-CoA) units that are used in the citric acid cycle to generate adenosine triphosphate (ATP), or are used in the synthesis of cholesterol of ketoacids that are released into the blood for use by other tissues as an energy source.

reductase inhibitors, or statins (fluvastatin, lovastatin, pravastatin, atorvastatin), are used to treat high cholesterol levels by inhibiting this step in cholesterol synthesis (see Chapter 22).

Almost all the fat synthesis in the body from carbohydrates and proteins occurs in the liver. Whenever a greater quantity of carbohydrates enters the body than can be immediately used, the excess is converted to triglycerides in the liver. The triglycerides formed in the liver are transported mainly in low-density lipoproteins (LDLs) to the adipose tissue, where they are stored.

Bile Production and Cholestasis

The secretion of bile is essential for digestion of dietary fats and absorption of fats and fat-soluble vitamins from the intestine. The liver produces approximately 600 to 1200 mL of yellow-green bile daily.[1] Bile contains water, bile salts, bilirubin, cholesterol, and certain byproducts of metabolism. Of these, only bile salts, which are formed from cholesterol, are important in digestion. The other components of bile depend on the secretion of sodium, chloride, bicarbonate, and potassium by the bile ducts.

Bile salts serve an important function in digestion; they aid in emulsifying dietary fats, and they are necessary for the formation of the micelles that transport fatty acids and fat-soluble vitamins to the surface of the intestinal mucosa for absorption.

Approximately 94% of bile salts that enter the intestine are reabsorbed into the portal circulation by an active transport process that takes place in the distal ileum. From the portal circulation, the bile salts move into the liver cells and are recycled. Normally, bile salts travel this entire circuit approximately 18 times before being expelled in the feces.[1] This system for recirculation of bile is called the *enterohepatic circulation.*

Cholestasis

Cholestasis represents a decrease in bile flow through the intrahepatic canaliculi and a reduction in secretion of water, bilirubin, and bile acids by the hepatocytes. As a result, the materials normally transferred to the bile, including bilirubin, cholesterol, and bile acids, accumulate in the blood.[3,4] The condition may be caused by intrinsic liver disease, in which case it is referred to as *intrahepatic cholestasis,* or by obstruction of the large bile ducts, a condition known as *extrahepatic cholestasis.*

A number of mechanisms are implicated in the pathogenesis of cholestasis. Primary biliary cirrhosis and primary sclerosing cholangitis are caused by disorders of the small intrahepatic canaliculi and bile ducts. In the case of extrahepatic obstruction, which can be caused by conditions such as cholelithiasis, common duct strictures, or obstructing neoplasms, the effects begin with increased pressure in the large bile ducts. Genetic disorders involving the transport of bile into the canaliculi also can result in cholestasis.

The morphologic features of cholestasis depend on the underlying cause. Common to all types of obstructive and hepatocellular cholestasis is the accumulation of bile pigment in the liver. Elongated green-brown plugs of bile are visible in the dilated bile canaliculi. Rupture of the canaliculi leads to extravasation of bile and subsequent degenerative changes in the surrounding hepatocytes. Prolonged obstructive cholestasis leads not only to fatty changes in the hepatocytes but to destruction of the supporting connective tissue, giving rise to bile lakes filled with cellular debris and pigment.[3] Unrelieved obstruction leads to biliary tract fibrosis and ultimately to end-stage biliary cirrhosis.

Pruritus is the most common presenting symptom in persons with cholestasis, probably related to an elevation in plasma bile acids. Skin xanthomas (focal accumulations of cholesterol) may occur, the result of hyperlipidemia and impaired excretion of cholesterol. A characteristic laboratory finding is an elevated serum alkaline phosphatase level, an enzyme present in the bile duct epithelium and canalicular membrane of hepatocytes. Other manifestations of reduced bile flow relate to intestinal absorption, including nutritional deficiencies of the fat-soluble vitamins A, D, and K.

Bilirubin Elimination and Jaundice

Bilirubin is the substance that gives bile its color. It is formed from senescent red blood cells. In the process of degradation, the hemoglobin from the red blood cell is broken down to form biliverdin, which is rapidly converted to free bilirubin (Fig. 38-7).

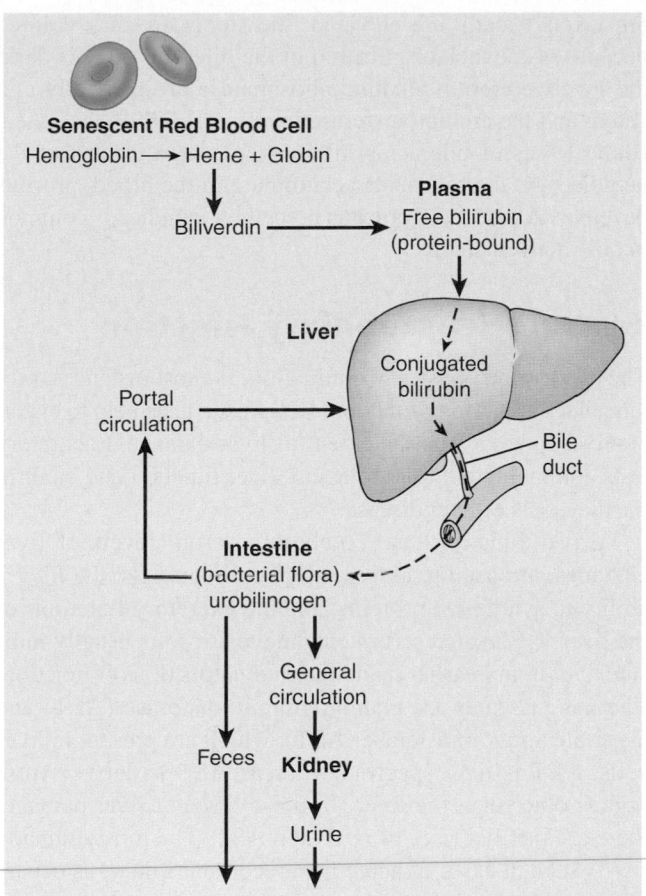

FIGURE 38-7 • The process of bilirubin formation, circulation, and elimination.

Free bilirubin, which is insoluble in plasma, is transported in the blood attached to plasma albumin. Even when it is bound to albumin, this bilirubin is still called *free bilirubin,* to distinguish it from conjugated bilirubin. As it passes through the liver, free bilirubin is absorbed through the hepatocytes' cell membrane and released from its albumin carrier molecule. Inside the hepatocytes, free bilirubin is converted to conjugated bilirubin, making it soluble in bile. Conjugated bilirubin is secreted as a constituent of bile, and in this form it passes through the bile ducts into the small intestine. In the intestine, approximately one half of the bilirubin is converted into a highly soluble substance called *urobilinogen* by the intestinal flora. Urobilinogen is either absorbed into the portal circulation or excreted in the feces. Most of the urobilinogen that is absorbed is returned to the liver to be reexcreted into the bile. A small amount of urobilinogen, approximately 5%, is absorbed into the general circulation and then excreted by the kidneys.

Usually, only a small amount of bilirubin is found in the blood; the normal level of total serum bilirubin is 0.1 to 1.2 mg/dL (17 to 21 μmol). Laboratory measurements of bilirubin usually measure the free and the conjugated bilirubin as well as the total bilirubin. These are reported as the direct (conjugated) bilirubin and the indirect (unconjugated or free) bilirubin.

Jaundice

Jaundice (*i.e.,* icterus) or a yellowish discoloration of the skin and deep tissues results from abnormally high levels of bilirubin in the blood. Jaundice becomes evident when the serum bilirubin levels rise above 2 to 2.5 mg/dL (34.2 to 42.8 μmol).[3,4] Because normal skin has a yellow cast, the early signs of jaundice often are difficult to detect, especially in persons with dark skin. Bilirubin has a special affinity for elastic tissue. The sclera of the eye, which contains a high proportion of elastic fibers, usually is one of the first structures in which jaundice can be detected (Fig. 38-8).

The four major causes of jaundice are excessive destruction of red blood cells, impaired uptake of bilirubin by the liver cells, decreased conjugation of bilirubin, and obstruction of bile flow in the canaliculi of the hepatic lobules or in the intrahepatic or extrahepatic bile ducts. From an anatomic standpoint, jaundice can be categorized as prehepatic, intrahepatic, and posthepatic. Chart 38-1 lists the common causes of prehepatic, hepatic, and posthepatic jaundice.

The major cause of prehepatic jaundice is excessive hemolysis of red blood cells. Hemolytic jaundice occurs when red blood cells are destroyed at a rate in excess of the liver's ability to remove the bilirubin from the blood. It may follow a hemolytic blood transfusion reaction or may occur in diseases such as hereditary spherocytosis, in which the red cell membranes are defective, or in hemolytic disease of the newborn (see Chapter 14). Neonatal hyperbilirubinemia results from increased production of bilirubin in newborn infants and their limited ability to excrete it.[5] Premature infants are at particular risk because their red cells have a shorter life span and higher turnover rate. In prehepatic jaundice, there is mild jaundice, the unconjugated bilirubin is elevated, the stools are of normal color, and there is no bilirubin in the urine.

Intrahepatic or hepatocellular jaundice is caused by disorders that directly affect the ability of the liver to remove

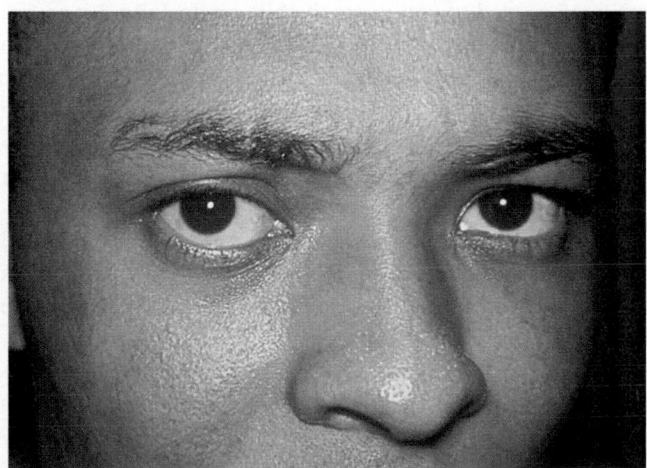

FIGURE 38-8 • Jaundice in a person with hepatitis A. (From Centers for Disease Control and Prevention. [2008]. Public Health Image Library. [Online.] Available: http://phil.cdc.gov/phil/home.asp.)

CAUSES OF JAUNDICE

Prehepatic (Excessive Red Blood Cell Destruction)
Hemolytic blood transfusion reaction
Hereditary disorders of the red blood cell
   Sickle cell disease
   Thalassemia
   Spherocytosis
Acquired hemolytic disorders
Hemolytic disease of the newborn
Autoimmune hemolytic anemias

Intrahepatic
Decreased bilirubin uptake by the liver
Decreased conjugation of bilirubin
Hepatocellular liver damage
   Hepatitis
   Cirrhosis
   Cancer of the liver
Drug-induced cholestasis

Posthepatic (Obstruction of Bile Flow)
Structural disorders of the bile duct
Cholelithiasis
Congenital atresia of the extrahepatic bile ducts
Bile duct obstruction caused by tumors

bilirubin from the blood or conjugate it so it can be eliminated in the bile. Gilbert disease is inherited as a dominant trait and results in a reduced removal of bilirubin from the blood; the disorder is benign and fairly common. Affected persons have no symptoms other than a slightly elevated unconjugated bilirubin and mild jaundice. Conjugation of bilirubin is impaired whenever liver cells are damaged, when transport of bilirubin into liver cells becomes deficient, or when the enzymes needed to conjugate the bile are lacking. Liver diseases such as hepatitis and cirrhosis are the most common causes of intrahepatic jaundice. Drugs such as the anesthetic agent halothane, oral contraceptives, estrogen, anabolic steroids, isoniazid, and chlorpromazine may also be implicated in this type of jaundice. Intrahepatic or hepatocellular jaundice usually interferes with all phases of bilirubin metabolism—uptake, conjugation, and excretion. Both conjugated and unconjugated bilirubin are elevated, the urine often is dark because of bilirubin in the urine, and the serum alkaline phosphatase is slightly elevated.

Posthepatic or obstructive jaundice, also called *cholestatic jaundice,* occurs when bile flow is obstructed between the liver and the intestine, with the obstruction located at any point between the junction of the right or left hepatic duct and the point where the bile duct opens into the intestine. Among the causes are strictures of the bile duct, gallstones, and tumors of the bile duct or the pancreas. Conjugated biliru-

bin levels usually are elevated; the stools are clay colored because of the lack of bilirubin in the bile; the urine is dark; the levels of serum alkaline phosphatase are markedly elevated; and the aminotransferase levels are slightly increased. Blood levels of bile acids often are elevated in obstructive jaundice. As the bile acids accumulate in the blood, pruritus develops. A history of pruritus preceding jaundice is common in obstructive jaundice.

Tests of Hepatobiliary Function

The history and physical examination, in most instances, provide clues about liver function. Diagnostic tests help to evaluate liver function and the extent of liver damage. Laboratory tests commonly are used to assess liver function and confirm the diagnosis of liver disease.

Liver function tests, including serum levels of liver enzymes, are used to assess injury to liver cells, the liver's ability to synthesize proteins, and the excretory functions of the liver.[6,7] Elevated serum enzyme test results usually indicate liver injury earlier than other indicators of liver function. The key enzymes are alanine aminotransferase (ALT) and aspartate aminotransferase (AST), which are present in liver cells. ALT is liver specific, whereas AST is derived from organs other than the liver. In most cases of liver damage, there are parallel rises in ALT and AST. The most dramatic rise is seen in cases of acute hepatocellular injury, as occurs with viral hepatitis, hypoxic or ischemic injury, acute toxic injury, or Reye syndrome.

The liver's synthetic capacity is reflected in measures of serum protein levels and prothrombin time (*i.e.,* synthesis of coagulation factors). Hypoalbuminemia due to depressed synthesis may complicate severe liver disease. Deficiencies of coagulation factor V and vitamin K–dependent factors (II, VII, IX, and X) may occur.

Serum bilirubin, γ-glutamyltransferase (GGT), and alkaline phosphatase measure hepatic excretory function. Alkaline phosphatase is present in the membranes between liver cells and the bile duct and is released by disorders affecting the bile duct.[6] GGT is thought to function in the transport of amino acids and peptides into liver cells; it is a sensitive indicator of hepatobiliary disease. Measurement of GGT may be helpful in diagnosing alcohol abuse.[6]

Ultrasonography provides information about the size, composition, and blood flow of the liver. It has largely replaced cholangiography in detecting stones in the gallbladder or biliary tree. Computed tomography (CT) scanning provides information similar to that obtained by ultrasonography. Magnetic resonance imaging (MRI) has proved to be useful in some disorders. Selective angiography of the celiac, superior mesenteric, or hepatic artery may be used to visualize the hepatic or portal circulation. A liver biopsy affords a means of examining liver tissue without surgery. There are several methods for obtaining liver tissue: percutaneous liver biopsy, which uses a suction, cutting, or spring-loaded cutting needle; laparoscopic liver biopsy; and fine-needle biopsy, which is performed under ultrasonographic or CT guidance.[8] The type of method used is based on the number of specimens needed and the amount of tissue required for evaluation. Laparoscopic liver biopsy provides the means for examining abdominal masses, evaluating ascites of unknown cause, and staging liver cancers.

IN SUMMARY, the hepatobiliary system consists of the liver, gallbladder, and bile ducts. The liver is the largest and, in functions, one of the most versatile organs in the body. It is located between the gastrointestinal tract and the systemic circulation; venous blood from the intestine flows through the liver before it is returned to the heart. In this way, nutrients can be removed for processing and storage, and bacteria and other foreign matter can be removed by Kupffer cells before the blood is returned to the systemic circulation.

The liver synthesizes fats, glucose, and plasma proteins. Other important functions of the liver include the deamination of amino acids, conversion of ammonia to urea, and the interconversion of amino acids and other compounds that are important to the metabolic processes of the body. The liver produces approximately 600 to 1200 mL of yellow-green bile daily. Bile serves as an excretory vehicle for bilirubin, cholesterol, and certain products of organic metabolism and it contains bile salts that are essential for digestion of fats and absorption of fat-soluble vitamins. The liver also removes, conjugates, and secretes bilirubin into the bile. Jaundice occurs when bilirubin accumulates in the blood. It can occur because of excessive red blood cell destruction, failure of the liver to remove and conjugate the bilirubin, or obstructed biliary flow.

Liver function tests, including serum aminotransferase levels, are used to assess injury to liver cells. Serum bilirubin, GGT, and alkaline phosphatase are used as measures of hepatic excretory function. Ultrasonography, CT scans, and MRI are used to evaluate liver structures. Angiography may be used to visualize the hepatic or portal circulation, and a liver biopsy obtains tissue specimens for microscopic examination. ■

DISORDERS OF HEPATIC AND BILIARY FUNCTION

After completing this section of the chapter, you should be able to meet the following objectives:

- State the three ways by which drugs and other substances are metabolized or inactivated in the liver and provide examples of liver disease related to the toxic effects of drugs and chemical agents.
- Compare hepatitis A, B, C, D, and E in terms of source of infection, incubation period, acute disease manifestations, development of chronic disease, and the carrier state.

- Define chronic hepatitis and compare the pathogenesis of chronic autoimmune and chronic viral hepatitis.
- Characterize the metabolism of alcohol by the liver and state metabolic mechanisms that can be used to explain liver injury.
- Summarize the three patterns of injury that occur with alcohol-induced liver disease.
- Describe the pathogenesis of intrahepatic biliary tract disease.
- Characterize the liver changes that occur with cirrhosis.
- Describe the physiologic basis for portal hypertension and relate it to the development of ascites, esophageal varices, and splenomegaly.
- Relate the functions of the liver to the manifestations of liver failure.
- Characterize etiologies of hepatocellular cancer and state the reason for the poor prognosis in persons with this type of cancer.

The structures of the hepatobiliary system are subject to many of the same pathologic conditions that affect other body systems: injury from drugs and toxins; infection, inflammation, and immune responses; metabolic disorders; and neoplasms. This section focuses on alterations in liver function due to drug-induced injury; viral and autoimmune hepatitis; intrahepatic biliary tract disorders; alcohol-induced liver disease; cirrhosis, portal hypertension, and liver failure; and cancer of the liver.

Hepatotoxic Disorders

By virtue of its many enzyme systems that are involved in biochemical transformations and modifications, the liver has an important role in the metabolism of many drugs and chemical substances. The liver is particularly important in terms of metabolizing lipid-soluble substances that cannot be directly excreted by the kidneys. Because the liver is central to the metabolic disposition of virtually all drugs and foreign substances, drug-induced liver toxicity is a potential complication of many medications.

Drug and Hormone Metabolism

Two major types of reactions are involved in the hepatic detoxification and metabolism of drugs and other chemicals: phase 1 reactions, which involve chemical modification or inactivation of a substance, and phase 2 reactions, which involve conversion of lipid-soluble substances to water-soluble derivatives.[9] Often, the two types of reactions are linked. Many phase 1 reactants are not water-soluble and must therefore undergo a subsequent phase 2 reaction to be eliminated. These reactions, which are called *biotransformations,* are important considerations in drug therapy.

Phase 1 reactions result in chemical modification of reactive drug groups by oxidation, reduction, hydroxylation, or other chemical reactions. Most drug-metabolizing enzymes are located in the lipophilic membranes of the smooth endoplasmic reticulum of liver cells (see Chapter 4). When these membranes are broken down and separated in the laboratory, they re-form into vesicles called *microsomes*. The enzymes in these membranes are often referred to as *microsomal enzymes*. The enzymes involved in most phase 1 oxidation–reduction processes are products of a gene superfamily that has nearly 300 members.[9] These genes code for a group of microsomal isoenzymes that make up the cytochrome (CYP) P450 system. (The name *cytochrome P450* is derived from the spectral properties [absorb light at 450 nm] of the hemoproteins that participate in oxidation–reduction processes.) The gene products of many of the *CYP* genes have been identified and traced to the metabolism of specific drugs and to potential interactions among drugs. Each family of genes is responsible for certain drug-metabolizing processes, and each member of the family undertakes specific drug-metabolizing functions. For example, the *CYP3* gene family contains an A subfamily and several genes numbered 1, 2, 3, and so forth. For example, the primary enzyme for the metabolism of erythromycin in humans is CYP 3A4.[9]

Many gene members of the *CYP* system can have their activity induced or suppressed as they undergo the task of metabolizing drugs. For example, drugs such as alcohol and barbiturates can induce certain members to increase enzyme production, accelerating drug metabolism and decreasing the pharmacologic action of the drug and of coadministered drugs that use the same member of the CYP system. In the case of drugs metabolically transformed to reactive intermediates, enzyme induction may exacerbate drug-mediated tissue toxicity. Enzymes in the cytochrome system also can be inhibited by drugs. For example, imidazole-containing drugs such as cimetidine (a histamine type 2 receptor blocking drug that is used to reduce gastric acid secretion) and ketoconazole (an antifungal agent) effectively inhibit the metabolism of testosterone.[9] Environmental pollutants also are capable of inducing *CYP* gene activity. For example, exposure to benzo[*a*]pyrene, which is present in tobacco smoke, charcoal-broiled meat, and other organic pyrolysis products, is known to induce members of the *CYP* family and alter the rates of metabolism of some drugs.

Phase 2 reactions, which involve the conversion of lipid-soluble derivatives to water-soluble substances, may follow phase 1 reactions or proceed independently. Conjugation, catalyzed by endoplasmic reticulum enzymes that couple the drug with an activated endogenous compound to render it more water soluble, is one of the most common phase 2 reactions. Although many water-soluble drugs and endogenous substances are excreted unchanged in the urine or bile, lipid-soluble substances tend to accumulate in the body unless they are converted to less active compounds or water-soluble metabolites. In general, the conjugates are more soluble than the parent compound and are pharmacologically inactive. Because the endogenous substrates used in the conjugation process are obtained from the diet, nutrition plays a critical role in phase 2 reactions.

An alternative cytochrome P450–dependent conjugation pathway is important in detoxifying reactive metabolic intermediates. This pathway uses a thiol, or sulfur-containing substance, called *glutathione,* which is used in conjugating drugs that form potentially harmful electrophilic groups. Glutathione is depleted in the detoxification process and must be constantly replenished by compounds from the diet or by cysteine-containing drugs such as *N*-acetylcysteine.[9] The glutathione pathway is central to the detoxification of a number of compounds, including the over-the-counter pain medication acetaminophen (*e.g.,* Tylenol). Acetaminophen metabolism involves a phase 2 reaction. Normally, the capacity of the phase 2 reactants is much greater than that required for metabolizing recommended doses of the drug. However, in situations of acetaminophen overdose, the capacity of the phase 2 system is exceeded and the drug is transformed into toxic metabolites that can cause necrosis of the liver if allowed to accumulate. In this situation, the glutathione pathway plays a critical role in the detoxification of these metabolites. Because the glutathione stores are rapidly depleted, the drug *N*-acetylcysteine, which serves as a glutathione substitute, is used as an antidote for acetaminophen overdose.[10] Chronic alcohol ingestion decreases glutathione stores and increases the risk of acetaminophen toxicity.

In addition to its role in metabolism of drugs and chemicals, the liver also is responsible for hormone inactivation or modification. Insulin and glucagon are inactivated by proteolysis or deamination. Thyroxine and triiodothyronine are metabolized by reactions involving deiodination. Steroid hormones such as the glucocorticoids are first inactivated by a phase 1 reaction and then conjugated by a phase 2 reaction.

Drug-Induced Liver Disease

As the major drug-metabolizing and detoxifying organ in the body, the liver is subject to potential damage from the enormous array of pharmaceutical and environmental chemicals. Many of the widely used therapeutic drugs, including over-the-counter "natural" products, can cause hepatic injury. Of the numerous remedies, medicinal agents, chemicals, and herbal remedies in existence, more than 600 are recognized as being capable of producing hepatic injury.[11]

Numerous host factors contribute to the susceptibility to drug-induced liver disease, including genetic predisposition, age differences, underlying chronic liver disease, diet and alcohol consumption, and the use of multiple interacting drugs. For unknown reasons, women generally predominate among persons with drug-induced liver disease. In one study, women accounted for 79% of reactions to acetaminophen and 73% of idiosyncratic drug reactions.[12] Early identification of drug-induced liver disease is important because withdrawal of the drug is curative in most cases.

Drugs and chemicals can exert their effects by causing hepatocyte injury and death or by cholestatic liver damage due to injury of biliary drainage structures.[13] Drug reactions can be predictable based on the drug's chemical structure and metabolites or unpredictable (idiosyncratic) based on individual characteristics of the person receiving the drug.

Direct Hepatotoxic Injury. Some drugs are known to have toxic effects on the liver based on their chemical structure and the way they are metabolized in the liver. Direct hepatic damage often is age and dose dependent. Direct hepatotoxic reactions usually are a recognized characteristic of certain drugs. They usually result from drug metabolism and the generation of toxic metabolites. Because of the greater activity of the drug-metabolizing enzymes in the central zones of the liver, these agents typically cause centrilobular necrosis. Examples of drugs that cause direct hepatotoxicity are acetaminophen, isoniazid, and phenytoin, as well as a number of chemical agents, including carbon tetrachloride. Acetaminophen toxicity produces the most common form of acute liver failure, accounting for 39% of cases in a recent survey of tertiary care centers.[11] The injury is characterized by marked elevations in ALT and AST values with minimally elevated alkaline phosphatase. Bilirubin levels invariably are increased, and the prognosis often is worse when hepatocellular necrosis is accompanied by jaundice.

Idiosyncratic Reactions. In contrast to direct hepatotoxic drug reactions, idiosyncratic reactions are unpredictable, not related to dose, and sometimes accompanied by features suggesting an allergic reaction. In some cases, the reaction results directly from a metabolite that is produced only in certain persons based on a genetic predisposition. For example, certain people are capable of rapid acetylation of isoniazid, an antituberculosis drug.

Cholestatic Reactions. Cholestatic drug reactions result in decreased secretion of bile or obstruction of the biliary tree. Acute intrahepatic cholestasis is one of the most frequent types of idiosyncratic drug reactions. Among the drugs credited with causing cholestatic drug reactions are estradiol; chlorpromazine, an antipsychotic drug; and some of the antibiotics, including amoxicillin/clavulanic acid, erythromycin, and nafcillin. Typically, cholestatic drug reactions are characterized by an early onset of jaundice and pruritus, with little alteration in the person's general feeling of well-being. Most instances of acute drug-induced cholestasis subside once the drug is withdrawn.

Chronic Hepatitis. Some drugs produce a more indolent form of liver damage that closely resembles autoimmune hepatitis. Early identification of drug-related chronic hepatitis often is difficult; cirrhosis may develop before the hepatitis is diagnosed. Identifying the responsible drug that caused the liver damage may be difficult retrospectively if the person has been consuming alcohol or taking several drugs.

Viral Hepatitis

Hepatitis refers to inflammation of the liver. It can be caused by hepatotropic viruses that primarily affect liver cells or hepatocytes, autoimmune mechanisms, or reactions to drugs and

---

> ## 🔑 DISEASES OF THE LIVER
>
> - Diseases of the liver can affect the hepatocytes or the biliary drainage system.
>
> - Diseases of hepatocytes impair the metabolic and synthetic functions of the liver, causing disorders in carbohydrate, protein, and fat metabolism; metabolism and removal of drugs, hormones, toxins, ammonia, and bilirubin from the blood; and the interconversion of amino acids and synthesis of proteins. Elevations in serum aminotransferase levels signal the presence of hepatocyte damage.
>
> - Diseases of the biliary drainage system obstruct the flow of bile and interfere with the elimination of bile salts and bilirubin, producing cholestatic liver damage because of the backup of bile into the lobules of the liver. Elevations in bilirubin and alkaline phosphatase signal the presence of cholestatic liver damage.

toxins, or be secondary to other systemic disorders. Viruses causing systemic disease that can involve the liver include Epstein-Barr virus (infectious mononucleosis), which may cause a mild hepatitis during the acute phase; cytomegalovirus (particularly in newborns and immunosuppressed persons); herpesviruses; and enteroviruses.

The known hepatotropic viruses include hepatitis A virus (HAV), hepatitis B virus (HBV), the hepatitis B–associated delta virus (HDV), hepatitis C virus (HCV), and hepatitis E virus (HEV). Although all of these viruses cause acute hepatitis, they differ in the mode of transmission and incubation period; mechanism, degree, and chronicity of liver damage; and ability to evolve to a carrier state. The presence of viral antigens and their antibodies can be determined through laboratory tests. Epidemiologic studies have indicated that some cases of infectious hepatitis are due to other agents. A viral agent similar to HCV has been cloned and identified as hepatitis G virus (HGV). Evidence of HGV has been found in 1% to 4% of blood donors in the United States. However, HGV does not appear to cause liver disease or exacerbations of liver disease.[3]

There are two mechanisms of liver injury in viral hepatitis: direct cellular injury and induction of immune responses against the viral antigens. The mechanisms of injury have been most closely studied in HBV. It is thought that the extent of inflammation and necrosis depends on the individual's immune response. Accordingly, a prompt immune response during the acute phase of the infection would be expected to cause cell injury but at the same time eliminate the virus. Thus, people who respond with fewer symptoms and a marginal immune response are less likely to eliminate the virus, and hepatocytes expressing the viral antigens persist, leading to the chronic or carrier state. Fulminant hepatitis would be explained in terms of an accelerated immune response with severe liver necrosis.

The clinical course of viral hepatitis involves a number of syndromes, including asymptomatic infection with only serologic evidence of disease; acute hepatitis; the carrier state without clinically apparent disease or with chronic hepatitis; chronic hepatitis with or without progression to cirrhosis; or fulminating disease (<1% to 3%) with rapid onset of liver failure. Not all hepatotoxic viruses provoke each of the clinical syndromes.

The manifestations of acute viral hepatitis can be divided into three phases: the prodromal or preicterus period, the icterus period, and the convalescent period. The manifestations of the prodromal period vary from abrupt to insidious, with general malaise, myalgia, arthralgia, easy fatigability, and severe anorexia out of proportion to the degree of illness. Gastrointestinal symptoms such as nausea, vomiting, and diarrhea or constipation may occur. Abdominal pain is usually mild and felt on the right side. Chills and fever may mark an abrupt onset. In persons who smoke, there may be a distaste for smoking that parallels the anorexia. Serum levels of AST and ALT show variable increases during the preicterus phase of acute hepatitis and precede a rise in bilirubin that accompanies the onset of the icterus or jaundice phase of infection. The icterus phase, if it occurs, usually follows the prodromal phase by 5 to 10 days. Jaundice is less likely to occur with HCV infection. The prodromal symptoms may become worse with the onset of jaundice, followed by progressive clinical improvement. Severe pruritus and liver tenderness are common during the icterus period. The convalescent phase is characterized by an increased sense of well-being, return of appetite, and disappearance of jaundice. The acute illness usually subsides gradually over a 2- to 3-week period, with complete clinical recovery by approximately 9 weeks in hepatitis A and 16 weeks in uncomplicated hepatitis B.

Infection with HBV and HCV can produce a *carrier state* in which the person does not have symptoms but harbors the virus and can therefore transmit the disease. Evidence also indicates a carrier state for HDV infection. There is no carrier state for HAV infection. There are two types of carriers: healthy carriers who have few or no ill effects, and those with chronic disease who may or may not have symptoms. Factors that increase the risk of becoming a carrier are age at time of infection and immune status. The carrier state for infections that occur early in life, as in infants of HBV-infected mothers, may be as high as 90% to 95%, compared with 1% to 10% of infected adults.[3] Other persons at high risk of becoming carriers are those with impaired immunity, those who have received multiple transfusions or blood products, those who are on hemodialysis, and drug addicts.

Hepatitis A

Hepatitis A is caused by the HAV, a small, unenveloped, single-stranded ribonucleic acid (RNA) virus. It usually is a benign, self-limited disease, although it can cause acute fulminant hepatitis and death from liver failure in rare cases.[3,14] The onset of symptoms usually is abrupt and includes fever, malaise, nausea, anorexia, abdominal discomfort, dark urine, and jaun-

dice. The likelihood of having symptoms is related to age.[14] Children younger than 6 years often are asymptomatic. The illness in older children and adults usually is symptomatic and jaundice occurs in approximately 70% of cases.[14] Symptoms usually last approximately 2 months but can last longer. HAV does not cause chronic hepatitis or induce a carrier state.

Hepatitis A is contracted primarily by the fecal-oral route.[14,15] It has a brief incubation period (15 to 50 days), with an average of 25 to 30 days. The virus replicates in the liver, is excreted in the bile, and shed in the stool. The fecal shedding of HAV occurs up to 2 weeks before the development of symptoms and ends as the immunoglobulin M (IgM) levels rise.[3,14] The disease often occurs sporadically or in epidemics. Drinking contaminated milk or water and eating shellfish from infected waters are fairly common routes of transmission. At special risk are persons traveling abroad who have not previously been exposed to the virus. Because young children are asymptomatic, they play an important role in the spread of the disease. Institutions housing large numbers of persons (usually children) sometimes are stricken with an epidemic of hepatitis A. Oral behavior and lack of toilet training promote viral infection among children attending preschool day care centers, who then carry the virus home to older siblings and parents. Hepatitis A usually is not transmitted by transfusion of blood or plasma derivatives, presumably because its short period of viremia usually coincides with clinical illness, so that the disease is apparent and blood donations are not accepted.

Serologic Markers. Antibodies to HAV (anti-HAV) appear early in the disease and tend to persist in the serum (Fig. 38-9). The IgM antibodies (see Chapter 17) usually appear during the first week of symptomatic disease and begin to decline in a few months.[3] Their presence coincides with a decline in fecal shedding of the virus. Peak levels of IgG antibodies occur after 1 month of illness and may persist for years; they provide long-term protective immunity against reinfection. The presence of

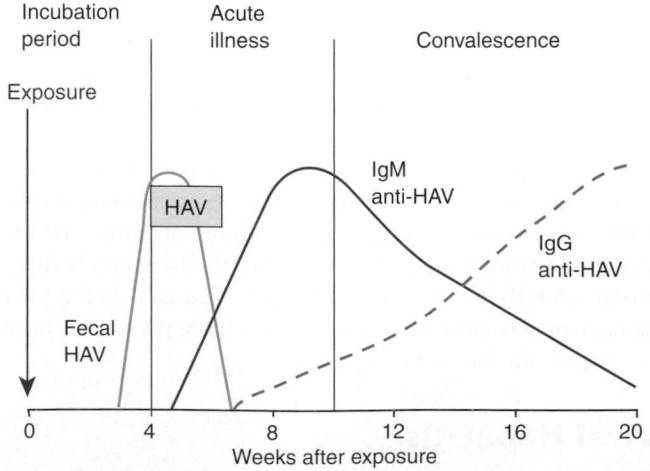

FIGURE 38-9 • The sequence of fecal shedding of the hepatitis A virus (HAV), HAV viremia, and HAV antibody (IgM and IgG anti-HAV) changes in hepatitis A.

IgM anti-HAV is indicative of acute hepatitis A, whereas IgG anti-HAV merely documents past infection.

Immunization.   A hepatitis A vaccine is available.[14-16] Immunization is intended to replace the use of immune globulin in persons at high risk for HAV exposure. These include international travelers to regions where sanitation is poor and endemic HAV infections are high, children living in communities with high rates of HAV infection, homosexually active men, and users of illicit drugs. Persons with preexisting chronic liver disease also may benefit from immunization. A public health benefit also may be derived from vaccinating persons with increased potential for transmitting the disease (*e.g.,* food handlers). The Centers for Disease Control and Prevention (CDC) has recently recommended vaccination of children in states, counties, and communities with high rates of infection.[16] Because the vaccine is of little benefit in prevention of hepatitis in persons with known HAV exposure, immune globulin (IgG) is recommended for these persons.

Hepatitis B

Hepatitis B is caused by the HBV, a double-stranded deoxyribonucleic acid (DNA) virus.[3,16] The complete virion, also called a *Dane particle,* consists of an outer envelope and an inner nucleocapsid that contains HBV DNA and DNA polymerase (Fig. 38-10). HBV infection can produce acute hepatitis, chronic hepatitis, progression of chronic hepatitis to cirrhosis, fulminant hepatitis with massive hepatic necrosis, and the carrier state. It also participates in the development of hepatitis D (delta hepatitis).

Hepatitis B affects more than 350 million people worldwide.[3,17] In the United States, the incidence of acute hepatitis B has declined steadily since the late 1980s, especially among vaccinated children.[18] In 2006, the overall incidence (1.6 cases per 100,000) was the lowest ever recorded and represents a decline of 81% since the national childhood vaccination strategy was implemented in 1991.[18] Although incidence has declined among persons aged 25 to 44 years, rates in this age group, particularly among males, still remains substantially higher than in other age groups, indicating a need for vaccination programs that target high-risk populations.

Hepatitis B has a longer incubation period and represents a more serious health problem than hepatitis A. The virus usually is transmitted through inoculation with infected blood or serum. However, the viral antigen can be found in most body secretions and can be spread by oral or sexual contact. In the United States, most persons with hepatitis B acquire the infection as adults or adolescents. The disease is highly prevalent among injecting drug users, heterosexuals with multiple sex partners, and men who have sex with men.[18,19] Health care workers are at risk owing to blood exposure and accidental needle injuries. Although the virus can be spread through transfusion or administration of blood products, routine screening methods have appreciably reduced transmission through this route. The risk of hepatitis B in infants born to HBV-infected mothers ranges from 10% to 85%, depending on the mother's HBV status. Infants who become infected

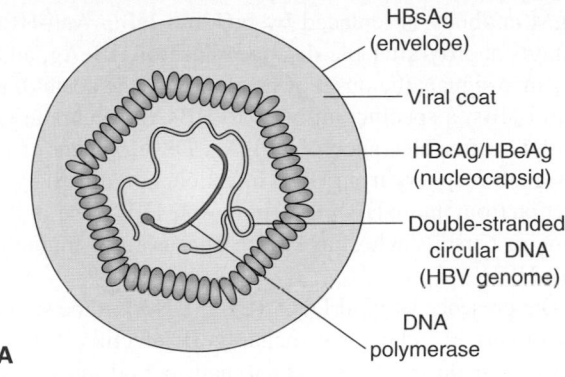

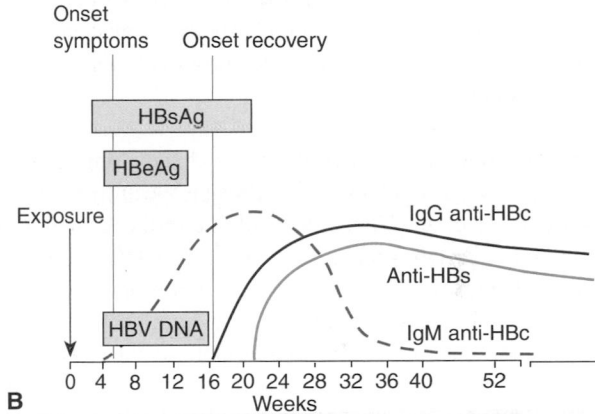

FIGURE 38-10 • **(A)** The hepatitis B virus. **(B)** The sequence of hepatitis B virus (HBV) viral antigens (HBsAg, HBeAg), HBV DNA, and HBV antibody (IgM, IgG, anti-HBc, and anti-HBs) changes in acute resolving hepatitis B.

have a 90% risk of becoming chronic carriers, and up to 25% will die of chronic liver disease as adults.[19]

Serologic Markers.   Three well-defined antigens are associated with the virus: a core antigen, HBcAg, which is contained in the nucleocapsid; a longer polypeptide transcript with precore and core regions, designated HBeAg; and a surface antigen, HBsAg, which is found in the outer envelope of the virus. The precore region directs the HBeAg polypeptide toward the blood, whereas the HBcAg remains in the hepatocytes to direct the assembly of new virions.

The HBV antigens evoke specific antibodies: anti-HBs, anti-HBc, and anti-HBe. These antigens (HBcAg does not circulate freely in the blood) and their antibodies serve as serologic markers for following the course of the disease[3,20] (see Fig. 38-10). The *HBsAg* is the viral antigen measured most routinely in blood. It appears before onset of symptoms, peaks during overt disease, and then declines to undetectable levels in 3 to 6 months. Persistence beyond 6 months indicates continued viral replication, infectivity, and risk of chronic hepatitis. HBeAg appears in the serum soon after HBsAg and signifies active viral replication. IgM anti-HBc becomes detectable shortly before the onset of symptoms, concurrent with onset of an elevation in serum transaminases. Over the months, the IgM antibody is replaced by IgG anti-HBc. Anti-HBe is detectable shortly after the disappearance of HBeAg, and its appearance signals the onset of resolution of the acute illness. IgG anti-HBs, a specific antibody to HBsAg, occurs in most individuals after clearance of HBsAg. Development of anti-HBs signals recovery from HBV infection, noninfectivity, and protection from future HBV infection. Anti-HBs is the antibody present in persons who have been successfully immunized against HBV.

The presence of viral DNA (HBV DNA) in the serum is the most certain indicator of hepatitis B infection. It is transiently present during the presymptomatic period and for a brief time during the acute illness. The presence of DNA polymerase, the enzyme used in viral replication, usually is transient but may persist for years in persons who are chronic carriers, and is an indication of continued infectivity.

Immunization. Hepatitis B vaccine provides long-term protection against HBV infection.[21] HBsAg is the antigen used for hepatitis B vaccines. Vaccines available in the United States use recombinant DNA technology to express HBsAg in yeast, which is then purified by biochemical and biophysical methods. The vaccine is available as a single-antigen formulation and also in fixed combination with other vaccines. The effectiveness of immunization was evidenced by a 75% decline in overall incidence of acute hepatitis B from 1990 to 2004, with the most drastic declines occurring in the cohort of children in whom recommendations for routine infant and adolescent vaccination were implemented. A hepatitis B immune globulin (HBIG) is available. Prepared from plasma donors with high concentrations of anti-HBs, it is used as an adjunct to hepatitis B vaccine for postexposure immunoprophylaxis to prevent HBV infection.

The CDC recommends vaccination of all children 0 to 18 years of age as a means of preventing HBV transmission.[22] The vaccine also is recommended for all unvaccinated adults (1) who are at high risk for infection by sexual exposure, including sex partners of HBsAg-positive persons, sexually active persons who are not in a long-term mutually monogamous relationship, persons seeking evaluation for treatment of sexually transmitted diseases, and men who have sex with men; (2) who are at high risk for infection by percutaneous or mucosal exposure to blood, including current and recent injecting drug abusers, household contacts of HBsAg-positive persons, residents and staff of institutions for the developmentally disabled, health care and public safety workers with reasonably anticipated risk for exposure to blood or blood-contaminated body fluids, and persons with chronic kidney disease (predialysis, hemodialysis, peritoneal dialysis; and home dialysis patients); and (3) *others,* including international travelers to regions with high or intermediate levels of endemic HBV infection, persons with chronic liver disease, persons with human immunodeficiency virus (HIV) infection, and all other persons seeking protection from HBV infection.[19] The CDC also recommends that all pregnant women be routinely tested for HBsAg during an early prenatal visit and that infants born to HBsAg-positive mothers receive appropriate doses of HBIG and hepatitis B vaccine.[21]

HBIG may be effective for unvaccinated persons who are exposed to the infection if given within 7 days of exposure. Hepatitis vaccination is recommended for pre-exposure and postexposure prophylaxis.

Hepatitis C

The HCV is the most common cause of chronic hepatitis, cirrhosis, and hepatocellular cancer in the world. Approximately 3.9 million Americans have antibodies against HCV, and 70% of these persons have evidence of chronic infection as determined by the presence of DNA in their serum.[3] Before 1990, the main route of transmission of HCV was through contaminated blood transfusions or blood products. With implementation of HCV testing in blood banks, the risk of HCV infection from blood transfusion is almost nonexistent in the United States and other developed countries.[23–25] However, unsafe medical procedures and unscreened blood transfusions may be the most important sources of HCV infections in less developed countries of the world. Currently, recreational injecting drug use is the most common mode of HCV transmission in the United States and Canada.[23–25] High-risk sexual behavior, defined as having sex with multiple sexual partners or sex with an HCV-infected partner, is currently the second most common risk factor in the United States. The rate of transmission to infants born to HCV RNA–positive mothers ranges from 4.6% to 10%.[23] HCV also can be spread through exposure in the health care setting, primarily through needle-stick injuries. There also is concern that transmission of small amounts of blood during tattooing, acupuncture, and body piercing may facilitate the transmission of HCV.

HCV is a single-stranded RNA virus with properties similar to those of the flaviviruses, a genus of the family of *Flaviviridae* that includes yellow fever and St. Louis encephalitis viruses.[25,26] The genome contains a single open reading frame that encodes a polyprotein of about 3000 amino acids.[26] The transcript is cleaved into single proteins, including three structural proteins (one core and two envelope proteins) and four nonstructural proteins. The virus is genetically unstable, which leads to multiple genotypes and subtypes. Six different genotypes and more than 50 subtypes of the virus have been recognized.[3,25] Genotype 1 accounts for 60% to 75% of all infections in the United States and Canada and is associated with the lower rate of response to therapy.[25,26] It is likely that the wide diversity of genotypes contributes to the pathogenicity of the virus, allowing it to escape the actions of host immune mechanisms and antiviral medications, and to difficulties in developing a preventive vaccine.[26] Development of a vaccine and treatment measures has also been hampered by the lack of a reliable, reproducible, and efficient culture system for propagating the virus.[25,26]

The incubation period for HCV infection ranges from 2 to 26 weeks (average, 6 to 12 weeks).[3] Children and adults who acquire the infection usually are asymptomatic (60% to 70%), or have a nonspecific clinical disease characterized by fatigue, malaise, anorexia, and weight loss. Jaundice is uncommon, and only 25% to 30% of symptomatic adults have jaundice.[27] These symptoms usually last for 2 to 12 weeks. Fulminant hepatic failure is rare and only a few cases have been reported. A minority of persons who are newly infected with HCV will clear the infection, but most (60% to 85%) go on to develop chronic hepatitis.[25] Factors associated with spontaneous clearing of HCV infection appear to include younger age, female sex, and certain histocompatibility genes. The most serious consequences of chronic HCV infection are progressive liver fibrosis leading to cirrhosis, end-stage liver disease, and hepatocellular cancer. Host factors that may exacerbate the progression of liver disease include older age at onset of infection, male sex, an immunosuppressed state, concurrent HBV infection, alcohol consumption, and hepatotoxic medications.

Serologic Markers. Both antibody and viral tests are available for detecting the presence of HCV infection (Fig. 38-11). False-negative results can occur in immunocompromised people and early in the course of the disease before antibodies develop. Direct measurement of HCV in the serum remains the most accurate test for infection. The viral tests are highly sensitive and specific, but more costly than antibody tests. With newer antibody testing methods, infection often can be detected as early as 6 to 8 weeks after exposure, and as early as 1 to 2 weeks with viral tests that use polymerase chain reaction methods (see Chapter 16). Unlike hepatitis A and B, antibodies to HCV are not protective, but they serve as markers for the disease.

Hepatitis D and E

Hepatitis D virus, or the delta hepatitis agent, is a defective RNA virus. It can cause acute or chronic hepatitis. Infection depends on concomitant infection with HBV, specifically the presence of HBsAg. Acute hepatitis D occurs in two forms: coinfection that occurs simultaneously with acute hepatitis B, and a superinfec-

tion in which hepatitis D is imposed on chronic hepatitis B or hepatitis B carrier state.[3,27] The delta agent often increases the severity of HBV infection. It can convert mild HBV infection into severe, fulminating hepatitis, cause acute hepatitis in asymptomatic carriers, or increase the tendency for progression to chronic hepatitis and cirrhosis.

The routes of transmission of hepatitis D are similar to those for hepatitis B. In the United States, infection is restricted largely to persons at high risk for HBV infection, particularly injecting drug users. The greatest risk is in HBV carriers; these persons should be informed about the dangers of HDV superinfection.

Hepatitis D is diagnosed by detection of antibody to HDV (anti-HDV) in the serum or HDV RNA in the serum. There is no specific treatment for hepatitis D. Because the infection is linked to hepatitis B, prevention of hepatitis D should begin with prevention of hepatitis B through vaccination.

HEV is an unenveloped, single-stranded RNA virus. It is transmitted by the fecal-oral route and causes manifestations of acute hepatitis that are similar to hepatitis A. It does not cause chronic hepatitis or the carrier state.[3] Its distinguishing feature is the high mortality rate (approximately 20%) among pregnant women, owing to the development of fulminant hepatitis. The infection occurs primarily in developing areas such as India, other Southeast Asian countries, parts of Africa, and Mexico. The only reported cases in the United States have been in persons who have recently been in an endemic area.

Chronic Viral Hepatitis

Chronic hepatitis is defined as a chronic inflammatory reaction of the liver of more than 3 to 6 months' duration. It is characterized by persistently elevated serum aminotransferase levels and characteristic histologic findings on liver biopsy. The clinical features of chronic viral hepatitis are highly variable and not predictive of outcome. The most common symptoms are fatigue, malaise, loss of appetite, and occasional bouts of jaundice. Elevation of serum aminotransferase concentrations depends on the level of disease activity.

Chronic viral hepatitis is the principal cause of chronic liver disease, cirrhosis, and hepatocellular cancer in the world and now ranks as the chief reason for liver transplantation in adults.[28] Of the hepatotropic viruses, only three are known to cause chronic hepatitis—HBV, HCV, and HDV. Hepatitis B, which is less likely than hepatitis C to progress to chronic infection, accounts for 5% to 10% of chronic liver disease and cirrhosis in the United States.[28] It is characterized by the persistence of HBV DNA and usually by HBeAg in the serum, indicating active viral replication. Many persons are asymptomatic at the time of diagnosis, and elevated serum aminotransferase levels are the first sign of infection. Chronic hepatitis D infection depends on concurrent infection with HBV.

Chronic hepatitis C accounts for most cases of chronic viral hepatitis. HCV infection becomes chronic in 60% to 85% of cases.[23] Chronic HCV infection often smolders over a period of years, silently destroying liver cells. Most persons with

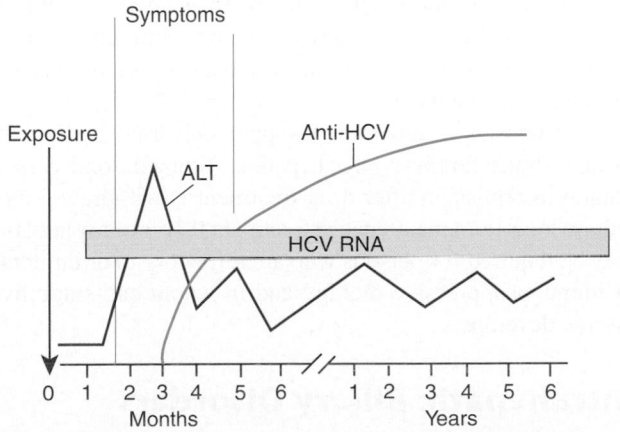

FIGURE 38-11 • The sequence of serologic changes in chronic hepatitis C, with persistence of hepatitis C virus (HCV) RNA and exacerbations and remissions of clinical symptoms indicated by changes in serum alanine aminotransferase (ALT) levels.

chronic hepatitis C are asymptomatic, and diagnosis usually follows a finding of elevated serum aminotransferase levels or complaints of fatigue or nonspecific weakness. Because the course of acute hepatitis C often is mild, many persons do not recall the events of the acute infection.

Treatment. There are no simple and effective treatment methods for chronic viral hepatitis. Drugs used in the treatment of chronic HBV include interferons (recombinant interferon-2α and peginterferon) and the nucleotide and nucleotide analog antiretroviral agents (lamivudine, entecavir, tentovir).[17,28,29] Persons with active viral replication may be treated with peginterferon (pegylated interferon alfa-2a). Peginterferons were developed by adding a polyethylene glycol (PEG) moiety to an interferon molecule (PEG-IFN), resulting in a prolonged serum half-life and the ability to administer the compound once weekly rather than three times a week.[29] Up to 40% of treated patients respond with sustained normalization of liver enzyme levels, disappearance of HBeAg and HBV DNA from the serum, appearance of anti-HBe, and improved survival.[28] Nucleoside and nucleotide analogs may be used instead of interferon for treatment of chronic HBV infection, and are better tolerated. Lamivudine can be given orally and usually is well tolerated, but has a higher rate of viral resistance, a lower durable rate of response, and a greater need for prolonged therapy compared with interferon. Entecavir, another nucleoside analog, can be used in the treatment of persons who are resistant to lamivudine or have cirrhosis. Tenofovir, a drug used for treatment of HIV infection, also has considerable activity against HBV. Other antiviral agents are under study, and strategies using multiple drugs are likely to be investigated. In persons with concurrent hepatitis D infection, interferon therapy may lead to normalization of aminotransferase levels, histologic improvement, and elimination of HDV RNA from the serum in approximately 50% of cases, but relapse is common after the therapy is stopped.[28] Lamivudine is not effective in chronic hepatitis D.

The current treatment for untreated persons with chronic hepatitis C is a combination of the new pegylated forms of interferon (alfa-2b or alfa-2a) plus ribavirin (a nucleoside analog).[28,30,31] Treatment with peginterferon and ribavirin is costly, and side effects, which include flulike symptoms, are almost universal. More serious side effects, which include psychiatric symptoms (depression), thyroid dysfunction, and bone marrow depression, are less common.[28] Although most persons with HCV infection are candidates for treatment, many have other health problems that are contraindications to therapy.

Liver transplantation is a treatment option for end-stage liver disease due to viral hepatitis. Liver transplantation has been more successful in persons with hepatitis C than those with hepatitis B. Although the graft often is reinfected, the disease seems to progress more slowly.

Autoimmune Hepatitis

Autoimmune hepatitis is a severe type of chronic hepatitis of unknown origin that is associated with high levels of serum immunoglobulins, including autoantibodies.[4,32,33] Although the disorder is usually seen in young women, it can occur in either sex at any age. In the United States, autoimmune hepatitis affects up to 200,000 people and accounts for 6% of liver transplantations.

Clinical and laboratory observations have led to the hypothesis that autoimmune hepatitis is a multifactorial disorder, with genetic and environmental factors playing important roles. Most knowledge of the genetics of the disease comes from the human leukocyte antigen (HLA) genes that reside in the major histocompatibility complex (MHC), located on the short arm of chromosome 6 (see Chapter 17). The environmental agents assumed to induce autoimmune hepatitis have not been delineated, but include viruses and chemical agents.

Two distinct types of autoimmune hepatitis have been identified. Type I autoimmune hepatitis, the most common form of the disease, is characterized by increased levels of anti–smooth muscle and antinuclear autoantibodies. Approximately 30% of cases occur in women younger than 40 years of age, a third of whom have other autoimmune diseases. Susceptibility to type I autoimmune hepatitis resides mainly with the *HLA-DRB1* gene. Type II autoimmune hepatitis occurs mainly in children 2 to 14 years of age and is characterized by the presence of antibody to liver and kidney microsomes and liver cytosol. The disorder is often accompanied by other autoimmune disorders, especially type 1 diabetes mellitus and thyroiditis. The genetic component for this type of autoimmune hepatitis is less well defined.

Clinical Manifestations. Clinical manifestations of the disorder cover a spectrum that extends from no apparent symptoms to the signs accompanying liver failure. Physical examination may reveal no abnormalities, but may also reveal hepatomegaly, splenomegaly, jaundice, and signs and symptoms of chronic liver disease. In asymptomatic cases, the disorder may be discovered when abnormal serum enzyme levels are identified during performance of routine screening tests.

Diagnosis and Treatment. The differential diagnosis includes measures to exclude other causes of liver disease, including hepatitis B and C. A characteristic laboratory finding is that of a marked elevation in serum gamma globulins. A biopsy is used to confirm the diagnosis.

Corticosteroid and immunosuppressant drugs are the treatment of choice for this type of hepatitis. Although some persons remain in remission after drug treatment is withdrawn, most require long-term maintenance treatment. Liver transplantation may be required for persons who are refractory to or intolerant of immunosuppressive therapy and in whom end-stage liver disease develops.

Intrahepatic Biliary Disorders

Intrahepatic biliary diseases disrupt the flow of bile through the liver, causing cholestasis and biliary cirrhosis. Among the causes of intrahepatic biliary disease are primary biliary cirrhosis and secondary biliary cirrhosis.

Primary Biliary Cirrhosis

Primary biliary cirrhosis is a chronic disease of the liver characterized by the autoimmune destruction of the small intrahepatic bile ducts and cholestasis.[34,35] The disease is seen most commonly in women 40 to 60 years of age. Familial occurrences of the disease are found between parents and children and among siblings. However, unlike other autoimmune disorders, there is little, if any, association with any particular MHC alleles. In addition, with the possible exception of a reportedly higher risk of a polymorphism of the gene for the vitamin D receptor, there are no clear genetic influences for the disorder. Antimitochondrial antibodies are found in approximately 98% of persons with the disease, but their role in the pathogenesis of the disease is unclear. As with other autoimmune disorders, possible environmental triggers include infectious and chemical agents.

Clinical Manifestations. The disorder is characterized by an insidious onset and progressive scarring and destruction of liver tissue. The liver becomes enlarged and takes on a green hue because of the accumulated bile. The earliest symptoms are unexplained pruritus or itching, weight loss, and fatigue, followed by dark urine and pale stools. Osteoporosis occurs in up to one third of persons with the disorder.[35] Jaundice is a late manifestation of the disorder, as are other signs of liver failure. Serum alkaline phosphatase levels are elevated in persons with primary biliary cirrhosis.

Treatment. Treatment is largely symptomatic. Cholestyramine, a bile acid–binding drug, may prove beneficial for treatment of pruritus. There is no generally accepted treatment for the underlying disease. Ursodeoxycholic acid (ursodiol), a drug that increases bile flow and decreases the toxicity of bile contents, has been shown to decrease the rate of clinical deterioration. Colchicine, which acts to prevent leukocyte migration and phagocytosis, and methotrexate, a drug with immunosuppressive properties, have also resulted in reported benefits in terms of symptom relief. However, liver transplantation remains the only treatment for advanced disease. Primary biliary cirrhosis does not recur after liver transplantation if appropriate immunosuppression is used.

Secondary Biliary Cirrhosis

Secondary biliary cirrhosis results from prolonged obstruction of the extrabiliary tree. The most common cause is cholelithiasis. Other causes of secondary biliary cirrhosis are malignant neoplasms of the biliary tree or head of the pancreas and strictures of the common duct caused by previous surgical procedures. Extrahepatic biliary cirrhosis may benefit from surgical procedures designed to relieve the obstruction.

Alcohol-Induced Liver Disease

The spectrum of alcoholic liver disease includes fatty liver disease, alcoholic hepatitis, and cirrhosis. About 2 million people in the United States are suspected of having alcoholic liver disease, and 14,000 die each year of cirrhosis[36] Most deaths from alcoholic cirrhosis are attributable to liver failure, bleeding esophageal varices, or kidney failure. It has been estimated that there are 14 million alcoholics in the United States. Only approximately 10% to 15% of alcoholics develop cirrhosis, however, suggesting that other conditions such as genetic and environmental factors contribute to its occurrence.[3]

Metabolism of Alcohol

Alcohol is absorbed readily from the gastrointestinal tract; it is one of the few substances that can be absorbed from the stomach. As a substance, alcohol fits somewhere between a food and a drug. It supplies calories but cannot be broken down or stored as protein, fat, or carbohydrate. As a food, alcohol yields 7.1 kcal/g, compared with the 4 kcal/g produced by metabolism of an equal amount of carbohydrate.[37,38] Between 80% and 90% of the alcohol a person drinks is metabolized by the liver. The rest is excreted through the lungs, kidneys, and skin.

Alcohol (ethyl alcohol or ethanol) metabolism proceeds simultaneously by two pathways: the alcohol dehydrogenase (ADH) system, located in the cytoplasm of the hepatocytes; and the microsomal ethanol-oxidizing system (MEOS), located in the endoplasmic reticulum.[37–40] The ADH and MEOS pathways produce specific metabolic and toxic disturbances. A third and minor pathway, the catalase pathway, located in the peroxisomes, can break down ethanol in unusual circumstances.[38]

The major pathway for ethanol metabolism involves ADH, an enzyme that catalyzes the conversion of alcohol to acetaldehyde. In the ADH-mediated oxidation of alcohol, both acetaldehyde and hydrogen are produced. The hydrogen (H^+) is transferred to the cofactor nicotinamide adenine dinucleotide (NAD), which is converted to its reduced form (NADH). The formed acetaldehyde again loses hydrogen and is metabolized to acetate, much of which is released in the bloodstream. As a result, ethanol metabolism generates an excess of NADH, which is thought to contribute to the liver damage that often accompanies excess alcohol consumption.

NAD is also necessary for many other metabolic processes, including the metabolism of pyruvates, urates, and fatty acids. Because alcohol competes for the use of NAD, it tends to disrupt other metabolic functions of the liver. The preferential use of NAD for alcohol metabolism can result in increased production and accumulation of lactic acid in the blood. By reducing the availability of NAD, alcohol also impairs the liver's ability to form glucose from amino acids and other glucose precursors. Alcohol-induced hypoglycemia can develop when excessive alcohol ingestion occurs during periods of depleted liver glycogen stores.

The MEOS pathway, which is located in the smooth endoplasmic reticulum, produces acetaldehyde and free radicals. Prolonged and excessive alcohol ingestion results in enzyme induction and increased activity of the MEOS. One of the most important enzymes of the MEOS, a member of the CYP P450 system, also oxidizes a number of other compounds, including various drugs (*e.g.,* acetaminophen, isoniazid), toxins (*e.g.,* carbon tetrachloride, halothane), vitamins A and D, and carcinogenic agents (*e.g.,* aflatoxin, nitrosamines). Increased activity of this system enhances the susceptibility of persons with heavy alcohol consumption to the hepatotoxic effects of industrial toxins, anesthetic agents, chemical carcinogens, vitamins, and the pain reliever acetaminophen.[38]

The metabolic end products of alcohol metabolism (*e.g.,* acetaldehyde, free radicals) are responsible for a variety of metabolic alterations that can cause liver injury. Acetaldehyde, for example, has multiple toxic effects on liver cells and liver function. Age and sex play a role in metabolism of alcohol and production of harmful metabolites. The ADH system is depressed by testosterone. Thus, women tend to produce greater amounts of acetaldehyde and are more predisposed to alcohol-induced liver damage than men.[38] Age also appears to affect the alcohol-metabolizing abilities of the liver and the resistance to hepatotoxic effects. Furthermore, genetic factors may influence the severity of alcohol-induced liver disease. ADH has multiple isoenzymes, the genetic polymorphism of which is now being studied in terms of possible clinical implications.[38]

Alcoholic Liver Disease

The metabolism of alcohol leads to chemical attack on certain membranes of the liver, but whether the damage is caused by acetaldehyde or other metabolites is unknown. Acetaldehyde is known to impede the mitochondrial electron transport system, which is responsible for oxidative metabolism and generation of ATP; as a result, the hydrogen ions that are generated in the mitochondria are shunted into lipid synthesis and ketogenesis.[38] Abnormal accumulations of these substances are found in hepatocytes (*i.e.,* fatty liver) and blood. Binding of acetaldehyde to other molecules impairs the detoxification of free radicals and synthesis of proteins. Acetaldehyde also promotes collagen synthesis and fibrogenesis. The lesions of hepatocellular injury tend to be most prevalent in the centrilobular area that surrounds the central vein, where the pathways for alcohol metabolism are concentrated. This is the part of the lobule that has the lowest oxygen tension; it is thought that the low oxygen concentration in this area of the liver may contribute to the damage.

The amount of alcohol required to produce chronic liver disease varies widely, depending on body size, age, sex, and ethnicity, but the lower range seems to be about 80 g/day (8 ounces of 86 proof [41% alcohol] whiskey, two bottles of wine, or six 12-ounce bottles of beer).[4] Even after alcohol intake has stopped and all alcohol has been metabolized, the processes that damage liver cells may continue for many weeks and months. Clinical and chemical effects often become worse before the disease resolves. The accumulation of fat usually disappears within a few weeks, and cholestasis and inflammation also subside with time. However, fibrosis and scarring remain. The liver lobules become distorted as new liver cells regenerate and form nodules.

Although the mechanism by which alcohol exerts its toxic effects on liver structures is somewhat uncertain, the changes that develop can be divided into three stages: fatty changes, alcoholic hepatitis, and cirrhosis.[3,4]

Fatty liver is characterized by the accumulation of fat in hepatocytes, a condition called *steatosis* (Fig. 38-12). The liver becomes yellow and enlarges owing to excessive fat accumulation. The pathogenesis of fatty liver is not completely understood and can depend on the amount of alcohol consumed, dietary fat content, body stores of fat, hormonal status, and other factors. There is evidence that ingestion of large amounts of alcohol can cause fatty liver changes even with an adequate diet. For example, young, nonalcoholic volunteers had fatty liver changes after 2 days of consuming an excess amount of alcohol, even though adequate carbohydrates, fats, and proteins were included in the diet.[41] The fatty changes that occur with ingestion of alcohol usually do not produce symptoms and are reversible after the alcohol intake has been discontinued.

Alcoholic hepatitis is the intermediate stage between fatty changes and cirrhosis. It often is seen after an abrupt increase in alcohol intake and is common in "spree" drinkers. Alcoholic hepatitis is characterized by inflammation and necrosis of liver cells. This stage usually is characterized by hepatic tenderness, pain, anorexia, nausea, fever, jaundice, ascites, and liver failure, but some individuals may be asymptomatic. The condition is always serious and sometimes fatal. The immediate prognosis correlates with severity of liver cell injury. In some cases, the disease progresses rapidly to liver failure and death. The mortality rate in the acute stage is about 10%.[4] In persons who survive and continue to drink, the acute phase often is followed

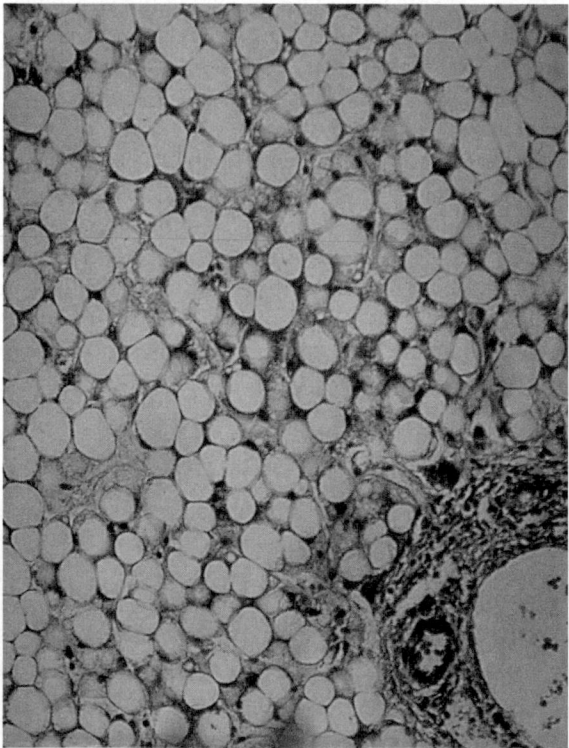

FIGURE 38-12 • Alcoholic fatty liver. A photomicrograph shows the cytoplasm of almost all the hepatocytes to be distended by fat, which displaces the nucleus to the periphery. Note the absence of inflammation and fibrosis. (From Rubin E., Farber J. L. [1999]. *Pathology* [3rd ed., p. 791]. Philadelphia: Lippincott-Raven.)

by persistent alcoholic hepatitis with progression to cirrhosis in a matter of 1 to 2 years.

Alcoholic cirrhosis is the end result of repeated bouts of drinking-related liver injury and designates the onset of end-stage alcoholic liver disease. The gross appearance of the early cirrhotic liver is one of fine, uniform nodules on its surface. The condition has traditionally been called *micronodular* or *Laennec cirrhosis*. With more advanced cirrhosis, regenerative processes cause the nodules to become larger and more irregular in size and shape. As this occurs, the nodules cause the liver to become relobulized through the formation of new portal tracts and venous outflow channels. The nodules may compress the hepatic veins, curtailing blood flow out of the liver and producing portal hypertension, extrahepatic portosystemic shunts, and cholestasis.

Nonalcoholic Fatty Liver Disease

The term *nonalcoholic fatty liver disease* (NAFLD) is often used to describe fatty liver disease with the potential for progression to cirrhosis and end-stage liver disease arising from causes other than alcohol.[42–45] The condition can range from simple steatosis (fatty infiltration of the liver) to nonalcoholic steatohepatitis (steatosis with inflammation and hepatocyte necrosis). Although steatosis alone does not appear to be progressive, approximately 20% of persons with nonalcoholic steatohepatitis progress to cirrhosis over the course of a decade.[44] Obesity, type 2 diabetes, the metabolic syndrome, and hyperlipidemia are coexisting conditions frequently associated with fatty liver disease (see Chapter 42). The condition is also associated with other nutritional abnormalities, surgical conditions, drugs, and occupational exposure to toxins. Both rapid weight loss and parenteral nutrition may lead to NAFLD. Jejunoileal bypass, a surgical procedure used for weight loss, has largely been abandoned for this reason.

Pathogenesis. The pathogenesis of NAFLD is thought to involve both lipid accumulation within hepatocytes and formation of free radicals, in a manner similar to that which occurs with alcohol metabolism. The primary metabolic abnormalities leading to lipid accumulation are poorly understood but are thought to include alterations in pathways for uptake, synthesis, degradation, or secretion of hepatic lipids resulting from insulin resistance. Obesity increases the synthesis and reduces the oxidation of free fatty acids. Type 2 diabetes or insulin resistance also increases adipose tissue lipolysis and the subsequent production of free fatty acids.[46] When the capacity of the liver to export triglyceride is exceeded, excess fatty acids contribute to the formation of fatty liver. Both ketones and free fatty acids are inducers of previously described CYP P450 enzymes of the MEOS pathway, which results in free radical formation, including hydrogen peroxide and superoxide (see Chapter 5). Abnormal lipid peroxidation ensues, followed by direct hepatocyte injury, release of toxic byproducts, inflammation, and fibrosis.

Clinical Manifestations. NAFLD is usually asymptomatic, although fatigue and discomfort in the right upper quadrant of the abdomen may be present. Mildly to moderately elevated serum levels of AST, ALT, or both are the most common and often the only abnormal laboratory findings. Other abnormalities, including hypoalbuminemia, a prolonged prothrombin time, and hyperbilirubinemia, may be present in persons with cirrhotic-stage liver disease. The diagnosis of NAFLD requires liver biopsy and exclusion of alcohol as a cause of the disorder.

Treatment. The aim of treatment is to slow progression of NAFLD and to prevent liver-related illness. Both weight loss and exercise improve insulin resistance and are recommended in conjunction with treatment of associated metabolic disturbances. Alcohol use should be avoided. Disease progression is slow and the magnitude of disease-related morbidity and mortality is uncertain. Liver transplantation is an alternative for some persons with end-stage liver disease, but NAFLD my recur or develop after liver transplantation.[44]

Cirrhosis, Portal Hypertension, and Liver Failure

Cirrhosis

Cirrhosis represents the end stage of chronic liver disease in which much of the functional liver tissue has been replaced by fibrous tissue. Although cirrhosis usually is associated with alcoholism, it can develop in the course of other disorders, including viral hepatitis, toxic reactions to drugs and chemicals, biliary obstruction, and NAFLD. Cirrhosis also accompanies metabolic disorders that cause the deposition of minerals in the liver. Two of these disorders are hemochromatosis (*i.e.,* iron deposition) and Wilson disease (*i.e.,* copper deposition).

Cirrhosis is characterized by diffuse fibrosis and conversion of normal liver architecture into nodules containing proliferating hepatocytes encircled by fibrosis. The formation of nodules, which vary in size from very small (<3 mm, micronodules) to large (several centimeters, macronodules), represents a balance between regenerative activity and constrictive scarring.[3,4] The fibrous tissue that replaces normally functioning liver tissue forms constrictive bands that disrupt flow in the vascular channels and biliary duct systems of the liver. The disruption of vascular channels predisposes to portal hypertension and its complications; obstruction of biliary channels and exposure to the destructive effects of bile stasis; and loss of liver cells, leading to liver failure.

Clinical Manifestations. The manifestations of cirrhosis are variable, ranging from asymptomatic hepatomegaly to hepatic failure (Fig. 38-13). Often there are no symptoms until the disease is far advanced.[47] The most common signs and symptoms of cirrhosis are weight loss (sometimes masked by ascites), weakness, and anorexia. Diarrhea frequently is present, although some persons may complain of constipation. Hepatomegaly and jaundice also are common signs of cirrhosis. There may be abdominal pain because of liver enlargement or stretching of the Glisson capsule. This pain is located in the epigastric area or in the upper right quadrant and is described as dull, aching, and causing a sensation of fullness.

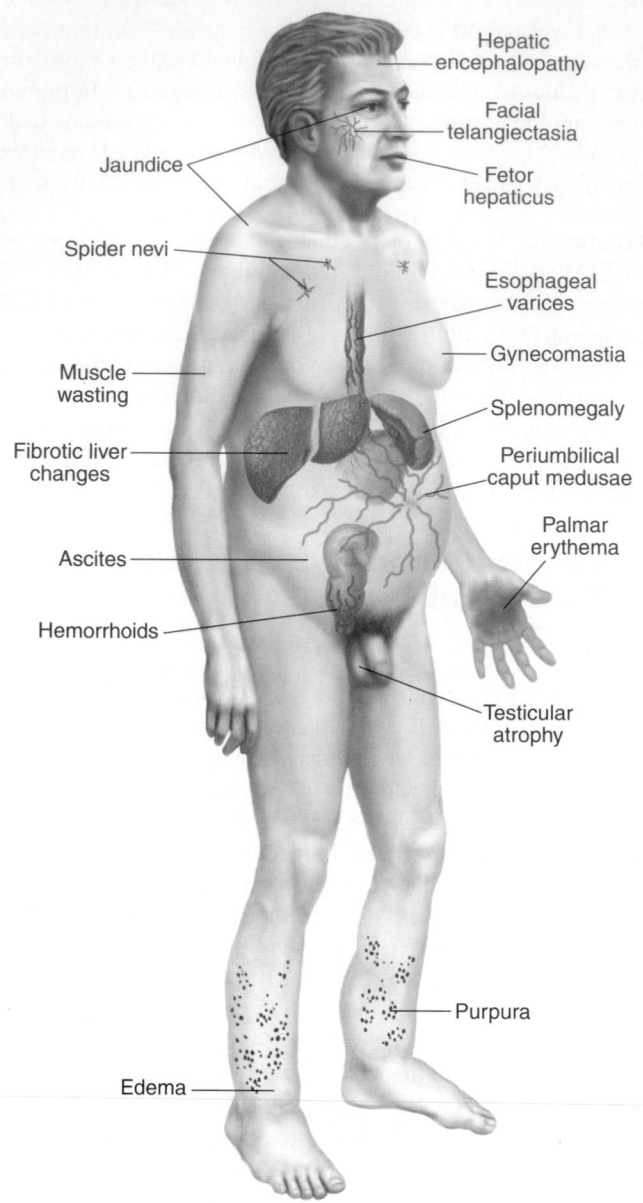

Hepatic encephalopathy
Facial telangiectasia
Jaundice
Fetor hepaticus
Spider nevi
Esophageal varices
Gynecomastia
Muscle wasting
Splenomegaly
Fibrotic liver changes
Periumbilical caput medusae
Palmar erythema
Ascites
Hemorrhoids
Testicular atrophy
Purpura
Edema

FIGURE 38-13 • Clinical manifestations of cirrhosis.

The late manifestations of cirrhosis are related to portal hypertension and liver cell failure. Splenomegaly, ascites, and portosystemic shunts (*i.e.,* esophageal varices, hemorrhoids, and caput medusae) result from portal hypertension.[48] Other complications include bleeding due to decreased clotting factors, thrombocytopenia due to splenomegaly, gynecomastia and a feminizing pattern of pubic hair distribution in men because of testicular atrophy, spider angiomas, palmar erythema, and encephalopathy with asterixis and neurologic signs.

Portal Hypertension

Portal hypertension is characterized by increased resistance to flow in the portal venous system and sustained portal vein pres-

> ### 🔑 PORTAL HYPERTENSION
>
> - Venous blood from the gastrointestinal tract empties into the portal vein and travels through the liver before moving into the general venous circulation.
> - Obstruction of blood flow in the portal vein produces an increase in the hydrostatic pressure within the peritoneal capillaries, contributing to the development of ascites, splenic engorgement with sequestration and destruction of blood cells and platelets, and shunting of blood to collateral venous channels causing varicosities of the hemorrhoidal and esophageal veins.

sure above 21 mm Hg (normal, 5 to 10 mm Hg).[4,49] Normally, venous blood returning to the heart from the abdominal organs collects in the portal vein and travels through the liver before entering the vena cava. Portal hypertension can be caused by a variety of conditions that increase resistance to hepatic blood flow, including prehepatic, posthepatic, and intrahepatic obstructions (with *hepatic* referring to the liver lobules rather than the entire liver).[4] Prehepatic causes of portal hypertension include portal vein thrombosis and external compression due to cancer or enlarged lymph nodes that produce obstruction of the portal vein before it enters the liver.

Posthepatic obstruction refers to any obstruction to blood flow through the hepatic veins beyond the liver lobules, either within or distal to the liver. It is caused by conditions such as thrombosis of the hepatic veins, veno-occlusive disease, and severe right-sided heart failure that impede the outflow of venous blood from the liver. *Budd-Chiari syndrome* refers to congestive disease of the liver caused by occlusion of the hepatic venules, large portal veins, the inferior vena cava, or the right atrium.[50] The principal cause of the Budd-Chiari syndrome is thrombosis of the hepatic veins, in association with diverse conditions such as polycythemia vera, hypercoagulability states associated with malignant tumors, pregnancy, bacterial infection, metastatic disease of the liver, and trauma. *Hepatic veno-occlusive disease* is a variant of the Budd-Chiari syndrome seen most commonly in persons treated with certain cancer chemotherapeutic drugs, hepatic irradiation, or bone marrow transplantation—possibly due to graft-versus-host disease in the latter instance.[4]

Intrahepatic causes of portal hypertension include conditions that cause obstruction of blood flow within the liver. In alcoholic cirrhosis, which is the major cause of portal hypertension, bands of fibrous tissue and fibrous nodules distort the architecture of the liver and increase the resistance to portal blood flow, which leads to portal hypertension.

Complications of portal hypertension arise from the increased pressure and dilation of the venous channels behind the obstruction (Fig. 38-14). In addition, collateral channels open that connect the portal circulation with the systemic circulation. The major complications of the increased portal vein

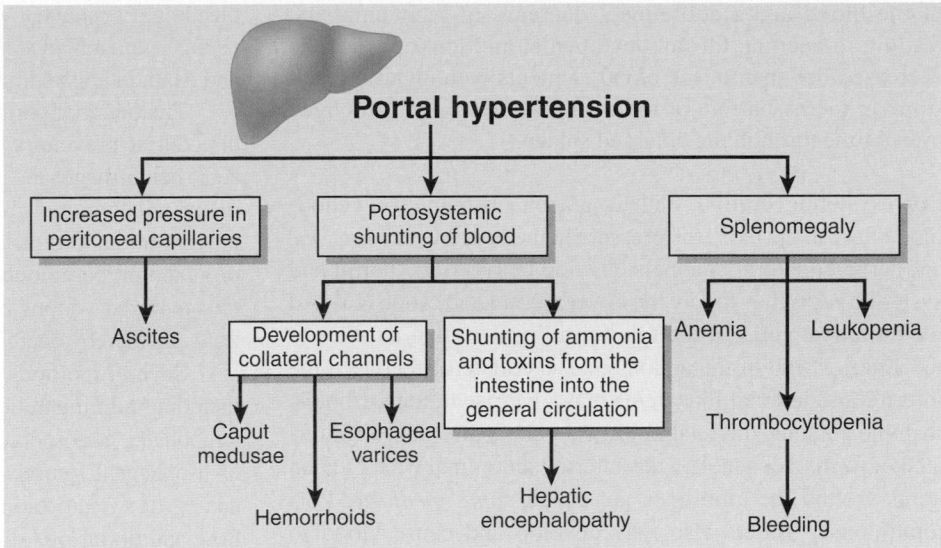

Portal hypertension

- Increased pressure in peritoneal capillaries
  - Ascites
- Portosystemic shunting of blood
  - Development of collateral channels
    - Caput medusae
    - Esophageal varices
    - Hemorrhoids
  - Shunting of ammonia and toxins from the intestine into the general circulation
    - Hepatic encephalopathy
- Splenomegaly
  - Anemia
  - Leukopenia
  - Thrombocytopenia
    - Bleeding

FIGURE 38-14 • Mechanisms of disturbed liver function related to portal hypertension.

pressure and the opening of collateral channels are ascites, splenomegaly, and the formation of portosystemic shunts with bleeding from esophageal varices.

Ascites. Ascites occurs when the amount of fluid in the peritoneal cavity is increased, and is a late-stage manifestation of cirrhosis and portal hypertension.[51–53] It is not uncommon for persons with advanced cirrhosis to present with an accumulation of 15 L or more of ascitic fluid. These persons often experience abdominal discomfort, dyspnea, and insomnia. They may also have difficulty walking or living independently.

Although the mechanisms responsible for the development of ascites are not completely understood, several factors seem to contribute to fluid accumulation, including an increase in capillary pressure due to portal hypertension and obstruction of venous flow through the liver, salt and water retention by the kidney, and decreased colloidal osmotic pressure due to impaired synthesis of albumin by the liver. Diminished blood volume (*i.e.,* underfill theory) and excessive blood volume (*i.e.,* overfill theory) have been used to explain the increased salt and water retention by the kidney. According to the underfill theory, a contraction in the effective blood volume constitutes an afferent signal that causes the kidney to retain salt and water. The effective blood volume may be reduced because of loss of fluid into the peritoneal cavity or because of vasodilation caused by the presence of circulating vasodilating substances. The overfill theory proposes that the initial event in the development of ascites is renal retention of salt and water caused by disturbances in the liver itself. These disturbances include failure of the liver to metabolize aldosterone, causing an increase in salt and water retention by the kidney. Another likely contributing factor in the pathogenesis of ascites is a decreased colloidal osmotic pressure, which limits reabsorption of fluid from the peritoneal cavity (see Chapter 31).

Treatment of ascites usually focuses on dietary restriction of sodium and administration of diuretics. Water intake also may

need to be restricted. Because of the many limitations in sodium restriction, the use of diuretics has become the mainstay of treatment for ascites. Two classes of diuretics are used: a diuretic that acts in the distal part of the nephron to inhibit aldosterone-dependent sodium reabsorption, and a loop diuretic such as furosemide (see Chapter 30). Oral potassium supplements often are given to prevent hypokalemia. The upright position is associated with the activation of the renin-angiotensin-aldosterone system; therefore, bed rest may be recommended for persons with a large amount of ascites.[53] Large-volume paracentesis (removal of 5 L or more of ascitic fluid) may be done in persons with massive ascites and pulmonary compromise. Because the removal of fluid produces a decrease in vascular volume along with increased plasma renin activity and aldosterone-mediated sodium and water reabsorption by the kidneys, a volume expander such as albumin usually is administered to maintain the effective circulating volume.[28] A transjugular intrahepatic portosystemic shunt may be inserted in persons with refractory ascites (to be discussed).[28]

Spontaneous bacterial peritonitis is a complication in persons with both cirrhosis and ascites. The infection is serious and carries a high mortality rate even when treated with antibiotics. Presumably, the peritoneal fluid is seeded with bacteria from the blood or lymph or from passage of bacteria through the bowel wall. Symptoms include fever and abdominal pain. Other symptoms include worsening of hepatic encephalopathy, diarrhea, hypothermia, and shock. It is diagnosed by a neutrophil count of 250/mm^3 or higher and a protein concentration of 1 g/dL or less in the ascitic fluid.[28]

Splenomegaly. The spleen enlarges progressively in portal hypertension because of shunting of blood into the splenic vein. The enlarged spleen often gives rise to sequestering of significant numbers of blood elements and development of a syndrome known as *hypersplenism*. Hypersplenism is characterized by a decrease in the life span of all the formed elements of the blood and a subsequent decrease in their numbers, leading to anemia, thrombocytopenia, and leukopenia. The decreased life span of the blood elements is thought to result from an increased rate of removal because of the prolonged transit time through the enlarged spleen.

Portosystemic Shunts. With the gradual obstruction of venous blood flow in the liver, the pressure in the portal vein increases, and large collateral channels develop between the portal and systemic veins that supply the lower rectum and esophagus and the umbilical veins of the falciform ligament that attaches to the anterior wall of the abdomen. The collaterals between the inferior and internal iliac veins may give rise to hemorrhoids. In some persons, the fetal umbilical vein is not totally obliterated; it forms a channel on the anterior abdominal wall. Dilated veins around the umbilicus are called *caput medusae*. Portopulmonary shunts also may develop and cause blood to bypass the pulmonary capillaries, interfering with blood oxygenation and producing cyanosis.

Clinically, the most important collateral channels are those connecting the portal and coronary veins that lead to reversal of flow and formation of thin-walled varicosities in the submucosa of the esophagus[54,55] (Fig. 38-15). These thin-walled *esophageal varices* are subject to rupture, producing massive and sometimes fatal hemorrhage. Impaired hepatic synthesis of coagulation factors and decreased platelet levels (*i.e.,* thrombocytopenia) due to splenomegaly may further complicate the control of esophageal bleeding. Esophageal varices develop in approximately 65% of persons with advanced cirrhosis and cause massive hemorrhage and death in approximately half of them.[3]

Treatment of portal hypertension and esophageal varices is directed at prevention of initial hemorrhage, management of acute hemorrhage, and prevention of recurrent hemorrhage. Pharmacologic therapy is used to lower portal venous pressure and prevent initial hemorrhage. β-Adrenergic blocking drugs (*e.g.,* propranolol) commonly are used for this purpose. These agents reduce portal venous pressure by decreasing splanchnic blood flow and thereby decreasing blood flow in collateral channels.

Several methods are used to control acute hemorrhage, including administration of octreotide or vasopressin, balloon tamponade, endoscopic injection sclerotherapy, vessel ligation, or esophageal transection. Octreotide, a long-acting synthetic analog of somatostatin, reduces splanchnic and hepatic blood flow and portal pressures in persons with cirrhosis. The drug, which is given intravenously, provides control of variceal bleeding in up to 80% of cases. Vasopressin, a hormone from the posterior pituitary, is a nonselective vasoconstrictor that also can be used to control variceal bleeding. Because octreotide has fewer side effects and appears to be more effective than vasopressin, it has become the drug of choice for pharmacologic management of acute variceal bleeding.[54] Balloon tamponade provides compression of the varices and is accomplished through the insertion of a tube with inflatable gastric and esophageal balloons. After the tube has been inserted, the balloons are inflated; the esophageal balloon compresses the bleeding esophageal veins, and the gastric balloon helps to maintain the position of the tube. During endoscopic sclerotherapy, the varices are injected with a sclerosing solution that obliterates the vessel lumen.

Prevention of recurrent hemorrhage focuses on lowering portal venous pressure and diverting blood flow away from the easily ruptured collateral channels. Two procedures may be used for this purpose: the surgical creation of a portosystemic shunt or a transjugular intrahepatic portosystemic shunt (TIPS). *Surgical portosystemic shunt* procedures involve the creation of an opening between the portal vein and a systemic vein. These shunts have a considerable complication rate, and TIPS has evolved as the preferred treatment for refractory portal hypertension. The TIPS procedure involves insertion of an expandable metal stent between a branch of the hepatic vein and the portal vein using a catheter inserted through the internal jugular vein. A limitation of the procedure is that stenosis and thrombosis of the stent occur in most cases over time, with consequent risk of rebleeding. A complication that is associated with the creation of a portosystemic shunt is hepatic encephalopathy, which is thought to result when ammonia and other neurotoxic substances from the gut pass directly into the systemic circulation without going through the liver.

Liver Failure

The most severe clinical consequence of liver disease is hepatic failure. It may result from sudden and massive liver destruction, as in fulminant hepatitis, or be the result of progressive

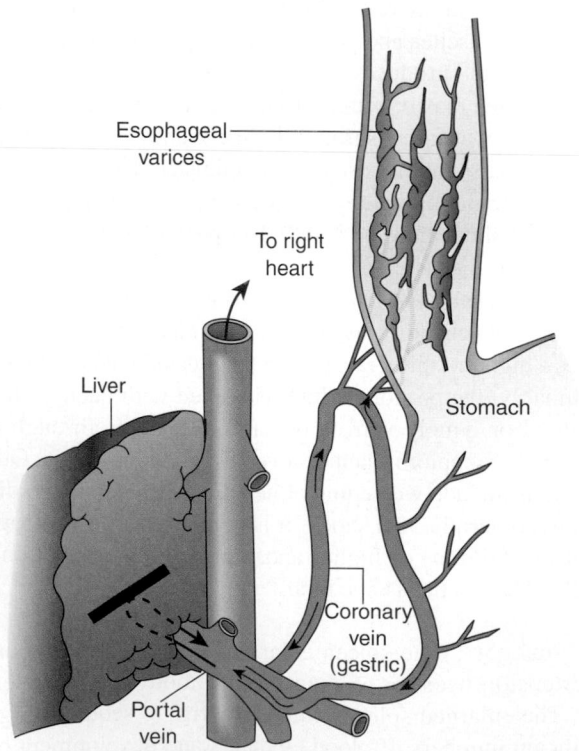

FIGURE 38-15 • Obstruction of blood flow in the portal circulation, with portal hypertension and diversion of blood flow to other venous channels, including the gastric and esophageal veins.

damage to the liver, as occurs in alcoholic cirrhosis. Whatever the cause, 80% to 90% of hepatic functional capacity must be lost before liver failure occurs.[3] In many cases, the progressive decompensating effects of the disease are hastened by intercurrent conditions such as gastrointestinal bleeding, systemic infection, electrolyte disturbances, or superimposed diseases such as heart failure.

Manifestations. The manifestations of liver failure reflect the various synthesis, storage, metabolic, and elimination functions of the liver (Fig. 38-16). *Fetor hepaticus* refers to a characteristic musty, sweetish odor of the breath in the patient in advanced liver failure, resulting from the metabolic byproducts of the intestinal bacteria.

Hematologic Disorders. Liver failure can cause anemia, thrombocytopenia, coagulation defects, and leukopenia. Anemia may be caused by blood loss, excessive red blood cell destruction, and impaired formation of red blood cells. A folic acid deficiency may lead to severe megaloblastic anemia. Changes in the lipid composition of the red blood cell membrane increase hemolysis. Because factors V, VII, IX, and X, prothrombin, and fibrinogen are synthesized by the liver, their decline in liver disease contributes to bleeding disorders. Malabsorption of the fat-soluble vitamin K contributes further to the impaired synthesis of these clotting factors. Thrombocytopenia often occurs as the result of splenomegaly. The person with liver failure is subject to purpura, easy bruising, hematuria, and abnormal menstrual bleeding, and

is vulnerable to bleeding from the esophagus and other segments of the gastrointestinal tract.

Endocrine Disorders. The liver metabolizes the steroid hormones. Endocrine disorders, particularly disturbances in gonadal (sex hormone) function, are common accompaniments of cirrhosis and liver failure. Women may have menstrual irregularities (usually amenorrhea), loss of libido, and sterility. In men, testosterone levels usually fall, the testes atrophy, and loss of libido, impotence, and gynecomastia occur. A decrease in aldosterone metabolism may contribute to salt and water retention by the kidney, along with a lowering of serum potassium resulting from increased elimination of potassium.

Skin Disorders. Liver failure brings on numerous skin disorders. These lesions, called variously *vascular spiders, telangiectases, spider angiomas,* and *spider nevi,* are seen most often in the upper half of the body. They consist of a central pulsating arteriole from which smaller vessels radiate. Palmar erythema is redness of the palms, probably caused by increased blood flow from higher cardiac output. Clubbing of the fingers may be seen in persons with cirrhosis. Jaundice usually is a late manifestation of liver failure.

Hepatorenal Syndrome. The hepatorenal syndrome refers to a functional renal failure sometimes seen during the terminal stages of liver failure with ascites.[56] It is characterized by progressive azotemia, increased serum creatinine levels, and oliguria. Although the basic cause is unknown, a decrease in renal

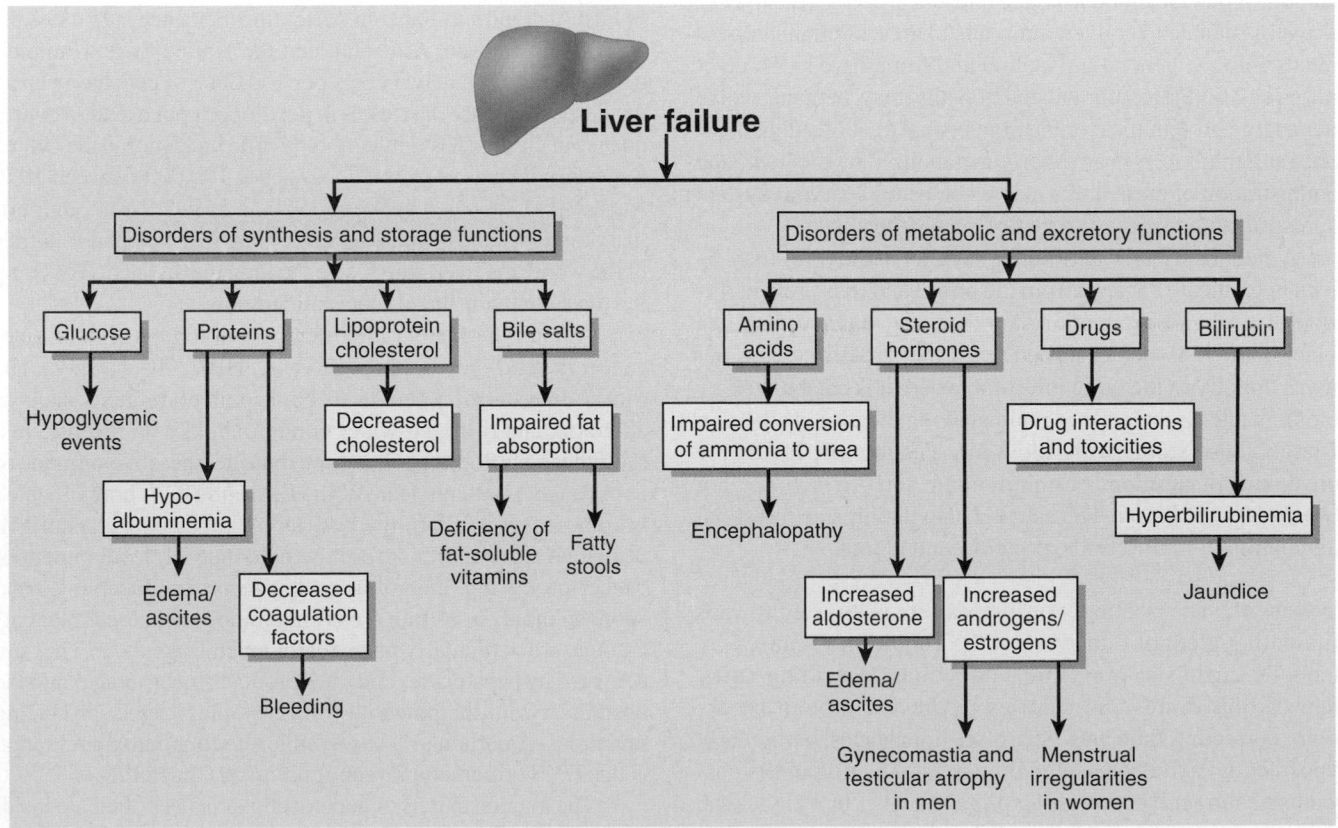

FIGURE 38-16 • Alterations in liver function and manifestations of liver failure.

blood flow is believed to play a part. Ultimately, when renal failure is superimposed on liver failure, azotemia and elevated levels of blood ammonia occur; this condition is thought to contribute to hepatic encephalopathy and coma.

Hepatic Encephalopathy. Hepatic encephalopathy refers to the totality of central nervous system manifestations of liver failure. It is characterized by neural disturbances ranging from a lack of mental alertness to confusion, coma, and convulsions. A very early sign of hepatic encephalopathy is a flapping tremor called *asterixis.* Various degrees of memory loss may occur, coupled with personality changes such as euphoria, irritability, anxiety, and lack of concern about personal appearance and self. Speech may be impaired, and the patient may be unable to perform certain purposeful movements. The encephalopathy may progress to decerebrate rigidity and then to a terminal deep coma.

Although the cause of hepatic encephalopathy is unknown, the accumulation of neurotoxins, which appear in the blood because the liver has lost its detoxifying capacity, is believed to be a factor. Hepatic encephalopathy develops in approximately 10% of persons with portosystemic shunts.

One of the suspected neurotoxins is ammonia. A particularly important function of the liver is the conversion of ammonia, a byproduct of protein and amino acid metabolism, to urea. The ammonium ion is produced in abundance in the intestinal tract, particularly in the colon, by the bacterial degradation of luminal proteins and amino acids. Normally, these ammonium ions diffuse into the portal blood and are transported to the liver, where they are converted to urea before entering the general circulation. When the blood from the intestine bypasses the liver or the liver is unable to convert ammonia to urea, ammonia moves directly into the general circulation and from there to the cerebral circulation. Hepatic encephalopathy may become worse after a large protein meal or gastrointestinal tract bleeding. Narcotics and tranquilizers are poorly metabolized by the liver, and administration of these drugs may cause central nervous system depression and precipitate hepatic encephalopathy.

A nonabsorbable antibiotic, such as neomycin, may be given to eradicate bacteria from the bowel and thus prevent this cause of ammonia production. Another drug that may be given is lactulose. It is not absorbed from the small intestine but moves directly to the large intestine, where it is catabolized by colonic bacteria to small organic acids that cause production of large, loose stools with a low pH. The low pH favors the conversion of ammonia to ammonium ions, which are not absorbed by the blood. The acid pH also inhibits the intestinal degradation of amino acids, proteins, and blood.

Treatment. The treatment of liver failure is directed toward eliminating alcohol intake when the condition is caused by alcoholic cirrhosis; preventing infections; providing sufficient carbohydrates and calories to prevent protein breakdown; correcting fluid and electrolyte imbalances, particularly hypokalemia; and decreasing ammonia production in the gastrointestinal tract by controlling protein intake. In many cases, liver transplantation remains the only effective treatment.

Liver transplantation rapidly is becoming a realistic form of treatment for many persons with irreversible chronic liver disease, fulminant liver failure, primary biliary cirrhosis, chronic active hepatitis, sclerosing cholangitis, and certain metabolic disorders that result in end-stage liver disease. Currently, 1-year survival rates approach 90%, and a 3-year survival rate of 80% is achieved at many transplantation centers in the United States.[57] In addition to longer survival, many liver recipients are now experiencing improved quality of life, including return to active employment. Unfortunately, the shortage of donor organs severely limits the number of transplantations that are done, and many persons die each year while waiting for a transplant. During the past several years a number of innovative methods have been developed to deal with the shortage, including split liver transplantation, in which a cadaver liver is split into two pieces and transplanted into two recipients, and living donor transplantation, in which a segment or lobe from the liver from a living donor is resected and grafted into a recipient.[57]

Cancer of the Liver

Primary Liver Cancers

There are two major types of primary liver cancer: hepatocellular carcinoma, which arises from the liver cells, and cholangiocarcinoma, which is a primary cancer of bile duct cells.[3]

Hepatocellular Carcinoma. Hepatocellular cancer, the most common form of liver cancer, is the fifth most common cancer and third leading cause of cancer-related mortality worldwide.[58,59] In East Asia and sub-Saharan Africa, the incidence is 15 cases per 100,000. In Europe, Australia, and the United States, the incidence is approximately 3 cases per 100,000.[59] There has been an increased incidence, however, in developed countries as a consequence of chronic HCV infection.[58,59] The incidence in the United States has increased from 1.4 cases per 100,000 between 1976 and 1980 to 2.4 cases between 1990 and 1995.[58] Although primary tumors of the liver are relatively rare in developed countries of the world, the liver shares with the lung the distinction of being the most common site of metastatic tumors.

Among the factors identified as etiologic agents in liver cancer are chronic viral hepatitis (*i.e.,* HBV, HCV, HDV), cirrhosis, long-term exposure to environmental agents such as aflatoxin, and drinking water contaminated with arsenic. Just how these etiologic agents contribute to the development of liver cancer is still unclear. With HBV and HCV, both of which become integrated into the host DNA, repeated cycles of cell death and regeneration afford the potential for development of cancer-producing mutations. Aflatoxins, produced by food spoilage molds in certain areas endemic for hepatocellular carcinoma, are particularly potent carcinogenic agents.[3,59] They are activated by hepatocytes and their products incorporated into the host DNA with the potential for developing cancer-producing mutations. A particularly susceptible site for aflatoxin mutation is the *TP53* tumor suppressor gene[59] (see Chapter 8).

The manifestations of hepatocellular cancer often are insidious in onset and masked by those related to cirrhosis or chronic hepatitis. The initial symptoms include weakness, anorexia, weight loss, fatigue, bloating, a sensation of abdominal fullness, and a dull, aching abdominal pain.[59,60] Ascites, which often obscures weight loss, is common. Jaundice, if present, usually is mild. There may be a rapid increase in liver size and worsening of ascites in persons with preexisting cirrhosis. Usually, the liver is enlarged when these symptoms appear. Various paraneoplastic syndromes (*e.g.*, disturbances due to ectopic hormone or growth factor production by the tumor [see Chapter 8]) have been associated with hepatocellular cancer, including erythrocytosis (erythropoietin), hypoglycemia (insulin-like growth factor), and hypercalcemia (parathyroid-related protein). Serum α-fetoprotein, which is present during fetal life but barely detectable in the serum after the age of 2 years, is present in 50% to 75% cases of hepatocellular carcinoma.[3] However, the test lacks specificity and is not very useful as a surveillance or diagnostic tool.[3,60] Diagnostic methods include ultrasonography, CT scans, and MRI. Liver biopsy may be used to confirm the diagnosis.

Primary cancers of the liver usually are far advanced at the time of diagnosis. The treatment of choice is subtotal hepatectomy, if conditions permit. Chemotherapy and radiation therapy are largely palliative. Although liver transplantation may be an option for people with well-compensated cirrhosis and small tumors, it often is impractical because of the shortage of donor organs.

Cholangiocarcinoma. Cholangiocarcinoma, with an incidence of 0.6 per 100,000 in North America, occurs much less frequently than hepatocellular carcinoma.[3] The etiology, clinical features, and prognosis vary considerably with the part of the biliary tree that is the site of origin. Cholangiocarcinoma is not associated with the same risk factors as hepatocellular carcinoma. Instead, most of the risk factors revolve around longstanding inflammation and injury of the bile duct epithelium. Cholangiocarcinoma often presents with pain, weight loss, anorexia, and abdominal swelling or awareness of a mass in the right hypochondrium. Tumors affecting the central or distal bile ducts may present with jaundice.

Metastatic Tumors

Metastatic tumors of the liver are much more common than primary tumors. Common sources include colorectal cancer and those spread from breast, lung, or urogenital cancer. In addition, tumors of neuroendocrine origin spread to the liver. It often is difficult to distinguish primary from metastatic tumors with the use of CT scans, MRI, or ultrasonography. Usually the diagnosis is confirmed by biopsy.

IN SUMMARY, the liver is subject to most of the disease processes that affect other body structures, such as vascular disorders, inflammation, metabolic diseases, toxic injury, and neoplasms. As the major drug-metabolizing and detoxifying organ in the body, the liver is subject to potential damage from the enormous array of pharmaceutical and environmental chemi-

cals. Drugs and chemicals can exert their effects by causing hepatocyte injury and death or by cholestatic liver damage due to injury of biliary drainage structures. Drug reactions can be predictable based on the drug's chemical structure and metabolites, or unpredictable (idiosyncratic) based on individual characteristics of the person receiving the drug. Early identification of drug-induced liver disease is important because withdrawal of the drug is curative in most cases.

Hepatitis is characterized by inflammation of the liver. Acute viral hepatitis is caused by hepatitis viruses A, B, C, D, and E. Although all these viruses cause acute hepatitis, they differ in terms of mode of transmission, incubation period, mechanism, degree and chronicity of liver damage, and the ability to evolve to a carrier state. HBV, HCV, and HDV infections have the potential for progression to the carrier state, chronic hepatitis, and hepatocellular carcinoma.

Intrahepatic biliary diseases disrupt the flow of bile through the liver, causing cholestasis and biliary cirrhosis. Among the causes of intrahepatic biliary diseases are primary biliary cirrhosis, primary sclerosing cholangitis, and secondary biliary cirrhosis. Because alcohol competes for use of intracellular cofactors normally needed by the liver for other metabolic processes, it tends to disrupt the metabolic functions of the liver. The spectrum of alcoholic liver disease includes fatty liver disease, alcoholic hepatitis, and cirrhosis.

Cirrhosis represents the end stage of chronic liver disease in which much of the functional liver tissue has been replaced by fibrous tissue. The fibrous tissue replaces normally functioning liver tissue and forms constrictive bands that disrupt flow in the vascular channels and biliary duct systems of the liver. The disruption of vascular channels predisposes to portal hypertension and its complications, loss of liver cells, and eventual liver failure. Portal hypertension is characterized by increased resistance to flow and increased pressure in the portal venous system; the pathologic consequences of the disorder include ascites, the formation of collateral bypass channels (*e.g.*, esophageal varices) from the portosystemic circulation, and splenomegaly. Liver failure represents the end stage of a number of liver diseases and occurs when less than 10% of liver tissue is functional. The manifestations of liver failure reflect the various functions of the liver, including hematologic disorders, disruption of endocrine function, skin disorders, hepatorenal syndrome, and hepatic encephalopathy.

There are two types of primary cancers of the liver: hepatocellular (the most common form, derived from hepatocytes and their precursors) and cholangiocarcinoma (bile duct cancer, arising from biliary epithelium). Hepatocellular carcinoma, which is associated with HBV and HCV hepatitis, alcoholic cirrhosis, and food contaminants (*e.g.*, aflatoxins), is the fifth most common cancer and third leading cause of cancer-related mortality worldwide. Cholangiocarcinoma occurs primarily in older persons with a history of chronic disorders of the bile ducts. Although primary tumors of the liver are relatively rare in developed countries of the world, the liver shares with the lung the distinction of being the most common site of metastatic tumors. ■

 CONCEPTS in action **ANIMATION**

DISORDERS OF THE GALLBLADDER AND EXOCRINE PANCREAS

After completing this section of the chapter, you should be able to meet the following objectives:

- Explain the function of the gallbladder in regulating the flow of bile into the duodenum and relate to the formation of cholelithiasis (gallstones).
- Describe the clinical manifestations of acute and chronic cholecystitis.
- Characterize the effects of choledocholithiasis and cholangitis on bile flow and the potential for hepatic and pancreatic complications.
- Cite the possible causes and describe the manifestations and treatment of acute pancreatitis.
- Describe the manifestations of chronic pancreatitis.
- State the reason for the poor prognosis in pancreatic cancer.

Disorders of the Gallbladder and Extrahepatic Bile Ducts

The so-called hepatobiliary system consists of the gallbladder, the left and right hepatic ducts, which come together to form the common hepatic duct, the cystic duct, which extends to the gallbladder, and the common bile duct, which is formed by the union of the common hepatic duct and the cystic duct (Fig. 38-17). The common bile duct descends posteriorly to the first part of the duodenum, where it comes in contact with the main pancreatic duct. These ducts unite to form the hepatopancreatic ampulla. The circular muscle around the distal end of the bile duct is thickened to form the sphincter of the bile duct.

The gallbladder is a distensible, pear-shaped muscular sac located on the ventral surface of the liver. It has an outer serous peritoneal layer, a middle smooth muscle layer, and an inner mucosal layer that is continuous with the linings of the bile duct. The function of the gallbladder is to store and concentrate bile. Bile contains bile salts, cholesterol, bilirubin, lecithin, fatty acids, and water and the electrolytes normally found in the plasma. The cholesterol found in bile has no known function; it is assumed to be a byproduct of bile salt formation, and its presence is linked to the excretory function of bile. Normally insoluble in water, cholesterol is rendered soluble by the action of bile salts and lecithin, which combine with it to form micelles. In the gallbladder, water and electrolytes are absorbed from the liver bile, causing the bile to become more concentrated. Because neither lecithin nor bile salts are absorbed in the gallbladder, their concentration

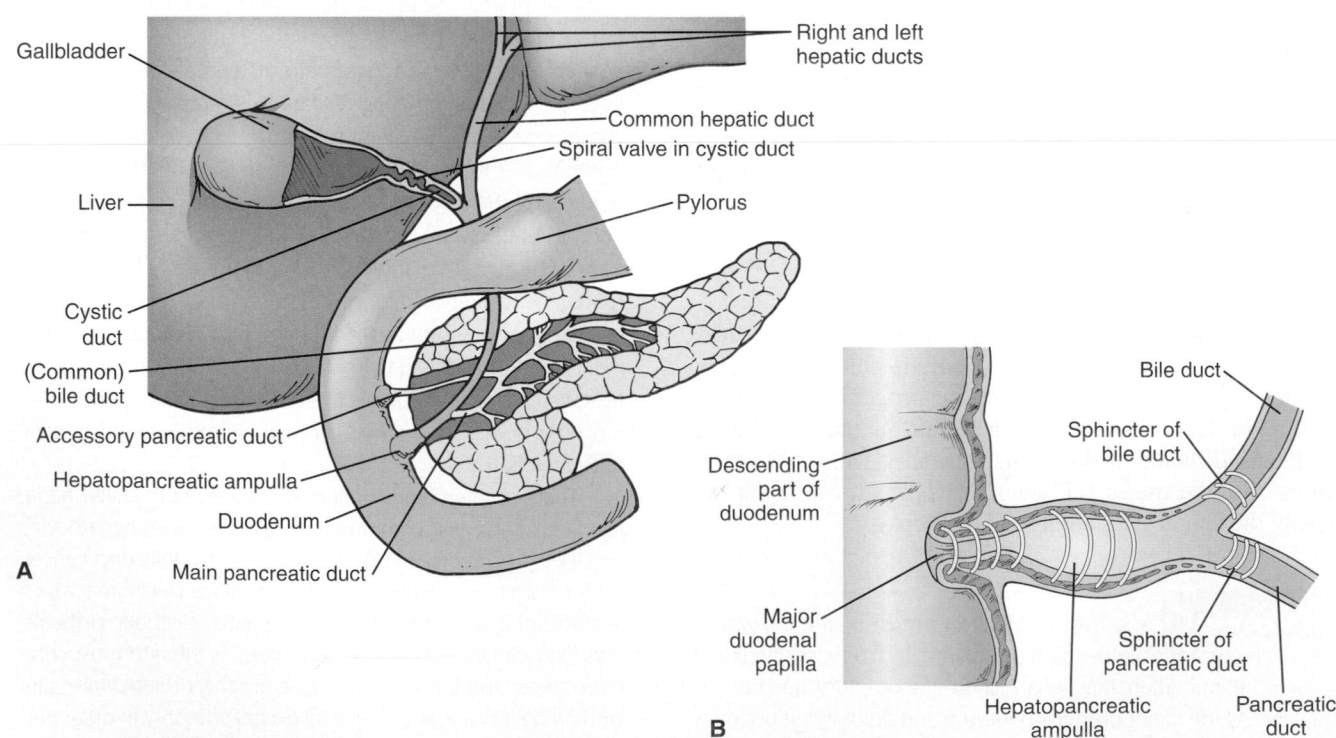

FIGURE 38-17 • **(A)** Extrahepatic bile passages, gallbladder, and pancreatic ducts. **(B)** Entry of bile duct and pancreatic duct into the hepatopancreatic ampulla, which opens into the duodenum.

increases along with that of cholesterol; in this way, the solubility of cholesterol is maintained.

Entrance of food into the intestine causes the gallbladder to contract and the sphincter of the bile duct to relax, such that bile stored in the gallbladder moves into the duodenum. The stimulus for gallbladder contraction is primarily hormonal. Products of food digestion, particularly lipids, stimulate the release of a gastrointestinal hormone called *cholecystokinin* from the mucosa of the duodenum. Cholecystokinin provides a strong stimulus for gallbladder contraction. The role of other gastrointestinal hormones in bile release is less clearly understood.

Passage of bile into the intestine is regulated largely by the pressure in the common duct. Normally, the gallbladder regulates this pressure. It collects and stores bile as it relaxes and the pressure in the common bile duct decreases, and it empties bile into the intestine as the gallbladder contracts, producing an increase in common duct pressure. After gallbladder surgery, the pressure in the common duct changes, causing the common duct to dilate. The flow of bile then is regulated by the sphincters in the common duct.

Two common disorders of the biliary system are cholelithiasis (*i.e.,* gallstones) and inflammation of the gallbladder (cholecystitis) or common bile duct (cholangitis). At least 10% of adults have gallstones.[3,4] There is an increased prevalence with age, and approximately twice as many white women as men have gallstones.[3] In both circumstances, hypersecretion of biliary cholesterol appears to play a major role.

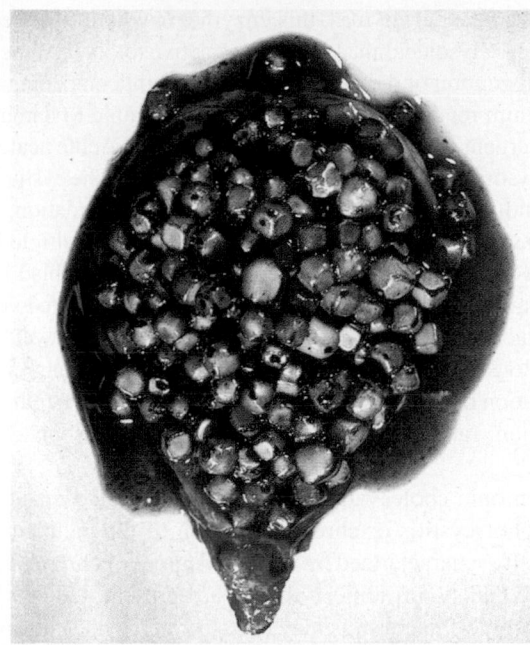

FIGURE 38-18 • Cholesterol gallstones. The gallbladder has been opened to reveal numerous yellow cholesterol gallstones (From Rubin R., Rubin E. [2008]. The liver and biliary system. In Rubin R., Strayer D. S. [Eds.], *Rubin's pathology: Clinicopathologic foundations of medicine* [5th ed., p. 668]. Philadelphia: Lippincott Williams & Wilkins.)

Cholelithiasis

Cholelithiasis or gallstones is caused by precipitation of substances contained in bile, mainly cholesterol and bilirubin. Approximately 80% of gallstones are composed primarily of cholesterol; the other 20% are black or brown pigment stones consisting of calcium salts with bilirubin.[3] Many stones have a mixed composition. Figure 38-18 shows a gallbladder with numerous cholesterol gallstones.

Three factors contribute to the formation of gallstones: abnormalities in the composition of bile, stasis of bile, and inflammation of the gallbladder.[3,4,61] The formation of cholesterol stones is associated with obesity and occurs more frequently in women, especially women who have had multiple pregnancies or who are taking oral contraceptives. All of these factors cause the liver to excrete more cholesterol into the bile. Estrogen reduces the synthesis of bile acid in women. Gallbladder sludge (thickened gallbladder mucoprotein with tiny trapped cholesterol crystals) is thought to be a precursor of gallstones. Sludge frequently occurs with pregnancy, starvation, and rapid weight loss. Drugs that lower serum cholesterol levels, such as clofibrate, also cause increased cholesterol excretion into the bile. Malabsorption disorders stemming from ileal disease or intestinal bypass surgery, for example, tend to interfere with the absorption of bile salts, which are needed to maintain the solubility of cholesterol. Inflammation of the gallbladder alters the absorptive characteristics of the mucosal layer, allowing excessive absorption of water and bile salts.

Cholesterol gallstones are extremely common among Native Americans, which suggests that a genetic component may have a role in gallstone formation. Pigment stones containing bilirubin are seen in persons with hemolytic disease (*e.g.,* sickle cell disease) and hepatic cirrhosis.

Clinical Manifestations. Many persons with gallstones have no symptoms. Gallstones cause symptoms when they obstruct bile flow.[61–63] Small stones (*i.e.,* <8 mm in diameter) pass into the common duct, producing symptoms of indigestion and biliary colic. Larger stones are more likely to obstruct flow and cause jaundice. The pain of biliary colic is usually located in the upper right quadrant or epigastric area and may be referred to the upper back, the right shoulder or midscapular region. Typically the pain is abrupt in onset, increases steadily in intensity, persists for 2 to 8 hours, and is followed by soreness in the upper right quadrant.

Acute and Chronic Cholecystitis

Acute cholecystitis is a diffuse inflammation of the gallbladder, usually secondary to obstruction of the gallbladder outlet. Most cases of acute cholecystitis (85% to 90%) are associated with the presence of gallstones (calculous cholecystitis).[3,4,62] The remaining cases (acalculous cholecystitis) are associated with sepsis, severe trauma, or infection of the gallbladder. It has been theorized that obstruction of the cystic duct by a gallstone leads to the release of phospholipase from the epithelium of the gallbladder. In turn, this enzyme may hydrolyze lecithin and release lysolecithin, a membrane-active toxin.[3,4] At the same time, disruption of the normally protective mucous lining of the epithelium renders the mucosal cells vulnerable to damage by the detergent action of concentrated bile salts. Acute acalculous cholecystitis is thought to result from ischemia. The cystic artery is an end artery with essentially no collateral circulation.[3] Contributing factors may include dehydration and multiple blood transfusions, leading to increased pigment load; gallbladder stasis, as might occur with hyperalimentation and assisted ventilation; and inflammation and edema of the gallbladder wall. Acute acalculous cholecystitis can rapidly progress to gangrene and perforation because the process appears to involve a transmural infarction, rather than inflammatory changes associated with stones.

Chronic cholecystitis results from repeated episodes of acute cholecystitis or chronic irritation of the gallbladder by stones. It is characterized by varying degrees of chronic inflammation. Gallstones almost always are present. Cholelithiasis with chronic cholecystitis may be associated with acute exacerbations of gallbladder inflammation, common duct stone, pancreatitis, and, rarely, carcinoma of the gallbladder.

Clinical Manifestations. Persons with acute cholecystitis usually experience an acute onset of upper right quadrant or epigastric pain, frequently associated with mild fever, anorexia, nausea, vomiting. Whereas in biliary colic the cystic duct obstruction is transient, in acute cholecystitis it is persistent. Persons with calculus cholecystitis usually, but not always, have experienced previous episodes of biliary pain. The pain may appear with remarkable suddenness and constitute a surgical emergency. In the absence of medical attention, the attack usually subsides in 7 to 10 days and frequently within 24 hours. In persons who recover, recurrence is common. The onset of acalculous cholecystitis tends to be more insidious because the manifestations are obscured by the underlying conditions precipitating the attack. In the severely ill patient, early recognition is crucial because a delay in treatment can prove life-threatening. Persons with acute cholecystitis usually have an elevated white blood cell count and many have mild elevations in AST, ALT, alkaline phosphatase, and bilirubin.

The manifestations of chronic cholecystitis are more vague than those of acute cholecystitis. There may be intolerance to fatty foods, belching, and other indications of discomfort. Often, there are episodes of colicky pain with obstruction of biliary flow caused by gallstones. The gallbladder, which in chronic cholecystitis usually contains stones, may be enlarged, shrunken, or of normal size.

Diagnosis and Treatment. The methods used to diagnose gallbladder disease include ultrasonography, cholescintigraphy (nuclear scanning), and CT scans.[62] Ultrasonography is widely used in diagnosing gallbladder disease and has largely replaced the oral cholecystogram in most medical centers. It can detect stones as small as 1 to 2 cm, and its overall accuracy in detecting gallbladder disease is high. In addition to stones, ultrasonography can detect wall thickening, which indicates inflammation. It also can rule out other causes of right upper quadrant pain such as tumors. Cholescintigraphy, also called a *gallbladder scan,* relies on the ability of the liver to extract a rapidly injected radionuclide, technetium-99m, bound to one of several iminodiacetic acids, that is excreted into the bile ducts. Serial scanning images are obtained within several minutes of the injection of the tracer and every 10 to 15 minutes during the next hour. The gallbladder scan is highly accurate in detecting acute cholecystitis. Although CT is not as accurate as ultrasonography in detecting gallstones, it can show thickening of the gallbladder wall or pericholecystic fluid associated with acute cholecystitis.

Gallbladder disease usually is treated by removing the gallbladder. The gallbladder stores and concentrates bile, and its removal usually does not interfere with digestion. Laparoscopic cholecystectomy has become the treatment of choice for symptomatic gallbladder disease.[62] The procedure involves insertion of a laparoscope through a small incision near the umbilicus, and surgical instruments are inserted through several stab wounds in the upper abdomen. Although the procedure requires more time than the older open surgical procedure, it usually requires only 1 night in the hospital. A major advantage of the procedure is that patients can return to work in 1 to 2 weeks, compared with 4 to 6 weeks after open cholecystectomy.

Choledocholithiasis and Cholangitis

Choledocholithiasis refers to stones in the common duct and *cholangitis* to inflammation of the common duct. Common duct stones usually originate in the gallbladder, but can form spontaneously in the common duct.

Clinical Manifestations. The manifestations of choledocholithiasis are similar to those of gallstones and acute cholecystitis. There is a history of acute biliary colic and right upper abdominal pain, with chills, fever, and jaundice associated with episodes of abdominal pain. Bilirubinuria and an elevated serum bilirubin are present if the common duct is obstructed. Complications include acute suppurative cholangitis accompanied by pus in the common duct. It is characterized by the presence of an altered sensorium, lethargy, and septic shock.[3] Acute suppurative cholangitis represents an endoscopic or surgical emergency. Common duct stones also can obstruct the outflow of the pancreatic duct, causing a secondary pancreatitis.

Diagnosis and Treatment. Ultrasonography, CT scans, and radionuclide imaging may be used to demonstrate dilation of bile ducts and impaired blood flow. Endoscopic ultrasonography and magnetic resonance cholangiography are used for detecting common duct stones. Both percutaneous transhepatic cholangiography (PTC) and endoscopic retrograde cholangiopancreatography (ERCP) provide a direct means for determining the cause, location, and extent of obstruction. PTC involves the injection of dye directly into the biliary tree. It requires the insertion of a thin, flexible needle through a small incision in the skin with advancement into the biliary tree. ERCP involves the passage of an endoscope into the duodenum and the passage of a catheter into the hepatopancreatic ampulla. ERCP can be used to enlarge the opening of the sphincter of the hepatopancreatic ampulla, which may allow the lodged stone to pass, or an instrument may be inserted into the common duct to remove the stone.

Common duct stones in persons with cholelithiasis usually are treated by stone extraction followed by laparoscopic cholecystectomy. Antibiotic therapy, with an agent that penetrates the bile, is used to treat the infection. Emergency decompression of the common duct, usually by ERCP, may be necessary for persons who are septic or fail to improve with antibiotic treatment.

Cancer of the Gallbladder

Cancer of the gallbladder is the fifth most common cancer of the gastrointestinal tract. It is slightly more common in women and occurs more often in the seventh decade of life. The onset of symptoms usually is insidious, and they resemble those of cholecystitis; the diagnosis often is made unexpectedly at the time of gallbladder surgery. About 80% to 85% of persons with gallbladder cancer have cholelithiasis.[62] Because of its ability to produce chronic irritation of the gallbladder mucosa, it is believed that cholelithiasis plays a role in the development of gallbladder cancer. It is seldom resectable at the time of diagnosis, and the mean 5-year survival rate has remained a dismal 1% for many years.[3]

Disorders of the Exocrine Pancreas

The pancreas lies transversely in the posterior part of the upper abdomen. The head of the pancreas is at the right of the abdomen; it rests against the curve of the duodenum in the area of the hepatopancreatic ampulla and its entrance into the duodenum. The body of the pancreas lies beneath the stomach. The tail touches the spleen. The pancreas is virtually hidden because of its posterior position; unlike many other organs, it cannot be palpated. Because of the position of the pancreas and its large functional reserve, symptoms from conditions such as cancer of the pancreas do not usually appear until the disorder is far advanced.

The pancreas is both an endocrine and exocrine organ. Its function as an endocrine organ is discussed in Chapter 42. The exocrine pancreas is made up of lobules that consist of acinar cells, which secrete digestive enzymes into a system of microscopic ducts. These ducts empty into the main pancreatic duct, which extends from left to right through the substance of the pancreas. The main pancreatic duct and the bile duct unite to the form hepatopancreatic ampulla, which empties into the duodenum. The sphincter of the pancreatic duct controls the flow of pancreatic secretions into duodenum (see Fig. 38-17).

The pancreatic secretions contain proteolytic enzymes that break down dietary proteins, including trypsin, chymotrypsin, carboxypolypeptidase, ribonuclease, and deoxyribonuclease. The pancreas also secretes pancreatic amylase, which breaks down starch, and lipases, which hydrolyze neutral fats into glycerol and fatty acids. The pancreatic enzymes are secreted in the inactive form and become activated in the intestine. This is important because the enzymes would digest the tissue of the pancreas itself if they were secreted in the active form. The acinar cells secrete a trypsin inhibitor, which prevents trypsin activation. Because trypsin activates other proteolytic enzymes, the trypsin inhibitor prevents subsequent activation of the other enzymes.

Two types of pancreatic disease are discussed in this chapter: acute and chronic pancreatitis and cancer of the pancreas.

Acute Pancreatitis

Acute pancreatitis represents a reversible inflammatory process of the pancreatic acini brought about by premature activation of pancreatic enzymes.[64-68] Although the disease process may be limited to pancreatic tissue, it also can involve peripancreatic tissues or those of more distant organs. In the United States, up to 220,000 persons are admitted to the hospital each year with acute pancreatitis.[66-67]

The pathogenesis of acute pancreatitis involves the autodigestion of pancreatic tissue by inappropriately activated pancreatic enzymes. The process is thought to begin with the activation of trypsin. Once activated, trypsin can then activate a variety of digestive enzymes that cause pancreatic injury, resulting in an intense inflammatory response. The acute inflammatory response itself causes substantial tissue damage and may progress beyond the pancreas to produce a systemic inflammatory response syndrome and multiorgan failure (see Chapter 26). Although a number of factors are associated with the development of acute pancreatitis, most cases result from gallstones (stones in the common duct) or alcohol abuse.[66-68] In the case of biliary tract obstruction due to gallstones, pancreatic duct obstruction or biliary reflux is believed to activate the enzymes in the pancreatic duct system. The precise mechanisms whereby alcohol exerts its action are largely unknown. Alcohol is known to be a potent stimulator of pancreatic secretions, and it also is known to cause partial obstruction of the sphincter of the pancreatic duct. Acute pancreatitis also is associated with hyperlipidemia, hypercalcemia, infections (particularly viral), abdominal and surgical trauma, and drugs such as thiazide diuretics.[64,67]

Clinical Manifestations. The manifestations of acute pancreatitis can range from mild with minimal organ dysfunction to severe and life-threatening. Overall, about 20% of persons with acute pancreatitis have a severe course, and 10% to 30% of those with severe pancreatitis die.[66,67] Abdominal pain is a cardinal manifestation of acute pancreatitis. The pain is usually located in the epigastric or periumbilical region and may radiate to the back, chest, or flank areas. Physical examination findings are variable and include fever, tachycardia, hypotension, severe abdominal tenderness, respiratory distress, and abdominal distention. Recognized markers of severe disease include laboratory values that measure the inflammatory response (e.g., C-reactive protein), scoring systems that assess inflammation or organ failure, and findings on imaging studies. Clinical findings such as thirst, poor urine output, progressive tachycardia, tachypnea, hypoxemia, agitation, confusion, a rising hematocrit level, and lack of improvement in symptoms within the first 48 hours are warning signs of impending severe disease. Complications include the systemic inflammatory response, acute respiratory distress syndrome, acute tubular necrosis, and organ failure. An important disturbance related to acute pancreatitis is the loss of a large volume of fluid into the retroperitoneal and peripancreatic spaces and the abdominal cavity. Signs of hypocalcemia may develop, probably as a result of the precipitation of serum calcium in the areas of fat necrosis.

Diagnosis and Treatment. Serum amylase and lipase are the laboratory markers most commonly used to establish a diagnosis of acute pancreatitis. The serum lipase may remain elevated slightly longer than amylase. However, the level of elevation of the serum amylase or lipase does not correlate with the severity of the disorder. The white blood cell count may be increased, and hyperglycemia and an elevated serum bilirubin level may be present. Determination of the cause is important in guiding the immediate management and preventing recurrence. Abdominal ultrasonography is usually performed to assess for gallstones. CT scans and dynamic contrast-enhanced CT of the pancreas are used to detect necrosis and fluid accumulation. Recent research has focused on potential biomarkers for predicting the severity and prognosis of pancreatitis. Trypsinogens and pancreatic proteases, enzymes involved in the autodigestive processes, appear promising. Other investigational serologic markers include trypsinogen activation peptide, C-reactive protein, procalcitonin, phospholipase A_2, and the cytokines interleukin-6 and interleukin-8.

Treatment measures depend on the severity of the disease. Persons who present with persistent or severe pain, vomiting, dehydration, or signs of impending severe acute pancreatitis require hospitalization. Treatment measures are directed at pain relief, "putting the pancreas to rest" by withholding oral foods and fluids, and restoration of lost plasma volume. Meperidine rather than morphine usually is given for pain relief because it causes fewer spasms of the sphincter of the pancreatic duct. Gastric suction is instituted to treat distention of the bowel and prevent further stimulation of the secretion of pancreatic enzymes. Intravenous fluids and electrolytes are administered to replace those lost from the circulation and to combat hypotension and shock. Intravenous colloid solutions are given to replace the fluid that has become sequestered in the abdomen and retroperitoneal space.

Complications. Sequelae in persons surviving an episode of severe acute pancreatitis include fluid collections and infection.[66] In 40% to 60% of persons with acute necrotizing pancreatitis, the necrotic debris becomes infected, usually by gram-negative organisms from the alimentary canal, further complicating the condition.[64] Fluid collections with a high level of pancreatic enzymes are usually associated with pancreatic duct disruptions and may eventually form pseudocysts

(a collection of pancreatic fluid enclosed in a layer of inflammatory tissue). A pseudocyst most often is connected to a pancreatic duct, so that it continues to increase in mass. The symptoms depend on its location; for example, jaundice may occur when a cyst develops near the head of the pancreas, close to the common duct. Pseudocysts may resolve or, if they persist, may require surgical intervention.

Chronic Pancreatitis

Chronic pancreatitis is characterized by progressive destruction of the exocrine pancreas, fibrosis, and in the later stages, by destruction of the endocrine pancreas.[69,70] Most factors that cause acute pancreatitis can also cause chronic pancreatitis. However, the chief distinction between the two conditions is the irreversibility of pancreatic function that is characteristic of chronic pancreatitis. By far the most common cause of chronic pancreatitis is long-term alcohol abuse. Less common causes are longstanding obstruction of the pancreatic duct by pseudocysts, calculi, or neoplasms; autoimmune chronic pancreatitis, which occurs in association with autoimmune disorders such as Sjögren syndrome, primary sclerosing cholangitis, and inflammatory bowel disease; idiopathic chronic pancreatitis, associated with cystic fibrosis (discussed in Chapter 29); and hereditary pancreatitis, a rare autosomal dominant disorder that is associated with both acute and chronic pancreatitis.

Clinical Manifestations. Chronic pancreatitis is manifested in episodes that are similar, albeit of lesser severity, to those of acute pancreatitis. Patients have persistent, recurring episodes of epigastric and upper left quadrant pain; the attacks often are precipitated by alcohol abuse or overeating. Anorexia, nausea, vomiting, constipation, and flatulence are common. Eventually the disease progresses to the extent that endocrine and exocrine pancreatic functions become deficient. At this point, signs of diabetes mellitus and the malabsorption syndrome (*e.g.,* weight loss, fatty stools [steatorrhea]) become apparent.

Treatment. Treatment consists of measures to treat coexisting biliary tract disease. A low-fat diet usually is prescribed. The signs of malabsorption may be treated with pancreatic enzymes. When diabetes is present, it is treated with insulin. Alcohol is forbidden because it frequently precipitates attacks. Because of the frequent episodes of pain, narcotic addiction is a potential problem in persons with chronic pancreatitis. Surgical intervention sometimes is needed to relieve the pain and usually focuses on relieving any obstruction that may be present. In advanced cases, a subtotal or total pancreatectomy may be necessary.[28]

Cancer of the Pancreas

Pancreatic cancer is now the fourth leading cause of death from cancer in the United States, with more than 30,000 new cases diagnosed each year.[64] Considered to be one of the most deadly malignancies, pancreatic cancer is associated with a 5-year survival rate of only 4% to 5%.[64,65,71,72] The incidence of pancreatic cancer seems to be increasing in all countries studied and has tripled in the United States over the past 50 years.[65]

The cause of pancreatic cancer is unknown. Age is a major risk factor. Pancreatic cancer rarely occurs in persons younger than 50 years of age, and the risk increases with age. The most significant and reproducible environmental risk factor is cigarette smoking.[64,65,71–73] The incidence of pancreatic cancer is twice as high among smokers than nonsmokers. Diabetes and chronic pancreatitis also are associated with pancreatic cancer, although neither the nature nor the sequence of the possible cause-and-effect relation has been established. There has been a recent focus on the molecular genetics of pancreatic cancer, and more insights into the genetic mechanisms involved in pancreatic cancer undoubtedly will be forthcoming.

Clinical Manifestations. Almost all pancreatic cancers are adenocarcinomas of the ductal epithelium, and symptoms are primarily caused by mass effect rather than disruption of exocrine or endocrine function. The clinical manifestations depend on the size and location of the tumor as well its metastasis. Pain, jaundice, and weight loss constitute the classic presentation of the disease. The most common pain is a dull epigastric pain often accompanied by back pain, often worse in the supine position, and relieved by sitting forward. Although the tumor can arise anywhere in the pancreas, the most frequent site is the head (60%), followed by the body (10%), and tail (5%). The pancreas is diffusely involved in the remaining 25%.[65] Because of the proximity of the pancreas to the common duct and the hepatopancreatic ampulla, cancer of the head of the pancreas tends to obstruct bile flow. Jaundice frequently is the presenting symptom of a person with cancer of the head of the pancreas, and it usually is accompanied by complaints of pain and pruritus. Cancer of the body of the pancreas usually impinges on the celiac ganglion, causing pain. The pain usually worsens with ingestion of food or assumption of the supine position. Cancer of the tail of the pancreas usually has metastasized before symptoms appear.

Migratory thrombophlebitis (deep vein thrombosis) develops in about 10% of persons with pancreatic cancer, particularly when the tumor involves the body or tail of the pancreas.[65] Thrombi develop in multiple veins, including the deep veins of the legs, the subclavian vein, the inferior and superior mesentery veins, and even the vena cava. It is not uncommon for the migratory thrombophlebitis to provide the first evidence of pancreatic cancer, although it may present in other cancers as well. The mechanism responsible for the hypercoagulable state is largely unclear, but may relate to activation of clotting factors by proteases released from the tumor cells.[65]

Diagnosis and Treatment. Patient history, physical examination, and elevated serum bilirubin and alkaline phosphate levels may suggest the presence of pancreatic cancer, but are not diagnostic.[71–73] The serum cancer antigen (CA) 19-9, a Lewis blood group antigen, may help confirm the diagnosis in symptomatic patients and may help predict prognosis and recurrence after resection. However, CA 19-9 lacks the sensitivity and specificity to screen asymptomatic patients effectively.[72] Ultrasonography and CT scanning are the most frequently used diagnostic methods to confirm the disease. Intravenous and oral contrast–enhanced spiral CT is the preferred method for imaging the pancreas. Percutaneous fine-needle aspiration cytology of the pancreas has been one of the major advances in the diagnosis of pancreatic cancer. Unfortunately, the smaller and more curable tumors are most likely to be missed by this procedure. ERCP may be used for evaluation of persons with suspected pancreatic cancer and obstructive jaundice.

Most cancers of the pancreas have metastasized by the time of diagnosis. Surgical resection of the tumor is done when the tumor is localized, or as a palliative measure. Radiation therapy may be useful when the disease is not resectable but appears to be localized. The use of irradiation and chemotherapy for pancreatic cancer continues to be investigated. Pain control is one of the most important aspects in the management of persons with end-stage pancreatic cancer.

IN SUMMARY, the biliary tract serves as a passageway for the delivery of bile from the liver to the intestine. This tract consists of the bile ducts and gallbladder. The most common causes of biliary tract disease are cholelithiasis and cholecystitis. Three factors contribute to the development of cholelithiasis: abnormalities in the composition of bile, stasis of bile, and inflammation of the gallbladder. Cholelithiasis predisposes to obstruction of bile flow, causing biliary colic and acute or chronic cholecystitis. Cancer of the gallbladder, which has a poor 5-year survival rate, occurs in 2% of persons with biliary tract disease.

The pancreas is an endocrine and exocrine organ. The exocrine pancreas produces digestive enzymes that are secreted in an inactive form and transported to the small intestine through the main pancreatic duct, which usually empties into the hepatopancreatic ampulla and then into the duodenum through the sphincter of the pancreatic duct. The most common diseases of the exocrine pancreas are acute and chronic forms of pancreatitis, and cancer. Acute and chronic pancreatitis are associated with biliary reflux and chronic alcoholism. Acute pancreatitis is an inflammatory condition of the pancreas due to inappropriate activation of pancreatic enzymes, with manifestations that can range from mild to severe and life-threatening. Chronic pancreatitis causes progressive destruction of the endocrine and exocrine pancreas. It is characterized by episodes of pain and epigastric distress that are similar to but less severe than those that occur with acute pancreatitis. Cancer of the pancreas is the fourth leading cause of cancer death in the United States. It usually is far advanced at the time of diagnosis, and the 5-year survival rate is 4% to 5%. ■

Review Exercises

1. A 24-year-old woman reports to her health care professional with complaints of a yellow discoloration of her skin, loss of appetite, and a feeling of upper gastric discomfort. She denies use of intravenous drugs and has not received blood products. She cannot recall eating uncooked shellfish or drinking water that might have been contaminated. She has a daughter who attends day care.

   A. What tests could be done to confirm a diagnosis of hepatitis A?

   B. What is the most common mode of transmission for hepatitis A? It is suggested that the source might be through the day care center that her daughter attends. Explain.

   C. What methods could be used to protect other family members from getting the disease?

2. A 56-year-old man with a history of heavy alcohol consumption and a previous diagnosis of alcoholic cirrhosis and portal hypertension is admitted to the emergency department with acute gastrointestinal bleeding due to a tentative diagnosis of bleeding esophageal varices and signs of circulatory shock.

   A. Relate the development of esophageal varices to portal hypertension in persons with cirrhosis of the liver.

   B. Many persons with esophageal varices have blood coagulation problems. Explain.

   C. What are the possible treatment measures for this man, both in terms of controlling the current bleeding episode and preventing further bleeding episodes?

3. A 40-year-old woman presents in the emergency department with a sudden episode of vomiting and severe right epigastric pain that developed after eating a fatty evening meal. Although there is no evidence of jaundice in her skin, the sclera of her eyes is noted to have a yellowish discoloration. Palpation reveals tenderness of the upper right quadrant with muscle splinting and rebound pain. Right upper quadrant abdominal ultrasonography confirms the presence of gallstones. The woman is treated conservatively with pain and antiemetic medications. She is subsequently scheduled for a laparoscopic cholecystectomy.

   A. Relate this woman's signs and symptoms to gallstones and their effect on gallbladder function.

   B. Explain the initial appearance of jaundice in the eyes as opposed to the skin. Which of the two laboratory tests for bilirubin would you expect to be elevated—direct (conjugated) or indirect (unconjugated or free)?

   C. What effect will removal of the gallbladder have on the storage and release of bile into the intestine, particularly as it relates to meals?

References

1. Guyton A., Hall J. E. (2006). *Textbook of medical physiology* (11th ed., pp. 799–804). Philadelphia: Elsevier Saunders.
2. Rose S. (1998). *Gastrointestinal and hepatic pathophysiology.* Madison, CT: Fence Creek.
3. Crawford J. M. (2005). Liver and biliary tract. In Kumar V., Abbas A. K., Fausto N. (Eds.), *Robbins and Cotran pathologic basis of disease* (7th ed., pp. 877–937). Philadelphia: Elsevier Saunders.
4. Rubin R., Rubin E. (2008). The liver and biliary system. In Rubin R., Strayer D. S. (Eds.), *Rubin's pathophysiology: Clinicopathologic foundations of medicine* (5th ed., pp. 617–673). Philadelphia: Lippincott Williams & Wilkins.
5. Denery P. A., Seidman D. S., Stevenson D. K. (2001). Neonatal hyperbilirubinemia. *New England Journal of Medicine* 344, 581–590.
6. Pratt D. S., Kaplan M. M. (2000). Evaluation of abnormal liver-enzyme results in asymptomatic patients. *New England Journal of Medicine* 342, 1266–1271.
7. Giannini E. G., Testa R., Savarino V. (2005). Liver enzyme alteration: A guide for clinicians. *Canadian Medical Association Journal* 172, 367–379.
8. Bravo A., Sheth S. G., Chopra S. (2001). Liver biopsy. *New England Journal of Medicine* 344, 495–500.
9. Katzung B. G. (2007). *Basic and clinical pharmacology* (10th ed., pp. 50–63). New York: McGraw-Hill Medical.
10. Navarro V. J., Senior J. R. (2006). Drug-related hepatotoxicity. *New England Journal of Medicine* 354, 731–739.
11. Lewis J. H. (2000). Drug-induced liver disease. *Medical Clinics of North America* 84, 1275–1311.
12. Ostapowicz G., Fontana F. J., Schiøtz F. V., et al. (2002). Results of a prospective study of acute liver failure at 17 tertiary care centers in the United States. *Annals of Internal Medicine* 137, 947–954.
13. Lee W. M. (2003). Drug-induced hepatotoxicity. *New England Journal of Medicine* 349, 474–485.
14. Brundage S., Fitzpatrick A. (2006). Hepatitis A. *American Family Physician* 73, 2162–2170.
15. Wasley A., Miller J. T., Finelli L. (2007). Surveillance for acute viral hepatitis—United States, 2005. *Morbidity and Mortality Weekly Report* 56(SS-3), 1–12.
16. Advisory Committee on Immunization Practices. (1999). Prevention of hepatitis A through active and passive immunization. *Morbidity and Mortality Weekly Report* 48(RR-12), 1–25.
17. Ghany M. G., Doo E. C. (2006). Assessment and management of chronic hepatitis B. *Infectious Disease Clinics of North America* 20, 63–69.
18. Wasley A., Grytdal S., Gallagher K. (2008). Surveillance for acute viral hepatitis—United States, 2006. *Morbidity and Mortality Weekly Report* 57(SS-02, 1–24).
19. Mast E. E., Weinbaum C. M., Fiore A. E., et al., Advisory Committee on Immunization Practices. (2006). A comprehensive strategy to eliminate transmission of hepatitis B virus infection in the United States: Recommendations of the Advisory Committee on Immunization Practices (ACIP) Part II: Immunization of adults. *Morbidity and Mortality Weekly Report* 55(RR-16), 1–28.
20. Servoss J. C., Friedman L. S. (2006). Serologic and molecular diagnosis of hepatitis B virus. *Infectious Disease Clinics of North America* 20, 47–61.

21. Yu A. S., Cheung R. C., Keeffe E. B. (2006). Hepatitis B vaccines. *Infectious Disease Clinics of North America* 20, 27–45.
22. Mast E. E., Margolis H. S., Fiore A. E., et al. (2005). A comprehensive immunization strategy to eliminate transmission of hepatitis B virus infection in the United States: Recommendations of the Advisory Committee on Immunization Practice (ACIP) Part I: Immunization of infants, children, and adolescents. *Morbidity and Mortality Weekly Report* 54(RR-16), 1–39.
23. Bialek S. R., Terrault N. A. (2006). The changing epidemiology and natural history of hepatitis C virus infection. *Clinics in Liver Disease* 10, 697–715.
24. Wong T., Lee S. S. (2006). Hepatitis C: A review for primary care physicians. *Canadian Medical Association Journal* 174, 649–659.
25. Seeff L. B., Hoofnagle J. H. (2003). Appendix: National Institutes of Health Consensus Development Conference Statement: Management of hepatitis C 2002. *Clinics in Liver Disease* 7, 261–287.
26. Glenn J. S. (2006). Molecular virology of the hepatitis C virus: Implications for novel therapies. *Infectious Disease Clinics of North America* 20, 81–98.
27. Hoofnagle J. H. (1989). Type D (delta) hepatitis. *Journal of the American Medical Association* 261, 1321–1325.
28. Friedman S. (2007). Liver, biliary tract and pancreas. In Tierney L. M., McPhee S. J., Papadakis M. A. (Eds.), *Current medical diagnosis and treatment* (46th ed., pp. 675–678, 644–651, 657–666). New York: Lange Medical Books/McGraw-Hill.
29. Davis G. L. (2002). Update on the management of chronic hepatitis B. *Reviews in Gastroenterological Disorders* 2(3), 106–115.
30. American Gastroenterological Association. (2006). American Gastroenterological Association medical position statement on management of hepatitis C. *Gastroenterology* 130, 225–230.
31. Russo M. W., Zacks S. L., Fried M. W. (2003). Management of newly diagnosed hepatitis C infection. *Cleveland Clinic Journal of Medicine* 70(Suppl. 4), S14–S20.
32. Krawitt E. L. (2006). Autoimmune hepatitis. *New England Journal of Medicine* 354, 54–66.
33. Alverez F. (2006). Autoimmune hepatitis and primary sclerosing cholangitis. *Clinics in Liver Disease* 10, 89–107.
34. Talwalker J. A. (2003). Primary biliary cirrhosis. *Lancet* 362, 53–61.
35. Kaplan M. M., Gershwin M. E. (2005). Primary biliary cirrhosis. *New England Journal of Medicine* 353, 1261–1273.
36. Wakim-Fleming J., Mullen K. D. (2005). Long-term management of alcoholic liver disease. *Clinics in Liver Disease* 9, 135–149.
37. Lieber C. S. (2000). Alcohol: Its metabolism and interaction with nutrients. *Annual Review of Nutrition* 20, 395–430.
38. Lieber C. S. (2005). Metabolism of alcohol. *Clinics in Liver Disease* 9, 1–35.
39. Alchord J. L. (1995). Alcohol and the liver. *Scientific American Science and Medicine* 2(2), 16–25.
40. Lieber C. S. (1994). Alcohol and the liver: 1994 update. *Gastroenterology* 106, 1085–1105.
41. Rubin E., Lieber C. S. (1968). Alcohol-induced hepatic injury in nonalcoholic volunteers. *New England Journal of Medicine* 278, 869–876.
42. Bayard M., Hot J., Boroughs E. (2006). Nonalcoholic fatty liver disease. *American Family Physician* 73, 1961–1969.
43. Adams L. A., Angulo P., Lindor K. D. (2005). Nonalcoholic fatty liver disease. *Canadian Medical Association Journal* 172, 899–904.
44. Angulo P. (2002). Nonalcoholic fatty liver disease. *New England Journal of Medicine* 346, 1221–1231.
45. Yu A. S., Keeffe E. B. (2002). Nonalcoholic fatty liver disease. *Reviews in Gastrointestinal Disorders* 2(1), 11–19.
46. Utzschneider K. M., Kahn S. E. (2006). Review: The role of insulin resistance in nonalcoholic fatty liver disease. *Journal of Clinical Endocrinology and Metabolism* 91, 4753–4761.
47. Heilelbaugh J. J., Bruderly M. (2006). Cirrhosis and chronic liver failure: Part I. Diagnosis and management. *American Family Physician* 74, 756–781.
48. Heilelbaugh J. J., Sherbondy M. (2006). Cirrhosis and chronic liver failure: Part II. Complications and treatment. *American Family Physician* 74, 756–781.
49. Trevillyan J., Carroll P. J. (1997). Management of portal hypertension and esophageal varices in alcoholic cirrhosis. *American Family Physician* 55, 1851–1858.
50. Menon K. V. N., Shah V., Karnath P. S. (2004). The Budd-Chiari syndrome. *New England Journal of Medicine* 350, 578–585.
51. Ginés P., Cárdenas A., Arroyo V., et al. (2004). Management of cirrhosis and ascites. *New England Journal of Medicine* 350, 1646–1654.
52. Sandhu B. S., Sanyal A. J. (2005). Management of ascites in cirrhosis. *Clinics in Liver Disease* 9, 715–732.
53. Garcia N., Sanyal A. J. (2001). Minimizing ascites: Complications of cirrhosis signals clinical deterioration. *Postgraduate Medicine* 109, 91–103.
54. Hegab A. M., Luketic V. A. (2001). Bleeding esophageal varices. *Postgraduate Medicine* 109, 75–89.
55. Longacre A. V., Garcia-Tsao G. (2006). A commonsense approach to esophageal varices. *Clinics in Liver Disease* 10, 613–625.
56. Brigalia A. E., Anania F. A. (2002). Hepatorenal syndrome: Definition, pathophysiology, and intervention. *Critical Care Clinics* 18, 345–373.
57. Weimer R. H., Rakela J., Ishitani M. B., et al. (2003). Recent advances in liver transplantation. *Mayo Clinic Proceedings* 78, 197–210.
58. Parikh S., Hyman D. (2007). Hepatocellular cancer: A guide for the internist. *American Journal of Medicine* 120, 194–202.
59. Ahn J., Flamm S. L. (2004). Hepatocellular carcinoma. *Disease of the Month* 50, 556–573.
60. Sherman M. (2004). Pathophysiology and screening for hepatocellular carcinoma. *Clinics in Liver Disease* 8, 419–443.
61. Johnston D. E., Kaplan M. M. (1993). Pathogenesis and treatment of gallstones. *New England Journal of Medicine* 328, 412–421.
62. Vogt D. P. (2002). Gallbladder disease. *Cleveland Clinic Journal of Medicine* 69, 977–984.
63. Bellows C. F., Berger D. H., Crass R. A. (2005). Management of gallstones. *American Family Physician* 72, 637–642.
64. Hruban R. H., Wilentz R. E. (2005). The pancreas. In Kumar V., Abbas A. K., Fausto N. (Eds.), *Robbins and Cotran pathologic basis of disease* (7th ed., pp. 939–963). Philadelphia: Elsevier Saunders.
65. Lauwers G. Y., Mino-Kenudson M., Rubin R. (2008). The pancreas. In Rubin R., Strayer D. S. (Eds.), *Rubin's pathophysiology: Clinicopathologic foundations of medicine* (5th ed., pp. 675–689). Philadelphia: Lippincott Williams & Wilkins.
66. Whitcomb D. C. (2006). Acute pancreatitis. *New England Journal of Medicine* 354, 2142–2150.
67. Carroll J. K., Herrick B., Gipson T., et al. (2007). Acute pancreatitis: Diagnosis, prognosis, and treatment. *American Family Physician* 75, 1513–1520.
68. Banks P. A., Freeman M. L., and the Practice Parameters Committee of the American College of Gastroenterologists. (2006). Practice guidelines for acute pancreatitis. *American Journal of Gastroenterology* 101, 2379–2400.
69. Steer M. L., Waxman L., Freeman S. (1995). Chronic pancreatitis. *New England Journal of Medicine* 332, 1482–1490.
70. Isla A. M. (2000). Chronic pancreatitis. *Hospital Medicine* 61, 386–389.
71. Freelove R., Walling A. D. (2006). Pancreatic cancer: Diagnosis and Management. *American Family Physician* 73, 485–492.
72. Brand R. (2004). Pancreatic cancer. *Disease of the Month* 50, 545–555.
73. Lillemoe K. D. (2000). Pancreatic cancer: State-of-the-art care. *CA: A Cancer Journal for Clinicians* 50, 241–268.

Visit thePoint **http://thePoint.lww.com for animations, journal articles, and more!**

Chapter 39

Alterations in Nutritional Status

JOAN PLEUSS AND GLENN MATFIN

Nutritional status describes the condition of the body related to the availability and use of nutrients. Nutrients that are taken into the body can be used to provide the energy needed to perform various body functions, or they can be stored for future use. The stability and composition of body weight over time require that a person's energy intake be balanced with energy expenditure. When a person is overfed, and nutrient intake consistently exceeds expenditure, most of the nutrients are stored and body weight increases; conversely, when energy expenditure exceeds nutrient intake, energy stores are lost and body weight decreases.

Also, because different foods contain different amounts of proteins, fats, carbohydrates, vitamins, and minerals, appropriate amounts of these dietary elements must be maintained to ensure that all parts of the body's metabolic systems can be supplied with requisite materials. This chapter discusses the regulation of energy expenditure and storage, nutritional needs, overnutrition and obesity, and undernutrition and eating disorders.

 **NUTRITIONAL STATUS**

After completing this section of the chapter, you should be able to meet the following objectives:

■ Define *nutritional status.*
■ Define *calorie* and state the number of calories derived from the oxidation of 1 g of protein, fat, or carbohydrate.
■ Explain the difference between anabolism and catabolism.
■ Relate the processes of glycogenolysis and gluconeogenesis to the regulation of blood glucose by the liver.
■ Define *basal metabolic rate* and cite factors that affect it.
■ Describe the function of adipose tissue in terms of energy storage and as an endocrine organ.

The nutrients that the body uses to maintain its nutritional status are derived from the digestive tract through the ingestion of foods or, in some cases, through liquid feedings that are delivered directly into the gastrointestinal tract by a synthetic tube (*i.e.,* tube feedings). The exception occurs in persons with certain illnesses in which the digestive tract is bypassed and the nutrients are infused directly into the circulatory system. Once inside the body, nutrients are used for energy or as the building blocks for tissue growth and repair. When excess nutrients are available, they frequently are stored for future use. If the required nutrients are unavailable, the body adapts by conserving and using its nutrient stores.

Energy Metabolism

Energy is measured in heat units called *calories.* A calorie, spelled with a small *c* and also called a *gram calorie,* is the amount of heat or energy required to raise the temperature of 1 g of water by 1°C. A *kilocalorie* (kcal) or *large Calorie,* which is equivalent to 1000 calories, is the amount of energy needed to raise the temperature of 1 kg of water by 1°C.[1] Because a gram calorie is so small, the kilocalorie or large Calorie, spelled with a capitol "C," is often used when discussing energy metabolism. The oxidation of proteins provides 4 kcal/g; fats, 9 kcal/g; carbohydrates, 4 kcal/g; and alcohol, 7 kcal/g.

⚡ ENERGY METABOLISM

- All body activities require energy, whether they involve a single cell, a single organ, or the entire body.

- Energy, which is measured in calories, is obtained from foods.

- Fats, which are a concentrated water-free energy source, contain 9 kcal/g. They are stored in fat cells as triglycerides, which are the main storage sites for energy.

- Carbohydrates are hydrated fuels, which supply 4 kcal/g. They are stored in limited quantities as glycogen and can be converted to fatty acids and stored in fat cells as triglycerides.

- Proteins are broken down into amino acids that generate 4 kcal/g. Amino acids are used in building body proteins. Amino acids in excess of those needed for protein synthesis are converted to fatty acids, ketones, or glucose and are stored or used as metabolic fuel.

Metabolism is the organized process through which nutrients such as carbohydrates, fats, and proteins are broken down, transformed, or otherwise converted into cellular energy. The process of metabolism is unique in that it enables the continual release of energy, and it couples this energy with physiologic functioning. For example, the energy used for muscle contraction is derived largely from energy sources that are stored in muscle cells and then released as the muscle contracts. Because most of our energy sources come from the nutrients in the food that is eaten, the ability to store energy and control its release is important.

Anabolism and Catabolism

There are two phases of metabolism: anabolism and catabolism. *Anabolism* is the phase of metabolic storage and synthesis of cell constituents. Anabolism does not provide energy for the body; it requires energy. *Catabolism* involves the breakdown of complex molecules into substances that can be used in the production of energy. The chemical intermediates for anabolism and catabolism are called *metabolites* (*e.g.,* lactic acid is a metabolite formed when glucose is broken down in the absence of oxygen). Both anabolism and catabolism are catalyzed by enzyme systems located in body cells. A *substrate* is a substance on which an enzyme acts. Enzyme systems selectively transform fuel substrates into cellular energy and facilitate the use of energy in the process of assembling molecules to form energy substrates and storage forms of energy.

Because body energy cannot be stored as heat, the cellular oxidative processes that release energy are low-temperature reactions that convert food components to chemical energy that can be stored or dissipated. The body transforms carbohydrates, fats, and proteins into the intermediary compound, *adenosine triphosphate* (ATP).[1] ATP is called the *energy currency of the cell* because almost all body cells store and use ATP as their energy source (see Chapter 4). The metabolic events involved in ATP formation allow cellular energy to be stored, used, and replenished. However, under some circumstances energy expenditure can be increased by decreasing metabolic efficiency: an uncoupling of ATP synthesis within the mitochondria results in a loss of energy as released heat. This process may have relevance to obesity (the more energy "wasted" as heat loss, the less weight gain), but is also important in maintaining body warmth in newborns. This is because the increased proportion of brown fat found in neonates is much less efficient at generating ATP than white fat, resulting in increased heat production (see subsequent discussion on brown and white fat).

Energy Expenditure

The expenditure of body energy results from five mechanisms of heat production (*i.e.,* thermogenesis): basal metabolic rate or resting energy equivalent, diet-induced thermogenesis, exercise-induced thermogenesis, nonexercise activity thermogenesis, and thermogenesis in response to changes in environmental conditions. The amount of energy used varies with age, body size, rate of growth, and state of health.

Basal Metabolic Rate

The *basal metabolic rate* (BMR) refers to the chemical reactions occurring when the body is at rest.[1] These reactions are necessary to provide energy for maintenance of normal body temperature, cardiovascular and respiratory function, muscle tone, and other essential activities of tissues and cells in the resting body. The BMR constitutes 50% to 70% of body energy needs.[1] The BMR is measured using an instrument called an *indirect calorimeter* that measures a person's rate of oxygen use. Oxygen consumption is measured under basal conditions: after a full night's sleep, after at least 8 hours without food, and while the person is awake and at rest in a warm and comfortable room. The BMR is then calculated in terms of calories per hour and normally averages approximately 65 to 70 calories per hour in an average 70-kg man.[1] Women in general have a 5% to 10% lower BMR than men because of their higher percentage of adipose tissue. Although much of the BMR is accounted for by essential activities of the central nervous system, kidneys, and other body organs, the variations in BMR among different individuals are related largely to skeletal muscle mass and body size. Under normal resting conditions, skeletal muscle accounts for 20% to 30% of the BMR.[1] For this reason, the BMR is commonly corrected for body size by expressing it as calories per hour per square meter of body surface area. Factors that affect the BMR are age, sex, physical state, and pregnancy. A progressive decline in the normal BMR occurs with aging[1] (Fig. 39-1). The BMR can be used to predict the calorie needs for maintenance of nutrition.

The *resting energy equivalent* (REE) is used for predicting energy expenditure. Several equations that determine REE have been published. Although the Harris-Benedict equation has been the most widely used, research indicates that the Mifflin-St. Jeor equation has better predictive value.[2] The most accurate way to determine REE is by indirect calorimetry. However, this is expensive and requires trained personnel. Multiplying the REE by a factor of 1.2 usually adequately predicts the caloric needs for maintenance of nutrition during health. A factor of 1.5 usually provides the needed nutrients during repletion and during illnesses such as pneumonia, long bone fractures, cancer, peritonitis, and recovery from most types of surgery.

Diet- and Exercise-Induced Thermogenesis

Diet-induced thermogenesis, or thermic effect of food, describes the energy used by the body for the digestion, absorption, and assimilation of food after its ingestion. It is energy expended over and above the caloric value of the food and accounts for approximately 10% of the total calories expended. When food is eaten, the metabolic rate rises and then returns to normal within a few hours. The amount of energy expended for physical activity is determined by the type of activity performed, the length of participation, and the person's weight and physical fitness.

Nonexercise Activity Thermogenesis

Energy expenditure can be increased by increasing voluntary physical activity and/or nonexercise activity thermogenesis. Nonexercise activity thermogenesis includes the energy expended in maintaining posture and in activities such as fidgeting.[3] This can range from 15% of total daily energy in very sedentary individuals to 50% or more in those who are more active. Nonexercise activity thermogenesis may be related to a propensity to gain weight—individuals with increased nonexercise activity thermogenesis may have less fat gain than those with decreased nonexercise activity thermogenesis.

Energy Storage
Adipose Tissue

More than 90% of body energy is stored in the adipose tissues of the body. *Adipocytes,* or fat cells, occur singly or in small groups in loose connective tissue. In many parts of the body, they cushion body organs such as the kidneys. In addition to isolated groups of fat cells, entire regions of fat tissue are committed to fat storage. Collectively, fat cells constitute a large body organ that is metabolically active in the uptake, synthesis, storage, and mobilization of lipids, which are the main source of stored fuel for the body. Some tissues, such as liver cells, are able to store small amounts of lipids, but when these lipids accumulate (so-called ectopic deposition, as occurs in fatty liver), they begin to interfere with normal cell function. Adipose tissue not only serves as a storage site for body fuels, it provides insulation for the body, fills body crevices, and protects body organs.

Studies of adipocytes in the laboratory have shown that fully differentiated cells do not divide. However, such cells have a long life span, and anyone born with large numbers of adipocytes runs the risk of becoming obese. Some immature adipocytes (termed *preadipocytes*) capable of division are present in postnatal life.[1] Fat deposition can result from proliferation of these existing immature adipocytes. Some medications can also have an important effect on fat cell numbers. The thiazolidinedione class of antidiabetic drugs can also stimulate the

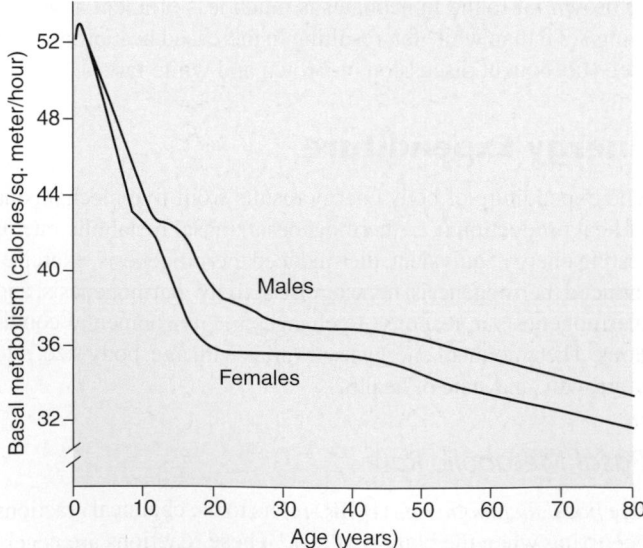

FIGURE 39-1 • Normal basal metabolic rates at different ages for each sex. From (Guyton A. C., Hall J. E. [2006]. *Textbook of medical physiology* [11th ed., p. 221]. Philadelphia: Elsevier Saunders.)

formation of new fat cells from preadipocytes, allowing increased uptake of glucose into these cells (and storage as fat) and resulting in the desired reduction in serum glucose levels, but with unwanted weight gain. In contrast, some drugs can cause loss of fat cells, resulting in lipodystrophy. This occurs in human immunodeficiency virus (HIV)–associated lipodystrophy in persons treated with highly active antiretroviral therapy (HAART). The mechanism of fat loss is unknown; however, it may be due to increased programmed cell death of the adipocytes (*i.e.*, increased apoptosis).

There are two types of adipose tissue: white fat and brown fat. White fat, which despite its name is cream-colored or yellow, is the prevalent form of adipose tissue in postnatal life. It constitutes 10% to 20% of body weight in adult men and 15% to 25% in adult women. At body temperature, the lipid content of fat cells exists as an oil. It consists of triglycerides, which are three molecules of fatty acids esterified to a glycerol molecule. Triglycerides, which contain no water, have the highest caloric content of all nutrients and are an efficient form of energy storage. Fat cells synthesize triglycerides, the major fat storage form, from dietary fats and carbohydrates. Insulin is required for transport of glucose into fat cells. When calorie intake is restricted for any reason, fat cell triglycerides are broken down, and the resultant fatty acids and glycerol are released as energy sources.

Brown fat differs from white fat in terms of its thermogenic capacity or ability to produce heat. Brown fat is found primarily in early neonatal life in humans and in animals that hibernate. In humans, brown fat decreases with age but is still detectable in the sixth decade. This small amount of brown fat has a minimal effect on energy expenditure.

Adipose Tissue as an Endocrine Organ

Adipose tissue is now recognized as an endocrine and paracrine organ that secretes a number of important factors.[4] These factors are termed *adipokines,* and include leptin, certain cytokines (*e.g.,* tumor necrosis factor-α [TNF-α]), growth factors, and adiponectin (important in insulin resistance).

Leptin. The discovery of leptin (from the Greek meaning "thin"), a peptide released from adipocytes, has led to renewed interest in adipose tissue and its role in energy homeostasis. Recent studies suggest that leptin acts at the level of the hypothalamus to decrease food intake and increase energy expenditure through an increase in thermogenesis and sympathetic nervous system activity. Leptin is also involved in glucose metabolism and normal sexual maturation and reproduction, and has interactions with the hypothalamic-pituitary-adrenal, thyroid, and growth hormones axes.

Leptin acts by binding to and activating specific leptin receptors found in several peripheral tissues and in many areas of the brain, including specific regions of the hypothalamus. Receptors in these hypothalamic regions are known to be involved in appetite, food intake, sympathetic nervous system activity, temperature regulation, and insulin release by the pan-

creatic beta cells. Leptin levels tend to rise after food intake and fall during fasting. Thus, leptin levels may be an important means by which adipose tissue signals the brain regarding the status of energy stores.

IN SUMMARY, nutritional status describes the condition of the body related to the availability and use of nutrients. Nutrients provide the energy and materials necessary for performing the activities of daily living and for the growth and repair of body tissues. Metabolism is the organized process whereby nutrients such as carbohydrates, fats, and proteins are broken down, transformed, or otherwise converted to cellular energy. Glucose, fats, and amino acids from proteins serve as fuel sources for cellular metabolism. These fuel sources are ingested during meals and stored for future use. Glucose is stored as glycogen or converted to triglycerides in fat cells for storage. Fats are stored in adipose tissue as triglycerides. Amino acids are the building blocks of proteins, and most of the stored amino acids are contained in body proteins and as fuel sources for cellular metabolism. Energy is measured in heat units called *calories.*

The expenditure of body energy results from heat production (*i.e.,* thermogenesis) associated with the BMR or basal energy equivalent, diet-induced thermogenesis, exercise-induced thermogenesis, nonexercise activity thermogenesis, and thermogenesis in response to changes in environmental conditions. ■

NUTRITIONAL NEEDS

After completing this section of the chapter, you should be able to meet the following objectives:

■ State the purpose of the Recommended Dietary Allowance of calories, proteins, fats, carbohydrates, vitamins, and minerals.

■ Describe methods used for a nutritional assessment.

■ State the factors used in determining body mass index and explain its use in evaluating body weight in terms of undernutrition and overnutrition.

Recommended Dietary Allowances and Dietary Reference Intakes

The *Dietary Reference Intakes* (DRIs) include a set of at least four nutrient-based reference values—the recommended dietary allowance, the adequate intake, the estimated average requirement, and the tolerable upper intake level, each of which has specific uses.[5] The DRIs, which are periodically updated, are published by the National Academy of Sciences. The DRIs are used in advising persons about the level of nutrient intake they need to decrease the risk of chronic disease. The current recommended DRIs for selected vitamins and minerals that have been released between 1997 and 2005 are cited in Appendix B (Tables B-1 and B-2). The Food and Nutrition Board also established acceptable macronutrient distribution ranges (AMDRs) as a percentage of energy intake for fat, carbohydrate, linoleic and α-linolenic acids, and protein[6] (see Appendix B, Table B-3).

The *recommended dietary allowance* (RDA) defines the intakes that meet the nutrient needs of almost all healthy persons in a specific age and sex group.[5] The *adequate intake* (AI) is set when there is not enough scientific evidence to estimate an average requirement. The AI is derived from experimental or observational data that show a mean intake that appears to sustain a desired indicator of health. An *estimated average requirement* is the intake that meets the estimated nutrient need of half of the persons in a specific group. This figure is used as the basis for developing the RDA and is expected to be used by nutrition policy makers in the evaluation of the adequacy of a nutrient for a specific group and for planning how much of the nutrient the group should consume. The *tolerable upper intake* level is the maximum intake that is judged unlikely to pose a health risk in almost all healthy persons in a specified group. It refers to the total intakes from food, fortified food, and nutrient supplements. This value is not intended to be a recommended level of intake, and there are no established benefits for persons who consume nutrients at the RDA or AI levels.

Food and supplement labels use *daily values* (DVs), which are set by the U.S. Food and Drug Administration (FDA). However, the DVs are based on data that are older than the data used to determine the DRIs. Percent daily value (%DV) tells the consumer what percentage of the DV one serving of a food or supplement supplies.

Proteins, fats, carbohydrates, vitamins, and minerals each have their own function in providing the body with what it needs to maintain life and health. Recommended allowances have not been established for every nutrient; some are given as a safe and adequate intake, but others, such as carbohydrates and fats, are expressed as a percentage of the calorie intake.

Nutritional Needs

Calories

Energy requirements are greater during growth periods. A person requires approximately 115 kcal/kg of body weight at birth, 105 kcal/kg at 1 year of age, and 80 kcal/kg from 1 to 10 years of age. During adolescence, boys require 45 kcal/kg of body weight and girls require 38 kcal/kg. During pregnancy, a woman needs an extra 300 kcal/day above her usual requirement, and during the first 3 months of breast-feeding, she requires an additional 500 kcal.[5] Table 39-1 provides examples of the estimated energy requirements (EER) at different activity levels for persons with a normal, overweight, and obese BMI.

Proteins

Proteins are required for growth and maintenance of body tissues, enzymes and antibody formation, fluid and electrolyte bal-

TABLE 39-1	**Estimated Energy Requirements (EER) at Different Activity Levels for Men and Women 30 Years of Age With a Normal (< 25), Overweight (25 to 29.9), and Obese (≥30) BMI**				
BMI	HEIGHT m (in)	WEIGHT kg (lb)	ACTIVITY LEVEL*	EER (kcal/d) MALE	EER (kcal/d) FEMALE
22.1 Normal	1.75 (69)	68 (150)	Rarely	2404	2055
			Low activity	2627	2285
			Active	2911	2571
			Very active	3378	2915
26.5 Overweight	1.75 (69)	77 (170)	Rarely	2620	2140
			Low activity	2867	2380
			Active	3182	2679
			Very active	3698	3038
31 Obese	1.75 (69)	95 (210)	Rarely	2837	2310
			Low activity	3108	2570
			Active	3452	2894
			Very active	4018	3284

*Activity level definitions:
Sedentary = rarely exercise
Low active = less 1 hour/day
Active = about 1 hour/day
Very active = more than 1 hour/day
Developed using "Adult Energy Needs and BMI Calculator" from USDA/ARS Children's Nutrition Center at Baylor College of Medicine. [Online.] Available: http://www.bcm.edu/cnrc/caloriesneed.htm. Accessed April 5, 2008.

ance, and nutrient transport. Proteins are composed of amino acids, nine of which are essential to the body (*i.e.,* these amino acids cannot be synthesized by the body and must be derived from dietary sources). These are leucine, isoleucine, methionine, phenylalanine, threonine, tryptophan, valine, lysine, and histidine. The foods that provide these essential amino acids in adequate amounts are milk, eggs, meat, fish, and poultry. Dried peas and beans, nuts, seeds, and grains contain all the essential amino acids but in less than adequate proportions. These proteins need to be combined with each other or with complete proteins to meet the amino acid requirements for protein synthesis. Diets that are inadequate in protein can result in kwashiorkor. If calories and protein are inadequate, protein-calorie malnutrition occurs.

The average protein consists of about 16% nitrogen. About 90% of this is excreted in the urine as urea, uric acid, creatinine, and other, less important nitrogen breakdown products, with the rest being excreted in the feces.[1] Therefore, the rate of protein breakdown can be estimated by measuring the amount of nitrogen in the urine. If the amount of nitrogen taken in as protein is equivalent to the nitrogen excreted, the person is said to be in nitrogen balance. A person is in positive nitrogen balance when the nitrogen consumed through protein is greater than the amount excreted. This occurs during growth, pregnancy, or healing after surgery or injury. A negative nitrogen balance often occurs with fever, illness, infection, trauma, or burns, when more nitrogen is excreted than is consumed.[1] It represents a state of tissue breakdown.

Fats

Dietary fats are composed primarily of triglycerides (*i.e.,* a mixture of fatty acids and glycerol). The fatty acids are saturated (*i.e.,* no double bonds), monounsaturated (*i.e.,* one double bond), or polyunsaturated (*i.e.,* two or more double bonds). The saturated fatty acids elevate blood cholesterol, whereas the monounsaturated and polyunsaturated fats lower blood cholesterol. Saturated fats usually are from animal sources and remain solid at room temperature. With the exception of coconut and palm oils (which are saturated), unsaturated fats are found in plant oils and usually are liquid at room temperature. *Trans fatty acids* are produced when unsaturated oils are partially hydrogenated and are called *artificial trans fats.* They are found primarily in vegetable shortenings and some margarines and in foods containing either of these. Natural sources of trans fatty acids include dairy products, some meats, and other animal-based foods. Trans fatty acids increase low-density lipoprotein (LDL) cholesterol and decrease high-density lipoprotein (HDL) cholesterol. However, the naturally occurring trans fats may have a beneficial effect. Dietary fats provide energy, function as carriers for the fat-soluble vitamins, serve as precursors of prostaglandins, and are a source of fatty acids. The polyunsaturated fatty acid, linoleic acid, is the only fatty acid that is required (*i.e.,* it is an essential fatty acid). A deficiency of linoleic acid results in

dermatitis. An AI has been set for both linoleic and α-linoleic acids[6] (see Appendix B, Table B-3). Because vegetable oils are rich sources of linoleic acid, this level can be met by including two teaspoons per day of vegetable oil in the diet.

Fat is the most concentrated source of energy. The Food and Nutrition Board has set an AMDR for fat of no less than 20% to prevent the fall of HDL cholesterol associated with very low-fat diets.[6] Guidelines from the National Cholesterol Education Program recommend that 25% to 35% of the calories in the diet should come from fats.[7] The daily dietary recommendation for cholesterol is less than 300 mg. The American Heart Association recommends limiting saturated fat to less than 7% and trans fatty acids to less than 1% of calories daily.[8]

Carbohydrates

Dietary carbohydrates are composed of simple sugars, complex carbohydrates, and undigestible carbohydrates (*i.e.,* fiber). Because of their vitamin, mineral, and fiber content, it is recommended that the bulk of the carbohydrate content in the diet be in the complex form rather than as simple sugars that contain few nutrients. Sucrose (*i.e.,* table sugar) is implicated in the development of dental caries.

There is no specific dietary requirement for carbohydrates. All of the energy requirements of the body can be met by dietary fats and proteins. Although some tissues, such as the nervous system, require glucose as an energy source, this need can be met through the conversion of amino acids and the glycerol part of the triglyceride molecule to glucose. The fatty acids from triglycerides are converted to ketones and used for energy by other body tissues. A carbohydrate-deficient diet usually results in the loss of tissue proteins and the development of ketosis. Because protein and fat metabolism increase the production of osmotically active metabolic wastes that must be eliminated through the kidneys, there is a danger of dehydration and electrolyte imbalances. The amount of carbohydrate needed to prevent tissue wasting and ketosis is 50 to 100 g/day. In practice, most of the daily energy requirement should be supplied by carbohydrate. This is because protein is an expensive source of calories and because it is recommended that dietary fat not exceed more than 35% of the calorie intake. The AMDR indicates that carbohydrate intake should be limited to no less than 45% of the calories in the diet to prevent high intakes of fat.[6]

Vitamins and Minerals

Vitamins. Vitamins are a group of organic compounds that act as catalysts in various chemical reactions. A compound cannot be classified as a vitamin unless it is shown that a deficiency of it causes disease. Contrary to popular belief, vitamins do not provide energy directly. As catalysts, they are part of the enzyme systems required for the release of energy from protein, fat, and carbohydrates. Vitamins also are necessary for the formation of red blood cells, hormones, genetic materials, and the nervous system. They are essential for normal growth and development.

There are two types of vitamins: fat soluble and water soluble. The four fat-soluble vitamins are vitamins A, D, E, and K. The nine required water-soluble vitamins are thiamine, riboflavin, niacin, pyridoxine (vitamin B_6), pantothenic acid, vitamin B_{12}, folic acid, biotin, and vitamin C. Because the water-soluble vitamins are excreted in the urine, they are less likely to accumulate in the body to toxic levels; however, the fat-soluble vi-

tamins are stored in the body and they may reach toxic levels. Table 39-2 lists sources and functions of vitamins.

Minerals. Minerals serve many functions. They are involved in acid-base balance and in the maintenance of osmotic pressure in body compartments. Minerals are components of vitamins, hormones, and enzymes. They maintain normal hemoglobin levels, play a role in nervous system function, and are involved in muscle contraction and skeletal development and maintenance. Minerals that are present in relatively large amounts in the body

TABLE 39-2 Sources and Functions of Vitamins

VITAMIN	MAJOR FOOD SOURCES	FUNCTIONS
Fat-Soluble Vitamins		
Vitamin A (retinol, provitamin, carotenoids)	Retinol: liver, butter, whole milk, cheese, egg yolk; provitamin A: carrots, green leafy vegetables, sweet potatoes, pumpkin, winter squash, apricots, cantaloupe, fortified margarine	Essential for normal retinal function; plays an essential role in cell growth and differentiation, particularly epithelial cells. Epidemiologic evidence suggests a role in preventing certain cancers
Vitamin D (calciferol)	Fortified dairy products, fortified margarine, fish oils, egg yolk	Increases intestinal absorption of calcium and promotes ossification of bones and teeth
Vitamin E (tocopherol)	Vegetable oil, margarine, shortening, green and leafy vegetables, wheat germ, whole-grain products, egg yolk, butter, liver	Functions as an antioxidant protecting vitamins A and C and fatty acids; prevents cell membrane injury
Water-Soluble Vitamins		
Vitamin C (ascorbic acid)	Broccoli, sweet and hot peppers, collards, brussel sprouts, kale, potatoes, spinach, tomatoes, citrus fruits, strawberries	Potent antioxidant involved in many oxidation–reduction reactions; required for synthesis of collagen; increases absorption of nonheme iron; is involved in wound healing and drug metabolism
Thiamin (vitamin B_1)	Pork, liver, meat, whole grains, fortified grain products, legumes, nuts	Coenzyme required for several important biochemical reactions in carbohydrate metabolism; thought to have an independent role in nerve conduction
Riboflavin (vitamin B_2)	Liver, milk, yogurt, cottage cheese, meat, fortified grain products	Coenzyme that participates in a variety of important oxidation–reduction reactions and an important component of a number of enzymes
Niacin (nicotinamide, nicotinic acid)	Liver, meat, poultry, fish, peanuts, fortified grain products	Essential component of the coenzymes nicotinamide adenine dinucleotide (NAD) and nicotinamide dinucleotide diphosphate (NADP), which are involved in many oxidative–reduction reactions
Folacin (folic acid)	Liver, legumes, green leafy vegetables	Coenzyme in amino acid and nucleoprotein metabolism; promotes red cell formation
Vitamin B_6 (pyridoxine)	Meat, poultry, fish, shellfish, green and leafy vegetables, whole-grain products, legumes	A major coenzyme involved in the metabolism of amino acids; required for synthesis of heme
Vitamin B_{12}	Meat, poultry, fish, shellfish, eggs, dairy products	Coenzyme involved in nucleic acid synthesis; assists in development of red cells and maintenance of nerve function
Biotin	Kidney, liver, milk, egg yolk, most fresh vegetables	Coenzyme in fat synthesis, amino acid metabolism, and glycogen formation
Pantothenic acid	Liver, kidney, meats, milk, egg yolk, whole-grain products, legumes	Coenzyme involved in energy metabolism

Data from *Vitamin facts,* National Dairy Council, and other sources.

are called *macrominerals.* These include calcium, phosphorus, sodium, chloride, potassium, magnesium, and sulfur. The remainder are classified as *trace minerals;* they include iron, manganese, copper, iodine, zinc, cobalt, fluorine, and selenium. Table 39-3 provides a list of mineral sources and their functions.

Fiber

Fiber, the carbohydrate portion of food that cannot be digested by the human gastrointestinal tract, increases stool bulk and facilitates bowel movements. Soluble fiber, the type that produces a gel in the intestinal tract, binds with cholesterol and prevents it from being absorbed by the body. Soluble fiber also lowers blood glucose. More studies are needed to establish whether fiber prevents colon cancer and promotes weight loss. In 2002, the Food and Nutrition Board gave its first recommended intake for fiber. Men and women who are 50 years of age and younger should

have 38 and 25 g, respectively, of fiber daily, whereas those older than 50 years should have 30 and 21 g, respectively, each day. The recommendation for children ranges from 19 to 31 g, and for teenagers is similar to that for adults.[6]

Regulation of Food Intake and Energy Storage

Stability of body weight and composition over time requires that energy intake matches energy utilization. Environmental, cultural, genetic, and psychological factors all influence food intake and energy expenditure. In addition, body weight is tightly controlled by various physiologic feedback control systems that contribute to the regulation of hunger and food intake.[1] We now appreciate that weight loss provokes counter-regulatory responses, resulting in major difficulties in maintaining long-term weight loss.

TABLE 39-3 Sources and Functions of Minerals

MINERAL	MAJOR SOURCES	FUNCTIONS
Calcium	Milk and milk products, fish with bones, greens	Bone formation and maintenance; tooth formation, vitamin B absorption, blood clotting, nerve and muscle function
Chloride	Table salt, meats, milk, eggs	Regulates pH of stomach, acid-base balance, osmotic pressure of extracellular fluids
Cobalt	Organ meats, meats	Aids in maturation of red blood cells (as part of B_{12} molecule)
Copper	Cereals, nuts, legumes, liver, shellfish, grapes, meats	Catalyst for hemoglobin formation, formation of elastin and collagen, energy release (cytochrome oxidase and catalase), formation of melanin, formation of phospholipids for myelin sheath of nerves
Fluoride	Fluorinated water	Strengthens bones and teeth
Iodine	Iodized salt, fish (saltwater and anadromous)	Thyroid hormone synthesis and its function in maintenance of metabolic rate
Iron	Meats, heart, liver, clams, oysters, lima beans, spinach, dates, dried nuts, enriched and whole-grain cereals	Hemoglobin synthesis, cellular energy release (cytochrome pathway), killing bacteria (myeloperoxidase)
Magnesium	Milk, green vegetables, nuts, bread, cereals	Catalyst of many intracellular nerve impulses, retention of reactions, particularly those related to intracellular enzyme reactions; low magnesium levels produce an increase in irritability of the nervous system, vasodilation, and cardiac arrhythmias
Phosphorus	Meats, poultry, fish, milk and cheese, cereals, legumes, nuts	Bone formation and maintenance; essential component of nucleic acids and energy exchange forms such as adenosine triphosphate (ATP)
Potassium	Oranges, dried fruits, bananas, meats, potatoes, peanut butter, coffee	Maintenance of intracellular osmolality, acid-base balance, transmission of nerve impulses, catalyst in energy metabolism, formation of proteins, formation of glycogen
Sodium	Table salt, cured meats, meats, milk, olives	Maintenance of osmotic pressure of extracellular fluids, acid-base balance, neuromuscular function; absorption of glucose
Zinc	Whole-wheat cereals, eggs, legumes	Integral part of many enzymes, including carbonic anhydrase, which facilitates combination of carbon dioxide with water in red blood cells; component of lactate dehydrogenase, which is important in cellular metabolism; component of many peptidases; important in digestion of proteins in gastrointestinal tract

Hunger, Appetite, and Food Intake

The sensation of *hunger* is associated with several sensory perceptions, such as the rhythmic contractions of the stomach and that "empty feeling" in the stomach that stimulates a person to seek food. A person's *appetite* is the desire for a particular type of food. It is useful in helping the person determine the type of food that is eaten. *Satiety* is the feeling of fullness or decreased desire for food.

The hypothalamus contains the feeding center for hunger and satiety (Fig. 39-2). It receives neural input from the gastrointestinal tract that provides information about stomach filling, chemical signals from nutrients (glucose, amino acids, and fatty

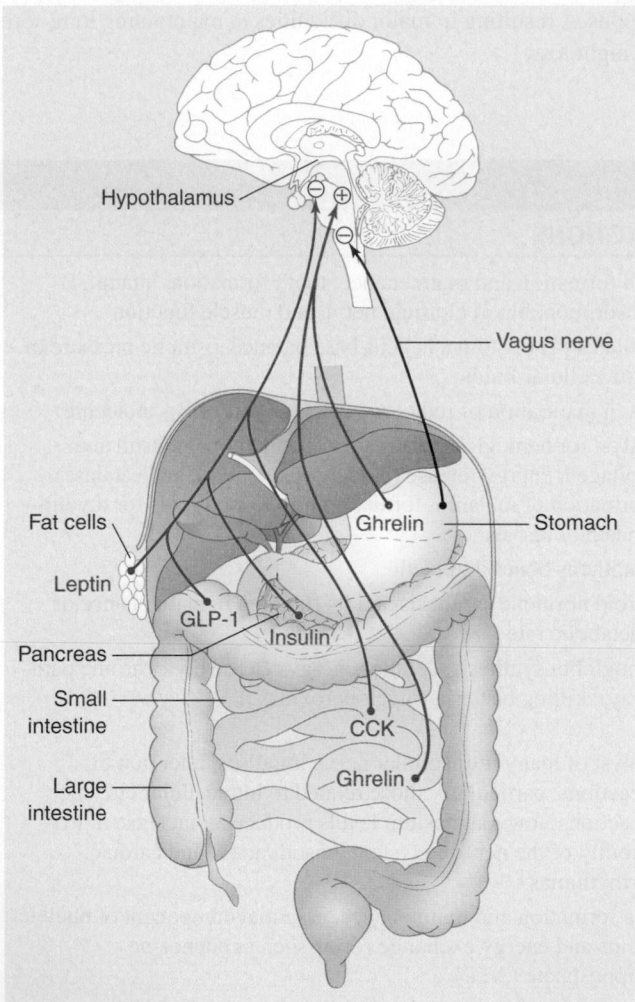

FIGURE 39-2 • Feedback mechanisms for control of food intake. Stretch receptors in the stomach activate sensory afferent pathways in the vagus and inhibit food intake. Insulin and the gastrointestinal hormones glucagon-like peptide-1 (GLP-1) and cholecystokinin (CCK) are released following ingestion of food and suppress further feeding. Ghrelin is released by the stomach and small intestine, especially during fasting, and stimulates appetite. Leptin is a hormone produced by fat cells as they increase in number and size; it inhibits food intake. (Modified from Guyton A. C., Hall J. E. [2006]. *Textbook of medical physiology* [11th ed., p. 868]. Philadelphia: Elsevier Saunders.)

acids) in the blood, and input from the cerebral cortex regarding the smell, sight, and taste of the food. Centers in the hypothalamus also control the secretion of several hormones (*e.g.*, thyroid and adrenocortical hormones) that regulate energy balance and metabolism.

The control of food intake is subject to short-term regulation, which is concerned with the amount of food that is consumed at a meal or snack, and intermediate and long-term regulation, which is concerned with the maintenance of energy stores over time.[1]

The short-term regulation of food intake provides a person with the feeling of satiety and turns off the desire for eating when adequate food has been consumed. It requires rapid feedback mechanisms that signal the adequacy of food intake before digestion has taken place and nutrients have been absorbed into the blood. These mechanisms include receptors that monitor filling of the gastrointestinal tract, gastrointestinal tract hormones, and oral receptors that monitor food intake. Stretch receptors in the gastrointestinal tract monitor gastrointestinal filling and send inhibitory impulses by way of the vagus nerve to the feeding center to suppress the desire for food.

The gastrointestinal hormones cholecystokinin (CCK), which is released in response to fat in the duodenum, and glucagon-like peptide-1 (GLP-1), which is released from the lower small bowel in response to nutrients, especially carbohydrates, have a strong suppressant effect on the hypothalamic feeding center. Ghrelin is a hormone released mainly by the stomach and to a lesser extent by the intestine. Its levels peak just before eating and then fall after a meal, suggesting that it may also stimulate eating.[9] The presence of food in the stomach increases the release of insulin and glucagon, both of which suppress the neurogenic feeding signals from the brain.[1] The act of tasting, chewing, and swallowing also appears to suppress the feeling of hunger.

The intermediate and long-term regulation of food intake is determined by the amount of nutrients that are in the blood and in storage sites. It has long been known that a decrease in blood glucose causes hunger. In contrast, an increase in breakdown products of lipids such as ketoacids produces a decrease in appetite. A ketogenic weight-loss diet (*e.g.*, the Atkins diet) relies partly on the appetite-suppressant effects of ketones in the blood.

Recent evidence suggests that the hypothalamus also senses the amount of energy that is stored in fat cells through a hormone called *leptin*. Increased amounts of leptin are released from the adipocytes when fat stores are increased. The stimulation of leptin receptors in the hypothalamus produces a decrease in appetite and food intake as well as an increase in metabolic rate and energy consumption. It also produces a decrease in insulin release from the beta cells, which decreases energy storage in fat cells.

Nutritional Assessment

The nutritional status can be assessed using the subjective global assessment (SGA). It includes weight status for the previous 6 months, dietary intake, gastrointestinal symptoms that affect food intake, functional capacity, and physical signs of fat loss and muscle wasting. Combined with objective measures such as albumin levels and body mass index, SGA accurately identifies malnourished individuals 90% of the time.[10]

Diet Assessment

A component of nutritional assessment is an evaluation of the person's diet. This can be accomplished by recording the food consumed or by 24-hour recall, and through the administration of a questionnaire or diet history. Each technique has its own shortcomings, such as the tendency to alter behavior when it is known that the behavior is being observed or reported.

Health Assessment

Health assessment, including a health history and physical examination, reveals weight changes, muscle wasting, fat stores, functional status, and nutritional status. Comparison of the person's current weight with previous weights identifies whether the person's weight is stable, changed drastically, or tends to fluctuate. For example, recent rapid weight loss can be a sign of cancer, an overactive thyroid gland, or self-imposed starvation. A history of fluctuating weight could be associated with bulimia. Degradation of muscle, or muscle wasting, is a serious sign of malnutrition. Decreased ability to initiate or complete activities of daily living could result from a decrease in energy caused by a poor diet, a neurologic malfunction such as multiple sclerosis, or symptoms related to chronic obstructive pulmonary disease. Changes in the quality of the hair or condition of the gums, absence of body hair, and presence of skin lesions could signal poor nutritional status.

Anthropometric Measurements

Anthropometric measurements provide a means for assessing body composition, particularly fat stores and skeletal muscle mass.[11] This is done by measuring height, weight, body circumferences, and thickness of various skinfolds. These measurements commonly are used to determine growth patterns in children and appropriateness of current weight in adults. Body weight is the most frequently used method of assessing nutritional status; it should be used in combination with measurements of body height to establish whether a person is underweight or overweight. For weight measurement, subjects should ideally be in light clothing and bare feet, fasting, and with an empty bladder. Repeat measurements are best made at the same time of the day.

An unintentional loss of 10% of body weight or more within the past 6 months usually is considered predictive of a poor clinical outcome, especially if weight loss is continuing.[12] The body mass index (BMI) uses height and weight to determine healthy weight (Table 39-4). It is calculated by dividing the weight in kilograms by the height in meters squared (BMI = weight [kg]/height [m^2]). A BMI between 18.5 and 24.9 has the lowest statistical health risk.[13] A BMI less than 18.5 is classified as being underweight, and one from 25 to 29.9 is considered overweight.[14] A BMI greater than 30 is diagnosed as obesity and is furthered classified into classes I (BMI 30 to 34.9), II (BMI 35 to 39.9), and III or extreme obesity (BMI >40). Body weight reflects both lean body mass and adipose tissue and cannot be used as a method for describing body composition or the percentage of fat tissue present. Statistically, the best percentage of body fat for men is between 12% and 20%, and for women, between 20% and 30%.[15] During physical training, body fat usually decreases and lean body mass increases.

Among the methods used to estimate body fat are skinfold thickness, body circumferences, bioelectrical impedance, air plethysmography, dual energy x-ray absorptiometry (DEXA), computed tomography (CT), and magnetic resonance imaging (MRI).[11] DEXA, CT, and MRI, are expensive and not portable, and usually are done in research settings.

TABLE 39-4 **Classification of Overweight and Obesity by BMI, Waist Circumference, and Associated Disease Risk***

| | BMI (kg/m²) | OBESITY CLASS | DISEASE RISK* RELATIVE TO NORMAL WEIGHT AND WAIST CIRCUMFERENCE | |
			Men ≤102 cm (≤40 in) Women ≤88 cm (≤35 in)	Men >102 cm (>40 in) Women >88 cm (>35 in)
Underweight	<18.5		—	—
Normal†	18.5–24.9		—	—
Overweight	25.0–29.9		Increased	High
Obesity	30.0–34.9	I	High	Very high
	35.0–39.9	II	Very high	Very high
Extreme obesity	≥40	III	Extremely high	Extremely high

BMI, body mass index.
*Disease risk for type 2 diabetes, hypertension, and cardiovascular disease.
†Increased waist circumference also can be a marker for increased risk, even in persons of normal weight.
Expert Panel. (1998). Clinical guidelines on the identification, evaluation, and treatment of overweight and obesity in adults.
National Institutes of Health. (Online.) Available: http://nhlbi.nih.gov/guidelines/ob_gdlns.htm.

Measurements of *skinfold thickness* can provide a reasonable assessment of body fat, particularly if taken at multiple sites. They can provide information about the location of the fat and can be used together with equations and tables to estimate the percentage of lean body mass and fat tissue. However, these measurements often are difficult to perform and subject to considerable variation between observers, and do not provide information about abdominal and intramuscular fat.

The measurement of *body circumferences* has received attention because excess visceral (or intra-abdominal) fat is closely associated with the metabolic syndrome. Also referred to as the *cardiometabolic syndrome*, the metabolic syndrome represents a collection of cardiovascular and metabolic risk factors, including dyslipidemia, glucose intolerance, and hyperinsulinemia (see Chapter 42).[16] The cause of the metabolic syndrome is unknown but is thought to be closely related to excess visceral fat. Studies have indicated that waist circumference at the abdomen (which is a surrogate measure of visceral fat) is highly correlated with insulin resistance, which is the other major association of the metabolic syndrome[16,17] (see Chapter 43).

Bioimpedance is performed by attaching electrodes at the wrist and ankle that send a harmless current through the body. The flow of the current is affected by the amount of water in the body. Because fat-free tissue contains virtually all the water and conducting electrolytes, measurements of the resistance (*i.e.,* impedance) to current flow can be used to estimate the percentage of body fat present.

Laboratory Studies

Various laboratory tests can aid in evaluating nutritional status. Some of the most commonly performed tests are serum albumin and prealbumin to assess the protein status, total lymphocyte count and delayed hypersensitivity reaction to assess cellular immunity, and creatinine–height index to assess skeletal muscle protein. Vitamin and mineral deficiencies can be determined by measurements of their levels in blood, saliva, and other body tissues or by measuring nutrient-specific chemical reactions. All of these tests are limited by confounding factors and therefore need to be evaluated along with other clinical data.

IN SUMMARY, the body requires more than 40 nutrients on a daily basis. Nutritional status reflects the continued daily intake of nutrients over time and the deposition and use of these nutrients in the body. The Dietary Reference Intakes (DRIs) classify the amounts of essential nutrients considered to be adequate to meet the known nutritional needs of healthy persons. The DRIs have 22 age and sex classifications and include recommendations for calories, proteins, fats, carbohydrates, vitamins, and minerals. The nutritional status of a person can be assessed by evaluation of dietary intake, anthropometric measurements, health assessment, and laboratory tests. Health assessment includes a health history and physical examination to determine weight changes, muscle wasting, fat stores, func-

tional status, and nutritional status. Anthropometric measurements are used for assessing body composition; they include height and weight measurements and measurements to determine the composition of the body in relation to lean body mass and fat tissue (*e.g.,* skinfold thickness, body circumferences, bioelectrical impedance, DEXA, and CT scans). ∎

OVERWEIGHT AND OBESITY

After completing this section of the chapter, you should be able to meet the following objectives:

■ Define and discuss the causes of obesity and health risks associated with obesity.
■ Differentiate upper and lower body obesity and their implications in terms of health risk.
■ Discuss the treatment of obesity in terms of diet, behavior modification, exercise, social support, pharmacotherapy, and surgical methods.
■ Explain the use of the body mass index in evaluating body weight in terms of overnutrition.

Obesity is defined as having excess body fat accumulation with multiple organ-specific pathologic consequences.[18,19] Clinically, obesity and overweight have been defined in terms of the BMI. Historically, various world bodies have used different BMI cutoff points to define obesity. In 1997, the World Health Organization (WHO) defined the various classifications of overweight (BMI ≥25) and obesity (BMI ≥30). This classification was subsequently adopted by the National Institutes of Health (NIH).[14] The use of a BMI cutoff of 25 as a measure of overweight raised some concern that the BMI of some men might be a function of muscle rather than fat weight. However, it has been shown that a BMI cutoff of 25 can sensitively detect most overweight people and does not erroneously detect over-lean people.

Overweight and obesity have become global health problems, increasing the risk of hypertension, hyperlipidemia, type 2 diabetes, coronary heart disease, and other health problems. According to recent worldwide estimates, 1.7 billion people are classified as overweight, greater than 1 billion have hypertension, and more than 500 million have either diabetes or impaired glucose tolerance.[20] In the United States, more than 65% of adults are currently either overweight or obese, and more than 30% of the population are obese, with obesity having an even higher prevalence in minority groups such as non-Hispanic blacks and those of Hispanic ethnicity.[21] The prevalence of overweight and obesity is alarming not only because of the number of people affected but because the prevalence continues to increase from previous surveys. The prevalence of severe obesity is increasing at an even faster rate; from 2000 to 2005, the number of persons self-reporting a BMI of 30 or more increased by

OVERWEIGHT AND OBESITY

- Obesity results from an imbalance between energy intake and energy consumption. Because fat is the main storage form of energy, obesity represents an excess of body fat.

- Overweight and obesity are determined by measurements of body mass index (BMI; weight [kg]/height [m²]) and waist circumference. A BMI of 25 to 29.9 is considered overweight; a BMI of 30 or greater as obese; and a BMI greater than 40 as very or morbidly obese.

- Waist circumference is used to determine the distribution of body fat. Central, or abdominal, obesity is an independent predictor of morbidity and mortality associated with obesity.

24%, those reporting a BMI of 40 or more increased by 50%, and those with a BMI of 50 or more increased by 75%.[22]

Causes of Obesity

The excess body fat of obesity often significantly impairs health, and as a result obesity is the second leading cause of preventable death in the United States.[23] It has been predicted that the health effects of obesity will result in a shorter life expectancy for today's youth.[24] This excess body fat is generated when the calories consumed exceed those expended through exercise and activity. Although factors that lead to the development of obesity are not understood, they are thought to involve the interaction of genotype and environmental factors, which include diet, physical activity, and early childhood factors.

Obesity is known to run in families, suggesting a hereditary component. The question that surrounds this observation is whether the disorder arises because of genetic endowment or environmental influences. Studies of twin and adopted children have provided evidence that heredity contributes to the disorder.[25] The most recent update of the human obesity gene map suggests that there are 20 to 30 candidate obesity genes that might contribute to the risk of obesity in humans.[26] It is unknown what combination of genes and mutations are involved in these risk factors and how environmental causes interact with them. There is also evidence that factors during pregnancy may affect the future weight of the child. These include gestational diabetes, smoking, and intrauterine undernutrition. Breast-fed infants may be less likely to be obese later in life.[27]

Although genetic factors may explain some of the individual variations in terms of excess weight, environmental influences are the major contributors. These influences include family eating patterns, inactivity because of labor-saving devices and time spent on the computer and watching television,[28] reliance on the automobile for transportation, easy access to food, higher energy density of food, increased consumption of sugar-sweetened beverages,[29] and increasing portion sizes.[30] The obese may be greatly influenced by the availability of food, the flavor of food, time of day, and other cues. The composition of the diet also may be a causal factor, and the percentage of dietary fat independent of total calorie intake may play a part in the development of obesity. Psychological factors include using food as a reward, comfort, or means of getting attention. Eating may be a way to cope with tension, anxiety, and mental fatigue. Some persons may overeat and use obesity as a means of avoiding emotionally threatening situations.

It has been suggested that the increased prevalence of obesity has resulted from increased caloric intake together with a sedentary lifestyle and energy-saving conveniences. In studies of persons who were overweight, the metabolic factors contributing to overweight were a low energy expenditure rate; a high respiratory quotient (RQ), which indicates the carbohydrate-to-fat oxidation ratio (suggesting that the person was oxidizing more carbohydrate than fat); and a low level of spontaneous physical activity.[31]

Epidemiologic surveys indicate that the prevalence of overweight may also be related to social and economic conditions. The second (1976 through 1980) National Health and Nutrition Examination Survey (NHANES II) has shown that if American women are divided into two groups according to economic status, the prevalence of obesity is much higher among those in the poverty group.[32] In contrast, men above the poverty level had a higher prevalence of overweight than men below the poverty level.

Types of Obesity

Two types of obesity based on distribution of fat have been described: upper body and lower body obesity. *Upper body obesity* is also referred to as *central, abdominal, visceral,* or *male ("android")* obesity. Lower body obesity is also known as *peripheral, gluteal-femoral,* or *female ("gynoid")* obesity. Subjects with upper body obesity are often referred to as being shaped like an "apple," compared with lower body obesity, which is more "pear" shaped (Fig. 39-3). In general, men have

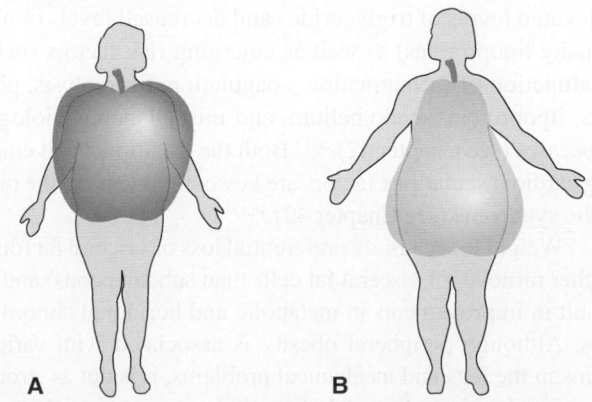

FIGURE 39-3 • Distribution of adipose tissue in (**A**) upper body or central (visceral) obesity and (**B**) lower body or peripheral (subcutaneous) obesity. People with upper body obesity are often described as having an "apple-shaped" body and those with lower body obesity as having a "pear-shaped" body.

more intra-abdominal fat and women more subcutaneous fat. As men age, the proportion of intra-abdominal fat to subcutaneous fat increases. After menopause, women tend to acquire more central fat distribution. Research suggests that fat distribution may be a more important factor for morbidity and mortality than BMI.[33]

The presence of excess fat in the abdomen out of proportion to total body fat is an independent predictor of risk factors and mortality. Both BMI and waist circumference are positively correlated with total body adipose tissue, but waist circumference is a better predictor of abdominal or visceral fat content than BMI.[33] The obesity type is determined by dividing the waist by the hip circumference. A waist circumference 88 cm (35 in) or greater in women and 102 cm (40 in) or greater in men has been associated with increased health risk[14] (see Table 39-4). A waist-hip ratio greater than 1.0 in men and 0.8 in women also indicates upper body or central obesity. Central obesity can be further differentiated into intra-abdominal adipose tissue (visceral fat) and subcutaneous abdominal adipose tissue by the use of CT or MRI scans.[34] Waist circumference, which is a measure of central fat distribution, measures both subcutaneous abdominal adipose tissue and intra-abdominal adipose tissue. One of the characteristics of visceral fat is the release of adipokines (such as TNF-α and adiponectin) and fatty acids directly to the liver before entering the systemic circulation, having a potentially greater impact on hepatic function (*e.g.,* the increased fatty acids are deposited in the liver, causing fatty liver, resulting in insulin resistance in the liver). Higher levels of these adipokines and circulating free fatty acids in obese persons, particularly those with upper body obesity, are thought to be associated with many of the adverse effects of obesity.[16]

Of particular importance is the effect excess abdominal fat has on cardiometabolic risk (Fig. 39-4). Cardiometabolic risk represents the overall risk of developing diabetes and/or cardiovascular disease (*e.g.,* coronary artery disease, stroke, peripheral vascular disease), which is due to a cluster of traditional risk factors such as obesity, hypertension, and dyslipidemia (elevated levels of triglycerides and decreased levels of high-density lipoproteins) as well as emerging risk factors such as dysfunction of inflammation, coagulation, fibrinolysis, platelets, lipoproteins, endothelium, and miscellaneous biological processes (see Chapter 42).[16,17] Both the traditional and emerging cardiovascular risk factors are key components of the metabolic syndrome (see Chapter 42).[16,17]

Weight loss causes a preferential loss of visceral fat (due to higher turnover of visceral fat cells than subcutaneous) and can result in improvements in metabolic and hormonal abnormalities. Although peripheral obesity is associated with varicose veins in the legs and mechanical problems, it is not as strongly associated with cardiometabolic risk. In terms of weight reduction, some studies have shown that persons with upper body obesity are easier to treat than those with lower body obesity. Other studies have shown no difference in terms of success with weight reduction programs between the two types of obesity.

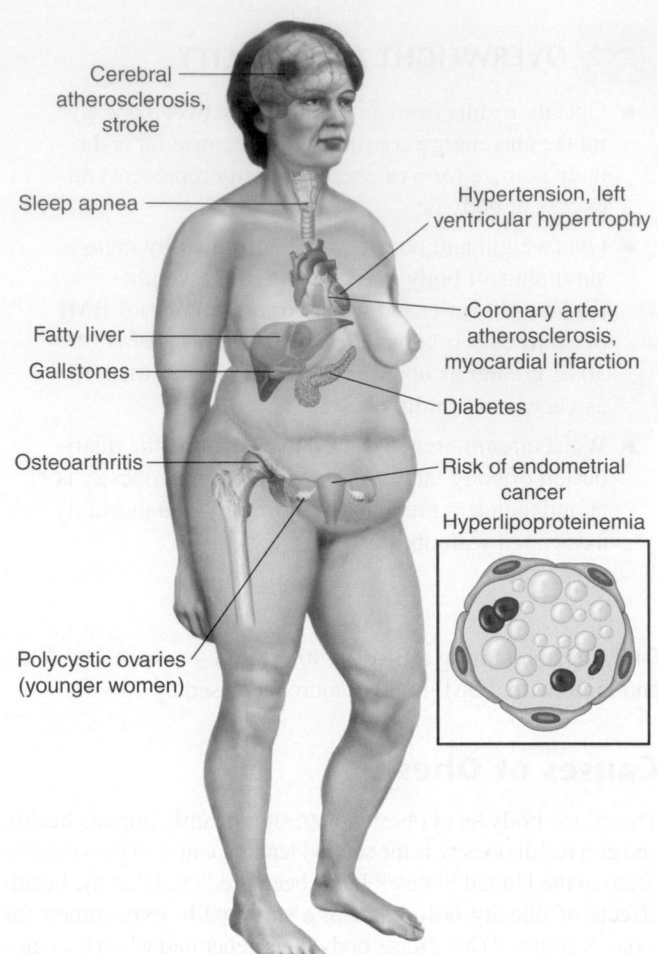

FIGURE 39-4 • Complications of obesity.

Weight cycling (the losing and gaining of weight) has been found to have little or no effect on metabolic variables, central obesity, or cardiovascular risk factors or future amount of weight loss.[35] More research is needed to determine its effect on dietary preference for fat, psychological adjustment, disordered eating, and mortality.[36] It is postulated that it is the underlying obesity and not the weight fluctuation that affects life expectancy.[37]

Health Risks Associated With Obesity

Obese individuals are at increased risk for developing many medical, psychosocial, and behavioral problems. In the United States as well as other countries, there are many negative stereotypes associated with obesity. People, especially women, are expected to be thin, and obesity may be seen as a sign of lack of self-control. Obesity may negatively affect employment and educational opportunities, as well as marital status. Obesity also may play a role in a person's treatment by health professionals.[38] Although nurses, physicians, and other health professionals are aware of the low success rate and difficulty in treating weight problems, they still may place the blame on the obese patient.

In addition to increased cardiometabolic risk (more likely to have high blood pressure, hyperlipidemia, prediabetes, insulin resistance, type 2 diabetes, cardiovascular disease, stroke, and peripheral vascular disease), obese people also have more gallbladder disease, infertility, and cancer of the endometrium, prostate, colon, uterus, ovaries, kidney, gallbladder, and, in postmenopausal women, the breast (see Fig. 39-4).[39] The increased weight associated with obesity stresses the bones and joints, increasing the likelihood of osteoarthritis. Other conditions associated with obesity include sleep apnea and pulmonary dysfunction, complications of pregnancy, menstrual irregularities, hirsutism, psychological distress, nonalcoholic fatty liver disease and nonalcoholic steatohepatitis (discussed in Chapter 38), carpal tunnel syndrome, venous insufficiency and deep vein thrombosis, and poor wound healing. Because some drugs are lipophilic and exhibit increased distribution in fat tissue, the administration of these drugs, including some anesthetic agents, can be more dangerous in obese persons. If surgery is required, the obese person heals more slowly than a nonobese person of the same age. Massive obesity, because of its close association with so many health problems, can be regarded as a disease in its own right. It is the second leading cause of preventable death.

Prevention and Treatment of Obesity

Prevention

Emphasis is being placed on the prevention of obesity. It has been theorized that obesity is preventable because the effect of hereditary factors is no more than moderate. A more active lifestyle together with a low-fat diet (<30% of calories) is seen as the strategy for prevention. The target audience should be young children, adolescents, and young adults.[40] Tools needed to achieve this goal include promotion of regular meals, increased intake of fruits and vegetables, substituting water for calorie-containing beverages, decreased television viewing time, and increased activity.[41] Other high-risk targeted periods include age 25 to 35 years, menopause, and the year after successful weight loss.

Treatment

The current recommendation is that treatment is indicated in all individuals who have a BMI of 30 or higher, or who have a BMI of 25 to 29.9 or a high waist circumference plus two or more risk factors.[42,43] Treatment should focus on individualized lifestyle modification through a combination of a reduced-calorie diet, increased physical activity, and behavior therapy. Pharmacotherapy and surgery are available as adjuncts to lifestyle changes in individuals who meet specific criteria. This was recently highlighted in a study showing that combining drugs and lifestyle counseling gives additive weight loss, compared with drugs alone.[44]

Before treatment begins, an assessment should be made of the degree of overweight and the overall risk status. This should include assessment of the following risk factors or complications

(as well as many other important considerations): coronary heart disease and other atherosclerotic diseases, sleep apnea, gynecologic abnormalities, osteoarthritis, gallstones, stress incontinence, cigarette smoking, hypertension, high LDL cholesterol levels, reduced HDL cholesterol levels, high triglyceride levels, prediabetes or type 2 diabetes, family history of premature coronary heart disease, and physical inactivity.[42]

It also is advisable to determine the person's barriers and readiness to lose weight. Several factors can be evaluated to make this assessment. These include reasons and motivations for weight loss, previous history of weight loss attempts, social support, attitude toward physical activity, ability to participate in physical activity, time available for attempting intervention, understanding the causes of obesity and its contribution to disease, and, finally, barriers the patient has for making changes.

The goals for weight loss are, at a minimum, prevention of further weight gain, but preferably reduction of current weight and maintenance of a lowered body weight indefinitely. An algorithm has been designed for use in treating overweight and obesity. The initial goal in treatment is to lower body weight by 5% to 10% from baseline over a 6-month period, with a 1- to 2-lb weight loss per week. Greater rates of weight loss do not achieve better long-term results.[40] This degree of weight loss requires a calorie reduction of 300 to 500 kcal/day in individuals with a BMI of 27 to 35. For those persons with a BMI greater than 35, the calorie intake needs to be reduced by 500 to 1000 kcal/day. After 6 months, the person should be given strategies for maintaining the new weight. Further weight loss can be considered after a period of weight maintenance. The person who is unable to achieve significant weight loss should be enrolled in a weight management program to prevent further weight gain.

Dietary Therapy. Dietary therapy should be individually prescribed based on the person's overweight status and risk profile.[41] The diet should be a personalized plan with realistic goals that are 500 to 1000 kcal/day less than the current dietary intake. Aim for weight loss initially, followed by strategy for weight maintenance. If the patient's risk status warrants it, the diet also should be decreased in saturated fat and contain 30% or less of total calories from fat. Reduction of dietary fat without a calorie deficit will not result in weight loss. Total caloric intake should be distributed in four or five meals or snacks throughout the day, including breakfast. The evidence also recommends teaching portion control. Meal replacements may be used as a substitute for one to two meals per day. Frequent contacts are required to provide ongoing support and give positive feedback to help motivate the patient.

Many popular diets exist, such as Atkins, Ornish, Weight Watchers, and South Beach. A recent study comparing several of these diets suggested that adherence to the diet and not the diet itself is most closely associated with weight loss (*i.e.*, the best diet is the one the patient likes best).[45]

Physical Activity. There is convincing evidence that increased physical activity decreases the risk of overweight and obesity.

In addition, it reduces cardiovascular and diabetes risk beyond that achieved by weight loss alone. Although physical activity is an important part of weight loss therapy and helps with maintaining weight loss, it does not independently lead to a significant weight loss.[46] It may, however, help reduce abdominal fat, increase cardiorespiratory fitness, and prevent the decrease in muscle mass that often occurs with weight loss. Exercise should be started slowly with the duration and intensity increased independently of each other. The goal should be 60 minutes or more of moderate to vigorous activity on most days of the week to maintain weight, and 60 to 90 minutes when trying to sustain weight loss.[47] The activity can be performed at one time or intermittently over the day.

Behavior Therapy. Techniques for changing behavior include self-monitoring of eating habits and physical activity, stress management, stimulus control, problem solving, contingency management, cognitive restructuring, social support, and relapse prevention.[41]

Pharmacotherapy. Drugs approved by the U.S. Food and Drug Administration (FDA) can be used as an adjunct to the aforementioned regimen in some patients with a BMI of 30 or more with no other risk factors or diseases, and for patients with a BMI of 27 or more with concomitant risk factors or diseases.[48] The risk factors and diseases defined as warranting pharmacotherapy are coronary heart disease, type 2 diabetes, metabolic syndrome, gynecologic abnormalities, osteoarthritis, gallbladder disease, stress incontinence, and sleep apnea.[49]

Two FDA-approved prescription drugs are available for long-term weight loss therapy—sibutramine (Meridia) and orlistat (Xenical). Another agent, rimonabant, is currently approved in several countries, but is awaiting U.S. approval due to safety concerns.[48] Sibutramine inhibits the reuptake of serotonin, norepinephrine, and dopamine. The drug produces weight loss by decreasing appetite. Orlistat is a lipase inhibitor that works by decreasing fat absorption in the intestine. Rimonabant is a cannabinoid type 1 receptor antagonist. The endocannabinoid system is a recently characterized physiologic system shown to influence appetite, mood, memory, cognition, and sleep, among others. Stimulation of the central and peripheral endocannabinoid system receptors can lead to weight gain, lipogenesis, insulin resistance, dyslipidemia, and impaired glucose homeostasis. Antagonizing some of these effects with rimonabant can lead to weight loss, decreased waist circumference, decreased blood glucose, decreased blood pressure, and improvements in lipids (these are all features of the metabolic syndrome).[48] All of these agents need careful monitoring for potential side effects. They also are contraindicated in certain patients.

Medication generally produces an increase in weight loss by about 4 to 6 kg beyond what can be achieved by diet alone. This will provide medical benefit, including improvement in cardiometabolic risk. Even after weight loss has stopped, the medication can be continued as a part of a weight maintenance program.

The FDA has recently approved the over-the-counter (OTC) sale of orlistat at half the prescription dosage. It is marketed under the trade name of Alli. The FDA states that it is to be used only in conjunction with a weight loss program that includes a low-fat, reduced-calorie diet and an exercise program. Like Xenical, it affects the absorption of fat and causes diarrhea, bloating, and stomach cramps. These can be avoided by eating a low-fat diet. Other OTC weight loss products are not FDA regulated. These usually contain ephedrine and caffeine. They should be used with extreme caution because of their adverse effects on blood pressure, heart rate, and glucose levels, and their potential to cause tremor.

Weight Loss (Bariatric) Surgery. In selected patients with acceptable operative risk factors, surgical therapy is currently the most effective treatment of obesity with respect to degree and duration of weight reduction achieved.[50] Bariatric surgery, although invasive, does afford significant weight loss, long-term weight loss maintenance, improved quality of life, decreased incidence of associated diseases, and decreased all-cause mortality (including mortality due to cardiovascular disease and cancer). This option is usually limited to persons with a BMI greater than 40; those with a BMI greater than 35 who have comorbid conditions and in whom efforts at medical therapy have failed; and those who have complications of extreme obesity. Approximately 66% of all bariatric procedures are done laparoscopically, with the remaining done by open method. The simplest operation is laparoscopic gastric banding, which obstructs food moving through the stomach, whereas more complicated procedures combine obstruction and bypass and are generally reserved for heavier patients. Bariatric surgery works by a variety of methods, including reduction in energy intake and absorption, and increased satiety or aversion to food. Adverse effects from surgery include those related to the operation itself (occurring in approximately 10%), and long-term effects, which include various mineral, vitamin, and protein deficiencies (occurring in approximately 20% to 30%). Persons who undergo surgical interventions also must continue in a program that provides guidance in nutrition and physical activity and behavioral and social support.

Childhood Obesity

Obesity is the most prevalent nutritional disorder affecting the pediatric population in the United States,[51] Canada,[52] and other industrialized countries in the world.[53] The definition for obesity in children is a BMI at or above the sex- and age-specific 95th percentile, whereas a BMI between the 85th and 95th percentiles is defined as being overweight.[51] These criteria have been selected because they correspond to adult BMIs of 30 and 25, respectively.[52] The findings from NHANES, conducted between 2003 and 2004, indicated that 18.8% of children from 6 to 11 years of age, and 17.4% of children 12 to 19 years of age were overweight[52] (Fig. 39-5). Obesity prevalence is higher among African American, Hispanic American, and Native American than white children.[52,54]

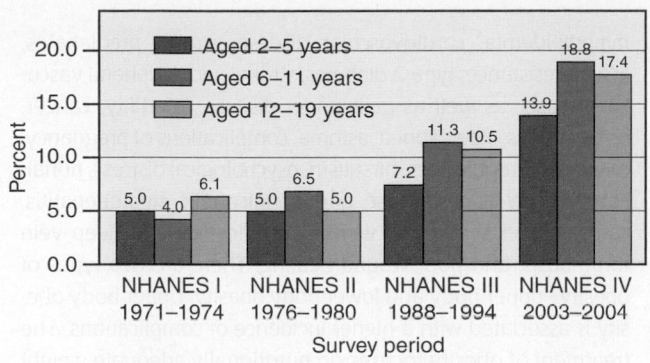

*Age-specific BMI ≥ 95th percentile based on the CDC growth charts.

FIGURE 39-5 • Prevalence of overweight among U.S. children and adolescents (aged 2 to 19 years). (Data from National Health and Nutrition Examination Surveys.)

The major concern of childhood obesity is that obese children will grow up to become obese adults. Pediatricians are now beginning to see hypertension, dyslipidemia, type 2 diabetes, and psychosocial stigma in obese children and adolescents. In North America, type 2 diabetes now accounts for half of all new diagnoses of diabetes (types 1 and 2) in some populations of adolescents.[55] In addition, there is a growing concern that childhood and adolescent obesity may be associated with negative psychosocial consequences, such as low self-esteem and discrimination by adults and peers.[51]

Childhood obesity is determined by a combination of hereditary and environmental factors. It is associated with obese parents, gestational diabetes and excessive weight gain during pregnancy, formula feeding, parenting style, parental eating, energy-dense food choices, erratic eating patterns, ethnicity, and sedentary lifestyle.[51–56] Children with overweight parents are at highest risk; in those with at least one overweight parent there is a 79% likelihood of being overweight as an adult.[54] One of the factors leading to childhood obesity is the increase in inactivity. Increasing perceptions that neighborhoods are unsafe has resulted in less time spent outside playing and walking and more time spent indoors engaging in sedentary activities such as television viewing and computer usage. Television viewing is associated with consumption of calorie-dense snacks and decreased indoor activity. Studies have shown a 10% decrease in obesity risk for each hour per day of moderate to vigorous physical activity, whereas the risk increased by 12% for each hour per day of television viewing.[55] Obese children also may have a deficit in recognizing hunger sensations, stemming perhaps from parents who use food as gratification. Fast food, increased portion sizes, increased energy density, sugar-sweetened soft drinks, and foods with a high glycemic index are all likely contributing to the increased weights in children and adolescents.

Assessment

Because of the enormity of the problem of overweight and obesity in children, the American Medical Association (AMA),

the U.S. Department of Health and Human Services' Health Resources and Services Administration (HRSA), and the Centers for Disease Control and Prevention (CDC) assembled an Expert Committee to develop recommendations for the assessment, prevention, and treatment of this public health problem.[57] Their recommendations include a yearly assessment of weight status in all children by measurement of height and weight to determine BMI for age and comparing it with standard growth charts (see Chapter 2). Children who are 2 to 18 years of age with a BMI in at least the 95th percentile for age and sex, or a BMI greater than 30 (whichever is smaller), should be classified as obese. Those children with a BMI in at least the 85th percentile, but less than the 95th percentile for age and sex, should be placed in the overweight category.

The Expert Committee recommends a qualitative assessment of dietary patterns of all pediatric patients at each well-child visit.[57] This assessment should include self-efficacy and readiness to change; frequency of eating at restaurants or fast food places; excessive consumption of sweetened beverages, 100% fruit juice, and foods high in energy density; consumption of excessive portion sizes for age; frequency and quality of breakfast and snacks; and low consumption of fruits and vegetables. The committee also recommends assessment of physical and sedentary activity at well-child visits to include environment, social support, and barriers to physical activity; and whether the child is getting a daily minimum of 60 minutes of moderate physical activity and spending less than 2 hours per day at sedentary activities such as video games, computer usage, or television viewing.[57]

Prevention and Treatment

Because adolescent obesity is predictive of adult obesity, treatment of childhood obesity is desirable.[53] The goals of therapy in uncomplicated obesity are directed toward healthy eating and activity, not achievement of ideal body weight. Families should be taught awareness of current eating habits, activity, and parenting behavior and how to modify them. For children with complications secondary to the obesity, the goal should be normalization of weight and treatment of the complications. The weight loss interventions should include all family members and caregivers; begin early at a point when the family is ready for change; assist the family to learn to monitor eating and activity patterns and make small and acceptable changes in these patterns; and should encourage and emphasize, not criticize. They should include information about the medical complications of obesity and be directed at permanent changes, not short-term diets or exercise programs aimed at rapid weight loss.

It is recommended that health care providers counsel parents and caregivers of children with a BMI between the 5th and 84th percentiles to limit sugar-sweetened beverages and encourage the recommended amount of fruits and vegetables, to limit screen time to no more than 2 hours daily, to remove television and computer screens from the child's sleeping area, to eat breakfast daily, to limit portion size and eating out, especially at fast food restaurants, and to encourage family meals where parents and children eat together.[57] The Expert Committee also recommends that the health care community advocate for the federal government to increase physical activity programs at school from grades 1 through 12 and to support initiatives in the community that would promote physical activity.[57]

The Expert Committee recommends that health care providers address weight and lifestyle with all patients regardless of their weight at least yearly, and that all children with a BMI between the 5th and 84th percentiles should follow recommendations for prevention.[57] Overweight children should be treated using a staged method based on their age, BMI, related comorbidities, weight status of parents, and progress in treatment, with the primary caregivers/families of the child being involved in the process. Dietary goals should focus on well-balanced, healthy meals with a healthy approach to eating. Specific strategies can include reduction of specific high-calorie foods or an appropriate balance of foods that are low, medium, and high calorie. Commercial diets should be used with caution. Pharmacologic therapy and bariatric surgery should be reserved for children with complications and for severe obesity, respectively.

For children between 2 and 19 years of age with a BMI >85th percentile, the expert committee outlines four stages of treatment.[57] Stage 1 recommendations, which are implemented by the primary care physician or allied care professional, involve counseling of children and their families in the eating of five or more servings of fruits and vegetables per day, elimination of sugar-sweetened beverages, limiting television or computer screen viewing to 2 or fewer hours per day with no television in the bedroom, and daily participation in 1 or more hours of physical activity. Children and their families should be encouraged to eat a daily breakfast, a limited number of meals outside of the home, and family meals 5-6 times per week and allow the child to self-regulate his or her meals. The goal should be weight maintenance so that BMI decreases as growth increases.

If no improvement is seen after 3 to 6 months in Stage 1, the Expert Committee recommends staged advancements based on readiness to change to a structured weight management protocol (Stage 2). If no improvement occurs in Stage 2, a comprehensive multidisciplinary protocol (Stage 3) should be implemented by a multidisciplinary obesity care team. In children with a BMI greater than the 95th percentile and significant comorbidities who have not improved during Stages 1 to 3, the Expert Committee recommends referral to a pediatric tertiary weight management center with expertise in childhood obesity and a designed protocol that includes continued diet and activity counseling and the consideration of meal replacement, very-low-calorie diet, medication, and surgery.[57]

IN SUMMARY, obesity is defined as having excess body fat accumulation with multiple organ-specific pathologic consequences. Genetic, socioeconomic, cultural, and environmental factors, psychological influences, and activity levels have been implicated as causative factors in the development of obesity. The health risks associated with obesity include increased cardiometabolic risk (*i.e.,* more likely to have high blood pressure,

hyperlipidemia, cardiovascular disease, stroke, prediabetes, insulin resistance, type 2 diabetes, stroke, and peripheral vascular disease), as well as gallbladder disease, infertility, cancer, osteoarthritis, sleep apnea, asthma, complications of pregnancy, menstrual irregularities, hirsutism, psychological distress, nonalcoholic fatty liver disease and nonalcoholic steatohepatitis, carpal tunnel syndrome, venous insufficiency and deep vein thrombosis, and poor wound healing. There are two types of obesity—upper body and lower body obesity. Upper body obesity is associated with a higher incidence of complications. The treatment of obesity focuses on nutritionally adequate weight loss diets, behavior modification, exercise, social support, and, in situations of marked obesity, pharmacotherapy and surgical methods.

Obesity is the most prevalent nutritional disorder affecting the pediatric population in the United States. Factors that predispose to childhood obesity include erratic eating patterns, dense calorie food choices, and lack of exercise and sedentary lifestyle. The major concern of childhood obesity is that obese children will grow up to become obese adults. Pediatricians are now beginning to see hypertension, dyslipidemia, type 2 diabetes, and psychosocial stigma in obese children and adolescents. Because of the scope of the problem, it is recommended that the weight status of all children be evaluated yearly and that measures to prevent and treat obesity be included in the health care plan for all children. ■

UNDERNUTRITION AND EATING DISORDERS

After completing this section of the chapter, you should be able to meet the following objectives:

- List the major causes of malnutrition and starvation.
- State the difference between protein-calorie starvation (*i.e.,* marasmus) and protein malnutrition (*i.e.,* kwashiorkor).
- Explain the effect of malnutrition on muscle mass, respiratory function, acid-base balance, wound healing, immune function, bone mineralization, the menstrual cycle, and testicular function.
- State the causes of malnutrition in severely ill or traumatized patients.
- Compare the eating disorders of anorexia and bulimia nervosa and the complications associated with each.

Undernutrition continues to be a major health problem throughout the world. Globally, nearly 852 million people were undernourished in 2000 to 2004.[58] Protein-energy malnutrition is most obvious in developing countries of the world, where it is indirectly responsible for half of all deaths of young children.[59] Even in developed nations, malnutrition remains a problem. In 1992, it was estimated that 12 million American children consumed diets that were significantly below the recommended allowances of the National Academy of Sciences.[60]

Malnutrition and Starvation

Malnutrition and starvation are conditions in which a person does not receive or is unable to use an adequate amount of nutrients for body function. An adequate diet should provide adequate energy in the form of carbohydrates, fats, and proteins; essential amino acids and fatty acids for use as building blocks for synthesis of structural and functional proteins and lipids; and vitamins and minerals, needed to function as coenzymes or hormones in vital metabolic processes, or, as in the case of calcium and phosphate, as important structural components of bone.[61]

Among the many causes of malnutrition are poverty and ignorance, acute and chronic illness, and self-imposed dietary restriction. Homeless people, the elderly, and children of the poor often demonstrate the effects of protein and energy malnutrition, as well as vitamin and mineral deficiencies. Even the affluent may fail to recognize that infants, adolescents, and pregnant women have increased nutritional needs. Some types of malnutrition are caused by acute and chronic illnesses, such as occurs in persons with Crohn disease who are unable to absorb nutrients from their food. Anorexia nervosa and less overt eating disorders affect a large population of persons who are concerned about body image or athletic performance.

Protein-Energy Malnutrition

Protein and energy (calorie) malnutrition represents a depletion of the body's lean tissues caused by starvation or a combination of starvation and catabolic stress. The lean tissues are the fat-free, metabolically active tissues of the body, namely, the skeletal muscles, viscera, and cells of the blood and immune system. Because lean tissues are the largest body compartment, their rate of loss is the main determinant of total body weight in most cases of protein-energy malnutrition.

Much of the literature on malnutrition and starvation has dealt with infants and children in underdeveloped countries in which food deprivation results in an inadequate intake of protein and calories to meet the body's energy needs. Protein-energy malnutrition in this population commonly is divided into two distinct conditions: marasmus (protein and calorie deficiency) and kwashiorkor (protein deficiency). The pathologic changes for both types of malnutrition include humoral and cellular immunodeficiencies resulting from protein deficiency and lack of immune mediators. There is impaired synthesis of pigments of the hair and skin (*e.g.,* hair color may change and the skin may become hyperpigmented) because of a lack of substrate (tyrosine) and coenzymes.

There are two functional compartments involved in the distribution of proteins within the body: the somatic compartment, represented by the skeletal muscles, and the visceral compartment, represented by protein stores in body organs, principally the liver.[61] These two compartments are regulated differently, with the somatic compartment being affected more severely in marasmus and the visceral compartment more severely in kwashiorkor.

Marasmus represents a progressive loss of muscle mass and fat stores due to inadequate food intake that is equally deficient in calories and protein.[61,62] It results in a reduction in body weight adjusted for age and size. The child with marasmus has a wasted appearance, with loss of muscle mass, stunted growth, and loss of subcutaneous fat; a protuberant abdomen (from muscular hypotonia); wrinkled skin; sparse, dry, and dull hair; and depressed heart rate, blood pressure, and body temperature. Diarrhea is common. Because immune function is impaired, concurrent infections occur and place additional stress on an already weakened body. An important characteristic of marasmus is growth failure; if sufficient food is not provided, these children will not reach their full potential stature.[62]

Kwashiorkor results from a deficiency in protein in diets relatively high in carbohydrates.[61,62] The term *kwashiorkor* comes from an African word meaning "the disease suffered by the displaced child," because the condition develops soon after a child is displaced from the breast after the arrival of a new infant and placed on a starchy gruel feeding. Kwashiorkor is a more severe form of malnutrition than marasmus. Unlike marasmus, severe protein deficiency is associated with extensive loss of the visceral protein compartment with a resultant hypoalbuminemia that gives rise to generalized or dependent edema. The child with kwashiorkor usually presents with edema, desquamating skin, discolored hair, anorexia, and extreme apathy (Fig. 39-6). There are "flaky paint" lesions of the skin on the face, extremities, and perineum and the hair becomes a sandy or reddish color, with linear depigmentation (flag sign).[62] There is generalized growth failure and muscle wasting as in marasmus, but subcutaneous fat is normal because calorie intake is adequate. Other manifestations include skin lesions, hepatomegaly and distended abdomen, cold extremities, and decreased cardiac output and tachycardia.

Marasmus-kwashiorkor is an advanced protein-energy deficit coupled with increased protein requirement or loss. This results in a rapid decrease in anthropometric measurements with obvious edema and wasting and loss of organ mass. One essential aspect of severe protein-energy malnutrition is fatty degeneration of such diverse organs as the heart and liver. This degeneration causes subclinical and overt cardiac dysfunction, especially when malnutrition is accompanied by edema. A second injurious aspect is the loss of subcutaneous fat, which markedly reduces the body's capacity for temperature regulation and water storage. As a consequence, malnourished children become dehydrated and hypothermic more quickly and more severely than normally nourished children.[58] Most children with severe protein-energy malnutrition have asymptomatic infections because their immune system fails to respond appropriately. So depressed is their immune system that many are unable to produce the fever that is typical of an acute infection.[58]

Malnutrition in Trauma and Illness

In industrialized societies, protein-energy malnutrition most often occurs secondary to trauma or illness. Kwashiorkor-like

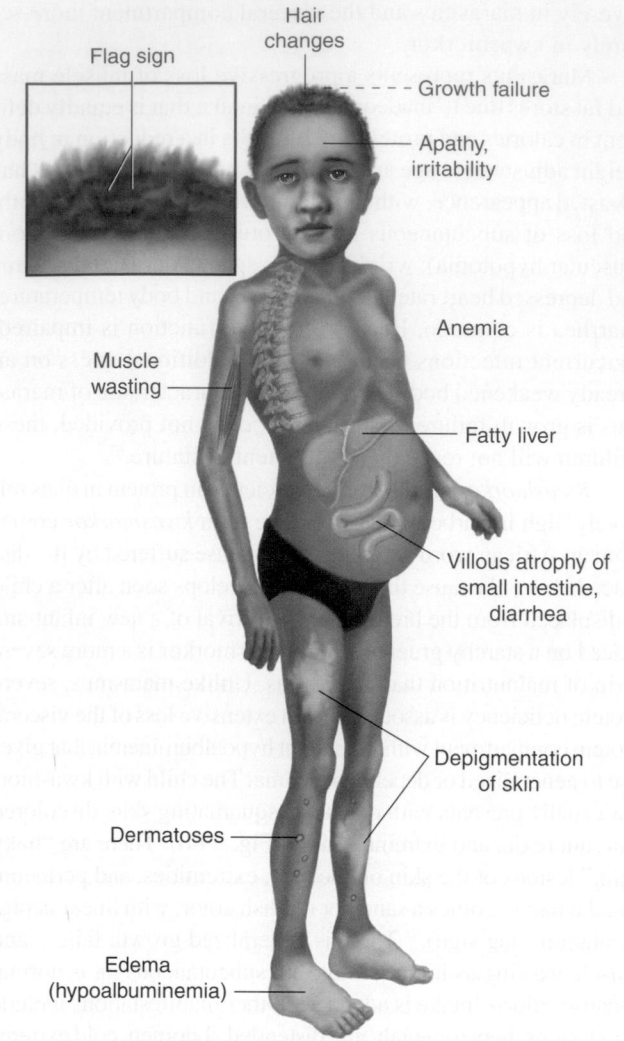

Flag sign

Hair changes

Growth failure

Apathy, irritability

Anemia

Muscle wasting

Fatty liver

Villous atrophy of small intestine, diarrhea

Depigmentation of skin

Dermatoses

Edema (hypoalbuminemia)

FIGURE 39-6 • Clinical manifestations of kwashiorkor.

protein malnutrition occurs most commonly in association with hypermetabolic acute illnesses, such as trauma, burns, and sepsis.[63] Marasmus-like secondary protein-energy malnutrition typically results from chronic illnesses such as chronic obstructive pulmonary disease, congestive heart failure, cancer, and HIV infection.[63] Approximately half of all persons with cancer experience tissue wasting, in which the tumor induces metabolic changes leading to a loss of adipose tissue and muscle mass.[64]

In healthy adults, body protein homeostasis is maintained by a cycle in which the net loss of protein in the postabsorptive state is matched by a net postprandial gain of protein.[65,66] In persons with severe injury or illness, net protein breakdown is accelerated and protein rebuilding disrupted. Protein mass is lost from the liver, gastrointestinal tract, kidneys, and heart. As protein is lost from the liver, hepatic synthesis of serum proteins decreases and decreased levels of serum proteins are observed. There is a decrease in immune cells. Wound healing is poor, and the body is unable to fight off infection because of multiple immunologic malfunctions. The gastrointestinal tract under-

goes mucosal atrophy with loss of villi in the small intestine, resulting in malabsorption. The loss of protein from cardiac muscle leads to a decrease in myocardial contractility and cardiac output. The muscles used for breathing become weakened, and respiratory function becomes compromised as muscle proteins are used as a fuel source. A reduction in respiratory function has many implications, especially for persons with burns, trauma, infection, or chronic respiratory disease, and for persons who are being mechanically ventilated because of respiratory failure.

In hospitalized patients, malnutrition increases morbidity and mortality rates, incidence of complications, and length of stay. Malnutrition may present at the time of admission or develop during hospitalization. The hospitalized patient often finds eating a healthful diet difficult and commonly has restrictions on food and water intake in preparation for tests and surgery. Pain, medications, special diets, and stress can decrease appetite. Even when the patient is well enough to eat, being alone in a room where unpleasant treatments may be given is not conducive to eating. Although hospitalized patients may appear to need fewer calories because they are on bed rest, their actual need for caloric intake may be higher because of other energy expenditures. For example, more calories are expended during fever, when the metabolic rate is increased. There also may be an increased need for protein to support tissue repair after trauma or surgery.

Diagnosis

No single diagnostic measure is sufficiently accurate to serve as a reliable test for malnutrition. Techniques of nutritional assessment include evaluation of dietary intake, anthropometric measurements, clinical examination, and laboratory tests.[63] Evaluation of weight is particularly important. Body weight can be assessed in relation to height using the BMI. Evaluation of body composition can be performed by inspection or using anthropometric measurements such as skinfold thickness. Serum albumin and prealbumin are used in the diagnosis of protein-calorie malnutrition. Albumin, which has historically been used as a determinant of nutrition status, has a relatively large body pool and a half-life of 20 days and is less sensitive to changes in nutrition than prealbumin, which has a shorter half-life and a relatively small body pool.[63]

Treatment

The treatment of severe protein-energy malnutrition involves the use of measures to correct fluid and electrolyte abnormalities and replenish proteins, calories, and micronutrients.[63] Treatment is started with modest quantities of proteins and calories based on the person's actual weight. Concurrent administration of vitamins and minerals is needed. Either the enteral or parenteral route can be used. The treatment should be undertaken slowly to avoid complications. The administration of water and sodium with carbohydrates can overload a heart that has been weakened by malnutrition and result in heart failure. Enteral feedings can result in malabsorptive symptoms due to abnormalities in the gastrointestinal tract. Refeeding edema is benign dependent edema that results from renal sodium reabsorption and poor skin and blood vessel integrity. It is treated by elevation of the dependent area and modest sodium restrictions. Diuretics are ineffective and may aggravate electrolyte deficiencies.

Eating Disorders

Eating disorders affect an estimated 5 million Americans each year.[67] These illnesses, which include anorexia nervosa, bulimia nervosa, and binge-eating disorder and their variants, incorporate serious disturbances in eating, such as restriction of intake and binging, with an excessive concern over body shape or body weight.[68–70] Eating disorders typically occur in adolescent girls and young women, although 10% of cases of anorexia nervosa and bulimia nervosa occur in boys and men.[71] However, binge-eating disorder is more prevalent in men than anorexia nervosa and bulimia combined. Compared with women, men tend to experience less pressure to engage in behaviors such as self-induced vomiting or laxative use when overeating, less of a sense of loss of control when binge eating, and a greater tendency to use compulsive exercise rather than purging for weight control.[71]

EATING DISORDERS

- Eating disorders are serious disturbances in eating, such as willful restriction of intake and binge eating, as well as excessive concern over body weight and shape.

- Anorexia nervosa is characterized by a refusal to maintain a minimally normal body weight (*e.g.,* at least 85% of minimal expected weight); an excessive concern over gaining weight and how the body is perceived in terms of size and shape; and amenorrhea (in girls and women after menarche).

- Bulimia nervosa is characterized by recurrent binge eating; inappropriate compensatory behaviors such as self-induced vomiting, fasting, or excessive exercise that follow the binge-eating episode; and extreme concern over body shape and weight.

- Binge eating consists of consuming unusually large quantities of food during a discrete period (*e.g.,* within any 2-hour period) along with lack of control over the binge-eating episode.

- Binge-eating disorders are characterized by eating behaviors such as eating rapidly, eating until becoming uncomfortably full, eating large amounts when not hungry, eating alone because of embarrassment, and disgust, depression, or guilt because of eating episodes.

Eating disorders are more prevalent in industrialized societies and occur in all socioeconomic and major ethnic groups. A combination of genetic, neurochemical, developmental, and sociocultural factors is thought to contribute to the development of the disorders.[68,69] The fourth edition of the American Psychiatric Association's *Diagnostic and Statistical Manual of Mental Disorders* (text revision [*DSM-IV-TR*]) has established criteria for the diagnosis of anorexia nervosa and bulimia nervosa. Although these criteria allow clinicians to make a diagnosis in persons with a specific eating disorder, the symptoms often occur along a continuum between those of anorexia nervosa and bulimia nervosa. Preoccupation with weight and excessive self-evaluation of weight and shape are common to both disorders, and persons with eating disorders may demonstrate a mixture of both disorders.[69,72] The female athlete triad, which includes disordered eating, amenorrhea, and osteoporosis, does not meet the strict *DSM-IV-TR* criteria for anorexia nervosa or bulimia nervosa, but shares many characteristics and therapeutic concerns with the two disorders[73] (see Chapter 58). Persons with eating disorders may require concomitant evaluation for psychiatric illness because eating disorders often are accompanied by mood, anxiety, and personality disorders. Suicidal behavior may accompany anorexia nervosa and bulimia nervosa and should be ruled out.[70]

Anorexia Nervosa

Anorexia nervosa is an eating disorder that usually begins in adolescence and is characterized by determined dieting, often accompanied by compulsive exercise and, in a subgroup of persons, purging behavior with or without binge eating, resulting in sustained low weight.[74] Other features include a disturbed body image, a pervasive fear of becoming obese, and an obsession with severely restricted caloric intake and frequently with excessive physical exercise. Anorexia nervosa is more prevalent among young women than men. The lifetime risk for the full disorder among women is estimated to be 0.3% to 1% (with a greater frequency of subclinical anorexia nervosa); the risk among men is about one tenth of the rate for women.[74]

The causes of anorexia appear to be multifactorial, with determinants that include genetic influence, personality traits of perfectionism and compulsiveness, anxiety disorders, family history of depression and obesity, and peer, familial, and cultural pressures with respect to appearance.[74] The *DSM-IV-TR* diagnostic criteria for anorexia nervosa are (1) a refusal to maintain a minimally normal body weight for age and height (*e.g.,* at least 85% of minimal expected weight or BMI ≥17.5); (2) an intense fear of gaining weight or becoming fat; (3) a disturbance in the way one's body size, weight, or shape is perceived; and (4) amenorrhea (in girls and women after menarche).[75] Other psychiatric disorders often coexist with anorexia nervosa, including major depression or dysthymia, and obsessive-compulsive disorder (see Chapter 53). Alcohol and substance abuse may also be present, more often among those with binging-purging type of anorexia nervosa.[74]

Many organ systems are affected by the malnutrition that accompanies anorexia nervosa. The severity of the abnormalities tends to be related to the degree of malnutrition and is reversed by refeeding. The most frequent complication of anorexia is amenorrhea and loss of secondary sex characteristics with decreased levels of estrogen, which can eventually lead to osteoporosis. Bone loss can occur in young women after as short a period of illness as 6 months.[69] Symptomatic compression fractures and kyphosis have been reported. Constipation, cold intolerance and failure to shiver in cold, bradycardia, hypotension, decreased heart size, electrocardiographic changes, blood and electrolyte abnormalities, and increased growth of lanugo (*i.e.,* fine hair) are common. Abnormalities in cognitive function may also occur. The brain loses both white and gray matter during severe weight loss; weight restoration results in return of white matter, but some loss of gray matter persists.[74] Unexpected sudden deaths have been reported; the risk appears to increase as weight drops to less than 35% to 40% of ideal weight. It is believed that these deaths are caused by myocardial degeneration and heart failure rather than arrhythmias.

The most exasperating aspect of the treatment of anorexia is the inability of the person with anorexia to recognize that there is a problem. However, persons with the disorder are usually willing to talk about their preoccupation with weight loss, food refusal and rituals about food, and excessive exercise routines; purging and laxative use; and withdrawal from activities and relationships.[76] Because anorexia is a form of starvation, it can lead to death if left untreated. A multidisciplinary approach appears to be the most effective method of treating persons with the disorder.[73] The goals of treatment are eating and weight gain, resolution of issues with the family, healing of pain from the past, and efforts to work on psychological, relationship, and emotional issues. Adults whose weight loss is more than 25% below the expected weight (or with less weight loss if there are coexisting medical or psychiatric conditions, or both), and children or adolescents who are losing weight rapidly, generally require hospitalization to ensure food intake and limit physical activity.[74]

Bulimia Nervosa

Bulimia nervosa is defined by recurrent binge eating and activities such as vomiting, fasting, excessive exercise, and use of diuretics, laxatives, or enemas to compensate for that behavior. Binge eating is characterized by the consumption of an unusually large quantity of food during a discrete time (*e.g.,* within a 2-hour period) along with lack of control over the binge-eating episode. Bulimia nervosa usually begins during adolescence, with a peak period of onset around 18 years of age.[76] The lifetime prevalence is 3%, and ratio of women to men ranges from 10:1 to 20:1.[77]

The *DSM-IV-TR* criteria for bulimia nervosa are (1) recurrent binge eating (at least two times per week for 3 months); (2) inappropriate compensatory behaviors such as self-induced vomiting, abuse of laxatives or diuretics, fasting, or excessive exercise that follow the binge-eating episode; (3) self-evaluation that is unduly influenced by body shape and weight; and (4) a determination that the eating disorder does not occur exclusively

during episodes of anorexia nervosa.[75] In contrast to anorexia nervosa, which is characterized by a weight that is less than 85% of the normal value, most persons with bulimia nervosa are of normal weight. The diagnostic criteria for bulimia nervosa now include subtypes to distinguish patients who compensate by purging (*e.g.,* vomiting or abuse of laxatives or diuretics) and those who use nonpurging behaviors (*e.g.,* fasting or excessive exercise).[75] The disorder may be associated with other psychiatric disorders such as anxiety disorder or depression. There is also an association with substance abuse and risky and self-destructive behaviors.[77]

The complications of bulimia nervosa include those resulting from overeating, self-induced vomiting, and cathartic and diuretic abuse.[59,77,78] Among the complications of self-induced vomiting are dental disorders, parotitis, and fluid and electrolyte disorders. Dental abnormalities, such as sensitive teeth, increased dental caries, and periodontal disease, occur with frequent vomiting because the high acid content of the vomitus causes tooth enamel to dissolve. Esophagitis, dysphagia, and esophageal strictures are common. With frequent vomiting, there often is reflux of gastric contents into the lower esophagus because of relaxation of the lower esophageal sphincter. Vomiting may lead to aspiration pneumonia, especially in intoxicated or debilitated persons. Potassium, chloride, and hydrogen are lost in the vomitus, and frequent vomiting predisposes to metabolic acidosis with hypokalemia (see Chapter 32). An unexplained physical response to vomiting is the development of benign, painless parotid gland enlargement.

The weights of persons with bulimia nervosa may fluctuate, although not to the dangerously low levels seen in anorexia nervosa. Their thoughts and feelings range from fear of not being able to stop eating to a concern about gaining too much weight. They also experience feelings of sadness, anger, guilt, shame, and low self-esteem.

Treatment strategies include psychological and pharmacologic treatments. Cognitive behavioral therapy is the psychosocial therapy predominantly used.[78] This therapy is designed to help the individual become aware of other ways to cope with the feelings that precipitate the desire to purge and to try to correct maladaptive beliefs regarding their self image. Unlike persons with anorexia nervosa, persons with bulimia nervosa or binge eating are upset by the behaviors practiced and the thoughts and feelings experienced, and they are more willing to accept help. Pharmacotherapeutic agents include the tricyclic antidepressants (*e.g.,* desipramine, imipramine), the selective serotonin reuptake inhibitors (*e.g.,* fluoxetine), and other antidepressant medications.[77]

Eating Disorder Not Otherwise Specified

Eating disorder not otherwise specified is a new diagnostic category for patients who have eating disorder symptoms but do not meet the full criteria for either anorexia nervosa or bulimia nervosa. This condition is diagnosed in 50% of primarily adolescent patients admitted to eating disorder programs. Within this group is subgroup, binge-eating disorder. These are usually obese patients who do not use behaviors to compensate for the binge eating. Many of these individuals are found in weight control programs.[78]

Binge-Eating. Binge eating is characterized by recurrent episodes of binge eating at least 2 days per week for 6 months and at least three of the following: (1) eating rapidly; (2) eating until becoming uncomfortably full; (3) eating large amounts when not hungry; (4) eating alone because of embarrassment; and (5) disgust, depression, or guilt because of eating episodes. The great majority of persons with binge-eating disorder are overweight, and in turn, obese persons have a higher prevalence of binge-eating disorder than the nonobese population.[78,79]

The primary goal of therapy for binge-eating disorder is to establish a regular, healthful eating pattern. Persons with binge-eating disorder who have been successfully treated for their eating disorder have reported that making meal plans, eating a balanced diet of three regular meals a day, avoiding high-sugar foods and other binge foods, recording food intake and binge-eating episodes, exercising regularly, finding alternative activities, and avoiding alcohol and drugs are helpful in maintaining their more healthful eating behaviors after treatment.

IN SUMMARY, undernutrition can range from a selective deficiency of a single nutrient to starvation, in which there is deprivation of all nutrients. Malnutrition and starvation are among the most widespread causes of morbidity and mortality in the world. Protein-energy malnutrition in this population commonly is divided into two distinct conditions: marasmus (protein and calorie deficiency) and kwashiorkor (protein deficiency). There are two functional compartments involved in the distribution of proteins within the body: the somatic compartment, represented by the skeletal muscles, and the visceral compartment, represented by protein stores in body organs, principally the liver. In marasmus, there is a greater loss of protein from the skeletal muscle compartment, and in kwashiorkor, a greater loss of visceral proteins, particularly those of the liver. Malnutrition is common during illness, recovery from trauma, and hospitalization. The effects of malnutrition and starvation on body function are widespread. They include loss of muscle mass, impaired wound healing, impaired immunologic function, decreased appetite, loss of calcium and phosphate from bone, anovulation and amenorrhea in women, and decreased testicular function in men.

Anorexia nervosa and bulimia nervosa are eating disorders that result in malnutrition. In anorexia nervosa, distorted attitudes about eating lead to determined dieting, weight loss to below 85% of normal body weight, and malnutrition. Bulimia nervosa is characterized by secretive episodes or binges of eating large quantities of easily consumed, high-calorie foods, followed by compensatory behaviors such as fasting, self-induced vomiting, or abuse of laxatives or diuretics.

Eating disorder not otherwise specified is a new diagnostic category for patients who have eating disorders such as binge-eating disorder, but do not meet the full criteria for either anorexia nervosa or bulimia nervosa. ∎

Review Exercises

1. A 25-year-old woman is 65 inches (165 cm) tall and weighs 300 pounds (136 kg). She works as a receptionist in an office, brings her lunch to work with her, spends her evenings watching television, and gets very little exercise. She reports that she has been fat ever since she was a little girl, has tried "every diet under the sun," and when she diets she loses some weight, but gains it all back again.

A. Calculate her BMI using the website referenced in Table 39-1.

B. How would you classify her obesity?

C. What are her risk factors for obesity?

D. What would be one of the first steps in helping her develop a plan to lose weight?

2. A 16-year-old high school student is brought into the physician's office by her mother, who is worried because her daughter insists on dieting because she thinks she is too fat. The daughter is 67 inches (170 cm) tall and weighs 96 pounds (43.5 kg). Her history reveals that she is a straight-A student, plays in the orchestra, and is on the track team. Although she had been having regular menstrual periods, she has not had a period in 4 months. She is given a tentative diagnosis of anorexia nervosa.

A. What are the criteria for a diagnosis of anorexia nervosa?

B. What is the physiologic reason for her amenorrhea?

C. What are some of the physiologic manifestations associated with malnutrition and severe weight loss?

References

1. Guyton A. C., Hall J. E. (2006). *Textbook of medical physiology* (10th ed., pp. 881–858, 865–879, 880–887). Philadelphia: Elsevier Saunders.
2. Frankenfield D., Roth-Yousey L., Compher C. (2005). Comparison of predictive equations for resting metabolic rate in healthy nonobese and obese adults: A systematic review. *Journal of the American Dietetic Association* 105, 775–789.
3. Levine J. A. (2004). Nonexercise activity thermogenesis (NEAT). *Nutritional Reviews* 62, S82–S97.
4. Kershaw E. E., Flier J. S. (2004). Adipose tissue as an endocrine organ. *Journal of Clinical Endocrinology and Metabolism* 89, 2548–2556.

5. Otten J. J., Hellwig J. P., Meyers L. D. (2006). *Dietary reference intakes: The essential guide to nutrient requirements.* Washington, DC: National Academy Press.

6. Trumbo P., Schlicker S., Yates A. A., et al. (2002). Dietary reference intakes for energy, carbohydrate, fiber, fat, fatty acids, cholesterol, protein, and amino acids. *Journal of the American Dietetic Association* 102, 1621–1630.

7. National Institutes of Health Expert Panel. (2002). *Third Report of the National Cholesterol Education Program (NCEP) Expert Panel on Detection, Evaluation, and Treatment of High Blood Cholesterol in Adults (Adult Treatment Panel III).* NIH publication no. 02–5215. Bethesda, MD: National Institutes of Health.

8. Lichtenstein A. L., Apple L. J., Brandis M., et al. (2006). AHA scientific statement: Diet and lifestyle recommendations revision 2006: A scientific statement from AHA Nutrition Committee. *Circulation* 114, 82–96.

9. Murphy K. G., Bloom S. R. (2006). Gut hormones and the regulation of energy homeostasis. *Nature* 444, 854–859.

10. Carney D. E., Meguid M. M. (2002). Current concepts in nutritional assessment. *Archives of Surgery* 137, 42–45.

11. Han T. S., Sattar N., Lean M. (2006). Assessment of obesity and its clinical implications. *British Medical Journal* 333, 695–698.

12. Detsky A. S., Smalley P. S., Chang J. (1994). Is this patient malnourished? *Journal of the American Medical Association* 271, 54–58.

13. World Health Organization. (1989). *Measuring obesity: Classification and description of anthropometric data.* Copenhagen: World Health Organization.

14. National Heart, Lung, and Blood Institute. (1998). Clinical guidelines on the identification, evaluation, and treatment of overweight and obesity in adults. NIH publication no. 98-4083. *Obesity Research* 6(Suppl. 2), 51S–209S.

15. Abernathy R. P., Black D. R. (1996). Healthy body weight: An alternative perspective. *American Journal of Clinical Nutrition* 63(Suppl.), 448S–451S.

16. Eckel R., Grundy S., Zimmet P. (2005). Metabolic syndrome. *Lancet* 365, 1415–28.

17. Scott M., Grundy J. I., Cleeman S. R., et al. (2005). Diagnosis and management of the metabolic syndrome: An American Heart Association/National Heart, Lung, and Blood Institute scientific statement. *Circulation* 112, 2735–2752.

18. Bray G. A. (2006). Obesity: The disease. *Journal of Medicinal Chemistry* 49, 4001–4007.

19. Bray G. A. (2004). Obesity is a chronic, relapsing neurochemical disease. *International Journal of Obesity* 28, 34–38.

20. Hossain P., Kawar B., El Nahas M. (2007). Obesity and diabetes in the developing world: A growing challenge. *New England Journal of Medicine* 356, 213–215.

21. Ogden C. L., Carroll M. D., Curtin L. R. (2006). Prevalence of overweight and obesity in the United States, 1999–2004. *Journal of the American Medical Association* 295, 1549–1555.

22. Sturm R. (2007). Increases in morbid obesity in the USA: 2000–2005. *Public Health* 121, 492–496.

23. Flegal K. M., Graubard B. I., Williamson D. F., et al. (2005). Excess deaths associated with underweight, overweight, and obesity. *Journal of the American Medical Association* 293, 1861–1867.

24. Olshansky S. J., Passaro D. J., Hershow R. C., et al. (2005). A potential decline in life expectancy in the United States in the 21st century. *New England Journal of Medicine* 352, 1138–1145.

25. Soreneson T. J., Holst C., Stunkard A. J., et al. (1992). Correlations of body mass index of adult adoptees and their biological and adoptive relatives. *International Journal of Obesity and Related Metabolic Disorders* 16, 227–236.

26. Rankinen T., Zuberi A., Chagnon Y. C., et al. (2006). The human obesity gene map: The 2005 update. *Obesity* 14, 529–644.

27. vonKries R., Koletzke B., Sauerwalk T., et al. (1999). Breast feeding and obesity: Cross sectional study. *British Medical Journal* 319, 147–150.

28. Gortmaker S. L., Must A., Sobol A. M., et al. (1996). Television viewing as a cause of increasing obesity among children in the United States, 1986–1990. *Archives of Pediatric and Adolescent Medicine* 150, 356–362.

29. Malik V. S., Schulze M. B., Hu F. B. (2006). Intake of sugar-sweetened beverages and weight gain: A systematic review. *American Journal of Clinical Nutrition* 84, 274–288.

30. Young L. R., Nestle M. (2002). The contribution of expanding portion sizes to U.S. obesity epidemic. *American Journal of Public Health* 92, 246–249.

31. Goran M. I. (2000). Energy metabolism and obesity. *Medical Clinics of North America* 84, 347–362.

32. McDowell A., Engel A., Massey J. T., et al. (1981). *Plan and operation of the National Health and Nutrition Examination Survey, 1976–1980.* Vital and Health Statistics Series 1(15), 1–144. Hyattsville, MD: National Center for Health Statistics.

33. Klein S., Allison D. B., Heymsfield S. B., et al. (2007). Waist circumference and cardiometabolic risk: A consensus statement from Shaping America's Health: Association for Weight Management and Obesity Prevention; NAASO, The Obesity Society; the American Society for Nutrition; and the American Diabetes Association. *American Journal of Clinical Nutrition* 85, 1197–1202.

34. Klein S., Allison D. B., Heymsfield S. B., et al. (2007). Waist circumference and cardiometabolic risk. A consensus statement from shaping America's health: Association for weight management and obesity prevention; NAASO, The Obesity Society; the American Society of Nutrition; and the American Diabetes Association. *Diabetes Care* 30(6), 1647–1652.

35. Jeffery R. W. (1996). Does weight cycling present a health risk? *American Journal of Clinical Nutrition* 63(Suppl.), 452S–455S.

36. Williamson D. F. (1996). "Weight cycling" and mortality: How do the epidemiologists explain the role of intentional weight loss? *Journal of the American College of Nutrition* 15, 6–13.

37. Garn S. M. (1996). Fractionating healthy weight. *American Journal of Clinical Nutrition* 63(Suppl.), 412S–414S.

38. The Obesity Society. (2007). Obesity, bias, and stigmatization. [Online.] Available: www.naaso.org. Accessed August 10, 2007.

39. Kushner R. F., Blatner D. J. (2005). Risk assessment of the overweight and obese patient. *Journal of the American Dietetic Association* 105, S53–S62.

40. Task Force on Prevention and Treatment of Obesity. (1994). Towards prevention of obesity: Research directives. *Obesity Research* 2, 571.

41. Avenell A., Sattar N., Lean M. (2006). Management: Part 1. Behaviour change, diet, and activity. *British Medical Journal* 333, 740–743.

42. U.S. Department of Health and Human Services. (2000). *The practical guide: Identification, evaluation, and treatment of overweight and obesity in adults.* NIH publication no. 00-4084. Rockville, MD: U.S. Department of Health and Human Services, National Institutes of Health; National Heart, Lung, and Blood Institute; North American Association of the Study of Obesity.

43. Pi-Sunyer F. X., Becker D. M., Bouchard C., et al. (1998). NHLBI Obesity Education Initiative Expert Panel on the Identification, Evaluation, and Treatment of Overweight and Obesity in Adults. *Obesity Research* 6(Suppl. 2), 51S–209S.

44. Wadden T. A., Berkowitz R. I., Womble L. G., et al. (2005). Randomized trial of lifestyle modification and pharmacotherapy for obesity. *New England Journal of Medicine* 353, 2111–2120.

45. Dalsinger M. L., Gleason J. A., Griffith J. L., et al. (2005). Comparison of the Atkins, Ornish, Weight Watchers, and Zone diets for weight loss and heart disease reduction. *Journal of the American Medical Association* 293, 43–53.

46. Jakicic J. M., Marcus B. H., Gallagher K. I., et al. (2003). Effect of exercise duration and intensity on weight loss in overweight, sedentary women: A randomized trial. *Journal of the American Medical Association* 290, 1323–1330.

47. U.S. Department of Health and Human Services and the U.S. Department of Agriculture. (2005). Dietary guidelines for Americans, 2005. [Online.] Available: www.health.gov/dietaryguidelines/dga2005/document/default.htm. Accessed April 16, 2008.

48. Lean M., Finer N. (2006). Management: Part 2. Drugs. *British Medical Journal* 333, 794–797.

49. Fujioka K. (2002). Management of obesity as a chronic disease: Nonpharmacologic, pharmacologic, and surgical options. *Obesity Research* 10, 116S–123S.

50. Kral J. G. (2006). Management: Part 3. Surgery. *British Medical Journal* 333, 900–903.

51. Centers for Disease Control and Prevention. (2007). Childhood overweight. [Online.] Available: www.cdc.gov/nccdphp/dnpa/obesity/childhood/index.htm. Accessed July 19, 2007.

52. Virani T., Lappan-Gracon S., McConnell H., et al. (2007). Primary prevention of childhood obesity. Ontario, Canada: Registered Nurses' Association of Ontario. [Online.] Available: http://www.rnao.org/bestpractices/PDF/BPG_childhood_obesity.pdf. Accessed April 16, 2008.

53. Reilly J. J., Wilson D. (2006). Childhood obesity. *British Medical Journal* 333, 1207–1210.

54. The Obesity Society. (2007). Childhood overweight. [Online.] Available: http://www.naaso.org. Accessed July 18, 2007.

55. Fagot-Campagna A., Pettitt D. J., Engelgau N. M., et al. (2000). Type 2 diabetes among North American children and adolescents: An epidemiologic review and a public health perspective. *Journal of Pediatrics* 136, 664–672.

56. Ebbeling C. B., Pawlak D. B., Ludwig D. S. (2002). Childhood obesity: Public-health crisis, common sense cure. *Lancet* 360, 473–482.

57. Expert Committee Recommendations on the Assessment, Prevention, and Treatment of Child and Adolescent Overweight and Obesity. (2007). [Online.] Available: www.ama-assn.org/ama1/pub/upload/mm/433/ped_obesity_recs.pdf. Accessed April 16, 2008.

58. Müller O., Krawinkel M. (2005). Malnutrition and health in developing countries. *Canadian Medical Association Journal* 173, 279–286.

59. Judge B. S., Eisenger B. H. (2005). Disorders of fuel metabolism: Medical complications associated with starvation, eating disorders, dietary fads, and supplements. *Emergency Medicine Clinics of North America* 23, 789–813.

60. Brown J. L., Pollitt E. (1996). Malnutrition, poverty, intellectual development. *Scientific American* 274(2), 38–43.

61. Kane A. B., Kumar V. (2005). Environmental and nutritional pathology. In Kumar V., Abbas A. K., Fausto N. (Eds.), *Robbins and Cotran pathologic basis of disease* (7th ed., pp. 442–450). Philadelphia: Elsevier Saunders.

62. Rubin R., Strayer D. E. (2008). Environmental and nutritional pathology. In Rubin R., Strayer D. E. (Eds.), *Rubin's pathology: Clinicopathologic foundations of medicine* (5th ed., pp. 277–278). Philadelphia: Lippincott Williams & Wilkins.

63. Baron R. B. (2007). Nutrition. In Tierney L. M., McPhee S. J., Papadakis M. A. (Eds.), *Current diagnosis and treatment* (46th ed., pp. 1289–1295). New York: McGraw-Hill.

64. Tisdale M. J. (1999). Wasting in cancer. *Journal of Nutrition* 129(IS Suppl.), 43S–46S.

65. Biolo G., Gabriele T., Ciccchi B., et al. (1999). Metabolic response to injury and sepsis: Changes in protein metabolism. *Journal of Nutrition* 129(IS Suppl.), 53S–57S.

66. Capra S. (2007). Nutrition assessment or nutrition screening—how much information is enough to make a diagnosis of malnutrition in acute care? *Nutrition* 23, 356–357.

67. Hudson J. I., Hiripi E., Pope H. G., et al. (2007). The prevalence and correlates of eating disorders in the National Comorbidity Survey Replication. *Biological Psychiatry* 61, 348–358.

68. Rome E. S., Ammerman S., Rosen D. S. (2003). Children and adolescents with eating disorders: The state of the art. *Pediatrics* 111, e98–e108.

69. Ricanati E. H. W., Rome E. S. (2005). Eating disorders: Recognizing early to prevent complications. *Cleveland Clinic Journal of Medicine* 72, 895–906.

70. Becker A., Grinspoon S. K., Klibanski A., et al. (1999). Eating disorders. *New England Journal of Medicine* 340, 1092–1098.

71. Weltzin T. E., Weisensel N., Franczyk D., et al. (2005). Eating disorders in men. *Journal of Men's Health and Gender* 2, 186–193.

72. American Psychiatric Association. (2006). *Practice guideline for the treatment of patients with eating disorders* (3rd ed.). [Online.] Available: http://www.psychiatryonline.com/content.aspx?aID=138722. Accessed April 29, 2008.

73. Brunet M. (2005). Female athlete triad. *Clinics in Sports Medicine* 24, 623–636.

74. Yager J., Anderson A. E. (2005). Anorexia nervosa. *New England Journal of Medicine* 353, 1481–1488.

75. American Psychiatric Association. (2000). *Diagnostic and statistical manual of mental disorders* (4th ed., text rev.). Washington, DC: Author.

76. Zerbe K. J. (1999). Eating disorders. In *Women's mental health in primary care* (pp. 109–137). Philadelphia: W. B. Saunders.

77. Mehler P. S. (2003). Bulimia nervosa. *New England Journal of Medicine* 349, 875–881.

78. Kondo D. G., Sokol M. S. (2006). Eating disorders in primary care. *Postgraduate Medicine* 119, 59–65.

79. Schneider M. (2003). Bulimia nervosa and binge-eating disorders in adolescents. *Adolescent Medicine* 14, 119–131.

Visit thePoint **http://thePoint.lww.com for animations, journal articles, and more!**

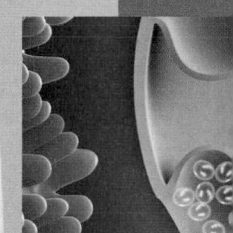

Disorders of Endocrine Function

By the end of the Middle Ages, a great storehouse of anatomic knowledge existed; however, this repository had been culled from a combination of incomplete observations, religious beliefs, extrapolation from animal structures, and philosophical guesswork. Scientists slavishly adhered to these teachings, many of which were the products of the early Greeks (such as Aristotle and Galen), even though personal experience provided them with contradictory evidence.

The endocrine system fell victim to the outdated theories postulated long before. Even when some of its parts were discovered, their importance went unrecognized. For example, the pituitary gland, first noted in 1524 by Jacob Berengar of Carpi, was considered to be necessary to the cooling function of the brain. The brain was thought to secrete *pituita,* phlegm (mucus), and discharge it from the nose as part of its cooling process. The gland received its name from Andreas Vesalius, who referred to it in his text *De Fabrica* (1543) as *glandula pituitam cerebri excipiens,* or the gland that receives the phlegm from the brain. It was not until the late 19th and early 20th centuries that the field of endocrinology had its beginnings. It was then that the importance of the pituitary gland was finally realized, and it was called the master endocrine gland.

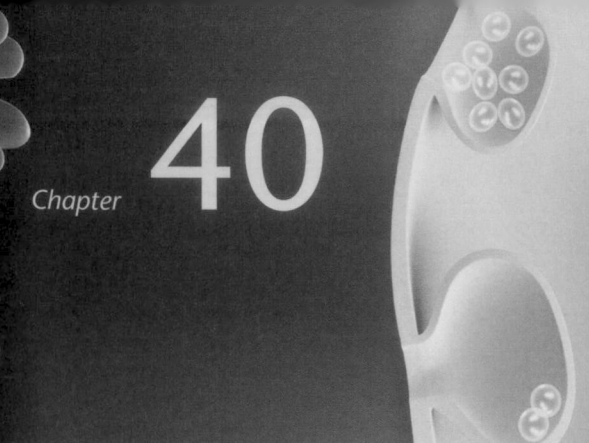

Chapter **40**

Mechanisms of Endocrine Control

GLENN MATFIN

➤ The endocrine system is involved in all of the integrative aspects of life, including growth, sex differentiation, metabolism, and adaptation to an ever-changing environment. This chapter focuses on general aspects of endocrine function, organization of the endocrine system, hormone receptors and hormone actions, and regulation of hormone levels.

THE ENDOCRINE SYSTEM

After completing this section of the chapter, you should be able to meet the following objectives:

- Characterize a hormone.
- Differentiate vesicle-mediated and non–vesicle-mediated mechanisms of hormone synthesis in terms of their stimuli for hormone synthesis and release.
- Describe mechanisms of hormone transport and inactivation.
- State the function of a hormone receptor and the difference between cell surface hormone receptors and intracellular hormone receptors.
- Describe the role of the hypothalamus in regulating pituitary control of endocrine function.
- State the major difference between positive and negative feedback control mechanisms.
- Describe methods used in diagnosis of endocrine disorders.

The endocrine system uses chemical substances called *hormones* as a means of regulating and integrating body functions. The endocrine system participates in the regulation of digestion and the usage and storage of nutrients, growth and development, electrolyte and water metabolism, and reproductive functions. Although the endocrine system once was thought to consist solely of discrete endocrine glands, it is now known that a number of other tissues release chemical messengers that modulate body processes. The functions of the endocrine system are closely linked with those of the nervous system and the immune system. For example, neurotransmitters such as epinephrine can act as neurotransmitters or as hormones. The functions of the immune system also are closely linked with those of the endocrine system. The immune system responds to foreign agents by means of chemical messengers (cytokines, such as interleukins, interferons) and complex receptor mechanisms (see Chapter 17). The immune system also is extensively regulated by hormones such as the adrenal corticosteroid hormones.

Hormones

Hormones generally are thought of as chemical messengers that are transported in body fluids. They are highly specialized organic molecules produced by endocrine organs that exert their action on specific target cells. Hormones do not initiate reactions but function as modulators of cellular and systemic responses. Most hormones are present in body fluids at all times, but in greater or lesser amounts depending on the needs of the body.

HORMONES

- Hormones function as chemical messengers, moving through the blood to distant target sites of action, or acting more locally as paracrine or autocrine messengers that incite more local effects.

- Most hormones are present in body fluids at all times, but in greater or lesser amounts depending on the needs of the body.

- Hormones exert their actions by interacting with high-affinity receptors, which in turn are linked to one or more effector systems in the cell. Some hormone receptors are located on the surface of the cell and act through second messenger mechanisms, and others are located in the cell, where they modulate the synthesis of enzymes, transport proteins, or structural proteins.

A characteristic of hormones is that a single hormone can exert various effects in different tissues or, conversely, a single function can be regulated by several different hormones. For example, estradiol, which is produced by the ovary, can act on the ovarian follicles to promote their maturation, on the uterus to stimulate its growth and maintain the cyclic changes in the uterine mucosa, on the mammary gland to stimulate ductal growth, on the hypothalamic-pituitary system to regulate the secretion of gonadotropins and prolactin, on the bone to maintain skeletal integrity, and on general metabolic processes to affect adipose tissue distribution. Lipolysis, which is the release of free fatty acids from adipose tissue, is an example of a single function that is regulated by several hormones, including the catecholamines, insulin, and glucagon, but also by the cytokine, tumor necrosis factor-α. Table 40-1 lists the major actions and sources of body hormones.

Paracrine and Autocrine Actions

In the past, hormones were described as chemical substances that were released into the bloodstream and transported to distant target sites, where they exerted their action. Although many hormones travel by this mechanism, some hormones and hormone-like substances never enter the bloodstream but instead act locally in the vicinity in which they are released (see Chapter 4, Fig. 4-8). When they act locally on cells other than those that produced the hormone, the action is called *paracrine*. The action of sex steroids on the ovary is a paracrine action. Hormones also can exert an *autocrine* action on the cells from which they were produced. For example, the release of insulin from pancreatic beta cells can inhibit its release from the same cells.

Structural Classification

Hormones, which have diverse structures ranging from single amino acids to complex proteins and lipids, are divided into three categories: (1) amines and amino acids; (2) peptides, polypeptides, proteins, and glycoproteins; and (3) steroids (Table 40-2). The first category, the amines, includes norepinephrine and epinephrine, which are derived from a single amino acid (*i.e.,* tyrosine), and the thyroid hormones, which are derived from two iodinated tyrosine amino acid residues. The second category, the peptides, polypeptides, proteins, and glycoproteins, can be as small as thyrotropin-releasing hormone (TRH), which contains 3 amino acids, and as large and complex as growth hormone (GH) and follicle-stimulating hormone (FSH), which have approximately 200 amino acids. Glycoproteins are large peptide hormones associated with a carbohydrate (*e.g.,* FSH). The third category consists of the steroid hormones, which are derivatives of cholesterol.

Synthesis and Release

The mechanisms for hormone synthesis and release vary with hormone structure. Hormones such as the protein and polypeptide hormones are synthesized and stored in vesicles in the cytoplasm of the endocrine cell until secretion is required. These hormones are released by fusion of the vesicle with the cell membrane. Their release may or may not be coupled with the stimulus for synthesis. Other hormones, such as the steroid hormones, are secreted upon synthesis. For these hormones, there typically is no distinction between the stimulus for synthesis and release.

The protein and polypeptide hormones comprise the most prominent class of hormones whose synthesis and release is vesicle mediated. These hormones are synthesized in the rough endoplasmic reticulum of the endocrine cell in a manner similar to the synthesis of other proteins (see Chapter 4). The appropriate amino acid sequence is dictated by messenger ribonucleic acids (mRNAs) from the nucleus. Usually, synthesis involves the production of a precursor hormone, which is modified by the addition of peptides or sugar units. These precursor hormones often contain extra peptide units that ensure proper folding of the molecule and insertion of essential linkages. If extra amino acids are present, as in insulin, the precursor hormone is called a *prohormone*. After synthesis and sequestration in the endoplasmic reticulum, the protein and peptide hormones move

TABLE 40-1 Major Action and Source of Selected Hormones

SOURCE	HORMONE	MAJOR ACTION

Hypothalamus	Releasing and inhibiting hormones
	    Corticotropin-releasing hormone (CRH)
	    Thyrotropin-releasing hormone (TRH)
	    Growth hormone-releasing hormone (GHRH)
	    Gonadotropin-releasing hormone (GnRH)
		Controls the release of pituitary hormones

	Somatostatin	Inhibits GH and TSH
Anterior pituitary	Growth hormone (GH)	Stimulates growth of bone and muscle, promotes protein synthesis and fat metabolism, decreases carbohydrate metabolism
	Adrenocorticotropic hormone (ACTH)	Stimulates synthesis and secretion of adrenal cortical hormones
	Thyroid-stimulating hormone (TSH)	Stimulates synthesis and secretion of thyroid hormone
	Follicle-stimulating hormone (FSH)	Female: stimulates growth of ovarian follicle, ovulation Male: stimulates sperm production
	Luteinizing hormone (LH)	Female: stimulates development of corpus luteum, release of oocyte, production of estrogen and progesterone Male: stimulates secretion of testosterone, development of interstitial tissue of testes
	Prolactin	Prepares female breast for breast-feeding
Posterior pituitary	Antidiuretic hormone (ADH)	Increases water reabsorption by kidney
	Oxytocin	Stimulates contraction of pregnant uterus, milk ejection from breasts after childbirth
Adrenal cortex	Mineralocorticosteroids, mainly aldosterone	Increases sodium absorption, potassium loss by kidney
	Glucocorticoids, mainly cortisol	Affects metabolism of all nutrients; regulates blood glucose levels, affects growth, has anti-inflammatory action, and decreases effects of stress
	Adrenal androgens, mainly dehydro-epiandrosterone (DHEA) and androstenedione	Have minimal intrinsic androgenic activity; they are converted to testosterone and dihydrotestosterone in the periphery
Adrenal medulla	Epinephrine Norepinephrine	Serve as neurotransmitters for the sympathetic nervous system
Thyroid (follicular cells)	Thyroid hormones: triiodothyronine (T_3), thyroxine (T_4)	Increase the metabolic rate; increase protein and bone turnover; increase responsiveness to catecholamines; necessary for fetal and infant growth and development
Thyroid C cells	Calcitonin	Lowers blood calcium and phosphate levels
Parathyroid glands	Parathyroid hormone (PTH)	Regulates serum calcium
Pancreatic islet cells	Insulin	Lowers blood glucose by facilitating glucose transport across cell membranes of muscle, liver, and adipose tissue
	Glucagon	Increases blood glucose concentration by stimulation of glycogenolysis and glyconeogenesis
	Somatostatin	Delays intestinal absorption of glucose
Kidney	1,25-Dihydroxyvitamin D	Stimulates calcium absorption from the intestine
Ovaries	Estrogen	Affects development of female sex organs and secondary sex characteristics
	Progesterone	Influences menstrual cycle; stimulates growth of uterine wall; maintains pregnancy
Testes	Androgens, mainly testosterone	Affect development of male sex organs and secondary sex characteristics; aid in sperm production

TABLE 40-2 Classes of Hormones Based on Structure

AMINES AND AMINO ACIDS	PEPTIDES, POLYPEPTIDES, AND PROTEINS	STEROIDS
Dopamine	Corticotropin-releasing hormone (CRH)	Aldosterone
Epinephrine	Growth hormone–releasing hormone (GHRH)	Glucocorticoids
Norepinephrine	Thyrotropin-releasing hormone (TRH)	Estrogens
Thyroid hormone	Adrenocorticotropic hormone (ACTH)	Testosterone
	Follicle-stimulating hormone (FSH)	Progesterone
	Luteinizing hormone (LH)	Androstenedione
	Thyroid-stimulating hormone (TSH)	1,25-Dihydroxyvitamin D
	Growth hormone (GH)	Dihydrotestosterone (DHT)
	Antidiuretic hormone (ADH)	Dehydroepiandrosterone (DHEA)
	Oxytocin	
	Insulin	
	Glucagon	
	Somatostatin	
	Calcitonin	
	Parathyroid hormone (PTH)	
	Prolactin	

into the Golgi complex, where they are packaged in vesicles. It is in the Golgi complex that prohormones are converted into hormones. Stimulation of the endocrine cell causes the vesicles to move to the cell membrane and release their hormones. The vesicle-mediated pathway is also used for secretion of a number of nonpolypeptide hormones and neurotransmitters such as the catecholamines (dopamine, epinephrine, and norepinephrine). However, these small molecules do not pass through the full range of intracellular mechanisms seen in the synthesis and secretion of the larger protein and polypeptide hormones.

Hormones synthesized by non–vesicle-mediated pathways include the glucocorticoids, androgens, estrogens, and mineralocorticoids—all steroids derived from cholesterol. These hormones are synthesized in the smooth endoplasmic reticulum, and steroid-secreting cells can be identified by their large amounts of smooth endoplasmic reticulum. Certain steroids serve as precursors for the production of other hormones. In the adrenal cortex, for example, progesterone and other steroid intermediates are enzymatically converted into aldosterone, cortisol, or androgens (see Chapter 41). The release of hormones synthesized by non–vesicle-mediated pathways is not fully understood. Historically it was thought to occur by simple diffusion. In recent years, however, specific transporters have been implicated in directing some of these classes of hormones out of the cell. Whether all hormones produced by non–vesicle-mediated pathways depend on transporters for their secretion remains a subject for further investigation.

Transport

Hormones that are released into the bloodstream circulate as either free or unbound molecules, or as hormones attached to transport carriers (Fig. 40-1). Peptide hormones and protein hormones usually circulate unbound in the blood. Steroid hormones and thyroid hormone are carried by specific carrier proteins synthesized in the liver. The extent of carrier binding influences the rate at which hormones leave the blood and enter the cells. The half-life of a hormone—the time it takes for the body to reduce the concentration of the hormone by one half—is positively correlated with its percentage of protein binding. Thyroxine, which is more than 99% protein bound, has a half-

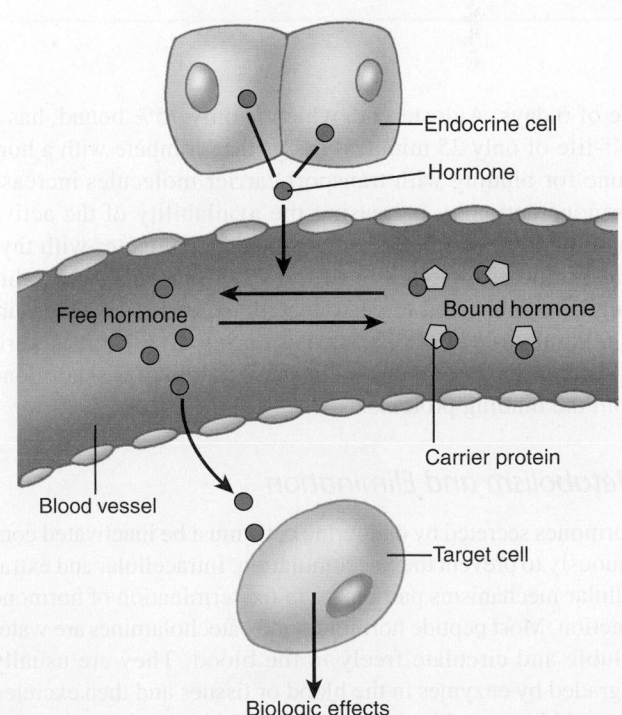

FIGURE 40-1 • Relationship of free and carrier-bound hormones.

Understanding • Hormone Receptors

Hormones bring about their effects on cell activity by binding to specific cell receptors. There are two general types of receptors: (1) cell surface receptors that exert their actions through cytoplasmic second messenger systems, and (2) intracellular nuclear receptors that modulate gene expression by binding to DNA or promoters of target genes.

❶ Cell Surface Receptors

Water-soluble peptide hormones, such as parathyroid hormone and glucagon, which cannot penetrate the lipid layer of the cell plasma membrane, exert their effects through intracellular second messengers. They bind to a portion of a membrane receptor that protrudes through the surface of the cell. This produces a structural change in the receptor molecule itself, causing activation of a hormone-regulated signal system located on the inner aspect of the cell membrane. This system allows the cell to sense extracellular events and pass this information to the intracellular environment. There are several types of cell surface receptors, including G-protein–coupled receptors that mediate the actions of catecholamines, prostaglandins, thyroid-stimulating hormone, and others. Binding of the hormone to the receptor activates a G protein, which in turn acts on an effector such as adenyl cyclase to generate a second messenger such as cyclic adenosine monophosphate (cAMP). The second messenger, in turn, activates other enzymes that participate in cellular secretion, gene activation, or other target cell responses.

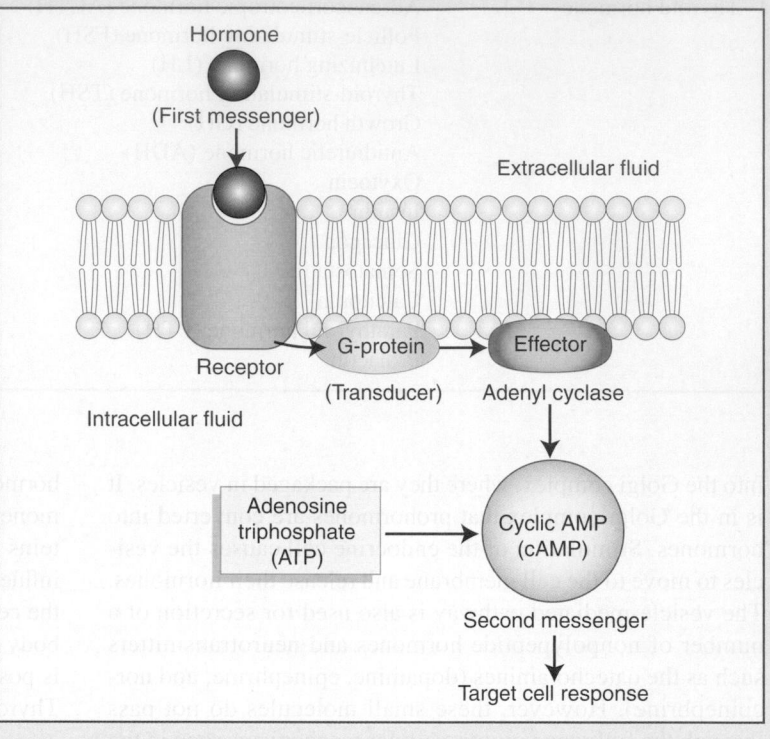

life of 6 days. Aldosterone, which is only 15% bound, has a half-life of only 25 minutes. Drugs that compete with a hormone for binding with transport carrier molecules increase hormone action by increasing the availability of the active unbound hormone. For example, aspirin competes with thyroid hormone for binding to transport proteins; when this drug is administered to persons with excessive levels of circulating thyroid hormone, such as during thyroid crisis, serious effects may occur due to the dissociation of free hormone from the binding proteins.

Metabolism and Elimination

Hormones secreted by endocrine cells must be inactivated continuously to prevent their accumulation. Intracellular and extracellular mechanisms participate in the termination of hormone function. Most peptide hormones and catecholamines are water soluble and circulate freely in the blood. They are usually degraded by enzymes in the blood or tissues and then excreted by the kidneys and liver. For example, the catecholamines are rapidly degraded by catechol-*O*-methyl transferase (COMT)

and monoamine oxidase (MAO). Because of their short half-life, their production is measured by some of their metabolites. In general, peptide hormones also have a short life span in the circulation. Their major mechanism of degradation is through binding to cell surface receptors, with subsequent uptake and degradation by peptide-splitting enzymes in the cell membrane or inside the cell. Steroid hormones are bound to protein carriers for transport and are inactive in the bound state. Their activity depends on the availability of transport carriers. Unbound adrenal and gonadal steroid hormones are conjugated in the liver, which renders them inactive, and then excreted in the bile or urine. Thyroid hormones also are transported by carrier molecules. The free hormone is rendered inactive by the removal of amino acids (*i.e.*, deamination) in the tissues, and the hormone is conjugated in the liver and eliminated in the bile.

Mechanisms of Action

Hormones produce their effects through interaction with high-affinity receptors, which in turn are linked to one or more effec-

❷   Nuclear Receptors

Steroid hormones, vitamin D, thyroid hormones, and other lipid-soluble hormones diffuse across the cell membrane into the cytoplasm of the target cell. Once inside, they bind to an intracellular receptor that is activated by the interaction. The activated hormone–receptor complex then moves to the nucleus, where the hormone binds to a hormone response element (HRE) in the promoters on a target gene or to another transcription factor. Attachment to the HRE results in transcription of a specific messenger RNA (mRNA). The mRNA then moves into the cytoplasm, where the "transcribed message" is translated and used by cytoplasmic ribosomes to produce new cellular proteins or changes in the production of existing proteins. These proteins promote a specific cellular response or, in some cases, the synthesis of a structural protein that is exported from the cell.

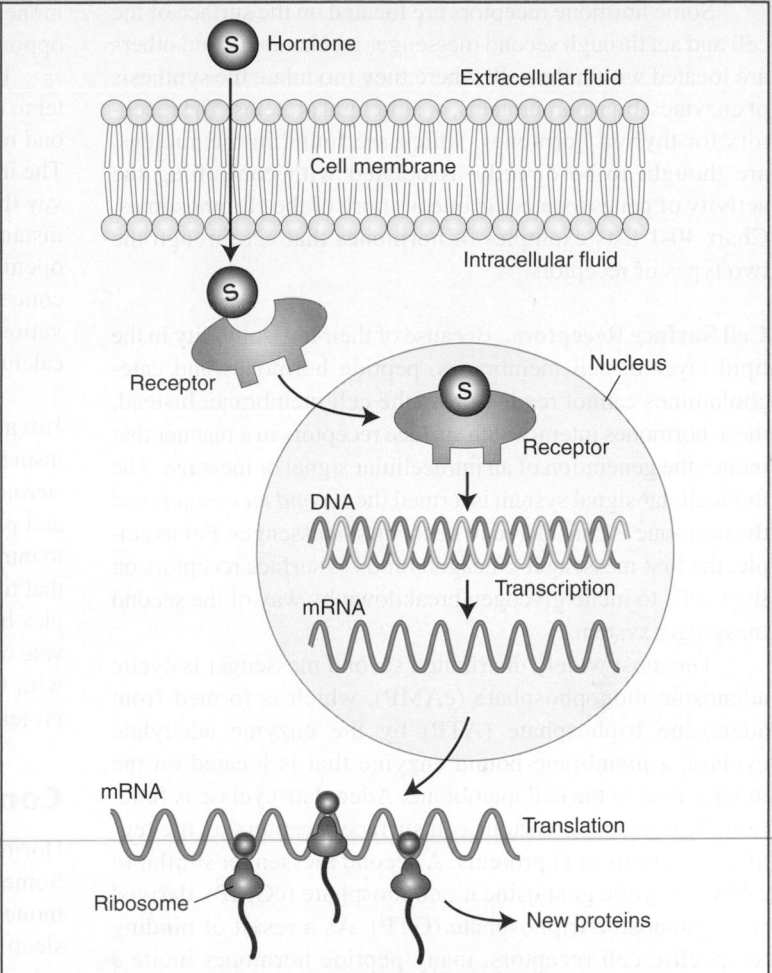

tor systems within the cell. These mechanisms involve many of the cell's metabolic activities, ranging from ion transport at the cell surface to stimulation of nuclear transcription of complex molecules. The rate at which hormones react depends on their mechanism of action. The neurotransmitters, which control the opening of ion channels, have a reaction time of milliseconds. Thyroid hormone, which functions in the control of cell metabolism and synthesis of intracellular signaling molecules, requires days for its full effect to occur.

Receptors. Hormone receptors are complex molecular structures that are located either on the surface or inside target cells. The function of these receptors is to recognize a specific hormone and translate the hormonal signal into a cellular response. The structure of these receptors varies in a manner that allows target cells to respond to one hormone and not to others. For example, receptors in the thyroid are specific for thyroid-stimulating hormone, and receptors on the gonads respond to the gonadotropic hormones.

The response of a target cell to a hormone varies with the *number* of receptors present and with the *affinity* of these recep-

tors for hormone binding. A variety of factors influence the number of receptors that are present on target cells and their affinity for hormone binding.

There are approximately 2000 to 100,000 hormone receptor molecules per cell. The number of hormone receptors on a cell may be altered for any of several reasons. Antibodies may destroy or block the receptor proteins. Increased or decreased hormone levels often induce changes in the activity of the genes that regulate receptor synthesis. For example, decreased hormone levels often produce an increase in receptor numbers by means of a process called *up-regulation;* this increases the sensitivity of the body to existing hormone levels. Likewise, sustained levels of excess hormone often bring about a decrease in receptor numbers by *down-regulation,* producing a decrease in hormone sensitivity. In some instances, the reverse effect occurs, and an increase in hormone levels appears to recruit its own receptors, thereby increasing the sensitivity of the cell to the hormone. The process of up-regulation and down-regulation of receptors is regulated largely by inducing or repressing the transcription of receptor genes.

Some hormone receptors are located on the surface of the cell and act through second messenger mechanisms, and others are located within the cell, where they modulate the synthesis of enzymes, transport proteins, or structural proteins. The receptors for thyroid hormones, which are found in the nucleus, are thought to be directly associated with controlling the activity of genes located on one or more of the chromosomes. Chart 40-1 lists examples of hormones that act through the two types of receptors.

Cell Surface Receptors. Because of their low solubility in the lipid layer of cell membranes, peptide hormones and catecholamines cannot readily cross the cell membrane. Instead, these hormones interact with surface receptors in a manner that incites the generation of an intracellular signal or message. The intracellular signal system is termed the *second messenger,* and the hormone is considered to be the first messenger. For example, the first messenger glucagon binds to surface receptors on liver cells to incite glycogen breakdown by way of the second messenger system.

The most widely distributed second messenger is cyclic adenosine monophosphate (cAMP), which is formed from adenosine triphosphate (ATP) by the enzyme adenylate cyclase, a membrane-bound enzyme that is located on the inner aspect of the cell membrane. Adenylate cyclase is functionally coupled to various cell surface receptors by the regulatory actions of G proteins. A second messenger similar to cAMP is cyclic guanosine monophosphate (cGMP), derived from guanosine triphosphate (GTP). As a result of binding to specific cell receptors, many peptide hormones incite a series of enzymatic reactions that produce an almost immediate increase in cAMP and target cell response. Some hormones act to decrease cAMP levels and have another or an opposite effect on cell responses.

In some cells, the binding of a hormone or neurotransmitter to a surface receptor acts directly, rather than through a second messenger, to open an ion channel in the cell membrane. The influx of ions then serves as an intracellular signal to convey the hormonal message to the interior of the cell. In many instances, the activation of hormone receptors results in the opening of calcium channels. The increasing cytoplasmic concentration of calcium ions may result in the direct activation of calcium-dependent enzymes or in the formation of calcium–calmodulin complexes with their attendant effects.

Intracellular Receptors. A second type of receptor mechanism is involved in mediating the action of hormones such as the steroid and thyroid hormones. These hormones are lipid soluble and pass freely through the cell membrane. They then attach to intracellular receptors and form a hormone–receptor complex that travels to the cell nucleus. The hormone–messenger complex binds to hormone response elements (HREs) that then activate or suppress intracellular mechanisms such as gene activity, with the subsequent production or inhibition of mRNA and protein synthesis.

Control of Hormone Levels

Hormone secretion varies widely over a 24-hour period. Some hormones, such as GH and adrenocorticotropic hormone (ACTH), have diurnal fluctuations that vary with the sleep–wake cycle. Others, such as the female sex hormones, are secreted in a complicated cyclic manner. The levels of hormones such as insulin and antidiuretic hormone (ADH) are regulated by feedback mechanisms that monitor substances such as glucose (insulin) and water (ADH) in the body. The levels of many of the hormones are regulated by feedback mechanisms that involve the hypothalamic-pituitary–target cell system.

Hypothalamic-Pituitary Regulation

The hypothalamus and pituitary (*i.e.,* hypophysis) form a unit that exerts control over many functions of several endocrine glands as well as a wide range of other physiologic functions. These two structures are connected by blood flow in the hypophysial portal system, which begins in the hypothalamus and drains into the anterior pituitary gland, and by the nerve axons that connect the supraoptic and paraventricular nuclei of the hypothalamus with the posterior pituitary gland (Fig. 40-2). The pituitary is enclosed in the bony sella turcica ("Turkish saddle") and is bridged over by the diaphragma sellae. Embryologically, the anterior pituitary gland developed from glandular tissue and the posterior pituitary developed from neural tissue.

Hypothalamic Hormones. The synthesis and release of anterior pituitary hormones are largely regulated by the action of

---

CHART 40-1   HORMONE–RECEPTOR INTERACTIONS

Second Messenger Interactions
Glucagon
Insulin
Epinephrine
Parathyroid hormone (PTH)
Thyroid-stimulating hormone (TSH)
Adrenocorticotropic hormone (ACTH)
Follicle-stimulating hormone (FSH)
Luteinizing hormone (LH)
Antidiuretic hormone (ADH)
Secretin

Intracellular Interactions
Estrogens
Testosterone
Progesterone
Adrenal cortical hormones
Thyroid hormones

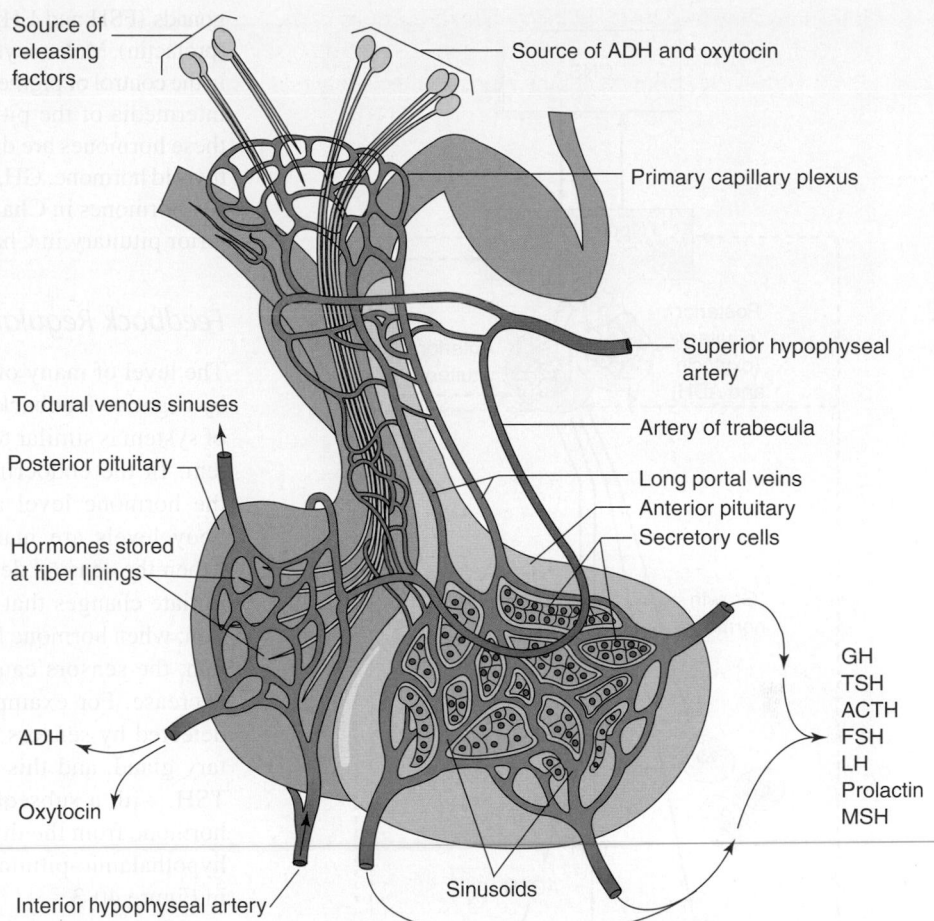

Source of releasing factors

Source of ADH and oxytocin

Primary capillary plexus

Superior hypophyseal artery

Artery of trabecula

To dural venous sinuses

Posterior pituitary

Long portal veins

Anterior pituitary

Secretory cells

Hormones stored at fiber linings

ADH

Oxytocin

Interior hypophyseal artery

Sinusoids

GH
TSH
ACTH
FSH
LH
Prolactin
MSH

FIGURE 40-2 • The hypothalamus and the anterior and posterior pituitary. The hypothalamic releasing or inhibiting hormones are transported to the anterior pituitary through the portal vessels. Antidiuretic hormone and oxytocin are produced by nerve cells in the supraoptic and paraventricular nuclei of the hypothalamus and then transported through the nerve axon to the posterior pituitary, where they are released into the circulation.

releasing or inhibiting hormones from the hypothalamus, which is the coordinating center of the brain for endocrine, behavioral, and autonomic nervous system function. It is at the level of the hypothalamus that emotion, pain, body temperature, and other neural input are communicated to the endocrine system (Fig. 40-3). The posterior pituitary hormones, ADH and oxytocin, are synthesized in the cell bodies of neurons in the hypothalamus that have axons that travel to the posterior pituitary. The release and function of ADH are discussed in Chapter 31.

The hypothalamic hormones that regulate the secretion of anterior pituitary hormones include GH-releasing hormone (GHRH), somatostatin, dopamine, TRH, corticotropin-releasing hormone (CRH), and gonadotropin-releasing hormone (GnRH). With the exception of GH and prolactin, most of the pituitary hormones are regulated by hypothalamic stimulatory hormones. GH secretion is stimulated by GHRH; thyroid-stimulating hormone (TSH) by TRH; ACTH by CRH; and luteinizing hormone (LH) and FSH by GnRH. Somatostatin functions as an inhibitory hormone for GH and TSH. Prolactin secretion is inhibited by dopamine; thus, persons receiving antipsychotic drugs that block dopamine often have increased prolactin levels.

The activity of the hypothalamus is regulated by both hormonally mediated signals (*e.g.,* negative feedback signals) and by neuronal input from a number of sources. Neuronal signals are mediated by neurotransmitters such as acetylcholine, dopamine, norepinephrine, serotonin, γ-aminobutyric acid (GABA), and opioids. Cytokines that are involved in immune and inflammatory responses, such as the interleukins, also are involved in the regulation of hypothalamic function (see Chapter 17). This is particularly true of the hormones involved in the hypothalamic-pituitary-adrenal axis. Thus, the hypothalamus can be viewed as a bridge by which signals from multiple systems are relayed to the pituitary gland.

Pituitary Hormones. The pituitary gland has been called the *master gland* because its hormones control the functions of many target glands and cells. The anterior pituitary gland contains five cell types: (1) thyrotrophs, which produce thyrotropin, also called *thyroid-stimulating hormone* (TSH); (2) corticotrophs, which produce corticotrophin, also called *adrenocorticotropic hormone* (ACTH); (3) gonadotrophs, which produce the gonadotropins, luteinizing hormone (LH) and follicle-stimulating hormone (FSH); (4) somatotrophs, which produce growth hormone (GH); and (5) lactotrophs, which produce prolactin. Hormones produced by the anterior pituitary control body growth and metabolism (GH), function of the thyroid gland (TSH), glucocorticoid hormone levels (ACTH), function of the

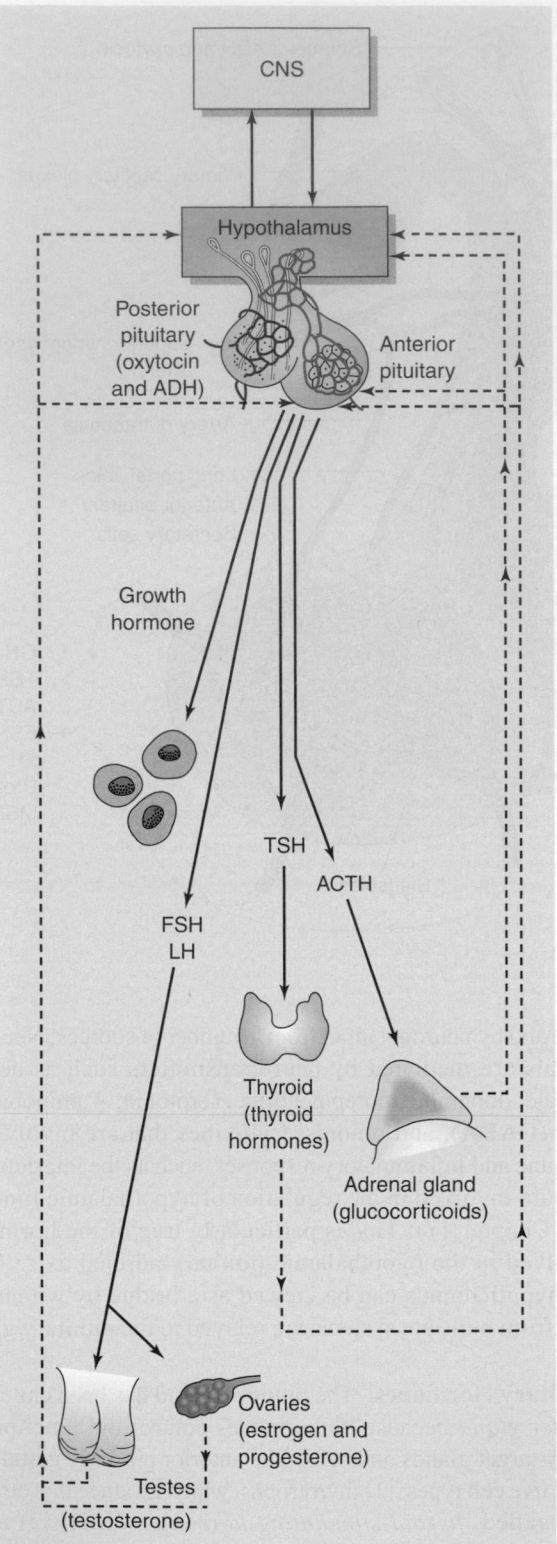

FIGURE 40-3 • Control of hormone production by the hypothalamic-pituitary–target cell feedback mechanism. Hormone levels from the target glands regulate the release of hormones from the anterior pituitary through a negative feedback system. The *dashed line* represents feedback control.

gonads (FSH and LH), and breast growth and milk production (prolactin). Melanocyte-stimulating hormone, which is involved in the control of pigmentation of the skin, is produced by the pars intermedia of the pituitary gland. The functions of many of these hormones are discussed in other parts of this book (*e.g.,* thyroid hormone, GH, and the corticosteroids in Chapter 41, the sex hormones in Chapters 44 and 46, and ADH from the posterior pituitary in Chapter 31).

Feedback Regulation

The level of many of the hormones in the body is regulated by negative feedback mechanisms. The function of this type of system is similar to that of the thermostat in a heating system. In the endocrine system, sensors detect a change in the hormone level and adjust hormone secretion so that body levels are maintained within an appropriate range. When the sensors detect a decrease in hormone levels, they initiate changes that cause an increase in hormone production; when hormone levels rise above the set point of the system, the sensors cause hormone production and release to decrease. For example, an increase in thyroid hormone is detected by sensors in the hypothalamus or anterior pituitary gland, and this causes a reduction in the secretion of TSH, with a subsequent decrease in the output of thyroid hormone from the thyroid gland. The feedback loops for the hypothalamic-pituitary feedback mechanisms are illustrated in Figure 40-3.

Exogenous forms of hormones (given as drug preparations) can influence the normal feedback control of hormone production and release. One of the most common examples of this influence occurs with the administration of the corticosteroid hormones, which causes suppression of the hypothalamic-pituitary–target cell system that regulates the production of these hormones.

Although the levels of most hormones are regulated by negative feedback mechanisms, a small number are under positive feedback control, in which rising levels of a hormone cause another gland to release a hormone that is stimulating to the first. There must, however, be a mechanism for shutting off the release of the first hormone, or its production would continue unabated. An example of such a system is that of the female ovarian hormone estradiol. Increased estradiol production during the follicular stage of the menstrual cycle causes increased gonadotropin (FSH) production by the anterior pituitary gland. This stimulates further increases in estradiol levels until the demise of the follicle, which is the source of estradiol, results in a fall in gonadotropin levels.

In addition to positive and negative feedback mechanisms that monitor changes in hormone levels, some hormones are regulated by the level of the substance they regulate. For example, insulin levels normally are regulated in response to blood glucose levels, and those of aldosterone in response to body levels of sodium and potassium. Other factors such as stress, environmental temperature, and nutritional status can alter feedback regulation of hormone levels.

Diagnostic Tests

Several techniques are available for assessing endocrine function and hormone levels. One technique measures the effect of a hormone on body function. Measurement of blood glucose, for example, is an indirect method of assessing insulin availability. The most common method is to measure hormone levels directly.

Blood Tests

Hormones circulating in the plasma were first detected by bioassays using the intact animal or a portion of tissue from the animal. However, most bioassays lack the precision, sensitivity, and specificity to measure low concentrations of hormones in plasma, and they are inconvenient to perform.

Blood hormone levels provide information about hormone levels at a specific time. For example, blood insulin levels can be measured along with blood glucose after administration of a challenge dose of glucose to measure the time course of change in blood insulin levels.

Real progress in measuring plasma hormone levels came more than 40 years ago with the use of competitive binding and the development of radioimmunoassay (RIA) methods. This method uses a radiolabeled form of the hormone and a hormone antibody that has been prepared by injecting an appropriate animal with a purified form of the hormone. The unlabeled hormone in the sample being tested competes with the radiolabeled hormone for attachment to the binding sites of the antibody. Measurement of the radiolabeled hormone–antibody complex then provides a means of arriving at a measure of the hormone level in the sample. Because hormone binding is competitive, the amount of radiolabeled hormone–antibody complex that is formed decreases as the amount of unlabeled hormone in the sample is increased. Newer techniques of RIA have been introduced, including the immunoradiometric assay (IRMA). IRMA uses two antibodies instead of one. These two antibodies are directed against two different parts of the molecule, and therefore IRMA assays are more specific. RIA has several disadvantages, including limited shelf life of the radiolabeled hormone and the cost for the disposal of radioactive waste.

Nonradiolabeled methods have been developed in which the antigen of the hormone being measured is linked to an enzyme-activated label (e.g., fluorescent label, chemiluminescent label) or latex particles that can be agglutinated with an antigen and measured. The enzyme-linked immunosorbent assays (ELISA) use antibody-coated plates and an enzyme-labeled reporter antibody. Binding of the hormone to the enzyme-labeled reporter antibody produces a colored reaction that can be measured using a spectrophotometer.

Other blood tests that are routinely measured in endocrine disorders include various autoantibodies. For example, anti-thyroid peroxidase (anti-TPO) antibodies are measured during the initial diagnostic work-up and subsequent follow-up of patients with Hashimoto thyroiditis. Other endocrine disorders that use autoantibody testing include type 1 diabetes, Graves disease, autoimmune hypoparathyroidism, and autoimmune Addison disease.

Urine Tests

Measurements of urinary hormone or hormone metabolite excretion often are done on a 24-hour urine sample and provide a better measure of hormone levels during that period than hormones measured in an isolated blood sample. The advantages of a urine test include the relative ease of obtaining urine samples and the fact that blood sampling is not required. The disadvantage is that reliably timed urine collections often are difficult to obtain. For example, a person may be unable to urinate at specific timed intervals, and urine samples may be accidentally discarded or inaccurately preserved. Because many urine tests involve the measurement of a hormone metabolite rather than the hormone itself, drugs or disease states that alter hormone metabolism may interfere with the test result. Some urinary hormone metabolite measurements include hormones from more than one source and are of little value in measuring hormone secretion from a specific source. For example, urinary 17-ketosteroids are a measure of both adrenal and gonadal androgens.

Stimulation and Suppression Tests

Stimulation tests are used when hypofunction of an endocrine organ is suspected. A tropic or stimulating hormone can be administered to test the capacity of an endocrine organ to increase hormone production. The capacity of the target gland to respond is measured by an increase in the appropriate hormone. For example, the function of the hypothalamic-pituitary-thyroid system can be evaluated through stimulation tests using TRH and measuring TSH response. Failure to increase TSH levels after a TRH stimulation test suggests an inadequate capacity to produce TSH by the pituitary (i.e., the pituitary is dysfunctional in some way).

Suppression tests are used when hyperfunction of an endocrine organ is suspected. When an organ or tissue is functioning autonomously (i.e., it is not responding to the normal negative feedback control mechanisms, and continues to secrete excessive amounts of hormone), a suppression test may be useful to confirm the situation. For example, when a GH-secreting tumor is suspected, the GH response to a glucose load is measured as part of the diagnostic work-up (see Chapter 41). Normally, a glucose load would suppress GH levels. However, in adults with GH-secreting tumors (a condition known as acromegaly), GH levels are not suppressed (and paradoxically increase in 50% of cases).

Genetic Tests

The diagnosis of genetic diseases using deoxyribonucleic acid (DNA) analysis is rapidly becoming a routine part of endocrine

Understanding • Feedback Regulation of Hormone Levels

Like many physiologic systems, the endocrine system is regulated by feedback mechanisms that enable the endocrine cells to change their rate of hormone secretion. Feedback can be negative or positive and may involve complex feedback loops involving hypothalamic-pituitary regulation.

❶ Negative Feedback

With negative feedback, the most common mechanism of hormone control, some feature of hormone action directly or indirectly inhibits further hormone secretion so that the hormone level returns to an ideal level or set point. In the simple negative feedback loop, the amount of hormone or its effect on a physiologic mechanism regulates the response of the endocrine gland. After a meal, for example, a rise in blood glucose stimulates the pancreas to secrete insulin; insulin acts on target cells to take up the glucose, thus lowering blood glucose. The lowered glucose levels, in turn, suppress insulin release, causing blood glucose to rise.

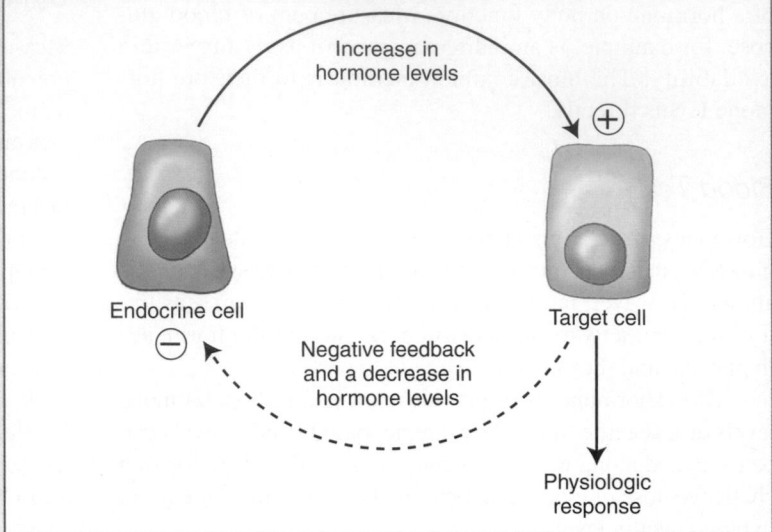

❷ Hypothalamic-Pituitary–Target Cell Feedback

Hormones of the thyroid, adrenal cortex, and the gonads are regulated by more complex loops involving the hypothalamus and anterior pituitary gland. The hypothalamus produces a releasing hormone that stimulates the production of a tropic hormone by the anterior pituitary. The tropic hormone then stimulates the peripheral target gland to secrete its hormone, which acts on target cells to produce a physiologic response. A rise in blood levels of the target gland hormone also feeds back to the hypothalamus and anterior pituitary gland, resulting in a decrease in tropic hormone secretion and a subsequent reduction in hormone secretion by the target gland. As a result, blood levels of the hormone vary only within a narrow range.

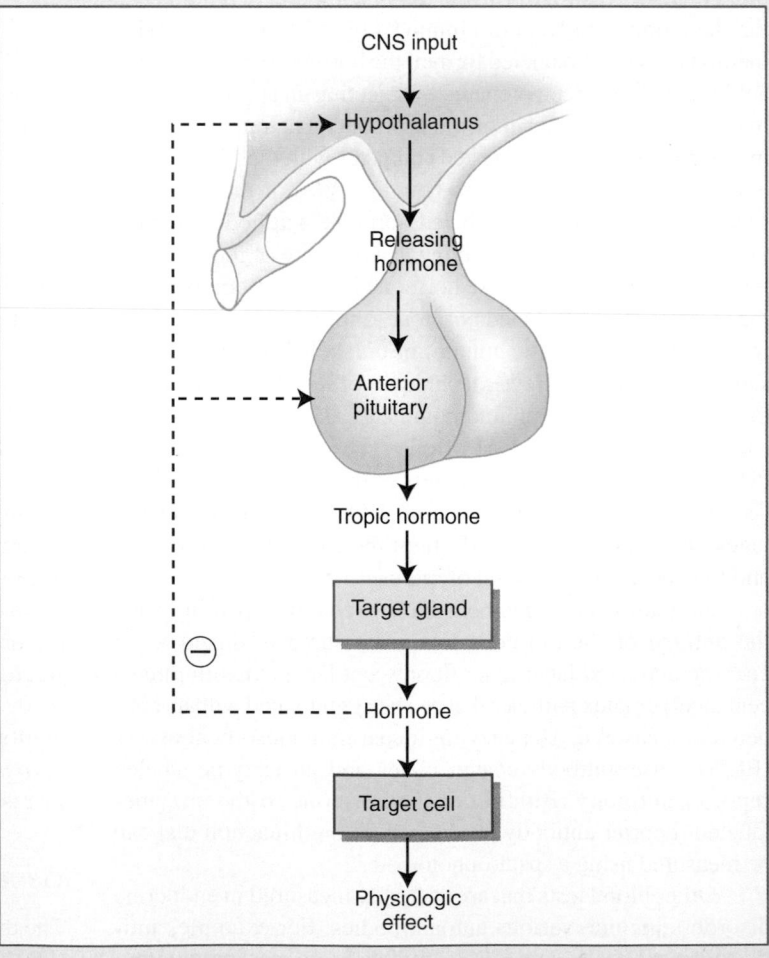

Positive Feedback

A small number of hormones are regulated by positive feedback. In this type of regulation, a hormone stimulates continued secretion until appropriate levels are reached. An example of positive feedback is the preovulatory surge in luteinizing hormone (LH) levels that trigger ovulation. At that time, an increase in estrogen levels exerts a positive feedback effect on the anterior pituitary secretion of LH.

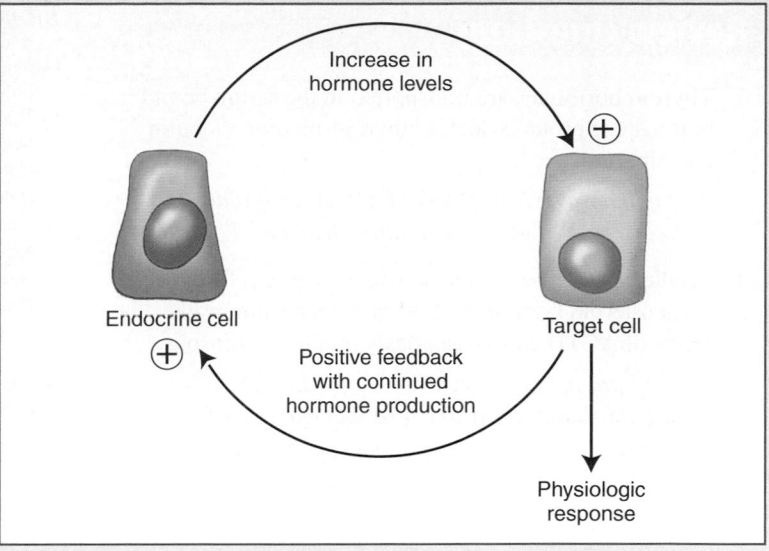

practice. Completion of the human genome sequence has revealed the presence of about 30,000 to 40,000 genes. The considerable interest in the field of genomics (*i.e.,* examination of the DNA) and transcriptomics (*i.e.,* examination of the mRNA) has been complemented by advances in proteomics (*i.e.,* examination of the proteome, which is all of the proteins expressed by a cell or tissue type). It is proposed that compared with the size of the genome, the proteome is far larger, with several hundred thousand to several million different protein forms possible. Analysis of the proteins produced by normal and abnormal endocrine cells, tissues, and organs will lead to a better understanding of the pathophysiologic processes of endocrine conditions. This may also lead to selective targeting for new drug development.

The cloning of many endocrine system genes has had an enormous impact on everyday clinical practice. For example, identification of a gene for a given disorder (*e.g.,* the *RET* proto-oncogene in certain multiple endocrine neoplasia syndromes) means that faster diagnosis and more appropriate management for the affected individual can occur, but also that screening of family members for kindred harboring a known mutation can also be undertaken.

Imaging

Imaging studies are important in the diagnosis and follow-up of endocrine disorders. Imaging modalities related to endocrinology can be divided into isotopic and nonisotopic types. Isotopic imaging includes radioactive scanning of the thyroid (*e.g.,* using radioiodine), parathyroids (*e.g.,* using sestamibi), and adrenals (*e.g.,* using MIBG to detect pheochromocytoma). Nonisotopic imaging includes magnetic resonance imaging (MRI), which is the preferred choice for pituitary and hypothalamic imaging, and computed tomography (CT) scanning, which

is preferred for adrenal lesions and abdominal endocrine lesions. Ultrasonographic scanning provides excellent and reproducible anatomic images for the thyroid, parathyroids, and neighboring structures. Thyroid ultrasonography is recommended for managing thyroid nodules and can aid in visualization of the nodule for biopsy (fine-needle aspiration), which is necessary to help distinguish benign from malignant etiology. Selective venography is usually accompanied by venous sampling to determine hormonal output from a gland or organ (*e.g.,* adrenal, pituitary, and kidney). Positron emission tomography (PET) scanning is being used more widely for evaluation of endocrine tumors. Dual electron x-ray absorptiometry (DEXA) is used routinely for the diagnosis and monitoring of osteoporosis and metabolic bone diseases.

IN SUMMARY, the endocrine system acts as a communication system that uses chemical messengers, or hormones, for the transmission of information from cell to cell and from organ to organ. Hormones act by binding to receptors that are specific for the different types of hormones. Many of the endocrine glands are under the regulatory control of other parts of the endocrine system. The hypothalamus and the pituitary gland form a complex integrative network that joins the nervous system and the endocrine system; this central network controls the output from many of the other glands in the body.

Endocrine function can be assessed directly by measuring hormone levels, or indirectly by assessing the effects that a hormone has on the body (*e.g.,* assessment of insulin function through blood glucose). Imaging techniques are increasingly used to visualize endocrine structures, and genetic techniques are used to determine the presence of genes that contribute to the development of endocrine disorders. ∎

Review Questions

1. Thyroid hormones are transported in the serum bound to transport proteins such as thyroid-binding globulin and albumin.

   A. *Explain why free thyroxine (T₄) levels are usually used to assess thyroid function rather than total T₄ levels.*

2. People who are being treated with exogenous forms of corticosteroid hormones often experience diminished levels of ACTH and exogenously produced cortisol.

   A. *Explain, using information regarding the hypothalamic-pituitary feedback control of cortisol production by the adrenal cortex.*

Bibliography

Gardner D. G. (Ed.). (2007). *Greenspan's basic and clinical endocrinology* (8th ed.). New York: Lange Medical Books/McGraw-Hill.

Griffin J. E., Sergio R. O. (2005). *Textbook of endocrine physiology* (5th ed.). New York: Oxford University Press.

Holt R. I. G., Hanley N. A. (2007). *Essential endocrinology and diabetes* (5th ed.). Malden, MA: Blackwell.

Molina P. E. (2006). *Endocrine physiology* (2nd ed.). New York: Lange Medical Books/McGraw-Hill.

Jameson J. L. (Ed.). (2006). *Harrison's endocrinology.* New York: McGraw-Hill.

Visit the Point http://thePoint.lww.com for animations, journal articles, and more!

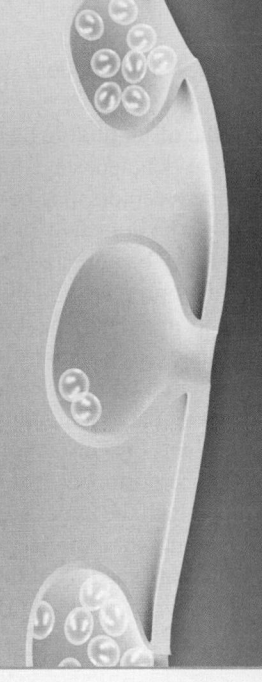

Chapter 41

Disorders of Endocrine Control of Growth and Metabolism

GLENN MATFIN

> The endocrine system affects all aspects of body function, including growth and development, energy metabolism, muscle and adipose tissue distribution, sexual development, fluid and electrolyte balance, and inflammation and immune responses. This chapter focuses on disorders of pituitary function, growth and growth hormone, thyroid function, and adrenal cortical function.

GENERAL ASPECTS OF ALTERED ENDOCRINE FUNCTION

After completing this section of the chapter, you should be able to meet the following objectives:

- Describe the mechanisms of endocrine hypofunction and hyperfunction.
- Differentiate among primary, secondary, and tertiary endocrine disorders.

Hypofunction and Hyperfunction

Disturbances of endocrine function usually can be divided into two categories: hypofunction and hyperfunction. Hypofunction of an endocrine gland can occur for a variety of reasons. Congenital defects can result in the absence or impaired development of the gland or the absence of an enzyme needed for hormone synthesis. The gland may be destroyed by a disruption in blood flow, infection, inflammation, autoimmune responses, or neoplastic growth. There may be a decline in function with aging, or the gland may atrophy as the result of drug therapy or for unknown reasons. Some endocrine-deficient states are associated with receptor defects: hormone receptors may be absent, the receptor binding of hormones may be defective, or the cellular responsiveness to the hormone may be impaired. It is suspected that in some cases a gland may produce a biologically inactive hormone or that an active hormone may be destroyed by circulating antibodies before it can exert its action.

Hyperfunction usually is associated with excessive hormone production. This can result from excessive stimulation and hyperplasia of the endocrine gland or from a hormone-producing tumor. A tumor can produce hormones that are not normally secreted by the tissue from which the tumor is derived (so-called ectopic hormone production); for example, certain bronchogenic tumors produce hormones such as antidiuretic hormone (ADH) and adrenocorticotropic hormone (ACTH).

Primary, Secondary, and Tertiary Disorders

Endocrine disorders in general can be divided into primary, secondary, and tertiary groups. *Primary defects* in endocrine function originate in the target gland responsible for producing the hormone. In *secondary disorders* of endocrine function, the target gland is essentially normal, but its function is altered by defective levels of stimulating hormones or releasing factors from the pituitary system. For example, total thyroidectomy produces a primary deficiency of thyroid hormones. Removal or destruction of the pituitary gland eliminates ACTH stimulation of the adrenal cortex and brings about a secondary deficiency. A *tertiary disorder* results from hypothalamic dysfunction (as may occur with craniopharyngiomas or cerebral irradiation); thus, both the pituitary and target organ are understimulated.

> **IN SUMMARY,** endocrine disorders are the result of hypofunction or hyperfunction of an endocrine gland. They can occur as a primary defect in hormone production by a target gland or as a secondary or tertiary disorder resulting from a defect in the hypothalamic-pituitary system that controls a target gland's function. ■

PITUITARY AND GROWTH DISORDERS

After completing this section of the chapter, you should be able to meet the following objectives:

- Discuss the classification of pituitary tumors.
- Describe the clinical features and causes of hypopituitarism.
- State the effects of a deficiency in growth hormone.
- Differentiate genetic short stature from constitutional short stature.

- State the mechanisms of short stature in hypothyroidism, poorly controlled diabetes mellitus, chronic treatment with excessive glucocorticoid hormones, malnutrition, and psychosocial dwarfism.
- List three causes of tall stature.
- Relate the functions of growth hormone to the manifestations of acromegaly and adult-onset growth hormone deficiency.
- Explain why children with isosexual precocious puberty are tall-statured children but short-statured adults.

The pituitary gland, or *hypophysis,* is a pea-sized gland located at the base of the brain, where it lies in a saddle-shaped depression in the sphenoid bone called the *sella turcica.* A short funnel-shaped stalk, the *infundibulum,* connects the pituitary gland with the hypothalamus (see Chapter 40, Fig. 40-2). The pituitary gland has two components: a posterior lobe (neurohypophysis) or neural component (discussed in Chapter 31) and an anterior lobe (adenohypophysis) or glandular component.

The anterior lobe of the pituitary gland produces ACTH, thyroid stimulating hormone (TSH), growth hormone (GH), the gonadotrophic hormones (follicle stimulating hormone [FSH] and luteinizing hormone [LH]), and prolactin (see Chapter 40, Fig 40-3).[1] Four of these, ACTH, TSH, LH, and FSH control the secretion of hormones from other endocrine glands. ACTH controls the release of cortisol from the adrenal gland, TSH the secretion of thyroid hormone from the thyroid gland, LH regulates sex hormones and FSH regulates fertility.

Pituitary Tumors

Pituitary tumors can be divided into primary or secondary tumors (*i.e.,* metastatic lesions). Tumors of the pituitary can be further divided into functional tumors that secrete pituitary hormones and nonfunctional tumors that do not secrete hormones. They can range in size from small lesions that do not enlarge the gland (microadenomas, <10 mm) to large, expansive tumors (macroadenomas, >10 mm) that erode the sella turcica and impinge on surrounding cranial structures.[1] Small, nonfunctioning tumors are found in up to 20% of adult autopsies. Benign adenomas account for most of the functioning anterior pituitary tumors. Carcinomas of the pituitary are less common tumors. Functional adenomas can be subdivided according to cell type and the type of hormone secreted (Table 41-1).

Hypopituitarism

Hypopituitarism, which is characterized by a decreased secretion of pituitary hormones, is a condition that affects many of the other endocrine systems.[1] Typically, 70% to 90% of the anterior pituitary must be destroyed before hypopituitarism becomes clinically evident. The cause may be congenital or result from a variety of acquired abnormalities (Chart 41-1). The manifestations of hypopituitarism usually occur gradually, but it can present as an acute and life-threatening condition. Patients usually complain of being chronically unfit, with weak-

TABLE 41-1 Frequency of Adenomas of the Anterior Pituitary

CELL TYPE	HORMONE	FREQUENCY (%)
Lactotrope	Prolactin (PRL)	32
Somatotrope	Growth hormone (GH)	21
Lactotrope/ somatotrope	Mixed PRL/GH	6
Corticotrope	Adrenocorticotropic hormone (ACTH)	13
Gonadotrope	Follicle-stimulating hormone (FSH)	
	Luteinizing hormone (LH)	<4
Thyrotrope	Thyroid-stimulating hormone (TSH)	
Nonfunctional tumors		25

ness, fatigue, loss of appetite, impairment of sexual function, and cold intolerance. However, ACTH deficiency (secondary adrenal insufficiency) is the most serious endocrine deficiency, leading to weakness, nausea, anorexia, fever, and postural hypotension. Hypopituitarism is associated with increased morbidity and mortality.

Anterior pituitary hormone loss tends to follow a typical sequence, especially with progressive loss of pituitary reserve due to tumors or previous pituitary radiation therapy (which may take 10 to 20 years to produce hypopituitarism). The sequence of loss of pituitary hormones can be remembered by the mnemonic "*Go Look For The Adenoma*," for *G*H (GH secretion typically is first to be lost), *L*H (results in sex hormone deficiency), *F*SH (causes infertility), *T*SH (leads to secondary hypothyroidism), and *A*CTH (usually the last to become deficient, results in secondary adrenal insufficiency).

Treatment of hypopituitarism includes treating any identified underlying cause. Hormone deficiencies should be treated as dictated by baseline hormone levels, and more sophisticated pituitary testing where appropriate (and safe). Cortisol replacement is started when ACTH deficiency is present; thyroid replacement when TSH deficiency is detected; and sex hormone replacement when LH and FSH are deficient. GH replacement is indicated for pediatric GH deficiency, and is being increasingly used to treat GH deficiency in adults.[1-3]

Assessment of Hypothalamic-Pituitary Function

The assessment of hypothalamic-pituitary function has been made possible by many newly developed imaging and radio-immunoassay methods. Assessment of the baseline status of the hypothalamic-pituitary target cell hormones involves measuring the following (ideally performed at 8:00 AM): (1) serum cortisol, (2) serum prolactin, (3) serum thyroxine and TSH, (4) serum testosterone (male)/serum estrogen (female) and serum LH/FSH, (5) serum GH/insulin-like growth factor-1, and (6) plasma osmolality and urine osmolality. Imaging studies (*e.g.,* magnetic resonance imaging [MRI] of the hypothalamus/pituitary) also should be performed as required. When further information regarding pituitary function is required, combined hypothalamic-pituitary function tests are undertaken (although these are performed less often today).[1] These tests consist mainly of hormone stimulation tests (*e.g.,* rapid ACTH stimulation test) or suppression tests (*e.g.,* GH suppression test).

It often is important to test pituitary function, especially if pituitary adenomas are discovered and surgery or radiation treatment is being considered. Diagnostic methods include both static and dynamic testing, and radiologic assessment as required. Any of the systems discussed previously may be affected by either deficiency or excess of the usual hormones secreted.

CHART 41-1   CAUSES OF HYPOPITUITARISM

- Tumors and mass lesions—pituitary adenomas, cysts, metastatic cancer, and other lesions
- Pituitary surgery or radiation
- Infiltrative lesions and infections—hemochromatosis, lymphocytic hypophysitis
- Pituitary infarction—infarction of the pituitary gland after substantial blood loss during childbirth (Sheehan syndrome)
- Pituitary apoplexy—sudden hemorrhage into the pituitary gland
- Genetic diseases—rare congenital defects of one or more pituitary hormones
- Empty sella syndrome—an enlarged sella turcica that is not entirely filled with pituitary tissue
- Hypothalamic disorders—tumors and mass lesions (*e.g.,* craniopharyngiomas and metastatic malignancies), hypothalamic radiation, infiltrative lesions (*e.g.,* sarcoidosis), trauma, infections

Growth and Growth Hormone Disorders

Several hormones are essential for normal body growth and maturation, including growth hormone (GH), insulin, thyroid hormone, and androgens.[3] In addition to its actions on carbohydrate and fat metabolism, insulin plays an essential role in growth processes. Children with diabetes, particularly those with poor control, often fail to grow normally even though GH levels are normal. When levels of thyroid hormone are lower than normal, bone growth and epiphyseal closure are delayed. Androgens such as testosterone and dihydrotestosterone exert anabolic growth effects through their actions on protein synthesis. Glucocorticoids at excessive levels inhibit growth, apparently because of their antagonistic effect on GH secretion.

8 GROWTH HORMONE

- Growth hormone (GH), which is produced by soma-totropes in the anterior pituitary, is necessary for linear bone growth in children. It also increases the rate at which cells transport amino acids across their cell membranes, and it increases the rate at which they utilize fatty acids and decreases the rate at which they use carbohydrates.

- The effects of GH on linear growth requires insulin-like growth factors (IGFs), which are produced mainly by the liver.

- GH (or IGF) deficiency in children interferes with linear bone growth, resulting in short stature or dwarfism.

- In children, GH excess results in increased linear growth or gigantism; in adults it results in overgrowth of the cartilaginous parts of the skeleton, enlargement of the heart and other organs, and metabolic disturbances in fat and carbohydrate metabolism.

Growth Hormone

Growth hormone, also called *somatotropin,* is a 191–amino-acid polypeptide hormone synthesized and secreted by spe-cial cells in the anterior pituitary called *somatotropes.* For many years, it was thought that GH was produced primarily during periods of growth. However, this has proved to be incorrect because the rate of GH production in adults is almost as great as in children. GH is necessary for growth and contributes to the regulation of metabolic functions (Fig. 41-1). All aspects of cartilage growth are stimulated by GH; one of the most striking effects of GH is on linear bone growth, resulting from its action on the epiphyseal growth plates of long bones. The width of bone increases because of enhanced periosteal growth; visceral and endocrine organs, skeletal and cardiac muscle, skin, and connective tissue all undergo increased growth in response to GH. In many instances, the increased growth of visceral and endocrine organs is accom-panied by enhanced functional capacity. For example, increased growth of cardiac muscle is accompanied by an increase in cardiac output.

In addition to its effects on growth, GH facilitates the rate of protein synthesis by all of the cells of the body; it enhances fatty acid mobilization and increases the use of fatty acids for fuel; and it maintains or increases blood glucose levels by decreasing the use of glucose for fuel. GH has an initial effect of increasing insulin levels. However, the predominant effect of prolonged GH excess is to increase glucose levels despite an insulin increase. This is because GH induces a resistance to insulin in the peripheral tissues, inhibiting the uptake of glucose by muscle and adipose tissues.[1]

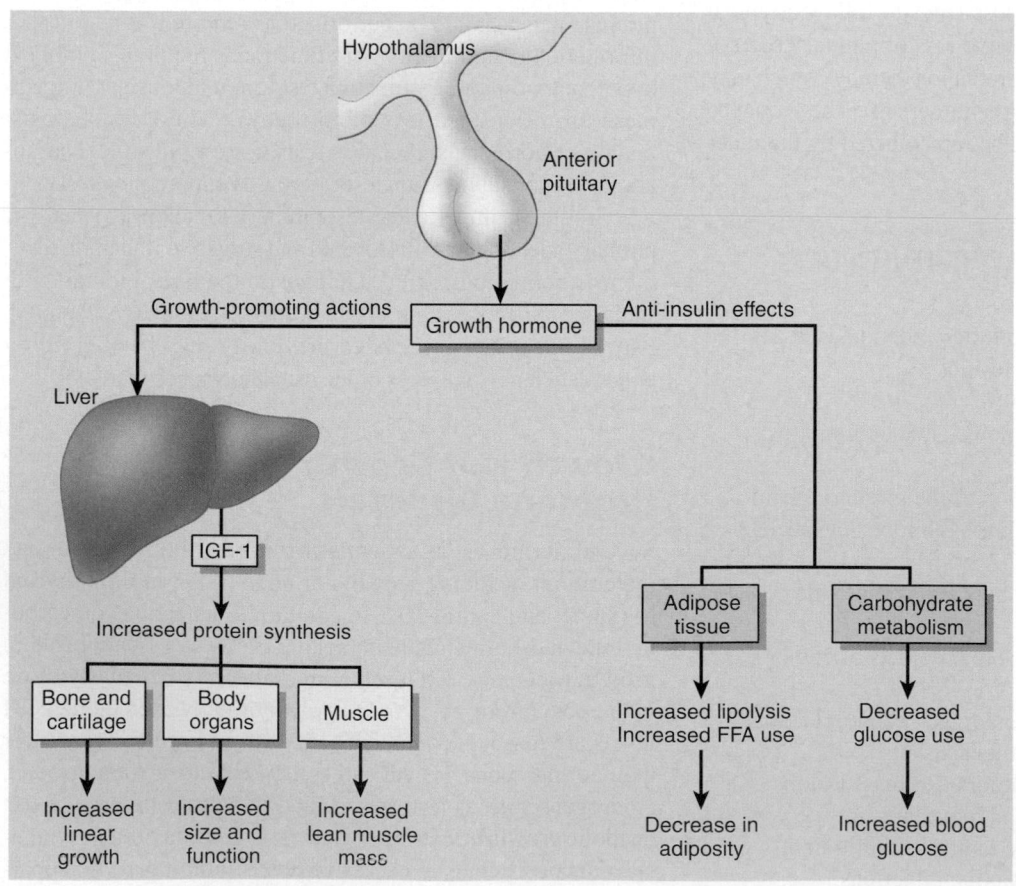

FIGURE 41-1 • Growth pro-moting and anti-insulin effects of growth hormone. FFA, free fatty acids; IGF-1, insulin-like growth factor-1.

Many of the effects of GH depend on a family of peptides called *insulin-like growth factors* (IGFs), also called *somatomedins,* which are produced mainly by the liver.[3] GH cannot directly produce bone growth; instead, it acts indirectly by causing the liver to produce IGF. These peptides act on cartilage and bone to promote their growth. At least four IGFs have been identified; of these, IGF-1 (somatomedin C) appears to be the more important in terms of growth, and it is the one that usually is measured in laboratory tests. The IGFs have been sequenced and have structures that are similar to those of proinsulin. This undoubtedly explains the insulin-like activity of the IGFs and the weak action of insulin on growth. IGF levels are themselves influenced by a family of at least six binding factors called *IGF-binding proteins* (IGFBPs).

GH is carried unbound in the plasma and has a half-life of approximately 20 to 50 minutes. The secretion of GH is regulated by two hypothalamic hormones: GH-releasing hormone (GHRH), which increases GH release, and somatostatin, which inhibits GH release. A third hormone, the recently identified ghrelin, also may be important. These hypothalamic influences (*i.e.,* GHRH and somatostatin) are tightly regulated by neural, metabolic, and hormonal factors. The secretion of GH fluctuates over a 24-hour period, with peak levels occurring 1 to 4 hours after onset of sleep (*i.e.,* during sleep stages 3 and 4 [see Chapter 52]). The nocturnal sleep bursts, which account for 70% of daily GH secretion, are greater in children than in adults.

GH secretion is stimulated by hypoglycemia, fasting, starvation, increased blood levels of amino acids (particularly arginine), and stress conditions such as trauma, excitement, emotional stress, and heavy exercise. GH is inhibited by increased glucose levels, free fatty acid release, cortisol, and obesity. Impairment of secretion, leading to growth retardation, is not uncommon in children with severe emotional deprivation.

Short Stature in Children

Short stature is a condition in which the attained height is well below the third percentile or linear growth is below normal for age and sex. Short stature, or growth retardation, has a variety of causes, including chromosomal abnormalities such as Turner syndrome (see Chapter 7), GH deficiency, hypothyroidism, and panhypopituitarism (*i.e.,* deficiency of *all* pituitary-derived hormones).[3] Other conditions known to cause short stature include protein-calorie malnutrition, chronic diseases such as chronic kidney disease and poorly controlled diabetes mellitus, malabsorption syndromes, and certain therapies such as excessive glucocorticoid administration. Emotional disturbances can lead to functional endocrine disorders, causing psychosocial dwarfism. The causes of short stature are summarized in Chart 41-2.

Accurate measurement of height is an extremely important part of the physical examination of children. Completion of the developmental history and growth charts is essential. Growth curves and growth velocity studies also are needed. Diagnosis of short stature is not made on a single measure-

---

CHART 41-2	**CAUSES OF SHORT STATURE**

Variants of Normal
Genetic or "familial" short stature
Constitutional short stature

Low Birth Weight (*e.g.,* **intrauterine growth retardation**)

Endocrine Disorders
Growth hormone (GH) deficiency
   Primary GH deficiency
      Idiopathic GH deficiency
      Pituitary agenesis
   Secondary GH deficiency (panhypopituitarism)
Biologically inactive GH production
Deficient IGF-1 production in response to normal or
   elevated GH (Laron-type dwarfism)
Hypothyroidism
Diabetes mellitus in poor control
Glucocorticoid excess
   Endogenous (Cushing syndrome)
   Exogenous (glucocorticoid drug treatment)
Abnormal mineral metabolism
   (*e.g.,* pseudohypoparathyroidism)

Chronic Illness and Malnutrition
Chronic organic or systemic disease (*e.g.,* asthma,
   especially when treated with glucocorticoids;
   heart or renal disease)
Nutritional deprivation
Malabsorption syndrome (*e.g.,* celiac sprue)

**Functional Endocrine Disorders
(Psychosocial Dwarfism)**

Chromosomal Disorders (*e.g.,* **Turner syndrome**)

Skeletal Abnormalities (*e.g.,* **achondroplasia**)

---

ment, but is based on sequential height measurements and on velocity of growth and parental height.[3]

The diagnostic procedures for short stature include tests to exclude nonendocrine causes. If the cause is hormonal, extensive hormonal testing procedures are initiated. Usually, GH and IGF-1 levels are determined (IGFBP-3 levels also are useful). Tests can be performed using insulin (to induce hypoglycemia), GHRH, levodopa, and arginine, all of which stimulate GH secretion so that GH reserve can be evaluated.[3] Because administration of pharmacologic agents can result in false-negative responses, two or more tests usually are performed. If a prompt rise in GH is realized, the child is considered normal. Physiologic tests of GH reserve (*e.g.,* GH response to exercise) also can be performed. Levels of IGF-1 usually reflect those of GH and may be used to indicate GH deficiency. Radiologic films are used to assess bone age, which most often is delayed. MRI of the hypothalamic-pituitary area is recommended if a lesion is clinically suspected. After the cause of short stature has been determined, treatment can be initiated.

Genetic and Constitutional Short Stature. Two forms of short stature, genetic short stature and constitutional short stature, are not disease states but variations from population norms. Genetically short children tend to be well proportioned and to have a height close to the mid-parental height of their parents. The mid-parental height for boys can be calculated by adding 13 cm (5 in) to the height of the mother, adding the father's height, and dividing the total by two. For girls, 13 cm (5 in) is subtracted from the father's height, the result is added to the mother's height, and the total is divided by two. Ninety-five percent of normal children are within 8 cm (*i.e.,* ± 2 standard deviations) of the mid-parental height.

Constitutional short stature is a term used to describe children (particularly boys) who have moderately short stature, thin build, delayed skeletal and sexual maturation, and absence of other causes of decreased growth. *Catch-up growth* is a term used to describe an abnormally high growth rate that occurs as a child approaches normal height for age. It occurs after the initiation of therapy for GH deficiency and hypothyroidism and the correction of chronic diseases.[3]

Psychosocial Dwarfism. Psychosocial dwarfism involves a functional hypopituitarism and is seen in some emotionally deprived children. These children usually present with poor growth, potbelly, and poor eating and drinking habits. Typically, there is a history of disturbed family relationships in which the child has been severely neglected or disciplined. Often, the neglect is confined to one child in the family. GH function usually returns to normal after the child is removed from the constraining environment. The prognosis depends on improvement in behavior and catch-up growth. Family therapy usually is indicated, and foster care may be necessary.

 Growth Hormone Deficiency in Children

There are several forms of GH deficiency that present in childhood. Children with idiopathic GH deficiency lack the hypothalamic GHRH but have adequate somatotropes, whereas children with pituitary tumors or agenesis of the pituitary lack somatotropes. The term *panhypopituitarism* refers to conditions that cause a deficiency of all of the anterior pituitary hormones. In a rare condition called *Laron-type dwarfism,* GH levels are normal or elevated, but there is a hereditary defect in IGF production that can be treated directly with IGF-1 replacement.[4]

Congenital GH deficiency is associated with decreased birth length, followed by a decrease in growth rate that can be identified by careful measurement during the first year and that becomes obvious by 1 to 2 years of age. Persons with classic GH deficiency have normal intelligence, short stature, obesity with immature facial features, and some delay in skeletal maturation (Fig. 41-2). Puberty often is delayed, and males with the disorder

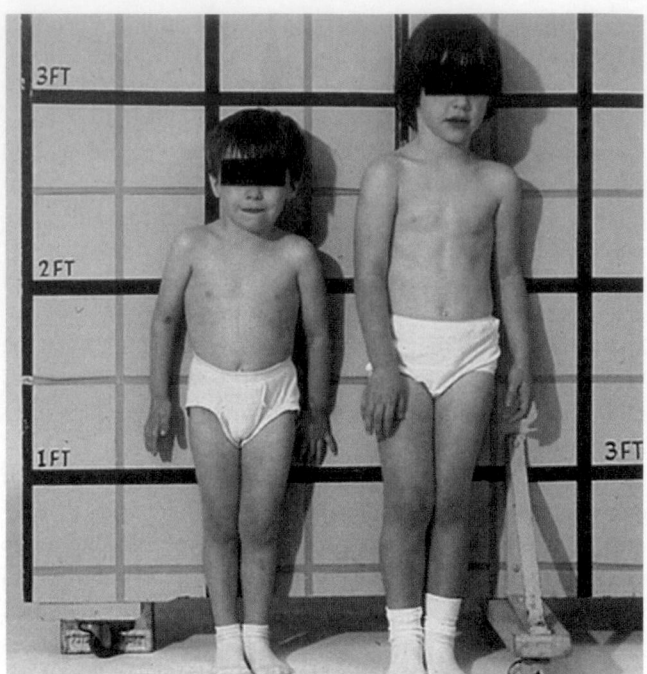

FIGURE 41-2 • Child with growth hormone deficiency. A 5.5-year-old boy (**left**) with growth hormone deficiency was significantly shorter than his fraternal twin sister (**right**), with the discrepancy beginning early in childhood. Notice his chubby, immature appearance compared with his sister. (From Shulman D., Bercu B. [2000]. *Atlas of clinical endocrinology, neuroendocrinology, and pituitary diseases.* Korenman S. [Series Ed.]. Philadelphia: Current Medicine.)

have microphallus (abnormally small penis), especially if the condition is accompanied by gonadotropin-releasing hormone (GnRH) deficiency. In the neonate, GH deficiency can lead to hypoglycemia and seizures; if ACTH deficiency also is present, the hypoglycemia often is more severe. Acquired GH deficiency develops in later childhood; it may be caused by a hypothalamic-pituitary tumor, particularly if it is accompanied by other pituitary hormone deficiencies.

When short stature is caused by a GH deficiency, GH replacement therapy is the treatment of choice. GH is species specific, and only human GH is effective in humans. GH previously was obtained from human cadaver pituitaries, but now is produced by recombinant DNA technology and is available in adequate supply. GH is administered by daily subcutaneous injection during the period of active growth, and can be continued into adulthood.[3]

Children with short stature due to Turner syndrome and chronic renal insufficiency also are treated with GH. GH therapy may be considered for children with short stature but without GH deficiency. Several studies suggest that short-term treatment with GH increases the rate of growth in these children. Although the effect of GH on adult height is not great, it can result in improved psychological well-being. There are concerns about misuse of the drug to produce additional growth in children with normal GH function who are of near-normal height. Guidelines for use of the hormone continue to be established.[3]

Growth Hormone Deficiency in Adults

There are two categories of GH deficiency in adults: (1) GH deficiency that was present in childhood, and (2) GH deficiency that developed during adulthood, mainly as the result of hypopituitarism resulting from a pituitary tumor or its treatment. GH levels also can decline with aging, and there has been interest in the effects of declining GH levels in the elderly (described as the *somatopause*). GH replacement obviously is important in the growing child; however, the role in adults (especially for the somatopause) is being assessed. Some of the differences between childhood and adult-onset GH deficiency are described in Table 41-2.

Several studies have shown that cardiovascular mortality is increased in GH-deficient adults. A higher prevalence of atherosclerotic plaques and endothelial dysfunction has been reported in both childhood and adult GH deficiency. The GH deficiency syndrome is associated with a cluster of cardiovascular risk factors, including central adiposity (associated with increased visceral fat), insulin resistance, and dyslipidemia. These features also are associated with the *metabolic syndrome* (see Chapter 42). In addition to these so-called traditional cardiovascular risk factors, nontraditional cardiovascular risk factors (*e.g.,* high-sensitivity C-reactive protein [hsCRP], which are markers of the inflammatory pathway) are also elevated. GH therapy can improve many of these factors.[3,5]

The diagnosis of GH deficiency in adults is made by finding subnormal serum GH responses to provocative stimuli. A low IGF-1 level in the presence of known pituitary disease may also indicate GH deficiency. Measurements of the basal GH levels do not distinguish reliably between normal and subnormal GH secretion in adults. Insulin-induced hypoglycemia is the gold standard test for GH reserve. The arginine plus GHRH test is probably the next best test. Other stimulation tests involve the use of arginine, L-dopa, clonidine (an α-adrenergic agonist), glucagon, or GHRH alone.

GH replacement therapy may lead to increased lean body mass and decreased fat mass, increased bone mineral density, increased glomerular filtration rate, decreased lipid levels, increased exercise capacity, and improved sense of well-being in GH-deficient adults. The most common side effects of GH treatment in adults with hypopituitarism are peripheral edema, arthralgias and myalgias, carpal tunnel syndrome, paresthesias, and decreased glucose tolerance. Side effects appear to be more common in people who are older and heavier and are overtreated, as judged by a high serum IGF-1 concentration during therapy. Women seem to tolerate higher doses better than men.[1,2]

 ## Tall Stature in Children

Just as there are children who are short for their age and sex, there also are children who are tall for their age and sex.[3,6] Normal variants of tall stature include genetic tall stature and constitutional tall stature. Children with exceptionally tall parents tend to be taller than children with shorter parents. The term *constitutional tall stature* is used to describe a child who is taller than his or her peers and is growing at a velocity that is within the normal range for bone age. Other causes of tall stature are genetic or chromosomal disorders such as Marfan syndrome or XYY syndrome (see Chapter 7). Endocrine causes of tall stature include sexual precocity because of early onset of estrogen and androgen secretion and excessive GH.

Exceptionally tall children (*i.e.,* genetic tall stature and constitutional tall stature) can be treated with sex hormones—estrogens in girls and testosterone in boys—to effect early epiphyseal closure. Such treatment is undertaken only after full consideration of the risks involved. To be effective, such treatment must be instituted 3 to 4 years before expected epiphyseal fusion.[3,6]

 ## Growth Hormone Excess in Children

Growth hormone excess occurring before puberty and the fusion of the epiphyses of the long bones results in *gigantism* (Fig. 41-3). Excessive secretion of GH by somatotrope adenomas causes gigantism in the prepubertal child. It occurs when the epiphyses are not fused and high levels of IGF-1 stimulate excessive skeletal growth. Fortunately, the condition is rare because of early recognition and treatment of the adenoma.

Growth Hormone Excess in Adults

When GH excess occurs in adulthood or after the epiphyses of the long bones have fused, the condition is referred to as *acromegaly*. Acromegaly results from excess levels of GH that stimulate the hepatic secretion of IGF-1, which causes most of the clinical manifestations of acromegaly. The annual incidence of acromegaly is 3 to 4 cases per 1 million people, with a mean age at the time of diagnosis of 40 to 45 years.[1,7]

TABLE 41-2 **Differences Between Childhood and Adult-Onset Growth Hormone Deficiency**		
CHARACTERISTIC	**CHILDHOOD ONSET**	**ADULT ONSET**
Adult height	↓	NL
Body fat	↑	↑
Lean body mass	↓↓	↓
Bone mineral density	↓	NL, ↓
Insulin-like growth factor (IGF)-1	↓↓	NL, ↓
IGF binding protein-3	↓	NL
Low-density lipoprotein cholesterol	↑	↑
High-density lipoprotein cholesterol	NL, ↓	↓

NL, normal

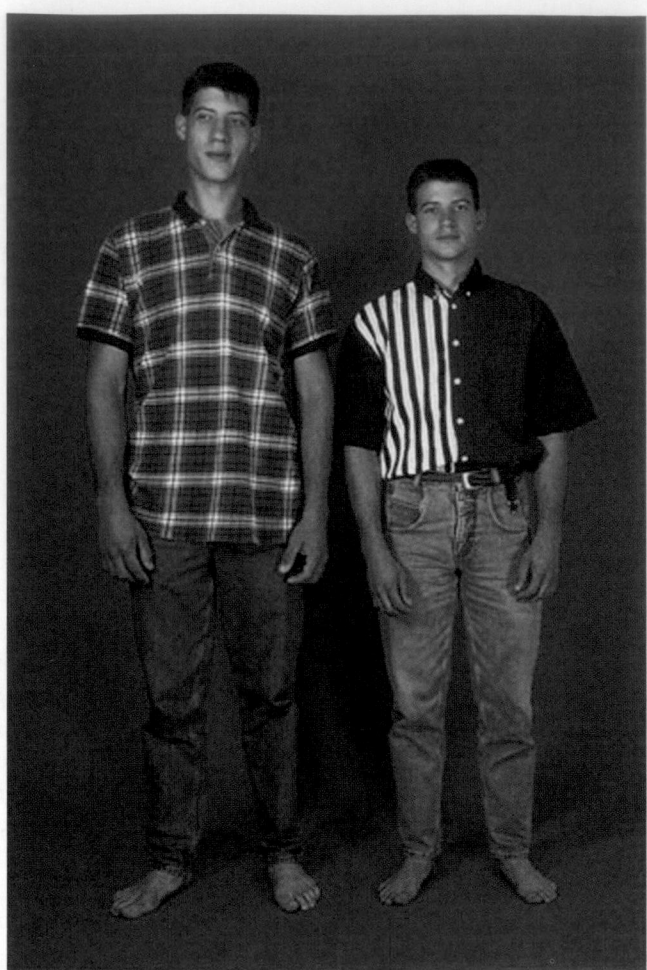

FIGURE 41-3 • Primary gigantism. A 22-year-old man with gigantism due to excess growth hormone is shown to the left of his identical twin. (From Gagel R. F., McCutcheon I. E. [1999]. Images in clinical medicine. *New England Journal of Medicine* 340, 524. Copyright © 2003. Massachusetts Medical Society.)

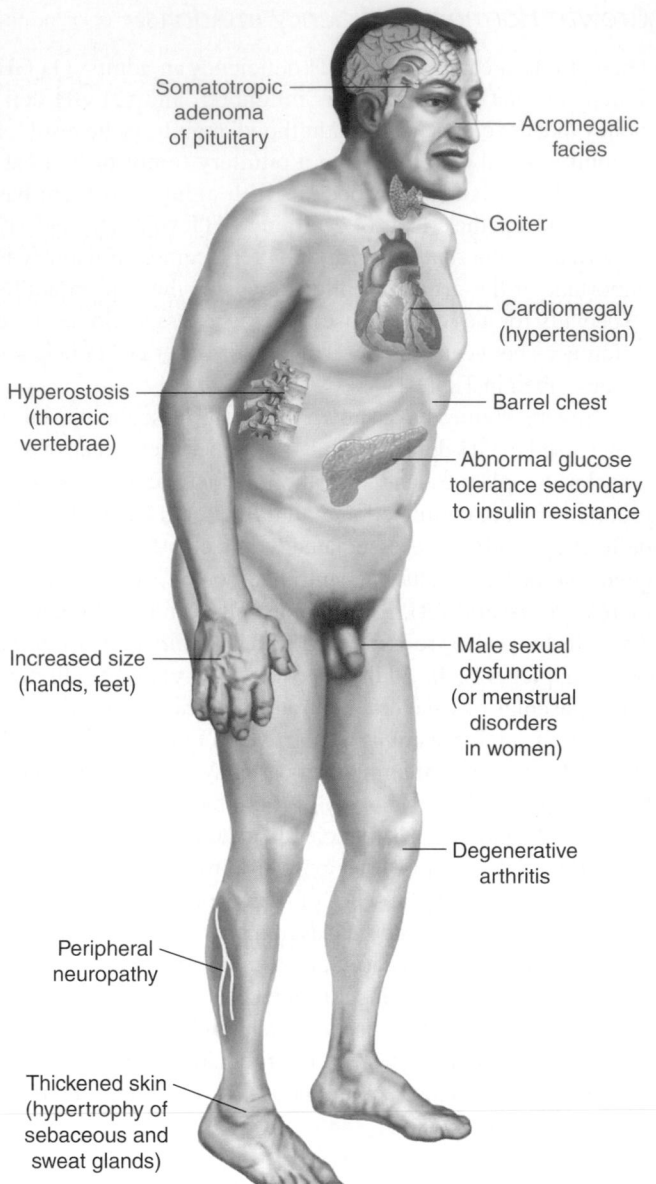

FIGURE 41-4 • Clinical manifestations of acromegaly.

The most common cause (95%) of acromegaly is a somatotrope adenoma. Approximately 75% of persons with acromegaly have a somatotrope macroadenoma at the time of diagnosis, and most of the remainder have microadenomas. The other causes of acromegaly (<5%) are excess secretion of GHRH by hypothalamic tumors, ectopic GHRH secretion by nonendocrine tumors such as carcinoid tumors or small cell lung cancers, and ectopic secretion of GH by nonendocrine tumors.[1,7]

The disorder usually has an insidious onset, and symptoms often are present for a considerable period before a diagnosis is made. When the production of excessive GH occurs after the epiphyses of the long bones have closed, as in the adult, the person cannot grow taller, but the soft tissues continue to grow. Enlargement of the small bones of the hands and feet and of the membranous bones of the face and skull results in a pronounced enlargement of the hands and feet, a broad and bulbous nose, a protruding lower jaw, and a slanting forehead (Fig. 41-4). The teeth become splayed, causing a disturbed bite and difficulty in chewing. The cartilaginous structures in the

larynx and respiratory tract also become enlarged, resulting in a deepening of the voice and tendency to develop bronchitis. Vertebral changes often lead to kyphosis, or hunchback. Bone overgrowth often leads to arthralgias and degenerative arthritis of the spine, hips, and knees. Virtually every organ of the body is increased in size. Enlargement of the heart and accelerated atherosclerosis may lead to an early death.

The metabolic effects of excess levels of GH include alterations in fat and carbohydrate metabolism. GH causes increased release of free fatty acids from adipose tissue, leading to increased concentration of free fatty acids in body fluids. In addition, GH enhances the formation of ketones and the use of free fatty acids for energy in preference to use of carbohydrates and proteins. GH exerts multiple effects on carbohydrate metabolism, including decreased glucose uptake by tissues such as skeletal muscle and adipose tissue, increased glucose production by the liver, and increased insulin secretion. Each of these changes results in GH-induced insulin resistance (see Chapter 42). This leads to glucose intolerance, which stimulates the beta cells of the pancreas to produce additional insulin. Long-term elevation of GH results in overstimulation of the beta cells, causing them literally to "burn out." Impaired glucose tolerance occurs in as much as 50% to 70% of persons with acromegaly; overt diabetes mellitus subsequently can result.

The pituitary gland is located in the pituitary fossa of the sphenoid bone (*i.e.,* sella turcica), which lies directly below the optic nerve. Enlargement of the pituitary gland eventually causes erosion of the surrounding bone, and because of its location, this can lead to headaches, visual field defects resulting from compression of the optic nerve (classically, bitemporal hemianopia), and palsies of cranial nerves III, IV, and VI. Compression of other pituitary structures can cause secondary hypothyroidism, hypogonadism, and adrenal insufficiency. The hypogonadism can result from direct damage to the hypothalamic or pituitary system, or indirectly because of hyperprolactinemia due to prevention of the prolactin inhibitory factor (dopamine) from reaching pituitary lactotropes (cells that secrete prolactin) because of damage by the pituitary tumor.

Other manifestations include excessive sweating with an unpleasant odor, oily skin, heat intolerance, moderate weight gain, muscle weakness and fatigue, menstrual irregularities, and decreased libido. Hypertension is relatively common. Sleep apnea syndrome is present in up to 90% of patients. The pathogenesis of the sleep apnea syndrome is obstructive in the majority of patients, due to increased pharyngeal soft tissue accumulation. Paresthesias may develop because of nerve entrapment and compression caused by excess soft tissue and accumulation of subcutaneous fluid (especially carpal tunnel syndrome). Acromegaly also is associated with an increased risk of colonic polyps and colorectal cancer. The mortality rate of patients with acromegaly is two to three times the expected rate, mostly from cardiovascular diseases and cancer. The cardiovascular disease results from the combination of cardiomyopathy, hypertension, insulin resistance and hyperinsulinemia, and hyperlipidemia.

Acromegaly often develops insidiously, and only a small number of persons seek medical care because of changes in appearance. The diagnosis of acromegaly is facilitated by the typical features of the disorder—enlargement of the hands and feet and coarsening of facial features. Laboratory tests to detect elevated levels of GH not suppressed by a glucose load are used to confirm the diagnosis. MRI scans can detect and localize the pituitary lesions. Because most of the effects of GH are mediated by IGF-1, IGF-1 levels may provide information about disease activity.

The treatment goals for acromegaly focus on the correction of metabolic abnormalities, and include normalization of the GH response to an oral glucose load; normalization of IGF-1 levels to age- and sex-matched control levels; removal or reduction of the tumor mass; relieving the central pressure effects; improvement of adverse clinical features; and normal-ization of the mortality rate.[7] Pituitary tumors can be removed surgically using the transsphenoidal approach or, if that is not possible, a transfrontal craniotomy. Radiation therapy may be used, but remission (reduction in GH levels) may not occur for several years after therapy. Radiation therapy also significantly increases the risk of hypopituitarism, leading to hypothyroidism, hypoadrenalism, and hypogonadism.

Medical therapy is usually given in an adjunctive role.[1,7] Somatostatin analogs (especially long-acting formulations of octreotide and lanreotide) produce feedback inhibition of GH, and are effective in the medical management of acromegaly. Dopamine agonists (*e.g.,* cabergoline) reduce GH levels and have been used with some success in the medical management of acromegaly. Growth hormone receptor antagonists (*e.g.,* pegvisomant) are analogs of human GH that have been structurally altered. GH receptor antagonists bind to GH receptors on the cell surfaces, where they block the binding of endogenous GH and thus interfere with GH signal transduction. This results in a decrease in serum IGF-1 levels in more than 90% of patients.[7]

 ## Isosexual Precocious Puberty

Isosexual precocious puberty is defined as early activation of the hypothalamic-pituitary-gonadal axis, resulting in the development of appropriate sexual characteristics and fertility.[8,9] Classically, sexual development was considered precocious and warranting investigation when it occurred before 8 years of age for girls and before 9 years of age for boys. However, these criteria were revised recently based on an office pediatric study of more than 17,000 American girls.[10] Precocious puberty is now defined as the appearance of secondary sexual development before the age of 7 years in white girls and 6 years in African American girls.[9] In boys of both races, the lower age limit remains 9 years; however, it is recognized that puberty can develop earlier in boys with obesity (an increasingly common problem).[9] Precocious sexual development may be idiopathic or may be caused by gonadal, adrenal, or hypothalamic disease.[8,9] Benign and malignant tumors of the central nervous system (CNS) can cause precocious puberty. These tumors are thought to remove the inhibitory influences normally exerted on the hypothalamus during childhood. CNS tumors are found more often in boys with precocious puberty than in girls. In girls, most cases are idiopathic.

Diagnosis of precocious puberty is based on physical findings of early thelarche (*i.e.,* beginning of breast development), adrenarche (*i.e.,* beginning of augmented adrenal androgen production), and menarche (*i.e.,* beginning of menstrual function) in girls. The most common sign in boys is early genital enlargement. Radiologic findings may indicate advanced bone age. Persons with precocious puberty usually are tall for their age as children but short as adults because of the early closure of the epiphyses. MRI or CT should be used to exclude intracranial lesions.

Depending on the cause of precocious puberty, the treatment may involve surgery, medication, or no treatment. Administration of a long-acting GnRH agonist results in a decrease in pituitary responsiveness to GnRH, leading to decreased secretion of gonadotropic hormones and sex steroids (*i.e.*, due to down-regulation of GnRH receptors). Parents often need education, support, and anticipatory guidance in dealing with their feelings and the child's physical needs and in relating to a child who appears older than his or her years.[9]

IN SUMMARY, pituitary tumors can result in deficiencies or excesses of pituitary hormones. Hypopituitarism, which is characterized by a decreased secretion of pituitary hormones, is a condition that affects many of the other endocrine systems. Depending on the extent of the disorder, it can result in decreased levels of GH, thyroid hormones, adrenal corticosteroid hormones, and testosterone in the male and estrogens and progesterone in the female.

A number of hormones are essential for normal body growth and maturation, including GH, insulin, thyroid hormone, and androgens. GH exerts its growth effects through IGF-1. GH also exerts an effect on metabolism and is produced in the adult and in the child. Its metabolic effects include a decrease in peripheral use of carbohydrates and an increased mobilization and use of fatty acids.

In children, alterations in growth include short stature, isosexual precocious puberty, and tall stature. Short stature is a condition in which the attained height is well below the third percentile or the linear growth velocity is below normal for a child's age or sex. Short stature can occur as a variant of normal growth (*i.e.*, genetic short stature or constitutional short stature) or as the result of endocrine disorders, chronic illness, malnutrition, emotional disturbances, or chromosomal disorders. Short stature resulting from GH deficiency can be treated with human GH preparations. In adults, GH deficiency represents a deficiency carried over from childhood or one that develops during adulthood as the result of a pituitary tumor or its treatment. GH levels also can decline with aging, and there has been interest in the effects of declining GH levels in the elderly (described as the *somatopause*).

Tall stature refers to the condition in which children are tall for their age and sex. It can occur as a variant of normal growth (*i.e.*, genetic tall stature or constitutional tall stature) or as the result of a chromosomal abnormality or GH excess. GH excess in adults results in acromegaly, which involves proliferation of bone, cartilage, and soft tissue along with the metabolic effects of excessive hormone levels. Isosexual precocious puberty defines a condition of early activation of the hypothalamic-pituitary-gonadal axis (*i.e.*, before 6 years of age in African American girls and 7 years in white girls, and before 9 years of age in boys of both races), resulting in the development of appropriate sexual characteristics and fertility. It causes tall stature during childhood but results in short stature in adulthood because of the early closure of the epiphyses. ■

THYROID DISORDERS

After completing this section of the chapter, you should be able to meet the following objectives:

■ Characterize the synthesis, transport, and regulation of thyroid hormone.

■ Diagram the hypothalamic-pituitary-thyroid feedback system.

■ Describe tests in the diagnosis and management of thyroid disorders.

■ Relate the functions of thyroid hormone to hypothyroidism and hyperthyroidism.

■ Describe the effects of congenital hypothyroidism.

■ Characterize the manifestations and treatment of myxedematous coma and thyroid storm.

Control of Thyroid Function

The thyroid gland is a shield-shaped structure located immediately below the larynx in the anterior middle portion of the neck (Fig. 41-5A). It is composed of a large number of tiny, saclike structures called *follicles* (see Fig. 41-5B). These are the functional units of the thyroid. Each follicle is formed by a single layer of epithelial (follicular) cells and is filled with a secretory substance called *colloid*, which consists largely of a glycoprotein–iodine complex called *thyroglobulin*.

The thyroglobulin that fills the thyroid follicles is a large glycoprotein molecule that contains 140 tyrosine amino acids. In the process of thyroid synthesis, iodine is attached to these tyrosine molecules. Both thyroglobulin and iodide are secreted into the colloid of the follicle by the follicular cells.

The thyroid is remarkably efficient in its use of iodide. A daily absorption of 150 to 200 μg of dietary iodide is sufficient to form normal quantities of thyroid hormone. In the process of removing it from the blood and storing it for future use, iodide is pumped into the follicular cells against a concentration gradient. Iodide (I^-) is transported across the basement membrane of the thyroid cells by an intrinsic membrane protein called the Na^+/I symporter (NIS).[11] At the apical border, a second I^- transport protein called *pendrin* moves iodine into the colloid, where it is involved in hormonogenesis. The NIS derives its energy from Na^+/K^+-ATPase, which drives the process. As a result, the concentration of iodide in the normal thyroid gland is approximately 40 times that in the blood.

The NIS is stimulated by both TSH and the TSH receptor–stimulating antibody found in Graves disease (to be discussed). Pendrin, encoded by the Pendred syndrome gene (*PDS*), is a transporter of chloride and iodide. Mutations in the *PDS* gene have been found in patients with goiter and congenital deafness (Pendred syndrome).

Once inside the follicle, most of the iodide is oxidized by the enzyme thyroid peroxidase (TPO) in a reaction that facilitates combination with a tyrosine molecule to form monoiodotyrosine

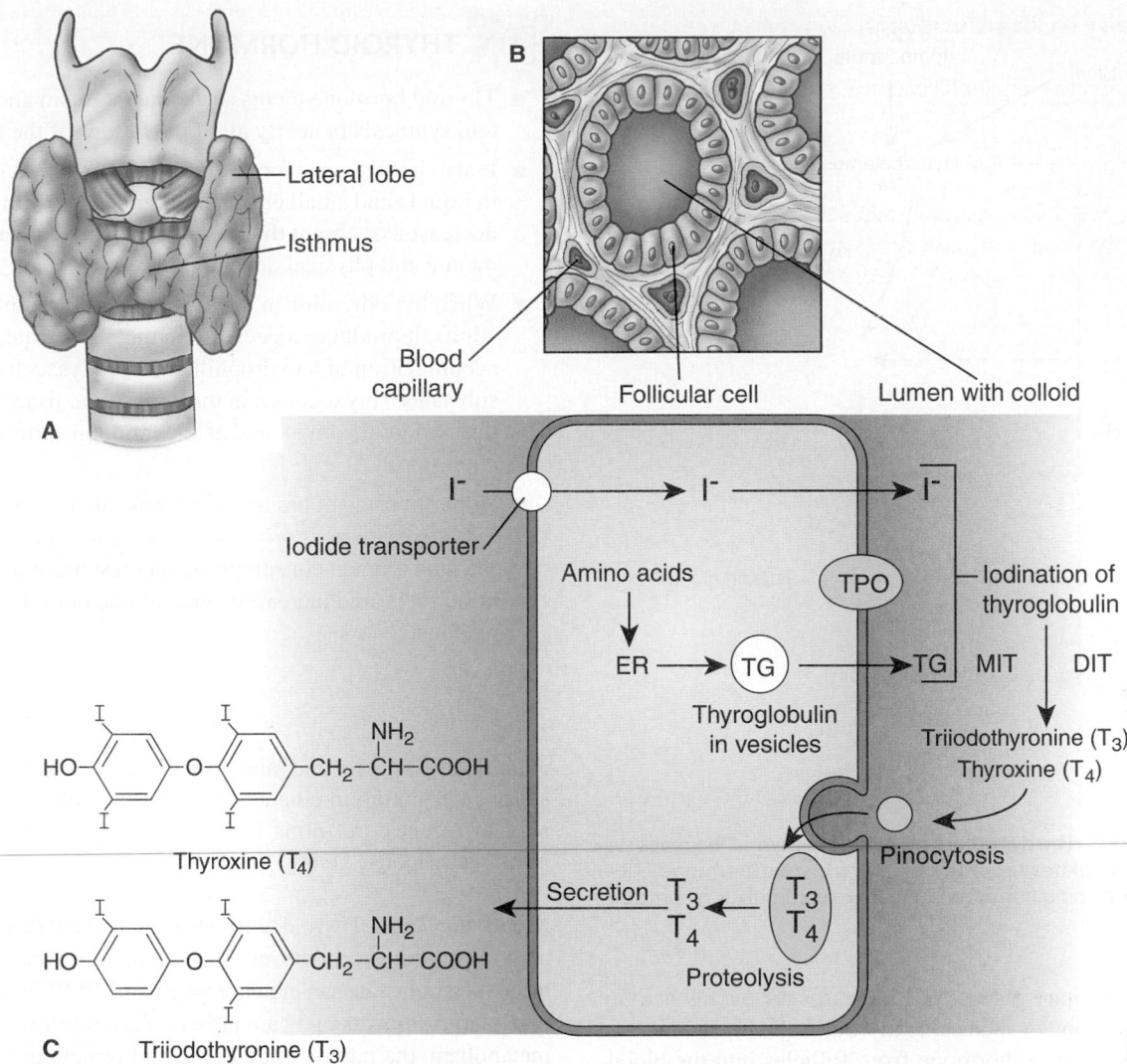

FIGURE 41-5 • (A) The thyroid gland. **(B)** Microscopic structure of thyroid follicles. **(C)** Cellular mechanisms for transport of iodide (I⁻), oxidation of I⁻ by thyroperoxidase (TPO), coupling of oxidized I⁻ with thyroglobulin to form thyroid hormones, and movement of T_3 and T_4 into the follicular cell by pinocytosis and release into the blood.

(MIT) and then diiodotyrosine (DIT). Two diiodotyrosine residues are coupled to form thyroxine (T_4), or a monoiodotyrosine and a diiodotyrosine are coupled to form triiodothyronine (T_3). Only T_4 (90%) and T_3 (10%) are released into the circulation (see Fig. 41-5C). There is evidence that T_3 is the active form of the hormone and that T_4 is converted to T_3 before it can act physiologically.

Thyroid hormones are bound to thyroxine-binding globulin (TBG) and other plasma proteins for transport in the blood. Only the free hormone enters cells and regulates the pituitary feedback mechanism. Protein-bound thyroid hormone forms a large reservoir that is slowly drawn on as free thyroid hormone is needed. There are three major thyroid-binding proteins: TBG, transthyretin (formerly known as thyroxine-binding prealbumin [TBPA]), and albumin. More than 99% of T_4 and T_3 is carried in the bound form. TBG carries approximately 70% of T_4 and

T_3; transthyretin binds approximately 10% of circulating T_4 and lesser amounts of T_3; and albumin binds approximately 15% of circulating T_4 and T_3.

A number of disease conditions and pharmacologic agents can decrease the amount of binding protein in the plasma or influence the binding of hormone. Congenital TBG deficiency is an X-linked trait that occurs in 1 of every 5000 live births. Glucocorticoid medications and systemic disease conditions such as protein malnutrition, nephrotic syndrome, and cirrhosis decrease TBG concentrations. Medications such as phenytoin, salicylates, and diazepam can affect the binding of thyroid hormone to normal concentrations of binding proteins.

The secretion of thyroid hormone is regulated by the hypothalamic-pituitary-thyroid feedback system (Fig. 41-6). In this system, thyrotropin-releasing hormone (TRH), which is produced by the hypothalamus, controls the release of TSH from

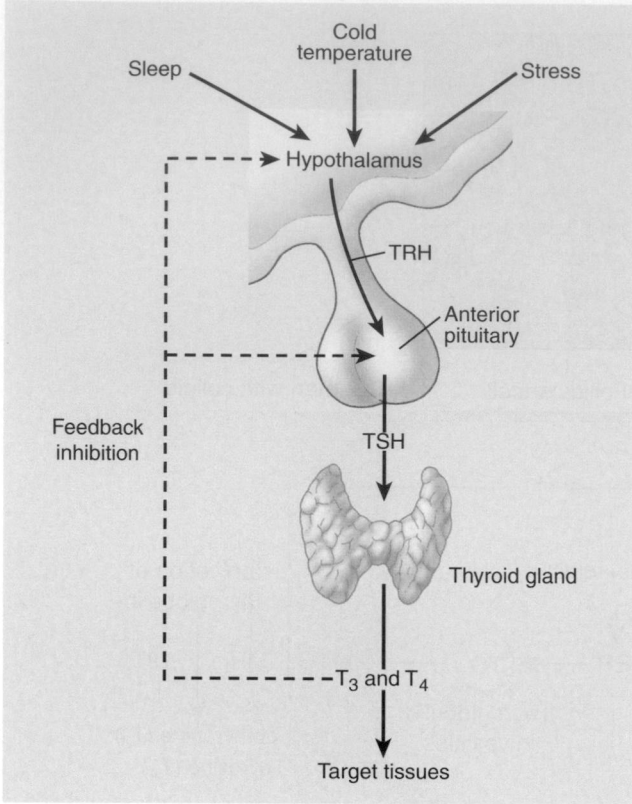

FIGURE 41-6 • The hypothalamic-pituitary-thyroid feedback system, which regulates the body levels of thyroid hormone. TRH, thyrotropin-releasing hormone, TSH, thyroid-stimulating hormone.

the anterior pituitary gland. TSH increases the overall activity of the thyroid gland by increasing thyroglobulin breakdown and the release of thyroid hormone from follicles into the bloodstream, activating the iodide pump (by increasing NIS activity), increasing the oxidation of iodide and the coupling of iodide to tyrosine, and increasing the number and the size of the follicle cells. The effect of TSH on the release of thyroid hormones occurs within approximately 30 minutes, but the other effects require days or weeks.

Increased levels of thyroid hormone act in the feedback inhibition of TRH or TSH. High levels of iodide (*e.g.,* from iodide-containing cough syrup or kelp tablets) also cause a temporary decrease in thyroid activity that lasts for several weeks, probably through a direct inhibition of TSH on the thyroid. Cold exposure is one of the strongest stimuli for increased thyroid hormone production and probably is mediated through TRH from the hypothalamus. Various emotional reactions also can affect the output of TRH and TSH and therefore indirectly affect secretion of thyroid hormones.

Actions of Thyroid Hormone

All the major organs in the body are affected by altered levels of thyroid hormone. Thyroid hormone has two major functions: it increases metabolism and protein synthesis, and it is necessary for growth and development in children, including

🖐 THYROID HORMONE

■ Thyroid hormone increases the metabolism and protein synthesis in nearly all of the tissues of the body.

■ It also is necessary for brain development and growth in infants and small children. Infants born with decreased or absent thyroid function have impaired mental and physical development.

■ When hypothyroidism occurs in older children or adults, it produces a decrease in metabolic rate, an accumulation of a hydrophilic mucopolysaccharide substance (myxedema) in the connective tissues throughout the body, and an elevation in serum cholesterol.

■ Hyperthyroidism has an effect opposite that of hypothyroidism. It produces an increase in metabolic rate and oxygen consumption, increased use of metabolic fuels, and increased sympathetic nervous system responsiveness.

mental development and attainment of sexual maturity. These actions are mainly mediated by T_3. In the cell, T_3 binds to a nuclear receptor, resulting in transcription of specific thyroid hormone response genes.[11]

Metabolic Rate. Thyroid hormone increases the metabolism of all body tissues except the retinas, spleen, testes, and lungs. The basal metabolic rate can increase by 60% to 100% above normal when large amounts of T_4 are present. As a result of this higher metabolism, the rate of glucose, fat, and protein use increases. Lipids are mobilized from adipose tissue, and the catabolism of cholesterol by the liver is increased. Blood levels of cholesterol are decreased in hyperthyroidism and increased in hypothyroidism. Muscle proteins are broken down and used as fuel, probably accounting for some of the muscle fatigue that occurs with hyperthyroidism. The absorption of glucose from the gastrointestinal tract is increased. Because vitamins are essential parts of metabolic enzymes and coenzymes, an increase in metabolic rate "speeds up" the use of vitamins and tends to cause vitamin deficiency.

Cardiovascular Function. Cardiovascular and respiratory functions are strongly affected by thyroid function. With an increase in metabolism, there is a rise in oxygen consumption and production of metabolic end products, with an accompanying increase in vasodilation. Blood flow to the skin, in particular, is augmented as a means of dissipating the body heat that results from the higher metabolic rate. Blood volume, cardiac output, and ventilation all are increased as a means of maintaining blood flow and oxygen delivery to body tissues. Heart rate and cardiac contractility are enhanced as a means of maintaining the needed cardiac output. On the other hand, blood pressure is likely to change little because the increase in vasodilation tends to offset the increase in cardiac output.

Gastrointestinal Function. Thyroid hormone enhances gastrointestinal function, causing an increase in motility and production of gastrointestinal secretions that often results in diarrhea. An increase in appetite and food intake accompanies the higher metabolic rate that occurs with increased thyroid hormone levels. At the same time, weight loss occurs because of the increased use of calories.

Neuromuscular Effects. Thyroid hormone has marked effects on neural control of muscle function and tone. Slight elevations in hormone levels cause skeletal muscles to react more vigorously, and a drop in hormone levels causes muscles to react more sluggishly. In the hyperthyroid state, a fine muscle tremor is present. The cause of this tremor is unknown, but it may represent an increased sensitivity of the neural synapses in the spinal cord that control muscle tone. In the infant, thyroid hormone is necessary for normal brain development. The hormone enhances cerebration; in the hyperthyroid state, it causes extreme nervousness, anxiety, and difficulty in sleeping.

Evidence suggests a strong interaction between thyroid hormone and the sympathetic nervous system. Many of the signs and symptoms of hyperthyroidism suggest overactivity of the sympathetic division of the autonomic nervous system, such as tachycardia, palpitations, and sweating. Tremor, restlessness, anxiety, and diarrhea also may reflect autonomic nervous system imbalances. Drugs that block sympathetic activity have proved to be valuable adjuncts in the treatment of hyperthyroidism because of their ability to relieve some of these undesirable symptoms.

Tests of Thyroid Function

Various tests aid in the diagnosis of thyroid disorders.[11,12] Measures of T_3, T_4, and TSH have been made available through immunoassay methods. The free T_4 test measures the unbound portion of T_4 that is free to enter cells to produce its effects. TSH levels are used to differentiate between primary and secondary thyroid disorders. T_3, T_4, and free T_4 levels are low in primary hypothyroidism, and the TSH level is elevated. The assessment of thyroid autoantibodies (*e.g.,* anti-TPO antibodies in Hashimoto thyroiditis) is important in the diagnostic work-up and consequent follow-up of patients with thyroid disorders.

The radioiodine (^{123}I) uptake test measures the ability of the thyroid gland to remove and concentrate iodine from the blood. Thyroid scans (^{123}I, ^{99m}Tc-pertechnetate) can be used to detect thyroid nodules and determine the functional activity of the thyroid gland. Ultrasonography can be used to differentiate cystic from solid thyroid lesions, and CT and MRI scans are used to demonstrate tracheal compression or impingement on other neighboring structures. Fine-needle aspiration biopsy of a thyroid nodule has proved to be the best method for differentiation of benign from malignant thyroid disease.

Alterations in Thyroid Function

An alteration in thyroid function can represent a hypofunctional or a hyperfunctional state. The manifestations of these two altered states are summarized in Table 41-3. Disorders of the

TABLE 41-3 Manifestations of Hypothyroid and Hyperthyroid States

LEVEL OF ORGANIZATION	HYPOTHYROIDISM	HYPERTHYROIDISM
Basal metabolic rate	Decreased	Increased
Sensitivity to catecholamines	Decreased	Increased
General features	Myxedematous features Deep voice Impaired growth (child)	Exophthalmos (in Graves disease) Lid lag Accelerated growth (child)
Blood cholesterol levels	Increased	Decreased
General behavior	Mental retardation (infant) Mental and physical sluggishness Somnolence	Restlessness, irritability, anxiety Hyperkinesis Wakefulness
Cardiovascular function	Decreased cardiac output Bradycardia	Increased cardiac output Tachycardia and palpitations
Gastrointestinal function	Constipation Decreased appetite	Diarrhea Increased appetite
Respiratory function	Hypoventilation	Dyspnea
Muscle tone and reflexes	Decreased	Increased, with tremor and twitching
Temperature tolerance	Cold intolerance	Heat intolerance
Skin and hair	Decreased sweating Coarse and dry skin and hair	Increased sweating Thin and silky skin and hair
Weight	Gain	Loss

thyroid may be due to a congenital defect in thyroid development, or they may develop later in life, with a gradual or sudden onset.

Goiter is an increase in the size of the thyroid gland. It can occur in hypothyroid, euthyroid, and hyperthyroid states. Goiters may be diffuse, involving the entire gland without evidence of nodularity, or they may contain nodules. Diffuse goiters usually become nodular. Goiters may be toxic, producing signs of extreme hyperthyroidism, or thyrotoxicosis, or they may be nontoxic. Diffuse nontoxic and multinodular goiters are the result of compensatory hypertrophy and hyperplasia of follicular epithelium from some derangement that impairs thyroid hormone output.

The degree of thyroid enlargement usually is proportional to the extent and duration of thyroid deficiency. Multinodular goiters produce the largest thyroid enlargements. When sufficiently enlarged, they may compress the esophagus and trachea, causing difficulty in swallowing, a choking sensation, and inspiratory stridor. Such lesions also may compress the superior vena cava, producing distention of the veins of the neck and upper extremities, edema of the eyelids and conjunctiva, and syncope with coughing.

Hypothyroidism

Hypothyroidism can occur as a congenital or an acquired defect. Congenital hypothyroidism develops prenatally and is present at birth. Acquired hypothyroidism develops later in life because of primary disease of the thyroid gland or secondary to disorders of hypothalamic or pituitary origin.

 *Congenital Hypothyroidism*

Congenital hypothyroidism is a common cause of preventable mental retardation. It affects approximately 1 of 5000 infants. Hypothyroidism in the infant may result from a congenital lack of the thyroid gland or from abnormal biosynthesis of thyroid hormone or deficient TSH secretion. With congenital lack of the thyroid gland, the infant usually appears normal and functions normally at birth because hormones have been supplied in utero by the mother. The manifestations of untreated congenital hypothyroidism are referred to as *cretinism*. However, the term does not apply to the normally developing infant in whom replacement thyroid hormone therapy was instituted shortly after birth.

Thyroid hormone is essential for normal growth and brain development, almost half of which occurs during the first 6 months of life. If untreated, congenital hypothyroidism causes mental retardation and impairs physical growth. Long-term studies show that closely monitored T_4 supplementation begun in the first 6 weeks of life results in normal intelligence. Fortunately, neonatal screening tests have been instituted to detect congenital hypothyroidism during early infancy. Screening usually is done in the hospital nursery. In this test, a drop of blood is taken from the infant's heel and analyzed for T_4 and TSH.

Transient congenital hypothyroidism has been recognized more frequently since the introduction of neonatal screening (accounting for approximately 25% of cases detected by screening). It is characterized by high TSH levels and low or normal thyroid hormone levels. The fetal and infant thyroids are sensitive to iodine excess. Iodine crosses the placenta and mammary glands and is readily absorbed by infant skin. Transient hypothyroidism may be caused by maternal or infant exposure to substances such as povidone-iodine used as a disinfectant (*i.e.*, vaginal douche or skin disinfectant, in the nursery). Antithyroid drugs such as propylthiouracil and methimazole can cross the placenta and block fetal thyroid function.

Congenital hypothyroidism is treated by hormone replacement. Evidence indicates that it is important to normalize T_4 levels as rapidly as possible because a delay is accompanied by poorer psychomotor and mental development. Dosage levels are adjusted as the child grows. Infants with transient hypothyroidism usually can have the replacement therapy withdrawn at 6 to 12 months. When early and adequate treatment regimens are followed, the risk of mental retardation in infants detected by screening programs essentially is nonexistent.

Acquired Hypothyroidism and Myxedema

Hypothyroidism in older children and adults causes a general slowing down of metabolic processes and myxedema. Myxedema implies the presence of a nonpitting mucous type of edema caused by an accumulation of a hydrophilic mucopolysaccharide substance in the connective tissues throughout the body. The hypothyroid state may be mild, with only a few signs and symptoms, or it may progress to a life-threatening condition called *myxedematous coma.* It can result from destruction or dysfunction of the thyroid gland (*i.e.*, primary hypothyroidism), or it can be a secondary disorder caused by impaired pituitary function or as a tertiary disorder caused by a hypothalamic dysfunction.

Primary hypothyroidism is much more common than secondary (and tertiary) hypothyroidism. It may result from thyroidectomy (*i.e.*, surgical removal) or ablation of the gland with radiation. Certain goitrogenic agents, such as lithium carbonate (used in the treatment of manic-depressive states), and the antithyroid drugs propylthiouracil and methimazole in continuous dosage can block hormone synthesis and produce hypothyroidism with goiter. Large amounts of iodine (*i.e.*, ingestion of kelp tablets or iodide-containing cough syrups, or administration of iodide-containing radiographic contrast media or the cardiac drug amiodarone, which contains 75 mg of iodine per 200-mg tablet) also can block thyroid hormone production and cause goiter, particularly in persons with autoimmune thyroid disease. Iodine deficiency, which can cause goiter and hypothyroidism, is rare in the United States because of the widespread use of iodized salt and other iodide sources. However, iodine deficiency affects an estimated 100 million people worldwide.

The most common cause of hypothyroidism is Hashimoto thyroiditis, an autoimmune disorder in which the thyroid gland may be totally destroyed by an immunologic process.[13] It is the major cause of goiter and hypothyroidism in children and adults. Hashimoto thyroiditis is predominantly a disease of women, with a female-to-male ratio of 5:1. The course of the disease varies. At the onset, only a goiter may be present. In time, hypothyroidism usually becomes evident. Although the disorder usually causes hypothyroidism, a hyperthyroid state may develop midcourse in the disease. The transient hyperthyroid state is caused by leakage of preformed thyroid hormone from damaged cells of the gland. Subacute thyroiditis, which can occur in up to 10% of pregnancies postpartum (postpartum thyroiditis), also can result in hypothyroidism.

Hypothyroidism may affect almost all body functions. The manifestations of the disorder are related largely to two factors: the hypometabolic state resulting from thyroid hormone deficiency, and myxedematous involvement of body tissues. The hypometabolic state associated with hypothyroidism is characterized by a gradual onset of weakness and fatigue, a tendency to gain weight despite a loss of appetite, and cold intolerance (Fig. 41-7). As the condition progresses, the skin becomes dry and rough and acquires a pale yellowish cast, which primarily results from carotene deposition, and the hair becomes coarse and brittle. The face becomes puffy with edematous eyelids, and there is thinning of the outer third of the eyebrows. Fluid may collect in almost any serous cavity and in the middle ear, giving rise to conductive deafness. Gastrointestinal motility is decreased, producing constipation, flatulence, and abdominal distention. Delayed relaxation of deep tendon reflexes and bradycardia are sometimes noted. Central nervous system involvement is manifested in mental dullness, lethargy, and impaired memory.

Although the myxedemous fluid is usually most obvious in the face, it can collect in the interstitial spaces of almost any body structure and is responsible for many of the manifestations of the severe hypothyroid state. The tongue is often enlarged, and the voice becomes hoarse and husky. Carpal tunnel and other entrapment syndromes are common, as is impairment of muscle function with stiffness, cramps, and pain. Pericardial or pleural effusion may develop. Mucopolysaccharide deposits in the heart cause generalized cardiac dilation, bradycardia, and other signs of altered cardiac function. The signs and symptoms of hypothyroidism are summarized in Table 41-3.

Diagnosis of hypothyroidism is based on history, physical examination, and laboratory tests. A low serum T_4, and elevated TSH levels are characteristic of primary hypothyroidism. The tests for antithyroid antibodies should be done when Hashimoto thyroiditis is suspected (anti-TPO antibody titers is the preferred test).

Hypothyroidism is treated by replacement therapy with synthetic preparations of T_3 or T_4. Most people are treated with T_4. Serum TSH levels are used to estimate the adequacy of T_4 replacement therapy. When the TSH level is normalized, the T_4 dosage is considered satisfactory (for primary hypothyroidism only). A "go-low and go-slow" approach should be considered in the treatment of elderly with hypothyroidism because of the risk of inducing acute coronary syndromes in the susceptible individual.

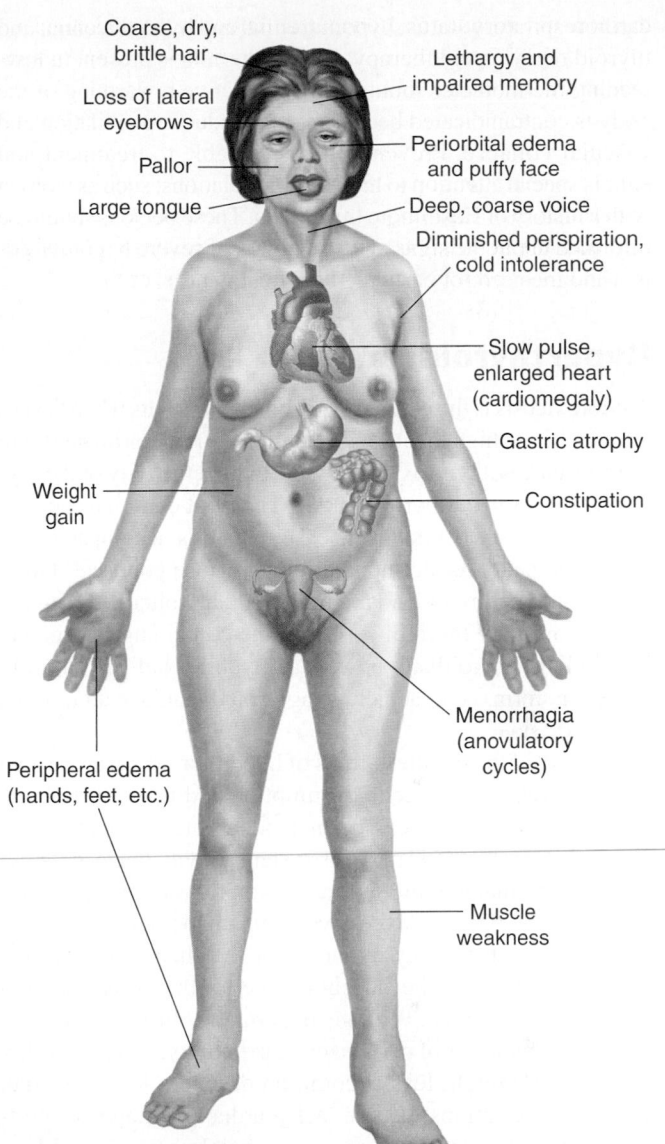

FIGURE 41-7 • Clinical manifestations of hypothyroidism.

Myxedematous Coma

Myxedematous coma is a life-threatening, end-stage expression of hypothyroidism. It is characterized by coma, hypothermia, cardiovascular collapse, hypoventilation, and severe metabolic disorders that include hyponatremia, hypoglycemia, and lactic acidosis. The pathophysiology of myxedema coma involves three major aspects: (1) carbon dioxide retention and hypoxia, (2) fluid and electrolyte imbalance, and (3) hypothermia.[11] It occurs most often in elderly women who have chronic hypothyroidism from a spectrum of causes. The fact that it occurs more frequently in winter months suggests that cold exposure may be a precipitating factor. The severely hypothyroid person is unable to metabolize sedatives, analgesics, and anesthetic drugs, and buildup of these agents may precipitate coma.

Treatment includes aggressive management of precipitating factors; supportive therapy such as management of cardiorespiratory status, hyponatremia, and hypoglycemia; and thyroid replacement therapy. If hypothermia is present (a low-reading thermometer should be used), active rewarming of the body is contraindicated because it may induce vasodilation and vascular collapse. Prevention is preferable to treatment and entails special attention to high-risk populations, such as women with a history of Hashimoto thyroiditis. These persons should be informed about the signs and symptoms of severe hypothyroidism and the need for early medical treatment.

Hyperthyroidism

Thyrotoxicosis is the clinical syndrome that results when tissues are exposed to high levels of circulating thyroid hormone.[11,14] In most instances, thyrotoxicosis is due to hyperactivity of the thyroid gland, or hyperthyroidism.[11,14] The most common cause of hyperthyroidism is Graves disease, which is accompanied by ophthalmopathy (or dermopathy) and diffuse goiter.[11,14] Other causes of hyperthyroidism are multinodular goiter, adenoma of the thyroid, and thyroiditis.[11,14] Iodine-containing agents can induce hyperthyroidism as well as hypothyroidism. Thyroid crisis, or storm, is an acutely exaggerated manifestation of the thyrotoxic state.

Many of the manifestations of hyperthyroidism are related to the increase in oxygen consumption and use of metabolic fuels associated with the hypermetabolic state, as well as to the increase in sympathetic nervous system activity that occurs.[11,14] The fact that many of the signs and symptoms of hyperthyroidism resemble those of excessive sympathetic nervous system activity suggests that thyroid hormone may heighten the sensitivity of the body to the catecholamines or that it may act as a pseudocatecholamine. With the hypermetabolic state, there are frequent complaints of nervousness, irritability, and fatigability (Fig. 41-8). Weight loss is common despite a large appetite. Other manifestations include tachycardia, palpitations, shortness of breath, excessive sweating, muscle cramps, and heat intolerance. The person appears restless and has a fine muscle tremor. Even in persons without exophthalmos (*i.e.,* bulging of the eyeballs seen in ophthalmopathy), there is an abnormal retraction of the eyelids and infrequent blinking such that they appear to be staring. The hair and skin usually are thin and have a silky appearance. About 15% of elderly individuals with new-onset atrial fibrillation have thyrotoxicosis.[14] The signs and symptoms of hyperthyroidism are summarized in Table 41-3.

The treatment of hyperthyroidism is directed toward reducing the level of thyroid hormone. This can be accomplished with eradication of the thyroid gland with radioactive iodine, through surgical removal of part or all of the gland, or the use of drugs that decrease thyroid function and thereby the effect of thyroid hormone on the peripheral tissues. Eradication of the thyroid with radioactive iodine is used more frequently than surgery. The β-adrenergic blocking drugs (propranolol, metoprolol, atenolol, and nadolol are preferred) are administered to block the effects of the hyperthyroid state on sympathetic nervous system function. They are given in conjunction with antithyroid drugs such as propylthiouracil and methimazole. These

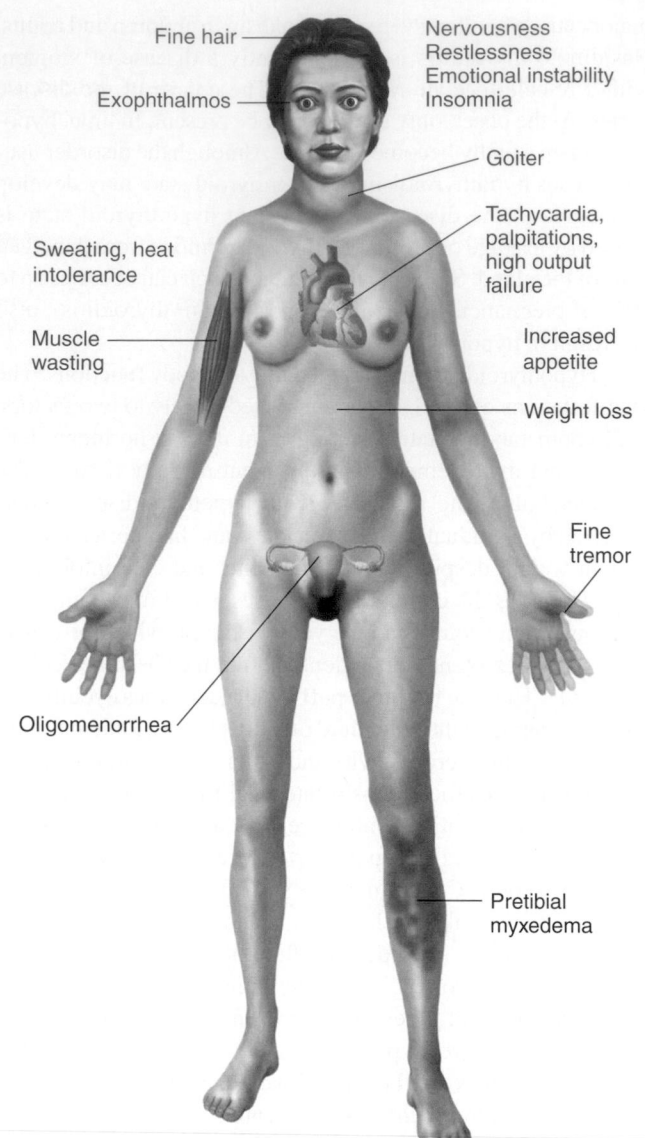

FIGURE 41-8 • Clinical manifestations of hyperthyroidism.

drugs prevent the thyroid gland from converting iodine to its organic (hormonal) form and block the conversion of T_4 to T_3 in the tissues (propylthiouracil only).

Graves Disease

Graves disease is a state of hyperthyroidism, goiter, and ophthalmopathy (or, less commonly, dermopathy).[11,14,15] The onset usually is between the ages of 20 and 40 years, and women are five times more likely to develop the disease than men. Graves' disease is an autoimmune disorder characterized by abnormal stimulation of the thyroid gland by thyroid-stimulating antibodies (TSH-receptor antibodies) that act through the normal TSH receptors. It may be associated with other autoimmune disorders such as myasthenia gravis and pernicious anemia. The disease is associated with human leukocyte antigen (HLA)-DR3 and HLA-B8, and a familial tendency is evident.

The ophthalmopathy, which occurs in up to one third of persons with Graves disease, is thought to result from a cytokine-mediated activation of fibroblasts in orbital tissue behind the eyeball.[11,14-16] Humoral autoimmunity also is important; an ophthalmic immunoglobulin may exacerbate lymphocytic infiltration of the extraocular muscles. The ophthalmopathy of Graves disease can cause severe eye problems, including tethering of the extraocular muscles resulting in diplopia; involvement of the optic nerve, with some visual loss; and corneal ulceration because the lids do not close over the protruding eyeball (due to the exophthalmos). The ophthalmopathy usually tends to stabilize after treatment of the hyperthyroidism. However, ophthalmopathy can worsen acutely after radioiodine treatment. Some physicians prescribe glucocorticoids for several weeks surrounding the radioiodine treatment if the person had signs of ophthalmopathy. Others do not to use radioiodine therapy under these circumstances, but prefer antithyroid therapy with drugs (which may decrease the immune activation in the condition). Unfortunately, not all of the ocular changes are reversible with treatment. Ophthalmopathy also can be aggravated by smoking, which should be strongly discouraged. Figure 41-9 shows a woman with Graves disease.

Thyroid Storm

Thyroid storm, or crisis, is an extreme and life-threatening form of thyrotoxicosis, rarely seen today because of improved diagnosis and treatment methods.[11,14] When it does occur, it is seen most often in undiagnosed cases or in persons with hyperthyroidism who have not been adequately treated. It often is precipitated by stress such as an infection (usually respiratory), by diabetic ketoacidosis, by physical or emotional trauma, or by manipulation of a hyperactive thyroid gland during thyroidectomy. Thyroid storm is manifested by a very high fever, extreme cardiovascular effects (*i.e.*, tachycardia, congestive failure, and angina), and severe CNS effects (*i.e.*, agitation, restlessness, and delirium). The mortality rate is high.

Thyroid storm requires rapid diagnosis and implementation of treatment. Peripheral cooling is initiated with cold packs and a cooling mattress. For cooling to be effective, the shivering response must be prevented. General supportive measures to replace fluids, glucose, and electrolytes are essential during the hypermetabolic state. A β-adrenergic blocking drug, such as propranolol, is given to block the undesirable effects of T_4 on cardiovascular function. Glucocorticoids are used to correct the relative adrenal insufficiency resulting from the stress imposed by the hyperthyroid state and to inhibit the peripheral conversion of T_4 to T_3. Propylthiouracil or methimazole may be given to block thyroid synthesis. Aspirin increases the level of free thyroid hormones by displacing the hormones from their protein carriers, and should not be used during thyroid storm.

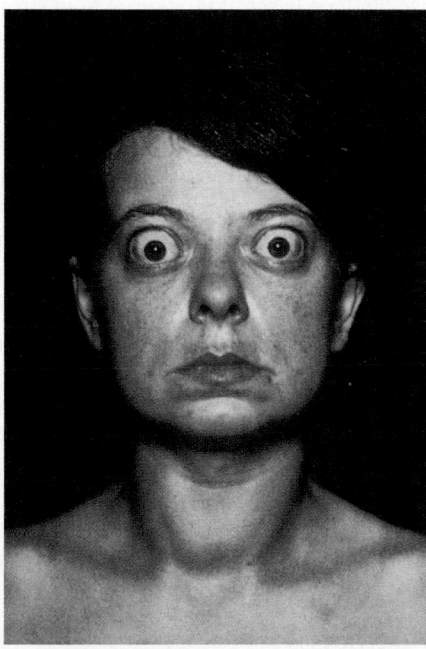

FIGURE 41-9 • Graves disease. A young woman with hyperthyroidism presented with a mass in the neck and exophthalmos. (From Merino M., Quezado M., Rubin E., et al. [2008]. The endocrine system. In Rubin E., Strayer D. [Eds.], *Rubin's pathology: Clinicopathologic foundations of medicine* [5th ed., p. 945]. Philadelphia: Lippincott Williams & Wilkins.)

IN SUMMARY, thyroid hormones play a role in the metabolic process of almost all body cells and are necessary for normal physical and mental growth in the infant and young child. Alterations in thyroid function can manifest as a hypothyroid or a hyperthyroid state. Hypothyroidism can occur as a congenital or an acquired defect. Congenital hypothyroidism leads to mental retardation and impaired physical growth unless treatment is initiated during the first months of life. Acquired hypothyroidism leads to a decrease in metabolic rate and an accumulation of a mucopolysaccharide substance in the intercellular spaces; this substance attracts water and causes a mucous type of edema called *myxedema*. Hyperthyroidism causes an increase in metabolic rate and alterations in body function similar to those produced by enhanced sympathetic nervous system activity. Graves disease is characterized by the triad of hyperthyroidism, goiter, and ophthalmopathy (or dermopathy). ∎

DISORDERS OF ADRENAL CORTICAL FUNCTION

After completing this section of the chapter, you should be able to meet the following objectives:

- Describe the function of the adrenal cortical hormones and their feedback regulation.
- State the underlying cause of congenital adrenal hyperplasia.
- Relate the functions of the adrenal cortical hormones to Addison disease (*i.e.*, adrenal insufficiency) and Cushing syndrome (*i.e.*, glucocorticoid excess).

Control of Adrenal Cortical Function

The adrenal glands are small, bilateral structures that weigh approximately 5 g each and lie retroperitoneally at the apex of each kidney (Fig. 41-10). The medulla or inner portion of the gland (which constitutes approximately 10% of each adrenal) secretes epinephrine and norepinephrine and is part of the sympathetic nervous system. The cortex forms the bulk of the adrenal gland (approximately 90%) and is responsible for secreting three types of hormones: the glucocorticoids, the mineralocorticoids, and the adrenal androgens.[17] Because the sympathetic nervous system also secretes epinephrine and norepinephrine, adrenal medullary function is not essential for life, but adrenal cortical function is. The total loss of adrenal cortical function is fatal in 4 to 14 days if untreated. This section of the chapter describes the synthesis and function of the adrenal cortical hormones and the effects of adrenal cortical insufficiency and excess.

Biosynthesis, Transport, and Metabolism

More than 30 hormones are produced by the adrenal cortex. Of these hormones, aldosterone is the principal mineralocorticoid,

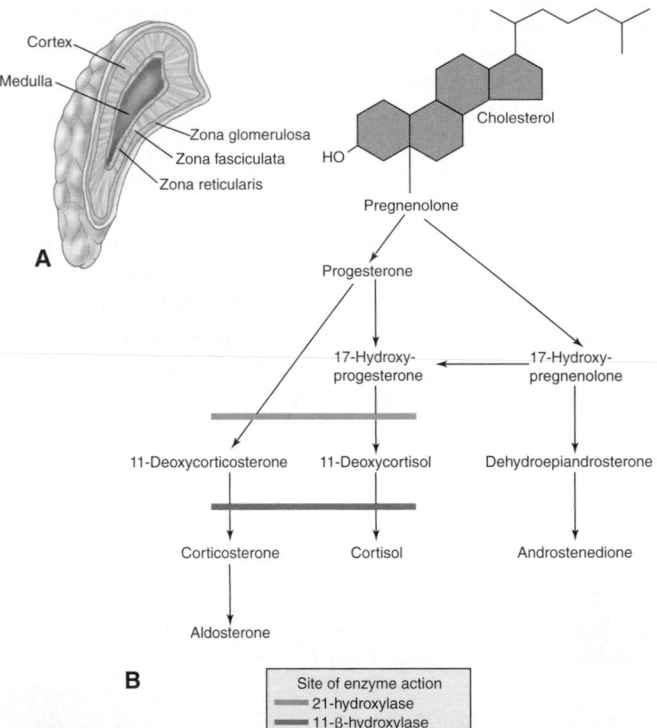

FIGURE 41-10 • **(A)** The adrenal gland, showing the medulla and the three layers of the cortex. The outer layer of the cortex (zona glomerulosa) is primarily responsible for mineralocorticoid production, and the middle layer (zona fasciculata) and the inner layer (zona reticularis) produce the glucocorticoids and the adrenal androgens. **(B)** Predominant biosynthetic pathways of the adrenal cortex. Critical enzymes in the biosynthetic process include 11-β-hydroxylase and 21-hydroxylase. A deficiency in one of these enzymes blocks the synthesis of hormones dependent on that enzyme and routes the precursors into alternative pathways.

cortisol (hydrocortisone) is the major glucocorticoid, and androgens are the chief sex hormones. All of the adrenal cortical hormones have a similar structure in that all are steroids and are synthesized from acetate and cholesterol. Each of the steps involved in the synthesis of the various hormones requires a specific enzyme (see Fig. 41-10). The secretion of the glucocorticoids and the adrenal androgens is controlled by the ACTH secreted by the anterior pituitary gland.

Cortisol, aldosterone, and the adrenal androgens are secreted in an unbound state and bind to plasma proteins for transport in the circulatory system. Cortisol binds largely to corticosteroid-binding globulin and to a lesser extent to albumin. Aldosterone and androgens circulate mostly bound to albumin. It has been suggested that the pool of protein-bound hormones may extend the duration of their action by delaying metabolic clearance.

The main site for metabolism of the adrenal cortical hormones is the liver, where they undergo a number of metabolic conversions before being conjugated and made water soluble. They are then eliminated in either the urine or the bile.

🔑 ADRENAL CORTICAL HORMONES

- The adrenal cortex produces three types of steroid hormones: the mineralocorticoids (principally aldosterone), which function in sodium, potassium, and water balance; the glucocorticoids (principally cortisol), which aid in regulating the metabolic functions of the body and in controlling the inflammatory response, and are essential for survival in stress situations; and the adrenal sex hormones (principally androgens), which serve mainly as a source of androgens for women.

- The manifestations of primary adrenal cortical insufficiency are related mainly to mineralocorticoid deficiency (impaired ability to regulate salt and water elimination) and glucocorticoid deficiency (impaired ability to regulate blood glucose and control the effects of the immune and inflammatory responses).

- Adrenal cortical excess results in derangements in glucose metabolism, disorders of sodium and potassium regulation (increased sodium retention and potassium loss), impaired ability to respond to stress because of inhibition of inflammatory and immune responses, and signs of increased androgen levels such as hirsutism.

Adrenal Androgens

The adrenal androgens are synthesized primarily by the zona reticularis and the zona fasciculata of the cortex (see Fig. 41-10A). These sex hormones probably exert little effect on normal sexual function. There is evidence, however, that the adrenal androgens (the most important of which is dehydroepiandrosterone [DHEA] and its sulfate [DHEAS]) contribute to the pubertal growth of body hair, particularly pubic and axillary hair in women. They also may play a role in the steroid hormone economy of the pregnant woman and the fetal-placental unit. DHEAS is increasingly being used in the treatment of both Addison disease (to be discussed) and adults who have decreased levels of DHEAS. Adrenal androgens are physiologically important in women with Addison disease, and replacement with 25 to 50 mg of DHEAS daily should be considered.[18] Because the testes produce these hormones, there is no rationale for using it in men. The levels of DHEAS decline to approximately one-sixth the levels of a 20-year-old by 60 years of age (the *adrenopause*). The value of routine replacement of DHEAS in the adrenopause is largely unproven, but replacement may improve general well-being and sexuality, and have other important effects in women.

Mineralocorticoids

The mineralocorticoids play an essential role in regulating potassium and sodium levels and water balance. They are produced in the zona glomerulosa, the outer layer of cells of the adrenal cortex. Aldosterone secretion is regulated by the renin-angiotensin mechanism and by blood levels of potassium. Increased levels of aldosterone promote sodium retention by the distal tubules of the kidney while increasing urinary losses of potassium. The influence of aldosterone on fluid and electrolyte balance is discussed in Chapter 31.

Glucocorticoids

The glucocorticoid hormones, mainly cortisol, are synthesized in the zona fasciculata and the zona reticularis of the adrenal gland. The blood levels of these hormones are regulated by negative feedback mechanisms of the hypothalamic-pituitary-adrenal (HPA) system (Fig. 41-11). Just as other pituitary hormones are controlled by releasing factors from the hypothalamus, corticotropin-releasing hormone (CRH) is important in controlling the release of ACTH. Cortisol levels increase as ACTH levels rise and decrease as ACTH levels fall. There is considerable diurnal variation in ACTH levels, which reach their peak in the early morning (around 6 to 8 AM) and decline as the day progresses. This appears to be due to rhythmic activity in the CNS, which causes bursts of CRH secretion and, in turn, ACTH secretion. This diurnal pattern is reversed in people who work during the night and sleep during the day. The rhythm also may be changed by physical and psychological stresses, endogenous depression, manic-depressive psychosis, and liver disease or other conditions that affect cortisol metabolism. One of the earliest signs of Cushing syndrome, a disorder of glucocorticoid excess, is the loss of diurnal variation in CRH and ACTH secretion.[19,20]

The glucocorticoids perform a necessary function in response to stress and are essential for survival. When produced as part of the stress response, these hormones aid in regulating the metabolic functions of the body and in controlling the inflam-

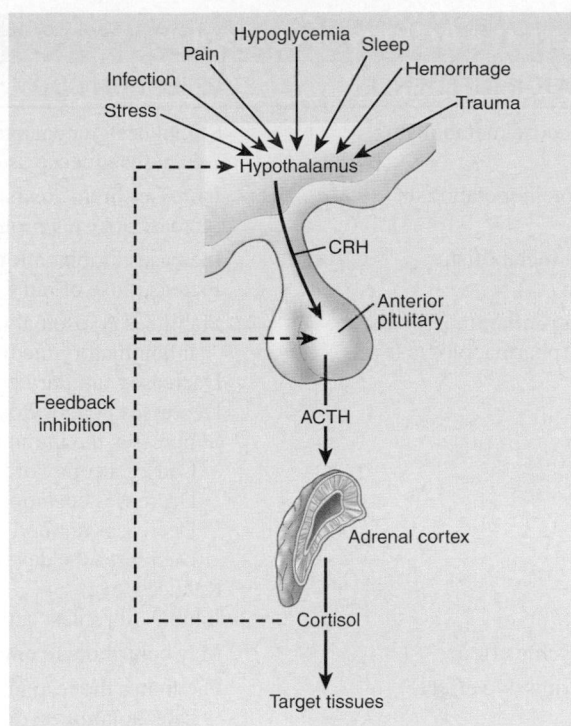

FIGURE 41-11 • The hypothalamic-pituitary-adrenal (HPA) feedback system that regulates glucocorticoid (cortisol) levels. Cortisol release is regulated by adrenocorticotropic hormone (ACTH). Stress exerts its effects on cortisol release through the HPA system and corticotropin-releasing hormone (CRH), which controls the release of ACTH from the anterior pituitary gland. Increased cortisol levels incite a negative feedback inhibition of ACTH release.

matory response. The actions of cortisol are summarized in Table 41-4. Many of the anti-inflammatory actions attributed to cortisol result from the administration of pharmacologic levels of the hormone.

Metabolic Effects. Cortisol stimulates glucose production by the liver, promotes protein breakdown, and causes mobilization of fatty acids. As body proteins are broken down, amino acids are mobilized and transported to the liver, where they are used in the production of glucose (*i.e.,* gluconeogenesis). Mobilization of fatty acids converts cell metabolism from the use of glucose for energy to the use of fatty acids instead. As glucose production by the liver rises and peripheral glucose use falls, a moderate resistance to insulin develops. In persons with diabetes and those who are diabetes prone, this has the effect of raising the blood glucose level.

Psychological Effects. The glucocorticoid hormones appear to be involved directly or indirectly in emotional behavior. Receptors for these hormones have been identified in brain tissue, which suggests that they play a role in the regulation of behavior. Persons treated with adrenal cortical hormones have been known to display behavior ranging from mildly aberrant to psychotic.

TABLE 41-4 **Actions of Cortisol**

MAJOR INFLUENCE	EFFECT ON BODY
Glucose metabolism	Stimulates gluconeogenesis Decreases glucose use by the tissues
Protein metabolism	Increases breakdown of proteins Increases plasma protein levels
Fat metabolism	Increases mobilization of fatty acids Increases use of fatty acids
Anti-inflammatory action (pharmacologic levels)	Stabilizes lysosomal membranes of the inflammatory cells, preventing the release of inflammatory mediators Decreases capillary permeability to prevent inflammatory edema Depresses phagocytosis by white blood cells to reduce the release of inflammatory mediators Suppresses the immune response Causes atrophy of lymphoid tissue Decreases eosinophils Decreases antibody formation Decreases the development of cell-mediated immunity Reduces fever Inhibits fibroblast activity
Psychic effect	May contribute to emotional instability
Permissive effect	Facilitates the response of the tissues to humoral and neural influences, such as that of the catecholamines, during trauma and extreme stress

Immunologic and Inflammatory Effects. Cortisol influences multiple aspects of immunologic function and inflammatory responsiveness. Large quantities of cortisol are required for an effective anti-inflammatory action. This is achieved by the administration of pharmacologic rather than physiologic doses of synthetic cortisol. The increased cortisol blocks inflammation at an early stage by decreasing capillary permeability and stabilizing the lysosomal membranes so that inflammatory mediators are not released. Cortisol suppresses the immune response by reducing humoral and cell-mediated immunity. With this lessened inflammatory response comes a reduction in fever. During the healing phase, cortisol suppresses fibroblast activity and thereby lessens scar formation. Cortisol also inhibits prostaglandin synthesis, which may account in large part for its anti-inflammatory actions.

Pharmacologic Suppression of Adrenal Function

A highly significant aspect of long-term therapy with pharmacologic preparations of the glucocorticoids is adrenal insufficiency on withdrawal of the drugs. The deficiency results from suppression of the HPA system. Chronic suppression causes atrophy of the adrenal gland, and the abrupt withdrawal of drugs can cause acute adrenal insufficiency. Recovery to a state of normal adrenal function may be prolonged, requiring up to 12 months or more.

Tests of Adrenal Function

Several diagnostic tests can be used to evaluate adrenal cortical function and the HPA system.[17] Blood levels of cortisol, aldo-sterone, and ACTH can be measured using immunoassay methods. A 24-hour urine specimen measuring the excretion of various metabolic end products of the adrenal hormones provides information about alterations in the biosynthesis of the adrenal cortical hormones. The 24-hour urinary free cortisol, late-night (between 11 PM and midnight) serum or salivary cortisol levels, and the overnight 1-mg dexamethasone suppression test (see later) are excellent screening tests for Cushing syndrome.[17,19,20]

Suppression and stimulation tests afford a means of assessing the state of the HPA feedback system. For example, a test dose of ACTH can be given to assess the response of the adrenal cortex to stimulation. Similarly, administration of dexamethasone, a synthetic glucocorticoid drug, provides a means of measuring negative feedback suppression of ACTH. Adrenal tumors and ectopic ACTH-producing tumors usually are unresponsive to ACTH suppression by dexamethasone. CRH tests can be used to diagnose a pituitary ACTH-secreting tumor (i.e., Cushing disease), especially when combined with inferior petrosal venous sampling (this allows the blood drainage of the pituitary to be sampled directly). Metyrapone blocks the final step in cortisol synthesis, resulting in the production of 11-dehydroxycortisol, which does not inhibit ACTH. This test measures the ability of the pituitary to release ACTH. The gold standard test for assessing the HPA axis is the insulin hypoglycemic stress test.

Congenital Adrenal Hyperplasia

Congenital adrenal hyperplasia (CAH), or the adrenogenital syndrome, describes a congenital disorder caused by an autosomal recessive trait in which a deficiency exists in any of the enzymes necessary for the synthesis of cortisol[21] (see Fig. 41-10). A common characteristic of all types of CAH is a defect in the synthesis of cortisol that results in increased levels of ACTH and adrenal hyperplasia. The increased levels of ACTH overstimulate the pathways for production of adrenal androgens. Mineralocorticoids may be produced in excessive or insufficient amounts, depending on the precise enzyme deficiency. Infants of both sexes are affected. Boys seldom are diagnosed at birth unless they have enlarged genitalia or lose salt and manifest adrenal crisis. In female infants, an increase in androgens is responsible for creating the virilization syndrome of ambiguous genitalia with an enlarged clitoris, fused labia, and urogenital sinus (Fig. 41-12). In male and female children, other secondary sex characteristics are normal, and fertility is unaffected if appropriate therapy is instituted.

The two most common enzyme deficiencies are 21-hydroxylase (accounting for >90% of cases) and 11-β-hydroxylase deficiency. The clinical manifestations of both deficiencies are largely determined by the functional properties of the steroid intermediates and the completeness of the block in the cortisol pathway.

A spectrum of 21-hydroxylase deficiency states exists, ranging from simple virilizing CAH to a complete salt-losing enzyme deficiency.[21,22] Simple virilizing CAH impairs the synthesis of cortisol, and steroid synthesis is shunted to androgen production. Persons with these deficiencies usually produce sufficient aldosterone or aldosterone intermediates to prevent signs and symptoms of mineralocorticoid deficiency. The salt-losing form is accompanied by deficient production of aldosterone and its intermediates. This results in fluid and electrolyte disorders after the fifth day of life (including hyponatremia, hyperkalemia, vomiting, dehydration, and shock).

The 11-β-hydroxylase deficiency is rare and manifests a spectrum of severity. Affected persons have excessive androgen production and impaired conversion of 11-deoxycorticosterone to corticosterone. The overproduction of 11-deoxycorticosterone, which has mineralocorticoid activity, is responsible for the hypertension that accompanies this deficiency. Diagnosis of CAH depends on the precise biochemical evaluation of metabolites in the cortisol pathway and on clinical signs and symptoms. Genetic testing is also invaluable; however, correlation between the phenotype and genotype is not always straightforward.[21,22]

Medical treatment of CAH includes oral or parenteral glucocorticoid replacement. Fludrocortisone acetate, a mineralocorticoid, also may be given to children who are salt losers. Depending on the degree of virilization, reconstructive surgery during the first 2 years of life is indicated to reduce the size of the clitoris, separate the labia, and exteriorize the vagina. Advances in surgical techniques have led to earlier use of single-stage surgery—between 2 and 6 months of life in girls with 21-hydroxylase deficiency, a time when the tissues are maximally pliable and psychological trauma to the child is minimized.[21] Surgery has provided excellent results and does not usually impair sexual function.

Adrenal Cortical Insufficiency

There are two forms of adrenal insufficiency: primary and secondary[23] (see Table 41-5 for distinguishing features). Primary adrenal insufficiency, or Addison disease, is caused by destruction of the adrenal gland. Secondary adrenal insufficiency results from a disorder of the HPA system.

Primary Adrenal Cortical Insufficiency

In 1855, Thomas Addison, an English physician, provided the first detailed clinical description of primary adrenal insufficiency, now called *Addison disease*. The use of this term is reserved for primary adrenal insufficiency in which adrenal cortical hormones are deficient and ACTH levels are elevated because of lack of feedback inhibition.

Addison disease is a relatively rare disorder in which all the layers of the adrenal cortex are destroyed. Autoimmune destruction is the most common cause of Addison disease in the United States. Before 1950, tuberculosis was the major cause of Addison disease in the United States and Canada, and it continues to be a major cause of the disease in countries where it is more prevalent. Rare causes include metastatic carcinoma, fungal infection (particularly histoplasmosis), cytomegalovirus infection, amyloid disease, and hemochromatosis. Bilateral adrenal hemorrhage may occur in persons taking anticoagulants, during open heart surgery, and during birth or major trauma. Adrenal insufficiency can be caused by acquired immunodeficiency syndrome, in which the adrenal gland is destroyed by a variety of opportunistic infectious agents. Drugs that inhibit synthesis or cause excessive breakdown of glucocorticoids can also result in adrenal insufficiency (*e.g.*, ketoconazole).

Addison disease, like type 1 diabetes mellitus, is a chronic metabolic disorder that requires lifetime hormone replacement therapy. The adrenal cortex has a large reserve capacity, and the manifestations of adrenal insufficiency usually do not become apparent until approximately 90% of the gland has been

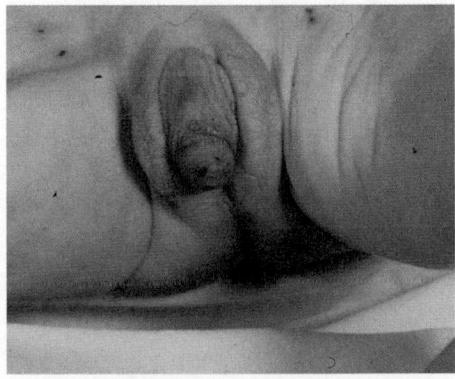

FIGURE 41-12 • A female infant with congenital adrenal hyperplasia demonstrating virilization of the genitalia with hypertrophy of the clitoris and partial fusion of labioscrotal folds. (From Merino M., Quezado M., Rubin E., et al. [2008]. The endocrine system. In Rubin E., Strayer D. [Eds.], *Rubin's pathology: Clinicopathologic foundations of medicine* [5th ed., p. 960]. Philadelphia: Lippincott Williams & Wilkins.)

TABLE 41-5 Clinical Findings of Adrenal Insufficiency

FINDING	PRIMARY	SECONDARY/TERTIARY
Anorexia and weight loss	Yes (100%)	Yes (100%)
Fatigue and weakness	Yes (100%)	Yes (100%)
Gastrointestinal symptoms, nausea, diarrhea	Yes (50%)	Yes (50%)
Myalgia, arthralgia, abdominal pain	Yes (10%)	Yes (10%)
Orthostatic hypotension	Yes	Yes
Hyponatremia	Yes (85%–90%)	Yes (60%)
Hyperkalemia	Yes (60%–65%)	No
Hyperpigmentation	Yes (>90%)	No
Secondary deficiencies of testosterone, growth hormone, thyroxine, antidiuretic hormone	No	Yes
Associated autoimmune conditions	Yes	No

destroyed. These manifestations are related primarily to mineralocorticoid deficiency, glucocorticoid deficiency, and hyperpigmentation resulting from elevated ACTH levels. Although lack of the adrenal androgens (*i.e.,* DHEAS) exerts few effects in men because the testes produce these hormones, women have sparse axillary and pubic hair.

Mineralocorticoid deficiency causes increased urinary losses of sodium, chloride, and water, along with decreased excretion of potassium (Fig. 41-13). The result is hyponatremia, loss of extracellular fluid, decreased cardiac output, and hyperkalemia. There may be an abnormal appetite for salt. Orthostatic hypotension is common. Dehydration, weakness, and fatigue are common early symptoms. If loss of sodium and water is extreme, cardiovascular collapse and shock ensue. Because of a lack of glucocorticoids, the person with Addison disease has poor tolerance to stress. This deficiency causes hypoglycemia, lethargy, weakness, fever, and gastrointestinal symptoms such as anorexia, nausea, vomiting, and weight loss.

Hyperpigmentation results from elevated levels of ACTH. The skin looks bronzed or suntanned in exposed and unexposed areas, and the normal creases and pressure points tend to become especially dark. The gums and oral mucous membranes may become bluish-black. The amino acid sequence of ACTH is strikingly similar to that of melanocyte-stimulating hormone; hyperpigmentation occurs in greater than 90% of persons with Addison disease and is helpful in distinguishing the primary and secondary forms of adrenal insufficiency.

The daily regulation of the chronic phase of Addison disease usually is accomplished with oral replacement therapy, with higher doses being given during periods of stress. The pharmacologic agent that is used should have both glucocorticoid and mineralocorticoid activity. Mineralocorticoids are needed only in primary adrenal insufficiency. Hydrocortisone usually is the drug of choice. In mild cases, hydrocortisone alone may be adequate. Fludrocortisone (a mineralocorticoid) is used for persons who do not obtain a sufficient salt-retaining effect from hydrocortisone. DHEAS replacement also may be helpful in the female patient.[18,23]

Because persons with the disorder are likely to have episodes of hyponatremia and hypoglycemia, they need to have a

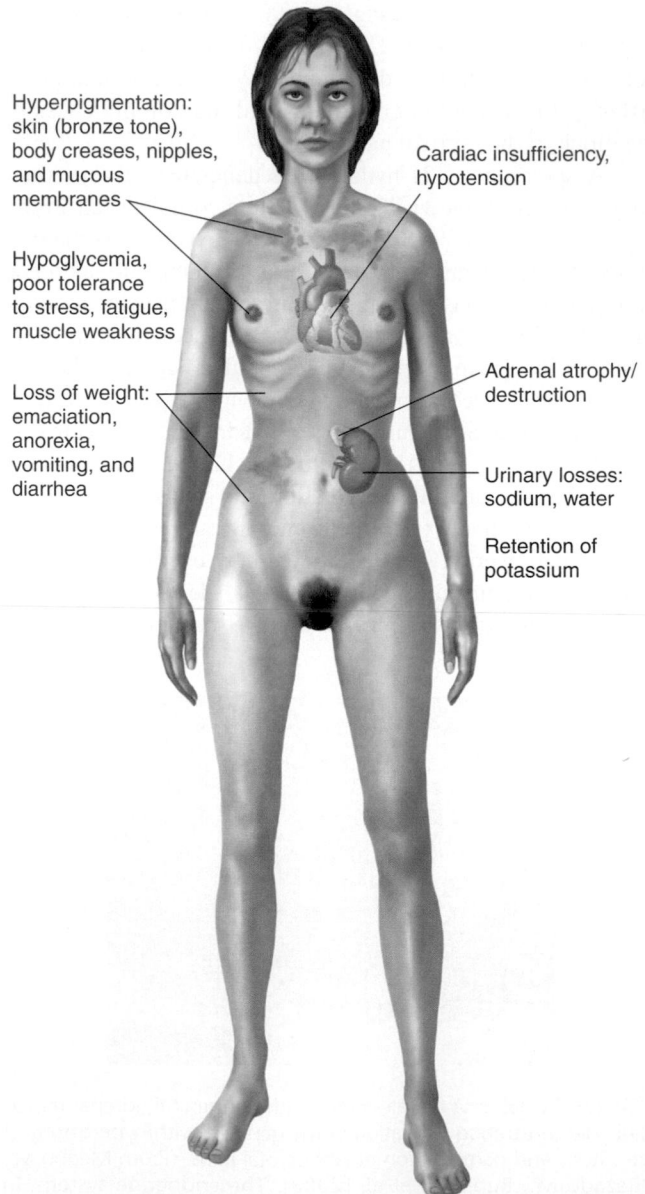

Hyperpigmentation: skin (bronze tone), body creases, nipples, and mucous membranes

Cardiac insufficiency, hypotension

Hypoglycemia, poor tolerance to stress, fatigue, muscle weakness

Adrenal atrophy/destruction

Loss of weight: emaciation, anorexia, vomiting, and diarrhea

Urinary losses: sodium, water

Retention of potassium

FIGURE 41-13 • Clinical manifestations of primary (Addison disease) and secondary adrenal insufficiency.

regular schedule for meals and exercise. Persons with Addison disease also have limited ability to respond to infections, trauma, and other stresses. Such situations require immediate medical attention and treatment. All persons with Addison disease should be advised to wear a medical alert bracelet or medal.

Secondary Adrenal Cortical Insufficiency

Secondary adrenal insufficiency can occur as the result of hypopituitarism or because the pituitary gland has been surgically removed. Tertiary adrenal insufficiency results from a hypothalamic defect. However, a far more common cause than either of these is the rapid withdrawal of glucocorticoids that have been administered therapeutically. These drugs suppress the HPA system, with resulting adrenal cortical atrophy and loss of cortisol production. This suppression continues long after drug therapy has been discontinued and can be critical during periods of stress or when surgery is performed.

Acute Adrenal Crisis

Acute adrenal crisis is a life-threatening situation.[23] If Addison disease is the underlying problem, exposure to even a minor illness or stress can precipitate nausea, vomiting, muscular weakness, hypotension, dehydration, and vascular collapse. The onset of adrenal crisis may be sudden, or it may progress over a period of several days. The symptoms may occur suddenly in children with salt-losing forms of CAH. Massive bilateral adrenal hemorrhage causes an acute fulminating form of adrenal insufficiency. Hemorrhage can be caused by meningococcal septicemia (i.e., Waterhouse-Friderichsen syndrome), adrenal trauma, anticoagulant therapy, adrenal vein thrombosis, or adrenal metastases.

Adrenal insufficiency is treated with hormone replacement therapy that includes a combination of glucocorticoids and mineralocorticoids. For acute adrenal insufficiency, the five S's of management should be followed: (1) Salt replacement, (2) Sugar (dextrose) replacement, (3) Steroid replacement, (4) Support of physiologic functioning, and (5) Search for and treat the underlying cause (e.g., infection). Extracellular fluid volume should be restored with several liters of 0.9% saline and 5% dextrose. Glucocorticoid replacement is accomplished through the intravenous administration of either dexamethasone or hydrocortisone. Dexamethasone is preferred acutely for two reasons: it is long acting (12 to 24 hours) and it does not interfere with measurement of serum or urinary steroids during subsequent corticotropin (ACTH) stimulation tests if diagnosis needs to be established. Thereafter, hydrocortisone often is given either intravenously or intramuscularly at 6-hour intervals and then tapered over 1 to 3 days to maintenance levels. Oral hydrocortisone replacement therapy can be resumed once the saline infusion has been discontinued and the person is taking food and fluids by mouth. Mineralocorticoid therapy is not required when large amounts of hydrocortisone are being given, but as the dose is reduced it usually is necessary to add fludrocortisone. Glucocorticoid and mineralocorticoid replacement therapy is moni-

tored using heart rate and blood pressure measurements; serum electrolyte values; and titration of plasma renin activity into the upper-normal range.

Glucocorticoid Hormone Excess (Cushing Syndrome)

The term *Cushing syndrome* refers to the manifestations of hypercortisolism from any cause.[17,19,20] Three important forms of Cushing syndrome result from excess glucocorticoid production by the body. One is a pituitary form, which results from excessive production of ACTH by a tumor of the pituitary gland. This form of the disease was the one originally described by Cushing; therefore, it is called *Cushing disease.* The second form is the adrenal form, caused by a benign or malignant adrenal tumor. The third form is ectopic Cushing syndrome, caused by a nonpituitary ACTH-secreting tumor. Certain extrapituitary malignant tumors such as small cell carcinoma of the lung may secrete ACTH or, rarely, CRH, and produce Cushing syndrome. Cushing syndrome also can result from long-term therapy with one of the potent pharmacologic preparations of glucocorticoids; this form is called *iatrogenic Cushing syndrome.*

The major manifestations of Cushing syndrome represent an exaggeration of the many actions of cortisol (see Table 41-4). Altered fat metabolism causes a peculiar deposition of fat characterized by a protruding abdomen; subclavicular fat pads or "buffalo hump" on the back; and a round, plethoric "moon face" (Figs. 41-14 and Fig 41-15). There is muscle weakness, and the extremities are thin because of protein breakdown and muscle wasting. In advanced cases, the skin over the forearms and legs becomes thin, having the appearance of parchment. Purple striae, or stretch marks, from stretching of the catabolically weakened skin and subcutaneous tissues are distributed over the breast, thighs, and abdomen. Osteoporosis may develop because of destruction of bone proteins and alterations in calcium metabolism, resulting in back pain, compression fractures of the vertebrae, and rib fractures. As calcium is mobilized from bone, renal calculi may develop.

Derangements in glucose metabolism are found in approximately 75% of patients, with clinically overt diabetes mellitus occurring in approximately 20%. The glucocorticoids possess mineralocorticoid properties; this causes hypokalemia as a result of excessive potassium excretion and hypertension resulting from sodium retention. Inflammatory and immune responses are inhibited, resulting in increased susceptibility to infection. Cortisol increases gastric acid secretion, which may provoke gastric ulceration and bleeding. An accompanying increase in androgen levels causes hirsutism, mild acne, and menstrual irregularities in women. Excess levels of the glucocorticoids may give rise to extreme emotional lability, ranging from mild euphoria and absence of normal fatigue to grossly psychotic behavior.

Diagnosis of Cushing syndrome depends on the finding of cortisol hypersecretion. The determination of 24-hour excretion of cortisol in urine provides a reliable and practical index of cortisol secretions. One of the prominent features of Cushing syndrome is loss of the diurnal pattern of cortisol secretion. This is

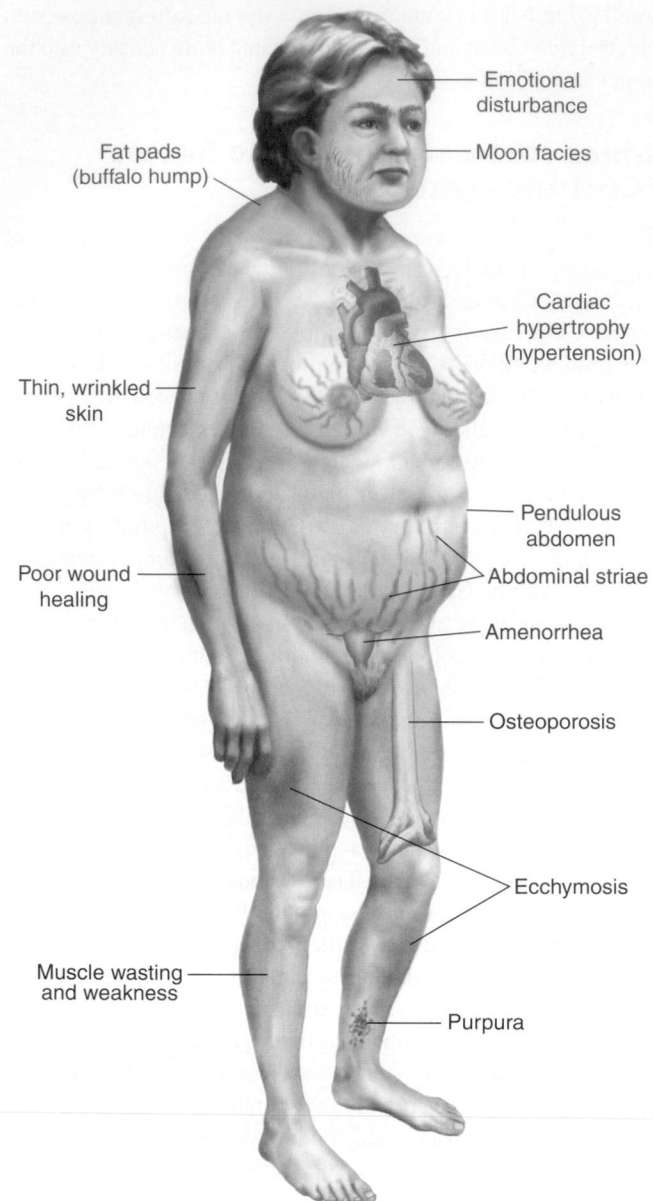

Emotional disturbance

Moon facies

Fat pads (buffalo hump)

Cardiac hypertrophy (hypertension)

Thin, wrinkled skin

Pendulous abdomen

Poor wound healing

Abdominal striae

Amenorrhea

Osteoporosis

Ecchymosis

Muscle wasting and weakness

Purpura

FIGURE 41-14 • Clinical features of Cushing syndrome.

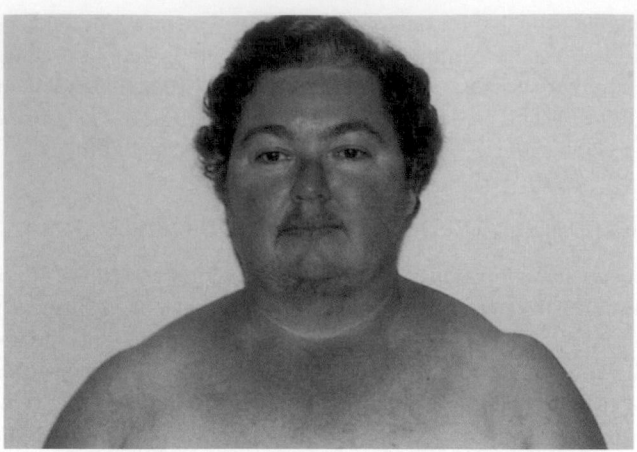

FIGURE 41-15 • Cushing syndrome. A woman who suffered from a pituitary adenoma that produced ACTH exhibits a moon face, buffalo hump, increased facial hair, and thinning of the scalp hair. (From Merino M., Quezado M., Rubin E., et al. [2008]. The endocrine system. In Rubin E., Strayer D. [Eds.], *Rubin's pathology: Clinicopathologic foundations of medicine* [5th ed., p. 966]. Philadelphia: Lippincott Williams & Wilkins.)

why late-night (between 11 PM and midnight) serum or salivary cortisol levels can be inappropriately elevated, aiding in the diagnosis of Cushing syndrome.[17,19,20] The overnight 1-mg dexamethasone suppression test is also used as a screening tool for Cushing syndrome.

Other tests include measurement of the plasma levels of ACTH.[17,19,20] ACTH levels should be normal or elevated in ACTH-dependent Cushing syndrome (Cushing disease and ectopic ACTH), and low in non–ACTH-dependent Cushing syndrome (adrenal tumors). Various suppression or stimulation tests of the HPA system are performed to delineate the cause further. MRI or CT scans afford a means for locating adrenal or pituitary tumors.

Untreated, Cushing syndrome produces serious morbidity and even death. The choice of surgery, irradiation, or pharmaco-

logic treatment is determined largely by the cause of the hypercortisolism. The goal of treatment for Cushing syndrome is to remove or correct the source of hypercortisolism without causing permanent pituitary or adrenal damage. Transsphenoidal removal of a pituitary adenoma or a hemihypophysectomy is the preferred method of treatment for Cushing disease. This allows removal of only the tumor rather than the entire pituitary gland. After successful removal, the person must receive cortisol replacement therapy for 6 to 12 months or until adrenal function returns. Patients also may receive pituitary radiation therapy, but the full effects of treatment may not be realized for 3 to 12 months. Unilateral or bilateral adrenalectomy may be done in the case of adrenal adenoma. When possible, ectopic ACTH-producing tumors are removed. Pharmacologic agents that block steroid synthesis (*i.e.,* mitotane, ketoconazole, and metyrapone) may be used to treat persons with ectopic tumors or adrenal carcinomas that cannot be resected.[17,19] Many of these patients also require *Pneumocystis jiroveci* (formerly known as *Pneumocystis carinii*) pneumonia prophylaxis because of the profound immunosuppression caused by the excessive glucocorticoid levels.

Incidental Adrenal Mass

An incidentaloma is a mass lesion found unexpectedly in an adrenal gland by an imaging procedure (done for other reasons), most commonly CT (but also MRI and ultrasonography). They have been increasingly recognized since the early 1980s. The prevalence of adrenal incidentalomas at autopsy is approximately 10 to 100 per 1000. In CT series, 0.4% to 0.6% are the usual figures published. Incidentalomas also can occur in other organs (*e.g.,* pituitary, thyroid). The two most important questions are (1) is the mass malignant, and (2) is the mass hormonally active (*i.e.,* is it functioning)?

Primary adrenal carcinoma is quite rare, but other cancers, particularly lung cancers, commonly metastasize to the adrenal gland (other cancers include breast, stomach, pancreas, colon, kidney, melanomas, and lymphomas). The size and imaging characteristics of the mass may help determine whether the tumor is benign or malignant. The risk of cancer is high in adrenal masses larger than 6 cm. Many experts recommend surgical removal of masses larger than 4 cm, particularly in younger patients.[24,25] Appropriate screening to exclude a hormonally active lesion includes tests to rule out pheochromocytoma, Cushing syndrome, and Conn syndrome (mineralocorticoid excess).

IN SUMMARY, the adrenal cortex produces three types of hormones: mineralocorticoids, glucocorticoids, and adrenal androgens. The mineralocorticoids, along with the renin-angiotensin mechanism, aid in controlling body levels of sodium and potassium. The glucocorticoids have anti-inflammatory actions and aid in regulating glucose, protein, and fat metabolism during periods of stress. These hormones are under the control of the HPA system. The adrenal androgens exert little effect on daily control of body function, but they probably contribute to the development of body hair in women. Congenital adrenal hyperplasia describes a genetic defect in the cortisol pathway resulting from a deficiency of one of the enzymes needed for its synthesis. Depending on the enzyme involved, the disorder causes virilization of female infants and, in some instances, fluid and electrolyte disturbances because of impaired mineralocorticoid synthesis.

Chronic adrenal insufficiency can be caused by destruction of the adrenal gland (Addison disease) or by dysfunction of the HPA system. Adrenal insufficiency requires replacement therapy with adrenal cortical hormones. Acute adrenal insufficiency is a life-threatening situation. Cushing syndrome refers to the manifestations of excessive glucocorticoid levels. This syndrome may be a result of pharmacologic doses of glucocorticoids, a pituitary or adrenal tumor, or an ectopic tumor that produces ACTH. The clinical manifestations of Cushing syndrome reflect the very high level of glucocorticoid that is present.

An incidentaloma is a mass lesion found unexpectedly in an adrenal gland (and other glands) by an imaging procedure done for other reasons. They are being recognized with increasing frequency, emphasizing the need for correct diagnosis and treatment. ∎

Review Exercises

1. A 59-year-old man was referred to a neurologist for evaluation of headaches. Subsequent MRI studies revealed a large suprasellar mass (2.5 × 2.4 cm), consistent with a pituitary tumor. His history is positive for hypertension and, on direct inquiry, he believes that his hands are slightly larger than previously, with increased sweating. Family history is negative, as are weight change, polyuria and polydipsia, visual disturbance, and erectile dysfunction. Subsequent laboratory findings reveal a baseline serum growth hormone (GH) of 8.7 ng/mL (normal is 0 to 5 ng/mL), which is unsuppressed after oral glucose tolerance testing; glucose intolerance; and increased insulin-like growth factor-1 (IGF-1) on two occasions (1044 and 1145 μg/L [upper limit of normal is 480 μg/L]). Other indices of pituitary function are within the normal range.

   A. *What diagnosis would this man's clinical features, MRI, and laboratory findings suggest?*

   B. *What is the reason for asking the patient about weight change, polyuria and polydipsia, visual disturbance, and erectile dysfunction?*

   C. *How would you explain his impaired glucose tolerance?*

   D. *What are the possible local effects of a large pituitary tumor?*

2. A 76-year-old woman presents with weight gain, subjective memory loss, dry skin, and cold intolerance. On examination she is found to have a multinodular goiter. Laboratory findings reveal a low serum T_4 and elevated TSH.

   A. *What diagnosis would this woman's history, physical, and laboratory tests suggest?*

   B. *Explain the possible relationship between the diagnosis and her weight gain, dry skin, cold intolerance, and subjective memory loss.*

   C. *What type of treatment would be indicated?*

3. A 45-year-old woman presents with a history of progressive weakness, fatigue, weight loss, nausea, and increased skin pigmentation (especially of creases, pressure areas, and nipples). Her blood pressure is 120/78 mm Hg when supine and 105/52 mm Hg when standing. Laboratory findings reveal a serum sodium of 120 mEq/L (normal is 135 to 145 mEq/L); potassium level of 5.9 mEq/L (normal is 3.5 to 5 mEq/L); and low plasma cortisol and high ACTH levels.

   A. *What diagnosis would this woman's clinical features and laboratory findings suggest?*

   B. *Would her diagnosis be classified as a primary or secondary endocrine disorder?*

   C. *What is the significance of her darkened skin?*

   D. *What type of treatment would be indicated?*

References

1. Aron D. C., Findling J. W., Tyrrell J. B. (2007). Hypothalamus and pituitary gland. In Gardner D. G., Shoback D. (Eds.), *Basic and clinical endocrinology* (8th ed., pp. 101–156). New York: Lange Medical Books/McGraw-Hill.

2. Molitch M. E., Clemmons D. R., Malzowski S., et al. (2006). Evaluation and treatment of adult growth hormone deficiency: An Endocrine Society clinical practice guideline. *Journal of Clinical Endocrinology and Metabolism* 91, 1621–1634.

3. Styne D. (2007). Growth. In Gardner D. G., Shoback D. (Eds.), *Basic and clinical endocrinology* (8th ed., pp. 171–208). New York: Lange Medical Books/McGraw-Hill.

4. Laron Z. (2004). Laron syndrome (primary GH resistance): The personal experience 1958–2003. *Journal of Clinical Endocrinology and Metabolism* 89, 1031–1044.

5. Sesmilo G., Biller B. M., Levadot J., et al. (2000). Effects of GH administration on inflammatory and other cardiovascular risk markers in men with GH deficiency. *Annals of Internal Medicine* 133, 111–122.

6. Root A. (2001). The tall, rapidly growing infant, child, and adolescent. *Current Opinion in Endocrinology and Diabetes* 8, 6–16.

7. Melmed S. (2006). Acromegaly. *New England Journal of Medicine* 355, 2558–2573.

8. Lebrethon M. C., Bourguignon J. P. (2001). Central and peripheral isosexual precocious puberty. *Current Opinion in Endocrinology and Diabetes* 8, 17–22.

9. Styne D. (2007). Puberty. In Gardner D. G., Shoback D. (Eds.), *Basic and clinical endocrinology* (8th ed., pp. 611–640). New York: Lange Medical Books/McGraw-Hill.

10. Kaplowitz P. B., Oberfield S. E. (1999). Reexamination of the age limit for defining when puberty is precocious in girls in the United States: Implications for evaluation and treatment. *Pediatrics* 104, 936–941.

11. Cooper D. S., Greenspan F. S., Ladenson P. W. (2007). The thyroid gland. In Gardner D. G., Shoback D. (Eds.), *Basic and clinical endocrinology* (8th ed., pp. 209–280). New York: Lange Medical Books/McGraw-Hill.

12. Dayan C. M. (2001). Interpretation of thyroid function tests. *Lancet* 357, 619–624.

13. Pearce E. N., Farwell A. P., Braverman L. E. (2003). Thyroiditis. *New England Journal of Medicine* 348, 2646–2655.

14. Cooper D. S. (2003). Hyperthyroidism. *Lancet* 362, 459–468.

15. McKenna T. J. (2001). Graves' disease. *Lancet* 357, 1793–1796.

16. Bahn R. (2003). Pathophysiology of Graves' ophthalmopathy: The cycle of disease. *Journal of Clinical Endocrinology and Metabolism* 88, 1939–1946.

17. Aron D. C., Findling J. W., Tyrrell J. B., et al. (2007). Glucocorticoids and adrenal androgens. In Gardner D. G., Shoback D. (Eds.), *Basic and clinical endocrinology* (8th ed., pp. 346–395). New York: Lange Medical Books/McGraw-Hill.

18. Ackermann J. C., Silverman B. L. (2001). Dehydroepiandrosterone replacement for patients with adrenal insufficiency. *Lancet* 357, 1381–1382.

19. Newell-Price J., Bertagna X., Grossman A. B., et al. (2006). Cushing's syndrome. *Lancet* 367, 1605–1617.

20. Raff H., Findling J. W. (2003). A physiological approach to the diagnosis of Cushing's syndrome. *Annals of Internal Medicine* 138, 980–991.

21. Speiser P. W., White P. C. (2003). Congenital adrenal hyperplasia. *New England Journal of Medicine* 349, 776–788.

22. Boos C. J., Rumsby G., Matfin G. (2002). Multiple tumors associated with late onset congenital hyperplasia due to aberrant splicing of adrenal 21-hydroxylase gene. *Endocrine Practice* 8, 470–473.

23. Arlt W., Allolio B. (2003). Adrenal insufficiency. *Lancet* 361, 1881–1893.

24. Gopan T., Remer E., Hamrahian A. H. (2006). Evaluating and managing adrenal incidentalomas. *Cleveland Clinic Journal of Medicine* 73, 561–568.

25. Grumbach M. M., Biller B. M. K., Braunstein G. D., et al. (2003). Management of the clinically inapparent adrenal mass ("incidentaloma"). *Annals of Internal Medicine* 138, 424–429.

Visit the Point. **http://thePoint.lww.com for animations, journal articles, and more!**

Diabetes Mellitus and the Metabolic Syndrome

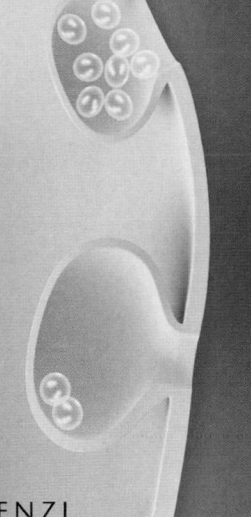

Chapter **42**

SAFAK GUVEN, GLENN MATFIN, AND JULIE A. KUENZI

➤ According to the American Diabetes Association, diabetes mellitus is a chronic health problem affecting 20.8 million people in the United States (approximately 7% of the population).[1] Type 1 diabetes accounts for 1 million of these people, with the remainder having type 2 diabetes. In addition, another 54 million people have been categorized with "prediabetes." Prediabetes and diabetes affects people in all age groups and from all walks of life. Diabetes is more prevalent among American Indians/Alaska Natives (15.1%), African Americans (13.3%), and Hispanic Americans (9.5%).[1]

The acute complications of diabetes are the most common causes of medical emergencies resulting from metabolic disease. Diabetes is a significant risk factor in coronary heart disease and stroke, and it is the leading cause of blindness and chronic kidney disease, as well as a major contributor to lower extremity amputations.

HORMONAL CONTROL OF GLUCOSE, FAT, AND PROTEIN METABOLISM

After completing this section of the chapter, you should be able to meet the following objectives:

- State the functions of glucose, fats, and proteins in meeting the energy needs of the body.
- Characterize the actions of insulin with reference to glucose, fat, and protein metabolism.
- Explain what is meant by *counter-regulatory hormones*, and describe the actions of glucagon, epinephrine, growth hormone, and the glucocorticoid hormones in regulation of blood glucose levels.

Glucose, Fat, and Protein Metabolism

The body uses glucose, fatty acids, and other substrates as fuel to satisfy its energy needs. Although the respiratory and circulatory systems combine efforts to furnish the body with the oxygen needed for metabolic purposes, it is the liver, in concert

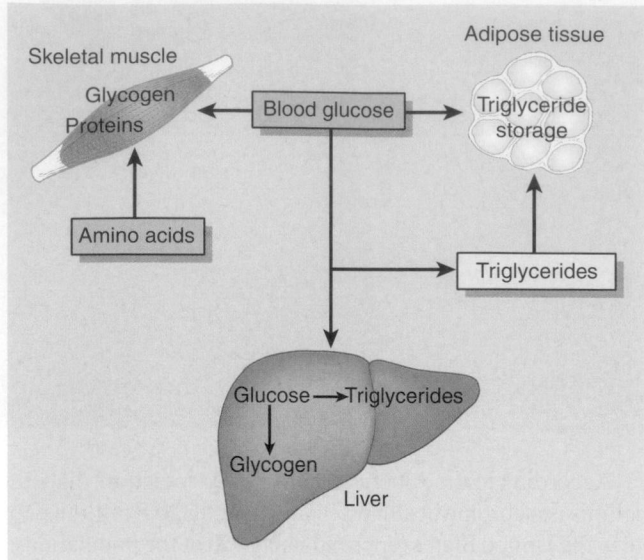

FIGURE 42-1 • Hormonal and hepatic regulation of blood glucose.

with hormones from the endocrine pancreas, that controls the body's fuel supply (Fig. 42-1).

Glucose Metabolism

Glucose is a six-carbon molecule; it is an efficient fuel that, when metabolized in the presence of oxygen, breaks down to form carbon dioxide and water. Although many tissues and organ systems are able to use other forms of fuel, such as fatty acids and ketones, the brain and nervous system rely almost exclusively on glucose as a fuel source. Because the brain can neither synthesize nor store more than a few minutes' supply of glucose, normal cerebral function requires a continuous supply from the circulation. Severe and prolonged hypoglycemia can cause brain death, and even moderate hypoglycemia can result in substantial brain dysfunction.

Body tissues obtain glucose from the blood. In individuals without diabetes, fasting blood glucose levels are tightly regulated between 80 and 90 mg/dL (4.4 to 5.0 mmol/L). After a meal, blood glucose levels rise, and insulin is secreted in response to this rise in glucose. Approximately two thirds of the glucose that is ingested with a meal is removed from the blood and stored in the liver as glycogen. Between meals, the liver releases glucose as a means of maintaining the blood glucose within its normal range.

Glucose that is not needed for energy is removed from the blood and stored as glycogen or converted to fat. When tissues such as those in the liver and skeletal muscle become saturated with glycogen, the additional glucose is converted into fatty acids by the liver and then stored as triglycerides in fat cells. When blood glucose levels fall below normal, as they do between meals, glycogen is broken down by a process called *glycogenolysis,* and glucose is released. Although skeletal muscle has glycogen stores, it lacks the enzyme glucose-6-phosphatase that allows

glucose to be broken down sufficiently to pass through the cell membrane and enter the bloodstream, limiting its usefulness to the muscle cell.

In addition to mobilizing its glycogen stores, the liver synthesizes glucose from amino acids, glycerol, and lactic acid in a process called *gluconeogenesis.* This glucose may be released directly into the circulation or stored as glycogen.

Fat Metabolism

Fat is the most efficient form of fuel storage, providing 9 kcal/g of stored energy, compared with the 4 kcal/g provided by carbohydrates and proteins. About 40% of the calories in the normal American diet are obtained from fats, which is about equal to the amount obtained from carbohydrates.[2] Therefore, the use of fats by the body for energy is as important as the use of carbohydrates. In addition, many of the carbohydrates consumed in the diet are converted to triglycerides for storage in adipose tissue.

A triglyceride contains three fatty acids linked by a glycerol molecule. The mobilization of fatty acids for use as an energy source is facilitated by the action of enzymes (lipases) that break triglycerides into a glycerol molecule and three fatty acids. The glycerol molecule can enter the glycolytic pathway and be used along with glucose to produce energy, or it can be used to produce glucose. The fatty acids are transported to tissues where they are used for energy. Almost all body cells, with the exception of the brain, nervous tissue, and red blood cells, can use fatty acids interchangeably with glucose for energy. Although many cells use fatty acids as a fuel source, fatty acids cannot be converted to the glucose needed by the brain for energy.

A large share of the initial degradation of fatty acids occurs in the liver, especially when excessive amounts of fatty acids are being used for energy. The liver uses only a small amount of the fatty acids for its own energy needs; it converts the rest into ketones and releases them into the blood. In situations that favor fat breakdown, such as diabetes mellitus and fasting, large amounts of ketones are released into the bloodstream. Because ketones are organic acids, they cause ketoacidosis when they are present in excessive amounts.

Protein Metabolism

Proteins are essential for the formation of all body structures, including genes, enzymes, contractile structures in muscle, matrix of bone, and hemoglobin of red blood cells.[2] Amino acids are the building blocks of proteins. Significant quantities of amino acids are present in body proteins. Unlike glucose and fatty acids, there is only a limited facility for the storage of excess amino acids in the body. Most of the stored amino acids are contained in body proteins. Amino acids in excess of those needed for protein synthesis are converted to fatty acids, ketones, or glucose and then stored or used as metabolic fuel. Because fatty acids cannot be converted to glucose, the body must break down proteins and use the amino acids as a major substrate for gluconeogenesis during periods when metabolic needs exceed food intake.

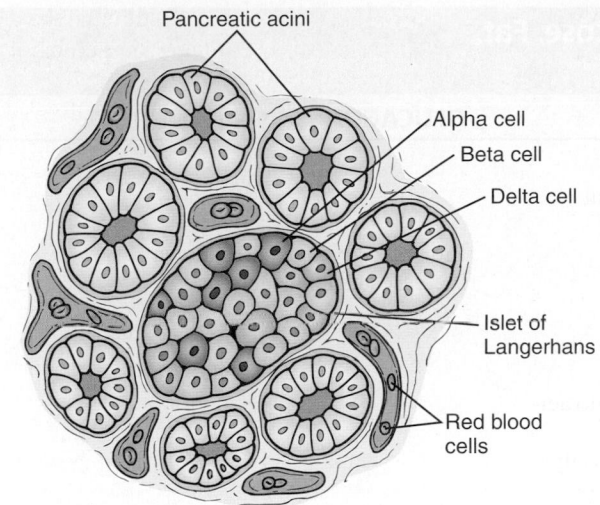

FIGURE 42-2 • Islet of Langerhans in the pancreas.

Glucose-Regulating Hormones

The hormonal control of blood glucose resides largely with the endocrine pancreas. The pancreas is made up of two major tissue types: the acini and the islets of Langerhans (Fig. 42-2). The acini secrete digestive juices into the duodenum, whereas the islets of Langerhans, which account for only about 1% to 2% of volume of the pancreas, secrete hormones into the blood. Each islet is composed of beta cells that secrete insulin and amylin, alpha cells that secrete glucagon, and delta cells that secrete somatostatin. In addition, at least one other type of cell, the PP cell, is present in small numbers in the islets and secretes a hormone of uncertain function called *pancreatic polypeptide*.[2,3] Blood glucose regulation is also influenced by several gut-derived hormones that increase insulin release after nutrient intake and by counter-regulatory hormones that help to maintain blood glucose levels during periods of limited glucose intake or excessive glucose use.

Insulin

Although several hormones are known to increase blood glucose levels, insulin is the only hormone known to have a direct effect in lowering blood glucose levels. The actions of insulin are threefold: (1) it promotes glucose uptake by target cells and provides for glucose storage as glycogen, (2) it prevents fat and glycogen breakdown, and (3) it inhibits gluconeogenesis and increases protein synthesis[2,3] (Table 42-1). Insulin acts to promote fat storage by increasing the transport of glucose into fat cells. It also facilitates triglyceride synthesis from glucose in fat cells and inhibits the intracellular breakdown of stored triglycerides. Insulin also inhibits protein breakdown and increases protein synthesis by increasing the active transport of amino acids into body cells; and it inhibits gluconeogenesis, or the building of glucose from new sources, mainly amino acids. When sufficient glucose and insulin are present, protein breakdown is minimal because the body is able to use glucose and fatty acids as a fuel source. In children and adolescents, insulin is needed for normal growth and development.

The active form of insulin is composed of two polypeptide chains—an A chain and a B chain (Fig. 42-3). Active insulin is formed in the beta cells from a larger molecule called *proinsulin*. In converting proinsulin to insulin, enzymes in the beta cell cleave proinsulin at specific sites to form two separate substances: active insulin and a biologically inactive C-peptide (connecting peptide) chain that joined the A and B chains before they were separated. Active insulin and the inactive C-peptide chain are packaged into secretory granules and released simultaneously from the beta cell. The C-peptide chains can be measured clinically, and this measurement can be used to study beta-cell function (*e.g.*, in patients with type 2 diabetes with very little or no remaining beta cell function, the patient will have very low or nonexistent levels of C-peptide in the blood, and thus will likely need insulin replacement for treatment).

The release of insulin from the pancreatic beta cells is regulated by blood glucose levels, increasing as blood glucose levels rise and decreasing when blood glucose levels decline. Blood glucose enters the beta cell by means of the glucose transporter, is phosphorylated by an enzyme called *glucokinase*, and metabolized to form the adenosine triphosphate (ATP) needed to close the potassium channels and depolarize the cell (Fig. 42-4). Depolarization, in turn, results in opening of the calcium channels and insulin secretion.[3] Secretion of insulin occurs in a pulsatile fashion. After exposure to glucose, which is a nutrient secretagogue, a first-phase release of stored preformed insulin occurs, followed by a second-phase release of newly synthesized insulin (Fig. 42-5). Diabetes may result from dysregulation or deficiency in any of the steps involved in this process (*e.g.*, impaired function of the glucose transporters, intracellular metabolic defects, glucokinase deficiency). Serum insulin levels begin to rise within minutes after a meal, reach a peak in approximately 3 to 5 minutes, and then return to baseline levels within 2 to 3 hours.

Insulin secreted by the beta cells enters the portal circulation and travels directly to the liver, where approximately 50% is used or degraded. Insulin, which is rapidly bound to peripheral tissues or destroyed by the liver or kidneys, has a half-life of approximately 15 minutes once it is released into the general circulation. To initiate its effects on target tissues, insulin binds to a membrane receptor. The insulin receptor is a combination of four subunits—a larger α subunit that extends outside the cell membrane and is involved in insulin binding, and a smaller β subunit that is predominantly inside the cell membrane and contains a kinase enzyme that becomes activated during insulin binding (Fig. 42-6). Activation of the kinase enzyme results in autophosphorylation of the β subunit itself. Phosphorylation of the β subunit in turn activates some enzymes and inactivates others, thereby directing the desired intracellular effect of insulin on glucose, fat, and protein metabolism.

Because cell membranes are impermeable to glucose, they require a special carrier, called a *glucose transporter*, to move glucose from the blood into the cell. These transporters move glucose across the cell membrane at a faster rate than would occur by diffusion alone. Considerable research has revealed a family of glucose transporters termed *GLUT-1, GLUT-2*, and so forth.[4] GLUT-4 is the insulin-dependent glucose transporter for skeletal

TABLE 42-1 Actions of Insulin and Glucagon on Glucose, Fat, and Protein Metabolism

	INSULIN	GLUCAGON
Glucose		
Glucose transport	Increases glucose transport into skeletal muscle and adipose tissue	
Glycogen synthesis	Increases glycogen synthesis	Promotes glycogen breakdown
Gluconeogenesis	Decreases gluconeogenesis	Increases gluconeogenesis
Fats		
Fatty acid and triglyceride synthesis	Promotes fatty acid and triglyceride synthesis by the liver	
Fat storage in adipose tissue	Increases the transport of fatty acids into adipose cells	
	Increases conversion of fatty acids to triglycerides by increasing the availability of a-glycerol phosphate through increased transport of glucose in adipose cells	
	Maintains fat storage by inhibiting breakdown of stored triglycerides by adipose cell lipase	Activates adipose cell lipase, making increased amounts of fatty acids available to the body for use as energy
Proteins		
Amino acid transport	Increases active transport of amino acids into cells	Increases amino acid uptake by liver cells and their conversion to glucose by gluconeogenesis
Protein synthesis	Increases protein synthesis by increasing transcription of messenger RNA and accelerating protein synthesis by ribosomal RNA	
Protein breakdown	Decreases protein breakdown by enhancing the use of glucose and fatty acids as fuel	

muscle and adipose tissue (Fig. 42-7). It is sequestered inside the membrane of these cells and thus is unable to function as a glucose transporter until a signal from insulin causes it to move from its inactive site into the cell membrane, where it facilitates glucose entry. GLUT-2 is the major transporter of glucose into beta cells and liver cells. It has a low affinity for glucose and acts as a transporter only when plasma glucose levels are relatively high, such as after a meal. GLUT-1 is present in all tissues. It does not require the actions of insulin and is important in transport of glucose into cells of the nervous system.

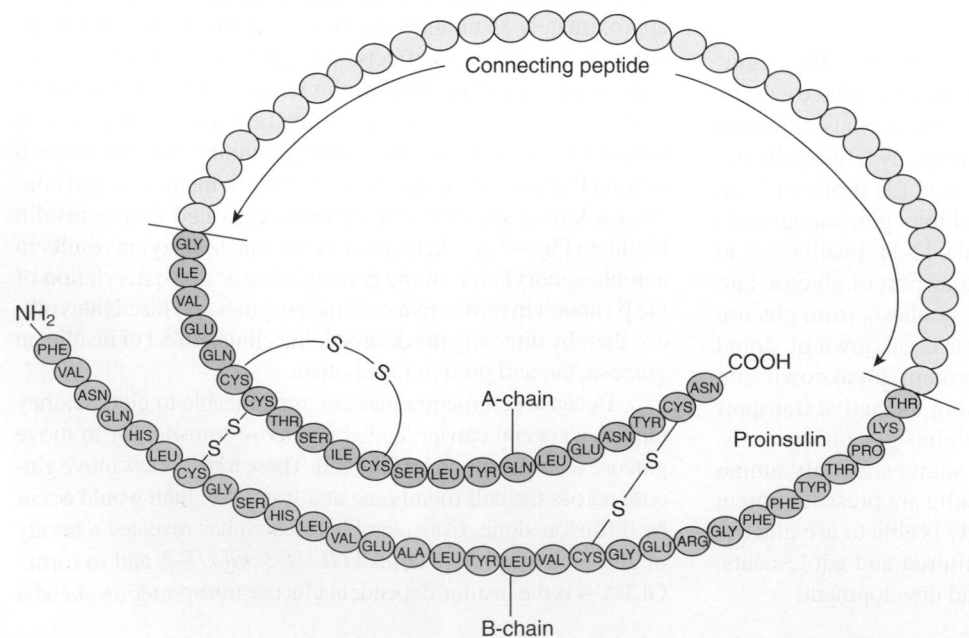

FIGURE 42-3 • Structure of proinsulin. With removal of the connecting peptide (C-peptide), proinsulin is converted to insulin.

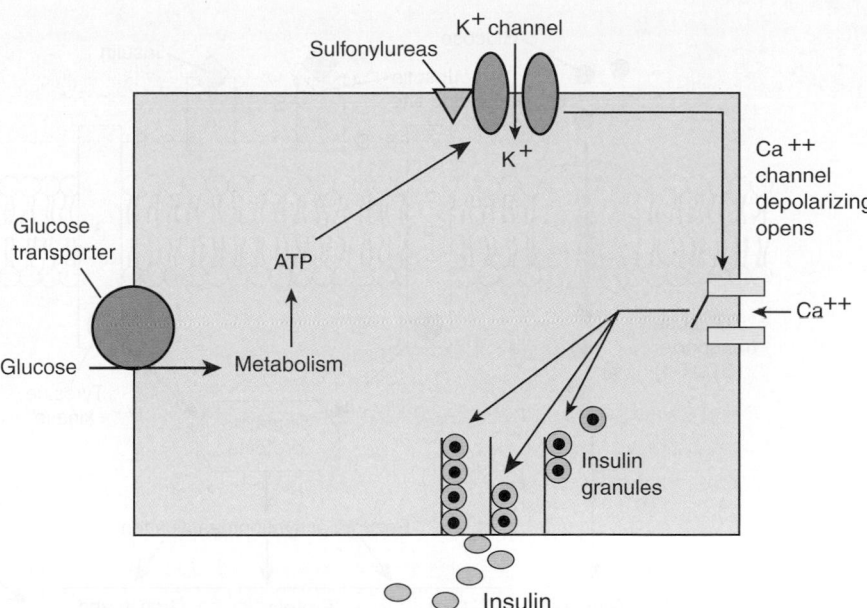

FIGURE 42-4 • One model of control of release of insulin by the pancreatic beta cells and the action of the sulfonylurea agents. In the resting beta cell with low ATP levels, potassium diffuses through the ATP-gated channels, maintaining the resting membrane potential. As blood glucose rises and is transported into the beta cell by the glucose transporter, ATP rises, causing the potassium channels to close and depolarization to occur. Depolarization results in opening of the voltage-gated calcium channels, which results in insulin secretion. (Modified from Karam J. H. [1992]. Type II diabetes and syndrome X. *Endocrinology and Metabolism Clinics of North America* 21, 339.)

Glucagon

Glucagon, a polypeptide molecule produced by the alpha cells of the islets of Langerhans, maintains blood glucose between meals and during periods of fasting.[2,3] Like insulin, glucagon travels through the portal vein to the liver, where it exerts its main action. Unlike insulin, glucagon produces an increase in blood glucose (see Table 42-1). The most dramatic effect of glucagon is its ability to initiate *glycogenolysis* or the breakdown of liver glycogen as a means of raising blood glucose, usually within a matter of minutes. Glucagon also increases the transport of amino acids into the liver and stimulates their conversion into glucose, a process called *gluconeogenesis*. Because liver glycogen stores are limited, gluconeogenesis is important in maintaining blood glucose levels over time. Other actions of glucagon occur only when the hormone is present in high concentrations, usually well above those normally present in the blood. At high concentrations, glucagon activates adipose cell lipase, making fatty acids available for use as energy.[2] At very high concentrations, glucagon can increase the strength of the heart, increase blood flow to some tissues, including the kidneys, enhance bile secretion, and inhibit gastric acid secretion.

As with insulin, glucagon secretion is regulated by blood glucose. A decrease in blood glucose concentration to a hypoglycemic level produces an immediate increase in glucagon secretion, and an increase in blood glucose to hyperglycemic levels produces a decrease in glucagon secretion. High concentrations of amino acids, as occur after a protein meal, also can stimulate glucagon secretion. In this way, glucagon increases the conversion of amino acids to glucose as a means of maintaining the body's glucose levels. Glucagon levels also increase during strenuous exercise as a means of preventing a decrease in blood glucose.

Amylin, Somatostatin, and Gut-Derived Hormones

Islet amyloid polypeptide, or *amylin*, was originally identified as a major constituent of pancreatic amyloid deposits in persons with type 2 diabetes and subsequently shown to be a polypeptide that is cosecreted with insulin from the beta cells in the pancreas.[3,5] Plasma levels of amylin increase in response to nutritional stimuli to produce inhibition of gastric emptying and glucagon secretion. As with insulin, the active monomeric form, amylin, is derived from a larger proamylin precursor. Although the active monomeric form of amylin is soluble and acts as a hormone, there has been renewed interest in the less soluble oligomeric and insoluble polymeric forms that may contribute to the pathogenesis of overt diabetes.[5]

Somatostatin is a polypeptide hormone containing only 14 amino acids that has an extremely short half-life.[2,3] Somatostatin acts locally in the islets of Langerhans to inhibit the release of insulin and glucagon. It also decreases gastro-

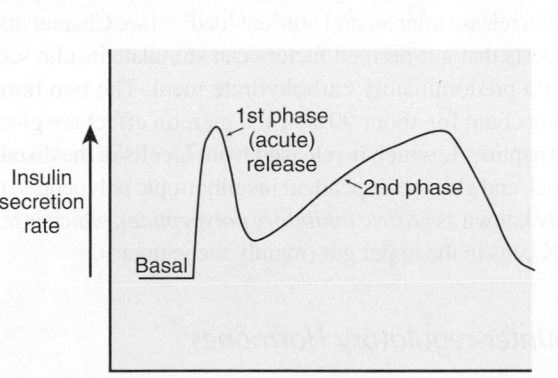

FIGURE 42-5 • Biphasic insulin response to a constant glucose stimulus. The peak of the first phase in humans is 3 to 5 minutes; the second phase begins at 2 minutes and continues to increase slowly for at least 60 minutes or until the stimulus stops. (From Ward W. K., Beard J. C., Halter J. B., et al. [1984]. Pathology of insulin secretion in non-insulin-dependent diabetes mellitus. *Diabetes Care* 7, 491–502. Used with permission.)

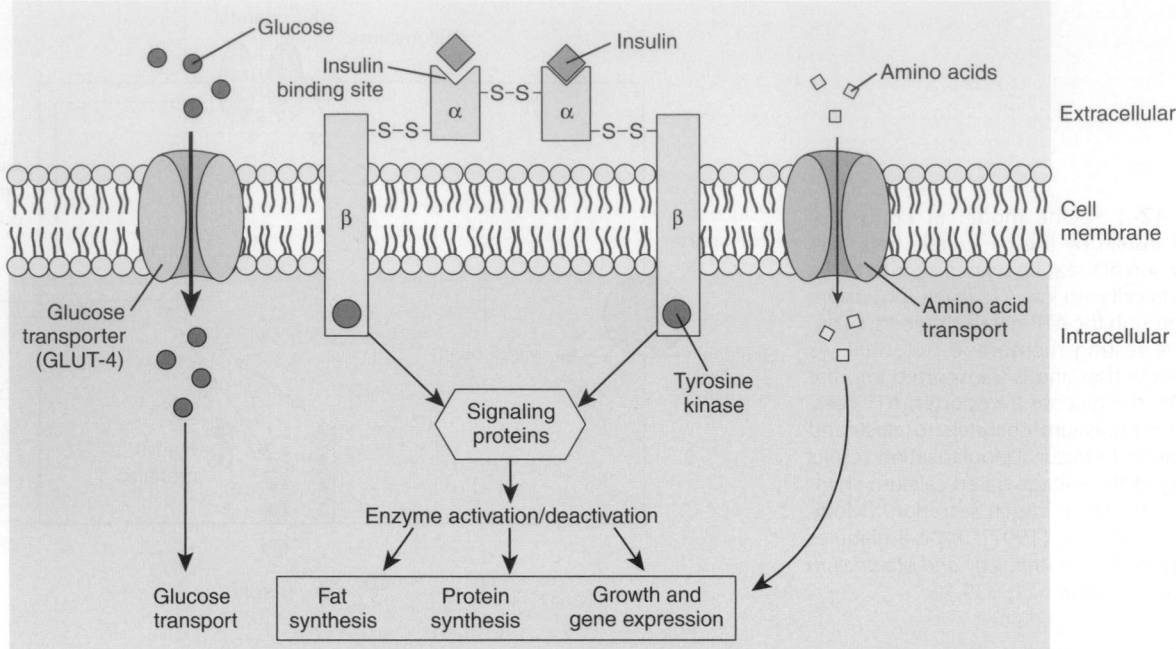

FIGURE 42-6 • Insulin receptor. Insulin binds to the α subunits of the insulin receptor, which increases glucose and amino acid transport and causes autophosphorylation of the β subunit of the receptor, which induces tyrosine kinase activity. Tyrosine phosphorylation, in turn, activates a cascade of intracellular signaling proteins that mediate the effects of insulin on glucose, fat, and protein metabolism.

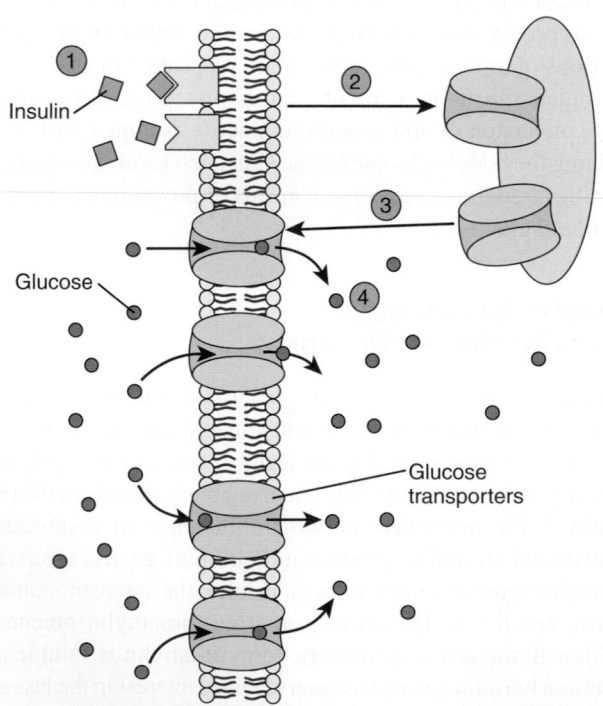

FIGURE 42-7 • Insulin-dependent glucose transporter (GLUT-4). (1) Binding of insulin to insulin receptor on the surface of the cell membrane, (2) generation of intracellular signal, (3) insertion of GLUT-4 receptor from its inactive site into the cell membrane, and (4) transport of glucose across the cell membrane.

intestinal activity after ingestion of food. Almost all factors related to ingestion of food stimulate somatostatin secretion. By decreasing gastrointestinal activity, somatostatin is thought to extend the time during which food is absorbed into the blood, and by inhibiting insulin and glucagon, it is thought to extend the use of absorbed nutrients by the tissues.[2]

Several *gut-derived hormones* have been identified as having what is termed an *incretin effect,* meaning that they increase insulin release after an oral nutrient load[2,3,6] (see Chapter 36). This suggests that gut-derived factors can stimulate insulin secretion after a predominantly carbohydrate meal. The two hormones that account for about 90% of the incretin effect are glucagon-like peptide-1, which is released from L cells in the distal small bowel, and glucose-dependent insulinotropic polypeptide (previously known as *gastric inhibitory polypeptide*), which is released by K cells in the upper gut (mainly the jejunum).

Counter-regulatory Hormones

Other hormones that can affect blood glucose include the catecholamines, growth hormone, and the glucocorticoids. These hormones, along with glucagon, are sometimes called *counter-regulatory hormones* because they counteract the storage functions of insulin in regulating blood glucose levels during periods of fasting, exercise, and other situations that either limit glucose intake or deplete glucose stores.

Epinephrine. *Epinephrine* from the adrenal medulla helps to maintain blood glucose levels during periods of stress. Epinephrine has the potent effect of causing glycogenolysis in the liver, thus causing large quantities of glucose to be released into the blood. It also inhibits insulin release from the beta cells and thereby decreases the movement of glucose into muscle cells, while at the same time increasing the breakdown of muscle glycogen stores. Although the glucose that is released from muscle glycogen cannot be released into the blood, the mobilization of these stores for muscle use conserves blood glucose for use by other tissues such as the brain and the nervous system. Epinephrine also has a direct lipolytic effect on adipose cells, thereby increasing the mobilization of fatty acids for use as an energy source. The blood glucose–elevating effect of epinephrine is also an important homeostatic mechanism during periods of hypoglycemia.

Growth Hormone. Growth hormone has many metabolic effects. It increases protein synthesis in all cells of the body, mobilizes fatty acids from adipose tissue, and antagonizes the effects of insulin. Growth hormone decreases cellular uptake and use of glucose, thereby increasing the level of blood glucose. The increased blood glucose level stimulates further insulin secretion by the beta cells. The secretion of growth hormone normally is inhibited by insulin and increased levels of blood glucose. During periods of fasting, when both blood glucose levels and insulin secretion fall, growth hormone levels increase. Exercise such as running and cycling, and various stresses, including anesthesia, fever, and trauma, increase growth hormone levels.

Chronic hypersecretion of growth hormone, as occurs in acromegaly (see Chapter 41), can lead to glucose intolerance and the development of diabetes mellitus. In people who already have diabetes, moderate elevations in growth hormone levels that occur during periods of stress and periods of growth in children can produce the entire spectrum of metabolic abnormalities associated with poor regulation, despite optimized insulin treatment.

Glucocorticoid Hormones. The glucocorticoid hormones, which are synthesized in the adrenal cortex along with other corticosteroid hormones, are critical to survival during periods of fasting and starvation. They stimulate gluconeogenesis by the liver, sometimes producing a 6- to 10-fold increase in hepatic glucose production. These hormones also moderately decrease tissue use of glucose. In predisposed persons, the prolonged elevation of glucocorticoid hormones can lead to hyperglycemia and the development of diabetes mellitus. In people with diabetes, even transient increases in cortisol can complicate control.

There are several steroid hormones with glucocorticoid activity; the most important of these is cortisol, which accounts for approximately 95% of all glucocorticoid activity (see Chapter 41). Almost any type of stress, whether physical or emotional, causes an immediate increase in adrenocorticotropic hormone (ACTH) secretion by the anterior pituitary gland, followed within minutes by greatly increased secretion of cortisol by the adrenal gland. Hypoglycemia is a potent stimulus for cortisol secretion. The excess cortisol secreted in persons with Cushing syndrome can also lead to prediabetes and development of diabetes mellitus.

IN SUMMARY, the body uses glucose, fatty acids, and other substrates as fuel to satisfy its energy needs. Body tissues, including the brain, which depends exclusively on glucose for its energy, obtain glucose from the blood. The liver stores excess glucose as glycogen and it uses gluconeogenesis to convert amino acids, lactate, and glycerol into glucose during fasting or when glucose intake does not keep pace with demand. Blood glucose levels reflect the difference between the amount of glucose released into the circulation by the liver and the amount of glucose removed from the blood by body tissues. Fats, which serve as an efficient source of fuel for the body, are stored in adipose tissue as triglycerides, which consist of three fatty acids linked to a glycerol molecule. In situations that favor fat breakdown, such as fasting or diabetes mellitus, the triglycerides in adipose tissue are broken down and the fatty acids are used as fuel or transported to the liver, where they are converted to ketones. Proteins, which are made up of amino acids, are essential for the formation of all body structures. Unlike glucose and fatty acids, there is only a limited facility for storage of excess amino acids in the body. Because fatty acids cannot be converted to glucose, the body must break down proteins and use the amino acids for gluconeogenesis.

Energy metabolism is controlled by a number of hormones, including insulin, glucagon, epinephrine, growth hormone, and the glucocorticoids. Of these hormones, only insulin has the effect of lowering the blood glucose level. Insulin's blood glucose–lowering action results from its ability to increase the transport of glucose into body cells and decrease hepatic production and release of glucose into the bloodstream. Insulin also has the effect of decreasing lipolysis and the use of fats as a fuel source. Other hormones—glucagon, epinephrine, growth hormone, and the glucocorticoids—maintain or increase blood glucose concentrations and are referred to as *counter-regulatory hormones*. Glucagon and epinephrine promote glycogenolysis. Glucagon and the glucocorticoids increase gluconeogenesis. Growth hormone decreases the peripheral use of glucose. Epinephrine and glucagon also increase the use of fat for energy by increasing the release of fatty acids from adipose cells. ∎

CONCEPTS in action **ANIMATI** **N**

DIABETES MELLITUS

After completing this section of the chapter, you should be able to meet the following objectives:

■ Compare the distinguishing features of type 1 and type 2 diabetes mellitus, list causes of other specific types of diabetes, and cite the criteria for gestational diabetes.
■ Describe what is meant by the term *prediabetes*.

(objectives continue)

- Relate the physiologic functions of insulin to the manifestations of diabetes mellitus.
- Define the metabolic syndrome and describe its associations with the development of type 2 diabetes.
- Discuss the role of diet and exercise in the management of diabetes mellitus.
- Characterize the blood glucose–lowering actions of the hypoglycemic agents used in treatment of type 2 diabetes.
- Name and describe the types (according to duration of action) of insulin.
- Differentiate between the causes and clinical manifestations of diabetic ketoacidosis and the hyperosmolar hyperglycemic state.
- Describe alterations in physiologic function that accompany diabetic peripheral neuropathy, retinopathy, and nephropathy.
- Describe the causes of foot ulcers in people with diabetes mellitus.
- Explain the relation between diabetes mellitus and infection.

The term *diabetes* is derived from a Greek word meaning "going through," and *mellitus* from the Latin word for "honey" or "sweet." Reports of the disorder can be traced back to the first century AD, when Aretaeus the Cappadocian described the disorder as a chronic affliction characterized by intense thirst and voluminous, honey-sweet urine: "the melting down of flesh into urine." It was the discovery of insulin by Banting and Best in 1922 that transformed the once-fatal disease into a manageable chronic health problem.[7]

Diabetes is a disorder of carbohydrate, protein, and fat metabolism resulting from an imbalance between insulin availability and insulin need. It can represent an absolute insulin deficiency, impaired release of insulin by the pancreatic beta cells, inadequate or defective insulin receptors, inadequate or defective insulin postreceptor regulation, or the production of inactive insulin or insulin that is destroyed before it can carry out its action. A person with uncontrolled diabetes is unable to transport glucose into fat and muscle cells; as a result, body cells are starved, and the breakdown of fat and protein is increased to generate alternative fuels.

Classification and Etiology

Although diabetes mellitus clearly is a disorder of insulin availability, it is not a single disease. A revised system for the classification of diabetes was developed in 1997 by the Expert Committee on the Diagnosis and Classification of Diabetes Mellitus[8] (Table 42-2). Type 2 diabetes currently accounts for about 90% to 95% of the cases of diabetes. Included in the classification system are the categories of gestational diabetes mellitus (*i.e.*, diabetes that develops during pregnancy) and other specific types of diabetes, many of which occur secondary to

other conditions (*e.g.*, Cushing syndrome, acromegaly, pancreatitis, hemochromatosis).

The revised classification system also includes a system for diagnosing diabetes according to stages of glucose intolerance[8] (Table 42-3). The revised criteria have retained the former category of *impaired glucose tolerance* (IGT) and have added a new category of *impaired fasting plasma glucose* (IFG). The categories of IFG and IGT refer to metabolic stages intermediate between normal glucose homeostasis and diabetes, and are labeled together as *prediabetes.* A fasting plasma glucose (FPG) of less than 100 mg/dL (5.5 mmol/L) or a 2-hour oral glucose tolerance test (OGTT) result of less than 140 mg/dL is considered normal. IFG is defined by an elevated FPG concentration (100 to 125 mg/dL [5.6 to 6.9 mmol/L]). IGT reflects abnormal plasma glucose measurements (140 to 199 mg/dL [7.8 to 11.0 mmol/L]) 2 hours after a 75-g oral glucose load.[8] IFG and IGT (*i.e.*, prediabetes) categories are associated with increased risk of atherosclerotic heart disease and increased risk of progression to type 2 diabetes. IFG and IGT have different rates of progression to diabetes because of different pathophysiologic mechanisms. Calorie restriction and weight reduction (even 5% to 10%) are important in overweight people with prediabetes.[9] Persons with an FPG of 126 mg/dL (6.9 mmol/L) or more, or a 2-hour OGTT of ≥200 mg/L (11.1 mmol/L) after a 75-g glucose load are considered to have *provisional diabetes.*[8] The criteria in Chart 42-1 are used to confirm the diagnosis of diabetes in persons with provisional diabetes.

Type 1 Diabetes Mellitus

Type 1 diabetes mellitus is characterized by destruction of the pancreatic beta cells.[10] Type 1 diabetes is subdivided into two types: type 1A immune-mediated diabetes, and type 1B idiopathic (non–immune-related) diabetes. In the United States and Europe, approximately 90% to 95% of people with type 1 diabetes mellitus have type 1A immune-mediated diabetes.

Type 1A Immune-Mediated Diabetes. Type 1A diabetes, commonly referred to simply as type 1 diabetes, is characterized by immune-mediated destruction of beta cells. This type of diabetes, formerly called *juvenile diabetes,* occurs more commonly in young persons but can occur at any age. The rate of beta cell destruction is quite variable, being rapid in some individuals and slow in others. The rapidly progressive form commonly is observed in children, but also may occur in adults. The slowly progressive form usually occurs in adults and is sometimes referred to as *latent autoimmune diabetes in adults* (LADA). LADA may account for up to 10% of adults who are currently classified as having type 2 diabetes.

Type 1 diabetes is a catabolic disorder characterized by an absolute lack of insulin, an elevation in blood glucose, and a breakdown of body fats and proteins. The absolute lack of insulin in people with type 1 diabetes mellitus means that they are particularly prone to the development of ketoacidosis. One of the actions of insulin is the inhibition of *lipolysis* (*i.e.*, fat breakdown) and release of free fatty acids (FFA) from fat cells. In the absence of insulin, ketosis develops when these fatty acids are released

TABLE 42-2 Etiologic Classification of Diabetes Mellitus

TYPE	SUBTYPES	ETIOLOGY OF GLUCOSE INTOLERANCE
I. Type 1*	Beta cell destruction usually leading to absolute insulin deficiency A. Immune mediated B. Idiopathic	 Autoimmune destruction of beta cells Unknown
II. Type 2*	May range from predominantly insulin resistance with relative insulin deficiency to a predominantly secretory defect with insulin resistance	
III. Other specific types	A. Genetic defects in beta cell function, *e.g.,* glucokinase	Dysregulation insulin secretion due to a defect in glucokinase generation
	B. Genetic defects in insulin action, *e.g.,* leprechaunism, Rabson-Mendenhall syndrome	Pediatric syndromes that have mutations in insulin receptors
	C. Diseases of exocrine pancreas, *e.g.,* pancreatitis, neoplasms, cystic fibrosis	Loss or destruction of insulin-producing beta cells
	D. Endocrine disorders, *e.g.,* acromegaly, Cushing syndrome	Diabetogenic effects of excess hormone levels
	E. Drug or chemical induced, *e.g.,* Vacor, glucocorticosteroids, thiazide diuretics, interferon-alfa	Toxic destruction of beta cells Insulin resistance Impaired insulin secretion Production of islet cell antibodies
	F. Infections, *e.g.,* congenital rubella, cytomegalovirus	Beta cell injury followed by autoimmune response
	G. Uncommon forms of immune-mediated diabetes, *e.g.,* "stiff man syndrome"	Autoimmune disorder of central nervous system with immune-mediated beta cell destruction
	H. Other genetic syndromes sometimes associated with diabetes, *e.g.,* Down syndrome, Klinefelter syndrome, Turner syndrome	Disorders of glucose tolerance related to defects associated with chromosomal abnormalities
IV. Gestational diabetes mellitus (GDM)	Any degree of glucose intolerance with onset or first recognition during pregnancy	Combination of insulin resistance and impaired insulin secretion

*Patients with any form of diabetes may require insulin treatment at some stage of the disease. Such use of insulin, does not, of itself, classify the patient.

Adapted from The Expert Committee on the Diagnosis and Classification of Diabetes Mellitus. (2004). Report of the Expert Committee on the Diagnosis and Classification of Diabetes Mellitus. Diabetes Care 27, S5–S10. Reprinted with permission from the American Diabetes Association. Copyright © 2004 American Diabetes Association.

TABLE 42-3 Expert Committee on the Diagnosis and Classification of Diabetes Mellitus Criteria for Classification of Diabetes Using Fasting* Plasma Glucose and Oral Glucose Tolerance Tests

TEST	NORMOGLYCEMIC	IFG†	IGT†	DIABETES MELLITUS‡
FPG	<100 mg/dL (5.6 mmol/L)	100–125 mg/dL (5.6–6.9 mmol/L)		≥126 mg/dL (7.0 mmol/L)
2-hr OGTT§	<140 mg/dL (7.8 mmol/L)		140–199 mg/dL (7.8–11.0 mmol/L)	≥200 mg/dL (11.1 mmol/L)
Other				Symptoms of diabetes mellitus and casual plasma glucose ≥200 mg/dL (11.1 mmol/L)

FPG, fasting plasma glucose; IFG, impaired fasting glucose; IGT, impaired glucose tolerance; OGGT, oral glucose tolerance test.

*Fasting is defined as no caloric intake for at least 8 hours.

†IFG and IGT are prediabetes states and can occur in isolation or together in a given subject.

‡In the absence of unequivocal hyperglycemia with acute metabolic decompensation, these criteria should be confirmed by repeat testing on a separate day.

§OGTT with 2-hr measurement of venous plasma or serum glucose after a 75-g carbohydrate load.

Developed from data in American Diabetes Association. (2007). Diagnosis and classification of diabetes mellitus. *Diabetes Care* 30(Suppl. 1), S42–S47.

CRITERIA FOR DIAGNOSIS OF DIABETES MELLITUS

1. Symptoms of diabetes plus casual plasma glucose concentration ≥200 mg/dL (11.1 mmol/L). "Casual" is defined as any time of the day without regard to time since last meal. The classic symptoms of diabetes include polyuria, polydipsia, and unexplained weight loss.

or

2. Fasting plasma glucose ≥126 mg/dL (7 mmol/L). "Fasting" is defined as no caloric intake for at least 8 h.

or

3. Two-hour postload glucose ≥200 mg/dL (11.1 mmol/L) during oral glucose tolerance test (OGTT). The test should be performed as described by the World Health Organization, using a glucose load containing the equivalent of 75 g anhydrous glucose dissolved in water.

In the absence of unequivocal hyperglycemia, these criteria should be confirmed by repeat testing on a different day. The third measure (OGTT) is not recommended for routine use.

Developed from data in American Diabetes Association. (2007). Diagnosis and classification of diabetes mellitus. *Diabetes Care* 30(Suppl. 1), S5–S10.

DIABETES MELLITUS

■ Diabetes mellitus is a disorder of carbohydrate, fat, and protein metabolism brought about by impaired beta cell synthesis or release of insulin, or the inability of tissues to use insulin.

■ Type 1 diabetes results from loss of beta cell function and an absolute insulin deficiency.

■ Type 2 diabetes results from impaired ability of the tissues to use insulin (insulin resistance) accompanied by a relative lack of insulin or impaired release of insulin in relation to blood glucose levels (beta cell dysfunction).

from fat cells and converted to ketones in the liver. Because of the loss of insulin response, all people with type 1A diabetes require exogenous insulin replacement to reverse the catabolic state, control blood glucose levels, and prevent ketosis.

Type 1A diabetes is thought to be an autoimmune disorder resulting from a genetic predisposition (*i.e.*, diabetogenic genes); an environmental triggering event, such as an infection; and a T-lymphocyte–mediated hypersensitivity reaction against some beta cell antigen (see Chapter 19). Much evidence has focused on the inherited major histocompatibility complex (MHC) genes on chromosome 6 that encode human leukocyte antigens HLA-DQ and HLA-DR, especially DR-3 and DR-4.[3] In addition to the MHC susceptibility genes for type 1 diabetes on chromosome 6, an insulin gene regulating

beta cell replication and function has been identified on chromosome 11.

Type 1A diabetes–associated autoantibodies may exist for years before the onset of hyperglycemia. There are two major types of autoantibodies: insulin autoantibodies (IAAs), and islet cell autoantibodies and antibodies directed at other islet autoantigens, including glutamic acid decarboxylase (GAD) and the protein tyrosine phosphatase IA-2.[6] Testing for antibodies to GAD or IA-2 and for IAAs using sensitive radiobinding assays can identify more than 85% of cases of new or future type 1 diabetes.[6] The appearance of IAAs may precede that of antibodies to GAD or IA-2, and IAAs may be the only antibodies detected at diagnosis in young children. These people also may have other autoimmune disorders such as Graves disease, rheumatoid arthritis, and Addison disease.

The fact that type 1 diabetes is thought to result from an interaction between genetic and environmental factors has led to research into methods directed at prevention and early control of the disease. These methods include the identification of genetically susceptible persons and early intervention in newly diagnosed persons with type 1 diabetes. After the diagnosis of type 1 diabetes, there often is a short period of beta cell regeneration, during which symptoms of diabetes disappear and insulin injections are reduced or not needed. This is sometimes called the *honeymoon period.* Immune interventions (immunomodulation) designed to interrupt the destruction of beta cells before development of type 1 diabetes are being investigated in various trials. Unfortunately, none of the interventions studied to date has shown real clinical utility. Modulation of environmental influences, such as infant diet and breast-feeding, has also led to conflicting results.[11]

Idiopathic Type 1B Diabetes. The term *idiopathic type 1B diabetes* is used to describe those cases of beta cell destruction in which no evidence of autoimmunity is present. Only a small number of people with type 1 diabetes fall into this category; most are of African or Asian descent. Type 1B diabetes is strongly inherited. People with the disorder have episodic ketoacidosis due to varying degrees of insulin deficiency with periods of absolute insulin deficiency that may come and go.

Type 2 Diabetes Mellitus and the Metabolic Syndrome

Type 2 diabetes mellitus is a heterogeneous condition that describes the presence of hyperglycemia in association with *relative* insulin deficiency. Most people with type 2 diabetes are older and overweight. Recently, however, type 2 diabetes has become a more common occurrence in obese adolescents and children.[12,13] Although type 1 diabetes remains the main form of diabetes in children worldwide, it seems likely that type 2 diabetes will become the predominant form within 10 years in some ethnic groups.[13]

A number of genetic and acquired pathogenic factors have been implicated in the progressive impairment of beta cell function in persons with prediabetes and type 2 diabetes. A positive family history confers a twofold to fourfold increased risk for type 2 diabetes, and 15% to 25% of first-degree relatives of persons with type 2 diabetes develop impaired glucose tolerance or diabetes.[14] Despite the strong familial predisposition, the genetics of type 2 diabetes is poorly defined. This is probably because of the heterogeneous nature of the disorder as well as the difficulty in sorting out the contribution of acquired factors affecting insulin action and glycemic control.[15]

The metabolic abnormalities that lead to type 2 diabetes include (1) insulin resistance, (2) deranged secretion of insulin by the pancreatic beta cells, and (3) increased glucose production by the liver[14–16] (Fig. 42-8). In contrast to type 1 diabetes, where *absolute* insulin deficiency is present, persons with type 2 diabetes can have high, normal, or low insulin levels. Insulin resistance initially stimulates an increase in insulin secretion, often to a level of modest hyperinsulinemia, as the beta cells attempt to maintain a normal blood glucose level. In time, the increased demand for insulin secretion leads to beta cell exhaustion and failure. This results in elevated postprandial blood glucose levels and an eventual increase in glucose production by the liver. Because people with type 2 diabetes do not have an absolute insulin deficiency, they are less prone to ketoacidosis than are people with type 1 diabetes.

Insulin resistance is said to be present when the biologic effects of insulin are less than expected for both glucose disposal in skeletal muscle and suppression of glucose production by the liver.[15] In the basal state, hepatic insulin resistance is manifested by overproduction of glucose despite fasting hyperinsulinemia, with the rate of glucose production being the primary determinant of the elevated FPG in persons with type 2 diabetes.[16] Although muscle glucose uptake is increased in absolute terms after a meal, the efficiency with which it is taken up (glucose clearance) is diminished, resulting in an increase in postprandial

blood glucose levels.[16] Although the insulin resistance seen in persons with type 2 diabetes can be caused by a number of factors, it is strongly associated with obesity and physical inactivity. A number of circulating hormones, cytokines, and metabolic fuels such as FFAs originate in adipose tissue and modulate insulin action.

Specific causes of beta cell dysfunction include an initial decrease in the beta cell mass related to genetic or prenatal factors (*e.g.,* intrauterine growth retardation; see Chapter 2); increased apoptosis or decreased beta cell regeneration; beta cell exhaustion due to long-standing insulin resistance; glucotoxicity (*i.e.,* glucose toxicity–induced beta cell desensitization); lipotoxicity (*i.e.,* toxic effects of lipids on beta cells); and amyloid deposition or other conditions that have the potential to reduce beta cell mass.[15] According to one study, beta cell function was reduced by 50% at the time of diagnosis in type 2 diabetes, and its progressive decrease (by approximately 4% per year) profoundly influenced the subsequent response to treatment (meaning that combination treatment with several agents is usually the "norm" to maintain glycemic goals as a result of progressive beta cell dysfunction).[17]

Insulin Resistance and the Metabolic Syndrome. There is increasing evidence to suggest that insulin resistance not only contributes to the hyperglycemia in persons with type 2 diabetes, but may play a role in other metabolic abnormalities. These include obesity, high levels of plasma triglycerides and low levels of high-density lipoproteins (HDL), hypertension, systemic inflammation (as detected by C-reactive protein [CRP] and other mediators), abnormal fibrinolysis, abnormal function of the vascular endothelium, and macrovascular disease (coronary artery, cerebrovascular, and peripheral arterial disease). This constellation of abnormalities often is referred to as the

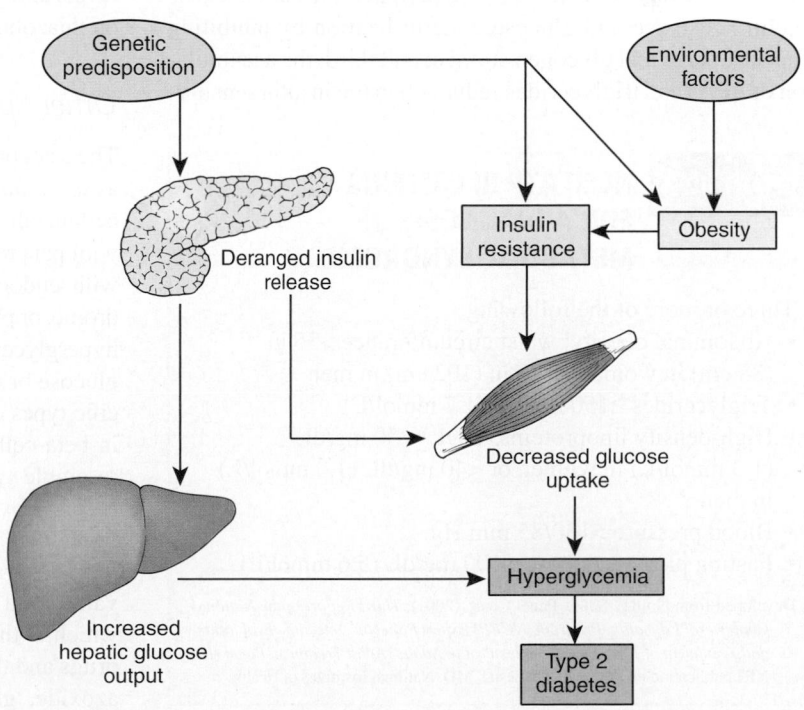

FIGURE 42-8 • Pathogenesis of type 2 diabetes mellitus.

insulin resistance syndrome, syndrome X, or, the preferred term, *metabolic syndrome.*[18] In clinical practice, the definition of metabolic syndrome given in the Third Report of the National Cholesterol Education Program (NCEP III) is widely used[19] (Chart 42-2). Insulin resistance and increased risk of developing type 2 diabetes are also seen in women with polycystic ovary syndrome[20] (see Chapter 46).

A major factor in persons with the metabolic syndrome that leads to type 2 diabetes is obesity.[14,15,21] Approximately 90% of persons with type 2 diabetes are overweight. Obese people have increased resistance to the action of insulin and impaired suppression of glucose production by the liver, resulting in both hyperglycemia and hyperinsulinemia.[15] The type of obesity is an important consideration in the development of type 2 diabetes. It has been found that people with upper body (or central) obesity are at greater risk for developing type 2 diabetes and metabolic disturbances than persons with lower body (or peripheral) obesity (see Chapter 39). The increased insulin resistance has been attributed to the increased visceral (intra-abdominal) fat that can be detected on computed tomography scan and other imaging modalities.[22] Waist circumference and waist–hip ratio (WHR), which are both surrogate measures of central obesity, have been shown to correlate well with insulin resistance. The new terminology that is emerging for persons with obesity and type 2 diabetes is *diabesity.* For management, weight loss with an initial loss of 5% to 10% of body weight should be incorporated into the treatment plan, as well as addressing the diabetes and other related metabolic abnormalities.

It has been theorized that the insulin resistance and increased glucose production in obese people with type 2 diabetes may stem from an increased concentration of FFAs.[15,23] This has several consequences: first, excessive and chronic elevation of FFAs can cause beta cell dysfunction (lipotoxicity); second, FFAs act at the level of the peripheral tissues to cause insulin resistance and glucose underutilization by inhibiting glucose uptake and glycogen storage; and third, the accumulation of FFAs and triglycerides reduces hepatic insulin sensitivity, leading to increased hepatic glucose production and hyperglycemia, especially in the fasting state. Thus, the increase in FFAs that occurs in obese individuals (especially visceral obesity) with a genetic predisposition to type 2 diabetes may eventually lead to beta cell dysfunction, increased insulin resistance, and greater hepatic glucose production. A further consequence is the diversion of excess FFAs to nonadipose tissues, including the liver, skeletal muscle, heart, and pancreatic beta cells.[18] In the liver, the uptake of FFAs from the portal blood can lead to hepatic triglyceride accumulation and nonalcoholic fatty liver disease (see Chapter 38).

Adipocytes are the source of a number of important factors (*e.g.,* adiponectin, leptin, FFAs) involved in a wide range of processes related to the features of the metabolic syndrome, including glucose and lipid metabolism, inflammation, and thrombosis.[15,18,24] In obesity and type 2 diabetes, there is a reduction in the production of some factors that are normally synthesized by adipocytes (*i.e.,* adiponectin), whereas there is an accelerated release of other factors such as angiotensinogen, plasminogen activator inhibitor-1, leptin, and proinflammatory cytokines (*e.g.,* tumor necrosis factor-α).[23] Adiponectin, which is secreted by adipocytes and circulates in the blood, is the only known adipocyte-secreted factor that increases tissue sensitivity to insulin.[23] It has been shown that decreased levels of adiponectin coincide with insulin resistance in patients with obesity and type 2 diabetes.[25] In skeletal muscle, adiponectin has been shown to decrease tissue triglyceride content by increasing the use of fatty acids as a fuel source.[25] Adiponectin also appears to have antidiabetes, anti-inflammatory, and antiatherogenic effects. Moreover, there is evidence that the secretion of adiponectin might be partially regulated by peroxisome proliferator–activated receptor gamma (PPAR-γ), a nuclear receptor that leads to the regulation of genes controlling FFA levels and glucose metabolism[24] (discussed later in the section on thiazolidinediones [oral antidiabetic agents]).

Other Specific Types of Diabetes

The category of other specific types of diabetes, formerly known as *secondary diabetes,* comprises diabetes that is associated with certain other conditions and syndromes. Such diabetes can occur with pancreatic disease or the removal of pancreatic tissue and with endocrine diseases, such as acromegaly, Cushing syndrome, or pheochromocytoma. Endocrine disorders that produce hyperglycemia do so by increasing the hepatic production of glucose or decreasing the cellular use of glucose. Several specific types of diabetes are associated with monogenetic defects in beta cell function. These specific types of diabetes, which resemble type 2 diabetes but occur at an earlier age (usually before 25 years of age), were formerly referred to as *maturity-onset diabetes of the young* (MODY).[3]

Several diuretics—thiazide and loop diuretics—can elevate blood glucose. These diuretics increase potassium loss, which is thought to impair beta cell release of insulin. Other drugs and therapies known to cause hyperglycemia include diazoxide, glucocorticoids, oral contraceptives, antipsychotic

---

CHART 42-2	**NCEP ATP III CRITERIA FOR A DIAGNOSIS OF METABOLIC SYNDROME**

Three or more of the following:

- Abdominal obesity: waist circumference >35 in (88 cm) in women or 40 in (102 cm) in men
- Triglycerides ≥150 mg/dL (1.7 mmol/L)
- High-density lipoproteins (HDL) <50 mg/dL (1.3 mmol/L) in women or <40 mg/dL (1.0 mmol/L) in men
- Blood pressure >130/85 mm Hg
- Fasting plasma glucose >100 mg/dL (5.6 mmol/L)

Developed from Grundy S. M., Panel Chair. (2001). *Third Report of the National Cholesterol Education Program (NCEP) Expert Panel on Detection, Evaluation, and Treatment of High Blood Cholesterol in Adults (Adult Treatment Panel III).* NIH publication no. 01-3670. Bethesda, MD: National Institutes of Health.

agents, and total parenteral nutrition (*i.e.,* hyperalimentation). Drug-related increases in blood glucose usually are reversed after the drug has been discontinued.

The advent of potent antiretroviral therapy (especially protease inhibitors) for the treatment of human immunodeficiency virus infection and acquired immunodeficiency syndrome has significantly improved survival in these conditions. However, these patients are now developing metabolic derangements with features similar to those seen in the metabolic syndrome (*i.e.,* insulin resistance, high levels of plasma triglycerides, low levels of HDLs, hypertension, obesity, systemic inflammation [as detected by elevated levels of CRP and other mediators], abnormal fibrinolysis, abnormal endothelial dysfunction, and macrovascular disease).[26] In addition, changes in fat distribution (peripheral lipoatrophy and visceral obesity), sometimes referred to as *lipodystrophy,* often occur (see Chapter 20). These people should be aggressively treated to prevent cardiovascular complications resulting from the abnormal risk factors.

TABLE 42-4 **Diagnosis of Gestational Diabetes Mellitus With a 100-g Glucose Load**	
BASELINE AND TIME AFTER ADMINISTRATION OF 100-g GLUCOSE LOAD	**PLASMA GLUCOSE LEVEL, mg/dL (mmol/L)**
Fasting	95 (5.3)
1 hr	180 (10.0)
2 hr	155 (8.6)
3 hr	140 (7.8)

Two more of the venous plasma concentrations must be met or exceeded for a positive diagnosis. The test should be done in the morning after an overnight fast of between 8 and 14 hr and after at least 3 days of unrestricted diet (>150 g carbohydrate/day) and unlimited physical activity. The subject should remain seated and should not smoke throughout the test.
Developed from data in American Diabetes Association. (2007). Diagnosis and classification of diabetes mellitus. *Diabetes Care* 30(Suppl. 1), S42–S27.

 *Gestational Diabetes*

Gestational diabetes mellitus (GDM) refers to any degree of glucose intolerance that is first detected during pregnancy. It occurs to various degrees in 1% to 14% of all pregnancies, depending on the population and diagnostic tests used.[27] It most frequently affects women with a family history of diabetes; with a history of stillbirth or spontaneous abortion, fetal anomalies in a previous pregnancy, or a previous large- or heavy-for-date infant; and who are obese, of advanced maternal age, or have had five or more pregnancies.

All pregnant women should undergo risk assessment for diabetes during their first prenatal visit to determine the need for additional screening tests. Women who are younger than 25 years of age, were of normal body weight before pregnancy, have no family history of diabetes or poor obstetric outcome, and are not members of a high-risk ethnic/racial group (*e.g.,* Hispanic, Native American, Asian, African American) may not need to be screened. Those with significant risk factors should undergo plasma glucose testing as soon as feasible. If they are found not to have GDM at the initial screening, they should be retested between 24 and 28 weeks. Women with average risk should be tested at 24 to 28 weeks' gestation. Women with an FPG greater than 126 mg/dL (7.0 mmol/L) or casual glucose greater than 200 mg/dL (11.1 mmol/L) meet the threshold for diabetes, if confirmed on a subsequent day, and do not need to undergo oral glucose tolerance testing.[27] Women with high or average GDM risk who do not demonstrate this degree of hyperglycemia on FPG testing should undergo further screening using the OGTT. This screening test consists of 50 g of glucose given without regard to the last meal, followed in 1 hour by a venous blood sample for glucose concentration. If the plasma glucose level is greater than 140 mg/dL (7.8 mmol/L), then a 100-g 3-hour OGTT is indicated to establish the diagnosis of GDM[27,28] (Table 42-4).

Diagnosis and careful medical management are essential because women with GDM are at higher risk for complications of pregnancy, mortality, and fetal abnormalities.[3] Fetal abnormalities include macrosomia (*i.e.,* large body size), hypoglycemia, hypocalcemia, polycythemia, and hyperbilirubinemia.

Treatment of GDM includes close observation of mother and fetus because even mild hyperglycemia has been shown to be detrimental to the fetus.[27] Maternal fasting and postprandial blood glucose levels should be measured regularly. Fetal surveillance depends on the degree of risk for the fetus. The frequency of growth measurements and determinations of fetal distress depends on available technology and gestational age. All women with GDM require nutritional guidance because nutrition is the cornerstone of therapy. The nutrition plan should provide the necessary nutrients for maternal and fetal health, result in normoglycemia and proper weight gain, and prevent ketosis.[3] If dietary management alone does not achieve a fasting blood glucose level no greater than 105 mg/dL (5.8 mmol/L) or a 2-hour postprandial blood glucose no greater than 120 mg/dL (6.7 mmol/L), the Third International Workshop on GDM recommends therapy with insulin.[27] Self-monitoring of blood glucose levels is essential.

Women with GDM have a 60% to 70% risk of developing type 2 diabetes within 5 to 15 years. Predictors of future diabetes or prediabetes include maternal obesity, elevated FBG on OGTT, and diagnosis of GDM early in gestation. Women in whom GDM is diagnosed should be followed after delivery to detect diabetes early in its course. These women should be evaluated during their first postpartum visit with a 2-hour OGTT with a 75-g glucose load.

Clinical Manifestations of Diabetes

Diabetes mellitus may have a rapid or an insidious onset. In type 1 diabetes, signs and symptoms often arise suddenly. Type 2 diabetes usually develops more insidiously; its presence may be detected during a routine medical examination or when a patient seeks medical care for other reasons.

The most commonly identified signs and symptoms of diabetes are referred to as the *three polys:* (1) polyuria (*i.e.,* excessive urination), (2) polydipsia (*i.e.,* excessive thirst), and (3) polyphagia (*i.e.,* excessive hunger). These three symptoms are closely related to the hyperglycemia and glycosuria of diabetes. Glucose is a small, osmotically active molecule. When blood glucose levels are sufficiently elevated, the amount of glucose filtered by the glomeruli of the kidney exceeds the amount that can be reabsorbed by the renal tubules; this results in glycosuria accompanied by large losses of water in the urine. Thirst results from the intracellular dehydration that occurs as blood glucose levels rise and water is pulled out of body cells, including those in the hypothalamic thirst center. This early symptom may be easily overlooked in people with type 2 diabetes, particularly in those who have had a gradual increase in blood glucose levels. Polyphagia usually is not present in people with type 2 diabetes. In type 1 diabetes, it probably results from cellular starvation and the depletion of cellular stores of carbohydrates, fats, and proteins.

Weight loss despite normal or increased appetite is a common occurrence in people with uncontrolled type 1 diabetes. The cause of weight loss is twofold. First, loss of body fluids results from osmotic diuresis. Vomiting may exaggerate the fluid loss in ketoacidosis. Second, body tissue is lost because the lack of insulin forces the body to use its fat stores and cellular proteins as sources of energy. In terms of weight loss, there often is a marked difference between type 2 diabetes and type 1 diabetes. Weight loss is a frequent phenomenon in people with uncontrolled type 1 diabetes, whereas many people with uncomplicated type 2 diabetes often have problems with obesity.

Other signs and symptoms of hyperglycemia include recurrent blurred vision, fatigue, paresthesias, and skin infections. In type 2 diabetes, these often are the symptoms that prompt a person to seek medical treatment. Blurred vision develops as the lens and retina are exposed to hyperosmolar fluids. Lowered plasma volume produces weakness and fatigue. Paresthesias reflect a temporary dysfunction of the peripheral sensory nerves. Chronic skin infections can occur and are more common in people with type 2 diabetes. Hyperglycemia and glycosuria favor the growth of yeast organisms. Pruritus and vulvovaginitis due to *Candida* infections are common initial complaints in women with diabetes. Balanitis secondary to *Candida* infections can occur in men.

Diagnostic Tests

The diagnosis of diabetes mellitus is confirmed through the use of laboratory tests that measure blood glucose levels (see Table 42-3). Testing for diabetes should be considered in all individuals 45 years of age and older. Testing should be considered at a younger age in people who are obese, have a first-degree relative with diabetes, are members of a high-risk group, have delivered an infant weighing more than 9 pounds or been diagnosed with GDM, have hypertension or hyperlipidemia, or have met the criteria for IGT or IFG (*i.e.,* prediabetes) on previous testing.[29]

Blood Tests

Blood glucose measurements are used in both the diagnosis and management of diabetes. Diagnostic tests include the FPG, casual plasma glucose, and the glucose tolerance test. Laboratory and capillary or finger-stick glucose tests are used for glucose management in people with diagnosed diabetes. Glycosylated hemoglobin (A1C, previously termed HbA_{1c}) provides a measure of glucose control over time. Table 42-5 lists whole-blood and plasma glucose, as well as A1C values for glycemic control for people with diabetes.[29]

Fasting Blood Glucose Test.   The FPG has been suggested as the preferred diagnostic test because of ease of administration, convenience, patient acceptability, and cost.[28] Glucose levels are measured after food has been withheld for at least 8 hours. An FPG level below 100 mg/dL (5.6 mmol/L) is considered normal (see Table 42-3). A level between 100 and 125 mg/dL (5.6 and 6.9 mmol/L) is significant and is defined as impaired fasting glucose. If the FPG level is 126 mg/dL (7.0 mmol/L) or more on two occasions, diabetes is diagnosed.

Casual Blood Glucose Test.   A casual plasma glucose is one that is done without regard to the time of the last meal. A casual plasma glucose concentration that is unequivocally elevated ($\geq$200 mg/dL [11.1 mmol/L]) in the presence of classic symptoms of diabetes such as polydipsia, polyphagia, polyuria, and blurred vision is diagnostic of diabetes mellitus at any age.

Oral Glucose Tolerance Test.   The OGTT is an important screening test for diabetes. The test measures the body's ability to store glucose by removing it from the blood. In men and women, the test measures the plasma glucose response to 75 g of concentrated glucose solution at selected intervals, usually 1 and 2 hours. In pregnant women, a glucose load of 100 g is given (see section on Gestational Diabetes, earlier) with an additional 3-hour plasma glucose determination. In people

TABLE 42-5 **Correlation Between Hemoglobin A1C Level and Mean Plasma Glucose Levels**	
HEMOGLOBIN A1C (%)	**MEAN PLASMA GLUCOSE, mg/dL (mmol/L)**
6	135 (7.5)
7	170 (9.4)
8	205 (11.4)
9	240 (13.3)
10	275 (13.3)
11	310 (17.2)
12	345 (19.2)

Adapted from The Expert Committee on the Diagnosis and Classification of Diabetes Mellitus. (1997). Report of the Expert Committee on the Diagnosis and Classification of Diabetes Mellitus. *Diabetes Care* 2007, Volume 30, S42–S47. Reprinted with permission from the American Diabetes Association. Copyright © 1997 American Diabetes Association.

with normal glucose tolerance, blood glucose levels return to normal within 2 to 3 hours after ingestion of a glucose load, in which case it can be assumed that sufficient insulin is present to allow glucose to leave the blood and enter body cells. Because a person with diabetes lacks the ability to respond to an increase in blood glucose by releasing adequate insulin to facilitate storage, blood glucose levels rise above those observed in normal people and remain elevated for longer periods (see Table 42-3).

Capillary Blood Glucose Monitoring. Technological advances have provided the means for monitoring blood glucose levels by using a drop of capillary blood. This procedure has provided health professionals with a rapid and economical means for monitoring blood glucose and has given people with diabetes a way of maintaining near-normal blood glucose levels through self-monitoring of blood glucose. These methods use a drop of capillary blood obtained by pricking the finger or forearm with a special needle or small lancet. Small trigger devices make use of the lancet virtually painless. The drop of capillary blood is placed on or absorbed by a reagent strip, and glucose levels are determined electronically using a glucose meter.

Laboratory tests that use plasma for measurement of blood glucose give results that are 10% to 15% higher than the fingerstick method, which uses whole blood.[29] Many blood glucose monitors approved for home use and some test strips now calibrate blood glucose readings to plasma values. It is important that people with diabetes know whether their monitors or glucose strips provide whole-blood or plasma test results.

Continuous glucose monitoring systems are becoming available to fine-tune glucose management. The various systems have small catheters implanted in the subcutaneous tissue to provide frequent samples. The variety and accuracy of these systems is continually improving. However, finger-stick glucose monitoring remains the standard of care.

Glycated Hemoglobin Testing. Glycated hemoglobin, also referred to as glycohemoglobin, glycosylated hemoglobin, HBA_{1c}, or A1C (the preferred term), is a term used to describe hemoglobin into which glucose has been incorporated. Hemoglobin normally does not contain glucose when it is released from the bone marrow. During its 120-day life span in the red blood cell, hemoglobin normally becomes glycated to form hemoglobins A_{1a} and A_{1b} (2% to 4%), and A1C (4% to 6%). Because glucose entry into red blood cells is not insulin dependent, the rate at which glucose becomes attached to the hemoglobin molecule depends on blood glucose levels. Glycosylation is essentially irreversible, and the level of A1C present in the blood provides an index of blood glucose levels over the previous 6 to 12 weeks. In uncontrolled diabetes or diabetes with hyperglycemia, there is an increase in the level of A1C. The American Diabetes Association (ADA) recommends initiating corrective measures for A1C levels greater than 7%. However, the goal has been redefined as lowering the A1C to less than 7.0%, or even achieving normal glycemic levels of less than 6.0%.[28]

Urine Tests

The ease, accuracy, and convenience of self-administered blood glucose monitoring techniques have made urine testing for glucose obsolete for most people with diabetes. These tests only reflect urine glucose levels and are influenced by such factors as the renal threshold for glucose, fluid intake and urine concentration, urine testing methodologies, and some drugs. It is recommended that all people with diabetes self-monitor their blood glucose. Urine ketone determinations remain an important part of monitoring diabetic control, particularly in people with type 1 diabetes who are at risk for development of ketoacidosis, and in pregnant diabetic women to check the adequacy of nutrition and glycemic control.[29]

Diabetes Management

The desired outcome of glycemic control in both type 1 and type 2 diabetes is normalization of blood glucose as a means of preventing short- and long-term complications. Treatment plans involve medical nutrition therapy, exercise, and antidiabetic agents. People with type 1 diabetes require insulin therapy from the time of diagnosis. Weight loss and dietary management may be sufficient to control blood glucose levels in people with type 2 diabetes. However, they require follow-up care because insulin secretion from the beta cells may decrease or insulin resistance may persist or worsen, in which case oral antidiabetic agents are prescribed.

Among the methods used to achieve these treatment goals are education in self-management and problem solving. Individual treatment goals should take into account the person's age and other disease conditions, the person's capacity to understand and carry out the treatment regime, and socioeconomic factors that might influence compliance with the treatment plan. Optimal control of both type 1 and type 2 diabetes is associated with prevention or delay of chronic diabetes complications.[28]

Dietary Management

Dietary management usually is prescribed to meet the specific needs of each person with diabetes.[30] The term *medical nutrition therapy,* which was introduced in 1994 by the ADA, is defined as the use of specific nutrition services to treat an illness, injury, or condition and involves both the assessment of the nutrition status and the treatment measure, including nutrition therapy, counseling, and use of specialized nutritional supplements.[31] The diabetic diet has undergone marked changes over the years, particularly in the recommendations for distribution of calories among carbohydrates, proteins, and fats. There no longer is a specific diabetic or ADA diet but rather a dietary prescription based on nutrition assessment and treatment goals. A coordinated team effort, including the person with diabetes, is needed to individualize the nutrition plan.

Goals and principles of diet therapy differ between type 1 and type 2 diabetes, as well as for lean and obese people. Integral to diabetes management is a prescribed plan for nutrition therapy.[30] Therapy goals include maintenance of near-normal blood glucose levels, achievement of optimal lipid levels, adequate calories to maintain and attain reasonable weights, prevention and treatment of chronic diabetes complications, and improvement of overall health through optimal nutrition. Initial guidelines may include 45% to 60% carbohydrate, 20% to 35% fat and 10% to 35% protein.[30]

For a person with type 1 diabetes, the usual food intake is assessed and used as a basis for adjusting insulin therapy to fit with the person's lifestyle. Eating consistent amounts and types of food at specific and routine times are encouraged. Home blood glucose monitoring is used to fine-tune the plan. Most people with type 2 diabetes are overweight. Nutrition therapy goals focus on achieving glucose, lipid, and blood pressure goals, and weight loss if indicated. Mild to moderate weight loss (5% to 10% of total body weight) has been shown to improve diabetes control, even if desirable weight is not achieved.

The registered dietitian plays an essential role in the diabetes care team and is able to select from a variety of methods such as carbohydrate counting, food exchanges, healthy food choices, glycemic index, and total available glucose to tailor the meal plan to meet individual needs. Simpler recommendations have been associated with improved client understanding and dietary adherence. Carbohydrate counting uses product label information that is easily available to people with diabetes.[30] Regardless of food source, total grams of carbohydrate are counted, placing an emphasis on the nutrient that most affects blood glucose control.

Medical nutrition therapy is also important in preventing, or at least slowing, the development of complications. Because diabetes is a risk factor for cardiovascular disease, it is recommended that less than 7% of daily calories should be obtained from saturated fat and that dietary cholesterol be limited to 200 mg or less, and intake of trans fats minimized. Periodic fasting lipid panels may identify concomitant lipid disorders. If lipid disorders are identified, appropriate modifications according to the NCEP III should be followed.[19] For people with diabetic nephropathy, studies suggest lowering the intake of protein to 0.8 to 1 g/kg body weight per day according to the degree of kidney impairment.[30] Recommendations for dietary sodium are the same as for the general population (2400 to 3000 mg/day), with a reduced sodium intake (<2300 mg/day) for people with mild to moderate hypertension and a moderate sodium restriction (<2000 mg/day) for those with severe hypertension, heart failure, and nephropathy.[30]

Exercise

The benefits of exercise include cardiovascular fitness and psychological well-being. For many people with type 2 diabetes, the benefits of exercise include a decrease in body fat, better weight control, and improvement in insulin sensitivity.[28,32] Exercise is so important in diabetes management that a planned program of regular exercise usually is considered an integral part of the therapeutic regimen for every person with diabetes. In general, sporadic exercise has only transient benefits; a regular exercise or training program is the most beneficial. It is better for cardiovascular conditioning and can maintain a muscle–fat ratio that enhances peripheral insulin receptivity.

In people with diabetes, the beneficial effects of exercise are accompanied by an increased risk of hypoglycemia. Although muscle uptake of glucose increases significantly, the ability to maintain blood glucose levels is hampered by failure to suppress the absorption of injected insulin and activate the counter-regulatory mechanisms that maintain blood glucose. Not only is there an inability to suppress insulin levels, but insulin absorption may increase. This increased absorption is more pronounced when insulin is injected into the subcutaneous tissue of the exercised muscle, but it occurs even when insulin is injected into other body areas. Even after exercise ceases, insulin's lowering effect on blood glucose continues. In some people with type 1 diabetes, the symptoms of hypoglycemia occur several hours after cessation of exercise, perhaps because subsequent insulin doses (in people using multiple daily insulin injections) are not adjusted to accommodate the exercise-induced decrease in blood glucose. The cause of hypoglycemia in people who do not administer a subsequent insulin dose is unclear. It may be related to the fact that the liver and skeletal muscles increase their uptake of glucose after exercise as a means of replenishing their glycogen stores, or that the liver and skeletal muscles are more sensitive to insulin during this time. People with diabetes should be aware that delayed hypoglycemia can occur after exercise and that they may need to alter their diabetes medication dose, their carbohydrate intake, or both.

Although of benefit to people with diabetes, exercise must be weighed on the risk–benefit scale. Before beginning an exercise program, persons with diabetes should undergo an appropriate evaluation for macrovascular and microvascular disease.[32] The goal of exercise is safe participation in activities consistent with an individual's lifestyle. As with nutrition guidelines, exercise recommendations need to be individualized. Considerations include the potential for hypoglycemia, hyperglycemia, ketosis, cardiovascular ischemia and arrhythmias (particularly silent ischemic heart disease), exacerbation of proliferative retinopathy, and lower extremity injury. For those with chronic diabetes, the complications of vigorous exercise can be harmful and cause eye hemorrhage and other problems. For people with type 1 diabetes who exercise during periods of poor control (*i.e.,* when blood glucose is elevated, exogenous insulin levels are low, and ketonemia exists), blood glucose and ketones rise to even higher levels because the stress of exercise is superimposed on preexisting insulin deficiency and increased counter-regulatory hormone activity.

Oral and Injectable Antidiabetic Agents

Historically, two categories of antidiabetic agents existed: insulin injections and oral medications. However, this classification has become somewhat blurred owing to the introduction of new injectable antidiabetic agents (*e.g.,* amylin analogs and glucagon-like peptide-1 [GLP-1] analogs). Because people with type 1 diabetes are deficient in insulin, they are in need of exogenous insulin replacement therapy from the start. People with type 2 diabetes can have increased hepatic glucose production; decreased peripheral utilization of glucose; decreased utilization of ingested carbohydrates; and, over time, impaired insulin secretion and excessive glucagon secretion from the pancreas (Fig. 42-9). The antidiabetic agents used in the treatment of type 2 diabetes attack each one of these areas and sometimes all.[33] If good glycemic control cannot be achieved with one or a combination of antidiabetic agents, insulin can be added or used by itself.

Oral antidiabetic agents fall into five categories: (1) insulin secretagogues (*i.e.,* sulfonylureas, repaglinide, and nateglinide), (2) biguanides, (3) α-glucosidase inhibitors, (4) dipeptidyl

peptidase-4 (DPP-4) enzyme inhibitors, and (5) thiazolidinediones (TZDs)[33,34] (Table 42-6). In addition, a GLP-1 agonist and amylin agonist in injectable formulations have been introduced.

Insulin Secretagogues: Sulfonylureas. The sulfonylureas were discovered accidentally in 1942, when scientists noticed that one of the sulfonamide drugs being developed at the time caused hypoglycemia. These drugs reduce blood glucose by stimulating the release of insulin from beta cells in the pancreas. These agents are effective only when some residual beta cell function remains. The sulfonylureas act by binding to a high-affinity sulfonylurea receptor on the beta cell that is linked to an adenosine triphosphate (ATP)–sensitive potassium channel (see Fig 42-4). Binding of a sulfonylurea closes

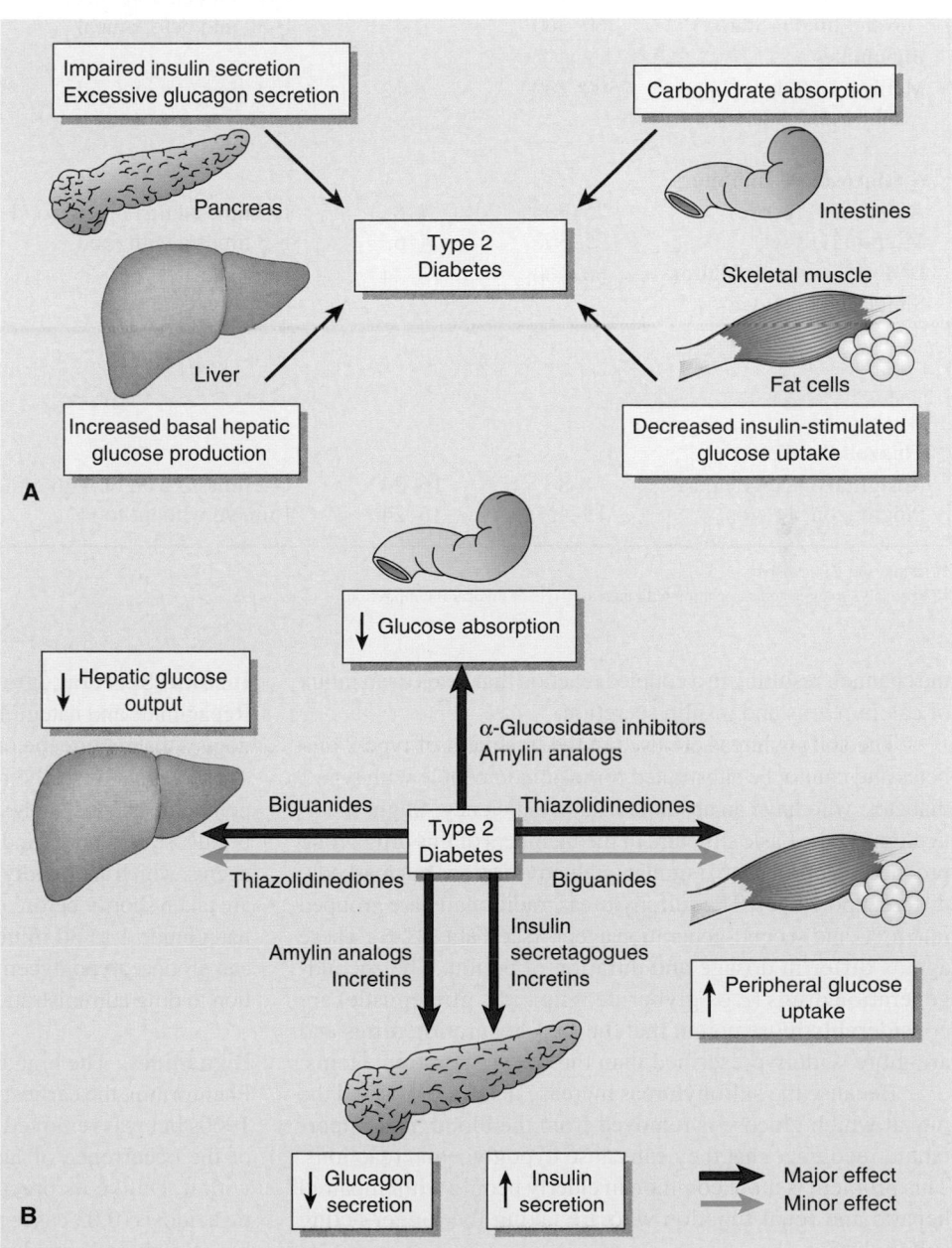

FIGURE 42-9 • **(A)** Mechanisms of elevated blood glucose in type 2 diabetes mellitus. **(B)** Action sites of hypoglycemic agents and mechanisms of lowering blood glucose in type 2 diabetes. The incretins are the dipeptidyl peptidase-4 (DPP-4) inhibitors and glucagon-like peptide-1 (GLP-1) agonists.

TABLE 42-6 Oral Antidiabetic Agents*

PHARMACOLOGIC AGENT	DOSAGE (mg/d)	DURATION OF ACTION (hr)	DOSING SCHEDULE	MECHANISM OF ACTION
Insulin Secretagogues				Stimulates release of insulin from beta cells in the pancreas
Sulfonylureas (first generation)				
Chlorpropamide (generic)	100–500	60	1 time/d	
Sulfonylureas (second generation)				
Glipizide (Glucotrol)	2.5–40	6–24	1–2 times/d, 30 min before meal	
Glyburide (Diabeta, Micronase)	1.25–20	16–24	1–2 times/d with meal	
Glimepiride (Amaryl)	1–8	18–24	1 time/d with first meal	
Nonsulfonylureas				
Repaglinide (Prandin)	0.5–16	5	15–30 min before meal	
Nateglinide (Starlix)	60–360	3–4	1–30 min before meal	
Biguanides				Decreases production and release of glucose by the liver
Metformin (Glucophage, Glucophage XR)	500–2000	7–12	1–3 times/d with food	
α-Glucosidase Inhibitors				Delays the breakdown and absorption of carbohydrates from the intestine
Acarbose (Precose)	25–300	4–6	1–3 times/d first bite of food	
Miglitol (Glyset)	25–300	4–6	1–3 times/d with food	
DDP-4 Enzyme Inhibitors Sitagliptin (Januvia)	50–100	18–24	1 time/d	Blocks enzyme DPP-4 (which breaks down GLP-1 and GIP), thereby increasing the release of insulin after blood glucose rises
Thiazolidinediones				Sensitizes body cells to the action of insulin
Rosiglitazone (Avandia)†	4–8	16–24	1–2 times/d with or without food	
Pioglitazone (Actos)	15–45	16–24	1 time/d without food	

*List may not be inclusive.
†2007 analysis suggested association with increased risk of myocardial infarction.

the channel, resulting in a coupled reaction that leads to an influx of calcium ions and insulin secretion.

The sulfonylureas are used in the treatment of type 2 diabetes and cannot be substituted for insulin in people with type 1 diabetes, who have an absolute insulin deficiency. Slight modifications in the basic structure of the members of this drug group produce agents that have similar qualitative actions but markedly different potencies. The sulfonylureas traditionally are grouped into first- and second-generation agents (see Table 42-6). These agents differ in dosage and duration of action. The second-generation drugs (*e.g.*, glyburide, glipizide, glimepiride) are considerably more potent that the first-generation drugs and are more widely prescribed than the first-generation agents.

Because the sulfonylureas increase insulin levels and the rate at which glucose is removed from the blood, it is important to recognize that they can cause hypoglycemic reactions. This problem is more common in elderly people with impaired hepatic and renal function who are taking the longer-acting sulfonylureas.

Insulin Secretagogues: Repaglinide and Nateglinide. Repaglinide and nateglinide are nonsulfonylurea insulin secretagogues that require the presence of glucose for their main action. These agents exert their action by closing the ATP-dependent potassium channel in the beta cells (see Fig. 41-4). Insulin release is glucose dependent and diminishes at low glucose levels. These agents, which are rapidly absorbed from the gastrointestinal tract, are taken shortly before meals (repaglinide 15 to 30 minutes and nateglinide 1 to 30 minutes). Both repaglinide and nateglinide can produce hypoglycemia; thus, proper timing of meals in relation to drug administration is essential.

Biguanides. The biguanides are older oral antidiabetic drugs. Phenformin, the earliest biguanide, was used extensively in the 1960s but was removed from the U.S. market in 1977 because of the occurrence of lactic acidosis in some patients treated with it. Unlike its precursor, metformin rarely results in lactic acidosis (0.03 cases per 1000 patients). Metformin inhibits hepatic glucose production and increases the sensitivity of peripheral tissues to the actions of insulin. Because metformin does not stimulate insulin secretion, it does not produce hypoglycemia as a side effect. Secondary benefits of metformin therapy include weight loss and improved lipid profiles. Whereas the primary action of the sulfonylurea drugs is to increase insulin secretion, metformin exerts its beneficial effects on glycemic control through increased peripheral use of glucose and decreased hepatic glucose production (main effect). To decrease the risk of lactic acidosis, metformin is contraindicated in people with elevated serum creatinine levels (a test of renal function), clinical and laboratory evidence of hepatic disease, and any condition associated with hypoxemia or dehydration.[33]

α-Glucosidase Inhibitors. In patients with type 2 diabetes, sulfonylureas, biguanides, or both may have beneficial effects on FPG levels. However, postprandial hyperglycemia persists in more than 60% of these patients and probably accounts for sustained increases in A1C levels. An alternative approach to the problem of postprandial hyperglycemia is the use of drugs such as acarbose and miglitol, inhibitors of α-glucosidase, which is a small intestine brush border enzyme that breaks down complex carbohydrates. By delaying the breakdown of complex carbohydrates, the α-glucosidase inhibitors delay the absorption of carbohydrates from the gut and blunt the postprandial increase in plasma glucose and insulin levels. Although not a problem with monotherapy or combination therapy with a biguanide, hypoglycemia may occur with concurrent sulfonylurea treatment. If hypoglycemia does occur, it should be treated with glucose (dextrose) and not sucrose (table sugar), whose breakdown may be blocked by the action of the α-glucosidase inhibitors.

Thiazolidinediones. The TZDs (or glitazones) are the only class of drugs that directly target insulin resistance, a fundamental defect in the pathophysiology of type 2 diabetes. The TZDs improve glycemic control by increasing insulin sensitivity in the insulin-responsive tissues—liver, skeletal muscle, and fat—allowing the tissues to respond to endogenous insulin more efficiently without increased output from already dysfunctional beta cells.[33–35] Pioglitazone and rosiglitazone are the most potent insulin sensitizers and were approved by the FDA in 1999. Another TZD, troglitazone, was approved in 1997, but because of hepatic safety concerns, it is no longer available, having been withdrawn worldwide in March 2000. Pioglitazone and rosiglitazone are both approved for use as monotherapy and in combination therapy. Because of the previous problem with liver toxicity in this class of drugs, liver enzymes should be monitored according to guidelines. In 2007, a published meta-analysis suggested that rosiglitazone may be associated with an increased risk of myocardial infarction.[36] This finding was not seen with pioglitazone. Both agents can cause fluid accumulation and are therefore contraindicated in patients with New York Heart Association stage III and IV heart failure (see Chapter 26, Table 26-2). In addition, an increased risk of bone fractures was recently observed in postmarketing studies of both compounds.

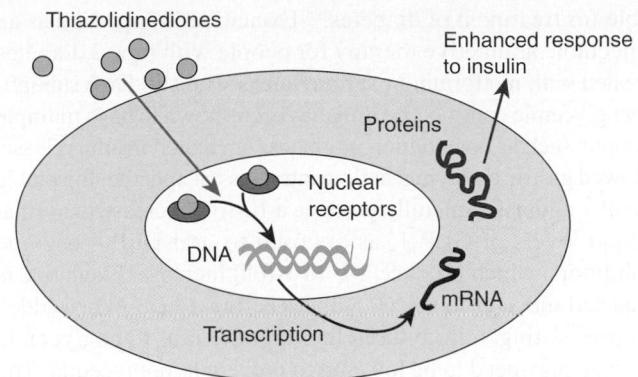

FIGURE 42-10 • Action of the thiazolidinediones on activation of the nuclear peroxisome proliferator–activated receptor gamma (PPAR-γ) that regulates gene transcription of proteins that regulate glucose uptake and reduce fatty acid release. mRNA, messenger ribonucleic acid.

The mechanism of action of the TZDs is complex and not fully understood. The action of the TZDs is associated with binding to the PPAR-γ nuclear receptor[35] (Fig. 42-10). Binding of the TZDs to the PPAR-γ receptor begins a cascade of events leading to regulation of genes involved in lipid and glucose metabolism. They result is an increase in the number of GLUT-4 transporters and increased insulin-mediated uptake of glucose in the peripheral tissues. *Adiponectin* is produced by adipocytes and directly sensitizes the body to the actions of insulin, may be a part of the missing link in explaining insulin resistance in persons with type 2 diabetes.[34] The TZDs are thought to decrease insulin resistance, at least in part, by increasing adipocyte production of adiponectin. Additional effects of TZDs are numerous, and include correction of many of the abnormal metabolic features associated with type 2 diabetes. This includes a decrease in FFA and triglycerides, microalbuminuria, blood pressure, inflammatory mediators (*e.g.*, fibrinogen and CRP), and procoagulation factors.[35]

Dipeptidyl Peptidase-4 Enzyme Inhibitors. Incretins are insulinotropic substances released into the circulation by the gastrointestinal tract after a meal, especially one high in carbohydrates.[37] Incretins act by stimulating insulin secretion by the beta cell. In normal individuals, incretins account for approximately 20% to 60% of insulin secretion after a meal. The main incretins secreted are *GLP-1* and *glucose-dependent insulinotropic polypeptide* (GIP). Both GLP-1 and GIP are rapidly degraded by the enzyme, DPP-4. DPP-4 enzyme inhibitors work by inhibiting the DPP-4 enzyme and increasing GLP-1 and GIP levels, which then increase insulin release. GLP-1 also helps to suppress glucagon release. The first oral agent of this category (sitagliptin) was introduced in 2006. These agents appear to be well tolerated.[38] Several other DPP-4 inhibitors (*e.g.*, alogliptin, vildagliptin) are currently in development.

Glucagon-like Polypeptide-1 Agonists. As a synthetic analog of GLP-1, exenatide was the first type of incretin to become available for treatment of diabetes.[38] Exenatide is approved as an injectable adjunctive therapy for people with type 2 diabetes treated with metformin or sulfonylureas who still have suboptimal glycemic control. The drug has been shown to have multiple actions such as potentiation of glucose-mediated insulin release, slowed gastric emptying, and a central loss of appetite. Injectable GLP-1 agonists generally produce a 10-fold increase in normal blood levels of GLP-1, as opposed to oral DPP-4 enzyme inhibitors, which produce a 2- to 3-fold increase. Exenatide is injected subcutaneously 60 minutes before a meal. When added to preexisting sulfonylurea therapy, the oral hypoglycemic dosage may need to be lowered to prevent hypoglycemia. The major side effects are nausea and weight loss.[38] Although exenatide was the first GLP-1 agonist to be developed and approved, other agents and formulations are in development.

Insulin

Type 1 diabetes mellitus always requires treatment with insulin, and many people with type 2 diabetes eventually require insulin therapy. Insulin is destroyed in the gastrointestinal tract and must be administered by injection or inhalation. All insulins are measured in units (the international unit of insulin is defined as the amount of insulin required to lower the blood glucose of a fasting 2-kg rabbit from 145 mg/dL to 120 mg/dL). Most types of insulin are available in U-100 strength (*i.e.,* 100 units of insulin/1 mL). Insulin preparations are categorized according to onset, peak, and duration of action. An inhaled form of insulin (Exubera) was on the market for a short time in the United States,

but was withdrawn for commercial reasons. Other inhaled insulin formulations are in clinical development.

During the past several decades, many pharmaceutical companies have entered the insulin manufacturing market. After much research, human insulin has become widely available, providing an alternative to previous forms of insulin that were obtained from bovine and porcine sources. The manufacture of human insulin uses recombinant deoxyribonucleic acid (DNA) technology. More recently, insulin analogs have become available that offer even better and more reproducible release characteristics.[39] In these agents, the human insulin sequence has been modified to improve their pharmacologic properties.

Insulin types are classified by length and peaking of action.[39] There are four principal types of insulin: rapid-acting, short-acting, intermediate-acting, and long-acting (Table 42-7). Short-acting insulin (regular) is a soluble crystalline insulin whose effects begin within 30 minutes after subcutaneous injection and generally last for 5 to 8 hours. The rapid-acting insulins (lispro, aspart, and glulisine) are produced by recombinant technology with an amino acid substitution. These insulins have a more rapid onset, peak, and duration of action than short-acting regular insulin. The rapid-acting insulins, which are used in combination with intermediate or long-acting insulins, are usually administered immediately before a meal. Intermediate- to long-acting insulins include NPH, glargine, and detemir. These insulins have slower onsets and a longer duration of action. They require several hours to reach therapeutic levels, so their use in type 1 diabetes requires supplementation with rapid- or short-acting insulin. Glargine and detemir have a slower, more

TABLE 42-7 **Activity Profiles of Insulin Preparations in the United States***			
TYPE (HUMAN INSULIN)	**ONSET**	**PEAK (hr)**	**DURATION (hr)**
Rapid-Acting			
Lispro (Humalog)	5–15 min	1–1.5	3–5
Aspart (Novalog)	5–15 min	1–1.5	3–5
Glulisine (Apidra)	5–15 min	1–1.5	3–5
Short-Acting			
Regular Insulin	0.5–1 h	2–4	5–8
Intermediate-Acting			
Isophane insulin suspension (NPH)	2–4 h	4–10	10–24
Long-Acting			
Detemir (Levemir)	2–4 h	No peak	6–23
Glargine (Lantus)†	2–4 h	No peak	20–24
Premixed			
70% NPH/30% regular	0.5–1 h	Dual	10–24
50% NPH/50% regular	0.5–1 h	Dual	10–24
75% NPL (insulin lispro protamine)/ 25% lispro	5–15 min	Dual	10–24
50% NPL/50% lispro	5–15 min	Dual	10–24
70% NPA (insulin aspart protamine)/ 30% aspart	5–15 min	Dual	10–24

*List may not be inclusive.
†Lantus insulin should never be mixed with or administered using the same syringe used to administer any other type of insulin.

prolonged absorption than NPH insulin and provide a relatively constant concentration over 12 to 24 hours. All forms of insulin have the potential to produce hypoglycemia or "insulin reaction" as a side effect (to be discussed).

Intensive Insulin Treatment Regimens. Two intensive treatment regimens—multiple daily injections and continuous subcutaneous infusion of insulin—closely simulate the normal pattern of insulin secretion by the body. With each method, a basal insulin level is maintained, and bolus doses of short- or rapid-acting insulin are delivered before meals. The choice of management is determined by the person with diabetes in collaboration with the health care team.

With *multiple daily injections* (MDI), the basal insulin requirements are met by an intermediate- or long-acting insulin administered once or twice daily. Boluses of rapid- or short-acting insulin are used before meals. The development of convenient injection devices (*e.g.,* pen injectors) has made it easier for people with diabetes to comply with algorithms for these insulins that are administered before meals.

The *continuous subcutaneous insulin infusion* (CSII) method uses an insulin pump. With this method, the basal insulin requirements are met by continuous infusion of subcutaneous insulin, the rate of which can be varied to accommodate diurnal variations.[40] The CSII technique involves the insertion of a small needle or plastic catheter into the subcutaneous tissue of the abdomen. Tubing from the catheter is connected to a syringe set into a small infusion pump worn on a belt or in a jacket pocket. The computer-operated pump then delivers one or more set basal amounts of insulin. In addition to the basal amount delivered by the pump, a bolus amount of insulin may be delivered when needed (*e.g.,* before a meal) by pushing a button.

Self-monitoring of blood glucose levels is a necessity when using the CSII method of management. Each basal and bolus dose is determined individually and programmed into the infusion pump computer. Although the pump's safety has been proven, strict attention must be paid to signs of hypoglycemia. However, investigations have found CSII therapy to be associated with a marked and sustained reduction in the rate of severe hypoglycemia. Ketotic episodes caused by pump failure, catheter clogging, and infections at the needle site also are possible complications. Candidate selection is crucial to the successful use of the insulin pump. Only people who are highly motivated to do frequent blood glucose tests and make daily insulin adjustments are candidates for this method of treatment.[40]

Amylin Analogs

Pramlintide, a synthetic analog of amylin, is an injectable antidiabetic agent that modulates postprandial glucose levels and is approved for use in type 1 and type 2 diabetes. Amylin is a 37-amino-acid peptide that is produced, stored, and cosecreted with insulin in response to glucose and other beta cell stimulators.[34] Therefore, in states of diabetes in which the beta cells and insulin secretion are largely depleted or dysfunctional, amylin secretion is also lost or dysfunctional. Pramlintide is injected (in a separate injection from insulin) before meals in those individuals who are unable to achieve their target postprandial blood glucose levels. Pramlintide, which has a rapid onset of action, suppresses glucagon release, slows gastric emptying, and tends to decrease appetite. The major side effects of pramlintide are hypoglycemia and gastrointestinal symptoms such as anorexia, nausea, and vomiting.

Pancreas or Islet Cell Transplantation

Pancreas or islet cell transplantation is not a lifesaving procedure. It does, however, afford the potential for significantly improving the quality of life. The most serious problems are the requirement for immunosuppression and the need for diagnosis and treatment of rejection. Investigators are looking for methods of transplanting islet cells and protecting the cells from destruction without the use of immunosuppressive drugs.[41]

Acute Complications

The three major acute complications of diabetes are diabetic ketoacidosis, hyperosmolar hyperglycemic state, and hypoglycemia. All are life-threatening conditions that demand immediate recognition and treatment.

Diabetic Ketoacidosis

Diabetic ketoacidosis (DKA) most commonly occurs in a person with type 1 diabetes, in whom the lack of insulin leads to mobilization of fatty acids from adipose tissue because of the unsuppressed adipose cell lipase activity that breaks down triglycerides into fatty acids and glycerol. The increase in fatty acid levels leads to ketone production by the liver (Fig. 42-11). It can occur at the onset of the disease, often before the disease has been diagnosed. For example, a mother may bring a child into the clinic or emergency department with reports of lethargy, vomiting, and abdominal pain, unaware that the child has diabetes. Stress increases the release of gluconeogenic hormones and predisposes the person to the development of ketoacidosis. DKA often is preceded by physical or emotional stress, such as infection, pregnancy, or extreme anxiety. In clinical practice, ketoacidosis also occurs with the omission or inadequate use of insulin.

The three major metabolic derangements in DKA are hyperglycemia, ketosis, and metabolic acidosis. The definitive diagnosis of DKA consists of hyperglycemia (blood glucose levels >250 mg/dL [13.8 mmol/L]), low serum bicarbonate (<15 mEq/L [15 mmol/L]), and low pH (<7.3), with ketonemia (positive at 1:2 dilution) and moderate ketonuria.[42,43] Hyperglycemia leads to osmotic diuresis, dehydration, and a critical loss of electrolytes. Hyperosmolality of extracellular fluids from hyperglycemia leads to a shift of water and potassium from the intracellular to the extracellular compartment. Extracellular sodium concentration frequently is low or normal despite enteric water losses because of the intracellular–extracellular fluid shift. This dilutional effect is referred to as *pseudohyponatremia*. Serum potassium levels may be normal or elevated, despite total potassium depletion resulting from protracted polyuria and vomiting. Metabolic acidosis is caused by the excess ketoacids that require buffering by bicarbonate ions; this leads to a marked decrease in serum bicarbonate levels.

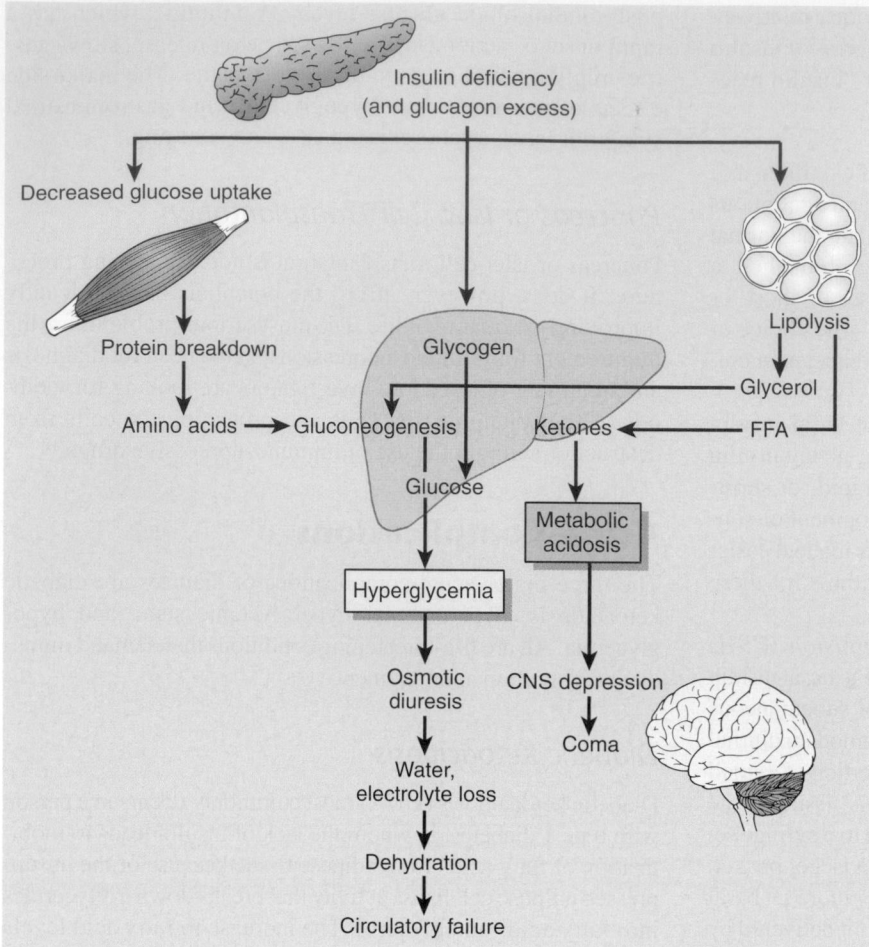

FIGURE 42-11 • Mechanisms of diabetic ketoacidosis. Diabetic ketoacidosis is associated with very low insulin levels and extremely high levels of glucagon, catecholamines, and other counter-regulatory hormones. Increased levels of glucagon and the catecholamines lead to mobilization of substrates for gluconeogenesis and ketogenesis by the liver. Gluconeogenesis in excess of that needed to supply glucose for the brain and other glucose-dependent tissues produces a rise in blood glucose levels. Mobilization of free fatty acids (FFA) from triglyceride stores in adipose tissue leads to accelerated ketone production and ketosis. CNS, central nervous system.

The appearance of DKA is commonly preceded by a day or more of polyuria, polydipsia, nausea, vomiting, and marked fatigue, with eventual stupor that can progress to coma. Abdominal pain and tenderness may be experienced without abdominal disease. The breath has a characteristic fruity smell because of the presence of the volatile ketoacids. Hypotension and tachycardia may be present because of a decrease in blood volume. A number of the signs and symptoms that occur in DKA are related to compensatory mechanisms. The heart rate increases as the body compensates for a decrease in blood volume, and the rate and depth of respiration increase (*i.e.,* Kussmaul respiration) as the body attempts to prevent further decreases in pH. Metabolic acidosis is discussed further in Chapter 32.

The goals in treating DKA are to improve circulatory volume and tissue perfusion, decrease blood glucose, correct the acidosis, and correct electrolyte imbalances. These objectives usually are accomplished through the administration of insulin and intravenous fluid and electrolyte replacement solutions. Because insulin resistance accompanies severe acidosis, low-dose insulin therapy is used. An initial loading dose of regular insulin often is given intravenously, followed by continuous low-dose infusion. Frequent laboratory tests are used to monitor blood glucose and serum electrolyte levels and to guide fluid and electrolyte replacement. It is important to replace fluid and electrolytes and correct pH while bringing the blood glucose concentration to a normal level. Too rapid a drop in blood glucose may cause hypoglycemia. A sudden change in the osmolality of extracellular fluid can also occur when blood glucose levels are lowered too rapidly, and this can cause cerebral edema. Serum potassium levels often fall as acidosis is corrected and potassium moves from the extracellular into the intracellular compartment. Thus, it may be necessary to add potassium to the intravenous infusion. Identification and treatment of the underlying cause, such as infection, also are important. With the better understanding of the pathogenesis of DKA and more uniform agreement on diagnosis and treatment, the mortality rate has been reduced to less than 5%.

Hyperosmolar Hyperglycemic State

The hyperosmolar hyperglycemic state (HHS) is characterized by hyperglycemia (blood glucose >600 mg/dL [33.3 mmol/L]), hyperosmolarity (plasma osmolarity >320 mOsm/L) and dehydration, the absence of ketoacidosis, and depression of the sensorium.[42] HHS may occur in various conditions, including type 2 diabetes, acute pancreatitis, severe infection, myocardial infarction, and treatment with oral or parenteral nutrition solutions. It is seen most frequently in people with type 2 diabetes.

A partial or relative insulin deficiency may initiate the syndrome by reducing glucose utilization while inducing hyperglucagonemia and increasing hepatic glucose output. With massive glycosuria, obligatory water loss occurs. If the person is unable to maintain adequate fluid intake because of associated acute or chronic illness or has excessive fluid loss, dehydration develops. As the plasma volume contracts, renal insufficiency develops and the resultant limitation of renal glucose losses leads to increasingly higher blood glucose levels and severity of the hyperosmolar state.

In hyperosmolar states, the increased serum osmolarity has the effect of pulling water out of body cells, including brain cells. The condition may be complicated by thromboembolic events arising because of the high serum osmolality. The most prominent manifestations are weakness, dehydration, polyuria, neurologic signs and symptoms, and excessive thirst. The neurologic signs include hemiparesis, Babinski reflexes, aphasia, muscle fasciculations, hyperthermia, hemianopia, nystagmus, visual hallucinations, seizures, and coma. The onset of HHS often is insidious, and because it occurs most frequently in older people, it may be mistaken for a stroke.

The treatment of HHS requires judicious medical observation and care as water moves back into brain cells, posing a threat of cerebral edema. Extensive potassium losses that also have occurred during the diuretic phase of the disorder require correction. Because of the problems encountered in the treatment and the serious nature of the disease conditions that cause HHS, the prognosis for this disorder is less favorable than that for ketoacidosis.

Hypoglycemia

Hypoglycemia, or an insulin reaction, occurs from a relative excess of insulin in the blood and is characterized by below-normal blood glucose levels.[44,45] It occurs most commonly in people treated with insulin injections, but prolonged hypoglycemia also can result from some oral hypoglycemic agents. There are many factors that can precipitate an insulin reaction in a person with type 1 diabetes, including error in insulin dose, failure to eat, increased exercise, decreased insulin need after removal of a stress situation, medication changes, and a change in insulin injection site. Alcohol decreases liver gluconeogenesis, and people with diabetes need to be cautioned about its potential for causing hypoglycemia, especially if it is consumed in large amounts or on an empty stomach.

Hypoglycemia usually has a rapid onset and progression of symptoms. The signs and symptoms of hypoglycemia can be divided into two categories: (1) those caused by altered cerebral function, and (2) those related to activation of the autonomic nervous system. Because the brain relies on blood glucose as its main energy source, hypoglycemia produces behaviors related to altered cerebral function. Headache, difficulty in problem solving, disturbed or altered behavior, coma, and seizures may occur. At the onset of the hypoglycemic episode, activation of the parasympathetic nervous system often causes hunger. The initial parasympathetic response is followed by activation of the sympathetic nervous system; this causes anxiety, tachycardia, sweating, and constriction of the skin vessels (*i.e.*, the skin is cool and clammy).

The signs and symptoms of hypoglycemia are highly variable, and not everyone manifests all or even most of the symptoms. The signs and symptoms are particularly variable in children and in elderly people. Elderly people may not display the typical autonomic responses associated with hypoglycemia but frequently develop signs of impaired function of the central nervous system, including mental confusion. Some people develop hypoglycemic unawareness. Unawareness of hypoglycemia should be suspected in people who do not report symptoms when their blood glucose concentrations are less than 50 to 60 mg/dL (2.8 to 3.3 mmol/L). This occurs most commonly in people who have a longer duration of diabetes and A1C levels within the normal range.[44] Some medications, such as β-adrenergic blocking drugs, interfere with the sympathetic response normally seen in hypoglycemia. If hypoglycemia occurs with α-glucosidase inhibitors, it should be treated with glucose (dextrose) and not sucrose (table sugar), whose breakdown may be blocked by the action of the α-glucosidase inhibitors.

The most effective treatment of an insulin reaction is the immediate administration of 15 to 20 g of glucose in a concentrated carbohydrate source, which can be repeated as necessary. Monosaccharides such as glucose, which can be absorbed directly into the bloodstream, work best. Complex carbohydrates can be administered after the acute reaction has been controlled to sustain blood glucose levels. It is important not to overtreat hypoglycemia and cause hyperglycemia.

Alternative methods for increasing blood glucose may be required when the person having the reaction is unconscious or unable to swallow. Glucagon may be given intramuscularly or subcutaneously. Glucagon acts by hepatic glycogenolysis to raise blood sugar. The liver contains only a limited amount of glycogen (approximately 75 g); glucagon is ineffective in people whose glycogen stores have been depleted. Some people report becoming nauseated after glucagon administration, which also could be in response to the severe hypoglycemia. A small amount of glucose gel (available in most pharmacies) may be inserted into the buccal pouch when glucagon is unavailable. In situations of severe or life-threatening hypoglycemia, it may be necessary to administer glucose (20 to 50 mL of a 50% solution) intravenously.

Counter-regulatory Mechanisms and the Somogyi Effect and Dawn Phenomenon

The Somogyi effect describes a cycle of insulin-induced posthypoglycemic episodes. In 1924, Joslin and associates noticed that hypoglycemia was associated with alternate episodes of hyperglycemia. It was not until 1959 that Somogyi presented the results of his 20 years of studies, which confirmed the observation that "hypoglycemia begets hyperglycemia."[46] In people with diabetes, insulin-induced hypoglycemia produces a compensatory increase in blood levels of catecholamines, glucagon, cortisol, and growth hormone. These counter-regulatory hormones cause blood glucose to become elevated and produce some degree of insulin resistance. The cycle begins when the increase in blood glucose and insulin resistance is treated with larger insulin doses. The hypoglycemic episode often occurs during the night or at a time when it is not recognized, rendering the diagnosis of the phenomenon more difficult.

Research suggests that even rather mild insulin-associated hypoglycemia, which may be asymptomatic, can cause hyperglycemia in people with type 1 diabetes through the recruitment of counter-regulatory mechanisms, although the insulin action does not wane. A waning of insulin's effects when it occurs (*i.e.,* end of the duration of action) causes an exacerbation of the posthypoglycemic hyperglycemia that occurs and accelerates its development. These findings may explain the labile nature of the disease in some people with diabetes. Measures to prevent hypoglycemia and the subsequent activation of counter-regulatory mechanisms include a redistribution of dietary carbohydrates and an alteration in insulin dose or time of administration.[47]

The dawn phenomenon is characterized by increased levels of fasting blood glucose or insulin requirements, or both, between 5 and 9 AM without antecedent hypoglycemia. It occurs in people with type 1 or type 2 diabetes. It has been suggested that a change in the normal circadian rhythm for glucose tolerance, which usually is higher during the later part of the morning, is altered in people with diabetes.[48] Growth hormone has been suggested as a possible factor. When the dawn phenomenon occurs alone, it may produce only mild hyperglycemia, but when it is combined with the Somogyi effect, it may produce profound hyperglycemia.

Chronic Complications

The chronic complications of diabetes include disorders of the microvasculature (*i.e.,* neuropathies, nephropathies, and retinopathies), macrovascular complications (*i.e.,* coronary artery, cerebral vascular, and peripheral vascular disease), and foot ulcers (Fig. 42-12). The level of chronic hyperglycemia is the best-established concomitant factor associated with diabetic complications.[49,50] The Diabetes Control and Complications Trial (DCCT), which was conducted with 1441 patients with type 1 diabetes, demonstrated that the incidence of retinopathy, nephropathy, and neuropathy can be reduced by intensive diabetic treatment.[50] Similar results have been demonstrated by the United Kingdom Prospective Diabetes Study (UKPDS) in 5000 patients with type 2 diabetes.[51]

Recent studies have also determined the positive benefits of excellent glycemic control during hospitalization, surgery, and acute illness states.[52] All patients with diabetes admitted to acute health care facilities need to be identified and have an order for blood glucose monitoring. Goals for blood glucose control for hospitalized patients are as close to 110 mg/dL (5.6 mmol/L) as possible, and generally less than 140 mg/dL (7.8 mmol/L) for critically ill patients and generally less than 180 mg/dL (10 mmol/L) for non–critically ill patients.

CHRONIC COMPLICATIONS OF DIABETES

- The chronic complications of diabetes result from elevated blood glucose levels and associated impairment of lipid and other metabolic pathways.

- Diabetic nephropathy, which is a leading cause of chronic kidney disease, is associated with the increased work demands and microalbuminuria imposed by poorly controlled blood glucose levels.

- Diabetic retinopathy, which is a leading cause of blindness, is closely linked to elevations in blood glucose and hyperlipidemia seen in persons with uncontrolled diabetes.

- Diabetic neuropathies, which can affect the somatic and autonomic nervous systems, result from the demyelinating effect of long-term uncontrolled diabetes.

- Macrovascular disorders such as coronary heart disease, stroke, and peripheral vascular disease reflect the combined effects of unregulated blood glucose levels, elevated blood pressure, and hyperlipidemia.

- The chronic complications of diabetes are best prevented by measures aimed at tight control of blood glucose levels, maintenance of normal lipid levels, and control of hypertension.

Theories of Pathogenesis

The interest among researchers in explaining the causes and development of chronic lesions in a person with diabetes has led to a number of theories. Several of these theories have been summarized to prepare the reader for understanding specific chronic complications.

Polyol Pathway. A polyol is an organic compound that contains three or more hydroxyl (OH) groups. The polyol pathway refers to the intracellular mechanisms responsible for changing the number of hydroxyl units on a glucose molecule. In the sorbitol pathway, glucose is transformed first to sorbitol and then to fructose. This process is activated by the enzyme aldose reductase.[49] Although glucose is converted readily to sorbitol, the rate at which sorbitol can be converted to fructose and then metabolized is limited. Sorbitol is osmotically active, and it has been hypothesized that the presence of excess intracellular amounts may alter cell function in those tissues that use this pathway (*e.g.,* lens, kidneys, nerves, blood vessels). In the lens, for example, the osmotic effects of sorbitol cause swelling and opacity. Increased sorbitol also is associated with a decrease in myoinositol and reduced adenosine triphosphatase activity. The reduction of these compounds may contribute to the pathogenesis of neuropathies caused by Schwann cell damage. Aldose reductase inhibitors are in development with the aim of reducing complications

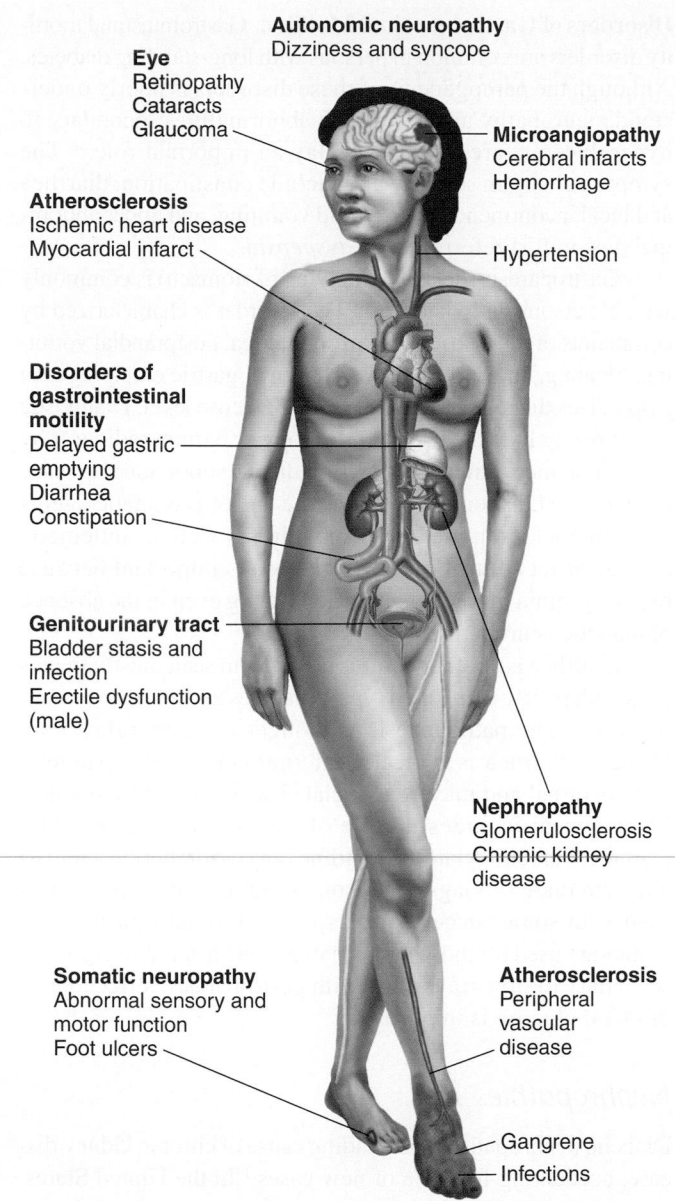

Autonomic neuropathy
Dizziness and syncope

Eye
Retinopathy
Cataracts
Glaucoma

Microangiopathy
Cerebral infarcts
Hemorrhage

Atherosclerosis
Ischemic heart disease
Myocardial infarct

Hypertension

Disorders of gastrointestinal motility
Delayed gastric emptying
Diarrhea
Constipation

Genitourinary tract
Bladder stasis and infection
Erectile dysfunction (male)

Nephropathy
Glomerulosclerosis
Chronic kidney disease

Somatic neuropathy
Abnormal sensory and motor function
Foot ulcers

Atherosclerosis
Peripheral vascular disease

Gangrene
Infections

FIGURE 42-12 • Long-term complications of diabetes mellitus.

resulting from this pathway; however, to date none of them has been successful for a variety of reasons.[49]

Formation of Advanced Glycation End Products. Glycoproteins, or what could be called *glucose proteins,* are normal components of the basement membrane in smaller blood vessels and capillaries. These glycoproteins are also termed *advanced glycation end products* (AGEs). It has been suggested that the increased intracellular concentration of glucose associated with uncontrolled blood glucose levels in diabetes favors the formation of AGEs. These abnormal glycoproteins are thought to produce structural defects in the basement membrane of the microcirculation and to contribute to eye, kidney, and vascular complications. Some of the altered cellular functions resulting from AGEs are due to binding to specific receptors for AGEs (RAGE).[49]

Problems With Tissue Oxygenation. Proponents of the tissue oxygenation theories suggest that many of the chronic complications of diabetes arise because of a decrease in oxygen delivery in the small vessels of the microcirculation. Among the factors believed to contribute to this inadequate oxygen delivery is a defect in red blood cell function that interferes with the release of oxygen from the hemoglobin molecule.[49]

Protein Kinase C. Diacylglycerol (DAG) and protein kinase C (PKC) are critical intracellular signaling molecules that can regulate many vascular functions, including permeability, vasodilator release, endothelial activation, and growth factor signaling.[38] Levels of DAG and PKC are elevated in diabetes. Activation of PKC in blood vessels of the retina, kidney, and nerves can produce vascular damage. A PKC inhibitor is currently in clinical trials for diabetic retinopathy and neuropathy, but has shown variable results.[38]

All of these various abnormalities discussed in the theories above can ultimately result from increased free reactive oxygen species (*i.e.,* free radicals) generation and disordered mitochondrial function in response to chronic hyperglycemia.

Neuropathies

Although the incidence of neuropathies is high among people with diabetes, it is difficult to document exactly how many people are affected by these disorders because of the diversity in clinical manifestations and because the condition often is far advanced before it is recognized. Results of the DCCT study showed that intensive diabetic therapy can reduce the incidence of clinical neuropathy by 60% compared with conventional therapy.[53]

Two types of pathologic changes have been observed in connection with diabetic neuropathies. The first is a thickening of the walls of the nutrient vessels that supply the nerve, leading to the assumption that vessel ischemia plays a major role in the development of these neural changes. The second finding is a segmental demyelinization process that affects the Schwann cell. This demyelinization process is accompanied by a slowing of nerve conduction.

Although there are several methods for classifying the diabetic neuropathies, a simplified system divides them into the somatic and autonomic nervous system neuropathies (Chart 42-3).

Somatic Neuropathy. A distal symmetric polyneuropathy, in which loss of function occurs in a stocking–glove pattern, is the most common form of peripheral neuropathy. Somatic sensory involvement usually occurs first and usually is bilateral and symmetric, and associated with diminished perception of vibration, pain, and temperature, particularly in the lower extremities.[54] In addition to the discomforts associated with the loss of sensory or motor function, lesions in the peripheral nervous system predispose a person with diabetes to other complications. The loss of feeling, touch, and position sense increases the risk of falling. Impairment of temperature and pain sensation increases the risk of serious burns and injuries to the feet. Denervation of the small muscles of the foot result in clawing of the toes and displacement of the submetatarsal fat pad anteriorly. These changes, together

CHART 42-3   CLASSIFICATION OF DIABETIC NEUROPATHIES

Somatic

Polyneuropathies (bilateral sensory)

   Paresthesias, including numbness and tingling

   Impaired pain, temperature, light touch, two-point discrimination, and vibratory sensation

   Decreased ankle and knee-jerk reflexes

Mononeuropathies

   Involvement of a mixed nerve trunk that includes loss of sensation, pain, and motor weakness

Amyotrophy

   Associated with muscle weakness, wasting, and severe pain of muscles in the pelvic girdle and thigh

Autonomic

Impaired vasomotor function

   Postural hypotension

Impaired gastrointestinal function

   Gastric atony

   Diarrhea, often postprandial and nocturnal

Impaired genitourinary function

   Paralytic bladder

   Incomplete voiding

   Erectile dysfunction

   Retrograde ejaculation

Cranial nerve involvement

   Extraocular nerve paralysis

   Impaired pupillary responses

   Impaired special senses

with joint and connective tissue changes, alter the biomechanics of the foot, increasing plantar pressure and predisposing to development of foot trauma and ulcers.[54]

Painful diabetic neuropathy involves the somatosensory neurons that carry pain impulses. This disorder, which causes hypersensitivity to light touch and occasionally severe "burning pain," particularly at night, can become physically and emotionally disabling.[54]

Autonomic Neuropathy. The autonomic neuropathies involve disorders of sympathetic and parasympathetic nervous system function. There may be disorders of vasomotor function, decreased cardiac responses, inability to empty the bladder, and sexual dysfunction.[55] Defects in vasomotor reflexes can lead to dizziness and syncope when the person moves from the supine to the standing position (see Chapter 23). Incomplete emptying of the bladder predisposes to urinary stasis and bladder infection and increases the risk of renal complications.

In the male, disruption of sensory and autonomic nervous system function may cause sexual dysfunction (see Chapter 44). Diabetes is the leading physiologic cause of erectile dysfunction, and it occurs in both type 1 and type 2 diabetes. Of the 7.8 million men with diabetes in the United States, 30% to 60% have erectile dysfunction.[55]

Disorders of Gastrointestinal Motility. Gastrointestinal motility disorders are common in persons with long-standing diabetes. Although the pathogenesis of these disorders is poorly understood, neuropathy and metabolic abnormalities secondary to hyperglycemia are thought to play an important role.[56] The symptoms vary in severity and include constipation, diarrhea and fecal incontinence, nausea and vomiting, and upper abdominal discomfort referred to as *dyspepsia.*

Gastroparesis (delayed emptying of stomach) is commonly seen in persons with diabetes.[56] The disorder is characterized by complaints of epigastric discomfort, nausea, postprandial vomiting, bloating, and early satiety. Abnormal gastric emptying also jeopardizes the regulation of the blood glucose level. Diagnostic measures include the use of endoscopy or barium radiography to exclude mechanical obstruction due to peptic ulcer disease or cancer. Management includes the use of prokinetic agents (*e.g.,* metoclopramide, erythromycin) as well as antiemetic agents. Strict control of blood glucose is important because hyperglycemia may slow gastric emptying even in the absence of diabetic neuropathy.

Diarrhea is another common symptom seen mostly in persons with poorly controlled type 1 diabetes and autonomic neuropathy.[57] The pathogenesis is thought to be multifactorial. Diabetic diarrhea is typically intermittent, watery, painless, and nocturnal and may be associated with fecal incontinence. Management includes the use of antidiarrheal agents (loperamide, diphenoxylate). Clonidine (an α_2-adrenergic agonist) and octreotide (a long-acting somatostatin analog) have been used with some success in persons with rapid transit. Antibiotics are used for those with small bowel bacterial overgrowth secondary to slow transit. As with gastroparesis, strict control of blood glucose is important.

Nephropathies

Diabetic nephropathy is the leading cause of chronic kidney disease, accounting for 40% of new cases.[1] In the United States, 40% of all people who seek renal replacement therapy (see Chapter 34) have diabetes.[58] The complication affects people with both type 1 and type 2 diabetes. According to the reports of the U.S. Renal Data System, the increase in chronic kidney disease since the early 1980s has been predominantly among people with type 2 diabetes.[59]

The term *diabetic nephropathy* is used to describe the combination of lesions that often occur concurrently in the diabetic kidney. The most common kidney lesions in people with diabetes are those that affect the glomeruli. Various glomerular changes may occur in people with diabetic nephropathy, including capillary basement membrane thickening, diffuse glomerular sclerosis, and nodular glomerulosclerosis (see Chapter 33). Changes in the capillary basement membrane take the form of thickening of basement membranes along the length of the glomeruli. Diffuse glomerulosclerosis consists of thickening of the basement membrane and the mesangial matrix. Nodular glomerulosclerosis, also called *intercapillary glomerulosclerosis* or *Kimmelstiel-Wilson syndrome,* is a form of glomerulosclerosis that involves the development of nodular lesions in the glomerular capillaries of the kidneys, causing impaired blood flow with progressive loss of kidney function and, eventually, renal failure. Nodular glomerulosclerosis is thought to occur only in people with diabetes. Changes in the basement membrane in diffuse glomerulosclerosis and Kimmelstiel-Wilson syndrome allow plasma proteins to escape in the urine, causing proteinuria and the development of hypoproteinemia, edema, and others signs of impaired kidney function.

Not all people with diabetes develop clinically significant nephropathy; for this reason, attention is focusing on risk factors for the development of this complication. Among the suggested risk factors are genetic and familial predisposition, elevated blood pressure, poor glycemic control, smoking, hyperlipidemia, and microalbumuria.[28,60] Diabetic nephropathy occurs in family clusters, suggesting a familial predisposition, although this does not exclude the possibility of environmental factors shared by siblings. The risk for development of kidney disease is greater among Native Americans, Hispanic Americans (especially Mexican Americans), and African Americans.[28,60]

Kidney enlargement, nephron hypertrophy, and hyperfiltration occur early in the disease, reflecting the increased work performed by the kidneys in reabsorbing excessive amounts of glucose. One of the first manifestations of diabetic nephropathy is an increase in urinary albumin excretion (*i.e.,* microalbuminuria), which is easily assessed by laboratory methods. Microalbuminuria is defined as a urine protein loss between 30 and 300 mg/day or an albumin-to-creatinine ratio (A/C ratio) between 30 and 300 μg/mg (normal <30 μg/mg) from a spot urine collection.[58] It is recommended that the A/C ratio be the preferred screen for microalbuminuria. Both systolic and diastolic hypertension accelerate the progression of diabetic nephropathy. Even moderate lowering of blood pressure can decrease the risk of chronic kidney disease.[28]

Measures to prevent diabetic nephropathy or its progression in persons with diabetes include achievement of glycemic control; maintenance of blood pressure (<130/80 mm Hg, or <125/75 mm Hg in the presence of significant proteinuria); prevention or reduction in the level of proteinuria (using angiotensin-converting enzyme inhibitors or angiotensin receptor blockers, or protein restriction in selected patients); treatment of hyperlipidemia; and smoking cessation in people who smoke.[28,61] Smoking increases the risk of chronic kidney disease in both persons with and without diabetes. People with type 2 diabetes who smoke have a greater risk of microalbuminuria, and their rate of progression to chronic kidney disease is approximately twice as rapid as in those who do not smoke.[28]

Retinopathies

Diabetes is the leading cause of acquired blindness in the United States. Although people with diabetes are at increased risk for development of cataracts and glaucoma, retinopathy is the most common pattern of eye disease. Diabetic retinopathy is estimated to be the most frequent cause of newly diagnosed blindness among Americans between the ages of 20 and 74 years.[62]

Diabetic retinopathy is characterized by abnormal retinal vascular permeability, microaneurysm formation, neovascularization and associated hemorrhage, scarring, and retinal detachment[62] (see Chapter 54). Twenty years after the onset of diabetes, nearly all people with type 1 diabetes and more than 60% of people with type 2 diabetes have some degree of retinopathy. Pregnancy, puberty, and cataract surgery can accelerate these changes.[62] Although there has been no extensive research on risk factors associated with diabetic retinopathy, they appear to be similar to those for other complications. Among the suggested risk factors associated with diabetic retinopathy are poor glycemic control, elevated blood pressure, and hyperlipidemia. The strongest case for control of blood glucose comes from the DCCT and UKPDS studies, which demonstrated a reduction in retinopathy with improved glucose control.[50,51]

Because of the risk of retinopathy, it is important that people with diabetes have regular dilated eye examinations. They should have an initial examination for retinopathy shortly after the diagnosis of diabetes is made. The recommendation for follow-up examinations is based on the type of examination that was done and the findings of that examination. People with persistently elevated glucose levels or proteinuria should be examined yearly.[62] Women who are planning a pregnancy should be counseled on the risk of development or progression of diabetic retinopathy. Women with diabetes who become pregnant should be followed closely throughout pregnancy. This does not apply to women in whom GDM develops because such women are not at risk for development of diabetic retinopathy.

People with macular edema, moderate to severe nonproliferative retinopathy, or any proliferative retinopathy should receive the care of an ophthalmologist who is knowledgeable and experienced in the management and treatment of diabetic retinopathy. Methods used in the treatment of diabetic retinopathy include the destruction and scarring of the proliferative lesions with laser photocoagulation. The use of antagonists to growth factors (*e.g.,* vascular endothelial growth factor) may also play a role in management.

Macrovascular Complications

Diabetes mellitus is a major risk factor for coronary artery disease, cerebrovascular disease, and peripheral vascular disease. The prevalence of these macrovascular complications is increased twofold to fourfold in people with diabetes. Approximately 50% to 75% of all people with type 2 diabetes will die of a macrovascular problem.

Multiple risk factors for macrovascular disease, including obesity, hypertension, hyperglycemia, hyperinsulinemia, hyperlipidemia, altered platelet function, endothelial dysfunction, systemic inflammation (as evidenced by increased CRP), and elevated fibrinogen levels, frequently are found in people with diabetes. There appear to be differences between type 1 and type 2 diabetes in terms of duration of disease and the development of macrovascular disease. In people with type 2 diabetes, macrovascular disease may be present at the time of diagnosis. Indeed, approximately 50% of people with type 2 diabetes have some form of complication at presentation (either microvascular or macrovascular). The reason for these discrepancies has been attributed to the associated cardiovascular risk factors that are part of the metabolic syndrome.[18,19]

Aggressive management of cardiovascular risk factors should include smoking cessation, hypertension, lipid lowering, diabetes control, and antiplatelet agents (aspirin or clopidogrel) if not contraindicated[18,17,28] (see Chapter 22). If treatment is warranted for peripheral vascular disease, the peroneal arteries between the knees and ankles commonly are involved in diabetes, making revascularization difficult.

Diabetic Foot Ulcers

Foot problems are common among people with diabetes and may become severe enough to cause ulceration, infection, and, eventually, the need for amputation. Foot problems have been reported as the most common complication leading to hospitalization among people with diabetes. In people with diabetes, lesions of the feet represent the effects of neuropathy and vascular insufficiency. Approximately 60% to 70% of people with diabetic foot ulcers have neuropathy without vascular disease, 15% to 20% have vascular disease, and 15% to 20% have neuropathy and vascular disease.[63]

Distal symmetric neuropathy is a major risk factor for foot ulcers. People with sensory neuropathies have impaired pain sensation and often are unaware of the constant trauma to the feet caused by poorly fitting shoes, improper weight bearing, hard objects or pebbles in the shoes, or infections such as athlete's foot. Neuropathy prevents people from detecting pain; they are unable to adjust their gait to avoid walking on an area of the foot where pressure is causing trauma and necrosis. Motor neuropathy with weakness of the intrinsic muscles of the foot may result in foot deformities, which lead to focal areas of high pressure. When the abnormal focus of pressure is coupled with loss of sensation, a foot ulcer can occur. Common sites of trauma are the back of the heel, the plantar metatarsal area, or the great toe, where weight is borne during walking (Fig. 42-13).

All persons with diabetes should receive a full foot examination at least once a year. This examination should include assessment of protective sensation, foot structure and biomechanics, vascular status, and skin integrity.[3,63] Evaluation of neurologic function should include a somatosensory test using either the Semmes-Weinstein monofilament or vibratory sensation. The Semmes-Weinstein monofilament is a simple, inexpensive device for testing sensory status (Fig. 42-14). The monofilament is held in the hand or attached to a handle at one end. When the unattached or unsupported end of the monofilament is pressed against the skin until it buckles or bends slightly, it delivers 10 g of pressure at the point of contact.[63] The test consists of having the person being tested report at which of two moments he or she is being touched by the monofilament. For example, the examiner will call out "one" and then "two" and briefly touch the monofilament to the site at one of the two test times. Between 4 and 10 sites per foot are

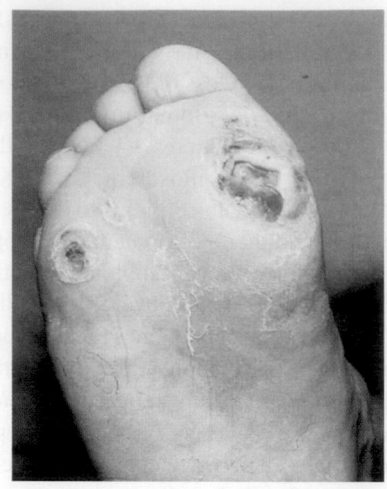

FIGURE 42-13 • Neuropathic ulcers occur on pressure points in areas with diminished sensation in diabetic polyneuropathy. Pain is absent (and therefore the ulcer may go unnoticed). (From Bates B. B. [1995]. *A guide to physical examination and history taking* [6th ed.]. Philadelphia: J. B. Lippincott.)

touched. An incorrect response at even one site indicates increased risk of neuropathy and foot complications.

Because of the constant risk of foot problems, it is important that people with diabetes wear shoes that have been fitted correctly and inspect their feet daily, looking for blisters, open sores, and fungal infection (*e.g.*, athlete's foot) between the toes. If their eyesight is poor, a family member should do this for them. In the event a lesion is detected, prompt medical attention is needed to prevent serious complications. Specially designed shoes have been demonstrated to be effective in preventing relapses in people with previous ulcerations.[63] Smoking should be avoided because it causes vasoconstriction and contributes to vascular disease. Because cold produces vasoconstriction, appropriate foot coverings should be used to keep the feet warm and dry. Toenails should be cut straight across

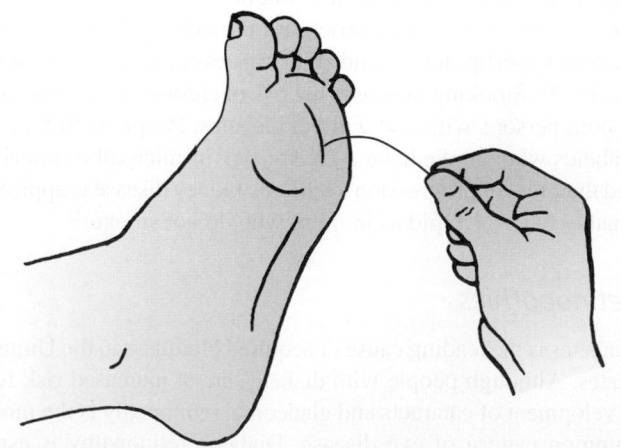

FIGURE 42-14 • Use of a monofilament in testing for impaired sensation in the foot of a person with diabetes.

to prevent ingrown toenails. The toenails often are thickened and deformed, requiring the services of a podiatrist.

Persons with diabetes mellitus develop more extensive and rapidly progressive peripheral vascular disease than do individuals without diabetes. Cardiovascular risk factors should be addressed in patients with diabetic ulcers and peripheral vascular disease. Ulcers that are resistant to standard therapy may respond to application of growth factors. Growth factors provide a means by which cells communicate with each other and can have profound effects on cell proliferation, migration, and extracellular matrix synthesis. Becaplermin, a topical preparation of recombinant human platelet-derived growth factor (PDGF), is used in treatment of neuropathic lower extremity ulcers.

Infections

Although not specifically an acute or a chronic complication, infections are a common concern of people with diabetes. Certain types of infections occur with increased frequency in people with diabetes: soft tissue infections of the extremities, osteomyelitis, urinary tract infections and pyelonephritis, candidal infections of the skin and mucous surfaces, dental caries and periodontal disease, and tuberculosis.[64] Controversy exists about whether infections are more common in people with diabetes or whether infections seem more prevalent because they often are more serious in people with diabetes.

Suboptimal response to infection in a person with diabetes is caused by the presence of chronic complications, such as vascular disease and neuropathies, and by the presence of hyperglycemia and altered neutrophil function. Sensory deficits may cause a person with diabetes to ignore minor trauma and infection, and vascular disease may impair circulation and delivery of blood cells and other substances needed to produce an adequate inflammatory response and effect healing. Pyelonephritis and urinary tract infections are relatively common in persons with diabetes, and it has been suggested that these infections may bear some relation to the presence of a neurogenic bladder or nephrosclerotic changes in the kidneys. Hyperglycemia and glycosuria may influence the growth of microorganisms and increase the severity of the infection. Diabetes and elevated blood glucose levels also may impair host defenses such as the function of neutrophils and immune cells. Polymorphonuclear leukocyte function, particularly adherence, chemotaxis, and phagocytosis, is depressed in persons with diabetes, particularly those with poor glycemic control.

IN SUMMARY, diabetes mellitus is a disorder of carbohydrate, protein, and fat metabolism resulting from an imbalance between insulin availability and insulin need. The disease can be classified as type 1 diabetes, in which there is destruction of beta cells and an absolute insulin deficiency, or type 2 diabetes, in which there is a lack of insulin availability or effectiveness. Type 1 diabetes can be further subdivided into type 1A immune-mediated diabetes, which is thought to be caused by autoimmune mechanisms, and type 1B idiopathic diabetes, for which the cause is unknown. Other specific types of diabetes include secondary forms of carbohydrate intolerance, which occur secondary to some other condition that destroys beta cells (*e.g.,* pancreatic disorders) or endocrine diseases that cause increased production of glucose by the liver and decreased use of glucose by the tissues (*e.g.,* Cushing syndrome). GDM develops during pregnancy, and although glucose tolerance often returns to normal after childbirth, it indicates an increased risk for the development of diabetes. The metabolic syndrome represents a constellation of metabolic abnormalities characterized by obesity, insulin resistance, high triglyceride levels and low HDL levels, hypertension, cardiovascular disease, insulin resistance, and increased risk for development of type 2 diabetes.

The most commonly identified symptoms of type 1 diabetes are polyuria, polydipsia, polyphagia, and weight loss despite normal or increased appetite. Although persons with type 2 diabetes may present with one or more of these symptoms, they are often asymptomatic initially. The diagnosis of diabetes mellitus is based on clinical signs of the disease, fasting blood glucose levels, random plasma glucose measurements, and results of the glucose tolerance test. Glycosylation involves the irreversible attachment of glucose to the hemoglobin molecule; the measurement of A1C provides an index of blood glucose levels over several months. Self-monitoring provides a means of maintaining near-normal blood glucose levels through frequent testing of blood glucose and adjustment of insulin dosage.

Dietary management focuses on maintaining a well-balanced diet, controlling calories to achieve and maintain an optimum weight, and regulating the distribution of carbohydrates, proteins, and fats. Two types of antidiabetic agents are used in the management of diabetes: injectable insulin (and newer injectable agents including amylin and GLP-1 analogs) and oral diabetic drugs. Type 1 diabetes, and sometimes type 2, requires treatment with injectable insulin. Oral antidiabetic drugs include the insulin secretagogues, biguanides, α-glucosidase inhibitors, TZDs, and DPP-4 enzyme inhibitors. These drugs require a functioning pancreas and may be used in the treatment of type 2 diabetes.

The metabolic disturbances associated with diabetes affect almost every body system. The acute complications of diabetes include diabetic ketoacidosis, hyperglycemic hyperosmolar state, and hypoglycemia in people with insulin-treated diabetes. The chronic complications of diabetes affect the microvascular system (including the retina, kidneys, and peripheral nervous system) and the macrovascular system (coronary, cerebrovascular, and peripheral arteries). The diabetic foot is usually a combination of both microvascular and macrovascular dysfunction. Infection is also a frequent cofactor in the diabetic foot. ■

CONCEPTS in action **ANIMATION**

Review Exercises

1. A 6-year-old boy is admitted to the emergency department with nausea, vomiting, and abdominal pain. He is very lethargic; his skin is warm, dry, and flushed; his pulse is rapid; and he has a sweet smell to his breath. His parents relate that he has been very thirsty during the past several weeks, his appetite has been poor, and he has been urinating frequently. His initial plasma glucose is 420 mg/dL (23.1 mmol/L), and a urine test for ketones is strongly positive.

   A. *What is the most likely cause of this boy's elevated blood glucose and ketonuria?*

   B. *Explain his presenting signs and symptoms in terms of the elevated blood glucose and metabolic acidosis.*

   C. *What type of treatment will this boy require?*

2. A 53-year-old accountant presents for his routine yearly examination. His history indicates that he was found to have a fasting glucose of 120 mg/dL (6.7 mmol/L) on two prior occasions. Currently, he is asymptomatic. He has no other medical problems and does not use any medications. He neither smokes nor drinks alcohol. His father had type 2 diabetes at age 60 years. His physical examination reveals a blood pressure of 125/80 mm Hg, BMI (body mass index) of 32 kg/m², and waist circumference of 45 in (114 cm). Laboratory study results are as follows: complete blood count (CBC), thyroid-stimulating hormone (TSH), and alanine aminotransferase (ALT) are within normal limits. The lipid panel shows that his HDL cholesterol (30 mg/dL [0.8 mmol/L]) and LDL cholesterol (136 mg/dL [3.5 mmol/L]) are within the normal range, and triglycerides are elevated (290 mg/dL [2.3 mmol/L]; normal is <165 mg/dL [1.9 mmol/L]).

   A. *What is this man's probable diagnosis?*

   B. *Based on this man's blood glucose level and the ADA diabetes classification system, what diabetic status would you place this man in? Does he need a 75-g oral glucose tolerance test (OGTT) for further assessment of his IFG?*

   C. *His OGTT test result reveals a 2-hour glucose value of 175 mg/dL (9.63 mmol/L). What is the diagnosis? What type of treatment would be appropriate for this man?*

References

1. American Diabetes Association. (2007). Diabetes facts and figures. [Online]. Available: www.diabetes.org. Accessed April 7, 2008.
2. Guyton A., Hall J. E. (2006). *Medical physiology* (11th ed., pp. 961–977). Philadelphia: Elsevier Saunders.
3. Masharani U., German M. S. (2007). Pancreatic hormones and diabetes mellitus. In Gardner D. G., Shoback D. (Eds.), *Greenspan's basic and clinical endocrinology* (8th ed., pp. 661–747). New York: Lange Medical Books/McGraw-Hill.
4. Shepard P. R., Kahn B. (1999). Glucose transporters and insulin action. *New England Journal of Medicine* 341, 248–256.
5. Riddle M. C., Drucker D. J. (2006). Emerging therapies mimicking the effects of amylin and glucagon-like peptide-1. *Diabetes Care* 29, 435–449.
6. Drucker D. J. (2006). The biology of incretin hormones. *Cell Metabolism* 3, 153–165.
7. Goldfine I. R., Youngren J. F. (1998). Contributions of the *American Journal of Physiology* to the discovery of insulin. *American Journal of Physiology: Endocrinology and Metabolism* 274, E207–E209.
8. Expert Committee on the Diagnosis and Classification of Diabetes Mellitus. (1997). Report of the Expert Committee on the Diagnosis and Classification of Diabetes Mellitus. *Diabetes Care* 20, 1183–1199.
9. Nathan, D. M., Davidson M. B., DeFronzo R. A., et al. (2007). Impaired fasting glucose and impaired glucose tolerance: Implications for care. *Diabetes Care* 30, 753–759.
10. Daneman D. (2006). Type 1 diabetes. *Lancet* 367, 847–858.
11. Atkinson M., Gale E. A. M. (2003). Infant diets and type 1 diabetes. *Journal of the American Medical Association* 290, 1771–1772.
12. Freemark M. (2003). Pharmacological approaches to the prevention of type 2 diabetes in high risk pediatric patients. *Journal of Clinical Endocrinology and Metabolism* 88, 3–13.
13. The International Diabetes Federation Consensus Workshop. (2004). Type 2 diabetes in the young: The evolving epidemic. *Diabetes Care* 27, 1798–1811.
14. Stumvolt M., Goldstein B. J., van Haeften T. W. (2005). Type 2 diabetes: Principles of pathogenesis and therapy. *Lancet* 365, 1333–1346.
15. Gerich J. E. (2003). Contributions of insulin-resistance and insulin-secretory defects to the pathogenesis of type 2 diabetes. *Mayo Clinic Proceedings* 78, 447–456.
16. DeFronzo R. A. (2004). Pathogenesis of type 2 diabetes mellitus. *Medical Clinics of North America* 88, 787–835.
17. Matthews D. R., Cull C. A., Stratton I. M., et al., United Kingdom Prospective Diabetes Study (UKPDS) Group. (1998). UKPDS 26: Sulfonylurea failure in non-insulin-dependent diabetic patients over six years. *Diabetes Medicine* 15, 297–303.
18. Matfin G. (2007). Challenges in developing drugs for the metabolic syndrome. *British Journal of Diabetes and Vascular Disease* 7, 152–156.
19. Grundy S. M., Panel Chair. (2001). *Third Report of the National Cholesterol Education Program (NCEP) Expert Panel on Detection, Evaluation, and Treatment of High Blood Cholesterol in Adults (Adult Treatment Panel III).* NIH publication no. 01-3670. Bethesda, MD: National Institutes of Health.
20. Ehrmann D. A. (2005). Polycystic ovary syndrome. *New England Journal of Medicine* 352, 1223–1236.
21. Kahn S. E., Hull R. L., Utzschneider K. M. (2006). Mechanisms linking obesity to insulin resistance and type 2 diabetes. *Nature* 444, 840–846.
22. Guven S., El-Bershawi A., Sonnenberg G. E., et al. (1999). Persistent elevation in plasma leptin level in ex-obese with normal body mass index: Relation to body composition and insulin sensitivity. *Diabetes* 48, 347–352.
23. Bays H., Mandarino L., DeFronzo R. A. (2004). Role of adipocyte, free fatty acid, and ectopic fat in pathogenesis of type 2 diabetes: Peroxisomal proliferator-activated receptor agonists provide a rationale therapeutic approach. *Journal of Clinical Endocrinology and Metabolism* 89, 463–478.
24. Kadowaki T., Yamauchi T., Kubota N., et al. (2006). Adiponectin and adiponectin receptors in insulin resistance, diabetes, and the metabolic syndrome. *Journal of Clinical Investigation* 116, 1784–1792.
25. Kissebah A. H., Sonnenberg G. F., Myklebust J., et al. (2000). Quantitative trait loci on chromosomes 3 and 17 influence phenotypes of metabolic syndrome. *Proceedings of the National Academy of Science of the U.S.A.* 97, 14478–14483.
26. Kuritzkes D. R., Currier J. (2003). Cardiovascular risk factors and antiretroviral therapy. *New England Journal of Medicine* 348, 679–680.
27. American Diabetes Association. (2004). Gestational diabetes mellitus. *Diabetes Care* 27(Suppl. 1), S88–S90.

28. American Diabetes Association. (2007). Standards of medical care for patients with diabetes mellitus. *Diabetes Care* 30(Suppl. 1), S4–S41.

29. American Diabetes Association. (2004). Tests of glycemia in diabetes. *Diabetes Care* 27(Suppl. 1), S91–S93.

30. Bantle J. P., Wylie-Rosett J., Albright A. L., et al. (2006). Nutritional recommendations and interventions for diabetes—2006: A position statement of the American Diabetes Association. *Diabetes Care* 29, 2140–2157.

31. Pastors J. G., Warshaw H., Daly A., et al. (2002). The evidence of the effectiveness of medical nutrition therapy in diabetes management. *Diabetes Care* 25, 608–613.

32. American Diabetes Association. (2004). Physical activity/exercise and diabetes mellitus. *Diabetes Care* 27(Suppl. 1), S55–S59.

33. Nathan D. M., Buse J. B., Davidson M. B., et al. (2006). Management of hyperglycemia in type 2 diabetes: A consensus algorithm for the initiation and adjustment of therapy. A consensus statement from the American Diabetes Association and the European Association for the Study of Diabetes. *Diabetes Care* 29, 1963–1972.

34. Nolte M. S., Karam J. H. (2007). Pancreatic hormones and antidiabetic drugs. In Katzung B. G. (Ed.), *Basic and clinical pharmacology* (10th ed., pp. 683–703). New York: McGraw-Hill Medical.

35. Zangeneh F., Kudva Y. C., Basu A. (2003). Insulin sensitizers. *Mayo Clinic Proceedings* 78, 471–479.

36. Nissen S. E., Wolski K. (2007). Effect of rosiglitazone on the risk of myocardial infarction and death from cardiovascular concerns. *New England Journal of Medicine* 356, 2457–2471.

37. Drucker D. J. (2007). Dipeptidyl peptidase-4 inhibition and the treatment of type 2 diabetes. *Diabetes Care* 30, 1335–1343.

38. Amori R. E., Lau J., Pittas A. G. (2007). Efficacy and safety of incretin therapy in type 2 diabetes. *Journal of the American Medical Association* 298, 194–206.

39. Hirsch I. (2005). Insulin analogs. *New England Journal of Medicine* 352, 174–183.

40. American Diabetes Association. (2004). Continuous subcutaneous insulin infusion. *Diabetes Care* 27(Suppl. 1), S110.

41. American Diabetes Association. (2004). Pancreas transplantation for patients with type 1 diabetes. *Diabetes Care* 27(Suppl. 1), S105.

42. American Diabetes Association. (2004). Hyperglycemic crises in patients with diabetes mellitus. *Diabetes Care* 27(Suppl. 1), S94–S102.

43. American Diabetes Association. (2006). Diabetic ketoacidosis in infants, children and adolescents. *Diabetes Care* 29, 1150–1159.

44. Masharani U., Gitelman S. E. (2007). Hypoglycemic disorders. In Gardner D. G., Shoback D. (Eds.), *Greenspan's basic and clinical endocrinology* (8th ed., pp. 748–769). New York: Lange Medical Books/McGraw-Hill.

45. American Diabetes Association Workgroup on Hypoglycemia. (2005). Defining and reporting hypoglycemia in diabetes: A report of the American Diabetes Association Workgroup on Hypoglycemia. *Diabetes Care* 28, 1245–1249.

46. Somogyi M. (1959). Exacerbation of diabetes in excess insulin action. *American Journal of Medicine* 26, 169–191.

47. Bolli G. B., Gotterman I. S., Campbell P. J. (1984). Glucose counterregulation and waning of insulin in the Somogyi phenomenon (posthypoglycemic hyperglycemia). *New England Journal of Medicine* 311, 1214–1219.

48. Bolli G. B., Gerich J. E. (1984). The dawn phenomenon: A common occurrence in both non-insulin and insulin dependent diabetes mellitus. *New England Journal of Medicine* 310, 746–750.

49. Sheetz M. J., King G. L. (2002). Molecular understanding of hyperglycemia's adverse effects for diabetic complications. *Journal of the American Medical Association* 288, 2579–2588.

50. The Diabetes Control and Complications Trial Research Group. (1993). The effect of intensified treatment of diabetes on the development and progression of long-term complications in insulin-dependent diabetes mellitus. *New England Journal of Medicine* 329, 955–977.

51. Stratton I. M., Adler A. I., Neil H. A., et al. (2000). Association of glycaemia with macrovascular and microvascular complications in type 2 diabetes (UKPDS 35): Prospective observational study. *British Medical Journal* 321, 405–412.

52. American College of Endocrinology and American Diabetes Association. (2006). Consensus statement on inpatient diabetes and glycemic control: A call to action. *Diabetes Care* 29, 1955–1962.

53. Boulton A. J. M., Vinik A. I., Arezzo J. C., et al. (2005). Diabetic neuropathies. *Diabetes Care* 28, 956–962.

54. Boulton A. J. M., Malik R. A. (2004). Diabetic somatic neuropathies. *Diabetes Care* 27, 1458–1486.

55. AACE Male Sexual Dysfunction Taskforce. (2003). AACE medical guidelines for clinical practice for the evaluation and treatment of male sexual dysfunction: A couple's problem—2003 update. *Endocrine Practice* 9, 77–95.

56. Camilleri M. (2007). Diabetic gastroparesis. *New England Journal of Medicine* 356, 820–829.

57. Lysy J., Israeli E., Goldin E. (1999). The prevalence of chronic diarrhea among diabetic patients. *American Journal of Gastroenterology* 94, 2165–2170.

58. American Diabetes Association. (2004). Diabetic nephropathy. *Diabetes Care* 27(Suppl. 1), S79–S83.

59. U.S. Renal Data System. (1998). *USRDS 1998 Annual Data Report.* National Institute of Diabetes and Digestive and Kidney Diseases. NIH publication no. 98:3176. Bethesda, MD: National Institutes of Health.

60. Barnett A. H. (2003). Adopting more aggressive strategies for the management of renal disease in type 2 diabetes. *Practical Diabetes International* 20, 186–190.

61. Chobanian A. V., Bakris G. L., Black H. R., et al. (2003). The seventh report of the Joint National Committee on Prevention, Detection, Evaluation, and Treatment of High Blood Pressure: The JNC 7 Report. *Journal of the American Medical Association* 289, 2560–2572.

62. American Diabetes Association. (2004). Diabetic retinopathy. *Diabetes Care* 27(Suppl. 1), S84–S87.

63. American Diabetes Association. (2004). Preventative foot care in people with diabetes. *Diabetes Care* 27(Suppl. 1), S63–S64.

64. Joshi N., Caputo G. M., Weitekamp M. R., et al. (1999). Infections in patients with diabetes mellitus. *New England Journal of Medicine* 341, 1906–1912.

Visit the**Point** http://thePoint.lww.com for animations, journal articles, and more!

Disorders of Genitourinary and Reproductive Function

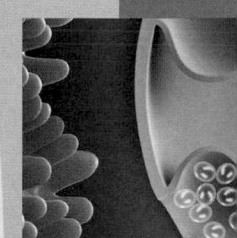

There is a long history of misunderstanding and myths about human reproduction, especially the female reproductive system. Early on, the uterus was deemed the most important structure of the female reproductive anatomy. One of the first representations of the uterus appears in ancient Egyptian hieroglyphs (c. 2900 BC). Its importance was a direct result of the understanding that it was from the uterus that a child was born. That a woman was the carrier of the next generation was enough to establish her importance to society. However, society also imposed harsh restrictions on women that made it difficult, if not impossible, for further understanding. Until the Renaissance, custom and manners dictated that a woman's body could not be represented unless it was fully clothed.

To a regrettable extent, the associations made in ancient times that surmised a destiny for women based on the anatomy peculiar to their sex still affect how women are viewed today. The Greek philosopher Plato (427?–347? BC) postulated that the unused womb became "indignant" and wandered around the body, inhibiting the body's "spirits," or life force, and causing disease. The reasonings of Aristotle (384–322 BC) were equally fanciful. It was he, believing as others of the time did that women were irrational and prone to emotional outbursts, who provided the nomenclature for the womb, naming it *hystera* (ustera). Their concept that emotional excitability or instability was the domain of women is confirmed by another word that was coined by the Greeks: hysteria.

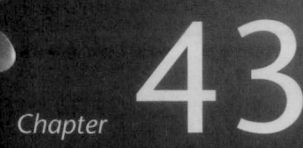

Chapter 43

Structure and Function of the Male Genitourinary System

GLENN MATFIN

➤ The male genitourinary system is composed of the paired gonads, or testes, genital ducts, accessory organs, and penis (Fig. 43-1). The dual function of the testes is to produce androgens (*i.e.,* male sex hormones), mainly testosterone, and spermatozoa (*i.e.,* male germ cells). The internal accessory organs produce the fluid constituents of semen, and the ductile system aids in the storage and transport of spermatozoa. The penis functions in urine elimination and sexual function. This chapter focuses on the structure of the male reproductive system, spermatogenesis and control of male reproductive function, neural control of sexual function, and changes in function that occur at puberty and as a result of the aging process.

STRUCTURE OF THE MALE REPRODUCTIVE SYSTEM

After completing this section of the chapter, you should be able to meet the following objectives:

■ Characterize the embryonic development of the male reproductive organs and genitalia.
■ Describe the structure and function of the testes and scrotum, the genital ducts, accessory organs, and penis.

Embryonic Development

The sex of a person is determined at the time of fertilization by the sex chromosomes. In the early stages of embryonic development, the tissues from which the male and female reproductive organs develop are undifferentiated. Until approximately the seventh week of gestation, it is impossible to determine whether an embryo is male or female unless the chromosomes are studied. Until this time, the male and female genital tracts consist of two wolffian ducts, from which the male genitalia develop, and two müllerian ducts, from which the female genital structures develop. During this period of gestation, the gonads (*i.e.,* ovaries and testes) also are undifferentiated.[1-3]

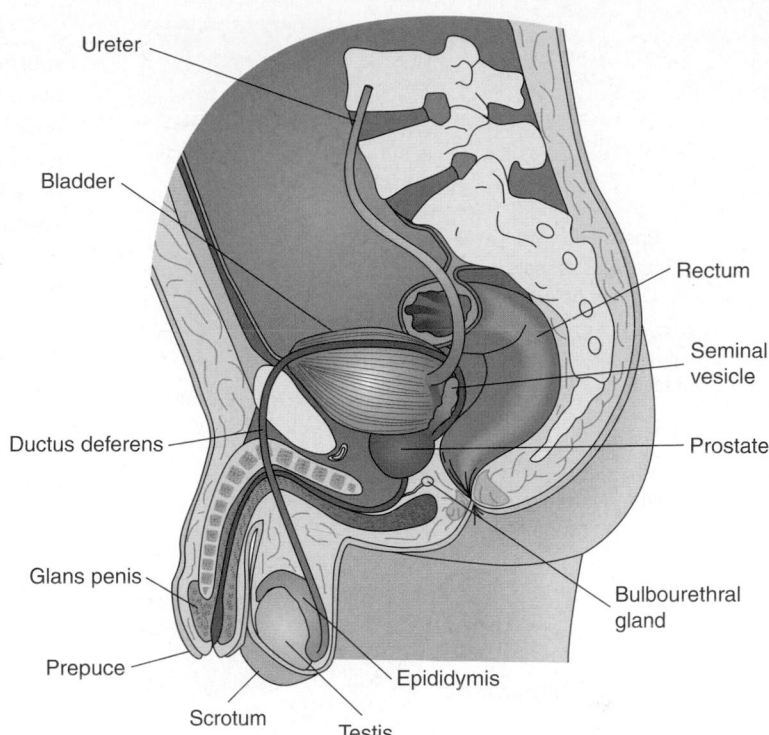

Ureter

Bladder

Rectum

Seminal vesicle

Ductus deferens

Prostate

Glans penis

Bulbourethral gland

Prepuce

Epididymis

Scrotum

Testis

FIGURE 43-1 • The structures of the male reproductive system, including the testes, the scrotum, and the excretory ducts.

Between the sixth and eighth weeks of gestation, the testes begin their development under the influence of the Y chromosome. Differentiation of the indifferent gonad into a testis is initiated by the actions of a single gene on the short arm of the Y chromosome. This gene is called the *sex-determining region of the Y chromosome (SRY)*.[1] In the presence of the *SRY* gene, the embryonic gonads develop into testes, and in its absence, the gonads develop into ovaries.

During this time, the testicular cells of the male embryo begin producing an anti-müllerian hormone (AMH) and testosterone. The AMH suppresses the müllerian ducts and prevents development of the uterus and fallopian tubes in the male. In parallel, testosterone stimulates the wolffian ducts to develop into the epididymis, vas deferens, and seminal vesicles. Testosterone also is the precursor of a third hormone, dihydrotestosterone (DHT), which functions in the formation of the male urethra, prostate, and external genitalia. The conversion of testosterone to DHT, predominantly in the peripheral tissues, is performed by the enzyme 5α-reductase. Although testosterone and DHT share the same nuclear androgen receptor, they have marked differences in tissue activity (DHT exerts most of its effects on the external genitalia, including the prostate, but is also subsequently important for the development of facial and body hair, including temporal hair recession). In the absence of testosterone (and DHT), a male embryo with an XY chromosomal pattern develops female external genitalia.[1]

Testes and Scrotum

The testes, or male gonads, are two egg-shaped structures located outside the abdominal cavity in the scrotum. The adult male testes are approximately 15 to 25 mL in volume (>4 mL indicates pubertal onset), with 80% of this volume being cells involved in spermatogenesis and 20% in testosterone production. Embryologically, the testes develop in the abdominal cavity and then descend through the inguinal canal into a pouch of peritoneum (which becomes the tunica vaginalis) in the scrotum. Testicular descent occurs in two stages. The first occurs between 7 and 12 weeks of fetal life, with AMH being responsible for descent to the inguinal region. The second occurs between 7 and 9 months of fetal life, with testosterone being responsible for descent into the scrotum. As they descend, the testes pull their arteries, veins, lymphatics, nerves, and conducting excretory ducts with them. These structures are encased by the cremaster muscle and layers of fascia that constitute the spermatic cord (Fig. 43-2A). After descent of the testes, the inguinal canal closes almost completely. Failure of this canal to close predisposes to the development of an inguinal hernia later in life (see Fig. 43-2B). An inguinal hernia or "rupture" is a protrusion of the parietal peritoneum and part of the intestine through an abnormal opening from the abdominal cavity. A loop of small bowel may become incarcerated in an inguinal hernia (strangulated hernia), in which case its lumen may become obstructed and its vascular supply compromised (see Chapter 37).

The testes are enclosed in a double-layered membrane, the tunica vaginalis, which is derived embryologically from the abdominal peritoneum[2,3] (see Fig. 43-2). An outer covering, the tunica albuginea, is a tough, white, fibrous sheath that resembles the sclera of the eye. The tunica albuginea protects the testes and gives them their ovoid shape. The cremaster muscles, which are bands of skeletal muscle arising from the internal oblique muscles of the trunk, elevate the testes. The testes receive their arterial blood supply from the long testicular arteries, which

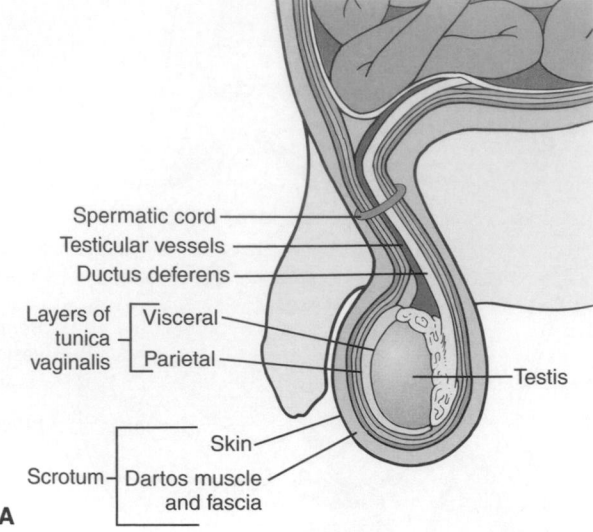

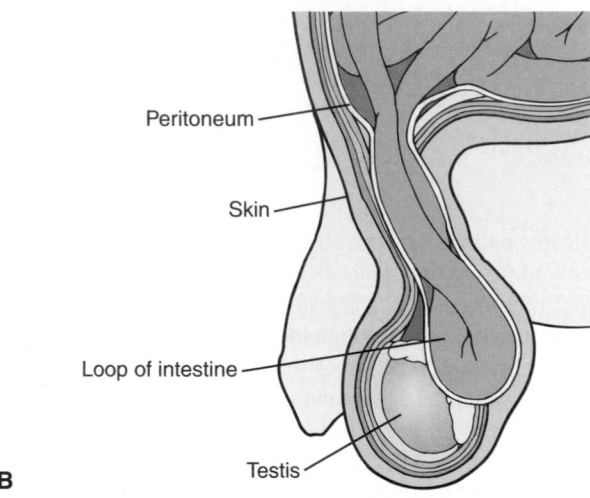

FIGURE 43-2 • **(A)** Anterior view of the spermatic cord and inguinal canal and coverings of the spermatic cord and testes. **(B)** Indirect inguinal hernia. (Adapted from Moore K. L., Agur A. M. [2002]. *Essentials of clinical anatomy* [2nd ed., pp. 130, 138]. Philadelphia: Lippincott Williams & Wilkins.)

branch from the abdominal artery. The testicular veins, which drain the testes, arise from a venous network called the *pampiniform plexus* that surrounds the testicular artery. The testes are innervated by fibers from both divisions of the autonomic nervous system. Associated sensory nerves transmit pain impulses, resulting in excruciating pain, especially when the testes are hit forcibly.

The scrotum, which houses the testes, is made up of a thin outer layer of skin that forms rugae, or folds, and is continuous with the perineum and outer skin of the groin. Under the outer skin lies a thin layer of fascia and smooth muscle (*i.e.,* dartos muscle). This layer contains a septum that separates the two testes. The dartos muscle responds to changes in temperature. When it is cold, the muscle contracts, bringing the testes closer to the body and the scrotum becomes shorter and heavily wrinkled. When it is warmer, the muscle relaxes, allowing the scrotum to fall away from the body.

The location of the testes in the scrotum is important for sperm production, which is optimal at 2°C to 3°C below body temperature. Two systems maintain the temperature of the testes at a level consistent with sperm production. One is the pampiniform plexus of testicular veins that surrounds the testicular artery. This plexus absorbs heat from the arterial blood, cooling it as it enters the testes. The other is the cremaster muscles, which respond to decreases in testicular temperature by moving the testes closer to the body. Prolonged exposure to elevated temperatures, as a result of prolonged fever or the dysfunction of thermoregulatory mechanisms, can impair spermatogenesis. Some tight-fitting undergarments hold the testes against the body and are thought to contribute to a decrease in sperm counts and infertility by interfering with the thermoregulatory function of the scrotum. Cryptorchidism, the failure of the testes to descend into the scrotum, also exposes the testes to the higher temperature of the body (see Chapter 44).

🔑 MALE REPRODUCTIVE SYSTEM

- The male genitourinary system functions in both urine elimination and reproduction.

- The testes function in both production of male germ cells (spermatogenesis) and secretion of the male sex hormone, testosterone.

- The ductile system (epididymides, vas deferens, and ejaculatory ducts) transports and stores sperm, and assists in their maturation; and the accessory glands (seminal vesicles, prostate gland, and bulbourethral glands) prepare the sperm for ejaculation.

- Sperm production requires temperatures that are 2°C to 3°C below body temperature. The position of the testes in the scrotum and the unique blood flow cooling mechanisms provide this environment.

- The urethra, which is enclosed in the penis, is the terminal portion of the male genitourinary system. Because it conveys both urine and semen, it serves both urinary and reproductive functions.

Genital Duct System

Internally, the testes are composed of several hundred compartments or lobules (Fig. 43-3). Each lobule contains one or more coiled seminiferous tubules. These tubules are the site of sperm production. As the tubules lead into the efferent ducts, the seminiferous tubules become the rete testis. From the rete testis, 10,000 to 20,000 efferent ducts emerge to join the epididymis, which is the final site for sperm maturation. Because the spermatozoa are not motile at this stage of development, peristaltic movements of the ductal walls of the epididymis aid

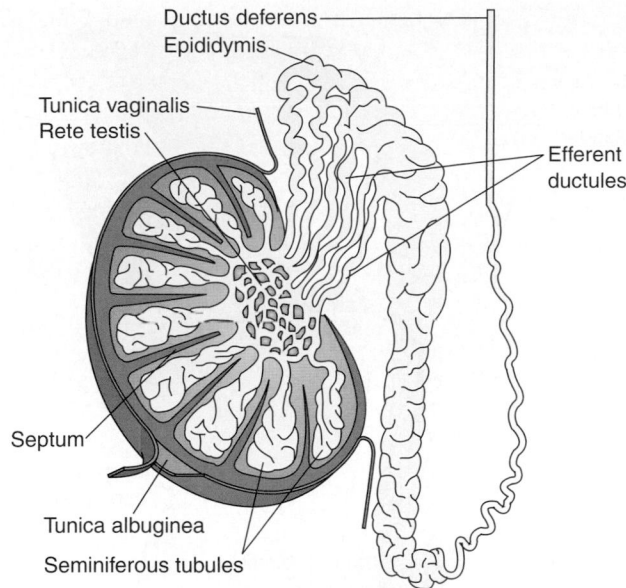

FIGURE 43-3 • The parts of the testes and epididymis.

in their movement. The spermatozoa continue their migration through the ductus deferens, also called the *vas deferens*. The ampulla of the vas deferens serves as a storage reservoir for sperm. Sperm are stored in the ampulla until they are released through the penis during ejaculation (Fig. 43-4). Spermatozoa can be stored in the genital ducts for as long as 42 days and still maintain their fertility. Surgical disconnection of the vas deferens in the scrotal area (*e.g.,* vasectomy) serves as an effective method of male contraception. Because sperm are stored in the ampulla, men can remain fertile for 4 to 5 weeks after performance of a vasectomy.

Accessory Organs

The male accessory organs consist of the seminal vesicles, the prostate gland, and the bulbourethral glands. Spermatozoa are transported through the reproductive structures by movement of the seminal fluid, which is combined with secretions from the genital ducts and accessory organs. The spermatozoa plus the secretions from the genital ducts and accessory organs make up the semen (from the Latin word meaning *seed*).

The seminal vesicles consist of two highly tortuous tubes that secrete fluid for the semen. Each of the paired seminal vesicles is lined with secretory epithelium containing an abundance of fructose, prostaglandins, and several other proteins. The fructose secreted by the seminal vesicles provides the energy for sperm motility. The prostaglandins are thought to assist in fertilization by making the cervical mucus more receptive to sperm and by causing peristaltic contractions in the uterus and fallopian tubes to move the sperm toward the ovaries.

Each seminal vesicle joins its corresponding vas deferens to form the ejaculatory duct, which enters the posterior part of the prostate and continues through until it ends in the prostatic portion of the urethra. During the emission phase of coitus, each vesicle empties fluid into the ejaculatory duct, adding bulk to the semen. Approximately 70% of the ejaculate originates in the seminal vesicles.

The prostate is a fibromuscular and glandular organ lying just inferior to the bladder. The prostate gland secretes a thin, milky, alkaline fluid containing citric acid, calcium, acid phosphate, a clotting enzyme, and a profibrinolysin. During ejaculation, the capsule of the prostate contracts and the added fluid increases the bulk of the semen. Both vaginal secretions and the fluid from the vas deferens are strongly acidic. Because sperm mobilization occurs at a pH of 6.0 to 6.5, the alkaline nature of

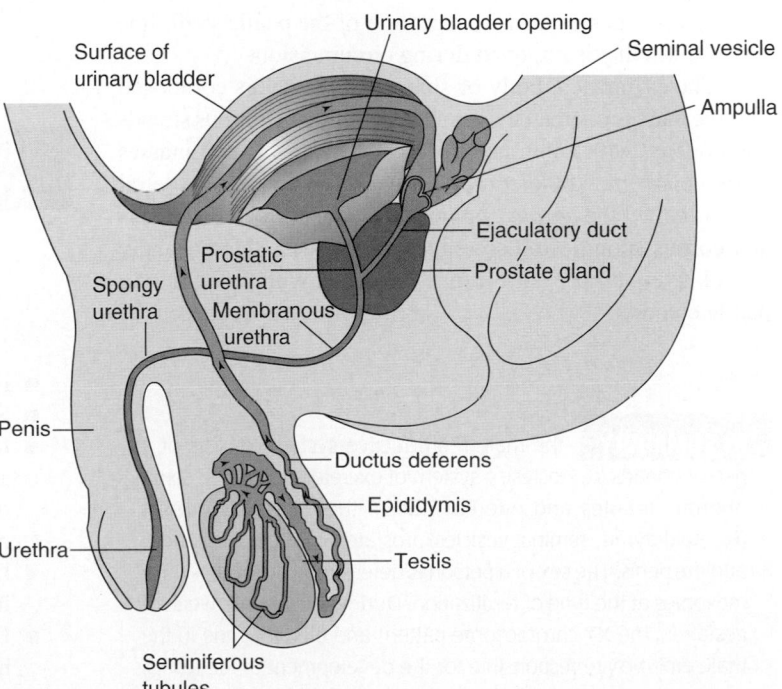

FIGURE 43-4 • The excretory ducts of the male reproductive system and the path that sperm follows as it leaves the testis and travels to the urethra.

the prostatic secretions is essential for successful fertilization of the ovum. The bulbourethral or Cowper glands lie on either side of the membranous urethra and secrete alkaline mucus, which further aids in neutralizing acids from the urine that remain in the urethra.

The prostate gland also functions in the elimination of urine and consists of a thin, fibrous capsule that encloses the circularly oriented smooth muscle fibers and collagenous tissue that surround the urethra where it joins the bladder. The segment of urethra that traverses the prostate gland is called the *prostatic urethra*. It is lined by a thin, longitudinal layer of smooth muscle that is continuous with the bladder wall. The smooth muscle incorporated with the prostate gland is derived primarily from the longitudinal bladder musculature. This smooth muscle represents the true involuntary sphincter of the male posterior urethra. Because the prostate surrounds the urethra, enlargement of the gland can produce urinary obstruction.

The prostate gland is made up of many secretory glands arranged in three concentric areas surrounding the prostatic urethra, into which they open. The component glands of the prostate include the small mucosal glands associated with the urethral mucosa, the intermediate submucosal glands that lie peripheral to the mucosal glands, and the large main prostatic glands that are situated toward the outside of the gland. It is the overgrowth of the mucosal glands that causes benign prostatic hyperplasia in older men (see Chapter 44).

Penis

The penis is the external genital organ through which the urethra passes. Anatomically, the external penis consists of a shaft that ends in a tip called the *glans* (Fig. 43-5). The loose skin of the penis shaft folds to cover the glans, forming the prepuce, or foreskin. The glans of the penis contains many sensory nerves, making this the most sensitive portion of the penile shaft. It is the foreskin that is removed during circumcision.

The cylindrical body or shaft of the penis is composed of three masses of erectile tissue held together by fibrous strands and covered with a thin layer of skin. The two lateral masses of tissue are called the *corpora cavernosa*. The third, ventral mass is called the *corpus spongiosum*. The corpora cavernosa and corpus spongiosum are cavernous sinuses that normally are relatively empty but become engorged with blood during penile erection.

IN SUMMARY,   the male reproductive system consists of a pair of gonads (*i.e.,* testes), a system of excretory ducts (*i.e.,* seminiferous tubules and efferent ducts), the accessory organs (*i.e.,* epididymis, seminal vesicles, prostate, and Cowper glands), and the penis. The sex of a person is determined by the sex chromosomes at the time of fertilization. During the seventh week of gestation, the XY chromosome pattern and the *SRY* gene in the male embryo are responsible for the development of the testes;

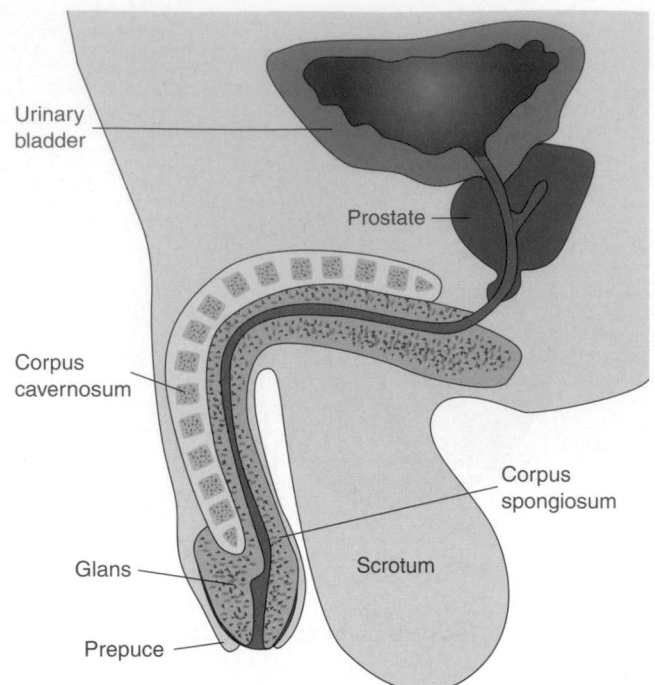

FIGURE 43-5 • Sagittal section of the penis, showing the prepuce, glans, corpus cavernosum, and corpus spongiosum.

with the subsequent production of AMH and testosterone, development of the internal and external male genital structures occurs. Before this period of embryonic development, the tissues from which the male and female reproductive structures develop are undifferentiated. In the absence of testosterone production (and its derivative DHT), the male embryo with an XY chromosomal pattern develops female external genitalia. ■

SPERMATOGENESIS AND HORMONAL CONTROL OF MALE REPRODUCTIVE FUNCTION

After completing this section of the chapter, you should be able to meet the following objectives:

- Describe the process of spermatogenesis.
- State the functions of testosterone.
- Draw a diagram illustrating the secretion, site of action, and feedback control of gonadotropin-releasing hormone, luteinizing hormone, follicle-stimulating hormone, and inhibin.
- Describe the function of follicle-stimulating hormone in terms of spermatogenesis.
- Describe the classification and clinical features of male hypogonadism.

During childhood, the gonads remain essentially quiescent. At puberty, the male gonads and testes begin to mature and to carry out spermatogenesis and hormone production. At approximately 10 or 11 years of age, the adenohypophysis, or anterior pituitary, under the control of the hypothalamus, begins to secrete the gonadotropins that stimulate testicular function and cause the interstitial Leydig cells to begin producing testosterone. At approximately the same time, hormonal stimulation induces mitotic activity of the germ cells that develop into sperm. After cell maturation has begun, the testes begin to enlarge rapidly as the individual tubules grow. Full maturity and spermatogenesis usually are attained by 15 or 16 years of age.

Spermatogenesis

Spermatogenesis refers to the generation of spermatozoa or sperm. It begins at an average age of 13 years and continues throughout the reproductive years of a man's life. Spermatogenesis occurs in the seminiferous tubules of the testes (see Fig 43-3). These tubules, if placed end to end, would measure approximately 750 feet. The outer layer of the seminiferous tubules is made up of connective tissue and smooth muscle; the inner lining is composed of Sertoli cells, which are embedded with sperm in various stages of development (Fig. 43-6A). Sertoli cells secrete a special fluid that contains nutrients to bathe and nourish the immature germ cells; they provide digestive enzymes that play a role in spermiation (*i.e.,* converting the spermatocytes to sperm); and they are thought to play a role in shaping the head and tail of the sperm. Sertoli cells also secrete several hormones, including AMH, which is secreted by the testes during fetal life to inhibit development of fallopian tubes; estradiol, the principal feminizing sex hormone, which seems to be required in the male for spermatogenesis; and inhibin, which controls the function of Sertoli cells through feedback inhibition of follicle-stimulating hormone (FSH) from the anterior pituitary gland.[4–6] For spermatogenesis to occur, FSH binds to specific receptors in Sertoli cells. A high concentration of intratesticular testosterone is also required.[4]

In the first stage of spermatogenesis, small and unspecialized diploid germinal cells located immediately adjacent to the tubular wall, called the *spermatogonia,* undergo rapid mitotic division and provide a continuous source of new germinal cells. As these cells multiply, the more mature spermatogonia divide into two daughter cells, which grow and become the primary spermatocytes—the precursors of sperm. Over several weeks, large primary spermatocytes divide by a process called *meiosis* to form two smaller secondary spermatocytes. Each of the secondary spermatocytes divides to form two spermatids, each containing 23 chromosomes. Meiosis is a unique form of cell division that occurs only in the gonads. It consists of two consecutive nuclear divisions with formation of four daughter cells, each containing a single set of 23 chromosomes rather than a pair of 46 chromosomes, as occurs during mitotic cell division in other body cells (see Chapter 6).

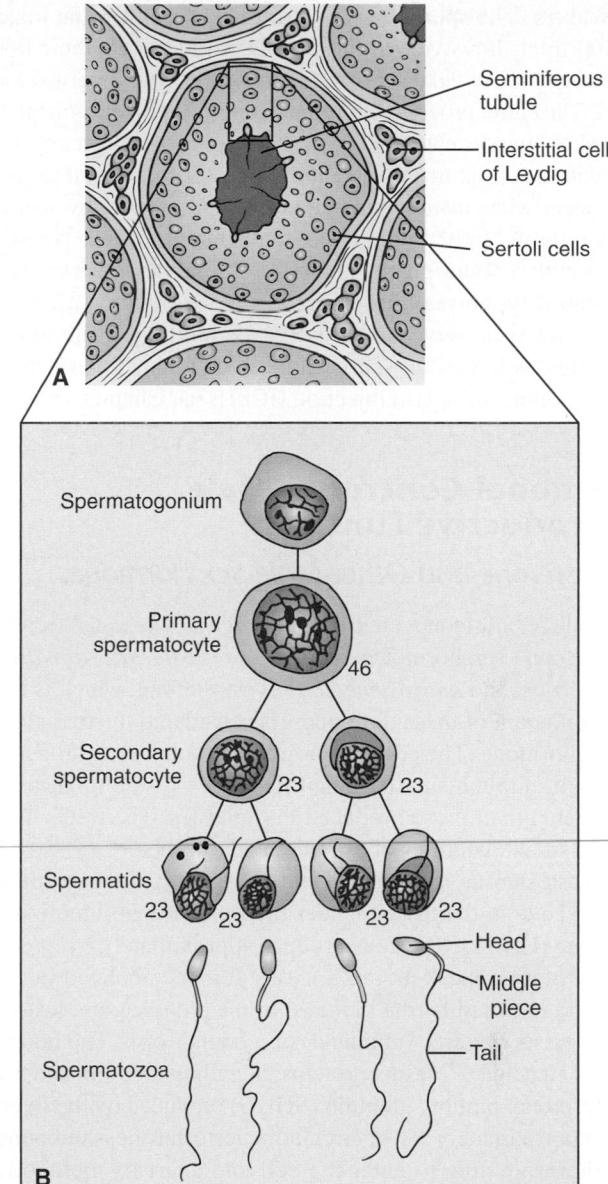

FIGURE 43-6 • The various stages of spermatogenesis. **(A)** Cross-section of seminiferous tubule. **(B)** Stages of development of spermatozoa.

The spermatid elongates into a spermatozoon, or mature sperm cell, with a head and tail (see Fig. 43-6B). The outside of the anterior two thirds of the head, called the *acrosome,* contains enzymes necessary for penetration and fertilization of the ovum. The to-and-fro flagellar motion of the tail imparts movement to the sperm. The energy for this process is supplied by the mitochondria in the tail. Normal sperm move in a straight line at a velocity of 1 to 4 mm/minute. This allows them to move through the female genital tract. As the sperm grow to full size, they move to the epididymis to mature further and gain mobility. A small quantity of sperm can be stored in the epididymis, but most are stored in the vas deferens or the ampulla of the vas deferens. With excessive sexual activity, storage may be no longer than a few days. The sperm can live for many weeks in the male genital tract; however, in the female genital tract, their life expectancy is 1 or 2 days. Frozen sperm have been preserved for years. The entire process of spermatogenesis and sperm maturation takes approximately 90 days. The sperm count in a normal ejaculate is approximately 100 million to 400 million. Infertility may occur when insufficient numbers of motile, healthy sperm are present. A "fertile sample" on seminal fluid analysis is associated with a count greater than 20 million/mL, greater than 50% motility, normal morphology, and a volume of 1.5 to 6 mL.[7] However, new reproductive technology techniques mean that as few as 20 sperm in the semen may be effective (intracytoplasmic sperm injection [ICSI]; see Chapter 46).

Hormonal Control of Male Reproductive Function

Testosterone and Other Male Sex Hormones

The male sex hormones are called *androgens*. The testes secrete several male sex hormones, including *testosterone, dihydrotestosterone,* and *androstenedione.* Testosterone, which is the most abundant of these hormones, is considered the main testicular hormone. The adrenal cortex also produces androgens, although in much smaller quantities (<5% of the total male androgens) than those produced in the testes. The testes also secrete small quantities of estradiol and estrone.[1,5,6]

Testosterone is produced and secreted by the interstitial Leydig cells in the testes. Under the influence of luteinizing hormone (LH), Leydig cells produce approximately 6 mg/day of testosterone (peak at 4 to 8 AM).[1,5] It is metabolized in the liver and excreted by the kidneys. In the bloodstream, testosterone exists in a free (unbound) or a bound form. The bound form is attached to plasma proteins, including albumin and the sex hormone–binding globulin (SHBG) produced by the liver. Only approximately 2% of circulating testosterone is unbound and therefore able to enter the cell and exert its metabolic effects. Much of the testosterone that becomes fixed to the tissues is converted to DHT by 5α-reductase, especially in certain target tissues such as the prostate gland. Some of the actions of testosterone depend on this conversion, whereas others do not.[1,5] Testosterone also can be aromatized or converted to estradiol in the peripheral tissues.

Testosterone (and DHT) exerts a variety of biologic effects in the male (Chart 43-1). In the male embryo, testosterone is essential for the appropriate differentiation of the internal and external genitalia, and it is necessary for descent of the testes in the fetus. Testosterone is essential to the development of primary and secondary male sex characteristics during puberty and for the maintenance of these characteristics during adult life.[1,6–8] It causes growth of pubic, chest, and facial hair; it produces changes in the larynx that result in the male bass voice; and it increases the thickness of the skin and increases the activity of the sebaceous glands, predisposing to acne.

All or almost all of the actions of testosterone and other androgens result from increased protein synthesis in target

---

CHART 43-1   MAIN ACTIONS OF TESTOSTERONE

Induces differentiation of the male genital tract during fetal development

Induces development of primary and secondary sex characteristics

    Gonadal function

    External genitalia and accessory organs

    Male voice timbre

    Male skin characteristics

    Male hair distribution

Anabolic effects

    Promotes protein metabolism

    Promotes musculoskeletal growth

    Influences subcutaneous fat distribution

Promotes spermatogenesis (in FSH-primed tubules) and maturation of sperm

Stimulates erythropoiesis

---

tissues. Androgens function as anabolic agents in males and females to promote metabolism and musculoskeletal growth. Testosterone and the androgens have a great effect on the development of increasing musculature during puberty, with boys averaging approximately a 50% increase in muscle mass compared with girls.

Action of the Hypothalamic and Anterior Pituitary Hormones

The hypothalamus and the anterior pituitary gland play an essential role in promoting spermatogenic activity in the testes and maintaining the endocrine function of the testes by means of the gonadotropic hormones. The synthesis and release of the gonadotropic hormones from the pituitary gland are regulated by gonadotropin-releasing hormone (GnRH), which is synthesized by the hypothalamus and secreted into the hypothalamic-hypophysial portal circulation (Fig. 43-7).

Two gonadotropic hormones are secreted by the pituitary gland: FSH and LH. The production of testosterone by the interstitial Leydig cells is regulated by LH (see Fig. 43-7). FSH binds selectively to Sertoli cells surrounding the seminiferous tubules, where it functions in the initiation of spermatogenesis. Under the influence of FSH, Sertoli cells produce androgen-binding protein, plasminogen activator, and inhibin. Androgen-binding protein binds testosterone and serves as a carrier of testosterone in Sertoli cells and as a storage site for testosterone. Although FSH is necessary for the initiation of spermatogenesis, full maturation of the spermatozoa requires testosterone (the intratesticular concentration of testosterone is 100-fold greater than serum levels). Androgen-binding protein also serves as a carrier of testosterone from the testes to the epididymis. Plasminogen activator, which converts plasminogen to plasmin, functions in the final detachment of mature spermatozoa from Sertoli cells.

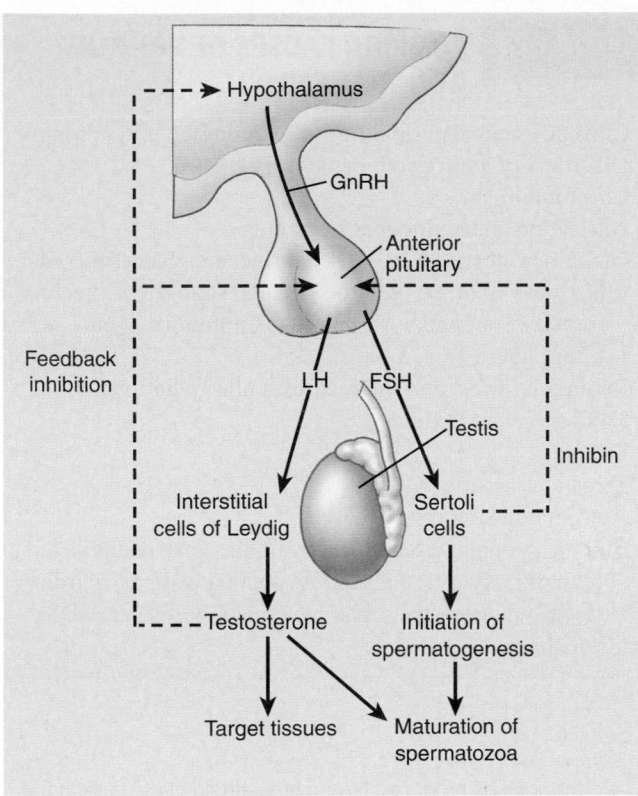

FIGURE 43-7 • Hypothalamic-pituitary feedback control of spermatogenesis and testosterone levels in the male. The *dashed line* represents negative feedback. FSH, follicle-stimulating hormone; GnRH, gonadotropin-releasing hormone; LH, luteinizing hormone.

ceased. Because testosterone can be aromatized to estradiol in the peripheral tissues, androgens can also produce gynecomastia (breast enlargement).

The undesired effects of androgens depend on the type and dose administered. Virtually all androgens produced for human and veterinary purposes have been taken by athletes. Occasionally, athletes take several medications simultaneously (termed "stacking") in an attempt to increase the overall effect on performance, or to counter a side effect of one medication. For example, an athlete may take human chorionic gonadotropin (hCG) for its LH-like action to counteract the decrease in testicular size resulting from high-dose androgen abuse, and take an antiestrogen to counteract the gynecomastia from administration of high doses of hCG and androgens.

Attention has also focused on androgen precursors, including oral androstenedione and dehydroepiandrosterone (DHEA) products that are available over the counter and often are marketed as safe natural alternatives to androgens for building muscle.[5,9] Androstenedione and DHEA exert only weak androgenic activity, but their main purpose is to act as a key precursor for testosterone after peripheral conversion. Whether large doses of these over-the-counter products can produce some of the serious side effects seen with standard anabolic steroids is largely unknown.

Other performance-enhancing agents can be used either alone or in combination with androgens or other agents in an attempt to improve performance. These include stimulants, erythropoietin (EPO), growth hormone, insulin-like growth factor-1 (IGF-1), insulin, and creatine.[9]

Circulating levels of the gonadotropic hormones are regulated in a negative feedback manner by testosterone. High levels of testosterone suppress LH secretion through a direct action on the pituitary and an inhibitory effect on the hypothalamus. FSH is thought to be inhibited by a substance called *inhibin,* produced by Sertoli cells. Inhibin suppresses FSH release from the pituitary gland. The pituitary gonadotropic hormones and Sertoli cells in the testes form a classic negative feedback loop in which FSH stimulates inhibin and inhibin suppresses FSH.[5,6] Unlike the cyclic hormonal pattern in females, in males, FSH, LH, and testosterone secretion and spermatogenesis occur at relatively unchanging rates during adulthood.[1]

Androgens and Athletic Performance

Because of the marked effect that testosterone and other androgens have on body musculature, synthetic androgens sometimes are used by athletes to improve their appearance and muscle performance.[9] Frequently, these agents are taken in doses that far exceed physiologic levels (typically up to 40 times the recommended therapeutic dosages). This practice has been strongly discouraged because of potential harmful effects. Among the undesired or harmful effects of supraphysiologic doses of androgens are acne, decreased testicular size, and azoospermia. These effects may persist for months after use of the agents has

Hypogonadism

Hypogonadism or androgen deficiency may be suspected by certain clinical features (*e.g.,* fatigue, depression, decreased libido); however, the diagnosis needs confirmation by appropriate laboratory testing. A measure of total testosterone is usually initially performed, and if low (generally <300 ng/dL; normal range 300 to 1000 ng/dL), the diagnosis of hypogonadism should be confirmed with either a repeat measure of total testosterone or a measure of "free testosterone" (not protein bound [especially to SHBG], and therefore available for binding to, and activating, androgen receptors).

Hypogonadism can be primary (testicular failure due to problem in the testes) or secondary (failure resulting from lack of stimulation by gonadotropins [LH and FSH] from the pituitary). Tertiary hypogonadism also occurs and is caused by lack of stimulation of LH and FSH secretion from the pituitary, due to decreased or absent GnRH secretion from the hypothalamus. In men, primary hypogonadism is characterized by low androgens and sperm count and is due to lack of negative feedback at the hypothalamic-pituitary level, coupled with high levels of gonadotropins (*i.e.,* low testosterone and high LH and FSH). This is termed *hypergonadotropic hypogonadism* ("hyper hypog"). Secondary (and tertiary) hypogonadism, which also is characterized by low androgens and sperm count, is due to lack of secretion of gonadotropins from the hypothalamic-pituitary level, coupled with low levels of gonadotropins (*i.e.*, low testosterone and low LH and FSH). This is termed *hypogonadotropic hypogonadism* ("hypog hypog").

The clinical features of male hypogonadism depend on whether the impairment involves only spermatogenesis (FSH increase reflects Sertoli cell damage) or if testosterone secretion is also impaired (LH increase reflects Leydig cell damage). There are only two clinical manifestations of impaired spermatogenesis: subfertility/infertility and decreased testicular size (80% of testicular size is related to sperm production and 20% to testosterone production). In contrast, there are several possible clinical manifestations of impaired testosterone secretion, which are determined by its time of onset. Onset occurring in the adult is associated with fatigue, depression, decreased sexual desire/activity, erectile dysfunction, loss of secondary sex characteristics, changes in body composition (including loss of muscle mass and increase in fat mass), osteoporosis, and subfertility/infertility.[8]

Diagnosis of hypogonadism includes measurement of total testosterone levels (ideally at 8:00 AM, when the testosterone level is at its peak) in the ambulatory man. If the initial total testosterone level is low, the diagnosis of hypogonadism should be confirmed with either a repeat measure of total testosterone or a measure of free (bioavailable) testosterone. Once the diagnosis of hypogonadism is established, the LH and FSH levels should also be measured. A subsequently high LH and FSH indicates a primary hypogonadism (hypergonadotropic hypogonadism), and low or inappropriately normal LH and FSH, a secondary or tertiary hypogonadism (hypogonadotropic hypogonadism). Seminal fluid analysis should be considered in both types of hypogonadism if fertility is a concern. In men with hypogonadotropic hypogonadism, other pituitary hormones should be assessed and a pituitary magnetic resonance imaging (MRI) scan done. In cases of hypergonadotropic hypogonadism, a karyotype (chromosome) analysis may be indicated because Klinefelter syndrome is the most common chromosomal abnormality associated with male hypogonadism (see Chapter 7). The usual karyotype is 47,XXY, although mosaicism or variants can present with a similar phenotype (the normal male is 46,XY and the normal female is 46,XX). Males with Klinefelter syndrome characteristically have small, firm testes (unlike many other cases of hypogonadism, in which the testicular consistency is soft). Other common causes of primary hypogonadism are listed in Chart 43-2.

Testosterone for treatment of androgen deficiency should be administered only to men with confirmed hypogonadism (as evidenced by a distinctly subnormal serum testosterone concentration). The principal goal of testosterone therapy is to restore the serum testosterone concentration to the normal range.[8]

IN SUMMARY, the function of the male reproductive system is under the negative feedback control of the hypothalamus and the anterior pituitary gonadotropic hormones FSH and LH. Spermatogenesis is initiated by FSH and the production of testosterone is regulated by LH. Testosterone, the major male

---

CHART 43-2   COMMON CAUSES OF PRIMARY GONADAL FAILURE

Chromosomal abnormalities (*e.g.*, Klinefelter syndrome)
Disorders of androgen biosynthesis
Cryptorchidism
Alkylating and antineoplastic agents
Other medications (*e.g.*, ketoconazole and glucocorticoids)
Infections—mumps orchitis (gonadal failure is a much more common manifestation when mumps occurs after puberty)
Radiation (direct and indirect testicular radiation)
Environmental toxins
Trauma
Testicular torsion
Autoimmune damage
Chronic systemic diseases (many of these can result in both primary and secondary hypogonadism, *e.g.*, cirrhosis, hemochromatosis, chronic renal failure, and AIDS)
Idiopathic

---

sex hormone, is produced by the interstitial Leydig cells in the testes. In addition to its role in the differentiation of the internal and external genitalia in the male embryo, testosterone is essential for the development of secondary male characteristics during puberty, the maintenance of these characteristics during adult life, and spermatozoa maturation.

Because of the marked effect that testosterone and other androgens have on body musculature, synthetic androgens sometimes are used by athletes to improve their appearance and muscle performance. Among the undesired or harmful effects of supraphysiologic doses of androgens are acne, decreased testicular size, azoospermia, and a change in libido (increase/decrease).

Hypogonadism refers to a decrease in testicular function. It can present as a primary hypogonadism originating in the testes; a secondary hypogonadism arising from lack of stimulation from the pituitary gonadotropins (LH and FSH); or as a tertiary hypogonadism due to decreased or absent GnRH secretion from the hypothalamus. ■

NEURAL CONTROL OF SEXUAL FUNCTION AND AGING CHANGES

After completing this section of the chapter, you should be able to meet the following objectives:

- Describe the autonomic and nonautonomic nervous systems' control of erection, emission, and ejaculation.
- Describe changes in the male reproductive system that occur with aging.

In the male, the stages of the sexual act involve erection, emission, ejaculation, and detumescence. The physiology of the sexual act involves a complex interaction between spinal cord reflexes, higher neural centers, the vascular system, and the endocrine system.

Neural Control

The most important source of impulse stimulation for initiating the male sexual act is the glans penis, which contains a highly organized sensory system. Afferent impulses from sensory receptors in the glans penis pass through the pudendal nerve to ascending fibers in the spinal cord by way of the sacral plexus. Stimulation of other perineal areas, such as the anal epithelium, the scrotum, and the testes, can transmit signals to higher brain centers, such as the limbic system and cerebral cortex, through the cord, adding to sexual arousal.

The psychic element to sexual stimulation, such as thinking sexual thoughts, can cause erection and ejaculation. Although psychic involvement and higher-center functions contribute to the sex act, they are not necessary for sexual performance. Genital stimulation can produce erection and ejaculation in some men with complete transection of the spinal cord (see Chapter 50).

Erection involves the shunting of blood into the corpus cavernosum. It is controlled by the sympathetic, parasympathetic, and nonadrenergic–noncholinergic (NANC) systems. Nitric oxide is the locally released NANC mediator that produces relaxation of vascular smooth muscle. In the flaccid or detumescent state, sympathetic discharge through α-adrenergic receptors maintains contraction of the arteries that supply the penis and vascular sinuses of the corpora cavernosa and corpus spongiosum (Fig. 43-8). Parasympathetic stimulation produces erection by inhibiting sympathetic neurons that cause detumescence and by stimulating the release of nitric oxide to effect a rapid relaxation of the smooth muscle in the sinusoidal spaces of the corpus cavernosum. During sexual stimulation, parasympathetic impulses also cause the urethral and bulbourethral glands to secrete mucus to aid in lubrication. Parasympathetic innervation is effected through the pelvic nerve and sacral segments of the spinal cord. Sympathetic innervation exits the spinal cord at the L1 and L2 levels. Erectile dysfunction can be caused by disease or dysfunction of the brain, spinal cord, cav-

ernous or pudendal nerves, or terminal nerve endings or receptors[10] (see Chapter 44).

Emission and ejaculation, which constitute the culmination of the male sexual act, are a function of the sympathetic nervous system. As with erection, emission and ejaculation are mediated through spinal cord reflexes. With increasing intensity of the sexual stimulus, reflex centers of the spinal cord begin to emit sympathetic impulses that leave the cord at the L1 and L2 levels and pass through the hypogastric plexus to the genital organs to initiate emission, which is the forerunner of ejaculation. Emission causes the sperm to move from the epididymis to the urethra. Efferent impulses from the spinal cord produce contraction of smooth muscle in the vas deferens and ampulla that move sperm forward and close the internal urethral sphincter to prevent retrograde ejaculation into the bladder.

Ejaculation represents the expulsion of the sperm from the urethra. It involves contraction of the seminal vesicles and prostate gland, which add fluid to the ejaculate and propel it forward. Ejaculation is accompanied by contraction of the ischiocavernous and bulbocavernous muscles at the base of the penis. The filling of the internal urethra elicits signals that are transmitted through the pudendal nerves from the spinal cord, giving the sudden feeling of fullness of the genital organs. Rhythmic increases in pressure in the urethra cause the semen to be propelled to the exterior, resulting in ejaculation. At the same time, rhythmic contractions of the pelvic and trunk muscles produce thrusting movements of the pelvis and penis, which help propel the ejaculate into the vagina.

The period of emission and ejaculation is called *male orgasm*. After ejaculation, erection ceases within 1 to 2 minutes. A man usually ejaculates approximately 2 to 5 mL of semen. The ejaculate may vary with frequency of intercourse. It is less with frequent ejaculation and may increase to two to four times its normal amount during periods of abstinence. The semen that is ejaculated is 98% fluid and approximately 2% sperm.

The role of circulating androgens in sexual function remains unclear.[8,10] It is apparent that sexual desire and performance depend on some threshold level of testosterone; however, this level varies from man to man. Studies of hypogonadal and castrated men show a variety of sexual behavior, ranging from complete loss of libido to normal sexual activity. It may be that the role of testosterone in male sexuality is in the area of sexual interest and motivation, with individual intrapsychic factors playing a significant role.

 Aging Changes

Like other body systems, the male reproductive system undergoes degenerative changes as a result of the aging process; it becomes less efficient with age. The declining physiologic efficiency of male reproductive function occurs gradually and involves the endocrine, circulatory, and neuromuscular systems. Compared with the marked physiologic changes in aging females, the changes in the aging male are more gradual and less drastic. Gonadal and reproductive failure usually are not

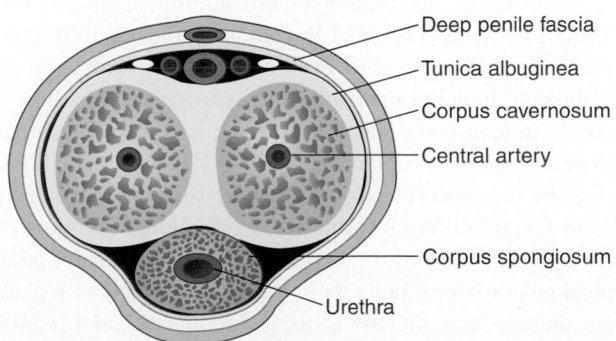

FIGURE 43-8 • Erectile tissue of the penis.

related directly to age because a man remains fertile into advanced age; 80- and 90-year-old men have been known to father children.[1]

As the male ages, his reproductive system becomes measurably different in structure and function from that of the younger male. Male sex hormone levels, particularly of testosterone, decrease with age, but the rate varies in different individuals and is affected by chronic disease and medications.[8] Beginning at about 25 to 30 years of age in healthy, nonobese men, testosterone levels gradually decrease at approximately 10% per decade. The term *andropause* has been used to describe an ill-defined collection of symptoms in aging men, typically those older than 50 years, who have a relative or absolute hypogonadism associated with aging.[8] The existence and significance of andropause has important public health implications given the current number of men older than 65 years of age, with the number expected to double over the next 30 years. One study reported a prevalence of hypogonadism (defined as serum total testosterone <325 ng/dL [normal is 300 to 1000 ng/dL]) in each decade as follows: 12% of men in their 50s, 19% in their 60s, 28% in their 70s, and 49% in their 80s.[11]

The sex hormones play a part in the structure and function of the reproductive system and other body systems from conception to old age; they affect protein synthesis, salt and water balance, bone growth, and cardiovascular function. Low testosterone levels have an atherogenic effect that may explain the higher incidence of heart disease in androgen-deficient men.[8,12] Decreasing levels of testosterone affect sexual energy, muscle strength, and the genital tissues. The testes become smaller and lose their firmness. The seminiferous tubules, which produce spermatozoa, thicken and begin a degenerative process that finally inhibits sperm production, resulting in a decrease in viable spermatozoa. The prostate gland enlarges and its contractions become weaker. The force of ejaculation decreases because of a reduction in the volume and viscosity of the seminal fluid. The seminal vesicle changes little from childhood to puberty. The pubertal increases in the fluid capacity of the gland remain throughout adulthood and decline after 60 years of age. After 60 years of age, the walls of the seminal vesicles thin, the epithelium shrinks, and the muscle layer is replaced by connective tissue. Age-related changes in the penis consist of fibrotic changes in the trabecula in the corpus spongiosum, with progressive sclerotic changes in arteries and veins. Sclerotic changes also follow in the corpora cavernosa, with the condition becoming generalized in 55- to 60-year-old men.

As a sexual partner, the aging male exhibits some differences in responsiveness and activity from his younger counterpart. Masters and Johnson studied the significant aging changes in the physiology of the sex act.[13] They observed that frequency of intercourse, intensity of sensation, speed of attaining erection, and force of ejaculation are all reduced.

Erectile dysfunction (see Chapter 44) in the elderly male often is directly related to the general physical condition of the person.[10] *Erectile dysfunction* (ED) has largely replaced the term *impotence*. It is defined as the persistent inability to achieve and maintain an erection sufficient to permit satisfactory sexual

intercourse. Aging is a major etiologic factor in this condition. However, even among younger men (those in their 40s), nearly 40% report at least occasional difficulty obtaining or maintaining an erection. This figure approaches 70% in 70-year-olds. In a large study of 31,742 men aged 50 to 93 years with no history of prostate cancer, 33% overall reported ED in the past 3 months. That number increased steadily with age: 26% of men aged 50 to 59, 40% aged 60 to 69, and 61% older than 70 years of age reported ED. However, men older than 50 years of age are less likely to suffer from ED if they avoid cigarettes and junk food, and spend less time watching television and more time in the gym.[14] Men who were more physically active (3 hours of running per week or the equivalent) had a 30% lower risk of ED compared with men who reported little or no physical activity. Conversely, watching television for more than 20 hours per week, smoking, and being overweight were associated with increased risk of ED.[14]

Diseases that accompany aging can have a direct bearing on male reproductive function. Various cardiovascular, respiratory, hormonal, neurologic, and hematologic disorders can be responsible for secondary impotence. For example, vascular disease affects male potency because it may impair blood flow to the pudendal arteries or their tributaries, resulting in loss of blood volume with subsequent poor distention of the vascular spaces of erectile tissue. Other diseases affecting potency include hypertension, diabetes, cardiac disease, and malignancies of the reproductive organs. In addition, certain medications can have an effect on sexual function.

One of the greatest inhibitors of sexual functioning in older men is the loss of self-esteem and the development of a negative self-image. The emphasis on youth pervades much of our society. The image of success for a man often involves qualities of masculinity and sexual attractiveness. When queried about success, men often mention such things as work, managing money well, participating in sports or other activities, discussing politics or world events, advising younger persons, and being attractive to women. When a man feels good about himself and expresses self-confidence, sexual attractiveness is communicated regardless of age. Many older men live in environments that are not sensitive to the importance of helping them maintain a positive self-image. Premature cessation of the aforementioned esteem-building activities can contribute to loss of libido and zest for life in the elderly man.

Testosterone and other synthetic androgens may be used in older men with confirmed low androgen levels to improve muscle strength and vigor. Preliminary studies of androgen replacement in aging men with low androgen levels show an increase in lean body mass and a decrease in bone turnover. Before testosterone replacement therapy is initiated, all men should be screened for prostate cancer. Testosterone is available in several different formulations, including an injectable form (administered every 1 to 3 weeks), transdermal patch, topical gel, or buccal delivery system. Side effects of replacement therapy may include acne, gynecomastia, and reduced high-density lipoprotein cholesterol levels. It also may contribute to a worsening of sleep apnea in men who are troubled by this problem.[8]

At present, it is not recommended that routine treatment of elderly men with testosterone should be undertaken. A trial of testosterone administration, however, might be warranted in an elderly man whose serum testosterone concentration is less than 300 ng/dL (although some believe it should be even lower, *i.e.*, <200 ng/dL) and who has manifestations of testosterone deficiency.[8] If treatment is undertaken, the man should be screened before treatment and monitored during therapy for evidence of testosterone-dependent diseases.

IN SUMMARY, the sex act involves erection, emission, ejaculation, and detumescence. The physiology of these functions involves a complex interaction between autonomic-mediated spinal cord reflexes, higher neural centers, and the vascular system. Erection is mediated by the parasympathetic nervous system and emission and ejaculation by the sympathetic nervous system. Like other body systems, the male reproductive system undergoes changes as a result of the aging process. The changes occur gradually and involve parallel changes in endocrine, circulatory, and neuromuscular function. Testosterone levels decrease (andropause), the size and firmness of the testes decrease, sperm production declines, and the prostate gland enlarges. There usually is a decrease in frequency of intercourse, intensity of sensation, speed of attaining erection, and force of ejaculation. However, sexual thought, interest, and activity usually continue into old age. ∎

Review Exercises

1. In the absence of the *SRY* gene on the Y chromosome, a developing embryo with an XY genotype will develop female genitalia.
   A. *Explain.*

2. Men who have had a vasectomy often remain fertile for 4 to 5 weeks after the procedure has been done.
   A. *Explain.*

3. A 55-year-old man presents with various vague symptoms (fatigue, depression). On examination, he is noted to have small testes (8 mL bilaterally), marked gynecomastia, and scanty body hair. He is obese at 122 kg, with a body mass index (BMI) of 34.2. Investigations reveal low testosterone and elevated gonadotropin (LH and FSH) levels.

   A. *What endocrine diagnosis is related to this phenotype and these biochemical manifestations?*

References

1. Federman D. D. (2006). The biology of human sex differences. *New England Journal of Medicine* 354, 1507–1514.
2. Tanagho E. A. (2004). Embryology of the genitourinary system. In Tanagho E. A., McAninch J. W. (Eds.), *Smith's general urology* (16th ed., pp. 18–30). New York: Lange Medical Books/McGraw-Hill.
3. Moore K. L., Persaud T. V. N. (2003). *The developing human: Clinically oriented embryology* (7th ed., pp. 304–328). Philadelphia: W. B. Saunders.
4. Guyton A. C., Hall J. (2006). *Textbook of medical physiology* (11th ed., pp. 996–1010). Philadelphia: Elsevier Saunders.
5. Griffin J. E., Wilson J. D. (2003). Disorders of the testes and the male reproductive tract. In Larsen P. R., Kronenberg H. M., Melmed S., et al. (Eds.), *Williams textbook of endocrinology* (10th ed., pp. 2143–2154). Philadelphia: W. B. Saunders.
6. Braunstein G. D. (2004). Testes. In Greenspan F. S., Gardner D. G. (Eds.), *Basic and clinical endocrinology* (7th ed., pp. 478–510). New York: Lange Medical Books/McGraw-Hill.
7. AACE Hypogonadism Taskforce. (2002). AACE medical guidelines for clinical practice for the evaluation and treatment of hypogonadism in adult male patients—2002 update. *Endocrine Practice* 8, 439–446.
8. Bhasin S., Cunningham G. R., Hayes F. J., et al. (2006). Testosterone therapy in adult men with androgen deficiency syndrome: An Endocrine Society Clinical Practice Guideline. *Journal of Clinical Endocrinology and Metabolism* 91, 1995–2010.
9. Saudan C., Baume N., Robinson N., et al. (2006). Testosterone and doping control. *British Journal of Sports Medicine* 40, 21–24.
10. Matfin G., Jawa A., Fonseca V. (2006). Erectile dysfunction in diabetes: An endothelial disorder. In Fonseca V. (Ed.), *Diabetes mellitus: Translating research to practice* (pp. 165–178). Philadelphia: Elsevier Saunders.
11. Harman S. M., Metter E. J., Tobin J., et al. (2001). Longitudinal effects of aging on serum total and free testosterone levels in healthy men. *Journal of Clinical Endocrinology and Metabolism* 86, 724–731.
12. Channer K. S., Jones T. H. (2003). Cardiovascular effects of testosterone: Implications of the "male menopause?" *Heart* 89, 121–122.
13. Masters W. H., Johnson V. (1970). *Human sexual inadequacy* (pp. 337–338). Boston: Little, Brown.
14. Bacon C. G., Mittleman M. A., Kawachi I., et al. (2003). Sexual function in men older than 50 years of age: Results from the Health Professionals follow-up study. *Annals of Internal Medicine* 139, 161–168.

Visit thePoint **http://thePoint.lww.com for animations, journal articles, and more!**

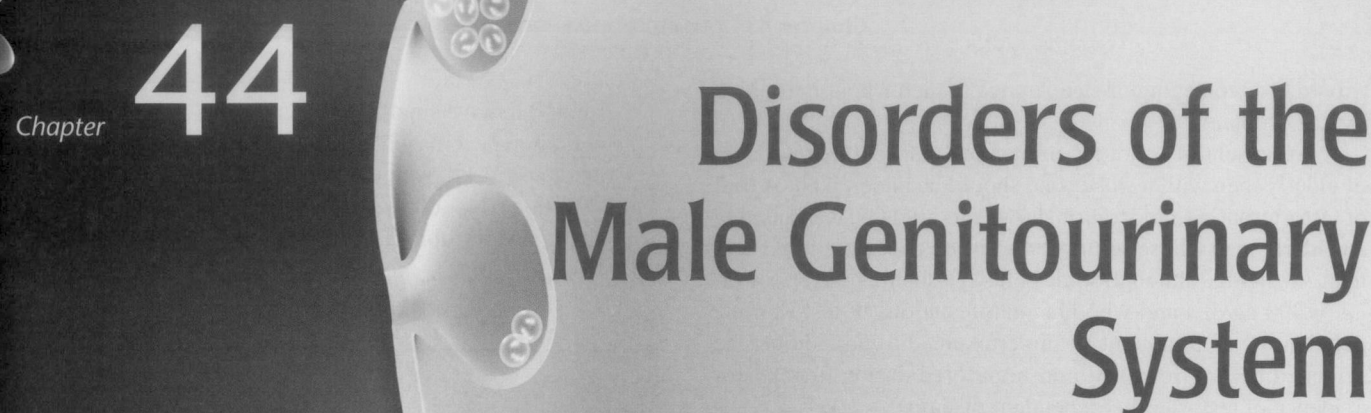

Chapter 44

Disorders of the Male Genitourinary System

GLENN MATFIN

> The male genitourinary system is subject to structural defects, inflammation, and neoplasms, all of which can affect urine elimination, sexual function, and fertility. This chapter discusses disorders of the penis, the scrotum and testes, and the prostate.

 **DISORDERS OF THE PENIS**

After completing this section of the chapter, you should be able to meet the following objectives:

■ State the difference between hypospadias and epispadias.
■ Cite the significance of phimosis.
■ Describe the anatomic changes that occur with Peyronie disease.
■ Explain the physiology of penile erection and relate it to erectile dysfunction and priapism.
■ Describe the appearance of balanitis xerotica obliterans.
■ List the signs of penile cancer.

The penis is the external male genital organ through which the urethra passes to the exterior of the body. It is involved in urinary and sexual function. Disorders of the penis include congenital and acquired defects, inflammatory conditions, and neoplasms.

Congenital and Acquired Disorders

 Hypospadias and Epispadias

Hypospadias and epispadias are congenital disorders of the penis resulting from embryologic defects in the development of the urethral groove and penile urethra (Fig. 44-1). In hypospadias, which affects approximately 1 in 300 male infants, the termination of the urethra is on the ventral surface of the penis.[1-3] It is common to categorize hypospadias as glandular

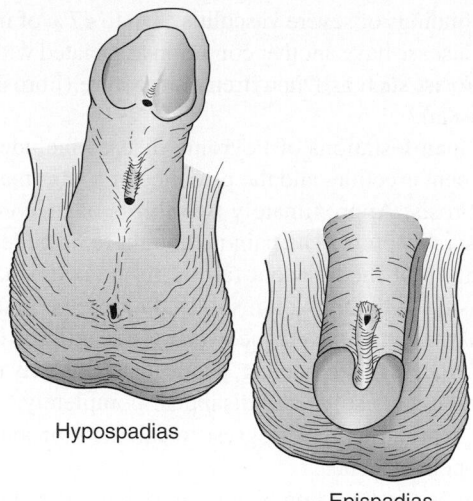

Hypospadias

Epispadias

FIGURE 44-1 • Hypospadias and epispadias.

(involving the glans penis), penile, or perineoscrotal. The etiology in most cases is unknown. Single-gene defects, chromosomal abnormalities, and maternal progestational drug ingestion in early pregnancy account for only about one fourth of cases. The testes are undescended in 10% of boys born with hypospadias and chordee (*i.e.,* ventral bowing of the penis), and inguinal hernia also may accompany the disorder. In the newborn with severe hypospadias and cryptorchidism (undescended testes), the differential diagnosis should consider ambiguous genitalia and masculinization that is seen in females with congenital adrenal hyperplasia (see Chapter 41). Recently, the term *disorders of sex development* (DSD) has been proposed to define congenital conditions in which development of chromosomal, gonadal, or anatomic sex is atypical.[3] Because many chromosomal aberrations result in DSD, chromosomal studies often are recommended for male infants with hypospadias and cryptorchidism.[1,3]

Surgery is the treatment of choice for hypospadias.[1,3] Circumcision is avoided because the foreskin is used for surgical repair. Factors that influence the timing of surgical repair include anesthetic risk, penile size, and the psychological effects of the surgery on the child. In mild cases, the surgery is done for cosmetic reasons only. In more severe cases, repair becomes essential for normal sexual functioning and to prevent the psychological sequelae of having malformed genitalia. In contrast to the practices of several decades ago, when surgical repair often was delayed until the child was 2 to 6 years of age, surgical repair is now done between the ages of 6 and 12 months. Judicious use of testosterone supplementation may also be warranted.[3]

Epispadias, in which the opening of the urethra is on the dorsal surface of the penis, is a less common defect. Although epispadias may occur as a separate entity, it often is associated with exstrophy of the bladder, a condition in which the abdominal wall fails to cover the bladder. The treatment depends on the extent of the developmental defect.

Phimosis and Paraphimosis

Phimosis refers to a tightening of the prepuce or penile foreskin that prevents its retraction over the glans. Embryologically, the foreskin begins to develop during the eighth week of gestation as a fold of skin at the distal edge of the penis that eventually grows forward over the base of the glans.[2] By the 16th week of gestation, the prepuce and the glans are adherent. Only a small percentage of newborns have a fully retractable foreskin. With growth, a space develops between the glans and foreskin, and by 3 years of age, approximately 90% of boys have retractable foreskins.

Because the foreskin of many boys cannot be fully retracted in early childhood, it is important that the area be cleaned thoroughly. There is no need to retract the foreskin forcibly because this could lead to infection, scarring, or paraphimosis. As the child grows, the foreskin becomes retractable, and the glans and foreskin should be cleaned routinely. If symptomatic phimosis occurs after childhood, it can cause difficulty with voiding or sexual activity. Circumcision is then the treatment of choice. Phimosis is also one of the most important predisposing factors for penile cancer.

In a related condition called *paraphimosis,* the foreskin is so tight and constricted that it cannot cover the glans. A tight foreskin can constrict the blood supply to the glans and lead to ischemia and necrosis. Many cases of paraphimosis result from the foreskin being retracted for an extended period, as in the case of catheterized uncircumcised males.

Balanitis and Balanoposthitis

Balanitis is an acute or chronic inflammation of the glans penis. *Balanoposthitis* refers to inflammation of the glans and prepuce. It usually is encountered in men with phimosis or a large, redundant prepuce that interferes with cleanliness and predisposes to bacterial growth in the accumulated secretions and smegma (*i.e.,* debris from the desquamated epithelia). If left untreated, the condition may cause ulcerations of the mucosal surface of the glans; these ulcerations may lead to inflammatory scarring of the prepuce and further aggravate the condition.

Acute superficial balanoposthitis is characterized by erythema of the glans and prepuce. An exudate in the form of malodorous discharge may be present. Extension of the erythema and edema may result in phimosis. The condition may result from infection, trauma, or irritation. Infective balanoposthitis may be caused by a wide variety of organisms. *Chlamydia* and mycoplasmas have been identified as causative organisms in this disease. Gonococcal balanitis may develop as a complication of infection in uncircumcised men. The inflammatory reaction is nonspecific, and correct identification of the specific organism requires microbial smears and cultures.

Balanitis due to candidal infection may be a presenting feature or result from poorly controlled diabetes mellitus. Balanitis also can result from noninfectious causes, such as circinate balanitis, which is seen in reactive arthritis (see

Chapter 59). Lesions are superficial, painless ulcers that heal without scarring.

Balanitis xerotica obliterans is a chronic, sclerosing, atrophic process of the glans penis that occurs in uncircumcised men. It is clinically and histologically similar to the lichen sclerosus that is seen in women (see Chapter 46). Typically, the lesions consist of whitish plaques on the surface of the glans penis and the prepuce. The foreskin is thickened and fibrous and is not retractable. Although balanitis xerotica obliterans was once considered a benign condition, it has been associated with several reports of penile cancer and is now recognized as a precancerous state. Treatment measures include circumcision and topical or intralesional injections of corticosteroids.[4]

Peyronie Disease

Peyronie disease involves a localized and progressive fibrosis of unknown origin that affects the tunica albuginea (*i.e.*, the tough, fibrous sheath that surrounds the corpora cavernosa) of the penis. It is named after Francois de la Peyronie, who in 1743 described a patient who had "rosary beads of scar tissue to cause upward curvature of the penis during erection."[5] The disorder is characterized initially by an inflammatory process that results in dense fibrous plaque formation. The plaque usually is on the dorsal midline of the shaft, causing upward bowing of the shaft during erection (Fig. 44-2). Some men may develop scarring on both the dorsal and ventral aspects of the shaft, causing the penis to be straight but shortened or have a lateral bend.[5] The fibrous tissue prevents lengthening of the involved area during erection, making intercourse difficult and painful. The disease usually occurs in middle-aged or elderly men. Although the cause of the disorder is unknown, the dense microscopic plaques are consistent with findings of severe vasculitis.[6] Up to 47% of men with Peyronie disease have another condition associated with fascial tissue fibrosis, such as Dupuytren contracture (fibrosis of the palmar fascia).[5]

The manifestations of Peyronie disease include painful erection, bent erection, and the presence of a hard mass at the site of fibrosis. Approximately two thirds of men complain of pain as a symptom. The pain is thought to be generated by inflammation of the adjacent fascial tissue and usually disappears as the inflammation resolves. During the first year or so after formation of the plaque, while the scar tissue is undergoing the process of remodeling, penile distortion may increase, remain static, or resolve and disappear completely.[5] In some cases, the scar tissue may progress to calcification and formation of bonelike tissue.

Diagnosis is based on history and physical examination. Doppler ultrasonography may be used to assess causation of the disorder. Although surgical intervention can be used to correct the disorder, it often is delayed because in many cases the disorder is self-limiting.[6] Indications for surgery include penile shortening, persistent pain, severe curvature, and penile narrowing or indentation. If surgery is required, satisfactory results have been obtained with various procedures with or without the use of an inflatable penile prosthesis.[7] Less invasive treatments include the administration of oral agents with antioxidant properties (*e.g.*, colchicine), and intralesional treatments such as corticosteroids or the calcium channel blocker, verapamil. Other therapies include low-dose radiation therapy and various modes of energy transfer, including ultrasound and short-wave diathermy. At present, these methods have been inadequately studied and most have met with variable degrees of success.[5]

Disorders of Erectile Function

Erection is a neurovascular process involving the autonomic nervous system, neurotransmitters and endothelial relaxing factors, the vascular smooth muscle of the arteries and veins supplying the penile tissue, and the trabecular smooth muscle of the sinusoids of the corpora cavernosa (Fig. 44-3). The penis is innervated by both the autonomic and somatic nervous systems. In the pelvis, the sympathetic and parasympathetic components of the autonomic nervous systems merge to form what are called the *cavernous nerves*. Erection is under the control of the parasympathetic nervous system, and ejaculation and detumescence (penile relaxation) are under sympathetic nervous system control. Somatic innervation, which occurs through the pudendal nerve, is responsible for penile sensation and contraction and relaxation of the extracorporeal striated muscles (bulbocavernous and ischiocavernous).

Penile erection is the first effect of male sexual stimulation, whether psychological or physical (Fig. 44-4). It involves increased inflow of blood into the corpora cavernosa due to relaxation of the trabecular smooth muscle that surrounds the sinusoidal spaces and compression of the veins controlling outflow of blood from the venous plexus. Erection is mediated by parasympathetic impulses that pass from the sacral segments

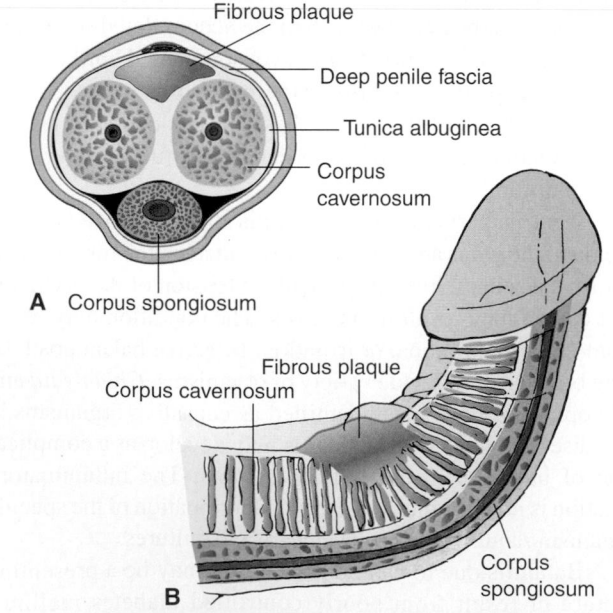

FIGURE 44-2 • Peyronie disease. **(A)** Penile cross-section showing plaque between the corpora. **(B)** Penile curvature.

🔑 DISORDERS OF PENILE ERECTION

- Erection is a neurovascular process involving the autonomic nervous system, the somatic nervous system by way of the pudendal nerve, the vascular system, and the sinusoidal spaces of the corpora cavernosa.

- Parasympathetic innervation through the pelvic nerves initiates relaxation of the trabecular smooth muscle of the corpora cavernosa through the action of nitric oxide, the inflow of arterial blood, and cessation of venous outflow.

- Erectile failure can result from disorders in one or a combination of the neural, vascular, or chemical mediator aspects of the erectile process.

- Priapism is an abnormal, painful, sustained erection that can lead to ischemic damage of penile structures. It can occur at any age and is one of the possible complications of sickle cell disease.

of the spinal cord through the pelvic nerves to the penis. Parasympathetic stimulation results in release of nitric oxide (a nonadrenergic–noncholinergic neurotransmitter), which causes relaxation of trabecular smooth muscle of the corpora cavernosa. This relaxation permits inflow of blood into the sinuses of the cavernosa at pressures approaching those of the arterial system. Because the erectile tissues of the cavernosa are

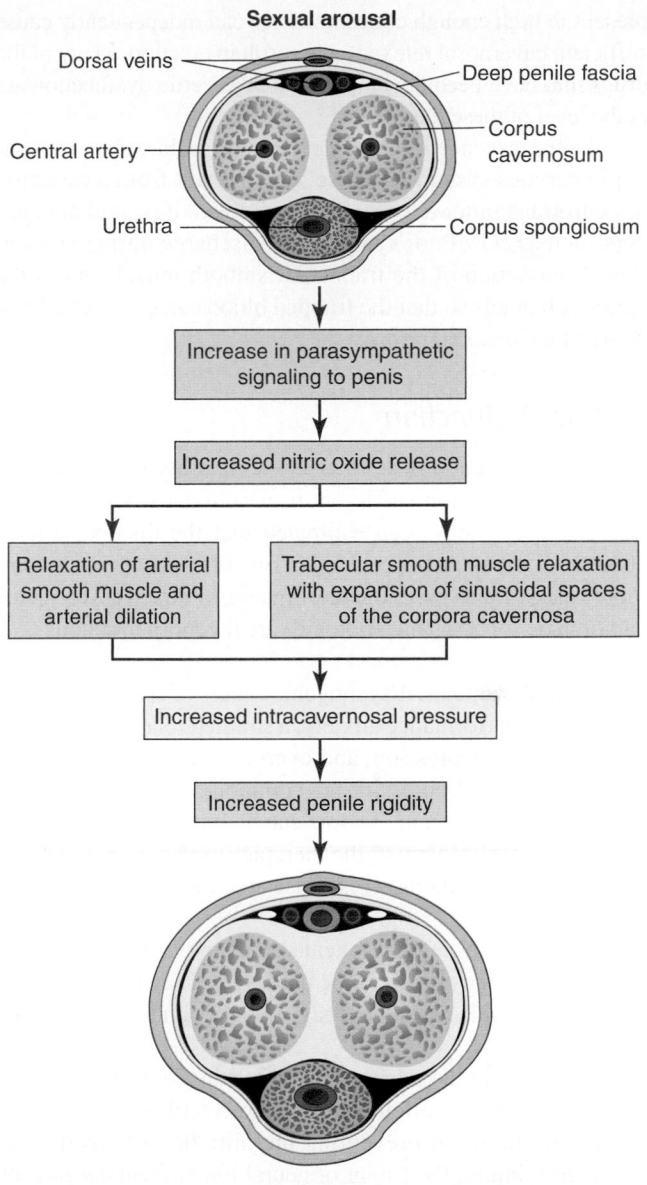

FIGURE 44-4 • Mechanisms of penile erection and sites of action of drugs, vacuum suction, and penile prosthesis used in treatment of erectile dysfunction.

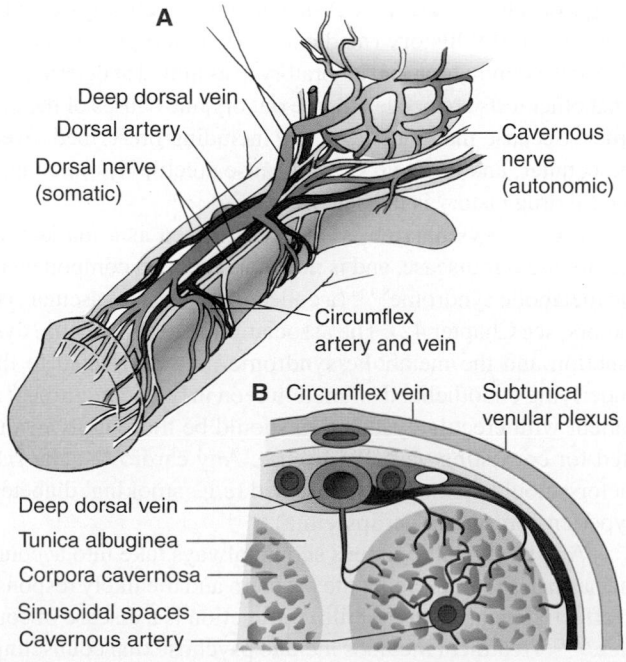

FIGURE 44-3 • Anatomy and mechanism of penile erection. **(A)** Innervation and arterial and venous blood supply to the penis. **(B)** Cross-section of the sinusoidal system of the corpora cavernosa.

surrounded by a nonelastic fibrous covering, high pressure in the sinusoids causes ballooning of the erectile tissue to such an extent that the penis becomes hard and elongated. At the same time, contraction of the somatically innervated ischiocavernous muscles forcefully compresses the blood-filled corpora cavernosa, producing a further rise in intercavernous pressures. During this phase of erection, inflow and outflow of blood cease.

Parasympathetic innervation must be intact and nitric oxide synthesis must be active for erection to occur. Nitric oxide activates guanyl cyclase, an enzyme that increases the concentration of cyclic guanosine monophosphate (cGMP), which in turn causes smooth muscle relaxation. Other smooth muscle relaxants (*e.g.*, prostaglandin E_1 analogs and α-adrenergic antagonists), if present in high enough concentrations, can independently cause sufficient cavernosal relaxation to result in erection. Many of the drugs that have been developed to treat erectile dysfunction act at the level of these mediators.[8,9]

Detumescence or penile relaxation is largely a sympathetic nervous system response. It can result from a cessation of neurotransmitter release, the breakdown of second messengers such as cGMP, or sympathetic discharge during ejaculation. Contraction of the trabecular smooth muscle opens the venous channels so that the trapped blood can be expelled and penile flaccidity can return.

Erectile Dysfunction

Erectile dysfunction is defined as the inability to achieve and maintain an erection sufficient to permit satisfactory sexual intercourse.[10] It has been estimated that the disorder affects about 150 million men worldwide.[9] Erectile dysfunction is commonly classified as psychogenic, organic, or mixed psychogenic and organic.[8,9,11] Organic etiologies are the most common.

Psychogenic Causes. Psychogenic causes of erectile dysfunction include performance anxiety, a strained relationship with a sexual partner, depression, and overt psychotic disorders such as schizophrenia. Depression is a common cause of erectile dysfunction.[8,11] Psychogenic factors can be further exacerbated by the side effects of many of the therapies used to treat these disorders, which can themselves cause erectile dysfunction.

Organic Causes. Organic causes of erectile dysfunction span a wide range of pathologic processes. They include neurogenic, hormonal, vascular, drug-induced, and penile-related etiologies.

Neurogenic disorders such as Parkinson disease, stroke, and cerebral trauma often contribute to erectile dysfunction by decreasing libido or preventing the initiation of erection. In spinal cord injury, the extent of neural impairment depends on the level, location, and extent of the lesion. Somatosensory involvement of the genitalia is essential to the reflex mechanisms involved in erection; this becomes important with aging and conditions such as diabetes that impair peripheral nerve function. Extensive pelvis surgery, especially radical prostatectomy (even so-called "nerve-sparing" procedures), are common causes of erectile dysfunction due to both direct and indirect nerve damage.

Hormonal causes of erectile dysfunction include a decrease in androgen levels because of both primary and secondary hypogonadism. Androgen levels may be decreased because of aging (andropause). Hyperprolactinemia from any cause interferes with both reproduction and erectile function. This is because prolactin acts centrally to inhibit the release of the hypothalamic gonadotropin-releasing hormone (GnRH) that controls the release of the pituitary gonadotropic hormones, luteinizing hormone (LH) and follicle-stimulating hormone (FSH). Elevated prolactin levels may also interfere with normal functioning at the level of the gonad.

Common risk factors for generalized penile arterial insufficiency include hypertension, hyperlipidemia, cigarette smoking, diabetes mellitus, and pelvic irradiation.[11] In hypertension, erectile function is impaired not so much by the increased blood pressure as by the associated stenotic arterial lesions. Focal stenosis of the common penile artery most often occurs in men who sustained blunt pelvic or perineal trauma (e.g., from bicycling accidents). Failure of the veins to close completely during an erection (veno-occlusive dysfunction) may occur in men with large venous channels that drain the corpora cavernosa. Other disorders that impair venous occlusion are degenerative changes involving the tunica albuginea, as in Peyronie disease.

Many drugs are reported to cause erectile dysfunction, including antidepressant, antipsychotic, antiandrogen, and antihypertensive medications.[8,9,11] Cigarette smoking can induce vasoconstriction and penile venous leakage because of its effects on cavernous smooth muscle and can double the risk of erectile dysfunction.[11] Alcohol in small amounts may increase libido and improve erection; however, in large amounts it can cause central sedation, decreased libido, and transient erectile dysfunction.

Aging is known to increase the risk of erectile dysfunction[12] (see Chapter 43). After 50 years of age, the overall prevalence of erectile dysfunction is reported to be greater than 50%.[13] Many of the pathologic processes that contribute to erectile dysfunction are more common in older men, including diabetes, hyperlipidemia, vascular disease, and the long-term effects of cigarette smoking. Age-related declines in testosterone may also play a role (andropause). Psychosocial problems such as depression, esteem issues, partner relationships, history of substance abuse, and anxiety and fear of performance failure also may contribute to erectile dysfunction in older men.[13]

Diagnosis and Treatment. A diagnosis of erectile dysfunction requires careful history (medical, sexual, and psychosocial), physical examination, and laboratory tests aimed at determining what other tests are needed to rule out organic causes of the disorder. Because many medications, including prescribed, over-the-counter, and illicit drugs, can cause erectile dysfunction, a careful drug history is indicated.

Erectile dysfunction is now recognized as a marker for cardiovascular disease, and is now considered a component of the metabolic syndrome[8,9,14] (a collection of cardiovascular risk factors; see Chapter 42). The association between erectile dysfunction and the metabolic syndrome may be related to the underlying endothelial dysfunction seen in both conditions.[9] A patient with erectile dysfunction should be thoroughly evaluated for coexisting vascular disease. Any cardiovascular risk factors should be modified or treated (e.g., smoking, diabetes, hypertension, and hyperlipidemia).[8,9,14]

Any treatment regimens should always take into account the partner's attitude about the problem and the likely response to effective treatment. Erectile dysfunction is a disease of couples.[8,9,11] Treatment methods include psychosexual counseling, androgen replacement therapy (when androgen deficiency is confirmed), oral and intracavernous drug therapy, vacuum constriction devices, and surgical treatment (prosthesis and vascular surgery).[8,9,11] Among the commonly prescribed drugs are sildenafil, vardenafil, tadalafil, alprostadil, papaverine, and phentolamine. Sildenafil (Viagra), vardenafil (Levitra), and tadalafil (Cialis) are selective inhibitors of phosphodiesterase type 5 (PDE-5), the enzyme that inactivates cGMP. This acts by facilitating corporeal smooth muscle relaxation in response to sexual stimulation (see Fig. 44-4). The concomitant use of PDE-5 inhibitors and nitrates (used, for example, in ischemic heart disease) is absolutely contraindicated because of the risk of profound hypotension.[14] The PDE-5 inhibitors are taken orally. Alprostadil, a prostaglandin E_1 analog, acts by producing relaxation of cavernous smooth muscle. It is either injected directly into the cavernosa (with diffusion into the opposite cavernosa) or placed in the urethra as a minisuppository. Phentolamine (an α_2-adrenergic receptor antagonist) and papaverine (smooth muscle relaxant) are also administered by intracavernous injection.

Priapism

Priapism is an involuntary, prolonged (>4 hours), abnormal and painful erection that continues beyond, or is unrelated to, sexual stimulation. Priapism is a true urologic emergency because the prolonged erection can result in ischemia and fibrosis of the erectile tissue with significant risk of subsequent impotence. Priapism can occur at any age, in the newborn as well as other age groups. Sickle cell disease or neoplasms are the most common cause in boys between 5 and 10 years of age.

Priapism is caused by impaired blood flow in the corpora cavernosa of the penis. Priapism is classified as primary (idiopathic) or secondary to a disease or drug effect. Secondary causes include hematologic conditions such as leukemia, sickle cell disease, and thrombocytopenia; neurologic conditions such as stroke, spinal cord injury, and other central nervous system lesions; and renal failure. Between 6% and 42% of males with sickle cell disease are affected at some stage by priapism.[15] The relative deoxygenation and stasis of cavernosal blood during erection is thought to increase sickling. Various medications, such as antihypertensive drugs, anticoagulant drugs, antidepressant drugs, alcohol, and marijuana, can contribute to the development of priapism. Currently, intracavernous injection therapy for erectile dysfunction is one of the more common causes of priapism.

The diagnosis of priapism usually is based on clinical findings. Color Doppler studies of penile blood flow, penile ultrasonography, and computed tomography (CT) scans may be used to determine intrapelvic pathology.

Initial treatment measures include analgesics, sedation, and hydration. Urinary retention may necessitate catheterization. Local measures include ice packs and cold saline enemas, aspiration and irrigation of the corpus cavernosum with plain or heparinized saline, or instillation of α-adrenergic drugs. If less aggressive treatment does not produce detumescence, a temporary surgical shunt may be established between the corpus cavernosum and the corpus spongiosum.

The prognosis for whether fibrosis or erectile failure will occur is determined by the severity and duration of blood stasis. Persistent stasis priapism is known to result in impaired erectile function and tissue fibrosis unless resolved within 24 to 48 hours of onset.[16]

Cancer of the Penis

Squamous cell cancer of the penis is most common in men between 45 and 60 years of age. Although relatively rare in developed countries (less than 1% of male genital tumors),[17–19] it may account for 10% to 20% of all malignant lesions in areas such as Africa and South America.[19] When it is diagnosed early, penile cancer is highly curable. The greatest hindrance to early diagnosis is a delay in seeking medical attention.

The cause of penile cancer is unknown. Several risk factors have been suggested, including increasing age, poor hygiene, smoking, human papillomavirus (HPV) infections, ultraviolet radiation exposure, and immunodeficiency states. There is an association between penile cancer and poor genital hygiene and phimosis. This type of cancer is rare in Jewish and Muslim men, who are circumcised routinely. One theory postulates that smegma accumulation under the phimotic foreskin may produce chronic inflammation, leading to carcinoma. The HPVs have been implicated in the genesis of several genital cancers, including cancer of the penis.[18] Ultraviolet radiation also is thought to have a carcinogenic effect on the penis.[18] Men who were treated for psoriasis with ultraviolet A radiation (i.e., PUVA) have had a reported increased incidence of genital squamous cell carcinomas. Because of this observation, it is suggested that men should shield their genital area when using tanning salons. Immunodeficiency states (e.g., acquired immunodeficiency syndrome) also may play a role in the pathogenesis of penile cancer.[18]

Dermatologic lesions with precancerous potential include balanitis xerotica obliterans and giant condylomata acuminata.[19] Giant condylomata acuminata are cauliflower-like lesions arising from the prepuce or glans that result from HPV infection.

Approximately 95% of penile cancers are squamous cell carcinoma.[18] It thought to progress from an in situ lesion to an invasive carcinoma. Penile lesions with histologic features of carcinoma in situ require careful follow-up because of their potential to progress to invasive carcinoma.

Invasive carcinoma of the penis begins as a small lump or ulcer. If phimosis is present, there may be painful swelling, purulent drainage, or difficulty urinating. Palpable lymph nodes may be present in the inguinal region. Diagnosis usually is based on physical examination and biopsy results. Cavernosonography, urethroscopy, CT scans, and magnetic resonance imaging (MRI) may be used in the diagnostic work-up.

Treatment options vary according to stage, size, location, and invasiveness of the tumor. Carcinoma in situ may be treated conservatively with fluorouracil cream application or laser treatment. Conservative treatment requires frequent follow-up examinations.[19] Surgery remains the mainstay of treatment for invasive carcinoma. Superficial primary lesions that are freely movable, do not invade the corpora, and show no evidence of metastatic disease can be treated with sleeve resection. Partial or total penectomy with appropriate lymph node dissection is indicated for invasive lesions.

Cumulative data reveal that men with penile cancer have an overall 5-year survival rate of 65% to 90%.[19] The most important prognostic indicator is the lymph node status. For men with tumor-positive inguinal lymph nodes, the 5-year survival rate is 30% to 50%, and with positive iliac nodes, it is 20%.[19]

IN SUMMARY, disorders of the penis can be congenital or acquired. Hypospadias and epispadias are congenital defects in which there is malpositioning of the urethral opening: it is located on the ventral surface in hypospadias and on the dorsal surface in epispadias. Phimosis is the condition in which the opening of the foreskin is too tight to permit retraction over the glans. Balanitis is an acute or chronic inflammation of the glans penis, and balanoposthitis is an inflammation of the glans and prepuce. Peyronie disease is characterized by the growth of a band of fibrous tissue on top of the penile shaft. Erectile dysfunction is defined as the inability to achieve and maintain an erection sufficient to permit satisfactory sexual intercourse. It can be caused by psychogenic factors, organic disorders, or mixed psychogenic and organic conditions. Priapism is a prolonged, painful erection that can lead to thrombosis with ischemia and necrosis of penile tissue. Cancer of the penis accounts for less than 1% of male genital cancers in developed countries. Although the tumor is slow growing and highly curable when diagnosed early, the greatest hindrance to successful treatment is a delay in seeking medical attention. ■

DISORDERS OF THE SCROTUM AND TESTES

After completing this section of the chapter, you should be able to meet the following objectives:

- State the physical manifestations and potential risks associated with uncorrected cryptorchidism.
- Compare the cause, appearance, and significance of hydrocele, hematocele, spermatocele, and varicocele.
- State the difference between extravaginal and intravaginal testicular torsion.
- Describe the symptoms of epididymitis.
- State the manifestations and possible complications of mumps orchitis.
- Relate environmental factors to development of scrotal cancer.
- State the cell types involved in seminoma, embryonal carcinoma, teratoma, and choriocarcinoma tumors of the testes.

The scrotum is a skin-covered pouch that contains the testes and their accessory organs. Defects of the scrotum and testes include cryptorchidism, disorders of the scrotal sac, vascular disorders, inflammation of the scrotum and testes, and neoplasms.

Congenital and Acquired Disorders

 Cryptorchidism

Cryptorchidism, or undescended testes, occurs when one or both of the testicles fail to move down into the scrotal sac. The condition usually is unilateral, but it may be bilateral in 25% of cases.[20] The testes develop intra-abdominally in the fetus and usually descend into the scrotum through the inguinal canal during the seventh to ninth months of gestation.[2,3] The undescended testes may remain in the lower abdomen or at a point of descent in the inguinal canal (Fig. 44-5).

The incidence of cryptorchidism is directly related to birth weight and gestational age; infants who are born prematurely or are small for gestational age have the highest incidence of the disorder. Up to one third of premature infants and 3% to 5% of full-term infants are born with undescended testicles.[21] The cause of cryptorchidism in full-term infants is poorly understood. Most cases are idiopathic, but some may result from genetic or hormonal factors.

The major manifestation of cryptorchidism is the absence of one or both testes from the scrotum. The testis either is not palpable or can be felt external to the inguinal ring. Spontaneous descent often occurs during the first 3 months of life, and by 6 months of age the incidence decreases to 0.8%.[1,21] Spontaneous descent rarely occurs after 6 months of age.[1]

In boys with cryptorchidism, histologic abnormalities of the testes reflect intrinsic defects in the testicle or adverse effects of the extrascrotal environment. The undescended testicle is normal at birth, but pathologic changes can be demonstrated at 6 to 12 months.[1] There is a delay in germ cell development, changes in the spermatic tubules, and a reduced number of Leydig cells.

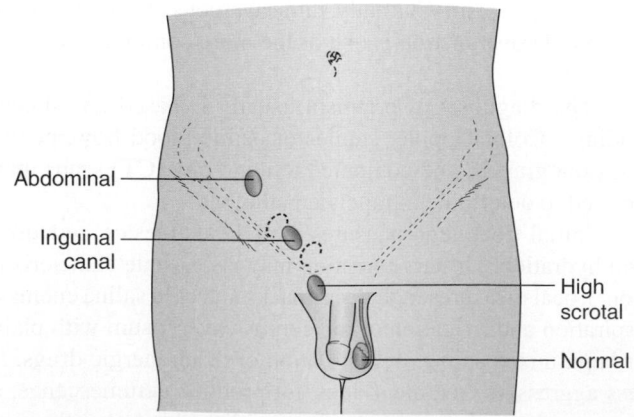

FIGURE 44-5 • Possible locations of undescended testes.

These changes are progressive over time if the testes remain undescended.

The consequences of cryptorchidism include infertility, malignancy, testicular torsion (10-fold increased risk), and the possible psychological effects of an empty scrotum. Indirect inguinal hernias usually accompany the undescended testis but rarely are symptomatic. Recognition of the condition and early treatment are important steps in preventing adverse consequences.

The risk of malignancy in the undescended testis is four to six times higher than in the general population.[1,21] The increased risk of testicular cancer is not significantly affected by orchiopexy, hormonal therapy, or late spontaneous descent after the age of 2 years. Orchiopexy, however, does allow for earlier detection of a testicular malignancy by positioning the testis in a more easily palpable location.

As a group, men with unilateral or bilateral cryptorchidism usually have decreased sperm counts, poorer-quality sperm, and lower fertility rates than men whose testicles descend normally. The likelihood of decreased fertility increases when the condition is bilateral. Unlike the risk of testicular cancer, there seems to be some advantage to early orchiopexy for protection of fertility.[1,21]

Diagnosis and Treatment. Diagnosis is based on careful examination of the genitalia in male infants. Undescended testes due to cryptorchidism should be differentiated from retractable testes that retract into the inguinal canal in response to an exaggerated cremaster muscle reflex. Retractable testes usually are palpable at birth but become nonpalpable later. They can be brought down with careful palpation in a warm room. Retractable testes usually assume a scrotal position during puberty. They have none of the complications associated with undescended testes due to cryptorchidism.[1]

Improved techniques for testicular localization include ultrasonography (*i.e.*, visualization of the testes by recording the pulses of ultrasonic waves directed into the tissues), gonadal venography and arteriography (*i.e.*, radiography of the veins and arteries of the testes after the injection of a contrast medium),

and laparoscopy (*i.e.*, examination of the interior of the abdomen using a visualization instrument). Adrenal hyperplasia in a genetic female should be considered in a phenotypically male infant with bilateral nonpalpable testes (see Chapter 41).

The treatment goals for the boys with cryptorchidism include measures to enhance future fertility potential, placement of the gonad in a favorable place for cancer detection, and improved cosmetic appearance. Regardless of the type of treatment used, it should be carried out between 6 months and 2 years of age.[1] Treatment modalities for children with unilateral or bilateral cryptorchidism include initial hormone therapy with human chorionic gonadotropin (hCG) or pulsatile GnRH, a hypothalamic hormone that stimulates production of the gonadotropic hormones (LH and FSH) by the anterior pituitary gland. For boys who do not respond to hormonal treatment, the surgical placement and fixation of the testes in the scrotum (*i.e.*, orchiopexy) has proved effective. Approximately 95% of infants who have orchiopexy for a unilateral undescended testis will be fertile, compared with a 30% to 50% fertility rate in uncorrected men.[22]

Treatment of males with undescended testes should include lifelong follow-up, considering the sequelae of testicular cancer and infertility. Parents need to be aware of the potential issues of infertility and increased risk of testicular cancer. On reaching puberty, boys should be instructed in the necessity of testicular self-examination.

Hydrocele

The testes and epididymis are completely surrounded by the tunica vaginalis, a serous pouch derived from the peritoneum during fetal descent of the testes into the scrotum. The tunica vaginalis has an outer parietal layer and a deeper visceral layer that adheres to the dense fibrous covering of the testes, the tunica albuginea. A space exists between these two layers that typically contains a few milliliters of clear fluid. A hydrocele forms when excess fluid collects between the layers of the tunica vaginalis (Fig. 44-6C). It may be unilateral or bilateral and can develop as a primary congenital defect or as a secondary

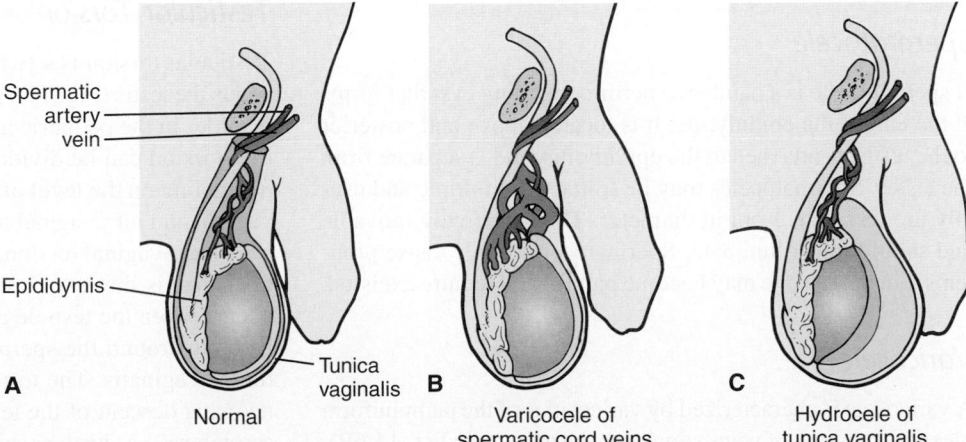

FIGURE 44-6 • **(A)** Normal testis and appendages, **(B)** varicocele, and **(C)** hydrocele.

Spermatic artery
vein

Epididymis

Tunica vaginalis   **A**   Normal

B   Varicocele of spermatic cord veins

C   Hydrocele of tunica vaginalis

condition. Acute hydrocele may develop after local injury, testicular torsion, epididymitis or orchitis, gonorrhea, lymph obstruction, or germ cell testicular tumor, or as a side effect of radiation therapy. Chronic hydrocele is more common; fluid collects about the testis and the mass grows gradually. Its cause is unknown, and it usually develops in men older than 40 years of age.

Most cases of hydrocele in male infants and children are caused by a patent processus vaginalis, which is continuous with the peritoneal cavity. There usually are reports that the mass increases in size during the day and decreases at night if the hydrocele communicates with the peritoneal cavity. In many cases they are associated with an indirect inguinal hernia.[23] Most hydroceles of infancy close spontaneously; therefore, they are not repaired before the age of 1 year. If the hydrocele persists beyond 2 years of age, surgical treatment usually is indicated.

Hydroceles are palpated as cystic masses that may attain massive proportions. If there is enough fluid, the mass may be mistaken for a solid tumor. Transillumination of the scrotum (*i.e.*, shining a light through the scrotum to visualize its internal structures) or ultrasonography can help to determine whether the mass is solid or cystic and whether the testicle is normal. A dense hydrocele that does not illuminate should be differentiated from a testicular tumor. If a hydrocele develops in a young man without apparent cause, careful evaluation is needed to exclude cancer or infection.

In an adult male, a hydrocele is a relatively benign condition. The condition often is asymptomatic, and no treatment is necessary. When symptoms do occur, the feeling may be that of heaviness in the scrotum or pain in the lower back. In cases of secondary hydrocele, the primary condition is treated. If the hydrocele is painful or cosmetically undesirable, surgical correction is indicated. Surgical repair may be done inguinally or transscrotally.

Hematocele

A hematocele is an accumulation of blood in the tunica vaginalis, which causes the scrotal skin to become dark red or purple. It may develop as a result of an abdominal surgical procedure, scrotal trauma, a bleeding disorder, or a testicular tumor.

Spermatocele

A spermatocele is a painless, sperm-containing cyst that forms at the end of the epididymis. It is located above and posterior to the testis, is attached to the epididymis, and is separate from the testes. Spermatoceles may be solitary or multiple and usually are less than 1 cm in diameter. They are freely movable and should transilluminate. Spermatoceles rarely cause problems, but a large one may become painful and require excision.

Varicocele

A varicocele is characterized by varicosities of the pampiniform plexus, a network of veins supplying the testes (see Fig. 44-6B).

The left side is more commonly affected because the left internal spermatic vein inserts into the left renal vein at a right angle, whereas the right spermatic vein usually enters the inferior vena cava. Incompetent valves are more common in the left internal spermatic veins, causing a reflux of blood back into the veins of the pampiniform plexus. The force of gravity resulting from the upright position also contributes to venous dilation. If the condition persists, there may be damage to the elastic fibers and hypertrophy of the vein walls, as occurs in formation of varicose veins in the leg. Sperm concentration and motility are decreased in men with varicocele.

Varicoceles rarely are found before puberty, and the incidence is highest in males between 15 and 35 years of age. Symptoms of varicocele include an abnormal feeling of heaviness in the left scrotum, although many varicoceles are asymptomatic. Usually, the varicocele is readily diagnosed on physical examination with the patient in the standing and recumbent positions. Typically, the varicocele disappears in the lying position because of venous decompression into the renal vein. Scrotal palpation of a varicocele has been compared to feeling a "bag of worms." Small varicoceles sometimes are difficult to identify. The Valsalva maneuver (*i.e.*, forced expiration against a closed glottis) may be used to accentuate small varicosities. If the varicocele is present, retrograde blood flow to the scrotum can be detected by color Doppler ultrasonography. Other diagnostic aids include radioisotope scanning and spermatic venography.

Treatment options include surgical ligation or sclerosis using a percutaneous transvenous catheter under fluoroscopic guidance. Both can be performed as outpatient procedures. The benefits of the percutaneous technique include a slightly lower recurrence rate and more rapid return to full physical activity. It has been suggested that men with abnormalities in their semen and a varicocele show some degree of improvement in fertility after obliteration of the dilated veins.[24] However, the effectiveness of varicocele treatment in men from subfertile couples is still debated, especially when other assisted reproductive techniques (*e.g.*, intracytoplasmic sperm injection [ICSI]) may be effective with as few as 20 sperm[24] (see Chapter 46). Aside from improving fertility, other reasons for surgery include the relief of the sensation of "heaviness" and cosmetic improvement.

Testicular Torsion

Testicular torsion is a twisting of the spermatic cord that suspends the testis (Fig. 44-7). It is the most common acute scrotal disorder in the pediatric and young adult population.[25] Testicular torsion can be divided into two distinct clinical entities, depending on the level of spermatic cord involvement: extravaginal and intravaginal torsion.[22,26]

Extravaginal torsion, which occurs almost exclusively in neonates, is the less common form of testicular torsion.[22] It occurs when the testicle and the fascial tunicae that surround it rotate around the spermatic cord at a level well above the tunica vaginalis. The torsion probably occurs during fetal or neonatal descent of the testes before the tunica adheres to the scrotal wall. At birth or shortly thereafter, a firm, smooth, pain-

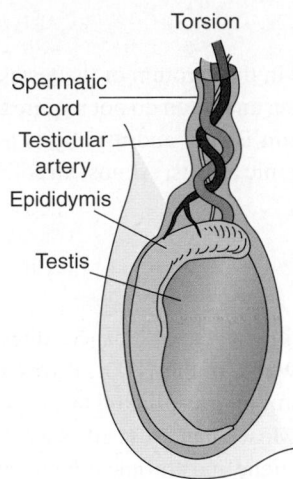

FIGURE 44-7 • Testicular torsion with twisting of the spermatic cord that suspends the testis and the spermatic vessels that supply the testis with blood.

less scrotal mass is identified. The scrotal skin appears red, and some edema is present. Differential diagnosis is relatively easy because testicular tumors, epididymitis, and orchitis are exceedingly rare in neonates; a hydrocele is softer and can be transilluminated, and physical examination can exclude the presence of hernia. The use of surgical treatment (orchiopexy and orchiectomy) is controversial. There are multiple animal studies indicating that failure to remove the torsed testis may produce an autoimmune response that affects the normal testis.[22,26]

Intravaginal torsion is considerably more common than extravaginal torsion. It occurs when the testis rotates on its long axis in the tunica vaginalis. In most cases, congenital abnormalities of the tunica vaginalis or spermatic cord exist. The tunica vaginalis normally surrounds the testis and epididymis, allowing the testicle to rotate freely in the tunica. Although anomalies of suspension vary, the epididymal attachment may be loose enough to permit torsion between the testis and the epididymis. More commonly, the testis rotates about the distal spermatic cord. Because this abnormality is developmental, bilateral anomalies are common.

Intravaginal torsion occurs most frequently between the ages of 8 and 18 years and rarely is seen after 30 years of age. Patients usually present in severe distress within hours of onset and often have nausea, vomiting, and tachycardia. The affected testis is large and tender, with pain radiating to the inguinal area. Extensive cremaster muscle contraction causes a thickening of the spermatic cord.

Testicular torsion must be differentiated from epididymitis, orchitis, and trauma to the testis. On physical examination, the testicle often is high in the scrotum and in an abnormal orientation. These changes are caused by the twisting and shortening of the spermatic cord. The degree of scrotal swelling and redness depends on the duration of symptoms. The testes are firm and tender. The cremasteric reflex, normally elicited by stroking the medial aspect of the thigh and observing testicular retraction, frequently is absent.[26] Color Doppler ultra-

sonography is increasingly used in the evaluation of suspected testicular torsion.[26]

Intravaginal testicular torsion is a true surgical emergency, and early recognition and treatment are necessary if the testicle is to be saved. Detorsion within 6 hours usually results in 100% viability of the testicle; this decreases to 20% at 12 hours, and 0% at 24 hours.[22] Treatment includes surgical detorsion and orchiectomy.[27] Orchiectomy is carried out when the testis is deemed nonviable after surgical detorsion. Testicular salvage rates are directly related to the duration of torsion.[27] Because the opposite testicle usually is affected by the same abnormal attachments, prophylactic fixation of that testis often is performed.

Infection and Inflammation

Epididymitis

Epididymitis is an inflammation of the epididymis, the elongated cordlike structure that lies along the posterior border of the testis, whose function is the storage, transport, and maturation of spermatozoa. There are two major types of epididymitis: sexually transmitted infections associated with urethritis and primary nonsexually transmitted infections associated with urinary tract infections and prostatitis. Most cases of epididymitis are caused by bacterial pathogens.

In primary nonsexual infections, the pressure associated with voiding or physical strain may force pathogen-containing urine from the urethra or prostate up the ejaculatory duct and through the vas deferens and into the epididymis. Infections also may reach the epididymis through the lymphatics of the spermatic cord. In rare cases, organisms from other foci of infection reach the epididymis through the bloodstream. In prepubertal children, the disorder usually is associated with congenital urinary tract abnormalities and infection with gram-negative rods. In postpubertal males, several factors may predispose to development of epididymitis, including sexual activity, heavy physical exertion, and bicycle or motorcycle riding. Sexually transmitted acute epididymitis occurs mainly in young men without underlying genitourinary disease and is most commonly caused by *Chlamydia trachomatis* and *Neisseria gonorrhoeae* (singly or in combination). In men older than 35 years of age, epididymitis often is associated with pathogens such as *Escherichia coli, Pseudomonas,* and gram-positive cocci.

Epididymitis is characterized by unilateral pain and swelling, accompanied by erythema and edema of the overlying scrotal skin that develops over a period of 24 to 48 hours. Initially, the swelling and induration are limited to the epididymis. However, the distinction between the testis and epididymis becomes less evident as the inflammation progresses, and the testis and epididymis become one mass. In contrast to patients with testicular torsion, patients with epididymitis usually have a normal cremasteric reflex. There may be tenderness over the groin (spermatic cord) or in the lower abdomen. Fever and complaints of dysuria occur in approximately one half of cases. Whether urethral discharge is present depends on the organism causing the infection; it usually accompanies gonorrheal infections, is common in chlamydial infections, and is less common in infections caused by gram-negative organisms.

Laboratory findings usually reveal an elevated white blood cell count. Urinalysis and urine culture are important in the diagnosis of epididymitis, with bacteriuria and pyuria suggestive of the disorder; however, the urinalysis may be normal. The cause of epididymitis can be differentiated by Gram stain examination or culture of a midstream urine specimen or a urethral specimen. If the diagnosis remains uncertain, color Doppler ultrasonography may be useful, revealing increased blood flow to the affected testis.

Treatment during the acute phase (which usually lasts for 3 to 4 days) includes bed rest, scrotal elevation and support, and antibiotics.[26] Bed rest with scrotal support improves lymphatic drainage. The choice of antibiotics is determined by age, physical findings, urinalysis, Gram stain results, cultures, and sexual history.[28] Oral analgesics and antipyretics usually are indicated. Sexual activity or physical strain may exacerbate the infection and worsen the symptoms, and should be avoided. If a sexually transmitted disease is suspected as an etiology, it is important to ensure that the sexual partner gets treatment[28] (see Chapter 47).

Orchitis

Orchitis is an infection of the testes. It can be precipitated by a primary infection in the genitourinary tract, or the infection can be spread to the testes through the bloodstream or the lymphatics. Epididymitis with subsequent infection of the testis is commonly related to genitourinary tract infections (cystitis, urethritis, genitoprostatitis) that travel to the epididymis and testis through the vas deferens or the lymphatics of the spermatic cord.

Orchitis can develop as a complication of a systemic infection, such as parotitis (*i.e.,* mumps), scarlet fever, or pneumonia. Probably the best known of these complications is orchitis caused by the mumps virus.[29] Mumps orchitis is the most common complication of mumps infection in the postpubertal male, occurring in approximately 20% to 35% of adolescent boys and young men with mumps. The onset of mumps orchitis is sudden; it usually occurs approximately 3 to 4 days after the onset of the parotitis and is characterized by fever, painful enlargement of the testes, and small hemorrhages into the tunica albuginea. Unlike epididymitis, the urinary symptoms are absent. The symptoms usually run their course in 7 to 10 days. Microscopically, an acute inflammatory response is seen in the seminiferous tubules, with proliferation of neutrophils, lymphocytes, and histiocytes causing distention of the tubules. The residual effects seen after the acute phase include hyalinization of the seminiferous tubules and atrophy of the testes (seen in half of affected men). Spermatogenesis is irreversibly impaired in approximately 30% of testes damaged by mumps orchitis. If both testes are involved (which occurs in fewer than 15% of cases), permanent sterility can result, but is rare. Androgenic hormone function is usually maintained in these cases.[29]

Neoplasms

Tumors can develop in the scrotum or the testes. Benign scrotal tumors are common and often do not require treatment. Carcinoma of the scrotum is rare and usually is associated with exposure to carcinogenic agents. Almost all solid tumors of the testes are malignant.

Scrotal Cancer

Cancer of the scrotum was the first cancer directly linked to a specific occupation when, in the 1800s, it was associated with chimney sweeps.[30] Studies have linked this cancer to exposure to tar, soot, and oils. Most squamous cell cancers of the scrotum are linked to poor hygiene and chronic inflammation. Exposure to PUVA or HPV also has been associated with the disease. The mean age of presentation with the disease is 60 years, often preceded by 20 to 30 years of chronic irritation.

In the early stages, cancer of the scrotum may appear as a small tumor or wartlike growth that eventually ulcerates. The thin scrotal wall lacks the tissue reactivity needed to block the malignant process; more than one half of the cases seen involve metastasis to the lymph nodes. Because this tumor does not respond well to chemotherapy or irradiation, the treatment includes wide local excision of the tumor with inguinal and femoral node dissection.[31] Prognosis correlates with lymph node involvement.

Testicular Cancer

Testicular cancer accounts for 1% of all male cancers and 3% of male urogenital cancers. Although relatively rare, it is the most common cause of cancer in the 15- to 35-year-old age group.[32,33] In the past, testicular cancer was a leading cause of death among men entering their most productive years. However, since the late 1970s, advances in therapy have transformed an almost invariably fatal disease into one that is highly curable. With the exception of men with advanced metastatic disease at the time of presentation or those who relapse after primary chemotherapy, most men with these tumors are cured with available therapy (>90% of all newly diagnosed patients will be cured). The prognosis and extent of treatment required for testicular cancer are related to the stage of the disease at the time of presentation.

Although the cause of testicular cancer is unknown, several predisposing influences may be important: cryptorchidism, genetic factors, and disorders of testicular development.[20] The strongest association has been with cryptorchid testis. Approximately 10% of testicular tumors are associated with cryptorchidism. The higher the location of the undescended testis, the greater the risk.[22] About 25% of these tumors occur in the contralateral, normally descended testicle, hence the need for regular follow-up of these individuals. Genetic predisposition also appears to be important. Family clustering of the disorder has been described, although a well-defined pattern of inheritance has not been established. An increased incidence of testicular germ cell tumors, particularly seminomas, has been described in human immunodeficiency virus–infected men. Men with disorders of testicular development, including those with Klinefelter syndrome and testicular feminization, have a higher risk of germ cell tumors.

Approximately 95% of malignant tumors arising in the testis are germ cell tumors.[22,33] Germ cell tumors can be classified as seminomas and nonseminomas based on their origin in primordial germ cells and their ability to differentiate in vivo. Because these tumors derive from germ cells in the testis, they are multipotential (able to differentiate into different tissue types) and often secrete polypeptide hormones or enzymes representing earlier stages of development.

Seminomas account for approximately 50% of germ cell tumors and are most frequent in the fourth decade of life.[33] They almost never occur in infants or small children.[22] Seminomas are thought to arise from the seminiferous epithelium of the testes and are the type of germ cell tumor most likely to produce a uniform population of cells.

The nonseminoma tumors include embryonal carcinoma, teratoma, choriocarcinoma, and yolk cell carcinoma derivatives. Nonseminoma tumors usually contain more than one cell type and are less differentiated than seminomas. Embryonal carcinomas are the least differentiated of the tumors, with the totipotential capacity to differentiate into other nonseminomatous cell types. They occur most commonly in the 20- to 30-year-old age group. Choriocarcinoma is a rare and highly malignant form of testicular cancer that is identical to tumors that arise in placental tissue. Yolk sac tumors mimic the embryonic yolk sac histologically. They are the most common type of testicular tumors in infants and children up to 3 years of age, and in this age group have a very good prognosis.[22] Teratomas are composed of somatic cell types from two or more germ-line layers (ectoderm, mesoderm, or endoderm). They constitute less than 2% to 3% of germ cell tumors and can occur at any age from infancy to old age. They usually behave as benign tumors in children; in adults, they often contain minute foci of cancer cells.

Often the first sign of testicular cancer is a slight enlargement of the testicle that may be accompanied by some degree of discomfort. This may be an ache in the abdomen or groin or a sensation of dragging or heaviness in the scrotum. Frank pain may be experienced in the later stages, when the tumor is growing rapidly and hemorrhaging occurs. Testicular cancer can spread when the tumor may be barely palpable. The presenting manifestations of testicular cancer can be attributed to metastasis in approximately 10% of cases. Signs of metastatic spread include swelling of the lower extremities, back pain, neck mass, cough, hemoptysis, or dizziness. Gynecomastia (breast enlargement) may result from hCG-producing tumors and occurs in about 5% of men with germ cell tumors. Regular self-examinations of the testes have not been studied enough to show that the practice lowers the death rate from this cancer. However, some health care professionals may think otherwise, and may advise their patients to do monthly self-examinations.[34]

The diagnosis of testicular cancer requires a thorough urologic history and physical examination. A painless testicular mass may be cancer. Conditions that produce an intrascrotal mass similar to testicular cancer include epididymitis, orchitis, hydrocele, or hematocele. The examination for masses should include palpation of the testes and surrounding structures, transillumination of the scrotum, and abdominal palpation. Testicular ultrasonography can be used to differentiate testicular masses. CT scans and MRI are used in assessing metastatic spread.

Tumor markers, assayed by immunoassay methods that measure protein antigens produced by malignant cells, provide information about the existence of a tumor and the type of tumor present. These markers may detect tumors that are too small to be found on physical examination or radiographs. Three tumor markers are useful in evaluating the tumor response to therapy: α-fetoprotein, a glycoprotein that normally is present in fetal serum in large amounts; hCG, a hormone that normally is produced by the placenta in pregnant women; and lactate dehydrogenase (LDH), a cellular enzyme normally found in muscle and the liver, kidneys, and brain. During embryonic development, the totipotential germ cells of the testes travel down normal differentiation pathways and produce different protein products. The reappearance of these protein markers in the adult suggests activity of undifferentiated cells in a testicular germ cell tumor.

The clinical staging (TNM classification) for testicular cancer is as follows: stage I, tumor confined to testes, epididymis, or spermatic cord; stage II, tumor spread to retroperitoneal lymph nodes below the diaphragm; and stage III, metastases outside the retroperitoneal nodes or above the diaphragm (see Chapter 8). Staging procedures include CT scans of the chest, abdomen, and pelvis; ultrasonography for detection of bulky inferior nodal metastases; and occasionally lymphangiography.

The basic treatment of all testicular cancers includes orchiectomy, which is done at the time of diagnostic exploration. The widely used surgical procedure is the unilateral radical orchiectomy through an inguinal incision. Surgical therapy is advantageous because it enables precise staging of the disease. Recommendations for further therapy (e.g., retroperitoneal lymph node dissection, chemotherapy, radiation therapy) are based on the pathologic findings from the surgical procedure.

Treatment after orchiectomy depends on the histologic characteristics of the tumor and the clinical stage of the disease. Seminomas are highly radiosensitive; the treatment of stage I or II seminoma is irradiation of the retroperitoneal and homolateral lymph nodes to the level of the diaphragm. Patients with bulky retroperitoneal or distant metastases often are treated with multi-agent chemotherapy. Seminoma is probably the most curable of all solid tumors. Men with nonseminomatous tumors usually are managed with observation, chemotherapy, or retroperitoneal lymph node dissection. Rigorous follow-up in all men with testicular cancer is necessary to detect recurrences, most of which occur within the 2 years of the end of treatment.[32,33] Testicular cancer is a disease in which even recurrence is highly treatable.

With appropriate treatment, the prognosis for men with testicular cancer is excellent. The 5-year survival rate for patients with stage I and II disease exceeds 95%.[32,33] Even patients with more advanced disease have excellent chances for long-term survival. Patients subsequently cured of testicular cancer are also at increased risk for the development of other cancers later in life.[32]

Therapy for testicular cancer can have potentially adverse effects on sexual functioning. Men who have retroperitoneal lymph node dissection may experience retrograde ejaculation or failure to ejaculate because of severing of the sympathetic plexus. Infertility may result from retrograde ejaculation, retroperitoneal lymph node dissection, or the toxic effects of chemotherapy or radiation therapy on the germ cells in the remaining testis.[32,33] Sperm banking should be considered for men undergoing these treatments.

> **IN SUMMARY,** disorders of the scrotum and testes include cryptorchidism (*i.e.,* undescended testes), hydrocele, hematocele, spermatocele, varicocele, and testicular torsion. Inflammatory conditions can involve the scrotal sac, epididymis, or testes. Tumors can arise in the scrotum or the testes. Scrotal cancers usually are associated with exposure to petroleum products such as tar, pitch, and soot. Testicular cancers account for 1% of all male cancers and 3% of cancers of the male genitourinary system. With current treatment methods, a large percentage of men with these tumors can be cured. ■

DISORDERS OF THE PROSTATE

After completing this section of the chapter, you should be able to meet the following objectives:

- Compare the pathology and symptoms of acute bacterial prostatitis, chronic bacterial prostatitis, and chronic prostatitis/pelvic pain syndrome.
- Describe the urologic manifestations and treatment of benign prostatic hyperplasia.
- List the methods used in the diagnosis and treatment of prostate cancer.

The prostate is a firm, glandular structure that surrounds the urethra. It produces a thin, milky, alkaline secretion that aids sperm motility by helping to maintain an optimum pH. The contraction of the smooth muscle in the gland promotes semen expulsion during ejaculation.

Infection and Inflammation

Prostatitis refers to a variety of inflammatory disorders of the prostate gland, some bacterial and some not. It may occur spontaneously, as a result of catheterization or instrumentation, or secondary to other diseases of the male genitourinary system. As an outcome of 1995 and 1998 consensus conferences, the National Institutes of Health has established a classification system with four categories of prostatitis syndromes: acute bacterial prostatitis, chronic bacterial prostatitis, chronic prostatitis/pelvic pain syndrome, and asymptomatic inflammatory prostatitis.[35] Men with asymptomatic inflammatory prostatitis have no subjective symptoms, and are detected incidentally on biopsy or examination of prostatic fluid. One U.S. community-based study (58,955 office-based physician visits by men older than 18 years of age) estimated that 9% of men have a diagnosis of chronic prostatitis at any one time.[36]

Acute Bacterial Prostatitis

Acute bacterial prostatitis often is considered a subtype of urinary tract infection. The most likely etiology of acute bacterial prostatitis is an ascending urethral infection or reflux of infected urine into the prostatic ducts. The most common organism is *E. coli*.[37,38] Other gram-negative bacteria (*Proteus, Klebsiella, Pseudomonas,* and *Serratia* species) and enterococci are less frequent pathogens. Anaerobic and gram-positive bacteria are rarely a cause of acute prostatitis. The manifestations of acute bacterial prostatitis include fever and chills, malaise, myalgia, arthralgia, frequent and urgent urination, dysuria, and urethral discharge.[37] Dull, aching pain often is present in the perineum, rectum, or sacrococcygeal region. The urine may be cloudy and malodorous because of urinary tract infection. Rectal examination reveals a swollen, tender, warm prostate with scattered soft areas. Prostatic massage produces a thick discharge with white blood cells that grows large numbers of pathogens on culture.

Treatment of acute bacterial prostatitis depends on the severity of symptoms. It usually includes antibiotics, bed rest, adequate hydration, antipyretics, analgesics (preferably nonsteroidal anti-inflammatory drugs) to alleviate pain, and stool softeners. Men who are extremely ill, such as those with sepsis, may require hospitalization. A suprapubic catheter may be indicated if voiding is difficult or painful.

Acute prostatitis usually responds to appropriate antimicrobial therapy chosen in accordance with the sensitivity of the causative agents in the urethral discharge. Depending on the urine culture results, antibiotic therapy usually is continued for at least 4 weeks. Because acute prostatitis often is associated with anatomic abnormalities, a thorough urologic examination usually is performed after treatment is completed.

A persistent fever indicates the need for further investigation for an additional site of infection or a prostatic abscess. CT scans and transrectal ultrasonography of the prostate are useful in the diagnosis of prostatic abscesses. Prostatic abscesses, which are relatively uncommon since the advent of effective antibiotic therapy, are found more commonly in men with diabetes mellitus.

Chronic Bacterial Prostatitis

In contrast to acute bacterial prostatitis, chronic bacterial prostatitis is a subtle disorder that is difficult to treat. Men with the disorder typically have recurrent urinary tract infections with persistence of the same strain of pathogenic bacteria in prostatic fluid and urine. Organisms responsible for chronic bacterial prostatitis usually are the gram-negative enterobacteria (*E. coli, Proteus,* or *Klebsiella*) or *Pseudomonas.*[37] Infected prostatic calculi may develop and contribute to the chronic infection.

The symptoms of chronic prostatitis are variable and include frequent and urgent urination, dysuria, perineal discomfort, and low back pain. Occasionally, myalgia and arthralgia accompany the other symptoms. Secondary epididymitis sometimes is associated with the disorder. Many men experience relapsing lower or upper urinary tract infections because of recurrent invasion of the bladder by the prostatic bacteria. Bacteria may exist in the prostate gland even when the prostatic fluid is sterile. The most accurate method of establishing a diagnosis is by localizing cultures. This method is based on sequential collections of the first part of the voided urine (urethral specimen), midstream specimen (bladder specimen), the expressed prostatic secretion (obtained by prostatic massage), and the urine voided after prostatic massage. The last two specimens are considered prostatic urine. A positive expressed prostatic specimen establishes the diagnosis of bacterial prostatitis, excluding nonbacterial prostatitis.

Even after an accurate diagnosis has been established, treatment of chronic prostatitis often is difficult and frustrating.[36] Unlike their action in the acutely inflamed prostate, antibacterial drugs penetrate poorly into the chronically inflamed prostate. Long-term therapy (3 to 4 months) with an appropriate low-dose oral antimicrobial agent often is used to treat the infection. Adding α_1-adrenergic blocking drugs (*e.g.,* prazosin, doxazosin) to antibacterial drugs may significantly improve symptoms and reduce recurrence.[35] Transurethral prostatectomy (TURP) has been used to treat men with refractory disease; however, the success rate has been variable and this approach is not generally recommended.[37]

Chronic Prostatitis/Chronic Pelvic Pain Syndrome

Chronic prostatitis/pelvic pain syndrome is both the most common and least understood of the prostatitis syndromes.[39] The category is divided into two types, inflammatory and noninflammatory, based on the presence of leukocytes in the prostatic fluid. The inflammatory type was previously referred to as *nonbacterial prostatitis,* and the noninflammatory type as *prostatodynia.*

Inflammatory Prostatitis. A large group of men with prostatitis have pains along the penis, testicles, and scrotum; painful ejaculation; low back pain; rectal pain along the inner thighs; urinary symptoms; decreased libido; and impotence, but they have no bacteria in the urinary system. Men with nonbacterial prostatitis often have inflammation of the prostate with an elevated leukocyte count and abnormal inflammatory cells in their prostatic secretions. The cause of the disorder is unknown, and efforts to prove the presence of unusual pathogens (*e.g.,* mycoplasmas, *Chlamydia,* trichomonads, viruses) have been largely unsuccessful. It also is thought that nonbacterial prostatitis may be an autoimmune disorder.

Noninflammatory Prostatitis. Men with noninflammatory prostatitis or prostatodynia have symptoms resembling those of nonbacterial prostatitis but have negative urine culture results and no evidence of prostatic inflammation (*i.e.,* normal leukocyte count). The cause of noninflammatory prostatitis is unknown, but because of the absence of inflammation, the search for the cause of symptoms has been directed toward extraprostatic sources. In some cases, there is an apparent functional obstruction of the bladder neck near the external urethral sphincter; during voiding, this results in higher-than-normal pressures in the prostatic urethra that cause intraprostatic urine reflux and chemical irritation of the prostate by urine. In other cases, there is an apparent myalgia (*i.e.,* muscle pain) associated with prolonged tension of the pelvic floor muscles. Emotional stress also may play a role.

Treatment. Treatment methods for chronic prostatitis/pelvic pain syndrome are highly variable and require further study. Antibiotic therapy is used when an occult infection is suspected. Treatment often is directed toward symptom control. Sitz baths and nonsteroidal anti-inflammatory drugs may provide some symptom relief. In men with irritative urination symptoms, anticholinergic agents (*e.g.,* oxybutynin) or α-adrenergic blocking agents may be beneficial. Reassurance can be helpful. It is important that these men know that the condition is neither infectious or contagious, nor is it known to cause cancer.[36,39]

Hyperplasia and Neoplasms

Benign Prostatic Hyperplasia

Benign prostatic hyperplasia (BPH) is an age-related, nonmalignant enlargement of the prostate gland (Fig. 44-8). It is characterized by the formation of large, discrete lesions in the periurethral region of the prostate rather than the peripheral zones, which commonly are affected by prostate cancer (Fig. 44-9). BPH is one of the most common diseases of aging men. It has been reported that more than 50% of men older than 60 years of age have BPH.[40] Between 15% and 30% of these men will develop lower urinary tract symptoms.

The exact cause of the BPH is unknown. Potential risk factors include age, family history, race, ethnicity, dietary fat and meat consumption, and hormonal factors. The incidence of BPH increases with advanced age and is highest in African Americans and lowest in native Japanese. Men with a family history of BPH are reported to have had larger prostates than those of control subjects, and higher rates of BPH were found in monozygotic twins than in dizygotic twins.

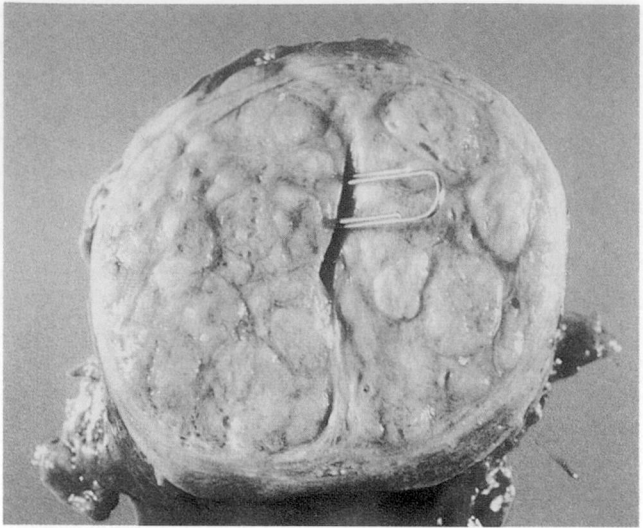

FIGURE 44-8 • Nodular hyperplasia of the prostate. Cut surface of a prostate enlarged by nodular hyperplasia shows numerous, well-circumscribed nodules of prostatic tissue. The prostatic urethra (paper clip) has been compressed to a narrow slit. (From Damjanov I. [2008]. The lower urinary tract and male reproductive system. In Rubin R., Strayer D. S. [Eds.], *Rubin's pathology: Clinicopathologic foundations of medicine* [5th ed., p. 774]. Philadelphia: Lippincott Williams & Wilkins.)

HYPERPLASIA AND CANCER OF THE PROSTATE

- The prostate gland surrounds the urethra and peri-urethral enlargement causes manifestations of urinary obstruction.

- Benign prostatic hyperplasia is an age-related enlargement of the prostate gland with formation of large, discrete lesions in the periurethral region of the prostate. These lesions compress the urethra and produce symptoms of dysuria or difficulty urinating.

- Prostate cancer begins in the peripheral zones of the prostate gland and usually is asymptomatic until the disease is far advanced and the tumor has eroded the outer prostatic capsule and spread to adjacent pelvic tissues or metastasized.

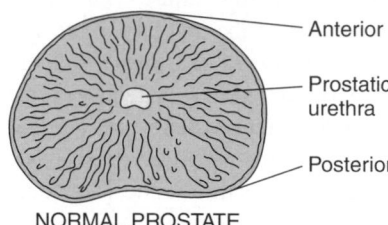

NORMAL PROSTATE

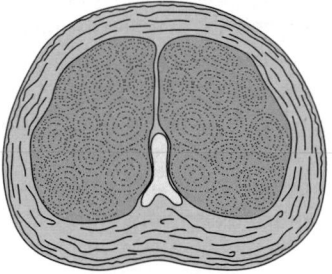

NODULAR PROSTATIC HYPERPLASIA

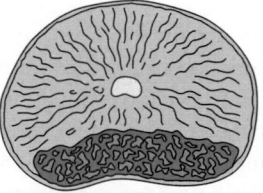

CARCINOMA OF PROSTATE

FIGURE 44-9 • Normal prostate, nodular benign prostatic hypertrophy, and cancer of the prostate. (From Damjanov I. [2008]. The lower urinary tract and male reproductive system. In Rubin R., Strayer D. S. [Eds.], *Rubin's pathology: Clinicopathologic foundations of medicine* [5th ed., p. 774]. Philadelphia: Lippincott Williams & Wilkins. Artist: Dmitri Karetnikov.)

Both androgens (testosterone and dihydrotestosterone) and estrogens appear to contribute to the development of BPH. The prostate consists of a network of glandular elements embedded in smooth muscle and supporting tissue, with testosterone being the most important factor for prostatic growth. Dihydrotestosterone (DHT), the biologically active metabolite of testosterone, is thought to be the ultimate mediator of prostatic hyperplasia, with estrogen serving to sensitize the prostatic tissue to the growth-producing effects of DHT. Free plasma testosterone enters prostatic cells, where at least 90% is converted into DHT by the action of 5α-reductase. The discovery that DHT is the active factor in BPH is the rationale for the use of 5α-reductase inhibitors (*e.g.*, finasteride, dutasteride) in the treatment of the disorder. Although the exact source of the estrogen is uncertain, small amounts of estrogen are produced in the male. It has been postulated that a relative increase in estrogen levels that occurs with aging may facilitate the action of androgens in the prostate despite a decline in testicular output of testosterone. Other hormonal factors that have been implicated include increased intraprostate levels of insulin-like growth factor-1 (IGF-1).[40]

The anatomic location of the prostate at the bladder neck contributes to the pathophysiology and symptomatology of BPH. There are two prostatic components to the obstructive properties of BPH and development of lower urinary tract symptoms: dynamic and static.[40] The static component of BPH is related to an increase in prostatic size and gives rise to symptoms such as a weak urinary stream, postvoid dribbling, frequency of urination, and nocturia. The dynamic component of BPH is related to prostatic smooth muscle tone. The α_1-adrenergic receptors are the main receptors for the smooth muscle component of the prostate. The recognition of the role of α_1-adrenergic receptors on neuromuscular function in the prostate is the basis for use of α_1-adrenergic receptor blockers in treating BPH. A third component, detrusor instability and impaired bladder contractility, may contribute to the symptoms of BPH independent of the outlet obstruction created by an enlarged prostate[40] (see Chapter 35). It has been suggested that some of the symptoms of BPH might be related to a decompensating or aging bladder rather than being primarily related to outflow obstruction. An example is the involuntary contraction that results in urgency and an attempt to void that occurs because of small bladder volume.[40]

The clinical significance of BPH resides in its tendency to compress the urethra and cause partial or complete obstruction of urinary outflow. As the obstruction increases, acute retention may occur with overdistention of the bladder. The residual urine in the bladder causes increased frequency of urination and a constant desire to empty the bladder, which becomes worse at night. With marked bladder distention, overflow incontinence may occur with the slightest increase in intra-abdominal pressure. The resulting obstruction to urinary flow can give rise to urinary tract infection, destructive changes of the bladder wall, hydroureter, and hydronephrosis. Hypertrophy and changes in bladder wall structure develop in stages. Initially, the hypertrophied fibers form trabeculations and then herniations, or sacculations; finally, diverticula develop as the herniations extend through the bladder wall (see Chapter 35, Fig. 35-4). Because urine seldom is completely emptied from them, these diverticula are readily infected. Back-pressure on the ureters and collecting system of the kidneys promotes hydroureter, hydronephrosis, and danger of eventual renal failure.

Diagnosis. It is now thought that the single most important factor in the evaluation and treatment of BPH is the man's own experiences related to the disorder. The American Urological Association Symptom Index consists of seven questions about symptoms regarding incomplete emptying, frequency, intermittency, urgency, weak stream, straining, and nocturia.[41] Each question is rated with a score of 0 (mild) to 7 (severe). A maximum score of 35 indicates severe symptoms. Total scores below 7 are considered mild; those between 8 and 20, moderate; and scores over 20, severe. A final question relates to quality of life due to urinary problems.

In 1994, the Agency for Health Care Policy and Research published clinical practice guidelines for management of BPH.[42] These guidelines suggest that the initial evaluation of men for a diagnosis of BPH includes history, physical examination, digital rectal examination, urinalysis, blood tests for serum creatinine and prostate-specific antigen (PSA), and urine flow rate. Blood and urine analyses are used as adjuncts to determine BPH complications. Urinalysis is done to detect bacteria, white blood cells, or microscopic hematuria in the presence of infection and inflammation. The serum creatinine test is used as an estimate of the glomerular filtration rate and renal function. The PSA test is used to screen for prostate cancer. These evaluation measures, along with the symptom index, are used to describe the extent of obstruction, determine if other diagnostic tests are needed, and establish the need for treatment.

The digital rectal examination is used to examine the external surface of the prostate. Enlargement of the prostate due to BPH usually produces a large, palpable prostate with a smooth, rubbery surface. Hardened areas of the prostate gland suggest cancer and should be sampled for biopsy. An enlarged prostate found during a digital rectal examination does not always correlate with the degree of urinary obstruction. Some men can have greatly enlarged prostate glands with no urinary obstruction, but others may have severe symptoms without a palpable enlargement of the prostate.

Residual urine measurement may be made by ultrasonography or postvoiding catheterization for residual urine volume. Residual urines greater than 100 mL are considered high. Uroflowmetry provides an objective measure of urine flow rate. The patient is asked to void with a relatively full bladder (at least 150 mL) into a device that electronically measures the force of the stream and urine flow rate. A urinary flow rate of greater than 15 mL/second is considered normal, and less than 10 mL/second is indicative of obstruction.

Transabdominal or transrectal diagnostic ultrasonography can be used to evaluate the kidneys, ureters, and bladder. Urethrocystoscopy is indicated in men with a history of hematuria, stricture disease, urethral injury, or prior lower urinary tract surgery. It is used to evaluate the length and diameter of the urethra, the size and configuration of the prostate, and bladder capacity. It also detects the presence of trabeculations, bladder stones, and small bladder cancers. CT scans, MRI studies, and radionuclide scans are reserved for rare instances of tumor detection.

Treatment. Treatment of BPH is determined by the degree of symptoms that the condition produces and complications due to obstruction. When a man develops mild symptoms related to BPH, a "watchful waiting" stance often is taken. The condition does not always run a predictable course; it may remain stable or even improve.

Until the 1980s, surgery was the mainstay of treatment to alleviate urinary obstruction due to BPH. Currently, there is an emphasis on less invasive methods of treatment, including use of pharmacologic agents. However, when more severe signs of obstruction develop, surgical treatment is indicated to provide comfort and avoid serious kidney damage.

Pharmacologic management includes the use of 5α-reductase inhibitors and α_1-adrenergic blocking drugs.[40] The 5α-reductase inhibitors such as finasteride reduce prostate size by blocking the effect of androgens on the prostate. Finasteride causes atrophy of the prostate glandular epithelial cells, which results in a 20% to 30% reduction in volume. The onset is slow (3 to 6 months), but long-lasting. The side effects of finasteride are minimal but include erectile dysfunction (4% to 16%) and decreased libido (1% to 10%).[39] The presence of α-adrenergic receptors in prostatic smooth muscle has prompted the use of α_1-adrenergic blocking drugs (*e.g.,* prazosin, terazosin) to relieve prostatic obstruction and increase urine flow. All α_1-adrenergic blocking drugs in current use have a rapid onset of action (within weeks), and similar effectiveness, producing a 40% increase in maximum urine flow rate with good symptom improvement.[40] Combinations of 5α-reductase inhibitors and α_1-adrenergic blocking agents seem to be more effective than either monotherapy.

Herbal therapies have been used for many years by men for the treatment of BPH and lower urinary tract symptoms. Several studies have looked at the effects of these agents, including the extract of the saw palmetto berry. Improvements in peak urine flow rates and nocturia can occur compared with placebo, but the durability of these effects is unproven. The long-term toxicity and mechanism of action of these agents remain unclear.[40] Standardization of these products is also worrisome (as with all herbal therapies).

The surgical removal of an enlarged prostate can be accomplished by the transurethral, suprapubic, or perineal approach. Currently, transurethral prostatectomy (TURP) is the most commonly used technique. With this approach, an instrument is introduced through the urethra, and prostate tissue is removed using a resectoscope and electrocautery. Immediate complications of TURP include the inability to urinate, postoperative hemorrhage or clot retention, and urinary tract infection. Late complications of TURP include erectile dysfunction, incontinence, and bladder neck contractures. Retrograde ejaculation is another problem that may occur because of resection of bladder neck tissue.

Many new and experimental techniques have also been used to treat BPH (*e.g.,* transurethral incision of the prostate [TUIP], laser surgery, transurethral vaporization, transurethral microwave therapy, transurethral needle ablation), and each has advantages and disadvantages when considered as an alternative treatment of BPH.

A balloon dilation approach for removing the obstruction is another new technique. Transrectal ultrasonography is used to monitor balloon dilation of the prostate. Although the procedure may improve symptom score and flow rates, the effects usually are transitory.

For men who have heart or lung disease or a condition that precludes major surgery, a stent may be used to widen and maintain the patency of the urethra. A stent is a device made of tubular mesh that is inserted under local or regional anesthesia. Within several months, the lining of the urethra grows to cover the inside of the stent.

Prostate Cancer

Prostate cancer is the most common nonskin cancer in the United States, and is third to lung cancer and colon/rectal cancer as a cause of cancer-related death in U.S. men.[17] The American Cancer Society estimates that during 2008, approximately 186,320 men in the United States were diagnosed with prostate cancer, and 28,660 men died of the disorder.[17] The increase in diagnosed cases is thought to reflect earlier diagnosis because

of the widespread use of PSA testing since the early 1990s. The incidence of prostate cancer varies markedly from country to country and varies among races in the same country.[43–45] African American men have the highest reported incidence for prostate cancer at all ages. Prostate cancer also tends to be diagnosed at a later stage in African American men. Asians and Native American men have the lowest rate.[45] Prostate cancer also is a disease of aging. The incidence increases rapidly after 50 years of age; more than 85% of all prostate cancers are diagnosed in men older than 65 years of age.[45]

The precise cause of prostate cancer is unclear. As with other cancers, it appears that the development of prostate cancer is a multistep process involving genes that control cell differentiation and growth.[44] Several risk factors, such as age, race, heredity, and environmental influences (*e.g.,* a high-fat diet), are suspected of playing a role.[43–45] Male hormone levels also play a role. There is insufficient evidence linking socioeconomic status, infectious agents, smoking, vasectomy, sexual behavior, or BPH to the pathogenesis of prostate cancer.

The incidence of prostate cancer appears to be higher in relatives of men with prostate cancer. It has been estimated that men who have an affected first-degree relative (*e.g.,* father, brother) and an affected second-degree relative (*e.g.,* grandfather, uncle) have an eightfold increase in risk.[45] It has been suggested that dietary patterns, including increased dietary fats, may alter the production of sex hormones and growth factors and increase the risk of prostate cancer.[44,45] Supporting the role of dietary fats as a risk factor for prostate cancer has been the observation that the diet of Japanese men, who have a low rate of prostate cancer, is much lower in fat content than that of U.S. men, who have a much higher incidence.

Several factors appear to be protective against the development of prostate cancer. These include dietary factors such as lycopene, selenium, and vitamin E.[44,45] Chemoprevention (using drugs to prevent disease) with the 5α-reductase inhibitor, finasteride, was shown to prevent the development of prostate cancer in men without BPH.[43] The role of these putative protective agents remains to be clarified.

In terms of hormonal influence, androgens are believed to play a role in the pathogenesis of prostate cancer.[43,45] Evidence favoring a hormonal influence includes the presence of steroid receptors in the prostate, the requirement of sex hormones for normal growth and development of the prostate, and the fact that prostate cancer almost never develops in men who have been castrated. The response of prostate cancer to estrogen administration or androgen deprivation further supports a correlation between the disease and testosterone levels. Other hormonal factors that have been implicated in prostate cancer include increased levels of IGF-1.[45]

Prostatic adenocarcinomas, which account for 98% of all primary prostate cancers, are commonly multicentric and located in the peripheral zones of the prostate (see Fig. 44-8). The high frequency of invasion of the prostatic capsule by adenocarcinoma relates to its subcapsular location. Invasion of the urinary bladder is less frequent and occurs later in the clinical course. Metastasis to the lung reflects lymphatic spread through the thoracic duct and dissemination from the prostatic venous plexus to the inferior vena cava. Bony metastases, particularly to the vertebral column, ribs, and pelvis, produce pain that often presents as a first sign of the disease.

Most men with early-stage prostate cancer are asymptomatic. The presence of symptoms often suggests locally advanced or metastatic disease. Depending on the size and location of prostate cancer at the time of diagnosis, there may be changes associated with the voiding pattern similar to those found in BPH. These include urgency, frequency, nocturia, hesitancy, dysuria, hematuria, or blood in the ejaculate. On digital rectal examination, the prostate can be nodular and fixed. Bone metastasis often is characterized by low back pain. Pathologic fractures can occur at the site of metastasis. Men with metastatic disease may experience weight loss, anemia, or shortness of breath.

Screening. Because early cancers of the prostate usually are asymptomatic, screening tests are important. The screening tests currently available are digital rectal examination, PSA testing, and transrectal ultrasonography. PSA is a glycoprotein secreted into the cytoplasm of benign and malignant prostatic cells that is not found in other normal tissues or tumors. However, a positive PSA test indicates only the possible presence of prostate cancer. It also can be positive in cases of BPH and prostatitis. It has been reported that one third of men with elevated PSA levels have prostate cancer determined by biopsy, and two thirds do not.[46] Measures to increase the specificity of PSA testing in terms of predicting prostate cancer are being developed and evaluated. For example, because PSA levels increase with age, age-specific ranges have been established.[47] PSA velocity (a change of PSA level over time) and PSA density (*i.e.,* PSA level/prostate volume as measured by rectal ultrasonography) are being evaluated as a method of predicting the presence of prostate cancer in men with a positive PSA test result.[47]

The American Cancer Society and the American Urological Association recommend that men 50 years of age or older should undergo annual measurement of PSA and digital rectal examination for early detection of prostate cancer.[48] Men at high risk for prostate cancer, such as African Americans and those with a strong family history, should undergo annual screening beginning at 45 years of age.[48] However, some controversy regarding the widespread use of PSA for screening remains. In 2002, the American College of Physicians and the U.S. Preventive Services Task Force emphasized the lack of reliable evidence for the benefits of screening.[49] Informed decision making regarding screening with PSA is warranted.

A new approach, transrectal ultrasonography, may detect cancers that are too small to be detected by physical examination. This method is not used for first-line detection because of its expense, but it may benefit men who are at high risk for development of prostate cancer.

Diagnosis. The diagnosis of prostate cancer is based on history and physical examination and confirmed through biopsy methods. Transrectal ultrasonography is used to guide a biopsy needle and document the exact location of the sampled tissue. It also is used for providing staging information. Newly developed small probes for transrectal MRI have been shown to be effective in detecting the presence of cancer in the prostate. Radiologic examination of the bones of the skull, ribs, spine, and pelvis can be used to reveal metastases, although radionuclide bone scans are more sensitive.

Staging. Cancer of the prostate, like other forms of cancer, is graded and staged (see Chapter 8). Prostatic adenocarcinoma commonly is classified using the Gleason grading system.[20] Well-differentiated tumors are assigned a grade of 1, and poorly differentiated tumors a grade of 5. In 2002, the American Joint Committee on Cancer updated the TNM system for staging.[50] Primary-stage tumors (T1) are asymptomatic and discovered on histologic examination of prostatic tissue specimens; T2 tumors are palpable on digital examination but are confined to the prostate gland; T3 tumors have extended beyond the prostate; and T4 tumors have pushed beyond the prostate to involve adjacent structures (Fig. 44-10). Regional lymph node (N) and distant metastases (M) are described as Nx or Mx (cannot be assessed), N0 or M0 (not present), and N1 or M1 (present).[50]

PSA levels are important in the staging and management of prostate cancer. In untreated cases, the level of PSA correlates with the volume and stage of disease. A rising PSA after treatment is consistent with progressive disease, whether it is locally recurring or metastatic. Measurement of PSA is used to detect recurrence after total prostatectomy. Because the prostate is the source of PSA, levels should drop to zero after surgery; a rising PSA indicates recurring disease.

Treatment. Cancer of the prostate is treated by surgery, radiation therapy, and hormonal manipulations.[51] Chemotherapy has shown limited effectiveness in the treatment of prostate cancer. Treatment decisions are based on tumor grade and stage and on the age and health of the man. Expectant therapy (watchful waiting) may be used if the tumor is not producing symptoms, is expected to grow slowly, and is small and contained in one area of the prostate. This approach is particularly suited for men who are elderly or have other health problems. Most men with an anticipated survival greater than 10 years are considered for surgical or radiation therapy.[51] Radical prostatectomy involves complete removal of the seminal vesicles, prostate, and ampullae of the vas deferens. Refinements in surgical techniques ("nerve-sparing" prostatectomy) have allowed maintenance of continence in most men and erectile function in selected cases. Radiation therapy can be delivered by a variety of techniques, including external-beam radiation therapy and transperineal implantation of radioisotopes (brachytherapy).

Metastatic disease often is treated with androgen deprivation therapy. Androgen deprivation may be induced at several levels along the pituitary-gonadal axis using a variety of methods or agents. Orchiectomy often is effective in reducing symptoms and extending survival. The GnRH analogs (*e.g.,* leuprolide, triptorelin) block LH (and FSH) release from the pituitary and reduce

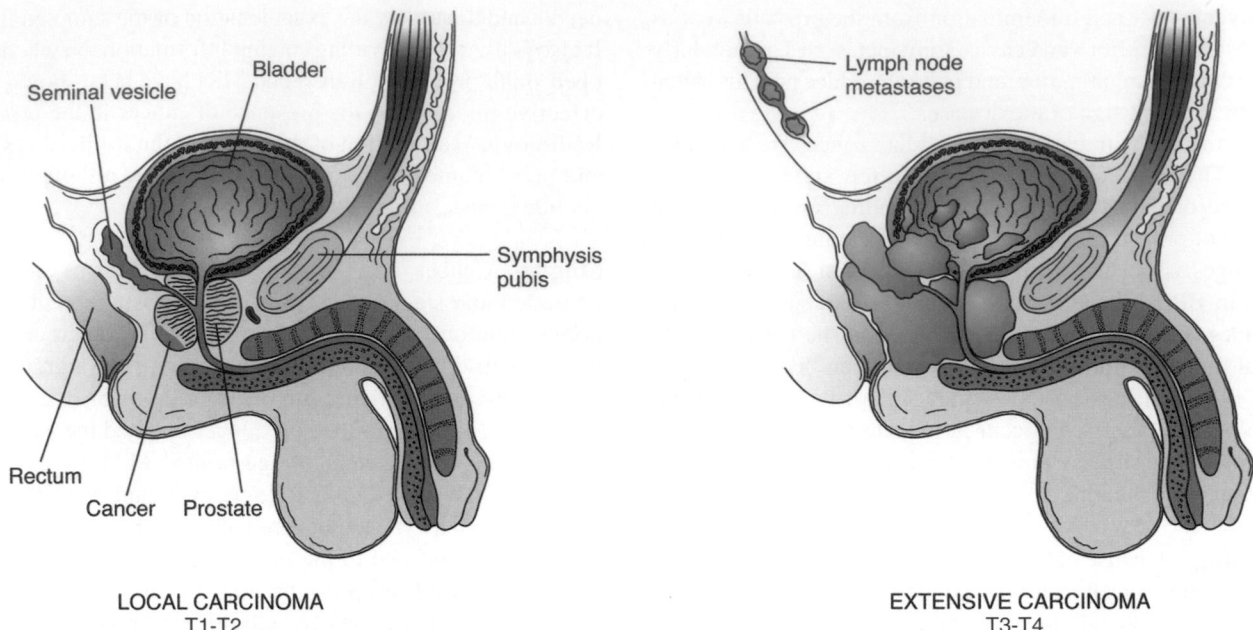

LOCAL CARCINOMA
T1-T2

EXTENSIVE CARCINOMA
T3-T4

FIGURE 44-10 • TNM staging for prostate cancer. (From Damjanov I. [2008]. The lower urinary tract and male reproductive system. In Rubin R., Strayer D. S. [Eds.], *Rubin's pathology: Clinicopathologic foundations of medicine* [5th ed., p. 778]. Philadelphia: Lippincott Williams & Wilkins.)

testosterone levels. When given continuously (as opposed to pulsatile, which is the normal physiologic secretory rhythm) and in therapeutic doses, these drugs desensitize GnRH receptors in the pituitary, thereby preventing the release of LH. However, initially, because these agents are GnRH *agonists*, LH and FSH rise and cause testosterone levels to increase. This can cause a clinical flare that can be especially important in certain circumstances, such as the presence of spinal cord compression due to metastatic disease.[51] This clinical flare can be decreased by pretreatment with antiandrogens. The nonsteroidal antiandrogens (*e.g.*, flutamide, bicalutamide) block the uptake and actions of androgens in the target tissues. Although testosterone is the main circulating androgen, the adrenal gland also secretes androgens. Complete androgen blockade can be achieved by blocking androgens of adrenal origin by combining an antiandrogen with a GnRH agent or orchiectomy. Inhibitors of adrenal androgen synthesis (*i.e.*, ketoconazole and aminoglutethimide) may also be used for treating men with advanced prostate cancer who present with spinal cord compression, bilateral ureteral obstruction, or disseminated intravascular clotting. This is because these men need rapid decreases in their testosterone levels (*i.e.*, ketoconazole can produce chemical castration within 24 hours). Palliative care includes adequate pain control and focal irradiation of symptomatic or unstable bone disease. In men with advanced prostate cancer, the bisphosphonates (*e.g.*, pamidronate, zoledronate), which act mainly by inhibiting osteoclastic activity (see Chapter 58), have several potential uses in prostate cancer. These include (1) prevention of osteopenia that accompanies the use of androgen deprivation therapy; (2) prevention and delay of skeletal complications (*e.g.*, the need for local radia-

tion treatment, fractures) in patients with metastatic bone involvement; (3) palliation of bone pain; and (4) treatment of hypercalcemia of malignancy.

IN SUMMARY, the prostate is a firm, glandular structure that surrounds the urethra. Inflammation of the prostate occurs as an acute or a chronic process. Chronic prostatitis probably is the most common cause of relapsing urinary tract infections in men. BPH is a common disorder in men older than 50 years of age. Because the prostate encircles the urethra, BPH exerts its effect through obstruction of urinary outflow from the bladder. Advances in the treatment of BPH include laser surgery, balloon dilation, prostatic stents, and pharmacologic treatment using 5α-reductase inhibitors such as finasteride, which reduce prostate size by blocking the effects of androgen on the prostate, and α₁-adrenergic receptor blockers, which inhibit contraction of prostatic smooth muscle.

Prostate cancer is the most common nonskin cancer in the United States and is third to lung cancer and colon/rectal cancer as a cause of cancer-related death in men. A recent increase in diagnosed cases is thought to reflect earlier diagnosis because of widespread use of PSA testing. The incidence of prostate cancer increases with age and is greater in African Americans of all ages. Most prostate cancers are asymptomatic and are incidentally discovered on rectal examination. Screening for prostate cancer has become recognized as a method for early identification of prostate cancer. The American Cancer Society suggests that every man 50 years of age or older should have a digital rectal examination and PSA test done as part of his annual physical examination. Cancer of the prostate, like other forms of cancer, is graded according to the histologic characteristics of the tumor and staged clinically using the TNM system. Treatment, which is based on the extent of the disease, includes surgery, radiation therapy, and hormonal manipulation. ∎

Review Exercises

1. A 64-year-old man presents to his family physician with erectile dysfunction. He is on multiple medications for his "heart disease." An initial physical examination is unremarkable.

   A. *What additional information should be obtained?*

   B. *Given his medical history, what are possible factors contributing to his problem?*

2. A 23-year-old man presents to the emergency department in severe distress. His left testicle is large and tender, and he has pain radiating to the inguinal area.

   A. *What would be a tentative diagnosis for this man?*

   B. *Why would this problem necessitate immediate diagnosis and surgical intervention?*

3. A 72-year-old man had a radical prostatectomy for localized prostate cancer. After surgery, his PSA level was undetectable. He presents 5 years later having been "lost to follow-up." He complains of pain in his hip and lower back. His PSA level is now markedly elevated.

   A. *What initial investigations are warranted?*

   B. *What therapies are available for this complication?*

References

1. Behrman R., Kliegman R. M., Jenson H. B. (2004). *Nelson textbook of pediatrics* (16th ed., pp. 1812–1815, 1817–1818). Philadelphia: Elsevier Saunders.
2. Moore K. L., Persaud T. V. N. (2003). *The developing human: Clinically oriented embryology* (7th ed., pp. 304–326). Philadelphia: W. B. Saunders.
3. Hughes I. A., Houk C., Ahmed S. F., et al. (2006). Consensus statement on management of intersex disorders. *Archives of Diseases of Childhood* 91, 554–563.
4. Edwards S. (1996). Balanitis and balanoposthitis: A review. *Genitourinary Medicine* 72, 155–159.
5. Fitkin J., Ho G. T. (1999). Peyronie's disease: Current management. *American Family Physician* 60, 549–554.
6. McAninch J. W. (2004). Disorders of the penis and male urethra. In Tanagho E. A., McAninch J. W. (Eds.), *Smith's general urology* (16th ed., pp. 612–626). New York: Lange Medical Books/McGraw-Hill.
7. Chaudary M., Sheikh N., Asterling S., et al. (2005). Peyronie's disease with erectile dysfunction: Modeling over inflatable penile prosthesis. *Urology* 65, 760–764.
8. Matfin G. (2005). Erectile dysfunction as a component of the metabolic syndrome. *Current Diabetes Reports* 5, 64–69.
9. Matfin G., Jawa G., Fonseca V. (2006). Erectile dysfunction in diabetes: An endothelial disorder. In Fonseca V. (Ed.), *Clinical diabetes: Translating research to practice* (pp. 165–178). Philadelphia: Elsevier Saunders.
10. NIH Consensus Development Panel on Impotence. (1993). NIH Consensus Conference: Impotence. *Journal of the American Medical Association* 270, 83–90.
11. AACE Male Sexual Dysfunction Taskforce. (2003). AACE medical guidelines for clinical practice for the evaluation and treatment of male sexual dysfunction: A couple's problem–2003 update. *Endocrine Practice* 9, 77–95.
12. Bacon C. G., Mittleman M. A., Kawachi I., et al. (2003). Sexual function in men older than 50 years of age: Results from the Health Professionals follow-up study. *Annals of Internal Medicine* 139, 161–168.
13. Feldman H. A., Goldstein J., Hatzichristou D. G., et al. (1994). Impotence and its medical and psychosocial effects: Results of the Massachusetts Male Aging Study. *Journal of Urology* 151, 54–61.
14. Rosen R. C., Jackson G., Kostis J. B. (2006). Erectile dysfunction and cardiac disease: Recommendations of the Second Princeton Conference. *Current Urology Reports* 7, 490–496.
15. Bruno D., Wigfall D. R., Zimmerman S. A., et al. (2001). Genitourinary complications of sickle cell disease. *Journal of Urology* 166, 803–811.
16. American Urological Association. (2003). Guidelines on the management of priapism. [Online.] Available: www.auanet.org/guidelines/priapism.cfm. Accessed March 20, 2008.
17. Jemal A., Seigel R., Ward E. (2008). Cancer statistics. *CA: A Cancer Journal for Clinicians* 58, 71–96.
18. Hamid R., Shergill I., Arya M., et al. (2002). Penile cancer: An overview. *Hospital Medicine* 63(12), 718–721.
19. Presti J. C. (2004). Genital tumors. In Tanagho E. A., McAninch J. W. (Eds.), *Smith's general urology* (16th ed., pp. 386–399). New York: Lange Medical Books/McGraw-Hill.
20. Epstein J. I. (2005). The lower urinary tract and male genital system. In Kumar V., Abbas A. K., Fausto N. (Eds.), *Robbins and Cotran pathologic basis of disease* (7th ed., pp. 1023–1058). Philadelphia: Elsevier Saunders.
21. Docimo S. G., Silver R. I., Cromie W. (2000). The undescended testicle: Diagnosis and management. *American Family Physician* 62, 2037–2048.
22. Pillai S. B., Besner G. E. (1998). Pediatric testicular problems. *Pediatric Clinics of North America* 45, 813–818.
23. Kapur P., Caty M. G., Glick P. L. (1998). Pediatric hernias and hydroceles. *Pediatric Clinics of North America* 45, 773–789.
24. Biyani C. S., Cartledge J., Janetschek G. (2006). Varicocele. *Clinical Evidence Concise* 15, 339–340.
25. Lavallee M. E., Cash J. (2005). Testicular torsion. *Current Sports Medicine Report* 4(2), 102–104.
26. Galejs L. E., Kass E. J. (1999). Diagnosis and treatment of acute scrotum. *American Family Physician* 59, 817–824.
27. Sessions A. E., Rabinowitz R., Hulbert W. C., et al. (2003). Testicular torsion: Direction, degree, duration, and disinformation. *Journal of Urology* 169, 663–665.
28. Centers for Disease Control and Prevention. (2006). Sexually transmitted diseases treatment guidelines. *Morbidity and Mortality Weekly Report* 51(RR-11), 1–94.
29. Gershon A. A. (2001). Mumps. In Kasper D. L. (Ed.), *Harrison's principles of internal medicine* (15th ed., pp. 1147–1148). New York: McGraw-Hill.
30. Mebcow M. M. (1975). Percivall Pott (1713–1788): 200th anniversary of first report of occupation-induced cancer of the scrotum in chimney sweeps (1745). *Urology* 6, 745.
31. Lowe F. C. (1992). Squamous cell carcinoma of the scrotum. *Urologic Clinics of North America* 19, 297–405.
32. Vaughn D. J., Gignac G. A., Meadows A. T. (2002). Long-term medical care of testicular cancer survivors. *Annals of Internal Medicine* 136, 463–470.
33. Motzer R. J., Bosl G. J. (2001). Testicular cancer. In Kasper D. L. (Ed.), *Harrison's principles of internal medicine* (15th ed., pp. 1147–1149). New York: McGraw-Hill.

34. American Cancer Society. (2006). What is testicular cancer? [Online.] Available: www.cancer.org. Accessed November 15, 2006.
35. Krieger J. N., Nyberg L., Nickel J. C. (1999). NIH consensus definition and classification of prostatitis. *Journal of the American Medical Association* 282, 721–725.
36. Erickson B. A., Jang T. L., Ching L., et al. (2006). Chronic prostatitis. *Clinical Evidence Concise* 15, 331–333.
37. Ngugen H. J. (2004). Bacterial infections of the genitourinary system. In Tanagho E. A., McAninch J. W. (Eds.), *Smith's general urology* (16th ed., pp. 203–237). New York: Lange Medical Books/McGraw-Hill.
38. Stevermer J. J., Easley S. K. (2000). Treatment of prostatitis. *American Family Physician* 61, 3015–3026.
39. Collins M. M., MacDonald R., Wilt T. J. (2000). Diagnosis and treatment of chronic abacterial prostatitis: A systemic review. *Annals of Internal Medicine* 133, 367–381.
40. Webber R. (2006). Benign prostatic hyperplasia. *Clinical Evidence Concise* 15, 324–326.
41. Barry M. J., Fowler F. J. Jr., O'Leary M. P., et al. (1992). The American Urological Association index of benign prostatic hypertrophy: The Measurement Committee of the American Urological Association. *Journal of Urology* 148, 1549–1557.
42. Agency of Health Care Policy and Research. (1994). *Clinical practice guidelines for benign prostatic hyperplasia.* AHCPR publication no. 94-0582. Rockville, MD: U.S. Department of Health and Human Services.
43. Scardino P. T. (2003). The prevention of prostate cancer: The dilemma continues. *New England Journal of Medicine* 349, 297–299.
44. Nelson W. G., De Manzo A. M., Isaacs W. B. (2003). Prostate cancer. *New England Journal of Medicine* 349, 366–381.
45. Gronberg H. (2003). Prostate cancer epidemiology. *Lancet* 361, 859–864.
46. Woolf S. H. (1995). Screening for prostate cancer with prostate specific antigen: An examination of the evidence. *New England Journal of Medicine* 333, 1401–1405.
47. Balk S. P., Ko Y. J., Bubley G. J. (2003). Biology of prostate-specific antigen. *Journal of Clinical Oncology* 21, 383–391.
48. American Cancer Society. (2008). Prostate cancer resource center. [Online.] Available: www.cancer.org. Accessed March 20, 2008.
49. U.S. Preventive Services Task Force. (2002). Screening for prostate cancer: recommendations and rationale. *Annals of Internal Medicine* 137, 915–916.
50. American Joint Committee on Cancer. (2002). *AJCC cancer staging manual: American Joint Committee on Cancer* (6th ed., pp. 310–311). New York: Springer-Verlag.
51. Scher H. I. (2001). Hyperplastic and malignant diseases of the prostate. In Kasper D. L. (Ed.), *Harrison's principles of internal medicine* (15th ed., pp. 608–616). New York: McGraw-Hill.

Visit the Point http://thePoint.lww.com for animations, journal articles, and more!

Chapter 45

Structure and Function of the Female Reproductive System

PATRICIA McCOWEN MEHRING

➤ The female genitourinary system consists of internal paired ovaries, fallopian or uterine tubes, the uterus, vagina, external mons pubis, labia majora, labia minora, clitoris, urethra, and perineal body. Although the female urinary structures are anatomically separate from the genital structures, their anatomic proximity provides a means for cross-contamination and shared symptomatology between the two systems (Fig. 45-1). This chapter focuses on the internal and external genitalia. It includes a discussion of hormonal and physical changes that occur throughout the life cycle in response to the gonadotropic hormones. The reader is referred to a specialty text for a discussion of pregnancy.

REPRODUCTIVE STRUCTURES

After completing this section of the chapter, you should be able to meet the following objectives:

- Describe the anatomic relationship of the structures of the external genitalia.
- Name the three layers of the uterus and describe their function.
- Cite the location of the ovaries in relation to the uterus, fallopian tubes, broad ligaments, and ovarian ligaments.
- Explain the function of the fallopian tubes.
- State the function of endocervical secretions.

External Genitalia

The external genitalia are located at the base of the pelvis in the perineal area and include the mons pubis, labia majora, labia minora, clitoris, and perineal body. The urethra and anus, although not genital structures, usually are considered in a discussion of the external genitalia. The external genitalia, also known collectively as the *vulva,* are diagrammed in Figure 45-2.

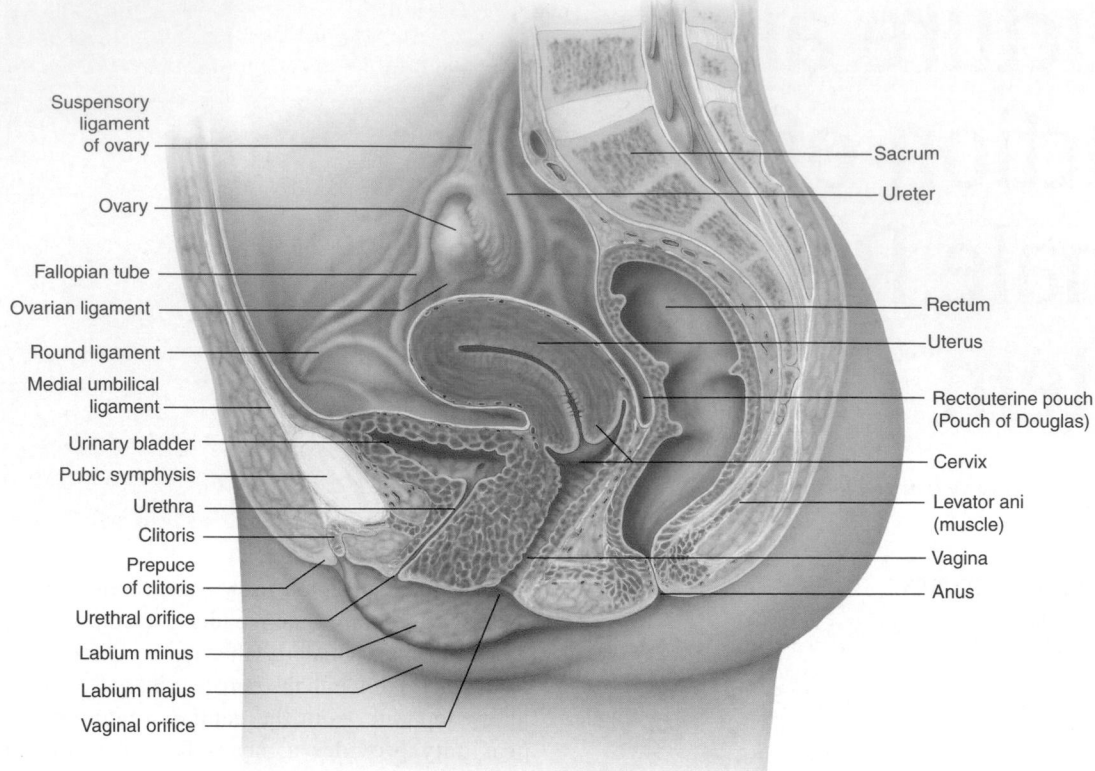

FIGURE 45-1 • Female reproductive system as seen in sagittal section. (Adapted from Anatomical Chart Company. [2001]. *Atlas of human anatomy* [p. 253]. Springhouse, PA: Springhouse.)

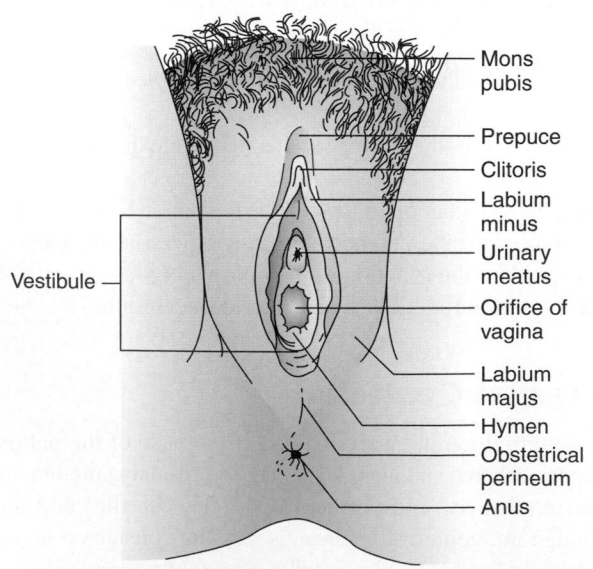

FIGURE 45-2 • External genitalia of the female.

The *mons pubis* is a rounded, skin-covered fat pad located anterior to the symphysis pubis. Puberty stimulates an increase in the amount of fat and the development of darker and coarser hair over the mons. Normal pubic hair distribution in the female follows an inverted triangle with the base centered over the mons. Hair color and texture varies from person to person and among racial groups. There is an abundance of sebaceous glands in the skin that can become infected owing to normal variations in glandular secretions or poor hygiene. The mons pubis is the most common site of pubic lice infestation in the female. The *labia majora* (singular, labium majus) are analogous to the male scrotum. These structures are the outermost lips of the vulva, beginning anteriorly at the base of the mons pubis and ending posteriorly at the anus. The labia majora are composed of folds of skin and fat and become covered with hair at the onset of puberty. Before puberty, the labia majora have a skin covering similar to that covering the abdomen. With sufficient hormonal stimulation, the labia of a mature woman close over the urethral and vaginal openings; this can change after childbirth or surgery.

The *labia minora* (singular, labium minus) are located between the labia majora. These delicate cutaneous structures are smaller than the labia majora and are composed of skin, fat, and some erectile tissue. Unlike the skin of the labia majora, that of the labia minora is hairless and usually light pink. The labia minora begin anteriorly at the hood of the clitoris and end posteriorly at the base of the vagina. During sexual arousal, the labia minora become distended with blood; with resolution, the labia throb and then return to normal size. The clitoris is located below the clitoral hood, or prepuce, which is formed by the joining of the two labia minora. The female clitoris is an erectile organ, rich in vascular and nervous sup-

THE FEMALE GENITOURINARY SYSTEM

■ The female reproductive system, which consists of the external and internal genitalia, has both sexual and reproductive functions.

■ The external genitalia (labia majora, labia minora, clitoris, and vestibular glands) surround the openings of the urethra and vagina. Although the female urinary and genital structures are anatomically separate, their close proximity provides a means for cross-contamination and shared symptomatology.

■ The internal genitalia of the female reproductive system are specialized to participate in sexual intercourse (the vagina), to produce and maintain the female egg cells (the ovaries), to transport these cells to the site of fertilization (the fallopian tubes), to provide a favorable environment for development of offspring (the uterus), and to produce the female sex hormones (the ovaries).

ply. Analogous to the male penis, it is a highly sensitive organ that becomes distended during sexual stimulation.

The area between labia minora is called the *vestibule.* Located in the vestibule are the urethral and vaginal openings and the Bartholin lubricating glands. The *urethra,* or urinary meatus, is the external opening of the internal urinary bladder. The urethra is located posterior to the clitoris and usually is closer to the vaginal opening than to the clitoris. The urethral opening is the site of the *Skene glands,* which have a lubricating function. The vaginal orifice, commonly known as the *introitus,* is the opening between the external and internal genitalia. The size and shape of the opening are determined by a connective tissue membrane called the *hymen* that surrounds the introitus. The opening may be oval, circular, or sievelike and may be partially or completely occluded. Occlusion may occur because of the presence of an intact or partially intact hymen. Contrary to popular notion, an intact hymen does not indicate virginity because this tissue can be stretched without tearing. At puberty, an intact hymen may require surgical intervention to permit discharge of menstrual fluids.

The *perineal body* is that tissue located posterior to the vaginal opening and anterior to the anus. It is composed of fibrous connective tissue and is the site of insertion of several perineal muscles.

Internal Genitalia

Vagina

Connecting the internal and external genitalia is a fibromuscular tube called the *vagina.* The vagina, which is essentially free of sensory nerve fibers, is located behind the urinary bladder and urethra and anterior to the rectum. The uterine cervix projects into the vagina at its upper end, forming recesses called

fornices (Fig. 45-3). The vagina functions as a route for discharge of menses and other secretions. It also serves as an organ of sexual fulfillment and reproduction.

The membranous vaginal wall forms two longitudinal folds and several transverse folds, or rugae. The vagina is lined with mucus-secreting stratified squamous epithelial cells. Vaginal tissue usually is moist, with a pH maintained within the bacteriostatic range of 3.8 to 4.2.

The epithelial cells of the vagina, like other tissues of the reproductive system, respond to changing levels of the ovarian sex hormones. Estrogen stimulates the proliferation and maturation of the vaginal mucosa; this results in a thickening of the vaginal mucosa and an increased glycogen content of the epithelial cells. The glycogen is fermented to lactic acid by the lactobacilli (*i.e.,* Döderlein bacilli) that are part of the normal vaginal flora, accounting for the mildly acid pH of vaginal fluid. The vaginal ecology can be disrupted at many levels, rendering it susceptible to infection. Pregnancy and the use of oral contraceptive agents increase the amount of estrogen in the system. Diabetes or a prediabetic state may increase the glycogen content of the cells. The use of systemic antibiotics may decrease the number of lactobacilli in the vagina.

Decreased estrogen stimulation after menopause causes the vaginal mucosa to become thin and dry, often resulting in dyspareunia (*i.e.,* painful intercourse), atrophic vaginitis, and occasionally in vaginal bleeding. Estrogen levels can be estimated by means of vaginal scrapings obtained during a routine pelvic examination. The scrapings are used for a test, the *mat-*

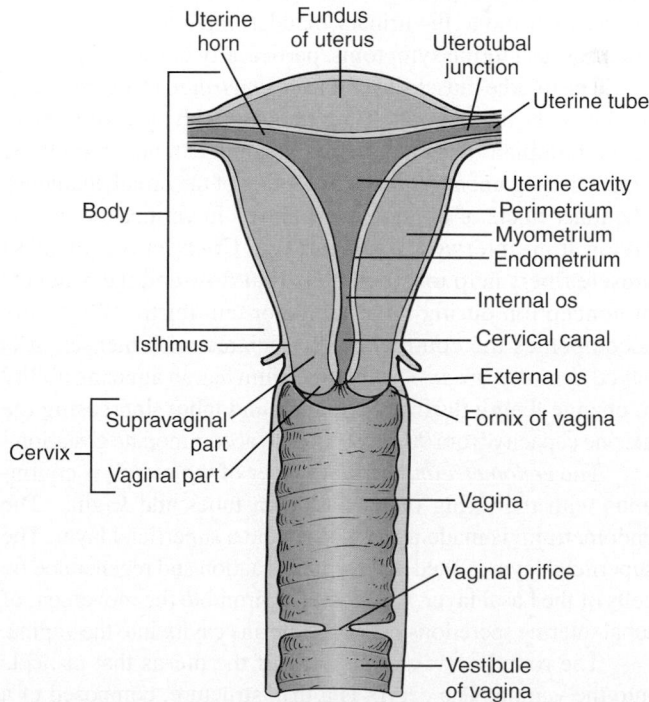

FIGURE 45-3 ● Median section of the vagina and uterus. (From Moore K. L., Agur A. M. R. [2002]. *Essential clinical anatomy* (2nd ed., p. 238). Philadelphia: Lippincott Williams & Wilkins.)

uration index, that examines the cellular structure and configuration of the vaginal epithelial cells. The maturation index determines the ratio of parabasal (least mature), intermediate, and superficial (most mature) cells. Typically, this index is 0-40-60 during the reproductive years. With diminished estrogen levels, there is a shift to the left, producing an index of 30-40-30 during the perimenopausal period and an index of 75-25-0 during the postmenopausal period.

Uterus and Cervix

The uterus is a thick-walled, muscular organ. This pear-shaped, hollow structure is located between the bladder and the rectum. The uterus can be divided into three parts: the portion above the insertion of the fallopian tubes, called the *fundus;* the lower, constricted part, called the *cervix;* and the portion between the fundus and the cervix, called the *body of the uterus.* The uterus is supported on both sides by four sets of ligaments: the *broad ligaments,* which run laterally from the body of the uterus to the pelvic side walls; the *round ligaments,* which run from the fundus laterally into each labium majus; the *uterosacral ligaments,* which run from the uterocervical junction to the sacrum; and the *cardinal* or *transverse cervical* ligaments.

The wall of the uterus is composed of three layers: the perimetrium, the myometrium, and the endometrium. The *perimetrium* is the outer serous covering that is derived from the abdominal peritoneum. This outer layer merges with the peritoneum that covers the broad ligaments. Anteriorly, the perimetrium is reflected over the bladder wall, forming the vesicouterine pouch; posteriorly, it extends to form the *cul-de-sac,* or *pouch of Douglas* (see Fig. 45-1). Because of the proximity of the perimetrium to the urinary bladder, infection of this organ often causes uterine symptoms, particularly during pregnancy.

The middle muscle layer, the *myometrium,* forms the major portion of the uterine wall. It is continuous with the myometrium of the fallopian tubes and the vagina and extends into all the supporting ligaments with the exception of the broad ligaments. The inner fibers of the myometrium run in various directions, giving it an interwoven appearance. Contractions of these muscle fibers help to expel menstrual flow and the products of conception during miscarriage or childbirth. When pain accompanies the contractions associated with menses, it is called *dysmenorrhea.* The myometrium has an amazing ability to change length during pregnancy and labor, increasing the uterine capacity from 90 g to 1000 g to accommodate gestation.[1]

The *endometrium,* the inner layer of the uterus, is continuous with the lining of the fallopian tubes and vagina. The endometrium is made up of a basal and a superficial layer. The superficial layer is shed during menstruation and regenerated by cells of the basal layer. Ciliated cells promote the movement of tubal–uterine secretions out of the uterine cavity into the vagina.

The round *cervix* is the neck of the uterus that projects into the vagina. The cervix is a firm structure, composed of a connective tissue matrix of glands and muscular tissue elements that become soft and pliable under the influence of hormones produced during pregnancy. Glandular tissue provides a rich supply of protective mucus that changes in character and quantity during the menstrual cycle and during pregnancy. The cervix is richly supplied with blood from the uterine artery and can be a site of significant blood loss during delivery.

The opening of the cervix, the os, forms a pathway between the uterus and the vagina. The vaginal opening is called the *external os* and the uterine opening is called, the *internal os* (see Fig. 45-3). The space between these two openings is the endocervical canal. Secretions from the columnar epithelium of the endocervix protect the uterus from infection, alter receptivity to sperm, and form a mucoid "plug" during pregnancy. The endocervical canal provides a route for menstrual discharge and sperm entrance.

Fallopian Tubes

The *fallopian,* or uterine, tubes are slender, cylindrical structures attached bilaterally to the uterus and supported by the upper folds of the broad ligament. The end of the fallopian tube nearest the ovary forms a funnel-like opening with fringed, finger-like projections, called *fimbriae,* that pick up the ovum after its release into the peritoneal cavity after ovulation (Fig. 45-4). The fallopian tubes are formed of smooth muscle and lined with a ciliated, mucus-producing epithelial layer. The beating of the cilia, along with contractile movements of the smooth muscle, propels the nonmobile ovum toward the uterus. If coitus has occurred recently, fertilization normally occurs in the middle to outer portion of the fallopian tube. Besides providing a passageway for ova and sperm, the fallopian tubes provide for drainage of tubal secretions into the uterus.

Ovaries

By the third month of fetal life, the *ovaries* have fully developed and descended to their permanent pelvic position. Remnants of the primitive genital system provide lateral supporting attachments to the uterus; in the mature female, these supporting structures evolve into the round and suspensory ligaments. Remnants that do not evolve may form cysts, which may become symptomatic later in life.

Oogenesis is the process of generation of ova by mitotic division that begins at the sixth week of fetal life. These primitive germ cells ultimately provide the 1 to 2 million oocytes that are present in the ovaries at birth. At puberty, this number is reduced through cell death to approximately 300,000.

The neonate's ovaries are smooth, pale, and elongated. They become shorter, thicker, and heavier before the onset of menarche, which is initiated by pituitary influence. The initial hormonal stimulus for this development is believed to come from ovarian rather than systemic estrogen.

In the adult, the ovaries are flat, almond-shaped structures that are 3 to 5 cm long and weigh 2 to 3 g. They are located on either side of the uterus below the fimbriated ends of the two oviducts, or fallopian tubes. The ovaries are attached to the posterior surface of the broad ligament and to the uterus by the ovarian ligament. They are covered with a thin layer of surface

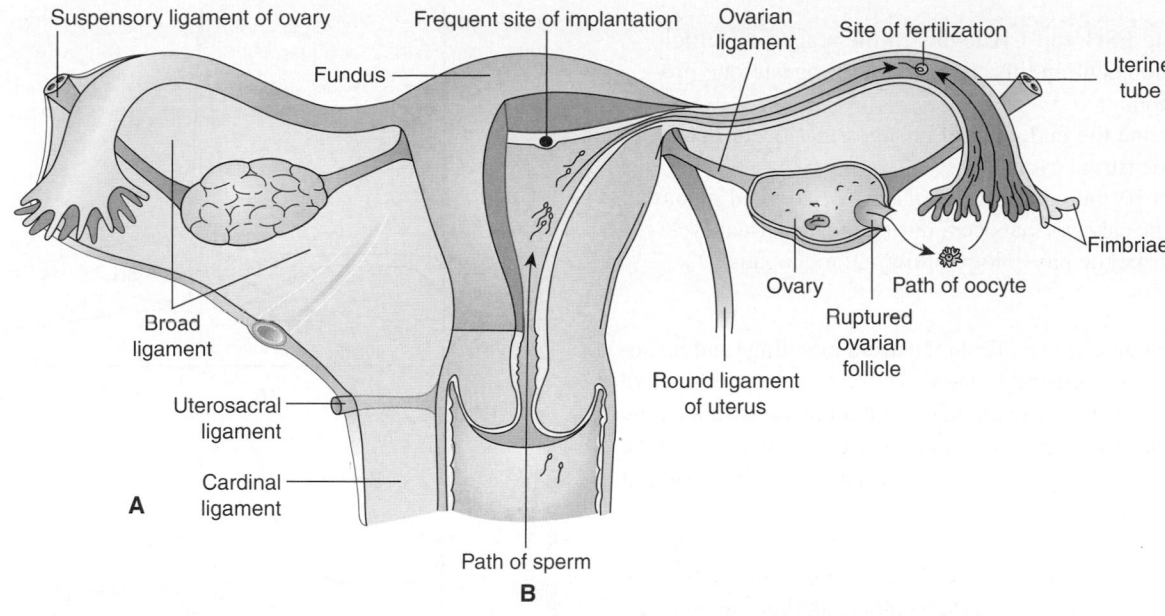

FIGURE 45-4 • Schematic drawing of female reproductive organs, showing **(A)** suspensory ligament of the ovary and the broad, uterosacral, and cardinal ligaments on the left, and **(B)** the path of the oocyte as it moves from the ovary into the fallopian (uterine) tube; the path of sperm is also shown, as is the usual site of fertilization.

epithelium that is continuous with the lining of the peritoneum. The integrity of this covering is periodically broken at the time of ovulation.

The ovaries, like the male testes, have a dual function: they store the female germ cells, or ova, and produce the female sex hormones, estrogen and progesterone. Unlike the male gonads, which produce sperm throughout a man's reproductive life, the female gonads contain a fixed number of ova at birth that diminishes throughout a woman's life.

Structurally, the mature ovary is divided into a highly vascular inner medulla, which contains supporting connective tissue, and an outer cortex of stroma and epithelial follicles (*i.e.*, vesicles), which contain the primary oocytes, or germ cells. After puberty, the pituitary gonadotropic hormones—follicle-stimulating hormone (FSH) and luteinizing hormone (LH)—stimulate the primordial follicles to develop into *mature graafian follicles*. The graafian follicle produces estrogen, which begins to stimulate the development of the endometrium in the uterus. Although several follicles begin to develop during each ovulatory cycle, only one or two complete the entire developmental process and rupture to release a mature ovum. After ovulation, the follicle becomes luteinized; as the corpus luteum, it produces estrogen and progesterone to support the endometrium until conception occurs or the cycle begins again.

IN SUMMARY, the female reproductive system consists of internal paired ovaries, fallopian or uterine tubes, uterus, vagina, external mons pubis, labia majora, labia minora, clitoris, urethra, and perineal body. The genitourinary system as a whole serves sexual and reproductive functions throughout the life cycle. The uterus is a thick-walled, muscular organ. The wall of the uterus is composed of three layers: the outer perimetrium; the myometrium or muscle layer, which is continuous with the myometrium of the fallopian tubes and the vagina; and the inner lining or endometrium, which is continuous with the lining of the fallopian tubes and vagina. The gonads, or ovaries, which are internal in the female (unlike the testes in the male), have the dual function of storing the female germ cells, or ova, and producing the female sex hormones. Through the regulation and release of sex hormones, the ovaries influence the development of secondary sexual characteristics, regulation of menstrual cycles, maintenance of pregnancy, and advent of menopause. ■

 MENSTRUAL CYCLE

After completing this section of the chapter, you should be able to meet the following objectives:

■ Describe the feedback control of estrogen and progesterone levels by means of gonadotropin-releasing hormone, LH, FSH, and ovarian follicle function.
■ List the actions of estrogen and progesterone.
■ Describe the four functional compartments of the ovary.

(objectives continue)

- Relate FSH and LH levels to the stages of follicle development and to estrogen and progesterone production.
- Describe the endometrial changes that occur during the menstrual cycle.
- Describe the composition of normal cervical mucus and the changes that occur during the menstrual cycle.
- Describe the physiology of normal menopause.

Between menarche (*i.e.,* first menstrual bleeding) and menopause (*i.e.,* last menstrual bleeding), the female reproductive system undergoes cyclic changes called the *menstrual cycle.* This includes the maturation and release of oocytes from the ovary during ovulation and periodic vaginal bleeding resulting from the shedding of the endometrial lining. It is not necessary for a woman to ovulate to menstruate; anovulatory cycles do occur. The menstrual cycle produces changes in the breasts, uterus, skin, ovaries, and perhaps other, unidentified tissues. The maintenance of the cycle affects biologic and sociologic aspects of a woman's life, including fertility, reproduction, sexuality, and femaleness.

🔑 MENSTRUAL CYCLE

- The menstrual cycle begins at menarche and continues until menopause. It includes the maturation and release of oocytes from the ovary during ovulation and periodic vaginal bleeding resulting from the shedding of the endometrial lining.

- The menstrual cycle is controlled by rhythmic synthesis and release of ovarian hormones (the estrogens and progesterone) under feedback control from the hypothalamic gonadotropin-releasing hormone and the anterior pituitary gonadotropic follicle-stimulating and luteinizing hormones.

Hormonal Control

Normal menstrual function results from interactions among the central nervous system, hypothalamus, anterior pituitary, ovaries, and associated target tissues (Fig. 45-5). Although each part of the system is essential to normal function, the ovaries are primarily responsible for controlling the cyclic changes and the length of the menstrual cycle. In most women in the middle reproductive years, menstrual bleeding occurs every 25 to 35 days, with a median length of 28 days.

The hormonal control of the menstrual cycle is complex. For example, the biosynthesis of estrogens that occurs in adipose tissue may be a significant source of the hormone. There is evidence that a certain minimum body weight (48 kg) and fat content (16% to 24%) are necessary for menarche to occur and

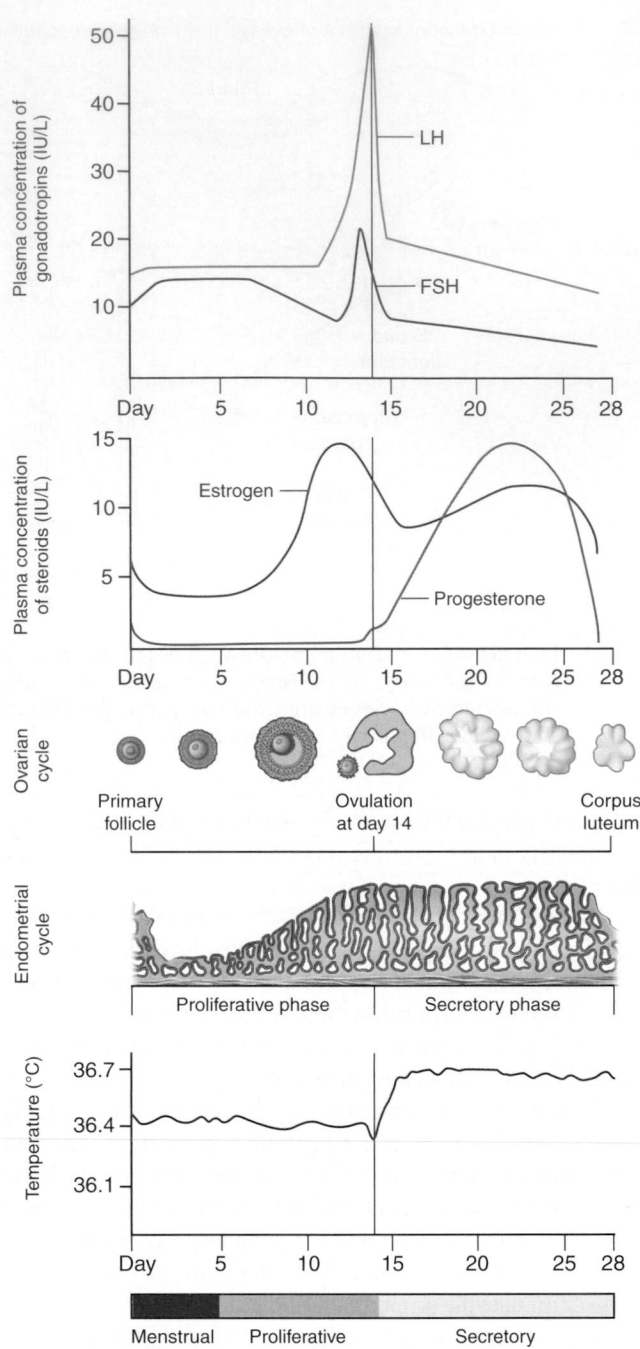

FIGURE 45-5 • Hormonal and morphologic changes during the normal menstrual cycle.

for the menstrual cycle to be maintained. This is supported by the observation of amenorrhea in women with anorexia nervosa, chronic disease, and malnutrition and in those who are long-distance runners. In women with anorexia nervosa, gonadotropin and estradiol secretion, including LH release and responsiveness to the hypothalamic gonadotropin-releasing hormone (GnRH), can revert to prepubertal levels. With resumption of weight gain and attainment of sufficient body mass, the normal hormonal pattern usually is reinstated. Obesity or significant weight gain also is associated with oligomenorrhea or amenorrhea and infertility, although the mechanism is not well understood.

Hypothalamic and Pituitary Hormones

Growth, prepubertal maturation, the reproductive cycle, and sex hormone secretion in males and females are regulated by FSH and LH from the anterior pituitary gland (Fig. 45-6). Because these hormones promote the growth of cells in the ovaries and testes as a means of stimulating the production of sex hormones, they are called the *gonadotropic hormones*. The secretion of LH and FSH is stimulated by GnRH from the hypothalamus. In addition to LH and FSH, the anterior pituitary secretes a third hormone called *prolactin*. The primary function of prolactin is the stimulation of lactation in the postpartum period. During pregnancy, prolactin, along with other hormones such as estrogen, progesterone, insulin, and cortisol, contributes to breast development in preparation for lactation. Although prolactin does not appear to play a physiologic role in ovarian function, hyperprolactinemia leads to hypogonadism. This may include an initial shortening of the luteal phase with subsequent anovulation, oligomenorrhea or amenorrhea, and infertility. The hypothalamic control of prolactin secretion is primarily inhibitory, and dopamine is the most important inhibitory factor. Hyperprolactinemia may occur as an adverse effect of drug treatment using phenothiazine derivatives (*i.e.,* antipsychotic drugs that block dopamine receptors).

Ovarian Hormones

The ovaries produce estrogens, progesterone, and androgens. Ovarian hormones are secreted in a cyclic pattern as a result of the interaction between the hypothalamic GnRH and the pituitary gonadotropic hormones, FSH and LH. The steroid sex hormones enter cells by passive diffusion, bind to specific receptor proteins in the cytoplasm, and then move to the nucleus, where they bind to specific sites on the chromosomes. These hormones exert their effects through gene–hormone interactions that stimulate the synthesis of specific messenger ribonucleic acid (mRNA). In addition, estrogen appears to have the ability to influence cell activity through other, nongenomic mechanisms. These nongenomic effects take place in cells that have no steroid receptors, possibly mediated by other membrane receptors. This may explain in part some of the nonreproductive effects of estrogen. An example of a nongenomic cardioprotective effect would be the antioxidant activity of estrogen in preventing endothelial injury that can lead to platelet adherence.[2] The number of hormonal receptor sites on a cell is not fixed; evidence suggests that they are constantly being removed and replaced. An increase or a decrease in the number of receptors can serve as a mechanism for regulating hormonal activity. For example, estrogen may induce the development of an increased number of estrogen receptors in some tissues and may stimulate the synthesis of progesterone receptors in others. In contrast, progesterone may cause a reduction in the number of estrogen and progesterone receptors.

The recent discovery of a second type of estrogen receptor (ER_2) that is different in structure, tissue distribution, and expression from ER_1 helps to expand our understanding of the mechanism of action of estrogen in the body. The ER_2 appears to be an activator of estrogen response, whereas the ER_1 appears to modulate or inhibit the action of estrogen.[3] Likewise, the progesterone receptor has two major forms (A and B), expressed by a single gene, but promoted differently in a complex system of transcription regulation.

Estrogens. Estrogens are a family of structurally related female sex hormones synthesized and secreted by cells in the ovaries and, in small amounts, by cells in the adrenal cortex. Androgens can be converted to estrogens peripherally, especially in fat tissue. Three estrogens occur naturally in humans: estrone (E_1), estradiol (E_2), and estriol (E_3). Of these, estradiol is the most biologically potent and the most abundantly secreted product of the ovary. Estrogens are secreted throughout the menstrual cycle. Two peaks occur: one before ovulation and one in the middle of the luteal phase. Estrogens are transported in the blood bound to specific plasma globulins (which can also bind testosterone), inactivated and conjugated in the liver, and then excreted in the bile.

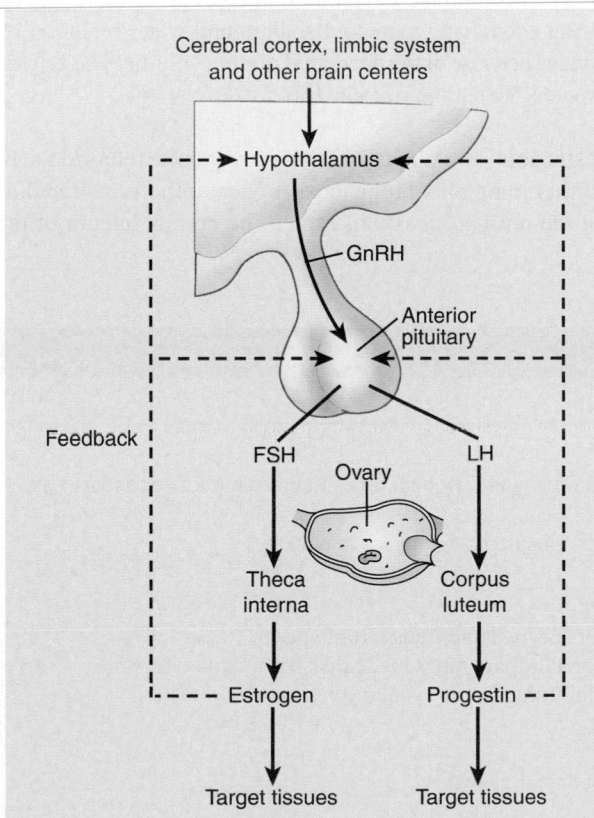

FIGURE 45-6 • Hypothalamic-pituitary feedback control of estrogen and progesterone levels in the female. The *dashed line* represents negative feedback.

Estrogens are necessary for normal female physical maturation. In concert with other hormones, estrogens provide for the reproductive processes of ovulation, implantation of the products of conception, pregnancy, parturition, and lactation by stimulating the development and maintaining the growth of the accessory organs. In the absence of androgens, estrogens stimulate the intrauterine development of the vagina, uterus, and uterine tubes from the embryonic müllerian system. They also stimulate the stromal development and ductal growth of the breasts at puberty, are responsible for the accelerated pubertal skeletal growth phase and for closure of the epiphyses of the long bones, contribute to the growth of axillary and pubic hair, and alter the distribution of body fat to produce the typical female body contours, including the accumulation of body fat around the hips and breasts. Larger quantities of estrogen stimulate pigmentation of the skin in the nipple, areolar, and genital regions.

In addition to their effects on the growth of uterine muscle, estrogens play an important role in the development of the endometrial lining. During anovulatory cycles, continued exposure to estrogens for prolonged periods leads to abnormal hyperplasia of the endometrium and abnormal bleeding patterns. When estrogen production is poorly coordinated during the normal menstrual period, inappropriate bleeding and shedding of the endometrium also can occur (see Chapter 46).

Estrogens have a number of important extragenital metabolic effects. They are responsible for maintaining the normal structure of skin and blood vessels in women. Estrogens decrease the rate of bone resorption by antagonizing the effects of parathyroid hormone on bone; for this reason, osteoporosis is a common problem in estrogen-deficient postmenopausal women. In the liver, estrogens increase the synthesis of transport proteins for thyroxine, estrogen, testosterone, and other hormones. Estrogens also affect the composition of the plasma lipoproteins. They produce an increase in high-density lipo-

proteins (HDLs), a slight reduction in low-density lipoproteins (LDLs), and a reduction in cholesterol levels (see Chapter 22).

Estrogens have additional cardioprotective actions, including direct antiatherosclerotic effects on the arterial wall (augmentation of vasodilating and antiplatelet aggregation factors such as nitric oxide and prostacyclin), vasodilation through endothelium-independent mechanisms, antioxidant activity, reduction of levels of angiotensin-converting enzyme and renin, reduction of homocysteine levels, improvement of peripheral glucose metabolism with subsequent decreased circulating insulin levels, and direct effects on cardiac function (i.e., increased left ventricular diastolic filling and stroke volume output). Estrogens increase plasma triglyceride levels and they enhance the coagulability of blood by effecting increased circulating levels of plasminogen and factors II, VII, IX, and X.

Estrogens appear to have both neurotropic and neuroprotective effects on cognitive function and memory. Observational studies indicate possible prevention of Alzheimer disease through anti-inflammatory mechanisms to prevent vascular injury, increased cerebral blood flow, and altered brain activation. Estrogens promote dendritic branching and enhance presynaptic and postsynaptic signal transmission through increased production of neurotransmitters and receptors.[4]

The estrogens cause moderate retention of sodium and water. Most women retain sodium and water and gain weight just before menstruation. This occurs because the estrogens facilitate the movement of intravascular fluids into the extracellular spaces, producing edema and increased sodium and water retention by the kidneys because of the decreased plasma volume. The actions of estrogens are summarized in Table 45-1.

Progesterone. Although the word *progesterone* refers to a substance that maintains pregnancy, progesterone is secreted as part of the normal menstrual cycle. The corpus luteum of the

TABLE 45-1 Actions of Estrogens

GENERAL FUNCTION	SPECIFIC ACTIONS
Growth and development	
Reproductive organs	Stimulate development of vagina, uterus, and fallopian tubes in utero and of secondary sex characteristics during puberty
Skeleton	Accelerate growth of long bones and closure of epiphyses at puberty
Reproductive processes	
Ovulation	Promote growth of ovarian follicles
Fertilization	Alter the cervical secretions to favor survival and transport of sperm
	Promote motility of sperm within the fallopian tubes by decreasing mucus viscosity
Implantation	Promote development of endometrial lining in the event of pregnancy
Vagina	Proliferate and cornify vaginal mucosa
Cervix	Increase mucus consistency
Breasts	Stimulate stromal development and ductal growth
General metabolic effects	
Bone resorption	Decrease rate of bone resorption
Plasma proteins	Increase production of thyroid and other binding globulins
Lipoproteins	Increase high-density and slightly decrease low-density lipoproteins

ovary secretes large amounts of progesterone after ovulation, and the adrenal cortex secretes small amounts. The hormone circulates in the blood attached to a specific plasma protein. It is metabolized in the liver and conjugated for excretion in the bile.

The local effects of progesterone on reproductive organs include the glandular development of the lobular and alveolar tissue of the breasts and the cyclic glandular development of the endometrium. Progesterone also can compete with aldosterone at the level of the renal tubule, causing a decrease in sodium reabsorption, with a resultant increase in secretion of aldosterone by the adrenal cortex, as occurs in pregnancy. Although the mechanism is uncertain, progesterone is responsible for the increase in basal body temperature that occurs with ovulation. Smooth muscle relaxation under the influence of progesterone plays an important role in maintaining pregnancy by decreasing uterine contractions, and is responsible for many of the common discomforts of pregnancy, such as edema, nausea, constipation, flatulence, and headaches. The increased progesterone present during pregnancy and the luteal phase of the menstrual cycle enhances the ventilatory response to carbon dioxide, leading to a measurable change in arterial and alveolar carbon dioxide (PCO_2) levels.

Androgens. The normal female produces androgens, estrogens, and progesterone. Approximately 25% of these androgens are secreted from the ovaries, 25% from the adrenal cortex, and 50% from ovarian or adrenal precursors. In the female, androgens contribute to normal hair growth at puberty and may have other important metabolic effects.

Ovarian Follicle Development and Ovulation

The tissues of the adult ovary can be conveniently divided into four compartments, or units: the stroma, or supporting tissue; the interstitial cells; the follicles; and the corpus luteum. The *stroma* is the connective tissue substance of the ovary in which the follicles are distributed. The *interstitial cells* are estrogen-secreting cells that resemble the Leydig cells, or interstitial cells, of the testes.

Beginning at puberty, a cyclic rise in the anterior pituitary hormones FSH and LH stimulates the development of several graafian, or mature, follicles. Follicles at all stages of development can be found in both ovaries, except in menopausal women (Fig. 45-7). Most follicles exist as primary follicles, each of which consists of a round oocyte surrounded by a single layer of flattened, epithelium-derived granulosa cells and a basement membrane. The primary follicles constitute an inactive pool of follicles from which all the ovulating follicles develop. Under the influence of endocrine stimulation, 6 to 12 primary follicles develop into secondary follicles once every ovulatory cycle. During the development of the secondary follicle, the primary

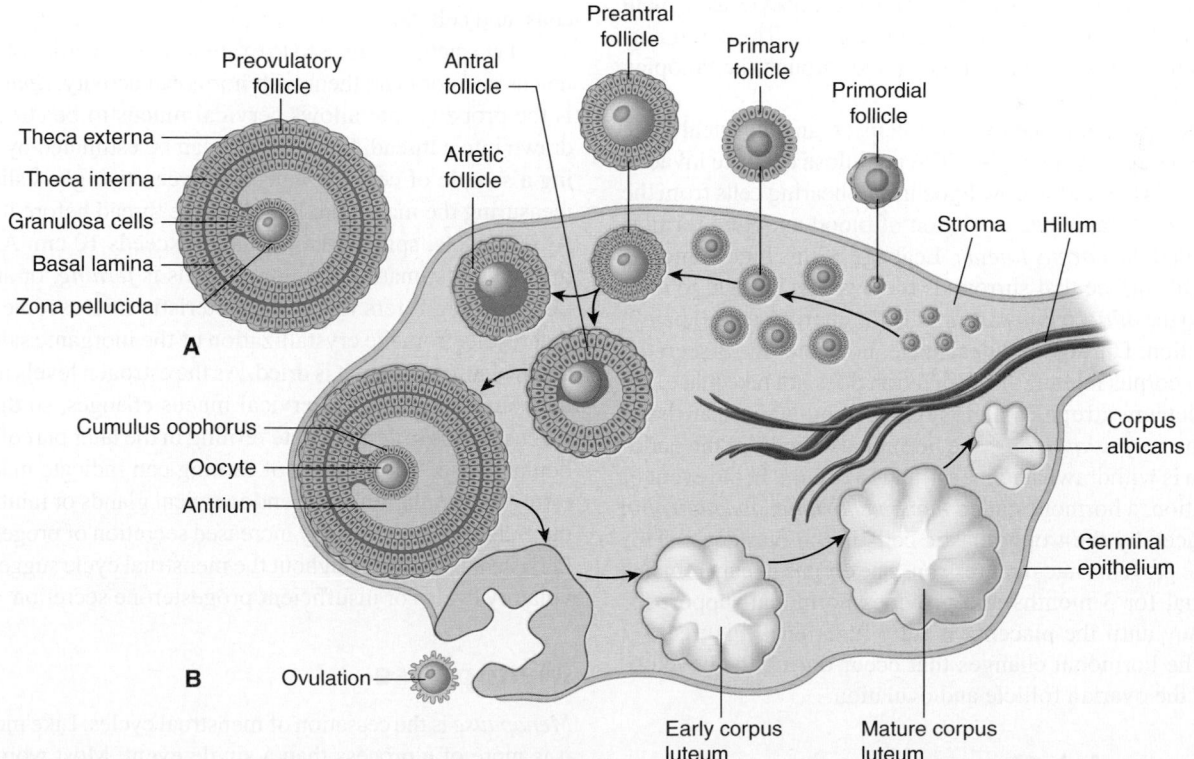

FIGURE 45-7 • **(A)** Cross-section of preovulatory follicle. **(B)** Schematic diagram of an ovary, showing the sequence of events in the origin, growth, and rupture of an ovarian follicle and the formation and retrogression of a corpus luteum. The atretic follicles are those that show signs of degeneration and death.

oocyte increases in size, and the granulosa cells proliferate to form a multilayered wall around it. During this time, a membrane called the *zona pellucida* develops and surrounds the oocyte and small pockets of fluid begin to appear between the granulosa cells. Blood vessels, however, do not penetrate the basement membrane; the granulosa cell layer remains avascular until after ovulation has occurred.

As the follicles mature, FSH stimulates the development of the cell layers. Cells from the surrounding stromal tissue align themselves to form a cellular wall called the *theca.* The cells of the theca become differentiated into two layers: an inner theca interna, which lies adjacent to the follicular cells, and an outer theca externa. As the follicle enlarges, a single large cavity, or *antrum,* is formed, and a portion of the granulosa cells and the oocyte are displaced to one side of the follicle by the fluid that accumulates. The secondary oocyte remains surrounded by a crown of granulosa cells, the corona radiata. As the follicle ripens, ovarian estrogen is produced by the granulosa cells. Selection of a dominant follicle occurs with the conversion to an estrogen microenvironment. The lesser follicles, although continuing to produce some estrogen, atrophy or become atretic. The dominant follicle accumulates a greater mass of granulosa cells, and the theca becomes richly vascular, giving the follicle a hyperemic appearance. High levels of estrogen exert a negative feedback effect on FSH, inhibiting multiple follicular development and causing an increase in LH levels. This represents the follicular stage of the menstrual cycle. As estrogen suppresses FSH, the actions of LH predominate, and the mature follicle (measuring approximately 20 mm) bursts; the oocyte, along with the corona radiata, is ejected from the follicle. The ovum normally is then picked up and transported through the fallopian tube toward the uterus.

After ovulation, the follicle collapses, and the luteal stage of the menstrual cycle begins. The granulosa cells are invaded by blood vessels and yellow lipochrome-bearing cells from the theca layer. A rapid accumulation of blood and fluid forms a mass called the *corpus luteum.* Leakage of this blood onto the peritoneal surface that surrounds the ovary is thought to contribute to the *mittelschmerz* ("middle [or intermenstrual] pain") of ovulation. During the luteal stage, progesterone is secreted from the corpus luteum. If fertilization does not take place, the corpus luteum atrophies and is replaced by white scar tissue called the *corpus albicans;* the hormonal support of the endometrium is withdrawn and menstruation occurs. In the event of fertilization, a hormone called *human chorionic gonadotropin* is produced by the trophoblastic cells in the blastocyst. This hormone prevents luteal regression. The corpus luteum remains functional for 3 months and provides hormonal support for pregnancy until the placenta is fully functional. Figure 45-7 shows the hormonal changes that occur during the development of the ovarian follicle and ovulation.

Endometrial Changes

The endometrium consists of two distinct layers, or zones, that are responsive to hormonal stimulation: a basal layer and a functional layer. The *basal layer* lies adjacent to the myo-

metrium and is not sloughed during menstruation. The *functional layer* arises from the basal layer and undergoes proliferative changes and menstrual sloughing. It can be subdivided into two components: a thin, superficial, compact layer and a deeper spongiosa layer that makes up most of the secretory and fully developed endometrium. The endometrial cycle can be divided into three phases: the proliferative, or preovulatory, phase, during which the glands and stroma of the superficial layer grow rapidly under the influence of estrogen; the secretory, or postovulatory, phase, during which progesterone produces glandular dilation and active mucus secretion and the endometrium becomes highly vascular and edematous; and the menstrual phase, during which the superficial layer degenerates and sloughs off (see Fig. 45-5).

Cervical Mucus Changes

Cervical mucus is a complex, heterogeneous secretion produced by the glands of the endocervix. It is composed of 92% to 98% water and 1% inorganic salts, mainly sodium chloride. The mucus also contains simple sugars, polysaccharides, proteins, and glycoproteins. Its pH usually is alkaline, ranging from 6.5 to 9.0. Its characteristics are strongly influenced by serum levels of estrogen and progesterone. Estrogen stimulates the production of large amounts of clear, watery mucus through which sperm can penetrate most easily. Progesterone, even in the presence of estrogen, reduces the secretion of mucus. During the luteal phase of the menstrual cycle, mucus is scant, viscous, and cellular.

Two methods are used to examine the properties of cervical mucus and correlate them with hormonal activity. *Spinnbarkeit* is the property that allows cervical mucus to be stretched or drawn into a thread. Spinnbarkeit can be estimated by stretching a sample of cervical mucus between two glass slides and measuring the maximum length of the thread before it breaks. At mid-cycle, spinnbarkeit usually exceeds 10 cm. A second method of estimating hormonal levels is *ferning,* or arborization. Ferning refers to the characteristic microscopic pattern that results from the crystallization of the inorganic salts in the cervical mucus when it is dried. As the estrogen levels increase, the composition of the cervical mucus changes, so that dried mucus begins to demonstrate ferning in the later part of the follicular phase. The absence of ferning can indicate inadequate estrogen stimulation of the endocervical glands or inhibition of the endocervical glands by increased secretion of progesterone. Persistent ferning throughout the menstrual cycle suggests anovulatory cycles or insufficient progesterone secretion.

Menopause

Menopause is the cessation of menstrual cycles. Like menarche, it is more of a process than a single event. Most women stop menstruating between 48 and 55 years of age. *Perimenopause* (the years immediately surrounding menopause) precedes menopause by approximately 4 years and is characterized by menstrual irregularity and other menopausal symptoms. *Climacteric* is a more encompassing term that refers to the entire transition to the nonreproductive period of life. Premature ovarian failure describes the approximately 1% of women who experience menopause before the age of 40 years. A woman who has not menstruated for a full year or who has a persistently elevated FSH level (>20 mIU/mL using newer, more sensitive assays) is considered menopausal.[4]

Functional Changes

Menopause results from the gradual cessation of ovarian function and the resultant diminished levels of estrogen. Although estrogens derived from the adrenal cortex continue to circulate in a woman's body, they are insufficient to maintain the secondary sexual characteristics in the same manner as ovarian estrogens. As a result, body hair, skin elasticity, and subcutaneous fat decrease. The breasts become pendulous with a decrease in tissue mass, leaving only the ducts, fat, and connective tissue. The ovaries and uterus diminish in size; and the cervix and vagina become pale and friable.

Problems that can arise as a result of urogenital atrophy include vaginal dryness, urinary stress incontinence, urgency, nocturia, vaginitis, and urinary tract infection (UTI). The woman may find intercourse painful and traumatic, although some type of vaginal lubrication may be helpful. A meta-analysis of studies published between 1969 and 1995 concluded that estrogen therapy is effective in the treatment of symptoms of genitourinary atrophy, including UTI.[5]

Systemically, a woman may experience significant vasomotor instability secondary to the decrease in estrogens and the relative increase in other hormones, including FSH, LH, GnRH, dehydroepiandrosterone, androstenedione, epinephrine, corticotropin, β-endorphin, growth hormone, and calcitonin gene–related peptide. This instability may give rise to "hot flashes," palpitations, dizziness, and headaches as the blood vessels dilate. Despite the association with these biochemical changes, the underlying cause of hot flashes is unknown.[6] Tremendous variation exists in the onset, frequency, severity, and length of time that women experience hot flashes. When they occur at night and are accompanied by significant perspiration, they are referred to as *night sweats*. Insomnia as well as frequent awakening because of vasomotor symptoms can lead to sleep deprivation. A woman may experience irritability, anxiety, and depression as a result of these uncontrollable and unpredictable events.

In addition to changes that closely follow the cessation of ovarian function, there are changes that over many years influence the health and well-being of postmenopausal women. Consequences of long-term estrogen deprivation include osteoporosis due to an imbalance in bone remodeling (*i.e.,* bone resorption occurs at a faster rate than bone formation), and an increased risk for cardiovascular disease (atherosclerosis is accelerated), which is the leading cause of death for women after menopause. Other potential health threats, which reflect both aging and cessation of ovarian function, are loss of vision due to macular degeneration, and cognitive impairment.

Hormone Therapy

Over the past four to five decades, hormone therapy (HT) became increasingly prescribed for postmenopausal women. Initially, hormone therapy was used only for symptom management, and later for prevention of osteoporosis. During the 1990s, hormone therapy evolved to the status of *replacement* for a vital hormone lost due to an endocrine organ failure (menopause). It was routinely offered to all postmenopausal women based on mounting evidence of preventive benefits in numerous areas. During this time, data from observational studies demonstrated a 50% reduction in coronary heart disease (CHD) mortality rates in women using HT.[7,8] Other reported advantages to HT included a reduced risk of Alzheimer disease,[9] decreased risk of colon cancer,[10] less tooth loss,[11] and lower incidence of macular degeneration.[12]

The type of HT prescribed was determined by whether the woman had an intact uterus. Women with an intact uterus received a combination of estrogen and progesterone (EPT), and those who had previously had their uterus removed received estrogen (ET) only. The addition of progesterone to HT was the established protocol for women with an intact uterus because the association between unopposed estrogen and the development of endometrial cancer was noted in the 1970s. Unopposed estrogen can lead to the development of endometrial hyperplasia, which in some cases can increase a woman's risk for endometrial cancer. HT that involves the use of both estrogen and progesterone is not associated with endometrial cancer. When used cyclically (continuous sequential estrogen–progesterone therapy [CSEPT]), progesterone is added for 12 to 14 days to mature any endometrium that has developed in response to the estrogen. Progesterone withdrawal results in endometrial shedding (*i.e.,* a cyclic bleeding episode). When used continuously, a small amount of progesterone is added to the daily estrogen regimen. This continuous exposure to progesterone inhibits endometrial development. Eventually, the combined continuous estrogen–progesterone therapy (CCEPT) results in no bleeding; however, it can be associated with irregular bleeding and spotting until the lining becomes atrophic. Prevention of endometrial hyperplasia either by shedding the endometrial build-up or by preventing its development minimizes the risk of endometrial cancer. This protection must now be considered when weighing the risks and benefits of HT.

Women's Health Initiative and Other Studies. With the current shift to evidence-based medicine, randomized, controlled trials were undertaken to confirm the reported benefits of HT using an experimental model and to demonstrate that the intervention (HT) was in fact responsible for the outcome, and not other variables. Several randomized, controlled trials have now demonstrated that HT does not prevent and can increase the likelihood of a cardiovascular event in women with established heart disease.[13–15] Other studies looking at the effect of HT on cognition and Alzheimer disease have failed to show benefit.[16,17]

The Women's Health Initiative (WHI) was planned as an 8- to 10-year nationwide research effort with an observational study component (93,700 women) and a multicenter, prospective, randomized, double-blind, placebo-controlled clinical trial component (68,000 women) to define the risks and benefits of strategies that could reduce the incidence of heart disease, breast and colorectal cancer, and fractures in postmenopausal women. Between 1993 and 1998, the WHI enrolled 161,809 mostly healthy postmenopausal women (50 to 79 years of age) into a set of clinical trials (trials of low-fat diet, calcium and vitamin D supplementation, and two parallel trials of postmenopausal HT).[15,18]

The two parallel trials of HT were undertaken to determine whether estrogen plus progestin (CCEPT; for women with an intact uterus) or estrogen alone (ET; for women with prior hysterectomy) would reduce the incidence of cardiovascular disease and lead to any change in risk for breast or colorectal cancer in postmenopausal women. A total of 16,608 women with an intact uterus were enrolled in the estrogen plus progestin arm, which was stopped in 2002, after 5.2 years of data analysis, when it was found that the risk of breast cancer crossed the predetermined safety boundary and it was determined that the risks of HT outweighed its benefits. In addition to breast cancer risk, the incidences of CHD, stroke, and venous thromboembolic disease were all increased. On the positive side, there was a reduction in colorectal cancer and hip fractures among the women using HT.[15] The ET-only clinical trial was also stopped prematurely, after 6.8 years.[18] It demonstrated no increased risk of breast cancer or heart disease, but a similar increased risk of stroke and venous thromboembolic disease.

Recent results from a 3-year follow-up study of women in the CCEPT arm of the WHI trial indicate that the increased cardiovascular risks observed at the time the intervention was stopped were not maintained, but a greater risk of fatal and nonfatal malignancies occurred (global risk index was 12% higher in women from the CCEPT group as compared with the placebo group).[19] The follow-up study also found that other effects of CCEPT, such as decreased risk of colorectal cancer and hip fractures, also stopped when therapy ended.[19]

Cardiovascular Risk. Subsequent critical reassessment and subgroup analyses of the WHI, as well as findings from other studies, have led to a reevaluation of some of the conclusions that were made. A complete review of the literature surrounding HT is beyond the scope of this chapter. However, the following summary statements represent some of the current thinking. First, the average age (63.7 years) and length of time since menopause (18 years) have been identified as indications that the women in WHI were already potentially predisposed to CHD and that the WHI may, in truth, have been a secondary prevention trial. Analyses of risk by age[20] and time since menopause[21] in the CCEPT trial reveal that the younger women (younger than 60 years of age) and those who started HT within 10 years of menopause demonstrated a trend toward lower rates of CHD. It has been hypothesized that HT, given during a "critical window" after menopause, may continue the cardioprotective actions provided by premenopausal levels of estrogen. However, when HT is started beyond this window period (when women may already have preexisting subclinical atherosclerosis), it may stimulate

inflammatory cytokines that predispose to atherosclerotic plaque rupture and development of symptomatic CHD.[22] The majority (70%) of the women in the WHI were in the age group that could be expected to have subclinical changes at the start of the study and therefore would be less likely to benefit from HT. Second, newly released data from the Nurses' Health Study[23] suggest that women starting HT near the onset of menopause had a significantly reduced risk (30%) of CHD. Third, a recently published meta-analysis[24] showed a 32% decrease in CHD in younger postmenopausal women. Although there was a reported initial increase in incidence of CHD during the first year in older postmenopausal women (those who started HT after age 60 years), there was a reduced incidence after 2 years. It is still a matter of debate whether the presence of the daily progestin contributed to the higher levels of CHD in the CCEPT group compared with the ET group.

The increased risk of venous thromboembolism does appear to be consistently associated with the use of HT. The absolute risk is low, appears to be greatest in the first 2 years of HT use, and declines thereafter. Women with a history of venous thromboembolism or who have a predisposition to clot formation as a result of coagulation defects such as factor V Leiden are generally advised to avoid the use of HT.

Breast Cancer Risk. The association with breast cancer has long been the other area of concern with HT. In evaluating the many studies reporting estimated risks of breast cancer associated with HT, most of the confidence intervals cross the relative risk of 1 and therefore are not statistically significant.[25] However, new studies linking estrogen and breast cancer continue to make front-page news, and consequently the worry persists. The WHI added to this concern by reporting a 26% increased risk of invasive breast cancer in the women using CCEPT.[16] In actual numbers this represented an additional 8 cases of breast cancer per 10,000 women using HT, a risk lower than that associated with postmenopausal obesity or daily alcohol consumption.[4] Results from a 3-year WHI follow-up study revealed that the breast cancer risk of women who stopped taking CCEPT continued at a rate similar to that observed during the intervention.[19] The use of ET alone did not increase breast cancer risk in the WHI, but it did appear to increase the need for additional follow-up mammograms due to the added density of the breasts in women using estrogen HT.[26]

An update from the Nurses' Health Study showed no increased risk of invasive breast cancer with estrogen HT until 20 years of use.[27] In contrast, another large European study recruited over 1 million women aged 50 to 64 years and analyzed the 80% who were postmenopausal for breast cancer incidence (2.6 years average follow-up) and mortality (4.1 years average follow-up). Approximately half the women had used HT at some time. Results of this observational study revealed increased risk among current users of HT. The largest increase in risk was associated with CCEPT, was slightly less with ET, and declined after discontinuation and returned to baseline within 5 years.[28]

Current thinking postulates that these studies may, in fact, constitute detection studies rather than incidence studies, because it is known that breast cancer cells can be present in the body for 8 to 10 years before the cancer can be detected by any currently available means. Estrogen may accelerate the growth of these cells to a point where the cancer can then be detected, which may explain why some studies show a positive correlation between estrogen and breast cancer and others do not. In this case, the increase in breast cancer detection may in fact be a positive outcome because it can be discovered while the cancer is still curable. Mortality studies to date show a lower death rate among women using hormones at the time of breast cancer diagnosis compared with those without HT. At present there is insufficient evidence to support estrogen as the cause (initiator) of breast cancer. Thus, a more reasonable approach may involve identifying predisposing factors for breast cancer and finding better ways for early detection. This would assist women in assessing their own risk–benefit ratio, taking into account their individual circumstances, when making decisions about HT.

Hip Fracture and Other Risks. The release of data from the other two clinical trials within the WHI (low-fat dietary patterns, calcium and vitamin D supplementation) has challenged conventional wisdom in other areas. The use of calcium (1000 mg/day) plus vitamin D (200 IU/day) was shown to result in a small but significant improvement in hip bone density, but failed to reduce the risk of hip fractures. Women using the supplements did have a slightly increased risk of kidney stones.[29] In addition, following a diet that is low in fat and plentiful in fruits, vegetables, and grains did not make a significant difference in the incidence of breast cancer, colorectal cancer, or heart disease.[30–32] Interestingly, there have been no sweeping recommendations for postmenopausal women regarding the discontinuation of calcium/vitamin D supplements or moving away from dietary modifications despite the lack of evidence to indicate effectiveness.

Current Recommendations. Although the average age of menopause has not changed substantially since 1900, life expectancy has increased dramatically. Today, the average woman will live almost one third of her life after menopause. Menopause now represents only the end of reproductive capability. Estrogen's role in many other bodily functions has been well documented, but its replacement after the ovary ceases production has become highly controversial. Although the U.S. Preventive Services Task Force has recommended against the routine use of HT for preventing chronic conditions in general,[33] statements from the North American Menopause Society (NAMS),[34] the American Society for Reproductive Medicine (ASRM),[35] the American College of Obstetricians and Gynecologists (ACOG),[36] and the National Institutes of Health (NIH) State-of-the-Science Conference Statement on Management of Menopause-Related Symptoms[37] all indicate that estrogen is the most consistently effective therapy for treating menopausal symptoms. Use of HT in younger, recently menopausal women appears less likely to result in the increased risks reported in the WHI and Heart and Estrogen/Progestin Replacement Study (HERS), which studied predominantly older, asymp-tomatic women who were on average 10 or more years beyond menopause.

Current recommendations for HT, in light of the findings of the WHI and other clinical trials, are to avoid HT for primary or secondary prevention of CHD; develop an individual risk profile for every woman contemplating HT and provide information regarding known risks; use HT only in those women who require relief from menopausal symptoms that affect quality of life; consider lower-than-standard doses and alternative routes of administration; limit the use of HT to the shortest duration consistent with goals, benefits, and risks of treatment for each woman; and because of the potential risks associated with HT products that are FDA-approved for the prevention of postmenopausal osteoporosis, consider alternative therapies if the woman is not symptomatic.[37]

The results of the WHI have also stimulated increased interest in alternative methods for management of postmenopausal symptoms, including the use of bio-identical hormones. Bio-identical hormone therapy uses "natural" substances derived from plant oils that are similar in structure to human steroid hormones,[38] and "phytoestrogens," substances occurring in nature with estrogen-like properties such as isoflavones (soy, red clover). To date, these agents, although widely used, have not demonstrated effectiveness in controlled trials.

Because the risk of osteoporosis remains high, there is a continued search for methods to prevent or decrease the rate of bone loss in postmenopausal women. At present, therapies with demonstrated effectiveness in treating osteoporosis include bisphosphonates, calcitonin, raloxifene (a selective estrogen receptor modulator [SERM] that works only on certain estrogen receptors, but not others), calcium, fluoride, and parathyroid hormone (see Chapter 59).

IN SUMMARY, between the menarche and menopause, the female reproductive system undergoes cyclic changes called the *menstrual cycle*. The normal menstrual cycle results from complex interactions among the hypothalamus, which produces GnRH; the anterior pituitary gland, which synthesizes and releases FSH, LH, and prolactin; the ovaries, which synthesize and release estrogens, progesterone, and androgens; and associated target tissues, such as the endometrium and the vaginal mucosa. Although each component of the system is essential for normal functioning, the ovarian hormones are largely responsible for controlling the cyclic changes and length of the menstrual cycle. Estrogens are necessary for normal female physical maturation, for growth of ovarian follicles, for generation of a climate that is favorable to fertilization and implantation of the ovum, and for promoting the development of the endometrium in the event of pregnancy. Estrogens also have a number of extragenital effects, including prevention of bone resorption and regulation of the composition of cholesterol-carrying lipoproteins (HDL and LDL) in the blood. The functions of progesterone include the glandular development of the lobular and alveolar tissue of the breasts, the cyclic glandular development of the endometrium, and maintenance of pregnancy. Androgens contribute to hair distribution in the female and may have important metabolic effects.

Menopause is the cessation of menstrual cycles. Systemically, a woman may experience significant vasomotor instability and "hot flashes" secondary to the decrease in estrogens and the relative increase in other hormones, including FSH, LH, GnRH, dehydroepiandrosterone, and androstenedione. The long-term effects of estrogen deprivation include osteoporosis due to an imbalance in bone remodeling (*i.e.,* bone resorption occurs at a faster rate than bone formation) and an increased risk for cardiovascular disease (atherosclerosis is accelerated), which is the leading cause of death in women after menopause. Hormone therapy, which was regarded as a hormone replacement therapy for postmenopausal women during the late 20th century, has come under scrutiny as a result of the WHI, which indicates that CCEPT (continuous-combined estrogen and progestin) may increase the risk for cardiovascular disease and breast cancer. ■

BREASTS

After completing this section of the chapter, you should be able to meet the following objectives:

- Describe the anatomy of the female breast.
- Describe the influence of hormones on breast development.
- Characterize the changes in breast structure that occur with pregnancy and lactation.

Although anatomically separate, the breasts are functionally related to the female genitourinary system in that they res-

pond to the cyclic changes in sex hormones and produce milk for infant nourishment. The breasts also are important for their sexual function and for cosmetic appearance. Breast cancer represents the most common malignancy among women in the United States. The high rate of breast cancer has drawn even greater attention to the importance of the breasts throughout the life span.

Structure and Function

The breasts, or mammary tissues, are located between the third and seventh ribs of the anterior chest wall and are supported by the pectoral muscles and superficial fascia. They are specialized glandular structures that have an abundant shared nervous, vascular, and lymphatic supply (Fig. 45-8). What are commonly called "breasts" are two parts of a single anatomic breast. This contiguous nature of breast tissue is important in health and illness. Men and women alike are born with rudimentary breast tissue, with the ducts lined with epithelium. In women, the pituitary release of FSH, LH, and prolactin at puberty stimulates the ovary to produce and release estrogen. This estrogen stimulates the growth and proliferation of the ductile system. With the onset of ovulatory cycles, progesterone release stimulates the growth and development of ductile and alveolar secretory epithelium. By adolescence, the breasts have developed characteristic fat deposition patterns and contours.

Structurally, the breast consists of fat, fibrous connective tissue, and glandular tissue. The superficial fibrous connective tissue is attached to the skin, a fact that is important in the visual observation of skin movement over the breast during breast self-examination. The breast mass is supported by the fascia of the pectoralis major and minor muscles and by the fibrous connective tissue of the breast. Fibrous tissue ligaments, called *Cooper ligaments,* extend from the outer boundaries of the breast to the nipple area in a radial manner, like the spokes on a wheel (see Fig. 45-8). These ligaments further support the

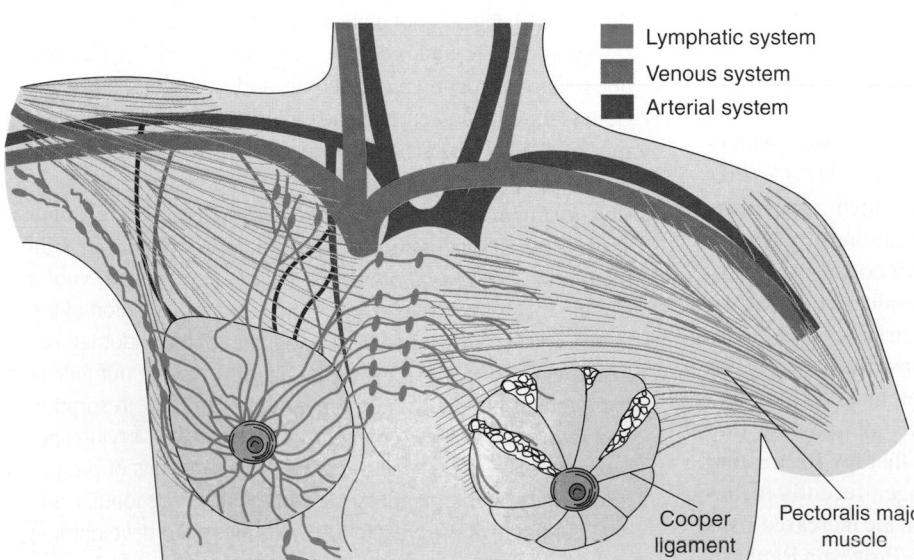

Lymphatic system
Venous system
Arterial system

Cooper ligament

Pectoralis major muscle

FIGURE 45-8 • The breasts, showing the shared vascular and lymphatic supply as well as the pectoral muscles.

breast and form septa that divide the breast into 15 to 25 lobes. Each lobe consists of grapelike clusters—alveoli or glands—that are interconnected by ducts. The alveoli are lined with secretory cells capable of producing milk or fluid under the proper hormonal conditions (Fig. 45-9). The route of descent of milk and other breast secretions is from alveoli to duct, to intralobar duct, to lactiferous duct and reservoir, to nipple. Breast milk is produced secondary to complex hormonal changes associated with pregnancy. Fluid is produced and reabsorbed during the menstrual cycle. The breasts respond to the cyclic changes in the menstrual cycle with fullness and discomfort.

The nipple is made up of epithelial, glandular, erectile, and nervous tissue. Areolar tissue surrounds the nipple and is recognized as the darker, smooth skin between the nipple and the breast. The small bumps or projections on the areolar surface known as *Montgomery tubercles* are sebaceous glands that keep the nipple area soft and elastic. At puberty and during pregnancy, increased levels of estrogen and progesterone cause the areola and nipple to become darker and more prominent and the Montgomery glands to become more active. The erectile tissue of the nipple is responsive to psychological and tactile stimuli, which contributes to the sexual function of the breasts.

There are many individual variations in breast size and shape. The shape and texture vary with hormonal, genetic, nutritional, and endocrine factors and with muscle tone, age, and pregnancy. A well-developed set of pectoralis muscles supports the breast mass higher on the chest wall. Poor posture, significant weight loss, and lack of support may cause the breasts to droop.

Pregnancy

During pregnancy, the breasts are significantly altered by increased levels of estrogen and progesterone. Estrogen stimulates increased vascularity of the breasts and the growth and extension of the ductile structures, causing "heaviness" of the breasts. Progesterone causes marked budding and growth of the alveolar structures. The alveolar epithelium assumes a secretory state in preparation for lactation. The progesterone-induced changes that occur during pregnancy may confer some protection against cancer. Cellular changes that occur in the alveolar lining are thought to change the susceptibility of these cells to estrogen-mediated changes later in life.

Lactation

During lactation, milk is secreted by alveolar cells, which are under the influence of the anterior pituitary hormone prolactin. Milk ejection from the ductile system occurs in response to the release of oxytocin from the posterior pituitary. The suckling of the infant provides the stimulus for milk ejection. Suckling produces feedback to the hypothalamus, stimulating the release of oxytocin from the posterior pituitary. Oxytocin causes contraction of the myoepithelial cells lining the alveoli and ejection of milk into the ductal system. A woman may have breast leakage for 3 months to 1 year after the termination of breast-feeding as breast tissue and hormones regress to the nonlactating state. Overzealous breast stimulation with or without pregnancy can likewise cause breast leakage.

IN SUMMARY, the breast is a complex structure of variable size, consistency, and composition. Although anatomically distinct, the breasts are functionally related to the female genitourinary system in that they respond to cyclic changes in sex hormones and produce milk for infant nourishment. ■

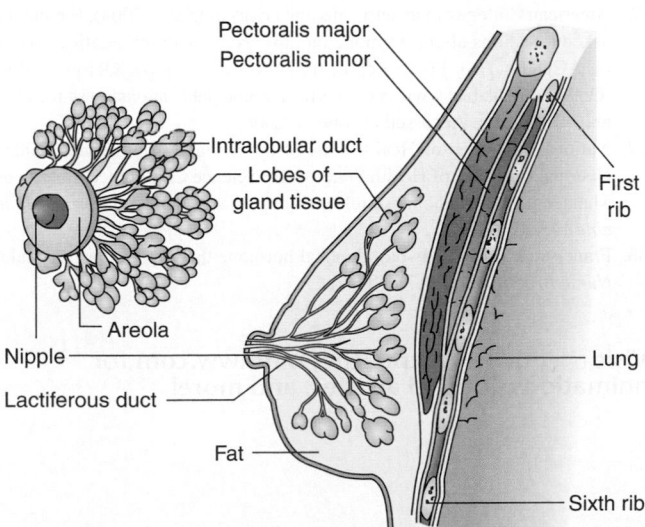

FIGURE 45-9 • The breast, showing the glandular tissue and ducts of the mammary glands.

Labels: Pectoralis major; Pectoralis minor; Intralobular duct; Lobes of gland tissue; First rib; Areola; Nipple; Lactiferous duct; Fat; Lung; Sixth rib

Review Exercises

1. Diabetes mellitus and treatment with broad-spectrum antibiotics increase the risk of vaginal infections.

   A. *Explain how these two conditions change the vaginal ecology, making it more susceptible to infection.*

2. Most oral contraceptive agents use low doses of estrogen and progestin to prevent conception.

   A. *Use Figure 45-4 to explain how these oral agents prevent ovulation and pregnancy.*

References

1. Pernoll M. L. (2001). *Benson and Pernoll's handbook of obstetrics and gynecology* (10th ed., p. 31). New York: McGraw-Hill.
2. Revelli A., Massobrio M., Tesarik J. (1998). Nongenomic actions of steroid hormones in reproductive tissue. *Endocrine Review* 19, 3–17.
3. Gruber C. J., Tschugguel W., Schneeberger C., et al. (2002). Production and actions of estrogens. *New England Journal of Medicine* 346, 340–352.

4. Speroff L. (2005). *Menopause: Guidelines for contemporary management* (pp. 83, 93). Montvale, NJ: Advastar Communications.

5. Maloney C. (2002). Estrogen and recurrent UTI in postmenopausal women. *American Journal of Nursing* 102(8), 47–52.

6. Dormire S. L. (2003). What we know about managing menopausal hot flashes: Navigating without a compass. *Journal of Obstetric, Gynecologic, and Neonatal Nursing* 32, 455–464.

7. Grodstein F., Manson J. E., Colditz G. A., et. al. (2000). A prospective, observational study of postmenopausal hormone therapy and primary prevention of cardiovascular disease. *Annals of Internal Medicine* 133, 933–941.

8. Speroff L., Fritz M. A. (2005). *Clinical gynecologic endocrinology and infertility* (7th ed., p. 724). Philadelphia: Lippincott Williams & Wilkins.

9. Seifer D. B., Kennard E. A. (1999). *Menopause: Endocrinology and management* (p. 100). Totowa, NJ: Humana Press.

10. Nanda K., Bostoc L. A., Hasselblad V., et al. (1999). Hormone replacement therapy and the risk of colorectal cancer: A meta-analysis. *Obstetrics and Gynecology* 93, 880–888.

11. Grodstein F., Colditz G. A., Stampfer M. J. (1996). Postmenopausal hormone use and tooth loss: A prospective study. *Journal of the American Dental Association* 127, 370–377.

12. The Eye Disease Case Control Study Group. (1992). Risk factors for neurovascular age-related macular degeneration. *Archives of Ophthalmology* 110, 1701–1708.

13. Hulley S., Grady D., Bush T., et al. (1998). Randomized trial of estrogen plus progestin for secondary prevention of coronary heart disease in postmenopausal women: Heart and Estrogen/Progestin Replacement Study (HERS) Research Group. *Journal of the American Medical Association* 280, 605–613.

14. Grady D., Herrington D., Bittner V., et al. (2002). Cardiovascular disease outcomes during 6.8 years of hormone therapy: Heart and Estrogen/Progestin Replacement Study Follow-up (HERS-II). *Journal of the American Medical Association* 288, 49–57.

15. Writing Group for the Women's Health Initiative Investigators. (2002). Risks and benefits of estrogen and progestin in healthy postmenopausal women: Principal results from the Women's Health Initiative randomized controlled trial. *Journal of the American Medical Association* 288, 321–333.

16. Grady D., Yaffe K., Kristof M., et al. (2002). Effect of postmenopausal hormone therapy on cognitive function: The Heart and Estrogen/Progestin Replacement Study. *American Journal of Medicine* 113, 543–548.

17. Mulnard R. A., Cotman C. W., Kawas C., et al. (2000). Estrogen replacement therapy for treatment of mild to moderate Alzheimer disease: A randomized controlled trial. Alzheimer Disease Cooperative Study. *Journal of the American Medical Association* 283, 1007–1015.

18. Anderson G. L., Limacher M., Assaf A. R., et al., The Women's Health Initiative Steering Committee. (2004). Effects of conjugated equine estrogen in postmenopausal women with hysterectomy. The Women's Heath Initiative randomized controlled trial. *Journal of the American Medical Association* 291, 1701–1712.

19. Heiss G., Wallace R., Anderson G. L. (2008). Health risks and benefits 3 years after stopping randomized treatment with estrogen and progestin. *JAMA* 299(9), 1036–1044.

20. Hsia J., Langer R. D., Manson J. E., et al. (2006). Conjugated equine estrogens and coronary heart disease: The Women's Health Initiative. *Archives of Internal Medicine* 166, 357–365.

21. Manson J. E., Hsia J., Johnson K. C., et al. (2003). Estrogen plus progestin and the risk of coronary heart disease. *New England Journal of Medicine* 349, 523–534.

22. Karas R. H., Clarkson T. B. (2003). Considerations in interpreting the cardiovascular effects of hormone replacement therapy observed in the WHI: Timing is everything. *Menopausal Medicine* 10, 8–12.

23. Grodstein F., Manson J. E., Stampfer M. J. (2006). Hormone therapy and coronary heart disease: The role of time since menopause and age at hormone initiation. *Journal of Women's Health* 15, 35–44.

24. Salpeter S. R., Walsh J. M. E., Greyber E., et al. (2006). Coronary heart disease events associated with hormone therapy in younger and older women: A meta-analysis. *Journal of General Internal Medicine* 21, 363–366.

25. Speroff L. (2000). Postmenopausal estrogen-progestin therapy and breast cancer: A clinical response to an epidemiologic report. *Contemporary Obstetrics/Gynecology* 3, 103–121.

26. Stefaniak M. L., Anderson G. L., Margolis K. L., et al. (2006). Effects of conjugated equine estrogens on breast cancer and mammography screening in postmenopausal women with hysterectomy. *Journal of the American Medical Association* 195, 1647–1657.

27. Chen W. Y., Manson J. E., Hankinson S. E., et al. (2006). Unopposed estrogen therapy and the risk of invasive breast cancer. *Archives of Internal Medicine* 166, 1027–1032.

28. Beral V. (2003). Current combined HRT use doubles risk of breast cancer. *Lancet* 362, 419–427.

29. Jackson R. D., LaCroix A. Z., Gass M., et al. (2006). Calcium and vitamin D supplementation and the risk of fracture. *New England Journal of Medicine* 364, 669–683.

30. Prentice R. L., Caan B., Chlebowski R. T., et al. (2006). Low-fat dietary pattern and risk of invasive breast cancer. *Journal of the American Medical Association* 295, 629–642.

31. Beresford S. A. A., Johnson K. C., Ritenbaugh C., et al. (2006). Low-fat dietary pattern and risk of colorectal cancer. *Journal of the American Medical Association* 295, 643–654.

32. Howard B. V., VanHorn L., Hsai J., et al. (2006). Low-fat dietary pattern and risk of cardiovascular disease. *Journal of the American Medical Association* 295, 655–666.

33. U.S. Preventive Services Task Force. (2003). Postmenopausal hormone replacement therapy for the primary prevention of chronic conditions: Recommendations and rationale. *American Journal of Nursing* 103, 83–91.

34. North American Menopause Society. (2004). Recommendations for estrogen and progesterone use in peri- and postmenopausal women: October 2004 position statement of the North American Menopause Society. *Menopause* 11, 589–600.

35. American Society of Reproductive Medicine Practice Committee. (2006). American Society for Reproductive Medicine Practice Committee opinion on estrogen and progesterone therapy in postmenopausal women. *Fertility & Sterility* 86(Suppl 4), S75–S88.

36. American College of Obstetricians and Gynecologists. (2004). Frequently asked questions about hormone therapy: New recommendations based on ACOG's Task Force Report on Hormone Therapy. October 2004. [Online.] Available: www.acog.org/from-home/publications/press-releases/nr10-01-04.cfm. Accessed October 4, 2006.

37. National Institutes of Health State-of-the-Science Conference. (2005). National Institutes of Health State-of-the-Science Conference Statement: Management of menopause-related symptoms. *Annals of Internal Medicine* 142, 1003–1013.

38. Francisco L. (2003). Is bio-identical hormone therapy fact or fairy tale? *Nurse Practitioner* 28(7), 39–47.

Visit the**Point** **http://thePoint.lww.com for animations, journal articles, and more!**

Disorders of the Female Reproductive System

PATRICIA McCOWEN MEHRING

➤ Disorders of the female genitourinary system have widespread effects on physical and psychological function, including general health status, sexuality, and reproductive potential. The reproductive structures are located close to other pelvic structures, particularly those of the urinary system, and disorders of the reproductive system may affect urinary function. This chapter focuses on infection and inflammation, benign conditions, and neoplasms of the female reproductive structures; disorders of pelvic support and uterine position; and alterations in menstruation. An overview of infertility also is included.

DISORDERS OF THE EXTERNAL GENITALIA AND VAGINA

After completing this section of the chapter, you should be able to meet the following objectives:

■ Compare the abnormalities associated with Bartholin cyst, non-neoplastic epithelial disorders, vulvodynia, and cancer of the vulva.
■ State the role of Döderlein bacilli in maintaining the normal ecology of the vagina.

(objectives continue)

■ Describe the conditions that predispose to vaginal infections and the methods used to prevent and treat these infections.

Disorders of the External Genitalia

Diseases of the external genitalia are similar to those that affect hair-bearing skin elsewhere in the body. Most skin cysts, nevi, and malignant neoplasms can occur on the skin of the external genitalia as well as on the skin in other parts of the body. The vulva is particularly prone to skin infections because it is constantly exposed to secretions and moisture. Nonspecific vulvitis is particularly common in women with diabetes, chronic kidney disease, blood dyscrasias, and malnutrition.

Bartholin Gland Cyst and Abscess

A Bartholin gland cyst is a fluid-filled sac that results from occlusion of the duct system in the Bartholin gland (Fig. 46-1). If the cyst becomes infected, an abscess may develop in the gland. Bartholin gland abscesses were formerly associated with gonorrhea, but are now more commonly caused by staphylococcal, chlamydial, and anaerobic infections.[1]

Acute symptoms are usually the result of infection and include pain, tenderness, and dyspareunia. The treatment of symptomatic cysts consists of the administration of appro-

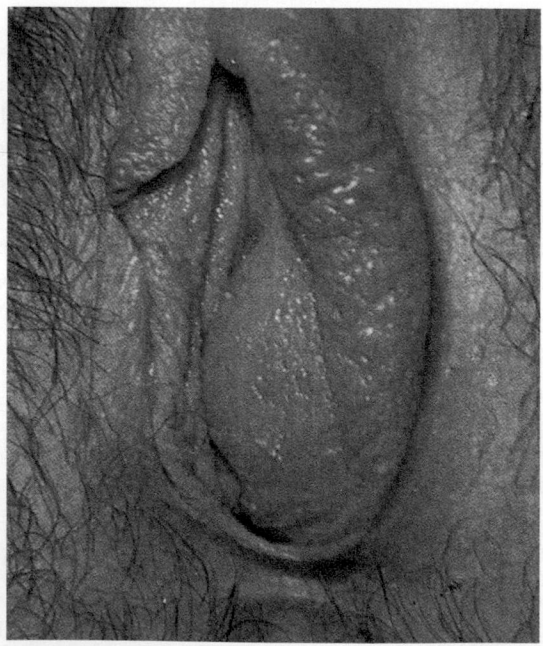

FIGURE 46-1 • Bartholin gland cyst. The 4-cm lesion is located to the right of and posterior to the vaginal introitus. (From Robboy S. J., Kurman R. J., Merino M. J. [2005]. The female reproductive system. In Rubin E., Gorstein F., Rubin R., et al. [Eds.], *Rubin's pathology: Clinicopathologic foundations of medicine* [4th ed., p. 935]. Philadelphia: Lippincott Williams & Wilkins.)

priate antibiotics, local application of moist heat, and incision and drainage. Cysts that frequently are abscessed or are large enough to cause blockage of the introitus may require surgical intervention (*i.e.,* marsupialization, a procedure that involves removal of a wedge of vulvar skin and the cyst wall).[1] Because the Bartholin glands usually shrink during menopause, a vulvar growth in postmenopausal women should be evaluated for malignancy.

Non-neoplastic Epithelial Disorders

The term *non-neoplastic epithelial disorders* refers to non-malignant atrophic and hyperplastic changes of the vulvar skin and mucosa.[2] The condition, commonly referred to as *leukoplakia,* presents as white lesions of the vulva. Itching is the most common symptom, and dyspareunia (painful intercourse) is common. Depending on clinical and histologic characteristics, the lesions can be further categorized as lichen simplex chronicus, lichen sclerosus, or other dermatoses such as psoriasis or chronic dermatitis.

Lichen simplex chronicus, or *chronic dermatitis,* presents as thickened, gray-white plaques with an irregular surface. Presumed to be a response of the genital skin to some type of irritant, this diagnosis is used only when human papillomavirus (HPV) infection, fungal infections, or other known causative conditions have been excluded.[3] Pruritus is the most common presenting complaint. Scaling is generally present, and excoriations due to recent scratching can often be seen.

Lichen sclerosus is an inflammatory disease of the vulva characterized by plaquelike areas that may progress to parchment-thin epithelium with focal areas of ecchymosis and superficial ulceration secondary to scratching. Atrophy and contracture of the vulvar tissues with eventual stenosis of the introitus are common when this condition becomes chronic. Itching is common and dyspareunia is frequent. The condition develops insidiously and is progressive.

Current treatment measures for lichen sclerosus favor the use of potent topical corticosteroids.[3] Hyperplastic areas respond well to a combination corticosteroid (betamethasone) and antipruritic cream (crotamiton). Lichen sclerosus frequently recurs, and lifetime maintenance therapy may be required. Hyperplastic areas that occur in the field of lichen sclerosus may be sites of malignant change and warrant close follow-up and possible biopsy.

Vulvodynia

Vulvodynia is a syndrome of unexplained vulvar pain, previously referred to as *vulvar pain syndrome* or *burning vulva syndrome.* The terminology and diagnostic criteria used for this chronic disorder remain in flux, but the most recent classification system of the International Society for the Study of Vulvovaginal Disorders (ISSVD) defines it as a condition characterized by "burning, stinging, irritation, soreness or rawness in the absence of relevant visible findings or a specific, clinically identifiable, neurological disorder."[4] Vulvodynia is further classified as localized or generalized, and as to whether it is provoked, unprovoked, or of mixed origin.

Localized vulvodynia or *vestibulodynia,* formerly referred to as *vulvar vestibulitis syndrome,* is characterized by pain at onset of intercourse (*i.e.,* insertional dyspareunia), localized point tenderness near the vaginal opening, and sensitivity to tampon placement, tight-fitting pants, bicycling, or prolonged sitting. It is the leading cause of dyspareunia in women younger than 50 years of age. The pain can be primary (present from first contact) or secondary (developing after a period of comfortable sexual relations). The etiology is unknown, but the problem may evolve from chronic vulvar inflammation or trauma. Nerve fibers that supply the vestibular epithelium may become highly sensitized, causing neurons in the dorsal horn of the spinal cord to respond abnormally, thus transforming the sensation of touch in the vestibule into pain (allodynia).[5] Surgical vestibulectomy may be necessary for symptom relief when medical management fails.

Generalized vulvodynia, formerly called *vulvar dysesthesia* or *essential vulvodynia,* involves severe, constant, widespread burning that interferes with daily activities. No abnormalities are found on examination, but there is diffuse and variable hypersensitivity and altered sensation to light touch. The quality of this unprovoked pain shares many of the features of other neuropathic pain disorders, particularly complex regional pain syndrome (see Chapter 49) or pudendal neuralgia. Although the cause of the neuropathic pain is unknown, it has been suggested that it may result from myofascial restrictions affecting the sacral and pelvic floor nerves. Surface electromyography-assisted pelvic floor muscle rehabilitation has been shown to be an effective primary therapy or adjunct to medical or surgical therapy for generalized vulvodynia.[4,5]

There are many proposed triggers for vulvodynia, including chronic recurrent vaginal infections; chemical irritation or drug effects, especially prolonged use of topical steroid creams; the irritating effects of elevated urinary levels of calcium oxalate; and immunoglobulin A deficiency or other disorders of immune regulation.[4,5] Often it is multifactorial in origin.

Careful history taking and physical assessment are essential for differential diagnosis and treatment. *Vulvodynia* is a diagnosis of exclusion after ruling out infections, such as candidiasis and genital herpes; inflammatory conditions, such as lichen simplex chronicus and lichen sclerosus; vulvar cancer; or neurologic disorders, such as herpes neuralgia or spinal nerve compression, as causes for the pain.

Treatment for this chronic, often debilitating problem is aimed at symptom relief, is frequently long term, and often needs to be managed from a multidimensional, chronic pain perspective.[4,5] Regimens can include long-term vaginal or oral antifungal therapy, avoidance of potential irritants, sitz baths with baking soda, emollients such as vitamin E or vegetable oil for lubrication, a low-oxalate diet plus calcium citrate supplements (calcium binds oxalate in the bowel and citrate inhibits the formation of oxalate crystals), anesthetic or steroid ointments, capsaicin cream (topical analgesic), physical therapy, and surgery. Oral medications, including tricyclic antidepressants,

other antidepressants (*e.g.,* selective serotonin receptor uptake inhibitors [SSRIs]), or gabapentin (an antiepileptic drug), are often used to treat the neuropathic pain associated with vulvodynia. Because this condition can cause strain in sexual, family, and work relationships, psychosocial support often is needed.

Cancer of the Vulva

Carcinoma of the vulva accounts for approximately 4% of all cancers of the female genitourinary system in the United States, occurring most often in women 50 years of age or older.[6] Approximately 90% of vulvar malignancies are squamous cell carcinomas, meaning they begin in squamous cells, the main type of skin cell.[7] Less common forms of vulvar cancer are malignant melanomas, adenocarcinoma, and basal cell carcinoma.[6]

🔑 GYNECOLOGIC CANCERS

- Cancers of the vulva, cervix, endometrium, and ovaries represent a spectrum of malignancies.

- Cancers of the vulva and cervix are mainly squamous cell carcinomas. Certain types of sexually transmitted human papillomaviruses are risk factors for cervical intraepithelial neoplasia, which can be a precursor lesion of invasive carcinoma.

- Endometrial cancers, which are seen most frequently in women 55 to 65 years of age, are strongly associated with conditions that produce excessive estrogen stimulation and endometrial hyperplasia.

- Ovarian cancer is the second most common female cancer and the most lethal. The most significant risk factors for ovarian cancer are the length of time that a woman's ovarian cycles are not suppressed by pregnancy, lactation, or oral contraceptive use, and family history.

In terms of etiology, pathogenesis, and clinical presentation, vulvar carcinoma can be divided into two general groups. The first group is associated with vulvar intraepithelial neoplasia (VIN), a precursor lesion of squamous cell carcinoma. One third to one half of VIN cases appear to be caused by the cancer-promoting potential of certain strains (subtypes 16 and 18) of HPV that are sexually transmitted and are associated with the type of vulvar cancer found in younger women (*i.e.,* younger than 40 years of age).[6] VIN lesions may take many forms. They may be singular or multicentric; macular or papular; red or white and plaquelike. VIN frequently is multicentric, and 10% to 30% of cases are associated with another squamous neoplasm in the vagina and cervix.[2] Microscopically, VIN presents as a proliferative process, characterized by epithelial cells with atypical nuclei, increased mitosis, and lack of surface differentiation. The same system that is used for grading cervical cancer is used for vulvar cancer.[2,3] The extent of replacement of epithelial cells by abnormal cells determines the grade of involvement (VIN I, II, or III). Full-thickness replacement (VIN III) is synonymous with carcinoma in situ. Spontaneous resolution of VIN lesions has occurred. The risk of progression to invasive cancer increases in older women and in women with suppressed immune function.

The second form of vulvar cancer, which is seen more often in older women, is generally preceded by vulvar non-neoplastic disorders such as chronic vulvar irritation or lichen sclerosus. The etiology of this group of vulvar cancers is unclear, but they are not typically associated with HPV. Neoplastic changes may arise from lichen sclerosus lesions or hyperplasia, leading directly to invasion, or through an intermediate step involving cellular atypia.[6]

The initial lesion of squamous cell vulvar carcinoma may appear as an inconspicuous thickening of the skin, a small raised area or lump, or an ulceration that fails to heal. It may be single or multiple and vary in color from white to velvety red or black. The lesions may resemble eczema or dermatitis and may produce few symptoms other than pruritus, local discomfort, and exudation. The symptoms frequently are treated with various home remedies before medical treatment is sought. The lesion may become secondarily infected, causing pain and discomfort. The malignant lesion gradually spreads superficially or as a deep furrow involving all of one labial side. Because there are many lymph channels around the vulva, the cancer metastasizes freely to the regional lymph nodes. The most common extension is to the superficial inguinal, deep femoral, and external iliac lymph nodes.[8]

Early diagnosis is important in the treatment of vulvar carcinoma. Because malignant lesions can vary in appearance and commonly are mistaken for other conditions, biopsy and treatment often are delayed. Any vulvar lesion that is increasing in size or has an unusual wartlike appearance should be biopsied.[8] Treatment is primarily wide surgical excision of the lesion for noninvasive cancer and radical excision or vulvectomy with node resection for invasive cancer. Postoperative groin and pelvic radiation is recommended when groin lymph nodes are involved. Nonsurgical treatment options such as photodynamic therapy or topical immunotherapy are currently under investigation for patients with early-stage vulvar cancer.[8] The 5-year survival rate for women with lesions less than 2 cm in diameter and minimal node involvement (stage I) is approximately 93% to 96% after surgical treatment.[6]

Disorders of the Vagina

The normal vaginal ecology depends on the delicate balance of hormones and bacterial flora. Normal estrogen levels maintain a thick, protective squamous epithelium that contains glycogen. Döderlein bacilli, part of the normal vaginal flora, metabolize glycogen, and in the process produce the lactic acid that normally maintains the vaginal pH of 3.8 to 4.5.[9] Disruptions in these normal environmental conditions predispose to infection.

Vaginitis

Vaginitis represents an inflammation of the vagina that is characterized by vaginal discharge and burning, itching, redness, and swelling of vaginal tissues. Pain often occurs with urination and sexual intercourse. Vaginitis may be caused by chemical irritants, foreign bodies, or infectious agents. The causes of vaginitis differ in various age groups. In premenarchal girls, most vaginal infections have nonspecific causes, such as poor hygiene, intestinal parasites, or the presence of foreign bodies. *Candida albicans, Trichomonas vaginalis,* and bacterial vaginosis are the most common causes of vaginitis in the childbearing years, and some of these organisms can be transmitted sexually[2,3,9] (see Chapter 47).

In postmenopausal women, atrophic vaginitis is the most common form. Atrophic vaginitis is an inflammation of the vagina that occurs after menopause or removal of the ovaries and their estrogen supply. Estrogen deficiency results in a lack of regenerative growth of the vaginal epithelium, rendering these tissues more susceptible to infection and irritation. Döderlein bacilli disappear, and the vaginal secretions become less acidic. The symptoms of atrophic vaginitis include itching, burning, and painful intercourse. These symptoms usually can be reversed by local application of estrogen.[2,3]

Every woman normally experiences vaginal discharge during the menstrual cycle, but it should not cause burning or itching or have an unpleasant odor. These symptoms suggest inflammation or infection. Because these symptoms are common to the different types of vaginitis, precise identification of the organism is essential for proper treatment. A careful history should include information about systemic disease conditions, the use of drugs such as antibiotics that foster the growth of yeast, dietary habits, stress, and other factors that alter the resistance of vaginal tissue to infections. A physical examination usually is done to evaluate the nature of the discharge and its effects on the genital structures. Microscopic examination of a saline wet-mount smear (prepared by placing a sample of vaginal mucus in one or two drops of normal saline) is the primary means of identifying the organism responsible for the infection.[9] Culture methods may be needed when the organism is not apparent on the wet-mount preparation.[3]

The prevention and treatment of vaginal infections depend on proper health habits and accurate diagnosis and treatment of ongoing infections (see Chapter 47). Measures to prevent infection include keeping the genital area clean and dry, maintaining normal vaginal flora and healthy vaginal mucosa, and avoiding contact with organisms known to cause vaginal infections. Perfumed products, such as feminine deodorant sprays, douches, bath powders, soaps, and even toilet paper, can be irritating and may alter the normal vaginal flora. Tight clothing prevents the dissipation of body heat and evaporation of skin moisture and promotes favorable conditions for irritation and the growth of pathogens. Cotton undergarments that can withstand hot water and bleach (a fungicide) may be preferable for women to prevent such infections. Avoiding sexual contact whenever an infection is known to exist or suspected should limit that route of transmission.

Cancer of the Vagina

Primary cancers of the vagina are extremely rare, accounting for approximately 1% of all cancers of the female reproductive system.[10] Like vulvar carcinoma, carcinoma of the vagina is largely a disease of older women. Approximately two thirds of women are 60 years of age or older at the time of diagnosis. The exception to that is the clear cell adenocarcinoma associated with diethylstilbestrol (DES) exposure in utero.[11] Vaginal cancers may result from local extension of cervical cancer, from exposure to sexually transmitted HPV, or rarely from local irritation such as occurs with prolonged use of a pessary. Smoking and human immunodeficiency virus (HIV) infection also increase the risk of vaginal cancer.

Approximately 85% to 90% of vaginal cancers are squamous cell carcinomas, with other common types being adenocarcinomas (5% to 10%), sarcomas (2% to 3%), and melanomas (2% to 3%).[10] Squamous cell carcinomas begin in the epithelium and progress over many years from precancerous lesions called *vaginal intraepithelial neoplasia* (VAIN), 65% to 80% of which contain HPV deoxyribonucleic acid (DNA). Maternal ingestion of DES in early pregnancy has been associated with the development of clear cell adenocarcinoma in female offspring who were exposed in utero. Between 1938 and 1971, DES, a nonsteroidal synthetic estrogen, commonly was prescribed to prevent miscarriage.[11] The incidence of clear cell adenocarcinoma of the vagina is low, approximately 0.1%, in young women who were exposed to DES in utero. Although only a small percentage of girls exposed to estrogen actually develop clear cell adenocarcinoma, 75% to 90% of them develop benign adenosis (*i.e.*, ectopic extension of cervical columnar epithelium into the vagina, which normally is stratified squamous epithelium), which may predispose to cancer. Most DES-exposed daughters are now between 40 and 60 years of age, so they are just entering the postmenopausal period when this malignancy develops in women who were not DES-exposed. Because the upper age limit for this type of cancer is unknown, there is no age at which a DES-exposed daughter can be considered risk free.[11]

The most common symptom of vaginal carcinoma is abnormal bleeding. Other signs or symptoms include an abnormal vaginal discharge, a palpable mass, or pain during intercourse. Most women with preinvasive vaginal carcinoma are asymptomatic, with the cancer being discovered during a routine pelvic examination. The anatomic proximity of the vagina to other pelvic structures (urethra, bladder, and rectum) permits early spread to these areas. Pelvic pain, dysuria, and constipation can be associated symptoms.

Since most preinvasive and early invasive cancers are silent, the use of the vaginal cytology (Papanicolaou [Pap] smear) is the most effective way to detect vaginal cancer. Women who have had a hysterectomy performed for reproductive cancer should continue to have vaginal cytologic studies every 3 to 5 years after surgery. Diagnosis requires biopsy of suspect lesions or areas.

Treatment of vaginal cancer must take into consideration the type of cancer, the size, location, and spread of the lesion, and the woman's age. Local excision, laser vaporization, or a loop electrode excision procedure (LEEP) can be considered with stage 0 squamous cell cancers. Radical surgery and radiation therapy are both curative with more advanced cancers. When there is upper vaginal involvement, radical surgery may be required. This includes a total hysterectomy, pelvic lymph node dissection, partial vaginectomy, and placement of a graft from the buttock to the area from which the vagina was excised. Vaginal reconstruction often is possible to allow for sexual intercourse. The ovaries usually are preserved unless they are diseased. Extensive lesions and those located in the middle or lower vaginal area usually are treated by radiation therapy, which can be intracavitary, interstitial, or external beam.

The prognosis depends on the stage of the disease, involvement of lymph nodes, and the degree of mitotic activity of the tumor. With appropriate treatment and follow-up, the 5-year survival rate for squamous cell carcinoma and adenocarcinoma confined to the vagina (stage I) is 73%, whereas it is only 36% for those with extensive spread (stages III and IV).[11]

IN SUMMARY, the surface of the vulva is affected by disorders that affect skin on other parts of the body. Bartholin cysts are the result of occluded ducts in Bartholin glands. They often are painful and can become infected. Non-neoplastic epithelial disorders are characterized by thinning or hyperplastic thickening of vulvar tissues. Vulvodynia is a chronic vulvar pain syndrome with several classifications and variable treatment results. Cancer of the vulva, which accounts for 4% of all female genitourinary cancers, is associated with HPV infections in younger women and lichen sclerosus in older women.

The normal vaginal ecology depends on the delicate balance of hormones and bacterial flora. Disruptions in these normal environmental conditions predispose to vaginal infections. Vaginitis or inflammation of the vagina is characterized by vaginal discharge and burning, itching, redness, and swelling of vaginal tissues. It may be caused by chemical irritants, foreign bodies, or infectious agents. Primary cancers of the vagina are relatively uncommon, accounting for 2% to 3% of all cancers of the female reproductive system. Daughters of women treated with DES to prevent miscarriage are at increased risk for development of adenocarcinoma of the vagina. ■

DISORDERS OF THE CERVIX AND UTERUS

After completing this section of the chapter, you should be able to meet the following objectives:

■ Describe the importance of the cervical transformation zone in the pathogenesis of cervical cancer.
■ Compare the lesions associated with nabothian cysts and cervical polyps.

(objectives continue)

- List the complications of untreated cervicitis.
- Describe the development of cervical cancer from the appearance of atypical cells to the development of invasive cervical cancer and relate to the importance of the Pap smear in early detection of cervical cancer.
- Cite the rationale for describing cervical cancer as a sexually transmitted infection and the rationale for use of the HPV vaccine in prevention of cervical cancer.
- Compare the pathology and manifestations of endometriosis and adenomyosis.
- Cite the major early symptom of endometrial cancer and describe the relationship between unopposed estrogen stimulation of the endometrium and development of endometrial cancer.
- Compare the location and manifestations of intramural and subserosal leiomyomas.

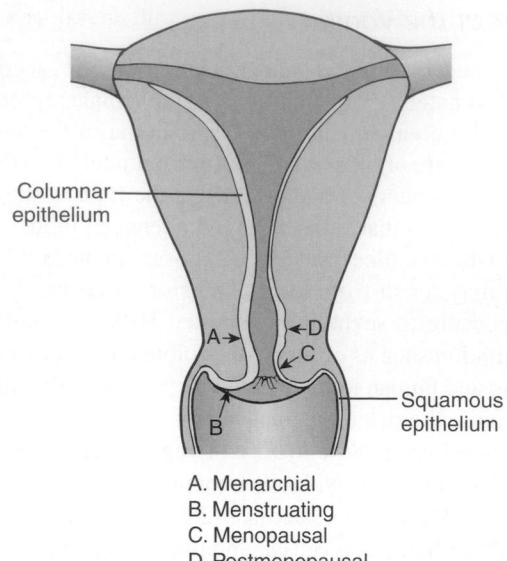

A. Menarchial
B. Menstruating
C. Menopausal
D. Postmenopausal

FIGURE 46-2 • Location of the squamocolumnar junction (transformation zone) in menarchial, menstruating, menopausal, and postmenopausal women.

Disorders of the Uterine Cervix

The cervix is composed of two distinct types of tissue. The exocervix, or visible portion, is covered with stratified squamous epithelium, which also lines the vagina. The endocervix is the canal that leads to the endometrial cavity. It is lined with columnar epithelium that contains large, branched mucus-secreting glands. During each menstrual cycle, the cervical glands undergo important functional changes related to the transport of spermatozoa within the cervical canal. The amount and properties of the mucus secreted by the gland cells vary during the menstrual cycle under the influence of the ovarian hormones. Blockage of the mucosal glands results in trapping of mucus in the deeper glands, leading to the formation of dilated cysts in the cervix called *nabothian cysts*. These are benign cysts that require no treatment unless they become so numerous that they cause cervical enlargement.

The junction of the squamous epithelium of the exocervix and mucus-secreting columnar epithelium of the endocervix (*i.e.,* squamocolumnar junction) appears at various locations on the cervix at different points in a woman's life (Fig. 46-2). During periods of high estrogen production, particularly fetal existence, menarche, and the first pregnancy, the cervix everts or turns outward, exposing the columnar epithelium to the vaginal environment. The combination of estrogen and low vaginal pH leads to a gradual transformation from columnar to squamous epithelium—a process called *metaplasia* (see Chapter 5). The dynamic area of change where metaplasia takes place is called the *transformation zone*.[2,10]

The transformation zone is a critical area for the development of cervical cancer. During metaplasia, the newly developed squamous epithelial cells are vulnerable to development of dysplasia and genetic change if exposed to cancer-producing agents. *Dysplasia* means disordered growth or development (see Chapter 5). Although initially a reversible cell change, untreated dysplasia can develop into carcinoma. The transformation zone is the area of the cervix that must be sampled

to have an adequate Pap smear and the area most carefully examined during colposcopy. Colposcopy is a vaginal examination using an instrument called a *colposcope* that affords a well-lit and magnified stereoscopic view of the cervix. During colposcopy, the cervical tissue may be stained with an iodine solution (*i.e.,* Schiller test) or acetic acid solution to accentuate topographic or vascular changes that can differentiate normal from abnormal tissue. A biopsy sample may be obtained from suspect areas and examined microscopically.

Cervicitis and Cervical Polyps

Cervicitis is an acute or chronic inflammation of the cervix. Acute cervicitis may result from the direct infection of the cervix or may be secondary to a vaginal or uterine infection. It may be caused by a variety of infective agents, including *C. albicans, T. vaginalis, Neisseria gonorrhoeae, Gardnerella vaginalis, Chlamydia trachomatis, Ureaplasma urealyticum,* and herpes simplex virus. *C. trachomatis* is the organism most commonly associated with mucopurulent cervicitis. With acute cervicitis, the cervix becomes reddened and edematous. Irritation from the infection results in copious mucopurulent drainage and leukorrhea. Depending on the causative agent, acute cervicitis is treated with appropriate antibiotic therapy.

Chronic cervicitis represents a low-grade inflammatory process. It is common in parous women and may be a sequela to minute lacerations that occur during childbirth, instrumentation, or other trauma. The organisms usually are nonspecific—often staphylococcal, streptococcal, or coliform bacteria. The symptoms of chronic cervicitis are less well defined than those of acute cervicitis. The cervix may be ulcerated or normal in appearance; it may contain nabothian cysts; the cervical os may be distorted by old lacerations or everted to expose areas of columnar epithelium; and a mucopurulent drainage may be present.

Untreated cervicitis may extend to include the development of pelvic cellulitis, low back pain, dyspareunia, cervical stenosis, dysmenorrhea, and ascending infection of the uterus or fallopian tubes. Diagnosis of chronic cervicitis is based on vaginal examination, colposcopy, cytologic (Pap) smears, and occasionally biopsy to exclude malignant changes. Treatment usually involves cryosurgery or cauterization, which causes the tissues to slough and leads to eradication of the infection. Colposcopically guided laser vaporization of the abnormal epithelium is the newest but most expensive treatment for cervicitis.

Polyps are the most common lesions of the cervix. They can be found in women of all ages, but their incidence is higher during the reproductive years. Polyps are soft, velvety, red lesions; they usually are pedunculated and often are found protruding through the cervical os. They usually develop as a result of inflammatory hyperplasia of the endocervical mucosa. Polyps typically are asymptomatic but may be associated with postcoital bleeding. Most are benign, but they should be removed and examined by a pathologist to exclude the possibility of malignant change.

Cancer of the Cervix

Cervical cancer is readily detected and, if detected early, is the most easily cured of all the cancers of the female reproductive system. According to the American Cancer Society, an estimated 11,150 cases of invasive cervical cancer were diagnosed in the United States in 2007, with approximately 3700 deaths from cervical cancer during the same period.[12] By comparison, there were four times as many new cases of cervical carcinoma in situ (i.e., precancerous lesion) diagnosed, indicating that a large number of potentially invasive cancers are cured by early detection and effective treatment. However, worldwide, the incidence of and mortality associated with cervical cancer are second only to breast cancer, and in parts of the developing world, cervical cancer is the major cause of death in women of reproductive age.[13]

Risk Factors and Pathogenesis. A preponderance of evidence suggests a causal link between HPV infection and cervical cancer. It is rare among celibate women. Risk factors include early age at first intercourse, multiple sexual partners, a promiscuous male partner, smoking, and a history of sexually transmitted infections (STIs). Specific strains of HPV have been associated with cervical cancer versus condylomata or genital warts (see Chapter 47). The strongest link with cervical cancer is with HPV types 16, 18, 31, 33, and 45.[14] Other factors such as smoking, nutrition, and coexisting sexual infections such as C. trachomatis, herpes simplex virus type 2, and HIV may play a contributing role in determining whether a woman with HPV infection develops cervical cancer.[2,14]

A quadrivalent vaccine (Gardisil) to prevent infection with the HPV subtypes 16, 18, 6, and 11 is now available. The vaccine targets the two strains of HPV (HPV 16 and 18) respon-

sible for 70% of cervical cancer, and the two most common benign strains (HPV 6 and 11), which account for up to 90% of genital warts. The target population for the vaccine is females between the ages of 9 and 26 years, optimally before initiation of sexual activity. Clinical studies have confirmed that the vaccine appears safe and effective in inducing long-term immunity to HPV.[15] Although its use in males and older women or those who have already become sexually active has not been studied, it may offer some protection.

Cervical Intraepithelial Neoplasia (Dysplasia of the Cervix). One of the most important advances in the early diagnosis and treatment of cancer of the cervix was made possible by the observation that this cancer arises from precancerous lesions that begin with the development of atypical cervical cells. Atypical cells differ from normal cervical squamous epithelium. There are changes in the nuclear and cytoplasmic parts of the cell and more variation in cell size and shape (i.e., dysplasia). These precancerous changes represent a continuum of morphologic changes with indistinct boundaries that may gradually progress to cancer in situ and then to invasive cancer, or they may spontaneously regress.[2]

A system of grading devised to describe the dysplastic changes of cancer precursors uses the term cervical intraepithelial neoplasia (CIN).[10] This histologic terminology system divides the precursors according to the thickness of cervical epithelial involvement (Table 46-1). Although previously presumed to represent a single progressive disease process, current understanding of the pathogenesis of cervical cancer precursors now suggests two distinct entities: (1) a productive HPV infection that can regress spontaneously (mild dysplasia or CIN 1); and (2) a true neoplastic process confined to the cervical squamous epithelium (CIN 2 or 3). CIN histologic terminology has been largely replaced with cytopathologic terms for these two biologic entities: low-grade squamous intraepithelial lesion (LSIL) and high-grade squamous intraepithelial lesion (HSIL).[2]

Studies of the natural history of cervical cancer precursor lesions have yielded variable rates of progression and regression. Generally, only a small percentage of lesions progress to invasive carcinoma. HSIL has a much greater potential for progressing than does LSIL. De novo development of HSIL has also been demonstrated, challenging the concept that LSIL is always a precursor to HSIL. Cancers of the cervix have a long latent period; untreated dysplasia gradually progresses to carcinoma in situ, which may remain static for 7 to 10 years before it becomes invasive. After the preinvasive period, growth may be rapid, and survival rates decline significantly depending on the extent of disease at the time of diagnosis.[2]

The accepted format for reporting cervical and vaginal cytologic diagnoses, called The Bethesda System (TBS), was developed during a National Cancer Institute Workshop in 1989 and updated in 1991 and 2001 (see Table 46-1). The TBS 2001 terminology includes the following components: specimen type (conventional versus liquid based); specimen adequacy; general

TABLE 46-1 Classification Systems for Papanicolaou Smears

DYSPLASIA/NEOPLASIA	CIN	BETHESDA SYSTEM
Benign	Benign	Negative for intraepithelial lesion or malignancy
Benign with inflammation	Benign with inflammation	Negative for intraepithelial lesion or malignancy, ASC-US
Mild dysplasia	CIN 1	Low-grade SIL, ASC-H
Moderate dysplasia	CIN 2	High-grade SIL
Severe dysplasia and carcinoma in situ (CIS)	CIN 3	High-grade SIL
Invasive cancer	Invasive cancer	Invasive cancer

CIN, cervical intraepithelial neoplasia; SIL, squamous intraepithelial lesion; ASC-US, atypical squamous cells of undetermined significance; ASC-H, cannot rule out high-grade SIL.

Adapted from information in Robboy S. J., Merino M. J., Mutter G. L. (2008). The female reproductive system. In Rubin R., Strayer D. S. (Eds.), *Rubin's pathology: Clinicopathologic foundations of medicine* (5th ed., p. 796). Philadelphia: Lippincott Williams & Wilkins. Solomon D., Davey D., Kurman R., et al., Forum Group Members and Bethesda 2001 Workshop. (2002). The 2001 Bethesda System. *Journal of the American Medical Association* 287(16), 2114–2119.

categorization (negative for intraepithelial lesion or malignancy versus epithelial cell abnormality); and interpretation/result.[16]

The atypical cellular changes that precede frank neoplastic changes consistent with cancer of the cervix can be recognized by a number of direct and microscopic techniques, including the Pap smear, colposcopy, and cervicography. Currently, Pap smears are used for cervical cancer screening. After an extensive review of the literature, the American Cancer Society in late 2002 released revised guidelines for cervical cancer screening[13] (Chart 46-1). The U.S. Preventive Services Task Force

CHART 46-1   GUIDELINES FOR CERVICAL CANCER SCREENING USING THE PAPANICOLAOU (PAP) SMEAR

• Screening should begin 3 years after first vaginal intercourse or after age 21, whichever comes first.
• Women 30 years of age and older may be screened at longer intervals after three consecutive normal/negative cytology results.
• Screening may be discontinued in women aged 65 years and older if they had adequate screening with normal Pap smears and are not otherwise at increased risk for cervical cancer.
• Women who have had a total hysterectomy with removal of the cervix do not need screening unless the surgery was performed to treat cervical cancer or a precancerous condition.
• If a woman has risk factors, such as HPV infection, DES exposure in utero, or strong family history of cervical cancer, more frequent Pap smears may be recommended.

Adapted from Smith R.A., Cokkinides V., von Eschenbach A.C., et al. (2002). American Cancer Society guideline for early detection of cervical neoplasia and cancer. *CA: A Cancer Journal for Clinicians* 52(1), 8–22; U.S. Preventive Services Task Force. (2002). Recommendations for Screening for Cervical Cancer. [Online.] Available: http://www.AHRQ.gov.

(USPSTF) screening guidelines were also updated in 2002.[17] Although many clinicians and women themselves are reluctant to move away from yearly Pap smears, the evidence about the natural progression of cervical cancer supports the position that the updated guidelines present a more cost-effective approach to screening.

It has been estimated that approximately 20% of women with intraepithelial lesions have normal Pap smear results, indicating that care must be taken to obtain an adequate smear from the transformation zone that includes endocervical cells and ensuring that the cytologic examination is done by a competent laboratory.[18] New techniques of specimen collection, slide preparation and processing, and computer-assisted evaluation of Pap smears are being evaluated and offer hope of improved accuracy in diagnosis of precancerous cervical changes. HPV DNA testing was approved by the FDA in 2003 as an adjunct to cervical cytologic screening for women older than 30 years of age, as well as in the management of women with questionable cytologic results.[19] It is not recommended as a screening tool for women younger than 30 years of age because the prevalence of HPV is quite high in this population.

The presence of normal endometrial cells in a cervical cytologic sample during the luteal phase of the menstrual cycle or during the postmenopausal period has been associated with endometrial disease and warrants further evaluation with endometrial biopsy. This demonstrates that shedding of even normal cells at an inappropriate time may indicate disease. Because adenocarcinoma of the cervix is being detected more frequently, especially in women younger than 35 years of age, a Pap smear result of atypical glandular cells warrants further evaluation by endocervical or endometrial curettage, hysteroscopy, or, ultimately, a cone biopsy if the abnormality cannot be located or identified through other means.[2,3]

In 2001, a task force comprising representatives of the Bethesda 2001 group members and the American Society of Colposcopy and Cervical Pathology (ASCCP) provided additional guidance regarding minimally abnormal Pap smear results.[20] Current guidelines indicate that the management of women with atypical squamous cells (ASC) depends on whether the Pap smear is subcategorized as "of undetermined significance (ASC-US)" or as "cannot exclude HSIL (ASC-H)." With a liquid-based Pap smear, a portion of the fluid can be sent for HPV DNA testing. If HPV testing is negative, the ASC-US is likely related to inflammation, atrophy, or other temporary or reversible processes, and the Pap smear can be repeated in 1 year. Referral for colposcopy or other definitive diagnostic measures is recommended for women with positive HPV DNA test results; ASC-H, LSIL, or HSIL lesions; or if compliance with follow-up observation is uncertain. Colposcopy can also be use if women have suspect findings on examination or are immunocompromised.[18,20]

Before the availability of colposcopy, many women with abnormal Pap smear results required surgical cone biopsy for further evaluation. Cone biopsy involves the removal of a cone-shaped wedge of cervix, including the entire transformation zone and at least 50% of the endocervical canal. Postoperative hemorrhage, infection, cervical stenosis, infertility, and incompetent cervix are possible sequelae that warrant avoidance of this procedure unless it is truly necessary. Diagnostic conization still is indicated when a lesion is partly or completely beyond colposcopic view or colposcopically directed biopsy fails to explain the cytologic findings.

The LEEP or LLETZ (large loop excision of the transformation zone), a refinement of loop diathermy techniques dating back to the 1940s, is quickly becoming the first-line management for SIL. This outpatient procedure allows for the simultaneous diagnosis and treatment of dysplastic lesions found on colposcopy. It uses a thin, rigid, wire loop electrode attached to a generator that blends high-frequency, low-voltage current for cutting and a modulated higher voltage for coagulation. In skilled hands, this wire can remove the entire transformation zone, providing adequate treatment for the lesion while obtaining a specimen for further histologic evaluation. Although data on long-term results are not available, this procedure, which requires only local anesthesia, appears to provide a lower-cost, office-based alternative to cone biopsy.

Diagnosis and Treatment of Cervical Cancer. In its early stages, cervical cancer often manifests as a poorly defined lesion of the endocervix. Frequently, women with cervical cancer present with abnormal vaginal bleeding, spotting, and discharge. Although bleeding may assume any course, it is reported most frequently after intercourse. Women with more advanced disease may present with pelvic or back pain that may radiate down the leg, hematuria, fistulas (rectovaginal or vesicovaginal), or evidence of metastatic disease to supraclavicular or inguinal lymph node areas.

Diagnosis of cervical cancer requires pathologic confirmation. Pap smear results demonstrating SIL often require further evaluation by colposcopy, during which a biopsy sample may be obtained from suspect areas and examined microscopically. An alternative diagnostic tool in areas where colposcopy is not readily available is a noninvasive photographic technique in which a cervicography camera is used to take photographs of the cervix. The projected cervicogram (a slide made from the film) is then sent for expert evaluation. In one study, the cervicogram was found to give a greater yield of CIN than Pap smear alone in patients with previous abnormal Pap smear results.[21]

Early treatment of cervical cancer involves removal of the lesion by one of various techniques. Biopsy or local cautery may be therapeutic in and of itself. Electrocautery, cryosurgery, or carbon dioxide laser therapy may be used to treat moderate to severe dysplasia that is limited to the exocervix (*i.e.,* squamo-columnar junction clearly visible). Therapeutic conization becomes necessary if the lesion extends into the endocervical canal and can be done surgically or with LEEP in the physician's office.[3]

Depending on the stage of involvement of the cervix, invasive cancer is treated with radiation therapy, surgery, or both. External-beam irradiation and intracavitary irradiation or *brachytherapy* (*i.e.,* insertion of radioactive materials into the body) can be used in the treatment of cervical cancer (see Chapter 8). Intracavitary radiation provides direct access to the central lesion and increases the tolerance of the cervix and surrounding tissues, permitting curative levels of radiation to be used. External-beam radiation eliminates metastatic disease in pelvic lymph nodes and other structures, as well as shrinking the cervical lesion to optimize the effects of intracavitary radiation. Surgery can include extended hysterectomy (*i.e.,* removal of the uterus, fallopian tubes, ovaries, and upper portion of the vagina) without pelvic lymph node dissection, radical hysterectomy with pelvic lymph node dissection, or pelvic exenteration (*i.e.,* removal of all pelvic organs, including the bladder, rectum, vulva, and vagina). The choice of treatment is influenced by the stage of the disease as well as the woman's age and health.[3]

Disorders of the Uterus

Endometritis

The endometrium and myometrium are relatively resistant to infections, primarily because the endocervix normally forms a barrier to ascending infections. Acute endometritis is uncommon and usually occurs after the cervical barrier is compromised by abortion, delivery, or instrumentation.[10,22] Curettage is diagnostic and often curative because it removes the necrotic tissue that has served as a site of infection.

Chronic inflammation of the endometrium is associated with intrauterine devices (IUD), pelvic inflammatory disease, and retained products of conception after delivery or abortion. The presence of plasma cells (which are not present in the normal endometrium) is required for diagnosis. The clinical picture is variable, but often includes abnormal vaginal bleeding, mild to severe uterine tenderness, fever, malaise, and foul-smelling discharge. Treatment involves oral or intravenous antibiotic therapy, depending on the severity of the condition.

Endometriosis

Endometriosis is the condition in which functional endometrial tissue is found in ectopic sites outside the uterus. The site may

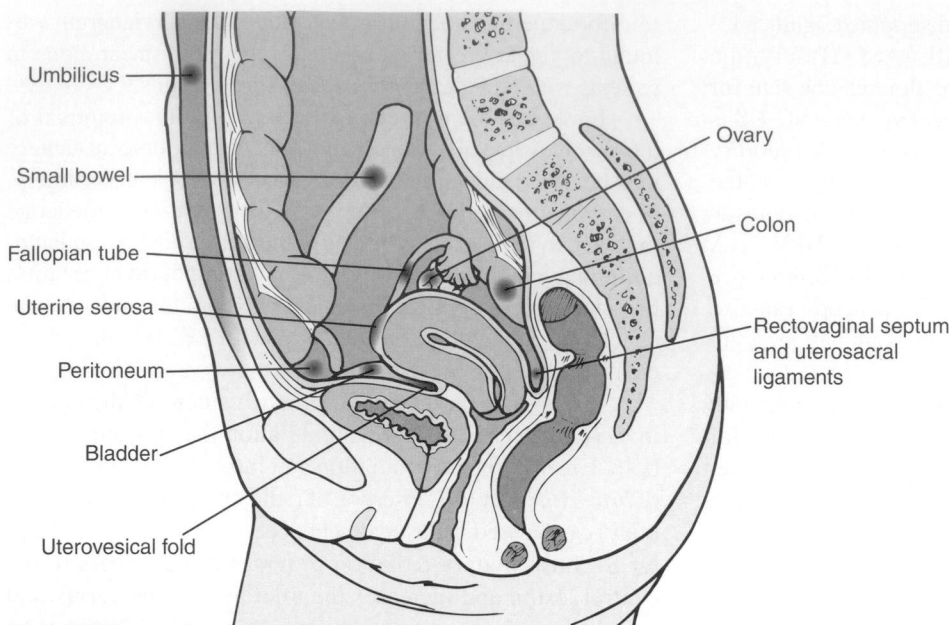

Umbilicus

Small bowel

Fallopian tube

Uterine serosa

Peritoneum

Bladder

Uterovesical fold

Ovary

Colon

Rectovaginal septum
and uterosacral
ligaments

FIGURE 46-3 • Common locations of endometriosis in the pelvis and abdomen.

be the ovaries, posterior broad ligaments, uterosacral ligaments, pouch of Douglas (cul-de-sac), pelvis, vagina, vulva, perineum, or intestines (Fig. 46-3). Rarely, endometrial implants have been found in the nostrils, umbilicus, lungs, and limbs.

The cause of endometriosis is unknown. There appears to have been an increase in its incidence in the developed Western countries during the past four to five decades. Approximately 10% to 15% of premenopausal women have some degree of endometriosis. The incidence may be higher in women with infertility (15% to 70%) or women younger than 20 years of age with chronic pelvic pain (47% to 73%).[23] It is also more common in women who have postponed childbearing. Risk factors for endometriosis may include early menarche; regular periods with shorter cycles (<27 days), longer duration (>7 days), or heavier flow; increased menstrual pain; and other first-degree relatives with the condition.

Several theories attempt to explain the origin of the dispersed endometrial lesions that occur in women with endometriosis.[10] One theory, the *regurgitation/implantation theory,* suggests that menstrual blood containing fragments of endometrium is forced upward through the fallopian tubes into the peritoneal cavity. Retrograde menstruation is not an uncommon phenomenon, and it is unknown why endometrial cells implant and grow in some women but not in others. A second theory, the *metaplastic theory,* proposes that dormant, immature cellular elements, spread over a wide area during embryonic development, persist into adult life and then differentiate into endometrial tissue. Another theory, the *vascular* or *lymphatic theory,* suggests that the endometrial tissue may metastasize through the lymphatics or vascular system. Genetic and immune factors also have been studied as contributing factors to the development of endometriosis.[2,3]

Endometriosis usually becomes apparent in the reproductive years when the lesions are stimulated by ovarian hormones

in the same way as normal endometrium, becoming proliferative, then secretory, and finally undergoing menstrual breakdown. Bleeding into the surrounding structures can cause pain and the development of significant pelvic adhesions. Symptoms tend to be strongest premenstrually, subsiding after cessation of menstruation. Pelvic pain is the most common presenting symptom; other symptoms include back pain, dyspareunia, and pain on defecation and micturition. Endometriosis is associated with infertility because of adhesions that distort the pelvic anatomy and cause impaired ovum release and transport.

The gross pathologic changes that occur in endometriosis differ with location and duration. In the ovary, the endometrial tissue may form cysts (*i.e.,* endometriomas filled with old blood that resembles chocolate syrup [chocolate cysts]). Rupture of these cysts can cause peritonitis and adhesions. Elsewhere in the pelvis, the tissue may take the form of small hemorrhagic lesions that may be black, bluish, red, clear, or opaque (Fig. 46-4). Some may be surrounded by scar tissue.

Endometriosis may be difficult to diagnose because its symptoms mimic those of other pelvic disorders and the severity of the symptoms does not always reflect the extent of the disease. Definitive diagnosis can be accomplished only through laparoscopy. This minimally invasive surgery allows direct visualization of pelvic organs to determine the presence and extent of endometrial lesions. Imaging techniques, including ultrasonography and magnetic resonance imaging (MRI), can be useful tools in evaluating endometriomas and deep endometriosis.[23] Serum cancer antigen 125 (CA-125), which is known for its use in diagnosis and monitoring of ovarian cancer, may be elevated in the presence of endometriosis. It has limitations as a screening tool, but can be useful in monitoring response to therapy and recurrence.

Treatment modalities fall into three categories: pain relief, endometrial suppression, and surgery. In young women, sim-

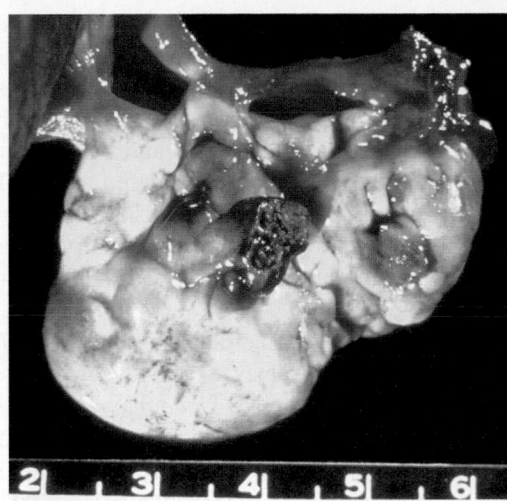

FIGURE 46-4 • Endometriosis. Implants of endometrium on the ovary appear as red-blue nodules. (From Robboy S. J., Merino M. J., Mutter G. L. (2008). The female reproductive system. In Rubin R., Strayer D. S. (Eds.), *Rubin's pathology: Clinicopathologic foundations of medicine* (5th ed., p. 829). Philadelphia: Lippincott Williams & Wilkins.)

ple observation and analgesics (nonsteroidal anti-inflammatory drugs [NSAIDs]) may be sufficient treatment. The use of hormones to induce physiologic amenorrhea is based on the observation that pregnancy and menopause afford pain relief by inducing atrophy of the endometrial tissue. This can be accomplished through administration of oral contraceptive pills, continuous progestogen agents (medroxyprogesterone acetate [oral or depot injection] or the levonorgestrel intrauterine system), danazol (a synthetic androgen), or long-acting gonadotropin-releasing hormone (GnRH) analogs that inhibit the pituitary gonadotropins and suppress ovulation.[3,23,24]

Surgery may offer more definitive therapy for women with large or symptomatic endometriomas, or those who have failed medical therapy for endometriosis. The goal of surgical treatment is to restore normal anatomic relationships, remove all visible lesions and slow progression of the disease—all done in a way that minimizes development of pelvic adhesions and avoids injury to normal surrounding structures. Laparoscopy is the preferred surgical approach today and has demonstrated equivalent pain relief with shorter perioperative recovery compared with laparotomy.[25] Laparoscopic treatment options include the use of cautery, laser ablation, and excision techniques. Advantages of laser surgery include better hemostasis, more precision in vaporizing lesions with less damage to surrounding tissue, and better access to areas that are not well visualized or would be difficult to reach with cautery. Electrosurgical, thermal, and ultrasonic ablation techniques are under investigation. Definitive treatment involves total hysterectomy and bilateral salpingo-oophorectomy when the symptoms are unbearable or the woman's childbearing is completed. Continuous combined estrogen–progestogen therapy is recommended to manage menopausal symptoms and minimize the risk of endometriosis recurrence.[24]

Treatment offers relief but not a cure. Recurrence of endometriosis is common, regardless of the treatment (except for radical surgery). Recurrence rates appear to correlate with severity of disease. With medical treatment, recurrence rates after 7 years ranged from 34% in women with mild disease to 74% in those with severe disease. Recurrence rates of 20% to 40% have been reported within 5 years after surgery.[26] Pregnancy may delay but does not preclude recurrence. Development of a lifelong management strategy is necessary for most women.

Adenomyosis

Adenomyosis is the condition in which endometrial glands and stroma are found within the myometrium, interspersed between the smooth muscle fibers. In contrast to endometriosis, which usually is a problem of young, infertile women, adenomyosis typically is found in multiparous women in their late fourth or fifth decade. It is thought that events associated with repeated pregnancies, deliveries, and uterine involution may cause the endometrium to be displaced throughout the myometrium. Adenomyosis frequently coexists with uterine myomas or endometrial hyperplasia. The diagnosis of adenomyosis often occurs as an incidental finding in a uterus removed for symptoms suggestive of myoma or hyperplasia. Heavy, painful periods with clots and painful intercourse are common complaints of women with adenomyosis. Although in the past the diagnosis was made primarily through careful history and the pelvic examination findings of an enlarged, boggy uterus, MRI is now considered an excellent diagnostic tool for confirming this condition. Color Doppler ultrasonography can be used to distinguish vascular patterns that may differentiate adenomyosis from uterine fibroids.[27] Adenomyosis resolves with menopause. Conservative therapy using oral contraceptives or GnRH agonists is the first choice for treatment. Hysterectomy (with preservation of the ovaries in premenopausal women) is considered when this approach fails.

Endometrial Cancer

Endometrial cancer is the most common cancer found in the female pelvis, occurring more than twice as often as cervical cancer. In 2007, the American Cancer Society estimated that approximately 39,200 women were diagnosed with endometrial cancer and 7400 died of the disorder.[12,28] Endometrial cancer occurs more frequently in older women (peak ages of 55 to 65 years), with only 8% occurring in women younger than 45 years of age.

Although the proportion of cases of endometrial cancer with a background of familial risk is low, endometrial cancer can develop as part of a hereditary cancer syndrome. Women with a family history of hereditary nonpolyposis colorectal cancer may have an inherited disorder in DNA mismatch repair genes that predisposes to endometrial and ovarian cancers, as well as colorectal cancer. This autosomal dominant disease carries an 80% risk of developing cancer of some type for those who inherit the mutation.[3]

Incidence and Pathogenesis. In terms of potential pathogenesis, two general groups of endometrial cancer can be identified. The first develops on a background of prolonged estrogen stimulation and endometrial hyperplasia, whereas the second is less commonly associated with hyperestrogenism and endometrial hyperplasia.

Most endometrial cancers (about 85%) are moderately well-differentiated adenocarcinomas that develop on a background of endometrial hyperplasia. These tumors, also known as *type 1 endometrial cancers,* are typically hormone sensitive, low grade, and have a favorable prognosis.[29] They are associated with long-duration unopposed estrogen stimulation and tend to be well differentiated, mimicking normal endometrial glands in histologic appearance, or display altered differentiation (mucinous, tubal, squamous differentiation).[10,29]

The endometrium undergoes structural modification and cellular changes in response to fluctuations in estrogen and progesterone levels that occur during the menstrual cycle. Prolonged unopposed estrogen stimulation leads to endometrial hyperplasia, which increases the chance of development of atypical hyperplasia and eventually type 1 endometrial cancer. Although the molecular basis for this process is still unknown, anovulatory cycles, disorders of estrogen metabolism, unopposed estrogen therapy, estrogen-secreting granulosa cell tumor, and obesity are all known to increase the risk of endometrial cancer.[2,3,29]

Ovulatory dysfunction that causes infertility at any age or occurs with declining ovarian function in perimenopausal women also can result in unopposed estrogen and increase the risk of endometrial cancer. A sharp rise in endometrial cancer was seen in the 1970s among middle-aged women who had received unopposed estrogen therapy (*i.e.,* estrogen therapy without progesterone) for menopausal symptoms. It was later determined that it was not the estrogen exposure that increased the risk of cancer, but that the hormone was administered without progesterone. It is the presence of progesterone in the second half of the menstrual cycle that matures the endometrium, and the withdrawal of progesterone that ultimately results in endometrial sloughing. Long-term unopposed estrogen exposure without periodic addition of progesterone allows for continued endometrial growth and hyperplasia, which increases the chance of development of atypical cells. Hyperplasia usually regresses after treatment with cyclic progesterone. Sequential oral contraceptives (estrogen alone for 15 days followed by 7 days of combined estrogen and progestin) were withdrawn from the market in the 1970s because of potential risk of endometrial hyperplasia. In contrast, combination oral contraceptives (estrogen and progestin in each pill) effectively prevent hyperplasia and decrease the risk of cancer by 50%.[3] Tamoxifen, a drug that blocks estrogen receptor sites and is used in treatment of breast cancer, exerts a weak estrogenic effect on the endometrium and represents another exogenous risk factor for endometrial cancer.

Diabetes mellitus, hypertension, and polycystic ovary syndrome are conditions that alter estrogen metabolism and elevate estrogen levels. Excessive fat consumption and overweight are important risk factors for endometrial cancer. In premenopausal women, overweight causes insulin resistance, ovarian androgen excess, anovulation, and chronic progesterone deficiency. In postmenopausal women, estrogens are synthesized in body fats from adrenal and ovarian androgen precursors. Because of its effect on insulin-like growth factor-1 (IGF-1) and its binding protein, obesity can be a risk factor even when circulating levels of estrogen are normal. Estrogen receptor transcriptional activity can be induced by IGF-1 signaling even in the absence of estrogen.

A second subset of endometrial cancers (about 10%) are high-grade tumors with a tendency to recur, even in early stages. These tumors, also known as *type 2 endometrial cancers,* are not estrogen driven, typically occur in women who acquire the disease at a somewhat older age, and are mostly associated with endometrial atrophy rather than hyperplasia.[29] Overall, this type of endometrial cancer usually has a poorer prognosis than that associated with prolonged estrogen stimulation and endometrial hyperplasia.

Clinical Course. The major symptom of endometrial hyperplasia or overt endometrial cancer is abnormal, painless bleeding. In menstruating women, this takes the form of bleeding between periods or excessive, prolonged menstrual flow. In postmenopausal women, any bleeding is abnormal and warrants investigation. Abnormal bleeding is an early warning sign of the disease, and because endometrial cancer tends to be slow growing in its early stages, the chances of cure are good if prompt medical care is sought. Later signs of uterine cancer may include cramping, pelvic discomfort, postcoital bleeding, lower abdominal pressure, and enlarged lymph nodes.

Although the Pap smear can identify a small percentage of endometrial cancers, it is not a good screening test for this type of gynecologic cancer. Endometrial biopsy (tissue sample obtained in an office procedure by direct aspiration of the endometrial cavity) is far more accurate. Dilation and curettage (D&C), which consists of dilating the cervix and scraping the uterine cavity, is the definitive procedure for diagnosis because it provides a more thorough evaluation. Transvaginal ultrasonography used to measure the endometrial thickness is being evaluated as an initial test for postmenopausal bleeding because it is less invasive than endometrial biopsy and less costly than D&C when biopsy is not possible.

The prognosis for endometrial cancer depends on the clinical stage of the disease when it is discovered and its histologic grade and type. Surgery and radiation therapy are the most successful methods of treatment for endometrial cancer. When used alone, radiation therapy has a 20% lower cure rate than surgery for stage I disease. It may be the best option, however, in women who are not good surgical candidates. Total abdominal hysterectomy with bilateral salpingo-oophorectomy plus sampling of regional lymph nodes and peritoneal washings for cytologic evaluation of occult disease is the treatment of choice whenever possible. Postoperative radiation therapy may be added in cases of advanced disease for more complete treatment and to prevent recurrence or metastasis, although the benefits of this as adjuvant therapy are still controversial. The 5-year relative survival rates are 96%, 66%, and 25% if the cancer is diagnosed at local, regional, and distant stages, respectively.[12]

Leiomyomas

Uterine leiomyomas (commonly called *fibroids*) are benign neoplasms of smooth muscle origin. These are the most common form of pelvic tumor and are believed to occur in one of every four or five women older than 35 years of age. They are seen more often and their rate of growth is more rapid in black women than in white women. Leiomyomas usually develop as submucosal, subserosal, or intramural tumors in the corpus of the uterus (Fig. 46-5). Intramural fibroids are embedded in the myometrium. They are the most common type of fibroid, and present as a symmetric enlargement of the nonpregnant uterus. Subserosal tumors are located beneath the perimetrium of the uterus. These tumors are recognized as irregular projections on the uterine surface; they may become pedunculated, displacing or impinging on other genitourinary structures and causing hydroureter or bladder problems. Submucosal fibroids displace endometrial tissue and are more likely to cause bleeding, necrosis, and infection than either of the other types.

Leiomyomas are asymptomatic approximately half of the time and may be discovered during a routine pelvic examination, or they may cause menorrhagia (excessive menstrual bleeding), anemia, urinary frequency, rectal pressure/constipation, abdominal distention, and infrequently pain. Their rate of growth is variable, but they may increase in size during pregnancy or with exogenous estrogen stimulation (*i.e.,* oral contraceptives or menopausal estrogen replacement therapy). Interference with pregnancy is rare unless the tumor is submucosal and interferes with implantation or obstructs the cervical outlet. These tumors may outgrow their blood supply, become infarcted, and undergo degenerative changes.

Most leiomyomas regress with menopause, but if bleeding, pressure on the bladder, pain, or other problems persist, hysterectomy may be required. Myomectomy (removal of just the tumors) can be done to preserve the uterus for future childbearing. Cesarean section may be recommended if the uterine cavity is entered during myomectomy. Hypothalamic GnRH agonists (*e.g.,* leuprolide) may be used to suppress leiomyoma growth before surgery. Uterine artery embolization done by an interventional radiologist is a nonsurgical therapy that has demonstrated significant reduction in bleeding and bulk symptoms, improvement in quality of life and uterine preservation with shorter hospitalization, quicker return to work, low complication rate, and financial savings for both patients and the health care system.[30]

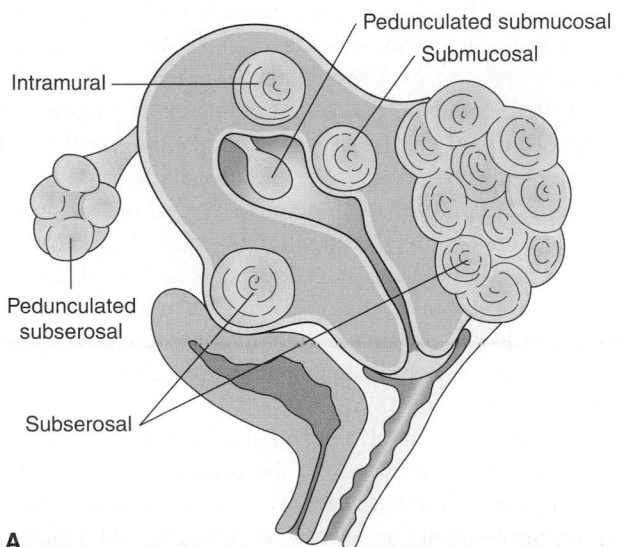

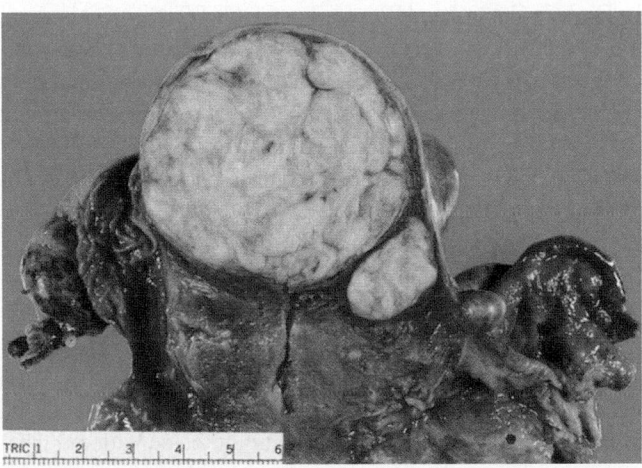

FIGURE 46-5 • **(A)** Submucosal, intramural, and subserosal leiomyomas. **(B)** A bisected uterus displays a prominent, sharply circumscribed, fleshy tumor. (From Robboy S. J., Merino M. J., Mutter G. L. (2008). The female reproductive system. In Rubin R., Strayer D. S. (Eds.), *Rubin's pathology: Clinicopathologic foundations of medicine* (5th ed., p. 813). Philadelphia: Lippincott Williams & Wilkins.)

IN SUMMARY, disorders of the cervix and uterus include inflammatory conditions (*i.e.,* cervicitis and endometritis), cancer (*i.e.,* cervical and endometrial cancer), endometriosis, and leiomyomas. Cervicitis is an acute or chronic inflammation of the cervix. Acute cervicitis may result from the direct infection of the cervix or may be secondary to a vaginal or uterine infection. It may be caused by a variety of infectious agents. Chronic cervicitis represents a low-grade inflammatory process resulting from trauma or nonspecific infectious agents. Cervical cancer arises from precursor lesions that can be detected on a Pap smear, and, if detected early, is the most easily cured of all the cancers of the female reproductive system. Evidence suggests a causal link between HPV infection and cervical cancer. A vaccine against several strains of the HPV is now available and shows promise for the prevention of cervical cancer.

Endometritis represents an ill-defined inflammation or infection of the endometrium that produces variable symptoms. Endometriosis is the condition in which functional endometrial tissue is found in ectopic sites outside the uterus, particularly in dependent parts of the pelvis and in the ovaries. It causes dysmenorrhea, dyspareunia, and infertility. Adenomyosis is the condition in which endometrial glands and stroma are found in the myometrium, interspersed between the smooth muscle fibers. Endometrial cancer is the most common cancer found in the female pelvis, occurring more than twice as often as cervical cancer. Prolonged estrogen stimulation with hyperplasia of the endometrium has been identified as a major risk factor for endometrial cancer.

Leiomyomas are benign uterine wall neoplasms of smooth muscle origin. They can develop in the corpus of the uterus and can be submucosal, subserosal, or intramural. Submucosal fibroids displace endometrial tissue and are more likely to cause bleeding, necrosis, and infection than either of the other types. ■

DISORDERS OF THE FALLOPIAN TUBES AND OVARIES

After completing this section of the chapter, you should be able to meet the following objectives:

- List the common causes and symptoms of pelvic inflammatory disease.
- Describe the risk factors and symptoms of ectopic pregnancy.
- State the underlying cause of ovarian cysts.
- Differentiate benign ovarian cyst from polycystic ovary syndrome.
- List the hormones produced by the three types of functioning ovarian tumors.
- State the reason that ovarian cancer may be difficult to detect in an early stage.

Pelvic Inflammatory Disease

Pelvic inflammatory disease (PID) is a polymicrobial infection of the upper reproductive tract (uterus, fallopian tubes, or ovaries) associated with the sexually transmitted organisms *N. gonorrhoeae* or *C. trachomatis* as well as endogenous organisms, including anaerobes, *Haemophilus influenzae,* enteric gram-negative rods, and streptococci.[31,32] The organisms ascend through the endocervical canal to the endometrial cavity, and then to the tubes and ovaries. The endocervical canal is slightly dilated during menstruation, allowing bacteria to gain entrance to the uterus and other pelvic structures. After entering the upper reproductive tract, the organisms multiply rapidly in the favorable environment of the sloughing endometrium and ascend to the fallopian tube (Fig. 46-6).

Factors that predispose women to the development of PID include an age of 16 to 24 years, nulliparity, history of multiple sexual partners, and previous history of PID. Although the use of an IUD has been associated with a three- to fivefold increased risk for development of PID, studies have shown that women with only one sexual partner who are at low risk of acquiring STIs have no significant risk for development of PID from using an IUD.

Clinical Course

The symptoms of PID include lower abdominal pain, which may start just after a menstrual period; dyspareunia; back pain; purulent cervical discharge; and the presence of adnexal tenderness and exquisitely painful cervix on bimanual pelvic examination. New-onset breakthrough bleeding in women who are on oral contraceptives or medroxyprogesterone contraceptive injection (Depo-Provera) has been associated with PID. Fever (>101°F), increased erythrocyte sedimentation rate, and an elevated white blood cell count (>10,000 cells/mL) commonly are seen, even though the woman may not appear acutely ill. Elevated C-reactive protein levels equate with inflammation and can be used as another diagnostic tool. Laparoscopy, which allows for direct visualization of the ovaries, fallopian tubes, and uterus, is one of the most specific procedures for diagnosing PID, but is costly and carries the inherent risks of surgery and anesthesia.[32] Minimal criteria for a presumptive diagnosis of PID require only the presence of lower abdominal pain, adnexal tenderness, and cervical motion tenderness on bimanual examination with no other apparent cause.[31]

Treatment may involve hospitalization with intravenous administration of antibiotics. If the condition is diagnosed early, outpatient antibiotic therapy may be sufficient. Antibiotic regimens should be selected according to STI treatment guidelines, which are published every 4 years by the Centers for Disease Control and Prevention (CDC).[32] Treatment is aimed at preventing complications, which can include pelvic adhesions, infertility, ectopic pregnancy, chronic abdominal pain, and tubo-ovarian abscesses. Accurate diagnosis and appropriate antibiotic therapy may decrease the severity and frequency of PID sequelae. The CDC recommends empiric treatment with a presumptive diagnosis of PID, while waiting for confirmation by culture or other definitive test results.

Ectopic Pregnancy

Although pregnancy is not discussed in detail in this text, it is reasonable to mention ectopic pregnancy because it represents a true gynecologic emergency and should be considered when a woman of reproductive age presents with the complaint of pelvic pain. Ectopic pregnancy occurs when a fertilized ovum implants outside the uterine cavity, the most common site being the fallopian tube (Fig. 46-7). According to the CDC, between 1970 and 1992, the number of ectopic pregnancies increased from 17,800 to 108,800, and the rate of occurrence among women aged 15 to 44 years rose from 4.5 to 19.7 per 1000 reported pregnancies (live births, abortions, and ectopic preg-

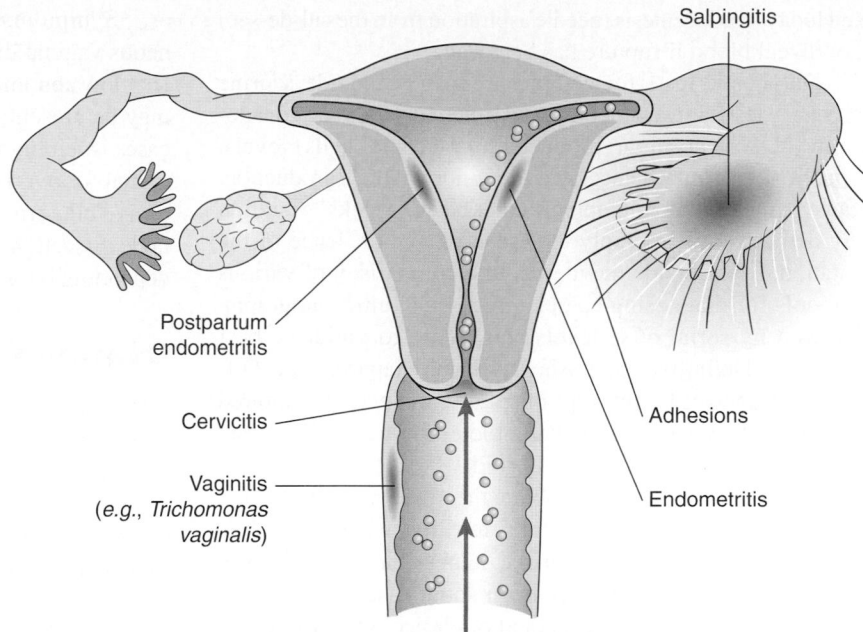

FIGURE 46-6 • Pelvic inflammatory disease. Microbial agents enter through the vagina and ascend to involve the uterus, fallopian tubes, and pelvic structures.

nancies).[33] Updated estimates for incidence rates are difficult to determine because many women are now treated on an outpatient basis, so data from hospital discharge records are no longer representative of the scope of the problem. Although ectopic pregnancy is the leading cause of maternal mortality

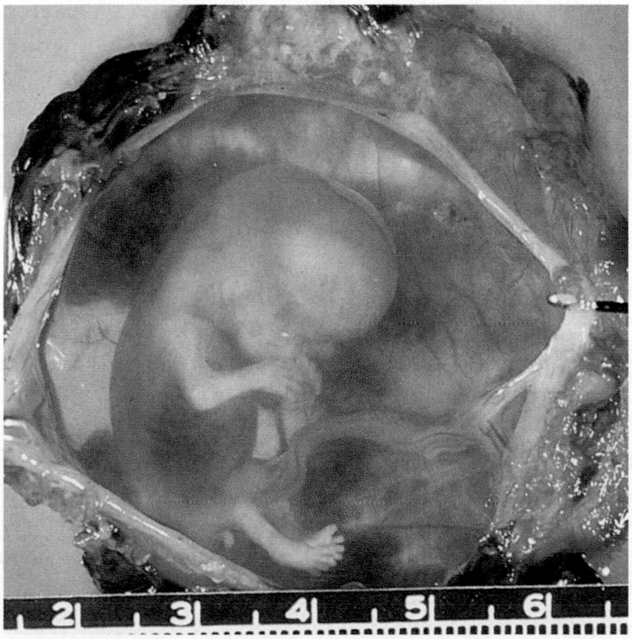

FIGURE 46-7 • Ectopic pregnancy. An enlarged fallopian tube has been opened to disclose a minute fetus. (From Robboy S. J., Kurman R. J., Merino M. J. [2005]. The female reproductive system. In Rubin E., Gorstein F., Rubin R., et al. [Eds.], *Rubin's pathology: Clinicopathologic foundations of medicine* [4th ed., p. 966]. Philadelphia: Lippincott Williams & Wilkins.)

in the first trimester and accounts for 6% of all maternal deaths in the United States, the death rate has steadily declined as a result of improved diagnostic methods. Earlier detection reduces the risk of tubal rupture, which could result in intra-abdominal hemorrhage, major complications, future infertility, or death.[34]

The cause of ectopic pregnancy is delayed ovum transport, which may result from decreased tubal motility or distorted tubal anatomy (*i.e.*, narrowed lumen, convolutions, or diverticula). Risk factors most strongly associated with ectopic pregnancy include previous tubal surgery, tubal ligation or reversal, previous ectopic pregnancy, and a tubal lesion or abnormality.[34–36] Smoking, current IUD use, history of PID or therapeutic abortion, and the use of fertility drugs to induce ovulation have also been associated with an increased risk for ectopic pregnancy.

Clinical Course

The site of implantation in the tube (*e.g.*, isthmus, ampulla) may determine the onset of symptoms and the timing of diagnosis. As the tubal pregnancy progresses, the surrounding tissue is stretched. The pregnancy eventually outgrows its blood supply, at which point the pregnancy terminates or the tube itself ruptures because it can no longer contain the growing pregnancy.

Symptoms can include lower abdominal discomfort—diffuse or localized to one side—that progresses to severe pain caused by rupture, spotting, syncope, referred shoulder pain from bleeding into the abdominal cavity, and amenorrhea. Physical examination usually reveals adnexal tenderness; an adnexal mass is found in only 50% of cases. Although rarely used today, culdocentesis (needle aspiration from the cul-de-sac) may reveal blood if rupture has occurred.

Diagnostic tests for ectopic pregnancy include a urine pregnancy test, ultrasonography, and β-human chorionic gonadotropin (hCG; a hormone produced by placental cells) levels. Serial hCG tests may detect lower-than-normal hCG production. Transvaginal ultrasonographic studies after 5 weeks' gestation may demonstrate an empty uterine cavity or presence of the gestational sac outside the uterus. In a comparison of various protocols for diagnosing ectopic pregnancy, ultrasonography followed by serial hCG levels was found to yield the best results.[34–36] Definitive diagnosis may require laparoscopy. Differential diagnosis for this type of pelvic pain includes ruptured ovarian cyst, threatened or incomplete abortion, PID, acute appendicitis, and degenerating fibroid.

Treatment is aimed at resolving the problem with minimal morbidity and protecting future fertility where possible. Advances in detection now make it possible to treat early ectopic pregnancies medically or in some cases expectantly. Surgical therapy is still the method of choice when rupture is imminent or has already occurred, when the woman has experienced pain for longer than 24 hours, or when the woman is hemodynamically unstable.[34,37] Laparoscopic treatment of ectopic pregnancy is well tolerated and more cost effective than laparotomy because of shorter convalescence and the reduced need for postoperative analgesia. Laparotomy, which involves an open incision into the abdominopelvic cavity, becomes necessary when there is uncontrolled internal bleeding, when the ectopic site cannot be visualized through the laparoscope, or when the surgeon is not trained in operative laparoscopy.

Methotrexate (an antimetabolite used in treatment of chronic inflammatory diseases and cancer) has been successfully used to eliminate residual ectopic pregnancy tissue after laparoscopy, and more recently as primary treatment in cases where the pregnancy is diagnosed early and tubal rupture has not occurred, or the pregnancy is not in an uncommon location such as one of the cornua of the uterus or the cervix. This folic acid antagonist interferes with DNA and ribonucleic acid (RNA) synthesis, thus inhibiting the growth of trophoblastic cells at the placental implantation site. The criteria for using methotrexate include hemodynamic stability, no symptoms of tubal rapture, hCG <5000 IU/L, extrauterine sac <4 cm when visible, and a willingness of the woman to return regularly for post-treatment monitoring. Adverse effects can include bone marrow depression, transient elevation of liver enzymes, anemia, and stomatitis. Close follow-up with weekly hCG levels is necessary until the pregnancy is completely resolved.[34,37]

Cancer of the Fallopian Tube

Although a common site of metastases, primary cancer of the fallopian tube is rare, accounting for less than 1% of all female genital tract cancers. Fewer than 3000 cases have been reported worldwide. Most primary tubal cancers are papillary adenocarcinomas, and these tumors develop bilaterally in 30% of patients with advanced disease.

Symptoms are uncommon, but intermittent serosanguineous vaginal discharge, abnormal vaginal bleeding, and colicky low abdominal pain have been reported. An adnexal mass may be present; however, the preoperative diagnosis in most cases is leiomyoma or ovarian tumor. Management is similar to that for ovarian cancer and usually includes total hysterectomy, bilateral salpingo-oophorectomy, and pelvic lymph node dissection. More extensive procedures may be warranted, depending on the stage of the disease.[2,38]

Ovarian Cysts and Tumors

The ovaries have a dual function: they produce germ cells, or ova, and they synthesize the female sex hormones. Disorders of the ovaries frequently cause menstrual and fertility problems. Benign conditions of the ovaries can present as primary lesions of the ovarian structures or as secondary disorders related to hypothalamic, pituitary, or adrenal dysfunction.

Ovarian Cysts

Cysts are the most common form of ovarian tumor. Many are benign. A follicular cyst is one that results from occlusion of the duct of the follicle. Each month, several follicles begin to develop and are blighted at various stages of development. These follicles form cavities that fill with fluid, producing a cyst. The dominant follicle normally ruptures to release the egg (*i.e.*, ovulation), but occasionally persists and continues growing. Likewise, a luteal cyst is a persistent cystic enlargement of the corpus luteum that is formed after ovulation and does not regress in the absence of pregnancy. Functional cysts are asymptomatic unless there is substantial enlargement or bleeding into the cyst. This can cause considerable discomfort or a dull, aching sensation on the affected side. These cysts usually regress spontaneously. Occasionally a cyst may become twisted or may rupture into the intra-abdominal cavity (Fig. 46-8).

Polycystic Ovary Syndrome

Polycystic ovary syndrome (PCOS) is a common endocrine disorder affecting 5% to 10% of women of reproductive age, and is a frequent source of chronic anovulation. The disorder is characterized by varying degrees of menstrual irregularity, signs of hyperandrogenism (acne, excess body hair [hirsutism], male-pattern hair loss), and infertility.[39–43] About 50% of women who are diagnosed with PCOS are obese, and most have polycystic ovaries. Hyperinsulinemia and insulin resistance have recently been hypothesized to play a role in the pathogenesis of the disorder.

The precise etiology of this condition is still being debated, but is probably multifactorial. A possible genetic basis has been suggested with an autosomal dominant mode of inheritance and premature balding as the phenotype in males.[39] There is increasing evidence that the disorder may begin before adolescence and that many of the manifestations of PCOS begin to make their appearance at that time. In fact, it has been suggested that the initial insult may begin in utero with changes in the

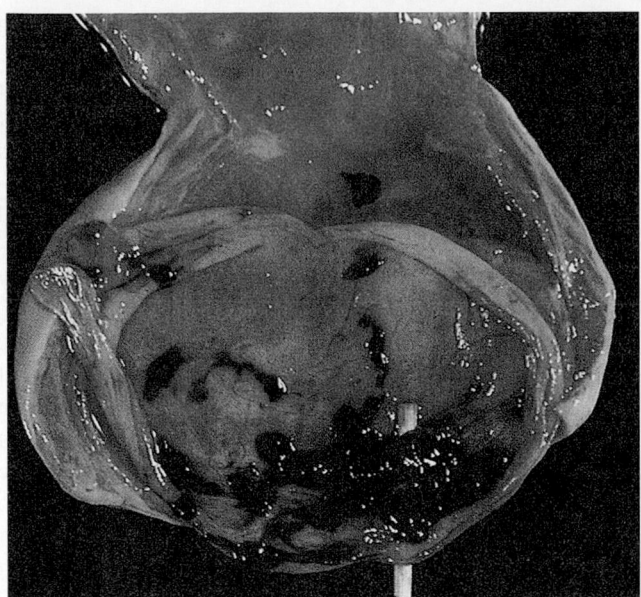

FIGURE 46-8 • Follicular cyst of the ovary. The rupture of this thin-walled follicular cyst (dowel stick) led to intra-abdominal hemorrhage. (From Robboy S. J., Merino M. J., Mutter G. L. [2008]. The female reproductive system. In Rubin R., Strayer D. S. [Eds.], *Rubin's pathology: Clinicopathologic foundations of medicine* [5th ed., p. 815]. Philadelphia: Lippincott Williams & Wilkins.)

fetal ovary that predispose to PCOS.[41] Because many of the symptoms common to PCOS, such as excess hair, acne, and obesity, can be detrimental to a teenage girl's health and self-esteem, early detection and treatment of PCOS in adolescents is essential.[44]

Although this syndrome has been the subject of considerable research, the underlying mechanisms remain unclear. Chronic anovulation is thought to be the underlying cause of the amenorrhea or irregular menses and enlarged, "polycystic" ovaries associated with this condition. Most women with PCOS have elevated luteinizing hormone (LH) levels with normal estrogen and follicle-stimulating hormone (FSH) production. Elevated levels of circulating total testosterone, free testosterone, and dehydroepiandrosterone sulfate (DHEAS) are not uncommon, and these women occasionally have hyperprolactinemia or hypothyroidism. Persistent anovulation results in an estrogen environment that alters the hypothalamic release of GnRH with a resultant increase in LH secretion and suppression of FSH release by the pituitary gland. This altered LH/FSH ratio often is used as a diagnostic criterion for this condition, but it is not universally present. Although the presence of some FSH allows for new follicular development, full maturation is not attained, and ovulation does not occur. The elevated LH level results in increased androgen production, which in turn prevents normal follicular development and contributes to the vicious cycle of anovulation.[39]

The association between hyperandrogenism and hyperinsulinemia is now well recognized.[41] It has been shown that the cause of hyperinsulinemia is insulin resistance. The frequency and degree of hyperinsulinemia in women with PCOS is often amplified by the presence of obesity. Insulin may cause hyperandrogenism in several ways, although the exact mechanism has not been well defined. It has been shown that the ovary possesses insulin receptors and there is evidence that insulin may act directly on the ovary. Several reports have shown that normal ovulation and sometimes pregnancy have occurred when women with hyperandrogenism were treated with insulin-sensitizing drugs.[39–41,43]

In addition to its clinical manifestations, long-term health problems including cardiovascular disease and diabetes have been linked to PCOS. There is also concern that women with PCOS who are anovulatory do not produce progesterone. This may, in turn, subject the uterine lining to an unopposed estrogen environment, which is a significant risk factor for development of endometrial cancer.[41] Although there also is a reported association with breast cancer and ovarian cancer, PCOS has not been conclusively shown to be an independent risk factor for either malignancy.

The diagnosis PCOS can be suspected from the clinical presentation. Although there is no consensus as to which tests should be used, laboratory evaluation to exclude hyperprolactinemia, late-onset adrenal hyperplasia, and androgen-secreting tumors of the ovary and adrenal gland is commonly done. Although a fasting blood glucose, 2-hour oral glucose tolerance test, and insulin levels are often measured to evaluate for hyperinsulinemia, this testing is not required prior to treatment as insulin resistance is almost universal in women with PCOS. Confirmation with ultrasonography or laparoscopic visualization of the ovaries is often done, but not required.[42]

The overall goal of treatment should be directed toward symptom relief, prevention of potential malignant endometrial sequelae, and reduction in risk for development of diabetes and cardiovascular disease. The preferred and most effective treatment for PCOS is lifestyle modification. Weight loss may be beneficial in restoring normal ovulation when obesity is present. Although numerous medications and protocols are available, the choice depends on the manifestations that are most bothersome to the woman and her stage in reproductive life. Combined oral contraceptive agents ameliorate menstrual irregularities and improve hirsutism and acne. The addition of spironolactone, an antimineralocorticoid that inhibits the production of androgens by the adrenal gland, may be beneficial to women with severe hirsutism.[41]

Metformin, an insulin-sensitizing drug, used with or without ovulation-inducing medications, is emerging as an important component of PCOS treatment.[45] In addition to expected improvements in insulin sensitivity and glucose metabolism, it has been associated with reductions in androgen and LH levels and is highly effective in restoring normal menstrual regularity and ovulatory cycles. The insulin-sensitizing thiazolidinediones (rosiglitazone and pioglitazone) have also shown promise in this area, but are not as well studied or used as often.[41] When medication is ineffective, laser surgery to puncture the multiple follicles may restore normal ovulatory function, although adhesion formation is a potential problem.

When fertility is desired, the condition usually is treated by the administration of the hypothalamic–pituitary–stimulating drug clomiphene citrate or injectable gonadotropins to induce ovulation. These drugs must be used carefully because they can induce extreme enlargement of the ovaries.

Benign and Functioning Ovarian Tumors

Ovarian tumors are common. Most are benign, but malignant ovarian tumors are the leading cause of death from reproductive cancers. Ovarian tumors can arise from any of the ovarian tissue types—serosal epithelium, germ cell layers, or gonadal stroma tissue[10,22] (Fig. 46-9). Serous and mucinous cystadenomas are the most common benign ovarian neoplasms. Endometriomas are the "chocolate cysts" that develop secondary to ovarian endometriosis. Ovarian fibromas are connective tissue tumors composed of fibrocytes and collagen. They range in size from 6 to 20 cm. Cystic teratomas, or dermoid cysts, are derived from primordial germ cells and are composed of various combinations of well-differentiated ectodermal, mesodermal, and endodermal elements. Not uncommonly, they contain sebaceous material, hair, or teeth.

Although most ovarian tumors are nonfunctional, some are hormonally active.[10] These tumors may be benign or cancerous. One such tumor, the granulosa cell tumor, is associated with excess estrogen production. When it develops during the reproductive period, the persistent and uncontrolled production of estrogen interferes with the normal menstrual cycle, causing irregular and excessive bleeding, endometrial hyperplasia, or amenorrhea and fertility problems. When it develops after menopause, it causes postmenopausal bleeding, stimulation of the glandular tissues of the breast, and other signs of renewed estrogen production. Androgen-secreting tumors (*i.e.,* Sertoli-Leydig cell tumor or androblastoma) inhibit ovulation and estrogen production. They tend to cause hirsutism and development of masculine characteristics, such as baldness, acne, oily skin, breast atrophy, and deepening of the voice.

Treatment for all ovarian tumors is surgical excision. Ovarian tissue that is not affected by the tumor can be left intact if frozen-section analysis does not reveal malignancy. When ovarian tumors are very large, as is frequently the case with serous or mucinous cystadenomas, the entire ovary must be removed.

Ovarian Cancer

Ovarian cancer is the second most common female genitourinary cancer and the most lethal. The rate of ovarian cancer has gone down by 0.7% per year since 1986; however, in 2007, there were still an estimated 22,400 new cases of ovarian cancer in the United States, with 15,300 deaths.[12] The incidence of ovarian cancer increases with age, being greatest between 65 and

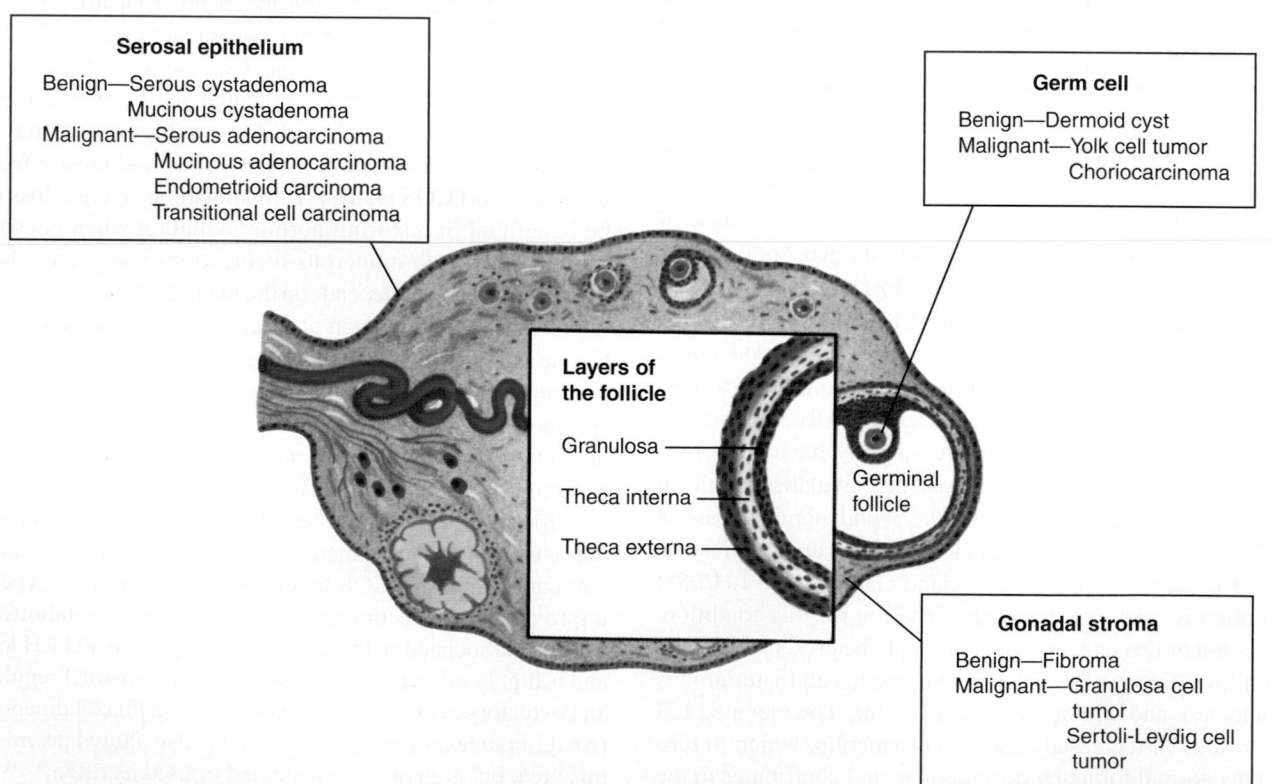

FIGURE 46-9 • Classification of ovarian neoplasms based on cell type. (From Robboy S. J., Merino M. J., Mutter G. L. [2008]. The female reproductive system. In Rubin R., Strayer D. S. [Eds.], *Rubin's pathology: Clinicopathologic foundations of medicine* [5th ed., p. 818]. Philadelphia: Lippincott Williams & Wilkins.)

84 years of age. Ovarian cancer is difficult to diagnose, and up to 75% of women have metastatic disease before the time of discovery.

The most significant risk factor for ovarian cancer appears to be ovulatory age—the length of time during a woman's life when her ovarian cycle is not suppressed by pregnancy, lactation, or oral contraceptive use. The incidence of ovarian cancer is much lower in countries where women bear numerous children. Family history also is a significant risk factor for ovarian cancer. Women with two or more first- or second-degree relatives who have had *site-specific ovarian cancer* have up to a 50% risk for development of the disease. There are two other types of inherited risk for ovarian cancer: *breast–ovarian cancer syndrome,* where both breast and ovarian cancer occur among first- and second-degree relatives; and *family cancer syndrome* or *Lynch syndrome II* (a subtype of hereditary nonpolyposis colon cancer), in which male or female relatives have a history of colorectal, endometrial, ovarian, pancreatic, or other types of cancer.[2,46,47] The breast cancer susceptibility genes, *BRCA1* and *BRCA2,* which are tumor suppressor genes (see Chapter 8), are incriminated in approximately 10% of hereditary ovarian cancers despite being identified as "breast cancer genes." Susceptibility to ovarian cancer is transmitted as an autosomal dominant characteristic; therefore, a mutated gene from either parent is sufficient to cause the problem. A high-fat Western diet and use of powders containing talc in the genital area are other factors that have been linked to the development of ovarian cancer.

Chemoprevention strategies that have been suggested include long-term oral contraceptive use, NSAIDs, acetaminophen, or retinoids.[48] Each of these agents acts in slightly different ways. The NSAIDs are thought to exert their protective effects through growth inhibition and increased apoptosis (programmed cell death) of ovarian cancer cell lines. The structure of acetaminophen bears a similarity to the sex hormones, suggesting a potential sex steroid–antagonist property. Support for the use of retinoids comes from experimental data in which retinoic acid was shown to induce the differentiation of cultured ovarian cancer cells. Additional clinical trials are needed to support the effectiveness of these chemoprevention agents. Surgical strategies that have reduced the risk of developing ovarian cancer include prophylactic removal of both fallopian tubes and ovaries. These strategies have generally been reserved for women at highest risk, and those who undergo surgical intervention must be counseled that there is still a small risk of developing peritoneal cancer.[46,48]

Cancer of the ovary is a complex neoplasm because of the diversity of tissue types that originate in the ovary. As a result of this diversity, there are several types of ovarian cancers. Malignant neoplasms of the ovary can be divided into three categories: epithelial tumors, germ cell tumors, and gonadal stromal tumors (see Fig. 46-9). Epithelial tumors account for approximately 90% of cases.[22] These different cancers display various degrees of virulence, depending on the type of tumor and degree of differentiation involved. A well-differentiated cancer of the ovary may have produced symptoms for many months and still be found to be operable at the time of surgery.

A poorly differentiated tumor may have been clinically evident for only a few days but found to be widespread and inoperable. Often no correlation exists between the duration of symptoms and the extent of the disease.

Clinical Course. Until recently it was believed that most cancers of the ovary produce no symptoms. Several studies have now established that symptoms are often present and reported by women before diagnosis, but are nonspecific and therefore difficult to distinguish from other problems presenting to a primary care provider. Symptoms that are believed to have a strong correlation to ovarian cancer include abdominal or pelvic pain, increased abdominal size or bloating, and difficulty eating or feeling full quickly after ingesting food. Because these gastrointestinal manifestations can occur for a variety of reasons, many women self-treat with antacids and other remedies for a time before seeking treatment, and health care providers may dismiss the woman's complaints as being caused by other conditions, further delaying diagnosis and treatment. Recent onset (<12 months) and frequent occurrence (>12 times per month) of these symptoms should increase the index of suspicion for ovarian cancer and suggest the need for further evaluation.[49] It is not fully understood why the initial symptoms of ovarian cancer are manifested as gastrointestinal disturbances. It is thought that biochemical changes in the peritoneal fluids may irritate the bowel or that pain originating in the ovary may be referred to the abdomen and be interpreted as a gastrointestinal disturbance. Clinically evident ascites (*i.e.,* fluid in the peritoneal cavity) is seen in approximately one fourth of women with malignant ovarian tumors and is associated with a worse prognosis.

No good screening tests or other early methods of detection exist for ovarian cancer.[50] The serum tumor marker CA-125 is a cell surface antigen; its level is elevated in 80% to 90% of women with stage II to IV nonmucinous ovarian epithelial cancers. The result is negative, however, for as much as 50% of women with stage I disease. In a postmenopausal woman with a pelvic mass, an elevated CA-125 has a positive predictive value of greater than 70% for cancer. It also can be used in monitoring therapy and recurrences when preoperative levels have been elevated. Despite its role in diagnostic evaluation and follow-up, CA-125 is not cancer or tissue specific for ovarian cancer. Levels also are elevated in the presence of endometriosis, uterine fibroids, pregnancy, liver disease, and other benign conditions and with cancers of the endometrium, cervix, fallopian tube, and pancreas. Because it lacks sensitivity and specificity, CA-125 has limited value as a single screening test.

Transvaginal ultrasonography (TVS) has been used to evaluate ovarian masses for malignant potential. Although TVS has demonstrated high sensitivity and specificity as a screening tool, cost precludes its use as universal screening method.[47] The National Institutes of Health Consensus Panel convened in 1995 recommended no widespread screening of women for ovarian cancer. CA-125 with TVS is suggested only for women who are part of a family with hereditary ovarian cancer syndrome (*i.e.,* two or more affected first-degree relatives).[51] This recommendation was further supported when the USPSTF updated guidelines were released in 2004.[52] Several large national studies are underway to determine the benefit of widespread population-based screening for ovarian cancer.[46,47] Molecular biologic studies have identified tumor suppressor genes that may play a role in the cause of ovarian cancer. Further evaluation in this area is ongoing and may eventually lead to identification of appropriate screening techniques for ovarian cancer.

When ovarian cancer is suspected, surgical evaluation is required for diagnosis, complete and accurate staging, and cytoreduction and debulking procedures to reduce the size of the tumor. The most common surgery involves removal of the uterus, fallopian tubes, ovaries, and omentum. The liver, diaphragm, retroperitoneal and aortic lymph nodes, and peritoneal surface are examined and biopsies are taken as needed. Cytologic washings are done to test for cancerous cells in the peritoneal fluid. Women with very early cancer who may wish to become pregnant will sometimes have only the affected ovary removed. Recommendations regarding treatment beyond surgery and prognosis depend on the stage of the disease. Women with limited disease (well-differentiated stage Ia or Ib) usually do not require adjuvant treatment; women with intermediate disease (stage Ib or II) or advanced disease (stage III or IV) can benefit from intravenous or intraperitoneal chemotherapy using a combination of a platinum compound (cisplatin or carboplatin) and a taxane (paclitaxel or docetaxel). When this combination therapy fails, salvage chemotherapy with newer drugs may prolong survival. Irradiation rarely plays a major role in treatment of ovarian cancer because of the difficulty in irradiating the entire abdomen without causing life-threatening damage to vital organs.[53]

The lack of accurate screening tools and the resistant nature of ovarian cancers significantly affect the success of treatment and survival. The 5-year survival rate is 94% for women whose ovarian cancer is detected and treated early; however, only 19% of all cases are detected at the localized stage. Overall, the 5-year survival rate is 45%.[53]

IN SUMMARY, PID is an inflammation of the upper reproductive tract that involves the uterus (endometritis), fallopian tubes (salpingitis), or ovaries (oophoritis). It is most commonly caused by *N. gonorrhoeae* or *C. trachomatis*. Accurate diagnosis and appropriate antibiotic therapy are aimed at preventing complications such as pelvic adhesions, infertility, ectopic pregnancy, chronic abdominal pain, and tubo-ovarian abscesses.

Ectopic pregnancy occurs when a fertilized ovum implants outside the uterine cavity; the most common site is the fallopian tube. Causes of ectopic pregnancy are delayed ovum transport resulting from complications of PID, therapeutic abortion, tubal ligation or tubal reversal, previous ectopic pregnancy, or other conditions such as use of fertility drugs to induce ovulation. It represents a true gynecologic emergency, often necessitating surgical intervention. Cancer of the fallopian tube is

rare; the diagnosis is difficult, and the condition usually is well advanced when diagnosed.

Disorders of the ovaries include benign cysts, functioning ovarian tumors, and cancer of the ovary; they usually are asymptomatic unless there is substantial enlargement or bleeding into the cyst, or the cyst becomes twisted or ruptures. PCOS is characterized by anovulation with varying degrees of menstrual irregularity and infertility; hyperandrogenism with hirsutism, acne, male-pattern of hair loss, and obesity; polycystic ovaries; and hyperinsulinemia with insulin resistance. Benign ovarian tumors consist of endometriomas (chocolate cysts that develop secondary to ovarian endometriosis); ovarian fibromas (connective tissue tumors composed of fibrocytes and collagen); and cystic teratomas or dermoid cysts (germ cell tumors composed of various combinations of ectodermal, mesodermal, and endodermal elements). Functioning ovarian tumors may be benign or malignant and are of three types: estrogen secreting, androgen secreting, and mixed estrogen–androgen secreting. Cancer of the ovary is the second most common female genitourinary cancer and the most lethal. It can be divided into three categories: epithelial tumors, germ cell tumors, and gonadal stromal tumors. There are no effective screening methods for ovarian cancer, and often the disease is well advanced at the time of diagnosis. ■

DISORDERS OF PELVIC SUPPORT AND UTERINE POSITION

After completing this section of the chapter, you should be able to meet the following objectives:

- Characterize the function of the supporting ligaments and pelvic floor muscles in maintaining the position of the pelvic organs, including the uterus, bladder, and rectum.
- Describe the manifestations of cystocele, rectocele, and enterocele.
- Explain how uterine anteflexion, retroflexion, and retroversion differ from normal uterine position.
- Describe the cause and manifestations of uterine prolapse.

Disorders of Pelvic Support

The uterus and the pelvic structures are maintained in proper position by the uterosacral ligaments, round ligaments, broad ligament, and cardinal ligaments. The two cardinal ligaments maintain the cervix in its normal position (see Chapter 45, Fig. 45-4). The uterosacral ligaments hold the uterus in a forward position and the broad ligaments suspend the uterus, fallopian tubes, and

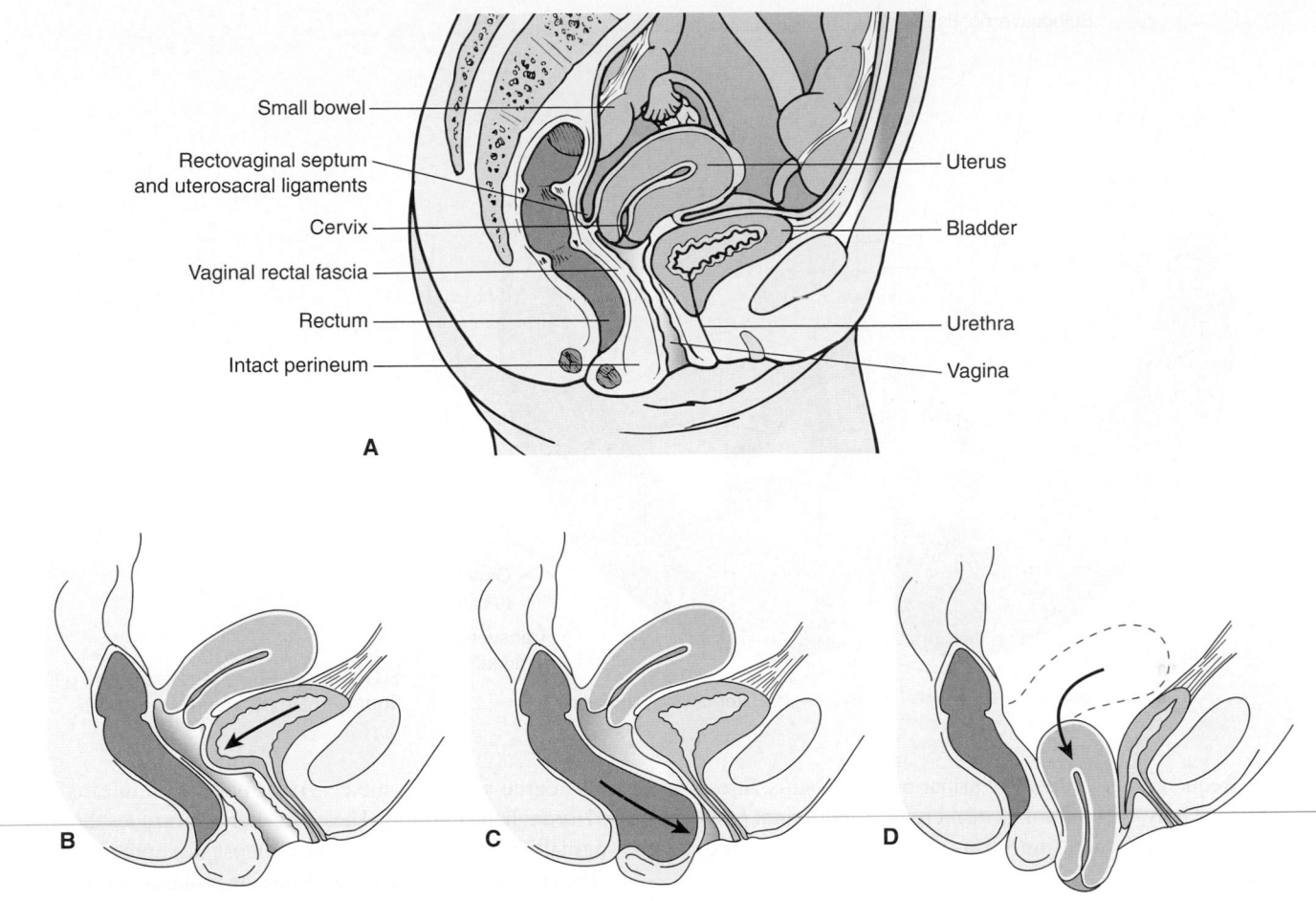

Small bowel

Rectovaginal septum and uterosacral ligaments

Cervix

Vaginal rectal fascia

Rectum

Intact perineum

Uterus

Bladder

Urethra

Vagina

A

B

C

D

FIGURE 46-10 • **(A)** Normal support of the uterus and vagina, **(B)** cystocele, **(C)** rectocele, and **(D)** uterine prolapse.

ovaries in the pelvis. The vagina is encased in the semirigid structure of the strong supporting fascia (Fig. 46-10A). The muscular floor of the pelvis is a strong, slinglike structure that supports the uterus, vagina, urinary bladder, and rectum (Fig. 46-11). In the female anatomy, nature is faced with the problems of supporting the pelvic viscera against the force of gravity and increases in intra-abdominal pressure associated with coughing, sneezing, defecation, and laughing while at the same time allowing for urination, defecation, and normal reproductive tract function, especially the delivery of an infant. Three supporting structures are provided for the abdominal pelvic diaphragm. The bony pelvis provides support and protection for parts of the digestive tract and genitourinary structures, and the peritoneum holds the pelvic viscera in place. The main support for the viscera, however, is the pelvic diaphragm, made up of muscles and connective tissue that stretch across the bones of the pelvic outlet. The openings that must exist for the urethra, rectum, and vagina cause an inherent weakness in the pelvic diaphragm. Congenital or acquired weakness of the pelvic diaphragm results in widening of these openings, particularly the vagina, with the possible herniation of pelvic viscera through the pelvic floor (*i.e.,* prolapse).

Relaxation of the pelvic outlet usually comes about because of overstretching of the perineal supporting tissues during pregnancy and childbirth. Although the tissues are stretched only during these times, there may be no difficulty until later in life, such as in the fifth or sixth decade, when further loss of elasticity and muscle tone occurs. Even in a woman who has not borne children, the combination of aging and postmenopausal changes may give rise to problems related to relaxation of the pelvic support structures. The three most common conditions associated with this relaxation are cystocele, rectocele, and uterine prolapse. These may occur separately or together.

Cystocele

Cystocele is a herniation of the bladder into the vagina. It occurs when the normal muscle support for the bladder is weakened, and the bladder sags below the uterus. This causes the anterior vaginal wall to stretch and bulge downward, allowing the bladder to herniate into the vagina due to the force of gravity and pressures from coughing, lifting, or straining at stool (see Fig. 46-10B). The symptoms of cystocele include an annoying bearing-down sensation, difficulty in emptying the

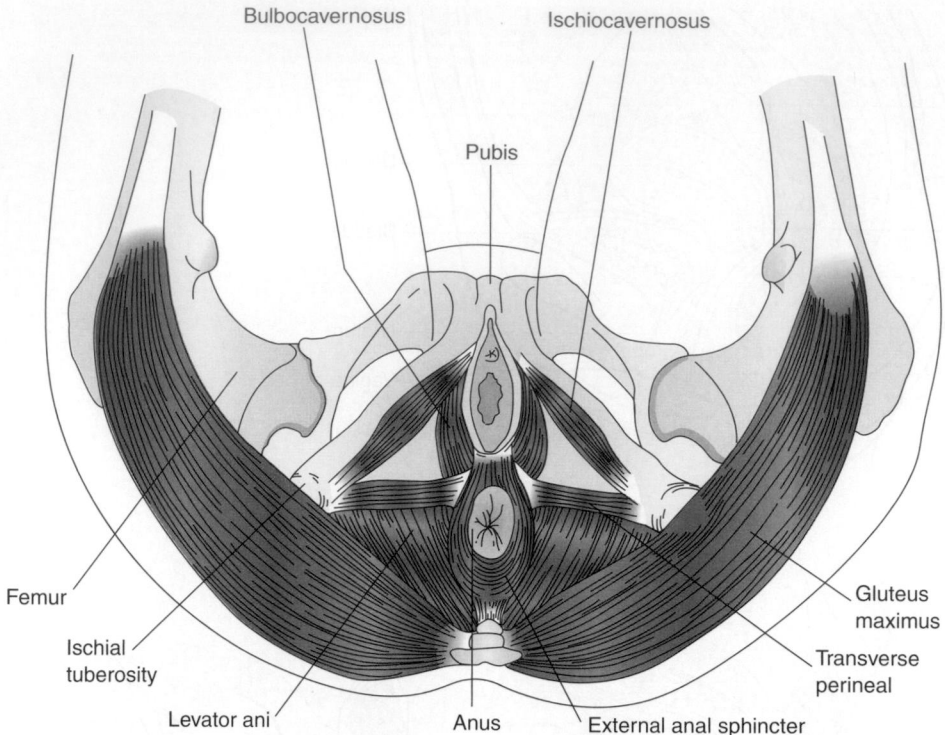

Bulbocavernosus   Ischiocavernosus

Pubis

Femur

Ischial
tuberosity

Levator ani   Anus   External anal sphincter

Gluteus
maximus

Transverse
perineal

FIGURE 46-11 • Muscles of the pelvic
floor (female perineum).

bladder, frequency and urgency of urination, and cystitis. Stress incontinence may occur at times of increased abdominal pressure, such as during squatting, straining, coughing, sneezing, laughing, or lifting.

Rectocele and Enterocele

Rectocele is the herniation of the rectum into the vagina. It occurs when the posterior vaginal wall and underlying rectum bulge forward, ultimately protruding through the introitus as the pelvic floor and perineal muscles are weakened. The symptoms include discomfort because of the protrusion of the rectum and difficulty in defecation (see Fig. 46-10C). Digital pressure (*i.e.,* splinting) on the bulging posterior wall of the vagina may become necessary for defecation. The area between the uterosacral ligaments just posterior to the cervix may weaken and form a hernial sac into which the small bowel protrudes when the woman is standing. This defect, called an *enterocele,* may extend into the rectovaginal septum. It may be congenital or acquired through birth trauma. Enterocele can be asymptomatic or cause a dull, dragging sensation and occasionally low backache.

Uterine Prolapse

Uterine prolapse is the bulging of the uterus into the vagina that occurs when the primary supportive ligaments (*i.e.,* cardinal ligaments) are stretched (see Fig. 46-10D). Prolapse is ranked as first, second, or third degree, depending on how far the uterus protrudes through the introitus. First-degree prolapse shows some descent, but the cervix has not reached the introitus. In

second-degree prolapse, the cervix or part of the uterus has passed through the introitus. The entire uterus protrudes through the vaginal opening in third-degree prolapse (*i.e.,* procidentia).

The symptoms associated with uterine prolapse result from irritation of the exposed mucous membranes of the cervix and vagina and the discomfort of the protruding mass. Prolapse often is accompanied by perineal relaxation, cystocele, or rectocele. Like cystocele, rectocele, and enterocele, it occurs most commonly in multiparous women because childbearing is accompanied by injuries to pelvic structures and uterine ligaments. It also may result from pelvic tumors and neurologic conditions, such as spina bifida and diabetic neuropathy, that interrupt the innervation of pelvic muscles. A pessary may be inserted to hold the uterus in place and may stave off surgical intervention in women who want to have children or in older women for whom the surgery may pose a significant health risk. A newer conservative approach to treatment involves use of a space-occupying device (Colpexin sphere) to elevate the prolapse while performing pelvic floor muscle contractions.[54]

Treatment of Pelvic Support Disorders

Most of the disorders of pelvic relaxation require surgical correction. These are elective surgeries and usually are deferred until after the childbearing years. The symptoms associated with the disorders often are not severe enough to warrant surgical correction. In other cases, the stress of surgery is contraindicated because of other physical disorders; this is particularly true of older women, in whom many of these disorders occur.

There are a number of surgical procedures for the conditions that result from relaxation of pelvic support structures.

Removal of the uterus through the vagina (vaginal hysterectomy) with appropriate repair of the vaginal wall (colporrhaphy) often is done when uterine prolapse is accompanied by cystocele or rectocele. A vesicourethral suspension may be done to alleviate the symptoms of stress incontinence. Repair may involve abdominal hysterectomy along with anteroposterior repair. Kegel exercises, which strengthen the pubococcygeus muscle, may be helpful in cases of mild cystocele or rectocele or after surgical repair to help maintain the improved function.

Variations in Uterine Position

Variations in the position of the uterus are common. Some variations are innocuous; others, which may be the result of weakness and relaxation of the perineum, give rise to various problems that compromise the structural integrity of the pelvic floor, particularly after childbirth.

The uterus usually is flexed approximately 45 degrees anteriorly, with the cervix positioned posteriorly and downward in the anteverted position. When the woman is standing, the angle of the uterus is such that it lies practically horizontal, resting lightly on the bladder.

Asymptomatic, normal variations in the axis of the uterus in relation to the cervix and physiologic displacements that arise after pregnancy or with pathology of the cul-de-sac include anteflexion, retroflexion, and retroversion (Fig. 46-12). An anteflexed uterus is flexed forward on itself. Retroflexion is flexion backward at the isthmus. Retroversion describes the condition in which the uterus inclines posteriorly while the cervix remains tilted forward. Simple retroversion of the uterus is the most common displacement, found in 30% of normal women. It usually is a congenital condition caused by a short anterior vaginal

wall and relaxed uterosacral ligaments; together, these force the uterus to fall back into the cul-de-sac. Retroversion also can follow certain diseases, such as endometriosis and PID, which produce fibrous tissue adherence with retraction of the fundus posteriorly. Large leiomyomas also may cause the uterus to move into a posterior position. Dyspareunia with deep penetration or low back pain with menses can be associated with retroversion. Most symptoms in these women are caused by the associated condition (*e.g.*, adhesions, fibroids) rather than congenital retroversion.

 **IN SUMMARY,** alterations in pelvic support frequently occur because of weaknesses and relaxation of the pelvic floor and perineum. Cystocele and rectocele involve herniation of the bladder or rectum into the vagina. Uterine prolapse occurs when the uterus bulges into the vagina. Pelvic relaxation disorders typically result from overstretching of the perineal supporting muscles during pregnancy and childbirth. The loss of elasticity in these structures that is a normal accompaniment of aging contributes to these problems. Variations in uterine position include anteflexion, retroflexion, and retroversion. These disorders, which often are innocuous, can be the result of a congenital shortness of the vaginal wall, development of fibrous adhesions secondary to endometriosis or PID, or displacement caused by large uterine leiomyomas. ■

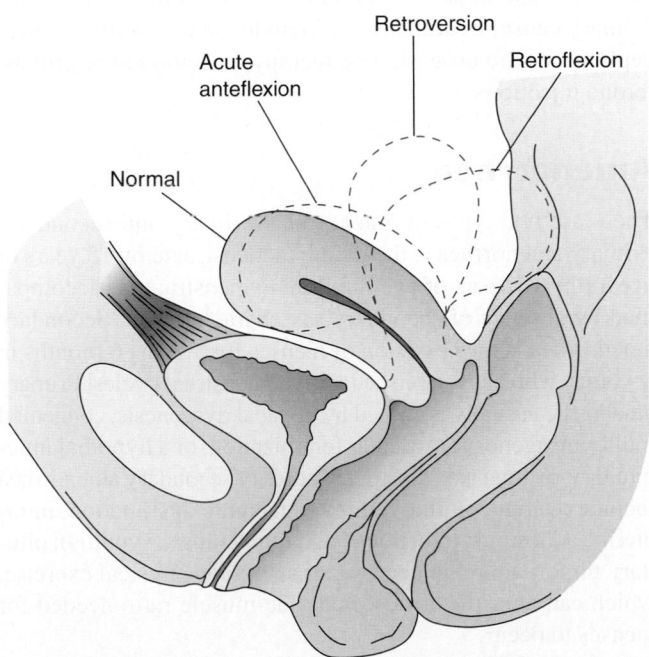

FIGURE 46-12 • Variations in uterine position.

MENSTRUAL DISORDERS

After completing this section of the chapter, you should be able to meet the following objectives:

- Define the terms amenorrhea, hypomenorrhea, oligomenorrhea, menorrhagia, metrorrhagia, and menometrorrhagia.
- Relate the alteration in estrogen and progesterone levels to the development of dysfunctional menstrual cycles.
- Differentiate between primary dysmenorrhea and secondary dysmenorrhea.
- Characterize the manifestations of the premenstrual syndrome, its possible causes, and the methods of treatment.

Dysfunctional Menstrual Cycles

Although unexplained uterine bleeding can occur for many reasons, such as pregnancy, abortion, bleeding disorders, and neoplasms, the most frequent cause in the nonpregnant woman is what is commonly called *dysfunctional menstrual cycles* or *bleeding.* Dysfunctional cycles may take the form of *amenorrhea* (absence of menstruation), *hypomenorrhea* (scanty menstruation), *oligomenorrhea* (infrequent menstruation, periods more than 35 days apart), *polymenorrhea* (frequent menstruation, periods less than 21 days apart), *menorrhagia* (excessive menstruation), or *metrorrhagia* (bleeding between periods). *Menometrorrhagia* is heavy bleeding during and between menstrual periods.

🔑 DYSFUNCTIONAL MENSTRUAL CYCLES

- The pattern of menstrual bleeding tends to be fairly consistent in most healthy women with regard to frequency, duration, and amount of flow.

- Dysfunctional bleeding in postpubertal women can take the form of absent or scanty periods, infrequent periods, excessive and irregular periods, excessive bleeding during periods, and bleeding between periods.

- When the basic pattern of bleeding is changed, it is most often due to a lack of ovulation and disturbances in the pattern of hormone secretion.

- When the basic pattern is undisturbed and there are superimposed episodes of bleeding or spotting, the etiology is more likely to be related to organic lesions or hematologic disorders.

Dysfunctional menstrual cycles are related to alterations in the hormones that support normal cyclic endometrial changes (see Chapter 45). Estrogen deprivation causes retrogression of a previously built-up endometrium and bleeding. Such bleeding often is irregular in amount and duration, with the flow varying with the time and degree of estrogen stimulation and with the degree of estrogen withdrawal. A lack of progesterone can cause abnormal menstrual bleeding; in its absence, estrogen induces development of a much thicker endometrial layer with a richer blood supply. The absence of progesterone results from the failure of any of the developing ovarian follicles to mature to the point of ovulation, with the subsequent formation of the corpus luteum and production and secretion of progesterone.

Periodic bleeding episodes alternating with amenorrhea are caused by variations in the number of functioning ovarian follicles present. If sufficient follicles are present and active and if new follicles assume functional capacity, high levels of estrogen develop, causing the endometrium to proliferate for weeks or even months. In time, estrogen withdrawal and bleeding develop. This can occur for two reasons: an absolute estrogen deficiency may develop when several follicles simultaneously degenerate, or a relative deficiency may develop as the needs of the enlarged endometrial tissue mass exceed the capabilities of the existing follicles, even though estrogen levels remain constant. Estrogen and progesterone deficiencies are associated with the absence of ovulation, hence the term *anovulatory*

bleeding. Because the vasoconstriction and myometrial contractions that normally accompany menstruation are caused by progesterone, anovulatory bleeding seldom is accompanied by cramps, and the flow frequently is heavy. Anovulatory cycles are common among adolescents during the first several years after menarche, when ovarian function is becoming established, and among perimenopausal women, whose ovarian function is beginning to decline.

Dysfunctional menstrual cycles can originate as a primary disorder of the ovaries or as a secondary defect in ovarian function related to hypothalamic–pituitary stimulation. The latter can be initiated by emotional stress, marked variation in weight (*i.e.*, sudden gain or loss), or nonspecific endocrine or metabolic disturbances. Nonhormonal causes of irregular menstrual bleeding include endometrial polyps, submucosal myoma (*i.e.*, fibroid), bleeding disorder (*e.g.*, von Willebrand disease, platelet dysfunction), infection, endometrial cancer, PCOS, and pregnancy.

The treatment of dysfunctional bleeding depends on what is identified as the probable cause. The minimum evaluation should include a detailed history with emphasis on bleeding pattern and a physical examination. Endocrine studies (*e.g.*, FSH/LH ratio, prolactin, testosterone, DHEAS levels), β-hCG pregnancy test, ultrasonography of the endometrium, endometrial biopsy, D&C with or without hysteroscopy, and progesterone withdrawal tests may be needed for diagnosis. Nonhormonal causes generally require surgical intervention. D&C can be therapeutic as well as diagnostic. Endometrial ablation (thinning or elimination of the basal layer of the endometrium from which the monthly buildup generates) has become a primary treatment strategy for heavy bleeding; it can be accomplished using heat, cold, microwave, chemicals, or radiofrequency energy sources.[55] If nonhormonal problems have been excluded and alterations in hormone levels are the primary cause, treatment may include the use of oral contraceptives, cyclic progesterone therapy, or long-acting progesterone injections.

Amenorrhea

There are two types of amenorrhea: primary and secondary. Primary amenorrhea is the failure to menstruate by 15 years of age, or by 13 years of age if failure to menstruate is accompanied by absence of secondary sex characteristics. Secondary amenorrhea is the cessation of menses for at least 6 months in a woman who has established normal menstrual cycles. Primary amenorrhea usually is caused by gonadal dysgenesis, congenital müllerian agenesis, testicular feminization, or a hypothalamic-pituitary-ovarian axis disorder. Causes of secondary amenorrhea include ovarian, pituitary, or hypothalamic dysfunction; intrauterine adhesions; infections (*e.g.*, tuberculosis, syphilis); pituitary tumor; anorexia nervosa; or strenuous physical exercise, which can alter the critical body fat–muscle ratio needed for menses to occur.[56]

Diagnostic evaluation resembles that for dysfunctional uterine bleeding, with the possible addition of a computed tomographic scan or MRI to exclude a pituitary tumor. Treatment is based on correcting the underlying cause and inducing menstruation with cyclic progesterone or combined estrogen-progesterone regimens.

Dysmenorrhea

Dysmenorrhea is pain or discomfort with menstruation. Although not usually a serious medical problem, it causes some degree of monthly disability for a significant number of women. There are two forms of dysmenorrhea: primary and secondary. Primary dysmenorrhea is menstrual pain that is not associated with a physical abnormality or pathologic process.[57] It usually occurs with ovulatory menstruation beginning 6 months to 2 years after menarche. Symptoms may begin 1 to 2 days before menses, peak on the first day of flow, and subside within several hours to several days. Severe dysmenorrhea may be associated with systemic symptoms such as headache, nausea, vomiting, diarrhea, fatigue, irritability, dizziness, and syncope. The pain typically is described as dull, lower abdominal aching or cramping, spasmodic or colicky in nature, often radiating to the lower back, labia majora, or upper thighs.

Secondary dysmenorrhea is menstrual pain caused by specific organic conditions, such as endometriosis, uterine fibroids, adenomyosis, pelvic adhesions, IUDs, or PID. Laparoscopy often is required for diagnosis of secondary dysmenorrhea if medication for primary dysmenorrhea is ineffective.

Treatment for primary dysmenorrhea is directed at symptom control. Although analgesic agents such as aspirin and acetaminophen may relieve minor uterine cramping or low back pain, prostaglandin synthetase inhibitors (*e.g.,* ibuprofen, naproxen, mefenamic acid, indomethacin) are more specific for dysmenorrhea and the treatment of choice if contraception is not desired. Ovulation suppression and symptomatic relief of dysmenorrhea can be instituted simultaneously with the use of oral contraceptives. Relief of secondary dysmenorrhea depends on identifying the cause of the problem. Medical or surgical intervention may be needed to eliminate the problem.

Premenstrual Symptom Disorders

According to surveys, 80% of women experience premenstrual emotional or physical changes, with 20% to 40% of the adult female population in the United States indicating these mild to moderate monthly symptoms cause some difficulty; only 3% to 8% report extreme or severe symptoms that have a negative impact on their life.[58,59] It appears there is a spectrum of premenstrual symptom disorders that runs from *premenstrual molimina* on the mild end; through *premenstrual syndrome* (PMS), which is characterized by mild to moderate physical and psychological symptoms limited to 3 to 14 days preceding menstruation and relieved by onset of the menses; to *premenstrual dysphoric disorder* (PMDD), which is the most severe form of premenstrual distress and generally is associated with mood disorders. How many of these women have symptoms that are severe enough to warrant treatment is unknown. The incidence of PMS seems to increase with age. It is less common in women in their teens and twenties, and most of the women seeking help for the problem are in their mid-thirties. The disorder is not culturally distinct; it affects both Westerners and non-Westerners. There is some dispute about whether PMS occurs more frequently in women who have had children or in those who have not.

Physical symptoms of PMS include painful and swollen breasts, bloating, abdominal pain, headache, and backache. Psychologically, there may be depression, anxiety, irritability, and behavioral changes. In some cases, there are puzzling alterations in motor function, such as clumsiness and altered handwriting. Women with PMS may report one or several symptoms, with symptoms varying from woman to woman and from month to month in the same patient. Signs and symptoms associated with this disorder are summarized in Table 46-2. PMS can significantly affect a woman's ability to perform at normal levels. Family responsibilities and relationships may suffer and she may lose time from or function ineffectively at work. Students have had lower grades during the premenstrual period. More crimes are committed by women during the premenstrual phase of the cycle, and more lives are lost to suicide during this period.

TABLE 46-2 **Symptoms of Premenstrual Syndrome (PMS) by System**	
BODY SYSTEM	**SYMPTOMS**
Cerebral	Irritability, anxiety, nervousness, fatigue, exhaustion, increased physical and mental activity, lability, crying spells, depression, inability to concentrate
Gastrointestinal	Craving for sweets or salt, lower abdominal pain, bloating, nausea, vomiting, diarrhea, constipation
Vascular	Headache, edema, weakness, fainting
Reproductive	Swelling and tenderness of the breasts, pelvic congestion, ovarian pain, altered libido
Neuromuscular	Trembling of the extremities, changes in coordination, clumsiness, backache, leg aches
General	Weight gain, insomnia, dizziness, acne

Although the causes of PMS are poorly documented, they probably are multifactorial. Like dysmenorrhea, it is only recently that PMS has been recognized as a bona fide disorder rather than merely a psychosomatic illness. There has been a tendency to link the disorder with endocrine imbalances such as hyperprolactinemia, estrogen excess, and alteration in the estrogen–progesterone ratio. Prolactin concentration affects sodium and water retention, is higher in the luteal phase than in the follicular phase, and can be increased by estrogens, stress, hypoglycemia, pregnancy, and oral contraceptives. Estrogens stimulate anxiety and nervous tension, and increased progesterone levels may produce depression. The role of hormonal factors in the cause of PMS is supported by two well-established phenomena. First, women who have undergone a hysterectomy but not an oophorectomy may have cyclic symptoms that resemble PMS. Second, PMS symptoms are rare in postmenopausal women. Research has failed, however, to confirm these theories. Because there appear to be no measurable differences in hormone levels between women with and without PMS, it is presumed that normal cyclic variation in the hormones is the trigger for symptoms in vulnerable or predisposed women.[59]

Other hypotheses suggest that increased aldosterone may contribute to symptoms associated with fluid retention (*e.g.,* headache, bloating, breast tenderness, weight gain); that pyridoxine (vitamin B_6) deficiency may lead to estrogen excess or decreased production of the neurotransmitters dopamine and serotonin, which may contribute to PMS symptoms; or that decreased prostaglandin E_1 concentrations can lead to abnormal sensitivity to prolactin, with associated fluid retention, irritability, and depression. In addition, increased appetite, binge eating, fatigue, and depression have been associated with altered endorphin activity and subclinical hypoglycemia. Learned beliefs about menstruation may also contribute to the development of PMS or at least affect the woman's response to the symptoms.

The most recent theory to emerge suggests a relationship between normal gonadal fluctuations and central neurotransmitter activity, particularly serotonin. It is unclear whether decreased levels of serotonin are present during the luteal phase, and only susceptible women respond with varying degrees of premenstrual symptoms, or if women with PMDD have a neurotransmitter abnormality.[3,58–61]

A complete history and physical examination are necessary to exclude other physical causes of the symptoms. Depending on the symptom pattern, blood studies, including thyroid hormones, glucose, and prolactin assays, may be done. Psychosocial evaluation is helpful to exclude emotional illness that is merely exacerbated premenstrually. In 2000, the American College of Obstetricians and Gynecologists (ACOG) published clinical management guidelines for PMS that included diagnostic criteria[61] (Table 46-3). Diagnosis focuses on identification of symptoms by means of a daily calendar on which the woman records her symptoms for 2 to 3 consecutive months. Although validated tools are available for recording symptoms, any calendar used for this purpose should include information regarding specific symptoms, severity, timing in relation to the

menstrual cycle, and baseline level of symptoms in the follicular phase.[3,58] PMDD is a psychiatric diagnosis that has been developed to distinguish those women whose symptoms are severe enough to interfere significantly with activities of daily living. It requires prospective symptom charting, and a minimum of 5 of the 11 symptom groups as described in the fourth edition of the *Diagnostic and Statistical Manual of Mental Disorders* (*DSM-IV*) to establish a diagnosis of PMDD (Box 46-1). Presence of a single symptom is sufficient for the diagnosis of PMS.[58,59]

TABLE 46-3 ACOG Diagnostic Criteria for Premenstrual Syndrome (PMS)

AFFECTIVE SYMPTOMS	SOMATIC SYMPTOMS
Irritability	Breast tenderness
Depression	Abdominal bloating
Angry outbursts	Headache
Anxiety	Swelling of the extremities
Confusion	
Social withdrawal	

PMS = one or more bothersome symptoms in either category occurring during the 5 days before menses in each of three consecutive menstrual cycles, must be relieved within 4 days of the onset of menses, and must not recur until at least cycle day 13.
Data from the American College of Obstetricians and Gynecologists (ACOG). (2000). Premenstrual syndrome. *ACOG practice bulletin no. 15* (pp. 1–9). Washington, DC: Author.

BOX 46-1 *DSM-IV-TR* CRITERIA FOR PREMENSTRUAL DYSPHORIC DISORDER (PMDD)

Core Symptoms

Depressed mood
Moodiness
Anxiety, edginess, nervousness
Anger, irritability

Other Symptoms

Fatigue, lethargy
Insomnia, hypersomnia
Difficulty concentrating
Appetite changes or cravings
Diminished interest in usual activities
Feeling overwhelmed or out of control
Physical symptoms (headache, breast tenderness or swelling, bloating, joint and muscle pain)

PMDD = patient must exhibit five or more symptoms, including at least one core symptom during the premenstrual period, confirmed by prospective charting during at least two consecutive menstrual cycles. Symptoms must cause marked impairment in the woman's ability to carry out her usual activities, must abate within a few days of the onset of menses, and not recur during the week after menses.
From American Psychiatric Association. (2000). Premenstrual dysphoric disorder. In *Diagnostic and statistical manual of mental disorders, fourth edition, text revision* (pp. 771–774). Washington, DC: Author.

Management of PMS/PMDD has been largely symptomatic and includes education and support directed toward lifestyle changes for women with mild symptoms. Treatment includes diuretics to reduce fluid retention; analgesics for pain, and anxiolytic drugs to treat mood changes. An integrated program of personal assessment by diary, regular exercise, avoidance of caffeine, and a diet low in simple sugars and high in lean proteins is often beneficial. Additional therapeutic regimens that have been used include vitamin or mineral supplements (particularly pyridoxine, vitamin E, and magnesium); evening primrose oil (which contains linoleic acid, a precursor of prostaglandin E_1); natural progesterone supplements; low-dose oral monophasic contraceptives; GnRH agonists; bromocriptine for prolactin suppression; danazol (a synthetic androgen); and spironolactone (an aldosterone antagonist and inhibitor of adrenal androgen synthesis).[58,59] Although a body of knowledge has evolved that offers a variety of therapeutic choices, few treatments have been adequately evaluated in randomized, controlled clinical trials. The SSRI antidepressants, however, have demonstrated significant improvement in overall symptoms compared with placebo, whether used continuously or only in the luteal phase, and are recommended by ACOG as first-line therapy for severe PMS or PMDD.[3,58–61] In addition, the FDA has approved an oral contraceptive pill containing drospirenone (a spironolactone derivative) for the treatment of the emotional and physical symptoms of PMS/PMDD.[58,59]

IN SUMMARY, menstrual disorders include dysfunctional menstrual cycles, dysmenorrhea, and PMS. Dysfunctional menstrual cycles, which involve amenorrhea, oligomenorrhea, metrorrhagia, or menorrhagia, occur when the hormonal support of the endometrium is altered. Estrogen deprivation causes retrogression of a previously built-up endometrium and bleeding. A lack of progesterone can cause abnormal menstrual bleeding; in its absence, estrogen induces development of a much thicker endometrial layer with a richer blood supply. The absence of progesterone results from the failure of any of the developing ovarian follicles to mature to the point of ovulation, with subsequent formation of the corpus luteum and production of progesterone.

Dysmenorrhea is characterized by pain or discomfort during menses. It can occur as a primary or secondary disorder. Primary dysmenorrhea is not associated with other disorders and begins soon after menarche. Secondary dysmenorrhea is caused by a specific organic condition, such as endometriosis or pelvic adhesions. It occurs in women with previously painless menses.

Premenstrual symptom disorders represent a spectrum from molimina, which is present to some degree in most ovulatory women, to PMS and PMDD. PMS represents a cluster of physical and psychological symptoms that precede menstruation by 1 to 2 weeks. PMDD describes the most severe, disabling form of PMS. The true incidence and nature of PMS has been recognized only recently, and its cause and methods for treatment are still under study. ■

DISORDERS OF THE BREAST

After completing this section of the chapter, you should be able to meet the following objectives:

- Describe changes in breast function that occur with galactorrhea, mastitis, and ductal ectasia.
- Describe the manifestations of fibrocystic breast changes.
- Cite the risk factors for breast cancer, the importance of clinical breast examination, and recommendations for mammography.
- Describe the methods used in the diagnosis and treatment of breast cancer.

Most breast disease may be described as benign or cancerous. Breast tissue is never static; the breast is constantly responding to changes in hormonal, nutritional, psychological, and environmental stimuli that cause continual cellular changes. Benign breast conditions are nonprogressive; some forms of benign disease, however, increase the risk of malignant disease. In light of this, strict adherence to a dichotomy of benign versus malignant disease may not always be appropriate. This dichotomy, however, is useful for the sake of simplicity and clarity.

Galactorrhea

Galactorrhea is the secretion of breast milk in a nonlactating breast. Galactorrhea may result from vigorous nipple stimulation during lovemaking, exogenous hormones, internal hormonal imbalance, or local chest infection or trauma. A pituitary tumor may produce large amounts of prolactin and cause galactorrhea. Galactorrhea occurs in men and women and usually is benign. Observation may be continued for several months before diagnostic hormonal screening. Spontaneous leaking from the breast (occurring without any type of stimulation) is pathologic and warrants investigation.[62]

Mastitis

Mastitis is inflammation of the breast. It most frequently occurs during lactation but may also result from other conditions. In the lactating woman, inflammation results from an ascending infection that travels from the nipple to the ductile structures. The most common organisms isolated are *Staphylococcus* and *Streptococcus*.[3] The offending organisms originate from the suckling infant's nasopharynx or the mother's hands. During the early weeks of nursing, the breast is particularly vulnerable to bacterial invasion because of minor cracks and fissures that occur with vigorous suckling. Infection and inflammation cause obstruction of the ductile system. The breast area becomes hard, inflamed, and tender if not treated early. Without treatment, the area becomes walled off and may abscess, requiring incision and drainage. It is advisable for the mother to continue breast-feeding during antibiotic therapy to prevent this.

Mastitis is not confined to the postpartum period; it can occur as a result of hormonal fluctuations, tumors, trauma, or skin infection. Cyclic inflammation of the breast occurs most frequently in adolescents, who commonly have fluctuating hormone levels. Tumors may cause mastitis secondary to skin involvement or lymphatic obstruction. Local trauma or infection may develop into mastitis because of ductal blockage of trapped blood, cellular debris, or the extension of superficial inflammation. Treatment for mastitis symptoms includes application of heat or cold, excision, aspiration, mild analgesics, antibiotics, and a supportive brassiere or breast binder.

Ductal Disorders

Ductal ectasia manifests in older women as a spontaneous, intermittent, usually unilateral, grayish-green nipple discharge. Palpation of the breast increases the discharge. Ectasia occurs during or after menopause and is symptomatically associated with burning, itching, pain, and a pulling sensation of the nipple and areola. The disease results in inflammation of the ducts and subsequent thickening. The treatment requires removal of the involved ductal mass.

Intraductal papillomas are benign epithelial tissue tumors that range in size from 2 mm to 5 cm. Papillomas usually manifest with a bloody nipple discharge. The tumor may be palpated in the areolar area. *Galactography,* a radiograph taken after dye is injected into the affected duct, is used for diagnosis.[62] The papilloma is probed through the nipple, and the involved duct is removed.

Fibroadenoma and Fibrocystic Changes

Fibroadenomas are seen in premenopausal women, most commonly in the third and fourth decades. The clinical findings include a firm, rubbery, sharply defined round mass. On palpation, the mass "slides" between the fingers and is easily movable. These masses usually are singular; only 15% are multiple or bilateral. Fibroadenomas are asymptomatic and usually found by accident. They are not thought to be precancerous. Treatment involves simple excision.

Fibrocystic changes is the most frequent lesion of the breast. It is most common in women 30 to 50 years of age and is rare in postmenopausal women not receiving hormone replacement.[62–64] Fibrocystic changes usually present as nodular (*i.e.,* "shotty"), granular breast masses that are more prominent and painful during the luteal or progesterone-dominant portion of the menstrual cycle. Discomfort ranges from heaviness to exquisite tenderness, depending on the degree of vascular engorgement and cystic distention.

Fibrocystic changes encompass a wide variety of lesions and breast changes. Microscopically, fibrocystic changes refer to a constellation of morphologic changes manifested by (1) cystic dilation of terminal ducts, (2) relative increase in fibrous tissue,

and (3) variable proliferation of terminal duct epithelial elements.[63] Autopsy studies have demonstrated some degree of fibrocystic change in 75% of adult women in the United States.[63] Symptomatic fibrocystic changes, in which large, clinically detectable cysts are present, is much less common, occurring in approximately 10% of adult women between 35 and 50 years of age.[63] Although fibrocystic changes have been thought to increase the risk of breast cancer, only certain variants in which proliferation of the epithelial components is demonstrated represent a true risk. Fibrocystic changes with giant cysts and proliferative epithelial lesions with atypia are more common in women who are at increased risk for development of breast cancer.[65] The nonproliferative form of fibrocystic changes that does not carry an increased risk for development of cancer is more common.

Diagnosis of fibrocystic changes is made by physical examination, mammography, ultrasonography, and biopsy (*i.e.,* aspiration or tissue sample). The use of mammography for diagnosis in high-risk groups younger than 35 years of age on a routine basis remains controversial. Mammography may be helpful in establishing the diagnosis, but increased breast tissue density in women with fibrocystic changes may make an abnormal or cancerous mass difficult to discern among the other structures. Ultrasonography is useful in differentiating a cystic from a solid mass. Because a mass caused by fibrocystic changes may be indistinguishable from carcinoma on the basis of clinical findings, suspect lesions should undergo biopsy. Fine-needle aspiration may be used, but if a suspect mass that was nonmalignant on cytologic examination does not resolve over several months, it should be removed surgically. Any discrete mass or lump on the breast should be viewed as possible carcinoma, and cancer should be excluded before instituting the conservative measures used to treat fibrocystic changes.

Treatment for fibrocystic changes is usually symptomatic. Mild analgesics (*e.g.,* aspirin, acetaminophen, or NSAIDs), vitamin E, evening primrose oil, and local application of heat or cold may be used for pain relief. Prominent or persistent cysts may be aspirated and any fluid obtained sent to the laboratory for cytologic analysis. Women should be encouraged to wear a good supporting brassiere, and are advised to avoid foods that contain xanthines (*e.g.,* coffee, cola, chocolate, and tea) in their daily diets, particularly premenstrually. Tamoxifen or danazol, a synthetic androgen, may be used for women with severe pain.[62]

Breast Cancer

Cancer of the breast is the most common female cancer. One in eight women in the United States will have breast cancer in her lifetime. In 2007, breast cancer affected an estimated 178,500 American women and killed an estimated 40,600 women.[12] Although the breast cancer mortality rate has shown a slight decline, it is second only to lung cancer as a cause of cancer-related deaths in women. An additional 450 deaths occurred from breast cancer in men.[12] Incidence rates for carcinoma in situ have increased dramatically since the mid-1970s because of recommendations regarding mammography screening. Death rates decreased approximately 2.3% per year between 1990 and 2002, particularly in women younger than 50 years of age. The decline in the breast cancer mortality rate since 1989 is due to earlier diagnosis through screening programs and increased awareness, as well as improvements in cancer treatments.[12]

Risk factors for breast cancer include sex, increasing age, personal or family history of breast cancer (*i.e.*, at highest risk are those with multiple affected first-order relatives), history of benign breast disease (*i.e.*, primary "atypical" hyperplasia), and hormonal influences that promote breast maturation and may increase the chance of cell mutation (*i.e.*, early menarche, late menopause, and no term pregnancies or first child after 30 years of age). Modifiable risk factors include obesity (particularly after menopause), physical inactivity, alcohol intake greater than one drink per day, and long-term use of postmenopausal hormone therapy (especially combined estrogen and progestin).[66] Most women with breast cancer have no identifiable risk factors.

Approximately 5% to 10% of all breast cancers are hereditary, with genetic mutations causing up to 80% of breast cancers in women younger than 50 years of age.[67] Two breast cancer susceptibility genes—*BRCA1* on chromosome 17 and *BRCA2* on chromosome 13—may account for most inherited forms of breast cancer (see Chapter 8). *BRCA1* is known to be involved in tumor suppression. A woman with known mutations in *BRCA1* has a lifetime risk of 60% to 85% for breast cancer and an increased risk of ovarian cancer. *BRCA2* is another susceptibility gene that carries an elevated cancer risk similar to that with *BRCA1*.[57,66,67] Guidelines have been established for when genetic counseling and testing should be offered.[67] Breast cancer risk reduction options available to known carriers of *BRCA1* and *BRCA2* mutations include surveillance and surgery. Breast evaluation using MRI is generally preferred over standard mammography for these women because of its enhanced sensitivity and lack of radiation exposure, which may be safer for them. Prophylactic surgery, in the form of bilateral mastectomy, bilateral oophorectomy, or both, has been shown to decrease the risk of developing cancer. These controversial surgeries can have physical and psychological side effects that warrant careful consideration before proceeding. The use of tamoxifen for prevention in these women is controversial because many cancers in these genetically susceptible women are estrogen-receptor negative.[66,67]

Detection

Cancer of the breast may manifest clinically as a mass, a puckering, nipple retraction, or unusual discharge. Many cancers are found by women themselves—sometimes when only a thickening or subtle change in breast contour is noticed. The variety of symptoms and potential for self-discovery underscore the need for all women to have an awareness of what their normal breast appearance and texture are like. In 2003, the American Cancer Society dropped its recommendation that all

women perform regular, systematic self-examination. Research has indicated that most women who discover their own cancer do so outside of a scheduled breast self-examination (BSE). American Cancer Society screening guidelines now place primary emphasis for breast cancer diagnosis on mammography and the clinical breast examination, while encouraging women in the area of self awarenenss.[66] Premenopausal women who do perform BSE should conduct the examination right after menses. This time is most appropriate in relation to cyclic breast changes that occur in response to fluctuations in hormone levels. Postmenopausal women and women who have had a hysterectomy can perform the examination any day of the month. Examination may be done in the shower or bath or at bedtime. The most important aspect of BSE is to devise a systematic, convenient, and consistent method of examination. Women should have a clinical examination by a trained health professional at least every 3 years between 20 and 40 years of age, and annually after 40 years of age.

Mammography is the only effective screening technique for the early detection of clinically inapparent lesions. Although there have been studies that brought into question the value of mammography, in 2002 the USPSTF issued new guidelines concluding that there were sufficient data to justify recommending mammography every 1 to 2 years in women older than 40 years of age.[68] A generally slow-growing form of cancer, breast cancer may have been present for 2 to 9 years before it reaches 1 cm, the smallest mass normally detected by palpation. Mammography can disclose lesions as small as 1 mm and the clustering of calcifications that may warrant biopsy to exclude cancer. The American Cancer Society recommends annual evaluation for women after 40 years of age.[69] Mammography has a sensitivity of 80% to 90% for the detection of breast cancer even when performed by the most capable institutions. Therefore, palpable masses need further evaluation and potentially biopsy even if the mammogram is negative.[66,70] Approximately 40% of breast cancers can be detected only by palpation and another 40% only by mammography.[12] The most comprehensive approach to screening is a combination of individual self-awareness, clinical breast evaluation by a health professional, and mammography.

Diagnosis and Classification

Procedures used in the diagnosis of breast cancer include physical examination, mammography, ultrasonography, percutaneous needle aspiration, stereotactic needle biopsy (*i.e.*, core biopsy), and excisional biopsy. Figure 46-13 illustrates the appearance of breast cancer on mammography. Breast cancer often manifests as a solitary, painless, firm, fixed lesion with poorly defined borders. It can be found anywhere in the breast but is most common in the upper outer quadrant. Because of the variability in presentation, any suspect change in breast tissue warrants further investigation. The diagnostic use of mammography enables additional definition of the clinically suspect area (*e.g.*, appearance, character, calcification). Placement of a wire marker under radiographic guidance can ensure accurate surgi-

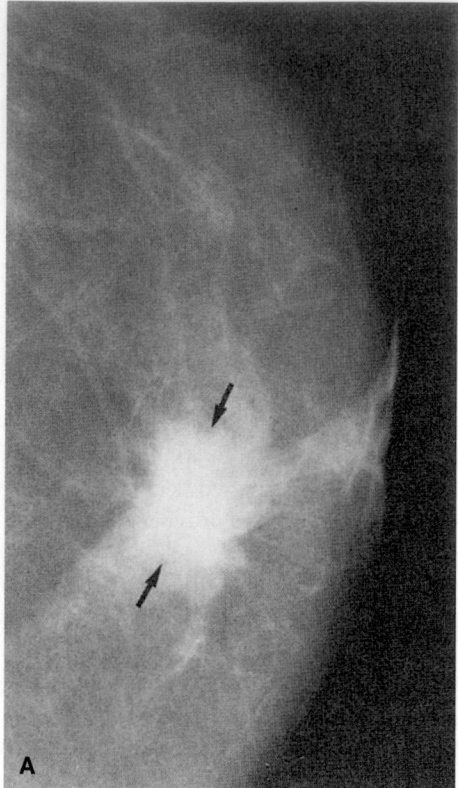
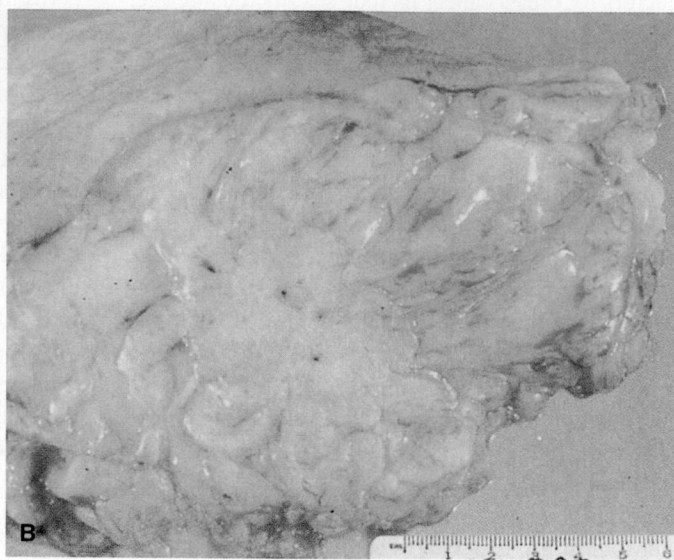

FIGURE 46-13 • Carcinoma of the breast. (**A**) Mammogram. An irregularly shaped, dense mass (*arrows*) is seen in this otherwise fatty breast. (**B**) Mastectomy specimen. The irregular white, firm mass in the center is surrounded by fatty tissue. (From Thor A. D., Osunkoya A. O. [2008]. The breast. In Rubin R., Strayer D. S. [Eds.], *Rubin's pathology: Clinicopathologic foundations of medicine* [5th ed., p. 851]. Philadelphia: Lippincott Williams & Wilkins.)

cal biopsy of nonpalpable suspect areas. Ultrasonography is useful as a diagnostic adjunct to differentiate cystic from solid tissue in women with nonspecific thickening.

Fine-needle aspiration is a simple in-office procedure that can be performed repeatedly in multiple sites and with minimal discomfort. It can be accomplished by stabilizing a palpable mass between two fingers or in conjunction with handheld sonography to define cystic masses or fibrocystic changes and to provide specimens for cytologic examination. Fine-needle aspiration can identify the presence of malignant cells, but it cannot differentiate in situ from infiltrating cancers. Stereotactic needle biopsy is an outpatient procedure done with the guidance of a mammography machine. After the lesion is localized radiologically, a large-bore needle is mechanically thrust quickly into the area, removing a core of tissue. Discomfort is similar to that with ear piercing, and even when multiple cores are obtained, healing occurs quite rapidly. Cells are available for histologic evaluation with 96% accuracy in detecting cancer. This procedure is less costly than excisional biopsy. Excisional biopsy to remove the entire lump provides the only definitive diagnosis of breast cancer, and often is therapeutic without additional surgery. MRI, positron emission tomography (PET), and computer-based or digital mammography are available as additional diagnostic modalities for breast cancer, and may be recommended to supplement conventional mammography in women with radiographically dense breasts or a strong family history of cancer, or who are known carriers of *BRCA1* or *BRCA2*.[70]

Tumors are classified histologically according to tissue characteristics and staged clinically according to tumor size, nodal involvement, and presence of metastasis. It is recommended that estrogen and progesterone receptor analysis be performed on surgical specimens. Information about the presence or absence of estrogen and progesterone receptors can be used in predicting tumor responsiveness to hormonal manipulation. High levels of both receptors improve the prognosis and increase the likelihood of remission.

Treatment

The treatment methods for breast cancer include surgery, chemotherapy, radiation therapy, and hormonal manipulation. Radical mastectomy (*i.e.*, removal of the entire breast, underlying muscles, and all axillary nodes) rarely is used today as a primary surgical therapy unless breast cancer is advanced at the time of diagnosis. Modified surgical techniques (*i.e.*, mastectomy plus axillary dissection or lumpectomy for breast conservation) accompanied by chemotherapy or radiation therapy have achieved outcomes comparable with those obtained with radical surgical methods and constitute the preferred treatment methods.

The prognosis is related more to the extent of nodal involvement than to the extent of breast involvement. Greater nodal involvement requires more aggressive postsurgical treatment, and many cancer specialists believe that a diagnosis of breast cancer is not complete until dissection and testing of the axillary lymph nodes has been accomplished. A newer technique for evaluating lymph node involvement is a sentinel lymph node (SLN) biopsy. A radioactive substance or dye is injected into the region of the tumor. In theory, the dye is carried to the first (sentinel) node to receive lymph from the tumor.[66] This would therefore be the node most likely to contain cancer cells if the cancer has spread. If the sentinel node biopsy is positive, more nodes are removed. If it is negative, further lymph node evaluation may not be needed. Successful identification of the SLN occurs 92% to 98% of the time, and when blue dye and isotope are used together, SLN has a positive predictive value approaching 100% and a negative predictive value near 95%.[3]

Systemic therapy refers to the administration of chemotherapy, biologic therapy, or hormonal therapy. Neoadjuvant therapy is given before surgery to shrink the tumor and make surgical removal more effective. Adjuvant therapy is given after surgery to women with and without detectable metastatic disease. The goal of this therapy depends on nodal involvement, menopausal status, and hormone receptor status. Systemic adjuvant therapy has been widely studied and has demonstrated benefits in reducing rates of recurrence and death from breast cancer.[3,66] Biologic therapy, using the drug trastuzumab (Herceptin), is used to stop the growth of breast tumors that express the HER2/neu receptor on their cell surface. The HER2/neu receptor binds an epidermal growth factor that contributes to cancer cell growth. Trastuzumab is a recombinant DNA-derived monoclonal antibody that binds to the HER2/neu receptor, thereby inhibiting proliferation of tumor cells that overexpress the receptor gene.[71]

Hormone therapy is used to block the effects of estrogen on the growth of breast cancer cells. Tamoxifen is a nonsteroidal antiestrogen that binds to estrogen receptors and blocks the effects of estrogens on the growth of malignant cells in the breast. Studies have shown decreased cancer recurrence, decreased mortality rates, and increased 5-year survival rates in women with estrogen receptor–positive tissue samples who have been treated with the drug. Aromatase inhibitors block the enzyme that converts androstenedione and testosterone to estrogen in the peripheral tissues. This reduces the circulating estrogen levels in postmenopausal women and is becoming the most effective adjuvant therapy for women with early-stage breast cancer.[72] Autologous bone marrow transplantation and peripheral stem cell transplantation are experimental therapies that may be used for treatment of advanced disease or in women at increased risk for recurrence.

The 5-year survival rate for localized cancer is 98%; with nodal involvement, it is approximately 81%; and it is approximately 26% with distant metastasis.[13] Five-year survival rates by age at diagnosis range from 82% for women younger than 40 years to 88% for women older than 75 years of age.[65]

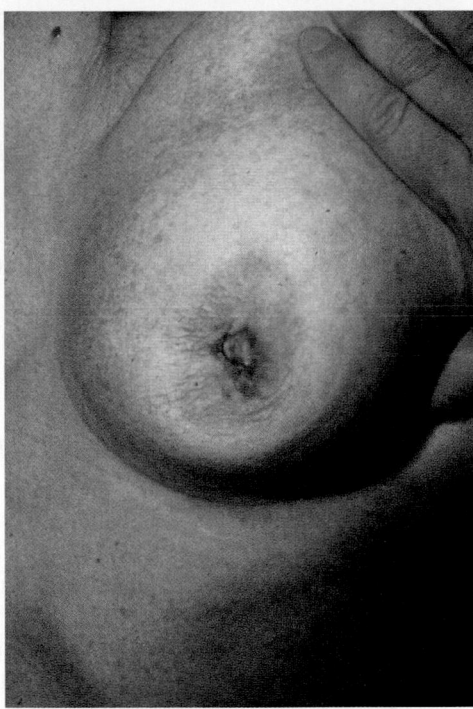

FIGURE 46-14 • Paget disease of the nipple. (From Thor A. D., Osunkoya A. O. [2008]. The breast. In Rubin R., Strayer D. S. [Eds.], *Rubin's pathology: Clinicopathologic foundations of medicine* [5th ed., p. 851]. Philadelphia: Lippincott Williams & Wilkins.)

Paget Disease

Paget disease accounts for 1% of all breast cancers. The disease presents as an eczematoid lesion of the nipple and areola (Fig. 46-14). Paget disease usually is associated with an infiltrating, intraductal carcinoma. When the lesion is limited to the nipple only, the rate of axillary metastasis is approximately 5%. Complete examination is required and includes a mammogram and biopsy. Treatment depends on the extent of spread.

IN SUMMARY, the breasts are subject to benign and malignant diseases. Mastitis is inflammation of the breast, occurring most frequently during lactation. Galactorrhea is an abnormal secretion of milk that may occur as a symptom of increased prolactin secretion. Ductal ectasia and intraductal papilloma cause abnormal drainage from the nipple. Fibroadenoma and fibrocystic changes are characterized by abnormal masses in the breast that are benign. By far the most important disease of the breast is breast cancer, which is a significant cause of death of women. Clinical breast examination and mammography afford a woman the best protection against breast cancer. They provide the means for early detection of breast cancer and, in many cases, allow early treatment and cure. ■

INFERTILITY

Infertility is the inability to conceive a child after 1 year of unprotected intercourse. Primary infertility refers to situations in which there has been no prior conception. Secondary infertility is infertility that occurs after one or more previous pregnancies. Sterility is the inability to father a child or to become pregnant because of congenital anomalies, disease, or surgical intervention. Approximately 15% of couples in the United States are affected by infertility and 1% to 2% by sterility.

The complexity of the process that must occur to achieve a pregnancy is taken for granted by most couples. For some couples, pregnancy occurs far too easily, whereas for others, no amount of money, hard work, love, patience, or medical resources seems to be able to bring about this amazing, desired event. Although a full discussion of the diagnosis and treatment of infertility is beyond the scope of this book, an overview of the areas in which problems can occur is presented.

The causes of infertility are almost equally divided between male factors (30% to 40%), female factors (30% to 40%), and combined factors (30% to 40%). In approximately 10% to 25% of infertile couples, the cause remains unknown even after a full work-up.

Male Factors

For pregnancy to occur, the man must be able to provide sperm in sufficient quantity, delivered to the upper end of the vagina, with adequate motility to traverse the female reproductive tract. The male contribution to this process is assessed by means of a semen analysis, which evaluates volume of semen (normally 2 to 5 mL), sperm density (20 million/mL), motility (50% good progressive), viability (50%), morphology (60% normal), and viscosity (full liquefaction within 20 minutes). The specimen is best collected by masturbation into a sterile container after 3 days of abstinence. Because of variability in specimens, abnormal results should lead to a repeat test before the need for treatment is presumed.

Azoospermia is the absence of sperm; *oligospermia* refers to decreased numbers of sperm; and *asthenospermia* refers to poor motility of sperm. Tests of sperm function include cervical mucus penetration tests (*e.g.*, postcoital test, Penetrak), sperm penetration assay (*i.e.*, Hamster Zona Free Ovum test), and

sperm antibody testing. None of these tests is included in the routine infertility evaluation.

The causes of male infertility include varicocele, ejaculatory dysfunction, hyperprolactinemia, hypogonadotropic hypogonadism, infection, immunologic problems (*i.e.*, antisperm antibodies), obstruction, and congenital anomalies. Risk factors for sperm problems include a history of mumps orchitis, cryptorchidism (*i.e.*, undescended testes), testicular torsion, hypospadias, previous urologic surgery, infection, and exposure to known gonadotoxins.[57] Treatment depends on the cause and may include surgery, medication, or the use of artificial insemination to deliver a more concentrated specimen directly to the cervical canal or uterine fundus. Artificial insemination with donor sperm can be offered if the man is sterile and this is an alternative acceptable to the husband and wife.

Female Factors

The female contribution to pregnancy is more complex, requiring production and release of a mature ovum capable of being fertilized; production of cervical mucus that assists in sperm transport and maintains sperm viability in the female reproductive tract; patent fallopian tubes with the motility potential to pick up and transfer the ovum to the uterine cavity; development of an endometrium that is suitable for the implantation and nourishment of a fertilized ovum; and a uterine cavity that allows for growth and development of a fetus. Each of these factors is discussed briefly, along with an overview of diagnostic tests and treatment.

Ovulatory Dysfunction

In a normally menstruating woman, ovulatory cycles begin several months to a year after menarche. Release of FSH from the pituitary causes the development of several primordial follicles in the ovary. At some point, a dominant follicle is selected and the remaining follicles undergo atresia. When the dominant follicle has become large enough to contain a mature ovum (16 to 20 mm in diameter) and is producing sufficient estradiol to ensure adequate proliferation of the endometrium, production of LH increases (*i.e.*, the LH surge), and the increased LH level induces release of the ovum from the follicle (*i.e.*, ovulation).

After ovulation, under the influence of LH, the former follicle luteinizes and begins producing progesterone in addition to estradiol. The progesterone stimulates the development of secretory endometrium, which has the capability to nourish a fertilized ovum if one should implant.

The presence of progesterone after ovulation causes a rise in the woman's basal body temperature (BBT). This thermogenic property of progesterone provides the basis for the simplest, most inexpensive beginning test of ovulatory function—the measurement of BBT. Women should be able to detect at least a 0.4°F rise in their BBT (at rest) after ovulation that should be maintained throughout the luteal phase. This biphasic temperature pattern demonstrates that ovulation has taken place, where in the cycle it occurred, and the length of the luteal phase. BBT can be influenced by many other factors, including restless sleep, alcohol intake, drug use, fever due to illness, and change in usual rising time. However, as an initial step in the infertility investigation, it can provide useful information to direct other forms of testing.

Endometrial biopsy, the removal of a sample of the endometrium during an office procedure, provides histologic evidence of secretory endometrium and the level of maturation of the lining. In a normal cycle, the luteal phase should be 14 days long. Without pregnancy and the subsequent secretion of hCG, the corpus luteum begins to degenerate 7 to 10 days after the LH surge. The luteal phase of the cycle is so consistent that a pathologist can tell by evaluating a section of endometrium that it is representative of a particular day of the luteal phase. The pathologist's assessment of maturation is compared with the arrival of the next menses. If a discrepancy of more than 2 days exists, the woman is said to have a luteal phase defect (LPD). This diagnosis indicates that, although ovulation is occurring, endometrial development is insufficient and implantation may not be possible. Pregnancy requires fertilization and implantation. LPD also can be suggested by an abnormal serum progesterone level 7 days after ovulation. It can be treated directly with supplemental progesterone after ovulation or with the use of clomiphene citrate to stimulate increased pituitary production of FSH and LH. Because this biopsy is painful and costly, many practitioners today still use history, with the possible addition of BBT charting, to assess ovulatory competence, and begin clomiphene citrate therapy without requiring biopsy.

Anovulation (no ovulation) and oligo-ovulation (irregular ovulation) are other forms of ovulatory dysfunction. These problems can be identified by the tests for LPD previously described, but are more often identified and treated based on a history of menstrual irregularity. Ovulatory problems can be primary problems of the ovary or secondary problems related to endocrine dysfunction. When disturbances in ovulation are confirmed, it is reasonable to rule out other endocrine system problems before initiating treatment. If the results of tests for pituitary hormones (*e.g.,* FSH, LH, prolactin), thyroid studies, and tests of adrenal function (*e.g.,* DHEAS, androstenedione) are normal, ovulatory dysfunction is primary and should respond to treatment. Abnormalities in any of the other endocrine areas should be further evaluated as needed and treated appropriately. Hyperprolactinemia responds well to bromocriptine or cabergoline (Dostinex), but pituitary microadenoma may need to be excluded first. Hypothyroidism requires thyroid replacement, and hyperthyroidism requires suppressive therapy and, sometimes, surgical intervention with thyroid replacement later. Adrenal suppression can be instituted with dexamethasone, a glucocorticoid analog. Normal ovulatory function may resume without further intervention; if not, treatment can be concurrent with management of other endocrine problems.

Cervical Mucus Problems

High preovulatory levels of estradiol stimulate the production of large amounts of clear, stretchy cervical mucus that aids the transport of sperm into the uterine cavity and helps to maintain an environment that keeps the sperm viable for up to 72 hours. Insufficient estrogen production (*i.e.,* inherent or secondary to treatment with clomiphene citrate, an antiestrogen), cervical abnormalities from disease or invasive procedures (*e.g.,* DES exposure, stenosis, conization), and cervical infection (*e.g.,* chlamydial infection, mycoplasmal infection, gonorrhea) can adversely affect the production of healthy cervical mucus.

A postcoital test (Sims-Huhner) involves evaluation of the cervical mucus 1 to 8 hours after intercourse within the 48 hours before ovulation. A sample of cervical mucus is obtained using a special syringe and evaluated grossly for amount, clarity, and stretch (*i.e.,* spinnbarkeit) and microscopically for cellularity, number and quality of motile sperm, and the presence of ferning after the sample has air dried on the slide. To obtain good-quality mucus, it is essential to obtain the sample within the 48 hours before ovulation. Tests may have to be repeated in the same cycle or in subsequent cycles to ensure appropriate timing. This can be a source of stress and frustration, as well as added cost to the couple. Intrauterine insemination (IUI) with the husband's sperm can bypass the cervical mucus, and is often offered empirically as an alternative to postcoital testing.

If inadequate estrogen effect is seen (poor-quality mucus), supplemental oral estrogen can be given in the first 9 days of the next cycle, and the test can be repeated. Administration of mucolytic expectorants (1 teaspoon four times daily, starting on day 10 and continuing until ovulation is confirmed) also may improve the quality of the mucus. If the quality of the mucus is good but sperm are inadequate in number or motility, further evaluation of the man may be needed. The man and woman can be tested for antisperm antibodies when repeated postcoital tests reveal that the sperm are all dead or agglutinated; however, IUI is the only effective treatment for sperm antibodies and is frequently offered without the need for further testing.

Cervical cultures for gonorrhea, chlamydial infection, and mycoplasmal infection should be obtained and treatment instituted as needed. Prophylactic treatment with antibiotics can be provided before IUI or other procedures that pass through the cervical canal as a more cost-effective alternative to obtaining cervical cultures.

Uterine Cavity Abnormalities

Alterations in the uterine cavity can occur because of DES exposure, submucosal fibroids, cervical polyps, bands of scar tissue, or congenital anomalies (*e.g.,* bicornuate septum, single horn). These defects may be suspected from the patient's history or pelvic examination but require hysterosalpingography (*i.e.,* x-ray study in which dye is placed through the cervix to outline the uterine cavity and demonstrate tubal patency) or hysteroscopy (*i.e.,* study in which a lighted fiberoptic endoscope placed through the cervix under general anesthesia allows direct visualization of the uterine cavity) for confirmation. Treatment is surgical when possible.

Tubal Factors

Tubal patency is required for fertilization and can be disrupted secondary to PID, ectopic pregnancy, large myomas, endometriosis, pelvic adhesions, and previous tubal ligation. Hysterosalpingography can reveal the location and type of any blockage, such as fimbrial, cornual, or hydrosalpinx. Microsurgical repair sometimes is possible.

Even when tubal patency is demonstrated, tubal disease may make ovum pickup impossible. Contrary to popular belief, the ovum is not extruded directly into the fallopian tube. The tube must be free to move to engulf the ovum after release. Pelvic adhesions from previous infection, surgery, or endometriosis can interfere with the tube's mobility. Laparoscopic evaluation of the pelvis is needed for diagnosis. Laser ablation or cautery can be used to lyse adhesions and remove endometriosis through the laparoscope or, if severe, by means of laparotomy.

Assisted Reproductive Technologies (ART)

In vitro fertilization (IVF) was developed in 1978 for women with significantly damaged or absent tubes to provide them with an opportunity for pregnancy where none normally exists. The ovaries are superstimulated to produce multiple follicles using clomiphene citrate, human menopausal gonadotropins (e.g., Repronex, Menopur) containing FSH and LH, pure FSH (e.g., Gonal F, Follistim, Bravelle), or a combination of these drugs. Follicular maturation is monitored by means of ultrasonography and assay of serum estradiol levels. When preovulatory criteria are met, an injection of hCG is given to simulate an LH surge; 35 hours later, the follicles are aspirated transvaginally using ultrasound guidance. The follicular fluid is evaluated microscopically for the presence of ova. When found, they are removed and placed into culture media in an incubator.

The eggs are inseminated with sperm from the husband that have been prepared by a washing technique that removes the semen, begins the capacitation process, and allows the strongest sperm to be used for fertilization. When very low numbers of normal motile sperm are available, microsurgical techniques can be used to assist with fertilization. Earlier procedures such as *partial zona dissection* (PZD), which involves the creation of a small opening in the layer (i.e., zona pellucida) that surrounds the egg, and subzonal insertion, where several sperm are inserted into the space just beneath the protective layer, are rarely used today. The most definitive form of micromanipulation is a procedure called *intracytoplasmic sperm injection* (ICSI), where a single spermatozoon is injected directly into the cytoplasm of the egg. More than half of all IVF procedures performed in 2004 used ICSI for fertilization.[73]

Between 12 and 24 hours after insemination, the ova are evaluated for signs of fertilization. If signs are present, the ova are returned to the incubator, and 48 to 72 hours after egg retrieval, the fertilized eggs are placed into the woman's uterus by means of a transcervical catheter. A procedure similar to

PZD can be performed just before embryo transfer to help the fertilized egg escape from the zona pellucida. This "assisted hatching" improves the chances of implantation. In an effort to reduce the number of multiple births resulting from this type of technology, the embryos may be grown to the blastocyst stage and transferred back to the uterus on the fifth day after fertilization. Because many embryos will not advance to the blastocyst stage in vitro, this therapy may be limited to those women who have produced a significant number of embryos. In 2004, 19% of embryos were transferred on day 5, compared with 72% transferred on day 3. In all age groups success rates were higher for day 5 transfers.[73]

Hormonal supplementation of the luteal phase is typically used to increase the possibility of implantation. The overall live delivery rate in 2004 for women using their own eggs, as reported by the Society for Assisted Reproductive Technology and CDC, was 34% per embryo transfer.[73] Indications for IVF have been expanded to include male factors (i.e., severe oligospermia or asthenospermia), ovulatory dysfunction, uterine factors, endometriosis, and idiopathic infertility (i.e., infertility of unknown cause). The substantial risk of multiple births with IVF procedures has been reduced with the availability of cryopreservation, which allows freezing of excess embryos and limits the number of fresh embryos transferred. The live delivery rate in 2004 after frozen embryo transfer was 27.7%.[73]

An outgrowth of IVF technology is gamete intrafallopian transfer (GIFT), which uses similar ovarian stimulation protocols and egg retrieval procedures but uses laparoscopy to place ovum and sperm directly into the fallopian tube. This procedure requires at least one patent fallopian tube and was developed primarily to increase the pregnancy rate in women with idiopathic infertility. The basic premises are that if a transportation problem is interfering with ovum pickup, GIFT could solve that problem, and that implantation may result more often if fertilization occurs in the body. Because of the added expense involving laparoscopy and the limited indications, GIFT procedures are used infrequently. In 2004, GIFT represented only 0.1% of all ART procedures performed, and demonstrated a 23.3% live delivery rate per retrieval.[73]

Alternatively, zygote intrafallopian transfer (ZIFT) proceeds like an IVF cycle through egg retrieval and fertilization in the laboratory, but the resulting embryo (zygote) is placed directly into the fallopian tube during laparoscopy. The theoretical advantage of this procedure involves tubal factors that may facilitate implantation. ZIFT accounted for only 0.3% of all ART procedures performed in 2004, with a 30% delivery rate.[73]

The use of donor gametes (eggs, sperm, embryos) provides an alternative for achieving pregnancy for those couples who are unable to use their own gametes and are comfortable raising a child that is not genetically related to them. Donor egg provides a much higher likelihood of success for women older than 40 years of age, when both egg numbers and egg quality decline. In 2004, there were over 9000 cycles using fresh embryos, with a 51% live birth rate per transfer.[73]

The number of ART cycles performed annually in the United States has almost doubled, from 64,681 cycles in 1996 to 127,977 cycles in 2004.[73] By 2003, more than 1 million infants had been born worldwide using some type of ART, with almost 100,000 births being made possible with the use of ICSI. Future research will focus on understanding and improving the implantation process in an effort to decrease the risk of multiple births while providing an optimal chance for pregnancy.

IN SUMMARY, infertility is the inability to conceive a child after 1 year of unprotected intercourse. Male factors are related to number and motility of sperm and their ability to penetrate the cervical mucus and the ovum. Causes of male infertility include varicocele, ejaculatory dysfunction, hyperprolactinemia, hypogonadotropic hypogonadism, infection, immunologic problems (*i.e.*, antisperm antibodies), obstruction, and congenital anomalies. Risk factors for sperm disorders include a history of mumps orchitis, cryptorchidism, testicular torsion, hypospadias, previous urologic surgery, infection, and exposure to known gonadotoxins.

The female contribution to pregnancy is more complex, requiring production and release of a mature ovum capable of being fertilized; production of cervical mucus that assists in sperm transport and maintains sperm viability in the female reproductive tract; patent fallopian tubes with the mobility potential to pick up and transfer the ovum to the uterine cavity; development of an endometrium that is suitable for the implantation and nourishment of a fertilized ovum; and a uterine cavity that allows for growth and development of a fetus.

Evaluation and treatment of infertility can be lengthy and highly stressful for the couple. Options for therapy continue to expand, but newer ART modalities are expensive, and financial resources can be strained while couples seek to fulfill their sometimes elusive dream of having a child. ■

Review Exercises

1. A 32-year-old woman has been told that the report of her annual Pap test revealed the presence of mild dysplasia.

   A. *What questions should this woman ask as a means of becoming informed about the significance of these findings?*

   B. *In obtaining additional information about the results of her Pap test, the woman is informed that dysplastic changes are consistent with a CIN 1 classification.*

      (1) *Does this mean that the woman has cervical cancer?*

      (2) *How would these findings translate into The Bethesda System for grading cervical cytology?*

      (3) *Cervical cancer is often referred to as a sexually transmitted infection. Explain.*

      (4) *What type of follow-up care would be indicated?*

2. A 30-year-old woman consults her gynecologist because of amenorrhea and an inability to become pregnant. Physical examination reveals an obese woman with hirsutism. The physician tells the woman that she might have a condition known as polycystic ovary syndrome and that further laboratory tests are indicated.

   A. *Among the tests ordered were fasting blood glucose, LH, FSH, and dehydroepiandrosterone levels. What information can these tests provide that would help in establishing a diagnosis of polycystic ovary syndrome?*

   B. *What is the probable cause of this woman's amenorrhea, hirsutism, and failure to become pregnant?*

   C. *What type of treatment might be used to help this woman become pregnant?*

3. A 45-year-old woman makes an appointment to see her physician because of a painless lump in her breast that she discovered while doing her routine monthly breast self-examination.

   A. *What tests should be done to confirm the presence or absence of breast cancer?*

   B. *During the removal of breast cancer, a sentinel lymph node biopsy is often done to determine whether the cancer has spread to the lymph nodes. Explain how this procedure is done and its value in determining lymph node spread.*

   C. *After surgical removal of breast cancer, tamoxifen may be used as an adjuvant systemic therapy for women without detectable metastatic disease. The presence or absence of estrogen receptors in the cytoplasm of tumor cells is important in determining the selection of an agent for use in adjuvant therapy. Explain.*

References

1. Omole F., Simmons B. J., Hacker Y. (2003). Management of Bartholin duct cyst and gland abscess. *American Family Physician* 68, 135–140.
2. Kurman R. J. (2002). *Blaustein's pathology of the female genital tract* (5th ed., pp. 53–55, 99, 109, 168, 216–222, 253–256, 327, 336, 502–503, 637–639, 746–749, 801–802). New York: Springer-Verlag.
3. Scott J. R., Gibbs R. S., Karlan B. Y., et al. (2003). *Danforth's obstetrics and gynecology* (9th ed., pp. 585–586, 591, 606–608, 653–662, 713–720, 727, 839, 898, 899, 906, 913, 927, 941–949, 953–963). Philadelphia: Lippincott Williams & Wilkins.

4. Jerzak L. A., Smith S. K. (2006). Vulvodynia: Diagnosis and treatment of a chronic pain syndrome. *Women's Health Care* 5(4), 29–50.

5. Cooper A. S., Boardman L. A. (2005). Diagnosing and treating vulvar pain syndromes. *Women's Health Gynecology Edition* 5(3), 153–162.

6. American Cancer Society. (2007). Cancer reference information. [Online.] Available: www.cancer.org/docroot/home/index.asp. Accessed February 21, 2007.

7. Canavan T. P., Cohen D. (2002). Vulvar cancer. *American Family Physician* 66, 1269–1274.

8. Tyring S. K. (2003). Vulvar squamous cell carcinoma: Guidelines for early diagnosis and treatment. *American Journal of Obstetrics and Gynecology* 189(3, Suppl. 1), S17–S23.

9. Eckert L. O. (2006). Acute vulvovaginitis. *New England Journal of Medicine* 355, 1244–1252.

10. Crum C. P. (2005). The female genital tract. In Kumar V., Abbas A. K., Fausto N. (Eds.), *Robbins and Cotran pathologic basis of disease* (7th ed., pp. 1059–1117). Philadelphia: Elsevier Saunders.

11. Hammes B., Laitman C. J. (2003). Diethylstilbestrol (DES) update: Recommendations for the identification and management of DES-exposed individuals. *Journal of Midwifery and Women's Health* 48(1), 19–29.

12. American Cancer Society. (2007). Cancer facts & figures 2006. [Online.] Available: www.cancer.org. Accessed February 28, 2007.

13. Saslow D., Runowicz C. D., Solomon D., et al. (2002). American Cancer Society guideline for the early detection of cervical neoplasia and cancer. *CA: A Cancer Journal for Clinicians* 52, 342–362.

14. Snyder U. (2003). A look at cervical cancer. *Medscape Obstetrics/Gynecology & Women's Health* 8(1). [Online.] Available: www.medscape.com/viewarticle/452727 print. Accessed November 7, 2003.

15. Saslow D., Castle P. E., Cox T., et al. (2007). American Cancer Society guideline for human papillomavirus (HPV) vaccine to prevent cervical cancer and its precursors. *CA: A Cancer Journal for Clinicians* 57, 7–28.

16. Solomon D., Davey D., Kurman R., et al., for the Forum Group Members and the Bethesda 2001 Workshop. (2002). The 2001 Bethesda System. *Journal of the American Medical Association* 287(16), 2114–2119.

17. U.S. Preventive Services Task Force. (2003). Screening for cervical cancer: Recommendations and rationale. *American Journal of Nursing* 103(11), 101–109.

18. Choma K. K. (2003). ASC-US HPV testing. *American Journal of Nursing* 103(2), 42–50.

19. Wright T. C., Schiffman M., Solomon D., et al. (2004). Interim guidance for the use of human papillomavirus DNA testing as an adjunct to cervical cytology for screening. *Obstetrics and Gynecology* 103, 304–309.

20. Wright T., Cox T., Massad L. S. J., et al., for the 2001 ASCCP-Sponsored Consensus Conference. (2002). 2001 consensus guidelines for the management of women with cervical cytological abnormalities. *Journal of the American Medical Association* 287, 2120–2129.

21. Eskridge C., Begneaud W. P., Landwehr C. (1998). Cervicography combined with repeat Papanicolaou test as triage for low grade cytologic abnormalities. *Obstetrics and Gynecology* 92, 351–355.

22. Robboy S. J., Kurman R. J., Merino M. J. (2005). The female reproductive system. In Rubin E., Gorstein F., Rubin R., et al. (Eds.), *Rubin's pathology: Clinicopathologic foundations of medicine* (4th ed., pp. 927–984). Philadelphia: Lippincott Williams & Wilkins.

23. Grow D. R., Hsu A. L. (2006). Endometriosis, part 1: Clinical diagnosis and analgesia. *Female Patient* 31(11), 62–29.

24. Practice Committee of the American Society for Reproductive Medicine. (2006). Treatment of pelvic pain associated with endometriosis. *Fertility and Sterility* 86(Suppl. 4), S18–S27.

25. Grow D. R., Hsu A. L. (2006). Endometriosis, part 2: Surgery for symptom relief and infertility. *Female Patient* 31(12), 54–59.

26. American College of Obstetricians and Gynecologists. (1999). Medical management of endometriosis. ACOG practice bulletin no. 11. In *2001 Compendium of selected publications* (pp. 982, 986). Washington, DC: Author.

27. Johnson K. (2003). Differentiating adenomyosis and fibroids. *Medscape Obstetrics/Gynecology & Women's Health* 8(2). [Online.] Available: www.medscape.com/viewarticle/459772. Accessed November 20, 2003.

28. Cancer Reference Information. (2006). Endometrial cancer. The American Cancer Society. [Online.] Available: www.cancer.org/docroot/CRI. Accessed January 3, 2007.

29. Amant F., Moeman P., Neven P., et al. (2005). Endometrial cancer. *Lancet* 366, 491–505.

30. Goldberg J. (2006). Uterine artery embolization for symptomatic leiomyomata. *Female Patient* 31(5), 45–50.

31. Crossman S. H. (2006). The challenge of pelvic inflammatory disease. *American Family Physician* 73, 859–864.

32. Centers for Disease Control and Prevention. (2006). Sexually transmitted diseases treatment guidelines, 2006. *Morbidity and Mortality Weekly Report* 55(30), 1–94.

33. Centers for Disease Control and Prevention. (1995). Current trends for ectopic pregnancy—United States, 1990–1992. *Morbidity and Mortality Weekly Report* 44(RR-3), 46–48.

34. Selway J. (2006). The challenge of ectopic pregnancy. *Journal for Nurse Practitioners* 2, 583–591.

35. Lozeau A.-M., Potter B. (2005). Diagnosis and management of ectopic pregnancy. *American Family Physician* 22, 1707–1720.

36. Kalyanakrishnan R., Scheid D. C. (2006). Ectopic pregnancy: Forget the "classic presentation" if you want to catch it sooner. *Journal of Family Practice* 55, 388–395.

37. Kalyanakrishnan R., Scheid D. C. (2006). Ectopic pregnancy: Expectant management or immediate surgery. *Journal of Family Practice* 55, 517–522.

38. Pectasides D., Pectasides E., Economopoulos T. (2006). Fallopian tube carcinoma: A review. *Oncologist* 11, 902–912.

39. Speroff L., Fritz M. A. (2004). *Clinical gynecologic endocrinology and infertility* (7th ed., pp. 472–476, 1119, 1187–1189). Philadelphia: Lippincott Williams & Wilkins.

40. Azziz R. (2005). Diagnostic criteria for polycystic ovary syndrome: A reappraisal. *Fertility and Sterility* 83, 1343–1346.

41. Rosen M., Cedars M. I. (2004). Female reproductive and endocrinology and infertility. In Greenspan F. S., Gardner D. G. (Eds.), *Basic and clinical endocrinology* (7th ed., pp. 530–535). New York: Lange Medical Books/McGraw-Hill.

42. Sheriff K. (2006). Polycystic ovary syndrome in primary care. *Female Patient* 31(2), 25–29.

43. Ehrmann D. A. (2005). Polycystic ovary syndrome. *New England Journal of Medicine* 352, 1223–1236.

44. Salmi D. J., Zisser H. C., Jovanovic L. (2004). Screening for and treatment of polycystic ovary syndrome in teenagers: A mini review. *Experimental Biology and Medicine* 229, 369–377.

45. Essah P. A., Apridonidze T. A., Iuorno M. J., et al. (2006). Effects of short-term and long-term metformin treatment on menstrual cyclicity in women with polycystic ovary syndrome. *Fertility and Sterility* 86, 230–232.

46. Cannistra S. A. (2004). Cancer of the ovary. *New England Journal of Medicine* 351, 2519–2529.

47. Rubin S. C., Sutton G. P. (2001). *Ovarian cancer* (2nd ed., pp. 167–177). Philadelphia: Lippincott Williams & Wilkins.

48. Barnes M. N., Grizzle W. E., Grubbs C. J., et al. (2002). Paradigms for primary prevention of ovarian carcinoma. *CA: A Cancer Journal for Clinicians* 52, 216–225.

49. Goff B. A., Mandel L. S., Drescher C. W., et al. (2006). Development of an ovarian cancer symptom index: Possibilities for earlier detection. *Cancer* 109, 221–227.

50. Goff B. A., Muntz H. G. (2005). Screening and early diagnosis of ovarian cancer. *Women's Health* 5(4), 194–206.

51. U.S. Preventive Services Task Force. (2005). Screening guidelines for ovarian cancer: Recommendation statement of the USPSTF. *American Family Physician* 71, 759–762.

52. National Institutes of Health Consensus Development Panel on Ovarian Cancer. (1995). Ovarian cancer: Screening and follow-up. *Journal of the American Medical Association* 273, 491–497.

53. Cancer Reference Information. (2006). Ovarian cancer. American Cancer Society. [Online.] Available: www.cancer.org/docroot/CRI. Accessed January 12, 2007.

54. Davila W. G. (2006). Treating genital prolapse. *American Journal for Nurse Practitioners* 10(5), 49–55.

55. Practice Committee of the American Society for Reproductive Medicine. (2006). Indications and options for endometrial ablation. *Fertility and Sterility* 86(Suppl. 4), S6–S10.

56. Practice Committee of the American Society for Reproductive Medicine. (2006). Current evaluation of amenorrhea. *Fertility and Sterility* 86(Suppl. 4), S148–S155.

57. Mishell D. R., Goodwin T. M., Brenner P. F. (2002). *Management of common problems in obstetrics and gynecology* (4th ed., pp. 236, 253, 260, 278, 395, 428, 431–435). Williston, VT: Blackwell Science.

58. Minkin M. J., Moore A. E. (2006). Identifying and managing premenstrual disorders: Putting strategies into practice. *Clinical Advisor* November (Suppl.), 4–15.

59. Steiner M., Pearlstein T., Cohen L. S., et al. (2006). Expert guidelines for the treatment of severe PMS, PMDD and co-morbidities: The role of SSRIs. *Journal of Women's Health* 15(1), 57–69.

60. Dickerson V. M. (2007). Premenstrual syndrome and premenstrual dysphoric disorder: Individualizing therapy. *Female Patient* 32(1), 38–46.

61. ACOG Practice Bulletin. (2000). Clinical management guidelines for obstetricians-gynecologists: Premenstrual syndrome. *Obstetrics and Gynecology* 95(4), 1–9.

62. Santen R. J., Mansel R. (2005). Benign breast disorders. *New England Journal of Medicine* 353, 275–285.

63. Lester S. C. (2005). The breast. In Kumar V., Abbas A. K., Fausto N. (Eds.), *Robbins and Cotran pathologic basis of disease* (7th ed., pp. 1119–1151). Philadelphia: Elsevier Saunders.

64. Thor A. D., Wang J., Bartows S. A. (2005). The breast. In Rubin E., Gorstein F., Rubin R., et al. (Eds.), *Rubin's pathology: Clinicopathologic foundations of medicine* (4th ed., pp. 997–1016). Philadelphia: Lippincott Williams & Wilkins.

65. Hartmann L. C., Sellers T. A., Tam Frost M. H., et al. (2005). Benign breast disease and the risk of breast cancer. *New England Journal of Medicine* 353, 229–237.

66. American Cancer Society. (2006). Breast cancer facts & figures 2005–2006. [Online.] Available: www.cancer.org. Accessed January 5, 2007.

67. Kolesar J. M. (2004). Clinical implications of BRCA1 and BRCA2 genes in hereditary breast and ovarian cancer. *Female Patient* 29(6), 39–45.

68. Humphrey L. L., Helfand M., Chan B. K. S., et al. (2002). Breast cancer screening: A summary of the evidence for the U.S. Preventive Service Task Force. *Annals of Internal Medicine* 137, 347–360.

69. Smith R. A., Saslow D., Sawyers K. A., et al. [2003]. American Cancer Society guidelines for breast cancer screening updated 2003. *CA: A Cancer Journal for Clinicians* 53, 141–169.

70. Pisano E. D., Gatsonis C., Hendrick E., et al. (2005). Diagnostic performance of digital versus film mammography for breast-cancer screening. *New England Journal of Medicine* 353, 1773–1783.

71. Piccart-Gehart M. J., Procter M., Leylan-Jones B., et al. (2005). Trastuzumab after adjuvant chemotherapy in Her2-positive cancer. *New England Journal of Medicine* 353, 1659–1672.

72. Geller M. L., Chlebowski R. T. (2006). The role of aromatase inhibitors in breast cancer therapy. *Female Patient* 31(1), 23–32.

73. CDC's Reproductive Health Information Source. (2006). 2004 Assisted reproductive technology success rates. Centers for Disease Control and Prevention. [Online.] Available: www.cdc.gov/ART/ART 2004. Accessed January 14, 2007.

Visit the Point. **http://thePoint.lww.com for animations, journal articles, and more!**

Chapter 47

Sexually Transmitted Infections

PATRICIA McCOWEN MEHRING

➤ Sexually transmitted infections (STIs), previously referred to as sexually transmitted diseases (STDs), encompass a broad range of infectious diseases that are spread by sexual contact. Although the incidence of syphilis and gonorrhea as reported in the professional literature and public health statistics has decreased slightly, the incidence of other STIs is increasing. The actual figures are probably much higher than those reported because many STIs are not reportable or not reported. The agents of infection include bacteria, *Chlamydia,* viruses, fungi, protozoa, parasites, and unidentified microorganisms (see Chapter 16). Portals of entry include the mouth, genitalia, urinary meatus, rectum, and skin. The rates of many STIs are highest among adolescents; all STIs are more common in persons who have more than one sexual partner; and it is not uncommon for a person to be concurrently infected with more than one type of STI.

There are many factors that contribute to the increased prevalence and the continued spread of STIs, including the fact that STIs are frequently asymptomatic, which promotes the spread of infection by persons who are unaware that they are carrying the infection. Furthermore, partners of infected persons are often difficult to notify and treat. Condoms could prevent the spread of many STIs, but they often are not used or are used improperly. In addition, there currently are no cures for viral STIs (*e.g.,* human immunodeficiency virus [HIV], herpes simplex virus); although there are drugs available that may help to manage the infections, they do not entirely control the spread. Also, drug-resistant microorganisms are rapidly emerging, making treatment of many STIs more difficult.

This chapter discusses the manifestations of STIs in men and women in terms of infections of the external genitalia, vaginal infections, and infections that have genitourinary as well as systemic manifestations. HIV infection is presented in Chapter 20.

INFECTIONS OF THE EXTERNAL GENITALIA

After completing this section of the chapter, you should be able to meet the following objectives:

■ Define what is meant by a sexually transmitted infection (STI).

- List common portals of entry for STIs.
- Name the organisms responsible for condylomata acuminata, genital herpes, molluscum contagiosum, chancroid, granuloma inguinale, and lymphogranuloma venereum.
- State the significance of being infected with high-risk strains of the human papillomavirus.
- Explain the pathogenesis of recurrent genital herpes infections.

Sexually transmitted infections can selectively infect the mucocutaneous tissues of the external genitalia, cause vaginitis in women, or produce both genitourinary and systemic effects. Some STIs may be transmitted by an infected mother to a fetus or newborn, causing congenital defects or death of the child. The discussion in this section of the chapter focuses on STIs that affect the mucocutaneous tissues of the oropharynx and external genitalia, and anorectal tissues. These infections include condylomata acuminata, genital herpes, molluscum contagiosum, chancroid, granuloma inguinale, and lymphogranuloma venereum.

SEXUALLY TRANSMITTED INFECTIONS

- Sexually transmitted infections (STIs) are spread by sexual contact and involve both male and female partners. Portals of entry include the mouth, genitalia, urinary meatus, rectum, and skin. All STIs are more common in persons who have more than one sexual partner, and it is not uncommon for a person to be concurrently infected with more than one type of STI.

- In general, STIs due to bacterial pathogens can be successfully treated and the pathogen eliminated by antimicrobial therapy. However, many of these pathogens are developing antibiotic resistance.

- STIs due to viral pathogens such as genital herpes simplex virus infections (HSV-1 and HSV-2) are not eliminated by current treatment modalities and persist with risk of recurrence (HSV infections).

- Untreated, STIs such as chlamydial infection and gonorrhea can spread to involve the internal genital organs with risk of complications and infertility.

- Intrauterine or perinatally transmitted STIs can have potentially fatal or severely debilitating effects on a fetus or an infant.

Condylomata Acuminata (Genital Warts)

Condylomata acuminata, or genital warts, are caused by the human papillomavirus (HPV). Although recognized for centuries, HPV-induced genital warts have become one of the fastest-growing STIs of the past decade. The Centers for Disease Control and Prevention (CDC) estimates that 20 million Americans carry the virus and up to 6.2 million new cases are diagnosed each year.[1] Risk factors for acquiring HPV include young age (<25 years), early age of first intercourse (<16 years), increased numbers of sex partners, and having a male partner with multiple sex partners. HPV infection can occur with any type of vaginal or anal penetration and is common in men having sex with men and women having sex with women. Oral–genital and manual–genital contact are less likely means of spreading this infection.[1] Most HPV infections are asymptomatic and transient, and resolve without treatment.[1-4] However, in some cases, HPV infection results in genital warts, Papanicolaou (Pap) test abnormalities, or, rarely, cervical cancer.

HPVs are nonenveloped, double-stranded deoxyribonucleic acid (DNA) viruses that cause proliferative lesions of the squamous epithelium.[5] More than 100 distinct HPV subtypes have been identified, over 40 of which affect the anogenital area.[1] These subtypes have been divided into three categories based on their likelihood of inducing dysplasia and carcinoma. HPV types 6 and 11 are considered low risk. They are found in most external genital warts but usually are benign, with only a low potential for dysplasia. Types 31, 33, 35, 39, 45, 51, 52, 56, and 58 are considered to be intermediate risk because they are common causes of intraepithelial neoplasia, but less common causes of squamous cell carcinoma. HPV types 16 and 18 are strongly associated with cervical dysplasia and anogenital cancers and are considered high risk. Only a subset of women infected with HPV go on to develop cervical cancer, however, suggesting that even the most virulent HPV strains may vary in terms of their oncogenic potential. Cofactors that may increase the risk for cancer include smoking, immunosuppression, and exposure to hormonal alteration (*e.g.,* pregnancy, oral contraceptives).[2-4]

HPV infection begins with viral inoculation into a stratified squamous epithelium, where infection stimulates replication of the squamous epithelium, producing the various HPV-proliferative lesions.[5] The incubation period for HPV-induced genital warts ranges from 6 weeks to 8 months, with a mean of 2 to 3 months. Genital warts typically present as soft, raised, fleshy lesions on the external genitalia, including the penis (Fig. 47-1), vulva, scrotum, perineum, and perianal skin. External warts may appear as small bumps, or they may be flat, rough surfaced, or pedunculated. Less commonly, they can appear as smooth reddish or brown raised papules or as dome-shaped lesions on keratinized skin. Internal warts are cauliflower-shaped lesions that affect the mucous membranes of the vagina, urethra, anus, or mouth. They may cause discomfort, bleeding, or painful intercourse.[6]

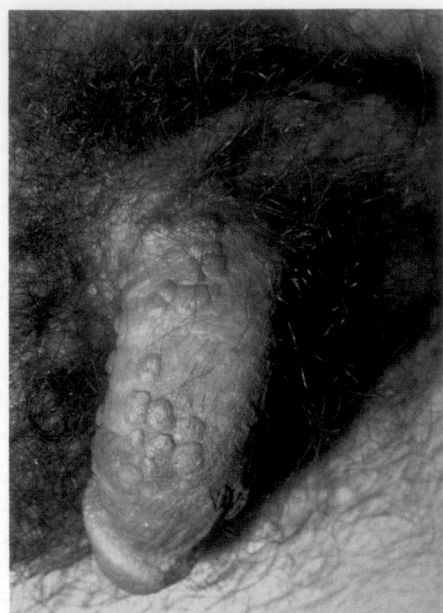

FIGURE 47-1 • Condylomata of the penis. Raised circumscribed lesions are seen on the shaft of the penis. (From Damjanov I. [2005]. The lower urinary tract and male reproductive system. In Rubin E., Gorstein F., Rubin R., et al. [Eds.], *Rubin's pathology: Clinicopathologic foundations of medicine* [4th ed., p. 904]. Philadelphia: Lippincott Williams & Wilkins.)

Subclinical infection occurs more frequently than visible genital warts. Both spontaneous resolution and infection with new HPV types are common. Approximately 70% of women with HPV become HPV DNA negative within 1 year, and as much as 91% become negative within 2 years.[1] Many women with transient HPV infections develop atypical squamous cells of undetermined significance (ASC-US) or low-grade squamous intraepithelial lesions (LSIL) of the cervix as detected on a Pap test, colposcopy, or biopsy (see Chapter 46). In men, transient HPV infection may be associated with intraepithelial neoplasia of the penis and anus. Development of an effective immune response helps clear the infection, but the virus can remain dormant for years and reactivate at a later time. Although reinfection from sexual partners has been considered a reason for the high prevalence of this disease, it is now thought that reinfection with the same HPV type is infrequent.

The association with premalignant and malignant changes has increased the concern regarding the diagnosis and treatment of this viral infection. Lack of regular cervical cancer screening (Pap test) is the primary risk factor for development of invasive cervical cancer.[1] There are no approved serologic tests for HPV or routine methods for culturing the virus. The only test that is currently approved by the U.S. Food and Drug Administration (FDA) is a solution hybridization method to test for high-risk HPV DNA.[1] The HPV DNA test detects whether one or more of the high-risk types of HPV is present; it does not identify the individual HPV type. HPV DNA testing is warranted with equivocal (ASC-US) Pap test results, and is now

recommended to determine which women older than 30 years of age need annual Pap smear screening (see Chapter 46).

The recent release of a quadrivalent vaccine to protect against HPV types 6, 11, 16, and 18 may eventually reduce the risk of cervical cancer associated with HPV.[1,7] Currently, however, there is no treatment to eradicate the virus once a person has become infected. Treatment goals are aimed at elimination of symptomatic warts, surveillance for malignancy and premalignant changes, and education and counseling to decrease psychosocial distress.[8] Prevention of HPV transmission through condom use has not been adequately demonstrated.

Genital condylomata should be considered in any woman who presents with the primary complaint of vulvar pruritus or who has had an abnormal Pap smear result. Microscopic examination of a wet-mount slide preparation and cultures are used to exclude associated vaginitis. Careful inspection of the vulva, with magnification as needed, generally reveals the characteristic lesions, and specimens for biopsy can be taken from questionable areas. Colposcopic examination of the cervix and vagina may be advised as a follow-up measure when there is an abnormal Pap smear result or when HPV lesions are identified on the vulva.

The choice of treatment is based on the number, size, site, and morphology of the lesions, as well the person's preference. Genital warts can resolve spontaneously, so expectant management is acceptable if the person is comfortable with this approach. Evaluation and treatment of sexual partners may be suggested, although this may be difficult considering that warts often do not become clinically apparent for several years after exposure.

The CDC identifies several pharmacologic treatments for symptomatic removal of visible genital warts, including patient-applied (podofilox and imiquimod) and provider-administered (podophyllin and trichloroacetic acid) therapies.[9] Podofilox is a topical antimitotic agent that results in visible necrosis of wart tissue. The safety of podofilox during pregnancy has not been established. Imiquimod cream is a new type of therapeutic agent that stimulates the body's immune system (*i.e.,* production of interferon-α and other cytokines). It is a category B drug and therefore potentially safe for use in pregnancy. Podophyllin, a topical cytotoxic agent, has long been used for treatment of visible external growths. Multiple applications may be required for resolution of lesions. The amount of drug used and the surface area treated should be limited with each treatment session to avoid systemic absorption and toxicity. This treatment is contraindicated in pregnancy for the same reason. An alternative therapy is the topical application of a solution of trichloroacetic acid. This weak destructive agent produces an initial burning in the affected area, followed in several days by a sloughing of the superficial tissue. Several applications at 1- to 2-week intervals may be necessary to eradicate the lesion. Sexual abstinence is suggested during any type of treatment to enhance healing.

Genital warts also may be removed using cryotherapy (*i.e.,* freezing therapy), surgical excision, laser vaporization, or electrocautery. Because it can penetrate deeper than other forms of therapy, cryotherapy often is the treatment of choice for cervical HPV lesions. Laser surgery can be used to remove large or widespread lesions of the cervix, vagina, or vulva, or lesions that have failed to respond to other first-line methods of treatment. Electrosurgical treatment has become more widespread for these types of lesions because it is more readily available in outpatient settings and is much less expensive than laser.

Genital Herpes

Genital herpes is one of the most common causes of genital ulcers in the United States. Because herpesvirus infection is not reportable in all states, reliable data on its true incidence (estimated number of new cases every year) and prevalence (estimated number of people currently infected) are lacking. From the late 1970s to early 1990s, genital herpes prevalence increased 30%. Incidence rates have been relatively stable since 1990, with an estimated 1 million new cases occurring each year. Recent estimates in the United States indicate 67 million people (1 in 4 adolescents or adults) are infected with genital herpes.[10] Women have a greater mucosal surface area exposed in the genital area and therefore are at greater risk of acquiring the infection.

Herpesviruses are large, encapsulated viruses with a double-stranded genome.[11] There are nine types of herpesviruses, belonging to three groups, that cause infections in humans: neurotropic α-group viruses, including herpes simplex virus type 1 (HSV-1; usually associated with cold sores) and HSV-2 (usually associated with genital herpes); varicella-zoster virus (causes chickenpox and shingles); and lymphotropic β-group viruses, including cytomegalovirus (causes cytomegalic inclusion disease), Epstein-Barr virus (causes infectious mononucleosis and Burkitt lymphoma), and human herpesvirus type 8 (the apparent cause of Kaposi sarcoma).[11]

HSV-1 and HSV-2 are genetically similar; both cause a similar set of primary and recurrent infections, and both can cause genital lesions.[11-13] These viruses replicate in the skin and mucous membranes at the site of infection (oropharynx or genitalia), where they cause vesicular lesions of the epidermis and infect the neurons that innervate the area. HSV-1 and HSV-2 are *neurotropic* viruses, meaning that they grow in neurons and share the biologic property of latency. Latency refers to the ability to maintain disease potential in the absence of clinical signs and symptoms. In genital herpes, the virus ascends through the peripheral nerves to the sacral dorsal root ganglia (Fig. 47-2). The virus can remain dormant in the dorsal root ganglia, or it can reactivate, in which case the viral particles are transported back down the nerve root to the skin, where they multiply and cause a lesion to develop. During the dormant or latent period, the virus replicates in a different manner so that the immune system or available treatments have no effect on it. It is not known what reactivates the virus. It may be that the body's defense mechanisms are altered. Numerous studies have shown that host responses to infection influence initial development of the disease, severity of infection, development and maintenance of latency, and frequency of HSV recurrences.

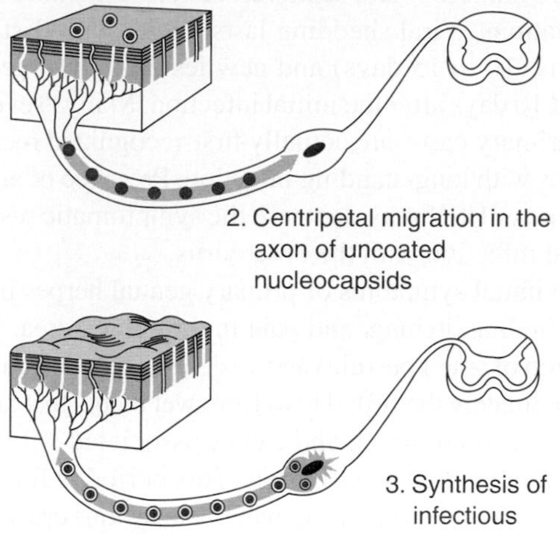

1. Penetration of virus into skin. Local replication and entry of virus into cutaneous neurons
2. Centripetal migration in the axon of uncoated nucleocapsids
3. Synthesis of infectious virions
4. Centrifugal migration of infectious virions to epidermis

FIGURE 47-2 • Pathogenesis of primary mucocutaneous herpes simplex virus infection. (From Corey L., Spear P. G. [1986]. Infections with herpes simplex viruses: Part 1. *New England Journal of Medicine* 314, 686.)

HSV is transmitted by contact with infectious lesions or secretions. HSV-1 is transmitted by oral secretions, and infections frequently occur in childhood. HSV-1 may be spread to the genital area by autoinoculation after poor handwashing or through oral–genital contact. Approximately 15% to 25% of new cases of genital herpes are caused by HSV-1,[14] and it has been estimated that among sexually active adults, new genital HSV-1 infections are almost as common as new HSV-2 infections.[3] HSV-2 usually is transmitted by sexual contact but can be passed to an infant during childbirth if the virus is actively being shed from the genital tract. Most cases of HSV-2 infection are subclinical, manifesting as truly asymptomatic or symptomatic but unrecognized infections. These subclinical infections can occur in people who have never had a symptomatic outbreak or they can occur between recognized clinical recurrences. Up to 70% of genital herpes is spread through asymptomatic shedding by people who do not realize they have the infection.[14] This "unknown" transmission of the virus to sex partners explains why this infection has reached epidemic proportions throughout the world. Because HSV is readily inactivated at room temperature and by drying, aerosol and fomite spread are unusual means of transmission.[15]

The incubation period for HSV is 2 to 10 days. Genital HSV infection may manifest as a first-episode or recurrent infection. There are two types of clinically apparent first-episode eruptions.[12] The first is a true primary infection that occurs in a person who is seronegative for antibodies to HSV-1 or HSV-2. The second is a nonprimary clinical eruption in a person who is seropositive for antibodies to the opposite HSV type (usually genital herpes in someone seropositive to HSV-1). Recurrent infections refer to the second or subsequent outbreak due to the same virus type. HSV-2 is responsible for greater than 90% of recurrent genital herpes infections.[8] First-episode infections have more numerous and scattered vesicles and more systemic manifestations. Viral shedding lasts longer with first-episode infections (10 to 15 days) and new lesions continue to form for about 10 days after the initial infection. Many "severe" presumed primary cases are actually first-recognized recurrences in persons with long-standing infection. Presence of antibodies to one type of HSV may decrease the symptomatic response to the initial infection with the other virus.

The initial symptoms of primary genital herpes infections include tingling, itching, and pain in the genital area, followed by eruption of small pustules and vesicles. These lesions rupture on approximately the fifth day to form wet ulcers that are excruciatingly painful to touch and can be associated with dysuria, dyspareunia, and urine retention. This period is followed by a 10- to 12-day interval during which the lesions crust over and gradually heal. Involvement of the cervix, vagina, urethra, and inguinal lymph nodes is common in women with primary infections. In men, the infection can cause urethritis and lesions of the penis and scrotum. Rectal and perianal infections are possible with anal contact. Systemic symptoms associated with primary infections include fever, headache, malaise, muscle ache, and lymphadenopathy. Primary infections may be debilitating enough to require hospitalization, particularly in women.

Recurrent HSV episodes are usually milder than the initial episode—there typically are fewer lesions, and viral shedding occurs at a lower concentration and for a shorter duration (about 3 days). However, the prodromal symptoms of itching, burning, and tingling at the lesion site are similar. Except for the greater tendency of HSV-2 to recur, the clinical manifestations of HSV-2 and genital HSV-1 infection are similar. The frequency and severity of recurrence vary from person to person. Numerous factors, including emotional stress, lack of sleep, overexertion, other infections, vigorous or prolonged coitus, and premenstrual or menstrual distress, have been identified as triggering mechanisms.

Diagnosis of genital herpes is based on the symptoms, appearance of the lesions, and identification of the virus from swab tests taken from the lesions for cell culture. Depending on the laboratory, a preliminary culture report takes from 2 to 5 days, and a final negative report takes from 10 to 12 days to establish. The stability of the virus in transport media is good for 48 to 72 hours, making mail transport possible. The likelihood of obtaining a positive culture decreases with each day that has elapsed after a lesion develops. The chance of obtaining a positive culture from a crusted lesion is slight, and persons suspected of having genital herpes should be instructed to have a culture within 48 hours of development of new lesions. Polymerase chain reaction (PCR) testing for HSV DNA is more sensitive than culture (see Chapter 16). Although PCR is more expensive than culture, even small amounts of the virus will result in a positive test, the results can be obtained more quickly (4 to 6 hours after reaching the laboratory), and the method can distinguish between HSV-1 and HSV-2. In many

clinics, PCR testing has become the preferred method of testing when active lesions are present, despite the fact that the method is not FDA approved for testing of genital specimens.[9]

Type-specific (HSV-1 and HSV-2) serologic tests are available for determining past infection. Because almost all HSV-2 infections are sexually acquired, the presence of type-specific HSV-2 antibodies usually indicates anogenital infection, whereas the presence of HSV-1 antibodies does not distinguish between anogenital and orolabial infections. The CDC recommends that type-specific glycoprotein G (gG) assays be requested when serologic testing is performed. This type of testing may prove useful in confirming infection in persons with recurrent genital symptoms and negative HSV cultures, or in establishing a clinical diagnosis of genital herpes without laboratory confirmation or in a partner of a person with genital herpes.[9]

There is no known cure for genital herpes, and the methods of treatment are largely symptomatic. The antiviral drugs acyclovir, valacyclovir, and famciclovir have become the cornerstone for management of genital herpes.[9,12] By interfering with viral DNA replication, these drugs decrease the frequency of recurrences, shorten the duration of active lesions, reduce the number of new lesions formed, and decrease viral shedding with primary infections. Valacyclovir, the active component of acyclovir, and famciclovir have greater bioavailability, which enables improved dosing schedules and increased compliance. Episodic intervention reduces the duration of viral shedding and the healing time for recurrent lesions. Continuous antiviral suppressive therapy may be advised when more than six outbreaks occur within 1 year.[9] These drugs are well tolerated, with few adverse effects. This long-term suppressive therapy does not limit latency, and reactivation of the disease frequently occurs after the drug is discontinued. In 2002, the FDA approved long-term suppressive therapy with valacyclovir for the prevention of HSV-2 transmission to an uninfected sexual partner.

Good hygiene is essential during HSV outbreaks to prevent secondary infections. Fastidious handwashing is recommended to avoid hand-to-eye spread of the infection. Sometimes symptomatic relief can be obtained with cool compresses (*i.e.,* Burow soaks), sitz baths, topical anesthetic agents, and oral analgesic drugs. Loose-fitting clothing and cotton undergarments are helpful. To prevent spread of the infection, intimate contact should be avoided until lesions are completely healed.

Current information indicates the risk of neonatal infection is very low when the mother has developed type-specific antibodies, which are then protective to the neonate. Newborns at highest risk are those born to women who shed the virus and have not developed antibodies from previous infections. Disseminated neonatal infection carries high mortality and morbidity rates. Active infection during labor may necessitate cesarean delivery, ideally before membranes rupture. Recommendations from the CDC direct care providers to obtain cultures only when a woman has active lesions during the third trimester. Vaginal delivery is acceptable if visible lesions are not present at the onset of labor.[9]

Molluscum Contagiosum

Molluscum contagiosum is a common viral disease of the skin that gives rise to multiple umbilicated papules. The infection is mildly contagious; it is transmitted by skin-to-skin contact, fomites, and autoinoculation. Lesions are domelike and have a dimpled appearance. A curdlike material can be expressed from the center of the lesion. Necrosis and secondary infection are possible. Diagnosis is based on the appearance of the lesion and microscopic identification of intracytoplasmic molluscum bodies. Molluscum is a benign and self-limited disease.

Spontaneous regression of mature lesions followed by continued emergence of new lesions is common with molluscum, and in the absence of therapy this cycle may persist for 6 months to 5 years. Recurrence is frequent after treatment; therefore, the goal of therapy is to hasten the resolution of individual lesions and reduce the likelihood of further spread.[15] When indicated, treatment consists of removing the top of the papule with a sterile needle or scalpel, expressing the contents of each lesion, and applying alcohol or silver nitrate to the base. Electrodesiccation, cryosurgery, laser ablation, and surgical biopsy are alternative treatments but seldom are needed unless lesions are large or extend over a wide area. A new approach to therapy is the application of imiquimod 1% cream to lesions. This self-applied therapy is the first to show efficacy in patients with immunosuppressive diseases such as acquired immunodeficiency syndrome (AIDS).[16]

Chancroid

Chancroid (*i.e.,* soft chancre) is a disease of the external genitalia and lymph nodes. The causative organism is the gram-negative bacterium *Haemophilus ducreyi,* which causes acute ulcerative lesions with profuse discharge. This disease has become uncommon in the United States, with only 17 reported cases in 2005.[17] It typically occurs in discrete outbreaks rather than as an endemic disease in this country. It is more prevalent in Southeast Asia, the West Indies, and North Africa. As a highly infectious disease, chancroid usually is transmitted by sexual intercourse or through skin and mucous membrane abrasions. Autoinoculation may lead to multiple chancres.

Lesions begin as macules, progress to pustules, and then rupture. This painful ulcer has a necrotic base and jagged edges. In contrast, the syphilitic chancre is nontender and indurated. Subsequent discharge can lead to further infection of self or others. On physical examination, lesions and regional lymphadenopathy may be found. Secondary infection may cause significant tissue destruction. Diagnosis usually is made clinically, but may be confirmed through culture. Gram stain rarely is used today because it is insensitive and nonspecific. PCR testing methods may soon be available commercially for definitive identification of *H. ducreyi.* The organism has shown resistance to treatment with sulfamethoxazole alone and to tetracycline. The CDC recommends treatment with azithromycin, erythromycin, or ceftriaxone.[9]

Granuloma Inguinale

Granuloma inguinale (*i.e.,* granuloma venereum) is caused by a gram-negative bacillus, *Klebsiella granulomatis* (previously known as *Calymmatobacterium* [*Donovania*] *granulomatis*), which is a tiny, encapsulated intracellular parasite. This disease is almost nonexistent in the United States. It is found most frequently in India, Brazil, the West Indies, and parts of China, Australia, and Africa.

Granuloma inguinale causes ulceration of the genitalia, beginning with an innocuous papule. The papule progresses through nodular or vesicular stages until it begins to break down as pink, granulomatous tissue. At this final stage, the tissue becomes thin and friable and bleeds easily. There are complaints of swelling, pain, and itching. Extensive inflammatory scarring may cause late sequelae, such as lymphatic obstruction with the development of enlarged and elephantoid external genitalia. The liver, bladder, bone, joint, lung, and bowel tissue may become involved. Genital complications include tubo-ovarian abscess, fistula, vaginal stenosis, and occlusion of vaginal or anal orifices. Lesions may become neoplastic.

Diagnosis is made through the identification of Donovan bodies (*i.e.,* large mononuclear cells filled with intracytoplasmic gram-negative rods) in tissue smears, biopsy samples, or culture. A minimum 3-week period of treatment with doxycycline, azithromycin, ciprofloxacin, or erythromycin is used in treating the disorder.[9]

Lymphogranuloma Venereum

Lymphogranuloma venereum (LGV) is an acute and chronic venereal disease caused by *Chlamydia trachomatis* types L1, L2, and L3. The disease, although found worldwide, has a low incidence outside the tropics. Most cases reported in the United States are in men. There appears to be a new variant, L2b, that is causing a resurgence of LGV in Europe and the United States, particularly in men who have sex with men.[18]

The lesions of LGV can incubate for a few days to several weeks and thereafter cause small, painless papules or vesicles that may go undetected. An important characteristic of the infection is the early (1 to 4 weeks later) development of large, tender, and sometimes fluctuant inguinal lymph nodes called *buboes.* There may be flulike symptoms with joint pain, rash, weight loss, pneumonitis, tachycardia, splenomegaly, and proctitis. In later stages of the disease, a small percentage of affected persons develop elephantiasis of the external genitalia, caused by lymphatic obstruction or fibrous strictures of the rectum or urethra from inflammation and scarring. Urethral involvement may cause pyuria and dysuria. Cervicitis is a common manifestation of primary LGV, and could extend to perimetritis or salpingitis, which are known to occur in other chlamydial infections.[15,18] Anorectal structures may be compromised to the point of incontinence. Complications of LGV may be minor or extensive, involving compromise of whole systems or progression to a cancerous state.

Diagnosis usually is accomplished by a complement fixation test for LGV-specific *Chlamydia* antibodies. High titers for this antibody differentiate this group from other chlamydial subgroups. PCR techniques, when more widely available, will provide a more practical, cost-effective tool for diagnosis.[18] Treatment involves 3 weeks of doxycycline, tetracycline, or erythromycin.[9] Surgery may be required to correct sequelae such as strictures or fistulas or to drain fluctuant lymph nodes.

> **IN SUMMARY,** STIs that primarily affect the external genitalia include HPV-induced genital warts, genital herpes, molluscum contagiosum, chancroid, granuloma inguinale, and LGV. The lesions of these infections occur on the external genitalia of male and female sexual partners. Of concern is the relation between HPV and genital neoplasms. Genital herpes is caused by a neurotropic HSV (HSV-2 and, sometimes, HSV-1) that ascends through the peripheral nerves to reside in the sacral dorsal root ganglia. The herpesvirus can be reactivated, producing recurrent lesions in genital structures that are supplied by the peripheral nerves of the affected ganglia. There is no permanent cure for herpes infections. Molluscum contagiosum is a benign and self-limited infection that is only mildly contagious. Chancroid, granuloma inguinale, and LGV produce external genital lesions with various degrees of inguinal lymph node involvement. These diseases are uncommon in the United States. ■

VAGINAL INFECTIONS

> *After completing this section of the chapter, you should be able to meet the following objectives:*
>
> ■ State the difference between wet-mount slide and culture methods of diagnosis of STIs.
> ■ Compare the signs and symptoms of infections caused by *Candida albicans, Trichomonas vaginalis,* and bacterial vaginosis.

Candidiasis, trichomoniasis, and bacterial vaginosis are vaginal infections that can be associated with sexual activity. Trichomoniasis is the only form of vaginitis that is known to be sexually transmitted and requires partner treatment. The male partner usually is asymptomatic.

Candidiasis

Also called *yeast infection, thrush,* and *moniliasis, candidiasis* is the second leading cause of vulvovaginitis in the United States. Approximately 75% of reproductive-age women in the United States experience one episode in their lifetime; 40% to 45% experience two or more infections.[19]

Candida albicans is the most commonly identified organism in vaginal yeast infections, but other *Candida* species, such as *Candida glabrata* and *Candida tropicalis,* may also be present. These organisms are present in 20% to 55% of healthy women without causing symptoms, and alteration of the host vaginal environment usually is necessary before the organism can cause pathologic effects.[19] Although vulvovaginal candidiasis usually is not transmitted sexually, it is included in the CDC STI treatment guidelines because it often is diagnosed in women being evaluated for STIs.[9] The possibility of sexual transmission has been recognized for many years; however, candidiasis requires a favorable environment for growth of the organism. The gastrointestinal tract also serves as a reservoir for this organism, and candidiasis can develop through autoinoculation in women who are not sexually active. Although studies have documented the presence of *Candida* on the penis of male partners of women with vulvovaginal candidiasis, few men develop balanoposthitis that requires treatment.

Reported risk factors for the overgrowth of *C. albicans* include recent antibiotic therapy, which suppresses the normal protective bacterial flora; high hormone levels owing to pregnancy or the use of oral contraceptives, which cause an increase in vaginal glycogen stores; and uncontrolled diabetes mellitus or HIV infection, because they compromise the immune system.[20,21] Women with vulvovaginal candidiasis commonly complain of vulvovaginal pruritus accompanied by irritation, erythema, swelling, dysuria, and dyspareunia. The characteristic discharge, when present, is usually thick, white, and odorless. In obese persons, *Candida* may grow in skin folds underneath the breast tissue, the abdominal flap, and the inguinal folds.

Accurate diagnosis is made by identification of budding yeast filaments (*i.e.,* hyphae) or spores on a wet-mount slide using 20% potassium hydroxide (Fig. 47-3). The pH of the discharge, which is checked with litmus paper, typically is less than 4.5. When the wet-mount technique is negative but the clinical manifestations are suggestive of candidiasis, a culture may be necessary.

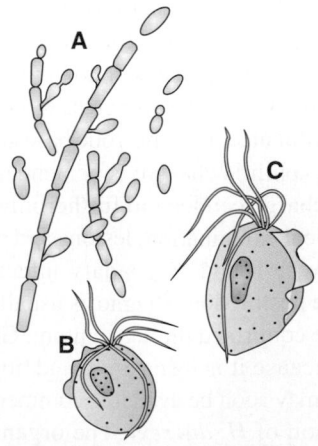

FIGURE 47-3 • Organisms that cause vaginal infections. **(A)** *Candida albicans* (blastospores and pseudohyphae). **(B, C)** *Trichomonas vaginalis.*

Antifungal agents such as clotrimazole, miconazole, butoconazole, and terconazole, in various forms, are effective in treating candidiasis. These drugs, with the exception of terconazole, are available without prescription for use by women who have had a previously confirmed diagnosis of candidiasis. Oral fluconazole has been shown to be as safe and effective as the standard intravaginal regimens.[9] Tepid sodium bicarbonate baths, clothing that allows adequate ventilation, and the application of cornstarch to dry the area may increase comfort during treatment. Chronic vulvovaginal candidiasis, defined as four or more mycologically confirmed episodes within 1 year, affects approximately 5% of women and is difficult to manage. Subsequent prophylaxis (maintenance therapy) often is required for long-term management of this problem.[19]

Candidiasis can be confused with Döderlein cytolysis—an excess of lactobacilli—which can present with a similar clinical picture but typically occurs during the 7 to 10 days before menses. In the case of Döderlein cytolysis, wet-mount and culture techniques show only excessive lactobacilli, but no yeast. Treatment for Döderlein cytolysis involves the use of a sodium bicarbonate douche two to three times in the week prior to menses to raise the vaginal pH and decrease the symptoms.

Trichomoniasis

Trichomoniasis is credited with being a far more prevalent STI than either chlamydial infection or gonorrhea.[22–24] In the United States, it has been estimated that 5 million new cases of trichomoniasis appear annually.[22] Epidemiologically, *Trichomonas vaginalis* infections are commonly associated with other STIs and are therefore a marker for high-risk sexual behavior. The majority of women with trichomoniasis also have other STIs, particularly gonorrhea.[24]

An anaerobic protozoan that can be transmitted sexually, *T. vaginalis* is shaped like a turnip and has three or four anterior flagella (see Fig. 47-3). Trichomonads can reside in the paraurethral glands of both sexes. Men harbor the organism in the urethra and prostate and are asymptomatic. Although 10% to 25% of women are asymptomatic, trichomoniasis is a common cause of vaginitis when some imbalance allows the protozoan to proliferate. This extracellular parasite feeds on the vaginal mucosa and ingests bacteria and leukocytes. The infection causes a copious, frothy, malodorous, green or yellow discharge. There commonly is erythema and edema of the affected mucosa, with occasional itching and irritation. Sometimes, small hemorrhagic areas, called *strawberry spots,* appear on the cervix (Fig. 47-4).

Trichomoniasis can cause a number of complications.[22–24] It is a risk factor for HIV transmission and infectivity in both men and women. In women, it increases the risk of tubal infertility and atypical pelvic inflammatory disease (PID; see Chapter 46), and it is associated with adverse outcomes such as premature birth in pregnant women. Trichomonads attach easily to mucous membranes. They may serve as vectors for the spread of other organisms, carrying pathogens attached to their surface into the fallopian tubes. In men, it is a common cause of nongonococcal urethritis and is a risk factor for

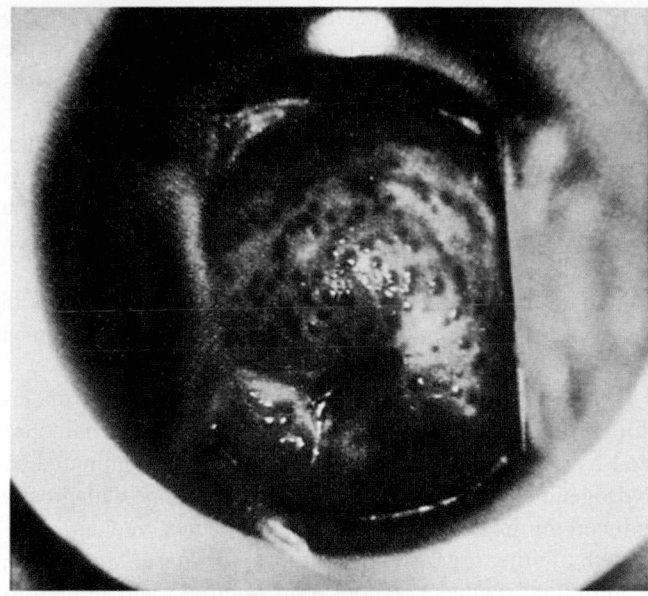

FIGURE 47-4 • Strawberry appearance of the cervix due to *Trichomonas vaginalis* infection, or trichomoniasis. The cervical mucosa reveals punctate hemorrhages along with accompanying vesicles and papules. (From the Centers for Disease Control and Prevention Public Health Image Library. [Online.] Available: http://phil.cdc.gov/phil/home.asp.)

infertility, altering sperm motility and viability.[22–24] It has also been associated with chronic prostatitis.

Diagnosis is made microscopically by identification of the motile protozoan on a wet-mount slide preparation. The pH of the discharge usually is greater than 6.0. Newer point-of-care tests include an antigen-based diagnostic test (OSOM *Trichomonas* Rapid Test) and a DNA probe test (Affirm VP III). Both tests have greater sensitivity than a vaginal mount and results can be available in less than an hour.[9,23] PCR-based tests for *T. vaginalis* are currently under development.

Because the organism resides in other urogenital structures besides the vagina, systemic treatment is recommended. The treatment of choice is oral metronidazole or tinidazole, medications that are effective against anaerobic protozoans.[9] Both drugs are chemically similar to disulfiram (Antabuse), a drug used in the treatment of alcohol addiction that causes nausea, vomiting, flushing of the skin, headache, palpitations, and lowering of the blood pressure when alcohol is ingested. Gastrointestinal disturbances and a metallic taste in the mouth are potential adverse effects of the drugs. Although metronidazole is considered safe for use during pregnancy, data on tinidazole use in pregnancy are limited. Sexual partners should be treated to avoid reinfection, and abstinence is recommended until the full course of therapy is completed.

Bacterial Vaginosis

Bacterial vaginosis is the most prevalent form of vaginal infection seen by health care professionals. The disorder is associated with having multiple sex partners, a new sex partner, douching, and a lack of vaginal lactobacilli. Its relation to sexual activity is not clear. Sexual activity is believed to be a catalyst rather than a primary mode of transmission, and endogenous factors may play a role in the development of symptoms.

The predominant symptom of bacterial vaginosis is a thin, grayish-white discharge that has a foul, fishy odor. Burning, itching, and erythema usually are absent because the bacteria have only minimal inflammatory potential. Because of the lack of inflammation, the term *vaginosis* rather than *vaginitis* is used to describe the condition. The organisms associated with bacterial vaginosis may be carried asymptomatically by men and women.

The pathogenesis of bacterial vaginosis is poorly understood. It is a complex polymicrobial disorder characterized by a shift in the vaginal flora from one dominated by hydrogen peroxide–producing lactobacilli to one with greatly reduced numbers of *Lactobacillus* species and an overgrowth of other organisms, including *Gardnerella vaginalis, Mobiluncus* species, *Mycoplasma hominis,* and numerous anaerobes.[20,21,23,25] The massive overgrowth of vaginal anaerobes is associated with increased conversion of vaginal peptides to a variety of amines that, in high pH, become volatile and malodorous. The amines are associated with increased vaginal transudation and squamous epithelial cell exfoliation, creating the typical discharge.[25] In conditions of elevated pH, *G. vaginalis* more efficiently adhere to the exfoliating epithelial cells, creating clue cells (squamous epithelial cells covered with masses of coccobacilli, often with large clumps of organisms floating free from the cell). Amines further provide a suitable substrate for *M. hominis* growth.

In addition to causing bothersome symptoms, bacterial vaginosis is associated with an increased risk of PID, preterm labor, premature rupture of membranes, chorioamnionitis, and postpartum endometritis linked to the organisms associated with bacterial vaginosis. Postoperative infections, including postabortion PID, posthysterectomy cuff cellulitis, and postcesarean endometritis, have been shown to be associated with asymptomatic bacterial vaginosis. Preoperative antibiotic prophylaxis that covers bacterial vaginosis–associated flora has been shown to reduce these complications.[25]

The diagnosis of bacterial vaginosis is made when at least three of the following characteristics are present: homogeneous, thin, white discharge; production of a fishy, amine odor when a 10% potassium hydroxide solution is dropped onto the secretions; vaginal pH above 4.5 (usually 5.0 to 6.0); and appearance of characteristic "clue cells" on wet-mount microscopic studies. Because *G. vaginalis* can be a part of the normal vaginal flora, cultures should not be done routinely.

When indicated, treatment is aimed at relieving the vaginal symptoms and signs of infection and reducing the risk of infectious complications after abortion or hysterectomy. All women who have symptomatic disease should be treated. Other potential benefits might include a reduction in the risk of other STIs. The CDC recommends treatment by oral metronidazole, metronidazole vaginal gel, or clindamycin vaginal cream. The same treatment regimens used for nonpregnant women can be used in pregnancy. Routine screening for bacterial vaginosis is not advocated, but all pregnant women with bacterial vaginosis should be treated, and women at increased risk for preterm labor should be screened during the first trimester.[9] Treatment of sexual partners is not recommended.[9]

IN SUMMARY, candidiasis, trichomoniasis, and bacterial vaginosis are common vaginal infections that become symptomatic because of changes in the vaginal ecosystem. Only trichomoniasis is spread through sexual contact. The infection, which is caused by the anaerobic protozoan *T. vaginalis,* incites the production of a copious, frothy, yellow or green, malodorous discharge. It is a risk factor for HIV transmission and infectivity in both men and women. In women, it increases the risk of tubal infertility and atypical PID and it is associated with adverse outcomes such as premature birth in pregnant women. Candidiasis, also called a *yeast infection,* is a frequent cause of vulvovaginitis. *Candida* can be present without producing symptoms; usually some host factor, such as altered immune status, contributes to the development of vulvovaginitis. It can be treated with over-the-counter medications. Bacterial vaginosis is the most common cause of vaginal discharge. It is a complex polymicrobial disorder characterized by a shift in the vaginal flora from one dominated by hydrogen peroxide–producing lactobacilli to one with greatly reduced numbers of lactobacilli and an overgrowth of other organisms, including *G. vaginalis, Mobiluncus* species, *M. hominis,* and numerous anaerobes. The predominant symptom of bacterial vaginosis is a thin, grayish-white discharge that has a foul, fishy odor. Because it does not produce inflammation, it is referred to as *vaginosis* rather than *vaginitis.* ■

VAGINAL-UROGENITAL-SYSTEMIC INFECTIONS

After completing this section of the chapter, you should be able to meet the following objectives:

- Compare the signs and symptoms of gonorrhea in the male and female.
- Describe the three stages of syphilis.
- State the genital and nongenital complications that can occur with chlamydial infections, gonorrhea, and syphilis.
- State the treatment for chlamydial urogenital infections, gonorrhea, nonspecific urogenital infections, and syphilis.

Some STIs infect male and female genital and extragenital structures. Among the infections of this type are chlamydial infections, gonorrhea, and syphilis. Many of these infections also pose a risk to infants born to infected mothers. Some infections, such as syphilis, may be spread to the infant while in utero, whereas others, such as chlamydial and gonorrheal infections, can be spread to the infant during the birth process.

Chlamydial Infections

Chlamydial infection is the most prevalent STI in the United States, with an incidence estimated to be more than twice that of gonorrhea. As of December 2000, chlamydial infections are reportable in all 50 states and the District of Columbia. According to CDC estimates, chlamydial infections occur at a rate of 2.8 million new cases each year, predominantly among individuals younger than 25 years of age. In 2005 there were 976,445 reported cases, with the remaining 60% of cases undiagnosed and untreated.[26] Rates for chlamydial infections have risen significantly over the past 15 years because of an increase in screening programs, improved sensitivity of diagnostic tests, and improved surveillance and reporting systems. Reported rates are higher in women largely because of screening efforts, although with the increasing availability of urine testing, reported infection rates in men have risen dramatically.[27–29]

Chlamydia trachomatis is an obligate intracellular bacterial pathogen that is closely related to gram-negative bacteria.[5,11] It resembles a virus in that it requires tissue culture for isolation, but like bacteria, it has ribonucleic acid (RNA) and DNA and is susceptible to some antibiotics. *C. trachomatis* causes a wide variety of genitourinary infections, including nongonococcal urethritis in men and PID in women. The closely related organisms *Chlamydia pneumoniae* and *Chlamydia psittaci* cause mild and severe pneumonia, respectively. *C. trachomatis* can be serologically subdivided into types A, B, and C, which are associated with trachoma and chronic keratoconjunctivitis; types D through K, which are associated with genital infections and their complications; and types L1, L2, and L3, which are associated with LGV. *C. trachomatis* can cause significant ocu-

lar disease in neonates; it is a leading cause of blindness in underdeveloped countries. In these countries, the organism is spread primarily by flies, fomites, and nonsexual personal contact. In industrial countries, the organism is spread almost exclusively by sexual contact and therefore affects primarily the genitourinary structures.

Chlamydiae exist in two forms: elementary bodies, which are the infectious particles capable of entering uninfected cells, and the initiator or reticulate bodies, which multiply by binary fission to produce the inclusions identified in stained cells.[11] The 48-hour growth cycle starts with attachment of the elementary body to the susceptible host cell, after which it is ingested by a process that resembles phagocytosis (Fig. 47-5). Once inside the cell, the elementary body is organized into the reticulate body, the metabolically active form of the organism that is capable of reproduction. The reticulate body is not infectious and cannot survive outside the body. The reticulate bodies divide in the cell for up to 36 hours and then condense to form new elementary bodies, which are released when the infected cell bursts.

The signs and symptoms of chlamydial infection resemble those produced by gonorrhea. The most significant difference between chlamydial and gonococcal salpingitis is that chlamydial infections may be asymptomatic or clinically nonspecific. In women, chlamydial infections may cause urinary frequency, dysuria, and vaginal discharge.[26–29] The most common symptom is a mucopurulent cervical discharge. The cervix itself frequently hypertrophies and becomes erythematous, edematous, and extremely friable. Seventy-five percent of women and 50% of men with chlamydial infection have no symptoms; therefore, most cases are undiagnosed, unreported, and untreated.[26] This can lead to greater fallopian tube damage and increase the reservoir for further chlamydial infections. Approximately 40% of women with an untreated chlamydial infection develop PID, and one in five of these women becomes infertile.[27] Research has identified a possible link between

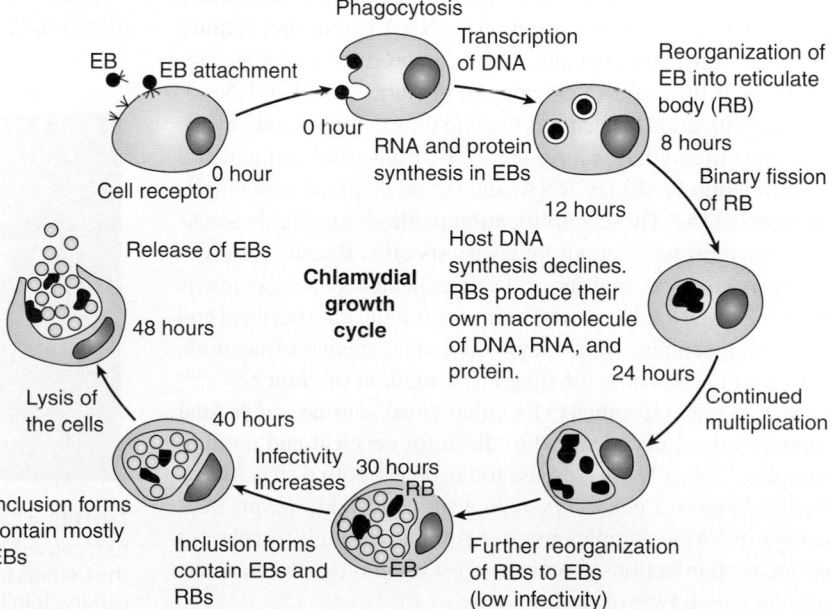

FIGURE 47-5 • Chlamydial growth cycle. EB, elementary body; RB, reticulate body. (From Thompson S. E., Washington A. E. [1983]. Epidemiology of sexually transmitted *Chlamydia trachomatis* infections. *Epidemiologic Reviews 5*, 96–123.)

three specific serotypes of chlamydiae and an increased risk for cervical cancer. The mechanism by which this occurs is unclear.[30]

In men, chlamydial infections cause urethritis, including meatal erythema and tenderness, urethral discharge, dysuria, and urethral itching. Prostatitis and epididymitis with subsequent infertility may develop. The most serious complication of untreated chlamydial infection is the development of Reiter syndrome, a reactive arthritis that includes the triad of urethritis, conjunctivitis, and painless mucocutaneous lesions[29] (see Chapter 59). Women can also develop reactive arthritis, but the male-to-female ratio for this complication is 5:1. The arthritis begins 1 to 3 weeks after the onset of chlamydial infection. The joint involvement is asymmetric, with multiple affected joints and a predilection for the lower extremities. The mucocutaneous lesions are papulosquamous eruptions that tend to occur on the palms of the hands and soles of the feet. Annual screening for sexually active adolescents and young adults has been suggested by the CDC and the U.S. Preventive Services Task Force (USPSTF) in an effort to minimize these serious sequelae of asymptomatic infection.[27] Between 25% and 50% of infants born to mothers with cervical chlamydial infections develop ocular disease (*i.e.*, inclusion conjunctivitis), and 10% to 20% develop chlamydial pneumonitis.[27]

Diagnosis of chlamydial infections takes several forms. The identification of polymorphonuclear leukocytes on Gram stain of penile discharge in the man or cervical discharge in the woman provides presumptive evidence. The direct fluorescent antibody test and the enzyme-linked immunosorbent assay that use antibodies against an antigen in the *Chlamydia* cell wall are rapid tests that are highly sensitive and specific. The positive predictive value of these tests is excellent among high-risk groups, but false-positive results occur more often in low-risk groups. The methodologic challenges of culturing this organism have led to the development of non–culture-based tests that amplify and detect *C. trachomatis*–specific DNA and RNA sequences.[29] One of the newest sets of nonculture techniques, the nucleic acid amplification tests (NAATs), do not require viable organisms for detection, and can produce a positive signal from as little as a single copy of the target DNA or RNA.[31] The amplification procedures that are now commercially available for chlamydial testing are PCR, transcription-mediated amplification (TMA) of RNA, and strand displacement amplification (SDA). These amplification methods are highly sensitive and, if properly monitored, very specific. Because NAATs can be performed on urine and self-collected swab specimens from the distal vagina as well as the traditional endocervical and urethral specimens, this easy, convenient means of accurate detection has become the diagnostic method of choice.[9,26,28,29] Detection rates (specificity) for chlamydiae in urine and vaginal samples are nearly identical to those for cervical and urethral samples.[31] Most NAATs in use today detect both *C. trachomatis* and *Neisseria gonorrhoeae* in a single test. However, PCR assays on urine samples are not reliable enough to rule out gonococcal infections in women. Cost often is a factor in determining which type of testing to use.

The CDC recommends the use of azithromycin or doxycycline in the treatment of chlamydial infection; penicillin is ineffective. Azithromycin or amoxicillin is the preferred choice in pregnancy.[9] Simultaneous antibiotic treatment of both sexual partners is recommended. Abstinence from sexual activity is encouraged to facilitate cure. Retesting all women with chlamydial infection 3 to 4 months after treatment has been recommended to rule out recurrence.[9]

Gonorrhea

Gonorrhea is a reportable STI caused by the bacterium *N. gonorrhoeae*. In 2005, there were 339,593 reported cases of gonorrhea in the United States. Of these reported cases, more than 90% involved persons between 15 and 44 years of age, with the heaviest concentration among young adults (15 to 24 years of age).[17] Like chlamydial infection, gonorrhea is frequently underdiagnosed: the CDC estimates there are 600,000 new cases every year.[9] Although the incidence of gonorrhea has declined steadily from its peak in 1975, rates in 2005 rose for the first time since 1999. Improved screening efforts as well as greater use of more sensitive nonculture methods of testing may have contributed to this trend. Rates in women have been higher than in men since 2001, with the highest being in 15- to 19-year-old African American women.[17]

The gonococcus is a pyogenic (*i.e.,* pus-forming), gram-negative diplococcus that evokes inflammatory reactions characterized by purulent exudates.[11] Humans are the only natural host for *N. gonorrhoeae*. The organism grows best in warm, mucus-secreting epithelia. The portal of entry can be the genitourinary tract, eyes, oropharynx, anorectum, or skin.

Transmission usually is by heterosexual or homosexual intercourse. Autoinoculation of the organism to the conjunctiva is possible. Neonates born to infected mothers can acquire the infection during passage through the birth canal and are in danger of developing gonorrheal conjunctivitis, with resultant blindness unless treated promptly (Fig. 47-6). An amniotic infection syndrome characterized by premature rupture of the

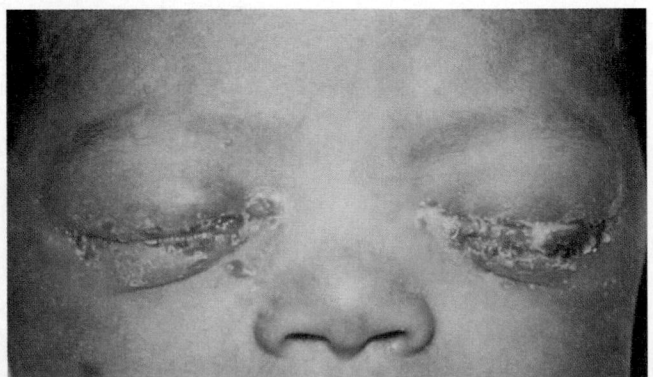

FIGURE 47-6 • Newborn with gonococcal ophthalmia neonatorum caused by maternally transmitted gonococcal infection. (From the Centers for Disease Control and Prevention Public Health Image Library. [Online.] Available: http://phil.cdc.gov/phil/home.asp.)

membranes, premature delivery, and increased risk of infant morbidity and mortality has been identified as an additional complication of gonococcal infections in pregnancy. Genital gonorrhea in young children should raise the possibility of sexual abuse.

The infection commonly manifests 2 to 7 days after exposure. It typically begins in the anterior urethra, accessory urethral glands, Bartholin or Skene glands, and the cervix. If untreated, gonorrhea spreads from its initial sites upward into the genital tract. In males, it spreads to the prostate and epididymis; in females, it commonly moves to the fallopian tubes[32] (Fig. 47-7). Pharyngitis may follow oral–genital contact. The organism also can invade the bloodstream (*i.e.,* disseminated gonococcal infection), causing serious sequelae such as bacteremic involvement of joint spaces, heart valves, meninges, and other body organs and tissues.

Persons with gonorrhea may be asymptomatic and may unwittingly spread the disease to their sexual partners. Men are more likely to be symptomatic than women.[32] In men, the initial symptoms include urethral pain and a creamy yellow, sometimes bloody, discharge (Fig 47-8). The disorder may become chronic and affect the prostate, epididymis, and periurethral glands. Rectal infections are common in homosexual men. In women, recognizable symptoms include unusual genital or urinary discharge, dysuria, dyspareunia, pelvic pain or tenderness, unusual vaginal bleeding (including bleeding after intercourse), fever, and proctitis. Symptoms may occur or increase during or immediately after menses because the bacterium is an intracellular diplococcus that thrives in men-

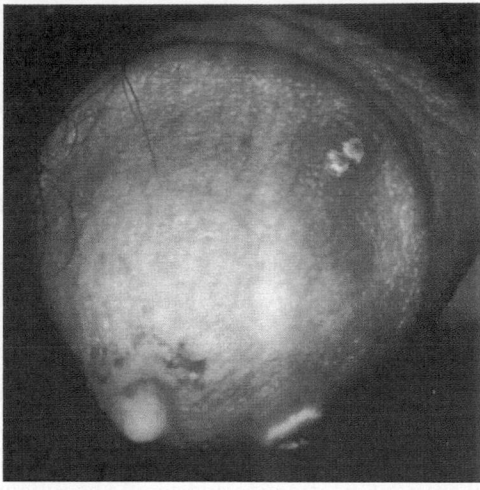

FIGURE 47-8 • Purulent penile discharge due to gonorrhea with overlying pyodermal lesions. (From the Centers for Disease Control and Prevention Public Health Image Library. [Online.] Available: http://phil.cdc.gov/phil/home.asp.)

strual blood but cannot survive long outside the human body. There may be infections of the uterus and development of acute or chronic infection of the fallopian tubes (*i.e.,* salpingitis), with ultimate scarring and sterility.

Diagnosis is based on the history of sexual exposure and symptoms. It is confirmed by identification of the organism on Gram stain or culture. A Gram stain usually is an effective means of diagnosis in symptomatic men (*i.e.,* those with discharge). In women and asymptomatic men, a culture usually is preferred because the Gram stain often is unreliable. Culture has been the gold standard, particularly when the Gram stain is negative. A specimen should be collected from the appropriate site (*i.e.,* endocervix, urethra, anal canal, or oropharynx), inoculated onto a suitable medium, and transported under appropriate conditions. *N. gonorrhoeae* is a fastidious organism with specific nutrient and environmental needs. Optimal growth requires a pH of 7.4, temperature of 35.5°C, and an atmosphere that contains 2% to 10% carbon dioxide.[4] The accuracy of culture results is affected if transport is delayed or growth requirements are not available. Culture detects more than 95% of male urethral gonorrhea and 80% to 90% of cervical, rectal, and pharyngeal infections.[6] An enzyme immunoassay for detecting gonococcal antigens (Gonozyme) is available but has several requirements that limit its usefulness. Detection by NAATs (PCR, SDA, TMA) is possible using urine and urethral swab specimens[31] (see information about NAATs in the previous section on Chlamydial Infections). The sensitivity of these tests is similar to that of culture, and they may be cost effective in high-risk populations. Men are often more willing to provide a urine specimen than to have a urethral swab done, and NAAT can be offered to women in locations where pelvic examination is not possible.

Updated recommendations from the USPSTF suggest that clinicians screen all sexually active men and women for gonorrhea who are at increased risk for infection (*i.e.,* younger

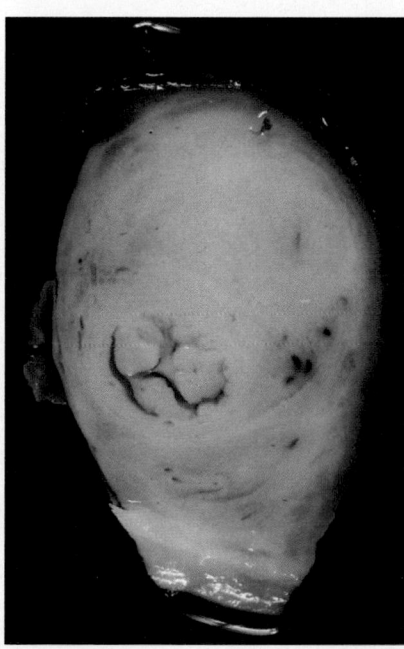

FIGURE 47-7 • Gonorrhea of the fallopian tube. Cross-section of a "pus tube" shows thickening of the wall and lumen swollen with pus. (From Schwartz D., Genta R. M., Conner D. H. [2005]. Infectious and parasitic diseases. In Rubin E., Gorstein F., Rubin R., et al. [Eds.], *Rubin's pathology: Clinicopathologic foundations of medicine* [4th ed., p. 386]. Philadelphia: Lippincott Williams & Wilkins.)

than 25 years of age, new or multiple sexual partners, inconsistent condom use, sex work or drug use).[33] Testing for other STIs, particularly syphilis and chlamydial infection, is suggested at the time of examination. Pregnant women are routinely screened at the time of their first prenatal visit; high-risk populations should have repeat cultures during the third trimester. Neonates are routinely treated with various antibacterial agents applied to the conjunctiva within 1 hour of birth to protect against undiagnosed gonorrhea and other diseases.

Penicillin-resistant strains of *N. gonorrhoeae* are prevalent worldwide and strains with other kinds of antibiotic resistance continue to evolve and spread. The current treatment recommendation to combat tetracycline- and penicillin-resistant strains of *N. gonorrhoeae* is ceftriaxone in a single injection or cefixime, ciprofloxacin, ofloxacin, or levofloxacin in a single oral dose.[9] All are equally effective and should be followed with azithromycin or doxycycline for chlamydiae. Quinolone-resistant strains are now common in Asia, the Pacific islands (including Hawaii), and California, so the CDC recommends avoiding the use of fluoroquinolones in those areas for infections in men who have sex with men or for individuals with a history of recent foreign travel. All sex partners within 60 days prior to discovery of the infection should be contacted, tested, and treated. Test of cure is not required with observed single-dose therapy. Patients are instructed to refrain from intercourse until therapy is completed and symptoms are no longer present.[9]

Syphilis

Syphilis is a reportable STI caused by a spirochete, *Treponema pallidum.* After declining every year from 1990 to 2000, the rate of primary and secondary syphilis increased every year since 2001. Increased rates were primarily in men, although in 2005 the rates in women increased as well.[17] In 2005, 8724 cases of syphilis were reported in the United States (3.0 per 100,000 population). Even though syphilis transmission occurred over a wider geographic area then in the past and there was a significant increase in the rates among whites, it continues disproportionately to affect minority populations. However, the rate for blacks increased by 11.4% over the previous year, only 5.4 times the rate reported in whites, reflecting an overall decrease in racial disparity. The rate for Hispanics increased by 6.5% and the rates for Asian/Pacific populations remained the same. The National Plan to Eliminate Syphilis was launched in 1999 with a goal of reducing primary and secondary syphilis to fewer than 1000 cases and increasing the number of syphilis-free counties to 90% by 2005. Greater than 75% of counties reached that goal, but efforts are still needed to combat the resurgence of this condition in some areas and populations. Federal funding continues to be available to support the revised effort.[17,34]

T. pallidum is spread by direct contact with an infectious moist lesion, usually through sexual intercourse. Bacteria-laden secretions may transfer the organism during kissing or intimate contact. Skin abrasions provide another possible portal of entry. There is rapid transplacental transmission of the organism from the mother to the fetus after 16 weeks' gestation, so that active infection in the mother during pregnancy can produce congenital syphilis in the fetus. Untreated syphilis can cause prematurity, stillbirth, and congenital defects and active infection in the infant. Because the manifestations of maternal syphilis may be subtle, testing for syphilis is mandatory in all pregnancies. Once treated for syphilis, a pregnant woman usually is followed throughout pregnancy by repeat testing of serum titers.

The clinical disease is divided into three stages: primary, secondary, and tertiary. Primary syphilis is characterized by the appearance of a chancre at the site of exposure.[11,35] Chancres typically appear within 3 weeks of exposure but may incubate for 1 week to 3 months. The primary chancre begins as a single, indurated, button-like papule up to several centimeters in diameter that erodes to create a clean-based ulcerated lesion on an elevated base. These lesions usually are painless and located at the site of sexual contact. Primary syphilis is readily apparent in the male, where the lesion is on the scrotum or penis (Fig. 47-9). Although chancres can develop on the external genitalia in females, they are more common on the vagina or cervix, and primary syphilis therefore may go untreated. There usually is an accompanying regional lymphadenopathy. The infection is highly contagious at this stage, but because the symptoms are mild, it frequently goes unnoticed. The chancre usually heals within 3 to 12 weeks, with or without treatment.

The timing of the second stage of syphilis varies even more than that of the first, lasting from 1 week to 6 months. The symptoms of a rash, (especially on the palms [Fig. 47-10] and soles), fever, sore throat, stomatitis, nausea, loss of appetite, and inflamed eyes may come and go for a year but usually last for 3 to 6 months. Secondary manifestations may include alopecia

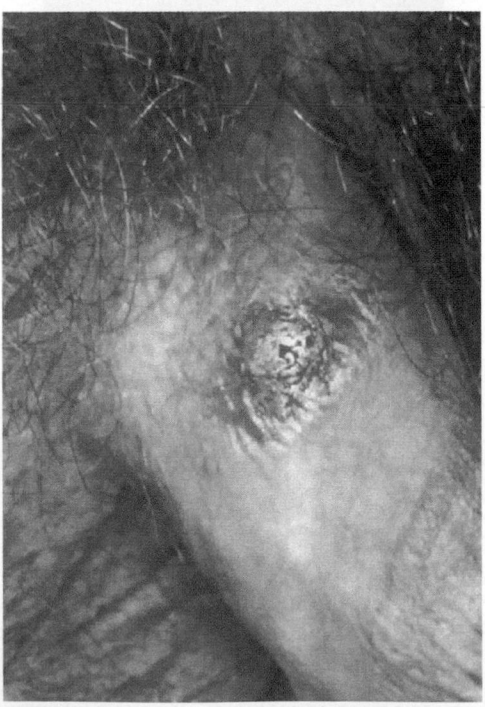

FIGURE 47-9 • Syphilitic chancre of the penis shaft. (From the Centers for Disease Control and Prevention Public Health Image Library. [Online.] Available: http://phil.cdc.gov/phil/home.asp.)

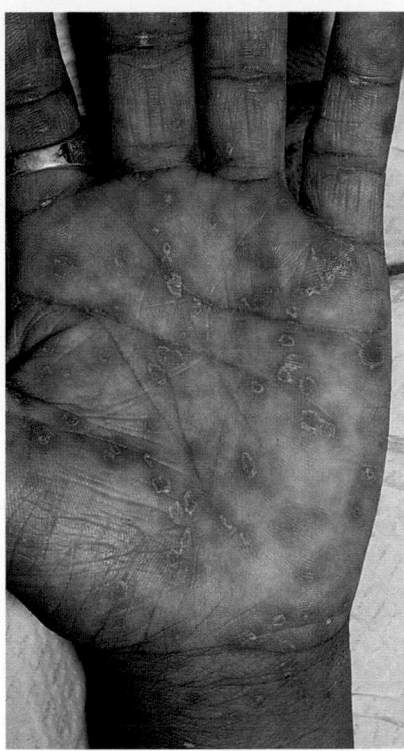

FIGURE 47-10 • Secondary syphilis. A maculopapular rash is present on the palm. (From Schwartz D., Genta R. M., Conner D. H. [2005]. Infectious and parasitic diseases. In Rubin E., Gorstein F., Rubin R., et al. [Eds.], *Rubin's pathology: Clinicopathologic foundations of medicine* [4th ed., p. 409]. Philadelphia: Lippincott Williams & Wilkins.)

and genital condylomata lata.[35] Condylomata lata are elevated, red-brown lesions that may ulcerate and produce a foul discharge. They are 2 to 3 cm in diameter, contain many spirochetes, and are highly infectious.

After the second stage, syphilis frequently enters a latent phase that may last the lifetime of the person or progress to tertiary syphilis at some point. Persons can be infective during the first 1 to 2 years of latency.

Tertiary syphilis is a delayed response to the untreated disease. It can occur as long as 20 years after the initial infection. Only approximately one third of those with untreated syphilis progress to the tertiary stage of the disease, and symptoms develop in approximately one half of these. Approximately one third undergo spontaneous cure, and the remaining one third continue to have positive serologic tests but do not develop structural lesions.[36] When syphilis does progress to the symptomatic tertiary stage, it commonly takes one of three forms: development of localized destructive lesions called *gummas,* development of cardiovascular lesions, or development of central nervous system lesions. The syphilitic gumma is a peculiar, rubbery, necrotic lesion that is caused by noninflammatory tissue necrosis. Gummas can occur singly or multiply and vary in size from microscopic lesions to large, tumorous masses. They most commonly are found in the liver, testes, and bone. Central nervous system lesions can produce dementia, blindness, or injury to the spinal cord, with ataxia and sensory

loss (*i.e.,* tabes dorsalis). Cardiovascular manifestations usually result from scarring of the medial layer of the thoracic aorta with aneurysm formation. These aneurysms produce enlargement of the aortic valve ring with aortic valve insufficiency.

T. pallidum cannot be cultured. It does, however, evoke a humoral immune response and production of antibodies that provide the basis for serologic tests. Although PCR tests have been developed for syphilis, serology remains the mainstay for diagnosis.[11] Because the disease's incubation period may delay test sensitivity, serologic tests usually are repeated after 6 weeks if the initial test results were negative.

Two types of antibodies—nonspecific and specific—are produced.[11] The nonspecific tests measure antibody to cardiolipin, a phospholipid that is present in both host cells and the *T. pallidum.* These antibodies are detected by flocculation tests such as the Venereal Disease Research Laboratory (VDRL) test or the rapid plasma reagin (RPR) test. Because these tests are nonspecific, positive results can occur with diseases other than syphilis. The tests are easy to perform, rapid, and inexpensive and frequently are used as screening tests for syphilis. Results become positive 4 to 6 weeks after infection or 1 to 3 weeks after the appearance of the primary lesion. Because these tests are quantitative, they can be used to measure the degree of disease activity or treatment effectiveness. The VDRL titer usually is high during the secondary stage of the disease and becomes less so during the tertiary stage. A falling titer during treatment suggests a favorable response. The fluorescent treponemal antibody absorption test or microhemagglutinin test is used to detect specific antibodies to *T. pallidum.* These qualitative tests are used to determine whether a positive result on a nonspecific test such as the VDRL is attributable to syphilis. The test results remain positive for life.

The treatment of choice for syphilis is penicillin.[9,35] Because of the spirochetes' long generation time, effective tissue levels of penicillin must be maintained for several weeks. Long-acting injectable forms of penicillin are used. Tetracycline or doxycycline is used for treatment in persons who are sensitive to penicillin. Pregnant patients should be desensitized and treated with penicillin because erythromycin does not treat fetal infection. Sexual partners should be evaluated and treated prophylactically even though they may show no sign of infection. All treated individuals should be reexamined clinically and serologically at 6 and 12 months after completing therapy; more frequent monitoring (3-month intervals) is suggested for individuals with HIV infection.[9]

IN SUMMARY, the vaginal-urogenital-systemic STIs—chlamydial infections, gonorrhea, and syphilis—can severely involve the genital structures and manifest as systemic infections. Gonorrheal and chlamydial infections can cause a wide variety of genitourinary complications in men and women, and both can cause ocular disease and blindness in neonates born to infected mothers. Syphilis is caused by a spirochete, *T. pallidum.* It can produce widespread systemic effects and is transferred to the fetus of infected mothers through the placenta. ■

Review Exercises

1. A 25-year-old woman has been told that her Pap test indicates infection with HPV type 16.

   A. *What are the possible implications of infection with HPV 16?*

   B. *How might she have acquired this infection?*

   C. *What treatments are currently available for treatment of this infection?*

2. A 35-year-old woman presents with vulvar pruritus, dysuria, dyspareunia, and an odorless, thick, cheesy vaginal discharge. She has diabetes mellitus and has recently recovered from a respiratory tract infection, which required antibiotic treatment.

   A. *Given that these manifestations are consistent with a* Candida *infection, what tests might be used to confirm the diagnosis?*

   B. *What risk factors does this woman have that predispose to this type of vaginitis?*

   C. *How might this infection be treated?*

References

1. Centers for Disease Control and Prevention. (2006). Human papillomavirus: HPV information for clinicians. [Online.] Available: www.cdc.gov/std/HPV/common-infection/cdc-HPV-clinicianbo-LR.pdf. Accessed February 7, 2007.
2. Kurman R. J. (2002). *Blaustein's pathology of the female genital tract* (5th ed., pp. 258–276). New York: Springer-Verlag.
3. Sweet R. L., Gibbs R. S. (2002). *Infectious diseases of the female genital tract* (4th ed., pp. 155–164). Philadelphia: Lippincott Williams & Wilkins.
4. Gunter J. (2003). Genital and perianal warts: New treatment opportunities for human papillomavirus infection. *American Journal of Obstetrics and Gynecology* 189, S3–S11.
5. Schwartz D., Centra R. M., Conner D. H. (2005). Infectious and parasitic diseases. In Rubin E., Gorstein F., Rubin R., et al. (Eds.) *Rubin's pathology: Clinicopathologic foundations of medicine* (4th ed., pp. 375–376, 408–411). Philadelphia: Lippincott Williams & Wilkins.
6. Kodner C. M., Nasraty S. (2004). Management of genital warts. *American Family Physician* 70, 2335–2342.
7. Moore S. L., Seybold V. K. (2007). HPV vaccine. *Clinician Reviews* 17(1), 36–41.
8. Handsfield H. H. (2001). *Color atlas and synopsis of sexually transmitted diseases* (pp. 13, 23, 71, 87, 163). New York: McGraw-Hill.
9. Centers for Disease Control and Prevention. (2006). Sexually transmitted diseases: Treatment guidelines 2006. *Morbidity and Mortality Weekly Report* 55(RR11), 1–94.
10. Baker D. A. (2006). Tip of the iceberg: The startling incidence and prevalence of HSV-2. *Primary Care Perspectives* March, 3–5.
11. McAdam A. J., Sharpe A. H. (2005). Infectious diseases. In Kumar V., Abbas A. K., Fausto N. (Eds.), *Robbins and Cotran pathologic basis of disease* (7th ed., pp. 365–371, 394–395). Philadelphia: Elsevier Saunders.
12. Beauman J. G. (2005). Genital herpes: A review. *American Family Physician* 72, 1527–1537, 1541–1542.
13. Kimberlin D. W., Rouse D. J. (2004). Genital herpes. *New England Journal of Medicine* 350, 1970–1977.
14. Burkhart C. G. (2006). A guide to recognizing and treating herpes. *The Clinical Advisor* November, 26–36.
15. Holmes K. K., Per-Anders M., Sparling P. F., et al. (1999). *Sexually transmitted diseases* (3rd ed., pp. 287, 290, 424, 563–564, 629, 820–821). New York: McGraw-Hill.
16. Turing S. K. (2003). Molluscum contagiosum: The importance of early diagnosis and treatment. *American Journal of Obstetrics and Gynecology* 189, S12–S16.
17. Centers for Disease Control and Prevention (2005). STD surveillance 2005. [Online.] Available: www.cdc/gov/std/stats. Accessed February 7, 2007.
18. Witt R. (2006). Emerging epidemic of lymphogranuloma venereum. *Clinician Reviews* 16(5), 56–64.
19. American College of Obstetricians and Gynecologists. (2006). ACOG practice bulletin: Vaginitis. *Obstetrics and Gynecology* 107, 1195–1205.
20. Owen M. K., Clenney T. L. (2004). Management of vaginitis. *American Family Physician* 70, 2125–2132, 2139–2140.
21. Eckert L. O. (2006). Acute vulvovaginitis. *New England Journal of Medicine* 355, 1244–1252.
22. Soper D. (2004). Trichomoniasis: Under control or undercontrolled? *American Journal of Obstetrics and Gynecology* 190, 281–290.
23. Sobel J. D. (2005). What's new in bacterial vaginosis and trichomoniasis? *Infectious Disease Clinics of North America* 19, 387–406.
24. Schwebke J. R., Burgess D. (2004). Trichomoniasis. *Clinical Microbiology Reviews* 17, 794–803.
25. Sobel J. D. (2000). Bacterial vaginosis. *Annual Review of Medicine* 51, 349–356.
26. Grimshaw-Mulcahy L. J. (2006). Chlamydia: Diagnosing the hidden STD. *The Clinical Advisor* March, 32–42.
27. U.S. Preventive Services Task Force. (2002). Screening for *Chlamydia* infection: Recommendations and rationale. *American Journal of Nursing* 102(10), 87–92.
28. Miller K. E. (2006). Diagnosis and treatment of *Chlamydia trachomatis* infection. *American Family Physician* 73, 1411–1416.
29. Peipert J. F. (2003). Genital chlamydial infections. *New England Journal of Medicine* 349, 2424–2430.
30. Antilla T., Saiku P., Koskela P., et al. (2001). Serotypes of *Chlamydia trachomatis* and risk for development of cervical squamous cell carcinoma. *Journal of the American Medical Association* 285, 47–51.
31. Cook R. L., Hutchison S. L., Ostergaard L., et al. (2005). Systematic review: Noninvasive testing for *Chlamydia trachomatis* and *Neisseria gonorrhoeae*. *Annals of Internal Medicine* 142, 914–925.
32. Miller K. E. (2006). Diagnosis and treatment of *Neisseria gonorrhoeae*. *American Family Physician* 73, 1779–1784, 1786.
33. U.S. Preventive Services Task Force. (2005). Screening for gonorrhea: Recommendation statement. *American Journal for Nurse Practitioners* 9(10), 35–40.
34. Centers for Disease Control and Prevention. (2003). Primary and secondary syphilis—United States, 2002. *Morbidity and Mortality Weekly Report* 52(46), 1117–1120.
35. Brown D. L., Frank J. E. (2003). Diagnosis and management of syphilis. *American Family Physician* 68, 283–290, 297.
36. Chapin K. (1999). Probing the STDs. *American Journal of Nursing* 99(7), 24AAA–24DDD.

Visit the Point. **http://thePoint.lww.com for animations, journal articles, and more!**

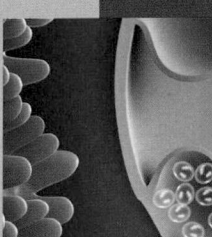

Disorders of
Neural Function

For centuries, the nervous system was ignored or even deemed unimportant. Aristotle (384–322 BC), the great Greek philosopher, decreed that the heart was the seat of the soul, whereas the brain—which he assumed was composed largely of water—simply cooled it. Although Galen (AD 130–200) was able to show that the spinal cord was essential to many sensations and movements, his experiments were conducted only on animals. Not until the 1500s, when the Flemish anatomist Andreas Vesalius (1514–1564) dissected "the heads of executed criminals . . . still warm," was the overarching importance of the human brain and spinal cord established.

Investigations continued with scientists debating whether the brain should be considered as a whole or as consisting of separate areas, each responsible for specific functions. Progress in brain research took an impressive, if accidental, leap in 1841, when an explosion at a railroad work site in Vermont shot an iron rod into the left cheek of Phineas Gage, through his brain, and out the top of his head. Gage survived the accident, but it became clear to all who knew him that he had changed greatly. Formerly a conscientious, hardworking man, he became fitful, obstinate, foul-mouthed, and capricious. Gage died in 1860, and an autopsy showed destruction of the left lobe of his brain and damage to his right lobe. Scientists concluded that his personality change was the result of the grievous damage to the frontal lobes, an observation that supported the then-emerging concept that different parts of the brain serve different functions.

Chapter 48

Organization and Control of Neural Function

EDWARD W. CARROLL AND ROBIN CURTIS

> The nervous system, in coordination with the endocrine system, provides the means by which cell and tissue functions are integrated into a solitary, surviving organism. It controls skeletal muscle movement and helps to regulate cardiac and visceral smooth muscle activity. The nervous system enables the reception, integration, and perception of sensory information; it provides the substratum necessary for intelligence, anticipation, and judgment; and it facilitates adjustment to an ever-changing external environment.

All portions of the nervous system can be divided into two basic components: the central nervous system (CNS) and the peripheral nervous system (PNS). The CNS consists of the brain and spinal cord, which are protected by the skull and vertebral column, whereas the PNS is found outside these structures. Inherent in the basic design of the nervous system is the provision for the concentration of computational and control functions in the CNS. In this design, the PNS functions as an input–output system for relaying information to the CNS and for transmitting output messages that control effector organs, such as muscles and glands.

This chapter is divided into five parts: (1) nervous tissue cells, (2) neurophysiology, (3) developmental organization of the nervous system, (4) the structure and function of the spinal cord and brain, and (5) the autonomic nervous system.

NERVOUS TISSUE CELLS

After completing this section of the chapter, you should be able to meet the following objectives:

■ Distinguish between the functions of the neurons and supporting cells of the nervous system.
■ List the three parts of a neuron and describe their structure and function.
■ Name the supporting cells in the central nervous system and peripheral nervous system and state their functions.
■ Describe the energy requirements of nervous tissue.

Nervous tissue contains two types of cells: neurons and supporting cells. The neurons are the functional cells of the nervous system. They exhibit membrane excitability and conductivity and secrete neurotransmitters and hormones, such as epinephrine and antidiuretic hormone. The supporting cells, such as Schwann cells in the PNS and the neuroglial cells in the CNS, protect the nervous system and provide metabolic support for the neurons.

THE STRUCTURAL ORGANIZATION OF THE NERVOUS SYSTEM

- The nervous system is divided into two parts: the central nervous system (CNS), consisting of the brain and spinal cord, which are located in the skull and spinal column, and the peripheral nervous system, which is located outside these structures.

- The nervous system contains two major types of cells: neurons, which are functioning cells of the nervous system, and supporting cells, which protect the nervous system and supply metabolic support.

- The neurons consist of a cell body with cytoplasm-filled processes, the dendrites, and the axons.

- There are two types of neurons: afferent neurons or sensory neurons, which carry information to the CNS, and efferent neurons or motoneurons, which carry information from the CNS to the effector organs.

Neurons

Neurons, which are the functioning cells of the nervous system, have three distinct parts: the cell body, and its cytoplasm-filled processes, the dendrites and axon. These processes form the functional connections, or synapses, with other nerve cells, with receptor cells, or with effector cells. Axonal processes are particularly designed for rapid communication with other neurons and the many body structures innervated by the nervous system. Afferent (sensory) neurons transmit information to the CNS, whereas efferent (motor) neurons carry information away from the CNS (Fig. 48-1). Interspersed between the afferent and efferent neurons is a network of interconnecting neurons (also called *interneurons* or *internuncial* neurons) that modulate and control the body's response to sensory input from the internal and external environments.

The cell body (soma) of a neuron contains a large, vesicular nucleus with one or more distinct nucleoli and a well-developed rough endoplasmic reticulum. A neuron's nucleus has the same deoxyribonucleic acid (DNA) and genetic code content present in other cells of the body, and its nucleolus, which is composed of portions of several chromosomes, produces ribonucleic acid (RNA) needed for protein synthesis. The cytoplasm contains large masses of ribosomes that are prominent in most neurons. These acidic RNA masses, which are involved in protein synthesis, stain as dark Nissl bodies with basic histologic stains (see Fig. 48-1).

Dendrites (*i.e.,* "treelike") are multiple, short, branched extensions of the nerve cell body; they conduct information toward the cell body and are the main source of information for

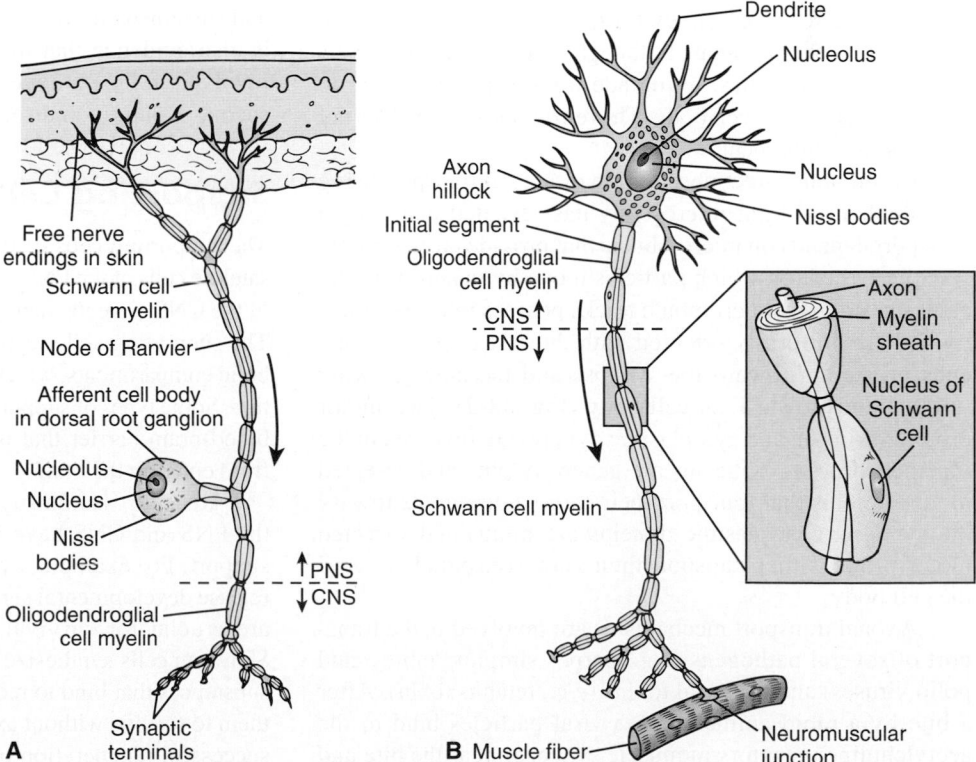

FIGURE 48-1 • Afferent (**A**) and efferent neurons (**B**), showing the soma or cell body, dendrites, and axon. *Arrows* indicate the direction for conduction of action potentials.

the neuron. The dendrites and cell body are studded with synaptic terminals that communicate with axons and dendrites of other neurons.

Axons are long efferent processes that project from the cell body. Most neurons have only one axon; however, axons may exhibit multiple branching that results in many axonal terminals. The axon of a neuron conducts nerve impulses from the cell body to its synapse. The axon also provides a physical conduit for the transport of materials between the cell body and the synaptic terminals of the axon. The cell body of the neuron is equipped for a high level of metabolic activity. This is necessary because the cell body must synthesize the cytoplasmic and membrane constituents required to maintain the function of the soma plus the many proteins and other cytoplasmic materials used by the axon and its synaptic terminals. Some of these axons extend for a distance of 1 to 1.5 m and have a volume that is 200 to 500 times greater than the cell body itself.

A bidirectional axonal transport system exists to carry materials to the nerve terminal (anterograde direction) and back to the cell body (retrograde direction). The anterograde component consists of fast and slow components. Fast anterograde systems transport molecules such as neurosecretory granules by an energy-dependent system at the rate of 200 to 400 mm/day. Another component of the fast anterograde system transports organelles, including mitochondria, at the rate of 50 to 100 mm/day. The antidiuretic hormone and oxytocin use the fast anterograde system to travel from hypothalamic neurons through their axons to the posterior pituitary, where the hormones are released into the blood. The slow anterograde component transports materials such as tubulin and cytoplasmic enzymes at a rate of 0.1 to 6 mm/day. A fast retrograde component of axonal transport carries materials that are shipped back to the cell body for degradation or reuse at the rate of 100 to 200 mm/day. Although much of this material is degraded in lysosomes, retrograde transport is also used to deliver signals to the cell body. The retrograde system does not have a slow component.

Continuous direct observation of axonal transport using video-enhanced light microscopy has revealed that axonal transport depends on microtubules that provide an essentially stationary track on which particles move by means of molecular motors. The microtubule tracks possess inherent polarity and are uniformly oriented with the fast-growing (plus) ends projecting toward the synapse and the slow-growing (minus) ends toward the cell body (Fig. 48-2). Two motor proteins (kinesin and cytoplasmic dynein) are involved in the transport process. Kinesins are generally plus-end–directed motor proteins that transport their cargo anterograde toward the synapse. Cytoplasmic dyneins are minus-end–directed motor proteins that transport their cargo retrograde toward the cell body.

Axonal transport mechanisms are involved in the transport of several pathogens (*e.g.,* herpes simplex, rabies, and polio viruses) and bacterial toxins (*e.g.,* tetanus toxin). After a bite by a rabid animal, rabies viral particles bind to the acetylcholine receptors in muscle synapses near the bite and

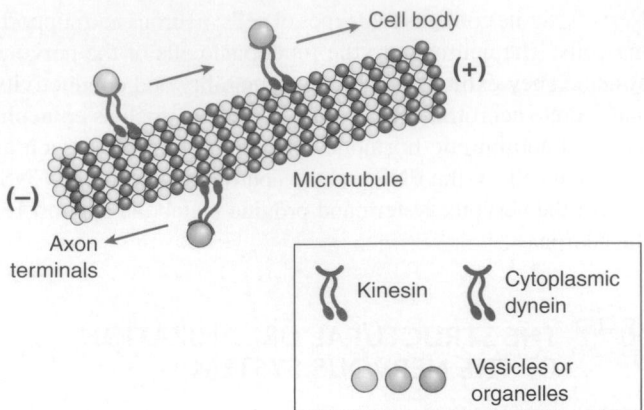

FIGURE 48-2 • The cellular mechanism for axonal transport. Two cellular motor proteins, kinesin and cytoplasmic dynein, are shown transporting vesicles or organelles in the anterograde (kinesin) and retrograde (cytoplasmic dynein) directions. Kinesin transports vesicles toward the rapidly forming (+) end of the microtubule, whereas cytoplasmic dynein transports toward the minus (–) or slower-growing end of the microtubule. (Courtesy of Edward W. Carroll.)

are carried by retrograde transport to the cell bodies of neurons living in the CNS. Affected neurons spread the rabies virus to other neurons throughout the CNS. Affected neurons then transport the virus particles along peripheral nerves by anterograde axonal transport to the salivary glands, where they can be transmitted by another bite. The retrograde axonal transport of the tetanus toxin produced by *Clostridium tetani* bacteria blocks the release of inhibitory substances at synapses, thereby permitting unopposed neural stimulation and sustained contraction of skeletal muscles (tetany). There is also evidence that disorders of axonal transport may be involved in the pathogenesis of neurodegenerative diseases such as Huntington disease and Alzheimer disease.

Supporting Cells

The supporting cells of the nervous system, the Schwann and satellite cells of the PNS and the several types of neuroglial cells of the CNS, give the neurons protection and metabolic support. The supporting cells segregate the neurons into isolated metabolic compartments, which are required for normal neural function. Some types of supporting cells (astrocytes) help to form the blood-brain barrier that prevents toxic materials in the blood from entering the brain.

Recent research suggests that many supporting cells of the PNS and CNS have functions other than protection and support. For example, evidence suggests that Schwann cells release developmental signals in embryonic nervous tissue that are crucial for survival of neonatal neurons. Postnatally, Schwann cells synthesize and release self-regulating autocrine substances that bind to receptors on their cell surface, enabling them to survive without axons, a feature that is essential for the successful regeneration of damaged peripheral nerves. Some supporting cells (Schwann cells and astrocytes) also respond to neuronal activity by triggering the release of communication molecules, thus influencing feedback regulation of neuronal function.

Two types of supporting cells (oligodendrocytes in the CNS and Schwann cells in the PNS) produce the myelin used to insulate nerve cell processes and increase the velocity of nerve impulse conduction. Myelin has a high lipid content, which gives it a whitish color, and the name *white matter* is given to the masses of myelinated fibers in the spinal cord and brain. Besides its role in increasing conduction velocity, the myelin sheath is essential for the survival of larger neuronal processes, perhaps by the secretion of neurotrophic compounds.

In some pathologic conditions, such as multiple sclerosis in the CNS and Guillain-Barré syndrome in the PNS, the myelin may degenerate or be destroyed. This leaves a section of the axonal process without myelin while leaving the nearby Schwann or oligodendroglial cells intact. Unless remyelination takes place, the axon eventually dies.

Supporting Cells of the Peripheral Nervous System

Schwann cells and satellite cells are the two types of supporting cells in the PNS. Normally, the nerve cell bodies in the PNS are collected into ganglia, such as the dorsal root and autonomic ganglia. Each of the cell bodies and processes of the peripheral nerves is separated from the connective tissue framework of the ganglion by a single layer of flattened capsular cells called *satellite cells*. Satellite cells secrete a basement membrane that protects the cell body from the diffusion of large molecules.

The processes of larger afferent and efferent neurons are surrounded by the cell membrane and cytoplasm of Schwann cells, which are close relatives of the satellite cells. During myelination, the Schwann cell wraps around each nerve process several times in a "jelly roll" fashion (Fig. 48-3). Schwann cells line up along the neuronal process, and each of these cells forms its own discrete myelin segment. The end of each myelin segment attaches to the cell membrane of the axon by means of intercellular junctions. Successive Schwann cells are separated by short extracellular fluid gaps, called the *nodes of Ranvier,* where the myelin is missing and voltage-gated sodium channels are concentrated (Fig. 48-4). The nodes of Ranvier increase nerve conduction by allowing the impulse to jump from node to node through the extracellular fluid in a process called *saltatory conduction* (from the Latin *saltare,* "to jump"). In this way, the impulse can travel more rapidly than it could if it were required to move systematically along the entire nerve process. This increased conduction velocity greatly reduces reaction time, or time between the application of a stimulus and the subsequent motor response. The short reaction time is especially important in peripheral nerves with long distances (sometimes 1 to 1.5 m) for conduction between the CNS and distal effector organs.

Each of the Schwann cells along a peripheral nerve is encased in a continuous tube of basement membrane, which in turn is surrounded by a multilayered sheath of loose connective

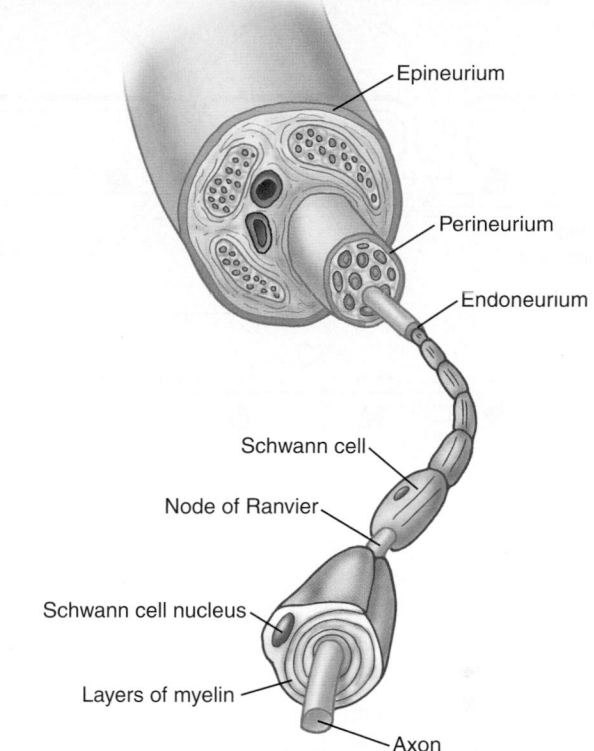

FIGURE 48-3 • Section of a peripheral nerve containing both afferent (sensory) and efferent (motor) neurons. Schwann cells form a myelin sheath around the larger nerve fibers in the peripheral nervous system. Successive Schwann cells are separated by short extracellular fluid gaps called the *nodes of Ranvier,* where the myelin is missing and the voltage-gated sodium channels are concentrated.

tissue known as the *endoneurium* (see Fig. 48-3). The endoneurial sheath, which is essential to the regeneration of peripheral nerves, provides a collagenous tube through which a regenerating axon can again reach its former target. The endoneurial sheath does not penetrate the CNS. The absence of the endoneurial sheaths is thought to be a major factor in the limited axonal regeneration of CNS nerves compared with those of the PNS.

The endoneurial sheaths are bundled with blood vessels into small bundles or clusters of nerves called *fascicles*. In the nerve, the fascicles consisting of bundles of nerve fibers are surrounded by another protective covering called the *perineurium.* Usually, several fascicles are further surrounded by the heavy, protective *epineurial sheath* of the peripheral nerve. The protective layers that surround the peripheral nerve processes are continuous with the connective tissue capsule of the sensory nerve endings and the connective tissue that surrounds the effector structures, such as the skeletal muscle cell. Centrally, the connective tissue layers continue along the dorsal and ventral roots of the nerve and fuse with the meninges that surround the spinal cord and brain.

Myelin formation is essentially the same in both the PNS and CNS; both contain myelin basic protein and both involve

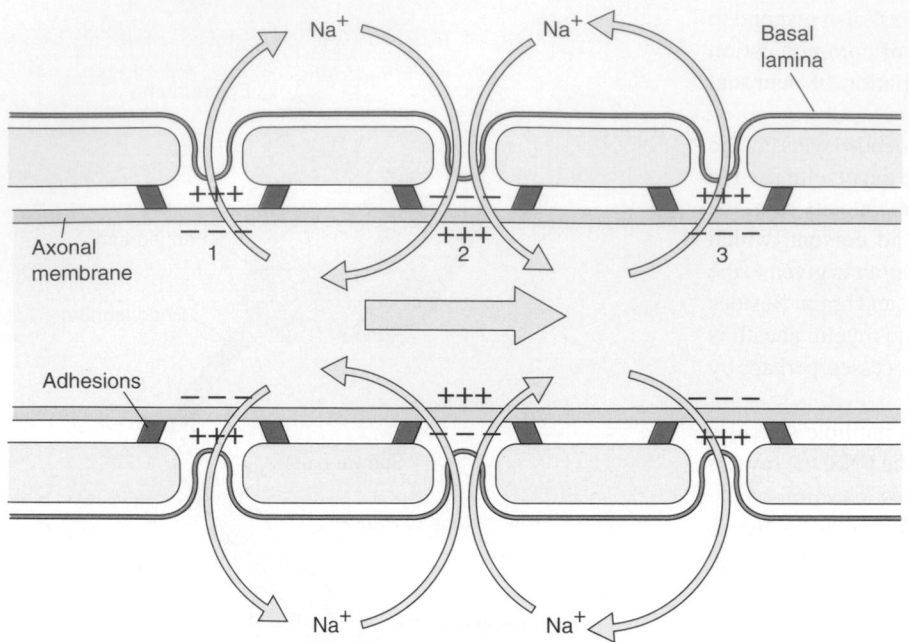

FIGURE 48-4 • Schematic drawing of a longitudinal section of a myelinated axon in the peripheral nervous system. Schwann cells insulate the axon, decreasing flow through the membrane. Action potentials occur at the nodes of Ranvier, which are unmyelinated areas of the basal lamina between the Schwann cells. The impulses jump from node to node in a process called *saltatory conduction,* which greatly increases the velocity of conduction. (*1*) represents the trailing hyperpolarized region behind the action potential, (*2*) the hypopolarized region at the action potential, and (*3*) the leading hyperpolarized area ahead of the action potential. The Schwann cell adhesions (*red*) to the plasma membrane of the axon block the leakage of current under the myelin.

the winding of plasma membranes around the nerve fiber. During the wrapping of myelin, the cytoplasm between two adjacent inner leaflets of the plasma membrane is expelled. The two adjacent inner leaflets and any remaining cytoplasm appear as a dark line called the *major dense line.* Likewise, during the wrapping of the plasma membranes to form myelin, adjacent outer plasma membrane leaflets become opposed, creating the interperiod or *minor dense line.* Linking proteins, *proteolipid protein* (PLP) found only in the CNS and *myelin protein zero*

(MPZ) found only in the PNS, help stabilize adjacent plasma membranes of the myelin sheath.

Supporting Cells of the Central Nervous System

Supporting cells of the CNS consist of the oligodendrocytes, astrocytes, microglia, and ependymal cells (Fig. 48-5). The *oligodendrocytes* form the myelin in the CNS. Instead of forming a myelin covering for a single axon, these cells reach out

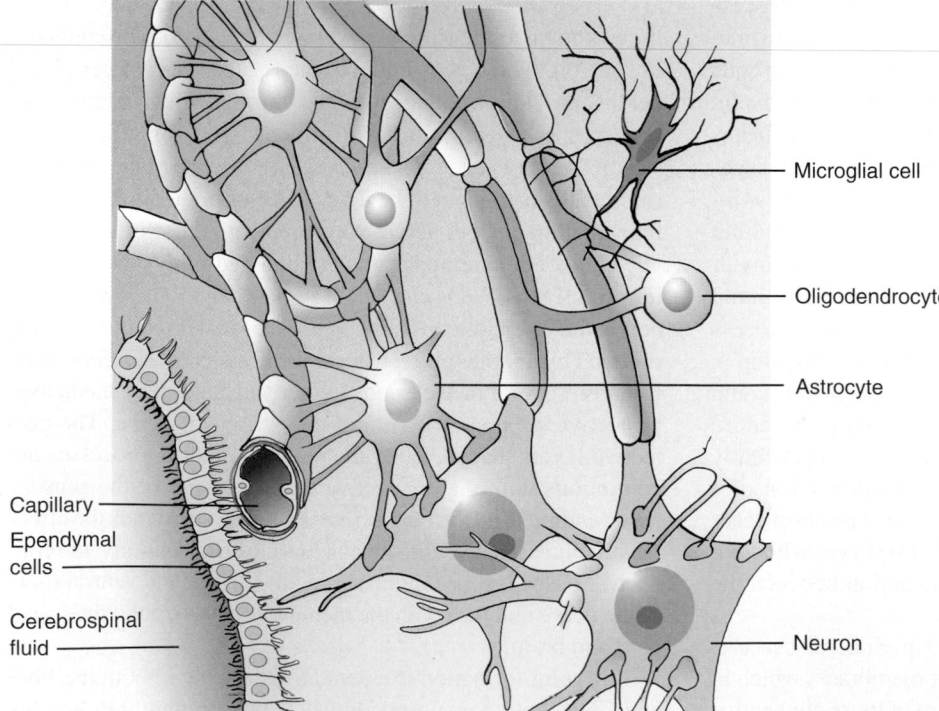

Microglial cell

Oligodendrocyte

Astrocyte

Capillary

Ependymal cells

Cerebrospinal fluid

Neuron

FIGURE 48-5 • The supporting cells of the central nervous system (CNS). Diagrammatic view of relationships between the glial elements (astrocyte, oligodendrocyte, microglial cell, and the ependymal cells), the capillaries, the cerebrospinal fluid, and the cell bodies of CNS neurons.

with several processes, each wrapping around and forming a multilayered myelin segment around several different axons. As with peripheral myelinated fibers, the covering of axons in the CNS increases the velocity of nerve conduction.

Astrocytes, the most numerous of neuroglial cells, are particularly prominent in the gray matter of the CNS. These large cells have many processes, some reaching to the surface of the capillaries, others reaching to the surface of the nerve cells, and still others filling most of the intercellular space within the CNS. Astrocytes maintain an important link between neurons, especially between synapses, and capillary blood flow. They also help to maintain the right potassium ion concentration in the extracellular space between neurons. Because astrocytes are highly permeable to potassium, they can take up excess potassium and so protect other neurons. In addition, astrocytes take up neurotransmitters from synaptic zones after their release and thereby help regulate synaptic activity. Recent studies suggest that astrocytes may also play an important role in the regulation of blood flow to the cerebral gray matter. Astrocytes are also the principal cells responsible for repair and scar formation in the brain. They can fill their cytoplasm with microfibrils (*i.e.,* fibrous astrocytes), and masses of these cells form the special type of scar tissue that develops in the CNS when tissue is destroyed, a process called *gliosis.*

A third type of neuroglial cell, the *microglia,* is a small phagocytic cell that is available for cleaning up debris after cellular damage, infection, or cell death. The fourth type of cell, the *ependymal cell,* forms the lining of the neural tube cavity, the ventricular system. In some areas, these cells combine with a rich vascular network to form the *choroid plexus,* where production of the cerebrospinal fluid (CSF) takes place.

Metabolic Requirements of Nervous Tissue

Nervous tissue has a high rate of metabolism. Although the brain comprises only 2% of the body's weight, it receives approximately 15% of the resting cardiac output and consumes 20% of its oxygen. Despite its substantial energy requirements, the brain cannot store oxygen or effectively engage in anaerobic metabolism. An interruption in the blood or oxygen supply to the brain rapidly leads to clinically observable signs and symptoms. Without oxygen, brain cells continue to function for approximately 10 seconds. Unconsciousness occurs almost simultaneously with cardiac arrest, and the death of brain cells begins within 4 to 6 minutes. Interruption of blood flow also leads to the accumulation of metabolic byproducts that are toxic to neural tissue.

Glucose is the major fuel source for the nervous system, but neurons have no provision for storing glucose. Ketones can provide for limited temporary energy requirements; however, these sources are rapidly depleted. Unlike muscle cells, neurons have no glycogen stores and must rely on glucose from the blood or the glycogen stores of supporting neuroglial cells. Persons receiving insulin for diabetes may experience signs of neural dysfunction and unconsciousness (*i.e.,* insulin reaction or shock) when blood glucose drops because of insulin excess (see Chapter 42).

IN SUMMARY, nervous tissue is composed of two types of cells: neurons and supporting cells. Neurons are composed of three parts: a cell body, which controls cell activity; the dendrites, which conduct information toward the cell body; and the axon, which carries impulses from the cell body. Axonal transport mechanisms provide the means to convey materials to and from the soma and axon terminals. The supporting cells consist of Schwann and satellite cells of the PNS and the neuroglial cells of the CNS. Supporting cells protect and provide metabolic support for the neurons, help to regulate blood flow, and aid in segregating them into isolated compartments, which is necessary for normal neuronal function. Nervous system function demands a high proportion of metabolic energy. Glucose is the major fuel for the nervous system. The brain comprises only 2% of body weight but receives 15% of the resting cardiac output. ■

CONCEPTS in action **ANIMATIN**

NEUROPHYSIOLOGY

After completing this section of the chapter, you should be able to meet the following objectives:

- Describe the three phases of an action potential and relate the functional importance of ion channels to the different phases.
- State the difference between electrical and chemical synapses.
- Describe the interaction of the presynaptic and postsynaptic terminals.
- Characterize the role of excitatory and inhibitory postsynaptic potentials as they relate to spatial and temporal summation of membrane potentials.
- Briefly describe how neurotransmitters are synthesized, stored, released, and inactivated.

Neurons are characterized by the ability to communicate with other neurons and body cells through electrical impulses or action potentials. The frequency and pattern of action potentials constitute the code used by neurons to transfer information from on location to another.

Action Potentials

The cell membranes of excitable tissue, including those of nerve and muscle cells, contain ion channels that are responsible for generating action potentials (see Chapter 4, Fig. 4-15). These membrane channels are guarded by voltage-dependent gates that open and close with changes in the membrane potential. Separate voltage-gated channels exist for the sodium, potassium, and calcium ions. Each type of ion channel has a characteristic membrane potential that opens and closes its channels. Also present are ligand-gated channels that respond to chemical messengers such as neurotransmitters, mechanically gated channels that respond to physical changes in the cell membrane, and light-gated channels that respond to fluctuations in light levels.

Nerve signals are transmitted by action potentials, which are abrupt, pulsatile changes in the membrane potential that last a few ten-thousandths to a few thousandths of a second. Action potentials can be divided into three phases: the resting or polarized state, depolarization, and repolarization (Fig. 48-6).

The *resting membrane potential* (approximately −90 mV for large nerve fibers) is the undisturbed period of the action potential during which the nerve is not transmitting impulses (discussed in Chapter 4). During this period, the membrane is said to be *polarized* because of the large separation of charge (*i.e.,* positive on the outside and negative on the inside). The resting phase of the membrane potential continues until some event causes the membrane to increase its permeability to sodium. A *threshold potential* (approximately −60 mV in large nerve fibers) represents the membrane potential at which neurons or other excitable tissues are stimulated to fire. When the threshold potential is reached, the gatelike structures in the ion channels open. Below the threshold potential, these gates remain tightly closed. The gates function on an all-or-none basis; they are either fully open or fully closed. Under ordinary circumstances, the threshold stimulus is sufficient to open many ion channels, triggering massive depolarization of the membrane (the action potential).

Depolarization is characterized by the flow of electrically charged ions. During the depolarization phase, the membrane suddenly becomes permeable to sodium ions; the rapid inflow of sodium ions produces local currents that travel through the adjacent cell membrane, causing the sodium channels in this part of the membrane to open. In neurons, sodium ion gates remain open for approximately a quarter of a millisecond. During this phase of the action potential, the inner face of the membrane becomes positive (approximately +30 to +45 mV).

Repolarization is the phase during which the polarity of the resting membrane potential is reestablished. This is accomplished with closure of the sodium channels and opening of the potassium channels. The outflow of positively charged potassium ions across the cell membrane returns the membrane potential to negativity. The sodium-potassium adenosine triphosphatase (Na^+/K^+-ATPase) pump gradually reestablishes the resting ionic concentrations on each side of the membrane. Membranes of excitable cells must be sufficiently repolarized before they can be reexcited. During repolarization, the membrane remains refractory (*i.e.,* does not fire) until repolarization is approximately one third complete. This period, which lasts approximately one half a millisecond, is called the *absolute refractory period.* During one portion of the recovery period, the membrane can be excited, although only by a stronger-than-normal stimulus. This period is called the *relative refractory period.*

The excitability of neurons can be affected by conditions that alter the resting membrane potential, moving it either closer to or further from the threshold potential. *Hypopolarization* increases the excitability of the postsynaptic neuron by bringing the membrane potential closer to the threshold potential so that a smaller subsequent stimulus is needed to cause the neuron to fire. *Hyperpolarization* brings the membrane potential further from the threshold and has the opposite, inhibitory effect, decreasing the likelihood that an action potential will be generated.

Synaptic Transmission

Neurons communicate with each other through structures known as *synapses.* Two types of synapses are found in the nervous system: electrical and chemical. *Electrical synapses* permit the passage of current-carrying ions through small openings called *gap junctions* that penetrate the cell junction of adjoining cells and allow current to travel in either direction. The gap junctions allow an action potential to pass directly and quickly from one neuron to another. They may link neurons having close functional relationships into circuits.

The most common type of synapse is the *chemical synapse.* Chemical synapses involve special presynaptic and post-

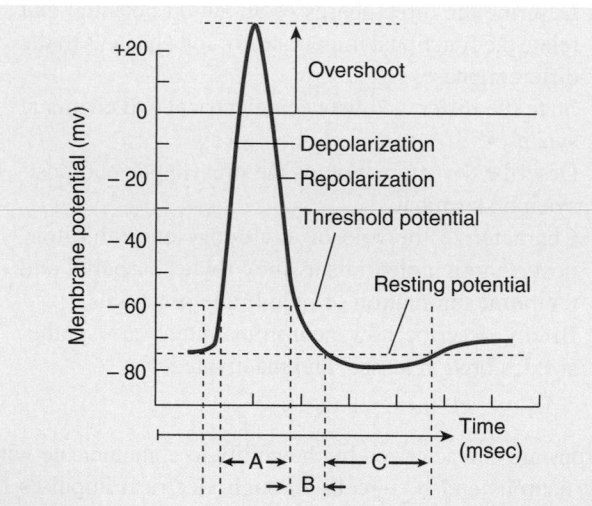

FIGURE 48-6 • Time course of the action potential recorded at one point of an axon with one electrode inside and one on the outside of the plasma membrane. The rising part of the action potential is called the *spike.* The rising phase plus approximately the first half of the repolarization phase is the absolute refractory period (**A**). The portion of the repolarization phase that extends from the threshold to the resting membrane potential represents the relative refractory period (**B**). The remaining portion of the repolarization phase to the resting membrane potential is the negative afterpotential (**C**). Relative refractory period is the period during which the membrane becomes hyperpolarized as the potential drops below the resting membrane potential.

synaptic membrane structures, separated by a synaptic cleft. The presynaptic terminal secretes one and often several chemical transmitter molecules (*i.e.,* neurotransmitters or neuromodulators). The secreted neurotransmitters diffuse into the synaptic cleft and bind to receptors on the postsynaptic membrane. In contrast to an electrical synapse, a chemical synapse serves as a rectifier, permitting only one-way communication. Chemical synapses are divided into two types: excitatory and inhibitory. In excitatory synapses, binding of the neurotransmitter to the receptor produces depolarization of the postsynaptic membrane. Binding of the neurotransmitter to the receptor in an inhibitory synapse reduces the postsynaptic neuron's ability to generate an action potential. Most inhibitory neurotransmitters induce hyperpolarization of the postsynaptic membrane by making the membrane more permeable to potassium or chloride, or both (see Chapter 31).

Chemical synapses are the slowest component in progressive communication through a sequence of neurons, such as in a spinal reflex. In contrast to the conduction of electrical action potentials, each successive event at the chemical synapse—transmitter secretion, diffusion across the synaptic cleft, interaction with postsynaptic receptors, and generation of a subsequent action potential in the postsynaptic neuron—consumes time.

A neuron's cell body and dendrites are covered by thousands of synapses, any or many of which can be active at any moment. Because of the interaction of this rich synaptic input, each neuron resembles a little integrator, in which circuits of many neurons interact with one another. It is the complexity of these interactions and the subtle integrations involved in producing behavioral responses that gives the system its intelligence.

Chemical synapses exhibit several relationships. Axons can synapse with dendrites (axodendritic), with the cell body (axosomatic), or with the axon (axoaxonic). Dendrites can synapse with axons (dendroaxonic), other dendrites (dendrodendritic), or the soma of other neurons (dendrosomatic). Synapses between the nerve cell body and axons (somatoaxonic synapses) also have been observed. Synapses occurring between the soma of neighboring neurons (somatosomatic) are uncommon, except between some efferent nuclei. The mechanism of communication between the presynaptic and the postsynaptic neuron is similar in all types of synapses; the action potential sweeps into the axonal terminals of the afferent neuron and triggers the rapid release of neurotransmitter molecules from the axonal, or presynaptic, surface.

Excitatory and Inhibitory Postsynaptic Potentials

Many CNS neurons possess thousands of synapses on their dendritic or somatic surfaces, each of which can produce partial excitation or inhibition of the postsynaptic neuron. When the combination of a neurotransmitter with a receptor site causes partial depolarization of the postsynaptic membrane, it is called an *excitatory postsynaptic potential* (EPSP). In other synapses, the combination of a transmitter with a receptor site is inhibitory in the sense that it causes the local nerve membrane to become hyperpolarized and less excitable. This is called an *inhibitory postsynaptic potential* (IPSP).

Action potentials do not begin in the membrane adjacent to the synapse. They begin in the initial segment of the axon, near the *axon hillock* (see Fig. 48-1), that lies just before the first myelin segment. The initial segment of the axon is more excitable than the rest of the neuron. The local currents resulting from an EPSP (sometimes called a *generator potential*) are usually insufficient to reach threshold and cause depolarization of the axon's initial segment. However, if several EPSPs occur simultaneously, the area of depolarization can become large enough and the currents at the initial segment can become strong enough to exceed the threshold potential and initiate an action potential. This summation of depolarized areas is called *spatial summation.* EPSPs also can summate and cause an action potential if they occur in rapid succession. This temporal aspect of the occurrence of two or more EPSPs is called *temporal summation.*

IPSPs also can undergo spatial and temporal summation with each other and with EPSPs, reducing the effectiveness of the latter by a roughly algebraic summation. If the sum of EPSPs and IPSPs keeps the depolarization at the initial segment below threshold levels, no action potential occurs.

Spatial and temporal summation during synaptic activity serves as a sensitive and complicated switch that requires the right combination of incoming activity before the cell can elicit an action potential. The occurrence and frequency of action potentials in axons constitute an all-or-none language (*i.e.,* a digital language), which varies only as to the presence or absence of such impulses and their frequency.

Messenger Molecules

The function of the nervous system relies on chemical messengers. These messengers include the neurotransmitters, neuromodulators, and neurotrophic or nerve growth factors.

Neurotransmitters

Neurotransmitters are small molecules that incorporate a positively charged nitrogen atom; they include several amino acids, peptides, and monoamines. *Amino acids* are the building blocks of proteins and are present in body fluids. The amino acids glutamine, glycine, and gamma-aminobutyric acid (GABA) serve as neurotransmitters at most CNS synapses. GABA mediates most synaptic inhibition in the CNS. Drugs such as the benzodiazepines (*e.g.,* the tranquilizer diazepam [Valium]) and the barbiturates exert their action by binding to their own distinct receptor on a GABA-operated ion channel. The drugs by themselves do not open the channel, but they change the effect that GABA has when it binds to the channel at the same time as the drug. *Peptides* are low–molecular-weight molecules that are made up of two or more amino acids. They include substance P and the endorphins and enkephalins, which are involved in pain

Understanding • Synaptic Transmission

Neurons communicate with each other through chemical synapses and the use of neurotransmitters. Chemical synapses consist of a presynaptic neuron, a synaptic cleft, and a postsynaptic neuron. The communication process relies on (1) synthesis and release of the neurotransmitter from a presynaptic neuron, (2) binding of the neurotransmitter to receptors in the postsynaptic neuron, and (3) removal of the neurotransmitter from the receptor site.

❶ Neurotransmitter Synthesis and Release

Neurotransmitters are synthesized in the presynaptic neuron, and then stored in synaptic vesicles. Communication between the two neurons begins with a nerve impulse that stimulates the presynaptic neuron, followed by movement of the synaptic vesicles to the cell membrane and release of neurotransmitter into the synaptic cleft.

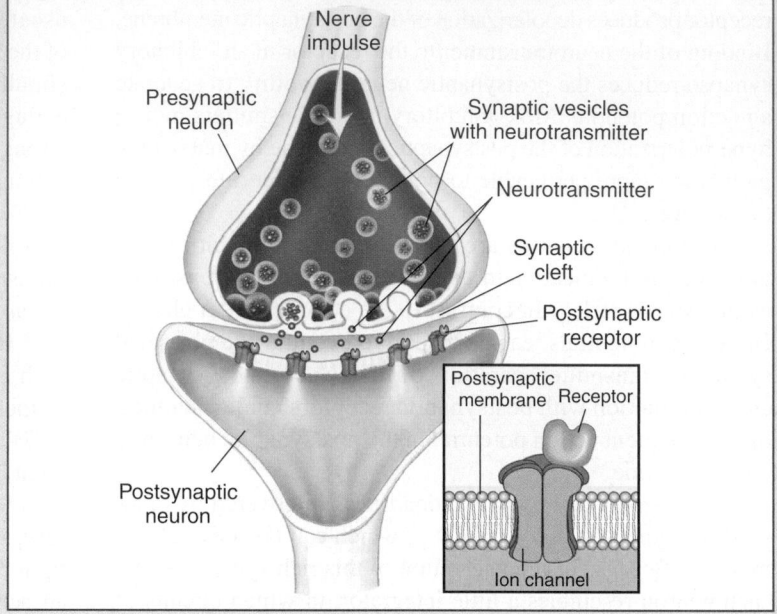

❷ Receptor Binding

Once released from the presynaptic neuron, the neurotransmitter moves across the synaptic cleft and binds to receptors on the postsynaptic neuron. The action of a neurotransmitter is determined by the type of receptor (excitatory or inhibitory) to which it binds. Binding of a neurotransmitter to a receptor with an excitatory function often results in the opening of an ion channel, such as the sodium channel. Many presynaptic neurons also have receptors to which a neurotransmitter binds. The presynaptic receptors function in a negative feedback manner to inhibit further release of the neurotransmitter.

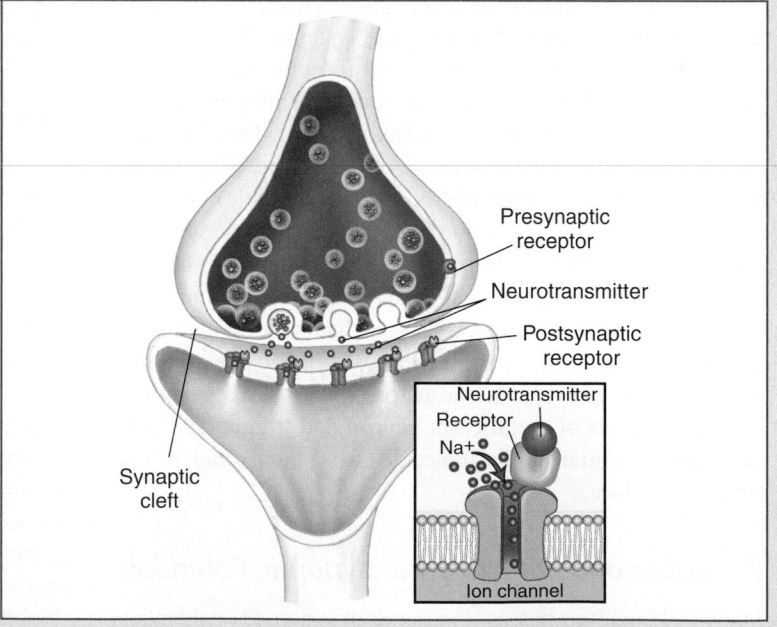

❸ Neurotransmitter Removal

Precise control of synaptic function relies on the rapid removal of the neurotransmitter from the receptor site. A released neurotransmitter can (1) be taken back up into the neuron in a process called reuptake, (2) diffuse out of the synaptic cleft, or (3) be broken down by enzymes into inactive substances or metabolites. The action of norepinephrine is largely terminated by the reuptake process, in which the neurotransmitter is taken back into the neuron in an unchanged form and reused. It can also be broken down by enzymes in the synaptic cleft or in the nerve terminals. The neurotransmitter acetylcholine is rapidly broken down by the enzyme acetylcholinesterase.

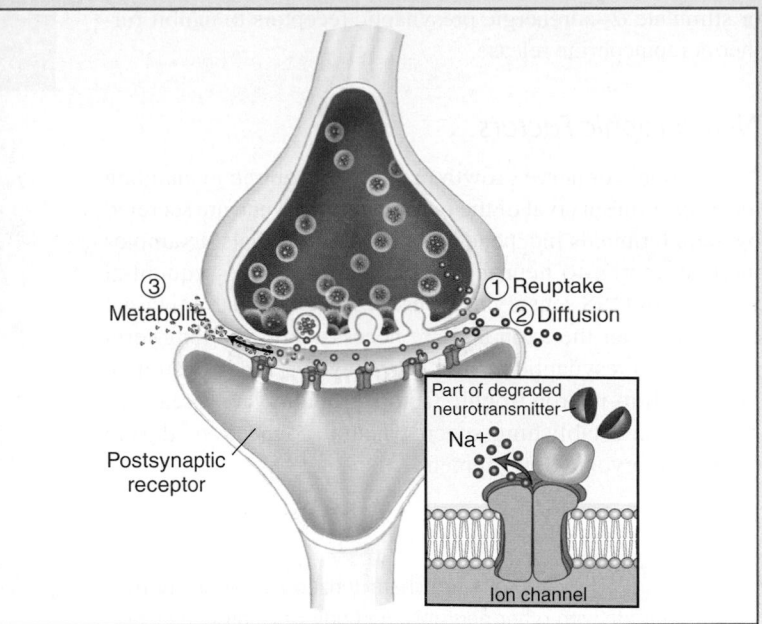

sensation and perception (see Chapter 49). A *monoamine* is an amine molecule containing one amino group (NH_2). Serotonin, dopamine, norepinephrine, and epinephrine are monoamines synthesized from amino acids. Fortunately, the blood-brain barrier protects the nervous system from circulating amino acids and other molecules with potential neurotransmitter activity.

The process of neurotransmission involves the synthesis, storage, and release of a neurotransmitter; the reaction of the neurotransmitter with a receptor; and termination of the receptor action. Neurotransmitters are synthesized in the cytoplasm of the axon terminal. The synthesis of transmitters may require one or more enzyme-catalyzed steps (*e.g.,* one for acetylcholine and three for norepinephrine). Neurons are limited as to the type of transmitter they can synthesize by their enzyme systems. After synthesis, the neurotransmitter molecules are stored in the axon terminal in tiny, membrane-bound sacs called *synaptic vesicles*. These vesicles protect the neurotransmitters from enzyme destruction in the nerve terminal. There may be thousands of vesicles in a single terminal, each containing 10,000 to 100,000 transmitter molecules. The arrival of an impulse at a nerve terminal causes the vesicles to move to the cell membrane and release their transmitter molecules into the synaptic space.

Neurotransmitters exert their actions through specific proteins, called *receptors,* embedded in the postsynaptic membrane. These receptors are tailored precisely to match the size and shape of the transmitter. In each case, the interaction between a transmitter and receptor results in a specific physiologic response. The action of a transmitter is determined by the type of receptor (excitatory or inhibitory) to which it binds. For example, acetylcholine is excitatory when it is released at a myoneural junction, and it is inhibitory when it is released at the sinoatrial node in the heart. Receptors are named according to the type of neurotransmitter with which they interact.

For example, a *cholinergic receptor* is a receptor that binds to acetylcholine.

Rapid removal of a transmitter, once it has exerted its effects on the postsynaptic membrane, is necessary to maintain precise control of neural transmission. A released transmitter can undergo one of three fates: (1) it can be broken down into inactive substances by enzymes; (2) it can be taken back up into the presynaptic neuron in a process called *reuptake;* or (3) it can diffuse into the intercellular fluid until its concentration is too low to influence postsynaptic excitability. For example, acetylcholine is rapidly broken down by acetylcholinesterase into acetic acid and choline, with the choline being taken back into the presynaptic neuron for reuse in acetylcholine synthesis. The catecholamines are largely taken back into the neuron in an unchanged form for reuse. Catecholamines also can be degraded by enzymes in the synaptic space or in the nerve terminals.

Neuromodulators

Other classes of messenger molecules, known as *neuromodulators,* also may be released from axon terminals. Neuromodulator molecules react with presynaptic or postsynaptic receptors to alter the release of or response to neurotransmitters. Neuromodulators may act on postsynaptic receptors to produce slower and longer-lasting changes in membrane excitability. This alters the action of the faster-acting neurotransmitter molecules by enhancing or decreasing their effectiveness. By combining with autoreceptors on its own presynaptic membrane, a transmitter can act as a neuromodulator to augment or inhibit further nerve activity. In some nerves, such as the peripheral sympathetic nerves, a messenger molecule can have both transmitter and modulator functions. For example, norepinephrine can activate α_1-adrenergic postsynaptic receptors to produce vasoconstriction or stimulate α_2-adrenergic presynaptic receptors to inhibit further norepinephrine release.

Neurotrophic Factors

Neurotrophic or nerve growth factors are required to maintain the long-term survival of the postsynaptic cell and are secreted by axon terminals independent of action potentials. Examples include neuron-to-neuron trophic factors in the sequential synapses of CNS sensory neurons. Trophic factors from target cells that enter the axon and are necessary for the long-term survival of presynaptic neurons also have been demonstrated. Target cell-to-neuron trophic factors probably have great significance in establishing specific neural connections during normal embryonic development.

IN SUMMARY, neurons are characterized by the ability to communicate with other neurons and body cells through electrical signals called *action potentials*. The cell membranes of neurons contain ion channels that are responsible for generating action potentials. These channels are guarded by voltage-dependent gates that open and close with changes in the membrane potential. Action potentials are divided into three parts: the resting membrane potential, during which the membrane is polarized but no electrical activity occurs; the depolarization phase, during which sodium channels open, allowing rapid inflow of the sodium ions that generate the electrical impulse; and the repolarization phase, during which the membrane is permeable to potassium ions, allowing for the efflux of potassium ions and the return to the resting membrane potential.

Synapses are structures that permit communication between neurons. Two types of synapses have been identified: electrical and chemical. Electrical synapses consist of gap junctions between adjacent cells that allow action potentials to move rapidly from one cell to another. Chemical synapses involve special presynaptic and postsynaptic structures, separated by a synaptic cleft. They rely on chemical messengers, released from the presynaptic neuron, that cross the synaptic cleft and then interact with receptors on the postsynaptic neuron.

Neurotransmitters are chemical messengers that control neural function; they selectively cause excitation or inhibition of action potentials. Three major types of neurotransmitters are known: amino acids such as glutamic acid and GABA, peptides such as the endorphins and enkephalins, and monoamines such as epinephrine and norepinephrine. Neurotransmitters interact with cell membrane receptors to produce either excitatory or inhibitory actions. Neuromodulators are chemical messengers that react with membrane receptors to produce slower and longer-acting changes in membrane permeability. Neurotrophic or growth factors, also released from presynaptic terminals, are required to maintain the long-term survival of postsynaptic neurons. ■

CONCEPTS in action **ANIMATION**

DEVELOPMENTAL ORGANIZATION OF THE NERVOUS SYSTEM

After completing this section of the chapter, you should be able to meet the following objectives:

■ Use the segmental approach to explain the development of the nervous system and the organization of the postembryonic nervous system.
■ Define the terms *afferent, efferent, ganglia, association neuron, cell column,* and *tract.*
■ State the origin and destination of nerve fibers contained in the dorsal and ventral roots.
■ State the structures innervated by general somatic afferent, special visceral afferent, general visceral afferent, special somatic afferent, general visceral efferent, pharyngeal efferent, and general somatic efferent neurons.

The organization of the nervous system can be described in terms of its development, in which newer functions and greater complexity resulted from the modification and enlargement of more primitive structures. Thus, the rostral or front end of the CNS became specialized, with the more ancient organization being retained in the brain stem and spinal cord. The dominance of the front end of the CNS is reflected in what has been termed a *hierarchy of control,* with the forebrain having control over the brain stem and the brain stem having control over the spinal cord. In the developmental process, newer functions were added to the surface of functionally older systems. As newer functions became concentrated at the rostral end of the nervous system, they also became more vulnerable to injury. Nothing exemplifies this principle better than the persistent vegetative state (discussed in Chapter 51) that occurs when severe brain injury causes irreversible damage to higher cortical centers, while lower stem centers such as those that control breathing remain functional.

Embryonic Development

All body tissues and organs have developed from the three embryonic layers (*i.e.,* endoderm, ectoderm, and mesoderm) that were present during the third week of embryonic life. The body is organized into the soma and viscera (see Chapter 4, Fig. 4-16). The *soma,* or body wall, includes all of the structures derived from the embryonic ectoderm, such as the epidermis of the skin and the CNS. Mesodermal connective tissues of the soma include the dermis of the skin, skeletal muscle, bone, and the outer lining of the body cavity (*i.e.,* parietal pleura and peritoneum). The nervous system innervates all somatic structures plus the internal structures making up the viscera. *Viscera* include the great vessels derived from the intermediate mesoderm, the urinary system, and the gonadal structures; it also includes the inner lining of the body cavities, such as the visceral pleura and peritoneum, and the mesodermal tissues that surround the endoderm-lined gut and its derivative organs (*e.g.,* lungs, liver, pancreas).

The nervous system appears very early in embryonic development (week 3). This early development is essential because it influences the development and organization of many other body systems, including the axial skeleton, skeletal muscles, and sensory organs such as the eyes and ears. Throughout life, the organization of the nervous system retains many patterns that were established during embryonic life. It is this early pattern of segmental development in the embryo that is presented as a framework for understanding the nervous system.

During the second week of development, embryonic tissue consists of two layers, the endoderm and the ectoderm. At the beginning of week 3, the ectoderm begins to invaginate and migrates between the two layers, forming a third layer called the *mesoderm* (Fig. 48-7). Mesoderm along the entire midline of the embryo forms a specialized rod of embryonic tissue called the *notochord.* The notochord and adjacent mesoderm provide the necessary induction signal for the overlying ectoderm to differentiate and form a thickened structure called the *neural plate,*

the primordium of the nervous system. Within the neural plate an axial groove (*i.e.,* neural groove) develops and sinks into the underlying mesoderm, allowing its walls to fuse across the top and form an ectodermal tube called the *neural tube.* This process, called *closure,* occurs during the later third and fourth weeks of gestation and is vital to the survival of the embryo.

During embryonic development, the neural tube develops into the CNS, while the notochord becomes the foundation around which the vertebral column ultimately develops. The surface ectoderm separates from the neural tube and fuses over the top to become the outer layer of skin. Initial closure of the neural tube begins at the cervical and high thoracic levels and zippers rostrally toward the cephalic end of the embryo and caudally toward the sacrum. Complete closure occurs at the rostral-most end of the brain (*i.e.,* anterior neuropore) around day 25, and about day 27 in the lumbosacral region (*i.e.,* posterior neuropore).

As the neural tube closes, ectodermal cells called *neural crest cells* migrate away from the dorsal surface of the neural tube to become the progenitors of the neurons and supporting cells of the PNS. During this period of embryonic development, neural cell adhesive molecules (N-CAMs) are produced to decrease migration of neural crest cells. In addition, fibronectin molecules are produced to increase the formation of pathways that guide the neural crest cells during their migration. Some of these cells gather into clusters to form the *dorsal root ganglia* at the sides of each spinal cord segment and the *cranial ganglia* that are present in most brain segments. Neurons of these ganglia become the afferent or sensory neurons of the PNS. Other neural crest cells become the pigment cells of the skin or contribute to the formation of the meninges, many structures of the face, and the peripheral ganglion cells of the autonomic nervous system, including those of the adrenal cortex.

During development, the more rostral portions of the embryonic neural tube—approximately 10 segments—undergo extensive modification and enlargement to form the brain (Fig. 48-8). In the early embryo, 3 swellings, or primary vesicles, develop, subdividing these 10 segments into the prosencephalon, or forebrain, containing the first 2 segments; the mesencephalon, or midbrain, which develops from segment 3; and the rhombencephalon, or hindbrain, which develops from segments 4 to 10. The brain stem is formed from modifications of the 10 rostral segments of the wall of the neural tube. In the prosencephalon or forebrain, two pairs of lateral outpouchings develop: the optic cup, which becomes the optic nerve and retina, and the telencephalic vesicles, which become the cerebral hemispheres. Within the prosencephalon, the hollow central canal expands to become enlarged CSF-filled cavities, the first and second (lateral) ventricles. The remaining diencephalic portion of the neural tube develops into the thalamus and hypothalamus. The neurohypophysis (posterior pituitary) grows as a midline ventral outgrowth at the junctions of segments 1 and 2. A dorsal outgrowth, the pineal body, develops between segments 2 and 3.

All brain segments, except segment 2, retain some portion of the basic segmental organization of the nervous system. The

 ## THE DEVELOPMENTAL ORGANIZATION OF THE NERVOUS SYSTEM

- Embryologically, the nervous system begins its development as a hollow tube, the cephalic portion of which becomes the brain and the more caudal part the spinal cord.

- In the process of development, the basic organizational pattern is that of a longitudinal series of segments, each repeating the same basic fundamental organizational pattern: a body wall or soma containing the axial skeleton and a neural tube, which develops into the nervous system.

- On cross-section, the embryonic neural tube develops into a central canal surrounded by gray matter or cellular portion (cell columns) and the white matter, or tract system of the central nervous system (CNS).

- As the nervous system develops, it becomes segmented, with a repeating pattern of afferent neuron axons forming the dorsal roots of each succeeding segmental nerve, and the exiting efferent neurons forming the ventral roots of each succeeding segmental nerve.

- The nerve cells in the gray matter are arranged longitudinally in cell columns, with afferent sensory neurons located in the dorsal columns and efferent motor neurons located in the ventral columns.

- The axons of the cell column neurons project out into the white matter of the CNS, forming the longitudinal tract systems.

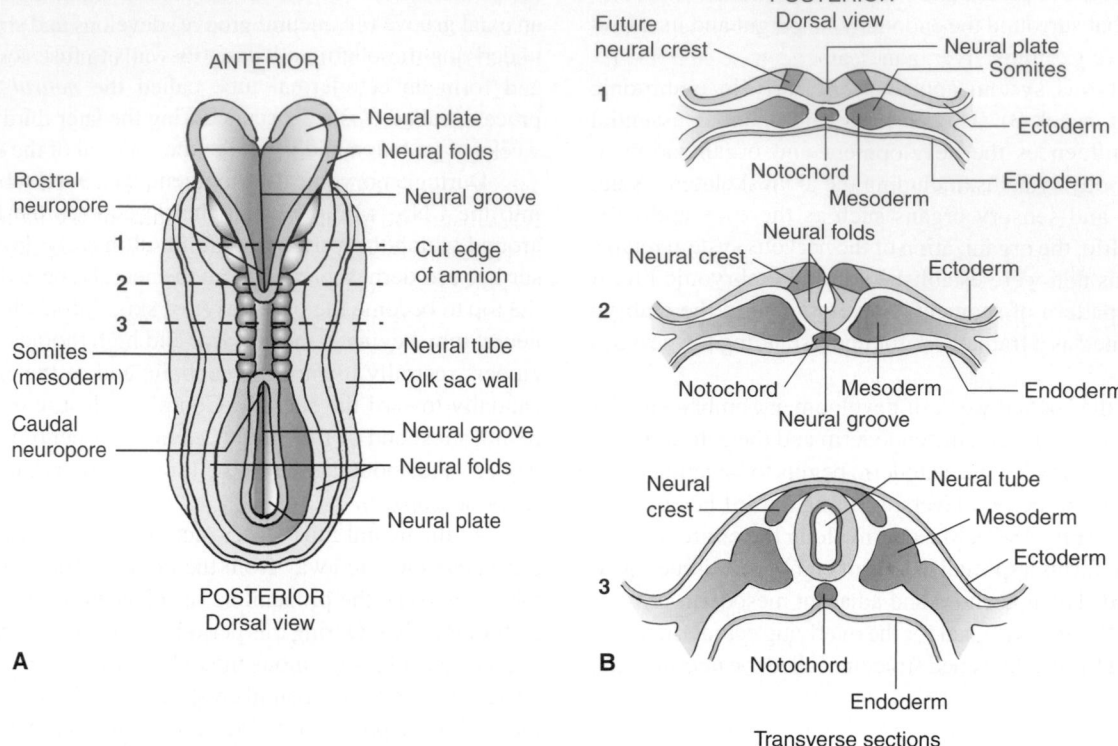

FIGURE 48-7 • Folding of the neural tube. **(A)** Dorsal view of a six-somite embryo (22 to 23 days) showing the neural folds, neural groove, and the fused neural tube. The anterior neuropore closes at about day 25 and the posterior neuropore at about day 27. **(B)** Three cross-sections taken at the levels indicated in **A**. The sections indicate where the neural tube is just beginning to form.

evolutionary development of the brain is reflected in the cranial and upper cervical paired segmental nerves. This reflects the original pattern of a segmented neural tube, each segment of which has multiple paired branches containing a grouping of component axons. One segment would have paired branches to body muscles and another set to visceral structures, and so on. The classic pattern of spinal nerve organization, which consists of a pair of dorsal and a pair of ventral roots, is a later evolutionary development that has not occurred in the cranial nerves. Consequently, the cranial nerves, which are arbitrarily numbered 1

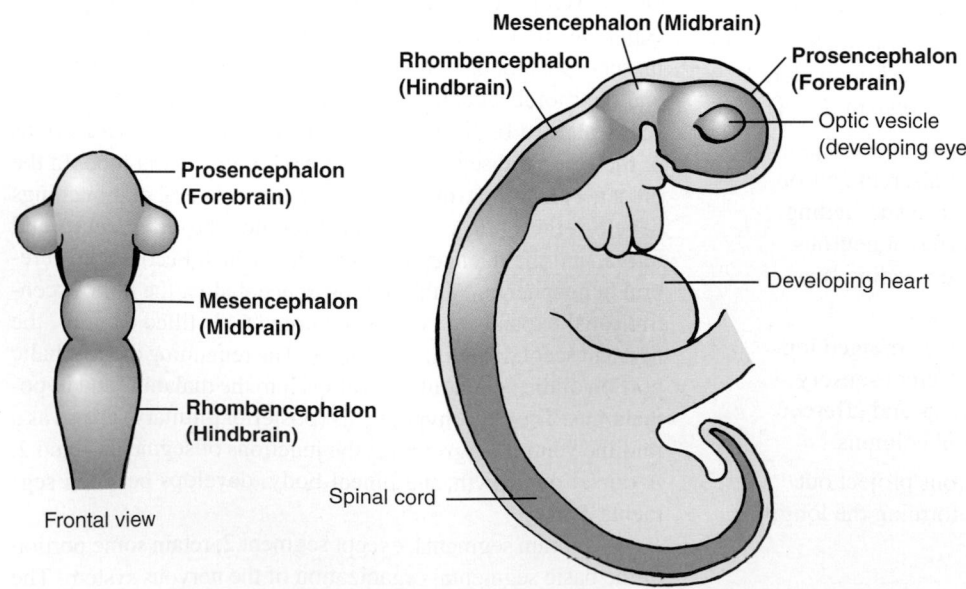

FIGURE 48-8 • Frontal and lateral views of a 5-week-old embryo showing the brain vesicles and three embryonic divisions of the brain and brain stem.

through 12, retain the ancient pattern, with more than one cranial nerve branching from a single segment. The truly segmental nerve pattern of the cranial nerves is altered because all branches from segment 2 and most of the branches from segment 1 are missing. Cranial nerve 2, also called the *optic nerve,* is not a segmental nerve. It is a brain tract connecting the retina (modified brain) with the first forebrain segment from which it developed.

 ## Neural Tube Defects

The major morphogenic defects of the spinal cord and brain are due to the abnormal formation or closure of the neural tube and surrounding tissues. These neural tube defects can involve neural tissue, the meninges, muscle tissue, skin, and the vertebral column. Severe neural tube defects occur in 1/1000 births. These defects fall into four main categories: spina bifida occulta, spina bifida with meningocele, spina bifida with meningomyelocele, and spina bifida with myeloschisis. In spina bifida occulta, the spinal cord and surrounding meninges lie within the incomplete vertebral column. Externally, a marked patch of hair in the lumbar region usually overlies the affected spinal region (Fig. 48-9A). In both spina bifida occulta and spina bifida cys-

tica (spina bifida with meningocele or meningomyelocele), the neural tube has closed but inductive messages fail to promote complete closure of the vertebral arches around the neural tube. In spina bifida with meningocele, the meninges protrude through the defect in the vertebral arch (see Fig. 48-9B). In a more severe situation, spina bifida with meningomyelocele, the spinal cord and the meninges protrude through the defect (see Fig. 48-9C). Nonclosure of the neural tube results in a condition called *myeloschisis* in which neither the vertebral arches nor the neural tube form. This severe condition leaves neural tissue exposed (see Fig. 48-9D).

Clinical neurologic dysfunction is related to abnormalities in the cord itself and to superimposed infections that extend from the thin overlying skin. Meningomyeloceles occur most commonly in the lumbosacral region and produce clinical deficits referable to motor and sensory function in the lower extremities as well as disturbances in bowel and bladder control (Fig. 48-10). The etiology of neural tube defects is unknown. Folate deficiency during the initial weeks of gestation has been implicated as a risk factor, possibly interacting with host and environmental factors. Antenatal diagnosis has been facilitated by ultrasonographic imaging and maternal blood sampling for elevated α-fetoprotein (see Chapter 7).

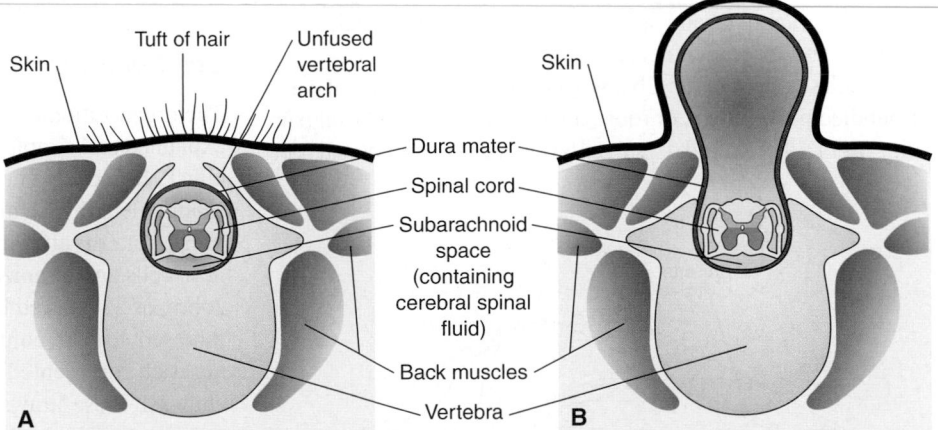

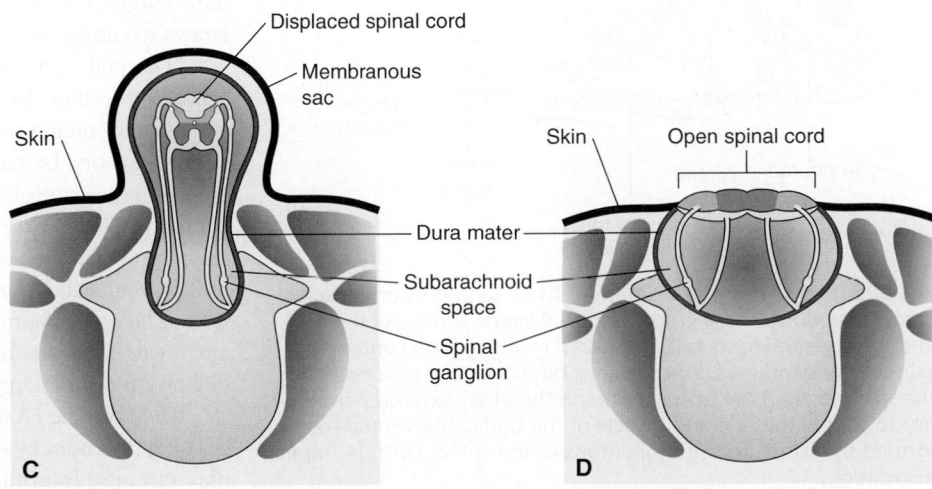

FIGURE 48-9 • Diagrammatic sketches illustrating various types of spina bifida and the commonly associated anomalies of the vertebral arch, spinal cord, and meninges. **(A)** Spina bifida occulta. Note the unfused vertebral arch. **(B)** Spina bifida with meningocele. **(C)** Spina bifida with meningomyelocele. **(D)** Spina bifida with myeloschisis. The types illustrated in **B** and **C** are referred to collectively as *spina bifida cystica* because of the cystlike sac associated with them. (From Moore K. L., Persaud T. V. N. [2003]. *The developing human* [7th ed., p. 437]. Philadelphia: Saunders.)

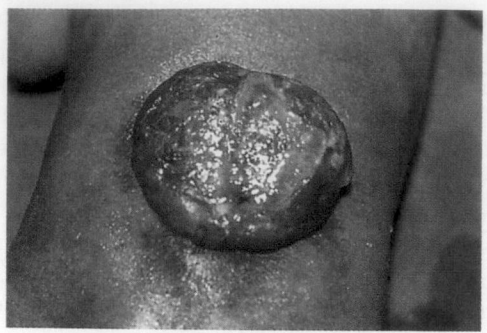

FIGURE 48-10 • Posterior view of spina bifida cystica. (From Moore K. L., Dalley A. F. [2006]. *Clinically oriented anatomy* [5th ed., p. 497]. Philadelphia: Lippincott Williams & Wilkins.)

Segmental Organization

Developmentally, the basic organizational pattern of the body is that of a longitudinal series of segments, each repeating the same fundamental pattern. Although the early muscular, skeletal, vascular, and excretory systems and the nerves that supply the somatic and visceral structures have the same segmental pattern, it is the nervous system that most clearly retains this organization in postnatal life. The CNS and its associated peripheral nerves consist of approximately 43 segments, 33 of which form the spinal cord and spinal nerves, and 10 of which form the brain and its cranial nerves.

Each segment of the CNS is accompanied by bilateral pairs of bundled nerve fibers, or roots, a ventral pair and a dorsal pair (Fig. 48-11). The paired dorsal roots connect a pair of dorsal root

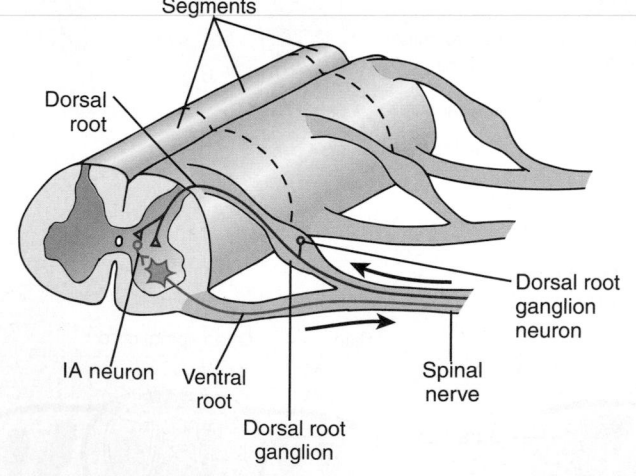

FIGURE 48-11 • In this diagram of three segments of the spinal cord, three dorsal roots enter the dorsal lateral surface of the cord, and three ventral roots exit. The dorsal root ganglion contains dorsal root ganglion cells, whose axons bifurcate: one process enters the spinal cord in the dorsal root, and the other extends peripherally to supply the skin and muscle of the body. The ventral root is formed by axons from motoneurons in the spinal cord. IA, input association.

ganglia and their corresponding CNS segment. The dorsal root ganglia contain many afferent nerve cell bodies, each having two axon-like processes—one that ends in a peripheral receptor and the other that enters the central neural segment. These axon-like processes that enter the central neural segment communicate with neurons called *input association* (IA) *neuron*s. Somatic afferent (SA) neurons transmit information from the soma to somatic IA (SIA) neurons, and visceral afferent (VA) neurons transmit information from the viscera to visceral IA (VIA) neurons. The paired ventral roots of each segment are bundles of axons that provide efferent output to effector sites such as the muscles and glandular cells of the body segment.

On cross-section, the hollow embryonic neural tube can be divided into a central canal, or ventricle, containing CSF and the wall of the tube. The latter develops into an inner gray cellular portion, which is functionally divided into longitudinal columns of neurons called the *cell columns*. These cell columns contain nerve cell bodies surrounded by a superficial white matter region containing the longitudinal tract systems of the CNS. These tract systems are composed of many nerve cell processes. The dorsal half, or *dorsal horn* of the gray matter, contains afferent neurons. The ventral portion, or *ventral horn*, contains efferent neurons that communicate by way of the ventral roots with effector cells of the body segment. Many CNS neurons develop axons that grow longitudinally as tract systems that communicate between neighboring and distal segments of the neural tube.

Cell Columns

The organizational structure of the nervous system can be best explained and simplified as a pattern in which functionally specific PNS and CNS neurons are repeated as parallel cell columns running lengthwise along the nervous system. In this organizational pattern, afferent neurons, dorsal horn cells, and ventral horn cells are organized as a bilateral series of 11 cell columns. A box of 22 colored beverage straws can be used as a model to represent the cell columns. In this model, the right and left sides are each represented in mirror fashion by a set of 11 colored straws. If these straws were cut crosswise (equivalent to a transverse section through the nervous system) at several places along their length, the spatial relations among the different colored straws would be repeated in each section.

The cell columns on each side can be further grouped according to their location in the PNS: four in the dorsal root ganglia that contain sensory neurons; four in the dorsal horn containing sensory IA neurons; and three in the ventral horn that contain motor neurons (Fig. 48-12). Each column of dorsal root ganglia projects to its particular column of IA neurons in the dorsal horn, which then distribute the afferent information to local reflex circuits and to more rostral and elaborate segments of the CNS. The ventral horns contain output association (OA) neurons and lower motor neurons (LMNs). The LMNs provide the final circuitry for organizing efferent nerve activity.

Between the IA neurons and the OA neurons are networks of small internuncial (interneuronal) neurons arranged in complex circuits. Internuncial neurons provide the discreteness,

FIGURE 48-12 • **(A)** Cell columns of the central nervous system. The cell columns in the dorsal horn contain input association (IA) neurons for the general visceral afferent (GVA), special visceral afferent (SVA), special sensory afferent (SSA), and general somatic afferent (GSA) neurons with cell bodies in the dorsal root ganglion. The cell columns in the ventral horn contain the general visceral efferent (GVE), pharyngeal efferent (PE), and general somite efferent (GSE) neurons and their output association (OA) neurons. **(B)** Schematic of the GVE cell column showing both parasympathetic and sympathetic components. The column is not continuous but is interrupted in the brain stem because only the nuclei of cranial nerves III, VII, IX, and X contain preganglionic parasympathetic neurons. The column again is interrupted until levels T1 to L1 or L2, where the preganglionic neurons of the sympathetic portion are found in the lateral horn of the spinal cord. Another gap is evident until the sacral portion of the parasympathetic nervous system.

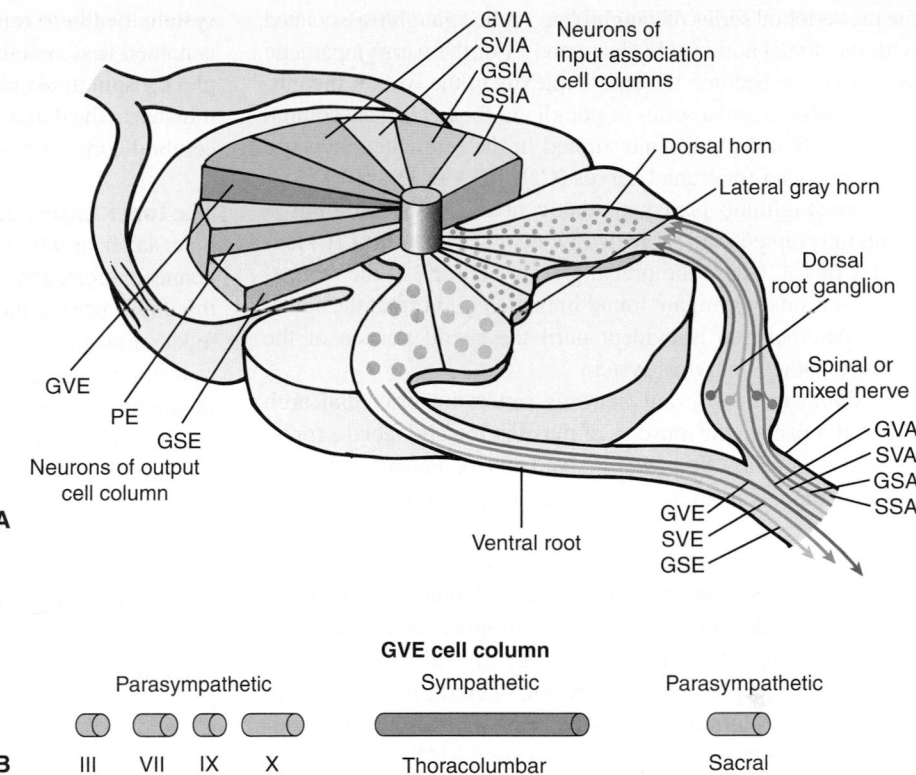

appropriateness, and intelligence of responses to stimuli. Most of the billions of CNS cells in the spinal cord and brain gray matter are internuncial neurons.

Dorsal Horn Cell Columns. Four columns of afferent (sensory) neurons in the dorsal root ganglia directly innervate four corresponding columns of IA neurons in the dorsal horn. These columns are categorized as special and general afferents: special somatic afferent, general somatic afferent, special visceral afferent, and general visceral afferent (see Fig. 48-12).

Special somatic afferent fibers are concerned with internal sensory information such as joint and tendon sensation (*i.e.,* proprioception). Neurons in the special SIA column cells relay their information to local reflexes concerned with posture and movement. These neurons also relay information to the cerebellum, contributing to coordination of movement, and to the forebrain, contributing to experience. Afferents innervating the labyrinth and derived auditory end organs of the inner ear also belong to the special somatic afferent category.

General somatic afferents innervate the skin and other somatic structures, and respond to stimuli such as those that produce pressure or pain. General SIA column cells relay the sensory information to protective and other reflex circuits and project the information to the forebrain, where it is perceived as painful, warm, cold, and the like.

Special visceral afferent cells innervate specialized gut-related receptors, such as the taste buds and receptors of the olfactory mucosa. Their central processes communicate with special VIA column neurons that project to reflex circuits pro-

ducing salivation, chewing, swallowing, and other responses. Forebrain projection fibers from these association cells provide sensations of taste and smell.

General visceral afferent neurons innervate visceral structures such as the gastrointestinal tract, urinary bladder, and heart and great vessels; they project to the general VIA column, which relays information to vital reflex circuits and sends information to the forebrain regarding visceral sensations such as stomach fullness, bladder pressure, and sexual experience.

Ventral Horn Cell Columns. The ventral horn contains three longitudinal cell columns: general visceral efferent, pharyngeal efferent, and general somatic efferent (see Fig. 48-12). Each of these cell columns contains OA and efferent neurons. The OA neurons coordinate and integrate the function of the efferent motor neurons cells of their column.

General visceral efferent neurons transmit the efferent output of the autonomic nervous system and are called *preganglionic neurons*. These neurons are structurally and functionally divided into either the sympathetic or the parasympathetic nervous systems. Their axons project through the segmental ventral roots (specifically from a group of neurons originating in the intermediolateral horn of the thoracolumbar cord) to innervate smooth and cardiac muscle and glandular cells of the body, most of which are in the viscera. In the viscera, three additional neural crest–derived cell columns are present on each side of the body. These become the postganglionic neurons of the autonomic nervous system. In the sympathetic nervous system, the columns are represented by paravertebral ganglia (sympathetic chain) and the prevertebral series of ganglia (*e.g.*, celiac ganglia) associated with the dorsal aorta (to be discussed). For the parasympathetic system, these become the enteric plexus in the wall of the gut-derived organs and a series of ganglia in the head. This column is not continuous but is interrupted in the brain stem because only the nuclei for cranial nerves (CN) III, VII, IX, and X contain preganglionic parasympathetic neurons. The column is again interrupted until thoracic (T) levels T1 to lumbar (L) levels L1 or L2, where the preganglionic neurons of the sympathetic nervous system are found in the lateral horn of the spinal cord. Another gap is evident until the sacral portion of the parasympathetic nervous system.

Pharyngeal efferent neurons innervate branchial arch skeletal muscles: the muscles of mastication and facial expression, and muscles of the pharynx and larynx. Pharyngeal efferent neurons also innervate muscles responsible for moving the head.

The *general somatic efferent* neurons supply somite-derived muscles of the body and head, which include the skeletal muscles of the body and limbs, the tongue, and extrinsic eye muscles. These efferent neurons transmit the commands of the CNS to peripheral effectors, the skeletal muscles. They are the "final common pathway neurons" in the sequence leading to motor activity. They are often called *LMNs* because they are under the control of higher levels of the CNS, including precise control by upper motor neurons (UMNs).

Peripheral Nerves. With rare exceptions, peripheral nerves, including the cranial nerves, contain afferent and efferent processes of more than one of the four afferent and three efferent cell columns. This provides the basis for assessing the function of any peripheral nerve. The functional components of each of the cranial nerves and spinal nerve roots are presented in Table 48-1.

Longitudinal Tracts

The gray matter of the cell columns in the CNS is surrounded by bundles of myelinated axons (*i.e.*, white matter) and unmyelinated axons that travel longitudinally along the length of the neural axis. This white matter can be divided into three layers: an inner, middle, and outer layer (Fig. 48-13). The inner layer, or *archilayer,* contains short fibers that project for a maximum of approximately five segments before reentering the gray matter. The middle layer, or *paleolayer,* projects to six or more segments. Archilayer and paleolayer fibers have many branches, or collaterals, that enter the gray matter of intervening segments. In the outer layer, or *neolayer,* are found large-diameter axons that can travel the entire length of the nervous system (Table 48-2). *Suprasegmental* is a term that refers to higher levels of the CNS, such as the brain stem and cerebrum and structures above a given CNS segment. Paleolayer and neolayer fibers have suprasegmental projections.

The longitudinal layers are arranged in bundles, or fiber tracts, that contain axons that have the same destination, origin, and function (Fig. 48-14). These longitudinal tracts are named systematically to reflect their origin and destination; the origin is named first, and the destination is named second. For example, the spinothalamic tract originates in the spinal cord and terminates in the thalamus. The corticospinal tract originates in the cerebral cortex and ends in the spinal cord.

The Inner Layer. Lying deep to the superficial gray matter, the inner layer of white matter contains the axons of neurons that connect neighboring segments of the nervous system. Axons of this layer permit motor neurons of several segments to work together as a functional unit. They also allow the afferent neurons of one segment to trigger reflexes that activate motor units in neighboring segments as well as in the same one. From the standpoint of evolutionary development, this is the oldest of the three layers, and it is sometimes called the *archilayer*. It is the first of the longitudinal layers to become functional, and its circuitry may be limited to reflex types of movements, including reflex movements of the fetus (*i.e.,* quickening) that begin during the fifth month of intrauterine life.

The inner layer of the white matter differs from the other two layers in one important aspect. Many neurons in the embryonic gray matter migrate out into this layer, resulting in a rich mixture of neurons and local fibers called the *reticular formation.* The circuitry of most reflexes is contained in the reticular formation. In the brain stem, the reticular formation becomes quite large and contains major portions of vital reflexes, such as those controlling respiration, cardiovascular function, swallowing, and vomiting. A functional system called the *reticular activating system* operates in the lateral portions of the reticular formation of the medulla, pons, and especially the midbrain. Information derived from all sensory modalities, including those of the somesthetic, auditory, visual, and visceral afferent nerves, bombards the neurons of this system.

The reticular activating system has descending and ascending portions. The descending portion communicates with all spinal segmental levels through paleolevel reticulospinal tracts and serves to facilitate many cord-level reflexes. For example, it speeds reaction time and stabilizes postural reflexes. The ascending portion accelerates brain activity, particularly thalamic and cortical activity. This is reflected by the appearance of awake-type patterns of brain wave activity. Sudden stimuli result in protective and attentive postures and increased awareness.

The Middle Layer. The middle layer of the white matter contains most of the major fiber tract systems required for sensation and movement, including the ascending spinoreticular and spinothalamic tracts. This layer consists of larger-diameter and longer suprasegmental fibers, which ascend to the brain stem and are largely functional at birth. These tracts are quite old from an evolutionary standpoint and, as such, this layer is sometimes called the *paleolayer.* It facilitates many primitive functions, such as the auditory startle reflex, which occurs in response to loud noises. This reflex consists of turning the head and body toward the sound, dilation of the pupils of the eyes, catching of the breath, and quickening of the pulse.

TABLE 48-1 The Segmental Nerves and Their Components

SEGMENT AND NERVE	COMPONENT	INNERVATION	FUNCTION
1. Forebrain			
I. Olfactory	SVA	Receptors in olfactory mucosa	Reflexes, olfaction (smell)
2. II. Optic nerve		Optic nerve and retina (part of brain system, not a peripheral nerve)	
3. Midbrain			
V. Trigeminal (V$_1$) ophthalmic division	SSA	Muscles: upper face: forehead, upper lid	Facial expression, proprioception
	GSA	Skin, subcutaneous tissue; conjunctiva; frontal/ethmoid sinuses	Somesthesia Reflexes (blink)
III. Oculomotor	GVE	Iris sphincter	Pupillary constriction
		Ciliary muscle	Accommodation
	GSE	Extrinsic eye muscles	Eye movement, lid movement
4. Pons			
V. Trigeminal (V$_2$) maxillary division	SSA	Muscles: facial expression	Proprioception Reflexes (sneeze), somesthesia
	GSA	Skin, oral mucosa, upper teeth, hard palate, maxillary sinus	
V. Trigeminal (V$_3$) mandibular division	SSA	Lower jaw, muscles: mastication	Proprioception, jaw jerk
	GSA	Skin, mucosa, teeth, anterior ⅔ of tongue	Reflexes, somesthesia
	PE	Muscles: mastication	Mastication: speech
		tensor tympani	Protects ear from loud sounds
		tensor veli palatini	Tenses soft palate
IV. Trochlear	GSE	Extrinsic eye muscle	Moves eye down and in
5. Caudal Pons			
VIII. Vestibular, cochlear (vestibulocochlear)	SSA	Vestibular end organs	Reflexes, sense of head position
		Organ of Corti	Reflexes, hearing
VII. Facial nerve, intermedius portion	GSA	External auditory meatus	Somesthesia
	GVA	Nasopharynx	Gag reflex: sensation
	SVA	Taste buds of anterior ⅔ of tongue	Reflexes: gustation (taste)
	GVE	Nasopharynx	Mucus secretion, reflexes
		Lacrimal, sublingual, submandibular glands	Lacrimation, salivation
Facial nerve	PE	Muscles: facial expression, stapedius	Facial expression
			Protects ear from loud sounds
VI. Abducens	GSE	Extrinsic eye muscle	Lateral eye deviation
6. Middle Medulla			
IX. Glossopharyngeal	SSA	Stylopharyngeus muscle	Proprioception
	GSA	Posterior external ear	Somesthesia
	SVA	Taste buds of posterior ⅓ of tongue	Gustation (taste)
	GVA	Oral pharynx	Gag reflex: sensation
	GVE	Parotid gland; pharyngeal mucosa	Salivary reflex: mucus secretion
	PE	Stylopharyngeus muscle	Assists swallowing
7,8,9,10. Caudal Medulla			
X. Vagus	SSA	Muscles: pharynx, larynx	Proprioception
	GSA	Posterior external ear	Somesthesia
	SVA	Taste buds, pharynx, larynx	Reflexes, gustation
	GVA	Visceral organs (esophagus to midtransverse colon, liver, pancreas, heart, lungs)	Reflexes, sensation
	GVE	Visceral organs as above	Parasympathetic efferent
	PE	Muscles: pharynx, larynx	Swallowing, phonation, emesis
XII. Hypoglossal	GSE	Muscles of tongue	Tongue movement, reflexes

(continued)

TABLE 48-1 **The Segmental Nerves and Their Components** (continued)

SEGMENT AND NERVE	COMPONENT	INNERVATION	FUNCTION
Spinal Segments			
C1–C4 Upper Cervical XI. Spinal accessory nerve	PE	Muscles: sternocleidomastoid, trapezius	Head, shoulder movement
Spinal nerves	SSA	Muscles of neck	Proprioception, DTRs
	GSA	Neck, back of head	Somesthesia
	GSE	Neck muscles	Head, shoulder movement
C5–C8 Lower Cervical	SSA	Upper limb muscles	Proprioception, DTRs
	GSA	Upper limbs	Reflexes, somesthesia
	GSE	Upper limb muscles	Movement, posture
T1–L2 Thoracic, *Upper Lumbar*	SSA	Muscles: trunk, abdominal wall	Proprioception
	GSA	Trunk, abdominal wall	Reflexes, somesthesia
	GVA	All of viscera	Reflexes and sensation
	GVE	All of viscera	Sympathetic reflexes, vasomotor control, sweating, piloerection
	GSE	Muscles: trunk, abdominal wall, back	Movement, posture, respiration
L2–S1 Lower Lumbar, *Upper Sacral*	SSA	Lower limb muscles	Proprioception, DTRs
	GSA	Lower trunk, limbs, back	Reflexes, somesthesia
	GSE	Muscles: trunk, lower limbs, back	Movement, posture
S2–S4 Lower Sacral	SSA	Muscles: pelvis, perineum	Proprioception
	GSA	Pelvis, genitalia	Reflexes, somesthesia
	GVA	Hindgut, bladder, uterus	Reflexes, sensation
	GVE	Hindgut, visceral organs	Visceral reflexes, defecation, urination, erection
S5–Co2 Lower Sacral, *Coccygeal*	SSA	Perineal muscles	Proprioception
	GSA	Lower sacrum, anus	Reflexes, somesthesia
	GSE	Perineal muscles	Reflexes, posture

Afferent (sensory) components: SSA, special somatic afferent; GSA, general somatic afferent; SVA, special visceral afferent;
GVA, general visceral afferent.
Efferent (motor) components: GVE, general visceral efferent (autonomic nervous system); PE, pharyngeal efferent; GSE, general
somatic efferent; DTRs, deep tendon reflexes.

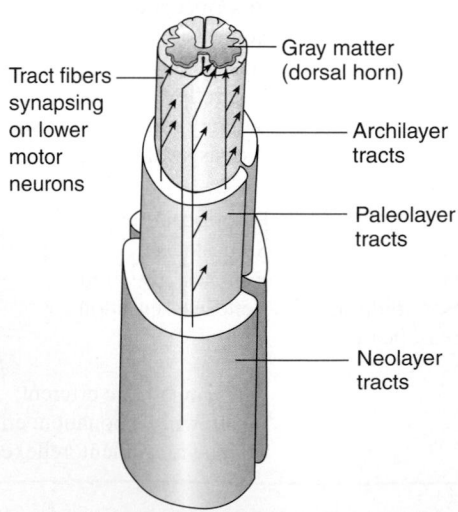

FIGURE 48-13 • The three concentric subdivisions of the tract
systems of the white matter. Migration of neurons into the archilayer converts it into the reticular formation of the white matter.

Gray matter
(dorsal horn)

Tract fibers
synapsing
on lower
motor
neurons

Archilayer
tracts

Paleolayer
tracts

Neolayer
tracts

The Outer Layer. The outer layer of the tract systems is the
newest of the three layers with respect to evolutionary development, and it is sometimes called the *neolayer*. It becomes
functional approximately the second year of life, and it includes
the pathways needed for bladder training. Myelination of these
suprasegmental tracts, which include many pathways required
for delicate and highly coordinated skills, is not complete
until approximately the fifth year of life. This includes the
development of tracts needed for fine manipulative skills, such
as the finger–thumb coordination required for using tools and
the toe movements needed for acrobatics. Neolayer tracts are
the most recently evolved systems and, because they are situated more superficially on the brain and spinal cord, are the
most vulnerable to injury. When neolayer tracts are damaged,
the paleolayer and archilayer tracts often remain functional,
and rehabilitation methods can result in effective use of the
older systems. Delicacy and refinement may be lost, but basic
function remains. For example, when the corticospinal system,
an important neolayer system that permits the fine manipulative control required for writing, is damaged, the remaining
paleolayer systems, if intact, permit the grasping and holding

TABLE 48-2 Characteristics of the Concentric Subdivisions of the Longitudinal Tracts in the White Matter of the Central Nervous System

CHARACTERISTICS	ARCHILAYER TRACTS	PALEOLAYER TRACTS	NEOLAYER TRACTS
Segmental span	Intersegmental (<5 segments)	Suprasegmental (≥5 segments)	Suprasegmental
Number of synapses	Multisynaptic	Multisynaptic but fewer than archilayer tracts	Monosynaptic with target structures
Conduction velocity	Very slow	Fast	Fastest
Examples of functional systems	Flexor withdrawal reflex circuitry	Spinothalamic tracts	Corticospinal tracts

of objects. The hand can still be used to perform basic functions, but the fine manipulative functions of the fingers are lost.

Collateral Communication Pathways. Axons in the archilayer and paleolayer characteristically possess many collateral branches that move into the gray cell columns or synapse with fibers of the reticular formation as the axon passes each succeeding CNS segment. Should a major axon be destroyed at some point along its course, these collaterals provide multisynaptic alternative pathways that bypass the local damage. Neolayer tracts do not possess these collaterals but instead project mainly to the target neurons with which they communicate. Because of this, damage to the neolayer tracts causes permanent loss of function. Damage to the archilayer or paleolayer systems is usually followed by a slow return of function, presumably through the collateral connections.

IN SUMMARY, development of the nervous system can be traced far back into evolutionary history. The CNS develops from the ectoderm of the early embryo by formation of a hollow tube that closes along its longitudinal axis and sinks below the surface. This hollow tube forms the ventricles of the brain and spinal canal, and the side wall develops to form the brain stem and spinal cord. Development of the CNS requires the coordinated production of many embryonic inductive factors. The brain stem and spinal cord are subdivided into the dorsal horn, which contains neurons that receive and process incoming or afferent information, and the ventral horn, which contains efferent motor neurons that handle the final stages of output processing. The PNS develops from ectodermal cells called *neural crest cells* that migrate away from the dorsal surface of the forming neural tube.

Throughout life, the organization of the nervous system retains many patterns established during early embryonic life. This segmental pattern of early embryonic development is retained in the fully developed nervous system. Each of the 43 or more body segments is connected to corresponding CNS or neural tube segments by segmental afferent and efferent neurons. Afferent neuronal processes enter the CNS through the dorsal root ganglia and the dorsal roots. Afferent neurons of the

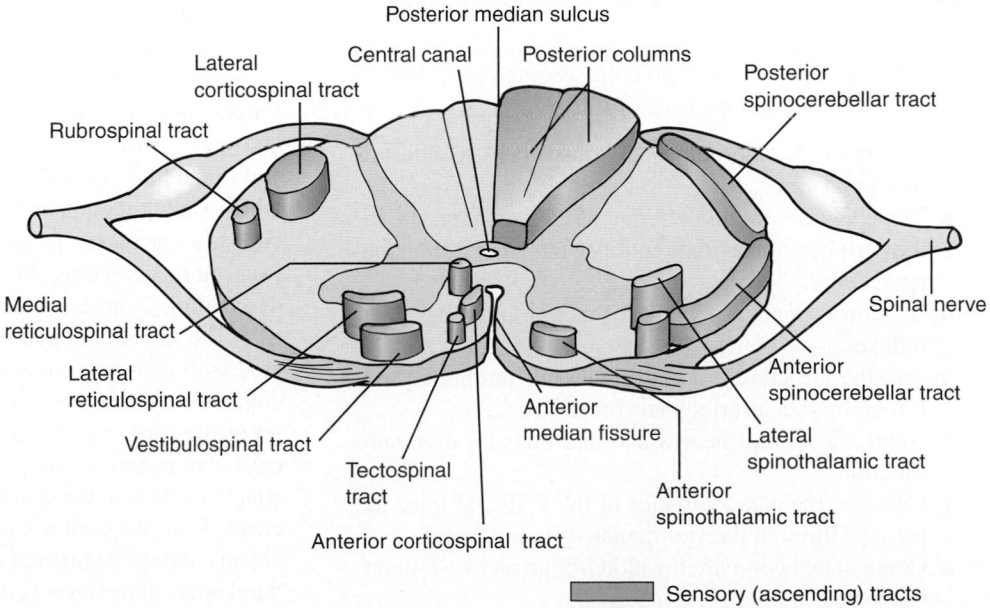

FIGURE 48-14 • Transverse section of the spinal cord showing selected sensory and motor tracts. The tracts are bilateral but are indicated only on one half of the cord.

dorsal root ganglia are of four types: general somatic afferent, special somatic afferent, general visceral afferent, and special visceral afferent. Each of these afferent neurons synapses with its appropriate IA neurons in the cell columns of the dorsal horn (*e.g.,* general somatic afferents synapse with neurons in the general somatic afferent IA cell column). Efferent fibers from motor neurons in the ventral horn exit the CNS in the ventral roots. General somatic efferent neurons are LMNs that innervate somite-derived skeletal muscles, and general visceral efferent neurons are preganglionic fibers that synapse with postganglionic fibers that innervate visceral structures. This pattern of afferent and efferent neurons, which is usually repeated in each segment of the body, forms parallel cell columns running lengthwise through the CNS and PNS.

Longitudinal communication between CNS segments is provided by neurons that send the axons into nearby segments by means of the innermost layer of the white matter, the ancient archilayer system of fibers. These cells provide coordination between neighboring segments. Neurons have invaded this layer, and the mix of these cells and axons is called the *reticular formation.* The reticular formation is the location of many important reflex circuits of the spinal cord and brain stem. Paleolayer tracts, located outside the archilayer, provide the longitudinal communication between more distant segments of the nervous system; this layer includes most of the important ascending and descending tracts. The recently evolved neolayer systems, which become functional during infancy and childhood, travel outside the white matter and provide the means for very delicate and discriminative function. The outer position of the neolayer tracts and their lack of collateral and redundant pathways make them the most vulnerable to injury. ■

STRUCTURE AND FUNCTION OF THE SPINAL CORD AND BRAIN

After completing this section of the chapter, you should be able to meet the following objectives:

- Describe the longitudinal and transverse structures of the spinal cord.
- Trace an afferent and efferent neuron from its site in the periphery through its entrance into or exit from the spinal cord.
- Explain the innervation and function of spinal cord reflexes.
- List the structures of the hindbrain, midbrain, and forebrain and describe their functions.
- Name the cranial nerves and cite their location and function.
- Describe the characteristics of the CSF and trace its passage through the ventricular system.
- Contrast and compare the blood-brain and CSF-brain barriers.

Spinal Cord

In the adult, the spinal cord is found in the upper two thirds of the spinal canal of the vertebral column (Fig. 48-15). It extends from the foramen magnum at the base of the skull to a cone-shaped termination, the conus medullaris, usually at the level of the first or second lumbar vertebra (L1 or L2) in the adult. Consequently, the dorsal and ventral roots of the more caudal portions of the cord elongate during development and angle downward from the cord, forming what is called the *cauda equina* (from the Latin for "horse's tail"). The filum terminale, which is composed of non-neural tissues and the pia mater, continues caudally and attaches to the second sacral vertebra (S2).

The spinal cord is somewhat oval on transverse section. Internally, the gray matter has the appearance of a butterfly or the letter "H" on cross-section (see Fig. 48-15). Some neurons that make up the gray matter of the cord have processes or axons that leave the cord, enter the peripheral nerves, and supply tissues such as autonomic ganglia or skeletal muscles. The white matter of the cord that surrounds the gray matter contains nerve fiber tracts of ascending and descending axons that transmit information between segments of the cord or from higher levels of the CNS, such as the brain stem or cerebrum.

Internally, the extensions of the gray matter that form the letter "H" are called the *horns.* Those that extend posteriorly are called the *dorsal horns,* and those that extend anteriorly are called the *ventral horns.* Dorsal horns contain IA neurons that receive afferent impulses through the dorsal roots and other connecting neurons. Ventral horns contain OA neurons and the efferent LMNs that leave the cord through the ventral roots. The central portion of the cord, which connects the dorsal and ventral horns, is called the *intermediate gray matter.* The intermediate gray matter surrounds the central canal. In the thoracic area, the small, slender projections that emerge from the intermediate gray matter are called the *intermediolateral columns* of the horns. These columns contain the visceral OA neurons and the efferent neurons of the sympathetic nervous system.

The amount of gray matter is proportional to how much tissue is innervated by a given segment of the cord (see Fig. 48-15). Larger amounts of gray matter are present in the lower lumbar and upper sacral segments, which supply the lower extremities, and in the fifth cervical segment to the first thoracic segment, which supply the upper limbs. The white matter in the spinal cord also increases progressively toward the brain because ever more ascending fibers are added and the number of descending axons is greater.

The spinal cord and the dorsal and ventral roots are covered by a connective tissue sheath, the pia mater, which also contains the blood vessels that supply the white and gray matter of the cord (Fig. 48-16). On the lateral sides of the spinal cord, extensions of the pia mater, the denticulate ligaments, attach the sides of the spinal cord to the bony walls of the spinal canal. Thus, the cord is suspended by both the denticulate ligaments and the segmental nerves. A fat- and vessel-filled epidural space intervenes between the spinal dura mater and the inner wall of the spinal canal.

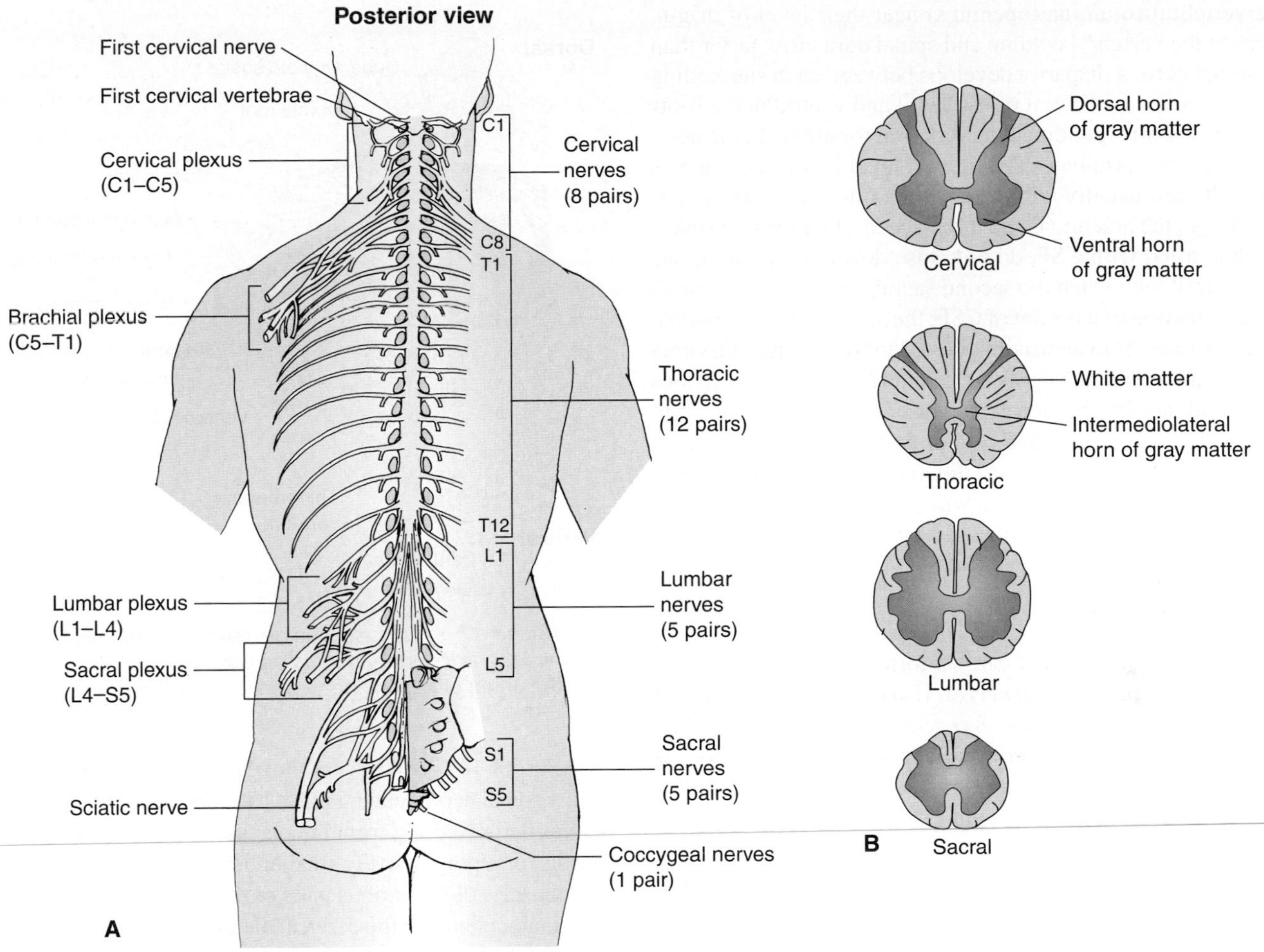

Posterior view

First cervical nerve

First cervical vertebrae

C1

Cervical plexus
(C1–C5)

Cervical
nerves
(8 pairs)

C8
T1

Brachial plexus
(C5–T1)

Thoracic
nerves
(12 pairs)

T12
L1

Lumbar plexus
(L1–L4)

Lumbar
nerves
(5 pairs)

L5

Sacral plexus
(L4–S5)

S1

Sacral
nerves
(5 pairs)

S5

Sciatic nerve

Coccygeal nerves
(1 pair)

A

Dorsal horn
of gray matter

Ventral horn
of gray matter

Cervical

White matter

Intermediolateral
horn of gray matter

Thoracic

Lumbar

B Sacral

FIGURE 48-15 • **(A)** Posterior view of the spinal cord, including portions of the major spinal nerves and some of the components of the major nerve plexuses. **(B)** Cross-sectional views of the spinal cord, showing regional variations in gray matter and increasing white matter as the cord ascends.

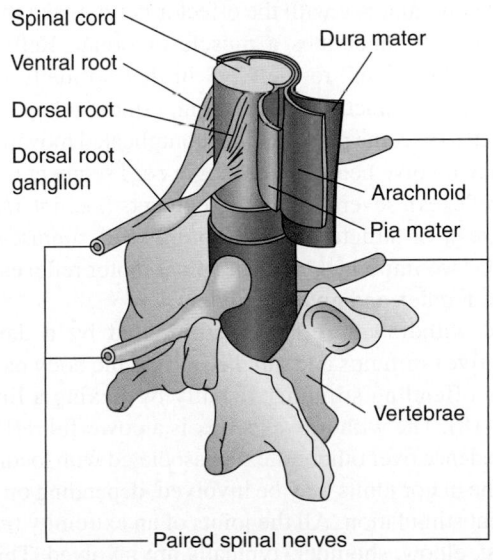

Spinal cord

Ventral root

Dorsal root

Dorsal root
ganglion

Dura mater

Arachnoid

Pia mater

Vertebrae

Paired spinal nerves

FIGURE 48-16 • Spinal cord and meninges.

The spinal cord and nerves and their supporting structures are protected by the vertebral column. The vertebral body is the anterior, more massive part of the bone that gives strength to the vertebral column and supports body weight. Each vertebral body has two pedicles that extend posteriorly and support the laterally oriented transverse processes of the laminae, which arch medially and fuse to continue as the spinal processes. The vertebral arch and posterior surface of the vertebral body form the wall of the vertebral foramen. The succession of vertebral foramina in the articulated spinal column forms the vertebral canal (spinal canal), which contains the spinal cord, meninges, fat, and spinal nerve roots. The spaces between the vertebral bodies are filled with fibrocartilaginous disks and stabilized with tough ligaments. A gap, the intervertebral foramen, occurs between each two succeeding pedicles, allowing for the exit of the segmental nerves and passage of blood vessels. Supporting structures of the spinal cord are discussed further in Chapter 50.

Early in fetal life, the spinal cord extends the entire length of the vertebral column and the spinal nerves exit through the intervertebral foramina (openings) near their level of origin. Because the vertebral column and spinal dura grow faster than the spinal cord, a disparity develops between each succeeding cord segment and the exit of its dorsal and ventral nerve roots through the corresponding intervertebral foramina. In the new-born, the cord terminates at vertebral level L2 or L3, whereas the adult cord usually terminates at the inferior border of L1. In addition, the arachnoid and its enclosed subarachnoid space, which is filled with CSF, do not close down on the filum ter-minale until they reach the second sacral vertebra. This results in the formation of a pocket of CSF, the *dural cisterna spinalis,* which extends from approximately L2 to S2. Because this area contains an abundant supply of CSF and the spinal cord does not extend this far, the area is often used for sampling the CSF. A procedure called a *spinal tap,* or puncture, can be done by inserting a special needle into the dural sac at L3 or L4. The spinal roots, which are covered with pia mater, are in little dan-ger of trauma from the needle used for this purpose.

Spinal Nerves

The peripheral nerves that carry information to and from the spinal cord are called *spinal nerves.* Usually, 32 or more pairs of spinal nerves are present (*i.e.,* 8 cervical, 12 thoracic, 5 lumbar, 5 sacral, and 2 or more coccygeal); each pair is named for the segment of the spinal cord from which it exits. Because the first cervical spinal nerve exits the spinal cord just above the first cer-vical vertebra (C1), the nerve is given the number of the bony vertebra just below it. The numbering is changed for all lower levels, however. Cervical nerve 8 (C8), exits above the T1 ver-tebra, and each subsequent nerve is numbered for the vertebra just above its point of exit (see Fig. 48-15).

Each spinal cord segment communicates with its corre-sponding body segment through the paired segmental spinal nerves (see Fig. 48-11). Each spinal nerve, accompanied by the blood vessels supplying the spinal cord, enters the spinal canal through an intervertebral foramen, where it divides into two branches, or roots. One branch enters the dorsolateral surface of the cord (*i.e.,* dorsal root), carrying the axons of afferent neurons into the CNS. The other branch leaves the ventrolateral surface of the cord (*i.e.,* ventral root), carrying the axons of efferent neurons into the periphery. These two branches or roots fuse at the intervertebral foramen, forming the mixed spinal nerve—"mixed" because it has both afferent and efferent axons.

After emerging from the vertebral column, the spinal nerve divides into two branches or *rami* (singular, *ramus*): a small dorsal primary ramus and a larger ventral primary ramus (Fig. 48-17). Thoracic and upper lumbar spinal nerves also pro-duce a third branch, the ramus communicans, which contains sympathetic axons supplying the blood vessels, the genitouri-nary system, and the gastrointestinal system. The dorsal pri-mary ramus contains sensory fibers from the skin and motor fibers to muscles of the back. The ventral primary ramus con-tains motor fibers that innervate the skeletal muscles of the ante-rior body wall and the legs and arms.

Spinal nerves do not go directly to skin and muscle fibers; instead, they form complicated nerve networks called *plexuses*

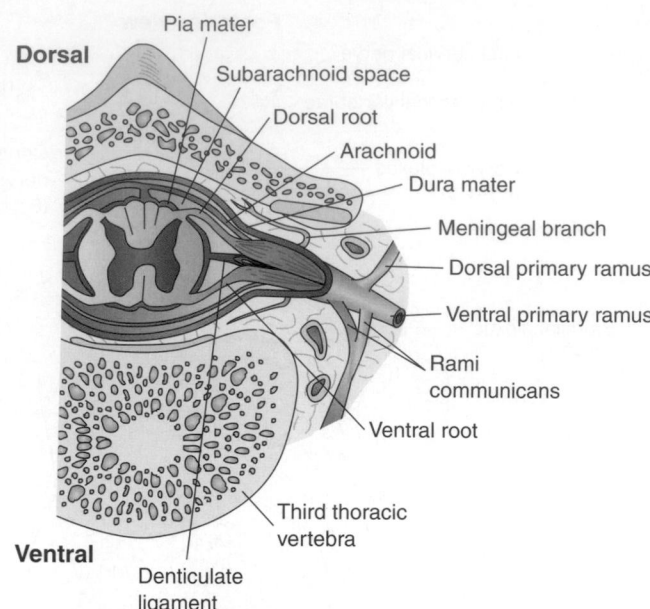

FIGURE 48-17 • Cross-section of vertebral column at the level of the third thoracic vertebra, showing the meninges, the spinal cord, and the origin of a spinal nerve and its branches or rami.

(see Fig. 48-14). A plexus is a site of intermixing nerve branches. Many spinal nerves enter a plexus and connect with other spinal nerves before exiting from the plexus. Nerves emerging from a plexus form progressively smaller branches that supply the skin and muscles of the various parts of the body. The PNS contains four major plexuses: the cervical plexus, the brachial plexus, the lumbar plexus, and the sacral plexus.

Spinal Reflexes

A *reflex* is a highly predictable relationship between a stimulus and an elicited motor response. Its anatomic basis consists of an afferent neuron, the connection or synapse with CNS interneu-rons that communicate with the effector neuron, and the effec-tor neuron that innervates a muscle or organ. Reflexes are essentially "wired in" to the CNS in that normally they are always ready to function; with training, most reflexes can be modulated to become parts of more complicated movements. A reflex may involve neurons in a single cord segment (*i.e.,* seg-mental reflexes), several or many segments (*i.e.,* intersegmen-tal reflexes), or structures in the brain (*i.e.,* suprasegmental reflexes). Two important types of spinal motor reflexes are the withdrawal reflex and myotatic reflex.

The withdrawal reflex is stimulated by a damaging (nociceptive) stimulus and quickly moves the body part away from the offending stimulus, usually by flexing a limb part (Fig. 48-18). The withdrawal reflex is a powerful reflex, tak-ing precedence over other reflexes associated with locomotion. Any of the major joints may be involved, depending on the site of afferent stimulation. All the joints of an extremity (*e.g.,* fin-ger, wrist, elbow, shoulder) typically are involved. This com-plex, polysynaptic reflex also shifts postural support to the

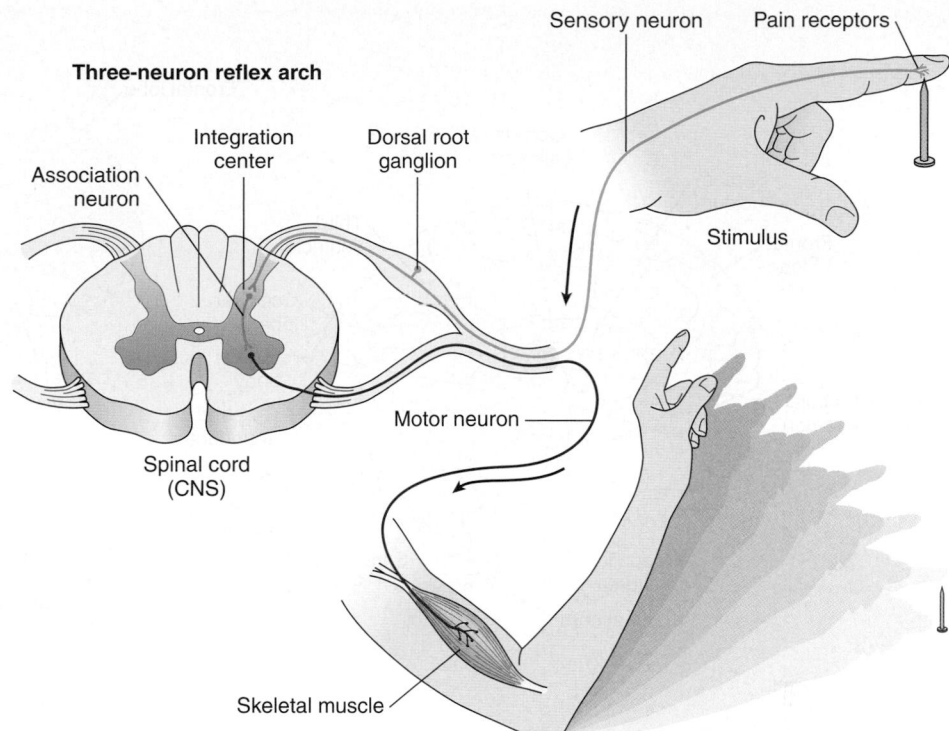

Three-neuron reflex arch

FIGURE 48-18 • Diagram of withdrawal reflex, showing the essential elements in a spinal reflex arc—a receptor in a sensory neuron, an integration center with an association neuron, and an effector (skeletal muscle).

opposite side of the body with a crossed extensor reflex and simultaneously alerts the forebrain to the offending stimulus event. The withdrawal reflex also can produce contraction of muscles other than the extremities. For example, irritation of the abdominal viscera may cause contraction of the abdominal muscles.

The myotatic or stretch reflex controls muscle tone and helps maintain posture. Specialized sensory nerve terminals in skeletal muscles and tendons relay information on muscle stretch and joint tension to the CNS (see Chapter 50). This information, which drives postural reflex mechanisms, also is relayed to the thalamus and the sensory cortex and is experienced as *proprioception,* the sense of body movement and position. To provide this information, the muscles and their tendons are supplied with two types of sensory receptors: muscle spindle receptors and Golgi tendon organs. *Muscle spindles* are stretch receptors distributed throughout the belly of a muscle that transmit information about muscle length and rate of stretch. The *Golgi tendon organs* are found in muscle tendons and transmit information about muscle tension or force of contraction at the junction of the muscle and the tendon that attaches to bone. A likely role of the tendon organs is to equalize the contractile forces of the separate muscle groups, spreading the load over all the fibers to prevent the local muscle damage that might occur when small numbers of fibers are overloaded.

The Brain

Based on its embryonic development, the brain can be divided into three regions: the hindbrain, the midbrain, and the forebrain (see Fig. 48-8). The hindbrain includes the medulla oblongata,

the pons, and its dorsal outgrowth, the cerebellum. Midbrain structures include two pairs of dorsal enlargements, the superior and inferior colliculi. The forebrain, which consists of two hemispheres and is covered by the cerebral cortex, contains central masses of gray matter, the basal ganglia, and the rostral end of the neural tube, the diencephalon, with its adult derivatives—the thalamus and hypothalamus.

An important concept is that the more rostral, recently developed parts of the neural tube gain dominance or control over regions and functions at lower levels. They do not replace the more ancient circuitry but merely dominate it. After damage to the more vulnerable parts of the forebrain, as occurs with brain death, a brain stem–controlled organism remains that is capable of breathing and may survive if the environmental temperature is regulated and nutrition and other aspects of care are provided. However, all aspects of intellectual function, experience, perception, and memory are usually permanently lost. The organization of content in this section moves from the more ancient circuitry of the hindbrain to the more dominant and recently developed structures of the forebrain.

Hindbrain

The term *brain stem* is often used to include the medulla, pons, and midbrain (Fig. 48-19B). These regions of the neural tube have the organization of spinal cord segments, except that more of the longitudinal cell columns are present, reflecting the increased complexity of the cranial segmental nerves. In the brain stem, the structure and function of the reticular formation have been greatly expanded. In the pons and medulla, the reticular formation contains networks controlling basic

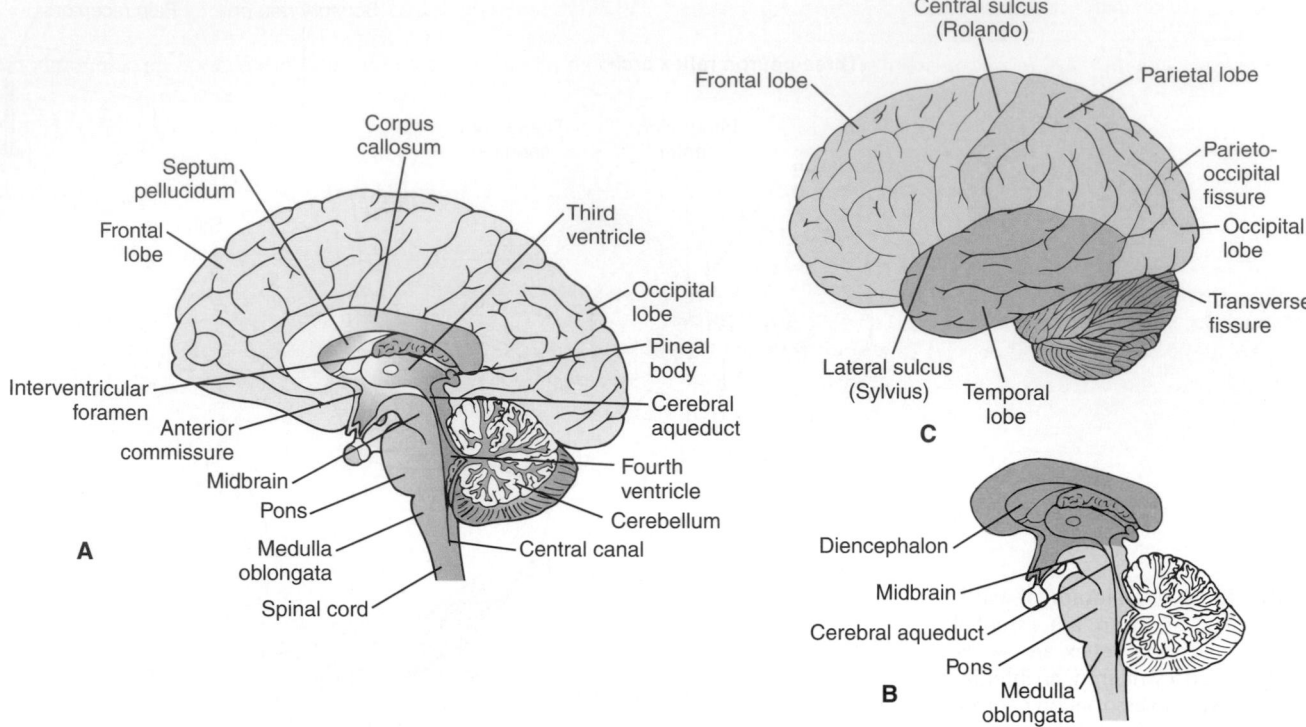

FIGURE 48-19 • **(A)** Mid-sagittal section of the brain, showing the structures of the forebrain, midbrain, and hindbrain. **(B)** Diencephalon, brain stem, and the cerebral aqueduct connecting the third and fourth ventricles. **(C)** Lateral view of the cerebral hemispheres.

breathing, eating, and locomotion functions. Higher-level integration of these functions occurs in the midbrain. The reticular formation is surrounded on the outside by the long tract systems that connect the forebrain with lower parts of the CNS.

Medulla. The *medulla oblongata* represents the caudal five segments of the brain part of the neural tube; the cranial nerve branches entering and leaving it have functions similar to the spinal segmental nerves. Although the ventral horn areas in the medulla are quite small, the dorsal horn areas are enlarged, processing a large amount of the information pouring through the cranial nerves. The segmental peripheral nerve components of the medulla can be divided into those leaving the neural tube ventromedially (*i.e.,* hypoglossal cranial nerve) or dorsolaterally (*i.e.,* vagus, spinal accessory, glossopharyngeal, and vestibulocochlear cranial nerves). Because pathologic signs and symptoms reflect the spatial segregation of brain stem components, neurologic syndromes resulting from trauma, tumors, aneurysms, and cerebrovascular accidents are often classified as ventral or dorsolateral syndromes.

The general somatic efferent LMNs of the lower segments of the medulla supply the extrinsic and intrinsic muscles of the tongue by means of the *hypoglossal nerve* (CN XII). Damage to the hypoglossal nerve results in weakness or paralysis of tongue muscles. When the tongue is protruded, it deviates toward the damaged and therefore weaker side because of the greater protrusion strength on the normal side. Axons of the hypoglossal

nerve exit the medulla adjacent to two long, longitudinal ridges along the medial undersurface of the medulla. These ridges, called the *pyramids,* contain the corticospinal fibers, most of which cross to descend in the lateral column to the opposite side of the spinal cord. Lesions of the ventral surface of the caudal medulla result in the syndrome of alternating hypoglossal hemiplegia. These lesions are characterized by signs of ipsilateral (*i.e.,* same side) denervation of the tongue and contralateral (*i.e.,* opposite side) weakness or paralysis of both the upper and lower extremities.

The *vagus nerve* (CN X) has several afferent (sensory) and efferent (motor) components. General somatic afferent neurons innervate the external ear, whereas special visceral afferent neurons innervate the pharyngeal taste buds. Sensory and motor components of the nerve innervate the pharynx, the gastrointestinal tract (from the laryngeal pharynx to the mid-transverse colon), the heart, the spleen, and the lungs. Initiation of many essential reflexes and normal functions depends on intact vagal innervation. For example, 80% of the fibers of the vagus nerve are afferents, some of which are involved in vomiting and hiccup reflexes and in ongoing feedback during swallowing and speech. The unilateral loss of vagal function can result in slowed gastrointestinal motility, a permanently husky voice, and deviation of the uvula away from the damaged side. Bilateral loss of vagal function can seriously damage reflex maintenance of cardiovascular and respiratory reflexes. Swallowing may become difficult and, occasionally, paralysis of laryngeal structures causes life-threatening airway obstruction.

The sternocleidomastoid, a powerful head-turning muscle, and the trapezius muscle, which elevates the shoulders, are innervated by the *spinal accessory nerve* (CN XI), with LMNs in the upper four cervical spinal segments. Intermediate rootlets from these segmental levels combine and enter the cranial cavity through the foramen magnum and exit the jugular foramen with CNs IX and X. Loss of spinal accessory nerve function results in drooping of the shoulder on the damaged side and weakness when turning the head to the opposite side.

The dorsolateral *glossopharyngeal nerve* (CN IX) contains the same components as the vagus nerve but for a more rostral segment of the gastrointestinal tract and the pharynx. This nerve provides the special visceral sensory innervation of the taste buds of the oral pharynx and the back of the tongue; the afferent innervation of the oral pharynx and the baroreceptors of the carotid sinus; the efferent innervation of the otic ganglion, which controls the salivary function of the parotid gland; and the efferent innervation of the stylopharyngeus muscles of the pharynx. This cranial nerve is seldom damaged, but when it is, anesthesia of the ipsilateral oral pharynx develops along with dry mouth resulting from reduced salivation.

The special sensory afferent *vestibulocochlear nerve* (CN VIII), formerly called the *auditory nerve,* is attached laterally at the junction of the medulla oblongata and the pons, often called the *caudal pons.* It consists of two distinct fiber divisions, the cochlear and vestibular divisions, both of which are sensory. Cell bodies in the cochlea of the inner ear produce fibers of the cochlear division. These fibers transmit impulses related to the sense of hearing. The vestibular division arises from two ganglia that innervate cell bodies in the utricle, saccule, and semicircular canals and transmit impulses related to head position and movement of the body through space. Irritation of the cochlear division results in tinnitus (*i.e.,* ringing of the ears); destruction of the nerve results in nerve deafness. Injury to the vestibular division leads to vertigo, nystagmus, and some postural instability (see Chapter 55).

The *facial nerve* (CN VII) and its intermediate component (the intermedius) is a mixed nerve that has both afferent and efferent components. It emerges from the junction of the pons and medulla. The nervus intermedius, containing the general somatic afferent, special visceral afferent, general visceral afferent, and general visceral efferent neurons, innervates the nasopharynx and taste buds of the palate. It also innervates the anterior two thirds of the tongue, the submandibular and sublingual salivary glands, the lacrimal glands, and the mucous membranes of the nose and roof of the mouth. Loss of this branch of the facial nerve can lead to eye dryness with risk of corneal scarring and blindness. The pharyngeal efferent LMNs of the facial nerve proper innervate muscles that control facial expression, such as wrinkling of the brow and smiling. Unilateral loss of facial nerve function results in flaccid paralysis of the muscles of half the face, a condition called *Bell palsy.*

Pons. The pons (from the Latin for "bridge") develops from the fifth neural tube segment. Internally, the central canal of the spinal cord, which is enlarged in the pons and rostral medulla,

forms the fourth ventricle (see Fig. 48-19B). An enlarged area on the ventral surface of the pons contains the pontine nuclei, which receive information from all parts of the cerebral cortex. Axons of these neurons form a massive bundle that swings around the lateral side of the fourth ventricle to enter the cerebellum. In the pons, the reticular formation is large and contains the circuitry for masticating food and manipulating the jaws during speech.

The *abducens nerve* (CN VI), which arises from the caudal pons, sends LMNs out ventrally on either side of the pyramids and then forward into the orbit to innervate the lateral rectus muscle of the eye. As the name suggests, the abducens nerve abducts the eye (lateral or outward rotation); peripheral damage to this nerve results in medial strabismus, which is a weakness or loss of eye abduction (see Chapter 54).

The *trigeminal nerve* (CN V), which has both sensory and motor subdivisions, exits the brain stem laterally on the forward surface of the pons. The trigeminal is the main sensory nerve conveying the modalities of pain, temperature, touch, and proprioception to the superficial and deep regions of the face. Regions innervated include the skin of the anterior scalp and face, the conjunctiva and orbit, the meninges, the paranasal sinuses, and the mouth, including the teeth and the anterior two thirds of the tongue. LMNs of the trigeminal nerve innervate skeletal muscles involved with mastication and contribute to swallowing and speech, movements of the soft palate, and tension of the tympanic membrane through the tensor tympani muscle. The tensor tympani muscle has a protective reflex function, dampening movement of the middle ear ossicles during high-intensity sound.

Cerebellum. The cerebellum is located in the posterior fossa of the cranium superior to the pons (see Fig. 48-19A). It is separated from the cerebral hemispheres by a fold of dura mater, the tentorium cerebelli. The cerebellum consists of a small unpaired median portion, called the *vermis,* and two large lateral masses, the *cerebellar hemispheres.* In contrast to the brain stem with its external white matter and internal gray nuclei, the cerebellum, like the cerebrum, has an outer cortex of gray matter overlying the white matter. Next to the fourth ventricle, several masses of gray matter, called the *deep cerebellar nuclei,* border the roof of the fourth ventricle. Cells of the cerebellar cortex and deep nuclei interact, and axons from the latter send information to many regions, particularly to the motor cortex by means of a thalamic relay. Synergistic functions of the cerebellum (*i.e.,* temporal and spatial smoothing) contribute to all movements of the limbs, trunk, head, larynx, and eyes, whether the movement is part of a voluntary movement or of a highly learned semiautomatic or automatic movement. During highly skilled movements, the motor cortex sends signals to the cerebellum, informing it about the movement that is to be performed. The cerebellum makes continuous adjustments, resulting in smoothness of movement, particularly during delicate maneuvers. Highly skillful movement requires extensive motor training, and considerable evidence suggests many of these learned movement patterns involve cerebellar circuits.

The cerebellum receives proprioceptor input from the vestibular system; feedback from the muscles, tendons, and joints; and indirect signals from the somesthetic, visual, and auditory systems that provide background information for on-going movement. Sensory and motor information from a given area of the body is sent to the same area in the cerebellum. In this way, the cerebellum can assess continuously the status of each body part—position, rate of movement, and forces such as gravity that are opposing movement. The cerebellum compares what is actually happening with what is intended to happen. It then transmits the appropriate corrective signals back to the motor system, instructing it to increase or decrease the activity of the participating muscle groups so that smooth and accurate movements can be performed.

Another function of the cerebellum is the dampening of muscle movement. All body movements are essentially pendular (*i.e.,* swinging back and forth). As movement begins, momentum develops and must be overcome before the movement can be stopped. This momentum would cause movements to overshoot if they were not dampened. In the intact cerebellum, automatic signals stop movement precisely at the intended point. The cerebellum analyzes proprioceptive information to predict the future position of moving parts, their rapidity of movement, and the projected time course of the movement. This allows the cerebellum to inhibit agonist muscles and excite antagonist muscles when movement approaches the intended target.

Midbrain

The midbrain develops from the fourth segment of the neural tube, and its organization is similar to that of a spinal segment. Internally, the central canal is reestablished as the cerebral aqueduct, connecting the fourth ventricle with the third ventricle (see Fig. 48-19B). Two general somatic efferent cranial nerves, the oculomotor nerve (CN III) and the trochlear nerve (CN IV), exit the midbrain.

Two prominent bundles of nerve fibers, the *cerebral peduncles,* pass along the ventral surface of the midbrain. These fibers include the corticospinal tracts and are the main motor pathways between the forebrain and the pons. On the dorsal surface, four "little hills," the *superior* and *inferior colliculi,* are areas of cortical formation. The inferior colliculi are involved in directional turning and, to some extent, in experiencing the direction of sound sources, whereas the superior colliculi are essential to the reflex mechanisms that control conjugate eye movements when the visual environment is surveyed.

The ventral central gray matter (*i.e.,* ventral horn) of the midbrain contains the LMNs that innervate most of the skeletal muscles that move the optic globe and raise the eyelids. These axons leave the midbrain through the oculomotor nerve (CN III). This nerve also contains the parasympathetic LMNs that control pupillary constriction and ciliary muscle focusing of the lens (see Table 48-1). Damage to the ventrally exiting CN III and to

the adjacent cerebral peduncle, which contains the corticospinal axon system on one side, results in paralysis of eye movement combined with contralateral hemiplegia.

A small group of cells in the ventral part of the caudal central gray matter contains the trochlear nerve (CN IV), which innervates the superior oblique eye muscle. This muscle moves the upper part of the eye downward and toward the nose when the eye is adducted, or turned inward. The trochlear nerve exits the dorsal surface of the midbrain and decussates (crosses over) before exiting the brain stem. Lesions of the trochlear nerve affect downward gaze on the side opposite the denervated muscle, producing diplopia, or double vision. Walking downstairs becomes particularly difficult. Because the superior oblique muscle has inward rotation of the optic globe as its major function, persons with trochlear nerve damage usually carry their heads tilted to the side of damage.

Forebrain

The most rostral part of the brain, the forebrain consists of the telencephalon, or "end brain," and the diencephalon, or "between brain." The diencephalon forms the core of the forebrain, and the telencephalon forms the cerebral hemispheres.

Diencephalon. Three of the most forward brain segments form an enlarged dorsal horn and ventral horn with a narrow, deep, enlarged central canal—the third ventricle—separating the two sides. This region is called the *diencephalon.* The dorsal horn part of the diencephalon is the thalamus and subthalamus, and the ventral horn part is the hypothalamus (Fig. 48-20). The optic nerve (CN II) and retina are outgrowths of the diencephalon. The structure and function of the optic nerve are presented in Chapter 54.

The thalamus consists of two large, egg-shaped masses, one on either side of the third ventricle. It is divided into several major parts, and each part is divided into distinct nuclei, which are the major relay stations for information going to and from the cerebral cortex. All sensory pathways have direct projections to thalamic nuclei, which convey the information to restricted areas of the sensory cortex. Coordination and integration of peripheral sensory stimuli occur in the thalamus, along with some crude interpretation of highly emotion-laden auditory experiences that not only occurs but can be remembered. For example, a person can recover from a deep coma in which cerebral cortex activity is minimal and remember some of what was said at the bedside.

The thalamus also plays a role in relaying critical information regarding motor activities to and from selected areas of the motor cortex. Two neuronal circuits are significant in this regard. One is the pathway from the cerebral cortex to the pons and cerebellum and then, by way of the thalamus, back to the motor cortex. The second is the feedback circuit that travels from the cortex to the basal ganglia, then to the thalamus, and from the thalamus back to the cortex. The subthalamus also contains movement control systems related to the basal ganglia.

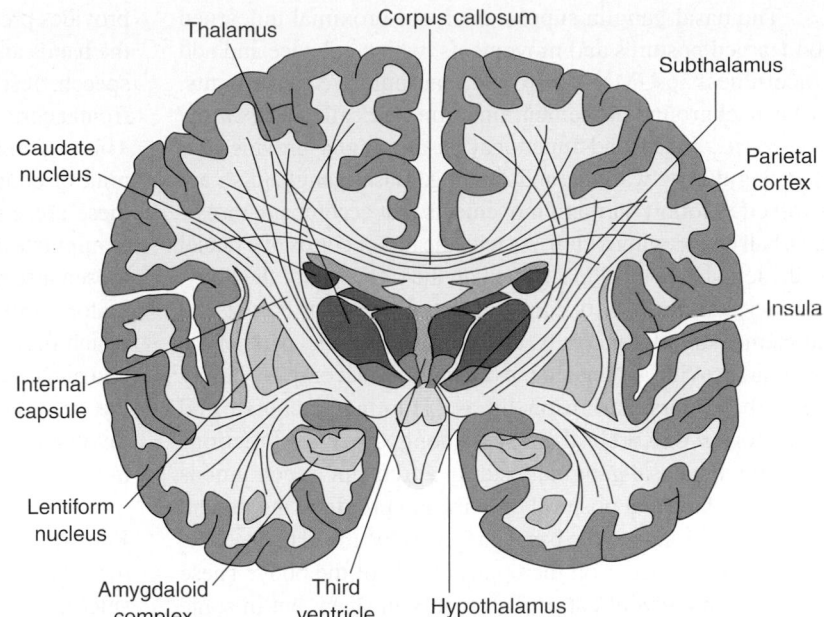

FIGURE 48-20 • Frontal section of the brain passing through the third ventricle, showing the thalamus, subthalamus, hypothalamus, internal capsule, corpus callosum, basal ganglia (caudate nucleus, lentiform nucleus), amygdaloid complex, insula, and parietal cortex.

Through its connections with the ascending reticular activating system, the thalamus processes neural influences that are basic to cortical excitatory rhythms (*i.e.*, those recorded on the electroencephalogram), to essential sleep–wakefulness cycles, and to the process of attending to stimuli. Besides their cortical connections, the thalamic nuclei have connections with each other and with neighboring nonthalamic brain structures such as the limbic system. Through their connections with the limbic system, some thalamic nuclei are involved in the relation between stimuli and the emotional responses they evoke.

Inferior to the thalamus and representing the ventral horn portion of the diencephalon is the hypothalamus. It also borders the third ventricle and includes a ventral extension, the neurohypophysis (*i.e.*, posterior pituitary). The hypothalamus is the area of master-level integration of homeostatic control of the body's internal environment. Maintenance of blood gas concentrations, water balance, food consumption, and major aspects of endocrine and autonomic nervous system control require hypothalamic function.

The internal capsule is a broad band of projection fibers that lies between the thalamus medially and the basal ganglia laterally (see Fig. 48-20). It contains all of the fibers that connect the cerebral cortex with deeper structures, including the basal ganglia, thalamus, midbrain, pons, medulla, and spinal cord.

Cerebral Hemispheres. The two cerebral hemispheres are lateral outgrowths of the diencephalon. Internally, the cerebral hemispheres contain the lateral ventricles (*i.e.*, ventricles I and II), which are connected to the third ventricle of the diencephalon by a small opening called the *interventricular foramen* (see Fig. 44-19A). Axons of the olfactory nerve (CN I) terminate in the most ancient portion of the cerebrum, the olfactory bulb, where initial processing of olfactory information occurs. Projection axons from the olfactory bulb relay information through the olfactory tracts to the thalamus and to other parts of the cerebral cortex (*i.e.*, orbital cortex), where olfactory-related reflexes and olfactory experience occur.

A massive commissure, or bridge, of myelinated axons called the *corpus callosum* connects the cerebral cortex of the two sides of the brain (see Fig. 48-20). Two smaller commissures, the anterior and posterior commissures, connect the two sides of the more specialized regions of the cerebrum and diencephalon.

The surfaces of the hemispheres are lateral (side), medial (area between the two sides of the brain), and basal (ventral). The cerebral cortex is the recently evolved six-layered neocortex. Many ridges and grooves are present on the surface of the hemispheres. A *gyrus* is the ridge between two grooves, and the groove is called a *sulcus* or *fissure*. The cerebral cortex is arbitrarily divided into lobes named after the bones that cover them: the frontal, parietal, temporal, and occipital lobes (see Fig. 48-19C).

Basal Ganglia. A section through the cerebral hemispheres reveals the surface of the cerebral cortex, a subcortical layer of white matter made up of masses of myelinated axons, and deep masses of gray matter: the basal ganglia that border the lateral ventricle (Fig. 48-20). The basal ganglia lie on either side of the internal capsule, just lateral to the thalamus. The basal ganglia consist of the comma-shaped *caudate* (tailed) *nucleus*, the shield-shaped *putamen*, and the *globus pallidus* ("pale globe"). The term *striatum* ("striped body") refers to the caudate plus the putamen. Together, the globus pallidus and putamen make up the *lentiform* (lens-shaped) *nucleus*.

The basal ganglia supply axial and proximal unlearned and learned postures and movements, which enhance and add gracefulness to UMN-controlled manipulative movements. These background movement functions are called *associated movements*. Intact and functional basal ganglia provide arm swinging during walking and running. Basal ganglia also are involved in follow-through movements that accompany throwing a ball or swinging a club. As with the motor cortex, the nuclei on the left side control movement on the right side of the body, and vice versa. Circuits connecting the premotor cortex and supplementary motor cortex, the basal ganglia, and parts of the thalamus provide associated movements that accompany highly skilled behaviors. Parkinson disease, Huntington chorea, and some forms of cerebral palsy, among other dysfunctions involving the basal ganglia, result in a frequent or continuous release of abnormal postural or axial and proximal movement patterns. If damage to the basal ganglia is localized to one side, the movements occur on the opposite side of the body. These automatic movement patterns stop only in sleep, but in some conditions, the movements are so violent that falling asleep becomes difficult.

Frontal Lobe. The frontal lobe extends from the frontal pole to the central sulcus (*i.e.,* fissure) and is separated from the temporal lobe by the lateral sulcus. Each frontal lobe can be subdivided rostrally into the frontal pole and laterally into the superior, middle, and inferior gyri, which continue on the undersurface over the eyes as the orbital cortex. These areas are associated with the medial thalamic nuclei, which also are related to the limbic system. Functionally, the prefrontal cortex is thought to be involved in anticipation and prediction of consequences of behavior.

The precentral gyrus (area 4), next to the central sulcus, is the *primary motor cortex* (Fig. 48-21). This area of the cortex provides precise movement control for distal flexor muscles of the hands and feet and of the phonation apparatus required for speech. Just rostral to the precentral gyrus is a region of the frontal cortex called the *premotor* or *motor association cortex.* This region (area 8 and rostral area 6) is involved in the planning of complex learned movement patterns, and damage to these areas results in dyspraxia or apraxia. Such people can manipulate a screwdriver, for instance, but cannot use it to loosen a screw. The primary motor cortex and the association motor cortex are connected with lateral thalamic nuclei, through which they receive feedback information from the basal ganglia and cerebellum. On the medial surface of the hemisphere, the premotor area includes a *supplementary motor cortex* involved in the control of bilateral movement patterns requiring great dexterity.

Parietal Lobe. The parietal lobe of the cerebrum lies behind the central sulcus (*i.e.,* postcentral gyrus) and above the lateral sulcus. A strip of cortex bordering the central sulcus is called the *primary somatosensory cortex* (areas 3, 1, and 2) because it receives very discrete sensory information from the lateral nuclei of the thalamus. Just behind the primary sensory cortex is the *somesthetic association cortex* (areas 5 and 7), which is connected with the thalamic nuclei and with the primary sensory cortex (see Fig. 48-21). This region is necessary for somesthetic perception (*i.e.,* appreciation of the meaningfulness of integrated sensory information from various sensory systems), especially concerning perception of "where" the stimulus is in space and in relation to body parts. Localized lesions of this region can result in the inability to recognize the meaningfulness of an object (a condition called *agnosia*). With the person's eyes closed, a screwdriver can be felt and described as to shape and texture. Nevertheless, the person cannot integrate the sensory information required to identify it as a screwdriver.

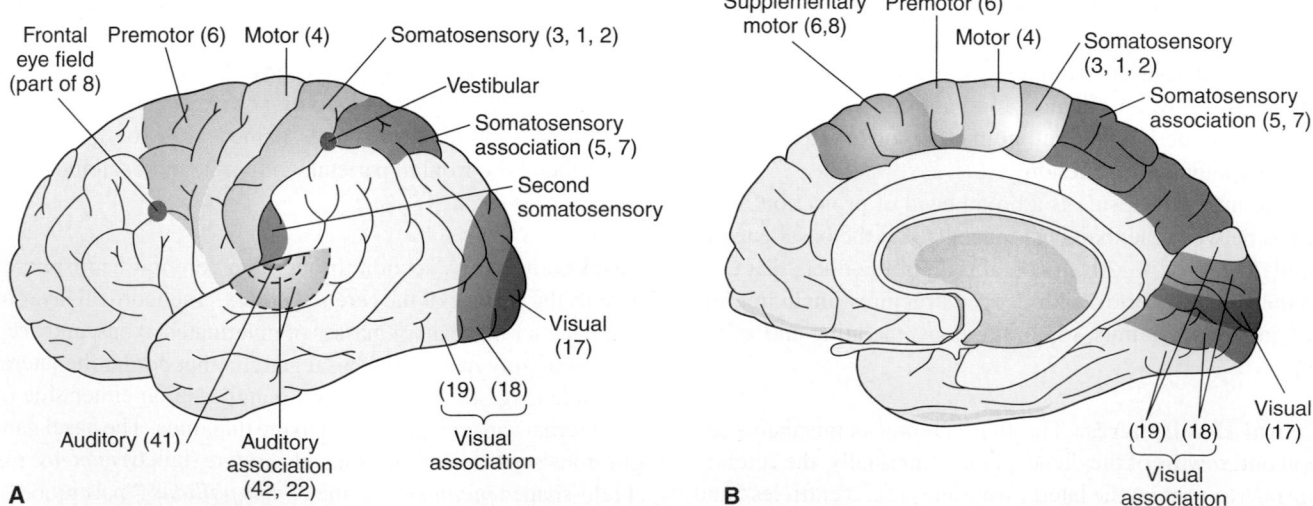

FIGURE 48-21 • Motor and sensory areas of the cerebral cortex. **(A)** Left lateral view of the cerebral cortex. **(B)** This diagram represents the areas in a brain that has been sectioned in the median plane.

Temporal Lobe. The temporal lobe lies below the lateral sulcus and merges with the parietal and occipital lobes. It includes the temporal pole and three primary gyri, the superior, middle, and inferior gyri. The primary auditory cortex (area 41) involves the part of the superior temporal gyrus that extends into the lateral sulcus (see Fig. 48-21). This area is particularly important in discrimination of sounds entering opposite ears. It receives auditory input projections through the inferior colliculus of the midbrain and a ventrolateral thalamic nucleus. The more exposed part of the superior temporal gyrus involves the auditory association or perception area (area 22). The aspects of hearing that attach meaning to certain sound patterns require that this area function properly. The remaining portions of the temporal cortex are less well defined, but apparently are important in long-term memory recall. This is particularly true with respect to perception and memory of complex sensory patterns such as geometric figures and faces (*i.e.,* recognition of "what" or "who" the stimulus is).

Occipital Lobe. The occipital lobe lies posterior to the temporal and parietal lobes and is arbitrarily separated from them (Fig. 48-21). The medial surface of the occipital lobe contains a deep sulcus extending from the limbic lobe to the occipital pole, the *calcarine sulcus,* which is surrounded by the primary visual cortex (area 17). Just superior and inferior and extending onto the lateral side of the occipital pole is the *visual association cortex* (areas 18 and 19). This area is closely connected with the primary visual cortex and with complex nuclei of the thalamus. Integrity of the association cortex is required for gnostic visual function, by which the meaningfulness of visual experience, including experiences of color, motion, depth perception, pattern, form, and location in space, takes place.

The neocortical areas of the parietal lobe, between the somesthetic and the visual cortices, have a function in relating the texture, or "feel," and location of an object with its visual image. Between the auditory and visual association areas, the *parieto-occipital region* is necessary for relating the meaningfulness of a sound and image to an object or person.

Limbic System. The medial aspect of the cerebrum is organized into concentric bands of cortex, the *limbic system* (from the Latin for "border"), which surrounds the connection between the lateral and third ventricles. The innermost band just above and below the cut surface of the corpus callosum is folded out of sight but is an ancient, three-layered cortex ending as the hippocampus in the temporal lobe. Just outside the folded area is a band of transitional cortex, which includes the cingulate and the parahippocampal gyri (Fig. 48-22). The limbic lobe has reciprocal connections with the medial and the intralaminar nuclei of the thalamus, with the deep nuclei of the cerebrum (*e.g.,* amygdaloid nuclei, septal nuclei), and with the hypothalamus. Overall, this region of the brain is involved in emotional experience and in the control of emotion-related behavior. Stimulation of specific areas in this system can lead to feelings of dread, high anxiety, or exquisite pleasure. It also can result in violent behaviors, including attack, defense, or explosive and emotional speech.

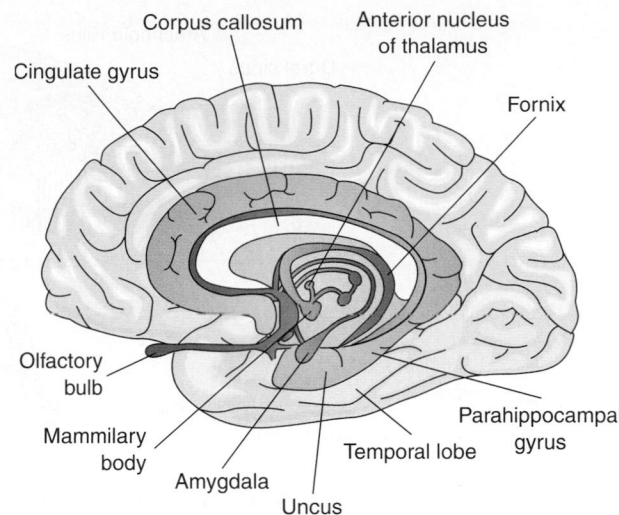

FIGURE 48-22 • The limbic system includes the limbic cortex (cingulate gyrus, parahippocampal gyrus, uncus) and associated subcortical structures (thalamus, hypothalamus, amygdala).

Meninges

Inside the skull and vertebral column, the brain and spinal cord are loosely suspended and protected by several connective tissue sheaths called the *meninges* (Fig. 48-23). All surfaces of the spinal cord, brain, and segmental nerves are covered with a delicate connective tissue layer called the *pia mater* (Latin for "delicate mother"). Surface blood vessels and those that penetrate the brain and spinal cord are encased in this protective tissue layer. A second, very delicate, nonvascular, and waterproof layer, called the *arachnoid,* encloses the entire CNS (Fig. 48-24). The arachnoid layer is named for its spider-web appearance. The CSF is contained in the subarachnoid space. Immediately outside the

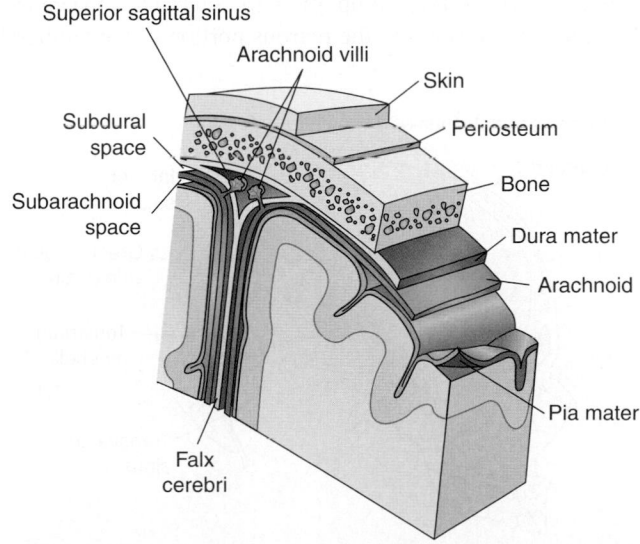

FIGURE 48-23 • The cranial meninges. Arachnoid villi, shown within the superior sagittal sinus, are one site of cerebrospinal fluid absorption into the blood.

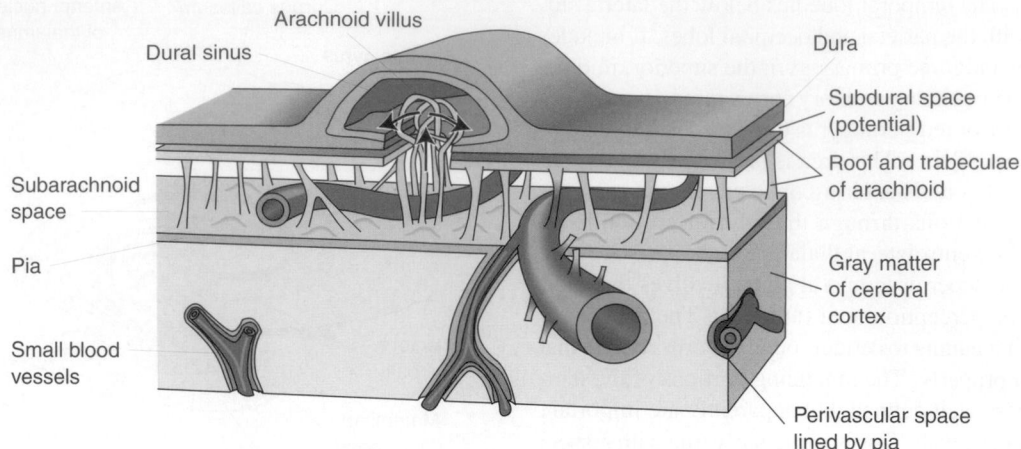

FIGURE 48-24 • Schematic diagram of the three connective tissue membranes (pia, arachnoid, and dura) constituting the meninges of the central nervous system. Cerebrospinal fluid is resorbed (*arrows*) through the arachnoid villi projecting into the dural sinuses. (From Cormack D. H. [1987]. *Ham's histology* [9th ed., p. 367]. Philadelphia: J.B. Lippincott.)

arachnoid is a continuous sheath of strong connective tissue, the *dura mater* (*i.e.,* "tough mother"), which provides the major protection for the brain and spinal cord. The cranial dura often splits into two layers, with the outer layer serving as the periosteum of the inner surface of the skull.

The inner layer of the dura forms two major infoldings: a longitudinal infolding called the *falx cerebri* and a transverse infolding called the *tentorium cerebelli* that anchor the brain to the skull (Fig. 48-25). The falx cerebri (from the Latin *falx,* "sickle-shaped") lies in the longitudinal fissure and separates the two cerebral hemispheres. It attaches to the crista of the ethmoid bone anteriorly and ends by becoming continuous with the tentorium cerebelli. The tentorium cerebelli is a wide crescentic septum that acts as a hammock, supporting the occipital lobes above the cerebellum. The falx cerebri attaches to the tentorium cerebri and holds it up, giving it a tentlike appearance. The tentorium attaches to the petrous portion of the temporal

bone and the dorsum sellae of the cranial floor, with a semicircular gap, or incisura, formed at the midline to permit the midbrain to pass forward from the posterior fossa. It also forms a tough septum, separating the anterior and middle cranial fossae, which contain the cerebral hemispheres, from the posterior fossa, found interiorly and containing the brain stem and cerebellum. This compartmentalization is the basis for the commonly used terms *supratentorial* (*i.e.,* above the tentorium) and *infratentorial* (*i.e.,* below the tentorium). The cerebral hemispheres and the diencephalon are supratentorial structures, and the pons, cerebellum, and medulla are infratentorial structures.

The tentorium and falx cerebri normally support and protect the brain, which floats in CSF within the enclosed space. During extreme trauma, however, the sharp edges of these folds can damage the brain. Space-occupying lesions such as enlarging tumors or hematomas can squeeze the brain against these edges or through the incisura of the tentorium (*i.e.,* herniation). As a result, brain tissue can be compressed, contused, or destroyed, often causing permanent deficits (see Chapter 51).

Ventricular System and Cerebrospinal Fluid

The ventricular system is a series of CSF-filled cavities in the brain (Fig. 48-26). The CSF provides a supporting and protective fluid in which the brain and spinal cord float. CSF helps maintain a constant ionic environment that serves as a medium for diffusion of nutrients, electrolytes, and metabolic end products into the extracellular fluid surrounding CNS neurons and neuroglia. Filling the ventricles, the CSF supports the mass of the brain. Because it fills the subarachnoid space surrounding the CNS, a physical force delivered to either the skull or spine is to some extent diffused and cushioned.

The ventricles and central canal of the spinal cord are lined by a thin layer of neuroglial cells collectively termed the *ependyma.* There is a tremendous expansion of the ependyma in the roof of the lateral, third, and fourth ventricles. The CSF

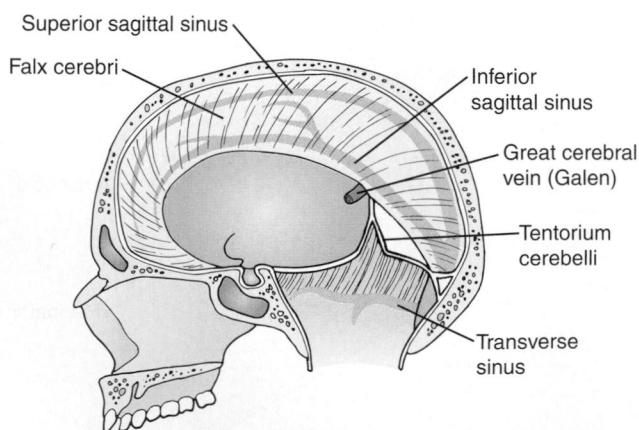

FIGURE 48-25 • Cranial dura mater. The skull is open to show the falx cerebri and the right and left portions of the tentorium cerebelli, as well as some of the cranial venous sinuses.

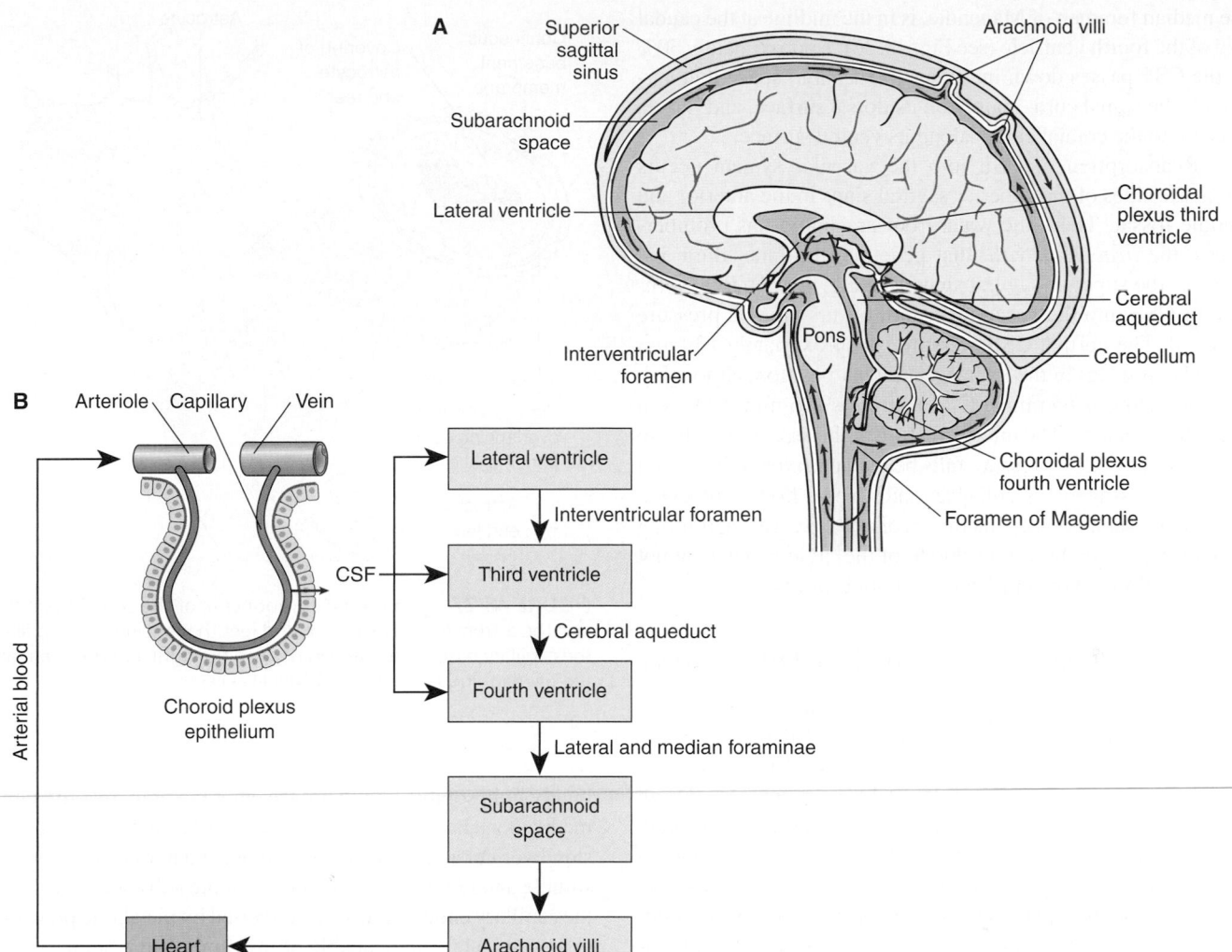

FIGURE 48-26 • **(A)** The flow of cerebrospinal fluid (CSF) from the time of its formation from blood in the choroid plexuses until its return to the blood in the superior sagittal sinus. Plexuses in the lateral ventricles are not illustrated. **(B)** CSF is a blood filtrate produced by the choroid plexus epithelium that is found in each brain ventricle. The flow of CSF from the lateral ventricles flows through the interventricular foramen (Monroe) into the third ventricle. From the third ventricle, CSF is conveyed to the fourth ventricle via the cerebral aqueduct (Sylvius). Three openings, a midline foramen of Magendie and two lateral foramina (Luschka), pass the CSF into the subarachnoid space, where it is returned to the venous circulation through the arachnoid villi.

is produced by tiny reddish masses of specialized ependymal cells and capillaries, called the *choroid plexus,* that project into the ventricles. CSF is an ultrafiltrate of blood plasma, composed of 99% water with other constituents, making it close to the composition of the brain extracellular fluid (Table 48-3). Humans secrete approximately 500 mL of CSF each day. However, only approximately 150 mL is in the ventricular system at any one time, meaning that the CSF is continuously being absorbed.

The CSF produced in the ventricles must flow through the interventricular foramen, the third ventricle, the cerebral aqueduct, and the fourth ventricle to exit from the ventricular system. Three openings, or foramina, allow the CSF to pass into the subarachnoid space. Two of these, the foramina of Luschka, are located at the lateral corners of the fourth ventricle. The third,

TABLE 48-3 Composition of Cerebrospinal Fluid Compared With Plasma

SUBSTANCE	PLASMA	CEREBROSPINAL FLUID
Protein mg/dL	6000.00	20.00
Na$^+$ mEq/L	145.00	141.00
CL$^-$ mEq/L	101.00	124.00
K$^+$ mEq/L	4.50	2.90
HCO$_3^-$ mEq/L	25.00	24.00
pH	7.4	7.32
Glucose mg/dL	92.00	61.00

the median foramen of Magendie, is in the midline at the caudal end of the fourth ventricle (see Fig. 48-26). Approximately 30% of the CSF passes down into the subarachnoid space that surrounds the spinal cord, mainly on its dorsal surface, and moves back up to the cranial cavity along its ventral surface.

Reabsorption of CSF into the vascular system occurs along the sides of the superior sagittal sinus in the anterior and middle fossae. Here, the waterproof arachnoid has protuberances, the *arachnoid villi,* that penetrate the inner dura and walls of the superior sagittal sinus (see Fig. 48-24). Reabsorption of CSF into the vascular system occurs along a pressure gradient. The normal CSF pressure is approximately 130 mm H_2O (10 mm Hg) in the lateral recumbent position, although it may be as low as 65 mm H_2O to as high as 195 mm H_2O, even in healthy persons. The microstructure of the arachnoid villi are such that if the CSF pressure falls below approximately 50 mm H_2O, the passageways collapse, and reverse flow is blocked. Thus, the arachnoid villi function as one-way valves, permitting CSF outflow into the venous blood of the sagittal sinus but not allowing blood to pass into the arachnoid spaces.

Blood-Brain and Cerebrospinal Fluid–Brain Barriers

Maintenance of a chemically stable environment is essential to the function of the brain. In most regions of the body, extracellular fluid undergoes small fluctuations in pH and concentrations of hormones, amino acids, and potassium ions during routine daily activities such as eating and exercising. If the brain were to undergo such fluctuations, the result would be uncontrolled neural activity because some substances such as amino acids act as neurotransmitters, and ions such as potassium influence the threshold for neural firing. Two barriers, the blood-brain barrier and the CSF-brain barrier, provide the means for maintaining the stable chemical environment of the brain. Only water, carbon dioxide, and oxygen enter the brain with relative ease; the transport of other substances between the brain and the blood is slower and more controlled.

The blood-brain barrier depends on the unique characteristics of the brain capillaries. Endothelial cells of brain capillaries are joined by continuous tight junctions. In addition, most brain capillaries are surrounded by a basement membrane and by the processes of supporting cells of the brain, called *astrocytes* (Fig. 48-27). The blood-brain barrier permits passage of essential substances while excluding unwanted materials. Reverse transport systems remove materials from the brain. Large molecules, such as proteins and peptides, are largely excluded from crossing the blood-brain barrier. Acute cerebral lesions, such as trauma and infection, increase the permeability of the blood-brain barrier and alter brain concentrations of proteins, water, and electrolytes.

The blood-brain barrier prevents many drugs from entering the brain. Most highly water-soluble compounds are excluded from the brain, especially molecules with high ionic charge such as many of the catecholamines. In contrast, many lipid-soluble molecules cross the lipid layers of the blood-brain barrier with ease. Some drugs, such as the antibiotic chloramphenicol, are

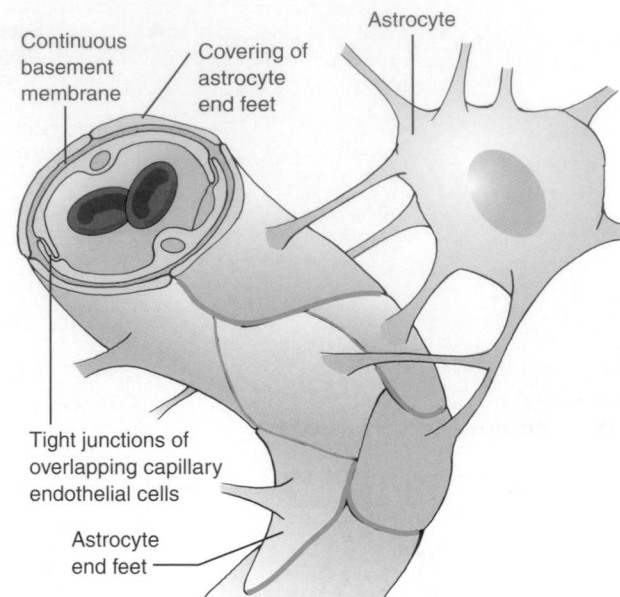

FIGURE 48-27 • The three components of the blood-brain barrier: the astrocyte and astrocyte end feet that encircle the capillary, the capillary basement membrane, and the tight junctions that join the overlapping capillary endothelial cells.

highly lipid soluble and therefore enter the brain readily. Other medications have a low solubility in lipids and enter the brain slowly or not at all. Alcohol, nicotine, and heroin are very lipid soluble and rapidly enter the brain. Some substances that enter the capillary endothelium are converted by metabolic processes to a chemical form incapable of moving into the brain.

The cerebral capillaries are much more permeable at birth than in adulthood, and the blood-brain barrier develops during the early years of life. In severely jaundiced infants, bilirubin can cross the immature blood-brain barrier, producing kernicterus and brain damage (see Chapter 14). In adults, the mature blood-brain barrier prevents bilirubin from entering the brain, and the nervous system is not affected.

The ependymal cells covering the choroid plexus are linked together by tight junctions, forming a blood-CSF barrier to diffusion of many molecules from the blood plasma of choroid plexus capillaries to the CSF. Water is transported through the choroid epithelial cells by osmosis. Oxygen and carbon dioxide move into the CSF by diffusion, resulting in partial pressures roughly equal to those of plasma. The high sodium and low potassium contents of the CSF are actively regulated and kept relatively constant. Lipids and nonpeptide hormones diffuse through the barrier rather easily, but most large molecules, such as proteins, peptides, many antibiotics, and other medications, do not normally get through. The choroid epithelium uses energy in the form of adenosine triphosphate (ATP) to actively secrete many components into the CSF, including proteins, sodium ions, and several micronutrients such as vitamins C, B_6 (pyridoxine), and folate. Because the resultant CSF has a relatively high sodium content, the negatively charged chloride and bicarbonate diffuse into the CSF along an ionic gradient. The choroid cells also generate bicarbonate from carbon dioxide in the blood. This bicarbonate is important to the regulation of the pH of the CSF.

Mechanisms exist that facilitate the transport of other molecules such as glucose without energy expenditure. Ammonia, a toxic metabolite of neuronal activity, is converted to glutamine by astrocytes. Glutamine moves by facilitated diffusion through the choroid epithelium into the plasma. This exemplifies a major function of the CSF, that of providing a means of removal of toxic waste products from the CNS. Because the brain and spinal cord have no lymphatic channels, the CSF serves this function.

Several specific areas of the brain do not have a blood-CSF barrier. One such area is at the caudal end of the fourth ventricle (*i.e.*, area postrema), where specialized receptors for the CSF carbon dioxide level influence respiratory function. Another area is the walls of the third ventricle, which permit hypothalamic neurons to monitor blood glucose levels. This permits hypothalamic centers to sense and respond to changes in blood glucose levels through hunger and eating behaviors. Although most of the cells lining the third ventricle are ependymal cells, modified ependymal cells called *tanycytes* are also present. Processes of tanycytes extend through the glial lining of the third ventricle to terminate on blood vessels, neurons, or glial cells of the surrounding brain tissue. Evidence suggests that tanycytes may have important neuroendocrine functions besides their function as barrier cells. For example, tanycytes express high levels of the enzyme needed to convert thyroxine (T_4) into the more potent triiodothyronine (T_3) form.

IN SUMMARY, in the adult, the spinal cord is in the upper two thirds of the spinal canal of the vertebral column. On transverse section, the spinal cord has an oval shape. Internally, the gray matter has the appearance of a butterfly or letter "H." The dorsal horns contain the IA neurons and receive afferent information from dorsal root and other connecting neurons. The ventral horns contain the OA neurons and efferent LMNs that leave the cord by the ventral roots. Thirty-two pairs of spinal nerves (*i.e.*, 8 cervical, 12 thoracic, 5 lumbar, 5 sacral, and 2 or more coccygeal) are present. Each pair communicates with its corresponding body segments. The spinal nerves and the blood vessels that supply the spinal cord enter the spinal canal through an intervertebral foramen. After entering the foramen, they divide into two branches, or roots, one of which enters the dorsolateral surface of the cord (*i.e.*, dorsal root), carrying the axons of afferent neurons into the CNS. The other root leaves the ventrolateral surface of the cord (*i.e.*, ventral root), carrying the axons of efferent neurons into the periphery. These two roots fuse at the intervertebral foramen, forming the mixed spinal nerve.

A reflex provides a highly reliable relation between a stimulus and a motor response. Its anatomic basis consists of an afferent neuron, the connection or synapse with CNS neurons that communicate with the effector neuron, and the effector

neuron that innervates a muscle or organ. Reflexes are essentially "wired in" to the CNS in that normally they are always ready to function; with training, most reflexes can be modulated to become parts of more complicated movements.

The brain can be divided into three parts, the hindbrain, midbrain, and forebrain. The hindbrain, consisting of the medulla oblongata, pons, and cerebellum, contains the neuronal circuits for the eating, breathing, and locomotive functions required for survival. Cranial nerves XII, XI, X, IX, VIII, VII, VI, and V are located in the hindbrain, and CNs III and IV arise from the midbrain. The forebrain is the most rostral part of the brain; it consists of the diencephalon and the telencephalon. The dorsal horn part of the diencephalon comprises the thalamus and subthalamus, and the ventral horn part is the hypothalamus. The cerebral hemispheres are lateral outgrowths of the diencephalon.

The cerebral hemispheres are arbitrarily divided into lobes—the frontal, parietal, temporal, and occipital lobes—named after the bones of the skull that cover them. Contained in the frontal lobe are the prefrontal premotor area and primary motor cortex; the primary sensory cortex and somesthetic association area are in the parietal cortex; the primary auditory cortex and the auditory association area are in the temporal lobe; and the primary visual cortex and association visual cortex are in the occipital lobe. The limbic system, which is involved in emotional experience and release of emotional behaviors, is located in the medial aspect of the cerebrum. These cortical areas are reciprocally connected with underlying thalamic nuclei through the internal capsule. Thalamic involvement is essential for normal forebrain function.

The brain is enclosed and protected by the pia mater, arachnoid, and dura mater. The protective CSF in which the brain and spinal cord float isolates them from minor and moderate trauma. CSF is secreted into the ventricles by the ependymal cells of the choroid plexus, circulates through the ventricular system, and is reabsorbed into the venous system through the arachnoid villi. The CSF-brain barrier and the blood-brain barrier protect the brain from substances in the blood that would disrupt brain function. ∎

THE AUTONOMIC NERVOUS SYSTEM

After completing this section of the chapter, you should be able to meet the following objectives:

■ Compare the sensory and motor components of the autonomic nervous system with those of the CNS.
■ Compare the anatomic location and functions of the sympathetic and parasympathetic nervous systems.
■ Describe neurotransmitter synthesis, release, and degradation, and receptor function in the sympathetic and parasympathetic nervous systems.

The ability to maintain homeostasis and perform the activities of daily living in an ever-changing physical environment is largely vested in the autonomic nervous system (ANS). This portion of the nervous system functions at the subconscious level and is involved in regulating, adjusting, and coordinating vital visceral functions such as blood pressure and blood flow, body temperature, respiration, digestion, metabolism, and elimination. The ANS is strongly affected by emotional influences and is involved in many of the expressive aspects of behavior. Blushing, pallor, palpitations of the heart, clammy hands, and dry mouth are several emotional expressions mediated through the ANS. Biofeedback and relaxation exercises have been used for modifying the subconscious functions of the ANS.

🔑 THE AUTONOMIC NERVOUS SYSTEM (ANS)

- The ANS functions at the subconscious level and is responsible for maintaining homeostatic functions of the body.

- The ANS has two divisions: the sympathetic and parasympathetic systems. Although the two divisions function in concert, they are generally viewed as having opposite and antagonistic actions.

- The sympathetic division functions in maintaining vital functions and responding when there is a critical threat to the integrity of the individual—the "fight-or-flight" response.

- The parasympathetic nervous system is concerned with conservation of energy, resource replenishment, and maintenance of organ function during periods of minimal activity.

- The outflow of both divisions of the ANS consists of a two-neuron pathway: a preganglionic and a postganglionic neuron. Acetylcholine is the neurotransmitter for the preganglionic neurons for both ANS divisions, as well as the postganglionic neurons of the parasympathetic nervous system. Norepinephrine and epinephrine are the neurotransmitters for most sympathetic postganglionic neurons.

As with the somatic nervous system, the ANS is represented in both the CNS and the PNS. Traditionally, the ANS has been defined as a general efferent system innervating visceral organs. The efferent outflow from the ANS has two divisions: the sympathetic nervous system and the parasympathetic nervous system. Afferent inputs to the ANS are provided by visceral afferent neurons and are not usually considered a part of the ANS.

The functions of the sympathetic nervous system include maintaining body temperature and adjusting blood flow and blood pressure to meet the changing needs of the body. These adjustments occur in response to changes in routine activities of daily living, such as moving from the supine to the standing position. The sympathoadrenal system also can discharge as a unit

when there is a critical threat to the integrity of the individual—the so-called fight-or-flight response. During a stress situation, the heart rate accelerates; blood pressure rises; blood flow shifts from the skin and gastrointestinal tract to the skeletal muscles and brain; blood sugar increases; the bronchioles and pupils dilate; the sphincters of the stomach and intestine and the internal sphincter of the urethra constrict; and the rate of secretion of exocrine glands involved in digestion diminishes. Emergency situations often require vasoconstriction and shunting of blood away from the skin and into the muscles and brain, a mechanism that, should a wound occur, provides for a reduction in blood flow and preservation of vital functions needed for survival. Sympathetic function is often summarized as "catabolic" in that its actions predominate during periods of pronounced energy expenditure, such as when survival is threatened.

In contrast to the sympathetic nervous system, the functions of the parasympathetic nervous system are concerned with conservation of energy, resource replenishment and storage, and maintenance of organ function during periods of minimal activity—the *rest-digest* response. The parasympathetic nervous system slows heart rate, stimulates gastrointestinal function and related glandular secretion, promotes bowel and bladder elimination, and contracts the pupil, protecting the retina from excessive light during periods when visual function is not vital to survival. The two divisions of the ANS are usually viewed as having opposite and antagonistic actions (*i.e.,* if one activates, the other inhibits a function). Exceptions are functions, such as sweating and regulation of arteriolar blood vessel diameter, controlled by a single division of the ANS, in this case the sympathetic nervous system.

The sympathetic and parasympathetic nervous systems are continually active. The effect of this continual or basal (baseline) activity is referred to as *tone*. The tone of an effector organ or system can be increased or decreased and is usually regulated by a single division of the ANS. For example, vascular smooth muscle tone is controlled by the sympathetic nervous system. Increased sympathetic activity produces local vasoconstriction from increased vascular smooth muscle tone, and decreased activity results in vasodilation due to decreased tone. In structures such as the sinoatrial node and atrioventricular node of the heart, which are innervated by both divisions of the ANS, one division predominates in controlling tone. In this case, the tonically active parasympathetic nervous system exerts a constraining or braking effect on heart rate, and when parasympathetic outflow is withdrawn, similar to releasing a brake, the heart rate increases. The increase in heart rate that occurs with vagal withdrawal can be further augmented by sympathetic stimulation. Table 48-4 describes the responses of effector organs to sympathetic and parasympathetic impulses.

Autonomic Efferent Pathways

The outflow of both divisions of the ANS follows a two-neuron pathway. The first motor neuron, called the *preganglionic neuron,* lies in the intermediolateral cell column of the spinal cord or its equivalent location in the brain stem. The second motor neuron, called the *postganglionic neuron,* synapses with a pre-

TABLE 48-4 **Characteristics of the Sympathetic and Parasympathetic Nervous Systems**		
CHARACTERISTIC	**SYMPATHETIC OUTFLOW**	**PARASYMPATHETIC OUTFLOW**
Location of preganglionic cell bodies	T1–T12, L1 and L2	Cranial nerves: III, VII (intermedius), IX, and X; sacral segments 2, 3, and 4
Relative length of preganglionic fibers	Short—to paravertebral chain of ganglia or to aortic prevertebral of ganglia	Long—to ganglion cells near or in the innervated organ
General function	Catabolic—mobilizes resources in anticipation of challenge for survival (preparation for "fight-or-flight" response)	Anabolic—concerned with conservation, renewal, and storage of resources
Nature of peripheral response	Generalized	Localized
Transmitter between preganglionic terminals and postganglionic neurons	ACh	ACh
Transmitter of postganglionic neuron	ACh (sweat glands and skeletal muscle vasodilator fibers); norepinephrine (most synapses); norepinephrine and epinephrine (secreted by adrenal gland)	ACh

ACh, acetylcholine.

ganglionic neuron in an autonomic ganglion in the PNS. The two divisions of the ANS differ as to location of their preganglionic cell bodies, the relative length of their preganglionic fibers, the nature of their peripheral responses, and their preganglionic and postganglionic neurotransmitters (see Table 48-4). This two-neuron pathway and the interneurons in the autonomic ganglia that add further modulation to ANS function are distinctly different from arrangements in the somatic nervous system.

Most visceral organs are innervated by both sympathetic and parasympathetic fibers. Exceptions include structures such as blood vessels and sweat glands that have input from only one division of the ANS. The fibers of the sympathetic nervous system are distributed to effectors throughout the body and, as a result, sympathetic actions tend to be more diffuse than those of the parasympathetic nervous system, in which there is a more localized distribution of fibers. The preganglionic fibers of the sympathetic nervous system may traverse a considerable distance and pass through several ganglia before synapsing with postganglionic neurons, and their terminals contact many postganglionic fibers. In some ganglia, the ratio of preganglionic to postganglionic cells may be 1:20; because of this, the effects of sympathetic stimulation are diffuse. Considerable overlap exists, and one ganglion cell may be supplied by several preganglionic fibers. In contrast to the sympathetic nervous system, the parasympathetic nervous system has its postganglionic neurons located very near or in the organ of innervation. Because the ratio of preganglionic to postganglionic communication is often 1:1, the effects of the parasympathetic nervous system are much more circumscribed.

Sympathetic Nervous System

The neurons of the sympathetic nervous system are located primarily in the intermediolateral cell column of the thoracic and upper lumbar segments (T1 to L2) of the spinal cord; hence, the sympathetic nervous system is often called the *thoracolumbar*

division of the ANS. These preganglionic neurons have axons that are largely myelinated and relatively short. Postganglionic neurons of the sympathetic nervous system are located in the paravertebral ganglia of the sympathetic chain of ganglia that lie on either side of the vertebral column, or in prevertebral sympathetic ganglia such as the celiac ganglia (Fig. 48-28). Besides postganglionic efferent neurons, the sympathetic ganglia contain neurons of the internuncial, short-axon type, similar to those associated with complex circuitry in the brain and spinal cord. Many of these inhibit and others modulate preganglionic-to-postganglionic transmission.

The axons of the preganglionic neurons leave the spinal cord through the ventral roots of the spinal nerves (T1 to L2), enter the ventral primary rami, and leave the spinal nerve through white rami of the rami communicantes to reach the paravertebral ganglionic chain (Fig. 48-29). In the sympathetic chain of ganglia, preganglionic fibers may synapse with neurons of the ganglion they enter, pass up or down the chain and synapse with one or more ganglia, or pass through the chain and move outward through a splanchnic nerve to terminate in prevertebral ganglia (*i.e.,* celiac, superior mesenteric, or inferior mesenteric) scattered along the dorsal aorta and its branches.

Preganglionic fibers from the thoracic segments of the cord pass upward to form the cervical chain connecting the inferior, middle, and superior cervical sympathetic ganglia with the rest of the sympathetic chain at lower levels (see Fig. 48-28). Postganglionic sympathetic axons of the cervical and lower lumbosacral chain ganglia spread further through nerve plexuses along continuations of the great arteries. Cranial structures, particularly blood vessels, are innervated by the spread of postganglionic axons along the external and internal carotid arteries into the face and the cranial cavity. The sympathetic fibers from T1 usually continue up the sympathetic chain into the head; those from T2 pass into the neck; those from T1 to T5 travel to the heart; those from T3, T4, T5, and T6 proceed to the thoracic viscera; those from T7, T8, T9, T10, and T11 pass to the abdominal

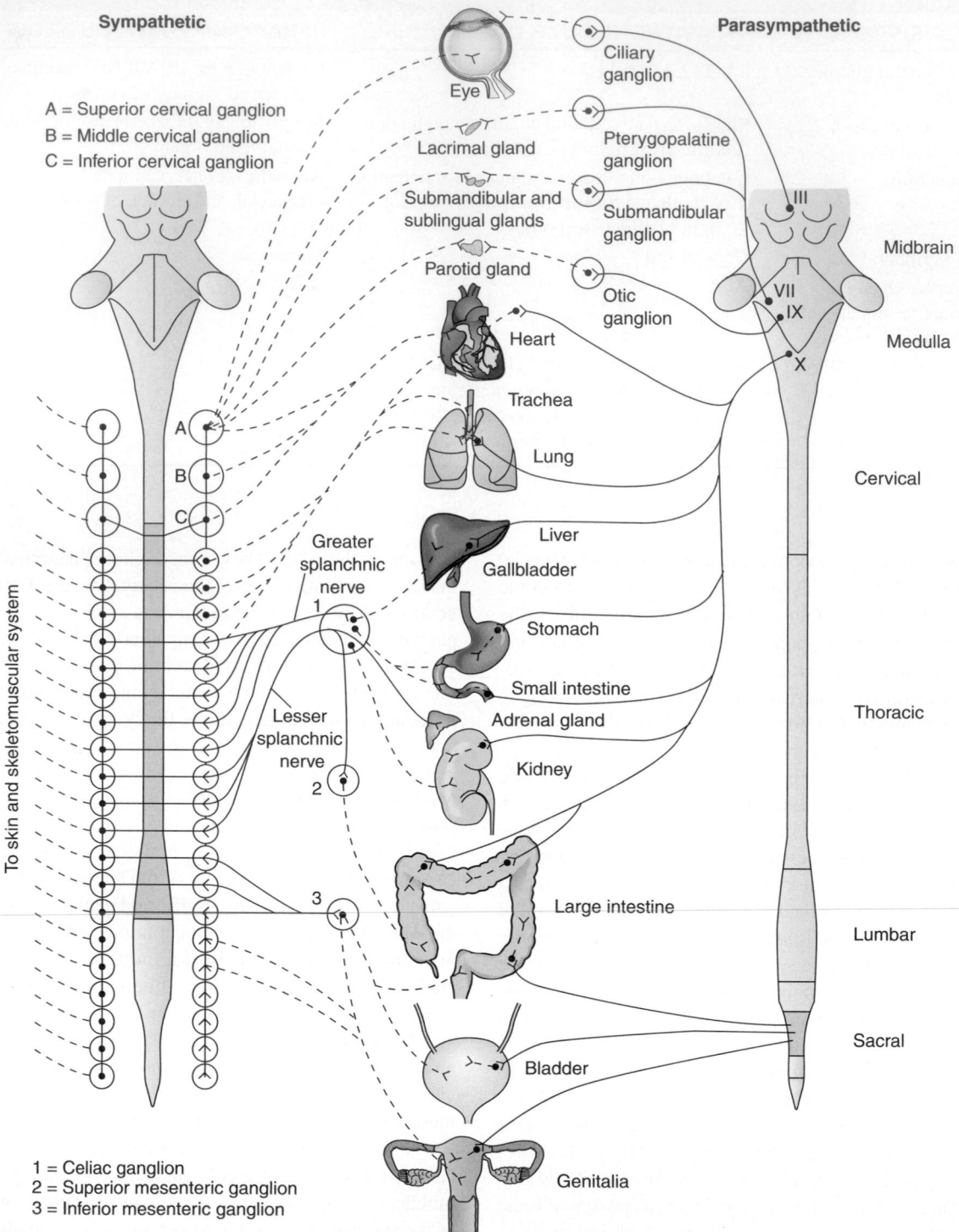

Sympathetic

A = Superior cervical ganglion
B = Middle cervical ganglion
C = Inferior cervical ganglion

Parasympathetic

Eye
Ciliary ganglion

Lacrimal gland
Pterygopalatine ganglion

Submandibular and sublingual glands
Submandibular ganglion

Parotid gland
Otic ganglion

Heart

Trachea

Lung

Liver

Gallbladder

Stomach

Small intestine

Adrenal gland

Kidney

Large intestine

Bladder

Genitalia

Greater splanchnic nerve

Lesser splanchnic nerve

To skin and skeletomuscular system

A
B
C

1
2
3

Midbrain
Medulla
Cervical
Thoracic
Lumbar
Sacral

III
VII
IX
X

1 = Celiac ganglion
2 = Superior mesenteric ganglion
3 = Inferior mesenteric ganglion

FIGURE 48-28 • The autonomic nervous system. The involuntary organs are depicted with their parasympathetic innervation (craniosacral) indicated on the right and sympathetic innervation (thoracolumbar) on the left. Preganglionic fibers are *solid lines;* postganglionic fibers are *dashed lines.* For purposes of illustration, the sympathetic outflow to the skin and skeletomuscular system is shown separately (to the far left); effectors include sweat glands, pilomotor muscles and blood vessels of the skin, and blood vessels of the skeletal muscles and bones. (Modified from Hemer L. [1983]. *The human brain and spinal cord: Functional neuroanatomy and dissection guide.* New York: Springer-Verlag.)

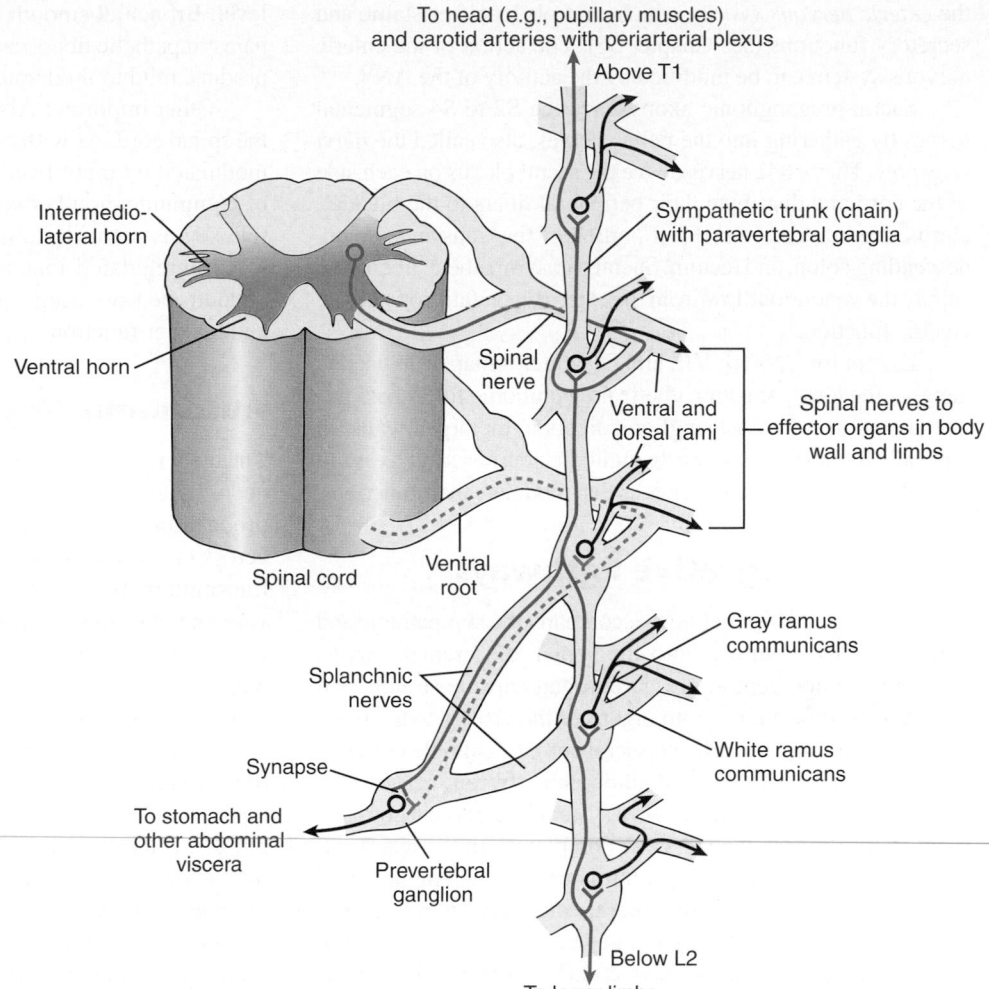

To head (e.g., pupillary muscles) and carotid arteries with periarterial plexus

Above T1

Intermedio-lateral horn

Sympathetic trunk (chain) with paravertebral ganglia

Ventral horn

Spinal nerve

Ventral and dorsal rami

Spinal nerves to effector organs in body wall and limbs

Spinal cord

Ventral root

Gray ramus communicans

Splanchnic nerves

White ramus communicans

Synapse

To stomach and other abdominal viscera

Prevertebral ganglion

Below L2

To lower limbs

FIGURE 48-29 • Sympathetic pathways. Sympathetic preganglionic fibers (*blue*) leave the spinal cord by way of the ventral root of the spinal nerves, enter the ventral primary rami, and pass through the white rami to the prevertebral or paravertebral ganglia of the sympathetic chain, where they synapse with postganglionic neurons (*black*). Other preganglionic neurons (*red dotted lines*) travel directly to their destination in the various effector organs.

viscera; and those from T12, L1, L2, and L3 pass to the kidneys and pelvic organs. Many preganglionic fibers from the fifth to the last thoracolumbar segments pass through the paravertebral ganglia to continue as the splanchnic nerves. Most of these fibers do not synapse until they reach the celiac or superior mesenteric ganglion; others pass to the adrenal medulla.

The adrenal medulla, which is part of the sympathetic nervous system, contains postganglionic sympathetic neurons that secrete sympathetic neurotransmitters directly into the bloodstream. Some postganglionic fibers, all of which are unmyelinated, exit the paravertebral ganglionic chain and reenter the segmental nerve through unmyelinated branches, called *gray rami*. These segmental nerves are then distributed to all parts of the body wall in the spinal nerve branches. These fibers innervate the sweat glands, piloerector muscles of the hair follicles, all blood vessels of the skin and skeletal muscles, and the CNS itself.

Parasympathetic Nervous System

The preganglionic fibers of the parasympathetic nervous system, also called the *craniosacral division* of the ANS, originate in some segments of the brain stem and sacral segments of the

spinal cord (see Fig. 48-28). The central regions of origin are the midbrain, pons, medulla oblongata, and the sacral spinal cord. The midbrain outflow passes through the oculomotor nerve (CN III) to the ciliary ganglion that lies in the orbit behind the eye; it supplies the pupillary sphincter muscle of each eye and the ciliary muscles that control lens thickness for accommodation. From the caudal pontine outflow originates the preganglionic fibers of the intermedius component of the facial nerve (CN VII) complex. This outflow synapses in the submandibular ganglion, which sends postganglionic fibers to supply the submandibular and sublingual glands. In addition, preganglionic fibers are distributed to the pterygopalatine ganglia to synapse on postganglionic neurons that supply the lacrimal and nasal glands. Fibers in the glossopharyngeal nerve (CN IX) synapse in the otic ganglia, which supply the parotid salivary glands. Approximately 75% of parasympathetic efferent fibers are carried in the vagus nerve (CN X). The vagus nerve provides parasympathetic innervation for the heart, trachea, lungs, esophagus, stomach, small intestine, proximal half of the colon, liver, gallbladder, pancreas, kidneys, and upper portions of the ureters. The gastrointestinal tract has its own intrinsic network of ganglionic cells located between the smooth muscle layers, called the *enteric nervous system,* which controls local peristaltic and secretory functions (see Chapter 36). The action of the enteric nervous system can be modified by the activity of the ANS.

Sacral preganglionic axons leave the S2 to S4 segmental nerves by gathering into the pelvic nerves, also called the *nervi erigentes.* The pelvic nerves leave the sacral plexus on each side of the cord and distribute their peripheral fibers to the bladder, uterus, urethra, prostate, distal portion of the transverse colon, descending colon, and rectum. Sacral parasympathetic fibers also supply the venous outflow from the external genitalia to facilitate erectile function.

Except for CNs III, VII, and IX, which synapse in discrete ganglia, the long parasympathetic preganglionic fibers pass uninterrupted to short postganglionic fibers in the organ walls. In the walls of these organs, postganglionic neurons send axons to smooth muscle and glandular cells that modulate their functions.

Central Integrative Pathways

General visceral afferent fibers accompany the sympathetic and parasympathetic outflow into the spinal and cranial nerves, bringing chemoreceptor, pressure, organ capsule stretch, and nociceptive information from organs of the viscera to the brain stem, thoracolumbar cord, and sacral cord. Local reflex circuits relating visceral afferent and autonomic efferent activity are integrated into a hierarchic control system in the spinal cord and brain stem. Progressively greater complexity in the responses and greater precision in their control occur at each higher level of the nervous system. Most visceral reflexes contain contributions from the LMNs that innervate skeletal muscles as part of their response patterns. The distinction between purely visceral and somatic reflex hierarchies becomes less and less meaningful at the higher levels of hierarchic control and behavioral integration.

For most autonomically mediated functions, the hypothalamus serves as the major control center. The hypothalamus, with connections to the cerebral cortex, the limbic system, and the pituitary gland, is in a prime position to receive, integrate, and transmit information to other areas of the nervous system. Signals from the hypothalamus can affect almost all the brain stem control centers. For example, stimulation of certain areas, mainly in the posterior hypothalamus, can cause the cardiovascular control centers to increase the arterial blood pressure to more than twice normal. Likewise, other hypothalamic centers control body temperature and increase salivation and gastrointestinal activity.

Reflex adjustments of cardiovascular and respiratory function occur at the level of the brain stem. A prominent example is the carotid sinus baroreflex. Increased blood pressure in the carotid sinus results in increased discharge from afferent fibers that travel by way of CN IX to cardiovascular centers in the brain stem. These centers increase the activity of descending efferent vagal fibers that slow heart rate, while inhibiting sympathetic fibers that increase heart rate and blood vessel tone. Striking features of the ANS are the rapidity and intensity with which it can change visceral function. Within 3 to 5 seconds, it can increase the heart rate to approximately twice its resting

level. Bronchial smooth muscle tone is largely controlled by parasympathetic fibers carried in the vagus nerve. These nerves produce mild to moderate constriction of the bronchioles.

Other important ANS reflexes are located at the level of the spinal cord. As with other spinal reflexes, these reflexes are modulated by input from higher centers. When there is a loss of communication between the higher centers and the spinal reflexes, as occurs in spinal cord injury, these reflexes function in an unregulated manner (see Chapter 50). This results in uncontrolled sweating, vasomotor instability, and reflex bowel and bladder function.

Autonomic Neurotransmission

The generation and transmission of impulses in the ANS occur in the same manner as in other neurons. There are self-propagating action potentials with transmission of impulses across synapses and other tissue junctions by neurohumoral transmitters. However, the somatic motor neurons that innervate skeletal muscles divide into many branches, with each branch innervating a single muscle fiber; in contrast, the distribution of postganglionic fibers of the ANS forms a diffuse neural plexus at the site of innervation. The membranes of the cells of many smooth muscle fibers are connected by conductive protoplasmic bridges, called *gap junctions,* that permit rapid conduction of impulses through whole sheets of smooth muscle, often in repeating waves of contraction. Autonomic neurotransmitters released near a limited portion of these fibers provide a modulating function extending to many effector cells. Smooth muscle layers of the gut and of the bladder wall are examples. Sometimes, isolated smooth muscle cells are individually innervated by the ANS, such as the piloerector cells that elevate the hair on the skin during cold exposure.

The main neurotransmitters of the autonomic nervous system are acetylcholine and the catecholamines, epinephrine and norepinephrine (Fig. 48-30). Acetylcholine is released at all preganglionic synapses in the autonomic ganglia of both sympathetic and parasympathetic nerve fibers and from postganglionic synapses of all parasympathetic nerve endings. It also is released at sympathetic nerve endings that innervate the sweat glands and cholinergic vasodilator fibers found in skeletal muscle. Norepinephrine is released at most sympathetic nerve endings. The adrenal medulla, which is a modified prevertebral sympathetic ganglion, produces epinephrine along with small amounts of norepinephrine. Dopamine, which is an intermediate compound in the synthesis of norepinephrine, also acts as a neurotransmitter. It is the principal inhibitory transmitter of internuncial neurons in the sympathetic ganglia. It also has vasodilator effects on renal, splanchnic, and coronary blood vessels when given intravenously and is sometimes used in the treatment of shock (see Chapter 26).

Acetylcholine and Cholinergic Receptors

Acetylcholine is synthesized in the cholinergic neurons from choline and acetyl coenzyme A (acetyl CoA; Fig. 48-31A). After acetylcholine is secreted by the cholinergic nerve endings, it is

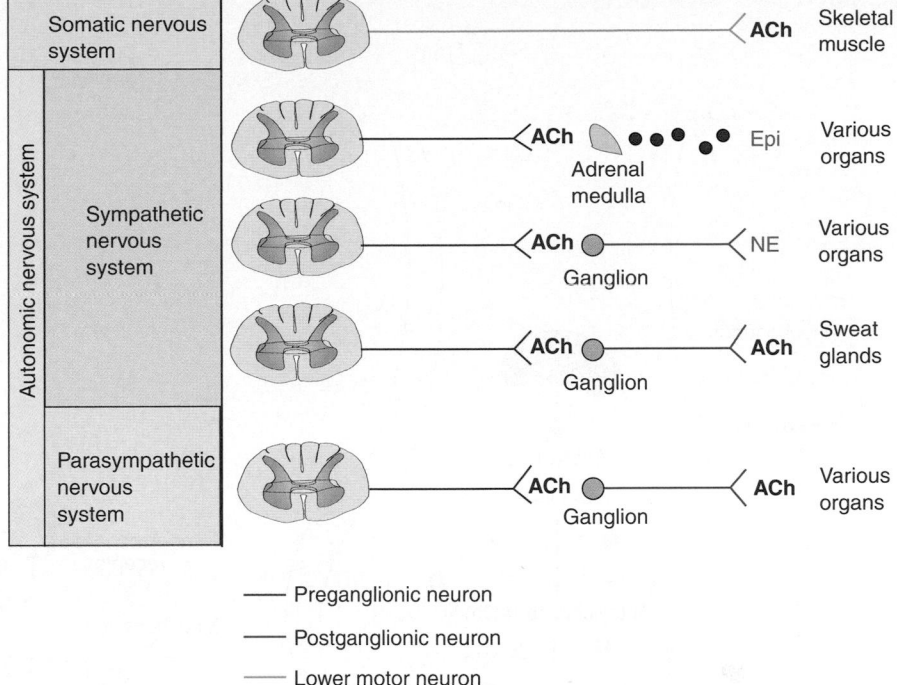

FIGURE 48-30 • Comparison of neurotransmission in the somatic and autonomic nervous systems. In the somatic nervous system, all lower motor neurons release acetylcholine (ACh) as their neurotransmitter. In the autonomic nervous system, both sympathetic and parasympathetic preganglionic neurons release ACh as their neurotransmitter. Parasympathetic postganglionic neurons release ACh at the site of organ innervation. Most postganglionic neurons of the sympathetic nervous system release norepinephrine (NE) at the site of organ innervation. The principal neurotransmitter released by the adrenal gland is epinephrine (Epi), which travels to the site of organ innervation through the bloodstream. The postganglionic neurons innervating the sweat gland are sympathetic fibers that use ACh as their neurotransmitter.

rapidly broken down by the enzyme acetylcholinesterase. The choline molecule is transported back into the nerve ending, where it is used again in the synthesis of acetylcholine.

Receptors that respond to acetylcholine are called *cholinergic receptors.* Two types of cholinergic receptors are known: muscarinic and nicotinic. Muscarinic receptors are present on the innervational targets of postganglionic fibers of the parasympathetic nervous system and the sweat glands, which are innervated by the sympathetic nervous system. Nicotinic receptors are found in autonomic ganglia and the end plates of skeletal muscle. Acetylcholine is excitatory to most muscarinic and nicotinic receptors, except those in the heart and lower esophagus, where it has an inhibitory effect. The drug atropine is an antimuscarinic or muscarinic cholinergic blocking drug that prevents the action of acetylcholine at excitatory and inhibitory muscarinic receptor sites. Because it is a muscarinic blocking drug, it exerts little effect at nicotinic receptor sites.

Catecholamines and Adrenergic Receptors

The catecholamines, which include norepinephrine, epinephrine, and dopamine, are synthesized in the axoplasm of sympathetic nerve terminal endings from the amino acid tyrosine (see Fig. 48-31B). During catecholamine synthesis, tyrosine is hydroxylated (*i.e.,* has a hydroxyl group added) to form DOPA, and DOPA is decarboxylated (*i.e.,* has a carboxyl group removed) to form dopamine. Dopamine in turn is hydroxylated to form norepinephrine. In the adrenal gland, an additional step occurs during which norepinephrine is methylated (*i.e.,* a methyl group is added) to form epinephrine.

Each step in sympathetic neurotransmitter synthesis requires a different enzyme, and the type of neurotransmitter produced depends on the types of enzymes that are available in a nerve terminal. For example, the postganglionic sympathetic neurons that supply blood vessels synthesize norepinephrine, but postganglionic neurons in the adrenal medulla produce epinephrine or norepinephrine. Epinephrine accounts for approximately 80% of the catecholamines released from the adrenal gland. The synthesis of epinephrine by the adrenal medulla is influenced by glucocorticoid secretion from the adrenal cortex. These hormones are transported through an intra-adrenal vascular network from the adrenal cortex to the adrenal medulla, where they cause the sympathetic neurons to increase their production of epinephrine through increased enzyme activity. Thus, any situation sufficiently stressful to evoke increased levels of glucocorticoids also increases epinephrine levels. As the catecholamines are synthesized, they are stored in vesicles. The final step of norepinephrine synthesis occurs in these vesicles. When an action potential reaches an axon terminal, the neurotransmitter molecules are released from the storage vesicles. The storage vesicles provide a means for concentrated storage of the catecholamines and protect the neurotransmitters from the cytoplasmic enzymes that degrade them.

Besides neuronal synthesis, a second major mechanism exists for the replenishment of norepinephrine in sympathetic nerve terminals. This mechanism consists of the active recapture or reuptake of the released neurotransmitter into the nerve terminal. Between 50% and 80% of the norepinephrine released during an action potential is removed from the synaptic area by an active reuptake process. This process stops the action of the neurotransmitter and allows it to be reused by the neuron. The remainder of the released catecholamines diffuses into the surrounding tissue fluids or is degraded by two special enzymes: catechol-*O*-methyltransferase, which is diffusely present in all tissues, and monoamine oxidase (MAO), which is found in the nerve endings. Some drugs, such as the tricyclic antidepressants,

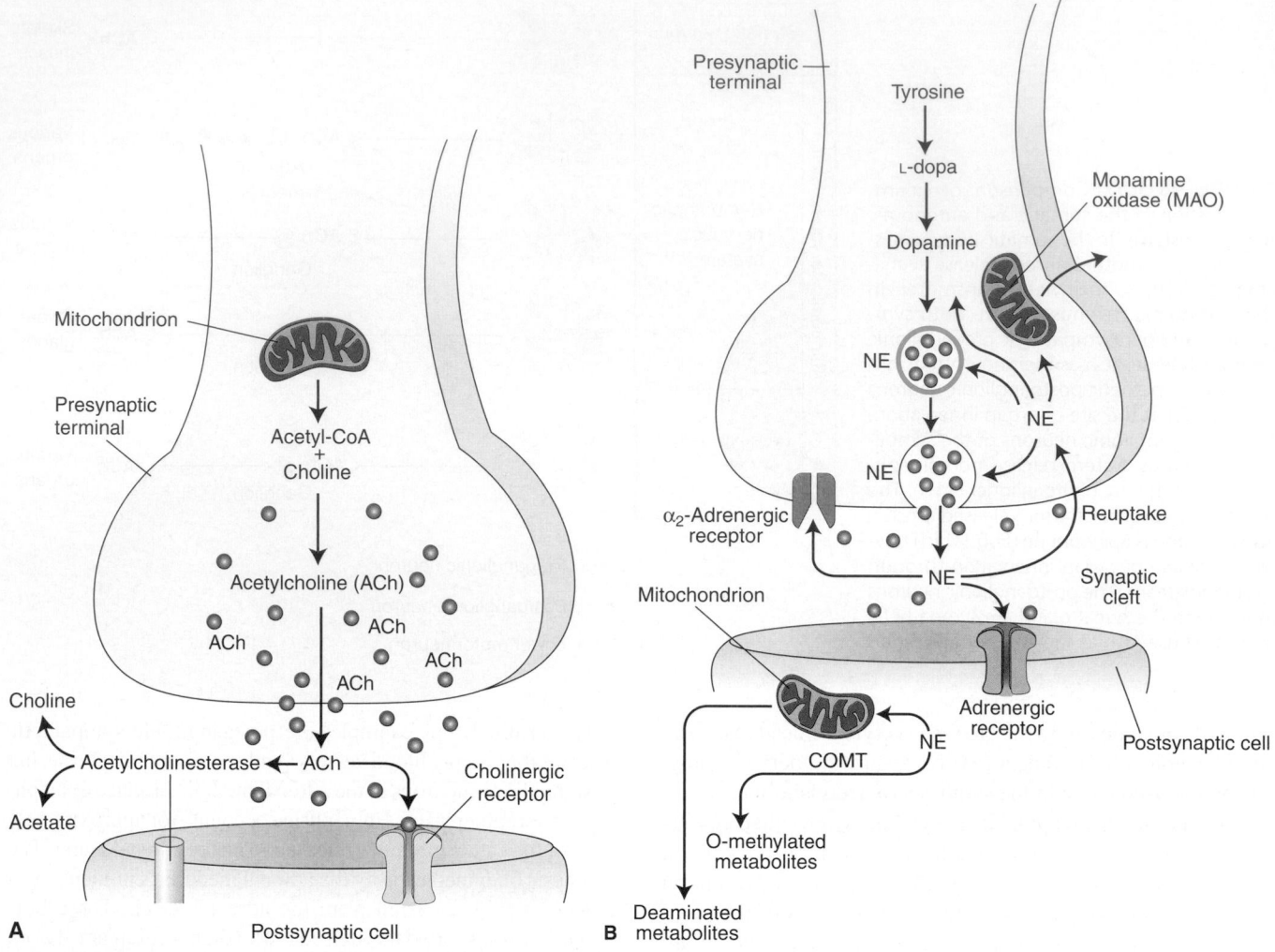

FIGURE 48-31 • Schematic illustration of cholinergic parasympathetic (**A**) and noradrenergic sympathetic (**B**) neurotransmitter synthesis, release, receptor binding, neurotransmitter degradation, and metabolite transport back into the presynaptic neuron (acetylcholine) and reuptake (norepinephrine). COMT, catechol-O-methyltransferase.

are thought to increase the level of catecholamines at the site of nerve endings in the brain by blocking the reuptake process. Others, such as the MAO inhibitors, increase the levels of neurotransmitters by decreasing their enzymatic degradation.

Catecholamines can cause excitation or inhibition of smooth muscle contraction, depending on the site, dose, and type of receptor present. Norepinephrine has potent excitatory activity and low inhibitory activity. Epinephrine is potent as both an excitatory and an inhibitory agent. The excitatory or inhibitory responses of organs to sympathetic neurotransmitters are mediated by interaction with special structures in the cell membrane called *receptors*. In 1948, Ahlquist proposed the designations α and β for the receptor sites where catecholamines produce their excitatory (α) and inhibitory (β) effects.

In vascular smooth muscle, excitation of α receptors causes vasoconstriction, and excitation of β receptors causes vasodilation. Endogenously and exogenously administered norepinephrine produces marked vasoconstriction of the blood vessels in

the skin, kidneys, and splanchnic circulation that are supplied with α receptors. The β receptors are most prevalent in the heart, the blood vessels of skeletal muscle, and the bronchioles. Blood vessels in skeletal muscle have α and β receptors. In these vessels, high levels of norepinephrine produce vasoconstriction; low levels produce vasodilation. The low levels are thought to have a diluting effect on norepinephrine levels in the arteries of these blood vessels so that the β effect predominates. With respect to vessels having few receptors, such as those that supply the brain, norepinephrine has little effect.

α-Adrenergic receptors have been further subdivided into α_1 and α_2 receptors, and β-adrenergic receptors into β_1 and β_2 receptors. β_1-Adrenergic receptors are found primarily in the heart and can be selectively blocked by β_1 receptor blocking drugs. β_2-Adrenergic receptors are found in the bronchioles and in other sites that have β-mediated functions. α_1-Adrenergic receptors are found primarily in postsynaptic effector sites; they mediate responses in vascular smooth muscle. α_2-Adrenergic receptors are mainly located presynaptically and can inhibit the release of norepinephrine from sympathetic nerve terminals. α_2-Adrenergic receptors are abundant in the CNS and are thought to influence the central control of blood pressure.

The various classes of adrenergic receptors provide a mechanism by which the same adrenergic neurotransmitter can have many selective effects on different effector cells. This mechanism also permits neurotransmitters carried in the blood-stream, whether from neuroendocrine secretion by the adrenal gland or from subcutaneously or intravenously administered drugs, to produce the same effects. The catecholamines produced and released from sympathetic nerve endings are called *endogenous neuromediators*. Sympathetic nerve endings also can be activated by exogenous forms of these neuromediators, which reach the nerve endings through the bloodstream after being injected into the body or administered orally. These drugs mimic the action of the neuromediators and are said to have a *sympathomimetic action*. Other drugs can selectively block the receptor sites on the neurons and temporarily prevent the neuro-transmitter from exerting its action.

IN SUMMARY, the ANS regulates, adjusts, and coordinates the visceral functions of the body. The ANS, which is divided into the sympathetic and parasympathetic systems, is an effer-ent system. It receives its afferent input from visceral afferent neurons. The ANS has CNS and PNS components. The outflow of the sympathetic and parasympathetic nervous systems fol-lows a two-neuron pathway, which consists of a preganglionic neuron in the CNS and a postganglionic neuron located outside the CNS. Sympathetic fibers leave the CNS at the thoraco-lumbar level, and the parasympathetic fibers leave at the cranial and sacral levels. Usually, the sympathetic and parasympathetic nervous systems have opposing effects on visceral function—if one excites, the other inhibits. The hypothalamus serves as the major control center for most ANS functions; local reflex circuits relating visceral afferent and autonomic efferent activity are integrated in a hierarchic control system in the spinal cord and brain stem.

The main neurotransmitters for the ANS are acetylcholine and the catecholamines, epinephrine and norepinephrine. Acetylcholine is the transmitter for all preganglionic neurons, for postganglionic parasympathetic neurons, and for selected postganglionic sympathetic neurons. The catecholamines are the neurotransmitters for most postganglionic sympathetic neu-rons. Neurotransmitters exert their target action through spe-cialized cell surface receptors—cholinergic receptors that bind acetylcholine and adrenergic receptors that bind the cate-cholamines. The cholinergic receptors are divided into nicotinic and muscarinic receptors, and adrenergic receptors are divided into α and β receptors. Different receptors for the same trans-mitter at various sites in the same tissue or in other tissues result in differences in tissue responses to the same transmit-ter. This arrangement also permits the use of pharmacologic agents that act at specific receptor types. ■

Review Exercises

1. Herpes zoster or shingles is a painful vesicular skin eruption involving the dermatomal distribution of a general somatic afferent nerve that is caused by reacti-vation of the chickenpox virus (varicella-zoster virus) that has remained dormant in the dorsal root ganglion since a childhood infection.

   A. *Explain.*

2. An event such as cardiac arrest, which produces global ischemia of the brain, can produce a selective loss of recent memory and cognitive skills, while the more vegetative and life-sustaining functions such as breathing are preserved.

   A. *Use principles related to the development of the nervous system and hierarchy of control to explain why.*

3. Usually spinal cord injury or disease produces both sensory and motor deficits. An exception is infection by the poliomyelitis virus, which produces weakness and paralysis without loss of sensation in the affected extremities.

   A. *Explain, using information on the cell column organization of the spinal cord.*

4. The functions of the sympathetic nervous system are often described in relation to the "fight-or-flight" response. Using this description, explain the physio-logic advantage for the following distribution of sym-pathetic nervous system receptors:

   A. *The presence of β_2 receptors on the blood vessels that provide blood flow to the skeletal muscles during "fight or flight," and the presence of α_1 receptors on the resistance vessels that control blood pressure.*

   B. *The presence of acetylcholine receptors on the sweat glands that allow for evaporative loss of body heat during "fight or flight," and the pres-ence of α_1 receptors that constrict the skin vessels that control blood flow to the skin.*

   C. *The presence of β_2 receptors that produce relax-ation in the detrusor muscle of the bladder during "fight or flight," and the presence of α_1 receptors that produce contraction of the smooth muscle in the internal sphincter of the bladder.*

Bibliography

Alberts B., Johnson A., Lewis J., et al. (2002). *Molecular biology of the cell* (4th ed., pp. 1227–1236). New York: Garland Science.

Bear M. F., Connors B. W., Paradiso M. A. (2001). *Neuroscience: Exploring the brain* (2nd ed.). Philadelphia: Lippincott Williams & Wilkins.

Brodal P. (1998). *The central nervous system: Structure and function* (2nd ed.). New York: Oxford University Press.

Carlson B. M. (2004). *Human embryology and developmental biology* (3rd ed., pp. 65–81, 103–127, 233–275, 277–290). St. Louis: C.V. Mosby.

Cochard L. R. (2002). *Netter's atlas of human embryology* (Chap. 3, pp. 51–81). Teterboro, NJ: Icon Learning Systems.

Filosa J. A., Bonev A. D., Straub S. V., et al. (2006). Local potassium signaling couples neuronal activity to vasodilation in the brain. *Nature Neuroscience* 9, 1397–1403.

Gartner L. P., Hiatt J. L. (2007). *Color textbook of histology* (3rd ed., pp. 185–218, 511–536). Philadelphia: Elsevier Saunders.

Haines D. E. (Ed.). (1997). *Fundamental neuroscience* (pp. 115–121, 126–127, 146–148, 443–454). New York: Churchill Livingstone.

Jung C., Chylinski T. M., Pimenta A., et al. (2004). Neurofilament transport is dependent on actin and myosin. *Journal of Neuroscience* 24, 9486–9496.

Kandel E. R., Schwartz J. H., Jessell T. M. (2000). *Principles of neural science* (4th ed.). New York: McGraw-Hill.

Kierszenbaum A. L. (2007). *Histology and cell biology: An introduction to pathology* (2nd ed., pp. 221–250, 251–290). St. Louis: Mosby.

Moore K. L., Dalley A. F. (2006). *Clinically oriented anatomy* (5th ed., pp. 885–955). Philadelphia: Lippincott Williams & Wilkins.

Moore K. L., Persaud T. V. N. (2003). *The developing human: Clinically oriented embryology* (7th ed., pp. 59–76, 427–463). Philadelphia: W. B. Saunders.

Parent A. (1996). *Carpenter's human neuroanatomy* (9th ed., pp. 186–192, 268–292, 748–756). Baltimore: Williams & Wilkins.

Rossi D. J. (2006). Another BOLD role for astrocytes: Coupling blood flow to neural activity. *Nature Neuroscience* 9, 159–160.

Sadler T. W. (2006). *Langman's medical embryology* (10th ed., pp. 5–10, 67–72, 285–316). Philadelphia: Lippincott Williams & Wilkins.

Sanes D. H., Reh T. A., Harris W. A. (2000). *Development of the nervous system.* San Diego: Academic Press.

Schliwa M. (2003). Kinesin: Walking or limping? *Nature Cell Biology* 5, 1043–1044.

Squire L. R., Bloom F. E., McConnell S. K., et al. (2003). *Fundamental neuroscience* (2nd ed., pp. 188–189, 391–416). New York: Academic Press.

Takano T., Tian G., Peng W., et al. (2006). Astrocyte-mediated control of cerebral blood flow. *Nature Neuroscience* 9, 260–267.

Tortora G. J., Derrickson B. (2009). *Principles of anatomy and physiology* (12th ed.). Hoboken, NJ: John Wiley & Sons.

Wong-Riley M. T. T. (2000). *Neuroscience secrets.* Philadelphia: Hanley & Belfus.

Zigmond M. J., Bloom E. F., Landis S. C., et al. (1999). *Fundamental neuroscience.* San Diego: Academic Press.

Visit the**Point** **http://thePoint.lww.com for animations, journal articles, and more!**

Chapter **49**

Somatosensory Function, Pain, and Headache

KIM LITWACK

Sensory mechanisms provide individuals with a continuous stream of information about their bodies, the outside world, and the interactions between the two. The somatosensory component of the nervous system provides an awareness of body sensations such as touch, temperature, limb position, and pain. Other sensory components of the nervous system include the special senses of vision, hearing, smell, and taste, which are discussed in other chapters. The sensory receptors for somatosensory function consist of discrete nerve endings in the skin and other body tissues. Between 2 and 3 million sensory neurons deliver a steady stream of encoded information. Only a small proportion of this information reaches awareness; most provides input essential for a myriad of reflex and automatic mechanisms that keep us alive and manage our functioning.

This chapter is organized into two distinct parts. The first part describes the organization and control of somatosensory function, and the second focuses on pain as a somatosensory modality.

ORGANIZATION AND CONTROL OF SOMATOSENSORY FUNCTION

After completing this section of the chapter, you should be able to meet the following objectives:

■ Describe the four major classes of somatosensory modalities.

(objectives continue)

1225

- Describe the organization of the somatosensory system in terms of first-, second-, and third-order neurons.
- Characterize the structure and function of the dorsal root ganglion neurons in terms of sensory receptors, conduction velocities, and spinal cord projections.
- Compare the discriminative pathway with the anterolateral pathway, and explain the clinical usefulness of this distinction.
- Compare the tactile, thermal, and position sense modalities in terms of receptors, adequate stimuli, ascending pathways, and central integrative mechanisms.
- Describe the role of clinical examination in assessing somatosensory function.

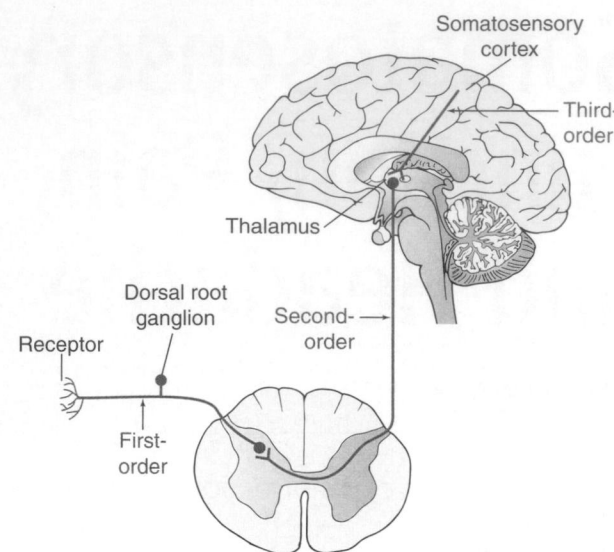

FIGURE 49-1 • Arrangement of first-order, second-order, and third-order neurons of the somatosensory system.

The somatosensory system is designed to provide the central nervous system (CNS) with information related to deep and superficial body structures as compared with the special senses such as sight and hearing. Sensory neurons can be divided into three types that vary in distribution and the type of sensation detected: general somatic, special somatic, and general visceral. *General somatic afferent neurons* have branches with widespread distribution throughout the body and with many distinct types of receptors that result in sensations such as pain, touch, and temperature. *Special somatic afferent neurons* have receptors located primarily in muscles, tendons, and joints. These receptors sense position and movement of the body. *General visceral afferent neurons* have receptors on various visceral structures that sense fullness and discomfort.

Sensory Systems

Sensory systems can be conceptualized as a serial succession of neurons consisting of first-order, second-order, and third-order neurons. *First-order neurons* transmit sensory information from the periphery to the CNS. *Second-order neurons* communicate with various reflex networks and sensory pathways in the spinal cord and travel directly to the thalamus. *Third-order neurons* relay information from the thalamus to the cerebral cortex (Fig. 49-1).

This organizing framework corresponds with the three primary levels of neural integration in the somatosensory system: the sensory units, which contain the sensory receptors; the ascending pathways; and the central processing centers in the thalamus and cerebral cortex. Sensory information usually is relayed and processed in a cephalad (toward the head) direction by the three orders of neurons. Many interneurons process and modify the sensory information at the level of the second- and third-order neurons, and many more participate before coordinated and appropriate learned-movement responses occur. The number of participating neurons increases exponentially from the primary through the secondary and the secondary through the tertiary levels.

THE SOMATOSENSORY SYSTEM

- The somatosensory system relays information about four major modalities: touch, temperature, pain, and body position.
- The system is organized segmentally into dermatomes, with each segment supplied by a single dorsal root ganglion that contains the neuronal cell bodies for the sensory units of the segment.
- Somatosensory information is sequentially transmitted over three types of neurons: first-order neurons, which transmit information from sensory receptors to dorsal horn neurons; second-order CNS association neurons, which communicate with various reflex circuits and transmit information to the thalamus; and third-order neurons, which forward the information from the thalamus to the sensory cortex.

The Sensory Unit

The somatosensory experience arises from information provided by a variety of receptors distributed throughout the body. These receptors monitor four major types or modalities of sensation: discriminative touch, which is required to identify the size and shape of objects and their movement across the skin; temperature sensation; sense of movement of the limbs and joints of the body; and nociception, or pain.

Each of the somatosensory modalities is mediated by a distinct system of receptors and pathways to the brain; however, all somatosensory information from the limbs and trunk shares a common class of sensory neurons called *dorsal root ganglion neurons.* Somatosensory information from the face and cranial structures is transmitted by the trigeminal sensory neurons, which function in the same manner as the dorsal root ganglion neurons. The cell body of the dorsal root ganglion neuron, its peripheral branch (which innervates a small area of periphery), and its central axon (which projects to the CNS) form what is called a *sensory unit.*

The fibers of different dorsal root ganglion neurons conduct impulses at varying rates, ranging from 0.5 to 120 m/second. This rate depends on the diameter of the nerve fiber. There are three types of nerve fibers that transmit somatosensory information: types A, B, and C. Type A fibers, which are myelinated, have the fastest rate of conduction.[1,2] Type A fibers convey cutaneous pressure and touch sensation, cold sensation, mechanical pain, and heat pain. Type B fibers, which also are myelinated, transmit information from cutaneous and subcutaneous mechanoreceptors. The unmyelinated type C fibers have the smallest diameter and the slowest rate of conduction. They convey warm–hot sensation and mechanical and chemical as well as heat- and cold-induced pain sensation.

Dermatomal Pattern of Dorsal Root Innervation

The somatosensory innervation of the body, including the head, retains a basic segmental organizational pattern that was established during embryonic development. Thirty-three paired spinal (*i.e.,* segmental) nerves provide sensory and motor innervation of the body wall, the limbs, and the viscera (see Chapter 48).

Sensory input to each spinal cord segment is provided by sensory neurons with cell bodies in the dorsal root ganglia.

The region of the body wall that is supplied by a single pair of dorsal root ganglia is called a *dermatome.* These dorsal root ganglion–innervated strips occur in a regular sequence moving upward from the second coccygeal segment through the cervical segments, reflecting the basic segmental organization of the body and the nervous system (Fig. 49-2). The cranial nerves that innervate the head send their axons to equivalent nuclei in the brain stem. Neighboring dermatomes overlap one another sufficiently so that a loss of one dorsal root or root ganglion results in reduced but not total loss of sensory innervation of a dermatome (Fig. 49-3). Dermatome maps are helpful in interpreting the level and extent of sensory deficits that are the result of segmental nerve and spinal cord damage.

Spinal Circuitry and Ascending Neural Pathways

On entry into the spinal cord, the central axons of the somatosensory neurons branch extensively and project to neurons in the spinal cord gray matter. Some branches become involved in local spinal cord reflexes and directly initiate motor reflexes (*e.g.,* flexor-withdrawal reflex). Two parallel pathways, the *discriminative pathway* and the *anterolateral pathway,* carry the information from the spinal cord to the thalamic level of sensation, each taking a different route through the CNS. The discriminative pathway crosses at the base of the medulla and the anterolateral path-

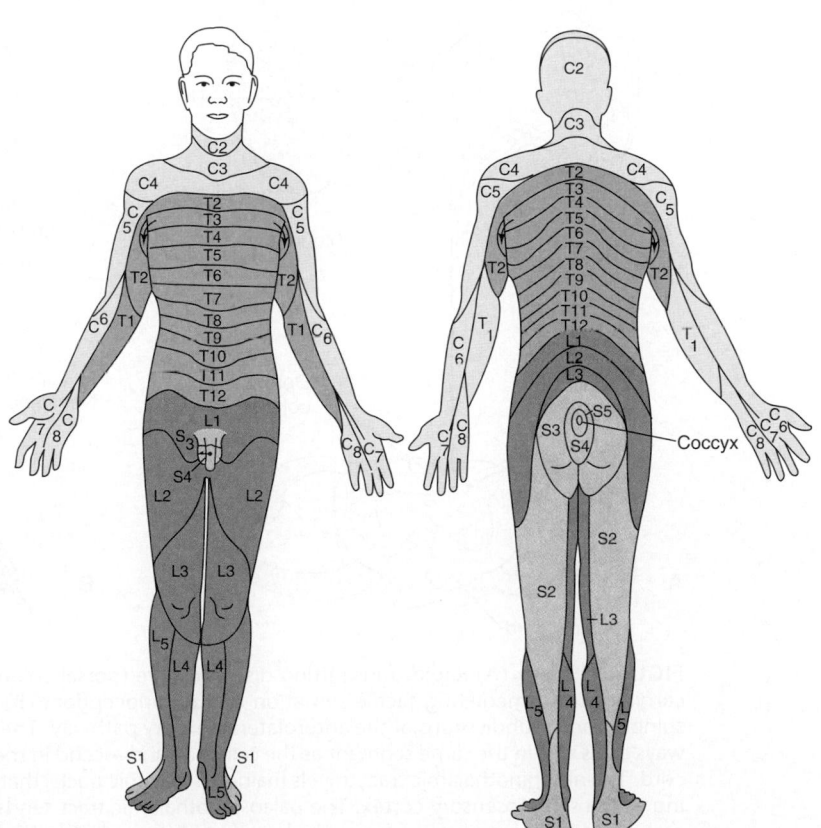

FIGURE 49-2 • Cutaneous distribution of spinal nerves (dermatomes). (From Barr M. [1993]. *The human nervous system.* New York: Harper & Row.)

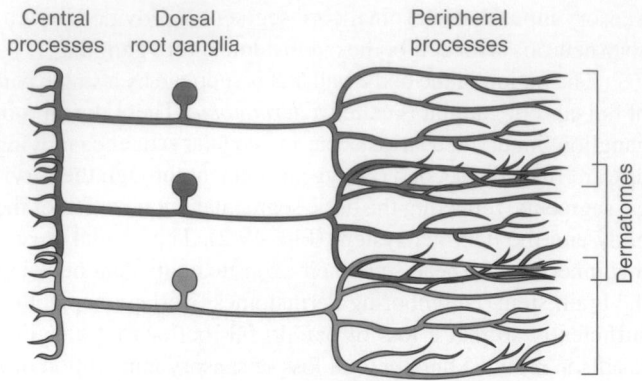

FIGURE 49-3 • The dermatomes formed by the peripheral processes of adjacent spinal nerves overlap on the body surface. The central processes of these fibers also overlap in their spinal distribution.

way crosses within the first few segments of entering the spinal cord. These pathways relay information to the brain for three purposes: perception, arousal, and motor control. Having a two-pathway system has several advantages. It adds richness to the sensory input by allowing sensory information to be handled in two different ways, and it ensures that if one pathway is damaged, the other still can provide input.

The Discriminative Pathway. The discriminative pathway, also known as the dorsal column–medial lemniscal pathway, is used for the rapid transmission of sensory information such as discriminative touch. It contains branches of primary afferent axons that travel up the ipsilateral (i.e., same side) dorsal columns of the spinal cord white matter and synapse with highly evolved somatosensory input association neurons in the medulla. The discriminative pathway uses only three neurons to transmit information from a sensory receptor to the somatosensory strip of parietal cerebral cortex of the opposite side of the brain: (1) the primary dorsal root ganglion neuron, which projects its central axon to the dorsal column nuclei; (2) the dorsal column neuron, which sends its axon through a rapid conducting tract, called the *medial lemniscus,* that crosses at the base of the medulla and travels to the thalamus on the opposite side of the brain, where basic sensation begins; and (3) the thalamic neuron, which projects its axons through the somatosensory radiation to the primary sensory cortex[1] (Fig. 49-4A). The medial lemniscus is joined by fibers from the sensory nucleus of the trigeminal nerve (cra-

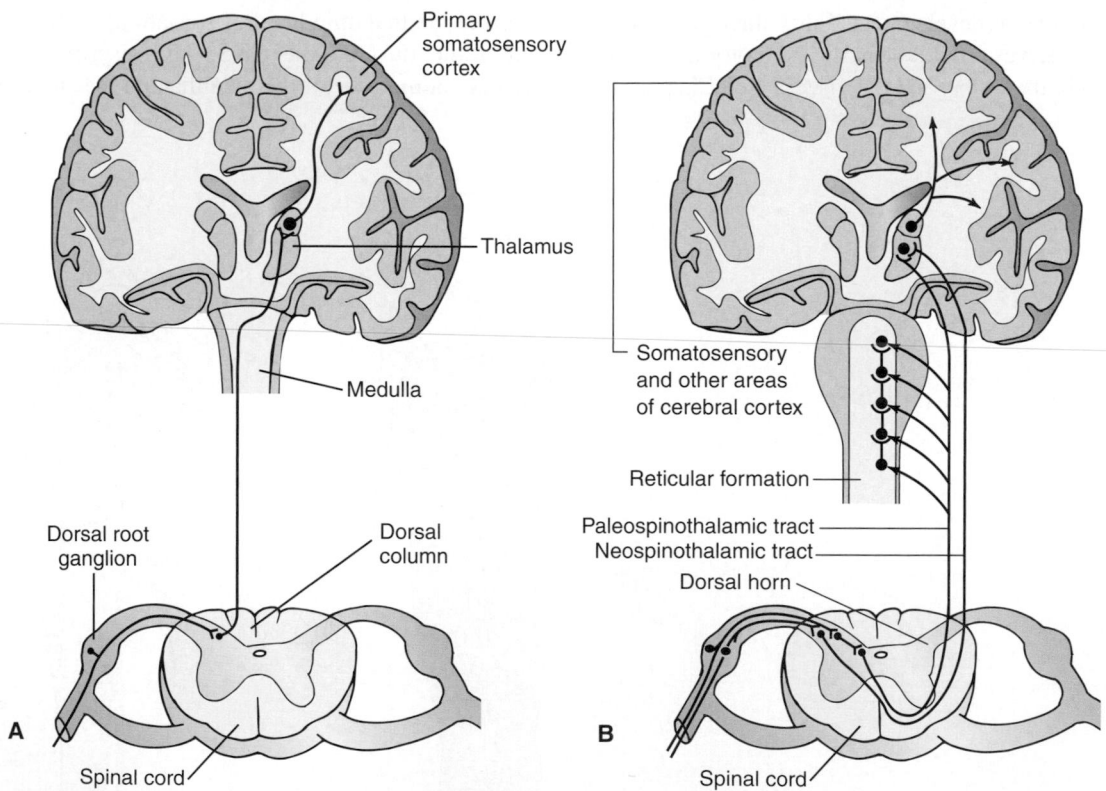

FIGURE 49-4 • **(A)** Rapid-transmitting discriminative (dorsal column–medial lemniscal) pathway carrying axons mediating tactile sensation and proprioception. **(B)** Neospinothalamic and paleospinothalamic subdivisions of the anterolateral sensory pathway. The neurons of anterolateral pathways cross within the same segment as the cell body and ascend in the contralateral side of the spinal cord. The neospinothalamic tract travels mainly to thalamic nuclei that have third-order fibers projecting to the somatosensory cortex. The paleospinothalamic tract sends collaterals to the reticular formation and other structures, from which further fibers project to the thalamus.

nial nerve V) that supplies the face. Sensory information arriving at the sensory cortex by this route can be discretely localized and discriminated in terms of intensity.

One of the distinct features of the discriminative pathway is that it relays precise information regarding spatial orientation. This is the only pathway taken by the sensations of muscle and joint movement, vibration, and delicate discriminative touch, as is required to differentiate correctly the location of touch on the skin at two neighboring points (*i.e.,* two-point discrimination). One of the important functions of the discriminative pathway is to integrate the input from multiple receptors. The sense of shape and size of an object in the absence of visualization, called *stereognosis,* is based on precise afferent information from muscle, tendon, and joint receptors. For example, a screwdriver is perceived as being different from a knife in terms of its texture (tactile sensibility) and shape based on the relative position of the fingers as they move over the object. This complex interpretive perception requires that both the discriminative system and the higher-order parietal association cortex are functioning properly. If the discriminative somatosensory pathway is functional but the parietal association cortex has become discretely damaged, the person can correctly describe the object but does not recognize that it is a screwdriver. This deficit is called *astereognosis.*

The Anterolateral Pathway. The anterolateral pathways (anterior and lateral spinothalamic pathways) consist of bilateral, multisynaptic, slow-conducting tracts (see Chapter 48, Fig. 48-14). These pathways provide for transmission of sensory information such as pain, thermal sensations, crude touch, and pressure that does not require discrete localization of signal source or fine discrimination of intensity. The fibers of the anterolateral pathway originate in the dorsal horns at the level of the segmental nerve, where the dorsal root neurons enter the spinal cord. They cross in the anterior commissure, within a few segments of origin, to the opposite anterolateral pathway, where they ascend upward toward the brain. The spinothalamic tract fibers synapse with several nuclei in the thalamus, but en route they give off numerous branches that travel to the reticular activating system of the brain stem. These projections provide the basis for increased wakefulness or awareness after strong somatosensory stimulation and for the generalized startle reaction that occurs with sudden and intense stimuli. They also stimulate autonomic nervous system responses, such as a rise in heart rate and blood pressure, dilation of the pupils, and the pale, moist skin that results from constriction of the cutaneous blood vessels and activation of the sweat glands.

There are two subdivisions in the anterolateral pathway: the *neospinothalamic tract* and the *paleospinothalamic tract*[1] (see Fig. 49-4B). The neospinothalamic tract consists of a sequence of at least three neurons with long axons. It provides for relatively rapid transmission of sensory information to the thalamus. The paleospinothalamic tract, which is phylogenically older than the neospinothalamic system, consists of bilateral, multisynaptic, slow-conducting tracts that transmit sensory signals that do not require discrete localization or discrimination of fine gradations in intensity. This slower-conducting pathway also projects into the intralaminar nuclei of the thalamus, which have close connections with the limbic cortical systems. This circuitry gives touch its affective or emotional aspects, such as the particular unpleasantness of heavy pressure and the peculiar pleasantness of the tickling and gentle rubbing of the skin.

Central Processing of Somatosensory Information

Perception, or the final processing of somatosensory information, involves awareness of the stimuli, localization and discrimination of their characteristics, and interpretation of their meaning. As sensory information reaches the thalamus, it begins to enter the level of consciousness. In the thalamus, the sensory information is roughly localized and perceived as a crude sense. The full localization, discrimination of the intensity, and interpretation of the meaning of the stimuli require processing by the somatosensory cortex.

The somatosensory cortex is located in the parietal lobe, which lies behind the central sulcus and above the lateral sulcus (Fig. 49-5). The strip of parietal cortex that borders the central sulcus is called the *primary somatosensory cortex* because it receives primary sensory information by direct projections from the thalamus. A distorted map of the body and head surface, called the *sensory homunculus,* reflects the density of cortical neurons devoted to sensory input from afferents in corresponding peripheral areas. As depicted in Figure 49-6, most of the cortical surface is devoted to areas of the body such as the thumb, forefinger, lips, and tongue, where fine touch and pressure discrimination are essential for normal function.

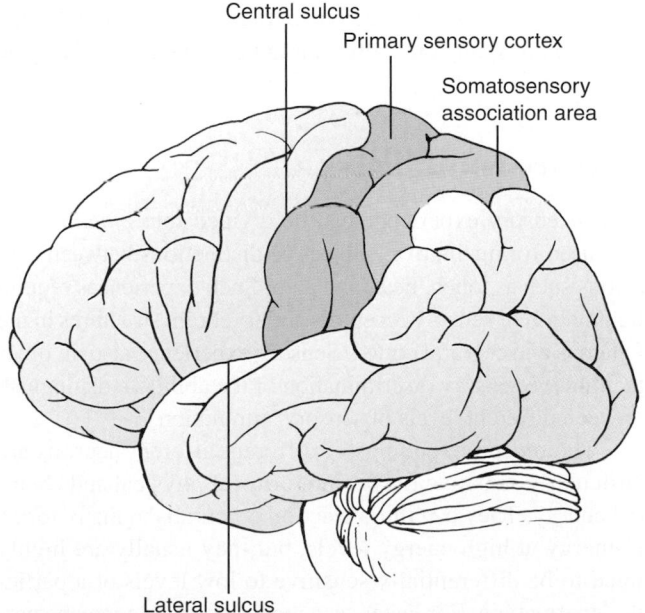

Central sulcus

Primary sensory cortex

Somatosensory association area

Lateral sulcus

FIGURE 49-5 • Primary somatosensory cortex and somatosensory association area.

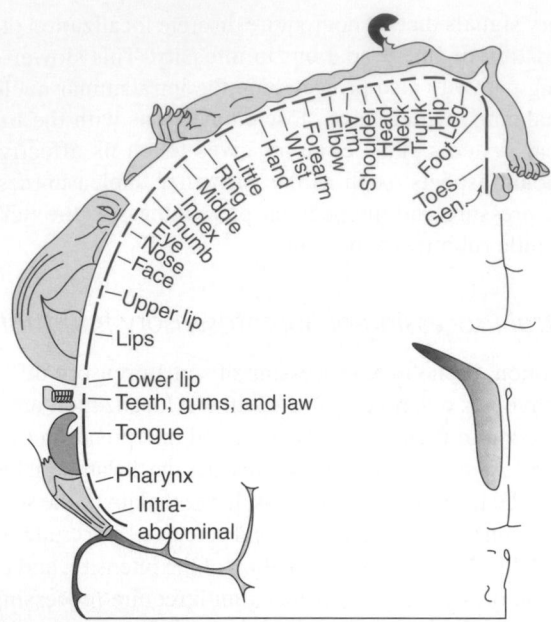

FIGURE 49-6 • Homunculus, as determined by stimulation studies on the human cortex during surgery. (From Penfield E., Rasmussen T. [1955]. *The cerebral cortex of man.* New York: Macmillan. Copyright © by Macmillan Publishing Co., Inc., renewed 1978 by Theodore Rasmussen.)

Parallel to and just behind the primary somatosensory cortex (*i.e.,* toward the occipital cortex) lie the somatosensory association areas, which are required to transform the raw material of sensation into meaningful learned perception. Most of the perceptive aspects of body sensation, or somesthesia, require the function of this parietal association cortex. The perceptive aspect, or meaningfulness, of a stimulus pattern involves the integration of present sensation with past learning. For instance, a person's past learning plus present tactile sensation provides the perception of sitting on a soft chair rather than on a hard bicycle seat.

Sensory Modalities

Somatosensory experience can be divided into *modalities,* a term used for qualitative, subjective distinctions between sensations such as touch, heat, and pain. Such experiences require the function of sensory receptors and forebrain structures in the thalamus and cerebral cortex. Sensory experience also involves quantitative sensory discrimination or the ability to distinguish between different levels of sensory stimulation.

The receptive endings of different afferent neurons are particularly sensitive to specific forms of physical and chemical energy. They can initiate action potentials to many forms of energy at high energy levels, but they usually are highly tuned to be differentially sensitive to low levels of a particular energy type. For instance, a receptive ending may be particularly sensitive to a small increase in local skin tempera-

ture. Stimulating the ending with electric current or strong pressure also can result in action potentials. The amount of energy required, however, is much greater than it is for a change in temperature. Other afferent sensory terminals are most sensitive to slight indentations of the skin, and their signals are subjectively interpreted as touch. Cool versus warm, sharp versus dull pain, and delicate touch versus deep pressure are all based on different populations of afferent neurons or on central integration of simultaneous input from several differently tuned afferents.

When information from different primary afferents reaches the forebrain, where subjective experience occurs, the qualitative differences between warmth and touch are called *sensory modalities.* Although the receptor-detected information is relayed to the thalamus and cortex over separate pathways, the experience of a modality, such as cold versus warm, is uniquely subjective.

Stimulus Discrimination

The ability to discriminate the location of a somesthetic stimulus is called *acuity* and is based on the sensory field in a dermatome innervated by an afferent neuron. High acuity (*i.e.,* the ability to make fine discriminations of location) requires a high density of innervation by afferent neurons. For example, acuity is highest on the lips and cheek but lower on the arm or back. High acuity also requires a projection system through the CNS to the forebrain that preserves distinctions between levels of activity in neighboring sensory fields. Receptors or receptive endings of primary afferent neurons differ as to the intensity at which they begin to fire. For instance, it is possible to assess two-point discrimination by using an open paperclip with its ends bent together to 5 mm apart. When placed on the lips or cheek, the person will readily detect two points of contact. On the back or arm, the ends of the paperclip must be moved progressively farther apart before two points of contact can be detected.

Tactile Sensation

The tactile system, which relays sensory information regarding touch, pressure, and vibration, is considered the basic somatosensory system. Loss of temperature or pain sensitivity leaves the person with no awareness of deficiency. If the tactile system is lost, however, total anesthesia (*i.e.,* numbness) of the involved body part results.

Touch sensation results from stimulation of tactile receptors in the skin and in tissues immediately beneath the skin, pressure from deformation of deeper tissues, and vibration from rapidly repetitive sensory signals. There are at least six types of specialized tactile receptors in the skin and deeper structures: free nerve endings,[1,2] Meissner corpuscles, Merkel disks, pacinian corpuscles, hair follicle end-organs, and Ruffini end-organs (Fig. 49-7).

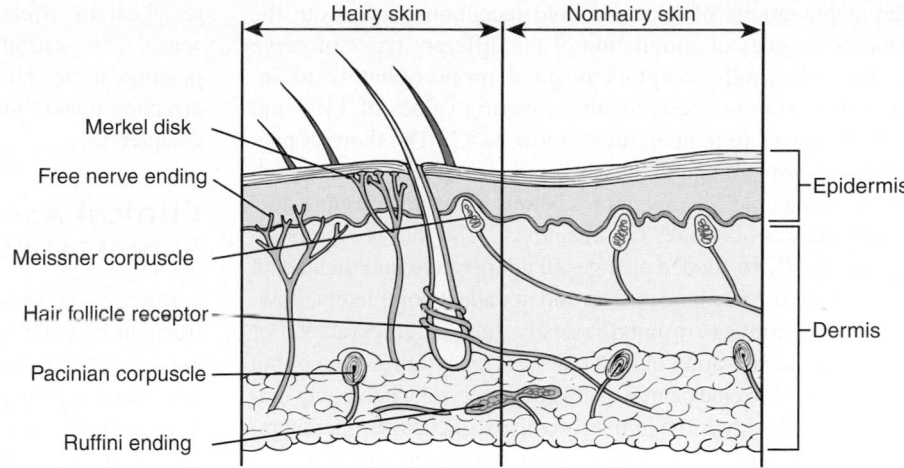

Hairy skin | Nonhairy skin

Merkel disk
Free nerve ending
Meissner corpuscle
Hair follicle receptor
Pacinian corpuscle
Ruffini ending

Epidermis
Dermis

FIGURE 49-7 • Somatic sensory receptors in the skin. Hairy and nonhairy skin have a variety of sensory receptors within the skin. (Adapted from Bear M. F., Connors B. W., Paradiso M. A. [1996]. *Neuroscience: Exploring the brain* [p. 311]. Baltimore: Williams & Wilkins.)

Free nerve endings are found in skin and many other tissues, including the cornea. They detect touch and pressure. *Meissner corpuscles* are elongated, encapsulated nerve endings present in nonhairy parts of the skin. They are particularly abundant in the fingertips, lips, and other areas where the sense of touch is highly developed. *Merkel disks* are dome-shaped receptors found in nonhairy areas and in hairy parts of the skin. In contrast to Meissner corpuscles, which adapt within a fraction of a second, Merkel disks transmit an initial strong signal that diminishes in strength but is slow in adapting. For this reason, Meissner corpuscles are particularly sensitive to the movement of very light objects over the surface of the skin and to low-frequency vibration. Merkel disks are responsible for giving steady-state signals that allow for continuous determination of touch against the skin.

The *pacinian corpuscle* is located immediately beneath the skin and deep in the fascial tissues of the body. This type of receptor, which is stimulated by rapid movements of the tissues and adapts within a few hundredths of a second, is important in detecting tissue vibration. The *hair follicle end-organ* consists of afferent unmyelinated fibers entwined around most of the length of the hair follicle. These receptors, which are rapidly adapting, detect movement on the surface of the body. *Ruffini end-organs* are found in the skin and deeper structures, including the joint capsules. These receptors, which have multibranched encapsulated endings, have very little adaptive capacity and are important for signaling continuous states of deformation, such as heavy and continuous touch and pressure.

Almost all the specialized touch receptors, such as Merkel disks, Meissner corpuscles, hair follicle end-organs, pacinian corpuscles, and Ruffini end-organs, transmit their signals in large myelinated nerve fibers (*i.e.,* types Aα, Aβ) that have transmission velocities ranging from 25 to 70 m/second. Most free nerve endings transmit signals by way of small myelinated fibers (*i.e.,* type Aδ) with conduction velocities of 10 to 30 m/second.

The sensory information for tactile sensation enters the spinal cord through the dorsal roots of the spinal nerves. All tactile sensation that requires rapid transmission is transmitted through the discriminative pathway to the thalamus by way of the medial lemniscus. This includes touch sensation requiring a high degree of localization or fine gradations of intensity, vibratory sensation, and sensation that signals movement against the skin. In addition to the ascending discriminative pathway, tactile sensation uses the more primitive and crude anterolateral pathway. The afferent axons that carry tactile information up the dorsal columns have many branches or collaterals, and some of these synapse in the dorsal horn near the level of dorsal root entry. After several synapses, axons are projected up both sides of the anterolateral aspect of the spinal cord to the thalamus. Few fibers travel all the way to the thalamus. Most synapse on reticular formation neurons that then send their axons on toward the thalamus. The lateral nuclei of the thalamus are capable of contributing a crude, poorly localized sensation from the opposite side of the body. From the thalamus, some projections travel to the somatosensory cortex, especially to the side opposite the stimulus.

Because of these multiple routes, total destruction of the anterolateral pathway seldom occurs. The only time this crude alternative system becomes essential is when the discriminative pathway is damaged. Then, despite projection of the anterolateral system information to the somatosensory cortex, only a poorly localized, high-threshold sense of touch remains. Such persons lose all sense of joint and muscle movement, body position, and two-point discrimination.

Thermal Sensation

Thermal sensation is discriminated by three types of receptors: cold, warmth, and pain. The cold and warmth receptors are located immediately under the skin at discrete but separate points, each serving an area of approximately 1 mm². In some areas, there are more cold receptors than warmth receptors. For example, the lips have 15 to 25 cold receptors per square centimeter, compared with 3 to 5 in the same-sized area of the finger.[1] Different gradations of heat and cold reception result from the relative degrees of stimulation of the different types of nerve endings. Warmth receptors respond proportionately to increases in skin temperature above resting values of 34°C and cold receptors to temperatures below 34°C.[2] The thermal pain receptors are stimulated only by extremes of temperature such as "freezing cold" (temperatures below 5°C) and "burning hot" (temperatures above 45°C) sensations.[2] Thermal receptors respond rapidly to sudden changes in temperature and then adapt over the next few minutes. They do not adapt completely, however, but continue to respond to steady states of temperature. For example, the sensation of heat one feels on entering a tub of hot water or the extreme degree of cold experienced when going outside on a cold day is the initial response to a change in temperature, followed by an adaptation in which one gets accustomed to the temperature change but still feels the heat or cold because the receptors have not adapted completely.

Thermal afferents, with receptive thermal endings in the skin, send their central axons into the segmental dorsal horn of the spinal cord. On entering the dorsal horn, thermal signals are processed by second-order input association neurons. These association neurons activate projection neurons whose axons then cross to the opposite side of the cord and ascend in the multisynaptic, slow-conducting anterolateral system to the opposite side of the brain. Thalamic and cortical somatosensory regions for temperature are mixed with those for tactile sensibility.

Conduction of thermal information through peripheral nerves is quite slow compared with the rapid tactile afferents that travel through the discriminative system. If a person places a foot in a tub of hot water, the tactile sensation occurs well in advance of the burning sensation. The foot has been removed from the hot water by the local withdrawal reflex well before the excessive heat is perceived by the forebrain. Local anesthetic agents block the small-diameter afferents that carry thermal sensory information before they block the large-diameter axons that carry discriminative touch information.

Position Sensation

Position sense refers to the sense of limb and body movement and position without using vision. It is mediated by input from proprioceptive receptors (muscle spindle receptors and Golgi tendon organs) found primarily in muscles, tendons, and joint capsules (see Chapter 50). There are two submodalities of proprioception: the stationary or static component (limb position sense) and the dynamic aspects of position sense (kinesthesia). Both of these depend on constant transmission of information to the CNS regarding the degree of angulation of all joints and the rate of change in angulation. In addition, stretch-sensitive receptors in the skin (Ruffini end-organs, pacinian corpuscles, and Merkel cells) also signal postural information. Signals from these receptors are processed through the dorsal column–medial lemniscus pathway. In addition to the transmission of signals from the periphery to the cerebral cortex, the signals are processed in the thalamus before reaching the cerebral cor-

tex. Lesions affecting the posterior column impair position sense. The vestibular system also plays an essential role in position sense. The vestibular system's role and the diseases affecting it and thus impairing position sense are discussed in Chapter 55.

Clinical Assessment of Somatosensory Function

Clinically, neurologic assessment of somatosensory function can be done by testing the integrity of spinal segmental nerves. A pinpoint pressed against the skin of the sole of the foot that results in a withdrawal reflex and a complaint of skin pain confirms the functional integrity of the afferent terminals in the skin, the entire pathway through the peripheral nerves of the foot, leg, and thigh to the sacral (S1) dorsal root ganglion, and through the dorsal root into the spinal cord segment. It confirms that the somatosensory input association cells receiving this information are functioning and that the reflex circuitry of the cord segments (L5 to S2) is functioning. In addition, the lower motor neurons of the L4 to S1 ventral horn can be considered operational, and their axons through the ventral roots, the mixed peripheral nerve, and the motor neuron to the muscles producing the withdrawal response can be considered intact and functional. The communication between the lower motor neuron and the muscle cells is functional, and these muscles have normal responsiveness and strength.

Testing is done at each segmental level, or dermatome, moving upward along the body and neck from coccygeal segments through the high cervical levels to test the functional integrity of all the spinal nerves. Similar dermatomes cover the face and scalp, and these, although innervated by cranial segmental nerves, are tested in the same manner.

Observation of a normal withdrawal reflex rules out peripheral nerve disease, disorders of the dorsal root and ganglion, diseases of the myoneural junction, and severe muscle diseases. Normal reflex function also indicates that many major descending CNS tracts are functioning within normal limits. If the person is able to report the pinprick sensation and accurately identify its location, many ascending systems through much of the spinal cord and brain also are functioning normally, as are basic intellect and speech mechanisms.

The integrity of the discriminative dorsal column–medial lemniscus pathway compared with the anterolateral tactile pathways is tested with the person's eyes closed by gently brushing the skin with a wisp of cotton, touching an area with one or two sharp points, touching corresponding parts of the body on each side simultaneously or in random sequence, and passively bending the person's finger one way and then another in random order. If only the anterolateral pathway is functional, the tactile threshold is markedly elevated, two-point discrimination and proprioception are missing, and the patient has difficulty discriminating which side of the body received stimulation.

IN SUMMARY, the somatosensory component of the nervous system provides an awareness of body sensations such as touch, temperature, position sense, and pain. There are three primary levels of neural integration in the somatosensory system: the sensory units containing the sensory receptors, the ascending pathways, and the central processing centers in the thalamus and cerebral cortex. A sensory unit consists of a single dorsal root ganglion neuron, its receptors, and its central axon that terminates in the dorsal horn of the spinal cord or medulla. The part of the body innervated by the somatosensory afferent neurons of one set of dorsal root ganglia is called a *dermatome.* Ascending pathways include the discriminative pathway, which crosses at the base of the medulla, and the anterolateral pathway, which crosses within the first few segments of entering the spinal cord. Perception, or the final processing of somatosensory information, involves centers in the thalamus and somatosensory cortex. In the thalamus, the sensory information is crudely localized and perceived. The full localization, discrimination of the intensity, and interpretation of the meaning of the stimuli require processing by the somatosensory cortex. A distorted map of the body and head surface, called the *sensory homunculus,* reflects the density of cortical neurons devoted to sensory input from afferents in corresponding peripheral areas.

The tactile system relays the sensations of touch, pressure, and vibration. It uses two anatomically separate pathways to relay touch information to the opposite side of the forebrain: the dorsal column discriminative pathway and the anterolateral pathway. Delicate touch, vibration, position, and movement sensations use the discriminative pathway to reach the thalamus, where third-order relay occurs to the primary somatosensory strip of the parietal cortex. Crude tactile sensation is carried by the bilateral slow-conducting anterolateral pathway. Temperature sensations of warm–hot and cool–cold are the result of stimulation to thermal receptors of sensory units projecting to the thalamus and cortex through the anterolateral system on the opposite side of the body. Proprioception is the sense of limb and body movement and position without using vision. Proprioceptive information is processed through the rapid-transmitting dorsal column–medial lemniscus pathway. Testing of the ipsilateral dorsal column (discriminative touch) system or the contralateral temperature projection system permits diagnostic analysis of the level and extent of damage in the somatosensory pathways. ■

PAIN

After completing this section of the chapter, you should be able to meet the following objectives:

- Differentiate among the specificity, pattern, gate control, and neuromatrix theories of pain.
- Characterize the response of nociceptors to stimuli that produce pain.

- State the difference between the Aδ- and C-fiber neurons in the transmission of pain information.
- Trace the transmission of pain signals with reference to the neospinothalamic, paleospinothalamic, and reticulospinal pathways, including the role of chemical mediators and factors that modulate pain transmission.
- Describe the function of endogenous analgesic mechanisms as they relate to transmission of pain information.
- Compare pain threshold and pain tolerance.
- Differentiate acute pain from chronic pain in terms of mechanisms, manifestations, and treatment.
- Describe the mechanisms of referred pain, and list the common sites of referral for cardiac and other types of visceral pain.
- Describe three methods for assessing pain.
- State the proposed mechanisms of pain relief associated with the use of heat, cold, transcutaneous electrical nerve stimulation, and acupuncture and acupressure.
- Cite the mechanisms whereby non-narcotic and narcotic analgesics, tricyclic antidepressants, and antiseizure drugs relieve pain.

Pain is an "unpleasant sensory and emotional experience associated with actual and potential tissue damage, or described in terms of such damage."[3] The early work by Sir Charles Sherrington[4] introduced the important concept that pain perception and reaction to pain can be separated. This is particularly important for clinical pain because suffering is more heavily influenced by the reaction to pain than by actual pain intensity. Attention, motivation, past experience, and the meaning of the situation can influence the individual's reaction to pain. Thus, pain involves anatomic structures and physiologic behaviors, as well as psychological, social, cultural, and cognitive factors.

Pain is a common symptom that varies widely in intensity and spares no age group. When pain is extremely severe, it disrupts a person's customary behavior and can consume all of a person's attention. It can be equally devastating for infants and children, young and middle-aged adults, as well as the young-old and the old-old. Both acute pain and chronic pain can be major health problems. Pain is the most common symptom for which patients seek medical attention. Acute pain often results from injury, surgery, or invasive medical procedures. It also can be a presenting symptom for some infections (*e.g.,* pharyngitis, appendicitis, otitis media). Chronic pain can be symptomatic of a wide range of health problems (*e.g.,* arthritis, back injury, cancer). Approximately 75 million people in the United States live in "serious pain" and nearly 50 million are partially or totally disabled by pain.[5,6]

The experience of pain depends on both sensory stimulation and perception. The perception of pain can be heavily influenced by the endogenous analgesia system that modulates the sensation of pain. This is perhaps most dramatically illustrated by the phenomenon of soldiers injured in battle or athletes injured during a game who do not perceive major injuries as painful until they leave the battlefield or the game.

Pain can be either nociceptive or neuropathic in origin. When nociceptors (pain receptors) are activated in response to actual or impending tissue injury, *nociceptive pain* is the consequence. *Neuropathic pain,* on the other hand, arises from direct injury or dysfunction of the sensory axons of peripheral or central nerves. Tissue and nerve injury can result in a wide range of symptoms. These include pain from noninjurious stimuli to the skin (*allodynia*), extreme sensitivity to pain (*hyperalgesia*), and the absence of pain from stimuli that normally would be painful (*analgesia*). The latter, although not painful, can be extremely serious (*e.g.,* in diabetic persons with peripheral neuropathy) because the normally protective early warning system for the presence of tissue injury is absent.

Pain Theories

Traditionally, two theories have been offered to explain the physiologic basis for the pain experience. The first, *specificity theory,* regards pain as a separate sensory modality evoked by the activity of specific receptors that transmit information to pain centers or regions in the forebrain where pain is experienced.[7] The second theory includes a group of theories collectively referred to as *pattern theory*. It proposes that pain receptors share endings or pathways with other sensory modalities, but that different patterns of activity (*i.e.,* spatial or temporal) of the same neurons can be used to signal painful and nonpainful stimuli.[7] For example, light touch applied to the skin would produce the sensation of touch through low-frequency firing of the receptor; intense pressure would produce pain through high-frequency firing of the same receptor. Both theories focus on the neurophysiologic basis of pain, and both probably apply. Specific nociceptive afferents have been identified; however, almost all afferent stimuli, if driven at a very high frequency, can be experienced as painful.

Gate control theory, a modification of specificity theory, was proposed by Melzack and Wall in 1965 to meet the challenges presented by the pattern theories. This theory postulated the presence of neural gating mechanisms at the segmental spinal cord level to account for interactions between pain and other sensory modalities.[8] The original gate control theory proposed a spinal cord–level network of transmission or projection cells and internuncial neurons that inhibits the transmission cells, forming a segmental-level gating mechanism that could block projection of pain information to the brain.

According to the gate control theory, the internuncial neurons involved in the gating mechanism are activated by large-diameter, faster-propagating fibers that carry tactile information. The simultaneous firing of the large-diameter touch fibers has the potential for blocking the transmission of impulses from the small-diameter myelinated and unmyelinated pain fibers. Pain therapists have long known that pain intensity can be temporarily reduced during active tactile stimulation. For example, repeated sweeping of a soft-bristled brush on the skin (*i.e.,* brush-

ing) over or near a painful area may result in pain reduction for several minutes to several hours.

Pain modulation is now known to be a much more complex phenomenon than that proposed by the original gate control theory. Tactile information is transmitted by small- and large-diameter fibers. Major interactions between sensory modalities, including the so-called gating phenomenon, occur at several levels of the CNS rostral to the input segment. Perhaps the most puzzling aspect of locally applied stimuli, such as brushing, that can block the experience of pain is the relatively long-lasting effect (minutes to hours) of such treatments. This prolonged effect has been difficult to explain on the basis of specificity theories, including the gate control theory. Other important factors include the effect of endogenous opioids and their receptors at the segmental and brain stem level, descending feedback modulation, altered sensitivity, learning, and culture. Despite this complexity, the Melzack and Wall theory has served a useful purpose. It sparked interest in pain and stimulated research and clinical activity related to the pain-modulating systems.

More recently, Melzack has developed the *neuromatrix theory* to address further the brain's role in pain as well as the multiple dimensions and determinants of pain.[9] This theory is particularly useful in understanding chronic pain and phantom limb pain, in which there is not a simple one-to-one relationship between tissue injury and pain experience. The neuromatrix theory proposes that the brain contains a widely distributed neural network, called the *body–self neuromatrix,* that contains somatosensory, limbic, and thalamocortical components. Genetic and sensory influences determine the synaptic architecture of an individual's neuromatrix that integrates multiple sources of input and yields the neurosignature pattern that evokes the sensory, affective, and cognitive dimensions of pain experience and behavior. These multiple sources include somatosensory inputs; other sensory inputs affecting interpretation of the situation; phasic and tonic inputs from the brain addressing such things as attention, expectation, culture, and personality; intrinsic neural inhibitory modulation; and various components of stress regulation systems. This theory may open entire new areas of research such as an understanding of the role that cortisol plays in chronic pain, the effect estrogen has on pain mediated through the release of peripheral cytokines, and the reported increase in chronic pain that occurs with age.

Pain Mechanisms and Pathways

Pain usually is viewed in the context of tissue injury. The term *nociception,* which means "pain sense," comes from the Latin word *nocere,* "to injure." Nociceptive stimuli are objectively defined as stimuli of such intensity that they cause or are close to causing tissue damage. Researchers often use the withdrawal reflex (*e.g.,* the reflexive withdrawal of a body part from a tissue-damaging stimulus) to determine when a stimulus is nociceptive. Stimuli used include pressure from a sharp object, strong electric current to the skin, or application of heat or cold of approximately 10°C above or below normal skin temperature.

At low levels of intensity these noxious stimuli do activate nociceptors (pain receptors), but typically are perceived as painful only when the intensity reaches a level where tissue damage occurs or is imminent.

The mechanisms of pain are many and complex. As with other forms of somatosensation, the pathways are composed of first-, second-, and third-order neurons (Fig. 49-8). The first-order neurons and their receptive endings detect stimuli that threaten the integrity of innervated tissues. Second-order neurons are located in the spinal cord and process nociceptive information. Third-order neurons project pain information to the brain. The thalamus and somatosensory cortex integrate and modulate pain as well as the person's subjective reaction to the pain experience.

Pain Receptors and Mediators

Nociceptors, or pain receptors, are sensory receptors that are activated by noxious insults to peripheral tissues. Structurally, the receptive endings of the peripheral pain fibers are free nerve endings. These receptive endings, which are widely distributed in the skin, dental pulp, periosteum, meninges, and some internal organs, translate the noxious stimuli into action potentials that are transmitted by a dorsal root ganglion to the dorsal horn of the spinal cord.

Nociceptive action potentials are transmitted through two types of afferent nerve fibers: myelinated Aδ fibers and unmyelinated C fibers.[1,2] The larger Aδ fibers have considerably greater conduction velocities, transmitting impulses at a rate of 10 to 30 m/second. The C fibers are the smallest of all peripheral nerve fibers; they transmit impulses at the rate of 0.5 to 2.5 m/second. Pain conducted by Aδ fibers traditionally is called *fast pain* or first pain and typically is elicited by mechanical or thermal stimuli. C-fiber pain often is described as *slow-wave pain* or second pain because it is slower in onset and longer in duration. It typically is incited by chemical stimuli or by persistent mechanical or thermal stimuli. The slow postexcitatory potentials generated in C fibers are now believed to be responsible for central sensitization to chronic pain.

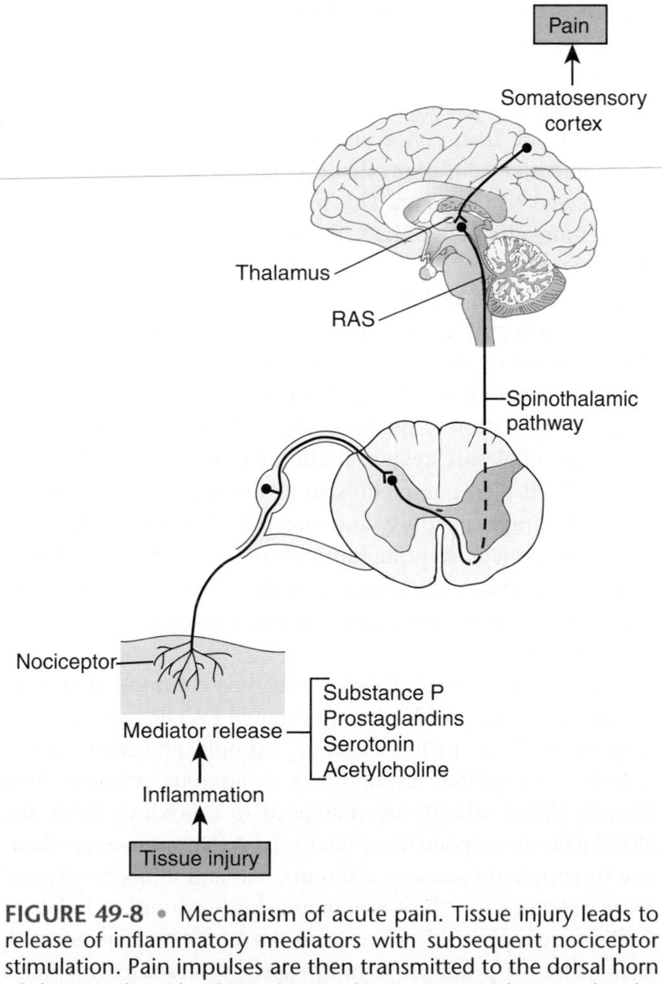

FIGURE 49-8 • Mechanism of acute pain. Tissue injury leads to release of inflammatory mediators with subsequent nociceptor stimulation. Pain impulses are then transmitted to the dorsal horn of the spinal cord, where they make contract with second-order neurons that cross to the opposite side of the cord and ascend by the spinothalamic tract to the reticular activating system (RAS) and thalamus. The localization and meaning of pain occur at the level of the somatosensory cortex.

PAIN SENSATION

- Pain is both a protective and an unpleasant physical and emotionally disturbing sensation originating in pain receptors that respond to a number of stimuli that threaten tissue integrity.

- There are two pathways for pain transmission:
  - The pathway for fast, sharply discriminated pain that moves directly from the receptor to the spinal cord using myelinated Aδ fibers and from the spinal cord to the thalamus using the neospinothalamic tract
  - The pathway for slow, continuously conducted pain that is transmitted to the spinal cord using unmyelinated C fibers and from the spinal cord to the thalamus using the more circuitous and slower-conducting paleospinothalamic tract

- The central processing of pain information includes transmission to the somatosensory cortex, where pain information is perceived and interpreted; the limbic system, where the emotional components of pain are experienced; and to brain stem centers, where autonomic nervous system responses are recruited.

- Modulation of the pain experience occurs by way of the endogenous analgesic center in the midbrain, the pontine noradrenergic neurons, and the nucleus raphe magnus in the medulla, which sends inhibitory signals to dorsal horn neurons in the spinal cord or trigeminal nerve.

Stimulation of Nociceptors. Unlike other sensory receptors, nociceptors respond to several forms of stimulation, including mechanical, thermal, and chemical. Some receptors respond to a single type of stimuli (mechanical or thermal) and others, called *polymodal receptors,* respond to all three types of stimuli (mechanical, thermal, and chemical). Mechanical stimuli can arise from intense pressure applied to skin or from the violent contraction or extreme stretch of a muscle. Both extremes of heat and cold can stimulate nociceptors. Chemical stimuli arise from a number of sources, including tissue trauma, ischemia, and inflammation. A wide range of chemical mediators are released from injured and inflamed tissues, including hydrogen and potassium ions, prostaglandins, leukotrienes, histamine, bradykinin, acetylcholine, and serotonin. These chemical mediators produce their effects by directly stimulating nociceptors or sensitizing them to the effects of nociceptive stimuli; perpetuating the inflammatory responses that lead to the release of chemical agents that act as nociceptive stimuli; or inciting neurogenic reflexes that increase the response to nociceptive stimuli. For example, bradykinin, histamine, serotonin, and potassium activate and also sensitize nociceptors.[10,11] Adenosine triphosphate, acetylcholine, and platelets act alone or in concert to sensitize nociceptors through other chemical agents such as prostaglandins. Aspirin and other nonsteroidal anti-inflammatory drugs (NSAIDs) are effective in controlling pain because they block the enzyme needed for prostaglandin synthesis.

Nociceptive stimulation that activates C fibers can cause a response known as *neurogenic inflammation* that produces vasodilation and an increased release of chemical mediators to which nociceptors respond.[11] This mechanism is thought to be mediated by a dorsal root neuron reflex that produces retrograde transport and release of chemical mediators, which in turn causes increasing inflammation of peripheral tissues. This reflex can set up a vicious cycle, which has implications for persistent pain and hyperalgesia.[10]

Mediators in the Spinal Cord. In the spinal cord, the transmission of impulses between the nociceptive neurons and the dorsal horn neurons is mediated by chemical neurotransmitters released from central nerve endings of the nociceptive neurons. Some of these neurotransmitters are amino acids (*e.g.,* glutamate), others are amino acid derivatives (*e.g.,* norepinephrine), and still others are low–molecular-weight peptides composed of two or more amino acids. The amino acid glutamate is a major excitatory neurotransmitter released from the central nerve endings of the nociceptive neurons. Substance P, a neuropeptide, also is released in the dorsal horn by C fibers in response to nociceptive stimulation. Substance P elicits slow excitatory potentials in dorsal horn neurons. Unlike glutamate, which confines its action to the immediate area of the synaptic terminal, some neuropeptides released in the dorsal horn can diffuse some distance because they are not inactivated by reuptake mechanisms. In persistent pain, this may help to explain the excitability and unlocalized nature of many painful conditions. Neuropeptides such as substance P also appear to prolong and enhance the action of glutamate. If these neurotransmitters are released in large quantities or over extended periods, they can lead to secondary hyperalgesia, a condition in which the second-order neurons are overly sensitive to low levels of noxious stimulation. Understanding how chemical mediators function in nociception is an active area of research that has implications for the development of new treatments for pain.

Spinal Cord Circuitry and Pathways

On entering the spinal cord through the dorsal roots, the pain fibers bifurcate and ascend or descend one or two segments before synapsing with association neurons in the dorsal horn. From the dorsal horn, the axons of association projection neurons cross through the anterior commissure to the opposite side and then ascend upward in the previously described neospinothalamic and paleospinothalamic pathways (Fig. 49-9).

The faster-conducting fibers in the neospinothalamic tract are associated mainly with the transmission of sharp–fast pain information to the thalamus. In the thalamus, synapses are made and the pathway continues to the contralateral parietal somatosensory area to provide the precise location of the pain. Typically, the pain is experienced as bright, sharp, or stabbing in nature.

The paleospinothalamic tract is a slower-conducting, multisynaptic tract concerned with the diffuse, dull, aching, and unpleasant sensations that commonly are associated with chronic and visceral pain. This information travels through the small, unmyelinated C fibers. Fibers of this system also project up the contralateral (*i.e.,* opposite) anterolateral pathway to terminate in several thalamic regions, including the intralateral nuclei, which project to the limbic system. It is associated with the emotional or affective–motivational aspects of pain. Spinoreticular fibers from this pathway project bilaterally to the reticular formation of the brain stem. This component of the paleospinothalamic system facilitates avoidance reflexes at all levels. It also contributes to an increase in the electroencephalographic activity associated with alertness and indirectly influences hypothalamic functions associated with sudden alertness, such as increased heart rate and blood pressure. This may explain the tremendous arousal effects of certain pain stimuli.

Dorsal horn (second-order) neurons are divided primarily into two types: wide–dynamic-range (WDR) neurons that respond to different low-intensity stimuli, and nociceptive-specific neurons that respond only to noxious or nociceptive stimuli. When stimuli are increased to a noxious level, the WDR neurons respond more intensely. After more severe damage to peripheral sensory afferents, Aδ and C fibers respond more intensely as they are increasingly stimulated. When C fibers are repetitively stimulated at a rate of once per second, each stimulus produces a progressively increased response from the WDR neurons. This phenomenon of amplification of transmitted signals has been called *windup* and may explain why pain sensation appears to increase with repeated stimulation. Windup and sensitization of dorsal horn neurons have

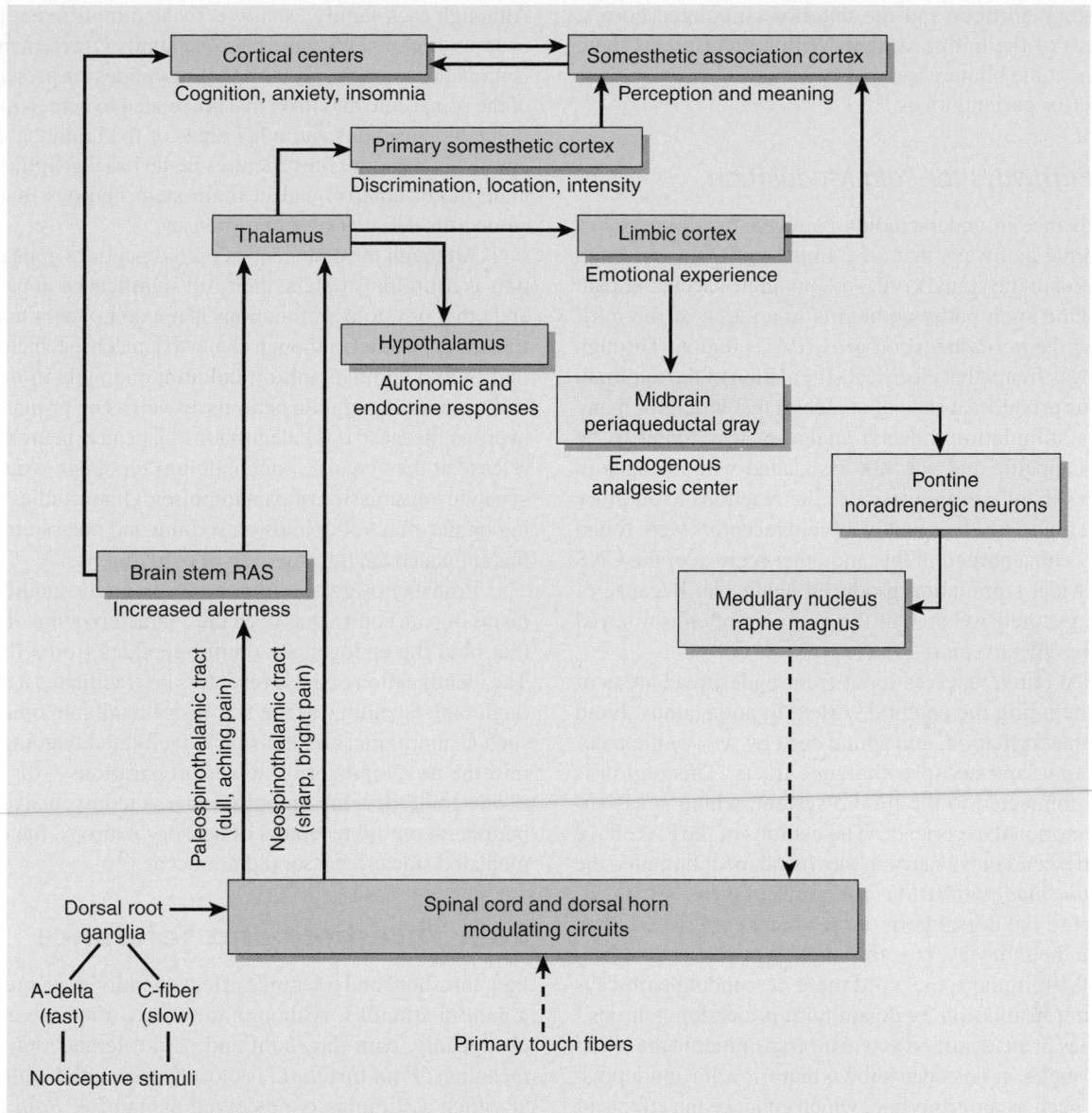

FIGURE 49-9 • Primary pain pathways. The transmission of incoming nociceptive impulses is modulated by dorsal horn circuitry that receives input from primary touch receptors and from descending pathways that involve the limbic cortical systems (orbital frontal cortex, amygdala, and hypothalamus), the periaqueductal endogenous analgesic center in the midbrain, pontine noradrenergic neurons, and the nucleus raphe magnus (NRM) in the medulla. *Dashed lines* indicate inhibition or modulation of pain transmission by dorsal horn projection neurons. RAS, reticular activating system.

implications for appropriate and early, or even preemptive, pain therapy to avoid the possibility of spinal cord neurons becoming hypersensitive or subject to firing spontaneously.[10,12]

Brain Centers and Pain Perception

Information from tissue injury is carried from the spinal cord to brain centers in the thalamus where the basic sensation of hurtfulness, or pain, occurs (See Fig. 49-9). In the neospinothalamic system, interconnections between the lateral thalamus and the somatosensory cortex are necessary to add precision,

discrimination, and meaning to the pain sensation. The paleospinothalamic system projects diffusely from the intralaminar nuclei of the thalamus to large areas of the limbic cortex. These connections probably are associated with the hurtfulness and the mood-altering and attention-narrowing effect of pain.

Recent research using magnetoencephalography has demonstrated cortical representation of first and second pain sensation in humans. In healthy adults, nociceptive Aδ afferent stimulation is related to activation in the contralateral primary somatosensory cortex in the parietal lobe, whereas C afferent stimulation is related to activation of the secondary somatosensory cortices and the anterior cingulated cortex, which is part of the limbic system. With both afferents there is activation of the bilateral secondary somatosensory cortices in the posterior parietal lobes.[13]

Central Pathways for Pain Modulation

A major advance in understanding pain was the discovery of neuroanatomic pathways that arise in the midbrain and brain stem, descend to the spinal cord, and modulate ascending pain impulses. One such pathway begins in an area of the midbrain called the *periaqueductal gray* (PAG) region. Through research it was found that electrical stimulation of the midbrain PAG regions produced a state of analgesia that lasted for many hours. This stimulation-induced analgesia was found to be remarkably specific and was not associated with changes in either the levels of consciousness or the reactions to auditory and visual stimuli.[2] Subsequently, opioid receptors were found to be highly concentrated in this and other regions of the CNS where electrical stimulation produced analgesia. Because of these findings, the PAG area of the midbrain often is referred to as the *endogenous analgesia center.*[1]

The PAG area receives input from widespread areas of the CNS, including the cerebral cortex, hypothalamus, brain stem reticular formation, and spinal cord by way of the pale-ospinothalamic and neospinothalamic tracts. This region is intimately connected to the limbic system, which is associated with emotional experience. The neurons of the PAG have axons that descend into an area in the rostral medulla called the *nucleus raphe magnus* (NRM). The axons of these NRM neurons project to the dorsal horn of the spinal cord, where they terminate in the same layers as the entering primary pain fibers (see Fig. 49-9). In the spinal cord these descending pathways inhibit pain transmission by dorsal horn projection neurons.[2] Serotonin has been identified as a neurotransmitter in the NRM medullary nuclei. It has been shown that tricyclic antidepressant drugs, such as amitriptyline, which enhance the effects of serotonin by blocking its presynaptic uptake, have been found to be effective in the management of certain types of chronic pain.[14] Additional inhibitory spinal projections arise from noradrenergic neurons in the pons and medulla, which also receive input from the PAG.[2] The discovery that norepinephrine can block pain transmission led to studies directed at the combined administration of opioids and clonidine, a central-acting α-adrenergic agonist, for pain relief.

Endogenous Analgesic Mechanisms

There is evidence that opioid receptors and endogenously synthesized opioid peptides, which are morphine-like substances, are found on the peripheral processes of primary afferent neurons and in many regions of the CNS.[15] Three families of endogenous opioid peptides have been identified—the enkephalins, endorphins, and dynorphins. Each family is derived from a distinct precursor polypeptide and has a characteristic anatomic distribution.

Although each family usually is located in different groups of neurons, occasionally more than one family is present in the same neuron. For example, proenkephalin peptides are present in areas of the spinal cord and PAG that are related to perception of pain, in the hippocampus and other areas of the brain that modulate emotional behavior, in structures in the basal ganglia that modulate motor control, and in brain stem neurons that regulate autonomic nervous system responses.

Although the endogenous opioid peptides appear to function as neurotransmitters, their full significance in pain control and other physiologic functions is not completely understood. Laboratory studies, although somewhat inconsistent, have found that opioid agonists inhibit calcium channels in dorsal root and trigeminal ganglion neurons as well as on primary afferent neurons. Because it is calcium ions that cause neurotransmitter release at the synapse, such calcium blockage would inhibit synaptic transmission of pain impulses. Other studies are focusing on the effect of opioids on sodium and potassium channels that influence the transmission of pain impulses.[15]

Probably of greater importance in understanding mechanisms of pain control has been the characterization of receptors that bind the endogenous opioid peptides (to be discussed). The identification of these receptors has facilitated a more thorough understanding of the actions of available opioid drugs, such as morphine, and it also has facilitated ongoing research into the development of newer preparations—for example, if one could develop an opioid that acted exclusively on the peripheral opioid receptors of sensory neurons, then centrally mediated side effects should not occur.[15]

Pain Threshold and Tolerance

Pain threshold and tolerance affect an individual's response to a painful stimulus. Although the terms often are used interchangeably, pain threshold and pain tolerance have distinct meanings. *Pain threshold* is closely associated with the point at which a stimulus is perceived as painful. *Pain tolerance* relates more to the total pain experience; it is defined as the maximum intensity or duration of pain that a person is willing to endure before the person wants something done about the pain. Psychological, familial, cultural, and environmental factors significantly influence the amount of pain a person is willing to tolerate. The threshold to pain is fairly uniform from one person to another, whereas pain tolerance is extremely variable.[10] Separation and identification of the role of each of these two aspects of pain continue to pose fundamental problems for the pain management team and for pain researchers.

Types of Pain

The most widely accepted classifications of pain are according to source or location, referral, and duration (acute or chronic). Classification based on associated medical diagnosis (*e.g.,* surgery, trauma, cancer, sickle cell disease, fibromyalgia) is useful in planning appropriate interventions.

TYPES OF PAIN

- Pain can be classified according to location (cutaneous or deep and visceral), duration (acute or chronic), and site of referral.
- Cutaneous pain is a sharp, burning pain that has its origin in the skin or subcutaneous tissues.
- Deep pain is a more diffuse and throbbing pain that originates in structures such as the muscles, bones, and tendons and radiates to the surrounding tissues.
- Visceral pain is a diffuse and poorly defined pain that results from stretching, distention, or ischemia of tissues in a body organ.
- Acute pain is a self-limiting pain that lasts less than 6 months.
- Chronic pain is persistent pain that lasts longer than 6 months, lacks the autonomic and somatic responses associated with acute pain, and is accompanied by loss of appetite, sleep disturbances, depression, and other debilitating responses.
- Referred pain is pain that originates at a visceral site but is perceived as originating in the part of the body wall that is innervated by neurons entering the same segment of the nervous system.

Cutaneous and Deep Somatic Pain

Cutaneous pain arises from superficial structures, such as the skin and subcutaneous tissues. A paper cut on the finger is an example of easily localized superficial, or cutaneous, pain. It is a sharp pain with a burning quality and may be abrupt or slow in onset. It can be localized accurately and may be distributed along the dermatomes. Because there is an overlap of nerve fiber distribution between the dermatomes, the boundaries of pain frequently are not as clear-cut as dermatome diagrams indicate.

Deep somatic pain originates in deep body structures, such as the periosteum, muscles, tendons, joints, and blood vessels. This pain is more diffuse than cutaneous pain. Various stimuli, such as strong pressure exerted on bone, ischemia to a muscle, and tissue damage, can produce deep somatic pain. This is the type of pain a person experiences from a sprained ankle. Radiation of pain from the original site of injury can occur. For example, damage to a nerve root can cause a person to experience pain radiating along its fiber distribution.

Visceral Pain

Visceral, or splanchnic, pain has its origin in the visceral organs and is one of the most common pains produced by disease. While similar to somatic pain in many ways, both the neurologic mechanisms and the perception of visceral pain differ from somatic pain. One of the most important differences between surface pain and visceral pain is the type of damage that causes pain. For example, "a surgeon can cut the bowel entirely in two in a patient who is awake without causing significant pain."[1] In contrast, strong contractions, distention, or ischemia affecting the walls of the viscera can induce severe pain. Also, visceral pain is not evoked from all viscera (e.g., the liver, lung parenchyma).[16] Another difference is the diffuse and poorly localized nature of visceral pain, its tendency to be referred to other locations and to be accompanied by symptoms associated with autonomic reflexes (e.g., nausea).[17] There are several explanations for this. There is a low density of nociceptors in the viscera compared with the skin. There is functional divergence of visceral input within the CNS, which occurs when many second-order neurons respond to a stimulus from a single visceral afferent. There is also convergence between somatic and visceral afferents in the spinal cord and in the supraspinal centers and possibly also between visceral afferents (e.g., bladder, uterus, cervix, and vagina).[17]

Visceral afferents are predominantly small, unmyelinated pain fibers that terminate in the dorsal horn of the spinal cord and express peptide neurotransmitters such as substance P.[16] There are thought to be two classes of nociceptive receptors that innervate the viscera: high-threshold and intensity-coding receptors.[16,17] High-threshold receptors have a high threshold for stimulation and respond only to stimuli within the noxious range. Intensity-coding receptors have a lower threshold for stimulation and an encoding function that incorporates the intensity of the stimulus into the magnitude of their discharge. Acute visceral pain, such as pain produced by intense contraction of a hollow organ, is thought to be triggered initially by high-threshold receptors. More extended forms of visceral stimulation, such as that caused by hypoxia and inflammation, often result in sensitization of the receptors. Once sensitized, these receptors begin to respond to otherwise innocuous stimuli (e.g., motility and secretory activity) that normally occur in the viscera. This sensitization may resolve more slowly than the initial injury and thus visceral pain may persist longer than expected based on the initial injury.[16]

Visceral nociceptive afferents from the thorax and abdomen travel along the cranial and spinal nerve pathways of the autonomic nervous system. For many years it was believed that the spinothalamic and spinoreticular tracts carried visceral nociceptive information. More recently, additional pathways have been identified: the dorsal column pathway, the spino(trigemino)-parabrachio-amygdaloid pathway, and the spinohypothalamic pathway.[16] Identification of new pathways is sometimes quite important clinically. For example, knowledge of the dorsal column pathway has led to new surgical approaches to visceral pain due to pelvic cancer, such as midline myelotomy.[17]

Referred Pain

Referred pain is pain that is perceived at a site different from its point of origin but innervated by the same spinal segment. It is

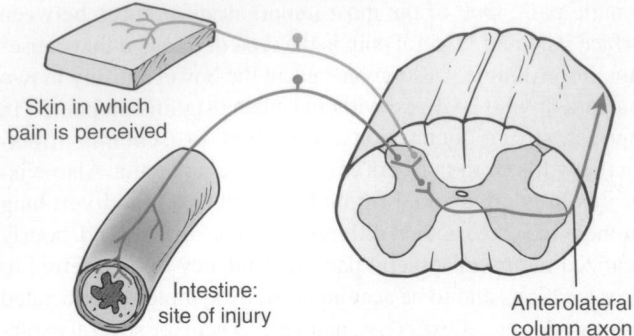

FIGURE 49-10 • Convergence of cutaneous and visceral inputs onto the same second-order projection neuron in the dorsal horn of the spinal cord. Although virtually all visceral inputs converge with cutaneous inputs, most cutaneous inputs do not converge with other sensory inputs.

hypothesized that visceral and somatic afferent neurons converge on the same dorsal horn projection neurons (Fig. 49-10). For this reason, it can be difficult for the brain to correctly identify the original source of pain. Pain that originates in the abdominal or thoracic viscera is diffuse and poorly localized and often perceived at a site far removed from the affected area. For example, the pain associated with myocardial infarction commonly is referred to the left arm, neck, and chest, which may delay diagnosis and treatment of a potentially life-threatening condition.

Referred pain may arise alone or concurrent with pain located at the origin of the noxious stimuli. This lack of correspondence between the location of the pain and the location of the painful stimuli can make diagnosis difficult. Although the term *referred* usually is applied to pain that originates in the viscera and is experienced as if originating from the body wall, it also may be applied to pain that arises from somatic structures. For example, pain referred to the chest wall could be caused by nociceptive stimulation of the peripheral portion of the diaphragm, which receives somatosensory innervation from the intercostal nerves. An understanding of pain referral is of great value in diagnosing illness. The typical pattern of pain referral can be derived from our understanding that the afferent neurons from visceral or deep somatic tissue enter the spinal cord at the same level as the afferent neurons from the cutaneous areas to which the pain is referred (Fig. 49-11).

The sites of referred pain are determined embryologically with the development of visceral and somatic structures that share the same site for entry of sensory information into the CNS and then move to more distant locations. For example, a person with peritonitis may complain of pain in the shoulder. Internally, there is inflammation of the peritoneum that lines the central part of the diaphragm. In the embryo, the diaphragm originates in the neck, and its central portion is innervated by the phrenic nerve, which enters the cord at the level of the third to fifth segments (C3 to C5). As the fetus develops, the diaphragm descends to its adult position between the thoracic and abdominal cavities, while maintaining its embryonic pat-

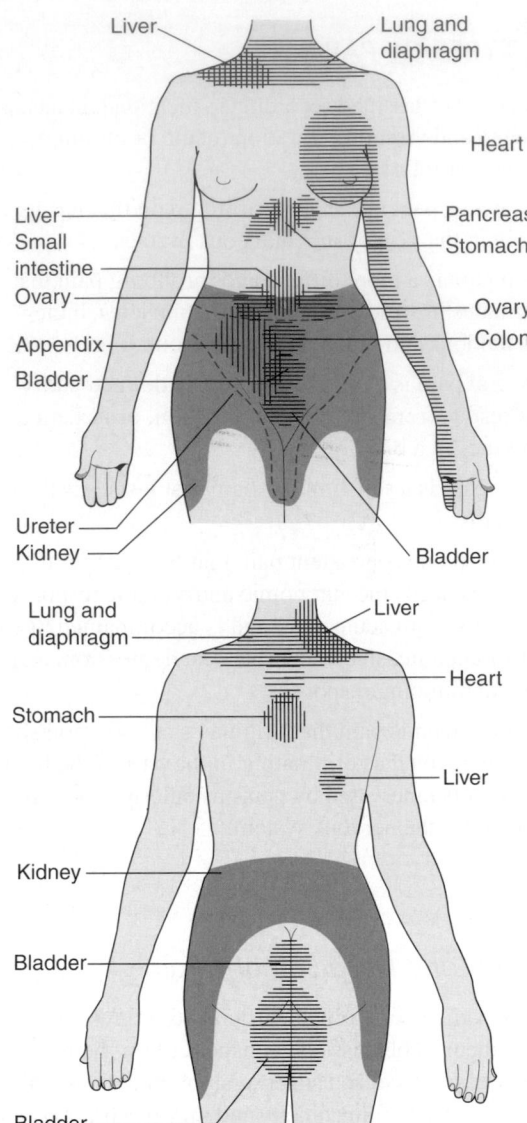

FIGURE 49-11 • Areas of referred pain. (**Top**) Anterior view. (**Bottom**) Posterior view.

tern of innervation. Thus, fibers that enter the spinal cord at the C3 to C5 levels carry information from both the neck area and the diaphragm, and the diaphragmatic pain is interpreted by the forebrain as originating in the shoulder or neck area.

Although the visceral pleura, pericardium, and peritoneum are said to be relatively free of pain fibers, the parietal pleura, pericardium, and peritoneum do react to nociceptive stimuli. Visceral inflammation can involve parietal and somatic structures, and this may give rise to diffuse local or referred pain. For example, irritation of the parietal peritoneum resulting from appendicitis typically gives rise to pain directly over the inflamed area in the lower right quadrant. Such stimuli can evoke pain referred to the umbilical area.

Muscle spasm, or *guarding,* occurs when somatic structures are involved. Guarding is a protective reflex rigidity; its purpose is to protect the affected body parts (*e.g.,* an abscessed appendix or a sprained muscle). This protective guarding may cause blood vessel compression and give rise to the pain of muscle ischemia, causing local and referred pain.

Acute and Chronic Pain

It is common to classify pain according to its duration. Pain research of the past three decades has emphasized the importance of differentiating acute pain from chronic pain. The diagnosis and therapy for each is distinctive because they differ in cause, function, mechanisms, and psychological sequelae (Table 49-1).

Traditionally, the distinction between acute and chronic pain has relied on a single continuum of time with some interval (*e.g.,* 6 months) since the onset of pain used to designate the onset of acute pain or the transition when acute pain became chronic.[18] A more recent conceptualization includes both time and pathophysiologic dimensions.[18,19] Some conditions such as osteoarthritis exhibit dimensions of both acute and chronic pain.

Acute Pain. Acute pain is pain that is elicited by injury to body tissues and activation of nociceptive stimuli at the site of local tissue damage.[20] It is generally of short duration and remits when the underlying pathologic process has resolved.[18] The purpose of acute pain is to serve as a warning system. Besides alerting the person to the existence of actual or impending tissue damage, it prompts a search for professional help. The pain's location, radiation, intensity, and duration, as well as those factors that aggravate or relieve it, provide essential diagnostic clues.

Acute pain can lead to anxiety and secondary reflex musculoskeletal spasms, which in turn tend to worsen the pain.[21] Interventions that alleviate the pain usually relieve the anxiety and musculoskeletal spasms as well. Inadequately treated pain can provoke physiologic responses that alter circulation and tissue metabolism and produce physical manifestations, such as tachycardia, reflective of increased sympathetic activity. Inadequately treated acute pain tends to decrease mobility and respiratory movements such as deep breathing and coughing to the extent that it may complicate or delay recovery.

Chronic Pain. Chronic pain is pain that persists longer than might be reasonably expected after an inciting event and is sustained by factors that are both pathologically and physically remote from the originating cause. Chronic pain continues for long periods and generally represents low levels of an underlying pathologic process that do not explain the presence or extent of the pain.[18] Chronic pain can be quite variable. It may be unrelenting and extremely severe, as in metastatic bone pain. It can be relatively continuous with or without periods of escalation, as with some forms of back pain. Some conditions with recurring episodes of acute pain are particularly problematic because they have characteristics of both acute and chronic pain. These include the pain associated with sickle cell crisis or migraine headaches.

Chronic pain is a leading cause of disability. Unlike acute pain, persistent chronic pain usually serves no useful function. To the contrary, it imposes physiologic, psychological, familial, and economic stresses and may exhaust a person's resources. In contrast to acute pain, psychological and environ-

TABLE 49-1 **Characteristics of Acute and Chronic Pain**		
CHARACTERISTIC	**ACUTE PAIN**	**CHRONIC PAIN**
Onset	Recent	Continuous or intermittent
Duration	Short (<6 months)	6 months or more
Autonomic responses	Consistent with sympathetic fight-or-flight response*	Absence of autonomic responses
	Increased heart rate	
	Increased stroke volume	
	Increased blood pressure	
	Increased pupillary dilation	
	Increased muscle tension	
	Decreased gut motility	
	Decreased salivary flow (dry mouth)	
Psychological component	Associated anxiety	Increased irritability
		Associated depression
		Somatic preoccupation
		Withdrawal from outside interests
		Decreased strength of relationships
Other types of response		Decreased sleep
		Decreased libido
		Appetite changes

*Responses are approximately proportional to intensity of the stimulus.

mental influences may play an important role in the development of behaviors associated with chronic pain.

The biologic factors that contribute to chronic pain include peripheral mechanisms, peripheral–central mechanisms, and central mechanisms.[19] Peripheral mechanisms result from persistent stimulation of nociceptors. They contribute to the pain associated with chronic musculoskeletal, visceral, and vascular disorders. Peripheral–central mechanisms involve abnormal function of the peripheral and central portions of the somatosensory system. These disorders include conditions such as those resulting from partial or complete loss of descending inhibitory pathways or spontaneous firing of regenerated nerve fibers. They include conditions such as causalgia, phantom limb pain, and postherpetic neuralgia. Central pain mechanisms are associated with disease or injury of the CNS. Central pain is characterized by burning, aching, hyperalgesia, dysesthesia, and other abnormal sensations. Central pain is associated with conditions such as thalamic lesions (thalamic pain), spinal cord injury, surgical interruption of pain pathways, and multiple sclerosis.

Persons with chronic pain may not exhibit the somatic, autonomic, or affective behaviors often associated with acute pain. As painful conditions become prolonged and continuous, autonomic nervous system responses tend to decrease. In addition, chronic pain often is associated with loss of appetite, sleep disturbances, and depression. Amazingly, depression commonly is relieved once the pain is removed. The link between depression and decreased pain tolerance may be explained by the similar manner in which both respond to changes in the biologic pathways of serotonergic and noradrenergic systems. Tricyclic antidepressants and other medications with serotonergic and noradrenergic effects have been shown to relieve a variety of chronic pain syndromes, lending credence to the theory that chronic pain and depression share a common biologic pathway.[22]

Assessment of Pain

Careful assessment of pain assists clinicians in diagnosing, managing, and relieving the patient's pain. Assessment includes such things as the nature, severity, location, and radiation of the pain. As with other disease states, eliminating the cause of the pain is preferable to simply treating the symptom. A careful history often provides information about the triggering factors (*i.e.,* injury, infection, or disease) and the site of nociceptive stimuli (*i.e.,* peripheral receptor or visceral organ). Clinical Practice Guideline No. 1, *Acute Pain Management: Operative and Medical Procedures and Trauma* (released in 1992 by the Agency for Health Care Policy and Research [AHCPR], currently the Agency for Healthcare Research and Quality, Public Health Service, U.S. Department of Health and Human Services) emphasizes that "the single most reliable indicator of the existence and intensity of acute pain—and any resultant affective discomfort or distress—is the patient's self report."[23] A comprehensive pain history should include pain onset; description, localization, radiation, intensity, quality,

and pattern of the pain; anything that relieves or exacerbates it; and the individual's personal reaction to the pain.

Unlike many other bodily responses, such as temperature and blood pressure, the nature, severity, and distress of pain cannot be measured objectively. To overcome this problem, various methods have been developed for quantifying a person's pain based on the patient's report. They include numeric pain intensity, visual analog, and verbal descriptor scales. Most pain questionnaires assess a single aspect of pain such as pain intensity. For example, a *numeric pain intensity* scale would have patients select which number best represents the intensity of their pain, where 0 represents no pain and 10 represents the most intense pain imaginable. A *visual analog* scale also can be used; it is a straight line, often 10 cm in length, with a word description (*e.g.,* "no pain" and "the most intense pain imaginable") at each of the ends of the line representing the continuum of pain intensity. Patients are asked to choose a point on the continuum that represents the intensity of their pain. The response can be quantified by measuring the line to determine the distance of the mark, measured in millimeters, from the "no pain" end of the line. *Verbal descriptor* scales consist of several numerically ranked choices of words such as none = 0, slight = 1, mild = 2, moderate = 3, and severe = 4. The word chosen is used to determine the numeric representation of pain severity on an ordinal scale.

Some pain questionnaires are multidimensional (*e.g.,* the McGill Pain Questionnaire) in that they include several sections or sets of questions that are scored into subscales that quantify various aspects of pain. The McGill Pain Questionnaire[24] is divided into four parts. The first part uses a drawing of the body on which the person indicates the location of pain. The second part uses a list of 20 words to describe the sensory, affective, evaluative, and other qualities of pain, with the selected words being given a numeric score (*e.g.,* words implying the least pain are assigned a value of 1, moderate pain a value of 2, and so on). The third part asks the person to select words such as *brief, momentary,* and *constant* to describe the pattern of pain. The fourth part of the instrument evaluates the present pain intensity on a scale with scores from 0 to 5. The Memorial Pain Assessment Card, another multidimensional instrument, can be used to determine the intensity of pain, mood, and effectiveness of analgesia.[23]

Scales developed for use in children rely on behavioral and physiologic signs for assessment of pain in preverbal children. The Objective Pain Scale was developed for use in children 6 months to 3 years of age, evaluating blood pressure, crying, movement, and agitation.[25] The CRIES scale was developed for use in neonates and infants up to 6 months of age, evaluating crying, need for oxygen to maintain saturation, vital signs, expression, and sleeplessness.[26]

Management of Pain

The therapeutic approaches to acute and chronic pain differ markedly. In acute pain, therapy is directed at providing pain relief by interrupting the nociceptive stimulus. Because the pain is self-limited, in that it resolves as the injured tissues heal, long-term therapy usually is not needed. Chronic pain management is much more complex and is based on multiple considerations, including life expectancy.

Acute Pain

Acute pain should be aggressively managed and pain medication provided before the pain becomes severe. This allows the person to be more comfortable and active and to assume a greater role in directing his or her own care. Part of the reluctance of health care workers to provide adequate relief for acute pain has been fear of addiction. However, addiction to opioid medications is thought to be virtually nonexistent when these drugs are prescribed for acute pain. Usually, less medication is needed when the drug is given before the pain becomes severe and the pain pathways become sensitized.

The AHCPR guideline, which addresses pain from surgery, medical procedures, and trauma, emphasizes the need for (1) a collaborative, interdisciplinary approach to pain control, which includes members of the health care team and input from the patient and the patient's family when appropriate; (2) an individualized, proactive pain control plan developed before surgery (if possible) by patients and providers; (3) the assessment and frequent reassessment of the patient's pain, facilitated by a pain management log or flow sheet; (4) the use of drug and nondrug therapies to control or prevent pain; and (5) a formal, institutional approach to management of acute pain with clear lines of responsibility.[23]

Chronic Pain

Management of chronic pain requires early attempts to prevent pain and adequate therapy for acute bouts of pain. Specific treatment depends on the cause of the pain, the natural history of the underlying health problem, as well as the life expectancy of the individual. If the organic illness causing the pain cannot be cured, then noncurative methods of pain control become the cornerstone of treatment. Treatment methods for chronic pain can include neural blockade, electrical modalities (e.g., transcutaneous electrical nerve stimulation), physical therapy, cognitive-behavioral interventions, and non-narcotic and narcotic medications. Non-narcotic medications such as tricyclic antidepressants, antiseizure medications, and NSAIDs serve as useful adjuncts to opioids for the treatment of different types of chronic pain. Chronic pain is best handled by a multidisciplinary team that includes specialists in areas such as anesthesiology, nursing, physical therapy, social services, and surgery.

Cancer is a common cause of chronic pain. The goal of chronic cancer pain management should be pain alleviation and prevention. Preemptive therapy tends to reduce sensitization of pain pathways and provides for more effective pain control. In 1994, the AHCPR published Clinical Practice Guideline No. 9, *Management of Cancer Pain.*[27] This guideline highlights the fact that pain control remains a significant problem despite the advances in understanding and management of pain. The report emphasizes that pain control merits high priority because it diminishes activity, appetite, and sleep and can further weaken a person already debilitated by cancer. It also emphasizes that pain interferes with productive employment, enjoying recreation, and taking an active part in family life. Like the AHCPR acute pain guideline, the cancer pain guideline emphasizes the need for a collaborative multidisciplinary approach to cancer pain management. Clinically useful interventions are described in the guideline. Some of these (e.g., analgesics, adjuvant drugs, cognitive or behavioral strategies, physical modalities, and nerve blocks) are used for many forms of chronic pain. Depending on the form and stage of the cancer, other treatments such as palliative radiation, antineoplastic therapies, and palliative surgery may help to control the pain. The AHCPR guideline also stresses that written patient education materials at an appropriate reading level should be provided. The World Health Organization has created an analgesic ladder for cancer pain that assists clinicians in choosing the appropriate analgesic.[28]

Nonpharmacologic Treatment

A number of nonpharmacologic methods of pain control often are used in pain management. These include cognitive-behavioral interventions, physical agents such as heat and cold, and electroanalgesia. Often these methods are used in addition to analgesics rather than as the only form of pain management.

Cognitive-Behavioral Interventions. Cognitive-behavioral interventions, which often are helpful for individuals experiencing acute as well as chronic pain, include relaxation, distraction, cognitive reappraisal, imagery, meditation, and biofeedback. If the person is having surgery or a painful procedure, it is ideal to teach these techniques before the pain begins (e.g., before surgery). If the person is already in severe pain, the use of cognitive-behavioral interventions should be based on the person's ability to master the technique as well as his or her response to the intervention. For example, it may be a more appropriate adjunct to analgesics for a terminally ill person in severe pain to use self-selected relaxing music rather than trying to teach that person an intervention requiring more attention (e.g., meditation or cognitive reappraisal).

Relaxation is one of the best-evaluated cognitive-behavioral approaches to pain relief. The relaxation method need not be complex. Relatively simple strategies, such as slow, rhythmic breathing and brief jaw relaxation procedures, have been successful in decreasing self-reported pain and analgesic use.

Distraction (i.e., focusing a person's attention on stimuli other than painful stimuli or negative emotions) does not eliminate pain, but it can make pain more tolerable. It may serve as a type of sensory shielding whereby attention to pain is sacrificed to pay attention to other stimuli that are easily perceived. Examples of distraction include counting, repeating phrases or poems, and engaging in activities that require concentration, such as projects, activities, work, conversation, or describing pictures. Television, adventure movies, music, and humor also can provide distraction. *Cognitive reappraisal* is a form of self-distraction or cognitive control in which individuals focus their attention on the positive aspects of the experience and away from their pain. Individuals using distraction may not appear to be in severe pain. Nonetheless, it is inappropriate to assume that a person who copes with pain by using distraction does not have pain. Prescribed analgesics should not be denied to patients simply because they appear to be coping with their pain without medication. Appropriate assessment is needed to determine the patient's level of pain and what other interventions for pain may be needed.

Imagery consists of using one's imagination to develop a mental picture. In pain management, therapeutic guided imagery (*i.e.,* goal-directed imaging) is used. It can be used alone or in conjunction with other cognitive behavioral interventions (*e.g.,* relaxation or biofeedback) to develop sensory images that may decrease the perceived intensity of pain. It also can be used to lessen anxiety and reduce muscle tension. *Meditation* also can be used, but it requires practice and the ability to concentrate to be effective.

Biofeedback is used to provide feedback to a person concerning the current status of some body function (*e.g.,* finger temperature, temporal artery pulsation, blood pressure, or muscle tension). It involves a process of learning designed to make the person aware of certain of his or her own body functions for the purpose of modifying these functions at a conscious level. Interest in biofeedback increased with the possibility of using this treatment modality in the management of migraine and tension headaches or for other pain that has a muscle tension component.

Physical Agents.   Heat and cold are physical agents that are used to provide pain relief. The choice of physical agent depends on the type of pain being treated and, in many cases, personal preference.

Heat has long been used to relieve pain. Heat dilates blood vessels and increases local blood flow; it also can influence the transmission of pain impulses and increase collagen extensibility. An increase in local circulation can reduce the level of nociceptive stimulation by reducing local ischemia caused by muscle spasm or tension, increase the removal of metabolites and inflammatory mediators that act as nociceptive stimuli, and help to reduce swelling and relieve pressure on local nociceptive endings. The heat sensation is carried to the posterior horn of the spinal cord and may exert its effect by modulating projection of pain transmission. It also may trigger the release of endogenous opioids. Heat also alters the viscosity of collagen fibers in ligaments, tendons, and joint structures so that they are more easily extended and can be stretched further before the nociceptive endings are stimulated. Thus, heat often is applied before therapy aimed at stretching joint structures and increasing range of motion. Care must be taken not to use excessive heat. When excessive heat is used, the heat itself becomes a noxious stimulus, which results in actual or impending tissue damage and pain. In certain conditions, the use of heat is controversial, and in some conditions (*e.g.,* peripheral vascular dis-

ease) where increased blood flow or metabolism would be detrimental, the use of heat is contraindicated.

Like heat, the application of *cold* may produce a dramatic reduction in pain. Cold exerts its effect on pain through circulatory and neural mechanisms. The initial response to local application of cold is sudden local vasoconstriction. This initial vasoconstriction is followed by alternating periods of vasodilation and vasoconstriction during which the body "hunts" for its normal level of blood flow to prevent local tissue damage. This gives rise to the so-called *hunting reflex* whereby the circulation to the cooled area undergoes alternating periods of pallor caused by ischemia and flushing caused by hyperemia.[29] The vasoconstriction is caused by local stimulation of sympathetic fibers and direct cooling of blood vessels, and the hyperemia by local autoregulatory mechanisms. In situations of acute injury, cold is used to produce vasoconstriction and prevent extravasation of blood into the tissues; pain relief results from decreased swelling and decreased stimulation of nociceptive endings. The vasodilation that follows can be useful in removing substances that stimulate nociceptive endings.

Cold also can have a marked and dramatic effect on pain that results from the spasm-induced accumulation of metabolites in muscle. In terms of pain modulation, cold may reduce afferent activity reaching the posterior horn of the spinal cord by modulating sensory input. The application of cold is a noxious stimulus and may influence the release of endogenous opioids from the PAG area. Cold packs should be flexible to conform to body parts easily, adequately wrapped to protect the skin, and applied no more than 15 to 20 minutes at a time. Cold should be used only with great caution in anyone whose circulation is compromised.

Stimulus-Induced Analgesia.   Stimulus-induced analgesia is one of the oldest known methods of pain relief. Historical references to the use of electricity to decrease or control pain date back to 46 AD, when a Roman physician, Scribonius Largus, described how the stimulus from an electric eel was able to provide pain relief for headache and gout.[30] Electrical stimulation methods of pain relief include transcutaneous electrical nerve stimulation (TENS), electrical acupuncture, and neurostimulation. TENS refers to the transmission of electrical energy across the surface of the skin to the peripheral nerve fibers. TENS units have been developed that are convenient, easily transported, and relatively economical to use. Most are approximately the size of a deck of cards. These battery-operated units deliver an electrical current to a target site.

The system usually consists of three parts: a pair of electrodes, lead wires, and a stimulator. The electrical stimulation is delivered in a pulsed waveform that can be varied in terms of pulse amplitude, width, and rate. The type of stimulation used varies with the type of pain being treated. Electrode placement is determined by the physiologic pathways and an understanding of the pain mechanisms involved. They may be placed on either side of a painful area, over an affected dermatome, over an affected peripheral nerve where it is most superficial, or over a nerve trunk. For example, the electrodes commonly are placed medial and lateral to the incision when treating post-operative pain.

There probably is no single explanation for the physiologic effects of TENS. Each specific type of stimulator may have different sites of action and may be explained by more than one theory. The gate control theory was proposed as one possible mechanism. According to this theory, pain information is transmitted by small-diameter Aδ and C fibers. Large-diameter afferent A fibers and small-diameter fibers carry tactile information mediating touch, pressure, and kinesthesia. TENS may function on the basis of differential firing of impulses in the large fibers that carry nonpainful information. Accordingly, increased activity in these larger fibers purportedly modulates transmission of painful information to the forebrain. A second possible explanation is that the high-frequency stimulation (50 to 60 Hz) produced by some units simply acts as a counterirritant.[31] A third possible explanation is that stimulators that produce strong rhythmic contractions may act through the release of endogenous analgesics such as the endorphins and enkephalins that suppress or modulate pain transmission. A fourth, and probably the best, explanation for quick analgesia with brief, intense stimulation is that it acts as a conduction block.[32,33] TENS has the advantage that it is noninvasive, easily regulated by the person or health professional, and effective in some forms of acute and chronic pain. Its use can be taught before surgery, affording a reduction in postoperative analgesic medication and, possibly, preventing the development of persistent pain.

Acupuncture. The practice of acupuncture involves introducing needles into specific points on the surface of the body. Charts are available that describe the points of needle placement that are used to relieve pain at certain anatomic sites. In addition to needles, sometimes palpation is used. The practice of acupuncture dates back thousands of years to ancient China, when the stimulation was achieved by using needles made of bone, stone, or bamboo. Annually, approximately 1 million individuals in the United States receive acupuncture, and pain is the major complaint for which they receive it.[34] Acupuncture is widely available in pain clinics even though large, high-quality, randomized studies on the effects of acupuncture for chronic pain are not plentiful. Various theories of how acupuncture achieves analgesia have been proposed, including the gate control theory and the neurohumoral theory, involving the cascade of endorphins and monoamines.[34]

Neurostimulation. Neurostimulation delivers low-voltage electrical stimulation to the spinal cord or targeted peripheral nerve to block the sensation of pain. Melzack and Wall (gate theory) proposed that neurostimulation activates the body's pain-inhibiting system.[8] The neurostimulation system implanted in the epidural space stimulates pain-inhibiting nerve fibers in the dorsal horn of the spinal cord, masking the sensation of pain with a tingling sensation (paresthesia).[35]

There are two types of neurostimulation systems: one that is completely internal (surgically implanted) and one that

has both internal and external components.[35] For a totally implantable system, the power source (battery) and lead(s) are surgically implanted. In the other type of system, the radio-frequency receiver and leads are implanted and the power source with an antenna is worn externally.

Pharmacologic Treatment

Analgesics have been used for many years to relieve pain of short duration, enabling the person to achieve mobility after surgery, for example, when exercises such as coughing and deep breathing may be required. The use of analgesics is only one aspect of a comprehensive pain management program with acute pain, and even more so with chronic pain. An analgesic drug is a medication that acts on the nervous system to decrease or eliminate pain without inducing loss of consciousness. Analgesic drugs do not cure the underlying cause of the pain, but their appropriate use may prevent acute pain from progressing to chronic pain. The AHCPR cancer pain guideline classifies pain medications into three categories: aspirin, other NSAIDs, and acetaminophen; opioid analgesics; and adjuvant analgesics.[27]

The ideal analgesic would be effective, nonaddictive, and inexpensive. In addition, it would produce minimal adverse effects and not affect the person's level of consciousness. Although long-term treatment with opioids can result in opioid tolerance (*i.e.,* more drug being needed to achieve the same effect) and physical dependence, this should not be confused with addiction. Long-term drug-seeking behavior is rare in persons who are treated with opioids only during the time that they require pain relief. The unique needs and circumstances presented by each person in pain must be addressed to achieve satisfactory pain management.

Non-narcotic Analgesics. Common non-narcotic oral analgesic medications include aspirin, other NSAIDs, and acetaminophen. Aspirin, or acetylsalicylic acid, acts centrally and peripherally to block the transmission of pain impulses. It also has antipyretic and anti-inflammatory properties. The action of aspirin and other NSAIDs is through the inhibition of the cyclooxygenase (COX) enzymes, which mediate the biosynthesis of prostaglandins. Prostaglandins (particularly, prostaglandin E_2) exert their effect through peripheral sensitization of nociceptors to chemical mediators such as bradykinin and histamine.[36] The NSAIDs also decrease the sensitivity of blood vessels to bradykinin and histamine, affect cytokine production by T lymphocytes, reverse vasodilation, and decrease the release of inflammatory mediators from granulocytes, mast cells, and basophils. Acetaminophen is an alternative to the NSAIDs. Although usually considered equivalent to aspirin as an analgesic and antipyretic agent, it lacks anti-inflammatory properties.

Opioid Analgesics. The term *opioid* or *narcotic* is used to refer to a group of medications, natural or synthetic, with morphine-like actions.[36] The older term *opiate* was used to designate drugs derived from opium—morphine, codeine, and many other semisynthetic congeners of morphine. Opioids are used for relief of short-term pain and for more long-term use in conditions such as cancer pain. When given for temporary relief of severe pain, such as that occurring after surgery, there is much evidence that opioids given routinely before the pain starts (preemptive analgesia) or becomes extreme are far more effective than those administered in a sporadic manner. Persons who are treated in this manner seem to require fewer doses and are able to resume regular activities sooner.

Opioids also are used for persons with limited life expectancy. Too often, because of undue concern about the possibility of addiction, many chronic pain sufferers with a short life expectancy receive inadequate pain relief. Most pain experts agree that it is appropriate to provide the level of opioid necessary to relieve the severe, intractable pain of persons whose life expectancy is limited. Addiction is not considered a problem in patients with cancer.[37,38] In persons with chronic cancer pain, morphine remains the most useful strong opioid. The World Health Organization has recommended that oral morphine be part of the essential medication list and be made available throughout the world as the medication of choice for cancer pain.[27,39] Oral forms of morphine are well absorbed from the gastrointestinal tract and have a half-life of approximately 2.5 hours and a duration of action of 4 to 6 hours. Liquid forms of the medication usually are given at 4-hour intervals to maintain an adequate blood level for analgesia, while minimizing the potential for toxic side effects. Controlled-release forms of the drug also are available, lasting 8 to 20 hours.

Although the analgesic and psychopharmacologic properties of morphine have been known for centuries, the fact that the brain contains its own endogenous opioid-like chemicals, the endorphins (enkephalins, endorphins, and dynorphins), has become known only within the last 40 to 50 years. It has been hypothesized that part of the pain-relieving properties of exogenous opioids such as morphine involves the release of these endogenous opioid peptides.[36]

The opioid analgesics are characterized by their interaction with three types of opioid receptors, designated mu (μ, for "morphine"), delta (δ), and kappa (κ).[36,40] Each receptor type has been cloned and subtypes have been identified using receptor binding and molecular studies. Morphine and most opioids that are used clinically exert their effects through the mu receptor. Kappa receptor opioids are effective analgesics, but their side effects have proven troublesome, and the clinical impact of delta receptor opioids has been negligible.

It is well documented that the mu receptors modulate both the therapeutic effect of analgesia, as well as the side effects of respiratory depression, miosis, reduced gastrointestinal motility (causing constipation), feelings of well-being or euphoria, and physical dependence. The mu receptors are found at presynaptic and postsynaptic sites in the spinal dorsal horn, and in the ascending pathways of the brain stem, thalamus, and cortex, as well as the descending inhibitory system

that modulates pain at the spinal cord. Their spinal location has been used clinically by direct application of opioid analgesics to the spinal cord by injection, infusion, or implantable intrathecal device (pump), which provides regional anesthesia while minimizing the unwanted respiratory depression, nausea and vomiting, and sedation that occur with systemically administered drugs that act at the brain level. Mu receptors are also found in peripheral sensory neurons after inflammation. This location supports the exploration and eventual clinical use of locally applied opioids (*e.g.,* intra-articular instillation of opioids after knee surgery).

As more information becomes available regarding the opioids and their receptors, it seems likely that pain medications can be developed that act selectively at certain receptor sites, providing more effective pain control while producing fewer adverse effects and affording less danger of addiction. For example, it might be possible to develop opioid drugs that produce effective analgesia but not undesirable adverse effects, such as respiratory depression and the most common complication, constipation.[41]

One of the problems with the need for long-term use of opioids, as in relief of cancer pain, is the development of tolerance or the need for larger and larger doses to achieve the same level of pain relief. Clinicians have long noted two important phenomena that suggest the possibility of multiple mu opioid receptor subtypes and support the importance of research in this area.[38] First, there are often noteworthy differences in patient responses to mu opioids. Patient-specific responses to these drugs include both the extent of relief obtained and the side effect profiles observed. Second, patients who become tolerant to one mu opioid are often far less tolerant to another mu opioid. The difference in tolerance across mu opioids is called *incomplete cross-tolerance.*[40]

Some clinicians use opioid rotation to improve analgesia once opioid tolerance becomes problematic. It is important to note that the standard equianalgesic conversion tables are based primarily on single-dose studies and as such do not account for incomplete cross-tolerance. When opioid rotation is used with patients demonstrating a tolerance to opioids, it is recommended that the new opioid be started at a fraction of the dosage that is predicted to be equivalent to the current opioid dosage.[40]

Adjuvant Analgesics. Adjuvant analgesics include medications such as tricyclic antidepressants, antiseizure medications, and neuroleptic anxiolytic agents. The fact that the pain suppression system has nonendorphin synapses raises the possibility that potent, centrally acting, nonopiate medications may be useful in relieving pain. Serotonin has been shown to play an important role in producing analgesia. The tricyclic antidepressant medications (*i.e.,* imipramine, amitriptyline, and doxepin) that block the removal of serotonin from the synaptic cleft have been shown to produce pain relief in some persons. These medications are particularly useful in some chronic painful conditions, such as postherpetic neuralgia.

Certain antiseizure medications, such as carbamazepine and gabapentin, have analgesic effects in some pain conditions. These medications, which suppress spontaneous neuronal firing, are particularly useful in the management of pain that occurs after nerve injury (neuropathic pain), including diabetic neuropathy and chronic regional pain syndrome. Other agents, such as the corticosteroids, may be used to decrease inflammation and the nociceptive stimuli responsible for pain.

Surgical Intervention

If surgery removes the problem causing the pain, such as a tumor pressing on a nerve or an inflamed appendix, it can be curative. In other instances, surgery is used for symptom management rather than for cure. However, with rare exceptions, noninvasive analgesic approaches should precede invasive palliative approaches.[20] Surgery for severe, intractable pain of peripheral or central origin has met with some success. It can be used to remove the cause or block the transmission of intractable pain from phantom limb pain, severe neuralgia, inoperable cancer of certain types, and causalgia.

IN SUMMARY, pain is an elusive and complex phenomenon; it is a symptom common to many illnesses. It is a highly individualized experience that is shaped by a person's culture and previous life experiences, and it is difficult to measure. Traditionally, there have been two principal theories of pain, specificity and pattern theories. Scientifically, pain is viewed within the context of nociception. Nociceptors are receptive nerve endings that respond to noxious stimuli. Pain receptors respond to mechanical, thermal, and chemical stimuli. Nociceptive neurons transmit impulses to the dorsal horn neurons using chemical neurotransmitters. The neospinothalamic and the paleospinothalamic pathways are used to transmit pain information to the brain. Several neuroanatomic pathways as well as endogenous opioid peptides modulate pain in the CNS.

Pain can be classified according to location, referral, and duration as well as associated medical diagnoses. Pain can arise from cutaneous, deep somatic, or visceral locations. Referred pain is pain perceived at a site different from its origin. Acute pain is self-limiting pain that ends when the injured tissue heals, whereas chronic pain is pain that lasts much longer than the anticipated healing time for the underlying cause of the pain. Pain threshold, pain tolerance, age, sex, and other factors affect an individual's reaction to pain.

Treatment modalities for pain include the use of physiologic, cognitive, and behavioral measures; heat and cold; stimulation-induced analgesic methods; and pharmacologic agents singly or in combination. It is becoming apparent that even with chronic pain, the most effective approach is early treatment or even prevention. After pain is present, the greatest success in pain assessment and management is achieved with the use of an interdisciplinary approach. ■

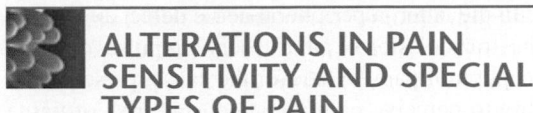

ALTERATIONS IN PAIN SENSITIVITY AND SPECIAL TYPES OF PAIN

After completing this section of the chapter, you should be able to meet the following objectives:

- Define allodynia, hypoesthesia, hyperesthesia, paresthesias, hyperpathia, analgesia, and hypoalgesia and hyperalgesia.
- Describe the cause and characteristics and treatment of neuropathic pain, trigeminal neuralgia, postherpetic neuralgia, and complex regional pain syndrome.
- Cite possible mechanisms of phantom limb pain.

Alterations in Pain Sensitivity

Sensitivity to and perception of pain vary among persons and in the same person under different conditions and in different parts of the body. Irritation, mild hypoxia, and mild compression of a peripheral nerve often result in hyperexcitability of the sensory nerve fibers or cell bodies. This is experienced as unpleasant hypersensitivity (*i.e., hyperesthesia*) or increased painfulness (*i.e., hyperalgesia*). Primary hyperalgesia describes pain sensitivity that occurs directly in damaged tissues. Secondary hyperalgesia occurs in the surrounding uninjured tissue. Possible causes of hyperalgesia include increased sensitivity to noxious stimuli, a decrease in the threshold of nociceptors, an increase in pain produced by suprathreshold stimuli, and the windup phenomenon. Hyperalgesia can also be induced by mediators released by immune cells during an inflammatory or allergic response that act directly on nociceptors or indirectly through the release of other mediators, such as the prostaglandins.[42]

Hyperpathia is a syndrome in which the sensory threshold is raised, but when it is reached, continued stimulation, especially if repetitive, results in a prolonged and unpleasant experience. This pain can be explosive and radiates through a peripheral nerve distribution. It is associated with pathologic changes in peripheral nerves, such as localized ischemia. Spontaneous, unpleasant sensations called *paresthesias* occur with more severe irritation (*e.g.*, the pins-and-needles sensation that follows temporary compression of a peripheral nerve). The general term *dysesthesia* is given to distortions (usually unpleasant) of somesthetic sensation that typically accompany partial loss of sensory innervation.

More severe pathologic processes can result in reduced or lost tactile (*e.g., hypoesthesia, anesthesia*), temperature (*e.g., hypothermia, athermia*), and pain sensation (*i.e., hypoalgesia*). *Analgesia* is the absence of pain on noxious stimulation or the relief of pain without loss of consciousness. The inability to sense pain may result in trauma, infection, and even loss of a body part or parts. Inherited insensitivity to pain may take the form of congenital indifference or congenital insensitivity to pain. In the former, transmission of nerve impulses appears normal but appreciation of painful stimuli at higher levels appears to be absent. In the latter, a peripheral nerve defect apparently exists such that transmission of painful nerve impulses does not result in perception of pain. Whatever the cause, persons who lack the ability to perceive pain are at constant risk of tissue damage because pain is not serving its protective function.

Allodynia (Greek *allo,* "other," and *odynia,* "painful") is the term used for the puzzling phenomenon of pain that follows a non-noxious stimulus to apparently normal skin. Non-noxious stimuli may include wind, touching sheets, and showering. This term is intended to refer to instances in which otherwise normal tissues may be abnormally innervated or may be referral sites for other loci that give rise to pain with non-noxious stimuli. It can result from increased responsiveness within the spinal cord (central sensitization) or a reduction in the threshold for nociceptor activation (peripheral sensitization). With central sensitization, activity in non-nociceptive nerve fibers can produce pain. With peripheral sensitization, tissue damage and inflammation (referred to as the "inflammatory soup") may cause the area to become hypersensitive, in which case a normally subthreshold stimulus is sufficient to trigger the sensation of pain.[12]

One type of allodynia involves *trigger points,* which are highly localized points on the skin or mucous membrane that can produce immediate intense pain at that site or elsewhere when stimulated by light tactile stimulation. Myofascial trigger points are foci of exquisite tenderness found in many muscles and can be responsible for pain projected to sites remote from the points of tenderness. Trigger points are widely distributed in the back of the head and neck and in the lumbar and thoracic regions. These trigger points cause reproducible myofascial pain syndromes in specific muscles. These pain syndromes are the major source of pain in clients at chronic pain treatment centers.

Special Types of Pain

Neuropathic Pain

"Neuropathic pain refers to pain that originates from pathology of the nervous system."[43] When peripheral nerves are affected by injury or disease, it can lead to unusual and sometimes intractable sensory disturbances. The notable features that point to neuropathic processes as a cause of pain include widespread pain that is not otherwise explainable, evidence of sensory deficit (*e.g.,* numbness, paresthesias), burning pain, pain that occurs with light stroking of the skin, and attacks of pain that occur without seeming provocation.[43] Depending on the cause, few or many axons could be damaged and the condition could be unilateral or bilateral. Neuropathic pain is distinguished from other pain conditions where the pain stimulus begins in non-neuronal tissues.

Causes of neuropathic pain can be categorized according to the extent of peripheral nerve involvement. Conditions that can lead to pain by causing damage to peripheral nerves in a single area include nerve entrapment, nerve compression from a tumor mass, and various neuralgias (*e.g.,* trigeminal, posther-

petic, and post-traumatic). Conditions that can lead to pain by causing damage to peripheral nerves in a wide area include diabetes mellitus, long-term alcohol use, hypothyroidism, renal insufficiency, and drug treatment with neurotoxic agents.[44] Diabetes often causes a length-dependent neuropathy (meaning that the longest axons in a peripheral nerve are most vulnerable). Injury to a nerve also can lead to a multisymptom, multisystem syndrome called *complex regional pain syndrome.* Nerve damage associated with amputation is believed to be a cause of phantom limb pain.

Neuropathic pain can vary with the extent and location of disease or injury. There may be allodynia or pain that is stabbing, jabbing, burning, or shooting. The pain may be persistent or intermittent. The diagnosis depends on the mode of onset, the distribution of abnormal sensations, the quality of the pain, and other relevant medical conditions (*e.g.,* diabetes, hypothyroidism, alcohol use, rash, or trauma). Injury to peripheral nerves sometimes results in pain that persists beyond the time required for the tissues to heal. Peripheral pathologic processes (*e.g.,* neural degeneration, neuroma formation, and generation of abnormal spontaneous neural discharges from the injured sensory neuron) and neural plasticity (*i.e.,* changes in CNS function) are the primary working hypotheses to explain persistent neuropathic pain.

Treatment methods include measures aimed at restoring or preventing further nerve damage (*e.g.,* surgical resection of a tumor causing nerve compression, improving glycemic control for diabetic patients with painful neuropathies), and interventions for the palliation of pain. Although many adjuvant analgesics are used for neuropathic pain, pain control often is difficult. The initial approach in seeking adequate pain control is to try these drugs in sequence and then in combination. The adjuvant analgesics can be divided into three general classes according to the pain they are used to treat: burning, tingling, or aching pain; stabbing or shooting pain; and neurogenic pain. For pain that is burning, tingling or aching, tricyclic antidepressants and the α_2-adrenergic agonist clonidine frequently are used. For the stabbing or shooting pain of neuralgias, antiseizure medications or baclofen, a drug used in treatment of spasticity, may be used.[44]

Poor pain control or unacceptable side effects may lead to a trial with other medications. If there has been a poor response to the adjuvant analgesics, opioids also can be used. However, concerns about side effects and the remote possibility of addiction must be considered. When opioids are used, the use of long-acting opioids with a plan for breakthrough pain is desirable because it addresses the typically continuous nature of neuropathic pain. Nonpharmacologic therapies also are used for neurogenic pain. Electrical stimulation of the peripheral nerve or spinal cord can be used for radiculopathies and neuralgias. As a last resort, neurolysis or neurosurgical blockade sometimes is used.

Neuralgia

Neuralgia is characterized by severe, brief, often repetitive attacks of lightning-like or throbbing pain. It occurs along the distribution of a spinal or cranial nerve and usually is precipitated by stimulation of the cutaneous region supplied by that nerve.

Trigeminal Neuralgia. Trigeminal neuralgia, or *tic douloureux*, is one of the most common and severe neuralgias. It is manifested by facial tics or spasms and characterized by paroxysmal attacks of stabbing pain that usually are limited to the unilateral sensory distribution of one or more branches of the trigeminal nerve, most often the maxillary or mandibular divisions.[44,45] Although intermittent, the pain often is excruciating and may be triggered by light touch, movement, drafts, and eating.[45] Considerable controversy remains regarding the pathophysiology of trigeminal neuralgia. One theory suggests that peripheral injury or disease of the trigeminal nerve increases afferent firing in the nerve. Failure of central inhibitory mechanisms may be involved as well.[45]

Treatment of trigeminal neuralgia includes pharmacologic and surgical modalities. Other interventions include avoidance of precipitating factors (*e.g.,* stimulation of trigger spots) and eye injury due to irritation; provision for adequate nutrition; and avoidance of social isolation. Carbamazepine, an antiseizure drug, is recognized as a first-line agent for treatment of trigeminal neuralgia.[45] Surgical release of vessels, dural structures, or scar tissue surrounding the semilunar ganglion or root in the middle cranial fossa often eliminates the symptoms. If not, percutaneous blocking or partial destruction of peripheral branches of the trigeminal nerve with heat, glycerol, or balloon compression may be used.[45] Gamma knife radiosurgery, a form of stereotactic radiosurgery, is one of the newest techniques for trigeminal neuralgia.[45] The procedure uses a stereotactic head frame, stereotactic imaging of the trigeminal nerve root entry zone, and radiation of the trigeminal nerve. There has also been recent interest in the use of botulinum toxin as a treatment modality.[45]

Postherpetic Neuralgia. Herpes zoster (also called *shingles*) is caused by the same herpes virus (varicella-zoster virus) that causes chickenpox and is thought to represent a localized recurrent infection by the varicella-zoster virus that has remained latent in the dorsal root ganglia since the initial attack of chickenpox[46,47] (see Chapter 61). Reactivation of viral replication is associated with a decline in cellular immunity, such as occurs with aging. Thus, the probability of developing herpes zoster increases strikingly with aging, and most cases occur in the elderly.[47] Impaired cellular immunity also increases the risk of herpes zoster.

During the acute attack of herpes zoster, the reactivated virus travels from the affected sensory ganglia and peripheral nerve to the skin of the corresponding dermatomes, causing a unilateral localized vesicular eruption and hyperpathia (*i.e.,* abnormally exaggerated subjective response to pain). In the acute infection, proportionately more of the large nerve fibers are destroyed. Regenerated fibers appear to have smaller diameters. Because there is a relative loss of large fibers with age, elderly persons are particularly prone to suffering because of the shift in the proportion of large- to small-diameter nerve fibers.

Most recent definitions of postherpetic neuralgia describe the presence of pain more than 90 to 120 days after the onset of the herpes rash, which eliminates pain from acute inflammation and ensures that the person has true chronic neuropathic pain.[46] Persons with postherpetic neuralgia may suffer from constant pain ("burning, aching, throbbing"), intermittent pain ("stabbing, shooting"), and stimulus-evoked pain (allodynia). Persons with allodynia often suffer from excruciating pain after the slightest touch to affected skin by such things as cold wind or clothing.[46] These subtypes of pain may interfere with sleep and basic activities of living, causing chronic fatigue, depression, anorexia, weight loss, and social isolation.

Early treatment of shingles with antiviral drugs such as acyclovir or valacyclovir that inhibit herpes virus deoxyribonucleic acid (DNA) replication may reduce the severity of herpes zoster. Initially, postherpetic neuralgia can be treated with a topical anesthetic agent, lidocaine–prilocaine cream or 5% lidocaine gel. A tricyclic antidepressant medication, such as amitriptyline or desipramine, may be used for pain relief. Regional nerve blockade (*i.e.,* stellate ganglion, epidural, local infiltration, or peripheral nerve block) has been used with limited success.

A recent trial investigating a new live attenuated herpes zoster vaccine among adults 60 years of age and older, designed to boost their cell-mediated immunity to the varicella-zoster virus, demonstrated dramatic decreases in the incidence of herpes zoster and postherpetic neuralgia.[48] In 2006, the vaccine was approved by the U.S. Food and Drug Administration (FDA) for prevention of herpes zoster in persons 60 years of age and older. It is not indicated for treatment of herpes zoster or postherpetic neuralgia.

Complex Regional Pain Syndrome

The complex regional pain syndrome (CRPS), formerly known as *reflex sympathetic dystrophy* (RSD), is a rare disorder of the extremities characterized by autonomic and vasomotor instability.[49–51] There are two forms of the CRPS: CRPS I (equivalent of RSD) and CRPS II, also known as *causalgia.* The International Association for the Study of Pain (IASP) lists the diagnostic criteria for CRPS I (RSD) as the presence of an initiating traumatic event, continuing pain, allodynia (perception of pain from a nonpainful stimulus), or hyperalgesia disproportionate to the inciting event with evidence at some time of edema, changes in skin blood flow, or abnormal sensorimotor activity in the area of pain. The diagnosis is excluded by the existence of any condition that would otherwise account for the degree of pain and dysfunction.[51]

According to the IASP, CRPS II (*i.e.,* causalgia) is diagnosed as the presence of continuing pain, allodynia, or hyperalgesia after a nerve injury, not necessarily limited to the distribution of the injured nerve with evidence at some time of edema, changes in skin blood flow, or abnormal sensorimotor activity in the region of pain.[51] The diagnosis is excluded by the existence of any condition that would otherwise account for the degree of pain and dysfunction. The primary difference between type I and type II is the identification of a definable nerve injury.

The hallmark of both types of CRPS is pain and mobility problems more severe than the injury warrants. Characteristically, the pain is severe and burning with or without deep aching. Usually, the pain can be elicited with the slightest movement or touch to the affected area, it increases with repetitive stimulation, and it lasts even after the stimulation has stopped. The pain can be exacerbated by emotional upsets or any increased peripheral sympathetic nerve stimulation. All the variations of CRPS include sympathetic components. These are characterized by vascular and trophic (*e.g.*, dystrophic or atrophic) changes to the skin, soft tissue, and bone, and can include rubor or pallor, sweating or dryness, edema (often sharply demarcated), and, with time, patchy osteoporosis.

The pathophysiologic process of CRPS remains obscure. In 1916, Leriche proposed that increased local sympathetic outflow in response to heightened afferent activity was the cause of symptoms such as pain, redness, heat, and edema. Although abnormalities in sympathetic activity are observed, recent experimental data suggest sensitization of small-diameter, polymodal C and Aδ fibers to noxious stimuli may be the basis for hyperalgia to heat and nociceptive stimuli.[52] There is also evidence that central mechanisms may play a role in sensitization of central neurons (the previously described dorsal horn WDR neurons) that occurs after intense peripheral mechanical stimuli or continuous activity in nociceptors. The role of the α_1-adrenergic receptors in sympathetic efferent or afferent coupling, either directly or indirectly through prostaglandin or α_1-adrenergic receptor activity, is considered to contribute to the excitation and sensitization of the nociceptive afferents. Other proposed mechanisms include neurogenic inflammation caused by the activation of neuromediators, such as substance P, calcitonin gene-related peptide, and histamine, which also mediates inflammation and vasodilation of microvessels.[49] Recent research demonstrated the presence of autoantibodies against autonomic nervous system structures in patients with CRPS, especially CRPS II, suggesting that the disorder may result from dysfunction of the autonomic nervous system caused by an autoimmune attack.[53]

Early mobilization after injury or surgery reduces the likelihood of developing the syndrome.[52] In addition to addressing the underlying disorder, treatment is directed at restoration of function. Physical therapy is a cornerstone of therapy. Pain management involves the use of standard pharmacologic agents used in the management of neuropathic pain, namely, antidepressants (*e.g.*, amitriptyline) and antiseizure drugs (*e.g.*, gabapentin). Short-term corticosteroid (prednisone) treatment may be used in resistant cases. If this does not lead to improvement, treatment by sympathetic blockade may provide relief from pain; it also determines the extent to which the pain is sympathetically maintained. The latter mechanism, when present, might respond to the use of an α_1-adrenergic receptor antagonist (*e.g.*, terazosin, phenoxybenzamine). Electrical neurostimulation of the spinal cord may also be considered. Neurostimulation not only may provide analgesia, it may reduce the burning dysesthesia of

which many patients complain. It may also improve circulation in the affected extremity by blocking the sympathetic efferent pathways.[52]

Phantom Limb Pain

Phantom limb pain, a type of neurologic pain, follows amputation of a limb or part of a limb. As many as 70% of amputees experience phantom limb pain.[54] The pain often begins as sensations of tingling, heat and cold, or heaviness, followed by burning, cramping, or shooting pain. It may disappear spontaneously or persist for many years. One of the more troublesome aspects of phantom pain is that the person may experience painful sensations that were present before the amputation, such as that of a painful ulcer or bunion.

Several theories have been proposed as to the causes of phantom limb pain.[54] One theory is that the end of a regenerating nerve becomes trapped in the scar tissue of the amputation site. It is known that when a peripheral nerve is cut, the scar tissue that forms becomes a barrier to regenerating outgrowth of the axon. The growing axon often becomes trapped in the scar tissue, forming a tangled growth (*i.e.*, neuroma) of small-diameter axons, including primary nociceptive afferents and sympathetic efferents. It has been proposed that these afferents show increased sensitivity to innocuous mechanical stimuli and to sympathetic activity and circulating catecholamines. A related theory moves the source of phantom limb pain to the spinal cord, suggesting that the pain is due to the spontaneous firing of spinal cord neurons that have lost their normal sensory input from the body. In this case, a closed self-exciting neuronal loop in the posterior horn of the spinal cord is postulated to send impulses to the brain, resulting in pain. Even the slightest irritation to the amputated limb area can initiate this cycle. Other theories propose that the phantom limb pain may arise in the brain itself. In one hypothesis, the pain is caused by changes in the flow of signals through somatosensory areas of the brain. In other words, there appears to be plasticity even in the adult CNS. Treatment of phantom limb pain has been accomplished by the use of sympathetic blocks, TENS of the large myelinated afferents innervating the area, hypnosis, and relaxation training.

> **IN SUMMARY,** pain may occur with or without an adequate stimulus, or it may be absent in the presence of an adequate stimulus—either of which describes a pain disorder. There may be analgesia (absence of pain), hyperalgesia (increased sensitivity to pain), hypoalgesia (a decreased sensitivity to painful stimuli), hyperpathia (an unpleasant and prolonged response to pain), hyperesthesia (an abnormal increase in sensitivity to sensation), hypoesthesia (an abnormal decrease in sensitivity to sensations), paresthesia (abnormal touch sensation such as tingling or "pins and needles" in the absence of external stimuli), or allodynia (pain produced by stimuli that do not normally cause pain).
>
> Neuropathic pain may be due to trauma or disease of neurons in a focal area or in a more global distribution (*e.g.*, from

endocrine disease or neurotoxic medications). Neuralgia is characterized by severe, brief, often repetitive attacks of lightning-like or throbbing pain that occurs along the distribution of a spinal or cranial nerve and usually is precipitated by stimulation of the cutaneous region supplied by that nerve. Trigeminal neuralgia, or tic douloureux, is one of the most common and severe neuralgias. It is manifested by facial tics or spasms. Postherpetic neuralgia is a chronic pain that can occur after shingles, an infection of the dorsal root ganglia and corresponding areas of innervation by the varicella-zoster virus. CRPS types I and II are severe pain syndromes characterized by severe pain or hyperalgesia, edema, changes in skin blood flow, and abnormal sensorimotor activity that typically follow an initiating traumatic event. The primary difference between CRPS I and II is the identification of a definable nerve injury. Phantom limb pain, a neurologic pain, can occur after amputation of a limb or part of a limb. ■

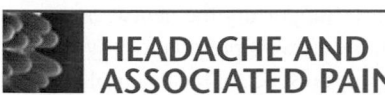

HEADACHE AND ASSOCIATED PAIN

After completing this section of the chapter, you should be able to meet the following objectives:

- State the importance of distinguishing between primary and secondary types of headache.
- Differentiate between the periodicity of occurrence and manifestations of migraine headache, cluster headache, tension-type headache, and headache due to temporomandibular joint syndrome.
- Characterize the nonpharmacologic and pharmacologic methods used in treatment of headache.
- Cite the most common cause of temporomandibular joint pain.

Headache

Headache is a very common health problem, with over 90% of adults reporting having a headache at least once. Seventy-six percent of women and 57% of men report at least one headache a month.[55] Twenty-five percent of adults report having recurrent severe headaches and 4% report having daily or nearly daily headaches.[56] Although head and facial pain have characteristics that distinguish them from other pain disorders, they also share many of the same features.

Headache is caused by a number of conditions. Some headaches represent primary disorders and others occur secondary to other disease conditions in which head pain is a symptom. The most common types of primary or chronic headaches are migraine headache, tension-type headache, cluster headache, and chronic daily headache. Although most causes of secondary headache are benign, some are indications of serious

disorders such as meningitis, brain tumor, or cerebral aneurysm. The sudden onset of a severe, intractable headache in an otherwise healthy person is more likely related to a serious intracranial disorder, such as subarachnoid hemorrhage or meningitis, than to a chronic headache disorder. Headaches that disturb sleep, exertional headaches (*e.g.*, triggered by physical or sexual activity or a Valsalva maneuver), and headaches accompanied by neurologic symptoms such as drowsiness, visual or limb disturbances, or altered mental status also are suggestive of underlying intracranial lesions or other pathologic processes. Other red flags for secondary headache disorder include a fundamental change or progression in headache pattern or a new headache in individuals younger than 5 or older than 50 years of age, or in individuals with cancer, immunosuppression, or pregnancy.[56]

The diagnosis and classification of headaches often is difficult. It requires a comprehensive history and physical examination to exclude secondary causes. The history should include factors that precipitate headache, such as foods and food additives, missed meals, and association with the menstrual period. A careful medication history is essential because many medications can provoke or aggravate headaches. Alcohol also can cause or aggravate headache. A headache diary in which the person records his or her headaches and concurrent or antecedent events may be helpful in identifying factors that contribute to headache onset. Appropriate laboratory and imaging studies of the brain may be done to rule out secondary headaches.

In 2004, the International Headache Society (IHS) published the second edition of *The International Classification of Headache Disorders* (ICHD-2). The classification system is divided into three sections: (1) primary headaches, (2) headaches secondary to other medical conditions, and (3) cranial neuralgias and facial pain.[57,58] Primary headaches include migraine, tension-type headache, cluster headache, and other trigeminal autonomic cephalalgias.

Migraine Headache

Migraine headaches affect approximately 20 million persons in the United States. They occur in about 18% of women and 6% of men and result in considerable time lost from work and other activities.[59] Migraine headaches tend to run in families and are thought to be inherited as an autosomal dominant trait with incomplete penetrance. It is noteworthy that the genetic influence is stronger for migraine with aura than for migraine without aura.[59]

The ICHD-2 classifies migraine headaches into five major categories, the two most important of which are migraine without aura, which accounts for approximately 85% of migraines, and migraine with aura, which accounts for most of the remaining migraines.[58] Migraine without aura is a pulsatile, throbbing, unilateral headache that typically lasts 1 to 2 days and is aggravated by routine physical activity. The headache is accompanied by nausea and vomiting, which often is disabling, and sensitivity to light and sound. Visual disturbances occur quite commonly and consist of visual hallucinations such as stars, sparks, and flashes of light. Migraine with aura has similar symptoms, but with the addition of reversible visual symptoms, including positive features (*e.g.,* flickering lights, spots, or lines) or negative features (loss of vision); fully reversible sensory symptoms, including positive features (feeling of pins or needles) or negative features (numbness); and fully reversible speech disturbances or neurologic symptoms that precede the headache.[58] The aura usually develops over a period of 5 to 20 minutes and lasts from 5 minutes to an hour. Although only a small percentage of persons with migraine experience an aura before an attack, many persons without aura have prodromal symptoms, such as fatigue and irritability, that precede the attack by hours or even days.

The other ICHD-2 migraine headache categories are retinal migraine, complications of migraine (*e.g.,* chronic migraine, migrainous infarction, and migraine-triggered seizures), and childhood periodic syndromes that are commonly precursors of migraine. Retinal migraines are a rare form of migraine characterized by recurrent attacks of fully reversible scintillations (visual sensation of sparks or flashes of light), scotomata (visual blind spots), or blindness affecting one eye, followed within an hour by migrainous headache. The ICHD-2 classifies chronic migraine when a headache meeting the criteria for migraine is present on 15 or more days per month for 3 months or more, in the absence of medication overuse. Migrainous infarction is an uncommon occurrence in which one or more otherwise typical aura symptoms persists beyond 1 hour and neuroimaging confirms ischemic infarction. Strictly applied, these criteria distinguish this disorder from stroke, which must be excluded.[58] Migraine headache also can present as a mixed headache, including symptoms typically associated with tension-type headache, sinus headache, or chronic daily headache. These are called *transformed migraine* and are difficult to classify. Although nasal symptoms are not one of the diagnostic criteria for migraine, they frequently accompany migraine and are probably due to cranial parasympathetic activation. Sinus pain may indicate either a headache due to sinus inflammation or migraine. In a recent study, 96% of those self-diagnosed with sinus headache in fact met the IHS criteria for migraine or migrainous headache.[60]

Migraine headaches occur in children as well as adults.[57,61,62] Before puberty, migraine headaches are equally distributed between the sexes. The essential diagnostic criterion for migraine in children is the presence of recurrent headaches separated by pain-free periods. Diagnosis is based on at least three of the following symptoms or associated findings: abdominal pain, nausea or vomiting, throbbing headache, unilateral location, associated aura (visual, sensory, motor), relief during sleep, and a positive family history.[62] Symptoms vary widely among children, from those that interrupt activities and cause the child to seek relief in a dark environment to those detectable only by direct questioning. A common feature of migraine in children is intense nausea and vomiting. The vomiting may be associated with abdominal pain and fever; thus, migraine may be confused with other conditions such as appendicitis. More

than half of children with migraine undergo spontaneous prolonged remission after their 10th birthday. Because headaches in children can be a symptom of other, more serious disorders, including intracranial lesions, it is important that other causes of headache that require immediate treatment be ruled out.

The pathophysiologic mechanisms of the pain associated with migraine headaches remain poorly understood. Although many alternative theories exist, it is well established that during a migraine the trigeminal nerve becomes activated.[63,64] Activation of the trigeminal sensory fibers may lead to the release of neuropeptides, causing painful neurogenic inflammation within the meningeal vasculature characterized by plasma protein extravasation, vasodilation, and mast cell degranulation.[64] Another possible mechanism implicates neurogenic vasodilation of meningeal blood vessels as a key component of the inflammatory processes that occur during migraine. Activation of trigeminal sensory fibers evokes a neurogenic dural vasodilation mediated by calcitonin gene-related peptide. It also has been observed that the calcitonin gene-related peptide level is elevated during migraine and is normalized after successful treatment with sumatriptan.[64] Supporting the neurogenic basis for migraine is the frequent presence of premonitory symptoms before the headache begins; the presence of focal neurologic disturbances, which cannot be explained in terms of cerebral blood flow; and the numerous accompanying symptoms, including autonomic and constitutional dysfunction.[55]

Hormonal variations, particularly in estrogen levels, play a role in the pattern of migraine attacks. For many women, migraine headaches coincide with their menstrual periods. The greater predominance of migraine headaches in women is thought to be related to the aggravating effect of estrogen on the migraine mechanism.[55] Dietary substances, such as monosodium glutamate, aged cheese, and chocolate, also may precipitate migraine headaches. The actual triggers for migraine are the chemicals in the food, not allergens.

Treatment. The treatment of migraine headaches includes preventive and abortive nonpharmacologic and pharmacologic treatment. In 2002, the American College of Physicians–American Society of Internal Medicine and the American Academy of Family Physicians produced a set of evidence-based guidelines for the nonpharmacologic and pharmacologic management and prevention of migraine headaches in primary care settings.[65]

Nonpharmacologic treatment includes the avoidance of migraine triggers, such as foods, that precipitate an attack. Many persons with migraines benefit from maintaining regular eating and sleeping habits. Measures to control stress, which also can precipitate an attack, also are important. During an attack, many persons find it helpful to retire to a quiet, darkened room until symptoms subside.

Pharmacologic treatment involves both abortive therapy for acute attacks and preventive therapy. A wide range of medications is used to treat the acute symptoms of migraine headache. Based on clinical trials, first-line agents include acetylsalicylic acid; combinations of acetaminophen, acetylsalicylic acid, and caffeine; NSAIDs (*e.g.*, naproxen sodium, ibuprofen); serotonin (5-HT$_1$) receptor agonists (*e.g.*, sumatriptan, naratriptan, rizatriptan, zolmitriptan); ergotamine derivatives (*e.g.*, dihydroergotamine); and antiemetic medications (*e.g.*, ondansetron, metoclopramide). Nonoral routes of administration may be preferred in individuals who develop severe pain rapidly or on awakening, or in those with severe nausea and vomiting. Both sumatriptan and dihydroergotamine have been approved for intranasal administration. For intractable migraine headache, dihydroergotamine may be administered parenterally with an antiemetic or opioid analgesic (transnasal butorphanol).[66] Frequent use of abortive headache medications may cause rebound headache.

Preventive pharmacologic treatment may be necessary if migraine headaches become disabling, if they occur more than two or three times a month, if abortive treatment is being used more than two times a week, or if the individual has hemiplegic migraine, migraine with prolonged aura, or migrainous infarction.[65] In most cases, preventative treatment must be taken daily for months to years. First-line agents include β-adrenergic blocking medications (*e.g.*, propranolol, atenolol), antidepressants (amitriptyline), and antiseizure medications (divalproex sodium, sodium valproate).[64] When a decision to discontinue preventive therapy is made, the medications should be gradually withdrawn.

Other effective medications are available, but they can have serious side effects in some individuals. For example, because of the risk of coronary vasospasm, the 5-HT$_1$ receptor agonists should not be given to persons with coronary artery disease. Ergotamine preparations can cause uterine contractions and should not be given to pregnant women. They also can cause vasospasm, and should be used with caution in persons with peripheral arterial disease.

Cluster Headache

Cluster headaches are relatively uncommon headaches that occur in about 1 in 1000 individuals, affecting men (80% to 85%) more frequently than women and typically beginning in the third decade of life and rarely beginning beyond age 70 years.[67] These headaches tend to occur in clusters over weeks or months, followed by a long, headache-free remission period. Cluster headache is a type of primary neurovascular headache that typically includes severe, unrelenting, unilateral pain located, in order of decreasing frequency, in the orbital, retro-orbital, temporal, supraorbital, and infraorbital region.[67-69] The pain is of rapid onset and builds to a peak in approximately 10 to 15 minutes, lasting for 15 to 180 minutes. The pain behind the eye radiates to the ipsilateral trigeminal nerve (*e.g.*, temple, cheek, gum). The headache frequently is associated with one or more symptoms such as restlessness or agitation, conjunctival redness, lacrimation, nasal congestion, rhinorrhea, forehead and facial sweating, miosis, ptosis, and eyelid edema. Because of their location and associated symptoms, cluster headaches are often mistaken for sinus infections or dental problems.

The underlying pathophysiologic mechanisms of cluster headaches are not completely known. Although recently it has been noted that heredity, through an autosomal dominant gene, plays some role in the pathogenesis of cluster headache. The most likely pathophysiologic mechanisms include the interplay of vascular, neurogenic, metabolic, and humoral factors. Activation of the trigemino-vascular system and the cranial autonomic parasympathetic reflexes is thought to explain the pain and autonomic symptoms. The hypothalamus is believed to play a key role. The possible role of the regulating centers in the anterior hypothalamus is implicated from observations of circadian biologic changes and neuroendocrine disturbances (*e.g.*, changes in cortisol, prolactin, and testosterone) that occur in both active periods and during clinical remission. The hypothalamic gray matter also has been implicated. Positron emission tomography (PET) scanning has demonstrated increased blood flow as well as structural changes in the hypothalamic gray area on the painful side during an attack.[67-69] Magnetic resonance imaging has demonstrated dilated intracranial arteries on the painful side. Loss of vascular tone is believed to result from a defect in the sympathetic perivascular innervation.

Treatment. Because of the relatively short duration and self-limited nature of cluster headache, oral preparations typically take too long to reach therapeutic levels. The most effective treatments are those that act quickly (*e.g.*, oxygen inhalation and subcutaneous sumatriptan). Intranasal lidocaine also may be effective.[68,69] Oxygen inhalation may be indicated for home use. Prophylactic medications for cluster headaches include ergotamine, verapamil, methysergide, lithium carbonate, corticosteroids, and sodium valproate. Deep-brain surgical neurostimulation is an experimental approach beginning to show promise in the elimination of cluster headaches.[68]

Tension-Type Headache

The most common type of headache is tension-type headache. Unlike migraine and cluster headaches, tension-type headache usually is not sufficiently severe that it interferes with daily activities. Tension-type headaches frequently are described as dull, aching, diffuse, nondescript headaches, occurring in a hat-band distribution around the head, and not associated with nausea or vomiting or worsened by activity. They can be infrequent, episodic, or chronic.

The exact mechanisms of tension-type headache are not known and the hypotheses of causation are contradictory. One popular theory is that tension-type headache results from sustained tension of the muscles of the scalp and neck; however, some research has found no correlation between muscle contraction and tension-type headache. Many authorities now believe that tension-type headaches are forms of migraine headache.[70] It is thought that migraine headache may be transformed gradually into chronic tension-type headache. Tension-type headaches also may be caused by oromandibular dysfunction, psychogenic stress, anxiety, depression, and muscular stress. They also may result from overuse of analgesics or caffeine. Daily use of caffeine, whether in beverages or medications, can produce addiction, and a headache can develop in such persons who go without caffeine for several hours.[71]

Treatment. Tension-type headaches often are more responsive to nonpharmacologic techniques, such as biofeedback, massage, acupuncture, relaxation, imagery, and physical therapy, than other types of headache. For persons with poor posture, a combination of range-of-motion exercises, relaxation, and posture improvement may be helpful.

The medications of choice for acute treatment of tension-type headaches are analgesics, including acetylsalicylic acid, acetaminophen, and NSAIDs.[71] Persons with infrequent tension-type headache usually self-medicate using over-the-counter analgesics to treat the acute pain, and do not require prophylactic medication. These agents should be used cautiously because rebound headaches can develop when the medications are taken regularly.

Because the "dividing lines" between tension-type headache, migraine, and chronic daily headache often are vague, addition of medications as well as the entire range of migraine medications may be tried in refractory cases. Other medications used concomitantly with analgesics include sedating antihistamines (*e.g.*, promethazine and diphenhydramine), antiemetics (*e.g.*, metoclopramide and prochlorperazine), or sedatives (*e.g.*, butalbital). Prophylactic treatment for chronic tension-type headaches can include antidepressants (*e.g.*, amitriptyline) and selective serotonin reuptake inhibitors (SSRIs; *e.g.*, paroxetine, venlafaxine, and fluoxetine).[71]

Chronic Daily Headache

The term *chronic daily headache* (CDH) is used to refer to headaches that occur 15 days or more a month, including those due to medication overuse.[72–74] Little is known about the prevalence and incidence of CDH. Diagnostic criteria for CDH are not provided in the IHS Classification System. The cause of CDH is unknown, although there are several hypotheses. They include transformed migraine headache, evolved tension-type headache, new daily persistent headache, and post-traumatic headache. In many persons, CDH retains certain characteristics of migraine, whereas in others it resembles chronic tension-type headache. CDH may be associated with chronic and episodic tension-type headache. New daily persistent headache may have a fairly rapidly onset, with no history of migraine, tension-type headache, trauma, or psychological stress. Although overuse of symptomatic medications (*e.g.*, analgesics, ergotamine) has been related to CDH, there is a group of patients in whom CDH is unrelated to excessive use of medications.

Treatment. For patients with CDH, a combination of pharmacologic and behavioral interventions may be necessary. As with tension-type headaches, nonpharmacologic techniques, such as biofeedback, massage, acupuncture, relaxation, imagery,

and physical therapy, may be helpful. Measures to reduce or eliminate medication, including caffeine, overuse may be helpful. If the patient is abusing medications, the overuse must be managed before prophylactic agents will be effective.[73] Most of the medications used for prevention of CDH have not been examined in well-designed, double-blind studies.

Temporomandibular Joint Pain

A common cause of head pain is temporomandibular joint (TMJ) syndrome. It usually is caused by an imbalance in joint movement because of poor bite, bruxism (*i.e.*, teeth grinding), or joint problems such as inflammation, trauma, and degenerative changes.[75] The pain almost always is referred and commonly presents as facial muscle pain, headache, neck ache, or earache. Referred pain is aggravated by jaw function. Headache associated with this syndrome is common in adults and children and can cause chronic pain problems.

Treatment of TMJ pain is aimed at correcting the problem, and in some cases this may be difficult. The initial therapy for TMJ should be directed toward relief of pain and improvement in function. Pain relief often can be achieved with use of the NSAIDs. Muscle relaxants may be used when muscle spasm is a problem. In some cases, the selected application of heat or cold, or both, may provide relief. Referral to a dentist who is associated with a team of therapists, such as a psychologist, physical therapist, or pain specialist, may be indicated.[75]

IN SUMMARY, head pain is a common disorder that is caused by a number of conditions. Some headaches represent primary disorders and others occur secondary to another disease state in which head pain is a symptom. Primary headache disorders include migraine headache, tension-type headache, cluster headache, and chronic daily headache. Although most causes of secondary headache are benign, some are indications of serious disorders such as meningitis, brain tumor, or cerebral aneurysm. TMJ syndrome is one of the major causes of headaches. It usually is caused by an imbalance in joint movement because of poor bite, teeth grinding, or joint problems such as inflammation, trauma, and degenerative changes. ∎

PAIN IN CHILDREN AND OLDER ADULTS

After completing this section of the chapter, you should be able to meet the following objectives:

- State how the pain response may differ in children and older adults.
- Explain how pain assessment may differ in children and older adults.
- Explain how pain treatment may differ in children and older adults.

Pain frequently is underrecognized and undertreated in both children and the elderly. In addition to the common obstacles to adequate pain management, such as concern about the effects of analgesia on respiratory status and the potential for addiction to opioids, there are additional deterrents to adequate pain management in children and the elderly. With regard to both children and the elderly, there are stereotypic beliefs that they feel less pain than other patients.[76–79] These beliefs may affect a clinician's opinion about the need for pain control. In very young children and confused elderly, there are several additional factors. These include the extreme difficulty of assessing the location and intensity of pain in individuals who are cognitively immature or cognitively impaired, and the argument that even if they feel pain, they do not remember it. Research during the past few decades has added a great deal to the body of knowledge about pain in children and the elderly.

 ## Pain in Children

Human responsiveness to painful stimuli begins in the neonatal period and continues through the life span. Although the specific and localized behavioral reactions are less marked in the younger neonate or the more cognitively impaired individual, protective or withdrawal reflexes in response to nociceptive stimuli are clearly demonstrated. Pain pathways, cortical and subcortical centers, and neurochemical responses associated with pain transmission are developed and functional by the last trimester of pregnancy.[77] Neonates clearly perceive pain, as demonstrated by their integrated physiologic response to nociceptive stimuli. In fact, pain may be accentuated because descending inhibitory pathways to the dorsal horn are not as well developed at birth.[80] Furthermore, dorsal horn neurons in neonates have a wider receptive field and lower excitatory threshold than those in older children.

As infants and children mature, their responses to pain become more complex and reflective of their maturing cognitive and developmental processes. Children do feel pain and have been shown to reliably and accurately report pain at as young as 3 years of age.[81] They also remember pain, as evidenced in studies of children with cancer, whose distress during painful procedures increases over time without intervention, and in neonates in intensive care units, who demonstrate protective withdrawal responses to a heel stick after repeated episodes.

Pain Assessment

To treat pain adequately, ongoing assessment of the presence of pain and response to treatment is essential.[77,78] Self-report is usually regarded as the most reliable estimate of pain. With children 8 years of age or older, numeric scales (*i.e.,* 1 to 10) and word graphic scales (*i.e.,* "none," "a little," "most I have ever experienced") can be used. With children 3 to 8 years of age, scales with faces of actual children or cartoon faces can be used to obtain a report of pain. Another supplementary strategy for assessing a child's pain is to use a body outline and ask the child to indicate where the hurt is located. Particular care must be taken in assessing children's reports of pain because their reports may be influenced by a variety of factors, including age, anxiety and fear levels, and parental presence. In very young children, infants, and neonates as well as in children with disabilities that impair cognition or communication, clinicians must rely on physiologic parameters or age/development-appropriate behavioral pain scales.[77] Some physiologic measures, such as heart rate, are convenient to measure and respond rapidly to brief nociceptive stimuli, but they are nonspecific. Relying on indicators of sympathetic nervous system activity and behaviors can also be problematic because they can be caused by things other than pain (*e.g.,* anxiety and activity) and they do not always accompany pain, particularly chronic pain.

Pain Management

The management of children's pain basically falls into two categories: pharmacologic and nonpharmacologic. In terms of pharmacologic interventions, many of the analgesics used in adults can be used safely and effectively in children and adolescents. However, it is critical when using specific medications to determine that the medication has been approved for use with children and that it is dosed appropriately according to the child's weight and level of physiologic development. Age-related differences in physiologic functioning, notably in neonates, will affect drug action. Neonates have decreased fat and muscle and increased water, which increases the duration of action for some water-soluble drugs; neonates also have decreased concentration of plasma proteins (albumin and α_1-glycoprotein), which increases the unbound concentration of protein-binding drugs.[80] Neonates and infants have decreased levels of the hepatic enzymes needed for metabolism of many analgesics. The levels of these hepatic enzymes quickly increase to adult levels in the first few months of life. Drug clearance in the 2- to 6-year-old age group is actually higher than adult levels because of the larger hepatic mass relative to body weight.[80,82] The renal excretion of drugs depends on renal blood flow, glomerular filtration rate, and tubular secretion, all of which are decreased in neonates, particularly premature neonates. Renal function reaches adult levels by 1 year of age.[80,82]

As with any person in pain, the type of analgesic used should be matched to the type and intensity of pain; and whether the patient is a child or adult, the management of chronic pain may require a multidisciplinary team.[82] The overriding principle in all pediatric pain management is to treat each child's pain on an individual basis and to match the analgesic agent with the cause and the level of pain. A second principle involves maintaining the balance between the level of side effects and pain relief such that pain relief is obtained with as little opioid and sedation as possible. One strategy toward this end is to time the administration of analgesia so that a steady blood level is achieved and, as much as possible, pain is prevented. This requires that the child receive analgesia on a regular dosing schedule, not "as needed." Also, most drugs are packaged primarily for adult use, and dose calculations and serial dilutions may predispose to medication errors. Common errors include milligram–microgram errors, decimal point errors, confusion between daily dose and fractional dose (*e.g.,* 100 mg per kilogram per day divided by 6 hours versus 100 mg per kilogram per dose every 6 hours), and dilution errors.[82]

Nonpharmacologic strategies can be very effective in reducing the overall amount of pain and amount of analgesia used. In addition, some nonpharmacologic strategies can reduce anxiety and increase the child's level of self-control during pain. In full-term infants, ingesting 2 mL of a sucrose solution has been found to relieve the pain from a heel stick.[83] Children as young as 4 years of age can use TENS,[84] and they can be taught to use simple distraction and relaxation and other techniques such as application of heat and cold.[85] Other nonpharmacologic techniques can be taught to the child to provide psychological preparation for a painful procedure or surgery. These include positive self-talk, imagery, play therapy, modeling, and rehearsal. The nonpharmacologic interventions must be developmentally appropriate and, if possible, the child and parent should be taught these techniques when the child is not in pain (*e.g.,* before surgery or a painful procedure) so that it is easier to practice the technique.

 Pain in Older Adults

Among adults, the prevalence of pain in the general population increases with age: 32% of those between 18 and 34 years of age report daily pain, whereas 55% of Americans aged 65 and older report daily pain. Among the elderly the most common self-attributed causes of pain are getting older (88%) and arthritis (69%).[86] In long-term care facilities, it has been estimated that 80% of individuals experience pain on a regular basis.[79] Research is inconsistent about whether there are age-related changes in pain perception. Some apparent age-related differences in pain may be due to differences in willingness to report the pain rather than actual differences in pain. The elderly may be reluctant to report pain so as not to be a burden or out of fear of the diagnoses, tests, medications, or costs that may result from an attempt to diagnose or treat their pain.

Pain Assessment

The assessment of pain in the elderly can range from relatively simple in a well-informed, alert, cognitively intact individual with pain from a single source and no comorbidities to extraordinarily difficult in a frail individual with severe dementia and many concurrent health problems.[87,88] When possible, a patient's report of pain is the gold standard, but behavioral signs of pain should be considered as well. Accurately diagnosing pain when the individual has many health problems or some decline in cognitive function can be particularly challenging. In recent years, there has been increased awareness of the need to address issues of pain in individuals with dementia. The Assessment for Discomfort in Dementia Protocol is one example of the efforts to improve assessment and pain

management in these individuals. It includes behavioral criteria for assessing pain and recommended interventions for pain. Its use has been shown to improve pain management.[89]

Pain Management

When prescribing pharmacologic and nonpharmacologic methods of pain management for the older population, care must be taken to consider the cause of the pain, the patient's health status, the concurrent therapies, and the patient's mental status. In the older population, where the risk of adverse events is higher, the nonpharmacologic options are usually less costly and cause fewer side effects.

Common nonpharmacologic interventions include application of cold (which suppresses the release of products from tissue damage) and heat (which promotes the release of endogenous endorphins).[79] The role of mental focus and anxiety is important, and relaxation techniques, massage, and biofeedback may be useful. Physical therapy and occupational therapy bring a variety of modalities, including the use of braces or splints, changes in biomechanics, and exercise, all of which have been shown to promote pain relief.

Although efficacy is important when considering the use of pharmacologic agents for pain relief in the elderly population, cost and safety must also be considered. Safety issues that must be considered among older adults include changes in drug metabolism, other disease comorbidity, and polypharmacy. The elderly may have physiologic changes that affect the pharmacokinetics of medications prescribed for pain management. These changes include decreased blood flow to organs, delayed gastric motility, reduced kidney function, and decreased albumin related to poor nutrition.[90] The elderly also often have many coexisting health problems, leading to polypharmacy. On the average, a 70-year-old takes seven different medications.[79] The addition of analgesics to a complex medication regimen is even more likely to cause drug interactions and complicate compliance in the elderly. However, these considerations should not preclude the appropriate use of analgesic drugs to achieve pain relief. Nonopioids are generally the first line of therapy for mild to moderate pain, and acetaminophen is usually the first choice because it is relatively safe for older adults.[79] Opioids are used for more severe pain and for palliative care. As with younger persons, adjuvant analgesics are effectively used for treatment of pain in older adults. The use of some assessment tool to evaluate the level of pain and effectiveness of treatment is essential. Monitoring for side effects is also critical.

IN SUMMARY, children experience and remember pain, and even fairly young children are able to accurately and reliably report their pain. Recognition of this has changed the clinical practice of health professionals involved in the assessment of children's pain. Pharmacologic (including opioids) and nonpharmacologic pain management interventions have been shown to be effective in children. Nonpharmacologic techniques must be based on the developmental level of the child and should be taught to both children and parents.

Pain is a common symptom in the elderly. Assessment, diagnosis, and treatment of pain in the elderly can be complicated. The elderly may be reluctant or cognitively unable to report their pain. Diagnosis and treatment can be complicated by comorbidities and age-related changes in cognitive and physiologic function. ■

Review Exercises

1. A 25-year-old man is admitted to the emergency department with acute abdominal pain that began in the epigastric area and has now shifted to the lower right quadrant of the abdomen. There is localized tenderness and guarding or spasm of the muscle over the area. His heart rate and blood pressure are elevated, and his skin is moist and cool from perspiring. He is given a tentative diagnosis of appendicitis and referred for surgical consultation.

   A. *Describe the origin of the pain stimuli and the neural pathways involved in the pain that this man is experiencing.*

   B. *Explain the neural mechanisms involved in the spasm of the overlying abdominal muscles.*

   C. *What is the significance of his cool, moist skin and increased heart rate and blood pressure?*

2. A 65-year-old woman with breast cancer is receiving hospice care in her home. She is currently receiving a long-acting opioid analgesic supplemented with a short-acting combination opioid and non-narcotic medication for breakthrough pain.

   A. *Explain the difference between the mechanisms and treatment of acute and chronic pain.*

   B. *Describe the action of opioid drugs in the treatment of pain.*

   C. *Define the terms* tolerance *and* cross-tolerance *as they refer to the use of opioids for treatment of pain.*

   D. *Describe the common side effects associated with the use of opioid drugs to relieve pain in persons with cancer.*

3. A 42-year-old woman presents with sudden, stabbing-type facial pain that arises near the right side of her mouth and then shoots toward the right ear, eye, and nostril. She is holding her hand to protect her face because the pain is "triggered by touch, movement, and drafts." Her initial diagnosis is trigeminal neuralgia.

   A. *Explain the distribution and mechanisms of the pain, particularly the triggering of the pain by stimuli applied to the skin.*

   B. *What are possible treatment methods for this woman?*

4. A 21-year-old woman presents to the student health center with complaints of a throbbing pain on the left side of her head, nausea and vomiting, and extreme sensitivity to light, noise, and head movement. She also tells you she had a similar headache 3 months ago that lasted for 2 days and states that she thinks she is developing migraine headaches like her mother. She is concerned because she has been unable to attend classes and has exams next week.

   A. *Are this woman's history and symptoms consistent with migraine headaches? Explain.*

   B. *Use the distribution of the trigeminal nerve and the concept of neurogenic inflammation to explain this woman's symptoms.*

5. A 72-year-old man presents to the emergency department after a fall with a complaint of the "worst headache ever experienced." He is able to answer your questions with increasing difficulty.

   A. *Differentiate primary headache from secondary headache.*

   B. *Given the information that you have, what type of headache do you suspect, and why?*

6. A 48-year-old man presents with complaints of severe pain in his right foot after a crush injury. He reports that although he had his ankle pinned surgically, it still causes severe pain now, almost 1 year after injury. He states that he cannot stand to have the sheets touch his foot, and even wearing shoes is painful. His physician has diagnosed chronic regional pain syndrome, type I.

   A. *Differentiate chronic regional pain syndrome type I from type II.*

   B. *Explain the proposed theories of why this pain syndrome develops.*

References

1. Guyton A., Hall J. E. (2006). *Textbook of medical physiology* (11th ed.). Philadelphia: Elsevier Saunders.
2. Kandel E. R., Schwartz J. H., Jessell T. M. (2007). *Principles of neural science* (5th ed.). New York: McGraw-Hill.
3. Merskey H., Bogduk N. (Eds.). (1994). *Classification of chronic pain: Description of chronic pain and definitions of pain terms* (2nd ed.). Seattle: IASP Publications.
4. Sherrington C. (1947). *The integrative action of the nervous system.* New Haven, CT: Yale University Press.
5. Crombie I., Croft P., Linton S., et al. (1999). *Epidemiology of pain.* Seattle: IASP Publications.
6. Carver A. (2000). Neurology: Pain. In Dale D. C., Federman D. D. (Eds.), *ACP Emedicine Online.* [Online.] Available: www.medscape.com/viewarticle/534649. Accessed March 8, 2008.

7. Bonica J. J. (1991). History of pain concepts and pain theory. *Mount Sinai Journal of Medicine* 58, 191–202.

8. Melzack R., Wall P. D. (1965). Pain mechanisms: A new theory. *Science* 150, 971–979.

9. Melzack R. (1999). From the gate to the neuromatrix. *Pain* 6(Suppl.), S121–S126.

10. Cross S. A. (1994). Pathophysiology of pain. *Mayo Clinic Proceedings* 69, 375–383.

11. Julius D., Basbaum A. I. (2001). Molecular mechanisms of nociception. *Nature* 413, 203–210.

12. Markenson J. A. (1996). Mechanisms of chronic pain. *American Journal of Medicine* 101(Suppl. 1A), 6S–18S.

13. Ploner M., Gross J., Timmerman L., et al. (2002). Cortical representation of first and second pain sensation in humans. *Proceedings of the National Academy of Sciences of the United States of America* 99, 12444–12448.

14. Fields H. L., Heinricher M. M., Mason P. (1991). Neurotransmitters in nociceptive modulatory circuits. *Review of Neuroscience* 14, 219–245.

15. Stein C. (2003). Opioid receptors on peripheral sensory neurons. In Machelska H., Stein C. (Eds.), *Immune mechanisms of pain and analgesia* (pp. 69–76). New York: Kluwer Academic/Plenum.

16. Cervero F., Laird J. M. (1999). Visceral pain. *Lancet* 353, 2145–2148.

17. Al-Chaer E. D., Traub R. J. (2002). Biological basis of visceral pain: Recent developments. *Pain* 96, 221–225.

18. Turk D. C., Okifuji A. (2001). Pain terms and taxonomies of pain. In Loser J. D. (Ed.), *Bonica's management of pain* (3rd ed., pp. 17–25). Philadelphia: Lippincott Williams & Wilkins.

19. Jacobson L., Mariano A. J. (2001). General considerations in chronic pain. In Loser J. D. (Ed.), *Bonica's management of pain* (3rd ed., pp. 241–254). Philadelphia: Lippincott Williams & Wilkins.

20. Fink W. A. (2005). The pathophysiology of acute pain. *Emergency Medicine Clinics of North America* 23, 277–284.

21. Grichnick K., Ferrante F. M. (1991). The difference between acute and chronic pain. *Mount Sinai Journal of Medicine* 58, 217–220.

22. Maizels M., McCarberg B. (2005). Antidepressant and antiepileptic drugs for chronic non-cancer pain. *American Family Physician* 71, 483–490.

23. Acute Pain Management Guideline Panel. (1992). *Clinical practice guideline no. 1. Acute pain management: Operative or medical procedures and trauma.* AHCPR publication no. 92-0032. Rockville, MD: Agency for Health Care Policy and Research, Public Health Service, U.S. Department of Health and Human Services.

24. Melzack R. (1975). The McGill Pain Questionnaire: Major properties and scoring methods. *Pain* 1, 277–299.

25. Norden J., Hanallah R. (1991). Reliability of an objective pain scale in children. *Journal of Pain and Symptom Management* 6, 196.

26. Krechel S. W., Bilder J. (1995). CRIES: A new neonatal postoperative pain management score: Initial testing of validity. *Pediatric Anesthesia* 5(1), 53–61.

27. Jacox A., Carr D. B., Payne R., et al. (1994). *Clinical practice guideline no. 9. Management of cancer pain.* AHCPR publication no. 94-0592. Rockville, MD: Agency for Health Care Policy and Research, Public Health Service, U.S. Department of Health and Human Services.

28. World Health Organization. (1990). *Cancer pain relief and palliative care: Report of the WHO Expert Committee* (Technical Report Series no. 804). Geneva, Switzerland: Author.

29. Shepard J. T., Rusch N. J., Vanhoutte P. M. (1983). Effect of cold on the blood vessel walls. *General Pharmacology* 14(1), 61–64.

30. Hymes A. (1984). A review of the historical area of electricity. In Mannheimer J. S., Lampe G. N. (Eds.), *Clinical transcutaneous electrical stimulation* (pp. 1–5). Philadelphia: F. A. Davis.

31. Anderson S. A. (1979). Pain control by sensory stimulation. In Bonica J. J., Liebeskind J. C., Albe-Fessard D. G. (Eds.), *Advances in pain research and therapy* (pp. 569–585). New York: Raven Press.

32. Ignelzi R. J., Nyquist J. K. (1979). Excitability changes in peripheral nerve fibers after repetitive electrical stimulation: Implications for pain modulation. *Journal of Neurosurgery* 51, 824–833.

33. Wolf S. L. (1984). Neurophysiologic mechanisms of pain modulation: Relevance to TENS. In Mannheimer J. S., Lampe G. N. (Eds.), *Clinical transcutaneous electrical stimulation* (pp. 41–55). Philadelphia: F. A. Davis.

34. Ezzo J., Berman B., Hadhazy A., et al. (2000). Is acupuncture effective for the treatment of chronic pain: A systematic review. *Pain* 86, 217–225.

35. Shealey C. N., Mortimer J. T., Reswick J. B. (2007). Electrical inhibition of pain by stimulation of the dorsal columns: Clinical report. *Anesthesia and Analgesia* 46, 489–491.

36. Katzung H. (Ed.). (2007). *Basic and clinical pharmacology* (10th ed., pp. 489–510, 575–583). New York: Lange Medical Books/McGraw-Hill.

37. Inturrisi C. E. (2002). Clinical pharmacology of opioids for pain. *Clinical Journal of Pain* 18(Suppl. 4), S3–S13.

38. Melzack R. (1990). The tragedy of needless pain. *Scientific American* 262(2), 2–8.

39. Kurz A., Sessler D. (2003). Opioid-induced bowel dysfunction: Pathophysiology and potential new therapies. *Drugs* 63, 649–671.

40. Pasternak G. W. (2001). The pharmacology of mu analgesics: From patients to genes. *The Neuroscientist* 7, 220–231.

41. Swerdlow M., Stjerward J. (1982). Cancer pain relief: An urgent problem. *World Health Forum* 3, 325–330.

42. Marchand F., Perretti D., McMahon S. B. (2005). Role of the immune system in chronic pain. *Nature Reviews Neuroscience* 6, 521–532.

43. Campbell J. N., Meyer R. A. (2006). Mechanisms of neuropathic pain. *Neuron* 52, 77–92.

44. Rozen T. D. (2004). Trigeminal neuralgia and glossopharyngeal neuralgia. *Neurologic Clinics* 22, 185–206.

45. Liu J. K., Apfelbaum R. I. (2004). Treatment of trigeminal neuralgia. *Neurosurgical Clinics of North America* 15, 319–334.

46. Kost R. G., Straus S. E. (1996). Postherpetic neuralgia: Pathogenesis, treatment and prevention. *New England Journal of Medicine* 335, 32–42.

47. Schmader K. (2007). Herpes zoster and postherpetic neuralgia in older adults. *Clinics in Geriatric Medicine* 23, 615–632.

48. Kimberlin D. W., Whitley R. J. (2007). Varicella-zoster vaccine for the prevention of herpes zoster. *New England Journal of Medicine* 356, 1338–1343.

49. Pham T., Lafforgue P. (2003). Reflex sympathetic dystrophy syndrome and neuromediators. *Joint, Bone, Spine* 70, 12–17.

50. Parillo S. J. (2007). Complex regional pain syndrome. Emedicine, Web MD. [Online.] Available: www.emedicine.com/emerg/topic497.htm. Accessed March 8, 2008.

51. Campell J., Basbaum A., Dray A., et al. (2006). *Emerging strategies for the treatment of neuropathic pain.* Seattle: IASP Publications.

52. Stanton-Hicks M. (2003). Complex regional pain syndrome. *Anesthesia Clinics of North America* 21, 733–744.

53. Blaes F., Schmitz K., Tschernatsch M. (2004). Autoimmune etiology of chronic regional pain syndrome. *Neurology* 63, 1734–1736.

54. Melzack R. (1992). Phantom limb. *Scientific American* 226, 120–126.

55. Saper J. R. (1999). Headache disorders. *Medical Clinics of North America* 83, 663–670.

56. Kaniecki R. (2003). Headache assessment and management. *Journal of the American Medical Association* 289, 1430–1433.

57. Headache Classification Subcommittee of the International Headache Committee. (2004). The International Classification of headache disorders, 2nd edition. *Cephalalgia* 24(Suppl. 1), 1–152.

58. Lipton R. B., Biglal M. E., Stiener T. J. et al. (2004). Classification of primary headaches. *Neurology* 63, 427–435.

59. Mathew N. T. (2001). Pathophysiology, epidemiology, and impact of migraine. *Clinical Cornerstone* 4, 1–17.

60. Cady R., Schreiber C. (2003). Sinus headache or migraine? Considerations in making a differential diagnosis. *Headache* 43, 305.

61. Lewis D. J. (2002). Headaches in children and adolescents. *American Family Physician* 65, 625–632.

62. Haslam R. H. A. (2004). Headaches. In Behrman R. E., Kliegman R. M., Jenson H. B. (Eds.), *Nelson textbook of pediatrics* (17th ed., pp. 2012–2015). Philadelphia: Elsevier Saunders.

63. Tepper S. J., Rapoport A., Sheftell F. (2001). The pathophysiology of migraine. *The Neurologist* 7, 279–786.

64. Williamson D. H., Hargreaves R. J. (2001). Neurogenic inflammation in the context on migraine. *Microscopy Research and Technique* 53, 167–178.

65. Snow V., Weiss K., Wall E. M., et al. (2002). Pharmacologic management of acute attacks of migraine and prevention of migraine headache. *Annals of Internal Medicine* 137, 840–849.

66. Silberstein S. D. (2000). Practice parameter: Evidence-based guidelines for migraine headache. *Neurology* 55, 754–763.

67. Ekbom K., Hardebo J. E. (2002). Cluster headache aetiology, diagnosis and management. *Drugs* 62, 61–69.

68. May A. (2005). Cluster headache: Pathogenesis, diagnosis, and management. *Lancet* 366, 843–855.

69. Beck E., Sieber W. J., Trejo R. (2005). Management of cluster headache. *American Family Physician* 71, 717–728.

70. Gladstein J. (2006). Headache. *Medical Clinics of North America* 90, 275–290.

71. Millea P. J., Brodie J. J. (2002). Tension-type headache. *American Family Physician* 66, 797–804.

72. Biondi D. M. (2005). Chronic daily headache. *Clinics in Family Practice* 7, 463–491.

73. Maizels M. (2004). The patient with daily headaches. *American Family Physician* 70, 2299–2306, 2313–2314.

74. Lake A., Saper J. (2002). Chronic headache: New advances in treatment strategies. *Neurology* 59(5 Suppl. 2), S8–S13.

75. Lobbezoo F. (2004). Topical review: New insights into the pathology and diagnosis of disorders of the temporomandibular joint. *Journal of Orofacial Pain* 18, 181–191.

76. Broome M., Richtsmeier A., Maikler V., et al. (1996). Pediatric pain practices: A survey of health professionals. *Journal of Pain and Symptom Management* 4, 315–319.

77. Howard R. F. (2003). Current status of pain management in children. *Journal of the American Medical Association* 290, 2464–2469.

78. Committee on Psychological Aspects of Child and Family Health. (2001). The assessment and management of acute pain in infants, children, and adolescents. *Pediatrics* 108, 793–797.

79. Gloth M. F. (2001). Pain management in older adults: Prevention and treatment. *Journal of the American Geriatrics Society* 49, 188–199.

80. Brislin R. P., Rose J. B. (2005). Pediatric acute pain management. *Anesthesia Clinics of North America* 23, 789–814.

81. Bursch B., Zeltzer L. K. (2004). Pediatric pain management. In Behrman R. E., Kliegman R. M., Jenson H. B. (Eds.), *Nelson textbook of pediatrics* (17th ed., pp. 358–366). Philadelphia: Elsevier Saunders.

82. Berde C. B., Sethna N. F. (2002). Analgesics for the treatment of pain in children. *New England Journal of Medicine* 347, 1094–1103.

83. Haouari N., Wood C., Griffiths G., et al. (1995). The analgesic effect of sucrose in full term infants: A randomized controlled trial. *British Medical Journal* 310, 1498–1500.

84. Merkel S. I., Gutstein H. B., Malviya S. (1999). Use of transcutaneous electrical nerve stimulation in a young child with pain from open perineal lesions. *Journal of Pain and Symptom Management* 18, 376–381.

85. Gold J., Kim S. H., Kant A. J., et al. (2006). Effectiveness of virtual reality for pediatric pain distraction during IV placement. *CyberPsychology & Behavior* 9, 207–212.

86. Gallup Survey, Conducted by the Gallup Organization from May 21 to June 9, 1999. Supported by the Arthritis Foundation and Merck & Company, Inc. [Online.] Available: www.arthritis.org/conditions/speaking ofpain/factsheet.asp. Accessed August 1, 2003.

87. Kovach C. R., Weissman, D. E., Griffie J., et al. (1999). Assessment and treatment of discomfort for people with late-stage dementia. *Journal of Pain and Symptom Management* 18, 412–419.

88. Hutt E., Pepper G. A., Vojir C., et al. (2006). Assessing the appropriateness of pain medication prescribing practices in nursing homes. *Journal of the American Geriatrics Society* 54, 231–239.

89. Barkin R. L., Barkin S. J., Barkin D. S. (2005). Perception, assessment, treatment, and management of pain in the elderly. *Clinics in Geriatric Medicine* 21, 465–490.

90. Katzung B. G. (2007). Special aspects of geriatric pharmacology. In Katzung H. (Ed.), *Basic and clinical pharmacology* (10th ed., pp. 983–990). New York: Lange Medical Books/McGraw-Hill.

Visit the Point. **http://thePoint.lww.com for animations, journal articles, and more!**

Chapter 50

Disorders of Motor Function

SERENA W. HUNG

> Just as our perceptual skills reflect the ability of our sensory systems to detect, analyze, and estimate the significance of our physical environment, the ability to carry out skilled movements requires skeletal muscles that contract and neural pathways that plan, coordinate, and execute these contractions in a manner that provides for smooth purposeful, and coordinated movement. In some cases, purposeless and disruptive movements can be almost as disabling as relative or complete absence of movement. This chapter provides an introduction to the organization and control of motor function, followed by a discussion of disorders of motor function, including muscular dystrophy and disorders of the neuromuscular junction, peripheral nerves, the basal ganglia and cerebellum, and upper motor neurons.

ORGANIZATION AND CONTROL OF MOTOR FUNCTION

After completing this section of the chapter, you should be able to meet the following objectives:

■ Relate the functional hierarchy of motor function to the performance of a complicated movement such as writing your name or throwing a ball.
■ Define the term *motor unit* and characterize its mechanism of controlling skeletal muscle movement.
■ Describe the distribution of upper and lower motor neurons in relation to the central nervous system.
■ Differentiate between the functions of the primary, premotor, and supplemental motor cortices.
■ Compare the effect of upper and lower motor neuron lesions on the spinal cord stretch reflex function and muscle tone.

Motor function, whether it involves walking, running, or precise finger movements, requires movement and maintenance of posture. Posture can be described as the relative position of various parts of the body with respect to one another (limb extension, flexion) or to the environment (standing, supine).[1] Posture also can be described as the active muscular resistance to the displacement of the body by gravity or acceleration. The structures that control posture and movement are located throughout the neuromuscular system. The system consists of the motor unit (motor neuron and the muscle fibers it innervates); the spinal cord, which contains the basic reflex circuitry for posture and movement; and the descending pathways from brain stem circuits, the cerebellum, basal ganglia, and the motor cortex.

MOTOR SYSTEMS

- Motor systems require upper motor neurons (UMNs) that project from the motor cortex to the brain stem or spinal cord, where they directly or indirectly innervate the lower motor neurons (LMNs) of the contracting muscles; sensory feedback from the involved muscles that is continuously relayed to the cerebellum, basal ganglia, and sensory cortex; and a functioning neuromuscular junction that links nervous system activity with muscle contraction.

- The pyramidal motor system originating in the motor cortex provides control of delicate muscle movement, and the extrapyramidal system originating in the basal ganglia provides the background for the more crude, supportive movement patterns.

- The efficiency of the movement by the motor system depends on a background of muscle tone provided by the stretch reflex and vestibular system input to maintain stable postural support.

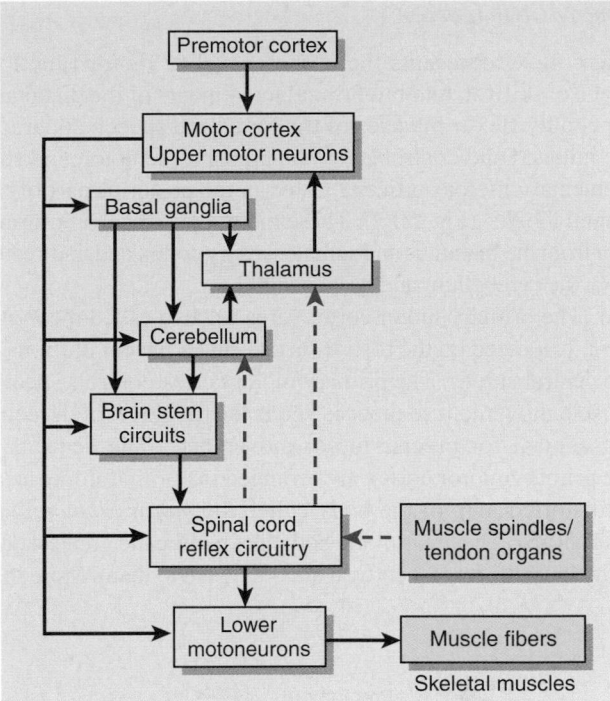

FIGURE 50-1 • The motor control system. The final common pathway transmits all central nervous system commands to the skeletal muscles. This path is influenced by sensory input from the muscle spindles and tendon organs (*dashed lines*) and descending signals from the cerebral cortex and brain stem. The cerebellum and basal ganglia influence the motor function indirectly, using brain stem and cortical pathways.

Organization of Movement

As with other parts of the nervous system, the motor systems are organized in a functional hierarchy, each concerned with increased levels of complexity[2] (Fig. 50-1). The lowest level of the hierarchy occurs at the spinal cord, which contains the basic reflex circuitry needed to coordinate the function of the motor units involved in the planned movement. Above the spinal cord is the brain stem, and above the brain stem are the cerebellum and basal ganglia, structures that modulate the actions of the brain stem systems. Overseeing these supraspinal structures are the motor centers in the cerebral cortex. The highest level of function, which occurs at the level of the frontal cortex, is concerned with the purpose and planning of the motor movement. The efficiency of movement depends on input from sensory systems that operate in parallel with the motor systems.

The Spinal Cord

The spinal cord is the lowest level of motor hierarchical organization.[2] It contains the neuronal circuits that mediate a variety of reflexes and automatic rhythmic movements. Similar circuits governing reflex movements of the face and mouth are located in the brain stem. The simplest circuits are monosynaptic, containing only a primary motor neuron. However, most reflexes are polysynaptic, involving one or more interposed interneurons. Interneurons and motor neurons also receive input from axons descending from higher centers. These supraspinal signals can modify reflex responses to peripheral stimuli by facilitating or inhibiting different populations of interneurons. They also coordinate movements through these interneurons.

The Brain Stem

The next level of motor hierarchy is in the brain stem. The brain stem contains, in addition to the facial nerves, many groups of neurons that project from the spinal gray matter. These projections are grouped into two main systems: the medial and lateral brain stem pathways.[2] The medial pathways provide for the basic postural control systems that the cortical motor areas use to organize highly differentiated movements. They consist of tracts that descend in the ipsilateral ventral columns of the spinal cord and terminate in interneurons that influence motor neurons of axial and proximal muscles that are responsible for postural reflexes such as those needed for pacing of steps during walking or running and recovery of posture when balance is disrupted. The lateral brain stem pathways are more concerned with goal-directed movements. They terminate on the interneurons in the dorsolateral part of the spinal gray matter and thus influence the motor neurons that control distal muscles of the limbs. These descending pathways modify the activity of extensor and flexor motor neurons to produce complex motor movements such as walking and running.

The Motor Cortex

The cortex represents the highest level of motor function. Precise, skillful, and intentional movements of the distal and especially flexor muscles of the limbs and speech apparatus are initiated and controlled by the primary, premotor, and supplementary motor cortices located in the posterior part of the frontal lobe[1,3,4] (Fig. 50-2). These motor areas receive information from the thalamus and somatosensory cortex and, indirectly, from the cerebellum and basal ganglia.

The primary motor cortex (area 4), also called the *motor strip,* is located on the rostral surface and adjacent portions of the central sulcus. The primary motor cortex controls specific muscle movement sequences and is the first level of descending control for precise motor movements. The neurons in the primary motor cortex are arranged in a somatotopic array or distorted map of the body called the *motor homunculus*[5] (Fig. 50-3). The areas of the body that require the greatest dexterity have the largest cortical areas devoted to them. More than

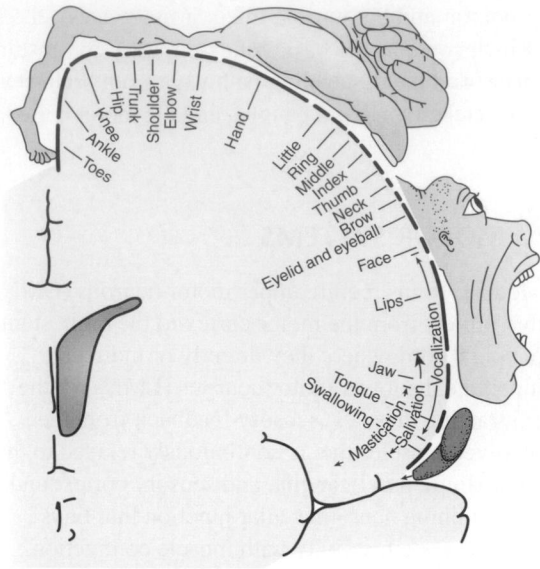

FIGURE 50-3 • Representation of the relative extent of motor cortical area 4 devoted to muscles of the various body regions. Medial surface is at the left, lateral fissure is at the right, with pharyngeal and laryngeal muscle representation extending toward the insula. (From Penfield E., Rasmussen T. [1968]. *The cerebral cortex in man: A clinical study of localization of function.* New York: Macmillan.)

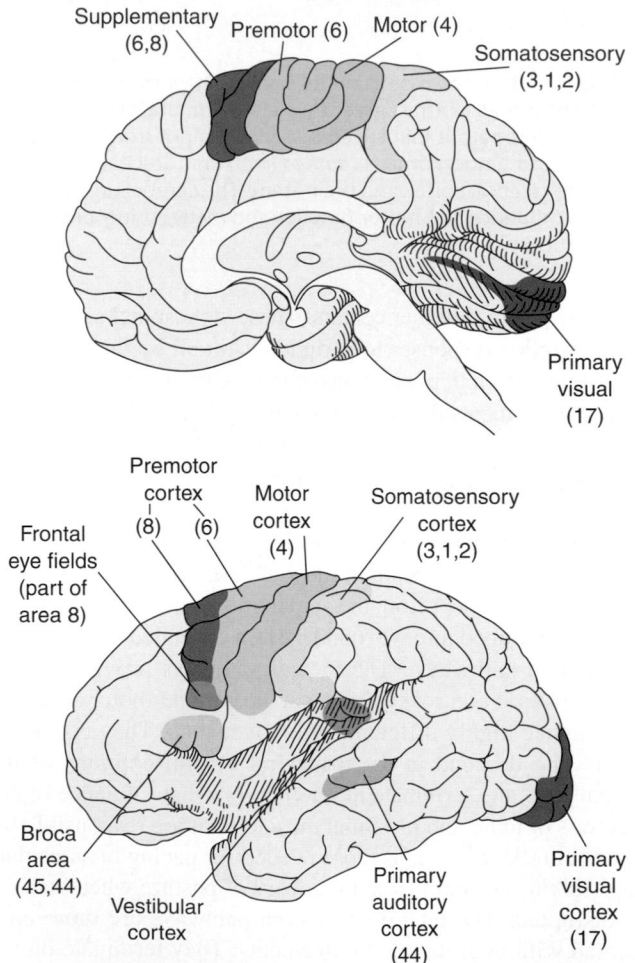

FIGURE 50-2 • Primary motor cortex. **(Top)** The location of the primary, premotor, and supplementary cortex on the medial surface of the brain. **(Bottom)** The location of the primary and premotor cortex on the lateral surface of the brain. (Courtesy of Carole Russell Hilmer, CMI.)

half of the primary motor cortex is concerned with controlling the muscles of the hands, of facial expression, and of speech.

The premotor cortex (areas 6 and 8), which is located just anterior to the primary motor cortex, sends some fibers into the corticospinal tract but mainly innervates the primary motor strip. Nerve signals generated by the premotor cortex produce much more complex "patterns" of movement than the discrete patterns generated by the primary motor cortex. For example, the movement pattern to accomplish a particular objective, such as throwing a ball or picking up a fork, is programmed by the prefrontal association cortex and associated thalamic nuclei.

The supplementary motor cortex, which contains representations of all parts of the body, is located on the medial surface of the hemisphere in the premotor region (areas 6 and 8). It is intimately involved in the performance of complex, skillful movements that involve both sides of the body.

The Cerebellum and Basal Ganglia

In addition to the brain stem and cerebral cortex, two other parts of the brain assist in the planning and execution of motor movements. The cerebellum and basal ganglia provide feedback circuits that regulate cortical and brain stem motor areas.[2] They receive inputs from various areas of the cortex and project to the motor cortex through the thalamus. The cerebellum and basal ganglia do not send significant output directly to the spinal cord, but act directly on motor neurons in the brain stem.

Although the precise contributions of the cerebellum and basal ganglia are still unclear, both are necessary for smooth movement and posture. The basal ganglia provide gracefulness to the performance as well the supportive posture for highly skilled movements. As will be discussed, degenerative diseases of the basal ganglia such as Parkinson disease produce involuntary movements and posture. Cerebellar circuits are involved with the timing and coordination of movements that are in progress, and with learning of motor skills. Damage to the cerebellum by vascular lesions of certain familial degenerative disorders produces cerebellar ataxia, a characteristic loss of coordination and accuracy of limb movement.

The Motor Unit

The neurons that control motor function are referred to as *motor neurons* or sometimes as *alpha motor neurons*.[3,6] The motor neuron and the group of muscle fibers it innervates in a muscle is called a *motor unit*. When the motor neuron develops an action potential, all of the muscle fibers in the motor unit it innervates develop action potentials, causing them to contract simultaneously. Thus, a motor neuron and the muscle fibers it innervates function as a single unit—the basic unit of motor control.

Each motor neuron undergoes multiple branchings, making it possible for a single motor neuron to innervate a few to thousands of muscle fibers. In general, large muscles—those containing hundreds or thousands of muscle fibers and providing gross motor movement—have large motor units. This contrasts sharply with those that control the hand, tongue, and eye movements, for which the motor units are small and permit very precise control.

The motor neurons supplying a motor unit are located in the ventral horn of the spinal cord and are called *lower motor neurons* (LMNs). Upper motor neurons (UMNs), which exert control over LMNs, project from the motor strip in the cerebral cortex to the ventral horn and are fully contained in the central nervous system (CNS; Fig. 50-4).

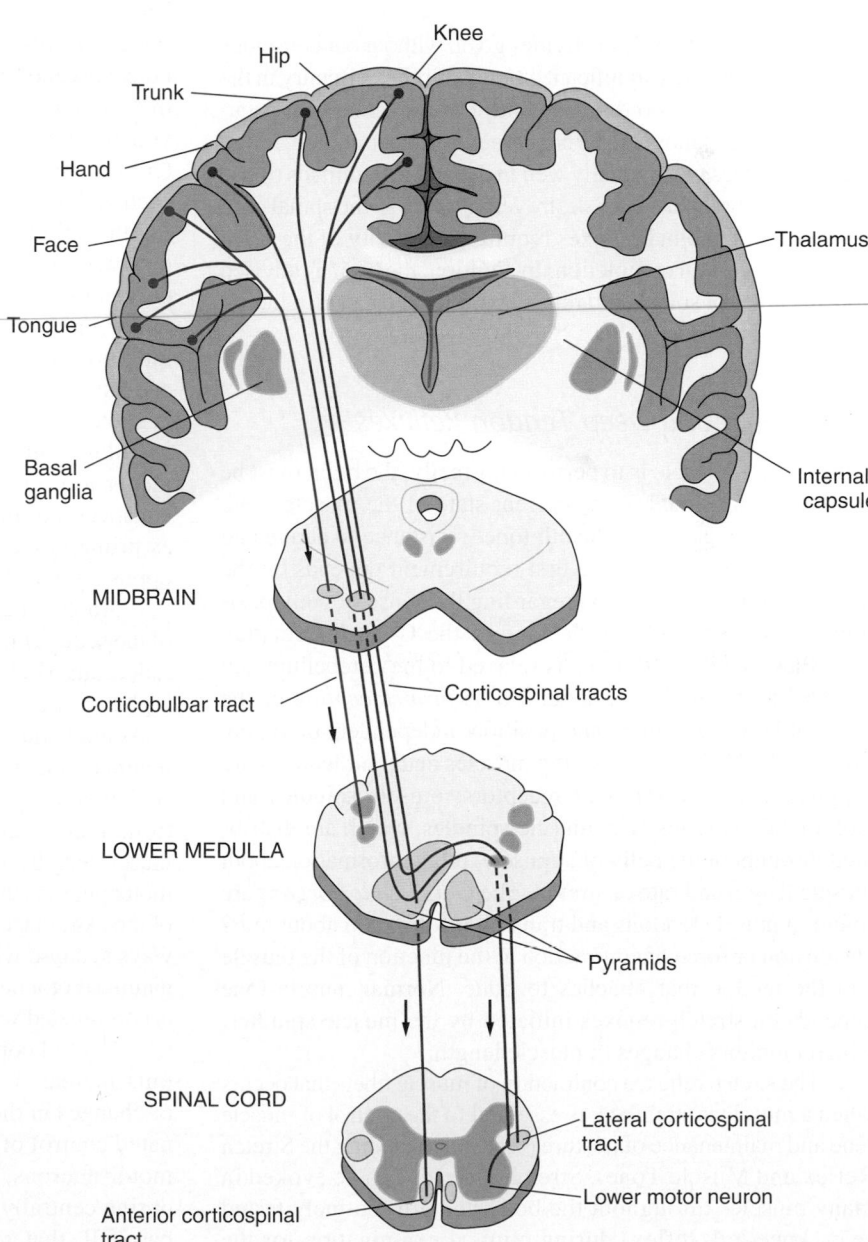

FIGURE 50-4 • Motor pathways: corticospinal and corticobulbar tracts (Modified from Bickley L. S. [2003]. *Bates' guide to physical examination and history taking* [8th ed., p. 543]. Philadelphia: Lippincott Williams & Wilkins.)

Spinal Reflexes

Reflexes are coordinated, involuntary motor responses that are initiated by a stimuli applied to peripheral receptors.[3,7] Some reflexes, such as the flexor-withdrawal reflex, initiate movements to avoid hazardous situations, whereas others, such as the stretch reflex or crossed-extensor reflex, serve to integrate motor movements so they function in a coordinated manner. The anatomic basis of a reflex consists of an afferent neuron that synapses either directly with an effector neuron that innervates a muscle, or with an interneuron that synapses with an effector neuron. Reflexes are essentially "wired into" the CNS so that they are always ready to function; with training, most reflexes can be modulated to become parts of more complicated movements. A reflex may involve neurons in a single cord segment (*i.e.,* segmental reflexes), several or many segments (*i.e.,* intersegmental reflexes), or structures in the brain (*i.e.,* suprasegmental reflexes).

In many cases, reflex activities go on without our conscious awareness. There is a significant amount of reflex circuitry in the spinal cord for the coordinated control of movements, particularly stereotyped movements concerned with locomotion. Many of these reflexes work equally well in decerebrate animals (those in which the brain has been destroyed) as long as the spinal cord is intact. Other spinal reflexes require the activity of the brain for their successful completion. In addition, the brain is advised of many types of spinal cord reflex activities and can then inhibit or facilitate them.

The Stretch and Deep Tendon Reflexes

If the skeletal muscle is to perform normally, the brain must be continually informed of the current state of the muscles, and the muscles must exhibit health tone (resistance to active and passive stretch at rest). The first requirement depends on the transmission of information regarding the sense of body position, movement, and muscle tone to the CNS. Information from these sensory afferents is relayed to the cerebellum and cerebral cortex and is experienced as *proprioception* or the sense of body movement and position, independent of vision. To provide this information, the muscles and their tendons are supplied with two types of receptors: muscle spindles and Golgi tendon organs. The muscle spindles, which are distributed throughout the belly of a muscle, relay information about muscle length and rate of stretch. The *Golgi tendon organs* are found in muscle tendons and transmit information about muscle tension or force of contraction at the junction of the muscle and the tendon that attaches to bone. Normal muscle tone depends on stretch reflexes initiated by the muscle spindles, which monitors changes in muscle length.

The stretch reflex, a contraction of muscle fibers that occurs when a muscle is stretched, is essential to the control of muscle tone and maintenance of posture (see Understanding the Stretch Reflex and Muscle Tone). Stretch reflexes can be evoked in many muscles throughout the body and are routinely tested (*e.g.,* knee-jerk reflex) during clinical examination for the diagnosis of neurologic conditions. Stretch reflexes tend to be hypoactive or absent in cases of peripheral nerve damage or ventral horn injury involving the test area. However, they are hyperactive when lesions of the corticospinal tract (*e.g.,* stroke or spinal cord injury) reduce or disrupt the inhibitory effect of the brain on the spinal cord.

The muscle spindles consist of a group of specialized miniature skeletal muscle fibers called *intrafusal fibers* that are encased in a connective tissue capsule and attached to the extrafusal fibers of a skeletal muscle. In the center of the receptor area, a large sensory neuron spirals around the intrafusal fiber, forming the so-called *primary* or *annulospiral ending*. The intrafusal muscle fibers function as stretch receptors. When a skeletal muscle is stretched, the spindle and its intrafusal fibers are stretched, resulting in increased firing of their afferent nerve fibers. Axons of these afferent neurons enter the spinal cord through several branches of the dorsal root. Some branches end in the segment of entry; others ascend to adjacent segments, influencing intersegmental reflex function; and still others ascend in the dorsal column of the cord to the medulla of the brain stem. Segmental branches make connections, along with other branches, that pass directly to the anterior gray matter of the spinal cord and establish monosynaptic contact with each of the LMNs that have motor units in the muscle containing the spindle receptor. This produces an opposing muscle contraction. Another segmental branch of the same afferent neuron innervates an internuncial neuron that is inhibitory to motor units of antagonistic muscle groups. This disynaptic inhibitory pathway is the basis for the reciprocal activity of agonist and antagonist muscles (*i.e.,* when an agonist muscle is stretched, the antagonists relax). Reciprocal innervation is useful not only for the stretch reflex, but for voluntary movements. Relaxation of the antagonist muscle during movements enhances the speed and efficiency because the muscles that act as prime movers are not working against the contraction of opposing muscle.[1]

Another function of the stretch reflex is to inform the CNS of the status of muscle length. Ascending fibers from the stretch reflex ultimately provide information about muscle length to higher centers in the cerebellum and cerebral cortex. When a skeletal muscle lengthens or shortens against tension, a feedback mechanism needs to be available for readjustment such that the spindle apparatus remains sensitive to moment-to-moment changes in muscle stretch, even while changes in muscle length are occurring. This is accomplished by the gamma motor neurons that adjust spindle fiber length to match the length of the extrafusal muscle fiber. Descending fibers of motor pathways synapse with and simultaneously activate both alpha and gamma motor neurons so that the sensitivity of the spindle fibers is coordinated with muscle movement.

Central control over the gamma motor neurons also permits increases or decreases in muscle tone in anticipation of changes in the muscle force. The CNS, through its coordinated control of the muscle's alpha and the spindle's gamma motor neurons, can suppress the stretch reflex. This occurs during centrally programmed movements, such as pitching a baseball, that require a muscle to produce a full range of unopposed motion. Without this programmed adjustability of the stretch reflex, any movement is immediately opposed and prevented.

Motor Pathways

The primary motor cortex contains many layers of pyramid-shaped output neurons that project to the premotor and somatosensory areas on same side of the cortex (*i.e.*, premotor and somesthetic cortices), project to the opposite side of the cortex, or descend to subcortical structures such as the basal ganglia and thalamus. The large pyramidal cells located in the fifth layer project to the brain stem and spinal cord. The axons of these UMNs project through the subcortical white matter and internal capsule to the deep surface of the brain stem, through the ventral bulge of the pons, and to the ventral surface of the medulla, where they form a ridge or pyramid (see Fig. 50-2). About 80% of the corticospinal UMNs cross the midline in the pyramidal decussation at the junction of the medulla and cervical spinal cord to form the lateral corticospinal tract in the lateral white matter of the spinal cord.[8] This tract extends throughout the spinal cord, with roughly 50% of the fibers terminating in the cervical segments, 20% in the thoracic segments, and 30% in the lumbosacral segments.[8] Most of the remaining uncrossed fibers travel down the ventral column of the cord, mainly to cervical levels, where they cross and innervate contralateral LMNs.

Traditionally, motor tracts have been classified as belonging to one of two motor systems: the pyramidal and extrapyramidal systems. According to this classification system, the pyramidal system consists of the motor pathways originating in the motor cortex and terminating in the corticobulbar fibers in the brain stem and the corticospinal fibers in the spinal cord. Other fibers from the cortex and basal ganglia project to the brain stem reticular formation and reticulospinal systems, following a more ancient pathway to LMNs of proximal and extensor muscles. These fibers do not decussate in the pyramids, hence the name *extrapyramidal system.* Disorders of the pyramidal tracts (*e.g.*, stroke) are characterized by spasticity and paralysis, whereas those affecting the extrapyramidal tracts (*e.g.*, Parkinson disease) result in involuntary movements, muscle rigidity, and immobility without paralysis. As increased knowledge regarding motor pathways has emerged, it has become evident that the extrapyramidal and pyramidal systems are extensively interconnected and cooperate in the control of movement.[1]

Assessment of Motor Function

Disorders of the motor system produce signs and symptoms that can be used in localizing the disorder. These signs and symptoms include changes in muscle characteristics (strength, bulk, and tone), spinal reflex activity, and motor coordination.[9] For diagnostic purposes, clinicians often use the terms *LMN*, referring to neurons that are located in the spinal cord and brain stem and directly innervate skeletal muscle, and *UMN*, refer-

ring to neurons that originate in higher regions of the brain, such as the motor cortex, and synapse with motor neurons. The distinction between LMNs and UMNs is important because either class of neurons produces distinctive symptoms.

Muscle Strength, Bulk, and Tone

Muscle Strength. Abnormalities in any part of the motor pathway can produce impaired strength or muscle weakness. *Paralysis* refers to loss of movement, and *paresis,* to weakness or incomplete loss of strength. The pattern of weakness may be helpful in the localization of the lesion. *Monoparesis* or *monoplegia* results from the destruction of pyramidal UMN innervation of one limb; *hemiparesis* or *hemiplegia,* both limbs on one side; *diparesis* or *diplegia* or *paraparesis* or *paraplegia,* both upper or lower limbs; and *tetraparesis* or *tetraplegia,* also called *quadriparesis* or *quadriplegia,* all four limbs (Fig. 50-5).

Paresis or paralysis can be further designated as of UMN or LMN origin. UMN lesions of the motor cortex or corticospinal tract typically affect the extensors in the upper extremities more than the flexors, whereas in the lower extremities, the flexors are more affected. In LMN or peripheral nerve disorders, the weakness is predominantly in the distal limb, whereas in muscle disorders, such as muscular dystrophy, proximal limb function may be affected sooner than distal limb function.

Muscle Bulk. The size of muscle (whether muscles are normal sized, enlarged, or atrophied) also helps localize the lesion, and sometimes provide helpful hints to the pathologic process. Muscular atrophy, or loss of muscle bulk, usually results from LMN lesions as well as diseases of the muscles themselves. Hypertrophy refers to an increase in muscle bulk with a proportionate increase in strength. Pseudohypertrophy, as occurs with Duchenne muscular dystrophy, refers to an increase in bulk without an accompanying increase in strength.

Fasciculations are visible squirming and twitching movements of muscle fibers that can be seen as flickers under the skin. They are caused by spontaneous contractions of all the muscle fibers in a motor unit due to irritation and hyperexcitability of the cell body and its motor neuron, and suggest LMN disease.

Muscle Tone. Muscle tone is the normal state of muscle tension. It is assessed by palpating the muscle while at rest and during passive stretching. With the person at rest, the joints are put through the normal range of motion (flexion and extension) by the examiner. Disorders of skeletal muscle tone are characteristic of many nervous system lesions. Any interruption of the myotatic or stretch reflex circuitry by peripheral nerve injury, pathologic process of the neuromuscular junction, injury to the spinal cord, or damage to the corticospinal system can result in disturbances of muscle tone.

Abnormalities of muscle tone may be described as hypotonia (less than normal), flaccidity (absent), or hypertonia, rigidity, spasticity, or tetany (all indicating higher-than-

Understanding • The Stretch Reflex and Muscle Tone

Muscle tone is controlled by the stretch reflex, which monitors changes in muscle length. The activity of the stretch reflex can be divided into three steps: (1) activation of the stretch receptors, (2) integration of the reflex in the spinal cord, and (3) regulation of reflex sensitivity by higher centers in the brain. Testing the (4) knee-jerk reflex provides a means of assessing that reflex.

❶ Stretch Reflex Receptors

Skeletal muscle is composed of two types of muscle fibers: a large number of extrafusal fibers, which control muscle movement, and a smaller number of intrafusal fibers, which control muscle tone. The intrafusal fibers are encapsulated in sheaths, forming a muscle spindle that runs parallel to the extrafusal fibers. Each intrafusal fiber is innervated by a large Ia sensory nerve fiber, which encircles the central noncontractile portion of the fiber to form the so-called *annulospiral ending*. Because the spindles are oriented parallel to the extrafusal muscle fibers, stretching of the extrafusal fibers also stretches the spindle fibers and stimulates the receptive endings of the Ia afferent neuron.

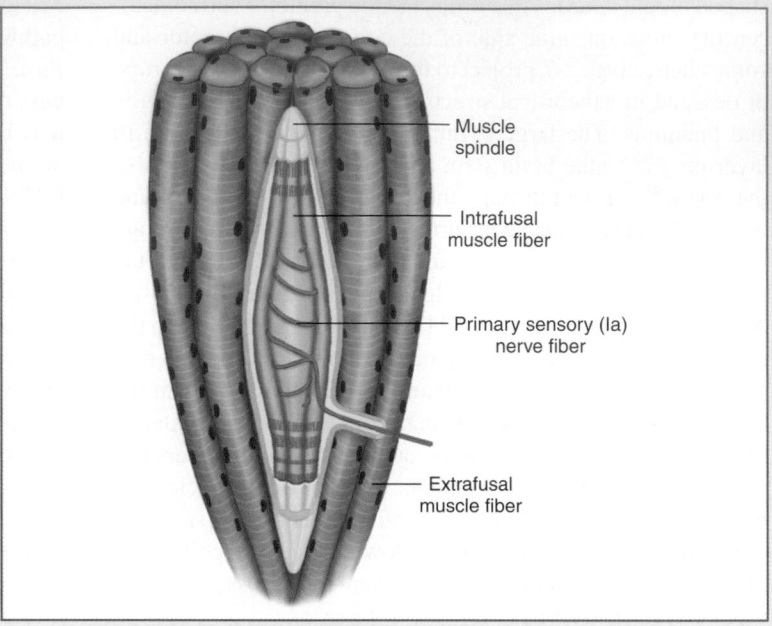

❷ Spinal Reflex Centers

Afferent impulses from the Ia sensory fiber of the muscle spindle are transmitted to the spinal cord, where they synapse with alpha motor neurons of the stretched muscle to form a monosynaptic reflex arc—"monosynaptic" because only one synapse separates the primary sensory input from the motor neuron output. The reflex muscle contraction that follows resists further stretching of the muscle. As this spinal reflex activity is occurring, impulses providing information on muscle length are transmitted to higher centers in the brain. It is the coordinated activity of all the monosynaptic reflexes supplying the extrafusal fibers in a skeletal muscle that provides the muscle tone needed for organized movement.

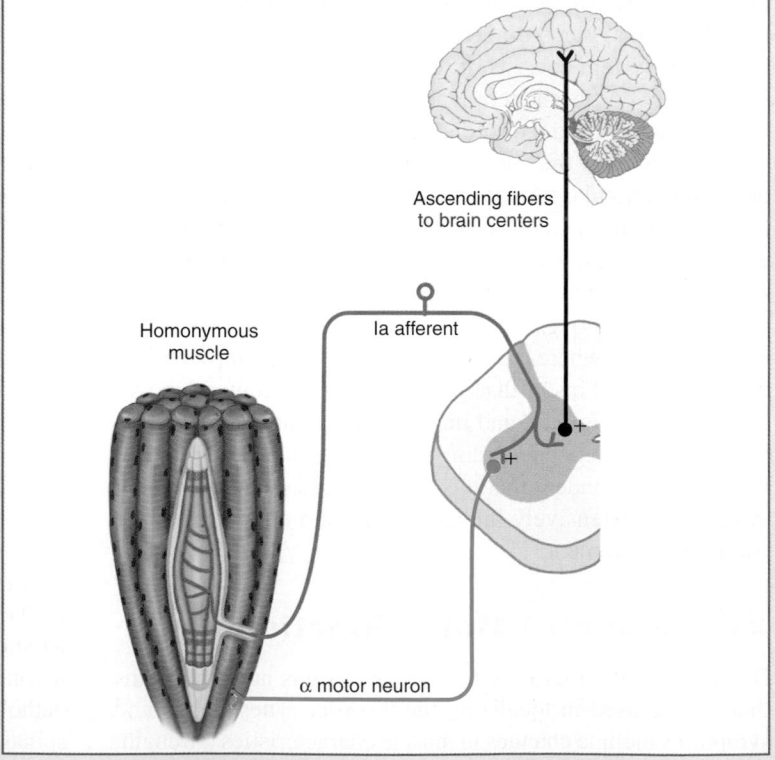

❸ Brain Center Connections

Although a spinal reflex can function independently, its sensitivity is adjusted by higher centers in the brain. Both types of muscle fibers are supplied with motor neurons—the extrafusal fibers with large alpha motor neurons, which produce muscle contraction; and the intrafusal fibers with smaller gamma motor neurons, which control the sensitivity of the stretch reflex. Descending fibers of motor pathways synapse with both alpha and gamma motor neurons, and the impulses are sent simultaneously to the large extrafusal fibers and to the intrafusal fibers to maintain muscle spindle tension (and sensitivity) during muscle contraction.

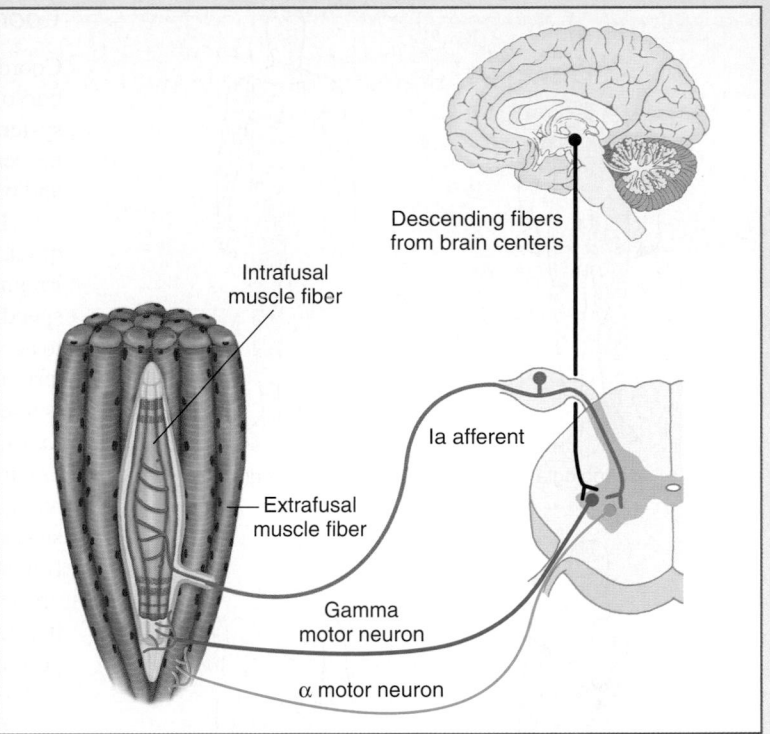

❹ The Knee-Jerk Reflex

The knee-jerk reflex that occurs when the knee is tapped with a reflex hammer tests for the intactness of the stretch reflex arc in the quadriceps muscle. Stretching of the extrafusal fibers by tapping with a reflex hammer leads to lengthening of the intrafusal fibers and increased firing of the type Ia afferent neuron. Impulses from the Ia fiber enter the dorsal horn of the spinal cord and make monosynaptic contact with the ventral horn alpha motor neuron supplying the extrafusal fibers in the quadriceps muscle. The resultant reflex contraction (shortening) of the quadriceps muscle is responsible for the knee jerk. These muscle reflexes are called *deep tendon reflexes* (DTRs). They can be checked at the wrists, elbows, knees, and ankles as a means of assessing the components of the stretch reflex at different spinal cord segments.

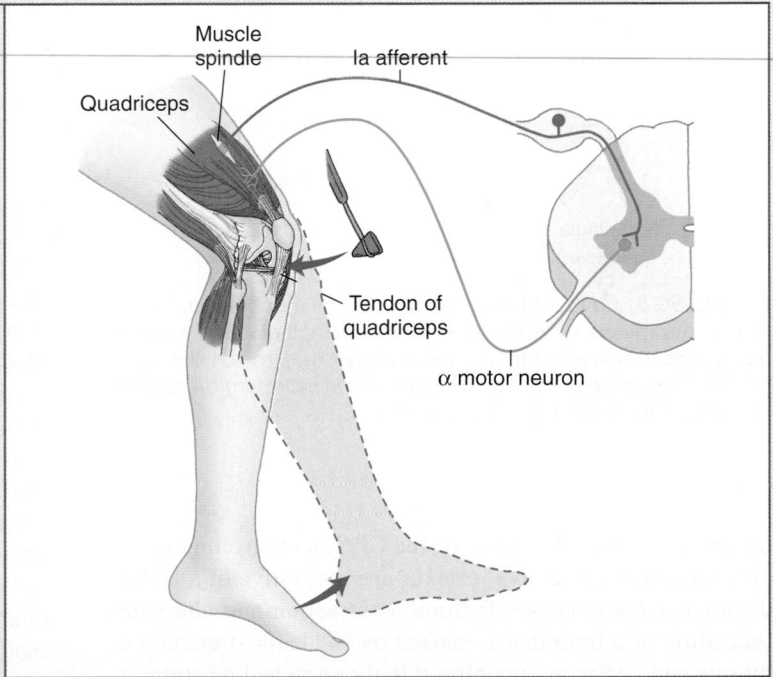

normal tone). Typically, UMN lesions produce increased tone, whereas LMN lesions produce decreased tone. Increased resistance that varies and commonly becomes worse at the extremes of the range of motion is called *spasticity*. Resistance that becomes worse throughout the range and in both directions is called *lead-pipe rigidity*. Decreased resistance suggests disease of the LMNs or the acute stages of spinal cord injury. Marked floppiness indicates hypotonic or flaccid muscles.

Spinal Reflex Activity

Testing of deep tendon reflexes (see Understanding the Stretch Reflex and Muscle Tone) can provide important

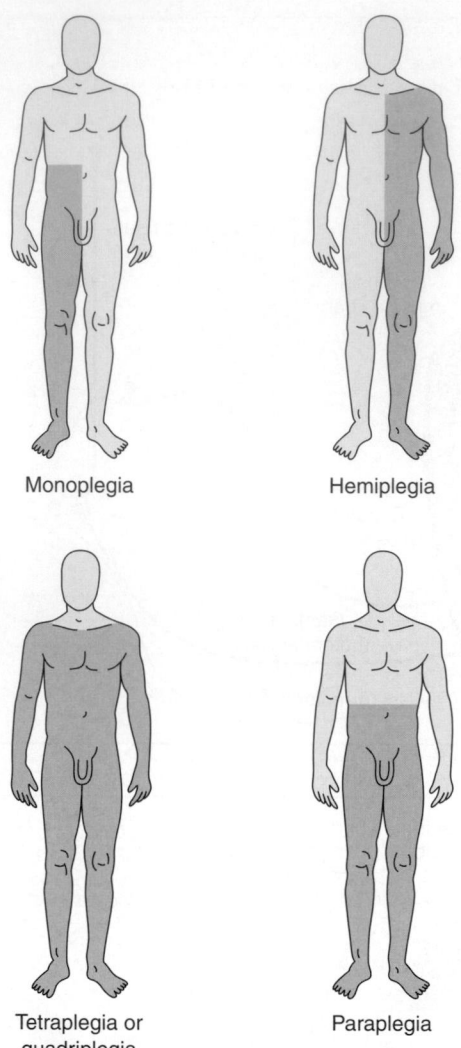

Monoplegia

Hemiplegia

Tetraplegia or
quadriplegia

Paraplegia

FIGURE 50-5 • Areas of the body affected by monoplegia, hemiplegia, tetraplegia or quadriplegia, and paraplegia. The *shaded area* shows the extent of motor and sensory loss. (From Hickey J. V. [1997]. *The clinical practice of neurological and neurosurgical nursing* [3rd ed.]. Philadelphia: J. B. Lippincott.)

information about the status of the CNS in controlling muscle function. Hyperactive reflexes are suggestive of a UMN disorder. *Clonus* is the rhythmic contraction and alternate relaxation of a limb that is caused by suddenly stretching a muscle and gently maintaining it in the stretched position. It is seen in the hypertonia of spasticity associated with UMN lesions, such as spinal cord injury. *Hyporeflexia* or *areflexia* suggests the presence of an LMN lesion. The distribution of abnormality in the reflexes is also helpful in determining the location of the lesion. For example, hyperreflexia in both lower extremities would suggest a lesion in the spinal cord, whereas hyperreflexia on one side of the body would suggest a lesion in the UMN along the motor pathway (*e.g.,* in the motor cortex or internal capsule).

Coordination of Movement

Coordination of muscle movement requires that four areas of the nervous system function in an integrated manner—the motor system for muscle strength, the cerebellar system for rhythmic movement and steady posture, the vestibular system for posture and balance, and the sensory system for position sense.

In cerebellar disease, one movement cannot be followed quickly by its opposite movement and movements are slow, irregular, clumsy, unsteady, and inappropriately varying in their speed, force, and direction. *Dysdiadochokinesia* is the failure to accurately perform rapid alternating movements. *Ataxia* is a term used to describe a wide-based, unsteady gait. *Dysmetria* is a term used to describe inaccuracies of movements leading to a failure to reach a specified target. This can be tested by having the person touch the examiner's finger and then alternately touch his or her finger. These movements are normally smooth and accurate. Asking the person to touch the examiner's finger with an outstretched arm and finger, first with the eyes open and then closed, provides a test for position sense. Repetitive and consistent deviation to one side (referred to as past pointing), which is worse with the eyes closed, suggests cerebellar or vestibular disease.

Chorea (abnormal writhing movements), *dystonia* (abnormal simultaneous contractions of agonist and antagonist muscles, leading to abnormal postures), *tremor* (rhythmic movements of a particular body part), *bradykinesia* (slowness of movements), and *myoclonus* (involuntary jerking movement) indicate abnormalities in the basal ganglia, although the exact localization may be difficult to determine.

IN SUMMARY, motor function, whether it involves walking, running, or precise finger movements, requires movement and maintenance of posture. The system consists of the LMNs, which are located in the ventral horn of the spinal cord and the group of muscle fibers it innervates in the muscle; spinal cord circuitry and reflexes; and the descending UMNs that project from the motor cortex to the opposite side of the medulla, where they form a pyramid before crossing the midline to form the lateral corticospinal tract in the spinal cord. Voluntary control of motor function is directed by the motor cortex, which consists of the primary, premotor, and supplementary motor cortex. The primary motor cortex is responsible for execution of a movement, the premotor cortex for generating a plan of movement, and the supplemental motor cortex for rehearsing the motor sequences of a movement, including those involving both sides of the body. As with other parts of the nervous system, the motor systems are organized in a functional hierarchy of, from bottom to top, the spinal cord, brain stem, and motor cortex, each with circuits that, through their input and output connections, can contribute to the organization and regulation of complex motor responses.

Proper control of muscle function requires not only excitation of the muscle by the LMNs located in the spinal cord but the function of reflex circuitry that monitors the functional status of the muscle fibers on a moment-by-moment basis. The muscle spindles of the stretch reflex function to monitor and correct for changes in muscle length when extrafusal fibers are either shortened (by contraction) or lengthened (by stretch).

Assessments of muscle strength and muscle bulk, muscle tone and motor reflexes, and patterns of motor movement and posture provide the means for determining the location of disorders of motor function. Paresis (weakness) and paralysis (loss of muscle movement) reflect a loss of muscle strength. UMN lesions tend to produce spastic paralysis and LMN lesions flaccid paralysis. Changes in muscle bulk are characterized by a loss of muscle mass (atrophy) or an increase in muscle mass (hypertrophy). Muscle tone is maintained through the combined function of the spinal cord stretch reflex, and higher centers monitor and buffer UMN innervation of the LMNs. Hypotonia is a condition of less-than-normal muscle tone, and hypertonia or spasticity is a condition of excessive tone. Abnormal and uncoordinated movements and postures are suggestive of a cerebellar or basal ganglia pathologic process. ■

DISORDERS OF THE MOTOR UNIT

After completing this section of the chapter, you should be able to meet the following objectives:

- Describe muscle atrophy and differentiate between disuse and degenerative atrophy.
- Relate the molecular changes in muscle structure that occur in Duchenne muscular dystrophy to the clinical manifestations of the disease.
- Describe the actions of *Clostridium botulinum* neurotoxins in terms of their pathologic and therapeutic potential.
- Relate the clinical manifestations of myasthenia gravis to its cause.
- Define the term *peripheral nervous system* and describe the characteristics of peripheral nerves.
- Trace the steps in regeneration of an injured peripheral nerve.
- Compare the cause and manifestations of peripheral mononeuropathies with polyneuropathies.
- Describe the manifestation of peripheral nerve root injury due to a ruptured intervertebral disk.

Most of the diseases of the motor unit cause weakness and wasting of skeletal muscles. The distinguishing features of these diseases vary depending on which of the components of the motor

unit is primarily affected: the cell body of the motor neuron, its axon, the neuromuscular junction, or the muscle fibers.[6,10,11] Disorders affecting the nerve cell body are often referred to as *lower motor neuron disorders;* those affecting the nerve axon as *peripheral neuropathies;* and primary disorders affecting the muscle fibers as *myopathies.*

Skeletal Muscle Disorders

Muscle Atrophy

Maintenance of muscle strength requires relatively frequent movements against resistance. Reduced use results in muscle atrophy, which is characterized by a reduction in the diameter of the muscle fibers because of a loss of protein filaments.[11] When a normally innervated muscle is not used for long periods, the muscle cells shrink in diameter, and although the muscle cells do not die, they lose much of their contractile proteins and become weakened. This is called *disuse atrophy,* and it occurs with conditions such as immobilization and chronic illness.

The most extreme examples of muscle atrophy are found in persons with disorders that deprive muscles of their innervation. This is called *denervation atrophy.* During early embryonic development, outgrowing skeletal nerves innervate partially mature muscle cells. If the developing muscle cells are not innervated, they do not mature and eventually die. In the process of innervation, randomly contracting muscle cells become enslaved by the innervating neurons, and from then on, the muscle cell contracts only when stimulated by that particular neuron. If the LMN dies or its axon is destroyed, the skeletal muscle cell is again free of neural domination. When this happens, it begins to have temporary spontaneous contractions, called *fibrillations.* In contrast to previously described fasciculations, fibrillations are not visible clinically and can be detected only by electromyography.[6] The muscle also begins to lose its contractile proteins and, after several months, if not reinnervated, it is replaced by fibrous connective tissue, which makes rehabilitation difficult. Atrophy of denervation can often be delayed by electrically stimulating the muscle periodically while waiting to determine if the damaged nerve fiber regenerates.

 ### Muscular Dystrophy

Muscular dystrophy is a term applied to a number of genetic disorders that produce progressive deterioration of skeletal muscles because of mixed muscle cell hypertrophy, atrophy, and necrosis. They are primary diseases of muscle tissue and probably do not involve the nervous system. As the muscle undergoes necrosis, fat and connective tissue replace the muscle fibers, which increases muscle size and results in muscle weakness. The increase in muscle size resulting from connective tissue infiltration is called *pseudohypertrophy.* The muscle weakness is insidious in onset but continually progressive, varying with the type of disorder.

The most common form of the disease is *Duchenne muscular dystrophy* (DMD), which occurs once in every 3500 live male births.[11,12] DMD is inherited as a recessive single-gene defect on the X chromosome and is transmitted from the mother to her male offspring (see Chapter 7). A spontaneous (mutation) form may occur in girls. Another form of dystrophy, *Becker muscular dystrophy,* is similarly X-linked but manifests later in childhood or adolescence and has a slower course of progression.

DMD is caused by mutations in a gene located on the short arm of the X chromosome that codes for a protein called *dystrophin.* Dystrophin is a large cytoplasmic protein located on the inner surface of the sarcolemma or muscle fiber membrane. The dystrophin molecules are concentrated over the Z-bands of the muscle, where they form a strong link between the actin filaments of the intracellular contractile apparatus and the extracellular connective tissue matrix[10,11] (see Chapter 4, Fig. 4-21). It is thought that abnormalities in the dystrophin-associated protein complex compromise sarcolemma integrity, particularly with sustained contractions. This disruption in integrity may be responsible for the observed increased fragility of dystrophic muscle, excessive influx of calcium ions, and release of soluble muscle enzymes such as creatine kinase into the serum. The degenerative process in DMD consists of a relentless necrosis of muscle fibers, accompanied by a continuous process of repair and regeneration, and progressive fibrosis. The degenerative process eventually outpaces the regenerative capacity of the muscle, causing a gradual replacement of muscle fibers by fibrofatty connective tissue. The end stage is characterized by almost complete loss of skeletal muscle fibers, with relative sparing of intrafusal fibers of the muscle spindles.[11]

Clinical Course. Children with DMD are usually asymptomatic at birth and during infancy.[13] Early gross movements such as rolling, sitting, and standing are usually achieved at the proper ages. The postural muscles of the hips and shoulders are usually the first to be affected. Pseudohypertrophy of the calf muscles eventually develops (Fig. 50-6). Signs of muscle weakness usually become evident beginning at 2 to 3 years, when frequent falling begins to occur. Imbalances between agonist and antagonist muscles lead to abnormal postures and the development of contractures and joint immobility. Scoliosis is common. Wheelchairs usually are needed at approximately 7 to 12 years of age.[13] Function of the distal muscles usually is preserved well enough that the child can continue to use eating utensils and a computer keyboard. Function of the extraocular muscles also is well preserved, as is the function of the smooth muscle controlling bladder and bowel activity. Incontinence is an uncommon and late event. Respiratory muscle involvement results in weak and ineffective cough, frequent respiratory infections, and decreasing respiratory reserve. DMD also affects cardiac muscle, and cardiomyopathy is a common feature of the disease. The severity of cardiac involvement, however, does not necessarily correlate with skeletal muscle weakness. Some patients die at an early age from severe cardiomyopathy, whereas others maintain adequate cardiac function until the terminal stages of the disease.

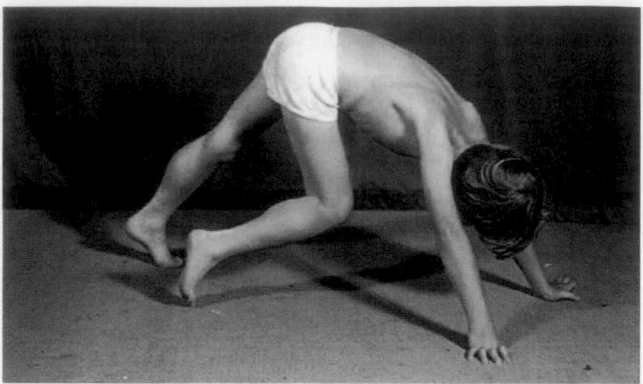

FIGURE 50-6 • A boy with Duchenne muscular dystrophy demonstrating pseudohypertrophy of his calves and climbing from a sitting position because of proximal muscle weakness. (From Bird T., Sumi S. [2002]. *Atlas of clinical neurology.* Edited by Roger N. Rosenberg. © Current Medicine, Inc.)

Death from respiratory and cardiac muscle involvement usually occurs in young adulthood.

Observation of the child's voluntary movements and a complete family history provide important diagnostic data for the disease. Serum levels of the enzyme creatine kinase, which leaks from damaged muscle fibers, can be used to assist the diagnosis. Muscle biopsy, which shows a mixture of muscle cell degeneration and regeneration and reveals fat and scar tissue replacement, is diagnostic of the disorder. Echocardiography, electrocardiography, and chest radiography are used to assess cardiac function. A specific molecular genetic diagnosis is possible by demonstrating defective dystrophin through the use of immunohistochemical staining of sections of muscle biopsy tissue or by polymerase chain reaction (PCR) analysis of genomic deoxyribonucleic acid (DNA) derived from leukocytes in a blood sample. The same methods of DNA analysis may be used on blood samples to establish carrier status in female relatives at risk, such as sisters and cousins. Prenatal diagnosis is possible as early as 12 weeks' gestation by sampling chorionic villi for DNA analysis[13] (see Chapter 7).

Management of the disease is directed toward maintaining ambulation and preventing deformities. Passive stretching, correct or counter posturing, and splints help to prevent deformities. Precautions should be taken to avoid respiratory infections. Although there have been exciting advances in identifying the gene and gene product involved in DMD, there is no known cure.

Disorders of the Neuromuscular Junction

The neuromuscular junction serves as a synapse between a motor neuron and a skeletal muscle fiber. It consists of the axon terminals of a motor neuron and a specialized region of the muscle membrane called the motor *end plate.* The transmission of impulses at the neuromuscular junction is mediated by the release of the neurotransmitter *acetylcholine* from the axon terminals. Acetylcholine binds to specific receptors in the end-plate region of the muscle fiber surface to cause muscle contraction (Fig. 50-7). Acetylcholine is active in the neuromuscular junction only for the brief period of time that it takes to generate an action potential in the innervated muscle cell. In the synaptic space are large quantities of the enzyme *acetylcholinesterase,* which destroy acetylcholine a few milliseconds after it has been released. The rapid inactivation of acetylcholine allows repeated muscle contractions and gradations of contractile force.

Drug- and Toxin-Induced Disorders

A number of drugs and agents can alter neuromuscular function by changing the release, inactivation, or receptor binding of acetylcholine. Curare acts on the postjunctional membrane of the motor endplate to prevent the depolarizing effect of the neurotransmitter. Blocking of neuromuscular transmission by curare-type drugs is used during many types of surgical procedures to facilitate relaxation of involved musculature. Drugs such as physostigmine and neostigmine inhibit the action of acetylcholinesterase and allow acetylcholine released from the motor neuron to accumulate and prolong its action. These drugs are used in the treatment of myasthenia gravis.

Neurotoxins from the botulism organism (*Clostridium botulinum*) produce paralysis by blocking acetylcholine release.[14] Clostridia are anaerobic, gram-positive, spore-forming bacilli found worldwide in soils, marine and fresh water sediments, and the intestines of many animals. Classic food-borne botulism occurs through ingestion of soil-grown foods that are not properly cooked or preserved.[15] Spores can be dormant, are resistant to heat, and germinate in low-acidity, and low-nitrate environments. Canned vegetables, items preserved in garlic oil, and soups are usually the cause of sporadic outbreaks. Ingestion of the spores leads to toxin synthesis and absorption of the toxins from the intestinal tract. Wound botulism occurs through colonization of wounds with *C. botulinum.* Although postsurgical cases were initially the cause of wound botulism, almost all recent adult cases have involved intravenously injected heroin users.[16]

Infant botulism, now the most commonly reported form of the disease, occurs through infant ingestion of *C. botulinum* spores.[17] An infant's immature gastrointestinal tract allows the spores to germinate and elaborate the botulinum toxins. Ninety percent of the world's cases of infant botulism are diagnosed in the United States (an estimated 250 cases/year), mainly because of increased awareness among health care professionals.[17] Infants who acquire botulism range in age from 6 weeks to 9 months, with peak incidence occurring from 2 to 3 months of age. Infants usually develop botulism by ingesting *C. botulinum* spores, which are found in the soil or in honey products. According to microbiologic studies, 25% of honey products have been found to contain spores.[16] Therefore, it is recommended that honey should not be given to infants younger than 1 year of age. The classic clinical features of the disorder include constipation, cranial nerve abnormalities, hypotonia, hyperreflexia, and respiratory distress. Constipation may be present in affected infants for a variable time and precede weakness by several weeks.

Pharmacologic preparations of the botulinum toxin (botulinum type A toxin [Botox] and botulinum type B toxin [Myobloc]) have become available for use in treating eyelid and eye movement disorders such as blepharospasm and strabismus.[15] It also is used for treatment of spasmodic torticollis, spasmodic dysphonias (laryngeal dystonia), and other dystonias. The drug is injected into the target muscle using the electrical activity recorded from the tip of a special electromyographic injection needle to guide the injection. The treatment is not permanent and usually needs to be repeated approximately every 3 months.

The aminoglycoside antibiotics (*e.g.,* gentamicin) may produce a clinical disturbance similar to botulism by preventing the release of acetylcholine from nerve endings. The symptoms usually subside rapidly once the drug is eliminated from the body. These drugs are particularly dangerous in persons with preexisting disturbances of neuromuscular transmission, such as myasthenia gravis.

The organophosphates that are used in some insecticides bind acetylcholinesterase to prevent the breakdown of acetylcholine. They produce excessive and prolonged acetylcholine action with a depolarization block of cholinergic receptors,

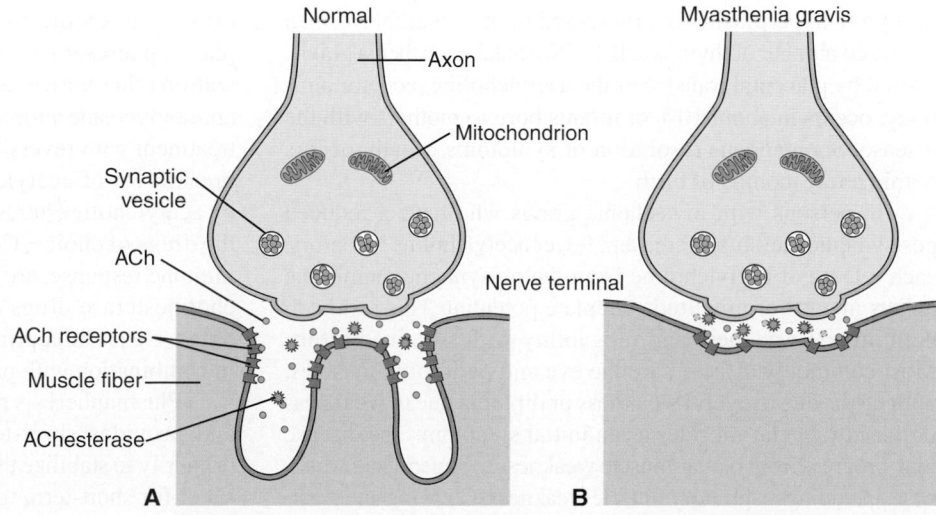

FIGURE 50-7 • Neuromuscular junction. **(A)** Acetylcholine (ACh) released from the motor neurons in the myoneural junction crosses the synaptic space to reach receptors that are concentrated in the folds of the endplate of the muscle fiber. Once released, ACh is rapidly broken down by the enzyme acetylcholinesterase (AChesterase). **(B)** Decrease in ACh receptors in myasthenia gravis.

including those of the neuromuscular junction.[15] The organophosphates are well absorbed from the skin, lungs, gut, and conjunctiva of the eye, making them particularly effective as insecticides but also potentially dangerous to humans. Malathion and certain other organophosphates are rapidly metabolized to inactive products in humans and are considered safe for sale to the general public. The sale of other insecticides, such as parathion, which is not effectively metabolized to inactive products, has been banned. Other organophosphate compounds were developed as "nerve gases" with military potential; if absorbed in high enough concentrations, they have lethal effects from depolarization block and loss of respiratory muscle function.

Myasthenia Gravis

Myasthenia gravis is a disorder of transmission at the neuromuscular junction that affects communication between the motor neuron and the innervated muscle cell. The disease may occur at any age, but the peak incidence occurs between 20 and 30 years of age, and the disease is approximately three times more common in women than men. A smaller, second peak occurs in later life and affects men more often than women.[18] The Lambert-Eaton myasthenic syndrome is a special type of myasthenic syndrome that develops in association with neoplasms, particularly small cell carcinoma of the lung (see Chapter 8).

Now recognized as an autoimmune disease, the disorder is caused by an antibody-mediated loss of acetylcholine receptors in the neuromuscular junction[18–20] (see Fig. 50-7). Although the exact mechanism that triggers the autoimmune response is unclear, it is thought to be caused by sensitized helper T cells and an antibody-directed attack on the acetylcholine receptor in the neuromuscular junction. The antibody attack leads to a shedding of the acetylcholine receptor—rich terminal portions of the folds in the endplate of the muscle fiber, a decreased number of receptors, and a widened synaptic space that impairs signal transmission.[12] The antibodies do not directly block binding of acetylcholine to prevent neuromuscular transmission. Approximately 75% of persons with myasthenia gravis also have thymic abnormalities, such as a thymoma (i.e., thymus tumor) or thymic hyperplasia (i.e., increased thymus weight from an increased number of thymus cells).[18] Neonatal myasthenia gravis, caused by placental transfer of the acetylcholine receptor antibody, occurs in about 10% of infants born to mothers with the disease. Spontaneous resolution of symptoms usually occurs within a few months of birth.

In persons with myasthenia gravis who have a reduced postsynaptic membrane area and fewer acetylcholine receptors, each release of acetylcholine from the presynaptic membrane results in a lower-amplitude endplate potential. This results in both muscle weakness and fatigability with sustained effort. Most commonly affected are the eye and periorbital muscles, with ptosis due to eyelid weakness or diplopia due to weakness of the extraocular muscles as an initial symptom. The disease may progress from ocular muscle weakness to generalized weakness, including respiratory muscle weakness. Chewing and swallowing may be difficult. Weakness in limb movement usually is more pronounced in proximal than in distal parts of the extremity, so that climbing stairs and lifting objects are difficult. As the disease progresses, the muscles of the lower face are affected, causing speech impairment. In most persons, symptoms are least evident when arising in the morning, but grow worse with effort and as the day proceeds.

Persons with myasthenia gravis may experience a sudden exacerbation of symptoms and weakness known as *myasthenic crisis*. Myasthenic crisis occurs when muscle weakness becomes severe enough to compromise ventilation to the extent that ventilatory support and airway protection are needed. This usually occurs during a period of stress, such as infection, emotional upset, pregnancy, alcohol ingestion, cold exposure, or surgery. It also can result from inadequate or excessive doses of the anticholinesterase drugs used in treatment of the disorder.

Diagnosis and Treatment. The diagnosis of myasthenia gravis is based on history and physical examination, the anticholinesterase test, nerve stimulation studies, and an assay for acetylcholine receptor antibodies. The anticholinesterase test uses a drug that inhibits acetylcholinesterase, the enzyme that breaks down acetylcholine. Edrophonium (Tensilon), a short-acting acetylcholinesterase inhibitor, commonly is used for the test. The drug, which is administered intravenously, decreases the breakdown of acetylcholine in the neuromuscular junction. When weakness is caused by myasthenia gravis, a dramatic transitory improvement in muscle function occurs. Electrophysiologic studies can be done to demonstrate a decremental muscle response to repetitive 2- or 3-Hz stimulation of motor nerves. An advance in diagnostic methods for myasthenia gravis is single-fiber electromyography, which is available in many medical centers. Single-fiber electromyography detects delayed or failed neuromuscular transmission in muscle fibers supplied by a single nerve fiber.[18–20] An immunoassay test can be used to detect the presence of antiacetylcholine receptor antibodies circulating in the blood.

Treatment methods include the use of pharmacologic agents; immunosuppressive therapy, including corticosteroid drugs; management of myasthenic crisis; thymectomy; and plasmapheresis or intravenous immunoglobulin.[18–20] Medications that may exacerbate myasthenia gravis, such as the aminoglycoside antibiotics, should be avoided. Pharmacologic treatment with reversible anticholinesterase drugs inhibits the breakdown of acetylcholine at the neuromuscular junction by acetylcholinesterase. Pyridostigmine and neostigmine are the drugs of choice. Corticosteroid drugs, which suppress the immune response, are used in cases of a poor response to anticholinesterase drugs and thymectomy. Immunosuppressant drugs (e.g., azathioprine, cyclosporine) also may be used, often in combination with plasmapheresis.

Plasmapheresis removes antibodies from the circulation and provides short-term clinical improvement. It is used primarily to stabilize the condition of persons in myasthenic crisis or for short-term treatment in persons undergoing thymectomy. Intravenous immunoglobulin also produces improvement in persons with myasthenia gravis. Although the effect is temporary, it may last for weeks to months. The indications for its use are similar to those for plasmapheresis. The mechanism of action of intravenous immunoglobulin is unknown. Intravenous immunoglobulin therapy is very expensive, which limits its use.

Thymectomy, or surgical removal of the thymus, may be used as a treatment for myasthenia gravis. Because the mechanism whereby surgery exerts its effect is unknown, the treatment is controversial. Thymectomy is performed in persons with thymoma, regardless of age, and in persons between puberty and 55 years age with generalized myasthenia gravis.[19]

Lower Motor Neuron Disorders

Lower motor neuron diseases are progressive neurologic illnesses that selectively affect the anterior horn cells of the spinal cord and cranial nerve motor neurons.[10,21] An example of a disorder that involves purely LMNs is a distinctive group of degenerative disorders that begin in childhood or adolescence called *spinal muscular atrophy* (SMA). Weakness and muscle atrophy are prominent findings in all forms of the disorder. This condition is likely to be inherited, usually in an autosomal recessive fashion, and is caused by the deletion of the survival motor neuron-1 gene (*SMN1*). Some forms of SMA result from degeneration of the anterior horn cells but are not caused by deletion of the *SMN1* gene. The most severe form may be symptomatic at birth or in the first months of life. In addition to hypotonia in the infant, patients frequently die from respiratory failure. More indolent forms may become symptomatic later in life, from infancy to as late as adolescence.[21]

Peripheral Nerve Disorders

The peripheral nervous system consists of the motor and sensory branches of the cranial and spinal nerves, the peripheral parts of the autonomic nervous system, and the peripheral ganglia. A peripheral neuropathy is any primary disorder of the peripheral nerves. The result usually is muscle weakness, with or without atrophy and sensory changes.

Unlike nerves in the CNS, peripheral nerves are fairly strong and resilient. They contain a series of connective tissue sheaths that enclose their nerve fibers. An outer fibrous sheath called the *epineurium* surrounds the medium-sized to large nerves; inside, a sheath called the *perineurium* invests each bundle of nerve fibers; and within each bundle, a delicate sheath of connective tissue known as the *endoneurium* surrounds each nerve fiber (see Chapter 48, Fig. 48-3). Inside the endoneurial sheath are the Schwann cells that produce the myelin sheath that surrounds the peripheral nerves. Each Schwann cell can myelinate only one segment of a single axon—the one that it covers—so that myelination of an entire axon requires the participation of a long line of these cells.

Peripheral Nerve Injury and Repair

There are two main types of peripheral nerve injury based on the target of the insult: segmental demyelination involving the Schwann cell and axonal degeneration involving the neuronal cell body or its axon.[10,11] The peripheral nerve disorders can affect a spinal nerve or nerve root, a nerve plexus, or peripheral nerve trunk (mononeuropathies), or multiple peripheral nerves (polyneuropathies).

Segmental Demyelination. Segmental demyelination occurs when there is a disorder of the Schwann cell (as in Guillain-Barré syndrome) or damage to the myelin sheath (*e.g.,* sensory neuropathies), without a primary abnormality of the axon. It typically affects some Schwann cells while sparing others. The denuded axon provides a stimulus for remyelination, and the population of cells in the endoneurium has the capacity to replace the injured Schwann cells. These cells proliferate and encircle the axon, and in time remyelinate the denuded portion. However, the new myelin sheath is thin in proportion to the axon, and over time, many chronic demyelinating neuropathies give way to axonal injury.

Axonal Degeneration. Axonal degeneration is caused by primary injury to a neuronal cell body or its axon. Damage to the axon may be due either to a focal event occurring at some point along the length of the nerve (*e.g.,* trauma or ischemia) or to a more generalized abnormality affecting the neuronal cell body (neuropathy).

Damage to a peripheral nerve axon, whether due to injury or neuropathy, results in degenerative changes, followed by breakdown of the myelin sheath and Schwann cells. In distal axonal degeneration, the proximal axon and neuronal cell body, which synthesizes the material required for nourishing and maintaining the axon, remain intact. In neuropathies and crushing injuries in which the endoneurial tube remains intact, the outgrowing fiber will grow down this tube to the structure that was originally innervated by the neuron (Fig. 50-8). However, it can take weeks or months for the regrowing fiber to reach its target organ and for communicative function to be reestablished. More time is required for the Schwann cells to form new myelin segments and for the axon to recover its original diameter and conduction velocity.

The successful regeneration of a nerve fiber in the peripheral nervous system depends on many factors. If a nerve fiber is destroyed relatively close to the neuronal cell body, the chances are that the nerve cell will die, and if it does, it will not be replaced. If a crushing type of injury has occurred, partial or often full recovery of function occurs. Cutting-type trauma to a nerve is an entirely different matter. Connective scar tissue forms rapidly at the wound site, and when it does, only the most rapidly regenerating axonal branches are able to get through to the intact distal endoneurial tubes. A number of scar-inhibiting agents have been used in an effort to reduce this hazard, but have met with only moderate success. In another attempt to improve nerve regeneration, various types

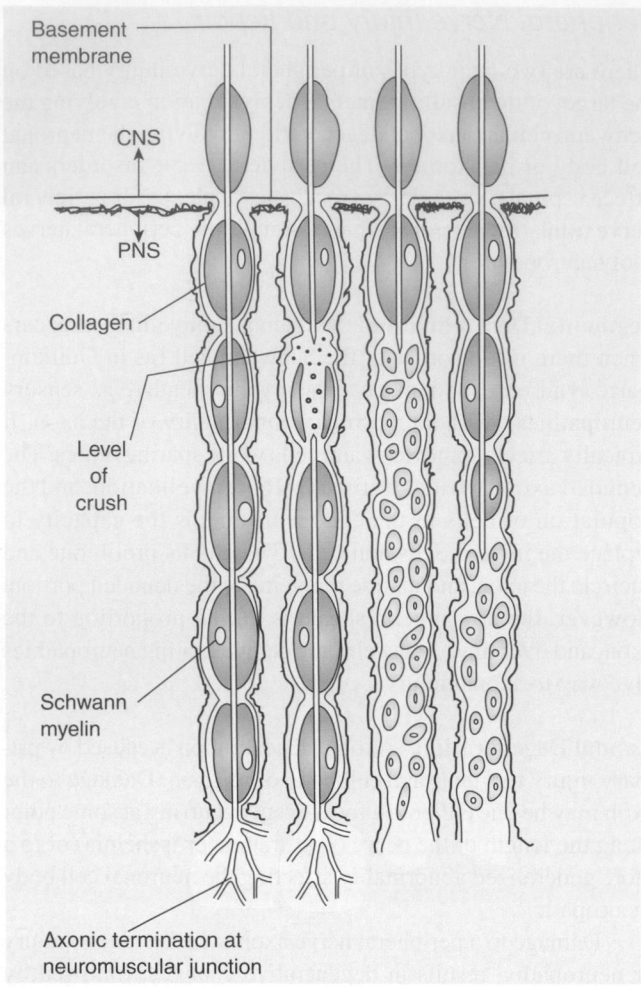

Basement
membrane

CNS

PNS

Collagen

Level
of
crush

Schwann
myelin

Axonic termination at
neuromuscular junction

FIGURE 50-8 • Sequential stages in efferent axon degeneration and regeneration within its endoneurial tube, after peripheral nerve crush injury. PNS, peripheral nervous system.

of tubular implants have been placed to fill longer gaps in the endoneurial tube.

Neuropathies involving the neuronal cell body are much less common than those affecting the axons. In these cases, there is little potential for recovery of function because death of the neuronal cells precludes axonal regeneration.

Mononeuropathies

Mononeuropathies usually are caused by localized conditions such as trauma, compression, or infection that affect a single spinal nerve, plexus, or peripheral nerve trunk. Fractured bones may lacerate or compress nerves; excessively tight tourniquets may injure nerves directly or produce ischemic injury; and infections such as herpes zoster may affect a single segmental afferent nerve distribution. Recovery of nerve function usually is complete after compression lesions and incomplete or faulty after nerve transection.

Carpal Tunnel Syndrome. Carpal tunnel syndrome is a relatively common compression-type mononeuropathy.[22–24] It is caused by compression of the median nerve as it travels with the flexor tendons through a canal made by the carpal bones and transverse carpal ligament (Fig. 50-9). The condition can be caused by a variety of conditions that produce a reduction in the capacity of the carpal tunnel (*i.e.*, bony or ligamentous changes) or an increase in the volume of the tunnel contents (*i.e.*, inflammation of the tendons, synovial swelling, or tumors). Carpal tunnel syndrome may be a feature of a number of systemic diseases, such as rheumatoid arthritis, hyperthyroidism, acromegaly, and diabetes mellitus.[22] However, most cases are due to repetitive use of the wrist (*i.e.*, flexion—extension movements and stress associated with pinching and gripping motions).

Carpal tunnel syndrome is characterized by pain, paresthesia, and numbness of the thumb and first two and one half digits of the hand; pain in the wrist and hand, which worsens at night; atrophy of the abductor pollicis muscle; and weakness in precision grip. All of these abnormalities may contribute to clumsiness of fine motor activity.

Diagnosis usually is based on sensory disturbances confined to median nerve distribution and a positive Tinel or Phalen sign.[23,24] The *Tinel sign* is the development of a tingling sensation radiating into the palm of the hand that is elicited by light percussion over the median nerve at the wrist. The *Phalen maneuver* is performed by having the person hold the wrist in complete flexion for approximately a minute; if numbness and paresthesia along the median nerve are reproduced or exaggerated, the test result is considered to be positive. Electromyog-

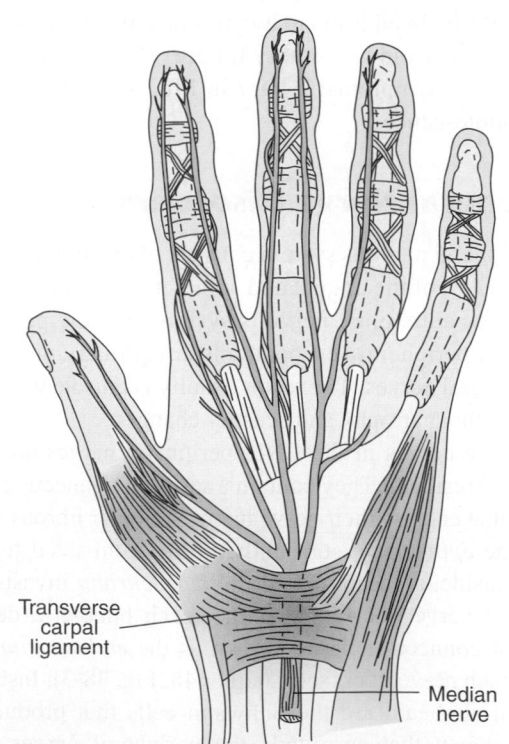

Transverse
carpal
ligament

Median
nerve

FIGURE 50-9 • Carpal tunnel syndrome: compression of the median nerve by the transverse carpal ligament. (Courtesy Carole Russell Hilmer, CMI.)

raphy and nerve conduction studies often are done to confirm the diagnosis and exclude other causes of the disorder.

Treatment includes avoidance of movements that cause nerve compression, splinting, and anti-inflammatory medications. Measures to decrease the causative repetitive movements should be initiated. Splints may be confined to nighttime use. When splinting is ineffective, corticosteroids may be injected into the carpal tunnel to reduce inflammation and swelling. Surgical intervention consists of operative division of the volar carpal ligaments as a means of relieving pressure on the median nerve.

Polyneuropathies

Polyneuropathies involve demyelination or axonal degeneration of multiple peripheral nerves that leads to symmetric sensory, motor, or mixed sensorimotor deficits. Typically, the longest axons are involved first, with symptoms beginning in the distal part of the extremities. If the autonomic nervous system is involved, there may be postural hypotension, constipation, and impotence. Polyneuropathies can result from immune mechanisms (*e.g.,* Guillain-Barré syndrome), toxic agents (*e.g.,* arsenic polyneuropathy, lead polyneuropathy, alcoholic polyneuropathy), and metabolic diseases (*e.g.,* diabetes mellitus, uremia). Different causes tend to affect axons of different diameters and to affect sensory, motor, or autonomic neurons to different degrees.

Guillain-Barré Syndrome. Guillain-Barré syndrome is an acute immune-mediated polyneuropathy.[25–28] The syndrome defines a clinical entity that is characterized by rapidly progressive limb weakness and loss of tendon reflexes. It has been described as the most common cause of acute, flaccid paralysis in developed countries, now that poliomyelitis has been eliminated. As a syndrome, there are several subtypes of the disorder, including pure motor axonal degeneration, axonal degeneration of both motor and sensory nerves, and a variant characterized by ophthalmoplegia, ataxia, and areflexia.[27]

The disorder is manifested by infiltration of mononuclear cells around the capillaries of the peripheral neurons, edema of the endoneurial compartment, and demyelination of ventral spinal roots. The cause of the Guillain-Barré syndrome probably has an immune component. Controlled epidemiologic studies have linked it to infection with *Campylobacter jejuni* in addition to other viruses, including cytomegalovirus and Epstein-Barr virus.[29] Approximately two thirds of patients report having had an acute, influenza-like illness before the onset of symptoms. About one third have antibodies against nerve gangliosides, which in some cases also react with constituents of the lipopolysaccharide of *C. jejuni*.[29]

The disorder is characterized by progressive ascending muscle weakness of the limbs, producing a symmetric flaccid paralysis. Symptoms of paresthesia and numbness often accompany the loss of motor function. The rate of disease progression varies, and there may be disproportionate involvement of the upper or lower extremities. Paralysis may progress to involve the respiratory muscles; approximately 30% of persons with the disorder require ventilatory assistance.[25] Auto-

nomic nervous system involvement that causes postural hypotension, arrhythmias, facial flushing, abnormalities of sweating, and urinary retention is common. Pain is another common feature of Guillain-Barré syndrome. It is most common in the shoulder girdle, back, and posterior thighs and occurs with even the slightest of movements.[26]

Guillain-Barré syndrome usually is a medical emergency. There may be a rapid development of ventilatory failure and autonomic disturbances that threaten circulatory function. Treatment includes support of vital functions and prevention of complications such as skin breakdown and thrombophlebitis. Clinical trials have shown the effectiveness of plasmapheresis in decreasing morbidity and shortening the course of the disease. Treatment is most effective if initiated early in the course of the disease. High-dose intravenous immunoglobulin therapy also has proved effective.[25] Approximately 80% to 90% of persons with the disease achieve a full and spontaneous recovery within 6 to 12 months.[26]

Back Pain and Herniated Intervertebral Disk

Low back pain is a common problem that affects an estimated two thirds of people at least once in their lifetime.[30] It has been reported that back pain is second only to upper respiratory problems as a symptom-related reason for a visit to a health care professional.[30–32] It affects men and women equally, with onset most often between the ages of 30 and 50 years.[31] Risk factors include heavy lifting, twisting, bodily vibration, obesity, and poor conditioning, but low back pain is common even in persons without these risk factors. Although acute low back pain resolves within 3 to 6 weeks in most persons, recurrences are common.[33]

Back pain can result from a number of interrelated problems involving spinal structures, including facet joints, the vertebral periosteum, ligaments, paravertebral musculature and fascia, and spinal nerve roots. Perhaps the most common are musculoligamentous injuries and age-related degenerative changes in the intervertebral disks and facet joints.[31] Other causes include disk herniation (to be discussed) and spinal stenosis. Spinal stenosis is characterized by narrowing of the central canal, typically from hypertrophic degenerative changes.

The diagnostic measures used in the evaluation of back pain include history and physical examination, including a thorough neurologic examination. Other diagnostic methods include radiographs of the back and magnetic resonance imaging (MRI). MRI or radiography early in the course of low back pain is not credited with improving clinical outcomes.[34] The diagnostic challenge is to identify those persons who require further evaluation for more serious problems.

Treatment of back pain usually is conservative and consists of analgesic medications, muscle relaxants, and instruction in the correct mechanics for lifting and methods of protecting the back.[31,34] Pain relief is usually provided using nonsteroidal anti-inflammatory drugs. Muscle relaxants may be used on a short-term basis. Bed rest does not increase the speed of recovery, and sometimes delays recovery.[31]

Herniated Intervertebral Disk. The intervertebral disk is considered the most critical component of the load-bearing structures of the spinal column. The intervertebral disk consists of a soft, gelatinous center called the *nucleus pulposus,* which is encircled by a strong, ringlike collar of fibrocartilage called the *annulus fibrosus.*[35] The structural components of the disk make it capable of absorbing shock and changing shape while allowing movement. With dysfunction, the nucleus pulposus can be squeezed out of place and herniate through the annulus fibrosus, a condition referred to as a *herniated* or *slipped disk* (Fig. 50-10A, B).

The intervertebral disk can become dysfunctional because of trauma, the effects of aging, or degenerative disorders of the spine. Trauma results from activities such as lifting while in the flexed position, slipping, falling on the buttocks or back, or suppressing a sneeze. With aging, the gelatinous center of the disk dries out and loses much of its elasticity, causing it to fray and tear. Degenerative processes such as osteoarthritis or ankylosing spondylitis predispose to malalignment of the vertebral column.

The cervical and lumbar regions are the most flexible areas of the spine and are most often involved in disk herniations. Usually, herniation occurs at the lower levels of the lumbar spine, where the mass being supported and the bending of the vertebral column are greatest. Approximately 90% to 95% of lumbar herniations occur in the L4 or L5 to S1 regions. With herniations of the cervical spine, the most frequently involved levels are C6 to C7 and C5 to C6. Protrusion of the nucleus pulposus usually occurs posteriorly and toward the intervertebral foramen and its contained spinal nerve root, where the annulus fibrosus is relatively thin and poorly supported by either the posterior or anterior ligaments[33,35] (see Fig. 50-10A).

The level at which a herniated disk occurs is important (see Fig. 50-10C). When the injury occurs in the lumbar area, only the nerve fibers of the cauda equina are involved. Because these elongated dorsal and ventral roots contain endoneurial tubes of connective tissue, regeneration of the nerve fibers is likely. However, several weeks or months are required for full recovery to occur because of the distance to the innervated muscle or skin of the lower limbs.

The signs and symptoms of a herniated disk are localized to the area of the body innervated by the nerve roots and include both motor and sensory manifestations (Fig. 50-11). Pain is the first and most common symptom of a herniated disk. The nerve roots of L4, L5, S1, S2, and S3 give rise to a syndrome of back pain that spreads down the back of the leg and over the

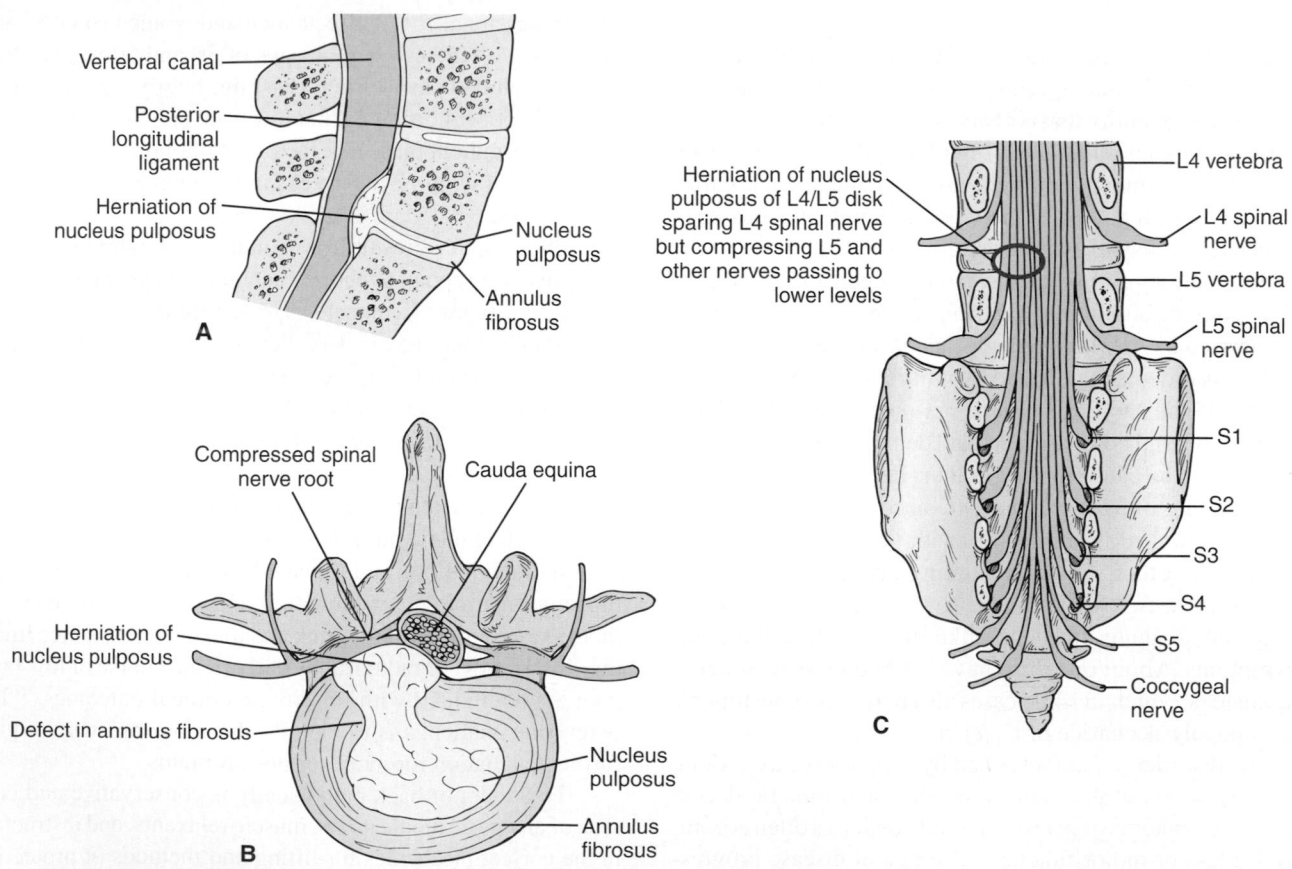

FIGURE 50-10 • Herniated intervertebral disk. **(A)** Longitudinal section. **(B)** Cross-section. **(C)** Location of L4–L5 and S1–S5 spinal nerves, with site of L4/L5 herniation of nucleus pulposus indicated. (Modified from Moore K. L. Dailey A. F. [1999]. *Clinically oriented anatomy* (4th ed., p. 452). Philadelphia: Lippincott Williams & Wilkins.)

include radiographs of the back, MRI, computed tomography (CT), and CT myelography.

Treatment usually is conservative and consists of analgesic medications and education on how to protect the back. Pain relief usually can be provided using nonsteroidal anti-inflammatory drugs, although short-term use of opioid pain medications may be required for severe pain. Muscle relaxants (*e.g.,* diazepam, cyclobenzaprine, carisoprodol, methocarbamol) may be used on a short-term basis. Conditioning exercises of the trunk muscles, particularly the back extensors, may be recommended. Surgical treatment may be indicated when there is documentation of herniation by an imaging procedure, consistent pain, or consistent neurologic deficit that has failed to respond to conservative therapy.

Back Pain Emergencies. Although acute back pain is usually a non–life-threatening condition, in 5% to 10% of persons it is a manifestation of a more serious pathologic process.[36] Vascular catastrophes (abdominal and dissecting aortic aneurysms), malignancy, spinal cord compression syndromes, and infectious processes may all present as acute back pain.

Clinical findings, commonly referred to as *red flags,* that indicate the possibility of more serious disease include gradual onset of pain; age younger than 20 years or older than 50 years; thoracic back pain; history of trauma, fever, chills, night sweats, immunosuppression, or malignancy; unintentional weight loss; recent procedure known to cause bacteremia; and history of intravenous drug use.[36] The gradual onset of pain may be indicative of malignancy or infection. Back pain that begins before 20 years of age suggests congenital or developmental disorders, and new-onset pain in persons 50 years of age or older is more likely to be a manifestation of serious conditions such as an aortic aneurysm, malignancy, or compression fracture. Pain that is aggravated by lying down is a red flag for malignancy or infection; and pain that improves with sitting or slight flexion of the spine suggests the presence of spinal stenosis. Reports of neurologic symptoms such as paresthesia, motor weakness, urinary or fecal incontinence, or gait abnormalities require additional diagnostic tests to rule out spinal cord compression.

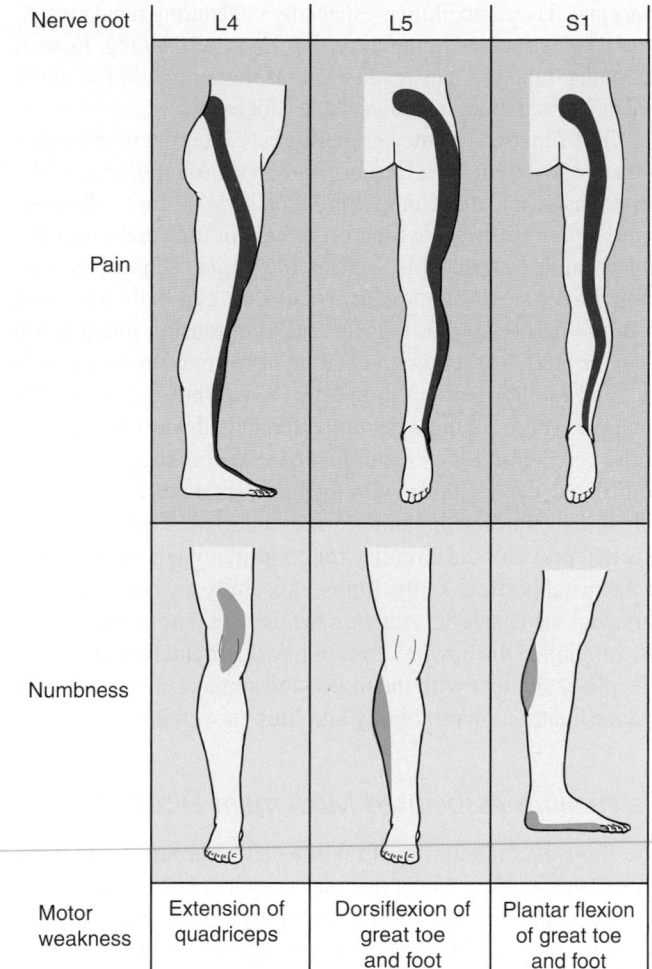

Nerve root	L4	L5	S1
Pain			
Numbness			
Motor weakness	Extension of quadriceps	Dorsiflexion of great toe and foot	Plantar flexion of great toe and foot

FIGURE 50-11 • Dermatomes of the leg (L1 through S5) where pain and numbness would be experienced with spinal root irritation.

sole of the foot. The pain is usually intensified with coughing, sneezing, straining, stooping, standing, and the jarring motions that occur during walking or riding. Slight motor weakness may occur, although major weakness is rare. The most common sensory deficits from spinal nerve root compression are paresthesias and numbness, particularly of the leg and foot. Knee and ankle reflexes also may be diminished or absent.

A herniated disk must be differentiated from other causes of acute back pain. Diagnostic measures include history and physical examination. Neurologic assessment includes testing of muscle strength and reflexes. The straight-leg test is an important diagnostic maneuver.[23,32] It is done in the supine position and is performed by passively raising the person's leg. The test can also be done by slowly extending the knee while the person sits on a table, with both hip and knee flexed at 90 degrees. The maneuver is designed to apply traction along the nerve root, which exacerbates pain if the nerve root is acutely inflamed. Normally, it is possible to raise the leg approximately 90 degrees without causing discomfort of the hamstring muscles. The test result is positive if pain is produced when the leg is raised to 60 degrees or less.[32] Other diagnostic methods

IN SUMMARY, the motor unit consists of the LMN, the neuromuscular junction, and the skeletal muscle that the nerve innervates. Disorders of the neuromuscular unit include muscular dystrophy and myasthenia gravis. *Muscular dystrophy* is a term used to describe a number of disorders that produce progressive deterioration of skeletal muscle due to necrosis followed by fibrofatty tissue replacement. One form, Duchenne muscular dystrophy, is inherited as an X-linked trait and transmitted by the mother to her male offspring. Myasthenia gravis is a disorder of the neuromuscular junction resulting from a deficiency of functional acetylcholine receptors, which causes weakness of the skeletal muscles. Because the disease affects the neuromuscular junction, there is no loss of sensory function. The most common manifestations are weakness of the eye muscles, with ptosis and diplopia.

Peripheral nerve disorders involve motor and sensory neurons outside the CNS. There are two main types of peripheral nerve injury based on target of the insult: segmental demyelination involving the Schwann cell, and axonal degeneration involving the nerve axon or cell body. Peripheral nerve disorders include mononeuropathies, involving a single spinal nerve, plexus, or peripheral nerve; and polyneuropathies that involve demyelination or axonal degeneration of multiple peripheral nerves that leads to symmetric sensory, motor, or mixed sensorimotor deficits. Carpal tunnel syndrome, a mononeuropathy, is caused by compression of the median nerve that passes through the carpal tunnel in the wrist. Guillain-Barré syndrome is a subacute polyneuropathy, probably due to immune mechanisms, that causes progressive ascending motor, sensory, and autonomic nervous system manifestations. Respiratory involvement may occur and necessitate mechanical ventilation.

Acute back pain is most commonly the result of conditions such as muscle strain; treatment focuses on measures to improve activity tolerance. A herniated intervertebral disk is characterized by protrusion of the nucleus pulposus into the spinal canal with irritation or compression of the nerve root. Usually, herniation occurs at the lower levels of the lumbar and sacral (L4 or L5 to S1) and cervical (C6 to C7 and C5 to C6) regions of the spine. The signs and symptoms of a herniated disk are localized to the area of the body innervated by the affected nerve roots and include pain and both motor and sensory manifestations. ■

DISORDERS OF THE CEREBELLUM AND BASAL GANGLIA

After completing this section of the chapter, you should be able to meet the following objectives:

- Relate the functions of the cerebellum to production of vestibulocerebellar ataxia, decomposition of movement, and cerebellar tremor.
- Describe the functional organization of the basal ganglia and communication pathways with the thalamus and cerebral cortex.
- State the possible mechanisms responsible for the development of Parkinson disease and characterize the manifestations and treatment of the disorder.

Disorders of the Cerebellum

The cerebellum is a cauliflower-shaped structure located in the posterior fossa and attached to the pons, medulla, and midbrain by the three paired cerebellar peduncles[3,37] (see Chapter 48). It has sometimes been referred to as the *silent area* of the brain because electrical stimulation does not produce any conscious sensation and rarely causes any motor movements.[3] However, removal or damage to the cerebellum causes movements to become highly abnormal. The cerebellum is especially vital during rapid muscular activities such as running, typing, and even talking. Loss of cerebellar function can result in total incoordination of these functions even though paralysis does not ensue.

The functions of the cerebellum are integrated into many connected afferent and efferent pathways throughout the brain. An extensive and important afferent pathway is the *corticopontocerebellar* pathway, which originates in the cerebral motor and premotor cortices as well as the somatosensory cortex. Other important afferent pathways link the cerebellum to input from the basal ganglia, muscle and joint tension information from the stretch receptors, visual input from the eyes, and balance and equilibrium sensation from the vestibular system in the inner ear. There are three general efferent pathways leading out of the cerebellum: the *vestibulocerebellar pathway* that functions in close association with the brain stem vestibular nuclei to maintain equilibrium and posture; the *spinocerebellar pathway* that provides the circuitry for coordinating the movements of the distal portions of the limbs, especially the hands and fingers; and the *cerebrocerebellar pathway* that transmits output information in the upward direction to the brain, functioning in a feedback manner with the motor and somatosensory systems to coordinate sequential body and limb movements.

Cerebellum-Associated Movement Disorders

The signs of cerebellar dysfunction can be grouped into three classes: vestibulocerebellar disorders, cerebellar ataxia or decomposition of movement, and cerebellar tremor. These disorders occur on the side of cerebellar damage, whether because of congenital defect, vascular accident, or growing tumor. Visual monitoring of movement cannot compensate for cerebellar defects, and the movement abnormalities occur whether the eyes are open or closed.

Damage to the part of the cerebellum associated with the vestibular system leads to difficulty or inability to maintain a steady posture of the trunk, which normally requires constant readjusting movements. This is seen as an unsteadiness of the trunk, called *truncal ataxia,* and can be so severe that standing is not possible. The ability to fix the eyes on a target also can be affected. Constant conjugate readjustment of eye position, called *nystagmus,* results and makes reading extremely difficult, especially when the eyes are deviated toward the side of cerebellar damage.

Cerebellar ataxia and tremor are different aspects of defects in the smooth, continuously correcting functions. Cerebellar dystaxia or, if severe, ataxia is characterized by a decomposition of movement, with each succeeding component of a complex movement occurring separately instead of being blended into a smoothly proceeding action. Because ethanol specifically affects cerebellar function, persons who are inebriated often walk with a staggering and unsteady gait. Rapid alternating movements such as supination—pronation—supination of the hands are jerky and performed slowly. Reaching to touch a target breaks down into small sequential components, each going too far, followed by overcorrection. The finger moves jerkily toward the target, misses, corrects in the other direction, and misses again, until the target is finally reached. This is called *over- and under-reaching* or *dysmetria*.

Cerebellar tremor is a rhythmic back-and-forth movement of a finger or toe that worsens as the target is approached. The tremor results from the inability of the damaged cerebellar system to maintain ongoing fixation of a body part and to make smooth, continuous corrections in the trajectory of the movement; overcorrection occurs, first in one direction and then the other. Often, the tremor of an arm or leg can be detected during the beginning of an intended movement. The common term for cerebellar tremor is *intention tremor*. Cerebellar function, as it relates to tremor, can be assessed by asking a person to touch one heel to the opposite knee, to gently move the toes along the back of the opposite shin, or to touch the nose with a finger.

Cerebellar function also can affect the motor skills of chewing and swallowing (dysphagia) and of speech (dysarthria). Normal speech requires smooth control of respiratory muscles and highly coordinated control of the laryngeal, lip, and tongue muscles. Cerebellar dysarthria is characterized by slow, slurred speech of continuously varying loudness. Rehabilitative efforts directed by speech therapists include learning to slow the rate of speech and to compensate as much as possible through the use of less-affected muscles.

Disorders of the Basal Ganglia

The basal ganglia are a group of deep, interrelated subcortical nuclei that play an essential role in control of movement. They function in the organization of inherited and highly learned and rather automatic movement programs, especially those affecting the trunk and proximal limbs. The basal ganglia are thought to be particularly important in starting, stopping, and monitoring movements ordered and executed by the cortex, especially those that are relatively slow and sustained, or stereotyped, such as arm-swinging during walking. They also help to regulate the intensity of these movements, and they act to inhibit antagonistic or unnecessary movements. The function of the basal ganglia is not limited to motor functions; they also are involved in cognitive and perceptual functions.

The structural components of the basal ganglia include the caudate nucleus, putamen, and the globus pallidus.[3,38] They are located lateral and caudal to the thalamus, occupying a large portion of the interior of both cerebral hemispheres. The caudate and putamen are collectively referred to as the *striatum*, and the putamen and the globus pallidus form a wedge-shaped region called the *lentiform nucleus*. Two other structures, the *substantia nigra* of the midbrain *and subthalamic nucleus* of the diencephalon, are considered part of the basal ganglia (Fig. 50-12). The dorsal part of the substantia nigra contains cells that use dopamine as a neurotransmitter and are rich in a black pigment called *melanin*. The high concentration of melanin gives the structure a black color, hence the name *substantia nigra*. The axons of the substantia nigra form the *nigrostriatal pathway,* which supplies dopamine to the striatum. The subthalamic nucleus lies just

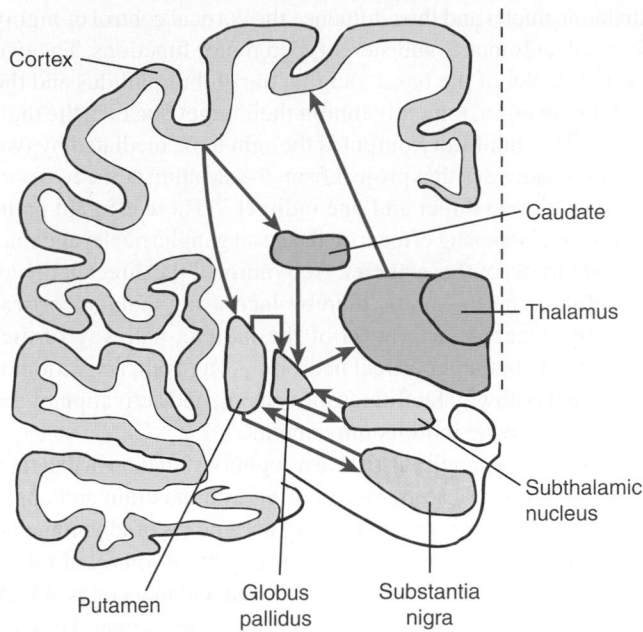

FIGURE 50-12 • Structures and basal neural circuitry of the basal ganglia.

below the thalamus and above the anterior portion of the substantia nigra. The glutaminergic cells of this nucleus are the only excitatory projections to the basal ganglia.

Associated with the basal ganglia are several thalamic nuclei. For the motor and premotor cortices, these nuclei are the ventral lateral (VL) and the ventral anterior (VA) nuclei. Each region of the cerebral cortex is interconnected with a corresponding region of the ventral row of thalamic nuclei. The cortex-to-thalamus and thalamus-to-cortex feedback circuitries are excitatory and, if unmodulated, would produce hyperactivity of the cortical area, causing stiffness and rigidity of the face, body, and limbs, and, if alternating, a continuous tremor (*i.e.,* tremor at rest). For many semiautomatic stereotyped movements, thalamic excitability is modulated through inhibition by the basal ganglia. The basal ganglia form a major component of an inhibitory loop from each specific cortical region. Discrete inhibitory cortex-to-basal ganglia and thalamus-to-cortex loops modulate the function of all cerebral cortex regions.

The basal ganglia have input structures that receive afferent information from outside structures, internal circuits that connect the various structures of the basal ganglia, and output structures that deliver information to other brain centers. The striatum represents the major input structure for the basal ganglia. Virtually all principal pathways for executing learned patterns of movement pass through the striatum. Other basal ganglia structures such as the substantia nigra and subthalamic nuclei are interconnected to one another or with the input and output nuclei, and are considered to be components of the internal structures.

The output functions of the basal ganglia are mainly inhibitory. Looping circuits from specific cortical centers pass through the basal ganglia to modulate the excitability of certain thalamic nuclei and thus influence the cortical control of highly learned, automatic, and stereotyped motor functions. The two output nuclei of the basal ganglia, the globus pallidus and the substantia nigra, tonically inhibit their target nuclei in the thalamus. This inhibitory output is thought to be mediated by two parallel pathways that project from the striatum to the two output nuclei: one direct and one indirect.[38] These efferent pathways have opposing effects on the basal ganglia nuclei and thus on the targets of these nuclei. Activation of the direct pathway disinhibits the thalamus, thereby increasing thalamocortical activity, whereas activation of the indirect pathway further inhibits the thalamocortical neurons. As a result, activation of the direct pathway facilitates movement, and activation of the indirect pathway inhibits movement.

The basal ganglia also have a cognitive function in that they monitor sensory information coming into the brain and apply it to information stored in memory as a means of planning and sequencing motor movements.[3] The cognitive control of motor activities determines, subconsciously and within seconds, which patterns of movement will be needed to achieve a goal. The caudate nucleus, which receives large amounts of input from the association areas of the brain, plays a major role in the cognitive control of motor activity.

Multiple pathways provide excitatory signals that balance the large number of inhibitory signals transmitted by GABA (γ-aminobutyric acid) ergic and dopaminergic neurons. One of these circuits involves a *neostriatal inhibitory projection* on the substantia nigra. The substantia nigra projects dopaminergic axons back on the striatum. A deficiency in the dopaminergic projection of this modulating circuit is implicated in parkinsonism. The function of the striatum also involves local cholinergic interneurons, and their destruction is thought to be related to the choreiform movements of Huntington disease, another basal ganglia—related syndrome (see Chapter 53).

Basal Ganglia–Associated Movement Disorders

Disorders of the basal ganglia comprise a complex group of motor disturbances characterized by tremor and other involuntary movements, changes in posture and muscle tone, and poverty and slowness of movement. They include tremors and tics, hypokinetic disorders, and hyperkinetic disorders[1] (Table 50-1).

Unlike disorders of the motor cortex and corticospinal (pyramidal) tract, lesions of the basal ganglia disrupt movement but do not cause paralysis. The various types of involuntary movements often occur in combination and appear to have a common underlying cause. Recent studies indicate that hypokinetic and hyperkinetic disorders can be explained as specific disturbances in the indirect and direct pathways that link the basal ganglia with the thalamocortical motor circuit.[38] Accordingly, overactivity of the indirect pathway relative

TABLE 50-1 **Characteristics of Basal Ganglia–Associated Movement Disorders**

MOVEMENT DISORDER	CHARACTERISTICS
Tremor	Involuntary, oscillating contractions of opposing muscle groups around a joint Usually fairly uniform in frequency and amplitude Can occur as resting tremors and postural tremors, which occur when the part is maintained in a stable position
Hypokinetic disorders	Slowness in initiating movement, and reduced range and force of the movement (bradykinesia)
Chorea	Irregular wriggling and writhing movements Accentuated by movement and by environmental stimulation; they often interfere with normal movement patterns May be grimacing movements of the face, raising the eyebrows, rolling of the eyes, and curling, protrusion, withdrawal of the tongue In the limbs, the movements largely are distal; there may be piano playing–type movements with alternating extension and flexion of the fingers
Athetosis	Continuous, wormlike, twisting and turning motions of the joints of a limb or the body
Ballismus	Violent, sweeping, flinging motions, especially of the limbs on one side of the body (hemiballismus)
Dystonia	Abnormal maintenance of a posture resulting from a twisting, turning movement of the limbs, neck, or trunk Often the result of simultaneous contraction of agonist and antagonist muscles Can result in grotesque and twisted postures
Dyskinesias	Bizarre wriggling and writhing movements Frequently involve the face, mouth, jaw, and tongue, causing grimacing, pursing of the lips, or protrusion of the tongue Limbs affected less often Tardive dyskinesia is an untoward reaction that can develop with long-term use of some antipsychotic medications

to the direct pathway would result in hypokinetic disorders such as Parkinson disease, and underactivity of the indirect pathway would result in hyperkinetic disorders such as chorea and ballismus.

Parkinson Disease

Parkinson disease is a degenerative disorder of basal ganglia function that results in variable combinations of tremor, rigidity, and bradykinesia. The disorder is characterized by progressive destruction of the nigrostriatal pathway, with subsequent reduction in striatal concentrations of dopamine. The prevalence of Parkinson disease in industrialized countries is estimated at 0.3% of the general population.[39–41] It usually begins after 50 years of age, with the prevalence increasing to 4% to 5% in those older than 85 years of age.[39]

The clinical syndrome arising from the degenerative changes in basal ganglia function often is referred to as *parkinsonism.* Parkinson disease, the most common form of parkinsonism, is named after James Parkinson, a British physician who first described the disease in a paper he published in 1817 on the "shaking palsy."[42] In Parkinson disease, also known as *idiopathic parkinsonism,* dopamine depletion results from degeneration of the dopamine nigrostriatal system. Parkinsonism can also develop as a postencephalitic syndrome, as a side effect of therapy with antipsychotic drugs that block dopamine receptors, as a toxic reaction to a chemical agent, or as an outcome of severe carbon monoxide poisoning. Postencephalitic parkinsonism was a particular problem in the 1930s and 1940s as a result of an outbreak of lethargic encephalitis (sleeping sickness) that occurred in 1914 to 1918.[43] Drug-induced parkinsonism can follow the administration of antipsychotic drugs in high doses (*e.g.,* phenothiazines, butyrophenones). These drugs block dopamine receptors and dopamine output by the cells of the substantia nigra. Symptoms of parkinsonism also may accompany conditions such as cerebral vascular disease, brain tumors, repeated head trauma, or degenerative neurologic diseases that structurally damage the nigrostriatal pathway.

The primary brain abnormality found in all persons with Parkinson disease is degeneration of the nigrostriatal dopamine neurons.[44,45] Other brain areas are affected to a lesser extent. On microscopic examination, there is loss of pigmented substantia nigra neurons. Some residual nerve cells are atrophic, and few contain *Lewy bodies,* which are visualized as spherical, eosinophilic cytoplasmic inclusions.

Although the cause of Parkinson disease is still unknown, it is widely believed that most cases are caused by an interaction of environmental and genetic factors. Over the past several decades, several pathologic processes (*e.g.,* oxidative stress, apoptosis, and mitochondrial disorders) that might lead to degeneration have been identified. Of interest in terms of research was the development of Parkinson disease in several persons who had attempted to make a narcotic drug and instead synthesized a compound called MPTP (1-methyl-phenyl-2,3,6-tetrahydropyridine).[43] This compound selectively destroys the dopaminergic neurons of the substantia nigra. This incident prompted investigations into the role of toxins that are produced by the body as a part of metabolic processes and those that enter the body from outside sources in the pathogenesis of Parkinson disease. One theory is that the autooxidation of catecholamines such as dopamine during melanin synthesis may injure neurons in the substantia nigra. There is increasing evidence that the development of Parkinson disease may be related to oxidative metabolites of this process and the inability of neurons to render these products harmless. MPTP is an inhibitor of the mitochondrial electron transport system that functions in the inactivation of these metabolites, suggesting that it may produce Parkinson disease in a manner similar to the naturally occurring disease.[43,45]

The recent discovery of inherited forms of Parkinson disease suggests that genetic factors play a role in the pathogenesis of early-onset Parkinson disease.[44–49] The first genetic mutation associated with Parkinson disease was found in the gene encoding α-*synuclein,* a member of a small family of proteins that are expressed preferentially in the substantia nigra.[44,45] Although mutations in this gene cause a very rare, autosomal dominant form of the disease, the mutation has received considerable attention because α-synuclein is one of the major components of the Lewy bodies that are found in brain tissue of persons with Parkinson disease.[44–46] Mutations in a second gene coding the protein *parkin* is associated with an autosomal recessive, early-onset form of Parkinson disease. The parkin protein acts as an enzyme (*i.e.,* ubiquitin ligase) in the ubiquitin-conjugating system that targets defective and abnormally folded proteins for destruction (see Chapter 5). Loss of normal parkin function is postulated to cause abnormal proteins to aggregate and cause neurodegenerative changes. Mutation in a third gene, coding for ubiquitin carboxyl-terminal hydrolase-L1 (UCH-L1), is thought to contribute to pathogenesis of Parkinson disease in a similar manner.[45] Numerous other genetic loci have been linked to Parkinson disease, but the genes remain to be mapped. Thus, the genetics of Parkinson disease are beginning to provide molecular clues that help explain the etiology of parkinsonism, just as epidemiologic studies have delineated an array of environmental modulators of susceptibility, which can now be explored in the context of gene expression.[46]

Clinical Manifestations. The cardinal manifestations of Parkinson disease are tremor, rigidity, and bradykinesia or slowness of movement.[39–41] Tremor is the most visible manifestation of the disorder. The tremor affects the distal segments of the limbs, mainly the hands and feet; head, neck, face, lips, and tongue; or jaw. It is characterized by rhythmic, alternating flexion and contraction movements (four to six beats per minute) that resemble the motion of rolling a pill between the thumb and forefinger. The tremor usually is unilateral, occurs when the limb is supported and at rest, and disappears with movement and sleep. The tremor eventually progresses to involve both sides of the body.

Rigidity is defined as resistance to movement of both flexors and extensors throughout the full range of motion. It is most evident during passive joint movement, and involves jerky, cogwheel-type or ratchet-like movements that require considerable energy to perform. Flexion contractions may develop as a result of the rigidity. As with tremor, rigidity usually begins unilaterally but progresses to involve both sides of the body.

Bradykinesia is characterized by slowness in initiating and performing movements and difficulty with sudden, unexpected stopping of voluntary movements. Unconscious associative movements occur in a series of disconnected steps rather than in a smooth, coordinated manner. This is the most disabling of the symptoms of Parkinson disease. Persons with the disease have difficulty initiating walking and difficulty turning. While walking, they may freeze in place and feel as if their feet are glued to the floor, especially when moving through a doorway or preparing to turn. When they walk, they lean forward to maintain their center of gravity and take small, shuffling steps without swinging their arms, and they have difficulty changing their stride (Fig. 50-13).

Manifestations of advanced-stage parkinsonism include falls, fluctuations in motor function, neuropsychiatric disorders, and sleep disorders. Loss of postural reflexes predisposes to falling, often backward. Emotional and voluntary facial movements become limited and slow as the disease progresses, and facial expression becomes stiff and masklike. There is loss of the blinking reflex and a failure to express emotion. The tongue, palate, and throat muscles become rigid; the person may drool because of difficulty in moving the saliva to the back of the mouth and swallowing it. The speech becomes slow and monotonous, without modulation, and poorly articulated.

Because the basal ganglia also influence the autonomic nervous system, persons with Parkinson disease often have excessive and uncontrolled sweating, sebaceous gland secretion, and salivation. Autonomic symptoms, such as lacrimation, dysphagia, orthostatic hypotension, thermal regulation, constipation, impotence, and urinary incontinence, may be present, especially late in the disease.

Cognitive dysfunction may also be an important feature associated with Parkinson disease. It occurs in approximately 20% of persons with the disease and develops late in the course of the disease.[50] Deficits in visuospatial discrimination, frontal lobe executive function, and memory retrieval (compared with formation of new memories, as seen in Alzheimer disease) are more typical of the cognitive dysfunction seen in persons with Parkinson disease than in other forms of dementia. Deficits in executive functioning may be among the earliest signs of cognitive decline, as evidenced by difficulty in planning, starting, and carrying out tasks. Dementia, when it does occur, is usually a late manifestation of the disease, and the rate of decline is slow compared with Alzheimer disease.

Treatment. The approach to treatment of Parkinson disease must be highly individualized. It includes nonpharmacologic, pharmacologic, and, when indicated, surgical methods.[39–41] Nonpharmacologic interventions offer group support, education, daily exercise, and adequate nutrition. Botulinum toxin injections may be used in the treatment of dystonias such as eyelid spasm and limb dystonias that frequently are associated with Parkinson disease. Persons with parkinsonism other than idiopathic Parkinson disease usually do not respond significantly to medications developed for Parkinson disease.

Pharmacologic treatment usually is determined by the severity of symptoms. Antiparkinson drugs act by increasing the functional ability of the underactive dopaminergic system, or by reducing the excessive influence of excitatory cholinergic neurons. Drugs that improve the function of the dopaminergic system include those that increase dopamine levels (levodopa), stimulate dopamine receptors (dopamine receptor agonists), or retard the breakdown of dopamine (monoamine oxidase inhibitors). Because dopamine transmission is disrupted in Parkinson disease, there is a preponderance of cholinergic activity, which may be treated with anticholinergic drugs.

Dopamine does not cross the blood-brain barrier. Administration of levodopa, a precursor of dopamine that does cross the blood-brain barrier, has yielded significant improvement in clinical symptoms of Parkinson disease and remains the most effective drug for treatment. The evidence of decreased

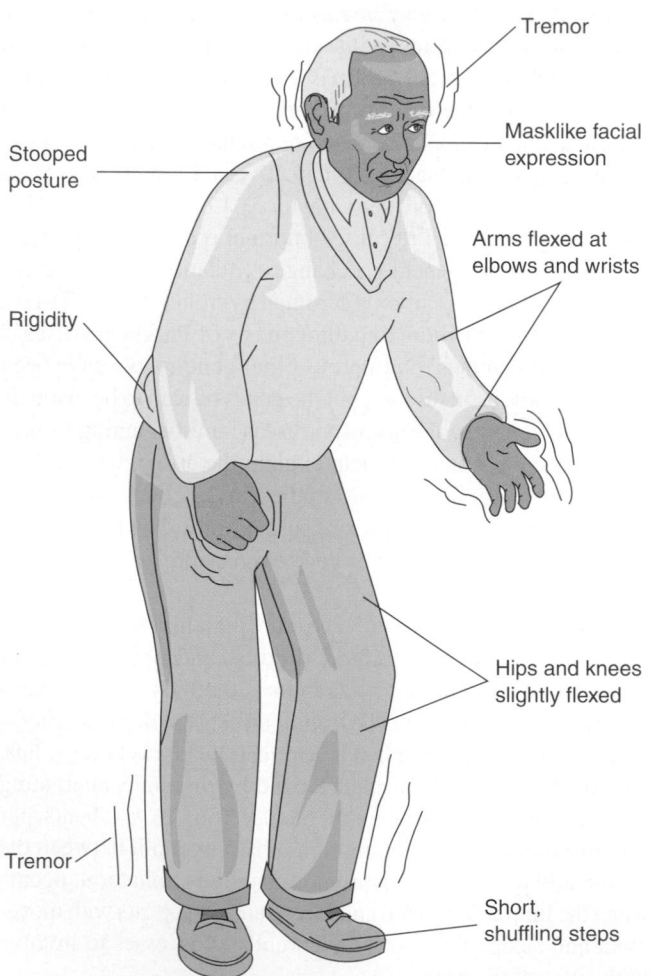

FIGURE 50-13 • The clinical features of Parkinson disease. (From Timby B. K., Smith N. E. [2003]. *Introductory medical–surgical nursing* [8th ed. p. 626]. Philadelphia: Lippincott Williams & Wilkins.)

Labels on figure: Tremor; Masklike facial expression; Arms flexed at elbows and wrists; Stooped posture; Rigidity; Hips and knees slightly flexed; Tremor; Short, shuffling steps

dopamine levels in the striatum in Parkinson disease led to the administration of large doses of the synthetic compound levodopa, which is absorbed from the intestinal tract, crosses the blood-brain barrier, and is converted to dopamine by centrally acting dopa decarboxylase. Unfortunately, only a small fraction of administered levodopa enters the brain unaltered; the remainder is metabolized outside the brain, predominantly by decarboxylation to dopamine, which cannot cross the blood-brain barrier.[15] However, when levodopa (a decarboxylase inhibitor) is given in combination with carbidopa, the peripheral metabolism of levodopa is reduced, plasma levels of levodopa are increased and its half-life is longer, more levodopa is available for entry into the brain, and a smaller dose is needed. A later adverse effect of levodopa treatment is the so-called *on–off phenomenon,* in which frequent, abrupt, and unpredictable fluctuations in motor performance occur during the day. These fluctuations include "on" periods without dyskinesia, "on" periods with dyskinesia, and periods of bradykinesia (the "off" response). Some fluctuations reflect the timing of drug administration, in which case the "on" response coincides with peak drug levels and the "off" response with low drug levels.

Bromocriptine, pramipexole, and ropinirole are dopamine agonists that act directly to stimulate dopamine receptors.[15] Rotigotine is a dopamine agonist that is supplied in a transdermal system. Apomorphine is another dopamine agonist that can be given intravenously. Bromocriptine, pramipexole, and ropinirole can be used as initial or adjunctive therapy in Parkinson disease. They can be given in combination with carbidopa/levodopa. Rotigotine is only approved by the U.S. Food and Drug Administration (FDA) for initial treatment of Parkinson disease, whereas apomorphine is used as a rescue medication in patients experiencing sudden "off" periods or delayed "on" periods.

Amantadine was introduced as an antiviral agent for prophylaxis of A_2 influenza and was unexpectedly found to cause symptomatic improvement in persons with Parkinson disease. Although the exact mechanism of action remains to be elucidated, it may augment release of dopamine from the remaining intact dopaminergic terminals in the nigrostriatal pathway of persons with Parkinson disease. It is used to treat persons with mild symptoms, but no disability.

Selegiline and rasagiline are monoamine oxidase type B inhibitors that inhibit the metabolic breakdown of dopamine. Selegiline and rasagiline may be used as adjunctive treatment to reduce mild on–off fluctuations in the responsiveness of persons who are receiving levodopa.

Anticholinergic drugs (*e.g.,* trihexyphenidyl, benztropine) are thought to restore a "balance" between reduced dopamine and uninhibited cholinergic neurons in the striatum. They are more useful in alleviating tremor and rigidity than bradykinesia. The anticholinergic drugs lessen the tremors and rigidity and afford some improvement of function. However, their potency seems to decrease over time, and increasing the dosage merely increases side effects such as blurred vision, dry mouth, bowel and bladder problems, cognitive dysfunction, and hallucinations.

Before the advent of deep brain stimulation, surgical treatment for Parkinson disease was limited to thalamotomy and pallidotomy performed using stereotactic surgery.[39–41] With these procedures, part of the thalamus or globus pallidus in the basal ganglia is destroyed using an electrical stimulator or supercooled tip of a metal probe (cryothalamotomy). Brain mapping is done during the surgery to identify and prevent injury to sensory and motor tracts. Thalamotomy and pallidotomy are generally confined to one side of the brain because of adverse effects associated with bilateral lesioning procedures. Surgical transplantation of adrenal medullary tissue or fetal substantia nigra tissue was studied in clinical trials, but neither was proven to be helpful.

Today, deep brain stimulation, which involves the implantation of electrodes into the subthalamic nuclei or the pars interna of the globus pallidus, is performed more frequently for treatment of Parkinson disease in the United States.[51] The electrodes are connected to a surgically implanted impulse generator that delivers electrical simulation to block the abnormal nerve activity that causes tremor and abnormal motor activity in Parkinson disease. The deep brain stimulation system allows the stimulation to be programmed to control the individual patient's symptoms, and the stimulation parameters can be changed over time as the disease progresses. Deep brain stimulation is used for persons with Parkinson disease who respond to levodopa but experience side effects associated with it (*e.g.,* motor fluctuation or dyskinesia). It is not a cure but serves to increase the duration of the "on" periods, allows for a reduction in medication dosages (in subthalamic nuclei stimulation), and improves function. Of note, other movement disorders can be treated by placing electrodes in different target sites (*e.g.,* thalamus for tremor and globus pallidus internus for dystonia).

IN SUMMARY, alterations in coordination of muscle movements and abnormal muscle movements result from disorders of the cerebellum and basal ganglia. The functions of the cerebellum, which are especially vital during rapid muscular movements, use afferent input from various sources, including the stretch receptors, proprioceptors, tactile receptors in the skin, visual input, and the vestibular system. Cerebellar disorders include vestibulocerebellar dysfunction, cerebellar ataxia, and cerebellar tremor.

The basal ganglia organize basic movement patterns into more complex patterns and release them when commanded by the motor cortex, contributing gracefulness to cortically initiated and controlled skilled movements. Disorders of the basal ganglia are characterized by involuntary movements, alterations in muscle tone, and disturbances in posture. These disorders include tremor, tics, hemiballismus, chorea, athetosis, dystonias, and dyskinesias.

Parkinsonism, a disorder of the basal ganglia, is characterized by destruction of the nigrostriatal pathway, with a subsequent reduction in striatal concentrations of dopamine. This results in an imbalance between the inhibitory effects of dopaminergic basal ganglia functions and an increase in the excitatory cholinergic functions. The disorder is manifested by resting tremor, increased muscle tonus and rigidity, slowness of movement (*i.e.*, bradykinesia), gait disturbances, and impaired autonomic postural responses. The disease usually is slowly progressive over several decades, but the rate of progression varies from 2 to 30 years. The tremor often begins in one or both hands and then becomes generalized. Postural changes and gait disturbances continue to become more pronounced, resulting in significant disability. ∎

UPPER MOTOR NEURON DISORDERS

After completing this section of the chapter, you should be able to meet the following objectives:

■ Relate the pathologic UMN and LMN changes that occur in amyotrophic lateral sclerosis to the manifestations of the disease.

■ Explain the significance of demyelination and plaque formation in multiple sclerosis.

■ Describe the manifestations of multiple sclerosis.

■ Relate the structures of the vertebral column to mechanisms of spinal cord injury.

■ Explain how loss of UMN function contributes to the muscle spasms that occur after recovery from spinal cord injury.

■ State the effects of spinal cord injury on ventilation and communication, the autonomic nervous system, cardiovascular function, sensorimotor function, and bowel, bladder, and sexual function.

Upper motor neuron disorders involve neurons that are fully contained within the CNS. They include the motor neurons arising in the motor areas of the cortex and their fibers as they project through the brain and descend in the spinal cord. Disorders that affect UMNs include multiple sclerosis and spinal cord injury. Stroke, which is a common cause of UMN damage, is discussed in Chapter 51. Amyotrophic lateral sclerosis is a mixed UMN and LMN disorder.

Amyotrophic Lateral Sclerosis

Amyotrophic lateral sclerosis (ALS), also known as *Lou Gehrig disease* after the famous New York Yankees baseball player, is a devastating neurologic disorder that selectively affects motor function. ALS has an annual incidence of 1 to 2 per 100,000 population.[44,52] ALS is primarily a disorder of middle to late adulthood, affecting persons between 55 and 60 years of age, with men developing the disease nearly twice as often as women. The disease typically follows a progressive course, with a mean survival period of 2 to 5 years from the onset of symptoms.

ALS affects motor neurons in three locations: the anterior horn cells (LMNs) of the spinal cord; the motor nuclei of the brain stem, particularly the hypoglossal nuclei; and the UMNs of the cerebral cortex.[44,45,52–55] The fact that the disease is more extensive in the distal parts of the affected tracts in the lower spinal cord rather than the proximal parts suggests that affected neurons first undergo degeneration at their distal terminals and that the disease proceeds in a centripetal direction until ultimately the parent nerve cell dies. A remarkable feature of the disease is that the entire sensory system, the regulatory mechanisms of control and coordination of movement, and the intellect remain intact. The neurons for ocular motility and the parasympathetic neurons in the sacral spinal cord also are spared.

The death of LMNs leads to denervation, with subsequent shrinkage of musculature and muscle fiber atrophy. It is this fiber atrophy, called *amyotrophy*, which appears in the name of the disease. The loss of nerve fibers in lateral columns of the white matter of the spinal cord, along with fibrillary gliosis, imparts a firmness or sclerosis to this CNS tissue; the term *lateral sclerosis* designates these changes.

The cause of LMN and UMN destruction in ALS is uncertain. Five percent to 10% of cases are familial; the others are believed to be sporadic, with no family history of the disease.[45] The gene for a subset of familial ALS has been mapped to superoxide dismutase 1 (*SOD1*) on chromosome 21. The mutation accounts for 20% of familial ALS, with the remaining 80% being caused by mutations in other genes.[53] Five percent of persons with sporadic ALS also have *SOD1* mutations. Possible targets of *SOD1*-induced toxicity include the neurofilament proteins, which function in the axonal transport of molecules necessary for the maintenance of axons[53] (see Chapter 48, Fig. 48-2). Other genetic loci for ALS have been mapped but not yet cloned. Another suggested mechanism of pathogenesis in ALS is exotoxic injury through activation of glutamate-gated ion channels, which are distinguished by their sensitivity to *N*-methyl-D-aspartic acid (see Chapter 51). The possibility of glutamate excitotoxicity in the pathogenesis of ALS was suggested by the finding of increased glutamine levels in the cerebrospinal fluid of patients with sporadic ALS.[53] Although autoimmunity has been suggested as a cause of ALS, the disease does not respond to the immunosuppressant agents that normally are used in treatment of autoimmune disorders.

The symptoms of ALS may be referable to UMN or LMN involvement. Manifestations of UMN lesions include weakness, spasticity or stiffness, and impaired fine motor control.[52–56] Dysphagia (difficulty swallowing), dysarthria (impaired articulation of speech), and dysphonia (difficulty making the sounds of speech) may result from brain stem LMN involvement or from dysfunction of UMNs descending to the brain stem. Manifestations of LMN destruction include fasciculations, weakness, muscle atrophy, and hyporeflexia. Muscle cramps involving the distal legs often are an early symptom. The most common clinical presentation is slowly progressive weakness and atrophy in distal muscles of one upper extremity. This is followed by regional spread of clinical weakness, reflecting involvement of neighboring areas of the spinal cord. Eventually, UMNs and LMNs involving multiple limbs and the head are affected. In the more advanced stages, muscles of the palate, pharynx, tongue, neck, and shoulders become involved, causing impairment of chewing, swallowing, and speech. Dysphagia with recurrent aspiration and weakness of the respiratory muscles produces the most significant acute complications of the disease. Death usually results from involvement of cranial nerves and respiratory musculature.

Currently, there is no cure for ALS. The treatment of persons with ALS, which requires management of medical problems, severe disability, and psychosocial problems, is best provided by a multidisciplinary team.[52–56] Measures to assist persons with the disorder to manage their symptoms (*e.g.,* weakness and muscle spasms, dysphagia, communication difficulty, excessive watery saliva, and emotional lability), nutritional status, and respiratory muscle weakness allow people with the disorder to survive longer than would otherwise have been the case. An antiglutamate drug, riluzole, is the only drug approved by the FDA and Health Canada for treatment of ALS.[52] The drug is designed to decrease glutamate accumulation and slow the progression of the disease.

Demyelinating Disorders of the Central Nervous System

Multiple Sclerosis

As with other demyelinating disorders, multiple sclerosis (MS) is characterized by inflammation and selective destruction of CNS myelin.[44,45,57–62] The peripheral nervous system is spared and there is usually no evidence of an associated systemic disease. MS is estimated to affect 1 to 2 million people worldwide.[62] The age of onset is typically between 20 and 40 years, with women being affected twice as frequently as men. In Western societies, MS is second only to trauma as a cause of

neurologic disability in early and young adulthood. As such, MS results in significant functional and often work-related disability in persons who are in the prime of their productivity.

Epidemiology and Genetics. Multiple sclerosis occurs more commonly in individuals of European ancestry and is uncommon in certain ethnic groups such as Inuits, Native Americans, and Africans. The highest known prevalence of MS occurs in the Orkney Islands, located north of Scotland, and similarly high rates are found throughout northern Europe, the northern United States, and Canada.[61] The prevalence is low in Japan, in other parts of Asia, in equatorial Africa, and in the Middle East. It has been observed that the disease is more common in northern latitudes, perhaps related to the selective migration of persons with a susceptible genetic background to these regions.

The risk for developing MS is 15-fold higher when the disease is present in a first-degree relative, and is even greater in monozygotic twins.[45] People with the human leukocyte antigen HLA-DR2 haplotype (see Chapter 17) are particularly susceptible. The molecular basis for the influence of this particular haplotype is unknown.

Pathogenesis. Multiple sclerosis is believed to be an immune-mediated disorder that occurs in genetically susceptible people. Although the target antigen has not been identified, the data suggest an immune response to a protein in the CNS.

The lesions of MS consist of hard, sharp-edged, demyelinated or sclerotic patches that are macroscopically visible throughout the white matter of the CNS[44,45,62–64] (Fig. 50-14). These lesions, which represent the end result of acute myelin breakdown, are called *plaques*. The lesions have a predilection for the optic nerves, periventricular white matter, brain stem, cerebellum, and spinal cord white matter. In an active plaque, there is evidence of ongoing myelin breakdown. The sequence of myelin breakdown is not well understood, although it is known that the lesions contain small amounts of myelin basic proteins

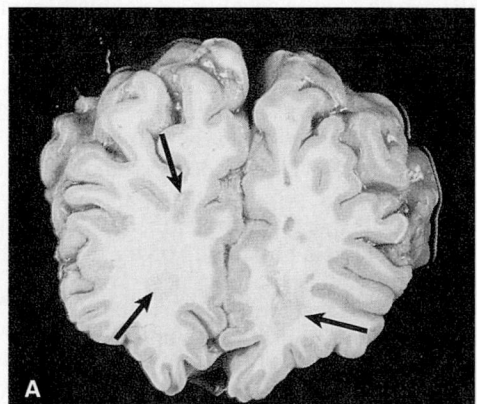
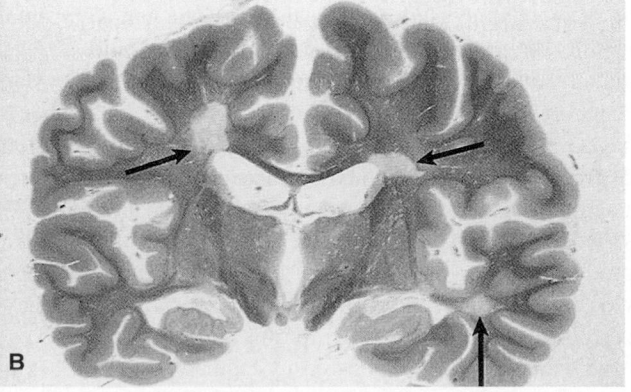

FIGURE 50-14 • Multiple sclerosis. **(A)** In this unfixed brain, the plaques of multiple sclerosis in the white matter (*arrows*) assume the darker color of the cerebral cortex. **(B)** A coronal section of the brain from a patient with long-standing multiple sclerosis, which has been stained for myelin, shows discrete areas of demyelination (*arrows*) with characteristic involvement of the superior angles of the lateral ventricles. (From Rubin E., Gorstein F., Rubin R., et al. [Eds.]. [2005]. *Rubin's pathology: Clinicopathologic foundations of medicine* [4th ed., p. 1464]. Philadelphia: Lippincott Williams & Wilkins.)

and increased amounts of proteolytic enzymes, macrophages, lymphocytes, and plasma cells. Oligodendrocytes are decreased in number and may be absent, especially in older lesions. Acute, subacute, and chronic lesions often are seen at multiple sites throughout the CNS.

MRI has shown that the lesions of MS may occur in two stages: a first stage that involves the sequential development of small inflammatory lesions, and a second stage during which the lesions extend and consolidate and when demyelination and gliosis (scar formation) occur. It is not known whether the inflammatory process, present during the first stage, is directed against myelin or against the oligodendrocytes that produce myelin. Remyelination of the nervous system was considered to be impossible until the late 1990s. Evidence now suggests that remyelination can occur in the CNS if the process that initiated the demyelination is halted before the oligodendrocyte dies.[65]

Manifestations and Clinical Course. The pathophysiology of MS involves the demyelination of nerve fibers in the white matter of the brain, spinal cord, and optic nerve. In the CNS, myelin is formed by the oligodendrocytes, chiefly those lying among the nerve fibers in the white matter. This function of the oligodendrocytes is equivalent to that of the Schwann cells in the peripheral nervous system (see Chapter 48). The properties of the myelin sheath—high electrical resistance and low capacitance—permit it to function as an electrical insulator. Demyelinated nerve fibers display a variety of conduction abnormalities, ranging from decreased conduction velocity to conduction blocks. The interruption of neural conduction in the demyelinated nerves is manifested by a variety of symptoms, depending on the location and extent of the lesion. Areas commonly affected by MS are the optic nerve (visual field), corticobulbar tracts (speech and swallowing), corticospinal tracts (muscle strength), cerebellar tracts (gait and coordination), spinocerebellar tracts (balance), medial longitudinal fasciculus (conjugate gaze function of the extraocular eye muscles), and posterior cell columns of the spinal cord (position and vibratory sensation). Typically, an otherwise healthy person presents with an acute or subacute episode of paresthesias, optic neuritis (*i.e.,* visual clouding or loss of vision in part of the visual field with pain on movement of the globe), diplopia, or specific types of gaze paralysis.

Paresthesias are evidenced as numbness, tingling, burning sensations, or pressure on the face or involved extremities, with symptoms ranging from annoying to severe. The *Lhermitte sign* is an electric shock–like tingling down the back and onto the legs that is produced by flexion of the neck. Pain from spasticity also may be a factor that can be alleviated by appropriate stretching exercises. Other common symptoms are abnormal gait, bladder and sexual dysfunction, vertigo, nystagmus, fatigue, and speech disturbance. These symptoms usually last for several days to weeks, and then completely or partially resolve. After a period of normal or relatively normal function, new symptoms appear. Psychological manifestations, such as mood swings, may represent an emotional reaction to the nature of the disease or, more likely, involvement of the white matter of the cerebral cortex. Depression, euphoria, inattentiveness, apathy, forgetfulness, and loss of memory may occur.

Fatigue is one of the most common problems for persons with MS. Fatigue often is described as a generalized low-energy feeling not related to depression and different from weakness. Fatigue has a harmful impact on activities of daily living and sustained physical activity. Interventions such as spacing activities and setting priorities often are helpful.

The course of the disease may fall into one of four categories: relapsing-remitting, secondary progressive, primary progressive, or progressive relapsing.[58–61] The *relapsing-remitting* form of the disease is characterized by episodes of acute worsening with recovery and a stable course between relapses. *Secondary progressive disease* involves a gradual neurologic deterioration with or without superimposed acute relapses in a person with previous relapsing-remitting disease. *Primary progressive disease* is characterized by nearly continuous neurologic deterioration from onset of symptoms. The *progressive relapsing* category of disease involves gradual neurologic deterioration from the onset of symptoms but with subsequent superimposed relapses.

Diagnosis. The diagnosis of MS is based on established clinical and, when necessary, laboratory criteria. Advances in cerebrospinal fluid analysis and MRI have greatly simplified the procedure. A definite diagnosis of MS requires evidence of one of the following patterns: two or more episodes of exacerbation separated by 1 month or more and lasting more than 24 hours, with subsequent recovery; a clinical history of clearly defined exacerbations and remissions, with or without complete recovery, followed by progression of symptoms over a period of at least 6 months; or slow and stepwise progression of signs and symptoms over a period of at least 6 months.[58–61] Primary progressive MS may be suggested by a progressive course that lasts longer than 6 months. A person who has not had a relapse or progression of symptoms is described as having stable MS.

MRI can be used as an adjunct to clinical diagnosis. MRI studies can detect lesions even when CT scans appear normal. A computer-assisted method of MRI can measure lesion size. Many new areas of myelin abnormality are asymptomatic. Serial MRI studies can be done to detect asymptomatic lesions, monitor the progress of existing lesions, and evaluate the effectiveness of treatment. Although MRI can be used to provide evidence of disseminated lesions in persons with the disease, normal findings do not exclude the diagnosis. Electrophysiologic evaluations (*e.g.,* evoked potential studies) and CT scans may assist in the identification and documentation of lesions.

Although no laboratory test can be used to diagnose MS, examination of the cerebrospinal fluid is helpful. A large percentage of patients with MS have elevated immunoglobulin G (IgG) levels, and some have oligoclonal patterns (*i.e.,* discrete electrophoretic bands) even with normal IgG levels. Total protein or lymphocyte levels may be mildly elevated in the cerebrospinal fluid. These test results can be altered in a variety of inflammatory neurologic disorders and are not specific for MS.

Treatment. Most treatment measures for MS are directed at modifying the course and managing the primary symptoms of the disease. The variability in symptoms, unpredictable course, and lack of specific diagnostic methods has made the evaluation and treatment of MS difficult. Persons who are minimally affected by the disorder require no specific treatment. The person should be encouraged to maintain as healthy a lifestyle as possible, including good nutrition and adequate rest and relaxation. Physical therapy may help maintain muscle tone. Every effort should be made to avoid excessive fatigue, physical deterioration, emotional stress, viral infections, and extremes of environmental temperature, which may precipitate an exacerbation of the disease.

The pharmacologic agents used in the treatment of MS fall into three categories: those used to (1) treat acute attacks or initial demyelinating episodes, (2) modify the course of the disease, and (3) treat symptoms of the disorder.[60–62] Corticosteroids are the mainstay of treatment for acute attacks of MS. These agents are thought to reduce the inflammation, improve nerve conduction, and have important immunologic effects. Long-term administration does not, however, appear to alter the course of the disease and can have harmful side effects. Adrenocorticotropic hormone (ACTH) also may be used in treatment of MS. Plasmapheresis has also proved beneficial in some cases.

The agents used to modify the course of the disease include interferon-beta, glatiramer acetate, and mitoxantrone.[65,66] These agents have shown some benefit in reducing exacerbations in persons with relapsing-remitting MS. Interferon-beta is a cytokine that acts as an immune enhancer. Two forms of recombinant interferon have been approved by the FDA for treatment of MS—interferon-beta-1a and interferon-beta-1b. Both types of interferon are administered by injection, and both are usually well tolerated. The most common side effects are flulike symptoms for 24 to 48 hours after each injection, and these usually subside after 2 to 3 months of treatment. Glatiramer acetate is a synthetic polypeptide that simulates parts of the myelin basic protein. Although the exact mechanism of action is unknown, the drug seems to block myelin-damaging T cells by acting as a myelin decoy. The drug is given daily by subcutaneous injection.

Mitoxantrone is an antineoplastic agent developed in the 1970s. It prevents the ligation of DNA strands and thus delays the cell-cycle progression. It also has immunomodulatory properties, inhibiting proliferation of macrophages and B and T lymphocytes.[67] Acute side effects of the drug include nausea and alopecia. Other immunomodulating agents such as azathioprine, methotrexate, and sirolimus have been suggested to delay progression of relapsing-remitting and secondary progressive MS.[67] Recently, natalizumab has also been approved for relapsing-remitting MS. Natalizumab is a monoclonal antibody against leukocyte $\alpha 4$ integrins, and its primary mechanism of action is suppression of leukocyte entry into the CNS.[67]

Among the medications used to manage the chronic problems associated with MS are dantrolene, baclofen, or diazepam for spasticity; cholinergic drugs for bladder problems; and antidepressant drugs for depression.

Vertebral and Spinal Cord Injury

Spinal cord injury (SCI) represents damage to the neural elements of the spinal cord. SCI is primarily a disorder of young people, with most injuries occurring in the 16- to 30-year age group.[68] The most common cause of SCI is motor vehicle accidents, followed by falls, violence (primarily gunshot wounds), and recreational sporting activities.[68] Life expectancy for persons with SCI continues to increase, but is somewhat below life expectancy for those without SCI. Mortality rates are significantly higher during the first year after injury than during subsequent years, particularly for severely injured persons.[68]

Most SCIs involve damage to the vertebral column or supporting ligaments as well as the spinal cord. Because of extensive tract systems that connect sensory afferent neurons and LMNs with high brain centers, SCIs commonly involve both sensory and motor function. Although the discussion in this section of the chapter focuses on traumatic SCI, much of the content is applicable to SCI caused by other disorders, such as congenital deformities (*e.g.,* spina bifida), tumors, ischemia and infarction, and bone disease with pathologic fractures of the vertebrae.

Injury to the Vertebral Column

Injuries to the vertebral column include fractures, dislocations, and subluxations. A fracture can occur at any part of the bony vertebrae, causing fragmentation of the bone. It most often involves the pedicle, lamina, or processes (*e.g.,* facets). Dislocation or subluxation (partial dislocation) injury causes the vertebral bodies to become displaced, with one overriding another and preventing correct alignment of the vertebral column. Damage to the ligaments or bony vertebrae may make the spine unstable. In an unstable spine, further unguarded movement of the spinal column can impinge on the spinal canal, causing compression or overstretching of neural tissue.

Most injuries result from some combination of compressive force or bending movements.[23] Flexion injuries occur when forward bending of the spinal column exceeds the limits of normal movement. Typical flexion injuries result, for example, when the head is struck from behind, as in a fall with the back of the head as the point of impact. Extension injuries occur with excessive forced bending (*i.e.,* hyperextension) of the spine backward. A typical extension injury involves a fall in which the chin or face is the point of impact, causing hyperextension of the neck. Injuries of flexion and extension occur more commonly in the cervical spine (C4 to C6) than in any other area. Limitations imposed by the ribs, spinous processes, and joint capsules in the thoracic and lumbar spine make this area less flexible and less susceptible to flexion and extension injuries than the cervical spine.

A compression injury, causing the vertebral bones to shatter, squash, or even burst, occurs when there is spinal loading from a high-velocity blow to the top of the head or when landing forcefully on the feet or buttocks[23] (Fig. 50-15A). This typically occurs at the cervical level (*e.g.,* diving injuries) or in the thoracolumbar area (*e.g.,* falling from a distance and landing on the buttocks). Compression injuries may occur when the vertebrae are weakened by conditions such as osteoporosis and cancer with bone metastasis. Axial rotation injuries can produce highly unstable injuries. Maximal axial rotation occurs in the cervical region, especially between C1 and C2, and at the lumbosacral joint[23] (see Fig. 50-15B). Coupling of vertebral motions is common in injury when two or more individual motions occur (*e.g.,* lateral bending and axial rotation).

Acute Spinal Cord Injury

Spinal cord injury involves damage to the neural elements of the spinal cord. The damage may result from direct trauma to the cord from penetrating wounds or indirect injury resulting from vertebral fractures, fracture-dislocations, or subluxations of the spine. The spinal cord may be contused, not only at the site of injury but above and below the trauma site[23] (Fig. 50-16). Traumatic injury may be complicated by the loss of blood flow to the cord, with resulting infarction.

Sudden, complete transection of the spinal cord results in complete loss of motor, sensory, reflex, and autonomic function below the level of injury. The immediate response to SCI is often referred to as *spinal cord shock.* It is characterized by flaccid paralysis with loss of tendon reflexes below the level of injury, absence of somatic and visceral sensations below the level of injury, and loss of bowel and bladder function. Loss of systemic sympathetic vasomotor tone may result in vasodilation, increased venous capacity, and hypotension. These

manifestations occur regardless of whether the level of the lesion eventually will produce spastic (UMN) or flaccid (LMN) paralysis. The basic mechanisms accounting for transient spinal shock are unknown. Spinal shock may last for hours, days, or weeks. Usually, if reflex function returns by the time the person reaches the hospital, the neuromuscular changes are reversible. This type of reversible spinal shock may occur in football-type injuries, in which jarring of the spinal cord produces a concussion-like syndrome with loss of movement and reflexes, followed by full recovery within days. In persons in whom the loss of reflexes persists, hypotension and bradycardia may become critical but manageable problems. In general, the higher the level of injury, the greater is the effect.

Pathophysiology. The pathophysiology of acute SCI can be divided into two types: primary and secondary.[69–74] The *primary neurologic injury* occurs at the time of mechanical injury and is irreversible. It is characterized by small hemorrhages in the gray matter of the cord, followed by edematous changes in the white matter that lead to necrosis of neural tissue. This type of injury results from the forces of compression, stretch, and shear associated with fracture or compression of the spinal vertebrae, dislocation of vertebrae (*e.g.,* flexion, extension, subluxation), and contusions due to jarring of the cord in the spinal canal. Penetrating injuries produce lacerations and direct trauma to the cord and may occur with or without spinal column damage. Lacerations occur when there is cutting or tearing of the spinal cord, which injures nerve tissue and causes bleeding and edema.

Secondary injuries follow the primary injury and promote the spread of injury. Although there is considerable debate about the pathogenesis of secondary injuries, the tissue destruction that occurs ends in progressive neurologic damage. After

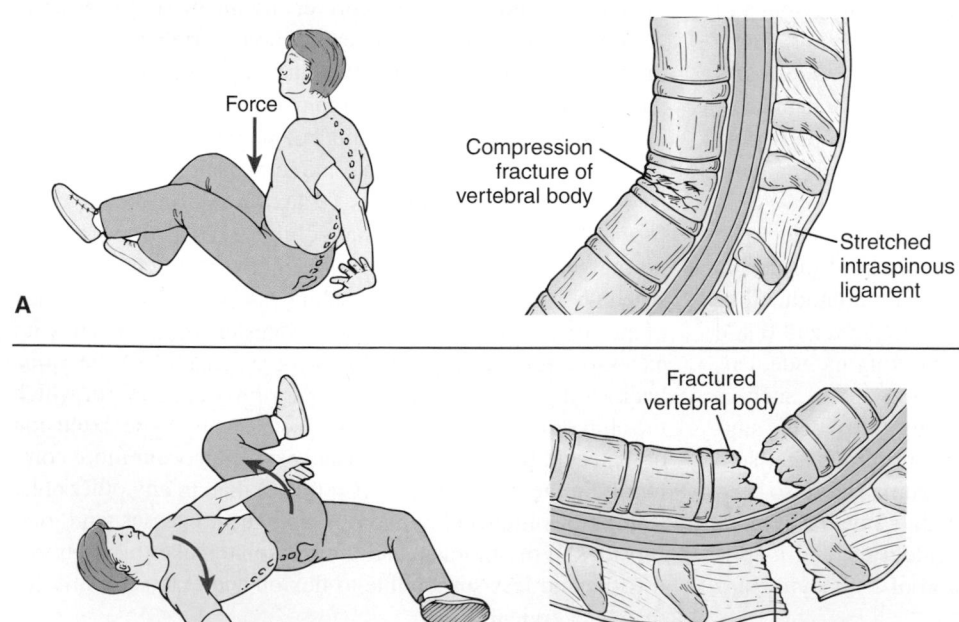

FIGURE 50-15 • **(A)** Compression vertebral fracture secondary to axial loading as occurs when a person falls from a height and lands on the buttocks. **(B)** Rotational injury, in which there is concurrent fracture and tearing of the posterior ligamentous complex, is caused by extreme lateral flexion or twisting of the head or neck. (Modified from Hickey J. V. [2003]. *The clinical practice of neurological and neurosurgical nursing.* [5th ed., pp. 411–412]. Philadelphia: Lippincott Williams & Wilkins.)

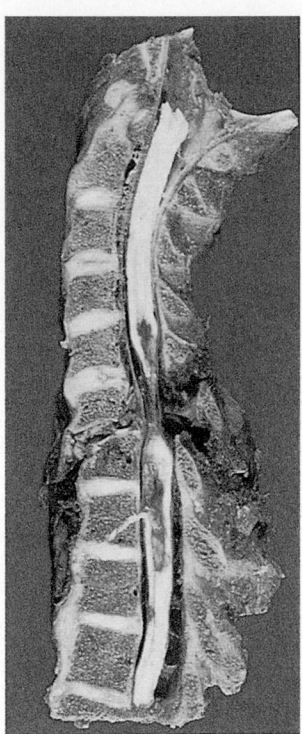

FIGURE 50-16 • Cervical contusion. Hyperflexion injury caused forward angulation of the cervical cord, with fracture of the anterior lip of the underlying vertebral body. The cord is angulated over the superior-posterior ridge of the fixed underlying cervical body. (From Rubin E., Farber J. L. [1999]. *Pathology* [3rd ed., p. 1465]. Philadelphia: Lippincott-Raven.)

SCI, several pathologic mechanisms come into play, including vascular damage, neuronal injury that leads to loss of reflexes below the level of injury, and release of vasoactive agents and cellular enzymes. Vascular lesions (*i.e.,* vessel trauma and hemorrhage) can lead to ischemia, increased vascular permeability, and edema. Blood flow to the spinal cord may be further compromised by spinal shock that results from a loss of vasomotor tone and neural reflexes below the level of injury. The release of vasoactive substances (*i.e.,* norepinephrine, serotonin, dopamine, and histamine) from the wound tissue causes vasospasm and impedes blood flow in the microcirculation, producing further necrosis of blood vessels and neurons. The release of proteolytic and lipolytic enzymes from injured cells causes delayed swelling, demyelination, and necrosis in the neural tissue in the spinal cord.

Management. The goal of management of acute SCI is to reduce the neurologic deficit and prevent any additional loss of neurologic function. The specific steps in resuscitation and initial evaluation can be carried out at the trauma site or in the emergency department, depending on the urgency of the situation.[23,75] Most traumatic injuries to the spinal column render it unstable, mandating measures such as immobilization with collars and backboards and limiting the movement of persons at risk for or with known SCI. Every person with multiple trauma or head injury, including victims of traffic and sporting accidents, should be suspected of having sustained an acute SCI. [23,75]

The nature of the injury determines further methods of stabilization and treatment. In unstable injuries of the cervical spine, cervical traction improves or restores spinal alignment, decompresses neural structures, and facilitates recovery. Fractures and dislocations of the thoracic and lumbar vertebrae may be initially stabilized by restricting the person to bed rest and turning him or her in a log-rolling manner to keep the spine rigid. Gunshot or stab wounds of the spinal column may not produce structural instability and may not require immobilization.

The goal of early surgical intervention for an unstable spine is to provide internal skeletal stabilization so that early mobilization and rehabilitation can occur. One of the more important aspects of early SCI care is the prevention and treatment of spinal or systemic shock and the hypoxia associated with compromised respiration. Correcting hypotension or hypoxia is essential to maintaining circulation to the injured cord.[75,76]

Early treatment with high-dose methylprednisolone is often used with the intent of improving neurologic recovery, based on recommendations from the Third National Acute Spinal Cord Injury Randomized Controlled Trial.[77] Methylprednisolone is a short-acting corticosteroid that has been used extensively in the treatment of inflammatory and allergic disorders. In acute SCI, it is thought to stabilize cell membranes, enhance impulse generation, improve blood flow, and inhibit free radical formation. However, methylprednisolone treatment remains controversial in many countries. Treatment with high-dose methylprednisolone is associated with complications such as increased frequency of gastric bleeding, wound infection, venous thrombosis, and steroid myopathy.[78,79] Other neuroprotective agents, including monosialoganglioside sodium (GM-1 ganglioside), naloxone, and tirilazad, have been tested in multicenter clinical trials, but primary end points have not been achieved.[79]

Types and Classification of Spinal Cord Injury

Alterations in body function that result from SCI depend on the level of injury and the amount of cord involvement. *Tetraplegia,* sometimes referred to as *quadriplegia,* is the impairment or loss of motor or sensory function (or both) after damage to neural structures in the cervical segments of the spinal cord.[23,80] It results in impairment of function in the arms, trunk, legs, and pelvic organs (see Fig. 50-5). *Paraplegia* refers to impairment or loss of motor or sensory function (or both) in the thoracic, lumbar, or sacral segments of the spinal cord from damage of neural elements in the spinal canal. With paraplegia, arm functioning is spared, but depending on the level of injury, functioning of the trunk, legs, and pelvic organs may be impaired. Paraplegia includes conus medullaris and cauda equina injuries (discussed later).

Further definitions of SCI describe the extent of neurologic damage as *complete* or *incomplete*[80] (Chart 50-1). Complete cord injuries can result from severance of the cord, disruption of nerve fibers although they remain intact, or interruption of

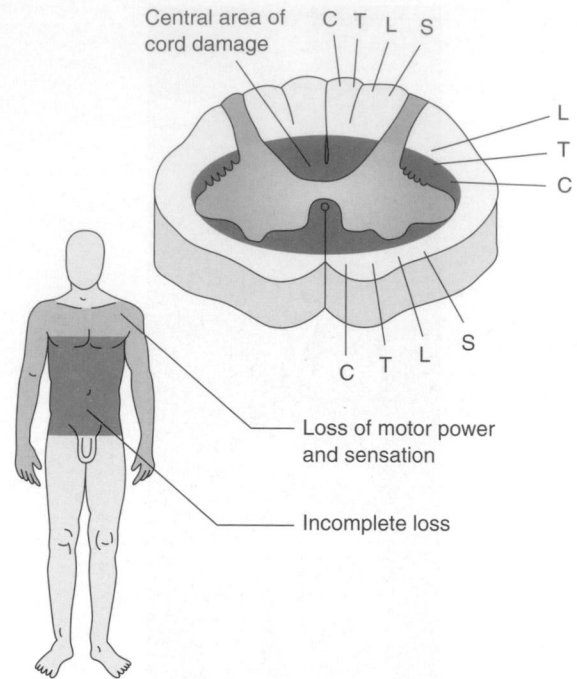

Central area of cord damage

C T L S

L
T
C

C T L S

Loss of motor power and sensation

Incomplete loss

FIGURE 50-17 • Central cord syndrome. A cross-section of the cord shows central damage and the associated motor and sensory loss. C, cervical; T, thoracic; L, lumbar; S, sacral. (From Kitt S., Kaiser J. [1990]. *Emergency nursing: A physiological and clinical perspective.* Philadelphia: W. B. Saunders.)

blood supply to that segment, resulting in complete destruction of neural tissue and UMN or LMN paralysis. With complete injuries, no motor or sensory function is preserved in sacral segments S4 to S6. Incomplete SCI implies there is some residual motor or sensory function below the level of injury. The prognosis for return of function is better in an incomplete injury because of preservation of axonal function. Incomplete injuries may manifest in a variety of patterns, but can be organized into certain patterns or "syndromes" that occur more frequently and reflect the predominant area of the cord that is involved. Types of incomplete lesions include the central cord syndrome, anterior cord syndrome, Brown-Séquard syndrome, and conus medullaris syndrome.

Central Cord Syndrome. A condition called *central cord syndrome* occurs when injury is predominantly in the central gray or white matter of the cord [23] (Fig. 50-17). Because the corticospinal tract fibers are organized with those controlling the arms located more centrally and those controlling the legs located more laterally, some external axonal transmission may remain intact. Motor function of the upper extremities is affected, but the lower extremities may not be affected or may be affected to a lesser degree, with some sparing of sacral sensation. Bowel, bladder, and sexual functions usually are affected to various degrees, and this may parallel the degree of lower extremity involvement. This syndrome occurs almost

exclusively in the cervical cord, rendering the lesion a UMN lesion with spastic paralysis. Central cord damage is more frequent in elderly persons with narrowing or stenotic changes in the spinal canal that are related to arthritis. Damage also may occur in persons with congenital stenosis.

Anterior Cord Syndrome. Anterior cord syndrome usually is caused by damage from infarction of the anterior spinal artery, resulting in damage to the anterior two thirds of the cord [23] (Fig. 50-18). The deficits include loss of motor function provided by the corticospinal tracts and loss of pain and temperature sensation from damage to the lateral spinothalamic tracts. The posterior one third of the cord is relatively unaffected, preserving the dorsal column axons that convey position, vibration, and touch sensation.

Brown-Séquard Syndrome. A condition called *Brown-Séquard syndrome* results from damage to a hemisection of the anterior and posterior cord [23] (Fig. 50-19). The effect is a loss of voluntary motor function from the corticospinal tract, proprioception loss from the ipsilateral side of the body, and contralateral loss of pain and temperature sensation from the lateral spinothalamic tracts for all levels below the lesion.

Conus Medullaris Syndrome. The conus medullaris syndrome involves damage to the conus medullaris or the sacral cord (*i.e.,* conus) and lumbar nerve roots in the neural canal. Func-

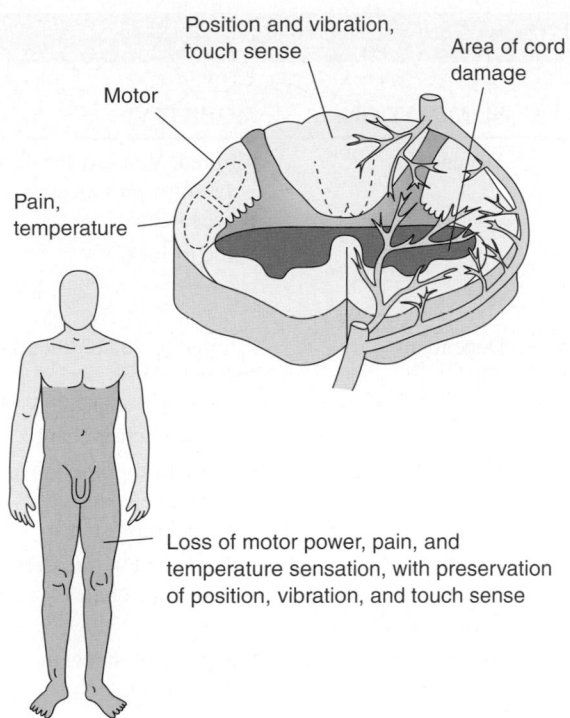

FIGURE 50-18 • Anterior cord syndrome. Cord damage and associated motor and sensory loss are illustrated. (From Kitt S., Kaiser J. [1990]. *Emergency nursing: A physiological and clinical perspective.* Philadelphia: W. B. Saunders.)

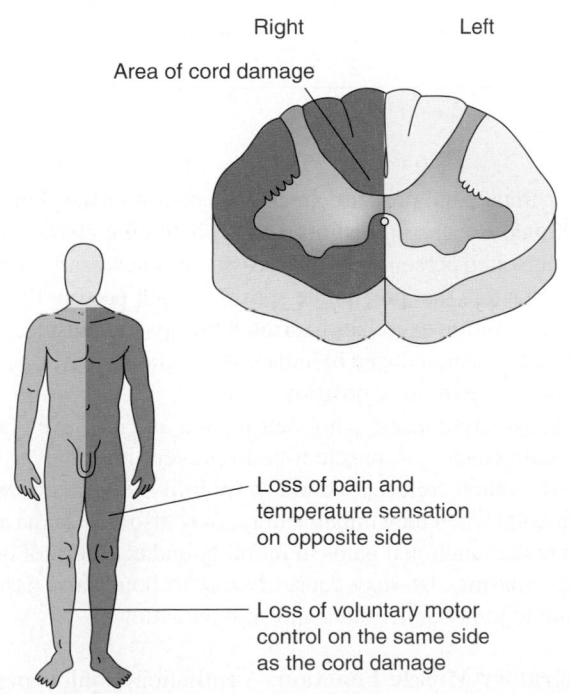

FIGURE 50-19 • Brown-Séquard syndrome. Cord damage and associated motor and sensory loss are illustrated. (From Kitt S., Kaiser J. [1990]. *Emergency nursing: A physiological and clinical perspective.* Philadelphia: W. B. Saunders.)

tional deficits resulting from this type of injury usually result in flaccid bowel and bladder and altered sexual function. Sacral segments occasionally show preserved reflexes if only the conus is affected. Motor function in the legs and feet may be impaired without significant sensory impairment. Damage to the lumbosacral nerve roots in the spinal canal usually results in LMN and sensory neuron damage known as *cauda equina syndrome.* Functional deficits present as various patterns of asymmetric flaccid paralysis, sensory impairment, and pain.

Disruption of Somatosensory and Skeletal Muscle Function

Functional abilities after SCI are subject to various degrees of somatosensory and skeletal muscle function loss and altered reflex activity based on the level of cord injury and extent of cord damage (Table 50-2).

Motor and Somatosensory Function. Motor function in cervical injuries ranges from complete dependence to independence with or without assistive devices in activities of mobility and self-care. The functional levels of cervical injury are related to C5, C6, C7, or C8 innervation. At the C5 level, deltoid and biceps function is spared, allowing full head, neck, and diaphragm control with good shoulder strength and full elbow flexion. At the C6 level, wrist dorsiflexion by the wrist extensors is functional, allowing tenodesis, which is the natural bending inward and flexion of the fingers when the wrist is extended and bent backward. Tenodesis is a key movement because it can be used to pick up objects when finger movement is absent. A functional C7 injury allows full elbow flexion and extension, wrist plantar flexion, and some finger control. At the C8 level, finger flexion is added.

Thoracic cord injuries (T1 to T12) allow full upper extremity control with limited to full control of intercostal and trunk muscles and balance. Injury at the T1 level allows full fine motor control of the fingers. Because of the lack of specific functional indicators at the thoracic levels, the level of injury usually is determined by sensory level testing.

Functional capacity in the L1 through L5 nerve innervations allows hip flexion, hip abduction (L1 to L3), movement of the knees (L2 to L5), and ankle dorsiflexion (L4 to L5). Sacral (S1 to S5) innervation allows for full leg, foot, and ankle control and innervation of perineal musculature for bowel, bladder, and sexual function.

Reflex Activity. Spinal cord reflexes are fully integrated in the spinal cord and can function independent of input from higher centers. Altered spinal reflex activity after SCI is essentially determined by the level of injury and whether UMNs or LMNs are affected. With UMN injuries at T12 and above, the cord reflexes remain intact, whereas communication pathways with higher centers have been interrupted. This results in spasticity of involved skeletal muscle groups and of smooth and skeletal muscles that control bowel, bladder, and sexual function. In LMN injuries at T12 or below, the reflex circuitry itself has been damaged at the level of the spinal cord or spinal nerve, resulting

TABLE 50-2 Functional Abilities by Level of Cord Injury

INJURY LEVEL	SEGMENTAL SENSORIMOTOR FUNCTION	DRESSING, EATING	ELIMINATION	MOBILITY*
C1	Little or no sensation or control of head and neck; no diaphragm control; requires continuous ventilation	Dependent	Dependent	Limited. Voice-controlled or sip-n-puff electric wheelchair
C2–C3	Head and neck sensation; some neck control. Independent of mechanical ventilation for short periods	Dependent	Dependent	Same as for C1
C4	Good head and neck sensation and motor control; some shoulder elevation; diaphragm movement	Dependent; may be able to eat with adaptive sling	Dependent	Limited to voice-, mouth-, head-, chin-, or shoulder-controlled electric wheelchair
C5	Full head and neck control; shoulder strength; elbow flexion	Independent with assistance	Maximal assistance	Electric or modified manual wheelchair, needs transfer assistance
C6	Fully innervated shoulder; wrist extension or dorsiflexion	Independent or with minimal assistance	Independent or with minimal assistance	Independent in transfers and wheelchair
C7–C8	Full elbow extension; wrist plantar flexion; some finger control	Independent	Independent	Independent; manual wheelchair
T1–T5	Full hand and finger control; use of intercostal and thoracic muscles	Independent	Independent	Independent; manual wheelchair
T6–T10	Abdominal muscle control, partial to good balance with trunk muscles	Independent	Independent	Independent; manual wheelchair
T11–L5	Hip flexors, hip abductors (L1–3); knee extension (L2–4); knee flexion and ankle dorsiflexion (L4–5)	Independent	Independent	Short distance to full ambulation with assistance
S1–S5	Full leg, foot, and ankle control; innervation of perineal muscles for bowel, bladder, and sexual function (S2–4)	Independent	Normal to impaired bowel and bladder function	Ambulate independently with or without assistance

*Assistance refers to adaptive equipment, setup, or physical assistance.

in a decrease or absence of reflex function. The LMN injuries cause flaccid paralysis of involved skeletal muscle groups and the smooth and skeletal muscles that control bowel, bladder, and sexual function. However, injuries near the T12 level may result in mixed UMN and LMN deficits (*e.g.*, spastic paralysis of the bowel and bladder with flaccid muscle tone).

After the period of spinal shock in a UMN injury, isolated spinal reflex activity and muscle tone that is not under the control of higher centers return. This may result in hypertonia and spasticity of skeletal muscles below the level of injury.[23] These spastic movements are involuntary instead of voluntary, a distinction that needs to be explained to persons with SCI and their families. The antigravity muscles, the flexors of the arms and extensors of the legs, are predominantly affected. Spastic movements are usually heightened initially after injury, reaching a peak and then becoming stable in approximately 1.5 to 2 years.[23]

The stimuli for reflex muscle spasm arise from somatic and visceral afferent pathways that enter the cord below the level of injury. The most common of these stimuli are muscle stretching, bladder infections or stones, fistulas, bowel disten-

tion or impaction, pressure areas or irritation of the skin, and infections. Because the stimuli that precipitate spasms vary from person to person, careful assessment is necessary to identify the factors that precipitate spasm in each person. Passive range-of-motion exercises to stretch the spastic muscles help to prevent spasm induced by muscle stretching, such as occurs with a change in body position.

Spasticity in itself is not detrimental and may even facilitate maintenance of muscle tone to prevent muscle wasting, improve venous return, and aid in mobility. Spasms become detrimental when they impair safety; they also reduce the ability to make functional gains in mobility and activities of daily living. Spasms also may cause trauma to bones and tissues, leading to joint contractures and skin breakdown.

Respiratory Muscle Function. Ventilation requires movement of the expiratory and inspiratory muscles, all of which receive innervation from the spinal cord.[81] The main muscle of ventilation, the diaphragm, is innervated by segments C3 to C5 through the phrenic nerves. The intercostal muscles, which function in elevating the rib cage and are needed for coughing and deep breathing, are innervated by spinal segments T1 through T7. The major muscles of expiration are the abdominal muscles, which receive their innervation from levels T6 to T12.

Although the ability to inhale and exhale may be preserved at various levels of SCI, functional deficits in ventilation are most apparent in the quality of the breathing cycle and the ability to oxygenate tissues, eliminate carbon dioxide, and mobilize secretions. Cord injuries involving C1 to C3 result in a lack of respiratory effort, and affected patients require assisted ventilation. Although a C3 to C5 injury allows partial or full diaphragmatic function, ventilation is diminished because of the loss of intercostal muscle function, resulting in shallow breaths and a weak cough. Below the C5 level, as less intercostal and abdominal musculature is affected, the ability to take a deep breath and cough is less impaired. Maintenance therapy consists of muscle training to strengthen existing muscles for endurance and mobilization of secretions. The ability to speak is compromised with assisted ventilation, whether continuous or intermittent. Thus, ensuring adequate communication of needs is also essential.

Disruption of Autonomic Nervous System Function

In addition to its effects on skeletal muscle function, SCI interrupts autonomic nervous system function below the site of injury.[82] This includes sympathetic outflow from the thoracic and lumbar cord and parasympathetic outflow from the sacral cord. Because of their sites of exit from the CNS, the cranial nerves, such as the vagus, are unaffected. Depending on the level of injury, the spinal reflexes that control autonomic nervous system function are largely isolated from the rest of the CNS. Afferent sensory input that enters the spinal cord is unaffected, as is the efferent motor output from the cord. Lacking are the regulation and integration of reflex function by centers in the brain and brain stem. This results in a situation in which the autonomic reflexes below the level of injury are uncontrolled, whereas those above the level of injury function in a relatively controlled manner.

Sympathetic nervous system regulation of circulatory function and body temperature (*i.e.*, thermoregulation) presents some of the most severe problems in SCI. The higher the level of injury and the greater the surface area affected, the more profound are the effects on circulation and thermoregulation. Persons with injury at the T6 level or above experience problems in regulating vasomotor tone; those with injuries below the T6 level usually have sufficient sympathetic function to maintain adequate vasomotor function. The level of injury and its corresponding problems may vary among persons, and some dysfunctional effects may be seen at levels below T6. With lower lumbar and sacral injuries, sympathetic function remains essentially unaltered.

Vasovagal Response.   The vagus nerve (cranial nerve X), which is unaffected in SCI, normally exerts a continuous inhibitory effect on heart rate. Vagal stimulation that causes a marked bradycardia is called the *vasovagal response*. Visceral afferent input to the vagal centers in the brain stem of persons with tetraplegia or high-level paraplegia can produce marked bradycardia when unchecked by a dysfunctional sympathetic nervous system. Severe bradycardia and even asystole can result when the vasovagal response is elicited by deep endotracheal suctioning or rapid position change. Preventive measures, such as hyperoxygenation before, during, and after suctioning, are advised. Rapid position changes should be avoided or anticipated, and anticholinergic drugs should be immediately available to counteract severe episodes of bradycardia.

Autonomic Dysreflexia.   Autonomic dysreflexia, also known as *autonomic hyperreflexia*, represents an acute episode of exaggerated sympathetic reflex responses that occur in persons with injuries at T6 and above, in which CNS control of spinal reflexes is lost (Fig. 50-20). It does not occur until spinal shock has resolved and autonomic reflexes return, most often within the first 6 months after injury. It is most unpredictable during the first year after injury, but can occur throughout the person's lifetime.

Autonomic dysreflexia is characterized by vasospasm, hypertension ranging from mild (20 mm Hg above baseline) to severe (as high as 240/120 mm Hg, or higher), skin pallor, and gooseflesh associated with the piloerector response.[83] Because baroreceptor function and parasympathetic control of heart rate travel by way of the cranial nerves, these responses remain intact. Continued hypertension produces a baroreflex-mediated vagal slowing of the heart rate to bradycardic levels. There is an accompanying baroreflex-mediated vasodilation, with flushed skin and profuse sweating above the level of injury, headache ranging from dull to severe and pounding, nasal stuffiness, and feelings of anxiety. A person may experience one, several, or all of the symptoms with each episode.

The stimuli initiating the dysreflexic response include visceral distention, such as a full bladder or rectum; stimulation of pain receptors, as occurs with pressure ulcers, ingrown toenails, dressing changes, and diagnostic or operative procedures; and visceral contractions, such as ejaculation, bladder spasms, or uterine contractions. In many cases, the dysreflexic response results from a full bladder.

Autonomic dysreflexia is a clinical emergency, and without prompt and adequate treatment, convulsions, loss of consciousness, and even death can occur. The major components of treatment include monitoring blood pressure while removing or correcting the initiating cause or stimulus. The person should be placed in an upright position, and all support hose or binders should be removed to promote venous pooling of blood and reduce venous return, thereby decreasing blood pressure. If the stimuli have been removed or the stimuli cannot be identified and the upright position is established, but the blood pressure remains elevated, drugs that block autonomic function are administered. Prevention of the type of stimuli that trigger the dysreflexic event is advocated.

Postural Hypotension.   Postural, or orthostatic, hypotension usually occurs in persons with injuries at T4 to T6 and above and

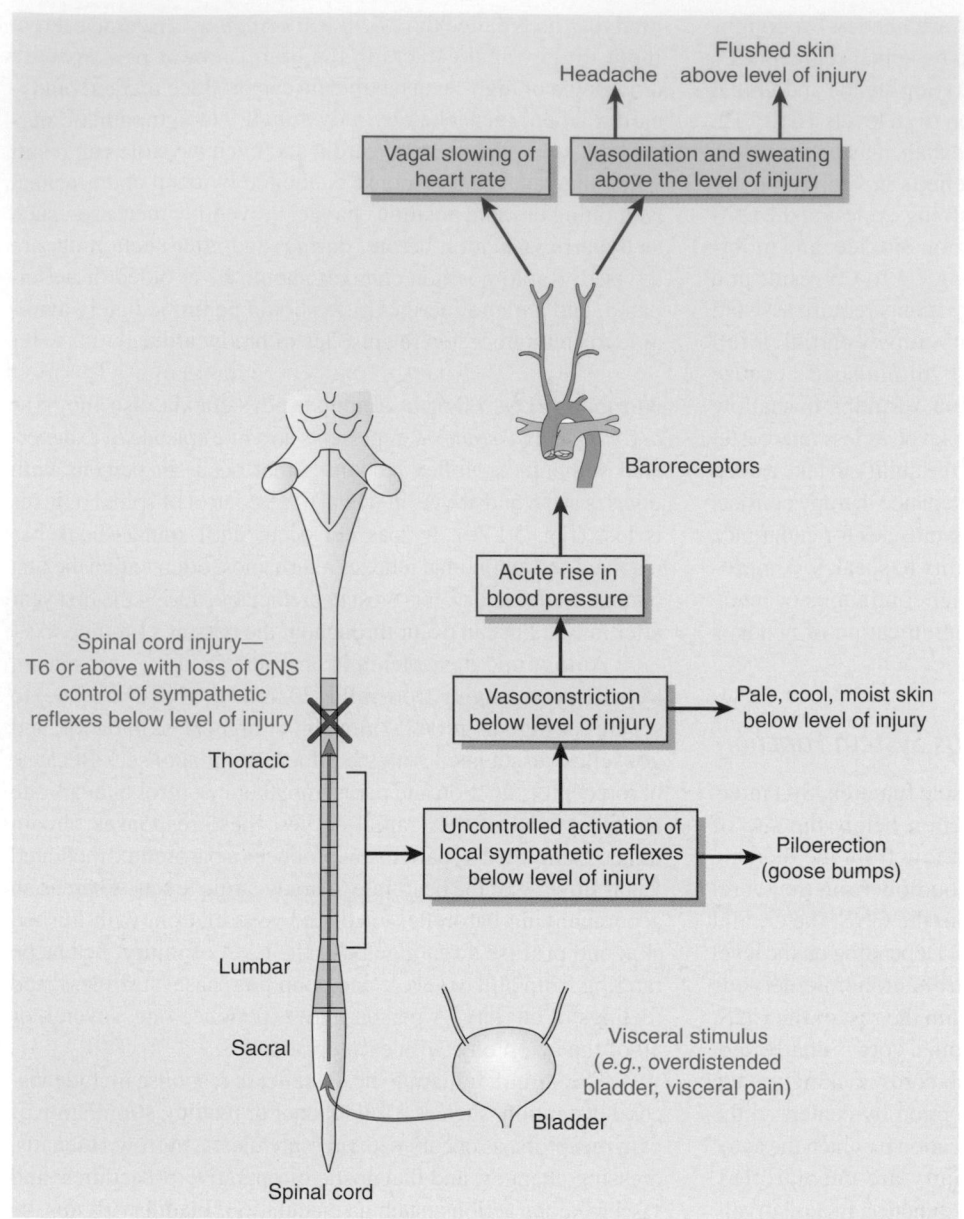

Headache

Flushed skin
above level of injury

Vagal slowing of
heart rate

Vasodilation and sweating
above the level of injury

Baroreceptors

Acute rise in
blood pressure

Spinal cord injury—
T6 or above with loss of CNS
control of sympathetic
reflexes below level of injury

Vasoconstriction
below level of injury

Pale, cool, moist skin
below level of injury

Thoracic

Uncontrolled activation of
local sympathetic reflexes
below level of injury

Piloerection
(goose bumps)

Lumbar

Sacral

Visceral stimulus
(*e.g.,* overdistended
bladder, visceral pain)

Bladder

Spinal cord

FIGURE 50-20 • Mechanisms of autonomic dysreflexia.

is related to the interruption of descending control of sympathetic outflow to blood vessels in the extremities and abdomen.[82] Pooling of blood, along with gravitational forces, impairs venous return to the heart, and there is a subsequent decrease in cardiac output when the person is placed in an upright position. The signs of orthostatic hypotension include dizziness, pallor, excessive sweating above the level of the lesion, complaints of blurred vision, and possibly fainting. Postural hypotension usually is prevented by slow changes in position and measures to promote venous return.

Disruption of Bladder, Bowel, and Sexual Function

Among the most devastating consequences of SCI is the loss of bowel, bladder, and sexual function.[63,84] Loss of bladder function results from disruption of neural pathways between the bladder and the reflex voiding center at the S2 to S4 level (*i.e.,* an LMN lesion) or between the reflex voiding center and higher brain centers for communication and coordinated sphincter control (*i.e.,* a UMN lesion). Persons with UMN lesions or spastic bladders lack awareness of bladder filling (*i.e.,* storage) and voluntary control of voiding (*i.e.,* evacuation). In LMN lesions or flaccid bladder dysfunction, lack of awareness of bladder filling and lack of bladder tone render the person unable to void voluntarily or involuntarily (see Chapter 35).

Bowel elimination is a coordinated function involving the enteric nervous system, the autonomic nervous system, and the CNS. Persons with SCI above S2 to S4 develop spastic functioning of the defecation reflex and loss of voluntary control of the external anal sphincter. Damage to the cord at the S2 to S4 level causes flaccid functioning of the defecation reflex and loss of anal sphincter tone. Even though the enteric nervous system innervation of the bowel remains intact, without the defecation reflex, peristaltic movements are ineffective in evacuating stool.

Sexual function, like bladder and bowel control, is mediated by the S2 to S4 segments of the spinal cord. The genital sexual response in SCI, which is manifested by an erection in men and vaginal lubrication in women, may be initiated by mental or touch stimuli, depending on the level of injury. The T11 to L2 cord segments have been identified as the mental-stimulus, or psychogenic, sexual response area, where autonomic nerve pathways in communication with the forebrain leave the cord and innervate the genitalia. The S2 to S4 cord segments have been identified as the sexual-touch reflex center. In T10 or higher injuries, reflex sexual response to genital touch may occur freely. However, a sexual response to mental stimuli (T11 to L2) does not occur because of the spinal lesion blocking the communication pathway. In an injury at T12 or below, the sexual reflex center may be damaged, and there may be no response to touch.

In men, the lack of erectile ability or inability to experience penile sensations or orgasm is not a reliable indicator of fertility, which should be evaluated by an expert. In women, fertility is parallel to menses; usually, it is delayed 3 months to 5 months after injury. There are hazards to pregnancy, labor, and use of birth control devices relative to SCI that require the input of knowledgeable health care providers.

Disruption of Other Functions

Temperature Regulation. The central mechanisms for thermoregulation are located in the hypothalamus (see Chapter 10). In response to cold, the hypothalamus stimulates vasoconstrictor responses in peripheral blood vessels, particularly those of the skin. This results in decreased loss of body heat. Heat production results from increased metabolism, voluntary activity, or shivering. To reduce heat, hypothalamus-stimulated mechanisms produce vasodilation of skin blood vessels to dissipate heat, and sweating to increase evaporative heat losses.

After SCI, the communication between the thermoregulatory centers in the hypothalamus and the sympathetic effector responses below the level of injury is disrupted; the ability to control blood vessel responses that conserve or dissipate heat is lost, as are the abilities to sweat and shiver. Higher levels of injury tend to produce greater disturbances in thermoregulation. In tetraplegia and high paraplegia, there are few defenses against changes in the environmental temperature, and body temperature tends to assume the temperature of the external environment, a condition known as *poikilothermy*. Persons with lower-level injuries have various degrees of thermoregulation. Disturbances in thermoregulation are chronic and may cause continual loss of body heat. Treatment consists of education in the adjustment of clothing and awareness of how environmental temperatures affect the person's ability to accommodate to these changes.

Deep Vein Thrombosis and Edema. Persons with SCI are at high risk for development of deep vein thrombosis (DVT) and

pulmonary embolism, particularly during the first 2 to 3 weeks after injury.[85] Fatal pulmonary embolism has been reported in 1% to 2% of all persons with SCI within the first 3 months of injury.[23] The high risk for DVT in patients with acute SCI is due to immobility, decreased vasomotor tone below the level of injury, and hypercoagulability and stasis of blood flow. Prevention strategies include the use of low–molecular-weight heparin, thigh-high graduated compression stockings, sequential compression boots, and early mobilization.[23,85] Electrical stimulation applied to the lower limbs has been reported to provide some benefit by achieving muscular contraction and improving venous flow. Local pain, a common symptom of DVT, is often absent because of sensory deficits. Thus, a regular schedule of visual inspection for local signs of DVT (*e.g.*, swelling) is important. Testing of persons at high risk for DVT includes plethysmography and duplex ultrasonography.

Edema is also a common problem in persons with SCI. The development of edema is related to decreased peripheral vascular resistance, decreased muscle tone in the paralyzed limbs, and immobility that causes increased venous pressure and abnormal pooling of blood in the abdomen, lower limbs, and upper extremities. Edema in the dependent body parts usually is relieved by positioning to minimize gravitational forces or by using compression devices (*e.g.*, support stockings, binders) that encourage venous return.

Skin Integrity. The entire surface of the skin is innervated by cranial or spinal nerves organized into dermatomes that show cutaneous distribution. The CNS and autonomic nervous system also play a vital role in skin function. The sympathetic nervous system, through control of vasomotor and sweat gland activity, influences the health of the skin by providing adequate circulation, excretion of body fluids, and temperature regulation. The lack of sensory warning mechanisms and voluntary motor ability below the level of injury, coupled with circulatory changes, place the spinal cord–injured person at major risk for disruption of skin integrity (see Chapter 61). Significant factors associated with disruption of skin integrity are pressure, shearing forces, and localized trauma and irritation. Relieving pressure, allowing adequate circulation to the skin, and skin inspection are primary ways of maintaining skin integrity. Of all the complications after SCI, skin breakdown is the most preventable.

Future Directions in Repair of the Injured Spinal Cord

There is a continued effort to determine new and innovative strategies for repairing the injured spinal cord.[86,87] At present, these strategies focus on promoting the regrowth of interrupted nerve fiber tracts, using nerve growth–stimulating factors or molecules that suppress inhibitors of neuronal extension; bridging spinal cord lesions with scaffolds that are impregnated with nerve growth factors, which promote axon growth and reduce the barriers caused by scar tissue; repairing damaged myelin and restoring nerve fiber conductivity in the lesion area; and enhancing CNS plasticity by promoting compensatory growth of spared, intact nerve fibers above and below the level of injury. Although these strategies may not allow for complete repair of the spinal cord so as to recreate what was present before the injury, even small successes may be useful for someone with SCI. For a person with an injury in the cervical region, "a return of function over even one spinal segment would improve the quality of life, while return to function over three or four segments would transform it."[87]

IN SUMMARY, UMN lesions are those involving neurons completely contained in the CNS. Amyotrophic lateral sclerosis is a progressive and devastating neurologic disorder that selectively affects motor function. It affects LMNs in the spinal cord as well as UMNs in the brain stem and cerebral cortex. Multiple sclerosis is a slowly progressive demyelinating disease of the CNS. The most common symptoms are paresthesias, optic neuritis, and motor weakness. The disease is usually characterized by exacerbations and remissions. Initially, near-normal function returns between exacerbations.

Spinal cord injury is a disabling neurologic condition most commonly caused by motor vehicle accidents, falls, and sports injuries. Dysfunctions of the nervous system after SCI comprise various degrees of sensorimotor loss and altered reflex activity based on the level of injury and extent of cord damage. Depending on the level of injury, the physical problems of SCI include spinal shock; ventilation and communication problems; autonomic nervous system dysfunction that predisposes to the vasovagal response, autonomic hyperreflexia, impaired body temperature regulation, and postural hypotension; impaired muscle pump and venous innervation leading to edema of dependent areas of the body and risk for deep vein thrombosis; altered sensorimotor integrity that contributes to uncontrolled muscle spasms, altered pain responses, and threats to skin integrity; alterations in bowel and bladder elimination; and impaired sexual function. ■

Review Exercises

1. A 32-year-old woman presents with complaints of drooping eyelids, difficulty chewing and swallowing, and weakness of her arms and legs that is less severe in the morning but becomes worse as the day progresses. She complains that climbing stairs and lifting objects are becoming increasingly difficult. Clinical examination confirms weakness of the eyelid and jaw muscles. She is told that she may have myasthenia gravis and is scheduled for a test using the short-acting acetylcholinesterase inhibitor edrophonium (Tensilon).

   A. *Explain the pathogenesis of this woman's symptoms as it relates to myasthenia gravis.*

   B. *Explain how information from the administration of the acetylcholinesterase inhibitor edrophonium can be used to assist in the diagnosis of the disorder.*

   C. *Explain the rationale for avoiding the use the aminoglycoside antibiotics for treatment of infections in this woman.*

2. A 16-year-old boy has approached you for assistance in preparing a poster for the science fair at his high school. He is interested in baseball and wants to focus his presentation on the neurophysiology of the pitching and catching of a baseball.

   A. *How would you go about helping him to outline the role of the cerebellum and basal ganglia in performing the motor movements associated with these maneuvers?*

3. A 20-year-old man suffered a spinal cord injury at the C2 to C3 level as the result of a motorcycle accident.

   A. *Explain the effects of this man's injury on ventilation and communication; sensorimotor function; autonomic nervous system function; bowel, bladder, and sexual function; and temperature regulation.*

   B. *Autonomic dysreflexia, which is a threat to persons with spinal cord injury at T6 or above, is manifested by hypertension, often to extreme levels, and bradycardia; constriction of skin vessels below the level of injury; and severe headache and nasal stuffiness. Explain the origin of the elevated blood pressure and bradycardia. The condition does not occur until after shock has resolved, and usually occurs only in persons with injuries at T6 and above. Explain.*

References

1. Jones G. M. (2000). Posture. In Kandel E. R., Schwartz J. H., Jessell T. M. (Eds.), *Principles of neural science* (4th ed., pp. 816–831). New York: McGraw-Hill.
2. Chez C., Krakauer J. (2000). The organization of movement. In Kandel E. R., Schwartz J. H., Jessell T. M. (Eds.), *Principles of neural science* (4th ed., pp. 653–672). New York: McGraw-Hill.
3. Guyton A., Hall J. E. (2006). *Medical physiology* (11th ed., pp. 673–684, 685–692, 698–713). Philadelphia: Elsevier Saunders.
4. Conn M. P. (1995). *Neuroscience in medicine* (pp. 312–317). Philadelphia: J. B. Lippincott.
5. Penfield W., Rasmussen T. (1950). *The cerebral cortex of man.* New York: Macmillan.
6. Rowland L. P. (2000). Diseases of the motor unit. In Kandel E. R., Schwartz J. H., Jessell T. M. (Eds.), *Principles of neural science* (4th ed., pp. 695–710). New York: McGraw-Hill.
7. Pearson K., Gordon J. (2000). Spinal reflexes. In Kandel E. R., Schwartz J. H., Jessell T. M. (Eds.), *Principles of neural science* (4th ed., pp. 713–735). New York: McGraw-Hill.
8. Noback C. R., Demarest R. J. (1981). *The human nervous system* (3rd ed., p. 197). New York: McGraw-Hill.

9. Bickley L. S., Szilagyi P. G. (2003). *Bates' guide to physical examination and history taking* (8th ed., pp. 571–592). Philadelphia: Lippincott Williams & Wilkins.

10. Anthony D. P., Frosch M. P. (2005). Peripheral nerve and skeletal muscle. In Kumar V., Abbas A. K., Fausto N. (Eds.), *Robbins and Cotran pathologic basis of disease* (7th ed., pp. 1335–1338). Philadelphia: Elsevier Saunders.

11. Kenyon L. C., Curtis M. T. (2008). Skeletal muscle. In Rubin R., Strayer D. S. (Eds.), *Rubin's Pathology: Clinicopathologic foundations of medicine* (5th ed., pp. 1153–1170). Philadelphia: Lippincott Williams & Wilkins.

12. Deconinck N., Dan B. (2007). Pathophysiology of Duchenne muscular dystrophy: Current hypothesis. *Pediatric Neurology* 36, 1–7.

13. Sarnat H. B. (2004). Muscular dystrophies. In Behrman R. E., Kliegman R. M., Jenson H. B. (Eds.), *Nelson textbook of pediatrics* (17th ed., pp. 1873–1877). Philadelphia: Elsevier Saunders.

14. Meiss R. A. (2003). Skeletal muscle and smooth muscle. In Rhoads R. A., Tanner G. A. (Eds.), *Medical physiology* (2nd ed., pp. 152–176). Philadelphia: Lippincott Williams & Wilkins.

15. Katzung B. G. (2007). *Basic and clinical pharmacology* (10th ed., pp. 92–102, 439, 442–456). New York: Lange Medical Books/McGraw-Hill.

16. Horowitz B. Z. (2005). Botulinum toxin. *Critical Care Clinics* 21, 825–839.

17. Cox N., Hinkle R. (2002). Infant botulism. *American Family Physician* 65, 1388–1392.

18. Vincent A., Palace J., Hilton-Jones D. (2001). Myasthenia gravis. *Lancet* 357, 2122–2128.

19. Drachman D. B. (2005). Myasthenia gravis and other diseases of the neuromuscular junction. In Kasper D. L., Braunwald E., Fauci A. S., et al. (Eds.), *Harrison's principles of internal medicine* (16th ed., pp. 2518–2523). New York: McGraw-Hill.

20. Kothari M. J. (2004). Myasthenia gravis. *Journal of the American Osteopathic Association* 104, 377–384.

21. Russman B. S. (2007). Spinal muscular atrophy: Clinical classification and disease heterogeneity. *Journal of Child Neurology* 22, 946–951.

22. Viera A. J. (2003). Management of carpal tunnel syndrome. *American Family Physician* 68, 265–272.

23. Hickey J. V. (2003). *Neurological and neurosurgical nursing* (5th ed., pp. 407–480). Philadelphia: Lippincott-Raven.

24. Katz J. N., Simmons B. P. (2002). Carpal tunnel syndrome. *New England Journal of Medicine* 346, 1807–1812.

25. Asbury A. K., Hauser S. L. (2005). Guillain-Barré syndrome. In Kasper D. L, Braunwald E., Fauci A., et al. (Eds.), *Harrison's principles of internal medicine* (16th ed., pp. 2513–2518). New York: McGraw-Hill.

26. Kuwabara S. (2004). Guillain-Barré syndrome. *Drugs* 64, 597–610.

27. Newswanger D. L., Warren C. R. (2004). Guillain-Barré syndrome. *American Family Physician* 69, 2405–2410.

28. Winer J. B. (2001). Guillain-Barré syndrome. *Molecular Pathology* 54, 381–385.

29. Rees J. H., Saudain S. E., Gregson N. A., et al. (1995). *Campylobacter jejuni* infection and Guillain-Barré syndrome. *New England Journal of Medicine* 333, 1374–1379.

30. McCamey K. M., Evans P. (2007). Low back pain. *Primary Care Clinics in Office Practice* 34, 71–82.

31. Deyo R. A., Weinstein J. N. (2001). Low back pain. *New England Journal of Medicine* 344, 363–370.

32. Harwood M. I., Smith B. J. (2005). Low back pain: A primary care approach. *Clinics in Family Practice* 7, 279–303.

33. Carragee E. J. (2005). Persistent low back pain. *New England Journal of Medicine* 352, 1891–1898.

34. Kinkade S. (2007). Evaluation and treatment of acute low back pain. *American Family Physician* 75, 1181–1192.

35. Moore K. L., Dalley A. F. (1999). *Clinically oriented anatomy* (4th ed., pp. 452–453). Philadelphia: Lippincott Williams & Wilkins.

36. Winters M. E., Kluetz P., Ziberstein J. (2006). Back pain emergencies. *Medical Clinics of North America* 90, 505–523.

37. Ghez C. (2000). The cerebellum. In Kandel E. R., Schwartz J. H., Jessell T. M. (Eds.), *Principles of neural science* (4th ed., pp. 832–852). New York. McGraw-Hill.

38. DeLong M. R. (2000). The basal ganglia. In Kandel E. R., Schwartz J. H., Jessell T. M. (Eds.), *Principles of neural science* (4th ed., pp. 853–867). New York. McGraw-Hill.

39. Guttman M., Kish S. J., Furukawa Y. (2003). Current concepts in the diagnosis and management of Parkinson disease. *Canadian Medical Association Journal* 168, 293–301.

40. Rao S. S., Hofmann L. A., Shakil A. (2006). Parkinson's disease: Diagnosis and treatment. *American Family Physician* 74, 2046–2055.

41. Samil A., Nutt J. G., Ransom B. R. (2004). Parkinson's disease. *Lancet* 363, 1783–1793.

42. Parkinson J. (1817). *An essay on the shaking palsy.* London: Sherwood, Nelley & Jones.

43. Youdim M. B. H., Riederer P. (1997). Understanding Parkinson disease. *Scientific American* 276, 52–59.

44. Trojanowski J. Q., Kenyon L. (2008). The nervous system. In Rubin R., Strayer D. S. (Eds.), *Rubin's pathology: Clinicopathologic foundations of medicine* (5th ed., 1211–1213, 1221–1224). Philadelphia: Lippincott Williams & Wilkins.

45. Frosch M. P., Anthony D. C., De Girolami U. (2005). The central nervous system. In Kumar V., Abbas A. K., Fausto N. (Eds.), *Robbins and Cotran pathologic basis of disease* (7th ed., pp. 1382–1384, 1391–1393). Philadelphia: Elsevier Saunders.

46. Klein C., Schlossmacher M. G. (2007). Parkinson disease, 10 years after its genetic revolution: Multiple clues to a complex disorder. *Neurology* 69, 2093–2104.

47. Ericksen J. L., Zbigniew W., Petrucelli L. (2005). Molecular pathogenesis of Parkinson disease. *Archives of Neurology* 62, 353–357.

48. Steece-Collier K., Maries E., Kordower J. H. (2002). Etiology of Parkinson disease: Genetics and environment revisited. *Proceedings of the National Academy of Science of the U.S.A.* 99, 1772–1774.

49. Siderowf A., Stern M. (2003). Update on Parkinson disease. *Annals of Internal Medicine* 138, 651–658.

50. Colcher A., Simuni T. (1999). Clinical manifestations of Parkinson's disease. *Medical Clinics of North America* 83, 327–327.

51. National Institute of Neurological Disorders and Stroke. (2007). Deep brain stimulation for Parkinson's disease. [Online.] Available: www.ninds.nih.gov/disorders/deep_brain_stimulation/deep_brain_stimulation.htm. Accessed January 29, 2008.

52. Shoesmith C. L., Strong M. J. (2006). Amyotrophic lateral sclerosis. *Canadian Family Physician* 52, 1563–1569.

53. Rowland L. P., Shneider N. A. (2001). Amyotropic lateral sclerosis. *New England Journal of Medicine* 344, 1688–1700.

54. Mackin G. A. (1999). Optimizing care of patients with ALS. *Postgraduate Medicine* 105, 143–146.

55. Walling A. D. (1999). Amyotropic lateral sclerosis: Lou Gehrig's disease. *American Family Practitioner* 59, 1489–1496.

56. Radunović A., Mitsumoto H., Leigh P. N. (2007). Clinical care of patients with amyotrophic lateral sclerosis. *Neurology: Lancet* 6, 913–925.

57. Noseworthy J. H., Lucchinetti C., Rodriguez M., et al. (2000). Multiple sclerosis. *New England Journal of Medicine* 343, 938–952.

58. Keegan B. M., Noseworthy J. H. (2002). Multiple sclerosis. *Annual Review of Medicine* 53, 285–302.

59. Frohman E. M. (2003). Multiple sclerosis. *Medical Clinics of North America* 87, 867–897.

60. Hawker K., Frohman E. (2004). Multiple sclerosis. *Primary Care Clinics in Office Practice* 31, 201–226.

61. Hauser S. L., Goodin D. S. (2005). Multiple sclerosis and other demyelinating diseases. In Kasper D. L, Braunwald E., Fauci A., et al. (Eds.), *Harrison's principles of internal medicine* (16th ed., pp. 2461–2471). New York: McGraw-Hill.

62. Peterson J. W., Trapp B. D. (2005). Neuropathobiology of multiple sclerosis. *Neurologic Clinics* 23, 107–129.

63. Lucchinetti C. F., Parisi J., Bruck W. (2005). The pathology of multiple sclerosis. *Neurologic Clinics* 23, 77–105.

64. Simon J. H. (2006). Update on multiple sclerosis. *Radiologic Clinics of North America* 44, 79–100.

65. Calabresi P. A. (2004). Diagnosis and management of multiple sclerosis. *American Family Physician* 70, 1935–1944.

66. Lubin D. D. (2005). Clinical features and diagnosis of multiple sclerosis. *Neurologic Clinics* 23, 1–15.
67. Neuhaus O., Kieseier B. L., Hartung H. P. (2007). Immunosuppressive agents in multiple sclerosis. *Neurotherapeutics* 4, 654–660.
68. National Spinal Cord Injury Statistical Center. (2007). Spinal cord injury: Facts and figures at a glance. Birmingham: University of Alabama. [Online]. Available: www.spinalcord.uab.edu/show.asp?durki=19775&site=1021&return=19679. Accessed January 29, 2008.
69. McDonald J. W. (2002). Spinal cord injury. *Lancet* 359, 417–425.
70. Dobkin B. H., Havton L. A. (2004). Basic advances and new avenues in therapy of spinal cord injury. *Annual Review of Medicine* 55, 255–282.
71. Branco F., Cardenas D. D., Svircev J. N. (2007). Spinal cord injury: A comprehensive review. *Physical Medicine and Rehabilitation Clinics of North America* 18, 651–679.
72. National Institute of Neurological Disorders and Stroke. (2007). Spinal cord injury: Hope through research. [Online.] Available: www.ninds.nih.gov/disorders/sci/detail_sci.htm. Accessed January 29, 2008.
73. Buckley D. A., Guanci M. K. (1999). Spinal cord trauma. *Nursing Clinics of North America* 34, 661–687.
74. Chiles B. W., Cooper P. R. (1996). Acute spinal cord injury. *New England Journal of Medicine* 334, 514–520.
75. Fehling M. G., Louw D. (1996). Initial stabilization and medical management of acute spinal cord injury. *American Family Physician* 42, 155–162.
76. Atkinson P. P., Atkinson J. L. D. (1996). Spinal shock. *Mayo Clinic Proceedings* 71, 384–389.
77. Bracken M. B., Shepard M. J., Collins W. F., et al. (1997). Administration of methylprednisolone for 24 or 48 hours or tirilazad mesylate for 48 hours in the treatment of acute spinal cord injury: Results of the Third National Acute Spinal Cord Injury Study. *Journal of the American Medical Association* 277, 1597–1604.
78. Hall E. D., Springer J. E. (2004). Neuroprotection and acute spinal cord injury: A reappraisal. *Neurotherapeutics* 1, 80–110.
79. Sipski M., Pearse D. D. (2006). Methylprednisone and other confounders to spinal cord injury trials. *Nature Clinical Practice: Neurology* 2, 402–403.
80. American Spinal Injury Association. (2002). *International standards for neurological classification of SCI, revised 2002*. Chicago: Author.
81. Zimmer M. B., Nantwi K., Goshgarian H. G. (2007). Effect of spinal cord injury on the respiratory system: Basic research and current clinical treatment options. *Journal of Spinal Cord Medicine* 30, 319–330.
82. Garstang S. V., Miller-Smith S. A. (2007). Autonomic nervous system dysfunction after spinal cord injury. *Physical Medicine and Rehabilitation Clinics of North America* 18, 275–296.
83. Blackner J. (2003). Rehabilitation medicine: Autonomic dysreflexia. *Canadian Medical Association Journal* 169, 931–935.
84. Benevento B. T., Sipski M. L. (2002). Neurogenic bladder, neurogenic bowel, and sexual dysfunction in people with spinal cord injury. *Physical Therapy* 62, 601–612.
85. Aito S., Pieri A., Marcelli F., et al. (2002). Primary prevention of deep venous thrombosis and pulmonary embolism in acute spinal cord injured patients. *Spinal Cord* 40, 300–303.
86. Schwab M. E. (2002). Repairing the injured spinal cord. *Science* 295, 1029–1031.
87. Fawcett J. (2002). Repair of spinal cord injuries: Where are we, where are we going? *Spinal Cord* 40, 615–623.

Visit the Point. **http://thePoint.lww.com for animations, journal articles, and more!**

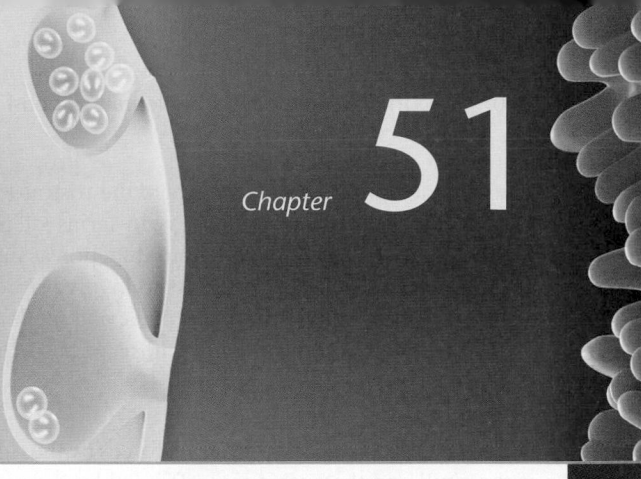

Disorders of Brain Function

DIANE S. BOOK

➤ Anatomically and functionally, the brain is the most complex structure in the body. It controls our ability to think, our awareness of things around us, and our interactions with the outside world. Brain functions are diverse and highly localized within the brain. Therefore, unlike other organs that have a global function, the brain is much more vulnerable to focal lesions. For example, an isolated renal infarct would not be expected to have a significant effect on kidney function, whereas an infarct of comparable size in the brain could have serious impact on brain function, such as complete paralysis on one side of the body.

MECHANISMS AND MANIFESTATIONS OF BRAIN INJURY

After completing this section of the chapter, you should be able to meet the following objectives:

■ Differentiate cerebral hypoxia from cerebral ischemia and focal from global ischemia.

■ Characterize the role of excitatory amino acids as a common pathway for neurologic disorders.

■ State the determinants of intracranial pressure and describe compensatory mechanisms used to prevent large changes in intracranial pressure when there are changes in brain, blood, and cerebrospinal fluid volumes.

■ Explain the causes of tentorial herniation of the brain and its consequences.

■ Compare the causes of communicating and non-communicating hydrocephalus.

■ Compare cytotoxic, vasogenic, and interstitial cerebral edema.

■ Differentiate primary and secondary brain injuries due to head trauma.

■ Describe the mechanism of brain damage in coup–contrecoup injuries.

■ List the constellation of symptoms involved in the postconcussion syndrome.

■ Differentiate among the location, manifestations, and morbidity of epidural, subdural, and intracerebral hematoma.

(objectives continue)

- Define consciousness and trace the rostral-to-caudal progression of consciousness in terms of pupillary changes, respiration, and motor function as the effects of brain dysfunction progress to involve structures in the diencephalon, midbrain, pons, and medulla.
- State two criteria for the diagnosis of brain death.

The brain is protected from external forces by the rigid confines of the skull and the cushioning afforded by the cerebrospinal fluid (CSF). The metabolic stability required by its electrically active cells is maintained by a number of regulatory mechanisms, including the blood-brain barrier and autoregulatory mechanisms that ensure its blood supply. Nonetheless, the brain remains remarkably vulnerable to injury by ischemia, trauma, tumors, degenerative processes, and metabolic derangements.

Mechanisms of Injury

Injury to brain tissue can result from a number of conditions, including trauma, tumors, stroke, metabolic derangements, and degenerative disorders. Brain damage resulting from these disorders involves several common pathways, including the effects of ischemia, excitatory amino acid injury, cerebral edema, and injury due to increased intracranial pressure (ICP). In many cases, the mechanisms of injury are interrelated.

Hypoxic and Ischemic Injury

The energy requirements of the brain are provided mainly by adenosine triphosphate (ATP); the ability of the cerebral circulation to deliver oxygen in sufficiently high concentrations to facilitate metabolism of glucose and generate ATP is essential to brain function. Although the brain makes up only 2% of the body's weight, it receives 15% of the resting cardiac output and accounts for 20% of the oxygen consumption.[1,2] Thus, deprivation of oxygen or blood flow can have a deleterious effect on brain structures.

By definition, hypoxia denotes a deprivation of oxygen with maintained blood flow (perfusion), whereas ischemia is a situation of greatly reduced or interrupted blood flow. The brain tends to have different sensitivities to the two conditions. Whereas hypoxia interferes with the delivery of oxygen, ischemia interferes with delivery of oxygen and glucose as well as the removal of metabolic wastes. Hypoxia usually is seen in conditions such as exposure to reduced atmospheric pressure, carbon monoxide poisoning, severe anemia, and failure to oxygenate the blood. Because hypoxia indicates decreased oxygen levels in all brain tissue, it produces a generalized depressant effect on the brain. Contrary to popular belief, neurons are capable of substantial anaerobic metabolism and are fairly tolerant of pure hypoxia; it commonly produces euphoria, listlessness, drowsiness, and impaired problem solving. Unconsciousness and convulsions may occur when hypoxia is sudden and severe. However, the effects of severe hypoxia (*i.e.,* anoxia) on brain function seldom are seen because the condition rapidly leads to cardiac arrest and ischemia.

Cerebral ischemia can be focal, as in stroke, or global, as in cardiac arrest. In global ischemia, the blood flow to the entire brain is compromised. In contrast, during focal ischemia, only a region of the brain is underperfused, as in ischemic stroke. Collateral circulation provides blood flow to uninvolved brain areas during focal ischemia. The collateral perfusion may even provide sufficient substrates to the borders of the focal ischemic region to maintain a low level of metabolic activity, thereby preserving membrane integrity. At the same time, interruption in delivery of glucose under these anaerobic conditions may result in additional lactic acid production and depletion of ATP stores.[2]

Global Ischemia. Global ischemia occurs when blood flow is inadequate to meet the metabolic needs of the entire brain. The result is a spectrum of neurologic disorders reflecting global brain dysfunction. Unconsciousness occurs within seconds of severe global ischemia, such as that resulting from complete cessation of blood flow, as in cardiac arrest, or with marked decrease in blood flow, as in serious cardiac arrhythmias. If cerebral circulation is restored immediately, consciousness is regained quickly. However, if blood flow is not promptly restored, severe pathologic changes take place. Energy sources, glucose and glycogen, are exhausted in 2 to 4 minutes, and cellular ATP stores are depleted in 4 to 5 minutes. Approximately 50% to 75% of the total energy requirement of neuronal tissue is spent on mechanisms for maintenance of ionic gradients across the cell membrane (*e.g.,* sodium-potassium pump), resulting in fluxes of sodium, potassium, and calcium ions[3] (Table 51-1). Excessive influx of sodium results in neuronal and interstitial edema. The influx of calcium initiates a cascade of events, including release of intracellular and nuclear enzymes that cause cell destruction (see section on Excitotoxic Injury). When ischemia is sufficiently severe or prolonged, infarction or death of all the cellular elements of the brain occurs. Even if

TABLE 51-1 **Pathophysiologic Consequences of Impaired Cerebral Perfusion**	
CONSEQUENCES	**TIMING**
Depletion of oxygen	10 sec
Depletion of glucose	2–4 min
Conversion to anaerobic metabolism	2–4 min
Exhaustion of cellular ATP	4–5 min
Consequences	
Efflux of potassium	
Influx of sodium	
Influx of calcium	

Adapted from Richmond T.S. (1997). Cerebral resuscitation after global brain ischemia: Linking research to practice. *AACN Clinical Issues* 8(2), 173.

blood flow is restored, if ischemic thresholds for injury were exceeded, then permanent cell death ensues. Furthermore, reperfusion of injured tissues can lead to secondary brain injury through the delivery of inflammatory cells and toxic byproducts, including excitatory amino acids. Such reperfusion injury compounds the initial ischemic damage.

The pattern of global ischemia reflects the anatomic arrangement of the cerebral vessels and the sensitivity of various brain tissues to oxygen deprivation[4] (Fig. 51-1). Selective neuronal sensitivity to a lack of oxygen is most apparent in the Purkinje cells of the cerebellum and neurons in the Sommer sector of the hippocampus, where cell death occurs earliest after global ischemia. The anatomic arrangement of the cerebral blood vessels predisposes to two types of injury: watershed infarcts and laminar necrosis.

Watershed infarcts are concentrated in anatomically vulnerable border zones between the overlapping territories supplied by the major cerebral arteries, notably the middle, anterior, and posterior cerebral arteries. The overlapping territory at the distal ends of these vessels forms extremely vulnerable areas in terms of global ischemia, called *watershed zones*. During events such as severe hypotension, these distal territories undergo a profound lowering of blood flow, predisposing to focal ischemia and infarction of brain tissues. Therefore, global ischemia can result in focal infarcts that occur in the border zones between major vascular territories. This is in contrast to primarily focal ischemia in which the pattern of infarction is within a vascular territory. Laminar necrosis refers to short, serpiginous segments of necrosis that occur within and parallel to the cerebral cortex, in areas supplied by the penetrating arteries. The gray matter of the cerebral cortex receives its major blood supply through short penetrating arteries that emerge at right angles from larger vessels in the pia mater and then form a cascade as they repeatedly branch, forming a rich capillary network. An abrupt loss of arterial blood pressure markedly diminishes flow through these capillary channels. Because the third cortical layer is most

sensitive to ischemia, the necrosis that develops is laminar and is most severe in this deep layer of the cortex.

The neurologic deficits that result from global ischemic injury vary widely. If the period of nonflow or low flow is minimal, the neurologic damage usually is minimal to nonexistent. When the period is extensive or resuscitation is lengthy, the early neurologic clinical picture is that of fixed and dilated pupils, abnormal motor posturing, and coma. If the victim survives, there may be gradual improvement in neurologic status, although permanent cognitive and focal deficits usually persist and can prevent a return to preischemic levels of functioning.

An exception to this time frame is the circumstance of cold-water drowning in which the person, especially a child, is submerged in cold water for longer than 10 minutes.[5] Hypothermia develops and reduces the cerebral metabolic requirements for oxygen, minimizes intracellular acidosis, and lessens the effects of excitotoxic byproducts.[6] In this case, recovery can be rapid and remarkable, and resuscitation efforts should not be discontinued precipitously.

Treatment of global cerebral ischemia varies with the underlying cause (*e.g.*, cardiac arrest, hanging, asthma attack). General goals common to all causes are aimed at providing oxygen to the troubled brain and decreasing the metabolic needs of brain tissue during the nonflow state. Hemodynamic support aimed at restoring systemic and cerebral perfusion is required. Respiratory support including mechanical ventilation and supplemental oxygen may be indicated. Methods that decrease brain temperature as a means of decreasing brain metabolism, as in cold-water drowning, are effective in certain patients after cardiac arrest.[7] Normovolemic hemodilution may be used to overcome sludging of cerebral blood flow during reperfusion. Because both hypoglycemia and hyperglycemia adversely affect the outcome in persons with global ischemia, control of blood glucose within a range of 100 to 200 mg/dL is appropriate, and even narrower targets have been advocated in acute stroke.[3,6,7] Recent interest has focused on other neuroprotective

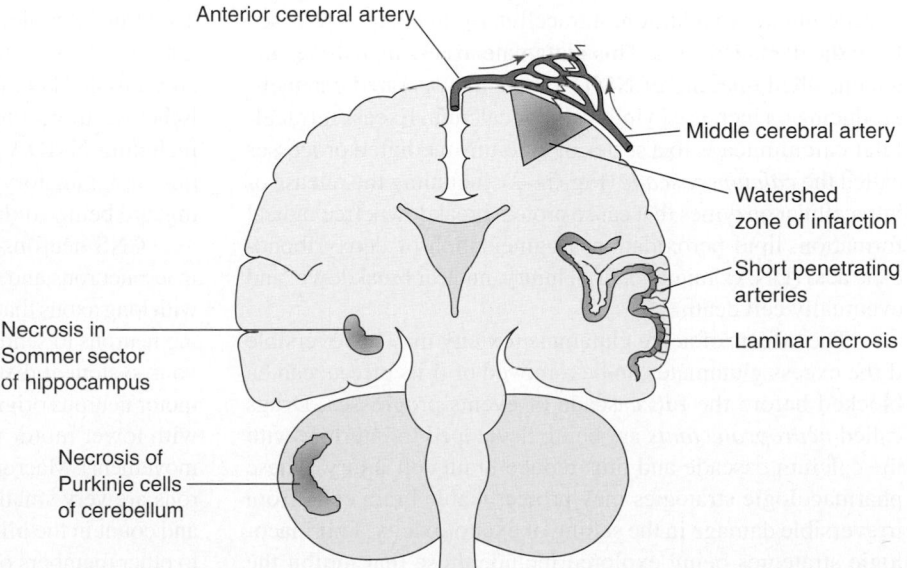

FIGURE 51-1 • Consequences of global ischemia. A global insult induces lesions that reflect the vascular architecture (watershed infarcts, laminar necrosis) and the sensitivity of individual neuronal systems (pyramidal cells of the Sommer section, Purkinje cells). (Courtesy of Dmitri Karetnikov, artist.) (From Trojanowsi J. Q., Kenyon L. [2008]. The central nervous system. In Rubin R., Strayer D. E. [Eds.], *Rubin's pathology: Clinicopathologic foundations of medicine* [5th ed., p. 1191]. Philadelphia: Lippincott Williams & Wilkins.)

therapies and pharmacologic agents that could minimize injury from free radicals, excitatory amino acids, and other forms of secondary injury.

Excitotoxic Brain Injury

In many neurologic disorders, injury to neurons may be caused by various mediators, including excitatory amino acids, catecholamines, nitric oxide, free radicals, inflammatory cells, apoptosis, and intracellular proteases.[8] The earliest and most studied of these is the overstimulation of receptors for specific amino acids, such as glutamate and aspartate, that act as excitatory neurotransmitters.[9] The neurologic conditions involved in excitotoxic injury range from acute insults such as stroke, hypoglycemic injury, and trauma to chronic degenerative disorders such as Huntington disease and possibly Alzheimer dementia. The term *excitotoxicity* has been coined for the final common pathway for neuronal cell injury and death triggered by excessive activity of the excitatory neurotransmitters and their receptor-mediated effects.

Glutamate is the principal excitatory neurotransmitter in the brain, and its interaction with specific receptors is responsible for many higher-order functions, including memory, cognition, movement, and sensation.[9] Many of the actions of glutamate are coupled with receptor-operated ion channels. One subtype in particular, the glutamate N-methyl-D-aspartate (NMDA) receptor, has been implicated in causing central nervous system (CNS) injury.[8,9] This subtype of glutamate receptor opens a large-diameter calcium channel that permits calcium and sodium ions to enter the cell and allows potassium ions to exit, resulting in prolonged (seconds) action potentials. The intracellular concentration of glutamate is approximately 16 times that of the extracellular concentration.[9] Normally, extracellular concentrations of glutamate are tightly regulated, with excess amounts removed and actively transported into astrocytes and neurons.

During prolonged ischemia, the glutamate transport mechanisms become immobilized, causing extracellular glutamate to accumulate. In addition, intracellular glutamate is released from the damaged cells. This glutamate excess then drives the uncontrolled opening of NMDA receptor–operated channels, producing an increase in intracellular calcium. Excess intracellular calcium leads to a series of calcium-mediated processes called the *calcium cascade* (Fig. 51-2), including the release of intracellular enzymes that cause protein breakdown, free radical formation, lipid peroxidation, fragmentation of deoxyribonucleic acid (DNA), mitochondrial injury, nuclear breakdown, and eventually cell death.

The effects of acute glutamate toxicity may be reversible if the excess glutamate can be removed or if its effects can be blocked before the full cascade of events progresses. Drugs called *neuroprotectants* are being developed to interfere with the calcium cascade and thus reduce brain cell injury. These pharmacologic strategies may protect viable brain cells from irreversible damage in the setting of excitotoxicity. Pharmacologic strategies being explored include those that inhibit the

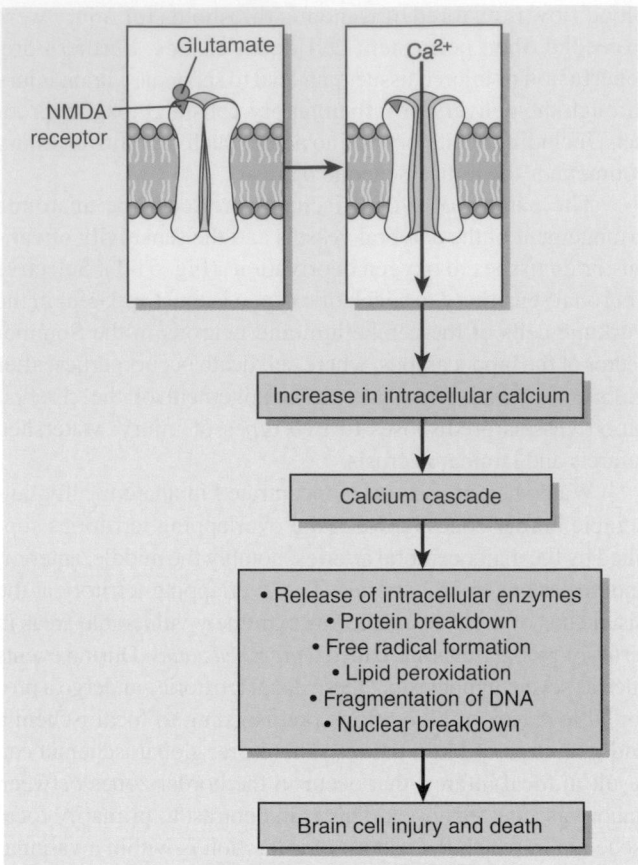

FIGURE 51-2 • The role of the glutamate-NMDA receptor in brain cell injury.

synthesis or release of excitatory amino acid transmitters; block the NMDA receptors; stabilize the membrane potential to prevent initiation of the calcium cascade using lidocaine and certain barbiturates; and specifically block certain intracellular proteases, endonucleases, and lipases that are known to be cytotoxic.[8,10,11] The drug riluzole, which acts presynaptically to inhibit glutamate release, currently is being used in the treatment of amyotrophic lateral sclerosis (see Chapter 50). In the setting of ischemic stroke, multiple mechanisms of pharmacologic action, including NMDA receptor blockade, nitric oxide manipulation, inflammatory suppression, and potassium channel opening, are being studied.[12]

CNS neurons can be divided into two major categories: macroneurons and microneurons. Macroneurons are large cells with long axons that leave the local network of intercommunicating neurons to send action potentials to other regions of the nervous system at distances of centimeters to meters (*e.g.,* upper motor neurons originating in the motor cortex that communicate with lower motor neurons of the spinal cord that control leg movement). Macroneurons number in the thousands. Microneurons are very small cells intimately involved in local circuitry, and count in the billions. Their axons transmit action potentials to other members of the same local network. It is the microneuron network that provides the analytic, integrative, and learning circuitry that is the basis for the higher-order function of the CNS. Many macroneurons use glutamate as a neurotransmitter in their excitatory communication with microneurons. The microneurons of the cerebral cortex and hippocampus are particularly vulnerable to excessive stimulation of the glutamate NMDA receptors and the neurotoxic effects of increased intracellular calcium levels. Because of their increased vulnerability, many of the small interneurons that make up essential parts of the complex control and memory functions of the brain are selectively damaged, even if the remainder of the brain survives the insult. This pattern may account for the long-term effects of brain insult, which frequently include subtle reductions in cognitive and memory functions.

Increased Intracranial Volume and Pressure

The brain is enclosed in the rigid confines of the skull, or cranium, making it particularly susceptible to increases in ICP. Increased ICP is a common pathway for brain injury from different types of insults and agents. Excessive ICP can obstruct cerebral blood flow, destroy brain cells, displace brain tissue (as in herniation), and otherwise damage delicate brain structures.

The cranial cavity contains blood (approximately 10%), brain tissue (approximately 80%), and CSF (approximately 10%) in the rigid confines of a nonexpandable skull.[13] Each of these three volumes contributes to the ICP, which normally is maintained within a range of 0 to 15 mm Hg when measured in the lateral ventricles. The volumes of each of these components can vary slightly without causing marked changes in ICP. This is because small increases in the volume of one component can be compensated for by a decrease in the volume of one or both of the other two components.[14] This association is called the *Monro-Kellie hypothesis.* Normal fluctuations in ICP occur with respiratory movements and activities of daily living such as straining, coughing, and sneezing.

Abnormal variation in intracranial volume with subsequent changes in ICP can be caused by a volume change in any of the three intracranial components. For example, an increase in tissue volume can result from a brain tumor, brain edema, or bleeding into brain tissue. An increase in blood volume develops when there is vasodilation of cerebral vessels or obstruction of venous outflow. Excess production, decreased absorption, or obstructed circulation of CSF affords the potential for an increase in the CSF component. When the change in volume is caused by a brain tumor, it tends to occur slowly and usually is localized to the immediate area, whereas the increase resulting from head injury usually develops rapidly.

According to the modified Monro-Kellie hypothesis, reciprocal compensation occurs among the three intracranial compartments.[13] Of the three intracranial volumes, tissue volume is relatively restricted in its ability to undergo change; CSF and blood volume are best able to compensate for changes in ICP. Initial increases in ICP are buffered by a translocation of CSF to the spinal subarachnoid space and increased reabsorption of CSF. The compensatory ability of the blood compartment is limited by the small amount of blood that is in the cerebral circulation. The cerebral blood vessels contain less than 10% of the intracranial volume, most of which is contained in the low-pressure venous system. As the volume-buffering capacity of this compartment becomes exhausted, venous pressure increases, and cerebral blood volume and ICP rise. Also, cerebral blood flow is highly controlled by autoregulatory mechanisms, which affect its compensatory capacity. Conditions such as ischemia and an elevated partial pressure of carbon dioxide (PCO_2) in the blood produce a compensatory vasodilation of the cerebral blood vessels. A decrease in PCO_2 has the opposite effect; for this reason, hyperventilation, which results in a decrease in PCO_2 levels, is sometimes used in the treatment of ICP.

The impact of increases in blood, brain tissue, or CSF volumes on ICP varies among individuals and depends on the amount of increase, effectiveness of compensatory mechanisms, and compliance of brain tissue. Compliance represents the ratio of change in volume to the resulting change in pressure (compliance = change in volume/change in pressure).[13] In the case of intracranial volumes and pressure, an increase in intracranial volume will have little, or no, effect on ICP as long as compliance is high. Factors that influence compliance include the amount of volume increase, the time frame for accommodation, and the size of the intracranial compartments. For example, small volume increments over long periods of time can be accommodated more easily than a comparable amount introduced over a short time.

The cerebral perfusion pressure (CPP), which represents the difference between the mean arterial blood pressure (MABP) and the ICP (CPP = MABP − ICP), is the pressure perfusing the brain.[13,14] CPP is determined by the pressure gradient between the internal carotid artery and the subarachnoid veins. The MABP and ICP are monitored frequently in persons with brain conditions that increase ICP and impair brain perfusion. Normal CPP ranges from 70 to 100 mm Hg. Brain ischemia develops at levels below 40 mm Hg.[13] When the pressure in the cranial cavity approaches or exceeds the MABP, tissue perfusion becomes inadequate, cellular hypoxia results, and neuronal death may occur. The highly specialized cortical neurons are the most sensitive to oxygen deficit; a decrease in the level of consciousness is one of the earliest and most reliable signs of increased ICP. The continued cellular hypoxia leads to general neurologic deterioration; the level of consciousness may deteriorate from alertness through confusion, lethargy, obtundation, stupor, and coma.

One of the late reflexes seen with a marked increase in ICP is the CNS ischemic response, which is triggered by ischemia of the vasomotor center in the brain stem. Neurons in the vasomotor center respond directly to ischemia by producing a marked increase in MABP in an attempt to increase CPP, sometimes to levels as high as 270 mm Hg, accompanied by a widening of the pulse pressure and reflex slowing of the heart rate. These three signs (*i.e.,* hypertension, bradycardia, and

Understanding • Intracranial Pressure

The intracranial pressure (ICP) is the pressure within the intracranial cavity. It is determined by (1) the pressure-volume relationships among the brain tissue, cerebrospinal fluid (CSF), and blood in the intracranial cavity; (2) the Monro-Kellie hypothesis, which relates to reciprocal changes among the intracranial volumes; and (3) the compliance of the brain and its ability to buffer changes in intracranial volume.

❶ Intracranial Volumes and Pressure

The ICP represents the pressure exerted by the essentially incompressible tissue and fluid volumes of the three compartments contained within the rigid confines of the skull—the brain tissue and interstitial fluid (80%), the blood (10%), and the CSF (10%).

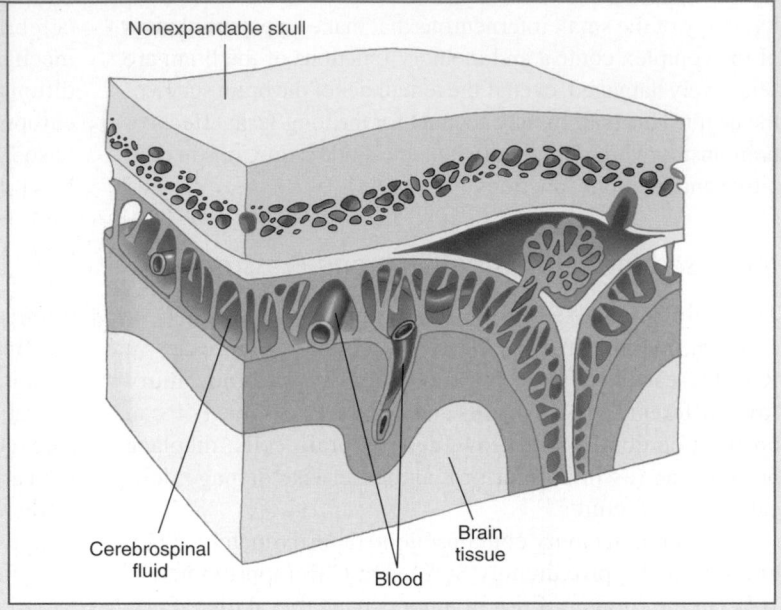

Nonexpandable skull

Cerebrospinal fluid

Blood

Brain tissue

❷ Monro-Kellie Hypothesis

Normally, a reciprocal relationship exists among the three intracranial volumes such that the ICP is maintained within normal limits. Because these volumes are practically incompressible, a change in one component must be balanced by an almost equal and opposite effect in one or both of the remaining components. This is known as the *Monro-Kellie hypothesis.*

Of the three intracranial volumes, the fluid in the CSF compartment is the most easily displaced. The CSF (**A**) can be displaced from the ventricles and cerebral subarachnoid space to the spinal subarachnoid space, and it can also undergo increased absorption or decreased production. Because most of the blood in the cranial cavity is contained in the low-pressure venous system, venous compression (**B**) serves as a means of displacing blood volume.

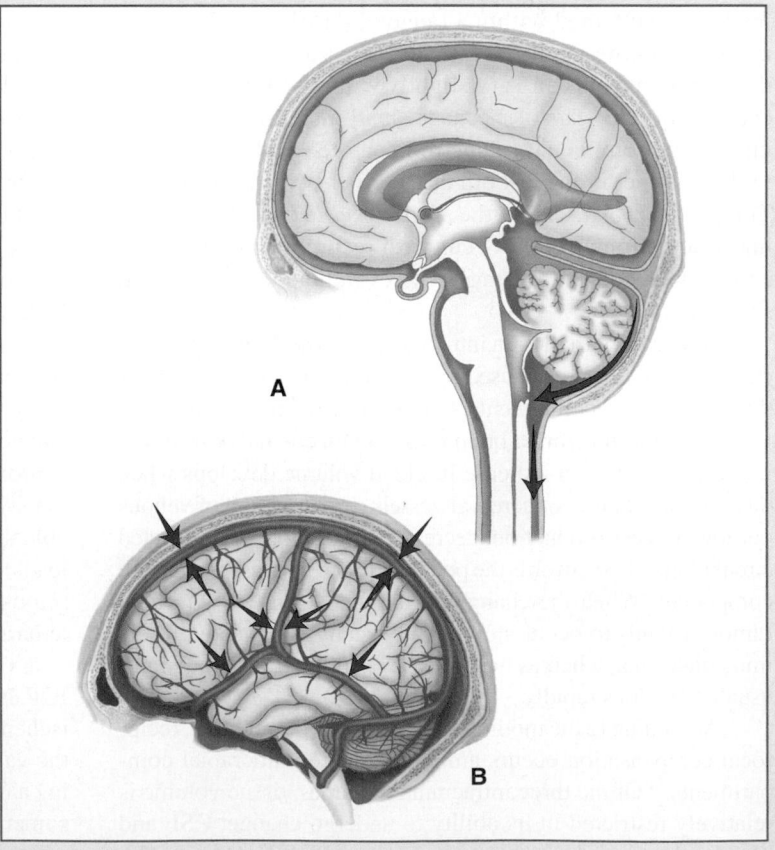

A

B

❸ Compliance and the Volume-Pressure Curve

Compliance, which refers to the ease with which a substance can be compressed or deformed, is a measure of the brain's ability to maintain its ICP during changes in intracranial volume. Compliance (C) represents the ratio of change (Δ) in volume (V) to change in pressure (P): $C = \Delta V/\Delta P$.

The dynamic effects of changes in intracranial volume and compliance on ICP can be illustrated on a graph with the volume represented on the horizontal axis and ICP on the vertical axis. The shape of the curve demonstrates the effect on ICP of adding volume to the intracranial cavity. From points A to B, the compensatory mechanisms are adequate, compliance is high, and the ICP remains relatively constant as volume is added to the intracranial cavity. At point B, the ICP is relatively normal, but the compensatory mechanisms have reached their limits, compliance is decreased, and ICP begins to rise with each change in volume. From points C to D, the compensatory mechanisms have been exceeded and ICP rises significantly with each increase in volume as compliance is lost.

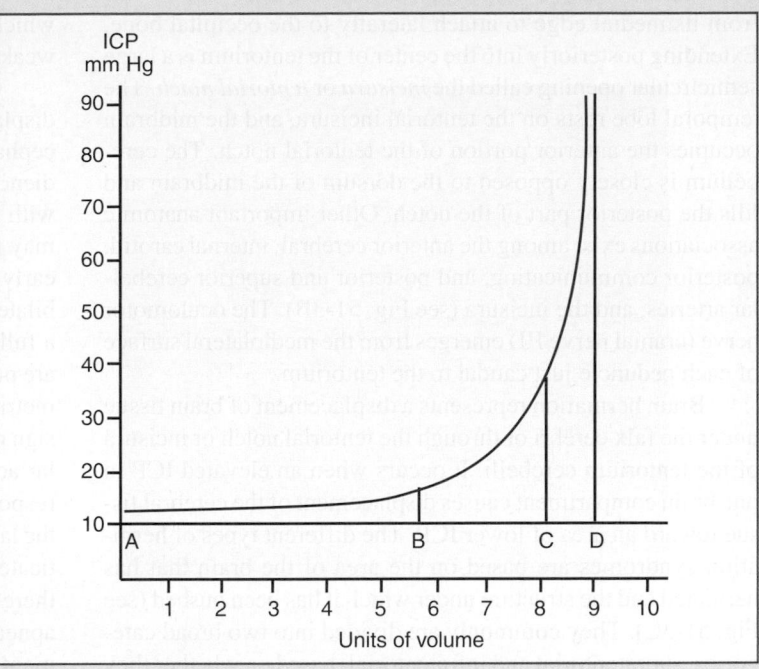

(From Hickey J.V. [2003]. *Neurological and neurosurgical nursing* [5th ed., p. 286]. Philadelphia. Lippincott Williams & Wilkins.)

widened pulse pressure), sometimes called the *Cushing reflex*, are important but late indicators of increased ICP.[15]

Brain Herniation

The brain is protected by the nonexpandable skull and supporting septa, the falx cerebri and the tentorium cerebelli, that divide the intracranial cavity into fossae or compartments that normally protect against excessive movement. The falx cerebri is a sickle-shaped septum that separates the two hemispheres. The tentorium cerebelli divides the cranial cavity into anterior and posterior fossae (Fig. 51-3A). This inflexible dural sheath extends posteriorly from the bony petrous ridges and anterior to the clinoid process, sloping downward and outward

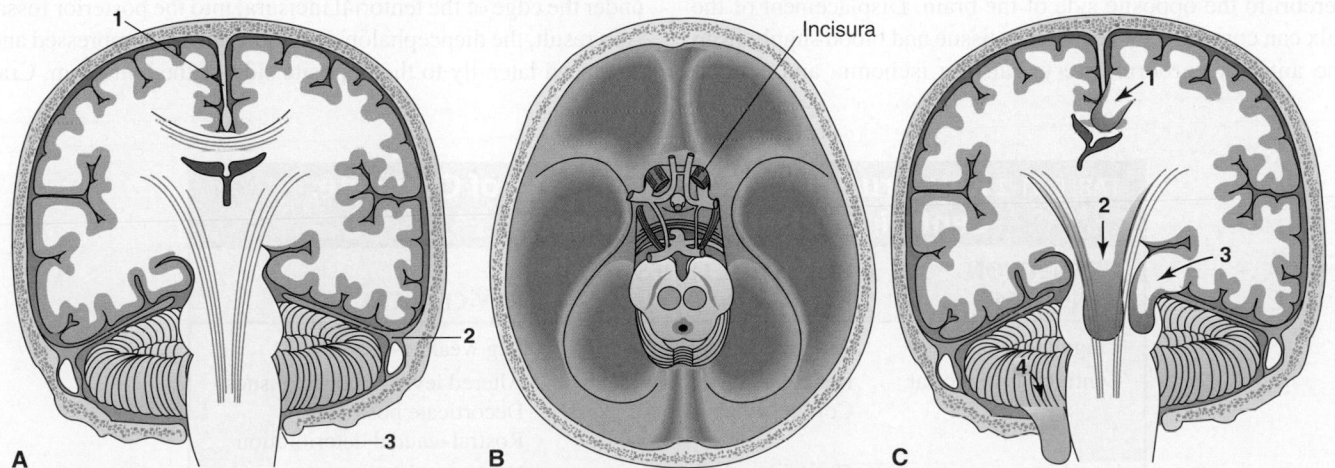

FIGURE 51-3 • Supporting septa of the brain and patterns of herniation. (**A**) The falx cerebri [1], tentorium cerebelli [2], foramen magnum [3]. (**B**) The location of the incisura or tentorial notch in relation to the cerebral arteries and oculomotor nerve. (**C**) Herniation of the cingulate gyrus under the falx cerebri [1], central or transtentorial herniation [2], uncal herniation of the temporal lobe into the tentorial notch [3], and infratentorial herniation of the cerebellar tonsils [4]. (Courtesy of Carole Hilmer, CMI.)

from its medial edge to attach laterally to the occipital bone. Extending posteriorly into the center of the tentorium is a large semicircular opening called the *incisura* or *tentorial notch.* The temporal lobe rests on the tentorial incisura, and the midbrain occupies the anterior portion of the tentorial notch. The cerebellum is closely opposed to the dorsum of the midbrain and fills the posterior part of the notch. Other important anatomic associations exist among the anterior cerebral, internal carotid, posterior communicating, and posterior and superior cerebellar arteries, and the incisura (see Fig. 51-3B). The oculomotor nerve (cranial nerve III) emerges from the mediolateral surface of each peduncle just caudal to the tentorium.

Brain herniation represents a displacement of brain tissue under the falx cerebri or through the tentorial notch or incisura of the tentorium cerebelli. It occurs when an elevated ICP in one brain compartment causes displacement of the cerebral tissue toward an area of lower ICP. The different types of herniation syndromes are based on the area of the brain that has herniated and the structure under which it has been pushed (see Fig. 51-3C). They commonly are divided into two broad categories, supratentorial and infratentorial, based on whether they are located above or below the tentorium.

Supratentorial Herniations. Three major patterns of supratentorial herniation were described by Plum and Posner in their classic work: cingulate, central transtentorial, and uncal transtentorial.[16] Table 51-2 describes the key structures and clinical signs of these three types of herniations. Of the three, cingulate herniation poses the less serious threat in terms of clinical outcomes.[13] Transtentorial herniations result in two distinct syndromes: an uncal syndrome and a central syndrome. Clinically, they display distinct patterns early in their course, but both merge in a similar pattern once they begin to involve the midbrain level and below (brain stem structures).

Cingulate herniation involves displacement of the cingulate gyrus and hemisphere beneath the sharp edges of the falx cerebri to the opposite side of the brain. Displacement of the falx can compress the local brain tissue and blood supply from the anterior cerebral artery, causing ischemia and edema, which further increase ICP levels. Unilateral or bilateral leg weakness is an early sign of impending cingulate herniation.

Central transtentorial herniations involve the downward displacement of the cerebral hemispheres, basal ganglia, diencephalon, and midbrain through the tentorial incisura. The diencephalon may be compressed tightly against the midbrain with such force that edema and hemorrhage result. It may or may not be associated with uncal or lateral herniation. In the early diencephalic stage, there is clouding of consciousness, bilaterally small pupils (approximately 2 mm in diameter) with a full range of constriction, and motor responses to pain that are purposeful or semipurposeful (localizing) and often asymmetric. The clouding of consciousness, which is often a first sign of central herniations, is caused by pressure on the reticular activating system (RAS) in the upper midbrain, which is responsible for wakefulness. As the herniation progresses to the late diencephalic stage, painful stimulation results in decorticate posturing, which may be asymmetric (Fig. 51-4A), and there is waxing and waning of respirations with periods of apnea (Cheyne-Stokes respirations). With midbrain involvement, the pupils are fixed and midsize (approximately 5 mm in diameter), and reflex adduction of the eyes is impaired; pain elicits decerebrate posturing (Fig. 51-4B); and respirations change from Cheyne-Stokes to neurogenic hyperventilation, in which the frequency may exceed 40 breaths per minute because of uninhibited stimulation of the inspiratory and expiratory centers. Progression to involve the lower pons and upper medulla produces fixed, midpoint (3- to 5-mm) pupils with loss of reflex abduction and adduction of the eyes, and absence of motor responses or only leg flexion on painful stimuli. Once the area of herniation has progressed beyond the diencephalon and into the midbrain and brain stem, the process is generally irreversible and the prognosis poor.[13]

Uncal herniation occurs when a lateral mass pushes the brain tissue centrally and forces the medial aspect of the temporal lobe, which contains the uncus and hippocampal gyrus, under the edge of the tentorial incisura, into the posterior fossa. As a result, the diencephalon and midbrain are compressed and displaced laterally to the opposite side of the tentorium. Cra-

TABLE 51-2 **Key Structures and Clinical Signs of Cingulate, Central, and Uncal Herniations**		
HERNIATION SYNDROME	**KEY STRUCTURES INVOLVED**	**KEY CLINICAL SIGNS**
Cingulate	Anterior cerebral artery	Leg weakness
Central transtentorial	Reticular activating system	Altered level of consciousness
	Corticospinal tract	Decorticate posturing
		Rostral–caudal deterioration
Uncal	Cerebral peduncle	Hemiparesis
	Oculomotor nerve	Ipsilateral pupil dilation
	Posterior cerebral artery	Visual field loss
	Cerebellar tonsil	
	Respiratory center	Respiratory arrest

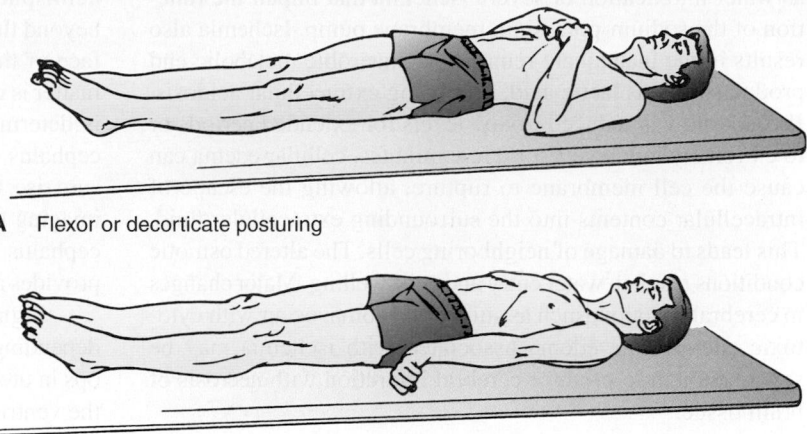

FIGURE 51-4 • Abnormal posturing. **(A)** Decorticate rigidity. In decorticate rigidity, the upper arms are held at the sides with elbows, wrists, and fingers flexed. The legs are extended and internally rotated. The feet are plantar flexed. **(B)** Decerebrate rigidity. In decerebrate rigidity, the jaws are clenched and neck extended. The arms are adducted and stiffly extended at the elbows with the forearms pronated and the wrists and fingers flexed. (From Fuller J., Schaller-Ayers J. [1994]. *Health assessment: A nursing approach* [2nd ed.]. Philadelphia: J. B. Lippincott.)

A Flexor or decorticate posturing

B Extensor or decerebrate posturing

nial nerve III (oculomotor nerve) and the posterior cerebral artery frequently are caught between the uncus and the tentorium. The oculomotor nerve controls pupillary constriction; entrapment of this nerve results in ipsilateral pupillary dilation, which usually is an early sign of uncal herniation. Consciousness may be unimpaired because the RAS has not yet been affected. However, after any signs of herniation or brain stem compression appear, deterioration may proceed rapidly—making it important to recognize the distinguishing early features of uncal herniations.

As uncal herniations progress, there are changes in motor strength and coordination of voluntary movements because of compression of the descending motor pathways. It is not unusual for initial changes in motor function to occur ipsilateral to the side of the brain damage because of compression of the contralateral cerebral peduncles. This may result in a false localizing sign of hemiparesis on the same side as cranial nerve III, rather than on the opposite side, which would be the case if a singular lesion in the midbrain were the cause. As the condition progresses, bilateral positive Babinski responses and respiratory changes (*e.g.,* Cheyne-Stokes respirations, ataxic patterns) occur. Decorticate and decerebrate posturing may develop, followed by dilated, fixed pupils, flaccidity, and respiratory arrest.

Infratentorial Herniation. Infratentorial herniation results from increased pressure in the infratentorial compartment. It often progress rapidly and can cause death because it is likely to involve the lower brain stem centers that control vital cardiopulmonary functions. Herniation may occur superiorly (upward) through the tentorial incisura or inferiorly (downward) through the foramen magnum.

Upward displacement of brain tissue can cause blockage of the aqueduct of Sylvius and lead to hydrocephalus and coma. Downward displacement of the midbrain through the tentorial notch or the cerebellar tonsils through the foramen magnum can interfere with medullary functioning and cause cardiac or respiratory arrest. In cases of preexisting ICP elevations, herniation

may occur when the pressure is released from below, such as in a lumbar puncture. If the CSF pathway is blocked and fluid cannot leave the ventricles, the volume expands, and fluid is displaced downward through the tentorial notch. The expanding volume causes all function at a given level to cease as destruction progresses in a rostral-to-caudal direction. The result of this displacement is brain stem ischemia and hemorrhage extending from the diencephalon to the pons. If the lesion expands rapidly, displacement and obstruction occur quickly, leading to irreversible infarction and hemorrhage.

Cerebral Edema

Cerebral edema, or brain swelling, is an increase in tissue volume secondary to abnormal fluid accumulation. There are two types of brain edema: vasogenic and cytotoxic.[1,17] Vasogenic edema occurs when integrity of the blood-brain barrier is disrupted, allowing fluid to escape into the extracellular fluid that surrounds brain cells. Cytotoxic edema involves the actual swelling of brain cells themselves. Brain edema may or may not increase ICP. The impact of brain edema depends on the brain's compensatory mechanisms and the extent of the swelling.

Vasogenic Edema. Vasogenic edema occurs with conditions that impair the function of the blood-brain barrier and allow transfer of water and protein from the vascular into the interstitial space. It occurs in conditions such as tumors, prolonged ischemia, hemorrhage, brain injury, and infectious processes (*e.g.,* meningitis). Vasogenic edema occurs primarily in the white matter of the brain, possibly because the white matter is more compliant than the gray matter. Vasogenic edema can displace a cerebral hemisphere and can be responsible for various types of herniation. The functional manifestations of vasogenic edema include focal neurologic deficits, disturbances in consciousness, and severe intracranial hypertension.

Cytotoxic Edema. Cytotoxic edema involves an increase in intracellular fluid. It can result from hypo-osmotic states such as water intoxication or severe ischemia that impair the function of the sodium-potassium membrane pump. Ischemia also results in the inadequate removal of anaerobic metabolic end products such as lactic acid, producing extracellular acidosis. If blood flow is reduced to low levels for extended periods or to extremely low levels for a few minutes, cellular edema can cause the cell membrane to rupture, allowing the escape of intracellular contents into the surrounding extracellular fluid. This leads to damage of neighboring cells. The altered osmotic conditions result in water entry and cell swelling. Major changes in cerebral function, such as stupor and coma, occur with cytotoxic edema. The edema associated with ischemia may be severe enough to produce cerebral infarction with necrosis of brain tissue.

Treatment. Although cerebral edema is viewed as a pathologic process, it does not necessarily disrupt brain function unless it increases the ICP. The localized edema surrounding a brain tumor often responds to corticosteroid therapy (*e.g.,* dexamethasone), but use of these drugs for generalized edema is controversial. The mechanism of action of the corticosteroid drugs in the treatment of cerebral edema is unknown, but in therapeutic doses, they seem to stabilize cell membranes and scavenge free radicals. Osmotic diuretics (*e.g.,* mannitol) may be useful in the acute phase of vasogenic and cytotoxic edema when hypo-osmolarity is present.

Hydrocephalus

Enlargement of the CSF compartment occurs with hydrocephalus, which is defined as an abnormal increase in CSF volume in any part or all of the ventricular system. The two causes of hydrocephalus are decreased absorption of CSF and overproduction of CSF. There are two types of hydrocephalus: noncommunicating and communicating.

Noncommunicating or obstructive hydrocephalus occurs when obstruction in the ventricular system prevents the CSF from reaching the arachnoid villi. CSF flow can be obstructed by congenital malformations, from tumors encroaching on the ventricular system, and by inflammation or hemorrhage. The ependyma (*i.e.,* lining of ventricles and CSF-filled spaces) is especially sensitive to viral infections, particularly during embryonic development; ependymitis is believed to be the cause of congenital aqueductal stenosis.[4]

Communicating hydrocephalus is caused by impaired reabsorption of CSF from the arachnoid villi into the venous system. Decreased absorption can result from a block in the CSF pathway to the arachnoid villi or a failure of the villi to transfer the CSF to the venous system. It can occur if too few villi are formed, if postinfective (meningitis) scarring occludes them, or if the villi become obstructed with fragments of blood or infectious debris. Adenomas of the choroid plexus can cause an overproduction of CSF. This form of hydrocephalus is much less common than that resulting from decreased absorption of CSF.

Similar pathologic patterns occur with noncommunicating and communicating types of hydrocephalus. The cerebral hemispheres become enlarged, and the ventricular system beyond the point of obstruction is dilated. The sulci on the surface of the brain become effaced and shallow, and the white matter is reduced in volume. The presence and extent of the ICP is determined by fluid accumulation and the type of hydrocephalus, the age at onset, and the rapidity and extent of pressure rise. Computed tomographic (CT) and magnetic resonance imaging (MRI) scans are used to diagnose all types of hydrocephalus. The usual treatment is a shunting procedure, which provides an alternative route for return of CSF to the circulation

Signs and symptoms of hydrocephalus vary greatly, depending on the rapidity of onset. When hydrocephalus develops in utero or before the cranial sutures have fused in infancy, the ventricles expand beyond the point of obstruction, the cranial sutures separate, the head expands, and there is bulging of the fontanels (Fig. 51-5). Because the skull is able to expand, signs of increased ICP may be absent, and intelligence spared. However, seizures are not uncommon, and in severe cases, optic nerve atrophy leads to blindness. Weakness and uncoordinated movement are common. Surgical placement of a shunt allows for diversion of excess CSF fluid, preventing extreme enlargement of the head and neurologic deficits.

In adults, head enlargement does not occur because the cranial sutures are fully fused. Thus, signs and symptoms are likely. Slowly developing hydrocephalus is unlikely to produce an increase in ICP, but it may still produce deficits such as progressive dementia and gait changes, as in normal-pressure hydrocephalus ("pseudotumor cerebri") in the elderly. In contrast, acute-onset hydrocephalus in adults usually is marked by symptoms of increased ICP, including headache, vomiting, and papilledema or lateral rectus palsy from pressure effects on the cranial nerves. If the obstruction is not relieved, progression to herniation ensues (see previous discussion of herniation). Treatment includes surgical decompression and shunting.

Head Injury

The brain is enclosed in the protective confines of the rigid bony skull. Although the skull generally affords protection to the soft tissues of the CNS from external forces, it also imposes risks as a source of injury from internal forces. The bony structures of the internal surface of the skull can induce traumatic and ischemic brain injuries when intracranial tissues increase in volume (swelling or bleeding) or shift (swelling or mechanical trauma). Furthermore, fractures of the skull can compress sections of the nervous system and cause penetrating wounds.

The term *head injury* is used to describe all structural damage to the head and has become synonymous with *traumatic brain injury*.[18,19] Head injury is the leading cause of death and disability among persons younger than 24 years of age. The main causes of head injury are road accidents, falls, and assaults, with the most common cause of fatal head injuries being road accidents involving vehicles and pedestrians.[20]

Head injuries can involve both closed injuries and open wounds. Skull fractures can be divided into three groups: simple, depressed, and basilar. A simple or linear skull fracture is

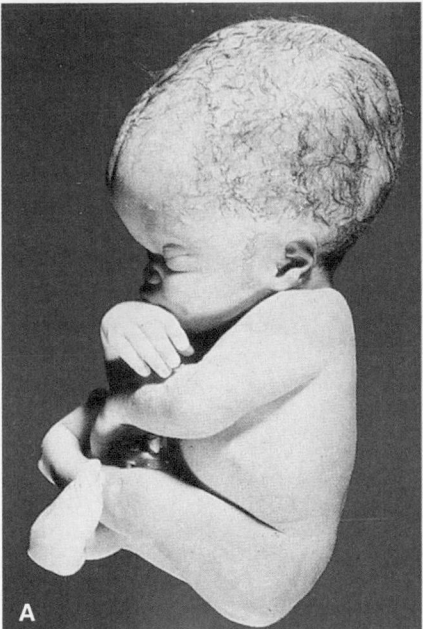 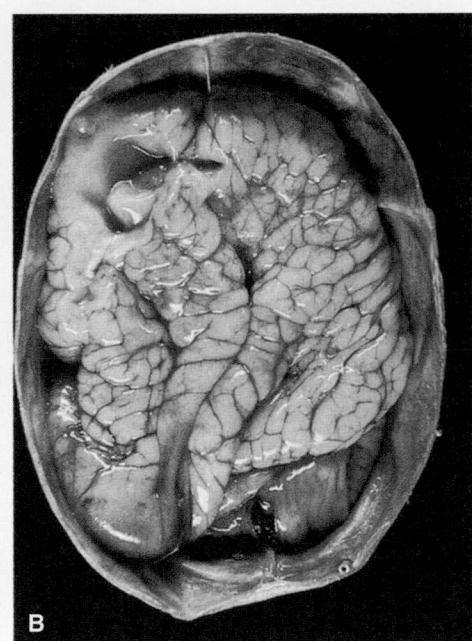

FIGURE 51-5 • Congenital hydrocephalus. (**A**) Hydrocephalus occurring before the fusion of the cranial sutures causes pronounced enlargement of the head. (**B**) Removal of the calvarium demonstrates an atrophic and collapsed cerebral cortex. (From Rubin E., Farber J. L. [1999]. *Pathology* [3rd ed., p. 1454]. Philadelphia: Lippincott-Raven.)

a break in the continuity of bone. A comminuted skull fracture refers to a splintered or multiple fracture line. When bone fragments are embedded into the brain tissue, the fracture is said to be depressed. A fracture of the bones that form the base of the skull is called a basilar skull fracture.

Radiologic examination usually is needed to confirm the presence and extent of a skull fracture. This evaluation is important because of the possible damage to the underlying tissues. The ethmoid cribriform plate, through which the olfactory fibers enter the skull, represents the most fragile portion of the neurocranium and is shattered in basal skull fractures. A frequent complication of basilar skull fractures is leakage of CSF from the nose (rhinorrhea) or ear (otorrhea); this occurs because of the proximity of the base of the skull to the nose and ears. This break in protection of the brain becomes a probable source of infection of the meninges or of brain substance. There may be lacerations to the vessels of the dura, with resultant intracranial bleeding. Skull fractures can damage the cranial nerves (I, II, III, VII, and VIII) as they exit the cranial vault.

Types of Brain Injuries

The effects of traumatic head injuries can be divided into two categories: primary or direct injuries, in which damage is caused by impact; and secondary injuries, in which damage results from the subsequent brain swelling, infection, or cerebral hypoxia. The direct brain injuries include diffuse axonal injury and the focal lesions of laceration, contusion, and hemorrhage. Secondary brain injuries are often diffuse or multifocal, including concussion, infection, and hypoxic brain injury. Although the skull and CSF provide protection for the brain, they also can contribute to trauma. When the mechanical forces inducing head injury cause bouncing of the brain in the closed confines

of the rigid skull, a coup–contrecoup injury occurs. Because the brain floats freely in the CSF, blunt force to the head accelerates the brain within the skull, and then the brain decelerates abruptly on hitting the inner skull surfaces (Fig. 51-6). The direct contusion of the brain at the site of external force is referred to as a *coup* injury, whereas the rebound injury on the opposite side of the brain is the *contrecoup* injury. As the brain strikes the rough surface of the cranial vault, brain tissue, blood vessels, nerve tracts, and other structures are bruised and torn, resulting in contusions and hematomas.

Ischemia is considered the most common cause of secondary brain injury. It can result from the hypoxia and hypotension that occur during the resuscitation process or from the impairment of regulatory mechanisms by which cerebrovascular responses maintain an adequate blood flow and oxygen supply.[21,22] Insults that occur immediately after injury or in the course of resuscitation efforts are important determinants of the outcome from severe brain injury. More than 25% of patients with severe head injury sustain one or more secondary insults in the time between injury and resuscitation, indicating the need for improved airway management and circulatory status.[21] The significance of secondary injuries depends on the extent of damage caused by the primary injury. Certain secondary injuries have been discussed, such as increased ICP, cerebral edema, and brain herniation.

In mild head injury, there may be momentary loss of consciousness without demonstrable neurologic symptoms or residual damage, except for possible residual amnesia. Microscopic changes usually can be detected in the neurons and glia within hours of injury, but brain imaging is negative. Concussion refers to "an immediate and transient loss of consciousness accompanied by a brief period of amnesia after a blow to the head."[23] Although recovery usually takes place within 24 hours,

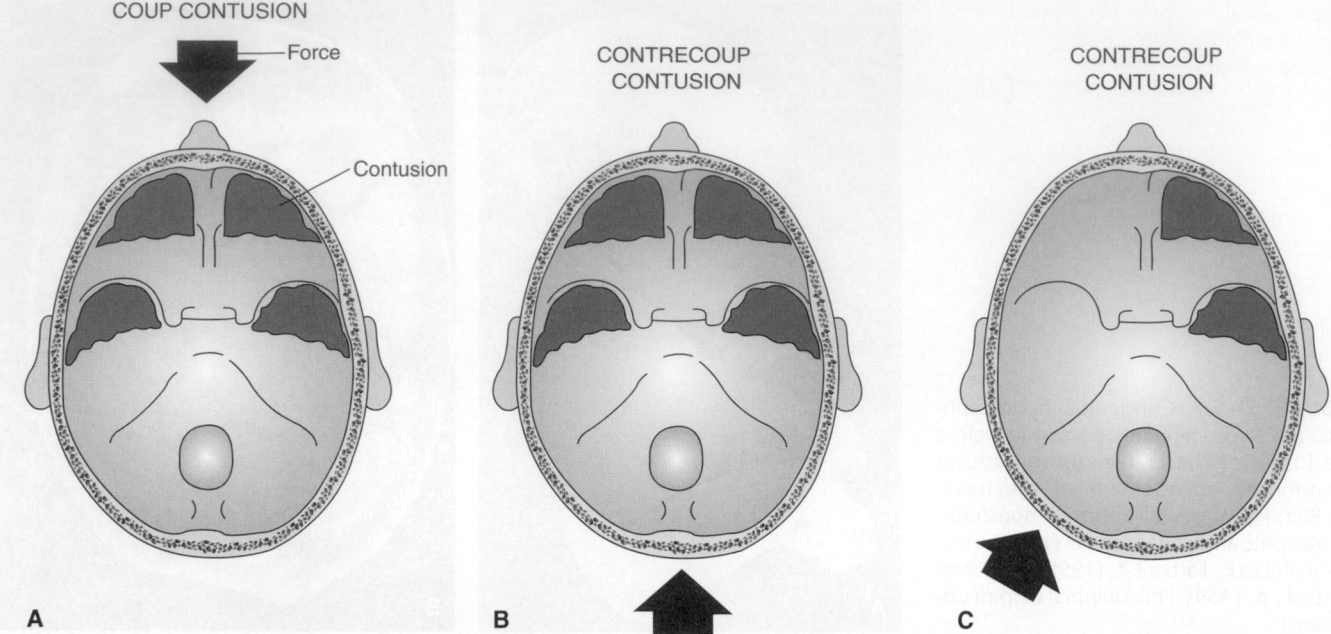

FIGURE 51-6 • Mechanisms of cerebral contusion in coup–contrecoup injuries. **(A)** A focal area of cerebral injury (coup contusion) at the point of impact. The cerebral hemispheres float in the cerebrospinal fluid. **(B)** Rapid deceleration or, less commonly, acceleration, causes the cortex to impact forcefully into the anterior and middle fossa, causing injury to the side of the brain opposite the site of injury (contrecoup contusion). **(C)** The position of a contrecoup contusion is determined by the direction of force and the intracranial anatomy. (Courtesy of Dmitri Karetnikov, artist.) (From Trojanowsi J. Q., Kenyon L. [2008]. The central nervous system. In Rubin R., Strayer D. E. [Eds.], *Rubin's pathology: Clinicopathologic foundations of medicine* [5th ed., p. 1186]. Philadelphia: Lippincott Williams & Wilkins.)

mild symptoms, such as headache, irritability, insomnia, and poor concentration and memory, may persist for months. This is known as the *postconcussion syndrome*. The memory loss usually includes an interval of time preceding the accident (retrograde amnesia) and after the injury (anterograde amnesia). The duration of retrograde amnesia correlates with the severity of the brain injury. Because these cognitive complaints are vague and subjective, they sometimes are regarded as being of psychological origin. Postconcussion syndrome can have a significant effect on activities of daily living and return to employment. Persons with postconcussion syndrome may need cognitive retraining, medications, or psychological support.

In moderate head injury, many small hemorrhages and some swelling of brain tissue occur. These contusions often are distributed along the rough, irregular inner surface of the brain and are more likely to occur in the frontal or temporal lobes, resulting in cognitive and motor deficits. Moderate head injury is characterized by a period of unconsciousness and may be associated with focal manifestations such as hemiparesis, aphasia, and cranial nerve palsy. In this type of injury, the contusions often can be visualized on CT scan.

Severe head injury involves extensive mechanical and secondary damage to brain structures and always deficits in arousal, usually coma. In severe head injury, the mechanical injury is instantaneous and irreversible, resulting from shearing and pressure forces that cause diffuse axonal injury, disruption of blood

vessels, and tissue damage. Contusions and intracerebral, subdural, epidural, and subarachnoid hemorrhages are often evident on CT scan. It often is accompanied by severe neurologic deficits such as coma, hemiplegia, and all the other signs of elevated ICP (see earlier). Severe head injuries often occur with injury to other parts of the body such as the extremities, chest, and abdomen, which often limits the examiner's ability to carefully assess the neurologic deficits.

Hematomas

Hematomas result from vascular injury and bleeding. Depending on the anatomic position of the ruptured vessel, bleeding can occur in any of several compartments, including the epidural, subdural, and subarachnoid spaces or into the brain itself (intracerebral hematoma).

Epidural Hematoma. Epidural hematomas usually are caused by head injury in which the skull is fractured. An epidural (extradural) hematoma is one that develops between the inner table of the bones of the skull and the dura (Fig. 51-7). It usually results from a tear in an artery, most often the middle meningeal, usually in association with a skull fracture.[1] Because bleeding is arterial in origin, rapid expansion of the hematoma compresses the brain. Epidural hematoma is more common in a young person because the dura is less firmly attached to the skull surface

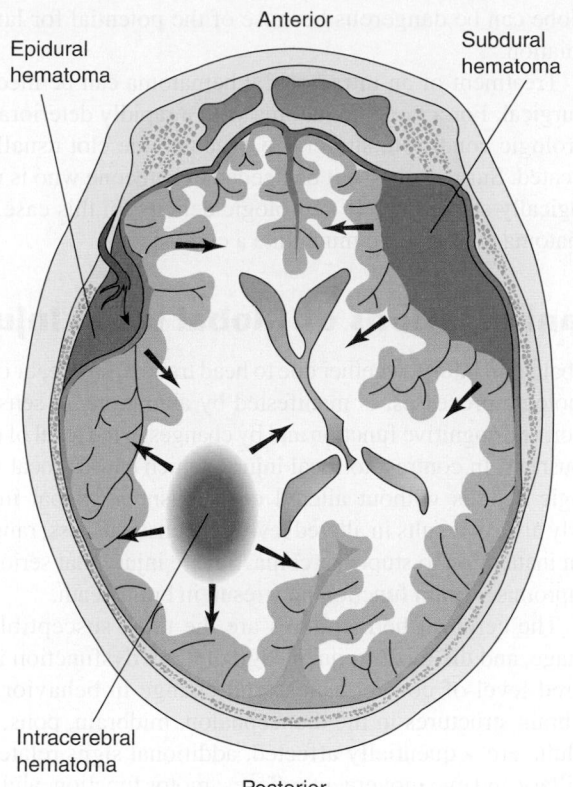

FIGURE 51-7 • Location of epidural, subdural, and intracerebral hematomas.

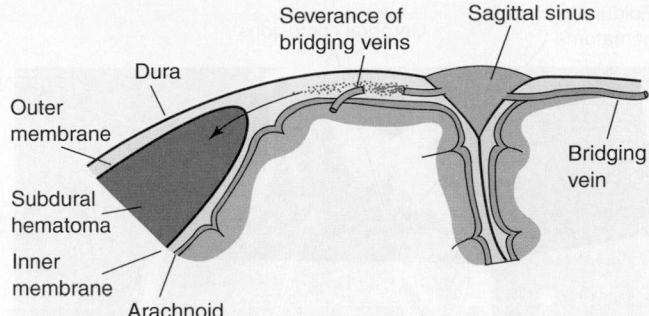

FIGURE 51-8 • Mechanism of bleeding in subdural hematoma. (Courtesy of Dmitri Karetnikov, artist.) (From Trojanowsi J. Q., Kenyon L. [2008]. The central nervous system. In Rubin R., Strayer D. E. [Eds.], *Rubin's pathology: Clinicopathologic foundations of medicine* [5th ed., p. 1184]. Philadelphia: Lippincott Williams & Wilkins.)

than in an older person; as a consequence, the dura can be easily separated from the inner surface of the skull, allowing the hematoma to grow.

Typically, a person with an epidural hematoma presents with a history of head injury and a brief period of unconsciousness followed by a lucid period in which consciousness is regained, followed by rapid progression to unconsciousness. The lucid interval does not always occur, but when it does, it is of great diagnostic value. With rapidly developing unconsciousness, there are focal symptoms related to the area of the brain involved. These symptoms can include ipsilateral (same side) pupil dilation and contralateral (opposite side) hemiparesis from uncal herniation. If the hematoma is not removed, the condition progresses, with increased ICP, tentorial herniation, and death. However, prognosis is excellent if the hematoma is removed before loss of consciousness occurs.

Subdural Hematoma. A subdural hematoma develops in the area between the dura and the arachnoid (subdural space) and usually is the result of a tear in the small bridging veins that connect veins on the surface of the cortex to dural sinuses. The bridging veins pass from the pial vessels through the CSF-filled subarachnoid space, penetrate the arachnoid and the dura, and empty into the intradural sinuses.[4] These veins are readily snapped in head injury when the brain moves suddenly in relation to the cranium (Fig. 51-8). Bleeding can occur between the dura and arachnoid (*i.e.*, subdural hematoma)

or into the CSF-filled subarachnoid space (*i.e.*, subarachnoid hematoma).

The venous source of bleeding in a subdural hematoma develops more slowly than the arterial bleeding in an epidural hematoma. Subdural hematomas are classified as acute, subacute, or chronic. This classification system is based on the approximate time before the appearance of symptoms. Symptoms of acute hematoma are seen within 24 hours of the injury, whereas subacute hematoma does not produce symptoms until 2 to 10 days after injury. Symptoms of chronic subdural hematoma may not arise until several weeks after the injury.

Acute subdural hematomas progress rapidly and have a high mortality rate because of the severe secondary injuries related to edema and increased ICP. The high mortality rate has been associated with uncontrolled ICP increase, loss of consciousness, decerebrate posturing, and delay in surgical removal of the hematoma. The clinical picture is similar to that of epidural hematoma, except that there usually is no lucid interval. Morbidity and mortality rates are higher with acute subdural hematoma than with epidural and intracerebral hematoma. By contrast, in subacute hematoma, there may be a period of improvement in the level of consciousness and neurologic symptoms, only to be followed by deterioration if the hematoma is not removed.

Symptoms of chronic subdural hematoma develop weeks after a head injury, so much later that the person may not remember having had a head injury. Chronic subdural hematoma is more common in older persons because brain atrophy causes the brain to shrink away from the dura and stretch fragile bridging veins. These veins rupture, causing slow seepage of blood into the subdural space. Fibroblastic activity causes the hematoma to become encapsulated. The sanguineous fluid in this encapsulated area has high osmotic pressure and draws in fluid from the surrounding subarachnoid space; the mass expands, exerting pressure on the cranial contents. In some instances, the clinical picture is less defined, with the most prominent symptom being a decreasing level of consciousness indicated by drowsiness, confusion, headache, and apathy.

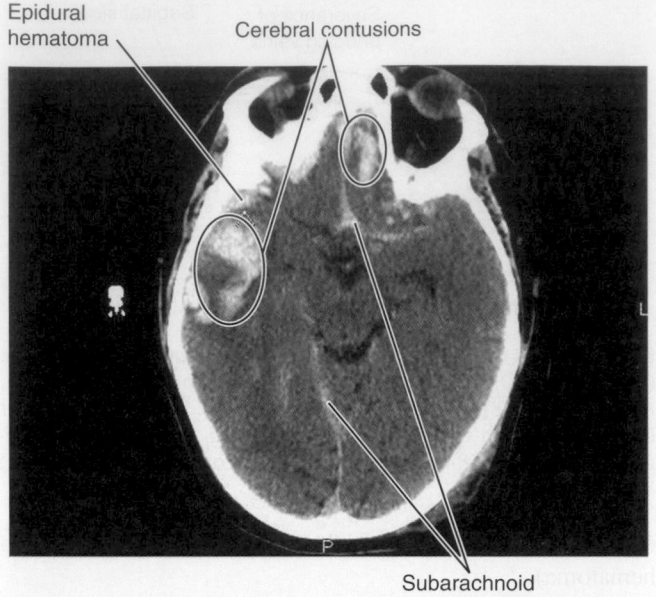

Epidural hematoma

Cerebral contusions

Subarachnoid hemorrhage

FIGURE 51-9 • Computed tomography scan of brain in traumatic brain injury, showing hemorrhagic cerebral contusions in right temporal and bifrontal lobes, subarachnoid hemorrhage, and epidural hematoma.

Traumatic Intracerebral Hematomas. Traumatic intracerebral hematomas may be single or multiple. They can occur in any lobe of the brain but are most common in the frontal or temporal lobes, related to the bony prominences on the inner skull surface (Fig. 51-9). They may occur in association with the severe motion that the brain undergoes during head injury, or a contusion can coalesce into a hematoma. Intracerebral hematomas occur more frequently in older persons and alcoholics, whose cerebral vessels are more friable.

The signs and symptoms produced by an intracerebral hematoma depend on its size and location in the brain. Signs of increased ICP can be manifested if the hematoma is large and encroaching on vital structures. A hematoma in the tempo-

ral lobe can be dangerous because of the potential for lateral herniation.

Treatment of an intracerebral hematoma can be medical or surgical. For a large hematoma with a rapidly deteriorating neurologic condition, surgery to evacuate the clot usually is indicated. Surgery may not be needed in someone who is neurologically stable despite neurologic deficits; in this case, the hematoma may resolve much like a contusion.

Manifestations of Global Brain Injury

Global brain injury, whether due to head trauma, stroke, or other pathologic processes, is manifested by alterations in sensory, motor, and cognitive function and by changes in the level of consciousness. In contrast to focal injury, which causes focal neurologic deficits without altered consciousness, global injury nearly always results in altered levels of consciousness, ranging from inattention to stupor or coma. Severe injury that seriously compromises brain function may result in brain death.

The cerebral hemispheres are the most susceptible to damage, and the most frequent sign of brain dysfunction is an altered level of consciousness and change in behavior. As the brain structures in the diencephalon, midbrain, pons, and medulla are sequentially affected, additional signs related to pupillary and eye movement reflexes, motor function, and respiration become evident (Table 51-3). Hemodynamic and respiratory instability are the last signs to occur because their regulatory centers are located low in the medulla.

In progressive brain deterioration, the person's neurologic capabilities appear to deteriorate in stepwise fashion. Similarly, as neurologic function returns, there appears to be stepwise progress to higher levels of consciousness. Deterioration of brain function from supratentorial lesions tends to follow a rostral-to-caudal stepwise progression, which is observed as the brain initially compensates for injury and subsequently decompensates with loss of autoregulation and cerebral perfusion. Infratentorial (brain stem) lesions may lead to an early, sometimes abrupt disturbance in consciousness without any orderly rostrocaudal progression of neurologic signs.

TABLE 51-3 **Key Signs in Rostral-to-Caudal Progression of Brain Lesions**	
LEVEL OF BRAIN INJURY	**KEY CLINICAL SIGNS**
Diencephalon	Impaired consciousness; small, reactive pupils; intact oculocephalic reflex; decorticate posturing; Cheyne-Stokes respirations
Midbrain	Coma; fixed, midsize pupils; impaired oculocephalic reflex; neurogenic hyperventilation; decerebrate posturing
Pons	Coma; fixed, irregular pupils; dysconjugate gaze; impaired cold caloric stimulation; loss of corneal reflex; hemiparesis/quadriparesis; decerebrate posturing; apneustic respirations
Medulla	Coma; fixed pupils, flaccidity, loss of gag and cough reflexes, ataxic/apneic respirations

BRAIN INJURY AND LEVELS OF CONSCIOUSNESS

- Consciousness is a global function that depends on a diffuse neural network that includes activity of the reticular activating system (RAS) and both cerebral hemispheres.

- Impaired consciousness implies diffuse brain injury to the RAS at any level (medulla through thalamus) or both cerebral hemispheres simultaneously.

- In contrast, local brain injury causes focal neurologic deficit but does not disrupt consciousness.

Altered Levels of Consciousness

All forms of brain injury and disease can lead to altered levels of consciousness. Consciousness is the state of awareness of self and the environment and of being able to orient to new stimuli.[16,24] It has traditionally been divided into two components: (1) arousal and wakefulness, and (2) content and cognition.[25] The content and cognition aspects of consciousness are determined by a functioning cerebral cortex. Arousal and wakefulness require the concurrent functioning of both cerebral hemispheres and an intact RAS in the brain stem.

Anatomic and Physiologic Basis of Consciousness. The reticular formation is a diffuse, primitive system of interlacing nerve cells and fibers in the brain stem that receive input from multiple sensory pathways (Fig. 51-10). Anatomically, the reticular formation constitutes the central core of the brain stem, extending from the medulla through the pons to the midbrain, which is

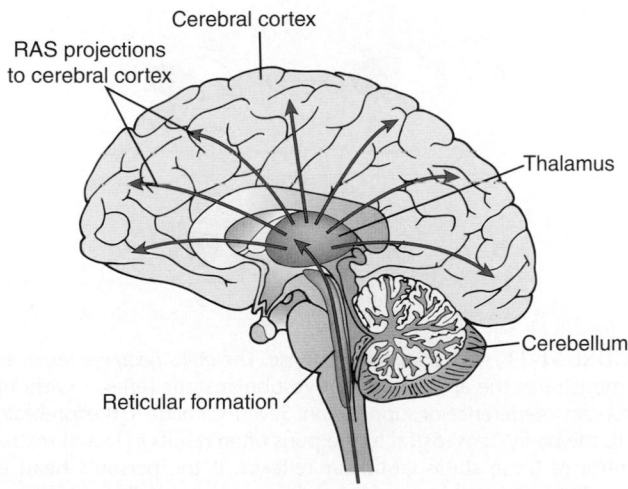

FIGURE 51-10 • The brain stem reticular formation and reticular activating system (RAS). Ascending sensory tracts send axon collateral fibers to the reticular formation. These give rise to fibers synapsing in the nonspecific nuclei of the thalamus. From there, the nonspecific thalamic projections influence widespread areas of the cerebral cortex and limbic system.

continuous caudally with the spinal cord and rostrally with the subthalamus, the hypothalamus, and the thalamus.[26] Fibers from the RAS also project to the autonomic nervous system and motor systems. The hypothalamus plays a predominant role in maintaining homeostasis through integration of somatic, visceral, and endocrine functions. Inputs from the reticular formation, vestibulospinal projections, and other motor systems are integrated to provide a continuously adapting background of muscle tone and posture to facilitate voluntary motor actions. Reticular formation neurons that function in regulation of cardiovascular, respiratory, and other visceral functions are intermingled with those that maintain other reticular formation functions.

Ascending fibers of the reticular formation, known as the ascending RAS, transmit activating information to all parts of the cerebral cortex. The flow of information in the ascending RAS activates the hypothalamic and limbic structures that regulate emotional and behavioral responses such as those that occur in response to pain and loud noises, and they exert facilitatory effects on cortical neurons. Without cortical activation, a person is less reactive to environmental stimuli, and the level of consciousness is reduced.

The pathways for the ascending RAS travel from the medulla through the midbrain, such that lesions of the brain stem can interrupt RAS activity, leading to altered levels of consciousness and coma. Any deficit in level of consciousness, from mild confusion to stupor or coma, indicates either direct injury to the RAS or to both cerebral hemispheres concurrently. For example, consciousness may decline owing to severe systemic metabolic derangements that affect both hemispheres, or from head trauma causing shear injuries to white matter of both the RAS and the cerebral hemispheres. Brain injuries that affect a hemisphere unilaterally and also spare the RAS, such as cerebral infarction, usually do not cause impaired consciousness.

Levels of Consciousness. Levels of consciousness reflect awareness and response to the environment. A fully conscious person is totally aware of her or his surroundings and able to react to stimuli in the environment.[16] Levels of consciousness exist on a continuum that includes consciousness, confusion, delirium, obtundation, stupor, and coma (Table 51-4).

The earliest signs of diminution in level of consciousness are inattention, mild confusion, disorientation, and blunted responsiveness. With further deterioration, the delirious person becomes markedly inattentive and variably lethargic or agitated. The person may progress to become obtunded and may respond only to vigorous or noxious stimuli.

Because of its simplicity of application, the Glasgow Coma Scale has gained almost universal acceptance as a method for assessing the level of consciousness in persons with brain injury[27,28] (Table 51-5). Numbered scores are given to responses of eye opening, verbal utterances, and motor responses. The total score is the sum of the best response in each category.

Other Manifestations of Deteriorating Brain Function

Additional elements in the initial neurologic evaluation of a person with brain injury include checking for abnormalities in

TABLE 51-4 Descending Levels of Consciousness and Their Characteristics

LEVEL OF CONSCIOUSNESS	CHARACTERISTICS
Confusion	Disturbance of consciousness characterized by impaired ability to think clearly, and to perceive, respond to, and remember current stimuli; also disorientation
Delirium	State of disturbed consciousness with motor restlessness, transient hallucinations, disorientation, and sometimes delusions
Obtundation	Disorder of decreased alertness with associated psychomotor retardation
Stupor	A state in which the person is not unconscious but exhibits little or no spontaneous activity
Coma	A state of being unarousable and unresponsive to external stimuli or internal needs; often determined by the Glasgow Coma Scale

Data from Bates D. (1993). The management of medical coma. *Journal of Neurology, Neurosurgery, and Psychiatry* 56, 590.

the size of the pupils and their reaction to light, evidence of decorticate or decerebrate posturing, and altered patterns of respiration.

Pupillary Reflexes and Eye Movements. Although the pupils may initially respond briskly to light, they become unreactive and dilated as brain function deteriorates. A bilateral loss of the pupillary light response is indicative of lesions of the brain stem. A unilateral loss of the pupillary light response may be due to a lesion of the optic or oculomotor pathways. The oculocephalic reflex (doll's-head eye movement) can be used to determine whether the brain stem centers for eye

movement are intact (Fig. 51-11). If the oculocephalic reflex is inconclusive, and if there are no contraindications, the oculovestibular test (*i.e.,* cold caloric test, in which cold water is instilled into the ear canal) may be used to elicit nystagmus (see Chapter 55).

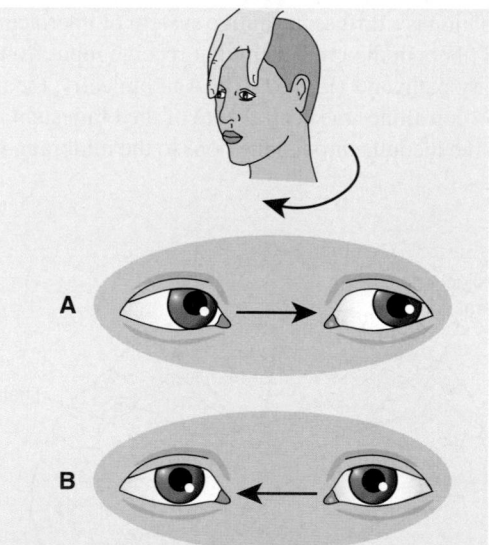

TABLE 51-5 The Glasgow Coma Scale

TEST	SCORE*
Eye Opening (E)	
Spontaneous	4
To call	3
To pain	2
None	1
Motor Response (M)	
Obeys commands	6
Localizes pain	5
Normal flexion (withdrawal)	4
Abnormal flexion (decorticate)	3
Extension (decerebrate)	2
None (flaccid)	1
Verbal Response (V)	
Oriented	5
Confused conversation	4
Inappropriate words	3
Incomprehensible sounds	2
None	1

*GCS Score = E + M + V. Best possible score = 15; worst possible score = 3.

FIGURE 51-11 • Doll's head response. The *doll's-head eye response* demonstrates the always-present vestibular static reflexes without forebrain interference or suppression. Severe damage to the forebrain or to the brain stem rostral to the pons often results in loss of rostral control of these static vestibular reflexes. If the person's head is moved from side to side or up and down, the eyes will move in conjugate gaze to the opposite side (**A**), much like those of a doll with counterweighted eyes. If the doll's-head phenomenon is observed, brain stem function at the level of the pons is considered intact (in a comatose person). In the unconscious person without intact brain stem function and vestibular static reflexes, the eyes stay in mid-position (fixed) or turn in the same direction (**B**) as the head is turned.

Decorticate and Decerebrate Posturing. With the early onset of unconsciousness, there is some combative and purposeful movement in response to pain. As coma progresses, noxious stimuli can initiate rigidity and abnormal postures if the motor tracts are interrupted at specific levels. These abnormal postures are classified as decorticate and decerebrate.[13] Decorticate (flexion) posturing is characterized by flexion of the arms, wrists, and fingers, with abduction of the upper extremities, internal rotation, and plantar flexion of the lower extremities (see Fig. 51-4A). Decorticate posturing results from lesions of the cerebral hemisphere or internal capsule. Decerebrate (extensor) posturing results from increased muscle excitability (see Fig. 51-4B). It is characterized by rigidity of the arms with palms of the hands turned away from the body and with stiffly extended legs and plantar flexion of the feet. This response occurs with rostral-to-caudal deterioration, when lesions of the diencephalon extend to involve the midbrain and upper brain stem. Both decerebrate and decorticate posturing are poor prognostic signs.

Respiratory Responses. Early respiratory changes include yawning and sighing, with progression to Cheyne-Stokes breathing. With progression of injury continuing to the midbrain, respirations change to neurogenic hyperventilation, in which the frequency of respirations may exceed 40 breaths per minute because of uninhibited stimulation of inspiratory and expiratory centers. With medullary involvement, respirations become ataxic (i.e., totally uncoordinated and irregular). Apnea may occur because of a lack of responsiveness to carbon dioxide stimulation. Complete ventilatory assistance is often required at this point.

Brain Death

Brain death is defined as the irreversible loss of function of the brain, including the brain stem.[29] Irreversibility implies that brain death cannot be reversed. Some conditions such as drug and metabolic intoxication can cause cessation of brain functions that is completely reversible, even when they produce clinical cessation of brain functions and electroencephalographic (EEG) silence. This needs to be excluded before declaring a person brain dead.

With advances in scientific knowledge and technology that have provided the means for artificially maintaining ventilatory and circulatory function, the definition of death has had to be continually reexamined. In 1995, the Quality of Standards Subcommittee of the American Academy of Neurology published the clinical parameters for determining brain death and procedures for testing persons older than 18 years of age.[30] According to these parameters, "brain death is the absence of clinical brain function when the proximate cause is known and demonstrably irreversible."[30] Clinical examination must disclose at least the absence of responsiveness, brain stem reflexes, and respiratory effort. Brain death is a clinical diagnosis, and a repeat evaluation at least 6 hours later is recommended.[30] Longer periods of observation of absent brain activity are required if the patient is a child, and in cases of drug overdose

(e.g., barbiturates, other CNS depressants), drug toxicity (e.g., neuromuscular blocking drugs, aminoglycoside antibiotics), and neuromuscular diseases such as myasthenia gravis, hypothermia, and shock. Medical circumstances may require use of confirmatory tests.

Medical documentation should include cause and irreversibility of the condition, absence of brain stem reflexes and motor responses to pain, absence of respiration with a PCO_2 of 60 mm Hg or more, and the justification for use of confirmatory tests and their results. Apnea is confirmed after ventilation with pure oxygen 10 minutes before withdrawal from the ventilator, followed by passive flow of oxygen. This method allows the PCO_2 to rise to 60 mm Hg after a 10-minute period of apnea, without hazardously lowering the oxygen content of the blood. If respiratory reflexes are intact, the hypercarbia that develops should stimulate ventilatory effort within 30 seconds. Spontaneous breathing efforts indicate that the brain stem is functioning. Confirmatory tests of brain death include conventional angiography (i.e., no intracerebral filling at the level of the carotid bifurcation or circle of Willis), transcranial Doppler ultrasonography, technetium-99m hexamethylpropyleneamine oxime brain scan (i.e., no uptake of isotope in brain parenchyma), somatosensory evoked potentials, and EEG. In the United States, EEG testing is often used to establish brain death. EEG testing should reveal no electrical activity during at least 30 minutes of recording that adheres to the minimal technical criteria for EEG recording in suspected brain death as adopted by the American Electroencephalographic Society (including 16-channel EEG instruments).

Persistent Vegetative State

Advances in the care of brain-injured persons during the past several decades have resulted in survival of many persons who previously would have died. Unfortunately, most persons in prolonged coma who survive evolve to what often is called the *persistent vegetative state*. The vegetative state is characterized by loss of all cognitive functions and the unawareness of self and surroundings. Reflex and vegetative functions remain, including sleep–wake cycles.[31] These individuals have spontaneous eye opening without concurrent awareness, often confusing hopeful families. Persons in the vegetative state require nonoral feeding and full nursing care.

The criteria for diagnosis of vegetative state include the absence of awareness of self and environment and an inability to interact with others; the absence of sustained or reproducible voluntary behavioral responses; lack of language comprehension; sufficiently preserved hypothalamic and brain stem function to maintain life; bowel and bladder incontinence; and variably preserved cranial nerve (e.g., pupillary, gag) and spinal cord reflexes.[31] The diagnosis of persistent vegetative state requires that the condition has continued for at least 1 month. The minimally conscious state has been more recently defined as a state of arousal similar to persistent vegetative state, but with the distinction of the objective presence of some awareness on the part of the patient.[32]

IN SUMMARY, many of the agents that cause brain damage do so through common pathways, including hypoxia or ischemia, accumulation of excitatory neurotransmitters, increased ICP, and cerebral edema. Deprivation of oxygen (*i.e.*, hypoxia) or blood flow (*i.e.*, ischemia) can have deleterious effects on the brain structures. Focal ischemia causes localized brain injury, as in stroke. Global ischemia, as in cardiac arrest, occurs when blood flow to the entire brain is inadequate, causing global deficits such as altered mental status.

The term *head injury* is used to describe all structural damage to the head and has become synonymous with *brain injury*. The effects of traumatic head injuries can be divided into two categories: primary and secondary injuries. Primary injuries result from direct impact, resulting in skull fracture, concussion, or contusion. In secondary injuries, damage results from the subsequent brain swelling; epidural, subdural, or intracerebral hematoma formation; infection; cerebral hypoxia; and ischemia. Even if there is no break in the skull, a blow to the head can cause severe and diffuse brain damage. Such closed injuries vary in severity and can be classified as focal or diffuse. Diffuse injuries include concussion and diffuse axonal injury. Focal injuries include contusion, laceration, and hemorrhage.

Brain injury is manifested by alterations in sensory and motor function and by changes in the level of consciousness. Consciousness is a state of awareness of self and environment. It exists on a continuum from normal wakefulness and sleep to the pathologic states of stupor and coma. In progressive brain injury, the onset of coma may follow a rostral-to-caudal progression with characteristic changes in levels of consciousness, respiratory activity, pupillary and oculovestibular reflexes, and muscle tone occurring as the diencephalon through the medulla are affected.

Brain death is defined as the irreversible loss of function of the brain, including that of the brain stem. Clinical examination must disclose at least the absence of responsiveness, brain stem reflexes, and respiratory effort. The vegetative state is characterized by loss of all cognitive functions and the unawareness of self and surroundings, whereas reflex and vegetative functions remain intact. ∎

CEREBROVASCULAR DISEASE

After completing this section of the chapter, you should be able to meet the following objectives:

■ List the major vessels in the cerebral circulation and state the contribution of the internal carotid arteries, the vertebral arteries, and the circle of Willis to the cerebral circulation.
■ Describe the autoregulation of cerebral blood flow.
■ Explain the substitution of "brain attack" for stroke in terms of making a case for early diagnosis and treatment.
■ Differentiate the pathologies of ischemic and hemorrhagic stroke.
■ Explain the significance of transient ischemic attacks, the ischemic penumbra, and watershed zones of infarction and how these conditions relate to ischemic stroke.
■ Cite the most common cause of subarachnoid hemorrhage and state the complications associated with subarachnoid hemorrhage.
■ Describe the alterations in cerebral vasculature that occur with arteriovenous malformations.
■ Describe the patterns of motor deficits and typical problems with speech and language that occur as a result of stroke.

Cerebrovascular disease encompasses a number of disorders involving vessels in the cerebral circulation. These disorders include stroke and transient ischemic attacks (TIAs), aneurysmal subarachnoid hemorrhage, and arteriovenous malformations.

Cerebral Circulation
Cerebral Blood Vessels

The blood flow to the brain is supplied by the two internal carotid arteries anteriorly and the vertebral arteries posteriorly (Fig. 51-12A). The internal carotid artery, a terminal branch of the common carotid artery, branches into several arteries: ophthalmic, posterior communicating, anterior choroidal, anterior cerebral, and middle cerebral (see Fig. 51-12 B). Most of the arterial blood in the internal carotid arteries is distributed through the anterior and middle cerebral arteries. The anterior cerebral arteries supply the medial surface of the frontal and parietal lobes and the anterior half of the thalamus, the corpus striatum, part of the corpus callosum, and the anterior limb of the internal capsule. The genu and posterior limb of the internal capsule and medial globus pallidus are fed by the anterior choroidal branch of the internal carotid artery. The middle cerebral artery passes laterally, supplying the lateral basal ganglia and the insula, and then emerges on the lateral cortical surface, supplying the inferior frontal gyrus, the motor and premotor frontal cortex concerned with delicate face and hand control. It is the major vascular source for the language cortices (frontal and superior temporal), the primary and association auditory cortex (superior temporal gyrus), and primary and association somesthetic cortex for the face and hand (postcentral gyrus, parietal). The middle cerebral artery is functionally a continuation of the internal carotid; emboli of the internal carotid most frequently become lodged in branches of the middle cerebral artery. The consequences of ischemia of these areas may be the most devastating, resulting in damage to the fine manipulative

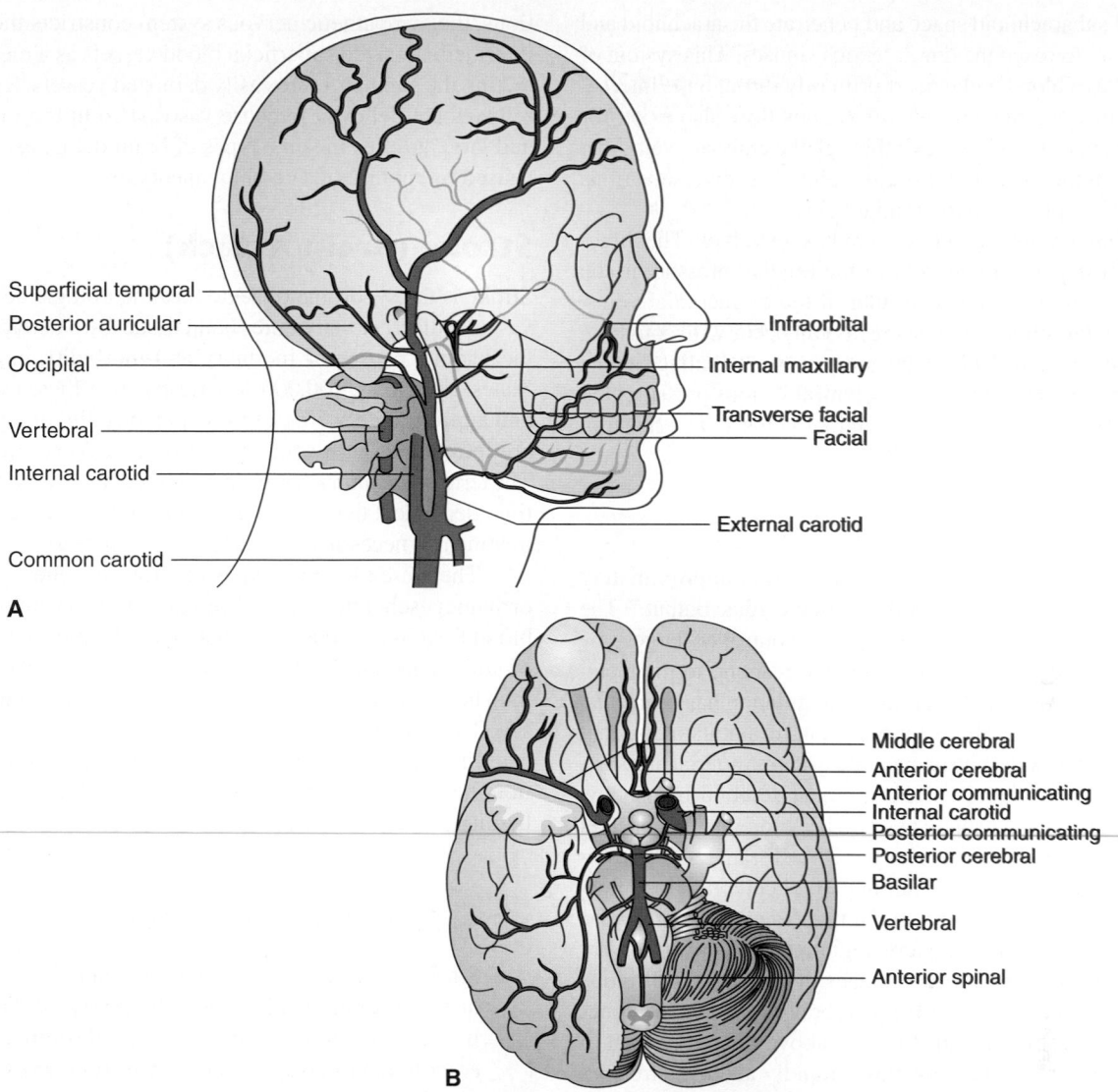

Superficial temporal
Posterior auricular
Occipital
Vertebral
Internal carotid
Common carotid

Infraorbital
Internal maxillary
Transverse facial
Facial
External carotid

A

Middle cerebral
Anterior cerebral
Anterior communicating
Internal carotid
Posterior communicating
Posterior cerebral
Basilar
Vertebral
Anterior spinal

B

FIGURE 51-12 • Cerebral circulation. **(A)** Branches of the right external carotid artery. The internal carotid artery ascends to the base of the brain. The right vertebral artery is also shown as it ascends through the transverse foramen of the cervical vertebrae. **(B)** The cerebral arterial circle (circle of Willis).

skills of the face and upper limbs and to receptive and expressive communication functions (*e.g.,* aphasia).

The two vertebral arteries arise from the subclavian artery and enter the foramina in the transverse spinal processes at the level of the sixth cervical vertebra and continue upward through the foramina of the upper six vertebrae; they wind behind the atlas and enter the skull through the foramen magnum and unite to form the basilar artery, which then diverges to terminate in the posterior cerebral arteries. Branches of the basilar and vertebral arteries supply the medulla, pons, cerebellum, midbrain, and caudal part of the diencephalon. The posterior cerebral arteries supply the remaining occipital and inferior regions of the temporal lobes and the thalamus.

The distal branches of the internal carotid and vertebral arteries communicate at the base of the brain through the circle of Willis; this anastomosis of arteries can provide contin-

ued circulation if blood flow through one of the main vessels is disrupted (see Fig. 51-12B). For instance, occlusion of one middle cerebral artery may have limited consequences if the anterior and posterior communicating arteries are patent, allowing collateral flow from the ipsilateral posterior cerebral and opposite carotid arteries. Without collateral input, cessation of blood flow in cerebral arteries results in ischemic neural damage as metabolic needs of electrically active cells exceed nutrient supply.

The cerebral circulation is drained by two sets of veins that empty into the dural venous sinuses: the deep (great) cerebral venous system and the superficial venous system. In contrast to the superficial cerebral veins that travel through the pia mater on the surface of the cerebral cortex, the deep system is well protected. These vessels connect directly to the sagittal sinuses in the falx cerebri by bridging veins. They travel through the

CSF-filled subarachnoid space and penetrate the arachnoid and then the dura to reach the dural venous sinuses. This system of sinuses returns blood to the heart primarily through the internal jugular veins. Alternate routes for venous flow also exist; for example, venous blood may exit through the emissary veins that pass through the skull and through veins that traverse various foramina to empty into extracranial veins.

The intracranial venous system has no valves. The direction of flow depends on gravity or the relative pressure in the venous sinuses compared with that of the extracranial veins. Increases in intrathoracic pressure, as can occur with coughing or performance of the Valsalva maneuver (*i.e.,* exhaling against a closed glottis), produce a rise in central venous pressure that is reflected back into the internal jugular veins and to the dural sinuses. This briefly raises the ICP.

Regulation of Cerebral Blood Flow

The blood flow to the brain is maintained at approximately 750 mL/minute or one sixth of the resting cardiac output.[15] The regulation of blood flow to the brain is controlled largely by autoregulatory or local mechanisms that respond to the metabolic needs of the brain. Cerebral autoregulation has been classically defined as the ability of the brain to maintain constant cerebral blood flow despite changes in systemic arterial pressure. This allows the cerebral cortex to adjust cerebral blood flow locally to satisfy its metabolic needs. The autoregulation of cerebral blood flow is efficient within a MABP range of approximately 60 to 140 mm Hg.[15] Although total cerebral blood flow remains relatively stable throughout marked changes in cardiac output and arterial blood pressure, regional blood flow may vary markedly in response to local changes in metabolism. If blood pressure falls below 60 mm Hg, cerebral blood flow becomes severely compromised, and if it rises above the upper limit of autoregulation, blood flow increases rapidly and overstretches the cerebral vessels. In persons with hypertension, this autoregulatory range shifts to higher MABP levels.

At least three metabolic factors affect cerebral blood flow: carbon dioxide, hydrogen ion, and oxygen concentration. Increased carbon dioxide provides a potent stimulus for vasodilation—a doubling of the PCO_2 in the blood results in a doubling of cerebral blood flow. Increased hydrogen ion concentrations also increase cerebral blood flow, serving to wash away the neurally depressive acidic materials.[15] Profound extracellular acidosis induces vasomotor paralysis, in which case cerebral blood flow may depend entirely on the systemic arterial blood pressure. Decreased oxygen concentration also increases cerebral blood flow.

The deep cerebral blood vessels appear to be completely controlled by autoregulation. However, the superficial and major cerebral blood vessels are innervated by the sympathetic nervous system. Under normal physiologic conditions, local regulatory and autoregulatory mechanisms override the effects of sympathetic stimulation. However, when local mechanisms fail, sympathetic control of cerebral blood pressure becomes important.[15] For example, when the arterial pressure rises to very high levels during strenuous exercise or in other conditions, the sympathetic nervous system constricts the large and intermediate-sized superficial blood vessels as a means of protecting the smaller, more easily damaged vessels. Sympathetic reflexes are believed to cause vasospasm in the intermediate and large arteries in some types of brain damage, such as that caused by rupture of a cerebral aneurysm.

Stroke (Brain Attack)

Stroke is the syndrome of acute focal neurologic deficit from a vascular disorder that injures brain tissue. Stroke remains one of the leading causes of mortality and morbidity in the United States. Each year, 700,000 Americans are afflicted with stroke, and approximately 20% of these persons die; many survivors are left with at least some degree of neurologic impairment.[33] The term *brain attack* has been promoted to raise awareness that time-dependent tissue damage occurs and that rapid emergency treatment is necessary, similar to that with heart attack.

There are two main types of strokes: ischemic and hemorrhagic. Ischemic strokes are caused by an interruption of blood flow in a cerebral vessel and are the most common type of stroke, accounting for 87% of all strokes.[33] The less common hemorrhagic strokes are caused by bleeding into brain tissue. This type of stroke usually is from a blood vessel rupture caused by hypertension, aneurysm, arteriovenous malformation, head injury, or blood dyscrasias and has a much higher fatality rate than ischemic strokes.

🔑 STROKE/BRAIN ATTACK

- Stroke is an acute focal neurologic deficit due to a disturbance in the blood vessels supplying the brain. It can be due to ischemia caused by thrombi or emboli that interrupt blood flow or rupture of a blood vessel with bleeding into brain tissue.

- The term *brain attack* as a description for stroke is intended to alert people to the need for immediate treatment at the first sign of a stroke.

- During the evolution of an ischemic stroke, there usually is a central core of dead or dying cells surrounded by an ischemic band of minimally perfused cells called a *penumbra*. Whether the cells of the penumbra continue to survive depends on the successful timely return of adequate circulation.

- The realization that there is a window of opportunity during which ischemic but viable brain tissue can be salvaged has led to the use of thrombolytic agents in the early treatment of ischemic stroke.

Risk Factors

Among the major risk factors for stroke are age, sex, race, family history, hypertension, smoking, diabetes mellitus, asymptomatic carotid stenosis, sickle cell disease, hyperlipidemia, and atrial fibrillation[34] (Box 51-1). The incidence of stroke increases with age, with men's stroke incidence rates being greater than women's at younger ages, but not at older ages. Because women live longer than men, more women die of stroke each year. Women accounted for 61% of U.S. stroke deaths in 2004.[33] African Americans have almost twice the risk of first-ever strokes as whites.[33] Blood pressure is a powerful determinant of stroke risk. Persons with a blood pressure less than 120/80 mm Hg have about half the lifetime risk of stroke compared with persons with hypertension.[33] Heart disease, particularly atrial fibrillation and other conditions that predispose to clot formation on the wall of the heart or valve leaflets, or to paradoxical embolism through right-to-left shunting, predisposes to cardioembolic stroke. Polycythemia, sickle cell disease (during sickle cell crisis), and blood disorders predispose to clot formation in the cerebral vessels.

Other, less well-documented risk factors include obesity, physical inactivity, alcohol and drug abuse, hypercoagulability disorders, hormone replacement therapy, and oral contraceptive use.[34] Clinical trial data indicate that estrogen plus progestin, as well as estrogen alone, increase stroke risk in postmenopausal, generally healthy women, and provide no protection for women with established heart disease.[33] Although extensively used in the past, the use for hormone therapy is no longer recommended (see Chapter 45). Alcohol can contribute to stroke in several ways: induction of cardiac arrhythmias and defects in ventricular wall motion that lead to cerebral embolism, induction of hypertension, enhancement of blood coagulation disorders, and reduction of cerebral blood flow.[35] Cocaine use causes both ischemic and hemorrhagic strokes by inducing vasospasm, enhanced platelet activity, and increased blood pressure, heart rate, body temperature, and metabolic rate. Cocaine stroke victims range in age from newborn (*i.e.,* from maternal cocaine use) to elderly.[36]

Elimination or control of risk factors for cerebrovascular disease (*e.g.,* use of tobacco, control of blood lipids and blood sugar, reduction of hypertension) offers the best opportunity to prevent cerebral ischemia from cerebral atherosclerosis. Primary prevention of stroke by early detection and treatment of modifiable risk factors offers significant advantages over waiting until a serious event has occurred.

Ischemic Stroke

Ischemic strokes are caused by cerebrovascular obstruction by thrombosis or emboli (Fig. 51-13). Various methods have been used to classify ischemic cerebrovascular disease. A common classification system identifies the five main mechanisms of stroke as stroke subtypes and their frequency: 20% large artery atherosclerotic disease (both thrombosis and arterial emboli); 25% small vessel or penetrating artery disease (so-called lacunar stroke); 20% cardiogenic embolism; 30% cryptogenic stroke (undetermined cause); and 5% other, unusual causes[37] (*i.e.,* migraine, vessel dissection, coagulopathy).

Ischemic Penumbra in Evolving Stroke. During the evolution of a stroke, there usually is a central core of dead or dying cells, surrounded by an ischemic band or area of minimally

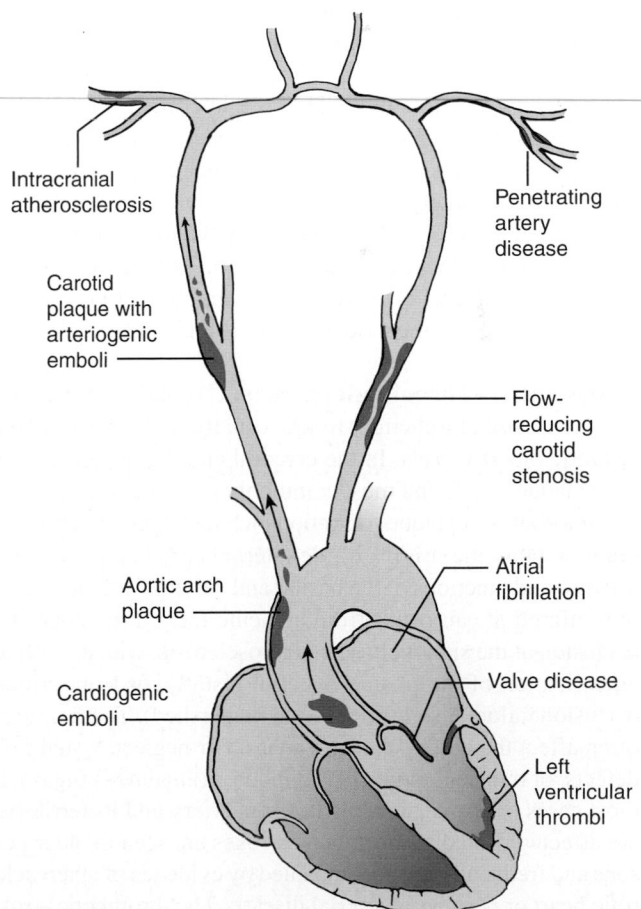

FIGURE 51-13 • The most frequent sites of arterial and cardiac abnormalities causing ischemic stroke. (From Albers G. W., Easton D., Sacco R. L., et al. [2001]. Antithrombotic and thrombotic therapy for ischemic stroke. *Chest* 119, 301S.)

perfused cells called the *penumbra* ("halo"). Brain cells of the penumbra receive marginal blood flow, and their metabolic activities are impaired; although the area undergoes an "electrical failure," the structural integrity of the brain cells is maintained.[38] Whether the cells of the penumbra continue to survive depends on the successful timely return of adequate circulation, the volume of toxic products released by the neighboring dying cells, the degree of cerebral edema, and alterations in local blood flow. If the toxic products result in additional death of cells in the penumbra, the core of dead or dying tissue enlarges, and the volume of surrounding ischemic tissue increases.

Transient Ischemic Attacks. Transient ischemic attacks are characterized by focal ischemic cerebral neurologic deficits that last for less than 24 hours (usually less than 1 to 2 hours).[39] A TIA or "ministroke" is equivalent to "brain angina" and reflects a temporary disturbance in focal cerebral blood flow, which reverses before infarction occurs, analogous to angina in relation to heart attack. The term *TIA* and the qualification of a deficit resolving within 24 hours were defined before the mechanisms of ischemic cell damage and the penumbra were known. A more accurate definition now is a deficit lasting less than 1 hour, and it may best be described as a zone of penumbra without central infarction. The causes of TIAs are the same as those of ischemic stroke and include atherosclerotic disease of cerebral vessels and emboli. TIAs are important because they may provide warning of impending stroke. In fact, the risk for stroke after a TIA is similar to the risk after a first stroke and is maximal immediately after the event: 4% to 8% risk for stroke within 1 month, 12% to 13% risk during the first year, and 24% to 29% risk over 5 years.[40] Diagnosis of TIA before a stroke may permit surgical or medical intervention that prevents an eventual stroke and the associated neurologic deficits.[40]

Large Vessel (Thrombotic) Stroke. Thrombi are the most common cause of ischemic strokes, usually occurring in atherosclerotic blood vessels. In the cerebral circulation, atherosclerotic plaques are found most commonly at arterial bifurcations. Common sites of plaque formation include larger vessels of the brain, notably the origins of the internal carotid and vertebral arteries, and junctions of the basilar and vertebral arteries. Cerebral infarction can result from an acute local thrombosis and occlusion at the site of chronic atherosclerosis, with or without embolization of the plaque material distally, or from critical perfusion failure distal to a stenosis (watershed). These infarcts often affect the cortex, causing aphasia or neglect, visual field defects, or transient monocular blindness (amaurosis fugax). In most cases of stroke, a single cerebral artery and its territories are affected. Usually, thrombotic strokes are seen in older persons and frequently are accompanied by evidence of atherosclerotic heart or peripheral arterial disease. The thrombotic stroke is not associated with activity and may occur in a person at rest.

Small Vessel Stroke (Lacunar Infarct). Lacunar infarcts are small (1.5- to 2-cm) to very small (3- to 4-mm) infarcts located in the deeper, noncortical parts of the brain or in the brain stem. They are found in the territory of single deep penetrating arteries supplying the internal capsule, basal ganglia, or brain stem. They result from occlusion of the smaller penetrating branches of large cerebral arteries, commonly the middle cerebral and posterior cerebral arteries. In the process of healing, lacunar infarcts leave behind small cavities, or *lacunae* ("lakes"). They are thought to result from arteriolar lipohyalinosis or microatheroma, commonly in the settings of chronic hypertension or diabetes. Six basic causes of lacunar infarcts have been proposed: embolism, hypertension, small vessel occlusive disease, hematologic abnormalities, small intracerebral hemorrhages, and vasospasm. Because of their size and location, lacunar infarcts usually do not cause cortical deficits like aphasia or apraxia. Instead, they produce classic recognizable "lacunar syndromes" such as pure motor hemiplegia, pure sensory hemiplegia, and dysarthria with the clumsy hand syndrome. Because CT scans are not sensitive enough to detect these tiny infarcts, diagnosis used to depend on clinical features alone. The use of MRI has allowed frequent visualization of small vessel infarcts and is obligatory to confirm such a lesion.

Cardiogenic Embolic Stroke. An embolic stroke is caused by a moving blood clot that travels from its origin to the brain. It usually affects the larger proximal cerebral vessels, often lodging at bifurcations. The most frequent site of embolic strokes is the middle cerebral artery, reflecting the large territory of this vessel and its position as the terminus of the carotid artery. Although most cerebral emboli originate from a thrombus in the left heart, they also may originate in an atherosclerotic plaque in the carotid arteries. The embolus travels quickly to the brain and becomes lodged in a smaller artery through which it cannot pass. Embolic stroke usually has a sudden onset with immediate maximum deficit.

Various cardiac conditions predispose to formation of emboli that produce embolic stroke, including rheumatic heart disease, atrial fibrillation, recent myocardial infarction, ventricular aneurysm, mobile aortic arch atheroma, and bacterial endocarditis. More recently, the use of transesophageal echocardiography, which better images the interatrial septum, has implicated a patent foramen ovale as a source for paradoxical venous emboli to the arterial system. Advances in the diagnosis and treatment of heart disease can be expected to alter favorably the incidence of embolic stroke.

Hemorrhagic Stroke

The most frequently fatal stroke is a spontaneous hemorrhage into the brain substance resulting in an intracerebral hemorrhage.[41–43] With rupture of a blood vessel, hemorrhage into the brain tissue occurs, resulting in a focal hematoma and sometimes intraventricular hemorrhage, edema, compression of the brain contents, or spasm of the adjacent blood vessels (Fig. 51-14). The most common predisposing factors are advancing age and hypertension. Other causes of hemorrhage are aneurysm, trauma, erosion of the vessels by tumors, arteriovenous malfor-

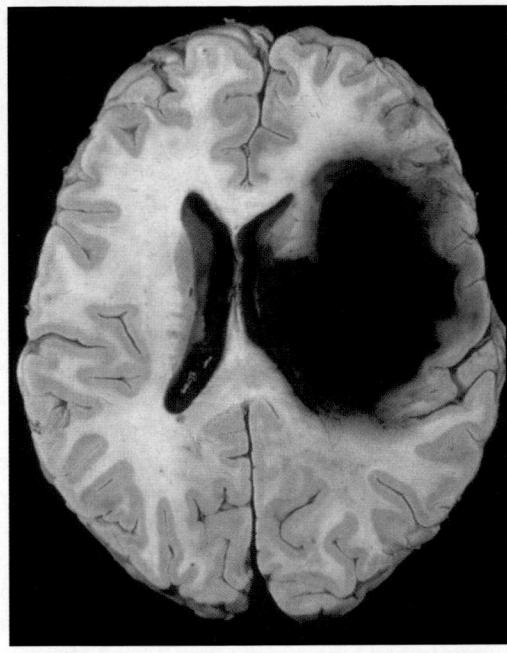

FIGURE 51-14 • Cerebral hemorrhage. A spontaneous cerebral hemorrhage began near the external capsule and produced a hematoma that threatened rupture of a lateral ventricle. (From Rubin E., Farber J. L. [1999]. *Pathology* [3rd ed., p. 1469]. Philadelphia: Lippincott-Raven.)

mations, blood coagulation disorders, vasculitis, and drugs. A cerebral hemorrhage occurs suddenly, usually when the person is active. Vomiting commonly occurs at the onset, and headache often occurs. Focal symptoms depend on which vessel is involved. In the most common situation, hemorrhage into the basal ganglia results in contralateral hemiplegia, with initial flaccidity progressing to spasticity. The hemorrhage and resultant edema exert great pressure on the brain substance, and the clinical course progresses rapidly to coma and frequently to death.

Manifestations of Acute Stroke

The specific manifestations of stroke or TIA are determined by the cerebral artery that is affected, by the area of brain tissue that is supplied by that vessel, and by the adequacy of the collateral circulation. Symptoms of stroke/TIA always are sudden in onset and focal, and usually are one-sided. The most common symptom is weakness of the face and arm, sometimes also of the leg. Other frequent stroke symptoms are unilateral numbness, vision loss in one eye (amaurosis fugax) or to one side (hemianopia), language disturbance (aphasia), slurred speech (dysarthria), and sudden, unexplained imbalance or ataxia. In the event of TIA, symptoms rapidly resolve spontaneously, usually within minutes, although the underlying mechanisms are the same as for stroke. The specific stroke signs depend on the specific vascular territory compromised (Table 51-6). As a generalization, carotid ischemia

CEREBRAL ARTERY	BRAIN AREA INVOLVED	SIGNS AND SYMPTOMS*
Anterior cerebral	Infarction of the medial aspect of one frontal lobe if lesion is distal to communicating artery; bilateral frontal infarction if flow in other anterior cerebral artery is inadequate	Paralysis of contralateral foot or leg; impaired gait; paresis of contralateral arm; contralateral sensory loss over toes, foot, and leg; problems making decisions or performing acts voluntarily; lack of spontaneity, easily distracted; slowness of thought; aphasia depends on the hemisphere involved; urinary incontinence; cognitive and affective disorders
Middle cerebral	Massive infarction of most of lateral hemisphere and deeper structures of the frontal, parietal, and temporal lobes; internal capsule; basal ganglia	Contralateral hemiplegia (face and arm); contralateral sensory impairment; aphasia; homonymous hemianopia; altered consciousness (confusion to coma); inability to turn eyes toward paralyzed side; denial of paralyzed side or limb (hemiattention); possible acalculia, alexia, finger agnosia, and left–right confusion; vasomotor paresis and instability
Posterior cerebral	Occipital lobe; anterior and medial portion of temporal lobe	Homonymous hemianopia and other visual defects such as color blindness, loss of central vision, and visual hallucinations; memory deficits, perseveration (repeated performance of same verbal or motor response)
	Thalamus involvement	Loss of all sensory modalities; spontaneous pain; intentional tremor; mild hemiparesis; aphasia
	Cerebral peduncle involvement	Oculomotor nerve palsy with contralateral hemiplegia
Basilar and vertebral	Cerebellum and brain stem	Visual disturbance such as diplopia, dystaxia, vertigo, dysphagia, dysphonia

TABLE 51-6 Signs and Symptoms of Stroke by Involved Cerebral Artery

*Depend on hemisphere involved and adequacy of collaterals.

causes monocular visual loss or aphasia (dominant hemisphere) or hemineglect (nondominant hemisphere), contralateral sensory or motor loss, or other discrete cortical signs such as apraxia and agnosia. Vertebrobasilar ischemia induces ataxia, diplopia, hemianopia, vertigo, cranial nerve deficits, contralateral hemiplegia, sensory deficits (either contralateral or crossed, *i.e.,* contralateral body and ipsilateral face), and arousal defects. Discrete subsets of these vascular syndromes usually occur, depending on which branches of the involved artery are blocked.

Stroke-Related Motor Deficits.   Motor deficits are most common, followed by deficits of language, sensation, and cognition. After a stroke affecting the corticospinal tract such as the motor cortex, posterior limb of the internal capsule, basis pontis, or medullary pyramids, there is profound weakness on the contralateral side (hemiparesis; see Chapter 50, Fig. 50-4). Involvement at the level of the motor cortex is most often in the territory of the middle cerebral artery, usually with a sparing of the leg, which is supplied by the anterior cerebral artery. Subcortical lesions of the corticospinal tracts cause equal weakness of the face, arm, and leg. Within 6 to 8 weeks, the initial weakness and flaccidity is replaced by hyperreflexia and spasticity. Spasticity involves an increase in the tone of affected muscles and usually an element of weakness. The flexor muscles usually are more strongly affected in the upper extremities and the extensor muscles more strongly affected in the lower extremities. There is a tendency toward foot drop; outward rotation and circumduction of the leg with gait; flexion at the wrist, elbow, and fingers; lower facial paresis; slurred speech; an upgoing toe to plantar stimulation (Babinski sign); and dependent edema in the affected extremities. A slight corticospinal lesion may be indicated only by clumsiness in carrying out fine coordinated movements rather than obvious weakness. Passive range-of-motion exercises help to maintain joint function and to prevent edema, shoulder subluxation (*i.e.,* incomplete dislocation), and muscle atrophy, and may help to reestablish motor patterns. If no voluntary movement or movement on command appears within a few months, significant function usually will not return to that extremity.

Stroke-Related Dysarthria and Aphasia.   Two key aspects of verbal communication are speech and language. Speech involves the mechanical act of articulating language, the "motor act" of verbal expression, whereas language involves the written or spoken use of symbolic formulations, such as words or numbers.[44] Dysarthria is a disorder of speech, manifest as the imperfect articulation of speech sounds or changes in voice pitch or quality. It results from a stroke affecting the muscles of the pharynx, palate, tongue, lips, or mouth and does not relate to the content of speech. A person with dysarthria may demonstrate slurred speech while still retaining language ability, or may have a concurrent language problem as well. *Aphasia* is a general term that encompasses varying degrees of inability to comprehend, integrate, and express language. Aphasia may be localized to the dominant cerebral cortex or thalamus, usually the left side in 95% of people who are right handed and 70% of

people who are left handed. In children, language dominance can readily shift to the unaffected hemisphere, resulting in more transient language deficits after stroke. A stroke in the territory of the middle cerebral artery is the most common aphasia-producing stroke.

Aphasia can be categorized as receptive or expressive, or as fluent or nonfluent. Fluency relates to the ease and spontaneity of conversational speech and is more strictly defined by the rate of speech, with "fluent" denoting many words, and "nonfluent," few words. Expressive or nonfluent aphasia is characterized by an inability easily to communicate spontaneously or translate thoughts or ideas into meaningful speech or writing. Speech production is limited, effortful, and halting and often may be poorly articulated because of a concurrent dysarthria. The person may be able, with difficulty, to utter or write two or three words, especially those with an emotional overlay. Comprehension is normal, and the person seems to be fully aware of his or her deficits but is unable to correct them. This often leads to frustration, anger, and depression. Expressive, nonfluent aphasia is associated with lesions of the Broca area at the dominant inferior frontal lobe cortex (areas 44 and 45).

Fluent speech requires little or no effort, is articulate, and is of increased quantity. The term *fluent* refers only to the ease and rate of verbal output, and does not relate to the content of speech or the ability of the person to comprehend what is being said. Verbal utterances are often paraphrasic, meaning that letters, syllables, or whole words are substituted for the target words. There are three categories of fluent aphasia: Wernicke, anomic, and conductive aphasia. Wernicke aphasia is characterized by an inability to comprehend the speech of others or to comprehend written material. Lesions of the posterior superior temporal or lower parietal lobe (areas 22 and 39) are associated with receptive, fluent aphasia. Anomic aphasia is speech that is nearly normal except for a difficulty with finding singular words. Conductive aphasia is manifest as impaired repetition and speech riddled with letter substitutions, despite good comprehension and fluency. Conductive aphasia (*i.e.,* disconnection syndrome) results from destruction of the fiber system under the insula that connects the Wernicke and Broca areas.

Stroke-Related Cognitive and Other Deficits.   Stroke can also cause cognitive, sensory, visual, and behavioral deficits. One distinct cognitive syndrome is that of hemineglect or hemiinattention. Usually caused by strokes affecting the nondominant (right) hemisphere, hemineglect is the inability to attend to and react to stimuli coming from the contralateral (left) side of space. Patients may not visually track, orient, or reach to the neglected side. They may neglect to use the limbs on that side, despite normal motor function, and may not shave, wash, or comb that side. Such persons are unaware of this deficit, which is another form of their neglect (*anosognosia*). Other cognitive deficits include apraxia (impaired ability to carry out previously learned motor activities despite normal sensory and motor function), agnosia (impaired recognition with normal sensory function), memory loss, behavioral syndromes, and depression. Sensory deficits affect the body contralateral to the lesion and can manifest as numbness, tingling paresthesias, or distorted sensations such as dysesthesia and neuropathic pain. Visual disturbances from stroke are diverse, but most common are hemianopia from a lesion of the optic radiations between the lateral geniculate body and the temporal or occipital lobes, or monocular blindness from occlusion of the ipsilateral central retinal artery, a branch of the internal carotid.

Diagnosis and Treatment

Diagnosis. Accurate diagnosis of acute stroke is based on a complete history and thorough physical and neurologic examination. A careful history, including documentation of previous TIAs, the time of onset and pattern and rapidity of system progression, the specific focal symptoms (to determine the likely vascular territory), and any coexisting diseases, can help to determine the type of stroke that is involved. The diagnostic evaluation should aim to determine the presence of hemorrhage or ischemia, identify the stroke or TIA mechanism (*i.e.,* large vessel or small vessel atherothrombotic, cardioembolic, hemorrhagic, other or cryptogenic), characterize the severity of clinical deficits, and unmask the presence of risk factors.

Brain imaging studies document the brain infarction, whereas vascular imaging reveals the anatomy and pathologic processes of the related blood vessels. CT scans and MRI have become essential brain imaging tools in diagnosing stroke, differentiating cerebral hemorrhage from ischemia and excluding intracranial lesions that mimic stroke clinically. CT scans are a necessary screening tool in the acute setting for rapid identification of hemorrhage, but are insensitive to ischemia within 24 hours and to any brain stem or small infarcts. MRI is superior for imaging ischemic lesions in all territories, and differentiating other nonstroke pathologic processes (*e.g.,* tumors, contusion, infection). Newer MRI techniques such as perfusion- and diffusion-weighted imaging (DWI) can reveal cerebral ischemia immediately after onset and identify areas of potentially reversible damage (*i.e.,* penumbra). Increasingly, fast MR DWI is used in settings of emergency stroke evaluation to rapidly identify the area and volume of ischemia, identifying candidates for emergency treatments.

Vascular imaging is accomplished with CT angiography (CTA), magnetic resonance angiography (MRA), catheter-based "conventional" arteriography, and ultrasonography. All except ultrasonography can demonstrate the site of vascular abnormality (intracranial and extracranial) and afford visualization of most intracranial vascular areas. However, each modality has relative strengths and weaknesses. MRA is noninvasive and most widely available, but less sensitive and specific than CTA or catheter angiography. CTA is exquisitely detailed for a noninvasive technique, but is limited in availability and requires iodinated contrast, which is nephrotoxic. Catheter angiography remains the gold standard in sensitivity, and allows visualization of dynamic patterns of collateral flow, but is invasive and requires significant contrast doses. CTA and MRA have largely replaced angiography as a screening tool for vascular lesions. Ultrasonographic techniques allow quick bedside assessment of the carotid bifurcation (duplex ultrasonography) or of flow velocities in the cerebral circulation (transcranial Doppler).

Treatment. Treatment of acute ischemic stroke has changed markedly since the early 1990s, with an emphasis on salvaging brain tissue, preventing secondary stroke, and minimizing long-term disability. The care of patients with stroke has shifted away from the "nearest hospital" to certified *stroke centers.* These are hospitals that have been certified by some external agency, most commonly the state or Joint Commission for the Accreditation of Healthcare Agencies, the federal agency overseeing all facilities that care for Medicare patients.[45] Certification establishes that a hospital can manage stroke patients with appropriate care throughout the continuum, from emergency treatments, through the inpatient stay, and into the rehabilitation phase. With this advancement, the medical and lay communities together acknowledge that care of the patient with stroke requires specialized personnel and resources to minimize the devastating costs to society from stroke, the leading cause of adult disability in the United States.

Stroke care begins with emergency treatments aimed at reversing the evolving ischemic brain injury. The realization that there is a window of opportunity during which ischemic but viable brain tissue can be salvaged has led to the use of reperfusion techniques and neuroprotective strategies in the early treatment of ischemic stroke. Although the results of emergent treatment of hemorrhagic stroke have been less dramatic, continued efforts to reduce disability have been promising. Reperfusion techniques include thrombolytic drugs (administered either intravenously or intra-arterially), catheter-directed mechanical clot disruption, and augmentation of CPP during acute stroke. The use of thrombolytic agents for treatment of stroke was first investigated in the late 1960s, but it was quickly abandoned because of hemorrhagic complications resulting from treatment many hours beyond the time window of penumbral cell viability and because exclusion of persons with hemorrhagic stroke was difficult before CT scanning was available. The interest in thrombolytic therapy has increased because of the development of new thrombolytic agents and the availability of rapid diagnostic scanning methods that are able to differentiate between ischemic and hemorrhagic stroke.

Thrombolytic agents include streptokinase, urokinase, recombinant tissue-type plasminogen activator (tPA), and p-anisoylated lys-plasminogen-streptokinase activator complex[46] (see Chapter 13). The first and only agent approved by the U.S. Food and Drug Administration (FDA) for treatment of acute ischemic stroke is tPA, which was approved in 1996. A subcommittee of the Stroke Council of the American Heart Association has developed guidelines for the use of tPA for acute stroke.[6] These guidelines recommend that in persons with suspected stroke, the diagnosis of hemorrhagic stroke be excluded through the use of CT scanning before administration of thrombolytic therapy, which must be administered within 3 hours of onset of symptoms. The major risk of treatment with thrombolytic agents is intracranial hemorrhage of the infarcted brain. A number of conditions, including therapeutic levels of oral anticoagulant medications, a history of gastrointestinal or urinary tract bleeding in the previous 21 days, prior stroke or head injury within 3 months, major surgery within the past 14 days, and a blood pressure greater than 185/110 mm Hg, are considered contraindications to intravenous thrombolytic therapy.[6]

Emerging experimental treatments for ischemic stroke are being increasingly used as alternative methods of reperfusion beyond intravenous thrombolysis. New catheter-based methods allow recanalization of a directly visualized cerebral clot with intra-arterial techniques. The interventional specialist might mechanically disrupt the clot, deliver thrombolytic drug intra-arterially at the clot surface, or urgently stent intracranial vessels to restore flow. Generally, although patient selection is more stringent for these invasive methods, patients can be treated past the 3-hour time window for intravenous tPA. However, these methods require an experienced interventional angiography team and extensive institutional infrastructure, and thus remain limited to tertiary care centers. Other experimental treatments include neuroprotection with drugs that limit the calcium cascade (see Fig. 51-2) and treatments like hypothermia that decrease brain metabolic demands in the setting of ischemia. All are being actively tested in clinical trials.

Poststroke treatment is aimed at preventing recurrent stroke and medical complications, while promoting the fullest possible recovery of function. The risk of stroke recurrence is highest in the first week after stroke or TIA, so the early implementation of antiplatelet agents in most cases, or warfarin (an anticoagulant) in cardioembolic stroke, is imperative. Long-term stroke recurrence is most effectively prevented with aggressive reduction of risk factors, primarily hypertension, diabetes, smoking, and hyperlipidemia. In cases of carotid territory stroke with carotid stenosis, revascularization with surgery or stenting should be considered. Early hospital care also requires careful prevention of aspiration, deep vein thrombosis, and falls. Recovery is maximized with early and aggressive rehabilitation efforts that include all members of the rehabilitation team—physician, nurse, speech therapist, physical therapist, and occupational therapist—and the family. Much research is ongoing into the determinants and mechanisms of stroke recovery.

The successful treatment of stroke depends on education of the public, paramedics, and health care professionals about the need for both early diagnosis and treatment and for risk factor reduction and prevention. As with heart attack, the message should be that prevention is the key, and to treat stroke symptoms as an emergency "brain attack." Effective medical and surgical procedures may preserve brain function and prevent disability.

Aneurysmal Subarachnoid Hemorrhage

Aneurysmal subarachnoid hemorrhage represents bleeding into the subarachnoid space caused by a ruptured cerebral aneurysm. Bleeding into the subarachnoid space can extend well beyond the site of origin, flooding the basal cistern, ventricles, and spinal subarachnoid space.[1,4,47,48] An aneurysm is a

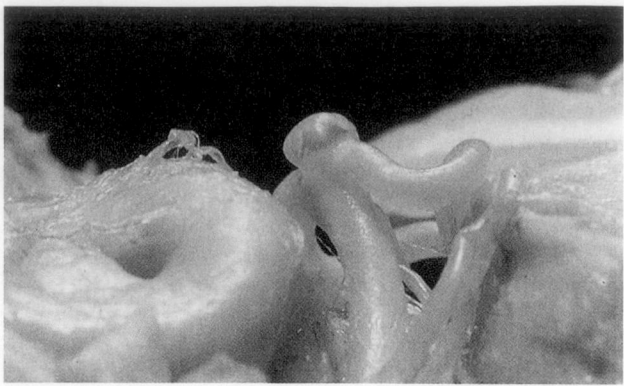

FIGURE 51-15 • Berry aneurysm. A thin-walled aneurysm protrudes from the arterial bifurcation in the circle of Willis. (From Rubin R., Strayer D. E. [Eds.], *Rubin's pathology: Clinicopathologic foundations of medicine* [4th ed., p. 1435]. Philadelphia: Lippincott Williams & Wilkins.)

bulge at the site of a localized weakness in the muscular wall of an arterial vessel. Most cerebral aneurysms are small saccular aneurysms called *berry aneurysms* (Fig. 51-15). They usually occur in the anterior circulation and are found at bifurcations and other junctions of vessels such as those in the circle of Willis (Fig. 51-16). They are thought to arise from a congenital defect in the media of the involved vessels. Their incidence is higher in persons with certain disorders, including polycystic kidney disease, fibromuscular dysplasia, coarctation of the aorta, and arteriovenous malformations of the brain.[1,4] Other causes of cerebral aneurysms are atherosclerosis, hypertension, and bacterial infections.

Rupture of a cerebral aneurysm results in subarachnoid hemorrhage.[47,48] The probability of rupture increases with the size of the aneurysm; aneurysms larger than 10 mm in diameter have a 50% chance of bleeding per year. Rupture often occurs with acute increases in ICP. Of the various environmen-

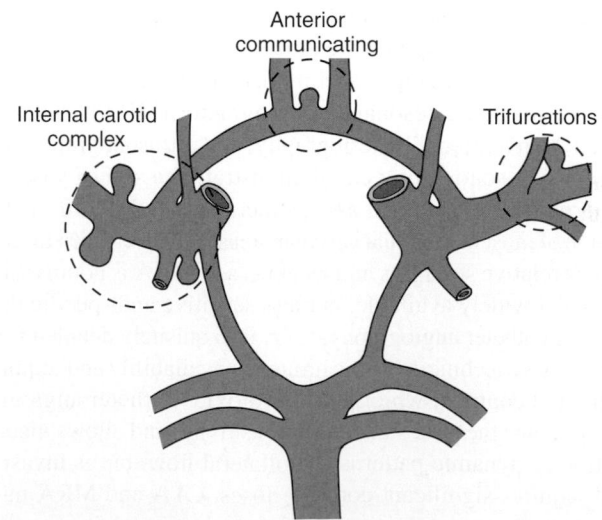

FIGURE 51-16 • Common sites of berry aneurysms.

tal factors that may predispose to aneurysmal subarachnoid hemorrhage, cigarette smoking, hypertension, and excessive alcohol intake appear to constitute the greatest threat.[49,50] Intracranial aneurysms are rare in children, and the mean age for subarachnoid hemorrhage is approximately 50 years. The mortality and morbidity rates with aneurysmal subarachnoid hemorrhage are high, with only one third of persons recovering without major disability.[50]

The signs and symptoms of cerebral aneurysms can be divided into two phases: those presenting before rupture and bleeding and those presenting after rupture and bleeding. Most small aneurysms are asymptomatic; intact aneurysms frequently are found at autopsy as an incidental finding.[1] Large aneurysms may cause chronic headache, neurologic deficits, or both.[47,48] Approximately 50% of persons with subarachnoid hemorrhage have a history of atypical headaches occurring days to weeks before the onset of hemorrhage, suggesting the presence of a small leak. These headaches are characterized by sudden onset and often are accompanied by nausea, vomiting, and dizziness. Persons with these symptoms may be mistakenly diagnosed as having tension or migraine headaches.

The onset of subarachnoid aneurysmal rupture often is heralded by a sudden and severe headache, described as "the worst headache of my life."[47,48] If the bleeding is severe, the headache may be accompanied by collapse and loss of consciousness. Vomiting may accompany the presenting symptoms. Other manifestations include signs of meningeal irritation such as nuchal rigidity (neck stiffness) and photophobia (light intolerance); cranial nerve deficits, especially cranial nerve II, and sometimes III and IV (diplopia and blurred vision); stroke syndromes (focal motor and sensory deficits); cerebral edema and increased ICP; and pituitary dysfunction (diabetes insipidus and hyponatremia). Hypertension, a frequent finding, and cardiac arrhythmias result from massive release of catecholamines triggered by the subarachnoid hemorrhage.

The diagnosis of subarachnoid hemorrhage and intracranial aneurysms is made by clinical presentation, CT scan, lumbar puncture, and angiography.[47,48] Lumbar puncture may reveal the presence of blood in the CSF, whereas CT may demonstrate the location and extent of subarachnoid blood. To identify the aneurysm at the source of bleeding, conventional angiography, MRA, and helical (spiral) CTA are used. Conventional catheter angiography is the definitive diagnostic tool for detecting the aneurysm. MRA is noninvasive and does not require the intravascular administration of contrast, but is less sensitive. Helical CTA does require intravenous contrast, but can be used in persons after aneurysmal clipping, when the use of MRI may be contraindicated.

The course of treatment after aneurysm rupture depends on the extent of neurologic deficit. The best outcomes are achieved when the aneurysm can be secured early and prevention of complications initiated.[50] Persons with mild to no neurologic deficits may undergo cerebral arteriography and early surgery, usually within 24 to 72 hours. Surgery involves craniotomy and inserting a specially designed silver clip that is tightened around the neck of the aneurysm. This procedure offers protection from rebleeding and may permit removal of the hematoma. The use of endovascular techniques such as balloon embolization and platinum coil electrothrombosis is emerging as an alternative to surgery, particularly in surgically inaccessible aneurysms or poor surgical candidates. Some persons with subarachnoid hemorrhage are managed medically for 10 days or more in an attempt to improve their clinical status before surgery.

The complications of aneurysmal rupture include rebleeding, vasospasm with cerebral ischemia, hydrocephalus, hypothalamic dysfunction, and seizure activity. Rebleeding and vasospasm are the most serious and most difficult to treat. Rebleeding, which has its highest incidence on the first day after the initial rupture, results in further and usually catastrophic neurologic deficits.

Vasospasm is a dreaded complication of aneurysmal rupture. The condition is difficult to treat and is associated with a high incidence of morbidity and mortality. Although the description of aneurysm-associated vasospasm is relatively uniform, its proposed mechanisms are controversial. Usually, the condition develops within 3 to 10 days (peak, 7 days) after aneurysm rupture and involves a focal narrowing of the cerebral artery or arteries that can be visualized on arteriography or by transcranial Doppler. The neurologic status gradually deteriorates as blood supply to the brain in the region of the spasm is decreased; this usually can be differentiated from the rapid deterioration seen in rebleeding. Vasospasm is treated by attempting to maintain adequate CPP through the use of vasoactive drugs or administration of large amounts of intravenous fluids to increase intravascular volume and produce hemodilution. There is risk for rebleeding from this therapy. Early surgery may provide some protection from vasospasm. Endovascular techniques, including balloon dilation, have been developed to treat spasmodic arterial segments mechanically. Nimodipine, a drug that blocks calcium channels and selectively acts on cerebral blood vessels, may be used to prevent or treat vasospasm.

Another complication of aneurysm rupture is the development of hydrocephalus. It is caused by plugging of the arachnoid villi with products from lysis of blood in the subarachnoid space. Hydrocephalus is diagnosed by serial CT scans showing increasing size of the ventricles and by the clinical signs of increased ICP. Hydrocephalus may respond to osmotic diuretics, but if neurologic deterioration is significant, surgical placement of a shunt is indicated.

Arteriovenous Malformations

Arteriovenous malformations are a complex tangle of abnormal arteries and veins linked by one or more fistulas[51,52] (Fig. 51-17). These vascular networks lack a capillary bed, and the small arteries have a deficient muscularis layer. Arteriovenous malformations are thought to arise from failure in development of the capillary network in the embryonic brain. As the child's brain grows, the malformation acquires additional arterial contri-

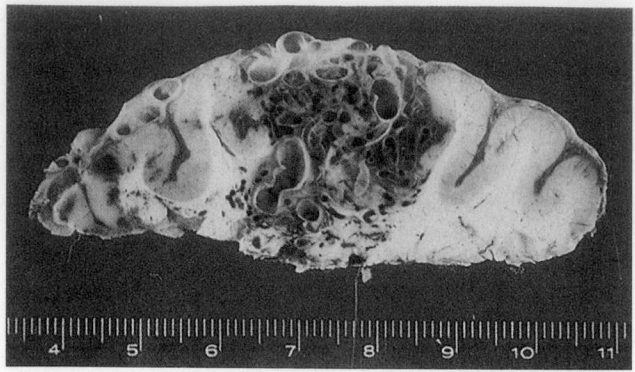

FIGURE 51-17 • Arteriovenous malformation. Abnormal blood vessels replace the cortical gray matter and extend deeply into the underlying white matter. (From Rubin R., Strayer D. E. [Eds.], *Rubin's pathology: Clinicopathologic foundations of medicine* [4th ed., p. 1435]. Philadelphia: Williams & Wilkins.)

butions that enlarge to form a tangled collection of thin-walled vessels that shunt blood directly from the arterial to the venous circulation. Arteriovenous malformations typically present before 40 years of age and affect men and women equally. Rupture of vessels in the malformation causing hemorrhagic stroke accounts for approximately 2% of all strokes.[52]

The hemodynamic effects of arteriovenous malformations are twofold. First, blood is shunted from the high-pressure arterial system to the low-pressure venous system without the buffering advantage of the capillary network. The draining venous channels are exposed to high levels of pressure, predisposing them to rupture and hemorrhage. Second, the elevated arterial and venous pressures divert blood away from the surrounding tissue, impairing tissue perfusion. Clinically, this is evidenced by slowly progressive neurologic deficits. The major clinical manifestations of arteriovenous malformations are intracerebral and subarachnoid hemorrhage, seizures, headache, and progressive neurologic deficits. Headaches often are severe, and persons with the disorder may describe them as throbbing and synchronous with their heartbeat. Other, focal symptoms depend on the location of the lesion and include visual symptoms (*i.e.,* diplopia and hemianopia), hemiparesis, mental deterioration, and speech deficits.

Definitive diagnosis often is obtained through cerebral angiography. Treatment methods include surgical excision, endovascular occlusion, and radiation therapy.[52] Because of the nature of the malformation, each of these methods is accompanied by some risk for complications. If the arteriovenous malformation is accessible, surgical excision usually is the treatment of choice. Endovascular treatment involves the insertion of microcatheters into the cerebral circulation for delivery of embolic materials (*e.g.,* microballoons, sclerosing agents, microcoils, or quick-drying glue) into the arteriovenous malformation vessels.[53] Radiation therapy (also known as *radiosurgery*) may involve the use of a gamma knife, proton beam, or linear accelerator.

IN SUMMARY, a stroke, or "brain attack," is an acute focal neurologic deficit caused by a vascular disorder that injures brain tissue. It is the third leading cause of death in the United States and a major cause of disability. There are two main types of stroke: ischemic and hemorrhagic. Ischemic stroke, which is the most common type, is caused by cerebrovascular obstruction by a thrombus or emboli. Hemorrhagic stroke, which is associated with greater morbidity and mortality, is caused by the rupture of a blood vessel and bleeding into the brain. The acute manifestations of stroke depend on the location of the blood vessel that is involved and can include motor, sensory, language, speech, and cognitive disorders. Early diagnosis and treatment with thrombolytic agents can prevent disabling brain injury from ischemic stroke. Treatment of long-term neurologic deficits from stroke is primarily symptomatic, involving the combined efforts of the health care team, the patient, and the family

A subarachnoid hemorrhage involves bleeding into the subarachnoid space. Most subarachnoid hemorrhages are the result of a ruptured cerebral aneurysm. Presenting symptoms include headache, nuchal rigidity, photophobia, and nausea. Complications include rebleeding, vasospasm, and hydrocephalus.

Arteriovenous malformations are congenital abnormal communications between arterial and venous channels that result from failure in development of the capillary network in the embryonic brain. The vessels in the arteriovenous malformations may enlarge to form a space-occupying lesion, become weak and predispose to bleeding, and divert blood away from other parts of the brain; they can cause brain hemorrhage, seizures, headache, and other neurologic deficits. ■

INFECTIONS AND NEOPLASMS

After completing this section of the chapter, you should be able to meet the following objectives:

- List the sequence of events that occur with meningitis.
- Describe the symptoms of encephalitis.
- List the major categories of brain tumors and interpret the meaning of benign and malignant as related to brain tumors.
- Describe the general manifestations of brain tumors.
- List the methods used in diagnosis and treatment of brain tumors.

Infections

Infections of the CNS may be classified according to the structure involved: the meninges, meningitis; the brain parenchyma, encephalitis; the spinal cord, myelitis; and the brain and spinal cord, encephalomyelitis. They also may be classified by the type of invading organism: bacterial, viral, or other. In general, the pathogens enter the CNS through the bloodstream by crossing the blood-brain barrier or by direct invasion through skull fracture or a bullet hole, or, rarely, by contamination during surgery or lumbar puncture.

Meningitis

Meningitis is an inflammation of the pia mater, the arachnoid, and the CSF-filled subarachnoid space. Inflammation spreads rapidly because of CSF circulation around the brain and spinal cord. The inflammation usually is caused by an infection, but chemical meningitis can occur. There are two types of acute infectious meningitis: acute purulent meningitis (usually bacterial) and acute lymphocytic (usually viral) meningitis.[1] Factors responsible for the severity of meningitis include virulence factors of the pathogen, host factors, brain edema, and the presence of permanent neurologic sequelae.

Bacterial Meningitis. Most cases of bacterial meningitis are caused by *Streptococcus pneumoniae* (the pneumococcus) or *Neisseria meningitidis* (the meningococcus), except in neonates (infected most by group B streptococci).[54] A leading cause of meningitis in decades past, the incidence of *Haemophilus influenzae* infection has declined dramatically during recent years because of vaccination against *H. influenza*. Epidemics of meningococcal meningitis occur in settings such as the military, where the recruits must reside in close contact. Other pathogens in adults are gram-negative bacilli and *Listeria monocytogenes*. The very young and the very old are at highest risk for pneumococcal meningitis. Risk factors associated with contracting meningitis include head trauma with basilar skull fractures, otitis media, sinusitis or mastoiditis, neurosurgery, dermal sinus tracts, systemic sepsis, or immunocompromise. Despite the use of antibiotics, morbidity and mortality rates remain high for bacterial meningitis. For adults, the overall mortality rate is 21% and the outcome is unfavorable in 34% of cases.[55]

In the pathophysiologic process of bacterial meningitis, the bacterial organisms replicate and undergo lysis in the CSF, releasing endotoxins or cell wall fragments. These substances initiate the release of inflammatory mediators, which set off a complex sequence of events permitting pathogens, neutrophils, and albumin to move across the capillary wall into the CSF. As the pathogens enter the subarachnoid space, they cause inflammation, characterized by a cloudy, purulent exudate. Thrombophlebitis of the bridging veins and dural sinuses or obliteration of arterioles by inflammation may develop, causing vascular congestion and infarction in the surrounding tissues. Ultimately, the meninges thicken and adhesions form. These adhesions may impinge on the cranial nerves, giving rise to cranial nerve palsies, or may impair the outflow of CSF, causing hydrocephalus.

The most common symptoms of acute bacterial meningitis are fever and chills; headache; stiff neck; back, abdominal, and extremity pains; and nausea and vomiting.[55,56] Other signs include seizures, cranial nerve palsies, and focal cerebral signs. Meningococcal meningitis causes a petechial rash with palpable purpura in most people. These petechiae vary in size from pinhead to large ecchymoses or even areas of skin gangrene that slough if the person survives. Other types of meningitis also may produce a petechial rash. Persons infected with *H. influenzae* or *S. pneumoniae* may present with difficulty in arousal and seizures, whereas those with *N. meningitidis* infection may present with delirium or coma.[56] The development of brain edema, hydrocephalus, or increased cerebral blood flow can increase ICP.

Meningeal signs (*e.g.*, photophobia and nuchal rigidity), such as those seen in subarachnoid hemorrhage, also may be present. Two assessment techniques can help determine whether meningeal irritation is present. The Kernig sign is resistance to extension of the knee while the person is lying with the hip flexed at a right angle. The Brudzinski sign is elicited when flexion of the neck induces flexion of the hip and knee. These postures reflect resistance to the painful stretching of the inflamed meninges from the lumbar level to the head. Cranial nerve damage (especially the eighth nerve, with resulting deafness) and hydrocephalus may occur as complications of pyogenic meningitis.

Diagnosis of bacterial meningitis is based on the history and physical examination, along with laboratory data. Lumbar puncture findings, which are necessary for accurate diagnosis, include a cloudy and purulent CSF under increased pressure. The CSF typically contains large numbers of polymorphonuclear neutrophils (up to 90,000/mm³), increased protein content, and reduced sugar content. Bacteria can be seen on smears and can easily be cultured with appropriate media. Occasionally, previous antibiotic use limits culture sensitivities, in which case latex agglutination can be used, or polymerase chain reaction (PCR) testing for *N. meningitidis, H. influenzae,* and *Listeria* species. Because complications associated with lumbar puncture include life-threatening cerebral herniation, at-risk patients (*i.e.,* those who are immunocompromised, had a seizure within a week, have papilledema, or have specific neurologic abnormalities) should have a CT scan before undergoing the procedure.

Treatment includes urgent antibiotics while diagnostic testing ensues.[54–56] Delay in initiation of antimicrobial therapy, most frequently because of performance of medical imaging before performance of lumbar puncture or transfer to another medical facility, can result in poor outcomes.[54,56] Initial choice of antibiotics includes broad-spectrum coverage with a third-generation cephalosporin, vancomycin, and sometimes ampicillin. Further adjustment of antibiotics is driven by results of CSF cultures. Effective antibiotics produce rapid lysis of the pathogen, which produces inflammatory mediators that have the potential for exacerbating the abnormalities of the blood-brain barrier. To suppress this pathologic inflammation, adjunctive corticosteroid therapy is increasingly administered with or just before the first dose of antibiotics in patients of all ages.[54,56]

Persons who have been exposed to someone with meningococcal meningitis should be treated prophylactically with antibiotics.[54] Effective polysaccharide vaccines are available to protect against meningococcal groups A, C, Y, and W-135. These vaccines are recommended for military recruits and college students, who are at increased risk for invasive meningococcal disease.

Viral Meningitis. Viral meningitis manifests in much the same way as bacterial meningitis, but the course is less severe and the CSF findings are markedly different. There are lymphocytes in the fluid rather than polymorphonuclear cells, the protein content is only moderately elevated, and the sugar content usually is normal. The acute viral meningitides are self-limited and usually require only symptomatic treatment, except for herpes simplex virus (HSV) type 2, which responds to intravenous acyclovir. Viral meningitis can be caused by many different viruses, most often enteroviruses, including coxsackievirus, poliovirus, and echovirus. Others include Epstein-Barr virus, mumps virus, HSV, and West Nile virus. Although often the virus cannot be identified, newer assays are emerging that allow in some circumstances for rapid identification of viral ribonucleic acid (RNA) in CSF.

Encephalitis

Encephalitis represents a generalized infection of the parenchyma of the brain or spinal cord. It usually is caused by a virus, but it also may be caused by bacteria, fungi, and other organisms. The nervous system is subject to invasion by many viruses, such as arbovirus, poliovirus, and rabies virus. The mode of transmission may be the bite of a mosquito (arbovirus), a rabid animal (rabies virus), or ingestion (poliovirus). Common causes of encephalitis in the United States are HSV and West Nile virus. Less frequent causes of encephalitis are toxic substances such as ingested lead and vaccines for measles and mumps. Encephalitis caused by human immunodeficiency virus (HIV) infection is discussed in Chapter 20.

The pathologic picture of encephalitis includes local necrotizing hemorrhage, which ultimately becomes generalized, with prominent edema. There is progressive degeneration of nerve cell bodies. The histologic picture, although rather general, may demonstrate some specific characteristics. For example, the poliovirus selectively destroys the cells of the anterior horn of the spinal cord.

Like meningitis, encephalitis is characterized by fever, headache, and nuchal rigidity, but more often patients also experience neurologic disturbances, such as lethargy, disorientation, seizures, focal paralysis, delirium, and coma. Diagnosis of encephalitis is made by clinical history and presenting symptoms, in addition to traditional CSF studies.

Brain Tumors

Primary brain tumors account for 2% of all cancer deaths. The American Cancer Society estimates that there were 20,500 new cases and more than 12,740 deaths from brain and CNS cancers in 2007.[57] Metastasis to the brain from other sites is even more common. One estimate suggests that more than 100,000 people per year die with symptomatic intracranial metastasis.[58] In children, primary brain tumors are second only to leukemia as a cause of death from cancer, with 2200 primary brain tumors being diagnosed each year. The mortality rate among this age group approaches 45%.[59]

Types of Tumors

The term *brain tumor* refers to a collection of intracranial neoplasms, each with its own histology, site of origin, prognosis, and treatment.[58,60,61] For most neoplasms, the term *malignant* is used to describe the tumor's lack of cell differentiation, its invasive nature, and its ability to metastasize. However, the terms *benign* and *malignant* do not apply to brain tumors in the same sense as they do to tumors in other parts of the body. In the brain, even a well-differentiated and histologically benign tumor may grow and cause death because of its location. Also, tumors in the brain are rarely benign because surgery rarely cures.[60] Most histologically benign tumors infiltrate the normal brain tissue, preventing total resection and allowing for tumor recurrence. Furthermore, brain tumors seldom metastasize, except within the CNS itself.[60] Because of difficulty with pathologic discrimination and absence of metastasis, the clinical staging systems used for other cancers are not used for describing brain tumors. Instead, the terms *low-grade tumors* and *high-grade tumors* are often used.[60]

Brain tumors can be divided into three basic types: primary intracranial tumors of neuroepithelial tissue (*e.g.,* neurons, neuroglia), primary intracranial tumors that originate in the skull cavity but are not derived from the brain tissue itself (*e.g.,* meninges, pituitary gland, pineal gland, primary CNS lymphoma), and metastatic tumors.[4] Collectively, neoplasms of astrocytic origin are the most common type of primary brain tumor in adults, followed by primary CNS lymphoma.

Glial Tumors. Glial tumors are divided into two main categories: astrocytic and oligodendroglial. For purposes of classification, astrocytic tumors can be subdivided into fibrillary (infiltrating) astrocytic tumors and pilocytic astrocytomas.

Fibrillary or diffuse astrocytomas account for 80% of adult primary brain tumors. They are most common in middle age, with the anaplastic astrocytomas having a peak incidence in the sixth decade. Although they usually are found in the cerebral hemispheres, they also can occur in the cerebellum, brain stem, or spinal cord. Astrocytomas of the cerebral hemispheres commonly are divided into three grades of increasing pathologic anaplasia and rapidity of progression: well-differentiated lesions, designated *astrocytomas;* intermediate-grade tumors, termed *anaplastic astrocytomas;* and the least differentiated and most aggressive, designated *glioblastoma multiforme.* Clinically, infiltrating astrocytic tumors present with symptoms of increased ICP (*e.g.,* headache) or focal abnormalities related to their position (*e.g.,* seizures).

Pilocytic astrocytomas are distinguished from other astrocytomas by their cellular appearance and their benign behavior. Typically, they occur in children and young adults and usually are located in the cerebellum, but they also can be found in the floor and walls of the third ventricle, in the optic chiasm and nerves, and occasionally in the cerebral hemispheres. The prognosis of persons with pilocytic astrocytomas is influenced primarily by their location. The prognosis is usually better for persons with surgically resectable tumors, such as those located in the cerebellar cortex, than for persons with less accessible tumors, such as those involving the hypothalamus or brain stem.

Oligodendrogliomas are tumors of the oligodendrocytes or their precursors, or with histologic features representing both oligodendrocytes and astrocytes.[58] They represent approximately 5% of glial tumors and are most common in middle life. The prognosis of persons with oligodendrogliomas is less predictable than for persons with infiltrating astrocytomas. It depends on the histologic grade of the tumor, its location, and, more recently, recognition of molecular features that can be linked to chemosensitivity.[58] The oligodendroglial tumors are prone to spontaneous hemorrhage owing to their delicate vasculature.

Ependymomas. Ependymomas are derived from the single layer of epithelium that lines the ventricles and spinal canal. Although they can occur at any age, they are most likely to occur in the first two decades of life and most frequently affect the fourth ventricle; they constitute 5% to 10% of brain tumors in this age group. The spinal cord is the most common site for ependymomas occurring in middle age. The clinical features depend on the location of the neoplasm. Intracranial tumors are often associated with hydrocephalus and evidence of increased ICP.

Meningiomas. Meningiomas develop from the meningothelial cells of the arachnoid and are outside the brain. They usually have their onset in the middle or later years of life and constitute approximately 20% of primary brain tumors in this age group. Meningiomas are slow growing, well circumscribed, and often highly vascular tumors. They usually are benign, and complete removal is possible if the tumor does not involve vital structures.

Primary Central Nervous System Lymphomas. Primary CNS lymphoma has increased in incidence by a factor of 10 in the past two decades. These deep, periventricular, and diffuse tumors are especially common in immunocompromised patients and are associated with the Epstein-Barr virus and derived from large B cells. Most are malignant, and recurrence is common despite treatment. Behavioral and cognitive changes, which are the most common presenting symptoms, occur in about 65% of patients; hemiparesis, aphasia, and visual field deficits in about 50%; and seizures in 15% to 20%.[58]

Etiology

The etiology of brain tumors is largely unknown. Although a large number of studies have examined the relationship between environmental and occupational factors, only two have shown a relationship to brain cancer: ionizing radiation and immunosuppression.[60] Irradiation given to treat intracranial and extracranial cancers, including prophylactic irradiation for leukemia, increases the incidence of gliomas. Immunosuppres-

sion, either congenital or acquired (*e.g.,* immunosuppression to prevent organ rejection, HIV infection), increases the risk of primary CNS lymphomas. There may also be a hereditary factor. A few inherited disorders predispose to the development of brain tumors. For example, neurofibromatosis (see Chapter 7) is associated with primary brain tumors. Some childhood tumors, such as medulloblastoma, are considered to be of embryonic origin.

Manifestations

Intracranial tumors give rise to focal disturbances in brain function and increased ICP. Focal disturbances occur because of brain compression, tumor infiltration, disturbances in blood flow, and brain edema.

Tumors may be located intra-axially (*i.e.,* within brain tissue) or extra-axially (*i.e.,* outside brain tissue, but within the cranium). Disturbances in brain function usually are greatest with fast-growing, infiltrative, intra-axial tumors because of compression, infiltration, and necrosis of brain tissue. Extra-axial tumors, such as meningiomas, may reach a large size without producing signs and symptoms. Cysts may form in tumors and contribute to brain compression. The clinical manifestations of brain tumors depend on the size and location of the tumor. General signs and symptoms include headache, nausea, vomiting, mental changes, papilledema, visual disturbances (*e.g.,* diplopia), alterations in sensory and motor function, and seizures. Because the volume of the intracranial cavity is fixed, brain tumors cause a generalized increase in ICP when they reach sufficient size or produce edema. Cerebral edema usually is of the vasogenic type, which develops around the tumors and is characterized by increased brain water and expanded extracellular fluid. The edema is thought to result from increased permeability of tumor capillary endothelial cells. Tumors can also obstruct the flow of CSF in the ventricular cavities and produce hydrocephalic dilation of the proximal ventricles and atrophy of the cerebral hemispheres. With very slow-growing tumors, complete compensation of ventricular volumes can occur, but with rapidly growing tumors, increased ICP is an early sign. Depending on the location of the tumor, brain displacement and herniation of the uncus or cerebellum may occur.

The brain itself is insensitive to pain. The headache that accompanies brain tumors results from compression or distortion of pain-sensitive dural or vascular structures. It may be felt on the same side of the head as the tumor, but more commonly is diffuse. In the early stages, the headache is mild and occurs in the morning on awakening and improves with head elevation. The headache becomes more constant as the tumor enlarges and often is worsened by coughing, bending, or sudden movements of the head.

Vomiting occurs with or without nausea, may be projectile, and is a common symptom of increased ICP and brain stem compression. Direct stimulation of the vomiting center, which is located in the medulla, may contribute to the vomiting that occurs with brain tumors. The vomiting is often associated with headache. Papilledema (edema of the optic disk) results from increased ICP and obstruction of the

CSF pathways. It is associated with decreased visual acuity, diplopia, and deficits in the visual fields. Visual defects associated with papilledema often are the reason that persons with brain tumor seek medical care.

Personality and mental changes are common with brain tumors. Persons with brain tumors often are irritable initially and later become quiet and apathetic. They may become forgetful, seem preoccupied, and appear to be psychologically depressed. Because of the mental changes, a psychiatric consultation may be sought before a diagnosis of brain tumor is made.

Focal signs and symptoms are determined by the location of the tumor. Tumors arising in the frontal lobe may grow to large size, increase the ICP, and cause signs of generalized brain dysfunction before focal signs are recognized. Tumors that impinge on the visual system cause visual loss or visual field defects long before generalized signs develop. Certain areas of the brain have a relatively low threshold for seizure activity. Temporal lobe tumors often produce seizures as their first symptom. Hallucinations of smell or hearing and déjà vu phenomena are common focal manifestations of temporal lobe tumors. Brain stem tumors commonly produce upper and lower motor neuron signs, such as weakness of facial muscles and ocular palsies that occur with or without involvement of sensory or long motor tracts. Cerebellar tumors often cause ataxia of gait.

Diagnosis and Treatment

The diagnosis of brain tumors in the modern era rests mainly on MRI. Gadolinium-enhanced MRI is the test of choice for identifying and localizing the presence and extent of tumor involvement. CT scans may fail to reveal certain mass lesions such as low-grade tumors or posterior fossa masses. Diagnostic maneuvers that suggest a possible tumor and indicate the need for MRI include physical and neurologic examinations, visual field and funduscopic examination, and sometimes EEG. Approximately 75% of persons with a brain tumor have an abnormal EEG, which can indicate an underlying structural lesion warranting MRI. Cerebral angiography can be used to visualize the tumor's vascular supply, information that is important when planning surgery. MRI may be supplemented with positron emission tomography to better characterize the metabolic properties of the tumor, useful in planning treatment.[58] MRA and CTA can be used to distinguish vascular masses from tumors.

The three general methods for treatment of brain tumors are surgery, irradiation, and chemotherapy. Surgery is part of the initial management of virtually all brain tumors; it establishes the diagnosis and achieves tumor removal in many cases. The development of microsurgical neuroanatomy, the operating microscope, and advanced stereotactic and ultrasonographic technology; the fusion of imaging systems with resection techniques; and the intraoperative monitoring of evoked potentials or the EEG have improved the effectiveness of surgical resection. However, the degree of removal may be limited by the location of the tumor and its invasiveness. Stereotactic surgery uses three-dimensional coordinates and CT and MRI to localize a brain lesion precisely. Ultrasonographic technology has been used for localizing and removing tumors. The ultrasonic aspirator, which combines a vibrating head with suction, permits atraumatic removal of tumors from cranial nerves and important cortical areas. Intraoperative monitoring of evoked potentials is an important adjunct to some types of surgery. For example, evoked potentials can be used to monitor auditory, visual, speech, or motor responses during surgery done under local anesthesia.

Most malignant brain tumors respond to external irradiation. Irradiation can increase longevity and sometimes can allay symptoms when tumors recur. The treatment dose depends on the tumor's histologic type, radioresponsiveness, and anatomic site and on the level of tolerance of the surrounding tissue. A newer technique called *gamma knife* combines stereotactic localization of tumor with radiosurgery, allowing delivery of high-dose radiation to deep tumors while sparing surrounding brain. Radiation therapy is avoided in children younger than 2 years of age because of the long-term effects, which include developmental delay, panhypopituitarism, and secondary tumors.

The use of chemotherapy for brain tumors is somewhat limited by the blood-brain barrier. Chemotherapeutic agents can be administered intravenously, intra-arterially, intrathecally (*i.e.*, into the spinal canal), as wafers impregnated with a drug and implanted into the tumor at the time of surgery, or intraventricularly. A recent advance in palliative therapy is the addition of the chemotherapeutic agent temozolomide for glioblastoma, a well-tolerated oral agent. Future agents being developed will target specific genetic features and molecular profiles of a tumor.

IN SUMMARY, infections of the CNS may be classified according to the structures involved (*e.g.*, meningitis, encephalitis) or the type of organism causing the infection. The damage caused by infection may predispose to hydrocephalus, seizures, or other neurologic defects.

Brain tumors account for 2% of all cancer deaths and are the second most common type of cancer in children. Brain tumors can arise primarily from intracranial structures, and tumors from other parts of the body often metastasize to the brain. Primary brain tumors can arise from any structure in the cranial cavity. Most begin in brain tissue, but the pituitary, the pineal region, and the meninges also are sites of tumor development. Brain tumors cause focal disturbances in brain function and increased ICP. Focal disturbances result from brain compression, tumor infiltration, disturbances in blood flow, and cerebral edema. The clinical manifestations of brain tumor depend on the size and location of the tumor. General signs and symptoms include headache, nausea, vomiting, mental changes, papilledema, visual disturbances, alterations in motor and sensory function, and seizures. Diagnostic tests include physical examination, visual field testing and funduscopic examination, CT scans, MRI studies, brain scans, EEG, and cerebral angiography. Treatment includes surgery, irradiation, and chemotherapy. ∎

SEIZURE DISORDERS

After completing this section of the chapter, you should be able to meet the following objectives:

- Explain the difference between a seizure and epilepsy.
- State four or more causes of seizures other than epilepsy.
- Differentiate between the origin of seizure activity in partial and generalized forms of epilepsy and compare the manifestations of simple partial seizures with those of complex partial seizures and major and minor motor seizures.
- Characterize status epilepticus.

A seizure represents the abnormal behavior caused by an electrical discharge from neurons in the cerebral cortex. A seizure is a discrete clinical event with associated signs and symptoms that vary according to the site of neuronal discharge in the brain. Manifestations of seizure generally include sensory, motor, autonomic, or psychic phenomena. A convulsion refers to the specific seizure type of a motor seizure involving the entire body. Approximately 2 million persons in the United States are subject to recurrent seizures.[62] Seizure activity is the most common disorder encountered in pediatric neurology, and among adults its incidence is exceeded only by cerebrovascular disorders. In most persons, the first seizure episode occurs before 20 years of age. After 20 years of age, a seizure is caused most often by a structural change, trauma, tumor, or stroke.

A seizure is not a disease but a symptom of underlying CNS dysfunction. Seizures may occur during almost all serious illnesses or injuries affecting the brain, including metabolic derangements, infections, tumors, drug abuse, vascular lesions, congenital deformities, and brain injury. A seizure represents the clinical manifestations of an abnormal, uncontrolled electrical discharge from a group of neurons. Seizures are one feature of epileptic syndromes. Epilepsy refers to the syndromes of associated seizure types, EEG patterns, examination findings, hereditary patterns, and precipitating factors. Patients with an epileptic syndrome may have several seizure types. The current classification system endorsed by the International League Against Epilepsy identifies both seizure type (generalized or partial), and epilepsy syndromes.

Etiology: Provoked and Unprovoked Seizures

Many theories have been proposed to explain the cause of the abnormal brain electrical activity that occurs with seizures. Seizures may be caused by alterations in cell membrane permeability or distribution of ions across the neuronal cell mem-

SEIZURES

- Seizures are paroxysmal motor, sensory, or cognitive manifestations of spontaneous, abnormally synchronous electrical discharges from collections of neurons in the cerebral cortex.
- Seizures are thought to result directly or indirectly from changes in excitability of single neurons or groups of neurons.
- The site of seizure generation and the extent to which the abnormal neural activity is conducted to other areas of the brain determine the type and manifestations of the seizure activity.
- Partial seizures originate in a small group of neurons in one hemisphere with secondary spread of seizure activity to other parts of the brain. Simple partial seizures usually are confined to one hemisphere and do not involve loss of consciousness. Complex partial seizures begin in a localized area, spread to both hemispheres, and involve impairment of consciousness.
- Generalized seizures show simultaneous disruption of normal brain activity in both hemispheres from the onset. They include unconsciousness and varying bilateral degrees of symmetric motor responses with evidence of localization to one hemisphere. Absence seizures are generalized nonconvulsive seizure events that are expressed mainly by brief periods of unconsciousness. Tonic-clonic seizures involve unconsciousness along with both tonic and clonic muscle contractions.

branes. Another cause may be decreased inhibition of cortical or thalamic neuronal activity or structural changes that alter the excitability of neurons. Neurotransmitter imbalances such as an acetylcholine excess or γ-aminobutyric acid (GABA, an inhibitory neurotransmitter) deficiency have been proposed as causes. Certain epilepsy syndromes have been linked to specific genetic mutations causing ion channel defects.[63]

Clinically, seizures may be categorized as unprovoked (primary or idiopathic) or provoked (secondary or acute symptomatic).[62–65] Unprovoked or idiopathic seizures are those for which no identifiable cause can be determined, and are thought to be genetic. Most unprovoked seizures occur in the setting of an epileptic syndrome. These patients usually require chronic administration of antiepileptic medications to limit seizure recurrences. Provoked or symptomatic seizures include febrile seizures, seizures precipitated by systemic metabolic conditions, and those that follow a primary insult to the CNS. Most provoked seizures are best prevented by treatment of the underlying cause. For example, the most common subgroup is that of febrile seizures in children.[66] In susceptible children, a high fever, usually over 104°F, will provoke a generalized seizure. Treatment includes aggressive use of antipyretics to prevent seizures during a febrile illness. Transient systemic metabolic disturbances may precipitate seizures. Examples include electrolyte imbalances, hypoglycemia, hypoxia, hypocalcemia, uremia, alkalosis, and rapid withdrawal of sedative drugs. Specific CNS injuries such as toxemia of pregnancy, water intoxication, meningoencephalitis, trauma, cerebral hemorrhage and stroke, and brain tumors may precipitate a seizure. In all cases of provoked seizures, treatment of the immediate underlying cause often results in their resolution.

Classification

The International Classification of Epileptic Seizures determines seizure type by clinical symptoms and EEG activity. It divides seizures into two broad categories: partial seizures, in which the seizure begins in a specific or focal area of one cerebral hemisphere, and generalized seizures, which begin simultaneously in both cerebral hemispheres[67,68] (Chart 51-1). Further classification of epileptic syndromes characterizes the underlying diseases that cause the seizures, and divides seizures into idiopathic (suspected to be genetic), symptomatic (resulting from some CNS injury), and cryptogenic (presumed to be symp-

tomatic of some unidentified cause).[65] The system also has categories for seizures of undetermined origin such as neonatal seizures and a category of special syndromes such as febrile seizures.

Partial Seizures

Partial or focal seizures are the most common type of seizure among newly diagnosed cases in all groups older than 10 years of age. Partial seizures can be subdivided into three major groups: simple partial (consciousness is not impaired), complex partial (impairment of consciousness), and secondarily generalized partial seizures. These categories are based primarily on current neurophysiologic theories related to seizure propagation and the extent of involvement of the brain's hemispheres.

Simple Partial Seizures. Simple partial seizures usually involve only one hemisphere and are not accompanied by loss of consciousness or responsiveness. These seizures also have been referred to as elementary partial seizures, partial seizures with elementary symptoms, or focal seizures. The 1981 Commission on Classification and Terminology of the International League Against Epilepsy classified simple partial seizures according to motor signs, sensory symptoms, autonomic manifestations, and psychic symptoms.[67]

The observed clinical signs and symptoms depend on the area of the brain where the abnormal neuronal discharge is taking place. If the motor area of the brain is involved, the earliest symptom is motor movement corresponding to the location of onset on the contralateral side of the body. The motor movement may remain localized or may spread to other cortical areas, with sequential involvement of body parts in an epileptic-type "march," known as a *Jacksonian seizure.* If the sensory portion of the brain is involved, there may be no observable clinical manifestations. Sensory symptoms correlating with the location of seizure activity on the contralateral side of the brain may involve somatic sensory disturbance (*e.g.,* tingling and crawling sensations) or special sensory disturbance (*i.e.,* visual, auditory, gustatory, or olfactory phenomena). When abnormal cortical discharge stimulates the autonomic nervous system, flushing, tachycardia, diaphoresis, hypotension or hypertension, or pupillary changes may be evident.

The term *prodrome* or *aura* traditionally has meant a stereotyped warning sign of impending seizure activity described by the affected person. The aura actually represents a simple partial seizure, reflecting only a small area of abnormal electrical activity in the brain. Simple partial seizures may progress to complex partial seizures or generalized tonic-clonic seizures that result in unconsciousness. Most patients perceive the aura as a warning sign of impending complex partial seizures or other generalized seizures.

Complex Partial Seizures. Complex partial seizures involve impairment of consciousness and often arise from the temporal lobe. The seizure begins in a localized area of the brain but may progress rapidly to involve both hemispheres. These

---

CHART 51-1	**CLASSIFICATION OF EPILEPTIC SEIZURES**

Partial Seizures
Simple partial seizures (no impairment of consciousness)
    With motor symptoms
    With sensory symptoms
    With autonomic signs
    With psychic symptoms
Complex partial seizures (impairment of consciousness)
    Simple partial onset followed by impaired
      consciousness
    Impairment of consciousness at onset
Partial seizures evolving to secondarily generalized seizures
    Simple partial leading to generalized seizures
    Complex partial leading to generalized seizures

Unclassified Seizures
Classification not possible because of inadequate or
    incomplete data

Generalized Seizures
Absence seizures (typical or atypical)
Atonic seizures
Myoclonic seizures
Clonic seizures
Tonic
Tonic-clonic seizures

Adapted from Commission on Classification and Terminology of the International League Against Epilepsy. (1981). Proposal for revised clinical and electroencephalographic classification of epileptic seizures. *Epilepsia* 22, 489.

seizures are sometimes referred to as *psychomotor seizures,* reflecting their typical manifestations.

Complex partial seizures often are accompanied by automatisms. Automatisms are repetitive, nonpurposeful activities such as lip smacking, grimacing, patting, or rubbing clothing. Confusion during the postictal state (after a seizure) is common. Hallucinations and illusional experiences such as déjà vu (familiarity with unfamiliar events or environments) or jamais vu (unfamiliarity with a known environment) have been reported. There may be overwhelming fear, uncontrolled forced thinking or a flood of ideas, and feelings of detachment and depersonalization. A person with a complex partial seizure disorder sometimes is misdiagnosed as having a psychiatric disorder.

Secondarily Generalized Partial Seizures.   These seizures are focal at onset but then become generalized as the ictal neuronal discharge spreads, involving deeper structures of the brain, such as the thalamus or the reticular formation. Discharges spread to both hemispheres, resulting in progression to tonic-clonic seizure activity. These seizures may start as simple or complex partial seizures and may be preceded by an aura. The aura, often a stereotyped peculiar sensation that precedes the seizure, is the result of partial seizure activity. A history of an aura is clinically useful to identify the seizure as partial and not generalized in onset. However, absence of an aura does not reliably exclude a focal onset because many partial seizures generalize too rapidly to generate an aura.

Generalized-Onset Seizures

Generalized-onset seizures are the most common type in young children. These seizures are classified as primary or generalized when clinical signs, symptoms, and supporting EEG changes indicate involvement of both hemispheres at onset. The clinical symptoms include unconsciousness and involve varying bilateral degrees of symmetric motor responses without evidence of localization to one hemisphere.

These seizures are divided into four broad categories: absence seizures (typical and atypical), atonic (akinetic) seizures, myoclonic seizures, and major motor (formerly grand mal) seizures, characterized by tonic, clonic, or tonic-clonic activity.[67,68]

Absence Seizures.   Absence seizures are generalized, nonconvulsive epileptic events and are expressed mainly as disturbances in consciousness. Formerly referred to as *petit mal seizures,* absence seizures typically occur only in children and cease in adulthood or evolve to generalized motor seizures. Children may present with a history of school failure that predates the first evidence of seizure episodes. Although typical absence seizures have been characterized as a blank stare, motionlessness, and unresponsiveness, motion occurs in many cases of absence seizures. This motion takes the form of automatisms such as lip smacking, mild clonic motion (usually in the eyelids), increased or decreased postural tone, and autonomic phenomena. There often is a brief loss of contact with the environment. The seizure usually lasts only a few seconds, and then the person is able to resume normal activity immediately. The manifestations often are so subtle that they may pass unnoticed. Because automatisms and unresponsiveness are common to complex partial seizures, the latter often are mistakenly labeled as "petit mal" seizures.

Atypical absence seizures are similar to typical absence seizures except for greater alterations in muscle tone and less abrupt onset and cessation. In practice, it is difficult to distinguish typical from atypical absence seizures without the benefit of supporting EEG findings. However, it is important to distinguish between complex partial and absence seizures because the drugs of choice for treatment are different. Medications that are effective for partial seizures may increase the frequency of absence seizures.

Atonic Seizures.   In akinetic or atonic seizures, there is a sudden, split-second loss of muscle tone leading to slackening of the jaw, drooping of the limbs, or falling to the ground. These seizures also are known as *drop attacks.*

Myoclonic Seizures.   Myoclonic seizures involve brief involuntary muscle contractions induced by stimuli of cerebral origin. A myoclonic seizure involves bilateral jerking of muscles, generalized or confined to the face, trunk, or one or more extremities. Tonic seizures are characterized by a rigid, violent contraction of the muscles, fixing the limbs in a strained position. Clonic seizures consist of repeated contractions and relaxations of the major muscle groups.

Tonic-Clonic Seizures.   Tonic-clonic seizures, formerly called *grand mal seizures,* are the most common major motor seizure. Frequently, a person has a vague warning (probably a simple partial seizure) and experiences a sharp tonic contraction of the muscles with extension of the extremities and immediate loss of consciousness. Incontinence of bladder and bowel is common. Cyanosis may occur from contraction of airway and respiratory muscles. The tonic phase is followed by the clonic phase, which involves rhythmic bilateral contraction and relaxation of the extremities. At the end of the clonic phase, the person remains unconscious until the RAS begins to function again. This is called the *postictal phase.* The tonic-clonic phases last approximately 60 to 90 seconds.

Unclassified Seizures

Unclassified seizures are those that cannot be placed in one of the previous categories. These seizures are observed in the neonatal and infancy periods. Determination of whether the seizure is focal or generalized is not possible. Unclassified seizures are difficult to control with medication.

Diagnosis and Treatment

The diagnosis of seizure disorders is based on a thorough history and neurologic examination, including a full description of the seizure. The physical examination and laboratory studies help exclude any metabolic disease (*e.g.,* hyponatremia) that could precipitate seizures. MRI scans are used to identify structural defects such as temporal lobe sclerosis or underlying congenital malformations causing the seizure. One of the most useful diagnostic tests is the EEG, which is used to record changes in the brain's electrical activity. It is used to support the clinical diagnosis of epilepsy, to provide a guide for prognosis, and to assist in classifying the seizure disorder.

The first rules of treatment are to protect the person from injury during a seizure, preserve brain function by aborting or preventing seizure activity, and treat any underlying disease. Persons with epilepsy should be advised to avoid situations that could be dangerous or life-threatening if seizures occur. Treatment of the underlying disorder may reduce the frequency of seizures.

After the underlying disease is treated, the aim of treatment is to bring the seizures under control with the least possible disruption in lifestyle and minimum side effects from medication. Since the late 1970s, the therapy for epilepsy has changed drastically because of an improved classification system, the ability to measure serum anticonvulsant levels, and the availability of potent new anticonvulsant drugs. With proper drug management, 60% to 80% of persons with epilepsy can obtain good seizure control.

Anticonvulsant Medications

More than 20 drugs are available for the treatment of epilepsy. Until 1990, approximately 16 antiseizure drugs were available including carbamazepine, phenytoin, ethosuximide, valproic acid, phenobarbital, primidone, and clonazepam.[69] Newer antiepileptic drugs that have been marketed since 1996 include gabapentin, lamotrigine, felbamate, topiramate, levetiracetam, tiagabine, oxcarbazepine, and vigabatrin.[69]

Choice of drugs used as first-line therapy for seizure disorders has changed since the newer drugs were introduced because they have much better side effect profiles.[70,71] Carbamazepine, gabapentin, lamotrigine, levetiracetam, oxcarbazepine, topiramate, valproic acid, and zonisamide are the drugs of choice in treating partial seizures or tonic-clonic seizures resulting from partial seizures. Ethosuximide or valproic acid is the drug of choice for absence seizures. Valproic acid, carbamazepine, oxcarbazepine, and lamotrigine are helpful for persons with many of the minor motor seizures and tonic-clonic seizures. Myoclonic seizures can be treated with valproic acid. Atonic seizures are highly resistant to therapy. Each of the new drugs—gabapentin, lamotrigine, topiramate, and oxcarbazepine—is approved for use as monotherapy in adults who have partial seizures alone or with secondarily generalized (grand mal) seizures. The other agents are approved as add-on therapy when the first-line agent is not fully effective. In all cases, side effect profiles and patient-specific factors affect choice of antiepileptic medications.

Women of childbearing age require special consideration concerning fertility, contraception, and pregnancy. Many of the drugs interact with oral contraceptives; some affect hormone function or decrease fertility. All such women should be advised to take folic acid supplementation. For women with epilepsy who become pregnant, antiseizure drugs increase the risk for congenital abnormalities and other perinatal complications. Carbamazepine, phenytoin, phenobarbital, primidone, and valproic acid can interfere with vitamin D metabolism and predispose to osteoporosis.

Whenever possible, a single drug should be used in epilepsy therapy. Monotherapy eliminates drug interactions and additive side effects. Determining the proper dose of the anticonvulsant drug is often a long and tedious process, which can be very frustrating for the person with epilepsy. Consistency in taking the medication is essential. Anticonvulsant drugs never should be discontinued abruptly; the dose should be decreased slowly to prevent seizure recurrence. The most frequent cause of recurrent seizures is patient noncompliance with drug regimens. Ongoing education and support are extremely important in the management of seizures. The psychosocial implications of a diagnosis of epilepsy continue to have a large impact on those affected with the disorder.

The neurologist and primary care physician must work together when a person on anticonvulsant medication becomes ill and must take additional medications. Some drugs act synergistically, and others interfere with the actions of anticonvulsant medications. This situation needs to be carefully monitored to avoid overmedication or interference with successful seizure control.

Surgical Therapy

Surgical treatment may be an option for persons with epilepsy that is refractory to drug treatment.[72] With the use of modern neuroimaging and surgical techniques, a single epileptogenic lesion can be identified and removed without leaving a neurologic deficit. The most common surgery consists of removal of the amygdala and an anterior part of the hippocampus and entorhinal cortex, as well as a small part of the temporal pole, leaving the lateral temporal neocortex intact. Another surgical procedure involves partial removal of the corpus callosum to prevent spread of a unilateral seizure to a generalized seizure. Some refractory patients benefit from an implantable electrical stimulator of the vagus nerve. Modern epilepsy surgery requires a multidisciplinary team of highly skilled surgeons and specialists working together in an epilepsy center. Most procedures require only a few hours in the operating room and a few days' stay in the hospital after surgery. Epilepsy surgery is increasingly considered a treatment modality for persons with medically intractable epilepsy.

Generalized Convulsive Status Epilepticus

Seizures that do not stop spontaneously or occur in succession without recovery are called *status epilepticus*. There are as many types of status epilepticus as there are types of seizures.

Tonic-clonic status epilepticus is a medical emergency and, if not promptly treated, may lead to respiratory failure and death.

The disorder occurs most frequently in the young and old. Morbidity and mortality rates are highest in elderly persons and persons with acute symptomatic seizures, such as those related to anoxia or cerebral infarction.[72] Approximately one third of patients have no history of a seizure disorder, and in another one third, status epilepticus occurs as an initial manifestation of epilepsy.[73] If status epilepticus is caused by neurologic or systemic disease, the cause needs to be identified and treated immediately because the seizures probably will not respond until the underlying cause has been corrected.

Treatment consists of appropriate life support measures. Medications are given to control seizure activity. Intravenously administered diazepam or lorazepam is considered first-line therapy for the condition. The prognosis is related to the underlying cause as well as the duration of the seizures themselves.

IN SUMMARY, seizures are caused by spontaneous, uncontrolled, paroxysmal, transitory discharges from cortical centers in the brain. Seizures may occur as a reversible symptom of another disease condition or as a recurrent condition called *epilepsy.* Epileptic seizures are classified as partial or generalized seizures. Partial seizures have evidence of local onset, beginning in one hemisphere. They include simple partial seizures, in which consciousness is not lost, and complex partial seizures, which begin in one hemisphere but progress to involve both. Generalized seizures involve both hemispheres from the start and include unconsciousness and rapidly occurring, widespread, bilateral symmetric motor responses. They include minor motor seizures such as absence and akinetic seizures, and major motor or grand mal seizures. Control of seizures is the primary goal of treatment and is accomplished with anticonvulsant medications. Anticonvulsant medications interact with each other and need to be monitored closely when more than one drug is used. ■

Review Exercises

1. A 20-year-man is an unbelted driver involved in a motor vehicle accident and presents in coma.

   A. *What are the clinical signs of coma?*

   B. *Where does the source of coma localize in the brain?*

   C. *Which complications of traumatic head injury might lead to coma?*

   D. *What are the key treatment options to manage elevated intracranial pressure?*

2. A 65-year-old woman presents with a 1-hour history of right-sided weakness and aphasia. An immediate CT scan of the brain is negative.

   A. *Where in the brain is the pathologic process?*

   B. *What are the indications to administer intravenous tissue plasminogen activator?*

   C. *What are the possible causes of this stroke, and what diagnostic tests would reveal the cause?*

3. A child is taken to the emergency department with lethargy, fever, and a stiff neck on examination.

   A. *What findings on initial lumbar puncture indicate bacterial versus viral meningitis?*

   B. *In the case of bacterial meningitis, what are the most likely organisms?*

4. A 60-year-old man develops involuntary shaking of his right arm, which spreads to the face; then he collapses with whole-body shaking and loss of consciousness. After 1 minute, the shaking stops, and he is confused and disoriented.

   A. *What type of seizure is suggested by the clinical manifestations?*

   B. *Assuming this is his first seizure, what diagnostic tests should be performed to identify a cause for the seizure?*

   C. *If he has a long history of similar recurrent seizures, what treatments should be instituted? What treatments should be considered if he has failed multiple adequate trials of anticonvulsant medications?*

References

1. Frosch M. P., Anthony D., DeGirofami U. (2005). The central nervous system. In Kumar V., Abbas A. K., Fausto N. (Eds.), *Robbins and Cotran pathologic basis of disease* (7th ed., pp. 1347–1419). Philadelphia: Elsevier Saunders.

2. Meyer F. B. (1992). Brain metabolism, blood flow, and ischemic thresholds. In Awad I. A. (Ed.), *Neurosurgical topics: Cerebrovascular occlusive disease and brain ischemia* (pp. 1–24). Cleveland: American Association of Neurological Surgeons.

3. Richmond T. S. (1997). Cerebral resuscitation after global brain ischemia: Linking research to practice. *AACN Clinical Issues* 8, 171–181.

4. Trojanowsi J. Q., Kenyon L. (2008). The central nervous system. In Rubin R., Strayer D. E. (Eds.), *Rubin's pathology: Clinicopathologic foundations of medicine* (5th ed., pp. 1171–1208). Philadelphia: Lippincott Williams & Wilkins.

5. Martin T. G. (1986). Drowning and near-drowning. *Hospital Medicine* 22(7), 53.

6. Adams H. P. Jr., del Zorro G., Alberts M. J., et al. (2007). Guidelines for the early management of adults with ischemic stroke. *Stroke* 38, 1655–1711.

7. American Heart Association. (2005). Guidelines for cardiopulmonary resuscitation and emergency cardiovascular care: Postresuscitation support. *Circulation* 112, IV-84–IV-88.

8. Harukuni I., Bhardwaj A. (2006). Mechanisms of brain injury after global cerebral ischemia. *Neurologic Clinics* 24, 1–21.

9. Lipton S. A., Rosenberg P. A. (1994). Excitatory amino acids as a final common pathway in neurologic disorders. *New England Journal of Medicine* 330, 613–622.

10. Feuerstein G., Hunter J., Barone F. C. (1992). Calcium blockers and neuroprotection. In Marangos P. J., Lal H. (Eds.), *Advances in neuroprotection: Emerging strategies in neuroprotection* (p. 129). Boston: Birkhauser.

11. Sauer D., Massiu L., Allegrini P. R., et al. (1992). Excitotoxicity, cerebral ischemia, and neuroprotection by competitive NMDA receptor antagonists. In Marangos P. J., Lal H. (Eds.), *Advances in neuroprotection: Emerging strategies in neuroprotection* (pp. 93–105). Boston: Birkhauser.

12. Albers G. W., Clark W. M., DeGraba T. J. (1998). *The evolving paradigm of neuronal protection following stroke.* Monograph. Englewood, CO: Postgraduate Institute for Medicine.

13. Hickey J. V. (2003). *The clinical practice of neurological and neurosurgical nursing* (5th ed., pp. 159–184, 295–327). Philadelphia: Lippincott-Raven.

14. Lang E. W., Chestnut R. M. (1995). Intracranial pressure and cerebral perfusion pressure in severe head injury. *New Horizons* 3, 400–409.

15. Guyton A. C., Hall J. E. (2006). *Textbook of medical physiology* (11th ed., pp. 192, 761–767). Philadelphia: Elsevier Saunders.

16. Plum F., Posner J. B. (1980). *The diagnosis of stupor and coma* (3rd ed.). Philadelphia: F. A. Davis.

17. Xao F. (2002). Bench to bedside: Brain edema and cerebral resuscitation: The present and the future. *Academy of Emergency Medicine* 9, 933–946.

18. Ghajar J. (2000). Traumatic brain injury. *Lancet* 356, 923–929.

19. White R. J., Likavec M. J. (1992). The diagnosis and initial management of head injury. *New England Journal of Medicine* 327, 1507–1511.

20. Jennett B. (1996). Epidemiology of head injury. *Journal of Neurology, Neurosurgery, and Psychiatry* 60, 362–369.

21. Chestnut R. M. (1995). Secondary brain insults after head injury: Clinical perspectives. *New Horizons* 3, 366–375.

22. Teasdale G. M. (1995). Head injury. *Journal of Neurology, Neurosurgery, and Psychiatry* 58, 526–539.

23. Ropper A. H., Gorson K. C. (2007). Concussion. *New England Journal of Medicine* 356, 166–172.

24. Alverzo J. P. (2006). A review of the literature on orientation as an indicator of level of consciousness. *Journal of Nursing Scholarship* 38, 159–170.

25. Stevens R. D., Bhardwaji A. (2006). Approach to the comatose patient. *Critical Care Medicine* 34, 31–41.

26. Rhoades R. A., Tanner G. A. (2003). *Medical physiology* (2nd ed., pp. 132–133). Philadelphia: Lippincott Williams & Wilkins.

27. Ingersoll G. L., Leyden D. B. (1987). The Glasgow Coma Scale for patients with head injuries. *Critical Care Nursing* 7(5), 26–32.

28. Teasdale G. M. (2000). Revisiting the Glasgow Coma Scale and Coma Score. *Intensive Care Medicine* 26, 153–154.

29. Wijdicks E. F. M. (2001). The diagnosis of brain death. *New England Journal of Medicine* 344, 1215–1221.

30. Quality Standards Subcommittee of American Academy of Neurology. (1995). Practice parameters for determining brain death in adults. *Neurology* 45, 1012–1014.

31. Quality Standards Subcommittee of American Academy of Neurology. (1995). Practice parameters: Assessment and management of patients with persistent vegetative state. *Neurology* 45, 1015–1018.

32. Giacino J. T., Ashwal S., Cranford R., et al. (2002). The minimally conscious state. *Neurology* 58, 349–353.

33. American Stroke Association. (2007). *Heart disease and stroke statistics—2007 update.* Dallas: Author.

34. Goldstein L. B., Chairperson, Stroke Council of American Heart Association. (2001). Primary prevention of ischemic stroke: A statement for health care professionals. *Circulation* 103, 163–182.

35. Gorelick P. B. (1987). Alcohol and stroke. *Current Concepts in Cerebrovascular Disease* 21(5), 21.

36. Blank-Reid C. (1996). How to have a stroke at an early age: The effects of crack, cocaine, and other illicit drugs. *Journal of Neuroscience Nursing* 28(1), 19–27.

37. Albers W. A., Chair. (1998). Antithrombotic and thrombolytic therapy for ischemic stroke. *Chest* 114, 683S–698S.

38. Zambramski J. M., Anson J. A. (1992). Diagnostic evaluation of ischemic cerebrovascular disease. In Awad I. A. (Ed.), *Neurosurgical topics: Cerebrovascular occlusive disease and brain ischemia* (pp. 73–101). Cleveland, OH: American Association of Neurological Surgeons.

39. Johnston S. C. (2002). Transient ischemic attack. *New England Journal of Medicine* 347, 1687–1692.

40. Gregory W., Chair, Ad Hoc Committee on Guidelines for Management of Transient Ischemic Attacks, Stroke Council, American Heart Association. (1999). Supplement to the guidelines for transient ischemic attacks. *Stroke* 30, 2502–2511.

41. Qureshi A. I., Tuhrim S., Broderick J. P., et al. (2001). Spontaneous intracerebral hemorrhage. *New England Journal of Medicine* 344, 1450–1460.

42. Fewel M. E., Thompson M. G., Hoff J. T. (2003). Spontaneous intracerebral hemorrhage: A review. *Neurosurgical Focus* 15, 1–17.

43. Broderick J. P., Adams H. P., Barson W., et al. (1999). American Heart Association Scientific Statement: Guidelines to the management of spontaneous intracerebral hemorrhage. *Stroke* 30, 905–915.

44. Bronstein K. S., Popovich J. M., Stewart-Amidei C. (1991). *Promoting stroke recovery: A research based approach for nurses* (p. 200). St. Louis: C. V. Mosby.

45. New Alberts M. J., Hademenos G., Latchaw R. E., et al. (2000). Recommendations for the establishment of primary stroke centers. *Journal of the American Medical Association* 283, 3102–3109.

46. Brott T., Bogousslavsy J. (2000). Treatment of acute ischemic stroke. *New England Journal of Medicine* 343, 709–721.

47. Brisman J. L., Song J. K., Newell D. W. (2006). Cerebral aneurysms. *New England Journal of Medicine* 355, 928–939.

48. Suarez J. I., Tarr R. W., Selman W. R. (2006). Aneurysmal subarachnoid hemorrhage. *New England Journal of Medicine* 354, 387–396.

49. Feigin V. L., Rinkel G. J. E., Lawes C. M. M., et al. (2005). Risk factors for subarachnoid hemorrhage: An updated systematic review of epidemiological studies. *Stroke* 36, 1773–2780.

50. Feigin V. L., Findlay M. (2006). Advances in subarachnoid hemorrhage. *Stroke* 37, 305–308.

51. Fleetwood I. G., Steinberg G. K. (2002). Arteriovenous malformations. *Lancet* 359, 893.

52. Friedlander R. M. (2007). Arteriovenous malformations of the brain. *New England Journal of Medicine* 356, 2704–2712.

53. Ogilvy C. S., Chair, Special Writing Group of the Stroke Council, American Heart Association. (2001). Recommendations for management of intracranial arteriovenous malformations. *Stroke* 32, 1458–1471.

54. van de Beek D., de Gans J., Tunkel A. R., et al. (2006). Community-acquired bacterial meningitis in adults. *New England Journal of Medicine* 354, 44–53.

55. van de Beek D., de Gans J., Spanjaard L., et al. (2004). Clinical features and prognostic factors in adults with bacterial pneumonia. *New England Journal of Medicine* 351, 1849–1859.

56. Tunkel A. R., Hartman B. J., Kaplan B. A., et al. (2004). Practice guidelines for management of bacterial meningitis. *Clinical Infectious Diseases* 39, 1267–1284.

57. American Cancer Society. (2007). *Cancer facts & figures: 2007.* [Online]. Available: www.cancer.org. Accessed April 11, 2008.

58. DeAngelis L. M. (2001). Brain tumors. *New England Journal of Medicine* 344, 114–123.

59. Kuttesch J. F. Jr., Ater J. L. (2004). Brain tumors in childhood. In Behrman R. E., Kliegman R. M., Jenson H. B. (Eds.), *Nelson textbook of pediatrics* (17th ed., pp. 1702–1711). Philadelphia: Elsevier Saunders.

60. DeAngelis L. M., Posner J. B. (2001). Cancer of the central nervous system and pituitary gland. In Lenhard R. E., Osteen R. T., Gansler T. (Eds.), *The American Cancer Society's clinical oncology* (pp. 655–703). Atlanta: American Cancer Society.

61. Behin A., Hoang-Xuan K., Carpenter A. F., et al. (2003). Primary brain tumors in adults. *Lancet* 361, 323–331.

62. Browne T. R., Holmes G. L. (2001). Epilepsy. *New England Journal of Medicine* 344, 1145–1151.

63. Chang B. S., Lowenstein D. H. (2003). Mechanisms of disease: Epilepsy. *New England Journal of Medicine* 349, 1257–1266.

64. Mosewich R. K., So E. L. (1996). The clinical approach to classification of seizures and epileptic syndromes. *Mayo Clinic Proceedings* 71, 405–441.

65. Benbadis S. (2001). Epileptic seizures and syndromes. *Neurology Clinics: Epilepsy* 19, 251–270.

66. Johnston M. V. (2004). Seizures in childhood. In Behrman R. E., Kliegman R. M., Jenson H. B. (Eds.), *Nelson textbook of pediatrics* (17th ed., pp. 1993–2009). Philadelphia: Elsevier Saunders.

67. Commission on Classification and Terminology of the International League Against Epilepsy. (1981). Proposal for revised clinical and electroencephalographic classification of epileptic seizures. *Epilepsia* 22, 489–501.

68. Commission on Classification and Terminology of the International League Against Epilepsy. (1989). Proposal for revised classification of epilepsies and epileptic syndromes. *Epilepsia* 30, 389–399.

69. Porter R. J., Meldrum M. B. (2007). Antiseizure drugs. In Katzung B. G. (Ed.), *Basic and clinical pharmacology* (10th ed., pp. 375–394). New York: McGraw-Hill Medical.

70. Nguyen D. K., Spencer S. S. (2003). Recent advances in the treatment of epilepsy. *Archives of Neurology* 60, 929–935.

71. Nardkarini S., LaJoie J., Devinsky O. (2005). Current treatments in epilepsy. *Neurology* 64(Suppl. 3), S2–S11.

72. Engel J. (1996). Surgery for seizures. *New England Journal of Medicine* 334, 647–652.

73. Cascino G. D. (1996). Generalized convulsive status epilepticus. *New England Journal of Medicine* 71, 787–792.

Visit the Point. **http://thePoint.lww.com for animations, journal articles, and more!**

Sleep and Sleep Disorders

CAROL M. PORTH

> As humans, we spend approximately a third of our lives asleep. We all know what sleep feels like. Yet defining sleep, describing what happens when we sleep, and explaining why we sleep are more difficult. Of equal concern is an understanding of factors that interfere with sleep. For many people, the inability to engage in appropriate periods of normal, restful sleep seriously impairs their functioning. The content in this chapter is divided into three parts: (1) the neurobiology of sleep, (2) sleep disorders, and (3) sleep and sleep disorders in children and the elderly.

NEUROBIOLOGY OF SLEEP

After completing this section of the chapter, you should be able to meet the following objectives:

- Cite the major brain structures that are involved in sleep.
- Describe the different stages of sleep in terms of the electroencephalogram tracing, eye movements, motor movements, heart rate, blood pressure, and cerebral activity.
- Characterize the circadian rhythm as it relates to sleep and wakefulness.
- Describe the possible role of melatonin in regulation of sleep.

Sleep is part of what is called the *sleep–wake cycle.* In contrast to wakefulness, which is a time of mental activity and energy expenditure, sleep is a period of inactivity and restoration of mental and physical function. It has been suggested that sleep provides time for entering information that has been acquired during periods of wakefulness into memory and for reestablishing communication between various parts of the brain. Sleep also is a time when other body systems restore their energy and repair their tissues. Muscle activity and digestion decrease and sympathetic nervous system activity is diminished. Many hormones, such as growth hormone, are produced in a cyclic manner correlating with the sleep–wake cycle, suggesting that growth and tissue repair may occur during sleep.

Neural Structures and Pathways

Anatomically, the sleep–wake cycle involves structures in the thalamus, associated areas of the cerebral cortex, and interneurons in the reticular formation of the midbrain, the pons, and the brain stem (Fig. 52-1A). The reticular formation of the midbrain, pons, and brain stem monitors and modulates the activity of various circuits controlling wakefulness. The thalamus and the cerebral cortex function in tandem, with all sensory information being relayed to the thalamus and from there to the cerebral cortex. For example, visual impulses from the retina go to the thalamus and are then relayed to the visual cortex. The pathways between each sensory area of the thalamus and the cortex form two-way communication loops called *thalamocortical loops*.[1] Communication between each sensory area of the thalamus and its companion area in the cortex is kept orderly by several neuronal control systems, including the midbrain reticular formation that controls the level of background activity so that external stimuli can be processed.

The Sleep–Wake Cycle

The sleep–wake cycle normally consists of a synchronous pattern of wakefulness and sleep. Wakefulness is a state of being aware of the environment—of receiving and responding to information arriving from all the senses, placing that information into memory, and recalling and integrating present experiences with previously stored memories. During wakefulness, both the thalamocortical loop and brain stem centers are active. A full repertoire of motor movements is made possible by corticospinal circuits that travel through the brain stem. Sleep represents a period of diminished consciousness from which a person can be aroused by sensory or other stimuli. It occurs in stages during which the brain remains active, but does not effectively process sensory information.

SLEEP–WAKE CYCLE

- The sleep–wake cycle normally consists of a synchronous pattern of wakefulness and sleep. Wakefulness is a state of being aware of the environment, receiving and responding to sensory input, recalling and integrating experiences into memory, and purposeful body movements.
- Sleep, which is a period of inactivity and restoration of mental and physical function, is characterized by alternations between non-REM and REM sleep.
- Non-REM sleep is a quiet type of sleep characterized by a relatively inactive, yet fully regulating brain, and fully movable body, whereas REM sleep is associated with rapid eye movements, loss of muscle movements, and vivid dreaming.

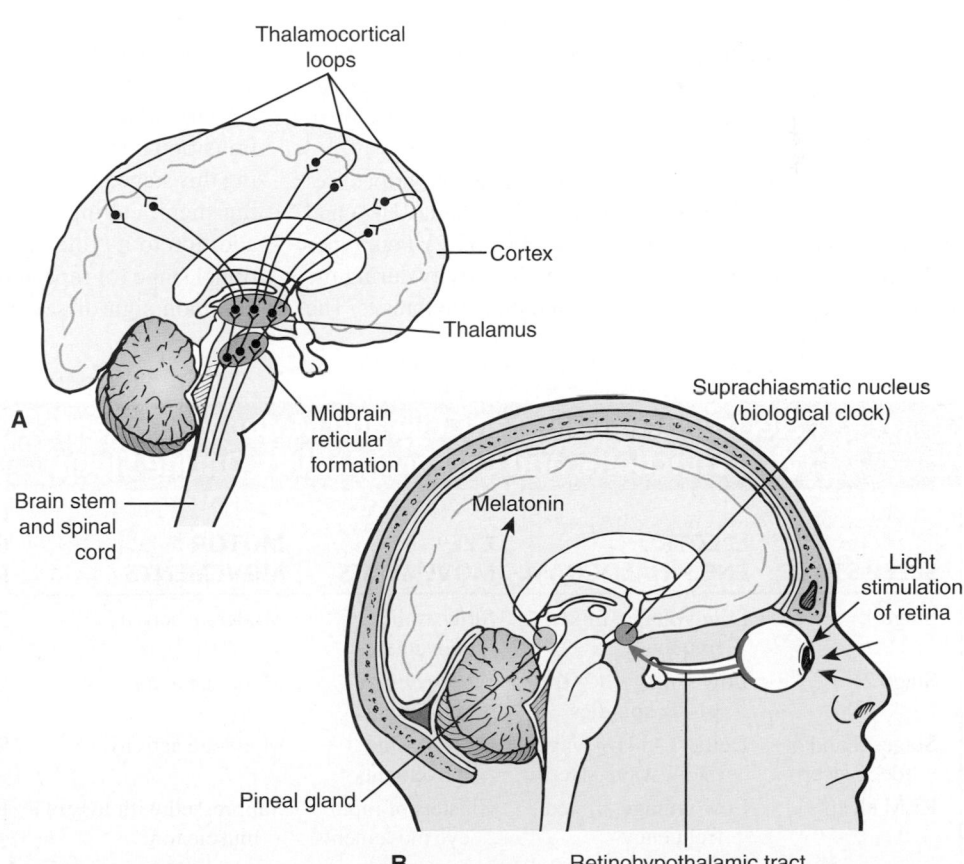

FIGURE 52-1 • (A) Brain structures involved in sleep. (B) Location of the suprachiasmatic nucleus (biologic clock) with input from the retina and its association with the pineal gland and melatonin production.

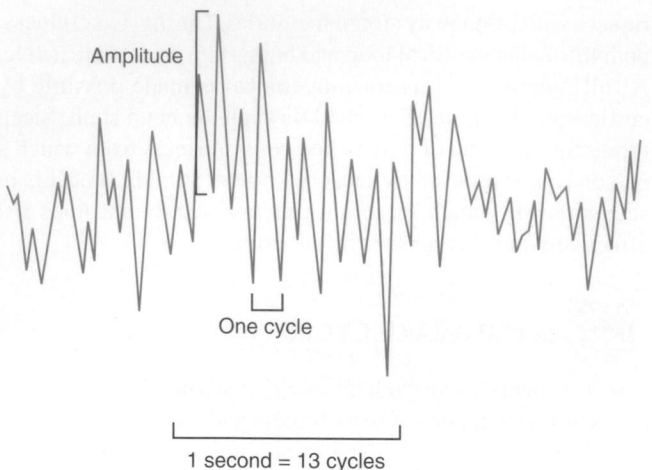

FIGURE 52-2 • The amplitude and frequency characteristics of an EEG tracing.

Brain Waves

Many of the advances in understanding the sleep–wake cycle have come about because of the ability to record brain waves through the use of the electroencephalogram (EEG). It was in 1928 that the German psychiatrist Hans Berger first successfully recorded continuous electrical activity from the scalp of human subjects.[1] The source of the brain waves is the alternating excitatory and inhibitory nerve activity in postsynaptic neurons.[2] During the recording of an EEG, the postsynaptic potentials are averaged and filtered to improve the quality of the signal. As such, the EEG does not measure the activity of a single neuron, but rather the combined activity and "crosstalk" among many hundreds of neurons responding to a given stimulus.

The normal EEG consists of brain waves of various frequencies (measured in cycles per second, or hertz [Hz]) and amplitude (measured in microvolts [μV]; Fig. 52-2). Four types of EEG rhythms are used to describe brain activity during the sleep–wake cycle: alpha, beta, delta, and theta rhythms.[2–4] The

alpha rhythm, which has a frequency of 7 to 13 Hz, occurs when a person is awake with eyes closed. When the eyes are open, the EEG becomes desynchronized and the dominant frequency changes to the low-amplitude *beta* rhythm with a frequency greater than 13 Hz. The increased frequency of the beta waves is thought to reflect a higher level of brain activity produced by firing of a large number of neurons, and the low amplitude a lack of synchronization resulting from nerve activity occurring in many different brain sites at the same time. The *delta* (0.5 to 4 Hz) and *theta* (4 to 7 Hz) rhythms are observed during sleep. The low-frequency, higher-amplitude waves that occur during sleep indicate that fewer neurons are firing and that those that are active are more highly synchronized and less affected by sensory stimulation.

Sleep Stages

There are two types of sleep: rapid eye movement (REM) and non-REM sleep.[2,4,5] These two types of sleep alternate with each other and are characterized by differences in eye movements, muscle tone and body movements, heart rate and blood pressure, breathing patterns, brain wave activity, and dreaming (Table 52-1).

Non–Rapid Eye Movement Sleep. Non-REM sleep is a quiet type of sleep characterized by a relatively inactive, yet fully regulating brain, and a fully movable body.[5] The brain stem coordinates activity between the spinal cord and various reflexes such as swallowing and chewing. Non-REM sleep normally is encountered when the person first becomes drowsy. It is divided into four stages that reflect an increasing depth of sleep (Fig. 52-3). *Stage 1* consists of low-voltage, mixed-frequency EEG activity. It occurs at sleep onset and is a brief (1 to 7 minutes) transitional stage between wakefulness and true sleep. During this stage, persons can be easily aroused simply by touching them, calling their name, or quietly closing a door. In addition to its role at sleep onset, stage 1 serves as a transitional stage for repeated sleep cycles throughout the night. A common sign of severely disrupted sleep is an increase or

TABLE 52-1 Electroencephalogram, Eye and Motor Movements, Vital Functions, and Cerebral Activity During Sleep

SLEEP STAGE	ELECTRO-ENCEPHALOGRAM	EYE MOVEMENTS	MOTOR MOVEMENTS	HEART RATE, BLOOD PRESSURE, RESPIRATIONS	CEREBRAL ACTIVITY
Stage 1	Low voltage, mixed frequency	Slow, rolling movements	Moderate activity	Slows	Decreases
Stage 2	Low voltage, 12- to 14-Hz spindles	Slow, rolling movements	Moderate activity	Slows	Decreases
Stages 3 and 4 (deep sleep)	Delta (1–3 Hz) waves (slow-wave sleep)	Slow, rolling movements	Moderate activity	Slows	Decreases
REM sleep	Low voltage, mixed frequency	Clusters of rapid eye movements	Suppressed with loss of muscle tone	Increases, variable	Increases

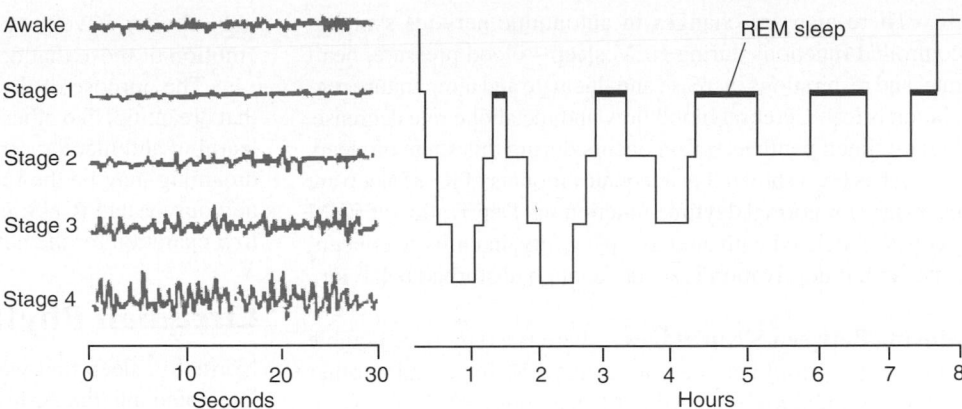

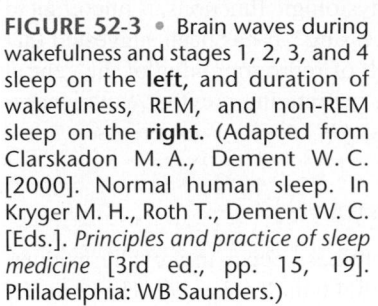

FIGURE 52-3 • Brain waves during wakefulness and stages 1, 2, 3, and 4 sleep on the **left**, and duration of wakefulness, REM, and non-REM sleep on the **right**. (Adapted from Clarskadon M. A., Dement W. C. [2000]. Normal human sleep. In Kryger M. H., Roth T., Dement W. C. [Eds.]. *Principles and practice of sleep medicine* [3rd ed., pp. 15, 19]. Philadelphia: WB Saunders.)

decrease in stage 1 sleep. *Stage 2,* which lasts approximately 10 to 25 minutes, is a deeper sleep during which EEG activity is interrupted by sleep spindles consisting of bursts of high-frequency (12 to 14 Hz) waves. *Stages 3* and *4* represent deep sleep and are dominated by high-voltage, low-frequency (1 to 3 Hz) waves. Stage 3 usually lasts only a few minutes and is transitional to stage 4, which lasts for approximately 20 to 40 minutes. During deep sleep, the muscles of the body relax and posture is adjusted intermittently. The heart rate and blood pressure decrease and gastrointestinal activity is slowed. An incrementally larger stimulus is required for arousal from slow-wave sleep.

Rapid Eye Movement Sleep. REM sleep is associated with rapid eye movements, loss of muscle movements, and vivid dreaming.[5] External sensory input is inhibited, whereas internal sensory circuits such as those of the auditory and visual systems are aroused. During this time, the brain can replay previous memories but cannot acquire new sensory information (Fig. 52-4). At the same time, motor systems that control body movements are inhibited. There is a loss of muscle movement and muscle tone. The result is an extraordinary set of paradoxes, in which people see things in their dreams, but cannot move. They imagine being engaged in activities such as running, flying, or dancing but are paralyzed.

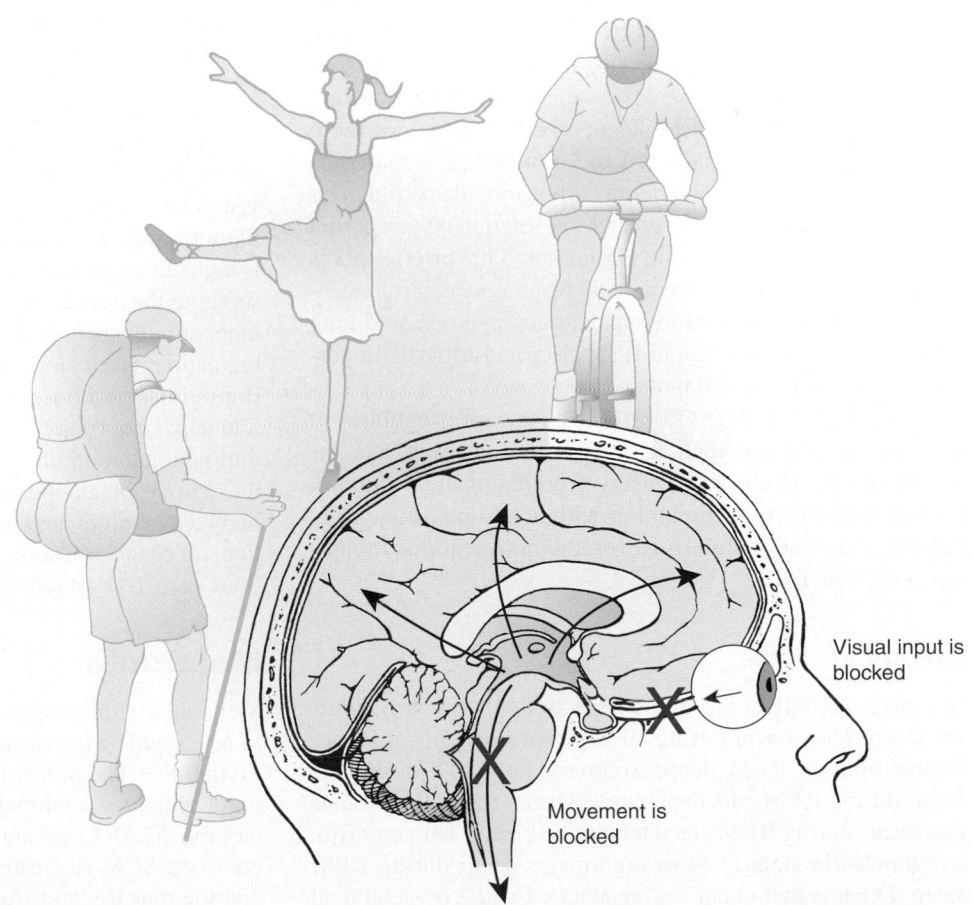

FIGURE 52-4 • Dreaming during REM sleep when sensory and motor activity are blocked.

There also are changes in autonomic nervous system–controlled functions during REM sleep—blood pressure, heart rate, and respirations increase and fluctuate and temperature regulation is lost. Cerebral blood flow and metabolic rate decrease. Sleep-related penile erection occurs during this stage of sleep.

It has been shown that adequate amounts of REM sleep are necessary for normal daytime functioning. Deprivation of REM sleep is associated with anxiety, irritability, inability to concentrate, and, if deprivation is severe enough, disturbed behavior.

Moving Between Sleep Stages.   There is a rather predictable pattern of shifting between one non-REM stage and another during a typical night's sleep.[4] At sleep onset, there is a stepwise descent from lighter stage 1 sleep to deeper stage 4 sleep, followed by an abrupt ascent back toward stage 1. However, in place of stage 1, the first REM episode usually occurs. REM sleep is comparatively short (1 to 5 minutes) during the first sleep cycle, but gradually becomes longer across the night. Stages 3 and 4 occupy less time in the second and subsequent sleep cycles and disappear altogether in later cycles.

Breathing During Sleep

Breathing normally changes during sleep. Stages 1 and 2 of non-REM sleep are characterized by a cyclic waning and waxing of the tidal volume and respiratory rate, which may include brief periods (5 to 15 seconds) of apnea. This pattern is called *periodic breathing.* Although the amount of periodic breathing that occurs during the first two stages of non-REM sleep differs among healthy persons, it is more common in persons older than 40 years of age.[6] After sleep has stabilized during stages 3 and 4 of non-REM sleep, breathing becomes more regular. Ventilation usually is 1 to 2 L/minute less than during quiet wakefulness; the arterial carbon dioxide partial pressure (PCO_2) is 2 to 8 mm Hg greater; the arterial oxygen partial pressure (PO_2) is 5 to 10 mm Hg less; and the arterial pH is 0.03 to 0.05 units lower.[7] Involuntary respiratory control mechanisms, such as responses to hypercapnia, hypoxia, and lung inflation, are intact during non-REM sleep and critically important to maintaining ventilation.

During REM sleep, respirations become irregular, but not periodic, and may include short periods of apnea. Breathing during REM sleep has many features of the voluntary control that integrates breathing with acts such as walking, talking, and swallowing. However, their influence on breathing is diminished.

Dreaming

Dreams are recollections of mental activity that occurred during sleep. They occur during all stages of sleep, but are more frequent during REM sleep. Approximately 80% of dreams occur during REM and sleep onset (stages 1 and 2).[8] Dreams that occur during REM sleep tend to be bizarre with colorful, storybook-like detail.[1] Most nightmares occur during REM sleep. Dreams that occur during stages 1 and 2 of sleep tend to be shorter, have fewer associations, and lack the color and emotion of those that occur during REM sleep.

The purpose of dreaming is unclear. Evidence suggests that dreaming, like other physiologic functions, is important to learning and memory processing.[8] It has been suggested that dreaming may be the result of reprogramming of the central nervous system (CNS; *i.e.,* rearranging previous experiences) in preparation for the next day's conscious experiences.

Circadian Rhythms

Normally, sleep and wakefulness occur in a cyclic manner, integrated into the 24-hour light–dark solar day. The term *circadian,* from the Latin *circa* ("about") and *dies* ("day"), is used to describe these 24-hour diurnal rhythms. The function of the circadian time system is to provide a temporal organization for physiologic processes and behaviors as a means of promoting effective adaptation to the environment. At the behavioral level, this is expressed in regular cycles of sleep and waking and body functions such as temperature regulation and hormone secretion based on changes in the 24-hour light–dark solar day.

The daily rhythm of the sleep–wake cycle is part of a timekeeping system created by an internal pacemaker or clock.[9,10] Time isolation experiments, in which people were placed in an environment without time cues, showed that the cycle length of the human internal clock is in general from 23.5 to 26.5 hours.[8] Because the intrinsic cycle tends to be longer than 24 hours, a daily resetting of the circadian clock is necessary to synchronize with the environmental day. This process is called *entrainment* and normally is accomplished by exposure to the light–dark changes of the solar day.

The circadian clock appears to be controlled by a small group of hypothalamic cells, called the *suprachiasmatic nucleus* (SCN), located just above the optic chiasm and lateral to the third ventricle[9–11] (see Fig. 52-1). The SCN, which receives light–dark input from the retina, exhibits a rhythm of neuronal firing that is high during the day and low during the night. Although light serves as the primary stimulus for resetting the circadian clock, other stimuli such as locomotion and activity contribute to its regulation. The major projections from the SCN are to the anterior pituitary, with lesser ones to the basal forebrain and midline thalamus. Projections to the anterior pituitary provide for diurnal regulation of growth hormone and cortisol secretion; those to hypothalamic centers, for changes in metabolism and body temperature; and those to the brain stem reticular formation, for changes in autonomic nervous system–regulated functions such as heart rate and blood pressure (Fig. 52-5).

Melatonin

Melatonin, a hormone produced by the pineal gland, is thought to help regulate the sleep–wake cycle and, possibly, circadian rhythm.[12–14] The pineal gland synthesizes and releases melatonin at night, a rhythm that is under direct control of the SCN (see Fig. 52-1). Large numbers of melatonin receptors are present in the SCN, suggesting a feedback loop between the SCN and the pineal gland. Administration of melatonin produces

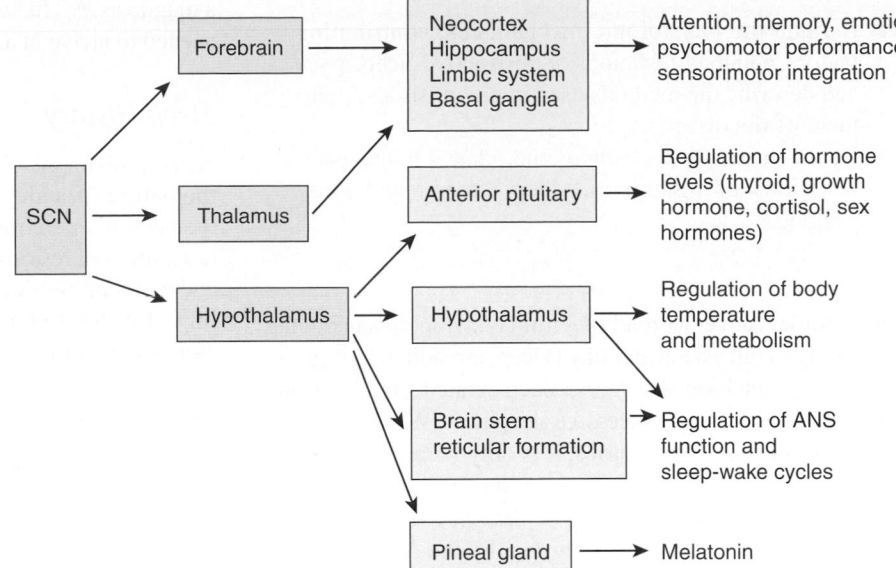

FIGURE 52-5 • Projections from the suprachiasmatic nucleus (SCN) to the forebrain, thalamus, and hypothalamus. ANS, autonomic nervous system

phase-shifting changes in the circadian rhythm, similar to those caused by light. There has been recent interest in the use of melatonin in treatment of various sleep disorders, particularly those related to a shift in the circadian rhythm. Although synthetic preparations are available without prescription in health food stores and pharmacies, their potency, purity, safety, and effectiveness cannot be ensured. There also is a lack of clinical trial evidence about appropriate dosage, adverse effects, drug interactions, and the effects of melatonin on various disease states.[13] A pharmacologic melatonin-receptor agonist has, however, become recently available as a prescription drug (to be discussed).

Normally, sleep and wakefulness occur in a cyclic manner, called the *circadian rhythm,* that is integrated into the 24-hour light–dark solar day. The circadian clock is thought to be controlled by the SCN in the hypothalamus. The SCN, which receives light–dark input from the retina, exhibits a rhythm of neuronal firing that is high during the day and low during the night. Melatonin, a hormone produced by the pineal gland, is thought to help regulate the sleep–wake cycle. ■

 SLEEP DISORDERS

IN SUMMARY, sleep is part of what is called the *sleep–wake cycle.* In contrast to wakefulness, which is a time of mental activity and energy expenditure, sleep is a period of inactivity and restoration of mental and physical function. There are two types of sleep: rapid eye movement (REM) and non-REM sleep. REM sleep is associated with rapid eye movements, loss of muscle movements, and vivid dreaming. External sensory input is inhibited, whereas internal sensory circuits such as those of the auditory and visual systems are aroused. Non-REM sleep is a quiet type of sleep characterized by a relatively inactive, yet fully regulating brain, and a fully movable body. It is divided into four stages that reflect an increasing depth of sleep. Stage 1 is a brief transitional stage that occurs at the onset of sleep, during which a person is easily aroused. Stage 2 is a deeper sleep, lasting approximately 10 to 25 minutes, during which EEG activity is interrupted by sleep spindles consisting of bursts of high-frequency waves. Stages 3 and 4 represent deep sleep, during which the muscles of the body relax, the heart rate and blood pressure decrease, and gastrointestinal activity is slowed.

After completing this section of the chapter, you should be able to meet the following objectives:

■ List the four categories of sleep disorders included in the *International Classification of Sleep Disorders.*

■ Describe the methods used in diagnosis of sleep disorders, including the sleep history, sleep diary, polysomnography, and wrist actigraphy.

■ Characterize the non–24-hour sleep–wake syndrome experienced by visually impaired individuals, sleep disorders associated with acute shifts in the sleep–wake cycle due to intercontinental travel and shift work, and advanced sleep phase and delayed sleep phase circadian rhythm sleep disorders.

■ Describe the causes, manifestations, diagnosis, and treatment of acute and chronic insomnia.

■ Differentiate periodic limb movement disorder and restless legs syndrome in terms of manifestations and treatment.

(objectives continue)

■ Explain the physiologic mechanisms, contributing factors, and manifestations of obstructive sleep apnea and describe the methods used in diagnosis and treatment of the disorder.

■ Define the term *parasomnias* and relate it to the manifestations of nightmare, sleep terrors, and sleep walking.

Sleep disorders cover a broad spectrum of symptoms including the inability to fall asleep and stay asleep, circadian rhythm and sleep–wake transition disorders, sleep-related breathing and movement disorders, and excessive sleepiness. While sleep disorders have existed for centuries, it is only within the last 3 to 4 decades that attention has focused on their diagnosis and classification. The development of the *Diagnostic Classification of Sleep and Arousal Disorders* by the Association of Sleep Disorders in 1979 heralded the emergence of the discipline of sleep medicine. This was followed by the *International Classification of Sleep Disorders* (ICSD), which was produced by the American Academy of Sleep Medicine, in association with the European Sleep Research Society, the Japanese Society of Sleep Research, and the Latin American Sleep Society. First produced in 1990, the ICSD was revised in 1997 and again in 2005 as ICSD-2.[15] ICSD-2 classifies sleep disorders into eight major categories, five of which—circadian rhythm disorders, insomnias, hypersomnias (*e.g.,* narcolepsy), sleep-related movement disorders, and sleep-related breathing disorders—were included under the category of dyssomnias in previous versions of the classification system (Chart 52-1).

Diagnostic Methods

The diagnosis of sleep disorders usually is based on an adequate sleep history and physical examination. A sleep diary or sleep log often is helpful in describing sleep problems and arriving at

---

CHART 52-1	**INTERNATIONAL CLASSIFICATION OF SLEEP DISORDERS**

- Insomnia
- Parasomnias
- Sleep-related breathing disorders
- Hypersomnia of central origin not due to circadian rhythm disorder or other cause of disturbed nocturnal sleep
- Sleep-related movement disorders
- Isolated symptoms, apparently related to normal variants and unresolved issues
- Circadian rhythm sleep disorders
- Other sleep disorders

Adapted from American Academy of Sleep Medicine. (2005). *International classification of sleep disorders: Diagnostic and coding manual* (2nd ed.). Westchester, IL: Author.

---

a diagnosis.[16,17] In some cases, sleep laboratory studies may be needed to arrive at an accurate diagnosis.

Sleep History

A sleep history is fundamental to the process of identifying the nature of a sleep disorder.[17] The history should include the person's perception of the sleep problem, sleep schedule (*e.g.,* times of retiring and arising), problems with falling asleep and maintaining sleep, quality of sleep, daytime sleepiness and impact of the sleep disorder on daytime functioning, general emotional and physical problems, sleep hygiene (*e.g.,* eating and drinking before retiring), and sleep environment (*e.g.,* bed comfort, room temperature, noise, light). Because drugs such as over-the-counter medications, herbal preparations, and prescription medications can influence sleep, a careful drug history is important. It also is important to obtain information about the use of alcohol, caffeine, tobacco, and illegal substances.

SLEEP DISORDERS

■ Circadian rhythm sleep disorders represent a misalignment between a person's sleep pattern and societal norms.

■ Hypersomnia (*e.g.,* narcolepsy) is characterized by excessive daytime sleepiness not related to disturbed nocturnal sleep or circadian rhythm disorders.

■ The insomnias represent a repeated difficulty with sleep initiation, duration, and quality of sleep.

■ The sleep-related breathing disorders are characterized by disordered respirations during sleep (sleep apnea) and sleep-related movement by disturbing limb movements (periodic limb movement and restless legs syndrome).

■ The parasomnias, which are undesirable physical phenomena that occur almost exclusively during sleep or are exaggerated by sleep, include nightmares, sleepwalking, and sleep terrors.

Sleep Log/Diary

A sleep log/diary is a person's written account of his or her sleep experience. It usually is recommended that the diary be kept for at least 2 weeks. The diary should record the person's account of their bedtime, wakeup time, total sleep time, time of sleep onset, time needed to prepare for bed and to fall asleep, use of sleep medications, number of awakenings, subjective assessment of sleep quality, time out of bed in the morning, and daytime naps and symptoms. A number of sample forms are available to health care professionals for distribution to their clients.

Actigraphy and Polysomnography

Actigraphy. Wrist actigraphy measures muscle motion and is used to obtain objective measurements of sleep duration and efficiency outside the sleep laboratory.[18] The actigraph is a compact device that is worn on the wrist and is used most often in conjunction with a sleep diary. Depending on the unit that is used, it can collect up to several week's worth of information.

Polysomnography. A typical sleep study, or *polysomnography,* involves use of the EEG, electro-oculogram (EOG), electromyogram (EMG), electrocardiogram (ECG), breathing movements, and pulse oximetry.[4] The EOG records eye movements. Because the eye is like a small battery with the retina negative to the cornea, an electrode placed on the skin near the eye records changes in voltage as the eye rotates in its socket. The EMG records the electrical activity from muscle movement. It is recorded from the surface of the skin. It typically is recorded from under the chin because muscles in this area of the body show very dramatic changes associated with the sleep cycle. The ECG is used to measure the heart rate and detect cardiac arrhythmias. The pulse oximeter (ear or finger) measures arterial oxygen saturation.

The multiple sleep latency test (MSLT) is used to evaluate daytime sleepiness. This test usually is completed the morning after a diagnostic sleep study. An average adult requires 10 or more minutes to fall asleep. An MSLT result of less than 5 minutes is considered abnormal. Polysomnographic recordings are made during three to five naps spaced 2 hours apart during the day. Special attention is paid to how much time elapses from when the lights go out to the first evidence of sleep. This interval is called *sleep latency.*

Circadian Rhythm Disorders

Circadian sleep disorders are characterized by a disturbance between an "individual's sleep pattern and that which is desired or considered to be within the societal norm."[19] Sleep problems due to alterations in circadian rhythm tend to fall into three categories: non–24-hour sleep–wake syndrome (disorders of visual input and SCN function); acute shifts in the sleep–wake cycle (jet lag and shift work); and changes in sleep phase disorders (advanced and delayed sleep phase disorders).[10,20–22]

Non–24-Hour Sleep–Wake Syndrome

The non–24-hour sleep–wake syndrome consists of a lack of synchronization between the internal sleep–wake rhythm and the external 24-hour day. Most persons with the disorder are blind or have brain lesions that affect the SCN. Studies have shown that 70% or more of blind persons have chronic sleep–wake complaints.[21]

The non–24-hour sleep–wake syndrome often goes unrecognized. In sighted persons, a neurologic examination, including magnetic resonance imaging to detect possible SNC lesions, often is indicated. The disorder usually is unresponsive to sedative and stimulant medications. Some blind people seem to respond to a schedule of strict 24-hour cues.

Acute Shifts in the Sleep–Wake Cycle

The normal diurnal clock is set for a 24-hour day and resists changes in its pattern by as little as 1 to 2 hours per day. This means that there is a limited range of day lengths to which humans can synchronize. Imposed sleep–wake schedules of less than 23 hours or more than approximately 26 hours, such as those that occur with intercontinental jet travel and switches in the work shift, produce increasing sleep difficulties.

Time Zone Change (Jet Lag) Syndrome. *Jet lag,* a popular term for symptoms of sleep disturbance that occur with air travel that crosses several time zones, is caused by the sudden loss of synchrony between a traveler's intrinsic circadian clock and the local time of the flight's destination. The severity and duration of symptoms vary depending on the number of times zones crossed, direction of travel (eastward versus westward), takeoff and arrival times, and age. Most people who cross three or four time zones experience some sleep disturbance, usually lasting two to four nights.

Circadian rhythms take longer to resynchronize to local time after eastward flights than westward flights, presumably because of the longer-than-24–hour intrinsic circadian period in most people.[21] Because the human time system seems to be less flexible in adjusting to sudden time changes after 35 years of age, age also affects adjustment to time zone changes.

Manifestations of jet lag syndrome include insomnia, daytime sleepiness, and decreased alertness and performance. Other symptoms, such as eye and nasal irritation, headache, abdominal distention, dependent edema, and intermittent dizziness, result from cabin conditions and usually remit sooner than symptoms of jet lag. Frequent travelers, such as airline personnel and business travelers, may develop chronic sleep disturbances accompanied by malaise, irritability, and performance impairment. Jet lag usually is milder in infrequent travelers, but may reduce the enjoyment of a vacation or effectiveness of business transactions. Persons with preexisting sleep disorders such as sleep apnea often experience a worsening of symptoms with jet travel.

Management of jet lag focuses on efforts either to maintain the home time schedule or to adapt to the new time zone schedule. For persons crossing four or fewer time zones for only a few days, trying to maintain a schedule that is nearer to the home time schedule may be helpful, especially with westward travel. For longer stays, adapting to the new time schedule as quickly as possible is probably a better strategy. Use of artificial light may enhance the adjustment to the time shift. Getting outdoors and engaging in local social events enhances resynchronization by providing social cues and increasing exposure to the new light–dark environment.[23]

Shift Work Sleep Disorder. The sleep disruption of night-shift work can be attributed to a clash between shift demands for wakefulness as part of the work environment and the sleep setting of the worker's intrinsic circadian clock.[24] Shift work usually creates an environment in which some circadian clock-setting cues (*e.g.,* artificial light and rest–activity) are shifted, whereas others (*e.g.,* natural light–dark schedule, family and social routines) are not. This situation almost never allows for a complete shift of the circadian system. To complicate the situation, most night-shift workers revert to a nighttime sleeping schedule on days off. The effect of abruptly attempting to sleep at normal hours after working nights and sleeping days is biologically equivalent to a 6- to 10-hour eastbound jet flight.

Manifestations of sleep disorders of night-shift workers include shortened and interrupted daytime sleep after the night shift, somnolence and napping at work, sleepiness while commuting home, and insomnia on the nights off from work. Shift workers usually sleep less per scheduled sleep period than daytime workers and therefore are in a condition of chronic sleep deprivation.[23,24] Permanent night workers report averaging 6 hours of sleep on work days, approximately an hour less than evening and day workers.[24]

Arriving at a sleep schedule that is most supportive of the worker's intrinsic circadian rhythm often is difficult for night-shift workers. Beginning sleep at noon rather than earlier in the morning may produce a more normal sleep period in relation to shift onset, but exacerbate insomnia on nights off. Sleeping in absolute darkness during daytime by using blackout shades or eye masks may benefit the night worker's sleep.

Change in Sleep Phase Disorders

Change in sleep phase disorders include delayed sleep phase syndrome and advanced sleep phase syndrome. The disorders may arise because of developmental changes in the sleep–wake cycle or because of poor sleep habits.

The main symptoms of *delayed sleep phase syndrome* (DSPS) are extreme difficulty falling asleep at a conventional hour of the night and awakening on time in the morning for school, work, or other responsibilities. Although most chronically sleep-deprived persons are sleepy in the late afternoon or evening, persons with DSPS report greatest alertness at these times of the day.[21]

The disorder is more common in adolescents and in persons older than 50 years of age.[21] In adults, there is evidence of association between some psychopathologic disorders and DSPS. Most cases are adolescents whose frustrated parents cannot wake them up in time for school and have trouble getting them to go to bed at night. Staying up late is fairly common among today's teenagers, who are strongly influenced by peer pressure, defiance of parental rules, and other pressures. It has been suggested that social pressure may contribute to, but may not be the only reason for, changes in a teenager's sleep pattern. Rather, puberty may be accompanied by a lengthening of the intrinsic circadian rhythm, with a corresponding increase in evening wakefulness, which in turn leads to later sleep onset and arising.

Diagnosis of DSPS usually can be made from information in a sleep history and confirmed with a 2-week sleep log or diary. The presence of concurrent psychopathologic disorders or chronic sedative or alcohol use should be considered. There are no quick remedies for DSPS. In adolescents, common-sense remedies such as setting earlier bedtimes and using multiple alarm clocks for waking up have been used, but with minimal success. The use of bright light may be helpful in maintaining morning wakefulness. For some people, engagement in a regular morning exercise program, such as taking a daily 20- to 30-minute walk outdoors as soon as possible after arising each morning, may prove beneficial. In persons with psychopathologic disorders or sedative abuse, treatment of the underlying disorder is indicated.[21]

Advanced sleep phase syndrome (ASPS) basically is the mirror image of DSPS—early sleep onset and early arising. People with ASPS have trouble staying awake in the evening and have to curtail evening activities to avoid falling asleep. Unlike persons with depression, who awaken early with feelings of hopelessness and sadness, the person with ASPS obtains a normal amount of consolidated sleep and wakes up feeling refreshed.[21] The pathophysiologic basis of ASPS is presumed to be a partial defect in phase delay capability, with the possibility that persons with the disorder have an inherently fast circadian timing system. This disorder often is found in the elderly. Time isolation studies in middle-aged and older subjects suggest that the circadian timing system shortens with aging, usually beginning sometime in the sixth decade of life.[21] Diagnosis of ASPS is based on history and information from a sleep log. Other pathologic causes, such as sleep apnea and depression, should be ruled out. The need for treatment depends on how disruptive a person perceives the problem to be. Current treatment methods, which focus largely on sleep schedule changes, are somewhat limited.

Insomnia

Insomnia has been defined as three or more of the following: difficulty initiating sleep, difficulty maintaining sleep, waking up too early, or sleep that is chronically nonrestorative or poor in quality.[25-28] To be classified as insomnia, these symptoms must be accompanied by at least one of the following forms of daytime impairment: fatigue or daytime sleepiness, impairment of attention, concentration, or memory; poor social, occupational, or academic performance; mood disturbance or irritability; proneness to errors or accidents at work or while driving; tension headaches or gastrointestinal distress due to sleep loss; or worries about sleep. Primary insomnia is sleep difficulty in which other causes of sleep disruption have been ruled out or treated, whereas secondary insomnia can be associated with medical conditions (*e.g.,* chronic pain), psychiatric disorders (*e.g.,* anxiety, depression, bipolar disorder), neurologic disorders (*e.g.,* Parkinson disease), primary sleep disorders (*e.g.,* sleep apnea, restless legs syndrome), and drugs.[25,27,28]

Estimates of the prevalence of insomnia vary depending on the method used in the diagnosis and monitoring of the condition. According to the fourth edition of the *Diagnostic and Statistical Manual of Mental Disorders,* 20% to 40% of adults in the United States have intermittent insomnia.[29] An estimated 10% to 15% of adults have chronic insomnia.[25,28,30,31] Chronic insomnia is more common in women, especially in the postmenopausal years; in older people, perhaps as a consequence of declining health and institutionalization; and in persons with psychological and other disease conditions.

Adjustment or Acute Insomnia

Adjustment or acute insomnia is characterized by short periods (days or weeks) of sleep difficulty that is expected to resolve with either adaptation or resolution of the stressor.[27,29] Acute insomnia often is caused by emotional and physical discomfort. Some common examples include an unfamiliar or nonconducive sleep environment, stress-related events, and sleep schedule problems. Probably one of the most common causes of acute insomnia is an unfamiliar sleep environment, such as that encountered when traveling.

Factors that contribute to a nonconducive sleep environment include excessive noise, extremes of temperature, an uncomfortable sleep surface, or being forced to sleep in an uncomfortable position. Hospital intensive care units with their noise, intensive lighting, and frequent interruptions for monitoring vital signs and providing treatments are excellent examples of nonconducive sleep environments. Common stress-related causes of insomnia are expected occurrences such as being on call or stressful life events. Sleep schedule changes include jet lag and sleep disruption due to shift work.

Chronic Insomnia

Chronic insomnia should be distinguished from acute insomnia. Accordingly, the National Institutes of Health (NIH) State-of-the-Science Conference on Manifestations and Management of Chronic Insomnia in Adults defined chronic insomnia as 30 days or more of the previously described symptoms.[25] Persons with chronic insomnia frequently complain of fatigue; mood changes, such as irritability and depression; difficulty concentrating; and impaired performance.

Chronic insomnia often is related to medical or psychiatric disorders. Factors such as pain, immobility, and hormonal changes associated with pregnancy or menopause also can cause insomnia. Interrupted sleep can accompany other sleep disorders such as restless legs syndrome and sleep apnea. Many health problems worsen during the night. Heart failure, respiratory disease, and gastroesophageal reflux can cause frequent awakening during the night. Mood and anxiety disorders are the most frequent cause of insomnia in persons with psychiatric diagnoses.

A number of drugs can lead to poor-quality sleep. Drugs commonly related to insomnia are caffeine, nicotine, stimulating antidepressants, alcohol, and recreational drugs. Although alcohol initially may induce sleep, it often causes disrupted and fragmented sleep. Sleep also is disrupted in persons undergoing alcohol or sleep medication withdrawal.

Diagnosis and Treatment

The diagnosis of insomnia is aided by a sleep history. Questions should address both sleep and daytime functioning. If the person has a bed partner, it is important to ask if the person snores, has unusual movement during sleep, or is excessively drowsy during the day.[28] Because sleep needs vary from person to person, a 1- to 2-week sleep diary can be useful in diagnosing the sleep problem and in serving as a baseline for treatment effects.[16,17,25] Other factors that need to be explored are the use of drugs such as caffeine, tobacco, and alcohol, as well as prescription and over-the-counter drugs that affect the sleep–wake cycle. Identification of physical and psychological factors that interfere with sleep also is important. Actigraphy or polysomnography may be used as diagnostic tools. Polysomnography is the most sensitive tool to evaluate sleep and wakefulness. However, it is expensive and because of the numerous monitoring electrodes can actually disrupt sleep. Its use as a diagnostic tool for insomnia is usually limited to causes in which other sleep disorders, such as sleep apnea, are suspected.[25]

Treatment of insomnia includes education and counseling regarding better sleep habits (sleep hygiene), behavioral therapy aimed at changing maladaptive sleep habits, and the judicious use of pharmacologic interventions. The cause and duration of insomnia are particularly important in deciding on a treatment strategy. With transient insomnia, treatment stresses the development of good sleep hygiene and judicious short-term use of sedatives or hypnotics. Long-term and chronic insomnia require careful assessment to determine the cause of the disorder. Depending on the findings, treatment options include behavioral strategies such as relaxation therapy, sleep restriction therapy, stimulus control therapy, and cognitive therapy. Sedatives and hypnotics, which tend to become less effective with time and may cause dependence, are used with caution.

Sleep hygiene refers to a set of rules and information about personal and environmental activities that affect sleep. These rules include establishing a regular wakeup time to help set the circadian clock and regularity of sleep onset; maintaining a practice of sleeping only as long as needed to feel refreshed; providing a quiet sleep environment that is neither too hot nor too cold; and avoiding the use of alcohol and caffeine (coffee, colas, tea, chocolate) before retiring for sleep. It is important that the bed and bedroom be identified with sleep and not with reading, watching television, or working. Persons who cannot fall asleep should be instructed to turn on the light and do something else outside the bed, preferably in another room.

Behavioral therapies include relaxation therapy, sleep restriction therapy, stimulus control therapy, and cognitive therapy.[25–28,30,31] Relaxation therapy is based on the premise that persons with insomnia tend to display high levels of physiologic, cognitive, and emotional arousal during both the day and the night. Sleep restriction therapy consists of curtailing the amount of time spent in bed in an effort to increase the sleep efficiency (time asleep/time in bed). People with insomnia often increase their time in bed in the misguided belief that it will provide more opportunity to sleep. Stimulus control therapy focuses on reassociating the bed and bedroom with sleep rather than sleeplessness. Cognitive therapy involves the identification of dysfunctional beliefs and attitudes about sleep and replacing them with more adaptive substitutes.

Pharmacologic treatment usually is reserved for short-term management of insomnia—either as the sole treatment or as adjunctive therapy until the underlying problem can be addressed. The most common type of agents used to promote sleep are the benzodiazepine receptor agonists and a new class of nonbenzodiazepine hypnotics (zolpidem, zaleplon, eszopiclone, ramelteon). The nonbenzodiazepines are often preferred because of their rapid onset and shorter duration of action. Ramelteon is the first and only nonscheduled drug approved by the U.S. Food and Drug Administration for treatment of insomnia. It was approved in 2005 for sleep-onset insomnia and can be prescribed for long-term use. Ramelteon is a melatonin receptor agonist with high selectivity for melatonin (MT)-1 and MT-2 receptors in the SCN of the hypothalamus, receptors that are believed to be involved in sleep promotion and maintenance of the circadian rhythm.[27] Ramelteon has no appreciable binding to gamma-aminobutyric acid (GABA) receptors, and hence no anxiolytic or abuse potential.

Sedating antidepressants also may be prescribed, particularly when insomnia is due to depression. Antihistamines have sedative effects and may be used to induce sleep. The most commonly used agents are diphenhydramine and doxylamine. Most over-the-counter sleep medications include an antihistamine. Adverse effects of antihistamines include daytime sleepiness, cognitive impairments, and anticholinergic effects. Falls and fractures are more frequent in persons using hypnotic or other psychotherapeutic agents. Melatonin, available in both natural and synthetic forms, is one of the most popular over-the-counter sleep aids. The pharmacokinetics of melatonin has not been established because of differences in dosing, large variations in absorption, and diversity of study subjects.[27]

Narcolepsy

Narcolepsy is a syndrome characterized by abnormal sleep tendencies, including excessive daytime sleepiness, disturbed nocturnal sleep, and manifestations related to REM sleep such as cataplexy (brief periods of muscle weakness), hypnagogic hallucinations, and sleep paralysis.[32–37] Daytime sleepiness is the most common initial symptom of narcolepsy. It is most apparent in boring, sedentary situations and often is relieved by movement. Although the sleepiness that occurs with narcolepsy is similar to that experienced after sleep deprivation, it is different in that no amount of nighttime sleep produces full alertness. The periods of daytime sleep usually are brief, lasting 30 minutes or less, and often are accompanied by brief interruptions of speech or irrelevant words, lapses in memory, and nonsensical activities. Cataplexy is characterized by brief periods of muscle weakness brought about by emotional reactions such as laughter, anger, or fear. Sleep paralysis is a terrifying experience that occurs on falling asleep or on awakening, during which persons find themselves unable to move, speak, or even breathe deeply.

Hypnagogic hallucinations are vivid hallucinations that occur at the onset of sleep. Similar hallucinations may occur on awakening (*i.e.,* hypnopompic hallucinations). Visual hallucinations, either simple or bizarre and fantastic, are the rule, although auditory and tactile components may occur.[34] The exact boundary between hypnagogic/hypnopompic hallucinations and dreams is not a clear one. Although the symptoms of narcolepsy generally begin in puberty, they have been reported in children and in adults up to 68 years of age. The impact of sleepiness is often underappreciated because persons with the disorder may be reluctant to report problems that may adversely affect their ability to work, drive, or obtain insurance.[36]

The mechanisms underlying the manifestations of narcolepsy appear to be linked to an abnormality in REM sleep regulation. The occurrence of REM sleep at sleep onset or within 10 to 15 minutes of sleep onset is the most characteristic and striking manifestation of the disorder. Periods of sleep-onset REM are thought to indicate impaired sleep–wake regulation rather than increased need for REM sleep. The sleep paralysis, dreamlike hallucinations, and the loss of muscle tone that occur during cataplexy are similar to behaviors that occur during REM sleep.

Although the cause of narcolepsy is unknown, there are indications that the disorder may have a genetic component. Persons with narcolepsy have been shown to have an unusually high rate of a specific human leukocyte antigen (HLA) subtype (HLA DQB1-0602).[34,37] This association is seen in approximately 90% of cases with cataplexy.[37] Importantly, this association is substantially lower in persons who have received the diagnosis of narcolepsy, but do not have cataplexy.[34,37] The strong association between HLA type and cataplexy raises the possibility that narcolepsy is an autoimmune disease.

Recent research has suggested a link between a newly identified group of neurotransmitters called *hypocretins* and narcolepsy. The hypocretins (hypocretin 1 and hypocretin 2) are secreted by cells in the area of the hypothalamus that is related to wakefulness.[33–37] A mutation in the hypocretin 2 receptor was shown to cause canine narcolepsy.[34] Although the role of the hypocretin transmitter system in human narcolepsy is unclear, a small preliminary study has shown a lack of hypocretin 1 in the cerebrospinal fluid of seven of nine patients with the disorder. Although these findings are preliminary, they suggest new avenues for research into the cause and possible treatment measures for narcolepsy.

Usually, sleep laboratory studies are required for accurate diagnosis of narcolepsy. Both daytime and nighttime studies usually are done.[32,36] Nighttime studies usually are performed after the person has been on a regular sleep schedule for 10 days or more to determine the presence and severity of sleep apnea, limb movement disorders, and nocturnal sleep disturbance. A daytime MSLT usually is done the next day. People with narcolepsy are observed to have a short period of sleep latency (2 to 4 minutes) during daytime studies, along with a rapid onset of REM sleep (usually within 10 minutes). A mean sleep latency of less than 5 minutes and two or more periods of sleep-onset REM during the repeated nap opportunities is considered diagnostic of narcolepsy.[32]

The treatment of narcolepsy focuses on the use of stimulant medications such as methylphenidate, methamphetamine, and modafinil to counteract daytime sleepiness.[34,36] Only modafinil, a nonamphetamine stimulant, has been studied and approved for use in treatment of narcolepsy. The mechanism of action of modafinil is unknown, although animal studies indicate the drug acts in areas of the brain involved in the sleep–wake cycle. Tricyclic antidepressants may be used to treat the cataleptic attacks.[36] Nonpharmacologic treatments include prevention of sleep deprivation, regular sleep and wake times, a stimulating work environment, and avoidance of shift work. Scheduled short naps may be effective in reducing day-time sleepiness.

Sleep-Related Movement Disorders

A variety of spontaneous limb movements occur during normal sleep. Many of these movements demonstrate characteristic rates and patterns during certain stages of sleep, with movements being minimal during non-REM sleep and maximal during REM sleep. Many movement disorders occur during stage 2 non-REM sleep. Some occur during normal sleep in all persons at some one time or another. Others are not part of normal sleep patterns and can be disruptive of sleep. Among the abnormal motor disorders are periodic limb movement disorder (PLMD) and restless legs syndrome (RLS).[38–42]

Periodic Limb Movement Disorder

PLMD is characterized by episodes of repetitive movement of the large toe with flexion of the ankle, knee, and hip during sleep.[38–42] It can occur simultaneously in both legs, alternate between legs, or occur unilaterally. The condition occurs most frequently during light (stages 1 and 2 non-REM) sleep compared with deep (stages 3 and 4 non-REM) sleep and REM sleep.

The incidence of the disorder, which occurs equally in men and women, increases with age. It may occur in as much as 29% of persons older than 50 years of age.[42] The disorder frequently accompanies RLS. It has been reported that approximately 80% of persons with RLS exhibit evidence of PLMD during polysomnographic studies.[40–42] Persons with PLMD are often unaware of periodic limb movements, but their bed partners may report the symptoms.

The cause of PLMD is largely unknown. It has been observed that the movements mimic the Babinski reflex, suggesting removal of an excitatory influence over a subcortical inhibitory system allowing for facilitation of abnormal movements during sleep.[40] Diagnosis of PLMD is facilitated with use of EMG recordings from both tibialis anterior muscles.[38,40] Four or more consecutive muscle contractions, each lasting 5 to 90 seconds (typically 20 to 40 seconds) and recurring at intervals of 5 to 90 seconds, is indicative of PLMD.

Restless Legs Syndrome

The NIH Consensus Panel recently characterized RLS as (1) an urge to move the limbs with or without sensations, (2) worsening at rest, (3) improving with activity, and (4) worsening in the evening or night.[43] The prevalence of the condition peaks in middle age and reportedly occurs in 2% to 15% of the elderly population. Although the prevalence increases with age, it has a variable age of onset and can even occur in children.

The disorder, which is thought to have its origin in the CNS, can occur as a primary or secondary disorder. There is a high familial incidence of primary RLS, suggesting a genetic disorder. Secondary causes of RLS include iron deficiency, neurologic disorders such as spinal cord and peripheral nerve lesions, pregnancy, uremia, and medications. Although the neurologic basis of RLS has not been determined, recent research suggests that it may involve homeostatic mechanisms that regulate the influx and efflux of iron from cells of the CNS that regulate motor movements.[42] Cerebrospinal fluid ferritin (the main iron storage molecules in the CNS) levels are lower in persons with RLS. Of interest is the role of iron in dopaminergic transmission in the CNS. Iron is an important cofactor for tyrosine hydroxylase, the rate-limiting enzyme in dopamine synthesis, and also plays a major role in the functioning of postsynaptic dopamine receptors.[38,42]

Diagnosis of RLS is based on a history of (1) a compelling urge to move the legs, usually associated with paresthesias; (2) motor restlessness, as seen by activities such as pacing, tossing and turning in bed, or rubbing the legs; (3) symptoms that become worse at rest and are relieved by activity; and (4) symptoms that are worse in the evening or at night.[43] Laboratory tests to determine secondary causes of RLS usually are done. Because RLS may be a symptom of iron deficiency, serum ferritin and iron saturation should be assessed. This is important because iron deficiency is frequently present in the absence of anemia. Sleep studies usually are not required because the condition can be diagnosed on the basis of history and clinical findings.

Treatment of RLS varies depending on the severity of symptoms. Dopaminergic agents are the first-line drugs for most persons with RLS.[38–42] These include precursors of dopamine (carbidopa-levodopa), dopamine agonists (pergolide, pramipexole, ropinirole), and facilitating agents (selegiline). Antiseizure agents (gabapentin), benzodiazepines (e.g., clonazepam, temazepam), and opioids (e.g., codeine, hydrocodone) are alternative agents.[38,42] Although pharmacologic treatment is helpful for many persons with RLS, those with mild symptoms may not require medications. For many persons, deliberate manipulation of the muscles through ambulation, kicking movements, stretching, or massage may provide relief. Good sleep habits are important. Because a high prevalence of iron deficiency has been found among persons with RLS, treatment of the deficiency may improve or resolve symptoms.

Sleep Apnea

Sleep apnea is sleep-disordered breathing, accompanied by daytime symptoms, most often excessive sleepiness. There are two types of sleep apnea: central and obstructive.[44,45] *Central sleep apnea,* which is caused by disorders affecting the respiratory center in the brain, is rare. It is characterized by a cessation or decrease in ventilatory effort during sleep and is usually associated with oxygen desaturation. *Obstructive sleep apnea,* which is caused by upper airway obstruction and characterized by snoring, disrupted sleep, and excessive daytime sleepiness, is the much more common type. Although airflow ceases, respiratory muscles continue to function. This is one of the features that distinguishes central from obstructive sleep apnea.

Obstructive Sleep Apnea

Apnea is defined as cessation of airflow through the nose and mouth for 10 seconds or longer.[44,45] The apneic periods typically last for 15 to 120 seconds, and some persons may have as many as 100 apneic periods per night. An accompanying reduction in tidal volume due to a decrease in the depth and rate of respiration (called *hypopnea*) is associated with a decrease in arterial oxygen saturation. The average number of apnea–hypopnea periods per hour is called the *apnea–hypopnea index* (AHI).[46,47] An adult may experience up to five events an hour without symptoms. As the AHI increases, so does the severity of symptoms. An AHI of five or greater in combination with reports of excessive daytime sleepiness is indicative of sleep apnea.[45,48]

A critical pathophysiologic feature of obstructive sleep apnea is sleep-related collapse of the upper airway at the level of the pharynx.[49] All skeletal muscles except the diaphragm undergo a decrease in tone during sleep. This loss of muscle tone is most pronounced during REM sleep. The loss of muscle tone in the upper airways predisposes to airway obstruction as the negative airway pressure produced by contraction of the diaphragm brings the vocal cords together, collapses the pharyngeal wall, and sucks the tongue back into the throat (Fig. 52-6). Airway collapse is accentuated in persons with conditions that cause narrowing of the upper airway or weakness of the throat muscles.

Conditions that predispose to sleep apnea include male gender, increasing age, and obesity. Alcohol and other drugs that depress the CNS tend to increase the severity of obstructive episodes. Most persons who develop sleep apnea are obese. Large neck girth in both male and female snorers is highly predictive of sleep apnea. Men with a neck circumference greater than 17 inches and women with a neck circumference greater than 16 inches are at higher risk for sleep apnea.[46] The pickwickian syndrome, named after the fat boy in Charles Dickens' *The Posthumous Papers of the Pickwick Club,* published in 1837, is characterized by obesity, hypersomnolence, periodic breathing, hypoxemia, and right-sided heart failure.[50] Men have a higher risk for obstructive sleep apnea than women. The reason for this is not entirely clear, but gonadal hormones may play a role.[44] Postmenopausal women are at higher risk than premenopausal women. Individuals with specific endocrine disorders, namely, acromegaly, Cushing syndrome, hypothyroidism, and diabetes mellitus, are at higher risk for obstructive sleep apnea. In each of these disorders, hormonal imbalances lead to structural distortion of the airways that leads to obstruction.[45]

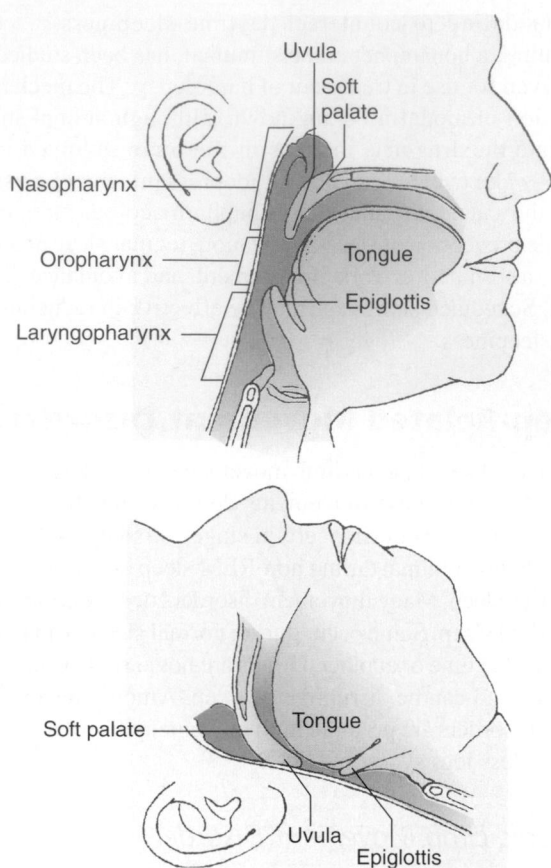

FIGURE 52-6 • Principal mechanism of obstructive sleep apnea. When the person is awake (**top**), the airway is kept open by the activity of the pharyngeal musculature. During sleep (**bottom**), this activity is decreased, causing airway obstruction, most commonly in the area behind the uvula, soft palate, and posterior tongue.

Obstructive sleep apnea is characterized by loud snoring interrupted by periods of silence. Abnormal gross motor movements during sleep are common. In many cases, the snoring precedes by many years the onset of other signs of sleep apnea. Persons with sleep apnea often complain of persistent daytime sleepiness, morning headache, memory and judgment problems, irritability, difficulty concentrating, and depression. They also are more likely to fall asleep at inappropriate times and have higher rates of automobile and work-related accidents. Men may complain of impotence. In children, a decline in school performance may be the only indication of the problem.

Sleep apnea also is associated with sleep-related cardiac arrhythmias and hypertension. Usually bradycardia is observed, but ventricular tachycardia may occur in situations of severe hypoxemia. Frequent apneic periods may result in increased systemic and pulmonary blood pressures. The morning blood pressure has been shown to increase almost linearly with increasing apnea episodes. In severe cases, pulmonary hypertension, polycythemia, and cor pulmonale may develop. The signs and symptoms of obstructive sleep apnea are summarized in Chart 52-2.

CHART 52-2 **SIGNS AND SYMPTOMS OF SLEEP APNEA**

- Noisy snoring
- Insomnia
- Abnormal movements during sleep
- Morning headaches
- Excessive daytime sleepiness
- Cognitive and personality changes
- Sexual impotence
- Systemic hypertension
- Pulmonary hypertension, cor pulmonale
- Polycythemia

Diagnosis and Treatment. Obstructive sleep apnea usually is suspected from a history of snoring, disturbed sleep, and daytime sleepiness. A definitive diagnosis is accomplished with sleep studies done in a sleep laboratory using polysomnography.[48,51] Currently, this procedure requires an overnight stay in a sleep laboratory. The procedure consists of EEG and EOG to determine the sleep stages; monitoring of the airflow; an ECG to detect arrhythmias; methods to measure ventilatory effort; and pulse oximetry to detect changes in oxygen saturation. An MSLT may be done to rule out narcolepsy in persons who exhibit excessive daytime sleepiness. Home evaluation using pulse oximetry and portable monitors may be used to screen for sleep apnea. This method is less expensive than laboratory sleep tests but often is less accurate.[48] It is most useful in persons with severe sleep apnea, in whom the results clearly are positive.

The treatment of obstructive sleep apnea is determined by the severity of the condition.[48,51] Behavioral measures may be the only treatment needed for persons with mild sleep apnea. These include weight loss, eliminating evening alcohol and sedatives, and proper bed positioning. Weight loss often is beneficial for persons with obstructive apnea. In many instances, the disordered breathing events are confined to the supine sleeping position, so that training the person to sleep in the lateral position may help to alleviate the problem.

Oral or dental appliances that displace the tongue forward and move the mandible to a more anterior and forward position may be an option for persons with mild to moderate sleep apnea. Persons who snore but do not have sleep apnea also may use these devices. They should be fitted by a dentist or orthodontist experienced in their use. Side effects of the devices include excessive salivation and temporomandibular joint discomfort.

The application of nasal continuous positive airway pressure (NCPAP) at night has proven helpful in treating obstructive sleep apnea. This method uses an occlusive nasal mask or a device that fits into the nares, an expiratory valve and tubing, and a blower system to generate positive pressure. The main difficulty with NCPAP is that many persons find it unacceptable. Common complaints include dryness of the mouth, claustrophobia, and noise.

Several surgical procedures have been used to correct airway obstruction, including nasal septoplasty (*i.e.,* repair of the nasal septum) and uvulopalatopharyngoplasty (*i.e.,* excision of excess soft tissue on the palate, uvula, and posterior pharyngeal wall). Both of these procedures have met with limited success. Severe cases of sleep apnea may require a tracheostomy (*i.e.,* surgical placement of a tube into the trachea for the purpose of maintaining an open airway). The tracheostomy tube remains occluded during the day and is opened during the night.

Parasomnias

The parasomnias are undesirable physical phenomena that occur almost exclusively during sleep or are exaggerated by sleep.[52–54] They include nightmares, sleepwalking (somnambulism) and sleep terrors, teeth grinding, and bed-wetting (enuresis). Sleepwalking, sleep terrors, and bed-wetting often are seen in children and may be considered normal to some degree at a certain age. They are less common in adults and may be indicative of other pathologic processes. For example, sleepwalking and sleep terrors may occur in persons with poorly controlled cardiac insufficiency after myocardial infarction. In rare cases, sleepwalking and sleep terrors may be the first sign of a slowly evolving brain tumor. Finally, sleepwalking and sleep terrors may be triggered by disorders interacting with the sleep–wake cycle. Particularly in the elderly, health problems such as a febrile illness may enhance non-REM sleep nightmares, sleep terrors, and sleepwalking.

Nightmares

Nightmares are vivid and terrifying nocturnal episodes in which the dreamer is abruptly awakened from sleep. Usually there is difficulty returning to sleep. Nightmares affect 20% to 39% of children between 5 and 12 years of age and 5% to 8% of adults.[53] Most nightmares occur during REM sleep. Most REM-altering disorders and medications that affect REM sleep affect dreaming.

Nightmares are a defining symptom of post-traumatic stress disorder[8] (PTSD; see Chapter 9). These nightmares occur after intensely frightening or highly emotional experiences and are associated with disturbed sleep and daytime hyperarousability. Persons with PTSD report awakening from dreams that involve reliving the trauma. The frequency of PTSD nightmares increases with the severity of trauma, and they can persist for long periods after the traumatic experience. It has been reported that 30% of veterans of the Vietnam War are affected by PTSD.[8,53] Among the civilian population, PTSD affects approximately 25% of persons who have experienced severe emotional and physical trauma or have had a severe medical illness.

Sleepwalking and Sleep Terrors

Sleepwalking and sleep terrors usually occur during stages 3 and 4 of non-REM sleep. Because stages 3 and 4 are more prolonged during the first third of the night, sleepwalking and sleep terrors usually occur during this time.[53–55] Sleep terrors are characterized by sudden, loud, terrified screaming and prominent autonomic nervous system activation (tachycardia, tachypnea, diaphoresis, and mydriasis). Sleepwalking is characterized by complex automatic behaviors, such as aimless wandering, furniture rearranging, urinating in closets, and going outdoors. During a typical episode, the sleepwalker appears dazed and relatively unresponsive to the communication efforts of others. On awakening, there may be a brief period of confusion or disorientation. The sleepwalker usually has no memory or only a vague awareness of what has happened.

Sleep terrors are more common in children and are discussed later in the chapter. In children, sleepwalking usually is a benign and self-limited disorder. In adults, sleepwalking occurs almost three times more often per year and persists for a longer period than in children. It often is associated with stress or major life events.[55] New-onset sleepwalking in older adults is uncommon and usually is a manifestation of another disorder such as delirium, drug toxicity, or seizure disorders.[55] Although rare, sleepwalking can occur during complex partial seizures.

Diagnosis and treatment of sleepwalking and sleep terrors depend on age. Because most children eventually outgrow the disorders, parents may simply need to be reassured and instructed in safety measures. Insufficient sleep may precipitate episodes of sleepwalking, so parents should make certain that the child goes to bed on time and gets enough sleep. In adults, a through medical, psychiatric, and sleep history should be done to eliminate other causes of the disorder. Because sleepwalking can be dangerous, it is important that the environment be safe. Dangerous objects should be removed and bolts should be placed on doors and windows. No attempt should be made to interrupt the sleepwalking event because such efforts may be frightening.

Pharmacologic treatment includes the selective use of the benzodiazepines (particularly diazepam and clonazepam) or the tricyclic antidepressant imipramine.[55] In elderly persons, treatment focuses on reversing the underlying causes of delirium. Because medications are a frequent cause of delirium in the elderly, a complete drug history should be done with the intent of eliminating medications that might be causing the disorder.

IN SUMMARY, sleep disorders include the circadian rhythm sleep disorders, insomnias, narcolepsy, sleep-related movement disorders, sleep apnea, and the parasomnias. Sleep problems due to *alterations in circadian rhythm* tend to fall into three categories: non–24-hour sleep–wake syndrome (disorders of visual input and SCN function); acute shifts in the sleep–wake cycle (jet lag and shift work); and changes in sleep phase disorders (advanced and delayed sleep phase disorders). *Insomnia* represents a subjective problem of insufficient or nonrestorative sleep despite an adequate opportunity to sleep. It includes transient and chronic problems in falling asleep and maintaining sleep, waking up too early, or nonrefreshing sleep.

Narcolepsy is a disorder of daytime sleep attacks, cataplexy, hallucinations occurring at the onset of sleep, and sleep paralysis. Among the *movement disorders* that occur during sleep are PLMD and RLS. PLMD is characterized by episodes of repetitive movement of the large toe with flexion of the ankle, knee, and hip during sleep, usually involving both legs. RLS is a neurologic disorder characterized by an irresistible urge to move the legs, usually owing to a "creeping," "crawling," or uncomfortable sensation. It usually is worse during periods of inactivity and often interferes with sleep.

Obstructive sleep apnea is a serious, potentially life-threatening disorder characterized by brief periods of apnea or breathing cessation during sleep, loud snoring interrupted by periods of silence, and abnormal gross motor movements. It is accompanied by complaints of persistent daytime sleepiness, morning headache, memory and judgment problems, irritability, difficulty concentrating, and depression. Sleep apnea also is associated with sleep-related cardiac arrhythmias and hypertension. The parasomnias are undesirable physical phenomena that occur almost exclusively during sleep or are exaggerated by sleep. They include nightmares, sleepwalking and sleep terrors, teeth grinding, and bed-wetting (enuresis). ■

SLEEP AND SLEEP DISORDERS IN CHILDREN AND THE ELDERLY

After completing this section of the chapter, you should be able to meet the following objectives:

- Characterize normal sleep patterns of the infant and small child and relate them to the development of sleep disorders.
- Describe the normal changes in sleep stages that occur with aging and relate them to sleep problems in the elderly.

It has been said that "sleep is of the brain, by the brain, and for the brain."[1] Thus, sleep changes as the brain develops in the fetus and neonate, matures during adolescence and early adulthood, and begins to decline with aging.

Sleep and Sleep Disorders in Children

Sleep Patterns in Children

A child's circadian rhythms and sleep patterns are established early in life. There is evidence that many of the sleep patterns in the newborn are present at birth.[1] The first behavioral manifestations of sleep patterns occur between 28 and 30 weeks of gestation, when movement of the fetus is interrupted by periods of quiet.[56] At 32 weeks, periods of quiescence begin to occur at regular intervals, suggesting the beginnings of a sleep–wake cycle.

An infant born at full term sleeps approximately 16 to 17 hours a day, half of which is spent in REM sleep. The other half of the infant's sleep resembles adult non-REM sleep.[1,57] Not only does the infant spend more time in REM sleep than adults, but the behavioral manifestations of REM sleep are more exaggerated. This probably is because inhibitory systems in the infant's brain are relatively immature. Thus, an infant's sleep behavior includes a wide range of physical behaviors such as changes in facial expression, cooing sounds, and movement and stretching of the extremities.

Although infants have some capacity to concentrate sleep in one part of the day, this capacity must be developed in the weeks after birth. As development progresses, the infant is able to concentrate sleep during the night and remain awake for longer periods during the day. By 5 to 6 months, the infant may sleep through the night and may nap at predictable times during the day. As the cyclic structure of the sleep–wake cycle progresses, the amount of time spent in REM sleep decreases. By the time the child is 8 months of age, the duration of sleep has decreased to approximately 13 hours and REM sleep occupies only approximately one third of that time. At 12 to 15 years of age, sleep has decreased to approximately 8 hours, with one fourth being spent in REM sleep.

Sleep Disorders in Children

Although sleep complaints are common among adults, children usually do not complain about sleep problems, although their parents might. The usual concerns of parents include irregular sleep habits, insufficient or too much sleep, nightmares, sleep terrors, sleepwalking, and bed-wetting. Complaints of excessive daytime sleepiness or sleep attacks not accounted for by an inadequate amount of sleep may be due to a more serious health or sleep problem (*e.g.,* narcolepsy), in which case a careful sleep history, physical examination, and other diagnostic tests may be needed. Three of the more common sleep problems of children are discussed in this section of the chapter: sleep terrors, confusional arousals, and sleepwalking.

Sleep Terrors. Sleep terrors are marked by repeated episodes of awakening from sleep. They usually occur during the first half of sleep in the first interval of non-REM sleep.[57–59] The age of onset usually is between 2 and 4 years of age.[59] The course is variable, usually occurring at intervals of days or weeks. The disorder gradually resolves in children and usually disappears during adolescence. In a typical episode, the child sits up abruptly in bed, appears frightened, and demonstrates signs of extreme anxiety, including dilated pupils, excessive perspiration, rapid breathing, and tachycardia. Until the agitation and confusion subside, efforts to comfort or help the child are futile. There usually is no memory of the episode. Occasionally, the child recounts a sense of terror on being aroused during a night terror, but there is only fragmentary recall of dreamlike images. Treatment consists primarily of educating and reassuring the family. The child should be assisted in settling down without awakening. The child must be protected if he or she gets up and walks about during the episodes.

Confusional Arousals. Confusional arousals are common in infants and toddlers.[58] They usually occur during the first third of the night when the brain is partially asleep while remaining partially awake. During these events, children present with marked confusion, slow and inappropriate responses to questions, and nonpurposeful activities. They do not express fear, terror, or panic. Children spontaneously return to sleep and have no recollection of the event in the morning. Recovery from sleep deprivation tends to increase the incidence of confusional arousals.

Sleepwalking. Sleepwalking involves repeated episodes of complex motor movements that lead to leaving the bed and walking without the child being conscious of the episode or remembering that it occurred. As with sleep terrors, it normally occurs in non-REM sleep stages 3 and 4 during the first third of the sleep period.

A sleepwalking episode typically lasts for a few minutes to half an hour, during which time the child sits up; makes purposeful movements such as picking at the bed coverings; then proceeds to semipurposeful movements such as getting out of bed, walking around, opening doors, dressing, or going to the bathroom. Often they end up in the parent's bedroom. Commonly, they are unresponsive to the efforts of others to communicate with them. Confusion and disorientation are typical of the events, and on awakening there is no memory of the event. There may be manifestations of extreme autonomic nervous system activity such as tachycardia, rapid breathing, perspiration, and urination.

Approximately 10% to 15% of children have had isolated sleepwalking events.[55] It occurs more commonly in boys than in girls and is more frequent in children in whom there is a family history of sleepwalking. The onset usually is between 4 and 8 years of age, and it lasts several years. Usually symptoms resolve by the end of the teens or in the early twenties. The primary concern is injury during an episode. Children may bump into things, fall down stairs, or even leave their home during an episode. Therefore, gates should be placed across stairs and windows and doors should be locked so the child cannot leave the house.

Sleep and Sleep Disorders in the Elderly

Complaints of difficulty sleeping increase with aging. In a National Institute of Aging Study of over 9000 persons aged 65 years and older, over one half of the men and women reported at least one chronic sleep complaint.[60] The consequences of chronic sleep problems in the elderly can be considerable. Left uncorrected, a sleep disorder affects the quality of life. Loss of sleep and use of sedating medications may lead to falls and accidents. Sleep-related disorders of breathing may have serious cardiovascular, pulmonary, and CNS effects.

There are a number of changes that occur in the sleep–wake cycle as a person ages. Elderly persons have more fragmented sleep and shorter duration of stages 3 and 4 sleep. Although REM sleep tends to be preserved, the deepest stages of non-REM sleep frequently are reduced or nonexistent.[61,62] Compared with younger persons, the elderly tend to achieve less total nighttime sleep. They often take longer to fall asleep, they awaken earlier, and they have more nighttime arousals. Environmental influences, particularly auditory stimuli, often are more disruptive in the elderly. With an increase in nighttime wakefulness, there is an increase in daytime fatigue and daytime napping. An often overlooked cause of nocturnal awakenings in the elderly population is nocturia or need to urinate during the night.[61]

The causes of sleep disorders in the elderly include age-related changes in sleep architecture, secondary sleep disturbances, primary sleep disorders, lack of exercise, and poor sleep habits. Factors that predispose to secondary sleep disturbances include physical and mental illness, medication effects, and emotional stress. A variety of medical illnesses contribute to sleep disorders in the elderly, including arthritic pain, respiratory problems and cardiac disease, and neurologic disorders. Nightmares and nighttime fears are common in elderly persons with Parkinson disease, particularly those who are receiving levodopa. Psychiatric illness, such as depression, is a common cause of disturbed sleep in this age group. Primary sleep disorders such as sleep apnea, RLS, and PLMD also increase in old age. Many medications have stimulating effects and interfere with sleep. These include some of the antidepressants, decongestants, bronchodilators, corticosteroids, and some antihypertensives. Alcohol use also may serve as a deterrent to sleep in the elderly. Sleep–wake problems may be compounded further by inappropriate interventions initiated by the older person, his or her family, or health care providers.

Sleep also is disturbed in disorders characterized by dementia. Episodes of nocturnal wandering, confusion, and delirium can occur despite normal daytime functioning. Persons with Alzheimer disease often have increased periods of nighttime awakening and daytime napping.

Diagnosis of sleep disorders in the elderly requires a comprehensive sleep history, inquiries about pain and anxiety or depression, review of current sleep hygiene practices, drug use history, spousal or bed partner reports, a comprehensive physical examination, and appropriate laboratory tests.[63,64] Treatment of a medical disorder and changes in medication regimes and timing of medication doses can often improve sleep. Avoidance of alcohol and stimulants before bedtime and improving sleep hygiene are other measures that can be used to improve sleep. Although hypnotics can be used to treat transient insomnia, they often fail to provide long-term relief of chronic sleep disturbances.

IN SUMMARY, circadian rhythms and sleep patterns are established early in life. In the newborn, REM sleep occurs at sleep onset, and periods of sleep and awakening are distributed throughout the day. As the cyclic structure of the sleep–wake cycle progresses, the amount of time spent in REM sleep decreases. By the time the child is 8 months of age, the duration of sleep has decreased to approximately 13 hours and REM sleep occupies only approximately one third of that time. At 12 to 15 years of age, sleep has decreased to approximately 8 hours, with one fourth being spent in REM sleep. Although sleep complaints are common among adults, children usually do not complain about sleep problems, although their parents might. The usual concerns of parents include irregular sleep habits, insufficient or too much sleep, nightmares, sleep terrors, sleepwalking, and bed-wetting.

Complaints of sleep disorders are common in the elderly. The sleep–wake cycle changes that occur with aging are evidenced by more fragmented sleep, shorter duration of stage 3 and 4 sleep, and reduced REM sleep. The circadian rhythm of a typical sleep period also changes; elderly persons tend to go to bed earlier in the evening and awaken earlier in the morning. Elderly persons also have more health problems that interrupt sleep, they are apt to be on medications that interfere with sleep, and they are more likely to have sleep disorders such as insomnia, RLS, and sleep apnea. Left uncorrected, sleep disorders in the elderly affect the quality of life. Loss of sleep and use of sedating medications may lead to falls and accidents. ∎

Review Exercises

1. A frustrated mother complains that her teenage son stays up at night and then has trouble waking up and getting to school on time.

   A. *Is there a developmental explanation for these behaviors?*

   B. *What suggestions would you make to this mother?*

2. A 30-year-old woman presents with complaints of fatigue, irritability, and difficulty concentrating. She relates that for the past 3 months or more, she has had difficulty falling asleep and staying asleep despite remaining in bed and focusing on measures to help her sleep. She laughingly tells you she has even tried counting sheep.

   A. *What type of diagnostic measure would prove useful in determining whether this woman's problem is related to insomnia?*

   B. *If the woman is diagnosed with insomnia, what type of treatment would be indicated?*

3. A 50-year-old man presents with hypertension, daytime sleepiness and difficulty concentrating, and injuries sustained from an automobile accident that occurred when he fell asleep at the wheel. He weighs 250 pounds, is 69 inches tall, and leads a sedentary lifestyle. He states that his wife has moved into the guest bedroom because his snoring disturbs his sleep.

A. *What is the possible cause of this man's problems?*

B. *What diagnostic tests could be used to confirm the diagnosis?*

C. *What type of lifestyle changes and other treatments might be used?*

References

1. Hobson J. A. (1989). *Sleep* (pp. 1–21, 74–78, 117–134, 159–169). New York: Scientific American Library.
2. McCarley R. W. (1995). Sleep, dreams, and states of consciousness. In Conn P. M. (Ed.), *Neuroscience in medicine* (pp. 537–583). Philadelphia: J. B. Lippincott.
3. Carskadon M. A., Dement W. C. (2005). Normal human sleep. In Kryger M. H., Roth T., Dement W. C. (Eds.), *Principles and practice of sleep medicine* (4th ed., pp. 13–23). Philadelphia: Elsevier Saunders.
4. Carskadon M. A., Rechtschaffen A. (2005). Monitoring and staging human sleep. In Kryger M. H., Roth T., Dement W. C. (Eds.), *Principles and practice of sleep medicine* (4th ed., pp. 1359–1377). Philadelphia: Elsevier Saunders.
5. Siegel J. M. (2005). REM sleep. In Kryger M. H., Roth T., Dement W. C. (Eds.), *Principles and practice of sleep medicine* (4th ed., pp. 120–135). Philadelphia: Elsevier Saunders.
6. Douglas N. J. (2005). Respiratory physiology: Control of ventilation. In Kryger M. H., Roth T., Dement W. C. (Eds.), *Principles and practice of sleep medicine* (4th ed., pp. 224–225). Philadelphia: Elsevier Saunders.
7. Strollo P. J., Rogers R. M. (1996). Obstructive sleep apnea. *New England Journal of Medicine* 334, 99–104.
8. Pagel J. F. (2000). Nightmares and disorders of dreaming. *American Family Physician* 61, 2037–2042, 2044.
9. Moore M. C., Czeisler C. A., Richardson G. S. (1983). Circadian timekeeping in health and disease. *New England Journal of Medicine* 309, 469–473.
10. Moore R. Y. (1997). Circadian rhythms: Basic neurobiology and clinical applications. *Annual Review of Medicine* 48, 253–266.
11. Czeisler C. A., Buxton O. M., Khalsa S. B. S. (2005). The human circadian timing system and sleep–wake regulation. In Kryger M. H., Roth T., Dement W. C. (Eds.), *Principles and practice of sleep medicine* (4th ed., pp. 375–394). Philadelphia: Elsevier Saunders.
12. Brzezinski A. (1997). Melatonin in humans. *New England Journal of Medicine* 336, 186–195.
13. Ahrendt J. (2000). Melatonin, circadian rhythms, and sleep. *New England Journal of Medicine* 343, 1114–1115.
14. Scheer F. A., Cojochen C., Turek F. W., et al. (2005). Melatonin in the regulation of sleep and circadian rhythms. In Kryger M. H., Roth T., Dement W. C. (Eds.), *Principles and practice of sleep medicine* (4th ed., pp. 395–404). Philadelphia: Elsevier Saunders.
15. American Academy of Sleep Medicine. (2005). *International classification of sleep disorders: Diagnostic and coding manual* (2nd ed.). Westchester, IL: Author.
16. Members of National Heart, Lung, and Blood Institute Working Group on Insomnia. (1998). *Insomnia: Assessment and management in primary care*. NIH publication no. 98-4088. Bethesda, MD: National Institutes of Health.
17. Epstein D. R., Bootzin R. R. (2002). Insomnia. *Nursing Clinics of North America* 37, 611–631.
18. Ancoli-Israel S. (2005). Actigraphy. In Kryger M. H., Roth T., Dement W. C. (Eds.), *Principles and practice of sleep medicine* (4th ed., pp. 1459–1467). Philadelphia: Elsevier Saunders.
19. Lu Brandon S., Zee P. S. (2006). Circadian rhythm sleep disorders. *Chest* 130(6), 1915–1923.
20. Reid K. J., Burgess H. J. (2005). Circadian rhythm sleep disorders. *Primary Care Clinics in Office Practice* 32, 449–473.
21. Fahey C. D., Zee P. C. (2006). Circadian rhythm sleep disorders and phototherapy. *Psychiatric Clinics of North America* 29, 989–1007.
22. Akerstedt T. (2005). Sleepiness and circadian rhythm sleep disorders. *Sleep Medicine Clinics* 1, 17–30.
23. Wagner D. R. (1996). Disorders of the circadian sleep–wake cycle. *Neurologic Clinics* 14, 651–669.
24. Pilcher J. J., Lambert B. J., Huffcutt A. I. (2000). Differential effects of permanent and rotating shifts on self-report sleep length: A meta-analytic view. *Sleep* 23, 155–163.
25. National Institutes of Health. (2005). Manifestations and management of chronic insomnia in adults. *NIH Consensus and State-of-the-Science Consensus Statements* 22(2), 1–30.
26. Summers M. O., Crisostomo M. I., Stephanski E. J. (2006). Recent developments in the classification, evaluation, and treatment of insomnia. *Chest* 130, 276–286.
27. Budur K., Rodriguez C., Foldvary-Schaefer N. (2007). Advances in treating insomnia. *Cleveland Clinic Journal of Medicine* 74, 251–266.
28. Silber M. H. (2005). Chronic insomnia. *New England Journal of Medicine* 353, 803–810.
29. American Psychiatric Society. (1999). Diagnostic criteria for primary insomnia. In *Diagnostic and statistical manual of mental disorders* (4th ed.). Washington, DC: Author.
30. Neubauer D. N. (2005). Insomnia. *Primary Care Clinics in Office Practice* 32, 375–388.
31. Sateia M. J., Nowell P. D. (2004). Insomnia. *Lancet* 364, 1959–1973.
32. Rogers A. E., Dreher H. M. (2002). Narcolepsy. *Nursing Clinics of North America* 37, 675–692.
33. Mignot E. (2005). Narcolepsy: Pharmacology and genetics. In Kryger M. H., Roth T., Dement W. C. (Eds.), *Principles and practice of sleep medicine* (4th ed., pp. 761–779). Philadelphia: Elsevier Saunders.
34. Guilleminault C., Fromherz S. (2005). Narcolepsy: Diagnosis and management. In Kryger M. H., Roth T., Dement W. C. (Eds.), *Principles and practice of sleep medicine* (4th ed., pp. 780–790). Philadelphia: Elsevier Saunders.
35. Krahn L. E., Black J. L., Silber M. H. (2001). Narcolepsy: A new understanding of irresistible sleep. *Mayo Clinic Proceedings* 76, 185–194.
36. Dyken M. E., Yamada T. (2005). Narcolepsy and disorders of excessive somnolence. *Primary Care Clinics in Office Practice* 32, 389–413.
37. Nishino S. (2006). Narcolepsy. *Sleep Medicine Clinics* 1, 47–61.
38. Monteplaisir J., Allen R. P., Walters A. S., et al. (2005). Restless legs syndrome and periodic limb movements during sleep. In Kryger M. H., Roth T., Dement W. C. (Eds.), *Principles and practice of sleep medicine* (4th ed., pp. 839–852). Philadelphia: Elsevier Saunders.
39. Earley C. J. (2003). Restless legs syndrome. *New England Journal of Medicine* 348, 2103–2109.
40. Trenkwalder C., Paulus W., Walters A. S. (2005). The restless legs syndrome. *Lancet Neurology* 4, 465–474.
41. Thorpy M. J. (2005). New paradigm in the treatment of restless legs syndrome. *Neurology* 64(Suppl. 3), S28–S33.
42. Ondo W. G. (2005). Restless legs syndrome. *Neurology Clinics* 23, 1165–1185.
43. National Center on Sleep Disorders Research. (2000). *Restless legs syndrome: Detection and management in primary care*. NIH publication no. 00-3788. Bethesda, MD: National Institutes of Health.
44. Guilleminault C., Stoohs R., Quera-Salva M. (1992). Sleep-related obstructive and nonobstructive apneas and neurological disorders. *Neurology* 42(Suppl. 6), 53–60.

45. Pashayan A. G., Passannante A. N., Rock P. (2005). Pathophysiology of obstructive sleep apnea. *Anesthesiology Clinics of North America* 23, 431–443.

46. Members of the National Heart, Lung, and Blood Institute Working Group on Sleep Apnea. (1995). *Sleep apnea: Is your patient at risk?* NIH publication no. 95-3803. Bethesda, MD: National Institutes of Health.

47. Caples S. M., Gami A. S., Somers V. K. (2005). Obstructive sleep apnea. *Annals of Internal Medicine* 142, 187–197.

48. Flemons W. W. (2002). Obstructive sleep apnea. *New England Journal of Medicine* 347, 498–504.

49. Ryan C. M., Bradley T. D. (2005). Pathogenesis of obstructive sleep apnea. *Journal of Applied Physiology* 99, 2240–2450.

50. Burwell C. S., Robin E. D., Whaley R. D., et al. (1956). Extreme obesity associated with alveolar hypoventilation: A pickwickian syndrome. *American Journal of Medicine* 21, 811–818.

51. Baldwin C. M., Quan S. F. (2002). Sleep disordered breathing. *Nursing Clinics of North America* 37, 633–654.

52. Schenck C. H., Mahowald M. W. (2000). Parasomnias. *Postgraduate Medicine* 107(3), 145–156.

53. Plante D. T., Winkleman J. W. (2006). Parasomnias. *Psychiatric Clinics of North America* 29, 969–987.

54. Mahowald M. W. (2004). Parasomnias. *Medical Clinics of North America* 88, 660–678.

55. Masand R., Popli A. P. (1995). Sleepwalking. *American Family Physician* 51, 649–653.

56. Graven S. (2006). Sleep and brain development. *Clinical Perinatology* 33, 693–706.

57. Ferber R. (1996). Childhood sleep disorders. *Neurologic Clinics* 14, 493–451.

58. Ward T., Mason T. B. A. (2002). Sleep disorders in children. *Nursing Clinics of North America 37,* 693–706.

59. Sheldon S. H. (2004). Parasomnias in childhood. *Pediatric Clinics of North America* 51, 69–88.

60. Foley D. J., Monjan A. A., Brown S. L., et al. (1995). Sleep complaints among elderly persons: An epidemiologic study of three communities. *Sleep 18,* 425–432.

61. Bliwise D. (2005). Normal aging. In Kryger M. H., Roth T., Dement W. C. (Eds.), *Principles and practices of sleep medicine* (4th ed., pp. 24–38). Philadelphia: Elsevier Saunders.

62. Avidan A. Y. (2005). Sleep disorders in the older patient. *Primary Care Clinics in Office Practice* 32, 563–586.

63. Neubauer D. N. (1999). Sleep problems in the elderly. *American Family Physician* 59, 2551–2559.

64. Vitello M. V. (1999). Effective treatments for age-related sleep disturbances. *Geriatrics* 54(11), 47–52.

Visit the Point http://thePoint.lww.com for animations, journal articles, and more!

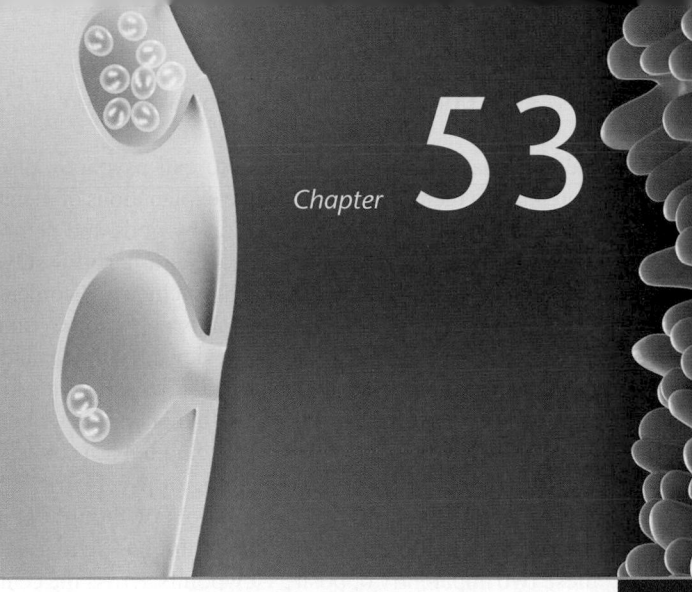

Disorders of Thought, Mood, and Memory

SANDRA KAWCZYNSKI PASCH

➤ Psychiatric disorders are characterized by changes in a person's thoughts, mood, or behaviors that preclude ordinary functioning in one or more spheres of life. Throughout the course of history, persons in the healing professions have tried to uncover the causes and find effective treatments for diseases that alter the way in which people experience the world and behave in it. Over the centuries, the pendulum has swung between those practitioners who espouse the view that mental disease arises from inadequate interpersonal relationships and those who espouse the view that mental disease arises from alterations in brain structure or activity. In the late 20th century, and now in the early years of the 21st, the conversation between these two apparently divergent philosophies continues, perhaps to conclude with a new synthesis of nurture versus nature and therefore new and effective therapies for those with mental illness.

The purpose of this chapter is to review the evolution in understanding of the pathogenesis and treatment of mental illness, and to relate the anatomy of the brain and its integrated regional functions to the causes, manifestations, and treatment of selected thought, mood, anxiety, and cognitive disorders.

 **EVOLUTION IN UNDERSTANDING OF MENTAL ILLNESS**

After completing this section of the chapter, you should be able to meet the following objectives:

- Define the terms *biologic psychiatry* and *psychosocial psychiatry* and compare them in terms of their definitions of the origins of mental disease.
- Describe the changes in the treatment of mental illness over the past three centuries.
- Explain the role that heredity plays in the epidemiology and development of mental illness.

Historical Perspectives

Psychiatry was not an organized specialty before the end of the 18th century, but mental disorders are as old as the human race. Artifacts and cave drawings from a half million years ago indicate that what we have come to call psychotic disorders were known then. Over the ages, the explanations of mental disorders have ranged from possession by gods and demons, to the breaking of taboos, to the idea that a harmful substance had entered the body. Persons with psychiatric disorders were treated with prayers, magic, and exorcisms. In some communities, people with mental illness were viewed with fear and often turned out of their homes, villages, and towns. In other communities, families took care of those with mental illness, but often these people were neglected or locked up in barns or cellars.[1]

The history of our understanding of psychiatric illnesses reveals a tension between two schools of thought as to the origin of mental disease. The pendulum has swung between these two apparently opposite viewpoints across the centuries. One view of psychiatric illness is that mental disorders are due to anatomic, developmental, and functional disorders of the brain, and is called *biologic psychiatry.* Another view is that mental disorders are due to impaired psychological development, a consequence of poor child rearing or environmental stress, and is called *psychosocial psychiatry.*[1] These differences of emphasis in terms of the pathogenesis of mental illness are important because the prevailing theory about the origins of mental disease influences what therapies for psychiatric illness predominate.

Early biologic psychiatry in the late 1800s to early 1900s emphasized the correlation of neurologic symptoms with postmortem microscopic study of anatomic changes in the brain. Although this research was of immense importance in terms of regional localization of brain functions (*e.g.,* Wernicke aphasia), it provided little help to the clinical psychiatrist of the time. Emil Kraepelin, a German psychiatrist, was the first to begin to classify psychiatric disorders by systematically studying the natural history of the disease. The intent was to be able to predict outcomes. In the sixth edition of his textbook, *Psychiatrie* (1899), Kraepelin laid the groundwork for the *Diagnostic and Statistical Manual of Mental Disorders* (*DSM;* the current 4th edition [text revision] is abbreviated *DSM-IV-TR*) of the American Psychiatric Association. He divided all mental disorders into 13 groups, including psychoses, which he divided into 2 distinct groups: those with an affective component, which he called *manic-depressive psychosis,* and those without, which he called *dementia praecox.*[1]

In the mid-20th century, the psychoanalytic view of mental disorders took hold, reaching its zenith in the 1950s and 1960s. Psychiatric illness was explained as the result of unconscious conflicts over events in an individual's past. Alterations in nurture, not nature, became the underlying cause of psychiatric illness.

In the last half of the 20th century, biologic psychiatry became important once again. During the 1970s, techniques of neuroimaging became available that allowed the neuroscientist to visualize brain structures and function.[1] The results of genetic studies examining the correlation between family relationships and incidence of psychiatric illness, in particular the studies of monozygotic and dizygotic twins, suggested that depression and schizophrenia had a strong genetic component.

The introduction of chlorpromazine (*i.e.,* Thorazine) as a treatment for schizophrenia revolutionized psychiatry because although it did not cure psychosis, it did control the symptoms of the disease, increasing the potential for more traditional therapies to work and allowing previously institutionalized individuals to lead much more normal lives. It also suggested strongly that mental illness had a biologic foundation. Chlorpromazine soon was followed by other drugs for psychosis and depression.

This move to biologic psychiatry, however, has not excluded the healing value of the therapist–client relationship. It appears that pharmacotherapy in conjunction with psychotherapy is of greater healing power than either alone. Perhaps the distinction drawn between biologic and psychosocial disease is arbitrary. Indeed, experiments indicate that learning and sensory stimulation or deprivation can in fact weaken or strengthen synaptic connections, which in turn could change brain function and thus behavior.[2]

Treatment of Mental Illness

Asylums have existed since the Middle Ages, but until the end of the 18th century, their only function was custodial. One of the oldest asylums was the Priory of St. Mary of Bethlehem, founded in London in the 13th century. Its name was eventually shortened to *Bedlam,* a term that has become synonymous with madness. The asylum as a therapeutic establishment did not become an important concept until the end of the 18th century.[1]

At this time, madness was viewed as an excessive irritation of the nerves, so establishing a calming environment was crucial. These asylums often had a very rigid schedule of daily activities meant to focus the patient and afford mental rest. It was also during this time that practitioners attempted to systematize the techniques known to establish a therapeutic relationship between the doctor and the patient.

In the 1800s, the number of patients in asylums was, at the most, in the hundreds. By the mid-1900s, the numbers were in the thousands. Unfortunately, by the early 1900s, asylums had become little more than warehouses for those living with chronic mental illness.[3] Whether this was due to the failure of asylums as a therapeutic environment or to the increased number of persons housed in them, overwhelming the available resources, remains a matter of debate. The reason for the increased numbers of persons in asylums in the 19th century also is debated. Was there an increased incidence of mental illness, or did society become increasingly intolerant of deviant behavior?

This debate exploded in the 1960s, during which time several writers suggested that there was no such thing as mental illness but rather a medicalizing of deviance, and that psychiatric institutions were evil. Schizophrenia in this view was a gifted and creative state of consciousness, not an illness. This antipsychiatry attitude, coupled with the advent of psychopharmacology, laid the foundations for the deinstitutionalization of the mentally ill and the move to community psychiatry. Unfortunately, deinstitutionalization was neither carefully planned nor adequately funded, leaving many mentally ill homeless and without proper care.[1]

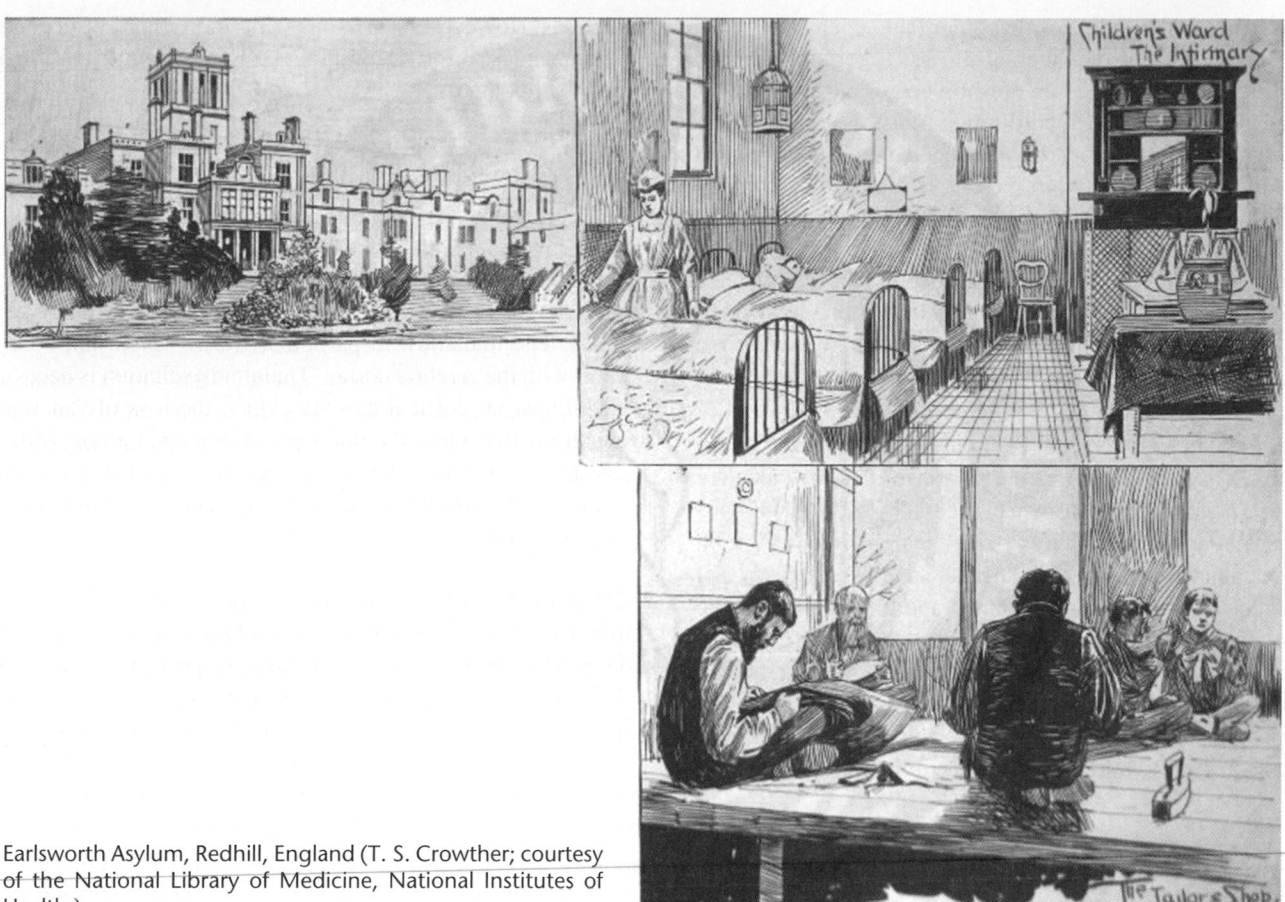

Earlsworth Asylum, Redhill, England (T. S. Crowther; courtesy of the National Library of Medicine, National Institutes of Health.)

The Role of Heredity in Mental Illness

Who we are and how we express ourselves through behavior depend on the complex influences of genetic and environmental factors on neural development and function. Since the early 1990s, the scientific knowledge base in genetics has grown exponentially and has created new tools to study the role of genetic inheritance in the development of mental illness. Research into the complexities of the regulation of gene expression can only deepen our understanding of the etiology of mental disorders, increase our ability to treat the disorders with more precisely targeted psychotherapeutic drugs, and ultimately lead to the discovery of ways to prevent the development of psychiatric illness.

Epidemiologic studies of twins, of adopted children, and of family histories or pedigrees have shed light on the debate over the relative influence of nurture versus nature in the development of mental illness. Twin studies compared the incidence of mental illness among monozygotic (identical) twins, dizygotic (fraternal) twins, and their siblings. If a disease were at all genetically determined, higher rates of coexistence of the disorder (concordance) would be expected among monozygotic twins compared with dizygotic twins, nontwin siblings, or the general population. Adoption studies questioned whether children with a genetic history of mental illness, adopted by parents with no history of psychiatric illness, had a greater risk of developing mental illness than children with no genetic history of mental illness who were adopted by parents with a psychiatric illness. Also, if a mental illness has a genetic component, it would be expected that higher numbers of persons in a family would have the disorder than would be found in the general population.[4-6] The overwhelming conclusions of these studies have been that both genetic vulnerability and environmental influences play significant roles in the development of mental illness.

For example, studies of twins have shown a 45% concordance for schizophrenia among monozygotic twins, compared with 15% for dizygotic twins or other siblings.[7] With bipolar depression, there is an 80% concordance in monozygotic twins, compared with 10% for siblings. In monozygotic twins living apart, the concordance rate for affective disorders is 40% to 60%.[8] Even the concordance rates among siblings for these two disorders is suggestive of a genetic influence because schizophrenia has approximately a 1% incidence and depression a 5% incidence among the general population.[7-9] The rate of occurrence of either disorder also is higher in the biologic families of adopted children than in the adoptive families. The incidence of suicide is six times higher among biologic relatives of adoptees with depressive illness than among the biologic relatives of adoptees without depression.

Although the evidence for a genetic basis for mental illness is compelling, the fact that the concordance among monozygotic twins is not 100% indicates that other factors may be involved in the development of a mental illness. It certainly is highly likely that mental illnesses are polygenic and multifactorial rather than simply inherited through transmission of a classic disordered dominant or recessive mendelian trait (see Chapter 6). In addition, mental disorders exhibit variable expressivity. It is possible that a person with the disease genotype needs to have the right environmental stressors (*e.g.*, viral illness, physical or emotional abuse, substance abuse) to express the disease phenotype, or that there are gene–gene interactions that influence the extent to which a mental illness is manifested.[4,5]

IN SUMMARY, psychiatric disorders are characterized by alterations in thought, mood, or behavior that may interfere with a person's ability to engage in ordinary social interactions and may in some instances require temporary or long-term institutionalization. Our understanding of the pathogeneses of mental disease is still in its infancy, and the historical debate over the relative importance of nurture and nature in the development of mental illness continues. It is likely that the cause of mental illness is multifactorial and includes a dynamic interplay among genetic predisposition, alterations in early neurodevelopment, and dysfunctional social interactions in a family. ∎

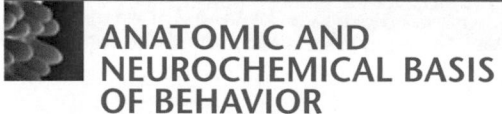

ANATOMIC AND NEUROCHEMICAL BASIS OF BEHAVIOR

After completing this section of the chapter, you should be able to meet the following objectives:

- Name the cerebral cortical structures and structures from the primitive brain involved in thought and emotion.
- Describe the major functions of each brain structure in terms of thought processes, learning, and emotion.
- Describe the cortical pathways by which learning and the development of memory occur.
- Define the terms *synapse, synaptic transmission,* and *neuromediators.*
- Name the major neuromediators in the brain, their major location and source, and possible involvement of each in the manifestations of mental illness.

Behavioral Anatomy of the Brain

There is scientific evidence that anatomic and biochemical alterations in the brain play a critical role in the behaviors observed in mental illness. The brain is extraordinarily complex, divided into several distinct groups of functional neurons that are highly interconnected and thus able to influence each other's activity.[10] Information processing occurs within nano-

seconds. However, for persons with brain injury or degenerative changes, information processing and cognitive function may be impaired.

Cerebral Cortical Structures

The cerebral cortex covers the outermost part of the brain. The cortex, which contains the centers for elaboration of thought, voluntary motor and sensory function, speech, and memory patterns, has extensive connections with deeper parts of the brain. The thalamus, in particular, forms important connections with the cerebral cortex. Thalamic excitation is necessary for almost all cortical activity. Thus, the loss of function is much greater when the thalamus is damaged along with the cerebral cortex than when damage is limited to the cortex. Table 53-1 summarizes the cerebral cortical structures and their functions.

Prefrontal Cortex. The frontal lobe is the largest lobe and often is referred to as the "chief administrator" of the brain (Fig. 53-1). It is responsible for planning, problem solving, intellectual insight, judgment, and expression of emotion. It is the function of the prefrontal areas to keep track of many bits of information simultaneously and then to recall this information as it is needed for subsequent intellectual tasks. Before the discovery of modern drugs to treat psychiatric conditions, some patients were treated surgically with a procedure called *prefrontal lobotomy* that severed the connections between the prefrontal areas of the brain and the remainder of the brain. Subsequent studies of these patients revealed a lack of ability to solve complex problems, link sequential tasks together, and learn to do parallel tasks at the same time. Their social responses were also inappropriate, and their levels of aggression were decreased to the point where they lost all ambition. They were, however, still able to perform at their previous level of motor function, talk, and comprehend language, but they were unable to carry through with any long-term trains of thought.

Temporal Lobe. The temporal lobe integrates and interprets somatic, visual, and auditory information that is critical for recognition of the familiar, as well as appropriate interpretation of and response to social contexts. The temporal lobe also contains the area of the brain (*Wernicke area*) that is responsible for language comprehension. It is one of the more important areas of the brain in terms of intellect because almost all intellectual functions depend on language.

Part of an appropriate social response is the accurate interpretation of emotions and the ability to respond with the socially appropriate level of emotionality and language. Impulse control, the management of aggression and sexual expression, including the culturally determined stereotypy of what it means to be male or female in a given society, also are temporal lobe functions. Emotion originates in the amygdala of the limbic system (discussed later), but the modulation and "fine-tuning" of that emotion to an appropriate level of intensity occur in the temporal lobe.

TABLE 53-1 Selected Functions of Several Brain Regions

FRONTAL LOBE	TEMPORAL LOBE	PARIETAL LOBE	OCCIPITAL LOBE
Abstract vs. concrete reasoning	Visual-spatial recognition	Sensory integration and spatial relations	Vision
Motivation–volition	Attention	Bodily awareness	Possible information holding area
Concentration	Motivation	Filtration of background stimuli	
Decision making	Emotional modulation and interpretation	Personality factors and symptom denial	
Purposeful behavior	Impulse and aggression control	Memory and nonverbal memory	
Memory and historical sense of self	Interpretation and meaning of social context	Concept formation	
Sequencing	Aspects of sexual action and meaning		
Making meaning of language			
Speech organization			
Speech production (Broca area)			
Aspects of emotional response—blunting			

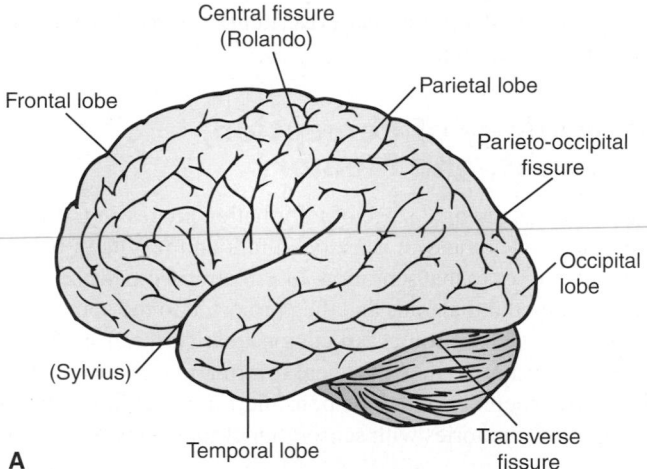

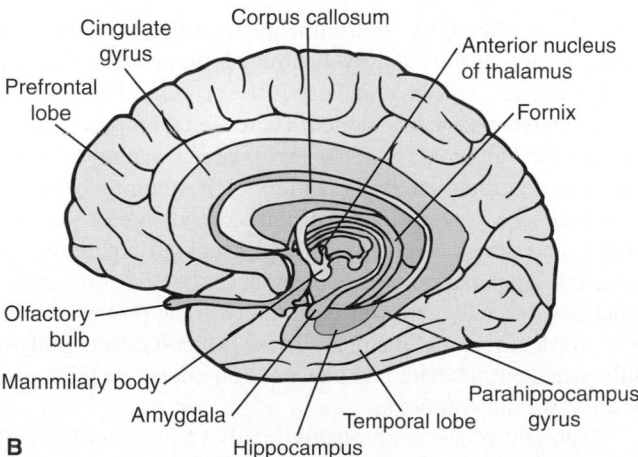

FIGURE 53-1 • **(A)** Lateral aspects of the cerebral hemispheres, including the frontal, temporal, parietal, and occipital lobes. **(B)** The structure of the limbic cortex, which includes the limbic cortex (cingulate gyrus, parahippocampal gyrus, hippocampus) and associated subcortical structures (thalamus, hypothalamus, amygdala).

Parietal Lobe. The parietal lobe is essential in the integration and processing of sensory (visual, tactile, and auditory) input. It is in the parietal lobe that sensory experiences first begin to coalesce into the cognitions we experience as thinking in the frontal lobes. The coordination of spatial awareness occurs in the parietal lobe and involves not only visual content, but the ability to experience, claim, and care for all of one's body. Another important parietal lobe function is to filter out extraneous information. The ability to filter out background and extraneous noise and sensations is critical to normal daily functioning.

Occipital Lobe. The occipital lobe is the most posterior of the lobes and is responsible for receiving visual information from the eyes. The visual association cortex of the occipital lobe is important for the interpretation of visual experiences, including depth perception and location in space.

Association Areas. A large part of the cerebral cortex forms association areas that add perception and meaning to incoming sensory information. The most important of these are the parieto-occipitotemporal association area, the prefrontal association area, and the limbic association area (Fig. 53-2).

The *parieto-occipitotemporal association area* lies in the large parietal-occipital cortical space bounded by the somatosensory cortex, the visual cortex, and the auditory cortex (see Chapter 48). This association area computes the coordinates of incoming visual, auditory, and somatosensory information, providing information about the location of body parts and their relationship to the environment. It also contains the major area for comprehending language, processing visual language (reading), and naming objects.

The *prefrontal association area* functions in close connection with the motor cortex to plan and execute complex motor movements. This area uses input from sensory receptors in muscles and joints, as well as sensory input from the skin and vestibular system. The prefrontal association area is also

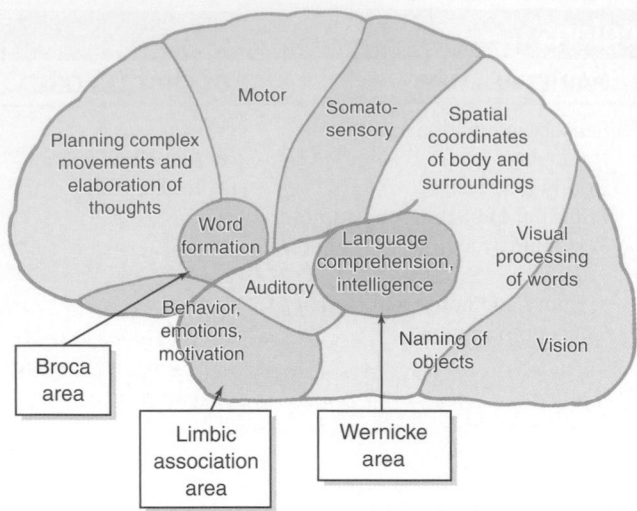

FIGURE 53-2 • Map of specific functional areas in the cerebral cortex, showing especially the Wernicke and Broca areas of language comprehension and speech production, which in 95% of all people are located in the left hemisphere. (Adapted from Guyton A. C., Hall J. E. [2006]. *Textbook of medical physiology* [11th ed., p. 717]. Philadelphia: Elsevier Saunders.)

important in carrying out thought processes that involve input from multiple sensory modalities. It is often described as being the area for short-term "working memories" that are used to analyze each new thought as it is entering the brain. A special area of the frontal cortex, called the *Broca area,* provides the neural circuitry for word formation.

The *limbic association area* is found in the anterior pole of the temporal lobe and in the cingulate gyrus on the medial aspect of the brain. It is concerned primarily with behavior, emotions, and motivation.

The Limbic System

The limbic system is a complex group of neurons that regulate our emotional behavior. It comprises several discrete structures in the deep part of the brain, including the hippocampus, parahippocampal gyrus, cingulate gyrus, amygdala, and a bridgelike structure called the *fornix,* which is a bundle of nerve fibers connecting the hippocampus with the hypothalamus (see Fig. 53-1). Higher and lower brain centers communicate with the limbic system to link thoughts and autonomic nervous system responses to emotions. The hippocampus, along with its adjacent temporal and parietal lobe structures, has numerous indirect connections with many portions of the cerebral cortex as well as other parts of the limbic system. The hippocampus plays a major role in the encoding, consolidation, and retrieval of memories. Almost all types of sensory information activate some part of the hippocampus. In turn, the hippocampus distributes information to the anterior thalamus, hypothalamus, and other parts of the limbic system. The hippocampus also groups and schematizes input in preparation for memory encoding. It plays a significant role in converting short-term

memory to long-term memory. Hippocampal atrophy has been noted in diseases in which memory problems play an important role, such as Alzheimer disease.

The amygdala is located deep in the medial temporal lobe. It receives neuronal signals from the temporal and occipital lobes of the cortex and has many bidirectional connections with the hypothalamus, as well as other parts of the limbic system. Through these connections, the amygdala helps a person relate to the surrounding environment and then pattern appropriate behavior. Because of the many connections, the amygdala has been called the "window" through which a person sees the world. The amygdala is important in emotional function and regulation and modulation of affective responses in social settings. Sexual arousal, aggression, and fear also are functions of the amygdala.

The hypothalamus, although not strictly an anatomic part of the limbic system, plays a critical role in it because of the extensive connections it has with the limbic system. The hypothalamus has a multitude of regulatory functions related to basic survival needs of the body, such as regulation of body temperature, sleep–rest patterns, hunger, sexual drive, and hormonal secretion.

Physiology of Perception, Thought, and Memory

Perception is the final stage of information processing. It is the conscious awareness of sensory stimuli and results in behavioral responses to that sensation. Information from the senses is received by the thalamus and then projected to the somatosensory cortex and prefrontal association area. The prefrontal association area keeps track of where information has been put in long-term memory and is responsible for retrieving and then integrating memories with sensory input for decision making.

Learning and Memory

Behavior is altered by environmental cues that are processed through learning and memory. Learning is the process of acquiring knowledge, whereas memory is the process of storing and retrieving what has been learned. There are two forms of memory: implicit memory, which is involved in learning reflexive motor and perceptual skills, and explicit memory, which is involved with processing the factual knowledge of persons, places, and things and its meaning.[11] Psychiatric patients and brain-injured persons not only experience specific cortical dysfunctions, but may experience difficulty in the proposed pathways for learning and memory. These difficulties are likely to influence their behavior and may have an impact on the design of effective interventions.

Thought processes probably involve a pattern of stimuli from many parts of the nervous system at the same time and in a definite sequence. Each thought requires simultaneous input from portions of the cerebral cortex, the thalamus, the limbic system, and the reticular formation in the brain stem. The prefrontal association cortex processes information from many areas of the brain and is necessary to achieve thinking. It has the ability to keep track of bits of information and recall them simultaneously from working memory. This allows us to plan, set goals, and solve problems. Thoughts are expressed in the form of language through the functions of the Broca area for word formation and the Wernicke area for language comprehension.

Physiologically, thought and memories are the result of synaptic transmission between neurons. During the process, new or reactivated pathways transmit neural circuits, sometimes called *memory traces,* through the brain.[12] Although we often think of memories as being positive recollections of past experiences, the greatest share of memories are probably negative encounters that the brain disregards as adverse or unimportant information. It is the basal regions of the limbic system that determine whether information is important and whether to store the thought as a memory trace or to suppress it. This aspect of memory selection is vital to the brain. Without it, the constant inundation of sensory information would exceed the capacity of the brain within minutes.

Memories can last minutes, hours, months, or years. For the purpose of classification, memory can be classified as short-term, intermediate-term, or long-term. Short-term memory is typically confined to the remembering of information for a period of several seconds to minutes (*e.g.,* 7 to 10 digits of a telephone number). It is thought that these memories involve nerve signals that travel around and around a temporary memory trace.[11] Intermediate-term memory involves the remembering of information for a period of many minutes to weeks. These memories become lost unless memory traces are established. Long-term memory, which lasts for years, is generally thought to result from actual structural changes in the synapses. For example, there might be an increase in the number of presynaptic structures responsible for neurotransmitter synthesis or release.

Disorders of Perception

Two disorders of information processing, hallucinations and delusional thoughts, are common symptoms of many psychiatric disorders. These symptoms may also occasionally occur in healthy persons, they may accompany other health problems, or they may be a side effect of drugs.

Hallucinations

Perception consists of the input of sensory information from the outside world and the processing of this information into meaning. All sensory information from the external world is transmitted to the thalamus; from there it is relayed to various parts of the brain and then transformed into meaningful experience. For example, visual stimuli from the retina are transmitted to centers in the thalamus through the optic nerve; from there, they are relayed to the primary visual cortex in the occipital lobe and then to the visual association cortex, where they gain meaning (see Chapter 54).

Hallucinations are described as "sensory perceptions with a compelling sense of reality."[10] Hallucinations should be differentiated from illusions, which are misinterpreted sensory perceptions that are stimulated by actual external stimuli. The pathophysiologic process of hallucinations can occur at several levels. The disorder may originate at the end organ, occur during sensory transmission, or be based on abnormal cortical reception, perception, or interpretation.

Hallucinations can be classified in several ways, such as by the structure or function involved, the etiology, or the affected sense perception. One functional method categorizes hallucinations as *release hallucinations* and *ictal hallucinations.* Release hallucinations occur when a normal sensory input is blocked and, as a replacement, stored images are experienced, whereas ictal hallucinations are produced by abnormal neuronal discharges. Visual ictal hallucinations tend to be of brief duration, stereotyped in content, and geometric in design. These are the types of hallucinations that occur during the aura in people with epilepsy. Hallucinations that are classified according to etiology may occur as the result of disorders of brain structure or function (brain tumors, epilepsy, metabolic disorders), drug reactions, sensory deprivation, sleep deprivation, or psychotic disorders. The type and content of hallucinations often provide insight into their etiology.

The most commonly used classification of hallucinations is based on the sensory perception involved (*e.g.,* visual, auditory, olfactory, tactile). Within this system, hallucinatory experiences involving the visual system are the most clearly categorized. Several types of visual hallucinations are normal life experiences (*e.g.,* images seen in a dream). Several ophthalmologic stimuli also are accompanied by visual hallucinations. Ocular phosphenes, which are produced by vigorous rubbing of the eye, are a form of visual hallucination. The Charles Bonnet syndrome is an organic disorder occurring in the elderly that is characterized by complex visual hallucinations. It is associated with loss of vision and is seen in older adults with preserved intellectual function.[13] In one study, 10% of persons (mean age of 75 years) with severe visual disability experienced visual hallucinations.[14] These persons retained insight into the problem and needed only reassurance that their hallucinations did not represent mental illness. Visual hallucinations associated with psychiatric disorders tend to be complex, may be enhanced by auditory hallucinations, and often lead to delusional beliefs.

Auditory hallucinations include misperceptions of sounds such as ringing and buzzing noises, music, and voices. Although they commonly occur in psychiatric disorders, particularly schizophrenia, they also occur in other disorders. Musical hallucinations featuring the perception of music without an external stimulus can be seen in disorders ranging from hearing impairment, especially in depressed elderly women, to temporal lobe lesions.[15] When associated with brain pathology, the lesion is usually on the right side of the brain. Auditory hallucinations are commonly reported as part of the aura of epilepsy. Tinnitus, the perception of ringing, buzzing, or whistling sounds, is often the result of disorders of the inner ear (Chapter 55). Withdrawal states, particularly from alcohol, are known to cause auditory hallucinations.

A variety of psychiatric disorders are accompanied by auditory hallucinations, such as the sound of voices. Often the source of the sound, which is sensed as occurring within the head, is difficult to localize. The voice often comments on the person's behavior and echoes his or her thoughts. Voices are rarely described as supportive; they are most often described as critical and negative in tone. Strategies of distraction used by persons hearing voices include listening to music, especially through headphones, or snapping rubber bands on their wrists. In addition, keeping a record helps to identify hallucinatory precipitants and thus helps individuals avoid those situations that act as precipitants.[16]

Hallucinations involving smell and taste are often the result of damage to the olfactory bulb. Tumors at the base of the brain that extend into the olfactory cortex can produce olfactory hallucinations. Persons with migraine headaches may also experience an aura consisting of olfactory or gustatory hallucinations. Somatosensory hallucinations, such as phantom limb pain, are discussed in Chapter 49.

Delusions

Delusions are characterized by a false belief and the persistent, unshakable acceptance of the false belief. In contrast to hallucinations, which are abnormalities of perception, delusions are abnormalities of thought. Delusions are formed from and colored by an individual's background, including personal, family, and social experiences; educational background; and cultural (including religious) influences. Delusional thinking may include, among others, delusions of persecution (*e.g.,* believing one's self or property is being threatened), influence (*e.g.,* believing thoughts can move through radio or atomic rays), ill health, grandeur (*e.g.,* believing oneself to be a great person, such as the King of England), poverty, and possession (*e.g.,* believing one's body is possessed by God or some great power).

The causes or mechanisms underlying delusional thinking are unclear. It has been suggested that delusional thinking is the product of repeated stress, rather than a disorder based on a single, acute situational problem. Interestingly, delusions have been associated with conditions that produce sensory deprivation, such as hearing loss. In one study that used a case-control method, elderly persons with late-life psychoses that included paranoid symptomatology were four times more likely to have hearing impairments than control subjects.[17]

Role of Neuromediators

Many of the new advances in the understanding and treatment of mental illness are derived from an increased understanding of how nerve cells in the brain communicate with one another. Nerve cells of discrete brain regions communicate with each other rapidly and over long distances by electrochemical signals that are propagated along the length of each neuron. The point at which two neurons meet is called a *synapse,* and the process by which the signal from one neuron to another is com-

municated is called *synaptic transmission* or *neurotransmission* (see Chapter 48). Chemical substances called *neurotransmitters* or *neuromediators* are released from the axonal terminal of one neuron (presynaptic cell), cross the synapse, bind to receptors on the postsynaptic cells, and cause excitatory or inhibitory actions.[18]

Neurotransmission involves several discrete steps: (1) the synthesis of a transmitter substance, (2) the storage and release of the transmitter, (3) binding of the transmitter to receptors on the postsynaptic membrane, and (4) removal of the transmitter from the synaptic cleft. The classic neurotransmitters include small-molecule transmitters and neuroactive peptides. These molecules typically are stored in vesicles in the presynaptic axonal terminal and released by the process of exocytosis[18] (see Chapter 48, section on Understanding Synaptic Transmission).

The substances generally agreed on to be neurotransmitters and that are implicated in mental illness include acetylcholine, the biogenic amines (dopamine, epinephrine, norepinephrine, and serotonin), and amino acids (gamma-aminobutyric acid [GABA], glutamate, glycine, and aspartate). Table 53-2 summarizes the major source and effect for each neurotransmitter.

Emergence of Psychotropic Medications

The treatment of many psychiatric disorders is based on pharmacologic interventions that alter neurotransmitter or receptor properties of the brain. In the 1950s, a French neurosurgeon, Henri Laborit, was searching for a drug that would reduce the affects of preoperative anxiety-induced histamine release in his patients. Through trial and error, he found chlorpromazine to be the most effective calming agent and recommended the drug to his psychiatric colleagues. It was subsequently found that high doses of chlorpromazine were efficacious in calming agitated persons with schizophrenia and bipolar disorders. It eventually became clear that chlorpromazine was not simply a tranquilizer but also had some specific antipsychotic effects. Chlorpromazine and related drugs in the phenothiazine class attenuated or abolished delusions, hallucinations, and disordered thinking.

There are now four major groups of antipsychotic agents used to treat schizophrenia, divided into two major categories: the typical and the atypical antipsychotics. The typical antipsychotics include the phenothiazines (*e.g.,* chlorpromazine [Thorazine]), butyrophenones (*e.g.,* haloperidol [Haldol]), and thioxanthenes (*e.g.,* thiothixene [Navane]). The atypical antipsychotics (*e.g.,* clozapine [Clozaril], risperidone [Risperdal], olanzapine [Zyprexa]) are more effective in treating the negative symptoms of schizophrenia (to be discussed) and produce fewer extrapyramidal effects. Both categories of drugs exert their effect by blocking dopamine receptors, although the atypical antipsychotics have a more refined blockade action. The atypical antipsychotics also exert some of their effects through blockade of serotonin (5-hydroxytryptamine [HT]) receptors.

Psychopharmacology has been particularly productive in developing highly effective treatments for affective disorders.

TABLE 53-2 **The Source and Effect of Brain Neuromediators**

NEUROMEDIATOR	MAJOR SOURCE IN THE BRAIN	EFFECT AND IMPLICATIONS FOR MENTAL ILLNESS
Acetylcholine (Ach)	Formed in many synapses of the brain; in high concentration in basal ganglia and motor cortex Derived from choline	Can be excitatory or inhibitory, depending on the area of the brain Underactivity implicated in Alzheimer disease
Dopamine (DA)	Substantia nigra and ventral segmental area in the midbrain Derived from tyrosine	Usually excitatory Involved in motivation, thought, and emotional regulation Overactivity thought to be involved in schizophrenia and other psychotic disorders
Norepinephrine (NE) and epinephrine (E)	Locus ceruleus in brain stem Derived from dopamine	Can be excitatory or inhibitory, depending on the area of the brain Noradrenergic pathways to cerebral cortex, limbic system, and brain stem Underactivity thought to be involved in some depressions
Serotonin (5-HT)	Raphe nucleus in the brain stem Derived from tryptophan	Involved in the regulation of attention and complex cognitive functions Pathways to cerebral cortex, limbic system, and brain stem Underactivity thought to be involved in some depressions and obsessive-compulsive disorder
γ-Aminobutyric acid (GABA), glutamate, aspartate, and glycine	No single major source	GABA and glycine usually are inhibitory; glutamate is excitatory Implicated in anxiety disorders

Antidepressants alleviate depressive symptoms by increasing the activity of norepinephrine and serotonin at postsynaptic membrane receptors. The most widely used antidepressants can be divided into four major categories: the monoamine oxidase (MAO) inhibitors, the tricyclic compounds, the serotonin reuptake inhibitors (SRIs), and the novel, or atypical antidepressants. MAO inhibitors (*e.g.,* phenelzine [Nardil], tranylcypromine [Parnate]) increase the concentration of serotonin and norepinephrine by reducing the degradation of these neurotransmitters by MAO. The tricyclic antidepressants (TCAs; *e.g.,* amitriptyline [Elavil], imipramine [Tofranil], nortriptyline [Aventyl, Pamelor]) block the reuptake of serotonin and norepinephrine by the presynaptic membrane, whereas the SRIs inhibit the reuptake of serotonin. Formulations of the SRIs vary and target different neurotransmitters. These include the selective serotonin reuptake inhibitors (SSRIs; *e.g.,* fluoxetine [Prozac], fluvoxamine [Luvox], paroxetine [Paxil], citalopram [Celexa]), the serotonin antagonist and reuptake inhibitors (SARIs; *e.g.,* nefazodone [Serzone]), and the serotonin and norepinephrine reuptake inhibitors (SNRIs; *e.g.,* venlafaxine [Effexor], duloxetine [Cymbalta]). The atypical antidepressants affect serotonergic and noradrenergic neurotransmission.

The therapeutic effect of the antipsychotic and antidepressant drugs probably is not entirely due to increasing or decreasing the neural levels of one or more neurotransmitters. For example, the clinical effect of the antidepressants typically is slow (weeks), even though the drugs rapidly block receptors. This suggests that the real mechanism of these drugs may be due to their effects on expression of receptors at the cellular membrane or on other intracellular pathways that regulate protein synthesis.[19]

Neuroimaging

Abnormalities in brain structure and function can contribute to the manifestations of mental illness. Since the early 1970s, imaging techniques have been developed that allow practitioners and researchers to map brain anatomy in exquisite detail and to estimate brain activity by measuring brain blood flow and metabolic rate. These imaging studies have suggested intriguing correlations between brain lesions and psychiatric manifestations that provide clues to the pathogenesis of mental disorders. Brain imaging techniques, however, remain research tools and have not yet been applied clinically, which means that imaging cannot be used to make a diagnosis of mental illness. The techniques include computed tomography (CT) scans, magnetic resonance imaging (MRI), magnetoencephalography (MEG), positron emission tomography (PET), and single-photon emission computed tomography (SPECT; Fig. 53-3).

A CT scan of the brain provides a three-dimensional view of brain structures that can differentiate fine densities. Abnormalities in a CT scan are not diagnostic of any particular mental illness; however, they suggest a brain-based problem. Structural abnormalities of the brain have been measured in people with schizophrenia, mood disorders, and dementias. MRI is used primarily for diagnosis of structural changes in the brain, although newer techniques are able to measure brain function as well. Unlike CT, MRI is able to distinguish between gray and white matter. MEG detects the minute magnetic fluctuations of

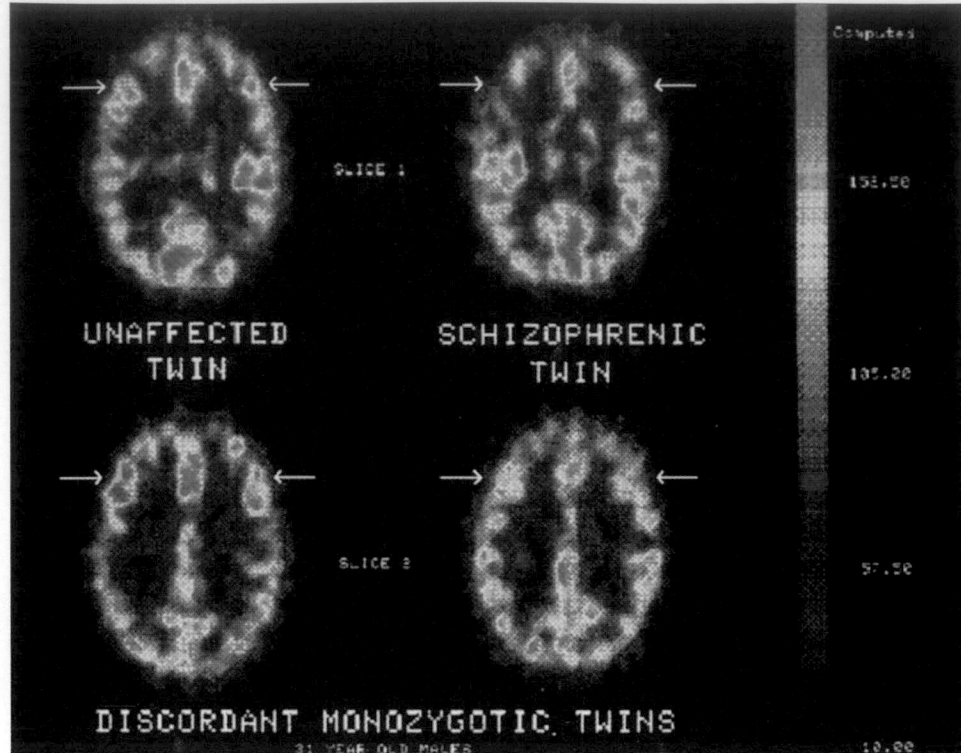

UNAFFECTED TWIN   SCHIZOPHRENIC TWIN

DISCORDANT MONOZYGOTIC TWINS

FIGURE 53-3 • Positron emission tomography (PET) scan showing differences in frontal lobe activity of a pair of twins, one with schizophrenia, and one who does not have the disorder. (From Boyd M. A. [2002]. *Psychiatric nursing: Contemporary practice* [2nd ed., p. 98]. Philadelphia: Lippincott Williams & Wilkins. Courtesy of Drs. K. F. Berman and D. R. Weinberger, Clinical Brain Disorders Branch, National Institutes of Health.)

regional brain activity.[20] The basis of PET is the variable brain tissue uptake of an infused radioactive substance. The tissue uptake of the substance depends on tissue type and metabolic activity. Labeled drugs can be infused to study neurotransmitter receptor activity or concentration in the brain. SPECT is similar to PET but is less expensive and uses more stable substances and different detectors to visualize blood flow patterns. This is useful for diagnosis of cerebrovascular accidents and brain tumors.[20,21]

IN SUMMARY, the symptoms of mental illness arise from alterations in neural functioning or from destruction of neurons in the brain. Because the brain integrates the processes of learning, memory, and emotions, the manifestations of mental disease may be primarily cognitive impairment, emotional impairment, or a combination of both. Psychiatric patients and brain-injured persons not only experience specific cortical dysfunctions but may experience difficulty in the proposed pathways for learning and memory. These difficulties are likely to influence behavior and may have an impact on the design of effective interventions.

Many of the new advances in the understanding and treatment of mental illness and symptoms such as hallucinations, mood disruptions, and cognitive dysfunction are derived from an increased understanding of how nerve cells in the brain communicate with one another. Neurotransmission involves several discrete steps: (1) the synthesis of a transmitter substance, (2) the storage and release of the transmitter, (3) the binding of the transmitter to receptors on the postsynaptic membrane, and (4) the removal of the transmitter from the

synaptic cleft. The substances generally agreed to be neurotransmitters and that are implicated in mental illness include acetylcholine, the biogenic amines, and amino acids.

New diagnostic tools, such as increasingly sophisticated neuroimaging techniques, may help in the development of more precise correlations between behavior, thought, and mood disorders and microscopic alterations in brain structure and neuron function. In addition, an increased understanding of the complex interactions among the different parts of the brain will assist in the development of more effective psychotherapies and more efficacious psychotropic drugs. ■

DISORDERS OF THOUGHT AND VOLITION

After completing this section of the chapter, you should be able to meet the following objectives:

■ Define the term *schizophrenia*.
■ Describe the epidemiology of schizophrenia.
■ Describe the manifestations of schizophrenia, both positive and negative symptoms, and their underlying neuropathophysiology.
■ Cite the diagnostic criteria for schizophrenia according to the *DSM-IV-TR* classification.
■ Describe the treatment for the positive and negative manifestations of schizophrenia.

Schizophrenia

Schizophrenia is a chronic debilitating psychotic disorder that involves the disconnection between thought and language. It affects a person's thoughts, feelings, perceptions, and overall behavior while interfering with filtering of stimuli from the environment.[22] Although the word *schizophrenia* means "splitting of the mind," it should not be confused with "split personality." The onset of the disorder typically occurs between 17 and 25 years of age. The peak age of onset for males is between 10 and 25 years of age, and for females between 25 and 35 years of age.[22] Ninety percent of those in treatment are between 15 and 55 years of age. Onset before 10 or after 60 years of age is rare. Men and women seem to be affected equally. Risk factors for schizophrenia include having a close relative with schizotypal personality disorder or schizophrenia (first-degree relatives of a person with schizophrenia have a 10-fold greater prevalence of the illness than the population at large), winter/spring birth date, second-trimester prenatal influenza infection, and early history of attentional deficits.[5,22]

SCHIZOPHRENIA

- Schizophrenia is a psychotic disorder of thought and language that is characterized by disorganized speech, delusions, visual and auditory hallucinations, and possible catatonic behavior.

- The positive symptoms of schizophrenia include delusions, or false beliefs, and hallucinations, or abnormal sensory perceptions, that occur without external visual or auditory input.

- The negative symptoms of schizophrenia reflect the absence of normal social and interpersonal relationships such as lack of motivation, apathy, and flattening of emotional expression.

Manifestations

Recent research and data concerning schizophrenia present a complex image of brain dysfunction with alterations in anatomic structures, biochemical variations, and functional disturbances.[10,22] The psychopathology of schizophrenia can be organized in various ways, but all such systems consider the positive and negative symptoms of the disease. *Positive* or *psychotic symptoms* reflect the presence of abnormal behaviors and include incomprehensible speech; delusions (*e.g.,* that one is being controlled by an outside force); hallucinations (hearing voices is the most common); and grossly disorganized or catatonic behavior. Alterations in speech patterns can include using invented words (neologisms), derailment (loose associations), tangentiality (inability to stick to the

original point), incoherence (loss of logical connections), or word salad (groups of disconnected words; Fig. 53-4). Frequently, persons with schizophrenia lose the ability to sort and interpret incoming stimuli, which impairs the ability to respond appropriately to the environment. An enhancement or a blunting of the senses is very common in the early stages of schizophrenia. Sounds may be experienced as louder and more intrusive; colors may be brighter and sharper. In addition, the person with schizophrenia often experiences sensory overload owing to a loss of the ability to screen external sensory stimuli.[23–26]

Delusions and hallucinations may be related to the inability of the person with schizophrenia to filter, interpret, and respond appropriately to stimuli. Delusions are false ideas believed by the affected person that cannot be corrected by reason. They range from simply believing that people are watching them to beliefs that they are being controlled and manipulated by others. Delusions of being a historical figure (*e.g.,* Jesus Christ or the President) also are common. Sometimes the delusions include a belief that the affected person is able to control others with his or her thoughts.[25]

Hallucinations are very common in schizophrenia, especially the auditory type. In these cases, the individual sees and hears things that are not in the external world but nevertheless are very real phenomena to the person experiencing them.

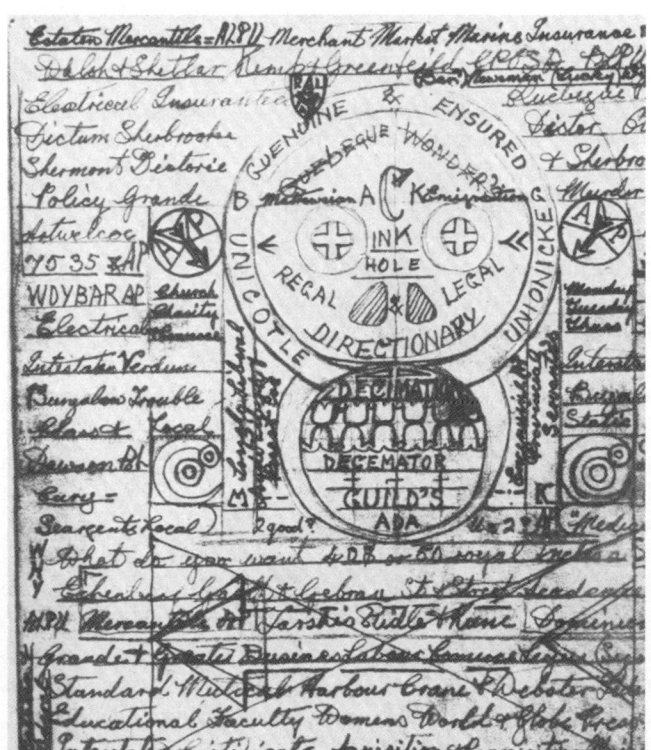

FIGURE 53-4 • A woman with schizophrenia expresses her incoherent thinking, combined with neologisms, in this drawing. (From Sadock B. J., Sadock V. A. [2003]. *Kaplan and Sadock's synopsis of psychiatry* [p. 494]. Philadelphia: Lippincott Williams & Wilkins [courtesy of Heinz E. Lehmann].)

Hallucinations may represent the end of the spectrum of increasing intensity of sensual stimuli. Auditory hallucinations range from simple repetitive sounds to many voices speaking at once. Sometimes the voices are pleasant, but often they accuse and curse. When visual hallucinations occur, they usually are in conjunction with auditory hallucinations.[22–25]

The *negative symptoms* of schizophrenia reflect the absence of normal social and interpersonal behaviors and include alogia (tendency to speak very little), avolition (lack of motivation for goal-oriented activity), apathy, affective flattening (lack of emotional expression), inappropriate affect, and anhedonia (an inability to experience pleasure in things that ordinarily are pleasurable). Some persons with schizophrenia have a blunted response to pain. Negative symptoms are the most difficult to treat, and often are severe and persistent between acute episodes of illness.[10]

Another component of schizophrenia concerns what is referred to alternatively as the *disorganized dimension, cognitive symptoms,* or *disorganization symptom cluster.*[10,26] It involves thought disorders and overlaps the categories of positive and negative symptoms. This component involves the disorganized speech and behavior described previously, and the incongruent mood and affect that interfere with relating to the environment.

These three dimensions of behavior—positive or psychotic symptoms, negative symptoms, and disorganization—are used in categorizing the various types of schizophrenia. They are also used in evaluating the neurocognitive impairment that occurs with schizophrenia. Studies have found less cognitive impairment when psychotic symptoms predominate, such as in paranoid schizophrenia. Conversely, there is more cognitive impairment related to negative and disorganized symptoms.[26]

Schizophrenia is divided into paranoid, disorganized, and catatonic subtypes, based on the presentation of behaviors and predominance of various symptom clusters. *Paranoid schizophrenia* manifests with persecutory or grandiose delusions. Auditory hallucinations are common. Interactions with others are rigid, intense, and controlled. It often has a sudden onset, and negative symptoms are not prominent. The prognosis of this form of schizophrenia seems to be better, with less evidence of disturbance in the anatomy of the brain and, as noted, fewer cognitive deficits than in those types in which negative symptoms predominate.[25,26]

Disorganized schizophrenia is characterized by a disintegration of the personality and a predominance of negative symptoms. Socially, the person is withdrawn and inept. Speech often is disorganized and incoherent. Personal grooming is neglected and because behavior is aimless, the person with this disorder often is not able to complete activities of daily living. The person also may have cognitive and psychomotor deficits. In general, the prognosis is not as good as for the paranoid schizophrenic type.[22]

Catatonic schizophrenia was common decades ago, but is now rare in developed countries of the world. This disorder is characterized by intense psychomotor disturbance (retardation or excitement), extreme negativism, and peculiar voluntary movements such as grimacing, posturing, and echolalia (repeating what is said by another) or echopraxia (imitating the movements of others).[25]

Neurophysiology of Symptoms

The exact pathogenesis of schizophrenia is unknown. No single lesion in the brain appears to be specific to schizophrenia or to the brain of all persons with schizophrenia.[27–29] With the advent of neuroimaging techniques of the 1960s, it became possible to document what had long been suspected: that schizophrenia was associated with brain abnormalities. These abnormalities are present at the first episode and in unmedicated persons. This suggests that the anatomic changes are not the result of progressive brain deterioration or the effects of psychiatric medications, but are caused by abnormalities in neurodevelopment that occur in prenatal or early postnatal life. There is an enlargement of the lateral and third ventricles; a reduction in frontal lobe, temporal lobe, and whole-brain volumes; and diminished neuronal content in both the thalamus and hippocampus.[5,27,28] Schizophrenia also is characterized by reduced metabolic activity in the frontal cortex on PET scan, although marked decreases in activity can be seen in almost every area of the brain, depending on the individual and the particular symptoms being experienced at the time of the scan[28] (see Fig. 53-3).

It is not known at what age these differences might be visible with imaging because children usually are not subjected to imaging techniques without a specific event indicating a clinical need for the procedure. Adolescents and young adults who are at high risk for development of schizophrenia because of a strong family history also have enlarged ventricles and smaller medial temporal lobes.[29] Studies have also found other brain abnormalities in nonpsychotic first-degree relatives of persons with schizophrenia. These were most pronounced in the hippocampus.[29]

An additional anatomic finding is an increased density of dopamine (D_2) receptor sites, particularly in the basal ganglia. With the finding that effective antipsychotic drugs are dopamine antagonists and that dopamine-releasing agents such as amphetamine can cause psychosis, the "dopamine hypothesis" was developed; it proposes that the symptoms of schizophrenia are due to dopaminergic overactivity. This hypothesis, however, cannot explain types of schizophrenia in which negative symptoms predominate, or the residual symptoms of an acute psychotic episode. In addition, it is possible that the increased density of dopamine receptors found in some studies is related to the effects of antipsychotic drugs. Other neurotransmitter changes implicated in the development of schizophrenia include a decreased activity of serotonin (through the 5-HT_{2A} receptor) and a decreased activity of glutamate through dysfunction of its *N*-methyl-D-aspartate receptor (see Chapter 51). Norepinephrine and GABA have also been implicated in the pathophysiology of schizophrenia.

Diagnostic Criteria

According to the *DSM-IV-TR* classification system, a diagnosis of schizophrenia requires that two or more of the following symptoms be present for a significant portion of 1 month: delusions, hallucinations, disorganized speech, grossly disorganized or catatonic behavior, or negative symptoms.[30] In addition, one or more areas of functioning must be significantly impaired compared with premorbid abilities, and continuous signs of the disturbance must persist for at least 6 months.[30]

Treatment

The goals of treatment for schizophrenia are to induce a remission, prevent a recurrence, and improve behavioral, cognitive, and psychosocial functions. Schizophrenia is a chronic illness, and for the person living with schizophrenia, the goal is *recovery*. According to the Substance Abuse and Mental Health Services Administration of the federal government, "mental health recovery is a journey of healing and transformation enabling a person with a mental health problem to live a meaningful life in a community of his or her choice while striving to achieve his or her full potential."[31] The implications and reality are that outcomes from this illness are varied, and some individuals function at a much higher level than originally thought.[32] Hospitalization may be indicated if the patient is a danger to self or others, is unable to provide basic care for self, or refuses to eat or drink.

Pharmacotherapy and psychosocial interventions, the latter of which include patient and family education, housing support, vocational rehabilitation, and case management, are components in the treatment of persons with schizophrenia. The positive symptoms of schizophrenia (delusions, hallucinations, agitation, thought broadcasting, loose associations, suspiciousness, and poor hygiene and dress) are most likely to respond to drug therapy. Both typical and atypical antipsychotic drugs address these positive symptoms. The negative symptoms of schizophrenia respond more favorably to the atypical antipsychotic drugs (*e.g.*, olanzapine, ziprasidone). Often antipsychotics are combined with benzodiazepines or antiparkinson agents during the acute phase of treatment to reduce the risk of extrapyramidal effects from large doses of antipsychotic agents.

Psychosocial interventions are important to help patients learn about and live successfully with their illness. Assistance with housing, employment or disability benefits, socialization, and co-occurring illnesses may be indicated and involves the role of a case manager. Family members may need assistance in learning about the illness and the best ways to support each other and their family member with schizophrenia. Maintenance of pharmacotherapy may be difficult for a variety of reasons, including side effects of medications, cost of medications, and beliefs that they are no longer necessary. Social support and nursing interventions aimed at identifying and assisting with noncompliance issues can lead to improved compliance.

IN SUMMARY, schizophrenia is a chronic psychotic disorder of thought and volition in which thought and language become disconnected. It is characterized by both positive symptoms and negative symptoms. Positive symptoms are abnormal behaviors (*e.g.*, incomprehensible speech), delusions, and auditory or visual hallucinations. Negative symptoms are the lack of normal social and interpersonal behaviors (*e.g.*, lack of emotional expression) and an inability to experience pleasure. The onset of the disorder typically occurs between the ages of 17 and 25 years, with an equal incidence in men and women. Risk factors for schizophrenia include having a close relative with schizotypal personality disorder or schizophrenia. The pathogenesis of schizophrenia is unknown, although neuroimaging studies reveal anatomic and functional changes in regions of the brain, including enlargement of the ventricles and diminished volumes in several areas of the brain, including the hippocampus and temporal cortex. Abnormalities in neurotransmission have been implicated, including changes in concentration and activity of the neurotransmitters dopamine, serotonin, norepinephrine, GABA, and glutamate. Treatment includes both psychosocial interventions and psychotropic medications. ■

DISORDERS OF MOOD

After completing this section of the chapter, you should be able to meet the following objectives:

- Define the terms *depression* and *mania*.
- Describe the epidemiology of major depression and bipolar depression.
- Describe the manifestations of major depression and bipolar depression.
- Cite the diagnostic criteria for depression according to the *DSM-IV-TR* classification.
- Describe the treatment modalities for depression.

Mood disorders are disorders of emotion (mania and depression) rather than disturbances of thought. Although relatively common, they are highly underdiagnosed and undertreated illnesses. Mood disorders include major depression and bipolar (manic-depressive) disorders. Depression is among the leading causes of disability worldwide, with a lifetime incidence in the United States of 20% in women and 12% in men.[33] The prevalence of major depression among women is double that in men. The prevalence of bipolar disorder is approximately 1.5% in the population at large, approximately equally distributed between men and women. Men more often have the manic phase in the initial episode, whereas women more often have the depressed phase as the initial episode.

Depressive Disorders

Approximately 20% to 40% of adolescents who present with major depression develop bipolar disorder within 5 years.[34] The average age of onset of bipolar disorder is the mid- to late twenties, and for depression, the mid-thirties; however, the age of onset of both disorders has been decreasing. In addition, the incidence of depression appears to be increasing. Prevalence of depression is higher in individuals from families with a history of mood disorders than in the population at large, indicating a genetic component to the etiology. Mood disorders are thought to occur with equal prevalence among races, although it is more frequently misdiagnosed as schizophrenia among nonwhite populations.[34,35] Depression rates are also higher among individuals living in or near poverty.

MOOD DISORDERS

- Mood disorders, which include depression and mania, represent a disturbance in emotion rather than thought.

- Major depression is characterized by feelings of worthlessness and guilt, decreased concentration, alterations in sleep and appetite, and possible suicidal ideation.

- Bipolar depression is characterized by alternating periods of depression and mania, during the latter of which there is a decreased need for food and sleep, racing thoughts, irritability, and high distractibility.

As with schizophrenia, genetic factors appear to play an important role in the development of mood disorders. Several studies have identified genetic loci that might contribute to the vulnerability to depression in families and individuals. However, the expression of affective disorders is not 100% in vulnerable families, and additional factors, such as environment, life history, development, and biologic challenges, likely interact to cause mood disorders.[36]

Major Depression and Dysthymia

Depression can vary in intensity and often is recurrent. The earlier and more frequent the onset of symptoms, the more likely it is that the affected individual will require medications for symptom relief. Depression in the elderly often appears with an element of confusion and often is left untreated. A first episode of depression that occurs after 65 years of age can be a precursor to dementia and should precipitate both assessment and treatment of the depression, as well as a thorough evaluation for dementia. Early intervention often greatly retards the progression of dementia, maintaining the individual's independence and quality of life.

Depressive disorders are commonly divided into two categories: major depressive disorder (characterized by a persis-

tent unpleasant mood) and dysthymia (characterized by chronic mild depressive symptoms).

Major Depressive Disorder. Major depressive disorder is characterized by the following: depressed mood, anhedonia (inability to experience pleasure), feelings of worthlessness or excessive guilt, decreased concentration, psychomotor agitation or retardation, insomnia or hypersomnia, decreased libido, change in weight or appetite, and thoughts of death or suicidal ideation.

Depression has various subclassifications distinguished by symptom patterns. Depression with *melancholic features* is characterized by depression that is worse in the morning, insomnia with early morning awakening, anorexia with significant weight loss, psychomotor retardation or agitation, excessive or inappropriate guilt, loss of interest in activity, inability to respond to pleasurable stimuli, and a complete loss of capacity for joy. The symptoms of *atypical* depression are opposite those of melancholic depression; it is characterized by a depression that becomes worse as the day progresses, overeating, and hypersomnia (excessive sleep). Depression with *psychotic features* involves the presence of delusions or hallucinations that may or may not be mood-congruent. The classification of depression with *catatonic features* is applied when symptoms include excessive mobility or motoric immobility, extreme negativism, repetitive speech, and peculiar voluntary movements. The *chronic* specifier is applied if symptoms of major depression persist for 2 or more years.

A *postpartum* specifier is included if the onset is within 6 weeks of childbirth. Most women experience some mild letdown of mood in the postpartum period. For some, the symptoms are more severe and similar to those seen in serious depression, with increased emphasis related to the infant (obsessive thoughts about harming it or an inability to care for it). When psychotic symptoms occur, there is frequently associated sleep deprivation, volatility of behavior, and manic-like symptoms. Biologic vulnerability with hormonal changes and psychological stressors all play a role.

Dysthymia. Dysthymia is characterized by the same symptoms as major depression, but in a milder form.[35-38] These include low self-esteem, sleep and energy problems, and appetite disturbances. The insidious and chronic nature of this disorder often makes it difficult for the person dealing with this illness to separate it from the usual manner of functioning and to recognize the symptoms as part of an illness. Persons with dysthymia are at risk for development of major depression and other psychiatric disorders, including substance abuse disorders.[36,37]

Bipolar Depression

Bipolar depression, or manic-depressive disorder, also has multiple subclassifications, all of which are usually characterized by episodes of elation and irritability (mania) with or without episodes of depression.[38] Although mania without associated depression (unipolar mania) can occur, it is rare. Mania, in persons with bipolar disorder, can be precipitated by antidepressant medications and the somatic therapies used to treat depression, such as electroconvulsive therapy.[39,40]

The manifestations of mania include decreased need for food and sleep, labile mood, irritability, racing thoughts, high distractibility, rapid and pressured speech, inflated self-esteem, and excessive involvement with pleasurable activities, some of which may be high risk. In its minor forms, the subjective experience of mania can be quite pleasurable to the individual, with a heightened sense of well-being and increased alertness.[41] The severity of manic symptoms runs the gamut from a condition called *cyclothymia,* in which mood fluctuates between mild elation and depression, to severe delusional mania. Mania may begin abruptly within hours or days, or develop over a few weeks. Mixed states with features of both mania and depression present at the same time often are not well recognized. Bipolar episodes, left untreated, become more severe with age. Rapid cycling is said to occur when an individual has four or more shifts in mood from normal within a 1-year period. Women are more likely than men to be rapid cyclers.[42]

Kindling is a hypothesized phenomenon in which a stressor creates an electrophysiologic vulnerability to future stressful events by causing long-lasting changes in neuronal function. This may be the basis for the phenomenon of rapid cycling in bipolar depression. The more frequently a person has a shift in mood, cycling into either mania or depression, the easier it becomes to have another episode. There now is evidence that many psychiatric disorders, not just bipolar disorder, are subject to this phenomenon. The better the control of the illness and the fewer cycles an individual has, the better his or her quality of life is likely to be.[43]

Neurophysiology of Symptoms

In some cases of familial major depressive disorder and bipolar disorder, PET and MRI studies have demonstrated a reduction in the volume of gray matter in the prefrontal cortex, with an associated decrease in activity in the region. Structural imaging studies have consistently found abnormalities in the subgenual prefrontal cortex in patients with familial bipolar disorder, a region related to responses to emotional experiences.[44] Clinical studies have suggested that this area of the brain is important for mood states and has extensive connections with the limbic system. Physiologically, there is evidence of decreased functioning in the frontal and temporal lobes, although it is not known if this is a cause or an effect of depression because the activity returns to normal with the resolution of the symptoms[44,45] (Fig. 53-5). The amygdala tends to have increased blood flow and oxygen consumption during depression.[38] Unlike those areas where function returns to normal with the resolution of depression, the amygdala continues to be excessively active for 12 to 24 months after the resolution of depression. It is hypothesized that relapse into depression is more likely to occur if medications are decreased or stopped before the amygdala returns to normal functioning. Other studies suggest abnormal neurodevelopment of the amygdala.[44] Neurologic disorders of the limbic system and basal ganglia are also involved in the development of mood disorders.[33,44]

A number of neurotransmitters, serotonin and norepinephrine in particular, are implicated in depression.[39,45,46] The biogenic amine hypothesis suggests that decreased levels of these neurotransmitters in the synaptic cleft, due either to decreased presynaptic release or decreased postsynaptic sensitivity, is the underlying pathologic process in depression. The hypothesis is

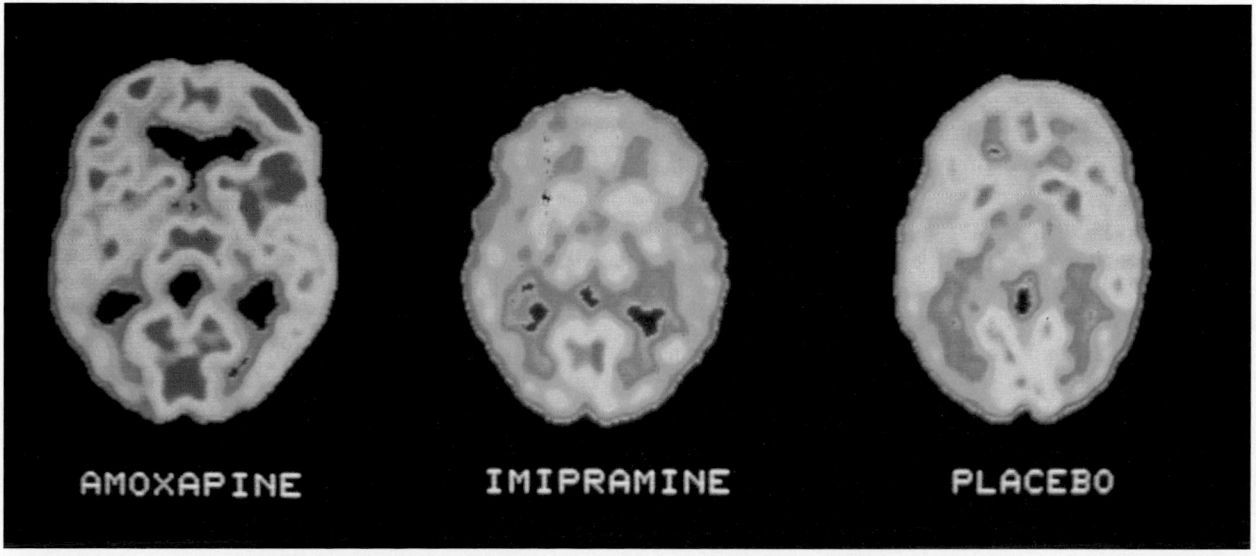

FIGURE 53-5 • Acute effects of antidepressant medications in patients with affective disorder showing widespread effects on the cortex that vary dramatically with the medication used. Positron emission tomography (PET) is useful in revealing specific patterns of metabolic change in the brain and in providing clues to the mechanisms of antidepressant response (Courtesy of Monte S. Buchsbaum, MD. The Mount Sinai Medical Center and School of Medicine, New York.)

derived from the fact that drugs that depleted brain serotonin and norepinephrine caused depression, and drugs that increased brain levels of norepinephrine and serotonin decreased depression. Dopamine activity has also been implicated in mood disorders, with decreased dopamine activity found in depression, and increased dopamine activity in mania.[45,46] It has become increasingly clear, however, that a simple decrease in the concentration of amines in neuronal synapses cannot entirely explain the complexities of depression. Neuromodulatory systems in the brain interact with each other in complex ways. For example, cholinergic and GABA-ergic pathways also may play a role in the development of depression because both of these pathways influence the activity of brain norepinephrine neurons.[44,45]

Disturbances in the function of the hypothalamic-pituitary-adrenal (HPA) axis also may play a critical role in depression. In the general population, cortisol levels usually are flat from late in the afternoon until a few hours before dawn, when they begin to rise. In persons with depression, cortisol levels spike erratically over the 24 hours of the day. Cortisol levels return to the normal pattern as depression resolves. In 40% of those diagnosed with depression, hypersecretion of cortisol is resistant to feedback inhibition by dexamethasone, indicating a dysfunction of the HPA axis.[45,46] About 5% to 10% of persons with depression have a decrease in thyroid function, in which case the person is less likely to have a vigorous response to medical intervention.

Alteration in the sleep–wake cycle is common in many mental illnesses and often is one of the prodromal signs of relapse. Researchers have found that the normal sleep cycle is reversed in depression. Persons with depression often have what is called *dream pressure sleep*. The depressed individual falls into light and dream-state sleep early in the sleep cycle and reaches deep stage 4 sleep only late in the sleep cycle. This finding helps explain why many inpatients report they did not sleep all night and the staff reports that the patient was asleep all night. Although the sleep cycle usually reverts to normal after the resolution of the depression, it may not be completely normal for weeks to months. Decreasing or halting medications before the sleep disturbances resolve may lead to a relapse of depressive symptoms. Fatigue and hypersomnia are common among individuals with depressive disorder, and individuals who complain of chronic fatigue are at risk for development of major depressive disorder.[47]

Circadian rhythms also are an area of serious research interest. A specific type of depression known as *seasonal affective disorder* (SAD) is triggered for persons in the winter by the shortening of daylight hours as fall commences, with symptoms of depression usually resolving in the spring when daylight hours again lengthen. Circadian rhythm considerations are also critical in symptom management for persons with bipolar depression. One of the fastest ways to precipitate a manic episode is for the individual to stay up all night. It is not unusual for a first manic episode to occur when someone "pulls an all-nighter" studying for final examinations. Persons with bipolar disorder should have a fairly rigid schedule for sleeping and awakening if cycling is to be minimized. Although exercise is important, the person with bipolar disorder should exercise before mid-afternoon to prevent the normal increase in metabolic rate from disrupting the sleep cycle.

Diagnostic Criteria

The *DSM-IV-TR* diagnostic criteria for a major depressive episode include the simultaneous presence of five or more of the aforementioned symptoms during a 2-week period, and these must represent a change from previous functioning.[30] Depression must be differentiated from grief reactions, medication side effects, and sequelae of medical illnesses. It should be noted, however, that depression often co-occurs with physical illnesses, notably myocardial infarction. It is estimated that 50% of hospitalized patients with coronary artery disease have some depressive symptoms, with up to 20% developing major depression.[48] Depression negatively impairs prognosis, affecting both behavioral and physiologic aspects of recovery, and increases the risk of death.[48]

Bipolar disorder is diagnosed on the basis of the pattern of occurrence of manic, hypomanic, and depressed episodes over time that are not due to medications or other therapies. The frequency, duration, and severity of the manic or depressive periods are unique to each individual. Mania, particularly in its severe delusional forms, also needs to be differentiated from schizophrenia or drug-induced states.

Treatment

Effective treatments exist for depression and bipolar disorders, including antidepressant drugs, electroconvulsive therapy (ECT), phototherapy, lithium, anticonvulsants, and psychotherapy.[38,41,42] The antidepressants most often used are SRIs, which inhibit the reuptake of serotonin; atypical antidepressants; MAO inhibitors, which block the degradation of norepinephrine and serotonin; and TCAs, which block the reuptake of norepinephrine and serotonin.[49] ECT, a procedure that electrically stimulates a generalized seizure, is a highly effective treatment for depression, with 70% to 90% of clients showing a good response.[49] Because the motor component of the seizure does not contribute to the therapeutic effects of the treatment, modern ECT is always given under general anesthesia with complete muscle relaxation.[35] On an average, six to eight treatments are given at 2-day intervals over a period of 2 to 4 weeks.

Phototherapy, or light therapy, uses artificial light to influence the production of melatonin and the function of the catecholamine systems. It is often a first-line treatment for depression associated with seasonal changes, such as SAD.[37]

Lithium and several anticonvulsant agents are used in the treatment of bipolar depression. Lithium's exact mechanism of action is unknown. It is known to inhibit the accumulation of cyclic adenosine monophosphatase (cAMP), and may down-regulate second-messenger systems that are associated with cAMP-linked receptors.[38] Anticonvulsant agents, especially carbamazepine and valproate, have also proved to be effective agents for treatment of bipolar depression. However, the mechanism by which these drugs act is not completely understood. One theory for the mechanism of action proposes blocked effects of the excitatory amino acid glutamate.[38]

Newer therapies, such as vagal nerve stimulation and transcranial magnetic stimulation, are being considered as treatment for depression that does not respond to pharmacologic interventions. The effectiveness of these treatments is still unclear.[50,51]

Psychotherapy is an important component of therapy for persons and families with major depressive disorders. Individuals and families can learn how to deal with stressful life events and heal disrupted interpersonal relationships.

Unfortunately, many people with bipolar disorder do not believe they need treatment, particularly during the manic phase of the illness, and tend to self-medicate with alcohol or recreational drugs. It is not unusual for people with bipolar depression to be diagnosed with substance abuse. When in the manic phase, they often feel exceptionally creative and talented. When helping people make the decision to enter treatment, it is important that they understand the treatment will not stop their creativity.

IN SUMMARY, mood disorders are disorders of emotion rather than disturbances of thought. Mood disorders include major depressive disorder (characterized by a persistent unpleasant mood), dysthymia (characterized by chronic mild depressive symptoms), and bipolar disorder (characterized by alternating periods of depression and mania). Depression is characterized by an inability to experience pleasure, feelings of worthlessness and excessive guilt, alterations in sleeping patterns and appetite, and thoughts of death or suicidal ideation. Mania is characterized by elation, irritability, high distractibility, and, often, engagement in high-risk pleasurable activities. As with schizophrenia, genetic factors appear to play an important role in the development of mood disorders. Neuroimaging techniques have revealed several anatomic and functional abnormalities in different regions of the brain. Abnormalities in neurotransmission also have been implicated in the development and maintenance of depression, including changes in concentration and activity of the neurotransmitters norepinephrine, serotonin, acetylcholine, and GABA. Treatment of depressive disorders includes the use of antidepressant medications, ECT, phototherapy, and psychotherapy. Bipolar disorders are usually treated with lithium or an anticonvulsant agent that has been shown to be effective in treating the disorder. ∎

ANXIETY DISORDERS

After completing this section of the chapter, you should be able to meet the following objectives:

- Define the terms *panic disorder, generalized anxiety disorder, social phobia,* and *obsessive-compulsive disorder.*
- Describe the epidemiology of panic disorder, generalized anxiety disorder, social phobia, and obsessive-compulsive disorder.

- Describe the manifestations of panic disorder, generalized anxiety disorder, social phobia, and obsessive-compulsive disorder and the underlying neuropathophysiology of each.
- Cite the diagnostic criteria for panic disorder, generalized anxiety disorder, social phobia, and obsessive-compulsive disorder according to the *DSM-IV-TR* classification.
- Describe the treatment for panic disorder, generalized anxiety disorder, social phobia, and obsessive-compulsive disorder.

Anxiety disorders are characterized by intense fearfulness that occurs without a precipitating potentially dangerous event, accompanied by subjective as well as objective manifestations. Just as grief is a normal response to personal loss, anxiety is a normal response to threatening situations. Anxiety disorders are the most prevalent of the psychiatric disorders. Anxiety disorders affect approximately 28.8% of all individuals, women more often than men.[52] Anxiety disorders have a higher rate of occurrence among family members, but there is not yet any clearly delineated genetic link.

A key component of anxiety disorders is increased fear accompanied by subjective as well as objective manifestations. The subjective manifestations range from heightened awareness to deep fear of impending disaster or death. The objective manifestations, which occur with activation of the sympathetic cascade through the HPA axis, include restlessness, sweating, palpitations, an increase in heart rate and blood pressure, dry mouth, and a desire to run and escape. According to the *DSM-IV-TR* classification system, anxiety is subdivided into five types, depending on clinical characteristics and response to pharmacologic agents: panic disorder, post-traumatic stress disorder (PTSD), generalized anxiety disorder, social phobia, and obsessive-compulsive disorder. PTSD is discussed in Chapter 9.

ANXIETY DISORDERS

- Anxiety disorders constitute a group of disorders that are characterized by intense episodes of fearfulness with symptoms related to activation of the sympathetic nervous system through the hypothalamic-pituitary-adrenal axis.
- Generalized anxiety disorder is characterized by excessive, uncontrollable worry.
- Obsessive-compulsive disorder is characterized by repetitive thoughts and actions.
- Panic disorder is characterized by an experience of intense fear with neurologic, cardiac, respiratory, and psychological symptoms.
- Social phobia is an intense fear reaction to social interaction.

Panic Disorder

Panic disorder is a disabling condition commonly seen in patients in the primary care setting.[53–55] The disorder has been reported to occur in 3% to 8% of persons seen by primary care physicians.[55] The disorder is twice as common in women as men, and there appears to be an apparent bimodal distribution in age of onset, with one peak in late adolescence and a second peak in the mid-thirties.[53] The diagnosis of panic disorder may be made more difficult by the presence of symptoms such as chest pain and shortness of breath that also are associated with potentially more serious conditions.

Persons with panic disorder typically have attacks characterized by neurologic symptoms (dizziness or lightheadedness, paresthesias, fainting), cardiac symptoms (tachycardia, chest pain, palpitations), respiratory symptoms (shortness of breath, feeling of smothering or choking), sweating, nausea or abdominal distress, and psychological symptoms (feelings of impending doom, fear of dying, and a sense of unreality). Panic attacks, which are unexpected and not related to external events, usually last 15 to 30 minutes, but sometimes continue for an hour. Depression may coexist in 40% to 80% of persons with panic disorder, and substance abuse disorders are not uncommon.[29]

Both biologic and environmental factors appear to be involved in the causation of panic attacks.[55,56] Monozygotic twins have a significantly higher concordance of the disorder than dizygotic twins.[55] First-degree relatives of persons with panic disorder have a 3- to 21-fold higher risk of developing panic disorder than unrelated persons. Approximately 80% of persons with panic disorder report major life stressors during the previous 12 months.[55] Persons with a history of sexual or physical abuse have a higher risk for panic disorder than those without such history.[55]

Neurophysiologic studies suggest that the attacks may result from an abnormally sensitive "fear network" that is centered in the amygdala and involves interactions with the hippocampus and prefrontal cortex.[56] Projections from the amygdala to hypothalamic and brain stem sites account for many of the observed signs (*e.g.*, sweating, increased heart rate, respiratory responses) of the fear response.[56] Responses to medications indicate that multiple mechanisms and neurotransmitters are involved in initiating the panic attack. Norepinephrine, serotonin, and GABA are the three neurotransmitters most associated with this disorder.[29] Persons experiencing panic attacks have been found to have somewhat lower levels of serotonin than do persons with no known mental illness, but the mechanism for that decrease is not known.

Treatment includes the use of behavioral, psychological, and drug therapies. All antidepressants, except bupropion, are effective in the treatment of panic disorders. There is growing evidence in the greater effectiveness of SSRIs in the treatment of panic, but full response to medication can take 12 or more weeks.[55,56] Many individuals may require the use of more than one class of medication for the management of panic attacks. However, treatment is most effective when psychotherapy focused on cognitive and behavioral changes is included as part of a comprehensive program. If inadequately treated, persons with panic disorder frequently develop phobias, particularly agoraphobia, which can be so debilitating that the person cannot leave his or her house.[56]

Generalized Anxiety Disorder

In 1980, generalized anxiety disorder was first recognized as a separate entity from panic disorder in the *DSM-III*. Since then, the diagnostic criteria have been sharpened in an attempt to improve the ability of practitioners to discriminate the disorder. The central characteristic of generalized anxiety disorder is prolonged (>6 months), excessive worry that is not easily controlled by the person. The characteristics of the disorder include muscle tension, autonomic hyperactivity, and vigilance and scanning (exaggerated startle response, inability to concentrate). The benzodiazepines (*e.g.*, chlordiazepoxide, diazepam) are particularly effective drugs in treating this disorder. These drugs increase the activity of the $GABA_A$ receptor, which increases the flow of chloride ions across the cell membrane, hyperpolarizing the membrane and thus inhibiting firing of target cells.[29]

Buspirone is another effective medication for treating generalized anxiety disorder, but may take up to 2 weeks to show antianxiety effects, and up to 6 weeks for maximum benefits. SSRIs are also used in the treatment of generalized anxiety disorder, and it is thought that they result in limbic, paralimbic, and frontal hyperactivity normalization. Other medications used in the treatment of generalized anxiety disorder include other antidepressants (tricyclic and atypical antidepressants) and β-adrenergic blockers, the latter of which block the symptoms of anxiety rather than treating the anxiety disorder itself.

Obsessive-Compulsive Disorder

Obsessive-compulsive disorder (OCD) is an anxiety disorder characterized by recurrent obsessions (repeated thoughts) and compulsions (repeated acts).[57–60] To be defined as compulsive, the behavior (activities such as handwashing, ordering, or checking, or mental activities such as praying, counting, or repeating words) must be repeated excessively and the repetition must not be related to any environmental condition. These behaviors are time consuming or distressing to the individual. Usually, the person experiencing the symptoms recognizes that the rituals are unreasonable. For instance, the person may have to recheck the stove many times before she is able to leave for work or may have to check the stairwells at work repeatedly for debris to ensure that no one is injured. Between 2% and 3% of the world's population has OCD, and OCD is the 10th most disabling disease worldwide.[57] This disorder is found with equal frequency among men and women, and there is a higher prevalence among family members. The average age of onset is approximately 20 years, although the disorder also may occur in children and, undiagnosed, may appear as behavior problems and angry outbursts that can seem impulsive and may be confused with attention deficit or hyperactivity disorders.[58]

Although the neurophysiology of OCD remains under investigation, the general anatomic model suggests dysfunction of the prefrontal cortex and structures of the basal ganglia, particularly the caudate nucleus and globus pallidus.[60] Studies have also suggested increased activity in the thalamus and the putamen of the basal ganglia, as well as a decrease in serotonin activity.[60] Several other neurologic syndromes that involve the basal ganglia, such as tic disorders, Sydenham chorea, post-encephalitic Parkinson disease, and Huntington disease, often are associated with a component of OCD.[60]

Diagnosis of OCD is based on the history and clinical observation. Treatment methods for OCD include behavioral therapy (involving exposure to feared situations and the prevention of compulsive behavior), cognitive therapy (in which maladaptive thoughts are challenged), and specific medications. About 50% to 60% of persons with OCD respond to SSRIs, but often require a higher dose than that prescribed for treatment of depression. The TCA clomipramine is sometimes prescribed if there is a poor response to SSRIs, and an atypical antipsychotic may be added in severe cases. This disorder is particularly amenable to cognitive-behavioral therapy, and for most persons with OCD, combining cognitive-behavioral therapy with medication is the best approach.[57]

Social Phobia

Social phobia, also called *social anxiety disorder,* is a generalized or specific, intense, irrational, and persistent fear of being scrutinized or negatively evaluated by others. Diagnostic criteria include the development of symptoms of anxiety when the person is exposed to the feared social situation, recognition by the person that the fear is irrational, avoidance by the person of the social situation, and interference of the anxiety or avoidance behavior with the person's normal routine. The fear must not be related to any physiologic effects of a substance and must be present for at least 6 months.[60]

Social phobia is a fairly common disorder with a lifetime prevalence of 12% and a slight tendency to occur more often in women than in men.[61] Typically, the onset occurs between 11 and 19 years of age. The major adverse effects of social phobia are felt in employment and school, causing a loss of earning power and socioeconomic status. In addition, approximately one half of persons with social phobia also have a drug or alcohol problem. Several drugs have proved efficacious for the treatment of social phobia, including SSRIs, benzodiazepines, and MAO inhibitors. β-Adrenergic blockers are useful in specific social performance situations. Social phobia also has been particularly responsive to behavioral and cognitive therapies.

> **IN SUMMARY,** anxiety disorders include generalized anxiety disorder, panic disorder, OCD, and social phobia. A common characteristic of the disorders is an intense fear that occurs in the absence of a precipitating dangerous event. The symptoms of anxiety disorders suggest an inappropriate and intense activation of the sympathetic nervous system. Panic disorder is characterized by neurologic, cardiac, respiratory, and psychological symptoms. The central characteristic of generalized anxiety disorder is excessive worry not easily controlled by the person and lasting more than 6 months. OCD is an anxiety disorder characterized by recurrent obsessions (repeated thoughts) and compulsions (repeated acts). Social phobia is a generalized or specific, intense, irrational, and persistent fear of being scrutinized or negatively evaluated by others. ■

DISORDERS OF ABUSE AND ADDICTION

After completing this section of the chapter, you should be able to meet the following objectives:

- Define substance dependence.
- Describe the epidemiology of addiction disorders.
- Describe the neurophysiologic alterations associated with substance dependence.
- Cite the actions of medications used in the treatment of substance dependence.

The *DSM-IV-TR* uses the term *substance use disorders* to include substance abuse and substance dependence.[30] *Substance abuse* refers to repeated use of alcohol or other drugs, resulting in functional problems.[62] *Dependence* refers to the behaviors exhibited when an individual is unable to control the use of drugs or alcohol and continues to use them in spite of negative consequences. *Addiction* is a difficult term to define; there is no clear consensus on a definition, nor is it defined in the *DSM-IV-TR*. Addiction usually describes a combination of craving, compulsive use, and high risk of relapse after withdrawal.

Problems related to alcohol and drug abuse exact a large toll on individuals and families, including financial, social, and physical. It is estimated that 14.6% of the U.S. adult population has substance abuse disorders, with addictions accounting for an estimated 8.5% of these numbers.[62] Although substance abuse is not a new problem—people have been abusing drugs and alcohol for thousands of years—our understanding of abuse and addiction as diseases is more recent. Although early understandings of these disorders attributed them to poor character and moral weakness, current and ongoing research has pointed to a neurophysiologic basis to addiction disorders, leading to a better understanding of the ongoing risk of relapse, even after a lengthy period of abstinence.

The vulnerability of certain individuals to substance abuse disorders appears to be multifactorial, involving a genetic disposition, environmental factors, and physiologic mechanisms resulting from repeated drug use. It has been suggested that self-medication of symptoms associated with psychiatric disorders provides another source for the initiation of drug abuse. Substance abuse disorders are more common among individuals with mood and anxiety disorders, and schizophrenia, all populations with altered levels of the neurotransmitter dopamine.[62,63] Epidemiologic data indicate that there is a high comorbidity between drug dependence and depression. Approximately 80% of alcoholics complain of depressive symptoms, and 30% meet the criteria for a depressive episode.[64] Research has also indicated that there is a high comorbidity between depression and cannabis use.[64]

Habitual use of drugs, including alcohol, is thought to induce adaptations in brain systems that alter the normal dopamine pathways and increase dopamine transmission. A neural pathway called the *mesolimbic dopamine system* is thought to gate signals that regulate biologic drives and motivation. These neurons send their axons to the nucleus accumbens, the striatum of the basal ganglia, and the frontal cortex. Drugs that facilitate dopamine transmission enhance the processes whereby otherwise neutral stimuli acquire incentive and reinforcing properties and facilitate drug-seeking behavior.[65] Some drugs, such as cocaine and amphetamines, raise the level of dopamine in the nucleus accumbens by blocking the dopamine transporter, thereby prolonging the time that dopamine remains in the synaptic cleft. Although many drugs of abuse alter dopamine levels, not all of them act by way of the dopamine transporter. Nicotine, perhaps the most addictive of all drugs, enhances the release of dopamine by acting on presynaptic cholinergic receptors.

The rewarding effect of drug abuse results not only from the release of dopamine; as addiction develops, behavior also is influenced by a glutamatergic pathway. Glutamine is the major excitatory transmitter in the brain and spinal cord. Animal studies focusing on stimuli for relapse have found that exposure to a cue associated with substance use (*i.e.*, stress, or a single dose of the substance) results in activation of glutamatergic projections from areas of the brain that stimulate dopamine release from the nucleus accumbens.[65,66] In addition, there is a reported increase in GABA (a neurotransmitter that activates inhibitory receptors) levels during alcohol intoxication and opiate use.[55,65] Opioid agonists appear to be rewarding because they inhibit GABA-ergic neurons that normally suppress dopaminergic neurons.

Treatment of addiction requires an understanding of physiologic alterations in brain function that can cause relapse, even years after abstinence. Precipitants for relapse include stress, environmental cues, and exposure to the substance. Relapses are not uncommon and should not be considered as failures in treatment, but rather as a reflection of the nature of the illness. Because there is a high comorbidity between depression and drug dependence, professional treatment of preexisting psychiatric problems may also decrease the use of illicit substances and help prevent relapse.[64]

Treatments are varied and include biologic, behavioral, and psychosocial interventions. Biologic interventions are used in the maintenance of recovery from alcohol and opiates, such as heroin. Methadone, used in opiate addictions, has the narcotic

properties of addiction and sedation, but lacks the euphoric effects of heroin and other opiates. Buprenorphine is a recently approved analgesic for treatment of opioid addictions with less euphoric and sedative properties than methadone. Naltrexone is used in treatment of alcohol and opiate addictions, and works by blocking the opioid receptors and euphoric effects. It does not, however, eliminate cravings. These medications work best in conjunction with other therapies, such as self-help groups (Alcoholics Anonymous), individual therapy, family therapy, behavioral contracting, and social skills training.[67]

IN SUMMARY, substance abuse refers to repeated use of alcohol or other drugs, resulting in functional problems; dependence refers to the behaviors exhibited when an individual is unable to control the use of drugs or alcohol; and addiction to a combination of craving, compulsive use, and high risk of relapse after withdrawal. Substance abuse disorders are more common among individuals with mood and anxiety disorders, and schizophrenia, all populations with altered levels of the neurotransmitter dopamine. The vulnerability of certain individuals to substance abuse disorders appears to be multifactorial, related to genetic disposition, environmental factors, and physiologic adaptations to repeated drug use. Habitual use of drugs, including alcohol, is thought to induce adaptations in brain systems that alter the normal dopamine pathways and increase dopamine transmission. Treatments are varied and include biologic, behavioral, and psychosocial interventions. ■

DISORDERS OF MEMORY AND COGNITION

After completing this section of the chapter, you should be able to meet the following objectives:

- State the criteria for a diagnosis of dementia.
- Compare the causes associated with Alzheimer disease, vascular dementia, frontotemporal dementia, Creutzfeldt-Jakob disease, Wernicke-Korsakoff syndrome, and Huntington disease.
- Describe the changes in brain tissue that occur with Alzheimer disease.
- Use the three stages of Alzheimer disease to describe its progress.
- Cite the difference between Wernicke disease and the Korsakoff component of the Wernicke-Korsakoff syndrome.

Cognition refers to all the processes by which the sensory input is transformed, reduced, elaborated, stored, recovered, and used. It involves the perception of sensory input and the ability to learn and manipulate new information, recognize familiar objects and recollect past experiences, solve problems, think abstractly, and make judgments. Dementia is a syndrome of deterioration in cognitive function severe enough to interfere with occupational or social performance.[68,69] It is a common and disabling disorder in the elderly and is becoming a growing public heath problem because of rapidly increasing numbers of elderly people in the developed countries of the world.

Normal Cognitive Aging

Memory shows a slow, progressive impairment over the life span, and it is important to differentiate what can be termed "normal cognitive aging" from disorders of memory and cognition. Many old people remain intellectually intact, and some even make outstanding contributions later in life.

Short-term memory typically is well preserved during normal cognitive aging unless there is a high demand placed on processing resources.[69] However, older persons may have greater difficulty than younger persons in manipulating the information that is held in short-term memory. With regard to long-term memory, age-related impairments in free recall of stories and word lists are evident by age 50 years. However, when structure is provided by the use of recognition cues, the age differences diminish, which suggests greater impairment of retrieval processes than of encoding and retrieval.[69]

Memory problems associated with normal aging tend to reflect a generalized decrease in the efficiency with which information is processed and retrieved. Memory of a past event can be based on retrieval that is accompanied by recollection of specific details or on the feeling that the event is old or new, based on its familiarity.[69] There is evidence that recollection is more dependent on the hippocampus, whereas familiarity is more dependent on the entorhinal cortex, and that healthy aging has greater effects on recollection than familiarity.[69]

Studies with human subjects and with experimental animals suggest that knowledge is first acquired through processing in one of the three polymodal association cortices (the prefrontal, limbic, and parieto-occipital-temporal cortices) that synthesize visual, auditory, and somatic sensory information[70] (Fig. 53-6). From there the information is conveyed to a series of parahippocampal and perirhinal cortices, then to the entorhinal cortex, dentate gyrus, hippocampus, and subiculum, and finally back to the entorhinal cortex. From the entorhinal cortex, the information is sent back to the parahippocampal cortices and finally back to the polymodal association areas of the neocortex.[70] Thus, in processing information for explicit memory storage, the entorhinal cortex has dual functions. It is the main input to the hippocampus and it is the major output to the hippocampus. With aging, there appears to be a reduced connectivity in the network that connects the hippocampus and association cortices but increased connectivity in the network that connects the entorhinal and association cortices.[69] This suggests that older adults may compensate for hippocampal deficits by relying more on the entorhinal cortex.

Originally, it was believed that the laying down and retrieval of memories was due primarily to action of a single neurotransmitter, acetylcholine. This led to the development of acetylcholinesterase inhibitors to treat cognitive impairment. The further recognition of the role of the glutamate N-methyl-D-aspartate receptor led to the development of memantine (discussed in the section on Alzheimer disease). More recently, it was recognized that several neuropeptides (*i.e.*, neuropeptide Y, orexin A, and the endogenous opioid peptides) also play an important role in memory.[69] Although these peptides have the

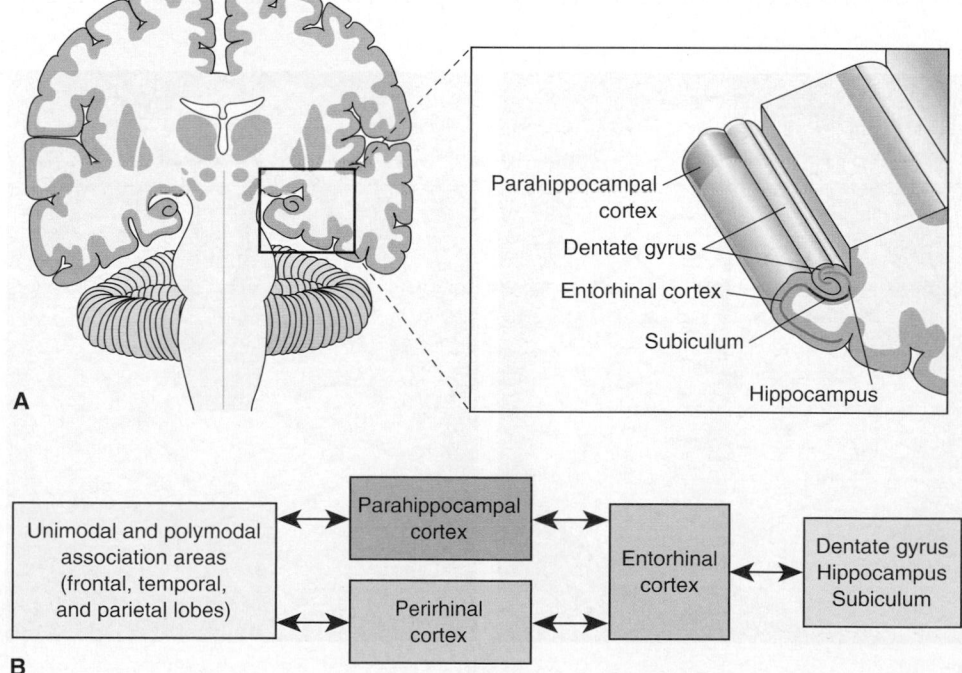

FIGURE 53-6 • **(A)** Key structures of the medial temporal lobe important for memory storage. **(B)** Input and output pathways for the hippocampal formation. (Adapted from Kandel E. R., Kupfermann I., Iverson S. [2000]. Learning and memory. In Kandel E. R., Schwartz J. H., Jessel T. M. [Eds.], *Principles of neural science* [4th ed., p. 1232]. New York: McGraw-Hill.)

potential for enhancing memory at low levels, they can inhibit memory at high levels. There is also emerging evidence that several gastrointestinal hormones may contribute to memory, as evidenced by the observation that tasks learned before a meal is ingested are recalled better at a later time.[69] This is thought to be related to the release of the gastrointestinal hormone cholecystokinin, which, through its stimulation of the vagus nerve, eventually leads to activation of neurons in the hippocampus. Another hormone, ghrelin, which is produced in the fundus of the stomach, has receptors in the hippocampus and is also thought to enhance memory.

Dementia

Dementia or non-normative cognitive decline can be caused by any disorder that permanently damages large association areas of the cerebral hemispheres or subcortical areas subserving memory and learning. Based on criteria in the third and fourth editions of the *DSM* (*DSM-III* and *DSM-IV*), the essential feature of dementia is impairment of short- and long-term memory, which is associated with deficits in abstract thinking, impaired judgment and other higher cortical functions, or personality change. The disturbance should be sufficiently severe as to interfere significantly with work or social activities.[71,72] Common causes of dementia are Alzheimer disease, vascular dementia, frontotemporal dementia, Creutzfeldt-Jakob disease, Wernicke-Korsakoff syndrome, and Huntington chorea.

The diagnosis of dementia is based on assessment of the presenting problem; history about the person that is provided by an informant (someone who has known the person, usually a family member); complete physical and neurologic examination; evaluation of cognitive, behavioral, and functional status; and laboratory and imaging studies. The American Academy of Neurology practice parameters recommend structural neuroimaging, which may include CT or MRI, and screening for depression, vitamin B_{12} deficiency, and hypothyroidism.[73] Depression is the most common treatable illness that may masquerade as dementia, and it must be excluded when a diagnosis of dementia is considered (see Chapter 3). This is important because cognitive functioning usually returns to baseline levels after depression is treated. Screening evaluations for subdural hematoma, cerebral infarcts, cerebral tumors, and normal-pressure hydrocephalus (discussed in Chapter 51) are also recommended. These and other reversible forms of dementia that should be ruled out can be remembered by the mnemonic DEMENTIA: *D*rugs (drugs with anticholinergic activity), *E*motional (depression), *M*etabolic (hypothyroidism), *E*yes and ears (declining vision and hearing), *N*ormal-pressure hydrocephalus, *T*umor or other space-occupying lesions; *I*nfection (human immunodeficiency virus infection or syphilis), *A*nemia (vitamin B_{12} or folate deficiency).[69]

Alzheimer Disease

Dementia of the Alzheimer type occurs in middle or late life and accounts for 60% to 80% of all cases of dementia. The disorder affects more than 4.5 million Americans and may be the fourth leading cause of death in the United States.[74] The risk for development of Alzheimer disease increases with age, and it is estimated that almost 50% of individuals 85 years of age and older live with this illness, which affects almost twice as many women as men. It is projected that, unless a cure or prevention is developed, there will be 14 million Americans with Alzheimer disease by the year 2050.[75]

Pathophysiology. The pathophysiologic aspects of Alzheimer disease involve neuropathologic and neurotransmitter changes. Alzheimer disease is characterized by cortical atrophy and loss of neurons, particularly in the parietal and temporal lobes[76,77] (Fig. 53-7). With significant atrophy, there is ventricular enlargement (*i.e.*, hydrocephalus) from the loss of brain tissue.

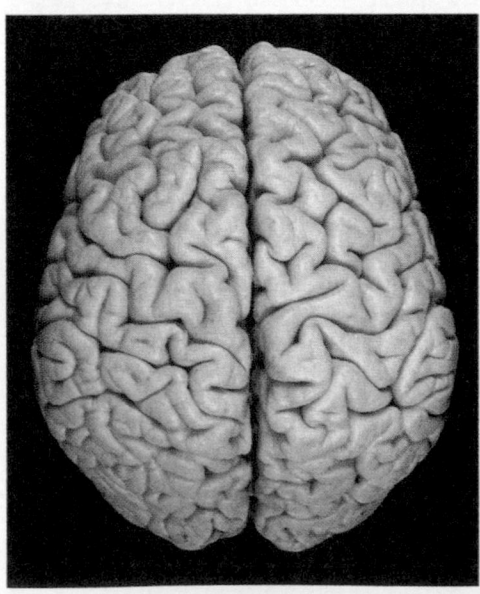

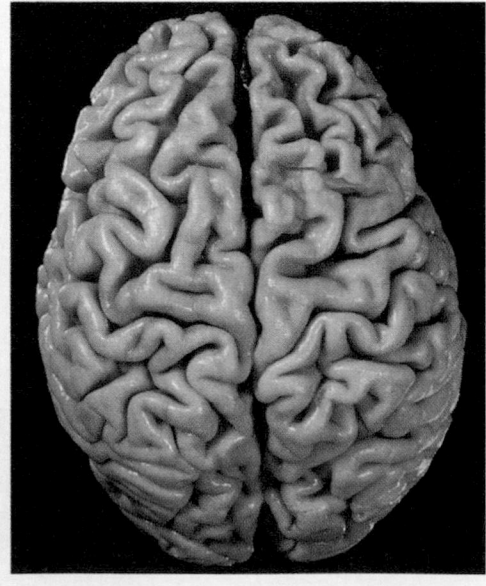

A

B

FIGURE 53-7 • Alzheimer disease. (**A**) Normal brain. (**B**) The brain of a patient with Alzheimer disease shows cortical atrophy, characterized by slender gyri and prominent sulci. (From Rubin E., Farber J. L. [Eds.]. [1999]. *Pathology* [3rd ed., p. 1511]. Philadelphia: Lippincott-Raven.)

The major microscopic features of Alzheimer disease are the presence of neuritic (senile) plaques, neurofibrillary tangles, and amyloid angiopathy.[77] The *neuritic plaques* are patches or flat areas composed of clusters of degenerating nerve terminals arranged around a central amyloid core.[77] The dominant component of the amyloid core is amyloid beta (Aβ), a peptide derived from the proteolysis of a larger membrane-spanning amyloid precursor protein (APP). There is increasing evidence that Aβ is the critical molecule in the pathogenesis of Alzheimer disease. Full-length APP has an intracellular region, a membrane-spanning sequence, and an extracellular region. The normal degradation of APP involves cleavage in the middle of the Aβ domain by a proteolytic α-secretase enzyme, with the release of two soluble nonamyloidogenic pieces. However, APP can also be cleaved at either end of the Aβ domain, leading to the release of intact and highly amyloidogenic Aβ that accumulates in senile plaques as amyloid fibrils. There are at least three distinct forms of secretase enzymes (α-, β-, γ-secretase). Evidence suggests that cleavage by the β- and γ-secretase leads to the generation of Aβ.[77] The *neurofibrillary tangles,* found in the cytoplasm of abnormal neurons, consist of fibrous proteins that are wound around each other in a helical fashion. These tangles are resistant to chemical or enzymatic breakdown, and they persist in brain tissue long after the neuron in which they arose has died and disappeared. A major component of the paired helical filaments is an abnormally hyperphosphorylated form of the protein *tau,* an axonal microtubule-associated protein that enhances microtubule assembly.[77]

Some plaques and tangles can be found in the brains of older persons who do not show cognitive impairment. The number and distribution of the plaques and tangles appear to contribute to the intellectual deterioration that occurs with Alzheimer disease. In persons with Alzheimer disease, the plaques and tangles and associated neuronal loss and glial reaction are evident earliest in the entorhinal cortex, then spread through the hippocampal formation and isocortex, and then extend to the neocortex.[77] Neurochemically, Alzheimer disease has been associated with a decrease in the level of choline acetyltransferase activity in the cortex and hippocampus. This enzyme is required for the synthesis of acetylcholine, a neurotransmitter that is associated with memory. The reduction in choline acetyltransferase is quantitatively related to the numbers of neuritic plaques and severity of dementia.

It is likely that Alzheimer disease is caused by several factors that interact differently in different persons. Progress on the genetics of inherited early-onset Alzheimer disease shows mutations in at least three genes—the *APP* gene on chromosome 21; presenilin-1 (*PS1*), a gene on chromosome 14; and presenilin-2 (*PS2*), a gene on chromosome 1—can cause Alzheimer disease in certain families.[68] The *APP* gene is associated with an autosomal dominant form of early-onset Alzheimer disease, and can be tested clinically. Persons with Down syndrome (trisomy 21) develop the pathologic changes of Alzheimer disease and a comparable decline in cognitive functioning at a relatively young age. Virtually all persons with Down syndrome exhibit the pathologic features of Alzheimer disease as they age. PS1 and PS2, both intracellular proteins, are components of γ-secretase and possibly part of a multiprotein complex containing the proteolytic site for breakdown of Aβ. A fourth gene, an allele (ε4) of the apolipoprotein E (ApoE) gene found on chromosome 19, increases the risk of Alzheimer disease and lowers the age of onset. ApoE can bind Aβ and is present in plaques, but how this allele increases the risk of Alzheimer disease has not been established.[77]

Although age is the greatest risk, additional factors have been identified as adding to the risks for development of Alzheimer disease. These include head trauma, inflammatory factors, and oxidative stress. Education has been identified as a protective factor, with suggestions that education can increase synaptic density.[78] Other studies have looked at exercise as a possible protective factor in maintaining hippocampal health.[79]

Manifestations. Alzheimer-type dementia follows an insidious and progressive course, with an average survival of 8 to 10 years after diagnosis.[74] The hallmark symptoms are loss of short-term memory and denial of such memory loss, with eventual disorientation, impaired abstract thinking, apraxias, and changes in personality and affect.[80] Various stages of the disease have been recognized, ranging from four to the more nuanced seven stages identified by the Alzheimer Association. All are characterized by progressive degenerative changes[81] (Chart 53-1). The initial change is subtle, characterized by short-term memory loss that often is difficult to differentiate from the normal forgetfulness that occurs in the elderly, and usually is reported by caregivers and denied by the patient. Although most elderly persons have trouble retrieving from memory incidental information and proper names, persons with Alzheimer disease randomly forget important and unimportant details. They forget where things are placed, get lost easily, and have trouble remembering appointments and performing novel tasks. Mild changes in personality, such as lack of spontaneity, social withdrawal, and loss of a previous sense of humor, occur during this stage.

As the disease progresses, the person with Alzheimer disease enters the moderate stage. This stage may last several years and is marked by a more global impairment of cognitive functioning. During this stage, there are changes in higher cortical functioning needed for language, spatial relationships, and problem solving. Depression may occur in persons who are aware of their deficits. There is extreme confusion, disorientation, lack of insight, and inability to carry out the activities of daily living. Personal hygiene is neglected, and language becomes impaired because of difficulty in remembering and retrieving words. Behavioral changes can include agitation, sleep problems, restlessness and wandering, aggression, and suspiciousness. Some persons may become hostile and abusive toward family members. Persons who enter this stage become unable to live alone and should be assisted in making decisions about supervised placement with family members or friends or in a community-based facility.

CHART 53-1   **STAGES OF ALZHEIMER DISEASE**

Stage 1: No impairment (normal function)

Stage 2: Very mild cognitive decline (may be normal age-related changes or earliest evidence of Alzheimer disease)
- Individuals may feel as if they have memory lapses, especially in forgetting everyday objects, but these problems are not evident during a medical examination.

Stage 3: Mild cognitive decline (early-stage Alzheimer disease)
- Early-stage Alzheimer disease can be diagnosed in some, but not all, individuals as friends, family, or coworkers begin to notice problems with word- or name-finding, performance issues in social or work settings, losing or misplacing a valuable object, and a decline in the ability to plan and organize.

Stage 4: Moderate cognitive decline (mild or early-stage Alzheimer disease)
- At this stage, a careful medical interview detects clearcut deficiencies in knowledge of recent occasions and current events, impaired ability to perform challenging mental arithmetic (*i.e.,* count backward from 75 by 7s),

decreased capacity to perform complex tasks, such as planning dinner for guests, paying bills, and managing finances, and reduced memory of personal history. The person may also seem subdued and withdrawn, especially in socially or mentally challenging situations.

Stage 5: Moderately severe cognitive decline (moderate or mid-stage Alzheimer disease)
- Major gaps in memory and deficits in cognitive function emerge. Some assistance with day-to-day activities becomes essential.

Stage 6: Severe cognitive decline (moderately severe or mid-stage Alzheimer disease)
- Memory difficulties continue to worsen, significant personality changes may emerge, and affected individuals need extensive help with customary daily activities.

Stage 7: Very severe cognitive decline (severe or late-stage Alzheimer disease)
- Final stage of the disease, when individuals lose the ability to respond to their environment, the ability to speak, and, ultimately, the ability to control movement.

Adapted from Alzheimer's Association. (2007). Stages of Alzheimer's. [Online.] Available: www.alz.org/alzheimers_disease_stages_of_alzheimers.asp#. Accessed March 25, 2008.

Severe Alzheimer disease is the last stage of the disease. It is characterized by a loss of ability to respond to the environment. Individuals in this stage require total care, and spend most of their time bedridden. Death can occur as a result of complications related to chronic debilitation.

Diagnosis and Treatment. Alzheimer disease is essentially a diagnosis of exclusion. There are no peripheral biochemical markers or tests for the disease. The diagnosis can be confirmed only by microscopic examination of tissue obtained from a cerebral biopsy or at autopsy. The diagnosis is based on clinical findings.

The diagnostic procedures for Alzheimer disease involve numerous steps, and a Differential Diagnosis in Alzheimer Algorithm has been developed.[81] A diagnosis of Alzheimer disease requires the presence of dementia established by clinical examination and documented by results of a Mini-Mental State Examination, Blessed Dementia Test, or similar mental status test; no disturbance in consciousness; onset between 40 and 90 years of age, most often after 65 years of age; and absence of systemic or brain disorders that could account for the memory or cognitive deficits. Brain imaging, CT scan, or MRI is done to exclude other brain disease. Metabolic screening should be done for known reversible causes of dementia such as vitamin B_{12} deficiency, thyroid dysfunction, and electrolyte imbalance.

There is no curative treatment for Alzheimer dementia. Drugs are used primarily to slow the progression and to control depression, agitation, or sleep disorders. Two major goals of care are maintaining the person's socialization and providing

support for the family. Self-help groups that provide support for family and friends have become available, with support from the Alzheimer Disease and Related Disorders Association. Day care and respite centers are available in many areas to provide relief for caregivers and appropriate stimulation for the patient.

Although there is no current drug therapy that is curative for Alzheimer disease, some show promise in terms of slowing the progress of the disease. Cholinesterase inhibitors have been shown to be effective in slowing the progression of the disease by potentiating the action of available acetylcholine.[80] These drugs—donepezil, rivastigmine, and galantamine—inhibit acetylcholinesterase, preventing the metabolism of endogenous acetylcholine, and are used in the early stages of the disease for mild cognitive impairment. Thus far, such therapy has not halted disease progression, but it can slow the disease progression by approximately 6 to 12 months. The therapeutic effects cease when the medication is discontinued.

Memantine, an *N*-methyl-D-aspartate antagonist, was recently approved by the FDA for treatment of moderate to severe Alzheimer disease.[80] This medication may act by interfering with the glutamatergic excitotoxicity (see Chapter 51, Fig. 51-2) caused by the ischemia and amyloid deposits associated with the disease, or it may provide symptomatic improvement through effects on the function of hippocampal neurons. This medication, like the cholinesterase inhibitors, does not reverse the disease, but does provide a modest delay in functional loss.

Other treatments for Alzheimer disease include agents that are thought to have a neuroprotective effect.[80] Aβ seems to exert its neurotoxic effects through a variety of secondary mechanisms, including oxidative injury and lipid peroxidation of cell membranes, and inflammation. Several strategies have involved the use of anti-inflammatory agents and antioxidants (vitamins E and C and *Ginkgo biloba*).[68,80] Several, but not all, epidemiologic studies provide evidence supporting the concept that vitamin E and vitamin C have a role in delaying the onset of Alzheimer disease. In some, but not all, trials, *G. biloba* had small but statistically significant effects compared with placebo in persons with Alzheimer disease.

Psychotropic medications, such as antipsychotics and mood stabilizers, may be used to assist in the behavioral management of the disease. Interventions also include environmental adjustments, behavioral intervention, and education and support for caregivers. Caregiver support is essential because they are responsible for supervising persons who live in the community and continue to visit and provide support after the person has been institutionalized. They are also responsible for administering medications, implementing nonpharmacologic treatments, and promoting the person's general health and well-being.

Current research efforts are focusing on aspects of amyloid production, which initiates neuronal dysfunction. The enzymes responsible for liberating $A\beta$ from APP are the β- and γ-secretases.[80] Inhibitors of these enzymes are under current study. Strategies aimed at reducing the aggregation of $A\beta$ offer another therapeutic avenue to be explored. The metabolism of cholesterol is intimately involved in the generation of $A\beta$, and preliminary evidence suggests that the statin drugs may be beneficial in reducing the accumulation of $A\beta$.[80] A program to vaccinate humans was implemented after the observation that immunization with $A\beta$ reduces pathologic signs of Alzheimer disease in transgenic mice with APP mutations. This clinical trial was terminated when encephalitis developed in 6% of the patients.[80] It has been suggested that passive immunization (*i.e.*, administration of $A\beta$ antibodies) represents an alternative and perhaps safer vaccination strategy.[80]

Vascular Dementia

Vascular dementia is caused by brain injury resulting from ischemic or hemorrhagic damage. Approximately 20% to 25% of dementias are vascular in origin, making it the second most common cause of dementia. The incidence is closely associated with hypertension, but also with arrhythmias, myocardial infarction, peripheral vascular disease, lipid abnormalities, diabetes mellitus, autoimmune and infectious vasculitis, and smoking.[68,76,82] The usual onset is between the ages of 55 and 70 years, and more men are affected than women.[68,76]

Vascular dementia differs from Alzheimer disease in its presentation and tissue abnormalities. Slowness in psychomotor functioning is a main clinical feature of this dementia, and symptoms of depression present in up to 60% of patients with this disease.[76] The onset may be gradual or abrupt, the course usually is a stepwise progression, and there are focal neurologic symptoms related to local areas of infarction.

Frontotemporal Dementia

Frontotemporal dementia (FTD) refers to a group of disorders associated with atrophy of the frontal and anterior temporal lobes of the brain.[83,84] Originally known as *Pick disease*, FTD now refers to a syndrome that includes primary progressive aphasia, corticobasal degeneration, progressive supranuclear palsy, and semantic dementias.[68,70] The disease occurs with the same frequency in men and women, with onset between 35 and 75 years of age.[68] The median age of onset for FTD is about 58 years, with 22% of persons with the disorder having onset after 65 years of age.

There are two distinct clinical presentations that reflect the symptoms of FTD: behavior and language. The former is more common, with behavioral presentations of disinhibited and impulsive actions or apathy, with inappropriate social behavior. The behavioral abnormalities can be quite extreme, and can be misdiagnosed as schizophrenia or psychotic depression. The second type of FTD involves disturbances in understanding or expressing language.

Diagnosis is based on evidence of cognitive impairment and exclusion of other illnesses that cause cognitive and behavioral deficits. Neuroimaging can be helpful in distinguishing FTD from other types of cognitive disorders. Typically, structural imaging shows anterior temporal and frontal lobe atrophy. The course of the disease is relentless, with death ensuing within 2 to 10 years. The immediate cause of death usually is infection.

Creutzfeldt-Jakob Disease

Creutzfeldt-Jakob disease (CJD) is a rare, rapidly degenerative form of dementia thought to be caused by an infective protein agent called a *prion*[85] (see Chapter 16). There are three categories of CJD: sporadic, hereditary, and acquired. Sporadic, in which the disease occurs without known risk factors, is the most common form, accounting for up to 85% of the cases. Familial or hereditary CJD represents 10% to 15% of cases, and acquired CJD is rare, representing less than 1% of cases. Variants of the disease occur in animals, including scrapie in sheep and goats and bovine spongiform encephalopathy (BSE; mad cow disease) in cattle.

CJD causes degeneration of the pyramidal and extrapyramidal systems and is distinguished most readily by its rapid course. Affected persons usually are demented within 6 months of onset. The disease is uniformly fatal, with death often occurring within months, although a few persons may survive for several years.[68] The early symptoms consist of abnormalities in personality and visual-spatial coordination, and impaired memory and judgment. Extreme dementia, insomnia, and ataxia follow as the disease progresses.[85] There is no medical treatment for the disease.

Wernicke-Korsakoff Syndrome

Wernicke-Korsakoff syndrome most commonly results from chronic alcoholism. Wernicke disease is characterized by acute weakness and paralysis of the extraocular muscles, nystagmus, ataxia, and confusion. The affected person also may have signs of peripheral neuropathy. The person has an unsteady gait and complains of diplopia. There may be signs attributable to alcohol withdrawal such as delirium, confusion, and hallucinations. This disorder is caused by a deficiency of thiamine (vitamin B$_{12}$), which directly interferes with production of glucose, the brain's main nutrient. Many of the symptoms are reversed when nutrition is improved with supplemental thiamine.

The Korsakoff component of the syndrome involves the chronic phase with severe impairment of recent memory. There often is difficulty in dealing with abstractions, and the person's capacity to learn is defective. Confabulation (*i.e.*, recitation of imaginary experiences to fill in gaps in memory) probably is the most distinctive feature of the disease. Polyneuritis also is common. Unlike Wernicke disease, Korsakoff psychosis does not improve significantly with treatment.

Huntington Disease

Huntington disease is a hereditary disorder characterized by chronic progressive chorea, psychological changes, and dementia. Although the disease is inherited as an autosomal dominant disorder, the age of onset most commonly is in the fourth and fifth decades. By the time the disease has been diagnosed, the person often has passed the gene on to his or her children. Approximately 10% of Huntington cases involve juvenile onset.[68,86] Children with the disease rarely live to adulthood.

Huntington disease produces localized death of brain cells. The first and most severely affected neurons are of the caudate nucleus and putamen of the basal ganglia. The neurochemical changes that occur with the disease are complex. The neurotransmitter GABA is an inhibitory neurotransmitter in the basal ganglia. Postmortem studies have shown a decrease of GABA and GABA receptors in the basal ganglia of persons with Huntington disease. Likewise, the levels of acetylcholine, an excitatory neurotransmitter in the basal ganglia, are reduced in persons with Huntington disease. The dopaminergic pathway of the nigrostriatal system, which is affected in Parkinson disease, is preserved in Huntington disease, suggesting that an imbalance in dopamine and acetylcholine may contribute to manifestations of the disease.

Depression and personality changes are the most common early psychological manifestations; memory loss often is accompanied by impulsive behavior, moodiness, antisocial behavior, and a tendency toward emotional outbursts.[68] An estimated 30% of persons with Huntington disease experience major depressive disorder or dysthymic disorder, with about 6% of deaths attributed to suicide.[68] Other early signs of the disease are lack of initiative, loss of spontaneity, and inability to concentrate. Fidgeting or restlessness may represent early signs of dyskinesia, followed by choreiform and some dystonic posturing. Eventually, progressive rigidity and akinesia (rather than chorea) develop in association with dementia. Symptoms of juvenile onset Huntington disease include Parkinson-like dystonias and seizures.

There is no cure for Huntington disease. The treatment is largely symptomatic. Drugs may be used to treat the dyskinesias and behavioral disturbances. Study of the genetics of Huntington disease led to the discovery that the gene for the disease is located on chromosome 4. The discovery of a marker probe for the gene locus has enabled testing that can predict whether a person will develop the disease.

IN SUMMARY, cognition refers to all the processes by which sensory input is transformed, reduced, elaborated, stored, recovered, and used. It is important to differentiate what can be termed "normal cognitive aging" from disorders of memory and cognition. Memory problems that are associated with normal aging tend to reflect a generalized decrease in the efficiency with which information is processed and retrieved. Memory of a past event can be based on retrieval that is accompanied by recollection of specific details, or on the feeling that the event is old or new based on its familiarity. There is evidence that recollection is more dependent on the hippocampus, whereas familiarity is more dependent on the entorhinal cortex, and that healthy aging has greater effects on recollection than familiarity.

Dementia represents a syndrome of deterioration in cognitive function severe enough to interfere with occupational or social performance. The diagnosis of dementia is based on history; complete physical and neurologic examination; evaluation of cognitive, behavioral, and functional status; and laboratory (particularly thyroid hormone and vitamin B$_{12}$) and neuroimaging studies. There are several potentially reversible causes of dementia that can be remembered by the mnemonic DEMENTIA: *D*rug (any drug with anticholinergic activity), *E*motional (depression), *M*etabolic (thyroid function), *E*yes and ears declining, *N*ormal-pressure hydrocephalus, *T*umor or other space-occupying lesion, *I*nfection (HIV or syphilis), *A*nemia (vitamin B$_{12}$ or folate deficiency).

The major syndromes of progressive dementia include Alzheimer disease, vascular dementia, frontotemporal dementia, Creutzfeldt-Jakob disease, Wernicke-Korsakoff syndrome, and Huntington disease. By far the most common cause of dementia (60% to 80%) is Alzheimer disease. The condition is a major health problem among the elderly. It is characterized by cortical atrophy and loss of neurons, and the presence of neuritic plaques, granulovacuolar degeneration, and cerebrovascular deposits of amyloid. The disease follows an insidious and progressive course that begins with memory impairment and terminates in an inability to recognize family or friends and the loss of control over bodily functions. Ischemic or hemorrhagic damage is associated with vascular dementia, and frontotemporal dementia with atrophy of the frontal and temporal lobes. Creutzfeldt-Jakob disease is a rare, rapidly progressive form of dementia. Wernicke-Korsakoff syndrome most often results from chronic alcoholism. Huntington disease is a hereditary disorder characterized by chronic and progressive chorea, psychological changes, and dementia. ∎

Review Exercises

1. A 45-year-old woman was brought to the emergency department after being picked up by the police. She was wandering in and out of traffic saying someone was after her and was recognized as a homeless person. Her appearance is dirty and disheveled and she is wearing several layers of clothing, although it is summer. She smacks her lips and at times does not seem to understand questions. Periodically she laughs for no apparent reason and often repeats the words of her questioner. She has a 20-year history of schizophrenia with multiple admissions.

   A. *List the positive and negative signs she exhibits.*

   B. *What are the brain areas and transmitters responsible for these signs?*

   C. *What are the DSM-IV-TR criteria that would have led to her diagnosis?*

2. A 35-year-old woman was recently admitted with suicidal tendencies shortly after a diagnosis of major depression. She had lost 40 pounds in the last 6 months. She appears tired and supplies only short answers to questions. She complains of dizziness and informs the nurse that it is not her business to discuss her suicidal thoughts. Her husband says she relies heavily on alcohol.

   A. *Describe some of her manifestations. Why is she using alcohol?*

   B. *Provide an explanation for her tiredness.*

   C. *What areas of the brain and neurotransmitters are involved in depression? How is it different from mania?*

   D. *What are the possible roles of thyroid and adrenal hormones?*

3. A 40-year-old woman is seen in the emergency department in a state of severe panic. She has had panic attacks for several months and had not sought treatment until her husband came home and found her sitting in the bedroom unable to move. She had been there all day and had soiled her clothing. In the emergency department she appeared frightened and paced in one area. She had difficulty understanding questions and cooperated only as long as she could pace. The husband relates that his wife had been under a lot of stress in her job and had recently lost some important clients.

   A. *What are some manifestations of her panic?*

   B. *What is the biologic cause of anxiety disorders (the brain structures and neurotransmitters)?*

   C. *Describe the physiologic manifestations of a panic attack.*

References

1. Shorter E. (1997). *A history of psychiatry: From the era of the asylum to the age of Prozac.* New York: John Wiley & Sons.
2. Kandel E. R. (2000). Cellular mechanisms of learning and biological basis of individuality. In Kandel E. R., Schwartz J. H., Jessel T. M. (Eds.), *Principles of neural science* (4th ed., pp. 1247–1277). New York: McGraw-Hill.
3. Grob G. N. (1994). *The mad among us: A history of the care of America's mentally ill.* New York: Macmillan.
4. Plomin R. (1996). Beyond nature vs. nurture. In Hall L. L. (Ed.), *Genetics and mental illness: Evolving issues for research and society* (pp. 29–50). New York: Plenum Press.
5. Walker E., Kestler L., Bollini A., et al. (2004). Schizophrenia: Etiology and course. *Annual Review of Psychology* 55, 401–430.
6. Hyman S. E. (1999). Looking to the future: The role of genetics and molecular biology in research on mental illness. In Weissman S., Sabshin M., Eist H. (Eds.), *Psychiatry in the new millennium* (pp. 97–117). Washington, DC: American Psychiatric Press.
7. Taylor C. J. A., Macdonald A. M., Murray R. M. (1992). The genetics of psychiatric syndromes. In Weller M., Eysenck M. (Eds.), *The scientific basis of psychiatry* (2nd ed., pp. 270–300). Philadelphia: W. B. Saunders.
8. Gottesman I. I. (1996). Blind men and elephants: Genetic and other perspectives on schizophrenia. In Hall L. L. (Ed.), *Genetics and mental illness: Evolving issues for research and society* (pp. 51–77). New York: Plenum Press.
9. Tsuang M. T., Faraone S. V. (1996). The inheritance of mood disorders. In Hall L. L. (Ed.), *Genetics and mental illness: Evolving issues for research and society* (pp. 79–109). New York: Plenum Press.
10. Mohr W. K. (2006). *Johnson's psychiatric-mental health nursing* (6th ed., p. 835). Philadelphia: Lippincott Williams & Wilkins.
11. Kandel E. R., Kupfermann I., Iverson S. (2000). Learning and memory. In Kandel E. R., Schwartz J. H., Jessell T. M. (Eds.), *Principles of neural science* (4th ed., pp. 1227–1246). New York: McGraw-Hill.
12. Guyton A. G., Hall J. E. (2006). *Textbook of medical physiology* (11th ed., pp. 714–727). Philadelphia: Elsevier Saunders.
13. Mojica T. R., Baily P. P. (2000). Hallucinations in the vision-impaired elderly: The Charles Bonnet syndrome. *Nurse Practitioner* 25(8), 74–76.
14. Teunisse R. J., Cruysberg J. R., Hoefnagels W. H., et al. (1996). Visual hallucinations in psychologically normal people: Charles Bonnet's syndrome. *Lancet* 347, 794–797.
15. Ovsiew F. (2004). Bedside neuropsychiatry: Eliciting the clinical phenomena of neuropsychiatric illness. In Yudofsky S. C., Hales R. E. (Eds.), *Essentials of neuropsychiatry and clinical neurosciences* (pp. 3–53). Washington, DC: American Psychiatric Publishing.
16. National Empowerment Center. (2006). Hearing voices that are distressing: Self-help resources. [Online.] Available: www.power2u.org/selfhep/voices.html. Accessed November 17, 2003.
17. Almedia O. P., Howard R. J., Levy R. (1995). Psychotic states arising in late life (late paraphrenia): The role of risk factors. *British Journal of Psychiatry* 166, 215–228.
18. Kandel E. R., Siegelbaum S. A. (2000). Overview of synaptic transmission. In Kandel E. R., Schwartz J. H., Jessel T. M. (Eds.), *Principles of neural science* (4th ed., pp. 175–185). New York: McGraw-Hill.
19. Kandel E. R. (2000). Neurotransmitters. In Kandel E. R., Schwartz J. H., Jessel T. M. (Eds.), *Principles of neural science* (4th ed., pp. 280–296). New York: McGraw-Hill.
20. Patterson J. C., Kotria K. J. (2004). Functional neuroimaging in psychiatry. In Yudofsky S. C., Hales R. E. (Eds.), *Essentials of neuropsychiatry and clinical neurosciences* (pp. 109–138). Washington, DC: American Psychiatric Publishing.
21. Callicott J. H., Weinberger D. R. (1999). Functional brain imaging: Future perspectives for clinical practice. In Weissman S., Sabshin M., Eist H. (Eds.), *Psychiatry in the new millennium* (pp. 119–135). Washington, DC: American Psychiatric Press.
22. Torrey E. F. (2006). *Surviving schizophrenia: A manual for families, patients, and providers.* New York: Harper & Row.

23. Tamminga C. A., Thaker G. K., Medoff D. R. (2004). Neuropsychiatric aspects of schizophrenia. In Yudofsky S. C., Hales R. E. (Eds.), *Essentials of neuropsychiatry and clinical neurosciences* (pp. 457–487). Washington, DC: American Psychiatric Publishing.

24. Cannon C., Clarke M. C. (2005). Risk for schizophrenia: Broadening the concepts, pushing back the boundaries. *Schizophrenia Research* 79, 5–13.

25. Varcarolis E. M. (2006). The schizophrenias. In Varcolis E. M., Carson V. B., Shoemaker N. C. (Eds.), *Foundations of psychiatric mental health nursing: A clinical approach* (5th ed., pp. 384–421). St. Louis: Elsevier Saunders.

26. Flashman L. A., Green M. F. (2004). Review of cognition and brain structure in schizophrenia: Profiles, longitudinal course, and effects of treatment. *Psychiatric Clinics of North America* 27, 1–18.

27. Freedman R. (2004). Schizophrenia. *New England Journal of Medicine* 349, 1738–1749.

28. Boos H. B. M., Aleman A., Cahn W., et al. (2007). Brain volumes in relatives of patients with schizophrenia. *Archives of General Psychiatry* 64, 297–304.

29. Sadock B. J., Sadock V. A. (Eds.). (2005). *Kaplan & Sadock's comprehensive textbook of psychiatry* (8th ed.). Philadelphia: Lippincott Williams & Wilkins.

30. American Psychiatric Association. (2000). *Diagnostic and statistical manual of mental disorders* (4th ed., text revision). Washington, DC: Author.

31. U.S. Department of Heath and Human Services. (2004). National Consensus Statement on Mental Health Recovery. [Online.] Available: http://mentalhealth.samhsa.gov/_scripts/printpage.aspx?FromPage=http%3A//mentalhealth.samhsa.gov/publications/allpubs/sma05-4129. Accessed May 28, 2007.

32. Diamond R. J. (2006). Recovery from a psychiatrist's viewpoint. New directions in schizophrenia: A Postgraduate Medicine Special Report. *Postgraduate Medicine* 8, 54–62.

33. Kessler R. C., Berglund P., Demler O., et al. (2003). The epidemiology of major depressive disorders. *Journal of the American Medical Association* 289, 3095–3105.

34. Brent D. A., Birmaher B. (2002). Adolescent depression. *New England Journal of Medicine* 347, 667–671.

35. Surgeon General's Report. (1999). Mental health for African Americans. [Online.] Available: http://mentalhealth.samhsa.gov/cre/ch3_appropriateness.asp. Accessed May 28, 2007.

36. Kandel E. R. (2000). Disorders of mood: Depression, mania, and anxiety disorders. In Kandel E. R., Schwartz J. H., Jessel T. M. (Eds.), *Principles of neural science* (4th ed., pp. 1209–1225). New York: McGraw-Hill.

37. Cornwall C. J. (2006). The client with a mood disorder. In Mohr W. K. (Ed.), *Johnson's psychiatric-mental health nursing* (6th ed., pp. 577–618). Philadelphia: Lippincott Williams & Wilkins.

38. Beimaker R. H. (2004). Bipolar disorder. *New England Journal of Medicine* 351(5), 476–486.

39. Varcarolis E. M. (2006). Mood disorders: Depression. In Varcarolis E. M., Carson V. B., Shoemaker N. C. (Eds.), *Foundations of psychiatric mental health nursing: A clinical approach* (5th ed., pp. 326–358). St. Louis: Elsevier Saunders.

40. Howland R. H. (2006). Challenges in the diagnosis and treatment of bipolar depression. Part two: Treatment options. *Journal of Psychosocial Nursing* 44, 9–12.

41. Daly I. (1997). Mania. *Lancet* 349, 1157–1160.

42. Kilzieh N., Akiskal H. S. (1999). Rapid-cycling bipolar disorder: An overview of research and clinical experience. *Psychiatric Clinics of North America* 22, 585–607.

43. Varcarolis E. M. (2006). Mood disorders: Bipolar. In Varcarolis E. M., Carson V. B., Shoemaker N. C. (Eds.), *Foundations of psychiatric mental health nursing: A clinical approach* (5th ed., pp. 359–383). St. Louis: Elsevier Saunders.

44. Hajek T., Carrey N., Alda M. (2005). Neuroanatomical abnormalities as risk factors for bipolar disorder. *Bipolar Disorders* 7, 393–403.

45. Mayberg H. S., Keightly M., Mahurin R. K., et al. (2004). Neuropsychiatric aspects of mood and affective disorders. In Yudofsky S. C., Hales R. E. (Eds.), *Essentials of neuropsychiatry and clinical neurosciences* (pp. 489–517). Washington, DC: American Psychiatric Publishing.

46. Brunswick D. J., Amsredam J. D., Mozley P. D., et al. (2003). Greater availability of brain dopamine transporters in major depression shown by [99mTc] TRODAT-1 SPECT imaging. *American Journal of Psychiatry* 160, 1836–1841.

47. Baldwin D. S., Psych F. R. C., Papakostas G. I. (2006). Symptoms of fatigue and sleepiness in major depressive disorder. *Journal of Clinical Psychiatry* 67(Suppl. 6), 9–15.

48. Agency for Healthcare Research and Quality. (May 2005). Post-myocardial infarction depression: Structured abstract. [Online.] Available: www.ahrq.gov/clinic/tp/mideptp.htm. Accessed May 28, 2007.

49. Williams J. W., Mulrow C. D., Chiquette E., et al. (2000). A systematic review of newer pharmacotherapies for depression in adults: Evidence report summary: Clinical guideline, part 2. *Annals of Internal Medicine* 132, 743–756.

50. Shuchman M. (2007). Approving the vagus-nerve stimulator for depression. *New England Journal of Medicine* 356, 1604–1607.

51. Academic Highlights. (2007). Transcranial magnetic stimulation: Potential new treatment for resistant depression. *Journal of Clinical Psychiatry* 68, 315–330.

52. Kessler R. C., Berglund P., Demler O., et al. (2005). Lifetime prevalence and age-of-onset distributions of DSM-IV disorders in the national comorbidity survey replication. *Archives of General Psychiatry* 62, 593–602.

53. Katon W. J. (2006). Panic disorder. *New England Journal of Medicine* 354, 2360–2367.

54. Diamond R. J. (2002). *Instant psychopharmacology* (2nd ed.). New York: W. W. Norton.

55. Stein D. J., Hugo M. B. (2004). Neuropsychiatric aspects of anxiety disorders. In Yudofsky S. C., Hales R. E. (Eds.), *Essentials of neuropsychiatry and clinical neurosciences* (pp. 519–533). Washington, DC: American Psychiatric Publishing.

56. Gorman J. M., Kent J. M., Sullivan G. M., et al. (2000). Neuroanatomical hypothesis of panic disorder, revised. *American Journal of Psychiatry* 157, 493–505.

57. Jenike M. A. (2004). Obsessive-compulsive disorder. *New England Journal of Medicine* 350, 259–265.

58. Tibbo P., Warneke L. (1999). Obsessive-compulsive disorder in schizophrenia: Epidemiologic and biologic overlap. *Journal of Psychiatry and Neuroscience* 24, 15–24.

59. Massachusetts General Hospital School Psychiatry Program & MADI Resource Center. (2006). Obsessive-compulsive disorder. [Online.] Available: www.massgeneral.org/schoolpsychiatry/info_ocd.asp. Accessed June 3, 2007.

60. Anderson K. E., Savage C. R. (2004). Cognitive and neurobiological findings in obsessive-compulsive disorder. *Psychiatric Clinics of North America* 27, 37–47.

61. Greene J. A. (2006). The client with an anxiety disorder. In Mohr W. K. (Ed.), *Johnson's psychiatric-mental health nursing* (6th ed., pp. 445–469). Philadelphia: Lippincott Williams & Wilkins.

62. Cornwell C. J., Lickteig M. K. (2006). The client who abuses drugs or alcohol. In Mohr W. K. (Ed.), *Johnson's psychiatric-mental health nursing* (6th ed., pp. 687–722). Philadelphia: Lippincott Williams & Wilkins.

63. Green A. I., Drake R. E., Brunette M. F., et al. (2007). Schizophrenia and co-occurring substance use disorder. *American Journal of Psychiatry* 163, 402–408.

64. Bruinjnzeel A. W., Repetto M., Gold M. (2004). Neurobiological mechanisms of addiction and psychiatric disorders. *Psychiatric Clinics of North America* 27, 661–674.

65. Kalivas P. W., Volkow N. D. (2005). The neural basis of addiction: A pathology of motivation and choice. *American Journal of Psychiatry* 162, 1403–1413.

66. Nestler E. J., Self D. W. (2004). Neuropsychiatric aspects of ethanol and other chemical dependencies. In Yudofsky S. C., Hales R. E. (Eds.), *Essentials of neuropsychiatry and clinical neurosciences* (pp. 399–419). Washington, DC: American Psychiatric Publishing.

67. Galanter M., Kleber H. D. (2004). *Textbook of substance abuse treatment* (3rd ed.). Arlington, VA: American Psychiatric Publishing.

68. Millsap P. (2007). Neurological system. In Linton A. D., Lach H. W. (Eds.), *Matteson & McConnell's gerontological nursing: Concepts and practice* (3rd ed., pp. 406–441). St. Louis: Elsevier Saunders.
69. Josshi S., Morley J. E. (2006). Cognitive impairment. *Medical Clinics of North America* 90, 769–787.
70. Kandel E. R., Kupfermann I., Iverson S. (2000). Learning and memory. In Kandel E. R., Schwartz J. H., Jessel T. M. (Eds.), *Principles of neural science* (4th ed., pp. 1231–1236). New York: McGraw-Hill.
71. American Psychiatric Association. (1993). *Diagnostic and statistical manual of mental disorders* (3rd ed.). Washington, DC: Author.
72. American Psychiatric Association. (1994). *Diagnostic and statistical manual of mental disorders* (4th ed.). Washington, DC: Author.
73. Knopman D. S., DeKosky S. T., Cummings J. L., et al. (2001). Practice parameter: Diagnosis of dementia (an evidence-based review). Report of the Quality Standards Subcommittee of the American Academy of Neurology. *Neurology* 56, 1143–1153.
74. Sadock B. J., Sadock V. A. (Eds.). (2005). *Kaplan & Sadock's comprehensive textbook of psychiatry* (8th ed., pp. 1076–1082). Philadelphia: Lippincott Williams & Wilkins.
75. Askin-Edgar S., White K. E., Cummings J. L. (2004). Neuropsychiatric aspects of Alzheimer's disease and other dementing illnesses. In Yudofsky S. C., Hales R. E. (Eds.), *Essentials of neuropsychiatry and clinical neurosciences* (pp. 421–456). Washington, DC: American Psychiatric Publishing.
76. Trojanowsky J. O., Kenyon L. (2008). The nervous system. In Rubin R., Strayer D. E. (Eds.), *Rubin's pathology: Clinicopathologic foundations of medicine* (5th ed., pp. 1212–1225). Philadelphia: Lippincott Williams & Wilkins.
77. Frosch M. P., Anthony D. C., DeGirolami U. (2005). The central nervous system. In Kumar V., Abbas A. K., Fausto N. (Eds.), *Robbins and Cotran pathologic basis of disease* (7th ed., pp. 1385–1394). Philadelphia: Elsevier Saunders.
78. National Institute of Aging. (2007). Alzheimer's disease general information. [Online.] Available: www.nia.nih.gov/Alzheimers/Alzheimers Information/GeneralInfo. Accessed June 16, 2007.
79. Kiraly M. A., Kiraly S. J. (2005). The effect of exercise on hippocampal integrity: Review of recent research. *International Journal of Psychiatry in Medicine* 35, 75–89.
80. Cummings J. L. (2004). Alzheimer disease. *New England Journal of Medicine* 351, 56–67.
81. Alzheimer's Association. (2007). Diagnostic procedures. [Online.] Available: www.alz.org/professionals_and_researchers_diagnostic_procedures.asp. Accessed June 18, 2007.
82. Fladd D. (2005). Subcortical vascular dementia. *Geriatric Nursing* 26, 117–121.
83. Weder N. D., Aziz R., Wilkins K., et al. (2007). Frontotemporal dementias: A review. *Annals of General Psychiatry* 6, 15.
84. National Institute of Neurologic Disorders and Stroke. (2008). Frontotemporal dementia information page. [Online.] Available: www.ninds.nih.gov/disorders/picks/picks.htm. Accessed June 18, 2007.
85. Prusiner S. B. (2001). Shattuck lecture: Neurodegenerative diseases and prions. *New England Journal of Medicine* 344, 1516–1526.
86. Huntington's Disease Society of America. (2000). Juvenile Huntington's disease. [Online.] Available: www.geocities.com/hdsarmc/juvenile_hd.htm. Accessed November 16, 2003.

Visit the Point http://thePoint.lww.com for animations, journal articles, and more!

Disorders of Special Sensory Function

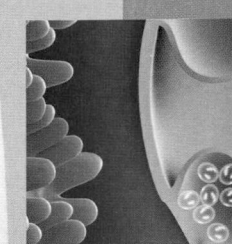

Of all the ancient civilizations, it was the Greeks who led the way in understanding the body and its workings. One of the earliest Greek anatomists was Alcmaeon of Croton (c. 500 BC). Through his animal dissections, Alcmaeon came to recognize many structures and was the first to mention the eye in his writings. He described the optic nerve and decided that three things were necessary for vision—external light, the "fire" in the eye (he assumed there must be fire in the eye because a blow to the eye produces sparks, or stars), and the liquid in the eyeball.

The Greeks also developed early surgical procedures, among them techniques for the removal of cataracts. However, it was the Roman encyclopedist, Aulus Cornelius Celsus (1st century AD), whose most important surviving works are concerned with medicine, who provided a vivid description of the procedure:

The needle is to be sharp enough to penetrate, yet not too fine; and this to be inserted straight through . . . at a spot between the pupil of the eye and the angle adjacent to the temple, away from the middle of the cataract, in such a way that no vein is wounded. The needle, however, should not be inserted timidly. When the spot is reached, the needle is to be sloped against the colored area [lens] itself and rotated gently, guiding it little by little below the pupil; when the cataract has passed below the pupil, it is pressed upon more firmly in order that it may settle below.

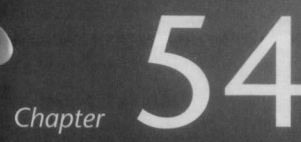

Chapter 54

Disorders of Visual Function

EDWARD W. CARROLL, SCOTT A. JENS, AND ROBIN CURTIS

> There are 161 million people worldwide who are visually impaired—37 million are blind and 124 million have partial vision loss that cannot be corrected, a visual impairment known as low vision. Without intervention, the number of people with impaired vision could double by 2020. The prevalence of vision impairment increases with age. An estimated 26% of persons 75 years of age and older report visual impairment severe enough to interfere with recognizing a friend across the room or reading newspaper print even when wearing glasses. At the other end of the age spectrum, an estimated 95,100 children younger than 18 years of age are severely visually impaired.[1]

Alterations in vision can result from disorders of the eyelids and optic globe (conjunctiva, cornea, and uvea), intraocular pressure (glaucoma), lens (cataract), vitreous humor and retina (retinopathy and macular degeneration), optic pathways and visual cortex, and extraocular muscles and eye movement (Fig. 54-1).

DISORDERS OF THE ACCESSORY STRUCTURES OF THE EYE

After completing this section of the chapter, you should be able to meet the following objectives:

- State the cause of eyelid weakness.
- Define the terms *entropion* and *ectropion*.

1388

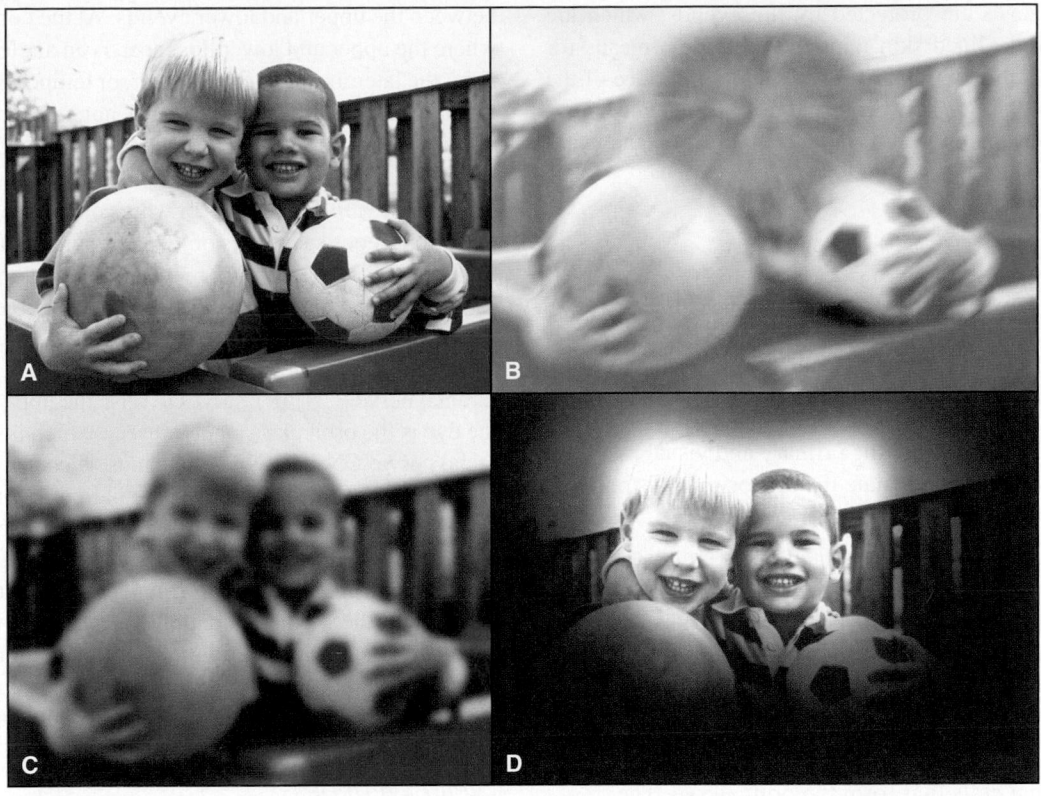

FIGURE 54-1 • A scene as it might be viewed by a person with (**A**) normal vision, (**B**) age-related macular degeneration, (**C**) cataract, and (**D**) glaucoma. (From National Eye Institute, National Institutes of Health. [Online.] Available: www.nei.nih.gov/photo.)

- Explain the differences between marginal blepharitis, a hordeolum, and a chalazion as to causes and manifestations.
- State the causes and treatment of dry eye.

The optic globe, commonly called the *eyeball,* is a remarkably mobile, nearly spherical structure contained in a pyramid-shaped cavity of the skull called the *orbit.* Only the anterior one fifth of the orbit is occupied by the eyeball; the remainder is filled with muscles, nerves, the lacrimal gland, and adipose tissue that support the normal position of the optic globe (Fig. 54-2). Exposed

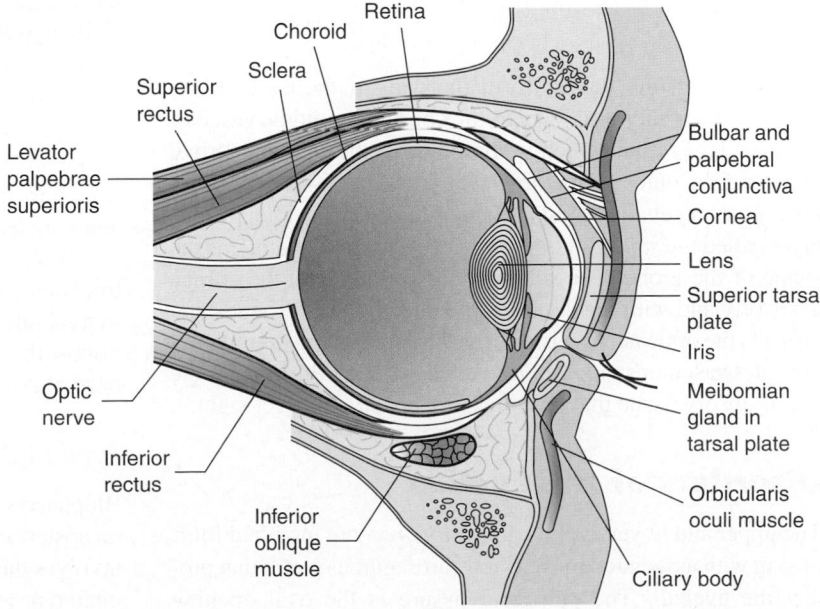

FIGURE 54-2 • The eye and its appendages: lateral view.

surfaces of the eyes are protected by the eyelids, which are mucous membrane–lined skin flaps that provide a means for shutting out most light. Tears bathe the anterior surface of the eye; they prevent friction between it and the lid, maintain hydration of the cornea, and protect the eye from infection and irritation by foreign objects.

🔑 VISION

- Vision is a special sensory function that incorporates the visual receptor functions of the eyeball, the optic nerve, and optic pathways that carry and distribute sensory information from the optic globe to the central nervous system, and the primary and visual association cortices that translate the sensory signals into visual images.

- The eyeball is a hollow spherical structure that functions in the reception of the light rays that provide the stimuli for vision. The refractive surface of the cornea and accommodative properties of the lens serve to focus the light signals from near and far objects on the photoreceptors in the retina.

- Visual information is carried to the brain by axons of the retinal cells that form the optic nerve. The two optic nerves fuse in the optic chiasm, where axons of the nasal retina of each eye cross to the contralateral side and travel with axons of the ipsilateral temporal retina to form the fibers of the optic radiations that travel to the visual cortex.

- Binocular vision depends on the coordination of three pairs of extraocular nerves that provide for the conjugate eye movements, with optical axes of the two eyes maintained parallel with one another as the eyes rotate in their sockets.

Three distinct layers form the wall of the eyeball: the sclera or outer supporting layer, the choroid or middle vascular layer, and the retina, which is composed of the neuronal retinal layer and the outer pigmented layer (see Fig. 54-2). The outer layer of the eyeball consists of a tough, opaque, white, fibrous layer called the *sclera*. It is strong yet elastic, and maintains the shape of the globe. The sclera is continuous with the cornea anteriorly and with the cranial dural sheath that surrounds and protects the optic nerve posteriorly. The choroid predominantly provides vascular support of the retina, whereas the retina is the neurosensory tissue that provides the sensory input for sight.

Disorders of the Eyelids

The upper and lower eyelids, the *palpebrae,* are modified folds of skin with associated muscle and cartilaginous plates that protect the eyeball. The palpebral fissure is the oval opening between the upper and lower eyelids. At the corners of the eye, where the upper and lower lids meet, is an angle called the *canthus;* the lateral canthus is the outer, or temporal, angle, and the medial canthus is the inner, or nasal, angle. In each lid, a tarsus, or plate of dense connective tissue, gives the lid its shape (Fig. 54-3). Each tarsus contains modified sebaceous glands, called *meibomian glands,* the ducts of which open onto the eyelid margins. Sebaceous secretions of the meibomian glands enable airtight closure of the lids and prevent rapid evaporation of tears.

Two striated muscles, the levator palpebrae superioris and the orbicularis oculi, provide for movement of the eyelids. The levator palpebrae superioris, innervated by the oculomotor nerve (cranial nerve [CN] III), serves to raise the upper lid. Encircling the eye is the orbicularis oculi muscle, which is supplied by the facial nerve (CN VII). When this muscle contracts, it closes the eyelids. Between the nose and medial angle of the eye is the medial palpebral ligament, which connects to the medial margin of the orbit (see Fig. 54-3). A similar palpebral ligament attaches to the lateral margin of the orbit. The orbicularis oculi nerve inserts into the medial palpebral ligament that passes through each eyelid and inserts into the lateral palpebral junction. The four recti and two oblique muscles provide for movement of the eyeball (discussed under disorders of eye movement).

Eyelid Weakness

Drooping of the eyelid is called *ptosis.* It can result from weakness of the levator muscle that elevates the upper lid in conjunction with the unopposed action of the orbicularis oculi that forcefully closes the eyelids. Weakness of the orbicularis oculi causes an open eyelid, but not ptosis. Neurologic causes of eyelid weakness include damage to the innervating cranial nerves or to the nerves' central nuclei in the midbrain and the caudal pons.

Normally, the edges of the eyelids, or palpebrae, are in such a position that the palpebral conjunctiva that lines the eyelids is not exposed and the eyelashes do not rub against the cornea. Turning in of the lid margin is called *entropion.* It is usually caused by scarring of the palpebral conjunctiva or degeneration of the fascial attachments to the lower lid that occurs with aging. Corneal irritation may occur as the eyelashes turn inward. *Ectropion* refers to eversion of the lower lid margin. The condition is usually bilateral and caused by relaxation of the orbicularis oculi muscle because of CN VII weakness or the aging process. Ectropion causes tearing and ocular irritation and may lead to inflammation of the cornea.

Entropion and ectropion can be treated surgically. Electrocautery penetration of the lid conjunctiva also can be used to treat mild forms of ectropion. After electrocautery, contraction of the resulting scar tissue usually draws the lid up to its normal position.

Eyelid Inflammation

Blepharitis is a common bilateral inflammation of the anterior or posterior structures of eyelid margins. *Anterior blepharitis* involves the eyelid skin, eyelashes, and associated glands. Two main types of anterior blepharitis occur: seborrheic and staphy-

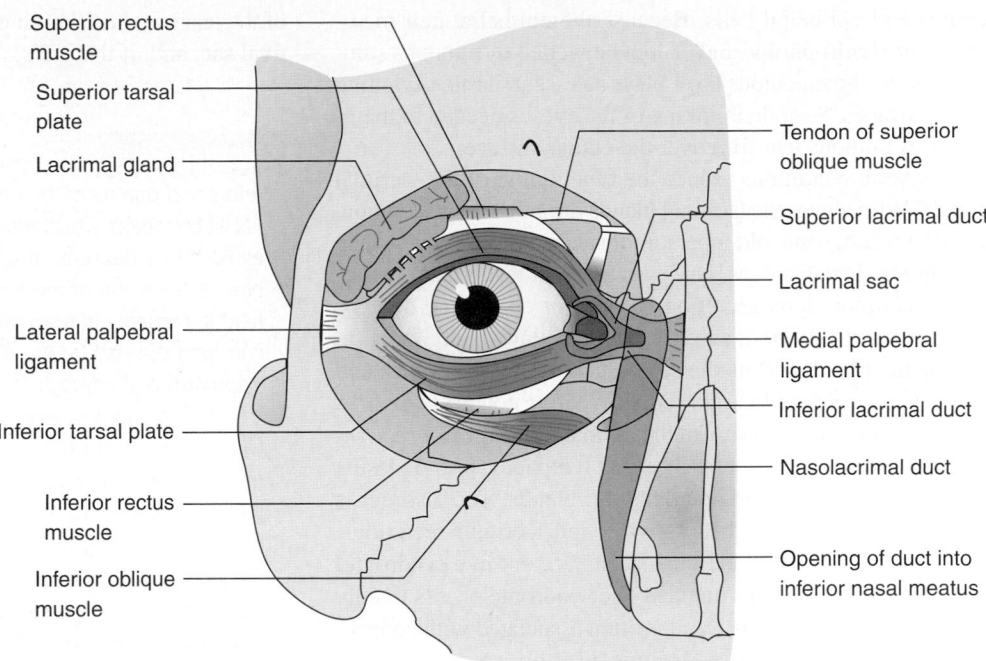

Superior rectus muscle
Superior tarsal plate
Lacrimal gland
Lateral palpebral ligament
Inferior tarsal plate
Inferior rectus muscle
Inferior oblique muscle

Tendon of superior oblique muscle
Superior lacrimal duct
Lacrimal sac
Medial palpebral ligament
Inferior lacrimal duct
Nasolacrimal duct
Opening of duct into inferior nasal meatus

FIGURE 54-3 • The eye and its appendages: anterior view.

lococcal.[2] The seborrheic form is usually associated with seborrhea (*i.e.,* dandruff) of the scalp or brows. Staphylococcal blepharitis may be caused by *Staphylococcus epidermidis* or *Staphylococcus aureus,* in which case the lesions are often ulcerative. The main symptoms of anterior blepharitis are irritation, burning, redness, and itching of the eyelid margins. Treatment includes careful cleaning with a damp applicator to remove the scales. When the disorder is associated with a microbial infection, an antibiotic ointment or drops is prescribed.

Posterior blepharitis is inflammation of the eyelids that involves the meibomian glands. It may result from a bacterial infection, particularly with staphylococci, or dysfunction of the meibomian glands, in which there is a strong association with acne rosacea[2,3] (see Chapter 61). The meibomian glands and their orifices are inflamed, with dilation of the glands, plugging of the orifices, and abnormal secretions. The tears may be frothy and abnormally greasy from the meibomian secretions. Treatment of posterior blepharitis is determined by associated conjunctival and corneal changes. Initial therapies can include warm compression of the lids, and use of flaxseed or fish oil tablets to provide omega-3 fatty acid benefits to meibomian oil secretions. Long-term, low-dose systemic antibiotic therapy guided by results of bacterial cultures along with short-term topical steroids may also be needed.

A *hordeolum,* or *stye,* is caused by infection of the sebaceous glands of the eyelid and can be internal or external. The main symptoms are pain, redness, and swelling. The treatment is similar to that for abscesses in other parts of the body. Heat such as a warm compress is applied, and short-term treatment with systemic antibiotics (*e.g.,* doxycycline) may be used to reduce or eliminate the infection. Incision or expression of the infectious contents of the abscess may be necessary.

A *chalazion* is a chronic inflammatory granuloma of a meibomian gland that may follow an internal hordeolum. It is characterized by a small, nontender nodule on the upper or lower lid. The conjunctiva around the chalazion is red and elevated. If the chalazion is large enough, it may press on the eyeball and distort vision. Treatment consists of surgical excision.

Disorders of the Lacrimal System

The lacrimal system includes the major lacrimal gland, which produces the tears, the puncta, canaliculi, and tear sac, which collect the tears, and the nasolacrimal duct, which empties the tears into the nasal cavity. The lacrimal gland lies in the orbit, superior and lateral to the eyeball (see Fig. 54-3). Approximately 12 small ducts connect the lacrimal gland to the superior conjunctival fornix. Tears contain approximately 98% water, 1.5% sodium chloride, and small amounts of potassium, albumin, and glucose. The function of tears is to provide a smooth optical surface by abolishing minute surface irregularities. Tears also wet and protect the delicate surface of the cornea and conjunctiva. They flush and remove irritating substances and microorganisms, and provide the cornea with necessary nutrient substances. Tears also contain lysozymes and immunoglobulin A (IgA), IgG, and IgE, which synergistically act to protect against infection. Although IgA predominates, IgE concentrations are increased in some allergic conditions.

Dry Eyes

The thin film of tears that covers the cornea is essential in preventing drying and damage of the outer layer of the cornea. This tear film is composed of three layers: (1) a superficial lipid layer, which is derived from the meibomian glands and thought to retard evaporation; (2) an aqueous layer, secreted by the lacrimal glands; and (3) a mucinous layer, which overlies the cornea and epithelial cells. Because the epithelial cell membranes are hydrophobic and cannot be wetted by aqueous solutions alone, the mucinous layer plays an essential role in wetting these surfaces. Periodic blinking of the eyes is needed to maintain a continuous tear film over the ocular surface.

Several conditions reduce the functioning of the lacrimal glands. With aging, the lacrimal glands diminish their secretion, and as a result, some older persons awaken from a night's sleep with highly irritated eyes. Dry eyes also can result from loss of reflex lacrimal gland secretion because of congenital defects, infection, irradiation, damage to the parasympathetic innervation of the gland, and medications such as antihistamines and drugs with an anticholinergic action. Wearing contact lenses can contribute to an interruption of the normal tear film. *Sjögren syndrome* is a systemic disorder in which lymphocytes and plasma cells infiltrate the lacrimal and parotid glands. The disorder is associated with diminished salivary and lacrimal secretions, resulting in keratoconjunctivitis sicca (*i.e.,* dry eye syndrome) and xerostomia (*i.e.,* dry mouth). The syndrome occurs mainly in women near menopause and is often associated with connective tissue disorders such as rheumatoid arthritis.

Persons with dry eyes complain of a dry or gritty sensation in the eye, burning and itching, inability to produce tears, photosensitivity, redness, pain, and difficulty in moving the eyelids.[3] Some persons experience excess tearing as the eyes attempt to react to dry symptoms. Dry eyes and the absence of tears can cause keratinization of the cornea and conjunctival epithelium. In severe cases, corneal ulcerations can occur.

The treatment of dry eyes includes frequent instillation of artificial tear solutions into the conjunctival sac.[3] More prolonged duration of action can be obtained from topical preparations containing methylcellulose or polyvinyl alcohol. An ointment is useful for prolonged lubrication. Overall, these artificial tear preparations are safe and without side effects. However, the preservatives necessary to maintain their sterility can be irritating to the cornea.[2] Further treatment can include occlusion of the lacrimal puncta with silicone plugs or use of therapeutic topical drugs to increase natural tear volume. Increased intake of omega-3 fatty acids has also been shown to provide improvement in dry eye symptoms.[3]

Dacryocystitis

Dacryocystitis is an infection of the lacrimal sac. It occurs most often in infants or in persons older than 54 years of age.[2,4] It is usually unilateral and most often occurs secondary to obstruction of the nasolacrimal duct. Often the cause of the obstruction is unknown, although there may be a history of severe trauma to the midface. The symptoms include tearing and discharge, pain, swelling, and tenderness. The treatment includes application of warm compresses and antibiotic therapy. In chronic forms of the disorder, surgical repair of the tear duct may be necessary.

In infants, dacryocystitis is usually caused by failure of the nasolacrimal ducts to open spontaneously before birth. When a duct fails to open, a secondary dacryocystitis may develop. These infants are usually treated with gentle massage

of the tear sac, instillation of antibiotic drops into the conjunctival sac, and, if that fails, probing of the tear duct.

IN SUMMARY, the eyelids serve to protect the eye. Ptosis refers to drooping of the upper lid, which is caused by injury to CN III. Entropion, which refers to turning in the upper eyelid and eyelashes, is discomforting and causes corneal irritation. Ectropion, or eversion of the lower eyelid, causes tearing and may lead to corneal inflammation. Marginal blepharitis is the most common disorder of the eyelids. It commonly is caused by a staphylococcal infection or seborrhea (*i.e.,* dandruff).

The lacrimal system includes the major lacrimal gland, which produces the tears, the puncta and tear sac, which collect the tears, and the nasolacrimal duct, which empties the tears into the nasal cavity. Tears protect the cornea from drying and irritation. Impaired tear production or conditions that prevent blinking and the spread of tears produce drying of the eyes and predispose them to corneal irritation and injury. Dacryocystitis is an infection of the lacrimal sac. ∎

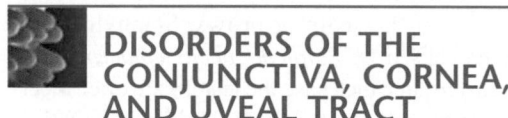

DISORDERS OF THE CONJUNCTIVA, CORNEA, AND UVEAL TRACT

After completing this section of the chapter, you should be able to meet the following objectives:

- Compare symptoms associated with red eye caused by conjunctivitis, corneal irritation, and acute glaucoma.
- Describe the appearance of corneal edema.
- Characterize the manifestations, treatment, and possible complications of bacterial, *Acanthamoeba,* and herpes keratitis.
- Describe the structures of the uveal tract.
- Describe tests used in assessing the pupillary reflex and cite the possible causes of abnormal pupillary reflexes.

Disorders of the Conjunctiva

The conjunctiva is a delicate mucous membrane that lines the anterior surface of both eyelids as the *palpebral conjunctiva* and folds back over the anterior surface of the optic globe as the *ocular* or *bulbar conjunctiva*[4] (see Fig. 54-2). The ocular conjunctiva covers only the sclera or white portion of the optic globe, not the cornea. When both eyes are closed, the conjunctiva lines the closed conjunctival sac. Although the conjunctiva protects the eye, its main function is the production of a lubricating mucus that bathes the eye and keeps it moist.

Conjunctivitis, or inflammation of the conjunctiva (*i.e.,* red or pink eye), is one of the most common forms of eye disease.[5-8] It may result from bacterial or viral infection, allergens, chemical agents, physical irritants, or radiant energy. Depending on the cause, conjunctivitis can vary in severity from a mild hyperemia (redness) with tearing to severe conjunctivitis with purulent drainage. The conjunctiva is extremely sensitive to irritation and inflammation. Symptoms of conjunctivitis are a foreign body sensation, a scratching or burning sensation, itching, and photophobia. Severe pain suggests corneal rather than conjunctival disease. A discharge, or exudate, may be present. It is usually watery when the conjunctivitis is caused by allergy, a foreign body, or viral infection, and mucopurulent in the presence of bacterial or fungal infection. A characteristic of many forms of conjunctivitis is papillary hypertrophy. This occurs because the palpebral conjunctiva is bound to the tarsus by fine fibrils. As a result, inflammation that develops between the fibrils causes the conjunctiva to be elevated in mounds called *papillae*. When the papillae are small, the conjunctiva has a smooth, velvety appearance. Red papillary conjunctivitis suggests bacterial or chlamydial conjunctivitis. In allergic conjunctivitis, the papillae often become flat-topped, polygonal, and milky in color and have a cobblestone appearance.

The diagnosis of conjunctivitis is based on history, physical examination, and microscopic and culture studies to identify the cause. Because a red eye may be the sign of several eye conditions, it is important to differentiate between redness caused by conjunctivitis and that caused by more serious eye disorders, such as corneal lesions and acute glaucoma. In contrast to corneal lesions and acute glaucoma, conjunctivitis produces injection (*i.e.*, enlargement and redness) of the peripheral conjunctival blood vessels rather than those radiating around the corneal limbus (Fig. 54-4). Conjunctivitis also produces only mild discomfort compared with the moderate to severe discomfort associated with corneal lesions or the severe and deep pain associated with acute glaucoma. Infectious forms of conjunctivitis are usually bilateral and may involve other family members and associates. Unilateral disease suggests sources of irritation such as foreign bodies or chemical irritation.

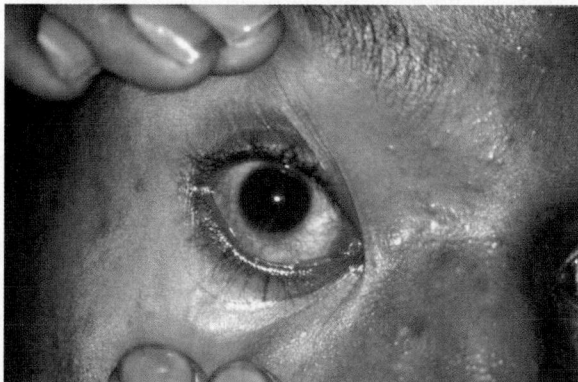

FIGURE 54-4 • Gonococcal conjunctivitis of right eye. Note injection of the peripheral conjunctival blood vessels. (From the Centers for Disease Control and Prevention Public Health Image Library. [Online.] Available: http://phil.cdc.gov/phil/home.asp.)

Allergic Conjunctivitis

Allergic conjunctivitis encompasses a spectrum of conjunctival conditions usually characterized by itching. The most common of these is seasonal allergic rhinoconjunctivitis, or hay fever. Seasonal allergic conjunctivitis is an IgE-mediated hypersensitivity reaction precipitated by small airborne allergens such as pollens.[9] It typically causes bilateral tearing, itching, and redness of the eyes.

The treatment of seasonal allergic rhinoconjunctivitis includes allergen avoidance and the use of cold compresses and eye washes with tear substitute. Allergic conjunctivitis also has been successfully treated with topical mast cell stabilizers, histamine type 1 (H_1) receptor antagonists, and topical nonsteroidal anti-inflammatory drugs.[7] Systemic antihistamines may be useful in prolonged allergic conjunctivitis. In severe cases, a short course of topical corticosteroids may be required to afford symptomatic relief.

Infectious Conjunctivitis

The agents of infectious conjunctivitis include bacteria, viruses, and chlamydiae. Infections may spread from areas adjacent to the conjunctiva or may be blood-borne, such as in measles or chickenpox. Newborns can contract conjunctivitis during the birth process.

Bacterial Conjunctivitis. Bacterial conjunctivitis may present as a hyperacute, acute, or chronic infection. *Hyperacute conjunctivitis* is a severe, sight-threatening ocular infection. The infection has an abrupt onset and is characterized by a copious amount of yellow-green drainage. The symptoms, which typically are progressive, include conjunctival redness, chemosis (swelling around the cornea), lid swelling, and tender, swollen preauricular lymph nodes. The most common causes of hyperacute purulent conjunctivitis are *Neisseria gonorrhoeae* and *Neisseria meningitidis*, with *N. gonorrhoeae* being the most common.[5–7] Gonococcal ocular infections left untreated result in corneal ulceration with ultimate perforation, and sometimes permanent loss of vision. Diagnostic methods include immediate Gram staining of ocular specimens and special cultures for *Neisseria* species. Treatment includes systemic antibiotics supplemented with ocular antibiotics. Because of the increasing prevalence of penicillin-resistant *N. gonorrhoeae*, antibiotic choice should be determined by current information regarding antibiotic sensitivity.

Acute bacterial conjunctivitis typically presents with burning, tearing, and mucopurulent or purulent discharge. Common agents of bacterial conjunctivitis are *Streptococcus pneumoniae, S. aureus,* and *Haemophilus influenzae*.[6] The eyelids are sticky, with possible excoriation of the lid margins. Treatment may include local application of antibiotics. The disorder is usually self-limited, lasting approximately 10 to 14 days if untreated. Scrupulous handwashing and prompt treatment of infected persons and their contacts are essential.

Chronic bacterial conjunctivitis most commonly is caused by *Staphylococcus* species, although other bacteria may be involved. It is often associated with blepharitis and bacterial colonization of eyelid margins. The symptoms of chronic bacterial conjunctivitis vary and can include itching, burning, foreign body sensation, and morning eyelash crusting. Other symptoms include flaky debris and erythema along the lid margins, eyelash loss, and eye redness. Some people with chronic bacterial conjunctivitis also have recurrent styes and chalazia of the lid margins. Treatment includes good eyelid hygiene and application of topical antibiotics.

Viral Conjunctivitis. Etiologic agents of viral conjunctivitis include adenoviruses, herpesviruses, and enteroviruses. One of the most common causes of viral conjunctivitis is adenovirus type 3.[5] The infection, which causes generalized conjunctival hyperemia, copious tearing, and minimal exudate, is usually accompanied by pharyngitis, fever, and malaise. Children are affected more often than adults. Swimming pools contaminated because of inadequate chlorination are common sources of infection.

Viral epidemic keratoconjunctivitis is caused by adenoviruses types 8, 19, 29, and 37.[5] It presents with marked discomfort and is highly contagious, with rapid spread from person to person. The disease lasts for at least 2 weeks and may be complicated by visual symptoms due to epithelial and subepithelial involvement. Topical antibiotics are ineffective in controlling the inciting viral agent, but may be used to prevent secondary bacterial infection. The most important aspect of treatment is education regarding the highly transmissible nature of the infection. Instructions should include the need for scrupulous handwashing and avoiding the shared use of eyedroppers, eye makeup, goggles, and towels. Persons who use contact lenses should avoid them and wear their prescription glasses instead.

Chlamydial Conjunctivitis. Chlamydial conjunctivitis is usually a benign suppurative conjunctivitis transmitted by the type of *Chlamydia trachomatis* (serotypes D through K) that causes venereal infections[10] (see Chapter 47). It is spread by contaminated genital secretions and occurs in newborns of mothers with *C. trachomatis* infections of the birth canal. It also can be contracted through swimming in unchlorinated pools. The incubation period varies from 5 to 12 days, and the disease may last for several months if untreated. The infection is usually treated with appropriate oral antibiotics.

A more serious form of infection is caused by a different strain of *C. trachomatis* (serotypes A, B, and C).[10] This form of chlamydial infection affects the conjunctiva and causes ulceration and scarring of the cornea. It is the leading cause of preventable blindness in the world. Although the agent is widespread, it is seen mostly in developing countries, particularly those of Africa, Asia, and the Middle East.[6,10] It is transmitted by direct human contact, contaminated objects (fomites), and flies.

Ophthalmia Neonatorum

Ophthalmia neonatorum is a form of conjunctivitis that occurs in newborns younger than 1 month of age and is usually contracted during or soon after vaginal delivery. Many causes are known, including *N. gonorrhoeae, Pseudomonas,* and *C. trachomatis.*[6,11] Epidemiologically, these infections reflect those sexually transmitted infections most common in a particular area. Once the most common form of conjunctivitis in the newborn, gonococcal ophthalmia neonatorum now has an incidence of 0.3 per 1000 live births in the United States. In comparison, *C. trachomatis* ophthalmia neonatorum has an incidence of 8.2 per 1000 live births.[11] To prevent gonococcal ophthalmia, 0.5% erythromycin ointment or 1% silver nitrate drops are applied immediately after birth. Silver nitrate instillation may cause mild, self-limited conjunctivitis.

Signs of ophthalmia neonatorum include redness and swelling of the conjunctiva, swelling of the eyelids, and discharge, which may be purulent. The conjunctivitis caused by silver nitrate occurs within 6 to 12 hours of birth and clears within 24 to 48 hours.[11] The incubation period for *N. gonorrhoeae* is 2 to 5 days and for *C. trachomatis,* 5 to 14 days.[11] Infection should be suspected when conjunctivitis develops 48 hours after birth. Ophthalmia neonatorum is a potentially blinding condition, and it can cause serious and potentially systemic manifestations. It requires immediate diagnosis and treatment.

Disorders of the Cornea

At the anterior part of the eyeball, the outer covering of the eye is modified to form the transparent cornea, which bulges anteriorly from its junction with the sclera (Fig. 54-5). A major part of the refraction (*i.e.,* bending) of light rays and focusing of vision occurs in the cornea. Three layers of tissue form the cornea: an extremely thin outer epithelial layer, which is continuous with the bulbar conjunctiva; a middle layer called the *substantia propria* or *stroma;* and an inner endothelial layer, which lies next to the aqueous humor of the anterior chamber.[4,12] The substantia propria is composed of regularly arranged collagen bundles embedded in a mucopolysaccharide matrix. This organization of the collagen fibers, which makes the substantia propria transparent, is necessary for light transmission. Hydration within a limited range is necessary to maintain the spacing of the collagen fibers and transparency. The three layers of the cornea are separated by two important basement membranes: Bowman and Descemet membranes. *Bowman membrane,* which lies between the corneal epithelium and stoma, acts as a barrier to infection. It does not regenerate; if damaged, an opaque scar forms that can impair vision. *Descemet membrane,* which lies between the corneal endothelium and stroma, has a felt-like appearance and consists of interwoven fibers and pores. Unlike Bowman membrane, it regenerates readily after injury.

The cornea is avascular and obtains its nutrient and oxygen supply by diffusion from blood vessels of the adjacent sclera, from the aqueous humor at its deep surface, and from tears.[12] The corneal epithelium is heavily innervated by sensory neurons

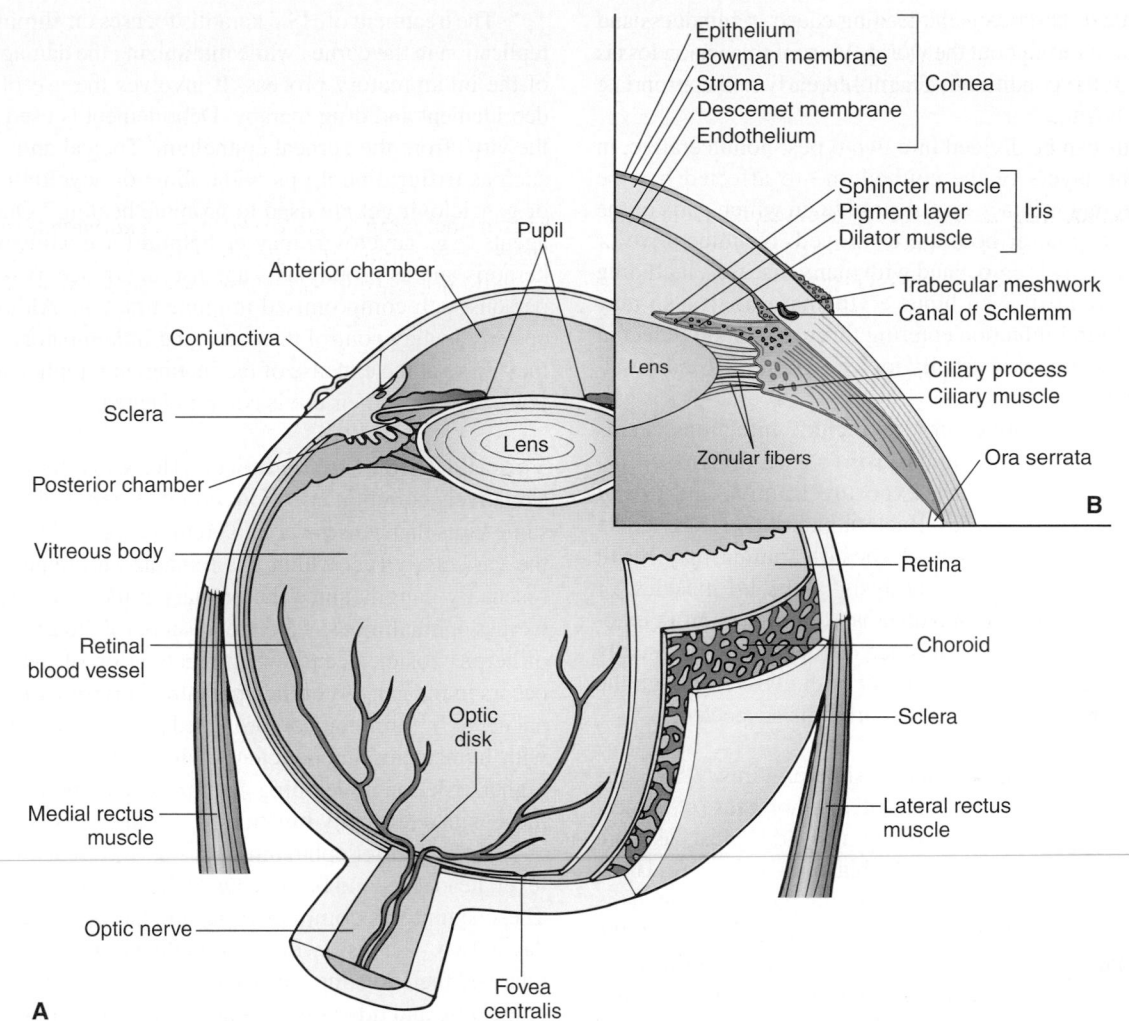

FIGURE 54-5 • **(A)** Transverse section of the eyeball. **(B)** Enlargement of the anterior and posterior chambers of the eye, showing the layers of the cornea, the structures of the iris, and aqueous drainage system (trabecular meshwork, canal of Schlemm), and the ciliary process and ciliary muscle.

(trigeminal nerve [CN V], ophthalmic division [CN V₁]). Epithelial damage causes discomfort that ranges from a foreign body sensation and burning of the eyes to severe, incapacitating pain. Reflex lacrimation is common.

Disorders of the cornea include trauma, inflammation and infection, abnormal corneal deposits, and degenerative processes such as arcus senilis. Diagnosis of corneal disorders is based on history of trauma, medication use, and signs and symptoms associated with corneal irritation and disease.[13] Because of the discomfort involved, examination of the eye is often eased by instillation of a local anesthetic agent. Fluorescein staining can be used to outline an ulcerated area. The biomicroscope (slit lamp) is used for proper examination of the cornea. In cases of an infectious etiology, scrapings from the ulcer are obtained for staining and culture studies.

Corneal Trauma

The integrity of the epithelium and the endothelium is necessary to maintain hydration of the cornea within a limited range. Damage to either structure leads to edema and loss of transparency.

Among the causes of corneal edema is the prolonged wearing of contact lenses, which can deprive the epithelium of oxygen, disrupting its integrity. Corneal edema also occurs after a sudden rise in intraocular pressure. With corneal edema, the cornea appears dull, uneven, and hazy; visual acuity decreases, and iridescent vision (*i.e.,* rainbows around lights) occurs.

Trauma that causes abrasions of the cornea can be extremely painful, but if minor, the abrasions usually heal in a few days. The epithelial layer can regenerate, and small defects heal without scarring. If the stroma is damaged, healing occurs more slowly, and the danger of infection is increased. Injuries to the Bowman membrane and the stromal layer heal with scar formation that impairs the transmission of light.

Keratitis

Keratitis refers to inflammation of the cornea. It can be caused by infections, misuse of contact lenses, hypersensitivity reactions, ischemia, trauma, defects in tearing, and interruption in sensory innervation, as occurs with local anesthesia. Scar tissue formation due to keratitis is the leading cause of blindness and impaired vision throughout the world. Most of this vision loss is preventable if the condition is diagnosed early and appropriate treatment is begun.

Keratitis can be divided into two types: nonulcerative, in which all the layers of the epithelium are affected but the epithelium remains intact, and ulcerative, in which parts of the epithelium, stroma, or both are destroyed. Nonulcerative or interstitial keratitis is associated with many diseases, including syphilis, tuberculosis, and lupus erythematosus. It also may result from a viral infection entering through a small defect in the cornea. Treatment is usually topical antibiotics and possibly anti-inflammatory agents.

Causes of ulcerative keratitis include infectious agents such as those causing conjunctivitis (*e.g., Staphylococcus, S. pneumoniae, Chlamydia*), exposure trauma, and use of extended-wear contact lenses. Bacterial keratitis is aggressive and demands immediate care. Exposure trauma may result from deformities of the lid, paralysis of the lid muscles, or severe exophthalmos. Mooren ulcer is a chronic, painful, indolent ulcer that occurs in the absence of infection. It is usually seen in older persons and may affect both eyes. Although the cause is unknown, an autoimmune origin is suspected.

Herpes Simplex Keratitis. Herpes simplex virus (HSV) keratitis with stromal scarring is the most common cause of corneal ulceration and blindness in the Western world.[13] Most cases are caused by HSV type 1, the cause of labial or lip infections. However, in neonatal infections acquired during passage through the birth canal, approximately 80% are caused by HSV type 2 (the cause of genital herpes). The disease can occur as a primary or recurrent infection.[13] Primary epithelial infections are the optical counterpart of labial herpes with similar immunologic and pathologic features as well as a similar time course. During childhood, mild primary HSV infection may go unnoticed. After the initial primary infection, the virus may persist in a quiescent or latent state in the trigeminal ganglion and possibly in the cornea without causing signs of infection.

Recurrent infection may be precipitated by various poorly understood, stress-related factors that reactivate the virus. Involvement is usually unilateral. The first symptoms are irritation, photophobia, and tearing. Some reduction in vision may occur when the lesion affects the central part of the cornea. Because corneal anesthesia occurs early in the disease, the symptoms may be minimal, and the person may delay seeking medical care. A history of fever blisters or other herpetic infection is often noted, but corneal lesions may be the only sign of recurrent herpes infection. Most typically, the corneal lesion involves the epithelium and has a typical branching pattern. These epithelial lesions heal without scarring. Herpetic lesions that involve the stromal layer of the cornea produce increasingly severe corneal opacities. Although previously thought to be a purely immunologic response to viral particles or virally induced cellular changes, there is increasing evidence that infection due to active viral particles can occur in stromal and possibly endothelial cells, as well as other tissues in the anterior segment such as the iris and trabecular endothelium.

The treatment of HSV keratitis focuses on eliminating viral replication in the cornea while minimizing the damaging effects of the inflammatory process. It involves the use of epithelial debridement and drug therapy. Debridement is used to remove the virus from the corneal epithelium. Topical antiviral agents such as trifluridine drops, vidarabine or acyclovir ointment, or ganciclovir gel are used to promote healing.[8] Oral antiviral agents (*e.g.,* acyclovir) may be helpful for treatment of severe keratitis and as prophylaxis against recurrence, particularly in persons with compromised immune function. Although corticosteroids may control the damaging inflammatory responses, they do so at the expense of facilitating viral replication. With a few exceptions, their use is contraindicated.

Varicella Zoster Ophthalmicus. Herpes zoster or shingles is a relatively common infection caused by herpesvirus type 3, the same virus that causes varicella (chickenpox).[14] It occurs when the varicella virus, which has remained dormant in the neurosensory ganglia since the primary infection, is reactivated. Herpes ophthalmicus, which represents 10% to 25% of all cases of herpes zoster, occurs when reactivation of the latent virus occurs in the ganglia of the ophthalmic division of the trigeminal nerve.[13,14] Immunocompromised persons, particularly those with human immunodeficiency virus (HIV) infection, are at higher risk for developing herpes zoster ophthalmicus than those with a normally functioning immune system.

Herpes zoster ophthalmicus usually presents with malaise, fever, headache, and burning and itching of the periorbital area. These symptoms commonly precede the ocular eruption by a day or two. The rash, which is initially vesicular, becomes pustular and then crusting (see Chapter 61). Involvement of the tip of the nose and lid margins indicates a high likelihood of ocular involvement. Ocular signs include conjunctivitis, keratitis, and anterior uveitis, often with elevated intraocular pressure. Persons with corneal disease present with varying degrees of decreased vision, pain, and sensitivity to light.

Treatment includes the use of high-dose oral antiviral drugs (*i.e.,* acyclovir, valacyclovir, famciclovir). Initiation of treatment within the first 72 hours after the appearance of the rash reduces the incidence of ocular complications but not the postherpetic neuralgia (see Chapter 49).

Acanthamoeba Keratitis. *Acanthamoeba* is a free-living protozoan that thrives in contaminated water.[12] *Acanthamoeba* keratitis is a rare but serious and sight-threatening complication of wearing soft contact lenses, particularly when they are worn overnight beyond doctor-recommended periods or when poor disinfection techniques are used. It also may occur in non–contact lens wearers after exposure to contaminated water or soil. It is characterized by pain that is disproportionate to the clinical manifestations, redness of the eye, and photophobia. The disorder commonly is misdiagnosed as herpes keratitis. Diagnosis is confirmed by scrapings and culture with specially prepared medium. In the early stages of infection, epithelial debridement may be beneficial. Treatment includes intensive use of topical antibiotics. However, the organism may encyst within the corneal stroma, making treatment more difficult. Keratoplasty may be necessary in advanced disease to arrest the progression of the infection.

Abnormal Corneal Deposits

The cornea frequently is the site for deposition of abnormal metabolic products. In hypercalcemia, calcium salts can precipitate in the cornea, producing a cloudy band keratopathy. Cystine crystals are deposited in cystinosis, cholesterol esters in hypercholesterolemia, and a golden ring of copper (*i.e.*, Kayser-Fleischer ring) in hepatolenticular degeneration due to Wilson disease. Pharmacologic agents, such as chloroquine, can result in crystal deposits in the cornea.

Arcus senilis is an extremely common, bilateral, benign corneal degeneration that may occur at any age, but is more common in the elderly. It consists of a grayish-white infiltrate, approximately 2 mm wide, that occurs at the periphery of the cornea. It represents an extracellular lipid infiltration and commonly is associated with hyperlipidemia. Arcus senilis does not produce visual symptoms, and there is no treatment for the disorder.

Corneal Transplantation

Advances in ophthalmologic surgery permit corneal transplantation using a cadaver cornea. Unlike kidney or heart transplantation procedures, which are associated with considerable risk of rejection of the transplanted organ (see Chapter 19), the use of cadaver corneas entails minimal danger of rejection. The low rejection rate is due to several factors: the cornea is avascular, including lymphatics, thereby limiting perfusion by immune elements; major histocompatibility complexes (class II) are virtually absent in the cornea; antigen-presenting cells are not present in great numbers; the cornea secretes immunosuppressive factors; and corneal cells secrete substances (*e.g.*, Fas ligand) that protect against apoptosis, thereby minimizing inflammation.[15]

Disorders of the Uveal Tract

The middle vascular layer, or uveal tract, is an incomplete ball with gaps at the pupil and the optic nerve. The pigmented uveal tract has three distinct regions: the choroid, ciliary body, and the iris. The *choroid* is a highly vascular, dark brown membrane that forms the posterior five-sixths of the uveal tract. Its blood vessels provide nourishment for the other layers of the eyeball. Its brown pigment, produced by melanocytes, absorbs light within the eyeball and light that penetrates the retina. The light absorptive function prevents the scattering of light and is important for visual acuity, particularly with high background illumination levels. The *ciliary body* is a thickened ring of tissue that encircles the lens. It has smooth muscle and secretory functions. Its smooth muscle function contributes to changes in lens shape and its secretory function to the production of aqueous humor.

The iris is an adjustable diaphragm that permits changes in pupil size and in the light entering the eye. The posterior surface of the iris is formed by a two-layer epithelium continuous with those layers covering the ciliary body. The anterior layer contains the dilator or radial muscles of the iris. Just anterior to these muscles is a layer of highly vascular connective tissue. Embedded in this layer are concentric rings of smooth muscle that compose the sphincter muscle of the pupil. The anterior layer of the iris forms an irregular anterior surface, containing many fibroblasts and melanocytes. Eye color differences result from the density of the pigment. The amount of pigment decreases from that found in dark brown eyes through shades of brown and green to that found in blue eyes.

Several mutations affect the pigment of the uveal tract, including albinism. *Albinism* is a genetic (autosomal recessive trait) deficiency of tyrosinase, the enzyme needed for the synthesis of melanin by the melanocytes. Tyrosinase-negative albinism, also called *classic albinism,* is characterized by an absence of tyrosinase; affected persons have white hair, pink skin, and light blue eyes. In these persons, excessive light penetrates the unpigmented iris and choroid, and, to some extent, the anterior sclera. Their photoreceptors are flooded with excess light, and visual acuity is markedly reduced. Excess stimulation of the photoreceptors at normal or high illumination levels is experienced as painful photophobia.

Uveitis

Inflammation of the entire uveal tract, which supports the lens and neural components of the eye, is called *uveitis.* It is one of several inflammatory disorders of ocular tissue with clinical features in common and an immunologically based cause.[8] A serious consequence of uveitis can be the involvement of the underlying retina. Parasitic invasion of the choroid can result in local atrophic changes that usually involve the retina; examples include toxoplasmosis and histoplasmosis.

The Pupil and Pupillary Reflexes

Changes in pupil size are controlled by contraction or relaxation of the sphincter and radial muscles of the iris. The pupillary reflex, which controls the size of the pupillary opening, is controlled by the autonomic nervous system, with the parasympathetic nervous system producing pupillary constriction or *miosis* and the sympathetic nervous system producing pupillary dilation or *mydriasis.* The sphincter muscle that produces pupillary constriction is innervated by postganglionic parasympathetic neurons of the ciliary ganglion and other scattered ganglion cells between the scleral and choroid layers. Part of the oculomotor (CN III) nucleus is called the *Edinger-Westphal nucleus.*[16] This autonomic nucleus, found in the midbrain, provides the preganglionic innervation for these parasympathetic axons. Pupillary dilation by the radial muscles is provided by sympathetic innervation under excitatory descending control from the hypothalamus. Innervation is derived from preganglionic neurons in the upper thoracic cord, which send axons along the sympathetic chain to synapse with postganglionic neurons in the superior ciliary ganglion (see Chapter 48, Fig. 48-28). Postganglionic fibers travel along the surfaces of the carotid and smaller arteries to reach the eye.

The pupillary reflex is controlled by a region in the midbrain called the *pretectum*. Pretectal areas on each side of the brain are connected, explaining the binocular aspect of the light reflex. The afferent stimuli for pupillary constriction arise in the ganglionic cells of the retina and are transmitted to the *pretectal nuclei* at the junction of the thalamus and the midbrain, and from there to preganglionic neurons in the oculomotor (CN III) nuclei (Fig. 54-6).

Normal function of the pupillary reflex mechanism can be tested by shining a penlight into one eye of the person being tested. To avoid a change in pupil size due to accommodation, the person is asked to stare into the distance. A rapid constriction of the pupil exposed to light should occur; this is called the *direct pupillary light reflex*. Because the reflex is normally bilateral, the contralateral pupil also should constrict, a reaction called the *consensual pupillary light reflex*. The circuitry of the light reflex is partially separated from the main optic pathway. This is illustrated by the fact that the pupillary reflex remains unaffected when lesions to the optic radiations or the visual cortex occur.

Integrity of the dual autonomic control of pupillary diameter is vulnerable to trauma, tumor enlargement, or vascular disease. With diffuse damage to the forebrain involving the thalamus and hypothalamus, the pupils are typically small but respond to light. Damage to the CN III nucleus results in permanent pupillary dilation in the affected eye. Lesions affecting the cervical spinal cord or the ascending sympathetic ganglionic chain in the neck or internal carotid artery (*e.g.*, Horner syndrome) can interrupt the sympathetic control of the iris dilator muscle, resulting in permanent pupillary constriction. Tumors of the orbit that compress structures behind the eye can eliminate all pupillary reflexes, usually before destroying the optic nerve.

Pupillary size can also be differentially affected by pharmacologic agents. Bilateral pupillary constriction is characteristic of opiate usage. Pupillary dilation results when topical parasympathetic blocking agents such as atropine are applied and sympathetic pupillodilatory function is left unopposed. Dilation can be enhanced by sympathomimetic agents. These medications are used by ophthalmologists and optometrists to facilitate the examination of the transparent media and fundus of the eye. Miotic drugs (*e.g.*, pilocarpine), which are used in the treatment of angle-closure glaucoma (to be discussed), produce pupil constriction and in that manner facilitate aqueous humor circulation.

IN SUMMARY, the conjunctiva lines the inner surface of the eyelids and covers the optic globe to the junction of the cornea and sclera. Conjunctivitis, also called *red eye* or *pink eye,* may result from bacterial or viral infection, allergens, chemical agents, physical agents, or radiant energy. It is important to differentiate between redness caused by conjunctivitis and that caused by more serious eye disorders, such as acute glaucoma or corneal lesions.

Keratitis, or inflammation of the cornea, can be caused by infections, hypersensitivity reactions, ischemia, trauma, defects in tearing, or trauma. Trauma or disease that involves the stromal layer of the cornea heals with scar formation and permanent opacification. These opacities interfere with the transmission of light and may impair vision.

The uveal tract is the middle vascular layer of the eye. It contains melanocytes that prevent diffusion of light through the wall of the optic globe. Inflammation of the uveal tract (uveitis) can affect visual acuity.

The pupillary reflex, which controls the size of the pupil, is controlled by the autonomic nervous system. The parasympathetic nervous system controls pupillary constriction, and the sympathetic nervous system controls pupillary dilation. ■

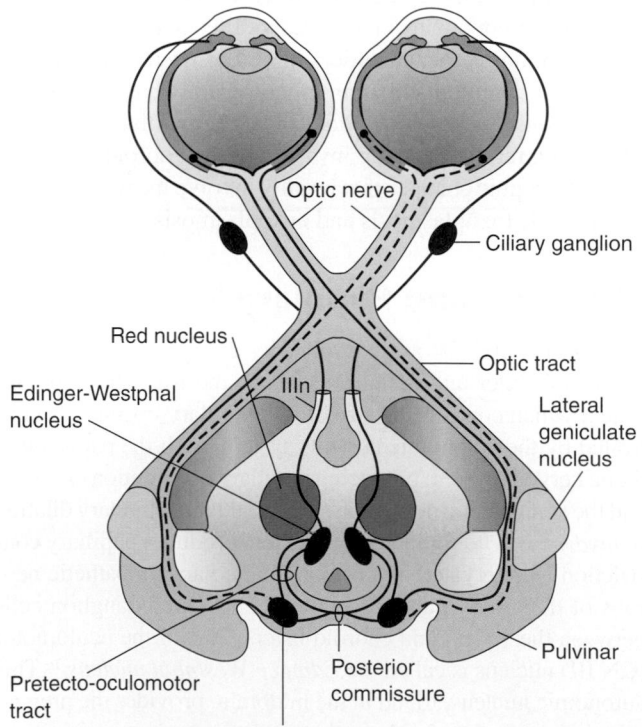

FIGURE 54-6 • Diagram of the path of the pupillary light reflex. (Reproduced with permission from Walsh F. B., Hoyt W. F. [1969]. *Clinical neuro-ophthalmology* [3rd ed., vol. 1]. Baltimore: Williams & Wilkins.)

Labels: Optic nerve; Ciliary ganglion; Red nucleus; Optic tract; Edinger-Westphal nucleus; IIIn; Lateral geniculate nucleus; Pretecto-oculomotor tract; Posterior commissure; Pulvinar; Pretectal nucleus

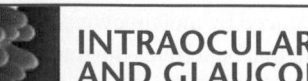

INTRAOCULAR PRESSURE AND GLAUCOMA

After completing this section of the chapter, you should be able to meet the following objectives:

■ Describe the formation and outflow of aqueous humor from the eye and relate to the development of glaucoma.

- Compare open-angle and angle-closure glaucoma in terms of pathology, symptomatology, and diagnosis and treatment.
- Explain why glaucoma leads to blindness.

Glaucoma comprises a group of conditions that produce an elevation in intraocular pressure. If left untreated, the pressure may increase sufficiently to cause ischemic and compressive degeneration of the optic nerve, leading to progressive blindness. It is one of the leading causes of blindness worldwide, and is second only to age-related macular degeneration as the leading cause of blindness in North America.[17,18] The condition is often asymptomatic, and a significant loss of peripheral vision may occur before medical attention is sought (see Fig. 54-1D).

Control of Intraocular Pressure

The intraocular pressure is largely regulated by the aqueous humor, which fills the anterior and posterior chambers of the eye. The aqueous humor is produced by the ciliary body and passes from the posterior chamber through the pupil into the anterior chamber[19,20] (Fig. 54-7A). Aqueous humor leaves through the iridocorneal angle between the anterior surface of the iris and the sclera. Here it filters through the trabecular meshwork and enters the canal of Schlemm for return to the venous circulation. The canal of Schlemm is actually a thin-walled vein that extends circumferentially around the iris of the eye. Its endothelial membrane is so porous that even large protein molecules up to the size of a red blood cell can pass from the posterior chamber into the canal of Schlemm.

The pressure of the aqueous humor results from a balance of several factors, including the rate of aqueous secretion, the resistance to flow between the iris and the ciliary body, and the resistance to resorption at the trabeculated region of the sclera at the iridocorneal angle. Normally, the rate of aqueous production is equal to the rate of aqueous outflow, and the intraocular pressure is maintained within a normal range of 9 to 21 mm Hg.[20]

Tonometry is the measurement of intraocular pressure. The most widely used instrument is the Goldman applanation tonometer, which is attached to a slit lamp and measures the force required to flatten a fixed area on the cornea. Central corneal thickness, which can be measured by either optical or ultrasonic methods, is thought to influence the accuracy of measurement, with intraocular pressure being overestimated in eyes with a thick cornea and underestimated in eyes with a thin cornea.[19] Another type of tonometer, the noncontact ("air-puff") tonometer, which uses the rebound force of a small puff of air blown against the cornea to estimate the intraocular pressure, is not as accurate as the applanation tonometer. However, this method does not require anesthetic drops because no instrument touches the eye. It is therefore more easily used by technicians and is useful in screening programs.[19]

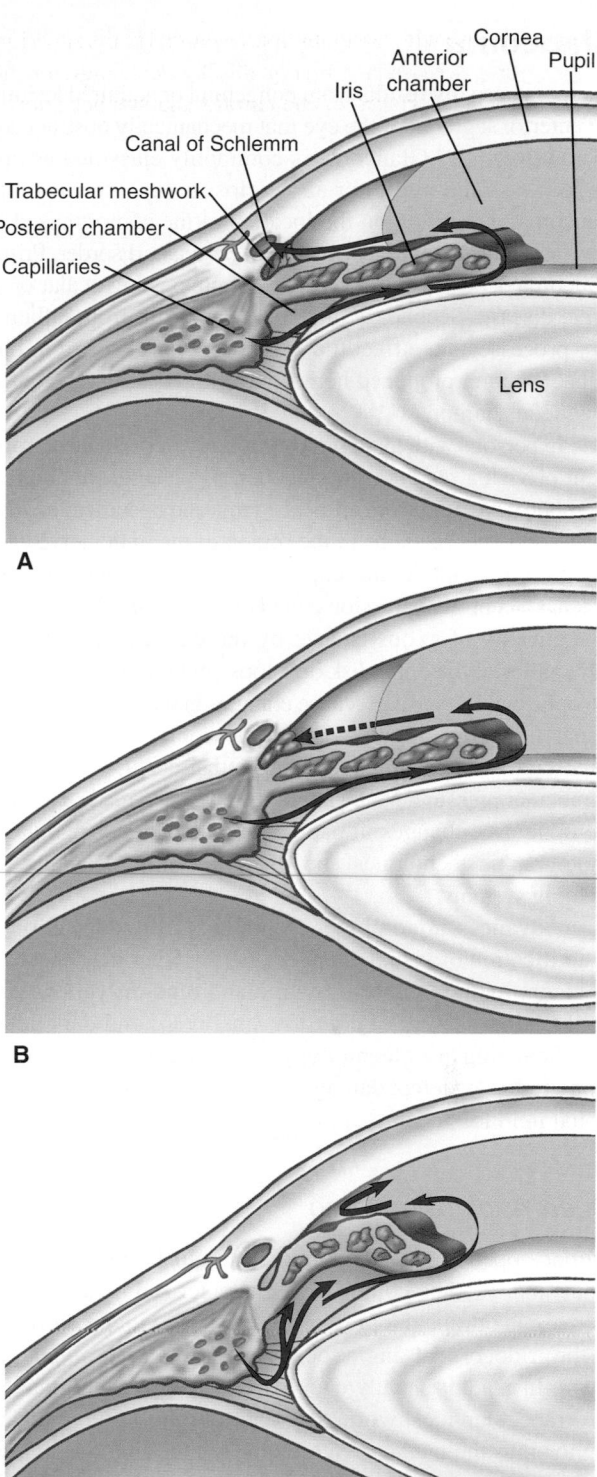

FIGURE 54-7 • **(A)** Normally, aqueous humor, which is secreted in the posterior chamber, gains access to the anterior chamber by flowing through the pupil. In the angle of the anterior chamber, it passes through the canal of Schlemm into the venous system. **(B)** In open-angle glaucoma, the outflow of aqueous humor is obstructed at the trabecular meshwork. **(C)** In angle-closure glaucoma, the aqueous humor encounters resistance to flow through the pupil. Increased pressure in the posterior chamber produces a forward bowing of the peripheral iris, so that the iris blocks the trabecular meshwork.

Glaucoma

Glaucoma usually results from congenital or acquired lesions of the anterior segment of the eye that mechanically obstruct aqueous outflow.[8,12,19] Glaucoma is commonly classified as open-angle (*i.e.,* wide-angle) or angle-closure (*i.e.,* narrow-angle) glaucoma, depending on the location of the compromised outflow, and may occur as a primary or secondary disorder. Primary glaucoma occurs without evidence of preexisting ocular or systemic disease. Secondary glaucoma can result from inflammatory processes that affect the eye, from tumors, or from blood cells of trauma-produced hemorrhage that obstruct the outflow of aqueous humor.

In persons with glaucoma, temporary or permanent impairment of vision results from degenerative changes in the retina and optic nerve and from corneal edema and opacification. Damage to optic nerve axons in the region of the optic nerve can be recognized on ophthalmoscopic examination. The normal optic disk has a central depression called the *optic cup*. With progressive atrophy of axons caused by increased intraocular pressure, pallor of the optic disk develops, and the size and depth of the optic cup increase. Because changes in the optic cup precede visual field loss, regular ophthalmoscopic examinations are important for detecting eye changes that occur with increased intraocular pressure. Many attempts have been made to quantify the optic disk changes in people with glaucoma using various photographic techniques and, more recently, scanning laser imaging systems.

Advances in computer technology allow detection and quantification of visual changes due to glaucoma. These tests of vision include white-on-white and blue-on-yellow visual field testing, testing of contrast sensitivity, and dark adaptation. Scanning laser technology and optical coherence tomography tests can detect damage to retinal ganglion axons before visual field loss occurs.

Open-Angle Glaucoma

Primary open-angle glaucoma is the most common form of glaucoma.[17–19] The condition is characterized by an abnormal increase in intraocular pressure that occurs without obstruction at the iridocorneal angle, hence the name *open-angle glaucoma*. Instead, it usually occurs because of an abnormality of the trabecular meshwork that controls the flow of aqueous humor into the canal of Schlemm[12,19] (see Fig. 54-7B). Secondary open-angle glaucoma occurs as a result of other conditions, including the formation of red cell fragments after trauma and iris pigment epithelial granules that may clog the trabecular meshwork.

The condition is usually asymptomatic and chronic, causing progressive damage to the optic nerve and visual field loss unless it is appropriately treated. Elevated intraocular pressure is a primary factor for open-angle glaucoma, but it is not the only diagnostic factor. Some people maintain a higher intraocular pressure without evidence of optic nerve damage or visual field loss, demonstrating a condition described as *glaucoma suspect* or *ocular hypertension.*[19] It is questionable whether damage to the optic nerve results from excessive intraocular pressure, decreased blood flow to the optic nerve, or both factors.

The etiology of primary open-angle glaucoma remains unclear. Major risk factors for this disorder include an age of 40 years and older, black race, a positive first-degree family history, myopia, and increased intraocular pressure.[17,18] Other risk factors with moderate to fair epidemiologic evidence include hypertension, type 2 diabetes, hyperthyroidism, migraine headaches, and sleep apnea.[18] In some persons, the use of moderate amounts of topical or inhaled corticosteroid medications can cause an increase in intraocular pressure. Sensitive persons also may sustain an increase in intraocular pressure with the use of systemic corticosteroid drugs. There is emerging evidence that central corneal thickness is also an important predictor for the development of primary open-angle glaucoma, and it may be a relevant predictor of both glaucoma progression and response to intraocular pressure–lowering drugs.[21]

Diagnostic methods include applanation tonometry, ophthalmoscopic visualization of the optic nerve, and central visual field testing. Measurement of intraocular pressures provides a means of assessing glaucoma risk. Because the condition is usually asymptomatic, persons at risk for open-angle glaucoma should have regular direct ophthalmoscopic examinations, on both eyes, concentrating on the optic disk. Optic disk changes frequently are noted before visual field defects become apparent. Periodic stereoscopic assessment of the optic disk by an eye care provider trained in the detection of glaucoma is strongly recommended for at-risk patients.

The elevation in intraocular pressure in persons with open-angle glaucoma is usually treated pharmacologically or, in cases where pharmacologic treatment fails, by increasing aqueous outflow through a surgically created pathway. Drugs used in the long-term management of glaucoma fall into five classes: β-adrenergic antagonists, prostaglandin analogs, adrenergic agonists, carbonic anhydrase inhibitors, and cholinergic agonists.[17,18] Most glaucoma drugs are applied topically. However, systemic side effects may occur. When treatment with one drug does not reduce the intraocular pressure to the target level, a drug from a different class may be used or a second medication may be added as adjunctive therapy.

Topical β-adrenergic antagonists are usually the drugs of first choice for lowering intraocular pressure. The β-adrenergic antagonists are thought to lower intraocular pressure by decreasing aqueous humor production in the ciliary body.[17] Systemic adsorption of these eye drops can cause bradycardia and bronchospasm in persons with asthma. Carbonic anhydrase inhibitors reduce the secretion of aqueous humor by the ciliary epithelium. The topical carbonic anhydrase inhibitors (dorzolamide and brinzolamide) are often used as adjunctive therapy, but rarely as initial therapy. Selective α_2-adrenergic agonists (*i.e.,* brimonidine and apraclonidine) increase aqueous outflow in addition to decreasing aqueous production. They are effective as an adjunctive, or occasionally as a primary treatment agent. Local ocular allergy often limits the usefulness of apraclonidine.

Several classes of drugs increase aqueous outflow. Prostaglandins are locally acting substances found in most tissues. At low concentrations, prostaglandin $F_{2\alpha}$ increases the outflow of aqueous humor through the iris root and ciliary body, either by decreasing the extracellular matrix or by relaxing the ciliary musculature. Latanoprost, a topical prostaglandin analog, is now one of the most frequently prescribed glaucoma drugs. Acetylcholine is the postganglionic neuromediator for the parasympathetic nervous system; it increases aqueous outflow through contraction of the ciliary muscle and pupillary constriction (miosis). Pilocarpine, a parasympathomimetic miotic and once the mainstay of treatment, has largely been replaced by newer and more effective drugs.

When a reduction in intraocular pressure cannot be maintained through pharmacologic methods, laser or surgical trabeculoplasty may become necessary. With laser trabeculoplasty, the microburns created by the laser treatment scar rather than penetrate the trabecular meshwork, a process thought to enlarge the outflow channels by increasing the tension exerted on the trabecular meshwork. Cryotherapy, diathermy, and high-frequency ultrasound may be used in some cases to destroy the ciliary epithelium and reduce aqueous humor production.

Angle-Closure Glaucoma

Angle-closure glaucoma results from occlusion of the anterior chamber angle by the iris (see Fig. 54-7C). It is most likely to develop in eyes with preexisting shallow anterior chambers. An acute attack is often precipitated by pupillary dilation, which causes the iris to thicken, thus blocking the circulation between the posterior and anterior chambers.[10,19] Approximately 10% to 15% of all cases of glaucoma fall into this category.[19] Angle-closure glaucoma usually occurs as the result of an inherited anatomic defect that causes a shallow anterior chamber. It is seen more commonly in people of Asian or Inuit (Eskimo) descent and in people with hypermetropic eyes. This defect is exaggerated by the anterior displacement of the peripheral iris that occurs in older persons because of the increase in lens thickness that occurs with aging.

The depth of the anterior chamber can be evaluated by side/shadow illumination or by a technique called *gonioscopy*. Gonioscopy uses a special contact lens and mirrors or prisms to view and measure the angle of the anterior chamber. The side/shadow illumination method uses only a penlight. The light source is held at the temporal side of the eye and directed horizontally across the iris. In persons with a normal-sized anterior chamber, the light passes through the chamber to illuminate both halves of the iris. In persons with a narrow anterior chamber, only the half of the iris adjacent to the light source is illuminated, whereas a shadow is cast on the half of the iris opposite the light source.

Symptoms of acute angle-closure glaucoma are related to sudden, intermittent increases in intraocular pressure. These occur after prolonged periods in the dark, emotional upset, and other conditions that cause extensive and prolonged dilation of the pupil. Administration of pharmacologic agents such as atropine that cause pupillary dilation (mydriasis) also can precipitate an acute episode of increased intraocular pressure in persons with the potential for angle-closure glaucoma. Attacks of increased intraocular pressure are manifested by ocular pain and blurred or iridescent vision caused by corneal edema.[19] The pupil may be enlarged and fixed. Symptoms are often spontaneously relieved by sleep and conditions that promote pupillary constriction. With repeated or prolonged attacks, the eye becomes reddened, and edema of the cornea may develop, giving the cornea a hazy appearance. A unilateral, often excruciating, headache is common. Nausea and vomiting may occur, causing the headache to be confused with migraine.

Some persons with congenitally narrow anterior chambers never develop symptoms, and others develop symptoms only in older age. Because of the dangers of vision loss, those with narrow anterior chambers should be warned about the significance of blurred vision, halos, and ocular pain. Sometimes, decreased visual acuity and an unreactive pupil may be the only clues to angle-closure glaucoma in the elderly.

Acute angle-closure glaucoma is an ophthalmic emergency. Treatment is initially directed at reducing the intraocular pressure, usually with pharmacologic agents. Once the intraocular pressure is under control, a laser peripheral iridotomy is performed to create a permanent opening between the anterior and posterior chambers, allowing the aqueous humor to bypass the pupillary block. The anatomic abnormalities responsible for angle-closure glaucoma are usually bilateral, and prophylactic surgery is often performed on the other eye.

Congenital and Infantile Glaucoma

There are several types of childhood glaucoma, including congenital glaucoma that is present at birth and infantile glaucoma that develops during the first 2 to 3 years of life. As with glaucoma in adults, childhood glaucoma can occur as a primary or secondary disorder.

Congenital glaucoma is caused by a disorder in which the anterior chamber retains its fetal configuration, with aberrant trabecular meshwork extending to the root of the iris, or is covered by a membrane. In general it has a much poorer prognosis than infantile glaucoma. Primary infantile glaucoma occurs in approximately 1 in 10,000 live births, but accounts for 2% to 15% of persons in institutions for the blind.[22] It is bilateral in 65% to 80% of cases, and occurs more commonly in boys than girls. About 10% of cases have a familial origin; and the rest are either sporadic or possibly multifactorial with reduced penetrance. The familial cases are usually transmitted as an autosomal dominant trait with potentially high penetrance. Recent studies suggest a mutation in chromosome 2 (2p21 region). This gene is expressed in the tissues of the anterior chamber of the eye and its protein product plays an important role in the metabolism of molecules that are used in signaling pathways during the terminal stages of anterior chamber development.[18]

The earliest symptoms of congenital or infantile glaucoma are excessive lacrimation and photophobia. Affected infants tend to be fussy, have poor eating habits, and rub their eyes frequently. Diffuse edema of the cornea usually occurs, giving the eye a grayish-white appearance. Chronic elevation of the intraocular pressure before the age of 3 years causes enlargement of the entire optic globe. Early surgical treatment is necessary to prevent blindness.

IN SUMMARY, glaucoma is a leading cause of blindness worldwide. It is characterized by conditions that cause an increase in intraocular pressure and that, if untreated, can lead to atrophy of the optic disk and progressive blindness. The aqueous humor is formed by the ciliary epithelium in the posterior chamber and flows through the pupil to the angle formed by the cornea and the iris. Here, it filters through the trabecular meshwork and enters the canal of Schlemm for return to the venous circulation. Glaucoma results from overproduction or impeded outflow of aqueous humor from the anterior chamber of the eye.

There are two types of glaucoma: open-angle and angle-closure. Open-angle glaucoma is caused by microscopic obstruction of the trabecular meshwork. Open-angle glaucoma is usually asymptomatic, and considerable loss of the visual field often occurs before medical treatment is sought. Routine screening by applanation tonometry provides one of the best means for early detection of glaucoma before vision loss has occurred. Angle-closure glaucoma is caused by a narrow anterior chamber and blockage of the outflow channels at the angle formed by the iris and the cornea. This occurs when the iris becomes thickened during pupillary dilation. Congenital glaucoma is caused by a disorder in which the anterior chamber retains its fetal configuration, with aberrant trabecular meshwork extending to the root of the iris, or is covered by a membrane. Early surgical treatment is necessary to prevent blindness. ■

DISORDERS OF THE LENS AND LENS FUNCTION

After completing this section of the chapter, you should be able to meet the following objectives:

- Describe changes in eye structure that occur with nearsighted and farsighted vision.
- Describe the changes in lens structure that occur with cataract.
- Cite risk factors and visual changes associated with cataract.
- Describe the treatment of persons with cataracts.

The function of the eye is to transform light energy into nerve signals that can be transmitted to the cerebral cortex for interpretation. Optically, the eye is similar to a camera. It contains a lens system that focuses an inverted image, an aperture (*i.e.,*

the pupil) for controlling light exposure, and a retina that corresponds to the film and records the image.

Disorders of Refraction and Accommodation

The lens is an avascular, transparent, biconvex body, the posterior side of which is more convex than the anterior side. A thin, highly elastic lens capsule is attached to the surrounding ciliary body by delicate suspensory radial ligaments called *zonules,* which hold the lens in place (see Fig. 54-5). The tough elastic sclera, in providing for a change in lens shape, acts as a bow, and the zonule and the lens capsule act as the bowstring. The suspensory ligaments and lens capsule are normally under tension, causing the lens to have a flattened shape for distant vision. Contraction of the muscle fibers of the ciliary body narrows the diameter of the ciliary body, relaxes the fibers of the suspensory ligaments, and allows the lens to relax to a more convex shape for near vision.

When light passes from one medium to another, its velocity is decreased or increased, and the direction of light transmission is changed. This change in direction of light rays is called *refraction.* When light rays pass through the center of a lens, their direction is not changed; however, other rays passing peripherally through a lens are bent (Fig. 54-8). The refractive power of a lens is usually described as the distance (in meters) from its surface to the point at which the rays come into focus (*i.e.,* focal length). Usually, this is reported as the reciprocal of this distance (*i.e.,* diopters).[20] For example, a lens that brings an object into focus at 0.5 m has a refractive power of 2 diopters (1/0.5 = 2). With a fixed-power lens, the closer an object is to the lens, the further behind the lens is its focus point. The closer the object, the stronger and more precise the focusing system must be.

In the eye, the major refraction of light begins at the convex corneal surface. Further refraction occurs as light moves from the posterior corneal surface to the aqueous humor, from the aqueous humor to the anterior lens surface, from the anterior lens surface to the posterior lens surface, and from the posterior lens surface to the vitreous humor.

Disorders of Refraction

A perfectly shaped optic globe and cornea result in optimal visual acuity, producing a sharp image in focus at all points on the retinal surface in the posterior part, or fundus, of the eye. Unfortunately, individual differences in formation and growth of the eyeball and cornea frequently result in inappropriate focal image formation. If the anterior-posterior dimension of the eyeball is too short, the image is theoretically focused posterior to (behind) the retina. This is called *hyperopia* or *farsightedness.* In such cases, the accommodative changes of the lens can bring distant images into focus, but near images become blurred. Hyperopia is corrected by appropriate convex-surface lenses. If the anterior-posterior dimension of the eyeball is too long, the focus point for an infinitely distant target is anterior to the retina.

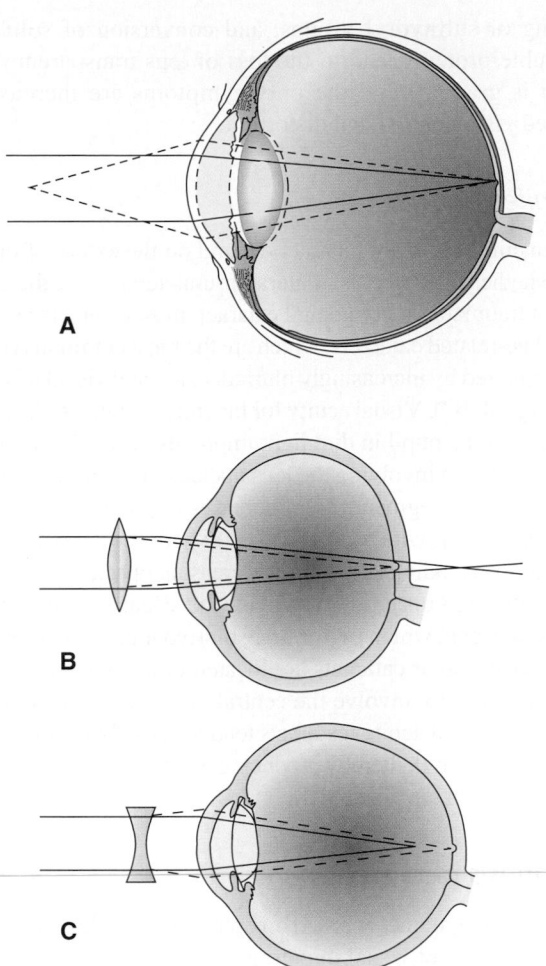

FIGURE 54.8 • **(A)** Accommodation. The *solid lines* represent rays of light from a distant object, and the *dotted lines* represent rays from a near object. The lens is flatter for the former and more convex for the latter. In each case, the rays of light are brought to a focus on the retina. **(B)** Hyperopia corrected by a biconvex lens, shown by the *dotted lines*. **(C)** Myopia corrected by a biconcave lens, shown by the *dotted lines*.

This condition is called *myopia* or *nearsightedness* (see Fig. 54-8C). Persons with myopia can see close objects without problems because accommodative changes in their lens bring near objects into focus, but distant objects are blurred. Myopia can be corrected with an appropriate concave-surface lens. Refractive corneal surgeries such as laser in situ keratomileusis (LASIK), photorefractive keratectomy, and radial keratotomy, can be performed to correct the corneal curvature to create accurate optical focus.[23,24]

Refractive defects of the corneal surface do not permit the formation of a sharp image. Nonuniform curvature of the refractive medium with regard to the horizontal and vertical planes is called *astigmatism*. Astigmatism is usually the result of an asymmetric bowing of the cornea, but it can result from defects in the cornea, lens, or the retina. Lens correction is available to sharpen focus in case of such refractive error.

Disorders of Accommodation

Because the retina is at a fixed distance from the lens, adjustability in the refractive power of the lens is needed so that a clear image is maintained as gaze is shifted from a far to a near object. The process by which the refractive power of the lens is increased, and the diverging light rays are bent more sharply, is called *accommodation*. Accommodation is neurologically associated with convergence of the eyes and pupillary constriction, and results from thickening of the lens through contraction of the ciliary muscle. Contraction of the ciliary muscles is controlled mainly by the parasympathetic fibers of the oculomotor cranial nerve (CN III). In near vision, pupillary constriction (*i.e.*, miosis) improves the clarity of the retinal image. This must be balanced against the resultant decrease in light intensity reaching the retina. During changes from near to far vision, pupillary dilation partially compensates for the reduced size of the retinal image by increasing the light entering the pupil. A third component of accommodation involves the reflex narrowing of the palpebral opening during near vision and widening during far vision.

Paralysis of the ciliary muscle, with loss of accommodation, is called *cycloplegia*. Pharmacologic cycloplegia is sometimes necessary to aid refractive examination of the eye, especially in small children who are unable to hold a steady degree of accommodation during the examination. Lens shape is totally controlled by the pretectal region and the parasympathetic pathways through the oculomotor nerve to the ciliary muscle. Accommodation is lost with destruction of this pathway.

The term *presbyopia* refers to a decrease in accommodation that occurs because of aging. The lens consists of transparent fibers arranged in concentric layers, of which the external layers are the newest and softest. No loss of lens fibers occurs with aging; instead, additional fibers are added to the outermost portion of the lens. As the lens ages, it thickens, and its fibers become less elastic, so that the range of focus or accommodation is diminished to the point where reading glasses become necessary for near vision.

Cataracts

A cataract is a lens opacity that interferes with the transmission of light to the retina. It has been estimated that 13 million persons in the United States 40 years of age or older are visually disabled because of cataracts.[1] Cataracts are the most common cause of age-related visual loss in the world; they are found in approximately 50% of those between 65 and 74 years of age, and in 70% of those older than 75 years.[1] Cataract surgery is the most common surgical procedure covered by Medicare, with more than 1 million procedures performed annually. More than 90% of persons undergoing cataract surgery experience visual improvement if there is no ocular comorbidity.[25]

Causes and Types of Cataracts

The cause of cataract development is thought to be multifactorial, with different factors being associated with different types of opacities.[26] The pathogenesis of cataracts is not completely understood. Several risk factors have been proposed, including the effects of aging, genetic influences, environmental and metabolic influences, drugs, and injury.[27] Metabolically induced cataracts are caused by disorders of carbohydrate metabolism (diabetes) or inborn errors of metabolism.[27] Long-term exposure to sunlight (ultraviolet B radiation) and heavy smoking have been associated with increased risk of cataract formation.[27] Occasionally, cataracts occur as a developmental defect (*i.e.,* congenital cataracts) or secondary to trauma or diseases.

Cataracts can result from several drugs. Corticosteroids drugs have been implicated as causative agents in cataract formation. Both systemic and inhaled corticosteroids have been cited as risk factors.[28,29] Other drugs associated with cataracts include the phenothiazines, amiodarone, and strong miotic ophthalmic drugs such as phospholine iodine.[27] Frequent examination of lens transparency should accompany the use of these and any other medications with potential cataract-forming effects.

Traumatic Cataract. Traumatic cataracts are usually caused by foreign body injury to the lens or blunt trauma to the eye. Foreign body injury that interrupts the lens capsule allows aqueous and vitreous humor to enter the lens and initiate cataract formation. Other causes of traumatic cataract are overexposure to heat (*e.g.,* glassblower cataract) or to ionizing radiation. The radiation dose necessary to cause a cataract varies with the amount and type of energy; younger lenses are most vulnerable.

Congenital Cataract. A congenital cataract is one that is present at birth. Among the causes of congenital cataracts are genetic defects, toxic environmental agents, and viruses such as rubella.[11] Cataracts and other developmental defects of the ocular apparatus depend on the total dose of the agent and the embryonic stage at the time of exposure. During the last trimester of fetal life, genetically or environmentally influenced malformation of the superficial lens fibers can occur. Congenital lens opacities may occur in children of diabetic mothers.

Most congenital cataracts are not progressive and are not dense enough to cause significant visual impairment. However, if the cataracts are bilateral and the opacity is significant, lens extraction should be done on one eye by the age of 2 months to permit the development of vision (see later section on amblyopia). If the surgery is successful, the contralateral lens should be removed soon after.

Senile Cataract. Cataracts are the most common cause of age-related vision loss in the world.[30] With normal aging, the nucleus and the cortex of the lens enlarge as new fibers are formed in the cortical zones of the lens. In the nucleus, the old fibers become more compressed and dehydrated. Metabolic changes occur and lens proteins become more insoluble, and concentrations of calcium, sodium, potassium, and phosphate increase. During the early stages of cataract formation, a yellow pigment and vacuoles accumulate in the lens fibers. The unfolding of protein molecules, cross-

linking of sulfhydryl groups, and conversion of soluble to insoluble proteins lead to the loss of lens transparency. The onset is gradual, and the only symptoms are increasingly blurred vision and visual distortion.

Manifestations

The manifestations of cataract depend on the extent of opacity and whether the defect is bilateral or unilateral. With the exception of traumatic or congenital cataract, most cataracts are bilateral. Age-related cataracts, which are the most common type, are characterized by increasingly blurred vision and visual distortion (see Fig. 54-1C). Visual acuity for far and near objects decreases. Dilation of the pupil in dim light improves vision. With nuclear cataracts (those involving the lens nucleus), the refractive power of the anterior segment often increases to produce an acquired myopia. Persons with hyperopia may experience a "second sight" or improved reading acuity until increasing opacity reduces acuity. Central lens opacities may divide the visual axis and cause an optical defect in which two or more blurred images are seen. Posterior subcapsular cataracts are located in the posterior cortical layer and usually involve the central visual axis. In addition to decreased visual acuity, cataracts tend to cause light entering the eye to be scattered, thereby producing glare or the abnormal presence of light in the visual field.

Diagnosis and Treatment

Diagnosis of cataract is based on ophthalmoscopic examination and the degree of visual impairment on the Snellen vision test. On ophthalmoscopic examination, cataracts may appear as a gross opacity filling the pupillary aperture or as an opacity silhouetted against the red background of the fundus. A Snellen test acuity of 20/50 is a common requirement for drivers of motor vehicles so tests of potential vision (*i.e.,* the ability to see well after surgery) may be done to ensure that the visual loss can be corrected to necessary functional levels if the cataract were removed.

There is no effective medical treatment for cataract. Strong bifocals, magnification, appropriate lighting, and visual aids may be used as the cataract progresses. Surgery is the only treatment for correcting cataract-related vision loss. Surgery usually involves lens extraction and intraocular lens implantation. It is commonly performed on an outpatient basis with the use of local anesthesia. The use of extracapsular surgery, which leaves the posterior capsule of the lens intact, has significantly improved the outcomes of cataract surgery. The cataract lens is usually removed using phacoemulsification techniques.[26] Phacoemulsification involves ultrasonic fragmentation of the lens into fine pieces, which then are aspirated from the eye.

One of the greatest advances in cataract surgery has been the development of reliable intraocular implants. Monofocal intraocular lenses that correct for distance vision are available, and eyeglasses may be needed for near vision, although this has been addressed by the recent introduction of multifocal intraocular lenses.[26]

IN SUMMARY, the lens is a biconvex, avascular, colorless, and almost transparent structure suspended behind the iris. The shape of the lens is controlled by the ciliary muscle, which contracts and relaxes the zonule fibers, thus changing the tension on the lens capsule and altering the focus of the lens. Refraction, which refers to the ability to focus an object on the retina, depends on the size and shape of the eyeball and the cornea and on the focusing ability of the lens. Errors in refraction occur when the visual image is not focused on the retina because of individual differences in the size or shape of the eyeball or cornea. In hyperopia, or farsightedness, the image theoretically falls behind the retina. In myopia, or nearsightedness, the image falls in front of the retina. Accommodation is the process by which a clear image is maintained as the gaze is shifted from a far to a near object. It is associated with convergence of the eyes and pupillary constriction, and thickening of the lens results from contraction of the ciliary muscle. Presbyopia is a change in the lens that occurs because of aging such that the lens becomes thicker and less able to change shape and accommodate for near vision.

A cataract is a lens opacity. It can occur as the result of congenital influences, metabolic disturbances, infection, injury, and aging. The most common type of cataract is the senile cataract that occurs with aging. The treatment for a totally opaque or mature cataract is surgical extraction. An intraocular lens implant may be inserted during the surgical procedure to replace the removed lens; otherwise, thick convex lenses or contact lenses are used to compensate for the loss of lens function. ∎

DISORDERS OF THE VITREOUS AND RETINA

After completing this section of the chapter, you should be able to meet the following objectives:

- Relate the phagocytic function of the retinal pigment epithelium to the development of retinitis pigmentosa.
- Cite the manifestations and long-term visual effects of papilledema.
- Describe the pathogenesis of background and proliferative diabetic retinopathies and their mechanisms of visual impairment.
- Relate the role of posterior vitreous detachment to the development of retinal tears and detachment.
- Explain the pathology and visual changes associated with macular degeneration.

The posterior segment, comprising five sixths of the eyeball, contains the transparent vitreous humor and the neural retina. The innermost layer of the eyeball, the fundus, is visualized through the pupil with an ophthalmoscope.

Disorders of the Vitreous

Vitreous humor (*i.e.*, vitreous body) is a colorless, amorphous biologic gel that fills the posterior cavity of the eye (see Fig. 54-5). It consists of approximately 99% water, some salts, glycoproteins, proteoglycans, and dispersed collagen fibrils. The vitreous is attached to the ciliary body and the peripheral retina in the region of the ora serrata and to the periphery of the optic disk.

Disease, aging, and injury can disturb the factors that maintain the water of the vitreous humor in suspension, causing liquefaction of the gel to occur. With the loss of gel structure, fine fibers, membranes, and cellular debris develop. When this occurs, floaters (images) can often be noticed as these substances move within the vitreous cavity during head movement. In disease, blood vessels may grow from the surface of the retina or optic disk onto the posterior surface of the vitreous, and blood may fill the vitreous cavity.

In a procedure called a *vitrectomy*, the removal and replacement of the vitreous with a balanced saline solution can restore sight in some persons with vitreous opacities resulting from hemorrhage or vitreoretinal membrane formations that cause legal blindness. Using this procedure, a small probe with a cutting tip is used to remove the opaque vitreous and membranes. The procedure is difficult and requires complex instrumentation. It is of no value if the retina is not functional.

Disorders of the Retina

The function of the retina is to receive visual images, partially analyze them, and transmit this modified information to the brain.[16] It is composed of two layers: the inner neural retina that contains the photoreceptors and an outer melanin-containing layer that rests on, and is firmly attached to the choriocapillaris, the capillary layer of the choroid. A non–light-sensitive portion of the retina, along with the retinal pigment epithelium, continues anteriorly to form the posterior surface of the iris. A wavy border called the *ora serrata* exists at the junction between the light-sensitive and the non–light-sensitive retinas. Separating the vascular portion of the choroid from pigmented cells of the retina is a thin layer of elastic tissue, the *Bruch membrane*, which contains collagen fibrils in its superficial and deep portions. Cells of the pigmented layer receive their nourishment by diffusion from the choriocapillaris.

Disorders of the retina and its function include derangements of the pigment epithelium (*e.g.*, retinitis pigmentosa); ischemic conditions caused by disorders of the retinal blood supply; disorders of the retinal vessels such as retinopathies that cause hemorrhage and the development of opacities; separation of the pigment and sensory layers of the retina (*i.e.*, retinal detachment); abnormalities of the Bruch membrane and choroid (*e.g.*, macular degeneration); and malignant tumors of the nuclear layer of the retina (*i.e.*, retinoblastoma). Because the retina has no pain fibers, most diseases of the retina are painless and do not cause redness of the eye.

The Neural Retina

The neural retina is composed of three layers of neurons: a posterior layer of photoreceptors, a middle layer of bipolar cells, and an inner layer of ganglion cells that communicate with the photoreceptors (Fig. 54-9). A pattern of light on the retina falls on a massive array of photoreceptors. These photoreceptors synapse with bipolar and other interneurons before action potentials in ganglion cells relay the message to specific regions of the brain and the brain stem associated with vision. For rods, this microcircuitry involves the convergence of signals from many rods on a single ganglion cell. This arrangement maximizes spatial summation and the detection of stimulated (light versus dark) receptors. The interneurons, composed of horizontal and amacrine cells, have cell bodies in the bipolar layer, and they play an important role in modulating retinal function. A superficial marginal layer contains the axons of the ganglion cells as they collect and leave the eye through the optic nerve. These fibers lie beside the vitreous humor. Light must pass through the transparent inner layers of the sensory retina before it reaches the photoreceptors.

Photoreceptors

Two types of photoreceptors are present in the retina: rods, capable of black–white discrimination, and cones, capable of color discrimination.[16] Both types of photoreceptors are thin, elongated, mitochondria-filled cells with a single, highly modified cilium (Fig. 54-10). The cilium has a short base, or inner segment, and a highly modified outer segment. The plasma membrane of the outer segment is tightly folded to form membranous disks (rods) or conical shapes (cones) containing visual pigment. These disks are continuously synthesized at the base of the outer segment and shed at the distal end. Discarded membranes are phagocytized by the retinal pigment cells. If this phagocytosis is disrupted, as in retinitis pigmentosa, the sensory retina degenerates.

Rods. Photoreception involves the transduction of light energy into an altered ionic membrane potential of the rod cell. Light passing through the eye penetrates the nearly transparent neural elements to produce decomposition of the photochemical substance (visual pigment) called *rhodopsin* in the outer segment of the rod. Light that is not trapped by a rhodopsin molecule is absorbed by the retinal pigment melanin or deeper choroid melanin. Rhodopsin consists of a protein called *opsin* and a vitamin A–derived pigment called *retinal*. During light stimulation, rhodopsin is broken down into its component parts, opsin and retinal; retinal subsequently is converted into vitamin A. The reconstitution of rhodopsin occurs during total darkness; vitamin A is transformed into retinal, and then opsin and retinal combine to form rhodopsin. Considerable stores of vitamin A are present in the retinal pigment cells and in the liver; therefore, a vitamin A deficiency must be present for weeks or months to affect the photoreceptive process. Reduced sensitivity to light, a symptom of vitamin A deficiency, initially affects night vision; however, this is quickly reversed by injection or ingestion of the vitamin.

Rod-based vision is particularly sensitive to detecting light, especially moving light stimuli, at the expense of clear pattern discrimination. Rod vision is particularly adapted for night and low-level illumination. Dark adaptation is the process by which rod sensitivity increases to the optimum level. This requires approximately 4 hours in total or near-total darkness and is referred to as scotopic vision (night vision). During daylight or high-intensity bombardment, the

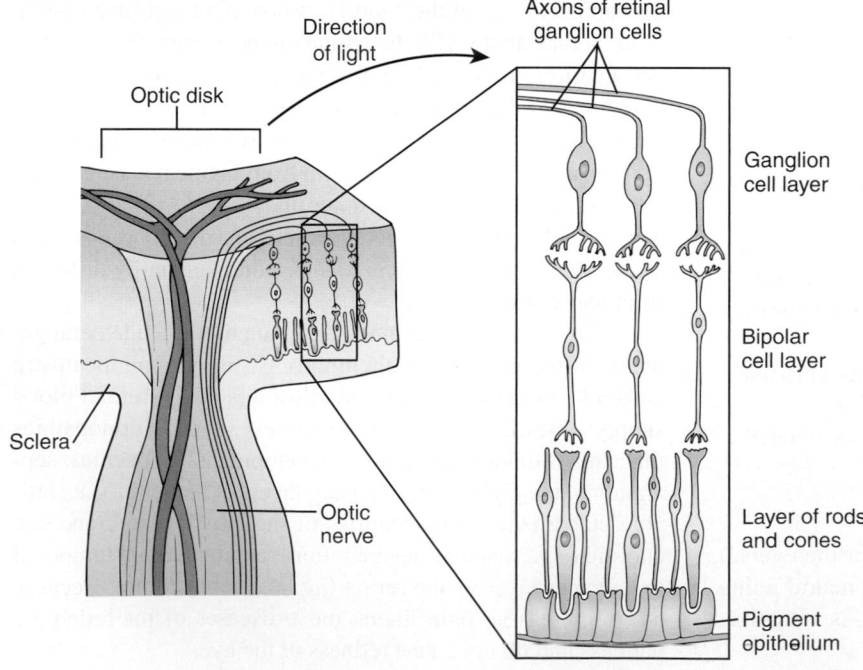

FIGURE 54-9 • Organization of the human retina. The optic pathway begins with photoreceptors (rods and cones) in the retina. The responses of the photoreceptors are transmitted by the bipolar cells to the ganglion cell layer of the retina.

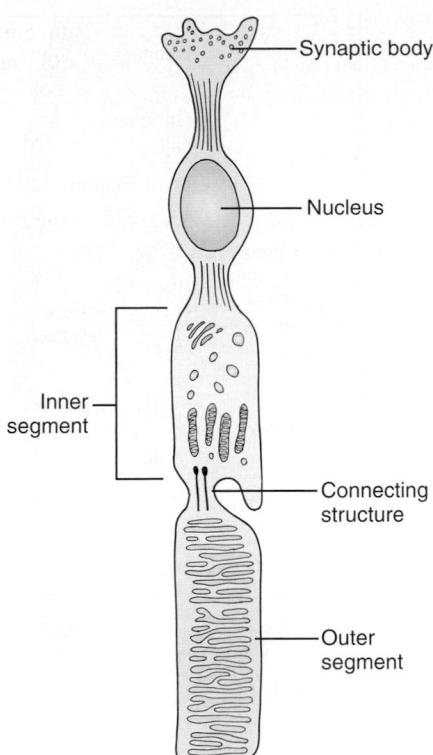

- Synaptic body
- Nucleus
- Inner segment
- Connecting structure
- Outer segment

FIGURE 54-10 • Retinal rod, showing its component parts and the distribution of its organelles. Its outer segment contains the disks (rods). The connecting structure joins the outer and inner segments. The inner segment contains the mitochondria, the ribosomal endoplasmic reticulum, the free ribosomes, and the Golgi saccules. The synaptic body is the site where the photoreceptor synapses with other nerve cells.

concentration of vitamin A increases, whereas the concentration of the photopigment retinal decreases. During dark adaptation, an increase in synthesis of retinal from vitamin A results in a higher concentration of rhodopsin available to capture light energy.

Cones and Color Sensitivity. Cone receptors that are selectively sensitive to different wavelengths of light provide the basis for color vision. Three types of cones, or cone-color systems, respond to the blue, green, and red portions of the visible electromagnetic spectrum. This selectivity reflects the presence of one of three color-sensitive molecules to which the photochemical substance (visual pigment) is bound. The decomposition and reconstitution processes of the cone visual pigments are believed to be similar to that of the rods. The color a person perceives depends on which set of cones or combination of sets of cones is stimulated in a given image.

Cones do not have the dark adaptation capability of rods. Consequently, the dark-adapted eye is a rod receptor eye with only black-gray-white discrimination (*scotopic* or *night vision*). The light-adapted eye (*photopic vision*) adds the capacity for color discrimination. Rhodopsin has its maximum sensitivity in the blue-green region of the electromagnetic spectrum. If red

lenses are worn in daylight, the red cones (and green cones to some extent) are in use, whereas the rods and blue cones are essentially in the dark, and therefore dark adaptation proceeds. This method is used by military and night-duty airport control tower personnel to allow adaptation to take place before they go on duty in the dark.

Macula and Fovea. An area approximately 1.5 mm in diameter near the center of the retina, called the *macula lutea* (*i.e.*, "yellow spot"), is especially adapted for acute and detailed vision.[16] This area is composed entirely of cones. In the central portion of the macula, the *fovea centralis* (foveola), the blood vessels and innermost layers are displaced to one side instead of resting on top of the cones (Fig. 54-11). This allows light to pass unimpeded to the cones without passing through several layers of the retina. Of the approximately 6.4 million cones in the retina, 200,000 are located in the fovea. The density of cones drops off rapidly away from the fovea. Rods are not present in the fovea, but their numbers increase as the cones decrease in density toward the periphery of the retina.

Color Blindness. "Color blindness" is a misnomer for a condition in which persons appear to confuse or mismatch colors, or experience reduced acuity for color discrimination. Such persons are often unaware of their defect until they attempt to discriminate between red and green traffic lights or show difficulty matching colors. Color blindness is inherited as an X-linked deficiency of a specific type of retinal photoreceptor. The most common abnormality is red-green color blindness. The deficiency is usually partial but can be complete. Rarely are two of the color mechanisms missing; when this occurs, usually red and green are missing. Complete lack of color discrimination is rare; for such people, the world is experienced entirely as black, gray, and white.

The genetically color-blind person has never experienced the full range of normal color vision and is unaware of what he or she is missing. Color discrimination is necessary for everyday living, and color-blind persons, knowingly or unknowingly, make color discriminations based on other criteria, such as brightness or position. For example, the red light of a traffic signal is always the upper light, and the green is the lower light. Color-blind persons experience difficulties when brightness differences are small and discrimination must be based on hue and saturation qualities.

Retinitis Pigmentosa. Retinitis pigmentosa represents a group of hereditary diseases that cause slow degenerative changes in the retinal photoreceptors. The disease can be inherited as an autosomal dominant (30% to 40% of cases), autosomal recessive (50% to 60%), or sex-linked (5% to 15%) trait. With advances in genetics technology, there are now 36 known or predicted retinitis pigmentosa genes.[31] The group of genes most commonly mutated encodes proteins in the visual cascade of the photoreceptor outer segment. Although retinitis pigmentosa is a disease usually confined to the eye, approximately 20% to

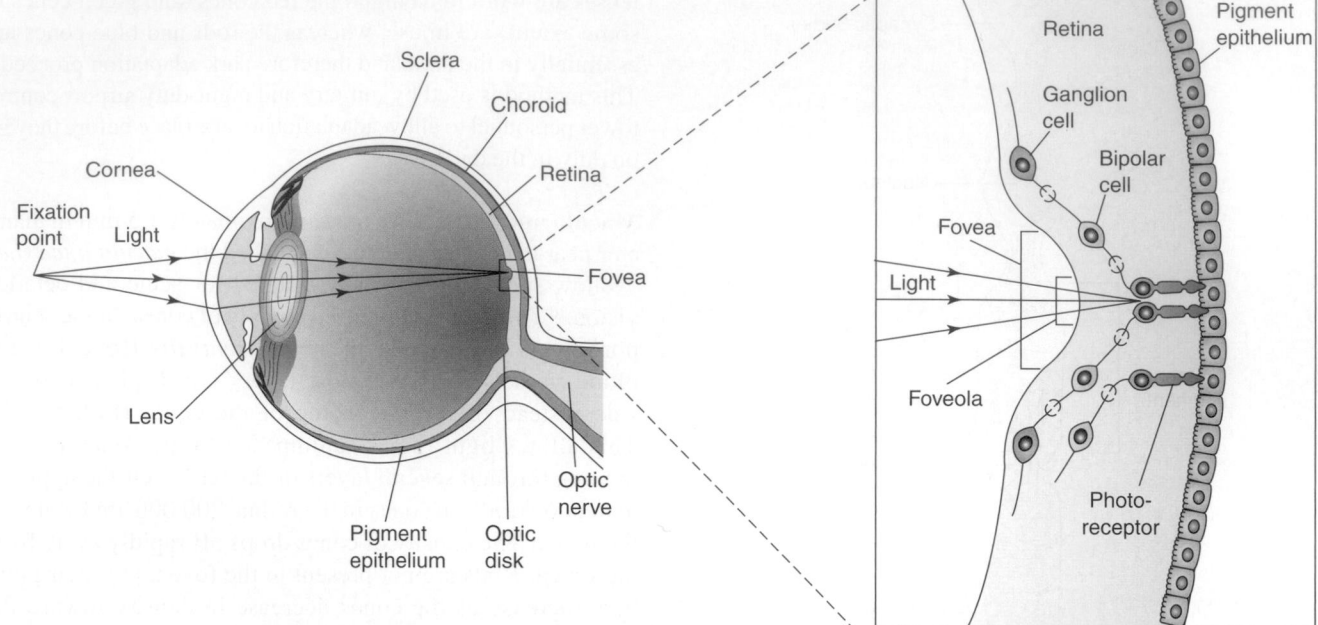

FIGURE 54-11 • Location of fovea in the retina. (From Kandel E. R., Schwartz J. H., Jessel T. M. [1991]. *Principles of neural science* [3rd ed.]. New York: Elsevier.)

30% of persons have associated nonocular disease. Usher syndrome, in which retinitis pigmentosa is associated with hearing impairment, is the most frequent of these combined syndromes.[31] The hearing loss can be either profound, present at birth, and associated with vestibular ataxia, or moderate to mild and nonprogressive.

In typical cases, known as *rod–cone retinitis pigmentosa*, the rods are the predominantly affected photoreceptor cells. This generally produces a number of characteristic clinical symptoms, including night blindness, which is usually an early symptom, and bilateral symmetric loss of mid-peripheral fields. Although there is relative preservation of macular vision, the visual field defects gradually increase both centrally and peripherally. With progression, cone photoreceptor cells are also affected and day vision and central visual acuity are compromised. The rate of visual failure is variable. Some people are severely visually handicapped before the age of 20 years, whereas others experience few symptomatic visual deficits even after 60 years of age.[31]

Disorders of Retinal Blood Supply

The blood supply for the retina is derived from two sources: the choriocapillaris (*i.e.,* the capillary layer of the choroid) and branches of the central retinal artery (Fig. 54-12). Oxygen and other nutritional substances needed by the retina and its component parts (pigment cells, rods, and cones) are supplied by diffusion from blood vessels in the choroid. Because the choriocapillaris provides the only blood supply for the fovea centralis (*i.e.,* foveola), detachment of this part of the sensory retina from the pigment epithelium causes irreparable visual loss.

 DISORDERS OF THE RETINAL BLOOD SUPPLY

■ The blood supply for the retina is derived from the central retinal artery, which supplies blood flow for the entire inside of the retina, and from vessels in the choroid, which supply the rods and cones.

■ The retinopathies, which are disorders of the retinal vessels, interrupt blood flow to the visual receptors, leading to visual impairment.

■ Retinal detachment separates the visual receptors from the choroid, which provides their major blood supply.

The bipolar, horizontal, amacrine, and ganglion cells, and the ganglion cell axons that gather at the optic disk, are supplied by branches of the retinal artery.[32] The central artery of the retina is a branch of the ophthalmic artery. It enters the globe through the optic disk. Branches of this artery radiate over the entire retina, except the central fovea, which is surrounded by, but is not crossed by, arterial branches. The central artery of the retina is an end artery, meaning that it does not anastomose with other arteries. This is critical because an infarct in this artery will totally deprive distal structures of their vascular supply. Retinal veins follow a distribution parallel to the arterial branches and carry venous blood

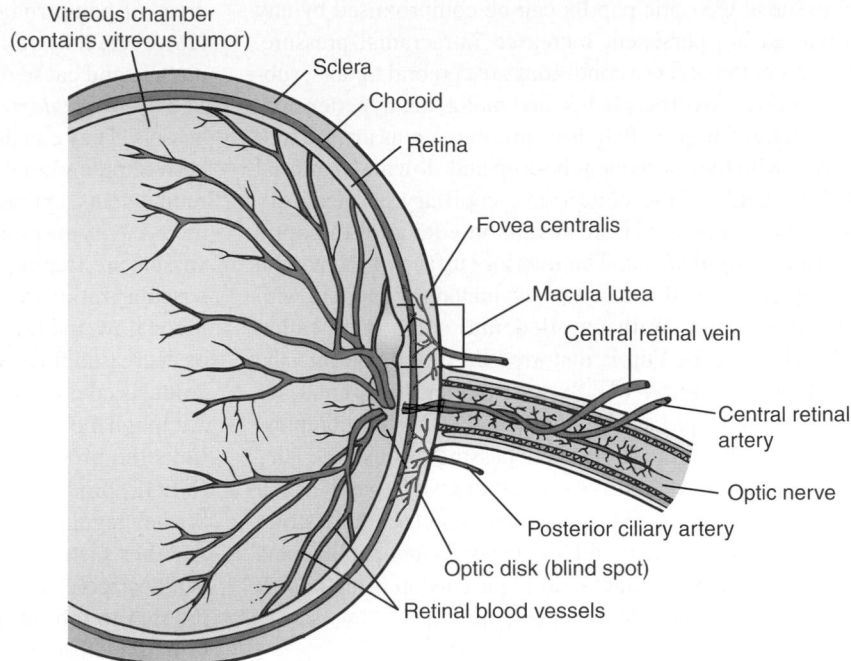

Vitreous chamber
(contains vitreous humor)

Sclera

Choroid

Retina

Fovea centralis

Macula lutea

Central retinal vein

Central retinal artery

Optic nerve

Posterior ciliary artery

Optic disk (blind spot)

Retinal blood vessels

FIGURE 54-12 • Retinal circulation.

to the central vein of the retina, which exits the back of the eye through the optic disk.

Funduscopic examination of the eye with an ophthalmoscope provides an opportunity to examine the retinal blood vessels and other aspects of the retina (Fig. 54-13). Because the retina is an embryonic outgrowth of the brain and the blood vessels are to a considerable extent representative of brain blood vessels, the ophthalmoscopic examination of the fundus of the eye permits the study and diagnosis of metabolic and vascular diseases of the brain as well as pathologic processes that are specific to the retina.

Functioning of the retina, like that of other cellular portions of the central nervous system (CNS), depends on an oxygen supply from the vascular system. One of the earliest signs of decreased perfusion pressure in the head region is a graying-out or blackout of vision, which usually precedes loss of consciousness. This can occur during large increases in intrathoracic pressure, which interfere with the return of venous blood to the heart, as occurs with the Valsalva maneuver; with systemic hypotension; and during sudden postural changes (*e.g.,* postural hypotension).

Ischemia of the retina occurs during general circulatory collapse. If a person survives cardiopulmonary arrest, for instance, permanently decreased visual acuity can occur as a result of edema and the ischemic death of retinal neurons. This is followed by primary optic nerve atrophy proportional to the extent of ganglionic cell death. The ophthalmic artery, the source of the central artery of the retina, takes its origin from the internal carotid artery.[32] Intermittent retinal ischemia can accompany internal carotid or common carotid stenosis. *Amaurosis fugax* is characterized by transient episodes of monocular visual loss lasting 5 to 10 minutes.[32] Persons with the disorder often describe a curtain coming down from above or across their vision, usually with complete return of vision within seconds or minutes. Besides the vision loss, contralateral hemiplegia or sensory deficits may accompany the episodes. The condition, commonly due to emboli, is most often the result of carotid artery disease.[32]

Papilledema. The central retinal artery enters the eye through the optic papilla in the center of the optic nerve. An accompanying vein exits the eye along the same path. The entrance and exit of the central retinal artery and vein through the tough

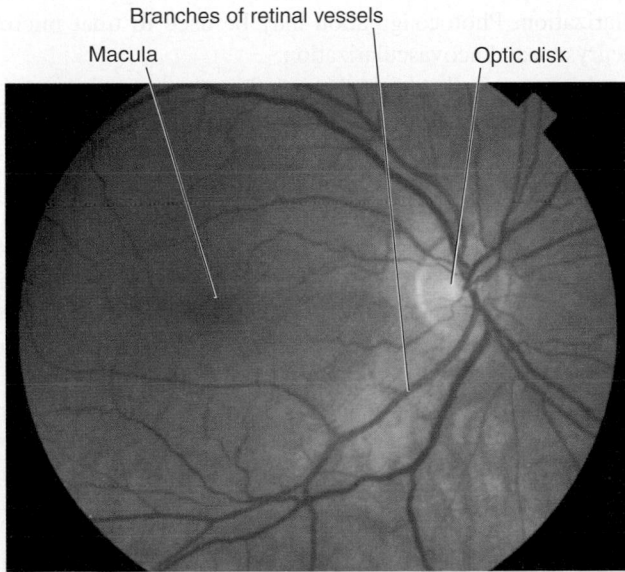

Branches of retinal vessels

Macula

Optic disk

FIGURE 54-13 • Funduscopic image of normal retina. (From Moore K. L., Dalley A. F. [2006]. *Clinically oriented anatomy* [5th ed., p. 967]. Philadelphia: Lippincott Williams & Wilkins.)

scleral tissue at the optic papilla can be compromised by any condition causing persistent increased intracranial pressure. The most common of these conditions are cerebral tumors, subdural hematomas, hydrocephalus, and malignant hypertension.

Usually, the thin-walled, low-pressure veins are the first to collapse, with the consequent backup and slowing of arterial blood flow. Under these conditions, capillary permeability increases and leakage of fluid results in edema of the optic papilla, called *papilledema.* The interior surface of the papilla is normally cup-shaped and can be evaluated for cupping with an ophthalmoscope. With papilledema, sometimes called *choked disk,* the optic cup is distorted by protrusion into the interior of the eye (Fig. 54-14). Because this sign does not occur until the intracranial pressure is significantly elevated, compression damage to the optic nerve fibers passing through the lamina cribrosa may have begun. As a warning sign, papilledema occurs quite late. Unresolved papilledema results in the destruction of the optic nerve axons and blindness. Pseudopapilledema can result from benign intracranial hypertension or optic disk drusen (calcified deposits in the optic papilla).

Retinopathies

Disorders of the retinal vessels can result in microaneurysms, neovascularization, hemorrhage, and formation of retinal opacities. *Microaneurysms* are outpouchings of the retinal vasculature. On ophthalmoscopic examination, they appear as minute, unchanging red dots associated with blood vessels. These microaneurysms tend to leak plasma, resulting in localized edema that gives the retina a hazy appearance. Microaneurysms can be identified with certainty using fluorescein angiography; the fluorescein dye is injected intravenously, and the retinal vessels subsequently are photographed using a special ophthalmoscope and fundus camera. The microaneurysms may bleed, but

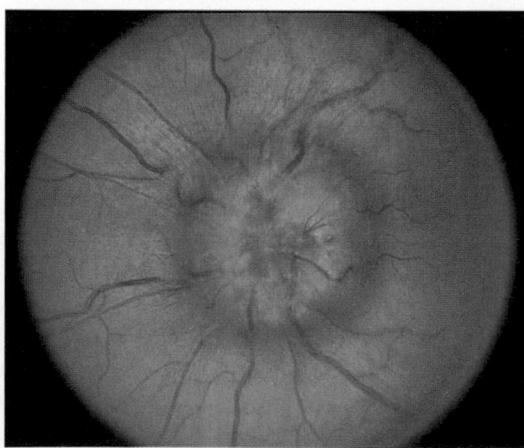

FIGURE 54-14 • Chronic papilledema. The optic nerve head is congested and protrudes anteriorly toward the interior of the eye. It has blurred margins, and vessels within it are poorly seen. (From Klintworth G. K. [2008]. The eye. In Rubin R., Strayer D. E. [Eds.], *Rubin's pathology: Clinicopathologic foundations of medicine* [5th ed., p. 1262]. Philadelphia: Lippincott-Williams & Wilkins.)

areas of hemorrhage and edema tend to clear spontaneously. However, they reduce visual acuity if they encroach on the macula and cause degeneration before they are absorbed.

Neovascularization involves the formation of new blood vessels. They can develop from the choriocapillaris, extending between the pigment layer and the sensory layer, or from the retinal veins, extending between the sensory retina and the vitreous cavity and sometimes into the vitreous. These new blood vessels are fragile, leak protein, and are likely to bleed. Neovascularization occurs in many conditions that impair retinal blood flow, including stasis because of hyperviscosity of blood or decreased flow, vascular occlusion, sickle cell disease, sarcoidosis, diabetes mellitus, and retinopathy of prematurity. Although the cause of neovascularization is uncertain, research links the process with a vascular endothelial growth factor (VEGF) produced by the lining of blood vessels.[33-35] Hypoxia is a key regulator of VEGF-induced retinal neovascularization. Another factor, pigment epithelium–derived factor (PEDF), synthesized elsewhere in the eye and throughout the body, is thought to inhibit neovascularization.[35] It is likely that other growth factors and signaling systems are also involved.

Hemorrhage can be preretinal, intraretinal, or subretinal. *Preretinal hemorrhages* occur between the retina and the vitreous. These hemorrhages are usually large because the blood vessels are only loosely restricted; they may be associated with a subarachnoid or subdural hemorrhage and are usually regarded as a serious manifestation of the disorder. They usually reabsorb without complications unless they penetrate into the vitreous. *Intraretinal hemorrhages* occur because of abnormalities of the retinal vessels, diseases of the blood, increased pressure in the retinal vessels, or vitreous traction on the vessels. Systemic causes include diabetes mellitus, hypertension, and blood dyscrasias. *Subretinal hemorrhages* are those that develop between the choroid and pigment layer of the retina. A common cause of subretinal hemorrhage is neovascularization. Photocoagulation may be used to treat microaneurysms and neovascularization.

Light normally passes through the transparent inner portions of the sensory retina before reaching the photoreceptors. *Opacities* such as hemorrhages, exudate, cotton-wool spots, edema, and tissue proliferation can produce a localized loss of transparency observable with an ophthalmoscope. Exudates are opacities resulting from inflammatory processes. The development of exudates often results in the destruction of the underlying retinal pigment and choroid layer. Deposits are localized opacities consisting of lipid-laden macrophages or accumulated cellular debris. Cotton-wool spots are retinal opacities with hazy, irregular outlines. They occur in the nerve fiber layer and contain cell organelles. Cotton-wool patches are associated with retinal trauma, severe anemia, papilledema, and diabetic retinopathy.

Diabetic Retinopathy. Diabetic retinopathy is the third leading cause of blindness for all ages in the industrialized countries of the world. It ranks first as the cause of newly reported cases of blindness in persons between the ages of 20 and 74 years. Advances in treatment have greatly reduced the risk of blindness from diabetes, but because diabetes is so common, retinopathy remains an important cause of visual impairment.

Diabetic retinopathy can be divided into two types: *nonproliferative* (*i.e.,* background) and *proliferative*.[35–38] Background or nonproliferative retinopathy is confined to the retina. It involves engorgement of the retinal veins, thickening of the capillary endothelial basement membrane, and development of capillary microaneurysms (Fig. 54-15A, B). Small intraretinal hemorrhages may develop and microinfarcts may cause cotton-wool spots and leakage of exudates. A sensation of glare (because of the scattering of light) is a common complaint. The most common cause of decreased vision in persons with background retinopathy is macular edema.[38] The edema is caused primarily by the breakdown of the inner blood-retina barrier at the level of the capillary endothelium, allowing leakage of fluid and plasma constituents into the surrounding retina.

Proliferative diabetic retinopathy represents a more severe retinal change than background retinopathy (Fig. 54-15C, D). It is characterized by formation of new, fragile blood vessels (*i.e.,*

neovascularization) at the disk and elsewhere in the retina. These vessels grow in front of the retina along the posterior surface of the vitreous or into the vitreous. They threaten vision in two ways. First, because they are abnormal, they often bleed easily, leaking blood into the vitreous cavity and decreasing visual acuity. Second, the blood vessels attach firmly to the retinal surface and posterior surface of the vitreous, such that normal movement of the vitreous may exert a pull on the retina, causing retinal detachment and progressive blindness. Because early proliferative diabetic retinopathy is likely to be asymptomatic, it must be identified early, before bleeding occurs and obscures the view of the fundus or leads to fibrosis and retinal detachment.

The cause of diabetic retinopathy is uncertain. Several biochemical mechanisms have been proposed as explanations for the development and progression of diabetic retinopathy and have led to exploration of possible treatments.[35] However, except for the demonstration that chronically elevated levels of blood glucose contribute to the development and progression of retinopathy and other complications of diabetes, no mechanism can be regarded as established. The increased expression

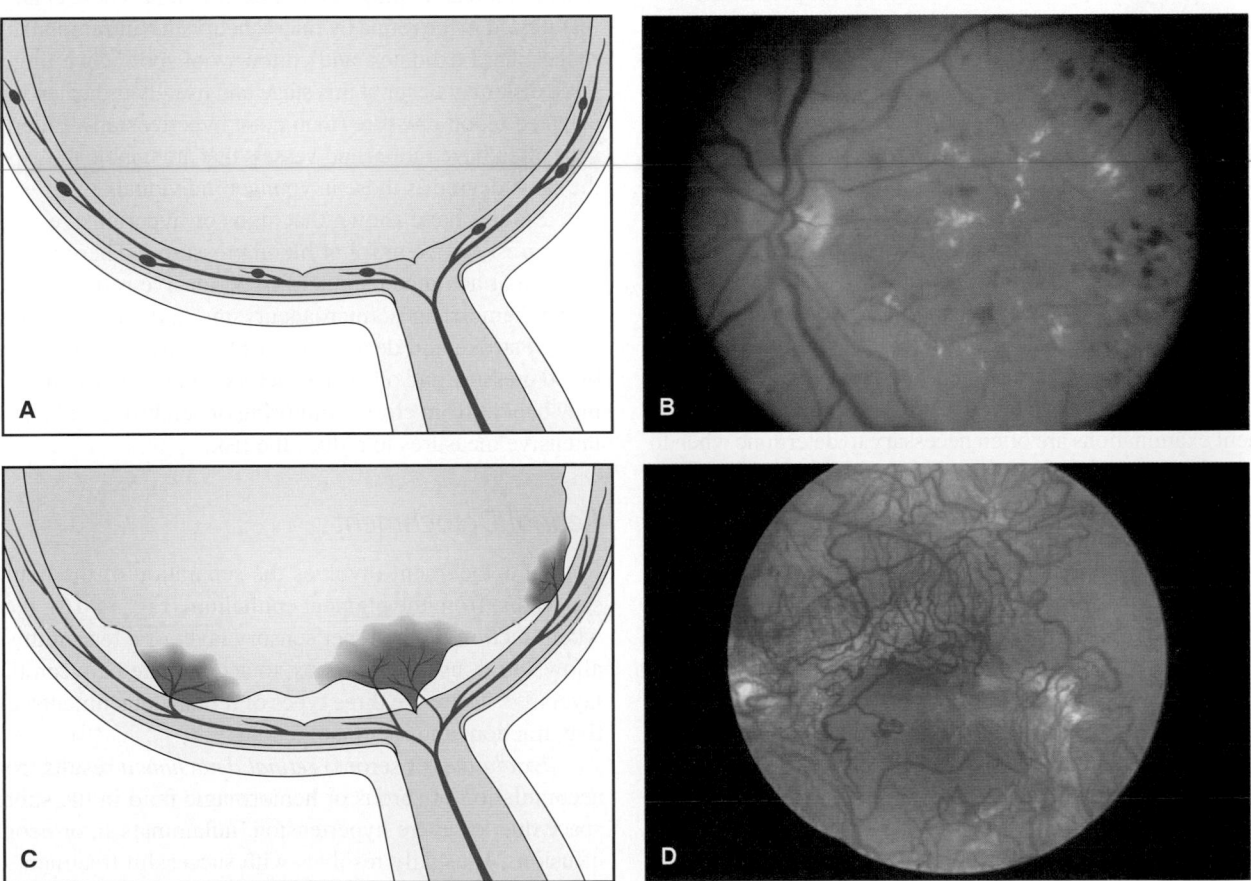

FIGURE 54-15 • (**A**) Nonproliferative (background) retinopathy showing microaneurysms. (**B**) Ocular fundus of a patient with background diabetic retinopathy. Several yellowish "hard" exudates (which are rich in lipids) and several relatively small retinal hemorrhages are present. (**C**) Proliferative retinopathy. (**D**) Ocular fundus in a patient with proliferative retinopathy. A vascular frond (branching pattern of preretinal neovascularization) has extended anterior to the retina. (**B** and **D** from Klintworth G. K. [2008]. The eye. In Rubin R., Strayer D. E. [Eds.], *Rubin's pathology: Clinicopathologic foundations of medicine* [5th ed., p. 1257]. Philadelphia: Lippincott-Williams & Wilkins.)

of VEGF has become a focus of current research on the patho-genesis of diabetic retinopathy as well as other retinal and choroidal vascular disorders. Hypertension is also thought to increase the risk for the development and progression of dia-betic retinopathy. Recent evidence suggests that the renin-angiotensin system is activated by chronically elevated levels of blood glucose. Angiotensin II increases vascular permeabil-ity and promotes angiogenesis, and it has been suggested that a relationship may exist between angiotensin II and VEGF in ocular tissues.[39] Accordingly, angiotensin-converting enzyme inhibitors or receptor blockers may be useful agents for pre-venting the progression of diabetic retinopathy. In addition to chronic hyperglycemia and hypertension, several studies have indicated the association of diabetic exudative retinopathy with hypercholesteremia and combined inflammatory mediators on the retinal microvasculature.[36]

Preventing diabetic retinopathy from developing or pro-gressing is considered the best approach to preserving vision. Growing evidence suggests that careful control of blood glu-cose levels in persons with diabetes mellitus may retard the onset and progression of retinopathy. The Diabetes Control and Complications Trial Research Group demonstrated that intensive management of persons with type 1 diabetes to main-tain blood glucose at near-normal levels reduced the risk of retinopathy by 76% in persons with no retinopathy and slowed the progress by 54% in persons with early disease.[40] There also is a need for intensive management of hypertension and hyper-lipidemia, both of which have been shown to increase the risk of diabetic retinopathy in persons with diabetes.[36]

Regular dilated eye examinations are an effective approach to detecting and treating vision-threatening diabetic retinopa-thy. Current guidelines recommend that persons with diabetes have yearly eye examinations, although deviations from this guideline are appropriate in certain low-risk groups.[37] For per-sons with moderate to severe nonproliferative retinopathy, more frequent examinations are often necessary to determine when to initiate treatment. Persons with any levels of macular edema, severe nonproliferative diabetic retinopathy, or any prolifera-tive retinopathy require the prompt care of an ophthalmologist who is knowledgeable and experienced in the management and treatment of diabetic retinopathy. Women with preexist-ing diabetes who plan to become pregnant should have a com-prehensive eye examination and be counseled about the risk for initiation or progression of diabetic retinopathy. Women with diabetes who become pregnant should have a comprehensive eye examination in the first trimester and close follow-up throughout pregnancy.

Photocoagulation using an argon laser provides the major direct treatment modality for diabetic retinopathy.[8,33] Treat-ment strategies include laser photocoagulation applied directly to leaking microaneurysms and grid photocoagulation with a checkerboard pattern of laser burns applied to diffuse areas of leakage and thickening.[33] Because laser photocoagulation destroys the proliferating vessels and the ischemic retina, it reduces the stimulus for further neovascularization. However, photocoagulation of neovascularization near the disk is not recommended.[33] Vitrectomy has proved effective in removing vitreous hemorrhage and severing vitreoretinal membranes that develop.[37]

Because of the limitations of current treatment measures, new pharmacologic therapies that target the underlying bio-chemical mechanisms that cause diabetic retinopathy are being investigated. Recent interest has focused on intravitreal corti-costeroid or VEGF inhibitor injections[37] (discussed in the sec-tion on Macular Degeneration).

Hypertensive Retinopathy. As with other blood vessels in the body, the retinal vessels undergo changes in response to chron-ically elevated blood pressure. In the initial, vasoconstrictor stage, there is vasospasm and an increase in retinal arterial tone because of local autoregulatory mechanisms. On ophthal-moscopy, this stage is represented by a general narrowing of the retinal arterioles. Persistently elevated blood pressure results in the compensatory thickening of arteriolar walls, which effec-tively reduces capillary perfusion pressure.[41] With severe, uncontrolled hypertension, there is disruption of the blood-retina barrier, necrosis of smooth muscle and endothelial cells, exuda-tion of blood and lipids, and retinal ischemia. These changes are manifested in the retina by microaneurysms, intraretinal hemor-rhages, hard exudates, and cotton-wool spots. Swelling of the optic disk may occur at this stage and usually indicates severely elevated blood pressure (malignant hypertension). Elderly per-sons often have more rigid vessels that are unable to respond to the same degree as those in younger individuals.

Studies have shown that signs of hypertensive retinopa-thy regress with control of blood pressure.[41] There is also evi-dence that advanced signs of hypertensive retinopathy (*e.g.,* retinal hemorrhages, microaneurysms, and cotton-wool spots) predict stroke and death from stroke independent of elevated blood pressure and other risk factors.[41] Persons with these signs may benefit from close monitoring of cerebrovascular risk and intensive measures to reduce the risk.

Retinal Detachment

Retinal detachment involves the separation of the neurosen-sory retina from the pigment epithelium (Fig. 54-16). It occurs when traction on the inner sensory layer or a tear in this layer allows fluid, usually vitreous, to accumulate between the two layers.[33,42] There are three types of retinal detachments: exuda-tive, traction, and rhegmatogenous.[42]

Exudative (or serous) *retinal detachment* results from the accumulation of serous or hemorrhagic fluid in the subretinal space due to severe hypertension, inflammation, or neoplastic effusions. It usually resolves with successful treatment of the underlying disease and without visual impairment. *Traction retinal attachment* occurs with mechanical forces on the retina, usually mediated by fibrotic tissue, resulting from previous hemorrhage (*e.g.,* from diabetic retinopathy), injury, infection, or inflammation. Intraocular surgery such as cataract extraction may produce traction on the peripheral retina that causes even-tual detachment months or even years after surgery. Correction

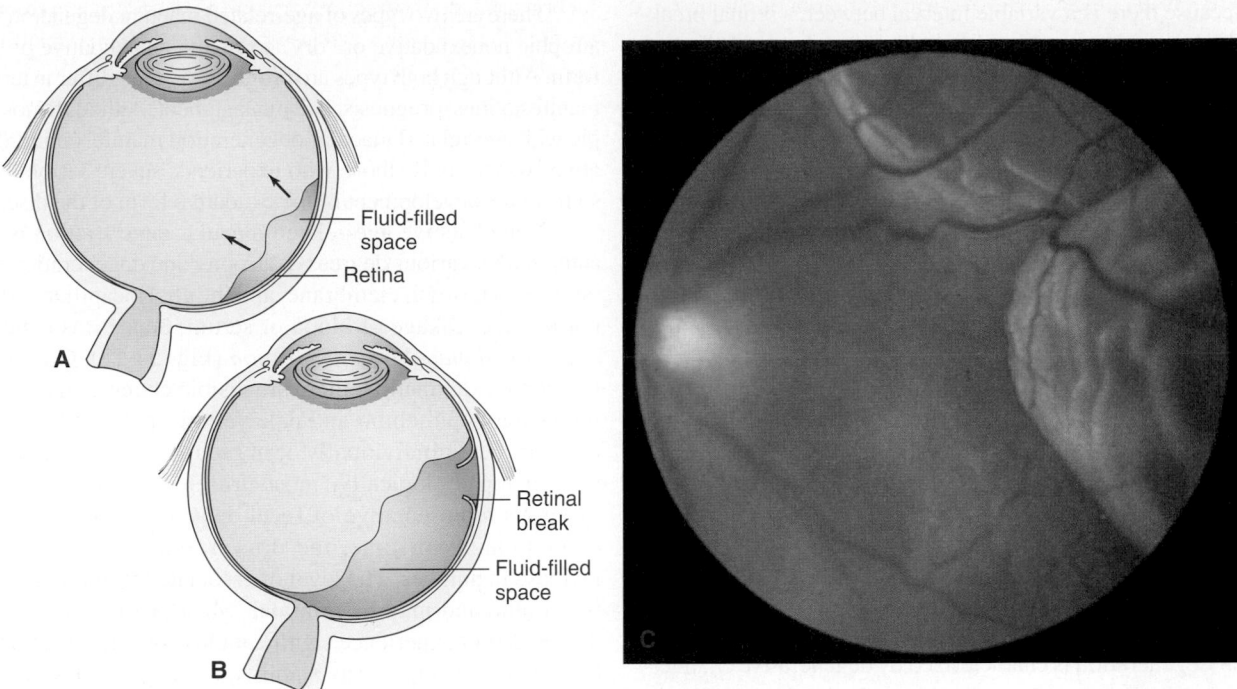

FIGURE 54-16 • Pathogenesis of rhegmatogenous retinal detachment. (**A**) Changes in the vitreous structure cause it to shrink and separate from the retina, causing posterior vitreous detachment; (**B**) sustained fluid collection and tractional forces cause the retina to tear (rhegmatogenous retinal detachment). (**C**) Ophthalmoscopic photograph of retinal detachment. (**C** From Moore K. L., Dalley A. F. [2006]. *Clinically oriented anatomy* [5th ed., p. 967]. Philadelphia: Lippincott Williams & Wilkins).

of traction retinal detachment requires disengaging scar tissue from the retinal surface, and vision outcomes are often poor.

Rhegmatogenous detachment (*rhegma* is the Greek for "rent" or "hole") is the most common type of retinal detachment. The vitreous is a hydrated gel whose structure is maintained by a collagenous and mucopolysaccharide matrix. As persons age, this macromolecular network begins to liquefy and collapse. As this occurs, the vitreous shrinks and partly separates from the retinal surface, a condition known as *posterior vitreous detachment* (see Fig. 54-16). Rhegmatogenous detachment occurs when the liquid vitreous enters the subretinal space through the retinal tear. Detachment of the neural retina from the retinal pigment layer separates the receptors from their major blood supply, the choroid. If retinal detachment continues for some time, permanent destruction and blindness of that part of the retina occur.

Risk factors for retinal detachment include advancing age and myopia. Approximately one in four persons between the ages of 61 and 70 years develops a posterior vitreous detachment. In about 10% to 15% of these persons, a retinal tear or hole forms as the vitreous pulls away from the retina, especially in the periphery where the retina is thinner.[42] Persons with high grades of myopia may have abnormalities in the peripheral retina that predispose to sudden detachment. In moderate to severe myopia or nearsightedness, the axial (anteroposterior) length of the eye is increased, resulting in an egg-shaped globe. As a result, there is greater vitreoretinal traction, and posterior

vitreous detachment may occur at a younger age than in persons without myopia. Also, the retina tends to be thinner and more prone to formation of a hole or tear.[42] Other, less common risk factors include a family history of retinal detachment, a history of congenital eye disease (glaucoma, cataracts), and hereditary vitreopathies with abnormal vitreous gel.

The primary symptom of retinal detachment consists of painless changes in vision. Commonly, flashing lights or sparks, followed by small floaters or spots in the field of vision, occur as the vitreous pulls away from the posterior pole of the eye. As detachment progresses, the person perceives a shadow or dark curtain progressing across the visual field. Because the process begins in the periphery and spreads circumferentially and posteriorly, initial visual disturbances may involve only one quadrant of the visual field. Large peripheral detachments may occur without involvement of the macula, so that visual acuity remains unaffected.

Diagnosis is based on a history of visual disturbances (*e.g.,* presence of floaters, luminous rays or light flashes) and the ophthalmoscopic appearance of the retina. The direct (hand-held) ophthalmoscope is useful in detecting an altered red reflex sometimes associated with retinal detachment. However, because the view is narrow, a negative examination with direct ophthalmoscopy cannot exclude the diagnosis of retinal detachment. Ophthalmologists and optometrists use indirect examination techniques that greatly enhance visualization of the peripheral retina.[42]

Because there is a variable interval between a retinal break and retinal detachment, treatment methods focus on early detection and prevention of further vitreous detachment and retinal tear formation. Symptomatic retinal breaks are usually treated with laser or cryotherapy to seal the retinal tears so that the vitreous can no longer leak into the subretinal space. The treatment is more than 95% effective in preventing progression of a retinal tear and preventing retinal detachment.[42] The primary treatment of traction retinal detachment is vitreoretinal surgery and may involve vitrectomy, membrane removal, scleral buckling, or pneumatic retinopexy. Scleral buckling is the primary surgical procedure performed to reattach the retina.[33,42] With scleral buckling, a piece of silicone (*i.e.,* the buckle) is sutured and infolded into the sclera, physically indenting the sclera so it contacts the separated pigment and retinal layers. A less invasive procedure, pneumatic retinopexy, involves the intraocular injection of an expandable gas instead of a piece of silicone to form the indentation.

Macular Degeneration

Macular degeneration is characterized by degenerative changes in the central portion of the retina (the macula) that result primarily in loss of central vision (see Fig. 54-1B). Age-related macular degeneration is the most common cause of reduced vision in the elderly population.[43–46] The causes of age-related macular degeneration are poorly understood. In addition to older age, identifiable risk factors include female sex, white race, and cigarette smoking. Increasing evidence suggests that genetic factors may also play a role.[47] Careful attention should be paid to cardiovascular risk factors, which appear to be more common in patients with age-related macular degeneration.

There are two types of age-related macular degeneration: an atrophic nonexudative or "dry" form and an exudative or "wet" form. Although both types are progressive, they differ in terms of manifestations, prognosis, and management. Although most people with age-related macular degeneration manifest nonproliferative changes only, those who experience severe vision loss do so from the development of the exudative form of the disease.[33]

Nonexudative age-related macular degeneration is characterized by various degrees of atrophy and degeneration of the outer retina, Bruch membrane, and the choriocapillaris. It does not involve leakage of blood or serum; hence it is called *dry age-related macular degeneration* (Fig. 54-17). On ophthalmoscopic examination, there are visible changes in the retinal pigmentary epithelium and pale yellow spots, called *drusen,* that may occur individually or in groups throughout the macula. Histopathologically, most drusen contain remnants of materials representative of focal detachment of the pigment epithelium. With time, the drusen enlarge, coalesce, and increase in number. The level of associated visual impairment is variable and may be minimal. Most people with macular drusen do not experience significant loss of central vision, and the atrophic changes may stabilize or progress slowly. However, people with the nonexudative form of age-related macular degeneration need to be followed closely because the exudative stage may develop suddenly, at any time. Careful monitoring for metamorphopsia, or distorted vision of straight lines, can aid in the early detection of retinal damage.

The exudative or "wet form" of macular degeneration is characterized by the formation of a choroidal neovascular membrane that separates the pigmented epithelium from the neuroretina. These new blood vessels have weaker walls than normal and are prone to leakage. The leakage of serous or

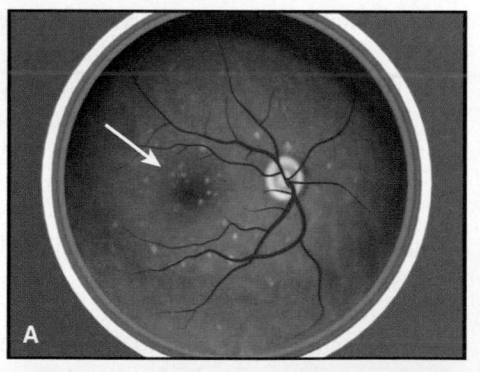
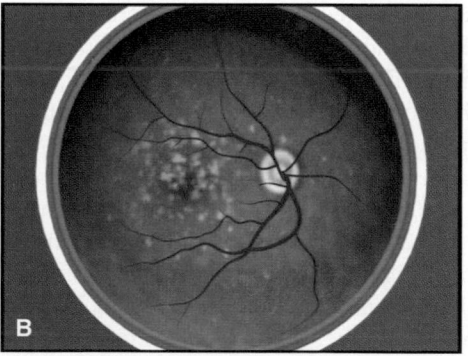
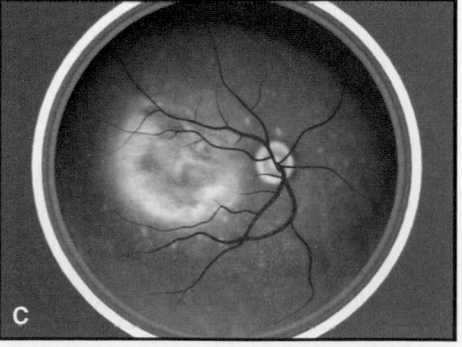

FIGURE 54.17 • Funduscopic view of different stages of age-related macular degeneration (AMD). (**A**) Early intermediate AMD (*white arrow*), (**B**) intermediate AMD, (**C**) advanced AMD with fibrosis. (From the National Eye Institute, National Institutes of Health.)

hemorrhagic fluid into the subretinal space causes separation of the pigmented epithelium from the neurosensory retina. Over time, the subretinal hemorrhages organize to form scar tissue, causing death of the underlying retinal tissue and loss of all visual function in the corresponding macular area (see Fig. 54-17). The early stages of subretinal neovascularization may be difficult to detect with an ophthalmoscope. Therefore, there is a need to be alert for recent or sudden changes in central vision, blurred vision, or scotomata in persons with evidence of age-related macular degeneration.

Although some subretinal neovascular membranes may regress spontaneously, the natural course of exudative macular degeneration is toward irreversible loss of central vision. Persons with late-stage disease often find it difficult to see at long distances (*e.g.*, in driving), do close work (*e.g.*, reading), see faces clearly, or distinguish colors. However, they may not be severely incapacitated because the peripheral retinal function usually remains intact. With the use of low-vision aids, many of them are able to continue many of their normal activities.

Effective therapies for exudative or wet-type macular degeneration include thermal laser photocoagulation, photodynamic therapy, intravitreal and periocular corticosteroid injections, and intravitreal injections of VEGF inhibitors.[48,49] The decision about specific therapies must take into account the likelihood of visual recovery, which is greater with smaller, more recent lesions, as well as the risks of the various therapies. Currently there is no established effective treatment for the dry form of macular degeneration, and most current therapies and new investigational treatments are directed at choroidal (or subretinal) neovascularization.

Photodynamic laser therapy, which involves the intravenous injection of a dye that is subsequently activated by retinal laser irradiation to produce selective vascular damage, is indicated when the neovascular membrane is well defined.[33] Conventional photocoagulation of subfoveal neovascular membranes is associated with an inevitable immediate reduction in vision because of associated retinal damage and thus is indicated only for extrafoveal membranes. Various surgical procedures to excise subfoveal neovascular membranes or position the macula away from them continue to be investigated.

The VEGF inhibitors that are administered by intravitreal injection include pegaptanib, ranibizumab, and bevacizumab.[49] Pegaptanib is a VEGF inhibitor that was approved by the U.S. Food and Drug Administration (FDA) in 2004 for the treatment of slow vision loss in eyes affected by all subtypes of age-related macular degeneration. Ranibizumab is a recombinant humanized monoclonal antibody with specificity for VEGF that was approved by the FDA in 2006 for the treatment of the wet form of age-related macular degeneration. Bevacizumab is approved in the United States as an intravenous infusion for treatment of colorectal cancer. Although bevacizumab has not been approved for ophthalmologic neovascular use, it can be used on an off-label basis. The corticosteroids have an angiostatic activity that appears to be independent of their hormone activity. The intravitreal injection of these agents bypasses the blood-ocular barrier, achieving therapeutic levels in the eye while avoiding systemic side effects.

In addition to currently used and forthcoming treatments, there is interest in the so-called preventative category of treatments. Tobacco smoking is consistently identified as a preventable age-related macular degeneration risk; thus, its elimination should be one the first therapeutic recommendations. Preventative recommendations also include dietary supplementation with antioxidants and minerals such as vitamin E (α-tocopherol), vitamin C (ascorbic acid), zinc, and β-carotene for persons at risk for developing macular degeneration and for slowing the progression of age-related macular degeneration in persons with the disease.[50] Although dietary supplements seems reasonable, more experimental data and randomized clinical trials are needed to support their therapeutic value and their most effective composition in terms of single- or multiple-supplement combinations, as well as dosing of particular supplements.

Retinoblastoma

Retinoblastoma is the most common intraocular malignant neoplasm of children, affecting 1 in 20,000.[50,51] The tumor occurs most frequently in children younger than 2 years of age and may even be found at birth. Retinoblastomas are related inherited or acquired mutations in the retinoblastoma (*Rb*) tumor suppressor gene, located on the long arm of chromosome 13 (13q14; see Chapter 8). If untreated, almost all children die of intracranial extension and disseminated disease. However, new diagnostic and treatment methods allow for a high rate of cure (93% survival in the United States).[51]

Leukokoria (*i.e.*, cat's-eye reflex, white reflex, or white pupil) is the most common presenting sign and is often noticed by the family; light entering the eye commonly reflects a yellowish-white color similar to that of the membranous covering of a cat's eye (Fig. 54-18). Strabismus (squint) is the second most common sign.[50–52] Red, tearing, and painful eyes are a late

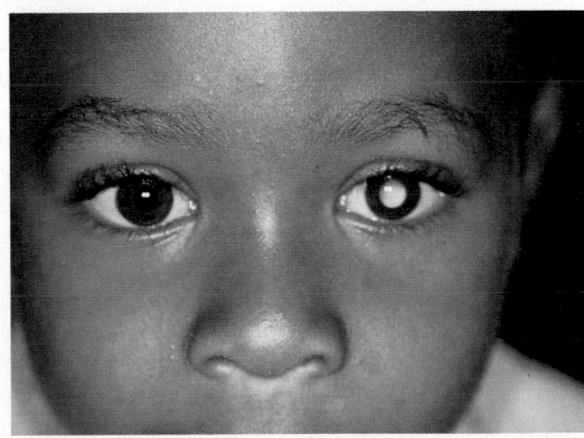

FIGURE 54-18 • The white pupil reflex (leukokoria) in the left eye of a child with retinoblastoma. (From Klintworth G. K. [2008]. The eye. In Rubin R., Strayer D. E. [Eds.], *Rubin's pathology: Clinicopathologic foundations of medicine* [5th ed., p. 1266]. Philadelphia: Lippincott-Williams & Wilkins.)

sign of the disorder. Limited or poor vision is also a late sign. Most retinoblastomas occur sporadically and are unilateral. Up to 25% of sporadic retinoblastomas and most inherited forms of the disorder are bilateral.

Diagnostic measures for detection of retinoblastoma are usually prompted by abnormal results of an eye examination in the hospital nursery or health care provider's office. All children with a family history of retinoblastoma should be screened soon after birth. Screening should be repeated every 4 to 6 weeks until 1 year of age, and then every 2 to 3 months until 3 years of age.[51] Congenital cataracts are an important cause of childhood leukokoria and should be ruled out. A definitive diagnosis usually requires ophthalmoscopic examination under general anesthesia by an ophthalmologist to obtain complete visualization of both eyes, which facilitates photographing and mapping of the tumors. CT or MRI scans are used to evaluate the extent of intraocular disease and extraocular spread.

The treatment of retinoblastoma has changed dramatically in recent years owing to the evolution of treatment options. The goals of treatment are primarily to save the child's life and secondarily to save the eye. Treatment options include laser thermotherapy, cryotherapy, chemotherapy, and enucleation (removal of the eye).[51] The choice of treatment is determined by the size of the tumor and its location and extension, as well as the visual potential and age of the child. Up to 45% of children treated with eye-preserving therapy may need subsequent therapy for recurrence of tumor, and up to 10% of children with unilateral tumors will develop a tumor in the contralateral eye.[51]

IN SUMMARY, the neural retina covers the inner aspect of the posterior two thirds of the eyeball and is continuous with the optic nerve. It contains the neural receptors for vision, and it is here that light energy of different frequencies and intensities is converted to graded local potentials, which then are converted to action potentials and transmitted to visual centers in the brain. The photoreceptors normally shed portions of their outer segments. These segments are phagocytized by cells in the pigment epithelium. Failure of phagocytosis, as occurs in one form of retinitis pigmentosa, results in degeneration of the pigment layer and blindness.

The retina receives its blood from two sources: the choriocapillaris, which supplies the pigment layer and the outer portion of the sensory retina adjacent to the choroid, and the branches of the retinal artery, which supply the inner half of the retina. Retinal blood vessels are normally apparent through the ophthalmoscope. Neovascularization involves the formation of new, fragile blood vessels that leak protein, and are likely to bleed. Although the cause of neovascularization is uncertain, research links the process with a vascular endothelial growth factor (VEGF) produced by the lining of blood vessels. Hypoxia is a key regulator of VEGF-induced retinal neovascularization.

Disorders of retinal vessels can result from many local and systemic disorders, including diabetes mellitus and hypertension. They cause vision loss through changes that result in hem-

orrhage, production of opacities, and separation of the pigment epithelium and sensory retina. Retinal detachment involves separation of the sensory receptors from their blood supply; it causes blindness unless reattachment is accomplished promptly. Macular degeneration is characterized by loss of central vision due to destructive changes of the macula of the retina. There are two types of age-related macular degeneration: a nonexudative "dry form" that causes atrophy and degeneration of the outer retina and an exudative "wet form" that results in formation of a choroidal neovascular membrane with vessels that leak blood and serum and predispose to separation of the pigmented epithelium from the neuroretina. Although there are currently no effective therapies for the dry form of age-related macular degeneration, effective forms of treatment for the wet form include photodynamic therapy, laser photocoagulation, and intravitreal injection of corticosteroids and VEGF inhibitors.

Retinoblastoma is an intraocular malignant neoplasm of children (most often those younger than 2 years of age) that is caused by inherited or acquired mutations in the retinoblastoma (*Rb*) tumor suppressor gene. The most common presenting sign is leukokoria (white reflex or white pupil), with strabismus being the second most common sign. With new diagnostic and treatment methods, nearly 95% of retinoblastomas are cured in the United States. ∎

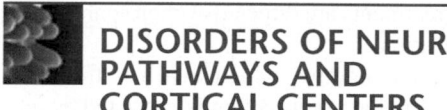

DISORDERS OF NEURAL PATHWAYS AND CORTICAL CENTERS

After completing this section of the chapter, you should be able to meet the following objectives:

- Characterize what is meant by a *visual field defect.*
- Explain the use of perimetry in the diagnosis of a visual field defect.
- Define the terms *hemianopia, quadrantanopia, heteronymous hemianopia,* and *homonymous hemianopia* and relate them to disorders of the optic pathways.
- Describe visual defects associated with disorders of the visual cortex and visual association areas.

Full visual function requires the normally developed brain-related functions of photoreception and the pupillary reflex. These functions depend on the integrity of all optic pathways, including retinal circuitry and the pathway from the optic nerve to the visual cortex and other visual regions of the brain and brain stem.

Optic Pathways

Visual information is carried to the brain by axons of the retinal ganglion cells, which form the optic nerve. Surrounded by

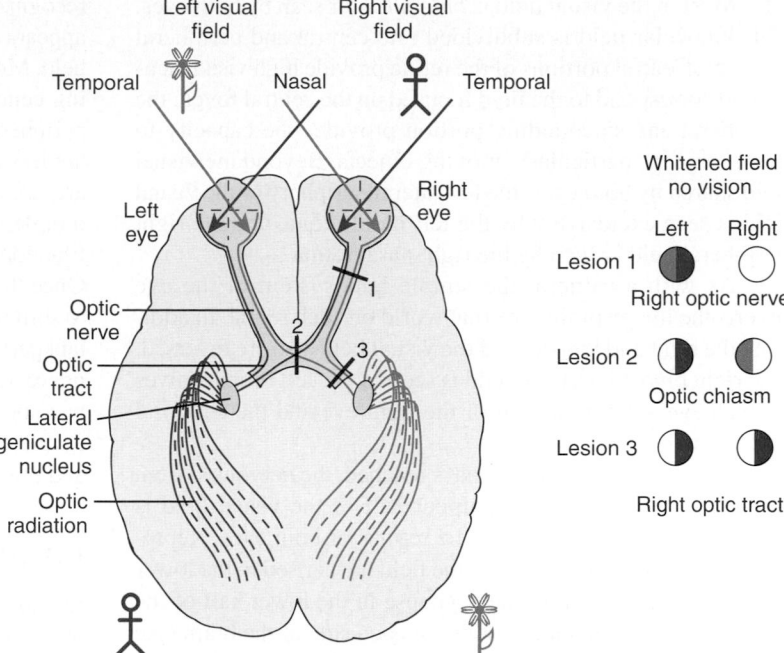

FIGURE 54-19 • Diagram of optic pathways. The *red lines* indicate the right visual field and the *blue lines* the left visual field. Note the crossing of fibers from the medial half of each retina at the optic chiasm. Lesion 1 (right optic nerve) produces unilateral blindness. Lesion 2 (optic chiasm) may involve only those fibers that originate in the nasal half of each retina and cross to the opposite side in the optic chiasm; visual loss involves the temporal half of each field (bitemporal hemianopia). Lesion 3 (right optic tract) interrupts fibers (and vision) originating on the same side of both eyes (homonymous) with loss of vision from half of each field (hemianopia).

pia mater, cerebrospinal fluid, arachnoid, and the dura mater, the optic nerve represents an outgrowth of the brain rather than a peripheral nerve. The optic nerve extends from the back of the optic globe through the orbit and the optic foramen, into the middle cranial fossa, and on to the optic chiasm at the base of the brain[16] (Fig. 54-19). Axons from the nasal portion of the retina remain medial, and those from the temporal retina remain lateral in the optic nerve.

The two optic nerves meet and fuse in the optic chiasm, beyond which they are continued as the optic tracts. In the optic chiasm, axons from the nasal retina of each eye cross to the opposite side and join with the axons of the temporal retina of the contralateral eye to form the optic tracts. Thus, one optic tract contains fibers from both eyes that transmit information from the same visual hemifield (half-field.)

Visual Cortex

The primary visual cortex (area 17) surrounds the calcarine fissure, which lies in the occipital lobe. It is at this level that visual sensation is first experienced (Fig. 54-20). Immediately surrounding area 17 are the visual association cortices (areas 18 and 19) and several other association cortices.[16] These association cortices, with their thalamic nuclei, must be functional to add meaningfulness to visual perception.

Circuitry in the primary visual cortex and the visual association areas is extremely discrete with respect to the location of retinal stimulation. For example, specific neurons respond to the particular orientation of a moving edge, specific colors, or familiar shapes. This elaborate organization of the visual cortex, with its functionally separate and multiple representations of the same visual field, provides the

major basis for visual sensation and perception. Because of this discrete circuitry, lesions of the visual cortex must be large to be detected clinically.

Visual Fields

The *visual field* refers to the area that is visible during fixation of vision in one direction. Because visual system deficits are often expressed as visual field deficits rather than as direct measures of neural function, the terminology for normal and abnormal visual characteristics usually is based on visual field orientation.

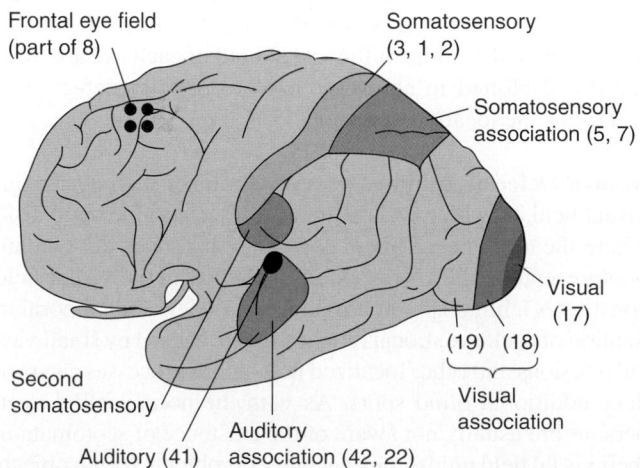

FIGURE 54-20 • Lateral view of the cortex illustrating the location of the visual, visual association, auditory, and auditory association areas.

Most of the visual field is *binocular,* or seen by both eyes. This binocular field is subdivided into central and peripheral portions. Central portions of the retina provide high visual acuity and correspond to the field focused on the central fovea; the peripheral and surrounding portion provides the capacity to detect objects, particularly moving objects. Beyond the visual field shared by both eyes, the left lateral periphery of the visual field is seen exclusively by the left nasal retina, and the right peripheral field is seen by the right nasal retina.

As with a camera, the simple lens system of the eye inverts the image of the external world on each retina. In addition, the right and left sides of the visual field also are reversed. The right binocular visual field is seen by the left retinal halves of each eye—the nasal half of the right eye and the temporal half of the left eye.

Once the level of the retina is reached, the nervous system plays a consistent role. The upper half of the visual field is received by the lower half of the retinas of both eyes. Representations of this upper half of the field are carried in the lower half of each optic nerve: they synapse in the lower half of the lateral geniculate nucleus (LGN) of each side of the brain (see Fig. 54-19). Neurons in this part of the LGN send their axons through the inferior half of the optic radiation, looping into the temporal lobe to terminate in the lower half of the primary visual cortex on each side of the brain.

Because of the lateral separation of the two eyes, each eye contributes a different image of the world to the visual field. This is called *binocular disparity.* Disparity between the laterally displaced images seen by the two eyes provides a powerful source of three-dimensional depth perception for objects within a distance of 30 m. Beyond that distance, binocular disparity becomes insignificant: depth perception is based on other cues (*e.g.,* the superimposition of the image of near objects over that of far objects, and the faster movement of near objects than of far objects).

Visual Field Defects

Visual field defects result from damage to the retina, optic pathways, or the visual cortex. Perimetry or visual field testing, in which the limits of the visual field of each eye are measured and plotted in an arc, is used to identify defects and determine the location of lesions.

Retinal Defects. All of us possess a hole, or *scotoma,* in our visual field, of which we are unaware. Because the optic disk, where the optic nerve fibers exit the retina, does not contain photoreceptors, the corresponding location in the visual field constitutes a blind spot approximately 15 degrees temporal to fixation of each eye. Local retinal damage caused by small vascular lesions and other localized pathologic processes can produce additional blind spots. As with the normal blind spot, persons are usually not aware of the existence of scotomata in their visual field unless they encounter problems seeing objects in certain restricted parts of the visual field.

Absences near or in the center of the bilateral visual field can be annoying and even disastrous. Although the hole is not recognized as such, the person finds that a part of a printed page appears or disappears, depending on where the fixation point is held. Most persons learn to position their eyes to use the remaining central foveal vision for high-acuity tasks. Defects in the peripheral visual field, including the monocular peripheral fields, are less annoying but potentially more dangerous. Persons who are unaware of the defect, when walking or driving an automobile, do not see cars or bicyclists until their image reaches the functional visual field—sometimes too late to avert an accident. Once these persons become aware of the defect, they can learn to shift their gaze constantly to obtain visual coverage of important parts of the visual field. If the damage is at the retinal or optic nerve level, only the monocular field of the damaged eye becomes a problem. A lesion affecting the central foveal vision of one eye can result in complaints of eyestrain during reading and other close work because only one eye is being used.

Disorders of the Optic Pathways

Localized damage to the optic tracts, LGN, optic radiation, or primary visual cortex affects corresponding parts of the visual fields of both eyes (see Fig. 54-19). Examination of visual system function is of particular importance because lesions at various points along the pathway have characteristic symptoms that assist in the localization of the lesion.

Among the disorders that can interrupt the optic pathway are vascular lesions, trauma, and tumors. For example, normal visual system function depends on adequate perfusion of the ophthalmic artery and its branches; the central artery of the retina; the anterior and middle cerebral arteries, which supply the intracranial optic nerve, chiasm, and optic tracts; and the posterior cerebral artery, which supplies the LGN, optic radiation, and visual cortex. The adequacy of posterior cerebral artery function depends on that of the vertebral and basilar arteries that supply the brain stem. Vascular insufficiency in any one of these arterial systems can seriously affect vision.

Visual field defects of each eye and of the two eyes together are useful in localizing lesions affecting the system. Blindness in one eye is called *anopia.* If half of the visual field for one eye is lost, the defect is called *hemianopia,* and if a quarter of the field is lost, it is called *quadrantanopia.* Enlarging pituitary tumors can produce longitudinal damage through the optic chiasm with loss of the medial fibers of the optic nerve representing both nasal retinas and both temporal visual half-fields. The loss of different half-fields in the two eyes is called a *heteronymous loss,* and the abnormality is called *heteronymous hemianopia.* Destruction of one or both lateral halves of the chiasm is common with multiple aneurysms of the circle of Willis (see Chapter 51). In this condition, the function of one or both temporal retinas is lost, and the nasal fields of one or both eyes are lost. The loss of the temporal fields (nasal retina) of both eyes is called *bitemporal heteronymous anopia.* With both eyes open, the person with bilateral defects still has the full binocular visual field.

Loss of the optic tract, LGN, full optic radiation, or complete visual cortex on one side results in loss of the corresponding visual half-fields in each eye. *Homonymous* means "the same" for both eyes. In left-side lesions, the right visual field is lost for each eye and is called *complete right homonymous hemianopia.* Partial injury to the left optic tract, LGN, or optic radiation can result in the loss of a quarter of the visual field in both eyes. This is called *homonymous quadrantanopia,* and depending on the lesion, it can involve the upper (superior) or lower (inferior) fields. Because the optic radiation fibers for the superior quarter of the visual field traverse the temporal lobe, superior quadrantanopia is more common.

Disorders of the Visual Cortex

Discrete damage to the binocular portion of the primary visual cortex also can result in scotomata in the corresponding visual fields. The central high-acuity portion of the visual field is located at the occipital pole. If the visual loss is in the central high-acuity part of the field, severe loss of visual acuity and pattern discrimination occurs. Mechanical trauma to the cortex results in firing of neurons, experienced as flashes of light or "seeing stars." Destruction of the polar visual cortex causes severe loss of visual acuity and pattern discrimination. Such damage is permanent and cannot be corrected with lenses.

The bilateral loss of the entire primary visual cortex, called *cortical blindness,* eliminates all visual experience. Crude analysis of visual stimulation at reflex levels, such as eye-orienting and head-orienting responses to bright moving lights, pupillary reflexes, and blinking at sudden bright lights, may be retained even though vision has been lost. Extensive damage to the visual association cortex (areas 18 and 19) that surrounds an intact primary visual cortex results in a loss of the learned meaningfulness of visual images (*i.e.,* visual agnosia). The person can see the patterns of color, shapes, and movement, but no longer can recognize formerly meaningful stimuli. Familiar objects can be described but not named or reacted to meaningfully. However, if other sensory modalities, such as hearing and touch, can be applied, full recognition occurs. This disorder represents a problem of recognition rather than intellect.

Testing of Visual Fields

Crude testing of the binocular visual field and the visual field of each individual eye (*i.e.,* monocular vision) can be accomplished without specialized equipment. In the confrontation method, the examiner stands or sits in front of the person to be tested and instructs the person to focus with one eye closed on the examiner's nose while random presentations of finger quantities are presented roughly three feet from the observer in each of the four major field quadrants to assess for the awareness of the finger quantities. In a kinetic assessment of the expansiveness of the gross visual field, an object such as a penlight is moved from the center toward the periphery of the person's visual field and from the periphery toward the center, and the person is instructed to report the presence or absence of the object. By moving the object through the vertical, horizontal, and oblique aspects of the visual field, a crude estimate can be made of the visual field. Large field defects can be estimated

by the confrontation method, and it may be the only way for testing young children and uncooperative adults.

Accurate determination of the presence, size, and shape of smaller holes, or scotomata, in the visual field of a particular eye can be demonstrated only by perimetry. This is done by having the person look with one eye toward a central spot directly in front of the eye while the head is stabilized by a chin rest or bite board. A small dot of light or a colored object is moved back and forth in all areas of the visual field. The person reports whether the stimulus is visible and, if a colored stimulus is used, what the perceived color is. A hemispheric support is used to control and standardize the movement of the test object, and a plot of radial coordinates of the visual field is made. Automated perimetry uses static dots of varying intensity and color, as well as flicker frequency stimuli, to assess higher levels of retinal cell function. Perimetry provides a means of determining alterations from normal and, with repeated testing, a way of following the progress of the condition causing the visual field defect or its treatment.

IN SUMMARY, visual information is carried to the brain by axons of the retinal ganglion cells that form the optic nerve. The two optic nerves meet and fuse in the optic chiasm. The axons of each nasal retina cross in the chiasm and join the uncrossed fibers of the temporal retina of the opposite eye in the optic tract to form the optic tracts. The fibers of each optic tract then synapse in the LGN, and from there, travel by way of the optic radiations to the primary visual cortex in the calcarine area of the occipital lobe. Damage to the visual association cortex can result in the phenomenon of seeing an object without the ability to recognize it (*i.e.,* visual agnosia). Optic pathway or visual cortex damage leads to visual field defects that can be identified through visual field testing. Perimetry, which maps the sensitivity contours of the visual field, can be used to determine the presence, size, and shape of smaller holes, or scotomata, in the visual field of an eye. ■

DISORDERS OF EYE MOVEMENT

After completing this section of the chapter, you should be able to meet the following objectives:

- Describe the function and innervation of the extraocular muscles.
- Recognize the use of smooth pursuit, saccadic, and vergence conjugate gaze movements in self or others.
- Explain the difference between paralytic and non-paralytic strabismus.
- Define *amblyopia* and explain its pathogenesis.
- Explain the need for early diagnosis and treatment of eye movement disorders in children.

For complete visual function, it is necessary that the two eyes focus on the same fixation point, that the image of the object falls simultaneously on the fovea of each eye, and that the retinal and CNS visual mechanisms are functional. It is through these mechanisms that an object is simultaneously imaged on the fovea of both eyes and perceived as a single image. Strabismus and amblyopia are two disorders that affect this highly integrated system.

Extraocular Eye Muscles and Their Innervation

Each eyeball can rotate around its vertical axis (lateral or medial rotation in which the pupil moves away from or toward the nose), its horizontal left-to-right axis (vertical elevation or depression, in which the pupil moves up or down), and longitudinal horizontal axis in which the top of the pupil moves toward or away from the nose.

Three pairs of extraocular muscles—the superior and inferior recti, the medial and lateral recti, and the superior and inferior obliques—control the movement of each eye (Fig. 54-21). The four rectus muscles are named according to where they insert into the sclera on the medial, lateral, inferior, and superior surfaces of each eye. The two oblique muscles insert on the lateral posterior quadrant of the eyeball—the superior oblique on the upper surface and the inferior oblique on the lower. Each of the three sets of muscles in each eye is reciprocally innervated so that one muscle relaxes when the other contracts. Reciprocal contraction of the medial and lateral recti moves the eye from side to side (adduction and abduction); the superior and inferior recti move the eye up and down (elevation and depression). The oblique muscles rotate (intorsion and extorsion) the eye around its optic axis. A seventh muscle, the levator palpebrae superioris, elevates the upper lid.

The extraocular muscles are innervated by three cranial nerves. The abducens nerve (CN VI) innervates the lateral rectus, the trochlear nerve (CN IV) innervates the superior oblique, and the oculomotor nerve (CN III) innervates the remaining four muscles (Table 54-1). The CN VI (abducens) nucleus, in the caudal pons, innervates the lateral rectus muscle, which rotates the ipsilateral (same-side) eye laterally (abduction). Partial or complete damage to this nerve results in weakness or complete paralysis of the muscle. Medial gaze is normal, but the affected eye fails to rotate laterally with an attempted gaze toward the affected side, a condition called *medial strabismus*. The CN IV (trochlear) nucleus, at the junction of the pons and midbrain, innervates the contralateral or opposite-side superior oblique muscle, which rotates the top of the globe inward toward the nose, a movement called *intorsion*. In combination with other muscles, it also contributes strength to movement of the innervated eye downward and inward.

The CN III (oculomotor) nucleus, which extends through a considerable part of the midbrain, contains clusters of lower motor neurons for each of the five eye muscles it innervates: inferior rectus, superior rectus, inferior oblique, medial rectus, and levator palpebrae superioris. The medial rectus, superior rectus, and inferior rectus rotate the eye in the directions shown in Table 54-1. The action of the inferior rectus is antagonistic to the superior rectus. Because of its plane of attachment to the globe, the inferior oblique rotates the eye in the frontal plane (*i.e.,* torsion), pulling the top of the eye laterally (*i.e.,* extorsion). CN III also innervates the levator palpebrae superioris muscle that elevates the upper eyelid and is involved in vertical gaze eye movements. As the eyes rotate upward, the upper eyelid is reflexively retracted and in the downward gaze it is lowered, restricting exposure of the conjunctiva to air and reducing the effects of drying.

Communication between the eye muscle nuclei of each side of the brain occurs primarily through the posterior commissure at the rostral end of the midbrain. Longitudinal communication among the three nuclei occurs along a fiber tract called the *medial longitudinal fasciculus* (MLF), which extends from the midbrain to the upper part of the spinal cord. Each pair of eye muscles is reciprocally innervated, by the

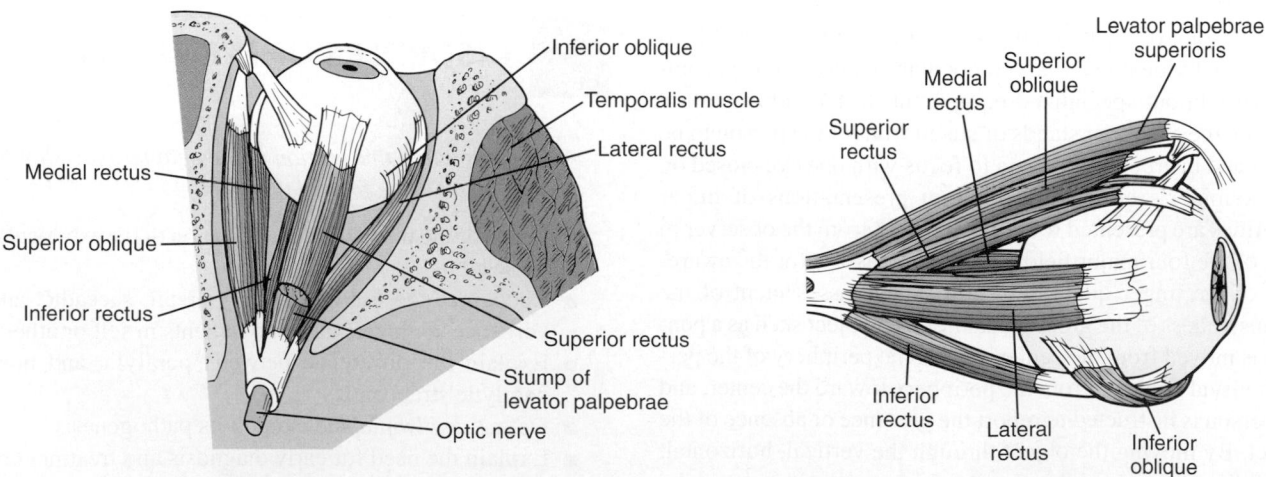

FIGURE 54-21 • Extraocular muscles of the right eye.

```
    3–SR        IO–3        3–IO        SR–3

 6–LR ─┤  ( )  ├─ MR   MR ─┤  ( )  ├─ LR–6
              │              │
              3              3

    3–IR        SO–4        4–SO        IR–3
```

TABLE 54-1 **Eye in Primary Position: Extrinsic Ocular Muscle Actions**				
MUSCLE*	**INNERVATION**	**PRIMARY**	**SECONDARY**	**TERTIARY**
MR: medial rectus	III	Adduction		
LR: lateral rectus	VI	Abduction		
SR: superior rectus	III	Elevation	Intorsion	Adduction
IR: inferior rectus	III	Depression	Extorsion	Adduction
SO: superior oblique	IV	Intorsion	Depression	Abduction
IO: inferior oblique	III	Extorsion	Elevation	Abduction

*In the schema of the functional roles of the six extraocular muscles, the major directional force applied by each muscle is indicated on the top. These muscles are arranged in functionally opposing pairs per eye and in parallel opposing pairs for conjugate movements of the two eyes. The numbers associated with each muscle indicate the cranial nerve innervation: 3, oculomotor (III) cranial nerve; 4, trochlear (IV) cranial nerve; 6, abducens (VI) cranial nerve.

MLF or other associated pathways, so that as one muscle contracts, the other relaxes. These MLF-linked communication paths are vulnerable to damage in the caudal midbrain and pons. Damage to the pontine MLF on one side of the brain results in loss of this linkage, such that lateral deviation of the ipsilateral eye is no longer linked to adduction on the contralateral side. If the MLF is damaged bilaterally, the linkage is lost for lateral gaze in either direction.

Eye Movements and Gaze

Conjugate movements are those in which the optical axes of the two eyes are kept parallel, sharing the same visual field. *Gaze* refers to the act of looking steadily in one direction. Eye movements can be categorized into smooth pursuit movements, saccadic movements, optic tremor, and vergence movements. Although the conjugate reflexes are essential to efficient visual function during head movement or target movement, their circuitry is so deeply embedded in CNS function that they are present and can be elicited when the eyes are closed, during sleep, and in deep coma, and they function normally and accurately in congenitally blind persons.

Smooth Pursuit Movements. Smooth pursuit movements are tracking movements that serve to maintain an object at a fixed point in the center of the visual fields of both eyes. The object may be moving with the eyes following, or the object may be stationary with the head moving. Normal eye posture is a conjugate gaze directed straight forward with the head held in a forward-looking posture. Smooth pursuit movements normally begin from this position. In fact, holding a strongly deviated gaze becomes tiring after about 30 seconds, and most people will make head and body rotation adjustments to bring the eyes to a central position within that time.

Voluntary pursuit movements are tested by asking the person to follow a finger or another object as it is moved slowly through the visual field. Successful conjugate following requires a functional optic system communicating to the superior colliculus and to the primary visual cortex.

Saccadic Eye Movements. Saccadic eye movements are sudden, jerky conjugate movements that quickly change the fixation point. During reading, the fixation pattern involves a focus on a word or short series of words and then a sudden jump of the eyes to a new fixation point on the next word or phrase. During the saccade, a person does not experience the blur of the rapidly moving visual field. Saccadic movements are automatic reflex movements that, in most situations, operate at the brain stem level. Saccadic shifts of a gaze toward the source of a sudden, unexpected visual, auditory, tactile, or painful stimulus are a component of the startle pattern. This is functionally a visual grasping reflex, redirecting conjugate gaze in the direction of the startle stimulus.

The frontal eye fields of the premotor cortex are important for voluntary saccadic movements such as reading. If this frontal premotor area is not functional, a person can describe objects in the visual field but cannot voluntarily search the visual environment.

Eye Tremor. An eye tremor refers to involuntary, rhythmic, oscillatory eye movements, occurring approximately 10 times per second. Small-range optical tremors are a normal and useful independent function of each eye. One function of the fine optic tremor is to constantly move a bright image onto a new bank of cones, permitting previously stimulated receptors quickly to recover from adaptation.

Vergence Eye Movements. Vergence eye movements are those that move the eyes in opposite directions to keep the image of an object precisely positioned on the fovea of each eye. Convergence and divergence, which assist in maintaining a binocularly fixed image in near vision, have a major role in accurate depth perception. The vergence system is driven by retinal disparity (*i.e.,* differential placement of an object's image on each retina). A nearby target (<30 ft) moving in the same dimension as the optical axis elicits a reflex mechanism that provides redirection of the optical axes of each eye away from parallel (*i.e.,* in opposite directions) in the horizontal plane. This process permits a continued binocular focus on the near target. Perception of depth is a higher-order function of the cortical visual system and is based on one or more of several classes of stimuli, such as superimposition and relative movement.

 **Strabismus**

Strabismus, or squint, refers to any abnormality of eye coordination or alignment that results in loss of binocular vision.[53–55] When images from the same spots in visual space do not fall on corresponding points of the two retinas, diplopia, or double vision, occurs. Strabismus affects approximately 4% of children younger than 6 years of age.[53–55] Because 30% to 50% of these children sustain permanent secondary loss of vision, or amblyopia, if the condition is left untreated, early diagnosis and treatment are essential.

In standard terminology, the disorders of eye movement are described according to the direction of movement. *Esotropia* refers to medial (inward) deviation, *exotropia* to lateral (outward) deviation, *hypertropia* to upward deviation, *hypotropia* to downward deviation, and *cyclotropia* to torsional deviation. The term *concomitance* refers to equal deviation in all directions of gaze. A nonconcomitant strabismus is one that varies with the direction of gaze. Strabismus may be divided into nonparalytic (concomitant) forms, in which there is no primary muscle impairment, and paralytic (nonconcomitant) forms, in which there is weakness or paralysis of one or more of the extraocular muscles. Strabismus is called *intermittent,* or *periodic,* when there are periods in which the eyes are parallel. It is monocular when the same eye always deviates and the opposite eye fixates. Figure 54-22 illustrates abnormalities in eye movement associated with esotropia and exotropia.

Nonparalytic Strabismus

Nonparalytic esotropia is the most common type of strabismus. The individual ocular muscles have no obvious defect and the amount of deviation is constant, or relatively constant in the various directions of gaze. With persistent deviation, secondary abnormalities may develop because of overactivity or underactivity of the extraocular muscles in some fields of gaze.

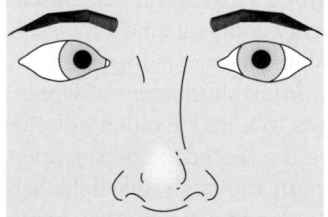

A   Primary position: right esotropia

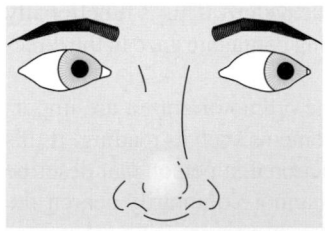

B   Left gaze: no deviation

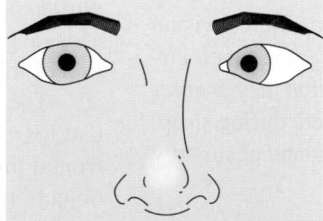

C   Right gaze: left esotropia

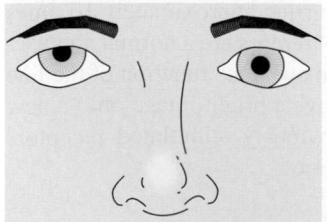

D   Right hypertropia

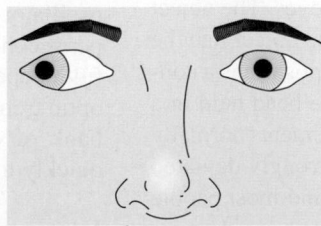

E   Right exotropia

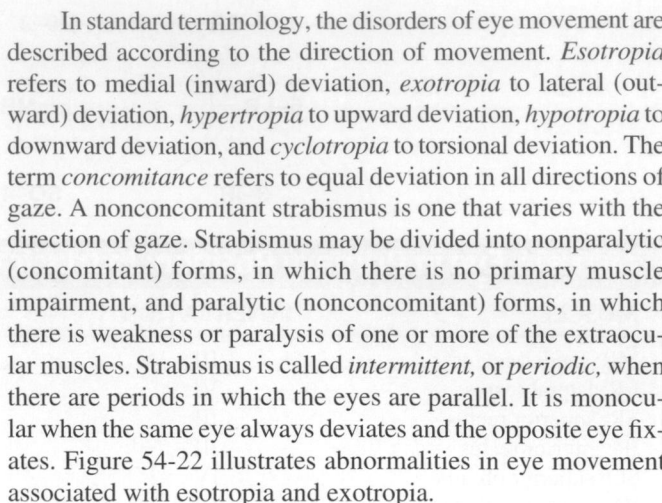

FIGURE 54-22 • **(A–C)** Paralytic strabismus associated with paralysis of the right lateral rectus muscle: **(A)** primary position of the eyes (looking straight ahead); **(B)** left gaze with no deviation; and **(C)** right gaze with left esotropia. **(D)** Primary position of the eyes with weakness of the right inferior rectus and right hypertropia. **(E)** Primary position of the eyes with weakness of the right medial rectus and right exotropia.

The disorder may be nonaccommodative, accommodative, or a combination of the two. Infantile esotropia is the most common cause of nonaccommodative strabismus. It occurs in the first 6 months of life, with large-angle deviations, in an otherwise developmentally and neurologically normal infant. Eye movements are full, and the child often uses each eye independently to alter fixation (cross-fixation). The cause of the disorder is unclear. Research suggests that idiopathic strabismus may have a genetic basis; siblings often present with similar disorders.

Accommodative strabismus is caused by disorders such as uncorrected hyperopia of a significant degree, in which the esotropia occurs with accommodation that is undertaken to focus clearly. Onset of this type of esotropia characteristically occurs between 18 months and 4 years of age because accommodation is not well developed until that time. The disorder most often is monocular but may be alternating.

Paralytic Strabismus

Paralytic strabismus results from paresis (*i.e.,* weakness) or plegia (*i.e.,* paralysis) of one or more of the extraocular muscles. When the normal eye fixates, the affected eye is in the position of primary deviation. In the case of esotropia, there is weakness of one of the lateral rectus muscles, usually due to a disorder of the abducens nerve (CN VI). When the affected eye fixates, the unaffected eye is in a position of secondary deviation. The secondary deviation of the unaffected eye is greater than the primary deviation of the affected eye. This is because the affected eye requires an excess of innervational impulse to maintain fixation; the excess impulses also are distributed to the unaffected eye, causing overaction of its muscles.[53]

Paralytic strabismus is uncommon in children but accounts for nearly all cases of adult strabismus; it can be caused by infiltrative processes (*e.g.,* Graves disease; see Chapter 41), myasthenia gravis, stroke, and direct optical trauma.[54] The pathway of the oculomotor, trochlear, and abducens nerves through the cavernous sinus and the back of the orbit make them vulnerable to basal skull fracture and tumors of the cavernous sinus or orbit.[56] In infants, paralytic strabismus can be caused by birth injuries affecting the extraocular muscles or the cranial nerves supplying these muscles. In general, paralytic strabismus in an older child or adult does not produce amblyopia, and binocular vision can be maintained when the strabismus is corrected. Most adult strabismus represents deterioration of childhood strabismus, which can occur even decades after good ocular alignment.

Treatment

Treatment of strabismus is directed toward the development of normal visual acuity, correction of the deviation, and superimposition of the retinal images to provide binocular vision. Early and adequate treatment is crucial because a delay in or lack of treatment can lead to amblyopia and permanent loss of vision. In addition to its effects on visual function, strabismus can have an adverse impact on interpersonal relationships, self-image, schoolwork, and participation in extracurricular activi-ties. Children begin to develop negative attitudes toward classmates with strabismus as early as 6 years of age.

Treatment includes both surgical and nonsurgical methods. Infantile esotropia is usually treated surgically by weakening the medial rectus muscle on each eye while the infant is under general anesthesia. Surgery in children with esotropia should be done as early as possible to preserve stereoptic acuity. Early surgical treatment also appears to result in better outcomes than later intervention. Recurrent strabismus is common with infantile esotropia, and multiple surgeries are often required.

Nonsurgical treatment includes glasses, occlusive patching, and eye exercises (*i.e.,* pleoptics). Glasses are often used in the treatment of accommodative esotropia that occurs with hypermetropia (farsightedness). Because accommodation is linked with convergence, focusing drives the eyes inward, producing esotropia. Intermittent exotropia is commonly treated with patching, use of over-minus glasses, and eye exercises. Although no appreciable deviation is present when the child with intermittent strabismus sees near objects, the deviation becomes obvious when the child views distant objects or is fatigued. Patching for 1 to 2 hours daily for several months works by preventing, rather than treating, suppression of an eye. Patching is most effective in infants, and the efficacy is limited in children older than 3 years of age. The use of over-minus glasses stimulates accommodative convergences, which contracts the exotropic drift. Vision therapy involves exercises to stimulate convergence (*e.g.,* focusing on reading-distance targets up to 30 minutes several times a day) and techniques to train the visual system to recognize the suppressed images. Surgical treatment of intermittent exotropia is indicted when conservative methods fail to correct the deviation. Early treatment of children with intermittent exotropia is not as crucial as it is for those for constant deviations because stereopsis can still develop.

A relatively new form of treatment involves the injection of botulinum toxin type A (Botox) into the extraocular muscle to produce a dose-dependent paralysis of that extraocular muscle. Paralysis of the muscle shifts the eye into the field of action of the antagonist muscle. During the time the eye is deviated the paralyzed muscle is stretched, whereas the antagonistic muscle is contracted. Usually two or more injections of the drug are necessary to obtain a lasting effect.

 ## Amblyopia

Amblyopia, sometimes called *lazy eye,* describes a decrease in visual acuity resulting from abnormal visual development in infancy or early childhood.[53,57–61] The vision loss ranges from mild (worse than 20/25) to severe (legal blindness, 20/200 or worse).[57] It is the leading cause of visual impairment, affecting 1% to 4% of the population. With early detection and treatment, most cases of amblyopia are reversible and the most severe forms of the condition can be prevented.[59]

Normal development of the thalamic and cortical circuitry necessary for binocular visual perception requires simultaneous binocular use of each fovea during a critical period early in life (0 to 5 years). Amblyopia can result from visual deprivation (*e.g.*, cataracts, ptosis) or abnormal binocular interactions (*e.g.*, strabismus, anisometropia) during visual immaturity. In infants with unilateral cataracts that are dense, central, and larger than 2 mm in diameter, this time is before 2 months of age.[53] In conditions causing abnormal binocular interactions, one image is suppressed to provide clearer vision. In esotropia, vision of the deviated eye is suppressed to prevent diplopia. A similar situation exists in anisometropia, in which the refractive indexes of the two eyes are different. Although the eyes are correctly aligned, they are unable to focus together, and the image of one eye is suppressed.

The reversibility of amblyopia depends on the maturity of the visual system at the time of onset and the duration of the abnormal experience. Occasionally in strabismus, some persons alternate eye fixation and do not experience deep amblyopia or diplopia. With late adolescent or adult onset, this habit pattern must be unlearned after correction. Amblyopia is remarkably responsive to treatment if the treatment is initiated early in life; thus, all infants and young children should be evaluated for visual conditions that could lead to amblyopia (see the section on Eye Examination in Infants and Children).

The treatment of children with the potential for development of amblyopia must be instituted well before the age of 6 years to avoid the suppression phenomenon. Surgery for congenital cataracts and ptosis should be done early. Severe refractive errors should be corrected. In children with strabismus, the alternate blocking of the vision in one eye and then the other forces the child to use both eyes for form discrimination. The duration of occlusion of vision in the good eye must be short (2 to 5 hours per day) and closely monitored, or deprivation amblyopia can develop in the good eye as well. Although amblyopia is not likely to occur after 8 or 9 years of age, some plasticity in central circuitry is evident even in adulthood. For example, after refractive correction for long-standing astigmatism in adults, visual acuity improves slowly, requiring several months to reach normal levels.

Eye Examination in Infants and Children

Early detection and prompt treatment of ocular disorders in children are important to prevent amblyopia and lifelong visual impairment. The American Academy of Pediatrics in association with the American Association of Certified Orthoptists, American Association of Pediatric Ophthalmology and Strabismus, and American Academy of Ophthalmology recommends that all newborn infants be examined in the nursery for structural abnormalities and have a red reflex test performed to check for abnormalities in the back of the eye (posterior segment) and opacities in the visual axis, such as cataracts or corneal opacity.[61] An infant with an abnormal red reflex requires immediate referral to an eye care specialist. Visual examinations should then be performed on all well-child visits. These should include age-appropriate evaluation

of visual acuity, ocular alignment, and ocular media clarity (cataracts, tumors).

Visual assessment of infants and children younger than 3 years of age is accomplished by determining whether each eye can fixate on an object, maintain fixation, and then follow the object in various gaze positions. Failure to perform these maneuvers indicates significant visual impairment. The assessment should be done binocularly and monocularly. If poor fixation is noted binocularly after 3 months of age, a significant bilateral eye or brain abnormality should be suspected and the child should be referred for further evaluation. Emphasis should be placed on screening for visual acuity as soon as the child is cooperative enough to complete the examination. Decreased vision in one eye requires evaluation for ocular deviation or other ocular abnormalities, which may be difficult to discern on screening examination.[61,62] Strabismus deviations of only a few degrees, too small to be detected by gross inspection, can lead to amblyopia and vision loss.

Every effort should be made to ensure that eye examinations are performed by properly prepared examiners, using appropriate testing conditions, instruments, and techniques (the reader is referred to an appropriate reference source for a detailed description of the various methods that are used).[61] The InfantSEE assessment program offers early detection of potential eye and vision problems as a complement to the eye screening provided in a pediatric well-care visit.[63]

The results of vision assessments and visual acuity measurements, along with instructions for follow-up care should be clearly communicated to the parents. Parent's observations are also important. Questions about whether the child's eyes seem straight or seem to cross or drift, or appear lazy; whether the child's eyelids droop or one eyelid tends to close; and, in older children, whether the child seems to see well or tends to hold objects close to his or her face when trying to focus, can provide helpful information.[61]

IN SUMMARY, binocular vision depends on the extraocular muscles and their innervating cranial nerves to move the eye up and down and rotate it around its optical axis. For full visual function, it is necessary that the two eyes point toward the same fixation point and the two images become fused. Binocular fusion is controlled by ocular reflex mechanisms that adjust the orientation of each eye to produce a single image. The term *conjugate gaze* refers to the use of both eyes to look steadily in one direction. During conjugate eye movements, the optical axes of the two eyes are maintained parallel with each other as the eyes rotate upward, downward, or from side to side in their sockets.

Strabismus refers to abnormalities in the coordination of eye movements, with loss of binocular eye alignment. This inability to focus a visual image on corresponding parts of the two retinas results in diplopia. Esotropia refers to medial deviation, exotropia to lateral deviation, hypertropia to upward deviation, hypotropia to downward deviation, and cyclotropia to torsional deviation. Paralytic strabismus is caused by weakness or paralysis of the extraocular muscles, whereas nonparalytic strabismus results from the inappropriate length or insertion of the extraocular muscles or from accommodation disorders.

Amblyopia (*i.e.,* lazy eye) is a decrease in visual acuity resulting from abnormal visual development in infancy and early childhood. It results from inadequately developed CNS circuitry because of visual deprivation (*e.g.,* cataracts) or abnormal binocular interactions (*e.g.,* strabismus) during visual immaturity. ■

Review Exercises

1. The mother of a 3-year-old boy notices that his left eye is red and watering when she picks him up from day care. He keeps rubbing his eye as if it itches. The next morning, however, she notices that both eyes are red, swollen, and watering. Being concerned, she takes him to the pediatrician in the morning and is told that he has "pink eye." She is told that the infection should go away by itself.

   A. *What part of the eye is involved?*

   B. *What type of conjunctivitis do you think this child has: bacterial, viral, or allergic?*

   C. *Why didn't the pediatrician order an antibiotic?*

   D. *Is the condition contagious? What measures should she take to prevent its spread?*

2. During a routine eye examination to get new glasses because she had been having difficulty with her distant vision, a 75-year-old woman is told that she is developing cataracts.

   A. *What type of visual changes occurs as the result of a cataract?*

   B. *What can the woman do to prevent the cataracts from getting worse?*

   C. *What treatment may she eventually need?*

3. A 50-year-old woman is told by her "eye doctor" that her intraocular pressure is slightly elevated and that although there is no evidence of damage to her eyes at this time, she is at risk for developing glaucoma and should have regular eye examinations.

   A. *Describe the physiologic mechanisms involved in the regulation of intraocular pressure.*

   B. *What are the risk factors for developing glaucoma?*

   C. *Explain how an increase in intraocular pressure produces its damaging effects.*

4. The parents of a newborn infant have been told that their son has congenital cataracts in both eyes and will require cataract surgery to prevent loss of sight.

   A. *Explain why the infant is at risk for losing his sight if the cataracts are not removed.*

   B. *When should this procedure be done to prevent loss of vision?*

References

1. Lighthouse International. About us. [Online]. Available: www.lighthouse.org. Accessed July 16, 2007.
2. Sullivan J. H., Shetlar D. J., Whitcher J. P. (2004). Lids, lacrimal apparatus and tears. In Riordan-Eva P. (Ed.), *Vaughan & Ashbury's general ophthalmology* (16th ed., pp. 80–99). New York: Lange Medical Books/McGraw-Hill.
3. Gilbard J. P. (2005). The diagnosis and management of dry eyes. *Otolaryngologic Clinics of North America* 38, 871–885.
4. Riordan-Eva P. (2004). Anatomy and embryology of the eye. In Riordan-Eva P. (Ed.), *Vaughan & Ashbury's general ophthalmology* (16th ed., pp. 1–28). New York: Lange Medical Books/McGraw-Hill.
5. Garcia-Ferrier F., Schwab J. R., Shetlar D. J. (2004). Conjunctivitis, lacrimal apparatus and tears. In Riordan-Eva P. (Ed.), *Vaughan & Ashbury's general ophthalmology* (16th ed., pp. 100–128). New York: Lange Medical Books/McGraw-Hill.
6. Pasternak A., Irish B. (2004). Ophthalmologic infections in primary care. *Clinics in Family Practice* 6(1), 19–33.
7. Leibowitz H. M. (2000). The red eye. *New England Journal of Medicine* 343, 345–351.
8. Riordan-Eva P. (2007). Eye. In Tierney L. M., McPhee S. J., Papadakis M. A. (Eds.), *Current medical diagnosis and treatment* (46th ed., pp. 151–173). New York: McGraw-Hill.
9. Ono S. J., Abelson M. B. (2006). Allergic conjunctivitis: Update on pathophysiology and prospects for future treatment. *Journal of Allergy and Clinical Immunology* 115, 118–122.
10. McAdam A. J., Sharpe A. H. (2005). Infectious diseases. In Kumar V., Abbas A. K., Fausto N. (Eds.), *Robbins and Cotran pathologic basis of disease* (7th ed., pp. 394–395). Philadelphia: Elsevier Saunders.
11. Olitsky S. E., Nelson L. (2004). Disorders of the eye. In Behrman R. E., Kliegman R. M., Jenson H. B. (Eds.), *Nelson textbook of pediatrics* (17th ed., pp. 2099–2102, 2105–2111). Philadelphia: Elsevier Saunders.
12. Folberg R. (2005). The eye. In Kumar V., Abbas A. K., Fausto N. (Eds.), *Robbins and Cotran pathologic basis of disease* (7th ed., pp. 1421–1447). Philadelphia: Elsevier Saunders.
13. Biswell R. (2004). Cornea. In Riordan-Eva P. (Ed.), *Vaughan & Ashbury's general ophthalmology* (16th ed., pp. 129–153). New York: Lange Medical Books/McGraw-Hill.
14. Shaikh S., Ta C. (2002). Evaluation and management of herpes zoster ophthalmicus. *American Family Physician* 66, 1723–1732.
15. Keirszenbaum A. L. (2007). *Histology and cell biology: An introduction to pathology* (2nd ed., p. 256). Philadelphia: Mosby-Elsevier
16. Kandel E. R., Schwartz J. H., Jessell T. M. (2000). *Principles of neural science* (4th ed., pp. 523–547). New York: McGraw-Hill.
17. Distellhorst J. S., Hughes G. M. (2003). Open-angle glaucoma. *American Family Physician* 67, 1937–1950.
18. Adatia F. A., Damji K. F. (2005). Chronic open-angle glaucoma. *Canadian Family Physician* 51, 1229–1237.
19. Riordan-Eva P. (2004). Glaucoma. In Riordan-Eva P. (Ed.), *Vaughan & Ashbury's general ophthalmology* (16th ed., pp. 212–229). New York: Lange Medical Books/McGraw-Hill.
20. Guyton A. C., Hall J. E. (2006). *Textbook of medical physiology* (11th ed., pp. 623, 616–617). Philadelphia: Elsevier Saunders.

21. Behki R., Damji K. F., Crichton A. (2007). Canadian perspectives in glaucoma management: The role of central corneal thickness. *Canadian Journal of Ophthalmology* 42, 66–74.

22. Kipp M. A. (2003). Childhood glaucoma. *Pediatric Clinics of North America* 50, 89–104.

23. Wilson S. E. (2004). Use of lasers for vision correction of nearsightedness and farsightedness. *New England Journal of Medicine* 351, 470–475.

24. Packer M., Fine H., Hoffman R. S. (2006). Refractive lens surgery. *Ophthalmology Clinics of North America* 19, 77–88.

25. Quillen D. A. (1999). Common causes of vision loss in elderly patients. *American Family Physician* 60, 99–108.

26. Harper R. A., Shock J. P. (2004). Lens. In Riordan-Eva P. (Ed.), *Vaughan & Ashbury's general ophthalmology* (16th ed., pp. 212–229). New York: Lange Medical Books/McGraw-Hill.

27. Schmitt C., Hockwin O. (1990). The mechanisms of cataract formation. *Journal of Inherited Metabolic Disease* 13, 501–508.

28. Chylack L. T. (1997). Cataracts and inhaled corticosteroids. *New England Journal of Medicine* 337, 44–48.

29. Jobling A. J., Augusteyn R. C. (2002). What causes steroid cataracts? A review of steroid-induced posterior subcapsular cataracts. *Clinical and Experimental Optometry* 852, 61–75.

30. Solomon B., Donnenfeld E. D. (2003). Recent advances and future frontiers in treating age-related cataracts. *Journal of the American Medical Association* 290, 248–251.

31. Harton D. T., Berson E. L., Dryja T. P. (2006). Retinitis pigmentosa. *Lancet* 368, 1795–1809.

32. Poole T. R. G., Graham E. M. (2004). Ocular disorders associated with systemic disease. In Riordan-Eva P. (Ed.), *Vaughan & Ashbury's general ophthalmology* (16th ed., pp. 307–342). New York: Lange Medical Books/McGraw-Hill.

33. Hardy R. A., Shetlar D. J. (2004). Retina. In Riordan-Eva P. (Ed.), *Vaughan & Ashbury's general ophthalmology* (16th ed., pp. 189–211). New York: Lange Medical Books/McGraw-Hill.

34. Shams N., Ianchuley T. (2006). Role of endothelial growth factor in ocular angiogenesis. *Ophthalmology Clinics of North America* 19, 335–344.

35. Frank R. N. (2004). Diabetic retinopathy. *New England Journal of Medicine* 350, 48–58.

36. Donaldson M., Dockson P. (2003). Medical treatment of diabetic neuropathy. *Eye* 17, 550–562.

37. Fong D. S., Aiello L., Ferris F. L., et al. (2004). Diabetic retinopathy. *Diabetes Care* 27, 2540–2553.

38. Cuilla T. A., Amador A. G., Zinman B. (2003). Diabetic retinopathy and diabetic macular edema. *Diabetes Care* 26, 2653–2664.

39. Funatsu H., Yamashita H. (2003). Pathogenesis of diabetic retinopathy and the renin-angiotensin system. *Ophthalmic and Physiological Optics* 23, 495–501.

40. Diabetes Control and Complications Trial Research Group. (1993). The effect of intensive treatment of diabetes on the development and progression of long-term complications in insulin-dependent diabetes mellitus. *New England Journal of Medicine* 329, 977–986.

41. Wong T. Y., Mitchell P. (2004). Hypertensive retinopathy. *New England Journal of Medicine* 351, 2310–2317.

42. Gariano R. F., Chang-Hee K. (2004). Evaluation and management of suspected retinal detachment. *American Family Physician* 69, 1691–1698.

43. de Jong P. T. V. M. (2006). Age-related macular degeneration. *New England Journal of Medicine* 355, 1474–1485.

44. Chopdar A., Chakravarthy U., Verma D. (2003). Age-related macular degeneration. *British Medical Journal* 326, 484–488.

45. Gottlieb J. L. (2002). Age-related macular degeneration. *Journal of the American Medical Association* 288, 2233–2236.

46. Nowak J. Z. (2006). Age-related macular degeneration (AMD): Pathogenesis and therapy. *Pharmacological Reports* 58, 353–363.

47. MacDonald I. M. (2005). Genetic aspects of age-related macular degeneration. *Canadian Journal of Ophthalmology* 40, 288–292.

48. Ng E. W. M., Adamis A. (2005). Targeting angiogenesis, the underlying disorder in neovascular age-related macular degeneration. *Canadian Journal of Ophthalmology* 40, 352–368.

49. Rothen M., Jablon E., Monares G., et al. (2005). Anti-macular degenerative agents. *Ophthalmology Clinics of North America* 18, 561–567.

50. Klintworth G. K. (2008). The eye. In Rubin R., Strayer D. E. (Eds.), *Rubin's pathology: Clinicopathologic foundations of medicine* (5th ed., pp. 1265–1266). Philadelphia: Lippincott Williams & Wilkins.

51. Melamud A., Palekar R., Singh A. (2006). Retinoblastoma. *American Family Physician* 73, 1039–1044.

52. Herzog C. (2004). Retinoblastoma. In Behrman R. E., Kliegman R. M., Jenson H. B. (Eds.), *Nelson textbook of pediatrics* (17th ed., pp. 1722–1723). Philadelphia: Elsevier Saunders.

53. Fredrick D. P., Asbury T. (2004). Strabismus. In Riordan-Eva P. (Ed.), *Vaughan & Ashbury's general ophthalmology* (16th ed., pp. 230–249). New York: Lange Medical Books/McGraw-Hill.

54. Donahue S. P. (2007). Pediatric strabismus. *New England Journal of Medicine* 356, 1040–1047.

55. Ticho B. H. (2003). Strabismus. *Pediatric Clinics of North America* 50, 173–188.

56. Kline L. B., Bajandas F. J. (1996). Neuro-ophthalmology review manual (Chapters 4–7). Thorofare, NJ: Slack.

57. Mittelman D. (2003). Amblyopia. *Pediatric Clinics of North America* 50, 189–196.

58. Doshi N. R., Rodriguez M. L. (2007). Amblyopia. *American Family Physician* 73, 361–367.

59. Wu C., Hunter D. G. (2006). Amblyopia: Diagnostic and therapeutic options. *American Journal of Ophthalmology* 141, 175–184.

60. Simon J. W., Kaw P. (2001). Commonly missed diagnoses in childhood eye exams. *American Family Physician* 64, 623–628.

61. American Academy of Pediatrics Committee on Practice and Ambulatory Medicine Section of Ophthalmology. (2003). Eye examination in infants, children, and young adults by pediatrician. *Pediatrics* 111, 902–907.

62. Olitsky S. E., Nelson L. B. (2004). Disorders of the eye. In Behrman R. E., Kliegman R. M., Jenson H. B. (Eds.), *Nelson textbook of pediatrics* (17th ed., pp. 2083–2095). Philadelphia: Elsevier Saunders.

63. InfantSEE. (2007). The InfantSEE assessment explained. [Online.] Available: http:www.infantsee.org. Accessed April 14, 2008.

Visit the Point. **http://thePoint.lww.com for animations, journal articles, and more!**

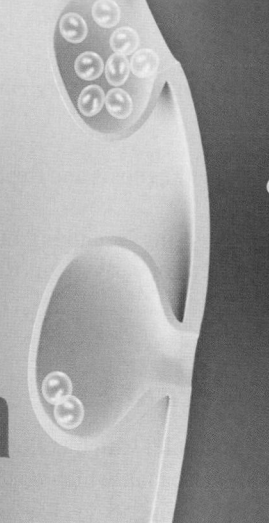

Disorders of Hearing and Vestibular Function

SUSAN A. FONTANA AND CAROL M. PORTH

➤ The ears are paired organs consisting of an external and middle ear, which function in capturing, transmitting, and amplifying sound, and an inner ear that contains the receptive organs that are stimulated by sound waves (*i.e.,* hearing) or head position and movement (*i.e.,* vestibular function). Acute otitis media, or inflammation of the middle ear, is a leading cause of primary care visits and the number one reason for antimicrobial prescriptions for children. Hearing loss is one of the most common disabilities experienced by people in the United States, particularly among the elderly. It is also a cause of impaired language development in children. Vertigo, a disorder of vestibular function, is also a common cause of disability among the elderly. This chapter is divided into two parts: the first focuses on disorders of the ear and auditory function, and the second on disorders of the inner ear and vestibular function.

DISORDERS OF THE AUDITORY SYSTEM

After completing this section of the chapter, you should be able to meet the following objectives:

- List the structures of the external, middle, and inner ear and cite their function.
- Describe two common disorders of the outer ear.
- Relate the functions of the eustachian tube to the development of middle ear problems, including acute otitis media and otitis media with effusion.
- Describe anatomic variations as well as risk factors that make infants and young children more prone to develop acute otitis media.
- List three common symptoms of acute otitis media.
- Describe the disease process associated with otosclerosis and relate it to the progressive conductive hearing loss that occurs.
- Characterize tinnitus.
- Differentiate between conductive, sensorineural, and mixed hearing loss and cite the more common causes of each.

(objectives continue)

■ Describe methods used in the diagnosis and treatment of hearing loss.
■ Characterize the causes of hearing loss in infants and children and describe the need for early diagnosis and treatment.

Disorders of the External Ear

The external ear consists of the auricle, which collects sound, and external acoustic meatus or ear canal, which conducts the sound to the tympanic membrane[1,2] (Fig. 55-1). The auricle, or pinna, is composed of an irregularly shaped plate of elastic cartilage that is covered by thin skin. Its rim is somewhat thicker, and its fleshy earlobe lacks surrounding cartilage. The funnel shape of the auricle concentrates high-frequency sound entering from the lateral-forward direction into the ear canal. This shape also helps to prevent front-to-back confusion of sound sources.

The external acoustic meatus, or ear canal, is S-shaped and spans 2 to 3 cm in adults. In infants and young children, the canal is relatively shorter so that extra care must be taken when inspecting it with an otoscope. A thin layer of skin containing fine hairs, sebaceous glands, and ceruminous glands lines the ear canal. These glands produce cerumen, or earwax, which has certain antimicrobial properties and is thought to serve a protective function.

The anterior portion of the auricle and external part of the ear canal are innervated by branches of the trigeminal nerve (cranial nerve [CN] V). The posterior portions of the auricle and the wall of the ear canal are innervated by auricular branches of the facial (CN VII), glossopharyngeal (CN IX), and vagus (CN X) nerves. Because of the vagal innervation, the insertion of a speculum or an otoscope into the external ear canal can stimulate coughing or vomiting reflexes, particularly in young children.

The tympanic membrane, approximately 1 cm in diameter, is a thin, transparent membrane that separates the external ear from the middle ear. The tympanic membrane is covered with thin skin externally and the mucous membrane of the middle ear internally. The tympanic membrane is attached in a manner that allows it to vibrate freely when audible sound waves enter the external auditory canal. Movements of the membrane are transmitted through the middle ear to the inner ear.

When viewed through an otoscope, the tympanic membrane appears as a shallow, oval cone pointing inward toward its apex, the umbo (Fig. 55-2). Landmarks include the lightened stripe over the handle of the malleus; the umbo at the end of the handle; the pars tensa (tense part), which constitutes most of the drum; a thinner membrane, the pars flaccida (flaccid part); and the small area above the malleus attachment. A bright light reflected from an otoscope's illuminator, called the *cone of light,* radiates anteroinferiorly from the umbo. The tympanic membrane is semitransparent, and a small, whitish cord, which traverses the middle ear from back to front, can be seen just under its upper edge. This is the *chorda tympani,* a branch of the intermedius component of the facial nerve (CN VII).

The function of the external ear is disturbed when sound transmission is obstructed by impacted cerumen, inflammation (*i.e.,* otitis externa), or drainage from the external ear (otorrhea).

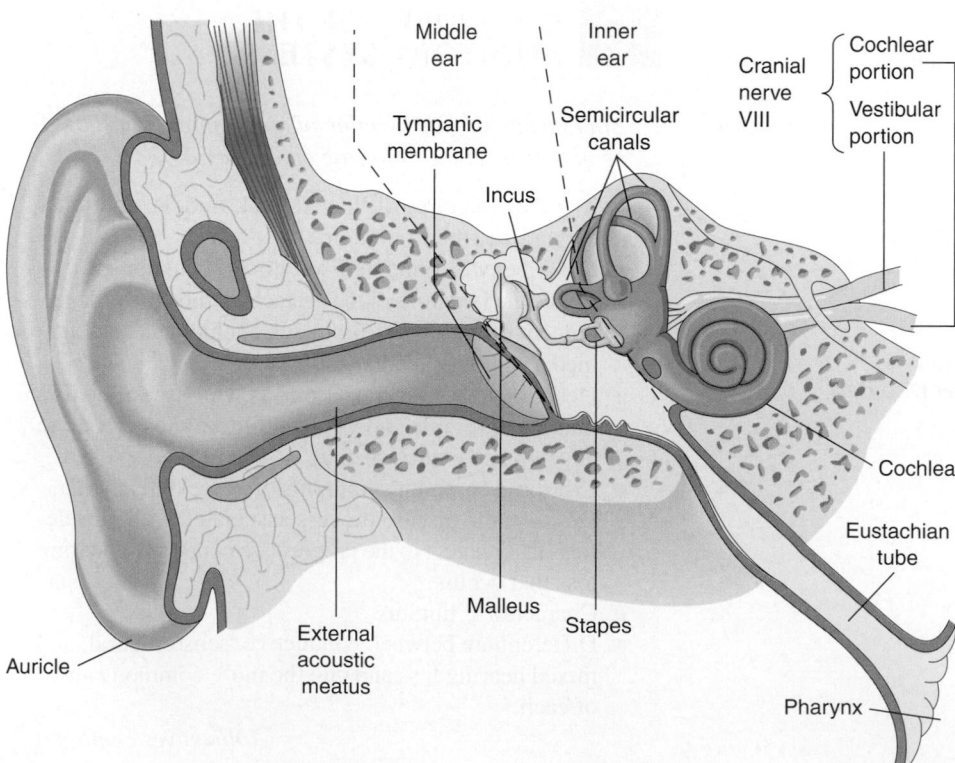

FIGURE 55-1 • External, middle, and internal subdivisions of the ear.

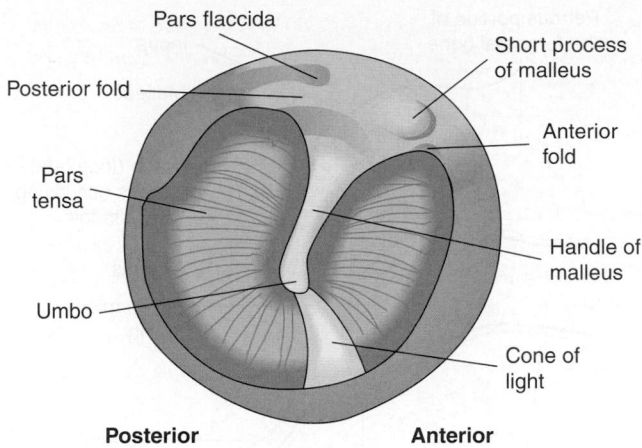

FIGURE 55-2 • Right eardrum.

Impacted Cerumen

Cerumen, or earwax, is a protective secretion produced by the sebaceous and ceruminous glands of the skin that lines the ear canal. Although the ear normally is self-cleaning, the cerumen can accumulate and narrow the canal, causing reversible hearing loss.[3,4]

Impacted cerumen usually produces no symptoms unless it hardens and touches the tympanic membrane, or the canal becomes irritated by a buildup of hardened cerumen. Clinical symptoms may include pain, itching, and a sensation of fullness. As the canal becomes completely occluded, a person may experience a feeling of fullness, a conductive hearing loss, and tinnitus (i.e., ringing in the ears). Because the external auditory canal is innervated by the auricular branch of the vagus nerve, coughing or even cardiac deceleration can result from stimulation of the canal by cerumen impaction or removal attempts.[3]

In most cases, cerumen can be removed by gentle irrigation using a bulb syringe and warm tap water. Warm water is used to avoid inducing a feeling of disequilibrium due to the vestibular caloric response. The ear canal should be dried thoroughly after irrigation to avoid introducing an infection. Irrigation should be avoided in an only-hearing ear or one that is postsurgical, prone to infection, or suspect for perforation of the tympanic membrane. Alternatively, health care professionals may remove cerumen using an otoscope and a metal curette.

Cerumen that has become hardened or impacted can be softened by instillation of a few drops of a ceruminolytic agent available commercially. Typically, these agents are instilled in the affected ear one or two times daily for up to 4 days before irrigation. Overuse should be avoided because this may make the condition worse. Ceruminolytic agents should not be used in ears that may have a perforated tympanic membrane.

Otitis Externa

Otitis externa is an inflammation of the external ear that can vary in severity from mild allergic dermatitis to severe cellulitis. It can be caused by infectious agents, irritation (e.g., wearing hearing aids or earphones), or allergic reactions. Predisposing factors include frequent exposure to moisture in the ear canal (i.e., swimmer's ear), trauma to the canal caused by cleaning or scratching, and allergies or skin conditions such as psoriasis. The most common bacterial pathogens are gram-negative rods (Pseudomonas aeruginosa, Proteus species) and fungi (Aspergillus) that grow in the presence of excess moisture.[5] Otitis externa commonly occurs in the summer and is manifested by itching, redness, tenderness, and narrowing of the ear canal because of swelling. Inflammation of the pinna or canal makes movement of the ear painful. There may be watery or purulent drainage and intermittent hearing loss.

Treatment usually includes the use of ear drops containing an appropriate antimicrobial or antifungal agent. For bacterial infections, a corticosteroid may be combined with an antimicrobial to reduce inflammation. Systemic oral agents are rarely needed. Protection of the ear from additional moisture (i.e., use of ear plugs) and avoidance of trauma from scratching with cotton-tipped applicators and other devices are important. Preventing recurrences is important, particularly in persons who swim frequently. Instillation of a dilute alcohol, acetic acid, or Burow otic solution (available in over-the-counter ear drops) immediately after contact with water is an effective prophylaxis.

Disorders of the Middle Ear and Eustachian Tube

The middle ear, or tympanic cavity, is a small, mucosa-lined cavity in the petrous portion of the temporal bone[1,6,7] (Fig. 55-3A). It is bounded laterally by the tympanic membrane and medially by a bony wall with two openings, the superior oval (vestibular) window and the round (cochlear) window. It is connected anteriorly with the nasopharynx by the eustachian tube, also called the pharyngotympanic tube. Posteriorly, it is connected with small air pockets in the temporal bone called mastoid air spaces or cells.

Three tiny bones, the auditory ossicles, are suspended from the roof of the middle ear cavity and connect the tympanic membrane with the oval window. They are connected by synovial joints and are covered with the epithelial lining of the cavity.[1,2] The malleus ("hammer") has its handle firmly fixed to the upper portion of the tympanic membrane. The head of the malleus articulates with the incus ("anvil"), which articulates with the stapes ("stirrup"), which is inserted and sealed into the oval window by an annular ligament. Arrangement of the ear ossicles is such that their lever movements transmit vibrations from the tympanic membrane to the oval window and from there to the fluid in the inner ear. Two tissue-covered openings in the medial wall, the oval and the round windows, provide for the transmission of sound waves between the air-filled middle ear and the fluid-filled inner ear. It is the piston-like action of the stapes footplate that sets up compression waves in the inner ear fluid.

DISORDERS OF THE MIDDLE EAR

- The middle ear is a small, air-filled compartment in the temporal bone. It is separated from the outer ear by the tympanic membrane; communication between the nasopharynx and the middle ear occurs through the eustachian tube; and tiny bony ossicles that span the middle ear transmit sound to the sensory receptors in the inner ear.

- Otitis media (OM) refers to inflammation of the middle ear. It can represent an acute otitis media (AOM) that has an abrupt onset and is usually related to bacterial infection, or otitis media with effusion (OME) that is associated with fluid in the middle ear without the manifestations of infection and which does not usually require treatment with antimicrobial agents.

- The function of the middle ear is to conduct sound waves from the external to the inner ear. Impaired conduction of sound waves and hearing loss occur when the tympanic membrane has been perforated; air in the middle ear has been replaced with fluid (OME); or the function of the bony ossicles has been impaired (otosclerosis).

Eustachian Tube Dysfunction

The eustachian tube, which connects the nasopharynx with the middle ear, is located in a gap in the bone between the anterior and medial walls of the middle ear (see Fig. 55-1). The eustachian tube serves three basic functions: (1) ventilation of the middle ear, along with equalization of middle ear and ambient pressures; (2) protection of the middle ear from unwanted nasopharyngeal sound waves and secretions; and (3) drainage of middle ear secretions into the nasopharynx.[5,6] The nasopharyngeal entrance to the eustachian tube, which usually is closed, is opened by the action of the trigeminal (CN V)–innervated *tensor veli palatini muscle.* Opening of the eustachian tube, which normally occurs with swallowing and yawning reflexes, provides the mechanism for equalizing the pressure of the middle ear with that of the atmosphere. This equalization ensures that the pressures on both sides of the tympanic membrane are the same, so that sound transmission is not reduced and rupture does not result from sudden changes in external pressure, as occurs during plane travel.

The eustachian tube is lined with a mucous membrane that is continuous with the pharynx and the mastoid air cells. Infections from the nasopharynx can travel from the nasopharynx along the mucous membrane of the eustachian tube to the middle ear, causing acute otitis media. Toward the nasopharynx, the eustachian tube becomes lined by columnar epithelium with mucus-secreting cells. Hypertrophy of the mucus-secreting cells is thought to contribute to the mucoid secretions that develop during certain types of otitis media.

Abnormalities in eustachian tube function are important factors in the pathogenesis of middle ear infections. There are

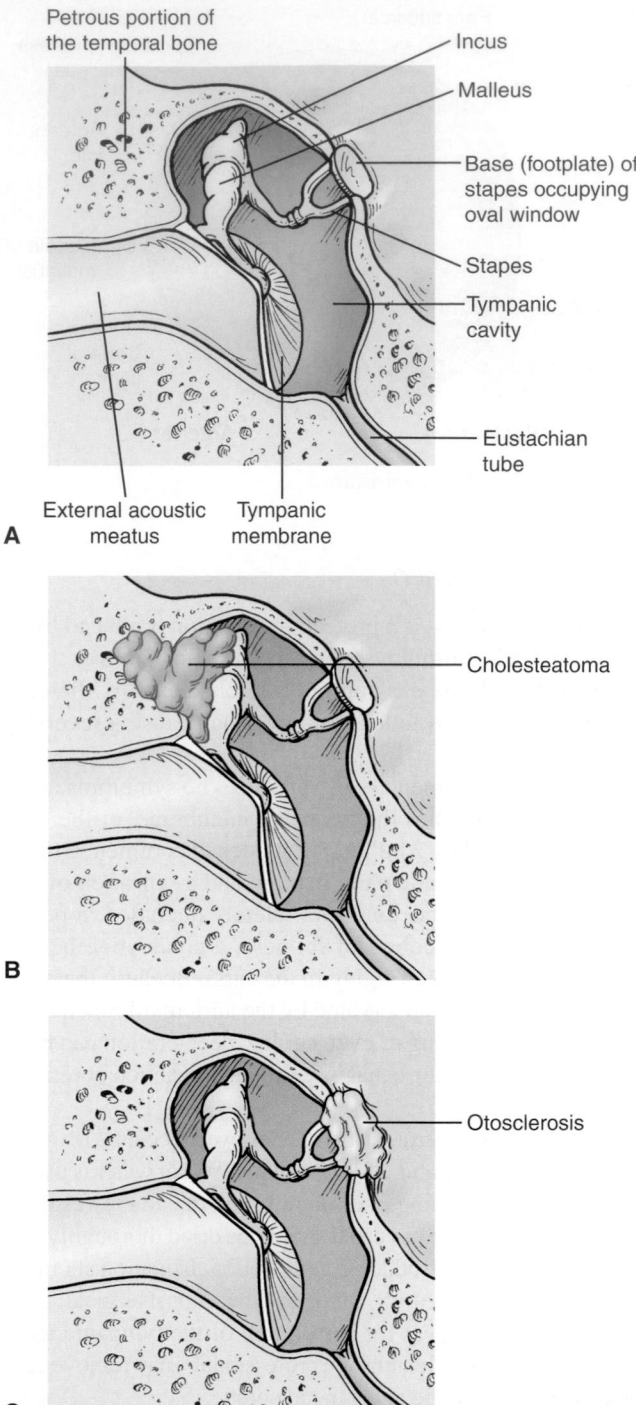

FIGURE 55-3 • Disorders of the middle ear. **(A)** Otitis media. Otitis involves inflammation of the tympanic cavity. Infection often enters through the eustachian tube. **(B)** Cholesteatoma, a cystlike mass of the middle ear that often extends to involve the temporal bone. **(C)** Otosclerosis involving formation of new, spongy bone around the stapes and oval window.

two important types of eustachian tube dysfunction: abnormal patency and obstruction (Fig. 55-4). The *abnormally patent tube* does not close or does not close completely. In infants and children with an abnormally patent tube, air and secretions often are pumped into the eustachian tube during crying and nose blowing.

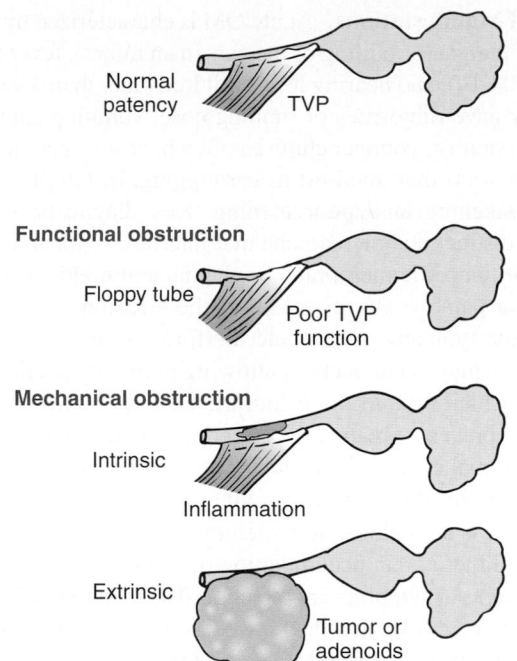

FIGURE 55-4 • Pathophysiology of the eustachian tube. TVP, tensor veli palatini. (Developed from Bluestone C. D. [1981]. Recent advances in the pathogenesis, diagnosis, and management of otitis media. *Pediatric Clinics of North America* 28, 737. With permission from Elsevier Science.)

Obstruction can be functional or mechanical. *Functional obstruction* results from the persistent collapse of the eustachian tube due to a lack of tubal stiffness or poor function of the tensor veli palatini muscle that controls the opening of the eustachian tube. It is common in infants and young children because the amount and stiffness of the cartilage supporting the eustachian tube are less than in older children and adults. Changes in the craniofacial base also render the tensor muscle less efficient for opening the eustachian tube in this age group. In addition, craniofacial disorders, such as a cleft palate, alter the attachment of the tensor muscle, producing functional obstruction of the eustachian tube.

Mechanical obstruction results from internal obstruction or external compression of the eustachian tube. Ethnic differences in the structure of the palate may increase the likelihood of obstruction. The most common internal obstruction is caused by swelling and secretions resulting from allergy and viral respiratory infections. External compression by prominent or enlarged adenoidal tissue surrounding the opening of the eustachian tube may make drainage less effective. Tumors also may obstruct drainage. With obstruction, air in the middle ear is absorbed, causing a negative pressure and the transudation of serous capillary fluid into the middle ear.

Barotrauma

Barotrauma represents injury resulting from the inability to equalize middle ear with ambient pressure during air travel or, less commonly, underwater diving. It occurs most often during air travel when there is a sudden change in atmospheric pressure. The pressure in the middle ear parallels atmospheric pressure; it decreases at high altitudes and increases at lower altitudes. The problem occurs during rapid airplane descent, when the negative pressure in the middle ear tends to cause the eustachian tube to collapse. If air cannot pass back through the eustachian tube, hearing loss and discomfort develop.

This most often occurs in persons who travel while suffering from an upper respiratory tract infection. Autoinflation measures such as yawning, swallowing, and chewing gum facilitate opening of the eustachian tube, which equalizes air pressure in the middle ear. Intranasal or systemic decongestants may be used to prevent symptoms. Acute negative middle ear pressure that persists on the ground is treated with decongestants and attempts at autoinflation. More severe hearing loss or discomfort may require that the person consult an otolaryngologist. Myringotomy (*i.e.*, surgical incision in the tympanic membrane) provides immediate relief and may be used in cases of acute otalgia and hearing loss. Placement of ventilation tubes may be considered for persons with repeated episodes of barotrauma related to frequent air travel.

Otitis Media

Otitis media (OM) refers to inflammation of the middle ear without reference to etiology or pathogenesis (see Fig. 55-3A). Acute OM is the most common infection for which antimicrobial agents are prescribed for children in the United States.[8] As such, the diagnosis and management of OM has a significant impact on the health of children, cost of providing care, and overall use of antimicrobial agents. During 2000, there were 16 million office visits for OM, with more than 13 million prescriptions for OM-related antimicrobial agents.[8]

Several terms are important in reference to OM. *Acute otitis media* (AOM) refers to an acute middle ear infection.[8] It usually has an abrupt onset of signs and symptoms related to middle ear inflammation and effusion. *Otitis media with effusion* (OME) refers to the presence of fluid in the middle ear without signs and symptoms of acute ear infection.[9] OME is more common than AOM.[8] It can develop spontaneously because of poor eustachian tube function, accompany a viral upper respiratory tract infection, or occur as a prelude or a sequela to AOM.[8,9] Because OME does not usually require treatment with antimicrobial agents, it is important to differentiate OME from AOM to avoid unnecessary use of antimicrobial agents.

Risk Factors. Although AOM may occur in any age group, it is the most frequent primary diagnosis in preschool-age children, and it accounts for almost 20% of ambulatory care visits in this age group.[10] Infants and young children between the ages of 3 months and 3 years are at highest risk for AOM, with the peak incidence between 6 and 11 months.[10] There is a second peak incidence at about 5 years of age that is believed to be associated with entrance into school.[10] Risk factors include premature birth, male gender, ethnicity (Native American, Inuit), family history of recurrent otitis media, presence of siblings in the household, genetic syndromes, and low socioeconomic status.[9,11,12] AOM is more frequent in children with orofacial abnormalities such as cleft lip and palate.

The most important factor that contributes to AOM is believed to be a dysfunction of the eustachian tube that allows reflux of fluid and bacteria into the middle ear space from the nasopharynx. There are two reasons for the increased risk of AOM in infants and young children: the eustachian tube is shorter, more horizontal, and wider in this age group than in older children and adults; and infection can spread more easily through the eustachian canal of infants who spend most of their day in the supine position.[8] Bottle-fed infants have a higher incidence of AOM than breast-fed infants, probably because they are held in a more horizontal position during feeding, and swallowing while in the horizontal position facilitates the reflux of milk into the middle ear. Breast-feeding also provides for the transfer of protective maternal antibodies to the infant.

Measures to reduce the risk for development of AOM during the first 6 months of life include breast-feeding and reduction or elimination of pacifier use.[8,13] Other ways to reduce the risk of developing AOM include minimal exposure to group settings and the avoidance or elimination of bottle-propping as well as exposure to passive tobacco smoke.[8,13] Efficacy in prevention of OM during the respiratory illness season has been demonstrated by immunoprophylaxis with killed and live-attenuated intranasal influenza vaccines.[8] The recent recommendation by the Advisory Committee on Immunization Practice to immunize children older than 6 months of age with influenza virus eliminates the specific need for using the vaccine in the prevention of OM.[14] Immunization with pneumococcal vaccine has also been shown to reduce the incidence of OM caused by vaccine-serotype *Pneumococcus,* but the overall effect has been small.[8]

Etiology. Acute OM may be of either bacterial or viral origin. The mucosal lining of the middle ear is continuous with the eustachian tube and nasopharynx, and most middle ear infections enter through the eustachian tube (see Fig. 55-1). Bacteria may replicate in fluid of the middle ear to cause bacterial OM; respiratory viruses may infect the middle ear mucosa, either alone, leading to viral OM, or in combination with bacteria. Most cases of AOM follow an uncomplicated upper respiratory tract infection that has been present for several days. Respiratory syncytial virus is the most common viral pathogen in middle ear fluid from children with AOM, although other viruses (*e.g.,* rhinovirus, parainfluenza virus, adenovirus) have been isolated.[10] The most common bacteria in AOM are *Streptococcus pneumoniae, Haemophilus influenzae,* and *Moraxella catarrhalis.*[10,12] Respiratory viruses (or virus-derived ribonucleic acid [RNA]) may also be found in the middle ear exudates of children with AOM, either alone or, more commonly, in association with pathogenic bacteria. Emergence of a multiple–drug-resistant strain of *S. pneumoniae* has led to increased numbers of treatment failures.[15] There is also evidence that the formation of bacterial biofilms may play a role in the pathogenesis of recurrent AOM that does not respond to antimicrobial therapy.[16] Biofilms consist of aggregated bacteria, usually adherent to a surface and surrounded by an extracellular matrix covering that isolates and protects them from antimicrobial agents (see Chapter 16).

Clinical Manifestations. Acute OM is characterized by acute onset of otalgia (or pulling of the ears in an infant), fever (up to 40°C [104°F]), and hearing loss. Children older than 3 years of age may have rhinorrhea or running nose, vomiting, and diarrhea. In contrast, younger children often have nonspecific signs and symptoms that manifest as ear tugging, irritability, nighttime awakening, and poor feeding. Key diagnostic criteria include distinct otalgia (earache that interferes with activity or sleep) or tympanic membrane erythema, and middle ear effusion.[8] Ear pain usually increases as the effusion accumulates behind the tympanic membrane. Perforation of the tympanic membrane may occur acutely, allowing purulent material from the eustachian tube to drain into the external auditory canal. This may prevent spread of the infection into the temporal bone or intracranial cavity. Healing of the tympanic membrane usually follows resolution of the middle ear infection.

OME is a condition in which the tympanic membrane is intact and there is an accumulation of fluid in the middle ear without signs or symptoms of infection. The duration of the effusion may range from less than 3 weeks to more than 3 months. The similarity between OME and AOM is that hearing loss may be present in both conditions. Many cases of OME resolve spontaneously, but 30% to 40% of patients have recurrent OME, and 5% to 10% of episodes last 1 year or longer.[9] Persistent middle ear fluid from OME results in decreased motility of the tympanic membrane and serves as a barrier to sound conduction.

Diagnosis. Distinguishing between AOM and OME on clinical grounds is often straightforward, but because each condition may evolve into the other without any clearly differentiating physical findings, any system for distinguishing between them is somewhat arbitrary. Because of the increasing antimicrobial resistance, distinguishing between AOM and OME has become increasingly important

Both AOM without otorrhea (drainage from the ear) and OME are accompanied by otoscopic signs of middle ear effusion, namely, the presence of at least two of three tympanic membrane abnormalities: white, yellow, amber (or occasionally blue) discoloration; opacification other than scarring; and decreased or absent motility. With OME the tympanic membrane is often cloudy with distinct impairment of mobility, and an air–fluid level or bubble may be visible in the middle ear.

A definitive diagnosis of AOM requires the following: history of acute onset of signs and symptoms, the presence of middle ear effusion, and signs and symptoms of middle ear inflammation.[8–13] Signs of middle ear inflammation include fullness or bulging of the tympanic membrane with or without erythema, limited or absent mobility of the tympanic membrane, a purulent (pus-containing) effusion, and ear pain that interferes with normal activity. Unless intense, erythema alone is insufficient to support a diagnosis of AOM because erythema without other abnormalities may result from crying or vascular flushing. The malleus may be obscured and the tympanic membrane may resemble a bagel without a hole, but with a central indentation.[11]

The diagnosis of AOM should be confirmed with pneumatic otoscopy and can be supplemented with tympanometry and acoustic reflectometry. The use of the pneumatic otoscope permits the introduction of air into the ear canal for the purpose of determining tympanic membrane flexibility. The movement of the tympanic membrane is decreased in some cases of AOM and absent in chronic middle ear infection. The diagnosis of AOM can also be confirmed using tympanometry or acoustic reflectometry. *Tympanometry* is helpful in detecting effusion in the middle ear or high negative middle ear pressure.[17] Portable tympanometers (resembling an otoscope) and desktop instruments are available. A tympanogram is obtained by using a small probe that is placed snugly into the external ear canal. A sound stimulus generator then transmits acoustic energy into the canal, while a vacuum pump introduces positive and negative pressures into the ear canal. A microphone in the instrument detects returning sound energy. The tympanogram provides a determination of the degree of negative pressure present in the middle ear. It detects disease when present but is less reliable when disease is absent. *Acoustic reflectometry* detects reflected sound waves from the middle ear and provides information on whether an effusion is absent or present. Increased reflected sound correlates with an increased likelihood of effusion. This technique is most useful in children older than 3 months, and its success depends on user technique.

Tympanocentesis (puncture of the tympanic membrane with a needle) may be done to relieve pain from an effusion or to obtain a specimen of middle ear fluid for culture and sensitivity testing. The procedure involves the insertion of a needle through the inferior part of the tympanic membrane. Because of the cost, effort, and lack of availability, it is not routinely used in management of AOM.[10] In selected cases of refractory or recurrent middle ear disease, tympanocentesis can help improve diagnostic accuracy, guide treatment, and avoid unnecessary medical or surgical interventions. In instances where the tympanic membrane has perforated with resultant drainage into the external ear, a specimen can be obtained and microbiologic studies can be done to identify the organism.

Treatment. The treatment of OM focuses on symptom control and management of the underlying pathologic process. A number of options for pain management are available, including the local application of heat and use of analgesic drugs such as acetaminophen, ibuprofen, and naproxen. Myringotomy (incision of the tympanic membrane) can be used for relief of pressure in the child who is in severe pain, providing almost immediate relief.[12]

The extensive use of antimicrobial agents contributes to the development of bacterial resistance, and evidence exists for the efficacy and safety of two alternative approaches to routine antibiotic prescription: delayed prescription and watchful waiting.[18,19] Observation without antimicrobial agents is an option in a child with uncomplicated AOM. These approaches involve waiting for 72 hours to see if symptoms improve before institution of antibiotic therapy. Factors to consider when deciding whether to defer treatment include the child's age, severity of illness, and certainty of the diagnosis. If observation is recommended, it is essential that the parent or caregiver have ready access to communication, follow-up, and a mechanism for obtaining medication if needed.

Most cases of OME resolve spontaneously within a 3-week to 3-month period. The management options for this duration include observation only, antibiotic therapy, or combination antibiotic and corticosteroid therapy. Topical and systemic decongestants usually are of little value in clearing middle ear effusion.[9] Referral to an otolaryngologist is indicated if the effusion persists for 4 months or longer. Because there is concern over hearing loss and its effect on learning and speech, a hearing evaluation is recommended when OME persists for 3 months or longer or at any time that language delay, learning problems, or a significant hearing loss is suspected.[9] Children with recurrent OM should be evaluated to rule out any anatomic variations (*e.g.,* enlarged adenoids), allergies, and immunologic abnormalities. Children with immunoglobulin G subclass deficiencies (see Chapter 21) and poor responses to polysaccharide vaccines are more likely to develop recurrent OM.[12]

Surgical treatment (*e.g.,* tympanostomy tubes, adenoidectomy) may be indicated if the effusion has persisted for 4 months or longer and is accompanied by persistent hearing loss and other manifestations; if recurrent or persistent effusion occurs in children at risk regardless of hearing status; or if there is structural damage to the tympanic membrane or middle ear.[9] Tympanostomy tube insertion is the preferred initial procedure and does not typically include the removal of adenoids unless the child has additional indications, such as postnasal obstruction from enlarged adenoids. The tubes usually are inserted under general anesthesia. The ears of children with tubes must be kept out of water. The adverse effects of tube placement include recurrent otorrhea; persistent perforation, scarring, and atrophy of the tympanic membrane; and cholesteatoma. Adenoidectomy plus myringotomy (without tube insertion) has been shown to have comparable efficacy in children 4 years of age or older, but is more invasive, with additional surgical and anesthetic risks.[9] Recent research indicates that prompt insertion of tympanostomy tubes for persistent OME in otherwise healthy children who were younger than 3 years of age did not improve developmental outcomes (*e.g.,* literacy, attention, social skills, and academic achievement) as compared with delayed insertion in children in whom effusion continued unremittingly.[20]

Complications of Otitis Media. The complications of OM include hearing loss, adhesive OM, cholesteatoma, mastoiditis, and intracranial complications such as otologic meningitis.

Hearing loss, which is a common complication of OM, usually is conductive and temporary based on the duration of the effusion. Hearing loss that is associated with fluid collection usually resolves when the effusion clears. Permanent hearing loss may occur as the result of damage to the tympanic membrane or other middle ear structures. Cases of sensorineural hearing loss are rare. Persistent and episodic conductive hearing loss in children may impair their cognitive, linguistic, and emotional development.[9,11] Children younger than 3 years of age with recurrent OME are at increased risk of impaired language development.

Additional studies indicate that before 3 years of age, time spent with middle ear effusion correlates with decreased cognitive development as measured by standardized inventories. However, the degree and duration of hearing loss required to produce such effects are unknown.

Adhesive OM involves an abnormal healing reaction in an inflamed middle ear.[11] It produces irreversible thickening of the mucous membranes and may cause impaired movement of the ossicles and possibly conductive hearing loss. Tympanosclerosis involves the formation of whitish plaques and nodular deposits on the submucosal surface of the tympanic membrane, with possible adherence of the ossicles and conductive hearing loss.

Cholesteatomas are cystlike lesions of the middle ear, usually associated with chronic otitis media[11] (see Fig. 55-3B). Measuring 1 to 4 cm in diameter, they are lined with keratinizing squamous epithelium or metaplastic mucus-secreting epithelium and filled with amorphous debris (derived largely from desquamated epithelium).[21–23] Sometimes they contain spicules of cholesterol. Although precise mechanisms involved in their development are unclear, it is proposed that chronic inflammation and perforation of the ear drum with ingrowth of squamous epithelium or metaplasia of the secretory epithelium of the middle are contributing factors. Sometimes the cyst ruptures, enhancing the inflammatory reaction. These lesions, by progressive enlargement, can erode the ossicles, the labyrinth, the adjacent mastoid bone, and the surrounding soft tissues. Although often thought of as a complication of otitis media, a cholesteatoma may also occur as a congenital condition. Symptoms commonly include painless drainage from the ear and hearing loss. Treatment involves microsurgical techniques to remove the cholesteatomatous material.

The mastoid antrum and air cells constitute a portion of the temporal bone and may become inflamed as an extension of acute or chronic OM.[21] The disorder causes necrosis of the mastoid process and destruction of the bony intercellular matrix, which are visible by radiologic examination. Mastoid tenderness and drainage of exudate through a perforated tympanic membrane can occur. Chronic mastoiditis can develop as the result of chronic middle ear infection. The usefulness of antimicrobial agents for this condition is limited. Mastoid or middle ear surgery, along with other medical treatment, may be indicated. The incidence of mastoiditis has markedly decreased compared with the pre-antimicrobial era. It remains uncertain whether this decrease is due to antimicrobial treatment, changes in the natural history of OM, changes in organism virulence, or increased host resistance.[21]

Intracranial complications are uncommon since the advent of antimicrobial therapy. Although rare, these complications can develop when the infection spreads through vascular channels, by direct extension, or through preformed pathways such as the round window.[21] These complications are seen more often with chronic suppurative OM and mastoiditis. They include otogenic meningitis, brain abscess, lateral sinus thrombophlebitis or thrombosis, labyrinthitis, and facial nerve paralysis. Any child who develops persistent headache, tinnitus, stiff neck, or visual or other neurologic symptoms should be investigated for possible intracranial complications.

Otosclerosis

Otosclerosis refers to the formation of new spongy bone around the stapes and oval window, which results in progressive deafness[24,25] (see Fig. 55-3C). In most cases, the condition is familial and follows an autosomal dominant pattern with variable penetrance. Otosclerosis may begin at any time in life but usually does not appear until after puberty, most frequently between the ages of 20 and 30 years. The disease process accelerates during pregnancy.

Otosclerosis begins with resorption of bone in one or more foci. During active bone resorption, the bone structure appears spongy and softer than normal (*i.e.,* osteospongiosis). The resorbed bone is replaced by an overgrowth of new, hard, sclerotic bone. The process is slowly progressive, involving more areas of the temporal bone, especially in front of and posterior to the stapes footplate. As it invades the footplate, the pathologic bone increasingly immobilizes the stapes, reducing the transmission of sound. Pressure of otosclerotic bone on middle ear structures or the vestibulocochlear nerve (CN VIII) may contribute to the development of tinnitus, sensorineural hearing loss, and vertigo.

The symptoms of otosclerosis involve an insidious hearing loss. Initially, the affected person is unable to hear a whisper or someone speaking at a distance. In the earliest stages, the bone conduction by which the person's own voice is heard remains relatively unaffected. At this point, the person's own voice sounds unusually loud, and the sound of chewing becomes intensified. Because of bone conduction, most of these persons can hear fairly well on the telephone, which provides an amplified signal. Many are able to hear better in a noisy environment, probably because the masking effect of background noise causes other persons to speak louder.

The treatment of otosclerosis can be medical or surgical. A carefully selected, well-fitting hearing aid may allow a person with conductive deafness to lead a normal life. Sodium fluoride has been used with some success in the medical treatment of osteospongiosis.[5] Because much of the conductive hearing loss associated with otosclerosis is caused by stapedial fixation, surgical treatment involves stapedectomy with stapedial reconstruction using the patient's own stapes or a stapedial prosthesis. The argon laser may be used in the surgical procedure.

Disorders of the Inner Ear

The inner ear contains a labyrinth or system of intercommunicating channels and the receptors for hearing and position sense.[1,2,26,27] Structurally, it consists of an outer bony labyrinth located in the otic capsule of the petrous part of the temporal bone and an inner membranous labyrinth (Fig. 55-5). The membranous labyrinth lies in the bony labyrinth and consists of a complex system of sacs and ducts (*i.e.,* semicircular ducts). The bony labyrinth, which occupies a space with a diameter less than 1.5 cm, is a series of cavities (the cochlea, vestibule, and semicircular canals). The receptors for hearing are contained in the cochlea and those for head position sense are con-

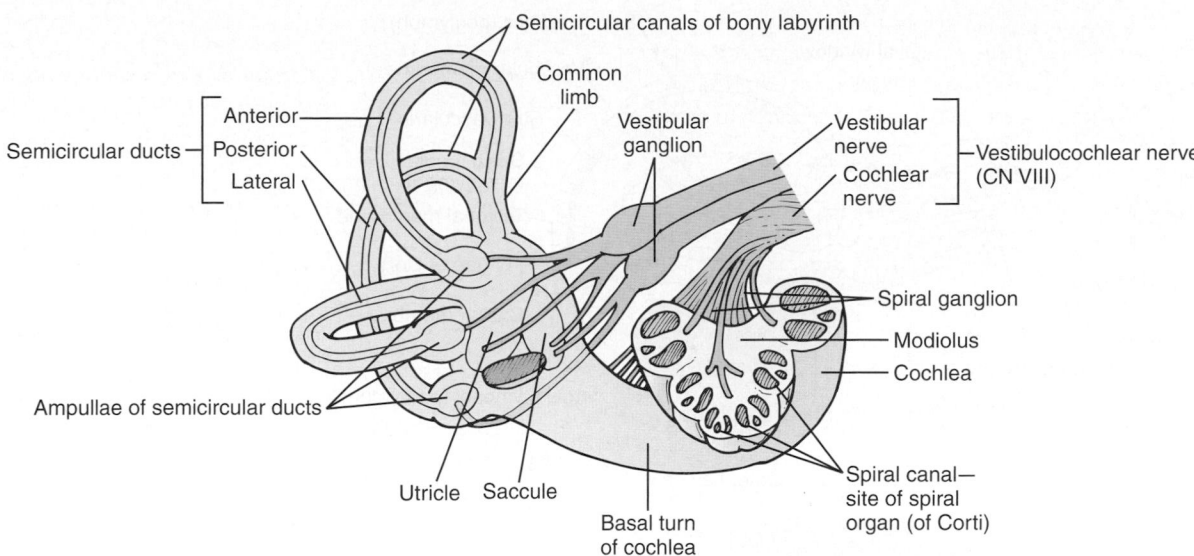

FIGURE 55-5 • Schematic lateral view of the bony canals of the vestibular system showing the membranous labyrinth in a closed system of ducts and chambers filled with endolymph and bathed in perilymph with the bony labyrinth. Observe the parts of the membranous labyrinth: the semi-circular ducts and the saccule and utricle within the vestibule. (Adapted from Moore K. L., Dalley A. F. [1999]. *Clinically oriented anatomy* [4th ed., p. 1102]. Philadelphia: Lippincott Williams & Wilkins.)

tained in the semicircular ducts, the utricle, and the saccule. The vestibule is the central egg-shaped cavity of the bony labyrinth that lies posterior to the cochlea and anterior to the semicircular canals. It contains the utricle and saccule and parts of the balancing apparatus (vestibular labyrinth). The vestibule features the oval window on its lateral wall, occupied by the base of the stapes.

The cochlea is the shell-shaped part of the bony labyrinth that contains the inner membranous cochlear duct, the part of the inner ear concerned with hearing. The spiral canal of the cochlea, which is shaped like a snail shell, begins at the vestibule and winds around a central core of spongy bone called the *modiolus* (see Fig. 55-5). The modiolus contains canals for blood vessels and for distribution of the cochlear nerve. The cochlea consists of three tubes coiled side-by-side: (1) the *scala vestibuli,* (2) the *scala media,* and (3) the *scala tympani* (see Fig. 55-5). The scala vestibuli and scala media are separated from each other by the vestibular membrane, also known as *Reissner membrane,* and the scala tympani is separated from the scala media by the basilar membrane. On the surface of the basilar membrane lies the spiral organ of Corti, which contains a series of electromechanically sensitive cells, the *hair cells.* They are the receptive organs that generate nerve impulses in response to sound vibrations.

Two separate fluids are found in the cochlea of the inner ear: the endolymph and perilymph. The scala vestibuli and scala tympani communicate directly with the subarachnoid space around the brain, so the perilymph is similar to cerebrospinal fluid.[26] The endolymph that fills scala media is an entirely different fluid that is secreted by the stria vascularis on the outer wall of the scala media (Fig. 55-6A). The perilymph

that fills the scala vestibuli and scala tympani has a high sodium (Na$^+$) concentration, whereas the endolymph that fills the scala media has a high potassium (K$^+$) content. A direct-current resting membrane potential of about +80 mV exists between the endolymph and perilymph, with positivity inside the scala media and negativity outside. This current, which is called the *endolymphatic potential,* is generated by the continual secretion of K$^+$ ions into the scala media by Na$^+$/K$^+$-adenosine triphosphatase (ATPase) pumps in the stria vascularis. This current is believed to sensitize the hair cells of the organ of Corti, increasing their ability to respond to the slightest sound. Degeneration of the stria vascularis, which has been called the "battery of the cochlea," and the resultant decline in the endolymphatic potential, is thought to be one of the causes of hearing loss that occurs with aging.[28]

Unlike light, which can be transmitted through a vacuum such as outer space, sound is a pressure disturbance originating from a vibrating object and propagated by the molecules of an elastic medium. Sound waves, which are delivered by the stapes footplate to the perilymph, travel throughout the fluid of the inner ear, including up the scala vestibuli, to the apex of the cochlea (see Fig. 55-6A). Because of the thinness of the vestibular membrane, sound vibrations from the scala vestibuli are readily transmitted into the scala media. Therefore, as far as sound conduction is concerned, the scala media and scala vestibuli function as a single chamber.

As the pressure wave descends through the endolymph of the scala media it sets the entire basilar membrane vibrating. The basilar membrane, which becomes progressively more massive from its base to its distal apex, resonates at higher frequencies near the base and at lower frequencies

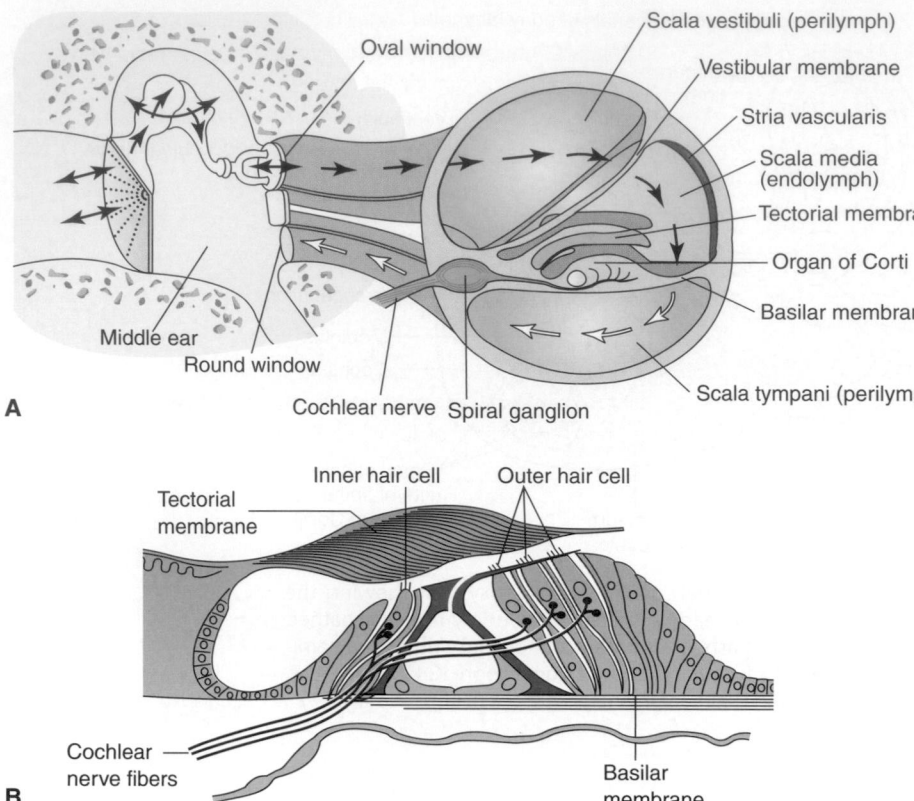

A

B

FIGURE 55-6 • **(A)** Path taken by sound waves reaching the inner ear. **(B)** Spiral organ of Corti has been removed from the cochlear duct and greatly enlarged to show the inner and outer hair cells, the basilar membrane, and cochlear nerve fibers.

toward its apex as the fluid pressure wave travels up the cochlear spiral. This "tuned" aspect of the basilar membrane results in increased amplitude of displacement at the resonant locations, responding to a particular sound frequency and greater firing of cochlear neurons innervating this region. This mechanism provides the major basis for the discrimination of sound frequency.

Perched on the basilar membrane and extending along its entire length is an elaborate arrangement of columnar epithelium called the *spiral organ of Corti* (see Fig. 55-6B). Continuous rows of hair cells separated into inner and outer rows can be found in the columnar arrangement of the spiral organ. The cells have hairlike cilia that protrude through openings in an overlying supporting reticular membrane into the endolymph of the cochlear duct. A gelatinous mass, the tectorial membrane, extends from the medial side of the duct to enclose the cilia of the outer hair cells. The hair cells in the organ of Corti are programmed to respond to deformation of the cochlear duct induced by compression waves moving through the perilymph, which ascend and descend in the surrounding scala vestibuli and scala tympani. Selective destruction of hair cells in a particular segment of the cochlea can lead to hearing loss of particular tones.

Neural Pathways

Information flows from the hair cells in the organ of Corti to neurons that have their cell bodies in the cochlear ganglion,

which follows a spiral course in the bony modiolus of the cochlear spiral. Afferent fibers from the spiral ganglion (*i.e.*, vestibulocochlear or auditory nerve [CN VIII]) travel to the cochlear nuclei in the caudal pons (see Fig. 55-5). Many secondary nerve fibers from the cochlear nuclei pass to the opposite side of the pons. These secondary fibers may project to such cell groups as the trapezoid or the superior olivary nucleus, or rostrally toward the inferior colliculus of the midbrain. Ipsilateral projections and interconnections between the nuclei of the two sides occur throughout the central auditory system. Consequently, impulses from either ear are transmitted through the auditory pathways to both sides of the brain stem.

From the inferior colliculus, the auditory pathway passes to the medial geniculate nucleus of the thalamus, where all the fibers synapse. From the medial geniculate nuclei, the auditory tract spreads through the auditory radiation to the primary auditory cortex (area 41), located mainly in the superior temporal gyrus and insula (see Chapter 48, Fig. 48-24). This area and its corresponding higher-order thalamic nuclei are required for high-acuity loudness discrimination and precise discrimination of pitch. The auditory association cortex (areas 42 and 22) borders the primary cortex on the superior temporal gyrus. This area and its associated higher-order thalamic nuclei are necessary for auditory gnosis, or the meaningfulness of sound, to occur. Experience and the precise analysis of momentary auditory information are integrated during this process.

Tinnitus

Tinnitus (from the Latin *tinniere,* meaning "to ring") is the perception of abnormal ear or head noises, not produced by an external stimulus.[29–32] Although it often is described as "ringing of the ears," it may also assume a hissing, roaring, buzzing, or humming sound. Tinnitus may be constant, intermittent, and unilateral or bilateral. According to the American Tinnitus Association, 50 million Americans have tinnitus, 12 million of whom seek medical care.[29] The condition affects both sexes equally, is most prevalent between 40 and 70 years of age, and occasionally affects children.[31]

Although tinnitus is subjective, for clinical purposes it is subdivided into objective and subjective tinnitus.[29] *Objective tinnitus* refers to those rare cases in which the sound is detected or potentially detectable by another observer. Typical causes of objective tinnitus include vascular abnormalities or neuromuscular disorders. In some vascular disorders, for example, sounds generated by turbulent blood flow (*e.g.,* arterial bruits or venous hums) are conducted to the auditory system. Vascular disorders typically produce a pulsatile form of tinnitus.

Subjective tinnitus refers to noise perception when there is no noise stimulation of the cochlea. A number of causes and conditions have been associated with subjective tinnitus. Intermittent periods of mild, high-pitched tinnitus lasting for several minutes are common in normal-hearing persons. Impacted cerumen is a benign cause of tinnitus, which resolves after the earwax is removed. Medications such as aspirin and stimulants such as nicotine and caffeine can cause transient tinnitus. Conditions associated with more persistent tinnitus include noise-induced hearing loss, presbycusis (sensorineural hearing loss that occurs with aging), hypertension, atherosclerosis, head injury, and cochlear or labyrinthine infection or inflammation.

The physiologic mechanism underlying subjective tinnitus is largely unknown. It seems likely that there are several mechanisms, including abnormal firing of auditory receptors, dysfunction of cochlear neurotransmitter function or ionic balance, damage to the auditory nerve, or alterations in central processing of the signal.

Because tinnitus is a symptom, the diagnosis relies heavily on the person's description of the problem, including onset, frequency, description, and location of the tinnitus; perceived cause; and the extent to which the person is bothered by the problem.[32] A history of medication or stimulant use and dietary factors that may cause tinnitus should be obtained. Tinnitus often accompanies hearing disorders, and tests of auditory function usually are done. Causes of objective tinnitus, such as serious vascular abnormalities, should be ruled out.

Treatment measures are designed to treat the symptoms rather than effect a cure.[29–31] They include elimination of drugs or other substances, such as caffeine, some cheeses, red wine, and foods containing monosodium glutamate, that are suspected of causing tinnitus. The use of an externally produced sound (*i.e.,* noise generators or tinnitus-masking devices) may be used to mask or inhibit the tinnitus. Medications, including antihistamines, anticonvulsant drugs, calcium channel blockers, benzodiazepines, and antidepressants, have been used for tinnitus alleviation, but most are not effective, and many produce undesirable side effects. For persistent tinnitus, psychological interventions may be needed to help the person deal with the stress and distraction associated with the condition. Tinnitus retraining therapy, which includes directive counseling and extended use of low-noise generators to facilitate auditory adaptation to the tinnitus, has met with considerable success. Surgical intervention (*i.e.,* cochlear nerve section, vascular decompression) is a last resort for persons in whom all other interventions have failed and in whom the disorder is disabling.

Disorders of the Central Auditory Pathways

The auditory pathways in the brain involve communication between the two sides of the brain at many levels. As a result, strokes, tumors, abscesses, and other focal abnormalities seldom produce more than a mild reduction in auditory acuity on the side opposite the lesion. For intelligibility of auditory language, lateral dominance becomes important. On the dominant side, usually the left side, the more medial and dorsal portion of the auditory association cortex is of crucial importance. This area is called the *Wernicke area,* and damage to it is associated with auditory receptive aphasia. Persons with damage to this area of the brain can speak intelligibly and read normally but are unable to understand the meaning of major aspects of audible speech.

Irritative foci that affect the auditory radiation or the primary auditory cortex can produce roaring or clicking sounds, which appear to come from the auditory environment of the opposite side (*i.e.,* auditory hallucinations). Focal seizures that originate in or near the auditory cortex often are immediately preceded by the perception of ringing or other sounds preceded by a prodrome (*i.e.,* aura). Damage to the auditory association cortex, especially if bilateral, results in deficiencies of sound recognition and memory (*i.e.,* auditory agnosia). If the damage is in the dominant hemisphere, speech recognition can be affected (*i.e.,* sensory or receptive aphasia).

Hearing Loss

Nearly 28 million Americans have hearing loss.[33] It affects persons of all age groups. Two to 3 of every 1000 children in the United States are born deaf or hard of hearing, and 9 of 10 children who are born deaf are born to parents who can hear.[33] Approximately 30% of people older than 65 years of age and 40% to 50% of those 75 years of age and older have a hearing loss.[33]

Hearing is a specialized sense that provides the ability to perceive vibration of sound waves. Functions of the ear include

🔑 HEARING LOSS

- Hearing is a special sensory function that incorporates the sound-transmitting properties of the external ear canal, the eardrum that separates the external and middle ear, the bony ossicles of the middle ear, the sensory receptors of the cochlea in the inner ear, the neural pathways of the vestibulocochlear or auditory nerve, and the primary auditory and auditory association cortices.

- Hearing loss represents impairment of the ability to detect and perceive sound.

- It can range from mild, affecting sounds of different tones and intensities, to moderate or profound.

- Hearing loss can be caused by conductive disorders, in which auditory stimuli are not transmitted through the structures of the outer and middle ears to the sensory receptors in the inner ear; by sensorineural disorders that affect the inner ear, auditory nerve, or auditory pathways; or by a combination of conductive and sensorineural disorders.

receiving sound waves, distinguishing their frequency, translating this information into nerve impulses, and transmitting these impulses to the central nervous system (CNS). The compression waves that produce sound have frequency and intensity. *Frequency* indicates the number of waves per unit time (reported in cycles per second [cps] or hertz [Hz]). The human ear is most sensitive to waves in the frequency range of 1000 to 3000 Hz. Most persons cannot hear compression waves that have a frequency higher than 20,000 Hz. Waves of higher frequency are called *ultrasonic waves,* meaning that they are above the audible range. In the audible frequency range, the subjective experience correlated with sonic frequency is the pitch of a sound. Waves below 20 to 30 Hz are experienced as a rattle or drum beat rather than a tone.

Wave intensity is represented by amplitude or units of sound pressure. By convention, the intensity (in power units or ergs per square centimeter) of a sound is expressed as the ratio of intensities between the sound and a reference value. A 10-fold increase in sound pressure is called a *bel,* after Alexander Graham Bell. Because this representation is too crude to be of use, the decibel (dB), or 1/10 of a bel, is used. For purposes of hearing evaluation, the threshold for perception of sound at a given frequency in persons with normal hearing is set at 0 dB.[30]

Hearing loss is classified as mild (26 to 40 dB), moderate (41 to 55 dB), severe (71 to 90 dB), or profound (91 dB or greater).[34] "Hard of hearing" is defined as hearing loss greater than 20 to 25 dB in adults and greater than 15 dB in children. Profound deafness is defined as hearing loss greater than 90 dB in adults[35] or 70 dB in children.[36]

There are many causes of hearing loss or deafness. Most fit into the categories of conductive, sensorineural, or mixed deficiencies that involve a combination of conductive and sensorineural function deficiencies of the same ear.[34–39] Hearing loss may be hereditary or acquired, sudden or progressive, unilateral or bilateral, partial or complete, reversible or irreversible. Age and suddenness of onset provide important clues as to the cause of hearing loss. Chart 55-1 summarizes common causes of conductive and sensorineural hearing loss.

Conductive Hearing Loss

Conductive hearing loss occurs when auditory stimuli are not adequately transmitted through the auditory canal, tympanic

---

CHART 55-1 **COMMON CAUSES OF CONDUCTIVE AND SENSORINEURAL HEARING LOSS**

Conductive Hearing Loss
- External ear conditions
  - Impacted earwax or foreign body
  - Otitis externa
- Middle ear conditions
  - Trauma
  - Otitis media (acute and with effusion)
  - Otosclerosis
  - Tumors

Sensorineural Hearing Loss
- Trauma
  - Head injury
  - Noise
- Central nervous system infections (*e.g.,* meningitis)
- Degenerative conditions
  - Presbycusis
- Vascular
  - Atherosclerosis
  - Sudden deafness
- Ototoxic drugs (*e.g.,* aminoglycosides, salicylates, loop diuretics)
- Tumors
  - Vestibular schwannoma (acoustic neuroma)
  - Meningioma
  - Metastatic tumors
- Idiopathic
  - Ménière disease

Mixed Conductive and Sensorineural Hearing Loss
- Middle ear conditions
  - Barotrauma
  - Cholesteatoma
  - Otosclerosis
- Temporal bone fractures

membrane, middle ear, or ossicle chain to the inner ear. Temporary hearing loss can occur as the result of impacted cerumen in the outer ear or fluid in the middle ear. Foreign bodies, including pieces of cotton and insects, may impair hearing. More permanent causes of hearing loss are thickening or damage of the tympanic membrane or involvement of the bony structures (ossicles and oval window) of the middle ear due to otosclerosis or Paget disease.

Sensorineural Hearing Loss

Sensorineural, or perceptive, hearing loss occurs with disorders that affect the inner ear, auditory nerve, or auditory pathways of the brain. With this type of deafness, sound waves are conducted to the inner ear, but abnormalities of the cochlear apparatus or auditory nerve decrease or distort the transfer of information to the brain. Tinnitus often accompanies cochlear nerve irritation. Abnormal function resulting from damage or malformation of the central auditory pathways and circuitry is included in this category.

Sensorineural hearing loss is usually irreversible and occurs most commonly in the higher frequencies. Sensorineural hearing loss may have a genetic cause or may result from intrauterine infections such as maternal rubella, or developmental malformations of the inner ear. Genetic hearing loss may result from mutation in a single gene (monogenetic) or from a combination of mutations in different genes and environmental factors (multifactorial). It has been estimated that 50% of profound deafness in children has a monogenetic basis.[33,34] The inheritance pattern for monogenetic hearing loss is autosomal recessive in approximately 75% of cases.[36] Hearing loss may begin before development of speech (prelingual) or after speech development (postlingual). Most prelingual forms are present at birth. Hereditary forms of hearing loss also can be classified as being part of a syndrome in which other abnormalities are present, or as nonsyndromic, in which deafness is the only abnormality.

Sensorineural hearing loss also can result from trauma to the inner ear, tumors that encroach on the inner ear or sensory neurons, vascular disorders with hemorrhage, or thrombosis of vessels that supply the inner ear. Other causes of sensorineural deafness are infections and drugs. Sudden sensorineural hearing loss represents an abrupt loss of hearing that occurs instantaneously or on awakening. It most commonly is caused by viral infections, circulatory disorders, or rupture of the labyrinth membrane that can occur during tympanotomy.

Environmentally induced deafness can occur through direct exposure to excessively intense sound, as in the workplace or at a concert. This is a particular problem in older adults who were working in noisy environments before the mid-1960s, when there were no laws mandating use of devices for protective hearing. Sustained or repeated exposure to noise pollution at sound intensities greater than 100 to 120 dB can cause corresponding mechanical damage to the organ of Corti. If the damage is severe, permanent sensorineural deafness to the corresponding sound frequencies occurs. Wearing earplugs or ear protection is impor-

tant under many industrial conditions and for musicians and music listeners exposed to high sound amplification.

A number of infections can cause hearing loss. Deafness or some degree of hearing impairment is the most common serious complication of bacterial meningitis in infants and children, reportedly resulting in sensorineural hearing loss in 5% to 35% of persons who survive the infection.[33] The mechanism causing hearing impairment seems to be a suppurative labyrinthitis or neuritis resulting in the loss of hair cells and damage to the auditory nerve. Untreated suppurative otitis media also can extend into the inner ear and cause sensorineural hearing loss through the same mechanisms.

Among the neoplasms that impair hearing are *acoustic neuromas*. Acoustic neuromas are benign Schwann cell tumors affecting CN VIII. These tumors usually are unilateral and cause hearing loss by compressing the cochlear nerve or interfering with blood supply to the nerve and cochlea. Other neoplasms that can affect hearing include meningiomas and metastatic brain tumors. The temporal bone is a common site of metastases. Breast cancer may metastasize to the middle ear and invade the cochlea.

Drugs that damage inner ear structures are labeled *ototoxic*. Vestibular symptoms of ototoxicity include lightheadedness, giddiness, and dizziness; if toxicity is severe, cochlear symptoms consisting of tinnitus or hearing loss occur. Hearing loss is sensorineural and may be bilateral or unilateral, transient or permanent. Several classes of drugs have been identified as having ototoxic potential, including the aminoglycosides and some other basic antimicrobial agents, antimalarial drugs, some chemotherapeutic drugs, loop diuretics, and salicylates (*e.g.,* aspirin). The symptoms of drug-induced hearing loss may be transient, as often is the case with salicylates and diuretics, or they may be permanent. The risk of ototoxicity depends on the total dose of the drug and its concentration in the bloodstream. It is increased in persons with impaired kidney function and in those previously or currently treated with another potentially ototoxic drug.

Diagnosis and Treatment

Diagnosis. Diagnosis of hearing loss is aided by careful history of associated otologic factors such as otalgia, otorrhea, tinnitus, and self-described hearing difficulties; physical examination to detect the presence of conditions such as otorrhea, impacted cerumen, or injury to the tympanic membrane; and hearing tests.[37,39] A history of occupational and noise exposure is important, as is the use of medications with ototoxic potential. Testing for hearing loss includes a number of methods, including a person's reported ability to hear an observer's voice, use of a tuning fork to test air and bone conduction, audioscopes, and auditory brain stem evoked responses (ABRs).

Tuning forks are used to differentiate conductive and sensorineural hearing loss. A 512-Hz or higher-frequency tuning fork is used because frequencies below this level elicit a tactile response. The Weber test evaluates conductive hearing loss by lateralization of sound. It is done by placing the lightly vibrating tuning fork on the forehead or vertex of the head. In persons with conductive losses, the sound is louder on the side with the hearing loss, but in persons with sensorineural loss, it radiates to the side with the better hearing. The Rinne test compares air and bone conduction. The test is done by alternately placing the tuning fork on the mastoid bone and in front of the ear canal. In conductive losses, bone conduction exceeds air conduction; in sensorineural losses, the opposite occurs.

An audioscope is a rechargeable battery–powered, hand-held instrument that combines a pure-tone screening audiometer and otoscope into a single unit. It produces pure sounds at 500, 1000, 2000, and 4000 Hz, at loudness levels of 20, 25, and 40 dB. If a person cannot hear pure tones at 1000 to 2000 Hz (usual speech frequencies), referral for a full audiogram is indicated. The audiogram is an important method of analyzing a person's hearing, and is generally considered the gold standard for diagnosis of hearing loss. It is done by an audiologist and requires highly specialized sound production and control equipment. Pure tones of controlled intensity are delivered, usually to one ear at a time, and the minimum intensity needed for hearing to be experienced is plotted as a function of frequency.

The ABR is a noninvasive method that permits functional evaluation of certain defined parts of the central auditory pathways. Electroencephalographic (EEG) electrodes and high-gain amplifiers are required to produce a record of the electrical wave activity elicited during repeated acoustic stimulations of either or both ears. ABR recording involves subjecting the ear to loud clicks and using a computer to pick up nerve impulses as they are processed in the midbrain. With this method, certain of the early waves that come from discrete portions of the pons and midbrain auditory pathways can be correlated with specific sensorineural abnormalities. Imaging studies such as computed tomography (CT) scans and magnetic resonance imaging (MRI) may be done to determine the site of a lesion and the extent of damage.[37]

Treatment. Hearing loss can have many consequences. It produces a loss of the important communicative function of auditory language. Social isolation and depressive disorders are common in hearing-impaired elderly. Safety issues, both in and out of the home, may become significant.

Treatment of hearing loss can range from simple removal of impacted cerumen in the external auditory canal to surgical procedures such as those used to reconstruct the tympanic membrane. For other people, particularly the frail elderly, hearing aids remain an option. Cochlear implants also are an option for some people. Although many assistive devices are available to persons with hearing loss, understanding on the part of family and friends is perhaps the most important. The interpretation of speech involves both visual and auditory clues. It is important that people speaking to persons with hearing impairment face the person and articulate so that lip reading cues can be used. Adequate lighting is important. Distractions such as background noise can make communication difficult and should be avoided when possible.

Hearing aids remain the mainstay of treatment for many persons with conductive and sensorineural hearing loss. With the advent of microcircuitry, hearing aids are now being designed with computer chips that allow multiple programs to be placed in a single hearing aid. The various programs allow the user to select a specific setting for different listening situations. The development of microcircuitry has also made it possible for hearing aids to be miniaturized to the point that, in many cases, they can be placed deep in the ear where they take advantage of the normal shape of the external ear and ear canal. Although modern hearing aids have improved greatly, they cannot replicate the hearing person's ability to hear both soft and loud noises. They also fail to consistently filter out distorted or background noise. Many persons who are fitted with hearing aids use them inconsistently, often because of social embarrassment, increase in background noise, or the sound of their own voice being transmitted through the hearing aid.[40] Other aids for the hearing impaired include alert and signal devices, assisted-listening devices from telephone companies, and dogs trained to respond to various sounds.

Surgically implantable cochlear prostheses for the profoundly deaf have been developed and are available for use in adults and children 1 year of age or older.[41] These prostheses are inserted into the scala tympani of the cochlea and work by providing direct stimulation to the auditory nerve, bypassing the stimulation that typically is provided by transducer cells but that is absent or nonfunctional in a deaf cochlea. For the implant to work, the auditory nerve must be functional. Although early implants used a single electrode, current implants use multielectrode placement, enhancing speech perception. Much of the progress in implant performance has been achieved through improvements in the speech processors that convert sound into electrical stimuli. Advances in the development of the multi-channel implant have improved performance such that cochlear implants have been established as an effective option for adults and children with profound hearing impairment.[41,42] Most persons who are deafened after learning speech derive substantial benefit when cochlear implants are used in conjunction with lip reading; some are able to understand some speech without lip reading; and some are able to communicate by telephone.

 Hearing Loss in Infants and Children

Even mild or unilateral hearing loss can have a detrimental effect on the language development and hearing-associated learning of the young child.[43–45] Although estimates vary depending on the group surveyed and testing methods used, from 1 to 2 per 1000 newborns have moderate (30 to 50 dB), severe (50 to 70 Db), or profound (≥70 dB) sensorineural hearing loss.[10] An additional 1 to 2 per 1000 may have milder or unilateral impairments. When considering less severe or transient conductive hearing loss that is commonly associated with middle ear disease in young children, the numbers are even greater.

The cause of hearing impairment in children may be conductive or sensorineural. Most conductive hearing loss is caused by middle ear infections. Causes of sensorineural hearing impairment include genetic, infectious, traumatic, and ototoxic factors. Genetic causes are probably responsible for as much as 50% of sensorineural hearing loss in children. The most common infectious cause of congenital sensorineural hearing loss is cytomegalovirus (CMV), which infects 1 of 100 newborns in the United States each year; of these, about 1200 to 2000 have sensorineural hearing loss.[10] Of particular concern is the fact that congenital CMV infection can cause both symptomatic and asymptomatic hearing loss in the newborn. Some children with congenital CMV infection, who were asymptomatic as newborns, have suddenly lost residual hearing at 4 to 5 years of age.[10] Postnatal causes of sensorineural hearing loss include beta-hemolytic streptococcal sepsis in the newborn and bacterial meningitis. *S. pneumoniae* is the most common cause of bacterial meningitis that results in sensorineural hearing loss after the neonatal period; this cause may become less frequent with the routine administration of the conjugate pneumococcal vaccine. Other causes of sensorineural hearing loss are toxins and trauma. Early in pregnancy, the embryo is particularly sensitive to toxic substances, including ototoxic drugs such as the aminoglycosides and loop diuretics. Trauma, particularly head trauma, may cause sensorineural hearing loss.

Hearing impairment can have a major impact on the development of a child; therefore, early identification through screening programs is strongly advocated. The American Academy of Pediatrics (AAP) and the Joint Commission on Infant Hearing (JCIH) published a position paper calling for universal screening of all infants by physiologic measurements before 3 months of age, with proper intervention no later than 6 months of age.[46,47] Many states have now enacted legislation supporting the position paper; as a result, newborn hearing screening programs have been implemented in newborn nurseries throughout the United States.[43] The currently recommended screening techniques are either the transient evoked otoacoustic emissions (TEOAE) or the ABR. Both methodologies are noninvasive, relatively quick (<5 minutes), and easy to perform. The TEOAE measures sound waves generated in the inner ear (cochlea) in response to clicks or tone bursts emitted and recorded by a minute microphone placed in the external ear canals of the infant. The ABR uses three electrodes pasted to the infant's scalp to measure the EEG waves generated by clicks. Because many children become hearing impaired after the neonatal period and are not identified by neonatal screening programs, the AAP and JCIH recommend that all infants with risk factors for delayed onset of progressive hearing loss receive ongoing audiologic and medical monitoring for 3 years and at appropriate intervals thereafter.[45]

Once hearing loss has been identified, a full developmental and speech and language evaluation is needed. Parental involvement and counseling are essential. Children with sensorineural hearing loss should be evaluated for possible hearing aid use by a pediatric audiologist.[48] Hearing aids may be fitted for infants as young as 2 months of age. The use of surgically implanted cochlear prostheses in children with profound hearing loss has currently been approved for children 2 years of age

and older.[41,42,49] One limitation is that the earliest age for implantation in children in the United States is no earlier than 2 years of age, which is beyond the critical period of auditory input for the acquisition of oral language. Because of the increased risk of pneumococcal meningitis, children who receive implants should receive age-appropriate immunization against pneumococcal disease.[10] At present, the best educational approach to children with significant hearing loss is open to controversy. Some members of the hearing-impaired community have objected to the use of cochlear implants in children, maintaining that the child can develop adequate communication skills using more conventional strategies such as sign language and lip reading.

Hearing Loss in the Elderly

The term *presbycusis* is used to describe degenerative hearing loss that occurs with advancing age.[28,50,51] Hearing loss is the third most prevalent chronic condition in older Americans, after hypertension and arthritis.[51] Between 25% and 40% of the population aged 65 years and older is hearing impaired.[51] Because of its high prevalence, presbycusis is a common social and health problem. People with the disorder have difficulty proportional to the degree of hearing impairment, in conversation, music appreciation, orientation to alarms, and participation in social activities.

The hearing loss associated with presbycusis is typically gradual, bilateral, and characterized by high-frequency hearing loss. It is further characterized by reduced hearing sensitivity and speech understanding in noisy environments, slowed central processing of acoustic information, and impaired localization of sound sources. The disorder first reduces the ability to understand speech and, later, the ability to detect, identify, and localize sounds. The most common complaint of persons with presbycusis is not that they cannot hear, but rather that they cannot understand what is being said. For example, they often confuse words like *mash* with *math, map* with *mat,* and *Sunday* with *some day.* High-frequency warning sounds, such as beepers, turn signals, and escaping steam, are not heard and localized, with potentially dangerous results.

Although the degeneration with aging of the sensory cells in the cochlea, supporting cells, and cochlear nerve are well described, the cause of presbycusis is largely unknown. Because of the age at which the problems occur varies widely, it seems likely that the disorder results from a mixture of acquired auditory stresses, trauma, and otologic diseases superimposed on an intrinsic, genetically controlled, aging process.

Given the high prevalence of presbycusis in people of retirement age and the adverse effects of hearing loss on well-being, screening for hearing loss should be performed at annual health care visits. The single question "do you have a hearing problem?" is usually an effective method of screening. The 10-item Hearing Handicap Inventory for the Elderly—Screening Version (HHIE-S) is also a widely used screening tool. Clinical measures for hearing loss such as whispered voice tests and finger friction tests are reportedly imprecise and are not reliable methods for screening. Screening audiometry administered by someone trained in its use is a practical and cost-effective method for detecting significant hearing loss. The equipment needed for screening audiometry is lightweight, low cost, and well accepted by persons being tested.

Several otologic abnormalities can be identified and treated. Cerumen impaction may result in substantial hearing loss and can be found in up to 30% of elderly persons with hearing loss. Many elderly persons are on multiple medications, some of which may possess ototoxic potential. A frequently overlooked ototoxic agent is aspirin. Little is known about what level of dosage causes ototoxicity, but it is generally believed that 81 mg of aspirin on a daily basis is safe. Fortunately, in most cases, the resulting tinnitus and hearing loss are temporary and reversible with cessation of the drug.

The majority of hearing loss in the elderly is sensorineural. In mild to severe loss, the most effective treatment is hearing amplification with hearing aids, speech reading, and assistive listening devices (*e.g.*, hearing aids with the telephone, captioning on televised programs, flashing alarms). Cochlear implants are indicated at any age for people with bilateral hearing losses not materially helped by hearing aids.

IN SUMMARY, hearing is a specialized sense whose external stimulus is the vibration of sound waves. Our ears receive sound waves, distinguish their frequencies, translate this information into nerve impulses, and transmit them to the CNS. Anatomically, the auditory system consists of the outer ear, middle ear, and inner ear, the auditory pathways, and the auditory cortex. The middle ear is a tiny, air-filled cavity in the temporal bone. A connection exists between the middle ear and the nasopharynx. This connection, called the *eustachian tube,* allows equalization of pressure between the middle ear and the atmosphere. The inner ear contains the receptors for hearing.

Disorders of the auditory system include infections of the external and middle ear, otosclerosis, and conduction and sensorineural deafness. Otitis externa is an inflammatory process of the external ear. Otitis media is an inflammation of the middle ear without reference to etiology or pathogenesis. Acute OM, which refers to an acute middle ear infection, is one of the most common illnesses in children. It usually follows an upper respiratory tract infection, has an abrupt onset, and is characterized by otalgia, fever, and hearing loss. OM with effusion refers to the presence of fluid in the inner ear without signs and symptoms of acute ear infection. The effusion that accompanies OM can persist for weeks or months, interfering with hearing and impairing speech development. It is important to differentiate OME from AOM to avoid unnecessary antimicrobial use. Otosclerosis is a familial disorder of the otic capsule. It causes bone resorption followed by excessive replacement with sclerotic bone. The disorder eventually causes immobilization of the stapes and conduction deafness.

Deafness, or hearing loss, can develop as the result of a number of auditory disorders. It can be conductive, sensorineural, or mixed. Conduction deafness occurs when transmission of sound waves from the external to the inner ear is impaired. Sensorineural deafness can involve cochlear structures of the inner ear or the neural pathways that transmit auditory stimuli. Sensorineural hearing loss can result from genetic or congenital disorders, trauma, infections, vascular disorders, tumors, or ototoxic drugs. Hearing loss in infants and young children impairs language and speech development. In the elderly, hearing loss is a common condition resulting in significant loss of social well-being. Treatment of hearing loss includes the use of hearing aids and, in some cases of profound deafness, implantation of a cochlear prosthesis. ■

CONCEPTSin action **ANIMATI🞶N**

 ## DISORDERS OF VESTIBULAR FUNCTION

After completing this section of the chapter, you should be able to meet the following objectives:

- Explain the function of the vestibular system with respect to postural reflexes and maintaining a stable visual field despite marked changes in head position.
- Relate the function of the vestibular system to nystagmus and vertigo.
- Differentiate the structures of peripheral and central vestibular function.
- Characterize the physiologic cause of motion sickness.
- Compare the manifestations and pathologic processes associated with benign paroxysmal positional vertigo and Ménière disease.
- Differentiate the manifestations of peripheral and central vestibular disorders.

The Vestibular System and Vestibular Reflexes

The vestibular receptive organs, which are located in the inner ear, and their connections to the CNS contribute to the reflex activity necessary for effective posture and movement in a physical world governed by momentum and a gravitational field. Because the vestibular apparatus is part of the inner ear and located in the head, it is head position and acceleration that is sensed. The vestibular system serves two general and related functions. It maintains and assists recovery of stable body and head position through control of postural reflexes, and it maintains a stable visual field despite marked changes in head position.

DISORDERS OF THE VESTIBULAR SYSTEM

■ The receptors concerned with the sense of balance and position in space are located in fluid (endolymph)-filled semicircular canals of the vestibular system of the inner ear.

■ The vestibular system has extensive interconnections with neural pathways controlling vision, hearing, and autonomic nervous system function. Disorders of the vestibular system are characterized by vertigo, nystagmus, tinnitus, nausea and vomiting, and autonomic nervous system manifestations.

■ Disorders of vestibular function can result from repeated stimulation of the vestibular system such as during car, air, and boat travel (motion sickness); acute infection of the vestibular pathways (acute vestibular neuritis); dislodgement of otoliths that participate in the receptor function of the vestibular system (benign paroxysmal positional vertigo); or distention of the endolymphatic compartment of the inner ear (Ménière disease).

Peripheral Vestibular Apparatus

The peripheral apparatus of the vestibular system is contained in the bony labyrinth of the inner ear next to and continuous with the cochlea of the auditory system. Like the cochlea, it consists of two fluid-filled compartments—an outer bony labyrinth that is filled with perilymph and an inner membranous labyrinth that is filled with endolymph[26,52] (Fig. 55-7A). The bony labyrinth is divided into three semicircular canals and a central vestibule or egg-shaped cavity that lies posterior to the cochlea and anterior to the semicircular canals. Suspended in the perilymph and united by a duct are two membranous labyrinth sacs, the saccule and utricle. The smaller saccule is continuous with the membranous labyrinth extending anteriorly into the cochlea through the ductus reuniens, which connects with the cochlear duct; whereas the utricle is continuous with the ducts extending into the semicircular canals posteriorly. The receptors of the vestibular system consist of small patches of hair cells located in membranous ampullae of three semicircular ducts and the maculae of the saccule and utricle.

The cavities of the three semicircular canals, the lateral, anterior, and posterior canals, are oriented in one of three planes of space. The lateral (horizontal) canals are in the same plane, whereas the anterior (superior) canal of one side is parallel with the posterior (inferior) canal on the other side, and the two function as a pair. Located in each semicircular canal is a corresponding semicircular duct, which communicates with the utricle. Each of these ducts has an enlarged swelling at one end called an *ampulla* (see Fig. 55-7A). The ampulla of each of the semicircular canals contains a ridge that is covered by a sensory epithelium with hair cells that are raised into a crest, called the *crista ampullaris,* which lies at a right angle to the duct (Fig. 55-7B). These hair cells are innervated by the primary afferents of the vestibular nerve, which is a subdivision of the eighth cranial nerve.

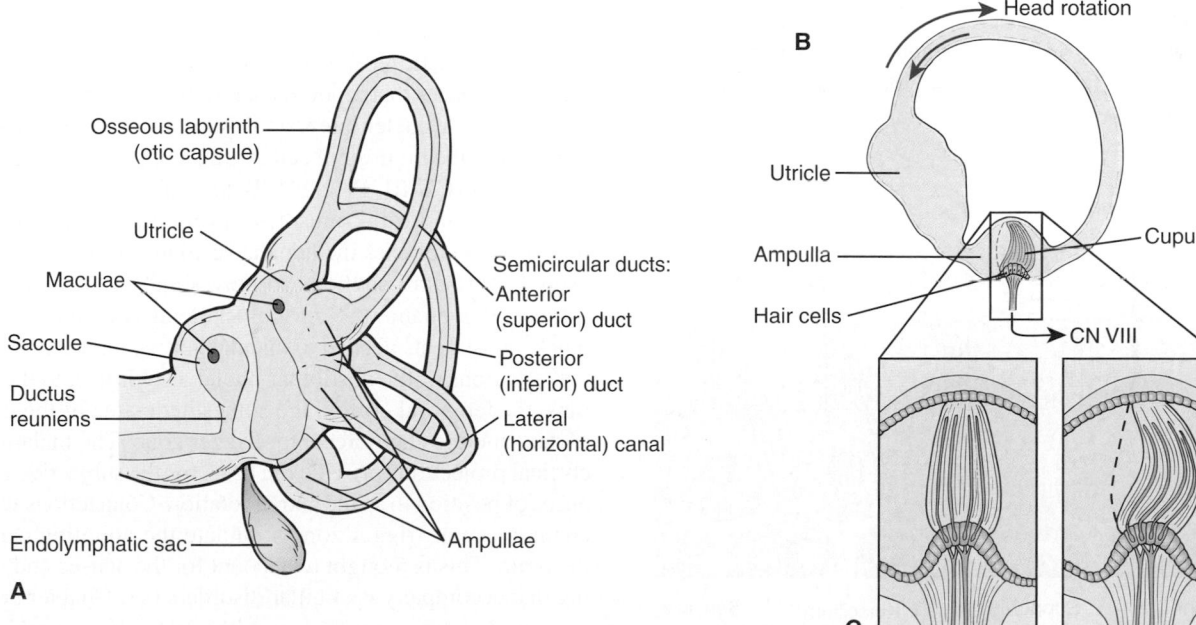

FIGURE 55-7 • **(A)** The osseous and membranous labyrinth of the left ear showing the utricle and saccule with their maculae and three semicircular canals and their ampullae. **(B)** Location of the crista ampullaris and its connection to the vestibular branch of CN VIII. **(C)** The location of the cupula and movement of hair cells of the crista ampullaris with head movement.

The hair cells of the crista ampullaris extend into a flexible gelatinous mass, called the *cupula*, which essentially closes off fluid flow through the semicircular ducts (see Fig. 55-7C). When the head begins to rotate around the axis of a semicircular canal (*i.e.,* undergoes angular acceleration), the momentum of the endolymph causes an increase in pressure on one side of the cupula. This is similar to the lagging behind of the water in a glass that is suddenly rotated, except that the endolymph cannot flow past the cupula. Instead, the endolymph applies a differential pressure to the two sides of the cupula, bending the hair bundles. Because all the hair cells in each semicircular canal share a common orientation, angular acceleration in one direction increases afferent nerve activity, whereas acceleration in the opposite direction diminishes nerve activity. Impulses from the semicircular ducts are particularly important in reflex movement of the eyes. Vestibular nystagmus (to be discussed) is a complex phenomenon that occurs during and immediately after rotational motion. As you rotate your head, your eyes slowly drift in the opposite direction and then jump rapidly back toward the direction of rotation to establish a new fixation point.

The saccule and utricle house equilibrium receptors called a *macula* that respond to the pull of gravity and head position. Each macula is a small, flat epithelial patch containing supporting cells and sensory hair cells, the sides and bases of which synapse with sensory endings of the vestibular nerve (Fig. 55-8). Each group of hair cells has a number of small cilia called *stereocilia,* plus one large cilium, the *kinocilium*. The kinocilium is located at one side of the cell, and the stereocilia become progressively shorter toward the other side of the cell. Minute filamentous attachments connect the tip of each stereocilium to the next longer stereocilium, and finally to the kinocilium. Movement of the head in one direction causes movement of the adjoined stereocilia and kinocilium and depolarization or activation of the receptor and movement of the head in the other direction causes hyperpolarization or inactivation of the receptor.

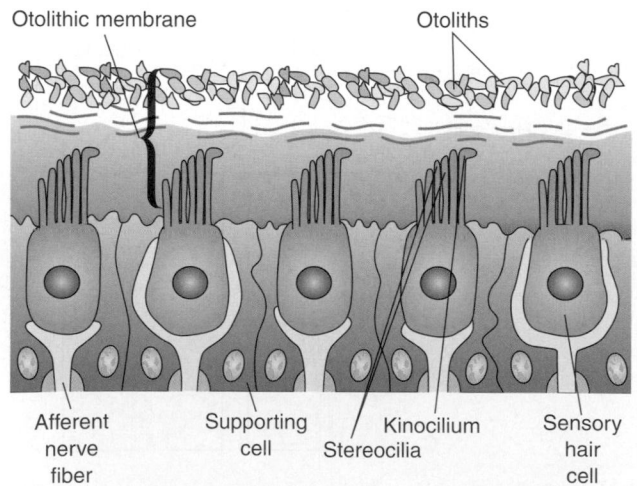

FIGURE 55-8 • The relation of the otoliths to the sensory cells in the maculae of the utricle and saccule. (From Ross M. H., Kaye G. I., Pawlina W. [2003]. *Histology* [4th ed., p. 829]. Philadelphia: Lippincott Williams & Wilkins.)

The hair cells in both the utricular and saccular maculae are embedded in a flattened gelatinous mass, the *otolithic membrane,* which is studded with tiny stones (calcium carbonate crystals) called *otoliths* (see Fig. 55-8). Although they are small, the density of the otoliths increases the membrane's weight and its resistance to change in motion. When the head is tilted, the gelatinous mass shifts its position because of the pull of the gravitational field, bending the stereocilia of the macular hair cells. Although each hair cell becomes more or less excitable depending on the direction in which the cilia are bending, the hair cells are oriented in all directions, making these sense organs sensitive to static or changing head position in relation to the gravitational field. In a condition called *benign paroxysmal positional vertigo* (sensation of whirling or spinning motion), the otoliths become dislodged from their gelatinous base, causing a vertigo that is precipitated by changes in the recumbent head position (to be discussed).

Neural Pathways

The response to body imbalance, such as stumbling, must be fast and reflexive. Hence, information from the vestibular system goes directly to reflex centers in the brain stem, rather than to the cerebral cortex. Ganglionic cells, homologous with dorsal root ganglion cells, form afferent ganglia: the superior and inferior vestibular ganglia that innervate the hair cells of the peripheral vestibular apparatus (see Fig. 55-5). The central axons of these ganglion cells become the superior and inferior vestibular nerves, which become part of the vestibulocochlear nerve (CN VIII).

Impulses from the vestibular nerves initially pass to one of two destinations: the vestibular nuclear complex in the brain stem, or the cerebellum. The vestibular nuclei, which form the main integrative center for balance, also receive input from visual and somatic receptors, particularly from proprioceptors in the neck muscles that report the angle or inclination of the head. The vestibular nuclei integrate this information and then send impulses to the brain stem centers that control the extrinsic eye movements (CN III, IV, and VI) and reflex movements of the neck, limb, and trunk muscles (through the vestibulospinal tracts). These reflexes include the vestibulo-ocular reflexes that keep the eyes still as the head moves and the vestibulospinal reflexes that enable the musculoskeletal system to make the quick adjustments needed to maintain or regain balance.

Neurons of the vestibular nuclei also project to the thalamus, the temporal cortex, the somesthetic area of the parietal cortex, and the chemoreceptor trigger zone. The thalamic and cortical projections provide the basis for the subjective experiences of position in space and of rotation. Connections with the chemoreceptor trigger zone stimulate the vomiting center in the brain. This is thought to account for the nausea and vomiting that accompany vestibular disorders (see Chapter 36).

Nystagmus

The term *nystagmus* refers to the involuntary rhythmic and oscillatory eye movements that preserve eye fixation on stable objects in the visual field during angular and rotational movements of the head.[26] The vestibulo-ocular reflexes produce slow compensatory conjugate eye rotations that occur in the direction precisely opposite to ongoing head rotation and provide for continuous, ongoing reflex stabilization of the binocular fixation point. This reflex can be demonstrated by holding a pencil vertically in front of the eyes and moving it from side to side through a 10-degree arc at a rate of approximately five times per second. At this rate of motion, the pencil appears blurred because a different and more complex reflex, smooth pursuit, cannot compensate quickly enough. However, if the pencil is maintained in a stable position and the head is moved back and forth at the same rate, the image of the pencil is clearly defined. The eye movements are the same in both cases. The reason that the pencil image remains clear in the second situation is because the vestibulo-ocular reflexes keep the image of the pencil on the retinal fovea. When compensatory vestibulo-ocular reflexes carry the conjugate eye rotations to their physical limit, a very rapid conjugate movement moves the eyes in the direction of head rotation to a new fixation point, followed by a slow

vestibulo-ocular reflex as the head continues to rotate past the new fixation point. This pattern of slow–fast–slow movements is called *nystagmus* (Fig. 55-9). Clinically, the direction of nystagmus is named for the fast phase of nystagmus.

Nystagmus can be classified according to the direction of eye movement: horizontal, vertical, rotary (torsional), or mixed. If head rotation is continued, friction between endolymph and semicircular duct walls results in endolymph rotating at the same velocity as the head, and nystagmus adapts to a stable eye posture. If rotation is suddenly stopped, vestibular nystagmus reappears in the direction precisely opposite to the angular accelerating nystagmus. This results because the inertia of the endolymph is again bending ampullary hair cells of a now stationary ampulla.

Spontaneous nystagmus that occurs without head movement or visual stimuli is always pathologic. It seems to appear more readily and more severely with fatigue and to some extent can be influenced by psychological factors. Nystagmus due to a CNS pathologic process, in contrast to vestibular end-organ or vestibulocochlear nerve sources, seldom is accompanied by vertigo. If present, the vertigo is mild. Nystagmus eye movements can be tested by caloric stimulation or rotation (to be discussed).

Vertigo

Disorders of vestibular function are characterized by a condition called *vertigo*, in which an illusion of motion occurs. With vertigo, the person may be stationary and the environment in motion (*i.e.*, objective vertigo) or the person may be in motion and the environment stationary (*i.e.*, subjective vertigo). Persons with vertigo frequently describe a sensation of spinning, "to-and-fro" motion, or falling.

Vertigo should be differentiated from lightheadedness, faintness, unsteadiness, or syncope[53–56] (loss of consciousness; Table 55-1). Presyncope, which is characterized by a feeling of lightheadedness or "blacking out," is commonly caused by postural hypotension (see Chapter 23) or a stenotic lesion in the cerebral circulation that limits blood flow. An inability to maintain normal gait may be described as dizziness despite the absence of objective vertigo. The unstable gait may be caused by disorders of sensory input (*e.g.*, proprioception), peripheral neuropathy, gait problems, or disorders other than vestibular function and usually is corrected by touching a stationary object such as a wall or table.

Vertigo or dizziness can result from central or peripheral vestibular disorders. Approximately 85% of persons with vertigo have a peripheral vestibular disorder, whereas only 15% have a central disorder.[53] Vertigo due to peripheral vestibular disorders tends to be severe in intensity and episodic or brief in duration. In contrast, vertigo due to central vestibular causes tends to be mild and constant and chronic in duration.

Motion Sickness

Motion sickness is a form of normal physiologic vertigo. It is caused by repeated rhythmic stimulation of the vestibular system, such as that encountered in car, air, or boat travel. Vertigo, malaise, nausea, and vomiting are the principal

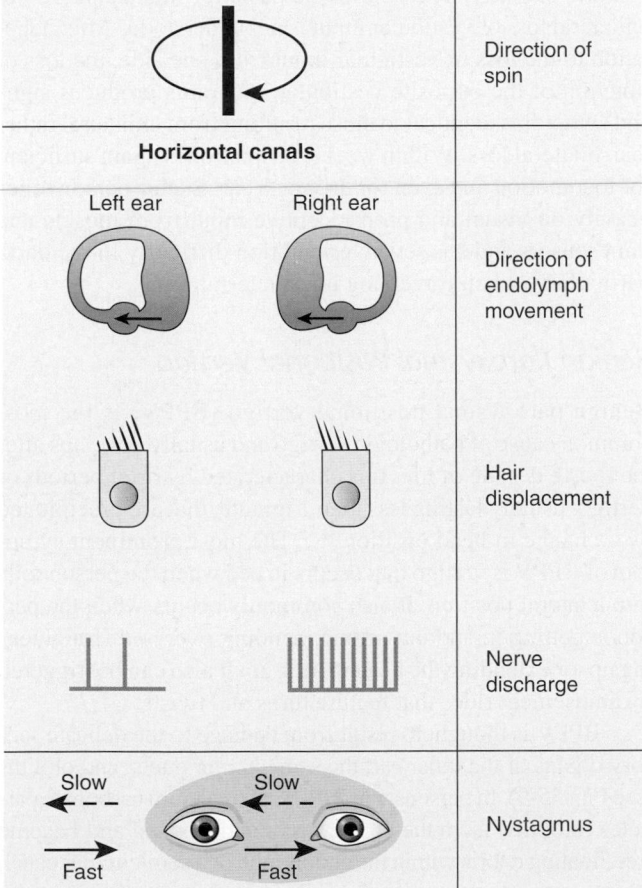

FIGURE 55-9 • Effect of spinning a subject clockwise. On acceleration, the endolymph in the horizontal canals will lag behind with respect to movement of the canal wall. The hairs of cristae will be displaced to the left. In the left semicircular canal, hair displacement is away from the kinocilium, leading to decreased nerve discharges below the resting level. On the right, hair displacement is toward the kinocilium, leading to an increase in nerve discharge above the resting level. (From Sekurt F. E. [1982]. *Basic physiology for the health professions* [2nd ed., p. 140]. Boston: Little, Brown.)

TABLE 55-1 Differences in Pathology and Manifestations of Dizziness Associated With Benign Paroxysmal Positional Vertigo, Presyncope, and Disequilibrium State

TYPE OF DISORDER	PATHOLOGY	SYMPTOMS
Benign paroxysmal positional vertigo	Disorder of otoliths	Vertigo initiated by a change in head position, usually lasts less than a minute
Presyncope	Orthostatic hypotension	Lightheadedness and feeling faint on assumption of standing position
Disequilibrium	Sensory (*e.g.,* vision, proprioception) deficits	Dizziness and unsteadiness when walking, especially when turning; relieved by additional proprioceptive stimulation such as touching wall or table

symptoms. Autonomic signs, including lowered blood pressure, tachycardia, and excessive sweating, may occur. Hyperventilation, which commonly accompanies motion sickness, produces changes in blood volume and pooling of blood in the lower extremities, leading to postural hypotension and sometimes to syncope. Some persons experience a variant of motion sickness, complaining of sensing the rocking motion of the boat after returning to ground. This usually resolves after the vestibular system becomes accustomed to the stationary influence of being back on land.

Motion sickness can usually be suppressed by supplying visual signals that more closely match the motion signals being supplied to the vestibular system. For example, looking out the window and watching the environment move when experiencing motion sickness associated with car travel provides the vestibular system with the visual sensation of motion, but reading a book provides the vestibular system with the miscue that the environment is stable. Motion sickness usually decreases in severity with repeated exposure. Anti–motion sickness drugs also may be used to reduce or ameliorate the symptoms. These drugs work by suppressing the activity of the vestibular system.

Disorders of Peripheral Vestibular Function

Disorders of peripheral vestibular function occur when signals from the peripheral vestibular apparatus are distorted, as in benign paroxysmal positional vertigo, or are unbalanced by unilateral involvement of one of the vestibular organs, as in Ménière disease. The inner ear is vulnerable to injury caused by fracture of the petrous portion of the temporal bones; by infection of nearby structures, including the middle ear and meninges; and by blood-borne toxins and infections. Damage to the vestibular system can occur as an adverse effect of certain drugs or from allergic reactions to foods. The aminoglycosides (*e.g.,* streptomycin, gentamicin) have a specific toxic affinity for the vestibular portion of the inner ear. Alcohol can cause transient episodes of vertigo. The cause of peripheral vertigo remains unknown in approximately half of the cases.

Severe irritation or damage of the vestibular end organs or nerves results in severe balance disorders reflected by instability of posture, ataxia, and falling accompanied by vertigo.

With irritation, falling is away from the affected side; with destruction, it is toward the affected side. Adaptation to asymmetric stimulation occurs within a few days, after which the signs and symptoms diminish and eventually are lost. After recovery, there usually is a slightly reduced acuity for tilt, and the person walks with a somewhat broadened base to improve postural stability. The neurologic basis for this adaptation to unilateral loss of vestibular input is not understood. After adaptation to the loss of vestibular input from one side, the loss of function of the opposite vestibular apparatus produces signs and symptoms identical to those resulting from unilateral rather than bilateral loss. Within weeks, adaptation is again sufficient for locomotion and even for driving a car. Such a person relies heavily on visual and proprioceptive input from muscle and joint sensors and has severe orientation difficulty in the dark, particularly when traversing uneven terrain.

Benign Paroxysmal Positional Vertigo

Benign paroxysmal positional vertigo (BPPV) is the most common cause of pathologic vertigo and usually develops after the fourth decade of life. It is characterized by brief periods of vertigo, usually lasting less than 1 minute, that are precipitated by a change in head position.[56,57] The most prominent symptom of BPPV is vertigo that occurs in bed when the person rolls into a lateral position. It also commonly occurs when the person is getting in and out of bed, bending over and straightening up, or extending the head to look up. It also can be triggered by amusement rides that feature turns and twists.

BPPV is thought to result from damage to the delicate sensory organs of the inner ear, the semicircular ducts, and otoliths (see Fig. 55-9). In persons with BPPV, the calcium carbonate particles (otoliths) from the utricle become dislodged and become free-floating debris within the endolymph of a semicircular canal, most commonly the posterior canal, which is the most dependent part of the inner ear.[56] Movement of the free-floating debris causes this portion of the vestibular system to become more sensitive, such that any movement of the head in the plane parallel to the posterior duct may cause vertigo and nystagmus. There usually is a several-second delay between head movement and onset of vertigo, representing the time it takes to generate the exaggerated endolymph activity. Symptoms usually subside with continued movement, probably because the movement causes the debris to be redistributed throughout the endolymph system and away from the posterior semicircular canal.

Diagnosis is based on tests that involve the use of a change in head position to elicit vertigo and nystagmus.[56,57] BPPV often is successfully treated with drug therapy to control vertigo-induced nausea. Nondrug therapies using habituation exercises and canalith repositioning are successful in many people.[57] Canalith repositioning involves a series of maneuvers in which the head is moved to different positions in an effort to reposition the free-floating debris in the endolymph of the semicircular canals.

Acute Vestibular Neuronitis

Acute vestibular neuronitis represents an inflammation of the vestibular nerve and is characterized by an acute onset (usually hours) of vertigo, nausea, and vomiting lasting several days and not associated with auditory or other neurologic manifestations. Most persons experience gradual improvement over 1 to 2 weeks, but some develop recurrent episodes.[58–60] A large percentage report an upper respiratory tract illness 1 to 2 weeks before onset of symptoms, suggesting a viral origin. The condition also can occur in persons with herpes zoster oticus. In some persons, attacks of acute vestibulopathy recur over months or years. There is no way to determine whether a person who experiences a first attack will have repeated attacks.

Ménière Disease

Ménière disease is a disorder of the inner ear due to distention of the endolymphatic compartment of the inner ear, causing a triad of hearing loss, vertigo, and tinnitus.[61–63] The primary lesion appears to be in the endolymphatic sac, which is thought to be responsible for endolymph filtration and excretion. A number of pathogenetic mechanisms have been postulated, including an increased production of endolymph, decreased production of perilymph accompanied by a compensatory increase in volume of the endolymphatic sac, and decreased absorption of endolymph caused by malfunction of the endolymphatic sac or blockage of endolymphatic pathways.

Ménière disease is characterized by fluctuating episodes of tinnitus, feelings of ear fullness, and violent rotary vertigo that often renders the person unable to sit or walk. There is a need to lie quietly with the head fixed in a comfortable position, avoiding all head movements that aggravate the vertigo. Symptoms referable to the autonomic nervous system, including pallor, sweating, nausea, and vomiting, usually are present. The more severe the attack, the more prominent are the autonomic manifestations. A fluctuating hearing loss occurs with a return to normal after the episode subsides. Initially the symptoms tend to be unilateral, resulting in rotary nystagmus caused by an imbalance in vestibular control of eye movements. Because initial involvement usually is unilateral and because the sense of hearing is bilateral, many persons with the disorder are not aware of the full extent of their hearing loss. However, as the disease progresses, the hearing loss stops fluctuating and progressively worsens, with both ears tending to be affected so that the prime disability becomes one of deafness.[63] The episodes of vertigo diminish and then disappear, although the person may be unsteady, especially in the dark.

The cause of Ménière disease is unknown. A number of conditions, such as trauma, infection (*e.g.,* syphilis), and immunologic, endocrine (*i.e.,* adrenal-pituitary insufficiency and hypothyroidism), and vascular disorders have been proposed as possible causes of Ménière disease.[63,64] The most common form of the disease is an idiopathic form thought to be caused by a single viral injury to the fluid transport system of the inner ear. One area of investigation has been the relation between autoimmune disorders and Ménière disease.

Methods used in the diagnosis of Ménière disease include audiograms, vestibular testing by electronystagmography, and petrous pyramid radiographs. The administration of hyperosmolar substances, such as glycerin and urea, often produces acute temporary hearing improvement in persons with Ménière disease and sometimes is used as a diagnostic measure of endolymphatic hydrops. The diuretic furosemide also may be used for this purpose.

The management of Ménière disease focuses on attempts to reduce the distention of the endolymphatic space, and can be medical or surgical. Pharmacologic management consists of suppressant drugs (*e.g.,* prochlorperazine, promethazine, diazepam), which act centrally to decrease the activity of the vestibular system. Diuretics are used to reduce endolymph fluid volume. Histamine analogs, which directly reduce inner ear fluid mainly by decreasing cochlear blood flow, are being studied.[62] A low-sodium diet is recommended in addition to these medications. The steroid hormone prednisone may be used to maintain satisfactory hearing and resolve dizziness. Intratympanic gentamicin therapy has been used for ablation of the vestibular system.[63,64] Persons who are candidates for intratympanic gentamicin infusion include those who have frequent attacks of Ménière disease, disease that involves one ear, good contralateral vestibular function, or normal or near-normal balance between episodes. This treatment is mainly effective in controlling vertigo and does not alter the underlying pathologic process.

Surgical methods include the creation of an endolymphatic shunt in which excess endolymph from the inner ear is diverted into the subarachnoid space or the mastoid (endolymphatic sac surgery), and vestibular nerve section. Advances in vestibular nerve section have facilitated the monitoring of CN VII and CN VIII potentials. These methods are used to prevent hearing damage. In unilateral cases, vestibular nerve section has a success rate of 90% to 95% in terms of providing complete relief of vertigo 2 years after surgery.[63,64] The surgery, however, involves an intracranial procedure with possible postoperative morbidity.

Disorders of Central Vestibular Function

Abnormal nystagmus and vertigo can occur as a result of CNS lesions involving the cerebellum and lower brain stem. Central causes of vertigo include brain stem ischemia, tumors, and multiple sclerosis. When brain stem ischemia is the cause of vertigo, it usually is associated with other brain stem signs such as diplopia, ataxia, dysarthria, or facial weakness. Compression of the vestibular nuclei by cerebellar tumors invading the fourth ventricle results in progressively severe signs and symptoms. In addition to abnormal nystagmus and vertigo, vomiting and a broad-based and dystaxic gait become progressively more evident. The central demyelinating effects of multiple sclerosis can present with vertigo up to 10% of the time, and up to one third of persons with multiple sclerosis experience vertigo and nystagmus some time in the course of the disease.[59]

Centrally derived nystagmus usually has equal excursion in both directions (*i.e.*, pendular). In contrast to peripherally generated nystagmus, CNS-derived nystagmus is relatively constant rather than episodic, can occur in any direction rather than being primarily in the horizontal or torsional (rotatory) dimensions, often changes direction through time, and cannot be suppressed by visual fixation. Repeated induction of nystagmus results in rapid diminution or "fatigue" of the reflex with peripheral abnormalities, but fatigue is not characteristic of central lesions. Abnormal nystagmus can make reading and other tasks that require precise eye positional control difficult.

Diagnosis and Treatment of Vestibular Disorders

Diagnostic Tests

Diagnosis of vestibular disorders is based on a description of the symptoms, a history of trauma or exposure to agents that are destructive to vestibular structures, and physical examination. Physical examination methods include use of the Romberg test, evaluation of gait, and observation for the presence of nystagmus. Other tests of vestibular function include electronystagmography and the caloric stimulation test.

In peripheral lesions, nystagmus is usually horizontal and with a rotary component; the fast beat usually beats away from the disease side (see Fig. 55-9). Several types of maneuvers can be used to provoke vertigo and observe for nystagmus. These tests usually have the person sitting upright on an examining table with the head turned toward the side being examined, and the eyes open and focused on the examiner's finger.[54] The person is then properly supported and lowered rapidly to the supine position with the head extending over the upper end of the examining table and placed about 30 degrees lower than the body. The person is observed for nystagmus for about 30 seconds while in that position. The test can be performed with the head turned to either side or with the person looking straight ahead.

Vertigo arising from central lesions tends to develop gradually, and nystagmus is not always present, can occur in any direction, and can be dissociated in the two eyes. The associated nystagmus is often nonfatigable, vertical rather than horizontal, and not suppressed by visual fixation.[54] Electronystagmography is often useful in documenting these characteristics. Further evaluation of central vertigo usually requires MRI.

Romberg Test. The Romberg test is used to demonstrate disorders of static vestibular function. The person being tested is requested to stand with feet together and arms extended forward so that the degree of sway and arm stability can be observed. The person then is asked to close his or her eyes. When visual clues are removed, postural stability is based on proprioceptive sensation from the joints, muscles, and tendons and from static vestibular reception. Deficiency in vestibular static input is indicated by greatly increased sway and a tendency for the arms to drift toward the side of deficiency.

If vestibular input is severely deficient, the subject falls toward the deficient side. Care must be taken because defects of proprioceptive projection to the forebrain also result in some arm drift and postural instability toward the deficient side. Only if two-point discrimination and vibratory sensation from the lower and upper limbs are bilaterally normal can the deficiency be attributed to the vestibular system.

Electronystagmography. Electronystagmography (ENG) is an examination that records eye movements in response to vestibular, visual, cervical (vertigo triggered by somatosensory input from head and neck movements), rotational, and positional stimulation. Electrodes are placed lateral to the outer canthus of each eye and above and below each eye. A ground electrode is placed on the forehead. With ENG, the velocity, frequency, and amplitude of spontaneous or induced nystagmus and the changes in these measurements brought by a loss of fixation, with the eyes open or closed, can be quantified. The advantages of ENG are that it is easily administered, is noninvasive, does not interfere with vision, and does not require head restraint.[65]

Caloric Stimulation. Caloric testing involves elevating the head 30 degrees and irrigating each external auditory canal separately with 30 to 50 mL of ice water. The resulting changes in temperature, which are conducted through the petrous portion of the temporal bone, set up convection currents in the endolymph that mimic the effects of angular acceleration. In an unconscious person with a functional brain stem and intact oculovestibular reflexes, the eyes exhibit a jerk nystagmus lasting 2 to 3 minutes, with the slow component toward the irrigated ear followed by rapid movement away from the ear (see Chapter 51, Fig, 51-11). With impairment of brain stem function, the response becomes perverted and eventually disappears. An advantage of the caloric stimulation method is the ability to test the vestibular apparatus on one side at a time. The test is never done on persons who do not have an intact eardrum or who have blood or fluid collected behind the eardrum.

Treatment

Pharmacologic Methods. Depending on the cause, vertigo may be treated pharmacologically. There are two types of drugs used in the treatment of vertigo.[66] The first type are the drugs used to suppress the illusion of motion. These include drugs such as antihistamines (*e.g.*, meclizine, cyclizine, dimenhydrinate, promethazine) and anticholinergic drugs (*e.g.*, scopolamine, atropine) that suppress the vestibular system. Although the antihistamines have long been used in treating vertigo, little is known about their mechanism of action. The second type includes drugs used to relieve the nausea and vomiting that commonly accompany the condition. Antidopaminergic drugs (*e.g.*, phenothiazines) and benzodiazepines commonly are used for this purpose.

Vestibular Rehabilitation Exercises. Vestibular rehabilitation, a relatively new treatment modality for peripheral vestibular disorders, has met with considerable success.[67,68] It commonly is done by physical therapists and uses a home exercise program that incorporates habituation exercises, balance retraining exercises, and a general conditioning program.[67] The habituation exercises take advantage of physiologic fatigue of the neurovegetative response to repetitive movement or positional stimulation and are done to decrease motion-provoked vertigo, lightheadedness, and unsteadiness. The exercises are selected to provoke the vestibular symptoms. The person moves quickly into the position that causes symptoms, holds the position until the symptoms subside (*i.e.*, fatigue of the neurovegetative response), relaxes, and then repeats the exercise for a prescribed number of times. The exercises usually are repeated twice daily. The habituation effect is characterized by decreased sensitivity and duration of symptoms. It may occur in as little as 2 weeks or take as long as 6 months.[69]

Balance-retraining exercises consist of activities directed toward improving individual components of balance that may be abnormal. General conditioning exercises, a vital part of the rehabilitation process, are individualized to the person's preferences and lifestyle. They should consist of motion-oriented activity that the person is interested in and should be done on a regular basis, usually four to five times per week.[69]

IN SUMMARY, the vestibular system plays an essential role in the equilibrium sense, which is closely integrated with the visual and proprioceptive (position) senses. Receptors in the semicircular canals, utricle, and saccule of the vestibular system, located in the inner ear, respond to changes in linear and angular acceleration of the head. The vestibular nerve fibers travel in CN VIII to the vestibular nuclei at the junction of the medulla and pons; some fibers pass through the nuclei to the cerebellum. Cerebellar connections are necessary for temporally smooth, coordinated movements during ongoing head movements, tilt, and angular acceleration. The vestibular nuclei also connect with nuclei of the oculomotor (CN III), trochlear (CN IV), and abducens (CN VI) nerves that control eye movement. *Nystagmus* is a term used to describe vestibular-controlled eye movements that occur in response to angular and rotational movements of the head. The vestibulospinal tract, which provides for the control of muscle tone in the axial muscles, including those of the back, provides the support for maintaining balance. Neurons of the vestibular nuclei also project to the thalamus, to the temporal cortex, and to the somesthetic area of the parietal cortex. The thalamic and cortical projections provide the basis for the subjective experiences of position in space and of rotation and vertigo.

Vertigo, an illusory sensation of motion of either oneself or one's surroundings, tinnitus, and hearing loss are common manifestations of vestibular dysfunction, as are autonomic manifestations such as perspiration, nausea, and vomiting. Common disorders of the vestibular system include motion sickness, BPPV, and Ménière disease.

BPPV is a condition believed to be caused by free-floating particles in the posterior semicircular canal. It presents as a sudden onset of dizziness or vertigo that is provoked by certain changes in head position. Ménière disease, which is caused by an overaccumulation of endolymph, is characterized by severe, disabling episodes of tinnitus; feelings of ear fullness; and violent rotary vertigo. The diagnosis of vestibular disorders is based on a description of the symptoms, a history of trauma or exposure to agents destructive to vestibular structures, and tests of eye movements (*i.e.*, nystagmus) and muscle control of balance and equilibrium. Among the methods used in treatment of the vertigo that accompanies vestibular disorders are habituation exercises and antivertigo drugs. These drugs act by diminishing the excitability of neurons in the vestibular nucleus. ■

Review Exercises

1. A mother notices that her 13-month-old child is fussy and tugging at his ear, and he refuses to eat his breakfast. When she takes his temperature, it is 37.8°C (100°F). Although the child attends day care, the mother has kept him home and made an appointment with the child's pediatrician. In the physician's office, his temperature is 37.9°C (100.2°F), he is somewhat irritable, and he has a clear nasal drainage. His left tympanic membrane shows normal landmarks and motility on pneumatic otoscopy. His right tympanic membrane is erythematous and there is decreased motility on pneumatic otoscopy.

   A. *What risk factors are present that predispose this child to the development of acute otitis media?*

   B. *Are his signs and symptoms typical of otitis media in a child this age?*

   C. *What are the most likely pathogens? What treatment would be indicated?*

   D. *Later in the week, the mother notices that the child does not seem to hear as well as he did before developing the infection. Is this a common occurrence and should the mother be concerned about transient hearing loss in a child of this age?*

2. A granddaughter is worried that her grandfather is "losing his hearing." Lately, he has been staying away from social gatherings that he always enjoyed, saying everybody mumbles. He is defiant in maintaining that there is nothing wrong with his hearing. However, he does complain that his ears have been ringing a lot lately.

   A. *What are common manifestations of hearing loss in the elderly?*

   B. *What type of evaluation would be appropriate for determining if this man has a hearing loss and the extent of his hearing loss?*

   C. *What are some things that the granddaughter might do so that her grandfather could hear her better when she is talking to him?*

3. A 70-year-old man complains that he gets this terrible feeling "like the room is moving around" and becomes nauseated when he rolls over in bed or bends over suddenly. It usually goes away once he has been up for a while. He has been told that his symptoms are consistent with benign paroxysmal positional vertigo.

   A. *What is the pathophysiology associated with this man's vertigo?*

   B. *Why do the symptoms subside once he has been up for a while?*

   C. *What methods are available for treatment of the disorder?*

References

1. Moore K. L., Dallen A. F. (2006). *Clinically oriented anatomy* (5th ed., pp. 1022–1043). Philadelphia: Lippincott Williams & Wilkins.

2. Rhoades R. A., Tanner G. A. (2003). *Medical physiology* (2nd ed., pp. 77–89). Philadelphia: Lippincott Williams & Wilkins.

3. McCarter D. F., Pollart S. M. (2007). Cerumen impaction. *American Family Physician* 75, 1523–1530.

4. Bagai A., Thavendiranathan P., Detsky A. S. (2006). Does this patient have hearing impairment? *Journal of the American Medical Association* 295, 416–428.

5. Jackler R. K., Kaplan M. J. (2007). Ear, nose and throat. In Tierney L. M., McPhee S. J., Papadakis M. A. (Eds.), *Current medical diagnosis and treatment* (46th ed., pp. 182–196). New York: McGraw-Hill Medical.

6. Licameli G. R. (2002). The eustachian tube: Update on anatomy, development and function. *Otolaryngologic Clinics of North America* 35, 803–809.

7. Danner C. J. (2006). Eustachian tube function and the middle ear. *Otolaryngologic Clinics of North America* 39, 1221–1235.

8. American Academy of Pediatrics and American Academy of Family Physicians. (2004). Diagnosis and management of acute otitis media. *Pediatrics* 113, 1451–1465.

9. American Academy of Pediatrics and American Academy of Family Physicians. (2004). Otitis media with effusion. *Pediatrics* 113, 1412–1429.

10. Bhetwal N., McConaghy J. R. (2007). The evaluation and treatment of children with acute otitis media. *Primary Care Clinics in Office Practice* 34, 59–70.

11. Haddad J., Jr. (2004). The ear. In Behrman R. E., Kliegman R. M., Jenson H. B. (Eds.), *Nelson textbook of pediatrics* (17th ed., pp. 2127–2152). Philadelphia: Elsevier Saunders.

12. Hendley J. O. (2002). Otitis media. *New England Journal of Medicine* 347, 1169–1174.

13. Marcy S. M. (2004). New guidelines for otitis media: An overview of their key principles for practice. *Cleveland Clinic Journal of Medicine* 71(Suppl. 4), S3–S9.

14. Advisory Committee on Immunization Practices. (2007). Recommendations of the Advisory Committee on Immunization Practices: Prevention and control of influenza. *Morbidity and Mortality Weekly Reports* 56(RR06), 1–54.

15. Pelton S. I. (2005). Otitis media: Re-evaluation of diagnosis and treatment in the era of antimicrobial resistance, pneumococcal conjugate vaccine, and evolving morbidity. *Pediatric Clinics of North America* 52, 711–728.

16. Hall-Stoodley L., Hu F. Z., Gieske A., et al. (2006). Direct detection of bacterial biofilms on the middle-ear mucosa of children with chronic otitis media. *Journal of the American Medical Association* 296, 202–211.

17. Onusko E. (2004). Tympanometry. *American Family Physician* 70, 1713–1720.

18. Dowell S. F., Butler J. C., Giebink G. S., et al. (1999). Acute otitis media: Management and surveillance in an era of pneumococcal resistance. A report from the Drug-Resistant *Streptococcus pneumoniae* Therapeutic Working Group. *Pediatric Infectious Disease Journal* 18, 1–9.

19. McCormick D. P., Chonmaitree T., Pittman C., et al. (2005). Nonsevere acute otitis media: A clinical trial comparing outcomes of watchful waiting versus immediate antibiotic treatment. *Pediatrics* 115, 1455–1465.

20. Paradise J. L., Feldman H. M., Campbell T. F., et al. (2007). Tympanostomy tubes and developmental outcomes at 9 to 11 years of age. *New England Journal of Medicine* 356 (3), 248–261.

21. Smith J. A., Danner C. J. (2006). Complications of chronic otitis media and cholesteatoma. *Otolaryngologic Clinics of North America* 39, 1237–1255.

22. Semann M. T., Mergerian C. A. (2006). The pathophysiology of cholesteatoma. *Otolaryngologic Clinics of North America* 39, 1143–1159.

23. Shohet J. A., deJong A. L. (2002). The management of pediatric cholesteatoma. *Otolaryngologic Clinics of North America* 35, 841–851.

24. National Institute of Deafness and Other Communication Disorders. (1999). Otosclerosis. [Online.] Available: www.nidcd.nih.gov/health/hearing/otosclerosis.asp. Accessed October 20, 2007.

25. Holt J. J. (2003). Cholesteatoma and otosclerosis. *Clinical Medicine and Research* 1, 151–154.

26. Guyton A. C., Hall J. E. (2006). *Textbook of medical physiology* (11th ed., pp. 651–662, 692–697). Philadelphia: Elsevier Saunders.

27. Kandel E. R., Schwartz J. H., Jessel T. M. (2000). *Principles of neural science* (pp. 591–624, 801–815). New York: McGraw-Hill.

28. Gates G. A., Mills J. H. (2005). Presbycusis. *Lancet* 366, 1111–1119.

29. Lockwood A. H. (2005). Tinnitus. *Neurologic Clinics* 23, 893–900.

30. Noell C. A., Meyerhoff W. L. (2003). Tinnitus: Diagnosis and treatment of this elusive symptom. *Geriatrics* 58(2), 28–34.

31. Lockwood A. H., Salvi R. J., Burckard R. F. (2002). Tinnitus. *New England Journal of Medicine* 347, 904–910.

32. Schwaber M. K. (2003). Medical evaluation of tinnitus. *Otolaryngologic Clinics of North America* 36, 287–292.

33. National Institute on Deafness and Other Communication Disorders. (2007). Statistics about hearing disorders, ear infections, and deafness. [Online.] Available: www.nidcd.nih.gov/health/statistics/hearing.asp. Accessed April 14, 2008.

34. Nadol J. G. (1993). Hearing loss. *New England Journal of Medicine* 329, 1092–1101.

35. American Speech–Language–Hearing Association. (2008). Type, degree, and configuration of hearing loss. [Online.] Available: http://www.asha.org/public/hearing/disorders/types.htm. Accessed April 22, 2008.

36. Willems P. J. (2000). Genetic causes of hearing loss. *New England Journal of Medicine* 342, 1101–1109.

37. Isaacson J. E., Vora N. M. (2003). Differential diagnosis and treatment of hearing loss. *American Family Physician* 68, 1125–1132.

38. Weissman J. L. (1996). Hearing loss. *Radiology* 199, 593–611.
39. Yueh B., Shapiro N., MacLean C. H., et al. (2003). Screening and management of hearing loss in primary care: Scientific review. *Journal of the American Medical Association* 289, 1976–1985.
40. Palmer C. V., Ortmann A. (2005). Hearing loss and hearing aids. *Neurologic Clinics* 23, 901–918.
41. Francis H. W., Niparko J. K. (2003). Cochlear implantation update. *Pediatric Clinics of North America* 50, 341–361.
42. National Institute of Deafness and Other Communication Disorders. (2007). Cochlear implants. [Online.] Available: http://www.nidcd.nih.gov/health/hearing/coch.asp. Accessed April 22, 2008.
43. Papsin B. C., Gordon K. A. (2007). Cochlear implants for children with severe-to-profound hearing loss. *New England Journal of Medicine* 357(23), 2380–2387.
44. Wrightson A. S. (2007). Universal newborn hearing screening. *American Family Physician* 75, 1349–1352.
45. Morton C. C., Nance W. E. (2006). Newborn hearing screening: A silent revolution. *New England Journal of Medicine* 354, 2151–2164.
46. Task Force on Newborn and Infant Hearing of the American Academy of Pediatrics. (1999). Newborn and infant hearing loss: Detection and intervention. *Pediatrics* 103, 527–530.
47. Joint Commission on Infant Hearing. (2000). Year 2000 position statement: Principles and guidelines for early hearing detection and intervention programs. *Pediatrics* 106, 798–817.
48. Johnson K. C. (2002). Audiologic assessment of children with suspected hearing loss. *Otolaryngologic Clinics of North America* 35, 711–732.
49. Rubinstein J. T. (2002). Paediatric cochlear implantation: Prosthetic hearing and language development. *Lancet* 360, 483–485.
50. Bance M. (2007). Hearing and aging. *Canadian Medical Association Journal* 176, 925–927.
51. Gates G. A., Murphy M., Rees T. S., et al. (2003). Screening for handicapping hearing loss in the elderly. *Journal of Family Practice* 52, 56–62.
52. Ross M. H., Kaye G. I., Pawlina W. (2003). *Histology: A text and atlas* (4th ed., pp. 824–833). Philadelphia: Lippincott Williams & Wilkins.
53. Chawla N., Olshaker J. S. (2006). Diagnosis and management of dizziness and vertigo. *Medical Clinics of North America* 90, 291–304.
54. Labuguen R. H. (2006). Initial evaluation of vertigo. *American Family Physician* 73, 244–254.
55. Schwartz R., Longwell B. (2005). Treatment of vertigo. *American Family Physician* 71, 1115–1130.
56. Furman J. M., Cass S. P. (1999). Benign paroxysmal positional vertigo. *New England Journal of Medicine* 341, 1590–1596.
57. Parnes L. S., Agrawal S. K., Atlas J. (2003). Diagnosis and management of benign paroxysmal positional vertigo (BPPV). *Canadian Medical Association Journal* 169, 681–693.
58. Hotson J. R., Baloh R. W. (1998). Acute vestibular syndrome. *New England Journal of Medicine* 339, 680–685.
59. Baloh R. W. (2003). Vestibular neuritis. *New England Journal of Medicine* 348, 1027–1032.
60. Savitz S. I., Caplan L. R. (2005). Vertebrobasilar disease. *New England Journal of Medicine* 352, 2618–2626.
61. Paparella M. M., Djalilian H. R. (2002). Etiology, pathophysiology of symptoms and pathogenesis of Ménière's disease. *Otolaryngologic Clinics of North America* 35, 529–545.
62. Dickins J. R. E., Graham S. S. (1990). Ménière's disease: 1983–1989. *American Journal of Otology* 11, 51–65.
63. Saeed S. R. (1998). Fortnightly review: Diagnosis and treatment of Ménière's disease. *British Medical Journal* 316, 368–372.
64. Hollis L., Bottrill I. (1999). Ménière's disease. *Hospital Medicine (London)* 60, 574–578.
65. Baloh R. W. (1989). Modern vestibular function testing. *Western Journal of Medicine* 150, 59–67.
66. Hain T. C., Yacovino D. (2005). Pharmacologic treatment of persons with vertigo. *Neurologic Clinics* 23, 831–853.
67. Horak F. B., Jones-Rycewicz C., Black F. W., et al. (1992). Effects of vestibular rehabilitation on dizziness and imbalance. *Otolaryngology–Head and Neck Surgery* 106, 175–180.
68. Smith-Whellock M., Shepard N. T., Telian S. A. (1991). Physical therapy program for vestibular rehabilitation. *American Journal of Otology* 12, 218–225.
69. Brandt T. (2000). Management of vestibular disorders. *Journal of Neurology* 247, 491–499.

Visit the Point. **http://thePoint.lww.com for animations, journal articles, and more!**

Disorders of Musculoskeletal and Integumentary Function

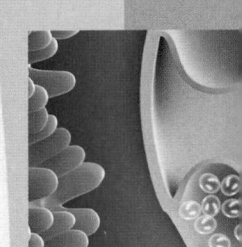

Some of the most significant investigations of the skeleton and muscles took place during the Renaissance—a time that celebrated the human body and lifted the knowledge of the body and its workings out of medieval murkiness.

The first comprehensive description of musculature was presented by Andreas Vesalius (1514–1564), a professor of anatomy and surgery at Padua. The product of his scrupulous dissections was the masterwork *De Humani Corporis Fabrica* (On the Structure of the Human Body), the second volume of which dealt with muscles and their structure. The work was beautifully illustrated with elegantly poised cadavers set against backgrounds of medieval Italy. Vesalius' effort successfully challenged many of the long-held pronouncements of Galen. The studies of artist Leonardo da Vinci (1452–1519) sought not to dispute or confirm previous teachings but to learn of the "divine form" so that it could be better rendered. A physician of the time wrote that "in order that he might be able to paint the various joints and muscles as they bend and extend according to the laws of nature, he [Leonardo] dissected in medical schools the corpses of criminals, indifferent to this inhuman and nauseating work." Although da Vinci was primarily a painter studying anatomy for the sake of art, there is little doubt that had his anatomic drawings been published during his lifetime or shortly after, science would have been advanced by years.

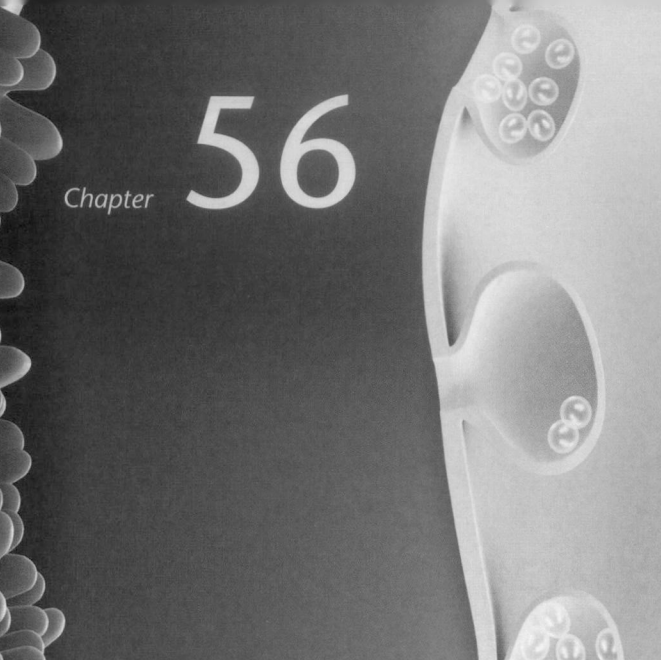

Chapter 56

Structure and Function of the Musculoskeletal System

CAROL M. PORTH

➤ Without the skeletal system, movement in the external environment would not be possible. The bones of the skeletal system serve as a framework for the attachment of muscles, tendons, and ligaments. The skeletal system protects and maintains soft tissues in their proper position, provides stability for the body, and maintains the body's shape. The bones act as a storage reservoir for calcium, and the central cavity of some bones contains the hematopoietic connective tissue in which blood cells are formed. Coordinated movement of the skeleton is made possible by the tendons and ligaments that join bones at joints.

For our purposes, the skeletal system is considered to include the bones and cartilage of the skeletal system, as well as the connective tissue structures (*i.e.*, ligaments and tendons) that connect the bones and join muscles to bone.

BONY STRUCTURES OF THE SKELETAL SYSTEM

After completing this section of the chapter, you should be able to meet the following objectives:

- Describe locations and characteristics of compact and cancellous bone.
- Describe the structure of a long bone.
- Cite the characteristics and name at least one location of elastic cartilage, hyaline cartilage, and fibrocartilage.
- Name and characterize the function of the four types of bone cells.
- State the function of parathyroid hormone, calcitonin, and vitamin D in terms of bone formation and metabolism.

The skeletal system consists of the axial and appendicular skeleton. The *axial skeleton,* which is composed of the bones of the skull, thorax, and vertebral column, forms the axis of the body. The *appendicular skeleton* consists of the bones of the upper and lower extremities, including the shoulder and hip. The skeletal system contains both bone and cartilage tissue. Bones provide protection for internal organs and rigid support for the extremities, whereas cartilage provides for flexibility and cushioning of bony structures and for skeletal development in both prenatal and postnatal life.

THE SKELETAL SYSTEM

- The skeletal system consists of the bones of the skull, thorax, and vertebral column, which form the *axial skeleton,* and the bones of the upper and lower extremities, which form the *appendicular skeleton.*

- Two types of connective tissue are found in the skeletal system: (1) cartilage, a semirigid and slightly flexible structure that plays an essential role in prenatal and childhood development of the skeleton and as a surface for the articulating ends of skeletal joints; and (2) bone, which provides for the firm structure of the skeleton and serves as a reservoir for calcium and phosphate storage.

- Both bone and cartilage tissue are composed of living cells and a nonliving intercellular matrix that is secreted by the living cells.

- Bone matrix is maintained by four types of cells: osteoblasts, which synthesize and secrete the constituents of bone; osteoclasts, which resorb surplus bone and are required for bone remodeling; osteocytes, which make up the osteoid tissue of bone; and osteoprogenitor cells, which are the source of all bone cells, except osteoclasts.

Bone Structures

There are two types of mature bones, compact and cancellous bone (Fig. 56-1). Cancellous (spongy) bone is found in the interior of bones and is composed of *trabeculae,* or *spicules,* of bone that form a lattice-like pattern. These lattice-like structures are lined with osteogenic cells and filled with red or yellow bone marrow. Cancellous bone is relatively light, but its structure is such that it has considerable tensile strength and weight-bearing properties. Compact (cortical) bone, which forms the outer shell of a bone, has a densely packed, calcified intercellular matrix that makes it more rigid than cancellous bone. Although bones contain both cancellous and compact elements, their proportions vary in different bones throughout the body and in different parts of the same bone, depending on the relative needs for strength and lightness. Compact bone is the major component of tubular bones. It is also found along the lines of stress on long bones and forms an outer protective shell on other bones.

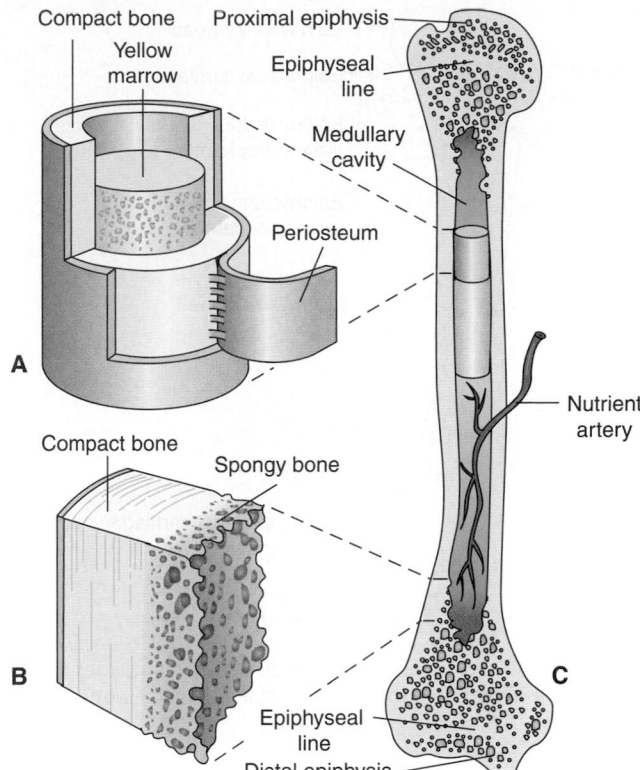

FIGURE 56-1 • A long bone shown in longitudinal section. **(A)** Periosteum and bone marrow, **(B)** compact and cancellous bone, **(C)** epiphysis and source of blood supply from epiphysial and nutrient arteries.

Types of Bones

Bones are classified by shape as long, short, flat, and irregular. Long bones are found in the upper and lower extremities. Short bones are irregularly shaped bones located in the ankle and the wrist. Except for their surface, which is compact bone, these bones are spongy throughout. Flat bones are composed of a layer of cancellous bone between two layers of compact bone. They are found in areas such as the skull and rib cage, where extensive protection of underlying structures is needed, or, as in the scapula, where a broad surface for muscle attachment must be provided. Irregular bones, because of their shapes, cannot be classified in any of the previous groups. This group includes bones such as the vertebrae and the bones of the jaw.

A typical long bone has a shaft, or *diaphysis,* and two ends, called *epiphyses* (Fig. 56-2). Long bones usually are narrow in the mid-portion and broad at the ends so that the weight they bear can be distributed over a wider surface. The shaft of a long bone is formed mainly of compact bone roughly hollowed out to form a marrow-filled medullary canal. The ends of long bones are covered with articular cartilage.

In growing bones, the part of the bone shaft that funnels out as it approaches the epiphysis is called the *metaphysis.* It is composed of bony trabeculae that have cores of cartilage. In the child, the epiphysis is separated from the metaphysis by the cartilaginous growth plate. After puberty, the metaphysis and epiphysis merge, and the growth plate is obliterated.

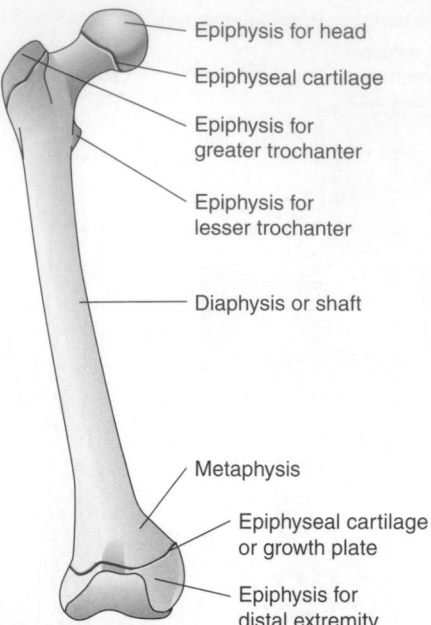

Epiphysis for head
Epiphyseal cartilage
Epiphysis for greater trochanter
Epiphysis for lesser trochanter
Diaphysis or shaft
Metaphysis
Epiphyseal cartilage or growth plate
Epiphysis for distal extremity

FIGURE 56-2 • A femur, showing epiphyseal cartilages for the head, metaphysis, trochanters, and distal end of the bone.

Periosteum and Endosteum

Bones are covered, except at their articular ends, by a membrane called the *periosteum* (see Fig. 56-1). The periosteum has an outer fibrous layer and an inner layer that contains the osteo-progenitor cells needed for bone growth and development. The periosteum contains blood vessels and acts as an anchorage point for vessels as they enter and leave the bone. The endosteum is the membrane that lines the spaces of spongy bone, the marrow cavities, and the haversian canals of compact bone. It is composed mainly of osteoprogenitor cells that contribute to the growth and remodeling of bone and are necessary for bone repair.

Bone Marrow

Bone marrow occupies the medullary cavities of the long bones throughout the skeleton and the cavities of cancellous bone in the vertebrae, ribs, sternum, and flat bones of the pelvis. The cellular composition of the bone marrow varies with age and skeletal location. Red bone marrow contains developing red blood cells and is the site of blood cell formation. Yellow bone marrow is composed largely of adipose cells. At birth, nearly all of the marrow is red and hematopoietically active. As the need for red blood cell production decreases during postnatal life, red marrow is gradually replaced with yellow bone marrow in most of the bones. In the adult, red marrow persists in the vertebrae, ribs, sternum, and ilia.

Blood Supply

The compact bone of long tubular bones is provided with blood supply from two sources, nutrient arteries and perforating arteries. The nutrient arteries enter the bone through a nutrient foramen and supply the marrow space and the internal one half of the cortex. The perforating arteries are small arteries that extend inward from the periosteal arteries on the external surface of the periosteum and anastomose in the cortex with branches of the nutrient arteries coming from the bone marrow. The distribution of blood in the cortex occurs through the haversian and Volkmann canals (Fig. 56-3). Haversian canals are spaces in the bone of the cortex that course parallel through the long axis of the bone for a short distance and then branch and communicate with other, similar canals. Each canal carries one or two blood vessels, lymphatics, and some nerve fibers. Volkmann canals, which also contain blood vessels, are spaces in the cortex that run perpendicular to the long axis of the cortex to connect adjacent haversian canals.

Cancellous bone is usually not penetrated by blood vessels. Instead, the bone cells of cancellous bone are nourished by diffusion from the endosteal surface through canaliculi, which interconnect their surrounding fluid-filled lacunae and extend to the bone surface.

Bone Tissue

Bone is connective tissue in which the intercellular matrix has been impregnated with inorganic calcium salts so that it has great tensile and compressive strength but is light enough to be moved by coordinated muscle contractions. The intercellular matrix is composed of two types of substances—organic matter and inorganic salts. The organic matter, including bone cells, blood vessels, and nerves, constitutes approximately one third of the dry weight of bone; the inorganic salts make up the other two thirds.

The organic matter consists primarily of collagen fibers embedded in an amorphous ground substance. The inorganic matter consists of hydroxyapatite, an insoluble macrocrystalline structure of calcium phosphate salts, and small amounts of calcium carbonate and calcium fluoride. Bone may also take up lead and other heavy metals, thereby removing these toxic substances from the circulation. This can be viewed as a protective mechanism. The antibiotic tetracycline is readily bound to calcium deposited in newly formed bones and teeth. When tetracycline is given during pregnancy, it can be deposited in the teeth of the fetus, causing discoloration and deformity. Similar changes can occur if the drug is given for long periods to children younger than 6 years of age.

Lamellar and Woven Bone

There are two types of bone tissue: lamellar bone and woven bone. Both forms of bone can be mineralized or unmineralized, the latter being referred to as *osteoid. Lamellar bone* is a strong, mature form of bone that is formed slowly and is highly organized. It is the mature bone found in the adult skeleton; anything other than lamellar bone in an adult skeleton is abnormal. Lamellar bone is composed largely of cylindrical units called *osteons* or *haversian systems.* The osteons consist of concentric lamellae of bone matrix, surrounding a central canal, called the

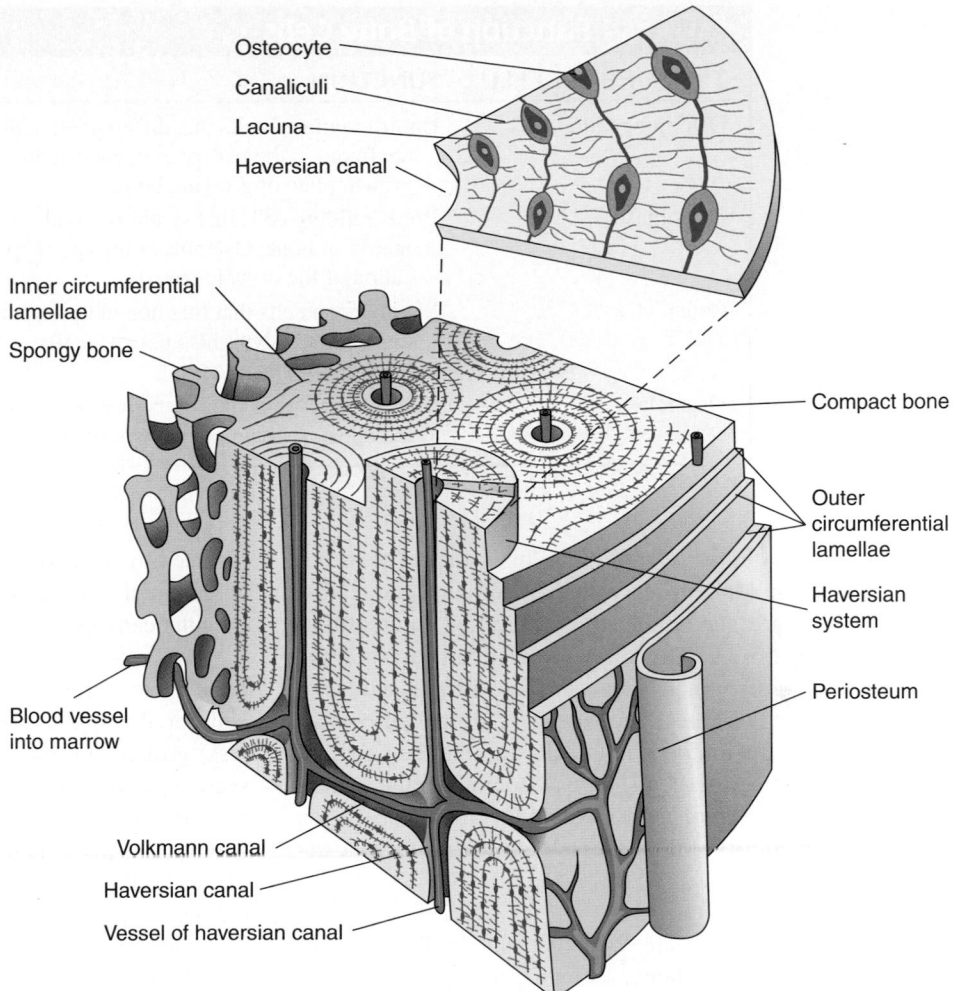

Osteocyte
Canaliculi
Lacuna
Haversian canal

Inner circumferential lamellae
Spongy bone

Compact bone

Outer circumferential lamellae

Haversian system

Periosteum

Blood vessel into marrow

Volkmann canal
Haversian canal
Vessel of haversian canal

FIGURE 56-3 • Haversian systems as seen in a wedge of compact bone tissue. The periosteum has been peeled back to show a blood vessel entering a Volkmann canal. **(Top)** Osteocytes lying within lacunae; canaliculi permit interstitial fluid to reach each lacuna.

haversian canal, that contains the blood vessels and nerve supply for the osteon (see Fig. 56-3). In compact bone, 4 to 20 lamellae are arranged concentrically around a central haversian canal, which runs essentially parallel to the long axis of the bone. Between the osteons are remnants of previous concentric lamellae, called the *interstitial lamella.* Circumferential lamellae follow the entire inner and outer shaft of a long bone, appearing much like the growth rings of a tree. Cancellous bone is also composed of lamellae, but, as mentioned previously, its trabeculae usually are not penetrated by blood vessels.

Woven bone is deposited more rapidly than lamellar bone. It is of low tensile strength, serving as temporary scaffolding for support. It is found in the developing fetus, in areas surrounding tumors and infections, and as part of a healing fracture.

Bone Cells

Four types of bone cells participate in the formation and maintenance of bone tissue: osteoprogenitor cells, osteoblasts, osteocytes, and osteoclasts (Table 56-1).

Osteoprogenitor Cells. The undifferentiated osteoprogenitor cells are found in the periosteum, endosteum, and epiphyseal plate of growing bone. These cells differentiate into osteoblasts and are active during normal growth; they may also be activated in adult life during healing of fractures and other injuries. Osteoprogenitor cells also participate in the continual replacement of worn-out bone tissue.

Osteoblasts. The osteoblasts, or bone-building cells, are responsible for the formation of the bone matrix. Bone formation occurs in two stages: ossification and calcification. Ossification involves the formation of osteoid, or prebone. Calcification of bone involves the deposition of calcium salts in the osteoid tissue. The osteoblasts synthesize collagen and other proteins that make up osteoid tissue. They also participate in the calcification process of the osteoid tissue, probably by controlling the availability of calcium and phosphate. Osteoblasts secrete the enzyme *alkaline phosphatase,* which is thought to act locally in bone tissue to raise calcium and phosphate levels to the point at which precipitation occurs. The activity of the osteoblasts undoubtedly contributes to the increase in serum levels of alkaline phosphatase that follows bone injury and fractures.

Osteocytes. The osteocytes are mature bone cells that are actively involved in maintaining the bony matrix. Death of the

TABLE 56-1 **Function of Bone Cells**	
TYPE OF BONE CELL	**FUNCTION**
Osteoprogenitor cells	Undifferentiated cells that differentiate into osteoblasts. They are found in the periosteum, endosteum, and epiphyseal growth plate of growing bones.
Osteoblasts	Bone-building cells that synthesize and secrete the organic matrix of bone. Osteoblasts also participate in the calcification of the organic matrix.
Osteocytes	Mature bone cells that function in the maintenance of bone matrix. Osteocytes also play an active role in releasing calcium into the blood.
Osteoclasts	Bone cells responsible for the resorption of bone matrix and the release of calcium and phosphate from bone.

osteocytes results in the resorption of this matrix. The osteocytes lie in a small lake filled with extracellular fluid, called a *lacuna,* and are surrounded by a calcified intercellular matrix (see Fig. 56-3). Extracellular fluid-filled passageways permeate the calcified matrix and connect with the lacunae of adjacent osteocytes. These passageways are called *canaliculi.* Because diffusion does not occur through the calcified matrix of bone, the canaliculi serve as communicating channels for the exchange of nutrients and metabolites between the osteocytes and the blood vessels on the surface of the bone layer.

Osteoclasts. Osteoclasts are "bone-chewing" cells that function in the resorption of bone, removing the mineral content and the organic matrix. They are large phagocytic cells of monocyte/macrophage lineage. Although the mechanism of osteoclast formation and activation remains elusive, it is known that parathyroid hormone increases the number and resorptive function of the osteoclasts. Calcitonin is thought to reduce the number and resorptive function of the osteoclasts. Estrogen also reduces the number and function of the osteoclasts; thus, the decrease in estrogen levels that occurs at menopause results in increased resorption of bone. The mechanism whereby osteoclasts exert their resorptive effect on bone is unclear. These cells may secrete an acid that removes calcium from the bone matrix, releasing the collagenic fibers for digestion by osteoclasts or mononuclear cells. Osteoclasts, by virtue of their phagocytic lineage, also imbibe minute particles of bone matrix and crystals, eventually dissolving and releasing them into the blood.

Cartilage

Cartilage is an essential part of the skeletal system. It constitutes the articular cartilage of joints; it is found in the tendinous and ligamentous insertions, menisci, the symphysis pubis, and insertions of joint capsules. It is also essential for growth before and after birth. In the embryo, most of the axial and appendicular skeleton is formed first as a cartilage model and then replaced by bone. In postnatal life, cartilage continues to play an essential role in the growth of long bones and persists as articular cartilage in the adult.

As a tissue, cartilage both resembles and differs from bone. Both of these connective tissue types consist of living cells, nonliving intercellular fibers, and an amorphous (shapeless) ground substance. The tissue cells are responsible for secreting and maintaining the intercellular substances in which they are housed. However, cartilage consists of more extracellular substance than bone, and its fibers are embedded in a firm gel rather than a calcified cement-like substance. Hence, cartilage has the flexibility of a firm plastic material rather than the rigid characteristics of bone.

There are three types of cartilage: elastic cartilage, hyaline cartilage, and fibrocartilage. *Elastic cartilage* contains some elastin in its intercellular substance. It is found in areas, such as the ear, where some flexibility is important. Pure cartilage is called *hyaline cartilage* (from a Greek word meaning "glass") and is pearly white. It is the type of cartilage seen on the articulating ends of fresh soup bones found in the supermarket. *Fibrocartilage* has characteristics that are intermediate between dense connective tissue and hyaline cartilage. It is found in the intervertebral disks, in areas where tendons are connected to bone, and in the symphysis pubis.

Hyaline cartilage is the most abundant type of cartilage. It forms much of the cartilage of the fetal skeleton. In the adult, hyaline cartilage forms the costal cartilages that join the ribs to the sternum and vertebrae, many of the cartilages of the respiratory tract, the articular cartilages, and the epiphyseal plates.

Cartilage cells, which are called *chondrocytes,* are located in lacunae. The lacunae are surrounded by an uncalcified, gel-like intercellular matrix of collagen fibers and ground substance. Cartilage is devoid of blood vessels and nerves. The free surfaces of most hyaline cartilage, with the exception of articular cartilage, are covered by a layer of fibrous connective tissue called the *perichondrium.*

It has been estimated that approximately 65% to 80% of the wet weight of cartilage is water held in its gel structure. Because cartilage has no blood vessels, this tissue fluid allows the diffusion of gases, nutrients, and wastes between the chondrocytes and blood vessels outside the cartilage. Diffusion cannot take place if the cartilage matrix becomes impregnated with calcium salts, and cartilage dies if it becomes calcified.

Hormonal Control of Bone Formation and Metabolism

The process of bone formation and mineral metabolism is complex. It involves the interplay among the actions of parathyroid hormone (PTH), calcitonin, and vitamin D. Other hormones, such as cortisol, growth hormone, thyroid hormone, and the sex hormones, also influence bone formation directly or indirectly (Table 56-2).

Parathyroid Hormone

Parathyroid hormone is one of the important regulators of calcium and phosphate levels in the blood. PTH prevents serum calcium levels from falling below and serum phosphate levels from rising above normal physiologic concentrations (see Chapter 41). The secretion of PTH is regulated by negative feedback; increased serum levels of ionized calcium inhibit PTH release. PTH maintains serum calcium levels by initiation of calcium release from bone, by conservation of calcium by the kidney, by enhanced intestinal absorption of calcium through activation of vitamin D, and by reduction of serum phosphate levels (Fig. 56-4). PTH also increases the movement of calcium and phosphate from bone into the extracellular fluid. Calcium is immediately released from the canaliculi and bone cells; a more prolonged release of calcium and phosphate is mediated by increased osteoclast activity. In the kidney, PTH stimulates tubular reabsorption of calcium while reducing the reabsorption of phosphate. The latter effect ensures that increased release of phosphate from bone during mobilization of calcium does not produce an elevation in serum phosphate levels. This is impor-

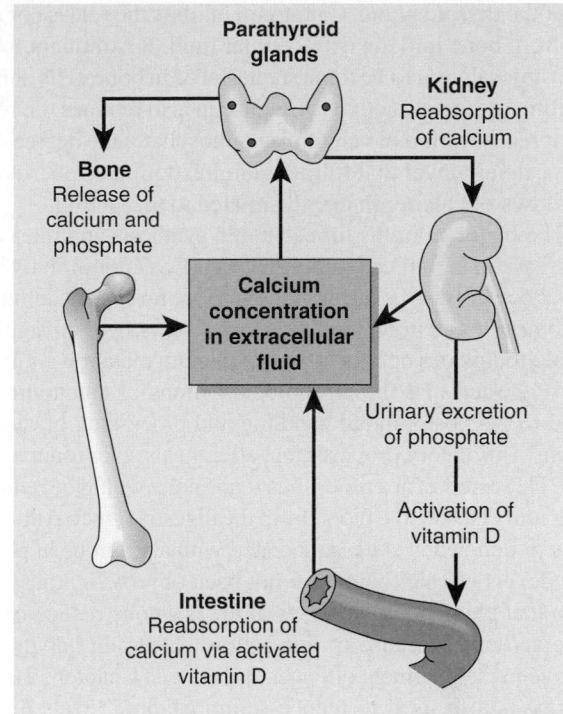

FIGURE 56-4 • Regulation and actions of parathyroid hormone.

tant because an increase in calcium and phosphate levels could lead to crystallization in soft tissues. PTH increases intestinal absorption of calcium because of its ability to stimulate activation of vitamin D by the kidney.

Calcitonin

Whereas PTH increases blood calcium levels, the hormone calcitonin lowers blood calcium levels. Calcitonin, sometimes called *thyrocalcitonin,* is secreted by the parafollicular, or C,

TABLE 56-2 Actions of Parathyroid Hormone, Calcitonin, and Vitamin D

ACTIONS	PARATHYROID HORMONE	CALCITONIN	VITAMIN D
Intestinal absorption of calcium	Increases indirectly through increased activation of vitamin D	Probably not affected	Increases
Intestinal absorption of phosphate	Increases	Probably not affected	Increases
Renal excretion of calcium	Decreases	Increases	Probably increases, but less effect than PTH
Renal excretion of phosphate	Increases	Increases	Increases
Bone resorption	Increases	Decreases	$1,25\text{-}(OH)_2D_3$ increases
Bone formation	Decreases	Uncertain	$24,25\text{-}(OH)_2D_3$ increases (?)
Serum calcium levels	Produces a prompt increase	Decreases with pharmacologic doses	No effect
Serum phosphate levels	Prevents an increase	Decreases with pharmacologic doses	No effect

cells of the thyroid gland. Calcitonin inhibits the release of calcium from bone into the extracellular fluid. It is thought to act by causing calcium to become sequestered in bone cells and by inhibiting osteoclast activity. Calcitonin also reduces the renal tubular reabsorption of calcium and phosphate; the decrease in serum calcium level that follows administration of pharmacologic doses of calcitonin may be related to this action.

The major stimulus for calcitonin synthesis and release is an increase in serum calcium. The role of calcitonin in overall mineral homeostasis is uncertain. There are no clearly definable syndromes of calcitonin deficiency or excess, which suggests that calcitonin does not directly alter calcium metabolism. It has been suggested that the physiologic actions of calcitonin are related to the postprandial handling and processing of dietary calcium. This theory proposes that after meals, calcitonin maintains PTH secretion at a time when it normally would be reduced by calcium entering the blood from the digestive tract. Although excess or deficiency states associated with alterations in physiologic levels of calcitonin have not been observed, it has been shown that pharmacologic doses of the hormone reduce osteoclastic activity. Because of this action, calcitonin has proved effective in the treatment of Paget disease (see Chapter 59). The hormone is also used to reduce serum calcium levels during hypercalcemic crises.

Vitamin D

Vitamin D and its metabolites are not true vitamins but steroid hormones. There are two forms of vitamin D: vitamin D_2 (ergocalciferol) and vitamin D_3 (cholecalciferol). The two forms differ by the presence of a double bond, but they have identical biologic activity. The term *vitamin D* is used to indicate both forms.

Vitamin D has little or no activity until it has been converted to physiologically active metabolized to compounds that mediate its activity. Figure 56-5 depicts sources of vitamin D and pathways for activation. The first step of the activation process occurs in the liver, where vitamin D is hydroxylated to form the metabolite 25-hydroxyvitamin D_3 [25-$(OH)D_3$]. From the liver, 25-$(OH)D_3$ is transported to the kidneys, where it undergoes conversion to 1,25-dihydroxyvitamin D_3 [1,25-$(OH)_2D_3$] or 24,25-dihydroxyvitamin D_3 [24,25-$(OH)_2D_3$]. Other metabolites of vitamin D have been and still are being discovered.

There are two sources of vitamin D: intestinal absorption and skin production. Intestinal absorption occurs mainly in the jejunum and includes vitamin D_2 and vitamin D_3. The most important dietary sources of vitamin D are fish, liver, and irradiated milk. Because vitamin D is fat soluble, its absorption is mediated by bile salts and occurs by means of the lymphatic vessels. In the skin, ultraviolet radiation from sunlight spontaneously converts 7-dehydrocholesterol D_3 to vitamin D_3. A circulating vitamin D–binding protein provides a mechanism to remove vitamin D from the skin and make it available to the rest of the body.

With adequate exposure to sunlight, the amount of vitamin D that can be produced by the skin is usually sufficient to meet physiologic requirements. The importance of sunlight

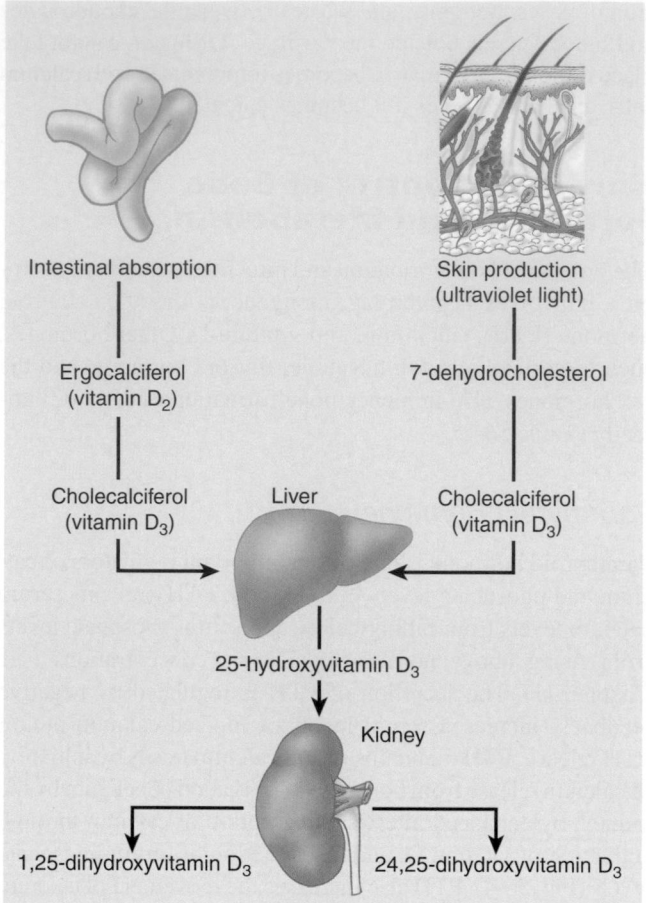

FIGURE 56-5 • Sources and pathways for activation of vitamin D.

exposure is evidenced by population studies that report lower vitamin D levels in countries, such as England, that have less sunlight than the United States. Elderly persons who are housebound or institutionalized frequently have low vitamin D levels. The deficiency often goes undetected until there are problems such as pseudofractures or electrolyte imbalances. Seasonal variations in vitamin D levels probably reflect changes in sunlight exposure.

The most potent of the vitamin D metabolites is 1,25-$(OH)_2D_3$. This metabolite increases intestinal absorption of calcium and promotes the actions of PTH on resorption of calcium and phosphate from bone. Bone resorption by the osteoclasts is increased, and bone formation by the osteoblasts is decreased; there is also an increase in acid phosphatase and a decrease in alkaline phosphatase. Intestinal absorption and bone resorption increase the amount of calcium and phosphorus available to the mineralizing surface of the bone. The role of 24,25-$(OH)_2D_3$ is less clear. There is evidence that 24,25-$(OH)_2D_3$, in conjunction with 1,25-$(OH)_2D_3$, may be involved in normal bone mineralization.

The regulation of vitamin D activity is influenced by several hormones. PTH and prolactin stimulate 1,25-$(OH)_2D_3$ production by the kidney. States of hyperparathyroidism are associated with increased levels of 1,25-$(OH)_2D_3$, and hypoparathyroidism leads to lowered levels of this metabolite. Prolactin may have an ancillary role in regulating vitamin D metabolism during pregnancy and lactation. Calcitonin inhibits 1,25-$(OH)_2D_3$ production by the kidney. In addition to hormonal influences, changes in the concentration of ions such as calcium, phosphate, hydrogen, and potassium exert an effect on 1,25-$(OH)_2D_3$ and 24,25-$(OH)_2D_3$ production. Under conditions of phosphate and calcium deprivation, 1,25-$(OH)_2D_3$ levels are increased, whereas hyperphosphatemia and hypercalcemia decrease the levels of metabolite.

IN SUMMARY, skeletal tissue consists of the bones and cartilage that form the appendicular and axial skeleton. There are two types of bone: compact bone, which forms the outer shell of a bone, and cancellous or spongy bone that forms the interior. The endosteum is the membrane that lines the spaces of spongy bone, the marrow cavities, and the haversian canals of compact bone. The periosteum, the membrane that covers bones, contains blood vessels and acts as an anchorage point for vessels as they enter and leave the bone. Mature bone is largely made up of cylindrical units called *osteons,* formed from concentric layers or lamellae of bone matrix and surrounding a central *haversian canal.* The haversian canals contain the blood vessels and nerve supply for the osteon. There are four types of bone cells: osteocytes, or mature bone cells; osteoblasts, or bone-building cells; osteoclasts, which function in bone resorption; and osteoprogenitor cells, which differentiate into osteoblasts.

Cartilage is a firm, flexible type of skeletal tissue that is essential for growth before and after birth. There are three types of cartilage: elastic, hyaline, and fibrocartilage. Hyaline cartilage, which is the most abundant type, forms the costal cartilages that join the ribs to the sternum and vertebrae, many of the cartilages of the respiratory tract, and the articular cartilages.

The process of bone formation and mineral metabolism involves the interplay among the actions of PTH, calcitonin, and vitamin D. PTH acts to maintain serum levels of ionized calcium; it increases the release of calcium and phosphate from bone, the conservation of calcium and elimination of phosphate by the kidney, and the intestinal reabsorption of calcium through vitamin D. Calcitonin inhibits the release of calcium from bone and increases renal elimination of calcium and phosphate, thereby serving to lower serum calcium levels. Vitamin D functions as a hormone in regulating body calcium. It increases absorption of calcium from the intestine and promotes the actions of PTH on bone. ■

ARTICULATIONS AND JOINTS

After completing this section of the chapter, you should be able to meet the following objectives:

- State the characteristics of tendons and ligaments.
- State the difference between synarthroses and synovial joints.

- Describe the source of blood supply to a synovial joint.
- Explain why pain is often experienced in all the joints of an extremity when only a single joint is affected by a disease process.
- Describe the structure and function of a bursa.
- Explain the pathology associated with a torn meniscus of the knee.

Articulations, or joints, are areas where two or more bones meet. The term *arthro* is the prefix used to designate a joint; for example, *arthrology* is the study of joints, and *arthroplasty* is the repair of a joint.

SKELETAL JOINTS

- Articulations, or joints, are sites where two or more bones meet to hold the skeleton together and give it mobility.
- There are two types of joints: synarthroses, which are immovable joints, and synovial joints, which are freely movable joints.
- All limb joints are synovial diarthroidal joints, which are enclosed in a joint cavity containing synovial fluid.
- The articulating surfaces of synovial joints are covered with a layer of avascular cartilage that relies on oxygen and nutrients contained in the synovial fluid.
- Regeneration of articular cartilage of synovial joints is slow, and healing of injuries often is slow and unsatisfactory.

Tendons and Ligaments

In the skeletal system, tendons and ligaments are dense connective tissue structures that connect muscles and bones. The dense connective tissue found in tendons and ligaments has a limited blood supply and is composed largely of intercellular bundles of collagen fibers arranged in the same direction and plane. Collagen is an inelastic and insoluble fibrous protein. Because of its molecular configuration, collagen has great tensile strength; the breaking point of collagenous fibers found in human tendons is reached with a force of several hundred kilograms per square centimeter. Fresh collagen is colorless, and tissues that contain large numbers of collagenous fibers generally appear white.

Tendons, which attach skeletal muscles to bone, are relatively inextensible because of their richness in collagen fibers. The collagen bundles of tendons aggregate into bundles that are enveloped by loose connective tissue, blood vessels, and nerves. Tendons that may rub against bone or other friction-generating surfaces are enclosed in double-layered sheaths. An outer connective tissue tube is attached to the structures surrounding the tendon, and an inner sheath encloses the tendon and is attached to it. The space between the inner and outer sheath is filled with a fluid similar to synovial fluid. Overuse can result in *tendonitis* or inflammation of the tendon.

Ligaments are fibrous thickenings of the articular capsule that join one bone to its articulating mate. They vary in size and shape depending on their specific role. Although most ligaments are considered inelastic, they are pliable enough to permit movement at the joints. However, ligaments tear rather than stretch when exposed to excess stress. Torn ligaments are extremely painful and accompanied by local swelling.

Types of Joints

Joints exhibit a variety of movements. Some joints have no movement; others allow only slight movement; and some are freely moveable, such as the shoulder joint. There are two classes of joints based on their movement and the presence or absence of a joint cavity: synarthroses and synovial joints.

Synarthroses

Synarthroses are joints that lack a joint cavity and move little or not at all. There are three types of synarthroses: synostoses, synchondroses, and syndesmoses. *Synostoses* are nonmovable joints in which the surfaces of the bones are joined by dense connective tissue or bone. The bones of the skull are joined by synostoses; they are joined by dense connective tissue in children and young adults and by bone in older persons. *Synchondroses* are joints in which bones are connected by hyaline cartilage and have limited motion. The ribs are attached to the sternum by this type of joint. *Syndesmoses* permit a certain amount of movement; they are separated by a fibrous disk and joined by interosseous ligaments. The symphysis pubis of the pelvis and the vertebral bodies joined by intervertebral disks are examples of syndesmoses.

Synovial (Diarthrodial) Joints

Synovial or diarthrodial joints are freely movable joints. Most joints in the body are of this type. Although they are classified as freely movable, their movement ranges from almost none (*e.g.*, sacroiliac joint), to simple hinge movement (*e.g.*, interphalangeal joint), to movement in many planes (*e.g.*, shoulder or hip joint). The bony surfaces of these joints are covered with thin layers of articular cartilage, and the cartilaginous surfaces of these joints slide past each other during movement. As discussed in Chapter 59, diarthrodial joints are the joints most frequently affected by rheumatic disorders.

In a diarthrodial joint, the articulating ends of the bones are not connected directly but are indirectly linked by a strong fibrous capsule (*i.e.*, joint capsule) that surrounds the joint and is continuous with the periosteum (Fig. 56-6). This capsule supports the joint and helps to hold the bones in place. Additional support may be provided by ligaments that extend between the bones of the joint.

The joint capsule consists of two layers: an outer fibrous layer and an inner membrane, the synovium. The synovium

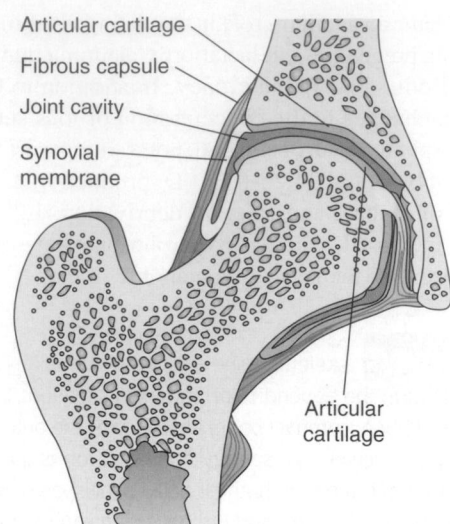

FIGURE 56-6 • Synovial (diarthrodial) joint, showing the articular cartilage, fibrous joint capsule, joint cavity, and synovial membrane.

surrounds the tendons that pass through the joints and the free margins of other intra-articular structures such as ligaments and menisci. The synovium forms folds that surround the margins of articulations but do not cover the weight-bearing articular cartilage. These folds permit stretching of the synovium so that movement can occur without tissue damage.

The synovium secretes a slippery fluid with the consistency of egg white called *synovial fluid*. This fluid acts as a lubricant and facilitates the movement of the articulating surfaces of the joint. Normal synovial fluid is clear or pale yellow, does not clot, and contains fewer than 100 cells/mm^3. The cells are predominantly mononuclear cells derived from the synovium. The composition of the synovial fluid is altered in many inflammatory and pathologic joint disorders. Aspiration and examination of the synovial fluid play an important role in the diagnosis of joint diseases.

The articular cartilage is an example of hyaline cartilage and is unique in that its free surface is not covered with perichondrium. It has only a peripheral rim of perichondrium, and calcification of the portion of cartilage abutting the bone may limit or preclude diffusion from blood vessels supplying the subchondral bone. Articular cartilage is apparently nourished by the diffusion of substances contained in the synovial fluid bathing the cartilage. Regeneration of most cartilage is slow; it is accomplished primarily by growth that requires the activity of perichondrium cells. In articular cartilage, which has no perichondrium, superficial injuries heal slowly.

Blood Supply and Innervation

All the tissues of synovial joints, except the articulating surfaces of the articulating cartilage, receive nourishment either directly or indirectly from blood vessels. The articulating areas are nourished indirectly by the synovial fluid that is distributed over the surface of the articular cartilage.

The blood supply to a joint arises from blood vessels that enter the subchondral bone at or near the attachment of the joint capsule and form an arterial circle around the joint. The synovial membrane has a rich blood supply, and constituents of plasma diffuse rapidly between these vessels and the joint cavity. Because many of the capillaries are near the surface of the synovium, blood may escape into the synovial fluid after relatively minor injuries. Healing and repair of the synovial membrane usually are rapid and complete. This is important because synovial tissue is injured in many surgical procedures that involve the joint.

The nerve supply to joints is provided by the same nerve trunks that supply the muscles that move the joints. These nerve trunks also supply the skin over the joints. As a rule, each joint of an extremity is innervated by all the peripheral nerves that cross the articulation; this accounts for the referral of pain from one joint to another. For example, hip pain may be perceived as pain in the knee.

The synovial membrane is innervated only by autonomic fibers that control blood flow. It is relatively free of pain fibers, as evidenced by the fact that surgical procedures on the joint are often done under local anesthesia. The joint capsule and the ligaments have pain receptors; these receptors are more easily stimulated by stretching and twisting than are other joint structures. Pain arising from the capsule tends to be diffuse and poorly localized.

The tendons and ligaments of the joint capsule are sensitive to position and movement, particularly stretching and twisting. These structures are supplied by the large sensory nerve fibers that form proprioceptor endings (see Chapter 48). The proprioceptors function reflexively to adjust the tension of the muscles that support the joint and are particularly important in maintaining muscular support for the joint. For example, when a weight is lifted, there is a proprioceptor-mediated reflex contraction and relaxation of appropriate muscle groups to support the joint and protect the joint capsule and other joint structures. Loss of proprioception and reflex control of muscular support leads to destructive changes in the joint.

Bursae

In some diarthrotic joints, the synovial membrane forms closed sacs that are not part of the joint. These sacs, called *bursae*, contain synovial fluid. Their purpose is to prevent friction on a tendon. Bursae occur in areas where pressure is exerted because of close approximation of joint structures (Fig. 56-7). Such conditions occur when tendons are deflected over bone or where skin must move freely over bony tissue. Bursae may become injured or inflamed, causing discomfort, swelling, and limitation in movement of the involved area. A bunion is an inflamed bursa of the metatarsophalangeal joint of the great toe.

Intra-articular Menisci

Intra-articular menisci are fibrocartilage structures that develop from portions of the articular disk that occupied the space between articular cartilage surfaces during fetal development. Menisci may extend part way through the joint and have a free inner border, as at the lateral and medial articular surfaces of the knee, or they may extend through the joint, separating it into two separate cavities, as in the sternoclavicular joint. The menisci of the knee joint may be torn as the result of an injury (see Chapter 57).

IN SUMMARY, articulations or joints are areas where two or more bones meet. Tendons and ligaments are dense connective tissue structures that connect muscles and bones. Tendons connect muscles to bones and ligaments connect the movable bones of joints.

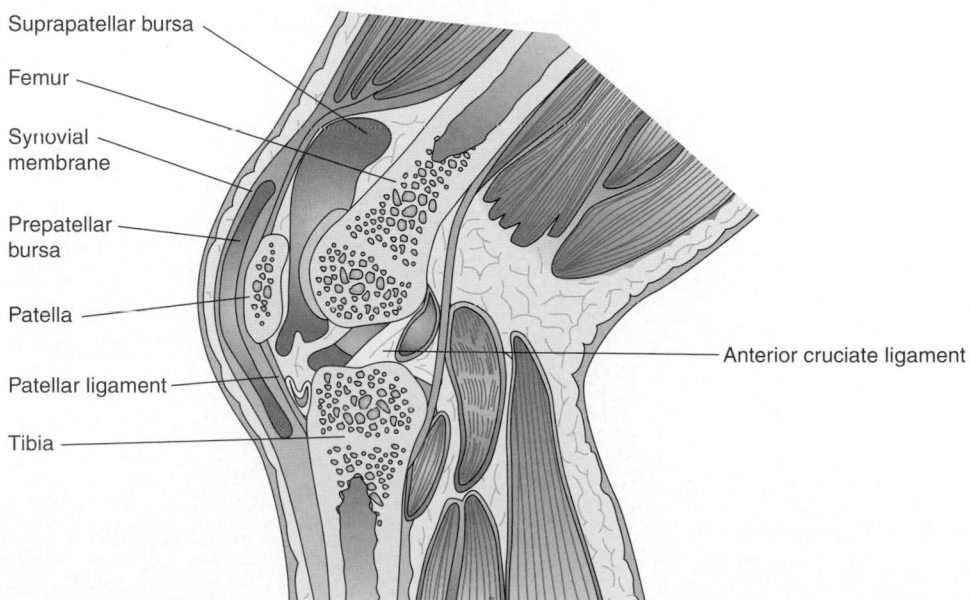

FIGURE 56-7 • Sagittal section of knee joint, showing prepatellar and suprapatellar bursae.

Synarthroses are joints in which bones are joined together by fibrous tissue, cartilage, or bone; they lack a joint cavity and have little or no movement. Synovial or diarthrodial joints are freely movable. The surfaces of the articulating ends of bones in synovial joints are covered with a thin layer of articular cartilage, and they are enclosed in a fibrous joint capsule. The joint capsule consists of two layers: an outer fibrous layer and an inner membrane, the synovium. The synovial fluid, which is secreted by the synovium into the joint capsule, acts as a lubricant and facilitates movement of the joint's articulating surfaces. Bursae, which are closed sacs containing synovial fluid, prevent friction in areas where tendons are deflected over bone or where skin must move freely over bony tissue.

Menisci are fibrocartilaginous structures that develop from portions of the articular disk that occupied the space between articular cartilage surfaces during fetal development. The menisci may have a free inner border, or they may extend through the joint, separating it into two cavities. The menisci in the knee joint may be torn as a result of injury. ■

CONCEPTSin action**ANIMATI⚙N**

Review Exercises

1. Often pain from injury to the knee is experienced as pain in the hip.

   A. *Explain why this might occur.*

2. Persons with end-stage kidney disease have a deficiency of activated vitamin D.

   A. *Explain why this occurs and what effect it would have on their bones.*

3. Recent studies have revealed that estrogen deficiency as well as normal aging may produce a decrease in osteoblast activity.

   A. *Explain how this would contribute to the development of osteoporosis.*

Bibliography

DeLuca H. F. (1988). The vitamin D story: A collaborative effort of basic science and clinical medicine. *FASEB Journal* 2, 236–242.

Guyton A. C., Hall J. E. (2006). *Textbook of medical physiology* (11th ed., pp. 980–989). Philadelphia: Elsevier Saunders.

Hoch B. L., Klein M. J., Schiller A. L. (2008). Bones and joints. In Rubin R., Strayer D. S. (Eds.), *Rubin's pathology: Clinicopathologic foundations of medicine* (5th ed., pp. 1084–1092). Philadelphia: Lippincott Williams & Wilkins.

Moore K. L., Dalley A. F. (2006). *Clinically oriented anatomy* (5th ed., pp. 16–30). Philadelphia: Lippincott Williams & Wilkins.

Rhoades R. A., Tanner G. A. (2003). *Medical physiology* (2nd ed., pp. 634–648). Philadelphia: Lippincott Williams & Wilkins.

Rosenberg A. (2005). Bones, joints, and soft tissue tumors. In Kumar V., Abbas A. K., Fausto N. (Eds.), *Robbins and Cotran pathologic basis of disease* (7th ed., pp. 1273–1288). Philadelphia: Elsevier Saunders.

Ross M. H., Kay G. I., Pawlina W. (2003). *Histology* (4th ed., pp. 180–213). Philadelphia: Lippincott Williams & Wilkins.

Visit the**Point** **http://thePoint.lww.com for animations, journal articles, and more!**

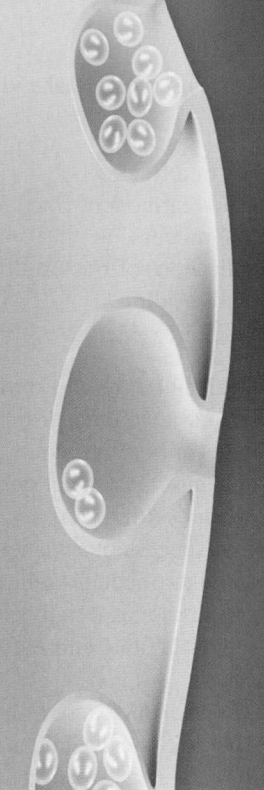

Disorders of Musculoskeletal Function: Trauma, Infection, and Neoplasms

Chapter **57**

KATHLEEN E. GUNTA

> The musculoskeletal system includes the bones, joints, and muscles of the body together with associated structures such as ligaments and tendons. This system, which constitutes more than 70% of the body's mass, is subject to a large number of disorders. These disorders affect persons in all age groups and walks of life, causing pain and disability. The discussion in this chapter focuses on the effects of trauma, infections, ischemia, and neoplasms on the musculoskeletal structures of the body.

INJURY AND TRAUMA OF MUSCULOSKELETAL STRUCTURES

After completing this section of the chapter, you should be able to meet the following objectives:

- Describe the physical agents responsible for soft tissue trauma.
- Differentiate among the three types of soft tissue injuries.
- Compare muscle strains and ligamentous sprains.
- Describe the healing process of soft tissue injuries.
- Differentiate open from closed fractures.

(objectives continue)

- List the signs and symptoms of a fracture.
- Explain the measures used in treatment of fractures.
- Describe the fracture healing process.
- Differentiate the early complications of fractures from later complications of fracture healing.

A broad spectrum of musculoskeletal injuries result from numerous physical forces, including blunt tissue trauma, disruption of tendons and ligaments, and fractures of bony structures. Many of the forces that cause injury to the musculoskeletal system are typical for a particular environmental setting, activity, or age group. Trauma resulting from high-speed motor vehicle accidents is ranked as the number one killer of adults younger than 45 years of age.[1] Motorcycle accidents are especially common in young men, with fractures of the distal tibia, midshaft femur, and radius occurring most often.

Unintentional falls are the number one cause of nonfatal injuries in all age groups in the United States.[1] Childhood falls cause approximately 3 million emergency department visits each year, and bicycle-related injuries, most of them involving the 5- to 14-year-old age group, account for another 50,000 visits.[1] More than 775,000 children younger than 15 years of age are treated each year in hospital emergency departments for sports injuries. About 80% of these injuries occur in football, basketball, baseball, and soccer.[2] Most injuries are strains and sprains. Teenage athletes get injured at about the same rate as professionals. Unfortunately, this is due in part to the increasing level of competition.[3]

Falls are the most common cause of injury in people 65 years of age and older. Current statistics indicate that 30% of persons in this age group experience at least one fall each year.[4] Impaired vision and hearing, dizziness, and unsteadiness of gait contribute to falls in the older person. Among older adults, the majority of fractures are caused by falls.[4] These falls often are compounded by osteoporosis, or bone atrophy, which makes fractures more likely. Fractures of the vertebrae, distal radius, and hip are particularly common in this age group. These injuries reduce mobility and independence and increase the risk for premature death.[5]

Athletic Injuries

Athletic injuries are either acute injuries or overuse injuries. Acute injuries are caused by sudden trauma and include injuries to soft tissues (contusion, strains, and sprains) and to bone (fractures). Overuse injuries have been described as chronic injuries, including stress fractures that result from constant high levels of physiologic stress without sufficient recovery time.[6] They commonly occur in the elbow ("Little League elbow" or "tennis elbow") and in tissue where tendons attach to the bone, such as the heel, knee, and shoulder. Contact sports pose a greater threat for injury to the neck, spine, and growth plates in children and adolescents, who have not yet reached maturity. Injuries can be prevented by proper training, use of

safety equipment, and limiting the level of competition according to skill and size rather than chronologic age. Adequate warm-up time, hydration, and proper nutrition are also key factors in injury prevention.[3]

Soft Tissue Injuries

Most skeletal injuries are accompanied by soft tissue (muscle, tendon, or ligament) injuries. These injuries include contusions, hematomas, and lacerations. They are discussed here because of their association with musculoskeletal injuries.

JOINT INJURIES

- Joints are the weakest part of the skeletal system and common sites for injury due to mechanical overloading or forcible twisting or stretching.
- Injury can include damage to the tendons, which connect muscle to bone; ligaments, which hold bones together; or the cartilage that covers the articular surface.
- Healing of the dense connective tissue involved in joint injuries requires time to restore the structures so that they are strong enough to withstand the forces imposed on the joint. Ligamentous injuries may require surgical intervention with approximation of many fibrous strands to facilitate healing.
- Injuries involving the articular cartilage may predispose to later joint disease.

A *contusion* is an injury to soft tissue that results from direct trauma and is usually caused by striking a body part against a hard object. With a contusion, the skin overlying the injury remains intact. Initially, the area becomes ecchymotic (*i.e.,* black and blue) because of local hemorrhage; later, the discoloration gradually changes to brown and then to yellow as the blood is reabsorbed. A large area of local hemorrhage is called a *hematoma*. Hematomas cause pain as blood accumulates and exerts pressure on nerve endings. The pain increases with movement or when pressure is applied to the area. The pain and swelling of a hematoma take longer to subside than those accompanying a contusion. A hematoma may become infected because of bacterial growth. Unlike a contusion, which does not drain, a hematoma may eventually split the skin because of increased pressures and produce drainage.

Treatment of a contusion and a hematoma consists of elevating the affected part and applying cold for the first 24 hours to reduce the bleeding into the area. A hematoma may need to be aspirated. After the first 24 hours, heat or cold should be applied intermittently for 20 minutes at a time.

A *laceration* is an injury in which the skin is torn or its continuity is disrupted. The seriousness of a laceration depends on the size and depth of the wound and on whether there is contamination from the object that caused the injury. Puncture wounds from nails or rusted material provide the setting for growth of anaerobic bacteria such as those that cause tetanus and gas gangrene.

Lacerations are usually treated by wound closure, which is done after the area is sufficiently cleaned; the closed wound is covered with a sterile dressing. It is important to minimize contamination of the wound and to control bleeding. Contaminated wounds and open fractures are copiously irrigated and debrided, and the skin usually is left open to heal to prevent the development of an anaerobic infection or a sinus tract. Antimicrobial agents are selectively used based on the suspected nature of the contaminants.

Joint (Musculotendinous) Injuries

Joints, or articulations, are sites where two or more bones meet. Joints (*i.e.,* diarthrodial joints) are supported by tough bundles of collagenous fibers called *ligaments* that attach to the joint capsule and bind the articular ends of bones together, and by *tendons* that join muscles to the periosteum of the articulating bones (see Chapter 56). Joint injuries involve mechanical overloading or forcible twisting or stretching.

Strains and Sprains

Strains. A *strain* is a stretching injury to a muscle or a musculotendinous unit caused by mechanical overloading. This type of injury may result from an unusual muscle contraction or an excessive forcible stretch. Although there usually is no external evidence of a specific injury, pain, stiffness, and swelling exist. The most common sites for muscle strains are the lower back and the cervical region of the spine. The elbow and the shoulder are also supported by musculotendinous units that are subject to strains. Foot strain is associated with the weight-bearing stresses of the feet; it may be caused by inadequate muscular and ligamentous support, overweight, or excessive exercise such as standing, walking, or running.

In the lumbar and cervical spine regions, muscle strains are more common than sprains. Mechanical low back pain is becoming increasingly common in the adolescent athlete. Overuse, especially hyperextension of the lumbar spine in such sports as track, wrestling, gymnastics, and diving, can tear the muscles, fascia, and ligaments. Careful diagnosis is necessary because chronic low back pain may indicate a stress fracture. Fractures near the top and bottom surface of the vertebrae can occur when the growing lumbar spine is overstressed, causing the disks to push into the spinal nerve roots. Early detection and treatment are important to prevent complications and disability. Treatment of back strains consists of a short period of rest and mild analgesics followed by a gradual return to activities. Cold should be used during the first 24 hours to reduce pain and swelling of the affected area. Exercises, correct posture, and good body mechanics help to reduce the risk for reinjury.

Sprains. A *sprain*, which involves the ligamentous structures (strong bands of connective tissue) surrounding the joint, resembles a strain, but the pain and swelling subside more slowly. It usually is caused by abnormal or excessive movement of the joint. With a sprain, the ligaments may be incompletely torn or, as in a severe sprain, completely torn or ruptured (Fig. 57-1). Occasionally, a chip of bone is evident when the entire ligament, including part of its bony attachment, has been ruptured or torn from the bone. The signs of sprain are pain, rapid swelling, heat, disability, discoloration, and limitation of function.

Any joint may be sprained, but the ankle joint is most commonly involved, especially in fast-moving injuries in which an ankle or knee can be suddenly twisted. Most ankle sprains occur in the lateral ankle when the foot is turned inward under a person, forcing the ankle into inversion beyond the structural limits. Other common sites of sprain are the knee (the collateral ligament and anterior cruciate ligament) and elbow (the ulnar side). As with a strain, the soft tissue injury that occurs with a sprain is not evident on the radiograph. Wrist sprains most often occur with a fall on an outstretched hand.

Healing. If properly treated, musculotendinous injuries usually heal with the restoration of the original tensile strength. Repair is accomplished by fibroblasts from the inner tendon sheath or, if the tendon has no sheath, from the loose connective tissue that surrounds the tendon. Capillaries infiltrate the

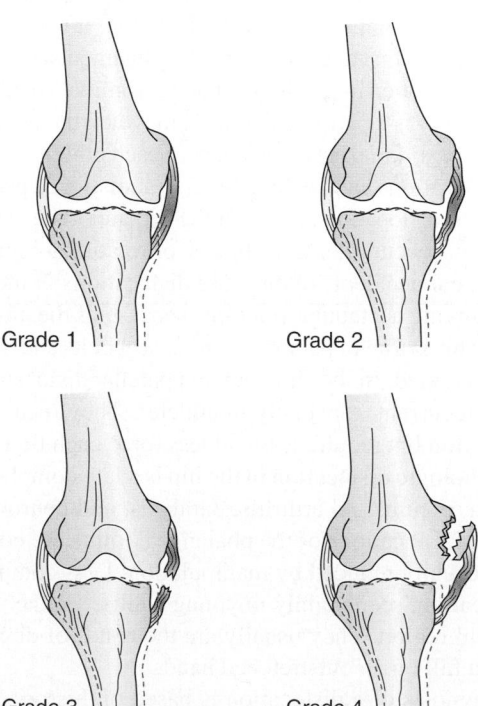

FIGURE 57-1 • Degrees of sprain on the medial side of the right knee: grade 1, mild sprain of the medial collateral ligament; grade 2, moderate sprain with hematoma formation; grade 3, severe sprain with total disruption of the ligament; and grade 4, severe sprain with avulsion of the medial femoral condyle at the insertion of the medial collateral ligament.

injured area during the initial healing process and supply the fibroblasts with the materials they need to produce large amounts of collagen. Formation of the long collagen bundles occurs within the first 2 weeks, and although tensile strength increases steadily thereafter, it is not sufficient to permit strong tendon pulls for 6 to 8 weeks.[7] During the healing process, there is a danger that muscle contraction will pull the injured ends apart, causing the tendon to heal in the lengthened position. There is also a danger that adhesions will develop in areas where tendons pass through fibrous channels, such as in the distal palm of the hands, rendering the tendon useless.

Treatment. The treatment of muscle strains and ligamentous sprains is similar in several ways. For an injured extremity, elevation of the part followed by local application of cold may be sufficient. Compression, accomplished through the use of adhesive wraps or a removable splint, helps reduce swelling and provides support. A cast is applied for severe sprains, especially those severe enough to warrant surgical repair. Immobilization for a muscle strain is continued until the pain and swelling have subsided. In a sprain, the affected joint is immobilized for several weeks. Immobilization may be followed by graded active exercises. Early diagnosis, treatment, and rehabilitation are essential in preventing chronic ligamentous instability.

Dislocations

A *dislocation* involves the displacement or separation of the bone ends of a joint with loss of articulation. It usually follows a severe trauma that disrupts the holding ligaments. Dislocations are seen most often in the shoulder and acromioclavicular joints. A *subluxation* is a partial dislocation in which the bone ends in the joint are still in partial contact with each other.

Dislocations can be congenital, traumatic, or pathologic. Congenital dislocations occur in the hip and knee. Traumatic dislocations occur after falls, blows, or rotational injuries. For example, car accidents often cause dislocations of the hip and accompanying acetabular fractures because of the direction of impact. This is true of persons wearing seat belts and those who are unrestrained. In the shoulder and patella, dislocations may become recurrent, especially in athletes. They recur with the same motion but require less and less force each time.

Pathologic dislocation in the hip is a late complication of infection, rheumatoid arthritis, paralysis, and neuromuscular diseases. Dislocations of the phalangeal joints are not serious and are usually reduced by manipulation. Less common sites of dislocation, seen mainly in young adults, are the wrist and mid-tarsal region. They usually are the result of direct force, such as a fall on an outstretched hand.

Diagnosis of a dislocation is based on history, physical examination, and radiologic findings. The symptoms are pain, deformity, and limited movement. With recurrent dislocations, the person often experiences apprehension during tests of joint rotation, fearing that the joint will slip out of place.

The treatment depends on the site, mechanism of injury, and associated injuries such as fractures. Dislocations that do not reduce spontaneously usually require manipulation or surgical repair. Various surgical procedures also can be used to prevent redislocation of the patella, shoulder, or acromioclavicular joints. Immobilization is necessary for several weeks after reduction of a dislocation to allow healing of the joint structures. In dislocations affecting the knee, alternatives to surgery are isometric quadriceps-strengthening exercises and a temporary brace.

Loose Bodies

Loose bodies are small pieces of bone or cartilage within a joint space. These can result from trauma to the joint or may occur when cartilage has worn away from the articular surface, causing a necrotic piece of bone to separate and become free floating. The symptoms are painful catching and locking of the joint. Loose bodies are commonly seen in the knee, elbow, hip, and ankle. The loose body repeatedly gets caught in the crevice of a joint, pinching the underlying healthy cartilage; unless the loose body is removed, it may cause osteoarthritis and restricted movement. The treatment consists of removal using operative arthroscopy.

Shoulder and Rotator Cuff Injuries

The shoulder is a complex series of joints that produce extraordinary range of motion. The extreme mobility is accomplished at the expense of relative instability. This instability, combined with its relatively exposed position, makes the shoulder extremely vulnerable to injuries such as sprains and dislocations and degenerative processes such as rotator cuff disorders.

The shoulder is composed of three bones: the scapula, the clavicle, and the humerus. The scapula is a thin bone that articulates widely and closely with the chest wall.[8] It also articulates with the humerus by way of the glenoid cavity and with the clavicle at the acromion process. Clavicle fractures are among the most common fractures of childhood.[9] The typical mechanism of fracture is a fall on the point of the shoulder.

Three articulations form the shoulder joint—the acromioclavicular joint that joins the clavicle to the acromion of the scapula, the sternoclavicular joint that joins the sternum to the clavicle, and the glenohumeral joint that connects the head of the humerus to the relatively shallow glenoid cavity in the scapula. The stability of these joints is provided by a series of muscles and tendons. Sprains of the acromioclavicular joint usually occur as a result of a blow to the top of the shoulder but are known to occur with a fall to the lateral or posterior aspects of the shoulder.[9] The most common site of shoulder dislocation is the glenohumeral joint.[9,10] Most acute dislocations involve anterior displacement of the humeral head with respect to the glenoid cavity, the result of the shoulder being abducted and forcefully extended and rotated. Other mechanisms include a fall on an outstretched arm or a blow to the posterior shoulder.

Motion of the arm involves the coordinated movement of muscles of the rotator cuff (supraspinous, teres minor, infraspinatus, subscapularis) and their musculotendinous attachments. These muscles are separated from the overlying cora-coacromial arch by two bursae, the subdeltoid and subcoracoid. These two bursae, sometimes referred to as the *subacromial bursae*, often communicate and are affected by lesions of the rotator cuff.

The rotator cuff is not unlike other muscle groups of the body in that its risk for injury increases when it is required to perform a high-stress function in an unconditioned state. Rotator cuff injuries and impingement disorders can result from a number of causes, including excessive use, a direct blow, or stretch injury, usually involving throwing or swinging, as with baseball pitchers or tennis players. Complete tears or rupture of the rotator cuff usually occur in young persons after severe trauma (Fig. 57-2).

Overuse and degenerative disorders have a slower onset and are seen in older persons with minor or no trauma. The tendons of the rotator cuff fuse together near their insertions into the tuberosities of the humerus to form the musculotendinous cuff. Degeneration of these tendons can result from a number of factors, including repetitive microtrauma, impairment of vascularity as a result of aging, or shoulder instability with secondary overload of the cuff. Degeneration is most severe near the tendon insertion, with the supraspinous being affected most often. Chronic irritation of the musculotendinous unit can lead to tendinitis with scarring and thickening of the tendon and secondary inflammation of the overlying bursae.[8] Thickening of these tissues decreases the distance between the cuff and the overlying coracoacromial arch. Pain and impingement may be noted when motions of the arm squeeze and pinch these tissues between the humerus and the overlying arch. Severe tendinitis also can cause either a partial or complete rotator cuff tear.

Several physical examination maneuvers are used to define shoulder pathologic processes.[11] The history and mechanism of injury are important. In addition to standard radiographs, arthrography, computed tomography (CT), or magnetic resonance imaging (MRI) may be used. Arthroscopic examination under anesthesia may be used for diagnostic purposes and operative arthroscopy may be done to repair severe tears. Conservative treatment with anti-inflammatory agents, corticosteroid injections, and physical therapy often is undertaken. A period of rest is followed by a customized exercise and rehabilitation program to improve strength, flexibility, and endurance.

Knee Injuries

The knee is a common site of injury, particularly sport-related injuries in which the knee is subjected to abnormal twisting and compression forces. These forces can result in injury to the menisci, patellar subluxation and dislocation, and chondromalacia. Knee injuries in young adulthood and both knee and hip injuries in middle age substantially increase the risk for osteoarthritis in the same joint later in life.

Meniscus Injuries. The menisci are C-shaped plates of fibrocartilage that are superimposed between the condyles of the femur and tibia. There are two menisci in each knee, a lateral and medial meniscus (Fig. 57-3). The menisci are thicker at their external margins and taper to thin, unattached edges at their interior margin. They are firmly attached at their ends to the intercondylar area of the tibia and are supported by the coronary and transverse ligaments of the knee. The menisci play a major role in load bearing and shock absorption. They also help to stabilize the knee by deepening the tibial socket and maintaining the femur and tibia in proper position. In addition, the meniscus

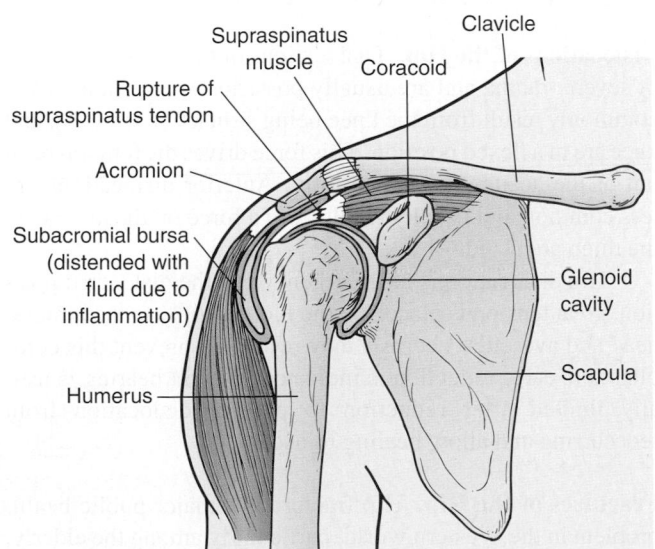

FIGURE 57-2 • Structures of the glenohumeral shoulder joint, showing the location of common rotator cuff injuries. The supraspinatus muscle is the most commonly injured part of the rotator cuff. (Adapted from Moore K. L., Dalley A. F. *Clinically oriented anatomy* [4th ed., p. 698]. Philadelphia: Lippincott Williams & Wilkins.)

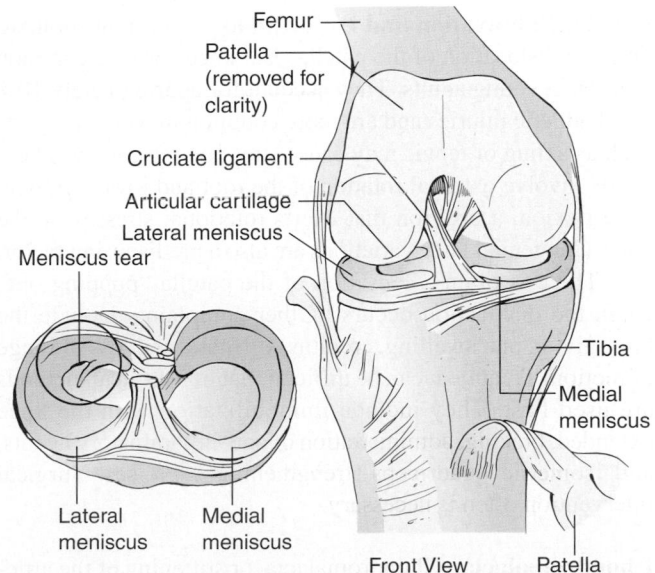

FIGURE 57-3 • The knee, showing the lateral and medial meniscus (with the patella removed for clarity). *Inset (lower left)* shows meniscus tear.

assists in joint lubrication and serves as source of nutrition for articular cartilage in the knee.

Meniscus injury commonly occurs as the result of a rotational injury from a sudden or sharp pivot or a direct blow to the knee, as in hockey, basketball, or football. It is often associated with other injuries, such as a torn anterior cruciate ligament (ACL).[12] The type and location of the meniscal tear are determined by the magnitude and direction of the force that acts on the knee and the position of the knee at the time of injury. Meniscus tears can be described by their appearance (*e.g.,* parrot-beak, bucket handle) or their location (*e.g.,* posterior horn, anterior horn). The injured knee is edematous and painful, especially with hyperflexion and hyperextension. A loose fragment may cause knee instability and locking.

Diagnosis is made by examination and confirmed by MRI. A regular radiograph may be needed to rule out osteoarthritis.[12] Initial treatment of meniscal injuries may be conservative. The knee may be placed in a removable knee immobilizer. Isometric quadriceps exercises may be prescribed. Activity usually is restricted until complete motion is recovered. Arthroscopic meniscectomy may be performed when there is recurrent or persistent locking, recurrent effusion, or disabling pain.

There is evidence that loss of meniscal function is associated with progressive deterioration of knee function.[13] Damaged articular cartilage has a limited capacity to heal because of its avascular nature and inadequate mobilization of regenerative cells. Meniscal reconstruction procedures have been developed to preserve these functions before significant degenerative changes develop, thus preventing a total joint replacement later in life. Among the reconstruction methods used is replacement of the damaged meniscus with a meniscal transplant (fresh, frozen, or cryopreserved allografts).[13,14] Use of a synthetic collagen scaffold that allows fibrochondrocyte ingrowth is being investigated.[13]

Patellar Subluxation and Dislocations. Recurrent subluxation and dislocation of the patella (*i.e.,* knee cap) are common injuries in young adults. They account for approximately 10% of all athletic injuries and are more common in women. Sports such as skiing or tennis may cause stress on the patella. These sports involve external rotation of the foot and lower leg with knee flexion, a position that exerts rotational stresses on the knee. Congenital knee variations are also a predisposing factor.

There is often a sensation of the patella "popping out" when the dislocation occurs.[8] Other complaints include the knee giving out, swelling, crepitus, stiffness, and loss of range of motion. Treatment can be difficult, but nonsurgical methods are used first. They include immobilization with the knee extended, bracing, administration of anti-inflammatory agents, and isometric quadriceps-strengthening exercises. Surgical intervention often is necessary.

Chondromalacia. Chondromalacia, or softening of the articular cartilage, is seen most commonly on the undersurface of the patella and occurs most frequently in young adults.[8] It can be the result of recurrent subluxation of the patella or overuse in strenuous athletic activities. Persons with this disorder typically complain of pain, particularly when climbing stairs or sitting with the knees bent. Occasionally, the person experiences weakness of the knee.

Treatment consists of rest, isometric exercises, and application of ice after exercise. Part of the patella may be surgically removed in severe cases. In less severe cases, the soft portion is shaved using a saw inserted through an arthroscope. Articular cartilage maintenance and repair is a complex process, currently under investigation. Polypeptide growth factors that direct cells to divide, differentiate, migrate, and produce matrix appear to have a role in the preservation and degradation of the articular cartilage matrix. Growth factors such as insulin-like growth factor (IGF), bone morphogenic proteins (BMP), and transforming growth factor-β (TGF-β) have been shown to affect chondrocyte growth and metabolism.[15]

Hip Injuries

The hip is a ball-and-socket joint in which the femoral head articulates deeply in the acetabulum.[4] The proximal part of the femur consists of a head, neck, and greater trochanter. The vascular anatomy of the femoral head is of critical importance in any disorder of the hip. The main sources of blood supply are the intramedullary vessels and the retinacular arteries arising from the circumflex femoral arteries, both of which course from the intertrochanteric region proximally to nourish the femoral head (Fig. 57-4). Disease or injuries that compromise the circulation may damage the viability of the femoral head and lead to avascular necrosis or osteonecrosis (to be discussed). Disorders of the hip include dislocations and fractures of the hip. Congenital dysplasia of the hip, Legg-Calvé-Perthes disease, and slipped capital femoral epiphysis are discussed in Chapter 58.

Dislocations of the Hip. Dislocations of the hip are the result of severe trauma and are usually posterior in direction.[8] They commonly result from the knee being struck while the hip and knee are in a flexed position. This force drives the femoral head out of the acetabulum posteriorly. Anterior dislocations are less common and usually result from a force on the knee with the thigh abducted.

Hip dislocation is an emergency.[8] In the dislocated position, great tension is placed on the blood supply to the femoral head and avascular necrosis may result. To prevent this complication, early reduction is indicated. Weight bearing is usually limited after reduction to prevent dislocation from reoccurring and allow healing to occur.

Fractures of the Hip. Hip fracture is a major public health problem in the Western world, particularly among the elderly. It results in hospitalization, disability, and loss of independence. The incidence of hip fractures increases with age, doubling for each decade after 50 years of age, and is two to three times higher in women than men.[16,17] The incidence is also higher in white women compared with nonwhite women. Risk factors for hip fracture include excessive consumption of

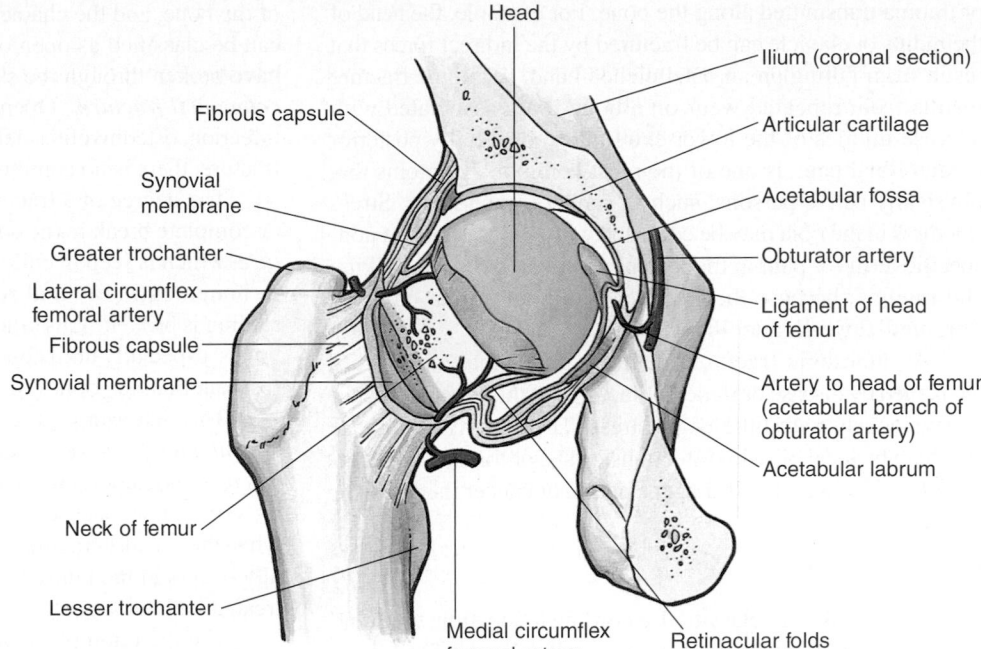

FIGURE 57-4 • Blood supply of the head and neck of the femur (anterior view). A section of the bone has been removed from the femoral neck. (Modified from Moore K., Agur A. M. R. [2002]. *Essential clinical anatomy* [2nd ed., p. 381]. Philadelphia: Lippincott Williams & Wilkins.)

Labels in figure: Head; Ilium (coronal section); Articular cartilage; Acetabular fossa; Obturator artery; Ligament of head of femur; Artery to head of femur (acetabular branch of obturator artery); Acetabular labrum; Retinacular folds; Medial circumflex femoral artery; Lesser trochanter; Neck of femur; Synovial membrane; Fibrous capsule; Lateral circumflex femoral artery; Greater trochanter; Synovial membrane; Fibrous capsule

alcohol and caffeine, physical inactivity, low body weight, tall stature, use of certain psychotropic drugs, residence in an institution, visual impairment, and dementia.[17] Osteoporosis is an important contributing factor.

Most hip fractures result from falls. Occasionally, the person may actually fracture the hip before falling, the fracture being caused by twisting or excessive force on a femur that has been weakened by osteoporosis or neoplasms. The characteristics of the fall (the direction, site of impact, and protective response) and environmental factors are important factors influencing the risk of hip fracture from a fall.

A hip fracture is generally a fracture of the proximal femur. Such fractures are commonly categorized according to the anatomic site in which they occur.[16,17] Femoral neck fractures are located in the area distal to the femoral head but proximal to the greater and lesser trochanters and are considered intracapsular because they are located within the capsule of the hip joint. Intertrochanteric fractures occur in the metaphyseal region between the greater and lesser trochanter. Subtrochanteric fractures are those that occur just below the greater trochanter. Femoral neck and intertrochanteric fractures account for over 90% of hip fractures, occurring in approximately equal proportions.[17]

The location of a hip fracture is important in terms of blood flow to the femoral head, which receives its blood supply from vessels that course proximally up the femoral neck (see Fig. 57-4). Subtrochanteric and intertrochanteric fractures that occur distal to these vessels do not usually disturb the blood supply to the femoral head, whereas femoral neck fractures, particularly those involving marked displacement, often disrupt the blood supply to the femoral head and are therefore associated with increased incidence of complications (nonunion and avascular necrosis).

Most hip fractures are diagnosed based on clinical findings and standard radiographs. A bone scan or MRI may be done when the radiograph is negative but the clinical findings support the diagnosis of hip fracture.

The primary goal of treatment is a return to preinjury level of function as soon as possible.[8] Undisplaced or impacted fractures have a better prognosis in terms of healing and are often treated nonoperatively or by simple internal fixation to provide stability. Displaced intracapsular fractures in the elderly are usually best treated by surgical hip replacement and early mobilization. Young, healthy people are treated by reduction of the fracture (if needed) and internal fixation. This method allows for preservation of the femoral head, which in this age group is desirable because the long-term results are better than with prosthetic replacement.[17] Intertrochanteric fractures are usually treated with open reduction and internal fixation. This allows for early ambulation by eliminating pain at the fracture site.[17] Nonunion in this type of fracture is much less common than with intracapsular fractures. Weight bearing, however, is usually restricted for 3 months until union of the fracture has occurred.

Fractures

Fracture, or discontinuity of the bone, is the most common type of bone lesion. Normal bone can withstand considerable compression and shearing forces and, to a lesser extent, tension forces. A fracture occurs when more stress is placed on the bone than it is able to absorb. Grouped according to cause, fractures can be divided into three major categories: fractures caused by sudden injury, fatigue or stress fractures, and pathologic fractures. The most common fractures are those resulting from sudden injury. The force causing the fracture may be direct, such as a fall or blow, or indirect, such as a massive muscle contraction or trauma transmitted along the bone. For example, the head of the radius or clavicle can be fractured by the indirect forces that result from falling on an outstretched hand. A fatigue fracture results from repeated wear on a bone. Pain associated with overuse injuries of the lower extremities, especially posterior medial tibial pain, is one of the most common symptoms that physically active persons, such as runners, experience. Stress fractures in the tibia may be confused with "shin splints," a nonspecific term for pain in the lower leg from overuse in walking and running, because they frequently do not appear on x-ray films until 2 weeks after the onset of symptoms.

A pathologic fracture occurs in bones that already are weakened by disease or tumors. Fractures of this type may occur spontaneously with little or no stress. The underlying disease state can be local, as with infections, cysts, or tumors, or generalized, as in osteoporosis, Paget disease, or cancer metastasis.

Classification

Fractures usually are classified according to location, type, and direction or pattern of the fracture line[8] (Fig. 57-5). A long bone is divided into three parts: proximal, midshaft, and distal. A fracture of the long bone is described in relation to its position in the bone. Other descriptions are used when the fracture affects the head or neck of a bone, involves a joint, or is near a prominence such as a condyle or malleolus.

The type of fracture is determined by its communication with the external environment, the degree of break in continuity

of the bone, and the character of the fracture pieces. A fracture can be classified as open or closed. When the bone fragments have broken through the skin, the fracture is called an *open* or *compound fracture.*[8] Open fractures often are complicated by infection, osteomyelitis, delayed union, or nonunion. In a closed fracture, there is no communication with the outside skin.

The degree of a fracture is described in terms of a partial or complete break in the continuity of bone. A *greenstick fracture,* which is seen in children, is an example of a partial break in bone continuity and resembles that seen when a young sapling is broken. This kind of break occurs because children's bones, especially until approximately 10 years of age, are more resilient than the bones of adults.

The character of a fracture is determined by its pieces. A *comminuted fracture* has more than two pieces. A *compression fracture,* as occurs in the vertebral body, involves two bones that are crushed or squeezed together. A fracture is called *impacted* when the fracture fragments are wedged together. This type usually occurs in the humerus, often is less serious, and usually is treated without surgery.

The direction of the trauma or mechanism of injury produces a certain configuration or pattern of fracture. The pattern of a fracture indicates the nature of the trauma and provides information about the easiest method for reduction. *Reduction* is the restoration of a fractured bone to its normal anatomic position. *Transverse fractures* are caused by simple angular forces. A *spiral fracture* results from a twisting motion, or torque. A transverse fracture is not likely to become displaced or lose its position after it is reduced. On the other hand, spiral, oblique, and comminuted fractures often are unstable and may change position after reduction.

Manifestations

The signs and symptoms of a fracture include pain, tenderness at the site of bone disruption, swelling, loss of function, deformity of the affected part, and abnormal mobility. The deformity varies according to the type of force applied, the area of the bone involved, the type of fracture produced, and the strength and balance of the surrounding muscles.

In long bones, three types of deformities—angulation, shortening, and rotation—are seen. Severely angulated fracture fragments may be felt at the fracture site and often push up against the soft tissue to cause a tenting effect on the skin. Bending forces and unequal muscle pulls cause angulation. Shortening of the extremity occurs as the bone fragments slide and override each other because of the pull of the muscles on the long axis of the extremity (Fig. 57-6).

Rotational deformity occurs when the fracture fragments rotate out of their normal longitudinal axis; this can result from rotational strain produced by the fracture or unequal pull by the muscles that are attached to the fracture fragments. A crepitus or grating may be felt as the bone fragments rub against each other. In the case of an open fracture, there is bleeding from the wound where the bone protrudes. Blood loss from a pelvic fracture or multiple long bone fractures can cause hypovolemic shock in a trauma victim.

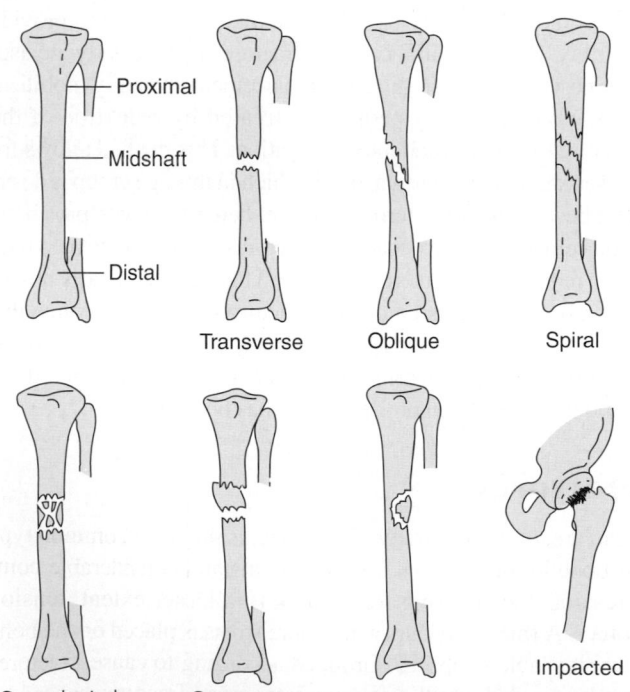

Proximal — Midshaft — Distal

Transverse   Oblique   Spiral

Comminuted   Segmental   Butterfly   Impacted

FIGURE 57-5 • Classification of fractures. Fractures are classified according to location (proximal, midshaft, or distal), the direction of fracture line (transverse, oblique, spiral), and type (comminuted, segmental, butterfly, or impacted).

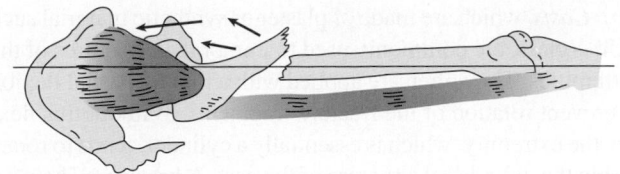

FIGURE 57-6 • Displacement and overriding of fracture fragments of a long bone (femur) caused by severe muscle spasm.

Shortly after the fracture has occurred, nerve function at the fracture site may be temporarily lost. The area may become numb, and the surrounding muscles may become flaccid. This condition has been called *local shock*. During this period, which may last for a few minutes to half an hour, fractured bones may be reduced with little or no pain. After this brief period, the pain returns and, with it, muscle spasms and contractions occur in the surrounding muscles.

The early complications of fractures are associated with loss of skeletal continuity, injury from bone fragments, pressure from swelling and hemorrhage, involvement of nerve fibers, or development of fat emboli. The extent of early complications depends on the severity of the fracture and the area of the body that is involved. For example, bone fragments from a skull fracture may cause injury to brain tissue, or multiple rib fractures may lead to a flail chest and respiratory insufficiency. With flail chest, the chest wall on the fractured side becomes so unstable that it may move in the opposite direction as the person breathes (*i.e.*, in during inspiration and out during expiration).

Diagnosis

Diagnosis is the first step in the care of fractures and is based on history and physical manifestations. X-ray examination is used to confirm the diagnosis and direct the treatment. The ease of diagnosis varies with the location and severity of the fracture. In the trauma patient, the presence of other, more serious injuries may make diagnosis more difficult. A thorough history includes the mechanism, time, and place of the injury; first recognition of symptoms; and any treatment initiated. A complete history is important because a delay in seeking treatment or a period of weight bearing on a fracture may cause further injury or displacement of the fracture. When a fracture is suspected, the injured part always should be splinted before it is moved.[8] This is essential for preventing further injury.

Determination of the severity of injury to soft tissue is an important component of assessment and management of closed fractures. The response of the soft tissue to blunt injury involves microvascular and inflammatory responses that produce localized tissue hypoxia and acidosis.[18] Incisions placed through such compromised tissue can lead to wound breakdown and infections. Therefore, recognizing the signs of soft tissue injury is the foundation for successful management of closed fractures. The classification of Oestern and Tscherne can be used to characterize the severity of closed fractures[18,19] (Table 57-1). This system remains the only published classification system for the soft tissue injury associated with closed fractures. Fractures are assigned one of four grades, from 0 to 3. The presence of deep skin abrasions, muscle contusion, fracture blisters, and massive soft tissue swelling suggests the need to use external fixation methods to limit further soft tissue injury and facilitate rapid recovery before surgical intervention.

Treatment

There are three objectives for treatment of fractures: reduction of the fracture, immobilization, and preservation and restoration of the function of the injured part.

Reduction and Internal Fixation. Reduction is directed at alignment of the bones in the angular and rotational planes, restoration of proper length, and restoration of apposition of the bone ends.[8] This can be accomplished by closed manipulation or surgical (open) reduction. Closed manipulation uses methods such as manual pressure and traction. Fractures are held in reduction by external or internal fixation devices. The benefits of internal fixation must be balanced against its associated risks. The advantages are precise restoration of the osseous anatomy and

TABLE 57-1 **Oestern and Tscherne Classification of Closed Fractures**		
GRADE	**SOFT TISSUE INJURY**	**BONY INJURY**
Grade 0	Minimal soft tissue damage Indirect injury to limb	Simple fracture pattern
Grade 1	Superficial abrasion/contusion	Mild fracture pattern
Grade 2	Deep abrasion with skin or muscle contusion Direct trauma to limb	Severe fracture pattern
Grade 3	Extensive skin contusion or crush Severe damage to underlying muscle Subcutaneous avulsion Compartmental syndrome may be present	Severe fracture pattern

From Bucholz R. W., Heckman J. D. (2006). *Rockwood & Green's fractures in adults* (6th ed., Vol. 1, p. 49). Philadelphia: Lippincott Williams & Wilkins.

early mobilization with at least partial weight bearing. The principal disadvantages are the increased risk of infection and the fact that healing may be impaired if a technique is not used properly. Patients are usually more comfortable after internal fixation than with a cast or external fixation device.[20] Surgical reduction involves the use of various types of hardware to accomplish internal fixation of the fracture fragments (Fig. 57-7).

Immobilization and External Fixation. Immobilization prevents movement of the injured parts and is the single most important element in obtaining union of the fracture fragments. Immobilization can be accomplished through the use of external devices, such as splints, casts, traction, or external fixation devices; or by internal fixation devices inserted during surgical reduction of the fracture.

Splints are made from many different materials. Metal splints or air splints may be used during transport to a health care facility as a temporary measure until the fracture has been reduced and another form of immobilization instituted. Plaster of Paris splints, which are molded to fit the extremity, work well. Splinting should be done if there is any suspicion of a fracture because motion of the fracture site can cause pain, bleeding, more soft tissue damage, and nerve or blood vessel compression. If the fracture has sharp fragments, movement can cause perforation of the skin and conversion of a closed fracture into an open one. When a splint is applied to an extremity, it should extend from the joint above the fracture site to the joint below it.

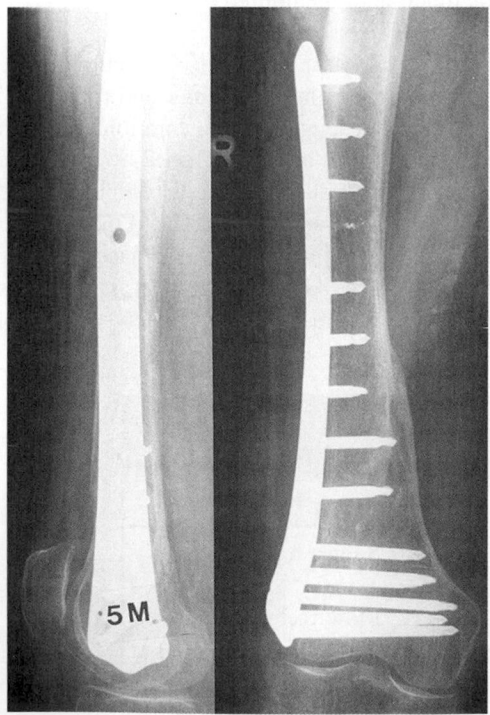

FIGURE 57-7 • Use of a locked screw plate to stabilize a supracondylar femoral fracture in an 89-year-old osteoporotic woman. The patient started immediate weight bearing. Fracture healing in good alignment was seen 5 months after the operation. (From Bucholz R. W., Heckman J. D. [2006]. *Rockwood & Green's fractures in adults* (6th ed., Vol. 1, p. 239). Philadelphia: Lippincott Williams & Wilkins.)

Casts, which are made of plaster or synthetic material such as fiberglass, are commonly used to immobilize fractures of the extremities. They often are applied with a joint in partial flexion to prevent rotation of the fracture fragments. Without this flexion, the extremity, which is essentially a cylinder, tends to rotate within the cylindrical structure of the cast. A brace may be used after a cast is removed or instead of a cast, as with a tibial stress fracture. The application of a cast carries the risk for impaired circulation to the extremity because of blood vessel compression. A cast applied shortly after a fracture may not be large enough to accommodate the swelling that inevitably occurs in the hours that follow. After a cast is applied, the peripheral circulation must be observed carefully until this danger has passed. If the circulation becomes inadequate, the parts that are exposed at the distal end of the cast (*i.e.,* the toes with a leg cast and the fingers with an arm cast) usually become cold and cyanotic or pale. An increase in pain may occur initially, followed by paresthesia (*i.e.,* tingling or abnormal sensation) or anesthesia as the sensory neurons that supply the area are affected. There is a decrease in the amplitude or absence of the pulse in areas where the arteries can be palpated. Capillary refill time, which is assessed by applying pressure to the fingernail and observing the rate of blood return, is prolonged to longer than 3 seconds. Signs of impaired circulation demand immediate measures, such as splitting the cast, to restore the circulation and prevent permanent damage to the extremity. A casted extremity should be elevated above the level of the heart for the first 24 hours to minimize swelling.

Traction is another method for achieving immobility, maintaining alignment of the bone ends, and maintaining the reduction, particularly if the fracture is unstable or comminuted. Traction is a pulling force applied to an extremity or part of the body while a counterforce, or countertraction, pulls in the opposite direction. The five goals of traction therapy are to correct and maintain the skeletal alignment of entire bones or joints; reduce pressure on a joint surface; correct, lessen, or prevent deformities such as contractures and dislocations; decrease muscle spasm; and immobilize the fracture site to promote healing. Traction may be used as a temporary measure before surgery or as a primary treatment method. There are three types of traction: manual traction, skin traction, and skeletal traction. *Manual traction* consists of a steady, firm pull that is exerted by the hands. It is a temporary measure used to manipulate a fracture during closed reduction, for support of a neck injury during transport when a cervical spine fracture is suspected, or for reduction of a dislocated joint. *Skin traction* is a pulling force applied to the skin and soft tissue. It is accomplished by strips of adhesive flannel or foam secured to the injured part. *Skeletal traction* is a pulling force applied directly to the bone. Pins, wires, or tongs are inserted through the skin and subcutaneous tissue into the bone distal to the fracture site. Skeletal traction provides an excellent pull and can be used for long periods with large amounts of weight. It is commonly used for fractures of the femur, the humerus, and the cervical spine (*e.g.,* Crutchfield tongs applied to the skull).

With *external fixation devices,* pins or screws are inserted directly into the bone above and below the fracture site. They are secured to a metal frame and adjusted to align the fracture.

This method of treatment is used primarily for open fractures, infections such as osteomyelitis and septic joints, unstable closed fractures, and limb lengthening.

Limb-Lengthening Systems. Limb-lengthening systems, such as the Ilizarov external fixator (Fig. 57-8), are used to lengthen or widen bones, correct angular or rotational defects, or immobilize fractures.[21] The apparatus is applied with a surgical technique called a *corticotomy,* which is a percutaneous osteotomy that preserves the periosteal and endosteal tissues. A circular external apparatus is attached to bone by tensioned Kirschner wires. The corticotomy site is gradually distracted or pulled apart by approximately 1 mm/day until the desired length is achieved. The continuous distraction activates regeneration of bone, soft tissue, nerves, and blood vessels. New bone forms in the distraction gap. This newly formed bone can fill post-traumatic defects or those formed after resection for osteomyelitis, consolidate nonunions, regenerate bone in limb lengthening, correct deformities, and eliminate the need for bone grafting. The apparatus is left on until the desired length is achieved and consolidation is complete.

Preservation and Restoration of Function. During the period of immobilization required for fracture healing, muscles tend to atrophy because of lack of use. Joints stiffen as muscles and tendons contract and shorten. The degree of muscle atrophy and joint stiffness depends on several factors. In adults, the degree of atrophy and muscle stiffness is directly related to the length of immobilization, with longer periods of immobility resulting in

greater stiffness. Children have a natural tendency to move on their own, and this movement maintains muscle and joint function. They usually have less atrophy and recover sooner after the source of immobilization has been removed. Associated soft tissue injury, infection, and preexisting joint disease increase the risk for stiffness. Although limbs are immobilized in a functional position, casts are removed as soon as fracture healing has taken place so that joint stiffness does not occur.

Exercises designed to preserve function, maintain muscle strength, and reduce joint stiffness in the unaffected and affected extremities should be started early. Active range of motion, in which the person moves the extremity, is done on unaffected extremities, and isometric, or muscle-tensing, exercises are done on the affected extremities. In some instances, an electrical muscle stimulator is applied directly to the skin to stimulate isometric muscle contraction as a means of preventing disuse atrophy. After the fracture has healed, a program of physical therapy may be necessary. However, the most important factor in restoring function is the person's own active exercises.

Bone Healing

Bone healing occurs in a manner similar to soft tissue healing. It is, however, a more complex process and takes longer. Although the exact mechanisms of bone healing are open to controversy, five stages of the healing process have been identified: hematoma formation, cellular proliferation, callus formation, ossification, and remodeling.[22,23,24] The degree of response during each of these stages is in direct proportion to the extent of trauma.

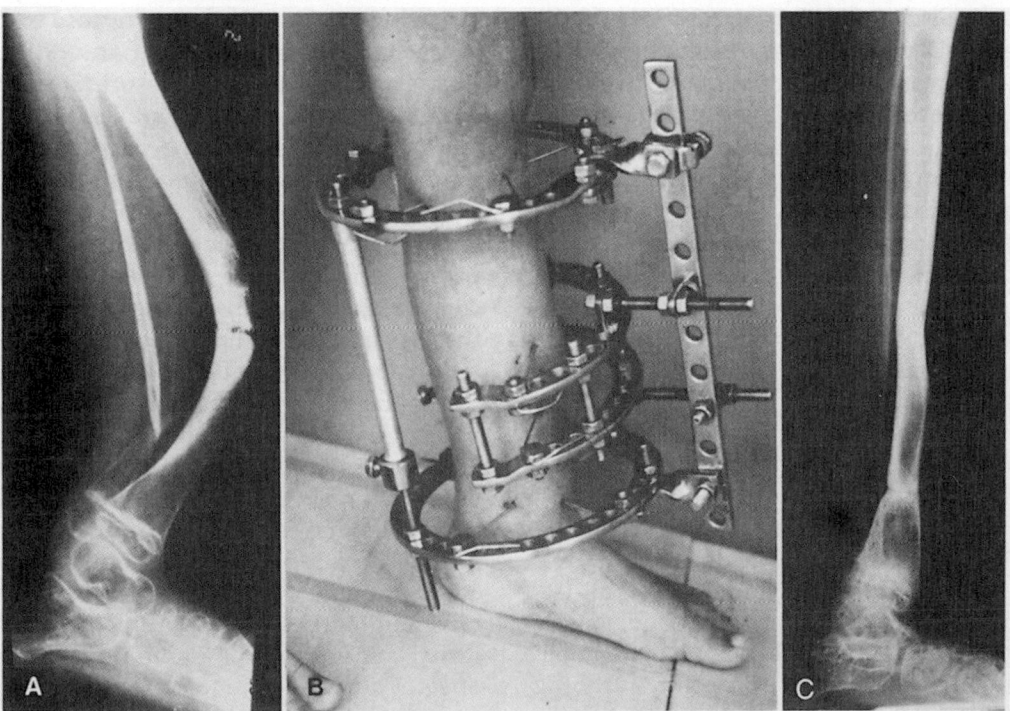

FIGURE 57-8 • Ilizarov device used to treat a tibial fracture with anterolateral bow and medullary sclerosis: before (**A**), with Ilizarov device in place (**B**), and 3-year follow-up lateral roentgenograph (**C**). (From Paley D., Catagni M., Argnani F., et al. [1992]. Treatment of congenital pseudoarthrosis of the tibia using Ilizarov technique. *Clinical Orthopaedics and Related Research, 280,* 84.)

Understanding • Fracture Healing

A fracture, which is any break in a bone, undergoes a healing process to reestablish bone continuity and strength. The repair of simple fractures is commonly divided into four phases: (1) hematoma formation, (2) fibrocartilaginous callus formation, (3) bony callus formation, and (4) remodeling.

❶ Hematoma Formation

When a bone breaks, blood vessels in the bone and surrounding tissues are torn and bleed into and around the fragments of the fractured bone, forming a blood clot, or hematoma. The hematoma facilitates the formation of the fibrin meshwork that seals off the fracture site and serves as a framework for the influx of inflammatory cells, the ingrowth of fibroblasts, and the development of new capillary buds (vessels). It is also the source of signaling molecules that initiate the cellular events that are critical to the healing process.

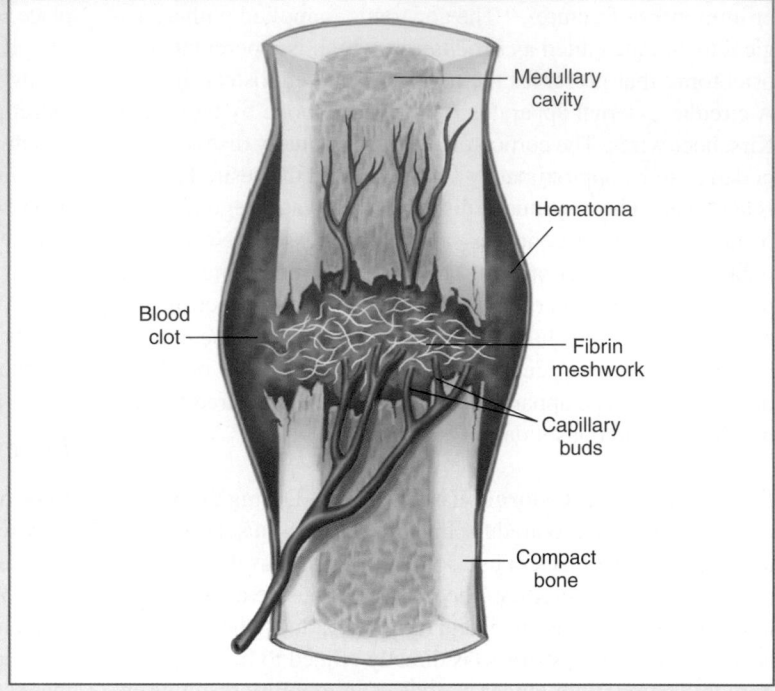

❷ Fibrocartilaginous Callus Formation

As new capillaries infiltrate the hematoma at the fracture site, it becomes organized into a form of granulation tissue, called *procallus*. Fibroblasts from the periosteum, endosteum, and red bone marrow proliferate and invade the procallus. The fibroblasts produce a fibrocartilaginous soft callus bridge that connects the bone fragments. Although this repair tissue usually reaches its maximum girth at the end of the second or third week, it is not strong enough for weight bearing.

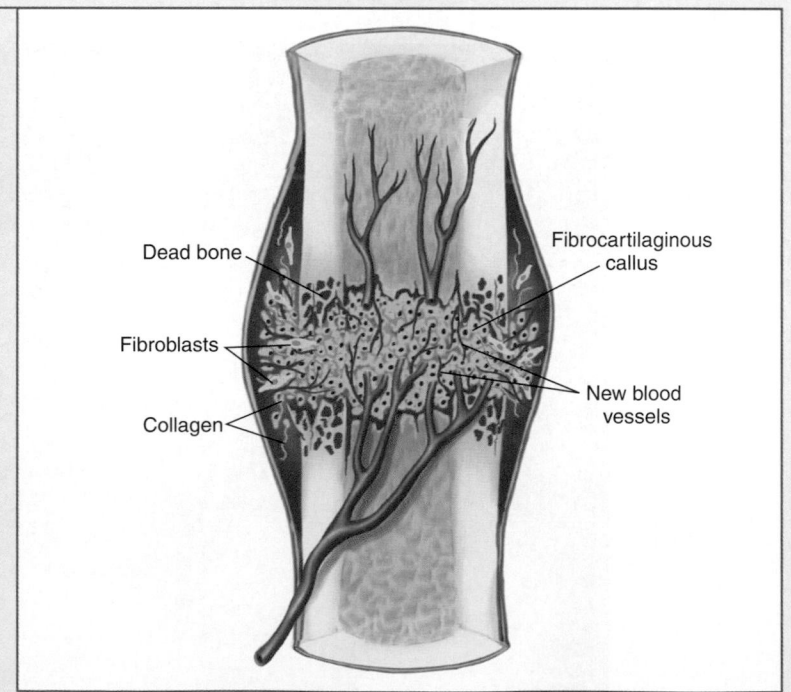

❸ Bony Callus Formation

Ossification represents the conversion of the fibro-cartilaginous cartilage to bony callus. In areas close to well-vascularized bone tissue, osteogenic cells develop into osteoblasts, or bone-building cells, which produce spongy bone trabeculae. The newly formed osteoblasts first deposit bone on the outer surface of the bone some distance from the fracture site. The formation of bone progresses toward the fracture site until a new bony sheath covers the fibrocartilaginous callus. In time, the fibrocartilage is converted to spongy bone, and the callus is then referred to as bony callus. Gradually, the bony callus calcifies and is replaced by mature bone. Bony callus formation begins 3 to 4 weeks after injury and continues until a firm bony union is formed months later.

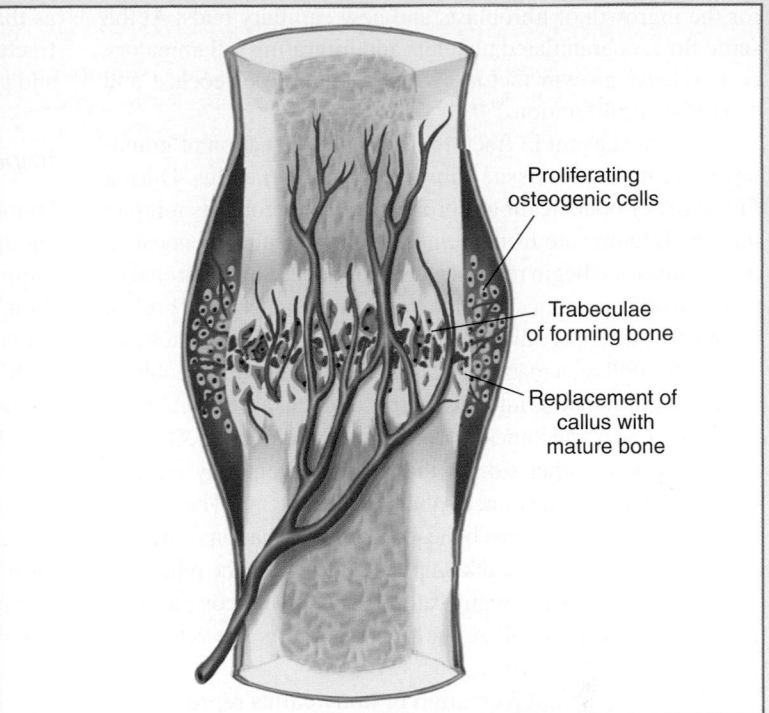

Proliferating osteogenic cells

Trabeculae of forming bone

Replacement of callus with mature bone

❹ Remodeling

During remodeling of the bony callus, dead portions of the bone are gradually removed by osteoclasts. Compact bone replaces spongy bone around the periphery of the fracture, and there is reorganization of mineralized bone along the lines of mechanical stress. During this period, the excess material on the outside of the bone shaft and within the medullary cavity is removed and compact bone is laid down to reconstruct the shaft. The final structure of the remodeled area resembles that of the original un-broken bone; however, a thickened area on the surface of the bone may remain as evidence of a healed fracture.

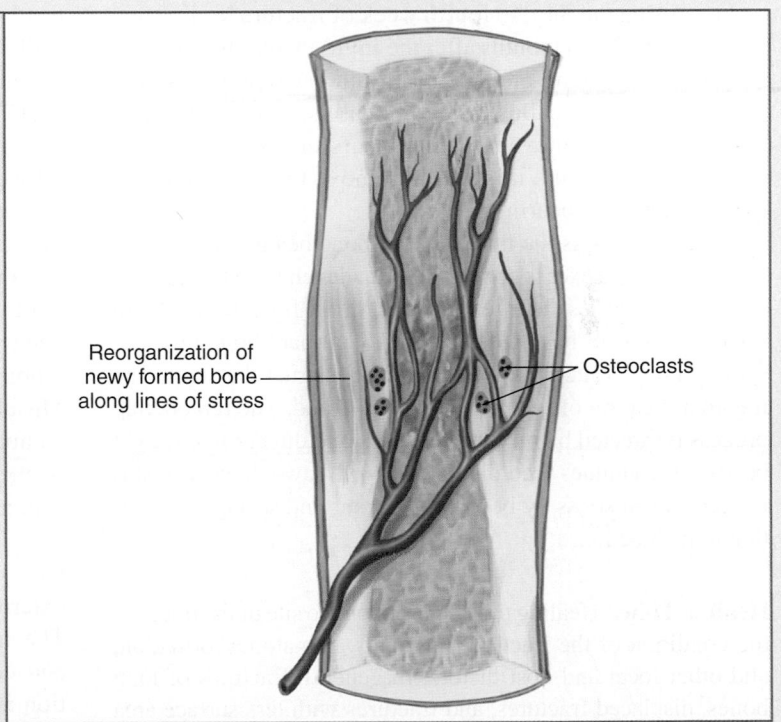

Reorganization of newy formed bone along lines of stress

Osteoclasts

Hematoma formation occurs during the first 1 to 2 days after fracture. It develops from torn blood vessels in the perios-teum and adjacent muscles and soft tissue. Disruption of blood vessels also leads to death of bone cells at the fracture site. In 2 to 5 days, the hemorrhage forms a large blood clot. Neovas-cularization begins peripheral to the blood clot. By the end of the first week, most of the clot is organized by invasion of blood vessels and early fibrosis. Hematoma formation is thought to be necessary for the initiation of the cellular events essential to bone healing.[24] As the result of hematoma forma-tion, clotting factors remain in the injured area to initiate the formation of a fibrin meshwork, which serves as a framework for the ingrowth of fibroblasts and new capillary buds. At the same time, degranulated platelets and migrating inflammatory cells release growth factors, which stimulate osteoclast and osteoblast proliferation.[22,24]

The next event in fracture healing is formation of granulation tissue or soft tissue (fibrocartilaginous) callus. During this stage of bone healing, fibroblasts and osteoblasts migrate into the fracture site from the nearby periosteal and endosteal membranes and begin reconstruction of bone. Some fibroblasts produce collagen that spans the break and connects the broken bone ends, whereas others differentiate into chondrocytes that secrete the collagen matrix. At about the same time, osteoblasts begin depositing bone into this matrix. After a few days, a fibrocartilage "collar" becomes evident around the fracture site. The collar edges on either side of the fracture eventually unite to form a bridge, which connects the bone fragments. The earliest bone, in the form of woven bone, begins its formation sometime after the first week. In an uncomplicated fracture, the repair tissue reaches its maximum girth at the end of the second to third week, which helps stabilize the fracture, but is not yet strong enough for weight bearing.

Ossification and formation of bony callus represent the deposition of mineral salts into the callus. This stage usually occurs during the third to fourth week of fracture healing and is prominent 2 to 3 months after the injury. Continued migration and multiplying of osteoblasts and osteocytes turns the fibrocartilaginous callus into bony callus. The fracture site feels firm and immovable and appears united on the radiograph. At this point, it is safe to remove the cast and allow increased weight bearing.

Remodeling is the final stage of bone healing. It involves resorption of the excess bony callus that develops in the marrow space and encircles the external aspect of the fracture site. Dead bone is removed by the osteoclasts. Compact bone replaces spongy bone around the fracture to reconstruct the shaft. The medullary cavity of the bone is also restored. The remodeling process is directed by mechanical stress and direction of weight bearing. It continues according to the Wolff law—bone responds to mechanical stress by becoming thicker and stronger in relation to its function.

Healing Time. Healing time depends on the site of the fracture, the condition of the fracture fragments, hematoma formation, and other local and host factors. In general, fractures of long bones, displaced fractures, and fractures with less surface area heal more slowly. Function usually returns within 6 months after union is complete. However, return to complete function may take longer. Stress fractures usually require less time to heal, usually 2 to 4 weeks, during which time a reduction in activity and protection of the area are needed.

Factors that influence bone healing are specific to the person, the type of injury sustained, and local factors that disrupt healing. Individual factors that may delay bone healing are the patient's age; current medications; debilitating diseases, such as diabetes and rheumatoid arthritis; local stress around the fracture site; circulatory problems and coagulation disorders; and poor nutrition.

Impaired Healing

Union of a fracture has occurred when the fracture is solid enough to withstand normal stresses and it is clinically and radiologically safe to remove the external fixation. In children, fractures usually heal within 4 to 6 weeks; in adolescents, they heal within 6 to 8 weeks; and in adults, they heal within 10 to 18 weeks.[25] The increased rate of healing among children compared with adults may be related to the increased cellularity and vascularity of the child's periosteum. A number of factors can contribute to impaired bone healing, including the nature and extent of the injury, the health of the person with the fracture and his or her responses to injury, the adequacy of initial treatment, and pharmacologic factors. For large bone defects caused by trauma or a tumor, bone regeneration may need enhancement. Various growth factors, such as BMP, are thought to induce bone formation and repair bone defects.[26]

Malunion is healing with deformity, angulation, or rotation that is visible on x-ray films. Early, aggressive treatment, especially of the hand, can prevent malunion and result in earlier alignment and return of function. Malunion is caused by inadequate reduction or alignment of the fracture. *Delayed union* is the failure of a fracture to unite within the normal period (*e.g.,* 20 weeks for a fracture of the tibia or femur in an adult). Intra-articular fractures (*i.e.,* those through a joint) may heal more slowly and may eventually produce arthritis. *Nonunion* is failure to produce union and cessation of the processes of bone repair. It is seen most often in the tibia, especially with open fractures or crushing injuries. It is characterized by mobility of the fracture site and pain on weight bearing. Muscle atrophy and loss of range of motion may occur. Nonunion usually is established 6 to 12 months after the time of the fracture. The complications of fracture healing are summarized in Table 57-2.

Treatment methods for impaired bone healing encompass surgical interventions, including bone grafts, bracing, external fixation, or electrical stimulation of the bone ends. The treatment for delayed union consists of determining and correcting the cause of the delay. Electrical stimulation is thought to stimulate the osteoblasts to lay down a network of bone. Three types of commercial bone growth stimulators are available: a noninvasive model, which is placed outside the cast; a semi-noninvasive model, in which pins are inserted around the fracture site; and a totally implantable type, in which a cathode coil is wound around the bone at the fracture site and operated by a battery pack implanted under the skin. The Ilizarov method of circular external fixation is used to treat nonunions, especially those that are infected.

TABLE 57-2 **Complications of Fracture Healing**		
COMPLICATION	**MANIFESTATIONS**	**CONTRIBUTING FACTORS**
Delayed union	Failure of fracture to heal within predicted time as determined by x-ray	Large displaced fracture Inadequate immobilization Large hematoma Infection at fracture site Excessive loss of bone Inadequate circulation
Malunion	Deformity at fracture site Deformity or angulation on x-ray	Inadequate reduction Malalignment of fracture at time of immobilization
Nonunion	Failure of bone to heal before the process of bone repair stops Evidence on x-ray Motion at fracture site Pain on weight bearing	Inadequate reduction Mobility at fracture site Severe trauma Bone fragment separation Soft tissue between bone fragments Infection Extensive loss of bone Inadequate circulation Malignancy Bone necrosis Noncompliance with restrictions

Complications of Fractures and Other Musculoskeletal Injuries

The complications of fractures and other orthopedic injuries are associated with loss of skeletal continuity, injury from bone fragments, pressure from swelling and hemorrhage (*e.g.,* fracture blisters, compartment syndrome), involvement of nerve fibers (*e.g.,* complex regional pain syndrome), or development of venous thromboembolism and fat embolism syndrome.

Fracture Blisters

Fracture blisters are skin bullae and blisters representing areas of epidermal necrosis with separation of epidermis from the underlying dermis by edema fluid. They occur when the intracompartmental pressure is too high to be relieved by normal means. They are seen with more severe, twisting types of injuries (*e.g.,* motor vehicle accidents and falls from heights), but can also occur after excessive joint manipulation, dependent positioning, and heat application, or from peripheral vascular disease. They can be solitary, multiple, or massive depending on the extent of injury. Most fracture blisters occur in the ankle, elbow, foot, knee, or areas where there is little soft tissue between the bone and the skin. The development of fracture blisters reportedly is reduced by early surgical intervention in persons requiring operative repair.[27] This probably reflects the early operative release of the fracture hematoma, reap-

proximation of the disrupted soft tissues, ligation of bleeding vessels, and fixation of bleeding fracture surfaces. Prevention of fracture blisters is important because they pose an additional risk for infection. They also constitute a warning sign of compartment syndrome.

Compartment Syndrome

The compartment syndrome has been described as a condition of increased pressure within a limited space (*e.g.,* abdominal and limb compartments) that compromises the circulation and function of the tissues in the space. The abdominal compartment syndrome alters cardiovascular hemodynamics, respiratory mechanics, and renal function. The discussion in this chapter is limited to a discussion of the limb compartment syndromes.

The muscles and nerves of an extremity are enclosed in a tough, inelastic fascial envelope called a *muscle compartment*[28–30] (Fig. 57-9). If the pressure in the compartment is sufficiently high, tissue circulation is compromised, causing death of nerve and muscle cells. Permanent loss of function may occur. The amount of pressure required to produce a compartment syndrome depends on many factors, including the duration of the pressure elevation, the metabolic rate of the tissues, vascular tone, and local blood pressure. Less tissue pressure is required to stop circulation when hypotension or vasoconstriction is present. Intracompartmental pressures greater than 30 mm Hg (normal is approximately 0 to 8 mm Hg) are considered sufficient to impair capillary blood flow.[28]

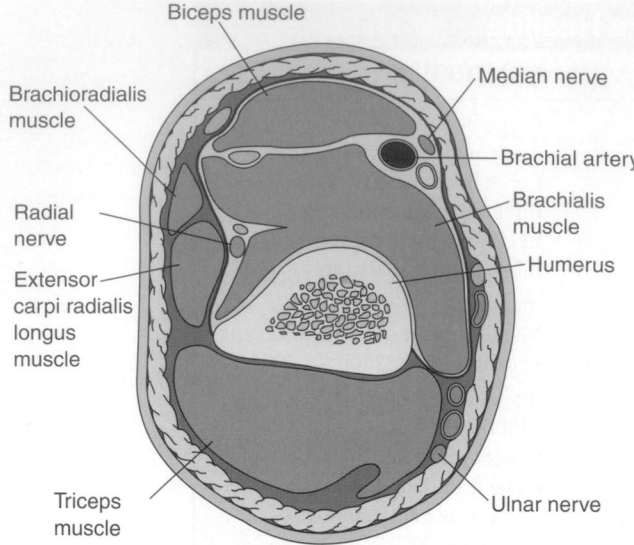

FIGURE 57-9 • The proximal muscle compartment of the arm, showing the location of fascia, muscles, nerves, and blood vessels.

Compartment syndrome can result from a decrease in compartment size, an increase in the volume of its contents, or a combination of the two factors. Among the causes of decreased compartment size are constrictive dressings and casts, closure of fascial defects, and burns. In persons with circumferential third-degree burns, the inelastic and constricting eschar decreases the size of the underlying compartments (see Chapter 61).

An increase in compartment volume can be caused by trauma, swelling, vascular injury and bleeding, and venous obstruction. One of the most important causes of compartment syndrome is bleeding and edema caused by fractures and bone surgery. Contusions and soft tissue injury also are common causes of compartment syndrome. Increased compartment volume may also follow ischemic events, such as arterial occlusion, that are of sufficient duration to produce capillary damage, causing increased capillary permeability and edema. Infiltration of intravenous fluids or bleeding from an arterial puncture can also cause compartment ischemia and postischemic swelling. During unattended coma caused by drug overdose or carbon monoxide poisoning, high compartment pressures are produced when an extremity is compressed by the weight of the overlying head or torso.

Compartment syndrome can be acute or chronic. Acute compartment syndrome can occur after a fracture or crushing injury, when excessive swelling around the site of injury results in increased pressure in a closed compartment. This increase in pressure occurs because fascia, which covers and separates muscles, is inelastic and unable to stretch and compensate for the extreme swelling. Chronic compartment syndrome may develop from exertion in long distance runners and others involved in a major change in activity level. Exertional compartment syndrome is an increase in compartment size and intramuscular pressure during exercise that causes ischemia, pain, and, rarely, neurologic symptoms and signs. The symptoms are less severe and tend to improve with rest, but may proceed to acute compartment syndrome if exercise continues.[31]

The hallmark symptom of an acute compartment syndrome is severe pain that is out of proportion to the original injury or physical findings. Nerve compression may cause changes in sensation (*e.g.,* paresthesias such as burning or tingling or loss of sensation), diminished reflexes, and eventually the loss of motor function. Symptoms usually begin within a few hours but can be delayed as long as 64 hours.[29]

Because muscle necrosis can occur in as little as 4 to 8 hours, it is important that persons at risk for compartment syndrome be identified and proper treatment methods instituted.[29] Assessment should include pain assessment, examination of sensory (*i.e.,* light touch and two-point discrimination) and motor function (*i.e.,* movement and muscle strength), as well as tests of passive stretch and palpation of the muscle compartments. Peripheral pulses frequently are normal in the presence of compartment syndrome because the major arteries are located outside the muscle compartments. Although edema may make it difficult to palpate the pulse, the increased compartment pressure seldom is sufficient to occlude flow in a major artery. Doppler methods usually confirm the existence of a pulse. Direct measurements of tissue pressure can be obtained using a needle or wick catheter inserted into the muscle compartment. This method is particularly useful in persons who are unresponsive and in those with nerve deficits.

Treatment consists of reducing compartmental pressures. This entails cast splitting or removal of restrictive dressings. These procedures often are sufficient to relieve most of the underlying pressure and symptoms. Elevating the extremity on pillows can help to reduce edema. However, excessive elevation should be avoided because the effects of gravity can lower the arterial pressure in the limb; thereby decreasing compartment perfusion. When compartment syndrome cannot be relieved by conservative measures, a fasciotomy may become necessary.[28–30] During this procedure, the fascia is incised longitudinally and separated so that the compartment volume can expand and blood flow can be reestablished. Because of potential problems with wound infection and closure, this procedure is usually performed as a last resort.

Complex Regional Pain Syndrome

The complex regional pain syndrome (CRPS), also referred to as *reflex sympathetic dystrophy* and *causalgia* (discussed in Chapter 49), represents soft tissue complications of musculoskeletal injuries that cause pain out of proportion to the injury, and autonomic nervous system dysfunction manifested by hyperhidrosis (increased sweating) and vasomotor instability (either flushed and warm or cold and pale).[27,32]

Pain, which is the prominent symptom of the disorder, is described as severe, aching, or burning. It usually increases in intensity with movement and with noxious and non-noxious stimuli. The pathophysiologic cause of the pain is unclear, but it is thought to have a sympathetic nervous system component. Muscle wasting, thin and shiny skin, and abnormalities of the nails and bone can occur. Decreased muscle strength and disuse can lead to contractures and osteoporosis. Treatment focuses on pain management and prevention of disability (see Chapter 49).

Thromboemboli

Because of inactivity and restrictions in weight bearing, the person with a lower extremity fracture is at risk for the development of venous thromboembolic disorders, which include pulmonary embolism and deep vein thrombosis (see Chapter 22). The Agency for Healthcare Research and Quality ranks prevention of venous thromboemboli as the first priority of 79 initiatives that can improve patient safety in health care settings.[33] The incidence of venous thromboemboli associated with hip fracture and surgery can be as high as 50%.[34] Fatal pulmonary embolism has an occurrence rate of 7.5% within 3 months of hip fracture surgery and is the fourth leading cause of death. Anticoagulant prophylaxis with unfractionated heparin or low–molecular-weight heparin is effective and safe for individuals with fracture or trauma.[34,35] For high-risk patients, the use of graduated compression stockings or intermittent pneumatic compression devices is regarded as the best practice.[34]

The majority of symptomatic venous thromboemboli associated with hospital admissions occur at least 2 months after hospital discharge.[34] Venous Doppler ultrasonography is the accepted test for the diagnosis of lower extremity deep vein thrombosis. A lung scan may be used in the diagnosis of a pulmonary embolus, but it may not differentiate between a thrombus and a fat embolus, especially in an individual with a long bone fracture.

Fat Embolism Syndrome

The fat embolism syndrome (FES) refers to a constellation of clinical manifestations resulting from the presence of fat droplets in the small blood vessels of the lung or other organs after a long bone fracture or other major trauma.[36–39] The fat emboli are thought to be released from the bone marrow or adipose tissue at the fracture site into the venous system through torn veins.

The pathophysiologic process of FES is unclear. Note that fat embolization and the fat emboli syndrome are not synonymous.[36] Fat embolization involves the presence of fat emboli in the circulation and fat embolism syndrome an identifiable clinical pattern of organ dysfunction associated with fat emboli in the circulation. One suggestion is that, when a bone is fractured, disruption of the venous sinusoids and fat cells allows fat globules to gain access to the venous circulation. The larger particles then become lodged in and block small pulmonary capillaries, whereas the smaller particles may pass through the lung capillaries and enter the systemic circulation. Although fat embolization occurs in many persons with fractures or operative fixation of fractures, FES occurs in only a small percentage of cases, supporting the hypothesis that factors other than fat embolization may be necessary for the development of FES.[36]

The main clinical features of FES are respiratory failure, cerebral dysfunction, and skin and mucosal petechiae. Cerebral manifestations include encephalopathy, seizures, and focal neurologic deficits unrelated to head injury. Initial symptoms of FES begin to develop within a few hours to 3 to 4 days after injury and do not appear beyond 1 week after the injury. The first symptoms include a subtle change in behavior and signs of disorientation resulting from emboli in the cerebral circulation combined with respiratory depression. There may be complaints of substernal chest pain and dyspnea accompanied by tachycardia and a low-grade fever. Diaphoresis, pallor, and cyanosis become evident as respiratory function deteriorates. A petechial rash that does not blanch with pressure often occurs 2 to 3 days after the injury. This rash usually is found on the anterior chest, axillae, neck, and shoulders. It also may appear on the soft palate and conjunctiva. The rash is thought to be related to embolization of the skin capillaries or thrombocytopenia.

An important part of the treatment of FES is early diagnosis. Arterial blood gases should be assayed immediately after recognition of clinical manifestations. Treatment is directed toward correcting hypoxemia and maintaining adequate fluid balance. Mechanical ventilation may be required. Corticosteroid drugs are administered to decrease the inflammatory response of lung tissues, decrease the edema, stabilize the lipid membranes to reduce lipolysis, and combat bronchospasm. Corticosteroids are also given prophylactically to high-risk persons. The only preventive approach to FES is early stabilization of the fracture.

IN SUMMARY, many external physical agents can cause trauma to the musculoskeletal system. Particular factors, such as environment, activity, or age, can place a person at greater risk for injury. Some soft tissue injuries, such as contusions, hematomas, and lacerations, are relatively minor and easily treated. Muscle strains and ligamentous sprains are caused by mechanical overload on the connective tissue. They heal more slowly than the minor soft tissue injuries and require some degree of immobilization. Healing of soft tissue begins within 4 to 5 days of the injury and is primarily the function of fibroblasts, which produce collagen. Joint dislocation is caused by trauma to the supporting structures. Repeated trauma to the joint can cause articular softening (i.e., chondromalacia) or the separation of small pieces of bone or cartilage, called loose bodies, in the joint.

Fractures occur when more stress is placed on a bone than the bone can absorb. The nature of the stress determines the type of fracture and the character of the resulting bone fragments. Healing of fractures is a complex process that takes place in five stages: hematoma formation, cellular proliferation, callus formation, ossification, and remodeling. For satisfactory healing to take place, the affected bone has to be reduced and immobilized. Immobilization is accomplished with the use of external devices, such as splints, casts, traction, or an external fixation apparatus, or with a surgically implanted internal fixation device. The complications associated with fractures can occur early because of soft tissue and nerve damage, or later when the healing process of the fracture is interrupted. The early complications of fractures and other orthopedic injuries are associated with swelling and hemorrhage (fracture blisters and compartment syndrome), involvement of nerve fibers (reflex sympathetic dystrophy and causalgia), and development of fat emboli. Impaired healing of a fracture can cause malunion with deformity, angulation, or rotation; delayed union, in which the healing process is prolonged; or nonunion, in which the fracture fails to heal. ■

BONE INFECTIONS

After completing this section of the chapter, you should be able to meet the following objectives:

- Explain the implications of bone infection.
- Differentiate among osteomyelitis due to spread from a contaminated wound, hematogenous osteomyelitis, and osteomyelitis due to vascular insufficiency in terms of etiologies, manifestations, and treatment.
- Cite the characteristics of chronic osteomyelitis.
- Describe the most common sites of tuberculosis of the bone.

Bone infections, including acute and chronic osteomyelitis, are known for their ability to cause pain, disability, and deformity. Despite the common use of antibiotics, they remain difficult to treat and eradicate. A resurgence of tubercular bone infections are occurring in industrialized parts of the world, attributed in part to immigration from developing countries and greater numbers of immunocompromised people.

BONE INFECTIONS

- Bone infections may be caused by a wide variety of microorganisms introduced during injury, during operative procedures, or from the bloodstream.
- Once localized in bone, the microorganisms proliferate, produce cell death, and spread within the bone shaft, inciting a chronic inflammatory response with further destruction of bone.
- Bone infections are difficult to treat and eradicate. Measures to prevent infection include careful cleaning and debridement of skeletal injuries and strict operating room protocols.

Osteomyelitis

Osteomyelitis represents an acute or chronic infection of the bone. *Osteo* refers to bone, and *myelo* refers to the marrow cavity, both of which are involved in this disease. The infection can be caused by direct penetration or contamination of an open fracture or wound (exogenous origin); seeding through the bloodstream (hematogenous spread); extension from a contiguous site; or skin infections in persons with vascular insufficiency. Osteomyelitis can occur as an acute, subacute, or chronic condition. All types of organisms, including viruses, parasites, fungi, and bacteria, can produce osteomyelitis, but infections caused by certain pyogenic bacteria and mycobacteria are the most common.

The specific agents isolated in pyogenic bacterial osteomyelitis are often associated with the age of the person or the inciting condition (*e.g.*, trauma or surgery). *Staphylococcus aureus* is the most common cause, but organisms such as *Escherichia coli, Neisseria gonorrhoeae, Haemophilus influenzae,* and *Salmonella* species are also seen.[22,24,40–42] *S. aureus* has two characteristics that favor its ability to produce osteomyelitis: (1) it has the ability to produce a collagen-binding adhesion molecule that allows it to adhere to the connective tissue elements of bone; and (2) it has the ability to be internalized and survive in osteoblasts, making the microorganism more resistant to antimicrobial (*e.g.*, antibiotic) therapy.[40]

Hematogenous Osteomyelitis

Hematogenous osteomyelitis originates with infectious organisms that reach the bone through the bloodstream. Acute hematogenous osteomyelitis occurs predominantly in children.[40–42] In adults, it is seen most commonly in debilitated persons and in those with a history of chronic skin infections, chronic urinary tract infections, and intravenous drug use and in those who are immunologically suppressed. Intravenous drug users are at risk for infections with *Streptococcus* and *Pseudomonas*.

Pathogenesis. The pathogenesis of hematogenous osteomyelitis differs in children and adults. In children, the infection usually affects the long bones of the appendicular skeleton. It starts in the metaphyseal region close to the growth plate, where termination of nutrient blood vessels and sluggish blood flow favor the attachment of blood-borne bacteria (Fig. 57-10). With advancement of the infection, purulent exudate collects in the rigidly enclosed bony tissue. Because of the bone's rigid structure, there is little room for swelling and the purulent exudate finds its way beneath the periosteum, shearing off the perforating arteries that supply the cortex with blood, thereby leading to necrosis of cortical bone. The necrotic bone that is formed may separate from the viable surrounding bone to form devascularized fragments, called *sequestra*.[22] Eventually, the purulent drainage may penetrate the periosteum and skin to form a draining sinus. In children 1 year of age and younger, the adjacent joint is often involved because the periosteum is not firmly

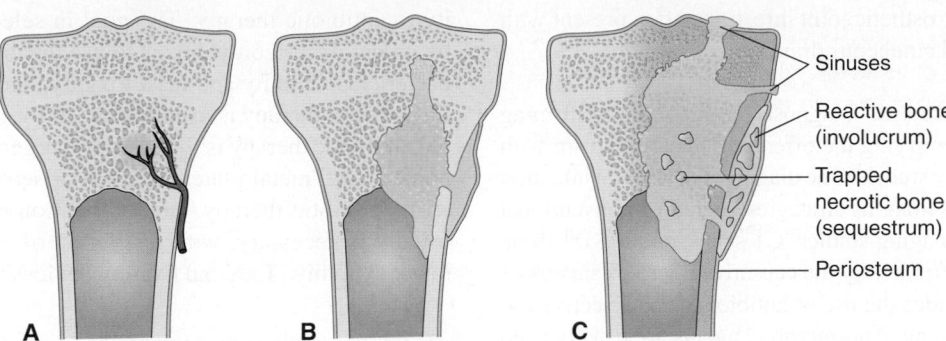

FIGURE 57-10 • Hematogenous osteomyelitis. **(A)** Infectious organisms reach the metaphysis through a nutrient blood vessel. **(B)** Bacterial growth results in bone destruction and abscess formation. From the abscess cavity, the infection spreads between the trabeculae into the medullary cavity of compact bone and then through the cortex to the outside. **(C)** The purulent exudate finds its way beneath the periosteum, shearing off the perforating arteries that supply the cortex with blood, thereby leading to necrosis of cortical bone and formation of devascularized fragments, called *sequestra*.

attached to the cortex.[22] From 1 year of age to puberty, subperiosteal abscesses are more common. As the process continues, periosteal new bone formation and reactive bone formation in the marrow tend to wall in the infection. *Involucrum* refers to a lesion in which bone formation forms a sheath around the necrotic sequestrum. It is seen most commonly in cases of chronic osteomyelitis (discussed later).

In adults, the long bone microvasculature no longer favors seeding, and hematogenous infection rarely affects the appendicular skeleton. Instead, vertebrae, sternoclavicular and sacroiliac joints, and the symphysis pubis are involved. Infection typically first involves subchondral bone, then spreads to the joint space.[43] With vertebral osteomyelitis, this causes sequential destruction of the endplate, adjoining disk, and contiguous vertebral body. Infection less commonly begins in the joint and spreads to the adjacent bone.

Manifestations. The signs and symptoms of acute hematogenous osteomyelitis are those of bacteremia accompanied by symptoms referable to the site of the bone lesion. Bacteremia is characterized by chills, fever, and malaise. There often is pain on movement of the affected extremity, loss of movement, and local tenderness followed by redness and swelling. X-ray studies may appear normal initially, but they show evidence of periosteal elevation and increased osteoclast activity after an abscess has formed. Changes are evident on a bone scan 10 to 14 days before any changes are seen on x-ray films.[42]

Treatment. The treatment of hematogenous osteomyelitis begins with identification of the causative organism through blood and bone aspiration cultures.[42] Antimicrobial agents are given first parenterally and then orally. The length of time the affected limb needs to be rested and pain control measures used is based on the person's symptoms. Debridement and surgical drainage also may be necessary.

Direct Penetration and Contiguous Spread Osteomyelitis

Direct penetration or extension of bacteria from an outside (exogenous) source is now the most common cause of osteomyelitis in the United States.[22] Bacteria may be introduced directly into the bone by a penetrating wound, an open fracture, or surgery. Inadequate irrigation or debridement, introduction of foreign material into the wound, and extensive tissue injury increase the bone's susceptibility to infection.

Iatrogenic bone infections are those inadvertently brought about by surgery or other treatments. These complications include pin tract infection in skeletal traction, septic (infected) joints in joint replacement surgery, and wound infections after surgery. Staphylococci and streptococci are still commonly implicated, but in 25% of postoperative infections, gram-negative organisms are detected.[22] Measures to prevent these infections include preparation of the skin to reduce bacterial growth before surgery or insertion of traction devices or wires; strict operating room protocols; prophylactic use of antibiotics immediately before and for 24 hours after surgery and as a topical wound irrigation; and maintenance of sterile technique after surgery when working with drainage tubes and dressing changes.

Pathogenesis. The pathogenesis of osteomyelitis resulting from direct penetration or contiguous spread differs from hematogenous infection in that virtually any traumatized bone may be involved. Although healthy bone is highly resistant to infection, injury from local inflammation and trauma may devitalize bone and surrounding tissue, providing an inert matrix on which microorganisms introduced during trauma thrive.

Manifestations. Osteomyelitis after trauma or bone surgery usually is associated with persistent or recurrent fever, increased pain at the operative or trauma site, and poor incisional healing, which often is accompanied by continued wound drainage and wound separation. Prosthetic joint infections often present with joint pain, fever, and cutaneous drainage.

Diagnosis and Treatment. Diagnosis requires both confirming the infection and identifying the offending microorganism with culture and sensitivity studies. The diagnosis of skeletal infection entails use of various imaging strategies, including conventional radiology, nuclear imaging studies, CT scans, and MRI.[42] Bone biopsy may be used to identify the causative microorganisms.

Treatment includes the use of antibiotics and selective use of surgical interventions. Antimicrobial agents are usually used prophylactically in persons undergoing bone surgery. However, prolonged use of prophylactic antimicrobial agents is associated with emergence of resistant bacterial strains.[44] For persons with osteomyelitis, early antimicrobial treatment, before there is extensive destruction of bone, produces the best results. The choice of agents and method of administration depend on the microorganisms causing the infection. Antimicrobial beads (*e.g.,* vancomycin, tobramycin, or other broad-spectrum antibiotics) can be embedded into the cement as part of the procedure for an infected hip arthroplasty or for a wound infection after spinal cord injury.[45] In acute osteomyelitis that does not respond to antibiotic therapy, surgical decompression is used to release intramedullary pressure and remove drainage from the periosteal area. Prosthesis removal may be necessary in cases of an infected prosthetic joint. The joint is left out while a 2- to 6-week course of therapy is given, after which another joint is implanted.[41]

Chronic Osteomyelitis

Chronic osteomyelitis usually occurs in adults. Generally, these infections occur secondary to an open wound, most often to the bone or surrounding tissue. Chronic osteomyelitis has long been recognized as a disease. However, the incidence has decreased in the past century because of improvements in surgical techniques and the advent of broad-spectrum antibiotic therapy. Chronic osteomyelitis includes all inflammatory processes of bone, excluding those in rheumatic diseases that are caused by microorganisms. It may be the result of delayed or inadequate treatment of acute hematogenous osteomyelitis or osteomyelitis caused by direct contamination of bone by exogenous organisms. Chronic osteomyelitis can persist for years; it may appear spontaneously, after a minor trauma, or when resistance is lowered.

The hallmark feature of chronic osteomyelitis is the presence of infected dead bone, a *sequestrum,* that has separated from the living bone.[22,24,41] A sheath of new bone, called the *involucrum,* forms around the dead bone. Radiologic techniques such as x-ray films, bone scans, and sinograms are used to identify the infected site. Chronic osteomyelitis or infection around a total joint prosthesis can be difficult to diagnose because the classic signs of infection are not apparent and the blood leukocyte count may not be elevated. A subclinical infection may exist for years. Bone scans are used with bone biopsy for a definitive diagnosis.

The treatment of chronic bone infections begins with wound cultures to identify the microorganism and its sensitiv-

ity to antibiotic therapy. The goal in selecting antimicrobial treatment for osteomyelitis is to use the drug with the highest bactericidal activity and least toxicity, and at the lowest cost. Intravenous therapy is usually needed for up to 6 weeks.[41] Initial antibiotic therapy is followed by surgery to remove foreign bodies (*e.g.,* metal plates, screws) or sequestra and by long-term antibiotic therapy. Immobilization of the affected part usually is necessary, with restriction of weight bearing on a lower extremity. External fixation devices are sometimes used.

Osteomyelitis With Vascular Insufficiency

In persons with vascular insufficiency, osteomyelitis may develop from a skin lesion. It is most commonly associated with chronic or ischemic foot ulcers in persons with long-standing diabetes. Neuropathy causes a loss of protective reflexes, and impaired arterial circulation and repetitive trauma are the major contributors to skin fissure and ulcer formation.

Persons with vascular insufficiency osteomyelitis often present with seemingly unrelated problems such as ingrown toenails, cellulitis, or a perforating foot ulcer, making diagnosis difficult. Furthermore, pain is often muted by peripheral neuropathy. Osteomyelitis is confirmed when bone is exposed in the ulcer bed or after debridement. Radiologic evidence is a late sign.

Treatment depends on the oxygen tension of the involved tissues. Debridement and antibiotic therapy may benefit persons who have good oxygen tension in the infected site. Hyperbaric oxygen therapy may be used as an adjunctive treatment. Amputation may be indicated when oxygen tension is inadequate.[43]

Tuberculosis of the Bone or Joint

A resurgence of tubercular osteomyelitis is occurring in industrialized countries, attributed to the influx of immigrants from developing countries and the greater numbers of immunocompromised people.[46] In developing countries, affected individuals are usually adolescents or young adults, whereas in the nonimmigrant population of developed countries, the victims tend to be older, except for those who are immunocompromised.

Tuberculosis can spread from one part of the body, such as the lungs or the lymph nodes, to the musculoskeletal system. Any bone, joint, or bursa may be affected, but the spine is the most common site, followed by the knees and hips.[24,47] Tubercular osteomyelitis tends to be more destructive and difficult to control than pyogenic osteomyelitis. The infection spreads through large areas of the medullary cavity and causes extensive necrosis. In tuberculosis of the spine, also known as *Pott disease,* the infection spreads through the intervertebral disks to involve multiple vertebrae and extends into the soft tissue, forming abscesses.

Local symptoms include pain, immobility, and muscle atrophy; joint swelling, mild fever, and leukocytosis also may occur. The most feared complication of spinal tuberculosis is neurologic compromise due to spinal deformity and epidural abscess formation. Because there are no specific radiographic findings in tubercular osteomyelitis, the diagnosis is usually made by tissue biopsy or culture findings. In spinal tuberculosis, a CT-guided biopsy is often used. The mainstay of treatment for tubercular osteomyelitis remains the appropriate three- or four-drug antimicrobial therapy based on current guidelines.[47] Conservative treatment is usually as effective as surgery, especially for earlier and milder cases.

IN SUMMARY, bone infections occur because of the direct or indirect invasion of the musculoskeletal system by microorganisms, most commonly *S. aureus*. Osteomyelitis, or infection of the bone and marrow, can be an acute or chronic disease. Acute osteomyelitis is seen most often as a result of the direct contamination of bone by a foreign object. Chronic osteomyelitis represents an infection that continues beyond 6 to 8 weeks and may persist for years. The incidence of all types of bone infection has been dramatically reduced since the advent of antibiotic therapy. Iatrogenic infections are those inadvertently brought about by surgery or other treatments. Tuberculosis of the bone, which is characterized by bone destruction and abscess formation, is caused by spread of the infection from the lungs or lymph nodes. ■

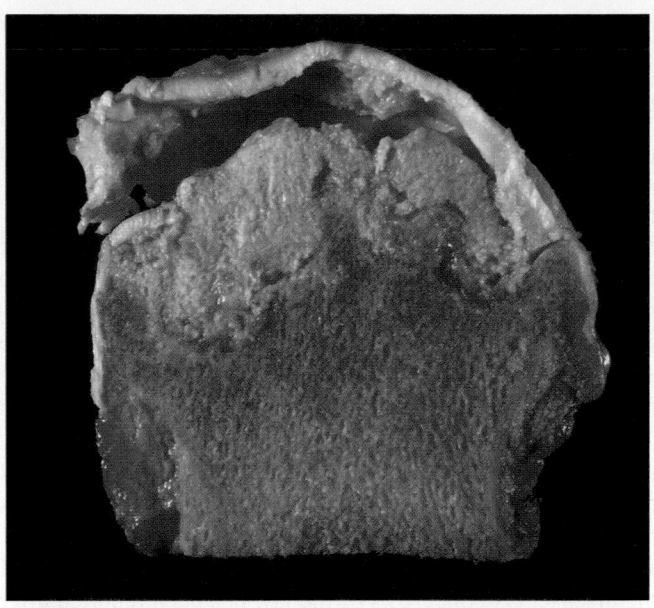

FIGURE 57-11 • Osteonecrosis of the head of the femur. A coronal section shows a circumscribed area of subchondral infarction with partial detachment of the overlying articular cartilage and subarticular bone. (From Hoch B. L., Klein M. J., Schiller A. L. [2008]. Bones and joints. In Rubin R., Strayer D. E. [Eds.], *Rubin's pathology: Clinicopathologic foundations of medicine* [5th ed., p. 1100]. Philadelphia: Lippincott Williams & Wilkins.)

OSTEONECROSIS

After completing this section of the chapter, you should be able to meet the following objectives:

■ Define *osteonecrosis*.
■ Cite four major causes of osteonecrosis.
■ Characterize the blood supply of bone and relate it to the pathologic features of the condition.
■ Describe the methods used in diagnosis and treatment of the condition.

Osteonecrosis, or death of a segment of bone, is a condition caused by the interruption of blood supply to the marrow, medullary bone, or cortex[22,24,47–50] (Fig. 57-11). It is a relatively common disorder and can occur in the medullary cavity of the metaphysis and the subchondral region of the epiphysis, especially in the proximal femur, distal femur, and proximal humerus. It is a common complicating disorder of Legg-Calvé-Perthes disease, slipped capital femoral epiphysis, sickle cell disease, steroid therapy, alcohol abuse, and hip trauma, fracture, or surgery. The rates of osteonecrosis among persons treated with corticosteroids range from 5% to 25%. More than 10% of the 500,000 joint replacements performed annually in the United States are for treatment of osteonecrosis.[47]

Although bone necrosis results from ischemia, the mechanisms producing the ischemia are varied and include mechanical vascular interruption such as occurs with trauma or a fracture; thrombosis and embolism (*e.g.*, sickle cell disease, nitrogen

bubbles caused by inadequate decompression during deep sea diving); and vessel injury (*e.g.*, vasculitis, radiation therapy). In many cases, the cause of the necrosis is uncertain. Other than fracture, the most common causes of bone necrosis are idiopathic (*i.e.*, those of unknown cause) and prior steroid therapy. Chart 57-1 lists disorders associated with osteonecrosis.

Bone has a rich blood supply that varies from site to site.[47] The flow in the medullary portion of bone originates in nutrient vessels from an interconnecting plexus that supplies the mar-

CHART 57-1	**CAUSES OF OSTEONECROSIS**

Mechanical disruption of blood vessels
 Fractures
 Legg-Calvé-Perthes disease
 Blount disease
Thrombosis and embolism
 Sickle cell disease
 Nitrogen bubbles in decompression sickness
Vessel injury
 Vasculitis
 Connective tissue disease
  Systemic lupus erythematosus
  Rheumatoid arthritis
 Radiation therapy
 Gaucher disease
Corticosteroid therapy

row, trabecular bone, and endosteal half of the cortex. The outer cortex receives its blood supply from periosteal, muscular, metaphyseal, and epiphyseal vessels that surround the bone. Some bony sites, such as the head of the femur, have only limited collateral circulation, so that interruption of the flow, such as with a hip fracture, can cause necrosis of a substantial portion of medullary and cortical bone and irreversible damage.

One of the most frequent causes of osteonecrosis is that associated with administration of corticosteroids.[16,20,47] Despite numerous studies, the mechanism of steroid-induced osteonecrosis remains unclear. The condition may develop after the administration of very high, short-term doses; during long-term treatment; or even from intra-articular injection. Although the risk increases with the dose and duration of treatment, it is difficult to predict who will be affected. The interval between corticosteroid administration and onset of symptoms rarely is less than 6 months and may be more than 3 years. There is no satisfactory method for preventing progression of the disease. Osteonecrosis of the jaw has been reported after long-term use of bisphosphonates.[51] The complication has mainly been reported in patients receiving the drugs intravenously for multiple myeloma and bone metastases from breast cancer.

The pathologic features of bone necrosis are the same, regardless of cause. The site of the lesion is related to the vessels involved. There is necrosis of cancellous bone and marrow. The cortex usually is not involved because of collateral blood flow. In subchondral infarcts (*i.e.,* ischemia below the cartilage), a triangular or wedge-shaped segment of tissue that has the subchondral bone plate as its base and the center of the epiphysis as its apex, undergoes necrosis. When medullary infarcts occur in fatty bone marrow, the death of bone cells causes calcium release and necrosis of fat cells, with the formation of free fatty acids. Released calcium forms an insoluble "soap" with free fatty acids. Because bone lacks mechanisms for resolving the infarct, the lesions remain for life.

The symptoms associated with osteonecrosis are varied and depend on the extent of infarction. Typically, subchondral infarcts cause chronic pain that is initially associated with activity but that gradually becomes more progressive until it is experienced at rest. Subchondral infarcts often collapse and predispose the patient to severe secondary osteoarthritis.

Diagnosis of osteonecrosis is based on history, physical findings, radiographic findings, and results of special imaging studies, including CT scans and technetium-99m bone scans. Treatment of osteonecrosis depends on the underlying pathologic process. In some cases, only short-term immobilization, nonsteroidal anti-inflammatory drugs, exercises, and limitation in weight bearing are used. Osteonecrosis of the hip is particularly difficult to treat. In persons with early disease, limitation of weight bearing through the use of crutches may allow the condition to stabilize. Although several surgical approaches have been used, the most definitive treatment of advanced osteonecrosis of the knee or hip is total joint replacement. Treatment with hyperbaric oxygenation can also be effective.[52]

IN SUMMARY, osteonecrosis is a common condition that has long been recognized but is not fully understood. Death of bone is caused by disruption of the blood supply from intravascular or extravascular processes. Sites with poor collateral circulation, such as the femoral head, are most seriously affected. Causative factors include corticosteroid therapy. Symptoms include pain that varies in severity, depending on the extent of infarction. Total joint replacement is the most frequently used treatment for advanced osteonecrosis. ■

NEOPLASMS

After completing this section of the chapter, you should be able to meet the following objectives:

- Differentiate between the properties of benign and malignant bone tumors.
- Contrast osteogenic sarcoma, Ewing sarcoma, and chondrosarcoma in terms of the most common age groups and anatomic sites that are affected.
- List the primary sites of tumors that frequently metastasize to the bone.
- State the three primary goals for treatment of metastatic bone disease.

Neoplasms in the skeletal system are referred to as *bone tumors.* Primary malignant tumors of the bone are uncommon, constituting less than 0.2% of all cancers.[53] Metastatic disease of the bone, however, is relatively common. Primary bone tumors may arise from any of the skeletal components, including osseous bone tissue, cartilage, and bone marrow. The discussion in this section focuses on primary benign and malignant bone tumors of osseous or cartilaginous origin and metastatic bone disease. Tumors of bone marrow origin (*i.e.,* leukemia and multiple myeloma) are discussed in Chapter 15.

Like other types of neoplasms, bone tumors may be benign or malignant. Benign tumors far outnumber malignant tumors. The benign types, such as osteochondromas, tend to grow rather slowly and usually do not destroy the supporting or surrounding tissue or spread to other parts of the body. Malignant tumors, such as osteosarcoma, grow rapidly and can spread to other parts of the body through the bloodstream or lymphatics. The two major forms of bone cancer in children and young adults are osteosarcoma and Ewing sarcoma. Both tumor types occur more frequently in the second decade of life.[24] Chondrosarcomas tend to occur during middle to late adulthood.[24] The classification of benign and malignant bone tumors is described in Table 57-3.

Characteristics of Bone Tumors

There are three major manifestations of bone tumors: pain, presence of a mass, and impairment of function. Pain is a feature common to almost all malignant tumors, but may or may

TABLE 57-3 **Classification of Primary Bone Neoplasms**		
TISSUE TYPE	**BENIGN NEOPLASM**	**MALIGNANT NEOPLASM**
Bone	Osteoid osteoma Benign osteo- blastoma	Osteosarcoma Parosteal osteo- genic sarcoma
Cartilage	Osteochondroma Chondroma Chrondroblastoma Chondromyxoid fibroma	Chondrosarcoma
Lipid	Lipoma	Liposarcoma
Fibrous and fibro-osseous tissue	Fibrous dysplasia	Fibrosarcoma Malignant fibrous histiocytoma
Miscellaneous	Giant cell tumor	Malignant giant cell Ewing sarcoma
Bone marrow		Multiple myeloma Reticulum cell sarcoma

not occur with benign tumors. For example, a benign bone cyst usually is asymptomatic until a fracture occurs. Pain that persists at night and is not relieved by rest suggests malignancy. A mass or hard lump may be the first sign of a bone tumor. A malignant tumor is suspected when a painful mass exists that is enlarging or eroding the cortex of the bone. The ease of discovery of a mass depends on the location of the tumor; a small lump arising on the surface of the tibia is easy to detect, whereas a tumor that is deep in the medial portion of the thigh may grow to a considerable size before it is noticed. Benign and malignant tumors may cause the bone to erode to the point at which it cannot withstand the strain of ordinary use. In such cases, even a small amount of bone stress or trauma precipitates a pathologic fracture. A tumor may produce pressure on a peripheral nerve, causing decreased sensation, numbness, a limp, or limitation of movement.

⚷ BONE NEOPLASMS

- Neoplasms of the skeletal system can affect bone tissue, cartilage, or bone marrow.

- Benign tumors tend to grow slowly, do not spread to other parts of the body, and exert their effects through the space-occupying nature of the tumor and their ability to weaken bone structures.

- Malignant bone tumors are rare before 10 years of age, have their peak incidence in the teenage years, tend to grow rapidly, and have a high mortality rate.

Benign Neoplasms

Benign bone tumors usually are limited to the confines of the bone, have well-demarcated edges, and are surrounded by a thin rim of sclerotic bone. The four most common types of benign bone tumors are osteoma, chondroma, osteochondroma, and giant cell tumor.[22,24] An *osteoma* is a small bony tumor found on the surface of a long bone, flat bone, or the skull. It usually is composed of hard, compact (ivory osteoma), or spongy (cancellous) bone. It may be excised or left alone.

A *chondroma* is a tumor composed of hyaline cartilage. It may arise on the surface of the bone (*i.e.,* ecchondroma) or in the medullary cavity (*i.e.,* endochondroma). These tumors may become large and are especially common in the hands and feet. A chondroma may persist for many years and then take on the attributes of a malignant chondrosarcoma. A chondroma usually is not treated unless it becomes unsightly or uncomfortable.

An *osteochondroma* is the most common form of benign tumor in the skeletal system, representing 50% of all benign bone tumors and approximately 15% of all primary skeletal lesions. It grows only during periods of skeletal growth, originating in the epiphyseal cartilage plate and growing out of the bone like a mushroom. An osteochondroma is composed of cartilage and bone and usually occurs singly, but may affect several bones in a condition called *multiple exostoses*. Malignant changes are rare, and excision of the tumor is done only when necessary.

A *giant cell tumor,* or *osteoclastoma,* is an aggressive tumor of multinucleated cells that often behaves like a malignant tumor, metastasizing through the bloodstream and recurring locally after excision. It arises most often in people in their 20s to 40s and is found most commonly in the knee, wrist, or shoulder. The tumor begins in the metaphyseal region, grows into the epiphysis, and may extend into the joint surface. Pathologic fractures are common because the tumor destroys the bone substance. Clinically, pain may occur at the tumor site, with gradually increasing swelling. X-ray films show destruction of the bone with expansion of the cortex.

The treatment of giant cell tumors depends on their location. If the affected bone can be eliminated without loss of function, such as the clavicle or fibula, the entire bone or part of it may be removed. When the tumor is near a major joint, such as the knee or shoulder, a local excision is done. Irradiation may be used to prevent recurrence of the tumor.

Malignant Bone Tumors

In contrast to benign tumors, primary malignant tumors tend to be ill defined, lack sharp borders, and extend beyond the confines of the bone. Primary bone tumors occur in all age groups and may arise in any part of the body. However, certain types of tumors tend to target certain age groups and anatomic sites (Fig. 57-12). For example, most osteogenic sarcomas occur in adolescents and are particularly common around the knee

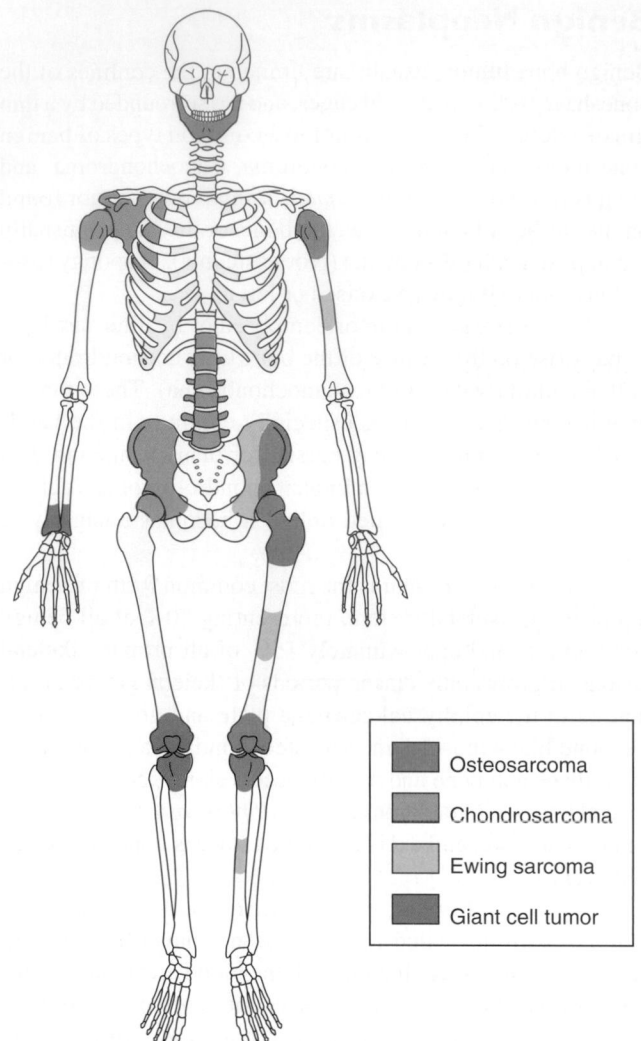

FIGURE 57-12 • Common sites of primary malignant bone tumors (chondrosarcoma, osteosarcoma, and Ewing sarcoma) and giant cell tumor, a locally aggressive benign tumor.

Osteosarcoma

Chondrosarcoma

Ewing sarcoma

Giant cell tumor

joint. Also, people with certain conditions such as Paget disease are at increased risk for development of bone cancer.

The diagnosis of bone tumors includes radiologic staging and biopsy.[51] Radiographs give the most general diagnostic information, such as malignant versus benign and primary versus metastatic status. The radiograph demonstrates the region of bone involvement, extent of destruction, and amount of reactive bone formed. Radioisotope scans are used to estimate the local intramedullary extent of the tumor and screen for other skeletal areas of involvement. CT scans further aid diagnosis and anatomic localization and can identify small pulmonary metastases not seen by conventional radiographs. MRI is the most accurate method of evaluating the intramedullary extent of bone tumor and can demarcate the soft structures in relation to neurovascular structures without the use of contrast media. It is best used in conjunction with a CT scan. Radionuclide bone scans are used to assess for metastasis. A biopsy also is done because the definitive treatment of most bone tumors is based on pathologic interpretation of the biopsy specimen.

Osteosarcoma

Osteosarcoma is an aggressive and highly malignant bone tumor. It is the most common primary malignant bone tumor, representing one fifth of all bone tumors.[22] Osteosarcoma is the most common bone tumor in children and the third most common cancer in children and adolescents.[22,24,54,55] Although osteosarcomas can develop in any bone, they most commonly arise in the vicinity of the knee (*e.g.,* lower femur or upper tibia or fibula). The proximal humerus is the second most common site. The hands, feet, skull, and jaw are less frequent sites for the disease, being affected most frequently in persons older than 25 years of age.[22]

The cause of osteosarcoma is unknown. The tumor has a bimodal distribution, with 75% occurring in persons younger than 20 years of age. A second peak occurs in the elderly with predisposing factors such as Paget disease, bone infarcts, or prior irradiation.[24] The correlation of age and location of most of the tumors with the period of maximum growth suggests some relation to increased osteoblastic activity. In younger persons, the primary tumor most often is located at the anatomic sites associated with maximum growth velocity—the distal femur, proximal tibia, and proximal humerus. Bone tumors in the elderly are more common in the humerus, pelvis, and proximal femur. Paget disease, which is linked to osteosarcoma in adults, also is associated with increased osteoblastic activity. Irradiation from an internal source, such as the radioactive pharmaceutical technetium used in bone scans, or an external source, such as x-ray films, also has been associated with osteosarcoma. There are known genetic factors associated with osteosarcoma. Mutations in two genes are reported to increase the susceptibility to the development of osteosarcoma: the retinoblastoma gene (*RB*) and the *TP53* tumor suppressor gene[18] (see Chapter 8).

Osteosarcomas are aggressive tumors that grow rapidly in a circular, ball-like mass in the bone tissue. They often are eccentrically placed in the bone and move from the metaphysis of the bone out into the periosteal surface, with subsequent spread to adjacent soft tissues (Fig. 57-13). The tumor infrequently metastasizes to the lymph nodes because the cells are unable to grow in the node. Nodal metastases usually occur only in the late course of disseminated disease. Most often, the tumor cells exit the primary tumor through the venous end of the capillary, and early metastasis to the lung is common. Lung metastases, even if massive, usually are relatively asymptomatic. The prognosis for a person with osteosarcoma depends on the aggressiveness of the disease, presence or absence of pathologic fractures, size of the tumor, and rapidity of tumor growth. Long-term survival is better in younger people with effective chemotherapy regimens and no metastases.[56] Despite advances in surgery and chemotherapy, the survival rate has remained unchanged at 55% to 70%.[57]

The primary clinical feature of osteosarcoma is deep, localized pain with nighttime awakening and swelling in the affected

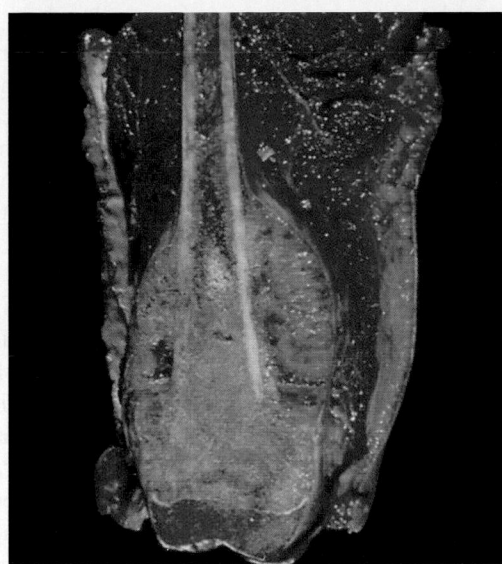

FIGURE 57-13 • Osteosarcoma. The distal femur contains a dense osteoblastic malignant tumor that extends through the center in the soft tissue and epiphysis. (From Hoch B. L., Klein M. J., Schiller A. L. [2008]. Bones and joints. In Rubin R., Strayer D. E. [Eds.], *Rubin's pathology: Clinicopathologic foundations of medicine* [5th ed., p. 1126]. Philadelphia: Lippincott Williams & Wilkins.)

bone. Because the pain is often of sudden onset, patients and their families often associate the symptoms with recent trauma.[54] The skin overlying the tumor may be warm, shiny, and stretched, with prominent superficial veins. The range of motion of the adjacent joint may be restricted.

History, physical examination, and radiographic studies are all part of the evaluation of a patient with osteosarcoma. Plain films of the primary site and of the chest are first obtained. MRI, CT scan, and full-body scan are required to evaluate the extent of the local disease and to determine the extent of metastasis if present. Radionuclide bone scans are done to evaluate for lung and bone metastasis. An open biopsy is required to confirm the diagnosis and to determine the histologic features and cell type of the tumor.

Osteosarcoma is treated by surgery in combination with multiagent chemotherapy used both before and after surgery.[53–55] In the past, treatment usually entailed amputation above the level of the tumor. Limb salvage surgical procedures, using a metal prosthesis or cadaver allograft, are now a standard alternative. Studies have shown that limb salvage surgery has no adverse effects on the long-term survival of persons with osteosarcoma. The success of limb salvage appears to depend on the use of a wide surgical margin, improved radiographic imaging studies, multiagent chemotherapy, and more refined surgical reconstructive techniques. Advanced imaging techniques, including serum thallium scans, and the use of angiography assist the surgeon in determining the best type of treatment. Chemotherapy using various drug combinations is the most effective treatment for metastatic osteosarcoma.[58,59] A preoperative regimen of intra-arterial cisplatin and infu-

sional doxorubicin is being used in combination with limb-sparing procedures.[55,57,58]

Amputation is another surgical option. It involves either the removal of expendable bones such as the fibula, ribs, toes, or ulna, or the complete removal of the tumor and the affected limb. The primary objective of overall treatment of patients with osteosarcoma is long-term disease-free survival or cure. Preserving limb function is a secondary objective. In cases in which adequate limb salvage surgery cannot be achieved, limb amputation may be necessary.

Ewing Sarcoma

Ewing sarcoma is a member of a group of small round cell, undifferentiated tumors thought to be of neural crest origin[16,24,54] (see Chapter 48). The family of tumors includes Ewing sarcoma of the bone and soft tissue and peripheral primitive neuroectodermal tumor (PPNET). Of the tumors in this family, Ewing sarcoma accounts for most cases. Ewing sarcoma and osteosarcoma occur in the same sex and age groups, but they can usually be distinguished radiographically and histologically. It can occur at any age, but is seen most commonly in patients 10 to 20 years of age. Males are affected slightly more frequently than females. There is a striking predilection for whites; black and Asian children are rarely affected.[24]

The most frequent site of Ewing sarcoma is the femur, usually in the diaphysis. The pelvis represents the second most common site; other sites include the pubis, sacrum, humerus, vertebrae, ribs, skull, and other flat bones. The characteristic pathologic findings of Ewing sarcoma include densely packed, regularly shaped, small cells with round or oval nuclei. A specific reciprocal translocation of chromosomes 11 and 22, or a variant thereof, is found in most of the Ewing sarcoma family of tumors.[22,54] Detection of the translocation by routine cytogenetic or polymerase chain reaction analysis can be helpful in confirming the diagnosis in highly undifferentiated tumors.[54]

Manifestations of Ewing tumor include bone pain, limitation of movement, and tenderness over the involved bone or soft tissue.[54] It often is accompanied by systemic manifestations such as fever or weight loss, which may serve to confuse the diagnosis. There may be a delay in diagnosis when the pain and swelling associated with the tumor are attributed to a sports injury or when the tumor is located in the pelvis and the pain is not localized and the mass is not apparent. Pathologic fractures are common because of bone destruction. The most common sites of metastasis are the lungs, bone marrow, and other bones.

Because Ewing sarcoma is a difficult diagnosis to establish, the diagnostic biopsy is very important. Clinical evaluations include MRI and CT scans of the primary tumor, chest radiographs, CT of the chest, bone scan, bilateral bone marrow aspiration, and biopsy of the primary tumor site.[54] The extent of disease at diagnosis is the most important prognostic factor. The presence of metastatic disease at diagnosis is a poor prognostic factor regardless of the site of the primary lesion.

Treatment methods incorporate a combination of multi-agent chemotherapy, surgery, and radiation therapy. Chemotherapy is important because it can shrink the tumor and improve overall survival rates from 10% to 70%.[54] It is generally given before local control measures are initiated. Ewing sarcoma is considered to be a radiosensitive tumor, and local control may be achieved through radiation, or surgery. Patients with small, nonmetastatic, distally located tumors generally have the best prognosis. Such patients have up to a 75% cure rate.[53] The presence of metastases at the time of diagnosis decreases the 3-year survival rate to 30% to 60%.[54]

Chondrosarcoma

Chondrosarcoma, a malignant tumor of cartilage that can develop in the medullary cavity or peripherally, is the second most common form of malignant bone tumor. It occurs primarily in middle or later life and slightly more often in men. The tumor arises from points of muscle attachment to bone, particularly the knee, shoulder, hip, and pelvis. Chondrosarcomas can arise from underlying benign lesions such as osteochondroma, chondroblastoma, or fibrous dysplasia.[24]

Chondrosarcomas are slow growing and metastasize late, and often are painless. They can remain hidden in an area such as the pelvis for a long time. This type of tumor, like many primary malignancies, tends to destroy bone and extend into the soft tissues beyond the confines of the bone of origin. Chondrosarcomas mainly affect the bones of the trunk, pelvis, or proximal femur and rarely develop in the distal portion of a bone. Irregular flecks and ringlets of calcification often are prominent radiographic findings.

Early diagnosis is important because chondrosarcoma responds well to early radical surgical excision. It usually is resistant to radiation therapy and available chemotherapeutic agents. Not infrequently, these tumors transform into a highly malignant tumor, mesenchymal chondrosarcoma, which requires a more aggressive treatment, including combination chemotherapy.

Metastatic Bone Disease

Skeletal metastases are the most common malignancy of osseous tissue.[60,61] Approximately half of all people with cancer have bone metastasis at some point in their disease. Metastatic lesions are seen most often in the spine, femur, pelvis, ribs, sternum, proximal humerus, and skull, and are less common in anatomic sites more distant from the trunk of the body. Tumors that frequently spread to the skeletal system are those of the breast, lung, prostate, kidney, and thyroid, although any cancer can ultimately involve the skeleton. More than 85% of bone metastases result from primary lesions in the breast, lung, or prostate.[60] The incidence of metastatic bone disease is highest in persons older than 40 years of age.

The major symptom of bone metastasis is pain with evidence of an impending pathologic fracture.[60,61] It usually develops gradually, over weeks, and is more severe at night. Pain is caused by stretching of the periosteum of the involved bone or by nerve entrapment, as when the nerve roots of the spinal cord are compressed by the vertebral body. Pathologic fractures occur in approximately 10% to 15% of persons with metastatic bone disease. The affected bone appears to be eaten away on x-ray images; in severe cases, it crumbles on impact, much like dried toast. Many pathologic fractures occur in the femur, humerus, and vertebrae.

Radiographic examinations are used along with CT or bone scans to detect, diagnose, and localize metastatic bone lesions. Approximately one third of persons with skeletal metastases have positive bone scans without radiologic findings. This is because 50% of the trabecular bone must be destroyed before a lesion is visible on plain radiographs.[61] Arteriography using radiopaque contrast media may be helpful in outlining the tumor margins. A bone biopsy usually is done when there is a question regarding the diagnosis or treatment. A closed-needle biopsy with CT localization is particularly useful with spine lesions. Serum levels of alkaline phosphatase and calcium often are elevated in persons with metastatic bone disease.

The primary goals in treatment of metastatic bone disease are to prevent pathologic fractures and promote survival with maximum functioning, allowing the person to maintain as much mobility and pain control as possible. Standard treatment methods include chemotherapy, irradiation, and surgical stabilization. Radiation therapy is primarily used as a palliative treatment to alleviate pain and prevent pathologic fractures. After a pathologic fracture has occurred, bracing, intramedullary nailing of the femur, or spine stabilization may be done. Because adequate fixation often is difficult in diseased bone, cement (*i.e.,* methylmethacrylate) often is used with internal fixation devices to stabilize the bone.

Recent research has focused on the role of osteoclastic and osteoblastic activity in the pathogenesis of metastatic bone disease and on the use of the bisphosphonates (*e.g.,* pamidronate disodium, zoledronic acid) for its treatment.[62,63] Bone tissue contains a rich environment of growth factors and cells of various embryonic origins, including hematopoietic, stromal, endothelial, and other cell types. The osteoclasts and osteoblasts, in particular, appear to play a dominant role in the pathogenesis of bone metastasis. Osteoclasts are involved in osteolytic or destructive bone lesions and osteoblasts in the excessive production of new and poor-quality bone.[60] The bisphosphonates, which are now well-established agents for the prevention and treatment of osteoporosis, have recently been shown to decrease symptoms associated with bone metastasis secondary to breast and prostate cancer. These agents bind preferentially to bone at sites of active bone metabolism, are released from the bone matrix during bone resorption, and potentially inhibit osteoclast activity and survival, thereby reducing osteoclast-mediated bone resorption. Recent studies suggest that besides their strong antiosteoclastic activity, these agents may also have some direct antitumor effects.[63]

IN SUMMARY, bone tumors, like any other type of neoplasm, may be benign or malignant. Benign bone tumors grow slowly and usually do not destroy the surrounding tissues. Malignant tumors can be primary or metastatic. Primary bone tumors are rare, grow rapidly, metastasize to the lungs and other parts of the body through the bloodstream, and have a high mortality rate. Metastatic bone tumors usually are multiple, originating primarily from cancers of the breast, lung, and prostate. The incidence of metastatic bone disease probably is increasing because improved treatment methods enable persons with cancer to live longer. Advances in chemotherapy, radiation therapy, and surgical procedures have substantially increased the survival and cure rates for many types of bone cancers. A primary goal in metastatic bone disease is the prevention of pathologic fractures. ■

knee playing football, his mother insists that he be seen by an orthopedic specialist, who raises the possibility that the boy may have an osteosarcoma.

A. *Use the theory that osteosarcoma has its origin in sites of maximal growth velocity to explain the site of this boy's possible tumor.*

B. *What diagnostic tests could be used to establish a diagnosis of osteosarcoma?*

C. *The boy and his family are concerned that he will require radical surgery with amputation of the leg. How would you explain possible treatment options to him?*

Review Exercises

1. A 39-year-old man is in intensive care after a motorcycle crash in which he skidded across the pavement on his right side. He has fractures of his right femur, pelvis, and several ribs on the right side. His leg was crushed beneath the motorcycle. He is beginning to lose movement in his leg.

   A. *What are the priorities in treating his orthopedic injuries? What are the options for stabilizing his leg?*

   B. *What risk factors for complications of fractures are present?*

   C. *What are the symptoms of compartment syndrome, and how is it treated?*

2. A 73-year-old woman sustained a comminuted fracture in the mid-diaphysis of her left humerus when her husband lifted her up in bed. She has multiple lucent lesions scattered throughout her proximal humerus, radius, and ulna. She was recently hospitalized for confusion and was found to have diffuse bone metastases. Her bone marrow biopsy showed adenocarcinoma. She has a history of breast cancer 30 years ago, but her most recent mammogram was negative.

   A. *What would you consider to be the most likely cause of her fracture?*

   B. *What are the most common sites for bone metastasis?*

   C. *Explain the treatment goals for persons with pathologic fractures.*

3. A 14-year-old boy has complained of recent pain and swelling of his knee, with some restriction in movement. Although he thinks he may have injured his

References

1. National Centers for Disease Control and Prevention, Centers for Disease Control and Prevention. CDC Web-based Injury Statistics Query and Reporting System (wisqars database). [Online.] Available: www.cdc.gov/ncipc/wisqars/. Accessed September 1, 2007.
2. Arthritis Foundation. (2007). Safe or sorry: A guide to sport injury preventions. [Online.] Available: www.arthritis.org/ja-guide-sports-injury-prevention.php. Accessed April 14, 2008.
3. American Academy of Orthopaedic Surgeons. (2003). Pay attention to high school sports injuries. [Online.] Available: http://orthoinfo.aaos.org. Accessed April 14, 2008.
4. American Academy of Orthopedic Surgeons. (2003). Don't let a fall be your last trip. [Online.] Available: http://orthoinfo.aaos.org. Accessed April 14, 2008.
5. Gourlay M., Richy F., Reginstar J. Y. (2003). Strategies for the prevention of hip fracture. *American Journal of Medicine* 115, 309–317.
6. Hogan K. A., Gross R. H. (2003). Overuse injuries in pediatric athletes. *Orthopedic Clinics of North America* 34, 405–415.
7. Weintraub W. (2003). *Tendons and ligament healing* (pp. 11–47). Brookline, MA: Paradigm Publications.
8. Mercier L. R. (2000). *Practical orthopedics* (5th ed., pp. 6–18, 48–74, 171–173). St. Louis: Mosby.
9. Gomez J. E. (2002). Upper extremity injuries in youth sports. *Pediatric Clinics of North America* 49, 593–626.
10. Hegenroeder A., Chorley J. N. (2004). Sports injuries. In Behrman R. E., Kliegman R. M., Jenson H. B. (Eds.), *Nelson textbook of pediatrics* (17th ed., pp. 2302–2314). Philadelphia: Elsevier Saunders.
11. Fongemie A. E., Buss D. D., Rolnick S. J. (2001). Management of shoulder impingement syndrome and rotator cuff tears. *American Family Physician* 57, 667–679.
12. American Association of Orthopedic Surgeons. (2002). Meniscal tears. *AAOS Bulletin* (June). [Online.] Available: http://www2.aaos.org/aaos/archives/bulletin/jun02/acdnw20.htm. Accessed September 1, 2007.
13. Maitra R. S., Miller M. D., Johnson D. L. (1999). Meniscal reconstruction: I. Indications, techniques, and graft considerations. *American Journal of Orthopedics* 28, 213–218.
14. Maitra R. S., Miller M. D., Johnson D. L. (1999). Meniscal reconstruction: II. Indications, techniques, and graft considerations. *American Journal of Orthopedics* 28, 280–286.
15. O'Connor W. J., Botti T., Khan S. N., et al. (2000). The use of growth factors in cartilage repair. *Orthopedic Clinics of North America* 31, 399–409.
16. Brunner L., Eshilian-Oats L. (2003). Hip fractures in adults. *American Family Physician* 67, 537–542.
17. Zuckerman J. D. (1996). Hip fracture. *New England Journal of Medicine* 334, 1519–1525.

18. Bucholz R. W., Heckman J. D. (2006). *Rockwood & Green's fractures in adults* (6th ed., Vol. 1, p. 49). Philadelphia: Lippincott Williams & Wilkins.

19. Tull F., Borrelli J., Jr. (2003). Soft-tissue injury associated with closed fractures: Evaluation and management. *Journal of the American Academy of Orthopedic Surgeons* 11, 431–438.

20. Kretlek C., Goasling T. (2006). Principles of internal fixation. In Rockwood C. A., Green D. P., Bucholz R. W. (Eds.), *Rockwood & Green's fractures in adults* (6th ed., vol. 1, pp. 209–255). Philadelphia: Lippincott Williams & Wilkins.

21. Paley D., Catagni M., Argnani F., et al. (1992). Treatment of congenital pseudoarthrosis of the tibia using Ilizarov technique. *Clinical Orthopaedics and Related Research* 280, 81.

22. Hoch B. J., Klein M. J., Schiller A. L. (2008). Bones and joints. In Rubin R., Strayer D. S. (Eds.), *Rubin's pathology: Clinicopathologic foundations of medicine* (5th ed., pp. 1098–1390). Philadelphia: Lippincott Williams & Wilkins.

23. Einhorn T. A. (1998). The cell and molecular biology of fracture healing. *Clinical Orthopaedics and Related Research* 355(Suppl.), S7–S21.

24. Rosenberg A. (2005). Bones, joints, and soft tissue tumors. In Kumar V. Abbas A. K., Fausto N. (Eds.), *Robbins and Cotran pathologic basis of disease* (7th ed., pp. 1288–1303). Philadelphia: Elsevier Saunders.

25. Hayda R. A., Brighton C. T., Esterhai J. L. (1998). Pathophysiology of delayed healing. *Clinical Orthopaedics and Related Research* 355(Suppl.), S31–S36.

26. Peng H., Wright V., Usas A., et al. (2002). Synergistic enhancement of bone formation and healing of stem cell-expressed VECF and bone morphogenetic protein-4. *Journal of Clinical Investigation* 110, 751–759.

27. Hoover T. J., Siefert J. A. (2000). Soft tissue complications of orthopedic emergencies. *Emergency Medicine Clinics of North America* 18, 115–139.

28. Edwards S. (2004). Acute compartment syndrome. *Emergency Nursing* 12(3), 32–38.

29. Kostler W. Strom P. C., Sudkamp N. P. (2004). Acute compartment syndrome of the limb. *Injury* 35, 1221–1227.

30. McQueen M. M. (2006). Acute compartment syndrome. In Rockwood C. A., Green D. P., Bucholz R. W. (Eds.), *Rockwood & Green's fractures in adults* (6th ed., Vol. 1, pp. 426–443). Philadelphia: Lippincott Williams & Wilkins.

31. Mohler L. R., Styf J. R., Pedowitz R., et al. (1997). Intramuscular deoxygenation during exercise in patients who have chronic anterior compartment syndrome of the leg. *Journal of Bone and Joint Surgery (American Volume)* 79, 844–849.

32. Schwartzman R. (2000). New treatments for reflex sympathetic dystrophy. *New England Journal of Medicine* 343, 654–656.

33. Shojania K. G., Duncan B. W., McDonald K. M., et al. (Eds.). (2001). *Making health care safer: A critical analysis of patient safety practices.* Evidence Report/Technology Assessment no. 43. AHRQP publication 01-E058. Rockville, MD: Agency for Healthcare Research and Quality; 2001. [Online.] Available: www.ahrq.gov/clinic/ptsafety/. Accessed September 1, 2007.

34. Geerts W. H., Pineo G. F., Bergqvist D., et al. (2004). Prevention of venous thromboembolism: The seventh ACCP conference on antithrombotic and thrombolytic therapy. *Chest* 126, 338S–400S.

35. Dentali F., Douketis J. D., Gianni M., et al. (2007). Meta-analysis: Anticoagulant prophylaxis to prevent symptomatic venous thromboembolism in hospitalized medical patients. *Annals of Internal Medicine* 146, 278–288.

36. Parisi D. M., Koval K., Egot K. (2002). Fat embolism syndrome. *American Journal of Orthopedics* 31, 507–512.

37. Richards R. R. (1997). Fat emboli syndrome. *Canadian Journal of Surgery* 40, 334–339.

38. Mellor A., Soni M. (2001). Fat embolism. *Anaesthesia* 56, 145–154.

39. Arai F., Kia T., Nakai T., et al. (2007). Histopathologic features of fat embolism in fulminant fat embolism syndrome. *Anesthesiology* 107, 509–511.

40. Green N. E., Nania J. J. (2005). Bone and joint infections in children. In Weinstein S. L., Buckwalter J. A. (Eds.), *Turek's orthopedics: Principles and their application* (6th ed., pp. 123–150). Philadelphia: Lippincott Williams & Wilkins.

41. Lew D. P., Waldvogel F. A. (2004). Osteomyelitis. *Lancet* 364, 369–379.

42. Carek P. J., Dickerson L. M., Sack J. L. (2001). Diagnosis and management of osteomyelitis. *American Family Physician* 63, 2413–2420.

43. Calhoun J. J., Manring M. M. (2005). Adult osteomyelitis. *Infectious Disease Clinics* 19, 765–786.

44. Bratzle D. W., Houck P. M. (2005). Antimicrobial prophylaxis for surgery: An advisory statement from the National Surgical Infection Prevention Project. *American Journal of Surgery* 189, 395–404.

45. Taggart T., Kerry R. M., Norman P., et al. (2002). The use of vancomycin-impregnated cement beads in the management of infection in prosthetic joints. *Journal of Bone and Joint Surgery (British Volume)* 84, 70–72.

46. Ludwig B., Lazarus A. A. (2007). Musculoskeletal tuberculosis. *Disease of the Month* 53, 39–45.

47. Assouline-Dayan Y., Chang C., Greenspan A., et al. (2002). Pathogenesis and history of osteonecrosis. *Seminars in Arthritis and Rheumatism* 32, 94–124.

48. Mankin H. J. (1992). Nontraumatic necrosis of bone (osteonecrosis). *New England Journal of Medicine* 326, 1475–1479.

49. Childs S. G. (2005). Osteonecrosis: Death of bone cells. *Orthopedic Nursing* 24, 295–301.

50. Johnson E. O., Soultanis K., Soucacos P. N. (2004). Vascular anatomy and microcirculation of skeletal zones vulnerable to osteonecrosis: Vascularization of the femoral head. *Orthopedic Clinics of North America* 35, 285–291.

51. Migliorati C. A., Siegel M. A., Elting L. S. (2006). Bisphosphonate-associated osteonecrosis: A long-term complication of bisphosphonate treatment. *Lancet Oncology* 7, 508–514.

52. Reis N. O., Schwartz D., Miltianu D., et al. (2003). Hyperbaric oxygen therapy as a treatment for stage I avascular necrosis of the femoral head. *Journal of Bone and Joint Surgery (British Volume)* 85, 371–375.

53. American Cancer Society. (2006). Bone cancer detailed guide. [Online.] Available: www.cancer.org/docroot/CRI/content/CRI_2_4_7x_CRC_Bone_Cancer_PDF.asp. Accessed April 14, 2008.

54. Arndt C. S. (2004). Neoplasms of bone. In Behrman R. E., Kliegman R. M., Jenson H. B. (Eds.), *Nelson textbook of pediatrics* (16th ed., pp. 1714–1723). Philadelphia: Elsevier Saunders.

55. Hayden J. B., Hoang B. H. (2006). Osteosarcoma: Basic science and clinical implications. *Orthopedic Clinics of North America* 37, 1–7.

56. Mankin H. J., Hornicek F. J., Rosenberg A. E., et al. (2004). Survival data for 648 patients with osteosarcoma treated at one institution. *Clinical Orthopaedics and Related Research* 429, 286–291.

57. Grimer R. J., Taminiau A. M., Cannon S. R. (2002). Surgical outcomes in osteosarcoma. *Journal of Bone and Joint Surgery (British Volume)* 84, 395–400.

58. Matthews E., Snell K., Coats H. (2006). Intra-arterial chemotherapy for limb preservation in patients with osteosarcoma: Nursing implications. *Clinical Journal of Oncology Nursing* 10, 581–589.

59. Longhi A., Setola E., Versari M., et al. (2005). The role of chemotherapy in the treatment of bone and soft tissue sarcomas. *Current Orthopaedics* 19, 119–126.

60. Roodman G. D. (2004). Mechanisms of bone metastasis. *New England Journal of Medicine* 350, 1655–1664.

61. O'Keefe R. J., Schwartz E. M., Boyce B. F. (2000). Bone metastasis: An update on bone resorption and therapeutic strategies. *Current Opinion in Orthopedics* 11, 353–359.

62. Juan J., Pollock C. B., Kelly K. (2005). Mechanisms of cancer metastasis to the bone. *Cell Research* 15, 57–62.

63. Hershey M. S. (2004). Toward new horizons: The future of bisphosphonate therapy. *The Oncologist* 9(Suppl. 4), 38–47.

Visit the**Point** **http://thePoint.lww.com for animations, journal articles, and more!**

Disorders of Musculoskeletal Function: Developmental and Metabolic Disorders

KATHLEEN E. GUNTA

➤ The development of skeletal structures begins in utero and continues to change throughout life. During childhood, skeletal structures grow in length and diameter and sustain a large increase in bone mass. The term *modeling* refers to the formation of the macroscopic skeleton, which ceases at maturity, usually between 18 and 20 years of age. Once skeletal growth has attained its adult size, the process of bone remodeling is responsible for skeletal maintenance. It involves bone resorption and formation and is responsible for skeletal maintenance at sites that require replacement or repair. With aging, bone resorption and formation are no longer perfectly coupled, and there is loss of bone.

Skeletal disorders may develop as a result of abnormal growth and developmental processes due to hereditary or congenital influences. Other skeletal disorders can occur later in life as a result of nutritional deficiencies, metabolic disorders, hormonal influences, or the aging process. This chapter is divided into two parts: the first part focuses on alterations in skeletal growth and development, and the second on metabolic bone disorders.

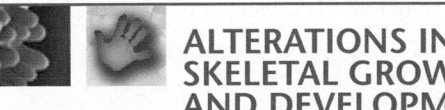

ALTERATIONS IN SKELETAL GROWTH AND DEVELOPMENT

After completing this section of the chapter, you should be able to meet the following objectives:

■ Describe the function of the epiphyseal growth plate in skeletal growth.
■ Describe common torsional deformities that occur in infants and small children, proposed mechanisms of development, diagnostic methods, and treatment.

(objectives continue)

- Define genu varum and genu valgum.
- List the problems that occur because of defective tissue synthesis in osteogenesis imperfecta.
- Characterize the abnormalities associated with developmental dysplasia of the hip and methods of diagnosis and treatment.
- Describe the treatment for a newborn with clubfoot.
- Define the term *osteochondroses* and describe the pathology and symptomatology of Legg-Calvé-Perthes disease and Osgood-Schlatter disease.
- Describe the pathology associated with a slipped capital femoral epiphysis and explain why early treatment is important.
- Differentiate between congenital, idiopathic, and neuromuscular scoliosis.

Bone Growth and Remodeling

Embryonic and Fetal Development

The skeletal system develops from the mesodermal and neural crest cells of the developing embryo[1] (see Chapter 48). Development of the vertebrae of the axial skeleton begins at approximately the fourth week in the embryo; during the ninth week, ossification begins with the appearance of ossification centers in the lower thoracic and upper lumbar vertebrae. The paddle-shaped limb buds of the lower extremities make their appearance late in the fourth week of development; the hand pads are developed by days 33 to 36; and the finger rays are evident on days 41 to 43.[1]

Abnormalities originating from the embryonic stage of development are relatively uncommon. When they do occur, they are usually limited to defined embryonic structures (*e.g.,* congenital absence of a phalanx; formation of extra bones [supernumerary digits], or fusion of adjacent digits [syndactylism]). The more common problems are caused by in utero positioning during fetal development. In the newborn, the imprint of in utero positioning may be evident and confused with an abnormality (to be discussed). The effects of in utero positioning are usually physiologic in origin, rather than anatomic. A child may be 3 to 4 years of age before the effects of in utero positioning resolve.

Bone Growth in Childhood

During the first two decades of life, the skeleton undergoes general overall growth. The long bones of the skeleton, which grow at a relatively rapid rate, are provided with a specialized structure called the *epiphyseal growth plate*. As long bones grow in length, the deeper layers of cartilage cells in the growth plate multiply and enlarge, pushing the articular cartilage farther away from the metaphysis and diaphysis of the bone.[2–4] As this occurs, the mature and enlarged cartilage cells at the meta-

physeal end of the plate become metabolically inactive and are replaced by bone cells (Fig. 58-1). This process allows bone growth to proceed without changing the shape of the bone or causing disruption of the articular cartilage. The cells in the growth plate stop dividing at puberty, at which time the epiphysis and metaphysis fuse.

Several factors can influence the growth of cells in the epiphyseal growth plate. Epiphyseal separation can occur in children as the result of trauma. The separation usually occurs in the zone of the mature enlarged cartilage cells, which is the weakest part of the growth plate. The blood vessels that nourish the epiphysis pass through the growth plate. These vessels are ruptured when the growth plate separates. This can cause cessation of growth and a shortened extremity. The growth plate also is sensitive to nutritional and metabolic changes. Scurvy (*i.e.,* vitamin C deficiency) impairs the formation of the organic matrix of bone, causing slowing of growth at the epiphyseal plate and cessation of diaphyseal growth. In rickets (*i.e.,* vitamin D deficiency), calcification of the newly developed bone on the metaphyseal side of the growth plate is impaired. Thyroid and growth hormones are required for normal growth. Alterations in these and other hormones can also affect growth (see Chapter 41).

Growth in the diameter of bones occurs as new bone is added to the outer surface of existing bone along with an accompanying resorption of bone on the endosteal or inner surface. Such oppositional growth allows for widening of the marrow cavity while preventing the cortex from becoming too thick and heavy. In this way, the shape of the bone is maintained. As a bone grows in diameter, concentric rings are added to the bone surface, much as rings are added to a tree trunk; these rings form the lamellar structure of mature bone. Osteocytes, which develop from osteoblasts, become buried in the rings. Haversian channels form as periosteal vessels running along the long axis become surrounded by bone (see Chapter 56, Fig. 56-2).

Alterations During Normal Growth Periods

Infants and children undergo changes in muscle tone and joint motion during growth and development. Toeing-in, toeing-out, bowlegs, and knock-knees occur frequently in infancy and childhood.[5] They usually cause few problems and are corrected during normal growth processes. The normal folded position of the fetus in utero causes physiologic flexion contractures of the hips and a froglike appearance of the lower extremities[6] (Fig. 58-2). The hips are externally rotated and the patellae point outward, whereas the feet appear to point forward because of the internal pulling force of the tibiae. During the first year of life, the lower extremities begin to straighten out in preparation for walking. Internal and external rotations become equal, and the hips extend.

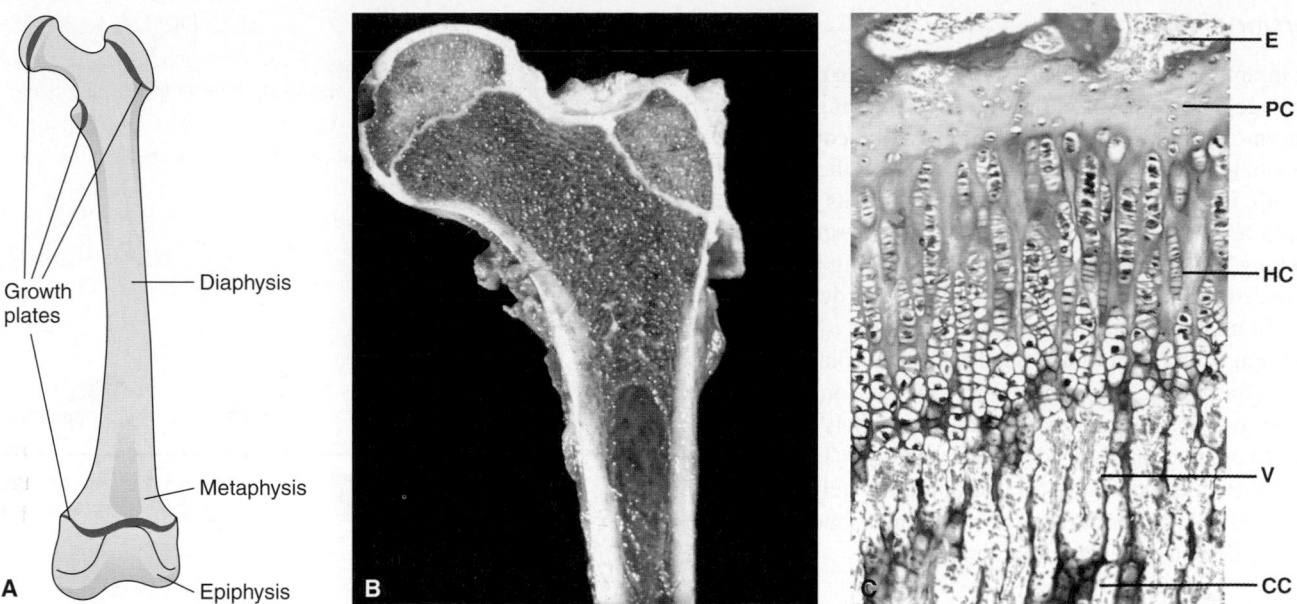

FIGURE 58-1 • Anatomy of long bone. **(A)** Diagram of femur illustrating the various compartments. **(B)** Coronal section of the proximal femur illustrates the various anatomic parts of a long bone. The epiphysis of the femoral head and the apophysis of the greater trochanter are separated from the metaphysis by their respective growth plates. The cortex and medullary cavity are well visualized. The medullary cavity contains cancellous bone until the metaphysis narrows into the diaphysis (shaft) of the bone, at which point the medullary cavity is completely devoid of bone and filled with marrow. **(C)** A section of the epiphysis with a zone of proliferating cartilage cells. Beneath this zone, the hypertrophic cartilage cells are arranged in columns. At the bottom, the calcifying matrix is invaded by blood vessels. E, epiphysis; PC, proliferative cartilage; HC, hypertrophic cartilage; V, vascular invasion; CC, calcified cartilage. (From Hoch B. J., Klein M. J., Schiller A. L. [2008]. Bones and joints. In Rubin R., Strayer D. S. [Eds.], *Rubin's pathology: Clinicopathologic foundations of medicine* [5th ed., p. 1086]. Philadelphia: Lippincott Williams & Wilkins.)

Musculoskeletal assessment of the newborn is important to identify abnormalities that require early intervention, facilitate treatment, establish baselines for future reference, and educate and counsel parents.[6–9] There are many clinical deviations that are easily correctable in a newborn. Many others correct spontaneously as the child grows.

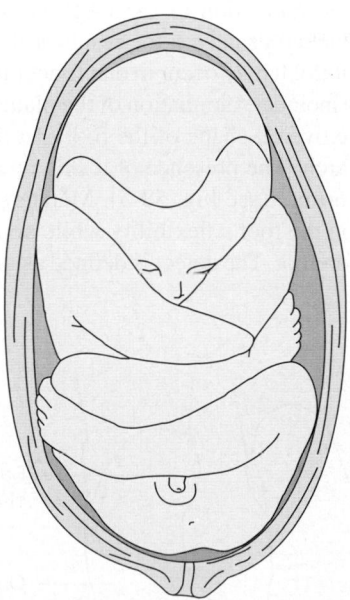

FIGURE 58-2 • Position of fetus in utero, with tibial bowing and legs folded. (From Dunne K. B., Clarren S. K. [1986]. The origin of prenatal and postnatal deformities. *Pediatric Clinics of North America* 33, 1282; with permission from Elsevier Science.)

 DEVELOPMENTAL SKELETAL DISORDERS

- Many disorders of early infancy are caused by intrauterine positions and resolve as the child grows.

- All infants and toddlers have lax ligaments that predispose to skeletal disorders caused by twisting or torsional forces.

- Bone growth in infants and children occurs at the epiphysis. Separation of the epiphyseal growth plate ruptures the blood vessels that nourish the epiphysis, causing cessation of growth and shortened extremity length.

- Nutritional and metabolic disorders can impair the formation of the organic matrix of bone, causing slowing of growth at the epiphyseal plate.

Torsional Deformities

All infants and toddlers have lax ligaments that become tighter with age and assumption of the weight-bearing posture. The hypermobility that accompanies joint laxity, coupled with the torsional (*i.e.*, rotational) forces exerted on the limbs during growth, is responsible for a number of variants seen in young children. Torsional forces caused by intrauterine positions or sleeping and sitting patterns twist the growing bones and can produce the deformities as a child grows and develops.

In infants, the femur normally is rotated to an anteverted position, with the femoral head and neck rotated anteriorly with respect to the femoral condyles. Femoral anteversion (*i.e.*, medial rotation) decreases from approximately 40 degrees at birth to approximately 15 degrees at maturity (Fig. 58-3). The normal tibia is externally rotated approximately 5 degrees at birth and 15 degrees at maturity. Torsional abnormalities frequently demonstrate a familial tendency.

Toeing-in and Toeing-out. The foot progression angle describes the angle between the axis of the foot and the line of progression. It is determined by watching the child walking and running, although it is usually less noticeable when the child is running or barefoot. Figure 58-4 illustrates the position of the foot in toeing-in and toeing-out, and the line of progression, when a child is walking.

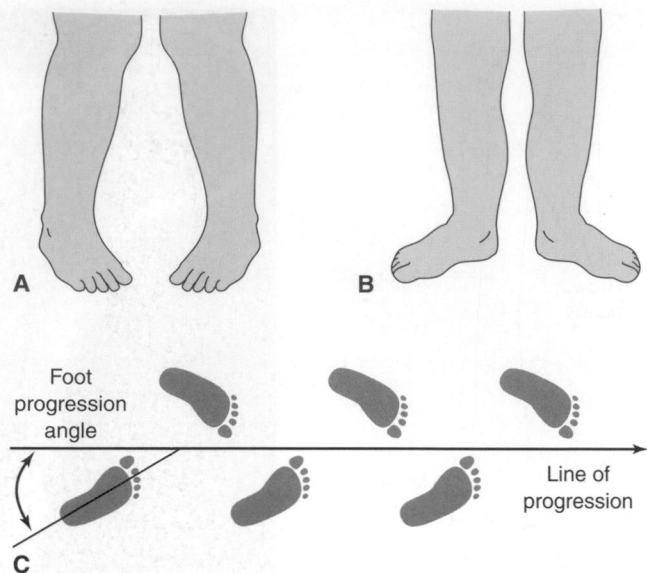

FIGURE 58-4 • (**A**) Toeing-in. (**B**) Toeing-out. (**C**) Toeing-in and toeing-out can be determined by watching a child walk and comparing the long axis of the foot with the direction in which the child is walking. If the foot is directed inward, the angle is negative and indicative of toeing-in; if it is positive, it is indicative of toeing-out.

Toeing-in (*i.e.*, metatarsus adductus) is the most common congenital foot deformity, with an incidence of approximately 1 to 2 per 1000, and it affects boys and girls equally.[7,8] The forefoot commonly is adducted and gives the foot a kidney-shaped appearance, whereas the hindfoot is normal[6–9] (Fig. 58-5). It can be caused by torsion in the foot, lower leg, or entire leg. Toeing-in due to adduction of the forefoot (*i.e.*, congenital metatarsus adductus) usually is the result of the fetal position maintained in utero. It may occur in one foot or both feet. Diagnostic methods include examination of the plantar aspect of the foot, noting the overall shape of the foot and the presence or absence of an arch. The presence of a skin crease indicates a congenital deformity (see Fig. 58-5). Metatarsus adductus is graded based on the foot's flexibility while applying pressure to the medial forefoot. The defect is defined as grade I, grade II,

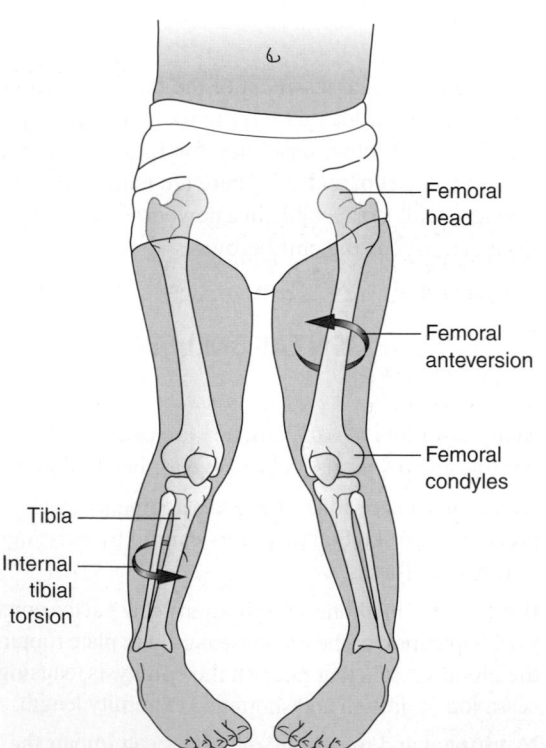

FIGURE 58-3 • Femoral anteversion and internal tibial rotation. Femoral anteversion normally decreases from about 40 degrees at birth to 15 degrees at maturity, and internal tibial rotation from 5 degrees at birth to 15 degrees at maturity.

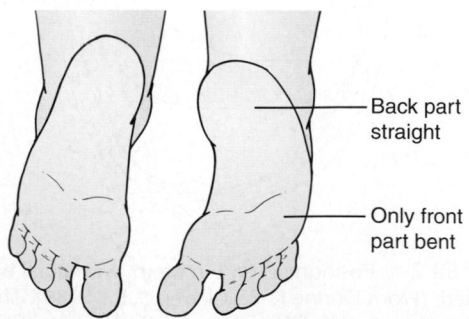

FIGURE 58-5 • Shape of foot. The left foot is normal, whereas the right foot has metatarsus adductus.

or grade III. Grade I is a supple deformity that can be passively manipulated into a straight position and requires no treatment. A grade II deformity corrects only to a straight lateral border, and a grade III deformity is more rigid and may require further treatment.[6] Treatment consisting of serial long leg casting or a brace that pushes the metatarsals (not the hindfoot) into abduction usually is required in a fixed (rigid) deformity (*i.e.,* one in which the forefoot cannot be passively manipulated into a straight position).

Toeing-out is a common problem in children and is caused by external femoral torsion. This occurs when the femur can be externally rotated to approximately 90 degrees but internally rotated only to a neutral position or slightly beyond. Because the femoral torsion persists when a child habitually sleeps in the prone position, an external tibial torsion also may develop. If external tibial torsion is present, the feet point lateral to the midline of the medial plane. External tibial torsion rarely causes toeing-out; it only intensifies the condition. Toeing-out usually corrects itself as the child becomes proficient in walking. Occasionally, a night splint is used.

Tibial Torsion. Tibial torsion is determined by measuring the thigh–foot angle, which is done with the ankle and knee positioned at 90 degrees (Fig. 58-6). In this position, the foot normally rotates outward. *Internal tibial torsion (i.e.,* bowing of the tibia) is a rotation of the tibia that makes the feet appear to turn inward (see Fig. 58-3). It is the most common cause of toeing-in in children younger than 2 years of age.[6] It is present at birth and may fail to correct itself if children sleep on their knees with the feet turned in, or sit on in-turned feet. It is thought to be caused by genetic factors and intrauterine compression, such as an unstretched uterus during a first pregnancy or intrauterine crowding with twins or multiple fetuses. Tibial torsion improves naturally with growth, but this may take years.[7]

External tibial torsion, a much less common disorder, is associated with calcaneovalgus foot and is caused by a normal variation of intrauterine positioning or a neuromuscular disorder. It is characterized by an abnormally positive thigh–foot angle of 30 to 50 degrees.[6] The condition corrects itself naturally, and treatment is observational. Significant improvement begins during the first year with the onset of ambulation, and usually is complete by 2 to 3 years of age.[6] The normal adult exhibits about 20 degrees of tibial torsion.

Femoral Torsion. *Femoral torsion* refers to abnormal variations in hip rotation. Hip rotation is measured at the pelvic level with the child in the prone position and the knees flexed at a 90-degree angle. In this position, the hip is in a neutral position. Rotating the lower leg outward produces internal or medial femoral rotation; rotating it inward produces external or lateral rotation. During measurement of hip rotation, the legs are allowed to fall to full internal rotation by gravity alone; lateral rotation is measured by allowing the legs to fall inward and cross. Hip rotation in flexion and extension also can be measured with computed tomography (CT). By 1 year of age, there is normally approximately 45 degrees of internal rotation and 45 degrees of external rotation.[6]

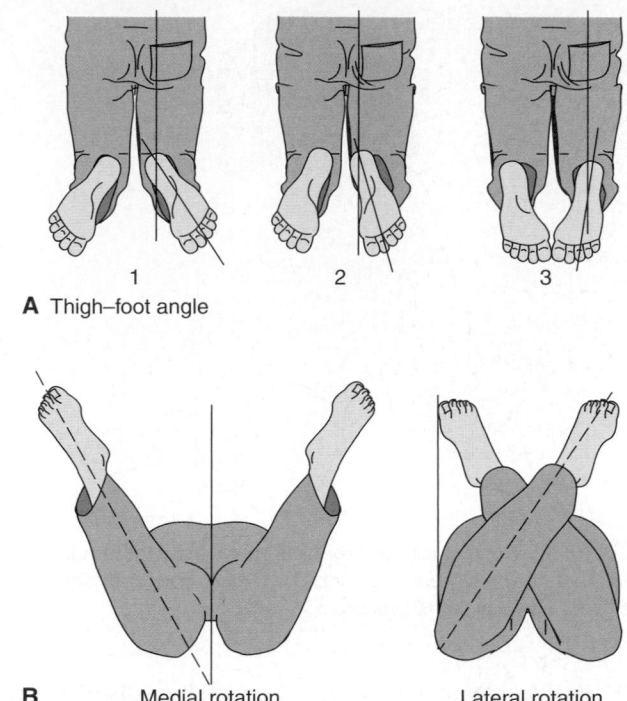

FIGURE 58-6 • **(A)** Assessment for tibial torsion using thigh–foot angle. When the child is in the prone position with the knee flexed, with normal alignment there is slight external rotation (2); internal tibial torsion produces inward rotation (3); external tibial torsion produces outward rotation (1). **(B)** Hip rotation is measured with the child prone and knees flexed at a 90-degree angle. On outward rotation the leg produces internal (medial) hip and femoral rotation; on inward rotation the leg produces external hip and femoral rotation. (Adapted from Staheli L. T. [1986]. Torsional deformity. *Pediatric Clinics of North America* 33, 1378; and Kliegman R. M., Neider M. I., Super D. M. [Eds.]. [1996]. *Practical strategies in pediatric diagnosis and therapy.* Philadelphia: W. B. Saunders.)

Internal femoral torsion, also called *femoral anteversion* (see Fig. 58-3), is a normal variant commonly seen during the first 6 years of life, especially in 3- and 4-year-old girls.[5] Characteristically, there is 80 to 90 degrees of internal rotation of the hip in the prone position.[7] The condition is thought to be related to increased laxity of the anterior capsule of the hip such that it does not provide the stable pressure needed to correct the anteversion that is present at birth. Children are most comfortable sitting in the "W" position, with their hips between their knees (Fig. 58-7). It is believed that this position allows the lower leg to act as a lever, producing torsional changes in the femur. When the child stands, the knees turn in and the feet appear to point straight ahead; when the child walks, the knees and toes point in. Children with this problem are encouraged to sit cross-legged or in the so-called *tailor position.* If left untreated, the tibiae compensate by becoming externally rotated so that by 8 to 12 years of age, the knees may turn in but the feet no longer do so. This can result in patellofemoral malalignment with patellar subluxation or dislocation and pain.[10] A derotational osteotomy may be done in severe cases or if there is functional disability.

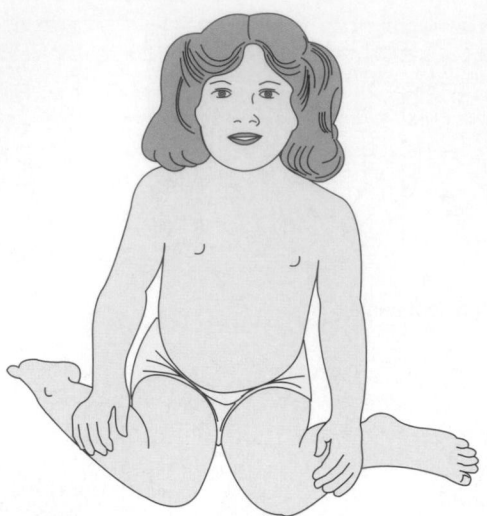

FIGURE 58-7 • Typical sitting position of child with femoral ante-version. (Adapted from Staheli L. T. [1986]. Torsional deformity. *Pediatric Clinics of North America* 33, 1382.)

External femoral torsion is an uncommon disorder characterized by excessive external rotation of the hip. Bilateral external torsion is usually a benign condition, and treatment is observational. When the disorder is unilateral, slipped capital femoral epiphysis should be excluded, particularly if the condition occurs in an obese child or young adolescent[6] (discussed later).

Genu Varum and Genu Valgum

Genu varum, or *bowlegs,* is an outward bowing of the knees greater than 1 inch when the medial malleoli of the ankles are touching. As children grow, lower limb alignment usually follows a predicable pattern (Fig. 58-8). Most infants and toddlers have some bowing of their legs up to 18 months of age. If there is a large separation between the knees (>15 degrees) after 2 years of age, the child may require bracing. The child also should be evaluated for diseases such as rickets or tibia vara (*i.e.,* Blount disease).[10]

Genu valgum, or *knock-knees,* is a deformity in which there is decreased space between the knees. The medial malleoli in the ankles cannot be brought in contact with each other when the knees are touching. Valgus gradually develops after age 24 months and is most apparent between 3 and 4 years of age (see Fig. 58-8). The condition usually is the result of lax medial collateral ligaments of the knee and may be exacerbated by sitting in the "M" position. By 7 years of age, the lower limb is in slight valgus and changes very little thereafter. Genu valgum can be ignored up to 7 years of age, unless it is more than 15 degrees, unilateral, or associated with short stature. It usually resolves spontaneously and rarely requires treatment. If genu varum or genu valgum persists and is uncorrected, osteoarthritis may develop in adulthood as a result of abnormal intra-articular stress. Genu varum can cause gait awkwardness and increased risk for sprains and fractures. Uncorrected genu valgum may cause subluxation and recurrent dislocation of the patella, with a predisposition to chondromalacia and joint pain and fatigue.

Idiopathic tibia vara, or *Blount disease,* is a developmental deformity of the medial half of the proximal tibial epiphysis that results in a progressive varus angulation below the knee[7,10,11] (Fig. 59-9). Onset can occur early in infancy, or later, during adolescence.[10,11] Untreated infantile tibia vera is almost always progressive, with evidence of outward angulation, flexion, internal rotation, and abnormal lateral knee laxity. There is radiographic evidence of progressive depression of the medial metaphysis, the growth plate, and the epiphysis. Fusion of the metaphysis to the epiphysis may occur in severe cases. Night-brace treatment is used for mild early-onset disease. Valgus rotational osteotomy of the tibia is usually indicated if angulation persists beyond 3 years of age. Persistent tibia vara leads to early degenerative changes of the knee.

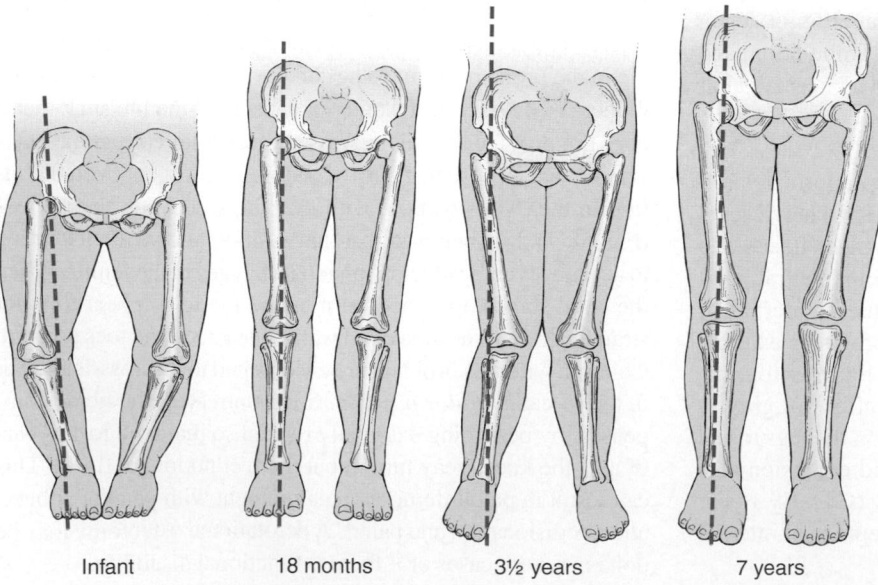

Infant   18 months   3½ years   7 years

FIGURE 58-8 • Lower limb alignment follows a predictable pattern. Infants typically have a gentle varus bow throughout the femur and tibia. By 18 to 24 months, the lower leg is nearly straight, with a neutral mechanical axis. Valgus gradually develops and is most apparent between 3 and 4 years of age. By 7 years of age, the lower limb is in slight valgus and changes very little thereafter. Varus should not recur, nor should valgus increase. (From Schoeneker P. L., Rich M. M. [2006]. The lower extremity. In Morissy R. T., Weinstein S. L. [Eds.], *Lovell & Winter's pediatric orthopaedics* [6th ed., pp. 1158–1213]. Philadelphia: Lippincott Williams & Wilkins.)

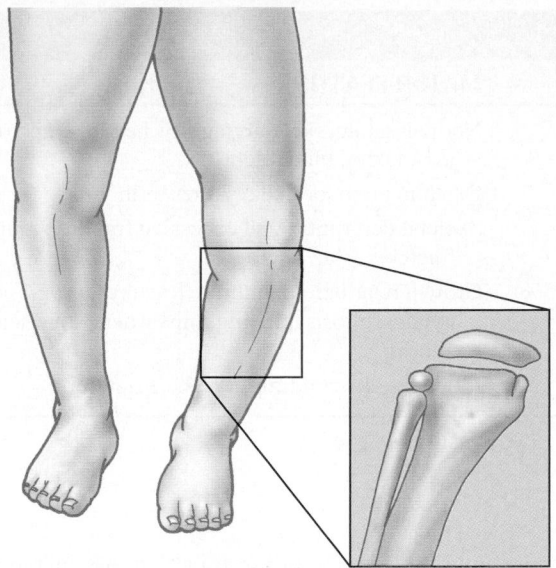

FIGURE 58-9 • Rotational deformity of the proximal tibia, especially when unilateral, suggests tibia vera (Blount disease).

Adolescent Blount disease occurs in the second decade of life, is seen in persons who are above the 95th percentile in height and weight, and is usually unilateral.[7] It is the most common cause of pathologic genu varum and is seen in obese boys.[10] Radiography shows medial femoral and tibial bowing. Bracing is not practical in obese adolescents. Treatment includes osteotomy to realign the limb or lateral growth plate closure to allow growth to "catch up" medially.

Flatfoot

Flatfoot (*i.e.,* pes planus) is a deformity characterized by the absence of the longitudinal arch of the foot. Infants normally have a wider and fatter foot than adults. The fat pads that normally are accentuated by pliable muscles create an illusion of fullness often mistaken for flatfoot. Until the longitudinal arch develops at 2 to 3 years of age, all children have flat feet. The true criterion for flatfoot is that the head of the talus points medially and downward, so that the heel is everted and the forefoot must be inverted (toed-in) for the metatarsal heads to be planted equally on the ground. Weight bearing may cause pain in the longitudinal arch and up the leg.

There are two types of flatfoot—flexible and rigid. Most children with flexible (or supple) flatfoot have loose ligaments, allowing the feet to sag when they gain weight. In supple flatfoot, the arch disappears only with weight bearing. No special treatment is needed for flexible flatfoot, and it usually is recommended that children with the disorder wear regular shoes.[6] People with flexible flatfoot are less prone to pain and injury than those with normal or high arches. The rigid flatfoot is fixed with no apparent arch in any position. It is seen in conjunction with congenitally tight heel cords, neuromuscular diseases such as cerebral palsy, or juvenile rheumatoid arthritis.[6]

In the adult, treatment of flatfoot is conservative and aimed at relieving fatigue, pain, and tenderness. Supportive, well-fitting shoes with arch supports may be helpful and prevent ligaments from becoming overstretched. Women may complain of pain in the forefoot when wearing poorly fitting high heels. Surgery may be done in cases of severe and persistent symptoms.

Hereditary and Congenital Deformities

Congenital deformities are abnormalities that are present at birth. They range in severity from mild limb deformities, which are relatively common, to major limb malformations, which are relatively rare. The most common anomaly of the toes or fingers is *polydactyly* or the presence of an extra digit on the hand or foot. Macrodactyly occurs when one or more toes or fingers are hypertrophied and are significantly larger than the surrounding toes or fingers.

There may also be a simple webbing of the fingers or toes (syndactyly), or the absence of a bone such as the phalanx, rib, or clavicle. Joint contractures and dislocations produce more severe deformity, as does the absence of entire bones, joints, or limbs. An epidemic of limb deformities occurred from 1957 to 1962 as a result of maternal ingestion of thalidomide. Surgery is done to relieve functional symptoms, such as pain or difficulty in fitting shoes. The cosmetic goal is to alter the grotesque appearance of the hand or foot and to achieve a similar size to the opposite extremity.

Congenital deformities are caused by many factors, some unknown. These factors include hereditary influences, external agents that injure the fetus (*e.g.,* radiation, alcohol, drugs, viruses), and intrauterine environmental factors. Many of the organic bone matrix components have been identified only recently, and their interactions were found to be more complex than originally thought. Hereditary disorders associated with abnormalities in bone matrix include those with deficient collagen synthesis and decreased bone mass.

Osteogenesis Imperfecta

Osteogenesis imperfecta is a hereditary disease characterized by defective synthesis of type I collagen.[4,12–14] It is one of the most common hereditary bone diseases, with an occurrence rate of approximately 1 case in 20,000 births.[12] Although it usually is transmitted as an autosomal dominant trait, a distinct form of the disorder with multiple lethal defects is thought to be inherited as an autosomal recessive trait.[14] In some cases, the defect is caused by a spontaneous mutation.

The clinical manifestations of osteogenesis imperfecta include a spectrum of disorders marked by extreme skeletal fragility. Four major subtypes of the disorder have been identified[4,12–14] (Table 58-1). The disorder is characterized by thin and poorly developed bones that are prone to multiple fractures. These children have short limbs and a soft, thin cranium with bifrontal prominences that give a triangular appearance to

TABLE 58-1 Types of Osteogenesis Imperfecta

TYPE	SUBTYPE	INHERITANCE	MAJOR FEATURES
I	Postnatal fractures, blue sclera	Autosomal dominant	Normal stature, skeletal fragility, hearing impairment, joint laxity, blue sclera
II	Perinatal, lethal	Autosomal recessive	Death in utero, or in days after birth
			Skeletal deformity with excessive fragility, multiple fractures, blue sclera
III	Progressive deformity	Autosomal dominant (75%) Autosomal recessive (25%)	Growth retardation, multiple fractures, progressive kyphoscoliosis, hearing impairment, blue sclera at birth
IV	Postnatal fractures, normal sclera	Autosomal dominant	Moderate skeletal fragility, short stature

Developed from Kumar V., Abbas A. K., Fausto N. (2005). *Robbins pathologic basis of disease* (7th ed., p. 1281). Philadelphia: Elsevier Saunders.

the face. Other problems associated with defective connective tissue synthesis include thin skin, blue or gray sclera, abnormal tooth development, hypotonic muscles, loose-jointedness, scoliosis, and a tendency toward hernia formation. Hearing loss due to otosclerosis of the tiny bones in the middle ear is common in affected adults.

The most serious defects occur when the disorder is inherited as a recessive trait (type II). Severely affected fetuses have multiple intrauterine fractures and bowing and shortening of the extremities. Many of these infants are stillborn or die during infancy. Less severe forms occur when the disorder is inherited as a dominant trait. The skeletal system is not as weakened, and fractures often do not appear until the child becomes active and starts to walk, or even later in childhood. These fractures heal rapidly, although with a poor-quality callus. In some cases, parents may be suspected of child abuse when the child is admitted to the health care facility with multiple fractures. There also is an increased incidence of complications such as hernias and congenital heart abnormalities.

There is no definitive treatment for correction of the defective collagen synthesis that is characteristic of osteogenesis imperfecta. However, the bisphosphonates (*e.g.,* pamidronate) have been shown to produce an increase in cortical bone width and cancellous bone volume, as well as increased bone strength and mineral content. In children treated with intravenous pamidronate, this has led to a decrease in fractures, improvements in mobility, and less pain.[12,13,15] Prevention and treatment of fractures is important. Precise alignment is necessary to prevent deformities. Nonunion is common, especially with repeated fractures. Surgical intervention often is needed to stabilize fractures and correct deformities (*e.g.,* internal fixation of long bones may be done with an intramedullary rod that "grows" with the child).

Developmental Dysplasia of the Hip

Developmental dysplasia of the hip (DDH), formerly known as *congenital dislocation of the hip,* is an abnormality in hip development that leads to a wide spectrum of hip problems in infants and children, including hips that are unstable, malformed, subluxated, or dislocated.[6,16–18] In less severe cases, the hip joint may be unstable, with excessive laxity of the joint capsule, or subluxated, so that the joint surfaces are separated and there is a partial dislocation (Fig. 58-10). With dislocated hips, the head of the femur is located outside of the acetabulum.

The results of newborn screening programs have shown that 1 of 100 infants have some evidence of hip instability, whereas dislocation of the hip is seen in 1 of every 1000 live births.[16] The left hip is involved more frequently than the right hip because of the left occipital intrauterine positioning of most infants.[10,16] The disorder occurs most frequently in first-born children and is six times more common in female than in male infants.[6] The cause of DDH is multifactorial, with heredity, environmental, and mechanical factors playing a role. A positive family history and generalized laxity of the ligaments are related. The increased frequency in girls is thought to result from their susceptibility to maternal estrogens and other hormones associated with pelvic relaxation. Dislocation also may result from environmental factors such as fetal position, a tight uterus that prevents fetal movement, and breech delivery. Approximately 30% to 50% of children with DDH have a history of breech presentation.[6] The presence of other congenital abnormalities is associated with an increased incidence of

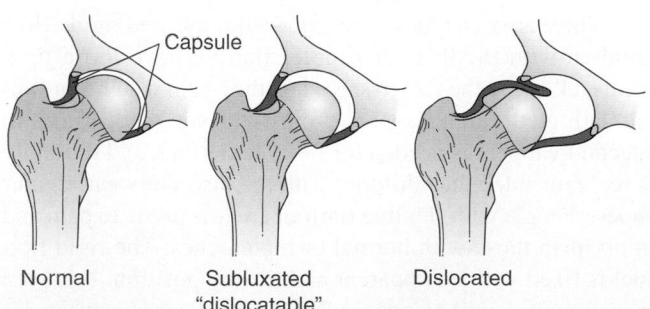

FIGURE 58-10 • Normal (**left**) and abnormal relationships of hip joint structure in subluxation (**middle**) and dislocation (**right**).

DDH. Thus, the hips of children presenting with congenital abnormalities should be examined carefully.

Early diagnosis of DDH is important because treatment is easiest and most effective if begun during the first 6 months of life. Also, repeated dislocations cause damage to the femoral head and the acetabulum. There is no uniformly accepted method for diagnosis of DDH during the newborn period, although clinical examination of the hips is recommended at birth and every several months during the first year of life.[17,18] Follow-up clinical examinations should be done in the presence of abnormality. In infants, signs of DDH include asymmetry of the hip or gluteal folds, shortening of the thigh so that one knee (on the affected side) is higher than the other hip, and limited abduction of the affected hip (Fig. 58-11). The asymmetry of gluteal folds is not definitive but indicates the need for further evaluation. The U.S. Preventive Services Task Force (USPSTF) recently concluded that evidence was insufficient to recommend routine screening of asymptomatic infants as a means of preventing adverse outcomes.[19]

Several examination techniques can be used to screen for a dislocatable hip.[16] Two specific maneuvers for assessing hip stability in the newborn are the Ortolani maneuver (for reducible dislocation) and the Barlow maneuver (for the dislocatable hip)[10,16–18] (Fig. 58-12). The Barlow maneuver involves a manual attempt to dislocate and reduce the abnormal hip while the infant is in the supine position with both knees flexed. With gentle downward pressure being applied to the knees, the knee and thigh are manually abducted as an upward and medial pressure is applied to the proximal thigh. In infants with the disorder, the initial downward pressure on the knee produces a dislocation of the hip, a positive Barlow sign. This is followed by a palpable or audible click (*i.e.*, Ortolani sign) as the hip is reduced and moves back into the acetabulum. The sensitivity of these tests is improved significantly with the use of trained and experienced examiners. The Galeazzi test is a measurement of the length of the femurs that is done by comparing the height at the knees while they are flexed at 90 degrees. An inequality in the height of the knees is a positive Galeazzi sign and is usually caused by hip dislocation or congenital femoral

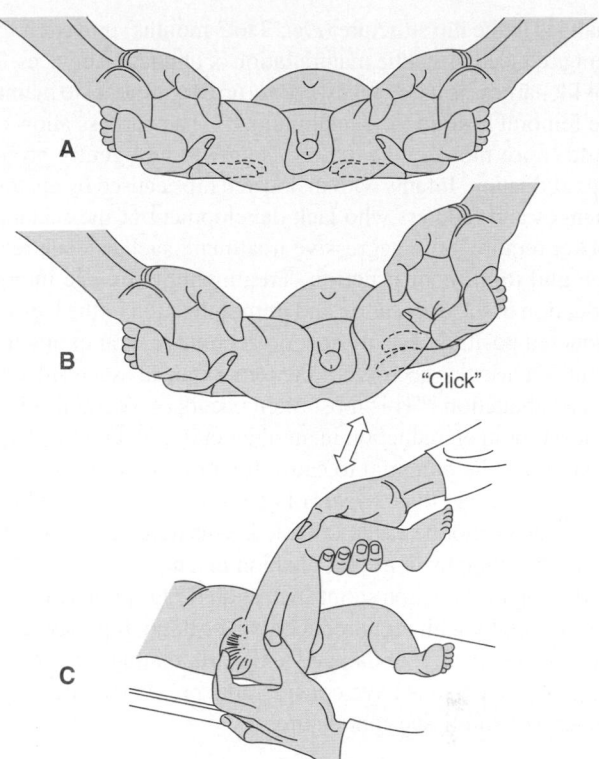

FIGURE 58-12 • Examination for developmental dysplasia of the hip. (**A**) In the newborn, both hips can be equally flexed, abducted, and externally rotated without producing a "click." (**B**) A diagnosis of congenital dislocation of the hip may be confirmed by the Ortolani "click" test. The involved hip cannot be abducted as far as the opposite one, and there is a "click" as the hip reduces. (**C**) Telescoping of the femur to aid in the diagnosis of a congenitally dislocated hip. (From Hoppenfeld S. [1976]. *Physical examination of the spine and extremities.* New York: Appleton-Century-Crofts.)

shortening. This test is not useful in detecting bilateral DDH because both leg lengths will be equal. In an older child, instability of the hip may produce a delay in standing or walking and eventually cause a characteristic waddling gait. When the thumbs are placed over the anterior iliac crest and the hands are placed over the lateral pelvis in examination, the levels of the thumbs are not even; the child is unable to elevate the opposite side of the pelvis (positive Trendelenburg test).

Diagnosis of DDH is confirmed by ultrasonography or radiography. Ultrasonography is used in infants with high risk factors (*e.g.*, female infants born in the breech position) or an abnormal result on examination.[10,16,17] Radiographs of newborns with suspected DDH are of limited value because the femoral heads do not ossify until 4 to 6 months of age. After 6 months of age, the increasing ossification of the femur renders ultrasonography less reliable, and radiographs are preferred.

Treatment of a DDH should be individualized and depends on whether the hip is subluxated or dislocated. Subluxation of the hip at birth often resolves without treatment and should be observed for 2 weeks. When subluxation persists beyond this time, treatment may be indicated and referral is recommended. The best results are obtained if the treatment is begun before

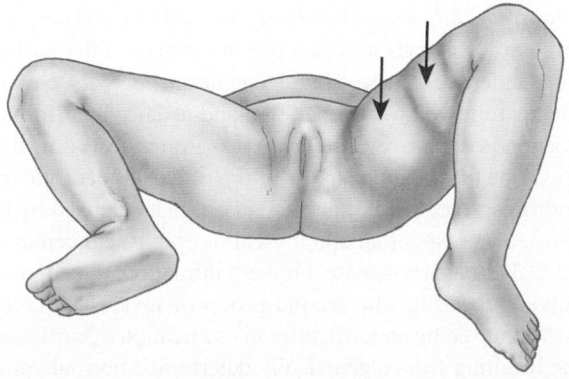

FIGURE 58-11 • Congenital dysplasia of the left hip with shortening of the femur, as indicated by legs in abduction and asymmetric gluteal and thigh folds (*arrows*).

changes in the hip structure (*e.g.,* 2 to 3 months) prevent it from being reduced by gentle manipulation or abduction devices. The Pavlik harness is used on newborns (up to 6 months) to maintain the femoral head in the acetabulum.[10,16] The harness allows the child more mobility as the leg is slowly and gently brought into abduction. Infants with dislocated hips caused by anatomic changes and toddlers who lack development of the acetabular socket require more aggressive treatment, such as open reduction and joint reconstruction. Treatment at any age includes reduction of the dislocation and immobilization of the legs in an abducted position. The most serious complication of any treatment is avascular necrosis of the femoral head as a result of the forced abduction.[16] This most often occurs as a complication of a closed or open reduction in an older child. In addition, hyperflexion has the potential to cause femoral nerve palsies. With children younger than 3 years of age, skin traction is used when reduction cannot be easily obtained. This treatment is followed by several months of immobilization in a hip spica cast, plaster splints, or an abduction splint such as an Ilfeld splint. Older children or adults with an unreduced dislocatable hip may require hip surgery because of damage to the articulating surface of the joint. These persons have considerable problems after surgery because of soft tissue contractures.

Congenital Clubfoot

Clubfoot, or talipes, is one of the most common pediatric orthopedic conditions. It has an incidence of approximately 1 to 2 cases per 1000 live births, is bilateral in about 50% of cases, and affects boys more often than girls.[6,20–22] Like congenital dislocation of the hip, its occurrence follows a multifactorial inheritance pattern. Clubfoot may be associated with chromosomal abnormalities or congenital syndromes that are transmitted by mendelian inheritance patterns. However, it is most commonly idiopathic and found in normal infants in whom no genetic or chromosomal abnormality or other extrinsic cause can be found. Maternal smoking is associated with occurrence of clubfoot, and the risk increases enormously in the presence of a family history.[23]

In forefoot adduction, which accounts for approximately 95% of idiopathic cases, the foot is plantar flexed and inverted. This is the so-called *equinovarus type* in which the foot resembles a horse's hoof (Fig. 58-13). The other 5% of cases are of the calcaneovalgus type, or reverse clubfoot, in which the foot is dorsiflexed and everted. The reverse clubfoot can occur as an isolated condition or in association with multiple congenital defects. At birth, the feet of many infants assume one of these two positions, but they can be passively overcorrected or brought back into the opposite position. If the foot cannot be overcorrected, some type of correction may be necessary.

Treatment of clubfoot is begun as soon as the diagnosis is made. When treatment is initiated during the first few weeks of life, a nonoperative procedure may be effective. Serial manipulations and casting are used gently to correct each component of the deformity. One method, called the *Ponseti method,* involves weekly gentle stretching and manipulation of the misaligned bones followed by application of a well-molded long leg plaster

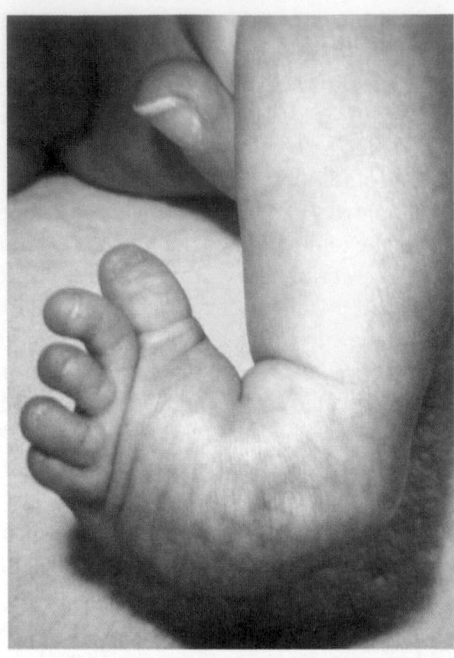

FIGURE 58-13 • Newborn with clubbing of the left foot. (Public Images Library, Centers for Disease Control and Prevention. ID#: 2632. Available at http://phil.cdc.gov/phil/detail.asp.)

cast with the knee held at a right angle.[22] The cast maintains the correction and allows for further relaxation of tight structures in anticipation of the next week's casting. Correction of the deformity is usually obtained within 6 to 8 weeks. Frequently, a percutaneous Achilles tendon lengthening is performed using a topical anesthetic cream before application of the final cast to allow for complete correction of the equinus deformity. The correction is maintained by full-time wear of a Denis Browne splint for 3 months and part-time night and nap wear for approximately 2 to 3 years.[22] Surgery may be required for severe deformities or when nonoperative treatment methods are unsuccessful. It is performed most commonly between 6 and 12 months of age.[6,10]

Juvenile Osteochondroses

The term *juvenile osteochondroses* is used to describe a group of children's diseases in which one or more growth ossification centers undergoes a period of degeneration, necrosis, or inactivity that is followed by regeneration and usually deformity. The osteochondroses are separated into two groups according to their causes. The first group consists of the true osteonecrotic osteochondroses, so called because the diseases are caused by localized osteonecrosis of an apophyseal or epiphyseal center (*e.g.,* Legg-Calvé-Perthes disease, Freiberg infraction, Panner disease, Kienböck disease). The second group of juvenile osteochondroses is caused by abnormalities in ossification of cartilaginous tissue resulting from a genetically determined normal variation or from trauma (*e.g.,* Osgood-Schlatter disease, Blount disease, Sever disease, Scheuermann disease). The discussion in this section focuses on Legg-Calvé-Perthes disease from the first group and Osgood-Schlatter disease from the second group. Slipped capital femoral epiphysis is a disorder of the growth plate.

Legg-Calvé-Perthes Disease

Legg-Calvé-Perthes disease is an idiopathic osteonecrotic disease of the proximal (capital) femoral epiphysis.[6,10] It occurs in 1 of 1200 children, affecting primarily those between ages 2 and 13 years, with a peak incidence between 3 and 9 years.[10,24] It occurs primarily in boys and is much more common in whites than African Americans. Although no definite genetic pattern has been established, it occasionally affects more than one family member.

The cause of Legg-Calvé-Perthes disease is unknown. The disorder usually is insidious in onset and occurs in otherwise healthy children. It may, however, be associated with acute trauma. Affected children usually have a shorter stature. Undernutrition has been suggested as a causative factor. When girls are affected, they usually have a poorer prognosis than boys because they are skeletally more mature and have a shorter period for growth and remodeling than boys of the same age. In most cases, only one leg is affected, but 10% to 20% of affected children have the condition in both legs.[25]

The primary pathologic feature of Legg-Calvé-Perthes disease is an avascular necrosis of the bone and marrow involving the epiphyseal growth center in the femoral head. The disorder may be confined to part of the epiphysis, or it may involve the entire epiphysis. In severe cases, there is a disturbance in the growth pattern that leads to a broad, short femoral neck. The necrosis is followed by slow absorption of the dead bone over 2 to 3 years. Although the necrotic trabeculae eventually are replaced by healthy new bone, the epiphysis rarely regains its normal shape. The process occurs in four predictable stages.[26] The *first stage,* which lasts for 6 to 12 months, is the avascular stage, during which the femoral head appears smaller and gradually increases in density. The ossification center becomes necrotic. Damage to the femoral head is determined by the degree of necrosis that occurs during this stage. The *second stage* is the regenerative or revascularization stage, during which resorption of the necrotic bone takes place. This stage usually lasts 1 to 3 years, during which the necrotic bone is gradually replaced by new immature bone cells and the contour of the bone is remodeled. The *third stage* is the reossification stage, during which radiolucent areas begin to ossify and become dense, while the shape of the femoral head improves. The *fourth stage,* which is the healed or residual stage, involves the formation and replacement of immature bone cells by normal bone cells and the resulting final shape of the femoral head.

The main symptoms of Legg-Calvé-Perthes disease are pain in the groin, thigh, or knee and difficulty in walking. The child may have a painless limp with limited abduction and internal rotation and a flexion contracture of the affected hip. The age of onset is important because young children have a greater capability for remodeling of the femoral head and acetabulum, and thus less flattening of the femoral head occurs. Early diagnosis is important and is based on correlating physical symptoms with radiographic findings that are related to the stage of the disease.

The goal of treatment is to reduce deformity and preserve the integrity of the femoral head. Conservative and surgical interventions are used in the treatment of Legg-Calvé-Perthes disease. Children younger than 4 years of age with little or no involvement of the femoral head may require only periodic observation. In all other children, some intervention is needed to relieve the force of weight bearing, muscular tension, and subluxation of the femoral head. It is important to maintain the femur in a well-seated position in the concave acetabulum to prevent deformity. This is done by keeping the hip in abduction and mild internal rotation. Treatment involves periods of rest, use of assistive devices for walking, non–weight bearing, and abduction braces to keep the legs separated in abduction with mild internal rotation. The Atlanta Scottish Rite brace, which does not extend below the knee, is the most widely used orthosis because it provides containment while allowing free knee motion and ambulation without crutches or external support[6,10] (Fig. 58-14). Surgery may be done to contain the femoral head in the acetabulum. This treatment usually is reserved for children older than 6 years of age who at the time of diagnosis have more serious involvement of the femoral head. The best surgical results are obtained when surgery is done early, before the epiphysis becomes necrotic.

Osgood-Schlatter Disease

Osgood-Schlatter disease involves microfractures in the area where the patellar tendon inserts into the tibial tubercle, which is an extension of the proximal tibial epiphysis.[6] This area is

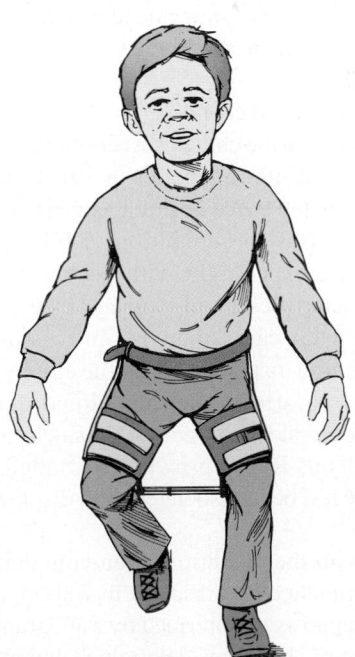

FIGURE 58-14 • Scottish Rite brace for Legg-Calvé-Perthes disease produces containment for abduction and allows free knee motion. (From Johnson K. B., Oski F. A. [1997]. *Oski's essential pediatrics.* Philadelphia: Lippincott-Raven.)

particularly vulnerable to injury caused by sudden or continued strain from the patellar tendon during periods of growth, particularly in athletic individuals. It occurs most frequently in boys between the ages of 11 and 15 years and in girls between 8 and 13 years.

The disorder is characterized by pain in the front of the knee that is associated with inflammation and thickening of the patellar tendon. The pain usually is associated with specific activities such as kneeling, running, bicycle riding, or stair climbing. There is swelling, tenderness, and increased prominence of the tibial tubercle. The symptoms usually are self-limiting. They may recur during growth periods, but usually resolve after closure of the tibial growth plate. In some cases, limitations on activity, tibial bands, or braces to immobilize the knee; anti-inflammatory agents; and application of cold are necessary to relieve the pain. The objective of treatment is to release tension on the quadriceps to permit revascularization and reossification of the tibial tubercle. Complete resolution of symptoms through healing (physical closure) of the tibial tubercle usually requires 12 to 24 months.[6] Occasionally, minor symptoms or an increased prominence of the tibial tubercle may continue into adulthood. In some cases, a high-riding patella can cause dislocation with chondromalacia of the patella and result in degenerative arthritis.

Slipped Capital Femoral Epiphysis

Slipped capital femoral epiphysis, or coxa vara, is a disorder of the growth plate that occurs near the age of skeletal maturity. It involves a three-dimensional displacement of the epiphysis (posteriorly, medially, inferiorly), meaning that the femur is rotated externally from under the epiphysis. The condition is rare, with an estimated frequency of between 1 in 100,000 and 1 in 800,000.[10]

The cause of slipped capital femoral epiphysis is obscure, but it may be related to the child's susceptibility to stress on the femoral neck as a result of genetics or structural abnormalities. Boys are affected twice as often as girls, and in approximately half of cases the condition is bilateral. Affected children often are overweight with poorly developed secondary sex characteristics, or, in some instances, are extremely tall and thin. In many cases, there is a history of rapid skeletal growth preceding displacement of the epiphysis. The condition also may be affected by nutritional deficiencies or endocrine disorders such as hypothyroidism, hypopituitarism, and hypogonadism. Rapid growth after administration of growth hormone has been associated with displacement of the epiphysis.

Children with the condition often complain of referred knee pain accompanied by difficulty in walking, fatigue, and stiffness. The diagnosis is confirmed by radiographic studies in which the degree of slipping is determined and graded according to severity (mild, <33%; moderate, 33% to 50%; and severe, >50%).[10] Early treatment is imperative to prevent lifelong crippling. Avoidance of weight bearing on the femur and bed rest are essential parts of the treatment. Traction or gentle manipulation

under anesthesia is used to reduce the slip. Surgical insertion of pins to keep the femoral neck and head of the femur aligned is a common method of treatment for children with moderate or severe slips. Crutches are used for several months after surgical correction to prevent full weight bearing until the growth plate closes.

Children with the disorder must be followed closely until the epiphyseal plate closes. Long-term prognosis depends on the amount of displacement that occurs. Complications include avascular necrosis, leg shortening, malunion, and problems with the internal fixation. Degenerative arthritis may develop, requiring joint replacement later in life.

Scoliosis

Scoliosis is a lateral deviation of the spinal column that may or may not include rotation or deformity of the vertebrae. The majority of scoliotic deformities are idiopathic. Others can be congenital, associated with neuromuscular disorders or intraspinal deformities, or are caused by compensation for leg-length discrepancy.[6] The estimated prevalence of scoliosis in the adolescent population is approximately 2%, using a definition of a spinal curve of greater than 10 degrees.[27] The prevalence of curves greater than 30 degrees is 0.1% to 0.2%.[28]

Scoliosis is classified as postural or structural. With postural scoliosis, there is a small curve that corrects with bending. It can be corrected with passive and active exercises. Structural scoliosis does not correct with bending. It is a fixed deformity classified according to the cause: congenital, neuromuscular, or idiopathic.

Congenital Scoliosis

Congenital scoliosis is caused by disturbances in vertebral development during the sixth to eighth weeks of embryologic development.[6,28,29] Congenital scoliosis may be divided into failures of formation and failures of segmentation. Failures of formation indicate the absence of a portion of the vertebra, such as hemivertebra (absence of a whole side of the vertebra) and wedge vertebra (missing only a portion of the vertebra). Failure of segmentation is the absence of the normal separation between the vertebrae.[6] The child may have other anomalies and neurologic complications if the spine is involved. Early diagnosis and treatment of progressive curves are essential for children with congenital scoliosis. Surgical intervention is the treatment of choice for progressive congenital scoliosis.[6]

Neuromuscular Scoliosis

Neuromuscular scoliosis develops from neuropathic or myopathic diseases. It is seen with cerebral palsy, myelodysplasia, and poliomyelitis. There is often a long, C-shaped curve from the cervical to the sacral region. In children with cerebral palsy, severe deformity may make treatment difficult. Myopathic neuromuscular scoliosis develops with Duchenne muscular dystrophy and usually is not severe.

Idiopathic Scoliosis

Idiopathic scoliosis is a structural spinal curvature for which no cause has been established. It occurs in healthy, neurologically normal children. Although the incidence is only slightly greater in girls than boys, it is more likely to progress and require treatment in girls.[6,28] The cause is most likely complex and multifactorial. It seems likely that heredity is involved because mother–daughter pairings are common, but identical twins are not uniformly affected. The magnitude of the curvature in an affected individual is not related to magnitude of curvature in relatives. A recent study of the melatonin receptor 1B (*MTNR1B*) gene in persons with adolescent idiopathic scoliosis suggests that *MTNR1B* may serve as a susceptibility gene for adolescent idiopathic scoliosis.[30]

Idiopathic scoliosis can be divided into three groups on the basis of age at onset: infantile (birth to 3 years), juvenile (4 to 10 years), and adolescent (11 years and older).[6,28] The infantile form is rare in the United States. It is seen primarily in the United Kingdom and Europe. It affects boys more often than girls, and the curvature usually is convex and to the left rather than to the right, as in other forms of scoliosis. Although most forms of juvenile scoliosis regress spontaneously, some progress and are difficult to treat effectively. Juvenile idiopathic scoliosis is uncommon. However, in many children with the diagnosis of adolescent scoliosis, the onset may have occurred when they were juveniles but was not diagnosed until later. Adolescent scoliosis is the most common type, accounts for approximately 80% of cases, and is seen most commonly in girls. An increase in joint laxity, which causes excessive joint motion and is found commonly in girls, has been associated with the development of idiopathic scoliosis. Delayed puberty and menarche are other risk factors for the development of adolescent scoliosis.[31]

Although a scoliotic curve may be present in any area of the spine, the most common curve is a right thoracic curve, which produces a rib prominence on the convex side and hypokyphosis from rotation of the vertebral column around its long axis as the spine begins to curve. A spinal curvature of less than 10 degrees is considered a normal variant, not scoliosis.[28] Curves greater than 40 degrees usually are considered severe.

Manifestations. Scoliosis usually is first noticed because of the deformity it causes. A high shoulder, prominent hip, or projecting scapula may be noticed by a parent or in a school-based screening program (Fig. 58-15). In girls, difficulty in hemming or fitting a dress may call attention to the deformity. Idiopathic scoliosis usually is a painless process, although pain may be present in severe cases, usually in the lumbar region. The pain may be caused by pressure on the ribs or on the crest of the ilium. There may be shortness of breath as a result of diminished chest expansion and gastrointestinal disturbances from crowding of the abdominal organs. Adults with less severe deformity may experience mild backache. If scoliosis is left untreated, the curve may progress to an extent that compro-

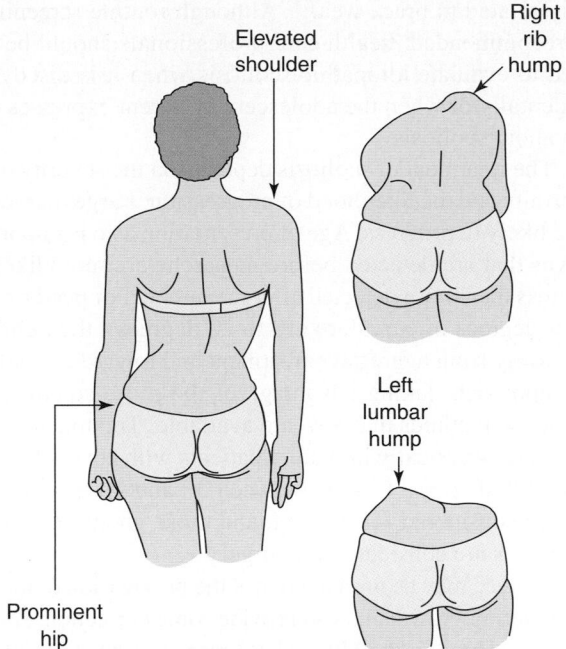

FIGURE 58-15 • Scoliosis: abnormalities to be determined at initial screening examination. (From Gore D. R., Passehl R., Sepic S., et al. [1981]. Scoliosis screening: Results of a community project. *Pediatrics 67*, 196–200. Copyright 1981 by the American Academy of Pediatrics.)

mises cardiopulmonary function and creates a risk for neurologic complications.

Diagnosis and Treatment. Early diagnosis of scoliosis can be important in the prevention of severe spinal deformity. The cardinal signs of scoliosis are uneven shoulders or iliac crest, prominent scapula on the convex side of the curve, malalignment of spinous processes, asymmetry of the flanks, asymmetry of the thoracic cage, and rib hump or paraspinal muscle prominence when bending forward (see Fig. 58-15). A complete physical examination is necessary for children with scoliosis because the defect may be indicative of other, underlying pathologic processes.

Diagnosis of scoliosis is made by physical examination and confirmed by radiography. A scoliometer should be used at the apex of the curvature to quantify a prominence; a scoliometer reading of greater than 10 degrees requires referral to a physician. The curve is measured by determining the amount of lateral deviation present on radiographs and is labeled "right" or "left" for the convex portion of the curve. Other radiographic procedures may be done, including CT scanning, magnetic resonance imaging (MRI), and myelography.

Although school screening continues to be mandated in a number of states, the USPSTF recommends against the routine screening of asymptomatic adolescents for idiopathic scoliosis, indicating that the potential harms from screening include unnecessary follow-up visits and evaluations due to false-positive results, and adverse psychological effects, especially related to brace wear.[32] Although routine screening is not recommended, health care professionals should be prepared to evaluate idiopathic scoliosis when it is discovered incidentally or when the adolescent or parent expresses concern about scoliosis.[32]

The treatment of scoliosis depends on the severity of the deformity and the likelihood of progression. Larger curves are more likely to progress. Age of presentation also is important. Curves that are detected before menarche are more likely to progress than those detected after menarche. For persons with lesser degrees of curvature (10 to 20 degrees), the trend has been away from aggressive treatment and toward a "wait and see" approach, taking advantage of the more sophisticated diagnostic methods that now are available. Treatment is considered for physically immature patients with curves between 20 and 30 degrees. Curves between 30 and 40 degrees usually are considered for bracing, and those greater than 40 to 45 degrees are considered for surgery.

A brace may be used to control the progression of the curvature during growth and can provide some correction. A commonly used brace is the Milwaukee brace, which was developed by Blount and Schmitt in the 1940s. This was the first brace to provide some degree of active correction. It involves a pelvic mold, various pads, and two metal upright supports around the throat. It is cumbersome, and compliance with wearing the brace has been shown to be poor. In an effort to improve compliance, a number of new bracing techniques have been developed. They include underarm or thoracolumbosacral orthoses. These orthoses consist of easily concealed, prefabricated forms that are modified to suit the patient.

Surgical intervention with instrumentation and spinal fusion is done in severe cases—when the curvature has progressed to 40 degrees or more at the time of diagnosis or when curves of a lesser degree are compounded with imbalance or rotation of the vertebrae. Unlike bracing, which is intended to halt progression of the curvature, surgical intervention is used to decrease the curve. Instrumentation helps correct the curve and balance, and spinal fusion maintains the spine in the corrected position.[6,28,29] Several methods of instrumentation (i.e., rods that attach to the vertebral column and posterior fusion) are used. Combined anterior and posterior surgery is used for more severe curvatures. The newer systems provide better sagittal control and more stable fixation, which allow earlier mobility. Despite great advances in spinal surgery, no one method seems to be the best for all cases. There is recent interest in growth modulation approaches using minimally invasive techniques, which will result in curve correction while maintaining spinal motion and disk and motion segment integrity.[33]

IN SUMMARY, skeletal disorders can result from congenital or hereditary influences or from factors that occur during normal periods of skeletal growth and development. Newborn infants undergo normal changes in muscle tone and joint motion, causing torsional conditions of the femur or tibia. Many of these conditions are corrected as skeletal growth and development take place. Osteogenesis imperfecta is a rare autosomal hereditary disorder characterized by defective synthesis of connective tissue, including bone matrix. It results in poorly developed bones that fracture easily. Developmental dysplasia of the hip includes a range of structural abnormalities. Dislocated hips are always treated to prevent changes in the anatomic structure. Other childhood skeletal disorders, such as the osteochondroses, slipped capital femoral epiphysis, and scoliosis, are not corrected by the growth process. These disorders are progressive, can cause permanent disability, and require treatment. Disorders such as developmental dysplasia of the hip and congenital clubfoot are present at birth. Both of these disorders are best treated during infancy. Regular examinations during the first year of life are recommended as a means of achieving early diagnosis of such disorders.

Scoliosis is a lateral deviation of the spinal column that may or may not include rotation or deformity of the vertebrae. Scoliosis is classified as postural, which corrects with bending, or structural, which does not. Structural scoliosis is a fixed deformity classified according to the cause: congenital, which results from defects in vertebral development; neuromuscular, which is caused by diseases such as cerebral palsy; and idiopathic, which is the most common form. Curves between 30 and 40 degrees usually are considered for bracing, and those greater than 40 to 45 degrees are considered for surgery. ■

METABOLIC BONE DISEASE

After completing this section of the chapter, you should be able to meet the following objectives:

■ Cite the origin of osteoclasts and osteoblasts and describe their functions in bone remodeling.

■ Describe the function of the RANK ligand/RANK receptor, and the osteoprotegerin-blocking molecule in the regulation of bone remodeling.

■ Describe risk factors that contribute to the development of osteoporosis and relate them to the prevention of the disorder.

■ Describe the primary features of osteoporotic bone.

■ Explain the methods used in the diagnosis of osteoporosis.

■ Describe the actions of medications used in the treatment of osteoporosis.

■ Compare the pathogenesis and manifestations of osteomalacia and rickets.

■ Characterize the cause and manifestations of Paget disease.

Bone is an admixture of inorganic elements and organic matrix that is in a constant state of bone resorption and bone formation. The inorganic elements include the calcium and phosphorus that mineralize bone, and the organic matrix includes bone cells and matrix proteins. The bone cells include the osteoprogenitor cells, the osteoblasts, and the osteoclasts[6,34–36] (see Chapter 56). The osteoprogenitor cells are pluripotent mesenchymal cells that are located in the vicinity of all bony surfaces. When appropriately stimulated by growth factors such as bone morphogenic proteins (BMPs), fibroblast growth factor (FGF), platelet-derived growth factor (PDGF), insulin-like growth factor, and transforming growth factor-β (TGF-β), they undergo cell division and differentiate into osteoblasts. The osteoblasts are the bone-forming cells. They also initiate the process of mineralization. Osteoblasts express cell surface receptors that bind a number of hormones (parathyroid hormone, vitamin D, estrogen), cytokines, and growth factors. The osteoclast is the cell responsible for bone resorption.[6,34–36] It is derived from the same hematopoietic precursor that gives rise to blood monocytes and tissue macrophages. The cytokines and growth factors crucial to osteoclast differentiation and maturation include the interleukins, tumor necrosis factor (TNF), and colony-stimulating factors (CSFs; discussed in Chapter 12). These factors function either by stimulating osteoclast progenitor cells or participating in a paracrine system in which osteoblasts and marrow stromal cells play a central role.

Osteoblasts and osteoclasts act in coordination and are considered the functional unit of bone, known as the *basic multicellular unit.* The processes of bone formation and resorption are tightly coupled, and their balance determines skeletal mass at any time. As the skeleton grows and enlarges during childhood, a process called *bone modeling* predominates. It results in a bone having adult form and shape. Peak bone mass is achieved during early adulthood after cessation of modeling. It is determined by a number of factors, including the type of vitamin D receptor inherited, nutrition, level of physical activity, age, and hormonal status. Once skeletal growth has attained its adult size, the breakdown and renewal of bone that is responsible for skeletal maintenance is initiated at sites that require replacement or repair. This process is called *bone remodeling.*

The sequence of bone resorption and bone formation begins with osteoclastic resorption of existing bone, during which the organic (protein matrix) and the inorganic (mineral) components are removed. The sequence proceeds to the formation of new bone by osteoblasts. In the adult, the length of one sequence (*i.e.,* bone resorption and formation) is approximately 4 months. Ideally, the replaced bone should equal the absorbed bone. If it does not, there is a net loss of bone. In the elderly, for example, bone resorption and formation no longer are perfectly coupled, and bone mass is lost.

It is only recently that significant progress has been made in understanding the phenomenon of bone remodeling as it relates to the coupling of bone resorption with bone formation. The pivotal paracrine pathway linking these two processes consists of three factors: the *r*eceptor *a*ctivator of *n*uclear factor κB *l*igand (RANKL); its receptor RANK; and a soluble inhibitor receptor for RANKL, osteoprotegerin (OPG).[6,34–36] RANKL is a member of the TNF superfamily and both RANK and OPG are members of the TNF receptor family. RANKL is expressed by osteoblasts and their immature precursors and is necessary for osteoclast differentiation and function. RANKL activates its receptor, RANK, which is expressed on osteoclasts and their precursors, thus promoting osteoclast differentiation and activation and prolonging osteoclast survival by suppressing apoptosis. The fact that RANKL is expressed on osteoblasts indicates that bone reabsorption and bone formation are linked through RANKL. The term *osteoprotegerin* was coined because of its protective effects against bone loss, detected in animal studies. The effects of RANKL are blocked by OPG, a soluble receptor protein, which acts as a decoy receptor that binds RANKL and prevents it from binding with RANK on osteoclasts.

It is now believed that dysregulation of the RANKL/RANK/OPG pathway plays a prominent role in the pathogenesis of bone diseases such as osteoporosis.[35] For example, it has been shown that postmenopausal women express higher levels of RANKL on their marrow stromal cells and lymphocytes than premenopausal women or postmenopausal women taking estrogen. It has also been shown that estrogens and the selective estrogen receptor modulator, raloxifene, stimulate OPG production in osteoblasts. Glucocorticoid exposure, which can contribute to steroid osteoporosis, enhances RANKL expression and suppresses OPG levels, thus elevating the RANKL-to-OPG ratio. There is also evidence linking the pathogenesis of inflammatory conditions such as rheumatoid arthritis to dysregulation of the RANKL/OPG system. Based on animal models of rheumatoid arthritis, cytokines differentially regulate RANKL and OPG, producing an enhanced RANKL-to-OPG ratio that favors skeletal damage. There is also evidence that RANKL is expressed on T cells, and in vitro studies have shown that activated T cells can regulate the development and activation of osteoclasts through RANKL.[35]

METABOLIC BONE DISORDERS

- Metabolic bone disorders have their origin in the bone remodeling process that involves an orderly sequence of osteoclastic bone reabsorption, the formation of new bone by the osteoblasts, and mineralization of the newly formed osteoid tissue.

- Osteoporosis represents an increased loss of total bone mass due to an imbalance between bone absorption and bone formation, most often related to the aging process and decreased estrogen levels in postmenopausal women.

- Osteomalacia and rickets represent a softening of bone due to inadequate mineralization of the bone matrix caused by a deficiency of calcium or phosphate.

- Paget disease is a disorder involving excessive bone destruction and repair, resulting in structural deformities of the long bones, spine, pelvis, and cranium.

Understanding • Understanding Bone Remodeling

Bone remodeling constitutes a process of skeletal maintenance once skeletal growth is complete. It takes place in the (1) osteons of mature bone and consists of a cycle of (2) bone resorption by osteoclasts, (3) followed by bone formation by osteoblasts. Bone remodeling is (4) controlled by cytokines and growth factors that interact with a paracrine system consisting of the RANK ligand (RANKL), the RANK receptor, and osteoprotegerin.

❶ Bone Remodeling Cycle

Mature bone is made up of osteons or units of concentric lamellae (bone layers) and the haversian canal they surround. Bone remodeling consists of a sequence of bone resorption within an osteon by osteoclasts, followed by new bone formation by osteoblasts. In the adult, the length of one sequence (*i.e.,* bone resorption and formation) is approximately 4 months. Ideally, the replaced bone should equal the resorbed bone. If it does not, there is net loss of bone. In the elderly, for example, bone resorption and formation no longer are perfectly coupled, and bone mass is lost.

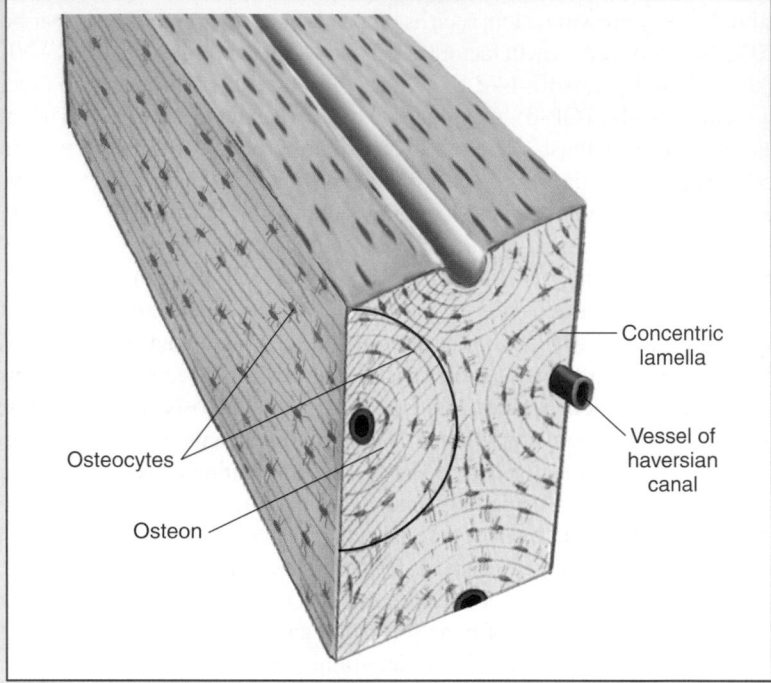

Concentric lamella

Vessel of haversian canal

Osteocytes

Osteon

❷ Bone Resorption

The osteoclasts, which are bone-resorbing cells derived from monocyte/macrophage precursors, are the cells involved in the initiation of bone remodeling. The sequence of bone resorption and bone formation is activated by many stimuli, including the action of parathyroid hormone and calcitonin. It begins with osteoclastic resorption of existing bone, during which the organic (protein matrix) and inorganic (mineral) components are removed, creating a tunnel-like space in the osteon. Soluble factors released during resorption aid in the recruitment of osteoblasts to the site, thereby linking bone resorption to bone formation.

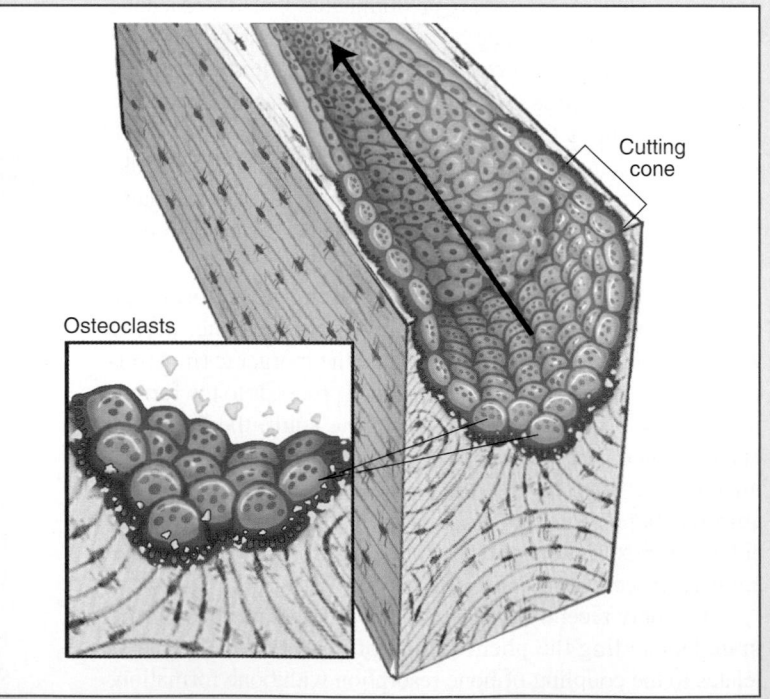

Cutting cone

Osteoclasts

Bone Formation

After osteoclastic activity has ceased, osteoblasts begin to deposit the organic matrix (osteoid) on the wall of the osteon canal. As successive lamellae of bone are deposited, the canal ultimately attains the relative proportions of the original osteon. In the formation and maintenance of bone, osteoblasts provide much of the local control because not only do they produce new bone matrix, they play an essential role in mediating osteoclast activity. Many of the primary stimulators of bone resorption, such as parathyroid hormone, have minimal or no direct effects on osteoclasts. Once the osteoblast, which has receptors for these substances, receives the appropriate signal, it releases a soluble mediator called *RANKL* that induces osteoclast activity.

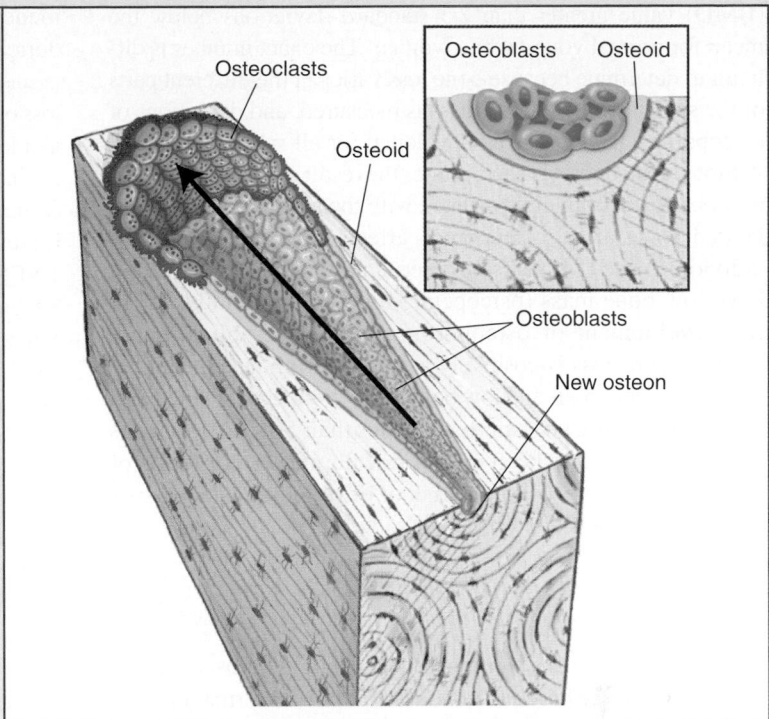

 Control of Bone Metabolism and Remodeling

The pivotal pathway linking osteoclast-mediated bone resorption with osteoblast-mediated bone formation consists of a paracrine system that includes RANKL, its receptor RANK, and a soluble protein called *osteoprotegerin* (OPG). RANKL, which is produced by osteoblasts and their precursors, binds to RANK, promoting osteoclast differentiation and proliferation. The soluble OPG molecule, which is produced by a number of tissues, acts as a decoy receptor to block the action of RANKL. This system ensures the tight coupling of bone formation and resorption, and provides a means whereby a wide variety of biologic mediators (*e.g.*, hormones, cytokines, growth factors) influence the homeostasis of bone.

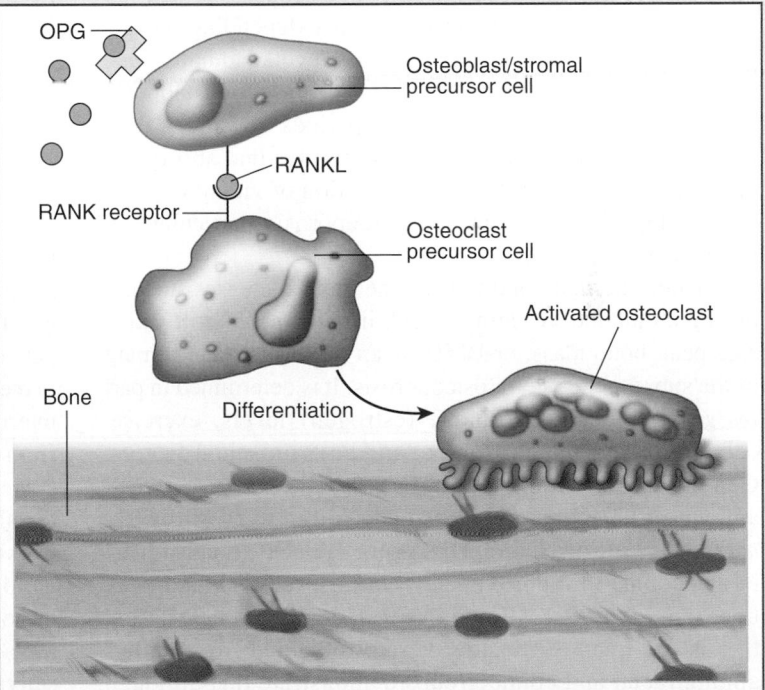

Osteopenia

Osteopenia is a condition that is common to all metabolic bone diseases. It is characterized by a reduction in bone mass greater than expected for age, race, or sex that occurs because of a decrease in bone formation, inadequate bone mineralization, or excessive bone deossification. *Osteopenia* is not a diagnosis but a term used to describe an apparent lack of bone seen on x-ray studies. The major causes of osteopenia are osteoporosis, osteo-malacia, malignancies such as multiple myeloma, and endocrine disorders such as hyperparathyroidism and hyperthyroidism.

Osteoporosis

Osteoporosis is a metabolic bone disease characterized by a loss of mineralized bone mass causing increased porosity of the skeleton and susceptibility to fractures.[37–40] The World Health Organization has defined osteoporosis as a bone mineral density

(BMD) value greater than 2.5 standard deviations below the mean for normal young white women. The exact number is difficult to determine because bone loss varies in the different parts of the skeleton where bone mass is measured, and definitions of osteoporosis have not been developed for all subpopulations.[41] Although osteoporosis can occur as the result of a number of disorders, it most often is associated with the aging process. In the United States alone, osteoporosis affects more than 10 million individuals aged 50 years or older; an additional 33.6 million have low bone mass (osteopenia) and are potentially at risk for development of osteoporosis and its complications.[42] Because bone loss is positively associated with age, the prevalence of osteoporosis and low bone mass is expected to increase. By 2020, one in two Americans older than 50 years of age is expected to have or be at risk of developing osteoporosis of the hip; even more will be at risk of developing osteoporosis at any site in the skeleton.[41]

Pathogenesis

The pathogenesis of osteoporosis is unclear, but most data suggest an imbalance between bone resorption and formation such that bone resorption exceeds bone formation. Although both of these factors play a role in most cases of osteoporosis, their relative contribution to bone loss may vary depending on age, gender, genetic predisposition, activity level, and nutritional status. Exercise may prevent or delay the onset of osteoporosis by increasing peak BMD during periods of growth. Poor nutrition or an age-related decrease in intestinal absorption of calcium because of deficient activation of vitamin D may contribute to the development of osteoporosis, particularly in the elderly.

Under normal conditions, bone mass increases steadily during childhood, reaching a peak in the young adult years. The peak bone mass, or BMD, is an important determinant of the subsequent risk for osteoporosis. It is determined in part by genetic factors, hormone (estrogen) levels, exercise, calcium intake and absorption, and environmental factors. Genetic factors are linked, in largest part, to the maximal amount of bone in a given person, referred to as *peak bone mass.* The type of vitamin D receptor molecule that is inherited accounts for approximately 75% of the maximal peak bone mass achieved.[14] Race is a key determinant of BMD and the risk of fractures. Incidence rates obtained from studies among racial and ethnic groups demonstrate that although women have higher fracture rates compared with men overall, these differences vary by race and age. White and Asian women had higher rates for all age groups older than 50 years.[38] The highest BMD values and lowest fracture rates have been reported for black women.[38] Body size is another factor affecting the risk of osteoporosis and risk of fractures. Women with smaller body builds are at increased risk of hip fracture because of lower hip BMD.

Hormonal factors play a significant role in the development of osteoporosis, particularly in postmenopausal women.[42,43] Post-

menopausal osteoporosis, which is caused by an estrogen deficiency, is manifested by a loss of cancellous bone and a predisposition to fractures of the vertebrae and distal radius. The loss of bone mass is greatest during early menopause, when estrogen levels are withdrawing. Several factors appear to influence the increased loss of bone mass associated with an estrogen deficiency. Decreased estrogen levels are associated with an increase in cytokines (*e.g.,* interleukin-1, interleukin-6, and TNF) that stimulate the production of osteoclast precursors. Recent studies indicate that estrogen deficiency also influences osteoclast differentiation through the RANK receptor pathways.[14] Estrogen stimulates the production of OPG and thus inhibits the formation of osteoclasts; it also blunts the responsiveness of osteoclast precursors to RANKL. With menopause and its accompanying estrogen deficiency, this inhibition of osteoclast production is lost.[14] Compensatory osteoblastic activity and new bone formation occurs, but it does not keep pace with the bone that is lost.

Sex hormone deficiency may contribute to bone loss in men with senile osteoporosis, although the effect is not of the same magnitude as that caused by estrogen deficiency. Unlike women, men do not have a midlife loss of sex hormone production.[44] Another factor that provides relative protection for men is the fact that they achieve 8% to 10% more peak bone mass than women. Although androgens have long been assumed to be critical for growth and maintenance of the male skeleton, it has recently been suggested that estrogens obtained from peripheral conversion of testicular and adrenal hormone precursors may be even more important than androgens in the maintenance of bone mass in men.

Age-related changes in bone density occur in all individuals and contribute to the development of osteoporosis in both sexes. After peak bone mass is attained at about 30 years of age, the rate of bone loss for both sexes is approximately 0.7% per year, and it increases to approximately 1% per year or more in menopausal women.[14] Age-related changes in bone cells and matrix have a strong impact on bone metabolism. Osteoblasts from elderly persons have reduced replicative and biosynthetic potential compared with those of younger persons. Growth factors that stimulate osteoblastic activity also lose their potential over time. The end result is a skeleton that has decreased ability to make bone. Reduced physical activity increases the rate of bone loss because mechanical forces are important stimuli for normal bone remodeling. Thus, the decreased physical activity that often accompanies aging may also contribute to the loss of bone mass in the elderly.

Secondary osteoporosis is associated with many conditions, including endocrine disorders, malabsorption disorders, malignancies, alcoholism, and certain medications.[45,46] Persons with endocrine disorders such as hyperthyroidism, hyperparathyroidism, Cushing syndrome, or diabetes mellitus are at high risk for development of osteoporosis. Hyperthyroidism causes an acceleration of bone turnover. Some malignancies (*e.g.,* multiple myeloma) secrete osteoclast-activating factor, causing significant bone loss. Alcohol is a direct inhibitor of osteoblasts and may also inhibit calcium absorption. Corticosteroid use is the most common cause of drug-related osteoporosis, and long-term corticosteroid use in the treatment of disorders such as rheumatoid arthritis and chronic obstructive lung disease is associated with a high rate of fractures. With the increased use of prednisone and other drugs that act like cortisol for the treatment of many inflammatory and autoimmune diseases, this form of bone loss has become a major clinical concern. The prolonged use of medications that increase calcium excretion, such as aluminum-containing antacids, corticosteroids, and anticonvulsants, also is associated with bone loss. Persons with human immunodeficiency virus (HIV) infection or acquired immunodeficiency syndrome (AIDS) who are being treated with antiretroviral therapy may develop a lower bone density and signs of osteopenia and osteoporosis.[47]

Several groups of children and adolescents are at increased risk for decreased bone mass, including premature infants and those with low birth weight who have lower-than-expected bone mass in the early weeks of life, children who require treatment with corticosteroid drugs (*e.g.,* those with childhood inflammatory diseases and transplant recipients), children with cystic fibrosis, and those with hypogonadal states (*e.g.,* anorexia nervosa and the female athlete triad).[40] Children with cystic fibrosis often have impaired gastrointestinal function that reduces the absorption of calcium and other nutrients, and many also require the frequent use of corticosteroid drugs.

Premature osteoporosis is increasingly being seen in female athletes owing to an increased prevalence of eating disorders and amenorrhea.[48-50] It most frequently affects women engaged in endurance sports, such as running and swimming; in activities where appearance is important, such as figure skating, diving, and gymnastics; or in sports with weight categories, such as horse racing, martial arts, and rowing. The *female athlete triad* refers to a pattern of disordered eating that leads to amenorrhea and eventually osteoporosis. Poor nutrition, combined with intense training, can decrease the critical body fat-to-muscle ratio needed for normal menses and estrogen production by the ovary. The decreased levels of estrogen combined with the lack of calcium and vitamin D from dietary deficiencies result in a loss of bone density and increased risk for fractures. There is a concern that athletes with low BMD will be at increased risk for fractures during their competitive years. It is unclear whether osteoporosis induced by amenorrhea is reversible. Data are emerging that even having only one or two elements of the triad greatly increases the risk of these women for long-term morbidity.[48]

Manifestations

Osteoporotic changes occur in the diaphysis and metaphysis of bone. In severe osteoporosis, the bones begin to resemble the fragile structure of a fine porcelain vase. There is loss of trabeculae from cancellous bone and thinning of the cortex to such an extent that minimal stress causes fractures. The changes that occur with osteoporosis have been explained by two distinct disease processes: postmenopausal and senile osteoporosis. In postmenopausal women, the increase in osteoclastic activity affects mainly bones or portions of bone that have increased surface area, such as the cancellous compartment of the vertebral bodies. The osteoporotic trabeculae become thinned and lose their interconnections, leading to microfractures and eventual vertebral collapse. In senile osteoporosis, the osteoporotic cortex is thinned by subperiosteal and endosteal resorption and the haversian systems are widened. In severe cases, the haversian systems are so enlarged that the cortex resembles cancellous bone (Fig. 58-16). Hip fractures, which are seen later in life, are more commonly associated with senile osteoporosis.

Osteoporosis is usually a silent disorder. Often, the first manifestations of the disorder are those that accompany a skeletal fracture—a vertebral compression fracture or fractures of the hip, pelvis, humerus, or any other bone (Fig. 58-17). Typically, the fractures occur with less force than usual, such as in a gymnast performing a common jump. Women who present with fractures are much more likely to sustain another fracture than are women of the same age without osteoporosis. Wedging and collapse of vertebrae cause a loss of height in the vertebral column and kyphosis, a condition commonly referred to as *dowager hump.* Usually, there is no generalized bone tenderness. When pain occurs, it is related to fractures. Systemic symptoms such as weakness and weight loss suggest that the osteoporosis may be caused by underlying disease.

Diagnosis and Treatment

An important advance in diagnostic methods used for the identification of osteoporosis has been the use of BMD assessment. The clinical method of choice for BMD studies is dual-energy x-ray absorptiometry (DXA) of the spine and hip.[51-55] Current

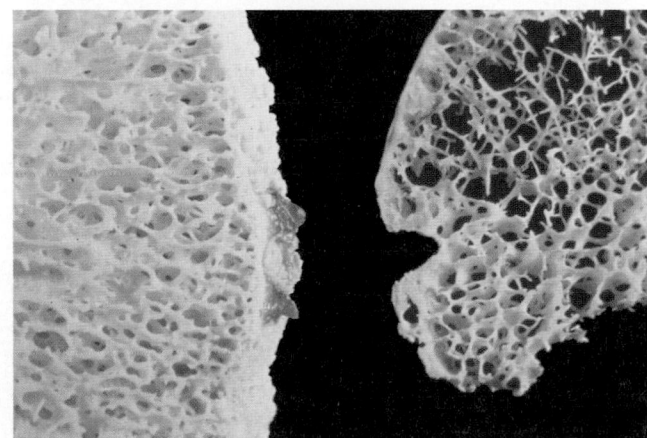

FIGURE 58-16 • Osteoporosis. Femoral head of an 82-year-old woman with osteoporosis and femoral neck fracture (**right**), compared with a normal control bone cut to the same thickness (**left**). (From Hoch B. J., Klein M. J., Schiller A. L. [2008]. Bones and joints. In Rubin R., Strayer D. S. [Eds.], *Rubin's pathology: Clinicopathologic foundations of medicine* [5th ed., p. 1109]. Philadelphia: Lippincott Williams & Wilkins.)

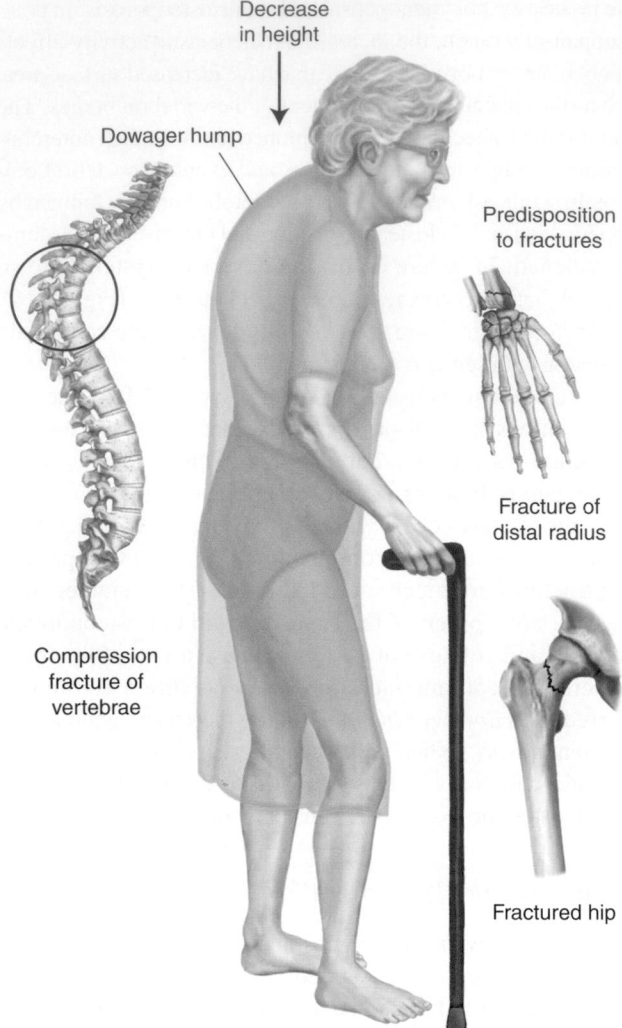

FIGURE 58-17 • Clinical manifestations of osteoporosis.

trauma fractures, have radiologic criteria consistent with low bone mass, have diseases that place them at risk for low BMD, or are receiving chronic glucocorticoid therapy.[56]

Prevention and early detection of osteoporosis are essential to the prevention of associated deformities and fractures. It is important to identify persons in high-risk groups so that treatment can begin early (Chart 58-1). Regular exercise and adequate calcium intake are important factors in preventing osteoporosis. Weight-bearing exercises such as walking, jogging, rowing, and weight lifting are important in the maintenance of bone mass. Studies have indicated that premenopausal women need more than 1000 mg/day of calcium, and postmenopausal women need 1500 mg of calcium daily.[57] Because most older American women do not consume a sufficient quantity of dairy products to meet their calcium needs, calcium supplementation is recommended. Calcium tablets vary in content of elemental calcium. Calcium carbonate contains 40% elemental calcium but requires normal stomach acidity to be absorbed. Calcium citrate is 21% elemental calcium but can be absorbed in the absence of acidity.[57] Vitamin D deficiency may be an important factor in the impaired intestinal absorption of calcium in the elderly. On the basis of this evidence, 1,25-dihydroxyvitamin D_3 is being studied as a treatment for osteoporosis. A daily intake of

practice is to perform DXA on the total hip, the femoral neck, and the anterior lumbar spine (L1 to L4).[53,54] The site with the lowest score should be used to make a diagnosis. Measurement of BMD has become increasingly common for early detection and fracture prevention. Measurement of serial heights in older adults is another simple way to screen for osteoporosis. A further advance in the diagnosis of osteoporosis is the refinement of risk factors, permitting better analysis of risk pertaining to particular persons. Testing for BMD should be performed based on the individual person's risk. The USPSTF and the National Osteoporosis Foundation have recommended that all women should have a measurement of BMD at 65 years of age.[53,54] Risk factors that may indicate a need for testing women at a younger age include a delayed menarche (*i.e.,* age 15 years or later), low body weight (*i.e.,* <21 kg/m², or 127 pounds at menopause), current smoker, history of fractures after menopause (other than skull, facial bone, ankle, finger, or toe), and history of a hip fracture in a parent.[52,56,57] Although there are no guidelines for BMD testing in men, it is recommended that it be considered for men who sustain low-

CHART 58-1   RISK FACTORS ASSOCIATED WITH OSTEOPOROSIS

Personal Characteristics
Advanced age
Female
White (fair, thin skin)
Small bone structure
Postmenopausal
Family history

Lifestyle
Sedentary
Calcium deficiency (long-term)
High-protein diet
Excessive alcohol intake
Excessive caffeine intake
Smoking

Drug and Disease Related
Aluminum-containing antacids
Anticonvulsants
Heparin
Corticosteroids or Cushing disease
Gastrectomy
Diabetes mellitus
Chronic obstructive lung disease
Malignancy
Hyperthyroidism
Hyperparathyroidism
Rheumatoid arthritis

400 to 800 IU of vitamin D is recommended because vitamin D optimizes calcium absorption and inhibits parathyroid secretion, which stimulates calcium resorption from bone.[57]

Active treatment of osteoporosis uses two main classes of drugs: antiresorptive agents (drugs that block bone resorption by osteoclasts) and anabolic agents (agents that stimulate bone formation by osteoblasts).[43]

There are three main types of antiresorptive agent: estrogens and selective estrogen receptor modulators, bisphosphonates, and calcitonin. Although estrogen is one of the most effective interventions for reducing the incidence and progression of osteoporosis in postmenopausal women, the use of hormone therapy (estrogen plus progestin) has come under scrutiny after the recent release of data from the Women's Health Initiative.[58,59] Raloxifene, a selective estrogen receptor modulator (SERM) that acts only on specific estrogen receptors has been approved by the U.S. Food and Drug Administration (FDA) for prevention and treatment of osteoporosis in postmenopausal women. The use of phytoestrogens, naturally occurring plant compounds, has gained popularity as an alternative to estrogens; however, information regarding their effect on bone health is conflicting and incomplete.[60]

Bisphosphonates are effective inhibitors of bone resorption and the most effective agents for prevention and treatment of osteoporosis. The bisphosphonates (*e.g.,* alendronate, risedronate, ibandronate) are analogs of endogenous inorganic pyrophosphate that the body cannot break down. In bone, they bind to hydroxyapatite and prevent bone resorption by inhibiting osteoclast activity. Bisphosphonates have been shown to reduce the risk of hip, vertebral, and nonvertebral fractures by up to 50%.[43] The most dramatic impact has been in the reduction of multiple spine fractures, showing that treatment can decrease progression of the disease.

Calcitonin is an endogenous peptide that partially inhibits osteoclastic activity. Nasal calcitonin and subcutaneous calcitonin have been approved for the treatment of postmenopausal osteoporosis. Teriparatide is an analog of parathyroid hormone recently approved by the FDA for the treatment of osteoporosis.[43] Unlike the antiresorptive drugs, parathyroid hormone stimulates bone remodeling by increasing osteoblast-mediated bone formation.

In men, testosterone appears to play an important role in bone homeostasis by stimulating osteoblasts and inhibiting osteoclasts. Testosterone can be administered by intramuscular injection, transdermal patch, or trans-scrotal patch.[61] The use of testosterone is contraindicated in men with prostate cancer. Men with osteoporosis may also benefit from bisphosphonate, calcitonin, or parathyroid hormone therapy. Like women, they have the same need for calcium and vitamin D supplementation.

Persons with osteoporosis have many special needs. Walking and swimming are encouraged. Unsafe conditions that predispose persons to falls and fractures should be corrected or avoided. In treating fractures, it is important to minimize immobility. Surgical intervention is done for stable fracture fixation that allows early restoration of mobility and function; for fractures of the lower extremities, this means early weight bearing.

Vertebral fractures are treated symptomatically. Conservative treatment with bracing is most often seen, especially in fractures of the thoracic verteba.[62] Vertebroplasty and kyphoplasty are minimally invasive spinal procedures that use bone cement to restore vertebral height and relieve pain (Fig. 58-18). Bone cement is instilled directly into the fractured vertebral body to restore height and shape. The procedure for kyphoplasty involves the use of a balloon as a tamp to create a void for the cement. Kyphoplasty seems to be associated with less cement extravasation and better restoration of vertebral height than vertebroplasty.[63]

Osteomalacia and Rickets

In contrast to osteoporosis, which causes a loss of total bone mass and results in brittle bones, osteomalacia and rickets produce a softening of the bones but do not involve a loss of bone matrix. Approximately 60% of bone is mineral content, approximately 30% is organic matrix, and the remainder is living bone cells. The organic matrix and the inorganic mineral salts are needed for normal bone consistency. The term *rickets* refers to

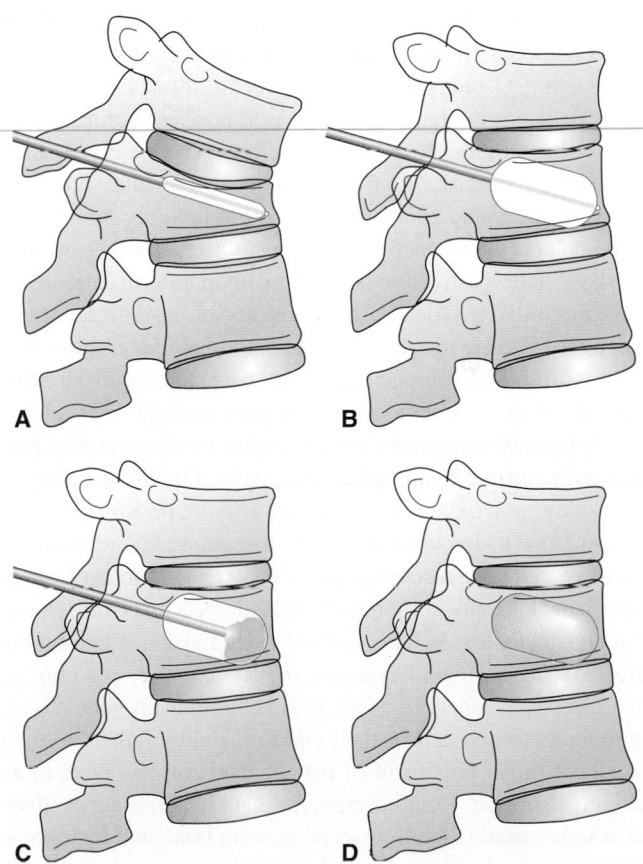

FIGURE 58-18 • Kyphoplasty. **(A)** Insertion of balloon tamp; **(B)** inflation of balloon tamp with collapsed vertebral bone being restored to normal height; **(C)** bone cavity being filled with cement; **(D)** cavity completely filled with cement. (Adapted from American Academy of Orthopedic Surgeons. Kyphoplasty. [Online.] Available: http://orthoinfo.aaos.org/fact/thr_report.cfm?Thread_ID =470&topcategory.)

the disorder in children in which changes in bone growth produce characteristic skeletal abnormalities, and *osteomalacia* is used in adults because the bone that forms during the remodeling process is undermineralized.[64]

Osteomalacia

Osteomalacia is a generalized bone condition in which there is inadequate mineralization of bone. There are two main causes of osteomalacia: (1) insufficient calcium absorption from the intestine because of a lack of dietary calcium or a deficiency of or resistance to the action of vitamin D; and (2) phosphate deficiency caused by increased renal losses or decreased intestinal absorption. Vitamin D deficiency is caused most commonly by reduced vitamin D absorption as a result of biliary tract or intestinal diseases that impair fat and fat-soluble vitamin absorption. Lack of vitamin D in the diet is rare in the United States because many foods are fortified with the vitamin. Anticonvulsant medications, such as phenobarbital and phenytoin, induce hepatic hydroxylases that accelerate breakdown of the active forms of vitamin D.

The incidence of osteomalacia is high among the elderly because of diets deficient in calcium and vitamin D, a problem often compounded by the intestinal malabsorption that accompanies aging. Osteomalacia often is seen in cultures in which the diet is deficient in vitamin D, such as in northern China, Japan, and northern India. Women in these areas have a higher incidence of the disorder than do men because of the combined effects of pregnancy, lactation, and more indoor confinement. Osteomalacia occasionally is seen in strict vegetarians, persons who have had a gastrectomy, and those on long-term anticonvulsant, tranquilizer, sedative, muscle relaxant, or diuretic drugs. There also is a greater incidence of osteomalacia in the colder regions of the world, particularly during the winter months, probably because of lessened exposure to sunlight.

A form of osteomalacia called *renal rickets* occurs in persons with chronic renal failure. It is caused by the inability of the kidney to activate vitamin D and excrete phosphate and is accompanied by hyperparathyroidism, increased bone turnover, and increased bone resorption (see Chapter 34). Another form of osteomalacia results from renal tubular defects that cause excessive phosphate losses. This form of osteomalacia is commonly referred to as *vitamin D–resistant rickets,* and often is a familial disorder.[14] It is inherited as an X-linked dominant gene passed by mothers to one half of their children and by fathers to their daughters only. This form of osteomalacia affects boys more severely than girls. Long-standing primary hyperparathyroidism causes increased calcium resorption from bone and hypophosphatemia, which can lead to rickets in children and osteomalacia in adults.

The clinical manifestations of osteomalacia are bone pain, tenderness, and fractures as the disease progresses. In severe cases, muscle weakness often is an early sign. The cause of muscle weakness is unclear. Osteomalacia predisposes a person to pathologic fractures in the weakened areas, especially in the distal radius and proximal femur. In contrast to osteoporosis, it is not a significant cause of hip fractures. There may be delayed healing and poor retention of internal fixation devices. Osteomalacia usually is accompanied by a compensatory or secondary hyperparathyroidism stimulated by low serum calcium levels. Parathyroid hormone reduces renal absorption of phosphate and removes calcium from the bone. Serum calcium levels are only slightly reduced in osteomalacia.

Diagnostic measures are directed toward identifying osteomalacia and establishing its cause. Diagnostic methods include x-ray studies, laboratory tests, bone scan, and bone biopsy. X-ray findings typical of osteomalacia are the development of transverse lines or pseudofractures called *Looser zones.* These apparently are caused by stress fractures that are inadequately healed, or by the mechanical inadequacy of penetrating nutrient vessels.[4] A bone biopsy may be done to confirm the diagnosis of osteomalacia in a person with nonspecific osteopenia who shows no improvement after treatment with exercise, vitamin D, and calcium.

The treatment of osteomalacia is directed at the underlying cause. If the problem is nutritional, restoring adequate amounts of calcium and vitamin D to the diet may be sufficient. The elderly with intestinal malabsorption also may benefit from vitamin D. The least expensive and most effective long-term treatment is a diet rich in vitamin D (*i.e.,* fish, dairy products, and margarine) along with careful exposure to the midday sun. Vitamin D is specific for adult osteomalacia and vitamin D–resistant rickets, but large doses usually are needed to overcome the resistance to calcium absorption action and to prevent renal loss of phosphate. The biologically active forms of vitamin D, 25-OH vitamin D (calciferol) or $1,25\text{-}(OH)_2$ vitamin D (calcitriol), are available for use in the treatment of osteomalacia resistant to vitamin D (*i.e.,* osteomalacia resulting from chronic liver disease and kidney failure). If osteomalacia is caused by malabsorption, the treatment is directed toward correcting the primary disease. For example, adequate replacement of pancreatic enzymes is of paramount importance in pancreatic insufficiency. In renal tubular disorders, the treatment is directed at the altered renal physiology.

 ## Rickets

Rickets is a metabolic bone disorder characterized by a failure or delay in calcification of the cartilaginous growth plate in children whose epiphyses have not yet fused.[4,14,64–66] It is also manifested by widening and deformation of the metaphyseal regions of long bones, and a delay in the mineralization of trabecular, endosteal, and periosteal bone surfaces. There are several forms of rickets, including nutritional rickets, vitamin D–dependent rickets, and vitamin D–resistant rickets. As with osteomalacia in the adult, rickets can result from kidney failure; malabsorptive syndromes such as celiac disease and cystic fibrosis; and medications such as anticonvulsants, which cause target organ resistance to vitamin D, and aluminum-containing antacids, which bind phosphorus and prevent its absorption.

Nutritional rickets results from inadequate sunlight exposure or inadequate intake of vitamin D, calcium, or phosphate. Nutritional rickets occurs primarily in underdeveloped areas of the world and among immigrants to developed countries. The causes are inadequate exposure to sunlight (*e.g.,* children are often kept clothed and indoors) and prolonged breast-feeding without vitamin D supplementation. Although the vitamin D content of human milk is low, the combination of breast milk and sunlight exposure usually provides sufficient vitamin D. Another cause of rickets is the use of commercial alternative milks (*e.g.,* soy or rice beverages) that are not fortified with vitamin D. Vitamin D–dependent rickets can result from abnormalities in the gene coding for the enzyme that converts inactive vitamin D to the active form of vitamin D, or from an autosomal disorder caused by mutations in the vitamin D receptor.[65] Vitamin D–resistant rickets involves hypophosphatemia or a decrease in serum phosphate levels, the most common form being caused by mutations of the phosphate-regulating gene on the X chromosome.[65] The gene mutation causes renal wasting of phosphate at the proximal tubular level of the kidney.

Rickets is characterized by changes in the growing bones of children with overgrowth of the epiphyseal cartilage due to inadequate provisional calcification and failure of the cartilage cells to disintegrate. Bones become deformed; ossification at the epiphyseal plates is delayed and disordered, resulting in widening of the epiphyseal cartilage plate. Any new bone that does grow is unmineralized. The conformation of the gross skeletal changes depends on the severity and duration of the rachitic process, and in particular on the stresses to which the individual bones are subjected.[4,14] During the nonmobile stage of infancy, the head and chest undergo the greatest stresses. The skull is enlarged and soft, and closure of the fontanels is delayed. Teeth are slow to develop, and the child may have difficulty standing. When an ambulating child develops rickets, deformities are likely to affect the spine, pelvis, and long bones (*i.e.,* tibia), causing, most notably, lumbar lordosis and bowing of the legs. The ends of long bones and ribs are enlarged. The thorax may be abnormally shaped, with prominent rib cartilage (*i.e.,* rachitic rosary). The child usually has stunted growth, with a height sometimes far below the normal range. Weight often is not affected so that the children, many of whom present with a protruding abdomen (*i.e.,* rachitic potbelly), have been described as presenting a Buddha-like appearance when sitting.

Nutritional rickets is treated with a balanced diet sufficient in calcium, phosphorus, and vitamin D. Exposure to sunlight also is important, especially for premature infants and those on artificial milk feedings. Supplemental vitamin D in excess of normal requirements is given for several months. Maintenance of good posture, positioning, and bracing in older children are used to prevent deformities. After the disease is controlled, deformities may have to be surgically corrected as the child grows.

Children with vitamin D–dependent and vitamin D–independent rickets require special treatment measures. Children with vitamin D–dependent rickets caused by lack of the enzyme needed to convert vitamin D to its active form are treated with calcitriol, the active form of vitamin D.[65] Vitamin D–resistant forms of rickets are treated with oral phosphorus or oral phosphorus and calcitriol.

Paget Disease

Paget disease (*i.e.,* osteitis deformans) is the second most common bone disease after osteoporosis.[4,14,67,68] The disease, which has been described as a "collage of matrix madness" is characterized by focal areas of excessive bone turnover and disorganized osteoid formation.[14] The disease usually begins during mid-adulthood and becomes progressively more common with increasing age. The disease is more common in older people and those of Northern European heritage. Men are about twice as likely as women to have the disease.[68]

Paget disease is a focal process with considerable variation in its stage of development in separate sites. At the onset, the disease is marked by regions of furious osteoclastic bone resorption, followed by a period of hectic bone formation with increased numbers of osteoblasts rapidly depositing bone in a chaotic fashion such that the newly formed bone is of poor quality and is disorganized rather than lamellar. The poor quality of bone accounts for the bowing and fractures that occur in bones affected by the disease. The bone marrow adjacent to the bone-forming surface is replaced by loose connective tissue that contains osteoprogenitor cells and numerous blood vessels, which transport blood to and from these metabolically active sites. The lesions of Paget disease may be solitary or may occur in multiple sites. They tend to localize to the bones of the axial skeleton, including the spine, skull, and pelvis. The proximal femur and tibia may be involved in more widespread forms of the disease. Histologically, Paget lesions show increased vascularity and bone marrow fibrosis with intense cellular activity. The bone has a somewhat mosaic-like pattern caused by areas of density outlined by heavy blue lines, called *cement lines* (Fig. 58-19).

Although the cause of Paget disease remains unclear, there is evidence of both genetic and environmental influences. It has been reported that 15% to 40% of persons with the disease have a first-degree relative with Paget disease, and numerous studies have described extended family members with the disease.[68] It is likely that factors other than genetics are also involved in the pathogenesis of the disease. Current evidence suggests a probable association with a virus, possibly a paramyxovirus.[14,68] This has been supported by the observation of viral particles resembling the paramyxovirus nucleocapsid in the cytoplasm of osteoclasts in persons with Paget disease.

In children, hyperostosis corticalis deformans juvenilis (a rare autosomal recessive disorder), hyperphosphatemia, and diseases that cause diaphyseal stenosis may mimic Paget disease and sometimes are referred to as *juvenile Paget disease.*[69] The disorder presents in infancy or early childhood with pain from debilitating fractures and deformities due to

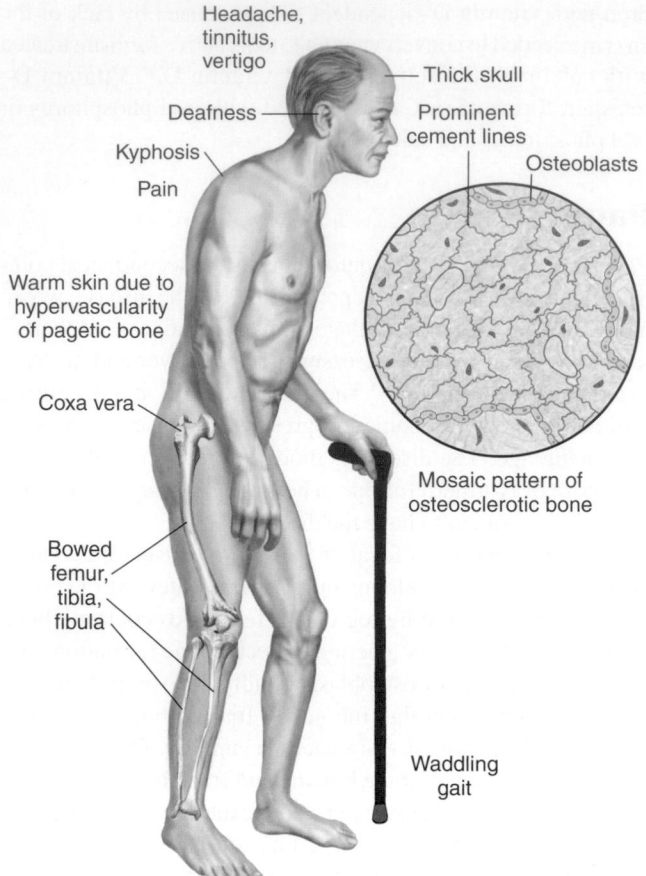

Headache, tinnitus, vertigo

Deafness

Kyphosis

Pain

Warm skin due to hypervascularity of pagetic bone

Coxa vera

Bowed femur, tibia, fibula

Thick skull

Prominent cement lines

Osteoblasts

Mosaic pattern of osteosclerotic bone

Waddling gait

FIGURE 58-19 • Clinical manifestations of Paget disease.

a markedly accelerated rate of bone remodeling throughout the skeleton.

Manifestations

The disease varies in severity from a simple lesion to involvement of many bones. It may be present long before it is detected clinically. The clinical manifestations of Paget disease depend on the specific area involved (see Fig. 58-19). Approximately 70% of persons with the disorder are totally asymptomatic, and the disease is discovered accidentally.[67] Involvement of the skull causes headaches, intermittent tinnitus, vertigo, and eventual hearing loss. In the spine, collapse of the anterior vertebrae causes kyphosis of the thoracic spine. The femur and tibia become bowed. Softening of the femoral neck can cause coxa vara (*i.e.,* reduced angle of the femoral neck). Coxa vara, in combination with softening of the sacral and iliac bones, causes a waddling gait. When the lesion affects only one bone, it may cause only mild pain and stiffness. Progressive deossification weakens and distorts the bone structure. The deossification process begins along the inner cortical surfaces and continues until the substance of the bone disappears. Pathologic fractures may occur, especially in the bones subjected to the

greatest stress (*e.g.,* upper femur, lower spine, pelvic bones). These fractures often heal poorly, with excessive and poorly distributed callus.

Other manifestations of Paget disease include nerve palsy syndromes from lesions in the upper extremities, mental deterioration, and cardiovascular disease. The hypervascularity of pagetic bone warms the overlying skin; in severe disease the increased blood flow acts as an arteriovenous shunt, leading to high-output heart failure or exacerbation of underlying cardiac disease.[14] Cardiovascular disease is the most serious complication and the most common cause of death in those with advanced generalized Paget disease. Calcific aortic stenosis may occur in severe cases. Ventilatory capacity may be limited by rib and spine involvement.

Osteogenic sarcomas occur in 5% to 10% of persons with severe polyostotic disease.[14] One fifth of all osteogenic sarcomas in persons 50 years of age or older originate in people with Paget disease.[70] The bones most often affected, in order of frequency, are the femur, pelvis, humerus, and tibia. There appears to be a close histopathogenic relationship between Paget disease and the associated sarcoma.[70]

Diagnosis and Treatment

Diagnosis of Paget disease is based on characteristic bone deformities and x-ray changes. Elevated levels of serum alkaline phosphatase and urinary hydroxyproline support the diagnosis, and continued surveillance of these levels may be used to monitor the effectiveness of treatment. Bone scans are used to detect the rapid bone turnover indicative of active disease and to monitor the response to treatment. The scan cannot identify bone activity resulting from malignant lesions. Bone biopsy may be done to differentiate the lesion from osteomyelitis or a primary or metastatic bone tumor.

The treatment of Paget disease is based on the degree of pain and the extent of the disease. Pain can be reduced with nonsteroidal or other anti-inflammatory agents. Suppressive agents such as the bisphosphonates and calcitonin are used to manage pain and prevent further spread of the disease and neurologic defects. Bisphosphonate therapy is the most effective way to control Paget disease.[70] These drugs act by binding directly to bone minerals, inhibiting bone loss by rapidly decreasing bone resorption, followed by a secondary, slower decrease in the rate of bone formation.[67] Treatment usually is continued for 3 to 4 months, although recent studies are evaluating shorter courses of treatment. Parenteral bisphosphonates are particularly useful in persons who cannot tolerate oral preparations. Calcitonin also inhibits bone resorption. It is available in injectable and nasal spray forms, but only the injectable form is approved by the FDA for treatment of Paget disease. Nasal-spray calcitonin, which is approved for other uses, is being studied for use in Paget disease. Persons with Paget disease should receive adequate doses of calcium and vitamin D. A recombinant form of osteoprotegerin is also being used to inhibit osteoclastogenesis in children, slowing the osteoclast activity. Juvenile Paget disease is being described as an osteoprotegerin deficiency.[69]

IN SUMMARY, in addition to its structural function, the skeleton is a homeostatic organ. Metabolic bone diseases such as osteoporosis, osteomalacia, rickets, and Paget disease are the result of a disruption in the equilibrium of bone formation and resorption. Osteoporosis, which is the most common of the metabolic bone diseases, occurs when the rate of bone resorption is greater than that of bone formation. It is seen frequently in postmenopausal women and is the major cause of fractures in persons older than 45 years of age. Osteomalacia and rickets are caused by inadequate mineralization of bone matrix, primarily because of a deficiency of vitamin D. Paget disease results from excessive osteoclastic activity and is characterized by the formation of poor-quality bone. The success rate of the various drugs and hormones that are used to treat metabolic bone diseases varies. Further research is needed to clarify the cause, pathologic process, and treatment of these diseases. ■

Review Exercises

1. A newborn girl was found to have developmental dysplasia of the hip (DDH) during a routine screening examination.

   A. *Describe the anatomic abnormalities that are present in the disorder.*

   B. *Explain the need for early treatment of DDH.*

2. A 12-year-old girl was noted to have asymmetry of the shoulders, scapular height, and pelvic height during routine physical examination. On x-ray examination, she is found to have a 30-degree curvature of the spine.

   A. *What possible treatments are available for this girl?*

   B. *Describe the physical problems associated with progressive scoliosis.*

3. A 60-year-old postmenopausal woman presents with a compression fracture of the vertebrae. She has also noticed increased backache and loss of height over the past few years.

   A. *Explain how the lack of estrogen and aging contribute to the development of osteoporosis.*

   B. *What other factors should be considered when assessing the risk for development of osteoporosis?*

   C. *What is the best way to measure bone density?*

   D. *Name the two most important factors in preventing osteoporosis.*

   E. *What medications might be used to treat this woman's condition?*

References

1. Moore K. L., Persaud T. V. N. (2003). *The developing human* (6th ed., pp. 382–399). Philadelphia: W. B. Saunders.
2. Ross M. H., Kaye G. I., Pawlina W. (2003). *Histology: A text and atlas* (4th ed., pp. 180–202). Philadelphia: Lippincott Williams & Wilkins.
3. Gartner L. P., Hiatt J. L. (2001). *Color textbook of histology* (2nd ed., pp. 129–154). Philadelphia: W. B. Saunders.
4. Hoch B. J., Klein M. J., Schiller A. L. (2008). Bones and joints. In Rubin R., Strayer D. S. (Eds.), *Rubin's pathology: Clinicopathologic foundations of medicine* (5th ed., pp. 1098–1390). Philadelphia: Lippincott Williams & Wilkins.
5. Schoeneker P. L., Rich M. M. (2006). The lower extremity. In Morissy R. T., Weinstein S. L. (Eds.), *Lovell & Winter's pediatric orthopaedics* (6th ed., pp. 1158–1213). Philadelphia: Lippincott Williams & Wilkins.
6. Thompson G. H. (2004). Bone and joint disorders. In Behrman R. E., Kliegman R. M., Jenson H. B. (Eds.), *Nelson textbook of pediatrics* (17th ed., pp. 2251–2290). Philadelphia: Elsevier Saunders.
7. Sass P., Hassan G. (2003). Lower extremity abnormalities in children. *American Family Physician* 68, 461–468.
8. Maher A. B., Salmond S. B., Pellino T. A. (2002). *Orthopaedic nursing* (3rd ed., pp. 552–568, 601–603). Philadelphia: W. B. Saunders.
9. Wall E. J. (2000). Practical primary pediatric orthopedics. *Pediatric Advanced Practice Nursing* 35(1), 95–113.
10. Crocetti M., Barone M. A. (2004). *Oski's essential pediatrics* (2nd ed., pp. 676–694). Philadelphia: Lippincott Williams & Wilkins.
11. Kim H. W., Park H. W. (2005). The pediatric leg and knee. In Weinstein S. L., Buckwalter J. A. (Eds.), *Turek's orthopaedics: Principles and their application* (6th ed., pp. 575–588). Philadelphia: Lippincott Williams & Wilkins.
12. National Institutes of Health. (2005). Osteogenesis imperfecta: A guide for nurses. [Online]. Available: www.niams.nih.gov/bone/hi/osteogenesis/OI_nurse_guide.pdf12. Accessed April 15, 2008.
13. Marini J. C. (2004). Osteogenesis imperfecta. In Behrman R. E., Kliegman R. M., Jenson H. B. (Eds.), *Nelson textbook of pediatrics* (17th ed., pp. 2336–2338). Philadelphia: Elsevier Saunders.
14. Rosenberg A. E. (2005). Bones, joints, and soft tissue tumors. In Kumar V., Abbas A. K., Fausto N. (Eds.), *Robbins and Cotran pathologic basis of medicine* (7th ed., pp. 1273–1314). Philadelphia: Elsevier Saunders.
15. Reid I. R. (2003). Bisphosphonates: New indications and methods of administration. *Current Opinion in Rheumatology* 15, 458–463.
16. Storer S., Skaggs D. L. (2006). Developmental dysplasia of the hip. *American Family Physician* 74, 1310–1316.
17. American Academy of Pediatrics, Committee on Quality Improvement, Subcommittee on Developmental Dysplasia of the Hip. (2000). Clinical practice guideline: Early detection of developmental dysplasia of the hip. *Pediatrics* 105, 896–905.
18. Patel H., with the Canadian Task Force on Preventive Health Care. (2001). Preventive health care, 2001 update: Screening and management of developmental dysplasia of the hip in newborns. [Online.] Available: www.ctfphc.org. Accessed April 15, 2008.
19. U.S. Preventive Services Task Force. (2006). Screening for developmental dysplasia of the hip: Recommendation statement. [Online.] Available: www.ahrq.gov/clinic/uspstf/uspshipd.htm. Accessed April 15, 2008.
20. Weinstein S. L. (2005). The pediatric foot. In Weinstein S. L., Buckwalter J. A. (Eds.), *Turek's orthopaedics: Principles and their application* (6th ed., pp. 633–670). Philadelphia: Lippincott Williams & Wilkins.
21. Gore A. I., Spencer J. (2004). The newborn foot. *American Family Physician* 69, 865–872.
22. Faulks S. (2005). Changing paradigm for treatment of clubfeet. *Orthopedic Nursing* 26(1), 25–30.
23. Honein M., Paulozzi L. J., Moore C. A. (2000). Family history, maternal smoking, and clubfoot: An indication of a gene–environment interaction. *American Journal of Epidemiology* 152, 658–665.
24. Alexander M. (2002). Congenital and developmental disorders In Maher A. B., Salmond S. W., Pellino T. A. (Eds.), *Orthopaedic nursing* (3rd ed., pp. 567–570). Philadelphia: W. B. Saunders.

25. Bronson W. E. (2001). The pediatric hip. *Current Opinion in Orthopaedics* 12, 470–479.

26. Herring J. A. (2002). Legg-Calvé-Perthes disease. In Herring A. J. (Ed.), *Tachdjian's pediatric orthopaedics* (3rd ed., Vol. 1, pp. 655–709). Philadelphia: W. B. Saunders.

27. Yawn B. P., Yawn R. A., Hodge D., et al. (1999). A population-based study of school scoliosis screening. *Journal of the American Medical Association* 282, 1427–1432.

28. Reamy B. V., Slakey J. B. (2001). Adolescent scoliosis: Review and current comments. *American Family Physician* 64, 111–116.

29. Weinstein S. (2005). The thoracolumbar spine. In Weinstein S. L., Buckwalter J. A. (Eds.), *Turek's orthopaedics: Principles and their application* (6th ed., pp. 477–518). Philadelphia: Lippincott Williams & Wilkins.

30. Qiu X. S., Tang N. L., Yeung H. Y., et al. (2007). Melatonin receptor 1B (MTNR1B) gene polymorphism is associated with occurrence of adolescent idiopathic scoliosis. *Spine* 32, 1748–1753.

31. Omey M. L., Micheli L. J., Gerbino P. G. (2000). Idiopathic scoliosis and spondylolysis in the female athlete: Tips for treatment. *Clinical Orthopaedics and Related Research* 372, 74–84.

32. U.S. Preventive Services Task Force. (2005). Screening for idiopathic scoliosis in adolescents: Recommendation statement. *American Family Physician* 71, 1975–1976.

33. Lonner B. S. (2007). Emerging minimally invasive technologies for management of scoliosis. *Orthopedic Clinics of North America* 38, 431–440.

34. Cohen S. (2006). Role of RANK ligand in normal and pathologic bone remodeling and therapeutic potential of novel inhibitory molecules in musculoskeletal disease. *Arthritis and Rheumatism* 55, 15–18.

35. Hofbauer L. C., Schoppet M. (2004). Clinical implications of osteoprotegerin/RANKL/RANK system for bone and vascular disease. *Journal of the American Medical Association* 292, 490–495.

36. Rogers A., Eastell R. (2005). Review: Circulating osteoprotegerin and receptor activator for nuclear factor κB ligand: Clinical utility in metabolic bone disease assessment. *Journal of Clinical Endocrinology and Metabolism* 90, 6323–6331.

37. Raisz L. G., Rodan G. A. (2003). Pathogenesis of osteoporosis. *Endocrinology Clinics of North America* 32, 15–24.

38. Lane N. E. (2006). Epidemiology, etiology, and diagnosis of osteoporosis. *American Journal of Obstetrics and Gynecology* 194, S3–S11.

39. Gass M., Dawson-Hughes B. (2006). Preventing osteoporosis-related fractures: An overview. *American Journal of Medicine* 119, 3S–11S.

40. Rodan G. A., Reska H. A. (2003). Osteoporosis and bisphosphonates. *Journal of Bone and Joint Surgery (American Volume)* 85(Suppl. 3), 8–12.

41. U.S. Department of Health and Human Services. (2004). *Bone health and osteoporosis: A report of the surgeon general.* Chapter 4: The frequency of bone disease [Online.] Available: www.surgeongeneral.gov/library/bonehealth/chapter_4.html#Prevalence. Accessed April 15, 2008.

42. Steinweg K. K. (2002). Menopause, bone physiology, and osteoporosis prevention. *Clinics in Family Practice* 4, 89–111.

43. Rosen C. J. (2005). Postmenopausal osteoporosis. *New England Journal of Medicine* 353, 595–603.

44. Gennari L., Bilezikian J. P. (2007). Osteoporosis in men. *Endocrinology and Metabolism Clinics of North America* 36, 399–419.

45. Stein E., Shane E. (2003). Secondary osteoporosis. *Endocrinology and Metabolism Clinics of North America* 32, 115–134.

46. Fitzpatrick L. A. (2007). Secondary causes of osteoporosis. *Mayo Clinic Proceedings* 77, 453–468.

47. Tebas P., Powderly W. G., Claxton S., et al. (2000). Accelerated bone mineral loss in HIV-infected patients receiving potent antiretroviral therapy. *AIDS* 14, F63–F67.

48. Beals K. A., Meyer N. L. (2007). Female athlete triad update. *Clinics in Sports Medicine* 26, 69–80.

49. Brunet M. (2005). Female athlete triad. *Clinics in Sports Medicine* 21, 623–636.

50. Kazis K., Iglesias E. (2003). Female athlete triad. *Adolescent Medicine* 14, 87–95.

51. Raisz L. C. (2005). Screening for osteoporosis. *New England Journal of Medicine* 353, 164–171.

52. Armstrong C. (2006). NAMS updates recommendations on diagnosis and management of osteoporosis in postmenopausal women. *American Family Physician* 74, 1631–1639.

53. U.S. Preventive Services Task Force (2002). Screening for osteoporosis in postmenopausal women: Recommendations and rationale. *Annals of Internal Medicine* 137, 526–528.

54. National Osteoporosis Foundation. (2003). *Physician's guide to prevention and treatment of osteoporosis.* Washington, DC: Author.

55. Rosen C. J. (2005). Screening for osteoporosis. *New England Journal of Medicine* 353, 164–171.

56. Brunader R., Shelton D. K. (2002). Radiologic bone assessment in the evaluation of osteoporosis. *American Family Physician* 65, 1357–1364.

57. Weinstein L., Ullery B. (2000). Age, weight, and estrogen use determine need for osteoporosis screen. *American Journal of Obstetrics and Gynecology* 183, 547–549.

58. Vogel R. A. (2003). The changing view of hormone replacement therapy. *Reviews in Cardiovascular Medicine* 4(2), 68–71.

59. Cauley J. A., Robbins J., Chen Z., et al. (2003). Effects of estrogen plus progestin on risk of fracture and bone mineral density. *Journal of the American Medical Association* 290, 1729–1738.

60. National Institutes of Health: Osteoporosis and Related Bone Diseases—National Resource Center. (2005). Phytoestrogens and bone health. [Online.] Available: www.niams.nih.gov/bone/hi/bone_phyto.htm. Accessed September 1, 2007.

61. Vondracek S. F., Hansen L. B. (2004). Current approaches to management of osteoporosis in men. *American Journal of Health-System Pharmacists* 61, 1801–1811.

62. Lavelle W., Lavelle E. D., Khaleel M. A. (2007). Vertebroplasty and kyphoplasty. *Medical Clinics of North America* 91, 299–314.

63. Pateder D. B., Khanna A. J., Lieberman I. H. (2007). Vertebroplasty and kyphoplasty for the management of osteoporotic vertebral compression fractures. *Orthopedic Clinics of North America* 38, 409–418.

64. Berg E. E. (2004). Rickets. *Orthopaedic Nursing* 23(1), 53–55.

65. Nield L. S., Mahajan P., Joshi A., et al. (2006). Rickets: Not a disease of the past. *American Family Physician* 74, 619–630.

66. Pttifor J. M. (2005). Rickets and vitamin D deficiency in children and adolescents. *Endocrinology and Metabolism Clinics of North America* 34, 537–553.

67. Schneider D., Hofmann M. T. (2002). Diagnosis and treatment of Paget's disease of bone. *American Family Physician* 65, 2069–2072.

68. Roodman G. D., Windle J. J. (2005). Paget disease of bone. *Journal of Clinical Investigation* 115, 200–208.

69. Cundy T., Davidson J., Rutland M. D., et al. (2005). Recombinant osteoprotegerin for juvenile Paget disease. *New England Journal of Medicine* 353, 918–923.

70. Drake W. M., Kendler D. L., Brown J. P. (2001). Consensus statement on the modern therapy of Paget's disease of bone from a Western Alliance Symposium. Biannual Foothills Meeting on Osteoporosis, Calgary, Alberta, Canada, September 9–10, 2000. *Clinical Therapeutics* 23, 620–626.

Visit the**Point** http://thePoint.lww.com for animations, journal articles, and more!

Disorders of Musculoskeletal Function: Rheumatic Disorders

Chapter 59

DEBRA BANCROFT RIZZO

SYSTEMIC AUTOIMMUNE RHEUMATIC DISEASES
Rheumatoid Arthritis
Etiology and Pathogenesis
Clinical Manifestations
Diagnosis and Treatment
Systemic Lupus Erythematosus
Etiology and Pathogenesis
Clinical Manifestations
Diagnosis and Treatment
Systemic Sclerosis/Scleroderma
Polymyositis and Dermatomyositis
SERONEGATIVE SPONDYLOARTHROPATHIES
Ankylosing Spondylitis
Etiology and Pathogenesis
Clinical Manifestations
Diagnosis and Treatment
Reactive Arthropathies
Reiter Syndrome
Enteropathic Arthritis
Psoriatic Arthritis
OSTEOARTHRITIS SYNDROME
Epidemiology and Risk Factors
Pathogenesis
Clinical Manifestations
Diagnosis and Treatment
CRYSTAL-INDUCED ARTHROPATHIES
Gout
Pathogenesis
Clinical Manifestations
Diagnosis and Treatment
RHEUMATIC DISEASES IN CHILDREN AND THE ELDERLY
Rheumatic Diseases in Children
Juvenile Idiopathic Arthritis
Systemic Lupus Erythematosus
Juvenile Dermatomyositis
Juvenile Spondyloarthropathies
Rheumatic Diseases in the Elderly
Rheumatoid Arthritis
Systemic Lupus Erythematosus
Osteoarthritis
Crystal-Induced Arthropathies

Polymyalgia Rheumatica
Management of Rheumatic Diseases in the Elderly

➤ *Arthritis* is a descriptive term applied to more than 100 rheumatic diseases, ranging from localized, self-limiting conditions to those that are systemic autoimmune processes. Arthritis affects persons in all age groups and is the second leading cause of disability in the United States.[1] Although arthritis cannot be cured, much can be done to control its progress.

The common use of the term *arthritis* oversimplifies the nature of the varied disease processes, the difficulty in differentiating one form of arthritis or rheumatic disease from another, and the complexity of treatment of these usually chronic conditions. These diverse conditions share inflammation of the joint as a prominent or accompanying symptom. In the systemic rheumatic diseases—those affecting body systems in addition to the musculoskeletal system—the inflammation is primary, resulting from an immune response. In rheumatic conditions limited to a single or few diarthrodial joints, the inflammation is secondary, resulting from a degenerative process and the resulting joint irregularities that occur as the bone attempts to remodel itself.

This chapter focuses on systemic autoimmune rheumatic diseases, arthritis associated with spondylitis, osteoarthritis syndrome, metabolic diseases associated with arthritis, and rheumatic disease in children and the elderly. A review of normal joint structures is presented in Chapter 56.

 SYSTEMIC AUTOIMMUNE
RHEUMATIC DISEASES

After completing this section of the chapter, you should be able to meet the following objectives:

■ Characterize the common characteristics of the different systemic autoimmune rheumatic disorders.

(objectives continue)

1519

- Describe the pathologic changes that may be found in the joint of a person with rheumatoid arthritis.
- List the extra-articular manifestations of rheumatoid arthritis.
- Describe the immunologic process that occurs in systemic lupus erythematosus.
- List four major organ systems that may be involved in systemic lupus erythematosus.
- Describe the manifestations of systemic sclerosis.

Systemic autoimmune rheumatic diseases are a group of chronic disorders characterized by diffuse inflammatory lesions and degenerative changes in connective tissue. These disorders share similar clinical features and may affect many of the same organs. Rheumatoid arthritis (RA), systemic lupus erythematosus (SLE), polymyalgia rheumatica, temporal arteritis, and juvenile arthritis and dermatomyositis, which share an autoimmune systemic pathogenesis, are discussed in this section.

Rheumatoid Arthritis

RA is a systemic inflammatory disease that affects 0.3% to 1.5% of the population, with women affected two to three times more frequently than men.[1] Although the disease occurs in all age groups, its prevalence increases with age. The peak incidence among women is between the ages of 40 and 60 years, with the onset at 30 to 50 years of age.

RHEUMATOID ARTHRITIS

- Rheumatoid arthritis is a chronic systemic inflammatory disease with bilateral involvement of synovial or diarthrodial joints.

- The initial joint changes involve the synovial cells lining the joint. Inflammatory cells accumulate, and angiogenesis and formation of pannus, which proceed to cover the articular cartilage and isolate it from its nutritional synovial fluid, take place.

Etiology and Pathogenesis

Although the cause of RA remains uncertain, evidence points to a genetic predisposition and the development of joint inflammation that is immunologically mediated. It has been suggested that the disease is initiated in a genetically predisposed individual by the activation of a T-cell–mediated response to an immunologic trigger, such as a microbial agent (Fig. 59-1). The importance of genetic factors in the pathogenesis of RA is supported by the increased frequency of the disease among first-degree relatives and monozygotic twins.[2] In addition, it is generally agreed that certain major histocompatibility complex (MHC) genes are expressed in a nonrandom manner in persons

with RA. An important genetic locus that predisposes to RA is present on the human leukocyte antigen (HLA) loci on the MHC class II molecules, with a specific set of HLA DR alleles (DR4, DR1, DR10, DR14) being consistently increased in persons with RA.[2] These alleles are thought to form a shared epitope in the hypervariable segment of the HLA-DRB1 gene, which forms a rheumatoid pocket on the HLA molecule (see Chapter 17). It seems likely that the binding properties of this pocket influence the types of peptides that can be bound by the RA-associated HLA-DR molecules, thereby affecting the immune response.[2]

The pathogenesis of RA can be viewed as an aberrant immune response that leads to synovial inflammation and destruction of the joint architecture. It has been suggested that the disease is initiated by the activation of helper T cells, release of cytokines (e.g., tumor necrosis factor [TNF], interleukin [IL]-1), and antibody formation. Approximately 70% to 80% of persons with the disease have a substance called the *rheumatoid factor* (RF), which is an autologous (self-produced) antibody (Ig RF) that reacts with a fragment of immunoglobulin G (IgG) to form immune complexes.[2,3] Immune complexes (Ig RF + IgG) and complement components are found in the synovium, synovial fluid, and extra-articular lesions of persons with RA. Although persons with RA may be seronegative (not have Ig RF in their serum), the presence of a high RF titer is frequently associated with severe and unremitting disease, mainly systemic complications.

The role of the autoimmune process in the joint destruction of RA remains obscure. At the cellular level, neutrophils, macrophages, and lymphocytes are attracted to the area. The neutrophils and macrophages phagocytize the immune complexes and, in the process, release lysosomal enzymes capable of causing destructive changes in the joint cartilage (see Fig. 59-1). The inflammatory response that follows attracts additional inflammatory cells, setting into motion a chain of events that perpetuates the condition. As the inflammatory process progresses, the synovial cells and subsynovial tissues undergo reactive hyperplasia. Vasodilation and increased blood flow cause warmth and redness. The joint swelling that occurs is the result of the increased capillary permeability that accompanies the inflammatory process.

Characteristic of RA is the development of an extensive network of new blood vessels in the synovial membrane that contributes to the advancement of the rheumatoid synovitis. This destructive vascular granulation tissue, which is called *pannus,* extends from the synovium to involve the "bare area," a region of unprotected bone at the junction between cartilage and subchondral bone. Pannus is a feature of RA that differentiates it from other forms of inflammatory arthritis[4] (Fig. 59-2C). The inflammatory cells found in the pannus have a destructive effect on the adjacent cartilage and bone. Eventually, pannus develops between the joint margins, leading to reduced joint motion and the possibility of eventual ankylosis. With progression of the disease, joint inflammation and the resulting structural changes lead to joint instability, muscle atrophy from disuse, stretching of the ligaments, and involvement of the ten-

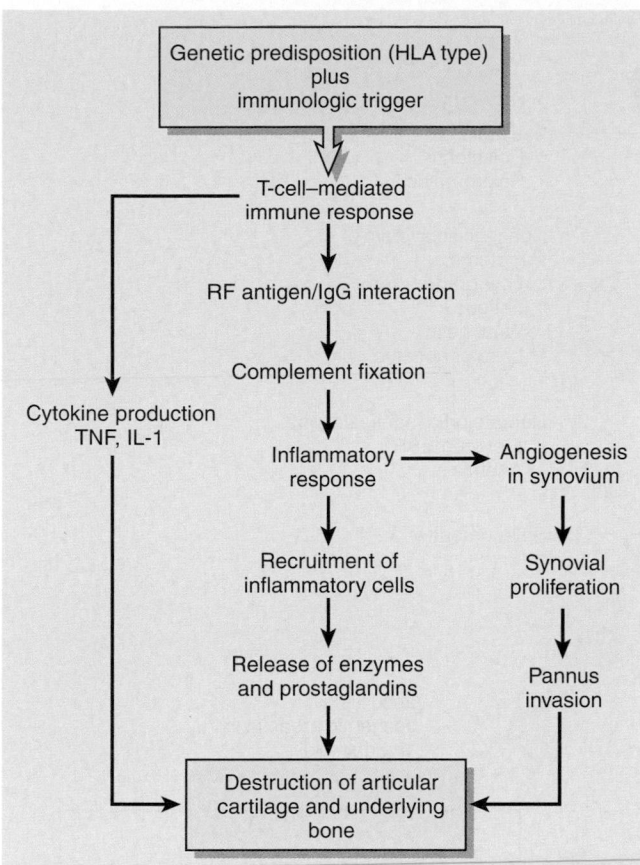

FIGURE 59-1 • Disease process in rheumatoid arthritis.

dons and muscles. The effect of the pathologic changes on joint structure and function is related to the degree of disease activity, which can change at any time. Unfortunately, the destructive changes are irreversible.

Clinical Manifestations

Rheumatoid arthritis often is associated with extra-articular as well as articular manifestations (see Fig. 59-2). It usually has an insidious onset marked by systemic manifestations such as fatigue, anorexia, weight loss, and generalized aching and stiffness. The disease, which is characterized by exacerbations and remissions, may involve only a few joints for brief durations, or it may become relentlessly progressive and debilitating. Approximately 3% of those with the disease have a progressive, unremitting form that does not respond to aggressive therapy.[4]

Joint Manifestations. Joint involvement usually is symmetric and polyarticular. Any diarthrodial joint can be involved. The person may complain of joint pain and stiffness that lasts for 30 minutes and frequently for several hours. The limitation of joint motion that occurs early in the disease usually is because of pain; later, it is because of fibrosis. The most frequently affected joints initially are the fingers, hands, wrists,

knees, and feet. Later, other diarthrodial joints may become involved. Spinal involvement usually is limited to the cervical region. In the hands, there usually is bilateral and symmetric involvement of the proximal interphalangeal (PIP) and metacarpophalangeal (MCP) joints in the early stages of RA; the distal interphalangeal (DIP) joints rarely are affected. The fingers often take on a spindle-shaped appearance because of inflammation of the PIP joints.

Progressive joint destruction may lead to subluxation (*i.e.,* dislocation of the joint resulting in misalignment of the bone ends) and instability of the joint and limitation of movement. Swelling and thickening of the synovium can result in stretching of the joint capsule and ligaments. When this occurs, muscle and tendon imbalances develop, and mechanical forces applied to the joints through daily activities produce joint deformities. In the MCP joints, the extensor tendons can slip to the ulnar side of the metacarpal head, causing ulnar deviation of the fingers (see Fig. 59-2A). Subluxation of the MCP joints may develop when this deformity is present. Hyperextension of the PIP joint and partial flexion of the DIP joint is called a *swan neck deformity.* After this condition becomes fixed, severe loss of function occurs because the person can no longer make a fist. Flexion of the PIP joint with hyperextension of the DIP joint is called a *boutonnière deformity.*

The knee is one of the most commonly affected joints and is responsible for much of the disability associated with the disease.[1] Active synovitis may be apparent as visible swelling that obliterates the normal contour over the medial and lateral aspects of the patella. The *bulge sign,* which involves milking fluid from the lateral to the medial side of the patella, may be used to determine the presence of excess fluid when it is not visible. Joint contractures, instability, and genu valgus (knock-knee) deformity are other possible manifestations. Severe quadriceps atrophy can contribute to the disability. A *Baker cyst* may develop in the popliteal area behind the knee. This is caused by enlargement of the bursa but does not usually cause symptoms unless the cyst ruptures, in which case symptoms mimicking thrombophlebitis appear.

Ankle involvement can limit flexion and extension, which can create difficulty in walking. Involvement of the metatarsophalangeal joints can cause subluxation, hallux valgus, and hammer toe deformities. Neck discomfort is common. In rare cases, long-standing disease can lead to neurologic complications such as occipital headaches, muscle weakness, and numbness and tingling in the upper extremities.

Extra-articular Manifestations. Although characteristically a joint disease, RA can affect a number of other tissues. Extra-articular manifestations probably occur with a fair degree of frequency but usually are mild enough to cause few problems. They are most likely to occur in persons who have the RF.

Because RA is a systemic disease, it may be accompanied by complaints of fatigue, weakness, anorexia, weight loss, and low-grade fever when the disease is active. The erythrocyte sedimentation rate (ESR), which commonly is elevated during

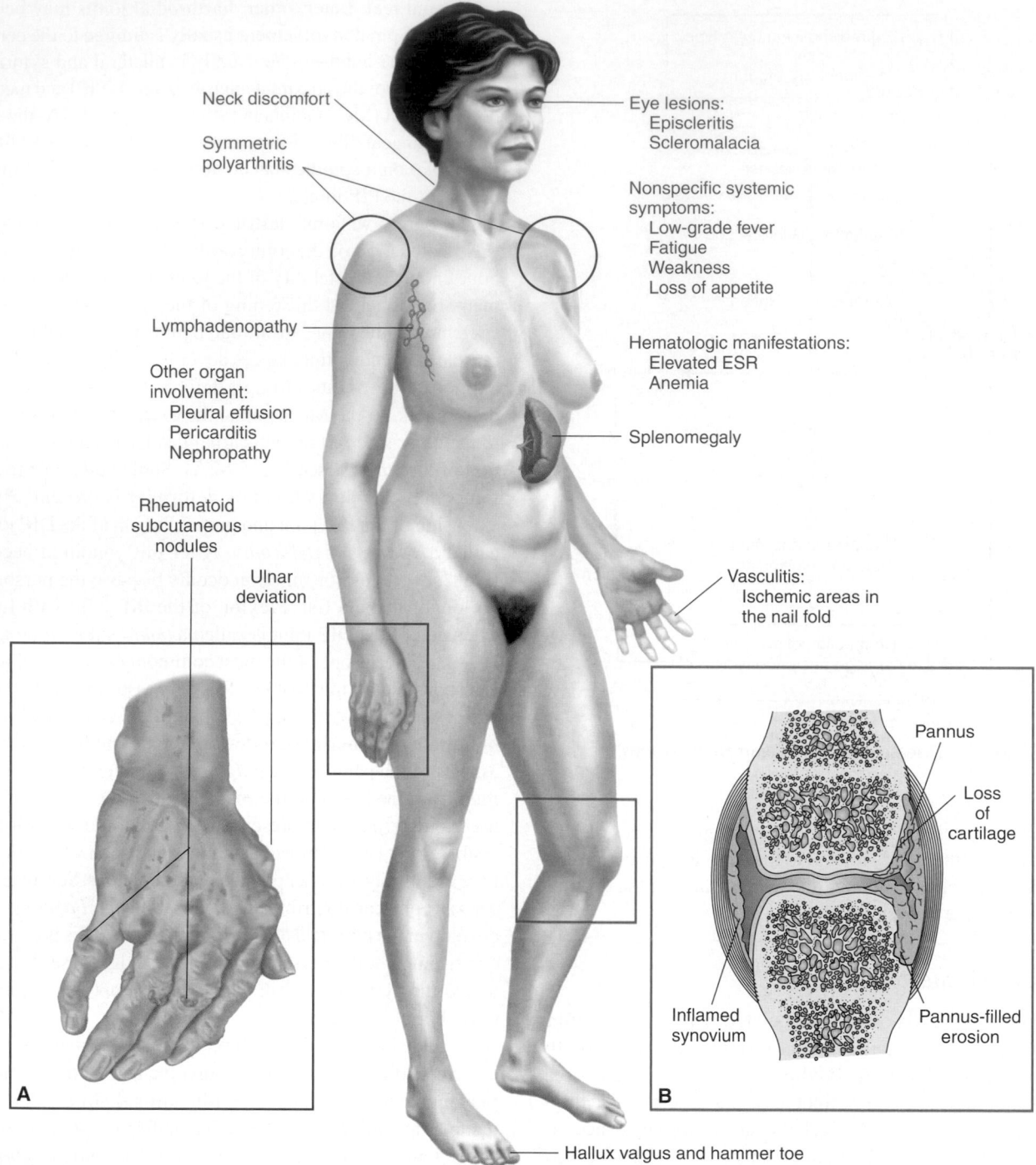

Neck discomfort

Symmetric
polyarthritis

Lymphadenopathy

Other organ
involvement:
    Pleural effusion
    Pericarditis
    Nephropathy

Rheumatoid
subcutaneous
nodules

Ulnar
deviation

Eye lesions:
    Episcleritis
    Scleromalacia

Nonspecific systemic
symptoms:
    Low-grade fever
    Fatigue
    Weakness
    Loss of appetite

Hematologic manifestations:
    Elevated ESR
    Anemia

Splenomegaly

Vasculitis:
    Ischemic areas in
    the nail fold

Pannus

Loss
of
cartilage

Inflamed
synovium

Pannus-filled
erosion

A

B

Hallux valgus and hammer toe

FIGURE 59-2 • Clinical manifestations of rheumatoid arthritis featuring (**A**) hand and finger manifestations and (**B**) destructive joint changes. ESR, erythrocyte sedimentation rate.

inflammatory processes, has been found to correlate with the
amount of disease activity.[5] Anemia associated with a low
serum iron level or low iron-binding capacity is common.[1] This
anemia usually is resistant to iron therapy.

Rheumatoid nodules are granulomatous lesions that
develop around small blood vessels. The nodules may be tender
or nontender, movable or immovable, and small or large. Typically, they are found over pressure points such as the extensor

surfaces of the ulna. The nodules may remain unless surgically
removed, or they may resolve spontaneously.

Vasculitis, or inflammation of small and medium-sized
arteries, is an uncommon manifestation of RA in persons with
a long history of active arthritis and high titers of RF (see
Chapter 22). Manifestations include ischemic areas in the nail
fold and digital pulp that appear as brown spots. Ulcerations
may occur in the lower extremities, particularly around the

malleolar areas. In some cases, neuropathy may be the only symptom of vasculitis. The visceral organs, such as the heart, lungs, and gastrointestinal tract, also may be affected.

Other extra-articular manifestations include eye lesions such as episcleritis, and scleromalacia, which is due to scleral nodules and is capable of causing retinal detachment, and pulmonary and cardiac complications (pleuritis and pericarditis). A small number of persons have splenomegaly and lymph node enlargement.

Diagnosis and Treatment

The diagnosis of RA is based on findings of the history, physical examination, and laboratory tests. Information should be elicited regarding the duration of symptoms, systemic manifestations, stiffness, and family history. The criteria for RA developed by the American Rheumatism Association are useful in establishing the diagnosis[5] (Chart 59-1). At least four of the criteria must be present to make a diagnosis of RA. Although these criteria were developed for use in epidemiologic studies and are designed for classification purposes, and not as diagnostic criteria, they can be used as guidelines for diagnosing the illness in individual patients.

In the early stages, the disease often is difficult to diagnose. On physical examination, the affected joints show signs of inflammation, swelling, tenderness, and possibly warmth and reduced motion. The joints have a soft, spongy feeling because of the synovial thickening and inflammation. Body movements may be guarded to prevent pain. Changes in joint structure usually are not visible early in the disease.

The RF test results are not diagnostic for RA, but they can be of value in differentiating RA from other forms of arthritis. Between 1% and 5% of healthy persons have the factor, and its presence seems to be more common with advancing age.[6] Also,

a person can have RA without the presence of RF. Disease severity and activity tend to correlate with RF levels; patients with high RF levels tend to have a significantly higher frequency of extra-articular involvement (*e.g.,* rheumatoid nodules, vasculitis, neuropathy).[6] The detection of anti–cyclic citrullinated peptide (CCP) antibodies may be more useful for diagnosing RA because of its higher specificity. Citrulline is an unusual amino acid that is generated by the enzymatic digestion of arginine. Recent research suggests that citrulline-containing proteins may serve as specific targets for the IgG antibody response in RA.[7,8] Anti-CPP antibodies, which have been detected very early in RA, appear to be a good prognostic marker for the disease and discriminate between erosive and nonerosive forms of the disease.[9] Radiologic findings also are not diagnostic in RA because joint erosions often are not seen on radiographic images in the early stages of the disorder. Synovial fluid analysis can be helpful in the diagnostic process. The synovial fluid has a cloudy appearance, the white blood cell count is elevated as a result of inflammation, and the complement components are decreased.

The treatment goals for a person with RA are to reduce pain, minimize stiffness and swelling, maintain mobility, and become an informed health care consumer. The treatment plan includes education about the disease and its treatment, rest, therapeutic exercises, and medications. Because of the chronicity of the disease and the need for continuous, long-term adherence to the prescribed treatment modalities, it is important that the treatment be integrated with the person's lifestyle.

Strategies to aid in symptom control also involve regulating activity by pacing, establishing priorities, and setting realistic goals. Support groups and group education experiences benefit some persons. The home and work environments should be assessed, and interventions should be incorporated as the situation warrants.

Both physical rest and emotional rest are important aspects of care.[1] Physical rest reduces joint stress. Rest of specific joints is recommended to relieve pain. For example, sitting reduces the weight on an inflamed knee, and the use of lightweight splints reduces undue movement of the hand or wrist. Emotional rest helps muscles relax and is often useful for persons who find that emotional stress increases discomfort. Although rest is essential, therapeutic exercises also are important in maintaining joint motion and muscle strength. Range-of-motion exercises involve the active and passive movement of joints. Isometric (muscle-tensing) exercises may be used to strengthen muscles. These exercises are usually taught by a physical therapist and performed daily at home. The difference between normal activity and therapeutic exercise should be emphasized. Aerobic exercise and muscle-strengthening exercises can be an important component of the treatment regimen of selected patients. Studies have shown that although persons with RA may have low levels of physical fitness, they can benefit from individualized exercise programs without experiencing joint damage or flare-ups of the disease.[10]

Instruction in the safe use of heat and cold modalities to relieve discomfort and in the use of relaxation techniques also is important. Proper posture, positioning, and body mechanics and the use of supportive shoes can provide further comfort. There often is a need for information about the principles of

---

CHART 59-1 | **CRITERIA FOR CLASSIFICATION OF RHEUMATOID ARTHRITIS**

Four or more of the following conditions must be present to establish a diagnosis of rheumatoid arthritis:

1. Morning stiffness for at least 1 hour and present for at least 6 weeks
2. Simultaneous swelling of three or more joints for at least 6 weeks
3. Swelling of wrist, metacarpophalangeal, or proximal interphalangeal joints for 6 or more weeks
4. Symmetric joint swelling for 6 or more weeks
5. Rheumatoid nodules
6. Serum rheumatoid factor identified by a method that is positive in less than 5% of normal subjects
7. Radiographic changes typical of rheumatoid arthritis on hand or wrist radiographs.

Adapted from Arnett F. C., Edworthy S. M., Block D. L., et al. (1988). The American Rheumatism Association 1987 revised criteria for the clarification of rheumatoid arthritis. *Arthritis and Rheumatism 31,* 315–324.

joint protection and work simplification. Some persons may need assistive devices to reduce pain and improve their ability to perform activities of daily living.

The goals of pharmacologic therapy for RA are to reduce pain, decrease inflammation, maintain or restore joint function, and prevent bone and cartilage destruction. Medications used to achieve these goals are classified as those that provide relief of arthritis symptoms and those that have the potential for modifying the course of the disease. The trend in RA management is toward a more aggressive pharmacologic approach at an earlier stage in the disease. Ideally, disease-modifying antirheumatic drug therapy should be used when the diagnosis of RA is established and before erosive changes appear on radiography.[1] Early treatment is based on the theory that T-cell–dependent pathways, which manifest early in the inflammatory process, are more responsive to treatment than later in the process, when disease progression is controlled by activated fibroblasts and macrophages, and the disease may be more resistant to treatment.

Nonsteroidal anti-inflammatory drugs (NSAIDs) usually are used early in the treatment of RA. The NSAIDs inhibit cyclooxygenase (COX)-mediated synthesis of prostaglandins, which have a damaging effect on joint structures. NSAIDs, including salicylates (*e.g.,* aspirin), provide analgesic and anti-inflammatory effects. Effectiveness, side effects, cost, and dosing schedules are considered when selecting an NSAID. There is a wide range of responses to the various NSAIDs, and the particular NSAID that works best for any one individual is not always predictable. The incidence of adverse reactions to the NSAIDs (*e.g.,* gastric irritation and bleeding, fluid retention, kidney damage) tends to increase with age and long-term use. The selective COX-2 inhibitors (*e.g.,* celecoxib) were developed with the goal of decreasing the gastrointestinal adverse effects seen with the traditional NSAIDs.[11] There are two COX isomers—COX-1 and COX-2. COX-1 is continuously expressed in many cells and is responsible for the general effects of prostaglandins, including protection of the gastric mucosa; whereas COX-2 is induced by cytokines and mainly expressed in inflammatory tissues.

Early treatment also includes the disease-modifying antirheumatic drugs (DMARDs). DMARDs include gold salts, hydroxychloroquine, sulfasalazine, methotrexate, and azathioprine. Methotrexate has become the drug of choice because of its potency, and it is relatively fast acting (*i.e.,* improvement is seen in 1 month) compared with the slower-acting DMARDs, which can take 3 to 4 months to work. Methotrexate is thought to interfere with purine metabolism, leading to the release of adenosine, a potent anti-inflammatory compound. All of the DMARDs can be toxic and require close monitoring for adverse effects, especially those related to bone marrow suppression.

Corticosteroid drugs may be used to reduce discomfort. These agents interrupt the inflammatory and immune cascade at several levels, such as interfering with inflammatory cell adhesion and migration, impairing prostaglandin synthesis, and inhibiting neutrophil superoxide production. To avoid long-term side effects, they are used only in specific situations for short-term therapy at a low dose level. They may be used for unremitting disease with extra-articular manifestations.

The corticosteroids do not modify the disease and are unable to prevent joint destruction. Intra-articular corticosteroid injections can provide rapid relief of acute or subacute inflammatory synovitis (after infection is excluded) in a few joints. They should not be repeated more than a few times each year.

Second-line antirheumatic drugs include leflunomide, etanercept, infliximab, and adalimumab.[12] Leflunomide is a pyrimidine synthesis inhibitor that blocks the expansion of T cells. Its efficacy is equal to that of methotrexate. Infliximab, etanercept, and adalimumab are biologic response–modifying agents that block TNF-α, one of the key proinflammatory cytokines in rheumatoid arthritis.[12] The anti-TNF-α agents have shown significant efficacy and favorable safety profiles. These agents have also been shown to inhibit radiologic disease progression and improve functional outcomes.[12]

Another approach to RA treatment is combination DMARD therapy.[13] This approach is a generally accepted one, and has been shown to be effective in several studies. Individual drugs with different mechanisms of action are given simultaneously to control the disease. The individual drugs are then tapered as symptoms subside and clinical remission is achieved.

Newer biologic response modifiers, abatacept and rituximab, have recently become available for treatment of persons with RA who have had an inadequate response to one or more of the DMARDs. Abatacept, a T-cell modulator, binds to CD80/CD86 on antigen-presenting cells, preventing the costimulatory signal that results in full T-cell activation.[14] Rituximab is a chimeric antibody that binds to the antigen CD20 on pre-B and mature B lymphocytes, causing their destruction. B-cell depletion is associated with reduction of markers of inflammation, including IL-6, C-reactive protein, anti-CCP, and RF.[14]

Surgery also may be a part of the treatment of RA.[1] Synovectomy may be indicated to reduce pain and joint damage when synovitis does not respond to medical treatment. The most common soft tissue surgery is tenosynovectomy (*i.e.,* repair of damaged tendons) of the hand to release nerve entrapments. Total joint replacements (*i.e.,* arthroplasty) may be indicated to reduce pain and increase motion. Arthrodesis (*i.e.,* joint fusion) is indicated only in extreme cases when there is so much soft tissue damage and scarring or infection that a replacement is impossible.

Although the course of RA is unpredictable, increasingly effective treatments for the disease have been developed since the late 1990s. Patients with arthritic symptoms are being diagnosed and treated earlier, and criteria have been developed for remission in RA.

Systemic Lupus Erythematosus

Systemic lupus erythematosus is a chronic inflammatory disease that can affect virtually any organ system, including the musculoskeletal system. It is a major rheumatic disease, with a prevalence of approximately 1 case per 2000 persons. Approximately 500,000 persons in the United States have this disease. There is a female predominance of 10 to 1, and this ratio is closer to 30 to 1 during the childbearing years. SLE is more common in

African Americans, Hispanics, and Asians than whites, and the incidence in some families is higher than in others.[15]

Etiology and Pathogenesis

The cause of SLE is unknown. It is characterized by the formation of autoantibodies and immune complexes. Persons with SLE appear to have B-cell hyperreactivity and increased production of antibodies against self (*i.e.,* autoantibodies) and nonself antigens. These B cells are polyclonal, each producing a different type of antibody. The autoantibodies can directly damage tissues or combine with corresponding antigens to form tissue-damaging immune complexes. Autoantibodies have been identified against an array of nuclear and cytoplasmic cell components (*e.g.,* microtubles, ribosomes, RNA). Some autoantibodies that have been identified in SLE are anti-nuclear antibodies (ANA), including anti-deoxyribonucleic acid (anti-DNA) antibodies. In addition to ANAs, persons with lupus have a host of other self-autoantibodies including those directed against elements of the blood (red cells, platelets, lymphocytes) and plasma proteins (clotting and complement factors).

The development of autoantibodies can result from a combination of factors, including genetic, hormonal, immunologic, and environmental factors.[16] Genetic predisposition is evidenced by the occurrence of familial cases of SLE, especially among identical twins. The increased incidence among African Americans compared with whites also suggests genetic factors. As many as four genes may be involved in the expression of SLE in humans. Genes linked to the HLA-DR and HLA-DQ loci in the MHC class II molecules show strong support for a genetic link in the development of SLE.[17] Studies also suggest that an imbalance in sex hormone levels may play a role in the development of the disease, especially because the disease is so prevalent among women. Androgens appear to protect against the development of SLE, whereas estrogens seem to favor its development. It has been suggested that an imbalance in sex hormone levels may lead to heightened helper T-cell and weakened suppressor T-cell immune responses that could in turn lead to the development of autoantibodies.[1]

Possible environmental triggers include ultraviolet (UV) light, chemicals (*e.g.,* drugs, hair dyes), some foods, and infectious agents.[16] UV light, specifically UVB associated with exposure to the sun or unshielded fluorescent bulbs, may trigger exacerbations. Photosensitivity occurs in approximately one third of patients with SLE. Certain drugs may also provoke a lupus-like disorder in susceptible persons, particularly in the elderly. The most common of these drugs are hydralazine and procainamide. Other drugs, such as quinidine, chlorpromazine, methyldopa, isoniazid, minocycline, and phenytoin, also have been known to produce this syndrome. The disease usually recedes when the drug is discontinued.[1]

Clinical Manifestations

Systemic lupus erythematosus can manifest in a variety of ways. The disease has been called the *great imitator* because it has the capacity for affecting many different body systems,

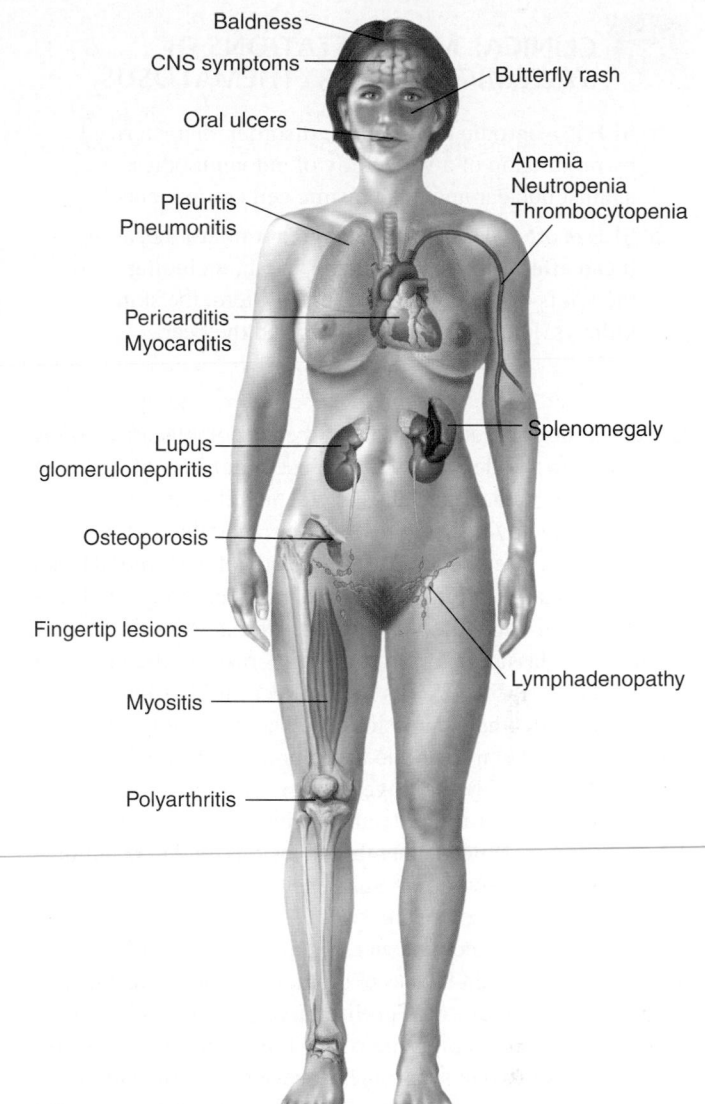

FIGURE 59-3 • Clinical manifestations of systemic lupus erythematosus.

including the musculoskeletal system, the skin, the cardiovascular system, the lungs, the kidneys, the central nervous system (CNS), and the red blood cells and platelets (Fig. 59-3). The onset may be acute or insidious, and the course of the disease is characterized by exacerbations and remissions. Rare cases result in death within weeks or months.

Arthralgias and arthritis are among the most commonly occurring early symptoms of SLE; approximately 90% of all persons with the disease complain of joint pain at some point during the course of their disease.[16] The polyarthritis of SLE initially can be confused with other forms of arthritis, especially RA, because of the symmetric arthropathy. However, on radiologic examination, articular destruction rarely is found. Ligaments, tendons, and the joint capsule may be involved, causing varied deformities in approximately 30% of persons with the disease. Flexion contractures, hyperextension of the interpha-

CLINICAL MANIFESTATIONS OF SYSTEMIC LUPUS ERYTHEMATOSUS

- SLE is a chronic autoimmune disorder characterized by production of a wide array of autoantibodies against nuclear and cytoplasmic cell components.
- SLE is often described as the great imitator because it can affect almost any organ system, including the joints of the musculoskeletal system, the skin, kidneys, lungs, nervous system, and the heart.

langeal joints, and subluxation of the carpometacarpal joints contribute to the deformity and subsequent loss of function in the hands. Other musculoskeletal manifestations of SLE include tenosynovitis, rupture of the intrapatellar and Achilles tendons, and avascular necrosis, frequently of the femoral head.

Skin manifestations can vary greatly and may be classified as acute, subacute, or chronic. The acute skin lesions include the classic malar or "butterfly" rash on the nose and cheeks (see Fig. 59-3). This rash is seen in SLE but may be associated with other skin lesions, such as hives or livedo reticularis (*i.e.,* reticular cyanotic discoloration of the skin, often precipitated by cold) and fingertip lesions, such as periungual erythema, nail fold infarcts, and splinter hemorrhages. Hair loss is common. Mucous membrane lesions tend to occur during periods of exacerbation. Sun sensitivity may occur in SLE even after mild sun exposure.

Renal involvement occurs in approximately 50% of persons with SLE. Several forms of glomerulonephritis may occur, including mesangial, focal proliferative, diffuse proliferative, and membranous (see Chapter 33). Interstitial nephritis also may occur. Nephrotic syndrome causes proteinuria with resultant edema in the legs and abdomen, and around the eyes. Renal failure may or may not be preceded by the nephrotic syndrome. Kidney biopsy is the best determinant of renal damage and the extent of treatment needed.

Pulmonary involvement in SLE occurs in 40% to 50% of patients and is manifested primarily by pleural effusions or pleuritis. Less frequently occurring pulmonary problems include acute pneumonitis, pulmonary hemorrhage, chronic interstitial lung disease, and pulmonary embolism.

Pericarditis is the most common of the cardiac manifestation, occurring in up to 30% to 40% of persons with SLE and often accompanied by pleural effusions. Myocarditis affects as much as 25% of those with SLE. Congenital heart block can occur in infants of mothers with SLE who have a specific type of ANA (anti-Ro) in their serum. Secondary heart disease also is a problem in those with SLE. Hypertension may be associated with lupus nephritis and long-term corticosteroid use. Ischemic heart disease can occur in older patients with longer-duration SLE. Infective endocarditis is rare but can occur with valvular lesions.[16]

The CNS is involved in 30% to 75% of persons with SLE. The pathologic basis for the CNS symptoms is not entirely clear. It has been ascribed to an acute vasculitis that impedes blood flow, causing strokes or hemorrhage; an immune response involving antineuronal antibodies that attack nerve cells; or production of antiphospholipid antibodies that damage blood vessels and cause blood clots in the brain. Seizures can occur and are more frequent when renal failure is present. Psychotic symptoms, including depression and unnatural euphoria, as well as decreased cognitive functioning, confusion, and altered levels of consciousness, may develop. More research is being done on the role of psychological factors in triggering the onset of SLE.

Hematologic disorders may manifest as hemolytic anemia, leukopenia, lymphopenia, or thrombocytopenia. Lymphadenopathy also may occur in 50% of all patients with SLE.[16] Discoid SLE (*i.e.,* chronic cutaneous lupus) involves plaque-like lesions on the head, scalp, and neck. These lesions first appear as red, swollen patches of skin, and later there can be scarring, depigmentation, and plugging of hair follicles. Ninety percent of patients with discoid lupus have disease that involves only the skin.

Subacute cutaneous lupus erythematosus (SCLE) is a less severe form of lupus. The skin lesions in this condition may resemble psoriasis. These lesions are found in sun-exposed areas such as the face, chest, upper back, and arms. Patients with SCLE may have mild systemic problems, which usually are limited to joint and muscle pains. There is a low incidence of lupus nephritis among those with SCLE.

Diagnosis and Treatment

The diagnosis of SLE can be complicated and difficult. The American College of Rheumatology has defined 11 criteria to be considered in the diagnosis of the disease, but these are intended for use in clinical trials rather than for individual diagnosis.[18] Diagnosis is based on a complete history, physical examination, and analysis of blood work. No single test can diagnose SLE in all persons.

The most common laboratory test performed is the immunofluorescence test for ANA. Ninety-five percent of persons with untreated SLE have high ANA levels. The ANA test is not specific for SLE, and positive ANA results may be found in healthy persons or may be associated with other disorders. The anti-DNA antibody test is more specific for the diagnosis of SLE.[18] Other serum tests may reveal moderate to severe anemia, thrombocytopenia, and leukocytosis or leukopenia. Additional immunologic tests may be done to give support to the diagnosis or to differentiate SLE from other connective tissue diseases.

Treatment of SLE focuses on managing the acute and chronic symptoms of the disease. Communication and trust between health care providers and the person with SLE are the basis for long-term disease management. The goals of treatment include preventing progressive loss of organ function, reducing the possibility of exacerbations, minimizing disability from the disease process, and preventing complications from medication therapy. Treatment with medications may be as simple as a drug to reduce inflammation, such as an NSAID. NSAIDs can control fever, arthritis, and mild pleuritis. An antimalarial drug (*e.g.*, hydroxychloroquine) may be the next medication considered to treat cutaneous and musculoskeletal manifestations of SLE. Corticosteroids are used to treat more significant symptoms of SLE, such as renal and CNS disorders. High-dose corticosteroid treatment is used for acute symptoms, and the drug is tapered to the lowest therapeutic dose as soon as possible to minimize the adverse effects. Immunosuppressive drugs are used in cases of severe disease. Cyclophosphamide, under closely monitored circumstances, has been found to be beneficial in the treatment of lupus nephritis.[19]

Systemic Sclerosis/Scleroderma

Systemic sclerosis, sometimes called *scleroderma,* is an autoimmune disease of connective tissue characterized by excessive collagen deposition in the skin and internal organs such as the lungs, gastrointestinal tract, heart, and kidneys. In this disorder, the skin is thickened through fibrosis, with an accompanying fixation of subdermal structures, including the sheaths or fascia covering tendons and muscles.[20] Systemic sclerosis affects women four times as frequently as men, with a peak incidence in the 35- to 50-year-old age group.[21] The cause of this rare disorder is poorly understood. There is evidence of both humoral and cellular immune system abnormalities.

Scleroderma presents as two distinct clinical entities: the diffuse or generalized form of the disease and the limited or CREST variant. In the CREST syndrome, hardening of the skin (scleroderma) is limited to the hands and face, whereas the skin changes in diffuse scleroderma also involve the trunk and proximal extremities. Almost all persons with scleroderma develop polyarthritis and Raynaud phenomenon, a vascular disorder characterized by reversible vasospasm of the arteries supplying the fingers (see Chapter 22).

Diffuse scleroderma is characterized by severe and progressive disease of the skin and the early onset of organ involvement. The typical person has a "stone facies" due to tightening of the facial skin with restricted motion of the mouth. Involvement of the esophagus leads to hypomotility and difficulty swallowing. Malabsorption may develop if the submucosal and muscular atrophy affect the intestine. Pulmonary involvement leads to dyspnea and eventually respiratory failure. Vascular involvement of the kidneys is responsible for malignant hypertension and progressive renal insufficiency. Cardiac problems include pericarditis, heart block, and myocardial fibrosis.

The CREST syndrome is manifest by *c*alcinosis (*i.e.,* calcium deposits in the subcutaneous tissue that erupt through the skin), *R*aynaud phenomenon, *e*sophageal dysmotility, *s*clerodactyly (localized scleroderma of the fingers), and *t*elangiectasia.[20]

Treatment of systemic sclerosis is largely symptomatic and supportive. Studies have indicated that if heart, lung, or kidney involvement is to become severe, it tends to do so early in the disease and is a predictor of shortened survival. Advances in treatment, primarily the use of angiotensin-converting enzyme (ACE) inhibitors in renal involvement, have led to a substantial decrease in the mortality from hypertensive renal disease.[21]

There is also some evidence that the ACE inhibitors may be disease modifying.[22] Cardiopulmonary manifestations of scleroderma, specifically pulmonary hypertension, can be treated with prostanoids (or endothelial receptor antagonists [bosentan]). Bosentan has been shown to improve survival in patients with scleroderma and pulmonary arterial hypertension.[23]

Polymyositis and Dermatomyositis

Polymyositis and dermatomyositis are chronic inflammatory myopathies. The pathogenesis is multifactorial and includes cellular and humoral immune mechanisms. Systemic manifestations are common, and cardiac and pulmonary complications often adversely affect the outcome. These conditions are characterized by symmetric proximal muscle weakness and occasional muscle pain and tenderness. Treatment for the inflammatory myopathies should seek to control inflammation and prevent long-term damage to muscles, joints, and internal organs. Corticosteroids are the mainstay of treatment for these conditions.

IN SUMMARY, rheumatoid arthritis is a systemic inflammatory disorder that affects 0.3% to 1.5% of the population. Women are affected more frequently than men. This form of arthritis, the cause of which is unknown, has a chronic course and usually is characterized by remissions and exacerbations. Joint involvement is symmetric and begins with inflammatory changes in the synovial membrane. As joint inflammation progresses, structural changes can occur, leading to joint instability and eventual deformity. Systemic manifestations include weakness, anorexia, weight loss, and low-grade fever. Some extra-articular features include rheumatoid nodules and vasculitis. The treatment goals include reducing pain, stiffness, and swelling; maintaining mobility; and assisting the person to become an informed health care consumer.

Systemic lupus erythematosus is a chronic autoimmune disorder that affects multiple body systems. There is no known cause of SLE, but the disease may result from an immunoregulatory disturbance brought about by a combination of genetic, hormonal, and environmental factors. Some drugs have been shown to induce SLE, especially in the elderly. There is an exaggerated production of autoantibodies, which interact with antigens to produce an immune complex. These immune complexes produce an inflammatory response in affected tissues. Treatment focuses on preventing loss of organ function, controlling inflammation, and minimizing complications of medication therapy.

Systemic sclerosis, often prefixed by the term *progressive,* is sometimes called *scleroderma.* In this disorder, the skin is thickened through fibrosis with an accompanying fixation to the subdermal structures, including the sheaths or fascia covering tendons and muscles. Polymyositis and dermatomyositis are chronic inflammatory myopathies. Its pathogenesis is multifactorial and includes cellular and humoral immune mechanisms. ■

SERONEGATIVE SPONDYLOARTHROPATHIES

After completing this section of the chapter, you should be able to meet the following objectives:

■ Cite a definition of the seronegative spondylo-arthropathies.
■ Cite the primary features of ankylosing spondylitis.
■ Describe how the site of inflammation differs in spondyloarthropathies from that in rheumatoid arthritis.
■ Contrast and compare ankylosing spondylitis, reactive arthritis, and psoriatic arthritis in terms of cause, pathogenesis, and clinical manifestations.

SERONEGATIVE SPONDYLOARTHROPATHIES

■ The seronegative spondyloarthropathies represent a group of related multisystem disorders that lack the RF.
■ The inflammatory process associated with the disorders commonly affects the axial skeleton, involving areas where ligaments and tendons attach to bone.
■ Although the cause of the disorders is unknown, there is a striking association between the HLA-B27 antigen and development of the spondyloarthropathies.

The *spondyloarthropathies* are an interrelated group of multisystem inflammatory disorders that primarily affect the axial skeleton, particularly the spine. Typically, the inflammation begins at sites where tendon and ligament insert into bone rather than in the synovium. Sacroiliitis is a pathologic hallmark of the disorders. Persons with the spondyloarthropathies may also have inflammation and involvement of the peripheral joints, in which case the signs and symptoms overlap with other inflammatory types of arthritis. Because there is an absence of the RF, these disorders often are referred to as *seronegative spondyloarthropathies.*

The seronegative spondyloarthropathies include ankylosing spondylitis, reactive arthritis, and psoriatic arthritis. Although they differ in terms of factors such as age and type of onset and extent of joint involvement, there is clinical evidence of overlap between the various seronegative spondyloarthropathies (Table 59-1). In none of these disorders is the cause or pathogenesis well understood. There is a striking association with the HLA-B27 antigen, but the presence of the HLA-B27 antigen by itself is neither necessary nor sufficient for the development of any of the diseases.[24]

Ankylosing Spondylitis

Ankylosing spondylitis is a chronic, systemic inflammatory disease of the joints of the axial skeleton manifested by pain and progressive stiffening of the spine. The disease is more common than once was believed, affecting approximately 2% to 8% of the HLA-B27–positive white population.[25] Clinical manifestations usually begin in late adolescence or early adulthood and are slightly more common in men than in women. The disease usually evolves more slowly and is less severe in women.

Ankylosing spondylitis produces an inflammatory erosion of the sites where tendons and ligaments attach to bone.[25] Typically, the disease process begins with bilateral involvement of the sacroiliac joints and then moves to the smaller joints of the posterior elements of the spine. The result is ultimate destruction of these joints with ankylosis or posterior fusion of the spine. The vertebrae take on a squared appearance and bone bridges fuse one vertebral body to the next across the intervertebral disks. Progressive spinal changes usually follow an ascending pattern beginning with the sacroiliac area and then moving up the spine to involve the costovertebral joints and cervical spine. Occasionally, large synovial joints (*i.e.,* hips, knees, and shoulders) may be

TABLE 59-1 **Comparison of the Spondyloarthropathies**				
CHARACTERISTIC	ANKYLOSING SPONDYLITIS	REITER SYNDROME	PSORIATIC ARTHRITIS	INFLAMMATORY BOWEL DISEASE
Age at onset	Young adult	Young to middle age	Any age	Any age
Type of onset	Gradual	Sudden	Variable	Gradual
Sacroiliitis	>95%	20%	20%	10%
Peripheral joint involvement	25%	90%	All (about 5% to 7% of those patients with psoriasis)	Occasional
HLA-B27 (in whites)	>90%	75%	<50%	<50%
Eye involvement	25% to 30%	Common	Occasional	Occasional

Adapted from Arnett F. C., Khan M. A., Willikens R. F. (1989). A new look at ankylosing spondylitis. *Patient Care 23*(19), 82–101.

involved. The small peripheral joints usually are not affected. The disease spectrum ranges from an asymptomatic sacroiliitis to a progressive disease that can affect many body systems.

Etiology and Pathogenesis

Although the pathogenesis of ankylosing spondylitis has not been established, the presence of mononuclear cells in the acutely involved tissue suggests an immune response. Epidemiologic findings indicate that genetic and environmental factors play a role in the pathogenesis of the disease. The HLA-B27 antigen remains one of the best-known examples of an association between a disease and a hereditary marker.[24] Although approximately 90% of those with ankylosing spondylitis possess the HLA-B27 antigen and nearly 100% of those who also have uveitis or aortitis have the marker, the HLA-B27 antigen also is present in approximately 8% of the normal population. Several theories have been advanced to account for the association between the HLA-B27 antigen and ankylosing spondylitis. One possibility is that the gene that determines the HLA-B27 antigen may be linked to other genes that determine the pathologic autoimmune phenomena or that lead to increased susceptibility to infections or environmental agents. A second theory postulates molecular mimicry; an autoimmune reaction to an antigenic determinant site in the host's tissues may occur as a consequence of an immunologic response to an identical or closely related antigen of a foreign agent, usually an infectious agent[25] (see Chapter 19).

Clinical Manifestations

The person with ankylosing spondylitis typically complains of low back pain, which may be persistent or intermittent. The pain, which becomes worse when resting, particularly when lying in bed, initially may be blamed on muscle strain or spasm from physical activity. Lumbosacral pain also may be present, with discomfort in the buttocks and hip areas. Sometimes, pain can radiate to the thigh in a manner similar to that of sciatic pain. Prolonged stiffness is present in the morning and after periods of rest. Mild physical activity or a hot shower helps reduce pain and stiffness. Sleep patterns frequently are interrupted because of these manifestations. Walking or exercise may be needed to provide the comfort needed to return to sleep. Muscle spasm also may contribute to discomfort.[25]

Loss of motion in the spinal column is characteristic of the disease (Fig. 59-4). The severity and duration of disease activity influence the degree of mobility. Loss of lumbar lordosis occurs as the disease progresses, and this is followed by kyphosis of the thoracic spine and extension of the neck. A spine fused in the flexed position is the end result in severe ankylosing spondylitis. A kyphotic spine makes it difficult for the patient to look ahead and to maintain balance while walking. The image is one of a person bent over looking at the floor and unable to straighten up. X-ray films show a rigid, bamboo-like spine. The heart and lungs are constricted in the chest cavity. Abnormal weight bear-

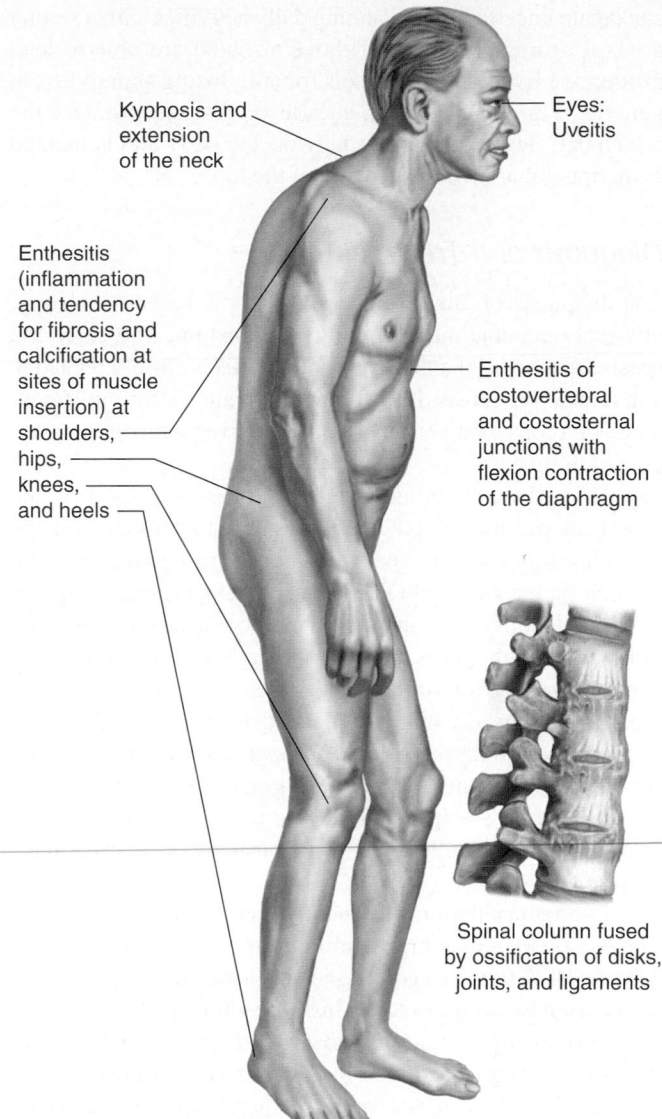

FIGURE 59-4 • Clinical manifestations of ankylosing spondylitis.

ing can lead to degeneration and destruction of the hips, necessitating joint replacement procedures. Peripheral arthritis is more common in the hips and shoulders. The incidence of hip joint involvement varies from 17% to 36% and potentially is more crippling than involvement in any other joint.[1]

The most common extraskeletal involvement is acute anterior uveitis, which occurs in 25% to 30% of patients sometime in the course of their disease.[1] Systemic features of weight loss, fever, and fatigue may be apparent. Sometimes, the fatigue is a greater problem than pain or stiffness. Osteoporosis can occur, especially in the spine, which contributes to the risk of spinal fracture. Fusion of the costovertebral joints can lead to reduced lung volume.

The disease process varies considerably among individuals. Exacerbations and remissions are common; their unpredictability can create uncertainty in planning daily activities and in setting goals. Fortunately, most of those affected are able to lead productive lives. The prognosis for ankylosing spondylitis in general is good. The first decade of disease predicts the remainder. Severe disease usually occurs early and is marked by peripheral arthritis, especially of the hip.

Diagnosis and Treatment

The diagnosis of ankylosing spondylitis is based on history, physical examination, and x-ray examination. The early and precise diagnosis of ankylosing spondylitis is closely related to a favorable prognosis. Early recognition allows for implementation of a conservative and usually effective treatment program on a lifelong basis.

Several methods are available to assess mobility and detect sacroiliitis. These methods include pressure on the sacroiliac joints with the person in a forward-bending position to elicit pain and muscle spasm, measurement of the distance between the tips of the fingers and the floor in a bent-over position with straight knees, and a modified Schober test in which contralateral flexion of the back is measured. Although these measures alone do not provide a diagnosis of ankylosing spondylitis or other spondyloarthropathies, they can provide useful measurements for monitoring the disease status. Measurement of chest expansion may be used as an indirect indicator of thoracic involvement, which usually occurs late in the disease course.

Laboratory findings frequently include an elevated ESR. The person also may have a mild normocytic normochromic anemia. HLA typing is not diagnostic of the disease and should not be used as a routine screening procedure. Radiologic evaluations help differentiate ankylosing spondylitis from sacroiliitis due to other diseases. However, x-ray images may be negative in early disease. Vertebrae normally are concave on the anterior border. In ankylosing spondylitis, the vertebrae take on a squared appearance (see Fig. 59-4).

Treatment of ankylosing spondylitis is directed at controlling pain and maintaining mobility by suppressing inflammation. Proper posture and positioning are important. This includes sleeping in a supine position on a firm mattress and using one small pillow or no pillow. A bed board may be used to supply additional firmness. Therapeutic exercises are important to assist in maintaining motion in peripheral joints and in the spine. Muscle-strengthening exercises for extensor muscle groups also are prescribed. Heat applications or a shower or bath may be beneficial before exercise to improve ease of movement. Swimming is an excellent general conditioning exercise that avoids joint stress and enhances muscle tone. Immobilizing joints is not recommended. Maintaining ideal weight reduces the stress on weight-bearing joints. Smoking should be discouraged because it can exacerbate respiratory problems. Occupational counseling or job evaluation may be warranted because of postural abnormalities.

Pharmacologic treatment includes the use of NSAIDs to reduce inflammation, relieve pain, and reduce muscle spasm.

DMARDs are potential second-line therapies, but their efficacy in ankylosing spondylitis is unproven. Sulfasalazine and methotrexate have not shown benefit for spondylitis-associated back pain, but have shown efficacy for the peripheral joint involvement. Anti–TNF-α therapies, including etanercept, infliximab, and adalimumab, have demonstrated rapid effectiveness in reducing both the axial and peripheral symptoms of ankylosing spondylitis, as well as improving quality-of-life measures.[26]

Reactive Arthropathies

The reactive arthropathies may be defined as sterile inflammatory joint disorders that are distant in time and place from the initial inciting infective process. The infecting agents cannot be cultured and are not viable once having reached the joints. The list of triggering agents is continuously increasing and may be divided into urogenic, enterogenic, and respiratory tract associated, and the idiopathic arthritides. In some cases, the identity of the causative agent is unknown.[27]

Commonly recognized forms of reactive arthritis include those involving *Chlamydia pneumoniae* infection and *Pseudomonas*. Additional and frequently occurring pathogens include *Chlamydia trachomatis, Salmonella, Shigella, Yersinia, Campylobacter,* and *Streptococcus*.[27] Reactive arthritis also has been observed in persons with acquired immunodeficiency syndrome (AIDS). Spondyloarthropathies such as Reiter syndrome and psoriatic arthritis are more severe and frequent in human immunodeficiency virus (HIV)–infected patients than in the general population. It is thought that the immune response to HIV infection is selective and largely spares the natural killer cells, which may be critical in the pathogenesis of these conditions.[27] This is in contrast to RA and SLE, which dramatically improve as immunodeficiency develops. Reactive arthritis may also result from the presence of a foreign substance in the joint tissue, as in silicone implants in the small joints of the hands or feet or after exposure to industrial gases and oils. However, there is no evidence of antigenicity of the causative substance.

In the strictest sense, the definition of reactive arthritis includes a possibility of immunologic sensitization before arthritic development.[27] Similarities exist between reactive arthritis and bacterial arthritis. Several bacteria cause both diseases. When cultured bacteria are isolated from the synovial fluid, the diagnosis is bacterial arthritis. When they cannot be isolated, even though there has been a preceding infection, the diagnosis of reactive arthritis is made.

Reactive arthritis may follow a self-limited course; it may involve recurrent episodes of arthritis; or, in a small number of cases, it may follow a continuous and unremitting course. The treatment is largely symptomatic. NSAIDs are used in treating the arthritic symptoms. Vigorous treatment of possible triggering infections is thought to prevent relapses of reactive arthritis, but in many cases the triggering infection passes unnoticed or is mild, and the patient contacts a physician only with the onset of definite arthritis. Short antibiotic courses at this time are not effective.

Reiter Syndrome

Reiter syndrome is considered to be a clinical manifestation of reactive arthritis that may be accompanied by extra-articular symptoms such as uveitis, bowel inflammation, and carditis. The disease develops in a genetically susceptible host after a bacterial infection due to *C. trachomatis* in the genitourinary tract or *Salmonella, Shigella, Yersinia,* or *Campylobacter* in the gastrointestinal tract.[28]

The term *Reiter syndrome* soon may be relegated to history as the pathogenesis becomes better understood. Alternative designations include SARA (sexually associated reactive arthritis) and the BASE syndrome (HLA-B27, arthritis, sacroiliitis, and extra-articular inflammation).[28] Reiter syndrome was the first rheumatic disease to be recognized in association with HIV infection. Symptoms of arthritis may precede any overt signs of HIV disease. Treatment with agents such as methotrexate and azathioprine may further suppress the immune response and provoke a full expression of AIDS.

Enteropathic Arthritis

Arthritis that is associated with an inflammatory bowel disease usually is considered an enteropathic arthritis because the intestinal disease is directly involved in the pathogenesis. Most cases of enteropathic arthritis are classified among the spondyloarthropathies. These include cases in which the arthritis is associated with inflammatory bowel disease (*i.e.,* ulcerative colitis and Crohn disease), the reactive arthritides triggered by enterogenic bacteria, some of the undifferentiated spondyloarthropathies, Whipple disease, and reactions after intestinal bypass surgery.[1] There is no direct relation between the activity of the bowel disease and the degree of arthritis activity.

Psoriatic Arthritis

Psoriatic arthritis is a seronegative inflammatory arthropathy that occurs in 5% to 7% of people with psoriasis. It is a heterogeneous disease with features of the spondyloarthropathies in some persons, RA in others, and features of both coexisting in yet others.

The etiology of psoriasis and psoriatic arthritis is unknown. Genetic, environmental, and immunologic factors appear to affect susceptibility and play a role in expression of the psoriatic skin disease and the arthritis. Environmental factors that may play a role in the pathogenesis of the disorder include infectious agents and physical trauma. T-cell–mediated immune responses seem to play an important role in the skin and joint manifestations of the disease, as indicated by the observation that there is improvement in disease status after treatment with immunosuppressant agents such as cyclosporine.

Although the arthritis can antedate a detectable skin rash, the definitive diagnosis of psoriatic arthritis cannot be made without evidence of skin or nail changes typical of psoriasis. Psoriatic arthritis falls into five subgroups: oligoarticular or asymmetric (48%); spondyloarthropathy (24%); polyarticular, or symmetric (18%); distal interphalangeal (8%); and mutilans (2%).[29] This heterogeneous clinical presentation suggests more than one dis-

ease is associated with psoriasis, or various clinical responses to a common cause. At least 20% of those with psoriatic arthritis have an elevated serum level of uric acid. The abnormally elevated serum uric acid level is caused by the rapid skin turnover of psoriasis and the subsequent breakdown of nucleic acid followed by its metabolism to uric acid. This finding may lead to a misdiagnosis of gout. Psoriatic arthritis tends to be slowly progressive, but has a more favorable prognosis than RA.

Basic management is similar to the treatment of RA. Suppression of the skin disease may be important in helping control the arthritis. Often, affected joints are surprisingly functional and only minimally symptomatic. The biologic response modifiers, specifically the TNF inhibitors (*e.g.,* etanercept, infliximab, and adalimumab), have been found to be beneficial in controlling the arthritis as well as the psoriasis in patients with psoriatic arthritis.[29]

IN SUMMARY, the seronegative arthropathies are a group of rheumatic disorders that lack the rheumatoid factor. The *seronegative spondyloarthropathies* affect the axial skeleton, particularly the spine. Inflammation develops at sites where tendons and ligaments insert into bone. They include ankylosing spondylitis, reactive arthritis, and psoriatic arthritis. Ankylosing spondylitis is considered a prototype of this classification category. Bilateral sacroiliitis is the primary feature of ankylosing spondylitis. The disease spectrum ranges from asymptomatic sacroiliitis to a progressive disorder affecting many body systems. The cause remains unknown; however, a strong association between the HLA-B27 antigen and ankylosing spondylitis has been identified. Loss of motion in the spinal column is characteristic of the disease. Peripheral arthritis may occur in some persons. Another form of spondyloarthritis is reactive arthritis. Although there are overlapping features for each of the spondyloarthropathies, identifying etiologic differences and clinical manifestations is important for determining treatment.

Psoriatic arthritis is a seronegative arthropathy that occurs in 5% to 7% of people with psoriasis. It is a heterogeneous disease with features of the spondyloarthropathies in some persons, RA in others, and features of both coexisting in yet others. ■

OSTEOARTHRITIS SYNDROME

After completing this section of the chapter, you should be able to meet the following objectives:

■ Compare rheumatoid arthritis and osteoarthritis in terms of joint involvement, level of inflammation, and local and systemic manifestations.

■ Describe the pathologic joint changes associated with osteoarthritis.

■ Characterize the treatment of osteoarthritis.

CHART 59-2	CAUSES OF OSTEOARTHRITIS

Postinflammatory disorders
    Rheumatoid arthritis
    Septic joint
Post-traumatic disorders
    Acute fracture
    Ligament or meniscal injury
    Cumulative occupational or recreational trauma
Anatomic or bony disorders
    Hip dysplasia
    Avascular necrosis
    Paget disease
    Slipped capital femoral epiphysis
    Legg-Calvé-Perthes disease
Metabolic disorders
    Calcium crystal deposition
    Hemochromatosis
    Acromegaly
    Wilson disease
    Ochronosis
Neuropathic arthritis
    Charcot joint
Hereditary disorders of collagen
Idiopathic or primary variants

 OSTEOARTHRITIS

- Often referred to as "wear-and-tear" arthritis, osteoarthritis is a slowly destructive disorder of the articular cartilage.

- It can present as a primary disease of unknown etiology or as a secondary disorder related to congenital or acquired defects that affect the distribution of joint stress.

- The pathogenesis of osteoarthritis includes the progressive disruption of the smooth surface of the articular cartilage with development of surface cracks that deepen to involve the subchondral bone, followed by complete erosion of the articular cartilage with exposure of ivory-like polished subchondral bone, dislodgment of fragments of free-floating osteocartilaginous bodies, development of bone cysts, and formation of abnormal bony spurs at the joint margins.

Osteoarthritis (OA), formerly called *degenerative joint disease,* is the most prevalent form of arthritis and is a leading cause of disability and pain in the elderly. OA is more of a disease process than a specific entity. The term encompasses a heterogeneous collection of syndromes, including OA of the hand, knee, hip, foot, and spine.[30] It can occur as a primary idiopathic disorder or as a secondary disorder, although this distinction is not always clear. Idiopathic or primary variants of OA occur as localized or generalized (*i.e.,* involvement of more than three joints) syndromes.[31] Secondary OA has a known underlying cause such as congenital or acquired defects of joint structures, trauma, metabolic disorders, or inflammatory diseases (Chart 59-2).

The joint changes associated with OA, which include a progressive loss of articular cartilage and synovitis, result from the inflammation caused when cartilage attempts to repair itself, creating osteophytes or spurs. These changes are accompanied by joint pain, stiffness, and limitation of motion, and in some cases by joint instability and deformity. Fortunately, changes in the traditional conservative management of this underemphasized condition are occurring. Attitudes regarding the inevitability of the limitations imposed by this condition are changing on the part of health care providers and persons with the disease.

Epidemiology and Risk Factors

Age, gender, and race interact to influence the time of onset and the pattern of joint involvement in OA. Men are affected more commonly at a younger age than women, but the rate of women affected exceeds that of men by middle age.[30] Heredity influences the occurrence of hand OA in the DIP joint. Hand OA is more likely to affect white women, whereas knee OA is more common in black women. The incidence of hip OA is lower among the Chinese than Europeans, perhaps representing the influence of other factors such as occupation, obesity, or heredity. Bone mass may also influence the risk of developing OA. In theory, thinner subchondral bone mass may provide a greater shock-absorbing function than denser bone, allowing less direct trauma to the cartilage.

Obesity is a particular risk factor for OA of the knee in women and a contributory biomechanical factor in the pathogenesis of the disease. Excess fat may have a direct metabolic effect on cartilage beyond the effects of excess joint stress. Weight loss reduces the risk of developing symptomatic arthritis of the knee.[30] Although the radiographic incidence of knee OA increases with advancing age, the incidence of symptomatic OA of the knee decreases.[30]

Pathogenesis

The pathogenesis of OA resides in the homeostatic mechanisms that maintain the articular cartilage. Articular cartilage plays two essential mechanical roles in joint physiology. First, the articular cartilage serves as a remarkably smooth weight-bearing surface. In combination with synovial fluid, the articular cartilage provides extremely low friction during movement of the joint. Second, the cartilage transmits the load down to the bone, dissipating the mechanical stress.[32] Thus, the subchondral bone protects the overlying articular cartilage, providing it with a pliable bed and absorbing the energy of the force (Fig. 59-5).

Cartilage is a specialized type of connective tissue. As with other types of tissue, it consists of cells (*i.e.,* chondro-

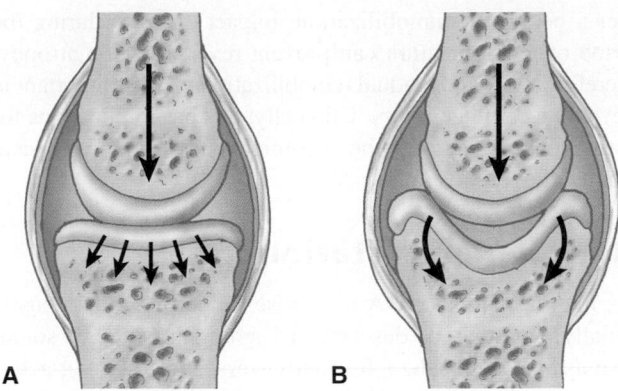

FIGURE 59-5 • (A) A joint normally undergoes deformation of the articular cartilage and the subchondral bone when carrying a load. This maximizes the contact area and spreads the force of the load. (B) If the joint does not deform with a load, the stresses are concentrated and the joint breaks down.

cytes) nested in an extracellular matrix. In articular cartilage, the extracellular matrix is composed of water, proteoglycans, collagen, and ground substance. The proteoglycans, which are large macromolecules made up of disaccharides and amino acids, afford elasticity and stiffness, permitting articular cartilage to resist compression. The ground substance constitutes a highly hydrated, semisolid gel. Collagen molecules consist of polypeptide chains that form long, fibrous strands. They provide form and tensile strength. The primary function of the collagen fibers is to provide a rigid scaffold to support the chondrocytes and ground substance of cartilage. The hydrated proteoglycan molecules, because of their size and charge, are trapped in the collagen meshwork of the extracellular matrix and prevented from expanding to their maximum size. This confers the high interstitial osmotic pressure and fluid volume that is needed for lubrication of the joint.[32] As in the case of adult bone, articular cartilage is not static; it undergoes turnover and its "worn out" matrix components are continually degraded and replaced. This turnover is maintained by the chondrocytes, which not only synthesize the matrix but secrete matrix-degrading enzymes. Thus, the health of the chondrocytes determines joint integrity. In OA, this integrity can be disturbed by a number of influences.

Popularly known as *wear-and-tear* arthritis, OA is characterized by significant changes in both the composition and mechanical properties of cartilage. Early in the course of the disease, the cartilage contains increased water and decreased concentrations of proteoglycans compared with healthy cartilage. In addition, there appears to be a weakening of the collagen network, presumably caused by a decrease in the local synthesis of new collagen and an increase in the breakdown of existing collagen. The articular cartilage injury that occurs in OA is thought to result from the release of cytokines such as IL-1 and TNF[32] (Fig. 59-6). These chemical messengers stimulate production and release of proteases (enzymes) that are destructive to joint structures.[32] The resulting damage predisposes the chondrocytes to more injury and impairs their ability

to repair the damage by producing new collagen and proteoglycans. The combined effects of inadequate repair mechanisms and imbalances between the proteases and their inhibitors contribute further to disease progression.

The earliest structural changes in OA include enlargement and reorganization of the chondrocytes in the superficial part of the articular cartilage. This is accompanied by edematous changes in the cartilaginous matrix, principally the intermediate layer. The cartilage loses its smooth aspect and surface cracks or microfractures occur, allowing synovial fluid to enter and widen the crack. As the crack deepens, vertical clefts form and eventually extend through the full thickness of the articular surface and into the subchondral bone.[32] Portions of the articular cartilage eventually become completely eroded and the exposed surface of the subchondral bone becomes thickened and polished to an ivory-like consistency (eburnation). Fragments of cartilage and bone often become dislodged, creating free-floating osteocartilaginous bodies ("joint mice") that enter the joint cavity. Synovial fluid may leak though the defects in the residual cartilage to form cysts within the bone.[32] As the disease progresses, the underlying trabecular bone becomes sclerotic in response to increased pressure on the surface of the joint, rendering it less effective as a shock absorber. Sclerosis, or formation of new bone and cysts, usually occurs at the joint margins, forming abnormal bony outgrowths called *osteophytes*, or *spurs* (Fig. 59-7). As the joint begins to lose its integrity, there is trauma to the synovial membrane, which results in nonspecific inflammation. Compared with RA, however, the changes in the synovium that occur in OA are not as pronounced, nor do they occur as early.

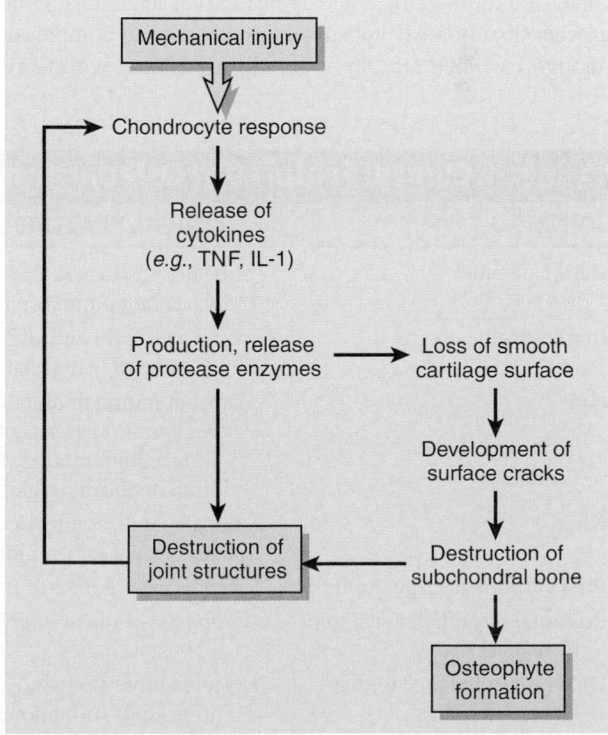

FIGURE 59-6 • Disease process in osteoarthritis.

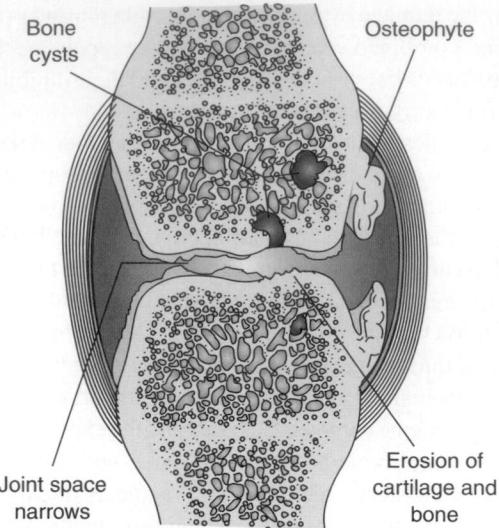

FIGURE 59-7 • Joint changes in osteoarthritis. The left side denotes early changes and joint space narrowing with cartilage breakdown. The right side shows more severe disease progression with lost cartilage and osteophyte formation.

In secondary forms of OA, repetitive impact loading contributes to joint failure, accounting for the high prevalence of OA specific to vocational or avocational sites, such as the shoulders and elbows of baseball pitchers, ankles of ballet dancers, and knees of basketball players. Immobilization also can produce degenerative changes in articular cartilage. Cartilage degeneration due to immobility may result from loss of the pumping action of lubrication that occurs with joint movement. These changes are more marked and appear earlier in areas of contact but occur also in areas not subject to mechanical compression. Although cartilage atrophy is rapidly reversible with activity after a period of immobilization, impact exercise during the period of remobilization can prevent reversal of the atrophy. Therefore, slow and gradual remobilization may be important in preventing cartilage injury. Clinically, this has implications for instructions concerning the recommended level of physical activity after removal of a cast.

Clinical Manifestations

The manifestations of OA may arise suddenly or insidiously. Initially, pain may be described as aching and may be somewhat difficult to localize. It usually worsens with use or activity and is relieved by rest. In later stages of disease activity, night pain may be experienced during rest. Pain can occur at rest, several hours after the use of the involved joints. Crepitus and grinding may be evident when the joint is moved. As the disease advances, even minimal activity may cause pain because of the limited range of motion resulting from intra-articular and periarticular structural damage.

The most frequently affected joints are the hips, knees, lumbar and cervical vertebrae, proximal and distal joints of the hands, the first carpometacarpal joint, and the first metatarsophalangeal joints of the feet. Table 59-2 identifies the joints that commonly are affected by OA and the common clinical features correlated with the disease activity of each particular joint. A single joint or several may be affected. Although a single weight-bearing joint may be involved initially, other joints often become affected because of the additional stress placed on them while trying to protect the initial joint. It is not unusual for a person having a knee replacement to discover soon after the surgery is done that the second knee also needs to be replaced. Other clinical features are limitations of joint motion and joint instability. Joint enlargement usually results from new bone formation; the joint feels hard, in contrast to the soft, spongy feeling character-

TABLE 59-2 Clinical Features of Osteoarthritis

JOINT	CLINICAL FEATURES
Cervical spine	Localized stiffness; radicular or nonradicular pain; posterior osteophyte formation may cause vascular compression
Lumbar spine	Low back pain and stiffness; muscle spasm; decreased back motion; nerve root compression causing radicular pain; spinal stenosis
Hip	Most common in older men; characterized by insidious onset of pain, localized to groin region or inner aspect of the thigh; may be referred to buttocks, sciatic region, or knee; reduced hip motion; leg may be held in external rotation with hip flexed and adducted; limp or shuffling gait; difficulty getting in and out of chairs
Knee	Localized discomfort with pain on motion; limitation of motion; crepitus; quadriceps atrophy due to lack of use; joint instability; genu varus or valgus; joint effusion
First carpometacarpal joint	Tenderness at base of thumb; squared appearance to joint
Proximal interphalangeal joint—Bouchard nodes	Same as for distal interphalangeal joint disease
Distal interphalangeal joint—Heberden nodes	Occurs more frequently in women; usually involves multiple DIPs, lateral flexor deviation of joint, spur formation at joint margins, pain and discomfort after joint use
First metatarsophalangeal joint	Insidious onset; irregular joint contour; pain and swelling aggravated by tight shoes

istic of the joint in RA. Sometimes, mild synovitis or increased synovial fluid can cause joint enlargement.

Diagnosis and Treatment

The diagnosis of OA usually is determined by history and physical examination, x-ray studies, and laboratory findings that exclude other diseases. Although OA often is contrasted with RA for diagnostic purposes, the differences are not always readily apparent. Other rheumatic diseases may be superimposed on OA. Psychological factors, severity of joint disease, and educational level affect the expression of symptoms.[31]

Characteristic radiologic changes initially include medial joint space narrowing, followed by subchondral bony sclerosis, formation of spikes on the tibial eminence, and osteophytes. The results of laboratory studies usually are normal because the disorder is not a systemic disease. The ESR may be slightly elevated in generalized OA or erosive inflammatory variations of the disease. If inflammation is present, there may be a slight increase in the white blood cell count. The synovial fluid usually is normal.

Because there is no cure, the treatment of OA is symptomatic and includes physical rehabilitative, pharmacologic, and surgical measures. Physical measures are aimed at improving the supporting structures of the joint and strengthening opposing muscle groups involved in cushioning weight-bearing forces. This includes a balance of rest and exercise, use of splints to protect and rest the joint, use of heat and cold to relieve pain and muscle spasm, and adjusting the activities of daily living. Weight reduction is helpful when the knee is involved. The involved joint should not be further abused, and steps should be taken to protect and rest it. These include weight reduction (when weight-bearing surfaces are involved) and the use of a cane or walker if the hips and knees are involved. Muscle-strengthening exercises may help protect the joint and decrease pain.[30]

Oral medications are aimed at reducing inflammation or providing analgesia. Popular medications used in the treatment of OA are the NSAIDs, many of which are available without a prescription. Ongoing research may confirm that some NSAIDs impede the repair mechanisms in early cartilage lesions. There is growing concern about the side effects of NSAIDs, and the newer COX-2–inhibiting agents also are indicated for the treatment of OA. However, studies have shown that the pain of OA may arise from factors other than an inflamed synovium. These factors include stretching of the joint capsule, ligaments, or nerve endings in the periosteum over osteophytes; nontrabecular microfractures; intraosseous hypertension; bursitis or tendinitis; and muscle spasm. In such cases, the pain may be relieved by an NSAID through the analgesic effect of the drug rather than its anti-inflammatory effect.[1] For many persons, acetaminophen may be as effective and less toxic than NSAIDs. The American College of Rheumatology (ACR) recommends the use of acetaminophen as the initial systemic treatment for OA.[33]

Intra-articular corticosteroid injections may be used when other treatment measures have been unsuccessful in adequately relieving symptoms. They are especially helpful in persons who have an effusion of the joint. Injections usually are limited to a total of four and not more than three within 1 year because their use is thought to accelerate joint destruction.

Viscosupplementation is a newer concept in treatment and is based on the hypothesis that joint lubrication is abnormal in OA. Hyaluronate is injected into the joint weekly for 3 to 5 weeks. Controlled studies have shown this approach to be equally as efficacious as NSAIDs.[34] Speculation that other agents (*i.e.*, glucosamine and chondroitin sulfate) may be chondroprotective has prompted other studies, some of which demonstrated greater pain relief with treatment with either compound than with placebo, and others finding little or no difference.[35,36] A recent multicenter trial funded by the National Institutes of Health found that glucosamine hydrochloride was no more efficacious than placebo.[35,36] It is interesting to note, however, that some studies that used glucosamine sulfate rather than glucosamine hydrochloride reported greater pain relief in their treatment group compared with their placebo group.[35] Other compounds with collagenase-inhibiting properties are being developed and investigated as structure- or disease-modifying agents for OA.[37]

Surgery is considered when the person is having severe pain and joint function is severely reduced. Procedures include arthroscopic lavage and debridement, bunion resections, osteotomies to change alignment of the knee and hip joints, and decompression of the spinal roots in osteoarthritic vertebral stenosis. Total hip replacements have provided effective relief of symptoms and improved range of motion for many persons, as have total knee replacements, although the latter procedure has produced less consistent results. Joint replacement is available for the first carpometacarpal joint. Arthrodesis (surgical stiffening of a joint) is used in advanced disease to reduce pain; however, this results in loss of motion.

Future management of OA lies in the development of techniques to identify and monitor cartilage lesions at an earlier stage. Potential approaches include bone scanning, magnetic resonance imaging, and arthroscopy.

IN SUMMARY, OA, the most common form of arthritis, is a localized condition affecting primarily the weight-bearing joints. Risk factors for OA progression include older age, OA in multiple joints, neuropathy, and for knees, obesity. The disorder is characterized by degeneration of the articular cartilage and subchondral bone. It has been suggested that the cellular events responsible for the development of OA begin with some type of abnormal mechanical insult or stimulus, including hormones and growth factors, drugs, mechanical stresses, and the extracellular environment. Studies also implicate immunologic factors in the perpetuation and acceleration of the osteoarthritic change. As cartilage ages, biochemical events such as collagen fatigue and fracture occur with less stress. Attempts at repair by increased matrix synthesis and cellular proliferation maintain the integrity of the cartilage until failure of reparative processes allows the degenerative changes to progress. Joint enlargement usually results from new bone formation, which causes the joint to feel hard. Pain and stiffness are primary features of the disease. Inflammatory mediators (*e.g.,* prostaglandins) may increase the inflammatory and degenerative response.

Treatment is directed toward the relief of pain and maintenance of mobility while preserving the articular cartilage. Although there is no known cure for OA, appropriate treatment can reduce pain, maintain or improve joint mobility, and limit functional disability. ■

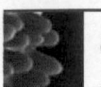

CRYSTAL-INDUCED ARTHROPATHIES

After completing this section of the chapter, you should be able to meet the following objectives:

- Relate the metabolism and elimination of uric acid to the pathogenesis of crystal-induced arthropathy.
- State why asymptomatic hyperuricemia is a laboratory finding and not a disease.
- Describe the clinical manifestations, diagnostic measures, and methods used in the treatment of gouty arthritis.

Metabolic bone and joint disorders result from biochemical and metabolic disorders that affect the joints. Metabolic and endocrine diseases associated with joint symptoms include amyloidosis, osteogenesis imperfecta, diabetes mellitus, hyperparathyroidism, thyroid disease, AIDS, and hypermobility syndromes. The discussion in this chapter is limited to the crystal-induced arthropathy caused by monosodium urate deposition, or gout.

Crystal deposition in joints produces arthritis. In gout, monosodium urate or uric acid crystals are found in the joint cavity. Another condition in which calcium pyrophosphate dihydrate crystals are found in the joints sometimes is referred to as *pseudogout* or *chondrocalcinosis*. A brief discussion of pseudogout is found in the section on rheumatic diseases in the elderly.

Gout

Gout is actually a group of diseases known as the *gout syndrome.*[38] It includes acute gouty arthritis with recurrent attacks of severe articular and periarticular inflammation; tophi or the accumulation of crystalline deposits in articular surfaces, bones, soft tissue, and cartilage; gouty nephropathy or renal impairment; and uric acid kidney stones.

The term *primary gout* is used to designate cases in which the cause of the disorder is unknown or an inborn error in metabolism and is characterized primarily by hyperuricemia and gout. Primary gout is predominantly a disease of men, with a peak incidence in the fourth to sixth decade.[1] In secondary gout, the cause of the hyperuricemia is known but the gout is not the main disorder. Asymptomatic hyperuricemia is a laboratory finding and not a disease. Most persons with hyperuricemia do not develop gout.

Pathogenesis

The pathogenesis of gout resides in an elevation of serum uric acid levels. Uric acid is the end product of purine (adenine and guanine from DNA and RNA) metabolism.[39] Two pathways are involved in purine synthesis: (1) a de novo pathway in which purines are synthesized from nonpurine precursors; and (2) the salvage pathway in which purine bases are recaptured from the breakdown of nucleic acids derived from exogenous (dietary) or endogenous sources. The elevation of uric acid and the subsequent development of gout can result from overproduction of purines, decreased salvage of free purine bases, augmented breakdown of nucleic acids as a result of increased cell turnover, or decreased urinary excretion of uric acid. Primary gout, which constitutes 90% of cases, may be a consequence of enzyme defects that result in an overproduction of uric acid; inadequate elimination of uric acid by the kidney; or a combination of the two.[39] In most cases, the reason is unknown. In secondary gout, the hyperuricemia may be caused by the increased breakdown of nucleic acids, as occurs with rapid tumor cell lysis during treatment for lymphoma or leukemia. Other cases of secondary gout result from chronic renal disease. Some of the diuretics, including the thiazides, can interfere with the excretion of uric acid.

An attack of gout occurs when monosodium urate crystals precipitate in the joint and initiate an inflammatory response. Synovial fluid is a poorer solvent for uric acid than plasma, and uric acid crystals are even less soluble at temperatures below 37°C. Crystal deposition usually occurs in peripheral areas of the body, such as the great toe, where the temperatures are cooler than other parts of the body. With prolonged hyperuricemia, crystals and microtophi (*i.e.,* small, hard nodules with irregular surfaces that contain crystalline deposits of monosodium urate) accumulate in the synovial lining cells and in the joint cartilage.[40] The released crystals are chemotactic to leukocytes and also activate complement. Phagocytosis of urate crystals by polymorphonuclear leukocytes occurs and leads to polymorphonuclear cell death with the release of lysosomal enzymes. As this process continues, the inflammation causes destruction of the cartilage and subchondral bone.

Repeated attacks of acute arthritis eventually lead to chronic arthritis and the formation of the large, hard nodules called *tophi*[39] (Fig. 59-8). They are found most commonly in the synovium, olecranon bursa, Achilles tendon, subchondral bone, and extensor surface of the forearm and may be mistaken for rheumatoid nodules. Tophi usually do not appear until 10 years or more after the first gout attack. This stage of gout, called *chronic tophaceous gout,* is characterized by more frequent and prolonged attacks, which often are polyarticular.

Clinical Manifestations

The typical acute attack of gout is monoarticular and usually affects the first metatarsophalangeal joint. The tarsal joints,

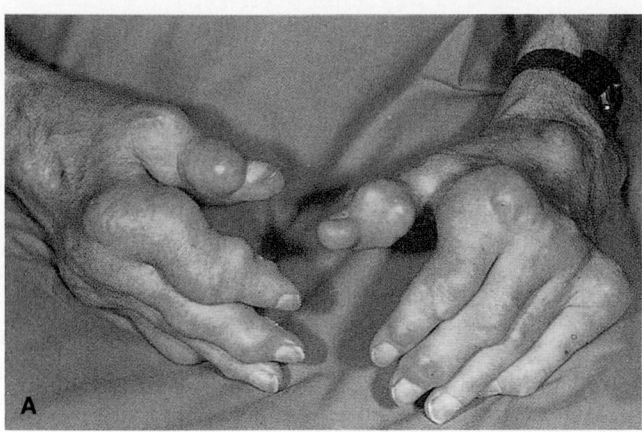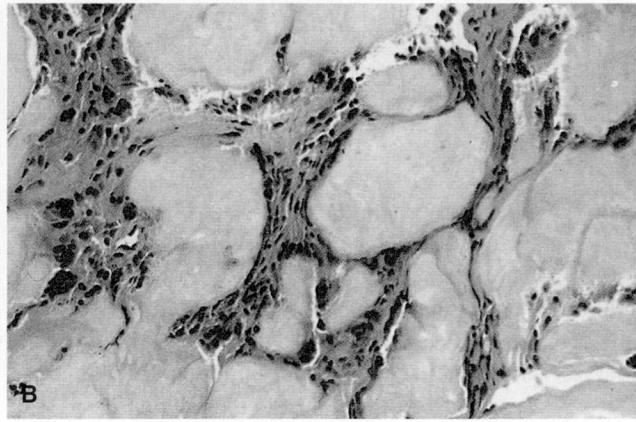

FIGURE 59-8 • Gout. (**A**) Gouty tophi project from the fingers as rubbery nodules. (**B**) A section from a tophus shows extracellular masses of urate crystals with accompanying foreign-body giant cells. (From Rubin E., Farber J. L. [Eds.]. [1999]. *Pathology* [3rd ed., p. 1404]. Philadelphia: Lippincott-Raven.)

insteps, ankles, heels, knees, wrists, fingers, and elbows also may be initial sites of involvement. Acute gout often begins at night and may be precipitated by excessive exercise, certain medications or foods, alcohol, or dieting. The onset of pain typically is abrupt, and redness and swelling are observed. The attack may last for days or weeks. Pain may be severe enough to be aggravated even by the weight of a bed sheet covering the affected area.

In the early stages of gout after the initial attack has subsided, the person is asymptomatic, and joint abnormalities are not evident. This is referred to as *intercritical gout.* After the first attack, it may be months or years before another attack. As attacks recur with increased frequency, joint changes occur and become permanent.

Diagnosis and Treatment

Although hyperuricemia is the biochemical hallmark of gout, the presence of hyperuricemia cannot be equated with gout because many persons with this condition never develop gout. A definitive diagnosis of gout can be made only when monosodium urate crystals are in the synovial fluid or in tissue sections of tophaceous deposits. Synovial fluid analysis is useful in excluding other conditions, such as septic arthritis, pseudogout, and RA. Diagnostic methods also include measures to determine if the disorder is related to overproduction or to underexcretion of uric acid. This is done through measurement of serum uric acid levels and collection of a 24-hour urine sample for determination of urate excretion in the urine.[39]

The objectives for treatment of gout include the termination and prevention of the acute attacks of gouty arthritis and the correction of hyperuricemia, with consequent inhibition of further precipitation of sodium urate and absorption of urate crystal deposits already in the tissues.

Pharmacologic management of acute gout is directed toward reducing joint inflammation. Hyperuricemia and

related problems of tophi, joint destruction, and renal problems are treated after the acute inflammatory process has subsided. NSAIDs, particularly indomethacin and ibuprofen, are used for treating acute gouty arthritis. Alternative therapies include colchicine and intra-articular deposition of corticosteroids. Treatment with colchicine is used early in the acute stage. Colchicine produces its anti-inflammatory effects by inhibition of leukocyte migration and phagocytosis. Although the drug usually is given orally, a more rapid response is obtained when colchicine is given intravenously. The acute symptoms of gout usually subside within 48 hours after treatment with oral colchicine has been instituted and within 12 hours after intravenous administration of the drug. The NSAIDs are also effective during the acute stage when used at their maximum dosage and sometimes are preferred to colchicine because they have fewer toxic side effects. The corticosteroid drugs have not been systemically studied, but can be useful in the treatment of acute gout limited to a single joint or bursa.

After the acute attack has been relieved, the hyperuricemia is treated. Treatment of hyperuricemia is aimed at maintaining normal uric acid levels and is lifelong. One method is to reduce hyperuricemia through the use of allopurinol or a uricosuric agent. Allopurinol inhibits xanthine oxidase, an enzyme needed for the conversion of hypoxanthine to xanthine and xanthine to uric acid.[40] The uricosuric drugs (*e.g.,* probenecid or sulfinpyrazone, a phenylbutazone derivative) prevent the tubular reabsorption of urate and increase its excretion in the urine. The serum urate concentrations are monitored to determine efficacy and dosage. Prophylactic colchicine or NSAIDs may be used between gout attacks.

Although gout can often be effectively controlled by nonpharmacologic methods, many persons with gout have a limited understanding of the disease and therefore a poor compliance with treatment. Thus, education about the disease and its management is fundamental to the treatment and management of gout. Some changes in lifestyle may be needed, such as maintenance of ideal weight, moderation in alcohol consumption, and avoidance of purine-rich foods (*e.g.*, liver, kidney, sardines, anchovies, and sweetbreads), particularly by patients with excessive tophaceous deposits.[40]

IN SUMMARY, crystal-induced arthropathy is characterized by crystal deposition in the joint. Gout is the prototype of this group. Acute attacks of arthritis occur with gout and are characterized by the presence of monosodium urate crystals in the joint. The disorder is accompanied by hyperuricemia, which results from overproduction of uric acid or from the reduced ability of the kidney to rid the body of excess uric acid. Management of acute gout is directed first toward the reduction of joint inflammation, after which the hyperuricemia is treated. Hyperuricemia is treated with uricosuric agents, which prevent the tubular reabsorption of urate, or with medication that inhibits the production of uric acid. Although gout is chronic, it can be controlled with appropriate lifestyle changes by most patients. ■

RHEUMATIC DISEASES IN CHILDREN AND THE ELDERLY

After completing this section of the chapter, you should be able to meet the following objectives:

■ List three types of juvenile arthritis and differentiate among their major characteristics.

■ Name one rheumatic disease that affects only the elderly population.

Rheumatic Diseases in Children

Children can be affected with almost all of the rheumatic diseases. In addition to disease-specific differences, these conditions affect not only the child but the family. Growth and development require special attention. Adherence to the treatment program requires intervention with the child and parents. School issues also must be addressed.

Juvenile Idiopathic Arthritis

Juvenile idiopathic arthritis (JIA) is a chronic disease that affects approximately 70,000 to 100,000 children younger than 16 years of age in the United States.[1] It is characterized by synovitis and can influence epiphyseal growth by stimulating growth of the affected side. Generalized stunted growth also may occur. JIA can be regarded not as a single disease, but as a category of diseases with three principal types of onset: (1) systemic-onset disease, (2) pauciarticular arthritis, and (3) polyarticular disease.

Systemic-onset disease affects approximately 10% of children with JIA.[1] The symptoms of systemic JIA include a daily intermittent high fever, which usually is accompanied by a rash, generalized lymphadenopathy, hepatosplenomegaly, leukocytosis, and anemia. Most of these children also have joint involvement, which develops concurrently with fever and rash. Systemic symptoms usually subside in 6 to 12 months. This form of JIA also can make an initial appearance in adulthood. Infections, heart disease, and adrenal insufficiency may cause death.

A second subgroup of JIA, pauciarticular arthritis, affects no more than four joints. This disease affects approximately 50% of children with JIA.[1] Pauciarticular arthritis affects two distinct groups. The first group generally consists of girls younger than 6 years of age with chronic uveitis. The results of ANA testing in this group usually are positive. The second group, characterized by late-onset arthritis, is made up mostly of boys. The HLA-B27 test results are positive in more than one half of this group. They are affected by sacroiliitis, and the arthritis usually occurs in the lower extremities.

The third subgroup, accounting for approximately 40% of the total cases of JIA, is polyarticular disease.[1] It affects five or more joints during the first 6 months of the disease. This form of arthritis more closely resembles the adult form of the disease than the other two subgroups. RF sometimes is present and may indicate a more active disease process. Systemic features include a low-grade fever, weight loss, malaise, anemia, stunted growth, slight organomegaly (*e.g.*, hepatosplenomegaly), and adenopathy.[1]

The prognosis for most children with JIA is good. NSAIDs are the first-line drugs used in treating JIA. Salicylates have been replaced by agents such as naproxen, ibuprofen, and ketoprofen. Second-line agents are low-dose methotrexate and, less often, sulfasalazine. Gold salts, hydroxychloroquine, and D-penicillamine rarely are used.[41] Biologic response modifiers are also being used in JIA, with etanercept being the first to get U.S. Food and Drug Administration approval.[42] Other aspects of treatment of children with JIA require careful attention to growth and development and nutritional issues. Children are encouraged to lead as normal a life as possible.

Systemic Lupus Erythematosus

The features of SLE in children are similar to those in adults. The incidence in children is 10 times lower, estimated at 1 in 167,000 children. The occurrence in the sexes is almost equal until puberty, after which it approaches the sex ratio seen in adults, which is predominantly female. The clinical manifestations of SLE in children reflect the extent and severity of systemic involvement. The best prognostic indicator in children is the extent of renal involvement, which is more common and more severe in children than in adults with SLE. Infectious complications are the most common cause of death (40%) in children with SLE.[1]

Children with SLE may present with constitutional symptoms, including fever, malaise, anorexia, and weight loss. Symptoms of the integumentary, musculoskeletal, central nervous, cardiac, pulmonary, and hematopoietic systems are similar to those of adults. Endocrine abnormalities include Cushing syndrome from long-term corticosteroid use and autoimmune thyroiditis. Adolescents often experience menstrual disturbances, which tend to resolve with disease remission.[1]

Treatment of SLE in children is similar to that in adults. The use of NSAIDs, corticosteroids, antimalarial drugs, and immunosuppressive agents depends on the symptoms. Corticosteroids may cause stunting of growth and necrosis of femoral heads and other joints. Immunization schedules should be maintained using attenuated rather than live vaccines. Rest periods should be balanced with exercise; children should be encouraged to maintain as normal a schedule as possible.[42] The diversity of the clinical manifestations of SLE in the young requires the establishment of a comprehensive treatment or management program.

Juvenile Dermatomyositis

Juvenile dermatomyositis (JDMS) is an inflammatory myopathy primarily involving skin and muscle and associated with a characteristic rash. JDMS can affect children of all ages, with a mean age at onset of 8 years. There is an increased incidence among girls. The cause is unknown. Symmetric proximal muscle weakness, elevated muscle enzymes, evidence of vasculitis, and electromyographic changes confirming an inflammatory myopathy are diagnostic for JDMS. Generalized vasculitis is not seen in the adult form of the disease. The rash may precede or follow the onset of proximal muscle weakness. Periorbital edema, erythema, and eyelid telangiectasia are common.

Calcifications can occur in 30% to 50% of children with JDMS and are by far the most debilitating symptom. The calcifications appear at pressure points or sites of previous trauma. JDMS is treated primarily with corticosteroids to reduce inflammation. Occasionally, immunosuppressives are used in cases of refractory disease.[1] Adjunct therapies include using sunblock with a sun protection factor (SPF) greater than 36, a calcium-sufficient diet, and vitamin D therapy.

Juvenile Spondyloarthropathies

Ankylosing spondylitis, reactive arthritis, psoriatic arthritis, and spondyloarthropathies associated with ulcerative colitis and regional enteritis can affect children as well as adults. In children, spondyloarthropathy manifests in peripheral joints first, mimicking pauciarticular JIA, with no evidence of sacroiliac or spine involvement for months to years after onset. The spondyloarthropathies are more common in boys and commonly occur in children who have a positive family history. HLA-B27 typing is helpful in diagnosing children because of the unusual presentation of the disease.

Management of the disease involves physical therapy, education, and attention to school and growth and development issues. Medication includes the use of salicylates or other NSAIDs such as tolmetin or indomethacin. More severe disease or symptoms may require systemic corticosteroids.[1] Etanercept and infliximab produce more dramatic improvement of disease activity; however, their long-term effects and toxicity are not yet known.[43]

 ## Rheumatic Diseases in the Elderly

Arthritis is the most common complaint of elderly persons. The pain, stiffness, and muscle weakness affect daily life, often threatening independence and quality of life. Symptoms of the rheumatic diseases can also have an indirect effect on and even threaten the duration of life for the elderly. The weakness and gait disturbance that often accompany the rheumatic diseases can contribute to the likelihood of falls and fracture, causing suffering, increased health care costs, further loss of independence, and the potential for a decreased life span.

The elderly cope less well with mild to moderately severe disease that in younger persons is less likely to lead to serious disability for the same degree of impairment. Unfortunately, the elderly and often their health care providers think the problems associated with arthritis are an inevitable consequence of aging and fail to take advantage of measures that can improve the quality of life.

Because arthritis is the leading cause of change in the functional status of older adults, a functional approach to the problems of the elderly is appropriate. Inactivity is a societal expectation of the elderly. What activity there is tends to be low impact (e.g., leisurely walking), and deconditioning occurs.

Older patients often have multiple problems complicating diagnosis and management. The diagnosis of an elderly patient with a musculoskeletal problem must consider a wide variety of disorders that usually are regarded as outside the range of typical rheumatic disease. Among these are metastatic malignancy, multiple myeloma, musculoskeletal disorders accompanying endocrine or metabolic disorders, orthopedic conditions, and neurologic disease. The diagnosis may be missed if the assumption is that musculoskeletal problems in the older person are caused by OA.

There is an increased incidence of false-positive test results for RF and ANA in the elderly population with or without rheumatic disease because older persons are better producers of autoantibodies than younger persons. There are differences in the manifestations, diagnosis, and treatment of some of the rheumatic diseases in the elderly. The usual presentation of these conditions was discussed earlier in this chapter. One form of rheumatic disease that has a predilection for the elderly is polymyalgia rheumatica.

Rheumatoid Arthritis

The prevalence of RA increases with advancing age, at least until 75 years of age.[44] Seropositive patients are more likely to have had an acute onset with systemic features and higher disease activity. Patients with seronegative, elderly-onset RA have a disease that usually follows a mild course. The close resemblance of the manifestations of seronegative RA in the elderly to those of polymyalgia rheumatica has led to speculation concerning the relationship of these syndromes.[44] It may be that RA in the elderly is a broad disorder that includes a number of distinct subsets with characteristic manifestations, courses, and outcomes.

Systemic Lupus Erythematosus

Systemic lupus erythematosus is another condition with different manifestations in the elderly. The disease is accompanied less frequently by renal involvement. However, pleurisy, pericarditis, arthritis, and symptoms closely resembling polymyalgia rheumatica are more common than in younger patients. The characteristics of SLE in the elderly closely resemble those of drug-induced SLE, leading to speculation that the syndrome may result from one of the multiple drugs that are taken by many elderly patients.[45]

Osteoarthritis

Osteoarthritis is by far the most common form of arthritis among the elderly. It is the greatest cause of disability and limitation of activity in older populations. It has been suggested that OA begins at a very young age, expressing itself in the elderly only after a long period of latency. Too often, it is accepted by the patient or expected by the physician. OA presents a major management problem, but there is much that can be done. Self-control by maintaining a positive attitude and sense of self-esteem is a frequent coping strategy.[46]

Crystal-Induced Arthropathies

Gout. The incidence of clinical gout increases with advancing age, in part because of the increased involvement of joints after years of continued hyperuricemia. High serum urate levels rarely occur in women before menopause; initial attacks of clinical gout occur around the age of 70 years, or 20 years after menopause.[38] Gouty attacks in elderly women may be precipitated by the use of diuretics. The treatment of gout is often more difficult in the elderly. Although colchicine may be effective in controlling the symptoms of chronic gout, it may cause diarrhea in some patients, limiting its effectiveness in maintenance therapy.

Pseudogout. As part of the tissue aging process, OA develops with associated cartilage degeneration and the shedding of calcium pyrophosphate crystals into the joint cavity. These crystals may produce a low-grade chronic inflammation—the chronic pseudogout syndrome. The accumulation of calcium pyrophosphate and related crystalline deposits in articular cartilage is common in the elderly. There are no medications that can remove the crystals from the joints. Although it may be asymptomatic, presence of the crystals may contribute to more

rapid cartilage deterioration. This condition may coexist with severe OA. Calcium pyrophosphate deposition disease may also present with proximal muscle pain mimicking polymyalgia rheumatica.[47]

Polymyalgia Rheumatica

Polymyalgia rheumatica is an inflammatory condition of unknown origin characterized by aching and morning stiffness in the cervical regions and shoulder and pelvic girdle areas.[48] Of the forms of arthritis affecting the elderly, it is one of the more difficult to diagnose and one of the most important to identify. Elderly women are especially at risk. Polymyalgia rheumatica is a common syndrome of older patients, rarely occurring before 50 years and usually after 60 years of age. The onset can be abrupt, with the patient going to bed feeling well and awakening with pain and stiffness in the neck, shoulders, and hips.

Diagnosis is based on the pain and stiffness persisting for at least 1 month and an elevated ESR. The diagnosis is confirmed when the symptoms respond dramatically to a small dose of prednisone, a corticosteroid. Biopsies have shown that the muscles are normal, despite the name, but that a nonspecific inflammation affecting the synovial tissue is present. It is possible that a number of patients are erroneously diagnosed as having RA or OA. For patients with an elevated ESR (0.5 mm), the diagnosis usually is based on a 3-day trial of prednisone treatment.[49] Patients with polymyalgia rheumatica typically exhibit striking clinical improvement approximately the second day. Patients with RA also show improvement, although usually days later.

Treatment with NSAIDs provides relief for some patients, but most require continuing therapy with prednisone, with gradual reduction of the dose over the course of 1.5 to 2 years, using the patient's symptoms as the primary guide. Patients need close monitoring during the maintenance phase with prednisone therapy. Because their symptoms are relieved, they often quit taking the prednisone and their symptoms recur, or doses are missed and the decreased dosage leads to an increase in symptoms. Unless careful assessment reveals the frequency of missed doses, the physician may be misled into increasing the dosage when it is not needed. Because of the side effects of the corticosteroids, the goal is to use the lowest dose of the drug necessary to control the symptoms. Weaning patients off low-dose prednisone therapy after this length of time can be a difficult and extended process.

A certain percentage of patients with polymyalgia rheumatica also develop giant cell arteritis (*i.e.,* temporal arteritis) with involvement of the ophthalmic arteries. The two conditions are considered to represent different manifestations of the same disease. Giant cell arteritis, a form of systemic vasculitis, is a systemic inflammatory disease of large and medium-sized arteries. The inflammatory response seems to be a T-cell response to an antigen.

Clinical manifestations of giant cell arteritis usually begin insidiously and may exist for some time before being recognized.[48] It is potentially dangerous if missed or mistreated, especially if the temporal artery or other vessels supplying the eye are involved, in which case blindness can ensue quickly without treatment. The condition is responsive to appropriate therapy. For those patients at risk, adherence to the medication program is critical, with preservation of sight being the goal. Because this complication can occur so quickly and is relatively asymptomatic, it is vital that the patient understand the importance of taking the correct dose regularly as prescribed. Initial treatment consists of large doses of prednisone. This dosage is continued for 4 to 6 weeks and then decreased gradually.

Management of Rheumatic Diseases in the Elderly

In addition to diagnosis-specific treatment, the elderly require special considerations. Management techniques that rely on modalities other than drugs are particularly important for the elderly. These include splints, walking aids, muscle-building exercise, and local heat. Muscle-strengthening and stretching exercises are particularly effective in the elderly person with age-related losses in muscle function and should be instituted early. Rest, the cornerstone of conservative therapy, is hazardous in the elderly, who can rapidly lose muscle strength.

In terms of medications, the selection of drugs used in the treatment of arthritic disorders and their dosages may need to be considered when prescribing for the elderly. For example, the NSAIDs may be less well tolerated by the elderly, and their side effects are more likely to be serious. In addition to bleeding from the gastrointestinal tract and renal insufficiency, there may be cognitive dysfunction manifested by forgetfulness, inability to concentrate, sleeplessness, paranoid ideation, and depression.

Joint arthroplasty can also be used for pain relief and increased function. Chronologic age is not a contraindication to surgical treatment of arthritis. In appropriately selected elderly candidates, survival and functional outcome after surgery are equivalent to those in younger age groups. The more sedentary activity level of the elderly makes them even better candidates for joint replacement because they put less stress and demand on the new joint.

IN SUMMARY, rheumatic diseases that affect children can be similar to the adult diseases, but there also are manifestations unique to the younger population. Children with chronic diseases also have to be approached with different priorities than adults. Managing rheumatic diseases in children requires a team approach to address issues of the family, school, growth and development, and coping strategies and requires a comprehensive disease management program.

Arthritis is the most common complaint of the elderly population. The pain, stiffness, and muscle weakness affect daily life, often threatening independence and quality of life. There is a difference in the manifestations, diagnosis, and treatment of some of the rheumatic diseases in the elderly compared with those in the younger population. Osteoarthritis is the most common form of arthritis among the elderly. The prevalence of rheumatoid arthritis and gout increases with advancing age. One form of rheumatic disease that has a predilection for the elderly is polymyalgia rheumatica. A certain percentage of patients with polymyalgia rheumatica also have giant cell arteritis, frequently with involvement of the ophthalmic arteries. If this condition is untreated, it carries a serious threat of blindness. ■

Review Exercises

1. A 30-year-old woman, recently diagnosed with rheumatoid arthritis (RA), complains of general fatigue and weight loss along with symmetric joint swelling, stiffness, and pain. The stiffness is more prominent in the morning and subsides during the day. Laboratory measures reveal a rheumatoid factor (RF) of 120 IU/mL (nonreactive, 0–39 IU/mL; weakly reactive, 40–79 IU/mL; reactive, >80 IU/mL).
   A. Describe the immunopathogenesis of the joint changes that occur with RA.
   B. How do these changes relate to this woman's symptoms?
   C. What is the significance of her RF test results?
   D. How do her complaints of general fatigue and weight loss relate to the RA disease process?

2. A 65-year-old obese woman with a diagnosis of osteoarthritis (OA) has been having increasing pain in her right knee that is made worse with movement and weight bearing and is relieved by rest. Physical examination reveals an enlarged joint with a varus deformity; coarse crepitus is felt over the joint on passive movement.
   A. Compare the pathogenesis and articular structures involved in OA with those of RA.
   B. What is the origin of the enlargement of the affected joint, the varus deformity, and the crepitus that is felt on movement of the affected knee?
   C. Explain the predilection for involvement of the knee in persons such as this woman.
   D. What types of treatment are available for this woman?

3. A 75-year-old woman is seen by her health care provider because of complaints of fever, malaise, and weight loss. She is having trouble combing her hair, putting on a coat, and getting out of chairs because of the stiffness and pain in her shoulders, hip, and lower back. Because of her age and symptoms, the health care provider suspects the woman has polymyalgia rheumatica.

A. *What laboratory test can be used to substantiate the diagnosis?*

B. *What other diagnostic strategies are used to confirm the diagnosis?*

C. *How is the disease treated?*

References

1. Klippel J. R. (Ed.). (2001). *Primer on the rheumatic diseases* (12th ed., pp. 209–235, 239–258, 285–298, 307–324, 329–351, 534–540). Atlanta: Arthritis Foundation.
2. Hoch B. L., Klein J. J., Schiller A. L. (2008). Bones and joints. In Rubin R., Strayer D. E. (Eds.), *Rubin's pathology: Clinicopathologic foundations of medicine* (5th ed., pp. 1131–1145). Philadelphia: Lippincott Williams & Wilkins.
3. Firestein G. S. (2005). Etiology and pathogenesis of rheumatoid arthritis. In Harris E. D., Budd R. C., Firestein G. S., et al. (Eds.), *Kelly's textbook of rheumatology* (7th ed., pp. 996–1042). Philadelphia: Elsevier Saunders.
4. Harris E. D. (2005). Clinical features of rheumatoid arthritis. In Harris E. D., Budd R. C., Firestein G. S., et al. (Eds.), *Kelly's textbook of rheumatology* (7th ed., pp. 1043–1078). Philadelphia: Elsevier Saunders.
5. American College of Rheumatology Subcommittee on Rheumatoid Arthritis Guidelines. (2002). Guidelines for the management of rheumatoid arthritis: 2002 update. *Arthritis and Rheumatism* 46, 328–346.
6. Rindfleisch J. A. (2005). Diagnosis and management of rheumatoid arthritis. *American Family Physician* 72, 1037–1047.
7. Turkiewicz A. M., Moreland L. W. (2006). Rheumatoid arthritis. In Bartlett S. J., Bingham C. O., Maricic M. J., et al. (Eds.), *Clinical care in the rheumatic diseases* (3rd ed., pp. 157–160). Atlanta: Association of Rheumatology Health Professionals.
8. Lee D. M., Schur P. H. (2003). The detection of anti-cyclic citrullinated peptides (CCP). *Annals of Rheumatic Disease* 62, 870–874.
9. Hill J. A., Southwood S., Sette A., et al. (2003). Cutting edge: The conversion of arginine to citrulline allows for high-affinity interaction between rheumatoid arthritis-associated HLA-DRB1*0401 class II molecule. *Journal of Immunology* 171, 538–541.
10. Munnek M., deJong Z., Zwinderman A. H., et al. (2005). Effect of a high intensity weight-bearing exercise program on radiologic damage progression of the large joints in subgroups of patients with rheumatoid arthritis. *Arthritis Care and Research* 53, 410–417.
11. Singh G., Fort J. G., Goldstein J. L., et al. (2006). Celecoxib versus naproxen and diclofenac in osteoarthritis patients: SUCCESS-1 Study. *American Journal of Medicine* 119, 255–266.
12. Olsen N. J., Stein C. M. (2004). New drugs for rheumatoid arthritis. *New England Journal of Medicine* 350, 2167–2179.
13. Suresh E., Lambert C. M. (2005). Combination treatment strategies in early rheumatoid arthritis. *Annals of Rheumatic Disease* 64, 1252–1256.
14. Calabrese L. H., Cohen M. D. (2006). *Targeting B cells in rheumatoid arthritis: Rationale and results* (pp. 1–21). Cleveland, OH: Cleveland Clinic Foundation for Continuing Education.
15. Petri M. A. (2005). Systemic lupus erythematosus. In Bartlett S. J., Bingham C. O., Maricic M. J., et al. (Eds.), *Clinical care in the rheumatic dis-*
eases (3rd ed., pp. 187–191). Atlanta: Association of Rheumatology Health Professionals.
16. Edworthy S. M. (2005). Clinical manifestations of systemic lupus erythematosus. In Harris E. D., Budd R. C., Firestein G. S., et al. (Eds.), *Kelly's textbook of rheumatology* (7th ed., pp. 1201–1219). Philadelphia: Elsevier Saunders.
17. James J. A., Dedeke A. B. (2007). How to diagnose and treat systemic lupus erythematosus. *Arthritis Practitioner* 3(1), 16–20.
18. Petri M. (2005). Review of classification criteria for systemic lupus erythematosus. *Rheumatic Disease Clinics of North America* 31, 245–254.
19. Ginzler E. M., Dooley M. A., Aranow C., et al. (2005). Mycophenolate mofetil or intravenous cyclophosphamide for lupus nephritis. *New England Journal of Medicine* 353, 2219–2228.
20. Seibold J. R. (2005). Scleroderma. In Harris E. D., Budd R. C., Firestein G. S., et al. (Eds.), *Kelly's textbook of rheumatology* (7th ed., pp. 1279–1299). Philadelphia: Elsevier Saunders.
21. Mayes M. D. (2003). Scleroderma epidemiology. *Rheumatic Disease Clinics of North America* 29, 240–254.
22. Lin A. T. H., Clements P. J., Furst D. E. (2003). Update on disease modifying antirheumatic drugs in the treatment of systemic sclerosis. *Rheumatic Disease Clinics of North America* 29, 409–426.
23. Williams M. H., Das C., Handler C. E., et al. (2005). Systemic sclerosis associated pulmonary hypertension: Improved survival in the current era. [Online.] Available: www.heartjnl.com.
24. Kuon W., Sieper J. (2003). Identification of HLA-B27 restricted peptides in reactive arthritis and other spondyloarthropathies. *Rheumatic Disease Clinics of North America* 29, 595–611.
25. Elyan M., Khan M. A. (2006). Diagnosing ankylosing spondylitis. *Journal of Rheumatology* 33(Suppl. 78), 12–23.
26. Clegg D. O. (2006). Treatment of ankylosing spondylitis. *Journal of Rheumatology* 33(Suppl. 78), 24–31.
27. Flores D., Marquez J., Garza M., et al. (2003). Reactive arthritis: Newer developments. *Rheumatic Disease Clinics of North America* 29, 37–59.
28. Klippel J. H. (2004). Reactive arthritis. In Lichtenstein L. M., Busse W. H., Geha R. S. (Eds.), *Current therapy in allergy, immunology and rheumatology* (6th ed., pp. 212–215). Philadelphia: Mosby.
29. Mease P. J. (2003). Current treatment of psoriatic arthritis. *Rheumatic Disease Clinics of North America* 29, 495–511.
30. Loeser R. F. (2003). A stepwise approach to the management of osteoarthritis. *Bulletin on the Rheumatic Diseases* 52(5).
31. Lozada C. J., Altman R. D. (2003). Osteoarthritis. In Koopman W., Boulware D. W., Heudebert G. R. (Eds.), *Clinical primer of rheumatology* (pp. 247–261). Philadelphia: Lippincott Williams & Wilkins.
32. Rosenberg A. E. (2005). Bones, joints, and soft tissue tumors. In Kumar V. Abbas A. K., Fausto N. (Eds.), *Robbins and Cotran pathologic basis of disease* (7th ed., pp. 1303–1314). Philadelphia: Elsevier Saunders.
33. American College of Rheumatology Subcommittee on Osteoarthritis Guidelines. (2000). Recommendations for the medical management of osteoarthritis of the hip and knee: 2000 update. *Arthritis and Rheumatology* 43, 1905–1915.
34. Lo G. H., LaValley M., McAllindon T., et al. (2003). Intra-articular hyaluronic acid in treatment of knee osteoarthritis: A meta-analysis. *Journal of the American Medical Association* 290, 3115–3121.
35. Hochberg M. C. (2006). Nutritional supplements for knee osteoarthritis: Still no resolution [editorial]. *New England Journal of Medicine* 354, 858–860.
36. Felson D. T. (2006). Osteoarthritis of the knee. *New England Journal of Medicine* 354, 841–848.
37. Ling S. M., Rudolph K. (2006). Osteoarthritis. In Bartlett S. J., Bingham C. O., Maricic M. J., et al. (Eds.), *Clinical care in the rheumatic diseases* (3rd ed., pp. 127–134). Atlanta: Association of Rheumatology Health Professionals.
38. Wortman R. L., Kelley W. N. (2005). Gout and hyperuricemia. In Harris E. D., Budd R. C., Firestein G. S., et al. (Eds.), *Kelly's textbook of rheumatology* (7th ed., pp. 1402–1425). Philadelphia: Elsevier Saunders.
39. Boulware D. W., Becker M. A., Edwards N. L. (2003). Gout and crystal induced synovitis. In Koopman W., Boulware D. W., Heudebert

G. R. (Eds.), *Clinical primer of rheumatology* (pp. 262–277). Philadelphia: Lippincott Williams & Wilkins.

40. Perez-Ruiz F., Atxotegl J., Hernando I., et al. (2006). Using serum urate levels to determine the period free of gouty symptoms after withdrawal of long-term urate lowering therapy: A prospective study. *Arthritis Care and Research* 55, 786–790.

41. Junnila J. L., Cartwright V. W. (2006). Chronic musculoskeletal pain in children: Part II. Rheumatic causes. *American Family Physician* 74, 293–300.

42. Milojevic D. S., Ilowite N. T. (2002). Treatment of rheumatic diseases in children: Special considerations. *Rheumatic Disease Clinics of North America* 28, 461–482.

43. Burgos-Vargas R. (2002). The juvenile-onset spondyloarthritides. *Rheumatic Disease Clinics of North America* 28, 531–560.

44. Yaziu Y., Paget S. A. (2000). Elderly-onset rheumatoid arthritis. *Rheumatic Disease Clinics of North America* 26, 517–526.

45. Kammer G. M., Misha N. (2000). Systemic lupus erythematosus in the elderly. *Rheumatic Disease Clinics of North America* 26, 475–492.

46. Rapp S. R., Rejeski W. J., Miller M. E. (2000). Physical function among older adults with knee pain: The role of coping skills. *Arthritis Care and Research* 13, 270–279.

47. Pego-Reigosa J. M., Rodriguez-Rodriguez M., Hurtado-Hernandez Z., et al. (2005). Calcium pyrophosphate deposition disease mimicking polymyalgia rheumatica: A prospective follow-up study of predictive factors for this condition in patients presenting with polymyalgia symptoms. *Arthritis Care and Research* 53, 931–938.

48. Weyand C. M., Goronzy J. J. (2003). Giant-cell arteritis and polymyalgia rheumatica. *Annals of Internal Medicine* 139, 505–515.

49. Frearson R., Cassidy T., Newton J. (2003). Polymyalgia rheumatica and temporal arteritis: Evidence and guidelines for diagnosis and management in older people. *Age and Ageing* 32, 370–374.

Visit thePoint **http://thePoint.lww.com for animations, journal articles, and more!**

Chapter 60

Structure and Function of the Skin

GLADYS SIMANDL

➤ The skin, also called the *integumentum,* is the largest and one of most versatile organs of the body, accounting for roughly 16% of the body's weight. It has a surface area of 1.5 to 2 m^2 and weighs approximately 4 kg (9 pounds) in the average adult, and forms the major interface between the internal organs and the external environment. As the body's first line of defense, the skin is continuously subjected to potentially harmful environmental agents, including solid matter, liquids, gases, sunlight, and microorganisms. Although it may become bruised, lacerated, burned, or infected, it has remarkable properties that allow for a continuous cycle of shedding, healing, and cell regeneration.

As the outer covering of the body, the skin may demonstrate outwardly what occurs inside the body. A number of systemic diseases are manifested by skin disorders (*e.g.,* rash associated with systemic lupus erythematosus and jaundice due to liver disease). Thus, it is important to recognize that although skin eruptions are frequently caused by primary disorders of the skin, they may also represent manifestations of systemic disease.

STRUCTURE AND FUNCTION OF THE SKIN

After completing this section of the chapter, you should be able to meet the following objectives:

- Describe the protective functions of skin.
- Characterize the changes in a keratinocyte from its inception in the basal lamina to its arrival on the outer surface of the skin.
- List the four specialized cells of the epidermis and describe their functions.
- Describe the structure and function of the dermis and subcutaneous layers of skin.
- Describe the following skin appendages and their functions: sebaceous gland, eccrine gland, apocrine gland, nails, and hair.
- Characterize the skin in terms of sensory and immune functions.

Functions of the Skin

The skin and its derivatives constitute a complex organ with many cell types. The diversity of cell types and their ability to

FUNCTIONS OF THE SKIN

- The skin is the largest organ of the body.

- As an interface between the internal and external environments, the skin prevents body fluids from leaving the body, protects the body from potentially damaging environmental agents, and serves as an area for heat exchange; in addition, cells of the skin immune system provide protection against invading microorganisms.

- Receptors in the skin relay touch, pressure, temperature, and pain sensation to the central nervous system for localization and discrimination.

Skin Structures

There are great variations in skin structure on different parts of the body; therefore, "normal skin" on any one surface of the body is difficult to describe. Variations are found in the properties of the skin, such as the thickness of skin layers, the distribution of sweat glands, and the number and size of hair follicles. For example, the epidermis is thicker on the palms of the hands and soles of the feet (0.8 mm) than elsewhere on the body (0.07 to 0.12 mm). The dermis, on the other hand, is thickest on the back, whereas the subcutaneous fat layer is thickest on the abdomen and buttocks. Hair follicles are densely distributed on the scalp, axillae, and genitalia, but they are sparse on the inner arms and abdomen. The apocrine sweat glands are confined to the axillae and the anogenital area.

Nevertheless, certain structural properties are common to all skin on all areas of the body. The skin is composed of three layers: the epidermis (outer layer), the dermis (inner layer), and the subcutaneous fat layer. The basement membrane divides the first two layers. The subcutaneous tissue, a layer of loose connective and fatty tissues, binds the dermis to the underlying tissues of the body (Fig. 60-1).

work together provide a number of ways of protecting a person from the elements in the external environment. As a barrier, microorganisms find it almost impossible to penetrate the skin from the outside, and water loss is limited from the inside. The skin surface is covered with a thin lipid film containing bactericidal fatty acids that protect against the entry of harmful microorganisms, and it harbors a constant flora of relatively harmless strains of microorganisms that protect against other, more virulent strains. The skin also plays an important role in immune regulation through skin-associated lymphoid tissues, including Langerhans cells, mast cells, and lymphocytes (see Chapter 17). Langerhans cells, the antigen-presenting cells of the skin, not only protect against harmful pathogens but also play an important role in the development of allergic skin conditions.

The skin serves several other vital functions, including somatosensory function, temperature regulation, and vitamin D synthesis. The skin is richly innervated with pain, temperature, and touch receptors. Skin receptors relay the numerous qualities of touch, such as pressure, sharpness, dullness, and pleasure to the central nervous system for localization and fine discrimination (see Chapter 49). Most of the heat produced in the body is generated by deep organs, such as the liver, heart, and skeletal muscles, and then transferred to the skin, where it is lost to the surrounding environment. The rate at which heat is dissipated from the body is determined by constriction or dilation of the arterioles that supply blood to the skin and through evaporation of moisture and sweat from the skin surface (see Chapter 10). The skin also functions as an endocrine organ, in which 7-dehydrocholesterol, a substance normally found in epidermal cells, is converted to cholecalciferol (an inactive form of vitamin D), by ultraviolet rays from the sun (discussed further in Chapter 56).

Although broken down into its constituent parts in this chapter, the skin is increasingly being understood as a complex and dynamic system involving neuroendocrine, immunologic, and cutaneous interactions.[1] Mind–body influences are bidirectional and the skin should be considered an "active neuro-immunoendocrine interface, where effector molecules such as neuropeptides act as common words used in a dynamic dialogue between brain, immune system, and skin."[2]

ORGANIZATION OF SKIN STRUCTURES

- The skin has two layers, an outer epidermis and an inner dermis, separated by a basement membrane.

- The epidermis, which is avascular, is composed of four to five layers of stratified squamous keratinized epithelial cells that are formed in the deepest layer of the epidermis and migrate to the skin surface to replace cells that are lost during normal skin shedding.

- The basement membrane is a thin adhesive layer that cements the epidermis to the dermis. This is the layer involved in blister formation.

- The dermis is a connective tissue layer that separates the epidermis from the underlying subcutaneous fat layer. It contains the blood vessels and nerve fibers that supply the epidermis.

Epidermis

The functions of the skin depend on the properties of its outermost layer, the epidermis. The epidermis covers the body, and it is specialized in areas to form the various skin appendages: hair, nails, and glandular structures.[3] The keratinocytes of the epidermis produce a fibrous protein called *keratin,* which is essential to the protective function of skin. In addition to the keratinocytes, the epidermis has three other types of cells that arise from its basal layer: melanocytes that produce a pigment called *melanin,* which is responsible for skin color, tanning, and protecting against ultraviolet radiation; Merkel cells that provide sensory information; and Langerhans cells that link the epidermis to the

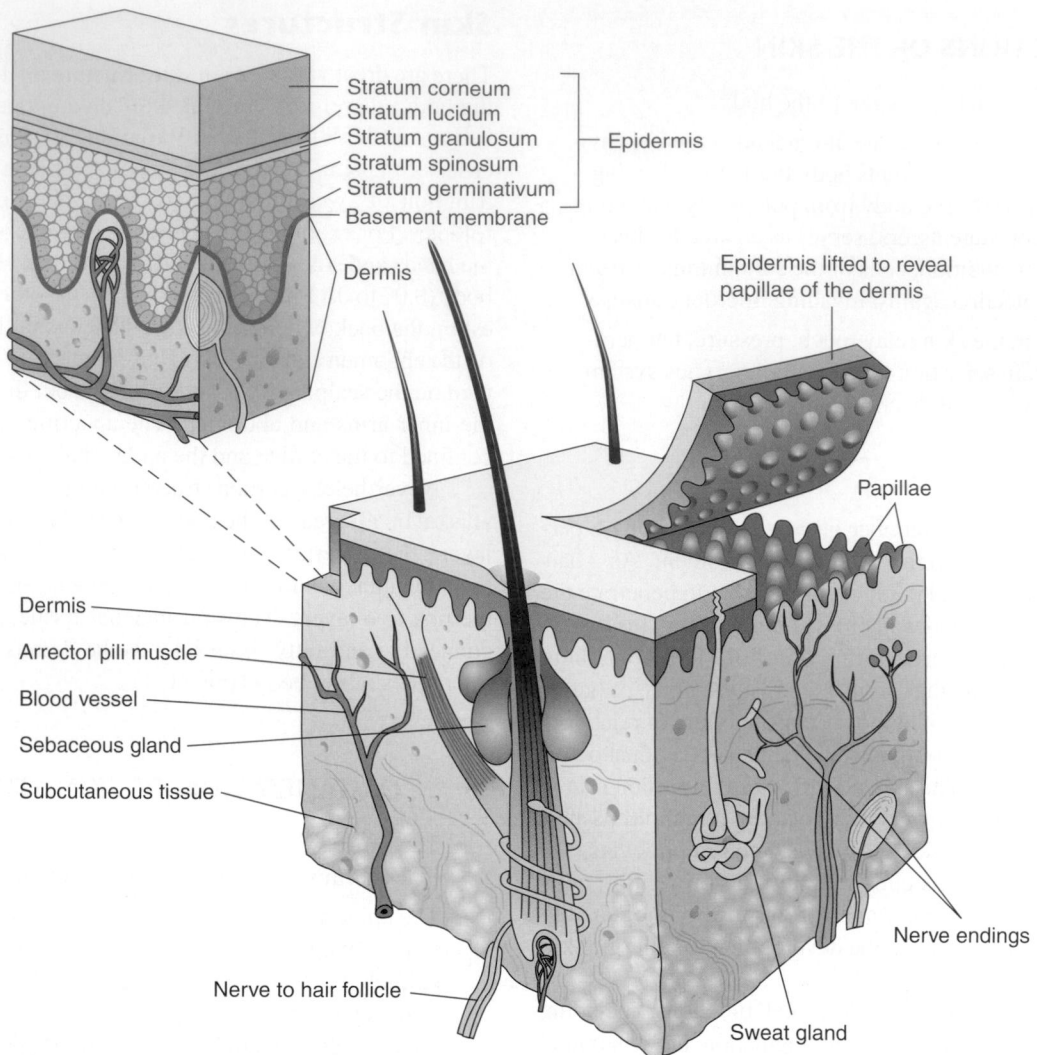

FIGURE 60-1 • Three-dimensional view of the skin.

immune system. The epidermis contains openings for two types of glands: sweat glands, which produce watery secretions, and sebaceous glands, which produce an oily secretion called *sebum.*

Keratinocytes

The *keratinocyte* is the major cell of the epidermis, comprising 95% of the cells of this layer. The epidermis is composed of stratified squamous keratinized epithelium, which, when viewed under the microscope, is seen to consist of five distinct layers, or strata, that represent a progressive differentiation or maturation of the keratinocytes: the stratum germinativum, or basal layer; the stratum spinosum; the stratum granulosum; the stratum lucidum; and the stratum corneum.

The deepest layer, the *stratum germinativum* or *stratum basale,* consists of a single layer of basal cells that are attached to the basal lamina. The basal cells, which are columnar, undergo mitosis to produce new keratinocytes that move toward the skin surface to replace cells lost during normal skin shedding. Unlike

the other layers of the epidermis, the basal cells do not migrate toward the skin surface, but remain stationary in the stratum germinativum.

The next layer, the *stratum spinosum,* is formed as the progeny of the basal cell layer move outward toward the skin surface. The stratum spinosum is two to four layers thick, and its cells become differentiated as they migrate outward. Because they develop a spiny appearance where their cell borders interconnect, the cells of this layer are commonly referred to as *prickle cells.*

The *stratum granulosum* is only a few cells thick; it consists of granular cells that are the most differentiated cells of the living skin. The cells in this layer are unique in that two opposing functions are occurring simultaneously: while some cells are losing cytoplasm and nuclear structures, others continue to synthesize keratin.

The *stratum lucidum,* which lies just superficial to the stratum granulosum, is a thin, transparent layer found primarily on the palms of the hands and soles of the feet. It consists of transitional cells that retain some of the functions of living skin cells from the layers below but otherwise resemble the cells of the stratum corneum.

The top or surface layer, the *stratum corneum,* consists of dead, keratinized cells. This layer contains the most cell layers and the largest cells of the epidermis. It ranges from 15 layers thick in areas such as the face to 25 layers or more on the arm. Specialized areas, such as the palms of the hands or soles of the feet, have 100 or more layers.

The keratinocytes that originate in the basal layer change morphologically as they are pushed toward the outer layer of the epidermis. For example, in the basal layer, the keratinocyte is round. As it is pushed into the stratum spinosum, the keratinocyte becomes multisided. It becomes flatter in the granular layer and is flattened and elongated in the stratum corneum (Fig. 60-2). Keratinocytes also change cytoplasmic structure and composition as they are pushed outward. This transformation from viable cells to the dead cells of the stratum corneum is called *keratinization.* The migration time of a keratinocyte from the basal layer to the stratum corneum is 20 to 30 days. The rate of production of new keratinocytes needs to be consistent with the rate of shedding old keratinocytes. When the rates are not in balance, skin anomalies occur.

The movement of the keratinocytes to the surface of the skin is best described as random or nonsynchronized. Keratinocytes pass other keratinocytes, melanocytes, and Langerhans cells as they migrate in a seemingly random fashion. However, the cells are connected by minute points of attachment called *desmosomes.* Desmosomes are localized patches or plaques that hold two cells tightly together. They are terminal end points on the cell walls of keratinocytes, made up of fibrous material that is bound into bundles, called *tonofilaments.* Desmosomes keep the cells from detaching and provide some structure to the skin while it is in perpetual motion. The basal layer provides the underlying structure and stability for the epidermis.

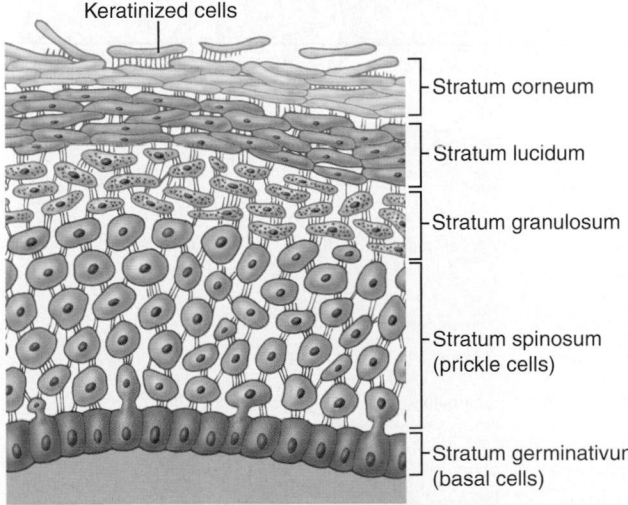

FIGURE 60-2 • Epidermal cells. The basal cells undergo mitosis, producing keratinocytes that change their size and shape as they move upward, replacing cells that are lost during normal cell shedding.

Besides desmosomes, there are three other types of cellular junctions that bind keratinocytes: adherens junctions, gap junctions, and tight junctions (see Chapter 4). *Adherens junctions* are specialized structures that provide strong mechanical connections between cells. They are responsible for adhesion between cells, communicate about the presence of neighboring cells, and anchor the skin cells. *Gap junctions* are cylindrical channels that permit ions and small molecules to pass between cells. They are composed of proteins called *connexins.* *Tight junctions* are sheets of cells that fill the spaces between cells. They prevent the passage of molecules and ions through the spaces between cells, thus controlling the substances that are allowed through. Hence, they are responsible for skin barrier integrity.[4]

Keratinocytes produce keratin, a complex protein that forms the surface of the skin and is also the structural protein of the hair and nails, Once believed to be passive cells passing through time while changing morphologically, keratinocytes are now known to be active secretory cells that play an important role in the immunobiology of the skin by communicating and regulating cells of the immune response and secreting cytokines and inflammatory mediators.

Melanocytes

Melanocytes are pigment-synthesizing cells that are located at or in the basal layer. They function to produce pigment granules called *melanin,* the substance that gives skin its color. There are two major forms of melanin: *eumelanin* and *pheomelanin.* The two forms of eumelanin are brown and black; pheomelanin is yellow to red. The type of melanin produced depends on the stimulation of specific hormones or proteins and the binding of these substances to receptors on the melanocyte. Eumelanin is the most abundant in humans. Exposure to the sun's ultraviolet rays increases the production of eumelanin, causing tanning to occur. The primary function of such melanin is to protect the skin by absorbing and scattering harmful ultraviolet rays, which are implicated in skin cancers. Localized concentrations of eumelanin are also responsible for the formation of freckles and moles.

Pheomelanin, the yellow to red pigment, is found in all humans. It is particularly concentrated in the lips, nipples, glans penis, and vagina. Besides the skin, it is found in hair, particularly red hair. It has been suggested that the reason fair-haired individuals are more susceptible to skin cancers may be due to the enhanced photoreactivity of pheomelanin, as compared with eumelanin.

The ability to synthesize melanin depends on the ability of the melanocytes to produce an enzyme called *tyrosinase,* which converts the amino acid tyrosine to a precursor of melanin. A genetic lack of this enzyme results in a clinical condition called *albinism.* Persons with this disorder lack pigmentation in the skin, hair, and iris of the eye. Tyrosinase is synthesized in the rough endoplasmic reticulum of the melanocytes and then routed to membranous vesicles in the Golgi complex called *melanosomes.* Melanin is subsequently synthesized in the melanosomes. Melanocytes have long, cytoplasm-filled dendritic processes that contain accumulated melanosomes and extend between the keratinocytes. Although the melanocytes remain in the basal layer, the melanosomes are transferred to the keratinocytes through their dendritic processes. The dendrite tip containing the melanosome is engulfed by a nearby keratinocyte, and the melanin is transferred (Fig. 60-3).

The amount of melanin in the keratinocytes determines a person's skin color. Dark-skinned and light-skinned people have approximately the same number of melanocytes, but the production and packaging of pigment is different. In dark-skinned people, *larger* melanin-containing melanosomes are produced and transferred individually to the keratinocyte, whereas in light-skinned people, *smaller* melanosomes are produced and then packaged together in a membrane before being transferred to the keratinocyte. All people, regardless of skin color, have relatively few or no melanocytes in the epidermis of the palms of the hands or soles of the feet. In light-skinned people, the number of melanocytes decreases with age; the skin becomes lighter and is more susceptible to skin cancer when exposed to ultraviolet light.

Merkel Cells

Merkel cells are clear cells found in the stratum basale of the epidermis; they are connected to other skin cells by desmosomes. Each Merkel cell is connected to an afferent nerve terminal, forming a structure known as a *Merkel disk*. They are the sparsest cells of the epidermis and are found over the entire body, but are most plentiful in the basal layer of the fingers, toes, lips, and oral cavity, and in the outermost sheath of hair follicles (*i.e.*, the touch areas). The exact function of Merkel cells is unclear, but they are believed to be neuroendocrine cells (*i.e.*, they release hormones into the blood in response to neural stimuli) and function as specific, slowly adapting sensory touch receptors. Merkel cells may also be involved in the metabolic

support of their associated neurons, neuron development and regeneration after injury, and neurotransmission for autonomic nerves, blood vessels, and inflammatory cells.

Langerhans Cells

Langerhans cells are scattered in the suprabasal layers of the epidermis among the keratinocytes. They are less numerous (3% to 5% of epidermal cells) than the keratinocytes. They are derived from precursor cells originating in the bone marrow, and continuously repopulate the epidermis. Like melanocytes, they have a dendritic shape and clear cytoplasm. *Birbeck granules* that often resemble tennis racquets are their most distinguishing characteristic microscopically.

Langerhans cells are the immunologic cells responsible for recognizing foreign antigens harmful to the body (Fig. 60-4). As such, Langerhans cells play an important role in defending the body against foreign antigens. Langerhans cells bind antigen to their surface and process it, and, bearing the processed antigen, migrate from the epidermis into lymphatic vessels and

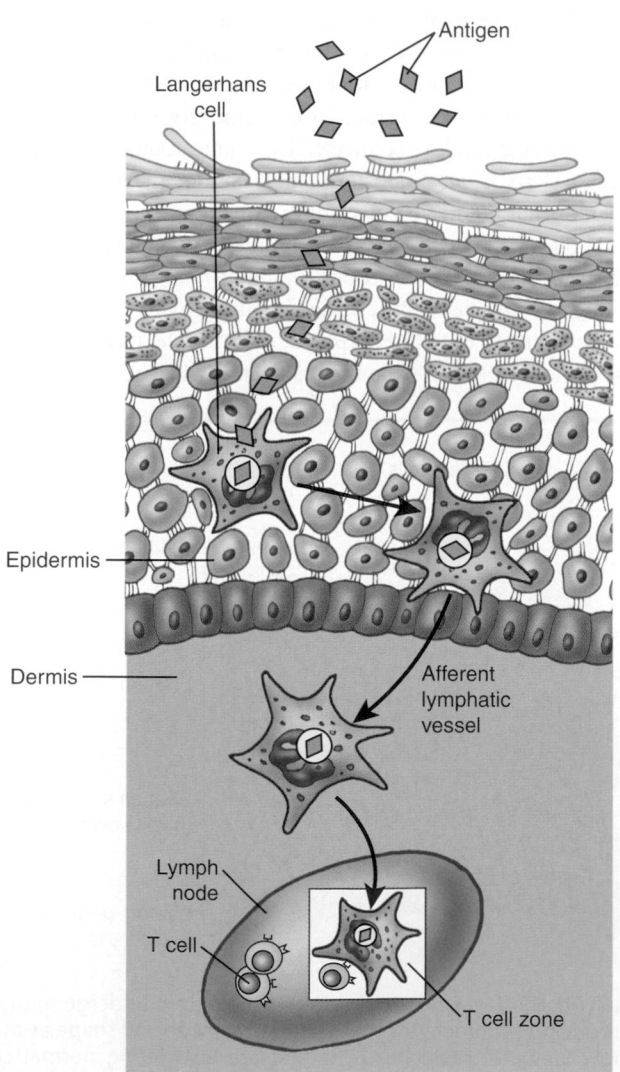

FIGURE 60-4 • Langerhans cells.

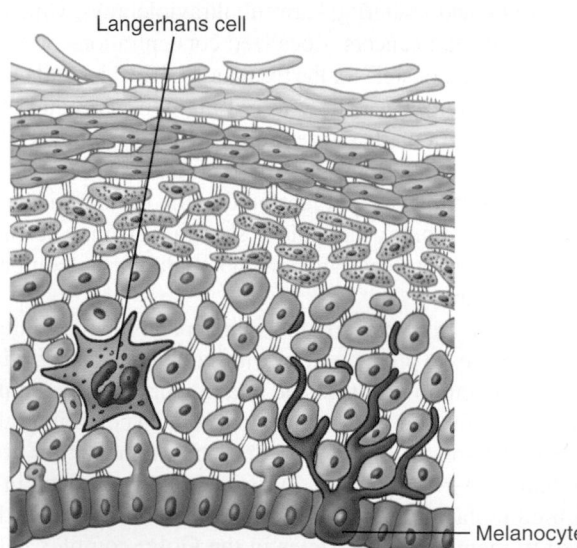

FIGURE 60-3 • The melanocytes, which are located in the basal layer of the skin, produce melanin pigment granules that give skin its color. The melanocytes have threadlike, cytoplasm-filled extensions that are used in passing the pigment granules to the keratinocytes.

then into regional lymph nodes, where they are known as *dendritic cells*. During their migration in the lymph system, the Langerhans cells become potent antigen-presenting cells (see Chapter 17). Langerhans cells are innervated by sympathetic nerve fibers, which may explain why the skin's immune system is altered under stress. An example of this is the exacerbations of acne seen in persons under stress. Langerhans cells and the keratinocytes produce a number of cytokines that stimulate maturation of skin-localizing T lymphocytes.

Basement Membrane

The terms *basement membrane* and *basal lamina* are often used interchangeably. Technically, however, the basal lamina is a component of the basement membrane. The basement membrane is a layer of intercellular and extracellular matrices that serves as an interface between the dermis and the epidermis (Fig. 60-5). It separates epithelium from the underlying connective tissue, it anchors the epithelium to the loose connective tissue underneath, and it serves as a selective filter for molecules moving between the two layers. It is also a major site of immunoglobulin and complement deposition in skin disease. The basement membrane is involved in skin disorders that cause bullae or blister formation.

The basement membrane consists of three distinct zones or layers—lamina lucida, lamina densa, and lamina fibroreticularis—all of which contribute to the adhesion of the two skin layers. The *lamina lucida* is an electron-lucent layer where adherence proteins are located. It consists of fine anchoring filaments and a cell adhesion glycoprotein, called *laminin,* that plays a role in the organization of the macromolecules in the basement membrane zone and promotes attachment of cells to the extracellular matrix. The *lamina densa* contains an adhe-

sive called *type IV collagen* as well as laminin. It is important in dermal–epidermal attachment. Combined, the lamina lucida and the lamina densa comprise what is known as the *basal lamina*. The *lamina fibroreticularis* then completes the basement membrane. This layer contains many anchoring microfibrils. These are short, curved structures that insert into the lamina densa and the upper part of the dermis (superficial dermis), where they are known as *anchoring fibrils*. Type VII collagen, another adherent substance, has been found in the anchoring fibrils and plaques. Another component of the lamina fibroreticularis are elastic fiber bundles that extend to the dermis.

Hemidesmosomes are like half-desmosomes in both structure and function. They lie immediately at the basal plasma membrane and form the site or source of tonofilaments, which attach the dermis and epidermis (see Fig. 60-5). Because they form a continuous link between the intracellular keratin filament network and the extracellular basement membrane, they are also involved in relaying signals between the skin systems.

Dermis

The dermis is the connective tissue layer that separates the epidermis from the subcutaneous fat layer (see Fig. 60-1). It supports the epidermis and serves as its primary source of nutrition. The two layers of the dermis, the papillary dermis and the reticular dermis, are composed of cells, fibers, ground substances, nerves, and blood vessels. The main component of the dermis is collagen, a group of fibrous proteins. Collagen represents 70% of dry skin weight and serves as the major stress-resistant material of the skin. Collagen is rich in amino acids. Collagen fibers are loosely arranged in the papillary dermis, but are tightly bundled in the reticular dermis.

The pilar (hair) and glandular structures are embedded in this layer and continue through the epidermis. In general, a dark dermis is more compact than the white dermis, and consequently darker-skinned people show less wrinkling.

Papillary Dermis

The *papillary dermis* (pars papillaris) is a thin, superficial layer that lies adjacent to the epidermis. It consists of collagen fibers and ground substance. This layer is densely covered with conical projections called *dermal papillae* (see Fig. 60-1). The basal cells of the epidermis project into the papillary dermis, forming *rete ridges*. Microscopically, the junction between the epidermis and the dermis appears like undulating ridges and valleys. It is believed that the dense structure of the dermal papillae serves to minimize the separation of the dermis and the epidermis. Dermal papillae contain capillaries, end arterioles, and venules that nourish the epidermal layers of the skin. This layer of the dermis is richly vascularized. Lymph vessels and nerve tissue also are found in this layer.

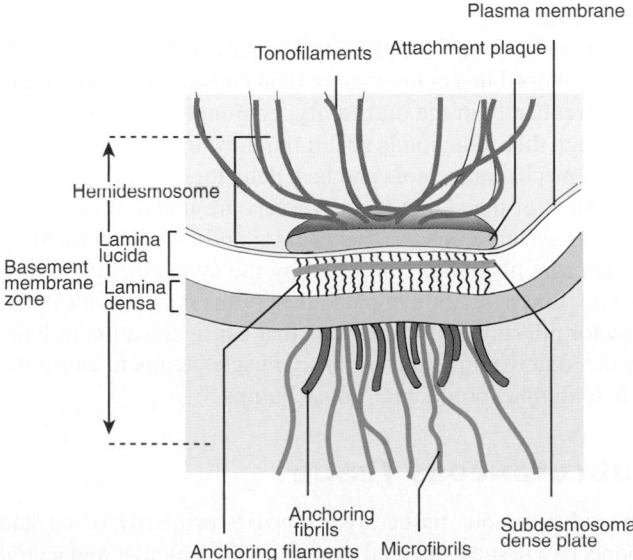

FIGURE 60-5 • The dermal–epidermal interface and basement membrane layers. (Adapted from Rubin R., Strayer D. E. [Eds.]. [2008]. *Rubin's pathology: Clinicopathologic foundations of medicine* [5th ed., p. 1004]. Philadelphia: Lippincott Williams & Wilkins.)

Reticular Dermis

The *reticular dermis* (pars reticularis) is the thicker area of the dermis and forms the bulk of the dermal layer. This is the tough layer in animal hides from which leather is made. The reticular dermis is characterized by a complex meshwork of three-dimensional collagen bundles interconnected with large elastic fibers and ground substance, a viscid gel that is rich in mucopolysaccharides. The collagen fibers are oriented parallel to the body's surface in any given area. Collagen bundles may be organized lengthwise, as on the abdomen, or in round clusters, as on the heel. The direction of surgical incisions is often determined by this organizational pattern.

Immune Cells. Over time, the reticular dermis has undergone much study. Once thought to be composed primarily of fibroblasts, it is now believed that the main cells of this layer are dendritic cells, called *dermal dendrocytes*. Dermal dendrocytes are spindle-shaped cells that have both phagocytic and dendritic properties. They are believed to possess antigen-presenting functions and play an important part in the immunobiology of the dermis. In addition, it is possible that dermal dendrocytes may be able either to initiate or respond to immunologic events in the epidermis. Dermal dendrocytes also are thought to be involved in processes such as wound healing, blood clotting, and inflammation.

Immune cells found in the dermis include macrophages, T cells, mast cells, and fibroblasts. Dermal macrophages and venular epithelial cells may present antigen to T cells in the dermis. Most of these T cells are previously activated or memory T cells. T-cell responses to macrophage- or endothelium-associated antigens in the dermis are probably more important in generating an immune response to antigen challenge in previously exposed persons than in initiating a response to a new antigen. The major type of T-cell–mediated immune response in the skin is delayed-type hypersensitivity (see Chapter 19).

Mast cells, which have a prominent role in immunoglobulin E–mediated immediate hypersensitivity, also are present in the dermis. These cells are strategically located at body interfaces such as the skin and mucous membranes and are thought to interact with antigens that come in contact with the skin.

Blood Vessels. The arterial vessels that nourish the skin form two plexuses (*i.e.,* collections of blood vessels), one located between the dermis and the subcutaneous tissue and the other between the papillary and reticular layers of the dermis. The pink color of light skin results primarily from blood in the vessels of this latter plexus. Capillary flow that arises from vessels in this plexus also extends up and nourishes the overlaying epidermis by diffusion. Blood leaves the skin through small veins that accompany the subcutaneous arteries. The lymphatic system of the skin, which aids in combating certain skin infections, also is limited to the dermis.

The skin is richly supplied with arteriovenous anastomoses in which blood flows directly between an artery and a vein, bypassing the capillary circulation. These anastomoses are important for temperature regulation. They can open up, letting blood flow through the skin vessels when there is a need to dissipate body heat, and close off, conserving body heat if the environmental temperature is cold.

Innervation. The innervation of the skin is complex. The skin, with its accessory structures, serves as an organ for receiving sensory information from the environment. The dermis is well supplied with sensory neurons as well as nerves that supply the blood vessels, sweat glands, and arrector pili muscles.

The receptors for touch, pressure, heat, cold, and pain are widely distributed in the dermis (see Chapter 49). The papillary layer of the dermis is supplied with free nerve endings that serve as nociceptors (*i.e.,* pain receptors) and thermoreceptors. The dermis also contains encapsulated pressure-sensitive receptors that detect pressure and touch. The largest of these are the *pacinian corpuscles,* which are widely distributed in the dermis and subcutaneous tissue. The afferent nerve endings of the pacinian corpuscle are surrounded by concentric layers of modified Schwann cells such that they resemble an onion when sectioned. Pacinian corpuscles are responsible for detecting gross pressure changes and vibrations. Pressure causes the pacinian corpuscle to change its shape, thereby triggering nerve impulses. Pacinian corpuscles are adaptive and they respond more to changes than to steady pressure or vibration.

Flat, encapsulated nerve endings found on the palmar surfaces of the fingers and hands and planter surfaces of the feet are called *Meissner corpuscles.* They are concentrated on the fingertips, palms, soles, lips, tongue, face, and genitalia. They are thick, laminated, ovoid capsules each containing up to six nerve endings. When the corpuscle is deformed by pressure, the nerve endings are stimulated, signaling the somatosensory portion of the cerebral cortex and informing the person about the location and strength of the stimulus. They are rapidly adapting and do not react to constant, steady stimulation.

The deep dermis is supplied with small, oval mechanoreceptors called *Ruffini corpuscles.* Ruffini corpuscles are located in the subcutaneous tissue of hairy and glabrous skin. Several expanded nerve endings branch from a single, myelinated afferent fiber. They are slowly adapting receptors, responding to heavy pressure and joint movement. They are also believed to detect cold.

The skin is also supplied by *Krause end bulbs*, nerve endings contained in a cylindrical or oval capsule. They are found most frequently in the oral cavity, conjunctiva, and genitalia. Although their function is uncertain, they are thought to function as mechanoreceptors and heat detectors.

Most of the skin's blood vessels are under sympathetic nervous system control. The sweat glands are innervated by cholinergic fibers but controlled by the sympathetic nervous system. Likewise, the sympathetic nervous system controls the arrector pili (pilomotor) muscles that cause elevation of hairs on the skin. Contraction of these muscles tends to cause the skin to dimple, producing "goose bumps."

Subcutaneous Tissue

The subcutaneous tissue layer consists primarily of fat and connective tissues that lend support to the vascular and neural structures supplying the outer layers of the skin. There is controversy about whether the subcutaneous tissue should be considered an actual layer of the skin. Because the eccrine glands and deep hair follicles extend to this layer and several skin diseases involve the subcutaneous tissue, the subcutaneous tissue may be considered part of the skin.

Skin Appendages

The skin houses a variety of appendages, including hair, nails, and sebaceous and sweat glands. The distribution and functions of the appendages vary.

Sweat Glands

There are two types of sweat glands: eccrine and apocrine. *Eccrine sweat glands* are simple tubular structures that originate in the dermis and open directly to the skin surface. They are numerous (several million), vary in density, and are located over the entire body surface. Their purpose is to transport sweat to the outer skin surface to regulate body temperature. *Apocrine sweat glands* are less numerous than eccrine sweat glands. They are larger and located deep in the dermal layer. They open through a hair follicle, even though a hair may not be present, and are found primarily in the axillae and groin. The major difference between these glands and the eccrine glands is that apocrine glands secrete an oily substance. In animals, apocrine secretions give rise to distinctive odors that enable animals to recognize the presence of others. In humans, apocrine secretions are sterile until mixed with the bacteria on the skin surface; they then produce what is commonly known as "body odor."

Sebaceous Glands

The sebaceous glands are located over the entire skin surface except for the palms, soles, and sides of the feet. They are part of the *pilosebaceous unit*. They secrete a mixture of lipids, including triglycerides, cholesterol, and wax. This mixture is called *sebum;* it lubricates hair and skin. Sebum is not the same as the surface lipid film. Sebum prevents undue evaporation of moisture from the stratum corneum during cold weather and helps to conserve body heat. Sebum production is under the control of genetic and hormonal influences. Sebaceous glands are relatively small and inactive until individuals approach adolescence. The glands then enlarge, stimulated by the rise in sex hormones. Gland size directly influences the amount of sebum produced, and the level of androgens influences gland size. The sebaceous glands are the structures that become inflamed in acne (see Chapter 61).

Hair

Hair is a structure that originates from hair follicles in the dermis. Most hair follicles are associated with sebaceous glands, and these structures combine to form the pilosebaceous unit. The entire hair structure consists of the hair follicle, sebaceous gland, hair muscle (arrector pili), and, in some instances, the apocrine gland (Fig. 60-6). Hair is a keratinized structure that is pushed upward from the hair follicle. Growth of the hair is

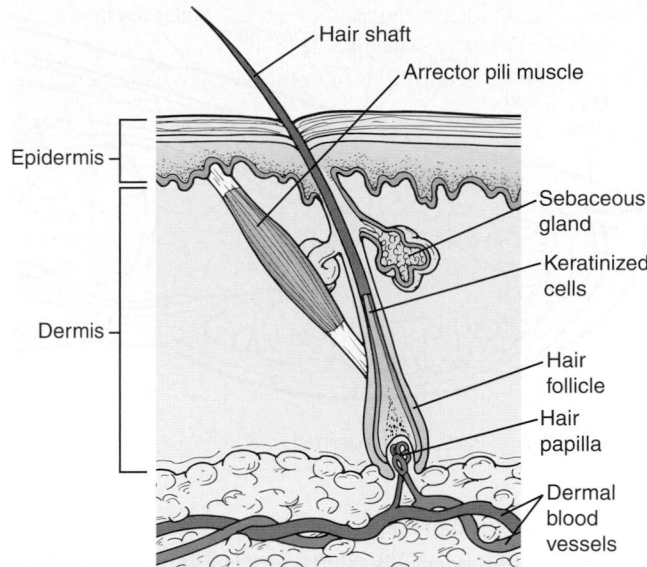

FIGURE 60-6 • Parts of a hair follicle.

centered in the bulb (*i.e.,* base) of the hair follicle, and the hair undergoes changes as it is pushed outward. Hair goes through three cyclic phases identified as anagen (the growth phase), catagen (the atrophy phase), and telogen (the resting phase, or no growth). Like most animals, human beings shed hair cyclically. However, human hair follicles work independently and therefore, unlike most animals, human beings shed hair asynchronously.

A vascular network at the site of the follicular bulb nourishes and maintains the hair follicle. Melanocytes in the bulb transfer melanosomes to the cells of the bulb matrix in much the same way as in the skin and are therefore responsible for the color of the hair. Similar to the skin, large melanosomes are found in the hair of darker-skinned persons; aggregated and encapsulated melanosomes are found in persons with light skin. Red hair has spherical melanosomes, whereas gray hair is the result of a decreased number of melanosome-producing melanocytes. The arrector pili muscle, located under the sebaceous gland, provides a thermoregulatory function by contracting to cause goose bumps, thereby reducing the skin surface area that is available for the dissipation of body heat.

Nails

The nails are hardened keratinized plates, called *fingernails* and *toenails,* that protect the fingers and toes and enhance dexterity. The nails grow out from a curved transverse groove called the *nail groove.* The floor of this groove, called the *nail matrix,* is the germinal region of the nail plate (Fig. 60-7). The underlying epidermis, attached to the nail plate, is called the *nail bed.* Like hair, nails are the end product of dead matrix cells that are pushed outward from the nail matrix. Unlike hair, nails grow continuously rather than cyclically, unless permanently damaged or diseased. The epithelium of the fold of skin

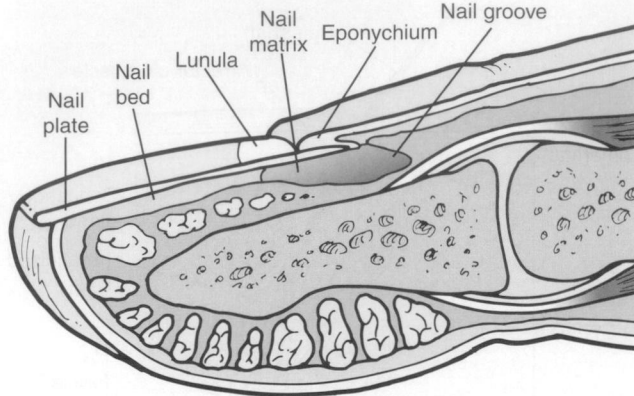

FIGURE 60-7 • Parts of a fingernail.

that surrounds the nail consists of the usual layers of skin. The stratum corneum forms the *eponychium* or cuticle. The nearly transparent nail plate provides a useful window for viewing the amount of oxygen in the blood, providing a view of the color of the blood in the dermal vessels. Changes or abnormalities of the nail can also serve to help diagnose skin or systemic diseases.

IN SUMMARY, the skin is primarily an organ of protection. It is the largest organ of the body and forms the major barrier between the internal organs and the external environment. The skin is richly innervated with pain, temperature, and touch receptors; it synthesizes vitamin D and plays an essential role in fluid and electrolyte balance. It contributes to glucose metabolism through its glycogen stores.

The skin is composed of two layers, the epidermis and the dermis, separated by a basement membrane. A layer of subcutaneous tissue binds the dermis to the underlying organs and tissues of the body. The epidermis, the outermost layer of the skin, contains four to five layers, or strata. The major cells of the epidermis are the keratinocytes, melanocytes, Langerhans cells, and Merkel cells. The stratum germinativum, or basal layer, is the source of the cells in all five layers of the epidermis. The keratinocytes, which are the major cells of the epidermis, are transformed from viable keratinocytes to dead keratin as they move from the innermost layer of the epidermis (*i.e.,* stratum germinativum) to the outermost layer (*i.e.,* stratum corneum). The melanocytes are pigment-synthesizing cells that give skin its color. The dermis provides the epidermis with support and nutrition and is the source of blood vessels, nerves, and skin appendages (*i.e.,* hair follicles, sebaceous glands, nails, and sweat glands). Sensory receptors for touch, pressure, heat, cold, and pain are widely distributed in the dermis. The skin serves as a first line of defense against microorganisms and other harmful agents. The epidermis contains Langerhans cells, which process foreign antigens for presentation to T cells, and the dermis contains macrophages, T cells, mast cells, and fibroblasts, all contributing to the body's immune defenses. ■

MANIFESTATIONS OF SKIN DISORDERS

After completing this section of the chapter, you should be able to meet the following objectives:

■ Describe the following skin rashes and lesions: macule, patch, papule, plaque, nodule, tumor, wheal, vesicle, bulla, and pustule.
■ Describe the characteristics and causes of blisters, calluses, and corns.
■ Cite two physiologic explanations for pruritus.
■ Describe the causes and treatment of dry skin.
■ State common variations found in dark skin.

No two skin disorders look exactly alike, nor are they necessarily caused by the same agents. The appearance of many skin disorders may be further influenced by excessive itching, infection, or the effects of self-treatment. Skin color also may influence the appearance. Nevertheless, most skin disorders have some common characteristics that can be used to describe them. This section of the chapter covers lesions and rashes, dry skin, pruritus, skin disorders due to mechanical forces, and variations in dark skin.

Lesions and Rashes

Rashes are temporary eruptions of the skin, such as those associated with childhood diseases, heat, diaper irritation, or drug-induced reactions. The term *lesion* refers to a traumatic or pathologic loss of normal tissue continuity, structure, or function. The components of a rash often are referred to as *lesions*. Rashes and lesions may range in size from a fraction of a millimeter (*e.g.,* the pinpoint spots of petechiae) to many centimeters (*e.g.,* pressure ulcer). They may be blanched (white), erythematous (reddened), hemorrhagic or purpuric (containing blood), or pigmented (colored). Repeated rubbing and scratching can lead to lichenification (thickened, leathery, and roughened skin characterized by prominent markings) or excoriation (a raw, denuded area caused by breakage of the epidermis). Skin lesions may occur as primary lesions arising in previously normal skin, or they may develop as secondary lesions resulting from other disease conditions. Figure 60-8 illustrates various types of skin lesions.

A *blister* is a vesicle or fluid-filled papule. Blisters of mechanical origin are caused by friction from repeated rubbing on a single area of the skin. Friction blisters most commonly occur on the palmar and plantar surfaces of the hands and feet where the skin is constantly exposed to mechanical trauma, such as from shoes and household tools and appliances. Blisters also develop in bullous skin disorders and from burns. Histologically, there is degeneration of the epidermal cells and a disruption of the intercellular junctions, causing the layers of the skin to separate. As a result, fluid accumulates and a noticeable

Circumscribed, flat, nonpalpable changes in skin color	Palpable elevated solid masses	Circumscribed superficial elevations of the skin formed by free fluid in a cavity within the skin layers
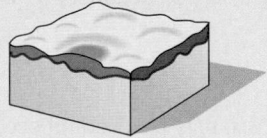	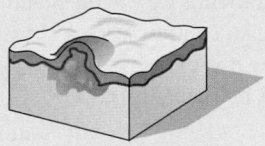	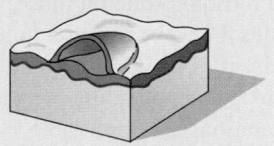
Macule—Small, up to 1 cm. Example: freckle, petechia *Patch*—Larger than 1 cm. Example: vitiligo	*Papule*—Up to 1 cm. Example: elevated nevus *Plaque*—A flat, elevated surface larger than 1 cm, often formed by the coalescence of papules *Nodule*—0.5 cm to 1–2 cm; often deeper and firmer than a papule *Tumor*—Larger than 1–2 cm *Wheal*—A somewhat irregular, relatively transient, superficial area of localized skin edema. Example: mosquito bite, hive	*Vesicle*—Up to 1 cm; filled with serous fluid. Example: herpes simplex *Bulla*—Greater than 1 cm; filled with serous fluid. Example: 2nd-degree burn *Pustule*—Filled with pus. Examples: acne, impetigo

FIGURE 60-8 • Primary lesions may arise from previously normal skin. Authorities vary somewhat in their definitions of skin lesions by size. Dimensions given should be considered approximate. (From Bates B. B. [1995]. *A guide to physical examination and history taking* [6th ed.]. Philadelphia: J. B. Lippincott.)

bleb forms on the skin surface. Friction blisters can be protected by adhesive bandages and gauze to prevent further irritation and rubbing. Breaking the skin of a blister to remove the fluid is inadvisable because of the risk of secondary infection.

A *callus* is a hyperkeratotic plaque of skin due to chronic pressure or friction. It represents hyperplasia of the dead, keratinized cells that make up the cornified or horny layer of the skin. Increased cohesion between cells results in hyperkeratosis and decreased skin shedding. A callus may be filed down but is likely to recur if pressure continues in the localized area.

Corns (helomas) are small, well-circumscribed, conical, keratinous thickenings of the skin. They usually appear on the toes from rubbing or ill-fitting shoes. The corn may be either hard (heloma durum) with a central hard, horny core, or soft (heloma molle), as commonly seen between the toes. They may appear on the hands as an occupational hazard. The hard tissue at the center of the corn looks like a funnel with a broad top and a pointed bottom, hence the name, "corn." Corns on the feet often are painful, whereas corns on the hands may be asymptomatic. Corns may be abraded or surgically removed, but they recur if the causative agent is not removed.

Pruritus

Pruritus, or the sensation of itch, is a common symptom of skin disorders. Symptoms of pruritus range from mild to severe. In some persons, the condition may be so severe that it interrupts sleep and the general quality of life. Although itching commonly occurs with skin disorders, it can also provide a valuable clue to internal disorders, such as chronic renal disease, diabetes, or biliary disease.

Despite the fact that almost all skin diseases manifest in pruritus, very little is known about it. It is generally agreed that itch is a sensation that originates in free nerve endings in the skin, is carried by small myelinated type C nerve fibers to the dorsal horn of the spinal cord, and is then transmitted to the somatosensory cortex through the spinothalamic tract (see Chapter 49). Until recently, it was believed that pain and itch traveled along the same nerve pathways and that itch was a low-level pain response. It has now been demonstrated through micrographic recordings that there are itch-specific neuronal pathways in the spinothalamic tract and central nervous system that process peripheral itch stimuli. Evidence over the years has supported this finding; for example, it has been shown that itch and pain are antagonistic—pain and peripheral inflammation suppress itch, whereas opioids often provoke itch. Further, itch induces scratching, whereas pain induces withdrawal, and itch and pain can be simultaneously perceived. Finally, the belief in polymodal pain–itch receptors may be discounted by the knowledge that massaging or rubbing the skin, which are sensations conducted by non-itch fibers, often results in the sensation of itch. In other words, although rubbing a painful area tends to decrease pain sensations, it increases itch sensations.

Specific afferent type C fibers, distinct from the polymodal nociceptors that are responsible for pain, may transmit itch sensations.[5–7] These specific itch neurons are believed to be sensitive to temperature, which explains why itch worsens in warm environments, including warm sleeping environments.

Given these new findings, it has been postulated that itch exists both locally and centrally, that in addition to localized itch, an "itch center" exists in the somatosensory cortex. For example, a mosquito bite on most people itches momentarily then subsides. However, central itch may be similar to central pain: that is, it is perceived by the brain but does not exist locally. This may explain the presence of localized itch when no skin alterations are observable.[8]

Advances have also been made in understanding peripheral mediators (*i.e.,* substances that cause itch) other than histamine. Mast cell tryptase may be an important itch mediator because it activates a specific receptor in the sensory nerves. Opioids operate centrally and peripherally in producing itch, whereas neuropeptides, such as substance P, induce itch by their effect on mast cells. Substances such as bradykinin and bile salts act locally to stimulate the itch sensation. Prostaglandins are modulators of the itch response, lowering the threshold for other mediators.

Scratching, the well-known response to itch, is a spinal reflex response that to varying degrees can be controlled by the individual. Many types of itch are not easily localized or relieved by scratching. Excoriations and thickened papular areas develop at the site of repeated scratching or rubbing, and in some skin conditions, such as dry skin, scratching further activates itch sensations. Chronic forms of pruritus can severely affect the quality of a person's life.

Most treatment measures for pruritus are nonspecific. Measures such as using the entire hand to rub over large areas and keeping the fingernails trimmed often can relieve itch and prevent skin damage. Self-limited or seasonal cases of pruritus may respond to treatment measures such as moisturizing lotions, bath oils, and the use of humidifiers. Because vasodilation tends to increase itching, cold applications may provide relief. Cool showers before bed, light sleepwear, and cool home temperatures also may be helpful. Topical corticosteroids may be helpful in some cases, such as itch related to allergy-mediated urticaria. However, unlike for some other skin problems, there is no armamentarium of effective antipruritic drugs available.

Mild cutaneous disorders, such as bug bites, are mediated by histamine; therefore, nonsedating antihistamines tend to be the treatment of choice. However, because most cases of pruritus are not histamine related, their management should be directed at the underlying cause. For example, systemic antihistamines and corticosteroids may be indicated for persons with severe pruritus or atopic dermatitis. Topical capsaicin cream and topical aspirin have been used for localized chronic pruritic disorders. Opioid antagonists may be used for pruritus caused by opioid medications such as morphine. Other modalities that have been used for all cases of pruritus with varying degrees of success are phototherapy, acupuncture,[9] vagus nerve stimulation,[10] antidepressant medications, behavior modification,[11] and alternative therapies (herbal, nutritional, and reflex therapies).[12] In persons with pruritus due to a systemic cause, itching gradually recedes as the primary condition improves.

Given the recent advances in the science of pruritus, it is anticipated that health care professionals will have available in the near future new, effective, and disease-specific antipruritic drugs. Classification schemes for pruritus may also be forthcoming. Similar to pain scales, visual analog scales may be developed and used in the diagnosis and treatment of pruritus.

Dry Skin

Dry skin, also called *xerosis,* may be a natural occurrence, as in the drying of skin associated with aging, or it may be symptomatic of an underlying systemic disease or skin disorder such as contact dermatitis. Most cases of dry skin are caused by dehydration of the stratum corneum. The effects of aging on skin dryness include a change in the composition of sebaceous gland secretions and a decrease in the secretion of moisture from the sweat glands. Aging is also accompanied by a decrease in skin capillaries as well as a flattening of the dermal rete ridges, resulting in less surface area for exchange of fluids between the dermis, epidermis, and skin surface.

Persons with dry skin often experience severe pruritus and discomfort, most commonly of the extremities. Other commonly involved areas include the back, abdomen, and waist. Dry skin appears rough and scaly; there may be increased wrinkles or lines. Skin drying also predisposes the skin to scratching, resulting in cracking, fissuring, and a number of other skin maladies.

Moisturizing agents are the cornerstone of treatment for dry skin. These agents exert their effects by repairing the skin barrier, increasing the water content of the skin, reducing transepidermal water loss, and restoring the lipid barrier's ability to attract, hold, and redistribute water. Moisturizing agents can be classified as emollients, humectants, and occlusives.[13] *Emollients* are fatty acid–containing lotions that replenish the oils on the skin surface, but usually do not leave a residue on the skin. They have a short duration of action and need to be applied frequently. *Humectants* are the additives in lotions, such as alpha-hydroxy acids and urea, that draw out water from the deeper skin layers and hold it on the skin surface. However, the water that is drawn to the skin is transepidermal water, not atmospheric water; thus, continued evaporation from the skin can actually exacerbate dryness. Alpha-hydroxy acids are derived from fruits, hence the abundance of fruit additives in shampoos and lotions in over-the-counter preparations. Urea is a nitrogenous substance that has been quite effective in reducing xerosis when combined with lotions. It is a humectant at lower concentrations (10%), but in higher concentrations (20% to 30%) it is mildly keratolytic. Clinical trials of urea have indicated its utility compared with ammonium lactate (lactic acid) lotion and glycerin.[14] *Occlusives* are thick creams that contain petroleum or some other moisture-proof material. They prevent water loss from the skin. They are the most effective agents for relieving skin dryness, but because of their greasiness and lack of cosmetic appeal, some people do not wish to use them.

Lotion or cream additives include corticosteroids or mild anesthetics, such as camphor, menthol, lidocaine, or benzocaine. These agents work by suppressing itching while moisturizing the skin. Using room humidifiers and keeping room temperatures as low as possible to prevent water loss from the skin also may be helpful. Soaps with moisturizers may be helpful. Glycerine soaps, although popular and visually appealing, are drying and can exacerbate the symptoms.

Variations in Dark-Skinned People

Some skin disorders common to people of African, Hispanic, or East Indian descent are not commonly found in those of European descent. Similarly, some skin disorders, such as skin cancers, affect light-skinned persons more commonly than dark-skinned persons. Because of these differences, serious skin disorders may be overlooked, and normal variations in darker skin may be mistaken for anomalies.

Skin color is determined by the melanin produced by the melanocytes. Although the number of melanosomes in dark and white skin is the same, black skin produces more melanin, and more quickly, than white skin. Because of their skin color, dark-skinned persons are better protected against skin cancer, premature wrinkling, and aging of the skin that occurs with sun exposure.

A condition common in people with dark skin is too much or too little color. Areas of the skin may darken after injury, such as a cut or scrape, or after disease conditions such as acne. These darkened areas may take many months or years to fade. Dry or "ashy" skin also can be a problem for people with dark skin. It often is uncomfortable, and it also is easily noticed because it gives the skin an ashen or grayish appearance. Although using a moisturizer may help relieve the discomfort, it may cause a worsening of acne in predisposed persons.

Normal variations in skin structure and skin tones often make evaluation of dark skin difficult. The darker pigmentation can make skin pallor, cyanosis, and erythema more difficult to observe. Therefore, verbal histories must be relied on to assess skin changes. The verbal history should include the client's description of her or his normal skin tones. Changes in skin color, in particular hypopigmentation and hyperpigmentation, often accompany disorders of dark skin and are very important signs to observe when diagnosing skin conditions. Common variations in dark skin and nails are described in Table 60-1.

IN SUMMARY, skin lesions and rashes are the most common manifestations of skin disorders. Rashes are temporary skin eruptions. Lesions result from traumatic or pathologic loss of the normal continuity, structure, or function of the skin. Lesions may be vascular in origin; they may occur as primary lesions in previously normal skin; or they may develop as secondary lesions resulting from primary lesions. Blisters, calluses, and corns result from rubbing, pressure, and frictional forces applied to the skin. Pruritus and dry skin are symptoms common to many skin disorders. Scratching because of pruritus can lead to excoriation, infection, and other complications. Normal variations in dark skin often make evaluation difficult and result in some disorders being overlooked. Changes in color, especially hypopigmentation or hyperpigmentation, often accompany the skin disorders of dark-skinned people. ■

TABLE 60-1 **Common Normal Variations in Dark Skin**	
VARIATION	**APPEARANCE**
Futcher (Voigt) line	Demarcation between darkly pigmented and lightly pigmented skin in upper arm; follows spinal nerve distribution; common in black and Japanese populations
Midline hypopigmentation	Line or band of hypopigmentation over the sternum, dark or faint, lessens with age; common in Latin American and black populations
Nail pigmentation	Linear dark bands down nails or diffuse nail pigmentation, brown, blue, or blue-black
Oral pigmentation	Blue to blue-gray pigmentation of oral mucosa; gingivae also affected
Palmar changes	Hyperpigmented creases, small hyperkeratotic papules, and tiny pits in creases
Plantar changes	Hyperpigmented macules, can be multiple with patchy distribution, irregular borders, and variance in color

Developed from information in Rosen T., Martin S. (1981). *Atlas of black dermatology.* Boston: Little, Brown

Review Exercises

1. Bullous pemphigoid is an autoimmune blistering disease caused by autoantibodies to constituents of the dermal–epidermal junction.

   A. *Explain how antibodies, which attack glycoproteins in the lamina lucida and their attachment to the hemidesmosomes, can cause blisters to form (hint: see Fig. 60-5).*

2. "Allergy tests" involve the application of an antigen to the skin, either through a small scratch or intradermal injection.

   A. *Explain how the body's immune system is able to detect and react to these antigens.*

References

1. Lotti T., Bianchi B., Ghersetich I., et al. (2002). Can the brain inhibit inflammation generated in the skin? The lesson of gamma-melanocyte-stimulating hormone. *International Journal of Dermatology* 41, 311–318.
2. Choung C. M., Nickoloff B. J., Elias P. M., et al. (2002). What is the "true" function of the skin? *Experimental Dermatology* 11, 159–187.
3. Hood A. F., Kwan T. H., Mihm M. C., et al. (2002). *Primer of dermatopathology* (3rd ed.). Philadelphia: Lippincott Williams & Wilkins.
4. McGrath J. A., Eady R. A. J., Pope F. M. (2004). Anatomy and organization of human skin. In Burns T., Breathnach S., Cox N., et al. (Eds.), *Rook's textbook of dermatology* (7th ed., pp. 3.1–3.84). Malden, MA: Blackwell.
5. Stander S., Steinhoff M., Luger T. A. (2002). Pathophysiology of pruritus. In Bieber T., Leung D. Y. M. (Eds.), *Atopic dermatitis* (pp. 183–216). New York: Marcel Dekker.
6. Greaves M. W. (2004). Pruritus. In Burns T., Breathnach S., Cox N., et al. (Eds.), *Rook's textbook of dermatology* (7th ed., vol. 1, pp. 16.1–16.5). Malden, MA: Blackwell.
7. Yosipovitch G., Fleischer A. B. (2003). Itch associated with skin disease: Advances in pathophysiology and emerging therapies. *American Journal of Clinical Dermatology* 4, 617–622.
8. Paus R., Schmelz M., Bíro T., et al. (2006). Frontiers in pruritus research: Scratching the brain for more effective itch therapy. *Journal of Clinical Investigation* 116, 1174–1186.
9. Charlesworth E. N., Beltrani V. S. (2002). Pruritic dermatoses: Overview of etiology and therapy. *American Journal of Medicine* 113(Suppl. 9A), 25S–33S.
10. Kirchner A., Stefan H., Schmelz M., et al. (2002). Influence of vagus nerve stimulation on histamine-induced itching. *Neurology* 59, 108–112.
11. Roebuck H. L. (2006). For pruritus, combination therapy works best. *American Journal of Primary Health Care* 31(3), 12–13.
12. Millikan L. E. (2003). Alternative therapy in pruritus. *Dermatologic Therapy* 16, 175–180.
13. Buchness M. R. (2006). A practical approach to basic skin care. *Women's Health in Primary Care* 9(8), 11–15.
14. Ademola J., Frazier C., Kim S. J., et al. (2002). Clinical evaluation of 40% urea and 12% ammonium lactate in the treatment of xerosis. *American Journal of Clinical Dermatology* 3, 217–222.

Visit the**Point** **http://thePoint.lww.com for animations, journal articles, and more!**

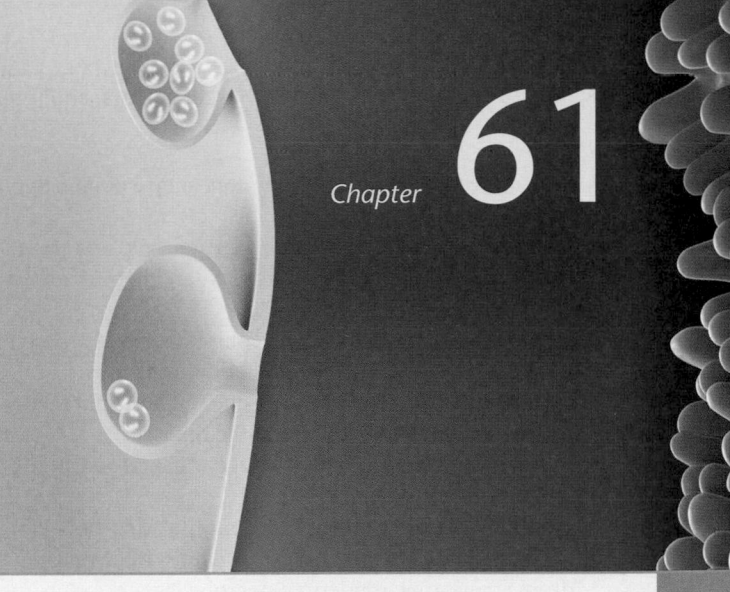

Chapter 61

Disorders of Skin Integrity and Function

GLADYS SIMANDL

➤ The skin is a unique organ in that numerous signs of disease or injury are immediately observable on the skin. The skin serves as the interface between the body's internal organs and the external environment. Therefore, skin disorders represent the culmination of environmental forces and the internal functioning of the body. Sunlight, insects, other arthropods, infectious organisms, chemicals, and physical agents all play a role in the pathogenesis of skin diseases. Although most disorders are intrinsic to skin, many are external manifestations of systemic disease. Thus, skin provides a valuable window for the recognition of many systemic disorders.

The skin also has an elusive property that reflects emotional states. It is through the skin that warmth and other responses are given and received. The skin conveys a sense of health, beauty, integrity, and emotion. Human beings emphasize the body and, in particular, the skin to the degree that even slight imperfections may evoke a wide variety of responses. With the wealth of scientific research and knowledge about the skin, it is extremely important that each person's emotional and psychological responses to her or his skin conditions be considered.

PRIMARY DISORDERS OF THE SKIN

After completing this section of the chapter, you should be able to meet the following objectives:

■ Describe common pigmentary disorders of the skin.
■ Relate the behavior of fungi to the production of superficial skin lesions associated with tinea or ringworm.

(objectives continue)

- State the cause and describe the appearance of impetigo and ecthyma.
- Compare the viral causes, manifestations, and treatments of verrucae, herpes simplex, and herpes zoster lesions.
- Compare acne vulgaris, acne conglobata, and rosacea in terms of appearance and location of lesions.
- Describe the pathogenesis of acne vulgaris and relate it to measures used in treating the disorder.
- Differentiate allergic and contact dermatitis and atopic and nummular eczema.
- Describe the differences and similarities between erythema multiforme minor, Stevens-Johnson syndrome, and toxic epidermal necrolysis.
- Define the term *papulosquamous* and use the term to describe the lesions associated with psoriasis, pityriasis rosea, and lichen planus.
- Relate the life cycle of *Sarcoptes scabiei* to the skin lesions seen in scabies.
- Use knowledge of the life cycles of *Pediculus humanus corporis* and *Pediculus humanus capitis* to explain the lesions associated with body, head, and pubic lice.

Primary skin disorders are those originating in the skin. They include pigmentary skin disorders, infectious processes, acne, rosacea, papulosquamous dermatoses, allergic disorders and drug reactions, and arthropod infestations. Although most of these disorders are not life-threatening, they can affect the quality of life.

🔑 PRIMARY SKIN DISORDERS

- Primary skin disorders originate in the skin.
- Pigmentary skin disorders involve increased, decreased, or absent melanocyte function.
- Infectious skin disorders are caused by viruses, bacteria, and fungi that invade the skin, incite inflammatory responses, and otherwise cause rashes and lesions that disrupt the skin surface.
- Acne involves occlusion of the pilosebaceous unit with noninflammatory and inflammatory lesions resulting from occlusion, inflammation due to the irritating effects of sebum, and infection caused by the *P. acnes* organism.
- Allergic and hypersensitivity responses are caused by antigen-antibody responses resulting from sensitization to topical or systemic antigens.
- The papulosquamous dermatoses constitute a group of disorders characterized by scaling papules and plaques that result from uncontrolled keratinocyte proliferation.
- Scabies and lice are arthropod skin infestations that are transmitted from person to person and from animals to humans.

Pigmentary Skin Disorders

Pigmentary skin disorders involve the melanocytes. In some cases, there is an absence of melanin production, as in vitiligo or albinism. In other cases, there is an increase in melanin or some other pigment, as in mongolian spots or melasma. In either case, the emotional impact can be devastating. Because pigmentary changes can result in social ostracism, it is also important to treat the physiologic, emotional, and social components of these skin disorders.

Vitiligo

Vitiligo is a pigmentary problem of concern to darkly pigmented persons of all races. It also affects white-skinned persons, but not as often, and the effects usually are not as socially problematic. The classic sign of vitiligo is the sudden appearance of white patches on the skin. The lesion is a depigmented macule with definite smooth borders on the face, axillae, neck, or extremities (Fig. 61-1). The patches vary in size from small macules to ones involving large skin surfaces. The large macular type is more common. Depigmented areas appear white, pale colored, or sometimes grayish-blue. Histologically, the depigmented areas may contain no melanocytes, greatly altered or decreased amounts of melanocytes, or, in some cases, melanocytes that no longer produce melanin. These areas sunburn easily and they enlarge over time. Vitiligo often is asymptomatic, although pruritus may occur.

Vitiligo appears at any age; roughly half of cases begin before the age of 20 years. Worldwide, it affects people of all races regardless of sex, with an incidence rate of 1% to 2%.[1] The cause is unknown, although several hypotheses have been postulated, including (1) a hereditary predisposition; up to 38% of people with vitiligo report a family history; (2) an autoimmune process in which there is immunologic destruction of the melanocytes; the disorder often accompanies other autoimmune

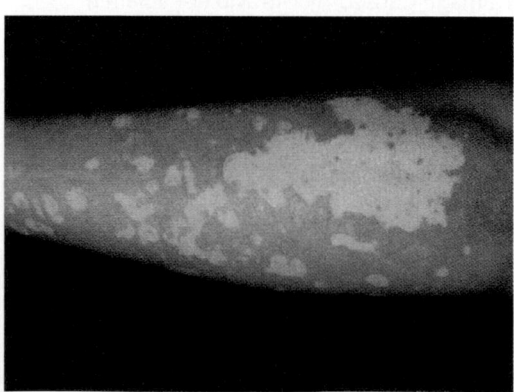

FIGURE 61-1 • Vitiligo of the forearm of a black person. (Neutrogena Skin Care Institute.) (From Sauer G. C., Hall J. C. [1996]. *Manual of skin diseases* [7th ed.]. Philadelphia: Lippincott-Raven.)

diseases, such as diabetes mellitus and pernicious anemia; (3) neural mechanisms in which the melanocytes are destroyed by a cytotoxic chemical secreted by nearby nerve endings; (4) a self-destruct phenomenon in which the melanocytes are preprogrammed for self-destruction; (5) a lack of melanocyte growth factors; or (6) a combination of factors in which multiple causes are involved and vary among individuals.[2] In some cases, vitiligo has been reportedly precipitated by emotional stress or physical trauma, such as sunburn.

Although there are many treatment regimens for vitiligo, none is curative. Self-tanning lotions, skin stains, and cosmetics are used for camouflage. Self-tanning compounds that contain a chemical such as *dihydroxyacetone* do not need melanocytes to color the skin. Corticosteroids administered topically, intralesionally, and orally have also been used successfully. Broad-band (large area) and narrow-band (focused) ultraviolet B (UVB) irradiation has also been used successfully in the treatment of vitiligo. The combination of psoralen and UVA (PUVA) treatment has also been successful in some people with large areas of skin involvement.[2]

A variety of skin grafting techniques have been used in persons unresponsive to other therapies. Successful skin grafting techniques vary from minigrafting (2-mm full-thickness punch grafts transplanted to involved areas) to grafting melanocytes into involved areas. Micropigmentation (tattooing) has been done on smaller, recalcitrant areas, but it is often difficult to attain a correct color match.

If extensive skin surfaces are involved, the treatment may be reversed and the pigmented areas bleached to match the remainder of the skin color. A melanocytotoxic agent is used to remove remaining melanocytes from skin areas. This process, which is called *depigmentation,* is permanent and irreversible; patients need to be apprised of this and their need to avoid the sun and use sunscreens for the remainder of their lives.

Albinism

Albinism, a genetic disorder in which there is complete or partial congenital absence of pigment in the skin, hair, and eyes, is found in all races. The prevalence is about 1 in 20,000 people world-wide, and 1 in 16,000 in the United States.[3] Although there are over 10 different types of albinism, the most common type is recessively inherited oculocutaneous albinism, in which there is a normal number of melanocytes but they lack tyrosinase, the enzyme needed for synthesis of melanin. It affects the skin, hair, and eyes. Individuals have pale or pink skin, white or yellow hair, and light-colored or sometimes pink eyes. Persons with albinism have ocular problems, such as extreme sensitivity to light, refractive errors, lack of stereopsis, and nystagmus. There is no cure for albinism. Treatment efforts for people with albinism are aimed at reducing their risk for cancer through protection from solar radiation and screening for malignant skin changes. Efforts to reduce the visual impact are important, such as glasses, preferential seating in classrooms, and large-

print books. Finally, public education regarding albinism is important to help integrate people with albinism into everyday society.

Melasma

Melasma is a disorder characterized by darkened macules on the face. It is common in all skin types, but most prominent in brown-skinned people from Asia, India, and South America. It occurs in men but is more common in women, particularly during pregnancy or while using oral contraceptives. It may or may not resolve after giving birth or discontinuing hormonal birth control. Melasma is exacerbated by sun exposure. Treatment measures are palliative, mostly consisting of limiting exposure to the sun and using sunscreens. Bleaching agents, containing 2% to 4% hydroquinone, are standard treatments. Tretinoin cream and azelaic acid have been useful in treating severe cases. Depending on the person's ability to tolerate topical treatments, triple combinations (hydroquinone, tretinoin, and fluocinolone acetonide) or double combinations (hydroquinone and tretinoin) have been highly successful, sometimes combined with glycolic acid.

Infectious Processes

The skin is subject to invasion by a number of microorganisms, including fungi, bacteria, and viruses. Normally, the skin flora, sebum, immune responses, and other protective mechanisms guard the skin against infection. Depending on the virulence of the infecting agent and the competence of the host's resistance, infections may result.

Superficial Fungal Infections

Fungi are free-living, saprophytic plantlike organisms, certain strains of which are considered part of the normal skin flora (see Chapter 16). There are two types of fungi, yeasts and molds. Yeasts, such as *Candida albicans,* grow as single cells and reproduce asexually. Molds grow in long filaments, called *hyphae.* There are thousands of known species of yeasts and molds, but only about 100 of them cause disease in humans and animals. Fungal or mycotic infections of the skin are traditionally classified as superficial or deep. The superficial mycoses, more commonly known as *tinea* or *ringworm,* invade only the superficial keratinized tissue (skin, hair, and nails). Deep fungal infections involve the epidermis, dermis, and subcutis. Infections that typically are superficial may exhibit deep involvement in immunosuppressed individuals.

Most of the superficial mycoses (or *dermatophytoses*) are caused by the dermatophytes, a group of closely related fungi classified into three genera: *Microsporum* (*M. audouinii, M. canis, M. gypseum*), *Epidermophyton* (*E. floccosum*), and *Trichophyton* (*T. schoenleinii, T. violaceum, T. tonsurans*). Another way of classifying the dermatophytes is according to their ecologic origin—human, animal, or soil. Anthropophilic species (*M. audouinii, M. tonsurans, T. violaceum*) are parasitic on humans and are spread by other infected humans. Zoophilic species (*M. canis* and *T. mentagrophytes*) cause parasitic infections in animals, some of which can be spread to humans. Geophilic species originate in the soil, but may infect animals, which in turn serve to infect humans.

The fungi that cause superficial mycoses live on the dead keratinized cells of the epidermis. They emit an enzyme that enables them to digest keratin, which results in superficial skin scaling, nail disintegration, or hair breakage, depending on the location of the infection. An exception to this is the invading fungus of tinea versicolor, which does not produce a keratolytic enzyme. Deeper reactions involving vesicles, erythema, and infiltration are caused by the inflammation that results from exotoxins liberated by the fungus. Fungi also are capable of producing an allergic or immune response. Superficial fungal infections affect various parts of the body, with the lesions varying according to site and fungal species. Tinea can affect the body (tinea corporis), face and neck (tinea faciale), scalp (tinea capitis), hands (tinea manus), feet (tinea pedis), nails (tinea unguium), or genitalia (tinea cruris).

Diagnosis of superficial fungal infections is primarily done by microscopic examination of skin scrapings for fungal spores, the reproducing bodies of fungi. Potassium hydroxide (KOH) preparations are used to prepare slides of skin scrapings. KOH disintegrates human tissue and leaves behind the threadlike filaments, or hyphae, that grow from the fungal spores. Cultures also may be done using a dermatophyte test medium or a microculture slide that produces color changes and allows for direct microscopic identification. The Wood light (UV light) is another method that can assist with the diagnosis of tinea. Some types of fungi (*e.g.,* *M. canis* and *M. audouinii*) fluorescence yellow-green when the light is directed onto the affected area.

Superficial fungal infections may be treated with topical or systemic antifungal agents. Treatment usually follows diagnosis confirmed by KOH preparation or culture, particularly if a systemic agent is to be used. Topical agents, both prescription and over-the-counter preparations, are commonly used in the treatment of tinea infections; however, success often is limited because of the lengthy duration of treatment, poor compliance, and high rates of relapse at specific body sites.

The oral systemic antifungal agents include griseofulvin, the azoles, and the allylamines. Griseofulvin is a fungicidal agent derived from a species of *Penicillium* that is used only in the treatment of dermatophytoses. It acts by binding to the keratin of newly forming skin, protecting the skin from new infection. Because its action is to prevent new infection, it must be administered for 2 to 6 weeks to allow for skin replacement. The azoles are a group of synthetic antifungal drugs that act by inhibiting the fungal enzymes needed for the synthesis of ergosterol, which is an essential part of fungal cell membranes. The azoles are classified as either imidazoles or triazoles. The imidazoles consist of ketoconazole, miconazole, and clotrimazole. The latter two drugs are used only in topical therapy. The triazoles include itraconazole and fluconazole, both of which are used for the systemic treatment of fungal infections. Terbinafine, a synthetic allylamine, acts by interrupting ergos-

terol synthesis, causing the accumulation of a metabolite that is toxic to the fungus. In contrast to griseofulvin, the synthetic agents are fungicidal (*i.e.,* kill the fungus) and therefore are more effective over shorter treatment periods. Some of the oral agents can produce serious side effects, such as hepatic toxicity, or interact adversely with other medications. A number of the synthetic fungicides (*e.g.,* ketoconazole, miconazole, clotrimazole, and terbinafine) are available as topical preparations that produce less severe side effects. Topical corticosteroids may be used in conjunction with antifungal agents to relieve itching and erythema secondary to inflammation.

Tinea of the Body or Face. *Tinea corporis* (ringworm of the body) can be caused by any of the fungi but is most frequently caused by *M. canis* in the United States and by *T. rubrum* worldwide. There has been an increase in *T. tonsurans* as the causative agent of tinea corporis as well. Although tinea corporis affects all ages, children seem most prone to infection. Transmission is most commonly from kittens, puppies, and other children who have infections.

The lesions vary, depending on the fungal agent. The most common types of lesions are oval or circular patches on exposed skin surfaces and the trunk, back, or buttocks (Fig. 61-2). Less common are foot and groin infections. The lesion begins as a red papule and enlarges, often with a central clearing. Patches have raised red borders consisting of vesicles, papules, or pustules. The borders are sharply defined, but lesions may coalesce. Pruritus, a mild burning sensation, and erythema frequently accompany the skin lesion.

Tinea faciale, or ringworm of the face (Fig. 61-3), is an infection caused by *T. mentagrophytes* or *T. rubrum.* Tinea faciale may mimic the annular, erythematous, scaling, pruritic lesions characteristic of tinea corporis. It also may appear as flat erythematous patches. Topical antifungal agents usually are effective in treating tinea corporis and tinea faciale. Oral antifungal agents may be used in resistant cases.

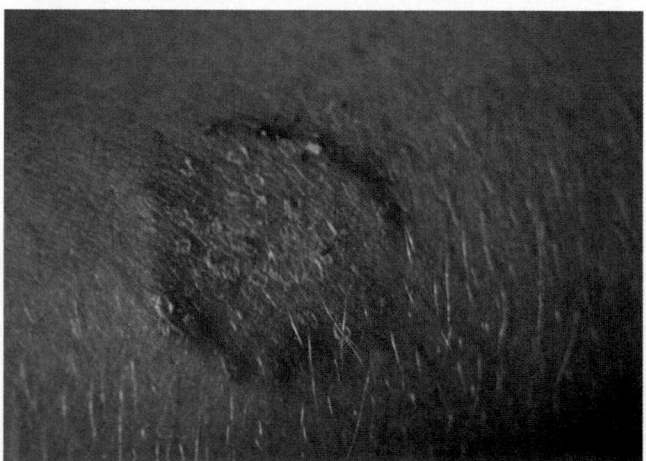

FIGURE 61-2 • Tinea corporis (ringworm) of the arm due to *Trichophyton mentagrophytes.* (Centers for Disease Control and Prevention Public Health Image Library. [Online.] Available: http://phil.cdc.gov/Phil/home.asp.)

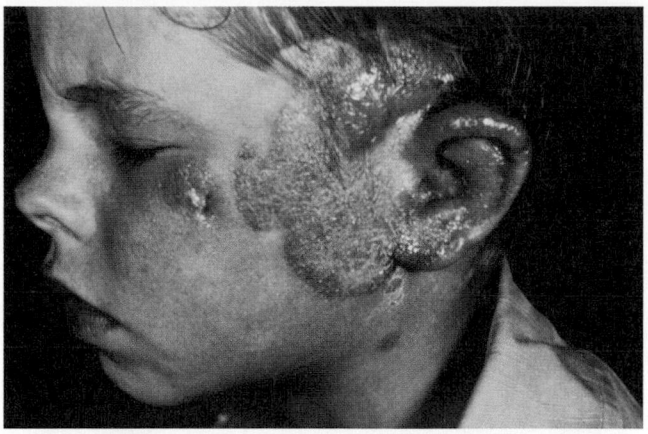

FIGURE 61-3 • Child with ringworm (tinea faciale) on the left side of his face and ear. Tinea faciale does not include the bearded areas (called *tinea barbae*). Tinea faciale infections are uncommon, and are often initially misdiagnosed. (Centers for Disease Control and Prevention Public Health Image Library. [Online.] Available: http://phil.cdc.gov/Phil/home.asp.)

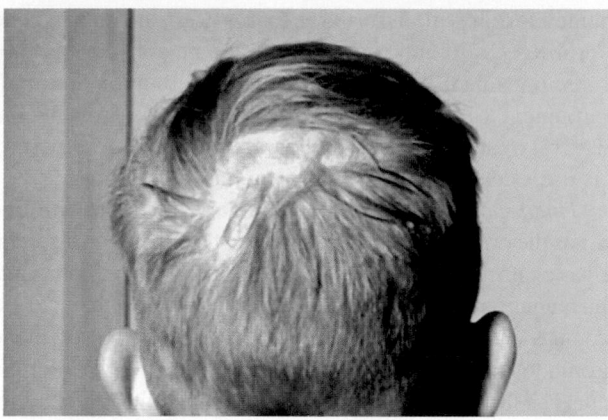

FIGURE 61-4 • Child with tinea capitis (ringworm of the scalp) caused by a *Microsporum* species. (Centers for Disease Control and Prevention Public Health Image Library. [Online.] Available: http://phil.cdc.gov/Phil/home.asp.)

Tinea of the Scalp. There are two common types of *tinea capitis* (ringworm of the scalp): primary (noninflammatory) and secondary (inflammatory). In the United States, 95% of the cases of noninflammatory tinea capitis are caused by *T. tonsurans;* however, forms commonly found in Africa and West Asia have been isolated.[4] *T. tonsurans* does not fluoresce green with a Wood lamp. Urban children between the ages of 3 and 14 years are primarily affected, with a higher incidence of tinea capitis among people of African American or Hispanic descent.[5] Although there is a lower incidence among adults attributed to the higher content of fatty acids in the sebum after puberty, increasing numbers of adults are being diagnosed. The infection is spread most often among household members who share combs and brushes on which the spores are shed and remain viable for long periods. Depending on the invading fungus, the lesions of the noninflammatory type can vary from grayish, round, hairless patches to balding spots, with or without black dots on the head. The lesions vary in size and are most commonly seen on the back of the head (Fig. 61-4). Mild erythema, crust, or scale may be present. The individual usually is asymptomatic, although pruritus may exist.

The inflammatory type of tinea capitis is caused by virulent strains of *T. mentagrophytes, T. verrucosum,* and *M. gypseum.* The onset is rapid, and inflamed lesions usually are localized to one area of the head. The inflammation is believed to be a delayed hypersensitivity reaction to the invading fungus. The initial lesion consists of a pustular, scaly, round patch with broken hairs. A secondary bacterial infection is common and may lead to a painful, circumscribed, boggy, and indurated lesion called a *kerion.* The highest incidence is among children and farmers who work with infected animals.

The treatment for both noninflammatory and inflammatory forms of tinea capitis is oral griseofulvin or synthetic antifungals. Griseofulvin has been the primary treatment for children because it was believed to have fewer side effects than the synthetic antifungals. However, terbinafine and other antifungals have had results comparable with griseofulvin and are therefore under investigation as replacement therapies.[6] Topical ointments or shampoos are sometimes indicated in addition to oral medications, both to decrease the spore population and protect household members. Because of the lower fatty acid content in the sebum of young children, several of the topical antifungal agents are prepared with fatty acid bases, or can be administered with high-fat meals. The antifungal agents have revolutionized treatment, replacing the old remedies in which children often were subjected to head shavings and the use of harsh shampoos and salves. Wet packs, medicated shampoos, steroids, and antibiotics may be prescribed for secondary infections that occur.

Tinea of the Foot and Hand. *Tinea pedis* (athlete's foot) is the most common fungal dermatosis, primarily affecting the spaces between the toes, the soles, or sides of the feet (Fig. 61-5). It is caused by *T. mentagrophytes* and *T. rubrum.* The lesions vary from a mildly scaling lesion to a painful, exudative, erosive,

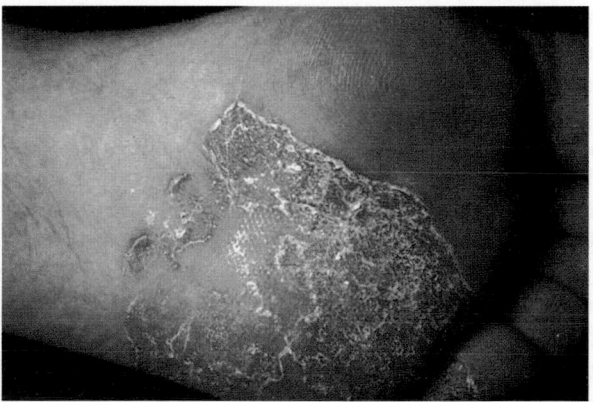

FIGURE 61-5 • Chronic tinea of the sole caused by *Trichophyton rubrum.* (Schering Corp.) (From Sauer G. C., Hall J. C. [1996]. *Manual of skin diseases* [7th ed.]. Philadelphia: Lippincott-Raven.)

inflamed lesion with fissuring. Lesions often are accompanied by pruritus, pain, and foul odor. Some persons are prone to chronic tinea pedis. Mild forms are more common during dry environmental conditions. Exacerbations occur as a result of hot weather, sweating, and exercise or when the feet are exposed to moisture, occlusive shoes, and communal swimming.

Tinea manus usually is a secondary infection with tinea pedis as the primary infection. In contrast to other skin disorders, such as contact dermatitis and psoriasis, which affect both hands, tinea manus usually occurs only on one hand. The characteristic lesion is a blister on the palm or finger surrounded by erythema. Chronic lesions are scaly and dry. Cracking and fissuring may occur. The lesions may spread to the plantar surfaces of the hand. If chronic, tinea manus may lead to tinea of the fingernails. Simple forms of tinea pedis and tinea manus are treated with topical applications of antifungals. Complex cases are treated with oral griseofulvin, ketoconazole, or terbinafine. Other treatment and preventive measures include careful cleaning and drying of affected areas. Persons with tinea pedis should wear clean, dry socks, changing them at least once daily. When bathed, the feet should be dried after other parts of the body or with a separate towel to prevent spread of the infection. Applying drying agents, such as medicated or nonmedicated powder or talc, directly on the feet or into socks, may be helpful in preventing excessive moisture, especially during sports or warm summer months. Some persons have found it helpful to dry the feet with hair blowers on cool cycles, being careful not to cause burns.

Tinea of the Nail. *Tinea unguium* is a dermatophyte infection of the nails. It is a subset of *onychomycosis,* which includes dermatophyte, nondermatophyte, and candidal infections of the nails. There is an increased incidence of fungal nail infections in recent years, probably reflecting better diagnostics, increased numbers of immunocompromised patients who have greater susceptibility, increased use of immunosuppressive drugs, increasing numbers of elderly people, worldwide travel, and increased use of communal bathing facilities.

Distal and lateral subungual onychomycosis, the most common form of tinea unguium, usually is caused by *T. rubrum* or *T. mentagrophytes.* Toenails are involved more commonly than fingernails because fingernails are more exposed to air. The infection often begins at the tip of the nail, where the fungus digests the nail keratin. In some cases, the infection may begin from a crushing injury to a toenail or from the spread of tinea pedis. Initially, the nail appears opaque, white, or silver (Fig. 61-6). The nail then turns yellow or brown. The condition often remains unchanged for years. During this time it may involve only one or two nails and may produce little or no discomfort. Gradually, the nail thickens and cracks as the infection spreads and includes the nail plate. Permanent discoloration and distortion result as the nail plate separates from the nail bed. Less common forms of tinea unguium are superficial white onychomycosis, in which areas of the nails become powdery white and erode, and proximal subungual onychomycosis, in which there is rapid invasion of the nail, leaving it white with no additional thickening of the nail. Although it is one of the

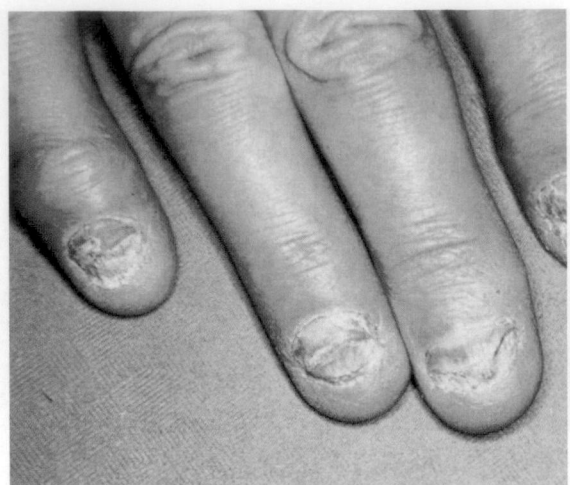

FIGURE 61-6 • Tinea of the fingernail caused by *Trichophyton rubrum.* (Duke Laboratories, Inc.) (From Sauer G. C., Hall J. C. [1996]. *Manual of skin diseases* [7th ed.]. Philadelphia: Lippincott-Raven.)

less common forms of tinea unguium, proximal subungual onychomycosis has increased among people with human immunodeficiency virus (HIV) infection.

Treatment of tinea unguium usually requires oral antifungal therapy. Toenail infections are usually treated with itraconazole and terbinafine. Terbinafine has been found to be highly effective,[7] cost effective,[8] and safe for vulnerable populations, such as children, the elderly, the immunocompromised, and people with diabetes.[7] Fluconazole has been effective, particularly if *Candida* is involved. Itraconazole is administered in pulses (intermittent weeks of therapy), whereas terbinafine or fluconazole is administered without interruption for 12 to 15 weeks. Fingernail infections are more easily treated, in part because the fingernails are more exposed to air. Itraconazole, terbinafine, and, to a lesser extent, griseofulvin have been effective in treating fingernail infections. All of the oral agents require careful monitoring for side effects. A nail lacquer containing the antifungal agent, ciclopirox, is available for use in the topical management of mild to moderate infections of the fingernails and toenails caused by *T. rubrum.* A new nail may require 3 to 12 months to grow. Thus, people being treated with antifungal agents need to be reminded that the resolution of the infection requires 4 to 6 months for fingernails and longer for toenails.

Although there has been an increase in the cure rate of toenail fungal infections, primarily because of the synthetic antifungals, recalcitrant cases remain. Some authorities recommend removal of the infected toenails. Many cases of tinea unguium would be prevented if primary infections of tinea pedis were diagnosed and treated promptly.

Tinea Versicolor. Tinea versicolor is a fungal infection involving the upper chest, the back, and sometimes the arms. The causative agent belongs to the *Malassezia* yeast genus, of which seven species are found on the human body. Until recently, *Malassezia furfur* was indicated as the cause; however, with genetic analysis, *Malassezia globosa* has now been identified as the cause.[9] The infection occurs primarily in young adults in tropical and temperate regions, but cases have been reported in the northern states. The characteristic lesion is a yellow, pink, or brown sheet of scaling skin. The name *versicolor* is derived from the multicolored variations of the lesion. The patches are depigmented and do not tan when exposed to UV light. The skin has an overall appearance of being "dirty." These cosmetic defects often bring the patient to the health care provider in the summer months. It is believed that the fungus filters the UV light, preventing tanning. In darker-skinned persons, the depigmented areas are more apparent.

Selenium sulfide, found in several shampoo preparations, has been an effective fungistatic treatment measure. Miconazole or ketoconazole creams or shampoos, because of their fungicidal properties, have become the drugs of choice. Oral antifungals are used for extensive cases. The infection may recur after drug therapy. Boiling or steam-pressing clothes may help prevent recurrence. Single applications of topical creams or shampoos every 30 to 60 days may be warranted in persons predisposed to this infection.

Tinea Incognito. Tinea incognito is a form of dermatophyte infection that developed with the widespread use of topical corticosteroids. It often is seen in cases where tinea infections are misdiagnosed as eczema and treated with corticosteroids. Because corticosteroids suppress inflammation, scaling and erythema may not be present or it may not resemble a fungal infection at all after several rounds of cortisone therapy. There has been an increased incidence of tinea incognito in persons with HIV infection. Persons with the disorder often present with thickened plaques with lichenification, papules, pustules, and nodules. Telangiectases, atrophy, and striae may be present. Tinea incognito is seen most often on the groin, the palms, or the dorsal aspect of the hand.

Treatment measures include discontinuing topical corticosteroids while using low-dose oral corticosteroids to prevent the flare-up associated with discontinuing potent topical steroids. Topical or oral antifungal agents are used, depending on the severity of the infection. Persons who must remain on potent topical corticosteroids are difficult to treat.

Dermatophytid Reaction. A secondary skin eruption may occur in persons allergic to the fungus responsible for the dermatophytosis. This dermatophytid or allergic reaction may occur during an acute episode of a fungal infection. The most common reaction occurs on the hands in response to tinea pedis. The lesions are vesicles with erythema extending over the palms and fingers, sometimes extending to other areas (Fig. 61-7). Less commonly, a more generalized reaction occurs in which papules or vesicles erupt on the trunk or extremities. These eruptions may resemble tinea corporis. Lesions may become excoriated and infected with bacteria. Treatment is directed at the primary site of infection. The intradermal reaction resolves in most cases without intervention if the primary site is cleared.

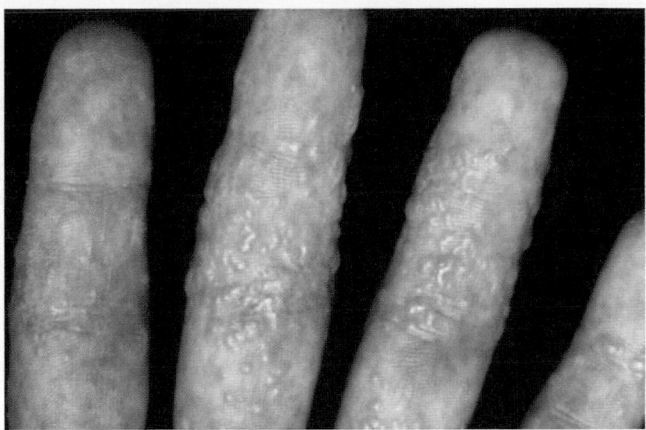

FIGURE 61-7 • Dermatophytid or id reaction on the fingers due to a tinea infection. An id immunologic reaction, also known as *autoeczematization,* is an itchy, vesicular rash produced in response to an intense inflammatory process that can be located in another region of the body. (Centers for Disease Control and Prevention Public Health Image Library. [Online.] Available: http://phil.cdc.gov/Phil/home.asp.)

Candidal Infections. Candidiasis (moniliasis) is a fungal infection caused by *C. albicans* and occasionally by a few other *Candida* species. This yeastlike fungus is a normal inhabitant of the gastrointestinal tract, mouth, and vagina (see Chapter 47). The skin problems result from the release of irritating toxins on the skin surface. *C. albicans* is found almost always on the surface of the skin; it rarely penetrates to the deeper layers of the skin. Some persons are predisposed to candidal infections by conditions such as diabetes mellitus, antibiotic therapy, pregnancy, oral contraceptive use, poor nutrition, and immunosuppressive diseases. Oral candidiasis may be the first sign of infection with HIV.

C. albicans thrives on warm, moist, intertriginous areas of the body. The rash is red with well-defined borders. Patches erode the epidermis, and there is scaling. Mild to severe itching and burning often accompany the infection. Severe forms of infection may involve pustules or vesiculopustules. In addition to microscopy, a candidal infection often can be differentiated from a tinea infection by the presence of satellite lesions. These satellite lesions are maculopapular and are found outside the clearly demarcated borders of the candidal infection. Satellite lesions often are diagnostic of diaper rash complicated by *Candida.* The appearance of candidal infections varies according to the site (see Chapter 47 for a discussion of vaginal candidiasis).

Diagnosis usually is based on microscopic examination of skin or mucous membrane scrapings placed in a KOH solution. Treatment measures vary according to the location. Preventive measures such as wearing rubber gloves are encouraged for persons with infections of the hands. Intertriginous areas often are separated with clean cotton cloth and allowed to air dry as a means of decreasing the macerating effects of heat and moisture. Topical and oral antifungal agents, such as clotrimazole, econazole, ketoconazole, and miconazole, are used in treatment depending on the site and extent of involvement.

Bacterial Infections

Bacteria are considered normal flora of the skin. Most bacteria are not pathogenic, but when pathogenic bacteria invade the skin, superficial or systemic infections may develop. Bacterial skin infections are commonly classified as primary or secondary infections. Primary infections are superficial skin infections such as impetigo or ecthyma. Secondary infections consist of deeper cutaneous infections, such as infected ulcers. Diagnosis usually is based on cultures taken from the infected site. Treatment measures include antibiotic therapy and measures to promote comfort and prevent the spread of infection.

Impetigo. Impetigo is a common, superficial bacterial infection caused by staphylococci or group A beta-hemolytic streptococci, or both. Impetigo is common among infants and young children, although older children and adults occasionally contract the disease. Its occurrence is highest during warm summer months or in warm, moist climates. Although overcrowded housing and poor hygiene contribute to its incidence, they are not causative. It is highly communicable in the younger population.

Impetigo initially appears as a small vesicle or pustule or as a large bulla on the face or elsewhere on the body. As the primary lesion ruptures, it leaves a denuded area that discharges a honey-colored serous liquid that hardens on the skin surface and dries as a honey-colored crust with a "stuck-on" appearance (Fig. 61-8). New vesicles erupt within hours. Pruritus often accompanies the lesions, and skin excoriations that result from scratching multiply the infection sites. Although a very low risk, a possible complication of untreated streptococcal impetigo is poststreptococcal glomerulonephritis (see Chapter 33). Topical mupirocin (Bactroban), which has few side effects, may be effective for limited infections. If the area is large or if there is concern about complications, systemic antibiotics are used.

Another form of impetigo exists, *bullous impetigo,* which is usually caused by *Staphylococcus aureus.* Bullous impetigo is common among children and occurs intermittently, with some cases transmitted among family members, but most often found among the institutionalized. Thin bullae erupt that appear clear to cloudy and coalesce. The bullae open, leaving the original bullous rim with central thin, flat, honey-colored crusts, or in some cases denuded areas. The face is often affected, but bullous impetigo may occur anywhere on the body. The treatment measures are the same as for nonbullous impetigo.

Ecthyma is an ulcerative form of impetigo, usually secondary to minor trauma. It is caused by group A beta-hemolytic streptococci, *S. aureus,* or *Pseudomonas* species. It frequently occurs on the buttocks and thighs of children (Fig. 61-9). The lesions are similar to those of impetigo. A vesicle or pustule ruptures, leaving a skin erosion or ulcer that weeps and dries to a crusted patch, often resulting in scar formation. With extensive ecthyma, there is a low-grade fever and extension of the infection to other organs. Treatment usually involves the use of systemic antibiotics.

A less common form of *S. aureus* infection, called *Ritter disease,* manifests with a diffuse, scarlet fever–like rash, followed by skin separation and sloughing (Fig. 61-10). It is also called *staphylococcal scalded skin syndrome* because the skin looks scalded. Ritter disease usually affects children younger than 5 years of age; immunosuppressed adults also are at risk. The disorder, which is considered a deeper skin infection because the superficial layers of the epidermis are separated and shed in sheets, is caused by the hematologic spread of toxins from a focal infection, such as the nasopharynx or a superficial skin abrasion. The onset of the rash may be preceded by malaise, fever, irritability, and extreme tenderness over the skin.

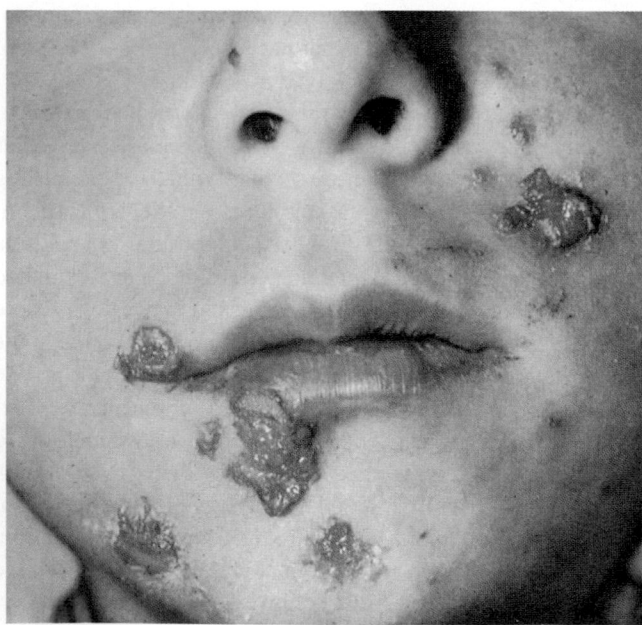

FIGURE 61-8 • Impetigo of the face. The lesions vary from small vesicles to large bullae that rupture and discharge a honey-colored serous liquid that hardens on the skin surface and dries as a honey-colored crust. (Abner Kurten, Folia Dermatologica. No. 2. Geigy Pharmaceuticals.) (From Sauer G. C., Hall J. C. [1996]. *Manual of skin diseases* [7th ed.]. Philadelphia: Lippincott-Raven.)

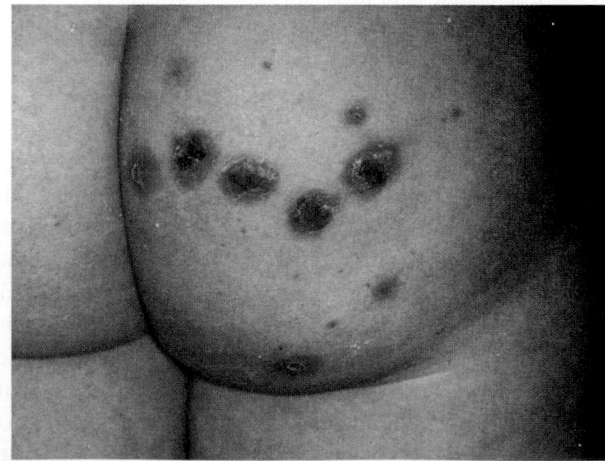

FIGURE 61-9 • Ecthyma on the buttocks of a 13-year-old boy. (Glaxo-Wellcome Co.) (From Sauer G. C., Hall J. C. [1996]. *Manual of skin diseases* [7th ed.]. Philadelphia: Lippincott-Raven.)

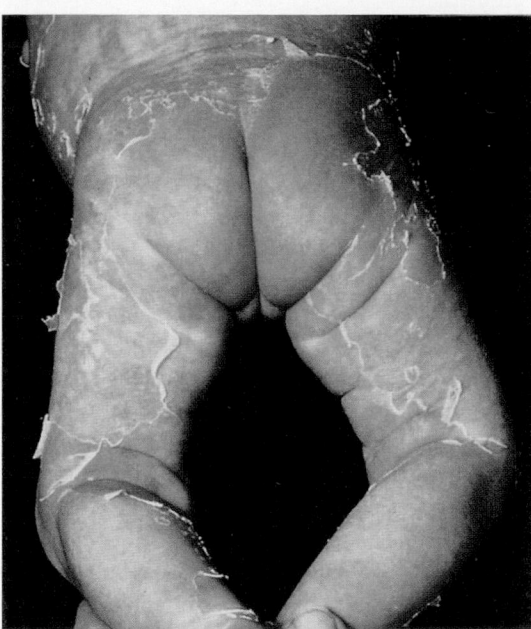

FIGURE 61-10 • Staphylococcal scalded-skin syndrome. (From Fitzpatrick T. B., Johnson R. A., Polono M. K., et al. [1992]. *Color atlas and synopsis of clinical dermatology* [2nd ed., p. 297]. New York: McGraw-Hill.)

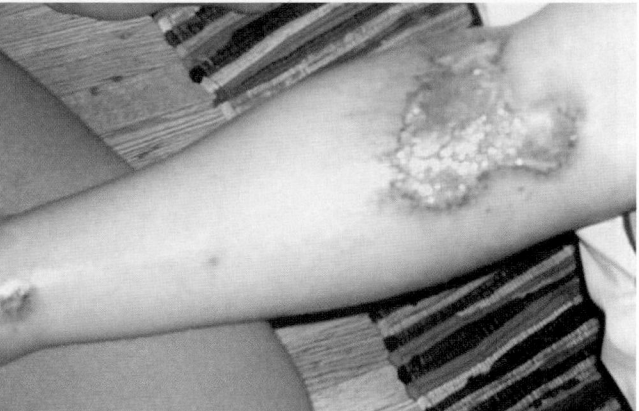

FIGURE 61-11 • Cellulitis on leg infected with *Staphylococcus aureus* and *Pseudomonas.*

The conjunctiva often is inflamed, with purulent drainage. Although the fluid in the unbroken bullae is sterile, cultures usually are obtained from suspected sites of local infection and from the blood. Systemic antibiotics, either oral or parenteral, are used to treat the disorder. Healing usually occurs in 10 to 14 days without scarring.

Cellulitis is a deeper infection affecting the dermis and subcutaneous tissues. It is usually caused by group A beta-hemolytic streptococci or *S. aureus,* but can be caused by bacteria specific to certain activities, such as fish handling, swimming in fresh water, or swimming in salt water, or from animal bites or scratches. Preexisting wounds (*e.g.,* ulcers, erosions) and tinea pedis are often portals of entry. Legs are the most common sites, followed by the hands and pinnae of the ears, but cellulitis may be seen on many body parts. The lesion consists of an expanding red, swollen, tender plaque with an indefinite border, covering a small to wide area (Fig. 61-11). Cellulitis is frequently accompanied by fever, erythema, heat, edema, and pain. Cellulitis often involves the lymph system and, once compromised, repeat infections may impair lymphatic drainage, leading to chronically swollen legs, and eventually dermal fibrosis and lymphedema. Incorrectly treated, it may result in septicemia, nephritis, or death. Treatment measures (oral and intravenous antibiotics) are aimed at the invasive organisms and the extent of the infection.

Viral Infections

Viruses are intracellular pathogens that rely on live cells of the host for reproduction. They have no organized cell structure but consist of a deoxyribonucleic acid (DNA) or ribonucleic acid (RNA) core surrounded by a protein coat. The viruses seen in skin lesion disorders tend to be DNA-containing viruses. Viruses invade the keratinocyte, begin to reproduce, and cause cellular proliferation or cellular death. The rapid increase in viral skin diseases has been attributed to the use of corticosteroid drugs, which have immunosuppressive qualities, and the use of antibiotics, which alter the bacterial flora of the skin. As the number of bacterial infections has decreased, there has been a proportional rise in viral skin diseases.

Verrucae. Verrucae, or warts, are common benign papillomas caused by the DNA-containing human papillomavirus (HPV). Transmission of HPV infection is largely by direct contact between individuals or by autoinoculation. As benign papillomas, warts represent an exaggeration of the normal skin structures. There is an irregular thickening of the stratum spinosum and greatly increased thickening of the stratum corneum. The classification of warts is based largely on morphology and location.

Although warts vary in appearance depending on their location, it is now recognized that the clinically distinct types of warts result not simply because of the anatomic sites in which they arise, but also because of the distinct types of HPV. There are more than 80 types of HPV found on the skin and mucous membranes of humans that cause several different kinds of warts, including skin warts and genital warts.[10] Many of the HPV types that cause genital warts are sexually transmitted, some of which (types 6, 11, 16, and 18) may increase the risk of cervical cancer (discussed in Chapter 47).

Nongenital warts often occur on the hands and feet. They are commonly caused by HPV types 1, 2, 3, 4, 27, and 57, and are not considered precancerous lesions. They are classified as common warts, flat warts, and plantar or palmar warts. Common warts, or verrucae vulgaris, are the most common type. The lesions can occur anywhere, but most frequently occur on dorsal surfaces of hands, especially the periungual area, where they appear as small, grayish-white to tan, flat to convex papules with a rough, pebble-like surface (Fig. 61-12). Verrucae plana, or flat warts, are common on the face or dorsal sur-

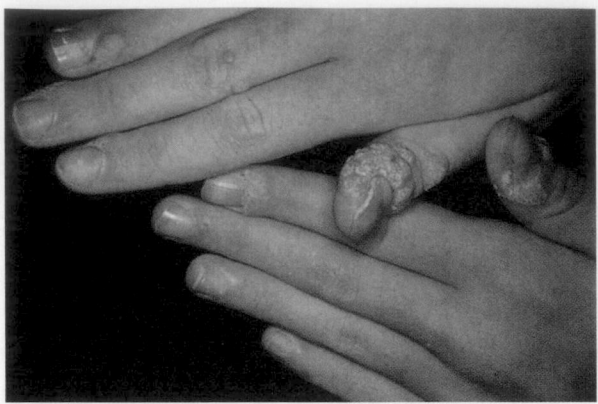

FIGURE 61-12 • Common and periungual warts. (Reed & Carnrick Pharmaceuticals.) (From Sauer G. C., Hall J. C. [1996]. *Manual of skin diseases* [7th ed.]. Philadelphia: Lippincott-Raven.)

faces of the hands. The warts are slightly elevated, flat, smooth, tan papules that are slightly larger than verrucae vulgaris. Verrucae plantaris and verrucae palmaris (*i.e.,* plantar and palmar warts, respectively) occur on the soles of the feet and palms of the hands, respectively. They appear as rough, scaly lesions that may reach 1 to 2 cm in diameter, coalesce, and be confused with ordinary calluses. HPV transmission usually occurs through breaks in skin integrity. For example, plantar warts, which occur on the soles of the feet, frequently are transmitted to the abraded, softened heels of children in swimming areas. Common hand warts can be transmitted by biting the cuticles surrounding the nail.

Treatment is usually directed at inducing a "wart-free" period without producing scarring. Warts resolve spontaneously when immunity to the virus develops. The immune response, however, may be delayed for years. Because of their appearance or discomfort, people usually desire their removal, rather than waiting for immunity to develop. Removal is usually done by applying a keratolytic agent, such as salicylic acid gel or plaster that breaks down the wart tissue, or by freezing with liquid nitrogen. Salicylic acid works by dissolving intercellular cement and producing desquamation of the horny layer of skin without affecting normal epidermal cells. Intralesional bleomycin injections have been effective for recalcitrant warts. Various types of laser surgery, electrosurgery, cryotherapy, immunotherapy (*e.g.,* oral zinc sulfate), and antiviral therapy (*e.g.,* cidofovir) also have been successful in wart eradication.

Occluding warts with duct tape has been a very effective treatment that is painless and inexpensive.[11,12] Duct tape is applied on warts for 6½ days, every 7 days, then repeated for up to 2 months. The mechanism of action for duct tape is unknown, but resolution of other untreated warts on the same person suggests that occluding the wart stimulates the immune response. Another possibility is that the tape debrides the skin surface while also removing the virus attached to it.

Herpes Simplex. Herpes simplex virus (HSV) infections of the skin and mucous membrane (*i.e.,* cold sore or fever blister) are

common. Two types of HSV infect humans: type 1 and type 2. HSV-1 is usually associated with oropharynx infections, and the organism is spread by respiratory droplets or by direct contact with infected saliva. HSV-1 may also be transmitted to other parts of the body through occupational hazards, such as skin contact athletics, dentistry, and medicine. Genital herpes usually is caused by HSV-2 (see Chapter 47). HSV-1 genital infections and HSV-2 oral infections are becoming more common, perhaps because of oral-genital sex.

Infection with HSV-1 may present as a primary or recurrent infection. Primary HSV-1 symptoms include fever, sore throat, painful vesicles, and ulcers of the tongue, palate, gingiva, buccal mucosa, and lips. Primary infection results in the production of antibodies to the virus so that recurrent infections are more localized and less severe. After an initial infection, the herpesvirus persists in the trigeminal and other dorsal root ganglia in the latent state, periodically reactivating in recurrent infections. This theory, however, is being questioned. It may be that reactivation of a herpes infection occurs both in the dorsal root ganglion and locally, where it has been found to exist in the epidermis and other organs. Further, it is believed that HSV infection imparts anticancer properties.[13] The symptoms of a primary HSV-1 infection most often occur in young children (1 to 5 years of age). It is likely that many adults were exposed to HSV-1 during childhood and therefore have antibodies to the virus.

The recurrent lesions of HSV-1 usually begin with a burning or tingling sensation. Umbilicated vesicles and erythema follow and progress to pustules, ulcers, and crusts before healing (Fig. 61-13). Lesions are most common on the lips, face, mouth, nasal septum, and nose. When a lesion is active, HSV-1 is shed and there is risk of transmitting the virus to others. Pain is common, and healing takes place within 10 to 14 days. Precipitating factors may be stress, menses, or injury. In particular, UVB exposure seems to be a frequent trigger for recurrence. Individuals who are immunocompromised may have severe attacks.

There is no cure for oropharyngeal herpes; most treatment measures are palliative. Penciclovir cream or docosanol cream,

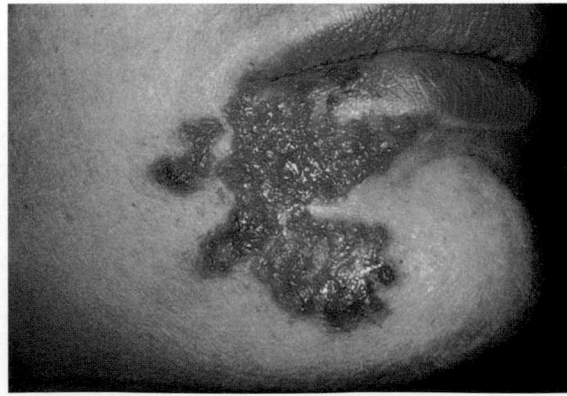

FIGURE 61-13 • Recurrent herpes simplex of the face. (Dermik Laboratories, Inc.) (From Sauer G. C., Hall J. C. [1996]. *Manual of skin diseases* [7th ed.]. Philadelphia: Lippincott-Raven.)

topical antiviral agents, applied at the first symptom and then several times daily, reduces the duration of an attack. Application of over-the-counter topical preparations containing antihistamines, antipruritics, and anesthetic agents along with aspirin or acetaminophen may be used to relieve pain. Oral acyclovir, an antiviral drug that inhibits herpesvirus replication, may be used prophylactically to prevent recurrences. The antiviral drugs valacyclovir and famciclovir also may be used for prophylaxis. Sunscreen preparations applied to the lips can prevent sun-induced herpes simplex. Efforts to develop vaccines to prevent HSV infections are in process. They may be the best hope for control of the disease.[14]

Herpes Zoster. Herpes zoster (shingles) is an acute, localized vesicular eruption distributed over a dermatomal segment of the skin. It is caused by the same herpesvirus, varicella-zoster, that causes chickenpox. It is believed to be the result of reactivation of a latent varicella-zoster virus infection that was dormant in the sensory dorsal root ganglia since a primary childhood infection. During an episode of herpes zoster, the reactivated virus travels from the ganglia to the skin of the corresponding dermatome. Although herpes zoster is not as contagious as chickenpox, the reactivated virus can be transmitted to nonimmune contacts.

Herpes zoster affects an estimated 1 million individuals in the United States annually, and more than half of the people who contract the disease are older than 60 years of age.[15,16] An age-related decline in varicella-zoster T-cell–mediated immunity is thought to account for the increased viral activation in this age group. The incidence is much less among African Americans. Other persons at risk because of impaired T-cell–mediated immunity are those with conditions such as HIV infection and certain malignancies, chronic corticosteroid users, and those undergoing chemotherapy and radiation therapy.

The lesions of herpes zoster typically are preceded by a prodrome consisting of a burning pain, a tingling sensation, extreme sensitivity of the skin to touch, and pruritus along the affected dermatome (see Chapter 49). Among the dermatomes, the most frequently involved are the thoracic (53%), the cervical (20%), the trigeminal (15%), and the lumbosacral (11%).[17] Prodromal symptoms may be present for 1 to 3 days or longer before the appearance of the rash. During this time, the pain may be mistaken for a number of other conditions, such as heart disease, pleurisy, musculoskeletal disorders, or gastrointestinal disorders.

The lesions appear as an eruption of vesicles with erythematous bases that are restricted to skin areas supplied by sensory neurons of a single or associated group of dorsal root ganglia (Fig. 61-14). In immunosuppressed persons, the lesions may extend beyond the dermatome. Eruptions usually are unilateral in the thoracic region, trunk, or face. New crops of vesicles erupt for 3 to 5 days along the nerve pathway. The vesicles dry, form crusts, and eventually fall off. The lesions usually clear in 2 to 3 weeks, although they can persist up to 6 weeks in some elderly persons.

Serious complications can accompany eruptions. Eye involvement can result in permanent blindness and occurs in a large percentage of cases involving the ophthalmic division of the trigeminal nerve (see Chapter 54). *Postherpetic neuralgia,* which is pain that persists longer than 1 to 3 months after the resolution of the rash, is an important complication of herpes zoster (discussed in Chapter 49). It is seen most commonly in persons older than 60 years of age, increasing age being the greatest risk factor. Given the aging population in the United States, the incidence of herpes zoster is expected to increase dramatically over the next two decades. Affected persons complain of sharp, burning pain that often occurs in response to non-noxious stimuli. Even the slightest pressure of clothing and bed

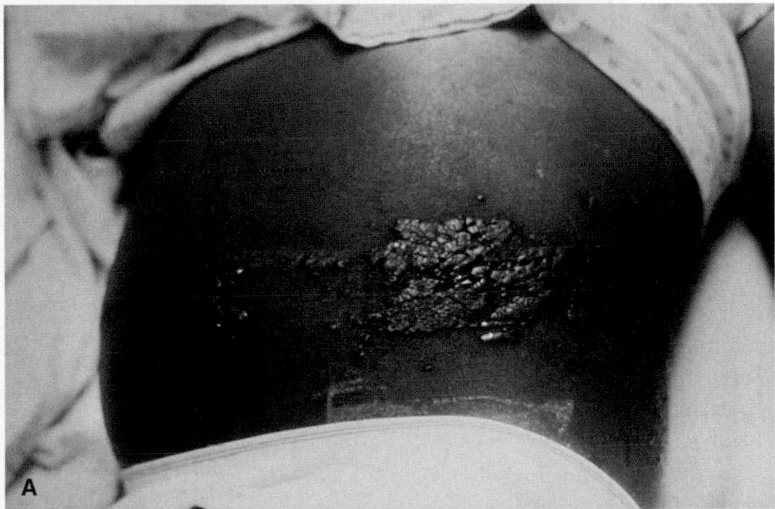
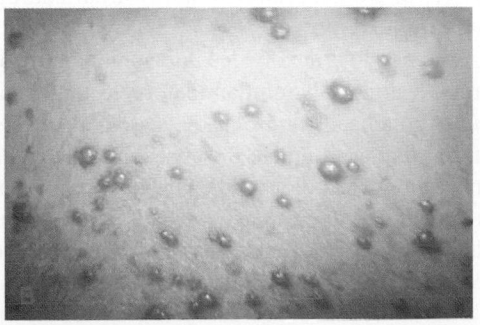

FIGURE 61-14 • **(A)** Dermatomal distribution of herpes zoster rash due to varicella-zoster virus in a child with a history of leukemia. **(B)** The pustulovesicular rash due to herpes zoster virus. (Centers for Disease Control and Prevention Public Health Image Library. [Online.] Available: http://phil.cdc.gov/Phil/home.asp.)

sheets may elicit pain. It usually is a self-limited condition that persists for months, with symptoms abating over time.

The treatment of choice for herpes zoster is the administration of an antiviral agent (*e.g.,* acyclovir, valacyclovir, famciclovir). The treatment is most effective when started within 72 hours of rash development. When given in the acute vesicular stage, the antiviral drugs have been shown to decrease the amount of lesion development and pain. Narcotic analgesics, tricyclic antidepressants, gabapentin, anticonvulsant drugs, and nerve blocks have been used for management of postherpetic neuralgia. Local application of capsaicin cream or lidocaine patches may be used in selected cases. Palliative treatments, such as heat and gentle pressure, may also be helpful. A vaccine for herpes zoster has been approved and recommended for use in people older than 60 years of age.[18] The vaccine has been found to reduce (1) the incidence of herpes zoster by 51.3%, and (2) the incidence of postherpetic neuralgia by 66.5%.[18]

Acne and Rosacea

Acne is a disorder of the pilosebaceous unit (hair follicle and sebaceous gland).[19–21] The hair follicle is a tubular invagination of the epidermis in which hair is produced (see Chapter 60, Fig. 60-7). The sebaceous glands empty into the hair follicle, and the pilosebaceous unit opens to the skin surface through a widely dilated opening called a *pore.* The sebaceous glands produce a complex lipid mixture called *sebum,* from the Latin word meaning "tallow" or "grease." Sebum consists of a mixture of free fatty acids, triglycerides, diglycerides, monoglycerides, sterol esters, wax esters, and squalene. Sebum production occurs through what is called a *holocrine process,* in which the sebaceous gland cells that produce the sebum are completely broken down and their lipid contents emptied through the sebaceous duct into the hair follicle. The amount of sebum produced depends on two factors: the size of the sebaceous gland and the rate of sebaceous cell proliferation. The sebaceous glands are largest on the face, scalp, and scrotum, but are present in all areas of the skin except for the soles and palms. Sebaceous cell proliferation and sebum production are uniquely responsive to direct hormonal stimulation by androgens. In men, testicular androgens are the main stimulus for sebaceous activity; in women, adrenal and ovarian androgens maintain sebaceous activity.

Acne lesions are divided into noninflammatory and inflammatory lesions.[22] Noninflammatory lesions consist of *comedones* (whiteheads and blackheads). *Blackheads* are plugs of material that accumulate in sebaceous glands that open to the skin surface. The color of blackheads results from melanin that has moved into the sebaceous glands from adjoining epidermal cells. *Whiteheads* are pale, slightly elevated papules with no visible orifice. Inflammatory lesions consist of papules, pustules, nodules, and, in severe cases, cysts. *Papules* are raised areas less than 5 mm in diameter. *Pustules* have a central core of purulent material. *Nodules* are larger than 5 mm in diameter and may become suppurative or hemorrhagic. Suppurative nodules often are referred to as *cysts* because of their resemblance to inflamed

epidermal cysts. The inflammatory lesions are believed to develop from the escape of sebum into the dermis and the irritating effects of the fatty acids contained in the sebum.

Two types of acne occur during different stages of the life cycle: acne vulgaris, which is the most common form among adolescents and young adults, and acne conglobata, which develops later in life. Other types of acne occur in association with various etiologic agents such as drugs (*e.g.,* steroids, iodides), occupational compounds, cosmetics, and other irritating agents. Treatment measures for these acnes depend on the precipitating agent and the extent of the lesions.

Acne Vulgaris

Acne vulgaris is a disorder of teenagers and young adults, affecting over 80% of persons aged 11 to 30 years.[21–23] In women, acne may begin earlier and persist longer; however, overall the incidence and severity are greater in men. Acne vulgaris lesions form primarily on the face and neck and, to a lesser extent, on the back, chest, and shoulders (Fig. 61-15). The lesions may consist of comedones (whiteheads and blackheads) or inflammatory lesions (pustules, nodules, and cysts).

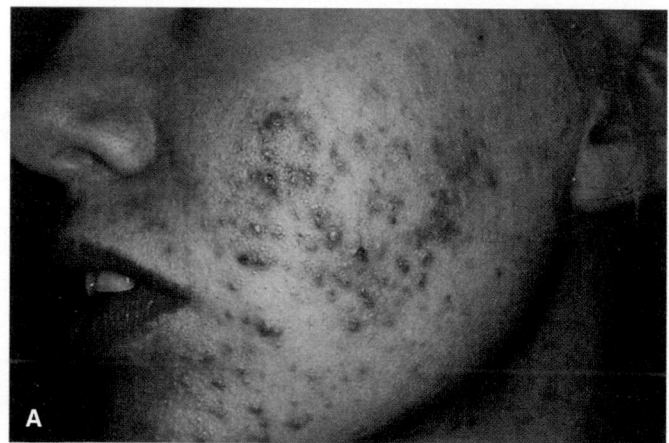
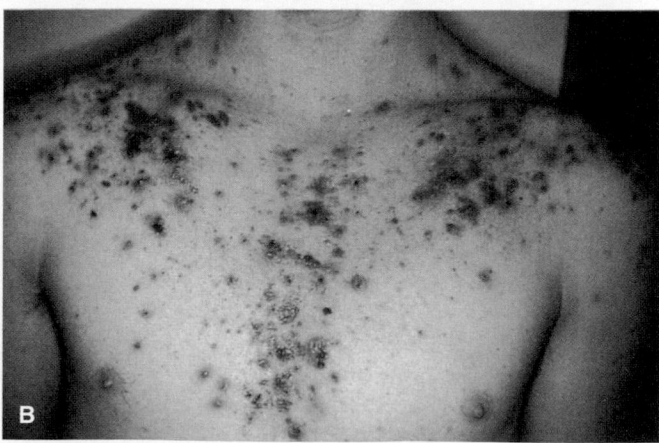

FIGURE 61-15 • (A) Acne of the face and (B) acne of the chest. (From Hall J. C. [1999]. *Sauer's manual of skin diseases* [8th ed., p. 118]. Philadelphia: Lippincott Williams & Wilkins.)

The cause of acne vulgaris remains unknown. It is considered a chronic inflammatory disease of the pilosebaceous unit. There is a hereditary factor; multiple generations of family members often experience it. Several factors are believed to contribute to acne, including (1) increased sebum production, (2) increased proliferation of the keratinizing epidermal cells that form the sebaceous cells, (3) the colonization and proliferation of *Propionibacterium acnes,* and (4) inflammation. These factors are probably interrelated. Increased androgen production results in increased sebaceous cell activity, with resultant plugging of the pilosebaceous ducts. The excessive sebum provides a medium for the growth of *P. acnes.* The *P. acnes* organism contains lipases that break down the free fatty acids that produce the acne inflammation. In addition, there have been new findings regarding the physiology of acne. One example is that *P. acnes* form a biofilm (an extracellular polysaccharide lining in which the bacteria are encased). The biofilm acts as a protective exoskeleton and as a physical barrier to antibiotic treatment, explaining why prolonged antibiotic treatments are necessary.[23] Given this and other discoveries, new drugs and therapies will emerge that selectively target such phenomena.

Over the years, several factors, such as poor hygiene, acne as an infectious process, diets high in fatty content, and certain foods (*e.g.,* chocolate) have been studied empirically and rejected as causal factors in the development of acne. Although general hygienic measures are important, obsessive scrubbing can traumatize the skin and worsen the condition. Instead, it is recommended that the affected areas are washed gently and patted dry. Water-based, rather than oil-based, cosmetics and moisturizers should be used. Mechanical trauma, such as squeezing, rubbing, or picking comedones, should be avoided. Even resting the chin, forehead, or cheek on a hand can exacerbate the condition. Hats, sweatbands, and shirt collars can also traumatize the skin and contribute to a worsening of acne. Although rigid dietary restrictions have not been shown to be beneficial in acne management, a balanced diet is recommended. Women should be informed that acne often becomes worse during the week before menses.

Diagnosis. The diagnosis of acne is based on history and physical examination. The severity of the acne is generally assessed by the number, type, and distribution of lesions.[19,23] *Mild acne* is usually characterized by the presence of a small number (generally <10) of open and closed comedones, with a few inflammatory papules; *moderate acne* by the presence of a moderate number (10 to 40) of erythematous papules and pustules, usually limited to the face; and *moderately severe* acne by the presence of numerous papules and pustules (40 to 100) and occasionally larger, deeper, nodular inflamed lesions involving the face, chest, and back. Acne conglobata (to be discussed) is a severe chronic form of acne.

Treatment. Treatment of acne focuses on clearing up existing lesions, preventing new lesions, and limiting scar formation. Depending on the extent of involvement and the types of lesions, treatment of acne may involve the use of topical or systemic agents.[20–23] Long-term treatment usually is required. Significant improvement may not be apparent for 3 to 6 weeks after initiation of treatment, and maximum effects may not be apparent for months. An important treatment measure is sensitivity to the client's emotional needs.

A number of topical agents are available for the treatment of acne, including retinoids, benzoyl peroxide, azelaic acid, and antibiotics. Topical retinoids, benzoyl peroxide, and azelaic acid are effective treatments for mild acne. Moderate to severe acne often requires combination therapy with a topical agent and systemic antibiotics. The type of vehicle (cream, gel, or lotion) may be an important consideration in the selection of an agent. Persons with drier skin may benefit from creams, whereas persons with oily skin may have better results using a gel or lotion. Many acne creams and lotions containing keratolytic agents such as sulfur, salicylic acid, phenol, and resorcinol are available as over-the-counter preparations. These agents act chemically to break down keratin, loosen comedones, and exert a peeling effect on the skin. With the advent of more effective products, these preparations are used less frequently than in the past.

Benzoyl peroxide is a topical agent that has both antibacterial and comedolytic properties. It is the topical agent most effective in reducing the *P. acnes* population. Bacterial proteins are oxidized by the oxygen free radicals released from the metabolism of benzoyl peroxide on the skin. Because of its mechanism of action, bacterial resistance does not develop to benzoyl peroxide. The irritant effect of the drug also causes vasodilation and increased blood flow, which may hasten resolution of the inflammatory lesions. *Azelaic acid,* derived from wheat, rye, and barley, has actions similar to benzoyl peroxide. It decreases the proliferation of keratinocytes and has antibacterial actions against *P. acnes.* Azelaic cream is moisturizing and causes only minimal skin irritation.

Topical tretinoin (Retin-A), an acid derivative of vitamin A, acts locally to decrease the cohesiveness of epidermal cells and increase epidermal cell turnover. This is thought to result in an increased extrusion of open comedones and a transformation of closed comedones into open ones. Tretinoin is inactivated by UV light and oxidized to benzoyl peroxide, and should be applied only at night and not with benzoyl peroxide. All tretinoin formulations are irritating to the skin, an effect that is increased with sun exposure. Another form of tretinoin, Retin-A Micro, works by entrapping the drug in microspheres that move into the follicle and serve as reservoirs for drug release. Other retinoid drugs, such as adapalene and tazarotene, have actions similar to tretinoin. Adapalene appears to be as effective as tretinoin, but may be less irritating to the skin.

Topical antibiotics also are effective in treating mild to moderate acne. Topical tetracycline, erythromycin, and clindamycin are used most commonly. They do not affect existing lesions but prevent future lesions by decreasing the amount of *P. acnes* on the skin, thereby reducing subsequent inflammation formed from the presence of sebaceous fatty acid metabolites. Treatment failure can result from development of antibiotic resistance. Combination drugs such as benzoyl peroxide and erythromycin also have been effective.

Oral antibiotics are indicated for moderate to severe disease, and for the treatment of acne on the chest, back, or shoulders. Low-dose tetracycline has been used effectively for many years. Tetracycline has no effect on sebum production, but it decreases bacterial growth and the amount of free fatty acids produced. Tetracycline requires a sufficient treatment period to establish effective blood levels. Side effects are minimal, which is why the drug has remained so useful. However, it does have teratogenic effects on skeletal and tooth development and should not be given to those who are pregnant or lactating, or to children. The tetracycline derivatives, minocycline and doxycycline, are better tolerated than tetracycline. Doxycycline may cause photosensitivity reactions. Erythromycin also is effective in acne treatment, especially when tetracycline and its derivatives cannot be used.

Isotretinoin (Accutane), an orally administered synthetic retinoid or acid form of vitamin A, revolutionized the treatment of recalcitrant cases of acne and cystic acnes. In carefully planned doses, oral isotretinoin has cleared major cases of acne and initiated long-term remissions of the disease. It is administered for 3- to 4-month treatment periods. Although the exact mode of action is unknown, it decreases sebaceous gland activity, prevents new comedones from forming, reduces the *P. acnes* count through sebum reduction, and has an anti-inflammatory effect. Because of its many side effects, it is used only in persons with severe acne. Side effects include dryness of the mouth and other mucous membranes, conjunctivitis, and musculoskeletal system abnormalities. Although not confirmed by population-based studies, there have been case reports of depression that occurred in the first 2 months after start of treatment, cleared after cessation of treatment, and recurred when the drug was restarted.[19] Careful clinical and laboratory monitoring is necessary because the drug can produce elevated serum lipid levels, abnormal liver enzyme test results, and hematologic disorders. Isotretinoin is a teratogen that causes brain, heart, and ear malformations. Women taking isotretinoin are strongly advised not to become pregnant.

Estrogens reduce the size and secretion of the sebaceous gland, but because of the high dosages required, they are contraindicated in men. In women, oral contraceptive agents that combine estrogen with a progestin that has low androgenic activity may be used.

Other treatment measures for acne include surgery, UV irradiation, cryotherapy (*e.g.,* freezing with carbon dioxide slushes, liquid nitrogen), laser therapy, and intralesional corticosteroid injection. Acne surgery involves the aspiration of comedones with small-bore needles or devices designed to extract comedonal contents.[24] Intralesional injection of corticosteroids using a syringe or needleless injector is limited to severe nodulocystic forms of acne. It has been effective in promoting cyst healing, but usually has to be repeated frequently.

Acne Conglobata

Acne conglobata occurs later in life and is a chronic form of acne. Comedones, papules, pustules, nodules, abscesses, cysts, and scars occur on the back, buttocks, and chest. Lesions occur to a lesser extent on the abdomen, shoulders, neck, face, upper arms, and thighs. The comedones or cysts have multiple openings, large abscesses, and interconnecting sinuses. Inflammatory nodules are not uncommon. Their discharge is odoriferous, serous or mucoid, and purulent. Healing often leaves deep keloidal lesions. Affected persons have anemia with elevated white blood cell counts, erythrocyte sedimentation rates, and neutrophil counts. The treatment is difficult and stringent. It often includes debridement, systemic corticosteroid therapy, oral retinoids, and systemic antibiotics.

Rosacea

Rosacea is a chronic inflammatory process that occurs in middle-aged and older adults. It is easily confused with acne and may coexist with it. Rosacea is more common in fair-skinned persons and has been called "the curse of the Celts." An early characteristic and diagnostic sign is seen in persons who "flush and blush." Rosacea affects an estimated 14 million people in the United States.[25] Most are white women older than 30 years of age.

The cause of rosacea is unknown; however, it is believed to be an inflammatory process accompanied by vascular instability with leakage of fluid and inflammatory mediators into the dermis. It often is accompanied by gastrointestinal symptoms, and *Helicobacter pylori* infection has been implicated as a possible cause.[26] In addition to microorganisms, other causes postulated have been genetic, environmental, and vascular.

Rosacea has now been classified into four types: (1) erythematotelangiectatic (flushing and persistent central facial erythema); (2) papulopustular (inflammatory); (3) phymatous (thickening of the skin with irregular surface nodularities and enlargement); and (4) ocular (involving the eyes).[27] In the early stage of rosacea development, there are repeated episodes of blushing. The blush eventually becomes a permanent dark red erythema on the nose and cheeks that sometimes extends to the forehead and chin. This stage often occurs before 20 years of age. Ocular problems occur in at least 50% of persons with rosacea, which may lead to visual losses. Prominent symptoms include eyes that are itchy, burning, or dry; a gritty or foreign body sensation; and erythema and swelling of the eyelid.[28] As the person ages, the erythema persists, and telangiectases with or without acne components (*e.g.,* comedones, papules, pustules, nodules, erythema, edema) develop. After years of affliction, acne rosacea may develop into an irregular bullous hyperplasia (thickening of the skin) of the nose, known as *rhinophyma* (Fig. 61-16). Rhinophyma is often considered the end stage of rosacea. The sebaceous follicles and openings of the nose enlarge, and the skin color changes to a purple-red, resulting in hypertrophy of the nose and impaired breathing. Although rosacea is more common in women, rhinophyma is more common in men.

Persons with rosacea are heat sensitive. They are instructed to avoid vascular stimulating agents such as heat, sunlight, hot liquids, foods, and alcohol. Treatment measures are similar to those used for acne vulgaris. Topical metronidazole and azelaic

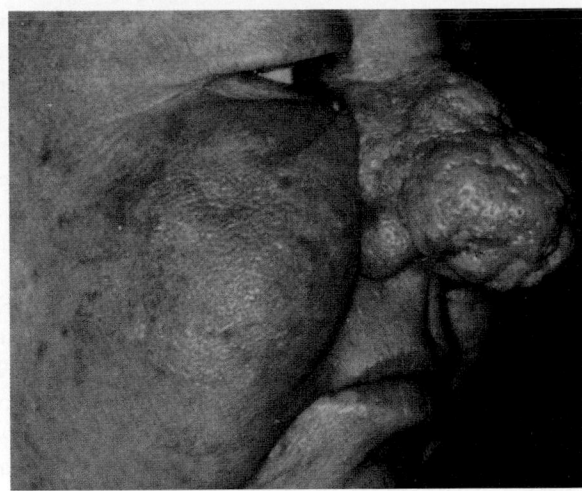

FIGURE 61-16 • Chronic rosacea with rhinophyma. (Hoechst Marion Roussel Pharmaceuticals, Inc.) (From Sauer G. C., Hall J. C. [1996]. *Manual of skin diseases* [7th ed.]. Philadelphia: Lippincott-Raven.)

acid have been effective. Topical antibiotics (*e.g.,* clindamycin, erythromycin) have been useful, as well as systemic antibiotics (*e.g.,* tetracycline and its derivatives). Light therapies, such as laser, have been recommended.[24] Rhinophyma can be treated by a number of surgical methods, including electrosurgery, laser ablation, dermabrasion, cryosurgery, and excision.

Allergic and Hypersensitivity Dermatoses

Allergic and hypersensitivity dermatoses involve the inflammatory response to multiple exogenous and endogenous agents. The disorders, which are usually characterized by epidermal edema with separation of epidermal cells, include irritant contact dermatitis, allergy contact dermatitis, atopic and nummular eczema, urticaria, and drug-induced skin eruptions.

Contact and Allergic Dermatitis

Contact dermatitis is a common inflammation of the skin. There are two types of contact dermatitis: allergic and irritant contact dermatitis. *Allergic contact dermatitis* results from a cell-mediated, type IV hypersensitivity response brought about by sensitization to an allergen (see Chapter 19). More than 2000 allergens have been identified as capable of producing an inflammatory skin response. Crude forms of many naturally occurring substances are in general less allergenic than alloys and synthetic products. Additives such as dyes and perfumes account for the major sources of known allergens. Some of the common topical agents causing allergic rashes are antimicrobial agents (especially neomycin), antihistamines, local anesthetic agents (benzocaine), preservatives (*e.g.,* parabens), and adhesive tape. Additional examples are poison ivy, poison oak, and metal alloys found in jewelry. Also of concern is the increased incidence of contact dermatitis from the heavy use of synthetic latex products, specifically latex gloves and condoms used to prevent communicable diseases. The top 10 causes of allergic contact dermatitis in order of frequency are nickel, gold (jewelry), balsam of Peru (perfume fragrance), thimerosal (preservative in cosmetics), neomycin sulfate, fragrance mix (eight fragrances used for testing fragrance allergies), formaldehyde (preservative in paper, paint, medications, fabrics), cobalt chloride (metal in medical products, hair dye, antiperspirants), bacitracin, and quaternium-15 (preservative in skin products similar to formaldehyde).[29]

The lesions of allergic contact dermatitis range from a mild erythema with edema to vesicles or large bullae (Fig. 61-17). Secondary lesions from bacterial infection may occur. Lesions can occur almost anywhere on the body and the many variations of eczema are often classified according to their location (*e.g.,* ear eczema, hand eczema). The location and pattern often help in identifying causative agents. For example, the typical poison ivy (or oak) lesion consists of vesicles or bullae in a linear pattern (from swiping the plant) on exposed areas. The vesicles and bullae break and weep, leaving an excoriated area.

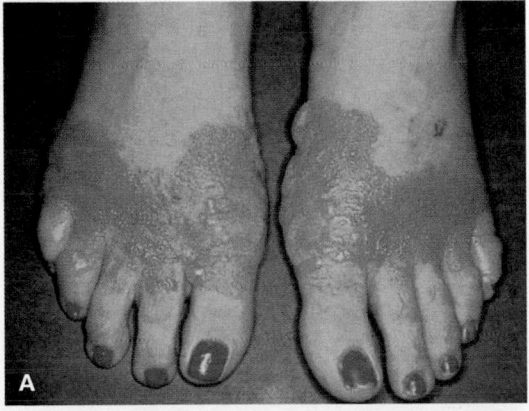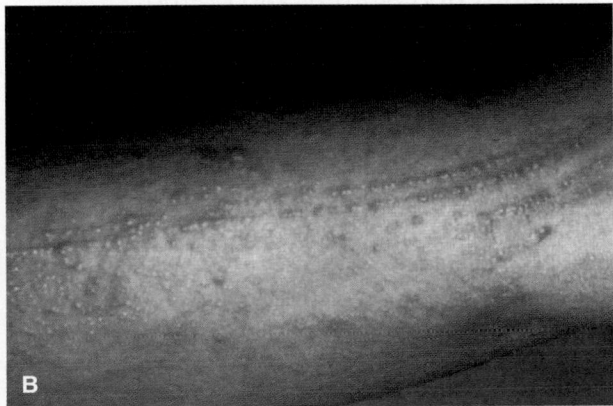

FIGURE 61-17 • (A) Contact dermatitis from shoe material. (Glaxo-Wellcome Co.) (From Sauer G. C., Hall J. C. [1996]. *Manual of skin diseases* [7th ed.]. Philadelphia: Lippincott-Raven. (B) Arm with a blistering oak rash. Note the linear pattern of the lesions. (Centers for Disease Control and Prevention Public Health Image Library. [Online.] Available: http://phil.cdc.gov/Phil/home.asp.)

Irritant contact dermatitis is caused by chemicals (soaps, detergents, organic solvents) that irritate the skin. It can occur from mechanical means such as rubbing (*e.g.,* wool, fiberglass), chemical irritants (*e.g.,* household cleaning products), or environmental irritants (*e.g.,* plants, urine). In contrast to allergic contact dermatitis, no allergens can be identified. A history of atopic dermatitis, either in the past or concurrent, is a major risk for the development of irritant contact dermatitis. Four types of irritant contact dermatitis exist: subjective, acute, chronic, and chemical burns. Subjective cases have no clinical manifestation, but the person reports burning or stinging sensations when exposed to the irritant, and the effect can be reproduced. Acute episodes are often due to single exposures to the irritant. There may be dryness and erythema or edema, inflammation, and vesicles. Chronic irritant dermatitis results from continued exposure to the irritant; even when the irritant is removed, the reaction may continue for several years. In addition to dryness and erythema, there may be scales, fissures, and vesicles. An example of the chemical burn type is the deep necrosis that occurs from contact with cement products.[30]

With both allergic and irritant contact dermatitis, the location of the lesions is of great benefit in diagnosing the causative agent. Patch testing, in which a small amount of the suspected antigen is applied to the skin, is used to identify the allergens.

Treatment measures for both types of contact dermatitis are aimed at removing the source of the irritant or allergen. This may mean that the person needs to modify his or her behavior. This may be particularly difficult for the person with hand eczema because it may mean changing employment to avoid contact with the irritant or allergen. Minor cases are treated by washing the affected areas to remove further contamination by the irritant or allergen, applying antipruritic creams or lotions, and bandaging the exposed areas. Topical corticosteroids may be helpful in these cases. Systemic treatment regimens differ according to the type of irritant or allergen and the severity of the reaction. Moderate to extreme cases are treated with wet dressings, oral antihistamines, and systemic corticosteroids.

Atopic Dermatitis and Nummular Eczema

Atopic Dermatitis. Atopic dermatitis (atopic eczema) is an itchy, inflammatory skin disorder that is characterized by poorly defined erythema with edema, vesicles, and weeping at the acute stage and skin thickening (lichenification) in the chronic stage.[30–33] Although often described as an immunoglobulin E (IgE)–mediated hypersensitivity (atopic) disease, allergic causation is difficult to document, and the disorder is increasingly viewed as a skin disease that predisposes to allergies. Greater than 50% of children with atopic dermatitis develop asthma and allergies in adolescence and adulthood.[32] There has been a two- to threefold increase in the prevalence of atopic dermatitis over the past 30 to 50 years in developed countries.[31] The reason for increased prevalence remains uncertain.

Atopic dermatitis presents differently at different ages (infantile and adult) and in people of different races. Approximately 70% of cases of atopic allergy start in children younger

than 5 years of age.[33] The infantile form of atopic dermatitis is characterized by vesicle formation, oozing, and crusting with excoriations. It usually begins on the cheeks and may progress to involve the scalp, arms, trunk, and legs (Fig. 61-18). The skin of the cheeks may be paler, with extra creases under the eyes, called *Dennie-Morgan folds.* The infantile form may become milder as the child ages, often disappearing by the age of 15 years. However, many individuals have resultant eczematous disorders and rhinitis symptoms throughout life.

Adolescents and adults usually have dry, red patches affecting the face, neck, and upper trunk, but without the thickening and discrete demarcation associated with psoriasis. The bends of the elbows and knees are usually involved. In chronic cases, the skin is dry, leathery, and lichenified. Persons with dark skin may have a papular eruption, and poorly demarcated hypopigmentation patches on the cheeks and extremities. In persons with black skin, pigmentation may be lost from lichenified skin. Acute flares may present with red patches that are weepy, shiny, or lichenified (*i.e.,* thickened, with more prominent markings), and with plaques and papules. Itching may be severe and prolonged with both childhood and adults forms of atopic dermatitis. Secondary infections are common.

Treatment of atopic eczema is designed to target the underlying abnormalities: dryness, pruritus, infection, and inflammation. The guidelines derived consensually from and endorsed by

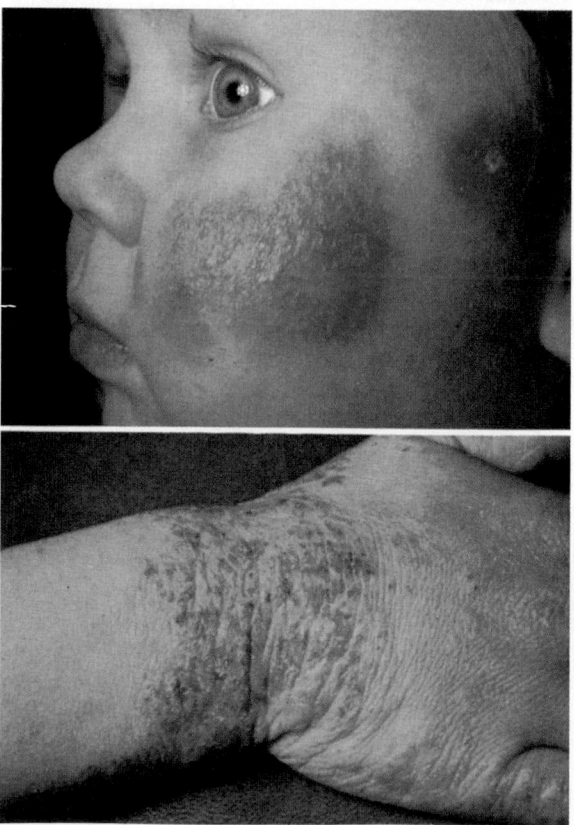

FIGURE 61-18 • Atopic eczema on an infant's face and wrist. (Dome Chemicals.) (From Sauer G. C., Hall J. C. [1996]. *Manual of skin diseases* [7th ed.]. Philadelphia: Lippincott-Raven.)

North American and European expert teams include a stepwise approach for the management of atopic dermatitis based on the intensity of the disease process.[34] Underlying all treatment measures is a comprehensive education program regarding the cause of the disorder, treatment measures, and avoidance of temperature changes and stress to minimize vascular and sweat responses. Basic therapy begins with optimal skin care, addressing the skin barrier defect with continuous use of emollients and skin hydration, along with avoiding exposure to environmental irritants and foods that cause exacerbations of the symptoms. Contacts with water should be minimized; the person should bathe with warm (not hot) water and mild soap. Bathing dries the skin, yet it is important to maintain a low level of microorganisms to prevent infection. Although there is no evidence that emollients improve atopic dermatitis directly, they are widely used to relieve the problem of dry skin and pruritus. A key feature of atopic dermatitis is severe dryness of the skin caused by dysfunction of the skin barrier with transepidermal water loss. This is accompanied by intense pruritus and inflammation.

Topical corticosteroids remain an important treatment for acute flare-ups but can cause local and systemic side effects. Potency of topical corticosteroids is classified by the potential for vasoconstriction. In general, only preparations that have weak or moderate potency are used on the face and genital areas, whereas those that have moderate or high potency are used on other areas of the body.[33] Lower-potency corticosteroids may be sufficient on all areas of the body in younger children. One of the main concerns of topical corticosteroid use is skin thinning. Another concern is secondary adrenal suppression and the suppression of growth in children resulting from systemic absorption.[33]

Topical immune modulators (i.e., tacrolimus and pimecrolimus) are demonstrating positive outcomes in atopic dermatitis without the side effect of cortisone therapy (dermal atrophy).[22-24] Immune modulators are immunosuppressive agents that have been used systemically for the prevention of organ rejection. Tacrolimus is believed to control atopic dermatitis by inhibiting activation of cells involved in atopic dermatitis: T lymphocytes, dendritic cells, mast cells, and keratinocytes.[33] In March 2005, the U.S. Food and Drug Administration (FDA) issued an alert to health care professionals concerning a potential link between topical tacrolimus and pimecrolimus and cancer (mainly lymphoma and skin cancer) based on animal studies, case reports, and knowledge of how these drugs work. The alert emphasizes the importance of using these drugs only as labeled and when first-line therapy has failed or cannot be tolerated.[33]

Wet-wrap therapy, in which a wet dressing is applied over emollients in combination with topical antiseptics (e.g., triclosan, chlorhexidine) or topical corticosteroids, has been shown to be beneficial in some cases of severe atopic dermatitis.[34] Secondary infection with S. aureus is common and usually treated with short courses of antibiotics.[33] Short-term corticosteroids are also used during acute flare-ups with adult patients. Cyclosporine and azathioprine, both immunosuppressive agents, may also be used, keeping in mind their potentially harmful effects. Antihistamines are useful for their sedative effects, and may be helpful during severe pruritus episodes. Phototherapy alone or in combination with corticosteroids during acute flares is often practiced, with beneficial results.

Less studied is the use of *probiotics,* foods containing live microorganisms, such as *Lactobacillus acidophilus* or *Bifidobacterium bifidum.* These foods include hydrolyzed cow's milk formula (predigested peptides of whey and casein), whey formulas, and yogurts. Probiotics are believed to reduce IgE-mediated reactions.[35]

Nummular Eczema. The lesions of nummular eczema are coin-shaped (hence its other name, *discoid eczema*), papulovesicular patches mainly involving the arms and legs (Fig. 61-19). Lichenification and secondary bacterial infections are common. It is not unusual for the initial lesions seemingly to heal, followed by a secondary outbreak of mirror-image lesions on the opposite side of the body. Nummular eczema is mostly chronic, with weeks to years between exacerbations. Exacerbations are more frequent in the cold winter months. The exact cause of nummular eczema is unknown, although many people have a history of atopy (allergy-related disorders), and there is heavy colonization of lesions with staphylococci. Ingestion of iodides and bromides usually aggravates the condition and should be avoided. Treatment is similar to that for other types of dermatitis. Frequent bathing and stress should be reduced, whereas environmental humidity should be increased. Topical emollients, corticosteroids, coal tar preparations, and UV light treatments may be prescribed as necessary.

Urticaria

Urticaria, or hives, is a common skin disorder characterized by the development of edematous wheals accompanied by intense itching.[36] The lesions typically appear as raised pink or red areas surrounded by a paler halo. They blanch with pressure and vary in size from a few millimeters to centimeters. Angioedema, which can occur alone or with urticaria, is characterized by non-

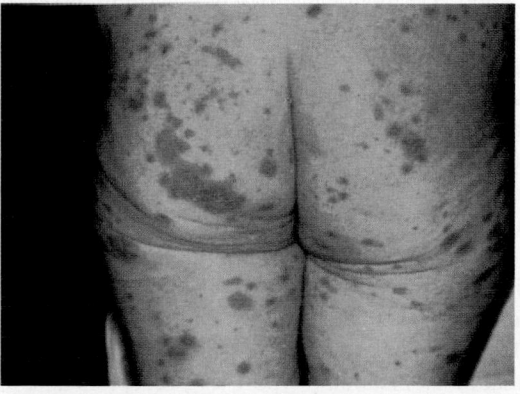

FIGURE 61-19 • Nummular eczema of the buttocks. (Johnson & Johnson.) (From Sauer G. C., Hall J. C. [1996]. *Manual of skin diseases* [7th ed.]. Philadelphia: Lippincott-Raven.)

pitting, nonpruritic, well-defined edematous swelling that involves subcutaneous tissues of the face, hands, feet, or genitals.[37] Occasionally there may be swelling of the tongue and upper airways. Angioedema tends to occur in the face and can cause significant disfigurement.

Urticaria can be acute or chronic and due to known or unknown causes. Numerous factors, both immunologic and nonimmunologic, can be involved in its pathogenesis. The urticarial wheal results from liberation of histamine from mast cells and basophils. Histamine causes hyperpermeability of the microvessels of the skin and surrounding tissue, allowing fluid to leak into the tissues, causing edema and wheal formation.

Acute immunologic urticaria is commonly the result of an IgE-mediated immune reaction that usually occurs within 1 hour of exposure to an antigen.[36] The most common causes of acute urticaria are foods or drinks, medications (most notably penicillin and cephalosporin), insect stings, viral infections, dust mites, and exposure to pollens or chemicals. Food is the most common cause of acute urticaria in children. Although nonsteroidal anti-inflammatory drugs, including aspirin, do not normally cause urticaria, they may exacerbate the preexisting disease.

Chronic urticaria affects primarily adults and is twice as common in women as in men. Usually its cause cannot be determined despite extensive laboratory tests. It appears to be an autoimmune disorder in a substantial number of persons. Approximately 40% to 50% of persons with chronic urticaria have circulating IgG antibodies to a subunit of the IgE receptor or to the IgE molecule. These antibodies activate basophils and mast cells to release histamine.[37] In rare cases, urticaria is a manifestation of underlying disease, such as certain cancers, collagen diseases, and hepatitis. There is an association between chronic urticaria and autoimmune thyroid disease (e.g., Hashimoto thyroiditis, Graves disease, toxic multinodular thyroiditis).[38] A hereditary deficiency of a C1 (complement 1) inhibitor also can cause urticaria and angioedema.

The physical urticarias constitute another form of chronic urticaria.[38] Physical urticarias are intermittent, usually last less than 2 hours, are produced by appropriate stimuli, have distinctive appearances and locations, and are seen most frequently in young adults. Dermographism, or skin writing, is one form of physical urticaria in which wheals appear in response to simple rubbing of the skin (Fig. 61-20). The wheals follow the pattern of the scratch or rubbing, appearing within 10 minutes and dissolving completely within 20 minutes. Other types of physical urticaria are induced by exercise (cholinergic), cold, delayed pressure, sunlight (solar), water (aquagenic), vibration, and heat (external localized). Appropriate challenge tests (e.g., application of an ice cube to the skin to initiate development of cold urticaria) are used to differentiate physical urticaria from chronic urticaria due to other causes.

Most types of urticaria are treated with antihistamines: drugs that block histamine type 1 (H_1) receptors and, less frequently, H_1 receptor blockers in combination with H_2 receptor blockers.[38,39] They control urticaria by inhibiting vasodilation and the escape of fluid into the surrounding tissues. Usually

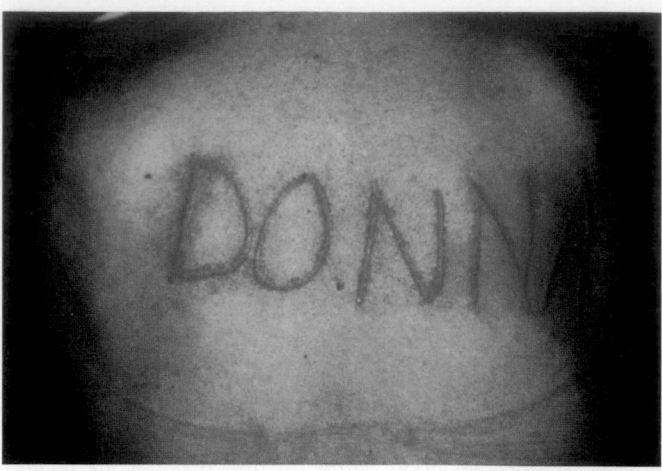

FIGURE 61-20 • Dermographism on a patient's back. (Dermik Laboratories, Inc.) (From Sauer G. C., Hall J. C. [1996]. *Manual of skin diseases* [7th ed.]. Philadelphia: Lippincott-Raven.)

nonsedating antihistamines that alleviate pruritus and decrease the incidence of hives, without producing drowsiness, are used. Leukotriene antagonists (zafirlukast and montelukast) may also be used.[38,39] Starch or colloid-type (e.g., Aveeno) baths may be used as comfort measures. Persons who experience angioedema of the larynx and pharynx can be counseled to carry a prescription of epinephrine in an autoinjectable instrument (e.g., EpiPen).[39] Oral corticosteroids may be used in the treatment of refractory urticaria. Tricyclic antidepressant drugs, particularly those with antihistamine actions, also may be used.

Drug-Induced Skin Eruptions

Most drugs can cause a localized or generalized skin eruption. Topical drugs are usually responsible for localized contact dermatitis types of rashes, whereas systemic drugs cause generalized skin lesions. Although many drug-induced skin eruptions are morbilliform (i.e., measles-like) or exanthematous, they may mimic most of the skin disorders described in this chapter. Because the lesions vary greatly, the diagnosis depends almost entirely on an accurate patient report, including a full drug history. Management of mild cases is aimed at eliminating the offending drug while treating the symptoms. Severe cases require prompt medical attention and treatment with systemic corticosteroids and antihistamines.

Some drug reactions result in epidermal skin detachment and formation of bullous lesions. Three types of drug reactions that result in bullous skin lesions are *erythema multiforme minor, Stevens-Johnson syndrome,* and *toxic epidermal necrolysis.* There is growing consensus that these three diagnoses are variants of the same disease with different severities.[40] There is also increasing agreement about the boundaries among the three diagnoses. Erythema multiforme minor is usually self-limiting. Cases involving less than 10% of the body surface area are called *Stevens-Johnson syndrome,* and detachment of more than 30% of the epidermis is labeled *toxic epidermal necrolysis,* with a 10% to 30% overlap of Stevens-Johnson syndrome and toxic epidermal necrolysis.[41]

Although the cause of erythema multiforme minor may be drug induced or unknown, it frequently occurs after infections, especially HSV infection. It is self-limiting, with a small amount of skin detachment at the lesion sites. Stevens-Johnson syndrome and toxic epidermal necrolysis are caused by hypersensitivity reaction to drugs, the most common being sulfonamides, anticonvulsants, nonsteroidal anti-inflammatory drugs, antimalarials, and allopurinol. Although rare, Stevens-Johnson and toxic epidermal necrolysis have an annual incidence rate of 0.4 to 7 per one million people and a high mortality rate.[41] Recovery is based upon the severity and quick, aggressive treatment.

The skin detachment seen with bullous skin lesions is different from the desquamation (*i.e.,* peeling) that occurs with other skin disorders. For example, with scarlet fever there is peeling of the dead keratinized layer of the stratum corneum. In the bullous disorders, there is full-thickness detachment of the entire epidermis from the dermis. This leaves the person vulnerable to multiple problems, including loss of body fluids and electrolytes, impaired body temperature control, and a greatly increased risk of infection.

The lesions of erythema multiforme minor and Stevens-Johnson syndrome are similar. The primary lesion of both is a round, erythematous papule, resembling an insect bite. Within hours to days, these lesions change into several different patterns. The individual lesions may enlarge and coalesce, producing small plaques, or they may change to concentric zones of color appearing as "target" or "iris" lesions (Fig. 61-21). The outermost rings of the target lesions usually are erythematous; the central portion usually is opaque white, yellow, or gray (dusky). In the center, small blisters on the dusky purpuric macules may form, giving them their characteristic target-like

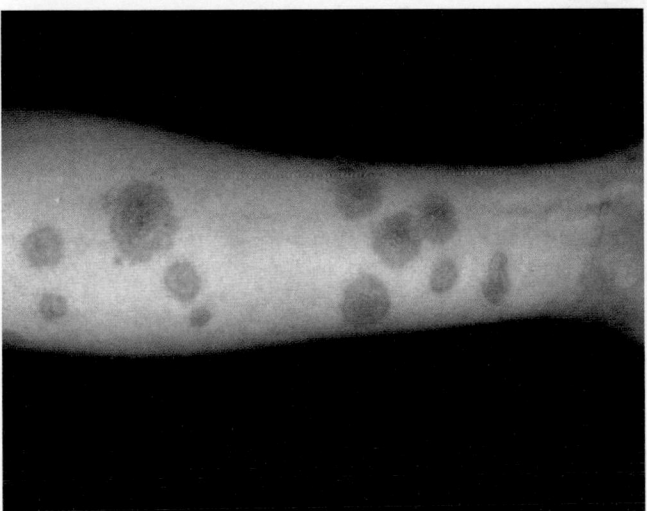

FIGURE 61-21 • Erythema-multiforme–like eruption on the patient's arm. Note the dusky, target-like appearance. (Dermik Laboratories, Inc.) (From Sauer G. C., Hall J. C. [1996]. *Manual of skin diseases* [7th ed.]. Philadelphia: Lippincott-Raven.)

appearance. Although there is wide distribution of lesions over the body surface area, there is a propensity for them to occur on the face and trunk.

Toxic epidermal necrolysis is the most serious drug reaction, with mortality rates of 25% to 35%.[41] The person experiences a prodromal period of malaise, low-grade fever, and sore throat. Within a few days, widespread erythema and large, flaccid bullae appear, followed by the loss of the epidermis, leaving a denuded and painful dermis. The skin surrounding the large denuded areas may have the typical target-like lesions seen with Stevens-Johnson syndrome. Lateral pressure causes the surrounding skin to separate easily from the dermis (*Nikolsky sign*). Usually, the epithelium of mucosal surfaces, especially the mouth and eyes, is also involved and may lead to blindness.

Treatment of erythema multiforme minor and less severe cases of Stevens-Johnson syndrome includes relief of symptoms using compresses, antipruritic drugs, and topical anesthetics. Recurrent cases of erythema multiforme have been prevented with continuous acyclovir therapy. Corticosteroid therapy may be indicated in moderate cases, although its use is controversial. For severe cases of Stevens-Johnson syndrome and toxic epidermal necrolysis, hospitalization is required for fluid replacement, respiratory care, administration of antibiotics and analgesics, and application of moist dressings. When large areas of skin are detached, the care is similar to that of thermal burn patients. Intravenous immunoglobulin may hasten the healing response of the skin. Generally, healing is a slow process, taking 6 weeks or more to regenerate skin. The mucous membranes heal slowly and follow-up treatment is often needed for ophthalmologic and mucous membrane sequelae. Avoidance of the responsible drug and chemically related compounds is essential.

Papulosquamous Dermatoses

Papulosquamous dermatoses are a group of skin disorders characterized by scaling papules and plaques. Among the major papulosquamous diseases are psoriasis, pityriasis rosea, and lichen planus, which are discussed in this section of the chapter.

Psoriasis

Psoriasis is a common, chronic inflammatory skin disease characterized by circumscribed, red, thickened plaques with an overlying silvery-white scale. Psoriasis occurs worldwide, although the incidence is lower in warmer, sunnier climates. In the United States and England, it affects 2% of the population.[42] The average age of onset is in the third decade; its prevalence increases with age. Approximately one third of patients have a genetic history, indicating a hereditary factor. Childhood onset of the disease is more strongly associated with a family history than psoriasis occurring in adults older than 30 years of age. The disease, which can persist throughout life and become exacerbated at unpredictable times, is classified as a chronic ailment. A few cases, however, have been known to clear and not recur. There appears to be an association between psoriasis and arthritis. Psoriatic arthritis occurs in 2% of the U.S. population and can account for a considerable amount of joint damage[43] (see Chapter 59).

The primary cause of psoriasis is uncertain. The unintended, yet dramatic, clearing of severe, disabling psoriasis with cyclosporine provided strong evidence that psoriasis may be an a T-cell–mediated autoimmune response to an unidentified antigen.[43] It is thought that activated T lymphocytes (mainly CD4+ helper cells) produce chemical messengers that stimulate abnormal growth of keratinocytes and dermal blood vessels. Accompanying inflammatory changes are caused by infiltration of neutrophils and monocytes. Skin trauma (*i.e.,* prepsoriasis) is a common precipitating factor in people predisposed to the disease. The reaction of the skin to an original trauma of any type is called the *Köbner reaction.* Stress, infections, trauma, xerosis, and use of medications such as angiotensin-converting enzyme inhibitors, β-adrenergic blocking drugs, lithium, and the antimalarial agent, hydroxychloroquine (Plaquenil), may precipitate or exacerbate the condition.

Histologically, psoriasis is characterized by increased epidermal cell turnover with marked epidermal thickening, a process called *hyperkeratosis.* The granular layer (stratum granulosum) of the epidermis is thinned or absent, and neutrophils are found in the stratum corneum. There also is an accompanying thinning of the epidermal cell layer that overlies the tips of the dermal papillae (suprapapillary plate), and the blood vessels in the dermal papillae become tortuous and dilated. These capillary beds show permanent damage even when the disease is in remission or resolved. The close proximity of the vessels in the dermal papillae to the hyperkeratotic scale accounts for multiple, minute bleeding points that are seen when the scale is lifted.

There are several variants or types of psoriasis, including plaque-type psoriasis, guttate psoriasis, pustular psoriasis (local-

ized and generalized), and erythrodermic psoriasis.[44] *Plaque-type psoriasis* (*psoriasis vulgaris*), which is the most common type, is a chronic stationary form of psoriasis. The lesions may occur anywhere on the skin, but most often involve the elbows, knees, and scalp (Fig. 61-22). The primary lesions are sharply demarcated, thick, red plaques with a silvery scale that vary in size and shape. In darker-skinned persons, the plaques may appear purple. There may be excoriation, thickening, or oozing from the lesions. A differential diagnostic finding is that the plaques bleed from minute points when removed, which is known as the *Auspitz sign.*

Guttate psoriasis is characterized by teardrop-shaped, pink to salmon, scaly lesions, and occurs in children and young adults. Its lesions are usually limited to the upper trunk and extremities. This form of psoriasis usually is brought on by a streptococcal infection. It generally responds to treatments such as UVB phototherapy, only to return with recurrent streptococcal infections. *Pustular psoriasis* is characterized by papules or plaques studded with pustules. Localized pustular psoriasis usually is limited to the palms of the hands and soles of the feet. Generalized pustular psoriasis is characterized by more general involvement and may be associated with systemic symptoms such as fever, malaise, and diarrhea. The person may or may not have had preexisting psoriasis.

Erythrodermic psoriasis is a rare form of psoriasis affecting all body surfaces, including the hands, feet, nails, trunk, and extremities. It is characterized by a process in which the lesions scale and become confluent, leaving much of the body surface bright red, with continuous skin shedding. Severe itching and pain often accompany it. Severe complications may develop related to loss of body fluids, proteins, and electrolytes and disturbances in temperature regulation. Without treatment,

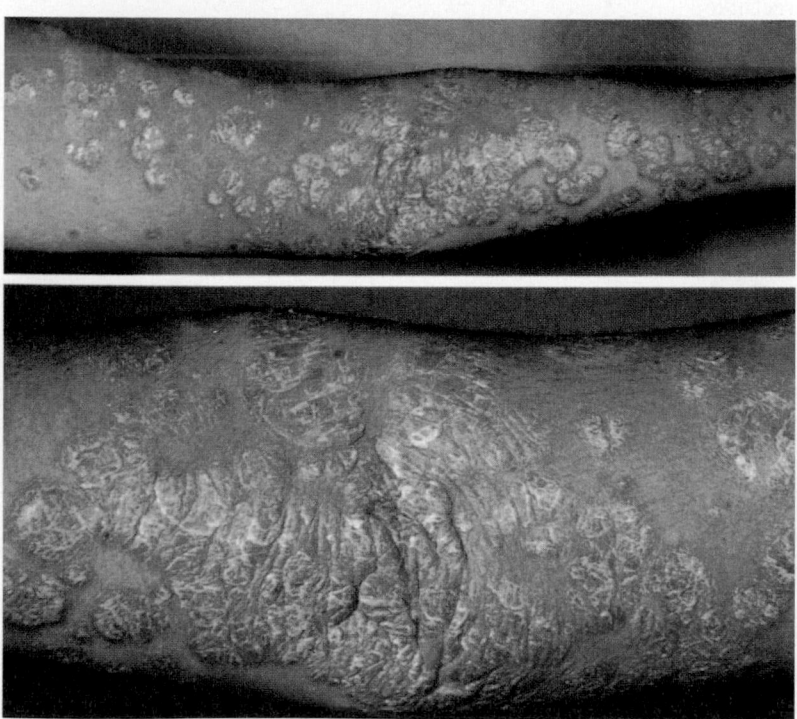

FIGURE 61-22 • Psoriasis on the elbows of a 17-year-old girl. (Roche Laboratories.) (from Sauer G. C., Hall J. C. [1996]. *Manual of skin diseases* [7th ed.]. Philadelphia: Lippincott-Raven.)

death from sepsis is a well-known complication of erythrodermic psorisasis.[44]

Treatment. There is no cure for psoriasis. The goal of treatment is to suppress the signs and symptoms of the disease: hyperkeratosis, epidermal inflammation, and abnormal keratinocyte differentiation. Treatment depends on the severity of the disease, as well as the person's age, sex, treatment history, and level of treatment compliance. Treatment measures are divided into topical and systemic approaches. Usually, topical agents are used first in any treatment regimen and when less than 20% of the body surface is involved. Combination therapies tailored to the needs of the client are most effective. Also, rotating various therapies may decrease the side effects of any one therapy.

Topical agents include emollients, keratolytic agents, coal tar products, anthralin, corticosteroids, and calcipotriene. Emollients hydrate and soften the psoriatic plaques. Petroleum-based products are more effective than water-based, but they are often less acceptable cosmetically to persons with psoriasis. Keratolytic agents are peeling agents. Salicylic acid is the most widely used. It softens and removes plaques. It has been used alone or in conjunction with other topical agents. Coal tar, the byproduct of the processing of coke and gas from coal, is one of the oldest yet more effective forms of treatment. The skin is covered with a film of coal tar for up to several weeks. The exact mechanism of action of tar products is unknown, but side effects of the treatment are few. Newer preparations of coal tar lotions and shampoos are more aesthetically pleasing, but the odor remains a problem.

Anthralin, a synthesized product of Goa powder from Brazilian araroba tree bark, has remained a topical treatment of choice. It has been effective in resolving lesions in approximately 2 weeks. A disadvantage to anthralin is that it stains the uninvolved skin and clothes brown or purple. A treatment variation, called the *Ingram method,* involves coal tar applications and UVB radiation, followed by anthralin paste application.

Topical corticosteroids are widely used and relatively effective. They are generally more acceptable because they do not stain and are easy to use. Topical corticosteroids are available as low-, medium-, and high-potency preparations. Treatment usually is started with a medium-potency agent. Low-potency drugs usually are used on the face and areas of the body, such as the groin and axillary areas, where the skin tends to be thinner. High-potency preparations are reserved for treatment of thick chronic plaques that do not respond to less potent preparations. Although the corticosteroids are rapidly effective in the treatment of psoriasis, they are associated with flare-ups after discontinuation and they have many potential side effects. Their effectiveness is increased when used under occlusive dressings, but there is an increase in side effects. *Calcipotriene,* a topical vitamin D derivative, has been effective for the treatment of psoriasis. It inhibits epidermal cell proliferation and enhances cell differentiation. *Tazarotene,* a synthetic retinoid, also has been effective, but it is teratogenic and should be avoided in women of childbearing age.

Systemic treatments include phototherapy, photochemotherapy, methotrexate, retinoids, corticosteroids, and cyclosporine. The positive effects of sunlight have long been established. Phototherapy with UVB is a widely used treatment. Newly developed narrow-band UVB radiation is reportedly more effective that broad-band UVB.[44] Photochemotherapy involves using a light-activated form of the drug methoxsalen. Methoxsalen, a psoralen, exerts its actions when exposed to UVA radiation in 320- to 400-nm wavelengths. The combination treatment regimen of psoralen and UVA is known by the acronym *PUVA.* Methoxsalen is given orally before UVA exposure. Activated by the UVA energy, methoxsalen inhibits DNA synthesis, thereby preventing cell mitosis and decreasing the hyperkeratosis that occurs with psoriasis. Although viewed as one of the safest therapies since its introduction in the 1970s, PUVA increases the risk for squamous cell carcinoma, and it may increase the risk for development of melanoma.

Systemic corticosteroids have been effective in treating severe or pustular psoriasis. However, they cause severe side effects, including Cushing syndrome. Intralesional injection of triamcinolone has proved effective in resistant lesions. The retinoids are another class of systemic psoriasis therapy. These drugs, which are derivatives of vitamin A, are only moderately effective as a monotherapy and are associated with numerous mucocutaneous side effects such as hair loss, cheilitis, and thinning of the nails. However, when used over the short term in combination with UVB phototherapy or PUVA, low-dose acitretin has been shown to be effective, allowing substantial clearing of lesions with fewer physician visits and fewer mucocutaneous side effects.[45] Teratogenicity limits use of retinoids in women of childbearing potential.

Methotrexate, which is used for cancer treatment, is an antimetabolite that inhibits DNA synthesis and prevents cell mitosis. Oral methotrexate has been effective in treating psoriasis when other approaches have failed. The drug has many side effects, including nausea, malaise, leukopenia, thrombocytopenia, and liver function abnormalities. Cyclosporine is a potent immunosuppressive drug used to prevent rejection of organ transplants. It suppresses inflammation and the proliferation of T cells in persons with psoriasis. Its use is limited to severe psoriasis because of serious side effects, including nephrotoxicity, hypertension, and increased risk of cancers. Intralesional cyclosporine also has been effective. Biologic agents (*e.g.,* infliximab, etanercept, efalizumab, and alefacept) that target the activity of T lymphocytes and cytokines responsible for the inflammatory nature of psoriasis have proven effective, not only with the skin lesions, but in halting the effects of the associated arthritis of psoriasis.[42,45]

Pityriasis Rosea

Pityriasis rosea is a rash that primarily affects children and young adults. The origin of the rash is unknown, but is thought to be caused by an infective agent. Numerous viruses have been investigated, thus far with no conclusive evidence. The incidence is highest in winter. Cases occur in clusters and among

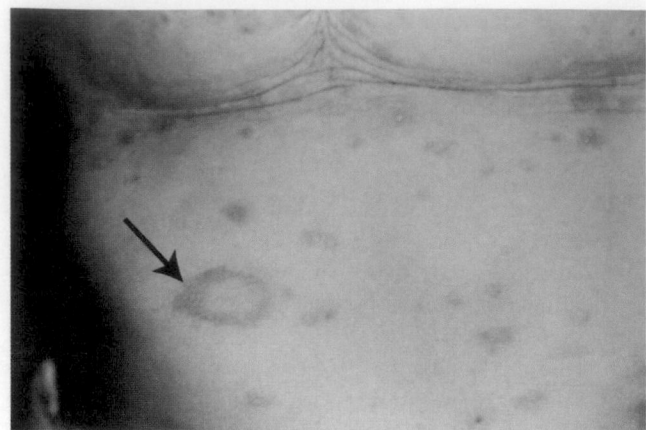

FIGURE 61-23 • Pityriasis rosea. Note oval herald patch (*arrow*) on the abdomen as well as a more generalized rash. (Centers for Disease Control and Prevention Public Health Image Library. [Online.] Available: http://phil.cdc.gov/Phil/home.asp.)

persons who are in close contact, indicating an infectious spread. However, there are no data to support communicability. It may be an immune response to any number of agents.

The characteristic lesion is an oval macule or papule with surrounding erythema (Fig. 61-23). The lesion spreads with central clearing, much like tinea corporis. This initial lesion is a solitary lesion called the *herald patch* and is usually on the trunk or neck. As the lesion enlarges and begins to fade (2 to 10 days), successive crops of lesions appear on the trunk and neck. The lesions on the back have a characteristic "Christmas tree" pattern. The extremities, face, and scalp may be involved. Mild to severe pruritus may occur. The disease is self-limited and usually disappears within 6 to 8 weeks. Treatment measures are palliative and include topical steroids, antihistamines, and colloid baths. Systemic corticosteroids may be indicated in severe cases.

Lichen Planus

The term *lichen* is of Greek origin and means "tree moss." The term is applied to skin disorders characterized by small (2 to 10 mm), flat-topped papules with irregular, angulated borders (Fig. 61-24). Lichen planus is a relatively common chronic pruritic disease. It involves inflammation and papular eruption of the skin and mucous membranes. There are variations in the pattern of lesions (*e.g.*, annular, linear) and differences in the sites (*e.g.*, mucous membranes, genitalia, nails, scalp). The characteristic lesion is a purple, polygonal papule covered with a shiny, white, lacelike pattern. The lesions appear on the wrist, ankles, and trunk of the body. Most persons who have skin lesions also have oral lesions, appearing as milky white lacework on the buccal mucosa or tongue. Other mucosal surfaces, such as the genital, nasal, laryngeal, otic, gastric, and anal areas may also be affected. As with psoriasis, lichen planus lesions can develop on scratches or skin injuries (Köbner phenomenon; see Fig. 61-24A).

The etiology of lichen planus is unknown, but it is believed to be an abnormal immune response in which epithelial cells are recognized as foreign. The disorder involves the epidermal–dermal junction with damage to the basal cell layer.

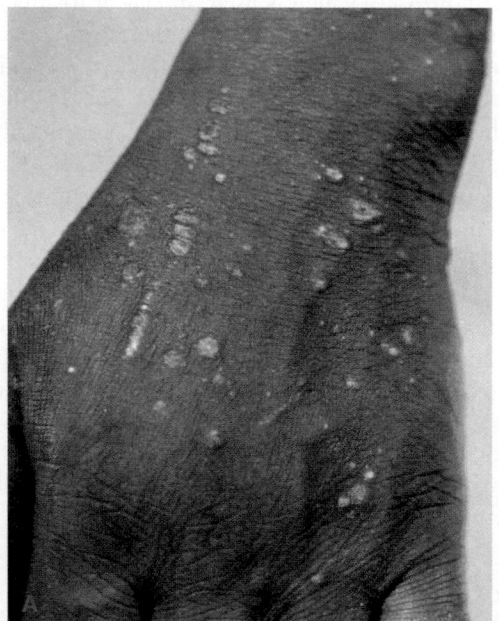

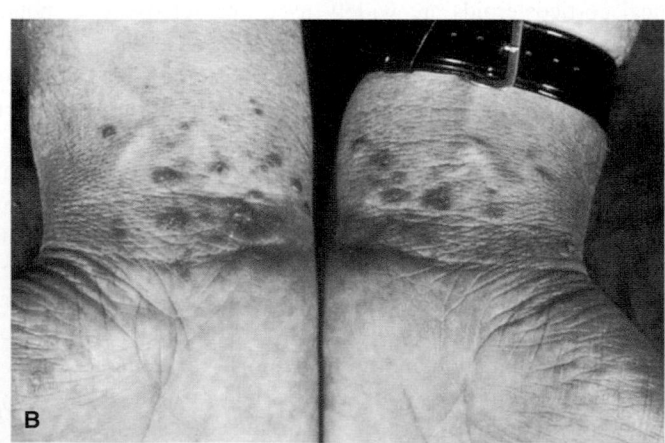

FIGURE 61-24 • (**A**) Lichen planus of the dorsum of the hand. Note the color of the plaques and the linear Köbner phenomenon. (E. R. Squibb.) (From Sauer G. C., Hall J. C. [1996]. *Manual of skin diseases* [7th ed.]. Philadelphia: Lippincott-Raven.) (**B**) Lichen planus affecting both wrists. (Centers for Disease Control and Prevention Public Health Image Library. [Online.] Available: http://phil.cdc.gov/Phil/home.asp.)

Some cases of lichen planus have been linked to hepatitis C virus infections or medication use. The most common medication agents include gold, antimalarial agents, thiazide diuretics, beta blockers, nonsteroidal anti-inflammatory agents, quinidine, and angiotensin-converting enzyme inhibitors. Some persons with oral lichen planus have reacted to the mercury in dental amalgams to the extent that when the dental fillings were replaced, the lesions healed.[46]

Diagnosis is based on the clinical appearance of the lesions and the histopathologic findings from a punch biopsy. For most persons, lichen planus is a self-limited disease. Treatment measures include discontinuation of all medications, followed by treatment with topical corticosteroids and occlusive dressings. Occlusion may be used to enhance the effect of topical medications. Antipruritic agents are helpful in reducing itch. Systemic corticosteroids may be indicated in severe cases. Intralesional corticosteroid injections also may be used. Acitretin, an orally administered retinoid agent, also may be effective. Because retinoids are teratogenic, they should be avoided in women of childbearing age. Cyclosporine, tacrolimus, and other immunosuppressive agents have been helpful.

Lichen Simplex Chronicus

Lichen simplex chronicus is a localized lichenoid pruritic dermatitis resulting from repeated rubbing and scratching. The term *lichen simplex* denotes the absence of a known predisposing skin disorder in the affected person. It is characterized by the occurrence of itchy, reddened, thickened, and scaly patches of dry skin (Fig. 61-25). Persons with the condition may have a single or, less frequently, multiple lesions. The lesions are seen most commonly at the nape of the neck, wrists, ankles, or anal area. The condition usually begins as a small pruritic patch, which after a repetitive cycle of itching and scratching develops into a chronic dermatosis. Because of the chronic itching and scratching, excoriations and lichenification with thickening of the skin develops, often giving the appearance of tree bark. Treatment consists of measures to decrease scratching of the area. A moderate-potency corticosteroid is often prescribed to decrease the itching and subsequent inflammatory process.

Arthropod Infestations

The skin is susceptible to a variety of disorders as a result of an invasion or infestation by arthropods, including mites and lice. The type of rash or sometimes singular lesion depends on the causative agent.

Scabies

A mite, *Sarcoptes scabiei,* which burrows into the epidermis, causes scabies. After a female mite is impregnated, she burrows into the skin and lays two to three eggs each day for 4 or 5 weeks. The eggs hatch after 3 to 4 days, and the larvae migrate to the skin surface. At this point, they burrow into the skin only for food or protection. The larvae molt and become nymphs;

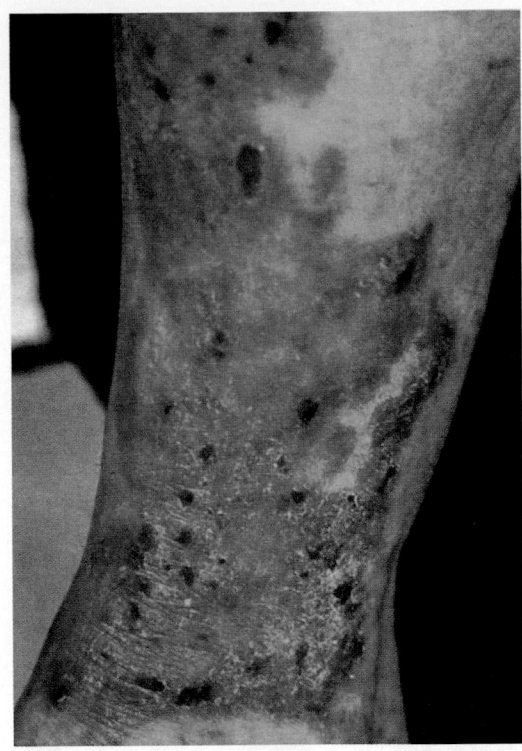

FIGURE 61-25 • Localized lichen simplex chronicus of the leg. (Duke Laboratories, Inc.) (from Sauer G. C., Hall J. C. [1996]. *Manual of skin diseases* [7th ed.]. Philadelphia: Lippincott-Raven.)

they molt once more to become adults. After the new adult females are impregnated, the cycle is repeated.

The characteristic lesion is a small burrow (*e.g.,* 2 mm) that may be red to reddish-brown. Small vesicles may cover the burrows. The areas most commonly affected are the interdigital web of the finger, flexor surface of the wrist, inner surface of the elbow, axilla, female nipple, penis, belt line, and gluteal crease (Fig. 61-26). Pruritus is common and may result from the burrows, the fecal material of the mite, or both. Excoriations may develop from scratching, leaving the host vulnerable to secondary bacterial infections and severe skin lesions if left untreated. A severe form of scabies that involves millions of mites is called *Norwegian* or *crusted scabies;* it differs from common scabies in the large number of mites living on the host and a crusting over of the infested region.

Scabies is transmitted by person-to-person contact, including sexual contact. It also is transmitted by contact with mite-infested sheets in hospitals and nursing homes because the mite can live up to 2 days on sheets or clothing. Scabies affects all people in all socioeconomic classes, although African Americans seem more resistant. Usually more prevalent in times of war and famine, scabies reached pandemic proportions in the 1970s, perhaps as a result of poverty, sexual promiscuity, and worldwide travel. Outbreaks continue to occur, but they are mostly sporadic and localized to nursing homes and families.

Diagnosis is done by skin scrapings. A positive diagnosis relies on the presence of mites, ova, or feces. The treatment is simple and curative. After bathing, permethrin, malathion, or

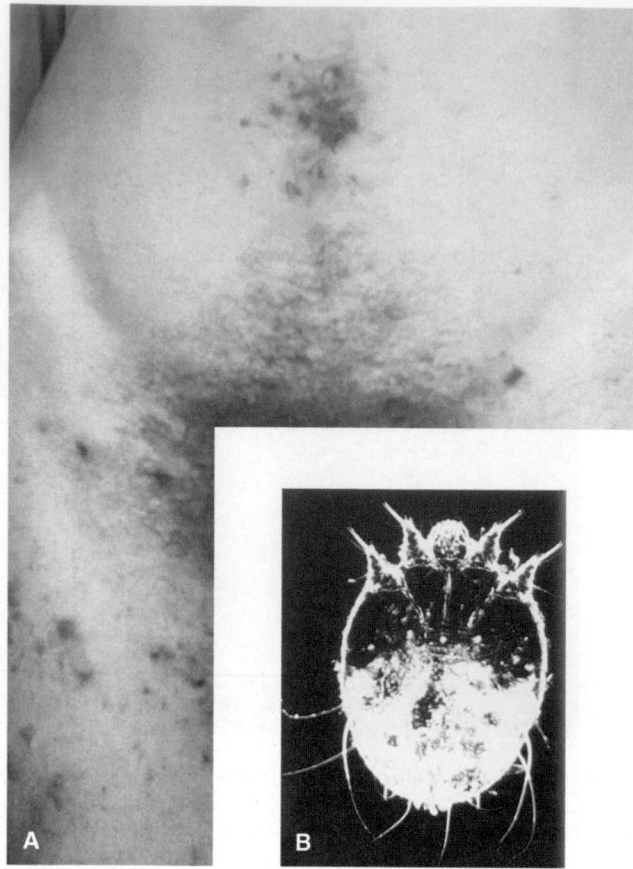

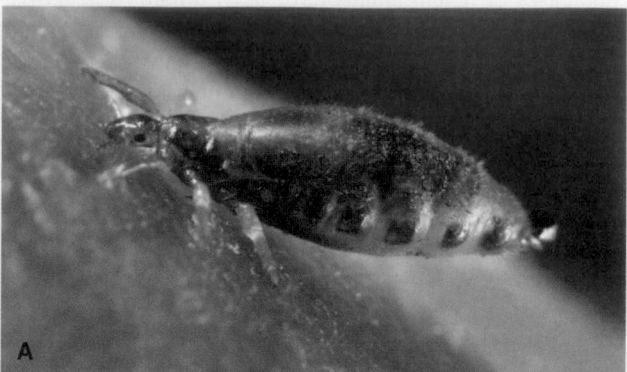

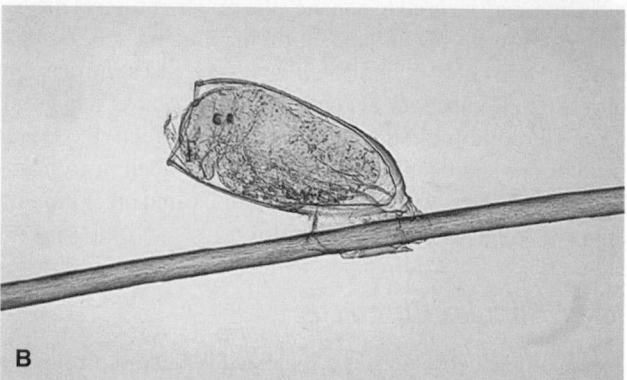

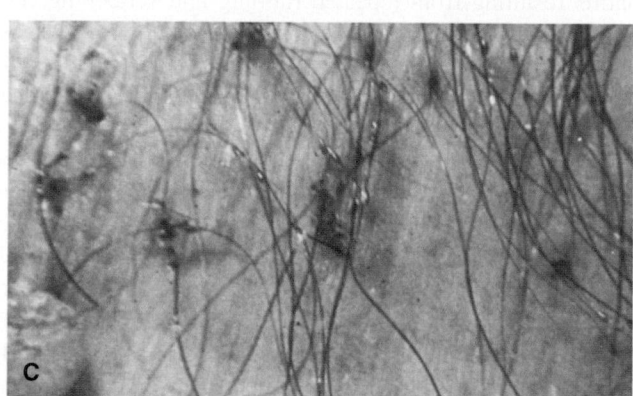

FIGURE 61-26 • **(A)** Pimple-like irritations, burrows, and rash of the skin due to infestation with **(B)** *Sarcoptes scabiei* var. *hominis,* or "itch mite." (Centers for Disease Control and Prevention Public Health Image Library. [Online.] Available: http://phil.cdc.gov/ Phil/home.asp.)

FIGURE 61-27 • **(A)** Female body louse, *Pediculus humanus corporis,* as it is obtaining a blood meal from a human host. **(B)** Unhatched nit of the head louse, *Pediculus humanus capitis,* attached to a human hair. **(C)** Pediculosis pubis infestation: erythematous lesions in the pubic region caused by *Phthirus pubis* (crab lice) bites. (Centers for Disease Control and Prevention Public Health Image Library. [Online.] Available: http://phil.cdc.gov/Phil/home.asp.)

other effective mite-killing agents are applied over the entire skin surface for 12 hours. Repeated applications may be recommended in certain cases, but one treatment usually is sufficient. Care must be taken to ensure that close contacts are treated. Clothes and towels are disinfected with hot water and detergent, or they can be isolated for 2 weeks. If symptoms persist after treatment, the patient should be advised not to re-treat the condition without consulting a health care provider. Oral ivermectin, a broad-spectrum antiparasitic agent, has been used for treatment-resistant scabies.[47] A red-brown nodule, thought to be an allergic response to the mite parts left on the skin, may form after treatment.

Pediculosis

Pediculosis is the term for infestation with lice (genus *Pediculus*). Lice are gray, gray-brown, or red-brown, oval, wingless insects that live off the blood of humans and animals (Fig. 61-27A). Lice are host specific; lice that live on animals do not transfer to humans, and vice versa. Lice also are host dependent; they cannot live apart from the host beyond a few hours. As with scabies, the incidence of pediculosis increased in the 1970s to pandemic levels, probably because of increases in poverty, sexual promiscuity, and worldwide travel.

Three types of lice affect humans: *Pediculus humanus corporis* (body lice), *Phthirus pubis* (pubic lice), and *Pediculus humanus capitis* (head lice). Although these three types differ biologically, they have similar life cycles. The life cycle of a louse consists of a "nit" or unhatched egg (see Fig. 61-27B), three molt stages, an adult reproductive stage, and death. Before adulthood, lice live off the host and are incapable of reproduction. After fertilization, the female louse lays her eggs along hair shafts. The nits appear pearl-gray to brown. Depending on the site, a female louse can lay between 150 and 300 nits in her life. The life span of a feeding louse is 30 to 50 days. Lice are equipped with stylets that pierce the skin. Their saliva contains an anticoagulant that prevents the host's blood from clotting while the louse is feeding. A louse takes up to 1 mL of blood during a feeding.

Pediculosis Corporis. Pediculosis corporis is infestation with *P. humanus corporis,* or body lice. The lice are transferred chiefly through contact with an infested person, clothing, or bedding. The lice live in clothes fibers, coming out only to feed—usually at night, causing nocturnal pruritus. Unlike pubic and head lice, the body louse can survive 10 to 14 days without the host.

The typical lesion is a macule at the site of the bite. Papules and wheals may develop. The infestation is pruritic and evokes scratching that brings about a characteristic linear excoriation. Eczematous patches are found frequently. Secondary lesions may become scaly and hyperpigmented and leave scars. Areas typically affected are the shoulders, trunk, and buttocks. The presence of nits in the seams of clothes confirms a diagnosis of body lice.

Treatment measures consist of eradicating the louse and nits on the body and on clothing. Dry-cleaning, washing in hot water, or steam pressing clothes are recommended methods. Special attention is given to the seams. Merely storing clothing in plastic bags for 2 weeks also rids clothes of lice. Many health care providers prefer not to treat the body unless nits are in evidence on hair shafts. If treatment is indicated, shampoos or topical preparations containing malathion or other pediculicides are recommended. Care must be taken to ensure that close contacts are treated.

Pediculosis Pubis. Pediculosis pubis, the infestation known as crabs or pubic lice, is a nuisance disease that is uncomfortable and embarrassing. The disease is spread by intimate contact with someone harboring *P. pubis.* The lice and nits are usually found in the pubic area of men and women, where their bites produce itching and erythematous lesions (see Fig. 61-27C). Occasionally, they may be found in sites of secondary sex characteristics, such as the beard in men or the axillae in both sexes. Symptoms include intense itching and irritation of the skin. Diagnosis is made on the basis of symptoms and microscopic examination. The treatment is the same as for head lice.

Pediculosis Capitis. Pediculosis capitis, or infestation with head lice, primarily affects white-skinned persons; it is relatively unknown in darker-skinned persons. The incidence is higher among girls, although hair length has not been indicated as a contributing factor. Infestations of head lice usually are confined to the nape of the neck and behind the ears. Less frequently, head lice are found on the beard, pubic areas, eyebrows, and body hairs. Although head lice can be transmitted by sharing combs and hats, they usually are spread from hair shaft to hair shaft through close personal contact. A positive

diagnosis depends on the presence of firmly attached nits or live adult lice on hair shafts. Pruritus and scratching of the head are the primary indicators that head lice may be present. The scalp may appear red and excoriated from scratching. In severe cases, the hair becomes matted together in a crusty, foul-smelling "cap." An occasional morbilliform rash, which may be misdiagnosed as rubella, may occur with lymphadenopathy.

Head lice are treated with permethrin or malathion shampoos or rinses. Repeated treatments may be needed to eliminate the hatching nits. Dead nits may be removed with a fine-toothed comb or over-the-counter nit removal hair rinses. Over the years, permethrin- and malathion-resistant lice have evolved. There is controversy over whether true resistance exists or other factors have an impact, such as not using the treatment measures correctly, not repeating the treatment measures, or misdiagnosing head lice.[48] There has been a resurgence of older remedies in response, such as asphyxiation with olive oil or petroleum products left on the hair from 24 hours to several months. Rotating therapies also may be helpful. "Bug busting" or removing nits by wet combing the hair every 3 to 4 days for 2 weeks as the only treatment measure, has proved ineffective.[48] Hot air applications have been effective.[49] Finally, studies on the physiology of the nit may reveal future options for lice control. For example, knowing that the nit sheath is composed of four bands of protein, similar in composition to human hair, may lead to a better understanding of these insect glues and provide avenues for treatment.[50]

The "no-nit" policies that had been adopted over the past several years have been rescinded. Both the National Association of School Nurses[51] and the American Academy of Pediatrics[52] recommend not excluding children from school because of residual nits. The primary goal is to control outbreaks and infestations; interventions beyond this are out of proportion to the medical significance of lice.

IN SUMMARY, primary disorders of the skin include pigmentary skin disorders, infectious processes, inflammatory conditions, immune disorders, allergic reactions, and arthropod infestations. Pigmentary skin disorders include vitiligo, albinism, and melasma. Although the causes of the disorders vary, all involve changes in the amount of melanin produced by the melanocytes. These disorders appear in people of every skin type; however, the manifestations of the disorders vary among light-skinned and dark-skinned persons.

Superficial fungal infections are called *dermatophytoses* and are commonly known as *tinea* or *ringworm.* Tinea can affect the whole body (tinea corporis), face and neck (tinea faciale), scalp (tinea capitis), hands (tinea manus), feet (tinea pedis), or nails (tinea unguium). The deep fungal infections invade the skin more deeply and go into living tissue, and are also capable of involving other organs. Impetigo, which is caused by staphylococci or beta-hemolytic streptococci, is the most common superficial bacterial infection. Viruses are responsible for verrucae (warts), herpes simplex type 1 lesions (cold sores or fever blisters), and herpes zoster (shingles).

Noninfectious inflammatory skin conditions, such as acne, lichen planus, psoriasis, and pityriasis rosea, are of unknown origin. They usually are localized to the skin and are rarely associated with a specific internal disease. Allergic skin responses involve the body's immune system and are caused by hypersensitivity reactions to allergens such as environmental agents, drugs, and other substances. They include contact dermatitis, atopic dermatitis, and drug-induced skin eruptions (erythema multiforme, Stevens-Johnson syndrome, and toxic epidermal necrolysis).

The skin is also subject to invasion or infestation by a number of arthropod species, including scabies, which is caused by a mite (*S. scabiei*), and pediculosis, which is caused by lice. There are three types of lice that affect humans: *Pediculus humanus corporis* (body lice), *Phthirus pubis* (pubic lice), and *Pediculus humanus capitis* (head lice). ■

ULTRAVIOLET RADIATION, THERMAL, AND PRESSURE INJURY

- Because the skin covers the body, it is exposed to a number of potentially damaging agents in the external environment.
- The ultraviolet rays of sunlight have the potential for directly damaging skin cells, accelerating the effect of aging on the skin, and predisposing to the development of skin cancer.
- Prolonged pressure can interrupt blood flow, causing pressure ulcers.
- Thermal injury can damage skin and subcutaneous tissue and destroy the barrier function of the skin in terms of preventing the loss of body fluids and protecting against the entry of infectious organisms.

ULTRAVIOLET RADIATION, THERMAL, AND PRESSURE INJURY

After completing this section of the chapter, you should be able to meet the following objectives:

- Describe the three types of ultraviolet radiation and relate them to sunburn, aging skin changes, and the development of skin cancer.
- Describe the manifestations and treatment of sunburn.
- State the properties of an effective sunscreen.
- Compare the tissue involvement in first-degree, second-degree full-thickness, and third-degree burns.
- State how the rule of nines is used in determining the body surface area involved in a burn.
- Cite the determinants for grading burn severity using the American Burn Association classification of burns.
- Describe the systemic complications of burns.
- Describe the major considerations in treatment of burn injury.
- Cite two causes of pressure ulcers.
- Explain how shearing forces contribute to ischemic skin damage.
- List four measures that contribute to the prevention of pressure ulcers.

Skin Damage Caused by Ultraviolet Radiation

The skin is the protective shield against harmful UV rays from the sun. Skin cancers and other skin disorders such as early wrinkling and aging of the skin have been attributed to the damaging effects of sunlight.

Sunlight is measured in wavelengths of nanometers (nm; one billionth of a meter) ranging from approximately 290 nm in the UV region up to approximately 2500 nm in the infrared region. UV radiation (UVR) is divided into three types: UVC, UVB, and UVA. UVC rays are short (100 to 290 nm) and do not pass through the earth's atmosphere. However, they can be produced artificially and are damaging to the eyes. UVB rays are 290 to 320 nm. Commonly referred to as *sunburn rays,* they are responsible for nearly all the skin effects of sunlight, including *photoaging*—the wrinkles, pigmentary changes, dryness, and loss of skin tone that occur with and are enhanced by exposure to sunlight. UVA rays are 320 to 400 nm, and can pass through window glass. They are further divided into UVA2 (320 to 339 nm) and UVA1 (340 to 400 nm) because the effects of UVA2 are now believed to be similar to UVB rays.[53] In general, it takes approximately 1000 times more UVA to match the untoward effects of UVB. Nonetheless, UVA, particularly UVA2, contributes greatly to skin alterations. Artificial sources of UVA, such as tanning salons and therapeutic solar interventions (PUVA) for certain skin conditions, also produce the same effects as UVB radiation.

The acute effects of UVA and UVB are short-lived and reversible. They include erythema, pigmentation, and injury to Langerhans cells and keratinocytes in the epidermis. These reactions differ depending on whether the inciting agent is UVA or UVB. For example, UVA-induced erythema occurs immediately, fades within 2 hours, and is believed to be due to the "heat load." UVB-induced erythema has a delayed response, peaking within 6 to 24 hours after exposure to sunlight and fading over 1 or 2 days. Pigmentation or tanning induced by UVA and UVB is due to a delayed increase in the number of melanocytes, elongation and extension of the dendritic processes, and transfer of melanin to keratinocytes (see Chapter 60, Fig. 60-4). For tanning to occur, there must be UVB-induced erythema. Small doses of UVA produce oxidation of melanin with transient, immediate darkening of the skin that fades within 2 hours, whereas higher doses of UVA can produce pigmentary changes lasting for several hours to days.[54] Tanning induced by UVB is protective against subsequent exposures, whereas tanning induced by UVA provides limited protection.

Skin damage induced by UVB is believed to be caused by the generation of reactive oxygen species and by damage to melanin. Cellular proteins and DNA are primarily damaged because of their abundance and ability to absorb UVR. Both UVA and UVB also deplete Langerhans cells and immune cells. It is believed that these effects prevent immune cells from detecting and removing sun-damaged cells with malignant potential.[55] Both UVA and UVB are now considered causes of cancer. UVA may actually be more carcinogenic than UVB. Although it causes less sunburn, UVA is present during all daylight hours, year-round. UVB, on the other hand, varies by season, location, and time of day. UVA penetrates deeply and causes greater damage in the keratinocytes, where most skin cancers arise.

Drug-Induced Photosensitivity

Some drugs are classified as photosensitive drugs because they produce an exaggerated response to UVR when the drug is taken in combination with sun exposure. Examples include some of the anti-infective agents (sulfonamides, tetracyclines, nalidixic acid), antihistamines (cyproheptadine, diphenhydramine), antipsychotic agents (phenothiazines, haloperidol), diuretics (thiazides, acetazolamide, amiloride), hypoglycemic agents (sulfonylureas), and nonsteroidal anti-inflammatory drugs (phenylbutazone, ketoprofen, naproxen).

Drug-induced photosensitivity, such as UVA photosensitivity induced by the psoralens, may be used in treating skin conditions, such as psoriasis, that respond well to UVR exposure. Because an increased incidence of cancerous lesions has been reported in people who have been treated with these agents, their use requires caution and careful surveillance.

Sunburn

Sunburn is caused by excessive exposure of the epidermal and dermal layers of the skin to UVR, resulting in an erythematous inflammatory reaction. Sunburn ranges from mild to severe. Mild sunburn consists of various degrees of skin redness. The burn continues to develop for 24 to 72 hours, occasionally followed by peeling skin in 3 to 8 days.[56] Some peeling and itching may continue for several weeks. Inflammation, blistering, weakness, chills, fever, malaise, and pain often accompany severe forms of sunburn. Scaling and peeling follow any overexposure to sunlight. Dark skin also burns and may appear grayish or gray-black. Severe sunburns are those that cover large portions of the body with blisters or are accompanied by a high fever or intense pain.

Mild to moderate sunburns are treated with anti-inflammatory medications, such as aspirin or ibuprofen, until redness and pain subside. Cold compresses, cool baths, and applying a moisturizing cream, such as aloe, to affected skin help treat the symptoms. Steroid and nonsteroidal agents are used depending on the severity of the burn.[55] Blisters should not be broken to preserve the protective layer of the skin, hasten the healing process, and decrease the risk of infection. Extensive second- and third-degree burns may require hospitalization and specialized burn care techniques, as described in the section on Thermal Injury.

Sunscreens and Other Protective Measures

The UV rays of sunlight or other sources can be completely or partially blocked from the skin by sunscreens. There are three primary types of sunscreens available on the market, those that reduce or prevent UV erythema chemically, physically, or biologically. Chemical agents absorb UVR, physical agents reflect UVR, whereas biologic agents reduce inflammation by either blocking the inflammatory response or by enhancing biologic repair.[57] Sunscreen agents no longer contain para-aminobenzoic acid (PABA), a chemical blocking agent that protects against UVB, because of its allergenic and staining properties. However, PABA derivatives, especially padimate O, are used widely, but protect only against UVB. Broad-spectrum suntan lotions protect against both UVA and UVB. These products contain a benzophenone, such as oxybenzone, dioxybenzone, or avobenzone. Newer agents, such as micronized titanium dioxide and microfine zinc, act by reflecting as well as absorbing sunlight. They protect against most of the UV spectrum. Anthelios SX (Mexoryl SX), a sunscreen that protects against both UVB and UVA, has also been recently approved for use.

Sunscreens are available as lotions, creams, oils, gels, and sprays. They also are incorporated into cosmetics and lip balms. Sunscreens should be used diligently and according to the person's tendency to burn rather than tan (Table 61-1). It is recommended that they be applied 30 minutes before sun exposure and reapplied every 2 hours. Water-resistant preparations maintain sunburn protection after being in the water for up to 40 min-

TABLE 61-1 Skin Phototypes

SKIN PHOTOTYPE	SUNTAN AND SUNBURN HISTORY
I	Very fair; always burns, never tans, sensitive to sun exposure Eyes blue or green; hair blond or red
II	Fair; burns easily, tans minimally Eyes blue, hazel, or brown; hair blond, red, or brown
III	Medium; burns moderately, tans gradually to light brown
IV	Olive; burns minimally, always tans well to moderately brown
V	Brown; rarely burns, tans profusely to dark
VI	Black; never burns, deeply pigmented, least sensitive

Adapted from Skin Cancer Foundation. (2007). Skin types and at risk groups. [Online.] Available: www.skincancer.org.

utes. Because many skin cancers are correlated with childhood sunburns, children younger than 18 years of age should use broad-spectrum (blocks UVA and UVB) sunscreens that have a Sun Protection Factor (SPF) of at least 15.

The FDA requires an SPF rating on all commercial suntan preparations based on their ability to obstruct UVR absorption. The ratings usually are on a scale of 1 to 30; higher ratings block more sunlight. SPFs are laboratory-measured proportions of how much UVR is needed to produce mild erythema in persons with protected versus unprotected skin. For example, an SPF of 8 means that a person needs eight times as much sun to elicit sunburn. Another way of stating it is an SPF of 8 filters out 88% of UVR. As seen in Table 61-2, an SPF of 16 blocks about 94% of the sun, with little gain in UVB protection as the SPF rises. Hence, an SPF of 15 is recommended for outdoor sun and tanning salon use.[57]

Sunless suntan creams, such as dihydroxyacetone, produce a tan without exposure to the sun. They come in various tones, with emollients or humectants added for moisturizing or gel or alcohol-based products for drying. Vitamins, herbal extracts, antioxidants, and α-hydroxy acids may be added as enhancers. It is important to avoid products that use the sun to create tans; they may exacerbate sun damage. Tanning pills contain the pigment, canthaxanthin, found in carrots and are especially dangerous because of their association with hepatitis and urticaria.

Sunscreens should be considered only one component of an overall program to reduce UVR exposure. The Centers for Disease Control and Prevention (CDC) recommends the following sun-protection behaviors: (1) wear a wide-brimmed hat; (2) cover up in the sun; (3) seek shade; (4) wear wrap-around sunglasses; and (5) avoid the sun during the hours of 10 AM to 4 PM, while using a broad-spectrum sunscreen with an SPF of 15 or higher.[58,59] It is also important to avoid tanning booths, perform a self-assessment of the skin every month, and obtain a professional skin examination every year. The *UV Index* was developed by the National Weather Service and the U.S. Environmental Protection Agency to predict the risk of overexposure to UVR. It helps people determine the degree to which they should take caution when outdoors. The index is based on a scale of 0 to 10+, with 0 being low risk and 10+ very high risk. It is calculated daily and is based on skin types of people who sunburn easily. For example, a UV Index value of 5 or 6 means there is a good possibility of UV overexposure.

Thermal Injury

About 1.2 million people in the United States require medical care for burns each year, with 51,000 requiring hospitalization. Between 30% and 40% of these are children younger than 15 years of age, with an average age of 32 months.[60]

The effects and complications of burns fully illustrate the essential function that the skin performs as it protects the body from the many damaging elements in the environment while serving to maintain the constancy of the body's internal environment. The massive loss of skin tissue not only predisposes to attack by microorganisms that are present in the environment, it allows for the massive loss of body fluids and their contents, it interferes with temperature regulation, it challenges the immune system, and it imposes excessive demands on the metabolic and reparative processes that are needed to restore the body's interface with the environment.

Burns are caused by a number of sources. Flame burns occur because of exposure to direct fire. Scald burns result from hot liquids spilled or poured on the skin surface. In a child, a scald burn may be indicative of child abuse. Chemical burns occur from industrial agents used in occupational sites. Electrical burns occur from contact with live electrical wires in fields or in the home. Electrical burns are usually more extensive because of internal tissue injury and the presence of entrance and exit wounds (see Chapter 5, Fig. 5-5). Lightning, electromagnetic radiation, and ionizing radiation also can cause skin burns.

Classification of Burns

Burns are typically classified according to the depth of involvement as first-degree, second-degree, and third-degree burns.[60–62] The depth of a burn is largely influenced by the duration of exposure to the heat source and the temperature of the heating agent. *First-degree burns* (superficial partial-thickness burns) involve only the outer layers of the epidermis. They are red or pink, dry, and painful. There usually is no blister formation. A mild sunburn is an example. The skin maintains its ability to function as a water vapor and bacterial barrier and heals in 3 to 10 days. First-degree burns usually require only palliative treatment, such as pain relief measures and adequate fluid intake. Extensive first-degree burns on infants, the elderly, and persons who receive radiation therapy for cancer may require more care.

Second-degree burns involve both the epidermis and dermis. *Second-degree partial-thickness burns* involve the epidermis and various degrees of the dermis. They are painful, moist, red, and blistered. Underneath the blisters is weeping, bright pink or red skin that is sensitive to temperature changes, air exposure, and touch. The blisters prevent the loss of body water and superficial dermal cells. Excluding excision of large

TABLE 61-2 **Percentage Reduction in Ultraviolet Radiation (UVR) With Increasing Sun Protection Factor (SPF) Number Showing an Exponential Relationship**	
SPF NUMBER	**REDUCTION IN UVR (%)**
2	30
4	75
8	87.5
16	93.75
32	96.88
64	98.14

From Marks R., Hill D. (2001). Prevention of skin cancer. In Sober A.J., Haluska F.G. (Eds.), *American Cancer Society atlas of clinical oncology: Skin cancer* (p. 326). Hamilton, Ontario: B.C. Decker.

burn areas, it is important to maintain intact blisters after injury because they serve as a good bandage and may promote wound healing. These burns heal in approximately 1 to 2 weeks.

Second-degree full-thickness burns involve the entire epidermis and dermis. Structures that originate in the subcutaneous layer, such as hair follicles and sweat glands, remain intact. These burns can be very painful because the pain sensors remain intact. Tactile sensation may be absent or greatly diminished in the areas of deepest destruction. These burns appear as mottled pink, red, or waxy white areas with blisters and edema. The blisters resemble flat, dry tissue paper, rather than the bullous blisters seen with superficial partial-thickness injury. After healing, in approximately 1 month, these burns maintain their softness and elasticity, but there may be the loss of some sensation. Scar formation is usual. These burns heal with supportive medical care aimed at preventing further tissue damage, providing adequate hydration, and ensuring that the granular bed is adequate to support reepithelialization.

Third-degree full-thickness burns extend into the subcutaneous tissue and may involve muscle and bone. Thrombosed vessels can be seen under the burned skin, indicating that the underlying vasculature is involved. Third-degree burns vary in color from waxy white or yellow to tan, brown, deep red, or black. These burns are hard, dry, and leathery. Edema is extensive in the burn area and surrounding tissues. There is no pain because the nerve sensors have been destroyed. However, there is no such thing as a "pure" third-degree burn. Third-degree burns are almost always surrounded by second-degree burns, which are surrounded by an area of first-degree burns. The injury sometimes has an almost target-like appearance because of the various degrees of burn. Full-thickness burns wider than 1.5 inches usually require skin grafts because all the regenerative (*i.e.,* dermal) elements have been destroyed.

Smaller injuries usually heal from the margins inward toward the center, the dermal elements regenerating from the healthier margins. However, regeneration may take many weeks and leave a permanent scar, even in smaller burns.

In addition to the depth of the wound, the extent of the burn also is important. Extent is measured by estimating the amount of total body surface area (TBSA) involved. Several tools exist for estimating the TBSA. For example, the *rule of nines* counts anatomic body parts as multiples of 9% (the head is 9%, each arm 9%, each leg 18%, anterior trunk 18%, posterior trunk 18%), with the perineum 1%. The Lund and Browder chart includes a body diagram table that estimates the TBSA by age and anatomic part.[60,63] Children are more accurately assessed using this method because it takes into account the difference in relative size of body parts. The estimates of TBSA are then converted to the American Burn Association Classification of Extent of Injury (Table 61-3).

Other factors, such as age, location, other injuries, and preexisting conditions, are taken into consideration for a full assessment of burn injury.[60–63] These factors can increase the assessed severity of the burn and the length of treatment. For example, a first-degree burn is reclassified as a more severe burn if other factors are present, such as burns to the hands, face, and feet; inhalation injury; electrical burns; other trauma; or existence of psychosocial problems. Genital burns almost always require hospitalization because edema may cause difficulty urinating and the location complicates maintenance of a bacteria-free environment.

Systemic Complications

Burn victims often are confronted with hemodynamic instability, impaired respiratory function, a hypermetabolic response,

TABLE 61-3 American Burn Association Grading System for Burn Severity and Disposition

| | TYPE OF BURN | | |
	Minor	Moderate	Major
Criteria	<10% TBSA in adult	10%–20% TBSA in adult	>20% TBSA in adult
	<5% TBSA in young (<10 years) or old (>50 years)	5%–10% TBSA in young or old	>10% TBSA in young or old
	<2% Full-thickness burn	2%–5% Full-thickness burn	>5% Full-thickness burn
		High-voltage injury	High-voltage burn
		Suspected inhalation injury	Known inhalation injury
		Circumferential burn	Any significant burn to face, eyes, ears, genitalia, hands, feet, or major joints
		Concomitant medical problem predisposing to infection (*e.g.*, diabetes, sickle cell disease)	Significant associated injuries (*e.g.*, major trauma)
Disposition	Outpatient management	Hospital admission	Referral to burn center

TBSA, total body surface area.
From American Burn Association. (1990). Hospital and prehospital resources for optimal care of patients with burn injury: Guidelines for development and operation of burn centers. *Journal of Burn Care and Rehabilitation* 11, 98–104.

major organ dysfunction, and sepsis.[64-66] The magnitude of the response is proportional to the extent of injury, usually reaching a plateau when approximately 60% of the body is burned. In addition to loss of skin, burn victims often have associated injuries or illnesses. The treatment challenge is to provide immediate resuscitation efforts and long-term maintenance of physiologic function. Pain and emotional problems are additional challenges faced by persons with burns.

Hemodynamic Instability. Hemodynamic instability begins almost immediately with injury to capillaries in the burned area and surrounding tissue. Fluid is lost from the vascular, interstitial, and cellular compartments. Because of a loss of vascular volume, major burn victims often present in the emergency department in a form of hypovolemic shock (Chapter 26) known as *burn shock*. The patient has a decrease in cardiac output, increased peripheral vascular resistance, and impaired perfusion of vital organs. Electrical injuries that cause burns can produce cardiac arrhythmias that require immediate attention.

Respiratory System Dysfunction. Another injury commonly associated with burns is smoke inhalation and postburn lung injury. Victims often are trapped in a burning structure and inhale significant amounts of smoke, carbon monoxide, and other toxic fumes. Water-soluble gases, such as ammonia, sulfur dioxide, and chlorine that are found in smoke from burning plastics and rubber react with mucous membranes to form strong acids and alkalis that induce ulceration of the mucous membrane, bronchospasm, and edema. Lipid-soluble gases, such as nitrous oxide and hydrogen chloride, are transported to the lower airways, where they damage lung tissue. There also may be thermal injury to the respiratory passages. Manifestations of inhalation injury include hoarseness, drooling, an inability to handle secretions, hacking cough, and labored and shallow breathing. Serial blood gases show a fall in the partial pressure of arterial oxygen (PO_2). Signs of mucosal injury and airway obstruction often are delayed for 24 to 48 hours after a burn. It is necessary continually to monitor the patient for early signs of respiratory distress. Other pulmonary conditions, such as pneumonia, pulmonary embolism, or pneumothorax, may occur secondarily to the burn.

Hypermetabolic Response. The stress of burn injury increases metabolic and nutritional requirements. Secretion of stress-related hormones such as catecholamines and cortisol is increased in an effort to maintain homeostasis. Heat production is increased in an effort to balance heat losses from the burned area. Hypermetabolism, characterized by increased oxygen consumption, increased glucose use, and protein and fat wasting, is a characteristic response to burn trauma and infection. The hypermetabolic state peaks at approximately 7 to 17 days after the burn, and tissue breakdown diminishes as the wounds heal. Nutritional support is essential to recovery from burn injury. Enteral and parenteral hyperalimentation may be used during this time to deliver sufficient nutrients to prevent tissue breakdown and postburn weight loss.

Dysfunction of Other Organ Systems. Burn shock results in impaired perfusion of vital organs. The patient may have impaired function of the kidneys, the gastrointestinal tract, and the nervous system. Although the initial insult often is one of hypovolemic shock and impaired organ perfusion, sepsis may contribute to impaired organ function after the initial resuscitation period.

Renal insufficiency can occur in burn patients as a result of the hypovolemic state, damage to the kidneys at the time of the burn, or from drugs that are administered. Immediately after the burn, a person goes into a short period of relative anuria, followed by a phase of hypermetabolism characterized by increased urine output and nitrogen loss.

The effects of burn injury on the gastrointestinal tract include gastric dilation and decreased peristalsis. These effects are compounded by immobility and narcotic analgesics. Burn victims are observed carefully for vomiting and fecal impaction. Acute ulceration of the stomach and duodenum (called *Curling ulcer*) is a potential complication in burn victims and is thought to be the result of stress and gastric ischemia. It is largely controlled by the prophylactic administration of histamine 2-receptor antagonists or proton pump inhibitors. Enteral feeding tubes are inserted almost immediately. Tube feeding is intended to mitigate ulcer formation, maintain the integrity of the intestinal mucosa, and provide sufficient calories and protein for the hypermetabolic state.

Neurologic changes can occur from periods of hypoxia. Neurologic damage may result from head injuries, drug or alcohol abuse, carbon monoxide poisoning, fluid volume deficits, and hypovolemia. With an electrical burn, the brain or spine can be directly injured. The responses to neurologic damage may include confusion, memory loss, insomnia, lethargy, and combativeness.

Musculoskeletal effects include fractures that occur at the time of the accident, deep burns extending to the muscles and bone, hypertrophic scarring, and contractures. The hypermetabolic state increases tissue catabolism and produces severe protein and fat wasting.

Sepsis. A significant complication of the acute phase of burn injury is sepsis. It may arise from the burn wound, pneumonia, urinary tract infection, infection elsewhere in the body, or the use of invasive procedures or monitoring devices. Immunologically, the skin is the body's first line of defense. When the skin is no longer intact, the body is open to bacterial infection. Destruction of the skin also prevents the delivery of cellular components of the immune system to the site of injury. There also is loss of normal protective skin flora and a shift to colonization by more pathogenic flora.

Emergency and Long-term Treatment

Regardless of the type of burn, the first step in any burn situation is to stop the burning process, cool the burn, provide pain relief, and cover the burn.[63-66] The heat source should be removed, and flames should be doused with water or smothered with a blanket. Active cooling removes the heat and prevents progression of the burn. Immersion or irrigation with lukewarm water for at least 20 minutes can be extremely helpful. This period should be increased for those with chemical burns. Immediate submersion is more important than removal of clothing, which may delay cooling the involved areas. The application of ice or cold water is not recommended because it can further limit blood flow to an area, turning a partial-thickness into a full-thickness burn.

Depending on the depth and extent of the burn, medical treatment is necessary. Emergency care consists of resuscitation and stabilization with intravenous fluids while maintaining cardiac and respiratory function. Once hospitalized, the immediate treatment regimen focuses on continued maintenance of cardiorespiratory function, pain alleviation, wound care, and emotional support. Intermediate and long-term treatments depend on the extent of injury.

After hemodynamic and pulmonary stability have been established, treatment is directed toward initial care of the wound. Treatment of the burn wound focuses on protection from desiccation and further injury of those burn areas that reepithelialize in 7 to 10 days (superficial second-degree burns). "Nature's own blister" is the best protection for these burns. Topical antimicrobial preparations (*e.g.,* silver sulfadiazine) and dressings are used to cover the wound when the blister has been broken. Wounds that will not heal spontaneously in 7 to 10 days (deep second-degree and third-degree burns) are usually treated by excision and skin grafts. The sloughed tissue, or *eschar,* produced by the burn is excised as soon as possible. This decreases the chance of infection and allows the skin to regenerate faster.

Burns that encircle the entire surface of the body or a body part (*e.g.,* arms, legs, torso) act like tourniquets and can cause major tissue damage to the muscles, tendons, and vasculature under the area of the leathery eschar skin. These burns are called *circumferential burns.* The eschar is incised longitudinally (escharotomy), and sometimes a fasciotomy (surgical incision through the fascia of the muscle) is performed. The timing of these incisions is important. Incision is done after the patient's circulatory condition stabilizes to some degree, thereby limiting some of the massive fluid loss. However, the incisions must be done before eschar formation can cause hypoxia and necrosis of the underlying tissues and organs. This is extremely important when torso burns occur because the pressure placed on the chest can result in an inability to breathe and decreased blood return to the heart.

Systemic infection remains a leading cause of morbidity among persons with extensive burns. Continuous microbiologic surveillance is necessary; protective isolation measures are often instituted. There is an increasing trend toward use of prophylactic antibiotic treatment in persons with major burns.

Skin grafts are surgically implanted as soon as possible, often at the same time the burn tissue is excised, to promote new skin growth, limit fluid loss, and act as a dressing. Skin grafts can be permanent or temporary, and split-thickness or full-thickness. Permanent skin grafts are used over newly excised tissue. Temporary skin grafts are used to cover a burned area until the tissue underneath it has healed.

Various sources of skin grafts exist: *autograft* (skin obtained from the person's own body), *homograft* (skin obtained from another human being, alive or recently dead), and *heterograft* (skin obtained from another species, such as pigs). The best choice is autografting when there is enough uninterrupted skin on the person's body. The thickness of these grafts depends on the donor site and the needs of the burn patient. A *split-thickness skin graft* is one that includes the epidermis and part of the dermis. A split-thickness skin graft can be sent through a skin mesher that cuts tiny slits into the skin, allowing it to expand up to nine times its original size. These grafts are used frequently because they can cover large surface areas and there is less autorejection. *Full-thickness skin grafts* include the entire thickness of the dermal layer. They are used primarily for reconstructive surgery or for deep, small areas. The donor site of a full-thickness skin graft requires a split-thickness skin graft to help it heal.

Two-layered synthetic skin grafts (*Apligraf, Integra*) are now available and approved by the FDA.[67] Synthetic skin grafts generally are composed of a layer of silicone, mimicking the properties of the epidermis, and a layer or matrix of fibers. Skin cells attach to the fibers, enabling dermal skin growth. Once the dermal skin has regenerated, the silicone layer is removed and a thin epidermal skin graft is applied, thus requiring less skin grafting overall.

Other treatment measures include positioning, splinting, and physical therapy to prevent contractures and maintain muscle tone. Because the normal body response to disuse is flexion, the contractures that occur with a burn are disfiguring and cause loss of limb or appendage use. Once the wounds have healed sufficiently, elastic pressure garments, sometimes for the full body, often are used to prevent hypertrophic scarring.

Pressure Ulcers

Pressure ulcers are ischemic lesions of the skin and underlying structures caused by unrelieved pressure that impairs the flow of blood and lymph. Pressure ulcers often are referred to as *decubitus ulcers* or *bedsores.* The word *decubitus* comes from the Latin term meaning "lying down." However, a pressure ulcer may result from pressure exerted in the seated or the lying position. Pressure ulcers are most likely to develop over a bony prominence, but they may occur on any part of the body that is subjected to external pressure, friction, or shearing forces. Several subpopulations are at particular risk, including persons with quadriplegia, elderly persons with restricted activity and hip fractures, and persons in the critical care setting.

Pressure ulcers are costly in terms of human suffering, financial expense, and allocation of health care resources.[68,69] The prevention and treatment of pressure ulcers is a public health issue and is addressed in *Healthy People 2010,* a national public health policy statement, which has set a target of a 50% decrease in the prevalence of pressure ulcers in nursing home residents.[70]

Mechanisms of Development

Four factors contribute to the development of pressure ulcers: (1) pressure (2) shearing forces, (3) friction, and (4) moisture.[68]

External pressures that exceed capillary pressure interrupt blood flow in the capillary beds. When the pressure between a bony prominence and a support surface exceeds the normal capillary filling pressure, capillary flow essentially is obstructed. If this pressure is applied constantly for 2 hours, oxygen deprivation coupled with an accumulation of metabolic end products leads to irreversible tissue damage. Although 32 mm Hg has been traditionally accepted as the amount of pressure necessary to compress capillaries and interrupt blood flow, this is highly variable among individuals.[68] Persons with impaired circulation require less pressure to interrupt circulation. The same amount of pressure causes more damage when it is distributed over a small area than over a larger area.

Whether a person is sitting or lying down, the weight of the body is borne by tissues covering the bony prominences. More than 95% of pressure ulcers are located on the lower part of the body, most often over the sacrum, the coccygeal area, the ischial tuberosities, and the greater trochanters.[69] Pressure over a bony area is transmitted from the surface to the underlying dense bone, compressing all of the intervening tissue. As a result, the greatest pressure occurs at the surface of the bone and dissipates outward in a conelike manner toward the surface of the skin (Fig. 61-28). Thus, extensive underlying tissue damage can be present when a small superficial skin lesion is first noticed.

Altering the distribution of pressure from one skin area to another prevents tissue injury. Pressure ulcers most commonly occur in persons with conditions such as spinal cord injury in which normal sensation and movement to effect redistribution of body weight are impaired. Normally, persons unconsciously shift their weight to redistribute pressure on the skin and underlying tissues. For example, during the night, people turn in their sleep, preventing ischemic injury of tissues that overlie the bony prominences that support the weight of the body; the same is true for sitting for any length of time. The movements needed to shift the body weight are made unconsciously, and only when movement is restricted do people become aware of discomfort.

Shearing forces are caused by the sliding of one tissue layer over another with stretching and angulation of blood vessels, causing injury and thrombosis. Shear occurs when the skeleton moves, but the skin remains fixed to an external surface, such as occurs with transfer from a stretcher to a bed or pulling a person up in bed. The same thing happens when the head of the bed is elevated, causing the torso to move toward the foot of the bed while friction and moisture cause the skin to remain fixed to the bed linens. *Friction* contributes to pressure ulceration by damaging the skin at the epidermal–dermal interface. It occurs as persons who are bedridden use their elbows and heels to aid in movement. *Moisture* contributes to pressure ulcer formation by weakening the cell wall of individual skin cells and by changing the protective pH of the skin. This makes the skin more susceptible to pressure, shear, and friction injury.

Prevention

The prevention of pressure ulcers is preferable to their treatment. In 1992, a special panel of the Agency for Health Care Policy and Research (AHCPR; now the Agency for Healthcare Research and Quality), the Panel for the Prediction and Prevention of Pressure Ulcers in Adults, released its clinical practice guideline, *Pressure ulcers in adults: Prediction and prevention.*[71] The panel recommended four overall goals: (1) identifying at-risk persons who need preventive measures and the specific factors placing them at risk; (2) maintaining and improving tissue tolerance to prevent injury; (3) protecting against the adverse effects of external mechanical forces (*i.e.,* pressure, friction, and shear); and (4) reducing the incidence of pressure ulcers through educational programs.[71] A 1994 publication of the AHCPR made specific recommendations for assessment of the person with pressure ulcers, management of tissue load, ulcer care, managing bacterial colonization and infection, operative repair, and education and quality control.[72]

Risk factors identified as contributing to the development of pressure ulcers were those related to sensory perception (*i.e.,* ability to respond meaningfully to pressure-related discomfort), level of skin moisture, urine and fecal continence, nutrition and hydration status, mobility, circulatory status, and presence of shear and friction forces.

Methods for preventing pressure ulcers include frequent position change, meticulous skin care, and frequent and careful observation to detect early signs of skin breakdown. Moisture macerates and injures skin. Sources of moisture include

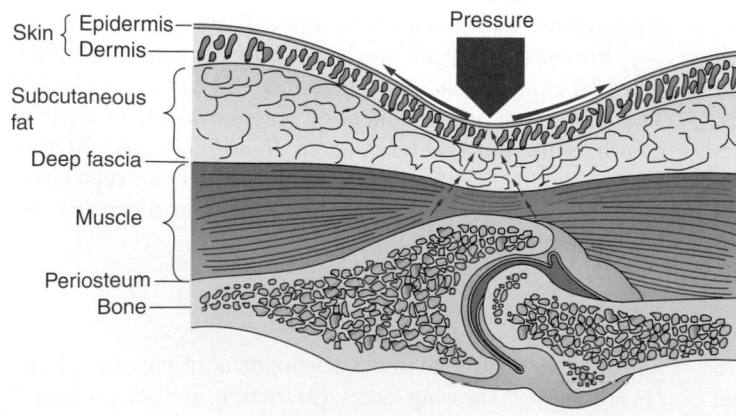

FIGURE 61-28 • Pressure over a bony prominence compresses all intervening soft tissue, with a resulting wide, three-dimensional pressure gradient that causes various degrees of tissue damage. (From Shea J. D. [1975]. Pressure sores: Classification and management. *Clinical Orthopedics and Related Research* 112, 90.)

sweat, wound drainage, urine and feces. Both urinary and fecal incontinence increase the risk of pressure ulcers. Food crumbs, intravenous tubing, and other debris in the bed can greatly increase local skin pressure points. Adequate hydration of the stratum corneum appears to protect the skin against mechanical insult.[71] The prevention of dehydration improves the circulation. It also decreases the concentration of urine, thereby minimizing skin irritation in persons who are incontinent, and it reduces urinary problems that contribute to incontinence. Maintenance of adequate nutrition is important. Anemia and malnutrition contribute to tissue breakdown and delay healing after tissue injury has occurred.

Staging and Treatment

Pressure ulcers can be staged using four categories.[72,73] *Stage I ulcers* are characterized by a defined area of persistent redness in lightly pigmented skin or an area of persistent redness with blue or purple hues in darker skin. *Stage II ulcers* represent a partial-thickness loss of skin involving the epidermis or dermis, or both. The ulcer is superficial and presents clinically as an abrasion, a blister, or a shallow crater. *Stage III ulcers* represent a full-thickness skin loss involving damage and necrosis of subcutaneous tissue that may extend down to but not through underlying fascia. The ulcer manifests as a deep crater with or without undermining of adjacent tissue. *Stage IV ulcers* involve full-thickness skin loss and necrosis with extensive destruction or damage to the underlying subcutaneous tissues that may extend to involve muscle, bone, and supporting structures (*e.g.,* tendon or joint capsule).

After skin breakdown has occurred, special treatment measures are needed to prevent further ischemic damage, reduce bacterial contamination and infection, and promote healing. Treatment methods are selected based on the stage of the ulcer.[68,69,72–74] Stage I ulcers usually are treated with frequent turning and measures to remove pressure. Stage II or III ulcers with little exudate are treated with semipermeable or occlusive dressings. Occlusive dressings are credited with preventing the loss of wound fluid and maintaining a moist environment that is necessary for epithelial cell migration.[75] Wound fluid is thought to contain a variety of growth factors that enhance wound healing. Occlusive dressings may also relieve wound pain and prevent bacterial contamination. There are several types of occlusive dressings available, including polymer films, hydrogels, hydrocolloids, biomembranes, and absorbing granules. The available products differ in their permeability to water vapor and wound protection, and each has advantages and disadvantages.

Necrotic debris increases the possibility of bacterial infection and delays wound healing. Stage III ulcers with exudate and necrotic debris and stage IV ulcers usually require debridement (*i.e.,* removal of necrotic tissue and eschar). This can be done surgically, with wet-to-dry dressings, or through the use of proteolytic enzymes. Stage IV wounds often require packing to obliterate dead space and are covered with nonadherent dressings. Stage IV ulcers may require surgical interventions, such as skin grafts or myocutaneous flaps.

IN SUMMARY, repeated exposure to the UV rays of the sun predisposes to sunburn, premature aging of the skin (wrinkling, solar elastosis, and irregularities in pigmentation), and skin cancer. Solar and artificial sources of UVR, such as from a tanning parlor, contribute to the amount of radiation to which human beings are exposed. Sunburn, which is caused by excessive exposure to UVR, is an erythematous inflammatory reaction, ranging from mild to severe. Photosensitive drugs can also produce an exaggerated response to UVR when they are taken in combination with sun exposure. Sunscreens are protective agents that work by either reflecting sunlight or preventing its absorption.

Burns cause damage to skin structures, ranging from first-degree burns, which damage the epidermis, to third-degree full-thickness burns, which extend into the subcutaneous tissue and may involve muscle and bone. The extent of injury is determined by the thickness of the burn and the total body surface area involved. In addition to skin involvement, burn injury can cause hemodynamic instability with hypovolemic shock, inhalation injury with respiratory involvement, a hypermetabolic state, organ dysfunction, immune suppression and sepsis, pain, and emotional trauma. Treatment methods vary with the severity of injury and include immediate resuscitation and maintenance of physiologic function, wound cleaning and debridement, application of antimicrobial agents and dressings, and skin grafting. Efforts are directed toward preventing or limiting disfigurement and disability.

Pressure ulcers are caused by ischemia of the skin and underlying tissues. They result from external pressure, which disrupts blood flow, or shearing forces, which cause stretching and injury to blood vessels. Pressure ulcers are divided into four stages, according to the depth of tissue involvement. The prevention of pressure ulcers is preferable to their treatment. The goals of prevention should include identifying at-risk persons who need prevention along with the specific factors placing them at risk; maintaining and improving tissue tolerance to pressure to prevent injury; and protecting against the adverse effects of external mechanical forces (*i.e.,* pressure, friction, and shear). ■

NEVI AND SKIN CANCERS

After completing this section of the chapter, you should be able to meet the following objectives:

- Describe the origin of nevi and state their relationship to skin cancers.
- Compare the appearance and outcome of basal cell carcinoma, squamous cell carcinoma, and malignant melanoma.

Nevi

Nevi, or moles, are common congenital or acquired tumors of the skin that are benign. Almost all adults have nevi, some in greater numbers than others. Nevi can be pigmented or nonpigmented, flat or elevated, and hairy or nonhairy.

Nevocellular nevi are pigmented skin lesions resulting from proliferation of melanocytes in the epidermis or dermis. Nevocellular nevi are tan to deep brown, uniformly pigmented, small papules with well-defined, rounded borders (Fig. 61-29A). They are formed initially by melanocytes with their long dendritic extensions that are normally interspersed among the basal keratinocytes (see Chapter 60, Fig. 60-3). The melanocytes are transformed into round or oval melanin-containing cells that grow in nests or clusters along the dermal–epidermal junction. Because of their location, these lesions are called *junctional nevi* (see Fig. 61-29B). Eventually, most junctional nevi grow into the surrounding dermis as nests or cords of cells. *Compound nevi* contain epidermal and dermal components. In older lesions, the epidermal nests may disappear entirely, leaving a *dermal nevi.* Compound and dermal nevi usually are more elevated than junctional nevi.

Another form of nevus, the *dysplastic nevus,* is important because of its capacity to transform into malignant melanoma. Although the association between nevocellular nevi and malignant melanoma was made over 175 years ago, it was not until 1978 that the role of dysplastic nevi as precursors to malignant melanoma was described in detail. Dysplastic nevi are usually larger than other nevi (often >5 mm in diameter). Their appearance is a flat, slightly raised plaque with a pebbly surface, or a target-like lesion with a darker, raised center and irregular border (Fig. 61-30). They vary in shade from brown and red to flesh tones. A person may have hundreds of these lesions. Unlike other moles or nevi, they occur on both sun-exposed and covered areas of the body. Dysplastic nevi have been documented in multiple members of families prone to development of malignant melanoma.

Because of the possibility of malignant transformation, any mole that undergoes a change warrants immediate medical attention. The changes to observe and report are changes in size, thickness, or color, itching, and bleeding.

Skin Cancer

There has been an alarming increase in skin cancers over the past several decades. Since the 1970s, the incidence of malignant melanoma, the most serious form of skin cancer, has increased significantly on an average of 6% per year from 1973 until the early 1980s. Since 1981, the rate has slowed to roughly 3% per year. In 2007, there were approximately 59,940 new cases and 8810 deaths from melanoma in the United States.[76] There were also approximately 1 million cases per year of highly curable nonmelanoma (basal cell and squamous cell) cancers.

SKIN CANCERS

- Increased and unprotected exposure to the ultraviolet rays of sunlight produces sunburn and increases the risk for development of skin cancer.

- The melanocytes, which protect against sunburn through increased production of melanin and suntanning, are particularly vulnerable to the adverse effects of unprotected exposure to ultraviolet light. Malignant melanoma, which is a malignant tumor of melanocytes, is a rapidly progressive and metastatic form of skin cancer.

- Basal cell carcinoma and squamous cell carcinoma, which also reflect the effects of increased sun exposure, are less aggressive forms of skin cancer and are more easily cured.

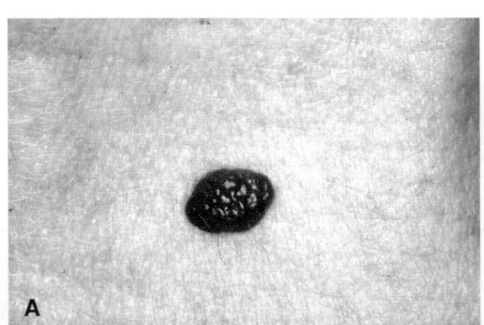
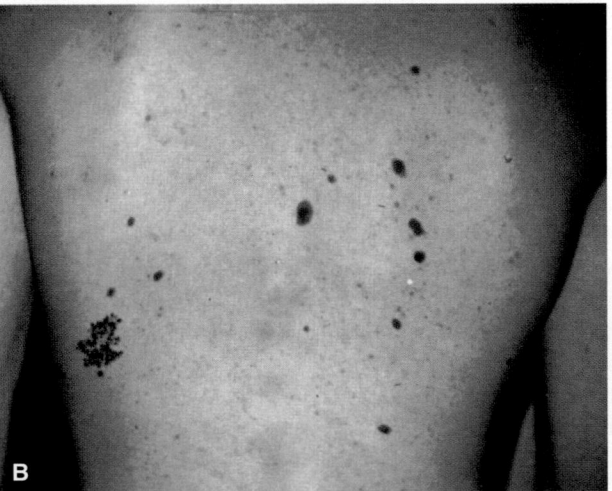

FIGURE 61-29 • **(A)** Normal mole, with no different shades of brown, black, or tan. (Centers for Disease Control and Prevention Public Health Image Library. [Online.] Available: http://phil.cdc.gov/Phil/home.asp.) **(B)** Junctional nevi on the back of a 16-year-old patient. (Owen Laboratories, Inc.) (From Sauer G. C., Hall J. C. [1996]. *Manual of skin diseases* [7th ed.]. Philadelphia: Lippincott-Raven.)

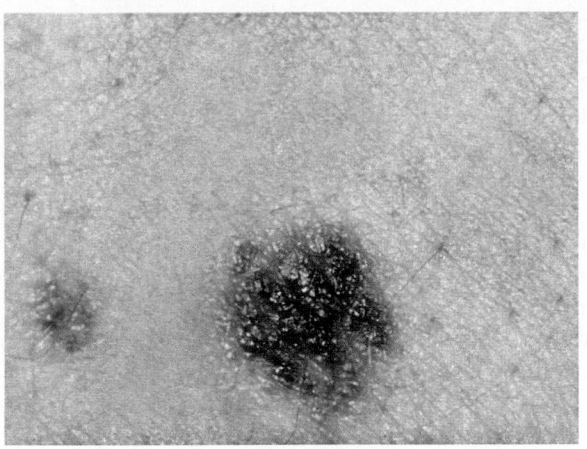

FIGURE 61-30 • Dysplastic nevi. Lesion has a dark brown "pebbly" elevated surface against a lighter tan, macular background. The irregular, indistinct margin helps to distinguish it from the small congenital-pattern nevus, which some dysplastic nevi closely resemble. Its distinct morphology, rather than its size (6 × 6 mm), identifies it as a dysplastic nevus. (National Cancer Institute Visuals. [Online.] Available: http://visualsonline.cancer.gov/browseaction. cfm?topicid=g11.)

The rising incidence of skin cancer has been attributed to increased sun exposure associated with social and lifestyle changes. The thinning of the ozone layer in the earth's stratosphere is thought to be another factor in this increased incidence. Society's emphasis on sun tanning also is implicated. People tend to have more leisure time and spend increasing amounts of time in the sun with uncovered skin.

Although the factors linking sun exposure to skin cancer are not completely understood, both total cumulative exposure and altered patterns of exposure are strongly implicated. Basal cell and squamous cell carcinomas are often associated with total cumulative exposure to UVR. Thus, basal cell and squamous cell carcinomas occur more commonly on maximally sun-exposed parts of the body, such as the face and back of the hands and forearms. Melanomas occur most commonly on areas of the body that are exposed to the sun intermittently, such as the back in men and the lower legs in women. They are more common in persons with indoor occupations whose exposure to sun is limited to weekends and vacations.

Malignant Melanoma

Malignant melanoma is a malignant tumor of the melanocytes. It is a rapidly progressing, metastatic form of cancer. The dramatic increase in the incidence of malignant melanoma over the past several decades has been credited to increased UVR exposure, including tanning salons. Fortunately, the mortality rate, which concomitantly increased, is now beginning to level off in the United States and many countries.[77] Public health screening measures, early diagnosis, increased knowledge of precursor lesions, and greater public knowledge of the disease may account for earlier intervention.

The risk is greatest in fair-skinned people, particularly those with blond or red hair who sunburn and freckle easily (see Table 61-1) African Americans, followed by Hispanics, and Asians/Pacific Islanders, have the lowest incidence rates.[77] Other risk factors include a family history of malignant melanoma, presence of marked freckling on the upper back, history of three or more blistering sunburns before 20 years of age, and presence of actinic keratoses. Still other significant risk factors for melanoma are atypical mole/dysplastic nevus syndrome, immunosuppression, and prior PUVA therapy.

Severe, blistering sunburns in early childhood and intermittent intense sun exposures (trips to sunny climates) contribute to increased susceptibility to melanoma in young and middle-aged adults. Roughly 90% of malignant melanomas in whites occur on sun-exposed skin. However, in darker-skinned people melanomas often occur on non–sun-exposed areas, such as the mucous membranes and subungual, palmar, and plantar surfaces.

Malignant melanomas differ in size and shape. Usually, they are slightly raised and black or brown. Borders are irregular and surfaces are uneven. Most seem to arise from preexisting nevi or new mole-like growths (Fig. 61-31). There may be

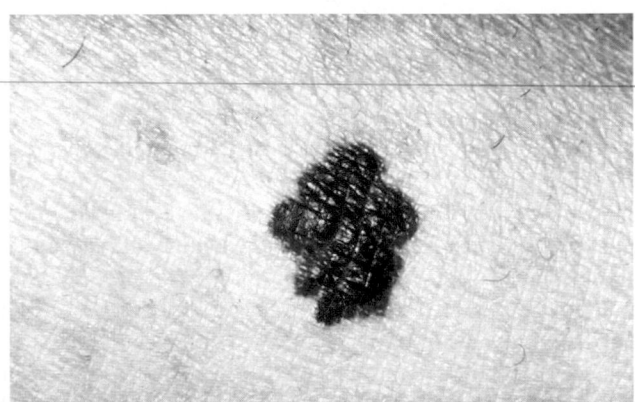

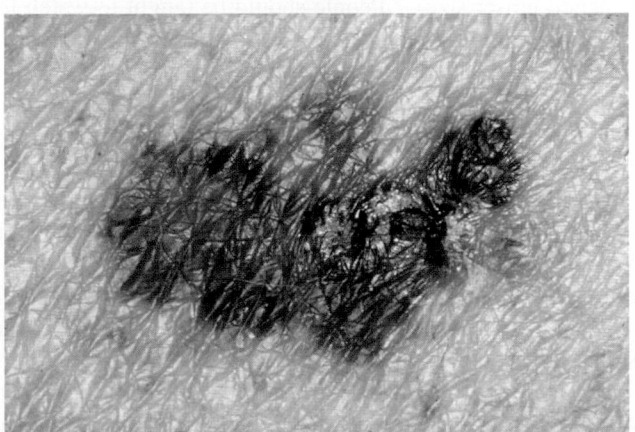

FIGURE 61-31 • Melanoma lesions, demonstrating the ABCD rule: A (asymmetry), B (irregular borders), C (different colors), and D (diameter change in size). (National Cancer Institute Visuals. [Online.] Available: http://visualsonline.cancer.gov/browseaction. cfm?topicid=g11.)

surrounding erythema, inflammation, and tenderness. Periodically, melanomas ulcerate and bleed. Dark melanomas are often mottled with shades of red, blue, and white. These three colors represent three concurrent processes: melanoma growth (blue), inflammation and the body's attempt to localize and destroy the tumor (red), and scar tissue formation (white).

Four types of melanomas have been identified: superficial spreading, nodular, lentigo maligna, and acral lentiginous.[78] *Superficial spreading melanoma* is characterized by a raised-edged nevus with lateral growth. It has a disorderly appearance in color and outline. This lesion tends to have biphasic growth, horizontally and vertically. It typically ulcerates and bleeds with growth. This type of lesion accounts for 70% to 80% of all melanomas and is most prevalent in persons who sunburn easily and have intermittent sun exposure. *Nodular melanomas,* which account for 10% to 15% of melanomas, are raised, dome-shaped lesions that can occur anywhere on the body. They are commonly a uniform blue-black color and tend to look like blood blisters. Nodular melanomas tend to rapidly invade the dermis from the start, with no apparent horizontal growth phase. *Lentigo maligna melanomas,* which account for 5% to 10% of all melanomas, are slow-growing, flat nevi that occur primarily on sun-exposed areas of elderly persons. Untreated lentigo maligna tends to exhibit horizontal and radial growth for many years before it invades the dermis to become lentigo maligna melanoma. *Acral lentiginous melanoma,* which accounts for 7% of melanomas, occurs primarily on the palms, soles, nail beds, and mucous membranes. It has the appearance of lentigo maligna.

Early detection is critical with malignant melanoma. Regular self-examination of the total skin surface in front of a well-lighted mirror provides a method for early detection. It requires that a person undress completely and examine all areas of the body using a full mirror, handheld mirror, and handheld hair dryer (to examine the scalp). An *ABCD* rule has been developed to aid in early diagnosis and timely treatment of malignant melanoma. The acronym stands for *a*symmetry, *b*order irregularity, *c*olor variegation, and *d*iameter greater than 6 mm (¼ inch or pencil eraser size).[79] People should be taught to watch for these changes in existing nevi or the development of new nevi, as well as other alterations such as bleeding or itching. Because of the existence of small-diameter melanomas (*i.e.,* <6mm in diameter), it has been suggested that people routinely screen their skin for all possible manifestations of skin cancer.

Diagnosis of melanoma is based on biopsy findings from a lesion. Consistent with other cancerous tumors, melanoma is commonly staged using the TNM (tumor, lymph node, and metastasis) staging system (see Chapter 8) or the 2002 American Joint Committee on Cancer Staging System for Cutaneous Melanoma, in which the tumor is rated 0 to 4, with further subclassifications depending on numerous factors, including extent of tumor invasion, ulceration, and metastasis.[80] Ulceration and invasion of the tumor into the deeper skin tissue result in a poorer prognosis. Although survival rates may vary with individual circumstances, the current 5-year survival rate for stage 0 melanoma is 100%; stage I melanoma, 89% to 95%; stage II melanoma, 45% to 77%; stage III melanoma, 27% to 63%; and

stage IV melanoma, 19%.[80] Early diagnosis and treatment are of extreme importance.

Treatment is usually surgical excision, the extent of which is determined by the thickness of the lesion, invasion into the deeper skin layers, and spread to the regional lymph nodes. Deep, wide excisions with elective removal of lymph tissue and the use of skin grafts were once the hallmarks of treatment.[81] When diagnosed in a premetastatic phase, melanoma is now treated in ambulatory settings, lessening the cost and inconvenience of care. Current capability allows for mapping lymph flow to a regional lymph node that receives lymphatic drainage from tumor sites on the skin. This lymph node, which is called the *sentinel lymph node,* is then sampled for biopsy. If tumor cells have spread from the primary tumor to the regional lymph nodes, the sentinel node will be the first node in which tumor cells appear. Therefore, sentinel node biopsy can be used to test for the presence of melanoma cells and determine if radical lymph node dissection is necessary. When nodes are positive, consideration is also given to systemic adjuvant therapy.

Routine cancer treatment, such as chemotherapy, is indicated when the disease becomes systemic. Despite many interventions used over the years, efforts to cure melanoma in its later stages have been disappointing. An area of active research in melanoma therapy is vaccine development or immunotherapy. Vaccines are targeted to prevent the recurrence of melanoma, especially in stages II and III. Several types of vaccines have been developed and are currently under investigation.[82]

Basal Cell Carcinoma

Basal cell carcinoma, which is a neoplasm of the nonkeratinizing cells of the basal layer of the epidermis, is the most common skin cancer in light-skinned people (Fig. 61-32). Like other skin cancers, basal cell carcinoma has increased in incidence over the past several decades. Fair-skinned persons with a history of significant long-term sun exposure are more susceptible.

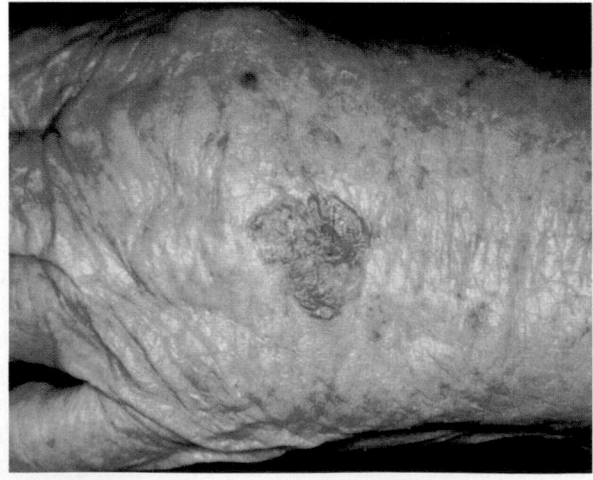

FIGURE 61-32 • Basal cell carcinoma and wrinkling of the hand. (Syntex Laboratories.) (From Sauer G. C., Hall J. C. [1996]. *Manual of skin diseases* [7th ed.]. Philadelphia: Lippincott-Raven.)

Black- and brown-skinned persons are affected occasionally. Basal cell carcinoma usually occurs in persons who were exposed to great amounts of sunlight. Of the 1,200,000 annually diagnosed skin cancers, 75% to 80% are basal cell carcinomas.[83] Basal cell carcinoma used to occur more frequently in men, but the sex difference has narrowed over recent years.[83]

Basal cell carcinoma usually is a nonmetastasizing tumor that extends wide and deep if left untreated. These tumors are most frequently seen on the head and neck, most often occurring on skin that has hair. They also occur on skin surfaces unexposed to the sun, although less frequently. Although there are several histologic types of basal cell carcinoma, nodular ulcerative and superficial basal cell carcinomas are the two most frequently occurring types. *Nodular ulcerative basal cell carcinoma* is the most common, accounting for 60% of all basal cell carcinomas.[83] It has a nodulocystic structure that begins as a small, flesh-colored or pink, smooth, translucent nodule that enlarges over time. Telangiectatic vessels frequently are seen beneath the surface. Over the years, a central depression forms that progresses to an ulcer surrounded by the original shiny, waxy border. Basal cell carcinoma in darker-skinned persons usually is darkly pigmented and frequently misdiagnosed as other skin diseases, including melanoma.

The second most common form is *superficial basal cell carcinoma,* which is seen most often on the chest or back. It begins as a flat, nonpalpable, erythematous plaque. The red, scaly areas slowly enlarge, with nodular borders and telangiectatic bases. This type of skin cancer is difficult to diagnose because it mimics other dermatologic problems.

Biopsies are obtained from all suspected basal cell carcinomas for diagnosis. It is highly curable if detected and treated early. The treatment depends on the site and extent of the lesion. The most important treatment goal is complete elimination of the lesion. Also important is the maintenance of function and optimal cosmetic effect. Curettage with electrodesiccation, surgical excision, irradiation, laser, cryosurgery, and chemosurgery are effective in removing all cancerous cells. Immune therapy, gene therapy, and photodynamic therapy are emerging treatments. Patients should be checked at regular intervals for recurrences.

Squamous Cell Carcinoma

Squamous cell carcinomas are the second most common malignant tumors of the outer epidermis and account for 10% to 20% of all skin cancers.[84] The increase in the incidence of squamous cell carcinomas is consistent with increased UVR exposure. There is also a strong occupational hazard link to the development of squamous cell carcinoma: persons exposed to arsenic (*i.e.,* Bowen disease), industrial tars, coal, and paraffin have an increased likelihood of contracting squamous cell carcinoma. Men are twice as likely as women to have squamous cell carcinoma. Black persons are rarely affected.

There are two types of squamous cell carcinoma: intraepidermal and invasive. *Intraepidermal squamous cell carcinoma* remains confined to the epidermis for a long time. However, at some unpredictable time, it penetrates the basement membrane to the dermis and metastasizes to the regional lymph nodes. It then converts to *invasive squamous cell carcinoma.* The invasive type can develop from intraepidermal carcinoma or from a premalignant lesion (*e.g.,* actinic keratoses). It may be slow growing or fast growing with metastasis.

Squamous cell carcinoma is a red-scaling, keratotic, slightly elevated lesion with an irregular border, usually with a shallow chronic ulcer (Fig. 61-33). The lesions usually lack the pearly rolled border and superficial telangiectases found on basal cell carcinomas. Later, lesions grow outward, show large ulcerations, and have persistent crusts and raised, erythematous borders. The lesions occur on sun-exposed areas of the skin, particularly the nose, forehead, helix of the ear, lower lip, and back of the hand. In dark-skinned black persons, the lesions may appear as hyperpigmented nodules and occur more frequently on non–sun-exposed areas. Metastasis is more common with squamous cell carcinoma than with basal cell carcinoma. The overall metastasis rate is 0.5% to 16%. With metastasis, the 5-year survival rate is 25%.[84]

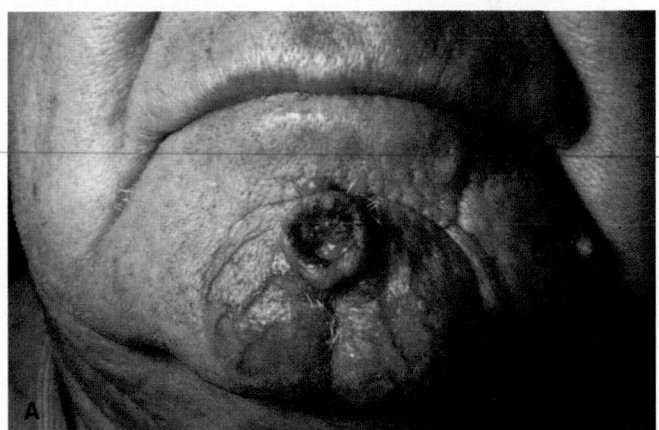

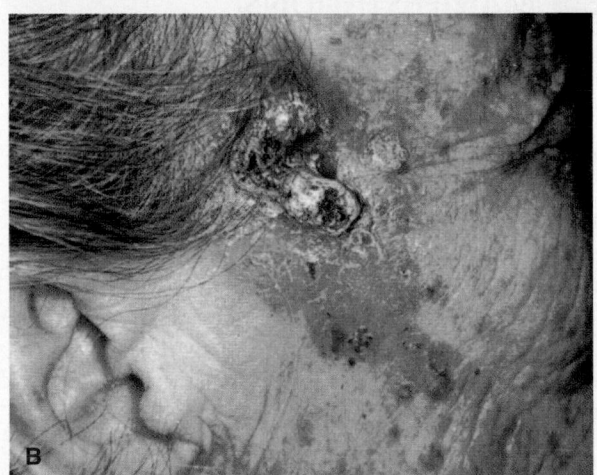

FIGURE 61-33 • **(A)** Squamous cell carcinoma of the chin. **(B)** Squamous cell carcinoma and keratosis of aged skin. (Syntex Laboratories, Westwood Pharmaceuticals.) (From Sauer G. C., Hall J. C. [1996]. *Manual of skin diseases* [7th ed.]. Philadelphia: Lippincott-Raven.)

Treatment measures are aimed at the removal of all cancerous tissue using methods such as electrosurgery, excision surgery, chemosurgery, or radiation therapy. After treatment, the person is observed for the remainder of his or her life for signs of recurrence.

IN SUMMARY, nevi or moles usually are benign. Because they may undergo cancerous transformation, any mole that undergoes a change warrants immediate medical attention. There has been an alarming increase in skin cancers over the past few decades. Repeated exposure to the UV rays of the sun has been implicated as the principal cause of skin cancer. Neoplasms of the skin include malignant melanoma, basal cell carcinoma, and squamous cell carcinoma.

Malignant melanoma is a malignant tumor of the melanocytes. It is a rapidly progressing, metastatic form of cancer. Clinically, malignant melanoma of the skin usually is asymptomatic. The most important clinical sign is the change in size, shape, and color of pigmented skin lesions, such as moles. As the result of increased public awareness, melanomas are being diagnosed earlier, when they can be cured surgically. Squamous cell carcinoma and basal cell carcinoma are of epidermal origin.

Basal cell carcinomas are the most common form of skin cancer among whites. They are slow-growing tumors that rarely metastasize. The two types of squamous cell carcinoma are intraepidermal and invasive. Intraepidermal squamous cell carcinoma remains confined to the epidermis for a long time. Invasive squamous cell carcinoma can develop from intraepidermal carcinoma or from premalignant lesions such as actinic keratoses. ■

AGE-RELATED SKIN MANIFESTATIONS

After completing this section of the chapter, you should be able to meet the following objectives:

- Differentiate a hemangioma of infancy from a port-wine stain in terms of appearance and outcome.
- Describe the manifestations and probable causes of diaper dermatitis, prickly heat, and cradle cap.
- Describe the distinguishing features of rashes associated with the following infectious childhood diseases: roseola infantum, rubeola, rubella, and varicella.
- Characterize the physiologic changes of aging skin.
- Describe the appearance of skin tags, keratoses, lentigines, and vascular lesions that are commonly seen in the elderly.

Many skin problems occur more commonly in certain age groups. Because of aging changes, infants, children, and elderly persons tend to have different skin problems.

Skin Manifestations of Infancy and Childhood

Skin Disorders of Infancy

Infancy connotes the image of perfect, unblemished skin. For the most part, this is true. However, several congenital skin lesions, such as mongolian spots, hemangiomas, and nevi, are associated with the early neonatal period. There are also several acquired skin conditions, including diaper dermatitis, prickly heat, and cradle cap, that are relatively common in infants.

Pigmented and Vascular Birthmarks. Pigmented and vascular lesions comprise most birthmarks. Pigmented birthmarks represent abnormal migration or proliferation of melanocytes. For example, *mongolian spots* are caused by selective pigmentation. They usually occur on the buttocks or sacral area and are seen commonly in Asian and black persons. *Nevi* or moles are small, tan to brown, uniformly pigmented solid macules. *Nevocellular nevi* are formed initially from aggregates of melanocytes and keratinocytes along the dermal–epidermal border. *Congenital melanocytic nevi* are collections of melanocytes that are present at birth or develop within the first year of life. They present as macular, papular, or plaquelike pigmented lesions of various shades of brown, with a black or blue focus. The texture of the lesions varies and they may be with or without hair. They usually are found on the hands, shoulders, buttocks, entire arm, or trunk of the body. Some involve large areas of the body in garment-like fashion. They usually grow proportionately with the child. Congenital melanocytic nevi are clinically significant because of their association with malignant melanoma.

Vascular birthmarks are cutaneous anomalies of angiogenesis and vascular development. Two types of vascular birthmarks commonly are seen in infants and small children: bright red, raised hemangiomas of infancy and flat, reddish-purple port-wine stains.

Hemangiomas of infancy (formerly called *strawberry hemangiomas*) are small, red lesions that are noticed shortly after birth. Hemangiomas of infancy are generally benign vascular tumors produced by proliferation of endothelial cells. Approximately 30% of these lesions are present at birth, and the remainder develop within a few weeks after birth.[85] They are seen in approximately 10% of children in the first year of life,[85] with about 60% located on the head and neck.[85] Girls are three times more likely to have hemangiomas than boys, and there is an increased incidence in premature infants (20%).[85] They also occur more frequently in white infants born to mothers of advanced maternal age, mothers with multiple gestations, and mothers with a history of chorionic villus sampling (21%).[86]

Hemangiomas of infancy typically undergo an early period of a proliferation during which they enlarge, followed by a period of slow involution where the growth is reversed until complete resolution. Hemangiomas of infancy can occur anywhere on the body; however, when they occur in the airway, they can be life-threatening. Ulceration, the most frequent complication, can be painful and carries the risk of infection, hemorrhage, and scarring. A small percentage of hemangiomas of infancy develop complications, such as infection or ulceration. Some hemangiomas of infancy are located in anatomic regions associated with other anomalies requiring careful monitoring and early intervention. Most hemangiomas of infancy disappear before 5 to 7 years of age without leaving an appreciable scar.

Port-wine stains are pink or red patches that can occur anywhere on the body and are very noticeable (Fig. 61-34). They represent slow-growing capillary malformations that grow proportionately with the child and persist throughout life. There is progressive dilation of the dermal capillaries, which initially is confined to the immediate epidermis, with gradual involvement of deeper dermal blood vessels, although the greater number is always in the upper dermis. Distribution of lesions on the face roughly corresponds to the sensory branches of the trigeminal nerve. The development of a port-wine stain may follow trauma. Port-wine stains usually are confined to the skin, but may be associated with vascular malformations of the eye, resulting primarily in glaucoma, or leptomeningeal involvement, leading to cognitive disorders, seizures, and other neurologic deficits (Sturge-Weber syndrome). Cover-up cosmetics are used in an attempt to conceal the disfiguring effects. Laser surgery has revolutionized the treatment of port-wine stains.

Diaper Dermatitis. Irritant diaper dermatitis, or *diaper rash*, is a form of contact dermatitis caused by the interaction of several factors, including prolonged contact of the skin with a mixture of urine and feces.[87,88] The wearing of diapers causes an increase in skin wetness and pH because of ammonia from urine. Prolonged wetness leads to softening and maceration of the skin, making it more susceptible to damage by friction from the surface of the diaper and local irritants. The contents of soiled diapers, if not changed frequently, can lead to contact dermatitis, bacterial infections, or other skin conditions. The proteases and lipases contained in feces are particularly irritating.

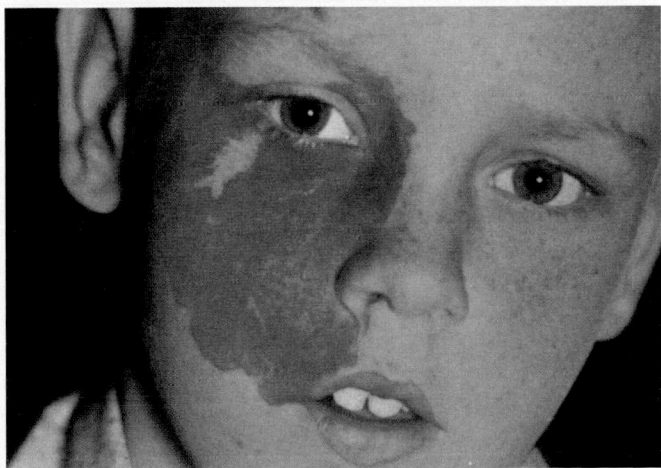

FIGURE 61-34 • Port-wine stain on the face of a boy. (Ortho Dermatology Corp.) (From Sauer G. C., Hall J. C. [1996]. *Manual of skin diseases* [7th ed.]. Philadelphia: Lippincott-Raven.)

The appearance of diaper rash ranges from simple (*i.e.,* widely distributed macules on the buttocks and anogenital areas) to severe (*i.e.,* beefy, red, excoriated skin surfaces in the diaper area). Secondary infections with bacteria and yeasts are common; discomfort may be marked because of intense inflammation. Such conditions as contact dermatitis, seborrheic dermatitis, candidiasis, and atopic dermatitis should be considered when the eruption is persistent and recalcitrant to simple therapeutic measures.

Diaper dermatitis often responds to simple measures, including frequent diaper changes with careful cleansing of the irritated area to remove all waste products. Feces in particular should be removed from the skin as soon as possible after the diaper has been soiled. Because soap and lipid solvents remove protective lipids from the stratum corneum, using water or an alcohol-free baby wipe is recommended. Exposing the irritated area to air is helpful. It has been shown that application of a barrier ointment after each diaper change is a valuable component of therapy. Topical corticosteroid therapy is usually effective, but should be used cautiously because infants absorb proportionately greater quantities through their skin than adults.[74] Antifungal therapy should not be used routinely, only when *Candida* infection is established or suspected. Antibacterial agents should not be used because it is known that bacterial infections are usually not involved in diaper dermatitis, and the normal microflora should be preserved.

Selection of a barrier preparation is important. It is now clear that the barrier function of the skin is provided by the stratum corneum, whose main function is to minimize water loss and prevent inward penetration of toxic substances and microorganisms. Ideally, a barrier should mimic the skin's natural function by forming a long-lasting barrier to increase protection against irritants and microorganisms and to maintain optimum moisture levels. Preparations should contain lipids similar to those naturally present in the stratum corneum. In general, water-in-oil formulations with a lipid content of at least 50% provide a superior moisture barrier compared with lighter oil-in-water products.[88] For this reason, ointments are generally more effective than creams and lotions. Products containing nonessential ingredients such as perfumes can cause allergic contact dermatitis and should be avoided. Inclusion of an antiseptic is not necessary or desirable. Ideally, the safety and effectiveness of a barrier product should be clinically proven.

There is controversy regarding the effects of cloth versus disposable diapers in preventing diaper rash. In the early days of disposable diapers, infants who wore cloth diapers without plastic pants had fewer diaper rashes than those who wore disposable diapers. It has been suggested that this may not be true with the newer disposable diapers that use absorbent gelling material.[87,88] These superabsorbent diapers have the smallest increase in skin wetness compared with conventional disposable diapers and cloth diapers. When cloth diapers are used, they should be washed in gentle detergent and thoroughly rinsed to remove all traces of waste products. Plastic pants should be discouraged.

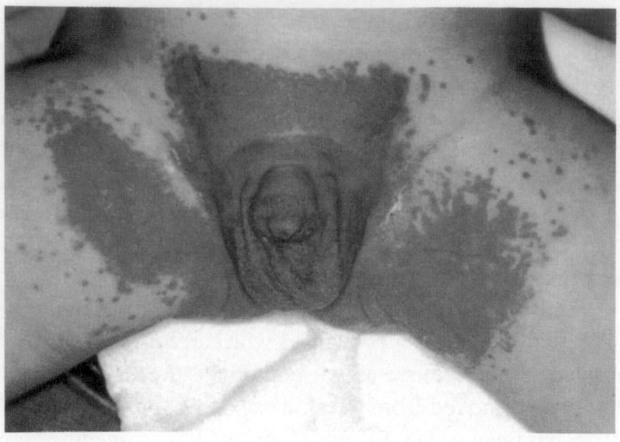

FIGURE 61-35 • Candidal intertrigo after a course of oral antibiotics in a 1-year-old child. (Owen Laboratories, Inc.) (From Sauer G. C., Hall J. C. [1996]. *Manual of skin diseases* [7th ed.]. Philadelphia: Lippincott-Raven.)

Intractable and severe cases of diaper dermatitis should be seen by a health care provider for treatment of any secondary infections. Secondary candidal (*i.e.,* yeast; Fig. 61-35) or other skin manifestations discussed in this chapter may occur in the diaper area. It is important to differentiate between normal diaper dermatitis and more serious skin problems.

Prickly Heat. Prickly heat (heat rash) results from constant maceration of the skin because of prolonged exposure to a warm, humid environment. Maceration leads to mid-epidermal obstruction and rupture of the sweat glands (Fig. 61-36). Although commonly seen during infancy, prickly heat may occur at any age. The treatment includes removing excessive clothing, cooling the skin with warm water baths, drying the skin with powders, and avoiding hot, humid environments.

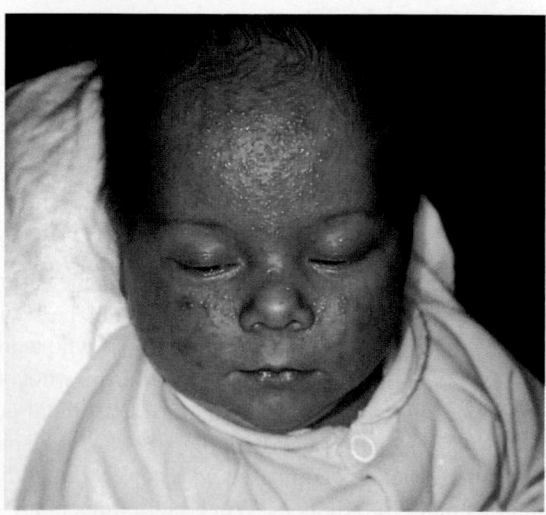

FIGURE 61-36 • Prickly heat in a 6-week-old infant. (From Hall J. C. [2000]. *Sauer's manual of skin diseases* [8th ed., p. 407]. Philadelphia: Lippincott Williams & Wilkins.)

Cradle Cap. Cradle cap is a greasy crust or scale formation on the scalp. It usually is attributed to infrequent and inadequate washing of the scalp. Cradle cap is treated using mild shampoo and gentle combing to remove the scales. Sometimes oil can be left on the head for minutes to several hours, softening the scales before scrubbing. Other emulsifying ointments or creams may be helpful in difficult cases. The scalp may need to be rubbed firmly to remove the buildup of keratinized cells. Recalcitrant cases need to be seen by a health care practitioner; serious or chronic forms of seborrheic dermatitis may exist.

Skin Manifestations of Common Infectious Diseases

Infectious childhood diseases that produce rashes include exanthem subitum, rubella, rubeola, varicella, and scarlet fever. Although these diseases are seen less frequently because of successful immunization programs and the use of antibiotics, they still occur.

Roseloa Infantum. Roseola infantum (exanthem subitum or sixth disease) is a contagious disease caused by human herpes virus type 6 (HHV-6). Because HHV-6 is the etiologic agent, the condition is often referred to as *sixth disease.* Primary HHV-6 infection occurs early in life. More than 95% of roseola cases occur in children younger than 3 years of age, with a peak at 6 to 15 months of age.[89] Transplacental antibodies likely protect most infants until 6 months of age. Roseola produces a characteristic maculopapular rash covering the trunk and spreading to the appendages. The rash is preceded by an abrupt onset of high fever ($\leq$105°F), inflamed tympanic membranes, and coldlike symptoms usually lasting 3 to 4 days. These symptoms improve at approximately the same time the rash appears. Because infants with roseola exhibit a unique constellation of symptoms over a short time, the infection may be confused with other childhood exanthems. Blood antibody titers may be taken to determine the actual diagnosis. In most cases, there are no long-term effects from this disease. Infants who spike high temperatures should be seen by their health care providers.

Rubella. Rubella (*i.e.,* 3-day measles or German measles) is a childhood disease caused by the rubella virus (a togavirus). It is characterized by a diffuse, punctate, macular rash that begins on the trunk and spreads to the arms and legs (Fig. 61-37). Mild febrile states occur (usually <100°F). Postauricular, suboccipital, and cervical lymph node adenopathy is common. Coldlike symptoms usually accompany the disease in the form of cough, congestion, and coryza (*i.e.,* nasal discharge).

Rubella usually has no long-lasting sequelae; however, the transmission of the disease to pregnant women early in their gestation periods may result in congenital rubella syndrome. Among the clinical signs of congenital rubella syndrome are cataracts, microcephaly, mental retardation, deafness, patent ductus arteriosus, glaucoma, purpura, and bone defects. Most states have laws requiring immunization to prevent transmission of rubella. Immunization is accomplished by live-virus injection. Rubella vaccination has close to a 100% immunity response in treated children.[90] Many states require a second preschool or later dose of rubella vaccine to increase immunity. Cases and outbreaks of rubella occur in the United States, especially among foreign-born unvaccinated adults.

Rubeola. Rubeola (measles, hard measles, 7-day measles) is an acute, highly communicable viral disease caused by a morbillivirus. The characteristic rash is macular and blotchy; sometimes the macules become confluent (Fig. 61-38). The rubeola rash usually begins on the face and spreads to the appendages. There are several accompanying symptoms: a fever of 100°F or greater, *Koplik spots* (*i.e.,* small, irregular red spots with a bluish-white speck in the center) on the buccal mucosa, and mild to severe photosensitivity. The patient commonly has coldlike symptoms, general malaise, and myalgia. In severe cases, the macules may hemorrhage into the skin tissue or onto the outer body surface. This form is called *hemorrhagic measles*. The course of measles is more severe in infants, adults, and malnourished children. The World Health Organization recommends vitamin A treatment for measles in developing countries to reduce morbidity and mortality. There may be severe complications, including otitis media, pneumonia, and encephalitis. Antibody titers are determined for a conclusive diagnosis of rubeola.

Measles is a disease preventable by vaccine, and immunization is required by law in the United States. Immunization is accomplished by the injection of a live-virus vaccine. Measles vaccination produces close to 100% immunity.[90]

Varicella. Varicella (chickenpox) is a common communicable childhood disease. It is caused by the varicella-zoster virus, which also is the agent in herpes zoster (shingles). The charac-

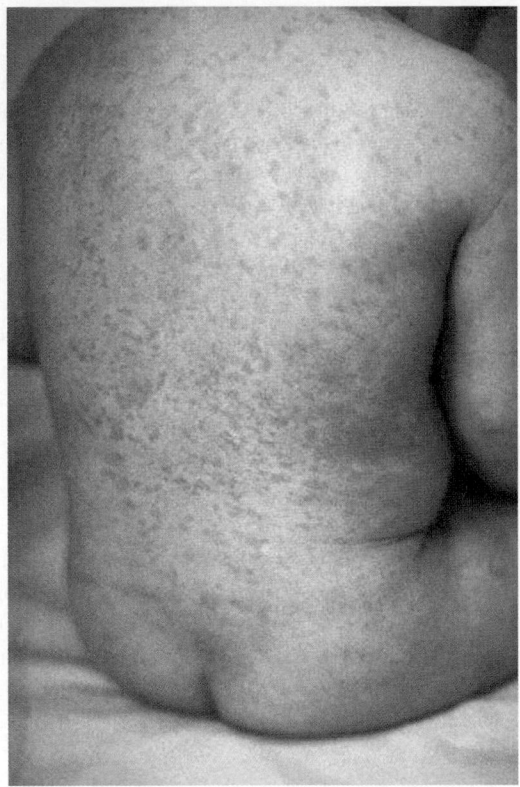

FIGURE 61-37 • Rash of rubella on a child's back. Distribution is similar to measles (rubeola), but not as intense. (Centers for Disease Control and Prevention Public Health Image Library. [Online.] Available: http://phil.cdc.gov/Phil/home.asp.)

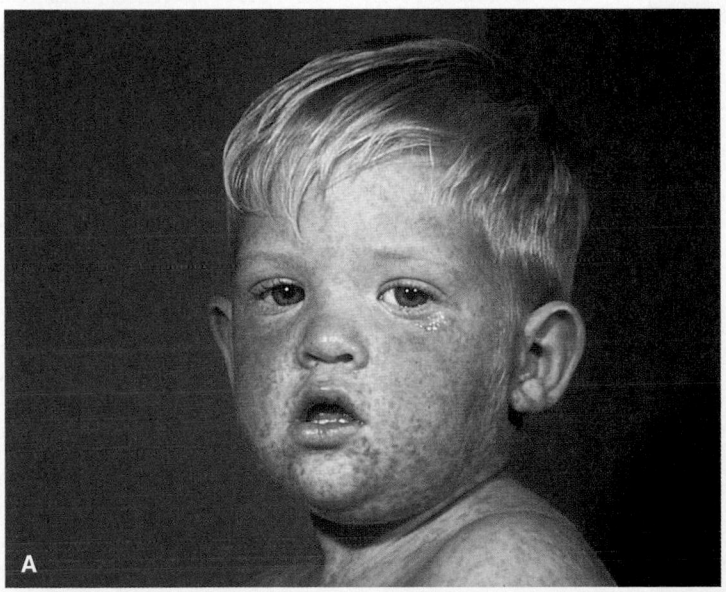
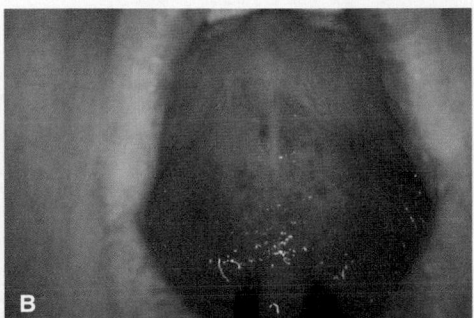

FIGURE 61-38 • (A) Child with measles (rubeola) showing the characteristic conjunctivitis, coryza, and red, blotchy rash that appear around day 3 of illness, first on the face and then becoming more generalized. (B) Koplik spots (irregularly shaped, bright red spots often with a bluish-white central dot), indicative of the beginning onset of rubeola. (Centers for Disease Control and Prevention Public Health Image Library. [Online.] Available: http://phil.cdc.gov/Phil/home.asp.)

teristic skin lesion occurs in three stages: macule, vesicle, and granular scab. The macular stage is characterized by development within hours of macules over the trunk, spreading to the limbs, buccal mucosa, scalp, axillae, upper respiratory tract, and conjunctiva. (Fig. 61-39). During the second stage, the macules form vesicles with depressed centers. The vesicles break open and a scab forms during the third stage. Crops of lesions occur successively, so that all three forms of the lesion usually are visible by the third day of the illness.

Mild to extreme pruritus accompanies the lesions, which can lead to scratching and subsequent development of secondary bacterial infections. Chickenpox also is accompanied by coldlike symptoms, including cough, coryza, and sometimes photosensitivity. Mild febrile states usually occur, typically beginning 24 hours before lesion outbreak. Side effects, such as pneumonia, septic complications, and encephalitis, are rare.

Varicella in adults may be more severe, with a prolonged recovery rate and greater chances for development of varicella pneumonitis or encephalitis. Immunocompromised persons may experience a chronic, painful form of the infection.

Live attenuated varicella vaccine has been demonstrated to have a lower efficacy (84%) than vaccines such as rubella and rubeola in preventing the disease.[90] There has been a dramatic decrease (71% to 84% decrease)[91] in varicella morbidity and mortality since 1995, when the varicella vaccine was intro-

duced in the United States. However, outbreaks of mild cases of varicella, called *breakthrough varicella,* have occurred in vaccinated populations. The breakthrough infection is difficult to diagnose because the maculopapular rash does not have the classic sign of vesicles. One dose of the vaccine is required by law in the United States; however, a second dose is now recommended to address what is called *primary vaccine failure.* Without a second dose, an estimated 200,000 vaccinees will remain susceptible annually, and 2 million adolescents and young adults will become susceptible in 10 years.[92] It is believed that a single dose of varicella vaccine may only prime the host response, without inducing protective immunity.[92]

Skin Manifestations and Disorders in the Elderly

Elderly persons experience a variety of age-related skin disorders and exacerbations of earlier skin problems. Aging skin is believed to involve a complex process of actinic (solar) damage, normal aging, and hormonal influences. Actinic changes primarily involve increased occurrence of lesions on sun-exposed surfaces of the body.

Normal Age-Related Changes

Normal skin changes associated with aging are seen on areas of the body that have not been exposed to the sun. They include thinning of the dermis and the epidermis, diminution in subcutaneous tissue, a decrease and thickening of blood vessels, and a decrease in the number of melanocytes, Langerhans cells, and Merkel cells. The keratinocytes shrink, but the number of dead keratinized cells at the surface increases. This results in less padding and thinner skin, with color and elasticity changes. The skin also loses its resistance to environmental and mechanical trauma. Tissue repair takes longer.

With aging, there is also less hair and nail growth, and there is permanent hair pigment loss. Hormonally, there is less sebaceous gland activity, although the glands in the facial skin may increase in size. Hair growth reduction also may be hormonally influenced. Although the reason is poorly understood, the skin in most elderly persons older than 70 years of age becomes dry, rough, scaly, and itchy. When there is no underlying pathologic process, it is called *senile pruritus.* Itching and dryness become worse during the winter, when the need for home heating lowers the humidity.

The aging of skin, however, is not just a manifestation of age itself. Most skin changes associated with the elderly are the result of cumulative actinic or environmental damage. For example, the wrinkled, leathery look of aged skin, as well as odd scars and ecchymotic spots, are due to solar elastotic degenerative change.

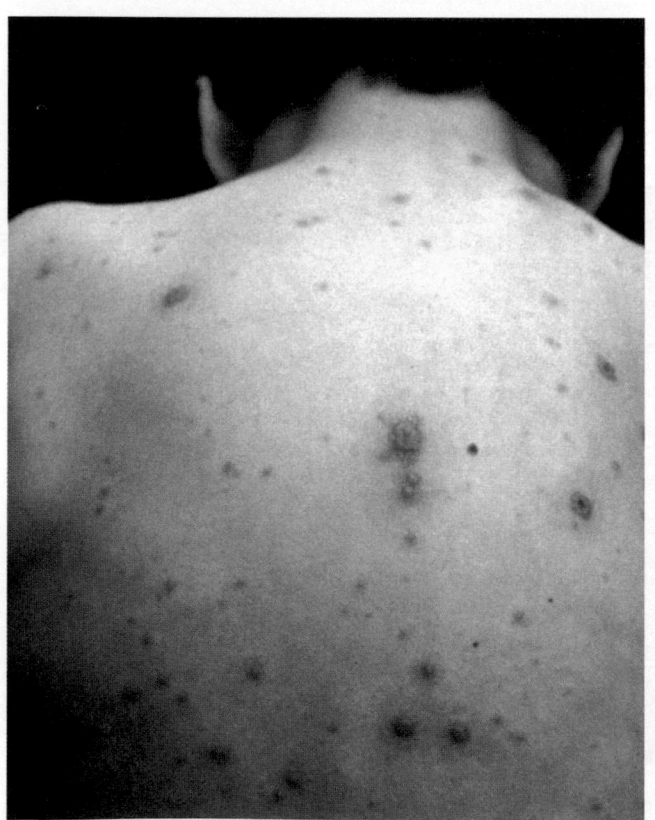

FIGURE 61-39 • Blister-like rash on the back of a person with varicella-zoster (*i.e.,* chickenpox). (Centers for Disease Control and Prevention Public Health Image Library. [Online.] Available: http://phil.cdc.gov/Phil/home.asp.)

Skin Lesions Common Among the Elderly

The most common skin lesions in the elderly are skin tags, keratoses, lentigines, and vascular lesions. Most are actinic manifestations; they occur as a result of exposure to sun and weather over the years.

Skin Tags. Skin tags are soft, brown or flesh-colored papules. They occur on any skin surface, but most frequently the neck, axilla, and intertriginous areas. They range in size from a pinhead to the size of a pea. Skin tags have the normal texture of the skin. They are benign and can be removed with scissors or electrodesiccation for cosmetic purposes.

Keratoses. A *keratosis* is a horny growth or an abnormal growth of the keratinocytes. A *seborrheic keratosis* (*i.e.,* seborrheic wart) is a benign, sharply circumscribed, wartlike lesion that has a stuck-on appearance (Fig. 61-40). They vary in size up to several centimeters. They are usually round or oval, tan, brown, or black lesions. Less pigmented ones may appear yellow or pink. Keratoses can be found on the face or trunk, as a solitary lesion or sometimes by the hundreds. Seborrheic keratoses are benign, but they must be watched for changes in color, texture, or size, which may indicate malignant transformation.

Actinic keratoses are the most common premalignant skin lesions that develop on sun-exposed areas. The lesions usually are less than 1 cm in diameter and appear as dry, brown, scaly areas, often with a reddish tinge. Actinic keratoses often are multiple and more easily felt than seen (Fig. 61-41). They often are indistinguishable from squamous cell carcinoma without biopsy. Actinic keratoses may accumulate dense scale on the surface of the skin and become hyperkeratotic (*i.e.,* developing cutaneous growths of fingernail-type tissue that grow into hornlike appendages). This form is more prominent and palpable. Often, there is a weathered appearance to the surrounding skin. Slight changes, such as enlargement or ulceration, may indicate malignant transformation. Roughly 20% of actinic keratoses convert to squamous cell carcinomas. There is controversy regarding the classification of actinic keratoses. Some believe them to be capable of converting to cancerous growths,[93] some

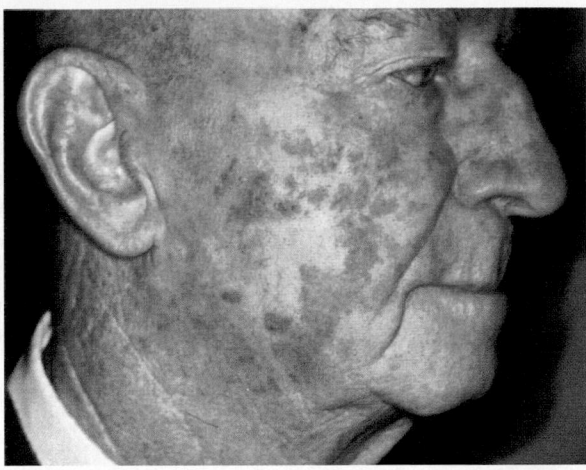

FIGURE 61-41 • Multiple actinic keratoses of the face of an 80-year-old man. (Dermik Laboratories, Inc.) (from Sauer G. C., Hall J. C. [1996]. *Manual of skin diseases* [7th ed.]. Philadelphia: Lippincott-Raven.)

believe them to be on a continuum of cancerous growth,[94] still others believe that actinic keratoses do not convert or progress to cancerous cells, but that they are actual early malignancies.[95,96] Actinic keratoses are removed with cryosurgery, electrodesiccation, or lasers. When surgery is not indicated they are treated with topical chemotherapy agents, like 5-fluorouracil or imiquimod creams, which erode the lesions.

Lentigines. A *lentigo* is a well-bordered, brown to black macule, usually less than 1 cm in diameter. *Solar lentigines* are tan to brown, benign spots on sun-exposed areas. Commonly referred to as *liver spots,* these lesions are considered risks for the development of skin cancers. Lentigines can be removed surgically (cryotherapy, laser therapy, liquid nitrogen). Topical creams and lotions containing adapalene or tretinoin have been used. Topical hydroquinone (*e.g.,* Eldoquin, Solaquin) temporarily bleaches the spots. These agents inhibit the synthesis of new pigment without destroying existing pigment. Higher concentrations are available by prescription. Successful treatment depends on avoiding sun exposure and consistently using sunscreens.

Lentigo maligna (*i.e.,* Hutchinson freckle) is a slowly progressive (≤20 years) preneoplastic disorder of melanocytes. It occurs on sun-exposed areas, particularly the face. The lesion is a pigmented macule with a well-defined border and grows to 5 cm or sometimes larger. As it grows over the years, it may become slightly raised and wartlike. If untreated, a true malignant melanoma often develops. Surgery, curettage, and cryotherapy have been effective at removing the lentigines. Careful monitoring for conversion to melanoma is important.

Vascular Lesions. Vascular lesions include angiomas, telangiectases, and venous lakes. *Cherry angiomas* are smooth, cherry-red or purple, dome-shaped papules that occur in nearly all people older than 30 years of age. They usually are found on the trunk and are generally benign unless there is a sudden appear-

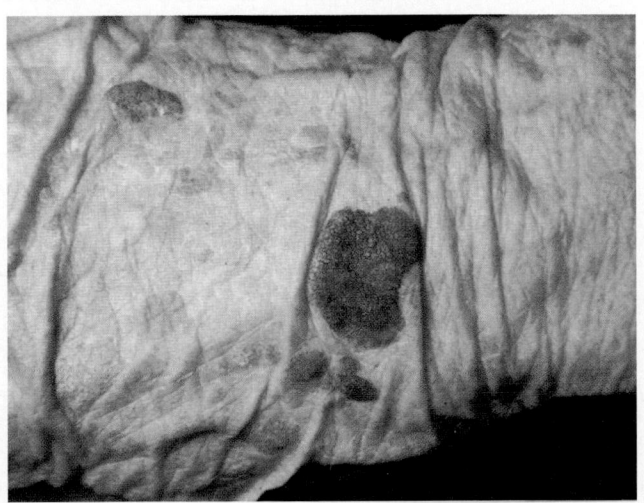

FIGURE 61-40 • Large seborrheic keratoses on the hand of an 84-year-old woman. (From Sauer G. C., Hall J. C. [1996]. *Manual of skin diseases* [7th ed.]. Philadelphia: Lippincott-Raven.)

ance of many cherry angiomas. *Telangiectases* are single dilated blood vessels, capillaries, or terminal arteries that appear on areas exposed to sun or harsh weather, such as the cheeks and the nose. They occur individually or in clusters, measure 1 cm or less, are nonpalpable, and easily blanch. They can become large and disfiguring. Pulsed dye lasers have been effective in removing them. *Venous lakes* are small, dark blue, slightly raised papules that have a lakelike appearance. They occur on exposed body parts, particularly the backs of the hands, ears, and lips. They are smooth and compressible. Venous lakes can be removed by electrosurgery, laser therapy, or surgical excision if a person desires.

IN SUMMARY, some skin problems occur in specific age groups. Common in infants are diaper rash, prickly heat, and cradle cap. Infectious childhood diseases that are characterized by rashes include roseola infantum, rubella, rubeola, varicella, and scarlet fever. Vaccines are available to protect against rubella, rubeola, and varicella.

With aging, there is thinning of the dermis and the epidermis, diminution in subcutaneous tissue, loss and thickening of blood vessels, and slowing of hair and nail growth. Dry skin is common among the elderly, becoming worse during the winter months. Among the skin lesions seen in the elderly are skin tags, keratoses, lentigines, and vascular lesions. ■

3. Psoriasis is a chronically recurring papulosquamous skin disorder, characterized by circumscribed red, thickened plaques with an overlying silvery-white scale.

   A. *Explain the development of the plaques in terms of epidermal cell turnover.*

   B. *Persons with psoriasis are instructed to refrain from rubbing or scratching the lesions. Explain the rationale for these instructions.*

   C. *Among the methods used in the treatment of psoriasis are the use of topical keratolytic agents and corticosteroid skin preparations. Explain how these two different types of agents exert their effect on the plaque lesions.*

4. During the past several decades there has been an alarming increase in the incidence of skin cancers, including malignant melanoma, that has been attributed to increased sun exposure.

   A. *Explain the possible mechanisms whereby ultraviolet radiation promotes the development of malignant skin lesions.*

   B. *Cite two important clinical signs that aid in distinguishing a dysplastic nevus from a malignant melanoma.*

Review Exercises

1. The mother of a 7-year-old boy notices that he is scratching his head frequently. On close examination she notices a grayish, round, and roughened area, where the hair has broken off. Examination by the child's pediatrician produces a diagnosis of tinea capitis.

   A. *Explain the cause of the infection and propose possible mechanisms for spread of this infection in school-age children, particularly during winter months.*

   B. *Referring to Chapter 16, explain the preference of the superficial mycoses (dermatophytoses) for the skin-covered areas of the body.*

   C. *What methods are commonly used in the diagnosis of superficial fungal infections?*

2. A 75-year-old woman presents with severe burning pain and a vesicular rash covering a strip over the rib cage on one side of the chest. She is diagnosed with herpes zoster or shingles.

   A. *What is the source of this woman's rash and pain?*

   B. *Explain the dermatomal distribution of the lesions.*

References

1. Taneja A. (2002). Treatment of vitiligo. *Journal of Dermatological Treatment* 13, 19–25.
2. Njoo D. M., Westerhof W. (2001). Vitiligo: Pathogenesis and treatment. *American Journal of Clinical Dermatology* 2, 167–181.
3. Okulicz J. F., Shah R. S., Schwartz R. A., et al. (2003). Oculocutaneous albinism. *Pigment Cell Research* 16, 307–311.
4. Magill S. S., Manfredi L., Swiderski A., et al. (2007). Isolation of *Trichophyton violaceum* and *Trichophyton soudanense* in Baltimore, Maryland. *Journal of Clinical Microbiology* 45, 461–465.
5. Habif T. P., Campbell J. L., Chapman M. S., et al. (Eds.). (2005). *Skin disease: Diagnosis and treatment* (pp. 258–261). Philadelphia: Mosby.
6. Roberts G. J., Friedlander S. F. (2005). Tinea capitis: A treatment update. *Pediatric Annals* 34, 191–200.
7. Gupta A. K., Ryder J. E., Lynch L. E., et al. (2005). The use of terbinafine in the treatment of onychomycosis in adults and special populations: A review of the evidence. *Journal of Drugs in Dermatology* 4, 302–308.
8. Warshaw E. M. (2006). Evaluating costs for onychomycosis treatments: A practitioner's perspective. *Journal of the American Podiatric Medical Association* 96, 38–52.
9. Hay R. J., Moore M. K. (2004). Mycology. In Burns T., Breathnach S., Cox N., et al. (Eds.), *Rook's textbook of dermatology* (7th ed., Vol. 2, pp. 31.1–31.101). Malden, MA: Blackwell.
10. Sterling J. C. (2004). Virus infections. In Burns T., Breathnach S., Cox N., et al. (Eds.), *Rook's textbook of dermatology* (7th ed., Vol. 2, p. 25.38). Malden, MA: Blackwell.
11. Lipke M. M. (2006). An armamentarium of wart treatments. *Clinical Medicine and Research* 4, 273–293.
12. Rudolph R. I. (2003). Warts and duct tape: A good combo! [Comment]. *Archives of Pediatric and Adolescent Medicine* 157, 489.

13. Burkhart C. G. (2005). Herpes acquisition and transmission. *Journal of Drugs in Dermatology* 4, 378–383.

14. Koelle D. M., Corey L. (2003). Recent progress in herpes simplex virus immunobiology and vaccine research. *Clinical Microbiology Reviews* 16, 96–113.

15. Weaver B. A. (2007). The burden of herpes zoster and postherpetic neuralgia in the United States. *Journal of the American Osteopathic Association* 107, S2–S7.

16. Holcomb K., Weinberg J. M. (2006). A novel vaccine (Zostavax) to prevent herpes zoster and postherpetic neuralgia. *Journal of Drugs in Dermatology* 5, 863–866.

17. Sterling J. C. (2004). Virus infections. In Burns T., Breathnach S., Cox N., et al. (Eds.), *Rook's textbook of dermatology* (7th ed., Vol. 2, pp. 25.25–25.26). Malden, MA: Blackwell.

18. Oxman M. N., Levin M. J., Johnson G. R., et al., Shingles Prevention Study Group. (2005). A vaccine to prevent herpes zoster and postherpetic neuralgia in older adults. *New England Journal of Medicine* 352, 2271–2284.

19. James W. D. (2005). Acne. *New England Journal of Medicine* 352, 1463–1472.

20. Feldman S., Careccia R. E., Barkham K. L. (2004). Diagnosis and treatment of acne. *American Family Physician* 69, 2123–2130, 2135–2136.

21. Yan A. C. (2006). Current concepts on acne management. *Adolescent Medicine Clinics* 17, 613–637.

22. Zaenglein A. L., Thiboutot D. M. (2006). Expert committee recommendations for acne management. *Pediatrics* 118, 1188–1199.

23. Burkhart C. N., Burkhart C. G. (2003). Microbiology's principle of biofilms as a major factor in the pathogenesis of acne vulgaris. *International Journal of Dermatology* 42, 925–927.

24. Ceilley R. I. (2004). Advances in the topical treatment of acne and rosacea. *Journal of Drugs in Dermatology* 3, S12–S22.

25. Del Rosso J. Q. (2004). Medical treatment of rosacea with emphasis on topical therapies. *Expert Opinion on Pharmacotherapy* 5, 5–13.

26. Szlachcic A. (2002). The link between *Helicobacter pylori* infection and rosacea. *Journal of the European Academy of Dermatology and Venereology* 16, 328–333.

27. Dahl M. V. (2004). Rosacea subtypes: A treatment algorithm. *Cutis* 74(3), 21–27.

28. Blount B. W., Pelletter A. L. (2002). Rosacea: A common, yet commonly overlooked, condition. *American Family Physician* 66, 435–442.

29. Davis M. (2007). Top 10 causes of allergic contact dermatitis. *Allergy & Asthma Today* 5(1), 44.

30. Lisby S., Baadsgaard O. (2006). Mechanisms of irritant contact dermatitis (pp. 69–82). In Frosch P. J., Menne T., Lepoittevin J. P. (Eds.), *Contact dermatitis* (4th ed.). New York: Springer.

31. Leung D. Y. M., Boguniewicz M., Howell M. D., et al. (2004). New insights into atopic dermatitis. *Journal of Clinical Investigation* 113, 651–657.

32. Boguniewicz M. (2005). Atopic dermatitis: Beyond the itch that rashes. *Immunology and Allergy Clinics of North America* 25, 333–351.

33. Williams H. C. (2005). Atopic dermatitis. *New England Journal of Medicine* 352, 2314–2324.

34. Akdis C. A., Akdis M., Bieber T., et al., PRACTALL Consensus Group. (2006). Diagnosis and treatment of atopic dermatitis in children and adults: European Academy of Allergology and Clinical Immunology/American Academy of Allergy, Asthma and Immunology/PRACTALL Consensus Report. *Allergy* 61, 969–987.

35. Schuerman G., Vezeau T. (2007). All bugs aren't bad: Probiotics in the treatment of pediatric atopic dermatitis. *American Journal for Nurse Practitioners* 11(4), 28–36.

36. Yates C. (2002). Parameters for the treatment of urticaria and angioedema. *Journal of the American Academy of Nurse Practitioners* 14, 478–747.

37. Kaplan A. P. (2002). Chronic urticaria and angioedema. *New England Journal of Medicine* 346, 175–179.

38. Kozel M. M. A., Sabroe R. A. (2004). Chronic urticaria. *Drugs* 64, 2615–2636.

39. Muller B. A. (2004). Urticaria and angioedema: A practical approach. *American Family Physician* 69, 1123–1128.

40. Letko E., Papaliodis D. N., Papaliodis G. N., et al. (2005). Stevens-Johnson syndrome and toxic epidermal necrolysis: A review of the literature. *Annals of Allergy, Asthma, & Immunology* 94, 419–436.

41. Khalili B., Bahna S. L. (2006). Pathogenesis and recent therapeutic trends in Stevens-Johnson syndrome and toxic epidermal necrolysis. *Annals of Allergy, Asthma, & Immunology* 97, 272–281.

42. Camisa C. (2004). *Handbook of psoriasis* (pp. 328–329). Malden, MA: Blackwell.

43. Galadari H., Fuchs B., Lebwohl M. (2003). Newly available treatments for psoriatic arthritis and their impact on skin psoriasis. *International Journal of Dermatology* 42, 231–237.

44. Lebwohl M. (2003). Psoriasis. *Lancet* 363, 1197–1204.

45. Galadari H., Fuchs B., Lebwohl M. (2003). Newly available treatments for psoriatic arthritis and their impact on skin psoriasis. *International Journal of Dermatology* 42, 231–237.

46. Wong L., Freeman S. (2003). Oral lichenoid lesions (OLL) and mercury in amalgam fillings. *Contact Dermatitis* 48, 74–79.

47. Cook A. M., Romanelli F. (2003). Ivermectin for the treatment of resistant scabies. *Annals of Pharmacotherapy* 37, 279–281.

48. Burgess I. F., Pollack R. J., Taplin D. (2003). *Cutting through controversy: Special report on the treatment of head lice* (pp. 10–11). Morristown, NJ: Premier Healthcare Resource.

49. Goates B. M., Atkin J. S., Wilding K. G., et al. (2006). An effective nonchemical treatment for head lice: A lot of hot air. *Pediatrics* 118, 1962–1970.

50. Burkhart C. N., Burkhart C. G. (2005). Head lice: Scientific assessment of the nit sheath with clinical ramifications and therapeutic options. *Journal of the American Academy of Dermatology* 53, 129–133.

51. Schoessler S. Z. (2004). Treating and managing head lice: The school nurse perspective. *American Journal of Managed Care* 10, S273–S276.

52. Frankowski B. L. (2004). American Academy of Pediatrics guidelines for the prevention and treatment of head lice infestation. *American Journal of Managed Care* 10, S269–S272.

53. Glogau R. G. (2004). *Photoaging and aging skin*. In Rigel D. S., Weiss R. A., Lim H. W., et al. (Eds.), *Photoaging* (pp. 65–72). New York: Marcel Dekker.

54. Moyal D., Fourtanier A. (2004). Acute and chronic effects of UV on skin: What are they and how to study them? In Rigel D. S., Weiss R. A., Lim H. W., et al. (Eds.), *Photoaging* (pp. 15–32). New York: Marcel Dekker.

55. Hawk J. L. M., Young A. R., Ferguson J. (2004). Cutaneous photobiology. In Burns T., Breathnach S., Cox N., et al. (Eds.), *Rook's textbook of dermatology* (7th ed., Vol. II, pp. 24.1–24.24). Malden, MA: Blackwell.

56. Saraiya M., Balluz L., Wen X. J., et al. (2007). Sunburn prevalence among adults: United States, 1999, 2003, and 2004. *Morbidity and Mortality Weekly Report* 56, 524–528.

57. Lim H. W., Thomas L., Rigel D. S. (2004). Photoprotection. In Rigel D. S., Weiss R. A., Lim H. W., et al. (Eds.), *Photoaging* (pp. 73–88). New York: Marcel Dekker.

58. Centers for Disease Control and Prevention. (2006). Skin cancer: Questions and answers. [Online.] Available: www.cdc.gov/cancer/skin/chooseyourcover/qanda.htm#how. Accessed April 18, 2008.

59. Morrison W. L. (2003). Photoprotection by clothing. *Dermatologic Therapy* 16, 16–22.

60. Behrman R. E., Kliegman R. M, Jenson H. B. (Eds.). (2004). *Nelson textbook of pediatrics* (17th ed., pp. 330–337, 1026–1034, 1057–1059, 1069–1072). Philadelphia: Elsevier Saunders.

61. Morgan E. D., Bledsoe S. C., Barker J. (2000). Ambulatory management of burns. *American Family Physician* 62, 2015–2026, 2029–2030.

62. Mertens D. M., Jenkins M. E., Warden G. D. (1997). Outpatient burn management. *Nursing Clinics of North America* 32, 343–346.

63. Benson A., Dickson W. A., Boyce D .E. (2006). ABC of wound healing: Burns. *BMJ* 332, 649–755.

64. Monafo W. W. (1996). Initial management of burns. *New England Journal of Medicine* 335, 1581–1585.

65. Allison K., Porter K. (2004). Consensus on the prehospital approach to burns: Patient management. *Emergency Medicine Journal* 21, 112–114.

66. Gordon M., Goodwin C. W. (1997). Initial assessment, management, and stabilization. *Nursing Clinics of North America* 32, 237–249.

67. Parenteau N. (1999). Skin: The first tissue-engineered products. *Scientific American* 280(4), 83–84.

68. Arnold M. C. (2003). Pressure ulcer prevention and management. *AACN Clinical Issues* 14, 411–428.

69. Maklebust J. (2005). Pressure ulcers: The great insult. *Nursing Clinics of North America* 40, 365–389.

70. National Institutes of Health. (2008). Healthy people 2010. [Online.] Available: www.health.gov/healthypeople. Accessed April 18, 2008.

71. Panel for the Prediction and Prevention of Pressure Ulcers in Adults. (1992). *Pressure ulcers in adults: Prediction and prevention.* Clinical practice guideline no. 3. AHCPR publication no. 92-0047. Rockville, MD: U.S. Department of Health and Human Services. Public Health Service, Agency for Health Care Policy and Research.

72. Bergstrom N., Bennett M. A., Carlson C. E., et al. (1994). *Treatment of pressure ulcers.* Clinical practice guideline no. 15. AHCPR publication no. 95-0652. Rockville, MD: U.S. Department of Health and Human Services. Public Health Service, Agency for Health Care Policy and Research.

73. National Pressure Ulcer Advisory Panel. (2003). Staging report. [Online.] Available: http://www.npuap.org/archive/positn6.htm. Accessed September 22, 2005.

74. Cannon B. C., Cannon J. P. (2004). Management of pressure ulcers. *American Journal of Health-System Pharmacists* 61, 1895–1905.

75. Thomas D. R. (2001). Prevention and treatment of pressure ulcers: What works? What doesn't? *Cleveland Clinic Journal of Medicine* 68, 704–722.

76. Jemad A., Murray T., Samuels A., et al. (2007). Cancer statistics, 2007. *CA: A Cancer Journal for Clinicians* 53, 5–26.

77. Eide M. J., Weinstock M. A. (2004). Epidemiology of skin cancer. In Rigel D. S., Friedman R. J., Dzubow L. M., et al. (Eds.), *Cancer of the skin* (pp. 47–48). Philadelphia: Elsevier Saunders.

78. Habif T. P., Campbell J. L., Chapman M. S., et al. (2005). Skin diseases: Diagnosis and treatment. In Rigel D. S., Friedman R. J., Dzubow L. M., et al. (Eds.), *Cancer of the skin* (pp. 472–485). Philadelphia: Elsevier Saunders.

79. Abbasi N. R., Shaw H. M., Rigel D. S., et. al. (2004). Early diagnosis of cutaneous melanoma. *Journal of the American Medical Association* 292, 2771–2776.

80. Balch C. M., Buzaid A. C., Soong S. J., et al. (2001). Final version of the American Joint Committee on Cancer Staging System for Cutaneous Melanoma. *Journal of Clinical Oncology* 19, 3635–3648.

81. Rhodes A. R. (2006). Cutaneous melanoma and intervention strategies to reduce tumor-related mortality: What we know, what we don't know, and what we think we know that isn't so. *Dermatologic Therapy* 19, 50–69.

82. Bystryn J. C., Reynolds S. R. (2005). Vaccine therapy for melanoma (pp. 607–618). In Rigel D. S., Friedman R. J., Dzubow L. M., et al. (Eds.), *Cancer of the skin.* Philadelphia: Elsevier Saunders.

83. Lang P. G., Maize J. C. (2005). Basal cell carcinoma (p. 101, 103). In Rigel D. S., Friedman R. J., Dzubow L. M., et al. (Eds.), *Cancer of the skin.* Philadelphia: Elsevier Saunders.

84. Nguyen T. H., Jaeyoung Y. (2005). Squamous cell carcinoma. In Rigel D. S., Friedman R. J., Dzubow L. M., et al. (Eds.), *Cancer of the skin* (pp. 133, 141). Philadelphia: Elsevier Saunders.

85. MacArthur C. J. (2006). Head and neck hemangiomas of infancy. *Current Opinion in Otolaryngology & Head & Neck Surgery* 14, 397–405.

86. Metry D. (2004). Update on hemangiomas of infancy. *Current Opinion in Pediatrics* 16, 373–377.

87. Kazaks E. L., Lane A. T. (2000). Diaper dermatitis. *Pediatric Clinics of North America* 47, 909–918.

88. Atherton D. J. (2004). A review of the pathophysiology, prevention and treatment of irritant diaper dermatitis. *Current Medical Research and Opinions* 20, 645–649.

89. Zerr D. M., Meier A. S., Selke S. S., et al. (2005). A population-based study of primary human herpesvirus 6 infection. *New England Journal of Medicine* 352, 753–755.

90. Zareba G. (2006). A new combination vaccine for measles, mumps, rubella and varicella. *Drugs of Today* 42, 321–329.

91. Hambleton S., Gershon A. A. (2005). Preventing varicella-zoster disease. *Clinical Microbiology Reviews* 18, 70–80.

92. Arvin A., Gershon A. (2006). Control of varicella: Why is a two-dose schedule necessary? *Pediatric Infectious Disease Journal* 25, 475–476.

93. Berman B., Villa A. M., Ramirez C. C. (2006). Mechanisms of action of new treatment modalities for actinic keratosis. *Journal of Drugs in Dermatology* 5, 167–173.

94. Gold M. H., Nestor M. S. (2006). Current treatments of actinic keratosis. *Journal of Drugs in Dermatology* 5(2 Suppl.), 17–25.

95. Lober B. A., Fenske N. A., Neil A. (2004). Optimum treatment strategies for actinic keratosis (intraepidermal squamous cell carcinoma). *American Journal of Clinical Dermatology* 5, 395–401.

96. Anwar J., Wrone D. A., Kimyai-Asadi A., et al. (2004). The development of actinic keratosis into invasive squamous cell carcinoma: Evidence and evolving classification schemes. *Clinics in Dermatology* 22, 189–196.

Visit the Point http://thePoint.lww.com for **animations, journal articles, and more!**

TABLE A-1 Prefixes Denoting Decimal Factors

PREFIX	SYMBOL	FACTOR
mega	M	10^6
kilo	k	10^3
hecto	h	10^2
deci	d	10^{-1}
centi	c	10^{-2}
milli	m	10^{-3}
micro	μ	10^{-6}
nano	n	10^{-9}
pico	p	10^{-12}
femto	f	10^{-15}

TABLE A-2 Hematology

TEST	CONVENTIONAL UNITS	SI UNITS
Erythrocyte count (RBC count)	M. $4.2–5.4 \times 10^6/\mu L$	M. $4.2–5.4 \times 10^{12}/L$
	F. $3.6–5.0 \times 10^6/\mu L$	F. $3.6–5.0 \times 10^{12}/L$
Hematocrit (Hct)	M. 40–50%	M. 0.40–0.50
	F. 37–47%	F. 0.37–0.47
Hemoglobin (Hb)	M. 14.0–16.5 g/dL	M. 140–165 g/L
	F. 12.0–15.0 g/dL	F. 120–150 g/L
Mean corpuscular hemoglobin (MHC)	27–34 pg/cell	0.40–0.53 fmol/cell
Mean corpuscular hemoglobin concentration (MCHC)	31–35 g/dL	310–350 g/L
Mean corpuscular volume (MCV)	80–100 fL/cell	
Reticulocyte count	1.0–1.5% total RBC	
Platelet count	$150–400 \times 10^3/\mu L$	$150–400 \times 10^9/L$
Leukocyte count (WBC count)	$4.8–10.8 \times 10^3/\mu L$	$4.8–10.8 \times 10^9/L$
Basophils	0–2%	
Eosinophils	0–3%	
Lymphocytes	24–40%	
Monocytes	4–9%	
Neutrophils (segmented [Segs])	47–63%	
Neutrophils (bands)	0–4%	

TABLE A-3 Blood Chemistry*

TEST	CONVENTIONAL UNITS	SI UNITS
Alanine aminotransferase (ALT, SGPT)	7–56 units/L[†]	0.12–0.93 µkat/L[†]
Alkaline phosphatase	41–133 units/L[†‡]	0.7–2.2 µkat/L[†‡]
Ammonia	18–60 µg/dL	11–35 µmol/L
Amylase	20–110 units/L[†]	0.33–1.83 µkat/L[†]
Aspartase aminotransferase (AST, SGOT)	0–35 units/L[†]	0–0.58 µkat/L[†]
Bicarbonate	24–31 mEq/L	24–31 mmol/L
Bilirubin (total)	0.1–1.2 mg/dL	17.1–21 µmol/L
Direct	0.1–0.5 mg/dL	<8 µmol/L
Indirect	0.1–0.7 mg/dL	<12 µmol/L
Blood urea nitrogen (BUN)	8–20 mg/dL	2.9–7.1 mmol/L
Calcium (Ca^{2+})	8.5–10.5 mg/dL	2.1–2.6 mmol/L
Chloride	98–106 mEq/L	98–106 mmol/L
Creatine kinase (CK, CPK)	32–267 units/L[†]	0.53–4.45 µkat/L[†]
Creatine kinase (MB)	<16 IU/L[†] or 4% of total CK	<0.27 µkat/L[†]
Creatinine (serum)	0.6–1.2 mg/dL[‡]	53–106 µmol/L[‡]
Gamma-glutamyl-transpeptidase (GGT)	9–85 units/L[†]	0.15–1.42 µkat/L[†]
Glucose (plasma, fasting)	<100 mg/dL	<5.5 mmol/L
Glycosylated hemoglobin (HbA$_{1c}$)	3.9–6.9%	
Lactate dehydrogenase (LDH)	88–230 units/L[†]	1.46–3.82 µkat/L[†]
Lipids		
Cholesterol	<200 mg/dL (optimal)	<5.2 mmol/L (optimal)
	200–239 mg/dL (borderline)	5.2–6.1 mmol/L (borderline)
	≥240 (high)	>6.2 mmol/L (high)
LDL cholesterol	<130 mg/dL	<3.37 mmol/L
HDL cholesterol	Male: 35–65 mg/dL	91–1.68 mmol/L
	Female: 35–80 mg/dL	0.91–2.07 mmol/L
Triglycerides	<165 mg/dL	<1.8 mmol/L (fasting)
Lipase	0–160 units/L[†]	0.266 µkat/L[†]
Magnesium	1.8–3.0 mg/dL	0.75–1.25 mmol/L
Osmolality	275–295 mOsm/kg H$_2$O	275–295 mmol/kg H$_2$O
pH (arterial)	7.35–7.45	
Phosphorus (inorganic)	2.5–4.5 mg/dL	0.80–1.45 mmol/L
Potassium	3.5–5.0 mEq/L	3.5–5.0 mmol/L
Prostate specific antigen (PSA)	0–4 ng/mL	0–4 µg/L
Protein total	6.0–8.0 g/dL	60–80 g/L
Albumin	3.4–4.7 g/dL	34–47 g/L
Globulin	2.3–3.5 g/dL	23–35 g/L
A/G ratio	1.0–2.2	1.0–2.2
Thyroid tests		
Thyroxine (T$_4$) total	5.0–11.0 µg/dL	64–142 nmol/L
Thyroxine, free (FT$_4$)	9–24 pmol/L[†]	
Triiodothyronine (T$_3$) total	95–190 ng/dL	1.5–2.9 nmol/L
Thyroid-stimulating hormone (TSH)	0.4–4.2 µU/mL	0.4–4.2 mU/L
Thyroglobin	3–42 ng/mL	3–42 µg/L
Sodium	135–145 mEq/L	135–145 mmol/L
Uric acid	Male: 2.4–7.4 mg/dL	Male: 143–440 µmol/L
	Female: 1.4–5.8 mg/dL	Female: 83–345 µmol/L

*Values may vary with laboratory. The values supplied by the laboratory performing the test should always be used since the ranges may be method specific.

[†]Laboratory and/or method specific

[‡]Varies with age and muscle mass

Values obtained from Tierney L. M., McPhee S. J., Papadakis M. A. (2007). *Current medical diagnosis and treatment* (46th ed., pp. 1769–1777). Stamford, CT: Appleton & Lange; Fischbach F. (2004). *A manual of laboratory and diagnostic tests* (7th ed.). Philadelphia: Lippincott Williams & Wilkins; and other sources.

Internet Sites

Labquest: Biochemistry Unit Conversion (site has calculator and conversion table for common laboratory tests)
http://www.vin.com/scripts/labquest/converthtml.pl

Northwestern University Medical Students by Dr. Al Telser, Department of Cell and Molecular Biology and the Galter Library (conventional and SI units for laboratory tests) http://www.galter.northwestern.edu/reftools/normals.html

University of Minnesota (Ward Manual/normal values for laboratory tests)
http://www.student.med.umn.edu/wardmanual/normallabs.php

APPENDIX B
Dietary Reference Intakes (DRIs)

TABLE B-1 Dietary Reference Intakes (DRIs): Recommended Intakes for Individuals, Vitamins Food and Nutrition Board, Institute of Medicine, National Academies

LIFE STAGE GROUP	VITAMIN A (μg/d)[a]	VITAMIN C (mg/d)	VITAMIN D (μg/d)[b,c]	VITAMIN E (mg/d)[d]	VITAMIN K (μg/d)	THIAMIN (mg/d)
Infants						
0–6 mo	400*	40*	5*	4*	2.0*	0.2*
7–12 mo	500*	50*	5*	5*	2.5*	0.3*
Children						
1–3 y	**300**	**15**	5*	**6**	30*	**0.5**
4–8 y	**400**	**25**	5*	**7**	55*	**0.6**
Males						
9–13 y	**600**	**45**	5*	**11**	60*	**0.9**
14–18 y	**900**	**75**	5*	**15**	75*	**1.2**
19–30 y	**900**	**90**	5*	**15**	120*	**1.2**
31–50 y	**900**	**90**	5*	**15**	120*	**1.2**
51–70 y	**900**	**90**	10*	**15**	120*	**1.2**
>70 y	**900**	**90**	15*	**15**	120*	**1.2**
Females						
9–13 y	**600**	**45**	5*	**11**	60*	**0.9**
14–18 y	**700**	**65**	5*	**15**	75*	**1.0**
19–30 y	**700**	**75**	5*	**15**	90*	**1.1**
31–50 y	**700**	**75**	5*	**15**	90*	**1.1**
51–70 y	**700**	**75**	10*	**15**	90*	**1.1**
>70 y	**700**	**75**	15*	**15**	90*	**1.1**
Pregnancy						
≤18 y	**750**	**80**	5*	**15**	75*	**1.4**
19–30 y	**770**	**85**	5*	**15**	90*	**1.4**
31–50 y	**770**	**85**	5*	**15**	90*	**1.4**
Lactation						
≤18 y	**1,200**	**115**	5*	**19**	75*	**1.4**
19–30 y	**1,300**	**120**	5*	**19**	90*	**1.4**
31–50 y	**1,300**	**120**	5*	**19**	90*	**1.4**

NOTE: This table (taken from the DRI reports, see www.nap.edu) presents Recommended Dietary Allowances (RDAs) in **bold type** and Adequate Intakes (AIs) in ordinary type followed by an asterisk (*) RDAs and AIs may both be used as goals for individual intake. RDAs are set to meet the needs of almost all (97 to 98 percent) individuals in a group. For healthy breastfed infants, the AI is the mean intake. The AI for other life stage and gender groups is believed to cover needs of all individuals in the group, but lack of data or uncertainty in the data prevent being able to specify with confidence the percentage of individuals covered by this intake.

[a] As retinol activity equivalents (RAEs). 1 RAE = 1 μg retinol, 12 μg β-carotene, 24 μg α-carotene, or 24 μg β-cryptoxanthin. The RAE for dietary provitamin A carotenoids is two-fold greater than retinol equivalents (RE), whereas the RAE for preformed vitamin A is the same as RE.

[b] Cholecalciferol. 1 μg cholecalciferol = 40 IU vitamin D.

[c] In the absence of adequate exposure to sunlight.

[d] As α-tocopherol. α-Tocopherol includes RRR-α-tocopherol, the only form of α-tocopherol that occurs naturally in foods, and the 2R-stereoisomeric forms of α-tocopherol (RRR-, RSR-, RRS-, and RSS-α-tocopherol) that occur in fortified foods and supplements. It does not include the 2S-stereoisomeric forms of α-tocopherol (SRR-, SSR-, SRS-, and SSS-α-tocopherol), also found in fortified foods and supplements.

RIBOFLAVIN (mg/d)	NIACIN (mg/d)[e]	VITAMIN B$_6$ (mg/d)	FOLATE (µg/d)[f]	VITAMIN B$_{12}$ (µg/d)	PANTOTHENIC ACID (mg/d)	BIOTIN (µg/d)	CHOLINE[g] (mg/d)
0.3*	2*	0.1*	65*	0.4*	1.7*	5*	125*
0.4*	4*	0.3*	80*	0.5*	1.8*	6*	150*
0.5	6	0.5	150	0.9	2*	8*	200*
0.6	8	0.6	200	1.2	3*	12*	250*
0.9	12	1.0	300	1.8	4*	20*	375*
1.3	16	1.3	400	2.4	5*	25*	550*
1.3	16	1.3	400	2.4	5*	30*	550*
1.3	16	1.3	400	2.4	5*	30*	550*
1.3	16	1.7	400	2.4[h]	5*	30*	550*
1.3	16	1.7	400	2.4[h]	5*	30*	550*
0.9	12	1.0	300	1.8	4*	20*	375*
1.0	14	1.2	400[i]	2.4	5*	25*	400*
1.1	14	1.3	400[i]	2.4	5*	30*	425*
1.1	14	1.3	400[i]	2.4	5*	30*	425*
1.1	14	1.5	400	2.4[h]	5*	30*	425*
1.1	14	1.5	400	2.4[h]	5*	30*	425*
1.4	18	1.9	600[j]	2.6	6*	30*	450*
1.4	18	1.9	600[j]	2.6	6*	30*	450*
1.4	18	1.9	600[j]	2.6	6*	30*	450*
1.6	17	2.0	500	2.8	7*	35*	550*
1.6	17	2.0	500	2.8	7*	35*	550*
1.6	17	2.0	500	2.8	7*	35*	550*

[e] As niacin equivalents (NE). 1 mg of niacin = 60 mg of tryptophan, 0–6 months = preformed niacin (not NE).

[f] As dietary folate equivalents (DFE). 1 DFE = 1 µg food folate = 0.6 µg of folic acid from fortified food or as a supplement consumed with food = 0.5 µg of a supplement taken on an empty stomach.

[g] Although AIs have been set for choline, there are few data to assess whether a dietary supply of choline is needed at all stages of the life cycle, and it may be that the choline requirement can be met by endogenous synthesis at some of these stages.

[h] Because 10 to 30 percent of older people may malabsorb food-bound B$_{12}$, it is advisable for those older than 50 years to meet their RDA mainly by consuming foods fortified with B$_{12}$ or a supplement containing B$_{12}$.

[i] In view of evidence linking folate intake with neural tube defects in the fetus, it is recommended that all women capable of becoming pregnant consume 400 µg from supplements or fortified foods in addition to intake of food folate from a varied diet.

[j] It is assumed that women will continue consuming 400 µg from supplements or fortified food until their pregnancy is confirmed and they enter prenatal care, which ordinarily occurs after the end of the periconceptional period—the critical time for formation of the neural tube.

TABLE B-2 Dietary Reference Intakes (DRIs): Recommended Intakes for Individuals, Elements Food and Nutrition Board, Institute of Medicine, National Academies

LIFE STAGE GROUP	CALCIUM (mg/d)	CHROMIUM (µg/d)	COPPER (µg/d)	FLUORIDE (mg/d)	IODINE (µg/d)	IRON (mg/d)
Infants						
0–6 mo	210*	0.2*	200*	0.01*	110*	0.27*
7–12 mo	270*	5.5*	220*	0.5*	130*	**11**
Children						
1–3 y	500*	11*	**340**	0.7*	**90**	**7**
4–8 y	800*	15*	**440**	1*	**90**	**10**
Males						
9–13 y	1,300*	25*	**700**	2*	**120**	**8**
14–18 y	1,300*	35*	**890**	3*	**150**	**11**
19–30 y	1,000*	35*	**900**	4*	**150**	**8**
31–50 y	1,000*	35*	**900**	4*	**150**	**8**
51–70 y	1,200*	30*	**900**	4*	**150**	**8**
>70 y	1,200*	30*	**900**	4*	**150**	**8**
Females						
9–13 y	1,300*	21*	**700**	2*	**120**	**8**
14–18 y	1,300*	24*	**890**	3*	**150**	**15**
19–30 y	1,000*	25*	**900**	3*	**150**	**18**
31–50 y	1,000*	25*	**900**	3*	**150**	**18**
51–70 y	1,200*	20*	**900**	3*	**150**	**8**
>70 y	1,200*	20*	**900**	3*	**150**	**8**
Pregnancy						
≤18 y	1,300*	29*	**1,000**	3*	**220**	**27**
19–30 y	1,000*	30*	**1,000**	3*	**220**	**27**
31–50 y	1,000*	30*	**1,000**	3*	**220**	**27**
Lactation						
≤18 y	1,300*	44*	**1,300**	3*	**290**	**10**
19–30 y	1,000*	45*	**1,300**	3*	**290**	**9**
31–50 y	1,000*	45*	**1,300**	3*	**290**	**9**

NOTE: This table presents Recommended Dietary Allowances (RDAs) in **bold type** and Adequate Intakes (AIs) in ordinary type followed by an asterisk (*). RDAs and AIs may both be used as goals for individual intake. RDAs are set to meet the needs of almost all (97 to 98 percent) individuals in a group. For healthy breastfed infants, the AI is the mean intake. The AI for other life stage and gender groups is believed to cover needs of all individuals in the group, but lack of data or uncertainty in the data prevent being able to specify with confidence the percentage of individuals covered by this intake.

SOURCES: Dietary Reference intakes for Calcium, Phosphorus, Magnesium, Vitamin D, and Fluoride (1997); Dietary Reference Intakes for Thiamin, Riboflavin, Niacin, Vitamin B$_6$, Folate, Vitamin B$_{12}$, Pantothenic Acid, Biotin, and Choline (1998); Dietary Reference Intakes for Vitamin C, Vitamin E, Selenium, and Carotenoids (2000); and Dietary Reference Intakes for Vitamin A, Vitamin K, Arsenic, Boron, Chromium, Copper, Iodine, Iron, Manganese, Molybdenum, Nickel, Silicon, Vanadium, and Zinc (2001). These reports may be accessed via www.nap.edu.

MAGNESIUM (mg/d)	MANGANESE (mg/d)	MOLYBDENUM (µg/d)	PHOSPHORUS (mg/d)	SELENIUM (µg/d)	ZINC (mg/d)
30*	0.003*	2*	100*	15*	2*
75*	0.6*	3*	275*	20*	3
80	1.2*	17	460	20	3
130	1.5*	22	500	30	5
240	1.9*	34	1,250	40	8
410	2.2*	43	1,250	55	11
400	2.3*	45	700	55	11
420	2.3*	45	700	55	11
420	2.3*	45	700	55	11
420	2.3*	45	700	55	11
240	1.6*	34	1,250	40	8
360	1.6*	43	1,250	55	9
310	1.8*	45	700	55	8
320	1.8*	45	700	55	8
320	1.8*	45	700	55	8
320	1.8*	45	700	55	8
400	2.0*	50	1,250	60	12
350	2.0*	50	700	60	11
360	2.0*	50	700	60	11
360	2.6*	50	1,250	70	13
310	2.6*	50	700	70	12
320	2.6*	50	700	70	12

TABLE B-3 Dietary Reference Intakes (DRIs): Recommended Intakes for Individuals, Macronutrients Food and Nutrition Board, Institute of Medicine, National Academies

LIFE STAGE GROUP	CARBOHYDRATE (g/d)	TOTAL FIBER (g/d)	FAT (g/d)	LINOLEIC ACID (g/d)	α-LINOLENIC ACID (g/d)	PROTEIN[a] (g/d)
Infants						
0–6 mo	60*	ND	31*	4.4*	0.5*	9.1*
7–12 mo	95*	ND	30*	4.6*	0.5*	**13.5**
Children						
1–3 y	**130**	19*	ND	7*	0.7*	**13**
4–8 y	**130**	25*	ND	10*	0.9*	**19**
Males						
9–13 y	**130**	31*	ND	12*	1.2*	**34**
14–18 y	**130**	38*	ND	16*	1.6*	**52**
19–30 y	**130**	38*	ND	17*	1.6*	**56**
31–50 y	**130**	38*	ND	17*	1.6*	**56**
51–70 y	**130**	30*	ND	14*	1.6*	**56**
>70 y	**130**	30*	ND	14*	1.6*	**56**
Females						
9–13 y	**130**	26*	ND	10*	1.0*	**34**
14–18 y	**130**	26*	ND	11*	1.1*	**46**
19–30 y	**130**	25*	ND	12*	1.1*	**46**
31–50 y	**130**	25*	ND	12*	1.1*	**46**
51–70 y	**130**	21*	ND	11*	1.1*	**46**
>70 y	**130**	21*	ND	11*	1.1*	**46**
Pregnancy						
14–18 y	**175**	28*	ND	13*	1.4*	**71**
19–30 y	**175**	28*	ND	13*	1.4*	**71**
31–50 y	**175**	28*	ND	13*	1.4*	**71**
Lactation						
14–18	**210**	29*	ND	13*	1.3*	**71**
19–30 y	**210**	29*	ND	13*	1.3*	**71**
31–50 y	**210**	29*	ND	13*	1.3*	**71**

NOTE: This table presents Recommended Dietary Allowances (RDAs) in **bold type** and Adequate Intakes (AIs) in ordinary type followed by an asterisk (*). RDAs and AIs may both be used as goals for individual intake. RDAs are set to meet the needs of almost all (97 to 98 percent) individuals in a group. For healthy breastfed infants, the AI is the mean intake. The AI for other life stage and gender groups is believed to cover needs of all individuals in the group but lack of data or uncertainty in the data prevent being able to specify with confidence the percentage of individuals covered by this intake.

[a]Based on 0.8g protein/kg body weight for reference body weight.

SOURCE: Dietary Reference Intakes for Energy, Carbohydrate, Fiber, Fat, Fatty Acids, Cholesterol, Protein, and Amino Acids (2002). This report may be accessed via www.nap.edu.

Abduction The act of abducting (moving or spreading away from a position near the midline of the body or the axial line of a limb) or the state of being abducted.

Abrasion The wearing or scraping away of a substance or structure, such as the skin, through an unusual or abnormal mechanical process.

Abscess A collection of pus that is restricted to a specific area in tissues, organs, or confined spaces.

Accommodation The adjustment of the lens (eye) to variations in distance.

Acromion The lateral extension of the spine of the scapula, forming the highest point of the shoulder. (Adjective: acromial)

Acuity The clearness or sharpness of perception, especially of vision.

Adaptation The adjustment of an organism to its environment, physical or psychological, through changes and responses to stress of any kind.

Adduction The act of adducting (moving or drawing toward a position near the midline of the body or the axial line of a limb) or the state of being adducted.

Adhesin The molecular components of the bacterial cell wall that are involved in adhesion processes.

Adrenergic Activated by or characteristic of the sympathetic nervous system or its neurotransmitters (*i.e.*, epinephrine and norepinephrine).

Aerobic Growing, living, or occurring only in the presence of air or oxygen.

Afferent Bearing or conducting inward or toward a center, as an afferent neuron.

Agglutination The clumping together of particles, microorganisms, or blood cells in response to an antigen–antibody reaction.

Agonist A muscle whose action is opposed by another muscle (antagonist) with which it is paired; or a drug or other chemical substance that has affinity for or stimulates a predictable physiologic function.

Akinesia An abnormal state in which there is an absence or poverty of movement.

Allele One of two or more different forms of a gene that can occupy a particular locus on a chromosome.

Alveolus A small saclike structure, as in the alveolus of the lung.

Amblyopia A condition of vision impairment without a detectable organic lesion of the eye.

Amine An organic compound containing nitrogen.

Amorphous Without a definite form; shapeless.

Amphoteric Capable of reacting chemically as an acid or a base.

Ampulla A saclike dilatation of a duct, canal, or any other tubular structure.

Anabolism A constructive metabolic process characterized by the conversion of simple substances into larger, complex molecules.

Anaerobic Growing, living, or occurring only in the absence of air or oxygen.

Analog A part, organ, or chemical having the same function or appearance but differing in respect to a certain component, such as origin or development.

Anaplasia A change in the structure of cells and in their orientation to each other that is characterized by a loss of cell differentiation, as in cancerous cell growth.

Anastomosis The connection or joining between two vessels; or an opening created by surgical, traumatic, or pathologic means.

Androgen Any substance, such as a male sex hormone, that increases male characteristics.

Anergy A state of absent or diminished reaction to an antigen or group of antigens.

Aneuploidy A variation in the number of chromosomes within a cell involving one or more missing chromosomes rather than entire sets.

Aneurysm An outpouching or dilation in the wall of a blood vessel or the heart.

Ankylosis Stiffness or fixation of separate bones of a joint, resulting from disease, injury, or surgical procedure. (Verb: ankylose)

Anorexia Lack or loss of appetite for food. (Adjective: anorexic)

Anoxia An abnormal condition characterized by the total lack of oxygen.

Antagonist A muscle whose action directly opposes that of another muscle (agonist) with which it is paired; or a drug or other chemical substance that can diminish or nullify the action of a neuromediator or body function.

Anterior Pertaining to a surface or part that is situated near or toward the front.

Antigen A substance that generates an immune response by causing the formation of an antibody or reacting with antibodies or T-cell receptors.

Apex The uppermost point, the narrowed or pointed end, or the highest point of a structure, such as an organ.

Aphagia A condition characterized by the refusal or the loss of ability to swallow.

Aplasia The absence of an organ or tissue due to a developmental failure.

Apnea The absence of spontaneous respiration.

Apoptosis A mechanism of programmed cell death, marked by shrinkage of the cell, condensation of chromatin, formation of cytoplasmic blebs, and fragmentation of the cell into membrane-bound bodies eliminated by phagocytosis.

Apraxia Loss of the ability to carry out familiar, purposeful acts or to manipulate objects in the absence of paralysis or other motor or sensory impairment.

Articulation The place of connection or junction between two or more bones of a skeletal joint.

Ascites An abnormal accumulation of serous fluid in the peritoneal cavity.

Asepsis The condition of being free or freed from pathogenic microorganisms.

Astereognosis A neurologic disorder characterized by an inability to identify objects by touch.

Asterixis A motor disturbance characterized by a hand-flapping tremor, which results when the prolonged contraction of groups of muscles lapses intermittently.

Ataxia An abnormal condition characterized by an inability to coordinate voluntary muscular movement.

Athetosis A neuromuscular condition characterized by the continuous occurrence of slow, sinuous, writhing movements that are performed involuntarily. (Adjective: athetoid)

Atopy Genetic predisposition toward the development of a hypersensitivity or an allergic reaction to common environmental allergens.

Atresia The absence or closure of a normal body orifice or tubular organ, such as the esophagus.

Atrophy A wasting or diminution of size, often accompanied by a decrease in function, of a cell, tissue, or organ.

Autocrine A mode of hormone action in which a chemical messenger acts on the same cell that secretes it.

Autophagy Segregation of part of the cell's own damaged cytoplasmic material within a vacuole and its disposal.

Autosome Any chromosome other than a sex chromosome.

Axillary Of or pertaining to the axilla, or armpit.

Bacteremia The presence of bacteria in the blood.

Bactericide An agent that destroys bacteria. (Adjective: bactericidal)

Bacteriostat An agent that inhibits bacterial growth. (Adjective: bacteriostatic)

Ballismus An abnormal condition characterized by violent flailing motions of the arms and, occasionally, the head, resulting from injury to or destruction of the subthalamic nucleus or its fiber connections.

Baroreceptor A type of sensory nerve ending such as those found in the aorta and the carotid sinus that is stimulated by changes in pressure.

Basal Pertaining to, situated at, or forming the base; or the fundamental or the basic.

Benign Not malignant; or of the character that does not threaten health or life.

Bipolar neuron A nerve cell that has a process at each end—an afferent process and an efferent process.

Bolus A rounded mass of food ready to swallow or such a mass passing through the gastrointestinal tract; or a concentrated mass of medicinal material or other pharmaceutical preparation injected all at once intravenously for diagnostic purposes.

Borborygmus The rumbling, gurgling, or tinkling noise produced by the propulsion of gas through the intestine.

Bruit A sound or murmur heard while auscultating an organ or blood vessel, especially an abnormal one.

Buccal Pertaining to or directed toward the inside of the cheek.

Buffer A substance or group of substances that prevents change in the concentration of another chemical substance.

Bulla A thin-walled blister of the skin or mucous membranes greater than 5 mm in diameter containing serous or seropurulent fluid.

Bursa A fluid-filled sac or saclike cavity situated in places in the tissues at which friction would otherwise develop, such as between certain tendons and the bones beneath them.

Cachexia A condition of general ill health and malnutrition, marked by weakness and emaciation.

Calculus A stony mass formed within body tissues, usually composed of mineral salts.

Capsid The protein shell that envelops and protects the nucleic acid of a virus.

Carcinogen Any substance or agent that causes the development or increases the incidence of cancer.

Carpal Of or pertaining to the carpus, or wrist.

Caseation A form of tissue necrosis in which the tissue is changed into a dry, amorphous mass resembling crumbly cheese.

Catabolism A metabolic process through which living organisms break down complex substances to simple compounds, liberating energy for use in work, energy storage, or heat production.

Catalyst A substance that increases the velocity of a chemical reaction without being consumed by the process.

Catecholamines Any one of a group of biogenic amines having a sympathomimetic action and composed of a catechol molecule and the aliphatic portion of an amine.

Caudal Signifying an inferior position, toward the distal end of the spine.

Cellulitis An acute, diffuse, spreading, edematous inflammation of the deep subcutaneous tissues and sometimes muscle, characterized most commonly by an area of heat, redness, pain, and swelling, and occasionally by fever, malaise, chills, and headache.

Cephalic Of or pertaining to the head, or to the head end of the body.

Cerumen The waxlike secretion produced by vestigial apocrine sweat glands in the external ear canal.

Cheilosis A noninflammatory disorder of the lips and mouth characterized by chapping and fissuring.

Chelate A chemical compound composed of a central metal ion and an organic molecule with multiple bonds, arranged in ring formation, used especially in treatment of metal poisoning.

Chemoreceptor A sensory nerve cell activated by chemical stimuli, as a chemoreceptor in the carotid artery that is sensitive to changes in the oxygen content in the blood and reflexly increases or decreases respiration and blood pressure.

Chemotaxis A response involving cell orientation or cell movement that is either toward (positive chemotaxis) or away from (negative chemotaxis) a chemical stimulus.

Chimeric Relating to, derived from, or being an individual possessing one's own immunologic characteristics and that of another individual; a phenomenon that can occur as the result of procedures such as a bone marrow graft.

Chondrocyte Any one of the mature polymorphic cells that form the cartilage of the body.

Chromatid One of the paired threadlike chromosome filaments, joined at the centromere, that make up a metaphase chromosome.

Chromosome Any one of the structures in the nucleus of a cell containing a linear thread of DNA, which functions in the transmission of genetic information.

Chyme The creamy, viscous, semifluid material produced during digestion of a meal that is expelled by the stomach into the duodenum.

Cilia A minute, hairlike process projecting from a cell, composed of nine microtubules arrayed around a single pair. Cilia beat rhythmically to move the cell around in its environment or they move mucus or fluids over the surface.

Circadian Being, having, pertaining to, or occurring in a period or cycle of approximately 24 hours.

Circumduction The active or passive circular movement of a limb or of the eye.

Cisterna An enclosed space, such as a cavity, that serves as a reservoir for lymph or other body fluids.

Clone One or a group of genetically identical cells or organisms derived from a single parent.

Coagulation The process of transforming a liquid into a semisolid mass, especially of blood clot formation.

Coarctation A condition of stricture or contraction of the walls of a vessel.

Cofactor A substance that must unite with another substance in order to function.

Colic Sharp, intermittent abdominal pain localized in a hollow or tubular organ, resulting from torsion, obstruction, or smooth muscle spasm. (Adjective: colicky)

Collagen The protein substance of the white, glistening, inelastic fibers of the skin, tendons, bone, cartilage, and all other connective tissue.

Collateral Secondary or accessory rather than direct or immediate; or a small branch, as of a blood vessel or nerve.

Complement Any one of the complex, enzymatic serum proteins that are involved in physiologic reactions, including antigen–antibody reaction and anaphylaxis.

Confluent Flowing or coming together; not discrete.

Congenital Present at, and usually before, birth.

Conjugate To pair and fuse in conjugation; or a form of sexual reproduction seen in unicellular organisms in which genetic material is exchanged during the temporary fusion of two cells.

Contiguous In contact or nearly so in an unbroken sequence along a boundary or at a point.

Contralateral Affecting, pertaining to, or originating in the opposite side of a point or reference.

Contusion An injury of a part without a break in the skin, characterized by swelling, discoloration, and pain.

Convolution An elevation or tortuous winding, such as one of the irregular ridges on the surface of the brain, formed by a structure being infolded upon itself.

Corpuscle Any small mass, cell, or body, such as a red or white blood cell.

Costal Pertaining to a rib or ribs.

Crepitus A sound or sensation that resembles a crackling or grating noise.

Cutaneous Pertaining to the skin.

Cyanosis A bluish discoloration, especially of the skin and mucous membranes, caused by an excess of deoxygenated hemoglobin in the blood.

Cytokine Any of a class of polypeptide immunoregulatory substances that are secreted by cells, usually of the immune system, that affect other cells.

Cytology The study of cells, including their origin, structure, function, and pathology.

Cytosol Cytoplasm exclusive of membranous components (*e.g.,* mitochondria, endoplasmic reticulum) and nonmembranous insoluble components.

Decibel A unit for expressing the relative power intensity of electric or acoustic signal power that is equal to one tenth of a bel.

Defecation The evacuation of feces from the digestive tract through the rectum.

Deformation The process of adapting in form or shape; also the product of such alteration.

Degeneration The deterioration of a normal cell, tissue, or organ to a less functionally active form. (Adjective: degenerative)

Deglutition The act or process of swallowing.

Degradation The reduction of a chemical compound to a compound less complex, usually by splitting off one or more groups.

Dehydration The condition that results from excessive loss of water from the body tissues.

Delirium An acute, reversible organic mental syndrome characterized by confusion, disorientation, restlessness, incoherence, fear, and often illusions.

Dendrite One of the branching processes that extends and transmits impulses toward a cell body of a neuron. (Adjective: dendritic)

Depolarization The reduction of a cell membrane potential to a less negative value than that of the potential outside the cell.

Dermatome The area of the skin supplied with afferent nerve fibers of a single dorsal root of a spinal nerve.

Desmosome A small, circular, dense area within the intercellular bridge that forms the site of adhesion between intermediate filaments and cell membranes.

Desquamation A normal process in which the cornified layer of the epidermis is shed in fine scales or sheets.

Dialysis The process of separating colloids and crystalline substances in solution, which involves the two distinct physical processes of diffusion and ultrafiltration; or a medical procedure for the removal of urea and other elements from the blood or lymph.

Diapedesis The outward passage of red or white blood corpuscles through the intact walls of the vessels.

Diaphoresis Perspiration, especially the profuse perspiration associated with an elevated body temperature, physical exertion, exposure to heat, and mental or emotional stress.

Diarthrosis A specialized articulation that permits, to some extent, free joint movement. (Adjective: diarthrodial)

Diastole The dilatation of the heart; or the period of dilatation, which is the interval between the second and the first heart sound and is the time during which blood enters the relaxed chambers of the heart from the systemic circulation and the lungs.

Differentiation The act or process in development in which unspecialized cells or tissues acquire more specialized characteristics, including those of physical form, physiologic function, and chemical properties.

Diffusion The process of becoming widely spread, as in the spontaneous movement of molecules or other particles in solution from an area of higher concentration to an area of lower concentration, resulting in an even distribution of the particles in the fluid.

Dimer A compound or unit formed by the combination of two identical molecules or radicals of a simpler compound. (Adjective: dimeric)

Diopter A unit of measurement of the refractive power of lenses equal to the reciprocal of the focal length in meters.

Diploid Pertaining to an individual, organism, strain, or cell that has two full sets of homologous chromosomes.

Disseminate To scatter or distribute over a considerable area.

Distal Away from or being the farthest from a point of reference.

Diurnal Of, relating to, or occurring in the daytime.

Diverticulum A pouch or sac of variable size occurring naturally or through herniation of the muscular wall of a tubular organ.

Dorsum The back or posterior. (Adjective: dorsal)

Dysgenesis Defective or abnormal development of an organ or part, typically occurring during embryonic development. (Also called dysgenesia.)

Dyslexia A disturbance in the ability to read, spell, and write words.

Dyspepsia The impairment of the power or function of digestion, especially epigastric discomfort following eating.

Dysphagia A difficulty in swallowing.

Dysphonia Any impairment of the voice that is experienced as a difficulty in speaking.

Dysplasia The alteration in size, shape, and organization of adult cell types.

Eburnation The conversion of bone or cartilage, through thinning or loss, into a hard and dense mass with a worn, polished, ivorylike surface.

Ecchymosis A small hemorrhagic spot, larger than a petechia, in the skin or mucous membrane caused by the extravasation of blood into the subcutaneous tissues.

Ectoderm The outermost of the three primary germ layers of the embryo, and from which the epidermis and epidermal tissues, such as nails, hair, and glands of the skin, develop.

Ectopic Relating to or characterized by an object or organ being situated in an unusual place, away from its normal location.

Edema The presence of an abnormal accumulation of fluid in interstitial spaces of tissues. (Adjective: edematous)

Efferent Conveyed or directed away from a center.

Effusion The escape of fluid from blood vessels into a part or tissue, as an exudation or a transudation.

Embolus A mass of clotted blood or other formed elements, such as bubbles of air, calcium fragments, or a bit of tissue or tumor, that circulates in the bloodstream until it becomes lodged in a vessel, obstructing the circulation. (Plural: emboli)

Empyema An accumulation of pus in a cavity of the body, especially the pleural space.

Emulsify To disperse one liquid throughout the body of another liquid, making a colloidal suspension, or emulsion.

Endocytosis The uptake or incorporation of substances into a cell by invagination of its plasma membrane, as in the processes of phagocytosis and pinocytosis.

Endoderm The innermost of the three primary germ layers of the embryo, and from which epithelium arises.

Endogenous Growing within the body; or developing or originating from within the body or produced from internal causes.

Endoscopy The visualization of any cavity of the body with an endoscope.

Enteropathic Relating to any disease of the intestinal tract.

Enzyme A protein molecule produced by living cells that catalyzes chemical reactions of other organic substances without itself being destroyed or altered.

Epiphysis The expanded articular end of a long bone (head) that is separated from the shaft of the bone by the epiphyseal plate until the bone stops growing, the plate is obliterated, and the shaft and the head become united.

Epithelium The covering of the internal and the external surfaces of the body, including the lining of vessels and other small cavities.

Epitope The simplest form of an antigenic determinant that combines with an antibody or a T-cell receptor to cause a specific reaction by an immunoglobulin.

Erectile Capable of being erected or raised to an erect position.

Erythema The redness or inflammation of the skin or mucous membranes produced by the congestion of superficial capillaries. (Adjective: erythematous)

Etiology The study or theory of all factors that may be involved in the development of a disease, including susceptibility of an individual, the nature of the disease agent, and the way in which an individual's body is invaded by the agent; or the cause of a disease.

Eukaryotic Pertaining to an organism with cells having a true nucleus; that is, a highly complex, organized nucleus surrounded by a nuclear membrane containing organelles and exhibiting mitosis.

Euploid Pertaining to an individual, organism, strain, or cell with a balanced set or sets of chromosomes, in any number, that is an exact multiple of the normal, basic haploid number characteristic of the species; or such an individual, organism, strain, or cell.

Evisceration The removal of the viscera from the abdominal cavity, or disembowelment; or the extrusion of an internal organ through a wound or surgical incision.

Exacerbation An increase in the severity of a disease as marked by greater intensity in any of its signs and symptoms.

Exfoliation Peeling and sloughing off of tissue cells in scales or layers. (Adjective: exfoliative)

Exocytosis The discharge of cell particles, which are packaged in membrane-bound vesicles, by fusion of the vesicular membrane with the plasma membrane and subsequent release of the particles to the exterior of the cell.

Exogenous Developed or originating outside the body, as a disease caused by a bacterial or viral agent foreign to the body.

Exophthalmos A marked or abnormal protrusion of the eyeball.

Extension A movement that allows the two elements of any jointed part to be drawn apart, increasing the angle between them, as extending the leg increases the angle between the femur and the tibia.

Extrapyramidal Pertaining to motor systems supplied by fibers outside the corticospinal or pyramidal tracts.

Extravasation A discharge or escape, usually of blood, serum, or lymph, from a vessel into the tissues.

Extubation The process of withdrawing a previously inserted tube from an orifice or cavity of the body.

Exudate Fluid, cells, or other substances that have been slowly exuded or have escaped from blood vessels and have been deposited in tissues or on tissue surfaces.

Fascia A sheet or band of fibrous connective tissue that may be separated from other specifically organized structures, as the tendons, the aponeuroses, and the ligaments.

Febrile Pertaining to or characterized by an elevated body temperature, or fever.

Fibrillation A small, local, involuntary contraction of muscle, resulting from spontaneous activation of a single muscle fiber or of an isolated bundle of nerve fibers.

Fibrin A stringy, insoluble protein formed by the action of thrombin on fibrinogen during the clotting process.

Fibrosis The formation of fibrous connective tissue, as in the repair or replacement of parenchymatous elements.

Filtration The process of passing a liquid through or as if through a filter, which is accomplished by gravity, pressure, or vacuum.

Fimbria Any structure that forms a fringe, border, or edge or the processes that resemble such a structure.

Fissure A cleft or a groove, normal or otherwise, on the surface of an organ or a bony structure.

Fistula An abnormal passage or communication from an internal organ to the body surface or between two internal organs.

Flaccid Weak, soft, and lax; lacking normal muscle tone.

Flatus Air or gas in the intestinal tract that is expelled through the anus. (Adjective: flatulent)

Flexion A movement that allows the two elements of any jointed part to be brought together, decreasing the angle between them, as bending the elbow.

Flora The microorganisms, such as bacteria and fungi, both normally occurring and pathologic, found in or on an organ.

Focal Relating to, having, or occupying a focus.

Follicle A sac or pouchlike depression or cavity.

Fontanel A membrane-covered opening in bones or between bones, such as the soft spot covered by tough membranes between the bones of an infant's incompletely ossified skull.

Foramen A natural opening or aperture in a membranous structure or bone.

Fossa A hollow or depressed area, especially on the surface of the end of a bone.

Fovea A small pit or depression in the surface of a structure or an organ.

Fundus The base or bottom of an organ or the portion farthest from the mouth of an organ.

Ganglion One of the nerve cell bodies, chiefly collected in groups outside the central nervous system. (Plural: ganglia)

Genotype The entire genetic constitution of an individual, as determined by the particular combination and location of the genes on the chromosomes; or the alleles present at one or more sites on homologous chromosomes.

Glia The neuroglia, or supporting structure of nervous tissue.

Globulin One of a broad group of proteins classified by solubility, electrophoretic mobility, and size.

Gluconeogenesis The formation of glucose from any of the substances of glycolysis other than carbohydrates.

Glycolysis A series of enzymatically catalyzed reactions, occurring within cells, by which glucose is converted to adenosine triphosphate (ATP) and pyruvic acid during aerobic metabolism.

Gonad A gamete-producing gland, as an ovary or a testis.

Gradient The rate of increase or decrease of a measurable phenomenon expressed as a function of a second; or the visual representation of such a change.

Granuloma A small mass of nodular granulation tissue resulting from chronic inflammation, injury, or infection. (Adjective: granulomatous)

Hapten A small, nonproteinaceous substance that is not antigenic by itself but that can act as an antigen when combined with a larger molecule.

Haustrum A structure resembling a recess or sacculation. (Plural: haustra)

Hematoma A localized collection of extravasated blood trapped in an organ, space, or tissue, resulting from a break in the wall of a blood vessel.

Hematopoiesis The normal formation and development of blood cells.

Hemianopia Defective vision or blindness in half of the visual field of one or both eyes.

Heterogeneous Consisting of or composed of dissimilar elements or parts; or not having a uniform quality throughout. (Noun: heterogeneity)

Heterophagy The taking into the cell of an exogenous substance by phagocytosis or pinocytosis and the subsequent digestion of the newly formed vacuole by a lysosome.

Heterozygous Having two different alleles at corresponding loci on homologous chromosomes.

Histology The branch of anatomy that deals with the minute (microscopic) structure, composition, and function of cells and tissue. (Adjective: histologic)

Homolog Any organ or part corresponding in function, position, origin, and structure to another organ or part, as the flippers of a seal that correspond to human hands. (Adjective: homologous)

Homozygous Having two identical alleles at corresponding loci on homologous chromosomes.

Humoral Relating to elements dissolved in the blood or body fluids.

Hybridoma A tumor of hybrid cells produced by fusion of normal lymphocytes and tumor cells.

Hydrolysis The chemical alteration or decomposition of a compound into fragments by the addition of water.

Hypercapnia Excess amounts of carbon dioxide in the blood.

Hyperemia An excess or engorgement of blood in a part of the body.

Hyperesthesia An unusual or pathologic increase in sensitivity of a part, especially the skin, or of a particular sense.

Hyperplasia An abnormal multiplication or increase in the number of normal cells of a body part.

Hypertonic A solution having a greater concentration of solute than another solution with which it is compared, hence exerting more osmotic pressure than that solution.

Hypertrophy The enlargement or overgrowth of an organ that is due to an increase in the size of its cells rather than the number of its cells.

Hypesthesia An abnormal decrease of sensation in response to stimulation of the sensory nerves. (Also called hypoesthesia.)

Hypocapnia A deficiency of carbon dioxide in the blood.

Hypotonic A solution having a lesser concentration of solute than another solution with which it is compared, hence exerting less osmotic pressure than that solution.

Hypoxia An inadequate supply of oxygen to tissue that is below physiologic levels despite adequate perfusion of the tissue by blood.

Iatrogenic Induced inadvertently through the activity of a physician or by medical treatment or diagnostic procedures.

Idiopathic Arising spontaneously or from an unknown cause.

Idiosyncrasy A physical or behavioral characteristic or manner that is unique to an individual or to a group. (Adjective: idiosyncratic)

Incidence The rate at which a certain event occurs (*e.g.*, the number of new cases of a specific disease during a particular period of time in a population at risk).

Inclusion The act of enclosing or the condition of being enclosed; or anything that is enclosed.

Indigenous Native, or natural, to the particular country or region where found.

Infarction Necrosis or death of tissues due to local ischemia resulting from obstruction of blood flow.

Inotropic Influencing the force or energy of muscular contractions.

In situ In the natural or normal place; or something, such as cancer, that is confined to its place of origin and has not invaded neighboring tissues.

Interferon Any one of a group of small glycoproteins (cytokines) produced in response to viral infection and which inhibit viral replication.

Interleukin Any of several multifunctional cytokines produced by a variety of lymphoid and nonlymphoid cells, including immune cells, that stimulate or otherwise affect the function of lympopoietic and other cells and systems in the body.

Interstitial Relating to or situated between parts or in the interspaces of a tissue.

Intramural Situated or occurring within the wall of an organ.

Intrinsic Pertaining exclusively to a part or situated entirely within an organ or tissue.

In vitro A biologic reaction occurring in an artificial environment, such as a test tube.

In vivo A biologic reaction occurring within the living body.

Involution The act or instance of enfolding, entangling, or turning inward.

Ionize To separate or change into ions.

Ipsilateral Situated on, pertaining to, or affecting the same side of the body.

Ischemia Decreased blood supply to a body organ or part, usually due to functional constriction or actual obstruction of a blood vessel.

Juxta-articular Situated near a joint or in the region of a joint.

Juxtaglomerular Near to or adjoining a glomerulus of the kidney.

Karyotype The total chromosomal characteristics of a cell; or the micrograph of chromosomes arranged in pairs in descending order of size.

Keratin A fibrous, sulfur-containing protein that is the primary component of the epidermis, hair, and horny tissues. (Adjective: keratinous)

Keratosis Any skin condition in which there is overgrowth and thickening of the cornified epithelium.

Ketosis A condition characterized by the abnormal accumulation of ketones (organic compounds with a carboxyl group attached to two carbon atoms) in the body tissues and fluid.

Kinesthesia The sense of movement, weight, tension, and position of body parts mediated by input from joint and muscle receptors and hair cells. (Adjective: kinesthetic)

Kyphosis An abnormal condition of the vertebral column, characterized by increased convexity in the curvature of the thoracic spine as viewed from the side.

Lacuna A small pit or cavity within a structure, especially bony tissue; or a defect or gap, as in the field of vision.

Lateral A position farther from the median plane or midline of the body or a structure; or situated on, coming from, or directed towards the side.

Lesion Any wound, injury, or pathologic change in body tissue.

Lethargy The lowered level of consciousness characterized by listlessness, drowsiness, and apathy; or a state of indifference.

Ligament One of many predominantly white, shiny, flexible bands of fibrous tissue that binds joints together and connects bones or cartilages.

Ligand A group, ion, or molecule that binds to the central atom or molecule in a chemical complex.

Lipid Any of the group of fats and fatlike substances characterized by being insoluble in water and soluble in nonpolar organic solvents, such as chloroform and ether.

Lipoprotein Any one of the conjugated proteins that is a complex of protein and lipid.

Lobule A small lobe.

Lordosis The anterior concavity in the curvature of the lumbar and cervical spine as observed from the side.

Lumen A cavity or the channel within a tube or tubular organ of the body.

Luteal Of or pertaining to or having the properties of the corpus luteum.

Lysis Destruction or dissolution of a cell or molecule through the action of a specific agent.

Maceration Softening of tissue by soaking, especially in acidic solutions.

Macroscopic Large enough to be visible with the unaided eye or without the microscope.

Macula A small, flat blemish, thickening, or discoloration that is flush with the skin surface. (Adjective: macular)

Malaise A vague feeling of bodily fatigue and discomfort.

Manometry The measurement of tension or pressure of a liquid or gas using a device called a manometer.

Marasmus A condition of extreme protein-calorie malnutrition that is characterized by growth retardation and progressive wasting of subcutaneous tissue and muscle and occurs chiefly during the first year of life.

Matrix The intracellular substance of a tissue or the basic substance from which a specific organ or kind of tissue develops.

Meatus An opening or passage through any body part.

Medial Pertaining to the middle; or situated or oriented toward the midline of the body.

Mediastinum The mass of tissues and organs in the middle of the thorax, separating the pleural sacs containing the two lungs.

Meiosis The division of a sex cell as it matures, so that each daughter nucleus receives one half of the number of chromosomes characteristic of the somatic cells of the species.

Mesoderm The middle layer of the three primary germ layers of the developing embryo, lying between the ectoderm and the endoderm.

Metabolism The sum of all the physical and chemical processes by which living organisms are produced and maintained, and also the transformation by which energy is provided for vital processes and activities.

Metaplasia Change in type of adult cells in a tissue to a form that is not normal for that tissue.

Metastasis The transfer of disease (*e.g.*, cancer) from one organ or part to another not directly connected with it. (Adjective: metastatic)

Miosis Contraction of the pupil of the eye.

Mitosis A type of indirect cell division that occurs in somatic cells and results in the formation of two daughter nuclei containing the identical complements of the number of chromosomes characteristic of the somatic cells of the species.

Molecule The smallest mass of matter that exhibits the properties of an element or compound.

Morbidity A diseased condition or state; the relative incidence of a disease or of all diseases in a population.

Morphology The study of the physical form and structure of an organism; or the form and structure of a particular organism. (Adjective: morphologic)

Mosaicism In genetics, the presence in an individual or in an organism of cell cultures having two or more cell lines that differ in genetic constitution but are derived from a single zygote.

Mutagen Any chemical or physical agent that induces a genetic mutation (an unusual change in form, quality, or some other characteristic) or increases the mutation rate by causing changes in DNA.

Mydriasis Physiologic dilatation of the pupil of the eye.

Myoclonus A spasm of a portion of a muscle, an entire muscle, or a group of muscles.

Myoglobin The oxygen-transporting pigment of muscle consisting of one heme molecule containing one iron molecule attached to a single globin chain.

Myopathy Any disease or abnormal condition of skeletal muscle, usually characterized by muscle weakness, wasting, and histologic changes within muscle tissue.

Myotome The muscle plate or portion of an embryonic somite that develops into a voluntary muscle; or a group of muscles innervated by a single spinal segment.

Necrosis Localized tissue death that occurs in groups of cells or part of a structure or an organ in response to disease or injury.

Neutropenia An abnormal decrease in the number of neutrophilic leukocytes in the blood.

Nidus The point where a morbid process originates, develops, or is located.

Nociception The reception of painful stimuli from the physical or mechanical injury to body tissues by nociceptors (receptors usually found in either the skin or the walls of the viscera).

Nosocomial Pertaining to or originating in a hospital, such as a nosocomial infection; an infection acquired during hospitalization.

Nystagmus Involuntary, rapid, rhythmic movements of the eyeball.

Oncogene A gene that is capable of causing the initial and continuing conversion of normal cells into cancer cells.

Oncotic Relating to, caused by, or marked by edema or any swelling.

Oocyte A primordial or incompletely developed ovum.

Oogenesis The process of the growth and maturation of the female gametes, or ova.

Opsonization The process of making cells, such as bacteria, more susceptible to the action of phagocytes.

Organelle Any one of the various membrane-bound particles of distinctive morphology and function present within most cells, as the mitochondria, the Golgi complex, and the lysosomes.

Orthopnea An abnormal condition in which a person must be in an upright position in order to breathe deeply or comfortably.

Orthosis An external orthopedic appliance or apparatus, as a brace or splint, used to support, align, prevent or correct deformities, or to improve the function of movable parts of the body.

Osmolality The concentration of osmotically active particles in solution expressed in osmols or milliosmols per kilogram of solvent.

Osmolarity The concentration of osmotically active particles in solution expressed in osmols or milliosmols per liter of solution.

Osmosis The movement or passage of a pure solvent, such as water, through a semipermeable membrane from a solution that has a lower solute concentration to one that has a higher solute concentration.

Osteophyte A bony project or outgrowth.

Palpable Perceptible by touch.

Papilla A small nipple-shaped projection, elevation, or structure, as the conoid papillae of the tongue.

Papule A small, circumscribed, solid elevation of the skin less than one centimeter in diameter. (Adjective: papular)

Paracrine A mode of hormone action in which a chemical messenger that is synthesized and released from a cell acts on nearby cells of a different type and affects their function.

Paralysis An abnormal condition characterized by the impairment or loss of motor function due to a lesion of the neural or muscular mechanism.

Paraneoplastic Relating to alterations produced in tissue remote from a tumor or its metastases.

Parenchyma The basic tissue or elements of an organ as distinguished from supporting or connective tissue or elements. (Adjective: parenchymal)

Paresis Slight or partial paralysis.

Paresthesia Any abnormal touch sensation, which can be experienced as numbness, tingling, or a "pins and needles" feeling, often in the absence of external stimuli.

Parietal Pertaining to the outer wall of a cavity or organ; or pertaining to the parietal bone of the skull or the parietal lobe of the brain.

Parous Having borne one or more viable offspring.

Pathogen Any microorganism capable of producing disease.

Pedigree A systematic presentation, such as in a table, chart, or list, of an individual's ancestors that is used in human genetics in the analysis of inheritance.

Peptide Any of a class of molecular chain compounds composed of two or more amino acids joined by peptide bonds.

Perfusion The process or act of pouring over or through, especially the passage of a fluid through a specific organ or an area of the body.

Peripheral Pertaining to the outside, surface, or surrounding area of an organ or other structure; or located away from a center or central structure.

Permeable A condition of being pervious, or permitting passage, so that fluids and certain other substances can pass through, as a permeable membrane.

Pervasive Pertaining to something that becomes diffused throughout every part.

Petechia A tiny, perfectly round, purplish red spot that appears on the skin as a result of minute intradermal or submucous hemorrhage. (Plural: petechiae)

Phagocytosis The process by which certain cells engulf and consume foreign material and cell debris.

Phalanx Any one of the bones composing the fingers of each hand and the toes of each foot.

Phenotype The complete physical, biochemical, and physiologic makeup of an individual, as determined by the interaction of both genetic makeup and environmental factors.

Pheresis A procedure in which blood is withdrawn from a donor, a portion (plasma, leukocytes, etc.) is separated and retained, and the remainder is reperfused into the donor. It includes plasmapheresis and leukopheresis.

Pili Hair; or in microbiology, the minute filamentous appendages of certain bacteria. (Singular: pilus)

Plethoric Relating to an excess of any of the body fluids, especially blood; the term used to describe the beefy red coloration of a newborn.

Plexus A network of intersecting nerves, blood vessels, or lymphatic vessels.

Polygene Any of a group of nonallelic genes that interact to influence the same character in the same way so that the effect is cumulative, usually of a quantitative nature, as size, weight, or skin pigmentation. (Adjective: polygenic)

Polymorph One of several, or many, forms of an organism or cell. (Adjective: polymorphic)

Polyp A small, tumor-like growth that protrudes from a mucous membrane surface.

Polypeptide A molecular chain of more than two amino acids joined by peptide bonds.

Presbyopia A visual condition (farsightedness) that commonly develops with advancing years or old age in which the lens loses elasticity causing defective accommodation and inability to focus sharply for near vision.

Prevalence The number of new and old cases of a disease that are present in a population at a given time or occurrences of an event during a particular period of time.

Prodrome An early symptom indicating the onset of a condition or disease. (Adjective: prodromal)

Prokaryotic Pertaining to an organism, such as bacterium, with cells lacking a true nucleus and nuclear membrane that reproduces through simple fission.

Prolapse The falling down, sinking, or sliding of an organ from its normal position or location in the body.

Proliferation The reproduction or multiplication of similar forms, especially cells.

Pronation Assumption of a position in which the ventral, or front, surface of the body or part of the body faces downward. (Adjective: prone)

Propagation The act or action of reproduction.

Proprioception The reception of stimuli originating from within the body regarding body position and muscular activity by proprioceptors (sensory nerve endings found in muscles, tendons, joints).

Prosthesis An artificial replacement for a missing body part; or a device designed and applied to improve function, such as a hearing aid.

Proteoglycans Any one of a group of polysaccharide-protein conjugates occurring primarily in the matrix of connective tissue and cartilage.

Proto-oncogene A normal cellular gene that with alteration, such as by mutation, becomes an active oncogene.

Proximal Closer to a point of reference, usually the trunk of the body, than other parts of the body.

Pruritus The symptom of itching, an uncomfortable sensation leading to the urge to rub or scratch the skin to obtain relief. (Adjective: pruritic)

Purpura A small hemorrhage, up to about 1 cm in diameter, in the skin, mucous membrane, or serosal surface; or any of several bleeding disorders characterized by the presence of purpuric lesions.

Purulent Producing or containing pus.

Quiescent Quiet, causing no disturbance, activity, or symptoms.

Reflux An abnormal backward or return flow of a fluid, such as stomach contents, blood, or urine.

Regurgitation A flow of material that is in the opposite direction from normal, as in the return of swallowed food into the mouth or the backward flow of blood through a defective heart valve.

Remission The partial or complete disappearance of the symptoms of a chronic or malignant disease; or the period of time during which the abatement of symptoms occurs.

Resorption The loss of substance or bone by physiologic or pathologic means, for example, the loss of dentin and cementum of a tooth.

Retrograde Moving backward or against the usual direction of flow; reverting to an earlier state or worse condition (degenerating); catabolic.

Retroversion A condition in which an entire organ is tipped backward or in a posterior direction, usually without flexion or other distortion.

Rhabdomyolysis Destruction or degeneration of muscle, associated with myoglobinuria (excretion of myoglobin in the urine).

Rostral Situated near a beak (oral or nasal region).

Sacroiliitis Inflammation in the sacroiliac joint.

Sclerosis A condition characterized by induration or hardening of tissue resulting from any of several causes, including inflammation, diseases of the interstitial substance, and increased formation of connective tissues.

Scotopic vision Describes vision, especially night vision, when the eye is dark adapted.

Semipermeable Partially but not wholly permeable, especially a membrane that permits the passage of some (usually small) molecules but not of other (usually larger) particles.

Senescence The process or condition of aging or growing old.

Sepsis The presence in the blood or other tissues of pathogenic microorganisms or their toxins; or the condition resulting from the spread of microorganisms or their products. (Adjective: septic)

Serous Relating to or resembling serum; or containing or producing serum, such as a serous gland.

Shunt To divert or bypass bodily fluid from one channel, path, or part to another; a passage or anastomosis between two natural channels, especially between blood vessels, established by surgery or occurring as an abnormality.

Soma The body of an organism as distinguished from the mind; all of an organism, excluding germ cells; the body of a cell.

Spasticity The condition characterized by spasms or other uncontrolled contractions of the skeletal muscles. (Adjective: spastic)

Spatial Relating to, having the character of, or occupying space.

Sphincter A ringlike band of muscle fibers that constricts a passage or closes a natural orifice of the body.

Stenosis An abnormal condition characterized by the narrowing or stricture of a duct or canal.

Stochastic Involving a random process.

Stria A streak or a linear scarlike lesion that often results from rapidly developing tension in the skin; or a narrow bandlike structure, especially the longitudinal collections of nerve fibers in the brain.

Stricture An abnormal temporary or permanent narrowing of the lumen of a duct, canal, or other passage, as the esophagus, because of inflammation, external pressure, or scarring.

Stroma The supporting tissue or the matrix of an organ as distinguished from its functional element, or parenchyma.

Stupor A lowered level of consciousness characterized by lethargy and unresponsiveness in which a person seems unaware of his or her surroundings.

Subchondral Beneath a cartilage.

Subcutaneous Beneath the skin.

Subluxation An incomplete or partial dislocation in which the relationship between joint surfaces is altered, but contact remains.

Sulcus A shallow groove, depression, or furrow on the surface of an organ, as a sulcus on the surface of the brain, separating the gyri.

Supination Assuming the position of lying horizontally on the back, or with the face upward. (Adjective: supine)

Suppuration The formation of pus, or purulent matter.

Symbiosis Mode of living characterized by close association between organisms of different species, usually in a mutually beneficial relationship.

Sympathomimetic An agent or substance that produces stimulating effects on organs and structures similar to those produced by the sympathetic nervous system.

Syncope A brief lapse of consciousness due to generalized cerebral ischemia.

Syncytium A multinucleate mass of protoplasm produced by the merging of a group of cells.

Syndrome A complex of signs and symptoms that occur together to present a clinical picture of a disease or inherited abnormality.

Synergist An organ, agent, or substance that aids or cooperates with another organ, agent, or substance.

Synthesis An integration or combination of various parts or elements to create a unified whole.

Systemic Pertaining to the whole body rather than to a localized area or regional portion of the body.

Systole The contraction, or period of contraction, of the heart that drives the blood onward into the aorta and pulmonary arteries.

Tamponade Stoppage of the flow of blood to an organ or a part of the body by pathologic compression, such as the compression of the heart by an accumulation of pericardial fluid.

Teratogen Any agent or factor that induces or increases the incidence of developmental abnormalities in the fetus.

Thrombus A stationary mass of clotted blood or other formed elements that remains attached to its place of origin along the wall of a blood vessel, frequently obstructing the circulation. (Plural: thrombi)

Tinnitus A tinkling, buzzing, or ringing noise heard in one or both ears.

Tophus A chalky deposit containing sodium urate that most often develops in periarticular fibrous tissue, typically in individuals with gout. (Plural: tophi)

Torsion The act or process of twisting in either a positive (clockwise) or negative (counterclockwise) direction.

Trabecula A supporting or anchoring stand of connective tissue, such as the delicate fibrous threads connecting the inner surface of the arachnoid to the pia mater.

Transmural Situated or occurring through the wall of an organ.

Transudate A fluid substance passed through a membrane or extruded from the blood.

Tremor Involuntary quivering or trembling movements caused by the alternating contraction and relaxation of opposing groups of skeletal muscles.

Trigone A triangular-shaped area.

Ubiquitous The condition or state of existing or being everywhere at the same time.

Ulcer A circumscribed excavation of the surface of an organ or tissue, which results from necrosis that accompanies some inflammatory, infectious, or malignant processes. (Adjective: ulcerative)

Urticaria A pruritic skin eruption of the upper dermis, usually transient, characterized by wheals (hives) of various shapes and sizes.

Uveitis An inflammation of all or part of the uveal tract of the eye.

Vector An invertebrate animal (*e.g.,* tick, mite, mosquito) that serves as a carrier, transferring an infective agent from one vertebrate host to another.

Ventral Pertaining to a position toward the belly of the body; or situated or oriented toward the front or anterior of the body.

Vertigo An illusory sensation that the environment or one's own body is revolving.

Vesicle A small bladder or sac, as a small, thin-walled, raised skin lesion, containing liquid.

Visceral Pertaining to the viscera, or internal organs of the body.

Viscosity Pertaining to the physical property of fluids, caused by the adhesion of adjacent molecules, that determines the internal resistance to shear forces.

Zoonosis A disease of animals that may be transmitted to humans from its primary animal host under natural conditions.

Index

Glipizide, for diabetes mellitus, 1064, 1064t
Glisson capsule, 950
Global brain injury, 1300–1302, 1300t, 1301f, 1312–1315, 1312t, 1313f, 1314f, 1314t
Global infections, 345
Globulins, 255, 255t, 768
Globus pallidus, 1209, 1279–1280, 1279f
Glomerular filtration rate, 745, 749, 752f
    in chronic kidney disease, 860–861, 860t, 871
    in elderly persons, 44, 871
    measurement of, 757
    in renal failure, 857
Glomerulus(i)
    anatomy of, 742–744, 743f–745f, 840, 841f
    function of, 840
Glomeruli, disorders of function, 840-848
    acute nephritic syndrome, 842–843, 842t, 843f
    acute postinfectious, 843, 843f
    in Alport syndrome, 846
    asymptomatic, 845–846
    chronic, 846
    etiology of, 841–842, 841f
    focal segmental, 845
    hematuria in, 845–846
    in Henoch-Schönlein purpura, 846
    in hypertension, 847
    in immunoglobulin A nephropathy, 845–846, 846f
    membranous, 845
    nephrotic syndrome, 843–845, 843t, 844f
    pathogenesis of, 841–842, 841f
    proteinuria in, 845–846, 846f
    rapidly progressive, 842t, 843, 844f
    in systemic lupus erythematosus, 846–847, 1526
Glomerulosclerosis
    in diabetes mellitus, 847, 1072–1073
    focal segmental, 845
Glossopharyngeal nerve (IX), 1199t, 1207, 1219
Glottis, 642, 643f
GLP-1 protein, 1065
Glucagon, 1010t, 1051
    actions of, 1050t
    in food intake regulation, 990, 990f
    for hypoglycemia, 1069
    receptors for, 1012
Glucagon-like peptide, 905, 906t, 1052
    agonists of, for diabetes mellitus, 1063f, 1065–1066
    in food intake regulation, 990, 990f
Glucocorticoids, 1010t, 1039–1040, 1039f, 1040t
    in glucose regulation, 1053
    in stress response, 202t, 203, 203f
    withdrawal of, 1043
Glucokinase, 1050
Gluconeogenesis, 71, 1048, 1048f, 1051
Glucosamine, for osteoarthritis, 1535
Glucose
    abnormal levels of. See Hyperglycemia; Hypoglycemia
    in brain metabolism, 1300
    in dialysis solutions, 868–869
    digestion and absorption of, 911, 911f, 911t
    metabolism of, 70–73, 71f, 1048, 1048f, 1050t
        in brain, 1187
        cortisol in, 1039
    osmotic activity of, 764
    regulation of, 1049–1053, 1049f–1052f, 1050t
    renal blood flow and, 751
    renal clearance of, 751
    storage of, 952, 953f
    tests for, 1060–1061, 1060t
    transport of, in renal tubules, 746, 746f, 747f
Glucose-dependent insulinotropic polypeptide, 903, 905, 906t, 1052, 1065
Glucose intolerance, categories of, 1054, 1055t

Glucose-6-phosphatase deficiency, 97, 289
Glucose transporters, 1051–1052, 1052f
Glulisine insulin, 1066, 1066t
Glutamate
    brain injury from, 1302–1303, 1302f, 1305
    in memory, 1377
    in mental illness, 1365t
    in pain mediation, 1236
Glutamic acid decarboxylase, antibodies to, 1056
Glutamine
    as neurotransmitter, 1189
    in substance abuse, 1376
Glutathione, in drug metabolism, 958
Gluteal-femoral obesity, 993–994, 993f
Gluteal fold, asymmetric, in hip dysplasia, 1501, 1501f
Gluten-sensitive enteropathy, 942–943, 943f
GLUTs (glucose transporters), 1049–1050, 1052f
Glyburide, for diabetes mellitus, 1064, 1064t
Glycated hemoglobin, in diabetes mellitus, 1061
Glycation end products, advanced, 1071
Glycine
    in mental illness, 1365t
    as neurotransmitter, 1189
Glycocalyx (cell coat), 65f, 66
Glycogen
    intracellular accumulation of, 97
    muscle, 236
Glycogenolysis, 1048, 1048f, 1052
Glycolysis, 70–72
Glycopeptides, 342t
Glycoproteins, on platelets, 263, 263f, 264, 271
Glycosaminoglycans, 91
Glycosides, cardiac, for arrhythmias, 602
Glycylcycline, 342t
GnRH (gonadotropin-releasing hormone), 1010t, 1015
Goblet cells, 84
Goiter, 1034, 1035
Goldman applanation tonometer, 1399
Golgi apparatus/complex, 59f, 61, 65–66, 65f, 1011
Golgi tendon organs, 1205, 1264
Gompertzian model, for tumor growth, 168, 168f
Gonad(s). See also Ovary; Testis
    embryology of, 1080–1081
Gonadotropes, 1009c, 1015
Gonadotropic hormones, in adolescents, 32
Gonadotropin(s), in males, 1086–1087, 1087f
Gonadotropin-releasing hormone (GnRH), 1010t, 1015, 1086–1087, 1087f
Gonadotropin-releasing hormone analogs, for cancer, 188
Gonioscopy, 1401
Gonorrhea, 1176–1178, 1176f, 1177f, 1393, 1393f, 1394
Goodpasture syndrome, 414, 843, 844f
Gout, 834, 1536–1538, 1537f, 1540
gp41 protein, HIV, 430, 431f
gp120 protein, HIV, 430–431, 431f
G proteins, receptors linked to, 68, 68f
Graafian follicles, 1116
Graft
    skin, for burns, 1587
    in transplantation, 419–420
Graft-versus-host disease, 420
Gram calorie, 983
Gram stain, 329, 1176
Grand mal (tonic-clonic) seizures, 1333
Granulation tissue, 391, 393, 394
Granules
    in basophils, 411
    in granulocytes, 256, 257f
    in mast cells, 411
    in platelets, 263–264, 263f

Granulocyte(s), 256–258, 257f, 302–303, 302f
    in inflammation, 379, 380f
    maturation of, 259f
    in phagocytosis, 349
Granulocyte colony-stimulating factor, 260
    action of, 352t, 353
    for neutropenia, 306
Granulocyte-monocyte colony-stimulating factor, 260, 303, 352t, 353
Granuloma(s), 258
    in Crohn disease, 930, 930f
    formation of, 388–389, 389f
    in sarcoidosis, 726–727
    in tuberculosis, 682
Granuloma inguinale, 1171
Granulomatosis, Wegener, 490t
Granulomatous disease, chronic, 409
Granulosa cells, 1121f, 1122
Graves disease, 422, 1036–1037, 1037f
Gravity
    physiologic effects of, 244–248, 244t, 245f, 246f
    pressure-volume distribution and, 452
    in varicose vein development, 499
    venous function and, 468
Gray hepatization, in pneumonia, 679
Gray matter
    astrocytes in, 1187
    of cerebellum, 1207
    intermediate, 1202
    of midbrain, 1208
    of spinal cord, 1202, 1203f
    tract systems of, 1198, 1200, 1200f
Gray rami, 1219
Great arteries, transposition of, 574f, 577
Greater omentum, 897–898, 898f
Griseofulvin, for fungal infections, 1560, 1561
Growth and development
    of adolescents, 32–33
    of bone, 1494, 1495f
    catch-up, 1026
    in chronic kidney disease, 871
    in early childhood, 27–28
    evaluation, standards for child(ren), 11, 12f
    hormones essential for, 1023
    of infants, 16–19, 17f
    iron requirements in, 290
    in middle to late childhood, 29
    prenatal, 11–15, 12f, 14f, 16f
    in thalassemia, 288
    thyroid hormone in, 1034
Growth factors
    cancer independence from, 165, 171, 172f
    in healing, 391–392
    receptors for, 68–69
Growth fraction, of tumors, 168, 168f
Growth hormone (GH), 1010t, 1023–1029
    actions of, 1024, 1024f
    in adolescents, 32
    deficiency of, 1023
        in adults, 1027, 1027t
        short stature in, 1025–1026, 1025c
    excess of
        in adults, 1027–1029, 1028f
        tall stature in, 1027
    in glucose regulation, 1053
    regulation of, 1016f
    replacement of, 1026
    secretion of, 1025
    in stress response, 204
    synthesis of, 1015f, 1024
    transport of, 1025
Growth hormone-releasing hormone (GHRH), 1010t, 1015, 1025, 1028
Growth plate, 1455, 1456f, 1494, 1495f

PREFIXES

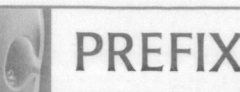

a-, an- without, lack of
apnea (without breath)
anemia (lack of blood)

ab- separation, away from
abductor (leading away from)
aberrant (away from the usual course)

ad- to, toward, near to
adductor (leading toward)
adrenal (near the kidney)

ana- up, again, excessive
anapnea (to breathe again)
anasarca (severe edema)

ante- before, in front of
antecubital (in front of the elbow)
antenatal (occurring before birth)

anti- against, counter
anticoagulant (opposing coagulation)
antisepsis (against infection)

ap-, apo- separation, derivation from
apocrine (type of glandular secretion
    that contains cast-off parts of the
    secretory cell)

aut-, auto- self
autoimmune (immunity to self)
autologous (pertaining to self graft or
    blood transfusion)

bi- two, twice, double
biarticulate (pertaining to two joints)
bifurcation (two branches)

brady- slow
bradyesthesia (slowness or dullness
    of perception)

cata- down, under, lower, negative, against
catabolism (breaking down)
catalepsy (diminished movement)

circum- around, about
circumflex (winding around)
circumference (surrounding)

contra- against, counter
contraindicated (not indicated)
contralateral (opposite side)

de- away from, down from, remove
dehydrate (remove water)
deaminate (remove an amino group)

dia- through, apart, across, completely
diapedesis (ooze through)
diagnosis (complete knowledge)

dis- apart, reversal, separation
discrete (made up of separated parts)
disruptive (bursting apart)

dys- difficulty, faulty, painful
dysmenorrhea (painful menstruation)
dyspnea (difficulty breathing)

e-, ex- out from, out of
enucleate (remove from)
exostosis (outgrowth of bone)

ec- out from
eccentric (away from center)
ectopic (out of place)

ecto- outside, situated on
ectoderm (outer skin)
ectoretina (outer layer of retina)

em-, en- in, on
empyema (pus in)
encephalon (in the brain)

endo- within, inside
endocardium (within heart)
endometrium (within uterus)

epi- upon, after, in addition
epidermis (on skin)
epidural (upon dura)

eu- well, easily, good
eupnea (easy or normal respiration)
euthyroid (normal thyroid function)

exo- outside
exocolitis (inflammation of outer coat
    of colon)
exogenous (originating outside)

extra- outside of, beyond
extracellular (outside cell)
extrapleural (outside pleura)

hemi- half
hemialgia (pain affecting only one side
    of the body)
hemilingual (affecting one side of
    the tongue)

hyper- extreme, above, beyond
hyperemia (excessive blood)
hypertrophy (overgrowth)

hypo- under, below
hypotension (low blood pressure)
hypothyroidism (underfunction of thyroid)

im-, in- in, into, on
immersion (act of dipping in)
injection (act of forcing fluid into)

im-, in- not
immature (not mature)
inability (not able)

infra- beneath
infraclavicular (below the clavicle)
infraorbital (below the eye)

inter- among, between
intercostal (between the ribs)
intervene (come between)

intra- within, inside
intraocular (within the eye)
intraventricular (within the ventricles)

intro- into, within
introversion (turning inward)
introduce (lead into)

iso- equal, same
isotonia (equal tone, tension, or activity)
isotypical (of the same type)

juxta- near, close by
juxtaglomerular (near an adjoining
    glomerulus in the kidney)
juxtaspinal (near the spinal column)

macro- large, long, excess
macrocephaly (excessive head size)
macrodystrophia (overgrowth of a part)

mal- bad, abnormal
maldevelopment (abnormal growth
    or development)
malfunction (to function imperfectly
    or badly)

mega- large, enlarged, abnormally large size
megaprosopous (having a large face)
megasoma (great size and stature)

meso- middle, intermediate, moderate
mesoderm (middle germ layer of embryo)
mesocephalic (pertaining to a skull with
    an average breadth–length index)

meta- beyond, after, accompanying
metacarpal (beyond the wrist)
metamorphosis (change of form)

micro- small size or amount
microbe (a minute living organism)
microtiter (a titer of minute quantity)

neo- new, young, recent
neoformation (a new growth)
neonate (newborn)

oligo- few, scanty, less than normal
oligogenic (produced by a few genes)
oligospermia (abnormally low number
    of spermatozoa in the semen)

para- beside, beyond
paracardiac (beside the heart)
paraurethral (near the urethra)

per- through
perforate (bore through)
permeate (pass through)

peri- around
peribronchia (around the bronchus)
periosteum (around bone)

poly- many, much
polyphagia (excessive eating)
polytrauma (occurrence of multiple
    injuries)

post- after, behind in time or place
postoperative (after operation)
postpartum (after childbirth)

pre-, pro- in front of, before in time or place
premaxillary (in front of the maxilla)
prognosis (foreknowledge)

pseud-, pseudo- false, spurious
pseudocartilaginous (made up of a
    substance resembling cartilage)
pseudopregnancy (false pregnancy)

retro- backward, located behind
retrocervical (located behind cervix)
retrograde (going backward)